FUNDAMENTAL IMMUNOLOGY

FIFTH EDITION

FUNDAMENTAL IMMUNOLOGY

FIFTH EDITION

Editor

WILLIAM E. PAUL, M.D.

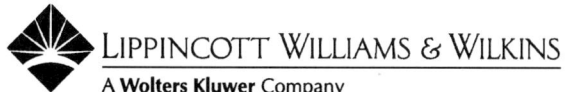 LIPPINCOTT WILLIAMS & WILKINS
A **Wolters Kluwer** Company

Philadelphia • Baltimore • New York • London
Buenos Aires • Hong Kong • Sydney • Tokyo

Acquisitions Editor: James Merritt
Developmental Editor: Julia Seto
Production Editor: Steven P. Martin
Manufacturing Manager: Colin J. Warnock
Cover Designer: Christine Jenny
Compositor: TechBooks
Printer: Quebecor/Versailles

© 2003 by LIPPINCOTT WILLIAMS & WILKINS
530 Walnut Street
Philadelphia, PA 19106 USA
LWW.com

Printed in the USA

Library of Congress Cataloging-in-Publication Data

Fundamental immunology / editor, William E. Paul.—5th ed.
   p. ; cm.
   Includes bibliographical references and index.
   ISBN 0-7817-3514-9
   1. Immunology.   I. Paul, William E.
   [DNLM: 1. Immunity.   QW 540 F981   2003]
   QR181.F84   2003
   616.07′9—dc21   2003044663

10 9 8 7 6 5 4 3 2 1

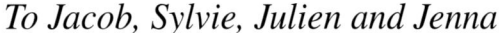

To Jacob, Sylvie, Julien and Jenna

Contents

Contributors xi

Acknowledgements.. xvii

Preface xix

Introduction

1. The Immune System: An Introuduction 1
William E. Paul

2. History of Immunology.. 23
Pauline M. H. Mazumdar

Immunoglobulins and B Lymphocytes

3. Immunoglobulins: Structure & Function..................................... 47
Grant R. Kolar and J. Donald Capra

4. Antigen-Antibody Interactions and Monoclonal Antibodies 69
Jay A. Berzofsky, Ira J. Berkower, and Suzanne L. Epstein

5. Immunoglobulins: Molecular Genetics 107
Edward E. Max

6. B-Lymphocyte Development and Biology 159
Richard R. Hardy

7. B-Cell Signaling Mechanisms and Activation................................ 195
Michael McHeyzer-Williams

T Cells & NK Cells

8. T-Cell Antigen Receptors.. 227
Mark M. Davis and Yueh-Hsiu Chien

9. T-Cell Developmental Biology 259
Ellen V. Rothenberg, Mary A. Yui, and Janice C. Telfer

10. Peripheral T-Lymphocyte Responses and Function 303
Marc K. Jenkins

11. T-Lymphocyte Activation.. 321
Arthur Weiss and Lawrence E. Samelson

12. Natural Killer Cells 365
David H. Raulet

13. Accessory Molecules and Co-Stimulation 393
Arlene H. Sharpe, Yvette Latchman, and Rebecca J. Greenwald

Organization and Evolution of the Immune System

14. Lymphoid Tissues & Organs 419
David D. Chaplin

15. Dendritic Cells 455
Muriel Moser

16. Macrophages and the Immune Response 481
Siamon Gordon

17. Innate Immune System 497
Ruslan Medzhitov

18. Evolution of the Immune System 519
Martin F. Flajnik, Kristina Miller, and Louis Du Pasquier

Antigen Processing and Presentation

19. The Major Histocompatibility Complex and its Encoded Proteins 571
David H. Margulies, and James McCluskey

20. The Biochemistry and Cell Biology of Antigen Processing 613
Peter Cresswell

Regulation of the Immune Response

21. Immunogenicity and Antigen Structure 631
Jay A. Berzofsky and Ira J. Berkower

22. Fc Receptors 685
Jeffrey V. Ravetch

23. Type I Cytokines and Interferons and Their Receptors 701
Warren J. Leonard

24. The Tumor Necrosis Factor Superfamily and its Receptors 749
Lyle L. Moldawer

25. Interleukin-1 Family of Ligands and Receptors 775
Charles A. Dinarello

26. Chemokines 801
Philip M. Murphy

27. Programmed Cell Death 841
Francis Ka-Ming Chan and Michael J. Lenardo

28. Immunologic Memory 865
David F. Tough and Jonathan Sprent

29. Immunological Tolerance 901
Ronald H. Schwartz and Daniel L. Mueller

30. Regulatory/Suppressor T Cells 935
Ethan M. Shevach

31. The Mucosal Immune System 965
Jiri Mestecky, Richard S. Blumberg, Hiroshi Kiyono, and Jerry R. McGhee

32. Neural Immune Interactions in Health and Disease 1021
Esther M. Sternberg and Jeanette I. Webster

33. Immunology of Aging 1043
Dan L. Longo

Effector Mechanisms of Immunity

34. Complement 1077
Wolfgang M. Prodinger, Reinhard Würzner, Heribert Stoiber, and Manfred P. Dierich

35. Phagocytosis 1105
Eric J. Brown and Hattie D. Gresham

36. Cytotoxic T Lymphocytes 1127
Pierre A. Henkart and Michail V. Sitkovsky

37. Inflammation 1151
Helene F. Rosenberg and John I. Gallin

Immunity to Infectious Agents

38. The Immune Response to Parasites 1171
Alan Sher, Thomas A. Wynn, and David L. Sacks

39. Viral Immunology 1201
Hildegund C. J. Ertl

40. Immunity to Intracellular Bacteria 1229
Stefan H. E. Kaufmann

41. Immunity to Extracellular Bacteria 1263
Moon H. Nahm, Michael A. Apicella, and David E. Briles

42. Immunology of HIV Infection 1285
Mark Dybul, Mark Connors, and Anthony S. Fauci

43. Vaccines 1319
G.J.V. Nossal

Immunologic Mechanisms in Disease

44. Systemic Autoimmunity 1371
Philip L. Cohen

45. Organ-Specific Autoimmunity 1401
Matthias G. von Herrath and Dirk Homann

46. Immunological Mechanisms of Allergic Disorders 1439
Marsha Wills-Karp and Gurjit K. Khurana Hershey

47. Transplantation Immunology 1481
Megan Sykes, Hugh Auchincloss Jr., and David H. Sachs

48. Tumor Immunology 1557
    Hans Schreiber

49. Primary Immunodeficiency Diseases 1593
    Rebecca H. Buckley

50. Immunotherapy 1621
    Ellen S. Vitetta, Elaine Coleman, Maria-Ana Ghetie, Victor Ghetie,
    Jaroslav Michálek, Laurentiu M. Pop, Joan E. Smallshaw, and
    Camelia Spiridon

Subject Index 1661

Contributors

Michael A. Apicella, M.D., *Professor and Head, Department of Microbiology, The University of Iowa College of Medicine, Iowa City, IA*

Hugh Auchincloss Jr., M.D., *Professor of Surgery (Immunology), Harvard Medical School, Department of Surgery, Boston, MA*

Ira J. Berkower, MD, Ph.D., *Chief, Laboratory of Immunogregulation, Office of Vaccines, Center for Biologics Evaluation and Research, Food and Drug Administration, Bethesda, MD*

Jay A. Berzofsky, MD, Ph.D., *Chief, Molecular Immunogenetics and Vaccine Research Section, Metabolism Branch, National Cancer Institute, National Institutes of Health, Bethesda, MD*

Richard S. Blumberg, M.D., *Associate Professor of Medicine, Brigham and Women's Hospital, Boston, MA*

David E. Briles, Ph.D., *Professor, Department of Microbiology, University of Alabama at Birmingham, Birmingham, AL*

Eric J. Brown, M.D., *Program in Host-Pathogen Interactions, University of California, San Francisco, San Francisco, CA*

Rebecca H. Buckley, M.D., *Professor, Departments of Pediatrics and Immunology, Duke University Durham, NC*

J. Donald Capra, M.D., *President and Program Head, Department of Molecular Immunogenetics, Oklahoma Medical Research Foundation, Oklahoma City, OK*

Francis Ka-Ming Chan, Ph.D., *Assistant Professor, Department of Pathology, University of Massachusetts Medical School, Worcester, MA*

David D. Chaplin, M.D., Ph.D., *Professor and Chairman, Department of Microbiology University of Alabama at Birmingham, Birmingham, AL*

Yueh-Hsiu Chen, Ph.D., *Professor, Department of Microbiology and Immunology, Stanford University, Stanford, CA*

Philip L. Cohen, M.D., *Professor, Department of Medicine, University of Pennsylvania, Philadelphia, PA*

Elaine Coleman, B.S., *Graduate Student, Cancer Immunobiology Center University of Texas Southwestern Medical Center, Dallas, TX*

Mark Connors, M.D., *Senior Investigator, Laboratory of Immunoregulation, National Institute of Allergy and Infectious Diseases, National Institutes of Health, Bethesda, MD*

Peter Cresswell, Ph.D., *Section of Immunobiology, Howard Hughes Medical Institute Yale University School of Medicine, New Haven, CT*

Mark M. Davis, Ph.D., *Professor, Microbiology and Immunology, Stanford University School of Medicine, Stanford CA*

Manfred P. Dierich, M.D., *Professor and Chairman, Institute of Hygiene, Medical University, Innsbruck, Austria*

Charles A. Dinarello, M.D., *Professor of Medicine, Department of Infectious Disease, University of Colorado Health Sciences Center, Denver, CO*

Mark Dybul, M.D., *Assistant Director for Medical Affairs, National Institute of Allergy and Infectious Diseases, The National Institutes of Health, Bethesda, MD*

Louis E. du Pasquier, Ph.D., *Professor, Department of Zoology, University of Basel, Basel, Switzerland*

Suzanne L. Epstein, Ph.D., *Chief, Laboratory of Immunology and Developmental Biology, Division of Cellular and Gene Therapies, Center for Biologics Evaluation and Research, Food and Drug Administration, Rockville, MD*

Hildegund C. J. Ertl, M.D., *Professor, The Wistar Institute, Philadelphia, PA*

Anthony S. Fauci, M.D., *Director, National Institute of Allergy and Infectious Diseases, National Institutes of Health, Bethesda, MD*

Martin F. Flajnik, Ph.D., *Professor, Department of Microbiology and Immunology, University of Maryland at Baltimore, Baltimore, MD*

John I. Gallin, M.D., *Laboratory of Host Defenses, National Institute of Allergy and Infectious Diseases, National Institutes of Health, Bethesda, MD*

Maria-Ana Ghetie, Ph.D., *Assistant Professor, Cancer Immunobiology Center, UT Southwestern Medical Center, Dallas, TX*

Victor F. Ghetie, Ph.D., *Professor, Cancer Immunobiology Center, UT Southwestern Medical Center, Dallas, TX*

Rebecca J. Greenwald, Ph.D., *Instructor, Department of Pathology, Harvard Medical School, Boston, MA*

Hattie D. Gresham, Ph.D., *Associate Professor, Department of Molecular Genetics and Microbiology, University of New Mexico, Albuquerque, NM*

Siamon Gordon, M.D., *Sir William Dunn School of Pathology, University of Oxford, Oxford, England*

Richard R. Hardy, Ph.D., *Institute for Cancer Research, Fox Chase Cancer Center, Philadelphia, PA*

Pierre A. Henkart, M.D., *Experimental Immunology Branch, National Cancer Institute, National Institutes of Health, Bethesda, MD*

Gurjit K. Khurana Hershey, M.D., Ph.D., *Assistant Professor, Department of Pediatrics, University of Cincinnati Hospital, Cincinnati, OH*

Dirk Homann, M.D., *Department of Neuropharmacology, The Scripps Research Institute, La Jolla, CA*

Marc K. Jenkins, Ph.D., *Professor, Department of Microbiology, Center for Immunology, University of Minnesota, Minneapolis, MN*

Stefan H. E. Kaufmann, Ph.D., *Director, Department of Immunology, Max-Planck-Institute for Infection Biology, Berlin, Germany*

Hiroshi Kiyono, D.D.S., Ph.D., *Professor and Director, Division of Mucosal Immunology, The University of Tokyo, Minato-ku, Tokyo*

Grant R. Kolar, B.S., *Graduate Student, Program in Molecular Immunogenetics, Oklahoma Medical Research Foundation, Oklahoma City, OK*

Yvette Latchman, Ph.D., *Department of Pathology, Brigham and Women's Hospital and Harvard Medical School, Boston, MA*

Michael J. Lenardo, M.D., *Chief, Molecular Development Section, Laboratory of Immunology, DIR, National Institute of Allergy and Infectious Diseases, National Institutes of Health, Bethesda, MD*

Warren J. Leonard, M.D., *Laboratory of Molecular Immunology, National Heart, Lung, and Blood Institute, National Institutes of Health, Bethesda, MD*

Dan L. Longo, M.D., *Scientific Director, National Institute on Aging, National Institutes of Health, Baltimore, MD*

David H. Margulies, M.D., Ph.D., *Chief, Molecular Biology Section, Laboratory of Immunology, National Institute of Allergy and Infectious Diseases, National Institutes of Health, Bethesda, MD*

Edward Ellis Max, M.D., Ph.D., *Associate Director for Research, Office of Therapeutics Research and Review, Center for Biologics Evaluation And Research, Food and Drug Administration, Bethesda, MD*

Pauline M. H. Mazumdar, M.B., B.S., Ph.D., *Department of History of Science and Technology, University of Toronto, Toronto, Ontario*

James McCluskey, M.D., *Department of Microbiology and Immunology, The University of Melbourne, Victoria, Australia*

Jerry R. McGhee, Ph.D., *Professor and Director, Department of Microbiology/Immunobiology Vaccine Center, University of Alabama at Birmingham, Birmingham, AL*

Michael G. McHeyzer-Williams, M.D., *Associate Professor, Department of Immunology, The Scripps Research Institute, La Jolla, CA*

Ruslan Medzhitov, Ph.D., *Assistant Professor, Department of Immunobiology, Yale University School of Medicine, New Haven, CT*

Jiri Mestecky, M.D., Ph.D., *Professor, Department of Microbiology, University of Alabama at Birmingham, Birmingham, AL*

Jaroslav Michálek, M.D., Ph.D., *Cancer Immunobiology Center, UT Southwestern Medical Center, Dallas, TX*

Kristina Miller, Ph.D., *Research Scientist, Department of Molecular Genetics, Pacific Biological Station, Fisheries and Oceans, Canada, Nanaimo, BC, Canada*

Lyle Moldawer, M.D., *Department of Surgery, College of Medicine, University of Florida, Shands Hospital, Gainesville, FL*

Muriel Moser, Ph.D., *Senior Research Assocaite, Institut de Biologie et Médecine Moléculaires, Université Libre de Bruxelles, Gosselies, Belgium*

Daniel L. Mueller, M.D., *Professor, Department of Medicine, University of Minnesota Medical School, Minneapolis, MN*

Philip M. Murphy, M.D., *Chief, Molecular Signaling Section, Laboratory of Host Defenses, National Institute of Allergy and Infectious Diseases, National Institutes of Health, Bethesda, MD*

Moon H. Nahm, M.D., *Professor, Departments of Pathology, University of Alabama at Birmingham, Birmingham, AL*

G.J.V. Nossal, M.D., Ph.D., *Professor Emeritus, Department of Pathology, The University of Melbourne, Australia*

William E. Paul, M.D., *Laboratory of Immunology, National Institute of Allergy and Infectious Diseases, Bethesda, MD*

Laurentiu M. Pop, M.D., *Postdoctoral Fellow, Cancer Immunobiology Center, University of Texas Southwestern Medical Center, Dallas, TX*

Wolfgang M. Prodinger, M.D., *Associate Professor, Institute for Hygiene and Social Medicine, University of Innsbruck, Innsbruck, Austria*

David H. Raulet, Ph.D., *Choh Hao Li Professor and Head, Division of Immunology, Department of Molecular and Cell Biology, University of California, Berkeley, Berkeley, CA*

Jeffrey V. Ravetch, M.D., Ph.D., *Theresa and Eugene M. Lang Professor and Head, Laboratory of Molecular Genetics and Immunology, The Rockefeller University, New York, NY*

Helene F. Rosenberg, M.D., Ph.D., *Chief, Eosinophil Pathophysiology Section, Laboratory of Host Defenses, National Institute of Allergy and Infectious Diseases, National Institutes of Health, Bethesda, Maryland*

Ellen V. Rothenberg, M.D., *Division of Biology 156-29, California Institute of Technology, Pasadena, CA*

David H. Sachs, M.D., *Professor of Surgery (Immunology), Harvard Medical School, and Director, Transplantation Biology Research Center, Massachusetts General Hospital, Boston, Massachusetts*

David L. Sacks, Ph.D., *Head, Intracellular Parasite Biology Section, Laboratory of Parasitic Diseases, National Institute of Allergy and Infectious Diseases, National Institutes of Health, Bethesda, MD*

Lawrence Samelson, M.D., *Chief, Laboratory of Cellular and Molecular Biology, Center for Cancer Research, National Cancer Institute, National Institutes of Health, Bethesda, MD*

Ronald H. Schwartz, M.D., Ph.D., *Chief, Laboratory of Cellular and Molecular Immunology, National Institute of Allergy and Infectious Diseases, National Institutes of Health, Bethesda, MD*

Hans Schreiber, M.D., Ph.D., *Department of Pathology, University of Chicago, IL*

Arlene H. Sharpe, M.D., Ph.D., *Associate Professor, Department of Pathology, Harvard Medical School, Boston, MA*

Alan Sher, Ph.D., *Acting Chief, Laboratory of Parasitic Diseases, National Institute of Allergy and Infectious Disease, National Institutes of Health, Bethesda, MD*

Ethan M. Shevach, M.D., *Chief, Cellular Immunology Section, Laboratory of Immunology, National Institute of Allergy and Infectious Diseases, National Institutes of Health, Bethesda, MD*

Michail V. Sitkovsky, Ph.D., *Laboratory of Immunology, National Institute of Allergy and Infectious Diseases, National Institutes of Health, Bethesda, MD*

Joan E. Smallshaw, Ph.D., *Postdoctoral Researcher, Cancer Immunobiology Center, University of Texas Southwestern Medical Center, Dallas, TX*

Camelia I. Spiridon, M.D., *Postdoctoral Researcher, Cancer Immunobiology Center, University of Texas Southwestern Medical Center, Dallas, TX*

Jonathan Sprent, M.D., Ph.D., *Department of Immunology, IMM4, The Scripps Research Institute, La Jolla, CA*

Esther M. Sternberg, M.D., *Director, Integrative Neural-Immune Program, National Institute of Mental Health, National Institutes of Health, Bethesda, MD*

Heribert Stoiber, M.D., *Associate Professor, Institute of Hygiene, University of Innsbruck, Innsbruck, Austria*

Megan Sykes, M.D., *Professor of Surgery and Medicine, Department of Immunology, Harvard Medical School, Boston, MA*

Janice C. Telfer, Ph.D., *Assistant Professor, Department of Veterinary and Animal Sciences, University of Massachusetts Amherst, Amherst, MA*

David F. Tough, Ph.D., *Senior Group Leader, The Edward Jenner Institute for Vaccine Research, Newbury, Berkshire, United Kingdom*

Ellen S. Vitetta, Ph.D., *Director, Cancer Immunobiology Center, University of Texas Southwestern Medical Center, Dallas, TX*

Matthias G. von Herrath, M.D., *Associate Professor, Department of Developmental Immunology, La Jolla Institute for Allergy and Immunology, San Diego, CA*

Jeanette I. Webster, Ph.D., *Research Fellow, Section of Neuroendocrine Immunology and Behavior, National Institute of Mental Health, National Institutes of Health, Bethesda, MD*

Arthur Weiss, M.D., Ph.D., *Ephraim P. Engleman Distinguished Professor, Investigator, Howard Hughes Medical Institute, Department of Medicine, University of California, San Francisco, San Francisco, CA*

Marsha Wills-Karp, Ph.D., *Professor and Director, Division of Immunobiology, Cincinnati Children's Hospital Medical Center, Cincinnati, OH*

Reinhard Würzner, M.D., Ph.D., *Professor, Institut für Hygiene und Sozialmedizin, University of Innsbruck, Innsbruck, Austria*

Thomas A. Wynn, Ph.D., *Senior Investigator, Immunopathogenesis Section, National Institute of Allergy and Infectious Disease, National Institutes of Health, Bethesda, MD*

Mary A. Yui, Ph.D., *Postdoctoral Scholar, Division of Biology, California Institute of Technology, Pasadena, CA*

Acknowledgements

The preparation of the *Fifth Edition of Fundamental Immunology* required the efforts of many individuals. I particularly wish to thank each of the authors. Their contributions, prepared in the midst of extremely busy schedules, are responsible for the value of this book. Julia Seto of Lippincott Williams & Wilkins saw that the process of receiving, editing and assembling the chapters went as smoothly as possible; without her work, the completion of the edition would have been immeasurably more difficult. Steven Martin saw that the complex process of preparing and revising proofs was done with admirable efficiency. I wish to gratefully acknowledge the efforts of each of the members of the editorial and production staffs of Lippincott Williams and Wilkins who participated in the preparation of this edition.

Preface

The fifth edition of *Fundamental Immunology* appears when the importance of the immune response in human health and the prevention of disease was never clearer. Bio-terrorism is a world-wide threat, with the possibility that one of the greatest achievements of mankind, the elimination of small pox, may be undone. The HIV pandemic shows no signs of abating and exacts an increasingly frightening toll. Tuberculosis and malaria continue to be major scourges of mankind. The number of infants and children that annually succumb to diarrheal infectious diseases is in the millions.

The true impact of autoimmunity is more fully appreciated than ever and we now recognize that inflammation plays a major role in many diseases, not the least of which is atherosclerosis. Childhood asthma and allergies have become a virtual epidemic, particularly in certain parts of the western world. The great promise of transplantation will only be fulfilled when we can induce specific tolerance and avoid the need for long-lasting immunosuppression. The possibility that the immune response can become a major modality for cancer therapy still remains to be determined.

These challenges demand a redoubled effort to more fully understand the basis of the immune response and to learn how it can be mobilized or inhibited. Innnovative approaches for the development of new vaccines are needed. A new generation of immunologists will be required to grapple with these issues. *Fundamental Immunology* and its sister publications play a key role in training those entering our field and in helping current immunologists to be as productive as possible.

Fundamental Immunology was first published in 1984; I began to work on it in late 1982. The *Fifth Edition* thus marks more than 20 years during which I have had the privilege of participating in the preparation of this book. My goal was, and continues to be, to make available to advanced students of immunology and to post-doctoral fellows in immunology and related fields an authoritative treatment of the major areas of immunology. *Fundamental Immunology* is also designed to provide my colleagues with a simple way to keep current in aspects of immunology outside their immediate area of expertise and to allow scientists in allied fields to rapidly inform themselves of the state of the art to aid them in aspects of their work that impinge on immunology.

In agreeing to take responsibility for editing an advanced text in immunology, I was motivated, in part, by my experience as a post-doctoral fellow working on the binding properties of antibodies when I made almost daily use of Kabat and Mayer's *Experimental Immunochemistry*. I hoped that *Fundamental Immunology* might serve a similar role for a new generation of immunologists. The degree to which I have succeeded must be judged by the readers.

What I failed to anticipate was the unremitting growth of our science. Indeed, immunology has been in a state of continuing revolution throughout my entire career. *Fundamental Immunology,* which was 809 pages in its first version, has more than doubled in size and a field that seemed almost too broad to be encompassed in a single volume in 1984 is now far broader.

I continue to be impressed with the vibrancy of immunology and with the upwelling of new subjects that gain center stage. Indeed, in the period since the *Fourth Edition*, virtually every area of immunology has seen major progress. Innate immunity and regulatory T cells, topics that had languished for years, have become the "hottest" of hot subjects. Of course, these are not new areas; the study of innate immunity and the inflammatory response have been central to our discipline since the 19th century. The competing ideas championed by Metchnikoff and by Ehrlich have always been in the minds of immunologists. Nonetheless, the thrust of innate immunity into the forefront of immunological science has been truly remarkable. Similarly, the re-emergence of the study of immunological suppression, with its new name, and the recognition of the central role that regulatory (suppressor) T cells play in control of autoimmunity has been nothing short of spectacular.

Fundamental Immunology has changed just as our field has changed. New chapters have been added to represent disciplines that have come to the fore and previous chapters have been dropped, with the material in them reassigned to other chapters. For the *Fifth Edition*, the previous organizational structure has been generally retained. The opening section, *Introduction*, provides an overview of contemporary immunology and a portrayal of the history of our field, prepared by a distinguished historian of immunology, so that those with a limited background in the field can productively read the subsequent chapters. The next three sections, *Immunoglobulins and B Lymphocytes, T Cells and NK Cells*, and *Organization and Evolution of the Immune System*, introduce the principal cellular components of the immune system and the context in which they act. Emphasizing the centrality of antigen-presentation and of major histocompatibility molecules in the process of T cell recognition of antigen, I have added the section *Antigen Processing and Presentation*. The book then considers the *Regulation of the Immune Response*, with 13 individual chapters detailing the critical aspects of this process. Among these are four separate chapters on the central regulatory molecules of the immune system, the cytokines. I then turn to consider how the immune system mediates its functions, deals with infectious agents, and participates in and may prevent or ameliorate a wide range of diseases. The chapters dealing with this are found in the sections *Effector Mechanisms of Immunity, Immunity to Infectious Agents* (a new section with five chapters) and *Immunologic Mechanisms in Disease.*

In the *Preface* to each of the previous editions, I reminded readers that *Fundamental Immunology* grapples with the most current of immunological subjects. In many areas, consensus may not yet have been reached. Each chapter has been written by a leader in the field, but inevitably there will be disagreement among them on certain issues. Rather than striving for an agreement where none yet exists, I ask the reader to take note of the differences and reach their own judgments in these contentious areas.

I welcome comments by readers of *Fundamental Immunology* for ways to improve the book and to increase its value. Such suggestions will be seriously considered in the preparation of subsequent editions.

William E. Paul
Bethesda, Maryland

From my teachers I have learned much, from my colleagues still more, but from my students most of all.

The Talmud

Discovery consists of seeing what everybody has seen and thinking what nobody has thought.

Albert Szent-Gyorgyi

. . .the clonal selection hypothesis. . .[SC]assumes that. . .[SC]there exist clones of mesenchymal cells, each carrying immunologically reactive sites. . .complementary. . .[SC]to one (or possibly a small number of) potential antigenic determinants.

Sir Macfarlane Burnet
The Clonal Selection Theory of Acquired Immunity

In the fields of observation, chance favors only the mind that is prepared.

Louis Pasteur
Address at the University of Lille

In all things of nature there is something of the marvelous.

Aristotle
Parts of Animals

CHAPTER 1

The Immune System: An Introduction

William E. Paul

Key Characteristics of the Immune System
    Innate Immunity · Primary Responses · Secondary Responses and Immunologic Memory · The Immune Response Is Highly Specific and the Antigenic Universe Is Vast · The Immune System Is Tolerant of Self-Antigens · Immune Responses Against Self-Antigens Can Result in Autoimmune Diseases · AIDS Is an Example of a Disease Caused by a Virus That the Immune System Generally Fails to Eliminate · Major Principles of Immunity

Cells of the Immune System and Their Specific Receptors and Products

B-Lymphocytes and Antibody
    B-Lymphocyte Development · B-Lymphocyte Activation · B-Lymphocyte Differentiation · B1 or CD5+ B-Lymphocytes · B-Lymphocyte Tolerance · Immunoglobulin Structure · Immunoglobulin Genetics · Class Switching · Affinity Maturation and Somatic Hypermutation

T-Lymphocytes
    T-Lymphocyte Antigen Recognition · T-Lymphocyte Receptors · T-Lymphocyte Activation · T-Lymphocyte Development · T-Lymphocyte Functions · T Cells That Help Antibody Responses · Induction of Cellular Immunity · Regulatory T Cells · Cytotoxic T Cells

Cytokines
    Chemokines

The Major Histocompatibility Complex and Antigen Presentation
    Class I MHC Molecules · Class II MHC Molecules · Antigen Presentation · T-Lymphocyte Recognition of Peptide/MHC Complexes Results in MHC-Restricted Recognition · Antigen-Presenting Cells

Effector Mechanisms of Immunity
    Effector Cells of the Immune Response · Monocytes and Macrophages · Natural Killer Cells · Mast Cells and Basophils · Granulocytes · Eosinophils · The Complement System · The Classical Pathway of Complement Activation · The Alternative Pathway of Complement Activation · The Terminal Components of the Complement System

Conclusion

The immune system is a remarkable defense mechanism. It provides the means to make rapid, specific, and protective responses against the myriad potentially pathogenic microorganisms that inhabit the world in which we live. The tragic example of severe immunodeficiencies, as seen in both genetically determined diseases and in acquired immunodeficiency syndrome (AIDS), graphically illustrates the central role the immune response plays in protection against microbial infection. The immune system also has a role in the rejection of tumors and may exert important effects in regulating other bodily systems, but most immunologists would agree that the evolutionary pressure that has principally shaped the immune system is the challenge to vertebrates of the microbial world.

Fundamental Immunology has as its goal the authoritative presentation of the basic elements of the immune system, of the means through which the mechanisms of immunity act in a wide range of clinical conditions, including recovery from infectious diseases, rejection of tumors, transplantation of tissue and organs, autoimmune and other immunopathologic conditions, and allergy; and how the mechanisms of

immunity can be martialed by vaccination to provide protection against microbial pathogens.

The purpose of this opening chapter is to provide readers with a general introduction to our current understanding of the immune system. It will thus be of particular importance for those with a limited background in immunology, providing them with the preparation needed for subsequent chapters of the book. Indeed, rather than providing extensive references in this chapter, each of the subject headings will indicate the chapters that deal in detail with the topic under discussion. Those chapters will not only provide an extended treatment of the topic but will also furnish the reader with a comprehensive reference list.

KEY CHARACTERISTICS OF THE IMMUNE SYSTEM

Innate Immunity (Chapter 17)

Most pathogenic microorganisms attempting to infect an individual encounter powerful nonspecific defenses. The epithelium provides both a physical barrier to the entry of microbes and produces a variety of antimicrobial factors. Microbes that penetrate the epithelium are met with macrophages and related cells that have receptors for cell-surface molecules found on many microbial agents. These interactions may lead to phagocytosis of the pathogen, activation of the macrophage so that it can destroy the agent and to the induction of an inflammatory response that recruits other cell types, including neutrophils, to the site. Microbial pathogens may also be recognized by components of the complement system leading to the enhanced phagocytosis of the agent and in some instances to its lysis as well as to independent activation of inflammatory responses.

The innate immune system also acts to recruit antigen-specific immune responses, not only by attracting cells of the immune system to the site of the infection, but also through the uptake of antigen by dendritic cells that transport antigen to lymphoid tissue where primary immune responses are initiated. Dendritic cells also produce cytokines that can regulate the quality of the immune response so that it is most appropriate to combating the pathogen.

Primary Responses (Chapters 6, 10, and 14)

Primary immune responses are initiated when a foreign antigenic substance interacts with antigen-specific lymphocytes under appropriate circumstances. The response generally consists of the production of antibody molecules specific for the antigenic determinants of the immunogen and of the expansion and differentiation of antigen-specific helper and effector T-lymphocytes. The latter include cells that produce cytokines and killer T cells, capable of lysing infected cells. Generally, the combination of the innate immune response and the primary response are sufficient to eradicate or to control the microbe. Indeed, the most effective function of the immune system is to mount a response that eliminates the infectious agent from the body.

Secondary Responses and Immunologic Memory (Chapters 6, 10, 14, and 28)

As a consequence of the initial encounter with antigen, the immunized individual develops a state of immunologic *memory*. If the same (or a closely related) microorganism is encountered again, a secondary response is made. This generally consists of an antibody response that is more rapid, greater in magnitude, and composed of antibodies that bind to the antigen with greater affinity and are more effective in clearing the microbe from the body. A more rapid and more effective T-cell response also ensues. One effect is that an initial infection with a microorganism initiates a state of immunity in which the individual is protected against a second infection. In the majority of situations, protection is provided by high-affinity antibody molecules that rapidly clear the reintroduced microbe. This is the basis of vaccination; the great power of vaccines is illustrated by the elimination of smallpox

from the world and by the complete control of polio in the Western Hemisphere.

The Immune Response Is Highly Specific and the Antigenic Universe Is Vast

The immune response is highly specific. Primary immunization with a given microorganism evokes antibodies and T cells that are specific for the antigenic determinants found on that microorganism but that fail to recognize (or recognize only poorly) antigenic determinants expressed by unrelated microbes. Indeed, the range of antigenic specificities that can be discriminated by the immune system is enormous.

The Immune System Is Tolerant of Self-Antigens (Chapter 29)

One of the most important features of the immune system is its ability to discriminate between antigenic determinants expressed on foreign substances, such as pathogenic microbes, and potential antigenic determinants expressed by the tissues of the host. The capacity of the system to ignore host antigens is an active process involving the elimination or inactivation of cells that could recognize self-antigens through a process designated immunologic *tolerance*.

Immune Responses Against Self-Antigens Can Result in Autoimmune Diseases (Chapters 44 and 45)

Failures in establishing immunologic tolerance or unusual presentations of self-antigens can give rise to tissue-damaging immune responses directed against antigenic determinants on host molecules. These can result in autoimmune diseases. It is now recognized that a range of extremely important diseases are caused by autoimmune responses or have major autoimmune components, including systemic lupus erythematosus, rheumatoid arthritis, insulin-dependent diabetes mellitus, multiple sclerosis, myasthenia gravis, and regional enteritis. Efforts to treat these diseases by modulating the autoimmune response are a major theme of contemporary medicine.

AIDS Is an Example of a Disease Caused by a Virus that the Immune System Generally Fails to Eliminate (Chapter 42)

Immune responses against infectious agents do not always lead to elimination of the pathogen. In some instances, a chronic infection ensues in which the immune system adopts a variety of strategies to limit damage caused by the organism or by the immune response. One of the most notable infectious diseases in which the immune response generally fails to eliminate the organism is AIDS, caused by the human immunodeficiency virus (HIV). In this instance, the principal infected cells are those of the immune system itself, leading to an eventual state in which the individual can no longer mount protective immune responses against other microbial pathogens.

Major Principles of Immunity

The major principles of the immune response are:

- Elimination of many microbial agents through the nonspecific protective mechanisms of the innate immune system
- Highly specific recognition of foreign antigens coupled with potent mechanisms for elimination of microbes bearing such antigens
- A vast universe of distinct antigenic specificities and a comparably vast capacity for the recognition of these antigens
- The capacity of the system to display immunologic memory
- Tolerance of self-antigens

The remainder of this introductory chapter will describe briefly the molecular and cellular basis of the system and how these central characteristics of the immune response may be explained.

CELLS OF THE IMMUNE SYSTEM AND THEIR SPECIFIC RECEPTORS AND PRODUCTS

The immune system consists of a wide range of distinct cell types, each with important roles. The lymphocytes occupy central stage because they are the cells that determine the specificity of immunity. It is their response that orchestrates the effector limbs of the immune system. Cells that interact with lymphocytes play critical parts both in the presentation of antigen and in the mediation of immunologic functions. These cells include dendritic cells, and the closely related Langerhans cells, monocyte/macrophages, natural killer (NK) cells, neutrophils, mast cells, basophils, and eosinophils. In addition, a series of specialized epithelial and stromal cells provide the anatomic environment in which immunity occurs, often by secreting critical factors that regulate migration, growth, and/or gene activation in cells of the immune system. Such cells also play direct roles in the induction and effector phases of the response.

The cells of the immune system are found in peripheral organized tissues, such as the spleen, lymph nodes, Peyer's patches of the intestine, and tonsils, where primary immune responses generally occur (see Chapter 14). A substantial portion of the lymphocytes and macrophages comprise a recirculating pool of cells found in the blood and lymph, as well as in the lymph nodes and spleen, providing the means to deliver immunocompetent cells to sites where they are needed and to allow immunity that is initiated locally to become generalized. Activated lymphocytes acquire the capacity to enter nonlymphoid tissues where they can express effector functions and eradicate local infections. Some memory lymphocytes are "on patrol" in the tissues, scanning for reintroduction of their specific antigens. Lymphocytes are also found in the central lymphoid organs, thymus, and bone marrow, where they undergo the developmental steps that equip them to mediate the responses of the mature immune system.

Individual lymphocytes are specialized in that they are committed to respond to a limited set of structurally related antigens. This commitment exists before the first contact of the immune system with a given antigen. It is expressed by the presence on the lymphocyte's surface membrane of receptors specific for determinants (epitopes) of the antigen. Each lymphocyte possesses a population of receptors, all of which have identical combining sites. One set, or clone, of lymphocytes differs from another clone in the structure of the combining region of its receptors and thus in the epitopes that it can recognize. The ability of an organism to respond to virtually any non-self antigen is achieved by the existence of a very large number of different lymphocytes, each bearing receptors specific for a distinct epitope. As a consequence, lymphocytes are an enormously heterogeneous group of cells. Based on reasonable assumptions as to the range of diversity that can be created in the genes encoding antigen-specific receptors, it seems virtually certain that the number of distinct combining sites on lymphocyte receptors of an adult human can be measured in the millions.

Lymphocytes differ from each other not only in the specificity of their receptors but also in their functions. There are two broad classes of lymphocytes: the B-lymphocytes, which are precursors of antibody-secreting cells, and the T- (thymus-derived) lymphocytes. T-lymphocytes express important helper functions, such as the ability to aid in the development of specific types of immune responses, including the production of antibody by B cells and the increase in the microbicidal activity of macrophages. Other T-lymphocytes are involved in direct effector functions, such as the lysis of virus-infected cells or certain neoplastic cells. Specialized T-lymphocytes (regulatory T cells) have the capacity to suppress specific immune responses.

B-LYMPHOCYTES AND ANTIBODY

B-Lymphocyte Development (Chapter 6)

B-lymphocytes derive from hematopoietic stem cells by a complex set of differentiation events (Fig. 1). A detailed picture has been obtained of the molecular mechanisms through which committed early members of the B lineage develop into mature B-lymphocytes. These events occur in the fetal liver and, in adult life, principally in the bone marrow. Interaction with specialized stromal cells and their products, including cytokines such as interleukin (IL)-7, are critical to the normal regulation of this process.

The key events in B-cell development occur in cells designated pro-B cells and pre-B cells. They center about the assembly of the genetic elements encoding the antigen-specific receptors of B cells, which are immunoglobulin (Ig) molecules specialized for expression on the cell surface. Igs are heterodimeric molecules consisting of heavy (H) and light

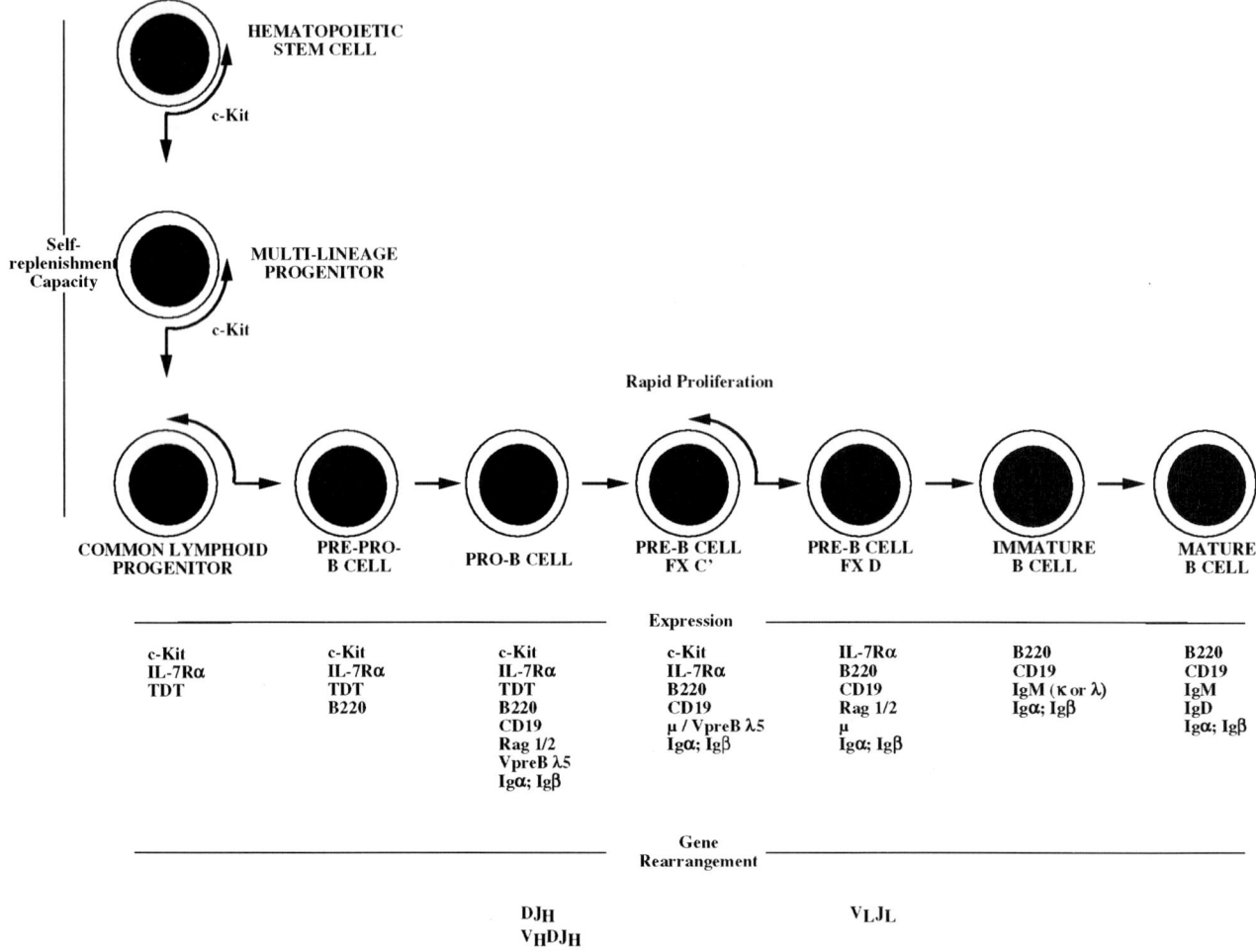

FIG. 1. The patterns of gene expression, timing of gene rearrangement events, capacity for self-replenishment and for rapid proliferation of developing B lymphocytes are indicated. Adapted from Hardy RR, Hayakawa K, B cell development pathways, *Annu Rev Immunol* 2001,19:595–621, with permission.

(L) chains, both of which have regions (variable [V] regions) that contribute to the binding of antigen and that differ in sequence from one Ig molecule to another (see Chapter 3) (Fig. 2). In addition, H and L chains contain regions that are nonvariable or constant (C regions).

The genetic elements encoding the variable portions of Ig H and L chains are not contiguous in germline DNA or in the DNA of nonlymphoid cells (see Chapter 5) (Fig. 3). In pro- and pre-B cells, these genetic elements are translocated to construct an expressible V-region gene. This process involves a choice among a large set of potentially usable variable (V), diversity (D), and joining (J) elements in a combinatorial manner. Such combinatorial translocation, together with a related set of events that add diversity in the course of the joining process, results in the generation of a very large number of distinct H and L chains. The pairing of H and L chains in a quasi-random manner further expands the number of distinct Ig molecules that can be formed.

The H-chain variable region is initially expressed in association with the product of the μ constant (C)-region gene.

Together these elements encode the μ IgH chain, which is used in Igs of the IgM class.

The successful completion of the process of Ig gene rearrangement and the expression of the resultant IgM on the cell surface marks the transition between the pre-B– and B–cell states (Fig. 1). The newly differentiated B cell initially expresses surface Ig solely of the IgM class. The cell completes its maturation process by expressing on its surface a second class of Ig composed of the same L chain and the same H chain variable (VDJ) region but of a different H-chain C region; this second Ig H chain is designated δ, and the Ig to which it contributes is designated IgD.

The differentiation process is controlled at several steps by a system of checks that determines whether prior steps have been successfully completed. These checks depend on the expression on the surface of the cell of appropriately constructed Ig or Ig-like molecules. For, example, in the period after a μ chain has been successfully assembled but before an L chain has been assembled, the μ chain is expressed on the cell surface in association with a surrogate light chain,

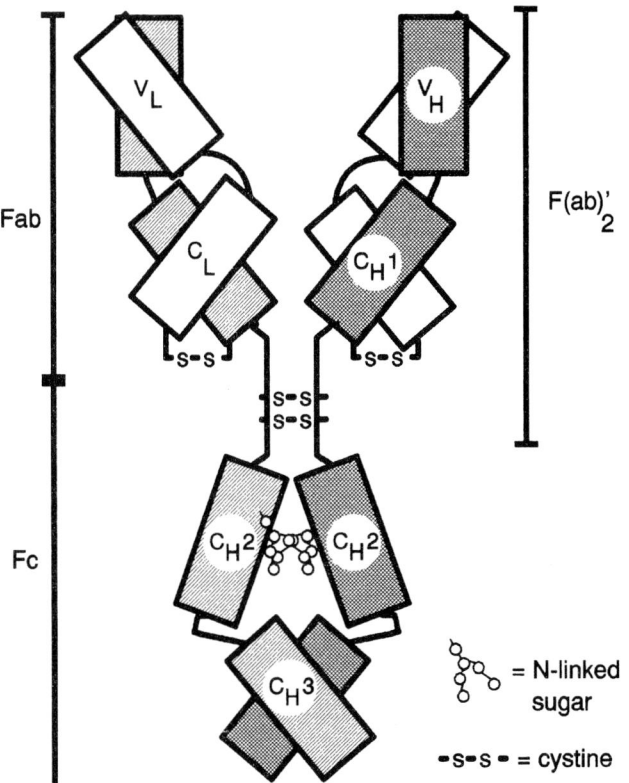

FIG. 2. A schematic representation of an Ig molecule indicating the means through which the V regions and the CH1 and CL regions of H and L chains pair with one another and how the CH2 and CH3 regions of the H chains pair.

consisting of VpreB and λ5. Pre-B cells that fail to express this μ/VpreB λ5 complex do not move forward to future differentiation states or do so very inefficiently.

B-Lymphocyte Activation (Chapter 7)

A mature B cell can be activated by an encounter with an antigen expressing epitopes that are recognized by its cell-surface Ig (Fig. 4). The activation process may be a direct one, dependent on cross-linkage of membrane Ig molecules by the antigen (*cross-linkage–dependent B-cell activation*), or an indirect one, occurring most efficiently in the context of an intimate interaction with a helper T cell, in a process often referred to as *cognate help*.

Because each B cell bears membrane Ig molecules with identical variable regions, cross-linkage of the cell-surface receptors requires that the antigen express more than one copy of an epitope complementary to the binding site of the receptor. This requirement is fulfilled by antigens with repetitive epitopes. Among these antigens are the capsular polysaccharides of many medically important microorganisms such as pneumococci, streptococci, and meningococci. Similar expression of multiple identical epitopes on a single immunogenic particle is a property of many viruses because they express multiple copies of envelope proteins on their surface. Cross-linkage–dependent B-cell activation is a major protective immune response mounted against these microbes. The binding of complement components (see Chapter 34) to antigen or antigen–antibody complexes can increase the magnitude of the cross-linkage–dependent B-cell activation due to the action of a receptor for complement, which, together with other molecules, increases the magnitude of a B-cell response to limiting amounts of antigen.

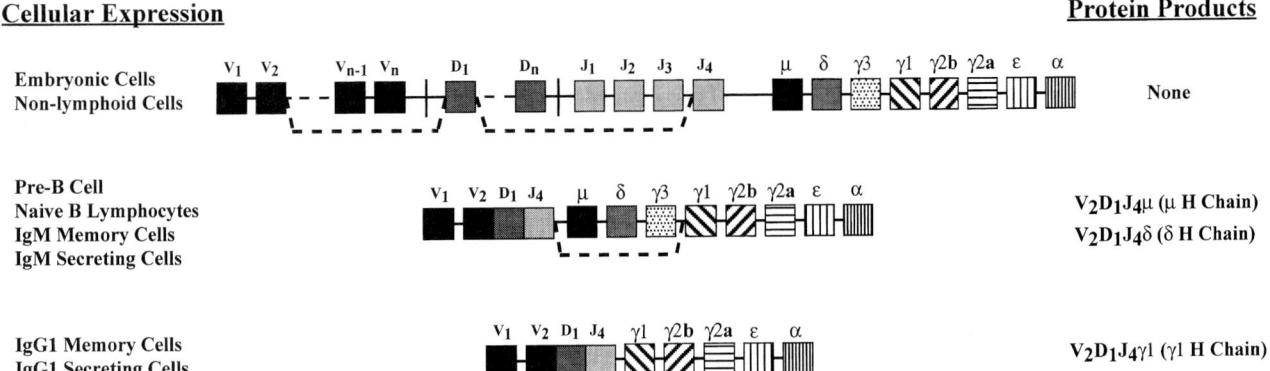

FIG. 3. Organization and translocation of mouse IgH genes. IgH chains are encoded by four distinct genetic elements: Igh-V (V), Igh-D (D), Igh-J (J), and Igh-C. The V, D, and J genetic elements together specify the variable region of the H chain. The Igh-C element specifies the C region. The same V region can be expressed in association with each of the C regions (μ, δ, γ3, γ1, γ2β, γ2α, ε, and α). In the germline, the V, D, and J genes are far apart and there are multiple forms of each of these genes. In the course of lymphocyte development, a VDJ gene complex is formed by translocation of individual V and D genes so that they lie next to one of the J genes, with excision of the intervening genes. This VDJ complex is initially expressed with μ and δ C genes, but may be subsequently translocated so that it lies near one of the other C genes (e.g. γ1) and in that case leads to the expression of a VDJ γ1 chain.

Cognate T Cell- B Cell Help

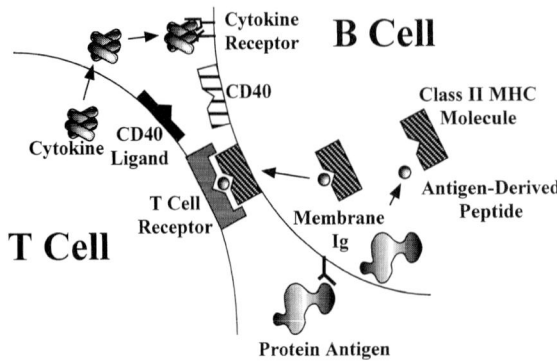

Cross-linkage-dependent B Cell Activation

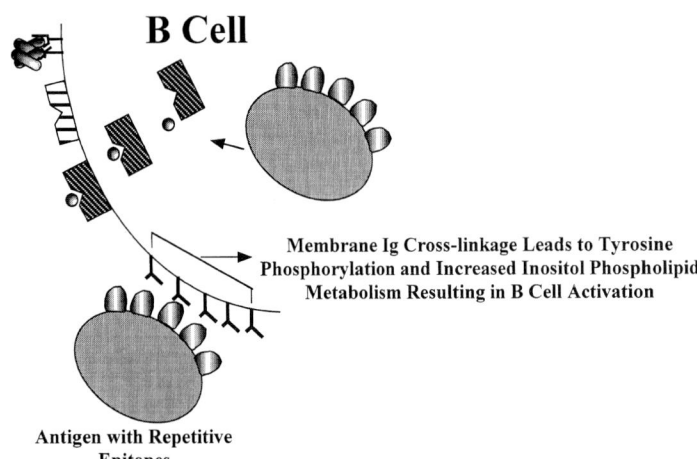

FIG. 4. Two forms of B-cell activation. **A:** Cognate T-cell/B-cell help. Resting B cells can bind antigens that bear epitopes complementary to their cell-surface Ig. Even if the antigen cannot cross-link the receptor, it will be endocytosed and enter late endosomes and lysosomes where it will be degraded to peptides. Some of these peptides will be loaded into class II MHC molecules and brought to the cell surface, where they can be recognized by CD4+ T cells that bear receptors specific for that peptide/class II complex. This interaction allows an activation ligand on the T cells (CD40 ligand) to bind to its receptor on B cells (CD40) and to signal B-cell activation. In addition, the T cells secrete several cytokines that regulate the growth and differentiation of the stimulated B cell. **B:** Cross-lineage–dependent B-cell activation. When B cells encounter antigens that bear multiple copies of an epitope that can bind to their surface Ig, the resultant cross-linkage stimulates biochemical signals within the cell leading to B-cell activation, growth, and differentiation. In many instances, B-cell activation events may result from both pathways of stimulation.

Cognate help allows B cells to mount responses against antigens that cannot cross-link receptors and, at the same time, provides co-stimulatory signals that rescue B cells from inactivation when they are stimulated by weak cross-linkage events. Cognate help is dependent on the binding of antigen by the B cell's membrane Ig, the endocytosis of the antigen, and its fragmentation into peptides within the endosomal/lysosomal compartment of the cell. Some of the resultant peptides are loaded into a groove in a specialized set of cell-surface proteins, the class II major histocompatibility complex (MHC) molecules (Fig. 5). The resultant class II/peptide complexes are expressed on the cell surface. As will be discussed below, these complexes are the ligands for the antigen-specific receptors of a set of T cells designated CD4+ T cells. CD4+ T cells that have receptors specific for the class II/peptide complex expressed on the B-cell surface recognize and interact with that B cell. That interaction results in the activation of the B cell through the agency of cell-surface molecules expressed by the T cells (e.g., the CD40 ligand [CD154]) and cytokines produced by the T cell (Fig. 4). The role of the B-cell receptor for antigen is to create the T-cell ligand on the surface of antigen-specific B cells;

activation of the B cell derives largely from the action of the T cell. However, in many physiologic situations, receptor cross-linkage stimuli and cognate help synergize to yield more vigorous B-cell responses.

B-Lymphocyte Differentiation (Chapter 5, 7, and 28)

Activation of B cells prepares them to divide and to differentiate either into antibody-secreting cells or into memory cells, so that there are more cells specific for the antigen used for immunization and these cells have new properties. Those cells that differentiate into antibody secreting cells account for primary antibody responses. Some of these antibody secreting cells migrate to the bone marrow where they may continue to produce antibody for an extended period of time and may have lifetimes in excess of 1 year.

Memory B cells give rise to antibody-secreting cells upon re-challenge of the individual. The hallmark of the antibody response to re-challenge (a secondary response) is that it is of greater magnitude, occurs more promptly, is composed of antibodies with higher affinity for the antigen, and is dominated by Igs expressing γ, α, or ϵ C regions (IgG, IgA, or IgE)

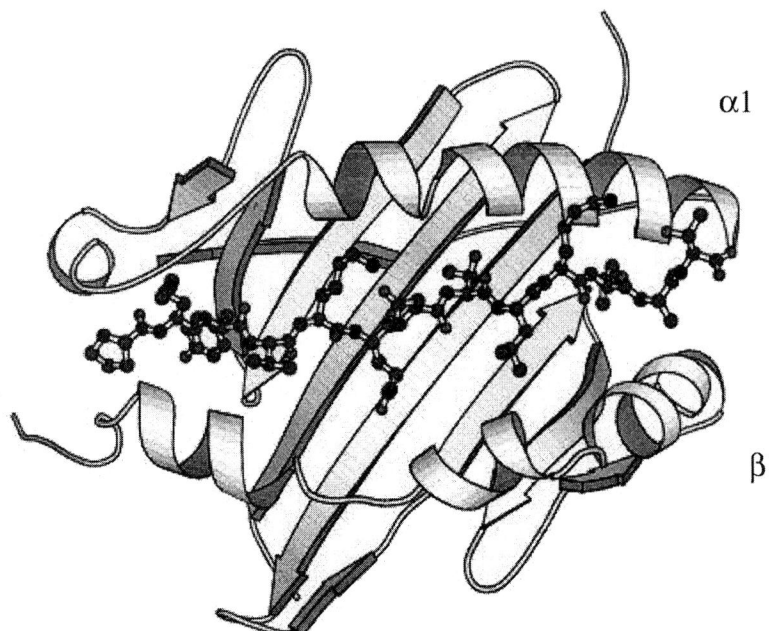

α1

β1

FIG. 5. Illustration of the structure of the peptide-binding domain (α1 and β1) of a class II MHC molecule (HLA-DR; protein data bank designation 1DLH) bound to an antigenic peptide from influenza hemagglutinin. Adapted by D.H. Margulies from Stern LJ et al., Crystal structure of the human class II MHC protein HLA-DR1 complexed with an influenza virus peptide, *Nature* 1994;368:215–221, with permission.

rather than by IgM, which is the dominant Ig of the primary response.

Division and differentiation of cells into antibody-secreting cells is largely controlled by the interaction of the activated B cells with T cells expressing CD154 and by their stimulation by T-cell–derived cytokines.

The differentiation of activated B cells into memory cells occurs in a specialized micro-environmental structure in the spleen and lymph nodes, the germinal center. The process through which increases in antibody affinity occurs also takes place within the germinal center. The latter process, designated *affinity maturation,* is dependent on somatic hypermutation. The survival of cells within the germinal center depends on the capacity to bind antigen so that as antigen availability diminishes, cells that have higher affinity receptors, either naturally or as a result of the hypermutation process, have a selective survival and growth advantage. Thus, such cells come to dominate the population.

The process through which a single H-chain V region can become expressed with genes encoding C regions other than μ and δ is referred to as Ig class switching. It is dependent on a gene translocation event through which the C-region genes between the genetic elements encoding the V region and the newly expressed C gene are excised, resulting in the switched C gene being located in the position that the Cμ gene formerly occupied (Fig. 3). This process also occurs in germinal centers.

B1 or CD5+ B-Lymphocytes (Chapter 6)

A second population of B cells (B1 cells) has been described that differs from the dominant B-cell population (sometimes designated B2 cells or conventional B cells) in several important respects. These cells were initially recognized because some express a cell-surface protein, CD5, not generally found on other B cells. In the adult mouse, B1 B cells are found in relatively high frequency in the peritoneal cavity but are present at low frequency in the spleen and lymph nodes. B1 B cells are quite numerous in fetal and perinatal life.

Whether B1 B cells derive from a separate set of stem cells found in the fetal liver but absent from (or present only at low frequency in) the adult bone marrow is still a matter of controversy. The alternative view is that B1 B cells are derived from conventional B cells as a result of cross-linkage–dependent B-cell activation. B1 B cells appear to be self-renewing, in contrast to conventional B cells, in which division and memory are antigen driven.

B1 B cells appear to be responsible for the secretion of the serum IgM that exists in nonimmunized mice, often referred to as natural IgM. Among the antibodies found in such "natural" IgM are molecules that can combine with phosphatidyl choline (a component of pneumococcal cell walls) and for lipopolysaccharide and influenza virus. B1 B cells also produce autoantibodies, although they are generally of low affinity and in most cases not pathogenic. It is believed that B1 B cells are important in resistance to several pathogens and may have a significant role in mucosal immunity.

B-Lymphocyte Tolerance (Chapter 29)

One of the central problems facing the immune system is that of being able to mount highly effective immune responses to the antigens of foreign, potentially pathogenic, agents while ignoring antigens associated with the host's own tissues. The mechanisms ensuring this failure to respond to self-antigens are complex and involve a series of strategies. Chief among them is elimination of cells capable of self-reactivity or the inactivation of such cells. The encounter of immature, naive B cells with antigens with repetitive epitopes capable of cross-linking membrane Ig can lead to elimination of the B cells, particularly if no T-cell help is provided at the time of the encounter. This elimination of potentially self-reactive cells is often referred to as clonal elimination. Some self-reactive cells, rather than dying upon encounter with self-antigens, may re-express the proteins needed for immunoglobulin gene rearrangement and undergo a further round of such rearrangement. This process, referred to as receptor editing, allows a self-reactive cell to substitute a new receptor and therefore to avoid elimination.

There are many self-antigens that are not encountered by the developing B-cell population or that do not have the capacity to cross-link B-cell receptors to a sufficient degree to elicit the clonal elimination/receptor editing process. Such cells, even when mature, may nonetheless be inactivated through a process that involves cross-linkage of receptors without the receipt of critical co-stimulatory signals. These inactivated cells may be retained in the body but are unresponsive to antigen and are referred to as anergic. When removed from the presence of the anergy-inducing stimulus, such cells may regain responsiveness.

Immunoglobulin Structure (Chapter 3)

The antigen-specific membrane receptors and secreted products of B cells are Ig molecules. Igs are members of a large family of proteins designated the immunoglobulin supergene family. Members of the Ig supergene family have sequence homology, a common gene organization, and similarities in

three-dimensional structure. The latter is characterized by a structural element referred to as the Ig fold, generally consisting of a set of seven β-pleated sheets organized into two apposing layers (Fig. 6). Many of the cell-surface proteins that participate in immunologic recognition processes, including the T-cell receptor (TCR), the CD3 complex, and molecules associated with the B-cell receptor (Igα and Igβ), are members of the Ig supergene family.

The Igs themselves are constructed of a unit that consists of two H chains and two L chains (Fig. 2). The H and L chains are composed of a series of domains, each consisting of approximately 110 amino acids.

The L chains, of which there are two types (κ and λ), consist of two domains. The carboxy-terminal domain is essentially identical among L chains of a given type and is referred to as the constant (C) region. As already discussed, the amino-terminal domain varies from L chain to L chain and contributes to the binding site of antibody. Because of its variability, it is referred to as the variable (V) region. The variability of this region is largely concentrated in three segments, designated as the hypervariable or complementarity-determining regions (CDRs). The CDRs contain the amino acids that are the L chain's contribution to the lining of the antibody's combining site. The three CDRs are interspersed among four regions of much lower degree of variability, designated framework regions (FRs).

The H chains of Ig molecules are of several classes (μ, δ, γ [of which there are several subclasses], α, and ε), as noted above. An assembled Ig molecule, consisting of one or more units of two identical H and L chains, derives its name from the H chain that it possesses. Thus, there are

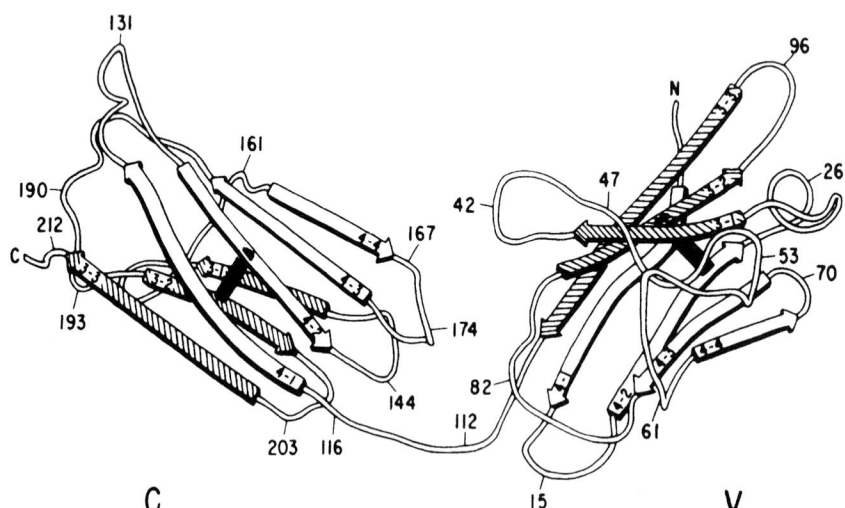

FIG. 6. Schematic drawing of the V and C domains of an Ig L chain illustrating the "Ig fold." The β strands participating in the antiparallel β-pleated sheets of each domain are represented as arrows. The β strands of the three-stranded sheets are shaded, whereas those in the four-stranded sheets are white. The intradomain disulfide bonds are represented as black bars. Selected amino acids are numbered with position 1 as the N terminus. From Edmundson AB, Ely KR, Abola EE, et al., Rotational allomerism and divergent evolution of domains in immunoglobulin light chains, *Biochemistry* 1975;14:3953–3961, with permission.

IgM, IgD, IgG, IgA, and IgE antibodies. The H chains each consist of a single amino-terminal V region and three or four C regions. In many H chains, a hinge region separates the first and second C regions and conveys flexibility to the molecule, allowing the two combining sites of a single unit to move in relation to one another so as to promote the binding of a single antibody molecule to an antigen that has more than one copy of the same epitope. Such divalent binding to a single antigenic structure results in a great gain in energy of interaction (see Chapter 4). The H-chain V region, like that of the L chain, contains three CDRs lining the combining site of the antibody and four FRs.

The C region of each H-chain class conveys unique functional attributes to the antibodies that possess it. Among the distinct biologic functions of each class of antibody are the following:

- IgM antibodies are potent activators of the complement system (Chapter 34).
- IgA antibodies are secreted into a variety of bodily fluids and are principally responsible for immunity at mucosal surfaces (Chapter 31).
- IgE antibodies are bound by specific receptors (FcϵRI) on basophils and mast cells. When cross-linked by antigen, these IgE/FcϵRI complexes cause the cells to release a set of mediators responsible for allergic inflammatory responses (Chapter 46).
- IgD antibodies act virtually exclusively as membrane receptors for antigen.
- IgG antibodies, made up of four subclasses in both humans and mice, mediate a wide range of functions including transplacental passage and opsonization of antigens through binding of antigen–antibody complexes to specialized Fc receptors on macrophages and other cell types (Chapters 22, 34, and 36).

IgD, IgG, and IgE antibodies consist of a single unit of two H and L chains. IgM antibodies are constructed of five or six such units, although they consist of a single unit when they act as membrane receptors. IgA antibodies may consist of one or more units. The antibodies that are made up of more than a single unit generally contain an additional polypeptide chain, the J chain, which plays an important role in the ability of these polymeric immunoglobulins to be secreted at mucosal surfaces.

Each of the distinct Igs can exist as secreted antibodies and as membrane molecules. Antibodies and cell-surface receptors of the same class made by a specific cell have identical structures except for differences in their carboxy-terminal regions. Membrane Ig possesses a hydrophobic region, spanning the membrane, and a short intracytoplasmic tail, both of which are lacking in the secretory form.

Immunoglobulin Genetics (Chapter 5)

The genetic makeup of the Ig H-chain gene has already been alluded to. The IgH-chain gene of a mature lymphocyte is derived from a set of genetic elements that are separated from one another in the germline. The V region is composed of three types of genetic elements: V_H, D, and J_H. More than 100 V_H elements exist; there are more than 10 D elements and a small number of J_H elements (4 in the mouse). An H-chain $V_H D J_H$ gene is created by the translocation of one of the D elements on a given chromosome to one of the J_H elements on that chromosome, generally with the excision of the intervening DNA. This is followed by a second translocation event in which one of the V_H elements is brought into apposition with the assembled $D J_H$ element to create the $V_H D J_H$ (V region) gene (Fig. 3). Although it is likely that the choice of the V_H, D, and J_H elements that are assembled is not entirely random, the combinatorial process allows the creation of a very large number of distinct H-chain V-region genes. Additional diversity is created by the imprecision of the joining events and by the deletion of nucleotides and addition of new, untemplated nucleotides between D and J_H and between V_H and D, forming N regions in these areas. This further increases the diversity of distinct IgH chains that can be generated from the relatively modest amount of genetic information present in the germline.

The assembly of L-chain genes follows generally similar rules. However, L chains are assembled from V_L and J_L elements only. Although there is junctional diversity, no N regions exist for L chains. Additional diversity is provided by the existence of two classes of L chains, κ and λ.

An Ig molecule is assembled by the pairing of IgH-chain polypeptide with an IgL-chain polypeptide. Although this process is almost certainly not completely random, it allows the formation of an exceedingly large number of distinct Ig molecules, the majority of which will have individual specificities.

The rearrangement events that result in the assembly of expressible IgH and IgL chains occur in the course of B-cell development in pro-B cells and pre-B cells, respectively (Fig. 1). This process is regulated by the Ig products of the rearrangement events. The formation of a μ chain signals the termination of rearrangement of H-chain gene elements and the onset of rearrangement of L-chain gene elements, with κ rearrangements generally preceding λ rearrangements. One important consequence of this is that only a single expressible μ chain will be produced in a given cell, since the first expressible μ chain shuts off the possibility of producing an expressible μ chain on the alternative chromosome. Comparable mechanisms exist to ensure that only one L-chain gene is produced, leading to the phenomenon known as allelic exclusion. Thus, the product of only one of the two alternative allelic regions at both the H- and L-chain loci are expressed. The closely related phenomenon of L-chain isotype exclusion ensures the production of either κ or λ chains in an individual cell, but not both. An obvious but critical consequence of allelic exclusion is that an individual B cell makes antibodies, all of which have identical H- and L-chain V regions, a central prediction of the clonal selection theory of the immune response.

Class Switching (Chapter 5)

An individual B cell can continue to express the same IgH-chain V region but, as it matures, can switch the IgH-chain C region that it uses (Fig. 3). Thus, a cell that expresses receptors of the IgM and IgD classes may differentiate into a cell that expresses IgG, IgA, or IgE receptors and then into a cell-secreting antibody of the same class as it expressed on the cell surface. This process allows the production of antibodies capable of mediating distinct biologic functions but that retain the same antigen-combining specificity. When linked with the process of affinity maturation of antibodies, Ig class switching provides antibodies of extremely high efficacy in preventing re-infection with microbial pathogens or in rapidly eliminating such pathogens. These two associated phenomena account for the high degree of effectiveness of antibodies produced in secondary immune responses.

The process of switching is known to involve a recombination event between specialized switch (S) regions, containing repetitive sequences, that are located upstream of each C region (with the exception of the δ C region). Thus, the S region upstream of the μ C_H region gene ($S\mu$) recombines with an S region upstream of a more 3' isotype, such as $S\gamma 1$, to create a chimeric $S\mu/S\gamma 1$ region resulting in the deletion of the intervening DNA (Fig. 7). The genes encoding the C regions of the various γ chains (in the human $\gamma 1$, $\gamma 2$, $\gamma 3$, and $\gamma 4$; in the mouse $\gamma 1$, $\gamma 2a$, $\gamma 2b$, and $\gamma 3$), of the α chain, and of the ϵ chain are located 3' of the $C\mu$ and $C\delta$ genes.

The induction of the switching process is dependent on the action of a specialized set of B-cell stimulants. Of these, the most widely studied are CD154, expressed on the surface of activated T cells, and bacterial lipopolysaccharide. The targeting of the C region that will be expressed as a result

of switching is largely determined by cytokines. Thus, IL-4 determines that switch events in the human and mouse will be to the ϵ C region and to the $\gamma 4$ (human) or $\gamma 1$ (mouse) C regions. In the mouse, interferon-gamma (IFN-γ) determines switching to $\gamma 2a$ and transforming growth factor-beta (TGF-β) determines switching to α. A major goal is to understand the physiologic determination of the specificity of the switching process. Because cytokines are often the key controllers of which Ig classes will represent the switched isotype, this logically translates into asking what regulates the relative amounts of particular cytokines that are produced by different modes of immunization.

The switching process depends on the RNA-editing, enzyme activation–induced cytidine deaminase (AID). Mice that lack AID fail to undergo immunoglobulin class switching. AID is also critical in the process of somatic hypermutation.

Affinity Maturation and Somatic Hypermutation (Chapter 5)

The process of generation of diversity embodied in the construction of the H- and L-chain V-region genes and of the pairing of H and L chains creates a large number of distinct antibody molecules, each expressed in an individual B cell. This primary repertoire is sufficiently large so that most epitopes on foreign antigens will encounter B cells with complementary receptors. Thus, if adequate T-cell help can be generated, antibody responses can be made to a wide array of foreign substances. Nonetheless, the antibody that is initially produced usually has a relatively low affinity for the antigen. This is partially compensated for by the fact that IgM, the antibody initially made, is a pentamer. Through multivalent binding, high avidities can be achieved even if individual combining sites have only modest affinity (see Chapter 4). In the course of T-cell–dependent B-cell stimulation, particularly within the germinal center, a process of somatic hypermutation is initiated that leads to a large number of mutational events, largely confined to the H-chain and L-chain V-region genes and their immediately surrounding introns.

During the process of somatic hypermutation, mutational rates of 1 per 1,000 base pairs per generation may be achieved. This implies that, with each cell division, close to one mutation will occur in either the H- or L-chain V region of an individual cell. This creates an enormous increase in antibody diversity. Although most of these mutations will either not affect the affinity with which the antibody binds its ligand or will lower that affinity, some will increase it. Thus, some B cells emerge that can bind antigen more avidly than the initial population of responding cells. Because there is an active process of apoptosis in the germinal center from which B cells can be rescued by the binding of antigen to their membrane receptors, cells with the most avid receptors should have an advantage over other antigen-specific B cells and should come to dominate the population of responding cells.

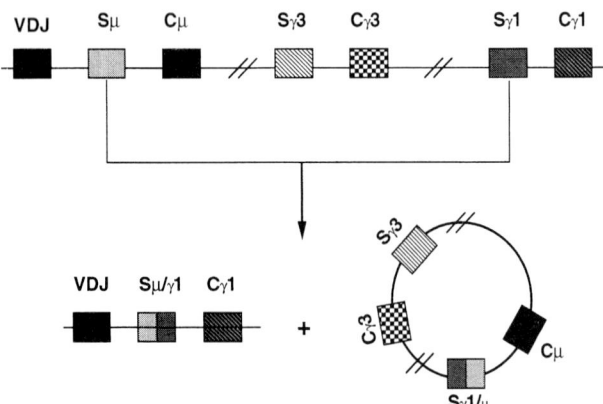

FIG. 7. Ig class switching. Illustrated here is the process through which a given VDJ gene in a stimulated B cell may switch the C-region gene with which it is associated from μ to another, such as $\gamma 1$. A recombination event occurs in which DNA between a cleavage point in $S\mu$ and one in $S\gamma 1$ forms a circular episome. This results in $C\gamma 1$ being located immediately downstream of the chimeric $S\mu/\gamma 1$ region, in a position such that transcription initiating upstream of VDJ results in the formation of VDJC$\gamma 1$ mRNA and $\gamma 1$ H-chain protein.

Thus, upon re-challenge, the affinity of antibody produced will be greater than that in the initial response. As time after immunization elapses, the affinity of antibody produced will increase. This process leads to the presence in immunized individuals of high-affinity antibodies that are much more effective, on a weight basis, in protecting against microbial agents and other antigen-bearing pathogens than was the antibody initially produced. Together with antibody class switching, affinity maturation results in the increased effectiveness of antibody in preventing re-infection with agents with which the individual has had a prior encounter.

T-LYMPHOCYTES

T-lymphocytes constitute the second major class of lymphocytes. They derive from precursors in hematopoietic tissue, undergo differentiation in the thymus (hence the name thymus-derived [T] lymphocytes), and are then seeded to the peripheral lymphoid tissue and to the recirculating pool of lymphocytes (see Chapter 14). T cells may be subdivided into two distinct classes based on the cell-surface receptors they express. The majority of T cells express antigen-binding receptors (TCRs) consisting of α and β chains. A second group of T cells express receptors made up of γ and δ chains. Among the α/β T cells are two important sublineages: those that express the co-receptor molecule CD4 (CD4+ T cells) and those that express CD8 (CD8+ T cells). These cells differ in how they recognize antigen and mediate different types of regulatory and effector functions.

CD4+ T cells are the major *helper* cells of the immune system. Their helper function depends both on cell-surface molecules such as CD154, induced upon these cells when they are activated, and on the wide array of cytokines they secrete when activated. CD4+ T cells tend to differentiate, as a consequence of priming, into cells that principally secrete the cytokines IL-4, IL-13, IL-5, IL-6, and IL-10 (T_{H2} cells) or into cells that mainly produce IL-2, IFN-γ, and lymphotoxin (T_{H1} cells). T_{H2} cells are very effective in helping B cells develop into antibody-producing cells, whereas T_{H1} cells are effective inducers of cellular immune responses, involving enhancement in the microbicidal activity of macrophages and consequent increased efficiency in lysing microorganisms in intracellular vesicular compartments.

T cells also mediate important effector functions. Some of these are determined by the patterns of cytokines they secrete. These powerful molecules can be directly toxic to target cells and can mobilize potent inflammatory mechanisms. In addition, T cells, particularly CD8+ T cells, can develop into cytotoxic T-lymphocytes (CTLs) capable of efficiently lysing target cells that express antigens recognized by the CTLs.

T-Lymphocyte Antigen Recognition (Chapters 8, 19, and 20)

T cells differ from B cells in their mechanism of antigen recognition. Immunoglobulin, the B-cell's receptor, binds to individual antigenic epitopes on soluble molecules or on particulate surfaces. B-cell receptors recognize epitopes expressed on the surface of native molecules. Antibody and B-cell receptors evolved to bind to and to protect against microorganisms in extracellular fluids.

By contrast, T cells invariably recognize cell-associated molecules and mediate their functions by interacting with and altering the behavior of these *antigen-presenting cells* (APCs). Indeed, the TCR does not recognize antigenic determinants on intact, undenatured molecules. Rather, it recognizes a complex consisting of a peptide, derived by proteolysis of the antigen, bound into a specialized groove of a class II or class I MHC protein. Indeed, what differentiates a CD4+ T cell from a CD8+ T cell is that the CD4+ T cells only recognize peptide/class II complexes, whereas the CD8+ T cells recognize peptide/class I complexes.

The TCR's ligand (i.e., the peptide/MHC protein complex) is created within the APC. In general, class II MHC molecules bind peptides derived from proteins that have been taken up by the APC through an endocytic process (Fig. 8). These endocytosed proteins are fragmented by proteolytic enzymes within the endosomal/lysosomal compartment, and the resulting peptides are loaded into class II MHC molecules that traffic through this compartment. These peptide-loaded, class II molecules are then expressed on the surface of the cell where they are available to be bound by CD4+ T cells with TCRs capable of recognizing the expressed cell-surface complex. Thus, CD4+ T cells are specialized to largely react with antigens derived from extracellular sources.

In contrast, class I MHC molecules are mainly loaded with peptides derived from internally synthesized proteins, such as viral gene products. These peptides are produced from cytosolic proteins by proteolysis within the proteasome and are translocated into the rough endoplasmic reticulum. Such peptides, generally nine amino acids in length, are bound by class I MHC molecules. The complex is brought to the cell surface, where it can be recognized by CD8+ T cells expressing appropriate receptors. This property gives the T-cell system, particularly CD8+ T cells, the ability to detect cells expressing proteins that are different from, or produced in much larger amounts than, those of cells of the remainder of the organism (e.g., viral antigens [whether internal, envelope, or cell surface] or mutant antigens [such as active oncogene products]), even if these proteins, in their intact form, are neither expressed on the cell surface nor secreted.

T-Lymphocyte Receptors (Chapter 8)

The TCR is a disulfide-linked heterodimer (Fig. 9). The constituent chains (α and β, or γ and δ) are members of the Ig supergene family. The TCR is associated with a set of transmembrane proteins, collectively designated the CD3 complex, that play a critical role in signal transduction. The CD3 complex consists of γ, δ (note that the CD3 γ and δ chains and the TCR γ and δ chains are distinct polypeptides that,

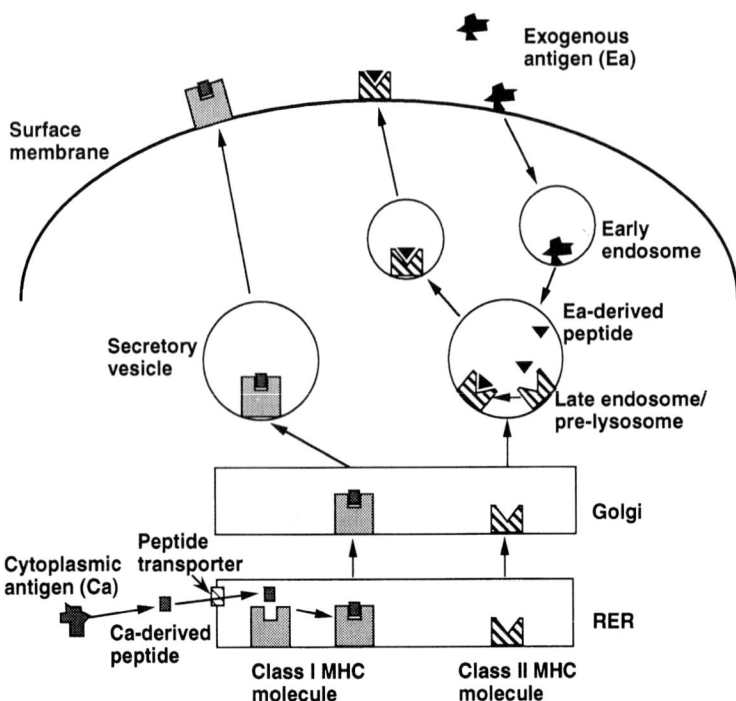

FIG. 8. Pathways of antigen processing. Exogenous antigen (Ea) enters the cell via endocytosis and is transported from early endosomes into late endosome or prelysosomes, where it is fragmented and where resulting peptides (Ea-derived peptides) may be loaded into class II MHC molecules. The latter have been transported from the rough endoplasmic reticulum (RER) through the Golgi apparatus to the peptide-containing vesicles. Class II MHC molecules/Ea-derived peptide complexes are then transported to the cell surface, where they may be recognized by TCR expressed on CD4+ T cells. Cytoplasmic antigens (Ca) are degraded in the cytoplasm and then enter the RER through a peptide transporter. In the RER, Ca-derived peptides are loaded into class I MHC molecules that move through the Golgi apparatus into secretory vesicles and are then expressed on the cell surface where they may be recognized by CD8+ T cells. From Paul WE, Development and function of lymphocytes, in Gallin JI, Goldstein I, Snyderman R, eds., *Inflammation*, New York: Raven, 1992, 776, with permission.

unfortunately, have similar designations), and ϵ chains, and is associated with a homodimer of two ζ chains or a heterodimer of ζ and η chains. CD3 γ, δ, and ϵ consist of extracellular domains that are family members of the Ig supergene. The cytosolic domains of CD3 γ, δ, and ϵ, and of

ζ and η, contain one or more copies of a signaling motif– the immunoreceptor tyrosine-based activation motif (ITAM) (D/ExxYxxLxxxxxxxYxxL/I)–that is found in a variety of chains associated with immune recognition receptors. This motif appears to be very important in the signal transduction process and provides a site through which protein tyrosine kinases can interact with these chains to propagate signaling events.

The TCR chains are organized much like Ig chains. Their N-terminal portions are variable and their C-terminal portions are constant. Furthermore, similar recombinational mechanisms are used to assemble the V-region genes of the TCR chains. Thus, the V region of the TCR β chain is encoded by a gene made of three distinct genetic elements (Vβ, D, and Jβ) that are separated in the germline. Although the relative numbers of Vβ, D, and Jβ genes differ from that for the comparable IgH variable-region elements, the strategies for creation of a very large number of distinct genes by combinatorial assembly are the same. Both junctional diversity and N-region addition further diversify the genes, and their encoded products. TCR β has fewer V genes than IgH but much more diversity centered on the D/J region, which encodes the equivalent of the third CDR of Igs. The α chain follows similar principles, except that it does not use a D gene.

The genes for TCR γ and δ chains are assembled in a similar manner except that they have many fewer V genes from which to choose. Indeed, γ/δ T cells in certain environments, such as the skin and specific mucosal surfaces, are exceptionally homogeneous. It has been suggested that the TCRs encoded by these essentially invariant γ and δ chains may

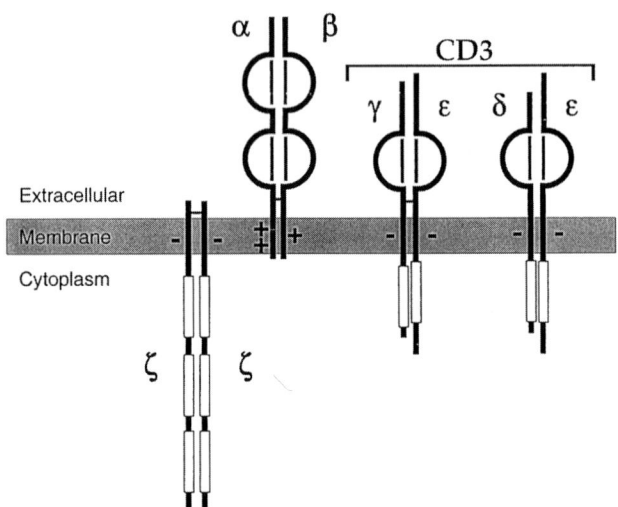

FIG. 9. The T-cell antigen receptor. Illustrated schematically is the antigen-binding subunit comprised of an $\alpha\beta$ heterodimer, and the associated invariant CD3 and ζ chains. Acidic (−) and basic (+) residues located within the plasma membrane are indicated. The open rectangular boxes indicate motifs within the cytoplasmic domains that interact with protein tyrosine kinases. (This figure also appears as in Chapter 11 as Fig. 2.)

be specific for some antigen that signals microbial invasion and that activation of γ/δ T cells through this mechanism constitutes an initial response that aids the development of the more sophisticated response of α/β T cells.

T-Lymphocyte Activation (Chapter 11)

T-cell activation is dependent on the interaction of the TCR/CD3 complex with its cognate ligand, a peptide bound in the groove of a class I or class II MHC molecule, on the surface of a competent antigen-presenting cell. Through the use of chimeric cell-surface molecules that possess cytosolic domains largely limited to the ITAM signaling motif alluded to above, it is clear that cross-linkage of molecules containing such domains can generate some of the signals that result from TCR engagement. Nonetheless, the molecular events set in motion by receptor engagement are complex ones. Among the earliest steps are the activation of tyrosine kinases leading to the tyrosine phosphorylation of a set of substrates that control several signaling pathways. Current evidence indicates that early events in this process involve the Src-family tyrosine kinases p56^{lck}, and p59^{fyn}, and ZAP-70, a Syk family tyrosine kinase, that binds to the phosphorylated ITAMs of the ζ chain, as well as the action of the protein tyrosine phosphatase CD45, found on the surface of all T cells.

A series of important substrates are tyrosine phosphorylated as a result of the action of the kinases associated with the TCR complex. These include (a) a set of adapter proteins that link the TCR to the Ras pathway; (b) phospholipase Cγ1, the tyrosine phosphorylation of which increases its catalytic activity and engages the inositol phospholipid metabolic pathway, leading to elevation of intracellular free-calcium concentration to the activation of protein, kinase C; and (c) a series of other important enzymes that control cellular growth and differentiation. Particularly important is the phosphorylation of LAT, a molecule that acts as an organizing scaffold to which a series of signaling intermediates bind and upon which they become activated and control downstream signaling.

The recognition and early activation events result in the reorganization of cell surface and cytosolic molecules on the T cell, and correspondingly, on the APC to produce a structure, the *immunological synapse*. The apposition of key interacting molecules involving a small segment of the membranes of the two cells concentrates these molecules in a manner that both strengthens the interaction between the cells and intensifies the signaling events. It also creates a limited space into which cytokines may be secreted to influence the behavior of cells. Indeed, the formation of the immunological synapse is one mechanism through which the recognition of relatively small numbers of ligands by TCRs on a specific T cell can be converted into a vigorous stimulatory process.

In general, normal T cells and cloned T-cell lines that are stimulated only by TCR cross-linkage fail to give complete responses. TCR engagement by itself may often lead to a response in which the key T-cell–derived growth factor, IL-2, is not produced and in which the cells enter a state of anergy such that they are unresponsive or poorly responsive to a subsequent competent stimulus (see Chapter 29). Full responsiveness of a T cell requires, in addition to receptor engagement, an accessory-cell–delivered co-stimulatory activity. The engagement of CD28 on the T cell by CD80 and/or CD86 on the APC (or the engagement of comparable ligand receptor pairs on the two cells) provides a potent co-stimulatory activity. Inhibitors of this interaction markedly diminish antigen-specific T-cell activation *in vivo* and *in vitro*, indicating that the CD80/86–CD28 interaction is physiologically very important in T-cell activation (see Chapter 13).

The interaction of CD80/86 with CD28 increases cytokine production by the responding T cells. For the production of IL-2, this increase appears to be mediated both by enhancing the transcription of the IL-2 gene and by stabilizing IL-2 mRNA. These dual consequences of the CD80/86–CD28 interaction cause a striking increase in the production of IL-2 by antigen-stimulated T cells.

CD80/86 has a second receptor on the T cell, CTLA-4, that is expressed later in the course of T-cell activation. The bulk of evidence indicates that the engagement of CTLA-4 by CD80/86 leads to a set of biochemical signals that terminate the T-cell response. Mice that are deficient in CTLA-4 expression develop fulminant autoimmune responses.

T-Lymphocyte Development (Chapter 9)

Upon entry into the thymus, T-cell precursors do not express TCR chains, the CD3 complex, or the CD4 or CD8 molecules (Fig. 10). Because these cells lack both CD4 and CD8, they are often referred to as double-negative (DN) cells. Thymocytes develop from this DN3 pool into cells that are both CD4+ and CD8+ (double-positive cells) and express low levels of TCR and CD3 on their surface. In turn, double-positive cells further differentiate into relatively mature thymocytes that express either CD4 or CD8 (single-positive cells) and high levels of the TCR/CD3 complex.

The expression of the TCR depends on complex rearrangement processes that generate TCR α and β (or γ and δ) chains. Once expressed, these cells undergo two important selection processes within the thymus. One, termed *negative selection,* is the deletion of cells that express receptors that bind with high affinity to complexes of self-peptides with self-MHC molecules. This is a major mechanism through which the T-cell compartment develops immunologic unresponsiveness to self-antigens (see Chapters 9 and 29). In addition, a second major selection process is *positive selection*, in which T cells with receptors with "intermediate affinity" for self-peptides bound to self-MHC molecules are selected, thus forming the basis of the T-cell repertoire for foreign peptides associated with self-MHC molecules. It appears that T cells that are not positively selected are eliminated in the thymic cortex

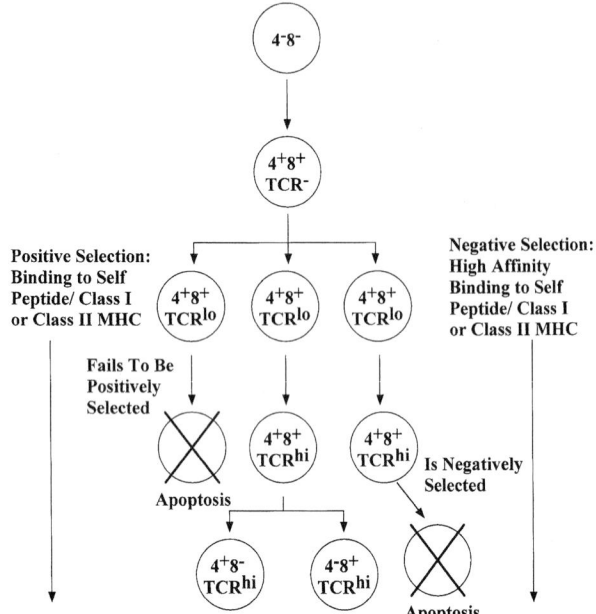

FIG. 10. Development of α/β T cells in the thymus. Double-negative T cells (4^-8^-) acquire CD4 and CD8 (4^+8^+) and then express α/β TCRs, initially at low levels. Thereafter, the degree of expression of TCRs increases and the cells differentiate into CD4 or CD8 cells and are then exported to the periphery. Once the T cells have expressed receptors, their survival depends on the recognition of peptide/MHC class I or class II molecules with an affinity above some given threshold. Cells that fail to do so undergo apoptosis. These cells have failed to be *positively selected*. Positive selection is associated with the differentiation of 4^+8^+ cells into CD4 or CD8 cells. Positive selection involving peptide/class I MHC molecules leads to the development of CD8 cells, whereas positive selection involving peptide/class II MHC molecules leads to the development of CD4 cells. If a T cell recognizes a peptide/MHC complex with high affinity, it is also eliminated via apoptosis (it is *negatively selected*).

by apoptosis. Similarly, T cells that are negatively selected as a result of high-affinity binding to self-peptide/self-MHC complexes are also deleted through apoptotic death. These two selection processes result in the development of a population of T cells that are biased toward the recognition of peptides in association with self-MHC molecules from which those cells that are potentially auto-reactive (capable of high-affinity binding of self-peptide/self-MHC complexes) have been purged.

One important event in the development of T cells is their differentiation from double-positive cells into CD4+ or CD8+ single-positive cells. This process involves the interaction of double-positive thymocytes with peptide bound to class II or class I MHC molecules on accessory cells. Indeed, CD4 binds to monomorphic sites on class II molecules, whereas CD8 binds to comparable sites on class I molecules. The capacity of the TCR and CD4 (or of the TCR and CD8) to bind to a class II MHC (or a class I MHC) molecule on an accessory cell leads either to the differentiation of double-

positive thymocytes into CD4+ (or CD8+) single-positive T cells or to the selection of cells that have "stochastically" differentiated down the CD4 (or CD8) pathway.

Less is understood about the differentiation of thymocytes that express TCRs composed of γ/δ chains. These cells fail to express either CD4 or CD8. However, γ/δ cells are relatively numerous early in fetal life; this, together with their limited degree of heterogeneity, suggests that they may comprise a relatively primitive T-cell compartment.

T-Lymphocyte Functions (Chapter 10)

T cells mediate a wide range of immunologic functions. These include the capacity to help B cells develop into antibody-producing cells, the capacity to increase the microbicidal action of monocyte/macrophages, the inhibition of certain types of immune responses, direct killing of target cells, and mobilization of the inflammatory response. In general, these effects depend on their expression of specific cell-surface molecules and the secretion of cytokines.

T Cells That Help Antibody Responses (Chapter 10)

Helper T cells can stimulate B cells to make antibody responses to proteins and other T-cell–dependent antigens. T-cell–dependent antigens are immunogens in which individual epitopes appear only once or only a limited number of times so that they are unable to cross-link the membrane Ig of B cells or do so inefficiently. B cells bind antigen through their membrane Ig, and the complex undergoes endocytosis. Within the endosomal and lysosomal compartments, antigen is fragmented into peptides by proteolytic enzymes and one or more of the generated peptides are loaded into class II MHC molecules, which traffic through this vesicular compartment. The resulting complex of class II MHC molecule and bound peptide is exported to the B-cell surface membrane. T cells with receptors specific for the peptide/class II molecular complex recognize that complex on the B cell.

B-cell activation depends not only on the binding of peptide/class II MHC complexes on the B cell surface by the TCR but also on the interaction of T-cell CD154 with CD40 on the B cell. T cells do not constitutively express CD154; rather, it is induced as a result of an interaction with an activated APC that expresses a cognate antigen recognized by the TCR of the T cell. Furthermore, CD80/86 are generally expressed by activated but not resting B cells so that interactions involving resting B cells and naïve T cells generally do not lead to efficient antibody production. By contrast, a T cell already activated and expressing CD154 can interact with a resting B cell, leading to its up-regulation of CD80/86 and to a more productive T-cell/B-cell interaction with the delivery of cognate help and the development of the B cell into an antibody-producing cell. Similarly, activated B cells expressing large amounts of class II molecules and CD80/86 can act as effective APC and can participate with T cells in efficient cognate help interactions. Cross-linkage of membrane Ig on the B cell, even if inefficient, may synergize with the CD154/CD40 interaction to yield vigorous B-cell activation.

The subsequent events in the B-cell response program, including proliferation, Ig secretion, and class switching either depend on or are enhanced by the actions of T-cell–derived cytokines. Thus, B-cell proliferation and Ig secretion are enhanced by the actions of several type I cytokines including IL-2 and IL-4. Ig class switching is dependent both on the initiation of competence for switching, which can be induced by the CD154/CD40 interaction, and on the targeting of particular C regions for switching, which is determined, in many instances, by cytokines. The best-studied example of this is the role of IL-4 in determining switching to IgG1 and IgE in the mouse and to IgG4 and IgE in the human. Indeed, the central role of IL-4 in the production of IgE is demonstrated by the fact that mice that lack the IL-4 gene or the gene for the IL-4 receptor α chain, as a result of homologous recombination-mediated gene knockouts, have a marked defect in IgE production.

Although CD4+ T cells with the phenotype of T_{H2} cells (i.e., IL-4, IL-13, IL-5, IL-6, and IL-10 producers) are efficient helper cells, T_{H1} cells also have the capacity to act as helpers. Because T_{H1} cells produce IFN-γ, which acts as a switch factor for IgG2a in the mouse, T_{H1}-mediated help often is dominated by the production of IgG2a antibodies.

Induction of Cellular Immunity (Chapter 10)

T cells also may act to enhance the capacity of monocytes and macrophages to destroy intracellular microorganisms. In particular, IFN-γ enhances several mechanisms through which mononuclear phagocytes destroy intracellular bacteria and parasites, including the generation of nitric oxide and induction of tumor necrosis factor (TNF) production. T_{H1}-type cells are particularly effective in enhancing microbicidal action because they produce IFN-γ. By contrast, two of the major cytokines produced by T_{H2} cells, IL-4 and IL-10, block these activities. Thus, T_{H2} cells often oppose the action of T_{H1} cells in inducing cellular immunity and in certain infections with microorganisms that are intracellular pathogens of macrophages, a T_{H2}-dominated response may be associated with failure to control the infection.

Regulatory T Cells (Chapter 30)

There has been a longstanding interest in the capacity of T cells to diminish as well as to help immune responses. Cells that mediate such effects are referred to as regulatory or suppressor T cells. Regulatory T cells may be identified by their constitutive expression of CD25, the IL-2 receptor alpha chain. These cells inhibit the capacity of both CD4 and CD8 T cells to respond to their cognate antigens. The mechanisms through which their suppressor function is mediated are still somewhat controversial. In some instances, it appears that cell–cell contact is essential for suppression,

whereas in other circumstances production of cytokines by the regulatory cells has been implicated in their ability to inhibit responses. Evidence has been presented for both IL-10 and TGFβ as mediators of inhibition.

Regulatory T cells have been particularly studied in the context of various autoimmune conditions. In the absence of regulatory cells, conventional T cells cause several types of autoimmune responses, including autoimmune gastritis and inflammatory bowel disease. Regulatory T cells express cell-surface receptors allowing them to recognize autoantigens and their responses to such recognition results in the suppression of responses by conventional T cells. Whether the T-cell receptor repertoire of the regulatory cells and the conventional T cells are the same has not been fully determined, nor it is completely clear whether regulatory (CD25+) T cells and conventional T cells derive from distinct T-cell lineages or whether regulatory T cells derive from conventional CD4+ T cells that may have been stimulated under certain conditions.

Cytotoxic T Cells (Chapter 36)

One of the most striking actions of T cells is the lysis of cells expressing specific antigens. Most cells with such cytotoxic activity are CD8+ T cells that recognize peptides derived from proteins produced within the target cell, bound to class I MHC molecules expressed on the surface of the target cell. However, CD4+ T cells can express CTL activity, although in such cases the antigen recognized is a peptide associated with a class II MHC molecule; often such peptides derive from exogenous antigens.

There are two major mechanisms of cytotoxicity. One involves the production by the CTL of perforin, a molecule that can insert into the membrane of target cells and promote the lysis of that cell. Perforin-mediated lysis is enhanced by a series of enzymes produced by activated CTLs, referred to as granzymes. Many active CTLs also express large amounts of Fas ligand on their surface. The interaction of Fas ligand on the surface of the CTL with Fas on the surface of the target cell initiates apoptosis in the target cell.

CTL-mediated lysis is a major mechanism for the destruction of virally infected cells. If activated during the period in which the virus is in its eclipse phase, CTLs may be capable of eliminating the virus and curing the host with relatively limited cell destruction. On the other hand, vigorous CTL activity after a virus has been widely disseminated may lead to substantial tissue injury because of the large number of cells that are killed by the action of the CTLs. Thus, in many infections, the disease is caused by the destruction of tissue by CTLs rather than by the virus itself. One example is hepatitis B, in which much of the liver damage represents the attack of HBV-specific CTLs on infected liver cells.

It is usually observed that CTLs that have been induced as a result of a viral infection or intentional immunization must be reactivated *in vitro* through the recognition of antigen on the target cell. This is particularly true if some interval has elapsed between the time of infection or immunization and the time of test. This has led to some question being raised as to the importance of CTL immunity in protection against re-infection and how important CTL generation is in the long-term immunity induced by protective vaccines. On the other hand, in active infections, such as seen in HIV+ individuals, CTL that can kill their targets cells immediately are often seen. There is much evidence to suggest that these cells play an active role in controlling the number of HIV+ T cells.

CYTOKINES (Chapters 23, 24, 25, and 26)

Many of the functions of cells of the immune system are mediated through the production of a set of small proteins referred to as cytokines. These proteins can now be divided into several families. They include the type I cytokines or hematopoietins that encompass many of the interleukins (i.e., IL-2, IL-3, IL-4, IL-5, IL-6, IL-7, IL-9, IL-11, IL-12, IL-13, IL-15, IL-21 and IL-23), as well as several hematopoietic growth factors; the type II cytokines, including the interferons and IL-10; the TNF-related molecules, including TNF, lymphotoxin, and Fas ligand; Ig superfamily members, including IL-1 and IL-18; and the chemokines, a growing family of molecules playing critical roles in a wide variety of immune and inflammatory functions.

Many of the cytokines are T-cell products; their production represents one of the means through which the wide variety of functions of T cells are mediated. Most cytokines are not constitutive products of the T cell. Rather, they are produced in response to T-cell activation, usually resulting from presentation of antigen to T cells by APCs in concert with the action of a co-stimulatory molecule, such as the interaction of CD80/86 with CD28. Although cytokines are produced in small quantities, they are very potent, binding to their receptors with equilibrium constants of approximately 10^{10} M^{-1}. In some instances, cytokines are directionally secreted into the immunological synapse formed between a T cell and an APC. In such cases, the cytokine acts in a paracrine manner. Indeed, many cytokines have limited action at a distance from the cell that produced them. This appears to be particularly true of many of the type I cytokines. However, other cytokines act by diffusion through extracellular fluids and blood to target cells that are distant from the producers. Among these are cytokines that have pro-inflammatory effects, such as IL-1, IL-6, and TNF, and the chemokines, which play important roles in regulating the migration of lymphocytes and other cell types.

Chemokines (Chapter 26)

A large family of small proteins that are *chemotactic cytokines* (chemokines) have been described. While members of this family have a variety of functions, perhaps the most dramatic is their capacity to regulate leukocyte migration and thus to act as critical dynamic organizers of cell distribution in the immune and inflammatory responses. The receptors for chemokines are seven transmembrane-spanning, G-protein coupled receptors.

The chemokines are subdivided based on the number and positioning of their highly conserved cysteines. Among chemokines with four conserved cysteines, the cysteines are adjacent in one large group (the CC chemokines) while in a second large group they are separated by one amino acid (CXC chemokines). There are also rare chemokines in which the cysteins are separated by three amino acids (CX3C) or in which there are only two conserved cysteins (C chemokines).

Individual chemokines may signal through more than one chemokine recptor and individual receptors may interact with more than one chemokine, producing a very complex set of chemokine/chemokine receptor pairs and providing opportunities for exceedingly fine regulation of cellular functions.

THE MAJOR HISTOCOMPATIBILITY COMPLEX AND ANTIGEN PRESENTATION (Chapters 19 and 20)

The MHC has already been introduced in this chapter in the discussion of T-cell recognition of antigen-derived peptides bound to specialized grooves in class I and class II MHC proteins. Indeed, the class I and class II MHC molecules are essential to the process of T-cell recognition and response. Nonetheless, they were first recognized not for this reason but because of the dominant role that MHC class I and class II proteins play in transplantation immunity (see Chapter 47).

When the genetic basis of transplantation rejection between mice of distinct inbred strains was sought, it was recognized that although multiple genetic regions contributed to the rejection process, one region played a dominant role. Differences at this region alone would cause prompt graft rejection, whereas any other individual difference usually resulted in a slow rejection of foreign tissue. For this reason, the genetic region responsible for prompt graft rejection was termed the major histocompatibility complex.

In all higher vertebrates that have been thoroughly studied, a comparable MHC exists. The defining features of the MHC are the transplantation antigens that it encodes. These are the class I and class II MHC molecules. The genes encoding these molecules show an unprecedented degree of polymorphism. This together with their critical role in antigen presentation explains their central role as the target of the immune responses leading to the rejection of organ and tissue allografts.

The MHC also includes other genes, particularly genes for certain complement components. In addition, genes for the cytokines TNF-α and lymphotoxin (also designated TNF-β) are found in the MHC.

Class I MHC Molecules (Chapter 19)

Class I MHC molecules are membrane glycoproteins expressed on most cells. They consist of an α chain of approximately 45,000 daltons noncovalently associated with β2-microglobulin, a 12,000-dalton molecule (Fig. 11). The gene for the α chain is encoded in the MHC, whereas that for β2-microglobulin is not. Both the α chain and β2-microglobulin are Ig supergene family members. The α chain is highly polymorphic, with the polymorphisms found mainly in the regions that constitute the binding sites for antigen-derived peptides and the contact sites for the TCR.

The class I α chain consists of three extracellular regions or domains, each of similar length, designated α1, α2, and α3. In addition, α chains have a membrane-spanning domain and a short carboxy-terminal cytoplasmic tail. The crystal structure of class I molecules indicates that the α1 and α2 domains form a site for the binding of peptides derived from antigens. This site is defined by a floor consisting of β sheets and bounded by α-helical walls. The polymorphisms of the class I molecule are mainly in these areas.

In the human, three loci encoding classical class I molecules have been defined; these are designated HLA-A, HLA-B, and HLA-C. All display high degrees of polymorphism. A similar situation exists in the mouse. In addition, there are a series of genes, defined principally in the mouse, that encode class I–like molecules (class Ib molecules). Recently, some of these also have been shown to have antigen-presenting activity for formylated peptides,

suggesting that they may be specialized to present certain prokaryotic antigens. In addition, the class Ib molecule CD1 has been shown to have antigen-presenting function for mycobacterial lipids, providing a mechanism through which T cells specific for such molecules can be generated. In the mouse, α-galactosylceramide bound to CD1 is recognized by a novel class of T cells (NK T cells) that produce large amounts of cytokines upon stimulation.

Class II MHC Molecules (Chapter 19)

Class II MHC molecules are heterodimeric membrane glycoproteins. Their constituent chains are designated α and β; both chains are immunoglobulin supergene family members, and both are encoded within the MHC. Each chain consists of two extracellular domains (α1 and α2; β1 and β2, respectively), a hydrophobic domain, and a short cytoplasmic segment. The overall conformation of class II MHC molecules appears to be quite similar to that of class I molecules. The peptide-binding site of the class II molecules is contributed to by the α1 and β1 domains (Fig. 5); it is within these domains that the majority of the polymorphic residues of class II molecules are found.

A comparison of the three-dimensional structures of class I and class II molecules indicates certain distinctive features that explain differences in the length of peptides that the two types of MHC molecules can bind. Class I molecules generally bind peptides with a mean length of nine amino acids, whereas class II molecules can bind substantially larger peptides.

In the mouse, class II MHC molecules are encoded by genes within the I region of the MHC. These molecules are often referred to as I region—associated (Ia) antigens. Two sets of class II molecules exist, designated I-A and I-E, respectively. The α and β chains of the I-A molecules (Aα and Aβ) pair with one another, as do the α and β chains of I-E (Eα and Eβ). In general, cross-pairing between I-A and I-E chains does not occur, although exceptions have been described. In heterozygous mice, α and β chains encoded on alternative chromosomes (i.e., Aα^b and Aβ^k) may cross-pair so that heterozygous mice can express both parental and hybrid class II molecules. However, the degree of cross-pairing is allele specific; not all hybrid pairs are formed with equal efficiency.

In the human, there are three major sets of class II molecules, encoded in the DR, DQ, and DP regions of the HLA complex.

Class II molecules have a more restricted tissue distribution than do class I molecules. Class II molecules are found on B cells, dendritic cells, epidermal Langerhans cells, macrophages, thymic epithelial cells, and, in the human, activated T cells. Levels of class II molecule expression are regulated in many cell types by interferons and in B cells by IL-4. Indeed, interferons can cause expression of class II molecules on many cell types that normally lack these cell-surface molecules. Interferons also can cause striking

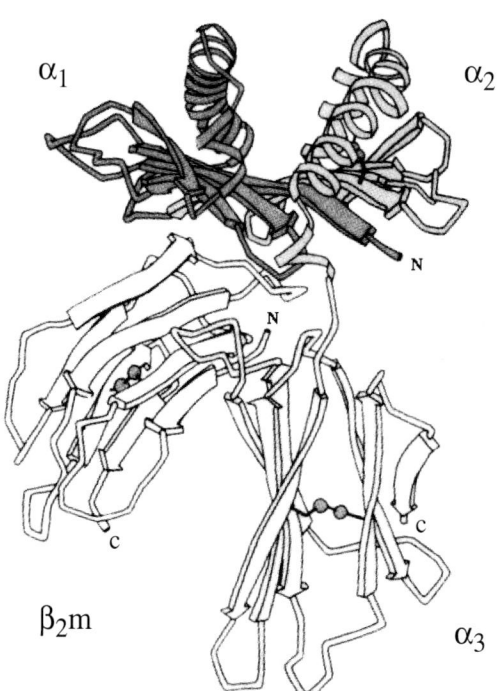

α_1 α_2

β_2m α_3

FIG. 11. Model of the class I IILA-A2 molecule. A schematic representation of the structure of the HLA-A2, class I MHC molecule. The polymorphic α1 and α2 domains are at the top. They form a groove into which antigen-derived peptides fit to form the peptide/MHC class I complex that is recognized by TCRs of CD8+ T cells. From Bjorkman PJ, Saper MA, Sauraomi B, et al., Structure of human class-I histocompatibility HLA-A. *Nature* 1987;329:506–512, with permission.

up-regulation in the expression of class I MHC molecules. Thus, immunologically mediated inflammation may result in aberrant expression of class II MHC molecules and heightened expression of class I molecules. Such altered expression of MHC molecules can allow cells that do not normally function as APCs for CD4+ T cells to do so and enhances the sensitivity of such cells to CD8+ T cells. This has important consequences for immunopathologic responses and for autoimmunity.

Antigen Presentation (Chapter 20)

As already discussed, the function of class I and class II MHC molecules is to bind and present antigen-derived peptides to T cells whose receptors can recognize the peptide/MHC complex that is generated. There are two major types of antigen-processing pathways, specialized to deal with distinct classes of pathogens that the T cell system must confront (Fig. 8).

Extracellular bacteria and extracellular proteins enter APCs by endocytosis or phagocytosis. Their antigens and the antigens of bacteria that live within endosomes or lysosomes are fragmented in these organelles and peptides derived from the antigen are loaded into class II MHC molecules as these proteins traverse the vesicular compartments in which the peptides are found. The loading of peptide is important in stabilizing the structure of the class II MHC molecule. The acidic pH of the compartments in which loading occurs facilitates the loading process. However, once the peptide-loaded class II molecules reaches neutral pH, such as at the cell surface, the peptide/MHC complex is stable. Peptide dissociation from such class II molecules is very slow, with a half-time measured in hours. The peptide/class II complex is recognized by T cells of the CD4 class with complementary receptors. As already pointed out, the specialization of CD4+ T cells to recognize peptide/class II complexes is due to the affinity of the CD4 molecule for monomorphic determinants on class II molecules. Obviously, this form of antigen processing can only apply to cells that express class II MHC molecules. Indeed, APCs for CD4+ T cells principally include cells that normally express class II MHC molecules, including dendritic cells, B cells, and macrophages.

T cells also can recognize proteins that are produced within the cell that presents the antigen. The major pathogens recognized by this means are viruses and other obligate intracellular (nonendosomal/lysosomal) microbes that have infected cells. In addition, proteins that are unique to tumors, such as mutant oncogenes, or are overexpressed in tumors also can be recognized by T cells. Endogenously produced proteins are fragmented in the cytosol by the proteases in the proteasome. The resultant peptides are transported into the rough endoplasmic reticulum, through the action of a specialized transport system. These peptides are then available for loading into class I molecules. In contrast to the loading of class II molecules, which is facilitated by the acid pH of the loading environment, the loading of class I

molecules is controlled by interaction of the class I α chain with β2-microglobulin. Thus, the bond between peptide and class I molecule is generally weak in the absence of β2-microglobulin, and the binding of β2-microglobulin strikingly stabilizes the complex. (Similarly, the binding of β2-microglobulin to the α chain is markedly enhanced by the presence of peptide in the α chain groove.) The peptide-loaded class I molecule is then brought to the cell surface. In contrast to peptide-loaded class II molecules, that are recognized by CD4+ T cells, peptide-loaded class I molecules are recognized by CD8+ T cells. This form of antigen processing and presentation can be performed by virtually all cells because, with a few exceptions, class I MHC molecules are universally expressed.

Although the specialization of class I molecules to bind and present endogenously produced peptides and of class II molecules to bind and present peptides derived from exogenous antigens is generally correct, there are exceptions, many of which have physiologic importance. Particularly important is the re-presentation by class II+ cells of antigens derived from class II− cells.

T-Lymphocyte Recognition of Peptide/MHC Complexes Results in MHC-Restricted Recognition (Chapter 8)

Before the biochemical nature of the interaction between antigen-derived peptides and MHC molecules was recognized, it was observed that T-cell responses displayed *MHC-restricted antigen recognition*. Thus, if individual animals were primed to a given antigen, their T cells would be able to recognize and respond to that antigen only if the APCs that presented the antigen shared MHC molecules with the animal that had been immunized. The antigen would not be recognized when presented by APCs of an allogeneic MHC type. This can now be explained by the fact that the TCR recognizes the peptide bound to an MHC molecule. MHC molecules display high degrees of polymorphism, and this polymorphism is concentrated in the regions of the class I and class II molecules that interact with the peptide and that can bind to the TCR. Differences in structure of the MHC molecules derived from different individuals (or different inbred strains of mice) profoundly affect the recognition process. Two obvious explanations exist to account for this. First, the structure of the grooves in different class I or class II MHC molecules may determine that a different range of peptides are bound or, even if the same peptide is bound, may change the conformation of the surface of the peptide presented to the TCR. Second, polymorphic sites on the walls of the α-helices that are exposed to the TCR can either enhance or diminish binding of the whole complex, depending on their structure. Thus, priming an individual with a given antigen on APCs that are syngeneic to the individual will elicit a response by T cells whose TCRs are specific for a complex consisting of a peptide derived from the antigen and the exposed polymorphic residues of the MHC molecule. When the same antigen is used with APCs of different MHC types, it is unlikely that the same peptide/MHC surface can be formed, and thus the primed T cells are not likely to bind and respond to such stimulation.

Indeed, this process also occurs within the thymus in the generation of the T-cell repertoire, as already discussed. T cells developing within the thymus undergo a positive selection event in which those T cells capable of recognizing MHC molecules displayed within the thymus are selected (and the remainder undergo programmed cell death). This leads to the skewing of the population of T cells that emerges from the thymus so that the cells are specialized to respond to peptides on self-MHC molecules. One of the unsolved enigmas of positive selection within the thymus is how the vast array of T cells with receptors capable of reacting with a very large set of foreign peptides associated with self-MHC molecules are chosen by self-MHC molecules that can only display self-peptides. It is believed that a high degree of cross-reactivity may exist so that T cells selected to bind a given class I (or class II) molecule plus a particular self-peptide can also bind a set of other (foreign) peptides bound to the same MHC molecule.

Furthermore, the affinity of an interaction required for positive selection in the thymus appears to be considerably lower that that required for full activation of peripheral T cells. Thus, thymocytes selected by a given self-peptide/self-MHC complex will generally not mount a full response when they encounter the same peptide/MHC complex in the periphery, although they will respond to a set of foreign peptide/MHC complexes to which they bind with higher affinity. Recognition of the self-peptide/self-MHC complex in the periphery may nonetheless have important consequences, such as sustaining the viability of resting lymphocytes.

Our modern understanding of T-cell recognition also aids in explaining the phenomenon of immune response (Ir) gene control of specific responses. In many situations, the capacity to recognize simple antigens can be found in only some members of a species. In most such cases, the genes that determine the capacity to make these responses have been mapped to the MHC. We would now explain Ir gene control of immune responses based on the capacity of different class II MHC molecules (or class I MHC molecules) to bind different sets of peptides. Thus, for simple molecules, it is likely that peptides can be generated that are only capable of binding to some of the polymorphic MHC molecules of the species. Only individuals that possess those allelic forms of the MHC will be able to respond to those antigens. Based on this, some individuals are nonresponders because of the failure to generate a peptide/MHC molecule complex that can be recognized by the T-cell system.

This mechanism also may explain the linkage of MHC type with susceptibility to various diseases. Many diseases show a greater incidence in individuals of a given MHC type. These include reactive arthritides, gluten-sensitive enteropathy, insulin-dependent diabetes mellitus, and rheumatoid arthritis (see Chapters 44 and 45). One explanation is that the MHC type that is associated with increased incidence

may convey altered responsiveness to antigens of agents that cause or exacerbate the disease. Indeed, it appears that many of these diseases may be due to enhanced or inappropriate immune responses.

Antigen-Presenting Cells (Chapter 15)

T cells recognize peptide/MHC complexes on the surface of other cells. Such cells are often referred to as antigen-presenting cells (APCs). Although effector cells can mediate their functions by recognizing such complexes on virtually any cell type, naïve cells are most efficiently activated by a set of specialized APCs, the dendritic cells (DCs). DCs are a multimember family whose complexity is only now being worked out. Both the common myeloid precursor and the common lymphoid precursor can give rise to immature DCs. In humans, there are two types of immature myeloid DCs emerging from the common myeloid precursor, CD11c+, CD14+ cells and CD11C+, CD14− cells. These cells become interstitial DCs and Langerhans cells. Common myeloid precursors also give rise to monocytes and plasmacytoid cells, which can act as DC precursors in the tissues. DCs can also arise from common lymphoid precursors. In the mouse, this has been demonstrated *in vivo*; in the human, *in vitro*.

In general, in their immature form, DCs are resident in the tissues where they are efficient at capturing and endocytosing antigen. Their antigen capture activity is dependent upon expression of several surface receptors including Fc receptors, receptors for heat shock proteins, and C-type lectins. If they receive signals, such as various inflammatory stimuli, often mediated by TLRs, they are stimulated to down-regulate the expression of these molecules but to increase their expression of surface MHC molecules and various co-stimulatory molecules such as CD80/86. In addition, such stimulation induces expression of chemokine receptors such as CCR2 and CCR7. The latter allows cells to follow signals from the chemokines SLC and ELC and to migrate into the T-cell zone of lymph nodes. As part of the maturation process, they may also acquire the capacity to produce cytokines that can aid in determining the polarization of T-cell priming. This includes the production of IL-12 p70 and the production of IFNγ itself. Such cells are highly efficient at priming naïve cells to develop into TH1 cells. Other sets of DCs have been reported to favor TH2 development and interaction of developing T cells with immature DCs may induce a state of peripheral tolerance.

One important function of DCs is the ability to acquire antigen from virally infected cells and to *cross-present* it through the class I pathway. This allows DCs to aid in the priming of precursors of cytotoxic T cells specific for viruses that do not infect the DCs themselves.

EFFECTOR MECHANISMS OF IMMUNITY

The ultimate purpose of the immune system is to mount responses that protect the individual against infections with pathogenic microorganisms by eliminating these microbes or, where it is not possible to eliminate infection, to control their spread and virulence. In addition, the immune system may play an important role in the control of the development and spread of some malignant tumors. The responses that actually cause the destruction of the agents that initiate these pathogenic states (e.g., bacteria, viruses, parasites, and tumor cells) are collectively the effector mechanisms of the immune system. Several have already been alluded to. Among them are the cytotoxic action of CTLs, which leads to the destruction of cells harboring viruses and, in some circumstances, expressing tumor antigens. In some cases, antibody can be directly protective by neutralizing determinants essential to a critical step through which the pathogen establishes or spreads an infectious process. However, in most cases, the immune system mobilizes powerful nonspecific mechanisms to mediate its effector function.

Effector Cells of the Immune Response

Among the cells that mediate important functions in the immune system are cells of the monocyte/macrophage lineage, NK cells, mast cells, basophils, eosinophils, and neutrophils. It is beyond the scope of this introductory chapter to present an extended discussion of each of these important cell types. However, a brief mention of some of their actions will help in understanding their critical functions in the immune response.

Monocytes and Macrophages (Chapter 16)

Cells of the monocyte/macrophage lineage play a central role in immunity. One of the key goals of cellular immunity is to aid the macrophages in eliminating organisms that have established such intracellular infections. In general, nonactivated macrophages are inefficient in destroying intracellular microbes. However, the production of IFN-γ and other mediators by T cells can enhance the capacity of macrophages to eliminate such microorganisms. Several mechanisms exist for this purpose, including the development of reactive forms of oxygen, the development of nitric oxide, and the induction of a series of proteolytic enzymes, as well as the induction of cytokine production. Macrophages can act as APCs and thus can enlist the "help" of activated, cytokine-producing CD4+ T cells in regulating their function.

Although macrophages function as APCs for attracting activated T cells, they do not appear to be particularly effective in the activation of naïve CD4 T cells. In instances in which they are the site of infection or have phagocytosed infectious agents or their proteins, antigens from these agents may be transferred to dendritic cells. In such cases the dendritic cells would be the principal antigen-presenting cells that activate naïve or possibly resting-memory CD4 T cells. This process is often described as cross-presentation. Such activated T cells would then be available to help infected macrophages.

Natural Killer Cells (Chapter 12)

Natural killer cells play an important role in the immune system. Indeed, in mice that lack mature T and B cells due to the *SCID* mutation, the NK system appears to be highly active and to provide these animals a substantial measure of protection against infection. NK cells are closely related to T cells. They lack conventional TCR (or Ig) but express two classes of receptors. They have a set of positive receptors that allow them to recognize features associated with virally infected cells or tumor cells. They also express receptors for MHC molecules that shut off their lytic activity. Thus, virally infected cells or tumor cells that escape the surveillance of cytotoxic T cells by down-regulating or shutting off expression of MHC molecules then become targets for efficient killing by NK cells, because the cytotoxic activity of the latter cells is no longer shut off by the recognition of particular alleles of MHC class I molecules.

In addition, NK cells express a receptor for the Fc portion of IgG (FcγRIII). Antibody-coated cells can be recognized by NK cells, and such cells can then be lysed. This process is referred to as antibody-dependent cellular cytotoxicity (ADCC).

NK cells are efficient producers of IFN-γ. A variety of stimuli, including recognition of virally infected cells and tumor cells, cross-linkage of FcγRIII and stimulation by the cytokines IL-12 and IL-18, cause striking induction of IFN-γ production by NK cells.

Mast Cells and Basophils (Chapter 46)

Mast cells and basophils play important roles in the induction of allergic inflammatory responses. They express cell-surface receptors for the Fc portions of IgE (FcϵRI) and for certain classes of IgG (FcγR). This enables them to bind antibody to their surfaces, and when antigens capable of reacting with that antibody are introduced, the resultant cross-linkage of FcϵRI and/or FcγR results in the prompt release of a series of potent mediators, such as histamine, serotonin, and a variety of enzymes that play critical roles in initiating allergic and anaphylactic-type responses. In addition, such stimulation also causes these cells to produce a set of cytokines, including IL-3, IL-4, IL-13, IL-5, IL-6, granulocyte–macrophage colony-stimulating factor (GM-CSF), and TNFα, which have important late consequences in allergic inflammatory responses.

Granulocytes (Chapter 37)

Granulocytes have critical roles to play in a wide range of inflammatory situations. Rather than attempting an extended discussion of these potent cells, it may be sufficient to say that in their absence it is exceedingly difficult to clear infections with extracellular bacteria and that the immune response plays an important role in orchestrating the growth, differentiation, and mobilization of these crucial cells.

Eosinophils (Chapters 38 and 46)

Eosinophils are bone marrow–derived myeloid cells that complete their late differentiation under the influence of IL-5. They migrate to tissue sites in response to the chemokine eotaxin and as a result of their adhesion receptors. Since TH2 cells can produce IL-5 and stimulate the production of eotaxin, eosinophil accumulation is often associated with TH2-mediated inflammation. Eosinophils store a series of proteins in their secondary granules, including major basic protein, eosinophil cationic protein and eosinophil peroxidase. When released, these proteins are responsible for much of the damage that eosinophils mediate, both to helminthic parasites and to the epithelium. They have been implicated as important in protective responses to helminths and in the tissue damage seen in allergic inflammation in conditions such as asthma. Eosinophils can also produce a set of cytokines.

The Complement System (Chapter 34)

The complement system is a complex system of proteolytic enzymes, regulatory and inflammatory proteins and peptides, cell-surface receptors, and proteins capable of causing the lysis of cells. The system can be thought of as consisting of three arrays of proteins. Two of these sets of proteins, when engaged, lead to the activation of the third component of complement (C3) (Fig. 12). The activation of C3 releases proteins that are critical for opsonization (preparation for phagocytosis) of bacteria and other particles and engages the third set of proteins that insert into biologic membranes and produce cell death through osmotic lysis. In addition, fragments generated from some of the complement components (e.g., C3a and C5a) have potent inflammatory activities.

The Classical Pathway of Complement Activation

The two activation systems for C3 are referred to as the classical pathway and the alternative pathway. The classical pathway is initiated by the formation of complexes of antigen with IgM or IgG antibody. This leads to the binding of the first component of complement, C1, and its activation, creating the C1 esterase that can cleave the next two components of the complement system, C4 and C2.

C4 is a trimeric molecule, consisting of α, β, and γ chains. C1 esterase cleaves the α chain, releasing C4b, which binds to surfaces in the immediate vicinity of the antigen/antibody/C1 esterase complex. A single C1 esterase molecule will cause the deposition of multiple C4b molecules.

C2 is a single polypeptide chain that binds to C4b and is then proteolytically cleaved by C1 esterase, releasing C2b. The resulting complex of the residual portion of C2 (C2a) with C4b (C4b2a) is a serine protease whose substrate is C3. Cleavage of C3 by C4b2a (also referred to as the classical pathway C3 convertase) results in the release of C3a and C3b. A single antigen–antibody complex and its associated C1 esterase can lead to the production of a large number of

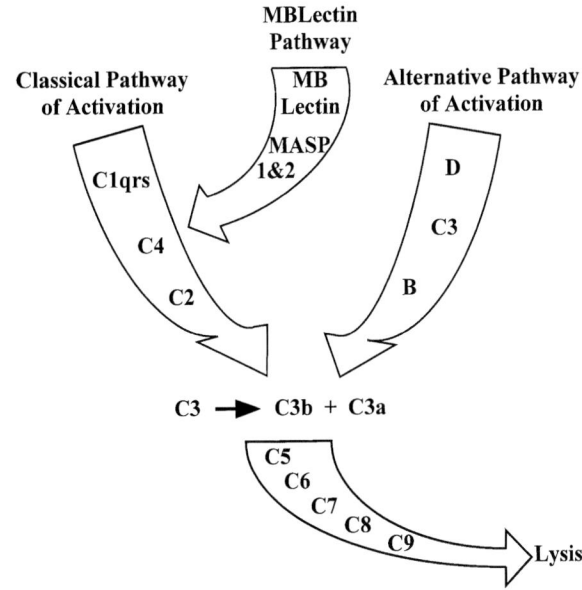

FIG. 12. The complement system. The classical pathway of complement activation, usually initiated by the aggregation of C1 by binding to antigen–antibody complexes, resulting in the formation of an enzyme, a C3 convertase, that cleaves C3 into two fragments, C3b and C3a. The classical pathway can also be initiated by the aggregation of MBLectin as a result of binding sugars expressed in the capsules of many pathogenic microbes. The components of the MBLectin pathway appear to mimic the function of C1qrs. The alternative pathway of complement activation provides a potent means of activating complement without requiring antibody recognition of antigen. It results in the formation of a distinct C3 convertase. The fragments formed by cleaving C3 have important biologic activities. In addition, C3b, together with elements of the classical pathway (C4b,C2a) or the alternative pathway (Bb, properdin), form enzymes (C5 convertases) that cleave C5, the initial member of the terminal family of proteins. Cleavage of C5 leads to the formation of the membrane attack complex that can result in the osmotic lysis of cells.

C3 convertases (i.e., C4b2a complexes) and thus to cleavage of a large number of C3 molecules.

The components of the classical pathway can be activated by a distinct, non–antibody-dependent mechanism. The mannose-binding lectin (MBL) is activated by binding to (and being cross-linked by) repetitive sugar residues such as N-acetylglucosamine or mannose. The activation of MBL recruits the MBL-associated serine proteases MASP-1 and MASP-2, which cleave C4 and C2 and lead to the formation of the classical pathway C3 convertase. Because the capsules of several pathogenic microbes can be bound by MBL, this provides an antibody-independent pathway through which the complement system can be activated by foreign microorganisms.

The Alternative Pathway of Complement Activation

Although discovered more recently, the alternative pathway is the evolutionarily more ancient system of complement activation. Indeed, this system, and the MBL activation of the classical pathway, can be regarded as providing individuals with an innate immune system. The alternative pathway can be activated by a variety of agents such as insoluble, yeast cell–wall preparations and bacterial lipopolysaccharide. Antigen–antibody complexes also can activate the alternative pathway. The C3 convertase of the alternative pathway consists of a complex of C3b (itself a product of cleavage of C3) bound to the b fragment of the molecule factor B. C3bBb is produced by the action of the hydrolytic enzyme, factor D, that cleaves factor B; this cleavage only occurs when factor B has been bound by C3b.

Apart from the importance of the alternative pathway in activating the complement system in response to nonspecific stimulants, it also can act to amplify the activity of the classical pathway because the C3 convertase of the classical system (C4b2a) provides a source of C3b that can strikingly enhance formation of the alternative pathway convertase (C3bBb) in the presence of factor D.

The Terminal Components of the Complement System

C3b, formed from C3 by the action of the C3 convertases, possesses an internal thioester bond that can be cleaved to form a free sulfhydryl group. The latter can form a covalent bond with a variety of surface structures. C3b is recognized by receptors on various types of cells, including macrophages and B cells. The binding of C3b to antibody-coated bacteria is often an essential step for the phagocytosis of these microbes by macrophages.

C3b is also essential to the engagement of the terminal components of the complement system (C5 through C9) to form the membrane attack complex that causes cellular lysis. This process is initiated by the cleavage of C5, a 200,000-dalton two-chain molecule. The C5 convertases that catalyze this reaction are C4b2a3b (the classical pathway C5 convertase) or a complex of C3bBb with a protein-designated properdin (the alternative pathway C5 convertase). Cleaved C5, C5b, forms a complex with C6 and then with C7, C8, and C9. This C5b–C9 complex behaves as an integral membrane protein that is responsible for the formation of complement-induced lesions in cell membranes. Such lesions have a donut like appearance, with C9 molecules forming the ring of the donut.

In addition to the role of the complement system in opsonization and cell lysis, several of the fragments of complement components formed during activation are potent mediators of inflammation. C3a, the 9,000-dalton fragment released by the action of the C3 convertases, binds to receptors on mast cells and basophils, resulting in the release of histamine and other mediators of anaphylaxis. C3a is thus termed an anaphylotoxin, as is C5a, the 11,000-dalton fragment released as a result of the action of the C5 convertases. C5a is also a chemoattractant for neutrophils and monocytes.

Finally, it is important to note that the process of activation of the complement cascade is highly regulated. Several regulatory proteins (e.g., C1 esterase inhibitor, decay accelerator factor, membrane cofactor protein) exist that function to prevent uncontrolled complement activation. Abnormalities in these regulatory proteins are often associated with clinical disorders such as hereditary angioedema and paroxysmal nocturnal hemoglobinuria.

CONCLUSION

This introductory chapter should provide the reader with an appreciation of the overall organization of the immune system and of the properties of its key cellular and molecular components. It should be obvious that the immune system is highly complex, that it is capable of a wide range of effector functions, and that its activities are subject to potent, but only partially understood, regulatory processes. As the most versatile and powerful defense of higher organisms, the immune system may provide the key to the development of effective means to treat and prevent a broad range of diseases. Indeed, the last two sections of this book deal with immunity to infectious agents and immunologic mechanisms in disease. The introductory material provided here should be of considerable help to the uninitiated reader in understanding the immunologic mechanisms brought into play in a wide range of clinical conditions in which immune processes play a major role either in pathogenesis or in recovery.

CHAPTER 2

History of Immunology

Pauline M. H. Mazumdar

Overview
Vaccination
The Age of Serology, 1890–1950
    The Side-Chain Theory of Antibody Production · Colloid Chemistry and the Template Theory of Antibody Production · Allergy and the Clinic · Serology at the League of Nations · Blood Groups and Transfusion
The Chemistry of the Antibody Globulins, 1930–1960
    Myeloma Proteins—A Model System
Cellular Immunology and the Selection Theories, 1950s to 1980s
    The Clonal Selection Theory · The Biology of the Thymus and the Dictatorship of the Lymphocyte · Monoclonal Antibodies
Molecular Immunology: Diversity, Histocompatibility, and the T-Cell Receptor, 1980–Present
AIDS: The Public Face of Immunology, 1986 to the Present
Conclusion
References

OVERVIEW

With the important exception of smallpox inoculation, immunology as modern science dates from the 1880s. Its history falls roughly into two periods, before and after World War II. It begins with serology: identification of bacteria, clinical application of vaccines and sera to infectious diseases, and the chemical problems of specificity and antibody diversity. Paul Erlich's side-chain theory of antibody production was replaced from about 1930 onward by Felix Haurowitz's template theory. Sources for this period are mainly German or French. After World War II, transplantation rather than infectious disease was paradigmatic. Unlike other biosciences, immunology was not reductionist: The newer work guided by the clonal selection theory concentrated on the activities of clones of cells and on experimental animals, rather than on chemistry. Major growth occurred in the 1960s and 1970s, and there are many memoirs by immunologists from that period. However, with the advent of monoclonal antibodies, interest in specificity was renewed, and serology entered a new period of growth powered by molecular biology and the pharmaceutical industry.

Most of the writing by historians dates from the 1990s and deals with social, scientific, and business history. New writing has emphasized the role of experimental systems, techniques, and instruments, as well as language. As Cambrosio (1) said, the history of science has as its object a cultural product: It is a history of culture not of nature. Until recently, however, there has been little emphasis on the interaction of the laboratory science with the clinic.

VACCINATION

The earliest known smallpox inoculation took place in China, perhaps as early as the 5th century AD. The Chinese method was reported to the Royal Society by an English merchant, John Lister, in 1700. A Jesuit priest, Father d'Entrecolles (2), provided details of the method, which he said was to collect scabs from the pustules, and blow a powder made from them into an infant's nose. The scabs or a thread imbibed with the pus could be stored, but the operation was usually done face-to-face with a sick patient. The same method was used in Japan beginning in 1747. In precolonial India, a *tika* or dot would be made on a child, usually on the sole of the foot, by traditional *tikadars* who were invited into a home (this professional niche was later blacklisted by colonial-era medical practitioners). The Turkish method was communicated to the Royal Society by Dr. Emmannuel Timoni in 1714. As commonly practiced in Constantinople, a small perforation was made in the skin, and a spot of pus from a benign case introduced with a needle. In 1715, the method famously came

23

to the notice of Lady Mary Montagu, wife of the English ambassador in Constantinople, who used it on her own son, and subsequently talked it up to great effect in aristocratic circles at home in England (3). Although nationalistic, ethical, and religious objections to this non-European folk practice abounded, the Royal Society with its interest in the empirical recorded many accounts of inoculation presented at its meetings. Dr. James Jurin, its secretary, an early user of the quantitative method, collected large numbers of cases in an effort to compare the risks from inoculation and from the disease. According to his figures, smallpox was both universal and often fatal: He assumed that almost everyone over the age of 2 had had it, and for every person who died, 7 or 8 recovered; inoculation, on the other hand, had a death rate of about 1 in 50. He had not, he said, been able to learn of any person either in England or Turkey, who had been inoculated but still took the disease in the natural way (4). The mathematician Daniel Bernoulli calculated similarly that if one neglected the point of view of the individual, inoculation would be useful to the state. In 18th-century France, according to Anne-Marie Moulin, the method was discussed, for instance by the *Encyclopédistes,* but not practiced; it was made illegal by a decree of 1763, and only permitted after the revolution. In England, on the other hand, it seems possible that it was used often enough by the end of the 18th century to affect the incidence and severity of smallpox (5).

The use of *Vaccinia* (cowpox) as inoculum was suggested several times in the late 1700s; the country doctor and inoculator Edward Jenner tried it out in 1798. He had heard it said that milkmaids who had had cowpox, never caught smallpox, and it struck him that he might be able to propagate the disease as he was accustomed to do with his usual inoculum. It is not clear whether in practice the material actually used was always *Vaccinia* (6). Vaccine production was unregulated; the operation was painful and sometimes did not "take." Nevertheless, public health authorities enforced it, for example, in Prussia and later under the British Compulsory Vaccination Act of 1853. Compulsion led to worldwide antivaccination movements with strong political and anticolonial overtones (7). However, the demographer Alex Mercer makes a strong case for its effectiveness: He argues that inoculation and subsequently vaccination were key in the general decline in death rates that took place from the late 18th through the 19th century, as the incidence of smallpox declined. With it went a network of linked respiratory diseases, late sequelae of the damage done by smallpox even when not fatal (8).

It should not be supposed, however, that because vaccination was accepted, an immune theory of disease resistance was an obvious conclusion. The experience of colonial troops in the tropics, where most of them died within a year or two of arrival throughout the 18th and 19th centuries, prompted a racial view of resistance, coupled with the development of acclimatization or seasoning in those few who survived. The constitution of the alien race soon broke down in the unfamiliar conditions of temperature and humidity; the expatriates felt themselves weakened by perspiration, tight clothes, and local miasmas that did not seem to affect the natives. There is a large 19th-century literature advising the displaced European on how to survive a posting to India, the Caribbean, or the Philippines, and on the tragic return home of the soldier or sailor broken in health by the tropics (9). The importation of Africans to work as slaves in the conditions that were so fatal to Europeans and white Americans was one of the results of the racial view of disease resistance. A theory with such significant historical connotations cannot be ignored (10).

The word vaccine originally applied only to *Vaccinia.* Anne-Marie Moulin points out that it was Louis Pasteur, who by claiming Jenner as his predecessor, metaphorically included in that word all prophylactic inoculation by attenuated *virus-vaccins,* organisms attenuated by passage through another species or by treatment with oxygen or antiseptics (11). Vaccines were prepared in this way against anthrax (1881), which was then a common agricultural problem, and rabies (1885) a frighteningly fatal result of the bite of a rabid animal. These vaccines were dramatically effective, although it was never clear whether the victim of a dog bite had in fact been infected. They led to a flood of donations from a hero-worshipping public, with which the Institut Pasteur was established in 1888.

In 1891, Robert Koch too had a dramatic announcement, which also paved the way for the establishment of an institute under his direction. "Koch's lymph" was a cure for tuberculosis, raising the hopes of sufferers who rushed to Berlin to be treated by the man who had discovered the tubercle bacillus. The reaction was acute and sometimes quite harmful to the patients, and the results were certainly not as good as expected. But it was not the debacle that has sometimes been thought. Koch's Old Tuberculin continued to be made until the 1940s for use as a treatment for chronic tuberculosis of bones, lymph nodes, and skin. The material was a protein extract of tubercle bacilli, which Koch regarded as an exotoxin similar to that produced by diphtheria bacilli. It was later used under the name of the Mantoux reaction as a skin test for tuberculosis (12).

In 1896, Sir Almroth Wright of St. Mary's Hospital in London and Richard Pfeiffer and Wilhelm Kolle in Berlin simultaneously prepared a vaccine against typhoid, an important disease in Europe and the colonies. Like the smallpox vaccine, it was very promising, but was attacked passionately by antivaccinationists. Their position was primarily political and ideological, but typhoid was a water-borne infection, and it was argued that improvements in sanitation and water supplies would eventually make vaccination unnecessary. Hostility focused on Wright's vaccine especially; it made its recipients feel very ill, and its effectiveness was statistically doubtful. Sir William Leishman of the Royal Army Medical Corps developed a vaccine incorporating typhoid and the newly defined paratyphoids A and B in 1909. Armies in France, Germany, and the United States were beginning to use the newer type, but in Britain compulsion was politically unacceptable, and when World War I came, the Royal Army Medical Corps depended upon pro-vaccination propaganda. As acceptance of the vaccine increased among the troops, the results became more obvious: Compared to dysentery, a disease that was similarly transmitted through infected water supplies, the numbers of enteric cases reported in the field fell steeply (13). Attempts to develop a dysentery vaccine were unsuccessful.

In the 1880s, germ theory had started to sound persuasive (14). In 1883, the Russian zoologist Élie Metchnikov had suggested that white blood cells attacked invaders from outside the body, an idea based on the Darwinian concept of interspecies struggle for existence, and which he saw as a form of "physiological inflammation" (15). Pasteur liked Metchnikov's idea, and invited him to Paris. Alfred Tauber sees Metchnikov's phagocytosis theory as the foundation of the self–not self concept, later to be central to immunology, and thinks that Metchnikov should be regarded as having founded the discipline (16). But as Anne-Marie Moulin points out, Metchnikov's phagocytes had neither specificity nor memory; they simply engulfed particles (17).

In the first half of the 20th century, the practical aspects of immunity, vaccination, and serum therapy defined research in the field. Serology and immunochemistry strove to provide a theoretical basis for these practices. Mechnikov's phagocytosis theory was briefly at center stage but was soon overtaken by a rush of publications from Koch and colleagues in Berlin—the Franco-Prussian war of 1870 was still being fought by other means (18). As bacteriologists, the Berlin group favored "humoral immunity" in preference to cellular: They focused on immune sera for their specificity to identify bacteria, and ignored the cells, which seemed to carry a taint of old-fashioned vitalism.

Cell-based vaccination systems, however, were to prove popular and very lucrative for their producers, especially in France. At the Institut Pasteur, Metchnikov's lineage of workers in the cellular style continued to flourish. Alexandre Besredka came to Paris in 1893; he was from Odessa, like Metchnikov, and found work in Metchnikov's laboratory. In 1918, he succeeded Metchnikov at its head. His interest centered on the then newly described phenomenon of anaphylaxis (19). He was concerned with sensitization and desensitization of the skin, an interest that was to evolve into his studies of natural resistance and acquired localized immunity. He proposed a system of specific dressings or local injections of a prepared antigen, a parallel to the local injections that desensitized animals to anaphylactic shock. The "terrain," the skin cells that allowed entry to the infection, was to be made resistant (20). Besredka's co-worker, Michel Bardach, was also from Odessa. He began work on an anti-reticuloendothelial serum along the lines suggested by a Russian researcher, Alexander Bogomoletz, who claimed that his serum was effective in a broad range of diseases involving

that system. After World War II, the serum was successfully and profitably marketed through the Institut Pasteur as a non-specific stimulator of immunity, only to be abandoned in the 1950s as ineffective, perhaps by contrast with the stunning success of penicillin.

A rather similar cell-based system had been developed in England. Sir Almroth Wright, originator of an early typhoid vaccine, linked cells with serum in an effort to boost immunity by the preparation of autovaccines from a patient's own lesion; they were thought to raise a patient's serum "opsonic index," and like Bardach's serum at a later date, to stimulate phagocytosis (21). Wright's slogan of 1909, "The physician of the future will be an immunisator," seems to have been perfectly true for the first decades of the 20th century (22). Wright's department at St. Mary's Hospital London made autovaccines and carried out thousands of index measurements yearly between 1908 and 1945. He built up a practice on a huge, even industrial, scale, out of which the department and the hospital itself were financed. As Wei Chen has commented, his laboratory was a vaccine factory, profitably manufacturing typhoid vaccine as well as the autovaccines that were Wright's specialty (23). The effectiveness of autovaccine therapy, like the effectiveness of his typhoid vaccine, was attacked by the statisticians. Even so, laboratory texts until the mid-1940s generally included a chapter on the technique of preparing an autovaccine (24). Wright's student George Ross carried both antityphoid and autovaccine manufacture with him to Canada in 1907, to an appointment at the Toronto General Hospital, where his techniques established and funded a new laboratory-based Department of Immunization and Medical Research, a precursor to the Connaught Laboratory, Toronto's serum institute (25). The use of Wright's autovaccines, along with Koch's Old Tuberculin, persisted more or less up to the appearance of penicillin on the therapeutic scene in 1945, when all such minimally effective treatments were swept away by the brilliance of the first antibiotics. Wei Chen has suggested that Wright's vaccine program provided a model and a financial goal for his junior colleague Alexander Fleming's "construction" of penicillin. She shows that penicillin was initially seen as a means of differentially culturing *Bacillus influenzae* from cases of influenza, and supporting Wright's claim that a vaccine made from that bacillus would be useful in the disease (26).

THE AGE OF SEROLOGY, 1890–1950

This period was characterized by the development of serum therapy, most famously diphtheria and tetanus antitoxins, the one affecting children, the other soldiers in the field, both powerfully evocative and important to governments. In its train came the network of serum institutes, problems of standardization, and, on the research front, an outgrowth of studies of the nature of specificity and the chemistry of the antigen–antibody reaction, which dominated the field until after World War II. As Frank Macfarlane Burnet realized in

1959, at a time when this era was giving way to another, very largely under his own influence,

> The subject matter of immunology has often been unconsciously confined to the high-titre antibodies produced by the immunization of horse or rabbit with diphtheria toxin or some other of the classical antigens. Such antisera react with the antigen by aggregation in the test tube and by neutralization of the biological function of the antigen.... Most of the practical applications of serology make use of such antisera, and all the classical work in immunology is based on their properties ... (27)

Animals were immunized at first with live organisms, then as the concept of immunity was generalized, with killed organisms, and later with tetanus or diphtheria toxin. It was found that antitoxic immunity could be transferred via serum to a second individual. Between 1888 and 1894, Emil von Behring and Shibasaburo Kitasato, working in Koch's Institute for Infectious Disease, laid the experimental foundations of serum therapy (28). Antitoxin proved itself clinically in cases of diphtheria in the winter of 1892 (29). Serum manufacture on a large scale using horses instead of the original guinea pigs and rabbits quickly began at the Institut Pasteur, and a global network soon followed: Instituts Pasteur appeared in the main cities of the French colonial empire. European countries followed by Canada set up their own publicly funded institutions dedicated to the production and distribution of therapeutic antisera: the serum institutes with their laboratories, stables and pastures—a horse-centered world—were to dominate medical research in the decades to come (30).

In Germany, four firms—Schering of Berlin; Meister, Lucius and Brüning, then of Berlin, later moving to Hoechst-am-Main; Merck of Darmstadt; and Ruete-Enoch of Hamburg—were licensed to produce antitoxin (31). They were soon joined by Burroughs-Wellcome of London. After the introduction of serum therapy, epidemics of diphtheria still continued, but the death rate from the disease dropped steeply.

Clinical results of serum therapy, however, were unpredictable. Reliable production required measurement: first the dose of immunizing toxin, and then quantification of the horse serum. A standardized antidiphtheria serum was first produced by Paul Ehrlich in the 1880s, when working in Berlin on the specificity of dyes in histology (32). The unit he devised, the first bioassay, was defined as the amount of antiserum that just neutralized 100 lethal doses (LDs) of a standard toxin. New batches of either toxin or antitoxin were compared with the old standards. The LD_{50} was the dose of toxin that was lethal to 50% of a batch of 250-gram guinea pigs within 4 days. The L_0 dose of a new toxin, L standing for *limes* or limit, was the number of lethal doses neutralized by one unit of the original antitoxin, and the L_+ dose of the new toxin was the number of LDs just not neutralized. In theory, $L_+ - L_0 = 1$ LD, but the difference in practice was always greater than 1, and as a toxin aged, the gap widened. Ehrlich

interpreted the stepped neutralization curve as evidence that toxin was composed of a group of discrete but unstable substances, all of which he named. All of them neutralized antibody irreversibly in proportions of simple chemical equivalence, but affected the toxicity of the mixture to different degrees (33).

> [T]he reaction between toxin and anti-toxin takes place in accordance with the proportions of simple equivalence.... A molecule of toxin combines with a definite and unalterable quantity of antitoxin. [Ehrlich's emphasis]
>
> It must be assumed that the ability of toxins to bind antibody must be due to a specific atom group of the toxin complex, which shows a maximum specific relationship to an atom group of the antitoxin complex. They fit together like lock and key, in the image suggested by Emil Fischer for the specific effect of the ferments (34).

It was typical of Ehrlich's way of thinking that he was prepared to postulate as many different substances as he needed to accord with the phenomena (Fig.1).

The Side-Chain Theory of Antibody Production

Ehrlich's vocabulary and his diagrams of the union of antibody and receptor, and his "side-chain theory" of immunity provided the first general theory for the new science of immunology. His system, modeled on a benzene ring with its attached side chains, linked immunity with nutrition. A cell was nourished by capturing nutrients with an array of different side chains, specific to each nutrient, which could be specifically blocked by toxin. The blocked side chains were shed by the cell, and then replaced by an excess of new ones as the cell repaired itself. The freed side chains were the antitoxins, released in great numbers into the serum (35). Later workers have pointed out that this implies a selection theory of immunity: Antigen selects the specific side chains to be released by the cell as antibody. Immunologists themselves have recognized Ehrlich's side-chain theory as a precursor of the clonal selection theory of antibody production, first introduced in 1957 (36) (Fig.2). Ehrlich himself did not pursue the chemistry of the antigen–antibody reaction, or the nature of the specificity that he postulated, except to claim that the reaction was like those of organic chemistry, firm and irreversible. In the early years of the century, he turned his attention to a new project, the development of chemotherapy, which eventuated in the Salvarsan treatment of syphilis in 1909 (37). But his cartoon-like diagrams of antigen and antibody oriented thinking around the visual metaphor of the receptor, providing a diagrammatic language for immunology that was to persist long after its supposed chemical basis had been dropped (38).

Ehrlich's work had immense heuristic power. His method of standardization formed the basis of the activities in the serum institutes over the next half-century. It also set off an era of serological reductionism, in which the chemical nature of the antigen–antibody reaction, rather than the resistance of

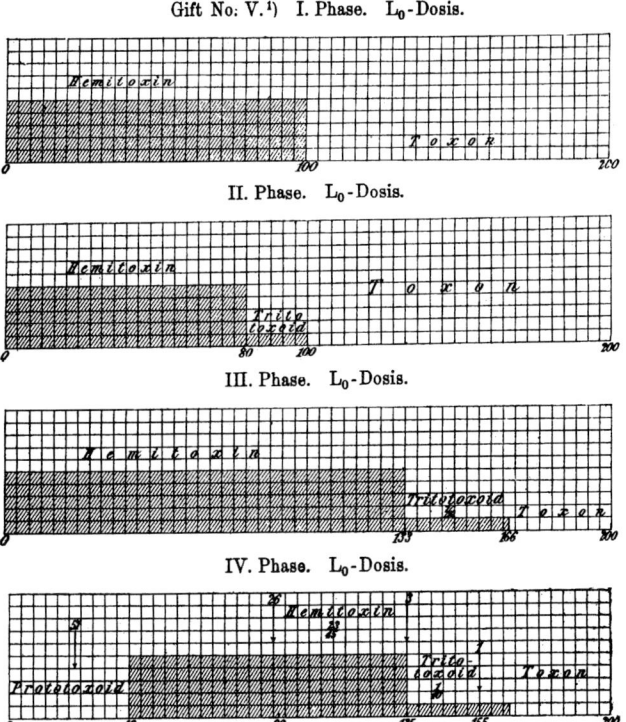

Gift No: V.¹)   I. Phase. L_0-Dosis.

II. Phase. L_0-Dosis.

III. Phase. L_0-Dosis.

IV. Phase. L_0-Dosis.

FIG. 1. Ehrlich's standardization of the antidiphtheria serum. Added antitoxin has little effect at first, then toxicity falls rapidly, then does not change any further. The relationships change as the toxin ages. Ehrlich sees the toxin as a mixture of different specific substances: he shows four phases in the breakdown of a single sample, "*Gift No. V.*" Each phase contains different breakdown products, which are supposed to react irreversibly with the antitoxin, in the manner of the reactions of organic chemistry. They react with the antitoxin in order of affinity; each substance is named according to its relative affinity and toxicity. Active toxins are *proto-, deutero-* and *trito-toxin,* in order of affinity; some, the *toxoids* and *tox-ones,* have lost the *toxophore* group, and are no longer toxic to guineapigs, but still neutralize antitoxin. The vocabulary is Ehrlich's own invention. From Paul Ehrlich, "Wertbemessung des Diphtherieheilserums und deren theoretische Grundlagen," (34).

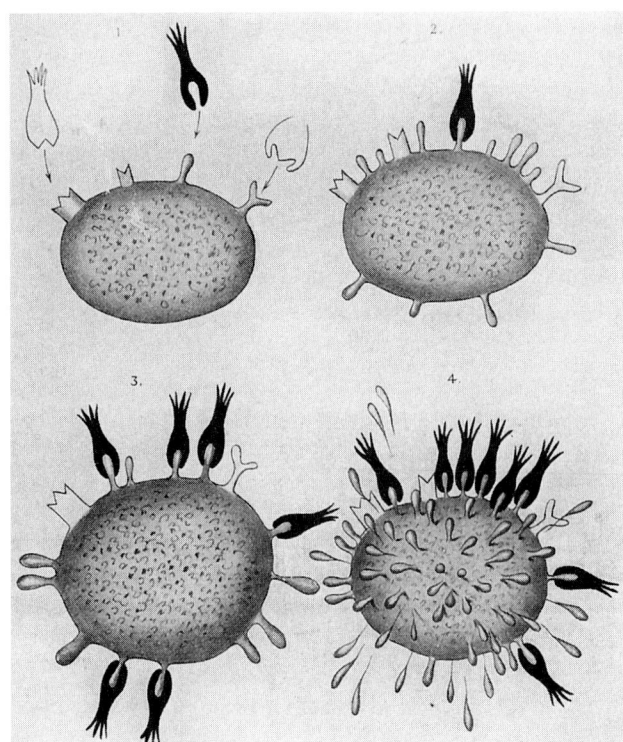

FIG. 2. Ehrlich's side-chain theory of antibody production. Antitoxin production is explained as a special case of cellular nutrition. The cell is equipped with *side-chains* or *receptors* to capture specific nutrients. A *receptor* can be blocked by a matching toxin; the cell then heals itself by shedding the blocked *receptors* and producing an excess of new ones. Some of the new side-chains are freed into the serum and constitute *antibodies* specific to the toxin. The vocabulary and the diagrams are Ehrlich's own invention. His conception of the antigen-antibody reaction is of a firm, specific, irreversible chemical binding. He uses the metaphor of a lock and key: another image suggested by his drawings is a snap-fastener or press-stud. On the influence of Ehrlich's diagrams and vocabulary, see Cambrosio *et al.* (n. 38). From Paul Ehrlich, "On immunity with special reference to cell life," (35).

the body to disease was at the center of interest (39). Opposition to his views stimulated representatives of other types of chemistry to propose alternative interpretations for the stepped neutralization spectrum. These other workers saw toxin–antitoxin neutralization not as a series of discontinuous steps, representing separate irreversible reactions, but as a smooth curve. The curve might represent either an acid-base type of reaction, in accordance with the dissociation theory of the Swedish chemist Svante Arrhenius, or a colloid reaction, according to Jules Bordet of Brussels and the Viennese immunochemist Karl Landsteiner (40). Both concepts postulated reversible reactions described by smooth curves, not discrete steps. Both allowed for variable proportions of antigen and antibody in the resulting complex that depended on the concentration of the reacting substances. Bordet said that

just because twice as much serum is needed to combine with two as with one dose of bacterial emulsion, some bacteriologists argue that antigen and antibody must combine according to a law of definite proportions. That, he said scornfully, was like claiming that paint must react in definite proportions with a wall (41). The regular chemical law of definite proportions need not apply.

Colloid Chemistry and the Template Theory of Antibody Production

All known antigens were proteins, and proteins were colloids. In 1912, the chemist Ernst Peter Pick of Vienna made this a slogan: "Kein Antigen ohne Eiweiss" (no antigen without protein) (42). The first decades of the century were a time of great excitement about colloid chemistry: This was the chemistry of life itself. It was not unexpected to find that this vital, even mystical, reaction did not obey the rules of ordinary chemistry (43).

Landsteiner's immunochemistry, and his lifelong opposition to Ehrlich and his theories, began in the early years of the century with an attempt to apply the new colloid chemistry to the problem of the relationship between antigen and antibody. Landsteiner argued that specificity could not be absolute: Ehrlich's pluralistic approach would require an absurd number of specific substances in the serum, whose significance for the animal body was unclear. In Landsteiner's words,

> According to the older view [i.e., Ehrlich's], for every single effect of a serum, there is a separate substance, or at least a particular chemical group.... A normal serum contained as many different haemagglutinins as it agglutinated different cells. The situation was undoubtedly made much simpler if, to use the Ehrlich terminology... the separate haptophore groups can combine with an extremely large number of receptors, in stepwise differing quantities as a stain does with different animal tissues.... A normal serum would therefore visibly affect such a large number of different blood cells, ... not because it contained countless special substances, but because of the colloids in the serum, [that is,] ... the agglutinins, by reason of their chemical constitution and the electrochemical properties resulting from it. That this manner of representation is a considerable simplification is clear; it also opens the way to direct experimental testing by the methods of structural chemistry (44).

Landsteiner's "simpler" view was that specificity was a matter of "more or less good fit," which he demonstrated through cross-reacting antibodies against a series of compounds of known structure. His key project began during the 1914–1918 war. Conditions were harsh in Vienna; food and heating were inadequate as the city administration crumbled around the researchers and the Donau monarchy came to its end. Many animals were needed for the project, immunized with many closely related antigens. The animals made low levels of antibody because they were cold and undernourished; the same was true of the researchers. But they were able to conclude that it was highly charged groups such as acid radicals that were most important in determining specificity, a finding that brought them closer to structural rather than colloid chemistry (45) (Fig. 3). Landsteiner was able to continue with these immunochemical studies of the antigen–antibody reaction at the Rockefeller Institute in New York, where he worked from 1922 to his death in 1946. Landsteiner and his mother had converted to Catholicism in the 1890s. He had left Vienna before the outpouring of anti-Semitism that led to the *Anschluss,* the unification of Austria with Nazi Germany, in 1938. He was already in New York, when many of the people he knew were desperately trying to emigrate, or to find jobs in a new and difficult country. Although he did not wish to be seen as Jewish, he was able to help some of them.

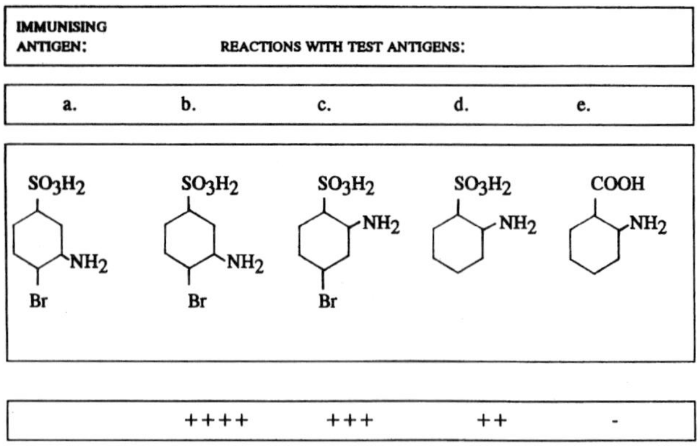

The Rockefeller Institute was a placement that was in many ways ideal for the man and for his program of research. It epitomizes in many ways the typically reductionist immunology carried on outside the ambit of the Institut

FIG. 3. Landsteiner's conception of specificity. The diagram shows a continuous spectrum of reactions to the benzene-sulphonic acid family of antigens. Starting from the immunizing antigen, stepwise small alterations in the chemistry of the test antigens reduce the strength of the reaction with the antiserum. It is the polar groups that have the most effect on specificity. According to Landsteiner, an antibody has a *graded quantitative affinity* with a range of different antigenic configurations. His conception of the reaction is one of a reversible, weak binding of broad specificity. Compared to Ehrlich's tightly bound snap-fastener receptors (Fig. 2 above), Landsteiner's view of the reaction suggests a silk scarf draped lightly over the charge outline of the antigen. This conception accords very well with the *template theory* of antibody production of Breinl and Haurowitz of 1930, in which the polar groups of the antigen control the assembly of antibody globulin (n. 47). Karl Landsteiner and Hans Lampl, "Ueber die Antigen-eigenschaften von Azoprotein: XI Mitteilung über Antigene," (45).

Pasteur. Writers such as George Corner and René Dubos, who experienced life and work in its laboratories, emphasize the role played by reductionist ideals at the Institute. Writing in 1976, Dubos says that the chemical approach is now more dominant than ever in fields such as cellular biology, genetics, immunology, and experimental pathology (46). In the 1940s at the Rockefeller Institute, there were six different laboratories working on protein chemistry.

Landsteiner's conception of specificity was that antibody draped itself over the charge outline of its antigen. The antigen–antibody reaction was a charge-based surface adsorption. This suggested to the Prague chemist Felix Haurowitz and his serologist colleague Friedrich Breinl, who had met Landsteiner in New York, that antibody formation might take place by the assembly of the globulin molecule on the antigen. The polarity of the antigenic groups served to orient the amino-acid building blocks of the nascent globulin. These concepts were later known as the template theory of antibody formation (47). Haurowitz fled from Prague to pass the Nazi period in Turkey, and then like Landsteiner, emigrated to the United States, where he settled in Indiana (48). He maintained his belief in the template theory to the end of his life.

The standardization of sera was key to research and theory building in immunochemistry and to the practical problems of serum production and utilization. It was the source

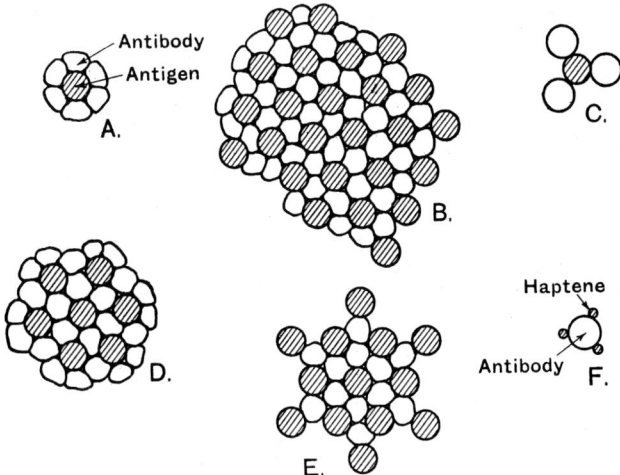

FIG. 4. Marrack's lattice theory of antigen–antibody precipitation. Marrack is explaining the *zoning phenomenon* whereby the precipitation of antigen by antibody depends on concentration. *Zoning,* as Ehrlich had found in the case of toxin neutralization (Fig. 1 above), made it difficult to standardize antisera for practical use. Increasing concentration of antibody leads to a crowding of antibody molecules around an antigen, forcing the polar groups of the antibody into such close contact that they attract each other instead of molecules of water, and precipitate out of solution. (A in the diagram). Differences in proportion of antigen and antibody in the complexes formed (C, D and E) account for differences between precipitates. If the antibody has more than one absorbing site, the complexes may form a large *lattice structure* (B). From: J. R. Marrack, *The Chemistry of Antigens and Antibodies* (49).

of Ehrlich's side-chain theory, Landsteiner's countervailing outline concept, Haurowitz's related template theory, and the lattice theory of the 1930s (Fig. 4). This last was proposed by the London serologist J.R. Marrack to account for the relation of antigen–antibody proportions to the appearance and disappearance of precipitation, the so-called zoning effect, which made it difficult to titrate antibody and antigen against each other by precipitation (49).

In Germany, the state guaranteed standards for the antisera produced there, based on Ehrlich's technique and on standards held at Ehrlich's laboratory in Frankfurt-am-Main (50). This hegemony was broken up by the outbreak of World War I, when other countries such as Britain found that they could not, indeed must not, rely on Frankfurt any more, and began to develop their own programs. Standardization was one of the first projects to be taken up by the new Medical Research Council of Britain. It was placed under the charge of the young Henry Dale, who had briefly studied under Ehrlich in Frankfurt, and had since been employed by Burroughs-Wellcome in serum manufacture. He was also delegated to supervise the testing of Ehrlich's Salvarsan and its substitutes, whose German patents had been abrogated at the outbreak of war. Interestingly, these toxic chemicals were treated as if they were bacterial toxins, and assayed by Ehrlich's LD_{50} method. It was a method that did not deal with the common problems that accompanied Salvarsan treatment, *Dermatitis*

exfoliativa, and sometimes sudden death, as well as *Icterus lueticus,* so-called, later shown to be syringe-transmitted hepatitis. At the time, these side effects were thought to be due to excess toxicity of the drug, but the batches always passed the LD_{50} test. In 1930, Henry Dale began to suspect that some of the cases of collapse during Salvarsan treatment were due to anaphylactic shock. Anaphylaxis had been described in 1902 by the eugenist Charles Richet in France. By 1913, when Richet received his Nobel Prize, he had come to see it as a mechanism of natural selection, which maintained the purity of races (51).

Allergy and the Clinic

Clinically, anaphylaxis was to be carefully distinguished from allergy and its relations, atopic eczema, asthma, and hay fever, although all of them were agreed to be mediated by substances known as reagins, presumed to be cell-bound antibodies. The earliest suggestion of that came in 1921, with the famous personal experiment of the German medical students Carl Prausnitz and Hans Küstner, who tried to exchange hypersensitivities by exchanging serum with each other in an immunological version of blood brotherhood. Both of them were allergic but only fish sensitivity was transferred. There was also the problem of serum sickness, a reaction to antitetanus and antidiphtheria sera, written up by Clemens von Pirquet and Béla Schick in 1905 (52).

In Britain, the first allergy clinic was set up in 1911, an offshoot of the vaccine department of St. Mary's Hospital under Sir Almroth Wright, following up on Wright's enthusiasm for autovaccines. Like Wright's immunizations, desensitization was both praised and attacked in the popular press, and in the medical journals. It was also a profitable enterprise, funded by a drug company, Parke Davis, which made the sets of allergens used. By the 1980s, the attacks had intensified: The method had had a longer run than most of the Wright-based procedures. But clinical allergists continued to offer desensitization treatments, in spite of warnings from the Committee on the Safety of Medicines in 1986 (53).

Allergy began to take shape in the United States as a clinical specialty in the course of the 1920s, the allergens here being ragweed and poison ivy. Private clinics were set up, societies were organized, and the clinical *Journal of Allergy* started in 1929. The more laboratory-oriented papers on the subject still appeared in the older *Journal of Immunology,* but in most cases, the allergists were not laboratory people, and it was felt that they could not come up to the standard demanded by the *Journal of Immunology.* In the course of the 1930s, the leaders of the profession began to fear that the specialty might gradually become a kind of medical quackery, focused on a single procedure, the skin test. The professional societies determined that clinics should be certified and controlled. In 1971, board certification was set up through a joint effort by the Boards of Internal Medicine and Pediatrics, and in 1973, the American Academy of Allergy was formed in succession to the two national societies. Founders were Robert Cooke, who had asthma attacks triggered by horses and cows, and Arthur Coca, who suffered from migraine and a large variety of food allergies (54). Coca was to become medical director at Lederle Laboratories, which was marketing sets of allergens for skin test diagnosis and desensitizing treatments, the clinical allergists' professional standby.

Serology at the League of Nations

Serology gained still more prestige during the First World War. In the mud of the trenches and battlefields of 1914–1918, tetanus antitoxin strikingly reduced the incidence of tetanus on both sides, but attempts by the German military to develop an antiserum for gas gangrene were not successful (55). Inoculation against typhoid had become increasingly accepted, and increasingly effective. After the war, the victorious Allies through the League of Nations and its Health Organization set up their own standardization project at the Statens Seruminstitut in Copenhagen. Postwar arrangements bypassed the German laboratories, which were then suffering under a boycott of all international contacts. However, the League's laboratories under Thorvald Madsen, a student of Ehrlich, still used the German techniques, and Madsen himself tried to make sure that science remained pure, protected from all national and political interference (56).

The League's program was a microcosm of practical serology. It began by working over the old sera such as diphtheria and tetanus, including the blood group antisera with their conflicting nomenclatures, and then attempted to add new ones of military importance, such as an antidysentery serum. It also worked at standardizing the serological test for syphilis: The Wassermann reaction was a two-stage complement-fixation test of the type introduced by Jules Bordet and applied by August von Wassermann to the diagnosis of syphilis in 1906 (57). Prodded by the international organizations and the requirements for a standard procedure for syphilis tracking in seamen under the Brussels Agreement of 1924, the League's scientists working through the Statens Seruminstitut began on this most difficult of projects (58). The Wassermann test had been accepted with great enthusiasm by clinical venereologists, but the laboratory workers saw it as unreliable and difficult to carry out. Newer, simpler versions, often based on colloid chemistry, were tested by the League (59). The most successful of the new colloid tests was probably the test designed by the American Rudolf Kahn (60). The Kahn test, however, never completely replaced the Wassermann, except in Kahn's own laboratory. Clinicians continued to ask for "WR and Kahn" on their patients until the late 1960s, when both tests gradually gave way to a more direct form of immunological screening, and finally to the ELISA test using monoclonal antibody (61).

Blood Groups and Transfusion

Karl Landsteiner described the human ABO blood groups in 1901 (62). For many years, however, he showed no great interest in his discovery. Blood groups probably seemed to be rather a dead end in terms of practice, and, possibly, to imply a sharp specificity rather too close to Ehrlich's for Landsteiner's comfort. Further work on blood group serology by the Polish serologist Ludwik Hirszfeld showed that they were inherited as Mendelian unit characters, which he interpreted as two pairs of alleles—A and not-A, B and not-B—along the lines of the then-current Mendelian "presence-and-absence hypothesis." Working at a front-line hospital in Macedonia during World War I, Hirszfeld and the bacteriologist Hanna Hirszfeld, his wife, were able to show that blood group distribution in the military units was linked to the place of origin of the people studied. These two discoveries rendered blood groups significant as forensic tests of paternity, and as race markers, and Hirszfeld himself tried to use them to elucidate the problem of resistance to disease (63). Felix Bernstein, a mathematician and director of the Institute for Mathematical Statistics in Göttingen, took up Hirszfeld's study of the inheritance of the ABO groups, then the only normal human trait for which there was enough family data to perform a satisfactory Mendelian analysis. He argued that the data showed them to be controlled by three alleles, all at the same locus, and not by paired alleles at two separate loci. The test case was that of the AB mother: According to his triple-allele hypothesis, an AB mother could not have an O child, whereas with Hirszfeld's two-locus hypothesis, such children should have been quite common. The literature was combed for cases in point—before Bernstein made his claim, there were quite a few, but as the triple-allele hypothesis took hold, they disappeared from published results (64).

A Nazi-oriented German Society for Blood Group Research founded in 1928 attempted to use Hirszfeld's results to define the Aryan race and to map its place in Europe. Official Nazidom, however, paid little attention to its findings. The Society excluded Jews from its membership; that meant that none of the leading researchers, such as Hirszfeld, Bernstein, or Landsteiner were members (65). Bernstein happened to be in the United States when the Nazi edict stripping him of his directorship arrived; he stayed there until after the war, but was never to reestablish himself and wrote no more after 1933. The Hirszfelds were in Warsaw where Ludwik was director of the State Epidemiological Institute; they managed to survive the Warsaw ghetto.

Landsteiner himself went back to the blood groups only when he reached the Rockefeller Institute in 1922. Over the next 20 years, he and his colleagues Philip Levine and Alexander S. Wiener described several more blood group systems, including M-N, P, and finally the rhesus system, establishing not only an expanded forensic tool, but also a causal mechanism for *Erythroblastosis fetalis,* hemolytic disease of the newborn (66). In spite of the efforts of the eugenics movement to show that feeblemindedness was inherited as a single-gene Mendelian recessive, blood groups were for decades the only normal human characteristic that was clearly Mendelian in its pattern of inheritance, and where the data were extensive and reliable enough to use in a mathematical approach to human genetics. For the geneticist, blood groups were the human equivalent of *Drosophila*.

In hindsight, one might have expected that blood grouping would have found immediate application as a condition for blood transfusion. But that was not the case. Transfusion itself was experimental rather than therapeutic, and technical problems abounded. George Crile, professor of surgery at Western Reserve Medical College, investigated the technique and its applications in 1909. Although Ludwig Hektoen had cited Landsteiner's work and had suggested that isoagglutination of human red corpuscles might be relevant to transfusion of blood, Crile's personal experience had shown that the occurrence of hemolysis *in vitro* did not necessarily indicate that it would occur in the vascular system of the recipient after transfusion (67). Crile's technique of transfer of blood involved the end-to-end anastomosis of the donor's and the recipient's veins, by cutting down and suturing the veins together, or joining them with a cannula. Just before the First World War, a method using a paraffin-coated intermediary bottle was introduced; but it was not until sodium citrate was suggested as anticoagulant that any quantity of blood could actually be transferred. Several individuals suggested it at about the same time, but in practice, it was not used until about 1916–1917, when the American Oswald Robertson and the Canadian Bruce Robertson introduced transfusion in the field (68). Soldiers who were checked out to act as "professional donors" were generally group O, a so-called universal donor. Grouping tests and cross-matching of donor and recipient were felt to take too long to do; group O donors continued to be the mainstay of transfusion into World War II. Only from about 1944, with the increased demand for blood by the Army, group-to-group transfusion began to take over (69). Landsteiner received a Nobel Prize in 1930 for his 1901 discovery of the ABO blood groups. It came only when it was clear that they had some practical use; he himself thought that his fundamental work on specificity was more important.

Until the outbreak of World War II, transfusions were usually organized on an individual basis. In Britain as in Canada, a service was set up through the Red Cross. A donor would be called to the hospital where the blood was needed, as stored blood even when properly refrigerated was felt to be unsafe (70). Elsewhere, stored blood was increasingly used. In the Soviet Union, the donors attended centers and blood was stored for use as needed. In the United States, Cook County Hospital of Chicago established a blood banking system in 1937, where a credit balance could be used for a given patient without necessarily using the bottle donated by the patient's own relatives (71).

Blood transfusion, like standardization, was driven by war and the interests of national governments. The technique was recognized as being of national and military importance following World War I, as military experience showed that blood could virtually resuscitate the dead. The British government, through the Medical Research Council became involved in developing blood transfusion, and the League of Nations in the interests of collective security put the stan-

dardization of grouping sera and of their confused terminology on its schedule. At the outbreak of a new war, the Red Cross Blood Transfusion Service became the state-supported National Blood Transfusion Service, with an expanded mandate to prepare and store sera and blood products, such as freeze-dried plasma, to deal with expected civilian casualties (72). In 1943, two British workers found that the addition of dextrose to the citrate anticoagulant solution made it possible to store refrigerated whole blood for as long as 21 days (73). This technique was quickly taken up by the Transfusion Service in wartime Britain, but only gradually adopted in the United States. The U.S. military preferred to use dried bovine albumin as an emergency lifesaver in the field. (See below.)

The new availability of stored blood was to make possible an era of large-scale surgery, including dialysis and open-heart surgery with extracorporeal circulation (74). It also facilitated the large-scale spread of serum hepatitis (hepatitis B) among patients, and technical, medical, nursing and cleaning personnel. In Britain, before the introduction of hepatitis testing in the 1960s, approximately 1 in 10 donated units were infected; in the United States, the numbers were higher (75). Pooled plasma, with material from several donors in a single bottle made things even worse. In a paragraph that looks forward to the AIDS problems of the 1980s, Vaughan and Panton wrote in 1952:

> Blood and blood products are highly dangerous materials.... False grouping, the transmission of infectious diseases other than jaundice, the use of the proper kinds and amounts of transfused fluid, the serious danger of infected material, can only be dealt with if the utmost care is taken. The prevention of jaundice is still under investigation and this unsolved problem serves as a reminder that blood transfusion is not in its final phase but is still in urgent need of further research.... The advances stimulated by war in this field have had profound repercussions in many fields of civilian medical practice and are likely to have more (76).

A marker for hepatitis B came in 1966, and a vaccine in 1982. Transfusion, in the course of the 1970s, came to be regarded as almost free of risk, on a par with vitamins. The AIDS crisis was to change that.

THE CHEMISTRY OF THE ANTIBODY GLOBULINS, 1930–1960

The history of protein chemistry is a sequence of developments in technology and instrumentation, each technical innovation opening the door to a new series of interpretations. The techniques centered around the separation of the protein mixtures found in nature, the drive to reduction first defining and naming individual proteins, then protein fragments and chains, and finally amino-acid sequences, focusing down on the nature of the antibody combining site.

Like the work on the antigen–antibody reaction, work on the proteins originated in colloid chemistry. In the first decade of the century, Swedish chemists using the ultramicroscope began differentiating inorganic colloids into separate molecules, arguing that colloids were in fact particulate and not homogeneous aggregates (77). Theodor (The) Svedberg's life work began with his project on Brownian motion, which he felt demonstrated *ad oculos* the reality of molecules. He was attacked from all sides, among others by Albert Einstein, but he stuck to his interpretation and in 1926 won a Nobel Prize. His work on proteins began in the early 1920s with the development of his ultracentrifuge, modified from a dairy cream separator. The addition of an oil turbine rotor gave a speed of 40,000 rpm and a force of 100,000 G, and an optical eyepiece made the boundary of the sedimenting material visible. The results persuaded a skeptical Svedberg that proteins too consisted of molecules, and that they had definite molecular weights. He gave each a sedimentation coefficient S that indicated a relative molecular weight, with serum globulin having a coefficient of 7S, corresponding to a molecular weight of about 15,000; there was also a small amount of a heavier 18S globulin (78). In fact, he went further and suggested that all proteins, like hemoglobin, might be aggregates of identical subunits with molecular weights of about 17,000. Joseph Fruton (79) ascribes this suggestion to the hypnotic power of numerology. I see it as an example of the need to find simple laws underlying complex phenomena, a principle of scientific research prominent in the work of others of the period, for example, Landsteiner (80). Svedberg saw ultracentrifugal analysis as classical colloid chemistry. Particle size, aggregation, and dispersal in a medium were central colloid problems, but the vitalistic tone of the earlier colloid enthusiasts was soon lost.

Svedberg's 1926 prize attracted enough government funding and Rockefeller grants to set up a new Institute of Physical Chemistry at Uppsala. Here ultracentrifuges of enormous size could be installed in a "building remarkable for its efficiency: no unnecessary, pointless fittings are to be found," says Arne Tiselius (81), in a reflection of the contemporary feeling for unity and simplicity in architecture as in science. Tiselius, Svedberg's erstwhile research assistant, wrote that the workshop with its highly skilled mechanics was "an increasingly important part of the Institute, for in many investigations, the building of the apparatus is perhaps the most important factor" (82). Several apparatuses were built for export to the United States and Britain. Tiselius himself followed in his senior's footsteps by developing another piece of industrial-sized equipment, the electrophoresis apparatus, based on a small-scale apparatus designed by Landsteiner and the colloid chemist Wolfgang Pauli. His apparatus was designed to separate serum proteins by charge, rather than by molecular weight. Tiselius too felt that the study of electrokinetic phenomena was among the most important tasks of colloid chemistry (83).

Lily Kay (84) has suggested that these large, complicated and very expensive pieces of equipment generated their own research programs as they diffused from Uppsala to other centers, beginning with the Rockefeller Institute in New York. Andrew Ede (85) goes further and suggests that colloid chemistry itself was a product of the original dialysis apparatus of 1849, the semipermeable membrane that separated colloids from crystalloids. These historians have put their finger on a feature that has been of singular importance in protein chemistry from its mid–19th-century origins to the mid–20th-century work that elucidated the structure of antibodies. At each stage, exploitation of a new separation technique revealed a broad new landscape for the explorers. Some, like the ultracentrifuge, were products of heavy industry, requiring factory-like laboratories. Others, like the starch-gel electrophoresis setup, were so simple that they could be made at home. All of them contributed to the drive to reduction: Every separation made the fragments smaller, until the smallest possible came into view, and with them, the secret of antibody specificity.

The earliest serum fractionation method was "salting out," by the addition of neutral salts, a technique dating to the mid-19th century, and still in use today for large-scale rough or preliminary separation of a bucket of serum. Here the antibody activity went down with the globulin fraction, leaving the albumin in solution. As late as 1930, however, it was still being argued that antibodies might not actually be globulins; they might simply be precipitated along with the globulins (86). In 1938, Tiselius collaborated with Elvin Kabat of Columbia University on the fractionation of immune sera, with the significant result that antibody was finally linked to the globulin fraction, which could be seen to separate into three bands, named by the discoverers the α, β, and γ globulin bands. Antibody activity was located in the γ band (87). By 1945, the first commercial version of the electrophoresis apparatus had appeared, cost and size were coming down, and the importance of the technique growing as it became more commonplace.

The tradition of large-scale fractionation was well established in Uppsala, but these were still analytic rather than preparative techniques. The new methods of the 1940s and 1950s allowed for the preparation of batches of material. Edwin Cohn's Plasma Fractionation Project, centered during the World War II in his laboratory at Harvard Medical School, reoriented his research on problems of protein structure to the large-scale preparation of plasma fractions for use in battlefield emergencies. Where others had organized a blood transfusion service or used whole plasma, the United States preferred albumin. Cohn's method was to isolate the albumin from bovine blood by fractionation with alcohol, not by salting out, and to freeze-dry it using a new commercial technique. Purity was guaranteed by inspection of the fractions in the Tiselius apparatus. He was later to change to human serum albumin, as bovine albumin could produce serum sickness. Serum globulin was a useful by-product: It could be used clinically as convalescent serum was used in childhood diseases, that is, as a source of antibodies against common infections, especially hepatitis. Cohn developed a small portable fractionator that could be attached to a donor's arm for plasmapheresis and the preparation of hyperimmune globulin. Angela Creager (88) has opened up an interesting pathway here in her studies of Cohn and his practical methods.

The name "chromatography" was introduced by the Russian botanist M. Tswett (89) in 1903 to describe his trick of separating colored plant materials by allowing a drop of the mixture to spread on a piece of blotting paper, producing concentric rings of distinct color. A.J.P. Martin (90) and his group at St. George's Hospital in London worked out the first good chromatographic method during the 1940s (90). They used a filter-paper sheet held vertically as the adsorbent, and allowed the test substance in solution to creep slowly upwards by capillary action, separating into smudges as it went. The separation could be made two-dimensional by turning the paper on its side and dipping it in another solvent, or using an electric current. The method was called "fingerprinting." It separated mixtures of differently charged peptide fragments, opening the way to protein genetics.

After the war, a new type of chromatography was worked out by Stanford Moore and William Stein at the Rockefeller Institute in New York (91). The adsorbent matrix this time was an insoluble resin, either acidic or basic, packed into a vertical column. A solvent carrying the mixture trickled down through it, leaving the oppositely charged components attached to the resin, while those with similar charge passed through unhindered. This ion-exchange chromatography was very effective as a preparative procedure, particularly when linked up with the automatic fraction collector that Moore and Stein designed that allowed the experimenters to run their columns overnight and read the results in the morning. But the rough treatment of the protein often resulted in the disappearance of biological activity, "lost on the column." The lab workers were proud of their sensitivity to the delicate treatment needed for the preservation of antibody. Rough handling that produced foaming often diminished antibody titer, or destroyed it altogether.

The "molecular sieve," another preparative technique from Uppsala, was developed by Jerker Porath in 1960 in collaboration with the Swedish firm Pharmacia. It consisted of a column of Sephadex™, a cross-linked dextran gel. Separation of the protein mixture was by molecular size, due probably, Porath thought, to steric hindrance as the molecules straggled through the maze of pores in the white fluffy gel (92). Its mate was the updated, and less destructive, ion-exchange method of column chromatography developed by the American Herbert Sober and his group in 1956 using charged forms of cellulose (diethyl aminoethyl or DEAE cellulose, and carboxymethyl or CM cellulose) and a buffer gradient (93). Here again separation of proteins and protein fragments was by charge. These two methods were complemented by the practical addition of an elegant Swiss-made automatic fraction collector.

Starch gel electrophoresis is a kind of counterexample to the power of the huge machines in creating and controlling their own program of research. A starch gel system could be set up by anyone with a flair for cutting perspex sheets neatly, and boiling up powdered starch and buffer solution in

a beaker (94). It cost virtually nothing, and could be shown to a visiting worker in a few hours. Like paper electrophoresis, it became a favorite in both research and clinical laboratories, partly perhaps because it allowed workers to feel very skilled and sensitive in controlling a simple apparatus that they had made themselves. Technically, starch gel stabilized confusing convection currents and combined charge and sieving properties in one. The thick gels could be stained and desiccated to form thin transparent films that were easy to photograph and store. It was a very effective means of separating complex mixtures such as serum proteins and protein fragments, and detecting genetically determined variants. Oliver Smithies (95) of the Connaught Laboratory in Toronto in his original paper of 1955 reports just such a finding.

One result of the separations was the increasing resolution of globulin types. IgG, IgM, and IgA were distinguished. The question of the nature of reagins was finally solved by the Ishizakas in 1966 as being none of the above, but a new globulin type that they named IgE (96). The time had come to standardize the nomenclature of the immunoglobulins. As the League of Nations under Madsen had done in the 1920s and 1930s, the World Health Organization under Howard Goodman applied its immunodiplomacy to come to a general agreement on terminology (97). It was not easy—I have been told that a scientist would rather use someone else's toothbrush than their terminology.

The accumulation of separation techniques now made it possible to work with fractions of serum and fractions of molecules. The British biochemist Rodney Porter working at the National Institute for Medical Research used DEAE to prepare a sample of immune globulin from whole rabbit serum, then digested it with the proteolytic enzyme papain, and separated the fragments on the ultracentrifuge. There was only one peak. His first stab at globulin structure followed the existing view of it as a long single chain folding on the antigen as a template, as Linus Pauling and Felix Haurowitz had taught (98). His next attempt involved opening the disulfide bonds of the molecule, adding the Sephadex column to his series of preparations. This produced a suggestion of two pieces, one light and one heavy, which would have normally been joined together by disulfide bonds (99). The relation of the pieces produced by opening the S–S bonds to the papain pieces was worked out immunologically, using goat precipitating sera raised against what now seemed to be two different fragments of the rabbit globulin. Porter then proposed a second model of the globulin molecule: a pair of heavy chains joined by disulphide bonds, each with a light chain attached, and with the antibody recognition site on papain fragment I, probably on the heavy chain. The model stood up well when new findings accumulated. Different types of heavy chain were found in different classes of immunoglobulin, and the light chains showed genetically determined polymorphisms (100). Recognition was prompt— in 1968, Porter was awarded the Karl Landsteiner Memorial Award, and in 1972, he shared a Nobel Prize. Porter's

Y-shaped model of the globulin molecule has come to be the symbol of immunology.

Myeloma Proteins—A Model System

Porter's model was built up on normal globulin fragments, with their heterogeneous collection of specificities and chain types. In 1965, the protein chemist Frank Putnam, then at the University of Florida could still write:

> The γ-globulins lack all the prerequisites needed to facilitate study of their primary structure. They are heterogeneous, non-crystallisable and not resolvable into pure components; they are antigenically diverse but share common determinants; many possess ... biological activity, but the site of activity has not been defined.... Yet the key question in immunology and protein biosynthesis today still hinges on the determination of whether antibodies of different specificity—or for that matter, antibodies of the same specificity—differ in amino-acid sequence (101).

A new opening was found when it turned out that the abnormal serum protein produced in such quantities by patients with multiple myeloma was a γ-globulin, but unlike the normal serum globulin, each one was absolutely homogeneous and could be resolved into pure components. Some of these globulins had antibody activity. With Smithies' starch gel separation technique, M.D. Poulik and Gerald Edelmann of the Rockefeller Institute had found in 1961 that if myeloma protein was reduced and alkylated, and the fragments separated, the pattern of components duplicated those of normal globulins, except that the bands that separated on starch gel were very much sharper (102). The Bence–Jones protein from the same patient's urine matched the bands for reduced and alkylated fragments of the parent protein, and corresponded to free light chains (103).

Myeloma proteins had antibody activity for a variety of antigens, but they did not have the heterogeneity of the normal protein, raising the possibility that they could be used for detailed studies of antibody chain structure. Human myeloma cells were difficult to grow in tissue culture, but Thelma Dunn, Ragna Rask-Nielsen, and Michael Potter found a way of growing mouse myelomas by transplanting them into inbred mice. Each myeloma derived from a single clone of cells, and produced a single homogeneous globulin. As Michael Potter (104) remarks, these were cancer workers for whom the idea of a tumor originating from a single cell was not new—the clone maintained its uniqueness through all its transplants. Many myeloma proteins were found later to have antidinitrophenyl activity, perhaps as a result of a cross-reaction with some gut antigen. Separations and amino-acid sequencing showed that all light chains of a given type shared a constant sequence of amino acids at one end, but were variable at the other, suggesting that antibody specificity was a result of a specific amino-acid sequence.

Parallel with the information that was building up through the 1950s on the sequence of amino acids in protein chains, there came evidence that the sequences appeared to be genetically controlled. Each amino-acid link in the chain was coded for in the nuclear deoxyribonucleic acid (DNA) and the coding transferred to a messenger ribonucleic acid (RNA), and transcribed as an addition to the chain. The system seemed to be strictly directional—the product could not affect the messenger. No protein could be formed by copying another. Francis Crick of Cambridge called this the "central dogma" of protein synthesis (105). If it was substantiated, it meant that the template theory of antibody synthesis could not stand. But the theory had deep roots and powerful supporters. American immunochemists such as Linus Pauling, Michael Heidelberger, and Felix Haurowitz, now in Indiana, still held to it. Haurowitz felt that fingerprinting had shown that globulins were all almost alike in sequence, and that even if the sequence was genetically determined, which he doubted, the folding of the chain might still depend on antigen. As he wrote in 1963,

> It is imaginable that the interference of a template with the folding pattern may affect the sequential pattern and thereby prevent or favour the incorporation of certain amino-acids into particular geometric patterns of the three-dimensional conformation of the globular molecule. The immunochemical observations show quite clearly that not all information required for biosynthesis of proteins is supplied by nucleic acids, and that proteins and other substances may act as templates. Life may then be more than merely the "expression of the chemistry of nucleic acids" (106).

Haurowitz was never to surrender. In fact, he felt that James Watson and Francis Crick's idea of the replication of DNA strands one from another was something that Watson had picked up while attending his, Haurowitz's, classes. The idea of a template for protein synthesis, disconnected from antigen, continued to appear from time to time like a ghost ship. Marshall Nirenberg (107), in his essay on protein synthesis of 1965, refers to messenger RNA and synthetic polyribonucleotides as "highly active templates," directing amino acids into nascent proteins.

CELLULAR IMMUNOLOGY AND THE SELECTION THEORIES 1950s TO 1980s

Antibiotics, beginning with the strategically important drug penicillin, came in with World War II. At first, it was a secret weapon reserved for the armed forces (108). New vaccines such as the polio vaccines of the 1950s, famously funded by the American charity March of Dimes, still appeared (109) (along with a revived antivaccinationist movement [110]) but the serological treatment of disease had lost its edge. In spite of all its successes, compared with the hopes raised by antibiotics, serology no longer seemed so powerful. Immunochemistry reached a climax with the Porter model of immunoglobulin of the 1960s, but from the 1950s onward, mainstream thinking in immunology became steadily more biological and less reductionist. Few immunologists were interested in both biology and chemistry. For instance, at the first meeting of the International Congress for Immunology, held in Washington, DC in 1971, cellular and chemical sessions ran simultaneously, making it impossible for adepts of either to attend the other's sessions (111). It was not the "central dogma" that turned immunologists away from the template theory of antibody production, but the new interest in immunologically competent cells and immunized animals.

The leading thinkers of the period, especially the Australian Sir Frank Macfarlane Burnet, saw themselves as biologists and drew on the ideas of contemporary biology, not chemistry. Burnet, a virologist with a childhood love of natural history and of Charles Darwin, took up the directorship of the Walter and Eliza Hall Institute in Melbourne in 1944. His colleague and successor, Sir Gus Nossal, remembered Burnet as having a fundamentally negative attitude to technology:

> Of course, Burnet was in many ways deeply correct to be mistrustful of technology. Sometimes scientists center their lives around an instrument, they become experts at running an electron microscope, ultracentrifuge or some more sophisticated piece of apparatus until they become prisoners of the instrument and cease asking deep, fact-finding questions. Burnet was wary of that behaviour (112).

In the 1960s, molecular biology was growing exponentially. It had already made its mark on immunology, first through immunochemistry and then through the proliferation of protein separation techniques. Standardization, reduction, and the ideal of molecularization had ruled immunology for decades, often in advance of the effective reduction of other biological sciences, except perhaps the pharmaceutical industry (113). But Macfarlane Burnet was uncomfortable with biochemistry and its sophisticated equipment, and he discouraged it in his institute. Under his leadership immunology moved in a different direction from most contemporary science, as it rejected reductionism and returned to the level of the immune animal and the cell.

Cellular immunology began in the late 1930s with the attempt to show that skin sensitivity to simple chemicals was due to antibodies or reagins (114). There was already a tradition of work on skin lesions, usually associated with infections—the tuberculin reaction was first mentioned by Robert Koch in 1891 (115). According to the Vienna pediatrician Clemens von Pirquet, this was the same reaction that followed smallpox vaccination and other skin infections (116). Landsteiner's artificial diazo-protein antigens provided the model: The diazo group would link to body protein, and stimulate antibody production, and hence skin contact sensitivity to the antigen. The elderly Landsteiner and his young colleague Merrill W. Chase at the Rockefeller Institute struggled with serum transfer experiments. Antibody could sometimes be found. Chase assumed that it must be cell bound, since contact sensitivity was not usually transferable by cell-free serum. The same was true of tuberculin hypersensitivity, also known as delayed hypersensitivity. That was usually contrasted with immediate hypersensitivity, in which a small amount of antigen introduced into the skin of a sensitized animal produced local swelling and redness within a few minutes. It could be transferred by serum from the sensitized individual to the normal. Histologically, immediate and delayed hypersensitivity seemed similar: Immediate hypersensitivity or local anaphylaxis was an acute inflammation, with edema, polymorphonuclear leukocytes, and a few lymphocytes, lasting roughly 24 hours. The tuberculin or delayed reaction was slower to develop, with many more lymphocytes and macrophages. It formed a solid red lump on the skin, often breaking down to a black, necrotic center and healing very slowly (117). It was only when some of the exudates that Landsteiner and Chase were using for transfer were incompletely cleared of cells, that it began to seem as if the transfer of skin hypersensitivity was mediated by the cells, not the serum. A serum factor, called "transfer factor" by New York immunologist Sherwood Lawrence, was mentioned in Chase's review of 1965, but it sounds from the text as if he did not believe in it. At the time, no one did. As Lawrence said in 1986 (118), after his factor seemed to have been justified, there was a subtle irony here—the emergence of cellular immunology as a scientific discipline was ushered in by the cataract of soluble factors it released.

Graft Rejection and Tolerance

The key practical problem of the period was graft rejection, which along with blood transfusion, was important in wartime. Sir Peter Medawar, a professor of zoology at University College, London, made his first attempts at grafting patients with burns in 1943. Comparison of the survival of grafts of the patients' own skin and skin from donors led him to suggest a genetically determined immune rejection mechanism. Like Landsteiner and Chase, he thought first of antibodies, a system like the blood groups perhaps, with "at least seven antigens" involved (119). As the surgeon Joseph Murray proved in 1954, between identical twins in the absence of an immunological barrier, a renal autograft could function permanently. He and the urological team at Peter Brent Brigham Hospital in Boston had bypassed the immunological problem, but at the same time, demonstrated its importance. Murray said that organ transplantation revitalized immunology (120).

Discussion centered on tolerance. In 1949, Frank Fenner and Macfarlane Burnet introduced the concept of self–not self discrimination by suggesting that tolerance for a range of self-markers developed in fetal life (121). They were able the cite the natural experiment of cattle twins, where exchange of blood precursor cells had taken place *in utero,* and gone on producing genetically foreign cells throughout life (122). Burnet's own attempt to induce tolerance failed, but the demonstration was carried out by Medawar and his colleagues Rupert E. Billingham and Leslie Brent, all three of them zoologists by training and practice. Tolerance could be induced experimentally in embryos, and it persisted after birth (123). Brent (124) said that it was only in the mid-1950s that the community of immunologists accepted that their work was relevant to the mainstream, and that they themselves began to regard themselves as immunologists. Burnet (125) saw the interest in the vital phenomenon of tolerance as one more justification for his view that the new immunology should be biological and not chemical.

Tolerance in theory did not solve the clinical problem of graft rejection, which Leslie Brent has called the "search for the holy grail." A temporary solution was achieved by Byron Waksman and his group with antilymphocyte serum, which suppressed delayed hypersensitivity and acute homograft rejection, though an antiglobulin was soon formed against it (126).

The importance of this work for skin and organ grafting is demonstrated in a peculiar way by the episode of the spotted mouse. William Summerlin, a young researcher at the Sloan–Kettering Institute in New York claimed in 1973 to have achieved a take of grafts between nonsyngeneic mice by culturing the graft cells before setting them. Medawar and colleagues and others tried and failed to replicate the results, and it appeared later that they had been faked. Medawar suggested that perhaps one such graft had taken—perhaps due to a mix-up of mice—and its importance was such that its author could not admit that his result was unrepeatable (127).

The first immunosuppressive drugs turned up initially in the early 1960s as antimitotic agents tested as chemotherapy for cancer, and it was the combination of these with corticosteroid hormones that finally made transplanted organs the commonplace they now are. The next generation of immunosuppressants was based on the cyclosporines, antilymphocytic agents first extracted from the fungus *Trichoderma polysporum*. They were detected in the laboratories of Sandoz in Basel, in the course of a broad pharmacological screening project that seems to have included all known fungi. Hartmann Stähelin (128) in discussing this sees it a serendipitous discovery, but it sounds more like the empiricism that once was the preferred program of science.

The success of organ grafting depended on the construction of a network of centers carrying waiting lists of patients ready to be correlated with available organs, so that a cadaver organ packed in ice could be rushed to a patient as quickly as possible. Initially, the patients were tissue typed, and organs sought that most nearly matched the antigens on the patients' leucocytes, the histocompatibility antigens. The mixed lymphocyte reaction, in which a culture of cells from two genetically different sources responded to each other's histocompatibility antigens, could be used as a kind of crossmatch of donor and patient on the blood transfusion model. A good match improved the survival of the graft, but perhaps not enough, it was argued, to justify the longer period that a patient would have to spend waiting for a matched transplant. From the early 1980s on, the use of cyclosporin improved graft survival so much that typing now seemed less important.

The Clonal Selection Theory

The insistent question of the generation of antibody diversity went through a biological metamorphosis too. The idea

that the sequence of amino acids in antibody globulin, or at least the folding of the chains, was directly molded on antigen had satisfied a generation of chemists and serologists brought up on Landsteiner's charge outline and more-or-less good fit picture of the antigen–antibody reaction. In 1955, however, Niels Kaj Jerne of the Statens Seruminstitut in Copenhagen had just finished a thesis on the old serological problem of antibody avidity (129). He now suggested something strikingly different as a theory of antibody production. He proposed that all possible specificities were randomly present in the serum as spontaneously synthesized natural antibodies, and antigen *selected*—not synthesized—its match from among these natural antibodies. Jerne called this a theory of natural selection. The antigen–antibody complex would be taken up by phagocytic cells, which would be "signaled" to reproduce that same antibody; the antigen, freed from its complex, could go back into circulation and do the same again. For Jerne, it is the antibody, not the antigen, which acts as a template.

> The crucial point of the natural-selection theory is the postulate that the introduction of antibody molecules into appropriate cells can be the signal for the production of more of their kind. This notion is unfamiliar. However, as nothing is known about the mechanism of antibody synthesis in a cell, it would seem a priori more reasonable to assume that an animal can translate a stimulus, introduced by protein molecules which it has itself at one time produced, into an increased synthesis of this same type of molecules, than to suppose that an animal can utilize all sorts of foreign substances and can build them functionally and semi-permanently into the most intimate parts of its globulin-synthesizing cells (130).

He suggests that the antibody protein can act as a template for the order of nucleotides in the synthesis of RNA, which in turn acts as a template for more of the same protein. Natural selection, he thinks, could account for the increased avidity of antibodies produced later on in the course of immunization. But as Thomas Söderqvist, Jerne's biographer, has said, for Jerne the expression "natural selection" had only the very faintest of Darwinian overtones (131).

Jerne's paper initiated a renewed discourse on antibody production. In 1957, two years after Jerne, David Talmage of the University of Colorado in a general review of immunology and its current problems and uncertainties, compared the theories with the available data. He recognized that the template theory was very widely held at the time. But it was beginning to seem strained. Jerne had shown in his thesis that antibody avidity increased during the secondary response when antibody was being most rapidly produced. Logically, increased avidity should have slowed release of new antibody from an antigen template. And Burnet in 1949 had found a logarithmic rise in antibody production, which suggested that antibody was being produced by something that was replicating, not just being recycled. Burnet, said Talmage, complains that a gap has grown up between immunology and existing knowledge of biology. He has pointed out that nowhere else in nature was there anything analogous to an antigen template. In fact, Burnet and Fenner were already stating programmatically in 1949 that they preferred to approach the problem "on biological rather than chemical or pseudo-chemical lines." It was a strange and surprising statement. The template theory's inventor, the chemist Felix Haurowitz, asked in a review of *The Production of Antibodies,*

> How can they hope to explain molecular phenomena taking place between molecules of the antigen, the antibody and possibly other substances, without invoking the principles of chemistry?... The words put by the reviewer in quotation marks [those quoted above] demonstrate that Burnet and Fenner use the strong language of men who know they are right (132).

Burnet at the time had a theory of antibody production linked to the enzyme induction well known in bacteria, which could adapt themselves to growing on different substrates. But it was soon abandoned.

Talmage welcomed Jerne's natural selection idea in that it offered an alternative to the template theory, but he proposed a major modification. He saw that it harked back to Ehrlich, and he suggested that, as in Ehrlich's theory, the recognizing antibody might be on a cell, rather than in the serum. This cellular version of the hypothesis would fit better with the long-continued production of antibody without any further stimulus, and with current views of protein synthesis. It took account of the transfer of active immunity by cells rather than by serum, as serum tended instead to suppress the immune response. Jerne explained by saying that an animal must be able to distinguish between its own globulin and that of another of the same species, or perhaps the globulin was somehow damaged in the course of the transfer. Talmage picked up the Darwinian suggestion in Jerne's title and gave it a more literally Darwinian content:

> The process of natural selection requires the selective multiplication of a few species out of a diverse population. As a working hypothesis it is tempting to consider that one of the multiplying units in the antibody response is the cell itself. According to this hypothesis, only those cells are selected for multiplication whose synthesized product has affinity for the antigen injected. This would have the disadvantage of requiring a different species of cell for each species of protein produced, but would not increase the total amount of information required of the hereditary process (133).

In the same year, after reading Talmage's critique, Burnet also modified Jerne's theory (134). It has been said that he purposely sent the paper to a modestly circulated journal, just in case it was embarrassingly dismissed by his colleagues. If that was so, this uncharacteristically tentative approach was soon dropped. Ten years later, he was to write confidently:

> It gradually dawned on me that Jerne's selection theory would make real sense if cells produced a characteristic pattern of globulin for genetic reasons and were stimulated to proliferate by contact with the corresponding antigenic determinant. This would demand a receptor on the cell with the same pattern as antibody and a signal resulting from contact of antigenic determinant and receptor that would initiate mitosis.... Once that central concept was clear, the other implications followed more or less automatically... (135)

Haurowitz had understood him very well: Burnet was a man who knew he was right.

Burnet defended his idea in *The Clonal Selection Theory of Acquired Immunity* of 1959. It is the clonal part that he is at pains to argue. There are many other examples of clones in biology; his models come from bacteriology and cancer research. The spread of the lethal myxomatosis epizootic in Australia, introduced in 1950 to control the rabbit population, provides one model. Here distinct clones of less virulent forms of virus multiplied to become the dominant, keeping the virus circulating as an epizootic. Mutation and selective survival were able to change the character of a population of cells (136). Another model is multiple myeloma:

> I hope it is not overstating the case to say that the multiple myeloma findings provide the best possible material for displaying the salient features of the clonal selection approach to the phenomena of antibody production and of malignancy.... The fact that each myeloma patient produces his own characteristic and individual serum protein, with its sharp spike evidence of homogeneity, provides support for what many workers might consider a weak point of the clonal selection theory, that each clone produces a specific antibody globulin whose pattern is genetically determined (137).

Like Burnet himself, contemporary commentators on Burnet's new approach underlined his Darwinism. According to Gordon Ada and Sir Gustav Nossal, younger colleagues of Burnet at the Walter and Eliza Hall Institute in Melbourne, for Burnet, the immune response was a Darwinian microcosm. Lymphocytes were the individuals in a particular ecological niche, mutating and being selected, like the myxomatosis virus. The fittest, in this case the variant that made rabbits sick but did not kill them outright, survived and kept the epidemic going. In the same way, the cells that made the fittest antibodies, those with the best fit to antigen, multiplied the most. In a Darwinian system, adaptation was not imposed from outside, but was favored by the multiplication of the best adapted (138). Burnet himself called the template theory "a grossly Lamarckian qualification on what might be described as a strictly Darwinian process at the cellular level" (139). He did not put his argument in terms of the so-called central dogma of molecular biology. In 1957, soon after the publication of his first statement of the theory, Burnet called his staff together and announced that the whole direction of the Hall Institute would change from virology to immunology. He saw virology as rapidly coming under biochemical influence, which, he said, he "preferred to eschew." He realized that his theory was the foundation of a fundamental change in immunology, and the Institute was to work out its implications (140).

Burnet had predicted that each cell would make only one antibody. The first experimental testing was done at the Hall Institute in 1958. Joshua Lederberg, who had arrived in Melbourne hoping to work on virology, joined up with Gus Nossal to develop a micromanipulation system where individual cells could be tested separately. Using rabbits immunized with two different antigens, they found that among 456 cells isolated, 62 made antibody, and each of them made one antibody only (141). Their system was difficult to reproduce, and only the authors and one or two others were truly able to handle it. But their result was confirmed by Jerne, who invented the ingenious and simple hemolytic plaque technique, something that could be easily learned from his published description (142). Other findings accumulated that made the template theory less likely, although there was in fact no final disproof. But as Talmage has said, the final acceptance of a theory only comes with utility (143). The development of hybridoma technology by Georges Köhler and César Milstein (see below), and the commercial production of monoclonal antibodies finally made the clonal selection theory irresistible (144).

The Biology of the Thymus and the Dictatorship of the Lymphocyte

As Burnet's views gained acceptance in the early 1960s, new work focused on populations of cells. The new theory released an avalanche of work. It coincided with the expansion of U.S. funding for science that followed the end of World War II. Clinical applications of cellular immunology included autoimmunity and transplantation surgery. Pharmaceutical companies, until then focused on vaccines and sera, began to develop and patent immunosuppressants, down-regulators of immunity. In the 1970s, with a new field to till the profession expanded, as journals proliferated, congresses national and international were initiated, and symposia and courses organized.

The Soviet immunologist Rem Viktorovich Petrov (145) called this the period of the dictatorship of the lymphocyte. Before the theory, lymphocytes had no known function. "Round cell infiltration" was pathologist's shorthand for reporting the nonspecific in a tissue section. Now, however, lymphocytes were seen as long-lived cells recirculating through the body's lymphatic tissue and carrying immune recognition and memory, including the recognition of self.

A new and revised anatomy gave a central place to the thymus, which until then was an organ whose histology was described in enormous detail, but whose function was completely blank (146). At this point, a link-up was made between the activities of cells and two much older fields within immunology, the tuberculin reaction and bacterial or delayed hypersensitivity. Each of these had been the product of a different technique, and had been investigated initially in a different context, but they now came to overlap each other. With the new emphasis on the cell, they appeared in a new light. Old cells-versus-serum controversies resolved as it appeared that T-lymphocytes, developing or maturing in the thymus, mediated cellular immunity, and interacted with B-lymphocytes from the bone marrow, producers of serum antibody.

Prepared mice came to be seen as the experimental system of choice—in studies of thymus function and of tolerance, the system was based on the neonatally thymectomized mouse (147). Indeed, the elucidation of thymus function depended on the mastery of the difficult technique of neonatal thymectomy: Jacques Miller at the Chester Beatty Research Institute in London found in 1961 that his thymectomized mice had fewer lymphocytes, made no antibody, and tolerated skin allografts. Other laboratories were close behind him. Here the inspiration was at least in part clinical, as the pediatrician Robert A. Good and his students at Minnesota worked through a family of patients with an X-linked absence of antibody globulins, and found that they all lacked plasma cells. They suffered from recurrent infections, but not from tuberculosis—cellular reactions seemed intact. Good could not reproduce the syndrome with thymectomized rabbits, but he and his students Bruce Glick and Timothy Chang found serendipitously that chicks that had had the bursa of Fabricius removed failed to make both antibody and plasma cells. In birds, they decided, the antibody side seemed to be controlled by the bursa, separately from cellular reactions. If thymectomy was carried out early enough in mice, in "hot little newborns," as Good called them, all immune reactions failed. This reproduced another clinical syndrome, that of the so-called "bubble boy," who spent his short life enclosed in a germ-free plastic bubble (148). Other laboratories were all on the same wavelength: Jacques Miller at the Chester Beatty Hospital; Byron Waksman at Harvard; and Delphine Parrott in John Humphrey's laboratory at the National Institute for Medical Research, Mill Hill. All worked to replicate the clinical syndromes of immune deficiency with thymectomized mice.

As immunobiology replaced immunochemistry in the mainstream, the laboratory turned to the inbred mouse as its key instrument (149). Ilana Löwy and Jean-Paul Gaudillière see genetically homogeneous mice as the equivalent of standardized, chemically pure compounds, produced on an industrial scale (150). By 1962, syngeneic mice were found to be capable of acting as a cell culture for transplanted clones of mouse myeloma cells, providing a library of monoclonal immunoglobulins for investigation.

Monoclonal Antibodies

Myelomas were potentially immortal in cell culture, but only about 5% of naturally occurring myeloma proteins had detectable antibody activity. Normal antibody-producing cells, on the other hand, quickly died out in culture. In 1975, this picture changed with Georges Köhler and César Milstein's fusion of myeloma cells with antibody-producing B cells from a mouse spleen, to produce immortalized cells that secreted monoclonal antibodies of any desired specificity (151). One lymphocyte clone produced one antibody. It was the epitome of the clonal selection theory: Milstein's articles include the experimental diagram showing a mouse with a syringe as the source of cells that has typified all cellular immunology since Burnet. But Milstein was an immunochemist, and he saw his invention as answering the questions left behind by the pre–World War II generation of chemists; he cited Ehrlich's introduction of the problem of diversity and specificity, and Marrack's lattice theory. One of his examples of a useful application is a superspecific anti-A, able to detect A_2B, an old blood-group serologist's problem. His true interest was not practice, however, but what he saw as the "more fundamental" use of monoclonal antibodies to define and characterize the antigenicity of cell membranes. Like Landsteiner, he was uninterested in the merely useful.

In the British tradition, and encouraged by the Medical Research Council, Milstein and Köhler refused to patent their invention. They had received mouse plasmacytoma cells from Michael Potter of the National Institutes of Health in Bethesda, Maryland, and they gave them away freely (152). But patents were quickly taken out by others—in 1979 for monoclonal antibodies against tumor cells, and 1980, for antibodies to viral antigens, in both cases including Hilary Koprowski of the Wistar Institute in Philadelphia among the patent holders. Legal struggles over the patents and the nature of the innovations patented were fought out through the courts by rival pharmaceutical companies.

Milstein and Köhler won their Nobel Prize for this work in 1984, shared with Niels Jerne. The prize was for "a methodological breakthrough that has profound practical significance," in the case of Milstein and Köhler, and "for theoretical advances that have shaped our concepts of the immune system," in Jerne's. Reporting on the prize, the immunologist Jonathan Uhr seemed to feel that the latter was of much more significance (153). Two of the prizewinners, Jerne and Köhler, were from the Basel Institute for Immunology. It had been funded by the pharmaceutical company Hoffman–La Roche as a vehicle for Jerne, and was the leading center for the fusion of the cellular style with molecular biology. Its reign lasted from 1969 to 2001, when the company decided to close it. Jerne retired in 1980.

Writing in 1997, Leslie Brent (154), an expert on transplantation, said that rarely has a technologic invention affected the course of immunology so dramatically; but that was in the future, and not immediately obvious to the inventors. Milstein and Köhler were to create an industry. By 1984, the date of the prize, the practical and commercial effects of having a purified source of antibody with a single defined specificity had become obvious. Cambrosio and Keating note that by then, according to *Index Medicus,* there were already 10,000 articles on the subject. The technique was difficult to master, and like much biological manipulation, required a good deal of tacit and local knowledge gained directly from a laboratory or an individual who could make it work. A careful protocol was not always enough (155).

The practical effect of monoclonal antibodies, apart from their many uses in research (156), was to retool tests for antigenic epitopes, including tumor antigens, viruses, and blood group antigens. The Wassermann test for syphilis, with its theoretical ambiguities, was replaced by a sandwich test, the enzyme-linked immunosorbent assay or ELISA. A similar test was devised for human immunodeficiency virus or HIV, used for both screening blood for transfusion and screening patients from early 1985. Convenient pocket-sized test kits for dozens of clinical problems appeared on the market—it

is safe to say that pharmaceutical companies, clinical pathologists and patients took full advantage of them. In blood transfusion, epitope-specific monoclonals elucidated the details of the Rhesus antigen, which turned out to be a mosaic of many epitopes, rather as Alexander Wiener, its discoverer and spokesman, had argued in Landsteiner's name in the 1940s (157). Different specificities of monoclonal anti-D identified nine critical residues of the protein molecule, protruding from the cell membrane on four loops. To produce recognizable binding, two to four residues were needed, either all on one loop, or on two, three, or four loops, so that there must be a very large number of possible combinations. No monoclonal anti-D will react with all of them. For blood donor typing, even the weak variants that could immunize an Rh-negative patient must be classed as Rh D positive. For pregnant women, on the other hand, weak variants and partial Ds should be classed as Rh negative, since they could be immunized by an Rh-positive fetus. The British Blood Transfusion Service, led by the Bristol Institute for Transfusion Sciences, adopted a saline-reactive monoclonal anti-D that detected the common epitopes, along with one that was specific for the subtype VI, whose cells lack most of them (158).

The example from blood-group serology shows monoclonal antibodies in action—older serological tests are refined and the molecular biology of the complex antigen is made visible by the extremely narrow and well-defined specificity of the antibodies. Clonal immunobiology has incorporated the molecular style, and returned to tease out the problems of the past.

MOLECULAR IMMUNOLOGY: DIVERSITY, HISTOCOMPATIBILITY, AND THE T-CELL RECEPTOR, 1980–PRESENT

Many years ago, I wrote a short paper, my first on the history of immunology. I used the occasion of the Tenth International Congress of Medicine, held in Berlin on 4 August 1880 as a cross-section of what was important in immunology on that date. It was an important meeting—there were 7,056 people present, a very large number for a meeting at that time. The issue debated was whether immunity was a matter of cells, or of serum (159). A hundred years later in 1980, the central matter of immunology was still cells and serum. They were now not alternative explanations of immunity, but linked together as part of a single interactive system, represented by T cells, B cells, and antibody. Descriptions of that relationship have surfaced and then disappeared (160). The current one, still under investigation as I write today, involves the genetics of the immune system, both cellular antigens and globulins. The new methods of the 1980s were those of molecular biology (161).

The elucidation of chain structure and amino-acid sequence by the separation methods of postwar biochemistry had not completely solved the problem of antibody diversity. If the template theory had collapsed, diversity must be genetically determined, but there were two schools of thought on that. If it had appeared far back in evolutionary time and was encoded in the germline, there must be a separate gene for each polypeptide fragment. But if the complete sequence was encoded, with one gene for every possible polypeptide chain, there would have to be an enormous number of genes to cover the enormous number of known and potential specificities, an echo of the problem that had divided Paul Ehrlich and Karl Landsteiner in the first decades of the century, and that was re-emphasized by Macfarlane Burnet in *The Clonal Selection Theory* of 1959. Another school of thought suggested that diversity might arise during the development of the individual, and might depend on somatic, not germline, inheritance. If diversification could be multiplied up in the somatic cells, for example, in B cells as they matured, fewer germline genes would be needed. But no other examples of non-germline inheritance were known, so that was a difficult position to support. The first hint of a solution came in 1976 from Susumu Tonegawa and colleagues at the Basel Institute for Immunology, who used restriction enzymes to dissect the DNA, and recombination to identify the fragments. Werner Arber and his group at Basel were to be awarded a Nobel Prize for the invention of genetic engineering—in fact, for the work on restriction enzymes—in 1978 (162). Recombination, joining the fragmented DNA across species, was introduced in 1972 (163). Morange sees this paper by Paul Berg as having a foundation value similar to that in 1953 of Watson and Crick on the double helix (164). However, public alarm was generated by the threat of such genes escaping into the environment, particularly since the Berg experiment was carried out using *E. coli,* a universal gut inhabitant, and a virus that might be a cause of cancer. Berg himself was well aware of the dangers. At a conference held in 1975, standard operating procedures for the confinement of these potential pathogens were laid out, and were converted into rules by the National Institutes of Health in 1976. Commercial exploitation of the recombination technique was quick to develop, at first by small start-up companies, and later by the well-established pharmaceutical industry. As this got under way, controls were to be loosened (165). But in the late 1970s, as Tonegawa remembers,

> Recombinant DNA was just becoming available and was the ideal means for this purpose. Debates on the possible hazards of this type of research were flaring, initially in the USA and shortly afterwards in European countries. In order to make sure that our research would not become a target of controversy, Charlie and I got in touch with Werner Arber at the University of Basel who was coordinating recombinant DNA research activities in Switzerland. A small informal work group was set up by the local researchers interested in this technique. The consensus of the group, which was supported by most of the other Swiss researchers, was that we should follow the practices and guidelines being adopted in the USA (166).

Tonegawa and his colleagues found that the V genes for light chains were split into two segments, separated by joining regions (167). The Leroy Hood group at the California

Institute of Technology found that there were several separate segments with their joining regions coding for the heavy chain. An examination of these regions in inbred BALB/c mice suggested that only one of the regions was always identical in all of them, and so must be the one represented in the germline. The rest differed by single-base changes. There were therefore two separate genetic mechanisms controlling immunoglobulin diversity. In Tonegawa's words, it turned out that an organism did not inherit even a single complete gene for antibody polypeptide chains. The genetic information was transmitted in the germline as a few hundred gene segments, then reshuffled into tens of thousands of complete genes. Further diversity resulted from hypermutation in these assembled genes. Tonegawa thinks that the initial rather low-affinity antibody response depends on pre-existing germline specificities. The later, higher-affinity antibody is produced by descendants of memory B cells through hypermutation, rearrangement, and splicing of germline genes in the course of B-cell maturation (168). Each generation of cells fits the antigen better and better—or as Niels Jerne noted in his thesis of 1954, antibody avidity increases with repeated exposure to antigen. In 1987, Susumu Tonegawa received a Nobel Prize for this work.

The field of histocompatibility was of practical importance with the rise of organ transplantation, but it soon grew beyond the practical boundaries of transplantation. A series of Histocompatibility Workshops beginning in 1964 took up the problems of typing and the formation of a nomenclature, hoping perhaps to forestall the bitter struggles over the terminology of the Rhesus blood group system, then still being fought out (169). New journals served the new field: *Transplantation* (1962), *Tissue Antigens* (1971), *Immunogenetics* (1971), and *Journal of Immunogenetics* (1974). By 1975, four loci each with a range of specificities had been worked out, and population studies had shown that distribution, as with the blood group antigens, varied globally. In the course of the 1980s, the histocompatibility site was shown to relate to immune response genes—with some simple antigens and some viruses, an all-or-none response can be detected differing between strains of an animal species. Ir gene control affected cellular immunity, and seemed to express itself through cells that collaborated with T cells (170). This is an area that is the subject of ongoing work, and it is treated elsewhere in this volume.

The molecular biology of these antigens was a matter of intense interest. Laboratories at California Institute of Technology under Leroy Hood, at Harvard under J.L. Strominger, and in Uppsala under P.A. Peterson competed to make use of amino-acid analyzers to sequence the molecules. This work led in 1987 to the determination of the sequence and the three-dimensional structure of the molecules. Crystallographic pictures by Pamela Bjorkman from Don Wiley's laboratory are summarized in her words as follows:

> The class I histocompatibility antigen ... [h]as two structural motifs: the membrane-proximal end of the glycoprotein

contains two domains with immunoglobulin folds that are paired in a novel manner, and the region distal from the membrane is a platform of eight anti-parallel β-strands topped by α-helices. A large groove between the α-helices provides a binding-site for foreign antigens ...

The groove is located on the top surface of the molecule, and is therefore a likely candidate for the binding site for the foreign antigen recognized by a T-cell receptor (171).

As Leslie Brent said recently, this was no longer the era of sole researchers working alone in their laboratories. These striking results were reached by competing teams of workers equipped with large grants, the heavy machinery of biomedical research. Equally, however, the inspiration for the problem was derived from the clinical importance, however brief, of the transplantation antigens, just as the work on immunochemistry of the 1920s and 1930s was derived ultimately from the requirements for a standardized diphtheria serum. Joseph Murray's claim that organ transplantation revitalized immunology was no exaggeration.

The importance of the thymus-dependent lymphocytes or T cells was first understood in the early 1960s. Several classes of T cell had been defined. They played a part in most immune reactions, turning on effector T and B cells against non-self antigens and suppressing activity directed against self. Since the 1970s, the T cells had been thought to work through the histocompatibility antigens recognized by the T-cell receptor. But the nature of this receptor was still unknown.

From the early 1980s, several groups of molecular immunologists collaborated, or competed, on the problem. They included teams under Ellis Reinherz and Stuart Schlossman at the Laboratory of Molecular Immunology at the Farber Cancer Institute and Medical School at Harvard, James Allison at the University of Texas, John Kappler and Philippa Marrack at the University of Colorado in Denver, Steve Hedrick and Mark Davis at the National Institutes of Health, and Tak Mak and his team at the Ontario Cancer Institute in Toronto. The newest techniques, such as monoclonal antibodies, gene hybridization, and DNA probes, drove the discoveries. First, the Harvard group in 1980 found a monoclonal antibody that blocked human T-cell function—it prevented the generation of cytotoxic T cells in a mixed lymphocyte culture, and stopped them from acting as helpers to B cells. The authors suggested that this might turn out to be useful in autoimmune disorders or in transplantation (172). In 1982, Allison and his group found another monoclonal antibody that identified a tumor-specific T-cell antigen in mice. The authors speculated that their antigen might be the T-cell equivalent of the B-cell idiotype, and that it might function as an antigen receptor (173). Also in 1982, Reinherz and his team at Harvard found a direct link between one of their monoclonal anti-T cell antibodies, and antigen recognition by T cells (174). The following year, John Kappler and Philippa Marrack (a hereditary immunochemist, since her father J.R. Marrack was the proposer of the lattice theory in 1934 [175]) in Denver, collaborating with Allison and McIntyre from Texas, used a fingerprinting technique to identify the peptides that con-

ferred specificity on the antigen receptor on T cells that recognized the major histocompatibility complex, the key to self–not self recognition. Like the immunoglobulins, the protein sequences showed variable and constant regions linked by joining segments. The T-cell receptor generally resembled a pair of immunoglobulin light chains, a heterodimer of α and β, joined by a disulfide bond, and with their −COOH ends buried in the cell membrane (176). By analogy to immunoglobulin, it was predicted that the DNA sequences coding for the T-cell receptor would be in separate regions in the genome, rearranging themselves somatically to form a complete gene. As Tak Mak explains, hybridization to a DNA probe complementary to a sequence encoding a T-cell receptor chain revealed different genomic hybridization patterns in different T-cell clones, all of them different again from the basic germ line pattern in non–T cells. The genetic reconstitution of a T-cell receptor by transfection of the DNA sequences into a recipient cell supported the hypothesis, and it was estimated that a total diversity of about 10^{10} could be achieved with combinatorial joining and somatic mutation together (177). A superfamily of Ig-like genetically determined proteins has been proposed. They include the immune globulins themselves, the T-cell receptors and other T markers defining different subsets of T cells, the histocompatibility antigens, some lymphoid–brain-associated antigens (in a piece of discreet advertising, one has been labeled MRC OX-2, associating it with the Medical Research Council's Immunology Research Unit at Oxford), and other neural-associated antigens. It has been suggested that they have all evolved from a single stable domain, which then produced various sequences ensconced in different cell lines. All are on cell membranes, and seem to be involved with cell recognition and interaction; perhaps they acquired immune functions at about the time of vertebrate evolution (178).

We are still fulfilling Macfarlane Burnet's ideal of the 1960s, an immunological theory based on the "simple concepts of biology—reproduction, mutation ... and selective survival," even though we have gone over to the chemical methods he so disliked (179). But biology itself is different now.

AIDS: THE PUBLIC FACE OF IMMUNOLOGY, 1986 TO THE PRESENT

The earliest cases of Acquired Immune Deficiency Syndrome (AIDS) appeared in 1982, as a series of otherwise unusual infections and malignancies in male homosexual patients. At first, it seemed to be a problem that concerned only the gay community; it was named Gay-Related Immunodeficiency, or GRID (180). Social change followed, as gays organized to deal with a sickness that was untreatable, progressive, and ultimately fatal in all cases. Groups such as ACT-UP of New York, an organization of HIV+ people in the arts, demonstrated to demand access to the newest drugs. They brought their anger into the AIDS congresses, to the surprise of the scientists expecting to address a quietly formal scientific meeting. Gay activism altered the image of the homosexual from irresponsible hedonist to that of a caring and politically active individual, and the image of the patient from a passive sufferer to an impatient, informed, and critical adversary (181).

Isolated in 1984, human immunodeficiency virus (HIV) was found to affect CD4 lymphocytes, key cells in the orchestration of the immune response (182). By the early 1990s, through the AIDS activist organizations, their outreach literature, and their brilliant posters, the immune system became part of popular discourse, as Emily Martin found in the streets of her home town. T cells entered the public domain as Mr. T, the killer cell (183). Historians, as well as their editors and publishers, began to see significance in immunology. A historiography of immunology appeared.

The style of the epidemic differed profoundly according to the community affected. The well-organized gay community took safer sex into its own hands; and antiviral drugs when they arrived were carefully studied and diligently taken, in spite of their unpleasant side effects. As a result, death rates dropped, followed by declining new infection rates. But other high-risk groups such as users of illegal intravenous drugs are notoriously difficult to reach. There were even ethical objections raised to so-called harm-reduction initiatives, such as providing the users with clean needles or bleach kits. As with hepatitis B, and later C, the infection was transmitted in transfused blood and blood products, affecting particularly hemophiliacs using concentrates of the blood-clotting Factors VIII and IX. These were made from very large pools of plasma, often from several thousand donors; 60% of the donors were from the United States, where infection rates at the time were the highest in the world. Hemophiliacs, their partners, and their children died in large numbers. In Montreal, 56% of hemophiliacs were infected by 1982; by 1988, 74%. By the time ELISA testing of donor blood began in 1985, 1 in 270 of the blood donors in Toronto were testing positive for HIV (184).

In every country, the seriousness of the epidemic was underestimated. The local blood transfusion organizations, including the trusted Red Cross, hesitated too long for reasons of economy to throw out products they knew were infected, even where heat-treated, infection-free materials were available. Everywhere legal remedies were demanded. In France, criminal proceedings against several senior members of the organizations resulted in prison sentences. The accusations reached beyond the serological establishment to three former ministers deemed politically responsible (185).

In South Africa, President Thabo Mbeki argued that the form of the epidemic in that country was more dependent on social factors such as poverty than on a virus. He invited a group of scientists who questioned the relevance of the virus, Peter Duesberg among them, to an open debate with a panel of mainstream thinkers. Arguments were presented to suggest that the increased death rates were due to a variety of infections, mainly linked to social stress, deprivation, and poverty. However, the statistician Malegapuru Makgoba of the South African Medical Research Council rejected that. He pointed to rising death rates among young adults of both sexes, beginning with the epidemic in the early 1990s. The significance of this is that a viral etiology makes it sensible to pressure drug companies to provide anti-virals or vaccines at low cost.

The numbers of people now infected or dead in Sub-Saharan Africa, as in the Black Death of 14th century Europe, has cut deeply into education, government, and medical services, leaving classes without teachers, government without administrators, hospitals without doctors or nurses, and children without parents (187). Life expectancy at birth has dropped to below 30 in some areas of Africa, and projections show that the epidemic is not yet leveling off. A vaccine is reported as being in the test phase, but testing is slow with a disease that takes 10 years to develop symptoms. For the present, healthcare activism, including improvements to the status of women and the use of condoms, remain the most effective means of controlling the disease.

CONCLUSION

Immunology is a laboratory science; individuals who call themselves immunologists are likely to work in a laboratory. This chapter treats immunology from their point of view, like most of the material on immunology and its history. But it is not a simple history of ideas. Between the lines, a careful reader can perceive that immunology is no abstract science that sets its own goals and wanders wherever science takes it. The force that directs its activities comes from the direction of clinical medicine and in turn, the scientific findings come back to the clinic and its ancillary, the pharmaceutical industry. Before World War II, the serologists responded to the need to understand and to standardize the antisera then in use—immunochemistry tried to answer questions posed by the diphtheria serum. During the 1940s, protein separation methods and plasma fractionation contributed to military medicine and later to civilian needs. After the war, the paradigm was set by transplantation. Work on tolerance and down-regulation succeeded work on immunization. New surgical procedures, the organization of organ supply networks, the development of immunosuppressive drugs, and the teasing out of the linked roles of transplantation antigens and cells were all part of a dialogue with the clinic. Monoclonal antibody research fed on the clinical opportunity, and supplied the pharmaceutical industry's appetite for neat and accurate test kits, as much as the abstract need to know about the details of epitopes and of the immunoglobulin molecule. Finally, the advent of the AIDS epidemic made immunology a household word, and released the interest of historians in the activities of lymp hocytes. It is to be hoped that a new generation of historians will analyze immunology as an applied clinical science. There is more to be said.

REFERENCES

1. Cambrosio A, Keating P, Tauber AI. Introduction: immunology as a historical object. *J Hist Biol* 1994;27:531–573.
2. Leung AKC. "Variolation" and vaccination in late imperial China, ca 1570–1911, in Plotkin S, Fantini B, eds, *Vaccinia, vaccination and vaccinology: Jenner, Pasteur and their successors,* Paris: Elsevier, 1996:65–71.
3. Miller G. *The adoption of inoculation for smallpox in France and England in the 18th century,* Philadelphia: Pennsylvania University Press, 1957.
4. Rusnock AA. The weight of evidence and the burden of authority: case histories, medical statistics and smallpox inoculation, *Clio Medica* 1995;29:289–314.
5. Moulin A-M. *Le dernier langage de la médecine: histoire de l'immunologie de Pasteur au SIDA,* Vendome: Presses Universitaires de France, 1991.
6. Razzell P. *Edward Jenner's cowpox vaccine: the history of a medical myth,* 2nd ed., Sussex: Caliban, 1980.
7. Arnold D. Smallpox and colonial medicine in nineteenth-century India, in Arnold D, ed., *Imperial medicine and indigenous societies,* Manchester: Manchester University Press, 1988:45–65.
8. Mercer AJ. *Disease, mortality and population in transition,* Leicester: University of Leicester Press. 1990.
9. Bewell A. *Romanticism and colonial disease,* Baltimore, MD: Johns Hopkins Press, 1999.
10. Anderson W, Jackson M, Rosenkrantz B. Towards an unnatural history of immunology. *J Hist Biol* 1994;27:575–594; Anderson W, Immunities of empire: race, disease and the new tropical medicine, 1900–1920, *Bull Hist Med* 1996;70:94–118.
11. Moulin A-M. La métaphore vaccine. De l'inoculation à la vaccinologie. *Hist Phil Life Sci* 1992;14:271–297. For a highly unflattering account of Pasteur's work on attenuation of organisms, see Geison GL, *The private science of Louis Pasteur,* Princeton, NJ: Princeton University Press, 1995, 145–176, 206–233.
12. Long ER. Tuberculin and the tuberculin reaction, in Jordan EO, Falk IS, eds., *The newer knowledge of bacteriology and immunology,* Chicago: University of Chicago Press, 1928:1016–1034.
13. Hardy A. Straight back to barbarism: anti-typhoid inoculation and the Great War. *Bull Hist Med* 2000;74:265–290.
14. Salomon-Bayet C, ed., *Pasteur et la révolution pastorienne,* Paris: Payot, 1986.
15. Metchnikov E. *Phagocytosis and immunity.* London: British Medical Association, 1891.
16. Tauber AI, Chernyak L. History of immunology. The birth of immunology: I. Metchnikoff and his critics, *Cell Immunol* 1989;121:447–473; Tauber AI. *The immune self: theory or metaphor?* Cambridge: Cambridge University Press, 1994. It is true that Macfarlane Burnet, who formally introduced the self–not self concept in 1949, referred both to Metchnikov and to Darwin as his predecessors.
17. Moulin. *Le dernier langage,* 49–66.
18. Mazumdar PMH. Immunity in 1890. *J Hist Med Allied Sci* 1972; 27:312–324; Besredka A, *Histoire d'une idée: l'oeuvre de Metchnikov,* Paris: Masson, 1921.
19. Portier C, Richet C. De l'action anaphylactique de certains venins, *Comptes Rendus de la Société de Biologie* 1902;54:170–172; Kröker K, Immunity and its other: the anaphylactic selves of Charles Richet, *Stud Hist Phil Biol Biomed Sci* 1999;30:273–296.
20. Besredka A. *Local immunization, specific dressings,* Baltimore: Williams, 1927, Plotz H, translator; Löwy I, "The terrain is all": Mechnikov's heritage at the Pasteur Institute, from Besredka's antivirus to Bardach's orthobiotic serum, in Lawrence C, Weisz G, eds., *Greater than the parts: holism in biomedicine 1920–1950,* Oxford: Oxford University Press, 1998:257–282.
21. Dunhill M. *The Plato of Praed Street: the life and times of Almroth Wright,* London: Royal Society of Medicine, 2000, 120–127; Keating P, Vaccine therapy and the problem of opsonins. *J Hist Med Allied Sci* 1988;43:275–296; Worboys M, Vaccine therapy and laboratory medicine in Edwardian England, in Pickstone J, ed., *Medical innovations in historical perspective,* Basingstoke: Macmillan, 1992:84–103.
22. Wright AE. *Studies on immunisation and their application to the diagnosis and treatment of bacterial infections,* London: Constable, 1909.
23. Chen W. The laboratory as business: Sir Almroth Wright and the construction of penicillin, in Cunningham A, Williams P, eds., *The laboratory revolution in medicine,* Cambridge: Cambridge University Press, 1992:245–292.
24. Panton PN, Marrack JR. *Clinical pathology* London: Churchill, 1st ed., 1913, 6th ed., 1951; Gillett HT. *Vaccine therapy in acute and chronic infections.* London: Lewis, 1933.
25. Connor JTH. *Doing good: the life of Toronto's General Hospital,* Toronto: University of Toronto Press, 2000.
26. Chen. The laboratory as business, 287–290.
27. Burnet FM. *The clonal selection theory of acquired immunity,* London: Cambridge University Press, 1959, 36.
28. Von Behring E, Kitasato S. Ueber das Zustandekommen der Diphtherieimmunität und der Tetanusimmunität beir Thieren, *Deutsche medizinische Wochenschrift* 1890;16:1113.
29. Weindling P. From medical research to clinical practice: serum therapy for diphtheria in the 1890s, in Pickstone JV, ed., *Medical innovations in historical perspective,* Basingstoke: Macmillan, 1992:72–83; Throm C, *Das Diphtherieserum: ein neues Therapieprinzip, seine Entwicklung und Markteinführung,* Stuttgart: Wissenschaftliche Verlagsgesellschaft, 1995, 50–52.
30. Madsen T. Institutets udvikling 1902–1927, in *Madsen. Statens Seruminstitut: Institutets Udvikling 1902–1940,* Copenhagen: Bianco Lunos, 1940:7–37; DeFries RD, The Connaught Medical Research Laboratories 1914–1948. *Can J Public Health* 1948;39:348–360.
31. Otto R. Die staatliche Prüfung der Heilsera, *Arbeiten aus dem königlichen Institut für experimentelle Therapie zu Frankfurt-a-M* 1906;2:7–86.
32. Bäumler E. *Paul Ehrlich: scientist for life,* New York: Holmes, 1984, Edwards G, translator.
33. Ehrlich P. The assay of the diphtheria-curative serum and its theoretical basis, 1897, translation in Himmelweit F, Marquardt M, Dale H, eds., *Collected papers of Paul Ehrlich,* vol. 2, London: Pergamon, 1957:107–125.
34. Ehrlich P. Die Wertbemessung des Diphtherieheilserums, und deren theoretische Grundlagen, 1897, translation in Himmelweit, Marquardt, Dale, eds., *Collected papers,* vol. 2, London: Pergamon, 1957:86–106 (German), 107–125 (English).
35. Ehrlich P. On immunity with special reference to cell life, The Croonian Lecture to the Royal Society of London, 1900, in Himmelweit, Marquardt, and Dale, eds., *Collected papers,* vol. 2, London: Pergamon, 1957:178–195.
36. Ada GL, Nossal GJV. The clonal selection theory. *Sci Am* 1987;257: 62–69.
37. Parascandola J. Jasensky R. Origins of the receptor theory of drug action, *Bull Hist Med* 1974;48:199–220.
38. Cambrosio A, Jacobi D, Keating P. Ehrlich's "beautiful pictures" and the controversial beginnings of immunologic imagery. *Isis* 1993;84: 662–699.
39. Silverstein A. A history of theories of antibody formation. *Cell Immunol* 1985;91:263–283.
40. Mazumdar PMH. *Species and specificity: an interpretation of the history of immunology,* Cambridge: Cambridge University Press, 1995, 202–213, 214–236.
41. Bordet J. Sur le mode d'action des antitoxines sur les toxines, 1903, in Gay FP, ed. and transl., *Studies in immunity by Professor Jules Bordet and his collaborators,* New York: Wiley, 1909:161–186.
42. Pick EP. Biochemie der Antigene, mit besonderer Berücksichtigung der chemischen Grundlagen der Antigenspezifität, in Kolle W, von Wassermann A, eds., *Handbuch der pathogenen Organismen,* 2nd ed., Jena, Austria: Fischer, 1912;685–868.
43. Mazumdar PMH. The antigen–antibody reaction and the physics and chemistry of life. *Bull Hist Med* 1974;48:1–21.
44. Landsteiner K. Die Theorien der Antikörperbildung, *Wiener klinische Wochenschrift* 1909;22:1623–1631.
45. Landsteiner K, Lampl H. Ueber die Antigen-eigenschaften von Azoprotein: XI. Mitteilung uber Antigene, *Zeitschrift f. Immuniyätsforschung* 1917;26:293–304.
46. Dubos RJ. Chemistry in medical research, in Dubos, *The professor, the Institute and DNA,* New York: Rockefeller University Press, 1976:35–46; Corner G, The laboratories are organised, in Corner, *A history of the Rockefeller Institute 1901–1953: origins and growth,* New York: Rockefeller Institute Press, 1964:56–87.

47. Mazumdar PMH. The template theory of antibody formation and the chemical synthesis of the twenties, in Mazumdar, ed., *Immunology 1930–1980: essays on the history of immunology,* Toronto: Wall & Thompson, 1989:13–32.

48. Putnam EW, Felix Haurowitz. in *Biographies of Members of the National Academy of Science,* Washington, DC: National Academy of Science, 1994;64:135–163.

49. Marrack JR. *The chemistry of antigens and antibodies,* London: HMSO, 1934, 113–123.

50. Throm C. *Das Diphtherie-serum: ein neues Therapieprinzip, seine Entwicklung und Markteinführung,* Stuttgart: Wissenschaftliche Verlagsgesellschaft, 1995. Ehrlich was never eligible for a university position, since he was a Jew. The offer by an institute came about because of the funding provided by an influential group of Frankfurt citizens.

51. Kröker K. Immunity and its other: the anaphylactic selves of Charles Richet. *Stud Hist Phil Biol Biomed Sci* 1999;30:273–296.

52. Prausnitz C. Küstner H, Studien über die Überempfindlichkeit, *Zentralblatt f. Bakt. Originalien)* 1921;86:160–169; von Pirquet CE, Schick B, *Die Serumkrankheit,* Leipzig: Deuticke, 1905.

53. Jackson M. Between scepticism and wild enthusiasm: the chequered history of allergen immunotherapy in Britain, in Moulin A-M, Cambrosio A, eds., *Singular selves: historical Issues and contemporary debates in immunology,* Amsterdam: Elsevier, 2001:155–164.

54. Chase MW. Irreverent recollections from Cooke and Coca, 1928–1978, *J Allergy Clin Immunol* 1979;64:306–320.

55. Linton DS. The obscure object of knowledge: German military medicine confronts gas gangrene during World War I. *Bull Hist Med* 2000;74:291–316.

56. Mazumdar PMH. "In the silence of the laboratory": the League of Nations standardises syphilis tests, *Social History of Medicine,* 2003 (*in press*). On the ban, see Schröder-Gudehus B, Deutsche Wissenschaft und internationale Zusammenarbeit 1914–1928: ein Beitrag zum Studium kultureller Beziehungen in politischen Krisenzeiten [thesis], University of Geneva, 1966.

57. Bordet J, Gengou O. Sur l'existence des substances sensibilatrices dans la plupart des sérums antimicrobiens, *Ann l'Inst Pasteur,* 1901, translated as On the existence of sensitising substances in the majority of antimicrobial sera, in Gay FP, ed., *Studies in immunity by Professor Jules Bordet and his collaborators,* New York: Wiley, 1909:217–227; Wassermann A, Neisser M, Brücke K, Eine serodiagnostisches Reaktion bei Syphilis, *Deutsche medizinische Wochenschrift* 1906; 32:745–746; Löwy I, Testing for a sexually transmissible disease, in Berridge V, Strong P, eds., *AIDS and contemporary history,* Cambridge: Cambridge University Press, 1993:74–92.

58. Weindling P. The politics of international co-ordination to combat sexually transmitted diseases, 1900–1890s, in Berridge V, Strong P, eds., *AIDS and contemporary history,* Cambridge: Cambridge University Press, 1993:93–107.

59. Fleck L. *Genesis and development of a scientific fact,* Chicago: University of Chicago Press, 1979, Trenn TJ, translator (of 1935 edition).

60. Kahn RL. *Serum diagnosis of syphilis by precipitation: governing principles, procedure and clinical application of the Kahn Precipitation Test,* Baltimore: Williams, 1926.

61. Slatkin M. Trends in the diagnosis and treatment of syphilis. *Med Clin North Am* 1965;49:823–847; Nicholas L, Beerman H, Present day serodiagnosis of syphilis: a review of some of the recent literature, *Am J Med Sci* 1965;249:466–483.

62. Landsteiner K. Ueber Agglutinationserscheinungen normalen menschlichen Blutes, *Wiener klinische Wochenschrift* 1901;14:1132–1134.

63. Hirszfeld L. *Konstitutionsserologie und Blutgruppenforschung,* Berlin: Springer, 1928; Keating P, Holistic bacteriology: Ludwik Hirszfeld's doctrine of serogenesis between the two world wars, in Lawrence C, Weisz G, eds., *Greater than the parts: holism in biomedicine 1920–1950,* Oxford: Oxford University Press, 1998:283–302.

64. Mazumdar PMH. Two models for human genetics: blood grouping and psychiatry between the wars, *Bull Hist Med* 1996;70:609–657.

65. Mazumdar PMH. Blood and soil: the serology of the Aryan racial state, *Bull Hist Med* 1990;64:187–219.

66. Zimmermann DR. *Rh: the intimate history of a disease and its conquest,* New York: Macmillan, 1973.

67. Crile GW. *Hemorrhage and transfusion: an experimental and clinical research,* New York: Appleton, 1909, 318–319, 323–324.

68. Robertson LB. The transfusion of whole blood, *BMJ* 1916;ǐ:38;

69. Robertson OH, A method of citrated blood transfusion, *BMJ* 1918;ǐ:477. For a conspectus of transfusion at the end of World War I, see Keynes G, *Blood transfusion,* London: Oxford University Press, 1922.

69. Vaughan JM, Panton PN. The civilian blood transfusion service, in Dunn CL, ed., *The emergency medical services,* vol. 1, London: HMSO, 1952:334–355; Medical Research Council, *War memorandum no. 9: determination of blood groups,* London: HMSO, 1943.

70. Riddell V. *Blood transfusion,* London: Oxford University Press, 1939,300–302.

71. Diamond LK. A short history of blood banking in the United States, *JAMA* 1965;193:128–132; Diamond LK, A history of blood transfusion, in Wintrobe MM, ed., *Blood pure and eloquent: a story of discovery, of people and of ideas,* New York: McGraw-Hill, 1980:659–688.

72. Vaughan JM, Panton PN. The civilian blood transfusion service, in Dunn CL, ed., *The emergency medical services,* London: HMSO, 1952, 1:334–355, 2:68–71.

73. Loutit JF, Mollison PL. Advantages of a disodium citrate–glucose mixture as blood preservative, *BMJ* 1943;ǐ:744–745.

74. Norris RF. Hospital programs of blood banking. *JAMA* 1965;193:133–135.

75. On the ethical problems and dangers of the U.S. system of paid donors from a British perspective, see Titmuss RM, *The gift relationship: from human blood to social policy,* London: Allen, 1970. On the political problems of vaccine development, see Muraskin W, *The war against hepatitis B,* Philadelphia: University of Pennsylvania Press, 1995.

76. Vaughan and Panton, Civilian blood transfusion service, 355.

77. Kerker M. The Svedberg and molecular reality. *Isis* 1976;67:190–216.

78. Rånby B, ed., *Physical chemistry of colloids and macromolecules,* Proceedings of the International Symposium on Physical Chemistry and Macromolecules to Celebrate the 100th Anniversary of the Birth of Professor Theodor Svedberg on 30 August 1884 ... Uppsala University, Sweden, 22–24 August 1984, Oxford: Blackwell, 1985. The proceedings contain several reminiscences and anecdotes by scientists who worked with Svedberg.

79. Fruton J. *Molecules and life: historical essays on the interplay of chemistry and biology* New York: Wiley, 1972:138–139.

80. Mazumdar. *Species and specificity,* 152–178.

81. Brohult S. Gralén N. The Institute of Physical Chemistry at the University of Uppsala: some notes on its history and activities, in Tiselius A, ed., [Festschrift for] *The Svedberg,* Uppsala: Almqvist, 1944:623–638. On unity and simplicity, see Mazumdar. *Species and specificity,* 152–178.

82. Brohult and Gralén. The Institute of Physical Chemistry, 629.

83. Tiselius A. Electrophoretische Messungen am Eiweiss, *Kolloid Zeitschrift* 1938;85:119–128.

84. Kay LE. Laboratory technology and biological knowledge: the Tiselius electrophoresis apparatus, 1930–1945. *Hist Phil Life Sci* 1988;10:51–72. See also Ede A, Colloids and quantification: the ultracentrifuge and its transformation of colloid chemistry. *Ambix* 1996;43:32–45.

85. Ede A. When is a tool not a tool? Understanding the role of equipment in the early colloidal laboratory. *Ambix* 1993;40:11–24.

86. Spiegel-Adolf M, *Die Globuline,* Leipzig: Steinkopf, 1930:422–429.

87. Kabat EA, Tiselius E. An electrophoretic study of immune sera and purified antibody preparations. *J Exper Med* 1939;69:119–131.

88. Creager ANH. Producing molecular therapeutics from human blood: Edwin Cohn's wartime enterprise, in de Chadarevian S, Kamminga H, eds., *Molecularizing biology and medicine,* Amsterdam: Harwood, 1998:107–138; Creager ANH, From blood fractions to antibody structure: gamma globulin research growing out of World War II, in Moulin A-M, Cambrosio A, eds., *Singular selves: historical issues and contemporary debates in immunology,* Amsterdam: Elsevier, 2000:140–154; Cohn EJ, The history of plasma fractionation, *Adv Mil Med* 1948;1:364–443.

89. Tswett M. Physikalisch-chemische Studien über Chlorophyll, *Berichte d. botanische Gesellschaft* 1906;24:316–323.

90. Consden R, Gordon AH, Martin AJP. Quantitative analysis of proteins: a partition chromatographic method using paper. *Biochem J* 1944;38:476–484.

91. Moore S, Stein WH. Chromatography of amino-acids on sulfonated polystyrene resins. *J Biol Chem* 1951;192:663–681.

92. Porath J. Gel filtration of proteins, peptides and amino-acids. *Biochim Biophys Acta* 1960;39:193–207.

93. Sober HA, Gutter FJ, Wyckoff MM, et al. Chromatography of proteins. II. Fractionation of serum protein on anion-exchange cellulose, *J Am Chem Soc* 1956;78:756–763; Sober R, Hartley W Jr, Carroll WR, et al., Fractionation of proteins, *The Proteins* 1965;3:1–97. For a contemporary overview of protein separation methods, see Morris CJOR, Morris P, *Separation methods in biochemistry,* London: Pitman, 1964, especially on the choice of separation methods, 838–853.

94. Morris and Morris, *Separation methods in biochemistry,* 701–705.

95. Smithies O. Grouped variations in the occurrence of new protein components in normal human serum. *Nature* 1955;175:307–308. Although this is the first publication to use a starch gel, Smithies does not describe the method, only the results.

96. Ishizaka K, Ishizaka T. Human reaginic antibodies and immunoglobulin E. *J Allergy* 1968;42:330–363. See Chase, Irreverent recollections, 315.

97. Goodman H. Immunodiplomacy: the story of the World Health Organisation's immunological research programme, in Mazumdar PMH, ed., *Immunology 1930–1980: essays on the history of immunology,* Toronto: Wall & Thompson, 1989:253–272.

98. Porter RR. The hydrolysis of rabbit γ-globulin and antibodies with crystalline papain. *Biochem J* 1959;73:119–127. See also Porter RR, Immunochemistry, *Annu Rev Biochem* 1962;31:625–652.

99. Porter RR. The structure of antibodies. *Scientific American,* 1967; 217:81–90.

100. Porter RR. Structural studies of immunoglobulins. *Science* 1973; 180:713–716.

101. Putnam FW. Structure and function of the plasma proteins. *The Proteins* 1965;3:153–267.

102. Poulik MD, Edelman GM. Comparison of reduced alkylated derivatives of some myeloma globulins and Bence–Jones proteins. *Nature* 1961;191:1274–1276.

103. Kunkel HG. Myeloma proteins and antibodies. *Harvey Lectures* 1965;59:219–242.

104. Potter M. Some reminiscences on the contributions of cancer research to immunology in the 1950s, in Mazumdar PMH, ed., *Immunology 1930–1980: essays on the history of immunology,* Toronto: Wall & Thompson, 1989:95–105.

105. Crick F. On protein synthesis. *Symp Soc Exp Biol* 1957;12:138–167.

106. Haurowitz F. *The chemistry and functions of proteins,* New York: Academic Press, 1963, 439. The quotation is from B. Commoner, in *Science* 1961;133:1747.

107. Nirenberg M. Protein synthesis and the RNA code. *Harvey Lectures* 1965;59:155–185.

108. Neushul P. Science, government and the mass production of penicillin. *J Hist Med Allied Sci* 1993;48:371–395.

109. Smith JS. *Patenting the sun: polio and the Salk vaccine,* New York: Morrow, 1990:279–312. On polio and other viral vaccines made in cell culture, see Beale AJ, The development of IPV, in Plotkin SA, Fantini B, *Vaccinia, vaccination, vaccinology: Jenner, Pasteur and their successors. International Meeting on the History of Vaccinology, December 1995,* Amsterdam: Elsevier, 1996:211–292.

110. Coulter HL, Fisher BL. *DPT: a shot in the dark,* New York: Harcourt, 1985.

111. Amos B, ed., *Progress in immunology: proceedings of the First International Congress of Immunology, Washington, DC, 1971,* New York: Academic Press, 1971. This arrangement of the sessions scuttled my attempt to use the congress to revise for my exam.

112. Nossal's statement dates from 1985. and is cited in Sexton C, *Burnet: a life,* 2nd ed., Melbourne: Oxford University Press, 1999:131–132.

113. Sturdy S. Reflections: molecularization, standardization and the history of science, in de Chadarevian S, Kamminga H, eds., *Molecularizing biology and medicine: new practices and alliances, 1910s–1970s,* Amsterdam: Harwood, 1998,273–292.

114. Chase MW. Hypersensitivity to simple chemicals. *The Harvey Lectures,* 1965–1966;61:169–203.

115. Koch R. Weitere Mittheilungen über das Tuberkulin. *Deutsche med Wschr* 1891;17:1189–1192.

116. von Pirquet CF. Quantitative experiments with the cutaneous tuberculin reaction, *J Pharm* 1909–1910;1:151–174; von Pirquet CF, Allergy. *Arch Int Med* 1911;7:259–288.

117. Humphrey JH, White RG. *Immunology for Students of Medicine,* 2nd ed., Oxford: Blackwell, 1963:337–377.

118. Lawrence HS. The early history of soluble factors, in Mazumdar PMH, ed., *Immunology 1930–1980: essays on the history of immunology,* Toronto: Wall and Thompson, 1989:221–230.

119. Brent L. *A history of transplantation immunology,* San Diego: Academic Press, 1997,70–115.

120. Murray JE. Organ transplantation and the revitalization of immunology, in Gallagher RB, Gilder J, Nossal GJV, et al., eds., *Immunology: the making of a modern science,* London: Academic Press, 1995:179–189.

121. Burnet FM, Fenner F. *The production of antibodies,* 2nd ed., New York: Macmillan, 1949:102–105; Tauber AI, Podolsky SH, Frank Macfarlane Burnet and the immune self. *J Hist Biol* 1994;27:531–573.

122. Own RD. Immunogenetic consequences of vascular anastomoses between bovine twins, *Science* 1945;102:400–401; Cinader BH, Down-regulation and tolerance: the trail from the past, in Mazumdar PMH, ed., *Immunology 1930–1980: essays on the history of immunology,* Toronto: Wall & Thompson, 1989:51–66.

123. Billingham RE, Brent L, Medawar PB. Actively acquired tolerance of foreign cells. *Nature* 1953;172:603–606.

124. Brent L. *History of transplantation immunology,* 73.

125. Burnet FM. A discussion of immunological tolerance under the leadership of Sir Frank Macfarlane Burnet. *Proc R Soc Lond B Biol Sci* 1957;146:1–92.

126. Brent. *History of transplantation,* 230–305.

127. Medawar PB. The strange case of the spotted mice, in *Medawar, The threat and the glory: reflections on science and scientists,* edited by D. Pyke, Oxford: Oxford University Press, 1991:71–82.

128. Stähelin H. The development of immunosuppressive agents from x-rays to cyclosporin, in Mazumdar PMH, ed., *Immunology 1930–1980: essays on the history of immunology,* Toronto: Wall & Thompson, 1989:185–201.

129. Jerne NK. A study of avidity. *Acta Pathol Microbiol Scand Suppl* 1951;87:1–183.

130. Jerne NK. The natural-selection theory of antibody formation, *Proc Nat Acad Sci* 1955;41:849–857.

131. Söderqvist T. Darwinian overtones: Niels K. Jerne and the origin of the clonal selection theory of antibody formation, *J Hist Biol* 27:481–529; Söderqvist T, *Hvilken Kamp for at Undslippe: en Biografi om Immunologen og Nobelpristrageren Niels Kaj Jerne,* Copenhagen: Borgens Forlag, 1998. Parabasis: the selection theory as a personal confession of its author, and Chapter 15, I just sit at my desk and think about life in general.

132. Haurowitz F. Review of *The production of antibodies,* 2nd ed., 1949. *J Immunol* 1951;66:485–486.

133. Talmage DW. Allergy and immunology. *Annu Rev Med* 1957;8:239–256.

134. Burnet FM. A modification of Jerne's theory of antibody formation, *Aust J Sci* 1957;20:67–68.

135. Burnet FM. The impact of ideas on immunology. *Cold Spring Harb Symp Quant Biol* 1967;32:1–8.

136. Burnet FM. *The clonal selection theory of acquired immunity,* Melbourne: Cambridge University Press, 1959:23–27.

137. Burnet. *Clonal selection theory,* 182–183.

138. Ada GL, Nossal GJV. How cells make antibody: the clonal selection theory of immunity. *Sci Am* 1987;257:62–69.

139. Burnet. *Clonal selection theory,* 64; Burnet FM, A Darwinian approach to immunity. *Nature* 1964;203:451–454.

140. Sexton, *Burnet: a life,* 134–141.

141. Nossal GJV, Lederberg J. Antibody production by single cells. *Nature* 1958;182:1383–1384.

142. Jerne NK, Noordin AA. Plaque formation in agar by single antibody producing cells. *Science* 1963;141:405.

143. Talmage DW. Is this theory necessary?, in Mazumdar PMH, ed., *Immunology 1930–1980: essays on the history of immunology,* Toronto: Wall & Thompson, 1989:67–72.

144. Cambrosio A, Keating P. *Exquisite specificity: the monoclonal antibody revolution,* (New York, NY: Oxford University Press 1995) 1995.

145. Petrov RV. *Me or not-me: immunological mobiles,* (Moscow: Mir Publishers, 1987) 1987, 99–110, Degtyaryova, GY, translator.

146. Gowans JL. The mysterious lymphocyte, in Gallagher RB, Gilder J, Nossal GJV, et al., eds., *Immunology: the making of a modern science,* London: Academic Press, 1992;65–74; Miller JFAP, The discovery of thymus function, in Gallagher RB, Gilder J, Nossal GJV, et al., eds., *Immunology: the making of a modern science,* London: Academic Press, 1995;75–84.

147. Stillwell CR. Thymectomy as an experimental system in immunology. *J Hist Biol* 1994;27:379–401.

148. Good RA. The Minnesota scene: a crucial portal of entry to modern cellular immunology, in Szentivanyi A, Friedman H, eds., *The immunologic revolution: facts and witnesses,* Boca Raton, FL: CRC Press, 1993:105–168.

149. Morse HC. *Origins of inbred mice,* New York: Academic Press, 1978; Foster J, Henry L, Small D, et al., *The mouse in biomedical research,* New York: Academic Press, 1981.

150. Löwy I, Gaudillière J-P. Disciplining cancer: mice and the practice of genetic purity, in Gaudillière J-P, Löwy I, eds., *The invisible industrialist: manufactures and the production of scientific knowledge,* Houndmills, Basingstoke, Hampshire: Macmillan Press; New York: St. Martin's Press, 1998:209–249.

151. Milstein C. Monoclonal antibodies. *Sci Am* 1980;243:66–74; Milstein, Monoclonal antibodies from hybrid myelomas, Wellcome Foundation Lecture, 1980. *Proc R Soc Lond B Biol Sci,* 211:393–412; Cambrosio A, Keating P, Between fact and technique: the beginnings of hybridoma technology. *J Hist Biol* 1992;25:175–230.

152. Potter M. Myeloma proteins, *Experientia* 1986;42:967–1068.

153. Uhr JW. The 1984 Nobel Prize for Medicine, *Science* 1984;226:1025.

154. Brent. *History of transplantation immunology,* 16–46.

155. Cambrosio A, Keating P. Going monoclonal: art, science and magic in the day-to-day use of hybridoma technology. *Soc Problems,* 1988; 35:244–260.

156. Springer TA. *Hybridoma technology in the biosciences and medicine.* New York: Plenum, 1985.

157. Mazumdar. *Species and specificity,* 337–378.

158. Scott ML, Voak D, Liu W, et al. Using monoclonal antibodies and site-directed mutagenesis to map the epitopes of the blood group D antigen, in Eibl M, Mayr WR, Thorbecke GJ, eds., *Epitope recognition since Landsteiner's discovery,* Berlin: Springer, 2002:83–102.

159. Mazumdar PMH. Immunity in 1890. *J Hist Med Allied Sci* 1972; 27:312–324.

160. Jerne NK. Towards a network theory of the immune system, *Ann d'Immunologie* 1974;125C:373–389; Moulin A-M, *Le dernier langage,* 333–339.

161. Morange M. *Histoire de la biologie moléculaire,* Paris: La Découverte, 1994, translated as *A history of molecular biology,* Cambridge, MA: Harvard University Press, 1998.

162. Arber W. Promotion and limitation of genetic exchange, *Science* 1979;205:361–365.

163. Jackson DA, Symons RH, Berg P. Biochemical method for inserting new genetic information into DNA of Simian Virus 40: circular SV40 molecules containing Lambda Phage genes and the galactose operon of *E. coli. Proc Nat Acad Sci USA* 1972;69:2904–2909.

164. Morange, *Histoire de la biologie moléculaire,* 241–245.

165. Morange, *Histoire de la biologie moléculaire,* 245–251; Krimsky S, *Genetic alchemy: the social history of the recombinant DNA controversy,* Cambridge, MA: MIT Press, 1982; Wright S, Recombinant DNA technology and its social transformation, 1972–1982, *Osiris* 2nd series, 1986;2:303–360.

166. Tonegawa S. Somatic generation of antibody diversity, in Gallagher RB, Gilder J, Nossal GJV, et al., eds., *Immunology: the making of a modern science,* London: Academic Press, 1995:145–161.

167. Tonegawa S, Maxam AM, Tizard R, et al. Sequence of a mouse germ line gene for a variable region of an immunoglobulin light chain. *Proc Nat Acad Sci USA* 1978;74:3171; Kurosawa Y, Tonegawa S, Organization, structure and assembly of the immunoglobulin heavy chain diversity DNA segments. *J Exp Med* 1982;155:201–218.

168. Tonegawa. Somatic generation, 159–160; Leder P, The genetics of antibody diversity. *Sci Am* 1982;246:102. For a contemporary textbook account of genetic control of diversity, see Hood LE, Weissman IL, Wood WB, et al., *Immunology,* 2nd ed., Menlo Park, CA: Benjamin, 1984:81–111.

169. Mazumdar. *Species and specificity,* 337–378.

170. Paul WE. *Immunogenetics* New York: Raven, 1984;151–167.

171. Bjorkman PJ, Saper MA, Samraoui B, et al. Structure of the human class I histocompatibility antigen, HLA-2, *Nature* 1987;329:506–512; Bjorkman PJ, Saper MA, Samraoui B, et al., The foreign antigen binding site and T cell recognition regions of class I histocompatibility antigens, *Nature* 1987;329:512–518. Also cited by Brent, *History of transplantation immunology,* 150–151.

172. Reinherz ER, Hussey RE, Schlossman SF. A monoclonal antibody blocking human T cell function. *Eur J Immunol* 1980;10:758–762.

173. Allison JP, McIntyre BW, Bloch D. Tumor-specific antigen of murine T-lymphoma defined with monoclonal antibody. *J Immunol* 1982;129:2293–2299.

174. Reinherz EL, Meuer S, Fitzgerald KA, et al. Antigen recognition by human T lymphocytes is linked to surface expression of the T3 molecular complex. *Cell* 1982;30:735–743.

175. Marrack. *The chemistry of antigens and antibodies,* 113–123.

176. Kappler J, Kubo R, Haskins K, et al. The major histocompatibility complex–restricted antigen receptor on T cells in mouse and man: identification of constant and variable peptides. *Cell* 1983;35:295–302.

177. Caccia N, Toyonaga B, Kimura N, et al. The α and β chains of the T-cell receptor, in Mak TW, ed., *The T-cell receptors,* New York: Plenum, 1988:9–51.

178. Barclay AN, Johnson P, McCaughan GW, et al. Immunoglobulin-related structures associated with vertebrate cell surfaces, in Mak TW, ed., *The T-cell receptors,* New York: Plenum, 1988:53–87.

179. Burnet FM. The impact of ideas on immunology, *Cold Spring Harb Symp Quant Biol* 1967;32:1–8.

180. Kahn AD. *AIDS: the winter war,* Philadelphia, PA: Temple University Press, 1993, 116–153.

181. Altman D. Legitimation through disaster: AIDS and the gay movement, in Fee E, Fox DM, *AIDS: the burdens of history,* Berkeley: University of California Press, 1988:301–315.

182. Nicholson JKA, Mawle AC, McDougal JS. The effects of HIV-1 on the immune system, in Madhok R, Forbes CD, Evatt BL, *Blood, blood products and HIV,* 2nd ed., London: Chapman, 1994:75–100.

183. Martin E. *Flexible bodies: tracking immunity in American culture from the days of polio to the age of AIDS,* Boston, MA: Beacon, 1993,23–112.

184. Gilmore N, Somerville MA. From trust to tragedy: HIV/AIDS and the Canadian blood system, in Feldman EA, Bayer R, *Blood feuds: AIDS, blood and the politics of medical disaster,* New York: Oxford University Press, 1999:127–159; Canadian Ministry of Public Works and Government Services, *Commission of inquiry on the blood system in Canada,* Commissioner Hon. Justice Horace Krever (Ottawa: Canadian Goverment Publishing 1997).

185. Steffen M. The nation's blood: medicine justice and the state in France, in Feldman EA, Bayer R, *Blood feuds: AIDS, blood and the politics of medical disaster,* New York: Oxford University Press, 1999:95–126.

186. South Africa. *Presidential AIDS Advisory Panel Report,* a synthesis report of the deliberations by the panel of experts invited by the President of the Republic of South Africa, the Hon. Mr Thabo Mbeki, March 2001.

187. Nolen S. Continent's educated can no longer run things: they're dead or can't cope, report datelined Nkhotakota, Malawi, *Globe and Mail* June 19, 2002, A13.

CHAPTER 3

Immunoglobulins: Structure and Function

Grant R. Kolar and J. Donald Capra

Introduction
A Historical Perspective
Introduction to Structure and Nomenclature
The Ig Domain
Fab Structure and Function
Antigen–Antibody Interactions
The Immunoglobulin Hinge
Fc Structure and Function
   IgM · IgD · IgA · IgE · IgG
Higher-Order Structure
An Evolutionary Perspective
Conclusion
References

INTRODUCTION

All who approach the study of the structure and function of immunoglobulins eventually marvel at the duality of the problem: There is variability and there is constancy, and an appreciation of both is critical to understand this class of proteins that are the prototypic members of the "immunoglobulin superfamily." Having co-authored this chapter in all previous editions of this volume, providing a fresh perspective may seem difficult, but it is not. The study of the structure and function of antibodies remains as fresh as it was three decades ago, as new and existing experiments continue to be published that provide critical new insights into these molecules.

The relationship between the structure and the function of the immunoglobulin molecule is a tribute to the power of molecular evolution. Via the duplication and diversification of the immunoglobulin homology domain, a family of molecules with diverse biological functions has been derived. The antibody molecule plays the central role in humoral immunity by attaching to pathogens and then recruiting effector systems to stem the invader. In doing so, as noted above, it embodies two antagonistic tendencies—diversify and commonality—since it must possess both a variable surface to recognize different foreign antigens, and a constant surface that its own effector systems can recognize.

The fundamental tertiary structure of antibodies is called the immunoglobulin fold—the basic three-dimensional structure that thematically describes the structure of both the variable and constant domains of an immunoglobulin, as well as other members of the immunoglobulin superfamily. It was the recognition of this repeating structure that many years ago led to one of the first descriptions of "families" of molecules, some of which bore only minimal amino-acid sequence similarity but at the same time had profound three dimensional structural homology. The major difference between the variable and constant domains from a structural perspective is the "loops" between the sandwich-like layers. In the variable domains these loops represent the amino acids, which by and large are in contact with antigen. As such they tend to be longer than the loops in the constant region where they serve, in general, as the structures that interact with certain effector molecules such as cell-surface receptors, or serum proteins such as certain complement components.

The antibody molecule is also called "the B-cell receptor," as at early stages of the immune response with a membrane exon at its carboxyl terminus, immunoglobulins serve as cell-surface receptors for antigen. Further stimulation of B cells with antigen leads to differentiation of the B cell such that antibody is secreted into the serum to make up the circulating antibody pool. Antibodies are one of the major plasma proteins and are often referred to as the "first line of defense" against infection. Additional stimulation of cell-surface antibodies leads to a "class switch" such that antibodies of different classes are produced, first as a cell-surface form and then as a secreted form. Thus, the antibody molecule has yet two other functions: to serve as a receptor molecule to transmit the signal from antigen capture to downstream signaling events that instruct the cell to perform such functions as division, secretion, and differentiation. Finally, a slightly modified immunoglobulin eventually enters the serum antibody pool.

This chapter will attempt to provide a framework for understanding the various structural elements of the immunoglobulin classes and subclasses and connect those structural elements with the discrete biologic functions commonly attributed to antibody molecules. Other chapters will deal with the molecular events leading to the formation of this remarkable set of molecules and yet others will deal with specific effector functions.

A HISTORICAL PERSPECTIVE

The structure and function of immunoglobulins is inexorably connected with the knowledge of the times in which discoveries were made in the field. Thus, in the 1940s and 1950s, when antibodies were known as "antitoxins" and "antisera" and the immune response was primarily studied as a serum response to antigenic challenge (largely from deliberate immunization although to some extent from response to disease) it was sufficient to label them simply as "antibodies." It is important to remember that until the 1950s, there were few ways to partition serum proteins, and most relied on techniques that separated albumins from globulins (in medicine this became known as the A/G ratio). In the 1960s, once electrophoresis became commonplace, the globulins were divided into α_1, α_2, β, and γ globulins. The connection between antibodies and γ globulins followed. "Sizing" columns were required to distinguish immunoglobulins into those that were "heavy" (IgM), "regular" (IgA, IgE, IgD, IgG), and "light" (light chain dimers). Only after immunoelectrophoresis was it clear that there were other "classes" of immunoglobulins. Finally, with the discovery of myeloma proteins as "gamma globulins" or "immunoglobulins," the clear class and subclass (isotype) distinctions that we know today became commonplace. When hybridomas and the immortalization of B cells became commonplace, further distinctions became evident. However, from a historical perspective it should be appreciated that significant "structure–function" issues were solved by biochemists. With the advent of molecular biology, we gained great insight into the genomic structure of antibodies, learned a great deal of how the information was stored for the variable regions and so on, but no new classes, subclasses, allotypes and the like were discovered. In addition, no new functions of antibodies were uncovered. Thus, we owe a great debt to the immunochemists of the 1940s through the 1960s for laying out the basic structure/function

relationship of arguably the most significant molecule of our field.

INTRODUCTION TO STRUCTURE AND NOMENCLATURE

The immunoglobulin molecule is a complex structure of four polypeptide chains. The central structural component of the molecule is the Ig domain. This key structure is discussed in a subsequent section. The four-polypeptide chains are organized as a homodimeric structure of a heterodimer between a heavy and light chain. Both chains contain variable and constant domains, with the heavy chain having two or three more constant domains than the light chain. Dimerization between the heavy and light chain variable domains and the first constant domain occurs as a result of hydrophobic interactions as well as a set of disulfide bonds at the carboxy-terminal end. A homodimer of this heavy–light chain configuration is then produced and held together by disulfide bonds in the hinge and tight hydrophobic interactions of the other constant domains. Therefore, an immunoglobulin contains two heavy chains (typically 55 kD each) and two light chains (25 kD each) (1). This forms an overall "Y" or "T" conformation that is the most widely recognized feature of immunoglobulin structure.

By enzymatic and/or chemical cleavage, the immunoglobulin molecule can be broken into a number of "sections" or "fragments." The experiments that created these fragments and later those that resulted in an understanding of these fragments are still among the most elegant experiments in our field. They continue to influence our descriptions of the molecule today and will be critical for understanding the structure/function issues discussed in this chapter. Porter (2) found that papain would cleave the antibody into two species of protein. The Fab (fragment antigen binding) portion acquired in this cleavage would monovalently bind to antigen. Two of these regions are produced per immunoglobulin as cleavage occurs N terminal to the disulfide bonds of the hinge (3,4). The remaining portion, the Fc (fragment crystallizable), was found to crystallize under low ionic conditions. Nisonoff et al. (5) and Palmer and Nisonoff (6) found that pepsin cleavage produced the bivalent F(ab)$_2$ that upon exposure to reducing conditions could be separated into Fab monomeric units. Further study revealed other subdivisions that are described in Table 1, Fig. 1, and Colorplate 1.

Immunoglobulins are glycosylated as they are secreted from the endoplasmic reticulum (ER). These glycosylation sites are illustrated (along with the most common disulfide bonds) in Fig. 2. Most immunoglobulins contain at least one asparagine (or N-linked glycosylation group), while others contain a significant amount of O-linked glycosylation particularly in the hinge. The N-linked glycosylation at Asn 267 is thought to have different orientations between various immunoglobulins (e.g., IgA and IgG) (7). As we discuss below, these features have important physiological consequences.

TABLE 1. *Definitions of key immunoglobulin structure nomenclature*

Fc	A constant region dimer lacking C_H1
Fab	A light chain dimerized to V_H-C_H1 resulting from papain cleavage; this is monomeric since papain cuts above the hinge disulfide bond(s)
$F(ab)'_2$	A dimer of Fab' resulting from pepsin cleavage below the hings disulfides; this is bivalent and can precipitate antigen
Fab'	A monomer resulting from mild reduction of $F(ab)'_2$: an Fab with part of the hinge
Fd	The heavy chain portion of Fab (V_H-C_H1) obtained following reductive denaturation of Fab
Fv	The variable part of Fab: a V_H-V_1 dimer
Fb	The constant par of Fab: a C_H1-C_1 dimer
pFc'	A C_H3 dimer

Transmembrane domains and cytoplasmic tails are present in membranous forms of antibodies. The extent of these structures varies with the immunoglobulin isotype. Finally, both IgM and IgA have a tailpiece important in polymerization that is present immediately carboxy terminal to the last constant region domain of the Fc ($C\mu4$ and $C\alpha3$, respectively).

The study of myeloma proteins led to a great leap in our understanding of immunoglobulin function. These "single" or "monoclonal" antibodies obtained from the sera of patients with the disease multiple myeloma were used in many of the serologic and biochemical studies of the 1950s and

1960s. They remained the major source of homogeneous immunoglobulins until the development of the hybridoma in 1974. The serologists injected them into animals and produced antisera that were used to detail some of the basic divisions of antibodies. For example, the immune sera were absorbed with other myeloma proteins and were used to identify isotypic, allotypic, and idiotypic specificities (8). The isotype of an antibody refers to the particular light or heavy chain-constant region that is used. Isotypes are present in all members of a species. The allotype refers to allelic differences in both the variable (particularly rabbit) and constant region. Allotypes are present in some but not all members of a species and are inherited in a simple Mendelian fashion. Idiotype refers to a specificity that is associated with the variable region and generally is a marker for the antigen-combining site (9). Anti-idiotypic antibodies generally prevent antigen–antibody interaction. Myeloma proteins were also used for the first amino acid sequencing of immunoglobulins and provided our first introduction to the idea of sequence variability (and indeed the definition of) the variable and the constant regions. Finally, myelomas were the first immunoglobulins that were subjected to crystallographic studies and provided the first glimpses of the domain structure of the prototypic immunoglobulin (10–12).

At first, immunologists thought of the antibody molecule in static terms, but increasingly there has been an appreciation of the motion of the immunoglobulin. The major motions of the Fab can be illustrated in Fig. 3. We now know that rotation about the hinge as well as segmental flexibility varies more than previously thought. The elbow peptide is important in the orientation of the Fv for antigen binding. Finally, flexibility in the Fc (fragment crystallizable) region, particularly between the constant domains as well as perpendicular to the plane of the constant region is increasingly appreciated in certain immunoglobulin–receptor interactions (particularly in IgE) (13).

The following sections focus on particular structural concepts important to understanding the functions of immunoglobulin beginning with Ig, the core domain of the immunoglobulin superfamily.

THE Ig DOMAIN

The immunoglobulin domain (Ig domain) is the central structural unit that defines members of the immunoglobulin superfamily (IgSF) (reviewed in Williams and Barclay [14] and Harpaz and Chothia [15]). This domain is composed of two sandwiched β pleated sheets. Each sheet is composed of an arrangement of β strands whose particular composition is based on the type of domain used in the molecule. There are two general types of domains in immunoglobulins, V and C. The β strand conformation in V-type domains consists of nine antiparallel strands with five strands in the first sheet and four strands in the second. C-type domains have seven antiparallel strands distributed as three strands in the first and four strands

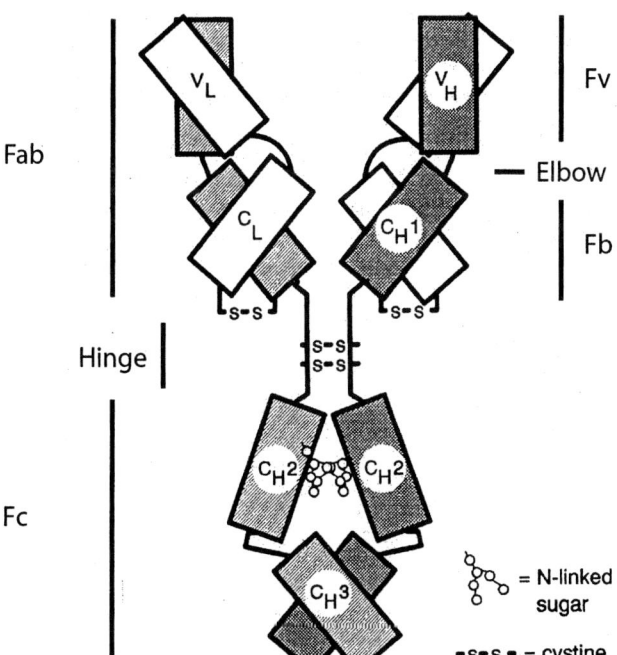

FIG. 1. Schematic representing the major features of a serum immunoglobulin (i.e., IgG). IgM and IgE have an extra CH domain in place of the hinge. Adapted from Carayannopoulos and Capra (153), with permission.

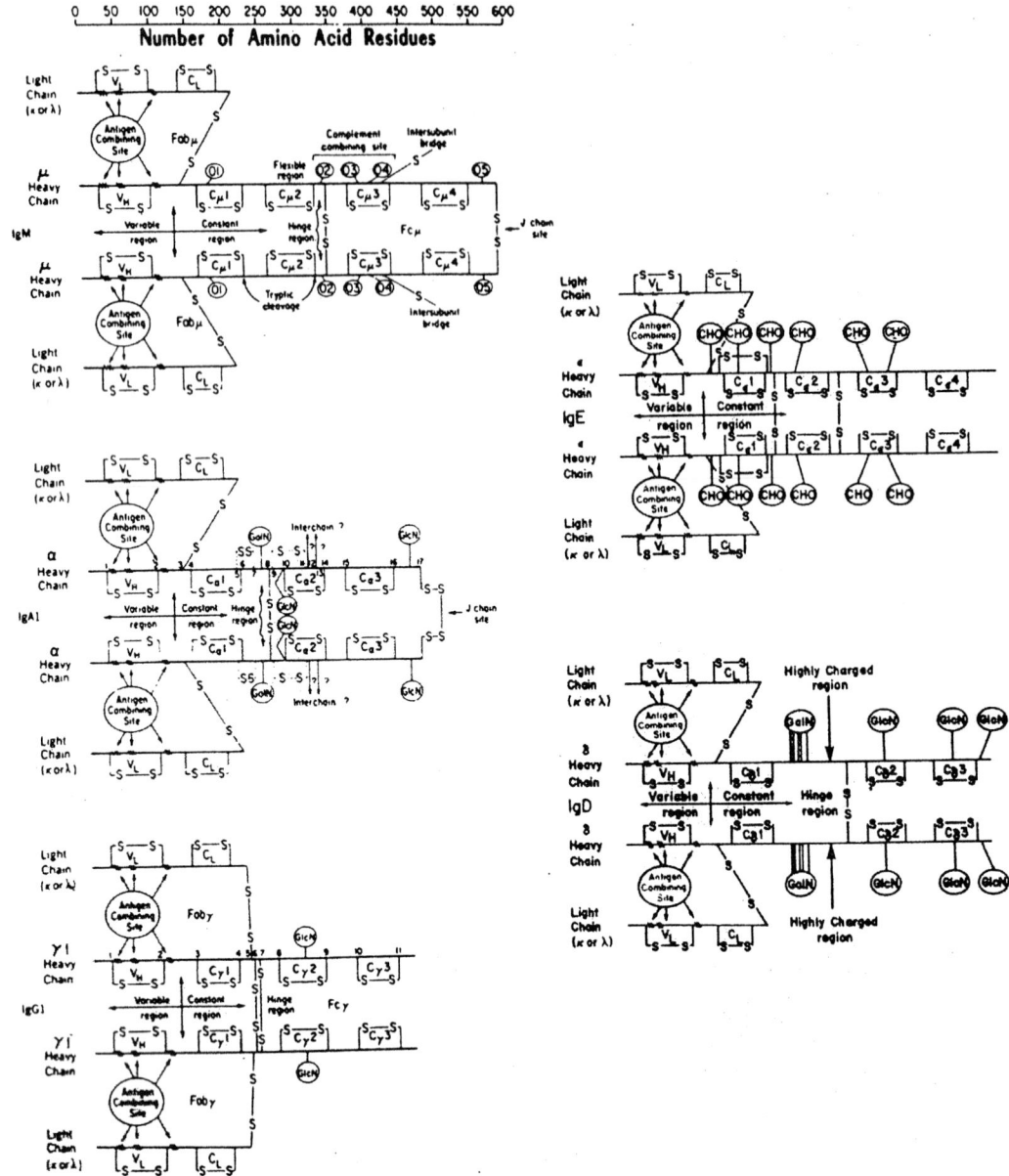

FIG. 2. Illustration of the potential glyosylation sites and disulfide bonds in immunoglobulin isotypes. From Putnam (158), with permission.

in the second sheet. The core of the domain is formed through the *b, c, e, f* and part of the *c'* or *c-d* loops. These portions comprise 31 amino acid residues. The edges formed of *a, g, c'*, and *c"* maintain conformational flexibility (see Fig. 4). Despite differences in conformation, these domains—in the case of most immunoglobulins—share a common set of cysteine residues that form a disulfide bridge linking the two sheets (see Colorplate 2). This disulfide bridge forms the nuclear portion of what is called "the pin region" and provides structural stability to the unit. Disulfide bridges are common to most of the IgSF members but vary in number and placement. Interestingly, in molecular biological experiments in which the disulfide bonds are removed (cysteines replaced by serines), there is remarkably little overall alteration in antibody

function. Thus, while almost universal among the domains of members of the IgSF, the disulfide bridges seem like evolutionary "add-ons." The tryptophan residue that packs against the disulfide bridge is also common to members of the IgSF. Beyond the common cysteine and tryptophan amino acids, the Ig domain can vary widely in the primary amino acid sequence. Despite this variability, however, a common secondary and tertiary structure characteristic to the Ig domain is preserved. The region between the two sheets maintains a hydrophobic character. Nonpolar amino acids occupy most of the positions where side chains are pointing into the domain. Other residues in this area participate in the formation of hydrogen bonds. Residues in the edges of the domain are solvent exposed. The variation among the size of residues that

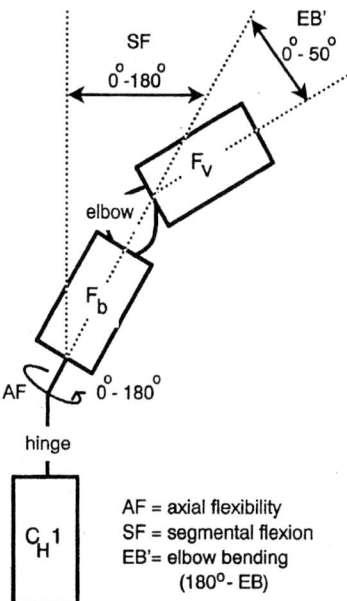

FIG. 3. Illustration of the motions and flexibility of the immunoglobulin. Axial and segmental flexibility are determined by the hinge. The switch peptide (elbow) also contributes flexibility to the Fab. The measure of its angle is defined as between the symmetry of the Fv and Fb axes. From Carayannopoulos and Capra (153), with permission.

occupy the central portion of the domain are considerable, but instead of being compensated strictly by local conformational changes and complementary mutations, the movement of the sheets relative to each other as well as the insertion of side chains from the periphery provide the majority of the changes required (16,17). These mechanisms allow considerable variation to occur, as in the process of somatic hypermutation while maintaining the structural conformation of the molecule. The Ig domain bears unusual functional properties by maintaining structural stability while providing extreme variability in binding specificity through its loops rather than secondary structural elements, as in the case of the binding

site formed by two V domains (heavy and light chains) for antigen. Usually binding domains of protein are considered the driving force of evolutionary conservation, unlike the Ig domain case.

FAB STRUCTURE AND FUNCTION

In order to combat a seemingly infinite range of potential pathogens, the humoral immune system is equipped with a highly structured yet extremely versatile weapon—the Fab domain of the immunoglobulin. This domain shows an amazing array of binding capabilities while maintaining a highly homologous scaffold. This section first describes the characteristics of this domain, the relationship of the variable segments, structurally important features, and finally, some of the important characteristics of the antigen interface.

The antigen-binding fragment (Fab) is comprised of heavy and light chains that are both divided into a constant region (Fb) and a variable region (Fv). Other than minor allotypic differences, the constant region does not vary for a given isotype in the heavy chain or for each class of light chain (κ or λ). However, the variable region exhibits significant plasticity. Gene segments are assembled in an ordered fashion by recombination to encode the Fv but these mechanisms are beyond the scope of this chapter (see Chapter 5). However, it is important, in the context of antibody structure and function to appreciate that two or more genes in virtually every species encode variable regions. Each variable region is approximately 120 to 130 amino acids long, and is generated by two light [L] chain and three heavy [H] chain gene segments. The "V gene segment" encodes the majority of the variable region while the D (H chain) and J (H or L chain) gene segments encode the rest. Multiple V, D, and J gene segments provide ample genetic information, which can be used in virtually every combination to provide the diversity required to respond to a limitless array of antigens (see Chapter 5).

When only a few amino acid sequences of Ig variable domains were available, a comparison of a number of sequences led to the observation that some regions of the

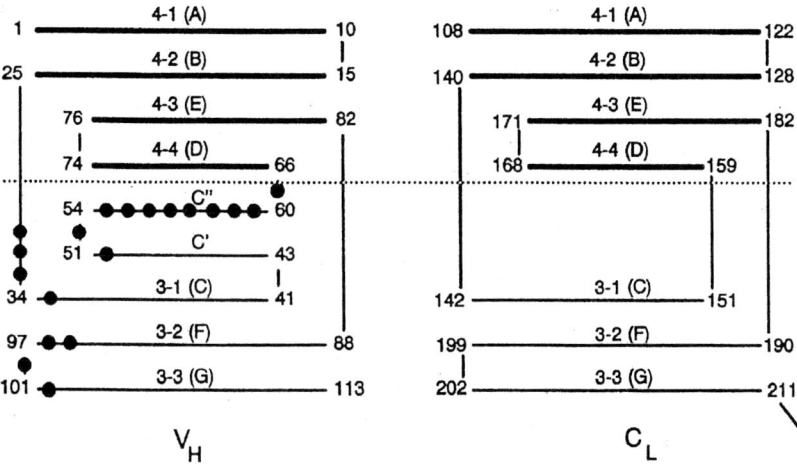

FIG. 4. Schematic of the secondary structural topology of the two major types of Ig domains present in the immunoglobulin (V and C). Horizontal lines are beta strands, and vertical lines are loops connecting them. Lines with large dots represent CDRs. C domains contain 7 strands and V domains contain 9 strands. Residue numbers are according to Kabat et al. (154). Numbering of beta strands (in parentheses) is according to Edmundson or Hood. From Carayannopoulos and Capra (153), with permission.

immunoglobulin sequence are more variable than others. A method of quantifying these differences was derived. Variability for a given residue is defined as the ratio of the number of different amino acids that are found at a given position to the frequency of the most common residue at that position. Thus, a residue that is always present will have a variability of 1, but variability at a position in which all amino acid residues are present at an equal frequency is 400 (18). By comparing regions of the immunoglobulin in this way, it was found that certain segments of the variable region varied more than others (see Fig. 5). From these early comparisons the concept of "framework" and "hypervariable" regions entered the lexicon of immunology (see Table 2). It was soon hypothesized that the hypervariable regions would play a prominent role in antigen recognition. In subsequent studies, most of the hypervariable regions were indeed the major antigen contact points and they were termed complementarity determining regions or "CDRs" (9).

Thus, molecular biology (showing that two or three gene segments generate variable regions), primary amino acid sequence analysis (revealing highly variable and reasonably constant areas within the variable region) and x-ray crystallography came together in the early 1970s to provide us with a view of the antibody variable regions that neither alone could provide: The framework regions determined by protein sequencing were seen to be the β strands forming the Ig domain of the Fv and are far less variable than the CDRs, which comprise the loops that make up the majority of the antigen-binding region of the Fab. Thus, three very different disciplines converged to provide an insight that has stood the test of 3 more decades of study largely intact; that is, the hypervariable regions represent those portions of the antibody molecule that directly interact with antigen and the framework regions provide the scaffold for the interaction to take place.

The variable regions of both the heavy and light chains are held together through the interaction of frameworks 2 and 4 of the heavy and light chains. Framework 2 in the heavy chain contains a specific sequence (Gly-Leu-Glu-Trp-hydrophobic) that interacts with a light-chain–specific stretch

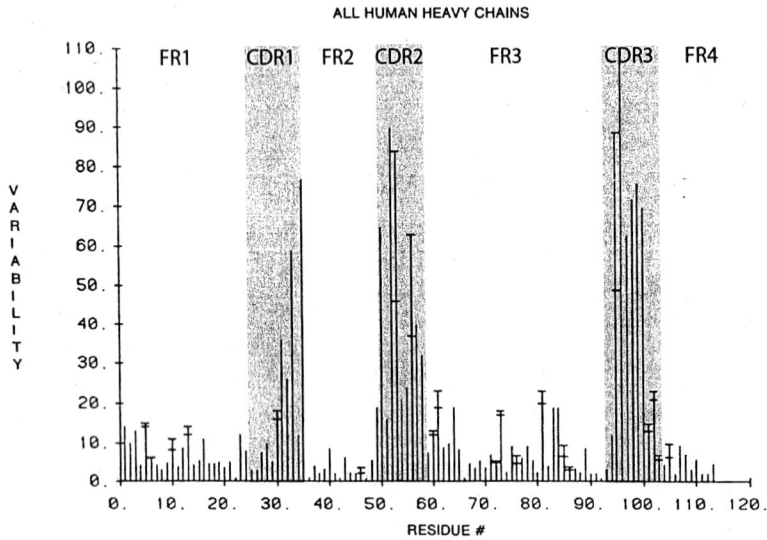

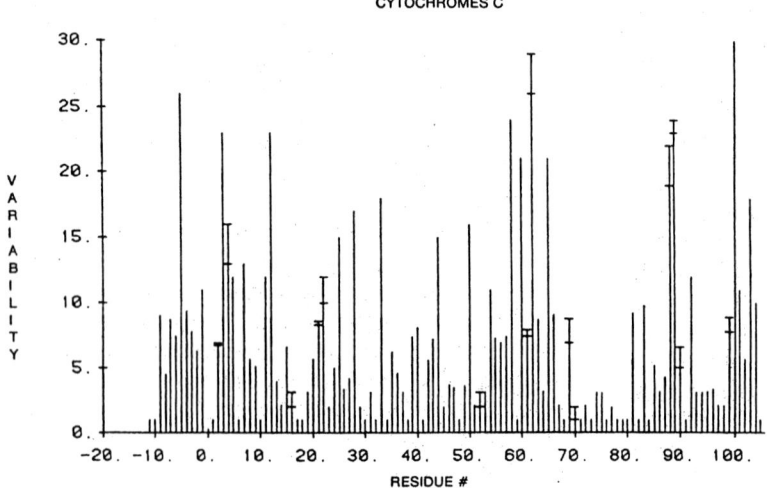

FIG. 5. Representation of the variability of amino acids in the primary sequence of the human heavy chain variable region. Framework and CDR regions are labeled. The hypervariable regions can be identified as the regions with large grouped peaks. For comparison, cytochrome C variability is also shown. Adapted from Kabat et al. (154), with permission.

TABLE 2. *Residues defining framework and CDR regions of immunoglobulin chains*

Subdomain region	Ig chain	Residue positions	Key residues
FR1	Heavy	1–26 (1–25)	Cys23 (22)
	Light	1–26 (1–26)	Cys23 (23)
CDR1	Heavy	27–38 (26–35)	
	Light	27–38 (27–32)	
FR2	Heavy	39–55 (35A–50)	Trp41 (36)
	Light	39–55 (33–49)	Trp41 (35)
CDR2	Heavy	56–65 (51–57)	
	Light	56–65 (50–52)	
FR3	Heavy	66–103 (58–91)	Leu89 (80)
	Light	66–103 (53–87)	Leu89 (73)
CDR3	Heavy	104–115 (92–95)	Cys104 (92)
	Light	104–111 (88–95 or 95D)	Cys104 (88)

Note: Numbering is according to the IMGT Unique Numbering System and the Kabat system (154) in parentheses. Key conserved residues are also listed. The IMGT Unique Numbering System assigns a designation for each residue in the primary sequence that allows direct correspondence between light and heavy chains. The Kabat system serves to optimally align conserved residues and accounts for evolutionary and junctional diversity by using lettered designations for additional residues. Compiled from Lefranc and Lefranc (155), with permission.

(Pro-hydrophobic-Leu-hydrophobic) in framework 2 as well, to help the two immunoglobulin folds of each chain to properly dimerize (19). In addition, the sequence Trp/Phe-Gly-X-Gly in framework 4 creates a beta bulge that is necessary for dimerization of the variable heavy- and light-chain domains (20). Regions in the CH1 domain are important for dimerization and effectively bind the Fab at the opposite end from the antigen-binding domain. The five-stranded, beta sheet face is used as the dimerization surface for the Fb region although only four of the strands participate (c″ is excluded). The three-stranded face generally participates in V-region dimerization (21). This orientation requires nearly a 180° rotation in comparison to the Fv region that is facilitated by the "elbow peptide" or "switch" region located as a spacer in between the Fv and Fb (22). Interactions between the Ig domains in both Fv and Fb regions of the Fab in addition to the CH3 or homologous structure have an interrupted alternating hydrophobic and hydrophilic residue patterns that are usually seen for other protein–protein interactions with Ig domains and replace it with hydrophobic residues that form a core for binding (10,22–24). Bulges in the g strand as well as the c′ strands of the variable regions protrude into the interior of the dimer and prevent tight adherence between the two variable regions. A hydrophilic groove is produced, which is lined by residues of the hypervariable region and other CDR loops forming the antigen-binding site. The core hydrophobic regions exist between contacts of frameworks 2 and 4 as mentioned previously, as well as between CDR3s of the heavy and light chain or between framework 2 and the CDR3 of the other variable region (25). These arrangements provide stable associations between the components of the Fab, maintaining structural integrity of the molecule, while at the same time allowing it the freedom to perform its antigen-binding function and conformational changes that might need to occur to facilitate this capacity. The tight interaction between

these roles is illustrated in the difficulty of successfully creating engineered antibodies with framework and CDR regions from separate species (26,27).

The sequence similarity among V regions can be used to place them into related groups. Framework-1 amino acid residues 6 to 24 divide them into three clans (see Fig. 6). In a further subdivision, framework 3 residues can be used to distinguish among family members within a clan (28–30). Families are then divided into individual members based on the rest of the differences in the germline repertoire that divide them (see Chapter 5). At the amino acid level, in general, different families display a similarity of 75% at the amino acid level, but between families display less than a 70% homology (31). There are seven families of VH genes, four families of Vκ genes, and ten families of Vλ genes in the human. In the mouse, these numbers are expanded to currently 14 VH and 20 Vκ families. The ability to group this large number of variable region structures into families and clans based on relatively strict similarity requirements reflects the concept that the origin of family members is likely to be through the duplication of an originally smaller set of genes.

While the framework regions exhibit high degrees of similarity, the CDR regions are characterized by their divergence. While some characteristics among families can be seen in parameters such as length, variability is the hallmark of the CDR. Many factors influence the construction of the CDRs. These include the length of the V gene used and the presence of somatic mutations and insertions or deletions that produce a sequence that differs from the germline. The latter two processes occur in the peripheral lymphoid compartments. The conformation of the CDR loops in a three-dimensional context is influenced by interactions that occur with neighboring framework residues (32,33), other CDRs from both the VH and VL chains, and even glycosylation that has been reported at CDR asparagines (34,35). As we will see, not only the

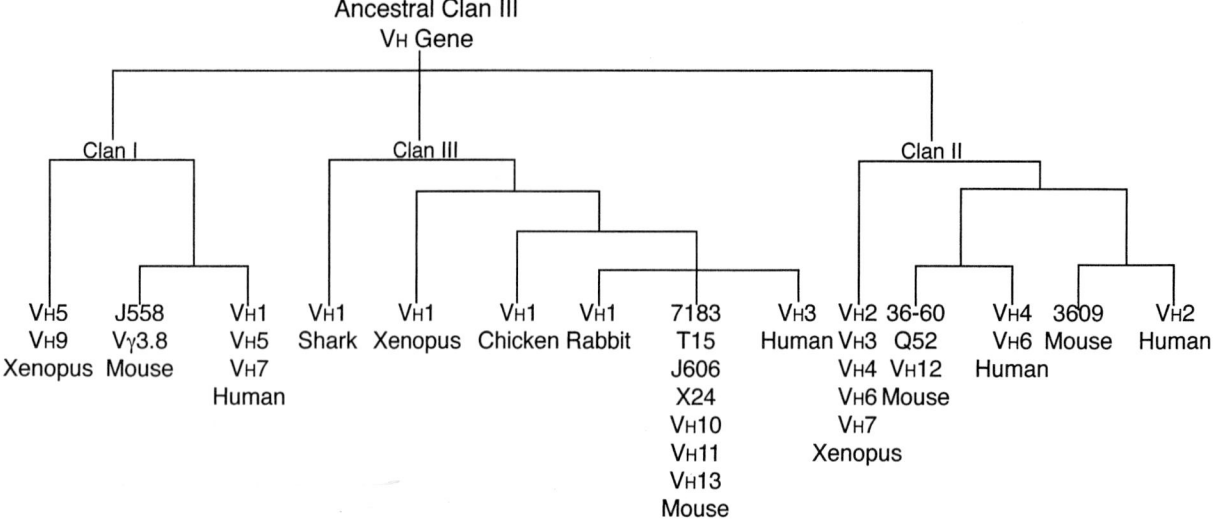

FIG. 6. Immunoglobulins can be organized into clans according to their amino acid homology. Clans can be further subdivided into families in different species as illustrated. Adapted from Kirkham and Schroeder (30), with permission.

immediate context of the antigen-binding region constructed by the CDR loops is important, but changes in the extended structure can also have profound influences upon the affinity of the antibody.

The third complementarity-determining region of the heavy chain, HCDR3, lies at the center of the classic antigen-binding site. HCDR3 is the direct product of nonhomologous gene rearrangement; D gene segments that have the potential to be read in any one of three reading frames; by deletion; and N addition, which has the potential to introduce a totally random sequence into the antigen-binding site (see Chapter 5). Together, these factors make HCDR3 the focus of somatic diversification of the antibody repertoire (36,37). In practice, however, as Schroeder and his group have shown (see Fig. 7), the sequence composition of HCDR3 is constrained, with a preference for tyrosine, glycine, and serine and underrepresentation of positively charged (Arg, Lys) and hydrophobic (e.g., Val, Ileu, Leu) amino acids (Fig. 7). Thus, the HCDR3 is enriched for neutral, hydrophilic sequences (38,39). In large part, these preferences reflect nonrandom representation of amino acids in D and J gene segment sequences. Whether these preferences reflect structural concerns or evolutionary selection for a specific range of antigen-binding sites remains a focus of active investigation (40).

Not only does the variable domain have the capacity to bind to antigens using its antigen-binding site using complementarity-determining regions, but the Fv can also bind bacterial virulence factors without the classical antigen–antibody interactions. Antigens that bind to immunoglobulins (and T-cell receptors) outside the classical binding sites, and therefore react with a large number of different antibodies, are referred to as "superantigens." Staphylococcal protein A (SpA) is an example of a B-cell superantigen that binds to human VH3-encoded immunoglobulins (Igs) independently of the D- and JH-encoded regions or light-chain sequences

(41). The exact SpA-binding structure formed by VH3-encoded Igs was first elucidated by work done in our laboratory in which we expressed a VH3-encoded Ab in baculovirus that bound SpA and then produced mutant Abs in which regions of the human VH3 Ab were exchanged with those from a mouse Ab of the J558 family—a family not associated with SpA binding. The pattern of SpA binding indicated not only that residues in FR1, CDR2, and FR3 were involved, but also that the three regions were required to interact simultaneously with SpA for binding to occur. When any one of the three regions was replaced with the corresponding region from the nonbinding Ab, SpA binding was severely disrupted. The data indicated that SpA required simultaneous interaction with three distinct regions of a VH3 structure, which together in three-dimensional space presumably formed an extended solvent-exposed surface (42). The crucial finding of these experiments was that framework residues played a central role in binding. Recent crystallographic studies have confirmed and extended these studies (43) (see Colorplate 3). Moreover, the VH surface-bound SpA seems to have been conserved in the B-cell repertoires of amphibian, avian, and mammalian species (44).

In the mouse, Fab-mediated SpA-binding interactions are commonly displayed by 5% to 10% of mature B cells, which express genes from the clan III set of related VH families (45,46). Of the murine analogs of human VH3 genes, certain J606-, 7183-, and DNA4-encoded VH regions commonly convey binding activity, while VH encoded by products of clan III/S107 VH genes commonly convey among the highest affinity for SpA, and this binding activity is independent of specific VL region usage (reviewed in Silverman and Goodyear [47]).

Thus, once again we see a duality in structure/function. A B-cell superantigen binds to certain VH genes primarily through interaction with framework residues, and at the same

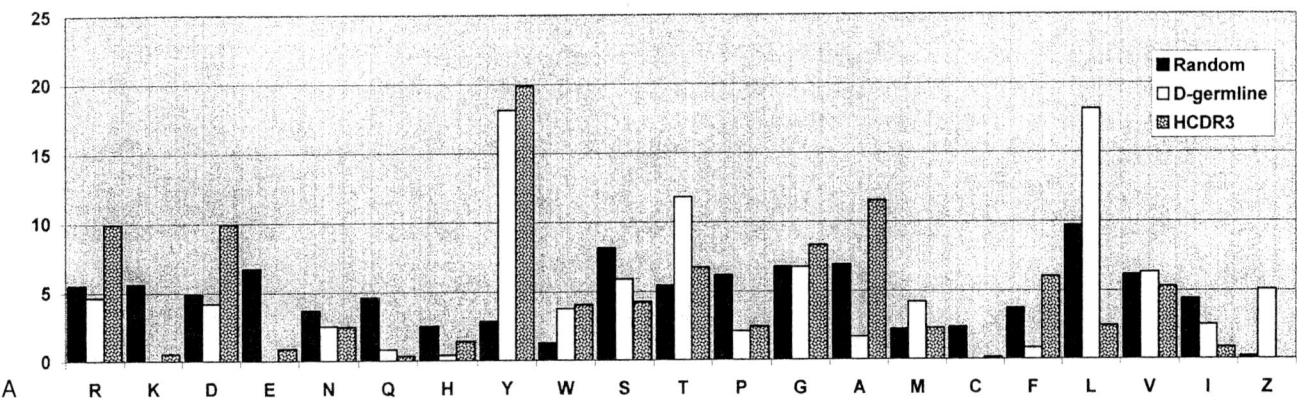

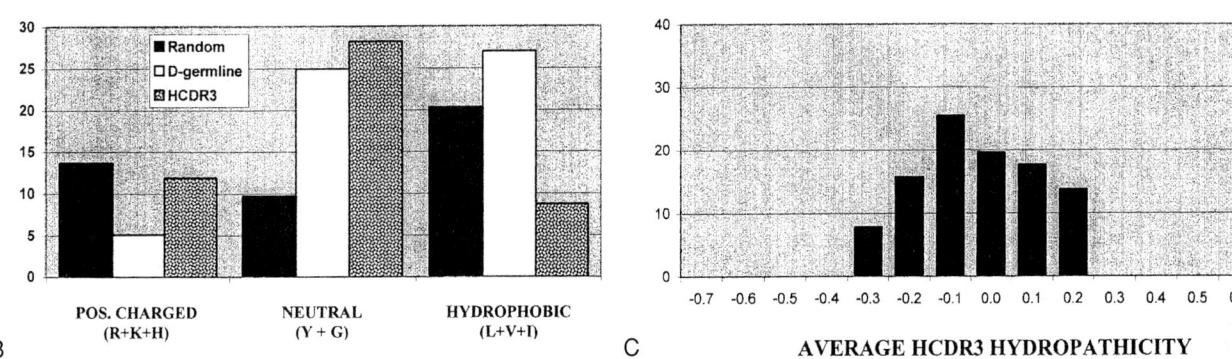

FIG. 7. A: Amino acid representation in the three deletional reading frames in mouse D segments and HCDR3. The first column for each amino acid corresponds to that amino acid's frequency of occurrence (in percentages) in all available Genbank protein sequences (36). The second column shows the amino acid content of the germline sequence of the D segments (in all three deletional RFs) (40). The third column shows the amino acid representation in adult mouse spleen HCDR3 (37). Z = Stop codons. **B:** Representation of three groups of amino acids (in percentages). Shading scheme as in **A. C:** Hydropathicity of HCDR3. Average hydropathicity of mouse HCDR3 intervals (40) and their frequency of occurrence (in percentages).

time, the same B-cell superantigen binds to the Fc region of certain immunoglobulins.

ANTIGEN–ANTIBODY INTERACTIONS

Recent studies have begun to refine our understanding of the types of interactions that occur at the antigen–antibody interface. These studies have come out of a body of work devoted to visualizing antigen–antibody complexes at resolutions down to 1.7 Å, at which levels the role of solvent is being elucidated. Some of these studies have been performed on monoclonal antibody interactions with their haptens in both complexed and uncomplexed states and with both germline and high-affinity configurations. In addition, stepwise manipulation of the antigen-binding sites by single and grouped sets of mutations has also been performed. The lessons learned through these studies are numerous and represent an exciting development in the study of antibody structure.

For example, the differences in antigen–antibody interactions in germline versus high-affinity, somatic, mutated counterparts provide a new glimpse into the nature of these interactions. The difference in the affinity between these two

forms has approached a 30,000-fold higher affinity in the mutated antibody than in the germline antibody. This enormous change for some antibodies in their affinity for antigen arises from the small additive changes that the mutations have contributed. Three common themes for the nature of the role of mutational differences in the forming of an affinity-matured antibody have arisen. The first is the contribution of direct interaction of the mutated base with the hapten. In some circumstances, a base-pair substitution contributes, for instance, a new hydrogen bond or creates a local hydrophobic region that is additive to the affinity. Furthermore, somatic mutation can result in an amino acid substitution that alters the flexibility of the antibody-binding site. This is illustrated in studies of both antigen-bound and antigen-unbound germline and high-affinity antibodies (48). Germline antibodies often undergo a localized antigen-combining, site-conformational change as antigen binds. The movement can approach the range of 4 to 5 Å for some antibodies. This is in contrast to what is seen with high-affinity antibodies to the same antigen in which the combining site has very little movement on binding. Finally, somatically mutated antibodies versus germline antibodies often show differences in the geometry of the hapten in relation to the antibody-combining site. These changes in orientation are the result of the addition, deletion, or replacement of interactions not only between the hapten and antibody but also between the peripheral loops and the most proximal loops to the hapten in the combining region (48–50). It should be noted, however, that some high-affinity antibodies have been reported that undergo exceptionally dramatic conformational changes upon binding to their ligand (51). Taken together, these studies reveal new depth to our ideas about antigen–antibody interactions. While we normally think of antibody–hapten complexes as a single hand-in-glove fit, this is not necessarily the case. Recent studies have also indicated that several high-affinity conformations are possible and occur for a given antigen–antibody interaction. In other words, redundancy can exist for high-affinity antibodies (52,53). In addition, there is some evidence for the ability of an antibody to bind to a region on antigen that is not necessarily solvent exposed. Small, localized conformational changes may therefore occur in antigen that allow these regions to be exposed perhaps for only brief periods of time (54). Such an activity is reinforced by the nature of catalytic antibodies.

At this point, there are over 20 different antigen–antibody crystal structures. While this represents one of the largest numbers of crystal structures within a family of proteins, few of the structures are at a resolution high enough to solve questions related to the role of water in the interaction with antigen as well as the thermodynamic questions that arise from its influence on the system. The recent publication of a few much-higher-resolution crystal structures is already beginning to demonstrate the role of water in these protein, carbohydrate, and DNA interactions.

The residues involved in the combining site include amphipathic amino acids such as Tyr and Trp at a high frequency. Water molecules in a number of studies have been shown to be present and involved with antigen interactions with the crystal structures. In general, water in areas where close protein–protein contacts are not occurring has been shown to participate in additional hydrogen bonds other than those that exist directly between antigen and antibody (55–57). The presence of water molecules in these areas then has the capacity to increase the interactions particularly for antigens that fit less well into the combining site. These interactions have been observed for both carbohydrate (58,59) and protein haptens (55). In other cases as well, water molecules bound to the surface of either antigens or antibodies are excluded. The release of these molecules participates to increase randomization in the solvent environment and provide for another means to enhance the affinity of antigen binding (57).

The primary view then of the role of water seems to be to provide a better "fit" for antigen by filling space in the binding region and to participate in extended hydrogen bonding. This contribution increases the enthalpy of the system and, in combination with hydrogen bonds between the interacting proteins as well as van der Waal forces, contributes to an enthalpy-driven antigen–antibody interaction. While this view of the presence of water contributing to an enthalpy-driven reaction is common to many studies, it should not be discounted that the exclusion of certain water molecules may play a role in driving the strength of affinity through entropic means. Studies of HIV protease inhibitors as well as some antibody–antigen interactions as indicated above suggest that the increase of randomization of the solution will contribute to the affinity of an antibody and may be worth pursuing as an additional strategy in antibody engineering studies (57).

Antigen recognition, as we have seen and as will be elaborated further in subsequent chapters, depends on diversification from a number of processes. V(D)J recombination, somatic hypermutation, gene conversion, and other such mechanisms generate nearly an infinite variety of molecules designed to *recognize antigen*. Class-switch recombination from "upstream" to "downstream" isotypes results in the generation of an antibody with the same antigen recognition capacity but different effector capacities to facilitate *antigen elimination*.

The various immunoglobulin classes have certain unique properties that when taken together allow for a wider range of host defenses than would be possible if only a single class of heavy chain constant regions existed. This is illustrated in the breakdown of immune defense as seen in hyper-IgM syndrome (the only isotype present in the patient is IgM) or IgA deficiency (the most common immunodeficiency in humans, complete absence of IgA). While many of the differences in Ig function can be localized to the CH2, CH3, or (if present) the CH4 domain, surprisingly, many of the structural properties of these classes can be attributed to the hinge region.

THE IMMUNOGLOBULIN HINGE

While not all immunoglobulin classes have a hinge that is separately encoded (see Chapter 5), all Ig classes have a structure that recognizably fulfills its function, albeit to various degrees. Classes that do not have genetic hinges use an extra C domain in its place. The genetic hinges that are encoded in the other classes have a great variety of lengths and structural properties. The most dramatic of these, IgG3, serves as an illustration of the construction of the hinge. The IgG3 hinge is divided into upper, middle, and lower regions that can be separated based on both structural (amino acid sequence) and genetic components. Structurally, the upper hinge (UH) stretches from the C terminal end of CH1 to the first hinge disulfide bond. The middle hinge (MH) stretches from the first cysteine to the last cysteine in the hinge. The lower hinge (LH) extends from the last cysteine to the glycine of CH2 (60). The cysteines present in the hinge form interchain disulfide bonds that link the two immunoglobulin monomers. Table 3 compares some of the structural features of hinges from various isotypes.

The structural differences among the hinges are reflected in the various properties of the heavy chains. In a simplistic way, one can think of the hinge as the structural unit that links the functions of the Fab and Fc fragments. With greater flexibility, antibodies can bind antigens on the surface of targets with varying degrees of distance between them. In addition, the

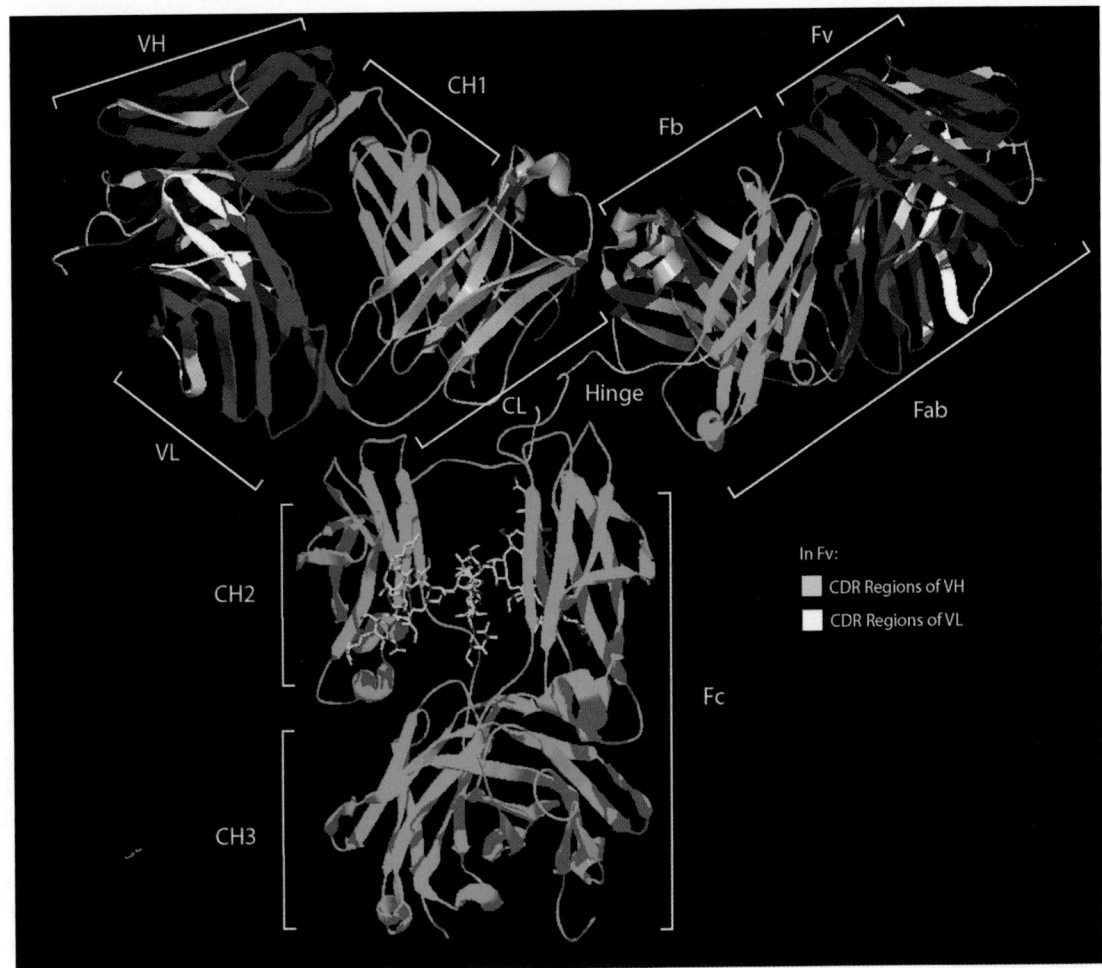

COLORPLATE 1. Ribbon diagram of a complete IgG1 crystal (1hzh in PDB from data of Harris et al. [119]). The major regions of the immunoglobulin are illustrated. The heavy-chain constant regions (green) also include the hinge (yellow) between the first two domains. Cγ2 is glycosylated (also seen in yellow). The heavy- and light-chain variable regions (red and dark blue, respectively) are N terminal to the heavy- (green) and light-chain (light blue) constant regions. CDR loops in the heavy- and light-chain variable regions (yellow and white) are illustrated as well.

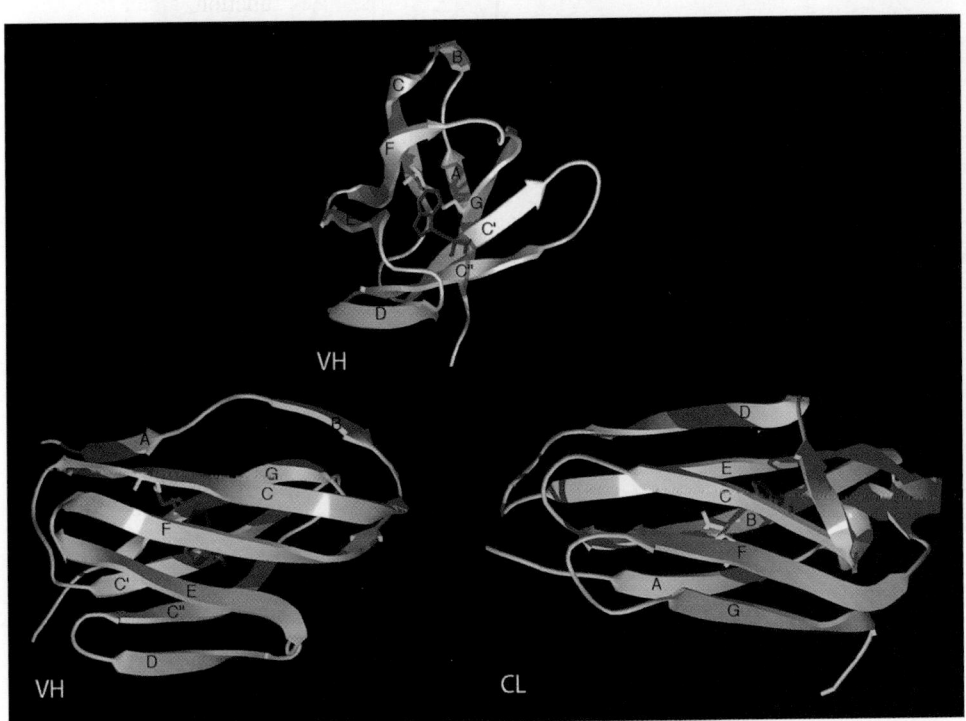

COLORPLATE 2. Ribbon diagrams of side and face on views of Ig domains from VH and Cλ regions. Strands are labeled according to Hood nomenclature. The "pin" composed of a disulfide bond between two cysteines is illustrated (yellow) along with the conserved tryptophan residue (red).

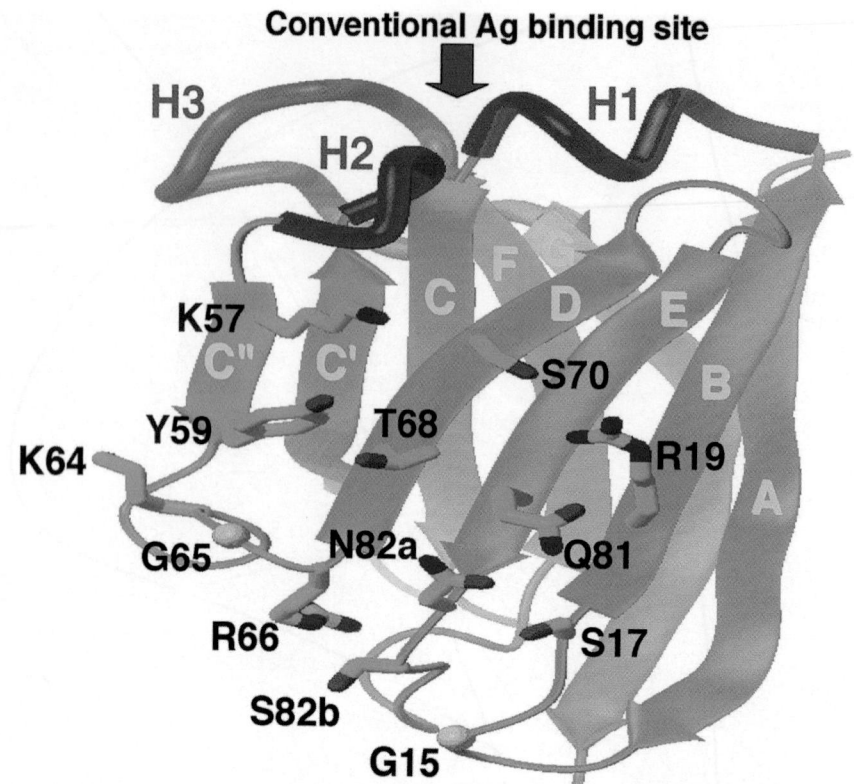

COLORPLATE 3. Schematic representation of the complex between SpA domain D and Fab 2A2 from a human IgM. A side view shows the peptide backbone of SpA domain D (red) bound to the framework region of the Fab heavy chain (cyan). The VL domain, which is not involved in this interaction, is shown in dark blue. The binding site for SpA is remote from the CDR loops, which are highlighted in magenta. This model is based on the superposition of helix I and II of SpA domains in the Fab-domain D complex reported here and in the previously determined Fcγ-domain B complex. From Graille et al. (43), with permission.

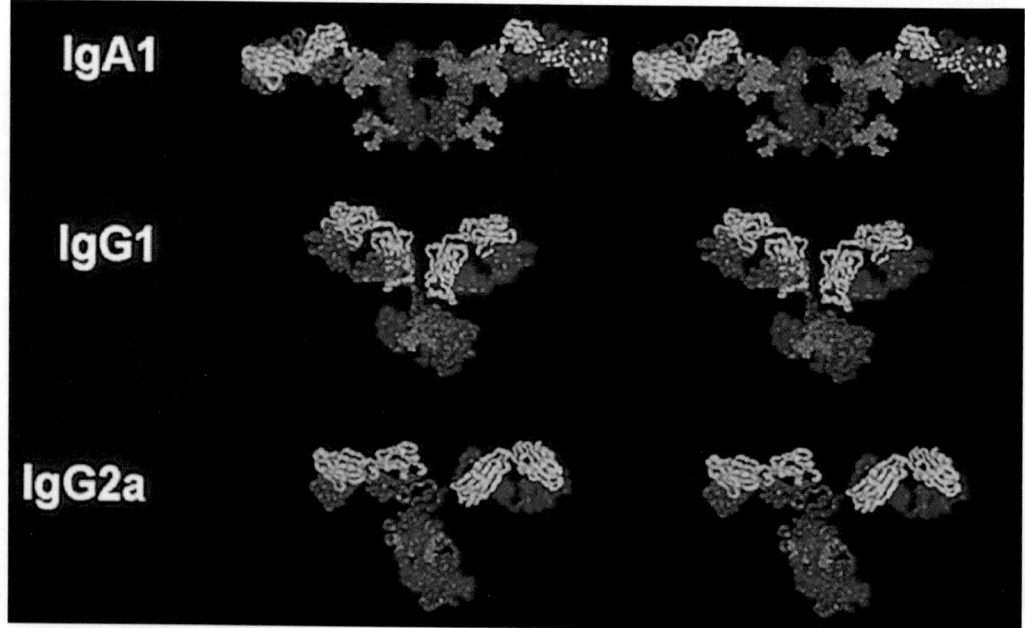

COLORPLATE 4. A comparison of an x-ray and neutron-solution–scattering theoretical model (human IgA1) and x-ray crystal (murine IgG1 and IgG2a) structures. Light chains (yellow), heavy chains (red and dark blue), and glycosylation (light blue) are illustrated. The extended length of IgA1 over that of IgG can be seen along with extensive glycosylation that characterizes this isotype. From Boehm et al. (66), with permission.

TABLE 3. *Properties of hinges in IgG, IgA, and IgD*

Ig type	Upper Hinge length	Middle Hinge length	Lower Hinge length	Genetic hinge configuration (amino acids/exon)	Susceptibility to proteolysis	Special features
IgG1	4	10	6	15		
IgG2	3	8	6	12		
IgG3	12	49	6	17-15-15-15		
IgG4	7	4	6	12		
IgA1	1	23	2	19	high	Heavily O-linked glycosylation
IgA2	1	10	2	6		
IgD				34-24	high	Extensive charged amino acids; heavy O-linked glycosylation at N terminus

Note: Lengths represent amino acids.

steric position of these two components may directly affect Fc binding to cellular receptors. Using a similar argument, the hinge may also be involved in the modulation of complement binding (see below). These hinge properties will be explored in more depth by focusing on the individual isotypes.

The motion about the IgG hinge has been extensively studied and serves as a basis of comparison for other isotypes (reviewed in Schumaker et al. [61]). With the exception of IgG3, IgG hinges are encoded by single exons (see Chapter 5). The upper and lower portions of the hinge are the most flexible and allow for motions such as bending between the Fc and Fab in both parallel and perpendicular planes. In contrast, the middle hinge is a rigid structure that is thought to provide spacing between the Fab and Fc domains. It can be seen from Table 3 that this structure is greatly extended in IgG3 compared to the other isotypes. It has been shown that for some functions, this large hinge region can even replace a missing CH domain.

In addition, rotation about the long axis of the Fab leads to additional levels of flexibility. A number of electron microscopic studies using immune complexes of IgG show that the Fab–Fab angles range from a very narrow "Y" with an apparent separation of 10° to a "T" with angles of 180°. An addition rotational flexibility of up to 180° is also required to account for some of the observed complexes (62). Thus, the remarkable conformational plasticity of the immunoglobulin molecule allows it to bind epitopes spaced at various distances on the surface of a target.

In addition to altering the Fab angles, the flexibility of the hinge plays a role in Fc function. While recent evidence suggests that other parts of the Ig constant region influence complement binding more than thought in the past, the role of the hinge still appears to be critical. In general, the more flexible hinges allow less steric hindrance and better binding of complement. The greater flexibility of some hinges allows them to either expose or sterically hinder certain complement-binding regions in CH2. While once thought to be a sequence-specific interaction between complement and portions of the CH2 domain, it has been recently shown that the accessibility of the site is more important for determining the activation ability of the various Ig subclasses. This can be illustrated by the trend of complement activation to follow the order of IgG3>IgG1>IgG4>IgG2 (reviewed in Brekke et al. [63] and

Feinstein et al. [64]) in the human (unless otherwise specified all subclass designations will refer to human immunoglobulins). Following a similar trend, hinge flexibility and relief of steric hindrance have also been shown to modulate to some degree the binding of the CH2 domain to certain Fc receptors (65).

While tip-to-tip separation of the Fabs in IgG structures varies from 13 to 16 nm, IgA1 has a spread of up to 23 nm. This additional distance that IgA1 is able to span may confer advantages for more efficient recognition of epitopes that are widely separated. IgA2, of decreased abundance in the serum (see below), has a hinge with a length equivalent to the shorter IgG subclasses. A study of the differences between IgA1 and the IgG subclasses is instructive about several aspects of the hinge. The extended structure of the IgA1 hinge is a combination of two properties: the abundance of O-linked glycosylation coupled with the location of the disulfide linkages between the Ig monomers near the top of the CH2 (Cα2) domain (66). Most other isotypes contain some N-linked glycosylation. In immunoglobulins, O-linked glycosylation is unique to IgA1 and IgD. This extensive glycosylation has two potential advantages for these molecules. The extended hinge of IgA1 is probably protected from proteolysis by many bacterial enzymes because of its glycosylation. There are several pathogenic bacteria that exploit two contiguous, repeating amino-acid octamers consisting of proline, serine, and threonine as a binding site for IgA1 proteases—an important virulence factor. It is thought that the resistance to common bacterial proteases allows IgA1 as a major secretory isotype to survive among the flora that also colonize the mucosa (reviewed in Kilian et al. [67]). Coupled with the separation of Fab arms, this extensive glycosylation most likely also aids in separating the Fab domains. Eliciting a similar effect, the disulfide bonds at the top of the CH2 domain rather than in the hinge itself allows the extended structure to give the molecule a greater spread than could be accomplished if disulfide bonds were contained within the hinge itself. The other IgA isotype, IgA2, lacks the extended hinge that IgA1 possesses and is also not heavily glycosylated (66). However, the smaller hinge in IgA2 does not contain the proteolytic motifs that are recognized by the enzymes produced by certain bacteria in IgA1 and may therefore be maintained in the isotype repertoire for this specialized niche. This may explain why, in serum, the ratio of IgA1:IgA2 is about 6:1, but in most secretions, it is close to 1:1.

The hinge of IgD, like IgA1, has extensive O-linked glycosylation on an extended hinge structure. The hinge is divided into two major subregions (and encoded by two exons) that are either rich in alanine and threonine or glutamate and lysine. This latter subregion is highly sensitive to proteolytic enzymes and is even sensitive to a yet unidentified enzyme and has thus been dubbed "spontaneously" proteolytic (68–71). Both IgA1 and IgD possess another characteristic that is linked to their O-linked glycosylation. Jacalin (jackfruit lectin) binds to these O-linked carbohydrates with high affinity and can be used to precipitate these specific isotypes. Interestingly, the cell-surface receptor for human IgD binds to these O-linked oligosaccharides. This receptor binds both IgD and IgA1 (72–74). Thus, this is an example of the hinge region and in particular the oligosaccharides of the hinge region playing a critical role in cellular binding.

Fc STRUCTURE AND FUNCTION

While the hinge is essential to modulate many properties of the immunoglobulin, the Fc portion is the primary effector domain of the molecule. While the antigen-binding function of the Fab domains allows the immunoglobulin to specifically recognize diverse antigens, the Fc domain allows an antibody at the same time to elicit host responses. This requires that the Fc region provide binding sites for both cellular receptors and complement—the two primary effector response types to antibody–antigen complexes. This property requires that the Fc domains maintain considerable conservation especially in structural support regions. While there is substantial conservation within species (some allotypes vary in function), many "Fc functions" seem to be conserved with only modest structural similarity—especially within the primary amino acid sequence. In humans, the subclasses are even closer in structure, being over 90% identical in amino acid sequences. (The degree of difference between the IgG isotypes varies widely in mammals—in the human, the IgG subclasses are among the most closely related and presumably are of very recent evolutionary origin.) However, the regions between the conserved Ig domain structures (generally small loops) also serve as a target region for the binding of certain bacterial and viral virulence factors and can be involved in binding to cell-surface receptors (see below).

Each constant region consists of 3 CH domains for IgM, IgA, and IgD or 4 CH domains in the case of IgM, and IgE. In the latter isotypes, the CH2 domain replaces the hinge structurally and to some degree functionally. Each CH domain contains a core of an Ig domain with 7 antiparallel beta sheets oriented by 3 in one direction and 4 in the opposite direction. This is in contrast to the structure of the Ig domain in the V region. Looking at all mammals, in general there is approximately 30% amino-acid sequence identity between the constant regions (IgM, IgD, IgG, IgA, IgE) and 60% to 90% homology among the subclasses. The majority of the homology is present in the β strands forming the Ig domains,

disulfide-bonding cysteines, and tryptophans. CH domains are numbered from the first domain located in the Fab and positioned above the hinge, to the CH2 and CH3 domains that are increasingly distal to the hinge.

The CH domains contain several general features that contribute to the structure of the Fc region. N-linked oligosaccharides are positioned in the middle of the CH2 domain that protect a hydrophobic patch in this region, and therefore increase the solubility of the molecule. For IgA, this N-linked glycosylation is thought to be located near the base of the CH2 domain (75). Longitudinal contact between CH2 and CH3 prevents binding between monomer chains at this junction. The CH3 domain uses 4 strands of the β sheet to dimerize between chains. In IgA and IgM, a tailpiece is added to this domain to create higher-order structures.

Glycosylation is an important component of immunoglobulin molecules and the isotypes vary in the extent and type of glycosylation present (see Fig. 2). Between 3% and 17% of the mass of an immunoglobulin is due to glycosylation. While the pattern of glycosylation varies among isotypes, certain conserved sites are preserved. The N-linked glycosylation on Asn297 is conserved for all mammalian IgGs and homologous portions of IgM, IgD, and IgE. This oligosaccharide is thought to project from the inner face of the CH2 domain (7). Major characteristics of the immunoglobulin isotypes are listed in Table 4.

IgM

IgM is the most versatile of the antibody classes. It is first expressed as a surface immunoglobulin on immature lymphocytes and as such is the first "B-cell receptor." B-cell maturation is critically dependent on the presence of immunoglobulin on the surface (76). The μ chain is the first to be produced upon heavy-chain rearrangement. Initially, the μ chain is expressed with a surrogate light chain, which allows a B cell to continue maturation in the bone marrow. Finally the μ chain is paired with a functional light chain and the naïve B cell leaves the bone marrow (77,78). In the periphery, IgM can be expressed by immature, mature, memory, and plasma cells. Of these, expression on immature and maturing cells is the most common where it remains as a surface receptor. Its presence on the surface of these cells provides a receptor for B-cell activation along with the Igα and Igβ accessory molecules (79). Following activation, the B cell undergoes the critical process of affinity maturation. As well, when these cells enter peripheral lymphoid tissues they also acquire IgD by differential RNA splicing. Thus, the two surface receptors (IgM and IgD) have the same antigen-binding capabilities. The Cμ4 domain contains the transmembrane and cytoplasmic regions of IgM that undergo RNA processing to be removed for the production of secreted IgM.

While the membrane-bound form of IgM is most common, IgM plasma cells secrete polymeric IgM that serves important functions as well. Polymeric IgM is an important complement activator, and thus participates in phagocytosis. IgM forms hexamers or pentamers, the latter upon the incorporation of

TABLE 4. Properties of immunoglobulin isotypes

Class or subclass properties	IgM	IgD	IgG1	IgG2	IgG3	IgG4	IgA1	IgA2	IgE
Molecular weight of secreted form (kDa)[a]	950(p)	175	150	150	160	150	160(m), 300(d)	160(m), 350(d)	190
Sedimentation coefficient	19S	7S	7S	6.6S	7S	7S	7S	11S	8S
Functional valency	5 or 10	2	2	2	2	2	2 or 4	2 or 4	2
Interheavy disulphide bonds per monomer	1	1	2	4	11	2	2	2	1
Membrane Ig cytoplasmic region	3	3	28	28	28	28	14	14	28
Secreted Ig tailpiece	20	9	2	2	2	2	20	20	2
Other chain	J chain (16 kDa)	—	—	—	—	—	J chain (16 kDa); secretory component (70 kDa)	secretory component (70 kDa)	—
N-glycosylation sites	5	3	1	1	2	1	2	4	7
O-glycosylation sites	0	7	0	0	0	0	8	0	0
Carbohydrate average (%)	10–12	9–14	2–3	2–3	2–3	2–3	7–11	7–11	12–13
Adult level range (age 16–60) in serum (mg/ml)[b]	0.25–3.1	0.03–0.4	5–12	2–6	0.5–1	0.2–1	1.4–4.2	0.2–0.5	0.0001–0.0002
Approximate % total Ig in adult serum	10	0.2	45–53	11–15	3–6	1–4	11–14	1–4	0.004
Synthetic rate (mg/kg weight/day)	3.3	0.2	33	33	33	33	19–29	3.3–5.3	0.002
Biological half-life (days)	5–10	2–8	21–24	21–24	7–8	21–24	5–7	4–6	1–5
Transplacental transfer	0	0	++	+	++	++	0	0	0
Complement activation classical pathway (C1q)	++++	0	+++	+	++++	0	0	0	0
Complement activation alternative pathway	0	0	0	0	0	0	+	0	0
Reactivity with protein A via Fc	0	0	++	++	+/-	++	0	0	0
Allotypes	—	—	G1m	G2m	G3m	—	—	A2m	Em
Biological properties	Primary antibody response, some binding to pIgR, some binding to phagocytes	Mature B cell marker	Placental transfer, secondary antibody for most responses to pathogen, binds macrophages and other phagocytic cells by FcγR				Secretory Ig, binds pIgR		Allergy and parasite reactivity, binds FcεR on mast cells and basophiles

[a]Light chain molecular weight is 25 kDa.
[b]Total = 9.5–21.7 mg/ml.
d, dimer; m, monomer; p, pentamer.
Compiled from Carayannopoulos and Capra (153), Lefranc and Lefranc (155), Kuby (156), and Janeway et al. (157), with permission.

a J chain, arranged in a star pattern with the Cμ4 domain at the center. Cμ4 and part of Cμ3 have been implicated in the formation of this structure, including certain aspartic acid, lysine, and histidine residues. (The next section on complex immunoglobulin structures contains further discussion of this structure.) While monomeric IgM itself has low affinity for antigen, in its polymeric form it has considerable avidity for antigen. It is this increased avidity that makes IgM an important complement activator and mediator of opsonization. The Cμ3 domain binds C1q with the essential participation of its carbohydrate residues (80). Aspartic acid, lysine, and proline residues in two clusters have been implicated for this activity in the mouse. However, the only homologous region to be shown with this activity between IgG and IgM is a single proline. Cμ1 as well interacts with the C3b (81) complement component and helps to mediate phagocytosis of opsonized antigens by macrophages.

IgM is second only to IgA in its contribution to mucosal immunity. It can be secreted through similar means by polymer association with a J chain, and like IgA, is transported by the polymeric Ig receptor (pIgR). In many patients with IgA deficiency, IgM adequately substitutes for IgA in mucosal protection.

IgD

IgD is perhaps the most enigmatic of the immunoglobulin isotypes. It is present on all naïve B cells and serves as a better receptor in terms of activation than IgM. It also requires the co-expression of Igα and Igβ to elicit a cellular signal due to its short lysine-valine-lysine cytoplasmic domain identical to that of IgM. However, other participating co-receptors differ between the two membrane-bound isotypes. Coexpression on naïve B cells of these two receptors occurs by differential mRNA splicing (82) (see Chapter 5). Two laboratories have made IgD knockouts and the phenotype is somewhat ambiguous. Although there are fewer lymphoid follicles and overall a slower process of affinity maturation, one does not see defects that would otherwise indicate an irreplaceable role (83–85). Yet at the same time, ligation of IgD can activate, delete, or anergize B cells independent of IgM (86–88). In mice, the overexpression of IgD creates a greater induction of APCs, upregulation of B7-1 and B7-2, and increased class switching.

Despite its short serum half-life and less abundant mRNA, membrane IgD density exceeds that of membrane IgM on naïve B cells. This phenomenon is thought to be due to a greater stability of IgD mRNA than IgM (85,89–91).

Through the process of maturation, most B cells lose IgD expression (92,93). However, there are notable exceptions. IgD-only plasma cells are present in various compartments and secrete IgD into the serum. These plasma cells are in high concentration in the nasal mucosa (94–97). The serum half-life of IgD is quite limited, however, being only about 2.8 days. As mentioned before, the extended hinge of IgD is prone to proteolytic enzyme activity and this sensitivity extends into the C terminus of the Cδ3 domain as well. While the Cδ1 and Cδ2 domains are similar in structure to that of

other isotypes, Cδ3 lacks several key proline residues that play structural roles in the loops between beta strands. In addition this domain contains two N-linked carbohydrates at asparagines 316 and 347 that are not present in other immunoglobulins in this location. These structural differences appear to play a role in binding of IgD to the IgD receptor, at least in the mouse (recognizing the N-linked sugars of Cδ1 and Cδ3 in a Ca^{2+}-dependent manner), but may have other functional properties in the human where the receptor binds to the Jacalin-binding domains (O-linked sugars) of the hinge without the requirement of calcium (reviewed in Preud'homme et al. [91]).

IgD plasma cells and a particular set of IgD+IgM− B cells from germinal centers exhibit an unusually high level of somatic hypermutation (98–100). In addition, it has recently been found that this population of cells is quite prone to a VH-region event called receptor revision (101).

IgA

IgA is the major isotype of mucosal secretions. In addition, it is also the most prominent isotype in colostrum and breast milk (102). A number of features make this molecule suitable to the mucosal environment. First, the secreted forms are dimerized by their tailpieces and stabilized by J chains. The polymeric Ig receptor (pIgR) transports dimeric IgA across the epithelial barrier where a portion of the pIgR is cleaved to result in the formation of the secretory component. Secretory component remains attached to dimeric IgA, and J chain dimerized IgA with a secretory component are called "secretory IgA." There are two subclasses or isotypes of IgA in humans (IgA1 and IgA2) (102). IgA2 is the main component of secreted IgA (103) and as noted earlier has a truncated hinge that is resistant to most bacterial proteases (104). IgA is an important component of the first line of defense from organisms entering by mucosal routes. While most secretory immunoglobulin is IgA, it also accounts for 10% to 15% of serum immunoglobulin, making it the third most plentiful. Serum IgA tends to be mostly IgA1 (103). As mentioned earlier, IgA1 has an extended hinge and can bind antigens at a variety of spacings. In addition, extensive O-linked glycosylation prevents cleavage by most bacterial proteases. Serum and secretory IgA are derived from separate pools of B cells, but antigenic exposure at any given site primes the development of both secretory and serum IgA (102). Inflammatory responses are not efficiently generated upon antigen binding with IgA. Such a response would most likely be damaging to the mucosa. Instead, IgA elicits protection primarily through exclusion, binding, and cross-linking of pathogens. As well, IgA has been shown to be able to fix the complement by the alternative pathway and most recently by the lectin-binding cascade.

Targets that are opsonized by IgA are removed by FcαR-mediated phagocytosis. FcαR, although more distantly related, is most similar in structure to the FcγRII and FcεRI receptors. However, its binding site on the IgA Fc does not follow the pattern in either of these other two receptors. It has

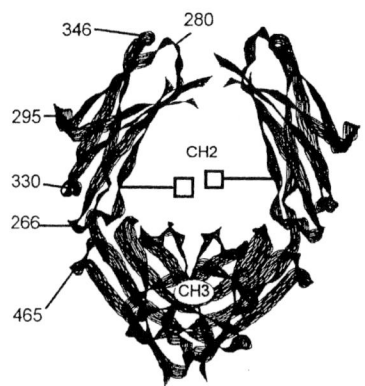

FIG. 8. Illustration of the residues essential for the binding of IgA to FcαR (CD89). Residues represent mutations made in IgA constant, heavy-chain regions as mapped on an Fcγ fragment. Of the residues, mutated L465 and L266 were found to be important for binding to CD89. From Carayannopoulos et al. (105), with permission.

been shown that the FcαR (CD89) binds to regions on the loops present between the Cα2 and Cα3 domains (105,106) (see Fig. 8). Mutation of certain residues in these regions eliminates FcαR binding. In addition, N-linked glycosylation at Asn263 appears necessary by some accounts for the interaction between IgA and its receptor (105). Others have found that this interaction may not be necessary (106). While we do not as yet have an x-ray structure of IgA, it has been postulated that the oligosaccharide at this location, unlike IgG, is oriented with the glycosylation pointing away from the cavity formed by the heavy chains and therefore released from protein interactions that otherwise would prevent its further modification. Indeed, these oligosaccharides exhibit more sialation than similar oligosaccharides in IgG (107).

An NMR solution structure of IgA1 has been obtained with molecular modeling to IgG and has provided some insights into the differences between the IgA1 hinge and the IgG1 hinge (murine) (66) (see Colorplate 4). The placement of interchain disulfide linkages between the immunoglobulin monomers is also a feature that sets IgA apart from other isotypes. Most isotopes contain interchain disulfide bonds in the hinge or, in the absence of the hinge, in the CH2 domain that replaces it. In IgA, however, these bonds are made at the top of Cα2 below (or carboxy-terminal to) the hinge. While it has been confirmed that the Cys241–Cys241 bridge is common among the IgA molecules studied, the other three or four cysteine–cysteine disulfide bonds that form out of a possible six candidates is unclear at the present time (66). Two cysteine residues remain exposed (one being Cys311), which are the likely to be covalently bonded with J chains. Cys471 forms another interchain disulfide bond between monomers outside of the cluster mentioned above (107).

IgE

IgE is the least abundant of all of the immunoglobulins. It is present 25-fold to 3,000-fold less than the other isotypes

and has the shortest free serum half-life. IgE is primarily produced in plasma cells in the lung and skin. It is quickly taken up by the high-affinity FcεRI. Thus, while the serum half-life of IgE is short, it remains for several weeks or months attached by this receptor to the surface of basophils and mast cells. Once a multivalent antigen is bound to the IgE–IgE receptor complex, the release of inflammatory mediators such as histamine and chemoattractants results in violent reactions (see Chapter 45). These reactions are involved in the clearance of parasites (108) and are intimately involved in allergy and anaphylaxis. People who suffer from atopy have an inappropriately high synthesis of IgE and almost always a high serum level of IgE.

Mast cells and basophiles express the high-affinity FcεRI receptor, as do Langerhans cells and eosinophils, although the reason for its presence on the latter two cell types is unknown (109,110). The interaction between IgE and the FcεR is among the strongest known with a k_d of 10^{-9} to 10^{-10} M. There are two distinct binding sites on IgE for its high-affinity receptor. They use identical residues from each Cε3 (111) with some involvement of Cε2 (112). The glycosylation status of IgE does not seem to play a role in this interaction. These bound regions of IgE are found on the surface loops of the Cε3 domain. Although there are two sites on the receptor, a 1:1 stoichiometry is maintained and both crystal structures of the interaction as well as biphasic dissociation rates in kinetic studies show that both sites are involved in IgE binding to its high-affinity receptor. Several aromatic amino acids as well as a buried interface surface contribute to the stability of this interaction (111). A large conformational change has been postulated to take place in the Cε3 domain as IgE is bound to its receptor (13,113).

Site 1 appears to provide specificity for IgE in binding to its receptor, while site 2 appears to contain certain conserved residues between IgG receptors and high-affinity IgE receptors. Pro426 from the IgE Fc is sandwiched between FcεRI residues Trp87 and Trp110. These three residues are absolutely conserved between IgG, IgE, and their receptors in the binding sites. Leu425 is also absolutely conserved. This illustrates the relation of the IgE and IgG receptors as well as the utility of the "proline" sandwich motif between the immunoglobulin and its receptor, which themselves are members of the Ig superfamily (111) (see Fig. 9).

IgE also binds to a low-affinity receptor, FcεRII (CD23). This receptor is a type-II integral-membrane glycoprotein that is involved in a number of activities. The low-affinity IgE receptor binds IgE with 1,000 times less affinity than the high-affinity receptor. Unlike the high-affinity receptor, the low-affinity receptor is expressed on monocytes (114). Cε3 is essential for binding of the low-affinity receptor, and a major determinant of binding appears to be Lys352 in the AB loop.

IgG

IgG is the most abundant isotype in the blood as well as in the lymph and peritoneal fluids. Seventy-five percent of the serum immunoglobulin is comprised of IgG. IgG has a long

Conservation of residues in site 1

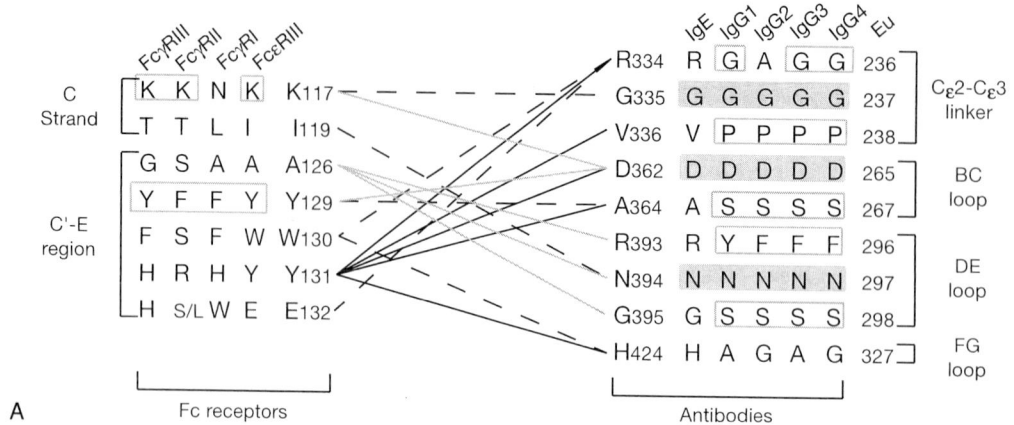

A   Fc receptors   Antibodies

Conservation of residues in site 2

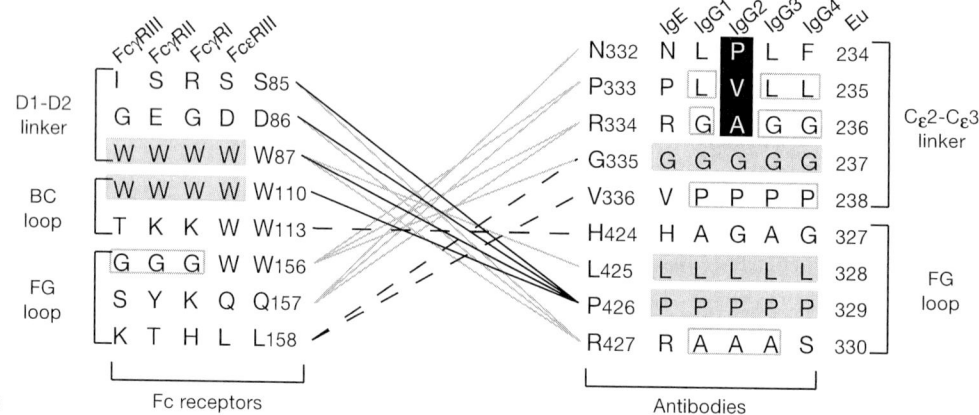

B   Fc receptors   Antibodies

FIG. 9. Certain residues are conserved between FcγRs and FcεRI as well as IgG and IgE that facilitate binding. Two sites participate: site 1 in (a) and site 2 in (b). Heavy lines indicate the highest number of contacts and dashed lines indicate the least. Of considerable note are residues W87 and W110 in site 2 of the receptors and P426 in the immunoglobulin that form a core "proline sandwich" in the interaction between immunoglobulin and receptor. From Garman (111), with permission.

half-life of 3 weeks in the serum. This makes it the most stable antibody in the serum (115). High-affinity IgG signifies the humoral immune response.

Among all isotypes, IgG may at first appear to be a bit bland in its function due to the absence of special properties, such as multimerization and secretion like IgM and IgA, or enigmatic roles like IgD, or extremely high-affinity interactions with receptors and unique modes of effect like IgE. But such a conclusion about this molecule would be an oversight. Of all isotypes, IgG has been the most studied structurally. This is the result of early crystal structures of two hinge-deletion mutants (116–118). More recently, two complete antibody structures have been reported of murine IgG1 and IgG2a (119,120). The most obvious lesson these structures have taught us is that the mobility of an otherwise perceived static molecule is quite striking. IgG must simultaneously bind with very high affinity to three independent sites in order to effect its immune response function. These

recent crystal structures will help us continue to refine our view of the immunoglobulin molecule and will serve as a basis of comparison for structures of immunoglobulins of other isotypes that are most likely not far from being solved.

IgG subclasses bind and activate the complement with different efficiencies, as discussed previously (121,122). However, all subclasses carry a core C1q binding motif at Glu337, Lys339, and Lys341 on the fairly mobile Cγ2 domain (123). This indicates that the variability is due rather to the steric properties that the various hinge conformations impart. The presence of carbohydrate on IgG has been shown to be absolutely necessary for complement activation (reviewed in Furukawa and Kobata [124]) and galactosylation has been shown to be especially important (125).

Bacterial proteins A and G have been classically known to bind IgG. This occurs at the Cγ2–Cγ3 junction involving residues 264 to 267 (24). These residues are consistently oriented between structures to Cγ3 in the same manner. In addition residues 330 and 465 are important as well. These regions overlap the binding site of the neonatal FcγRn and, in addition, may produce inhibition of other FcγRs (120).

Fc Receptors

IgG can bind to four types of receptors. These receptors vary in their affinity for IgG as well as their expressed location. We will discuss the receptors as two major groups. The first group consists of the high-affinity and lower-affinity receptors that are IgSF members. These receptors are the FcγRI (high affinity), FcγRII, and FcγRIII. The second contains the neonatal IgG receptor (FcγRn) that is related to the MHC class I.

The IgSF family of receptors, although differing in portions of their binding sites, shares an important motif. A "proline sandwich" is produced between Pro329 and two tryptophans in the receptor. This motif is even shared with the homologous high-affinity IgE receptor described previously in this chapter (see Fig. 9). In addition, the IgG receptors show a dependence on residues Leu234–Pro238 of the lower hinge (126). Although the individual amino acids involved vary between the receptors, this appears to be another common interaction. These lower-hinge residues account for four of the six hydrogen-bond interactions in crystal structures depicting FcγRIII interactions with IgG1 (127). Van der Waal interactions are plentiful between the receptor and the Fc. Finally, all receptors are dependent as well on the presence of a carbohydrate at Asn297 although the interaction is not direct. This carbohydrate is thought to stabilize the lower hinge by producing a hydrophobic core in the (Cγ2) domain by filling its cavity (126–129). Elimination of the branching mannose residues from the glycosylated IgG Fc produce a linear trisaccharide core that severely decreases affinity for the FcγRII, indicating the importance of this structure for proper conformation of the Fc (126).

The other regions involved in binding with these receptors are varied but important to the individual receptors. FcγRI binds to IgG1 Fc with 100 times greater affinity than the other IgG receptors. Residues within the stretch Gly316–Ala339 have been mapped with differential importance to binding interaction. In addition, a separate chain on the FcγRI receptor is involved in augmenting the binding chains of the receptor without making direct contact with the IgG1 Fc. While the FcγRI receptor uses essentially the same region for binding as the other receptors, the difference in affinity may be attributable to either conformational changes that are made, or differences in particular amino acids used for the actual binding of the receptor. FcγRII has been shown to require the presence of two identical IgG heavy chains in order to elicit binding. Residues in the loops of the Cγ2 domain are important for this interaction in addition to the lower hinge. For FcγRIII there are two important binding regions. The first are the class-1 residues of the hinge proximal region of Cγ2. The second is the Cγ2–Cγ3 interface. For both FcγRII and FcγRIII, several residues at the "bottom" of the Cγ3 domain influence the binding to IgG (126).

The FcγRn (neonatal receptor) has the interesting property of binding maternal IgG and transporting it across the epithelia of the placenta (115). Binding of the IgG occurs in the cells of this barrier at a pH of 6.5. Then the Fc is released by the receptor into the blood at a pH of 7.4. This sharp pH dependence is a function of the titration of ligand residues on the Fc of IgG. Several histidine residues in the Cγ2 and Cγ3 interface are involved that bind negatively charged residues at acidic but not basic pH. A further interesting element is the structural relationship of this receptor to the MHC class-I molecule (130).

HIGHER-ORDER STRUCTURE

While IgM and IgA have activities as monomeric immunoglobulins, both have the ability to form multimeric structures that fill yet other biological niches. IgA usually forms dimers through its tailpiece, an extra 18 amino acids at the end of the Cα2 domain, and, as noted above, is complexed with another B-cell protein, the J chain (131). This complex can then be bound by the polymeric Ig receptor (pIgR) and transported across the mucosal epithelial layers to provide important primary immune defense roles (132). This dimeric IgA can then bind with greater avidity to polymeric epitopes to increase its effectiveness in eliminating these targets from the mucosal surface. Similarly, IgM also forms a polymer, but is most commonly in the form of a pentamer. This configuration allows IgM to bind polymeric low-affinity epitopes and efficiently activate the complement to opsonize and eliminate its target. While the J chain is present in most IgM pentamers and binding to the pIgR is possible, dimeric IgA is the primary antibody of most mucosal surfaces. Polymeric IgM has significant activity in the serum.

The J chain is a 137 amino acid/15kDa protein that serves to link two immunoglobulin monomers covalently (133). It contains eight cysteine residues that participate in a disulfide bond with each tailpiece in addition to stabilizing its own structure (134). Whether the J chain forms other disulfide bonds with the immunoglobulins is still not clear. The J chain is a highly conserved molecule among a range of species and even predates the presence of the antibody (135–138). While thought to be arranged as a single domain in a beta barrel formation, it has not yet been crystallized and does not show sequence homology to an immunoglobulin domain. The J chain is proteolytically labile and contains a high amount of negatively charged residues (134).

Both tailpieces of each IgM and IgA carboxy-terminal domain contain a cysteine (the penultimate cysteine residues 575 and 495, respectively) that are involved in multimerization. One of these residues from each immunoglobulin is paired "at the tail" to form a direct disulfide bond between the monomers. The other two residues (one from each monomer) bind to separate cysteines in the J chain (139–142). The tailpieces are thought to form two extra beta strands on one face of the terminal domain that facilitate this interaction (143). In addition, there is evidence that Cμ3 and Cμ4 of

IgM, as well as the homologous regions in IgA, are also required for interaction with the J chain (144). The structure of the carbohydrate at Asn563 (in IgM and at the homologous region in IgA) is also important. Usually this carbohydrate contains a large amount of high mannose glycans, which indicates that it is protected by polymerization occurring before exposure to the Golgi-complex enzyme, mannosidase II (145).

In the case of IgA, the J chain is required for polymerization, although some reports of multimers in its absence have been reported. It exists in all forms of IgA polymers (not just dimers), including, as well, some reports of the secreted monomers. Domain-swapping experiments have shown that the propensity for IgA dimer formation and its binding by the J chain is due to the presence of the IgA tailpiece in the context of its own heavy chain. Tailpieces spliced to IgA from the μ chain result in higher-order multimers than the simple dimer (144).

IgM, unlike IgA, has no requirement for the J chain in its polymeric forms, although J chain is often present and essential for secretion. Two other disulfides besides the penultimate disulfide mentioned above are involved in the formation of multimers. Like Cys575, Cys414 forms intermonomeric disulfide bonds. Cys377 is most likely to form intramonomeric bonds. While pentameric IgM is the most common form of IgM, there are many reports of IgM hexamers (146). The latter almost never have incorporated the J chain, but are highly dependent on Cys414–Cys414 bonds between monomers. Hexameric IgM is rarely found *in vivo* except in the case of cold agglutinin disease and Waldenstrom's macroglobulinemia (147–149). Hexameric IgM has been reported to be far more efficient at complement activation than pentameric IgM (146). Pentameric IgM is regularly associated with one or more J chains. It has been hypothesized that pentameric IgM with J chains is more thermodynamically favorable than hexameric IgM as a possible explanation of why it is more common.

Thus, for the formation of multimeric immunoglobulin, we see that the presence and sequence of the tailpiece is important in the context of the proper heavy chain. IgM tailpieces incorporated into IgA will cause higher numbers of IgA multimers, but the reverse substitution does not induce dimers in IgM. It has therefore been proposed that IgM polymerization is more efficient than IgA (143).

As mentioned above, a J chain is essential for the secretion of IgA and IgM. The pIgR receptor binds to the J chain, and through clathrin-coated vesicle transport, moves dimeric IgA across the epithelial cell barrier of the mucosa (150). This receptor contains seven domains with five extracellular regions similar to the V regions of the immunoglobulin, a sixth transmembrane domain, and a seventh cytoplasmic domain (151). pIgR is synthesized on epithelial cells of respiratory, gastrointestinal, and genitourinary tracts, and is expressed on the basolateral aspect. Tight interactions with the J chain and the IgA Fc occur. Cys309 of IgA (homologous to Cys414 in

IgM) forms a disulfide bond with the receptor (152). After transcytosis, the pIgR is cleaved between its fifth and sixth domains to release dimeric IgA, J chain, and the rest of the receptor referred to as the secretory component (SC) as a complex (150). The remaining SC helps to provide protection for the secreted immunoglobulin from proteolysis on the mucosal surfaces.

AN EVOLUTIONARY PERSPECTIVE

From an evolutionary perspective, antibodies are easily traceable to the beginnings of the vertebrate radiation well over 400 million years ago. While the molecular biological events that bring VDJ and VJ together, and bring V domains in the context of C domains, have varied greatly over evolutionary time, the basic structure of the Ig fold and the concept of a variable and a constant region remain intact. Indeed, with the exception of the myriad ways in which diversity is generated within the V domain (somatic hypermutation, multiple germline genes, a variety of gene segments, and the like), the most profound events are rather remarkably similar: Proteins are required to splice various sections of the molecule together, and the hinge region seems required to transmit signals from one part of the molecule to another. Indeed, the functions we attribute to the Fc region—complement binding and binding to phagocytic cells—are very old in evolutionary time.

In essence, once evolution solved the problem of linking a common biologic function (recruiting proteins—like complement; and cells—like neutrophils) to an inflammatory site by a *specific* molecule (and Fv domain), the system seems to have been duplicated over and over, with remarkable constancy by a variety of vertebrates and perhaps some invertebrates.

CONCLUSION

Immunoglobulins are extremely versatile molecules that carry out many biological activities simultaneously. The duality of the structure between preparation to recognize unique antigen structures *a priori* and maintenance of host cell receptor or complement recognition properties presents a truly unique task for the system. As has been described, many varieties of antibodies have different biological niches, but the overall design for these molecules is the same.

As the science of our field progresses, attention will be given ever more closely to the engineering of antibodies for multiple tasks. Many therapeutic applications are already in various stages of development and various parts of immunoglobulins are being used for biotechnology applications. Thus, there has been a resurgence of interest in the structure–function aspects of antibodies as we approach "designer antibodies." It is reasonable to assume that at some point in time, therapeutics will be designed with, for example, the same variable region but with different constant regions depending on the desired effector function (complement binds vs. phagocytosis). Indeed, some effector function could be engineered out of antibody molecules as the need develops. Thus, the study of the structure and function of antibodies is ever more urgent as we take fundamental principles of protein chemistry to the bedside.

REFERENCES

1. Hill RL, Delaney R, Fellows RE, et al. The evolutionary origins of the immunoglobulins. *Proc Natl Acad Sci USA* 1966;56:1762–1769.
2. Porter RR. Separation and isolation of fractions of the rabbit gamma-globulin containing the antibody and antigenic combining sites. *Nature* 1958;182:670–671.
3. Plaut AG, Wistar R Jr, Capra JD. Differential susceptibility of human IgA immunoglobulins to streptococcal IgA protease. *J Clin Invest* 1974;54:1295–1300.
4. Plaut AG, Gilbert JV, Artenstein MS, et al. Neisseria gonorrhoeae and neisseria meningitidis: extracellular enzyme cleaves human immunoglobulin A. *Science* 1975;190:1103–1105.
5. Nisonoff A, Wissler FC, Lipman LN. Properties of the major component of a peptic digest of rabbit antibody. *Science* 1960;132:1770–1771.
6. Palmer JL, Nisonoff A. Dissociation of rabbit gamma-globulin into half-molecules after reduction of one labile disulfide bond. *Biochemistry* 1964;3:863–869.
7. Beale D, Feinstein A. Structure and function of the constant regions of immunoglobulins. *Q Rev Biophys* 1976;9:135–180.
8. Kindt TJ, Capra JD. *The Antibody Enigma.* New York: Plenum Press, 1984.
9. Capra JD, Kehoe JM. Hypervariable regions, idiotypy, and the antibody-combining site. *Adv Immunol* 1975;20:1–40.
10. Davies DR, Padlan EA, Segal DM. Three-dimensional structure of immunoglobulins. *Annu Rev Biochem* 1975;44:639–667.
11. Edmundson AB, Wood MK, Schiffer M, et al. A crystallographic investigation of the Mcg myeloma protein. *ANL Rep* 1969:283–185.
12. Edmundson AB, Schiffer M, Wood MK, et al. Crystallographic studies of an IgG immunoglobulin and the Bence–Jones protein from one patient. *Cold Spring Harb Symp Quant Biol* 1972;36:427–432.
13. Wurzburg BA, Garman SC, Jardetzky TS. Structure of the human IgE-Fc Cepsilon 3-Cepsilon4 reveals conformational flexibility in the antibody effector domains. *Immunity* 2000;13:375–385.
14. Williams AF, Barclay AN. The immunoglobulin superfamily—domains for cell surface recognition. *Annu Rev Immunol* 1988;6:381–405.
15. Harpaz Y, Chothia C. Many of the immunoglobulin superfamily domains in cell adhesion molecules and surface receptors belong to a new structural set which is close to that containing variable domains. *J Mol Biol* 1994;238:528–539.
16. Bork P, Holm L, Sander C. The immunoglobulin fold: structural classification, sequence patterns and common core. *J Mol Biol* 1994;242:309–320.
17. Lesk AM, Chothia C. Evolution of proteins formed by beta-sheets. II. The core of the immunoglobulin domains. *J Mol Biol* 1982;160:325–342.
18. Wu TT, Kabat EA. An analysis of the sequences of the variable regions of Bence Jones proteins and myeloma light chains and their implications for antibody complementarity. *J Exp Med* 1970;132:211–250.
19. Chothia C, Novotny J, Bruccoleri R, et al. Domain association in immunoglobulin molecules: the packing of variable domains. *J Mol Biol* 1985;186:651–663.
20. Colman PM. Structure of antibody–antigen complexes: implications for immune recognition. *Adv Immunol* 1988;43:99–132.
21. Saul FA, Amzel LM, Poljak RJ. Preliminary refinement and structural analysis of the Fab fragment from human immunoglobulin new at 20 A resolution. *J Biol Chem* 1978;253:585–597.
22. Edmundson AB, Ely KR, Girling RL, et al. Binding of 2,4-dinitrophenyl compounds and other small molecules to a crystalline lambda-type Bence–Jones dimer. *Biochemistry* 1974;13:3816–3827.
23. Amzel LM, Poljak RJ. Three-dimensional structure of immunoglobulins. *Annu Rev Biochem* 1979;48:961–997.
24. Deisenhofer J. Crystallographic refinement and atomic models of a human Fc fragment and its complex with fragment B of protein A from Staphylococcus aureus at 2.9- and 2.8-A resolution. *Biochemistry* 1981;20:2361–2370.
25. Padlan EA. Anatomy of the antibody molecule. *Mol Immunol* 1994; 31:169–217.
26. Jones PT, Dear PH, Foote J, et al. Replacing the complementarity-determining regions in a human antibody with those from a mouse. *Nature* 1986;321:522–525.
27. Foote J, Winter G. Antibody framework residues affecting the conformation of the hypervariable loops. *J Mol Biol* 1992;224:487–499.
28. Schroeder HW Jr, Hillson JL, Perlmutter RM. Structure and evolution of mammalian VH families. *Int Immunol* 1990;2:41–50.
29. Kirkham PM, Mortari F, Newton JA, et al. Immunoglobulin VH clan and family identity predicts variable domain structure and may influence antigen binding. *Embo J* 1992;11:603–609.
30. Kirkham PM, Schroeder HW Jr. Antibody structure and the evolution of immunoglobulin V gene segments. *Semin Immunol* 1994;6:347–360.
31. Pascual V, Capra JD. Human immunoglobulin heavy-chain variable region genes: organization, polymorphism, and expression. *Adv Immunol* 1991;49:1–74.
32. Chothia C, Lesk AM, Tramontano A, et al. Conformations of immunoglobulin hypervariable regions. *Nature* 1989;342:877–883.
33. Strong RK, Campbell R, Rose DR, et al. Three-dimensional structure of murine anti-p-azophenylarsonate Fab 36-71.1. X-ray crystallography, site-directed mutagenesis, and modeling of the complex with hapten. *Biochemistry* 1991;30:3739–3748.
34. Wright A, Tao MH, Kabat EA, et al. Antibody variable region glycosylation: position effects on antigen binding and carbohydrate structure. *Embo J* 1991;10:2717–2723.
35. Middaugh CR, Litman GW. Atypical glycosylation of an IgG monoclonal cryoimmunoglobulin. *J Biol Chem* 1987;262:3671–3673.
36. Nakamura Y, Gojobori T, Ikemura T. Codon usage tabulated from international DNA sequence databases: status for the year 2000. *Nucleic Acids Res* 2000;28:292.
37. Feeney AJ. Lack of N regions in fetal and neonatal mouse immunoglobulin V-D-J junctional sequences. *J Exp Med* 1990;172:1377–1390.
38. Kyte J, Doolittle RF. A simple method for displaying the hydropathic character of a protein. *J Mol Biol* 1982;157:105–132.
39. Eisenberg D. Three-dimensional structure of membrane and surface proteins. *Annu Rev Biochem* 1984;53:595–623.
40. Inanov I, et al. Constraints on the hydropathicity and sequence composition of HCDR3 are conserved evolution. In: *The antibodies.* New York: Taylor and Francis, 2002;43–68.
41. Sasso EH, Silverman GJ, Mannik M. Human IgM molecules that bind staphylococcal protein A contain VHIII H chains. *J Immunol* 1989;142:2778–2783.
42. Potter KN, Li Y, Capra JD. Staphylococcal protein A simultaneously interacts with framework region 1, complementarity-determining region 2, and framework region 3 on human VH3-encoded Igs. *J Immunol* 1996;157:2982–2988.
43. Graille M, Stura EA, Corper AL, et al. Crystal structure of a Staphylococcus aureus protein A domain complexed with the Fab fragment of a human IgM antibody: structural basis for recognition of B-cell receptors and superantigen activity. *Proc Natl Acad Sci USA,* 2000;97:5399–5404.
44. Cary SP, Lee J, Wagenknecht R, et al. Characterization of superantigen-induced clonal deletion with a novel clan III-restricted avian monoclonal antibody: exploiting evolutionary distance to create antibodies specific for a conserved VH region surface. *J Immunol* 2000;164:4730–4741.
45. Cary S, Krishnan M, Marion TN, et al. The murine clan V(H) III related 7183, J606 and S107 and DNA4 families commonly encode for binding to a bacterial B cell superantigen. *Mol Immunol* 1999;36:769–776.
46. Silverman GJ, Nayak JV, Warnatz K, et al. The dual phases of the response to neonatal exposure to a VH family–restricted staphylococcal B cell superantigen. *J Immunol* 1998;161:5720–5732.
47. Silverman GJ, Goodyear CS. A model B-cell superantigen and the immunobiology of B lymphocytes. *Clin Immunol* 2002;102:117–134.
48. Yin J, Mundorff EC, Yang PL, et al. A comparative analysis of the immunological evolution of antibody 28B4. *Biochemistry* 2001;40:10764–10773.

49. Mundorff EC, Hanson MA, Varvak A, et al. Conformational effects in biological catalysis: an antibody-catalyzed oxy-cope rearrangement. *Biochemistry* 2000;39:627–632.

50. Romesberg FE, Spiller B, Schultz PG, et al. Immunological origins of binding and catalysis in a Diels–Alderase antibody. *Science* 1998;279:1929–1933.

51. Guddat LW, Shan L, Anchin JM, et al. Local and transmitted conformational changes on complexation of an anti-sweetener Fab. *J Mol Biol* 1994;236:247–274.

52. Decanniere K, Transue TR, Desmyter A, et al. Degenerate interfaces in antigen–antibody complexes. *J Mol Biol* 2001;313:473–478.

53. Tribbick G, Edmundson AB, Mason TJ, et al. Similar binding properties of peptide ligands for a human immunoglobulin and its light chain dimer. *Mol Immunol* 1989;26:625–635.

54. Afonin PV, Fokin AV, Tsygannik IN, et al. Crystal structure of an anti-interleukin-2 monoclonal antibody Fab complexed with an antigenic nonapeptide. *Protein Sci* 2001;10:1514–1521.

55. Bhat TN, Bentley GA, Boulot G, et al. Bound water molecules and conformational stabilization help mediate an antigen–antibody association. *Proc Natl Acad Sci USA* 1994;91:1089–1093.

56. Li Y, Li H, Smith-Gill SJ, et al. Three-dimensional structures of the free and antigen-bound Fab from monoclonal antilysozyme antibody HyHEL-63. *Biochemistry* 2000;39:6296–6309.

57. Faelber K, Kirchhofer D, Presta L, et al. The 1.85 A resolution crystal structures of tissue factor in complex with humanized Fab D3h44 and of free humanized Fab D3h44: revisiting the solvation of antigen combining sites. *J Mol Biol* 2001;313:83–97.

58. Sigurskjold BW, Altman E, Bundle DR. Sensitive titration microcalorimetric study of the binding of Salmonella O-antigenic oligosaccharides by a monoclonal antibody. *Eur J Biochem* 1991;197:239–246.

59. Kelley RF, O'Connell MP, Carter P, et al. Antigen binding thermodynamics and antiproliferative effects of chimeric and humanized anti-p185HER2 antibody Fab fragments. *Biochemistry* 1992;31:5434–5441.

60. Roux KH, Strelets L, Brekke OH, et al. Comparisons of the ability of human IgG3 hinge mutants, IgM, IgE, and IgA2, to form small immune complexes: a role for flexibility and geometry. *J Immunol* 1998;161:4083–4090.

61. Schumaker VN, Phillips ML, Hanson DC. Dynamic aspects of antibody structure. *Mol Immunol* 1991;28:1347–1360.

62. Wade RH, Taveau JC, Lamy JN. Concerning the axial rotational flexibility of the Fab regions of immunoglobulin G. *J Mol Biol* 1989;206:349–356.

63. Brekke OH, Michaelsen TE, Sandlie I. The structural requirements for complement activation by IgG: does it hinge on the hinge? *Immunol Today* 1995;16:85–90.

64. Feinstein A, Richardson N, Taussig MJ. Immunoglobulin flexibility in complement activation. *Immunol Today* 1986;7:169–174.

65. Canfield SM, Morrison SL. The binding affinity of human IgG for its high affinity Fc receptor is determined by multiple amino acids in the CH2 domain and is modulated by the hinge region. *J Exp Med* 1991;173:1483–1491.

66. Boehm MK, Woof JM, Kerr MA, et al. The Fab and Fc fragments of IgA1 exhibit a different arrangement from that in IgG: a study by x-ray and neutron solution scattering and homology modelling. *J Mol Biol* 1999;286:1421–1447.

67. Kilian M, Reinholdt J, Lomholt H, et al. Biological significance of IgA1 proteases in bacterial colonization and pathogenesis: critical evaluation of experimental evidence. *Apmis* 1996;104:321–338.

68. Griffiths RW, Gleich GJ. Proteolytic degradation of IgD and its relation to molecular conformation. *J Biol Chem* 1972;247:4543–4548.

69. Lin LC, Putnam FW. Structural studies of human IgD: isolation by a two-step purification procedure and characterization by chemical and enzymatic fragmentation. *Proc Natl Acad Sci USA* 1979;76:6572–6576.

70. Goyert SM, Hugli TE, Spiegelberg HL. Sites of "spontaneous" degradation of IgD. *J Immunol* 1977;118:2138–2144.

71. Ishioka N, Takahashi N, Putnam FW. Analysis of the mechanism, rate, and sites of proteolytic cleavage of human immunoglobulin D by high-pressure liquid chromatography. *Proc Natl Acad Sci USA* 1987;84:61–65.

72. Aucouturier P, Mihaesco E, Mihaesco C, et al. Characterization of jacalin, the human IgA and IgD binding lectin from jackfruit. *Mol Immunol* 1987;24:503–511.

73. Aucouturier P, Pineau N, Brugier JC, et al. Jacalin: a new laboratory tool in immunochemistry and cellular immunology. *J Clin Lab Anal* 1989;3:244–251.

74. Zehr BD, Litwin SD. Human IgD and IgA1 compete for D-galactose–related binding sites on the lectin jacalin. *Scand J Immunol* 1987;26:229–236.

75. Deisenhofer J, Colman PM, Epp O, et al. Crystallographic structural studies of a human Fc fragment.II. A complete model based on a Fourier map at 3.5 A resolution. *Hoppe Seylers Z Physiol Chem* 1976;357:1421–1434.

76. Williams GT, Venkitaraman AR, Gilmore DJ, et al. The sequence of the mu transmembrane segment determines the tissue specificity of the transport of immunoglobulin M to the cell surface. *J Exp Med* 1990;171:947–952.

77. Karasuyama H, Kudo A, Melchers F. The proteins encoded by the VpreB and lambda 5 pre–B cell-specific genes can associate with each other and with mu heavy chain. *J Exp Med* 1990;172:969–972.

78. Tsubata T, Reth M. The products of pre–B cell-specific genes (lambda 5 and VpreB) and the immunoglobulin mu chain form a complex that is transported onto the cell surface. *J Exp Med* 1990;172:973–976.

79. Ishihara K, Wood WJ Jr, Damore M, et al. B29 gene products complex with immunoglobulins on B lymphocytes. *Proc Natl Acad Sci USA* 1992;89:633–637.

80. Arya S, Chen F, Spycher S, et al. Mapping of amino acid residues in the C mu 3 domain of mouse IgM important in macromolecular assembly and complement-dependent cytolysis. *J Immunol* 1994;152:1206–1212.

81. Du Pasquier L, Wabl MR. Antibody diversity in amphibians: inheritance of isoelectric focusing antibody patterns in isogenic frogs. *Eur J Immunol* 1978;8:428–433.

82. Forster I, Vieira P, Rajewsky K. Flow cytometric analysis of cell proliferation dynamics in the B cell compartment of the mouse. *Int Immunol* 1989;1:321–331.

83. Roes J, Rajewsky K. Cell autonomous expression of IgD is not essential for the maturation of conventional B cells. *Int Immunol* 1991;3:1367–1371.

84. Roes J, Rajewsky K. Immunoglobulin D (IgD)-deficient mice reveal an auxiliary receptor function for IgD in antigen-mediated recruitment of B cells. *J Exp Med* 1993;177:45–55.

85. Nitschke L, Kosco MH, Kohler G, et al. Immunoglobulin D-deficient mice can mount normal immune responses to thymus-independent and -dependent antigens. *Proc Natl Acad Sci USA* 1993;90:1887–1891.

86. Brink R, Goodnow CC, Crosbie J, et al. Immunoglobulin M and D antigen receptors are both capable of mediating B lymphocyte activation, deletion, or anergy after interaction with specific antigen. *J Exp Med* 1992;176:991–1005.

87. Morris SC, Lees A, Finkelman FD. In vivo activation of naive T cells by antigen–presenting B cells. *J Immunol* 1994;152:3777–3785.

88. Brink R, Goodnow CC, Basten A. IgD expression on B cells is more efficient than IgM but both receptors are functionally equivalent in up-regulation CD80/CD86 co-stimulatory molecules. *Eur J Immunol* 1995;25:1980–1984.

89. Havran WL, DiGiusto DL, Cambier JC. mIgM:mIgD ratios on B cells: mean mIgD expression exceeds mIgM by 10- fold on most splenic B cells. *J Immunol* 1984;132:1712–1716.

90. Finkelman FD, Holmes JM, Dukhanina OI, et al. Cross-linking of membrane immunoglobulin D, in the absence of T cell help, kills mature B cells in vivo. *J Exp Med* 1995;181:515–525.

91. Preud'homme JL, Petit I, Barra A, et al. Structural and functional properties of membrane and secreted IgD. *Mol Immunol* 2000;37:871–887.

92. Black SJ, van der Loo W, Loken MR, et al. Expression of IgD by murine lymphocytes. Loss of surface IgD indicates maturation of memory B cells. *J Exp Med* 1978;147:984–996.

93. McHeyzer-Williams MG, Nossal GJ, Lalor PA. Molecular characterization of single memory B cells. *Nature* 1991;350:502–505.

94. Surjan L Jr, Brandtzaeg P, Berdal P. Immunoglobulin systems of human tonsils.II. Patients with chronic tonsillitis or tonsillar hyperplasia: quantification of Ig-producing cells, tonsillar morphometry and serum Ig concentrations. *Clin Exp Immunol* 1978;31:382–390.

95. Korsrud FR, Brandtzaeg P. Quantitative immunohistochemistry of immunoglobulin- and J-chain–producing cells in human parotid and submandibular salivary glands. *Immunology* 1980;39:129–140.

96. Korsrud FR, Brandtzaeg P. Immunohistochemical evaluation of J-chain expression by intra- and extra-follicular immunoglobulin-producing human tonsillar cells. *Scand J Immunol* 1981;13:271–280.

97. Brandtzaeg P. Overview of the mucosal immune system. *Curr Top Microbiol Immunol* 1989;146:13–25.

98. Liu YJ, de Bouteiller O, Arpin C, et al. Normal human IgD+IgM− germinal center B cells can express up to 80 mutations in the variable region of their IgD transcripts. *Immunity* 1996;4:603–613.

99. Billian G, Bella C, Mondiere P, et al. Identification of a tonsil IgD+ B cell subset with phenotypical and functional characteristics of germinal center B cells. *Eur J Immunol* 1996;26:1712–1719.

100. Arpin C, de Bouteiller O, Razanajaona D, et al. The normal counterpart of IgD myeloma cells in germinal center displays extensively mutated IgVH gene, Cmu-Cdelta switch, and lambda light chain expression. *J Exp Med* 1998;187:1169–1178.

101. Wilson PC, Wilson K, Liu YJ, et al. Receptor revision of immunoglobulin heavy chain variable region genes in normal human B lymphocytes. *J Exp Med* 2000;191:1881–1894.

102. Lehner T, Bergmeier LA, Tao L, et al. Targeted lymph node immunization with simian immunodeficiency virus p27 antigen to elicit genital, rectal, and urinary immune responses in nonhuman primates. *J Immunol* 1994;153:1858–1868.

103. Mestecky J, McGhee JR. Immunoglobulin A (IgA): molecular and cellular interactions involved in IgA biosynthesis and immune response. *Adv Immunol* 1987;40:153–245.

104. Qiu J, Brackee GP, Plaut AG. Analysis of the specificity of bacterial immunoglobulin A (IgA) proteases by a comparative study of ape serum IgAs as substrates. *Infect Immun* 1996;64:933–937.

105. Carayannopoulos L, Hexham JM, Capra JD. Localization of the binding site for the monocyte immunoglobulin (Ig) A-Fc receptor (CD89) to the domain boundary between Calpha2 and Calpha3 in human IgA1. *J Exp Med* 1996;183:1579–1586.

106. Pleass RJ, Dunlop JI, Anderson CM, et al. Identification of residues in the CH2/CH3 domain interface of IgA essential for interaction with the human Fc alpha receptor (FcalphaR) CD89. *J Biol Chem* 1999; 274:23508–23514.

107. Mattu TS, Pleass RJ, Willis AC, et al. The glycosylation and structure of human serum IgA1, Fab, and Fc regions and the role of N-glycosylation on Fc alpha receptor interactions. *J Biol Chem* 1998;273:2260–2272.

108. Gounni AS, Lamkhioued B, Ochiai K, et al. High-affinity IgE receptor on eosinophils is involved in defence against parasites. *Nature* 1994;367:183–186.

109. Wang B, Rieger A, Kilgus O, et al. Epidermal Langerhans cells from normal human skin bind monomeric IgE via Fc epsilon RI. *J Exp Med* 1992;175:1353–1365.

110. Bieber T, de la Salle H, Wollenberg A, et al. Human epidermal Langerhans cells express the high affinity receptor for immunoglobulin E (Fc epsilon RI). *J Exp Med* 1992;175:1285–1290.

111. Garman SC, Wurzburg BA, Tarchevskaya SS, et al. Structure of the Fc fragment of human IgE bound to its high-affinity receptor Fc epsilonRI alpha. *Nature* 2000;406:259–266.

112. McDonnell JM, Calvert R, Beavil RL, et al. The structure of the IgE Cepsilon2 domain and its role in stabilizing the complex with its high-affinity receptor Fc epsilonRI alpha. *Nat Struct Biol*, 2001;8:437–441.

113. Sayers I, Helm BA. The structural basis of human IgE-Fc receptor interactions. *Clin Exp Allergy* 1999;29:585–594.

114. Hashimoto S, Koh K, Tomita Y, et al. TNF-alpha regulates IL-4–induced Fc epsilon RII/CD23 gene expression and soluble Fc epsilon RII release by human monocytes. *Int Immunol* 1995;7:705–713.

115. Saji F, Koyama M, Matsuzaki N. Current topic: human placental Fc receptors. *Placenta* 1994;15:453–466.

116. Guddat LW, Herron JN, Edmundson AB. Three-dimensional structure of a human immunoglobulin with a hinge deletion. *Proc Natl Acad Sci USA* 1993;90:4271–4275.

117. Silverton EW, Navia MA, Davies DR. Three-dimensional structure of an intact human immunoglobulin. *Proc Natl Acad Sci USA* 1977;74:5140–5144.

118. Sarma VR, Davies DR, Labaw LW, et al. Crystal structure of an immunoglobulin molecule by x-ray diffraction and electron microscopy. *Cold Spring Harb Symp Quant Biol* 1972;36:413–419.

119. Harris LJ, Skaletsky E, McPherson A. Crystallographic structure of an intact IgG1 monoclonal antibody. *J Mol Biol* 1998;275:861–872.

120. Harris LJ, Larson SB, Hasel KW, et al. Refined structure of an intact IgG2a monoclonal antibody. *Biochemistry* 1997;36:1581–1597.

121. Tan LK, Shopes RJ, Oi VT, et al. Influence of the hinge region on complement activation, C1q binding, and segmental flexibility in chimeric human immunoglobulins. *Proc Natl Acad Sci USA* 1990;87:162–166.

122. Sandlie I, Michaelsen TE. Engineering monoclonal antibodies to determine the structural requirements for complement activation and complement mediated lysis. *Mol Immunol* 1991;28:1361–1368.

123. Duncan AR, Winter G. The binding site for C1q on IgG. *Nature* 1988;332:738–740.

124. Furukawa K, Kobata A. IgG galactosylation—its biological significance and pathology. *Mol Immunol* 1991;28:1333–1340.

125. Tsuchiya N, Endo T, Matsuta K, et al. Effects of galactose depletion from oligosaccharide chains on immunological activities of human IgG. *J Rheumatol* 1989;16:285–290.

126. Shields RL, Namenuk AK, Hong K, et al. High resolution mapping of the binding site on human IgG1 for Fc gamma RI, Fc gamma RII, Fc gamma RIII, and FcRn and design of IgG1 variants with improved binding to the Fc gamma R. *J Biol Chem* 2001;276:6591–6604.

127. Sondermann P, Huber R, Oosthuizen V, et al. The 3.2-A crystal structure of the human IgG1 Fc fragment–Fc gammaRIII complex. *Nature* 2000;406:267–273.

128. Radaev S, Motyka S, Fridman WH, et al. The structure of a human type III Fcgamma receptor in complex with Fc. *J Biol Chem* 2001; 276:16469–16477.

129. Radaev S, Sun PD. Recognition of IgG by Fcgamma receptor: the role of Fc glycosylation and the binding of peptide inhibitors. *J Biol Chem* 2001;276:16478–16483.

130. Martin WL, West AP Jr, Gan L, et al. Crystal structure at 2.8 A of an FcRn/heterodimeric Fc complex: mechanism of pH-dependent binding. *Mol Cell* 2001;7:867–877.

131. Davis AC, Roux KH, Shulman MJ. On the structure of polymeric IgM. *Eur J Immunol* 1988;18:1001–1008.

132. Brandtzaeg P, Prydz H. Direct evidence for an integrated function of J chain and secretory component in epithelial transport of immunoglobulins. *Nature* 1984;311:71–73.

133. Mole JE, Bhown AS, Bennett JC. Primary structure of human J chain: alignment of peptides from chemical and enzymatic hydrolyses. *Biochemistry* 1977;16:3507–3513.

134. Koshland ME. The coming of age of the immunoglobulin J chain. *Annu Rev Immunol* 1985;3:425–453.

135. Max EE, Korsmeyer SJ. Human J chain gene. Structure and expression in B lymphoid cells. *J Exp Med* 1985;161:832–849.

136. Cann GM, Zaritsky A, Koshland ME. Primary structure of the immunoglobulin J chain from the mouse. *Proc Natl Acad Sci USA* 1982;79:6656–6660.

137. Hughes GJ, Frutiger S, Paquet N, et al. The amino acid sequence of rabbit J chain in secretory immunoglobulin A. *Biochem J* 1990;271:641–647.

138. Mikoryak CA, Margolies MN, Steiner LA. J chain in Rana catesbeiana high molecular weight Ig. *J Immunol* 1988;140:4279–4285.

139. Mestecky J, Schrohenloher RE, Kulhavy R, et al. Site of J chain attachment to human polymeric IgA. *Proc Natl Acad Sci USA* 1974;71:544–548.

140. Mestecky J, Schrohenloher RE. Site of attachment of J chain to human immunoglobulin M. *Nature* 1974;249:650–652.

141. Bastian A, Kratzin H, Fallgren-Gebauer H, et al. Intra- and interchain disulfide bridges of J chain in human S-IgA. *Adv Exp Med Biol* 1995;581–583.

142. Frutiger S, Hughes GJ, Paquet N, et al. Disulfide bond assignment in human J chain and its covalent pairing with immunoglobulin M. *Biochemistry* 1992;31:12643–12647.

143. Sorensen V, Sundvold V, Michaelsen TE, et al. Polymerization of IgA and IgM: roles of Cys309/Cys414 and the secretory tailpiece. *J Immunol* 1999;162:3448–3455.

144. Sorensen V, Rasmussen IB, Sundvold V, et al. Structural requirements for incorporation of J chain into human IgM and IgA. *Int Immunol* 2000;12:19–27.

145. Cals MM, Guenzi S, Carelli S, et al. IgM polymerization inhibits the Golgi-mediated processing of the mu- chain carboxy-terminal glycans. *Mol Immunol* 1996;33:15–24.

146. Randall TD, King LB, Corley RB. The biological effects of IgM hexamer formation. *Eur J Immunol* 1990;20:1971–1979.

147. Hughey CT, Brewer JW, Colosia AD, et al. Production of IgM hexamers by normal and autoimmune B cells: implications for the physiologic role of hexameric IgM. *J Immunol* 1998;161:4091–4097.

148. Metzger H. Structure and function of gamma M macroglobulins. *Adv Immunol* 1970;12:57–116.

149. Eskeland T, Christensen TB. IgM molecules with and without J chain in serum and after purification, studied by ultracentrifugation, electrophoresis, and electron microscopy. *Scand J Immunol* 1975;4:217–228.

150. Mostov KE, Blobel G. A transmembrane precursor of secretory component. The receptor for transcellular transport of polymeric immunoglobulins. *J Biol Chem* 1982;257:11816–11821.

151. Mostov KE, Friedlander M, Blobel G. The receptor for transepithelial transport of IgA and IgM contains multiple immunoglobulin-like domains. *Nature* 1984;308:37–43.

152. Fallgren-Gebauer E, Gebauer W, Bastian A, et al. The covalent link-age of the secretory component to IgA. *Adv Exp Med Biol* 1995:625–628.

153. Carayannopoulos L, Capra JD. Immunoglobulins: structure and function. In: *Fundamental Immunology.* Paul WE, ed. New York: Raven Press, 1993:283–314.

154. Kabat EA, Wu TT, Perry HM, et al. Sequences of proteins of immunological interest. Washington, DC: U.S. Department of Health and Human Services, 1991.

155. Lefranc MP, Lefranc G. *The Immunoglobulin Factsbook.* FactsBook Series. San Diego: Academic Press, 2001.

156. Kuby J. *Immunology,* 3rd ed. New York: W.H. Freeman and Company, 1997.

157. Janeway CA Jr, Travers P, Walport M, et al. *Immunobiology,* 4th ed. New York: Garland Publishing, 1999.

158. Putnam FW. *The Plasma Proteins: Structure, Function, and Genetic Control,* 2nd ed., vol. 3. New York: Academic Press, 1977.

CHAPTER 4

Antigen–Antibody Interactions and Monoclonal Antibodies

Jay A. Berzofsky, Ira J. Berkower, and Suzanne L. Epstein

Thermodynamics and Kinetics
 The Thermodynamics of Affinity · Kinetics of Antigen–Antibody Reactions
Affinity
 Interaction in Solution with Monovalent Ligand · Two-Phase Systems
Radioimmunoassay and Related Methods
 Separation of Bound and Free Antigen · Optimization of Antibody and Tracer Concentrations for Sensitivity · Analysis of Data: Graphic and Numerical Representation · Nonequilibrium Radioimmunoassay · Enzyme-Linked Immunosorbent Assay · Enzyme-Linked Immunospot Assay
Specificity and Cross-Reactivity
 Multispecificity
Other Methods
 Quantitative Precipitin · Immunodiffusion and the Ouchterlony Method · Immunoelectrophoresis · Hemagglutination and Hemagglutination Inhibition · Immunoblot (Western Blot) · Surface Plasmon Resonance
Monoclonal Antibodies
 Derivation of Hybridomas · Applications of Monoclonal Antibodies · Specificity and Cross-Reactivity
Conclusion
Acknowledgments
References

The basic principles of antigen–antibody interaction are those of any bimolecular reaction. Moreover, the binding of antigen by antibody can, in general, be described by the same theories and studied by the same experimental approaches as the binding of a hormone by its receptor, of a substrate by enzyme, or of oxygen by hemoglobin. There are several major differences, however, between antigen–antibody interactions and these other situations. First, unlike most enzymes and many hormone-binding systems, antibodies do not irreversibly alter the antigen they bind. Thus, the reactions are, at least in principle, always reversible. Second, antibodies can be raised, by design of the investigator, with specificity for almost any substance known. In each case, it is possible to find antibodies with affinities as high as and specificities as great as those of enzymes for their substrates and receptors for their hormones. The interaction of antibody with antigen can thus be taken as a prototype for interactions of macromolecules with ligands in general. In addition, the same features of reversibility and availability of a wide variety of specificities have made antibodies invaluable reagents for identifying, quantitating, and even purifying a growing number of substances of biological and medical importance. One other feature of antibodies that in the past created difficulty in studying and using them—in comparison with, say, enzymes—is their enormous heterogeneity. Even "purified" antibodies from an immune antiserum, all specific for the same substance and sharing the same overall immunoglobulin structure (see Chapter 9), are a heterogeneous mixture of molecules of different subclass, different affinity, and different fine specificity and ability to discriminate among cross-reacting antigens. The advent of hybridoma monoclonal antibodies (1–3) has made available a source of homogeneous antibodies to almost anything to which antisera can be raised. Nevertheless, heterogeneous antisera are still in widespread use and even have advantages for certain purposes, such as precipitation reactions. Therefore, it is critical to keep in mind throughout this chapter, and indeed much of this book, that the principles derived for the interaction of one antibody with one antigen must be modified and extended to cover the case of heterogeneous components in the reaction.

In this chapter, we examine the theoretical principles necessary for analyzing, in a quantitative manner, the interaction of antibody with antigen and the experimental techniques that have been developed both to study these interactions and to make use of antibodies as quantitative reagents. Furthermore, we discuss the derivation, use, and properties of monoclonal antibodies.

THERMODYNAMICS AND KINETICS

The Thermodynamics of Affinity

The basic thermodynamic principles of antigen–antibody interactions, as indicated previously, are the same as those for any reversible bimolecular binding reaction. We review these as they apply to this particular immunological reaction.

Chemical Equilibrium in Solution

For this purpose, S is the antibody binding sites, L is the ligand (antigen) sites, and SL is the complex of the two. Then for the reaction

$$S + L \rightleftharpoons SL \qquad [1]$$

according to the mass action law,

$$K_A = \frac{[SL]}{[S][L]} \qquad [2]$$

where K_A is the association constant (or affinity) and square brackets in the equation indicate molar concentration of the reactants enclosed. The importance of this equation is that, for any given set of conditions such as temperature, pH, and salt concentration, the ratio of the concentration of the complex to the product of the concentrations of the reactants at equilibrium is always constant. Thus, changing the concentration of either the antibody or the ligand invariably causes change in the concentration of the complex, provided that neither reactant is limiting—that is, neither has already been saturated—and provided that sufficient time is allowed to reach a new state of equilibrium. Moreover, because the concentrations of antibody and ligand appear in this equation in a completely symmetrical manner, doubling either the antibody concentration or the antigen concentration results in a doubling of the concentration of the antigen–antibody complex, provided that the other reactant is in sufficient excess. This proviso, an echo of the first one mentioned previously, is inherent in the fact that $[S]$ and $[L]$ refer to the concentrations of free S and free L, respectively, in solution, not the total concentration, which would include that of the complex. Thus, if L is not in great excess, doubling $[S]$ results in a decrease in $[L]$, because some of it is consumed in the complex; therefore, the net result is less than a doubling of $[SL]$. Similarly, halving the volume results in a doubling of the total concentration of both antibody and ligand. If the fraction of both reactants tied up in the complex is negligibly small (as

might be the case for low-affinity binding), the concentration of the complex quadruples. However, in most practical cases, the concentration of complex is a significant fraction of the total concentration of antigen or antibody or both; therefore, the net result is an increase in the concentration of complex, but by a factor of less than 4. The other important, perhaps obvious, but often forgotten principle to be gleaned from this example is that, because it is concentration, not amount, of each reactant that enters into the mass action law (Equation 2), putting the same amount of antigen and antibody in a smaller volume increases the amount of complex formed, and diluting them in a larger volume greatly decreases the amount of complex formed. Moreover, these changes occur approximately as the square of the volume; therefore, volumes are critical in the design of an experiment.

The effect of increasing free ligand concentration $[L]$, at constant total antibody concentration, on the concentration of complex, $[SL]$, is illustrated in Fig. 1. The mass action law (Equation 2) can be rewritten

$$[SL] = K_A[S][L] = K_A([S]_t - [SL])[L] \qquad [3]$$

or

$$[SL] = \frac{K_A[S]_t[L]}{(1 + K_A[L])} \qquad [3']$$

where $[S]_t$ = total antibody site concentration: that is, $[S]$ + $[SL]$. Initially, when the complex $[SL]$ is a negligible fraction of the total antibody $[S]_t$, the concentration of complex increases nearly linearly with increasing ligand. However, as a larger fraction of antibody is consumed, the slope tapers off, and the concentration of complex, $[SL]$, asymptotically approaches a plateau value of $[S]_t$ as all the antibody becomes saturated. Thus, the concentration of antibody-binding sites can be determined from such a saturation binding curve (Fig. 1), in which the concentration of (radioactively or otherwise labeled) ligand bound at saturation is a measure of the

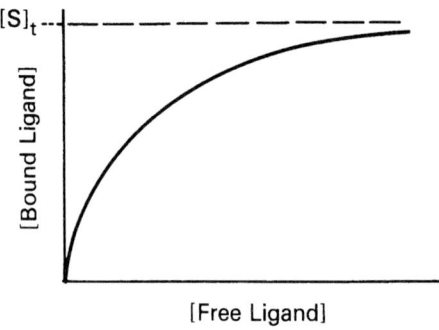

FIG. 1. Schematic plot of bound ligand concentration as a function of free ligand concentration at a constant total concentration of antibody combining sites, $[S]_t$. The curve asymptotically approaches a plateau at which [bound ligand] = $[S]_t$.

concentration of antibody sites.[1] This measurement is sometimes referred to as *antigen-binding capacity.*

The total concentration of ligand at which the antibody begins to saturate is a function not only of the antibody concentration but also of the association constant, K_A, also called the *affinity*. This constant has units of M^{-1}, or L/mol, if all the concentrations in Equation 2 are molar. Thus, the product $K_A[L]$ is unitless. The value of this product relative to 1 determines how saturated the antibody is, as can be seen from Equation 3'. For example, an antibody with an affinity of 10^7 M^{-1} is not saturated if the ligand concentration is 10^{-8} M (product $K_A[L] = 0.1$) even if the total amount of ligand is in great excess over the total amount of antibody. According to Equation 3', the fraction of antibody occupied would be only 0.1/1.1, or about 9%, in this example. These aspects of affinity and the methods for measuring affinity are analyzed in greater detail in the next section.

Free Energy

With regard to thermodynamics, the affinity, K_A, is also the central quantity, because it is directly related to the free energy, ΔF, of the reaction by the equations

$$\Delta F^\circ = -RT \ln K_A \qquad [4]$$

and

$$K_A = e^{-\Delta F^\circ / RT} \qquad [4']$$

where R is the so-called gas constant (1.98717 cal/$^\circ$K · mol), T is the absolute temperature (in degrees Kelvin), ln is the natural logarithm, and e is the base of the natural logarithms. The minus sign is introduced because of the convention that a negative change in free energy corresponds to positive binding. ΔF° is the standard free-energy change defined as the ΔF for 1 mol antigen + 1 mol antibody sites combining to form 1 mol of complex, at unit concentration.

It is also instructive to note an apparent discrepancy in Equations 4 and 4'. As defined in Equation 2, K_A has dimensions of M^{-1} (i.e., L/mol), whereas in Equation 4' it is dimensionless. The reason is that for Equation 4' to hold strictly, K_A must be expressed in terms of mole fractions rather than concentrations. The mole fraction of a solute is the ratio of moles of that solute to the total number of moles of all components in the solution. Because water (55 M) is by far the predominant component of most aqueous solutions, for practical purposes, K_A can be converted into a unitless ratio of mole fractions by dividing all concentrations in Equation 2 by 55 M. This transformation makes Equation 4' strictly correct, but it introduces an additional term, $-RT \ln 55$ (corresponding to the entropy of dilution), into Equation 4. This constant term cancels out when ΔF values are subtracted out, but not in ratios of ΔF values.

An important rule of thumb can be extracted from these equations. Because $\ln 10 = 2.303$, a 10-fold increase in affinity of binding corresponds to a free-energy change ΔF of only 1.42 kcal/mol at 37°C (310.15°K). (The corresponding values for 25°C and 4°C are 1.36 and 1.27 kcal/mol, respectively.) This is less than one-third the energy of a single hydrogen bond (about 4.5 kcal/mol). Looked at another way, a very high affinity of $10^{10} M^{-1}$ corresponds to a ΔF of only 14.2 kcal/mol, approximately the bonding energy of three hydrogen bonds. (Of course, because hydrogen bonds with water are broken during the formation of hydrogen bonds between antigen and antibody, the net energy per hydrogen bond is closer to 1 kcal/mol.) It is apparent from this example that of the many interactions (hydrophobic and ionic as well as hydrogen bonding) that occur between the contact residues in an antibody-combining site and the contacting residues of an antigen (such as a protein), almost as many are repulsive as attractive. It is this small difference of a few kilocalories between much larger numbers corresponding to the total of attractive interactions and the total of repulsive interactions that leads to net "high-affinity" binding. If ΔF were any larger, binding reactions would be of such high affinity as to be essentially irreversible. Viewed in this way, it is not surprising that a small modification of the antigen can result in an enormous change in affinity. A single hydrogen bond can change the affinity many-fold, and similar arguments apply to hydrophobic interactions and other forms of bonding. This concept is important in later discussions of specificity and antigen structure.

Effects of Temperature, pH, and Salt Concentration

It was mentioned earlier that K_A is constant for any given set of conditions such as temperature, pH, and salt concentration. However, it varies with each of these conditions. We have already seen that the conversion of free energy to affinity depends on temperature. However, the free energy itself is also a function of temperature:

$$\Delta F^\circ = \Delta H^\circ - T \Delta S^\circ \qquad [5]$$

where ΔH is change in enthalpy (the heat of the reaction)[2] and ΔS is the entropy (the change in disorder produced by the reaction),[2] and T is the absolute temperature (in degrees Kelvin).

It can be shown that the association constant K_A will thus vary with temperature as follows:

$$\frac{d \ln K_A}{dT} = \frac{\Delta H^\circ}{RT^2} \qquad [6]$$

or, equivalently,

$$\frac{d \ln K_A}{d(1/T)} = \frac{-\Delta H^\circ}{R} \qquad [6']$$

---

[1] This point is strictly true only for univalent ligands, but most multivalent ligands behave as effectively univalent at large antigen excess, at which this plateau is measured.

[2] For a more complete description of these concepts, see a physical chemistry text such as Moore's (4).

The derivation of these equations is beyond the scope of this book [see Moore (4)]. However, the practical implications are as follows. First, the standard enthalpy change $\Delta H°$ of the reaction can be determined from the slope of a plot of $\ln K_A$ versus $1/T$. Second, for an interaction that is primarily exothermic (i.e., driven by a large negative ΔH, such as the formation of hydrogen bonds and polar bonds), the affinity decreases with increasing temperature. Thus, many antigen–antibody interactions have a higher affinity at $4°C$ than at $25°C$ or $37°C$, and so maximum binding for a given set of concentrations can be achieved in the cold. In contrast, apolar or hydrophobic interactions are driven largely by the entropy term, $T\Delta S$, and $\Delta H°$ is near zero. In this case, there is little effect of temperature on the affinity.

As for the effects of pH and salt concentration (or ionic strength) on the affinity, these vary depending on the nature of the interacting groups. Most antigen–antibody reactions are studied at a pH near neutral and at physiologic salt concentrations (0.15 M NaCl). If the interaction is dominated by ionic interactions, high salt concentration lowers the affinity.

Kinetics of Antigen–Antibody Reactions

A fundamental connection between the thermodynamics and kinetics of antigen–antibody binding is expressed by the relationship

$$K_A = \frac{k_1}{k_{-1}} \qquad [7]$$

where k_1 and k_{-1} are the rate constants for the forward (association) and backward (dissociation) reactions.

The forward reaction is determined largely by diffusion rates (theoretical upper limit, 10^9 L/mol·sec) and by the probability that a collision will result in binding: that is, largely the probability that both the antigen and the antibody will be oriented in the right way to produce a good fit, as well as the activation energy for binding. The diffusive rate constant can be shown (5) to be approximated by the Smoluchowski equation:

$$k_{dl} = 4\pi a D(6 \times 10^{20}) \qquad [7a]$$

where a is the sum of the radii in centimeters of the two reactants, D is the sum of the diffusion constants in cm²/sec for the individual reactants, and the constant 6×10^{20} is necessary to convert the units to $M^{-1} \cdot sec^{-1}$. For example, if $a = 10^{-6}$ cm and $D = 10^{-7}$ cm²/sec, then $k_{dl} \sim 7.5 \times 10^8$ $M^{-1} \cdot sec^{-1}$. Association rates are generally slower for large protein antigens than for small haptens. This observation may be due to the smaller value of D, to the orientational effects in the collision, and to other nondiffusional aspects of protein–protein interactions. Therefore, association rates for protein antigens are more frequently on the order of 10^5 to 10^6 $M^{-1} \cdot sec^{-1}$ (see later discussion). However, this observation can also be partly understood from diffusion-limited rates alone. If the radii of hypothetically spherical reactants are r_1 and r_2, then

in Equation 7a, $a = r_1 + r_2$, whereas D is proportional to $1/r_1 + 1/r_2$. The diffusive rate constant is therefore proportional to

$$(r_1 + r_2) \left(\frac{1}{r_1} + \frac{1}{r_2} \right) = \frac{(r_1 + r_2)^2}{r_1 r_2} \qquad [7b]$$

From this result, it can be seen that if $r_1 = r_2 = r$, then r cancels out and the whole term in Equation 7b is simply equal to 4. Thus, for the interaction between two molecules of equal size, the diffusive rate constant is the same regardless of whether those molecules are large or small (6). However, if one molecule is large and the other small, the rate is greater than if both molecules are large. This difference occurs because reducing the radius r_1 while keeping r_2 constant (and larger than r_1) has a greater effect on increasing the diffusion constant term D, proportional to $1/r_1 + 1/r_2$, in which the smaller radius produces the larger term, than it has on the term a, which is still dominated by the larger radius r_2. For example, if $r_2 = r$, as previously, but $r_1 = 0.1r$, then the numerator in Equation 7b is reduced only from $4r^2$ to $1.21r^2$, whereas the denominator is reduced from $1r^2$ to $0.1r^2$. Thus, the ratio is increased from 4 to 12.1. Viewed another way, the greater diffusive mobility of the small hapten outweighs its diminished target area relative to a large protein antigen, inasmuch as the larger target area of the antibody is available to both.

The dissociation rate (or "off rate") k_{-1} is determined by the strength of the bonds (as it affects the activation energy barriers for dissociation) and the thermal energy kT (where k is Boltzmann's constant), which provides the energy to surmount this barrier. The activation energy for dissociation is the difference in energy between the starting state and the transition state of highest energy to which the system must be raised before dissociation can occur.

As pointed out by Eisen (7), if one of a series of related antigens, of similar size and other physical properties, is compared for binding to an antibody, all the association rates are very similar. The differences in affinity largely correspond to the differences in dissociation rates.

A good example is that of antibodies to the protein antigen staphylococcal nuclease (8). Antibodies to native nuclease were fractionated on affinity columns of peptide fragments to isolate a fraction specific for residues 99 through 126. The antibodies had an affinity of 8.3×10^8 M^{-1} for the native antigen and an association rate constant, k_{on}, of 4.1×10^5 $M^{-1} \cdot sec^{-1}$. This k_{on} was several orders of magnitude lower than had been observed for small haptens (9), as discussed previously. A value of k_{off} of 4.9×10^{-4} sec^{-1} was calculated by using these results in Equation 7. This is a first-order rate constant from which it is possible to calculate a half-time for dissociation (based on $t_{1/2} = \ln 2/k_{off}$) of 23 minutes. These rates are probably typical for high-affinity ($K_A \sim 10^9$ M^{-1}) antibodies to small protein antigens such as nuclease (molecular weight $\sim 17,000$). The dissociation rate is important to know in designing experiments to measure binding, because if the act of measurement perturbs the equilibrium, the time for making the measurement (e.g., to separate bound and free) is determined by this half-time for dissociation. For instance, a 2-minute procedure that involves dilution of the antigen–antibody mixture can be completed before significant dissociation has occurred if the dissociation half-time is 23 min. However, if the "on" rate is the same but the affinity is 10-fold lower, still a respectable 8×10^7 M^{-1}, then the complex could be 50% dissociated in the time required to complete the procedure. This caution is very relevant in the later discussion of methods of measuring binding and affinity.

Because knowledge of the dissociation rate can be very important in the design of experiments, techniques to measure it should be understood. Perhaps the most widely applicable one is the use of radiolabeled antigen. After equilibrium is reached and the equilibrium concentration of bound radioactivity determined, a large excess of unlabeled antigen is added. Because any radioactive antigen molecule that dissociates is quickly replaced by an unlabeled one, the probability that a radioactive molecule will associate again is very low. Therefore, the decrease in radioactivity bound to antibody with time can be measured to determine the dissociation rate.[3]

AFFINITY

It is apparent from the preceding discussion that a lot of information about an antigen–antibody reaction is packed into a single value: its affinity. In this section, we examine affinity more closely, including methods for measuring affinity and the heterogeneity thereof, the effects of multivalency of antibody and of antigen, and the special effects seen when the antigen–antibody interaction occurs on a solid surface (two-phase systems).

Interaction in Solution with Monovalent Ligand

The simplest case is that of the interaction of antibody with monovalent ligand. This category may include both antihapten antibodies reacting with truly monovalent haptens and antimacromolecule antibodies, which have been fractionated to obtain a population that reacts only with a single, nonrepeating site on the antigen.[4] In the latter case, the antigen behaves as if monovalent in its interaction with the particular antibody population under study. The proviso that the site recognized (antigenic determinant) be nonrepeating—that is, it occurs only once per antigen molecule—is, of course, critical.

---

[3] In this method, it is assumed that all binding sites are independent, as is generally true for antibodies and monovalent ligands. If there were either negative or positive cooperativity in binding, then the change in receptor occupancy that occurs when a large excess of unlabeled antigen is added would probably perturb the dissociation rate of radiolabeled antigen molecules already bound to other sites.

[4] Such fractionated antibodies may contain mixtures of antibodies to overlapping sites within a domain on the antigen, but as long as no two antibody molecules (or combining sites) can bind to the same antigen molecule simultaneously, the antigen still behaves as effectively monovalent.

If the combining sites on the antibody are independent (i.e., display no positive or negative cooperativity for antigen binding), then for many purposes these combining sites, reacting with monovalent ligands, can be treated as if they were separate molecules. Thus, many, but not all, of the properties we discuss can be analyzed in terms of the concentration of antibody-combining sites, independent of the number of such sites per antibody molecule [two for immunoglobulins G and A (IgG and IgA), 10 for immunoglobulin M (IgM)].

In general, to determine the affinity of an antibody, the equilibrium concentrations of bound and free ligand are determined, at increasing total ligand concentrations but at constant antibody concentration. Alternatively, the antibody concentration can be varied, but then the analysis is slightly more complicated. Perhaps the theoretically most elegant experimental method to determine these quantities is equilibrium dialysis (10,11), depicted and explained in Fig. 2, in which ligand (antigen) is allowed to equilibrate between two chambers, only one of which contains antibody, separated by a semipermeable membrane impermeable to antibody. The important feature of this method, as opposed to most others, is that the concentrations of ligand in each chamber can be determined without perturbing the equilibrium. The disadvantage of this method is that it is applicable only to antigens small enough to freely permeate a membrane that will exclude antibody. Another technical disadvantage is that bound antigen, determined as the difference between bound plus free antigen

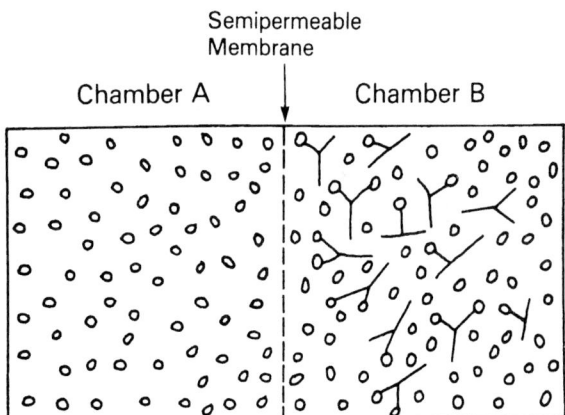

FIG. 2. Equilibrium dialysis. Two chambers are separated by a semipermeable membrane that is freely permeable to ligand but not at all to antibody. Antibody is placed in one chamber (chamber B), and ligand in one or both chambers. Regardless of how the ligand is distributed initially, after sufficient time to reach equilibrium, it is distributed as follows. The concentration of free ligand is identical in both chambers, but chamber B has additional ligand bound to antibody. The concentration of bound ligand is thus the difference between the ligand concentrations in the two chambers, whereas the free concentration is the concentration in chamber A. Because these concentrations must obey the mass action law, Equation 2, they can be used to determine the affinity K_A, from Equation 3 or 3′, by any of several graphical procedures, such as Scatchard analysis (described in the text).

in one chamber and free antigen in the other, is not measured independently of free antigen.

Another category of method involves using radiolabeled ligand in equilibrium with antibody and then physically separating free antigen bound to antibody and quantitating each separately. The methods used to separate bound and free antigen are discussed later in the section on radioimmunoassay. These methods generally allow independent measurement of bound and free antigen but may perturb the equilibrium.

Scatchard Analysis

Once data are obtained, there are a number of methods of computing the affinity, of which we shall discuss two. Perhaps the most widely used is that described by Scatchard (12) [Fig. 3; see Berzofsky et al. (13)]. The mass action equilibrium law is plotted in the form of Equation 3,

$$[SL] = K_A([S]_t - [SL])[L] \qquad [3]$$

and B is substituted for $[SL]$ and F for $[L]$, referring to bound and free ligand, respectively. Then the Scatchard equation is

$$\frac{B}{F} = K_A([S]_t - B) \qquad [8]$$

Note that a critical implicit assumption was made in this seemingly very simple conversion. The $[SL]$ within the parentheses in Equation 3 was intended to be the concentration of bound antibody sites, so that $([S]_t - [SL]) = $ free $[S]$. However, in Equation 8, we have substituted B, the concentration of bound ligand. If the ligand behaves as if it were monovalent, then this substitution is legitimate, because every bound ligand molecule corresponds to an occupied antibody site. However, if the ligand is multivalent and can bind more than one antibody site, then Equation 8 is valid only in ligand excess, in which the frequency of ligands with more than

one antibody bound is very low. In this section, we are discussing only monovalent ligands, but this proviso must be kept in mind when the Scatchard analysis is applied in other circumstances.

From Equation 8, we see that a plot of B/F versus B should yield a straight line (for a single affinity), with a slope of $-K_A$ and an intercept on the abscissa corresponding to antibody-binding site concentration (Fig. 3). This is the so-called Scatchard plot. An alternative version that is normalized for antibody concentration is especially useful if the data were obtained at different values of total antibody concentration, $[A]_t$, instead of constant $[A]_t$. However, for this version, an independent measure of total antibody concentration, other than the intercept of the plot, is required. Then Equation 8 is divided by the total concentration of antibody molecules (with no assumptions about the number of sites per molecule) to obtain

$$\frac{r}{c} = K_A(n - r) \qquad [9]$$

where r is defined as the number of occupied sites per antibody molecule, n is defined as the total number of sites per antibody molecule, and c is free ligand concentration; that is, $c = F$. Thus,

$$r = \frac{B}{[\text{total antibody}]} = \frac{B}{[A]_t}$$

and

$$n = \frac{[\text{total sites}]}{[\text{total antibody}]} = \frac{[S]_t}{[A]_t}$$

where $[A]_t = $ total molar antibody concentration. In this form of the Scatchard plot, r/c versus r, the slope is still $-K_A$ and the intercept on the r axis is n. Thus, the number of sites per molecule can be determined. Of course, if $[S]_t$ is determined

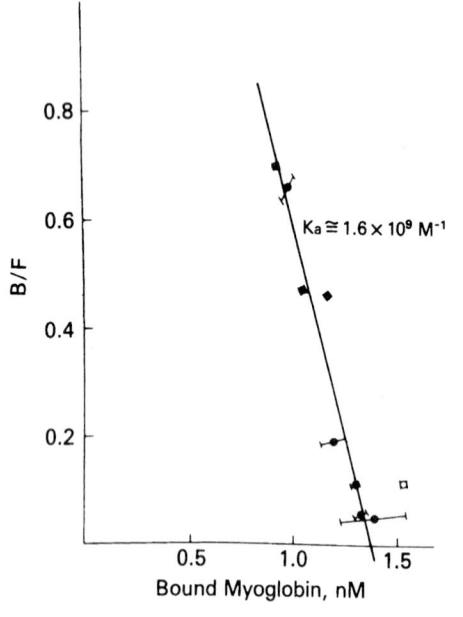

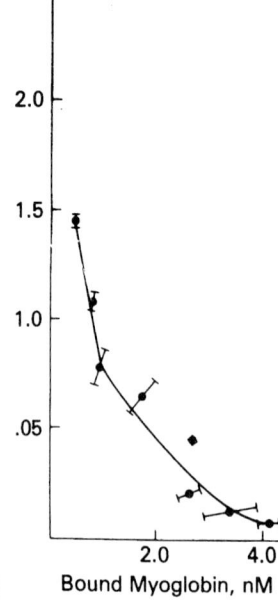

FIG. 3. Scatchard analysis of the binding of [^3H]–sperm whale myoglobin by a monoclonal antibody to myoglobin **(A)** and by the serum antibodies from the same mouse whose spleen cells were fused to prepare the hybridoma **(B)**. The monoclonal antibody (clone HAL 43-201E11, clone 5) produces a linear Scatchard plot, whose slope, -1.6×10^9 M^{-1}, equals $-K_A$ and whose intercept on the abscissa indicates the concentration of antibody-binding sites. In contrast, the serum antibodies produce a curved (concave-up) Scatchard plot, indicative of heterogeneity of affinity. From (13), with permission.

from the intercept of Equation 8, the number of sites per molecule by dividing $[S]_t$ can also be calculated by any independent measure of antibody concentration. Thus, the only advantage of normalizing all the data points first to plot the r/c form arises when the data were obtained at varying antibody concentrations. If the antibody concentration is unknown but held constant, then the B/F form is more convenient and actually provides one measure of antibody (site) concentration. Because today the value of n for each class of antibody is known (two for IgG and serum IgA, 10 for IgM), the concentration of sites and that of antibody are easily converted in many cases.

Heterogeneity of Affinity

The next level of complexity involves a mixture of antibodies of varying affinity for the ligand. This is the rule, rather than the exception, with antibodies from immune serum, even if they are fractionated to be monospecific: that is, all specific for the same site on the antigen. Contrast, for example, the linear Scatchard plot for a homogeneous monoclonal antibody to myoglobin (Fig. 3A) with the curved Scatchard plot for the serum antibodies from the same mouse used to prepare the hybridoma monoclonal antibody (Fig. 3B). This concave-up Scatchard plot is typical for heterogeneous antibodies. In a system such as hormone receptor–hormone interaction, in which negative cooperativity can occur between receptor sites (i.e., occupation of one site lowers the affinity of its neighbor), a concave-up Scatchard plot can be produced by negative cooperativity in the absence of any intrinsic heterogeneity in affinity. However, in the case of antibodies, for which no such allosteric effect has been demonstrated, a concave-up Scatchard plot indicates heterogeneity of affinity.

Ideally, the tangents all along the curve correspond (in slope) the affinities of the many subpopulations of antibodies. Mathematically, this is not strictly correct, but it is true that the steeper part of the curve corresponds to the higher affinity antibodies and the shallower part of the curve to the lower affinity antibodies. Graphical methods have been developed to analyze more quantitatively the components of such curves (14,15), and a very general and versatile computer program (LIGAND), developed by Munson and Rodbard (16), can fit such curves when any number of subpopulations of different affinity is used. For purposes of this chapter, we discuss only the case of two affinities and then examine the types of average affinities that have been proposed for much greater heterogeneity. We also examine mathematical estimates of the degree of heterogeneity (analogous to a variance).

When an antibody population consists of only two subpopulations of different affinities, K_1 and K_2, the component Equation 3' can be added to obtain

$$r = r_1 + r_2 = \frac{n_1 K_1 c}{(1 + K_1 c)} + \frac{n_2 K_2 c}{(1 + K_2 c)} \qquad [10]$$

so that

$$\frac{r}{c} = \frac{n_1 K_1}{(1 + K_1 c)} + \frac{n_2 K_2}{(1 + K_2 c)} \qquad [10']$$

where the subscripts correspond to the two populations. Then the graph of r/c versus r can be shown to be a hyperbola whose asymptotes are, in fact, the linear Scatchard plots of the two components (Fig. 4). This situation was analyzed graphically by Bright (17). If the limits are $c \to 0$ and $c \to \infty$, it can easily be shown that the intercept on the abscissa is just $n_1 + n_2$ (or, in the form B/F vs. B, the intercept is the total concentration of binding sites $[S]_t$), and the intercept on the ordinate is $n_1 K_1 + n_2 K_2$. Thus, it is still possible to obtain the total value of n or $[S]_t$ from the intercept on the abscissa. The problem is in obtaining the two affinities, K_1 and K_2, and the concentrations of the individual antibody subpopulations (corresponding to n_1 and n_2). If K_1 is greater than K_2, the affinities can be approximated from the slopes of

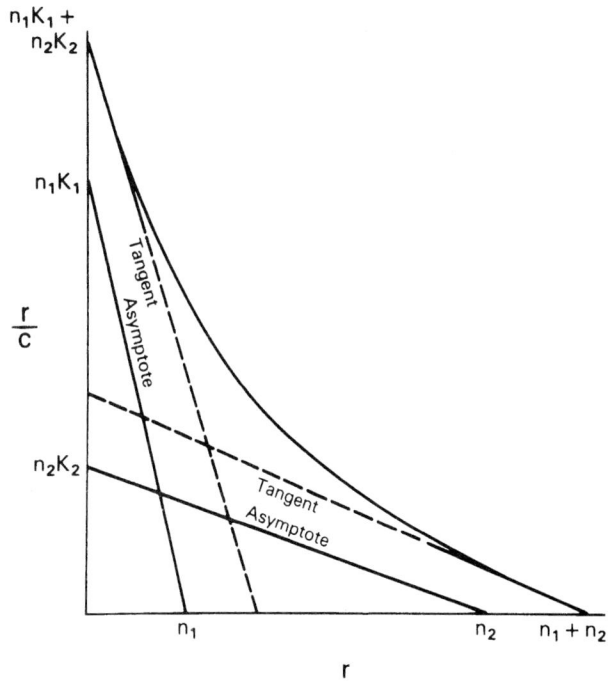

FIG. 4. Analysis of a curved Scatchard plot produced by a mixture of two antibodies with different affinities. The antibodies have affinities K_1 and K_2 and have n_1 and n_2 binding sites per molecule, respectively. r is the concentration of bound antigen divided by the total antibody concentration (i.e., bound sites per molecule), and c is the free antigen concentration. The curve is a hyperbola that can be decomposed into its two asymptotes, which correspond to the linear Scatchard plots of the two components in the antibody mixture. The tangents to the curve at its intercepts only approximate these asymptotes, so that the slopes of the tangents provide an estimate of but do not accurately correspond to the affinities of the two antibodies. However, the intercept on the r axis corresponds to $n_1 + n_2$. Note that in this case n_1 and n_2 must be defined in terms of the total antibody concentration, not that of each component.

the tangents at the two intercepts (Fig. 4); however, these are not, in general, exactly parallel to the two asymptotes, which give the true affinities, and so some error is always introduced, depending on the relative values of n_1, n_2, K_1, and K_2. A graphical method for solving for these exactly was worked out by Bright (17), and computer methods were worked out by Munson and Rodbard (16).

Average Affinities

In practice, of course, it is rarely known that exactly two subpopulations are involved, and most antisera are significantly more heterogeneous than that. Therefore, the case just discussed is more illustrative of principles than of practical value. When faced with a curved Scatchard plot, the investigator usually asks what the average affinity is, and perhaps some measure of the variance of the affinities, without being able to define exactly how many different affinity populations exist.

Suppose there are m populations each with site concentration $[S_i]$ and affinity K_i, so that at free ligand concentration $[L]$, the fraction of each antibody that has ligand bound is given by an equation of the form of Equation 3':

$$B_i = \frac{K_i[S_i]_t[L]}{(1 + K_i[L])} \quad [11]$$

Then the bound concentrations sum as follows:

$$B = \sum_{i=1}^{m} B_i = \sum_{i=1}^{m} \frac{K_i[S_i]_t[L]}{(1 + K_i[L])} \quad [11']$$

Substituting F for $[L]$ and dividing through by this quantity yields

$$\frac{B}{F} = \sum_{i=1}^{m} \frac{K_i[S_i]_t}{(1 + K_i F)} \quad [12]$$

or, equivalently,

$$\frac{r}{c} = \sum_{i=1}^{m} \frac{K_i n_i}{(1 + K_i c)} \quad [12']$$

These can be seen to be generalizations of Equations 10 and 10'. If the limits are $F \to 0$ and $F \to \infty$,

$$\text{intercept on ordinate} = \sum_{i=1}^{m} K_i[S_i]_t \quad [13]$$

and

$$\text{intercept on abscissa} = \sum_{i=1}^{m}[S_i]_t = [S]_t \quad [14]$$

Therefore, it is still possible to obtain the total antibody site concentration from the intercept on the abscissa (Fig. 5) (18).

Two types of average affinity can be obtained graphically from the Scatchard plot (18). A term perhaps the more widely used, K_0, is actually more accurately a median affinity rather than a mean affinity. It is defined as the slope of the tangent at

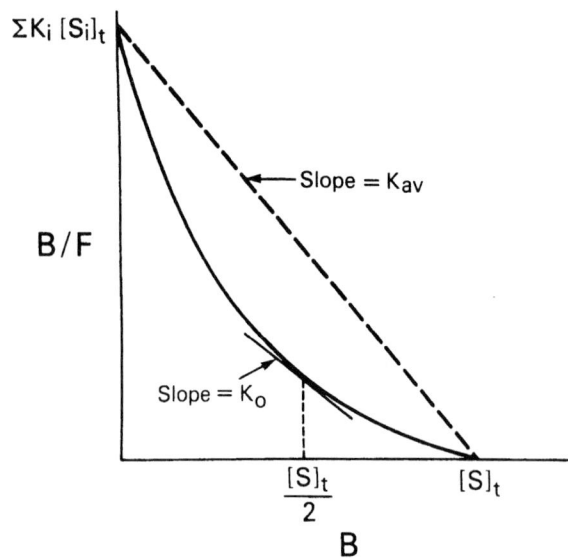

FIG. 5. Types of average affinities for a heterogeneous population of antibodies, as defined on a Scatchard plot. K_0 is the slope of the tangent to the curve at a point where $B = [S]_t/2$: that is, where half the antibody sites are bound. Thus, K_0 corresponds to a median affinity. K_{av} is the slope of the chord between the intercepts and corresponds to a weighted average of the affinities, weighted by the concentrations of the antibodies with each affinity. Adapted from (18), with permission.

the point on the curve where half the sites are bound: that is, where $B = [S]_t/2$ (Fig. 5). A second type of average affinity, which we call K_{av}, is a weighted mean of the affinities, each affinity weighted by its proportional representation in the antibody population. Thus, the ratio is

$$K_{av} = \sum_{i=1}^{m} \frac{K_i[S_i]_t}{[S]_t} \quad [15]$$

From Equations 13 and 14, it is apparent that K_{av} is simply the ratio of the two intercepts on the B/F and B axes: that is, the slope of the chord (Fig. 5). This type of weighted mean affinity, K_{av}, is therefore actually easier to obtain graphically in some cases than is K_0, and it is useful in other types of plots as well.

Indices of Heterogeneity: the Sips Plot

For a heterogeneous antiserum, it is desirable to have some idea of the extent of heterogeneity of affinity. For instance, if the affinities are distributed according to a normal (gaussian) distribution, it is helpful to know the variance (19,20). More complex analyses have been developed that do not require as many assumptions about the shape of the distribution (21–23), but the first and most widely used index of heterogeneity arbitrarily assumes that the affinities fit a distribution, first described by Sips (24), which is similar in shape to a normal distribution. This was applied to the case of antibody heterogeneity by Nisonoff and Pressman (25) and was summarized by Karush and Karush (26). The data are fit to the assumed binding function

$$r = \frac{n(K_0c)^a}{(1 + (K_0c)^a)} \qquad [16]$$

which is analogous to Equations 3′ and 11 (the Langmuir adsorption isotherm) except for the exponent a, which is the index of heterogeneity. This index, a, is allowed to range from 0 to 1. For $a = 1$, Equation 16 is equivalent to Equation 3 and there is no heterogeneity. As a decreases toward 0, the heterogeneity increases. To obtain a value for a graphically, the algebraic rearrangement of Equation 16 is plotted as follows:

$$\log \left(\frac{r}{n - r} \right) = a \log c + a \log K_0 \qquad [17]$$

so that the slope of log $[r/(n - r)]$ versus log c is the heterogeneity index a.

C. DeLisi (personal communication) derived the variance (second moment) of the Sips distribution in terms of the free energy $RT \ln K_0$, about the mean of free energy. The result (normalized to RT) gives the dispersion or width of the distribution as a function of a:

$$\frac{\sigma^2_{\text{Sips}}}{R^2 T^2} = \frac{\pi^2(1 - a^2)}{3a^2} \qquad [18]$$

This is useful for determining a quantity, σ_{Sips}, which can be thought of as analogous to a standard deviation, if one keeps in mind that this is not a true gaussian distribution. In addition, as noted previously, the use of the Sips distribution requires the assumption that the affinities (really the free energies) are continuously distributed symmetrically about a mean, approximating a gaussian distribution. This assumption frequently is not valid.

The Plot of B/F Versus F or T

Another graphical method that is useful for estimating affinities is the plot of bound/free versus free or total ligand concentration, denoted F and T, respectively (18) (Fig. 6). To simplify the discussion, we define the bound/free ratio, B/F, as R and define R_0 as the intercept, or limit, as free ligand $F \to 0$. First, for the case of a homogeneous antibody, from Equation 3′,

$$R = \frac{B}{F} = \frac{K[S]_t}{(1 + KF)} \qquad [19]$$

and

$$R_0 = \lim_{F \to 0} \frac{B}{F} = K[S]_t \qquad [20]$$

We define the midpoint of the plot (Fig. 6) as the point at which R decreases to half its initial value, R_0: that is, at which $R = K[S]_t/2$. For the case of homogeneous antibody (i.e., a single affinity), simple algebraic manipulation (18), substi-

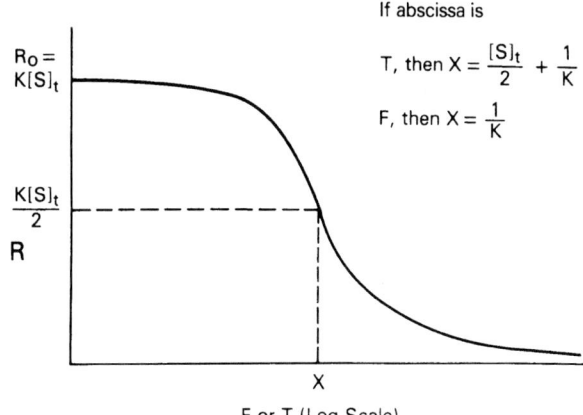

FIG. 6. Schematic plot of R, the bound/free ratio, as a function of free (F) or total (T) antigen concentration. The curves have a similar sigmoidal shape, but the midpoint (where $R = R_0/2$) of the plot of R versus T has a term dependent on antibody site concentration ($[S]_t$), whereas the midpoint of the plot of R versus F is exactly $1/K$, independent of antibody concentration. Adapted from (18), with permission.

tuting $K[S]_t/2$ (i.e., $R_0/2$) for B/F in Equation 8, will show that at this midpoint[5]

$$F = \frac{1}{K} \qquad [21]$$

and

$$B = [S]_t/2 \qquad [22]$$

so that the total concentration, T, is

$$T = B + F = \frac{[S]_t}{2} + \frac{1}{K} \qquad [23]$$

Thus, if B/F versus F is plotted, the midpoint directly yields $1/K$. However, it is frequently more convenient experimentally to plot B/F versus T. In this case, the midpoint is no longer simply the reciprocal of the affinity. As seen from Equation 23, the assumption that the midpoint is $1/K$ will result in an error equal to half the antibody-binding site concentration. Thus, in plots of B/F versus T, the midpoint is a good estimate of the affinity only if $[S]_t/2 << 1/K$: that is, if the antibody concentration is low in comparison with the dissociation constant. In fact, if the affinity is so high that $1/K << [S]_t/2$, then only the antibody concentration, not the affinity, is being measured (18) (Fig. 6).

In the case of a heterogeneous antiserum, we have already shown that

$$R_0 = \sum_i K_i[S_i]_t \qquad [13]$$

---

[5] It is important to note that R_0 must be the limit of B/F as F truly approaches zero. In a radioimmunoassay in which the concentration of tracer is significant compared to $1/K$, reducing the unlabeled ligand concentration all the way to zero will still not yield the true limit R_0. The tracer concentration must also be negligible. If not, R_0 will be estimated falsely low, and the affinity will also be underestimated.

Therefore, at the midpoint, when $B/F = R_0/2$, it is easy to see from equation 15 that

$$K_{av} = \left(\frac{B}{F}\right)\left(\frac{2}{[S]_t}\right) = \frac{R_0}{[S]_t} \qquad [24]$$

Thus, it is still possible to obtain the average affinity, as defined previously (18).

Regardless of average affinities, the effect of affinity heterogeneity is to broaden the curve or to make the slope shallower. This can be seen by visualizing the curve of B/F versus F as a step function. Each antibody subpopulation of a given affinity, K_i, will be titrated to 50% of its microscopic B/F at a free ligand concentration $F = 1/K_i$. The high-affinity antibodies will be titrated at low F, but the low-affinity antibodies will require much higher F to be titrated. The resulting step function is analogous to the successive transitions corresponding to different pK values in a pH titration.

Intrinsic Affinity

The affinity, K_A, that we have been discussing so far is what has been termed the *intrinsic affinity:* that is, the affinity of each antibody-combining site treated in isolation. We have been able to do this, regardless of the valence of the antibodies, by using the concentration of combining sites, $[S]$, in our equations rather than the concentration of antibody molecules, $[A]$, which may have more than one site. Even without any cooperativity between combining sites, there is a statistical effect that makes the actual affinity different from the intrinsic affinity if the antibody is multivalent and if whole antibody concentration rather than site concentration is used. The way this difference arises can best be seen by examining the case of a bivalent antibody, such as IgG. We assume that the two sites are equivalent and that neither is affected by events at the other. The ligand, as in this whole section, is monovalent. Then there are two binding steps,

$$A + L \overset{K_1}{\rightleftharpoons} AL, \qquad AL + L \overset{K_2}{\rightleftharpoons} AL_2 \qquad [25]$$

and the corresponding actual affinities are

$$K_1 = \frac{[AL]}{[A][L]}, \qquad K_2 = \frac{[AL_2]}{[AL][L]} \qquad [26]$$

If the intrinsic affinity of both equivalent sites is K, then K_1 is actually twice K, because the concentration of available sites, $[S]$, is twice the antibody concentration when the first ligand is about to bind, in step 1. However, once one site is bound, the reverse (dissociation) reaction of step 1 can occur from only one site—namely, the one that is occupied. Conversely, for the second step, the forward reaction has only one remaining available site; however, in the reverse reaction, $AL_2 \rightarrow AL + L$, either site can dissociate to go back to the AL state. The second site bound need not be the first to dissociate, and because the sites are identical, it is impossible to tell the difference. Thus, for step 2, the apparent concentration of sites for the reverse reaction is twice that available

for the forward reaction, and so the affinity K_2 for the second step is only half the intrinsic affinity, K.

It is easy to see how this statistical effect can be extrapolated to an antibody with n sites (27):

$$K_1 = nK \qquad \text{and} \qquad K_n = \frac{1}{n}K \qquad [27]$$

For the steps in between, two derivations are available (7,27), which yield

$$K_i = \frac{n - i + 1}{i}K \qquad [28]$$

The actual affinity, rather than the intrinsic affinity, is important with monovalent ligands in regard to the effective affinity (based on a molar antibody concentration) under conditions in which $[L]$ is so low that only one site can bind antigen. Therefore, for IgG or IgM (with 2 or 10 sites per molecule, respectively), the apparent affinity is theoretically 2 or 10 times the intrinsic affinity. For most purposes, it is easier to use site concentrations and intrinsic affinities. The analyses given previously, such as B/F versus F or the Scatchard plot, either B/F versus B or r/c versus r, all yield intrinsic affinities. The intrinsic affinity provides information about the nature of the antibody–ligand interaction.

With regard to multivalent ligands, the actual affinity or effective affinity involving multipoint binding between multivalent antibody molecule and multivalent ligand molecule can be much greater than the intrinsic affinity for binding at each site. This case is the subject of the next section.

Interaction with Multivalent Ligands

So far, we have discussed only situations in which the ligand is monovalent or effectively monovalent with regard to the particular antibody under study. However, in many situations, the ligand molecule has multiple repeating identical determinants, each of which can bind independently to the several identical combining sites on a divalent or multivalent antibody.[6] Although the intrinsic affinity for the interaction of any single antibody-combining site with any single antigenic determinant may be the same as that discussed in the preceding section, the apparent or effective affinity may be much higher, because of the ability of a single antibody molecule to bind more than one identical determinant of a multivalent antigen molecule. Karush (28) termed this phenomenon *monogamous bivalency.* Such monogamous binding can occur between two molecules in solution or between a molecule in solution and one on a solid surface, such as a cell membrane or microtiter plate. We first discuss the situation in solution and then discuss the additional considerations that apply when one of the reactants is bound to a solid surface.

---

[6] If only the antigen is multivalent and the antibody is monovalent, such as an Fab, the situation can be analyzed with the same statistical considerations discussed previously.

Monogamous Bivalency

Suppose that a divalent antibody molecule reacts with antigen that has two identical determinants. This situation was treated in detail by Crothers and Metzger (29) and by Karush (28). The two antibody sites are called S and S', and the antigenic determinants are called D and D', with the understanding that, in actuality, we cannot distinguish S from S' or D from D'. The interaction can be broken up into two steps: a bimolecular reaction,

$$\begin{array}{ccc} S & D & S-D \\ | + | & \stackrel{K_1}{\rightleftharpoons} & |\quad| \\ S' & D' & S'\quad D' \end{array} \qquad [29]$$

followed by an intramolecular reaction,

$$\begin{array}{ccc} S-D & & S-D \\ |\quad| & \stackrel{K_2}{\rightleftharpoons} & |\quad| \\ S'\quad D' & & S'-D' \end{array} \qquad [30]$$

The association constant for the first step, K_1, is related to the intrinsic affinity, K, simply by a statistical factor of 4 because of the degeneracy (equivalence) between S and S' and between D and D'. This is a typical second-order reaction between antigen and antibody. However, the second step (Equation 30) is a first-order reaction, inasmuch as it is effectively an interconversion between two states of a single molecular complex, the reactants S' and D' being linked chemically (albeit noncovalently) through the S—D bond formed in the first step. Thus, the first-order equilibrium constant, K_2, is not a function of the concentrations of S—S and D—D in solution, as K_1 would be. Rather, the forward reaction depends on the geometry of the complex and the flexibility of the arms; in other words, the probability that S' and D' will encounter each other and be in the right orientation to react if they do come in contact depends on the distances and freedom of motion along the chain S'—S—D—D' rather than on the density of molecules in solution (i.e., concentration).

The reverse reaction for step 2, on the other hand, will have a rate constant similar to that for the simple monovalent S—$D \rightarrow S + D$ reaction, because the dissociation reaction depends on the strength of the S'—D' (or S—D) bond and is not influenced by the other S—D interaction unless there is strain introduced by the angles required for simultaneous bonds between S and D and between S' and D'. Note that K_2 inherently has a statistical factor of 1/2 in comparison with the intrinsic K'_2 for the analogous reaction if the S'—S—D—D' link is all covalent, because in the forward reaction of Equation 30, only one pair can react, whereas in the reverse reaction, either S'—D' or S—D could dissociate to produce the equivalent result.

We would like to know the apparent or observed affinity for the overall reaction

$$\begin{array}{ccc} S & D & S-D \\ | + | & \stackrel{K_{obs}}{\rightleftharpoons} & |\quad| \\ S & D & S-D \end{array} \qquad [31]$$

Because the free energies, ΔF_1 and ΔF_2, for the two steps

are additive, the observed affinity is the product of K_1 and K_2:

$$K_{obs} = K_1 K_2 \qquad [32]$$

where we have defined K_1 and K_2 to include the statistical degeneracy factors.[7] The equilibrium constants K_1 and K_2 are the ratios of forward and reverse rate constants, as in Equation 7. All four rate constants are directly related to the corresponding terms for the intrinsic affinity between S and D except for the intramolecular forward reaction of step 2, as noted previously. Thus, the difficulty in predicting K_{obs} is largely a problem of analyzing the geometric (steric) aspects of K_2, if the intrinsic affinity, K, is already known. Crothers and Metzger (29) analyzed this problem for particular situations. Qualitatively, whether K_2 is larger or smaller than K depends on factors such as the enforced proximity of S' and D' in step 2 and the distance between D and D' in comparison with the possible distances accessible between S and S', which in turn depend on the length of the antibody arms and the flexibility of the hinge between them (see Chapter 9). Thus, since K_1 can be approximated by K, except for statistical factors, the apparent affinity for this "monogamous bivalent" binding interaction, K_{obs}, may range from significantly less than to significantly greater than K^2. If K_2 is of the same order of magnitude as K, then K_{obs} is of the order of K^2, which can be huge (e.g., if $K \sim 10^9$ M^{-1}, K_{obs} could be $\sim 10^{18}$ M^{-1}). The half-time for dissociation would be thousands of years. It is easy to see how such monogamous bivalent interactions can appear to be irreversible, even though in practice the observed affinity is rarely more than a few orders of magnitude larger than the K for a single site, possibly because of structural constraints (30).

If apparent affinities this high can be reached by monogamous bivalency, even greater ones should be possible for the multipoint binding of an IgM molecule to a multivalent ligand. Although IgM is decavalent for small monovalent ligands, steric restrictions often make it behave as if it is pentavalent for binding to large multivalent ligands. However, even five-point binding can lead to enormously tight interactions. Therefore, even though the intrinsic affinity of IgM molecules tends to be lower than that of IgG molecules for the same antigen (28), the apparent affinity of IgM can be quite high.

Two-Phase Systems

The same enhanced affinity seen for multipoint binding applies to two-phase systems. Examples include the reaction of multivalent antibodies with antigen attached to a cell surface or an artificial surface (such as Sepharose or the plastic walls of a microtiter plate), the reaction of a multivalent ligand with antibodies on the surface of a B cell, a Sepharose bead, or a plastic plate, and the reaction of either component with an

---

[7] In some treatments in which these statistical factors are not included in K_1 and K_2, the equivalent equation may be given as $K_{obs} = 2K_1K_2$.

antigen–antibody precipitate. For the reasons outlined previously, "monogamous" binding can cause the apparent affinity of a multivalent antibody or antigen for multiple sites on a solid surface to be quite large, to the point of effective irreversibility.

However, another effect also increases the effective affinity in a two-phase system. This effect applies even for monovalent antibodies [antigen-binding fragments (Fab)] or monovalent ligands. The effect arises from the enormously high effective local concentration of binding sites at the surface, in comparison with the concentration if the same number of sites were distributed in bulk solution (31). Looked at another way, the effect is caused by the violation, at the liquid–solid interface, of the basic assumption in the association constants, K_A, discussed previously, that all the reactants are distributed randomly in the solution. (To some extent, the latter is involved in the enhanced affinity of multivalency as well.) This situation was analyzed by DeLisi (32) and DeLisi and Wiegel (33), who broke the reaction down into two steps: (a) the diffusive process necessary to bring the antigen and antibody into the right proximity and orientation to react and (b) the reactive process itself. The complex between antigen and antibody, when positioned but when it has not yet reacted, is called the *encounter complex*. The reaction can then be written

$$S + D \underset{k_-}{\overset{k_+}{\rightleftharpoons}} S \cdots D \underset{k_{-1}}{\overset{k_1}{\rightleftharpoons}} SD \qquad [33]$$

where S is antibody site, D is antigenic determinant, k_+ and k_- are the forward and reverse diffusive rate constants, and k_1 and k_{-1} are the forward and reverse reactive rate constants once the encounter complex is formed. If the encounter complex is in a steady state, the overall rate constants are given by

$$k_f = \frac{k_1 k_+}{(k_1 + k_-)} \qquad [34]$$

and

$$k_r = \frac{k_{-1} k_-}{(k_1 + k_-)} \qquad [35]$$

where subscripts f and r stand for forward and reverse (32). The association constant, according to Equation 7, is the ratio of these two, or

$$K_A = \frac{k_1 k_+}{k_{-1} k_-} \qquad [36]$$

The relative magnitudes of k_1 and k_- determine the probable fate of the encounter complex. Is it more likely to react to form SD or to break up as the reactants diffuse apart?

Now suppose that k_- is slow in comparison with k_1. Then the SD-bound complex and the encounter complex, $S \cdots D$, may interconvert many times before the encounter complex breaks up and one of the reactants diffuses off into bulk solution. If the surface has multiple antigenic sites, D, then even a monovalent antibody (Fab) may, when SD dissociates to $S \cdots D$, be much more likely to rereact with the same or nearby sites than to diffuse away into bulk solution, again

depending on the relative magnitudes of these rate constants. This greater probability to rereact with the surface rather than diffuse away is the essence of the effect we are describing. A more extensive mathematical treatment of reactions with cells was provided by DeLisi (32) and DeLisi and Wiegel (33).

A somewhat different and very useful analysis of the same or a very similar effect was given by Silhavy et al. (34). These authors studied the case of a ligand diffusing out of a dialysis bag containing a protein for which the ligand had a significant affinity. Once the ligand concentration became low enough that there was an excess of free protein sites, the rate of exit of ligand from the dialysis bag was no longer simply its diffusion rate; nor was it simply the rate of dissociation of protein–ligand complex. These authors showed that, under these conditions, the exit of ligand followed quasi–first-order kinetics but with a half-life longer than the half-life in the absence of protein by a factor of $(1 + [P]K_A)$:

$$t_+ = t_-(1 + [P]K_A) \qquad [37]$$

where $[P]$ is the protein site concentration, K_A is the affinity, and t_+ and t_- are the half-lives in the presence and absence of protein in the bag.

In this case, the protein was in solution, and so the authors could use the actual protein concentration and the actual intrinsic affinity, K_A. In the case of protein on a two-dimensional surface, it is harder to know what to use as the effective concentration. However, the high local concentration of protein compartmentalized in the dialysis bag is analogous to the high local concentration attached to the solid surface. The underlying mechanisms of the two effects are essentially the same, and so are the implications. For instance, in the case of dialysis, a modest 10-μM concentration of antibody sites with an affinity of 10^8 M^{-1} can reduce the rate of exit of a ligand 1000-fold. A dialysis that would otherwise take 3 hours would take 4 months! It is easy to see how this "retention effect" can make even modest affinities appear infinite (i.e., the reactions appear irreversible). This retention effect applies not only to immunological systems but also to other interactions at a cell surface or between cell compartments, where the local concentration of a protein may be high. In particular, these principles of two-phase systems should also govern the interaction between antigen-specific receptors on the surface of T cells and antigen–major histocompatibility complex (MHC) molecule complexes on the surface of antigen-presenting cells, B cells, or target cells.

One final point is useful to note. Because these retention effects depend on a localized abundance of unoccupied sites, addition of a large excess of unlabeled ligand to saturate these sites will diminish or abolish the retention effect and will greatly accelerate the dissociation or exit of labeled ligand. This effect of unlabeled ligand can be used as a test for the retention effect, although in certain cases the same result can be an indication of negative cooperativity among receptor sites.

RADIOIMMUNOASSAY AND RELATED METHODS

Since it was first suggested in 1960 by Yalow and Berson (35), radioimmunoassay (RIA) has rapidly become one of the most widespread, most widely applicable, and most sensitive techniques for assessing the concentration of a whole host of biological molecules. Most of the basic principles necessary to understand and apply RIA have been covered earlier in this chapter. In this section, we examine the concepts and methodological approaches used in RIA. For detailed books on methods, we refer the reader to Chard (36), Rodbard (37), and Yalow (38).

The central concept of RIA is that the binding of an infinitesimal concentration of highly radioactive tracer antigen to low concentrations of a high-affinity specific antibody is very sensitive to competition by unlabeled antigen and is also very specific for that antigen. Thus, concentrations of antigen in unknown samples can be determined by their ability to compete with tracer for binding to antibody. The method can be used to measure very low concentrations of a molecule, even in the presence of the many impurities in biological fluids. Accomplishment of this requires an appropriate high-affinity antibody and radiolabeled antigen, a method to distinguish bound from free labeled antigen, optimization of concentrations of antibody and tracer-labeled antigen to maximize sensitivity, and generation of a standard curve, through the use of known concentrations of competing unlabeled antigen, from which to read off the concentrations in unknown samples, as well as the best method for representing the data. We review all these steps and the pitfalls in this procedure except the preparation of antibodies and labeled antigens.

Separation of Bound and Free Antigen

Regardless of which parameter is used to assess the amount of competition by the unlabeled antigen in the unknown sample to be tested, it is always a function of bound versus free, radiolabeled antigen. Therefore, one of the most critical technical requirements is the ability to distinguish clearly between antibody-bound radioactive tracer and free radioactive tracer. This distinction usually requires physical separation of bound and free ligand. If the bound fraction is contaminated by free ligand, or vice versa, enormous errors can result, depending on the part of the binding curve on which the data fall.

Solution Methods

Solution RIA methods have the advantage that binding can be related to the intrinsic affinity of the antibody. However, bound and free antigen must be separated by a method that does not perturb the equilibrium. Three basic types of approaches have been used: precipitate the antibody with bound antigen, leaving free antigen in solution; precipitate the free antigen, leaving antibody and bound antigen in solution; or separate free from antibody-bound antigen molecules in solution on the basis of size by gel filtration. The last method is too cumbersome to use for large numbers of samples and is too slow, in general, to ensure the equilibrium is not perturbed in the process. Therefore, gel filtration columns are not widely used for RIA.

Methods that precipitate antibody are probably the most widely used. If the antigen is sufficiently smaller (molecular weight < 30,000) than the antibody that it will remain in solution at concentrations of either ammonium sulfate (39) or polyethylene glycol, with a molecular weight of 6,000 (10% W:W) (40), which will precipitate essentially all the antibody, then these two reagents are frequently the most useful. Precipitation with polyethylene glycol and centrifugation can be accomplished before any significant dissociation has occurred as a result of dilutional effects (41). However, if the antigen is much larger than about 30,000 to 40,000 of molecular weight, then these methods will produce unacceptably high background control values in the absence of specific antibody. If the antibody is primarily of a subclass of IgG that binds to staphylococcal protein A or protein G, it is possible to take advantage of the high affinity of protein A or G for IgG by using either protein A (or G)–Sepharose or formalin-killed staphylococcal organisms (Cowan I strain) to precipitate the antibody (42). Finally, it is possible to precipitate the antibody by using a specific second antibody, an anti-immunoglobulin raised in another species. Maximal precipitation occurs not at antibody excess but at the "point of equivalence" in the middle of the titration curve where antigen (in this case, the first antibody) and the (second) antibody are approximately equal in concentration. Thus, carrier immunoglobulin must be added to keep the immunoglobulin concentration constant and the point of equivalence is determined by titrating with the second antibody. Even worse, the precipitin reaction is much slower than the antigen–antibody reaction itself, allowing reequilibration of the antigen–antibody interaction after dilution by the second antibody. Some of these problems can be reduced by enhancing precipitation with low concentrations of polyethylene glycol.

The other type of separation method is adsorption of free antigen to an agent, such as activated charcoal or talc, that leaves antigen bound to antibody in solution. Binding of antigen by these agents depends on size and hydrophobicity. Although these methods are inexpensive and rapid, careful adjustment and monitoring of pH, ionic strength, and temperature are necessary to obtain reproducible results and to avoid adsorption of the antigen–antibody complex. Furthermore, because these agents have a high affinity for antigen, they can compete with a low-affinity antibody and alter the equilibrium. Also, because charcoal quenches beta scintillation counting, it can be used only with gamma-emitting isotopes such as iodine 125.

Solid-Phase Methods

Solid-phase RIA methods have the advantages of high throughput and increased apparent affinity because of the effects at the solid-liquid interface noted previously. However, they have the concomitant disadvantage that the true intrinsic affinity is not measured because of these same effects. The method itself is fairly simple. The antibody is bound in advance to a solid surface such as a Sepharose bead or the walls of a microtiter plate well. To avoid competition from other serum proteins for the solid phase, purified antibody must be used in this coating step. Once the wells (or Sepharose beads) are coated, they can be incubated with labeled tracer antigen, with or without unlabeled competitor, and be washed, and the radioactivity bound to the plastic wells or to the Sepharose can be counted directly. The microtiter plate method is particularly useful for processing large numbers of samples. However, because the concentration, or even the amount, of antibody coating the surface is unknown, and because the affinity is not the intrinsic affinity, these methods cannot be used for studying the chemistry of the antigen–antibody reaction itself. A detailed analysis of the optimum parameters in this method is given by Zollinger et al. (41).

A variation that does allow determination of affinity, based on the enzyme-linked immunosorbent assay (ELISA), described later but equally applicable to RIA, was described by Friguet et al. (43). This method involves the use of antigen-coated microtiter wells and free antibody, but competition by free antigen is measured to prevent the antibody in solution from binding to the antibody on the plate (see Fig. 9B later). Thus, the antibody bound to the plastic is antibody that was free in the solution equilibrium. The affinity measured is that between the antibody and antigen in solution, not that on the plastic, and so it is not directly influenced by the multivalency of the surface. However, as pointed out by Stevens (44), the determination of affinity is strictly accurate only for monovalent Fab, because a bivalent antibody with only one arm bound to the plastic and one bound by antigen in solution is still counted as free. Therefore, the ligand occupancy of the antibody combining sites will be underestimated, and thus affinity will be underestimated. To correct for this error, Stevens also pointed out a method based on binomial analysis. Subsequently, Seligman (45) showed that the nature and density of the antigen on the solid surface can also influence the estimate of affinity.

Optimization of Antibody and Tracer Concentrations for Sensitivity

The primary limitations on the sensitivity of the assay are the antibody affinity and concentration, the tracer concentration, and the precision (reproducibility) of the data. In general, the higher the affinity of the antibody, the more sensitive the assay can be made. Once the highest affinity antibody available is prepared, this parameter limits the extent to which the other parameters can be manipulated. For instance, because the unlabeled antigen in the unknown sample is going to compete against labeled tracer antigen, the lower the tracer concentration is, the lower the concentration of the unknown, which can be measured up to a point. That point is determined by the affinity, K_A, as can be seen from the theoretical considerations discussed previously (36). The steepest part of the titration curve occurs in the range of concentrations around $1/K_A$. Concentrations of ligand much lower than $1/K_A$ leave most of the antibody sites unoccupied, so that competition is less effective. Thus, there is no value in reducing the tracer concentration more than a few-fold lower than $1/K_A$. Therefore, although it is generally useful to increase the specific radioactivity of the tracer and reduce its concentration, it is important to be aware of this limit of $1/K_A$. Increasing the specific activity more than necessary can result in denaturation of antigen.

Similarly, lowering the antibody concentration also increases sensitivity up to a point. This limit also depends on $1/K_A$ and on the background "nonspecific binding." Decreasing the antibody concentration to the point that binding of tracer is too close to background results in loss of sensitivity because of loss of precision. In general, the fraction of tracer bound in the absence of competitor should be kept greater than 0.2 and, in general, closer to 0.5 [see Ekins (46)].

A convenient procedure to follow to optimize tracer and antibody concentrations is first to choose the lowest tracer concentration that results in convenient counting times and counting precision for bound values of only one-half to one-tenth the total tracer. Then, with this tracer concentration constant, the antibody is diluted out until the bound/free antigen ratio is close to 1.0 (bound/total = 0.5) in the absence of competitor. This antibody concentration in conjunction with this tracer concentration generally yields near-optimal sensitivities, within the limits noted previously. It is important to be aware that changing the tracer concentration requires readjusting the antibody concentration to optimize sensitivity.

Analysis of Data: Graphic and Numerical Representation

We have already examined the Scatchard plot (bound/free vs. bound) and the plot of bound/free versus free or total antigen concentration as methods of determining affinity. The latter lends itself particularly to the type of competition curves that constitute a RIA. In fact, the independent variable must always be antigen concentration, because that is the known quantity that is varied to generate the standard curve. We use B, F, and T to represent the concentrations of bound, free, and total antigen, respectively. We have shown previously that the plot of B/F versus F is more useful for determining the affinity, K_A, than is the plot of B/F versus T. However, in RIA, the quantity to be determined is T, and, correspondingly, the known independent variable in generating the standard curve is T. Another difference between the situation in RIA and that discussed earlier is that, in RIA, both labeled and unlabeled antigen are available. The dependent variable, such as B/F, is the ratio of bound tracer over free tracer, because only radioactive antigen is counted. B/F for the unlabeled antigen is the same at equilibrium, if labeled and unlabeled antigen bind the antibody equivalently—that is, with the same K_A.

This assumption is not always valid and requires experimental testing.

The sigmoidal shape of B/F versus F or T, when F or T (the "dose") is plotted on a log scale, is shown in Fig. 6. The shape for B/T versus F or T would be similar. Note that because $B + F = T$,

$$\frac{B}{F} = \frac{B}{T - B} = \frac{B/T}{(1 - B/T)} \quad [38]$$

and

$$\frac{B}{T} = \frac{B/F}{(1 + B/F)} \quad [39]$$

These transformations can be useful. If B/F or B/T versus F or T is plotted on a linear scale, then the shape is approximately hyperbolic, as in Fig. 7. The plot of B/F versus T (log scale) was one of the first methods used to plot RIA data and is still among the most useful. The most sensitive part of the curve is the part with the steepest slope.

It has been shown by probability analysis that if the antigen has multiple determinants, each capable of binding antibody molecules simultaneously and independently of one another, then the more such determinants capable of being recognized by the antibodies in use there are, the steeper the slope will be (47). This effect of multideterminant binding on steepness arises because, in RIA, an antigen molecule is scored as bound whether it has one or several antibody molecules attached. It is scored as free only if no antibody molecules are attached. Thus, the probability that an antigen molecule is scored as free is the product of the probabilities that each of its determinants is free. The effect can lead to quite steep slopes and has been confirmed experimentally (47).

A transform that allows linearization of the data in most cases is the logit transform (48,49). To use this, the data are first expressed as B/B_0, where B_0 is the concentration of bound tracer in the absence of competitor. This ratio is then subjected to the logit transform, defined as

$$\text{logit} (Y) = \ln \left[\frac{Y}{(1 - Y)} \right] \quad [40]$$

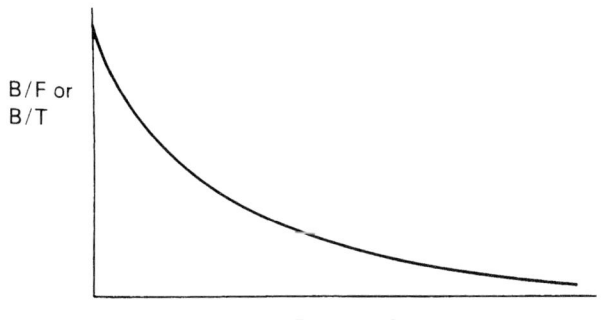

FIG. 7. Schematic plot of B/F or B/T (the bound over free or total antigen concentration) as a function of free (F) or total (T) antigen concentration, when plotted on a linear scale. Contrast with similar plot on a log scale in Fig. 6.

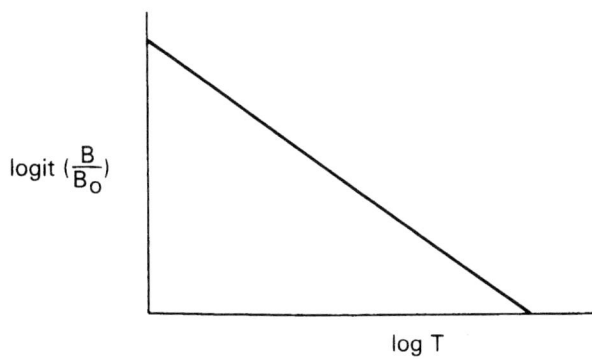

FIG. 8. Schematic logit–log plot used to linearize radioimmunoassay data. B and T are bound tracer and total antigen concentration, respectively, and B_0 is the value of B when no unlabeled antigen is added to tracer. The logit function is defined by Equation 40, logit $(Y) = \ln [Y/(1 - Y)]$.

where ln means the natural log (log to the base e). The plot of logit (B/B_0) versus ln T is usually a straight line (Fig. 8). The slope is usually -1 for the simplest case of a monoclonal antibody binding a monovalent antigen. The linearity of this plot obviously makes it very useful for graphical interpolation, which is desirable for reading antigen concentration off a standard curve. One additional advantage is that linearity facilitates tests of parallelism. If the unknown under study is identical to the antigen used to generate the standard curve, then a dilution curve of the unknown should be parallel to the standard curve in this logit-log coordinate system. If it is not, the assay is not valid.

These and other methods of analyzing the data, including statistical treatment of data, were discussed further by Feldman and Rodbard (50) and Rodbard (37). Although a number of computer programs have become available for rapid analysis of RIA data without the use of manual plots of standard curves, all are based on these and similar methods, and their accurate interpretation depends on an understanding of these concepts.

Corrections for B, F, and T

In conclusion of this section on analysis of RIA data, a few controls and corrections to the data, without which the results may be fallacious, must be mentioned.

First, in any method that precipitates antibody and bound antigen (or entails the use of a solid-phase antibody), there may always be a fraction of antigen that precipitates or binds nonspecifically in the absence of specific antibody. Thus, controls with normal serum or immunoglobulin must be used to determine this background. The nonspecific binding usually increases linearly with antigen dose; that is, it does not saturate. This control value should be subtracted from B but does not affect F when measured independently; it affects only F determined as T minus B. The total antigen that is meaningful is the sum of antigen that is specifically bound and antigen that is free. Nonspecifically bound antigen should be deleted from any term in which it appears.

A second correction is that for immunologically inactive radiolabel: that which is either free radioisotope or isotope coupled to an impurity or to denatured antigen. The fraction of radioactive material that is immunologically reactive with the antibodies in the assay can be determined by using a constant, low concentration of labeled antigen and adding increasing concentrations of antibody. If there is no contamination with inactive material, all the radioactivity should be able to be bound by sufficient antibody. If the fraction of tracer bound reaches a plateau at less than 100% bound, then only this fraction is active in the assay. The importance of this correction can be seen from the example in which the tracer is only 80% active. Then, when the true B/F is 3 ($B/T = 0.75$), applying only to the active 80% of the tracer, the remaining 20%—which can never be bound—will mistakenly be included in the free tracer, doubling the amount that is measured as free. Thus, the measured B/F is only 1.5 (i.e., 0.6/0.4) instead of the true value of 3 (i.e., 0.6/0.2). This factor of 2 makes a serious difference in the calculation of affinity, for instance, from a Scatchard plot. Also, it results in a plateau in the Scatchard plot at high values of B/F, because with 20% of the tracer obligatorily free, B/F can never exceed 4 (i.e., 0.8/0.2). To correct for this potentially serious problem, the inactive fraction must always be determined when subtracted from both F and T.

Nonequilibrium Radioimmunoassay

So far, we have assumed that tracer and unlabeled competitor are added simultaneously and that sufficient incubation time is allowed to achieve equilibrium. To measure the affinity, of course, equilibrium must be ensured. However, suppose the investigator's sole purpose is to measure the concentration of competitor by RIA. Then the sensitivity of the assay can actually be increased by adding the competitor first, allowing it to react with the antibody, and then intentionally adding the tracer for too short a time to reach a new equilibrium. Essentially, the competitor is being given a competitive advantage. It can be shown that the slope of the dose-response curve, B/T versus total antigen added, is increased in the low-dose range—a mathematical measure of increased sensitivity. A detailed mathematical analysis of this procedure was given by Rodbard et al. (51). Note, however, that use of such nonequilibrium conditions requires very careful control of time and temperature.

Enzyme-Linked Immunosorbent Assay

An alternative solid-phase readout system for the detection of antigen–antibody reactions is the ELISA (52). In principle, the only difference from RIAs is that antibodies or antigen are covalently coupled to an enzyme instead of a radioisotope, so that bound enzyme activity instead of bound counts per minute is measured. In practice, the safety and convenience

of nonradioactive materials and the commercial availability of plate readers that can measure the absorbance of 96 wells in a few seconds account for the widespread use of ELISA. Because both ELISA and RIA are governed by the same thermodynamic constraints, and because the enzyme can be detected in the same concentration range as can commonly used radioisotopes, the sensitivity and specificity are comparable. We consider three basic strategies for using ELISA to detect specific antibody or antigen.

As shown in Fig. 9A, the direct binding method is the simplest way to detect and measure specific antibody in an unknown antiserum. Antigen is noncovalently attached to each well of a plastic microtiter dish. For this purpose, it is fortunate that most proteins bind nonspecifically to plastic. Excess free antigen is washed off, and the wells are incubated with an albumin solution to block the remaining nonspecific protein binding sites. The test antiserum is then added, and any specific antibody binds to the solid-phase antigen. Washing removes unbound antibodies. Enzyme-labeled anti-immunoglobulin is added. This binds to specific antibody already bound to antigen on the solid phase, bringing along covalently attached enzyme. Unbound antiglobulin-enzyme conjugate is washed off; then substrate is added. The action of bound enzyme on substrate produces a colored product, which is detected as increased absorbance in a spectrophotometer.

Although this method is quick and very sensitive, it is often difficult to quantitate. Within a defined range, the increase in optical density is proportional to the amount of specific antibody added in the first step. However, the amount of antibody bound is not measured directly. Instead, the antibody concentration of the sample is estimated by comparing it with a standard curve for a known amount of antibody. It is also difficult to determine affinity by this method, because the solid-phase antigen tends to increase the apparent affinity. The sensitivity of this assay for detecting minute amounts of antibody is quite good, especially when affinity-purified antiglobulins are used as the enzyme-linked reagent. A single preparation of enzyme-linked antiglobulin can be used to detect antibodies to many different antigens. Alternatively, class-specific antiglobulins can be used to detect how much of a specific antibody response is caused by each immunoglobulin class. Obviously, reproducibility of the assay depends on uniform antigen coating of each well (which can vary), and the specificity depends on using purified antigen to coat the wells.

Figure 9B shows the competition technique for detecting antigen. Soluble antigen is mixed with limiting amounts of specific antibody in the first step. Then the mixture is added to antigen-coated wells and treated as described in Fig. 9A. Any antigen–antibody complexes formed in the first step reduce the amount of antibody bound to the plate and hence reduce the absorbance measured in the final step. This method permits the estimate of affinity for free antigen, which is related to the half-inhibitory concentration of antigen. Mathematical analysis of affinity by this approach was described by Friguet et al. (43) with modification by Stevens (44), as discussed

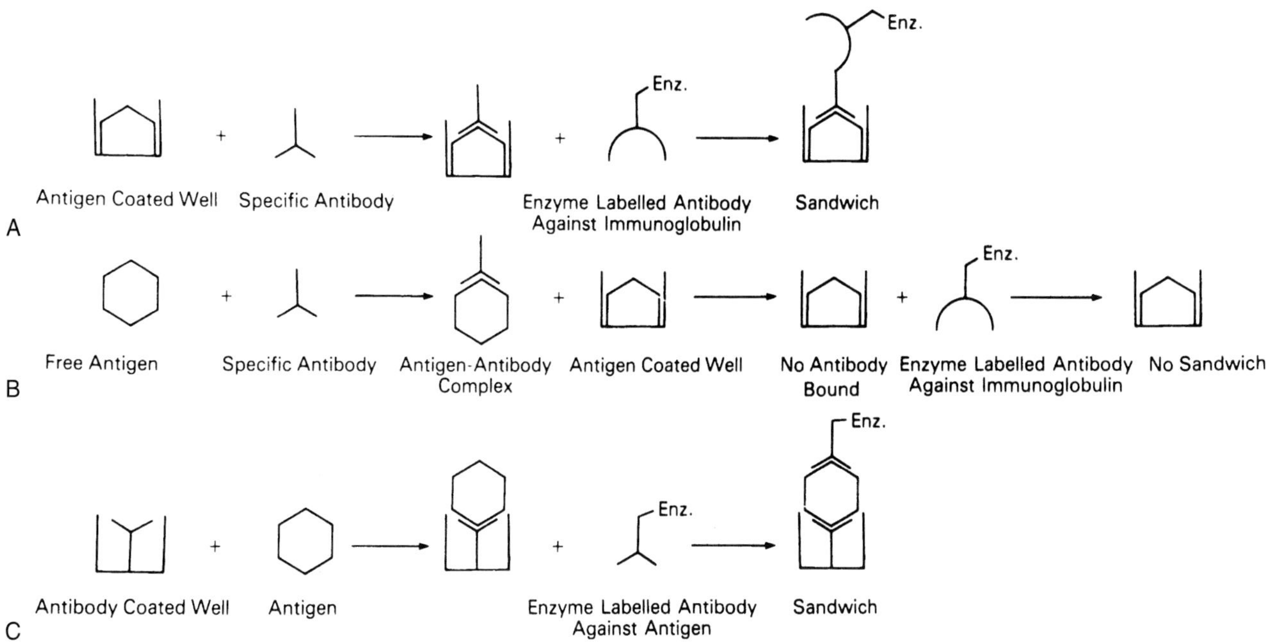

FIG. 9. Three strategies for the detection of specific antibody–antigen reactions by the ELISA technique. **A:** Direct binding. **B:** Hapten inhibition. **C:** Antigen sandwich. (Fig 9. A-C only)

previously in the RIA section on solid phase methods. In addition, some estimate of cross-reactivity between the antigen in solution and that on the plate can be obtained.

Figure 9C shows the sandwich technique for detecting antigen. Specific antibody is used to coat the microtiter wells. Antigen is then captured by the solid-phase antibody. Finally, a second antibody, linked to enzyme, is added. This binds to the solid-phase antigen–antibody complex, carrying enzyme along with it. Excess second antibody is washed off, and substrate is added. The absorbance produced is a function of the antigen concentration of the test solution, which can be determined from a standard curve. Specificity of the assay depends on the specificity of the antibodies used to coat the plate and detect antigen. Sensitivity depends on affinities and on the amount of the first antibody bound to the well, which can be increased by using affinity-purified antibodies or monoclonal antibodies in the coating step. The binding of both antibodies of the sandwich depends on divalency of the antigen, or else the two antibodies must be specific for different antigenic determinants on the same antigen molecule. If the antibodies are two different monoclonal antibodies that bind to the same monomeric antigen, this technique can be used to ascertain whether the two antibodies can bind simultaneously to the same molecule or whether they compete for the same site or sites close enough to cause steric hindrance (53).

When antibodies are serially diluted across a plate, the last colored well indicates the titer. Specificity of binding can be demonstrated by coating wells with albumin and measuring antibody binding in parallel with the antigen-coated wells. Because it can be used to test many samples in a short time, ELISA is often used to screen culture supernatants in the

production of hybridoma antibodies. The sensitivity of the method allows detection of clones producing specific antibodies at an early stage in cell growth.

An important caution when using native protein antigens to coat solid-phase surfaces (Fig. 9A) is that binding to a surface can alter the conformation of the protein. For instance, using conformation-specific monoclonal antibodies to myoglobin, Darst et al. (54) found that binding of myoglobin to a surface altered the apparent affinity of some antibodies more than that of others. This problem may be avoided by using the methods of Fig. 9C.

Enzyme-Linked Immunospot Assay

The normal ELISA assay can be modified to measure antibody production at the single-cell level. In the enzyme-linked immunospot (ELIspot) method, tissue culture plates are coated with antigen, and various cell populations are cultured on the plate for 4 hours. During that time, B cells settle to the bottom and secrete antibodies, which bind antigen nearby and produce a footprint of the antibody-secreting cell. The cells are then washed off, and a second antibody, such as enzyme-labeled goat antihuman IgG, is added. Finally, unbound antibody is washed off, and enzyme substrate is added in soft agar. Over the next 10 minutes, each footprint of enzyme activity converts the substrate to a dark spot of insoluble dye, corresponding to the localized zone where the B cell originally secreted its antibody.

Through this method, it is possible to detect as few as 10 to 20 antibody-producing B cells in the presence of 10^6 spleen cells, and typical results for immunized mice range from 200 to 500 spot-forming cells per 10^6 spleen cells (55,56).

Clearly, to work at all, this assay must be capable of detecting the amount of antibody secreted by a single immune B cell and specific enough to exclude nonspecific antibodies produced by the other nonimmune B cells. Sensitivity depends on the affinity and the amount of antibodies secreted, and it may be optimized by titering the amount of antigen on the plate.

This type of assay is useful in analyzing the cellular requirements for antibody production *in vitro,* because the number of responding B cells is measured directly. It can also be used to detect antibodies made in the presence of excess antigen. For example, in acute infections (57) and in autoimmunity (58), when antigen may be present in excess over antibody, this assay makes it possible to measure antibody-producing B cells, even though free antibody may not be detectable in circulation. It can also be used to measure local production of self-reactive antibodies in a specific tissue, such as synovium. Through the use of two detecting antibodies, each specific for a different immunoglobulin class and coupled to a different enzyme, and two substrates producing different colored dyes, cells secreting IgA and IgG simultaneously can be detected (59). ELIspot has been used to show that bacterial deoxyribonucleic acid (DNA) containing unmethylated CpG sequences is a polyclonal B cell mitogen (60).

ELIspot can also detect secreted antigens, as opposed to antibodies, by coating the plate with a capture antibody and detecting antigen with an enzyme-coupled second antibody (as in a sandwich ELISA) (Fig. 9C). For example, using plates coated with monoclonal antibody to interleukin-4, T cells secreting interleukin-4 could be detected (61). In this way, T helper 2 cells can be measured, even though a specific antibody for a marker on these cells is currently not available.

SPECIFICITY AND CROSS-REACTIVITY

The specificity of an antibody or antiserum is defined by its ability to discriminate between the antigen against which it was made (called the homologous antigen, or immunogen) and any other antigen that may be tested. In practice, it is possible to test not the whole universe of antigens but only selected antigens. In this sense, specificity can be defined experimentally only within the set of antigens being compared. Karush (28) defined a related term, *selectivity,* as the ability of an antibody to discriminate, in an all-or-none manner, between two related ligands. Thus, selectivity depends not only on the relative affinity of the antibody for the two ligands but also on the experimental lower limit for detection of reactivity. For instance, an anticarbohydrate antibody with an affinity of 10^5 M^{-1} for the immunogen may appear to be highly selective, inasmuch as reaction with a related carbohydrate with a 100-fold lower affinity, 10^3 M^{-1}, may be undetectable. On the other hand, an antibody with an affinity of 10^9 M^{-1} for the homologous ligand may appear to be less selective because any reaction with a related ligand with a 100-fold lower affinity would still be quite easily detectable.

Conversely, cross-reactivity is defined as the ability to react with related ligands other than the immunogen. More usually, this is examined from the point of view of the ligand. Thus, antigen Y may be said to cross-react with antigen X because it binds to anti-X antibodies. Note that in this sense, the two antigens, not the antibody, are cross-reactive. However, the cross-reactivity of two antigens, X and Y, can be defined only with regard to a particular antibody or antiserum. For instance, a different group of anti-X antibodies may not react at all with Y, and so, with regard to these antibodies, Y would not be cross-reactive with X. The term may be used in a different sense: that some anti-X antibodies cross-react with antigen Y.

In most cases, cross-reactive ligands have lower affinity than the immunogen for a particular antibody. However, exceptions can occur, in which a cross-reactive antigen binds with a higher affinity than the homologous antigen itself. This phenomenon is called *heterocliticity,* and the antigen that has a higher affinity for the antibody than does the immunogen is said to be *heteroclitic.* Antibodies that manifest this behavior are also described as heteroclitic antibodies. A good example is the case of antibodies raised in C57BL/10 mice against the hapten nitrophenyl acetyl (NP). These antibodies have been shown by Mäkelä and Karjalainen (62) to bind with higher affinity to the cross-reactive hapten nitroiodophenyl acetyl than to the immunogen itself. Another example is the case of retro-inverso or retro-D peptides (63–67). By reversing the chirality from L to D amino acids, and simultaneously reversing the sequence of amino acids, it is possible to produce a peptide that is resistant to proteolysis and has its side chains approximately in the same position as the original L amino acid peptide, with the exception of some amino acids with secondary chiral centers such as Thr and Ile. However, the backbone NH and CO moieties are reversed. Antibodies that interact with only the side chains might not distinguish these peptides, whereas antibodies that interact with the main chain as well as side chains may distinguish them and may have potentially higher or lower affinity. In a study of monoclonal antibodies to a hexapeptide from histone H3, some bound the retro-D form with higher affinity than the native sequence, and some did not (65,66). The former are an example of heterocliticity. In addition to greater binding affinity, the retro-D peptides may have even greater activity *in vivo* because of their resistance to proteolysis (63–67). This stability makes them more useful as drugs as well (63,64,68).

Cross-reactivity has often been detected by methods such as the Ouchterlony test, hemagglutination (see later descriptions of both of these), or similar methods, which have in common the fact that they do not distinguish well between differences in affinity and differences in concentration. This practical aspect, coupled with the heterogeneity of immune antisera, has led to ambiguities in the usage of the terms *cross-reactivity* and *specificity.* With the advent of RIA and ELISA techniques, this ambiguity in the terminology, as well as in the interpretation of data, has become apparent.

For these reasons, Berzofsky and Schechter (69) defined two forms of cross-reactivity and, correspondingly, two forms

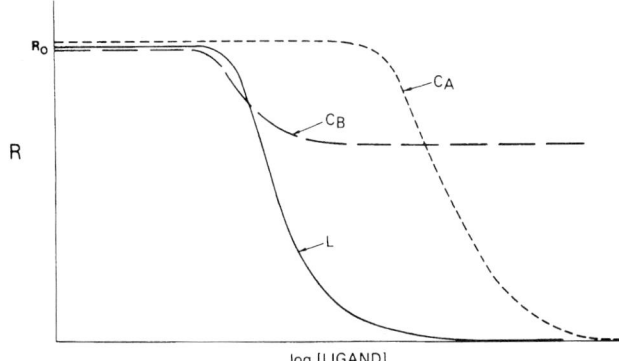

FIG. 10. Schematic radioimmunoassay binding curves for homologous ligand L and cross-reacting ligands. Cross-reacting ligand C_A manifests type 1 or true cross-reactivity, demonstrated by complete inhibition of tracer ligand binding, and a lower affinity. Ligand C_B displays type 2 cross-reactivity or determinant sharing, as recognized from the plateau at less than 100% inhibition, but not necessarily a lower affinity. The ordinate R is the ratio of bound/free radiolabeled tracer ligand, and R_0 is the limit of R as the concentration of all ligands, including tracer, approaches zero. From (69), with permission.

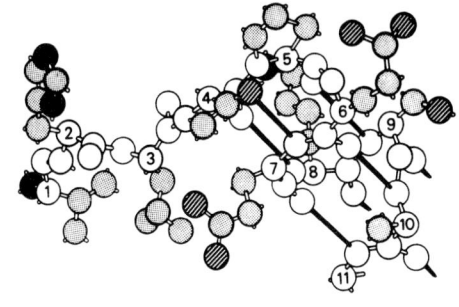

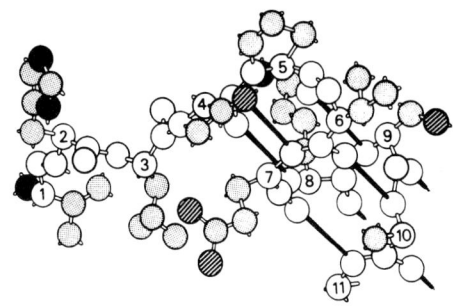

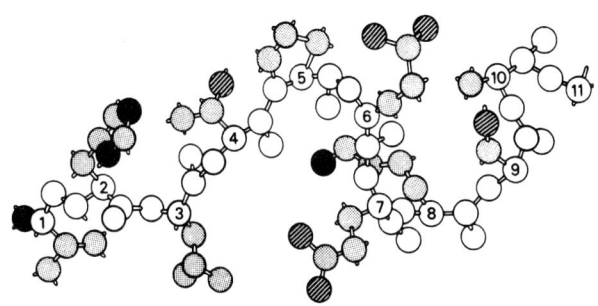

of specificity. These two forms of cross-reactivity are illustrated by the two prototype competition RIA curves in Fig. 10. In reality, most antisera display both phenomena simultaneously.

Type 1, or true, cross-reactivity is defined as the ability of two ligands to react with the same site on the same antibody molecule, possibly with different affinities. For example, the related haptens dinitrophenyl and trinitrophenyl may react with different affinity for antibodies raised to dinitrophenyl hapten. In protein antigens, such differences could occur with small changes in primary sequence (e.g., the conservative substitution of threonine for serine) or with changes in conformation, such as the cleavage of the protein into fragments (Fig. 11) (69–73). If a peptide fragment contained all the contact residues in an antigenic determinant (i.e., those that contact the antibody-combining site), it may cross-react with the native determinant for antibodies against the native form but with lower affinity, because the peptide would not retain the native conformation (see Chapter 8). This type of affinity difference is illustrated by competitor C_A in Fig. 10, in which complete displacement of tracer can be achieved at high enough concentrations of C_A, but higher concentrations of C_A than of the homologous ligand, L, are required to produce any given degree of inhibition.

A separate issue from affinity differences is the issue of whether the cross-reactive ligand reacts with all or only a subpopulation of the antibodies in a heterogeneous serum. This second type of cross-reactivity—type 2 cross-reactivity, or shared reactivity—can therefore occur only when the antibody population is heterogeneous, as in most conventional antisera. In this case, the affinity of the cross-reactive ligand may be greater than, less than, or equal to that of the homologous ligand for those antibodies with which it inter-

FIG. 11. An artist's drawing of the amino terminal region of the ß chain of hemoglobin. **A:** The first 11 residues of the β^A chain. **B:** The comparable regions of the β^S chain. The substitution of valine for the normal glutamic acid at position 6 makes a distinct antigenic determinant to which a subpopulation of antibodies may be isolated (70,71). **C:** A schematic diagram of the sequence in **A** unfolded as occurs when the protein is denatured. This region may be cleaved from the protein, or the peptide may be synthesized (72), which would result in changed antigenic reactivity. An antiserum to hemoglobin (or the ß chain thereof) may exhibit cross-reactivity with the structures shown in **B** and **C**, but the molecular mechanisms would be different. Polypeptide backbone atoms are in *white* in the side chains, oxygen atoms are *hatched*, nitrogen atoms are *black*, and carbon atoms are *lightly stippled*. Adapted from (69,73), with permission.

acts. Therefore, the competition curve is not necessarily displaced to the right, but the inhibition reaches a plateau at less than complete inhibition, as illustrated by competitor C_B in Fig. 10. As an example, consider the case of a protein with determinants X and Y and an antiserum against this protein containing both anti-X and anti-Y antibodies. A mutant

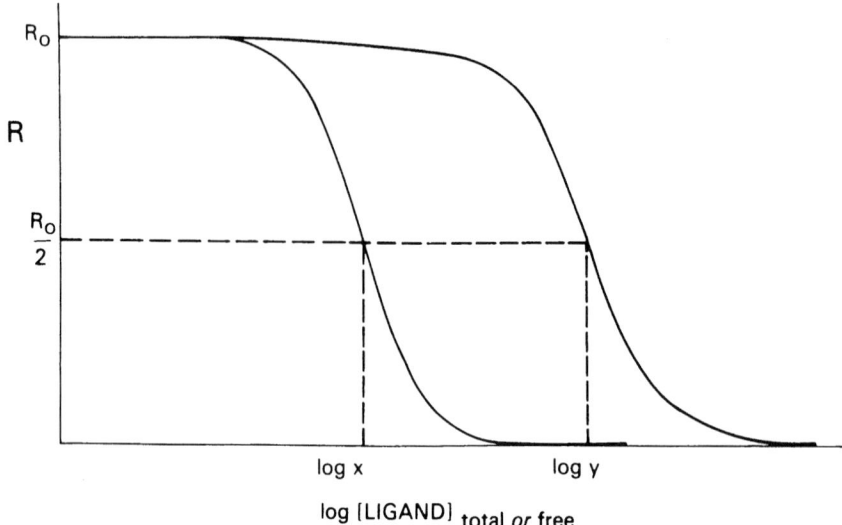

FIG. 12. Schematic radioimmunoassay binding curves showing (a) the effect of affinity on both the midpoint and the slope at the midpoint and (b) the value of using free [ligand] rather than total [ligand]. Ordinate R is the ratio of bound/free radiolabeled tracer ligand, and R_0 is the limit of R as all ligand concentrations approach zero. If x and y are the concentrations of ligands X and Y that reduce R to exactly $R_0/2$, then if the abscissa is total ligand concentration, $x = 1/K_X + [S]_t/2$ and $y = 1/K_Y + [S]_t/2$, where $[S]_t$ is the concentration of antibody binding sites and K_X and K_Y are the affinities of the antibody for the respective ligands. However, if the abscissa is free ligand concentration, $x = 1/K_X$ and $y = 1/K_Y$ so that the ratio x/y (or the difference $\log x - \log y$ on a log plot) corresponds to the ratio of affinities K_Y/K_X. Note that the slopes at the midpoints are the same on a log scale, but that for Y would be only K_Y/K_X that for X on a linear scale. From (69), with permission.

protein in which determinant Y was so altered as to be unrecognizable by anti-Y, but determinant X was intact, would manifest type 2 cross-reactivity. It would compete with the wild-type protein only for anti-X antibodies (possibly even with equal affinity) but not for anti-Y antibodies.

Of course, both types of cross-reactivity could occur simultaneously. A classic example is the peptide fragment discussed in the case of type I cross-reactivity previously. Suppose the fragment contained the residues of determinant X, albeit not in the native conformation, but did not contain the residues of a second determinant, Y, which was also expressed on the native protein. If the antiserum to the native protein consisted of anti-X and anti-Y, the peptide would compete only for anti-X antibodies (type 2 cross-reactivity) but would have a lower affinity than the native protein even for these antibodies. Thus, the competition curve would be shifted to the right and would plateau before reaching complete inhibition.[8]

In the case of a homogeneous (e.g., monoclonal) antibody in which only type 1 cross-reactivity can occur, the differences in affinity for different cross-reactive ligands can be

quantitated by a method analogous to the B/F versus F method described previously. Suppose that ligands X and Y cross-react with homologous ligand L for a monoclonal antibody. If the bound/free ($B/F = R$) ratio for radiolabeled tracer ligand L is plotted as a function of the log of the concentration of competitors X and Y, two parallel competition curves are obtained (Fig. 12) (69) under the appropriate conditions (discussed later). The first condition is that the concentration of free tracer be less than $1/K_L$, the affinity for tracer. In this case, it can be shown (69) that

$$K_X \simeq \frac{1}{[X]_{\text{free}}} \qquad [41]$$

at the midpoint where $R = R_0/2$, where K_X is the affinity for X. This is analogous to Equation 21 for the case in which unlabeled homologous ligand is the competitor. Also, in analogy with Equation 23, it can be shown that if the total concentration of competitor, $[X]_t$, is used instead of the free concentration, $[X]_{\text{free}}$, an error term will arise, yielding

$$[X]_t \text{ (at } R = R_0/2) = \frac{1}{K_X} + \frac{[S]_t}{2} \qquad [42]$$

Thus, with the competitor on a linear scale, the difference in midpoint for competitors X and Y correspond to the difference $1/K_X - 1/K_Y$ regardless of whether the free or total competitor is plotted, but the ratio of midpoint concentrations equals KX/KY only if the free concentrations are used. This last point is important if the log of competitor concentration

---

[8] An ambiguous case in which the distinction between the two types of cross-reactivity would be blurred could occur experimentally. For example, in the case of antibodies that all react with determinant X but have a very wide range of affinities for X, some such antibodies may have such a low affinity for cross-reactive determinant X' that they would appear not to bind X' at all. Then a competition curve with X' might appear to reach a plateau at incomplete inhibition even though all the antibodies were specific for X and the only difference between X and X' was affinity.

is plotted, as is usually done, because the horizontal displacement between the two curves on a log scale corresponds to the ratio $[X]/[Y]$, not the difference (69).

If a second condition also holds—namely, that the concentration of bound tracer is small in comparison with the antibody site concentration $[S]_t$—then the slopes (on a linear scale) of the curves at their respective midpoints (where $R = R_0/2$) are proportional to the affinity for that competitor, K_X or K_Y (69). (Both conditions can be met by keeping tracer L small relative to both KL and $[S]_t$.) When $[X]_{free}$ and $[Y]_{free}$ are plotted on a log scale, the slopes appear to be equal (i.e., the curves appear parallel), because a parallel line shifted m-fold to the right on a log scale is actually $1/m$ as steep, at any point, in terms of the antilog, as the abscissa.

When the antibodies are heterogeneous in affinity, the curves are broadened and are generally not parallel. When heterogeneity of specificity is present and type 2 cross-reactivity occurs, the fractional inhibition achieved at the plateau in a B/F versus free competitor plot is not proportional to the fraction of antibodies reacting with that competitor, but it is proportional to a weighted fraction, for which the antibody concentrations are weighted by their affinity for the tracer (69).

These two types of cross-reactivity lead naturally to two definitions of specificity (69). The overall specificity of a heterogeneous antiserum is a composite of both of these facets of specificity. Type 1 specificity is based on the relative affinities of the antibody for the homologous ligand and any cross-reactive ligands. If the affinity is much higher for the homologous ligand than for any cross-reactive ligand tested, then the antibody is said to be highly specific for the homologous ligand; that is, it discriminates very well between this ligand and the others. If the affinity for cross-reactive ligands is below the threshold for detection in an experimental situation, then type 1 specificity gives rise to selectivity, as discussed previously [cf. Karush (28)]. The specificity can even be quantitated in terms of the ratio of affinities for the homologous ligand and a cross-reactive ligand [cf. Johnston and Eisen (74)]. This type 1 specificity is what most immunochemists would call true specificity, just as we have called type 1 cross-reactivity true cross-reactivity.

The common use of the term *cross-reactivity* to include type 2 or partial reactivity leads to a second definition of specificity, which applies only to heterogeneous populations of antibodies such as antisera. We call this *type 2 specificity*. If all the antibodies in the mixture react with the immunogen but only a small proportion react with any single cross-reactive antigen, then the antiserum would be said to be relatively specific for the immunogen. Note that it does not matter whether the affinity of a subpopulation that reacts with a cross-reactive antigen is high or low (type 1 cross-reactivity). As long as that subpopulation is a small fraction of the antibodies, the mixture is specific. Thus, type 2 specificity depends on the relative concentrations of antibodies in the heterogeneous antiserum, not just on their affinities. Also, these relative concentrations of antibody subpopulations can be used to compare the specificity of a single antiserum for two cross-reactive ligands. However, it would not be meaningful to compare the specificity of two different antisera for the same ligand by comparing the fraction of antibodies in each serum that reacted with that ligand. Although type 2 specificity may appear a less classic concept of specificity than type 1, it is type 2 specificity that is primarily measured in such assays as the Ouchterlony double immunodiffusion test, and it carries equal weight with type 1 specificity in such assays as hemagglutination, discussed later. Type 2 specificity also leads naturally to the concept of "multispecificity" described as follows.

Multispecificity

The theory of multispecificity, introduced and analyzed by Talmadge (75) and Inman (76,77) and discussed on a structural level by Richards et al. (78), suggests a mechanism by which the great diversity and specificity of antisera can be explained without the need for a correspondingly large repertoire of antibody structures (or structural genes). The idea is that each antibody may actually bind, with high affinity, a wide variety of quite diverse antigens. When immunogen A is used for immunization, the clinician selects for many distinct antibodies, which have in common only that they all react with A. In fact, each antibody may react with other compounds, but if fewer than 1% of the antibodies bind B, and fewer than 1% bind C, and so on, then in accordance with type 2 specificity, the whole antiserum appears to be highly specific for A. The subpopulation that binds B may react with an affinity for B as high as or higher than that for A, so that the population would not have type 1 specificity for A. The same population would presumably be selected if B were used in immunization, as well as with perhaps hundreds of other immunogens with which these antibodies react. The net result would be that the diversity of highly (type 2) specific antisera that an organism could generate would be much greater than the diversity of B cell clones (or antibody structures) that it would require. This principle can explain how polyclonal antisera can sometimes appear paradoxically more specific than a monoclonal antibody.

OTHER METHODS

We mention only a few of the other methods for measuring antigen–antibody interactions. Useful techniques include quenching of the tryptophan fluorescence of the antibody by certain antigens on binding (79) (a sensitive method useful for such experiments as fast kinetic studies); antibody-dependent cellular cytotoxicity; immunofluorescence, including flow cytometry; immunohistochemistry; and inhibition by antibody of plaque formation by antigen-conjugated bacteriophage (80) (a method as sensitive as RIA because inhibition of even a few phage virions can be detected).

Quantitative Precipitin

Among the earliest known properties of antibodies were their ability to neutralize pathogenic bacteria and their ability to form precipitates with bacterial culture supernatants. Both activities of the antiserum were highly specific for the bacterial strain against which the antiserum was made. The precipitates contained antibody protein and bacterial products. The supernatants contained decreased amounts of antibody protein and, under the right conditions, had lost the ability to neutralize bacteria. However, quantitation of the antibody precipitated was difficult, because the precipitate contained antigen protein as well as antibody protein. Heidelberger and Kendall (81,82) solved this problem when they found that purified pneumococcal cell wall polysaccharide could precipitate with antipneumococcal antibodies. In this case, the amount of protein nitrogen measured in the precipitate was entirely attributable to antibody nitrogen, and the amount of reducing sugar was mostly attributable to the antigen. Plotting the amount of antibody protein precipitated from a constant volume of antiserum by increasing amounts of carbohydrate antigen yields the curve shown in Fig. 13.

As shown in Fig. 13A, the amount of antibody precipitated rises initially, reaches a plateau, then declines. The point of

maximum precipitation was found to coincide with the point of complete depletion of neutralizing antibodies and is called the *equivalence point.* The amount of antibody protein in the precipitate at equivalence is considered to equal the total amount of specific antibody in that volume of antiserum. The rising part of the curve is called the *antibody excess zone* (antigen limiting), and the part of the curve beyond the equivalence point is called the *antigen excess zone.*

Supernatants and precipitates were carefully analyzed for each zone of antibody or antigen excess, as shown in Fig. 13B. When antigen was limiting, the precipitate contained high ratios of antibody to antigen. The supernatant in this zone contained free antibody with no detectable antigen. As more antigen was added, the amount of antibody in the precipitate rose, but the ratio of antibody to antigen fell. At equivalence, no free antibody or antigen could be detected in the supernatant. As more antigen was added, the precipitate contained less antibody, but the ratio of antibody to antigen remained constant. The supernatant now contained antigen–antibody complexes, inasmuch as the complexes at antigen excess were small enough to remain in solution. No unbound antibody was detected.

The lattice theory (81,82) is a model of the precipitation reaction that explains these observations. It is assumed that antibodies are multivalent and antigens are bivalent or polyvalent. Thus, long chains consisting of antibody linked to antigen linked to antibody, and so on, can form. The larger the size of the aggregate, the less soluble the product is, until a precipitate is formed. In the antibody excess zone, branch points can form wherever three antibodies bind to a single antigen, yielding a large and insoluble product. For example, at the antibody-to-antigen ratio 3:1, every antigen molecule can bind three antibody molecules in a three-dimensional lattice structure. However, when equimolar amounts of antibody and antigen are mixed (the equivalence zone), the likelihood that more than two antibodies will bind each antigen molecule decreases. Thus, the number of branch points decreases, and the product consists of longer chains of alternating antibody and antigen molecules with fewer branches. As the antigen concentration reaches excess, the precipitate approaches linear chains with a molar ratio of 1:1. At even higher antigen ratios, more antigen molecules will have no or one antibody bound. One antibody bound is equivalent to a chain termination, and so shorter chain lengths are found until the product is small enough to remain soluble. Such soluble antigen–antibody "immune complexes" are detectable in the antigen excess zone, in which no free antibody is found.

Besides explaining the observed precipitation phenomena on a statistical basis, the lattice theory made the important prediction that antibodies are bivalent or multivalent. The subsequent structural characterization of antibodies (Chapter 9) revealed their molecular weight and valency. Antibodies are indeed bivalent, except for IgM, which is functionally pentavalent and forms precipitates even more efficiently.

Antigens can be polyvalent either by having multiple copies of the same determinant or by having many different

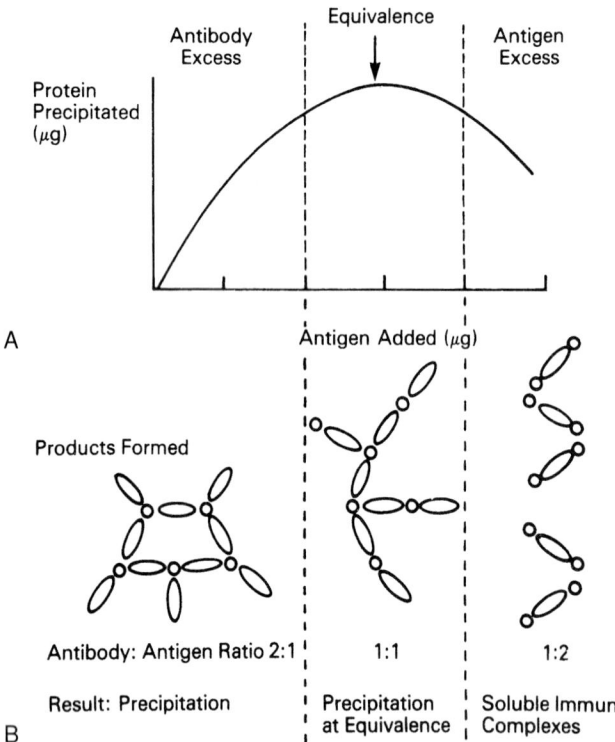

FIG. 13. Quantitative immunoprecipitation. Increasing amounts of nonprotein antigen are added to a fixed amount of specific antibody. The figure shows the amount of antibody protein **(A)** and the ratio of antibody to antigen **(B)** found in the precipitate. At antigen excess, soluble immune complexes are found in the supernatant, and the precipitate is decreased.

determinants, each of which reacts with different antibodies in a polyclonal antiserum. A good example of the former case was described in Chapter 21. The predominant antigenic determinants of polysaccharides are often the nonreducing end of the chain. Branched-chain polysaccharides have more than one end and are polyvalent. Nonbranched chains such as dextran (polymer of glucose) are monovalent for end-specific antidextran antibodies and do not precipitate them (83). However, a second group of antidextran antibodies is specific for internal glucose moieties. Because each dextran polymer consists of many of these internal units, it is polyvalent for internal $\alpha(1 \rightarrow 6)$–linked glucose-specific antibodies. Thus, unbranched dextran polymer can be used to distinguish between end-specific and internal specific antibodies, as it will precipitate with the latter antibodies but not with the former (83,84). Monomeric protein antigens, such as myoglobin (see Chapter 21) or lysozyme, are examples of the second case because they behave as if they are polyvalent for heterogeneous antisera but as if they are monovalent for monoclonal antibodies. This results from the fact that each antigen molecule has multiple antigenic determinants but only one copy of each determinant. Thus, a polyspecific antiserum can bind more than one antibody to different determinants on the same molecule and form a lattice. However, when antibodies directed against a single determinant (such as a monoclonal antibody) are used, no precipitate will form. In this case, antigen–antibody reactions must be measured by some other binding assay, such as RIA or ELISA.

Immunodiffusion and the Ouchterlony Method

One of the most useful applications of immunoprecipitation is in combination with a diffusion system (85). Diffusion could be observed by gently adding a drop of protein solution to a dish of water, without disturbing the liquid. The rate of migration of protein into the liquid is proportional to the concentration gradient multiplied by the diffusion coefficient of the protein according to Fick's law,

$$\frac{dQ}{dt} = -DA\frac{dc}{dx} \qquad [43]$$

where Q is the amount of substance that diffuses across an area A per unit time t; D is the diffusion coefficient, which depends on the size of the molecule; and dc/dx is the concentration gradient. Because antibody molecules are so large, their diffusion coefficients are quite low, and diffusion often takes 1 day or more to cover the 5 to 20 mm required in most systems. In order to stabilize the liquid phase for such long periods, a gel matrix is added to provide support without hindering protein migration. In practice, 0.3% to 1.5% agar or agarose permits migration of proteins up to the size of antibodies while preventing mechanical and thermal currents. With careful adjustment of the concentration of antibody and antigen, these systems can provide a simple analysis of the number of antigenic components and the concentration of a given component. With adjustment of the geometry of the

reactants entering the gel, immunodiffusion can provide useful information concerning antigenic identity or difference, or partial cross-reaction, as well as the purity of antigens and the specificity of antibodies.

In single diffusion methods (86–89), antibody is incorporated in the gel, and antigen is allowed to diffuse from one end of a tube gel or from a hole in a gel in a Petri dish in one or two dimensions, respectively. Over time, the antigen concentration reaches equivalence with the antibody in the gel, and a precipitin band forms. As more antigen diffuses, antigen excess is achieved at this position, and so the precipitate dissolves and the boundary of equivalence moves farther. By integrating Fick's law, we find that the distance moved is proportional to the square root of time. If two species of antigen a and b are diffusing and the antiserum contains antibodies to both, two independent bands form. These move at independent rates, depending on antigen concentration in the sample, diffusion coefficient (size), and antibody concentration in the agar. Similarly, in the two-dimensional method, at a given radius of diffusion, antigen concentration is equivalent to the antibody in the gel, and a precipitin ring forms. The higher the initial antigen concentration, the farther the antigen diffuses before precipitating and the wider the area of the ring is. The area of the ring is directly proportional to the initial antigen concentration. This method provides a convenient quantitative assay that can be used to measure immunoglobulin classes, by placing test serum in the well and antiserum to each class of human immunoglobulin in the agar. Sensitivity can be increased by lowering the concentration of antiserum in the gel, producing wider rings, because the antigen must reach a lower concentration to be at equivalence. However, if the antiserum is diluted too much, no precipitate will form.

The double diffusion methods are based on the same principles, except that instead of having one reactant incorporated in the gel at a constant concentration, both antigen and antibody are loaded some distance apart in a gel of pure agarose alone and allowed to diffuse toward each other. At some point in the gel, antigen diffusion and antibody diffusion provide sufficient concentrations of both reactants for immunoprecipitation to occur. The line of precipitation becomes a barrier for the further diffusion of the reactants, and so the precipitin band is stable. If the antigen preparation is heterogeneous and the antiserum is a heterogeneous mixture of antibodies, different bands form for each pair of antigen and antibody reacting, at positions dependent on concentration and molecular weight of each. The number of lines indicates the number of antigen–antibody systems reacting in the gel. The ability of immunodiffusion to separate different antigen–antibody systems yields a convenient estimate of antigen purity or antibody specificity.

In the most widely used Ouchterlony method of double diffusion in two dimensions (85), three or more wells are cut in an agarose gel in a dish in the pattern shown in Fig. 14. Antigen a or b is placed in the upper wells, whereas antiserum containing anti-a or anti-b antibody is placed in the lower well. Each antigen–antibody reaction system forms its

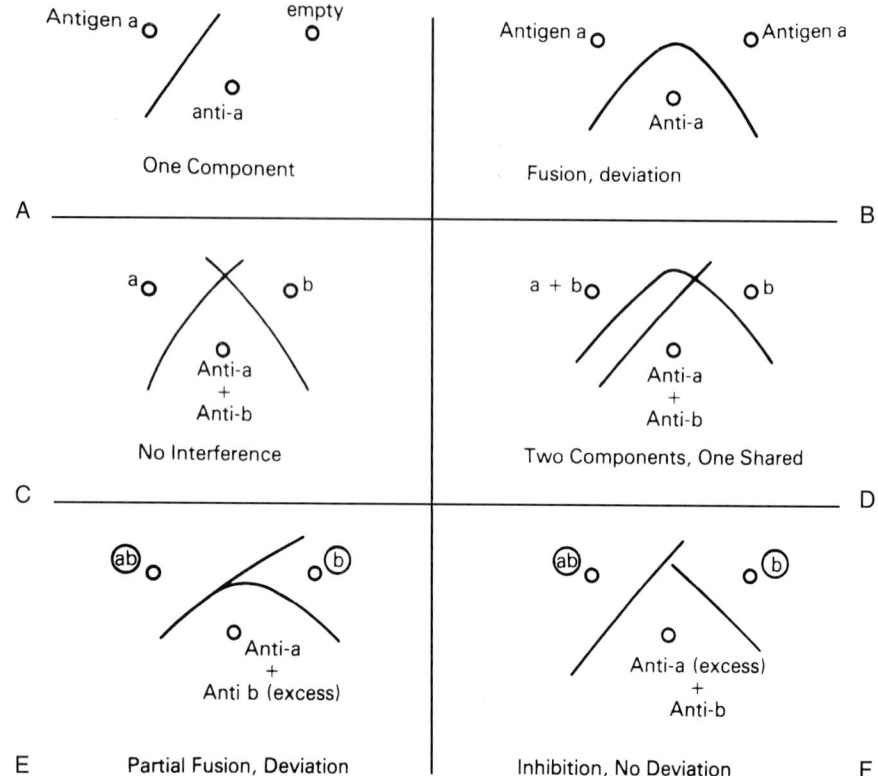

FIG. 14. Immunodiffusion of two components in two dimensions. Cross-reactions produce inhibition (*shortened bands*) or deviation (*curved bands*). Lines of identity are shown in **B** and **D**. From Ouchterlony O, Nilsson LA. Immunodiffusion and Immunoelectrophoresis. In Weir DM, ed. *Handbook of experimental immunology*. Oxford, UK: Blackwell Science, 1978:19.1–19.44. (85), with permission.

own precipitin line between the wells. As shown in Fig. 14A, this should extend an equal length on both sides of the wells. When different antigens are present in different wells (Fig. 14C), the precipitating systems do not interact immunochemically, and so the precipitin lines cross. However, when the same antigen is present in both wells (Fig. 14B), each line of precipitation becomes a barrier for the antigen and antibody involved, preventing them from diffusing past the precipitin line. This shortens the precipitin line on that side of the well. In addition, antigen diffusion from the neighboring wells shifts the zone of antigen excess, causing the equivalence line to deviate downward and meet between the two wells. Complete fusion of precipitin lines with no spurs is called a *line of identity,* which indicates that the antigen in each well reacts with all the antibody capable of reacting with antigen in the other well.

The great analytical power of this method is shown in Fig. 14D. When a mixed antigen sample is placed in one well and pure antigen b is placed in the other well, antiserum to a plus b gives the pattern shown. Two precipitin lines form with the left well and one precipitin line with the right well. The line of complete fusion allows the investigator to identify the second band as antigen b; the first band is antigen a. From their relative distance of migration, we can conclude that antigen a is in excess over antigen b, if their diffusion coefficients are comparable and both antibodies are present in equal amounts.

Finally, because the precipitin line of antigen a–anti-a is not shortened at all, there is no contamination of the right sample with antigen a, and the two antigens do not cross-react.

It is worth reemphasizing at this point that the type of cross-reactivity detected by this Ouchterlony double immunodiffusion in agar is what we have defined previously as type 2 cross-reactivity. The method is not really suitable for measuring affinity differences, which are required for quantitating type 1 cross-reactivity. Also, note that sensitivity can be increased by use of radioactive antigen and detection of the precipitate by autoradiography.

Immunoelectrophoresis

Some antigen–antibody systems are too complex for double immunodiffusion analysis, either because there are too many bands or because the bands are too close together. Immunoelectrophoresis combines electrophoresis in one dimension (Fig. 15) with immunodiffusion in the perpendicular direction. In the first step, electrophoresis separates the test antigens according to charge and size—in effect, separating the origin of diffusion of different antigens. This is equivalent to having each antigen start in a different well, as shown in Fig. 15A. A horizontal trough is then cut into the agar and filled with antiserum to all the components. Immunodiffusion occurs between the separated antigens and the linear

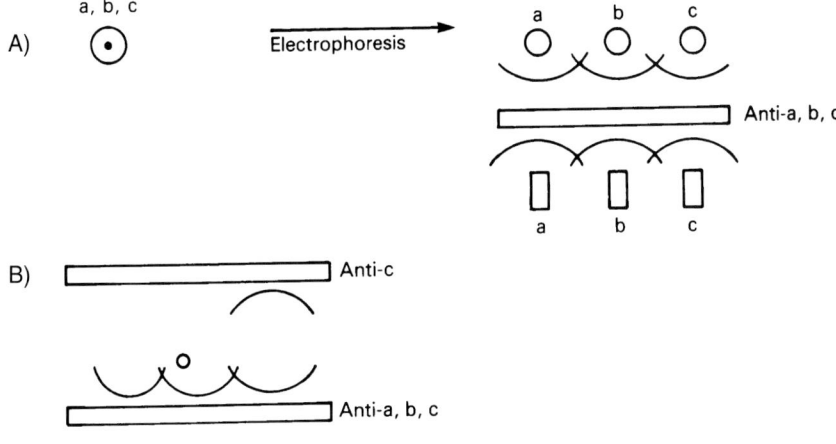

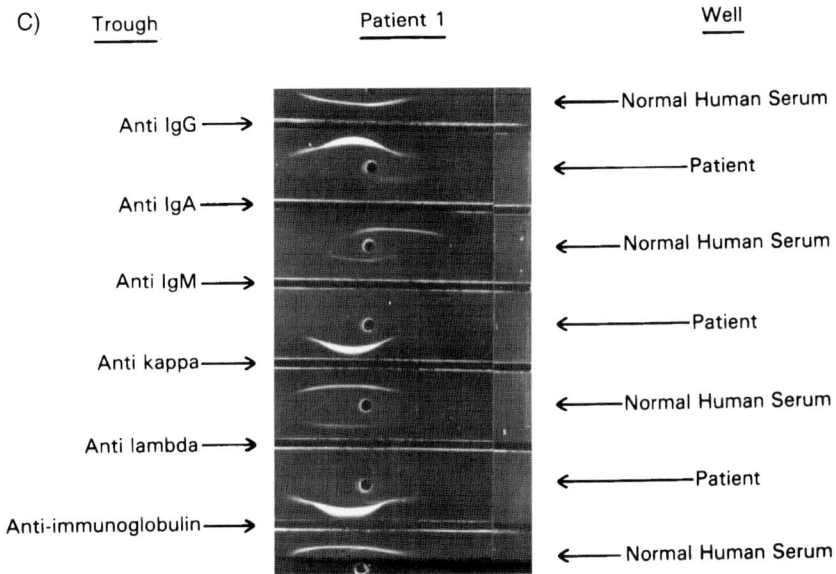

FIG. 15. Immunoelectrophoresis. A sample containing multiple components is electrophoresed in an agarose gel, which separates the antigens in the horizontal dimension. Then a horizontal trough is cut into the gel, and antiserum is added. Immunodiffusion between the separated antigens and the trough is equivalent to having separate wells, each with a different antigen (85). This technique is used to identify a myeloma protein in human serum. Sera from the patient or normal individual were placed in the circular wells and electrophoresed. Antisera were then placed in the rectangular troughs, and immunodiffusion proceeded perpendicular to the direction of electrophoresis. The abnormally strong reaction with anti–immunoglobulin G (IgG) and anti-κ, but no reaction with anti-λ antibodies, indicates a monoclonal protein (IgG, κ), because polyclonal immunoglobulin should react with both anti–light-chain antisera. Failure to form a band with anti-IgM and a reduced band with anti–immunoglobulin A show typical reduction of normal immunoglobulins in this disease. (Photograph courtesy of Theresa Wilson, National Institutes of Health, Clinical Chemistry Section.)

source of antibody. The results for a mixture of three antigens after electrophoresis approximate those shown for three antigens in separate wells (85). Fusion, deviation, and inhibition between precipitin lines can be analyzed as described previously. The resolution of each band is somewhat decreased, because of widening of the origin of diffusion during electrophoresis. However, the immunodiffusion of unseparated

human serum proteins, for example, is greatly facilitated by prior electrophoresis. Starting from a single well, only the heavier bands would be visible. However, prior electrophoresis makes it possible for each electrophoretic species to make its own precipitin line. Monospecific antiserum can be placed in a parallel horizontal trough, so that each band of precipitation can be identified (Fig. 15B). Immunoelectrophoresis is commonly used to diagnose myeloma proteins in human serum. The unknown serum is placed in wells and electrophoresed; this is followed by immunodiffusion against antihuman serum, antihuman κ antiserum, or antihuman λ antiserum. A widening in the arc of IgG precipitation with antiserum specific for IgG, A or M heavy chains or for κ or λ light chains human immunoglobulin serum suggests the presence of an abnormal immunoglobulin species. At this same electrophoretic mobility, a precipitin line with anti-κ reactivity but not anti-λ reactivity, or vice versa, strongly suggests the diagnosis of myeloma or monoclonal gammopathy, because these proteins are known to arise from a single clone that synthesizes only one or the other light chain. All normal electrophoretic species of human immunoglobulins contain both light chain isotypes, although κ exceeds λ by the ratio of 2:1 in humans. As shown in Fig. 15C, the abnormal arc with γ mobility reacts with anti-IgG and anti-κ antiserum but not with anti-λ antiserum. Thus, it is identified as an IgG-κ monoclonal protein.

Hemagglutination and Hemagglutination Inhibition

Hemagglutination

A highly sensitive technique yielding semiquantitative values for the interaction of antibody with antigen involves the agglutination by antibodies of red blood cells coated with the antigen (90). Because the antigen is not endogenous to the red blood cell surface, the reaction is called *passive hemagglutination.* Untreated red blood cells are negatively charged, and electrostatic forces oppose agglutination. After treatment with tannic acid (0.02 mg/mL for 10 minutes at 37°C), however, they clump readily.

Untreated red blood cells are easily coated with polysaccharide antigens, which they adsorb readily. After tanning, the uptake of some protein antigens is good, resulting in a sensitive reagent, whereas for others it tends to be quite variable; this has been the limiting factor in the usefulness of this method for certain antigens. Apparently, slightly aggregated or partially denatured protein antigens are adsorbed preferentially (90).

The test for specific antibodies is done by serially diluting the antiserum in the U-shaped wells of a microtiter plate and adding antigen-coated red blood cells. In the presence of specific antibodies, agglutinated cells settle into an even carpet covering the round bottom of the well. Unagglutinated red blood cells slide down the sides and form a button at the very bottom of the well. The titer of a sample is the highest dilution at which definite agglutination occurs. With hyperimmune antisera, inhibition of agglutination is observed at high doses of antibody; this is termed a *prozone effect.* Two interpretations have been offered: one is that, at great antibody excess, each cell is coated with antibody, so cross-linking by the same antibody molecule becomes improbable. The second interpretation is the existence of some species of inefficient or "blocking" antibodies that occupy antigen sites without causing aggregation of cells (7). To ensure antigen speci-

ficity, the antiserum should be absorbed against uncoated red blood cells before the assay, and an uncoated red blood cell control should be included with each assay.

The advantage of this test is its greater sensitivity, inasmuch as molecular events are amplified by the agglutination of an entire red blood cell. Antigen specificity is the same as for immunoprecipitation. IgM is up to 750 times more efficient than IgG at causing agglutination, which may affect interpretation of data based on titration. The titer may vary by a factor of 2 simply because of subjective estimates of the endpoint.

Hemagglutination Inhibition

Once the titer of an antiserum is determined, its interaction with antigen-coated red blood cells can be used as a sensitive assay for antigen. Varying amounts of free antigen are added to constant amounts of antibody (diluted to a concentration twofold higher than the limiting concentration producing agglutination). Agglutination is inhibited when half or more of the antibody sites are occupied by free antigen. In a similar manner, the assay can be used for the detection and quantitation of anti-idiotype antibodies that react with the variable region of antibodies and sterically block antigen binding.

Immunoblot (Western Blot)

A most useful technique in the analysis of proteins is polyacrylamide gel electrophoresis (PAGE), in which charged proteins migrate through a gel in response to an electric field. When ionic detergents such as sodium dodecyl sulfate are used, the distance traveled is inversely proportional to the logarithm of molecular weight. The protein components of complex structures, such as viruses, appear as distinct bands, each at its characteristic molecular weight. Because antibodies may be unable to diffuse into the gel, it is necessary to transfer the protein bands onto a nitrocellulose membrane support first, so they can be detected by specific antibodies. The locations of the antigens on the membrane are a faithful reproduction of the locations in the gel, and now it is easy to detect antibody binding to the specific bands that correspond to protein antigens (91).

The immunoblot is often used to detect viral proteins with specific antibodies that bind to these proteins on the nitrocellulose blot. Then a second antibody, which is either enzyme conjugated or radiolabeled, is used to detect the antigen–antibody band. The enzyme causes a localized color reaction that reveals the location of the antigen band, or the radiolabel is detected by exposing the nitrocellulose to photographic film. Crude viral antigen preparations can be used, because only bands that correspond to viral antigens are detected by antibodies, and this accounts for the specificity of the assay.

Typical results are shown in Fig. 16. Human immunodeficiency virus type 1 (HIV-1) was cultured in susceptible H9 cells, and the virus concentrated from the cell supernatant

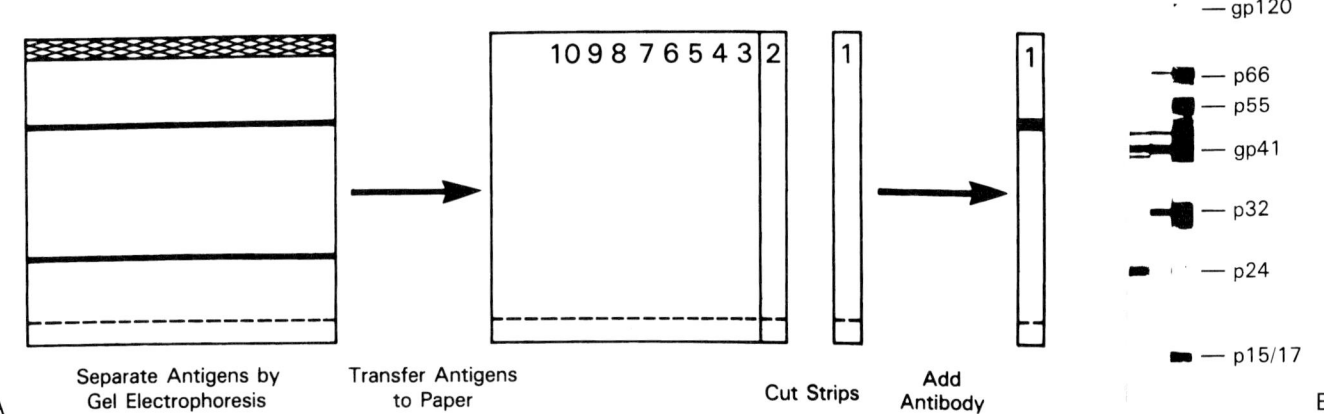

FIG. 16. A: Western blot technique. The antigen preparation is run through a polyacrylamide gel, which separates its components into different bands. These bands are then transferred to paper by electrophoresis in the horizontal dimension. The paper is cut into strips. Each strip is incubated with test antibodies, followed by further incubation with enzyme-labeled second antibodies. If the test antibodies bind to the component antigens, they will produce discrete dark bands at the corresponding positions on the strip. **B:** Clinical specimens from patients with acquired immunodeficiency syndrome tested on strips bearing human immunodeficiencyvirus–1 viral antigens, showing antibodies to viral gag (p15/17, p24, and p55 precursor), pol (p66 and possibly p32), and env (gp41 and gp120) proteins. *Lane 1* is the negative control, and *lanes 2 to 4* are sera from three different patients.

by sedimentation. The viral proteins were separated by PAGE and detected by immunoblot, using the serum of infected patients. Each antigen band recognized by the antiserum has been identified as a viral component or precursor protein. With monospecific antisera, it can be shown that the glycoprotein (gp) 160 precursor is processed to the gp120 and gp41 envelope proteins, a p66 precursor is processed to the p51 mature form of reverse transcriptase, and a p55 precursor becomes the p24 and p17 core antigens of the virus (92). The practical uses of the HIV Western blot include diagnosing infection, screening blood units to prevent HIV transmission, and testing new vaccines.

Surface Plasmon Resonance

In surface plasmon resonance (SPR), the electromagnetic properties of light are used to measure the binding affinity of a variety of biological molecules, including antigen–antibody pairs. In this method, polarized light passes through a glass plate coated on the back surface with a thin metal film, usually gold. Biological materials binding to the metal film behind the plate can alter its refractive index in ways that affect the angle and intensity of reflected light.

At angles close to perpendicular, light passes through the glass, although it bends at the interface because of differences in the refractive index of glass and what is behind it. Above a certain angle, called the *critical angle,* bending is so great that total internal reflection occurs. Small changes in refractive index behind the glass can be detected as significant changes in the critical angle, where light reflection occurs, and in the intensity of reflected light at this angle. By reading the

reflected light intensity in a diode array detector, the critical angle and intensity can be determined simultaneously.

Because of the wave nature of light, the effect of refractive index in the gold film extends about one wavelength beyond the glass, or about 300 to 700 nm (93). Within this layer, if an antigen is covalently attached to the gold, then antibody binding can be detected as a change in refractive index, resulting in a different critical angle and a different intensity of the reflected light.

SPR systems have three essential features (94): an optical system that allows determination of the critical angle and light intensity at the same time; a coupling chemistry that links antigen or antibody to the gold surface; and a flow system that rapidly delivers the complete molecule in the mobile phase. Therefore, SPR can measure the rate of binding, rather than the rate of diffusion. Because binding causes a physical change in the gold film, there is no need to label the antibody with radioactivity or to detect binding with an enzyme conjugated to a second antibody. Under optimal conditions, molecular binding interactions can be followed in real time.

A typical SPR experiment is shown in Fig. 17. HIV gp120 of type IIIB (left panel) or MN (right panel) were fixed to the gold layer, and various concentrations of monoclonal antibody to gp120 were added to the flow cell (95). Over the first 1,000 seconds, antibody binding was measured as a change in reflected light (in response units), allowing a calculation of the rate constant for the forward reaction of antibody binding. Once the signal reached a plateau, antibody was washed out of the flow cell, and the decrease in SPR signal over time indicated the rate at which antibody came off the antigen. The

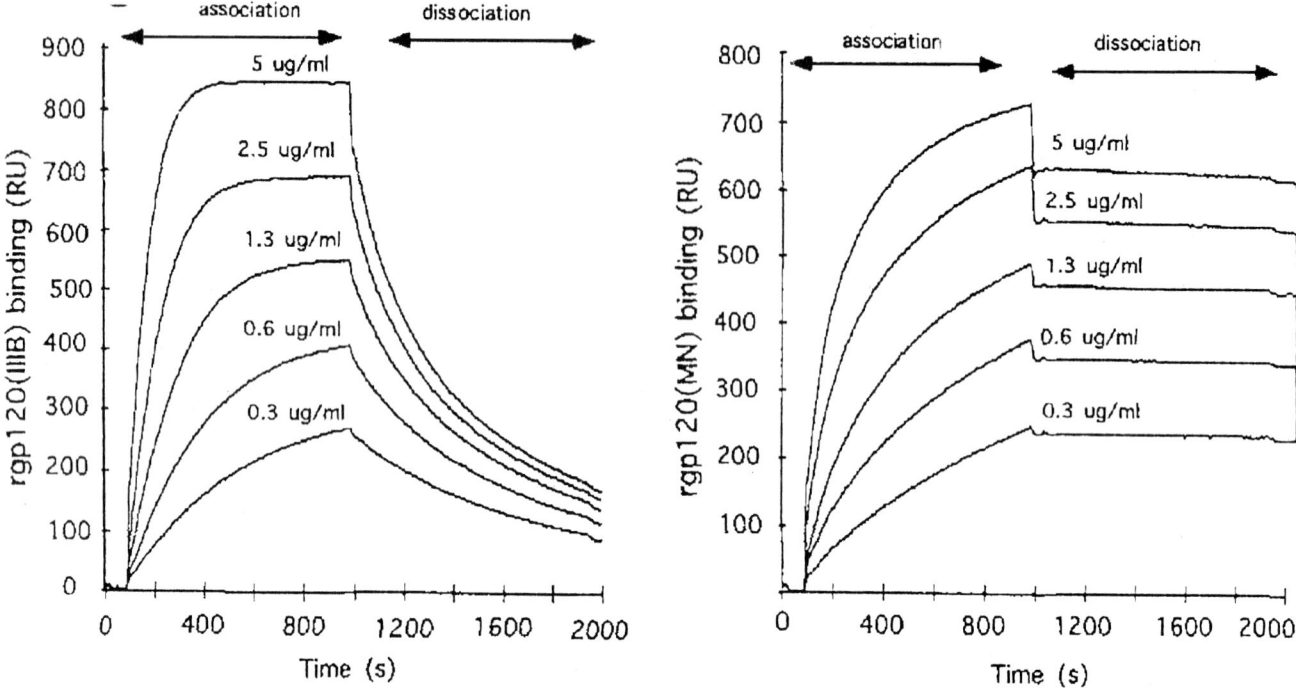

FIG. 17. Monoclonal antibody to glycoprotein 120 was introduced into the flow cell at time 0, and antibody binding was monitored over time as a change in the critical angle, measured in response units. After 1,000 seconds, free antibody was washed out, and the release of bound antibody was measured as a decrease in refractive index. Lower affinity binding to glycoprotein 120 from the IIIB strain (*left*) was shown as a faster "off rate," in comparison with the very slow rate of antibody release from the MN strain (*right*). These results, obtained under nonequilibrium conditions, provide direct measurement of the forward and reverse rate constants for antibody binding, and the ratio of these two provides the affinity constant. Modified from (95), with permission.

"on rate" for antibody binding to IIIB gp120 (left) was about twice as fast as for MN at each antibody concentration. However, the "off rate" was about 50-fold slower for MN than for IIIB. Combining these kinetic results indicates much greater binding affinity for gp120 of MN type, which may explain the observation that MN type virus was 10-fold more sensitive to neutralization by this antibody than was the IIIB strain.

MONOCLONAL ANTIBODIES

Homogeneous immunoglobulins have long played important roles in immunological research. Starting in the 1950s, Kunkel and colleagues studied sera from human patients with multiple myeloma and recognized the relationship between abnormal myeloma proteins and normal serum globulins (96). Potter and colleagues characterized numerous mouse myeloma tumors and identified the antigenic specificities of some of them (97). Human and mouse myeloma proteins were studied as representative immunoglobulins and recognized for the advantages they had with proteins as diverse as antibodies in studies of immunoglobulin structure, function, and genetics. It was not yet possible, however, to induce monoclonal immunoglobulins of desired specificity.

This goal was achieved by the introduction of hybridoma technology by Köhler and Milstein (1,98) and by Margulies et al. (99) in the 1970s. Since that time, monoclonal antibodies

have come to play an enormous role in biological research and applications. They offer as advantages the relative ease of the production and purification of large quantities of antibody, the uniformity of antibody batches, and the ready availability of immunoglobulin messenger RNA and DNA from the hybrid cell lines.

Derivation of Hybridomas

Hybridomas producing monoclonal antibodies are generated by the somatic cell fusion of two cell types: antibody-producing cells from an immunized animal, which by themselves die in tissue culture in a relatively short time, and myeloma cells, which contribute their immortality in tissue culture to the hybrid cell. The myeloma cells are variants carrying drug selection markers, so that only the myeloma cells that have fused with spleen cells providing the missing enzyme will survive under selective conditions. In initial work, researchers used myeloma cells that secreted their own immunoglobulin products, but later such fusion partners were replaced by myeloma variants that fail to express immunoglobulin (100,101), so that the fused cell secretes exclusively antibody of the desired specificity. Successful hybridoma production is influenced by the characteristics of the cell populations (immune lymphocytes and myeloma fusion partner), the fusion conditions, and the subsequent

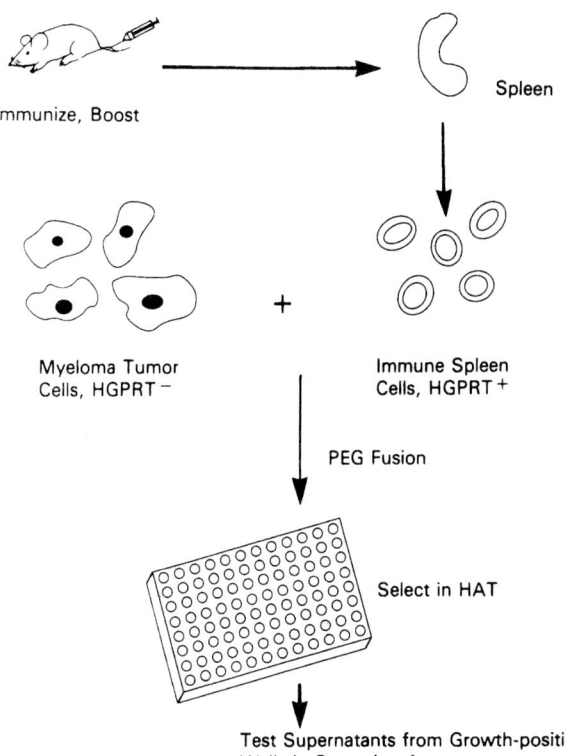

FIG. 18. Production of hybridomas. Steps in the derivation of hybridomas can be outlined as shown. Spleen cells from immunized donors are fused with myeloma cells bearing a selection marker. The fused cells are then cultured in selective medium until visible colonies grow, and their supernatants are then screened for antibody production.

selection and screening of the hybrids. A diagrammatic version of the overall process of hybridoma derivation is presented in Fig. 18.

In this section, we do not attempt to provide a detailed, step-by-step protocol for laboratory use. For that purpose, the reader is referred to monographs and reviews on the subject, including a detailed laboratory protocol with many hints and mention of problems to avoid (102).

Hybridomas Derived from Species Other than Mice

Laboratory mice are the species most commonly immunized for hybridoma production, but for a variety of reasons, other animal species often have advantages. If an antigen of interest is nonpolymorphic in the mouse, the mouse component might be immunogenic in other species, whereas mice would be tolerant to it. In the case of hybridomas for clinical use, mouse antibodies have the drawback of inducing antimouse immunoglobulin immune responses with possible deleterious effects; therefore, derivation of human hybridomas is important.

Several approaches to the derivation of hybridomas in species other than mouse have been taken. First, interspecies hybridization can be performed with mouse myeloma fusion partners. The resulting hybrids are often unstable and

throw off chromosomes, but it is sometimes possible to select clones that produce antibody in a stable manner. Examples of this include rat-mouse fusion to produce antibody to the mouse crystallizable fragment (Fc) receptor (103), and hamster-mouse fusion to produce antibody to the mouse CD3 equivalent (104). Rabbit-mouse hybridomas have also been described (105).

A second approach is the use of fusion partner cells from the desired species. Myeloma variants carrying drug selection markers are available in a number of species. A rat myeloma line adapted for this purpose, IR983F, was described by Bazin (106). This approach avoids some of the instability in interspecies hybrids and allows ascites production in homologous hosts.

Production of human hybridomas is of special importance, because their use in therapies would avoid the problem of human immune responses to immunoglobulin derived from other animal species. Because of its clinical importance, this subject is discussed in detail in the later section on applications.

Use of Gene Libraries to Derive Monoclonal Antibodies

Monoclonal antibodies produced by hybridoma technology are derived from B cells of immunized animals. An alternative technology entails the use of gene libraries and expression systems instead. This approach has the advantages of avoiding labor-intensive immunizations of animals and the screening of antibody-containing supernatants. Another advantage of the approach is circumventing tolerance. It is possible to derive monoclonal antibodies to antigens expressed in the animal species that donated the gene library, including highly conserved antigens for which there may be no available responder that does not express the antigen.

The first version of such an approach involved preparation of V_H and V_L libraries and expression of the libraries in bacteria. Further development of the system led to use of V_H and V_L libraries made separately and then to preparation of a combinatorial library by cleaving, mixing, and religating the libraries at a restriction site (107,108). A linker can be used so that both V_H and V_L can be expressed on one covalent polypeptide; the flexibility of the linker allows association of the V_H and V_L in a normal three-dimensional configuration and thus formation of an antigen-binding site (108).

Another innovation involves expression of V_H and $V\kappa$ genes on the surface of bacteriophage as fusion proteins with a phage protein, to permit rapid screening of large numbers of sequences (108–110). Adsorption of antibody-bearing phage on antigen-coated surfaces allows positive selection of phage containing DNA that encodes the desired variable reginal fragment (Fv). This technique can be applied to combinatorial variable region gene libraries (109,110).

Human antibody gene sequences can be recovered by polymerase chain reaction from peripheral blood cells (111), bone marrow (112), or human cells reimmunized in mice with severe combined immunodeficiency disease (113). The phage display technique can then be used to select antigen-binding clones and derive human reagents of desired specificity, such as antibody to hepatitis surface antigen (111) or HIV envelope (112).

One limitation in the phage library technique initially was low affinity of the monoclonal antibodies derived. Because they were generated by a random process and not subject to further somatic mutation, they did not achieve the exquisite fit of antibodies produced *in vivo*. Several approaches have since been used to improve affinities. Hypermutation and selection has been achieved *in vitro* through the use of a bacterial mutator strain (114). The process involves multiple rounds of mutation, followed by growth in nonmutator bacteria; selection for high-affinity binding then leads to an overall 100-fold increase in affinity (114). Improved affinity has also been achieved by use of site-directed mutagenesis to alter residues in hypervariable regions affecting dissociation rates (115).

Because arbitrary combinatorial possibilities of V_H and V_L can occur in the various libraries discussed previously, the antibodies generated do not reflect the combinations actually selected and expressed in immune responses (107). It has been suggested (109) that a "natural library" could be recovered by recovering variable region genes from individual cells through polymerase chain reaction. However, recovering genes from a large enough number of representative cells does not seem a reasonable or efficient approach to repertoire studies. Thus, the combinatorial library technology does not replace hybridoma technology for many immunological studies, including studies of the immune repertoire and patterns of its expression in immune responses. What combinatorial gene libraries do provide is a powerful way to derive antibody reagents of desired specificity, including some that would not occur naturally and thus could not be derived by other means.

Applications of Monoclonal Antibodies

Since monoclonal antibodies can be made easily and reproducibly in large quantities, they allow many experiments that were not possible or practical before. Affinity chromatography based on monoclonal antibodies can be used as a step in purification of molecular species that are difficult to purify chemically. Homogeneous antibody can be crystallized and can also be crystallized together with antigen to permit the study of the structure of antibody and of antigen–antibody complexes by x-ray diffraction. Homogeneous antibodies are also very valuable in the study of antibody diversity. Such analyses have revealed much about the roles of somatic mutation, changes in affinity, and changes in clonal dominance in antibody responses.

Catalytic Antibodies

One area of interest is the use of antibody molecules to catalyze chemical reactions (116). In this role, antibodies serve as an alternative to enzymes, an alternative that can be customized and manipulated more easily in some cases.

Enzymes can also be custom designed by site-directed mutagenesis of genes for natural enzymes and selection of ones with altered properties. However, the enormous diversity of the immune repertoire provides a huge pool of possible structures that do not require individual laboratory synthesis.

The concept of antibodies as catalysts was proposed in 1952 by D. W. Woolley [cited by Lerner et al. (116)]. Use of homogeneous antibodies permitted identification of some with significant catalytic effects; MOPC167 accelerates the hydrolysis of nitrophenyl-phosphorylcholine by 770-fold (117). Polyclonal antibodies have also been reported to possess detectable enzymatic activity (118). With the advent of hybridoma technology, purposeful selection of antibodies with potent enzymatic function became possible. Antibodies have been characterized that catalyze numerous chemical reactions, with rates nearing 10^8-fold above the spontaneous rate [reviewed by Lerner et al. (116)]. One common strategy for elicitation of such antibodies is immunization with transition state analogs (119), although there are other strategies (120). Antibodies function as catalysts in a stereospecific manner (121), a valuable property.

Why would binding of an antibody to a compound catalyze covalent bond changes? The possibilities are similar to those for enzymes. To accelerate a reaction, an antibody has to lower the activation energy barrier to the reaction, which means lowering the energy of the transition state by stabilizing it. This can be achieved because of the contribution of the binding energy to the overall energy of the transition state. For this reason, an antibody that recognizes the transition state is favorable, and immunizations with analogues of the transition state have advantages.

Antibodies can serve as what has been termed an *entropy trap* (116): Binding to the antibody "freezes out" the rotational and translational degrees of freedom of the substrate and thus makes a chemical reaction far more favorable energetically. Interactions with chemical groups on the antibody can neutralize charges or bury hydrophobic groups, thereby stabilizing a constrained transition state. Molecular mechanisms of antibody-mediated catalysis vary, as do enzymatic reactions (120,122).

Discovery of such catalytic antibodies opens practical opportunities: antibodies can be customized for an application by appropriate selection, produced relatively cheaply, and purified easily. Catalytic antibodies can be developed to perform chemical reactions for which no enzyme is available. They can shield intermediates from solvent: for example, allowing reactions that do not occur in aqueous solution (123). They can form peptide bonds (124), which suggests a new approach to polypeptide synthesis. Thus, catalytic antibodies will probably have many practical applications.

Bispecific and Bifunctional Antibodies

Antibodies produced naturally by a single B cell have only one binding site specificity, and their effector functions are determined by the structure of the Fc domain. The availability of monoclonal antibodies made possible the generation of many artificial antibodies as cross-linking reagents, by linking binding sites of two specificities to form bispecific antibodies. Various techniques have been used to prepare such hybrid or bispecific antibodies, and they have been put to a variety of uses. In addition, antibody binding sites can be linked to other functional domains such as toxins, enzymes, or cytokines to create "bifunctional antibodies" (125).

One of the most powerful uses of hybrid antibodies is in redirecting cytolytic cells to targets of a defined specificity. In one early demonstration of this use (126), a monoclonal antibody specific for the $Fc\gamma$ receptor and another specific for the hapten dinitrophenyl were chemically cross-linked. In the presence of this hybrid antibody, $Fc\gamma$ receptor–bearing cells were able to lyse haptenated target cells specifically. The $Fc\gamma$ receptor played a critical role; antibody to MHC class I antigens on the cell could not be substituted. Antibody to the T cell receptor complex has also been used extensively to redirect T cell lysis to desired targets. For example, anti-CD3 was cross-linked to antitumor antibodies and mixed with effector cells. These "targeted T cells" were able to inhibit the growth of human tumor cells *in vivo* in nude mice (127). Bispecific antibodies have also been used to alter the tropism of a viral gene therapy vector to target specific cells (128).

Cumbersome cross-linking chemistry can now be replaced by genetic engineering for creation of designer antibodies (125). Bifunctional and bispecific antibodies can be engineered as single chain variable fragment (scFv) constructs or by specialized strategies with two chains. Many different configurations are possible and can be used to make multivalent reagents as well as reagents with one site of each specificity. Tags can be built in by fusion of additional sequence such as streptavidin, or, as mentioned previously, antibody domains can be combined with other functional domains such as toxins, enzymes, or cytokines.

Clinical Applications

The possible clinical uses of monoclonal antibodies are many. *In vitro,* they are widely used in RIA and ELISA measurements of substances in biological fluids, from hormones to toxins. They are also extremely valuable in flow cytometric assays of cell populations using antibodies specific for differentiation antigens expressed on cell surfaces. Monoclonal antibodies plus complement or toxin-conjugated monoclonal antibodies have also been used to remove T cells from bone marrow before transplantation (129).

In vivo, monoclonal antibodies are already in use or in trials for a variety of purposes [reviewed by Waldmann (130) and Berkower (131)]. Monoclonal antibody OKT3 directed to a marker on human T-lymphocytes is used as a treatment for rejection reactions in patients with kidney transplants (132). Other monoclonal antibodies—for example, indium 111–labeled CYT-103, referred to as Oncoscint (133)—are used as diagnostic tumor imaging reagents. Monoclonal antibodies have now been approved for a variety of therapeutic

uses (134). Cancer therapies use either unconjugated monoclonal antibody (130,135–139) or toxin-coupled (140,141) or radiolabeled monoclonal antibody (135,139,142). Other therapies studied include anti-lipopolysaccharide for treatment of sepsis, anti–interleukin-6 receptor for treatment of multiple myeloma, anti–immunoglobulin E for treatment of allergy [surveyed by Berkower (131)], anti–tumor necrosis factor for treatment of arthritis (143,144), anti–respiratory syncytial virus for prevention of the disease-related morbidity and mortality in infants (145,146), and anti–interleukin-2 receptor for prevention of graft rejection (139).

In the specialized case of B cell lymphoma, monoclonal anti-idiotypes against the idiotype expressed by the patient's tumor have been tested as a "magic bullet" therapy (147). Active immunization of the patient with idiotype has the advantage that escape mutants (148) are less likely to emerge because multiple idiotopes are recognized. Another approach under study is immunization with not idiotype as protein but plasmid DNA encoding patient idiotype (149). This approach would have additional advantages, such as ease of preparing customized reagents for each patient.

Production of Human or Humanized Monoclonal Antibodies

Many of the side effects of monoclonal antibodies in clinical use originate from the foreign immunoglobulin constant regions. Recognition of foreign immunoglobulin epitopes can lead to sensitization and thereby preclude subsequent use of different monoclonal antibodies in the same individual. Thus, monoclonal antibodies with some or all structure derived from human immunoglobulin have advantages. Several approaches have been taken: fusion of human cells with animal myelomas or with human tumor cells of various kinds (150,151) and use of the Epstein-Barr virus to immortalize antibody-producing cells (152). Production of populations of sensitized human cells to be fused presents another special problem, because the donors cannot be immunized at will. In one example, *in vitro* stimulation of lymphocytes with antigen followed by fusion with mouse myeloma cells has been used to generate a series of antibodies to varicella zoster (153).

Another approach to production of monoclonal antibodies with human characteristics involves application of genetic engineering. The part of the antibody structure recognized as foreign by humans can be minimized by combining human constant regions with mouse variable regions (154,155) or even just mouse hypervariable segments (156) by molecular genetic techniques. Antigen-binding specificity is retained in some cases, and the "humanized" chimeric molecules have many of the advantages of human hybridomas.

Production of fully human monoclonal antibodies in transgenic mice has now been achieved by multiple laboratories. The strategy has involved insertion into the mouse germline of constructs containing clusters of human immunoglobulin V, D, J, and C genes to generate one transgenic line and targeted disruption of the mouse heavy chain and κ chain loci to generate another transgenic line. From these two lines, mice that express only human antibodies are then bred.

To show feasibility of this approach, cosmids carrying parts of the human heavy chain locus were used to make transgenic mice (157). The next step was to produce mice carrying human genes for both heavy and light chains to generate a functional human repertoire. Several groups using different technologies constructed heavy chain mini-loci containing functional V segments representing several major V region families, D and J segments, constant and switch regions, and enhancers. The researchers made κ chain constructs that contained multiple functional Vκ segments, the J segments, Cκ, and enhancers (158,159). Mice that were homozygous both for the transgene loci and for disruption of the mouse heavy chain and κ light chain loci were bred; the mouse λ locus was left intact. The human immunoglobulin genes could rearrange in the mouse genome, and expression of human immunoglobulin resulted. If these mice were immunized with a fragment of tetanus toxin, resulting antibodies included some that were fully human (159). In one of the studies (158), serum contained human μ, $\gamma 1$, and κ, as well as mouse λ and γ. Immunization of such mice with various antigens led to class switching, somatic mutation, and production of human antibodies with affinities of almost 10^8.

Immunoglobulin expression in these mice demonstrates cross-species compatibility of the components involved in antibody gene rearrangement and diversification. The mice also provide a responder able to provide fully human antibodies to clinically important antigens, and they have the advantage that they are not tolerant to human antigens, such as the human immunoglobulin E and human CD4 used by Lonberg et al. (158).

Nucleotide Aptamers: an Alternative to Monoclonal Antibodies

Antibodies are not the only biological macromolecules that have evolved to permit an enormous range of specific structures. Oligonucleotides selected for the ability to bind a ligand with high affinity and specificity are termed *aptamers* and can be used in many of the ways that antibodies have been used. Selection, properties, and uses of aptamers have been reviewed (160). Aptamers have the advantage that their production does not require animals or cell culture. These well-defined reagents may be used increasingly in diagnostic testing and are also being tested in clinical trials for use as imaging agents or therapeutics.

Specificity and Cross-Reactivity

Specificity of Monoclonal Antibodies

Because all the molecules in a sample of monoclonal antibody have the same variable region structure, except for variants

arising after cloning, they all have the same specificity. This uniformity has the advantage that batches of monoclonal antibody do not vary in specificity, as polyclonal sera often do. The most obvious fact about cross-reactions of monoclonal antibodies is that they are characteristic of all molecules and cannot be removed by absorption without removing all activity. An exception would be an apparent cross-reaction resulting from a subset of denatured antibody molecules, which could be removed on the basis of that binding. The homogeneity of monoclonal antibodies allows refinement of specificity analysis that was not possible with polyclonal sera. A few examples follow.

First, monoclonal antibodies can be used to distinguish closely related ligands in cases in which most antibodies in a polyclonal serum would cross-react, and thus absorption of a serum would not leave sufficient activity to define additional specificities. This ability is useful in, for example, designing clinical assays for related hormones. Such fine discrimination also allows the definition of new specificities on complex antigens. When large numbers of monoclonal antibodies specific for class I and class II MHC antigens were analyzed, some possessed specificities that could not be defined with existing polyclonal antisera (161–163).

On the other hand, monoclonal antibodies are also a powerful tool for demonstrating similarities rather than distinctions between two antigens. In some cases, only a minor portion of an antibody response detects a cross-reaction, and so it is not detected by polyclonal reagents. For example, determinants shared by the I-A and I-E class II MHC antigens in the mouse were demonstrated with monoclonal antibodies (163), whereas they had been suspected but were difficult to demonstrate with polyclonal sera.

Another type of fine specificity analysis possible only with monoclonal antibodies is the discrimination of spatial sites (epitope clusters) by competitive binding. In some cases, such epitope clusters correspond to specificities that are readily distinguished by other means. However, in other cases, the epitope clusters may not be distinguishable by any serologic or genetic means. An example is the splitting of the classical specificity Ia.7 into three epitope clusters by competitive binding with monoclonal antibodies (163). The epitopes cannot be distinguished genetically, because all three are expressed on cells of all Ia.7-positive mouse strains. Thus, polyclonal sera cannot be absorbed to reveal the different specificities. Only with the use of monoclonal antibodies were the epitopes distinguished from each other.

The importance of this type of analysis is shown by another example, the definition of epitope clusters on CD4, a surface molecule on a subset of human T cells that also functions as the receptor for HIV. Monoclonal antibodies to CD4 can be divided into several groups on the basis of competitive inhibition (164). The cluster containing the site recognized by OKT4A is closely related to virus infection, because antibodies to this site block syncytium formation. The cluster recognized by OKT4, however, is not related to infection since antibodies to it do not block syncytium formation (164), and cells expressing variant forms of the CD4 molecule lacking the OKT4 epitope can still be infected by HIV (165). This information about the sites on the molecule is important in understanding the molecular interactions of virus with its receptor and may be useful in designing vaccine candidates.

Although most antibodies are not MHC-restricted in their recognition of antigens, which distinguishes them from T-cell receptors, it is possible to select antibodies that recognize peptide-MHC complexes (166–168) (MHC-restricted antipeptide antibodies or peptide-dependent anti-MHC class I antibodies). Several monoclonal antibodies that require both a certain MHC class I antigen and a particular peptide for reactivity have been selected. Such monoclonal antibodies are useful reagents capable of detecting cells that present the appropriate peptide-MHC complexes on their surfaces (166). Such monoclonal antibodies may also be useful in dissection of T-cell responses. In one study, the monoclonal antibodies could inhibit interleukin-2 secretion by a T-cell hybridoma of corresponding specificity and could also block induction of cytotoxic T-lymphocytes, recognizing that epitope, when given in vivo during priming (168). Such monoclonal antibodies have been used to address structural questions about antigen recognition by T and B cells (167). Such antibodies also appeared to skew the repertoire of T cells for this particular HIV peptide-MHC complex to specific T-cell antigen receptor $V\beta$ types and T-cell avidities (169). However, only very rare monoclonal antibodies have this type of specificity, they were purposely selected in the fusions, and so they do not provide a general comparison of T-cell antigen receptor and antibody characteristics.

Cross-Reactions of Monoclonal Antibodies

Monoclonal antibodies display many type 1 cross-reactions, which emphasizes that antibody cross-reactions represent real similarities among the antigens, not just an effect of heterogeneity of serum antibodies. Even antigens that differ for most of their structure can share one determinant, and a monoclonal antibody recognizing this site would then give a 100% cross-reaction.

It should be emphasized that sharing a "determinant" does not mean that the antigens contain identical chemical structures; rather, it means that they bear a chemical resemblance that may not be well understood, such as a distribution of surface charges. Antibodies to the whole range of antigens can react with immunoglobulins in idiotype–anti-idiotype reactions, showing a cross-reactivity of the same antibodies with proteins (the anti-idiotypes) and with the carbohydrates, nucleic acids, lipids, or haptens against which they were raised.

Polyclonal Versus Monoclonal Antibodies

When monoclonal antibodies first became available, some people expected that they would be exquisitely specific and would be superior to polyclonal sera for essentially all pur-

poses. Further thought about the issues discussed previously, however, suggests that this is not always the case, and their superiority depends on the intended use of the antibodies. Not only do monoclonal antibodies cross-react, but when they do, the cross-reaction is not minor and cannot be removed by absorption. A large panel of monoclonal antibodies may be needed before one is identified with the precise range of reactivity desired for a study.

In polyclonal sera, on the other hand, each different antibody has a distinct range of reactivity, and the only common feature would be detectable reactivity with the antigen used for immunization or testing. Thus, the serum as a whole may show only a low-titered cross-reaction with any particular other antigen, and that cross-reaction can be removed by absorption, leaving substantial activity against the immunizing antigen. For the purposes of an experiment, a polyclonal serum may be "more specific" than any one of its clonal parts and may be more useful. This concept is the basis of the theory of multispecificity (see previous discussion).

Polyclonal sera also have advantages in certain technical situations, such as immunoprecipitation, in which multivalency is important. Many antigens are univalent with regard to monoclonal antibody binding but display multiple distinct sites that can be recognized by different components of polyclonal sera. Thus, a greater degree of cross-linking can be achieved.

The ultimate serological reagent in many cases may well be a mixture of monoclonal antibodies that have been chosen according to their cross-reactions. The mixture would be better defined and more reproducible than a polyclonal antiserum and would have the same advantage of overlapping specificities.

CONCLUSION

In conclusion, antibodies, whether monoclonal or polyclonal, provide a unique type of reagent that can be made with high specificity for almost any desired organic or biochemical structure, often with extremely high affinity. These can be naturally divalent, as in the case of IgG, or multivalent, as in the case of IgM, or they can be made as monovalent molecules such as Fab or recombinant variable fragments. They serve not only as a major arm of host defense, playing a major role in the protective efficacy of most existing antiviral and all antibacterial vaccines, but also as very versatile tools for research and clinical use. RIAs and ELISAs have revolutionized the detection of minute quantities of biological molecules, such as hormones and cytokines, and thus have become indispensable for clinical diagnosis and monitoring of patients as well as for basic and applied research. Current solid-phase versions of these take advantage not only of the intrinsic affinity and specificity of the antibodies but also of the implicit multivalency and local high concentration on a solid surface. Cross-reactivity of antibodies often provides the first clue to relationships between molecules that might not otherwise have been compared. Conversely, methods in which antigens are used to detect the presence of antibodies in serum have become widespread in testing for exposure to a variety of pathogens, such as HIV. Antibodies also provide specific reagents invaluable in the rapid purification of many other molecules by affinity chromatography. They have also become indispensable reagents for other branches of biology, such as in histocompatibility typing and phenotyping of cells with a myriad of cell-surface markers that were themselves discovered with monoclonal antibodies, and for separating these cells by fluorescence-activated cell sorting, panning, or chromatographic techniques. Monoclonal antibodies have also emerged as clinically important therapeutics in cancer, arthritis, organ graft rejection, and infectious diseases. Thus, antibodies are among the most versatile and widely used types of reagents today, and their use is constantly increasing. Understanding the fundamental concepts in antigen–antibody interactions therefore has become essential not only for an understanding of immunology but also for the effective use of these valuable molecules in many other fields.

ACKNOWLEDGMENTS

We thank Drs. Charles DeLisi, Elvin A. Kabat, and Henry Metzger for their detailed critique of the manuscript, as well as many helpful discussions, and Dr. Fred Karush for valuable suggestions.

REFERENCES

1. Köhler G, Milstein C. Derivation of specific antibody-producing tissue culture and tumor lines by cell fusion. *Eur J Immunol* 1976;6:511–519.
2. Melchers F, Potter M, Warner NC. *Lymphocyte hybridomas.* Berlin: Springer-Verlag, 1978.
3. Kennett RH, McKearn TJ, Bechtol KB. *Monoclonal antibodies. Hybridomas: A new dimension in biological analyses.* New York: Plenum Press, 1980.
4. Moore WJ. *Physical chemistry,* 3rd ed. Englewood Cliffs, NJ: Prentice-Hall, 1962.
5. DeLisi C. The biophysics of ligand-receptor interactions. *Q Rev Biophys* 1980;13:201–230.
6. Fersht A. *Enzyme structure and mechanisms.* New York: Freeman, 1977.
7. Eisen HN. *Immunology,* 2nd ed. Baltimore: Harper & Row, 1980.
8. Sachs DH, Schechter AN, Eastlake A, et al. Inactivation of staphylococcal nuclease by the binding of antibodies to a distinct antigenic determinant. *Biochemistry* 1972;11:4268–4273.
9. Hammes GG. Relaxation spectrometry of biological systems. *Adv Protein Chem* 1968;23:1–57.
10. Eisen HN, Karush F. The interaction of purified antibody with homologous hapten.Antibody valence and binding constant. *J Am Chem Soc* 1949;71:363–364.
11. Pinckard RN. Equilibrium dialysis and preparation of hapten conjugates. In: Weir DM, ed. *Handbook of experimental immunology.* Oxford: Blackwell Science 1978;17·1–17·23.
12. Scatchard G. The attractions of proteins for small molecules and ions. *Ann N Y Acad Sci* 1949;51:660–672.
13. Berzofsky JA, Hicks G, Fedorko J, et al. Properties of monoclonal antibodies specific for determinants of a protein antigen, myoglobin. *J Biol Chem* 1980;255:11188–11191.
14. Rodbard D, Munson PJ, Thakur AK. Quantitative characterization of hormone receptors. *Cancer* 1980;46:2907–2918.
15. Thakur AK, Jaffe ML, Rodbard D. Graphical analysis of ligand-binding systems: evaluation by Monte Carlo studies. *Anal Biochem* 1980;107:279–295.
16. Munson PJ, Rodbard D. LIGAND: a versatile computerized approach for characterization of ligand-binding systems. *Anal Biochem* 1980;107:220–239.
17. Bright DS. *On interpreting spectrophotometric measurements of two quinoline-DNA complexes* [Doctoral dissertation]. Fort Collins, CO: Colorado State University, 1974.
18. Berzofsky JA. The assessment of antibody affinity from radioimmunoassay. *Clin Chem* 1978;24:419–421.
19. Pauling L, Pressman D, Grossberg AL. Serological properties of simple substances.VII. A quantitative theory of the inhibition by haptens of the precipitation of heterogeneous antisera with antigens, and comparison with experimental results for polyhaptenic simple substances and for azoproteins. *J Am Chem Soc* 1944;66:784–792.
20. Karush F. The interaction of purified antibody with optically isomeric haptens. *J Am Chem Soc* 1956;78:5519–5526.
21. Thakur AK, DeLisi C. Theory of ligand binding to heterogeneous receptor populations: characterization of the free-energy distribution function. *Biopolymers* 1978;17:1075–1089.
22. DeLisi C. Characterization of receptor affinity heterogeneity by Scatchard plots. *Biopolymers* 1978;17:1385–1386.
23. Thakur AK, Munson PJ, Hunston DL, et al. Characterization of ligand-binding systems by continuous affinity distributions of arbitrary shape. *Anal Biochem* 1980;103:240–254.
24. Sips R. On the structure of a catalyst surface. *J Chem Phys* 1948;16:490–495.
25. Nisonoff A, Pressman D. Heterogeneity and average combining site constants of antibodies from individual rabbits. *J Immunol* 1958;80:417–428.
26. Karush F, Karush SS. Equilibrium dialysis. 3. Calculations. In: Williams CA, Chase MW, eds. *Methods in immunology and immunochemistry.* New York: Academic Press, 1971:389–393.
27. Klotz IM. Protein interactions. In: Neurath H, Bailey K, eds. *The proteins.* New York: Academic Press, 1953:727–806.
28. Karush F. The affinity of antibody: range, variability, and the role of multivalence. In: Litman GW, Good RA, eds. *Comprehensive Immunology.* New York: Plenum Publishing. 1978:85–116.
29. Crothers DM, Metzger H. The influence of polyvalency on the binding properties of antibodies. *Immunochemistry* 1972;9:341–357.
30. Hornick CL, Karush F. Antibody affinity—III. The role of multivalence. *Immunochemistry* 1972;9:325–340.
31. DeLisi C, Metzger H. Some physical chemical aspects of receptor-ligand interactions. *Immunol Commun* 1976;5:417–436.
32. DeLisi C. The effect of cell size and receptor density on ligand-receptor reaction rate constants. *Mol Immunol* 1981;18:507–511.
33. DeLisi C, Wiegel FW. Effect of nonspecific forces and finite receptor number on rate constants of ligand-cell bound-receptor interactions. *Proc Natl Acad Sci U S A* 1981;78:5569–5572.
34. Silhavy TJ, Szmelcman S, Boos W, et al. On the significance of the retention of ligand by protein. *Proc Natl Acad Sci U S A* 1975;72:2120–2124.
35. Yalow RS, Berson SA. Immunoassay of endogenous plasma insulin in man. *J Clin Invest* 1960;39:1157–1175.
36. Chard T. *An introduction to radioimmunoassay and related techniques.* Amsterdam: North Holland, 1978.
37. Rodbard D. Mathematics and statistics of ligand assays: an illustrated guide. In: Langan J, Clapp JJ, eds. *Ligand assay: analysis of international developments on isotopic and nonisotopic immunoassay.* New York: Masson, 1981:45–101.
38. Yalow R. Radioimmunoassay. *Rev Biophys Bioeng* 1980;9:327–345.
39. Farr RS. A quantitative immunochemical measure of the primary interaction between I*BSA and antibody. *J Infect Dis* 1958;103:239–262.
40. Desbuquois B, Aurbach GD. Use of polyethylene glycol to separate free and antibody-bound peptide hormones in radioimmunoassays. *J Clin Endocrinol Metab* 1971;33:732–738.
41. Zollinger WD, Dalrymple JM, Artenstein MS. Analysis of parameters affecting the solid phase radioimmunoassay quantitation of antibody to meningococcal antigens. *J Immunol* 1976;117:1788–1798.
42. Kessler SW. Rapid isolation of antigens from cells with a staphylococcal protein-A-antibody adsorbent: parameters of the interaction of antibody-antigen complexes with protein A. *J Immunol* 1975;115:1617–1624.
43. Friguet B, Chaffotte AF, Djavadi-Ohaniance L, et al. Measurements of the true affinity constant in solution of antigen–antibody

complexes by enzyme-linked immunosorbent assay. *J Immunol Methods* 1985;77:305–319.

44. Stevens FJ. Modification of an ELISA-based procedure for affinity determination: correction necessary for use with bivalent antibody. *Mol Immunol* 1987;24:1055–1060.

45. Seligman SJ. Influence of solid-phase antigen in competition enzyme-linked immunosorbent assays (ELISAs) on calculated antigen-antibody dissociation constants. *J Immunol Methods* 1994;168:101–110.

46. Ekins RP. Basic principles and theory. *Br Med Bull* 1974;30:3–11.

47. Berzofsky JA, Curd JG, Schechter AN. Probability analysis of the interaction of antibodies with multideterminant antigens in radioimmunoassay: application to the amino terminus of the beta chain of hemoglobin S. *Biochemistry* 1976;15:2113–2121.

48. von Krogh M. Colloidal chemistry and immunology. *J Infect Dis* 1916;19:452–477.

49. Rodbard D, Lewald JE. Computer analysis of radioligand assay and radioimmunoassay data. *Acta Endocrinol* 1970;64:79–103.

50. Feldman H, Rodbard D. Mathematical theory of radioimmunoassay. In: Odell WD, Daughaday WH, eds. *Principles of competitive protein-binding assays.* Philadelphia: JB Lippincott, 1971:158–203.

51. Rodbard D, Ruder JH, Vaitukaitis J, et al. Mathematical analysis of kinetics of radioligand assays: improved sensitivity obtained by delayed addition of labeled ligand. *J Clin Endocrinol Metab* 1971;33:343–355.

52. Voller A, Bidwell D, Bartlett A. Enzyme-linked immunosorbent assay. In: Rose NR, Friedman H, eds. *Manual of clinical immunology.* Washington, DC: American Society of Microbiology, 1980:359–371.

53. Kohno Y, Berkower I, Minna J, et al. Idiotypes of anti-myoglobin antibodies: shared idiotypes among monoclonal antibodies to distinct determinants of sperm whale myoglobin. *J Immunol* 1982;128:1742–1748.

54. Darst SA, Robertson CR, Berzofsky JA. Adsorption of the protein antigen myoglobin affects the binding of conformation-specific monoclonal antibodies. *Biophysical J* 1988;53:533–539.

55. Sedgwick J. A solid phase immunoenzymatic technique for the enumeration of specific antibody-secreting cells. *J Immunol Methods* 1983;57:301–309.

56. Czerkinsky CC, Nilsson L, Nygren H, et al. A solid-phase enzyme-linked immunospot (ELISPOT) assay for enumeration of specific antibody-secreting cells. *J Immunol Methods* 1983;65:109–121.

57. Bocher WO, Herzog-Hauff S, Herr W, et al. Regulation of the neutralizing anti-hepatitis B surface (HBs) antibody response *in vitro* in HBs vaccine recipients and patients with acute or chronic hepatitis virus (HBV) infection. *Clin Exp Immunol* 1996;105:52–58.

58. Ronnelid J, Huang YH, Norrlander T, et al. Short-term kinetics of the humoral anti-C1q response in SLE using the ELIspot method: fast decline in production in response to steroids. *Scand J Immunol* 1994;40:243–250.

59. Czerkinsky C, Moldoveanu Z, Mestecky J, et al. A novel two colour ELISPOT assay I. Simultaneous detection of distinct types of antibody-secreting cells. *J Immunol Methods* 1988;115:31–37.

60. Krieg AM, Yi A, Matson S, et al. CpG motifs in bacterial DNA trigger direct B-cell activation. *Nature* 1995;374:546–549.

61. Ronnelid J, Klareskog L. A comparison between ELISPOT methods for the detection of cytokine producing cells: greater sensitivity and specificity using ELISA plates as compared to nitrocellulose membranes. *J Immunol Methods* 1997;200:17–26.

62. Mäkelä O, Karjalainen K. Inherited immunoglobulin idiotypes of the mouse. *Immunol Rev* 1977;34:119–138.

63. Jameson BA, McDonnell JM, Marini JC, et al. A rationally designed CD4 analogue inhibits experimental allergic encephalomyelitis. *Nature* 1994;368:744–746.

64. Brady L, Dodson G. Reflections on a peptide. *Nature* 1994;368:692–693.

65. Guichard G, Benkirane N, Zeder-Lutz G, et al. Antigenic mimicry of natural L-peptides with retro-inverso-peptidomimetics. *Proc Natl Acad Sci U S A* 1994;91:9765–9769.

66. Benkirane N, Guichard G, Van Regenmortel MHV, et al. Cross-reactivity of antibodies to retro-inverso peptidomimetics with the parent protein histone H3 and chromatin core particle. *J Biol Chem* 1995;270:11921–11926.

67. Briand J, Guichard G, Dumortier H, et al. Retro-inverso peptidomimetics as new immunological probes. *J Biol Chem* 1995;270:20686–20691.

68. Häyry P, Myllärniemi M, Aavik E, et al. Stabile D-peptide analog of insulin-like growth factor-1 inhibits smooth muscle cell proliferation after carotid ballooning injury in the rat. *FASEB J* 1995;9:1336–1344.

69. Berzofsky JA, Schechter AN. The concepts of cross-reactivity and specificity in immunology. *Mol Immunol* 1981;18:751–763.

70. Young NS, Curd JG, Eastlake A, et al. Isolation of antibodies specific to sickle hemoglobin by affinity chromatography using a synthetic peptide. *Proc Natl Acad Sci U S A* 1975;72:4759–4763.

71. Young NS, Eastlake A, Schechter AN. The amino terminal region of the sickle hemoglobin beta chain.II. Characterization of monospecific antibodies. *J Biol Chem* 1976;251:6431–6435.

72. Curd JG, Young N, Schechter AN. Antibodies to an amino terminal fragment of beta globin. II. Specificity and isolation of antibodies for the sickle mutation. *J Biol Chem* 1976;251:1290–1295.

73. Dean J, Schechter AN. Sickle-cell anemia: molecular and cellular bases of therapeutic approaches. *N Engl J Med* 1978;299:752–763.

74. Johnston MFM, Eisen HN. Cross-reactions between 2,4-dinitrophenyl and nemadione (vitamin K3) and the general problem of antibody specificity. *J Immunol* 1976;117:1189–1196.

75. Talmadge D. Immunological specificity. *Science* 1959;129:1643–1648.

76. Inman JK. Multispecificity of the antibody combining region and antibody diversity. In: Sercarz EE, Williamson AR, Fox CF, eds. *The immune system: genes, receptors, signals.* New York: Academic Press, 1974:37–52.

77. Inman JK. The antibody combining region: speculations on the hypothesis of general multispecificity. In: Bell GI, Perelson AS, Pimbley GH Jr, eds. *Theoretical immunology.* New York: Marcel Dekker, 1978:243–278.

78. Richards FF, Konigsberg WH, Rosenstein RW, et al. On the specificity of antibodies. *Science* 1975;187:130–137.

79. Parker CW. Spectrofluorometric methods. In: Weir DM, ed. *Handbook of experimental immunology.* Oxford, UK: Blackwell Science, 1978:18.1–18.25.

80. Haimovich J, Hurwitz E, Novik N, et al. Preparation of protein-bacteriophage conjugates and their use in detection of antiprotein antibodies. *Biochim Biophys Acta* 1970;207:115–124.

81. Heidelberger M, Kendall FE. The precipitin reaction between type III pneumococcus polysaccharide and homologous antibody. *J Exp Med* 1935;61:563–591.

82. Heidelberger M, Kendall FE. A quantitative theory of the precipitin reaction. II. A study of an azoprotein-antibody system. *J Exp Med* 1935;62:467–483.

83. Kabat EA. *Structural concepts in immunology and immunochemistry,* 2nd ed. New York: Hold, Rinehart, & Winston, 1976.

84. Cisar J, Kabat EA, Dorner MM, et al. Binding properties of immunoglobulin containing sites specific for terminal or nonterminal antigenic determinants in dextran. *J Exp Med* 1975;142:435–459.

85. Ouchterlony O, Nilsson LA. Immunodiffusion and immunoelectrophoresis. In: Weir DM, ed. *Handbook of experimental immunology.* Oxford, UK: Blackwell Science, 1978:19.1–19.44.

86. Feinberg JG. Identification, discrimination and quantification in Ouchterlony gel plates. *Int Arch Allergy* 1957;11:129–152.

87. Tomasi TB Jr, Zigelbaum S. The selective occurrence of gamma 1A globulins in certain body fluids. *J Clin Invest* 1963;42:1552–1560.

88. Fahey JL, McKelvey EM. Quantitative determination of serum immunoglobulins in antibody-agar plates. *J Immunol* 1965;94:84–90.

89. Mancini G, Carbonara AO, Heremans JF. Immunochemical quantitation of antigens by single radial immunodiffusion. *Immunochemistry* 1965;2:235–254.

90. Herbert WJ. Passive haemagglutination with special reference to the tanned cell technique. In: Weir DM, ed. *Handbook of experimental immunology.* Oxford, UK: Blackwell Science, 1978:20.1–20.20.

91. Towbin H, Staehelin T, Gordon J. Electrophoretic transfer of proteins from polyacrylamide gels to nitrocellulose sheets: Procedure and some applications. *Proc Natl Acad Sci U S A* 1979;76:4350–4354.

92. Schupbach J, Popovic M, Gilden RV, et al. Serological analysis of a subgroup of human T-lymphotropic retroviruses (HTLV-III) associated with AIDS. *Science* 1984;224:503–505.

93. Feynman RP, Leighton RB, Sands M. *The Feynman lectures on physics,* Vol. II. Reading, MA: Addison-Wesley, 1964.

94. Mullett WM, Lai EP, Yeung JM. Surface plasmon resonance-based immunoassays. *Methods* 2000;22:77–91.

95. VanCott TC, Bethke FR, Polonis VR, et al. Dissociation rate of antibody-gp120 binding interactions is predictive of V3-mediated neutralization of HIV-1. *J Immunol* 1994;153:449–459.

96. Slater RJ, Ward SM, Kunkel HG. Immunological relationships among the myeloma proteins. *J Exp Med* 1955;101:85–108.

97. Potter M. Immunoglobulin-producing tumors and myeloma proteins of mice. *Physiol Rev* 1972;52:631–719.

98. Köhler G, Milstein C. Continuous cultures of fused cells secreting antibody of predefined specificity. *Nature* 1975;256:495–497.

99. Margulies DH, Kuehl WM, Scharff MD. Somatic cell hybridization of mouse myeloma cells. *Cell* 1976;8:405–415.

100. Shulman M, Wilde CD, Köhler G. A better cell line for making hybridomas secreting specific antibodies. *Nature* 1978;276:269–270.

101. Kearney JF, Radbruch A, Liesegang B, et al. A new mouse myeloma cell line that has lost immunoglobulin expression but permits the construction of antibody-secreting hybrid cell lines. *J Immunol* 1979; 123:1548–1550.

102. Yokoyama WM. Production of monoclonal antibodies. In: Coligan JE, Kruisbeek AM, Margulies DH, et al., eds. *Current protocols in immunology*, vol I. New York: John Wiley and Sons, 2001:2.5.1.

103. Unkeless JC. Characterization of monoclonal antibody directed against mouse macrophage and lymphocyte Fc receptors. *J Exp Med* 1979;150:580–596.

104. Leo O, Foo M, Sachs DH, et al. Identification of a monoclonal antibody specific for a murine T3 polypeptide. *Proc Natl Acad Sci U S A* 1987;84:1374–1378.

105. Yarmush ML, Gates FT, Weisfogel DR, et al. Identification and characterization of rabbit-mouse hybridomas secreting rabbit immunoglobulin chains. *Proc Natl Acad Sci U S A* 1980;77:2899–2903.

106. Bazin H. Production of rat monoclonal antibodies with the Lou rat non-secreting IR983F myeloma cell line. *Prot Biol Fluids* 1981;29:615–618.

107. Huse WD, Sastry L, Iverson SA, et al. Generation of a large combinatorial library of the immunoglobulin repertoire in phage lambda. *Science* 1989;246:1275–1281.

108. Clackson T, Hoogenboom HR, Griffiths AD, et al. Making antibody fragments using phage display libraries. *Nature* 1991;352:624–628.

109. McCafferty J, Griffiths AD, Winter G, et al. Phage antibodies: filamentous phage displaying antibody variable domains. *Nature* 1990;348:552–554.

110. Kang AS, Barbas CF, Janda KD, et al. Linkage of recognition and replication functions by assembling combinatorial antibody Fab libraries along phage surfaces. *Proc Natl Acad Sci U S A* 1991;88:4363–4366.

111. Zebedee SL, Barbas CF III, Hom Y, et al. Human combinatorial antibody libraries to hepatitis B surface antigen. *Proc Natl Acad Sci U S A* 1992;89:3175–3179.

112. Burton DR, Barbas CF III, Persson MAA, et al. A large array of human monoclonal antibodies to type 1 human immunodeficiency virus from combinatorial libraries of asymptomatic seropositive individuals. *Proc Natl Acad Sci U S A* 1991;88:10134–10137.

113. Duchosal MA, Eming SA, Fischer P, et al. Immunization of hu-PBL-SCID mice and the rescue of human monoclonal Fab fragments through combinatorial libraries. *Nature* 1992;355:258–262.

114. Low NM, Holliger P, Winter G. Mimicking somatic hypermutation: affinity maturation of antibodies displayed on bacteriophage using a bacterial mutator strain. *J Mol Biol* 1996;260:359–368.

115. Thompson J, Pope T, Tung J, et al. Affinity maturation of a high-affinity human monoclonal antibody against the third hypervariable loop of human immunodeficiency virus: use of phage display to improve affinity and broaden strain reactivity. *J Mol Biol* 1996;256:77–88.

116. Lerner RA, Benkovic SJ, Schultz PG. At the crossroads of chemistry and immunology: catalytic antibodies. *Science* 1991;252:659–667.

117. Pollack SJ, Jacobs JW, Schultz PG. Selective chemical catalysis by an antibody. *Science* 1986;234:1570–1573.

118. Shuster AM, Gololobov GV, Kvashuk OA, et al. DNA hydrolyzing autoantibodies. *Science* 1992;256:665–667.

119. Tramontano A, Janda KD, Lerner RA. Catalytic antibodies. *Science* 1986;234:1566–1570.

120. Shokat KM, Leumann CJ, Sugasawara R, et al. A new strategy for the generation of catalytic antibodies. *Nature* 1989;338:269–271.

121. Pollack SJ, Hsiun P, Schultz PG. Stereospecific hydrolysis of alkyl esters by antibodies. *J Am Chem Soc* 1989;111:5961–5962.

122. Wirsching P, Ashley JA, Benkovic SJ, et al. An unexpectedly efficient catalytic antibody operating by ping-pong and induced fit mechanisms. *Science* 1991;252:680–685.

123. Shabat D, Itzhaky H, Reymond J, et al. Antibody catalysis of a reaction otherwise strongly disfavoured in water. *Nature* 1995;374:143–146.

124. Hirschmann R, Smith AB, Taylor CM, et al. Peptide synthesis catalyzed by an antibody containing a binding site for variable amino acids. *Science* 1994;265:234–237.

125. Kriangkum J, Xu BW, Nagata LP, et al. Bispecific and bifunctional single chain recombinant antibodies. *Biomol Eng* 2001;18:31–40.

126. Karpovsky B, Titus JA, Stephany DA, et al. Production of target-specific effector cells using hetero-cross-linked aggregates containing anti-target cell and anti-Fcγ receptor antibodies. *J Exp Med* 1984;160:1686–1701.

127. Titus JA, Garrido MA, Hecht TT, et al. Human T cells targeted with anti-T3 cross-linked to antitumor antibody prevent tumor growth in nude mice. *J Immunol* 1987;138:4018–4022.

128. Wickham TJ, Segal DM, Roelvink PW, et al. Targeted adenovirus gene transfer to endothelial and smooth muscle cells by using bispecific antibodies. *J Virol* 1996;70:6831–6838.

129. Vallera DA, Ash RC, Zanjani ED, et al. Anti-T-cell reagents for human bone marrow transplantation: ricin linked to three monoclonal antibodies. *Science* 1983;222:512–515.

130. Waldmann TA. Monoclonal antibodies in diagnosis and therapy. *Science* 1991;252:1657–1662.

131. Berkower I. The promise and pitfalls of monoclonal antibody therapeutics. *Curr Opin Biotechnol* 1996;7:622–628.

132. A randomized clinical trial of OKT3 monoclonal antibody for acute rejection of cadaveric renal transplants. Ortho Multicenter Transplant Study Group. *N Engl J Med* 1985;313:337–342.

133. Collier BD, Abdel-Nabi H, Doerr RJ, et al. Immunoscintigraphy performed with In-111–labeled CYT-103 in the management of colorectal cancer: comparison with CT. *Radiology* 1992;185:179–186.

134. Ezzell C. Magic bullets fly again. *Sci Am* 2001;285:34–41.

135. Sears HF, Herlyn D, Steplewski Z, et al. Effects of monoclonal antibody immunotherapy on patients with gastrointestinal adenocarcinoma. *J Biol Response Mod* 1984;3:138–150.

136. Baselga J, Tripathy D, Mendelsohn J, et al. Phase II study of weekly intravenous recombinant humanized anti-p185HER2 monoclonal antibody in patients with HER2/neu-overexpressing metastatic breast cancer. *J Clin Oncol* 1996;14:737–744.

137. Baselga J, Norton L, Albanell J, et al. Recombinant humanized anti-HER2 antibody (Herceptin) enhances the antitumor activity of paclitaxel and doxorubicin against HER2/neu overexpressing human breast cancer xenografts. *Cancer Res* 1998;58:2825–2831.

138. Maloney DG, Grillo-Lopez AJ, Bodkin DJ, et al. IDEC-C2B8: results of a phase I multiple-dose trial in patients with relapsed non-Hodgkin's lymphoma. *J Clin Oncol* 1997;15:3266–3274.

139. Morris JC, Waldmann TA. Advances in interleukin 2 receptor targeted treatment. *Ann Rheum Dis* 2000;59(Suppl 1):i109–i114.

140. Frankel AE, Houston LL, Issell BF. Prospects for immunotoxin therapy in cancer. *Annu Rev Med* 1986;37:125–142.

141. Kreitman RJ, Wilson WH, Bergeron K, et al. Efficacy of the anti-CD22 recombinant immunotoxin BL22 in chemotherapy-resistant hairy-cell leukemia. *N Engl J Med* 2001;345:241–247.

142. Carrasquillo JA, Krohn JA, Beaumier P, et al. Diagnosis and therapy for solid tumors with radiolabeled antibodies and immune fragments. *Cancer Treat Rep* 1984;68:317–328.

143. Lipsky PE, van der Heijde DM, St. Clair EW, et al. Infliximab and methotrexate in the treatment of rheumatoid arthritis. Anti-Tumor Necrosis Factor Trial in Rheumatoid Arthritis with Concomitant Therapy Study Group. *N Engl J Med* 2000;343:1594–1602.

144. Pisetsky DS. Tumor necrosis factor blockers in rheumatoid arthritis. *N Engl J Med* 2000;342:810–811.

145. Johnson S, Oliver C, Prince GA, et al. Development of a humanized monoclonal antibody (MEDI-493) with potent *in vitro* and *in vivo* activity against respiratory syncytial virus. *J Infect Dis* 1997;176:1215–1224.

146. Palivizumab, a Humanized Respiratory Syncytial Virus Monoclonal Antibody, Reduces Hospitalization From Respiratory Syncytial Virus Infection in High-risk Infants. The IMpact-RSV Study Group. *Pediatrics* 1998;102:531–537.

147. Miller RA, Maloney DG, Warnke R, et al. Treatment of B-cell lymphoma with monoclonal anti-idiotype antibody. *N Engl J Med* 1982; 306:517–522.

148. Meeker T, Lowder J, Cleary ML, et al. Emergence of idiotype variants during treatment of B-cell lymphoma with anti-idiotype antibodies. *N Engl J Med* 1985;312:1658–1665.

149. Hakim I, Levy S, Levy R. A nine-amino acid peptide from IL-1β augments antitumor immune responses induced by protein and DNA vaccines. *J Immunol* 1996;157:5503–5511.

150. Cole RJ, Morrisey DM, Houghton AN, et al. Generation of human monoclonal antibodies reactive with cellular antigens. *Proc Natl Acad Sci U S A* 1983;80:2026–2030.

151. Olsson L, Kaplan HS. Human–human monoclonal antibody-producing hybridomas: technical aspects. *Methods Enzymol* 1983;92:3–16.

152. Seigneurin JM, Desgranges C, Seigneurin D, et al. Herpes simplex virus glycoprotein D: human monoclonal antibody produced by bone marrow cell line. *Science* 1983;221:173–175.

153. Sugano T, Matsumoto Y, Miyamoto C, et al. Hybridomas producing human monoclonal antibodies against varicella-zoster virus. *Eur J Immunol* 1987;17:359–364.

154. Morrison SL. Transfectomas provide novel chimeric antibodies. *Science* 1985;229:1202–1207.

155. Morrison SL, Johnson MJ, Herzenberg LA, et al. Chimeric human antibody molecules: mouse antigen-binding domains with human constant region domains. *Proc Natl Acad Sci U S A* 1984;81:6851–6855.

156. Jones PT, Dear PH, Foote J, et al. Replacing the complementarity-determining regions in a human antibody with those from a mouse. *Nature* 1986;321:522–525.

157. Brüggemann M, Spicer C, Buluwela L, et al. Human antibody production in transgenic mice: expression from 100 kb of the human IgH locus. *Eur J Immunol* 1991;21:1323–1326.

158. Lonberg N, Taylor LD, Harding FA, et al. Antigen-specific human antibodies from mice comprising four distinct genetic modifications. *Nature* 1994;368:856–859.

159. Green LL, Hardy MC, Maynard-Currie CE, et al. Antigen-specific human monoclonal antibodies from mice engineered with human Ig heavy and light chain YACs. *Nature Genet* 1994;7:13–21.

160. Jayasena SD. Aptamers: an emerging class of molecules that rival antibodies in diagnostics. *Clin Chem* 1999;45:1628–1650.

161. Klein J, Huang HS, Lemke H, Hämmerling GJ, et al. Serological analysis of H-2 and Ia molecules with monoclonal antibodies. *Immunogenetics* 1979;8:419–432.

162. Ozato K, Mayer N, Sachs DH. Hybridoma cell lines secreting monoclonal antibodies to mouse H-2 and Ia antigens. *J Immunol* 1980;124:533–540.

163. Pierres M, Devaux C, Dosseto M, et al. Clonal analysis of B- and T-cell responses to Ia antigens. I. Topology of epitope regions on I-A^k and I-E^k molecules analyzed with 35 monoclonal alloantibodies. *Immunogenetics* 1981;14:481–495.

164. Sattentau QJ, Dalgleish AG, Weiss RA, et al. Epitopes of the CD4 antigen and HIV infection. *Science* 1986;234:1120–1123.

165. Hoxie JA, Flaherty LE, Haggarty BS, et al. Infection of T4 lymphocytes by HTLV-III does not require expression of the OKT4 epitope. *J Immunol* 1986;136:361–363.

166. Porgador A, Yewdell JW, Deng YP, et al. Localization, quantitation, and *in situ* detection of specific peptide MHC class I complexes using a monoclonal antibody. *Immunity* 1997;6:715–726.

167. Messaoudi I, LeMaoult J, Nikolic-Zugic J. The mode of ligand recognition by two peptide:MHC class I–specific monoclonal antibodies. *J Immunol* 1999;163:3286–3294.

168. Polakova K, Plaksin D, Chung DH, et al. Antibodies directed against the MHC-I molecule H-2D^d complexed with an antigenic peptide: similarities to a T cell receptor with the same specificity. *J Immunol* 2000;165:5703–5712.

169. Chung DH, Belyakov IM, Derby MA, et al. Competitive inhibition *in vivo* and skewing of the T cell repertoire of antigen-specific CTL priming by an anti-peptide-MHC mAb. *J Immunol* 2001;167:699–707.

Immunoglobulins: Molecular Genetics

Edward E. Max

Overview of Immunoglobulin V Gene Assembly
  Evidence from Southern Blotting and Gene Cloning · How Recombination Contributes to Diversity · Recombination Signal Elements
The Three Immunoglobulin Gene Loci
  Heavy-Chain Genes · κ Light-Chain Genes · λ Light-Chain Genes · λ-Related "Surrogate" Light Chains
V Gene Assembly Recombination
  Topology of V Assembly Recombination · Mechanism of V assembly recombination · Regulation of V(D)J Recombination · Germline Diversity
  · Combinatorial Diversity Estimates
Regulation of Immunoglobulin Gene Expression
Immunoglobulin Gene Alterations in Germinal Centers
  Heavy-Chain Switch · Somatic Mutation
Conclusion
References

The unique mysteries of antibody genes lie in the diversity of proteins that they encode. This diversity exists at several levels.

1. Most striking is the diversity of antigen-combining sites of these molecules. The classic studies of Karl Landsteiner suggested that the repertoire of binding specificities of antibodies is essentially unlimited. The diversity of binding specificities is explained by the diversity of amino acid sequences found in the N-terminal domain of both light and heavy chains: the variable (V) region. Each V region contains three subregions of especially high variability (hypervariable regions), which correspond to the loops of the protein that contact antigen, or complementarity-determining regions (CDRs), as discussed in Chapter 3. However, on the C-terminal end, the single domain of the light chain and the three (or four, depending on isotype) domains of heavy chains were found to be invariant within each class of light or heavy chains; these segments are designated constant (C) regions. As an explanation for the strict dichotomy between the diverse V regions and singular C region sequences, Dreyer and Bennett (1) proposed in 1965 that, for each class of immunoglobulin (Ig) genes, there might be only a single C region gene, which was encoded in the germline separately from the multiple V region genes; during the development of an antibody-producing cell, one of the V region sequences would

become associated with the C region sequence, leading to a complete (V + C) gene, which the cell could then express. Thus, mechanisms that increase diversity in the isolated V region genes might leave the single C region gene at its distant locus untouched. This model, with its proposal of gene rearrangement occurring independently in each lymphocyte, was revolutionary in that it violated the then-accepted notion that deoxyribonucleic acid (DNA) is the same in all cells of the organism. There were two additional mysteries: In view of the fact that each B lymphocyte should contain two copies of each gene locus (i.e., from the maternally and paternally derived chromosomes), why does the cell express only a single light chain and a single heavy chain, as if the locus on the nonexpressed chromosome were somehow silenced (the phenomenon known as *allelic exclusion*)? And how can the fact that affinity of serum antibodies for antigen increases over a period of weeks after antigen exposure (the phenomenon of *affinity maturation*) be explained?

2. Apart from the diversity of V regions in both light and heavy chains, heavy chains exhibit a different sort of diversity that also deserves a molecular biological explanation: all developing B cells synthesize immunoglobulin M (IgM) initially and can switch heavy-chain isotype from μ to γ, ε, or α only later in their maturation. As the expressed C region "switches," the cell continues to express the same light and heavy-chain V regions, so that

antigen specificity remains unchanged. Thus, in addition to understanding how, in different cells, a single C region can become associated with multiple different V regions (V-C recombination), we need to understand the molecular mechanism by which, within one lymphocyte, a single V region may become associated sequentially with several C regions (heavy-chain switch) must be understood.

3. A final level of diversity exhibited by Ig heavy chains is represented by the alternative forms of Ig found embedded in the membrane of B cells versus those in blood and secretions. Membrane immunoglobulins have C-terminal extensions containing hydrophobic amino acids that associate with membrane lipids, whereas secreted immunoglobulins lack this C-terminal piece but are otherwise identical to the membrane counterparts. Analysis of Ig genes has revealed how these two forms are encoded in the genome.

This chapter begins with a brief discussion of V gene assembly in heavy- and light-chain genes. The heavy-chain locus—including molecular explanations for the membrane forms of immunoglobulin—is then described, followed by descriptions of the J ("joining") and C regions of the κ and λ loci. Next, the DNA recombination events underlying V gene assembly and the regulation of this process to maintain allelic exclusion are considered in detail. The chapter continues with a discussion of the germline repertoire of immunoglobulin genes of humans and mice and the combinatorial expansion of the repertoire resulting from V assembly recombination. A short discussion of the regulation of immunoglobulin gene expression follows. The chapter concludes with a discussion of the two alterations in Ig gene structure that occur in mature B cells stimulated in the germinal center environment: isotype switching and somatic hypermutation.

The investigations described in this chapter have been chosen from the literature to facilitate a clear exposition of the important issues rather than to provide a comprehensive compendium of data and references on Ig genes. In these descriptions, most of the discussion focuses on murine and human immunoglobulin genes. Murine genes were studied first because of the availability of pristane-induced murine myelomas of BALB/c mice, which served as convenient monoclonal sources of Ig protein for early structural studies. The same myelomas then provided messenger ribonucleic acid (mRNA) and DNA for molecular biology analysis. This work was greatly facilitated by the fact that these myelomas derived from the same genetic background: the inbred BALB/c strain. More recently, strains of mice carrying transgenes or strains engineered with targeted gene replacements or deletions have been valuable in understanding the function of various genes related to Ig function. Human Ig gene loci show many fundamental similarities to murine Ig gene loci, whereas some other mammalian orders show surprisingly significant differences.

OVERVIEW OF IMMUNOGLOBULIN V GENE ASSEMBLY

In the late 1970s, experiments on light-chain genes established that the Dreyer-Bennett hypothesis was fundamentally correct: Each lymphocyte expresses only a single Ig molecule encoded by one VL gene and one VH gene, each having been "activated" by a recombination event that brings the V gene near its respective C region gene. This conclusion was supported by comparisons of Ig genes from B lymphoid cells, particularly murine myelomas, and the corresponding gene loci from "germline" DNA. (Although true germline DNA can experimentally be obtained only from sperm, any nonlymphoid DNA is assumed to be representative of germline DNA, because the rearrangements of Ig genes occur only in lymphoid cells. When DNA from sperm versus other nonlymphoid tissues have been compared by Southern blotting, the results have been identical. Therefore, despite the risk of some imprecision, nonlymphoid DNA samples are conventionally referred to as germline, regardless of whether the DNA is from sperm, whole embryo, liver, placenta, or other nonlymphoid sources.)

Evidence from Southern Blotting and Gene Cloning

Myeloma and germline DNA were initially compared by Southern blotting with hybridization probes derived from myeloma complementary DNAs (cDNAs). As schematically shown in Fig. 1 for an analysis of κ light-chain genes, a Cκ probe detects only a single band in germline DNA, consistent with a single Cκ gene. A probe representing an expressed Vκ gene detects several bands, as though hybridizing to a family of related sequences. Moreover, although this is not shown in Fig. 1, probes representing different expressed Vκ genes are found to hybridize to a different set of bands, representing a different family of related Vκ genes. These observations support the multiple V genes, single C gene component of the Dreyer-Bennett model. The hypothesis that recombination occurs between V and C genes is supported by the different bands observed when these probes are hybridized to myeloma DNA instead of germline DNA. As shown in Fig. 1, the recombination bringing a V gene close to a C gene can cause an alteration in size of the Cκ-hybridizing restriction fragment. The new rearranged band may be larger, smaller, or, fortuitously, the same size as the germline band, depending on the location of the restriction sites flanking the V and C genes. Similarly, one of the V region bands may be expected to be rearranged in the myeloma so as to lie on a different-sized fragment, the same fragment that hybridizes to the Cκ probe. Results like these for κ and λ genes strongly supported the Dreyer-Bennett hypothesis and forcefully challenged the concept that every cell in the body has identical genes (2,3). In panels of myelomas analyzed for Cκ recombination by Southern blotting, many showed evidence of DNA rearrangement on both allelic chromosomes. This result contradicted the possibility that allelic exclusion might be explained by a

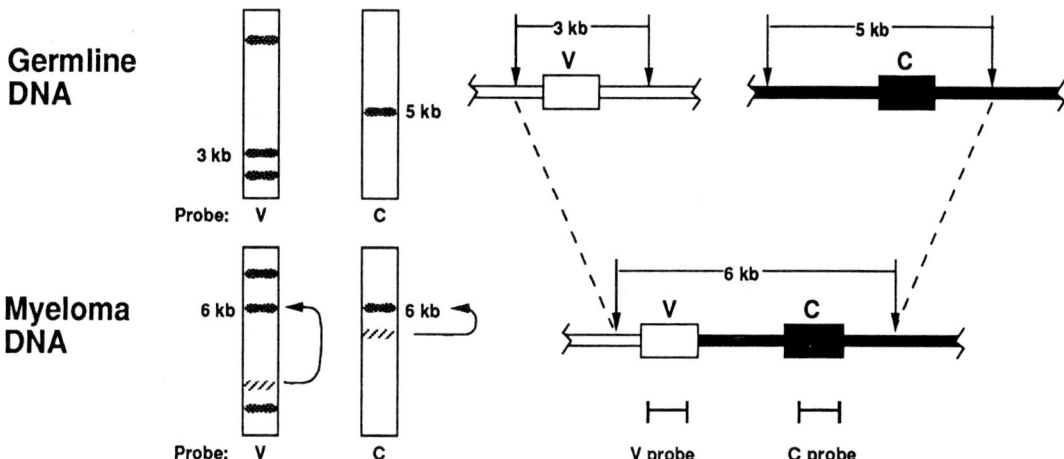

FIG. 1. Southern blot demonstration of rearrangement of immunoglobulin V and C region genes. EcoRI sites in this hypothetical example are indicated by *arrows*. In germline DNA (*upper drawings*), V and C are an unknown distance apart and are found by Southern blot hybridization (*left*) to lie on EcoRI fragments of 3 and 5 kb, respectively. The V region probe hybridizes to a family of related genes (shown by bands above and below the 3-kb band). In myeloma DNA (*lower panel*), V and C genes have been brought into close proximity and, in this example, are no longer separated by EcoRI sites; both genes are found on the same EcoRI fragment of 6 kb, which is thus identified by either probe. The germline-sized fragments (hatched bands in the Southern blots) may or may not be preserved in the myeloma, depending on whether the nonexpressed homologous chromosome has remained in its germline (unrearranged) state. In many myelomas, both chromosomes are present and both are rearranged.

mechanism that allowed recombination on only one chromosome, and it raised questions about the nature of the "second" gene rearrangement in these cells, as discussed later in this chapter.

A more complete understanding of recombination of Ig genes developed from sequence analysis of cloned myeloma versus germline DNA. The general structures of the germline V genes are similar for the three Ig loci: heavy chain, κ, and λ. Each V gene begins with sequence encoding a signal peptide of about 22 amino acids. (Signal peptides are found at the N-terminal of most proteins destined for secretion or expression on the cell membranes; after "routing" the protein to the endoplasmic reticulum, the peptide is generally removed by specific peptidases.) Within codon −4 (numbering backwards from the beginning of the mature protein sequence), the coding sequence is interrupted by an intron, usually roughly 0.1 to 0.3 kb long. What was unanticipated was the discovery that each V region gene as it exists in the germline is incomplete and that recombination is necessary to assemble a complete V gene. For example, most murine κ chains have V regions 108 amino acids in length, but murine germline Vκ genes encode only about 95 of these. The remaining 13 amino acids are encoded by segments known as J regions that lie upstream of the C region gene. An assembled Vκ gene thus results from recombination that joins one of many germline Vκ genes to one of five Jκ gene segments (Fig. 2A). A similar recombination event is necessary to assemble a complete Vλ chain sequence from germline Vλ and Jλ genes. For heavy chains, recombination assembles a V region from three types of germline elements; between the residues

encoded by germline VH and JH elements are interposed variable numbers of amino acids—commonly from zero to eight residues—encoded by a diversity (D) region. The assembly of a complete heavy-chain V region occurs in two separate steps (Fig. 2B): Initially, one of several germline DH regions joins with one of the JH regions; then a germline VH region is added to complete the assembled V-D-J heavy-chain gene.

How Recombination Contributes to Diversity

The V assembly recombination contributes in two significant ways to the diversity of antigen-binding specificities. First, because there are multiple germline V regions and multiple D and J regions, the number of possible combinations of VL, JL, VH, DH, and JH is the multiplication product of the numbers of each of these five classes of germline sequence elements. This repertoire is vastly larger than could be achieved by devoting the same total lengths of DNA sequence to preassembled V regions. A second factor that increases diversity was recognized from comparisons of nucleotide sequences of various myeloma genes to their germline precursors. For example, as shown in Fig. 3A, a comparison between the Vκ gene expressed in the murine myeloma MOPC41 and the corresponding germline Vκ and Jκ genes shows that the myeloma gene matches the germline precursor through the second nucleotide of codon 95; the V-J recombination junction clearly occurs at this point, inasmuch as sequence beyond this position in the myeloma gene clearly derives from Jκ1. Similar analyses of other myelomas reveal that the

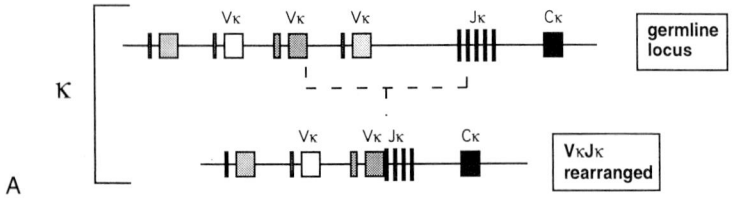

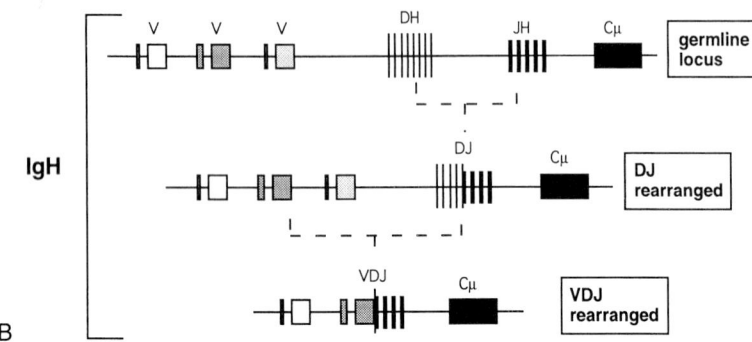

FIG. 2. V assembly recombination. **A:** In the κ locus, a single recombination event joins a germline Vκ region with one of the Jκ segments. **B:** In the heavy immunoglobulin locus, an initial recombination joins a D segment to a J segment. A second recombination completes the V assembly by joining a VH segment to D-JH.

recombination junctions can occur at several different positions within codon 95 or 96. As shown in Fig. 3B, this "flexibility" of the position of the recombination junction increases the diversity of the affected codons. Heavy-chain V regions exhibit this flexibility at both V-D and D-J junctions. In addition, many heavy-chain V-D-J junctions (and a smaller percentage of light-chain V-J junctions) contain insertions of a few extra nucleotides not present in the germline precursors; the mechanism of these insertions—known as N regions—is discussed later in this chapter. Of significance is that the three-dimensional structure of immunoglobulins established from x-ray crystallography reveals that both the VL-JL junction

and the VH-DH-JH junction form CDR3 loops that can contact antigen; thus this junctional diversity is functionality relevant for diversifying antigen binding. The important role of D junctional amino acids for antigen binding has been verified by mutational analysis (4).

When the "flexibility" of the position of recombination was initially discovered, it was hard to understand how the germline elements could be joined with such variability and yet maintain the correct triplet reading frame between V and J. (An out-of-frame recombination would cause the entire C region to be read in a nonsense reading frame, and so the gene would be nonfunctional.) It soon became clear, however,

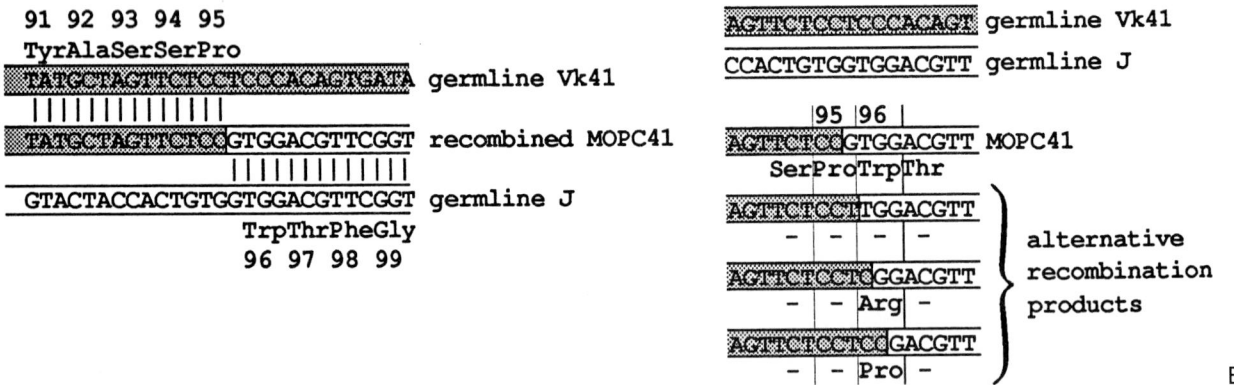

FIG. 3. Vκ-Jκ recombination at single-base resolution. **A:** The sequence of the recombined MOPC41 κ gene around the V-J junction is shown (*center*) with the sequences of the two germline precursors (Vκ41 and Jκ1) shown above and below. The germline origins of the recombined gene are indicated by the *vertical lines* and the *shading* of the V-derived sequence. **B:** The consequences of joining the same germline sequences (from part **A**) at four different positions are shown. Of the four alternative recombination products illustrated, the top one is that actually found in MOPC41. The second example has a single nucleotide difference but no change in encoded amino acid sequence. The third and fourth alternatives yield arginine or proline at position 96; both of these amino acids have been found at this position in sequenced murine κ chains.

that many assembled V genes could be found with out-of-frame recombination junctions (5). Indeed, in unselected V-J recombinations, the frequency of in-frame junctions is about 1/3, just as predicted for a recombination mechanism insensitive to reading frame. In myelomas with rearrangements on both allelic copies of an immunoglobulin gene locus, the unexpressed recombination is generally out-of-frame, or "nonproductive." For heavy-chain V-D-J recombination, it is theoretically possible to retain the correct reading frame between V and J while allowing the interposed D region segments to be used in all three reading frames. In murine heavy chains, however, only a single D region reading frame is generally found, and several mechanisms prevent expression of antibodies with D regions in the other two reading frames (6). In human antibodies, this intense selection against variant reading frames is not found (7), which allows for additional sequence diversity. The generation of V region diversity in the three–Ig gene loci (heavy, κ, and λ) is considered in more detail in a later section.

Recombination Signal Elements

Analysis of DNA sequences flanking the germline V, D, and J region sequences revealed two conserved sequence elements that have subsequently been shown to define targets for V(D)J recombination: a heptamer adjacent to the coding sequence and a more distal nonamer. (These sequences are diagrammed in Fig. 4.) For example, in the κ locus, the consensus heptamer CACTGTG occurs 5′ of the Jκ coding sequences, and its (reverse) complement CACAGTG appears 3′ to Vκ coding sequences. The consensus nonamer GGTTTTTGT appears about 23 nucleotides 5′ of the Jκ heptamer, and its complement ACAAAAACC appears about 12 nucleotides 3′ of the Vκ heptamer. Similar sequences flank Vλ and Jλ, as well as VH, DH, and JH (as shown in Fig. 4). These recombination signal sequences (RSSs) have been shown to be critical in the recombination, serving as recognition sequences for the

recombination activating gene (RAG) products RAG1 and RAG2, as discussed later in this chapter. Similar RSSs are present flanking light and heavy-chain Ig genes throughout phylogeny, as well as in T-cell receptor genes (see Chapter 8), which undergo similar V assembly recombinations. In all of these systems, the length of the spacer between the heptamer and nonamer (Fig. 4) appears significant. Recombination apparently occurs almost exclusively between one coding sequence associated with an approximately 12-bp spacer and another coding sequence with an approximately 23-bp spacer, a requirement referred to as the *12/23 rule.* This requirement may serve to prevent futile recombinations, such as between two Vκ or two Jκ gene segments. Although the heptamer and nonamer are the primary elements necessary for V(D)J recombination, a computerized alignment of several hundred spacer sequences has detected some preferred nucleotides at specific positions (8), and different spacer sequences can affect recombination frequency (9).

THE THREE IMMUNOGLOBULIN GENE LOCI

This section presents an overview of the three Ig loci: heavy chain, κ, and λ. The V regions of these loci are described in a later section on germline diversity.

Heavy-Chain Genes

Genomic clones encoding CH genes were obtained in the early 1980s by screening genomic DNA libraries with cDNA probes derived from myeloma mRNA. One striking characteristic of CH genes is that the approximately 100 to 110 amino acid domains—identified by internal homologies of amino acid sequences and by three-dimensional structural analysis (x-ray crystallography)—are encoded as intact exons, separated from other domain segments by introns of approximately 0.1 to 0.3 kb. Thus, for example, the murine γ2b protein has three major domains (CH1, CH2, and CH3)

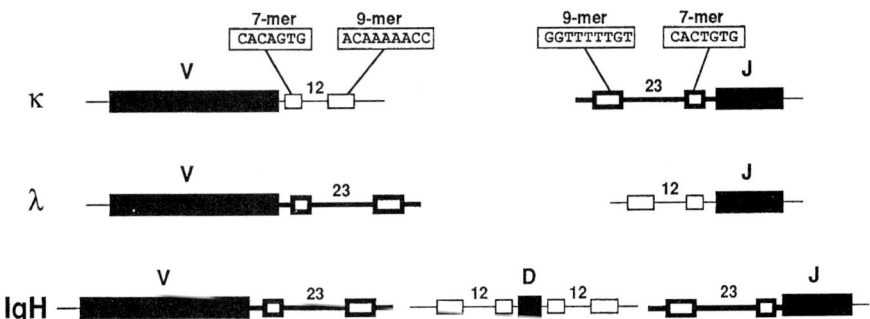

FIG. 4. Conserved elements flank germline V, D, and J region genes. Conserved heptamer and nonamer recombination signal sequences (RSSs) lie adjacent to V, D, and J coding sequences and are important for targeting V(D)J recombination. The heptamer and nonamer elements are separated by spacer regions of about 12 bp (illustrated by *thin lines*) or 23 bp (*thick lines*). Depending on the locus, V regions may be flanked by 12- or 23-bp RSSs; a similar situation exists for J regions. However, one of each type of element must be present for recombination to occur; this requirement prevents futile recombination events (e.g., J to J).

with a small hinge domain between CH1 and CH2. The gene structure may be summarized as follows:

CH1—intron—**hinge**—intron—**CH2**—intron—**CH3**
(292)   (314)   (64)   (106)   (328)   (119)   (322)

where the numbers in parentheses represent the number of nucleotides in each segment. As an interesting contrast, the hinge region of the α gene is encoded contiguously with the CH2 domain with no intervening intron, whereas the unusually long human $\gamma 3$ hinge is encoded by three or four hinge exons. Sequence analyses of genomic CH genes have led to speculations that the evolutionary history of heavy-chain genes may have included mutations that created or destroyed RNA splice sites and thereby converted portions of intron sequence into exon and vice versa. For example, the sequence of the intron $5'$ to the hinge of the murine $\gamma 2b$ gene shows a surprising degree of similarity with the sequence of CH1; this observation led to the speculation (10) that the hinge exon may have originated from a full Ig domain that became foreshortened either by the destruction of the RNA splice site at the $5'$ end of the domain or the creation of a new splice site within the domain.

About 7 kb upstream from the murine $C\mu$ gene lies a cluster of four JH segments (six JH segments in human) that participate in V-D-J recombination. Further upstream lie 13 D segments (about 27 in human) and beyond them the VH regions. V and D regions are described later in this chapter in the section on V region diversity.

In the development of a B lymphocyte, the cell initially produces IgM with a binding specificity determined by the productively rearranged VH and VL regions. Subsequently, the progeny cells deriving from that B cell synthesize antibodies with the same light- and heavy-chain V regions; however, they generally switch the isotype of the heavy chain to immunoglobulins G, A, or E (IgG, IgA, or IgE). Early evidence for this developmental scheme included the isotype switch seen during the course of an immune response and *in vivo* ablation studies that suggested that IgM-producing cells are the precursors of IgG producers (11). Many laboratories have subsequently found that IgM-producing resting B cells isolated from mouse spleen or human peripheral blood can be induced to switch isotype expression *in vitro* by appropriate culture conditions, including specific cytokines. The molecular mechanism by which one part of a protein can change while another part remains unchanged has generated considerable interest.

Several groups demonstrated that active rearranged α, $\gamma 2b$, and $\gamma 1$ genes isolated from myelomas expressing the respective heavy chains contain—between their V and C regions—DNA sequence derived from the DNA upstream of the germline $C\mu$ gene, including one or more JH sequences. These observations led to the model that the VH region rearranges initially to a position $5'$ to the $C\mu$ gene (leading to IgM production). Then, when a cell expresses a new isotype, a recombination event brings the C gene encoding that isotype immediately downstream of the expressed V-D-J gene by deleting $C\mu$ and the other intervening C genes, as shown in Fig. 5. Isotype switch recombination [also called *class switch recombination* (CSR)] is discussed later in this chapter.

Membrane Versus Secreted Immunoglobulin

Studies of heavy Ig gene and cDNA structure have provided an explanation for the alternative membrane and secreted forms of the heavy chain. As noted earlier, the membrane-bound forms of Ig heavy chains are slightly larger than the secreted forms owing to an additional C-terminal hydrophobic segment that anchors the protein in membrane lipids. In the case of the μ chain, the membrane and secreted forms are products of two different mRNAs of 2.7 and 2.4 kb, which can be separated by gel electrophoresis. Sequence comparisons between a genomic μ clone and μ cDNA clones corresponding to these two RNA species demonstrated that the two RNAs represent transcripts of the identical gene that have been spliced differently at their $3'$ or C-terminal ends (Fig. 6). The nucleotide sequence encoding the 20 C-terminal residues of the secretory (μs) form is derived from DNA contiguous with the CH4 domain of the μ gene, whereas in the membrane mRNA (μm), the sequence following CH4 derives from two exons (M1 and M2) about 2 kb further $3'$. These membrane exons encode 41 residues, including a stretch of 26 uncharged residues that span the membrane to fix the Ig to the cell surface. The same general gene structure has been found for the other CH genes, which suggests that the differential splicing mechanism accounts for the two forms of Ig of all isotypes.

Early B cells make roughly similar quantities of both μm and μs, whereas maturation to the plasma cell stage is associated with strong predominance of μs production, which is consistent with the function of such cells in generating the pool of circulating immunoglobulin. The balance between the two RNA splice forms of μ has been interpreted as a competition between CH4-M1 splicing and the cleavage/

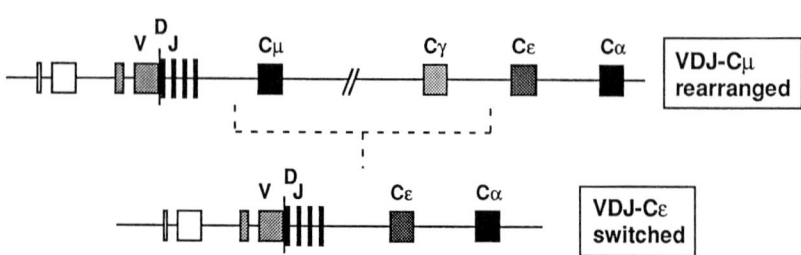

FIG. 5. Deletional isotype switch recombination. The expression of "downstream" heavy-chain genes is accomplished by a recombination event that replaces the $C\mu$ gene with the appropriate heavy-chain C gene ($C\epsilon$ in the figure), deleting the DNA between the recombination breakpoints.

antigen specificity remains unchanged. Thus, in addition to understanding how, in different cells, a single C region can become associated with multiple different V regions (V-C recombination), we need to understand the molecular mechanism by which, within one lymphocyte, a single V region may become associated sequentially with several C regions (heavy-chain switch) must be understood.

3. A final level of diversity exhibited by Ig heavy chains is represented by the alternative forms of Ig found embedded in the membrane of B cells versus those in blood and secretions. Membrane immunoglobulins have C-terminal extensions containing hydrophobic amino acids that associate with membrane lipids, whereas secreted immunoglobulins lack this C-terminal piece but are otherwise identical to the membrane counterparts. Analysis of Ig genes has revealed how these two forms are encoded in the genome.

This chapter begins with a brief discussion of V gene assembly in heavy- and light-chain genes. The heavy-chain locus—including molecular explanations for the membrane forms of immunoglobulin—is then described, followed by descriptions of the J ("joining") and C regions of the κ and λ loci. Next, the DNA recombination events underlying V gene assembly and the regulation of this process to maintain allelic exclusion are considered in detail. The chapter continues with a discussion of the germline repertoire of immunoglobulin genes of humans and mice and the combinatorial expansion of the repertoire resulting from V assembly recombination. A short discussion of the regulation of immunoglobulin gene expression follows. The chapter concludes with a discussion of the two alterations in Ig gene structure that occur in mature B cells stimulated in the germinal center environment: isotype switching and somatic hypermutation.

The investigations described in this chapter have been chosen from the literature to facilitate a clear exposition of the important issues rather than to provide a comprehensive compendium of data and references on Ig genes. In these descriptions, most of the discussion focuses on murine and human immunoglobulin genes. Murine genes were studied first because of the availability of pristane-induced murine myelomas of BALB/c mice, which served as convenient monoclonal sources of Ig protein for early structural studies. The same myelomas then provided messenger ribonucleic acid (mRNA) and DNA for molecular biology analysis. This work was greatly facilitated by the fact that these myelomas derived from the same genetic background: the inbred BALB/c strain. More recently, strains of mice carrying transgenes or strains engineered with targeted gene replacements or deletions have been valuable in understanding the function of various genes related to Ig function. Human Ig gene loci show many fundamental similarities to murine Ig gene loci, whereas some other mammalian orders show surprisingly significant differences.

OVERVIEW OF IMMUNOGLOBULIN V GENE ASSEMBLY

In the late 1970s, experiments on light-chain genes established that the Dreyer-Bennett hypothesis was fundamentally correct: Each lymphocyte expresses only a single Ig molecule encoded by one VL gene and one VH gene, each having been "activated" by a recombination event that brings the V gene near its respective C region gene. This conclusion was supported by comparisons of Ig genes from B lymphoid cells, particularly murine myelomas, and the corresponding gene loci from "germline" DNA. (Although true germline DNA can experimentally be obtained only from sperm, any nonlymphoid DNA is assumed to be representative of germline DNA, because the rearrangements of Ig genes occur only in lymphoid cells. When DNA from sperm versus other nonlymphoid tissues have been compared by Southern blotting, the results have been identical. Therefore, despite the risk of some imprecision, nonlymphoid DNA samples are conventionally referred to as germline, regardless of whether the DNA is from sperm, whole embryo, liver, placenta, or other nonlymphoid sources.)

Evidence from Southern Blotting and Gene Cloning

Myeloma and germline DNA were initially compared by Southern blotting with hybridization probes derived from myeloma complementary DNAs (cDNAs). As schematically shown in Fig. 1 for an analysis of κ light-chain genes, a Cκ probe detects only a single band in germline DNA, consistent with a single Cκ gene. A probe representing an expressed Vκ gene detects several bands, as though hybridizing to a family of related sequences. Moreover, although this is not shown in Fig. 1, probes representing different expressed Vκ genes are found to hybridize to a different set of bands, representing a different family of related Vκ genes. These observations support the multiple V genes, single C gene component of the Dreyer-Bennett model. The hypothesis that recombination occurs between V and C genes is supported by the different bands observed when these probes are hybridized to myeloma DNA instead of germline DNA. As shown in Fig. 1, the recombination bringing a V gene close to a C gene can cause an alteration in size of the Cκ-hybridizing restriction fragment. The new rearranged band may be larger, smaller, or, fortuitously, the same size as the germline band, depending on the location of the restriction sites flanking the V and C genes. Similarly, one of the V region bands may be expected to be rearranged in the myeloma so as to lie on a different-sized fragment, the same fragment that hybridizes to the Cκ probe. Results like these for κ and λ genes strongly supported the Dreyer-Bennett hypothesis and forcefully challenged the concept that every cell in the body has identical genes (2,3). In panels of myelomas analyzed for Cκ recombination by Southern blotting, many showed evidence of DNA rearrangement on both allelic chromosomes. This result contradicted the possibility that allelic exclusion might be explained by a

CHAPTER 5

Immunoglobulins: Molecular Genetics

Edward E. Max

Overview of Immunoglobulin V Gene Assembly
Evidence from Southern Blotting and Gene Cloning · How Recombination Contributes to Diversity · Recombination Signal Elements
The Three Immunoglobulin Gene Loci
Heavy-Chain Genes · κ Light-Chain Genes · λ Light-Chain Genes · λ-Related "Surrogate" Light Chains
V Gene Assembly Recombination
Topology of V Assembly Recombination · Mechanism of V assembly recombination · Regulation of V(D)J Recombination · Germline Diversity · Combinatorial Diversity Estimates
Regulation of Immunoglobulin Gene Expression
Immunoglobulin Gene Alterations in Germinal Centers
Heavy-Chain Switch · Somatic Mutation
Conclusion
References

The unique mysteries of antibody genes lie in the diversity of proteins that they encode. This diversity exists at several levels.

1. Most striking is the diversity of antigen-combining sites of these molecules. The classic studies of Karl Landsteiner suggested that the repertoire of binding specificities of antibodies is essentially unlimited. The diversity of binding specificities is explained by the diversity of amino acid sequences found in the N-terminal domain of both light and heavy chains: the variable (V) region. Each V region contains three subregions of especially high variability (hypervariable regions), which correspond to the loops of the protein that contact antigen, or complementarity-determining regions (CDRs), as discussed in Chapter 3. However, on the C-terminal end, the single domain of the light chain and the three (or four, depending on isotype) domains of heavy chains were found to be invariant within each class of light or heavy chains; these segments are designated constant (C) regions. As an explanation for the strict dichotomy between the diverse V regions and singular C region sequences, Dreyer and Bennett (1) proposed in 1965 that, for each class of immunoglobulin (Ig) genes, there might be only a single C region gene, which was encoded in the germline separately from the multiple V region genes; during the development of an antibody-producing cell, one of the V region sequences would

become associated with the C region sequence, leading to a complete (V + C) gene, which the cell could then express. Thus, mechanisms that increase diversity in the isolated V region genes might leave the single C region gene at its distant locus untouched. This model, with its proposal of gene rearrangement occurring independently in each lymphocyte, was revolutionary in that it violated the then-accepted notion that deoxyribonucleic acid (DNA) is the same in all cells of the organism. There were two additional mysteries: In view of the fact that each B lymphocyte should contain two copies of each gene locus (i.e., from the maternally and paternally derived chromosomes), why does the cell express only a single light chain and a single heavy chain, as if the locus on the nonexpressed chromosome were somehow silenced (the phenomenon known as *allelic exclusion*)? And how can the fact that affinity of serum antibodies for antigen increases over a period of weeks after antigen exposure (the phenomenon of *affinity maturation*) be explained?

2. Apart from the diversity of V regions in both light and heavy chains, heavy chains exhibit a different sort of diversity that also deserves a molecular biological explanation: all developing B cells synthesize immunoglobulin M (IgM) initially and can switch heavy-chain isotype from μ to γ, ϵ, or α only later in their maturation. As the expressed C region "switches," the cell continues to express the same light and heavy-chain V regions, so that

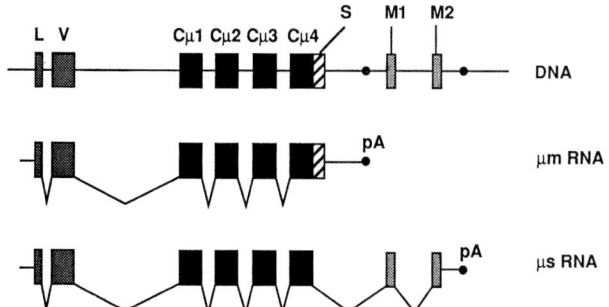

FIG. 6. Two RNAs generated from the μ gene by alternative processing. The exons of the μ gene (*black rectangles*) are illustrated (*top*) in an expressed, rearranged μ gene. A primary transcript that includes all the exons present in the DNA can be processed as shown to yield either μs RNA [containing a C-terminal "secreted" (S) sequence] or μm RNA [containing the two membrane (M) exons].

polyadenylation at the upstream μs poly(A) addition site. These processes are mutually exclusive because CH4-M1 splice removes the μs poly(A) site, whereas cleavage at the μs poly(A) site removes the membrane exons. The factors influencing the balance between these processes have been studied by transfecting either early or late B cells (or nonlymphoid cells) with μ gene sequences or constructs in which the splice sites, coding exons, or cleavage/polyadenylation sites have been mutated, placed different distances apart, or replaced with other sequences. The μm poly(A) site appears to be intrinsically more active than the μs poly(A) site when tested in separate plasmids, and some evidence suggests competition between these sites (12,13). The relative utilization of these two sites is influenced by cis-acting features of the RNA structure, including the length of RNA between the two sites (13) and the integrity of a guanine/uracil-rich sequence that forms a stem-loop downstream of the polyadenylation signal AAUAAA of the μs site (14). In addition, features of the mRNA that affect CH4-M1 splicing efficiency may also affect the μs/μm ratio, perhaps including the size of the CH4 exon (15). Other cis-acting sequences affecting the ratio of alternative splice forms have been described for other isotypes besides Cμ [e.g., Coyle and Lebman (16)]. Changes in *trans*-acting factors control the developmental shift toward greater secretory mRNA in Ig-secreting plasma cells. For the μ isotype, these factors include increasing content of the polyadenylation factor CstF-64 (a 64-kD subunit of the heterotrimeric cleavage stimulation factor), which binds to the guanine/uracil-rich sequence near the μs site. When levels of this protein were artificially increased in a B cell line, the μs/μm ratio was increased (17). The binding of this protein to the μs guanine/uracil-rich sequence may also be reduced before the secretory stage of B lymphoid development by inhibitory factors such as hnRNP F (18).

Membrane Ig serves as the antigen-specific component of the B-cell receptor (BCR) that is critical for initiating the signal for lymphocyte activation on contact with anti-

gen, as described in Chapter 7. The segments of membrane immunoglobulins (of all isotypes) that penetrate into the cytoplasm are too short to encode functional signal transduction domains. Instead, transduction is mediated by an associated protein dimer composed of the BCR components Igα and Igβ (CD79a and CD79b), whose cytoplasmic domains contain immunoreceptor tyrosine-based activation motifs (ITAMs) similar to those found in the CD3 chains mediating T-cell receptor (TCR) signaling. The Igα-Igβ dimer also plays important signaling roles during B cell development before the mature BCR is assembled, as discussed later in this chapter.

Organization of CH Gene Loci

The murine heavy-chain genes were cloned by a variety of investigators, and all eight CH genes—spanning about 200 kb of DNA on chromosome 12—were linked by contiguous clones in 1982 (19). These clones define the general structure of the region as shown in Fig. 7, in which the numbers indicate the distance in kilobases between the genes. All the CH genes are oriented in the same 5'–3' direction. Analysis by high-throughput sequencing has revealed several γ pseudogenes within the clustered γ genes (20). The sequence of the murine heavy Ig locus is now available online at www.ncbi.nlm.nih.gov.

The human CH genes have also been cloned and localized to chromosome 14q32 but were not completely linked unit the Human Gerome Project sequenced the entire locus. The human heavy Ig locus contains a large duplication, with two copies of a γ-γ-ϵ-α unit separated by a γ pseudogene (Fig. 7). One of the duplicated ϵ sequences is also a pseudogene, in which the CH1 and CH2 domains have been deleted. In addition, the human genome contains a third closely homologous ϵ-related sequence: a "processed" pseudogene retroposed to chromosome 9. The map presented in Fig. 7 is based on partial contiguous overlaps and Southern blot studies of large fragments separated by pulsed-field gel electrophoresis (PFGE). This map is consistent with the known deletions in the heavy-chain locus, as diagrammed in Fig. 7 and with sequence contigs in GenBank.

The heavy Ig locus has also been examined in several other species besides mouse and human, and several notable differences have been observed. Rabbits, for example, have 13 Cα sequences and only a single Cγ gene (21); this unusual expansion of genes contributing to mucosal immunity may be related to the peculiar habit of coprophagy in these animals. In contrast to the multiplicity of rabbit Cα genes, pigs have only one Cα gene and eight Cγ genes. Camels are unusual in having heavy chains that function in the absence of light chains (22). Heavy-chain Ig genes (VH or CH) have been cloned from a number of other species, including the rat (which is highly homologous with the mouse), cow, chicken, horse, shark, bony fish, crocodile, frog, and axolotl.

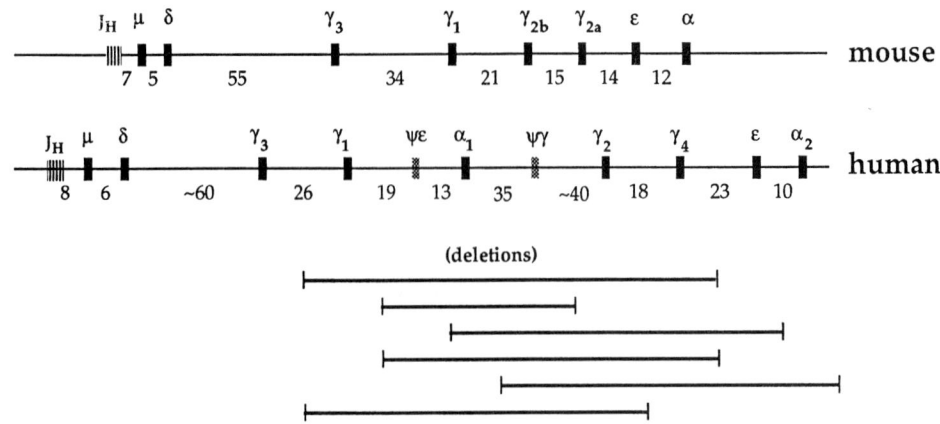

FIG. 7. Heavy-chain constant region loci of mouse and man. The murine locus has been cloned in its entirety (19); the constant region genes are diagrammed with the approximate intergene distance indicated below (in kb). The human locus shows a large duplication of γ-γ-ϵ-α sequences; the indicated order has been supported by cloned contigs, by the deletions observed in various individuals, and by PFGE mapping. High through-put sequences (available at www.ncbi.nlm.nih.gov) confirm both maps, though there are some differences in distances, possibly due to allelic polymorphisms.

κ Light-Chain Genes

In comparison to the heavy-chain genes, the κ locus is relatively simple. A single Cκ gene with a single exon and no reported alternative splice products is found in both mouse and human. Upstream of the murine Cκ gene lie five Jκ gene segments spaced about 0.3 kb apart. The third of these Jκ segments encodes an amino acid sequence never observed in κ chains and that is believed to be nonfunctional owing to a defect in the splice donor site that would join the corresponding RNA sequence to Cκ. The human locus is quite similar, with five Jκ regions upstream of Cκ; however, no homolog of the defective murine Jκ3 is present in the human Jκ cluster, whereas an additional Jκ sequence lies downstream of the sequence homologous to murine Jκ5. Upstream of the Jκ segments in both species lie the Vκ genes, which are described later in this chapter.

Apart from Vκ-Jκ rearrangement, an additional recombination event occurs in this locus, a recombination unique to κ genes and apparently mediated by the same heptamer/nonamer signal elements involved in V(D)J recombination. This event, which involves deletion of the Cκ gene segment, was initially suggested by the observation that Southern blots of DNA from λ-expressing human lymphoid cells generally show no detectable Cκ sequence (23). Apparently, in most B cells, the Cκ genes are deleted from both chromosomes before λ gene rearrangement begins. When the boundaries of the deleted segment of DNA were examined in several human and murine cell lines, a common sequence element was found at the downstream boundary; this element was designated RS (recombining sequence) in the mouse studies (24) and kde (κ-deleting element) in the human studies (25). The human kde in germline DNA is located 24 kb downstream of the Cκ gene and is flanked by a heptamer/nonamer RSS similar to that found flanking the Jκ regions: that is, with a 23-bp spacer. The similar murine RS is about 25 kb downstream

from murine Cκ. The kde element can apparently recombine either with a Vκ gene segment (leading to a deletion of the entire Jκ-Cκ locus) or with an isolated heptamer element that is located in the Jκ-Cκ intron (leading to deletion of Cκ but retention of the Jκ locus). The heptamer in the Jκ-Cκ intron is 30 bp 5′ from a poorly conserved nonamer-like sequence, a spacing that seems to violate the usual 12/23 rule. The significance of this unusual spacer is not understood, but possibly the heptamer in these recombinations is active without a functional nonamer, as seems to be the case for secondary VH recombinations (discussed in a later section).

A comparison between the murine RS and human kde sequences shows that the recombination signals are highly conserved and that, downstream of these elements, a region of about 500 bp is partially conserved (about 50% sequence identity). The latter region includes open reading frames of 127 (murine) or 102 (human) codons. It is not known whether these reading frames are ever expressed as protein as a consequence of the RS/kde recombination events, but the fact that the recombination may occur with either a Vκ region or intron sequence suggests that the sequences joined by the event may be less important than the sequences deleted. RS/kde elements are most often found to be rearranged in cells in which Cκ is deleted and λ rearrangements are present; this observation led to the speculation that the RS/kde recombination event may mediate the developmental switch from κ to λ gene rearrangement, perhaps by deleting a gene for a negative regulator of λ gene rearrangement. However, current evidence argues against this view, as discussed later.

λ Light-Chain Genes

Murine λ Locus

In laboratory mouse strains, λ chains represent only about 5% of light chains, and this diminished abundance is associated with remarkably meager diversity. In contrast to the κ system with its multiple V region families, amino acid sequence analysis of monoclonal λ chains detected only two sequences that appeared to represent germline Vλ regions. Furthermore, in contrast to the single murine Cκ region, three nonallelic murine isotypes are known from secreted λ chains; these are designated $\lambda1$, $\lambda2$, and $\lambda3$, in decreasing order of abundance.

Cloning and long-range mapping studies by PFGE led to a substantial understanding of the murine λ locus (Fig. 8). There are four Cλ genes, each with its own Jλ region gene located about 1.3 kb 5' of the C. The J-Cλ3 and J-Cλ1 genes are arranged in one cluster about 3 kb apart with the Vλ1 gene lying about 19 kb upstream. A second Cλ cluster lying about 130 kb upstream of the Cλ3–Cλ1 locus contains J-Cλ2 and an unexpressed gene J-Cλ4. (At the 3' end of Jλ4, a mutation has destroyed the "GT..." found at almost all known "donor" splice sites, so that an RNA transcript of this gene would not be properly processed; this is reminiscent of the murine Jκ3.) The gene order (V2-Vx-JC2-JC4-V1-JC3-JC1) explains the common expression of Vλ2 (or Vx) in association with Cλ2, and Vλ1 with Cλ1 or Cλ3. The Vλ2 has been found in rare association with the 190-kb distant Cλ1 locus, but the "backwards" recombination of Vλ1 with Cλ2 has not been observed. The similarities between the four J-C genes suggest that the two clusters arose by a duplication of an ancestral V-J-Cλx–J-Cλy unit that in turn was the result of a prior J-Cλ duplication event. The ancestry of the Vx gene is uncertain, inasmuch as this gene is rather dissimilar to the other Vλ genes; indeed, it resembles Vκ as much as Vλ. Anti-Vλx antisera detect expression of this Vλ in all

laboratory mice tested, but it may have a particular restricted function. Analyses of λ genes in wild mice by Southern blot tests have indicated more complex and varied loci than those seen in typical laboratory strains.

The Jλ gene segments are all flanked on their 5' side by sequences similar to the nonamer and heptamer signal elements observed in the heavy-chain and κ system. The 12/23 rule, discussed in relation to spacing between the signal elements, applies as well to λ, but in the λ locus, the RSS elements are spaced about 23 bp apart for V regions and about 12 bp apart for J regions (the opposite of the arrangement in κ genes), as shown in Fig. 4. The decreased abundance of λ2 and λ3 in comparison with λ1 may be related to discrepancies between their nonamer homology elements and the consensus nonamer element.

Human λ Locus

Lambda light chains are much more abundant in the human than in the mouse (about 40% of human light chains vs. about 5% in murine light chains). Four forms of human λ chains have been characterized serologically; differences reside in a small number of amino acids in the C region. The serological classification of Kern+ depends on Gly at position 152 versus Ser in Kern−. The Oz+ designation depends on Lys at position 190 versus Arg on Oz−. And Mcg+ λ chains (vs. Mcg−) depend on Asn112 (vs. Ala), Thr114 (vs. Ser), and Lys163 (vs. Thr).

Seven human Jλ-Cλ segments are clustered within an approximately 33-kb region of DNA that has been entirely

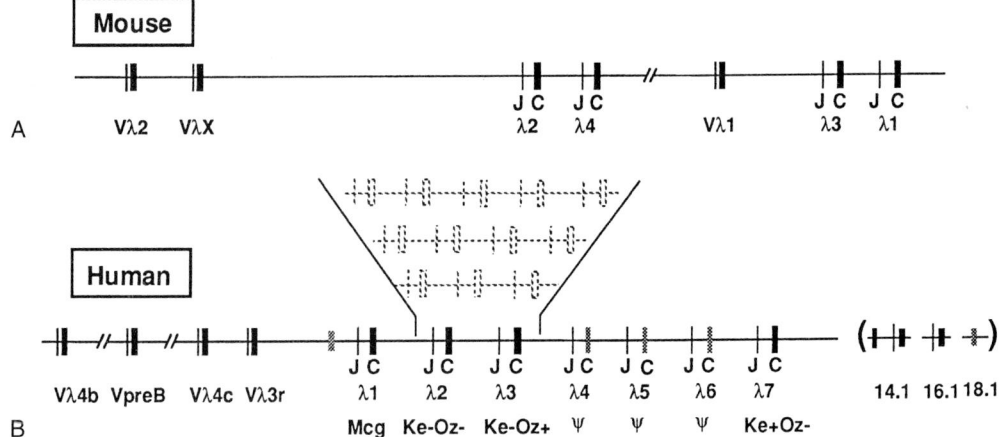

FIG. 8. Germline λ genes. The maps are schematic (i.e., not to scale). A: The murine λ gene system includes four J-C complexes and three V genes, which have been characterized in two unlinked contigs (sets of overlapping clones) as shown. B: The human λ locus has been characterized by complete sequence analysis. The human VpreB "surrogate" light-chain gene is located within the Vλ cluster. The Cλ locus includes a segment of seven J-C complexes plus three additional unlinked sequences. The hatched J-C complexes diagrammed above the seven linked λ sequences represent polymorphic variants with additional duplications of the J-C unit as deduced from Southern blots. The 14.1 sequence—the human λ5 "surrogate" light-chain homolog—lies downstream of the J-C cluster, but its location in relation to the other λ-like sequences is not known. Exon 1 of the 14.1 gene is homologous to an exon upstream of Jλ1 (as indicated by *gray rectangle*).

sequenced (26). As shown in Fig. 8, genes for four major expressed human λ isotypes have been localized within the major cluster and correspond to JCλ1, JCλ2, JCλ3 and JCλ7. JCλ7 was originally interpreted as encoding the Kern+Oz− serologic form of λ, but more recent data suggest that the latter is an allele of Cλ2 and that JCλ7 encodes an isotype provisionally designated Mcp (27). The other three homologous J-C segments found in most haplotypes are apparently pseudogenes, with either in-frame stop codons or frame-shifting deletions. However, JCλ6 may be functional in some individuals, and the common allele—which has a 4-bp insertion, leading to a deletion of the C-terminal third of the Cλ region—can nevertheless undergo Vλ-Jλ recombination, encoding a truncated protein that can associate with heavy chains. Various polymorphic variants of the human λ locus have been detected, apparently the result of gene duplication; as shown in Fig. 8, one to three extra λ segments have been detected on Southern blots of human DNA.

Three Cλ-related sequences have been discovered near the major Jλ-Cλ cluster. One of these, designated λ14.1, represents the human homolog of the murine "surrogate" light-chain λ5 (see the following discussion). Finally, an additional weakly hybridizing DNA segment outside the linked cluster has been characterized as a "processed" pseudogene. V genes of the human λ system have been completely characterized, as discussed in a later section.

λ-Related "Surrogate" Light Chains

In mature B cells, Ig heavy chains cannot reach the cell surface if light-chain synthesis is interrupted. However, immunoglobulin μ heavy chains can be detected on the surface of pre–B cells that do not make light chains. In these cells, a "surrogate light chain" (SLC) composed of two smaller proteins facilitates the surface expression of μ protein. One component of SLC was identified as a gene product expressed exclusively in pre–B cells and that showed high sequence similarity to the J and C regions of the λ locus. It was designated λ5, because four murine Cλ genes were already known (28). The genomic λ5 gene includes three exons: exon 1, which appears to encode a signal peptide; exon 2, whose 3′ end is homologous to Jλ; and exon 3, homologous to Cλ. The second component of SLC was found as a transcribed segment about 4.7 kb 5′ of λ5. Sequence analysis of the latter region revealed similarities to both Vλ and Vκ; for this reason (and because of its expression in pre–B cells), it is called VpreB1. A second, nearly identical sequence in the murine genome is named VpreB2 and appears to be functional (29), and a less similar VpreB3 has also been described. Neither λ5 nor VpreB genes show evidence of gene rearrangement in B or pre–B cells. Both genes appear functional, and homologs have been found in every mammalian species examined.

Evidence strongly supports the notion that these two SLC proteins associate with μ heavy chains to permit surface μ expression before the availability of light chains. Thus, when a μ heavy-chain gene was transfected into an Ig-negative myeloma line, no surface μ expression was observed unless λ5 and VpreB genes were also transfected (30). The surface μ chains were found to be covalently linked to the 22-kD product of the λ5 gene, whereas the 16-kD VpreB product was noncovalently associated. A similar complex is observed in pre–B cell lines and in normal bone marrow pre–B cells. The V-like VpreB gene product apparently associates with the Cλ-like λ5 product to form a light chain–like heterodimer that is able to fulfill some functions of a true light chain.

One likely role for a μ-SLC complex is suggested by the observation that most Vκ-Jκ recombination occurs only in cells expressing a functional μ heavy chain [as discussed more fully in the section on regulation of V(D)J recombination]; apparently, μ-SLC expression on the cell surface can trigger the onset of Vκ-Jκ rearrangement. Evidence for this view comes from experiments in which a pre–B cell line that normally does not rearrange its κ locus was transfected with a construct encoding the membrane form of μ heavy chain (31); when the transfected μ gene was expressed in a complex containing VpreB and λ5, Vκ rearrangement was induced. Further support for a role of the SLC in regulating B cell development has come from studies on mice or humans lacking functional λ5 or VpreB genes, as discussed later in this chapter.

Human homologs of both λ5 and VpreB have been cloned. As mentioned previously, three λ5-like sequences are located downstream of the human Cλ cluster on chromosome 22 (Fig. 8), but only one—designated 14.1—appears to be functional, possessing the three-exon structure of λ5. Interestingly, a sequence upstream of Jλ1 is homologous to exon 1 of 14.1/λ5, which suggests that 14.1 and Jλ-Cλ1 may have had a common ancestral gene that was capable of being expressed in either of two ways: (a) by rearranging its J-like exon 2 with a V region gene, like modern λ genes, or (b) without rearrangement, using exon 1, with the encoded protein assembling with a noncovalently linked VpreB-like subunit. The human VpreB homolog lies within the Vλ cluster (32); murine VpreB, in contrast, lies close upstream of λ5.

V GENE ASSEMBLY RECOMBINATION

The mechanism by which germline V region constituents (VL and JL, or VH, D, and JH) assemble in the DNA to form a complete active V gene has been pursued ever since Ig gene recombination was first discovered. This section addresses (a) the topology of the recombinations from a "macro" viewpoint, (b) the components of the recombinase machinery (a "micro" view), and (c) the regulation of that machinery in B cell development.

Topology of V Assembly Recombination

Deletion Versus Inversion

In the earliest model for Vκ-Jκ rearrangement, it was assumed that V segments and J segments were all oriented in the same direction of transcription and that the DNA between the recombining V and J segments would be simply excised. According to this model, and the supposition that the excised DNA would lack a replication origin, the excised DNA should be absent from long-cultured myeloma lines. However, Southern blot testing of a panel of myelomas and normal κ-bearing lymphocytes showed that some cells had retained the DNA just upstream of Jκ1, a region that should have been absent from all chromosomes that underwent deletional recombination. The reason for these retained regions is that some Vκ genes of both mouse and human are oriented in the opposite direction from the Jκ-Cκ region. This topology would allow the V-J recombination to occur by an inversion of the DNA between the recombining V and J segments (Fig. 9B), leaving the DNA upstream of Jκ1 retained on the chromosome. The same recombinase machinery can presumably rearrange the germline elements by either inversion or deletion—depending on the relative orientations of the sequences—because this enzymatic machinery detects only the DNA in the immediate vicinity of the recombination site (circled in Fig. 9) and is insensitive to the topology of the DNA strands far from this site. As shown in Fig. 9B, cells that have undergone an inversional Vκ-Jκ recombination should retain on the chromosome a recombination joint with two sets of signal sequences—the RSS from downstream of the Vκ and the RSS from upstream of the Jκ segment—joined together. Indeed, such "signal joints" (also known as "flank products" and "reciprocal joints") have been detected in several cell lines. In contrast to the "flexibility" observed in the position of the recombination breakpoint in the V-J segment (the "coding joint"), the sequences of signal joints usually show the J-derived heptamer joined directly to the V-derived heptamer, without even a single intervening nucleotide between them. The signal joints retained on the expressed chromosome have almost always been derived from Jκ1 (see later discussion). In contrast to the κ system, in the heavy-chain or λ loci, there is no evidence for inverted V genes or retained

signal joints, and so these loci apparently recombine only by deletion (and this is also true for all the T-cell receptor gene loci).

The model of Fig. 9A suggests that when the recombination occurs by deletion, a signal joint is formed on a circular DNA molecule; such a DNA circle would not be attached to the main chromosome and, failing to replicate, would be expected to be diluted out as cells divide after V(D)J recombination. By isolating circular DNA from cells that were undergoing Vκ-Jκ rearrangement, it was possible to clone the predicted molecules bearing signal joints (33), which supported the model. More recent experiments have used polymerase chain reaction (PCR) testing to detect signal joints, especially those generated by V(D)J recombination of T-cell receptor genes; a high content of TCR excision circles in a population has been interpreted as reflecting "recent" V(D)J recombination with relatively little subsequent proliferation (34).

Secondary Recombinations

A final issue for consideration of V assembly topology at the macro level concerns secondary V gene recombinations. As discussed in an earlier section, the flexibility of V-J or V-D-J joining causes nonproductive out-of-frame recombination with high frequency. A B lymphocyte that rearranged its κ genes nonproductively on both parental chromosomes might be thought to have no further avenue for making a functional light chain; however, the availability of upstream V genes and downstream J segments could allow additional recombinations to occur, as shown in Fig. 10A. More complex events are possible as a consequence of the inverted orientation of some Vκ genes. The occurrence of such secondary recombinations has in fact been reported for κ genes and would be implied by the recovery of chromosomal signal joints that are not reciprocal to coding joints in the same cells. The preponderance of Jκ1-derived nonreciprocal flank products

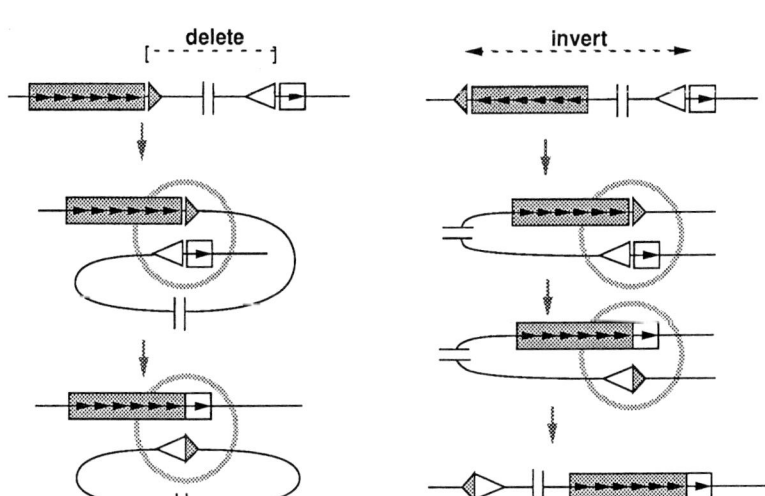

FIG. 9. The same "micro" mechanism of recombination can join Vκ and Jκ by deletion or inversion, depending on the relative orientation of the two precursors in germline DNA. **A:** When V coding sequence (*shaded rectangle*) and J coding sequence (*white rectangle*) are oriented in the same 5'→3' direction in germline DNA (as indicated by the *internal arrowheads*), the recombination yields a V-J coding joint plus a DNA circle containing the signal joint (*apposed triangles*). **B:** If V is oriented in the opposite direction in germline DNA, then an identical recombination reaction at the "micro" level (*inside shaded circle*) leaves the signal joint linked to the recombined V-J coding joint.

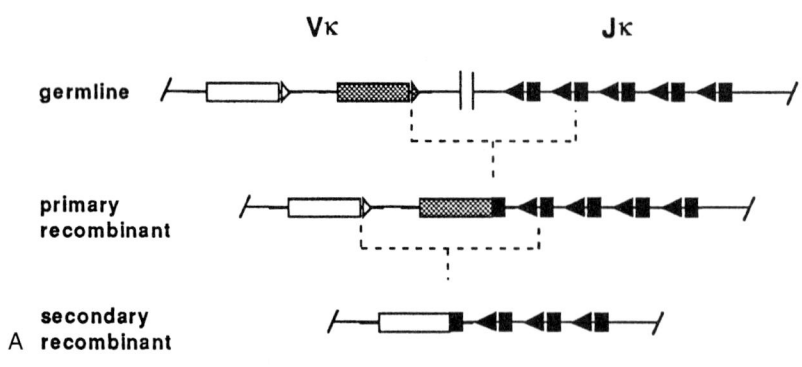

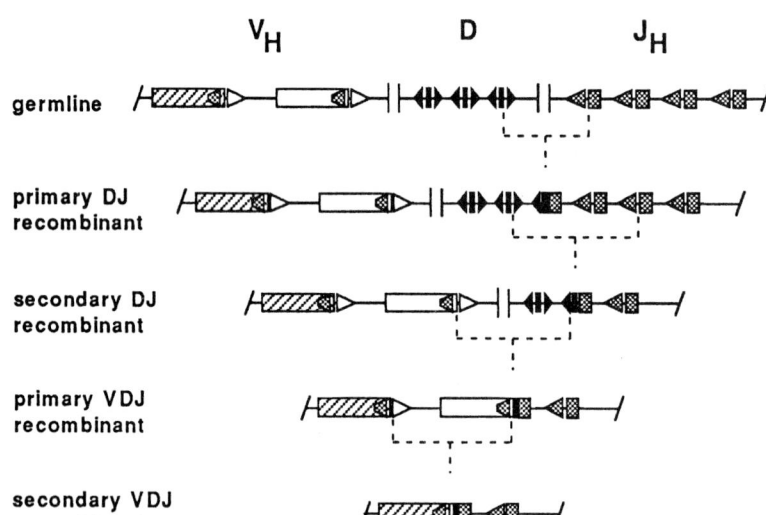

FIG. 10. Secondary recombinations. **A:** In the κ light-chain system, a primary recombination can be followed by recombination between an upstream V and a downstream J. **B:** Analogous secondary recombinations can occur in the heavy-chain system between upstream D and downstream J segments. After V-D-J recombination eliminates all "short spacer" signal elements from the chromosome, secondary recombination can still occur between VH (long spacer signal) and an internal heptamer within the VH coding sequence of the V-D-J unit.

observed in myelomas may result from initial nonproductive recombinations between this J segment and inverted V genes, followed by successive recombinations involving more downstream J segments; by the time a productive rearrangement occurs, many myelomas carry signal joint relics of earlier recombinations involving Jκ1. Secondary recombination may also occur in cells that have assembled a productive Vκ-Jκ joint if the resulting VH-VL pair recognizes an autoantigen; this type of secondary recombination, known as "receptor editing," is considered in more detail later in this chapter.

For heavy-chain genes, the possibility of secondary recombination might appear to be ruled out by the fact that a V-D-J rearrangement must eliminate all the 12-bp–spaced signal elements from the VH locus, because these elements are deleted on both sides of the D region that is retained in the recombined V-D-J unit and from all the germline D segments eliminated by the V-D and D-J recombination events (Fig. 10B). Secondary D-J rearrangements should be possible before VH-D recombination removes unrearranged upstream DH segments (Fig. 10B), and, indeed, this has been shown to occur. Of greater functional interest has been the demonstration (35)

that upstream germline VH genes can recombine with an established V-D-J unit, displacing the originally assembled V gene. This type of recombination is apparently mediated by a sequence that closely matches the consensus signal heptamer and that appears near the 3′ end of the coding region in about 70% of VH genes (Fig. 10B). The internal heptamer is not generally found in light-chain genes. After VH replacement, the few nucleotides remaining from the originally assembled VH could potentially contribute to diversity; such nucleotides would be difficult to distinguish from N-region nucleotides. Secondary recombination thus represents an escape mechanism for cells with nonproductive rearrangements on both heavy-chain chromosomes or, as alluded to previously, for cells whose antibody encodes an autoantigen; it is not known how frequently such escapes occur, as opposed to the alternative path of cell death. The fact that the isolated heptamer is apparently able to function in VH replacement recombinations without an associated nonamer again suggests that the heptamer is the more critical recombination signal, although it has been suggested that an additional consensus sequence upstream of the internal heptamer may contribute to VH replacement recombination (36).

Mechanism of V Assembly Recombination

As mentioned earlier, the same recombination machinery mediates all four types of immunoglobulin V gene assembly recombinations (Vκ-Jκ, Vλ-Jλ, VH-D, and D-JH), as well as similar recombinations in the four T-cell receptor gene loci; this fact has allowed investigators to pool mechanistic knowledge from studies of B-cell and T-cell systems. On the other hand, the assumption of a common recombinase raises the question of how B cells preferentially rearrange Ig genes (and how T cells rearrange TCR genes) when both gene systems are available to be rearranged by the common recombinase in both cell lineages; this issue is addressed later in this section.

Recombination Model

A model for the detailed mechanism of the recombination event must account for the observed features of the recombination products—namely, the coding and signal joints—and of their germline precursors. In the germline precursors, the heptamer and nonamer RSS with appropriate spacing (12 and 23 bp) are necessary and sufficient to create efficient recombination targets; as discussed later, model substrates containing these elements are competent to undergo recombination even in the absence of normal V, D, or J coding regions. However, the efficiency of recombination can be influenced by features of the sequences replacing the coding regions. As for the products, the features of the signal joints are relatively simple: the heptamers are joined "back-to-back," with only rare additions or deletions. The features of the coding joints are more complex, because of the "flexibility" of junctions as discussed earlier: (a) A variable number of bases are deleted from the ends of the coding regions (in comparison to the "complete" sequence in the germline precursor). (b) Nongermline nucleotides (N regions) unrelated to the germline precursor sequences are added in some coding joints; these are generally rich in guanine and cytosine nucleotides. (c) Less frequently, extra bases that can be interpreted as P nucleotides are added; these are nucleotides that are joined to the end of an undeleted coding sequence and that form a palindrome (hence, "P") with the end of that sequence (37). P nucleotides are generally only 1 or 2 bp, but they can be longer, especially in mice with the severe combined immunodeficiency defect (SCID) disorder, as discussed later.

The model shown in Fig. 11 can serve as a framework for consideration of the recombination mechanism. The recombination is thought to begin with binding of the RAG1 and RAG2 proteins to the heptamer-nonamer RSS adjacent to the two segments to be recombined. Both DNA segments are then cleaved at the border of the two heptamers, and the two heptamer ends are joined together without modification. In contrast, the ends bearing the coding sequences form transient "hairpin" loops, which are then nicked open and digested to varying extents by an exonuclease activity. Variable numbers of nucleotides may be added to the 3′ ends through the action of terminal deoxynucleotide transferase (TdT). Then the

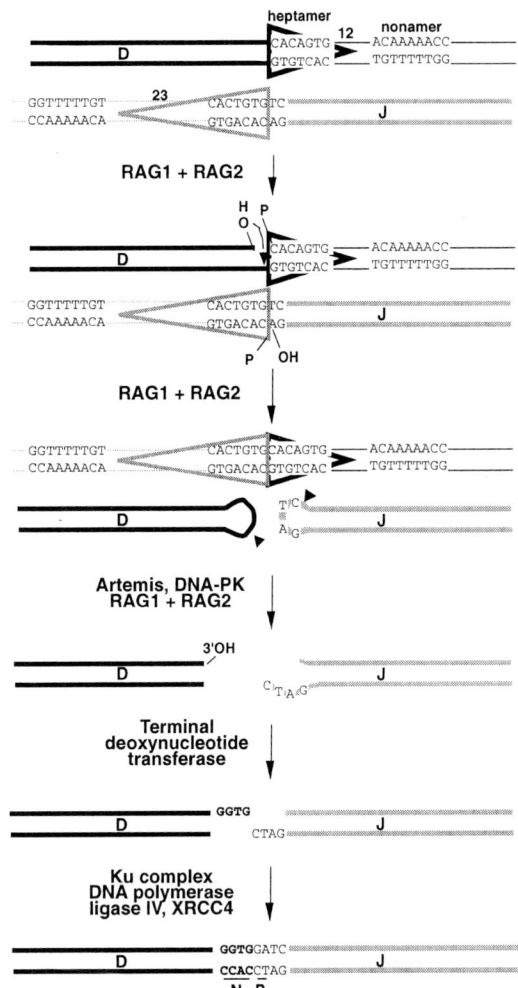

FIG. 11. Model for V assembly recombinations. All V assembly recombination reactions (in immunoglobulin and T-cell receptor genes) may proceed by a common mechanism, illustrated here by D-J recombination. The recombination signal sequences (RSSs) are included in *triangles,* which is the conventionally used RSS graphic. Hairpin loops are created on coding ends dependent on the action of recombination activating genes 1 and 2. After the opening of the hairpin loops, the pictured D coding sequence shows the effects of "nibbling" by exonuclease, but the J coding sequence is spared and shows P nucleotide generation; N region addition is pictured in this example as occurring only on the D region end. In reality, exonuclease digestion and N nucleotide addition can occur on either end or both ends. The steps in the proposed mechanism are discussed in the text.

5′ ends are filled in by a DNA polymerase, and the resulting flush ends are ligated together, which completes the recombination event.

Experiments to Investigate Substrates and Products

Investigations of the recombination mechanism have been advanced by the development of methods for monitoring these events *in vitro.* Some experiments have exploited the ability of the Abelson murine leukemia virus (AMuLV) to selectively transform pre–B cells without abolishing active

V gene assembly characteristic of this stage of lymphoid development. Particularly valuable information has been gained by transfecting AMuLV lines, as well as other lymphoid and nonlymphoid cells, with artificial gene constructs capable of undergoing V(D)J recombination. Several such constructs have been designed with selectable markers whose expression depends on a recombination event. For example, Lieber et al. (38) transfected various cell lines with a plasmid containing an ampicillin resistance gene (Amp^r) plus a chloramphenicol resistance gene (Cam^r) whose expression was blocked by a stop codon flanked by two V(D)J recombination signal sequences. In B cells, recombination between the two signal sequences deletes the stop codon, allowing expression of the Cam^r gene. When extrachromosomal plasmid circles are recovered from the cells and transfected into bacteria, the extent of recombination can be determined by the ratio of transformed Amp^r bacteria that are Cam^r. Depending on the orientation of the signal sequences in the starting construct, the recovered recombination products represent coding or signal joints, which can be recovered efficiently from the Cam^r colonies for analysis. The sequences of these joints were found to have all the characteristics of natural recombination products. One interesting outcome from such experiments was the discovery that pre–B and pre–T cells from SCID mice were capable of recombination to form signal joints but were markedly defective in their ability to join coding ends to form coding joints.

From recombined engineered substrates, certain nonstandard joints have also been recovered; although they do not contribute to physiological V gene assembly, they may reflect features of the recombination mechanism (39). These nonstandard joints can be understood by appreciating that there are three topologies in which DNA that has been cut twice—generating four ends—can be rejoined. If the four ends are coding (V), signal (V), signal (J), and coding (J), the three possibilities can be defined by considering the three different ends that may join to the coding (V) end (if it is assumed that the remaining two ends must join to each other). The possibilities are as follows:

1. Coding (V)–coding (J) plus signal (V)–signal (J): This is the standard reaction product in which the coding (V)–coding (J) product encodes the assembled V-J gene and the signal (V)–signal (J) represents the signal joint.
2. Coding (V)–signal (V) plus signal (J)–coding (J): These products ("open and shut joints") look like the starting DNAs, but can be distinguished from them if nucleotides have been added or deleted at the junctions so that they no longer hybridize to oligonucleotide probes specific for the coding/signal junction
3. Coding (V)–signal (J) plus signal (V)–coding (J): These are "hybrid joints," in which the signal ends have switched places.

So-called hybrid and open-and-shut joints have also been observed to form in endogenous immunoglobulin loci *in vivo* (40).

The critical characteristics of the recombination signal sequences have been explored through the use of transfected constructs carrying various mutations. These experiments have verified the importance of the heptamer/nonamer sequences and have shown that the spacer sequences are not critical as long as the spacer length—12 or 23 bp—is maintained. The heptamer appears especially important, with the 3 bp closest to the coding sequence being most critical for signaling recombination. Recombination activity could be detected in a variety of pro–B and pre–B cells as well as pre–T lines, but it was virtually absent in mature B and T cells and in cells of nonlymphoid lineages.

Recombination Intermediates: Hairpins and P Nucleotides

To study intermediates in V(D)J recombination, Roth et al. (41,42) designed a Southern blot strategy to detect double-strand breaks in the TCR δ locus between D and J and applied this strategy to DNA from newborn murine thymus cells, which actively rearrange the TCR δ locus. In comparison with DNA from adult liver cells, additional bands were found in the newborn thymus DNA, representing DNA fragments extending from a D-derived heptamer on one end to a J-derived heptamer on the other end. To characterize the sequence of the signal ends in detail, several laboratories have employed ligation-mediated PCR (LM-PCR). This technique involves ligating the blunt genomic signal ends with a double-stranded oligonucleotide, followed by amplification extending from a primer sequence near the genomic signal end to the ligated oligonucleotide sequence; amplified products can then be cloned and their sequence determined. LM-PCR analyses of both TCR and immunoglobulin genes have defined the signal ends as blunt-ended cuts, usually exactly at the heptamer border, leaving 5′ phosphate and 3′ hydroxyl groups (43).

In their original Southern blot assays, Roth et al. (41,42) detected the signal ends from these cuts at levels representing about 2% of the thymus DNA; however, the coding ends could not be visualized at all, perhaps because of rapid processing of these ends into coding joints. On the basis of the known defect of SCID lymphocytes in forming coding joints, Roth et al. (41) reasoned that SCID thymocytes might accumulate the cut coding ends that could not be visualized in normal thymocytes. Indeed, coding ends were detected in the SCID thymocyte DNA and, moreover, were found to have several properties suggestive of a hairpinlike structure. First, the coding ends in SCID thymocyte DNA were resistant to exonuclease treatment. Furthermore, restriction fragments bearing these *in vivo*-generated ends on one side were found to move on a denaturing electrophoresis gel as if they were twice as long as predicted from the size of the double-stranded fragment before denaturation. Finally, LM-PCR experiments failed to detect the coding ends unless they were pretreated with a single-strand–specific endonuclease, which was consistent with the impossibility of ligation to a hairpin unless it was first opened. The sequences of LM-PCR products obtained after endonuclease treatment suggested that the hairpins contained the entire sequence of the coding element, usually without loss or gain of a single nucleotide (44).

These hairpin ends apparently represent normal V(D)J recombination intermediates that, in wild-type cells, are opened at variable positions within the hairpin loop by an endonuclease activity that is dependent on the normal allele of the SCID gene. P nucleotides could then result from opening the loop at an asymmetric position (Fig. 11); this model would explain the absence of P nucleotides from coding ends that have been "nibbled" after opening of the hairpin. The unusually long P nucleotide segments observed in the rare coding joints assembled in SCID mice might then be interpreted as resulting from resolution of hairpins by nonspecific nicking enzymes that, unlike the exonuclease activity dependent on the normal allele of the SCID gene, do not focus on the hairpin loops but nick in variable positions in the double-stranded hairpin "stem" (41).

In support of the notion that the hairpin coding ends are intermediates in normal V-J recombination, hairpins have been found in vivo in a non-SCID B lymphoid line engineered to sustain a high level of κ gene recombination (45). In this line, broken Jκ1 signal ends were detectable in amounts corresponding to 30% to 40% of the κ loci present. Coding ends were observed at 10- to 100-fold lower abundance, including both hairpin and open ends. The observed kinetics were consistent with simultaneous production of signal ends and hairpin coding ends, with rapid processing of hairpins to open coding ends and then to coding joints but slower ligation of signal ends. This model is further supported by the observation that linear DNA molecules with hairpins at both ends can, after transfection into B cell lines, be recovered as recircularized molecules, with the frequent creation of P insertions (46). Interestingly, SCID B cells perform about as well as normal B cells in this assay, which suggests that the protein missing in SCID cells is not the hairpin nicking enzyme itself but rather an activity that makes natural endogenous hairpin coding ends available to the enzyme; these endogenous ends may require such an activity because of their association with recombinase or other chromosomal proteins, whereas transfected hairpins free of attached proteins may be accessible independently of the protein missing in SCID. The molecular basis of the SCID defect is considered in more detail in the following discussion.

Recombination Activating Gene Proteins: Mediators of Early Steps in V(D)J Recombination

A major advance in the investigation of V(D)J recombination was the identification of two genes whose products are critical for this process in B and T lineages. In the pioneering experiments, Schatz and Baltimore (47) stably transfected fibroblasts with a construct containing a selectable marker whose expression was dependent on V(D)J recombination; as expected, no measurable recombination occurred in this nonlymphoid cell. However, when either human or murine genomic DNA was transfected into these fibroblasts, a small fraction of recipient cells stably expressed recombinase activity, activating the selectable marker. This suggested that a single transfected genomic DNA fragment was able confer recombinase activity in a fibroblast. (Presumably, the fibroblast contained endogenous copies of the same genes, but their expression was repressed by mechanisms that could not repress the transfected genes.) After successive rounds of transfection and selection for recombinase activity, the critical genomic fragment was identified. This fragment turned out to contain two genes, designated RAG1 and RAG2. These genes are not homologous to each other, and neither is very similar to any other known genes, although weak similarities have been noted between RAG1 and a topoisomerase, and a shark RAG1 gene shows some similarity to a bacterial integrase. Both RAG1 and RAG2 are required for recombination; therefore, these genes would not have been discovered by this transfection technique if they had lain too far apart in the genome for both to be transferred on a single DNA fragment. The genes are notable for having no introns in most species (certain fish are exceptions) and for their close association and opposite transcriptional orientation in all species examined. The close proximity of these two genes related by function but not by sequence has led to the speculation that they might have arisen from a more primitive viral or fungal transposition system.

A crucial role for the RAG genes in V assembly recombination was supported by the conservation of these genes in a variety of immunoglobulin-producing vertebrate species from humans through sharks, whereas RAG homologs have not been identified in any species that does not demonstrate Ig V gene assembly recombination. RAG1 and RAG2 are expressed together in pre–B and pre–T cells, specifically at the stages expressing V(D)J recombinase activity. Moreover, mouse strains in which either gene has been eliminated by homologous recombination (gene "knockouts") have no mature B or T cells, as the apparent result of abrogation of V(D)J recombination (48,49). A subset of human patients with a SCID syndrome and no T- or B-lymphocytes has been found to have null mutations in RAG genes (50). Patients with less complete defects often have a complex of features (oligoclonal T cells, hepatosplenomegaly, eosinophilia, decreased serum immunoglobulin but elevated IgE) known as the Omenn syndrome (51). The same RAG mutation can in different patients cause either Omenn syndrome or SCID, depending on unknown factors (52). Many of the RAG2 mutations map to regions of the protein important for interaction with RAG1 (53).

Murine RAG1 is a 1,040-residue protein, with a central core (residues 384 to 1,008) that includes all the known enzymatic activities of the whole protein as well as a nuclear localization signal, although the addition of the N-terminal residues can increase V(D)J recombination frequency of transfected cells (54,55). The protein exists as a dimer, which shows intrinsic binding affinity for the RSS nonamer sequence in the absence of RAG2. This binding is dependent on residues 389 to 486, known as the nonamer-binding domain (56). Mutational analysis has revealed regions of the protein necessary for binding to RAG2, as well as three amino acids critical for enzymatic activity: D600, D708, and E962 (57–59). Murine RAG2 is a 527–amino acid protein, with a core (residues 1 to 382) sufficient for activity. This protein has little intrinsic binding affinity for RSS elements, but it improves the strength and specificity of RAG1 binding (60–62). The binding of RAG2 also extends the nucleotide sequence over which DNA–protein interactions can be detected (by DNA footprinting or ethylation interference experiments) beyond the nonamer and into the heptamer (63). In the presence of divalent cations, the two RAG proteins can form a stable signal complex with an RSS that has a 12-bp spacer (12-RSS), but efficient complex formation with a 23-RSS requires the addition of a high mobility group (HMG) protein, either HMG1 or HMG2 (64,65). These abundant and ubiquitous proteins are known to bind DNA in a non–sequence-specific manner and to cause a local bend in DNA. They apparently facilitate RAG1/RAG2 binding by stabilizing bending induced by the RAG proteins themselves (66).

Attempts to demonstrate activities of the RAG proteins on recombination substrates *in vitro* were hampered by poor solubility of the proteins, but functional analyses of truncated RAG genes—with the use of RAG expression vectors cotransfected with recombination substrate plasmids into fibroblasts—revealed that surprisingly large segments of both proteins can be deleted without eliminating recombinase activity; some of the deleted proteins were soluble and could be handled relatively easily as fusion proteins. This work allowed the demonstration that, in a cell-free *in vitro* system, the two RAG proteins together are capable of carrying out cleavage of substrate DNAs as well as hairpin formation on the coding end (67).

The RAG-induced cleavage occurs in two steps: First, a nick occurs on one strand adjacent to the heptamer (the top strand as drawn in Fig. 11); then the 3′-hydroxyl created at the nick causes transesterification by nucleophilic attack on the phosphodiester bond adjacent to the heptamer on the bottom strand (Fig. 11), yielding a hairpin on the coding end and a new 3′-hydroxyl on the 3′ end of the bottom heptamer strand (68). This transesterification mechanism is consistent with the observation that the formation of the new phosphodiester bond in the hairpin occurs in the absence of an external energy source such as adenosine triphosphate (ATP); the energy required for hairpin formation apparently derives from the phosphodiester bond broken in nucleophilic attack. The stereochemistry observed in the reaction suggests that no phosphodiester linkage to protein occurs as an intermediate, such as occurs in bacteriophage lambda integration; instead the direct transesterification mechanism resembles the mu transposition and retroviral integration, which can both produce hairpins under certain experimental conditions (68). Although the RAG proteins may not form a covalent intermediate to generate the hairpin, they apparently participate in the reaction, inasmuch as some RAG1 mutants can nick at the heptamer efficiently but show impaired hairpin formation under certain conditions (69). After DNA cleavage, the RAG proteins remain in a complex with the DNA (70). In this complex, the RAG proteins may participate in hairpin opening of the coding ends, inasmuch as this activity has been observed with *in vitro* reactions (71,72); however, the hairpin cleavage by RAG proteins requires nonphysiological conditions (Mn^{2+} rather than Mg^{2+}) that argue against its physiologic importance. The signal ends have also been found to remain tightly bound in a complex with the RAG proteins (73). A role for RAG proteins at steps beyond cleavage and hairpin formation is also suggested by the identification of mutant forms of RAG1 or RAG2 that are competent for cleavage but show impairment in coding or signal joint formation (74,75).

The actions of the RAG proteins were found to be dependent on divalent ions in the medium (61,76). In Mn^{2+}, the RAG proteins catalyze cleavage of substrates with a single RSS, but in Mg^{2+}, cleavage requires two RSSs and occurs most efficiently if the substrates conform to the 12/23 rule regarding the spacing between heptamer and nonamer elements. Thus, this rule may be enforced by the RAG proteins, although other proteins, including HMG1/HMG2, seem to contribute to 12/23 specificity, perhaps by promoting an optimal molecular architecture (77). In Ca^{2+}, the RAG proteins and a radiolabeled DNA substrate containing an RSS formed a stable complex that was apparent in an electrophoretic mobility shift assay (EMSA) and was stable to competition with unlabeled substrate, but the substrate was not nicked or cleaved. However, when Mg^{2+} was added to the stable complex, substrate cleavage occurred. The Ca^{2+}-mediated binding of RAG proteins to substrate DNA was significantly decreased 10-fold by the elimination of the nonamer from the RSS. In contrast, mutations in the heptamer that altered the nucleotides closest to the coding region—residues known to be critical for supporting cleavage—had minimal effect on binding. This is consistent with other evidence (78,79) that suggests that the heptamer may contribute to the sequence specificity of cleavage less by promoting RAG binding than by creating a local alteration in DNA helix structure that is important for the cleavage reactions.

In addition to the activities of RAG proteins already discussed, *in vitro* experiments have documented that these proteins can catalyze the insertion of a DNA fragment with signal ends into foreign DNA, acting essentially like a transposase (80,81). This transposase activity lends support to the early speculation (82) that the V(D)J recombination system may have originated by insertion of transposon-like DNA with signal ends into a primordial V region, thereby separating J region sequence from the remainder of the V sequence upstream. This model is consistent with the many mechanistic similarities between V(D)J recombination and transposition [reviewed by Roth and Craig (83)] and the unusual organization of the RAG genes, which presumably would have been carried on the original transposon to allow for subsequent rejoining of V and J. The transposase activity may also be the cause of certain translocations in lymphoid malignancies.

Double-strand DNA breaks catalyzed by the RAG proteins could be potentially deleterious if they occurred during DNA synthesis or mitosis, but this problem appears to be mitigated by tight post-transcriptional regulation of RAG2 protein levels across the cell cycle. Although the RAG1 protein and mRNA transcripts of both RAG genes vary little across the cell cycle, a phosphorylation-dependent degradation signal mediates destruction of the RAG2 protein (84), thereby preventing double-strand DNA breaks in the heavy-chain JH locus from occurring during M, G2 and S stages (43). The phosphorylation site, a threonine at amino acid 490, falls in a region of the sequence that is highly conserved across species and contains a consensus sequence characteristic of targets of cyclin-dependent kinases; this regulatory region is dispensable for enzymatic activity. In RAG2 knockout mice carrying a transgenic RAG2 gene with an alanine replacing the phosphorylatable threonine, RAG2 protein and double-stranded DNA breaks were found throughout the cell cycle, demonstrating the importance of the RAG2 degradation signal in cell-cycle control of V(D)J recombination (85).

Apart from the obvious importance of the RAG proteins in understanding the initial steps of V(D)J recombination, knowledge of these proteins and their genes has allowed two major technical advances that have opened the way to many additional experiments. First, various nonlymphoid cell lines with known defects in various DNA repair genes have been transfected with the RAG genes to determine whether these gene defects impair V(D)J recombination; these experiments have revealed several other proteins required for V(D)J recombination, as described later. The second major technical consequence from the RAG genes has been the availability of the RAG1 and RAG2 knockout mice. These mice have no functional B cells or T cells and are not "leaky" like SCID mice, which develop some functional B and T cells, especially as the animals age. The RAG knockouts can be used to study the importance of the "innate" immune system (i.e., responses that occur in the absence of antigen-specific lymphocytes) in particular immune responses. The knockout mice can be used as recipients for various lymphocyte subsets to explore the roles of different cell types. They can be used to study the signals for B cell development by introducing transgenes with specific functionally recombined Ig genes and characterizing the phenotypes of lymphocytes that develop (as discussed later). Finally, they can be used in "RAG complementation" experiments designed to assess the phenotype—in lymphocytes—of various other gene knockouts (86). In RAG complementation, embryonic stem cells in which the gene of interest has been knocked out by homologous recombination are injected into homozygous RAG knockout (RAG −/−) blastocysts. This procedure yields chimeric mice in which all B and T cells derive from the embryonic stem cells deleted for the gene of interest, because these are the only source of intact RAG genes to support lymphocyte development. Such animals can be bred more easily than a knockout mouse line and can be used to study the effect of gene deletion in lymphocytes independently of effects the deletion may have in other cells. In particular, for cases in which the gene knockout causes embryonic lethality because of effects on nonlymphoid cells, RAG complementation allows the selective knockout in lymphocytes to be studied in the background normal gene expression in nonlymphoid cells.

Components of Later Steps in V(D)J Recombination

Ku, DNA-PK, and XRCC4

The RAG genes are clearly critical for the first steps in V(D)J recombination (recognition of RSS, cleavage, hairpin formation, and perhaps hairpin cleavage), but additional components are required to complete the reaction. Most of the other known components function not only in V(D)J recombination but also in the ubiquitous DNA repair pathway known as nonhomologous end joining (NHEJ), which promotes the repair of double-strand DNA breaks such as those induced by ionizing radiation.

The first clear example of such a component to be recognized was the murine SCID mutation mentioned previously. This mutation was originally identified in a mouse strain that was immunodeficient as a result of a marked impairment in V(D)J recombination of both Ig and T-cell receptor genes; SCID lymphocytes are able to perform the RAG-mediated reactions of cleavage and hairpin formation and can form signal joints but are markedly defective in coding joint formation. Subsequently, it was found that the SCID mutation also impairs NHEJ, causing radiosensitivity. To test whether other DNA repair components participated in V(D)J recombination, Taccioli et al. (87) screened panels of radiosensitive Chinese hamster ovary cell lines for their ability to carry out V(D)J recombination after transfection with the RAG genes. These radiosensitive lines had previously been classified into x-ray cross-complementation (XRCC) groups by investigating the outcome when two mutant cell lines are combined to make a somatic hybrid. If such a hybrid shows no DNA repair defect, this implies that the two original cell lines carry mutations of different genes in such a way that the hybrid received at least one normal copy of each gene (the mutant cell lines "cross-complemented" one another); conversely, by definition, cells in the same cross-complementation group are unable to complement each other. Of eight XRCC groups of ionizing radiation-sensitive rodent cell lines, three were known to be defective in repair of double-strand breaks in DNA—XRCC groups 4, 5, and 7—and all three of these groups were found to be impaired in V(D)J recombination after RAG transfection.

The genes mutated in XRCC5 and XRCC7 turned out to encode two components of a three-polypeptide complex known as the Ku complex. Originally characterized as the autoantigen recognized by a patient antiserum, Ku is composed of an approximately 70-kD protein (Ku70) and an approximately

86-kD protein (Ku86, often called Ku80). Together, these two proteins form a heterodimer that can bind to DNA. The DNA-Ku heterodimer complex can then recruit the third component: DNA-PK, an approximately 460-kD protein with a protein kinase activity that is dependent on binding to DNA. [In an alternative terminology, the Ku-DNA-PK complex is designated DNA-PK, and the 460-kD kinase is designated DNA-PK$_{CS}$ (catalytic subunit).] Ku genes are conserved in *Drosophila* species, yeast, and even bacteria (88), which is consistent with a function in NHEJ not restricted to V(D)J recombination. The gene defective in the XRCC5 group encodes Ku80, whereas the gene defective in XRCC7—which corresponds to the gene mutated in murine SCID—encodes the 460-kD DNA-PK. An equine DNA-PK mutation (89) impairs both coding and signal joint formation, but targeted DNA-PK murine knockout strains show a phenotype resembling the original SCID mutation: that is, defective coding but not signal joint formation (90,91); the reason for this difference in phenotype is not clear. Ku80 mutant cell lines are also defective in both signal and coding joint formation, and mice with a knockout of the Ku80 gene are severely impaired in B and T cell development (92). Ku70 mutants were not detected in panels of existing XRCC mutants, but cells with homozygous disruption of Ku70 are also defective in V(D)J recombination induced by RAG gene transfection (93).

The Ku complex had previously been studied as an activity with an unusual DNA binding specificity: Rather than recognizing particular nucleotide sequences, it recognizes particular topological features of DNA, particularly double-stranded DNA ends such as might be generated by x-rays or by recombinases. Indeed, Ku may be the primary detector of broken DNA. Once bound to an end, Ku can translocate down the length of the DNA. These properties can be interpreted in light of the three-dimensional structure of the protein (94). DNA bound to the heterodimer resembles a finger wearing two adjacent engagement rings, with—in lieu of diamonds—two marshmallows squashed together. The Ku heterodimer shows limited interaction with the nucleotides in the major or minor groove of the DNA, but the internal channel of the heterodimer contacts the negatively charged DNA backbone over about 14 bp on one side of the double helix and includes several positively charged amino acid residues that undoubtedly contribute to the tight but non–sequence-specific binding. The other side of the DNA helix is open except for the narrow "ring" structures, allowing accessibility of the DNA to repair enzymes. In an unbound Ku heterodimer, these rings would block access of continuous DNA to the positively charged surface of the internal channel, but a DNA end could be threaded into the ring, which could then slide along the DNA axis. The three-dimensional structure of DNA-PK (95) includes a groove large enough to contain double-stranded DNA and an internal channel that might enclose single-strand DNA. This model would be consistent with binding studies that reveal a binding site for duplex DNA and a second site that binds single-strand DNA and

activates the kinase (96). The Ku complex has been reported to have an ATP-dependent helicase (DNA-unwinding) activity, and it may also influence recombination through DNA-PK–induced phosphorylation of other proteins involved in the recombination (e.g., Artemis, as described below).

Another important function of the Ku complex is to bind to the product of the XRCC4 gene (97). XRCC4 encodes a ubiquitously expressed protein of about 38 kD in predicted size that is not homologous to any known protein. The crystal structure of XRCC4 homodimers resembles a two-headed golf club, with the handle represented by two parallel alpha helices (98). The XRCC4 protein binds binds tightly to and activates DNA ligase IV, which is probably the ligase that seals the signal and coding joints in V(D)J recombination (99,100). In addition, the XRCC4 protein product interacts with DNA-PK and is phosphorylated by this kinase (101). In contrast to Ku or DNA-PK knockouts, which have relatively mild phenotypes apart from impaired NHEJ and V(D)J recombination, disruption of either the XRCC4 (102) or the ligase IV (103) genes in mice causes embryonic lethality associated with neuronal apoptosis. Humans with ligase IV mutations have also been reported but with a milder neurological defect (104). The neuronal phenotype of ligase IV mutations fueled speculation that the complexities of neural development might include DNA recombination events, an idea originally sparked by the observation of RAG1 and RAG2 expression in central nervous system and neuronal cell lines and by a single report of somatic DNA recombination in mouse brain. However, the embryonic lethality and neurodevelopmental abnormalities of XRCC4 −/− (105) or ligase IV −/− mice (106) were reversed by concomitant defects in p53, which suggests that neuronal cells do not require recombination for normal development but may be unusually susceptible to apoptosis induced by DNA damage, such as that caused by oxygen or its metabolites (107).

Artemis

In a group of human SCID patients without evidence of abnormalities in genes for the known V(D)J recombination proteins, a defect was mapped to chromosome 10, subsequently leading to the identification of a gene that has been designated Artemis (108). The gene shows no strong similarity to other known proteins, although weak similarity was noted to two yeast proteins involved in repair of DNA interstrand cross-linking reagents (but not of double-strand breaks). Patients with homozygous null mutations of Artemis survive (no embryonic lethality) and show radiosensitivity as well as defects in coding joint—but not signal joint—formation. *In vitro* experiments with purified recombinant Artemis protein (109) have demonstrated that this protein binds to DNA-PK, whereupon, in an ATP-dependent step, it gains an endonucleolytic activity that can cleave synthetic and RAG-generated hairpin ends under physiological conditions (Mg^{2+} buffers). Because a homozygous point mutation that abolishes this activity confers the SCID phenotype, it is likely that Artemis is responsible for hairpin cleavage *in vivo*.

N Regions and Terminal Deoxynucleotide Transferase

TdT, the apparent source of N region additions, is an enzyme found in the thymus and bone marrow; its expression is a distinguishing characteristic of lymphoid leukemias, as opposed to myeloid leukemias. It catalyzes the addition of nucleotides onto the 3′ end of DNA strands. Although no template specificity determines the nucleotides added, the enzyme adds deoxyguanosine residues preferentially. This fact is consistent with a role for this enzyme in the origin of N regions found at the V-D and D-J junctions because these N nucleotides tend to be guanosine-rich at the 3′ ends of both the upstream coding strand and the downstream noncoding strand. Both N region addition and TdT are characteristically absent from fetal lymphocytes (110). N region addition is common in heavy-chain genes but rare in murine light-chain genes, although perhaps less rare in human (111).

As evidence that TdT is the primary source of N nucleotides, lymphocytes with engineered defects in their TdT genes produced rearranged Ig V regions with almost no N additions. Conversely, when TdT expression was engineered in cells undergoing κ or λ light-chain rearrangement, the normally low level of N region insertion in these recombinations was dramatically increased. This result suggests that the low frequency of N region sequences in normal κ or λ recombinations is not a result of the inability of these coding sequences to accept N region nucleotides. Instead, the preferential occurrence of N regions in heavy- versus light-chain genes (in the mouse, at least) reflects TdT levels that are higher in early B lineage cells undergoing heavy-chain rearrangement than in the later stage of light-chain recombination (see later discussion); indeed, mice with an engineered mutation that allows premature Vκ-Jκ joining in pro–B cells show an increased frequency of N region nucleotides in their recombined Vκ genes (112). In normal mice, the expression of a μ heavy chain may down-regulate TdT expression (113), contributing to the reduced level during the stage of light-chain recombination.

In TdT mutant mice, as well as in normal fetal lymphocytes low in TdT activity, absence of N region addition is associated with an increase in the frequency of recombination junctions in which short stretches of nucleotides could have derived from either germline element because of an overlap of identical sequences at the coding ends. These junctions suggest a recombination intermediate in which the complementary single-stranded regions from the two coding ends hybridize to each other, much as sticky ends generated by restriction endonucleases can facilitate ligation of DNA fragments. Such "homology-mediated" recombination may restrict the diversity of neonatal antibodies; it is possible that the resulting antibodies are enriched in specificities for commonly encountered pathogens or have broadened specificity, as has been

reported for TCRs lacking N regions (114). Decreased N region nucleotides and a high incidence of homology-mediated recombination have also been found in the rare coding joints formed in Ku80 knockout mice, which suggests that Ku80 may be required for recruiting TdT or supporting its action (115).

Proteins that Bind to DNA Breaks

Cells protect themselves against gene loss by a complex mechanism; DNA breaks are detected and initiate signals that halt cell division, induce repair, and in some cases trigger apoptosis. One important intermediate in this process is γ-H2AX, a phosphorylated histone that is rapidly localized to domains of DNA near chromosome breaks. Within minutes of exposure to ionizing radiation, immunostaining reveals discrete foci of γ-H2AX that appear to be necessary for later recruitment of other proteins (including Rad50, Rad51, and Brca1) into foci (116). The phosphorylation of the H2AX protein has been reported to be mediated by ATM, the product of the gene mutated in the disease ataxia telangiectasia (117); ATM colocalizes with foci of γ-H2AX after induction of double-strand breaks (118). The foci also contain Nbs1 (or nibrin), the product of the gene mutated in Nijmegen breakage syndrome; this protein is a component of the Mre11-Rad50-Nbs1 complex involved in double-strand break repair and activation of the S-phase checkpoint. RAG-mediated DNA cleavage has been found to induce foci containing Nbs1 and γ-H2AX by immunostaining (119), and ATM has been detected near RAG-induced breaks by chromatin immunoprecipitation and LM-PCR (120). The significance of these findings for the mechanism of V(D)J recombination is not clear because defects in all three proteins are compatible with near normal V(D)J recombination, possibly because of compensation by related proteins. *In vitro* recombination experiments may be necessary to sort out the roles of these proteins.

Exonuclease

Many recombined V regions are found to be missing variable numbers of nucleotides at the recombination junctions, in comparison with the coding sequences present in their respective germline V, D, or J precursors. This observation has been proposed to result from exonuclease-induced "nibbling" of the cut double-strand DNA ends during the time between cleavage near the heptamer RSS and rejoining of the cut DNA ends. Although the responsible exonuclease has been searched for and several exonucleases are known to exist in mammalian cells, no enzyme that "nibbles" the ends of V, D, and J segments has been definitively identified. It is possible that the loss of nucleotides at the coding joints results from nicks that open the hairpin loops at a distance from the symmetry axis of the loop—followed by exonuclease-catalyzed trimming of the single-strand overhang—rather than from "nibbling" of double-stranded DNA.

Further clarification of the V(D)J recombination should result from studies of completely cell-free recombination, which has been achieved in several laboratories with a combination of crude nuclear extracts plus purified RAG and other proteins.

Regulation of V(D)J Recombination

The recombination events that occur between Ig gene segments are carefully regulated so that most B cells express only one light-chain isotype (isotype exclusion) and use only one of the two homologous chromosomal loci for heavy- and light-chain genes (allelic exclusion). Isotype and allelic exclusion ensure that each lymphocyte expresses a single H_2L_2 combination and thus a single antigen binding specificity, a crucial feature of the clonal selection model of the immune response. Current evidence suggests that V-D-J recombination is controlled at two levels: regulation of the RAG protein levels and regulation of accessibility of the recombinase machinery to the germline substrates of rearrangement. Both of these factors are affected by the stage of B cell development; and, conversely, the expression of immunoglobulin provides a signal critical for regulating maturation of B cells.

A brief scheme of B cell development is presented as follows as background; a detailed account is in Chapter 6.

B-Lymphocyte Development

As shown in Fig. 12, B- and T-lymphocytes differentiate from pluripotent hematopoietic stem cells in the fetal liver and bone marrow. The primordial lymphoid progenitor has the potential to differentiate into B- or T-lymphocytes or natural killer cells. Among the earliest markers that indicate B lineage specificity are the non-Ig components of the pre–B-cell receptor (pre-BCR): Igα, Igβ, and λ5. CD19, which functions as a co-receptor in signal transduction, first appears in large proliferating "pro–B" cells, which also express several other distinguishing surface markers, including c-kit (receptor for the stem cell factor SCF), B220 (a B-lineage form of the phosphatase CD45), TdT, and CD43 (a sialoglycoprotein known as leukosialin). In the absence of heavy-chain protein, most of the SLC protein remains cytoplasmic, but some SLC is displayed on the surface membrane in association with a complex of glycoproteins (represented by a hook shape in Fig. 12), which has sometimes been called a surrogate heavy chain. This complex includes a cadherin-related

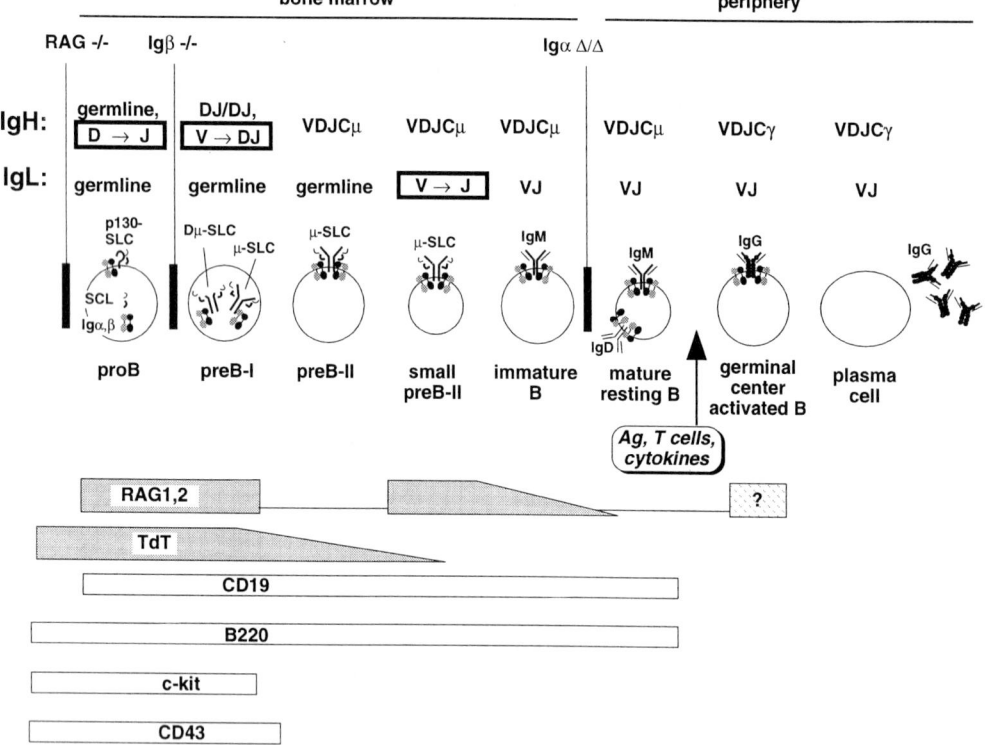

FIG. 12. Immunoglobulin (Ig) gene recombination in B-cell development. A simplified scheme of B-cell development is presented as a background for discussion of Ig gene recombination. The stages occurring in the bone marrow versus in the periphery (e.g., lymph nodes, spleen) are shown, along with the status of heavy and light Ig genes at each stage. A graphic depicting the Ig-related proteins displayed on the surface at each stage is presented; and, at the bottom, the stage-dependent expression of recombination activating genes and terminal deoxynucleotide transferase—both important in V(D)J recombination—is schematically depicted, as is the expression of several other marker proteins.

normal pre-BCR–induced shutoff may be mediated in part by down-regulation of RAG gene expression (141). This view would be consistent with the fact that in flow-sorted bone marrow cells, RAG1 and RAG2 mRNAs were detectable in pro–B and early pre–B cells (corresponding to cells undergoing D→J and V→D-J recombination) but undetectable in the large proliferating pre–B-II cells expressing μ-SLC. RAG gene expression then becomes detectable again in the small pre–B-II cells undergoing light-chain V→J recombination. In addition to effects on RAG activity, the pre-BCR may also down-regulate further V-D-J recombination by reducing "accessibility" of the heavy-chain locus, as indicated by reduced sterile VH gene transcription (142) and by reduced ability of RAG proteins to produce broken signal ends in nuclei incubated *in vitro,* as determined by LM-PCR (143). Diminished accessibility of the heavy Ig locus would prevent further V→D-J recombination during the subsequent stage when RAG proteins are up-regulated to activate light-chain V-J recombination.

The hypothesis that μ protein can activate κ chain recombination (effect ② in Fig. 13) was originally deduced from the fact that κ-expressing cells without heavy-chain gene rearrangement and expression are rare, as though heavy-chain expression were a prerequisite for κ expression. This view has been supported by observation of AMuLV-transformed lines and normal B-cell precursors developing *in vitro:* These lines consistently rearrange heavy-chain genes before κ genes. Furthermore, in a variety of experiments in which a μ heavy chain was absent in early B lineage cells, the introduction of a functional μ gene caused sterile κ gene transcription or Vκ-Jκ rearrangement. Although the evidence for pre-BCR stimulation of light-chain recombination seems strong, a small number of cells are apparently able to initiate light-chain recombination in the absence of heavy-chain synthesis. This has been demonstrated (a) by light-chain recombination in mice whose heavy-chain loci were rendered nonproductive by gene targeting and (b) by single-cell PCR analysis of normal B cell progenitors (144). Such precocious light-chain recombination may be a consequence of some "leakiness" of the controls on light-chain recombination in early B lymphopoiesis, or it may reflect a separate developmental lineage in which Vκ-Jκ recombination is activated earlier than VH-D-JH recombination. There is no known mechanism by which productive in-frame light-chain recombination could, in the absence of heavy chain, prevent continuing light-chain recombination from violating allelic exclusion, but the low incidence of this "premature" Vκ-Jκ recombination would keep the frequency of light-chain double-producers below 1%.

When κ recombination begins in μ-expressing cells, the possibilities for functional and nonfunctional V-J rearrangements resemble those discussed previously for the heavy chain. As soon as κ gene rearrangement leads to expression of a functional κ chain that can associate with μ to form a surface-expressed IgM molecule—that is, a mature BCR—then further κ rearrangement will be suppressed (effect ③ in Fig. 13). This regulatory influence would explain the observation of allelic exclusion in κ-expressing myelomas, and it has been supported by the finding that functional rearranged V-J-Cκ transgenes can suppress rearrangement of endogenous κ genes. Furthermore, in murine B lymphoma lines expressing RAG proteins, cross-linking of surface IgM with an anti-μ antibody was found to rapidly suppress RAG gene expression (145). It is possible that a ligand might deliver a corresponding signal in physiological circumstances, but this is not clear, especially because, under some conditions, cross-linking the BCR of pre–B cells—as might occur on binding of a self-antigen—can actually up-regulate RAG gene expression to activate "receptor editing," as described later.

Regulatory effect ④ in Fig. 13 is hypothetical, as little is known about regulation of λ gene rearrangement. The idea that λ recombination is somehow triggered by nonfunctional κ rearrangements on both chromosomes derives from the observations that most B cells show isotypic exclusion (i.e., they express either κ or λ but not both) and that κ rearrangement seems to occur before λ. Thus, in normal and malignant human B lymphoid cells (146), κ-expressing cells generally have their λ genes in germline configuration, whereas λ-expressing cells, κ genes are either rearranged (rarely) or deleted (commonly). The κ deletions reflect the RS recombination event discussed earlier in this chapter. These results suggest that λ genes may be held in germline configuration until κ genes rearrange nonproductively or are deleted (effect ④). An alternative possibility is that κ and λ rearrangement occur independently, but in the B lineage developmental program, κ is simply activated for recombination earlier than the λ locus (147).

The model of Fig. 13 assumes that membrane expression of a μ-λ IgM would shut off all further light-chain gene recombination by a mechanism similar to that in the κ locus (as illustrated by effect ③ in the figure), an idea supported by suppression of κ gene expression in λ transgenic mice. However, this suppression is somewhat "leaky," especially in older mice, and even in normal splenocytes, a small population of cells expresses both isotypes. These observations have led to the speculation that certain B-lymphocytes are not programmed for strict isotype exclusion. It is also possible that in some cells expressing both κ and λ, one of the isotype light chains has such a greater affinity for the expressed heavy-chain protein (on the basis of VH-VL compatibility) that the other isotype does not functionally contribute to surface Ig and is thus allelically excluded at the protein level.

Although this scheme of regulatory pathways may seem sufficient to explain allelic exclusion, an additional level of control is suggested by the observation that, in developing B cells, only a single allele of the κ locus is initially demethylated, and that allele is the target for Vκ-Jκ recombination (148). In this study, DNA from bone marrow B cells was used for a Southern blot similar to that of Fig. 1. DNA isolated from the gel at the position of the germline κ band was found to be methylated (i.e., resistant to a restriction enzyme inhibited by methylation of its CpG-containing recognition sequence), whereas DNA isolated from the region of the gel corresponding to rearranged bands was unmethylated. Other experiments suggested that demethylation occurs before recombination and requires the presence of the κ gene enhancers. Presumably, if the first allele to be demethylated is unsuccessful in recombining productively, the second allele could eventually become demethylated and undergo rearrangement. Which mechanism selects a particular chromosome for demethylation while leaving the homologous chromosome methylated is unknown, but it may be similar to the mechanism causing monoallelic expression of other genes such as interleukin-2, interleukin-4 (IL-4), and odorant receptor genes [reviewed by Schimenti (149)]. The demethylation of one Ig allele may also be related to mechanisms governing nonequivalent nuclear localization (150) and asynchronous replication (151) of Ig genes.

B-Cell Receptor Regulation of B-Cell Maturation

The signals mediated by the pre-BCR (μ-SLC) and the mature BCR (IgM) are critical not only for regulating V-D-J recombination but also as checkpoints controlling other features of B-lymphocyte differentiation. Thus, in the bone marrow of RAG or JH knockout mice, the absence of BCR signaling leaves B lymphopoiesis blocked at the earliest pro–B stage—large cells staining positive for B220, CD43, and c-kit—and cells with surface markers typical of mature B cells are absent from the periphery. When a recombined V-D-J-Cμ heavy-chain transgene is introduced into a RAG knockout background (152), the resulting μ protein allows the progression of B lineage cells to the stage of small pre–B-II cells, in which light-chain recombination would normally occur. These cells cannot undergo VL→JL recombination in the absence of RAG proteins, but they do show up-regulation of sterile κ transcription, an apparent reflection of regulatory effect ② in Fig. 13. If, in addition to the μ gene, a complete recombined light-chain transgene is also added to the genome of the RAG knockout mice, then B cell development is restored, with normal numbers of B cells in the periphery, expressing mature B cell surface markers. The developmental block in RAG knockouts is similar to that seen in mice with knockouts of λ5 or a double knockout of both VpreB1 and VpreB2. The λ5 knockout cells could be rescued from their developmental arrest by a productively rearranged κ transgene expressed in pre–B cells, indicating that a κ chain can substitute for the SLC in mediating maturation signals (153). Indeed, even without the κ transgene, some maturation occurs in the λ5 knockout mice, a presumed result of small amounts of Vκ-Jκ recombination occurring before V-D-JH recombination and thus providing a κ chain that allows surface IgM expression and signaling. The permissive effect of the pre-BCR or BCR on developmental progression appears to be mediated by the Igα-Igβ heterodimer, according to results with the mutant or chimeric μ transgenes linked to Igα or Igβ cytoplasmic domains, as described previously (139,140). The role of the SLC is apparently simply to facilitate surface expression of

μ heavy chain rather than directly advancing B cell development, inasmuch as a truncated μ heavy chain that was expressed on the surface membrane but could not associate with the SLC was still able to induce developmental progression (154). Ligand-dependent cross-linking of the pre-BCR is not necessary for inducing maturation; when a chimeric molecule containing the cytoplasmic signaling domains of Igα and Igβ without an extracellular domain was targeted to the inner leaflet of the plasma membrane, it was capable of driving developmental maturation beyond the pro–B stage, apparently through a basal unstimulated level of signaling (155). Even in mature circulating B cells, the BCR apparently provides a tonic signal necessary for survival of B cells, inasmuch as in vivo ablation of the BCR of adult mice by inducible Cre-lox gene targeting induces rapid B cell death (156).

Late Recombination Activating Gene Expression: Receptor Editing and Receptor Revision

Although the RAG genes are generally down-regulated by a signal mediated by the appearance of IgM at the end of the pre–B cell stage, RAG gene expression and V(D)J recombination can recur later during "receptor editing" of autoreactive B cells in the bone marrow and possibly during B cell maturation in germinal centers. Evidence for such secondary rearrangements was first observed for the κ locus. After production of an initial IgM-κ protein, receptor editing by light-chain rearrangement can take three forms: An initial Vκ-Jκ junction could be deleted by recombination between an upstream V and downstream J on the same chromosome; Vκ-Jκ recombination could occur on the other chromosome; or Vλ-Jλ recombination could be activated. V gene replacement of the heavy chain is less frequently observed, probably because it depends on an incomplete RSS, a lone heptamer embedded in the 3' end of some VH coding regions, as described in an earlier section. Most replacement of productively rearranged light- or heavy-chain genes probably serves to abort production of an antibody that was autoreactive. Thus, receptor editing might complement two other mechanisms for preventing autoantibodies: anergization and cell deletion by apoptosis.

Several researchers have studied receptor editing by using mice carrying rearranged genes expressing autoreactive antibodies inserted as either transgenes or "knocked-in" genes: that is, pre-recombined Vκ-Jκ genes engineered to replace the germline locus through homologous recombination in embryonic stem cells. In one study, the germline JH locus was replaced with the 3H9 recombined V-D-J gene encoding a heavy chain that, in combination with most (but not all) κ light chains, is capable of binding to DNA, a self-antigen (36). In such mice, most B cells have replaced the 3H9 gene by an upstream VH gene. When inserted as a transgene (which cannot undergo VH replacement because the transgene is inserted randomly distant from the VH locus), 3H9 stimulates light-chain editing, as evidenced by increased frequency of Jκ5 usage and reduced diversity of Vκ genes expressed by the

B cells displaying the 3H9 heavy chain (157). These results are consistent with the interpretation that primary rearrangements, yielding Vκ proteins capable of supporting DNA binding, were edited by secondary rearrangements joining downstream Jκ to Vκ regions incompatible with DNA binding. In a similar system, efficient receptor editing was observed in mice with knocked-in heavy- and light-chain genes encoding a self MHC class I specificity (158). Receptor editing appears to occur in the immature B cell population in the bone marrow (159) and is associated with increased RAG gene expression. Indeed, *in vitro* BCR ligation of cultured immature bone marrow B cells was found to up-regulate RAG gene expression and induce κ and λ recombinations (160). However, as previously discussed, BCR ligation has also been reported to terminate RAG gene expression of sIGM+ immature B cells to mediate allelic exclusion (145), and in immature B cells that have advanced to leave the bone marrow, BCR ligation causes apoptosis. How the same stimulus of BCR ligation can trigger RAG down-regulation to mediate allelic exclusion, RAG up-regulation to mediate receptor editing, and apoptosis in later stages is not currently understood. Possible explanations lie in developmentally regulated differences in receptor density on the cell surface (161), in affinity for the ligand (162), in developmentally regulated antiapoptotic proteins (163), in environmental co-stimulatory signals (164), and in BCR signal transduction machinery (165).

Although most studies on receptor editing have been carried out on mice engineered with genes encoding autoantibodies, receptor editing appears to affect a significant fraction of the normal repertoire. Casellas et al. (166) engineered mice with a pre-recombined Vκ-Jκ knock-in gene with no known autoantigen specificity on one chromosome, and an unrearranged κ locus with a human Cκ gene on the homologous chromosome. The rearranged knock-in κ gene could associate with the full repertoire of VH genes, some of which might encode an autoantigen. In these mice, about 22% of the B cells showed evidence of light-chain receptor editing, including secondary recombinations on the targeted chromosome, recombination of the other κ chromosome, or λ recombination. In another study (167), a high frequency of light-chain receptor editing was suggested by an analysis of IgMλ+ B cells from mice with a normal germline κ locus on one chromosome and a deleted κ locus on the other; almost half the RS deletions in these cells involved Vκ-Jκ junctions that were in-frame and presumably functional but were apparently edited by RS deletion and subsequent λ rearrangement. Apart from its role in normal B cell development, receptor editing as also been associated with pathological processes. An unusual population of B cells expressing both conventional light chains and SLCs and showing evidence of receptor editing was found in the blood of normal donors and accumulating in the joints of patients with rheumatoid arthritis (168). Rheumatoid joints were also found to harbor an unexpectedly high frequency of heavy-chain genes with evidence of VH replacement (169). These and other studies

suggest that dysregulated receptor editing may contribute to pathological processes of some autoimmune diseases.

In addition to receptor editing of bone marrow immature B cells, a second scenario of "late" RAG expression has been reported in germinal center (GC) B cells (170,171). RAG1 and RAG2 mRNA transcripts were detected by reverse transcriptase PCR in GC cells from immunized mice purified by fluorescence-activated cell sorting; the RAG proteins were detected in GC cells by immunofluorescence; and evidence of V(D)J recombination was found in GC cells (172). RAG expression was also observed constitutively in Peyer's patch GCs (which are maintained by food antigens in the absence of intentional immunization) and in splenic B cells cultured with IL-4 plus lipopolysaccharide (LPS). The RAG+ GC cells appear to recapitulate expression of several surface markers characteristic of early B lineage cells, including heat-stable antigen (CD24) and λ5; therefore, it is possible that the RAG gene expression may be just one aspect of a GC-induced reversion to a primitive phenotype. Could RAG expression in GC B cells be necessary for isotype switching or somatic mutation, both of which are Ig gene alterations that occur in GCs? The answer is probably not, because both processes occur in B cells of RAG −/− mice. One speculation is that RAG-dependent receptor revision may be turned on during somatic mutation, either to replace mutated V regions that have become autoreactive or to expand the potential repertoire of cells undergoing affinity maturation. However, an alternative interpretation of RAG+ GC B cells is that they do not reflect reexpression of RAG genes by mature cells; rather, they reflect an increase in the number of immature B cells that have left the bone marrow and lodged in GCs after immunization. To explore whether mature cells that have extinguished RAG expression can become RAG+ again, Yu et al. (173) engineered mice in which a green fluorescent protein coding sequence replaced one RAG2 allele, so that sorting for green fluorescent protein–positive (GFP+) cells could be used to select RAG2-expressing cells. When GFP+ splenic B cells from RAG2/GFP mice were adoptively transferred into RAG1 −/− mice along with primed T cells, GFP+ RAG2-expressing cells were observed in the spleen of immunized recipients, with expression declining over several days after transfer. However, if the recipients received only sorted GFP− cells, which had apparently already extinguished their RAG2 and GFP genes, no RAG2 expression was observed in the donor spleens. This observation suggests that RAG2 expression, once extinguished, cannot be reactivated in mature B cells in the GC and that RAG2 expressing GC B cells are immature B-cell immigrants from bone marrow. Similar conclusions were reported by another laboratory (174) [see also Nagaoka et al. (175)], but other results, such as a report of receptor editing in a cell that had undergone somatic mutation (176), seem to support the concept of receptor revision of mature cells. Further investigations are needed to clarify the role of receptor revision and to understand the regulation of RAG expression. This work should be aided by investigations of the transcriptional control of RAG genes. As of this writing, the promoters of RAG1 (177,178) and RAG2 (179) have been described, and a regulatory region upstream of RAG2 that coordinately controls both RAG genes has been deduced (180), but little is known about the detailed function of these regions.

GERMLINE DIVERSITY

A comprehensive evaluation of the germline repertoire of V gene segments requires an examination of the sequences of all germline V regions, a daunting task. However, targeted sequencing with modern molecular biology techniques—including cloning vectors that allow long genomic inserts and large-scale sequencing with fluorescent dyes and automated sample preparation—have enabled achievement of this goal for the human κ, λ, and heavy-chain loci; non-targeted (whole genome) sequencing has completed the murine κ and heavy-chain loci. (The tiny V repertoire of the murine λ loci has already been discussed in the section on λ genes.)

Several World Wide Web resources are devoted to providing convenient updated access to Ig germline gene sequences. The IMGT (international ImMunoGeneTics) database (http://imgt.cnusc.fr:8104/home.html), coordinated by Marie-Paule Lefranc, includes a database for Ig and T-cell receptor genes from a variety of species and includes maps, sequences, lists of chromosomal translocations, and multiple helpful links. IgBLAST (http://imgt.cnusc.fr/igblast/) is a service of the National Center for Biotechnology Information (NCBI) and allows a submitted sequence to be searched against germline V, D, and J sequences. V Base Gold available as a datbase at http://www.mrc-cpe.cam.ac.uk is an online catalog of human V gene segments and alleles coordinated by Ian M. Tomlinson.

Germline Diversity of the Murine VH Locus

Attempts to analyze the murine VH repertoire began before the gene cloning era with study of VH amino acid sequences from murine myelomas. Initial attempts to classify the observed VHs into related groups were based on limited amino acid sequence analysis, primarily of N-terminals of myeloma proteins. The current scheme classifies two V gene sequences as being in the same group or family if they show more than about 80% nucleotide sequence identity and as being in different families if their sequences are less than 70% identical. (Empirically, few VH comparisons yield identities between 70% and 80%.) These criteria for sequence similarity correspond well with the degree of similarity that allows Southern blot hybridization between a V probe and members of the same family under conditions of moderate stringency. Fifteen families are now recognized, and these apparently contribute to the bulk of the immune response. When 2,000 cDNA clones hybridizing to both Cμ and JH probes were analyzed, all were found to have V regions from the 15 families, according to hybridization or sequence analysis, except for about 2% of the clones, which represented truncated or aber-

rant cDNA synthesis (181). The families have been further classified into three groups, or "clans," on the basis of sequence conservation in the framework I region (FR1; codons 6 to 24) and FR3 (codons 67 to 85). (Framework amino acids are the non-CDR parts of the Ig V region that hold the CDR loops in position to contact antigen.) The clans are conserved among human, mouse, and frog, which suggests that several fundamental steps in germline VH diversification preceded the amphibian–reptile divergence (182). One interesting feature of the murine VH locus is that, unlike the organization of the human VH locus, members of a given murine VH family tend to be clustered together on the chromosome (although some interdigitation occurs). The map order (Fig. 14) has been studied in several laboratories by a variety of methods, including PFGE and Southern blot analysis of genomic DNA, and deletion mapping of VH regions in B-cell clones. The best consensus from different laboratories is on the families closest to Cμ: S107—Q52—7183—D—J—Cμ, with some overlap between these three families, as shown in the figure. This order is of special interest because the most proximal family cluster (designated 7183), particularly its most proximal member (designated VH81X), is the V region that is significantly overrepresented in the V-D-J rearrangements occurring in fetal liver pre–B cells. This observation was earlier taken as evidence favoring a "tracking" model of V gene rearrangement (i.e., that a recombinase would engage DNA near the J regions and slide 5' to find V regions to recombine); however, alternative interpretations have been proposed on the basis of more recent data (183,184).

The VH families differ widely in complexity. Several families have only a few members. For example, the VH S107 family yields four Southern blot bands, and extensive cloning with a probe for this family has in fact detected only four germline members (of which one is apparently a pseudogene). At the other extreme, the VH J558 family may contain several hundred members in the BALB/c mouse, although many of these may reflect recent duplications in the VH locus and would be expected to encode minimally diverged VH sequences. Other strains of mice besides BALB/c seem to have smaller J558 families, which is consistent with the notion of a recent expansion of J558 VH genes in BALB/c.

Mouse Germline JH and DH Regions

Four germline JH sequences were identified about 5 kb upstream of the murine Cμ gene. All appear to be functional in that the sequences they encode are found in secreted heavy chains. Upstream of each JH lies a typical RSS with 22- to 23-bp spacers.

D regions were initially hypothesized on the basis of the highly diverse amino acid sequences in myeloma proteins between the V and J regions, as briefly discussed earlier in this chapter. Because both VH and JH were known to be flanked by signal elements of the long space type (~23 bp), it was predicted that a germline D region would be flanked on both sides by short signal element spaces, so that both V-D and D-J

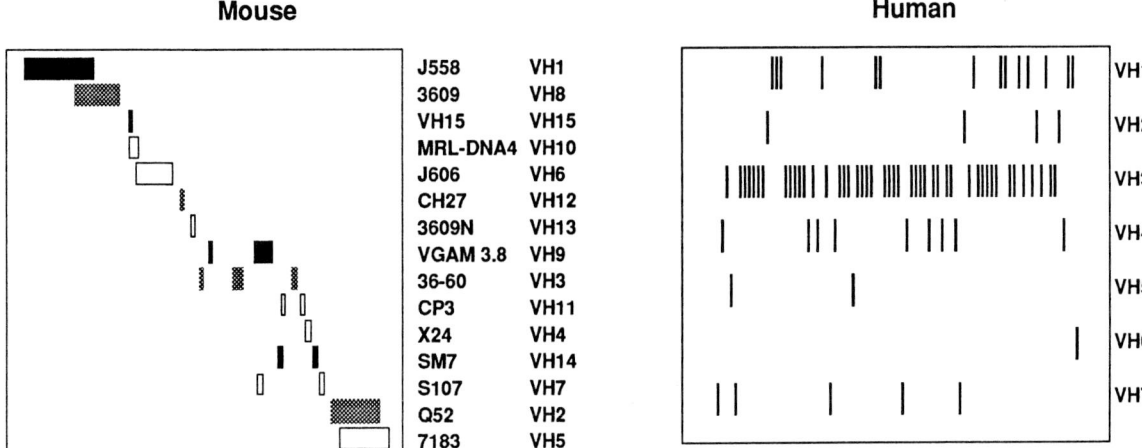

FIG. 14. Maps of the murine and human VH loci. The 15 known murine VH gene families are shown in their approximate map positions. Each *rectangle* represents a cluster of VH genes of the indicated family; the clan identification (358) of the VH families is indicated by the color of the rectangle: black for clan I, gray for clan II, and white for clan III. Although some interdigitation is shown by overlapping families (e.g., the Q52 and 7183 families), the families are largely clustered. In contrast, all human VH genes (*vertical lines*) of a prototypic haplotype are shown on the *right* and are based on the formulation by Cook and Tomlinson (359); extensive interdigitation of families is apparent.

recombination would conform to the 12/23 spacer rule. This is precisely what was found when germline D regions were cloned from murine DNA. The 13 murine D regions span about 80 kb upstream of the four JH segments. Eleven of the genes fall into two families: SP2 (nine Ds) and FL16 (two Ds). The most 3′ D region, DQ52, lies only 0.7 kb upstream of JH1. The final murine D region to be discovered, DST4, was identified through the recognition of a recurring nucleotide sequence observed between V and J in recombined V-D-J regions that was not accounted for by the previously known D sequences (185).

D regions contribute to Ig diversity by their ability to join with different combinations of VH and JH regions; in addition, the "flexibility" of the recombination junction (i.e., N region addition, "nibbled" coding sequences) applies on both ends of the D region. An out-of-frame recombination at the V-D junction may be compensated by the frame of the D-J junction, so that a particular D element could theoretically be read in all three frames in different V-D-J recombinants. As mentioned previously, this extra source of diversity is used by human heavy chains (7), but the murine system has evolved mechanisms that strongly favor the reading frame (RF) known as RF1 (6). D-J rearrangement in RF3 is counterselected, owing to frequent internal stop codons. When D-J recombination has occurred in RF2, the resulting transcripts can encode a D-J-Cμ protein (designated the Dμ protein), which can be expressed on the surface of a pre–B cell in association with the products of the VpreB and λ5 genes. Murine cells expressing Dμ protein cannot progress to normal Ig production, perhaps because the Dμ protein triggers the shut-off of V-D-J recombination before V assembly is complete; therefore, expressed heavy-chain V regions rarely include a D-J junction in RF2 (6). This unusual model is

supported by the observation that RF2 suppression is not observed in λ5 knockout mice (which fail to express Dμ protein on the cell surface). In humans, this mechanism is not operative because ATG initiation codons are not generally present 5′ of D regions to encode a Dμ protein. Some rearranged V-D-J sequences seem to be interpretable as V-D-D-J products, even though D-D recombination appears to violate the 12/23 rule (186).

Murine Germline Vκ Locus

Although murine light-chain genes were among the first Ig genes studied by molecular biology techniques, the organization of the murine germline Vκ locus has been less thoroughly characterized than the human version. The latest classification, based on the nucleotide sequence criteria described previously, recognizes about 20 families. As described, for VH genes, some Vκ families are shared by human and mouse, which suggests that the family divisions preceded primate–rodent species divergence. The murine locus has been cloned on a series of overlapping bacterial artificial chromosome (BAC) and yeast artificial chromosome (YAC) clones and spans about 3.5 Mb upstream of the Cκ gene on chromosome 6 (187). In addition, a few Vκ sequences have been localized to other chromosomes (chromosome 16 and 19), where they cannot contribute to diversity and are thus considered orphons. In the functional Vκ locus on chromosome 6, many related Vκ sequences are found to lie clustered together, although some interspersion of families also exists. Of the 140 Vκ sequences in the locus, 75 are known to be functional as their mRNA or protein products have been detected. Of the remaining sequences, 44 are clearly pseudogenes, 21 are apparently free of defects but have not been demonstrated to be expressed, and the rest have minor defects that might not preclude function (188).

Human Germline VH Locus

The human VH locus spans 1.1 Mb at the telomeric end of chromosome 14 (14q32.33). Essentially the entire locus (957 kb) was sequenced in 1998 (189), and overlapping sequence has more recently become available through the public database of the Human Genome Project. The original sequence includes 123 VH segments, including about 40 functional genes whose mRNA or protein products have been identified. Of the remaining sequences, 79 are clearly pseudogenes, and four show no apparent defect but have not been documented to be expressed. Many of these sequences were previously identified by large-scale mapping efforts. The human VH sequences fall into seven families that are extensively interdigitated, in contrast to the family clusters characteristic of the murine locus (Fig. 14). The sequence shows evidence of nine internal duplications, whose ages (spanning from about 10 to 130 million years) can be approximately estimated on the basis of the number of sequence differences accumulated between different copies. Some VH sequences are polymorphic, owing to VH insertions or deletions in different allelic chromosomes. All the VH regions share the same orientation characteristic of the JH regions, which is consistent with V-D-J recombination by deletion rather than inversion. With the availability of the complete sequence of the locus, the VH genes have been given systematic names that reflect both their family and their position in the locus; for example IGHV4-39 is the 39th VH gene in the locus (counting from the 5′ end) and is in family 4. In addition to the VH sequences on chromosome 14, 24 additional germline VH sequences have been mapped to chromosomes 15 and 16 and represent nonfunctional orphons that were apparently duplicated from the functional locus on chromosome 14; these sequences contributed to earlier overestimates of the length of the functional human VH locus. Scattered in the chromosome 14 VH locus are eight gene-like sequences that are unrelated to immunoglobulin and that probably represent ancient pseudogenes, as well as 722 inserted retroposed elements that constitute about 42% of the DNA. The complete sequence of the human VH locus offers clues to its evolution and to the conserved sequences (e.g., promoters, RSSs) necessary for function, as well as defining the repertoire of germline VH diversity available to the immune system.

Human JH and DH Regions

Upstream of the human Cμ gene lie six functional JH regions interspersed with three JH pseudogenes. The pseudogenes encode amino acid sequences never found in human heavy chains and lack the RNA splice signal found at the 3′ end of all active JH genes. All of the JH genes and pseudogenes demonstrate approximately 23-bp RSS spacing (as in the mouse).

The human D region locus has been defined by complete sequence analysis of a 92-kb region spanning the human D regions (7). One germline D gene is located in a position approximately homologous to that of the murine DQ52: that is, 5′ to the human JHI. This human D gene, initially designated DHQ52, bears striking homology to its murine counterpart but is the only human D segment showing such human/murine homology. All of the other human D regions belong to six families and lie in a cluster of duplicated domains beginning about 22 kb upstream of JH1. There are 27 D regions. Of these, 24 are accounted for by four tandem approximate duplications of a 9.5-kb segment containing a representative of the six D families. In addition to these 24 D regions, three more D regions result from (a) an additional partial duplication of 2.8 kb, including one D; (b) an internal duplication creating one D; and (c) DHQ52, which is in a family of its own, distinct from the six duplicated families. The D regions have been renamed according to a scheme similar to that used for the VH genes: A first number identifies the family, and a second identifies the sequential position in the locus. The locus starts with the 5′ most D region, D1-1, and ends with D7-27 (DHQ52). Three D regions are apparently nonfunctional as a result of mutations in RSS heptamers, and there are two pairs of D regions with identical coding sequences (including one of the D segments with a heptamer mutation); thus, there are 23 distinct D regions that can contribute to human immunoglobulin diversity. All of these sequences appear in the expressed Ig V-D-J regions, many in all three reading frames. In general, one reading frame encodes primarily hydrophilic residues, one encodes hydrophobic residues, and one includes frequent stop codons. (Some D regions that contain stop codons can be used if these codons are removed by nuclease trimming before V-D-J assembly is complete.) Additional human D segments originally thought to lie upstream of the main cluster apparently lie on the duplicated orphon cluster on chromosome 15 and are thus nonfunctional.

Human Germline Vκ Locus

The human Vκ locus is located on the short arm of chromosome 2 (2p11-2). Zachau and colleagues have carried out an extensive investigation of the human locus by cloning, PFGE, and sequence analysis, culminating in the complete sequence of about 1 Mb (10^6 bp) of DNA (190). This is composed of a proximal segment, which includes the Jκ-Cκ region and extends about 500 kb upstream, and a distal segment of about 430 kb. These two segments are separated by a spacer of about 0.8 Mb that is apparently devoid of Vκ sequences. The distal and proximal segments represent a large inverted repeat, and so most Vκ sequences on the proximal segment have duplicate copies in the opposite orientation on the distal segment. The average sequence similarity between the duplicated sequences is 98.9%, which suggests a recent (<5 million years old) duplication event. In accordance with this, the locus is not duplicated in chimpanzees, a species that is estimated to have diverged from the human lineage approximately 6 million years ago. About 5% of human alleles also lack the distal duplication.

The sequenced region contains 132 Vκ sequences, including 87 unambiguous pseudogenes and 46 open reading frames. Of these, 29 Vκ genes have been found expressed in proteins; these 29 include 25 unique genes and four that derive from identical gene pairs. In all B lymphoid cell lines examined, those with Vκ-Jκ rearrangements involving the distal inverted Vκ segments contained retained signal joints, which is consistent with Vκ-Jκ recombination by inversion. The two Vκ genes closest to Jκ1 are also in inverted orientation (and are not within the duplicated region). The locus additionally contains numerous insertions of retroposed elements (about 35% of the sequence) but no recognized interspersed non-Ig genes or pseudogenes. Multiple internal repeats suggest ancient duplications.

Apart from the Vκ sequences in the cluster near the Jκ-Cκ locus, Zachau and colleagues have identified at least 25 orphons (190). One orphon cluster is located in the long arm of chromosome 2; perhaps it was separated from the major locus—on the short arm of this chromosome—by a pericentric inversion (which must have occurred rather recently in evolution, inasmuch as it is absent from the chimpanzee and gorilla). Other orphons are located on chromosomes 1 and 22, and at least one probably nonfunctional Vκ lies about 1.5 Mb downstream from Cκ.

Human Germline Vλ Locus

The human Vλ has also been characterized by intensive cloning, sequencing, and mapping of Vλ regions and ultimately by the complete sequence analysis of 1,025,415 bp covering the entire locus (26). The locus contains about 36 potentially functional Vλ genes (in 10 families), 56 pseudogenes, and 13 "relics," containing less than 200 bp of Vλ-like sequences. (As noted for other loci, exact numbers may differ, depending on the haplotype and method of analysis.) Of the potentially functional genes, only about 30 have been documented to be expressed by comparison with cDNA sequences. Within the clustered Vλ sequences lies the human VpreB gene, as well as several genes and pseudogenes unrelated to the λ system. All the Vλ sequences (except a few pseudogenes) are in the same transcriptional orientation as the J-C cluster. Analysis of the approximately 1-Mb sequence reveals several segments of internal duplications, some including Vλ regions. The largest and most frequently expressed Vλ gene families lie relatively close to the J-C cluster, mostly within the proximal 400 kb.

Combinatorial Diversity Estimates

Before the era of recombinant DNA technology, the source of antibody diversity was so mysterious that it was whimsically referred to as the problem of G.O.D. (generation of diversity). Knowledge of antibody genes gained since the early 1980s

has elucidated the diversity inherent in the germline V repertoire and the diversity contributed by recombinational mechanisms (combinatorial multiplication, "flexibility" of recombination site, N and P nucleotides), as already discussed. Together, these diversity elements provide an immense potential repertoire, one so large that to some investigators it seemed unnecessary to postulate that diversity was further increased by somatic mutation. As an exercise in estimating the contribution of germline and recombinational diversity in the human, consider the number of different antibodies that could be formed from the germline V, D, and J sequences that are known to be functional. From 40 VH regions, 27 D regions, and 6 JH regions, it is possible to obtain 6,480 combinations; however, if the three reading frames available for the D regions are taken into account, the total comes to 19,440 combinations of amino acid sequences. For the light chain, there are the 145 κ combinations (29 Vκ × 5 Jκ) plus the 120 λ combinations (30 Vλ × 4 Jλ), or 265 total light-chain combinations. If H$_2$L$_2$ pairing occurs randomly, a total of 19,440 × 265, or more than 5 million combinations, can be calculated. This estimate has neglected additional sources of diversity that are substantial but difficult to quantitate: the "nibbling" of coding sequences and the insertion of N and P nucleotides. Even without these factors, however, the exercise demonstrates how nature has greatly enlarged the potential sequence diversity available from a limited number of total nucleotides by allowing flexible recombination between different classes of sequence elements.

Although it is clear that these mechanisms imply a vast repertoire, it is worth considering some qualifications that tend to reduce the actual combinatorial diversity, especially early in ontogeny. It seems unlikely, for example, that every possible combination of light and heavy chains yields a functional antibody molecule, because *in vitro* light- and heavy-chain reassociation experiments show that certain hybrid molecules (formed from light and heavy chains derived from different antibodies) are relatively unstable. Similarly, association of V and J (or V, D, and J) is conceivably not completely random. Evidence of striking bias in the selection of VH genes in fetal pre–B hybridomas has been mentioned, and other biases have been reported in J usage. In addition, fetal and newborn V-D-J junctions show a paucity of N nucleotides and a tendency to form V-D-J junctions across short stretches of sequence identity between the recombining sequences ("homology mediated" recombination, discussed earlier in this chapter). Effects that reduce diversity in early V(D)J recombination may facilitate the production of certain antibodies that are advantageous for young individuals.

REGULATION OF IMMUNOGLOBULIN GENE EXPRESSION

A detailed discussion of immunoglobulin gene regulation is beyond the scope of this chapter [for reviews, see Ernst and Smale (191) and Henderson and Calame (192)]. However, several regulatory features are worth mentioning because of their relevance to topics covered in this chapter, including V(D)J recombination, isotype switching, and somatic hypermutation. Three major classes of eukaryotic cis-regulatory elements have been defined. A promoter is a DNA segment that is located near the transcriptional initiation site and that promotes the initiation of RNA transcription in a specific direction: toward the coding sequence of the gene. An enhancer is a DNA segment that can stimulate transcription when positioned at variable distances from the transcription initiation site and in either orientation. A silencer down-regulates transcription, operating (like an enhancer) in both orientations and over variable distances via mechanisms not thoroughly understood. All three kinds of elements are generally active in only certain cell types and thus participate in regulating the tissue-specific expression of the associated gene. Two other types of cis-regulatory elements have been studied in eukaryotic chromosomes and but are less well understood than those just described. Matrix attachment regions attach DNA to the chromosomal "scaffold" proteins and may promote local unpairing of the DNA strands. Locus control regions (LCRs), first discovered in the β-globin locus, are complex regulatory regions that are composed of smaller elements that individually have enhancer function. LCRs affect chromatin structure and gene activity over longer distances than enhancers are thought to act. Operationally, they are defined by their ability—when tested in transgenic constructs—to program associated reporter genes for expression independent of the position of integration into chromosomal DNA; in contrast, constructs without LCRs generally are expressed at widely different levels in different transgenic mouse strains, depending on integration site.

Figure 15 provides a schematic overview of the currently known regulatory sequences of the Ig loci in the mouse (similar regions have been reported for most of the homologous human loci). Promoters are present in the flanking DNA just upstream of each V gene in all three loci: κ, λ, and heavy chain. In plasmacytomas, only the promoter of the rearranged V region that has undergone V(D)J recombination is active, whereas similar promoters of unrearranged upstream Vκ or VH regions are inactive. The selective activity of the promoter of the rearranged V is mediated by enhancers found in the J-C introns of both loci. (The J-C introns of λ loci apparently lack enhancers.) Near the intronic enhancers of the κ and heavy Ig loci, silencer regions that may inhibit the activity of the associated enhancers in non-B cells have been reported. After the discovery of intron enhancers, subsequent investigation

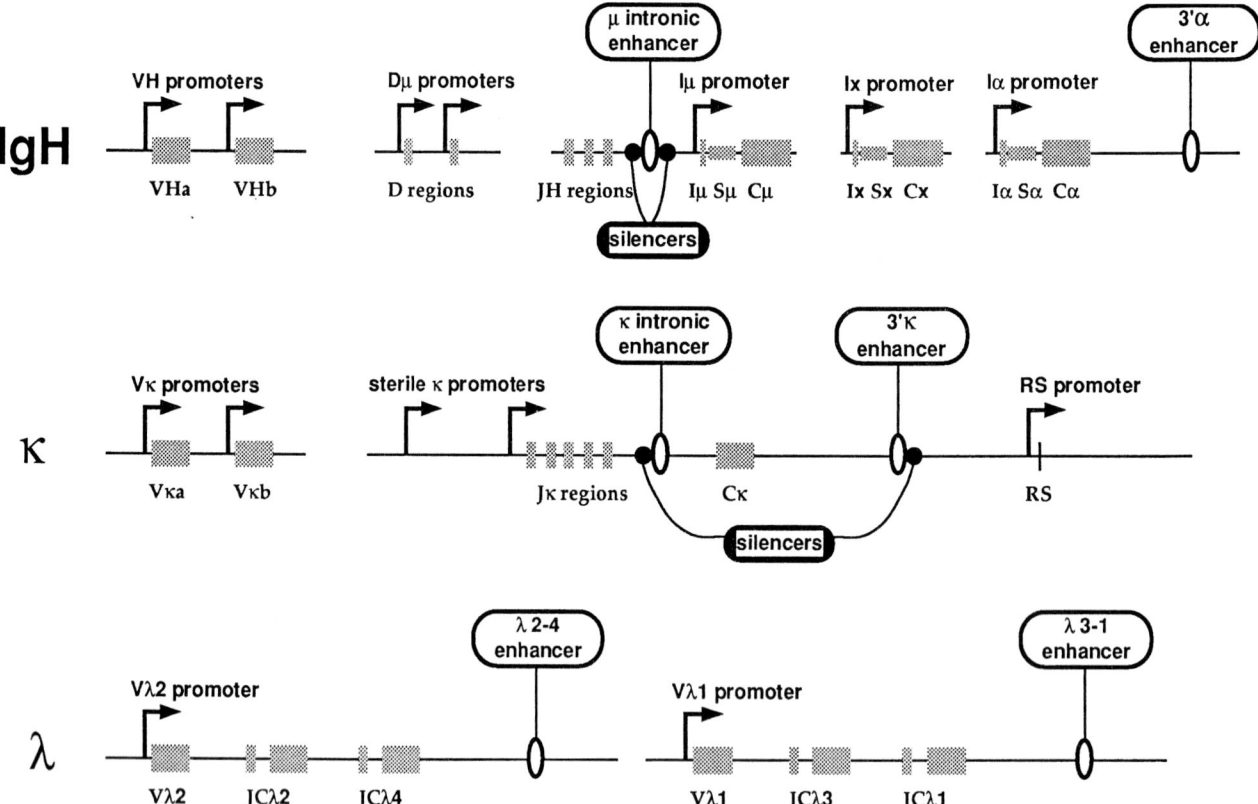

FIG. 15. Enhancers and promoters of the murine immunoglobulin (Ig) loci. Schematic maps (not to scale) of the three murine Ig loci are shown: heavy (*top*), κ (*middle*) and λ (*bottom*). The six known Ig enhancers are shown as *vertical ellipses,* the four silencer regions by *black circles,* and the various promoters by *arrows* indicating the direction of transcription.

uncovered enhancers 3' of κ and λ C region genes. In addition, a complex of enhancers, which together may function as an LCR, lies 3' of the murine Cα gene. This complex includes four separate enhancers that coincide with deoxyribonuclease I hypersensitivity sites. Strongest enhancer, corresponding to two closely spaced hypersensitivity sites designated HS12, is flanked by a long inverted repeat, at both ends of which lie the nearly identical enhancers designated HS3a and HS3b. Finally, HS4 lies at the 3' end of the complex. In the human locus, nearly identical enhancer complexes lie downstream of the duplicated Cα1 and Cα2 genes. More recently reported regulatory regions include an enhancer located upstream of murine DQ52 (193), a sequence between Cδ and Cγ3 (designated Eδ-γ3) that shows enhancer activity in early B lineage cells (194), a region between Eμ and Sμ that seems to affect expression in transgenes (195), and a sequence in an analogous region near Sγ1 that seems to act as an LCR (196).

Apart from the transcripts of functional Ig genes, additional "germline" or "sterile" transcripts are transcribed from Ig C region genes that are being activated for V assembly or isotype switch rearrangements. These transcripts are also controlled by promoters (Fig. 15), which in some cases have been found to be critical for regulation of the corresponding isotype switch rearrangement, as described later.

The activity of all these regulatory sequences is dependent on the nuclear content of specific transcription factors that bind to short DNA motifs within these regions; these factors are regulated by the developmental stage and the environmental milieu of the cell. For example, Eμ (the enhancer between JH and Cμ) functions primarily in early B cell development, whereas the HS12 enhancer of the 3'α complex functions later; and these differences have been attributed to the differential expression of specific transcription factors (197). Many transcription factors have been extensively studied as regulators of Ig gene expression [reviewed by Ernst and Smale (191) and Henderson and Calame (192)]. In addition to the local effects of factor binding, regulatory regions are affected by their chromatin context. For example, methylation of CpG dinucleotides of promotors or enhancers tends to down-regulate their expression, and so gene activation is often associated with demethylation. Gene expression can also be affected by various covalent modifications of the histone proteins that package DNA into nucleosomes. The binding of transcription factors and the control of chromatin responsiveness (e.g., methylation status, histone modification) interact in complex ways that are critical for understanding Ig gene expression but are outside the scope of this chapter.

IMMUNOGLOBULIN GENE ALTERATIONS IN GERMINAL CENTERS

Several days after exposure to an antigen, B cells accumulate in local lymph nodes, gut-associated lymphoid tissue,

and the spleen and begin additional maturation steps in GCs. During the GC response, antigen-driven B cells undergo cycles of proliferation, and their Ig genes undergo two unique alterations: CSR and affinity maturation through somatic hypermutation (SHM) and selection. Until recently, these two processes were considered to be mechanistically unrelated; but current evidence, although not completely clarifying either process, has suggested mechanistic similarities between them. These similarities are discussed in more detail later but are briefly mentioned here. First, although double-strand DNA breaks are expected intermediates for DNA recombinations such as CSR, such breaks have also been detected as likely intermediates in SHM. Second, transcription is required for both processes. Third, mutations have been observed not only in V regions where they underlie affinity maturation allowed by SHM, but also surrounding the recombination junctions of CSR. Fourth, evidence suggests that palindromic DNA structures may be important for targeting both CSR and SHM to specific sequences.

A fifth and dramatic link between CSR and SHM is the discovery that both processes require the product of a gene known as activation-induced deaminase (AID). This gene was discovered (198) by a subtractive strategy designed to screen for transcripts that were expressed in the murine B cell line CH12F3-2 when activated to undergo CSR but that were not expressed by the same cells uninduced. AID is expressed exclusively in GC B cells and in B cells activated *in vitro*. As translated from the cDNA, AID is a 198–amino acid protein showing 34% amino acid identity with the RNA editing enzyme APOBEC-1. The latter protein catalyzes the conversion of a cytosine to uracil residue in a specific position in the mRNA encoding apolipoprotein B. (This change produces a UAA stop codon that shortens the translated protein to yield apoB48.) The human APOBEC and AID genes appear to be linked, both lying at chromosome 12p13. APOBEC-1 by itself is unable to bind to its target RNA but must interact with a protein known as APOBEC complementation factor (ACF). Like APOBEC, recombinant AID protein has a cytidine deaminase activity *in vitro,* and it is possible that its function *in vivo* is to edit one or more specific RNAs, perhaps in association with an ACF-like protein, but this remains to be demonstrated. An alternate possibility, discussed later in this chapter, is that AID acts directly to decimate DNA in the Ig loci. Mice engineered with a targeted defect in the AID gene show profound defects in both CSR and SHM. Identical defects are seen in patients with a homozygous defect in the human AID gene, a condition known as the hyper-IgM syndrome 2 (HIGM2) (199). Affected patients have elevated serum levels of IgM because their B cells are profoundly impaired in CSR. Discriminating between various models for CSR and SHM should be facilitated by recent achievement of both processes in AID-transfected fibroblasts or T cells (200), as discussed later.

Heavy-Chain Switch

Switch Junctions and Switch Regions

As briefly mentioned earlier in this chapter, isotype switching involves removal of $C\mu$ from downstream of the rearranged heavy-chain V-D-J gene and its replacement by a new downstream CH region. This occurs by a deletional recombination between repetitive DNA sequences known as switch (S) regions that lie 5' of each CH region (except $C\delta$). The S region of the murine μ gene, $S\mu$, is located about 1 to 2 kb 5' to the $C\mu$ coding sequence and is composed of numerous tandem repeats of sequences of the form (GAGCT)n(GGGGT), where n is usually 2 to 5 but can range as high as 17. All of the S regions include pentamers similar to GAGCT and GGGGT that are the basic repeated elements of the $S\mu$ gene; in the other S regions, these pentamers are not precisely repeated tandemly as in $S\mu$ but instead are embedded in larger repeat units. The 10-kb $S\gamma 1$ region has an additional higher order structure: Two direct repeat sequences flank each of two clusters of 49-bp tandem repeats. Because of the apparent importance of the repeats in S regions, it was surprising to learn that mice with a complete deletion of the repetitive region of $S\mu$ were nonetheless able to accomplish CSR, although at a reduced level (201). (These mice still retained a few scattered guanine-rich pentamers that flank the tandem repeat region.)

A switch recombination between, for example, μ and ϵ genes produces a composite $S\mu$-$S\epsilon$ sequence (Fig. 16). By examination of the germline $S\mu$ and $S\epsilon$ sequences in comparison with the myeloma- or hybridoma-derived $S\mu$-$S\epsilon$ composite switch region, it has been possible to localize the exact recombination sites between $S\mu$ and $S\epsilon$ that occurred in dif-ferent cells; similar analyses have been performed with cells producing other isotypes. These studies have indicated that there is no specific site, either in $S\mu$ or in any other S region, where the recombination always occurs, although clusters of recombination sites have been reported at two specific regions within the tandem repeats of the murine $S\gamma 3$ region (202). Although most switch junctions fall in the S regions, some are in the flanking nonrepetitive region. Thus, unlike the enzymatic machinery of V-J recombination, the switch machinery can join sequences in a broad target region. Many composite switch junction sequences show evidence of mutations near the recombination breakpoint in comparison with the corresponding germline switch sequences; these mutations have been interpreted as reflecting an error-prone DNA synthesis step that may be a component of the switch recombination mechanism (203).

DNA fragments excised by switch recombination have been cloned from fractions of circular DNA isolated from cells actively undergoing isotype switch recombination. Thus, at least some of the excised DNA segments ligate their ends to form "switch circles"; these contain composite switch junctions that are, in theory, reciprocal to the composite switch junction retained on chromosomal DNA (Fig. 16). Because switch circles are not linked to centromeres and may not contain origins of replication, they not are efficiently replicated. Therefore, they are not found in cells that have divided multiple times after switching, like myelomas or hybridomas. As in the case of V(D)J recombination, another potential fate for the excised DNA is inversion rather than deletion. Inversional switch recombination has been detected in murine and human systems (204). Such inversion would prevent heavy-chain synthesis because the switched

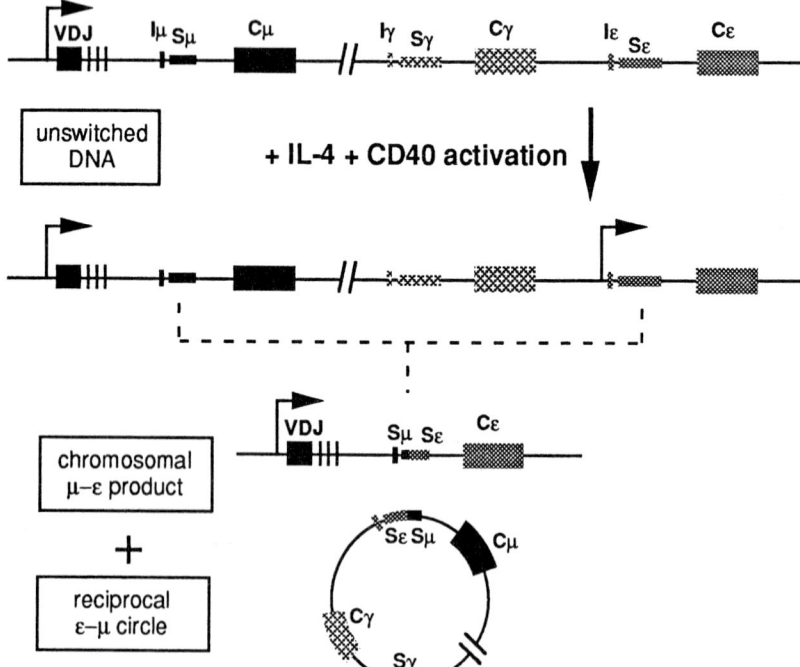

FIG. 16. Switch regions and composite switch junctions. The recombination breakpoints in isotype switch recombination fall within repetitive "switch" (S) regions. Stimuli that activate switch recombination (interleukin-4 and CD40 activation in the example shown) generally promote transcription across the target S region, initiating just upstream at the "I" exon. Recombination between $S\mu$ and $S\epsilon$ produces two composite switch junctions: an $S\mu$-$S\epsilon$ junction retained in chromosomal DNA and a reciprocal $S\epsilon$-$S\mu$ junction found in fractions of circular DNA. Polymerase chain reaction amplification across either composite junction can be used to study switch recombination.

CH gene would be in the wrong orientation, but inversional CSR would be required for expression of the chicken $C\alpha$ gene, which lies in reversed orientation in the germline (205).

Methods of Assaying Switch Recombination

In stable myelomas or hybridomas expressing switched isotypes, evidence of switch recombination can be obtained by gene cloning or Southern blot testing. However, studies of the regulation and mechanism of switch recombination require assays that can detect switch recombination in a minority population of cells switching in culture. Some laboratories assess switching by simply measuring Ig protein of the switched isotype appearing in the culture supernatant. Alternatively, reverse transcriptase PCR can be used to detect mRNA corresponding to the mature V-D-J-C RNA transcripts of the switched isotype. However, because the culture conditions favoring isotype switching may also influence transcription or protein synthesis rates independently of switch recombination, assays of RNA or protein may not faithfully reflect the DNA recombination events. Furthermore, "switched" RNA or protein cannot be assumed to reflect DNA recombination in the exploration of one of several models for nonrecombinational mechanisms for isotype switching, as discussed at the end of this section. Therefore, PCR strategies have been developed to assess switch recombination at the DNA level.

In one strategy, PCR primers are designed to amplify across the composite switch region of interest. A related strategy is to amplify the reciprocal switch junctions found on circular DNA (206,207); these junctions can be used to "count" recombination events independently of proliferation if it is assumed that each circle is produced as a byproduct of a single switch recombination event and, failing to replicate as the cells divide, is randomly partitioned to daughter cells at successive divisions after the recombination event. Because the efficiency of amplification varies for different composite switch junctions—smaller templates are amplified more efficiently, and the largest may not amplify at all—the PCR strategy just described cannot easily be adapted to assay switch recombination quantitatively.

For this reason, a second strategy known as digestion-circularization PCR was developed (208). In this approach, DNA from switching cells is digested with a restriction enzyme, and the resulting restriction fragments—including the ones bearing a composite $S\mu$-$S\epsilon$ junction—are ligated to form circles. Primers designed to amplify across the restriction site generated by ligation of the $S\mu$-$S\epsilon$ fragment ends yield a consistent product whose size depends only on the distance between primers and the restriction site. From unswitched DNA, no product is amplified, because the two primers can never hybridize simultaneously to the same ligated DNA circle. Therefore, with appropriate calibration (209), the amount of digestion-circularization PCR product formed can be used as a semiquantitative measure of the amount of composite switch junctions in a DNA sample.

Two other assays are based on the observation of "sterile" or "germline" RNA transcripts that initiate upstream of each S region, extending downstream through the associated C region; splicing of these transcripts removes the S region, leaving a small upstream "I" region ("intron") fused to the C region RNA. After switch recombination, transcription initiation continues from the $I\mu$ promoter through the C region of the new "switched" isotype; therefore, $I\mu$-Cx transcripts detected by reverse transcriptase PCR represent evidence of switch recombination (210). Transcripts of the reciprocal circle—that is, Ix-$C\mu$ (designated circle transcripts)—may be a marker for recent CSR, inasmuch as these transcripts disappear from cells after switch recombination more rapidly than the switch circles (211).

In order to determine which structures are necessary for CSR, some investigators have constructed transgenic animals carrying two S regions that might undergo CSR and have studied the effects of altering the S regions. Alternatively, the technology of homologous recombination has been used to target endogenous heavy-chain gene loci with various structural changes or to target the genes encoding candidate mediators of CSR. Particularly useful have been strategies for transfecting cell lines with switch substrate constructs containing a reporter gene whose expression requires recombination between two S regions in the plasmid.

Regulation of Isotype Switching by CD40

Isotype switching occurs physiologically in animals about 1 week after immunization with T-cell–dependent antigens, at about the same time that somatic mutation of Ig genes begins. Somatic mutation (discussed later in this chapter) clearly occurs in GCs of lymphoid organs, a location that facilitates T cell–B cell interaction, and evidence suggests that GCs are a major site for isotype switching as well. As demonstrated by in vitro switching experiments, T cells promote switching by secretion of cytokines—especially IL-4 and transforming growth factor β (TGFβ)—as well as by cell-to-cell contact.

A major component of the cell contact signal is mediated by an interaction between the B-cell surface marker CD40 and its ligand—designated CD40L, CD154, or gp39—expressed on activated T cells (primarily CD4$^+$). CD40 is a member of the tumor necrosis factor receptor family, whereas CD40L belongs to the tumor necrosis factor ligand family. The dependence of switching on the CD40–CD40L interaction is highlighted by the genetic disease known as the X-linked hyper-IgM syndrome 1 (HIGM1), which was found to be caused by a defect in the gene encoding CD40L/gp39 (212). Like AID-deficient patients with HIGM2 described previously, patients with HIGM1 have elevated concentrations of IgM in their serum and almost no immunoglobulins of other isotypes. In addition, their antibodies fail to show affinity maturation or evidence of B-cell memory responses. Similar defects are seen in humans with mutations in the CD40 gene, an autosomal recessive disease (213), and in mouse strains with engineered defects in CD40. The CD40 knockout mice respond with normal isotype switching to T-cell–independent antigens (214); little is known about this T-cell–independent switching pathway. The discovery of the importance of the CD40–CD40L interaction has facilitated *in vitro* switching experiments in which B cells are incubated with stimuli designed to engage their CD40 molecules: i.e., CD40L$^+$ T cells, nonlymphoid cells engineered to express surface CD40L or antibodies to CD40. One role of the CD40 engagement is to induce B cell proliferation. Indeed, other proliferative stimuli—such as LPS or IgM or IgD cross-linking—can support cytokine-induced isotype switching *in vitro* in the absence of T cells and CD40 activation. Switching may be related to the cell cycle (215) and to the number of cell divisions after stimulation (216). However, CD40 has additional effects, including up-regulation of IL-4 responsiveness and IL-4 receptor number (217) that may facilitate switching. CD40 signaling is mediated in part by activation of NFκB, a transcription factor that up-regulates many inflammatory reactions. Activated B cells also express CD40L, which not only can trigger CD40 signaling but also can transduce a "reverse" signal affecting B cell function (218).

The CD40–CD40L interaction appears to be counteracted by an interaction between two other members of the same protein families: CD30 and its ligand CD153. CD30 expression on B cells is induced by CD40L but inhibited by ligation of the BCR (219). Engagement of CD30 by its ligand down-regulates several of the effects of CD40 ligation, apparently by inhibiting the action of NFκB (220). This effect may represent a feedback mechanism to limit the activation of B cells that have not been stimulated effectively through their BCR by antigen. "Reverse" signaling by B cell–expressed CD153 has also been reported as an additional inhibitory influence on CSR (221). Pathological activation of CD30–CD153 signaling in chronic lymphocytic leukemia may contribute to the impairment in IgG and IgA production that leads to infection in these patients (222).

Despite the importance of CD40 for most CSR, switching to IgA occurs in lamina propria B cells of the gut independently of CD40L or T cells (223). Gut B cells appear to have an unusual developmental program in that they can switch to IgA even in mice that cannot develop normally because a stop codon in the first Cμ membrane exon prevents surface expression of IgM (224).

Isotype-Specific Regulation of Germline Transcripts

Different isotypes are known to predominate in different immune responses, depending on the antigen, route of antigen administration, and several other parameters. These different parameters act in part by influencing the cytokine milieu of the B cells. IL-4, for example, promotes the expression of IgE (and IgG1 in the mouse), whereas transforming growth factor β promotes switching to IgA. These lymphokines have been proposed to act by making the C region of the target isotype "accessible" to switch recombinase machinery that may

be non–isotype specific. The accessibility is associated with expression of "sterile" RNA transcript that initiates upstream of a target S region and extends through the target C region (Fig. 16), as discussed previously. The same experimental conditions—including the specific cytokines—that favor the accumulation of sterile transcripts from a particular isotype also favor switch recombination involving the corresponding S region. In some cases, the signals transduced by the cytokine receptor have been elucidated. For example, IL-4 stimulates transcription by activating the transcription factor STAT6, which attaches to one of several nuclear protein binding motifs in the promoter region upstream of Iϵ and Iγ1. CD40 engagement also acts in part through NFκB-mediated binding to I region promoters (225).

Apart from I region promoters, sterile transcription and isotype switching are also regulated by heavy Ig enhancers. Mice in which the HS12 enhancer from the $3'\alpha$ enhancer complex was replaced by a neomycin resistance gene in all B cells (226) were impaired in switching to IgE and several IgG isotypes but not to IgG1. This effect turned out to result not from the loss of HS12 but the presence of the neo^r gene, because CSR was normal in mice with a Cre-lox–generated deletion of HS12 (227); a deletion of HS3a was also without effect. However, a combined deletion of HS3b and HS4 was found to cause a significant impairment in switching to most isotypes, although switching to IgG1 was unaffected (and switching to IgA was only moderately decreased) (228). The diminished switching was associated with diminished sterile transcription of the same isotypes, which suggests that one major function of the enhancers in CSR is to increase sterile transcription. The relative independence of γ1 from regulation by enhancers may be related to the putative LCR region associated with that gene (196), which was mentioned previously. The intronic enhancer also seems to play a role in CSR because heavy Ig loci with a targeted deletion of the Eμ enhancer showed decreased switching when tested in RAG-complemented mice (229).

The importance of sterile transcription for CSR has been highlighted by experiments in which investigators constructed an artificial switch substrate bearing an Sμ sequence, an Sα sequence whose transcription was driven by a tetracycline-regulatable promoter, and a GFP gene whose expression required recombination between the two S regions (230). When this plasmid was stably transfected into the switch-competent cell line CH12F3-2, and transcription across the Sα sequence was manipulated by adjusting the tetracycline concentration, transcription levels were associated with higher CSR efficiency.

Although cytokines and CD40 ligation clearly affect CSR by regulating sterile transcription, it is likely that cytokines regulate other aspects of the switching mechanism as well, because several examples of cytokines up- or down-regulating switch recombination without a parallel effect on sterile transcripts have been reported (231). Furthermore, certain cell lines transfected with plasmid CSR substrates appear to support switching to only certain isotype S regions despite strong transcription through all S regions of the engineered constructs; this observation suggests the possibility that the CSR machinery might show isotype specificity based on recognition of features specific to certain S region sequences (232). In principle, the specificity of such recognition might also be regulatable by cytokines or other factors.

Role of Sterile Transcription in Class Switch Recombination

Gene targeting experiments have shown that mouse strains lacking the I region of a particular isotype do not switch to that isotype, which reinforces the idea that sterile transcription is necessary for CSR (reviewed by Stavnezer (233)]. The low extent of sequence conservation of the I exons and the lack of consistent open reading frames suggest that these transcripts do not encode a functional protein. Indeed, the exact sequence of the I region may be irrelevant because an I region can be replaced by an irrelevant sequence and still support CSR (234). However, the transcribed exon upstream of the S region apparently needs a splice donor site that allows the S region to be removed from the transcript, because targeted constructs lacking such a splice donor site could not support CSR even though transcription through the S region occurred (235).

One possible role for sterile transcripts in CSR involves the formation of an RNA:DNA triple helix or an R-loop. (An R-loop is a structure in which RNA complementary to one strand of a DNA molecule binds to that strand with Watson-Crick base pairing, displacing the other DNA strand, which forms a single-strand loop.) In support of the R-loop model, cell-free transcription of switch regions was found to lead to a stable association of the transcript RNA with the template DNA (236,237); significant association occurred only with RNA transcribed from switch region DNA and only when the RNA was transcribed in the physiological orientation. The displaced DNA strand in the R loops was susceptible to cleavage *in vitro* by nucleases that recognize single-strand DNA or junctions between single- and double-strand DNA; *in vivo* such cleavage could be a step in CSR. Although the R-loop concept provides a rationale for the requirement of sterile transcripts in CSR, the requirement for splicing in this model is harder to understand. Furthermore, as of this writing, there is no evidence in the literature for the formation of S region R-loops *in vivo*.

Critical Features that Target Class Switch Recombination to Switch Regions

Mammalian heavy Ig switch regions are guanine-rich on the transcribed strand and have been noted to contain palindromic sequences that could potentially form stem-loop structures if the normal double-helical structure were disrupted. To determine which of these characteristics might be critical in targeting CSR, Tashiro et al. (238) designed constructs in which a starting $S\mu$-$S\alpha$ CSR substrate was altered by replacing one

of the murine S regions with a variety of other sequences. All the plasmids were designed for constitutive transcription across the S regions (or their substitutes) and contained donor and acceptor splice sites that would allow the S regions of transcripts to be spliced out, as in normal sterile transcripts. The constructs included a GFP gene that could be expressed only after CSR had occurred, which allowed assessment of CSR by flow cytometry. CSR could be verified by diagnostic reverse transcriptase PCR and by sequence analysis of CSR junctions. The constructs were transfected into the murine B cell line CH12F3-2; stable transfectant cells were isolated and then incubated under conditions that promote CSR of endogenous genes. The original $S\mu$-$S\alpha$ construct supported robust CSR, but replacement of one of the switch regions with either an unrelated nonrepetitive intron-derived sequence or a guanine-rich telomeric sequence abolished CSR, whereas the AT-rich palindromic $S\mu$ sequence from a frog was able to support low but significant CSR. Guanine richness is thus apparently not necessary or sufficient for targeting CSR. Most surprisingly, a tandem repeat of the multiple cloning site from the commercial Bluescript plasmid (which contains palindromic recognition sites for restriction enzymes) was able to support substantial CSR. Sequence analysis of amplified junctions showed that breakpoints were preferentially located near the junction between single- and double-strand regions of potential stem-loop structures. The possible targeting of CSR to stem-loops has also been suggested by breakpoint analysis in other CSR constructs (239), by the location of double-strand DNA breaks in an endogenous $S\gamma3$ region undergoing CSR (as determined by LM-PCR) (240) and by the location of hotspots for insertion of exogenous DNA (241). The existence of some breakpoints at a distance from the nearest stem-loop does not argue against stem-loops as the target of a CSR endonuclease, because processing of DNA ends before ligation may obscure the location of the initial cleavage.

If stem-loops are the initial cleavage target, it is likely that staggered DNA ends would be produced, because the most thermodynamically favored stem-loops do not necessarily form at corresponding positions on complementary DNA strands. Evidence consistent with staggered cuts has been obtained from an analysis of the reciprocal products of CSR in single cells (239). Chen et al. (239) designed an artificial switch substrate so that GFP was expressed only if switch recombination occurred by inversion rather than by deletion; as a result of this strategy, both products of a single recombination were retained on the same chromosome, on which they could be amplified from single cells and then sequenced. Many recombinations were found with DNA deletions at the breakpoints, but a few involved duplications, which could have derived only from filling in of staggered DNA breaks. (Interestingly, many of the junctions recovered from this artificial switch construct showed mutations within about 10 bp of the junctions, similar to what has been reported in endogenous switch junctions, as mentioned previously.) At present, it is not clear whether the rare instances of staggered ends reported from these experiments or the blunt double-strand breaks detected by LM-PCR are more representative of CSR intermediates.

B-Cell–Specific versus Ubiquitously Expressed Components of Class Switch Recombination Machinery

An expression vector for AID (discussed previously) was introduced into fibroblasts transfected with an artificial $S\mu$-$S\alpha$ switch construct and was found to induce CSR of the construct at levels similar to that observed in stimulated B cells (200). Like physiological CSR, the induced recombination was dependent on switch region transcription and yielded breakpoint-associated mutations. (CSR was not observed at the endogenous heavy Ig locus.) This striking result implies that AID is the only B cell–specific factor required to trigger CSR between switch regions, other than factors that open the loci to transcription. In this regard, AID resembles the RAG proteins in V(D)J reactions.

If AID triggers cleavage at switch regions, ubiquitous DNA repair and ligation enzymes may accomplish the subsequent steps of CSR as in V(D)J recombination. This possibility has been tested for several proteins whose role in V(D)J recombination was discussed earlier in this chapter. Both SCID mice, which are natural mutants of DNA-PK, and homozygous RAG2 knockout mice are impaired in developing mature B-lymphocytes because of their inability to assemble V genes efficiently; however, when pro–B cells from these mice were allowed to proliferate in vitro and were then treated with IL-4 and anti-CD40, switch recombination occurred in the RAG2 knockout cells but not in the SCID cells (242). This result suggests that CSR is independent of RAG2 but requires DNA-PK [although one report suggested that switching to $C\gamma1$ may be spared in DNA-PK–deficient B cells (243)]. Ku70 and Ku80 knockout mice have also been tested for their CSR capacity through the use of mice expressing immunoglobulin from "knocked-in" productively rearranged heavy- and light-chain genes. Whereas "knock-in" mice with intact Ku genes switched to downstream isotypes, the corresponding Ku-deficient mice were impaired in CSR (244,245). A role for the Ku complex in CSR is also suggested by the fact that incubation conditions favoring CSR (IL-4 and CD40 engagement) increased the amount of Ku complex detectable in nuclear extracts of splenic B cells (246). This effect is apparently caused by migration of preformed cytoplasmic Ku into the nucleus, associated with loss of specific binding affinity between Ku and the cytoplasmic domain of CD40 (247). Treatment with IL-4 plus CD40 engagement also increased the level of nuclear DNA-PK.

Other Possible Class Switch Recombination Components

Despite the importance of AID as the only B cell–specific component required for CSR, other more widely distributed cellular components undoubtedly participate in this process. In an effort to identify components of the CSR machinery,

several laboratories have investigated proteins that cleave or bind to switch region DNAs in a sequence-specific manner in vitro or that are associated with chromosome breaks or repair of DNA damage. A few examples are described as follows, but none of the components discussed in this section has been unequivocally demonstrated to participate in switch recombination.

1. Nijmegen breakage syndrome is an autosomal recessive disease associated with immunodeficiency, chromosomal instability, and other defects. As discussed previously in the context of V(D)J recombination, the normal product of the mutant gene for this syndrome (Nbs1) associates with Mre11 and Rad50 to form a complex that rapidly accumulates at double-strand breaks, apparently recruited by the modified histone γ-H2AX. Experimenters have explored possible roles for Nbs1 and γ-H2AX in CSR. Like the RAG-dependent nuclear foci containing Nbs1 and γ-H2AX that are observed in B cells undergoing V(D)J recombination, AID-dependent nuclear foci of Nbs1 and γ-H2AX are observed in B cells undergoing CSR (248). Although Nbs1 is not required for V(D)J recombination, patients with Nijmegen breakage syndrome were found to have somewhat low levels of IgG and IgA associated with normal levels of IgM, which suggests the possibility of a very mild CSR defect (249). H2AX knockout mice were found to have modest impairment in CSR despite normal B-cell proliferation and sterile transcription (248). Thus, neither Nbs1 nor γ-H2AX appear to be absolutely required for CSR, although they may improve its efficiency.

2. Two proteins that bind within $S\gamma$ regions to subsequences associated with a high frequency of recombination breakpoints have been designated SNIP and SNAP and apparently correspond (respectively) to the transcription factors NFκB/p50 and E47, one of the proteins encoded by the E2A gene (250,251). A role for NFκB in switching is supported by experiments in B cells from a p50 knockout mouse strain. In these p50 knockout mice, isotype switching to IgE and IgG3 secretion was markedly reduced; however, reduced expression of the corresponding germline transcripts could indicate that the p50 was required for activating I region promoters rather than for the actual recombination event (252). In addition, human patients with an X-linked HIGM syndrome associated with ectodermal dysplasia have been found to have a defect in the gene encoding IKKγ (also known as NEMO), a protein required for efficient NFκB signaling (253). B cells from these patients are defective in CSR when cultured in vitro.

3. A role for the E2A transcription factors in CSR is further supported by experiments in which Id proteins, which antagonize E2 action, were found to inhibit CSR in the murine cell line CH12.LX2 and in splenic B cells (254). Although some decrease in sterile transcription was noted, it was not believed to account for the dramatic decrease in

CSR. Furthermore, culturing B cells with IL-4 plus CD40 engagement was found to induce increases in E2A protein levels.

4. The major role of mismatch repair (MMR) proteins is to recognize and repair DNA at positions that do not contain normal Watson-Crick base pairs. Investigations by several laboratories have shown that mice with defects in several MMR genes are able to perform CSR, but various subtle defects have been observed in the efficiency of switching to specific isotypes, in CSR breakpoint locations, and in the extent of microhomologies at breakpoints (255,256).

5. LR1 is a protein found in nuclear extracts from murine splenic B-lymphocytes after induction with LPS; it binds to Sγ1, Sγ3, and Sα, as well as to the heavy-chain enhancer (257). The protein is a heterodimer containing nucleolin and hnRNP D. Both of these proteins can bind with high affinity to "G4" DNA, a structure in which four DNA strands (parallel or antiparallel) containing runs of three or more guanine nucleotides can form stable complexes (258). (In this work, binding was studied through the use of a G4 structure formed by an oligonucleotide matching the murine Sγ2b sequence.)

6. G4 structures are the target for a specific nuclease designated G quartet nuclease 1 (GQN1), which has been proposed as a mediator of CSR (259).

7. Two laboratories have reported detecting cell-free CSR of plasmid substrates by nuclear extracts (261,262). The first group used their assay to purify an active complex composed of four proteins, including a novel 70-kD protein designated SWAP-70, which does not appear related to any other known protein (262). SWAP-70 is highly expressed in B cells that have been activated for switch recombination. SWAP-70 knockout mice show no dramatic impairment in CSR except for a decrease in switching of splenic B cells to Cϵ in vitro and a decrease serum IgE levels (263).

8. Spo11 is a protein that catalyzes double-strand breaks in yeast meiotic recombination. A murine Spo11 homolog was found to be modestly up-regulated in B cells undergoing CSR, and an antisense oligonucleotide was reported to reduce CSR efficiency. However, Spo11 knockout mice were found to be normal in CSR and SHM (264).

Non-"standard" Isotype Switching

Thus far, isotype switching has been considered to involve a simple deletion (or inversion) of the DNA between Sμ and a downstream switch region; although this is the most common scenario, three variant schemes are considered as follows.

1. Sequential switching. Several switch recombination events can occur sequentially on a given chromosome. One well-studied example involves sequential switching to γ1 followed by ϵ in murine B-lymphocytes. The same cytokine, IL-4, promotes switching to both isotypes. After an initial switch recombination generating a composite Sμ-Sγ1 junction (leading to IgG1 expression), this composite switch region can undergo a secondary switch recombination with Sϵ, which lies downstream. In IgE-expressing cells, evidence of the initial recombination to γ1 can be revealed by the presence of a composite Sμ-Sγ1-Sϵ junction or by the detection of the Sϵ-Sγ1 reciprocal switch circle product. To assess the quantitative importance of this pathway in IgE generation, resting B cells stimulated with IL-4 plus LPS were treated with an anti-IgG1 antibody to eliminate cells expressing this isotype from the culture; IgE secretion was inhibited about 70%, which suggests that most murine B cells expressing IgE have undergone an intermediate stage in which they expressed IgG1 (265). However, in mutant mice with a block in γ1 switching caused by a targeted deletion in the γ1 locus, the frequency of switching to ϵ is normal, which suggests that the sequential switching results from the sequential accessibility of both Sγ1 and Sϵ, rather than an obligatory sequential switch program (266). Sequential switching to IgE expression via IgG also occurs in human B cells (267,268), but the quantitative significance of this pathway is not known.

2. Trans-switching. Although most switch recombinations involve a single chromosome, transchromosomal switching (trans-switching) between allelic chromosomes has been detected in rabbit at a frequency of about 5% (269). The detection of trans-switching in rabbit was facilitated by the availability of allotypic markers of constant and V regions in this species; the frequency of trans-switching in other species is not known. Trans-switching may also explain certain cases in which myeloma cells producing IgG gave rise to "backwards switch" progeny producing IgM (270).

3. Switched isotypes without switch recombination. Several laboratories have reported detection of B cells expressing immunoglobulin of more than one isotype. Such "double-producing" cells may reflect a normal transient intermediate stage when a "switched" isotype may be expressed (after normal switch recombination) along with IgM that persists in the cells because of long half-life of the protein or its mRNA. However, this model would not explain reports of stable cell lines expressing IgM along with another isotype encoded by a distant CH region. If such double producers represent alternative splicing of long transcripts (the accepted explanation for IgM+-IgD+ double producers), such transcripts would have to be on the order of 100 kb. This is longer than RNAs that can be easily isolated with current laboratory methods, although precedents for genes whose exons are spread over similar distances are known, and early evidence for a long heavy Ig transcript has been reported (271). An alternative explanation is that separate short transcripts of V-D-J and a downstream CH gene (i.e., a "sterile" transcript) could be joined by a trans-splicing mechanism similar to that documented for trypanosomes and certain viruses (272). Mizuta et al. (273) described a nonphysiological mechanism that could

account for some cases of double isotype production in cell lines as a consequence of duplication of the heavy Ig locus followed by CSR on one copy. Stable double-isotype production appears to be common in hairy cell leukemia (274). At present, it is not clear whether this phenotype reflects a normal maturation stage or a B-cell subset. It is likely that most normal isotype switching is associated with switch recombination rather than nonrecombinational mechanisms, because the amount of IgG1 expression observed in a population of murine B-cell switching *in vitro* to IgG1 could be accounted for by the amount of switch recombination measured in these cells (209).

In summary, a possible (but by no means validated) model for CSR would be that cytokines and CD40 ligation trigger AID expression and isotype-specific sterile transcription. DNA strands in S regions become separated (either by a helicase activity associated with transcription or perhaps as a result of R-loop formation), allowing stem-loop structures to form on individual strands. These are recognized by a nuclease (perhaps targeted AID-induced deamination, or encoded by a transcript that must be edited by AID), which cuts the two strands, forming double-strand breaks. Alternatively, isotype-specific S region binding proteins may facilitate such breaks. These breaks are repaired by ubiquitous repair machinery, including the Ku-DNA-PK complex, perhaps aided by other proteins such as Nbs1 and γ-H2AX. Mutations surrounding the breakpoints suggest that repair enzymes include error-prone polymerases, such as are discussed later.

Somatic Mutation

Early Evidence for Somatic Mutation

Analyses of amino acid sequences of murine $\lambda 1$ chains from myeloma antibodies provided the first strong support for SHM even before the era of recombinant DNA analysis. When the amino acid sequences of $\lambda 1$ chains produced by 21 independently derived myelomas were analyzed (275,276), 12 were found to be identical, representing a prototype V$\lambda 1$ sequence. The remaining variants were each unique, generally differing from the prototype sequence by single amino acid substitutions that could be accounted for by single base changes. Significantly, all but one of the amino acid substitutions were unique to a single variant sequence. The investigators concluded that the prototype sequence corresponded to a single germline gene, whereas the variants arose by somatic mutation of this gene. This interpretation seemed consistent with the observation that each variant sequence occurred only once, whereas several occurrences of the same sequence might have been expected if there were several germline V$\lambda 1$ genes. Now that gene cloning has confirmed that there is only a single V$\lambda 1$ gene, the identification of the variants as products of somatic mutation has been verified.

Subsequent studies led to similar conclusions for murine Vκ or VH systems involving small V families whose germline

members could be readily cloned so that sequences of the corresponding expressed and germline (i.e., nonmutated) V gene could be compared. An example of such a system is the relatively restricted murine antibody response to phosphorylcholine. Sequence analysis of a panel of phosphorylcholine-binding hybridomas and myelomas expressing a similar VH sequence revealed that all IgM antibodies shared a single prototype sequence. In contrast, some IgA and most IgG VH regions showed scattered amino acid substitutions with respect to the prototype sequence. All of the sequence variants were unique to single cell lines. By analogy to the Vλ system discussed previously, these comparisons suggested that the prototype sequences reflected a germline gene, whereas the variants were products of diverse somatic mutations. A search of the four germline VH region genes homologous to the prototype expressed VH gene revealed only one gene that could have served as precursor for the phosphorylcholine-binding VH regions; this one matched the prototype sequence exactly (277). The fact that the variant VH sequences were seen only in IgA and IgG, not in IgM, is consistent with the fact that IgM is characteristically produced early in the immune response, whereas somatic mutation occurs later in the response, overlapping the stage of isotype switching (see following section); other studies have shown that somatic mutation can be seen in IgM at a low frequency, which indicates that the CSR and SHM occur independently, without an obligatory order.

Role of Hypermutation in Immune Responses

To understand the role of somatic mutation in the antibody response, several researchers have studied the extent of somatic mutation at different times after the immunization of mice. Studies of the responses to *p*-azophenylarsonate, phosphorylcholine, influenza hemagglutinin, oxazolone, and several other antigens have all indicated that the initial response after primary immunization is contributed by antibodies showing no somatic mutation. About 1 week after immunization, mutated sequences begin to be observed, increasing during the next week or so. Booster immunizations yield sequences showing additional mutations.

Many hybridomas made late in the immune response produce mutated antibodies with a higher antigen affinity than the unmutated (sometimes loosely called "germline") antibodies made early after immunization. The shift to higher affinity is a phenomenon long recognized at the level of (polyclonal) antisera and has been termed *affinity maturation*. This phenomenon can now be explained as the result of an "evolutionary" mechanism selecting antibodies of progressively higher affinity from the pool of randomly mutated V sequences. According to this model, at the time of initial antigen exposure, an animal has a set of B-lymphocytes expressing germline (unmutated) versions of Ig sequences resulting from gene rearrangements that occurred before immunization. Because of the diversity of available VH, D, JH, VL, and JL sequences, as well as the impressive recombinational potential described earlier, some B cells express Ig molecules capable of binding the antigen with modest affinity. These cells are stimulated—by antigen binding—to proliferate and to secrete antibody. Activated B cells located in lymphoid follicles also bind antigen and receive T cell help; at some point in the response, the SHM machinery is activated in these cells, generating random mutations in the Ig genes of stimulated cells in the GCs. Many of these mutations can be expected to reduce the resulting affinity of the encoded antibody for antigen; indeed, such mutated antibodies with markedly reduced affinity have been demonstrated (278), as have mutated antibodies that have acquired autoantibody specificity (279). As antigen clearance reduces antigen concentrations seen by the lymphocytes, only the cells displaying high affinity antibody are effectively stimulated by antigen; cells displaying lower affinity antibodies or antibodies with affinity for self-antigens may be subjected to programmed cell death (apoptosis) (280,281). The preferential proliferation of the high-affinity cells and their maturation to secreting plasma cells cause an increase in the average affinity of the antibodies in the serum. These high-affinity cells are left as the predominant population to be represented as memory cells when antigen exposure ceases; they thus can induce the rapid, high-affinity antibody response on secondary antigen exposure. In this model, the driving force for affinity maturation—analogous to natural selection in the evolution of species—is selection for high antibody affinity in the presence of low antigen concentration. The importance of this selective force is suggested by the observation that affinity maturation can be inhibited by repeated injection of antigen (which removes the selective pressure for high affinity) (282) or by overexpression of the antiapoptotic protein Bcl-XL (which allows survival of B cells expressing low affinity antibody) (283).

Cellular Context of Somatic Mutation

Somatic mutation occurs primarily in B cells of the GCs of lymphoid tissues, particularly in a subpopulation of B cells known as centroblasts. These cells proliferate in the "dark zone" of the GC and bear characteristic surface markers, including IgD, CD38, and the receptor for peanut agglutinin (PNA) (284). Each GC appears to be populated by a small number of antigen-specific founder B cells (285) and an unusual Thy-1 negative T cell population, also antigen-specific (286). The GC environment promotes contact between the B cell and both follicular dendritic cells, which store, process, and present antigen, and T-lymphocytes, which activate somatic mutation in part via CD40-CD40L interaction (287). Other critical signals promoting SHM have been investigated with *in vitro* systems, which implicate CD80:CD28 engagement (288) and cytokines (289). Proliferating GC centroblasts give rise to centrocytes in the "light zone" of the GC; there, centrocytes are programmed for apoptosis unless they are rescued by follicular dendritic cell–presented antigen and T cell activation via CD40 engagement (280,290). At this stage, positive selection for high affinity antibodies

occurs via apoptosis of cells expressing low-affinity antibodies; paradoxically, however, apoptosis is also promoted by soluble antigen, perhaps functioning to select against autoantibodies (291). As mentioned earlier, receptor editing may be another fate for autoantibody-producing cells in GCs. The features of antigen signaling that select for survival versus apoptosis or editing are not fully understood. Susceptibility of GC cell populations to apoptosis is correlated with their expression of Fas, Bax, p53 and c-myc, all of which promote apoptosis, and with down-regulation of the apoptosis suppressors Bcl-2 and c-FLIP (281). B cells of mice with engineered overexpression of Bcl-2 or Bcl-XL expression can escape selection against autoreactivity (283).

SHM is apparently unusually active in IgM−IgD+ cells, inasmuch as this subset of GC B cells from human tonsils was found to accumulate extremely high numbers of somatic mutations (292). An important role for IgD in somatic mutation is also suggested by the observation that mice with a homozygous targeted disruption of their Cδ gene were impaired in affinity maturation (293).

GC B cells may undergo several successive cycles of mutation and proliferation followed by selection. Such a scheme has been supported by the sequence analysis of mutated Ig genes amplified by PCR from single cells microdissected from a histologic section of a GC (294) or from mutations in copies of an engineered transgene that is unusually susceptible to SHM (295); in these and other systems, the mutated sequences can be organized into genealogical trees consistent with several cycles of somatic mutation followed by proliferation. Cyclical movement of the B cells from the dark zone to the light zone of the GC may be mediated by cyclically changing chemotactic responses to chemokines (296). A computer simulation has affirmed the high efficiency of alternating periods of somatic mutation and mutation-free selection as a strategy for generating high-affinity antibodies (297). Despite the evidence that somatic mutation occurs normally in GCs, the GC environment is apparently not obligatory, because mice lacking histologically detectable GCs as a result of lymphotoxin-α deficiency are capable of SHM and affinity maturation (298). T-cell–independent antigens can undergo a low level of SHM (299).

Targeting and Distribution of Mutations

The mutation rate of Ig genes undergoing SHM may reach as high as 10^{-3} mutations per base pair per generation, or about 10^6 times higher than the normal genomic mutation rate (300), a rate that could be lethal if it were not carefully targeted specifically to Ig genes. The molecular nature of this targeting is a critical question closely related to understanding the molecular mechanism of SHM.

Exactly what feature of the V(D)J locus targets the hypermutation machinery to the expressed V(D)J gene is not understood. Unrearranged Vκ, VH, and D-J regions are generally not mutated, which suggests that the V(D)J recombination generates a hypermutation target from elements contributed by both V and J, possibly by moving the V region promoters close to enhancers lying in the J-C intron. [In contrast to the κ and heavy-chain loci, the λ locus lacks an enhancer between J and C; unrearranged Vλ regions are transcribed in B cells (301) and can be mutated (302).] The specific chromosomal location of Ig genes does not seem to be necessary for hypermutation, because transgenic mice carrying a rearranged expressible Ig gene—presumably inserted randomly in the genome—show somatic mutations. This fact has allowed examination of the sequence requirements for mutation by studying the how engineered alterations in transgene structure affect the SHM rate.

Because somatic mutations of Ig genes are not confined to hypervariable (CDR) regions and sometimes even occur in introns, it is apparent that the hypermutation mechanism does not distinguish coding from noncoding regions, let alone hypervariable regions from framework. The apparent clustering of mutations in the CDRs of sequenced immunoglobulins may be partly a result of selection for cells expressing primarily CDR mutations, either because framework alterations interfere with the basic folding of the protein or because CDR mutations can lead to higher affinity for antigen and thus stronger activation to clonal expansion, as discussed previously. However, in Ig genes that are not selected for function—such as nonproductively rearranged V-D-J alleles or "passenger" transgenes engineered with stop codons to prevent expression as a protein—mutational "hot spots" as well as "cold spots" have been recognized, apparently resulting from local DNA features that may promote or suppress somatic mutation. For example, the consensus sequence RGYW—that is, (G/A)(G)(C/T)(A/T)—is a consistent hot spot for mutation (302), and different triplet codons are mutation targets at differing but largely consistent frequencies. It is possible that evolution has selected for sequences that create mutational hot spots in CDR regions to enhance the potential for diversity generation in the parts of the protein critical for antigen contact (303).

The importance of transcription in targeting hypermutation is reinforced by studies of transgenic constructs engineered with or without transcriptional enhancers from the Ig loci. Rearranged transgenes, including intronic and 3′Eκ enhancers, were more highly transcribed and better somatic mutation targets than similar constructs lacking these regions (304). Mutations in either of two transcription factor–binding motifs in the 3′Eκ enhancer were found to impair transcription and SHM (305). In contrast to these transgene experiments, a milder defect in SHM was seen in mice with a targeted deletion of the endogenous 3′Eκ enhancer (306). In a heavy-chain construct, SHM was stimulated by HS3 and HS4 from the downstream enhancer complex (307), and SHM of a λ transgene was supported by a λ enhancer (308).

Although enhancers are clearly required, the complete criteria for targeting SHM have not been defined. Ig promoters are not required for SHM, because replacement of the Vκ promoter with the β-globin promoter did not abolish hypermutation (309); non-Ig enhancers can also promote hypermutation

(310). Furthermore, the V coding sequence can be replaced by a human β-globin gene or prokaryotic neo or gpt gene without affecting the hypermutation rate downstream of the promoter (311)]. However, for unknown reasons, a similar transgenic construct in which the Vκ gene was replaced by the CD72 gene was not targeted for hypermutation despite high levels of transcription (312), and even a highly expressed Vλ-Cλ transgene was not mutated (313). To summarize, it appears that transcription is necessary but not sufficient for targeting hypermutation, and additional requirements have not been defined as of this writing [although gene demethylation may be one such requirement (314)]. One striking confirmation of the correlation between transcription and SHM derives from experiments in which the SHM-competent murine pre–B line 18-81 was stably transfected with a tetracycline-inducible GFP reporter gene engineered with a stop codon. Expression of the GFP gene could occur only after the stop codon was reverted by SHM, and the rate of this reversion, as measured by flow cytometric analysis of GFP fluorescence, was found to be directly related to the transcription rate induced by increasing concentrations of the tetracycline analogue doxycycline (315).

Targeting of V genes for somatic mutation is not completely specific in that some non-Ig genes that are transcribed in GC B cells may be also subject to mutation (316). Somatic mutations observed in the BCL6 (317) and CD95 (318) genes may represent examples of this phenomenon, although several other genes expressed in GC B cells at comparable levels are not targeted for SHM (319). One possible interpretation is that, although Ig and non-Ig enhancers share the ability to confer transcriptional stimulation, additional sequences that can target SHM are found only in immunoglobulin and a few exceptional other enhancers. The dissociation of transcriptional enhancement and SHM targeting is suggested by one report that reversing the orientation of an enhancer in an SHM reporter plasmid caused a 10-fold difference in mutation frequency without an apparent effect on transcription (320). Several non-Ig genes, including some proto-oncogenes, have been found to harbor mutations in B-cell–diffuse large-cell lymphomas; these mutations show many features of Ig SHM and seem to result from pathological dysregulation of that process, inasmuch as these genes are not mutated in normal GC B cells (321).

Several groups have studied mutational targeting by examining the distribution of mutations around Ig genes. When somatically mutated rearranged genes have been compared with their germline precursors, mutations have been found to occur not only in sequence derived from the germline V coding sequence but also in the J region and nearby flanking intron sequence. The somatic mutations seem to cluster in the V(D)J region, extending upstream no farther than the RNA initiation site (with few exceptions) and tapering off downstream to define a mutation target domain of about 1.5 kb. Therefore, for V-D-J units involving the downstream JH5 segment, mutations extend further towards the Cμ region than for units involving JH1. This distribution has suggested a model (322) in which a "mutator factor" is loaded onto the transcription initiation complex as transcription begins. The mutator factor then remains attached to the transcription machinery—and competent to induce mutations—for a period of time as this machinery moves downstream to extend the transcript; eventually, however, the mutator factor falls off, so that further transcription proceeds without mutations. In accordance with this model, a VκJκ-Cκ transgene in which a second Vκ promoter was engineered upstream of the Cκ region was found to incur mutations over a second domain extending into the Cκ region, in addition to the usual V region mutations (322). Conversely, the insertion of an irrelevant 2-kb DNA fragment between a Vκ promoter and the leader (signal peptide) exon prevented mutation within the Vκ transgene, which now apparently lay downstream of the mutational domain (323). However, according to an alternative model consistent with these results, targeting is achieved by some epigenetic change in a domain downstream of the promoter that makes the region amenable to mutation, and transcription is another consequence of this change but one independent of mutation. This interpretation is supported by a preliminary report (324) that insertion of a transcriptional terminator between the leader and V exon of a transgene prevented transcription into the V region but nonetheless allowed substantial somatic mutation to occur there. If verified, this result would argue against the model of a mutator factor that travels with the transcription machinery.

Molecular Mechanism of Hypermutation

The observed mutations have revealed little about what may have caused them. All four nucleotides are targets for mutation, and all are found as products. Transitions (purine–purine and pyrimidine–pyrimidine interchanges) are somewhat more frequent than transversions (purine–pyrimidine interchanges), with apparent preferential targeting of G-C base pairs (325). Small insertions and deletions rarely occur. In an unselected passenger Vκ transgene, adenine and guanine nucleotides were mutated more frequently on the coding strand than on the noncoding strand (326). This "strand polarity" was also observed in human VH regions (327) but is not universally found. Such polarity suggests that the mutation mechanism may be affected by a process that can distinguish between the strands, such as transcription through the V region.

The unexpected dependence of SHM on expression of the AID gene, discussed previously, presents a provocative mechanistic clue. Complementing the initial reports that defects in the human and murine AID genes prevent SHM, Martin et al. (328) showed that introduction of the AID gene can induce mutation in hybridomas representing late B lineage cells that do not normally undergo SHM. Strikingly, AID-transfected fibroblasts are also capable of SHM: A highly transcribed GFP gene introduced as a reporter for CSR was found to contain numerous mutations in cells expressing AID, which implies that AID may be the only B-cell–specific

factor required for SHM as well as for CSR (329). AID may act by editing specific mRNA(s), leading to new proteins mediating CSR and SHM, as discussed earlier. However, the following recent evidence suggests that AID deaminates cytosine residues in DNA of the Ig loci. If such deamination occurred, it would generate uracil, which would be an abnormal base for DNA, and would be excised by the enzyme uracil DNA glycosylase (UNG). Neuberger's lab (325A) found that UNG knockout mice show abnormal patterns of SHM and defects in CSR, consistent with a role for UNG in mediating AID action. This suggests a role for deamination of DNA cytosines in CSR and SHM, presumably by AID, though the mechanistic consequences of such deamination are not clear at this writing.

As a framework for considering the mechanism of SHM, it is useful to consider the two mechanisms that nonlymphoid cells use to constrain normal genomic mutation to an extremely low level. First, highly accurate DNA polymerases with intrinsic proofreading capability copy DNA sequences with high fidelity. Second, several independent high-efficiency mechanisms recognize abnormalities in DNA structure—including mismatches introduced by rare polymerase mistakes—and repair them before they can lead to replicated errors. These two strategies for normal suppression of mutation have led to two suggestions for SHM mechanisms. Brenner and Milstein (330) proposed in 1966 that Ig V region genes might be cleaved by a specific endonuclease and that these defects might then be repaired by an "error-prone" polymerase that introduced mutations into the DNA. Strong support for this mechanism has been obtained, as discussed in the following section. In addition, several investigators have explored the alternative possibility that SHM may result from targeted abrogation of normal DNA repair mechanisms.

DNA Breaks in V Regions

Recent evidence supports Brenner and Milstein's (330) speculation that double-strand DNA breaks are associated with SHM. DNA breaks are suggested by the occurrence of insertions and deletions in about 5% of V regions undergoing SHM in normal human GC B cells isolated by flow cytometry (331). Furthermore, transfection of the SHM-competent human Burkitt lymphoma line Ramos with TdT was found to lead to many insertions in mutated immunoglobulin VH genes, insertions that were found (like typical somatic mutations) in the V but not C region (332). These insertions are most easily interpreted as the result of TdT-catalyzed nucleotide addition at double-strand DNA breaks. More direct evidence for such breaks has come from two analyses in which LM-PCR was used to amplify blunt DNA ends within Ig genes undergoing SHM (333,334). Both of these studies found evidence for breaks occurring in VH regions, but not the nearby Cμ region, and preferentially in the same RGYW consensus identified as a hot spot for somatic mutations. In Ramos cells transfected with GFP constructs, efficient production of double-strand DNA breaks occurred with a construct containing the Igκ enhancers but not when these enhancers were omitted. In the presence of these enhancers, increasing transcription across the reporter by a tetracycline-regulatable promoter caused an increase in the frequency of double-strand DNA breaks. Thus, in their location and regulation, these breaks showed many of features associated with SHM, supporting their role as intermediates in the mutational process. Ends were amplified from the downstream side of the VH regions with much lower efficiency than those from the upstream ends, as though the downstream ends were modified in some way as to be unavailable for ligation. To determine in which part of the cell cycle the double-strand DNA breaks occurred, Ramos cells were separated into G1 and G2 pools by propidium iodine staining and were assessed for breaks with the LM-PCR assay (333). Most double-strand DNA breaks were found in G2, in which double-strand DNA breaks are repaired primarily by homologous recombination, rather than in G1, in which nonhomologous end joining is the major repair mechanism. This is consistent with the observations that a targeted knockout of the NHEJ component DNA-PK does not significantly impair SHM (335). Mutations observed near CSR breakpoints may be caused by the same machinery responsible for SHM of V regions. AID-dependent mutations have even been found in the Sμ regions of B cells that have not undergone CSR (248,336). However, whereas double-strand DNA breaks associated with CSR [as detected by foci of γH2AX and Nbs1 staining in splenic B cells incubated under conditions promoting CSR (248)] were dependent on AID, double-strand DNA breaks in V regions of GC B cells (as detected by LM-PCR) were not dependent on AID (336A,336B), even though somatic mutation in V regions is AID dependent. One interpretation of these results is that AID is necessary for the error-prone repair of double-strand DNA breaks in V regions but not for their formation.

Error-Prone Polymerases

Although avoidance of error is a high priority for most DNA replication, error-prone DNA synthesis existed long before immunoglobulins evolved; indeed, error-prone polymerases have been most thoroughly studied in *Escherichia coli* and yeast. These polymerases are useful for replication of DNA with focal lesions that would block replication of high-fidelity polymerases. The individual polymerases have evolved to handle different aspects of "lesion bypass" and have differing types of infidelity in replication of normal DNA. For example, polymerase ι usually inserts the correct deoxynucleotide opposite guanine, adenine, and cytosine, but opposite a thymine, it misincorporates guanine or cytosine more efficiently than it adds the complementary adenine nucleotide. This polymerase can insert nucleotides opposite highly distorting DNA lesions such as a T-T photoproduct or an abasic site, but it is not efficient at polymerization beyond a mismatch. Polymerase ζ, in contrast, is inefficient at inserting a nucleotide opposite a lesion, but it efficiently extends beyond mismatched bases (337). Thus, polymerase ι may initiate repair and then polymerase ζ finishes it. This is consistent with the low processivity of polι: that is, its propensity to dissociate from the DNA after incorporation of only a few nucleotides. Lesion bypass may be a joint effort of several polymerases, and the same may be true for SHM.

Several experiments have suggested a role for polymerase ζ in SHM. Homozygous knockout of the polζ gene was found to induce embryonic lethality, and so effects on SHM could not be directly tested. However, the polζ gene was found to be up-regulated in sorted human tonsillar BC B cells and was induced in the GC-like B cell line CL01 when the cells were incubated under conditions that initiate SHM (BCR engagement and addition of activated CD4+ T cells). Significantly, transfection of the CL01 cells with antisense oligonucleotides directed against the polζ mRNA reduced the frequency of mutations observed in the expressed VH gene and in the BCL6 gene by about 70%, in comparison with cells transfected with control oligonucleotides (338). *In vivo* SHM was suppressed by about 40% in mice transgenic for high-level expression of an antisense mRNA (339); these mice also showed delayed generation of high-affinity antibody. The residual mutations in antisense-treated cells may have resulted from incomplete suppression of polζ expression and showed a normal pattern for SHM, including a preference for RGYW.

As of this writing, polymerase η is the only other error-prone polymerase for which genetic defects have been correlated with alterations in SHM. The polη gene is known to be defective in patients with xeroderma pigmentosum variant disease, who are susceptible to sunlight-induced skin cancers. When SHM was examined in such patients by PCR amplification of rearranged VH6 genes from peripheral blood, normal rates of SHM were found, but a striking decrease in mutations from an adenine target was observed (340); because the known preference of this polη is for mutating adenine nucleotides, the abnormal adenine targeting in patients with xeroderma pigmentosum variant disease supports a role for this enzyme in SHM. The question of whether polη expression is up-regulated in SHM-competent cells is controversial.

Two other error-prone polymerases have been mentioned as candidates for mediators of SHM. Pol-μ shows sequence similarity to TdT and *in vitro* has a TdT-like template-independent polymerase activity in the presence of Mn²⁺. In the presence of Mg²⁺, the enzyme has a template-dependent error-prone polymerase activity (341). A possible role for this enzyme in SHM is suggested by its preferential expression in GC B cells, although it is also expressed in thymus (342). However, a polμ knockout showed no apparent abnormality in SHM (343). Polymerase ι is a polη homolog (both being related to the yeast enzyme RAD30), which has an extremely low fidelity, as described previously. It is expressed primarily in the testis and ovary, but in the spleen its expression is somewhat higher in GC B cells (B220+, PNA+)

than in non-GC B cells (B220+, PNA−) (344). Other lesion bypass polymerases have been considered unlikely candidates as mediators of SHM for a variety of reasons: for example, polκ (makes deletions uncharacteristic of SHM), polβ (knockout shows normal SHM), and polλ (expressed mainly in the testis; knockout is normal for SHM). If the lesion bypass polymerases cooperate in mediating SHM, it may be necessary to examine double or triple knockouts to observe a loss of SHM.

Mismatch Repair (MMR) in Somatic Hypermutation

Several investigators have studied a possible role for MMR components in SHM. The speculation that SHM might be caused by abrogation of MMR has been investigated by one group who found that GC centroblasts have an intact MMR system, as judged by an *in vitro* MMR assay and Western blot for MMR components (345). Most other studies on MMR in SHM have involved examining the effects of gene knockouts. MMR might correct some mismatches introduced by an error-prone polymerase, and so an MMR gene knockout might be expected to increase the frequency of observed somatic mutations, but this has not been found.

As a framework for considering MMR in SHM, a brief introduction to bacterial and mammalian MMR is useful. The well-studied *E. coli* MMR system has three main components. MutS binds tightly and specifically to mismatches caused by the incorporation of an incorrect nucleotide during DNA replication. MutL then binds and recruits MutH. At the mismatch, MutH distinguishes the newly copied (presumably erroneous) strand from the original correct strand by the absence of methylation on the new strand (the old strand has had time to be methylated by the Dam methyltransferase system of *E. coli*). The Mut complex then activates a latent nuclease activity that removes a segment of the newly synthesized strand, including the mismatched base; this gapped strand is then resynthesized by a DNA polymerase. Mammals have several MutS homologs, including three reported in somatic cells—MSH2, MSH3, and MSH6—that have some specificity for recognizing different kinds of mismatches. The two known mammalian homologs of MutL are MLH1 and PMS2. Mammals distinguish new from old DNA strands by a poorly understood mechanism that does not involve methylation, and there is no mammalian counterpart to MutH. (Mutations in the human MMR genes, especially MSH2 and MLH1, underlie hereditary nonpolyposis colorectal cancer.)

The first report relating an MMR defect to SHM involved a VH knock-in mouse (designated the quasi-monoclonal mouse) with a PSM2 knockout (346). In comparison with PSM2 heterozygous knockouts, homozygous animals showed a 6- to 20-fold decrease in the number of mutations observed in the knocked in VH gene in peripheral B cells of unimmunized mice. The investigators proposed an active role for PMS2 in SHM: namely, that the normal choice to correct the mismatched nucleotide on the newly synthe-

sized strand is reversed in SHM, so that MMR reconciles the mismatch by preserving the mutated nucleotide and "correcting" the old DNA strand. Subsequent studies of PSM2 knockout mice have reported much smaller or no decreases in mutation rates in these animals or decreased mutation only in young but not older mice [reviewed by Reynaud et al. (347)]. These differing observations may result from different experimental protocols and different genetic backgrounds for the PSM2 knockout (the quasi-monoclonal mice may, for example, be unusual because of the intense selective pressure for mutating the knocked in VH gene). Similar results (i.e., normal or modestly reduced SHM rates) have also been found in knockouts of the other MutL homolog, MLH1, and in knockouts of the MutS homolog MSH2. Some differences in the patterns of mutation have been observed in the knockouts, which suggests that MSH2 may play a role in creating mutations outside the usual hot spots (348) or in preferentially correcting mismatches at G:C pairs. However, the bottom line is that none of these experiments has documented a critical role for MMR components in SHM. If MMR is at all involved in SHM, it is not apparently by the original model that local MMR suppression increases observed mutation; rather, the trend for MMR knockouts to show decreased SHM suggests that activity of the MMR system modestly increases the mutational frequency. This might happen if resynthesis of the MMR-dependent gapped DNA strand is accomplished by an error-prone DNA polymerase. In evaluating the current evidence, it should be noted that only one of the human MutS homologs has been targeted in gene knockouts and that, given the overlapping function of these proteins, a significant role for MMR in SHM might be overlooked unless a double or triple knockout is examined.

A model for SHM consistent with much of the data in this section has been proposed (333) on the basis of the putative mechanism for repair of double-strand DNA breaks in yeast by homologous recombination, a process also associated with a high rate of mutation (349). Figure 17 illustrates some features of this model and incorporates other clues about SHM discussed in this section. However, as of this writing, the detailed mechanism of SHM is not clearly understood. Good evidence supports roles in SHM for transcription, immunoglobulin enhancers, AID, double-strand DNA breaks, and error-prone polymerases, but these factors cannot yet be linked into a coherent and convincing model. In view of the flurry of interest in error-prone polymerases and the advances anticipated from tracking down the role of AID, it seems likely that a much clearer understanding of SHM will be available in the near future.

CONCLUSION

Recombinant DNA technology has revolutionized the study of the antibody response. Initial investigations used powerful cloning and sequencing methods to define the structure of the Ig genes as they exist in the germline and in actively secreting B-lymphocytes. Subsequent experiments have begun to shed

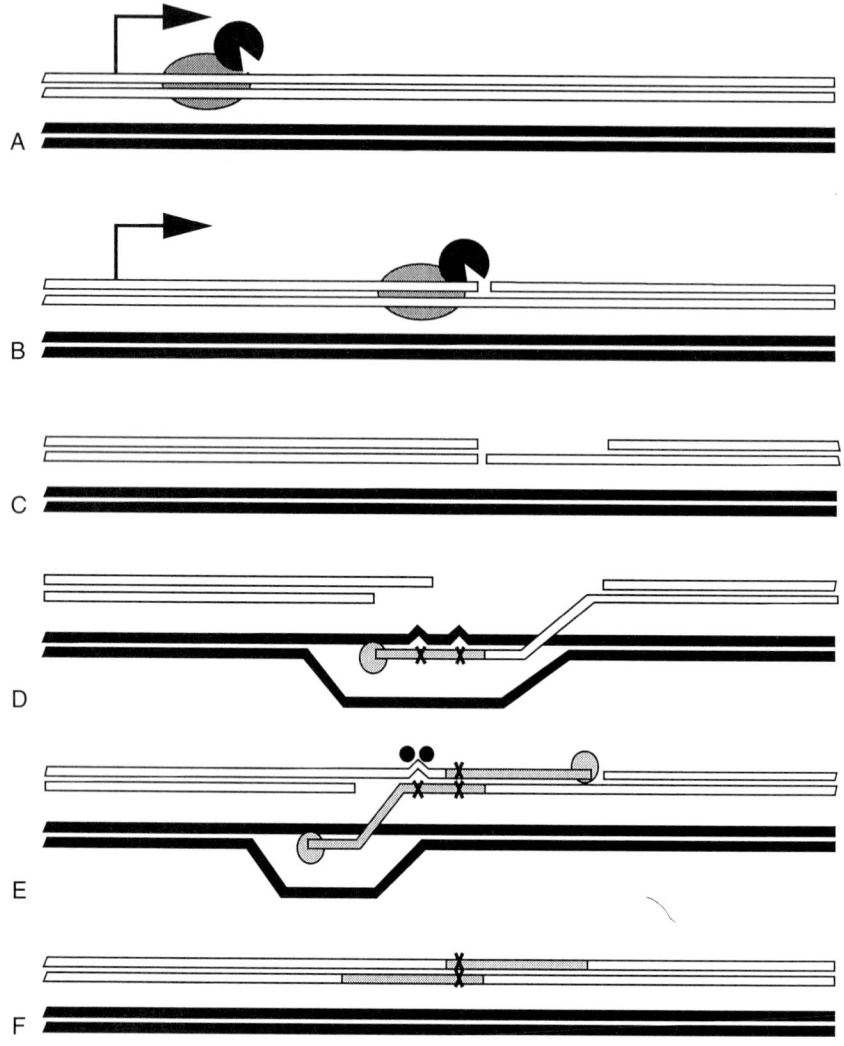

FIG. 17. Speculative model for the mechanism of somatic hypermutation. **A:** In this model, a mutation factor (*black "Pac-Man" graphic*) loads onto the transcription initiation complex about to transcribe across an immunoglobulin V region on one of two sister chromatids shown by *white and black double strands*. **B:** The mutation factor reveals itself to be an endonuclease, about to create a double-strand DNA break in the white chromatid. **C:** After DNA cleavage, a blunt end is seen on the upstream fragment; the downstream end is drawn with a 3′ overhang, to accord with the difficulty of detecting blunt ends on the downstream fragment and to suggest a source for a single strand end that could invade the homologous region of black chromatid. **D:** The 3′ overhang from the previous step has invaded its sister chromatid and has been extended (*gray DNA strand*) by an error-prone polymerase (*gray circle*), leading to two mismatched nucleotides (shown as *Xs*). **E.** The newly extended strand returns to the white chromatid, which has been shortened by nucleases and gets extended by error-prone polymerases. This extension leads to replication of one of the polymerase errors, leaving a permanent mutation. The other polymerase error is recognized by the mismatch repair complex (*small black circles*) and is repaired. **F:** The final V region sequence has acquired a single mutation.

light on the mechanisms of the processes unique to these genes: rearrangements and somatic mutation.

The knowledge of Ig genes gained so far has answered some of the most puzzling mysteries about antibody diversity and has also led to many practical ramifications involving these genes that are beyond the scope of this chapter. For example, cloned Ig genes have allowed the production of recombinant monoclonal antibodies in bacteria and the bioengineering of Ig-fusion proteins that exploit the exquisite specificity of antibody V region binding (e.g., antibody-toxin fusions) or the ability of Ig C region domains to extend serum half-life (e.g., immunoadhesins). Other engineered derivatives utilizing Ig genes include single-chain antibodies (350), bispecific antibodies (351), and "intrabodies" designed not to be secreted from a cell but rather to bind to intracellular targets (352). Ig V gene fragments cloned into bacteriophage so as to express single-chain V regions on the phage surface (phage display libraries) can be used to obtain specific monoclonal antibodies without immunization or use of mammalian cells, and *in vitro* mutation and selection protocols can mimic

affinity maturation to yield high-affinity antibodies [reviewed by Hoogenboom (353)]. Even Ig gene regulatory regions have been exploited, to achieve B-cell–specific expression of oncogenes (354) and of intracellular toxins that could be used to target B lymphomas (355). Apart from these biotechnological applications, Ig gene probes of Southern blot results and library clones from lymphomas have led to the identification of numerous proto-oncogenes that become activated by translocation into Ig gene loci (reviewed by Sarris and Ford (356)]. For instance, Bcl2 was initially discovered as the target of Ig heavy-chain translocation in follicular lymphoma and provided an entry into an entire family of apoptosis-related genes. A final example of medical benefit from Ig gene technology has been the use of patient-specific Ig gene rearrangements of leukemias or lymphomas to monitor disease status by PCR (357).

Further practical applications of Ig genes can be anticipated in the future, as can a deeper scientific understanding of their molecular biology and their contribution to the immune system.

REFERENCES

1. Dreyer WJ, Bennett JC. The molecular basis of antibody formation. *Proc Natl Acad Sci U S A* 1965;54:864–869.
2. Rabbitts TH. Evidence for splicing of interrupted immunoglobulin variable and constant region sequences in nuclear RNA. *Nature* 1978;275:291–296.
3. Brack C, Hirama M, Lenhard SR, et al. A complete immunoglobulin gene is created by somatic recombination. *Cell* 1978;15:1–14.
4. Parhami SB, Margolies MN. Contribution of heavy chain junctional amino acid diversity to antibody affinity among *p*-azophenylarsonate-specific antibodies. *J Immunol* 1996;157:2066–2072.
5. Fang W, Mueller DL, Pennell CA, et al. Frequent aberrant immunoglobulin gene rearrangements in pro–B cells revealed by a bcl-xL transgene. *Immunity* 1996;4:291–299.
6. Gu H, Kitamura D, Rajewsky K. B cell development regulated by gene rearrangement: arrest of maturation by membrane-bound D mu protein and selection of DH element reading frames. *Cell* 1991;65:47–54.
7. Corbett S, Tomlinson I, Sonnhammer E, et al. Sequence of the human immunoglobulin diversity (D) segment locus: A systematic analysis provides no evidence for the use of DIR segments, inverted D segments, "minor" D segments or D-D recombination. *J Molec Biol* 1997;271:597.
8. Ramsden DA, Baetz K, Wu GE. Conservation of sequence in recombination signal sequence spacers. *Nucleic Acids Res* 1994;22:1785–1796.
9. Nadel B, Tang A, Escuro G, et al. Sequence of the spacer in the recombination signal sequence affects V(D)J rearrangement frequency and correlates with nonrandom Vkappa usage *in vivo*. *J Exp Med* 1998;187:1495–1503.
10. Tucker PW, Marcu KB, Newell N, et al. Sequence of the cloned gene for the constant region of murine gamma 2b immunoglobulin heavy chain. *Science* 1979;206:1303–1306.
11. Kincade PW, Lawton AR, Bockman DE, et al. Suppression of immunoglobulin G synthesis as a result of antibody mediated suppression of immunoglobulin M synthesis in chickens. *Proc Natl Acad Sci U S A* 1970;67:1918–1925.
12. Fasel NJ, Deglon N, Beghdadi-Rais C, et al. Minimal membrane and secreted mu poly(A) signals specify developmentally-regulated immunoglobulin heavy chain mRNA ratios without RNA splicing. *Mol Immunol* 1994;31:563–566.
13. Galli G, Guise JW, McDevitt MA, et al. Relative position and strengths of poly(A) sites as well as transcription termination are critical to membrane versus secreted mu-chain expression during B-cell development. *Genes Dev* 1987;1:471–481.
14. Phillips C, Kyriakopoulou CB, Virtanen A. Identification of a stem-loop structure important for polyadenylation at the murine IgM secretory poly(A) site. *Nucleic Acids Res* 1999;27:429–438.
15. Peterson ML, Bryman MB, Peiter M, et al. Exon size affects competition between splicing and cleavage-polyadenylation in the immunoglobulin mu gene. *Mol Cell Biol* 1994;14:77–86.
16. Coyle JH, Lebman DA. Correct immunoglobulin alpha mRNA processing depends on specific sequence in the C alpha 3-alpha M intron. *J Immunol* 2000;164:3659–3665.
17. Takagaki Y, Seipelt RL, Peterson ML, et al. The polyadenylation factor CstF-64 regulates alternative processing of IgM heavy chain pre-mRNA during B cell differentiation. *Cell* 1996;87:941–952.
18. Veraldi KL, Arhin GK, Martincic K, et al. hnRNP F influences binding of a 64-kilodalton subunit of cleavage stimulation factor to mRNA precursors in mouse B cells. *Mol Cell Biol* 2001;21:1228–1238.
19. Shimizu A, Takahashi N, Yaoita Y, et al. Organization of the constant-region gene family of the mouse immunoglobulin heavy chain. *Cell* 1982;28:499–506.
20. Akahori Y, Kurosawa Y. Nucleotide sequences of all the gamma gene loci of murine immunoglobulin heavy chains. *Genomics* 1997;41:100–104.
21. Knight KL, Becker RS. Isolation of genes encoding bovine IgM, IgG, IgA and IgE chains. *Vet Immunol Immunopathol* 1987;17:17–24.
22. Hamers-Casterman C, Atarhouch T, Muyldermans S, et al. Naturally occurring antibodies devoid of light chains. *Nature* 1993;363:446–448.
23. Hieter PA, Korsmeyer SJ, Waldmann TA, et al. Human immunoglobulin kappa light-chain genes are deleted or rearranged in lambda-producing B cells. *Nature* 1981;290:368–372.
24. Durdik J, Moore MW, Selsing E. Novel kappa light-chain gene rearrangements in mouse lambda light chain-producing B lymphocytes. *Nature* 1984;307:749–752.
25. Siminovitch KA, Bakhshi A, Goldman P, et al. A uniform deleting element mediates the loss of kappa genes in human B cells. *Nature* 1985;316:260–262.
26. Kawasaki K, Minoshima S, Nakato E, et al. One-megabase sequence analysis of the human immunoglobulin lambda gene locus. *Genome Res* 1997;7:250–261.
27. Niewold TA, Murphy CL, Weiss DT, et al. Characterization of a light chain product of the human JC lambda 7 gene complex. *J Immunol* 1996;157:4474–4477.
28. Kudo A, Sakaguchi N, Melchers F. Organization of the murine Ig-related lambda 5 gene transcribed selectively in pre-B lymphocytes [published erratum appears in *EMBO J* 1987;6:4242]. *EMBO J* 1987;6:103–107.
29. Dul JL, Argon Y, Winkler T, et al. The murine VpreB1 and VpreB2 genes both encode a protein of the surrogate light chain and are co-expressed during B cell development. *Eur J Immunol* 1996;26:906–913.
30. Tsubata T, Reth M. The products of pre–B cell–specific genes (lambda 5 and VpreB) and the immunoglobulin mu chain form a complex that is transported onto the cell. *J Exp Med* 1990;172:973–976.
31. Tsubata T, Tsubata R, Reth M. Crosslinking of the cell surface immunoglobulin (mu-surrogate light chains complex) on pre–B cells induces activation of V gene rearrangements at the immunoglobulin kappa locus. *Int Immunol* 1992;4:637–641.
32. Frippiat JP, Williams SC, Tomlinson IM, et al. Organization of the human immunoglobulin lambda light-chain locus on chromosome 22q11.2. *Hum Mol Genet* 1995;4:983–991.
33. Shimizu T, Iwasato T, Yamagishi H. Deletions of immunoglobulin C kappa region characterized by the circular excision products in mouse splenocytes. *J Exp Med* 1991;173:1065–1072.
34. Douek DC, McFarland RD, Keiser PH, et al. Changes in thymic function with age and during the treatment of HIV infection. *Nature* 1998;396:690–695.
35. Reth M, Gehrmann P, Petrac E, et al. A novel VH to VHDJH joining mechanism in heavy-chain-negative (null) pre–B cells results in heavy-chain production. *Nature* 1986;322:840–842.
36. Chen C, Nagy Z, Prak EL, et al. Immunoglobulin heavy chain gene replacement: a mechanism of receptor editing. *Immunity* 1995;3:747–755.
37. McCormack WT, Tjoelker LW, Carlson LM, et al. Chicken IgL gene rearrangement involves deletion of a circular episome and addition of single nonrandom nucleotides to both coding segments. *Cell* 1989;56:785–791.
38. Lieber MR, Hesse JE, Mizuuchi K, et al. Developmental stage specificity of the lymphoid V(D)J recombination activity. *Genes Dev* 1987;1:751–761.
39. Lewis SM, Hesse JE, Mizuuchi K, et al. Novel strand exchanges in V(D)J recombination. *Cell* 1988;55:1099–1107.
40. Lew S, Franco D, Chang Y. Activation of V(D)J recombination induces the formation of interlocus joints and hybrid joints in SCID pre–B-cell lines. *Mol Cell Biol* 2000;20:7170–7177.
41. Roth DB, Menetski JP, Nakajima PB, et al. V(D)J recombination: broken DNA molecules with covalently sealed (hairpin) coding ends in SCID mouse thymocytes. *Cell* 1992;70:983–991.
42. Roth DB, Nakajima PB, Menetski JP, et al. V(D)J recombination in mouse thymocytes: double-strand breaks near T cell receptor delta rearrangement signals. *Cell* 1992;69:41–53.
43. Schlissel M, Constantinescu A, Morrow T, et al. Double-strand signal sequence breaks in V(D)J recombination are blunt, 5′-phosphorylated, RAG-dependent, and cell cycle regulated. *Genes Dev* 1993;7:2520–2532.
44. Zhu C, Roth DB. Characterization of coding ends in thymocytes of SCID mice: implications for the mechanism of V(D)J recombination. *Immunity* 1995;2:101–112.
45. Ramsden DA, Gellert M. Formation and resolution of double-strand break intermediates in V(D)J rearrangement. *Genes Dev* 1995;9:2409–2420.
46. Lewis SM. P nucleotide insertions and the resolution of hairpin

DNA structures in mammalian cells. *Proc Natl Acad Sci U S A* 1994;91:1332–1336.

47. Schatz DG, Baltimore D. Stable expression of immunoglobulin gene V(D)J recombinase activity by gene transfer into 3T3 fibroblasts. *Cell* 1988;53:107–115.

48. Shinkai Y, Rathbun G, Lam KP, et al. RAG-2-deficient mice lack mature lymphocytes owing to inability to initiate V(D)J rearrangement. *Cell* 1992;68:855–867.

49. Mombaerts P, Iacomini J, Johnson RS, et al. RAG-1–deficient mice have no mature B and T lymphocytes. *Cell* 1992;68:869–877.

50. Schwarz K, Gauss GH, Ludwig L, et al. RAG mutations in human B cell–negative SCID. *Science* 1996;274:97–99.

51. Villa A, Santagata S, Bozzi F, et al. Partial V(D)J recombination activity leads to Omenn syndrome. *Cell* 1998;93:885–896.

52. Corneo B, Moshous D, Gungor T, et al. Identical mutations in RAG1 or RAG2 genes leading to defective V(D)J recombinase activity can cause either T-B–severe combined immune deficiency or Omenn syndrome. *Blood* 2001;97:2772–2776.

53. Corneo B, Moshous D, Callebaut I, et al. Three-dimensional clustering of human RAG2 gene mutations in severe combined immune deficiency. *J Biol Chem* 2000;275:12672–12675.

54. McMahan CJ, Difilippantonio MJ, Rao N, et al. A basic motif in the N-terminal region of RAG1 enhances V(D)J recombination activity. *Mol Cell Biol* 1997;17:4544–4552.

55. Roman CA, Cherry SR, Baltimore D. Complementation of V(D)J recombination deficiency in RAG-1(−/−) B cells reveals a requirement for novel elements in the N-terminus of RAG-1. *Immunity* 1997;7:13–24.

56. Difilippantonio MJ, McMahan CJ, Eastman QM, et al. RAG1 mediates signal sequence recognition and recruitment of RAG2 in V(D)J recombination. *Cell* 1996;87:253–262.

57. Landree MA, Wibbenmeyer JA, Roth DB. Mutational analysis of RAG1 and RAG2 identifies three catalytic amino acids in RAG1 critical for both cleavage steps of V(D)J recombination. *Genes Dev* 1999;13:3059–3069.

58. Kim DR, Dai Y, Mundy CL, et al. Mutations of acidic residues in RAG1 define the active site of the V(D)J recombinase. *Genes Dev* 1999;13:3070–3080.

59. Fugmann SD, Villey IJ, Ptaszek LM, et al. Identification of two catalytic residues in RAG1 that define a single active site within the RAG1/RAG2 protein complex. *Mol Cell* 2000;5:97–107.

60. Akamatsu Y, Oettinger MA. Distinct roles of RAG1 and RAG2 in binding the V(D)J recombination signal sequences. *Mol Cell Biol* 1998;18:4670–4678.

61. Hiom K, Gellert M. A stable RAG1-RAG2-DNA complex that is active in V(D)J cleavage. *Cell* 1997;88:65–72.

62. Mo X, Bailin T, Sadofsky MJ. RAG1 and RAG2 cooperate in specific binding to the recombination signal sequence *in vitro*. *J Biol Chem* 1999;274:7025–7031.

63. Swanson PC, Desiderio S. V(D)J recombination signal recognition: distinct, overlapping DNA-protein contacts in complexes containing RAG1 with and without RAG2. *Immunity* 1998;9:115–125.

64. van Gent DC, Hiom K, Paull TT, et al. Stimulation of V(D)J cleavage by high mobility group proteins. *EMBO J* 1997;16:2665–2670.

65. Hiom K, Gellert M. Assembly of a 12/23 paired signal complex: a critical control point in V(D)J recombination. *Mol Cell* 1998;1:1011–1019.

66. Aidinis V, Bonaldi T, Beltrame M, et al. The RAG1 homeodomain recruits HMG1 and HMG2 to facilitate recombination signal sequence binding and to enhance the intrinsic DNA-bending activity of RAG1-RAG2. *Mol Cell Biol* 1999;19:6532–6542.

67. McBlane JF, van GD, Ramsden DA, et al. Cleavage at a V(D)J recombination signal requires only RAG1 and RAG2 proteins and occurs in two steps. *Cell* 1995;83:387–395.

68. van Gent DC, Mizuuchi K, Gellert M. Similarities between initiation of V(D)J recombination and retroviral integration. *Science* 1996;271:1592–1594.

69. Kale SB, Landree MA, Roth DB. Conditional RAG-1 mutants block the hairpin formation step of V(D)J recombination. *Mol Cell Biol* 2001;21:459–466.

70. Agrawal A, Schatz DG. RAG1 and RAG2 form a stable postcleavage synaptic complex with DNA containing signal ends in V(D)J recombination. *Cell* 1997;89:43–53.

71. Shockett PE, Schatz DG. DNA hairpin opening mediated by the RAG1 and RAG2 proteins. *Mol Cell Biol* 1999;19:4159–4166.

72. Besmer E, Mansilla-Soto J, Cassard S, et al. Hairpin coding end opening is mediated by RAG1 and RAG2 proteins. *Mol Cell* 1998; 2:817–828.

73. Jones JM, Gellert M. Intermediates in V(D)J recombination: a stable RAG1/2 complex sequesters cleaved RSS ends. *Proc Natl Acad Sci U S A* 2001;98:12926–12931.

74. Qiu JX, Kale SB, Yarnell Schultz H, et al. Separation-of-function mutants reveal critical roles for RAG2 in both the cleavage and joining steps of V(D)J recombination. *Mol Cell* 2001;7:77–87.

75. Yarnell Schultz H, Landree MA, Qiu JX, et al. Joining-deficient RAG1 mutants block V(D)J recombination *in vivo* and hairpin opening *in vitro*. *Mol Cell* 2001;7:65–75.

76. van Gent DC, Ramsden DA, Gellert M. The RAG1 and RAG2 proteins establish the 12/23 rule in V(D)J recombination. *Cell* 1996;85:107–113.

77. Sawchuk DJ, Weis GF, Malik S, et al. V(D)J recombination: modulation of RAG1 and RAG2 cleavage activity on 12/23 substrates by whole cell extract and DNA-bending proteins. *J Exp Med* 1997;185:2025–2032.

78. Ramsden DA, McBlane JF, van Gent DC, et al. Distinct DNA sequence and structure requirements for the two steps of V(D)J recombination signal cleavage. *EMBO J* 1996;15:3197–3206.

79. Cuomo CA, Mundy CL, Oettinger MA. DNA sequence and structure requirements for cleavage of V(D)J recombination signal sequences. *Mol Cell Biol* 1996;16:5683–5690.

80. Agrawal A, Eastman QM, Schatz DG. Transposition mediated by RAG1 and RAG2 and its implications for the evolution of the immune system. *Nature* 1998;394:744–751.

81. Hiom K, Melek M, Gellert M. DNA transposition by the RAG1 and RAG2 proteins: a possible source of oncogenic translocations. *Cell* 1998;94:463–470.

82. Sakano H, Huppi K, Heinrich G, et al. Sequences at the somatic recombination sites of immunoglobulin light-chain genes. *Nature* 1979;280:288–294.

83. Roth DB, Craig NL. VDJ recombination: a transposase goes to work. *Cell* 1998;94:411–414.

84. Lin WC, Desiderio S. Cell cycle regulation of V(D)J recombination-activating protein RAG-2. *Proc Natl Acad Sci U S A* 1994;91:2733–2737.

85. Li Z, Dordai DI, Lee J, et al. A conserved degradation signal regulates RAG-2 accumulation during cell division and links V(D)J recombination to the cell cycle. *Immunity* 1996;5:575–589.

86. Chen J, Lansford R, Stewart V, et al. RAG-2-deficient blastocyst complementation: an assay of gene function in lymphocyte development. *Proc Natl Acad Sci U S A* 1993;90:4528–4532.

87. Taccioli GE, Rathbun G, Oltz E, et al. Impairment of V(D)J recombination in double-strand break repair mutants. *Science* 1993;260:207–210.

88. Aravind L, Koonin EV. Prokaryotic homologs of the eukaryotic DNA-end–binding protein Ku, novel domains in the Ku protein and prediction of a prokaryotic double-strand break repair system. *Genome Res* 2001;11:1365–1374.

89. Shin EK, Perryman LE, Meek K. A kinase-negative mutation of DNA-PK(CS) in equine SCID results in defective coding and signal joint formation. *J Immunol* 1997;158:3565–3569.

90. Gao Y, Chaudhuri J, Zhu C, et al. A targeted DNA-PKcs-null mutation reveals DNA-PK-independent functions for KU in V(D)J recombination. *Immunity* 1998;9:367–376.

91. Taccioli GE, Amatucci AG, Beamish HJ, et al. Targeted disruption of the catalytic subunit of the DNA-PK gene in mice confers severe combined immunodeficiency and radiosensitivity. *Immunity* 1998;9:355–366.

92. Zhu C, Bogue MA, Lim DS, et al. Ku86-deficient mice exhibit severe combined immunodeficiency and defective processing of V(D)J recombination intermediates. *Cell* 1996;86:379–389.

93. Gu Y, Jin S, Gao Y, et al. Ku70-deficient embryonic stem cells have increased ionizing radiosensitivity, defective DNA end-binding activity, and inability to support V(D)J recombination. *Proc Natl Acad Sci U S A* 1997;94:8076–8081.

94. Walker JR, Corpina RA, Goldberg J. Structure of the Ku heterodimer bound to DNA and its implications for double-strand break repair. *Nature* 2001;412:607–614.

95. Leuther KK, Hammarsten O, Kornberg RD, et al. Structure of DNA-dependent protein kinase: implications for its regulation by DNA. *EMBO J* 1999;18:1114–1123.

96. Hammarsten O, DeFazio LG, Chu G. Activation of DNA-dependent protein kinase by single-stranded DNA ends. *J Biol Chem* 2000;275:1541–1550.

97. Li Z, Otevrel T, Gao Y, et al. The XRCC4 gene encodes a novel protein involved in DNA double-strand break repair and V(D)J recombination. *Cell* 1995;83:1079–1089.

98. Junop MS, Modesti M, Guarne A, et al. Crystal structure of the Xrcc4 DNA repair protein and implications for end joining. *EMBO J* 2000;19:5962–5970.

99. Critchlow SE, Bowater RP, Jackson SP. Mammalian DNA double-strand break repair protein XRCC4 interacts with DNA ligase IV. *Curr Biol* 1997;7:588–598.

100. Grawunder U, Wilm M, Wu XK, et al. Activity of DNA ligase IV stimulate by complex formation with XRCC4 in mammalian cells. *Nature* 1997;388:492.

101. Leber R, Wise TW, Mizuta R, et al. The XRCC4 gene product is a target for and interacts with the DNA-dependent protein kinase. *J Biol Chem* 1998;273:1794–1801.

102. Frank KM, Sekiguchi JM, Seidl KJ, et al. Late embryonic lethality and impaired V(D)J recombination in mice lacking DNA ligase IV. *Nature* 1998;396:173–177.

103. Barnes DE, Stamp G, Rosewell I, et al. Targeted disruption of the gene encoding DNA ligase IV leads to lethality in embryonic mice. *Curr Biol* 1998;8:1395–1398.

104. O'Driscoll M, Cerosaletti KM, Girard PM, et al. DNA ligase IV mutations identified in patients exhibiting developmental delay and immunodeficiency. *Mol Cell* 2001;8:1175–1185.

105. Gao Y, Ferguson DO, Xie W, et al. Interplay of p53 and DNA-repair protein XRCC4 in tumorigenesis, genomic stability and development. *Nature* 2000;404:897–900.

106. Sekiguchi JM, Gao Y, Gu Y, et al. Nonhomologous end-joining proteins are required for V(D)J recombination, normal growth, and neurogenesis. *Cold Spring Harb Symp Quant Biol* 1999;64:169–181.

107. Karanjawala ZE, Murphy N, Hinton DR, et al. Oxygen metabolism causes chromosome breaks and is associated with the neuronal apoptosis observed in DNA double-strand break repair mutants. *Curr Biol* 2002;12:397–402.

108. Moshous D, Callebaut I, de Chasseval R, et al. Artemis, a novel DNA double-strand break repair/V(D)J recombination protein, is mutated in human severe combined immune deficiency. *Cell* 2001;105:177–186.

109. Ma Y, Pannicke U, Schwarz K, et al. Hairpin opening and overhang processing by an Artemis/DNA-dependent protein kinase complex in nonhomologous end joining and V(D)J recombination. *Cell* 2002;108:781–794.

110. Feeney AJ. Lack of N regions in fetal and neonatal mouse immunoglobulin V-D-J junctional sequences. *J Exp Med* 1990;172:1377–1390.

111. Victor KD, Capra JD. An apparently common mechanism of generating antibody diversity: length variation of the VL-JL junction. *Mol Immunol* 1994;31:39–46.

112. Hiramatsu R, Akagi K, Matsuoka M, et al. The 3' enhancer region determines the B/T specificity and pro–B/pre–B specificity of immunoglobulin V kappa–J kappa joining. *Cell* 1995;83:1113–1123.

113. Wasserman R, Li YS, Hardy RR. Down-regulation of terminal deoxynucleotidyl transferase by Ig heavy chain in B lineage cells. *J Immunol* 1997;158:1133–1138.

114. Gavin MA, Bevan MJ. Increased peptide promiscuity provides a rationale for the lack of N regions in the neonatal T cell repertoire. *Immunity* 1995;3:793–800.

115. Bogue MA, Wang C, Zhu C, et al. V(D)J recombination in Ku86-deficient mice: distinct effects on coding, signal, and hybrid joint formation. *Immunity* 1997;7:37–47.

116. Paull TT, Rogakou EP, Yamazaki V, et al. A critical role for histone H2AX in recruitment of repair factors to nuclear foci after DNA damage. *Curr Biol* 2000;10:886–895.

117. Burma S, Chen BP, Murphy M, et al. ATM phosphorylates histone H2AX in response to DNA double-strand breaks. *J Biol Chem* 2001;276:42462–42467.

118. Andegeko Y, Moyal L, Mittelman L, et al. Nuclear retention of ATM at sites of DNA double strand breaks. *J Biol Chem* 2001;276:38224–38230.

119. Chen HT, Bhandoola A, Difilippantonio MJ, et al. Response to RAG-mediated VDJ cleavage by NBS1 and gamma-H2AX. *Science* 2000;290:1962–1965.

120. Perkins EJ, Nair A, Cowley DO, et al. Sensing of intermediates in V(D)J recombination by ATM. *Genes Dev* 2002;16:159–164.

121. Ohnishi K, Shimizu T, Karasuyama H, et al. The identification of a nonclassical cadherin expressed during B cell development and its interaction with surrogate light chain. *J Biol Chem* 2000;275:31134–31144.

122. Yancopoulos GD, Alt FW. Developmentally controlled and tissue-specific expression of unrearranged VH gene segments. *Cell* 1985;40:271–281.

123. Angelin-Duclos C, Calame K. Evidence that immunoglobulin VH-DJ recombination does not require germ line transcription of the recombining variable gene segment. *Mol Cell Biol* 1998;18:6253–6264.

124. Stanhope-Baker P, Hudson KM, Shaffer AL, et al. Cell type–specific chromatin structure determines the targeting of V(D)J recombinase activity *in vitro*. *Cell* 1996;85:887–897.

125. Sakai E, Bottaro A, Davidson L, et al. Recombination and transcription of the endogenous Ig heavy chain locus is effected by the Ig heavy chain intronic enhancer core region in the absence of the matrix attachment regions. *Proc Natl Acad Sci U S A* 1999;96:1526–1531.

126. Golding A, Chandler S, Ballestar E, et al. Nucleosome structure completely inhibits *in vitro* cleavage by the V(D)J recombinase. *EMBO J* 1999;18:3712–3723.

127. Kwon J, Imbalzano AN, Matthews A, et al. Accessibility of nucleosomal DNA to V(D)J cleavage is modulated by RSS positioning and HMG1. *Mol Cell* 1998;2:829–839.

128. Marmorstein R. Protein modules that manipulate histone tails for chromatin regulation. *Nat Rev Mol Cell Biol* 2001;2:422–432.

129. Agata Y, Katakai T, Ye SK, et al. Histone acetylation determines the developmentally regulated accessibility for T cell receptor gamma gene recombination. *J Exp Med* 2001;193:873–880.

130. McBlane F, Boyes J. Stimulation of V(D)J recombination by histone acetylation. *Curr Biol* 2000;10:483–486.

131. Kwon J, Morshead KB, Guyon JR, et al. Histone acetylation and hSWI/SNF remodeling act in concert to stimulate V(D)J cleavage of nucleosomal DNA. *Mol Cell* 2000;6:1037–1048.

132. Chowdhury D, Sen R. Stepwise activation of the immunoglobulin mu heavy chain gene locus. *EMBO J* 2001;20:6394–6403.

133. Bird A. DNA methylation patterns and epigenetic memory. *Genes Dev* 2002;16:6–21.

134. Hsieh CL, Lieber MR. CpG methylated minichromosomes become inaccessible for V(D)J recombination after undergoing replication. *EMBO J* 1992;11:315–325.

135. Engler P, Haasch D, Pinkert CA et al. A strain-specific modifier on mouse chromosome 4 controls the methylation of independent transgene loci. *Cell* 1991;65:939–947.

136. Cherry SR, Beard C, Jaenisch R, et al. V(D)J recombination is not activated by demethylation of the kappa locus. *Proc Natl Acad Sci U S A* 2000;97:8467–8472.

137. Alt FW, Enea V, Bothwell AL, et al. Activity of multiple light chain genes in murine myeloma cells producing a single, functional light chain. *Cell* 1980;21:1–12.

138. Nussenzweig MC, Shaw AC, Sinn E, et al. Allelic exclusion in transgenic mice that express the membrane form of immunoglobulin mu. *Science* 1987;236:816–819.

139. Papavasiliou F, Jankovic M, Suh H, et al. The cytoplasmic domains of immunoglobulin (Ig) alpha and Ig beta can independently induce the precursor B cell transition and allelic exclusion. *J Exp Med* 1995;182:1389–1394.

140. Papavasiliou F, Misulovin Z, Suh H, et al. The role of Ig beta in precursor B cell transition and allelic exclusion. *Science* 1995;268:408–411.

141. Grawunder U, Leu TM, Schatz DG, et al. Down-regulation of RAG1 and RAG2 gene expression in preB cells after functional immunoglobulin heavy chain rearrangement. *Immunity* 1995;3:601–608.

142. Schlissel MS, Morrow T. Ig heavy chain protein controls B cell development by regulating germ-line transcription and retargeting V(D)J recombination. *J Immunol* 1994;153:1645–1657.

143. Constantinescu A, Schlissel MS. Changes in locus-specific V(D)J

recombinase activity induced by immunoglobulin gene products during B cell development. *J Exp Med* 1997;185:609–620.

144. Novobrantseva TI, Martin VM, Pelanda R, et al. Rearrangement and expression of immunoglobulin light chain genes can precede heavy chain expression during normal B cell development in mice. *J Exp Med* 1999;189:75–88.

145. Ma A, Fisher P, Dildrop R, et al. Surface IgM mediated regulation of RAG gene expression in E mu-N-myc B cell lines. *EMBO J* 1992;11:2727–2734.

146. Brauninger A, Goossens T, Rajewsky K, et al. Regulation of immunoglobulin light chain gene rearrangements during early B cell development in the human. *Eur J Immunol* 2001;31:3631–3637.

147. Engel H, Rolink A, Weiss S. B cells are programmed to activate kappa and lambda for rearrangement at consecutive developmental stages. *Eur J Immunol* 1999;29:2167–2176.

148. Mostoslavsky R, Singh N, Kirillov A, et al. Kappa chain monoallelic demethylation and the establishment of allelic exclusion. *Genes Dev* 1998;12:1801–1811.

149. Schimenti J. Monoallelic gene expression in mice: who? When? How? Why? *Genome Res* 2001;11:1799–1800.

150. Skok JA, Brown KE, Azuara V, et al. Nonequivalent nuclear location of immunoglobulin alleles in B lymphocytes. *Nat Immunol* 2001;2:848–854.

151. Mostoslavsky R, Singh N, Tenzen T, et al. Asynchronous replication and allelic exclusion in the immune system. *Nature* 2001;414:221–225.

152. Spanopoulou E, Roman CA, Corcoran LM, et al. Functional immunoglobulin transgenes guide ordered B-cell differentiation in Rag-1–deficient mice. *Genes Dev* 1994;8:1030–1042.

153. Pelanda R, Schaal S, Torres RM, et al. A prematurely expressed Ig(kappa) transgene, but not V(kappa)J(kappa) gene segment targeted into the Ig(kappa) locus, can rescue B cell development in lambda5-deficient mice. *Immunity* 1996;5:229–239.

154. Shaffer AL, Schlissel MS. A truncated heavy chain protein relieves the requirement for surrogate light chains in early B cell development. *J Immunol* 1997;159:1265–1275.

155. Bannish G, Fuentes-Panana EM, Cambier JC, et al. Ligand-independent signaling functions for the B lymphocyte antigen receptor and their role in positive selection during B lymphopoiesis. *J Exp Med* 2001;194:1583–1596.

156. Lam KP, Kuhn R, Rajewsky K. In vivo ablation of surface immunoglobulin on mature B cells by inducible gene targeting results in rapid cell death. *Cell* 1997;90:1073–1083.

157. Radic MZ, Erikson J, Litwin S, et al. B lymphocytes may escape tolerance by revising their antigen receptors. *J Exp Med* 1993;177:1165–1173.

158. Pelanda R, Schwers S, Sonoda E, et al. Receptor editing in a transgenic mouse model: site, efficiency, and role in B cell tolerance and antibody diversification. *Immunity* 1997;7:765–775.

159. Hertz M, Nemazee D. BCR ligation induces receptor editing in IgM+IgD− bone marrow B cells in vitro. *Immunity* 1997;6:429–436.

160. Verkoczy LK, Stiernholm BJ, Berinstein NL. Up-regulation of recombination activating gene expression by signal transduction through the surface Ig receptor. *J Immunol* 1995;154:5136–5143.

161. Pogue SL, Goodnow CC. Gene dose-dependent maturation and receptor editing of B cells expressing immunoglobulin (Ig)G1 or IgM/IgG1 tail antigen receptors. *J Exp Med* 2000;191:1031–1044.

162. Tze LE, Baness EA, Hippen KL, et al. Ig light chain receptor editing in anergic B cells. *J Immunol* 2000;165:6796–6802.

163. Fang W, Weintraub BC, Dunlap B, et al. Self-reactive B lymphocytes overexpressing Bcl-xL escape negative selection and are tolerized by clonal anergy and receptor editing. *Immunity* 1998;9:35–45.

164. Sandel PC, Gendelman M, Kelsoe G, et al. Definition of a novel cellular constituent of the bone marrow that regulates the response of immature B cells to B cell antigen receptor engagement. *J Immunol* 2001;166:5935–5944.

165. Benschop RJ, Brandl E, Chan AC, et al. Unique signaling properties of B cell antigen receptor in mature and immature B cells: implications for tolerance and activation. *J Immunol* 2001;167:4172–4179.

166. Casellas R, Shih TA, Kleinewietfeld M, et al. Contribution of receptor editing to the antibody repertoire. *Science* 2001;291:1541–1544.

167. Retter MW, Nemazee D. Receptor editing occurs frequently during normal B cell development. *J Exp Med* 1998;188:1231–1238.

168. Meffre E, Davis E, Schiff C, et al. Circulating human B cells that express surrogate light chains and edited receptors. *Nat Immunol* 2000;1:207–213.

169. Itoh K, Meffre E, Albesiano E, et al. Immunoglobulin heavy chain variable region gene replacement as a mechanism for receptor revision in rheumatoid arthritis synovial tissue B lymphocytes. *J Exp Med* 2000;192:1151–1164.

170. Han S, Zheng B, Schatz DG, et al. Neoteny in lymphocytes: Rag1 and Rag2 expression in germinal center B cells. *Science* 1996;274:2094–2097.

171. Hikida M, Mori M, Takai T, et al. Reexpression of RAG-1 and RAG-2 genes in activated mature mouse B cells. *Science* 1996;274:2092–2094.

172. Papavasiliou F, Casellas R, Suh H, et al. V(D)J recombination in mature B cells: a mechanism for altering antibody responses. *Science* 1997;278:298–301.

173. Yu W, Nagaoka H, Jankovic M, et al. Continued RAG expression in late stages of B cell development and no apparent re-induction after immunization. *Nature* 1999;400:682–687.

174. Gartner F, Alt FW, Monroe RJ, et al. Antigen-independent appearance of recombination activating gene (RAG)-positive bone marrow B cells in the spleens of immunized mice. *J Exp Med* 2000;192:1745–1754.

175. Nagaoka H, Gonzalez-Aseguinolaza G, Tsuji M, et al. Immunization and infection change the number of recombination activating gene (RAG)-expressing B cells in the periphery by altering immature lymphocyte production. *J Exp Med* 2000;191:2113–2120.

176. de Wildt RM, Hoet RM, van Venrooij WJ, et al. Analysis of heavy and light chain pairings indicates that receptor editing shapes the human antibody repertoire. *J Mol Biol* 1999;285:895–901.

177. Brown ST, Miranda GA, Galic Z, et al. Regulation of the RAG-1 promoter by the NF-Y transcription factor. *J Immunol* 1997;158:5071–5074.

178. Fuller K, Storb U. Identification and characterization of the murine Rag1 promoter. *Mol Immunol* 1997;34:939–954.

179. Wang QF, Lauring J, Schlissel MS. c-Myb binds to a sequence in the proximal region of the RAG-2 promoter and is essential for promoter activity in T-lineage cells. *Mol Cell Biol* 2000;20:9203–9211.

180. Yu W, Misulovin Z, Suh H, et al. Coordinate regulation of RAG1 and RAG2 by cell type-specific DNA elements 5′ of RAG2. *Science* 1999;285:1080–1084.

181. Mainville CA, Sheehan KM, Klaman LD, et al. Deletional mapping of fifteen mouse VH gene families reveals a common organization for three Igh haplotypes. *J Immunol* 1996;156:1038–1046.

182. Nei M, Gu X, Sitnikova T. Evolution by the birth-and-death process in multigene families of the vertebrate immune system [In Process Citation]. *Proc Natl Acad Sci U S A* 1997;94:7799–7806.

183. Williams GS, Martinez A, Montalbano A, et al. Unequal VH gene rearrangement frequency within the large VH7183 gene family is not due to recombination signal sequence variation, and mapping of the genes shows a bias of rearrangement based on chromosomal location. *J Immunol* 2001;167:257–263.

184. Larijani M, Yu CC, Golub R, et al. The role of components of recombination signal sequences in immunoglobulin gene segment usage: a V81x model. *Nucleic Acids Res* 1999;27:2304–2309.

185. Feeney AJ, Riblet R. DST4: a new, and probably the last, functional DH gene in the BALB/c mouse. *Immunogenetics* 1993;37:217–221.

186. Kompfner E, Oliveira P, Montalbano A, et al. Unusual germline DSP2 gene accounts for all apparent V-D-D-J rearrangements in newborn, but not adult, MRL mice. *J Immunol* 2001;167:6933–6938.

187. Schupp IW, Schlake T, Kirschbaum T, et al. A yeast artificial chromosome contig spanning the mouse immunoglobulin kappa light chain locus. *Immunogenetics* 1997;45:180–187.

188. Roschenthaler F, Hameister H, Zachau HG. The 5′ part of the mouse immunoglobulin kappa locus as a continuously cloned structure. *Eur J Immunol* 2000;30:3349–3354.

189. Matsuda F, Ishii K, Bourvagnet P, et al. The complete nucleotide sequence of the human immunoglobulin heavy chain variable region locus. *J Exp Med* 1998;188:2151–2162.

190. Kawasaki K, Minoshima S, Nakato E, et al. Evolutionary dynamics of the human immunoglobulin kappa locus and the germline repertoire of the Vkappa genes. *Eur J Immunol* 2001;31:1017–1028.

191. Ernst P, Smale ST. Combinatorial regulation of transcription II: the immunoglobulin mu heavy chain gene. *Immunity* 1995;2:427–438.

192. Henderson AJ, Calame KL. Lessons in transcriptional regulation learned from studies on immunoglobulin genes. *Crit Rev Eukaryot Gene Expr* 1995;5:255–280.

193. Kottmann AH, Zevnik B, Welte M, et al. A second promoter and enhancer element within the immunoglobulin heavy chain locus. *Eur J Immunol* 1994;24:817–821.

194. Mundt CA, Nicholson IC, Zou X, et al. Novel control motif cluster in the IgH delta-gamma 3 interval exhibits B cell–specific enhancer function in early development. *J Immunol* 2001;166:3315–3323.

195. Luby TM, Sigurdardottir D, Berger ED, et al. Sequences associated with the mouse Smu switch region are important for immunoglobulin heavy chain transgene expression in B cell development. *Eur J Immunol* 2001;31:2866–2875.

196. Adams K, Ackerly H, Cunningham K, et al. A DNase I hypersensitive site near the murine gamma1 switch region contributes to insertion site independence of transgenes and modulates the amount of transcripts induced by CD40 ligation. *Int Immunol* 2000;12:1705–1713.

197. Arulampalam V, Eckhardt L, Pettersson S. The enhancer shift: a model to explain the developmental control of IgH gene expression in B-lineage cells. *Immunol Today* 1997;18:549–554.

198. Muramatsu M, Sankaranand VS, Anant S, et al. Specific expression of activation-induced cytidine deaminase (AID), a novel member of the RNA-editing deaminase family in germinal center B cells. *J Biol Chem* 1999;274:18470–18476.

199. Revy P, Muto T, Levy Y, et al. Activation-induced cytidine deaminase (AID) deficiency causes the autosomal recessive form of the hyper-IgM syndrome (HIGM2). *Cell* 2000;102:565–575.

200. Okazaki IM, Kinoshita K, Muramatsu M, et al. The AID enzyme induces class switch recombination in fibroblasts. *Nature* 2002;416:340–345.

201. Luby TM, Schrader CE, Stavnezer J, et al. The mu switch region tandem repeats are important, but not required, for antibody class switch recombination. *J Exp Med* 2001;193:159–168.

202. Du J, Zhu Y, Shanmugam A, et al. Analysis of immunoglobulin Sgamma3 recombination breakpoints by PCR: implications for the mechanism of isotype switching. *Nucleic Acids Res* 1997;25:3066–3073.

203. Dunnick W, Hertz GZ, Scappino L, et al. DNA sequences at immunoglobulin switch region recombination sites [published erratum appears in *Nucleic Acids Res* 1993;21:2285]. *Nucleic Acids Research* 1993;21:365–372.

204. Laffan M, Luzzatto L. Anomalous rearrangements of the immunoglobulin heavy chain genes in human leukemias support the loop-out mechanism of class switch. *J Clin Invest* 1992;90:2299–2303.

205. Zhao Y, Rabbani H, Shimizu A, et al. Mapping of the chicken immunoglobulin heavy-chain constant region gene locus reveals an inverted alpha gene upstream of a condensed upsilon gene. *Immunology* 2000;101:348–353.

206. Zhang K, Mills FC, Saxon A. Switch circles from IL-4–directed epsilon class switching from human B lymphocytes. Evidence for direct, sequential, and multiple step sequential switch from mu to epsilon Ig heavy chain gene. *J Immunol* 1994;152:3427–3435.

207. Malisan F, Briere F, Bridon JM, et al. Interleukin-10 induces immunoglobulin G isotype switch recombination in human CD40-activated naive B lymphocytes. *J Exp Med* 1996;183:937–947.

208. Chu CC, Paul WE, Max EE. Quantitation of immunoglobulin mu-gamma 1 heavy chain switch region recombination by a digestion-circularization polymerase chain reaction method. *Proc Natl Acad Sci U S A* 1992;89:6978–6982.

209. Chu CC, Max EE, Paul WE. DNA rearrangement can account for in vitro switching to IgG1. *J Exp Med* 1993;178:1381–1390.

210. Li SC, Rothman PB, Zhang J, et al. Expression of I mu-C gamma hybrid germline transcripts subsequent to immunoglobulin heavy chain class switching. *Int Immunol* 1994;6:491–497.

211. Kinoshita K, Harigai M, Fagarasan S, et al. A hallmark of active class switch recombination: transcripts directed by I promoters on looped-out circular DNAs. *Proc Natl Acad Sci U S A* 2001;98:12620–12623.

212. Allen RC, Armitage RJ, Conley ME, et al. CD40 ligand gene defects responsible for X-linked hyper-IgM syndrome. *Science* 1993;259: 990–993.

213. Ferrari S, Giliani S, Insalaco A, et al. Mutations of CD40 gene cause an autosomal recessive form of immunodeficiency with hyper IgM. *Proc Natl Acad Sci U S A* 2001;98:12614–12619.

214. Xu J, Foy TM, Laman JD, et al. Mice deficient for the CD40 ligand. *Immunity* 1994;1:423–431.

215. Hodgkin PD, Lee JH, Lyons AB. B cell differentiation and isotype switching is related to division cycle number. *J Exp Med* 1996; 184:277–281.

216. McCall MN, Hodgkin PD. Switch recombination and germ-line transcription are division-regulated events in B lymphocytes. *Biochim Biophys Acta* 1999;1447:43–50.

217. Siepmann K, Wohlleben G, Gray D. CD40-mediated regulation of interleukin-4 signaling pathways in B lymphocytes. *Eur J Immunol* 1996;26:1544–1552.

218. Grammer AC, McFarland RD, Heaney J, et al. Expression, regulation, and function of B cell–expressed CD154 in germinal centers. *J Immunol* 1999;163:4150–4159.

219. Cerutti A, Schaffer A, Shah S, et al. CD30 is a CD40-inducible molecule that negatively regulates CD40-mediated immunoglobulin class switching in non–antigen-selected human B cells. *Immunity* 1998;9:247–256.

220. Kehry MR. CD40-mediated signaling in B cells. Balancing cell survival, growth, and death. *J Immunol* 1996;156:2345–2348.

221. Cerutti A, Schaffer A, Goodwin RG, et al. Engagement of CD153 (CD30 ligand) by CD30$^+$ T cells inhibits class switch DNA recombination and antibody production in human IgD+ IgM+ B cells. *J Immunol* 2000;165:786–794.

222. Cerutti A, Kim EC, Shah S, et al. Dysregulation of CD30$^+$ T cells by leukemia impairs isotype switching in normal B cells. *Nat Immunol* 2001;2:150–156.

223. Fagarasan S, Kinoshita K, Muramatsu M, et al. In situ class switching and differentiation to IgA-producing cells in the gut lamina propria. *Nature* 2001;413:639–643.

224. Macpherson AJ, Lamarre A, McCoy K, et al. IgA production without mu or delta chain expression in developing B cells. *Nat Immunol* 2001;2:625–631.

225. Mao CS, Stavnezer J. Differential regulation of mouse germline Ig gamma 1 and epsilon promoters by IL-4 and CD40. *J Immunol* 2001;167:1522–1534.

226. Cogne M, Lansford R, Bottaro A, et al. A class switch control region at the 3' end of the immunoglobulin heavy chain locus. *Cell* 1994;77:737–747.

227. Manis JP, van der Stoep N, Tian M, et al. Class switching in B cells lacking 3' immunoglobulin heavy chain enhancers. *J Exp Med* 1998;188:1421–1431.

228. Pinaud E, Khamlichi AA, Le Morvan C, et al. Localization of the 3' IgH locus elements that effect long-distance regulation of class switch recombination. *Immunity* 2001;15:187–199.

229. Sakai E, Bottaro A, Alt FW. The Ig heavy chain intronic enhancer core region is necessary and sufficient to promote efficient class switch recombination. *Int Immunol* 1999;11:1709–1713.

230. Lee CG, Kinoshita K, Arudchandran A, et al. Quantitative regulation of class switch recombination by switch region transcription. *J Exp Med* 2001;194:365–374.

231. Snapper CM, Marcu KB, Zelazowski P. The immunoglobulin class switch: beyond "accessibility". *Immunity* 1997;6:217–223.

232. Ma L, Wortis HH, Kenter AL. Two new isotype-specific switching activities detected for Ig class switching. *J Immunol* 2002;168:2835–2846.

233. Stavnezer J. Antibody class switching. *Adv Immunol*, 1996;61:79–146.

234. Qiu G, Harriman GR, Stavnezer J. Ialpha exon-replacement mice synthesize a spliced HPRT-C(alpha) transcript which may explain their ability to switch to IgA. Inhibition of switching to IgG in these mice. *Int Immunol* 1999;11:37–46.

235. Hein K, Lorenz MG, Siebenkotten G, et al. Processing of switch transcripts is required for targeting of antibody class switch recombination. *J Exp Med* 1998;188:2369–2374.

236. Tian M, Alt FW. Transcription-induced cleavage of immunoglobulin switch regions by nucleotide excision repair nucleases in vitro. *J Biol Chem* 2000;275:24163–24172.

237. Daniels GA, Lieber MR. RNA:DNA complex formation upon

transcription of immunoglobulin switch regions: implications for the mechanism and regulation of class switch recombination. *Nucleic Acids Res* 1995;23:5006–5011.

238. Tashiro J, Kinoshita K, Honjo T. Palindromic but not G-rich sequences are targets of class switch recombination. *Int Immunol* 2001;13:495–505.

239. Chen X, Kinoshita K, Honjo T. Variable deletion and duplication at recombination junction ends: implication for staggered double-strand cleavage in class-switch recombination. *Proc Natl Acad Sci U S A* 2001;98:13860–13865.

240. Wuerffel RA, Du J, Thompson RJ, Kenter AL. Ig Sgamma3 DNA-specific double strand breaks are induced in mitogen-activated B cells and are implicated in switch recombination. *J Immunol* 1997;159:4139–4144.

241. Baar J, Pennell NM, Shulman MJ. Analysis of a hot spot for DNA insertion suggests a mechanism for Ig switch recombination. *J Immunol* 1996;157:3430–3435.

242. Rolink A, Melchers F, Andersson J. The SCID but not the RAG-2 gene product is required for S mu-S epsilon heavy chain class switching. *Immunity* 1996;5:319–330.

243. Manis JP, Dudley D, Kaylor L, et al. IgH class switch recombination to IgG1 in DNA-PKcs-deficient B cells. *Immunity* 2002;16:607–617.

244. Manis JP, Gu Y, Lansford R, et al. Ku70 is required for late B cell development and immunoglobulin heavy chain class switching. *J Exp Med* 1998;187:2081–2089.

245. Casellas R, Nussenzweig A, Wuerffel R, et al. Ku80 is required for immunoglobulin isotype switching. *EMBO J* 1998;17:2404–2411.

246. Zelazowski P, Max EE, Kehry MR, et al. Regulation of Ku expression in normal murine B cells by stimuli that promote switch recombination. *J Immunol* 1997;159:2559–2562.

247. Morio T, Hanissian SH, Bacharier LB, et al. Ku in the cytoplasm associates with CD40 in human B cells and translocates into the nucleus following incubation with IL-4 and anti-CD40 mAb. *Immunity* 1999;11:339–348.

248. Petersen S, Casellas R, Reina-San-Martin B, et al. AID is required to initiate Nbs1/gamma-H2AX focus formation and mutations at sites of class switching. *Nature* 2001;414:660–665.

249. van Engelen BG, Hiel JA, Gabreels FJ, et al. Decreased immunoglobulin class switching in Nijmegen breakage syndrome due to the DNA repair defect. *Hum Immunol* 2001;62:1324–1327.

250. Ma L, Hu B, Kenter AL. Ig S-gamma-specific DNA binding protein SNAP is related to the helix-loop-helix transcription factor E47. *Int Immunol* 1997;9:1021–1029.

251. Kenter AL, Wuerffel R, Sen R, et al. Switch recombination breakpoints occur at nonrandom positions in the S gamma tandem repeat. *J Immunol* 1993;151:4718–4731.

252. Snapper CM, Zelazowski P, Rosas FR, et al. B cells from p50/NF-kappa B knockout mice have selective defects in proliferation, differentiation, germ-line CH transcription, and Ig class switching. *J Immunol* 1996;156:183–191.

253. Jain A, Ma CA, Liu S, et al. Specific missense mutations in NEMO result in hyper-IgM syndrome with hypohydrotic ectodermal dysplasia. *Nat Immunol* 2001;2:223–228.

254. Quong MW, Harris DP, Swain SL, et al. E2A activity is induced during B-cell activation to promote immunoglobulin class switch recombination. *EMBO J* 1999;18:6307–6318.

255. Ehrenstein MR, Neuberger MS. Deficiency in Msh2 affects the efficiency and local sequence specificity of immunoglobulin class-switch recombination: parallels with somatic hypermutation. *EMBO J* 1999;18:3484–3490.

256. Schrader CE, Vardo J, Stavnezer J. Role for mismatch repair proteins Msh2, Mlh1, and Pms2 in immunoglobulin class switching shown by sequence analysis of recombination junctions. *J Exp Med* 2002;195:367–373.

257. Williams M, Maizels N. LR1, a lipopolysaccharide-responsive factor with binding sites in the immunoglobulin switch regions and heavy-chain enhancer. *Genes Dev* 1991;5:2353–2361.

258. Dempsey LA, Sun H, Hanakahi LA, et al. G4 DNA binding by LR1 and its subunits, nucleolin and hnRNP D, A role for G-G pairing in immunoglobulin switch recombination. *J Biol Chem* 1999;274:1066–1071.

259. Sun H, Yabuki A, Maizels N. A human nuclease specific for G4 DNA. *Proc Natl Acad Sci U S A* 2001;98:12444–12449.

260. Reference deleted in text.

261. Zhang K, Cheah HK. Cell-free recombination of immunoglobulin switch-region DNA with nuclear extracts. *Clin Immunol* 2000;94:140–151.

262. Borggrefe T, Wabl M, Akhmedov AT, et al. A B-cell–specific DNA recombination complex. *J Biol Chem* 1998;273:17025–17035.

263. Borggrefe T, Keshavarzi S, Gross B, et al. Impaired IgE response in SWAP-70–deficient mice. *Eur J Immunol* 2001;31:2467–2475.

264. Klein U, Esposito G, Baudat F, et al. Mice deficient for the type II topoisomerase–like DNA transesterase Spo11 show normal immunoglobulin somatic hypermutation and class switching. *Eur J Immunol* 2002;32:316–321.

265. Mandler R, Finkelman FD, Levine AD, et al. IL-4 induction of IgE class switching by lipopolysaccharide-activated murine B cells occurs predominantly through sequential switching. *J Immunol* 1993;150:407–418.

266. Jung S, Siebenkotten G, Radbruch A. Frequency of immunoglobulin E class switching is autonomously determined and independent of prior switching to other classes. *J Exp Med* 1994;179:2023–2026.

267. Mills FC, Mitchell MP, Harindranath N, et al. Human Ig S gamma regions and their participation in sequential switching to IgE. *J Immunol* 1995;155:3021–3036.

268. Baskin B, Islam KB, Evengard B, et al. Direct and sequential switching from mu to epsilon in patients with *Schistosoma mansoni* infection and atopic dermatitis. *Eur J Immunol* 1997;27:130–135.

269. Knight KL, Kingzette M, Crane MA, et al. Transchromosomally derived Ig heavy chains. *J Immunol* 1995;155:684–691.

270. Bakkus MH, Asosingh K, Vanderkerken K, et al. Myeloma isotype-switch variants in the murine 5T myeloma model: evidence that myeloma IgM and IgA expressing subclones can originate from the IgG expressing tumour. *Leukemia* 2001;15:1127–1132.

271. Perlmutter AP, Gilbert W. Antibodies of the secondary response can be expressed without switch recombination in normal mouse B cells. *Proc Natl Acad Sci U S A* 1984;81:7189–7193.

272. Fujieda S, Lin YQ, Saxon A, et al. Multiple types of chimeric germline Ig heavy chain transcripts in human B cells: evidence for trans-splicing of human Ig RNA. *J Immunol* 1996;157:3450–3459.

273. Mizuta TR, Suzuki N, Shimizu A, et al. Duplicated variable region genes account for double isotype expression in a human leukemic B–cell line that gives rise to single isotype-expressing cells. *J Biol Chem* 1991;266:12514–12521.

274. Forconi F, Sahota SS, Raspadori D, et al. Tumor cells of hairy cell leukemia express multiple clonally related immunoglobulin isotypes via RNA splicing. *Blood* 2001;98:1174–1181.

275. Weigert M, Riblet R. Genetic control of antibody variable regions. *Cold Spring Harb Symp Quant Biol* 1977;2:837–846.

276. Cohn M, Blomberg B, Geckler W, et al. First order considerations in analyzing the generator of diversity. In: Secarz EE, Williamson AR, Fox CF, eds. *The immune system—genes, receptors, signals*. New York: Academic Press, 1974:89–93.

277. Crews S, Griffin J, Huang H, et al. A single VH gene segment encodes the immune response to phosphorylcholine: somatic mutation is correlated with the class of the antibody. *Cell* 1981;25:59–66.

278. Manser T, Parhami SB, Margolies MN, et al. Somatically mutated forms of a major anti—p-azophenylarsonate antibody variable region with drastically reduced affinity for p-azophenylarsonate. By-products of an antigen-driven immune response? *J Exp Med* 1987;166:1456–1463.

279. Ray SK, Putterman C, Diamond B. Pathogenic autoantibodies are routinely generated during the response to foreign antigen: a paradigm for autoimmune disease. *Proc Natl Acad Sci U S A* 1996;93:2019–2024.

280. Choe J, Kim HS, Zhang X, et al. Cellular and molecular factors that regulate the differentiation and apoptosis of germinal center B cells. Anti-Ig down-regulates Fas expression of CD40 ligand-stimulated germinal center B cells and inhibits Fas-mediated apoptosis. *J Immunol* 1996;157:1006–1016.

281. Hennino A, Berard M, Krammer PH, et al. FLICE-inhibitory protein is a key regulator of germinal center B cell apoptosis. *J Exp Med* 2001;193:447–458.

282. Eisen HN, Siskind GW. Variations in affinities of antibodies during the immune response. *Biochemistry* 1964;3:996–1008.

283. Takahashi Y, Cerasoli DM, Dal Porto JM, et al. Relaxed negative selection in germinal centers and impaired affinity maturation in bcl-xL transgenic mice. *J Exp Med* 1999;190:399–410.

284. Lebecque S, de Bouteiller BO, Arpin C, et al. Germinal center founder cells display propensity for apoptosis before onset of somatic mutation. *J Exp Med* 1997;185:563–571.

285. Jacob J, Kelsoe G. *In situ* studies of the primary immune response to (4-hydroxy-3-nitrophenyl)acetyl. II. A common clonal origin for periarteriolar lymphoid sheath-associated foci and germinal centers. *J Exp Med* 1992;176:679–687.

286. Zheng B, Han S, Kelsoe G. T helper cells in murine germinal centers are antigen-specific emigrants that downregulate Thy-1. *J Exp Med* 1996;184:1083–1091.

287. Razanajaona D, van Kooten C, Lebecque S, et al. Somatic mutations in human Ig variable genes correlate with a partially functional CD40-ligand in the X-linked hyper-IgM syndrome. *J Immunol* 1996;157:1492–1498.

288. Zan H, Cerutti A, Dramitinos P, et al. Induction of Ig somatic hypermutation and class switching in a human monoclonal IgM+ IgD+ B cell line *in vitro*: definition of the requirements and modalities of hypermutation. *J Immunol* 1999;162:3437–3447.

289. Dahlenborg K, Pound JD, Gordon J, et al. Signals sustaining human immunoglobulin V gene hypermutation in isolated germinal centre B cells. *Immunology* 2000;101:210–217.

290. Casamayor PM, Khan M, MacLennan IC. A subset of CD4+ memory T cells contains preformed CD40 ligand that is rapidly but transiently expressed on their surface after activation through the T cell receptor complex. *J Exp Med* 1995;181:1293–1301.

291. Pulendran B, Kannourakis G, Nouri S, et al. Soluble antigen can cause enhanced apoptosis of germinal-centre B cells. *Nature* 1995;375:331–334.

292. Liu YJ, de Bouteiller BO, Arpin C, et al. Normal human IgD+IgM− germinal center B cells can express up to 80 mutations in the variable region of their IgD transcripts. *Immunity* 1996;4:603–613.

293. Roes J, Rajewsky K. Immunoglobulin D (IgD)–deficient mice reveal an auxiliary receptor function for IgD in antigen-mediated recruitment of B cells. *J Exp Med* 1993;177:45–55.

294. Kuppers R, Zhao M, Hansmann ML, et al. Tracing B cell development in human germinal centres by molecular analysis of single cells picked from histological sections. *EMBO J* 1993;12:4955–4967.

295. Michael N, Martin TE, Nicolae D, et al. Effects of sequence and structure on the hypermutability of immunoglobulin genes. *Immunity* 2002;16:123–134.

296. Casamayor-Palleja M, Mondiere P, Verschelde C, et al. BCR ligation reprograms B cells for migration to the T zone and B-cell follicle sequentially. *Blood* 2002;99:1913–1921.

297. Kepler TB, Perelson AS. Cyclic re-entry of germinal center B cells and the efficiency of affinity maturation. *Immunol Today* 1993;14:412–415.

298. Matsumoto M, Lo SF, Carruthers CJ, et al. Affinity maturation without germinal centres in lymphotoxin-alpha–deficient mice. *Nature* 1996;382:462–466.

299. Toellner KM, Jenkinson WE, Taylor DR, et al. Low-level hypermutation in T cell–independent germinal centers compared with high mutation rates associated with T cell–dependent germinal centers. *J Exp Med* 2002;195:383–389.

300. Rajewsky K. Clonal selection and learning in the antibody system. *Nature* 1996;381:751–758.

301. Picard D, Schaffner W. Unrearranged immunoglobulin lambda variable region is transcribed in kappa-producing myelomas. *EMBO J* 1984;3:3031–3035.

302. Rogozin IB, Kolchanov NA. Somatic hypermutagenesis in immunoglobulin genes. II. Influence of neighbouring base sequences on mutagenesis. *Biochim Biophys Acta* 1992;1171:11–18.

303. Shapiro GS, Aviszus K, Murphy J, et al. Evolution of Ig DNA sequence to target specific base positions within codons for somatic hypermutation. *J Immunol* 2002;168:2302–2306.

304. Klix N, Jolly CJ, Davies SL, et al. Multiple sequences from downstream of the J kappa cluster can combine to recruit somatic hypermutation to a heterologous, upstream mutation domain. *Eur J Immunol* 1998;28:317–326.

305. Kodama M, Hayashi R, Nishizumi H, et al. The PU.1 and NF-EM5 binding motifs in the Igkappa 3′ enhancer are responsible for directing somatic hypermutations to the intrinsic hotspots in the transgenic Vkappa gene. *Int Immunol* 2001;13:1415–1422.

306. van der Stoep N, Gorman JR, Alt FW. Reevaluation of 3′Ekappa

307. Terauchi A, Hayashi K, Kitamura D, et al. A pivotal role for DNase I-sensitive regions 3b and/or 4 in the induction of somatic hypermutation of IgH genes. *J Immunol* 2001;167:811–820.

308. Klotz EL, Storb U. Somatic hypermutation of a lambda 2 transgene under the control of the lambda enhancer or the heavy chain intron enhancer. *J Immunol* 1996;157:4458–4463.

309. Betz AG, Milstein C, Gonzalez FA, et al. Elements regulating somatic hypermutation of an immunoglobulin kappa gene: critical role for the intron enhancer/matrix attachment region. *Cell* 1994;77:239–248.

310. Bachl J, Wabl M. Enhancers of hypermutation. *Immunogenetics* 1996;45:59–64.

311. Yelamos J, Klix N, Goyenechea B, et al. Targeting of non-Ig sequences in place of the V segment by somatic hypermutation. *Nature* 1995;376:225–229.

312. Tumas-Brundage K, Vora KA, Giusti AM, et al. Characterization of the cis-acting elements required for somatic hypermutation of murine antibody V genes using conventional transgenic and transgene homologous recombination approaches. *Semin Immunol* 1996;8:141–150.

313. Hengstschlager M, Williams M, Maizels N. A lambda 1 transgene under the control of a heavy chain promoter and enhancer does not undergo somatic hypermutation. *Eur J Immunol* 1994;24:1649–1656.

314. Jolly CJ, Neuberger MS. Somatic hypermutation of immunoglobulin kappa transgenes: association of mutability with demethylation. *Immunol Cell Biol* 2001;79:18–22.

315. Bachl J, Carlson C, Gray-Schopfer V, et al. Increased transcription levels induce higher mutation rates in a hypermutating cell line. *J Immunol* 2001;166:5051–5057.

316. Storb U. The molecular basis of somatic hypermutation of immunoglobulin genes. *Curr Opin Immunol* 1996;8:206–214.

317. Migliazza A, Martinotti S, Chen W, et al. Frequent somatic hypermutation of the 5′ noncoding region of the BCL6 gene in B-cell lymphoma. *Proc Natl Acad Sci U S A* 1995;92:12520–12524.

318. Muschen M, Re D, Jungnickel B, et al. Somatic mutation of the CD95 gene in human B cells as a side-effect of the germinal center reaction. *J Exp Med* 2000;192:1833–1840.

319. Shen HM, Michael N, Kim N, et al. The TATA binding protein, c-Myc and survivin genes are not somatically hypermutated, while Ig and BCL6 genes are hypermutated in human memory B cells. *Int Immunol* 2000;12:1085–1093.

320. Bachl J, Olsson C, Chitkara N, et al. The Ig mutator is dependent on the presence, position, and orientation of the large intron enhancer. *Proc Natl Acad Sci U S A* 1998;95:2396–2399.

321. Pasqualucci L, Neumeister P, Goossens T, et al. Hypermutation of multiple proto-oncogenes in B-cell diffuse large-cell lymphomas. *Nature* 2001;412:341–346.

322. Peters A, Storb U. Somatic hypermutation of immunoglobulin genes is linked to transcription initiation. *Immunity* 1996;4:57–65.

323. Winter DB, Sattar N, Mai JJ, et al. Insertion of 2 kb of bacteriophage DNA between an immunoglobulin promoter and leader exon stops somatic hypermutation in a kappa transgene. *Mol Immunol* 1997;34:359–366.

324. Reynaud CA, Frey S, Aoufouchi S, et al. Transcription, beta-like DNA polymerases and hypermutation. *Philos Trans R Soc Lond B Biol Sci* 2001;356:91–97.

325. Bachl J, Wabl M. An immunoglobulin mutator that targets G.C base pairs. *Proc Natl Acad Sci U S A* 1996;93:851–855.

325a. Rada C, Williams GT, Nilsen H, et al. Immunoglobulin isotype switching is inhibited and somatic hypermutation perturbed in UNG-deficient mice. *Curr Biol* 2002;12:1748–1756.

326. Betz AG, Rada C, Pannell R, et al. Passenger transgenes reveal intrinsic specificity of the antibody hypermutation mechanism: clustering, polarity, and specific hot spots. *Proc Natl Acad Sci U S A* 1993;90:2385–2388.

327. Insel RA, Varade WS. Bias in somatic hypermutation of human VH genes. *Int Immunol* 1994;6:1437–1443.

328. Martin A, Bardwell PD, Woo CJ, et al. Activation-induced cytidine deaminase turns on somatic hypermutation in hybridomas. *Nature* 2002;415:802–806.

329. Yoshikawa K, Okazaki I, Eto T, et al. AID enzyme–induced hypermutation in an actively transcribed gene in fibroblasts. *Science* 2002;296:2033–2036.

330. Brenner S, Milstein C. Origin of antibody variation. *Nature* 1966; 211:242–243.

331. Goossens T, Klein U, Kuppers R. Frequent occurrence of deletions and duplications during somatic hypermutation: implications for oncogene translocations and heavy chain disease. *Proc Natl Acad Sci U S A* 1998;95:2463–2468.

332. Sale JE, Neuberger MS. TdT-accessible breaks are scattered over the immunoglobulin V domain in a constitutively hypermutating B cell line. *Immunity* 1998;9:859–869.

333. Papavasiliou FN, Schatz DG. Cell-cycle-regulated DNA double-stranded breaks in somatic hypermutation of immunoglobulin genes. *Nature* 2000;408:216–221.

334. Bross L, Fukita Y, McBlane F, et al. DNA double-strand breaks in immunoglobulin genes undergoing somatic hypermutation. *Immunity* 2000;13:589–597.

335. Bemark M, Sale JE, Kim HJ, et al. Somatic hypermutation in the absence of DNA-dependent protein kinase catalytic subunit (DNA-PK(cs)) or recombination-activating gene (RAG)1 activity. *J Exp Med* 2000;192:1509–1514.

335a. Bross L, Muramatsu M, Kinoshita K, et al. DNA double-strand breaks: prior to but not sufficient in targeting hypermutation. *J Exp Med* 2002; 195:1187–1192.

335b. Papavasiliou FN, Schatz D. The activation-induced deaminase funtions in a postcleavage step of the somatic hypermutation process. *J Exp Med* 2002;195:1193–1198.

336. Nagaoka H, Muramatsu M, Yamamura N, et al. Activation-induced deaminase (AID)–directed hypermutation in the immunoglobulin Smu region: implication of AID involvement in a common step of class switch recombination and somatic hypermutation. *J Exp Med* 2002;195:529–534.

337. Johnson RE, Washington MT, Haracska L, et al. Eukaryotic polymerases iota and zeta act sequentially to bypass DNA lesions. *Nature* 2000;406:1015–1019.

338. Zan H, Komori A, Li Z, et al. The translesion DNA polymerase zeta plays a major role in Ig and bcl-6 somatic hypermutation. *Immunity* 2001;14:643–653.

339. Diaz M, Verkoczy LK, Flajnik MF, et al. Decreased frequency of somatic hypermutation and impaired affinity maturation but intact germinal center formation in mice expressing antisense RNA to DNA polymerase zeta. *J Immunol* 2001;167:327–335.

340. Zeng X, Winter DB, Kasmer C, et al. DNA polymerase eta is an A-T mutator in somatic hypermutation of immunoglobulin variable genes. *Nat Immunol* 2001;2:537–541.

341. Dominguez O, Ruiz JF, Lain de Lera T, et al. DNA polymerase mu (Pol mu), homologous to TdT, could act as a DNA mutator in eukaryotic cells. *EMBO J* 2000;19:1731–1742.

342. Aoufouchi S, Flatter E, Dahan A, et al. Two novel human and mouse DNA polymerases of the polX family. *Nucleic Acids Res* 2000;28: 3684–3693.

343. Bertocci B, De Smet A, Flatter E, et al. Cutting edge: DNA polymerases mu and lambda are dispensable for Ig gene hypermutation. *J Immunol* 2002;168:3702–3706.

344. Frank EG, Tissier A, McDonald JP, et al. Altered nucleotide misinsertion fidelity associated with poliota-dependent replication at the end of a DNA template. *EMBO J* 2001;20:2914–2922.

345. Park K, Kim J, Kim HS, et al. Isolated human germinal center centroblasts have an intact mismatch repair system. *J Immunol* 1998; 161:6128–6132.

346. Cascalho M, Wong J, Steinberg C, et al. Mismatch repair co-opted by hypermutation. *Science* 1998;279:1207–1210.

347. Reynaud CA, Bertocci B, Frey S, et al. Mismatch repair and immunoglobulin gene hypermutation: did we learn something? *Immunol Today* 1999;20:522–527.

348. Rada C, Ehrenstein MR, Neuberger MS, et al. Hot spot focusing of somatic hypermutation in MSH2-deficient mice suggests two stages of mutational targeting. *Immunity* 1998;9:135–141.

349. Strathern JN, Shafer BK, McGill CB. DNA synthesis errors associated with double-strand–break repair. *Genetics* 1995;140:965–972.

350. Bird RE, Hardman KD, Jacobson JW, et al. Single-chain antigen-binding proteins. *Science* 1988;242:423–426.

351. Merchant AM, Zhu Z, Yuan JQ, et al. An efficient route to human bispecific IgG. *Nat Biotechnol* 1998;16:677–681.

352. Mhashilkar AM, Bagley J, Chen SY, et al. Inhibition of HIV-1 Tat-mediated LTR transactivation and HIV-1 infection by anti-Tat single chain intrabodies. *EMBO J* 1995;14:1542–1551.

353. Hoogenboom HR. Overview of antibody phage-display technology and its applications. *Methods Mol Biol* 2002;178:1–37.

354. Schmidt EV, Pattengale PK, Weir L, et al. Transgenic mice bearing the human c-myc gene activated by an immunoglobulin enhancer: a pre-B–cell lymphoma model. *Proc Natl Acad Sci U S A* 1988;85:6047–6051.

355. Maxwell IH, Glode LM, Maxwell F. Expression of the diphtheria toxin A-chain coding sequence under the control of promoters and enhancers from immunoglobulin genes as a means of directing toxicity to B-lymphoid cells. *Cancer Res* 1991;51:4299–4304.

356. Sarris A, Ford R. Recent advances in the molecular pathogenesis of lymphomas. *Curr Opin Oncol* 1999;11:351–363.

357. Sievers EL, Radich JP. Detection of minimal residual disease in acute leukemia. *Curr Opin Hematol* 2000;7:212–216.

358. Schroeder HWJ, Hillson JL, Perlmutter RM. Structure and evolution of mammalian VH families. *Int Immunol* 1990;2:41–50.

359. Cook GP, Tomlinson IM. The human immunoglobulin VH repertoire. *Immunol Today* 1995;16:237–242.

CHAPTER 6

B-Lymphocyte Development and Biology

Richard R. Hardy

Introduction
B-Cell Development in Mice
  Early Development · Bone Marrow Developmental Stages · Peripheral Maturation Stages and Functional Subsets
B-Cell Development in Humans—Similarities and Differences with Mice
  Fetal Development · Bone Marrow Development · Germinal Center Differentiation · Abnormalities of Development · New Insights into Treatment of B-Cell Malignancies
Alternative Strategies for B-Cell Development
  Chicken · Rabbit · Two B-Cell Developmental Pathways?
Concluding Remarks
Acknowledgments
References

INTRODUCTION

B-lymphocytes constitute one of the major arms of the immune system, being responsible for humoral immunity. B cells in humans and mice are produced throughout life, primarily in the fetal liver before birth and in the bone marrow afterwards. Their development from hematopoietic stem cells has been extensively characterized in mice, and the generation of numerous gene-targeted and transgenic lines in many cases has provided crucial information on the role of transcription factors, cellular receptors, and interactions that are critical in their generation. The complexity of this process is now apparent and their differentiation into multiple peripheral subsets with distinctive functions is also widely appreciated. This chapter focuses on B-cell development and function in the mouse, touching briefly on aspects of human B cells that are similar or distinctive with a focus on immunodeficiency. I conclude with a brief description of novel aspects of B-lymphocyte development in other species, highlighting differences from development in mouse and human.

B-CELL DEVELOPMENT IN MICE

In mice, B cells are produced from hematopoietic stem cells through a complex process of differentiation that is gradually becoming understood. One of the goals of classical hematology is the delineation of differentiation pathways for different lineages of blood cells, and this is rapidly being achieved.

Over the past decade there has been considerable progress in utilizing the ordered expression of a diverse set of cell surface and internal proteins, some with known functions and others whose roles are only suspected, to construct a description of the intermediate stages that cells transit as they develop into B-lymphocytes. A simplified example of such a description is presented in Fig. 1. Thus, uncommitted hematopoietic stem cells generate more restricted progeny, recognizable (in this example) by expression of IL-7Rα and these in turn produce B-lineage–restricted cells identified by expression of CD45R/B220 (and, importantly, by absence of CD19).

This kind of pathway is constructed based on isolation and short-term culture of intermediate stages; progression is allowed, which helps to define the order. This framework for development serves as a starting point for analysis of the effects of transcription factors, microenvironmental interactions, cytokines, and natural or engineered mutations. It can also be extended by analysis of gene or protein expression at distinct intermediate stages. Critical processes, such as D-J rearrangement and Ig heavy-chain expression can also be mapped onto this framework. Progress in this work allows additional questions to be approached, such as key regulatory interactions, developmental checkpoints, and the mechanism of B-lineage commitment.

In this chapter, I first discuss sites of B-lineage development at different stages of ontogeny, and then focus on what is known about their development in the bone marrow of adult mice, highlighting the function of the pre–B-cell receptor and

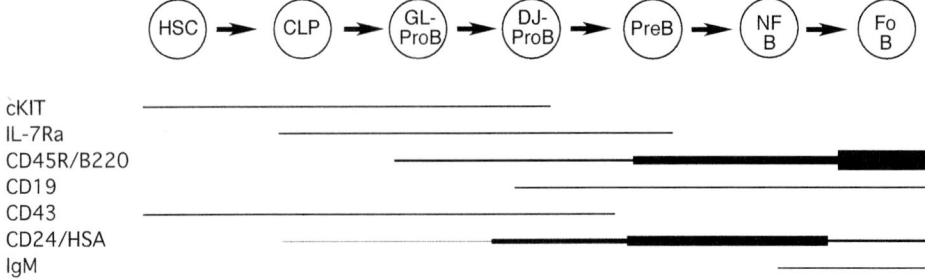

FIG. 1. Simplified differentiation diagram for development of B cells from hematopoietic stem cells. Expression of the each surface protein is indicated by a line. For CD45R/B220 and CD24/HSA, the distinct levels of expression are also indicated. HSC, hematopoietic stem cell; CLP, common lymphoid progenitor; GL-ProB, germline pro–B; DJ-ProB, DJ-rearranged Pro-B; NF B, newly formed B; Fo B, follicular B.

the crucial role of immunoglobulin heavy and light chains in guiding development. In later sections I consider their differentiation into various specialized peripheral populations and emphasize insights into B-cell selection gained from various transgenic models of tolerance.

Early Development

Sites of B-Lymphopoiesis During Ontogeny

In the mouse, hematopoiesis occurs predominantly in the fetal liver prior to birth, in the spleen just prior to and shortly after birth, and in the bone marrow thereafter. Prior to liver hematopoiesis, the blood islands of the yolk sac (YS) contain the first identifiable hematopoietic cells, nucleated erythrocytes with embryonic forms of hemoglobin (1). However, these early YS precursors appear incapable of generating other blood cell lineages and generation of all blood cell types, including lymphocytes (2,3), initiates at around 9 to 10 days post coitum (dpc) in an embryonic region referred to as the splanchnopleura/AGM (or simply Sp/AGM). Cells from this site are capable of long-term repopulation of lethally irradiated adult recipients with all blood lineages (4,5). These cells colonize the fetal liver at about 11 dpc, initiating hematopoiesis there. Thus, there are two sites of very early hematopoietic precursors, with one in the YS largely limited to erythropoiesis and the other in the Sp/AGM capable of complete (referred to as "definitive") hematopoiesis. However, it may be that precursors in the YS have a broader lineage potential in the fetal microenvironment, as when they are injected directly into the newborn liver (6).

Hematopoietic stem cells (HSCs) capable of developing into all the blood cell types are produced in the Sp/AGP and migrate to the fetal liver at about day 10. Thereafter, B-lineage cells develop largely in a wave, with earlier stages present at earlier times and later stages predominating at later times, close to (and shortly after) birth (7,8). This progression with gestation day is easily visualized by staining with antibodies that delineate B-cell development as shown in Fig. 2. Early precursors can also be found in the fetal omentum (9). In contrast with the bone marrow, cells at most differentiation stages in the fetal liver appear to be rapidly proliferating,

so that larger and larger numbers of B-lineage cells are detected at progressive days of gestation. Another distinction with bone marrow development in the adult is the absence of terminal deoxynucleotidyl transferase (TdT) (10,11), an enzyme that mediates the nontemplated addition of nucleotides at the D-J and V-D junctions of the Ig heavy chain (12–14). Therefore, heavy chains produced during fetal development have little or no N-region addition, and CDR3 diversity is constrained even further by favoring of short stretches of homology at the V-D and D-J junctions (15,16). Rearrangement of certain V or D elements may also differ between fetal and adult development, as for example, the reported high utilization of the DFL16.1 segment in fetal liver (17). Differential expression of genes other than TdT also distinguishes B-cell development during fetal life from that in the adult, including the precursor lymphocyte regulated myosin light chain like PLRLC transcripts (11,18) and MHC class II (19,20). There is a recent report that ablation of the cytokine IL-7 completely eliminates bone-marrow B-lineage development while sparing fetal development (21), suggesting a difference in growth requirements. The details of lineage-restricted progenitors may also differ (22). The B-cell progeny of this early fetal wave may largely consist of B cells quite distinct from adult-derived cells, which populate the B-1 subset (23).

At birth, B-cell development can also be detected in the spleen, but development at this site gradually decreases to very low levels by 2 to 4 weeks of age. Over this same period, B-cell development shifts to the bone marrow, and thereafter it continues for the life of the animal. B-lymphopoiesis decreases in aged mice and this may be due to diminished responsiveness of precursors to IL-7 (24,25). Early B-lineage cells from bone marrow of aged (2-year-old) mice also show distinctively decreased expression of surrogate light chain, possibly due to lower levels of the E2A transcriptional activator (26,27).

Stem Cells, Commitment, and Early B-Cell Progenitors in Bone Marrow

B cells are continually generated from hematopoietic stem cells (HSCs) in the bone marrow of adult mice. Considerable

Fetal Liver Gestation Day

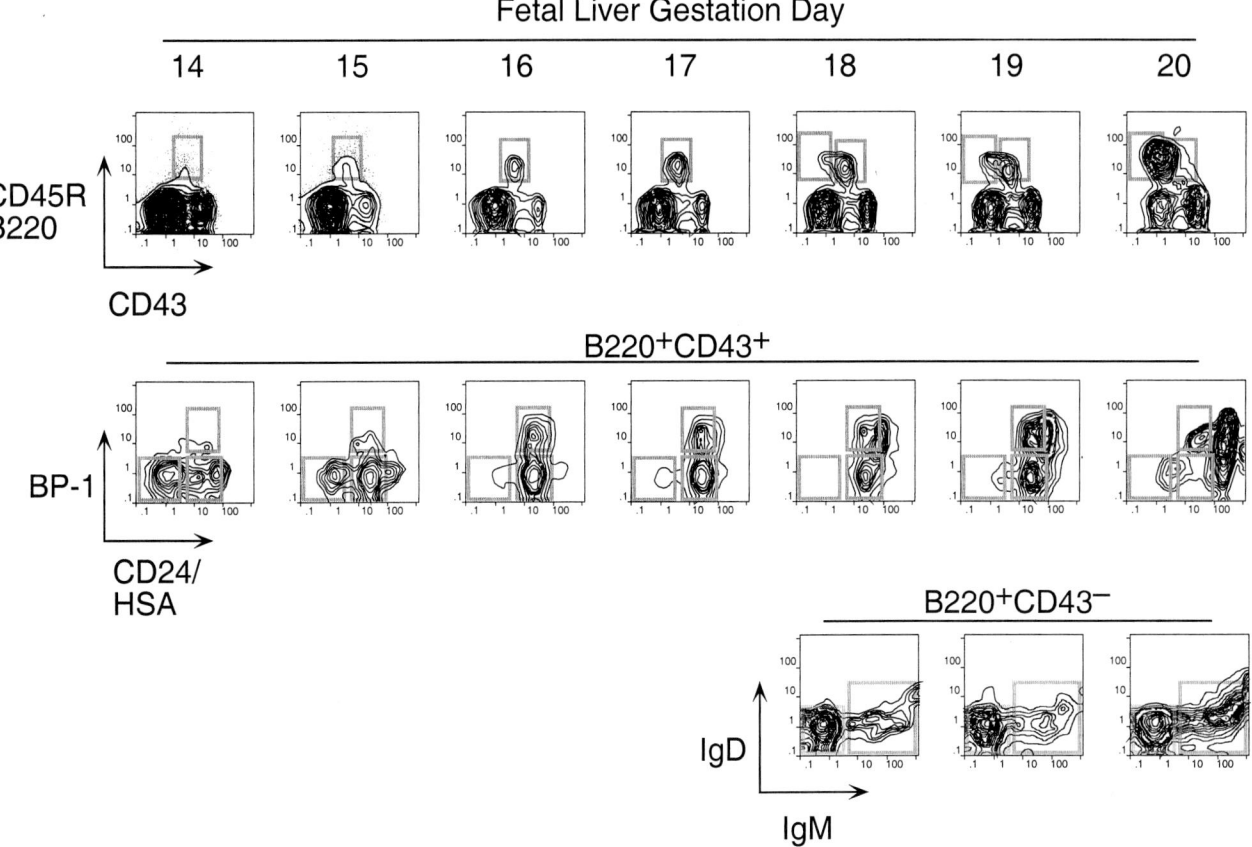

FIG. 2. Phenotypic progression of developing B-lineage cells in mouse fetal liver analyzed at different days of gestation. Note that B220$^+$CD43$^+$ cells precede B220$^+$CD43$^-$ cells and that within the B220$^+$CD43$^+$ fraction, HSA$^-$ cells precede HSA$^+$ cells, and BP-1$^-$ cells precede BP-1$^+$ cells. Within the B220$^+$CD43$^-$ fraction, the IgM$^+$ percentage increases until birth (at about day 20).

effort has focused on evaluating the functional capacity of fractions of bone marrow cells to repopulate diverse lineages of blood cells and this work has progressed to the stage of defining a phenotype for such cells, with expression of c-kit constituting an important marker in the so-called "lineage-negative" subset (28,29). This is the small fraction of bone marrow cells (less than 5%) that lacks expression of a panel of "differentiation markers," cell surface molecules that are expressed on later stages of various hematopoietic cell lineages. Careful analysis of this HSC fraction using additional markers has shown that it represents perhaps 1/30,000 of nucleated bone-marrow cells with as few as 10 mediating multilineage repopulation in cell transfer assays (30–32). An important capacity of "true" or "long-term repopulating" HSCs is their ability to give rise to cells in a recipient mouse that can also repopulate all the blood cell lineages upon re-transfer into a second host, indicating a capacity for extensive self-renewal without differentiation into more restricted progenitors.

Recently, a great deal of interest has focused on defining and characterizing lineage-restricted progenitors, such as the common myeloid and common lymphoid progenitors (33–35). The common lymphoid progenitor (CLP) is a cell fraction lacking a panel of lineage markers, but expressing the IL-7Rα chain and also bearing lower levels of c-kit com-

pared to the HSCs. Analysis in a variety of functional assays suggests that these cells can generate B, T, NK, and a subset of dendritic cells, but no other blood-cell lineages. The reason for this restriction is under intensive study and down-regulation of the receptor for granulocyte–myeloid-stimulating factor may be a key event in this process (36). Cells with the CLP phenotype constitute about 1/3000 of bone marrow cells.

CLP cells can give rise in short-term cultures to cells of the B lineage, naturally raising the issue of when cells become restricted to the B lineage. The majority of cells growing in stromal cultures give rise only to B cells upon transfer into mice, and the phenotype of these cells has been well characterized (37). Most have at least some heavy-chain rearrangement and bear the B-lineage marker CD19 (38,39). There is less certainty concerning the cells isolated directly from primary lymphoid tissues, as such cells will undoubtedly be quite rare, similar to the CLP and HSC. Most of the CD45R/B220$^+$ cells in bone marrow are also CD19$^+$, and the earliest of these already show extensive D-J rearrangement (see below). However, a subset of B220$^+$ cells lack detectable CD19 expression and cells within this fraction can generate CD19$^+$ cells in a short-term stromal culture with IL-7. Such cells are found within the CD43$^+$CD24^{low} fraction (Fr A, 1%

of bone marrow) of B220$^+$ cells in bone marrow, but this fraction also contains other cell types, including NK-lineage precursors (39,40). Thus, it is necessary to exclude cells lacking AA4.1 (about half) (39), and recent analysis (41) suggests that exclusion of Ly6c$^+$ cells (about half of the AA4.1$^+$ cells) is another useful criterion for purifying this subset. Many of these Ly6c$^+$ cells also express CD4, and recent work suggests that these are plasmacytoid dendritic cells (42,43). A phenotypic approach for enriching the B-lineage subset is shown in Fig. 3A. Such cells, constituting about 1/500 of bone marrow, express readily detectable levels of TdT (as do the CLP precursors), but have little if any rearrangement. Nevertheless, cells in this fraction are largely B-lineage restricted, failing to generate other blood lineages and, importantly, not repopulating T cells in intrathymic injection assays (Fig. 3B).

Interesting issues remain with regard to the extent of lineage restriction of cells at these early stages in B-cell development. For example, there is evidence that cells restricted to generating B and myeloid/macrophage lineages

exist, at least in the fetal liver (44). There are also clear data demonstrating that suppression of other blood-cell lineages in D-J–rearranged (pro–B stage) bone-marrow cells is dependent on the Pax-5 gene that encodes the BSAP transcription factor (45,46), yet CD19 is a well-established target of BSAP (47) and the pro–B-stage cells of the B-lineage–restricted germline clearly lack CD19 (48). There is also apparently a different dependence of fetal liver B-lymphopoiesis on BSAP compared with that in bone marrow, as determined in analysis of Pax-5–null mice (49). Thus, an important priority for further investigation in this area will be determining the mechanism of commitment at this cell stage, in bone marrow and fetal liver.

Transcription Factors Important in B-Lineage Development

The GATA-2 and Runx1/AML1 transcription factors are required for the development of hematopoietic stem cells that are the precursors of all blood-cell lineages, including B cells

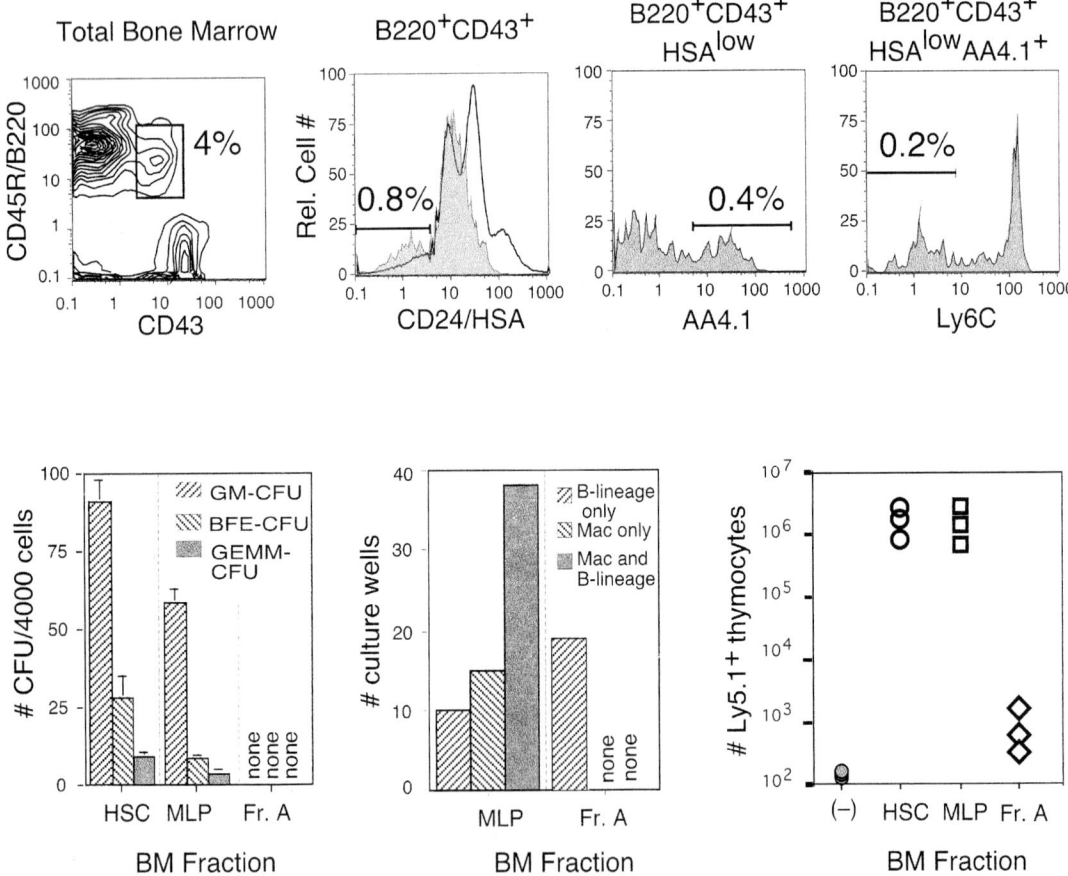

FIG. 3. A: One approach for purifying the earliest stage of B-lineage cells in mouse bone marrow. B220$^+$CD43$^+$ cells are restricted to low-level expression of CD24/HSA. This fraction, shown in the third panel is then restricted to only cells expressing AA4.1, and finally, these cells are restricted to the portion lacking Ly6C expression. The resulting fraction, germline pro–B cells, is referred to as Fr A. **B:** Functional analysis of early B-lineage cells, showing absence of myeloid, erythroid, or T-lineage generation, but production of B-lineage cells. HSC fraction is lineage-marker negative, c-kit$^+$. MLP (multilineage progenitor) is lineage negative, CD43$^+$, CD24/HSA^{low}, CD4^{low}. Fr A as described in **(A)**.

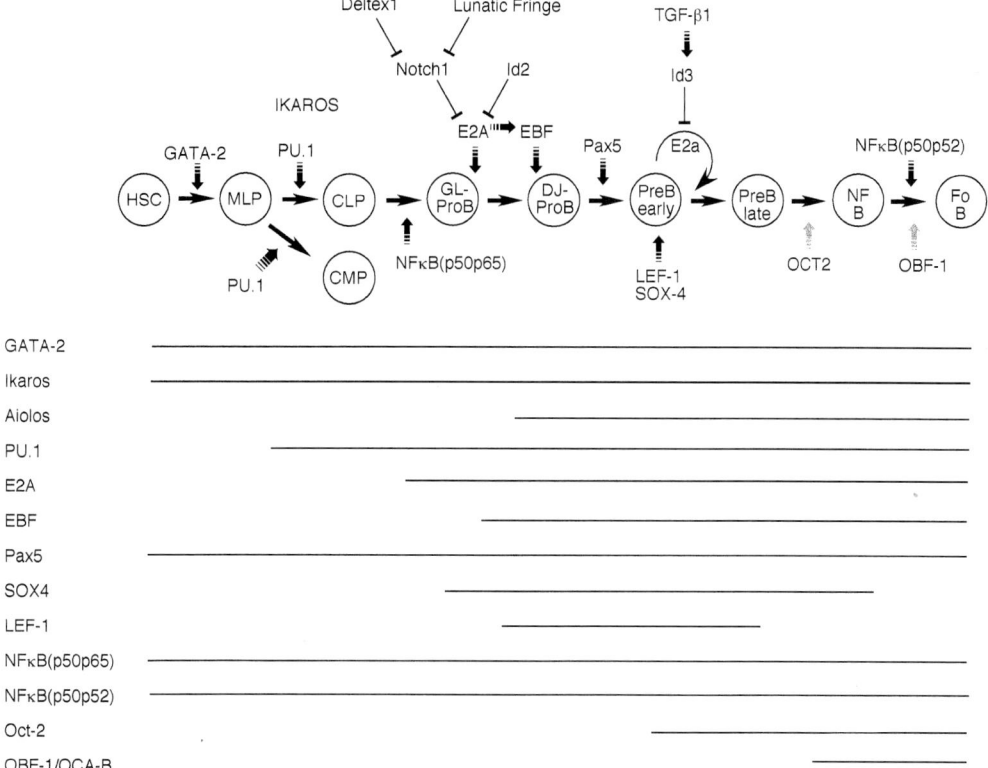

FIG. 4. Transcription factors important at different stages in B-cell development in mouse bone marrow. Positive/activating activity *(arrows)* and negative or blocking activity *(bars)* are shown. Rapidly cycling stage, early pre-B, is also indicated. Predominant stages of expression are indicated below the diagram.

(50–54) (Fig. 4). Somewhat later acting, but still very early in development is the Ikaros transcription factor (55–57). Ikaros and the related transcription factor Aiolos (58) play important roles in lymphocyte development. Ikaros is expressed very early in hematopoietic precursors. Ikaros-null mice lack B-lineage cells (57) and a different Ikaros mutant that acts as a dominant negative completely blocks lymphoid development (55). Ikaros activates numerous early B-lineage genes, including TdT, RAG1, λ5, and VpreB. Aiolos is detected somewhat later in development, at about the stage of B-lineage commitment, and its expression increases further at later stages.

PU.1, an Ets-family transcription factor, is critical for progression to the earliest stage of lymphoid development, as demonstrated by the inability of PU.1-null precursors to generate lymphocytes (59,60). An important target of PU.1 for B-lineage development is the gene for Ig-β, known as MB-1. The level of PU.1 appears to be critical for development along the B lineage—while low-level expression induced in PU.1null mice allowed B-lineage development, high-level expression blocked this and fostered myeloid lineage development (61), likely due to differential induction of the IL-7Rα and M-CSF receptor chains (62). In fact, retroviral mediated expression of the IL-7Rα chain complements defective B-lymphopoiesis in PU.1-null bone-marrow hematopoietic precursor cells (63).

E2A codes for two proteins, E12 and E47, members of the basic helix-loop-helix family of transcription factors, and its induction is crucial from the earliest stages of B-lineage development, since all stages after CD19 expression are absent from E2A-null mice (64,65). These mice lack detectable D-J rearrangements and, interestingly, such rearrangements can be induced in nonlymphoid cells by introduction of the RAG genes and ectopic expression of E2A (66), implicating this transcription factor in the process of chromatin remodeling of the Ig heavy-chain locus that permits accessibility by the recombinase machinery. The regulation of E2A is crucial for B-lineage development, as negative regulators such as Notch1 and ID2 have been shown to block this lineage and to induce alternate cell fates to the T and NK lineages (67–70). Consistent with this picture, ectopic expression of genes that negatively regulate Notch1, Lunatic fringe, and Deltex1, induce the B-cell fate (71,72).

Expression of the early B-cell factor (EBF), a member of the O/E-protein transcription-factor family, is requisite for progression of early B-lineage progenitors to the D-J–rearranged pro–B stage (Fr B), as shown in EBF-null mice (73). EBF and E2A act at a similar stage in early B-lineage development, and these two transcription factors can act together to up-regulate a family of early B-lineage–specific genes, including Ig-α/β, VpreB/λ5, and RAG1/2 (74,75). There is evidence that E2A up-regulates expression of EBF, found by transfection of E2A in a macrophage cell line (76), suggesting an ordering of these two in development.

BSAP, the product of the Pax-5 gene, is expressed throughout B-cell development until the plasma cell stage (77). Pax-5/BSAP transcriptional targets include CD19 and BLNK, and expression of this transcription factor acts to up-regulate V to D-J heavy-chain rearrangement (49). Pax-5–null mutant mice show arrest in bone marrow development at the pro–B stage, likely due to the lack of complete heavy-chain rearrangements and also due to the absence of the critical B-cell adaptor protein, BLNK, which serves to link the pre-BCR to the intracellular signaling pathway via the tyrosine kinase Syk (78). BSAP/Pax-5 also acts to repress alternate cell fates, since pro–B phenotype cells isolated from Pax-5–null bone marrow can generate diverse hematopoietic cell lineages, in contrast with such cells from wild-type mice that are B-lineage restricted (45,46). Finally, as mentioned above, in contrast with bone marrow, the absence of BSAP/Pax-5 arrests B-cell development prior to the B220$^+$ stage in fetal liver, suggesting a crucial difference in the early dependence on this transcription factor (49).

Lymphoid-enhancer binding factor (LEF-1) shows a pattern of expression restricted to the pro–B and pre–B stages of B-cell development (79). Targeted inactivation of the LEF-1 gene allows B-cell development, but with reduced numbers (80). This is because LEF-1 regulates transcription of the Wnt/β-catenin signaling pathway whose activation increases proliferation and decreases apoptosis of early B-lineage cells. In fact, exposure of normal pro–B cells to Wnt protein induces their proliferation (80). Interestingly, there is a counter-proliferative signal that can act at the pre–B proliferative stage, mediated by TGF-β1 (81). It appears that this occurs due to induction of the Id-3 inhibitor that negatively regulates the activity of E2A (82). Another transcription factor whose expression is similar to LEF-1 is SOX-4, and its inactivation also results in the inability of normal early B-lineage cell expansion and a block at the pro–B stage (83).

Several forms of NFκb subunits are expressed throughout B-cell development and this transcription factor can regulate kappa light-chain expression and also growth factor signaling (84). Mice lacking the p65 subunit die before birth and so development must be analyzed by transfer of fetal liver precursors into wild-type recipients. Such experiments showed diminished B-lineage cell numbers, but the major defect was in mature B-cell mitogenic responses (85). Mice lacking the p50 subunit showed relatively normal B-cell development, but again poor response to mitogen by mature B cells (85). However, mice lacking both the p50 and p65 subunits failed to generate any B220$^+$ B-lineage cells. Curiously, when mixed with wild-type fetal liver cells, normal numbers of mature B cells could be generated from the double-defective precursors, suggesting that the defect could be overcome by secreted or membrane-bound signals provided by the wild-type precursors. Another double mutant, p50p52, showed a late-stage

defect in B-cell development, with a failure to generate mature B cells in the spleen (86).

Inactivation of the Oct-2 transcription factor results in neonatal lethality, but transfers of fetal precursors can reconstitute lymphoid cells in wild-type recipients, allowing assessment of effects on the B lineage. Such studies have shown that fewer mature follicular B cells are generated in these mice, and B-1 (CD5$^+$) B cells are completely eliminated (87–89). Similarly, the Oct binding factor, OBF-1, also known as OCA-B and BOB-1, appears to function in the maturation of newly formed B cells in the bone marrow to become follicular B cells in the periphery, since inactivation of this gene resulted in a significant deficit in mature B cells (90–92). Both of these transcription factors have been shown to regulate the follicular B-cell chemokine receptor CXCR5 and this may explain at least part of the defect (93). Curiously, unlike Oct-2–null mice, there was reportedly no deficit in B-1 B cells in OBF-1–null mice. Interestingly, when the OBF-1 mutant mouse is crossed with Btk-deficient mice, then there is a complete lack of peripheral B-cell generation (94), suggesting that this transcription factor may function in the BCR-mediated selection of mature B cells.

Bone Marrow Developmental Stages

Functional Definition

Distinct stages of developing B-lineage cells can be delineated based on their capacity for growth under different culture conditions. That is, the earliest precursors require cell contact with the stromal microenvironment, in addition to specific cytokines, notably IL-7 (81,95). Later-stage cells do not require cell contact, but maintain a need for cytokines (96,97). Either cell type undergoes considerable cell proliferation under such culture conditions. Interestingly, the difference between cell contact requirement and independence appears to be linked to the expression of heavy-chain protein (96,98). Finally, there is a population of more mature surface-Ig negative B lineage cells expressing cytoplasmic heavy chain that does not proliferate in culture. These are sometimes referred to as "late" or "small" pre-B cells and likely require different culture conditions for survival, as they usually do not persist for extended periods, but rather die with a half-life of less than 24 hours, unless protected from apoptosis by a Bcl-2 transgene (99).

Phenotypic Definition

Further clarification of the heterogeneity in bone marrow can be achieved by analysis using fluorescent staining reagents and either microscopic or flow cytometric analysis. For example, the earliest determination that there were both heavy-chain surface-positive B-cell and cytoplasmic-positive pre–B cells was through microscopic examination using anti–Ig staining (100,101). Later studies in mice showed that there were specific surface proteins or "markers" that could be useful in identifying these populations, notably a restricted isoform (CD45Ra) of the common leukocyte antigen, CD45 (102). This largely B-lineage–restricted, 200-kDa–molecular mass isoform is often referred to as "B220." Some highly B-lineage–restricted monoclonal antibodies, such as RA3-6B2, recognize a specific glycosylation of the CD45Ra isoform (103). However, as described above, even highly specific antibodies such as 6B2 may also recognize other cell types, such as particular differentiation stages or subsets of NK or dendritic cells.

The application of multiparameter/multicolor flow cytometry and additional monoclonal antibodies specific for other cell surface proteins differentially expressed during B-lineage development has facilitated delineation of multiple additional intermediate stages in this pathway (97). For example, the B220$^+$ population in bone marrow can be further fractionated into an earlier subset expressing CD43 (about 3% to 5% of marrow cells) and a later fraction with much lower CD43 expression (20% to 30% of marrow). The precursor/progeny relationship of cells in these two fractions can be readily demonstrated by short-term culture, with CD43$^+$ cells giving rise to CD43$^-$ cells. These two populations can be further subfractionated based on additional developmentally regulated surface proteins, such as CD24/HSA (heat-stable antigen); BP-1 (a zinc-dependent surface metallopeptidase also known as aminopeptidase A) (104); and the surface Ig molecules IgM and IgD (97). This is shown in Fig. 5. Again, these cell populations can be isolated and short-term culture used to determine their order in the pathway. Alternative approaches based on other developmental markers can be correlated with this framework of cell stages, notably the system developed by Melchers' group using expression of CD45R/B220, CD19, c-kit, and the IL-2 receptor alpha

chain (105). A diagram summarizing this type of phenotypic subdivision and relating different nomenclatures is shown in Fig. 6.

Culture Systems and Critical Microenvironmental Interactions

The combination of phenotypic characterization coupled with analysis of growth and differentiation in culture has provided a very powerful approach for the further understanding of B-cell development, as employed by many different investigators. Bone marrow cultures developed by Whitlock and Witte (106–108) and fetal liver cultures developed by Melchers' group (109,110) have allowed determination of the critical cytokines and some of the cell adhesion molecules important in the *in vivo* development of these cells. Many of these are summarized in Table 1. A typical B-lineage colony proliferating on S17 stromal cells in the presence of IL-7 is shown in Fig. 7.

Survival and growth of the earliest stages of developing B-lineage cells require cell contact with non–lymphoid-adherent cells that can be isolated from bone marrow, cells referred to generically as "stromal cells." A number of lines have been derived from primary cultures of bone-marrow adherent cells and characterized in terms of their capacity to support B-lymphopoiesis *in vitro* (111). This work has led to the discovery of adhesion molecules that play important roles in mediating the organization of clusters of developing B-lineage cells on stromal layers, including CD44 interacting with hyaluronate and VLA-4 interacting with VCAM-1 (112–115). Both of these interactions could be disrupted by addition of blocking antibodies to CD44 and VLA-4 on B-cell precursors, resulting in a disruption of normal pre–B

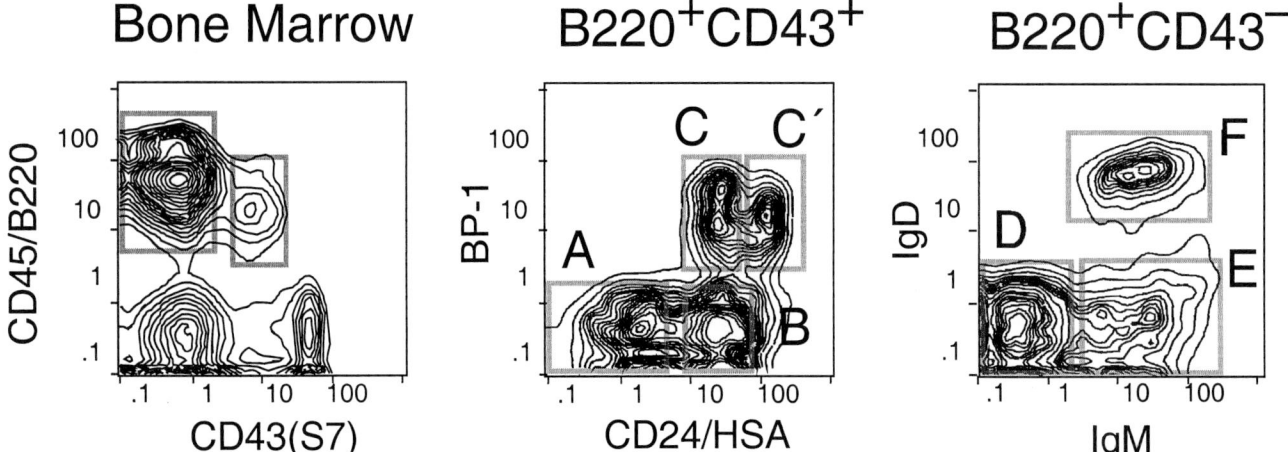

FIG. 5. Flow-cytometry approach for analyzing different stages of B-cell development in mouse bone marrow. Note that the antibody used for CD34/HSA staining, 30F1, is important, as other monoclonal antibodies that recognize HSA do not resolve high- from low-level expression as well. Also, level of antibody used is carefully titrated to avoid cell aggregation commonly encountered with anti-HSA antibodies.

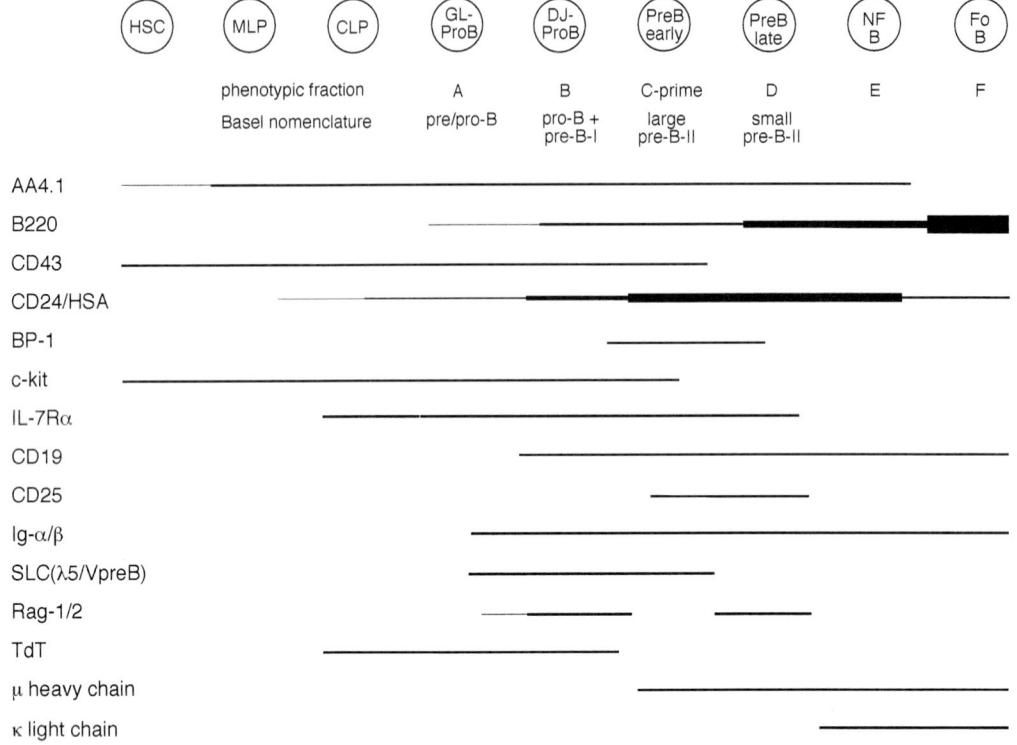

FIG. 6. Distinct phenotypic stages and characterization for surrogate light-chain expression, biphasic RAG expression, and TdT expression. Expression of heavy chain and light chain is also shown. The cell-type descriptions are cross-referenced to the alphabetic phenotypic fraction nomenclature and also to the Basel nomenclature.

proliferation *in vitro* (116). Such adhesion interactions may serve to transmit signals directly to the stromal cells or B precursors or both. There is some evidence that stromal cells are induced to elaborate specific growth mediators after interaction with B-cell precursors or soluble regulators (117).

Another function of the stromal cells is to produce growth factors critical to B-lineage survival, proliferation, and differentiation, and the most important of these for mouse B-cell development is IL-7 (81,95,118,119). IL-7 promotes the survival and proliferation of pro–B and pre–B stage cells, both

in vivo and *in vitro* (120,121). Neutralizing antibody to IL-7 can block B-cell development *in vitro* (97) and IL-7 expressed as a transgene can deregulate normal B-cell development, leading to B-cell lymphadenopathy (122). The IL-7 receptor consists of a unique IL-7Rα chain (123) paired with the common gamma chain (γc) that is also found in the receptors for IL-2, IL-4, IL-9, and IL-15 (124). IL-7Rα–null mice have a severe deficit of both B and T cells in the periphery and lack most B-lineage cells in bone marrow (125). Mice with targeted inactivation of the γc or IL-7 do have some

TABLE 1. *Regulators of growth of early B-lineage cells*

Mediator	Effect	Reference
IL-7	Stimulates CLP and B-precursor proliferation	81,118,119,489
TSLP	Alternate IL-7–like cytokine	126,127
IGF-1	Stimulates accumulation of cμ^+ cells in culture	152
FLT-3/FLK2-L	Critical for earliest stages of B-lineage development	135,139,490,491
c-KIT-L	Synergizes in IL-7 induced proliferation	28,133
IL-3	Substitute for IL-7 in proliferation of pre-B clones	143
CXCL12/CXCR4	Crucial chemokine interaction for early B-lineage precursors	161,163,165,166
Hemokinin	Novel regulator of B lymphopoiesis	154
VLA4/VCAM-1	Adhesive interaction; antibodies to either block B-lymphopoiesis	113,114,492
CD44/hyaluronate	Adhesive interaction; mediates association of B-lineage/stromal cells	112,116
TGF-β	Inhibits proliferation stimulated by IL-7	81
Sex steroids	Decrease B-lineage precursors in bone marrow	493,494
Growth hormones	Required for normal B-lymphopoiesis	155,156,495

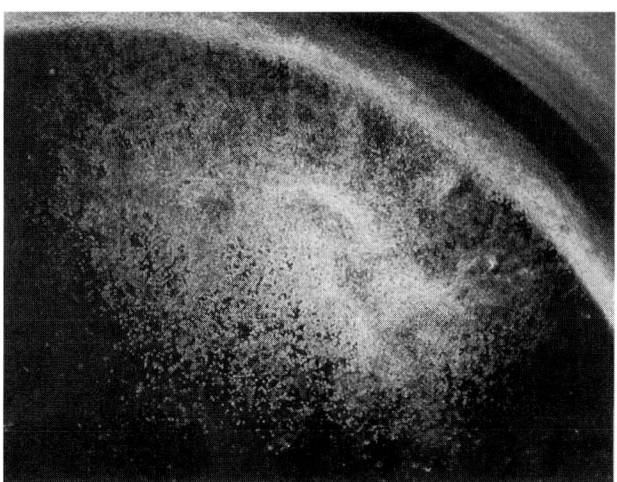 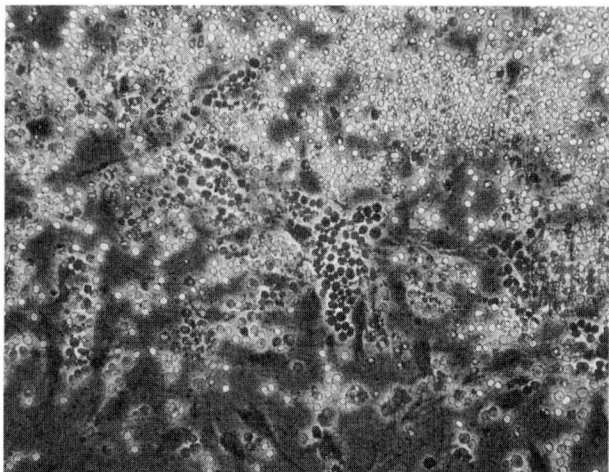

FIG. 7. Photomicrographs of B-lineage colony proliferating on S17 stromal layer (in the well of a 96-well microplate) in the presence of IL-7. Day 10 colony derived from a single Fr A phenotype (Fig. 3A) cell, including low- and high-power views. All of these cells now express CD19 and many have progressed to BP-1$^+$.

B-lineage development, suggesting an alternate cytokine, and this appears to be TSLP. This protein was first identified as a pre–B-cell growth factor produced by a thymic stromal line (126) and shows some of the same effects in culture as IL-7, although possibly inducing less proliferation and more differentiation (127). Its receptor has been cloned and requires the IL-7Rα chain for function (128). It shares both sequence homology and genomic exon organization with the common gamma chain (129). Signaling through the IL-7 receptor requires JAK3 and activates the transcription factor STAT5, whereas signaling through TSLP is JAK3 independent, but also activates STAT5 (127,130).

The earliest precursors in the B-lineage pathway, probably including cells that are not B-lineage committed but that can efficiently give rise to B cells in a short time *in vitro,* have receptors for SCF/c-kit-ligand (28,29,131–134) and FLK2/FLT3-ligand (135–139). Thus, the most permissive cultures for expanding precursors of B-lineage cells will include these cytokines, in addition to IL-7 and a stromal-adherent cell layer, such as S17 (140–142). IL-3 has also occasionally been suggested as playing a support role for pre–B cells *in vitro* (143), although its role *in vivo* may be at a much earlier stage. While culture conditions have been reported that can support B-lineage development in the absence of stromal cells (144,145), the clear-cut alteration of contact dependence prior and post heavy-chain expression (96–98,146,147) argues that the most physiological model for early B-lineage growth will include stromal cells. Besides providing important cell–cell contacts that may signal survival, proliferation, and differentiation, it is also likely that stromal cells bind at least some cytokines to their surface, providing higher local concentrations to the clusters of B-lineage precursors that adhere (148,149).

B-lineage development may be modified by exposure to hormones and considerable interest has focused on sex

steroids released during pregnancy that serve to depress B-lymphopoiesis, particularly the pre–B-cell pool (150). This may be important to avoid autoimmune responses by the mother, but could have negative consequences due to possible transient immunodeficiency. Interestingly, fetal B-lymphopoiesis is not similarly depressed, due to the absence of hormone receptors on fetal B-lineage cells (151). Insulin-like growth factor (IGF-1) has been reported to potentiate progression *in vitro* to the cμ^+ stage (152,153) and, more recently, there is a report of a bioactive peptide, a type of tachykinin, that synergizes with IL-7 to enhance the growth of IL-7 dependent cultures (154). Besides IGF-1, other pituitary hormones, thyroxine and growth hormone (GH), have effects on B-lymphopoiesis (155). For example, thyroxine treatment can restore normal B-cell development in dwarf Pit-1 mutant mice with deficient pituitary function (156). Thus, it is likely that more detail remains to be filled in to complete our picture of the growth requirements and modulating influences of B-lineage cells in mouse bone marrow.

Another function of cell–cell interaction is cell fate determination during the lineage commitment stage, very early in development of B-lineage cells. The Notch signaling pathway is implicated in cell fate determination in invertebrates and more recently has been shown to function in lymphoid lineage specification (67,157). Notch-family transmembrane receptors regulate transcription by being cleaved upon ligand binding to release an intracellular cytoplasmic domain that translocates to the nucleus where it interacts with the transcriptional repressor CSL (158). Recent studies have shown that Notch1 can play a pivotal role in commitment of common lymphoid progenitors to the T-cell lineage (67). That is, expression of Notch1 by retroviral transduction has been shown to re-direct B-lineage differentiation in bone marrow along the T lineage. Furthermore, a reciprocal result was found in conditional Notch1-null mice, blocking T-cell development in the thymus, to be replaced by B-cell development (159). Finally, altering the Notch1 modifier, Lunatic fringe, by over-expressing this molecule under regulation of an Lck promoter resulted in B-cell development in the thymus (71). Differentiation of lymphoid precursors to NK or dendritic cell lineages was unaffected in Notch1-null CLP cells, so Notch apparently affects only the B/T lineage decision.

Role of Chemokines in Migration of B-Cell Precursors

One of the most distinctive features of B-cell development in bone marrow is the migration of developing precursors from early stages nearest the bone endosteum layer to latter stages progressively closer to the central arteriole, where they will eventually exit (160). This migration is likely due to differential expression of specific adhesion molecules and also to expression of chemokine receptors. Analysis of B-cell migration has identified a critical chemokine that is important in this process, SDF-1, now known as CXCL12 (161,162), and its receptor CXCR4 (163). CXCL12 is expressed by fetal-liver and bone-marrow stromal cells, while CXCR4 is found on hematopoietic precursors and B-cell progenitors (164). Deletion of either the receptor or ligand results in severely impaired B-lymphopoiesis (165–167). Interestingly, the critical defect appears to be failure to retain precursors in the primary lymphoid organ, as progenitors and precursors can be found in the blood of mutant mice (168).

Gene Expression and Ig Rearrangement (See Fig. 8)

In addition to delineation of developmental stages based on changes in protein surface expression, B-lineage cells can also be characterized for expression of internal proteins related to critical processes in their progression along this pathway, specifically those related to rearrangement and expression of the B-cell antigen receptor. Thus, expression of μ heavy-chain constant region, prior to Ig rearrangement, from a cryptic promoter generates a "sterile transcript" that likely reflects an open chromatin structure important for the onset of rearrangement (169–171). Thus, analysis of sterile μ expression can be used to investigate very early stages of B-cell development. Classical Northern analysis can be done with transformed lines, but much work analyzing RNA levels in B-lineage cell fractions, whether directly isolated or cultured, has depended on PCR amplification of cDNA (39). For example, using this approach, sterile μ can be detected in a very early fraction of $B220^+CD43^+CD19^-$ (Fr A) cells, prior to high-level expression of the recombinase-activating genes, RAG1 and RAG2, that make the double-strand breaks in Ig rearrangement (172,173). Expression of RAG1 and RAG2 is up-regulated sharply in the early-stage $B220^+CD43^+CD19^+$ (Fr B) cells, which also have high levels of terminal deoxynucleotidyl transferase (TdT), the enzyme responsible for adding nontemplated nucleotides at the D-J and V-D junctions of the heavy chain (12,174).

The extent of heavy- or light-chain rearrangement can also be probed in these fractions of cells, either in bulk isolated populations (97) or in individual cells (48,105,175). At the heavy-chain locus, D-J rearrangement occurs prior to V-D-J rearrangement, and cells with extensive D-J, but little V-D-J rearrangement can be detected at the $B220^+CD43^+CD19^+$ (Fr B) stage, where RAG1/2 and TdT are strongly expressed. Little D-J rearrangement is detected at the earlier Fr A stage, even when individual cells are analyzed (48).

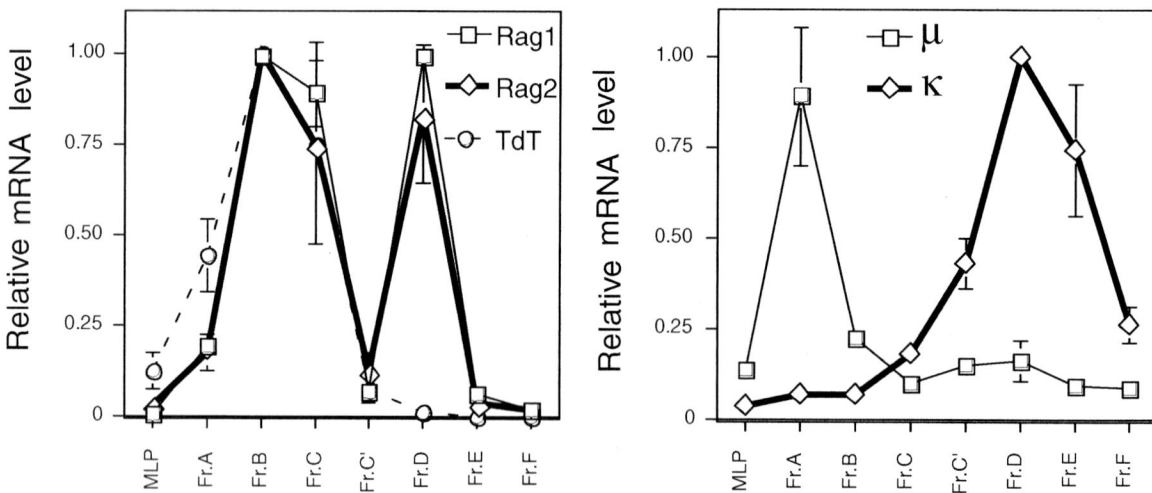

FIG. 8. Profile of Ig rearrangement–related gene expression. Cells isolated following fractionation scheme shown in Fig. 5. Relative mRNA levels assessed by performing semiquantitative RT-PCR using limited number of cycled, blotting, and then probing and quantitating the probe signal. Note the biphasic expression of RAG genes and the early expression of sterile μ during the first wave, where heavy chain rearranges, and the up-regulation of sterile kappa transcripts during the second wave, when most light-chain rearrangement takes place.

V-D-J rearrangements are readily detected in the abundant B220$^+$CD43$^-$ (Fr D)–stage of small pre–B cells, although productive rearrangement has already completed by the large pre–B (Fr C-prime) stage (see below). Single-cell PCR analysis of rearrangements in Fr C–stage cells shows a large proportion with nonproductive rearrangements on both chromosomes, suggesting that this may represent a dead-end fraction (175). Some light-chain rearrangement is detectable in early-stage B220$^+$CD43$^+$ (Fr B) cells, and this is consistent with the observation that some kappa light-chain rearrangement is detectable in bone marrow of mice where μ heavy chain has been crippled by deletion of the membrane exon (176). However, much higher levels of kappa rearrangement are found in the B220$^+$CD43$^-$ (Fr D) stage cells, consistent with the finding of sterile-kappa mRNA increase just prior to this stage likely induced by pre–BCR signaling (see below).

Role of Ig Heavy Chain and Pre–BCR

Careful analysis of SCID mouse (177) bone marrow revealed the presence of a population of B220$^+$ cells, all with a very early CD43$^+$ phenotype, suggesting a block in B-cell development at this stage (178). SCID mice a defect in the catalytic subunit of the DNA-dependent protein kinase DNA-PKcs (179,180), and as a result B-lineage cells in these mice are very ineffective at completing even initial D-J rearrangements at the heavy-chain locus. This block could be overcome by introduction of an Ig heavy-chain transgene, supporting the model of a critical role for μ protein in progressing past an early developmental checkpoint (181). An early gene-targeting experiment eliminated the membrane exon of μ heavy chain (μ-mt) and such mice also showed a block at this stage (182,183).

The μ heavy chain can be shown in co-immunoprecipitation experiments to associate with a set of B-cell–specific peptides at the early pre–B-cell stage (184), and this complex is referred to as the pre–B-cell receptor (pre–BCR). It seems clear that this complex mediates a type of signaling function analogous to the B-cell antigen receptor (BCR) in mature B cells. Prior to light-chain expression, two peptides known as λ5 and VpreB, originally isolated as B-lineage–specific cDNAs (185,186), associate with heavy chain. The λ5 shows homology to a lambda-constant region, and VpreB is so termed because it has homology to a variable-region domain, so together these peptides constitute a pseudo or surrogate light chain (SLC). The critical role of λ5 was demonstrated unambiguously in gene-targeted mice, where B-cell development was blocked at the B220$^+$CD43$^+$ stage (187). The production of some mature cells that accumulate in this mutant is likely due to early kappa rearrangement, with light chain substituting for SLC, as demonstrated in light-chain transgenic experiments (188).

The μ heavy chain has a very short cytoplasmic region consisting of only three amino acids, and an important finding has been that signal transduction through the BCR is mediated by accessory peptides, similar to the CD3 components

of the T-cell receptor, known as Ig-α and Ig-β (189–192). As predicted by the pre–BCR signaling, developmental checkpoint hypothesis, inactivation of Ig-β (193) results in a block at the B220$^+$CD43$^+$ stage in mouse bone marrow, similar to the μ-mt and λ5-null mice. Finally, the Syc tyrosine kinase plays a critical role in transducing BCR cross-linking signals in mature B cells and inactivation of this gene results in a "leaky" block at this same stage (194,195). Thus, any mutation that affects this pre–BCR complex (Fig. 9A) precludes efficient progression past the earliest stages of B-cell development.

Careful examination of B-cell development in normal mice shows that heavy chain is first expressed at a late fraction of the B220$^+$CD43$^+$ stage, termed Fr C-prime (Fig. 10A). This fraction is also interesting because it shows a much higher proportion of cells in cycle (revealed by a high frequency of cells with greater than 2N DNA content; Fig. 10B), compared with any other B220$^+$ stage in bone marrow (97). Mice unable to assemble a pre-BCR, due to inability to rearrange heavy chain (RAG1 null), show a block in development at the CD43$^+$ stage that can be complemented by introduction of a functionally rearranged μ heavy chain as a transgene (147) (Fig. 10C). Analysis of several types of pre–BCR defective mutant mice shows a complete absence of Fr C-prime stage cells, suggesting that pre–BCR signaling results in the up-regulation of CD24/HSA and also entry into rapid cell proliferation. Thus, a model of pre–BCR function is that it signals the clonal expansion phase of pre–B-cell development, amplifying cells with in-frame V-D-J rearrangements capable of making heavy-chain protein.

The precise nature of pre–BCR signaling remains to be completely understood. An early model suggested that cross-linking of heavy chain was mediated through interaction of SLC with a bone marrow–expressed ligand. However, subsequent experiments showed that normal light chain could substitute for SLC and that even a V$_H$ truncated μ heavy chain could mediate progression past this stage. Furthermore, intensive searches for the putative ligand over a 10-year period have been fruitless, leading to the model that pre–BCR signaling is more akin to "tonic" signaling in mature B cells (196,197). That is, simple assembly of the complex (or possibly some degree of multimerization fostered by the self-aggregating nature of SLC) (198) probably is sufficient for the cell to pass this developmental checkpoint (Fig. 9B). One clear-cut finding is that pre–BCR signaling in a transformed pro–B-cell model system can occur in the absence of any additional cell type, suggesting that if a ligand exists, it must be expressed on B-lineage cells, rather than stromal cells (199).

Mutations in other molecules in the pre–BCR signaling pathway have been shown to affect B-cell development and pre–B-cell clonal expansion. While the Btk mutation is less severe in mouse than in human, there nevertheless is an alteration in pre–B-cell expansion in Btk-deficient mice (200). Also, X-linked immunodeficient (Xid) B cells (deficient in Btk) have been reported to proliferate more in stromal cell cultures, possibly due to decreased differentiation to later

μ Heavy Chain Expression

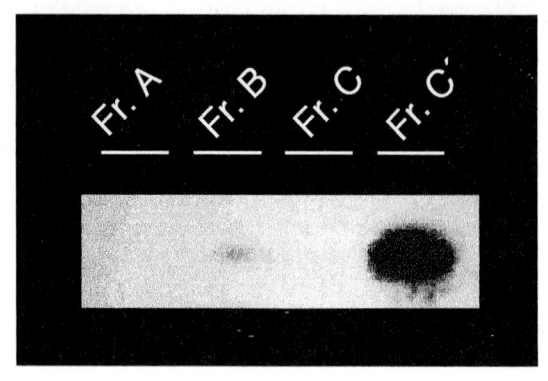

Cell Cycle Analysis

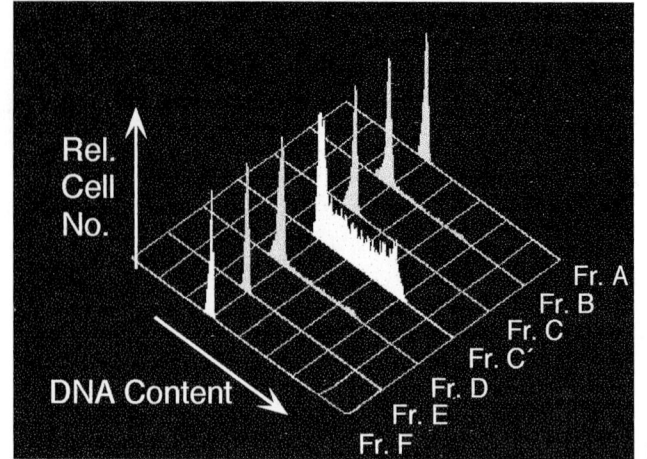

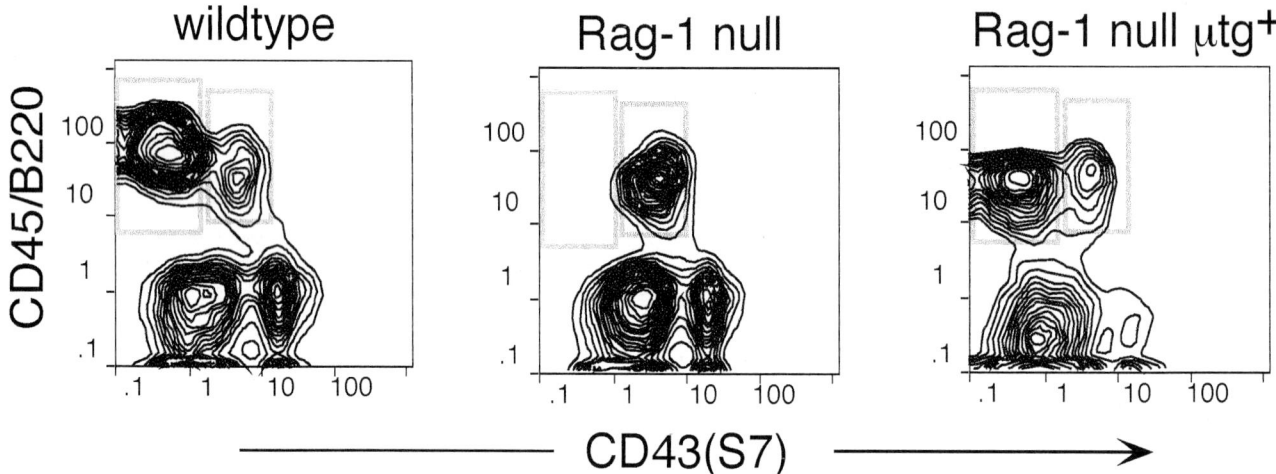

FIG. 9. A: Western blot of Ig μ heavy-chain expression showing high-level expression in Fr C-prime. **B:** Cell-cycle analysis of individual fractions shows that most cells in Fr C-prime are cycling. Propidium iodide staining of permeabilized sorted cells allows determination of DNA content per cell using flow cytometry. **C:** Block in B-cell development in RAG-1–deficient mice can be overcome by introduction of an Ig μ heavy-chain transgene.

nonproliferative stages (201,202). The role of Btk is thought to modulate BCR signaling strength (203) and this is probably also the case for pre–BCR signaling, allowing only strongly signaling pre-BCRs to progress in the mutant mice. BLNK serves to link the pre-BCR to the Syk kinase, critical in BCR signaling (204,205). Mutant mice lacking BLNK show a partial block in B-cell development at the pro–B to pre–B transition (206). Curiously, while pre–BCR signaling is thought to mediate allelic exclusion (expression of a single heavy-chain allele), this remains intact in BLNK-deficient mice (207). Syk-deficient mice show a more severe block at the pro–B to pre–B transition and a lack of allelic exclusion (194,195, 207).

Outcomes of pre–BCR signaling, in addition to pre–B proliferation, are down-regulation of the RAG genes (208), down-regulation of TdT (199) and transcriptional activation of the kappa locus, detected as up-regulation of sterile kappa transcripts (209). Extinction of recombinase activity

is probably important for chromosomal stability during the clonal burst period of B-cell development (210–212) and is also at least a part of the mechanism that ensures allelic exclusion, which is the expression of a single heavy chain by any given B-cell (213). There is evidence that pre–BCR selection requires low levels of IL-7 (214), and probably occurs naturally as the developing precursors migrate through different stromal cell microenvironments in bone marrow.

The function of the pre-BCR may be more complex than simply to sense whether an in-frame V-D-J rearrangement has occurred. This possibility is suggested by the observation that heavy chains with different V-D-J segments vary in their capacity to assemble with SLC components (215–218). V regions are classified into families based on sequence homology and many members of two of these families, the 7183 and Q52, appear to frequently generate heavy chains that assemble poorly with surrogate light chain (217). A consequence of this will likely be poor pre–BCR signaling and

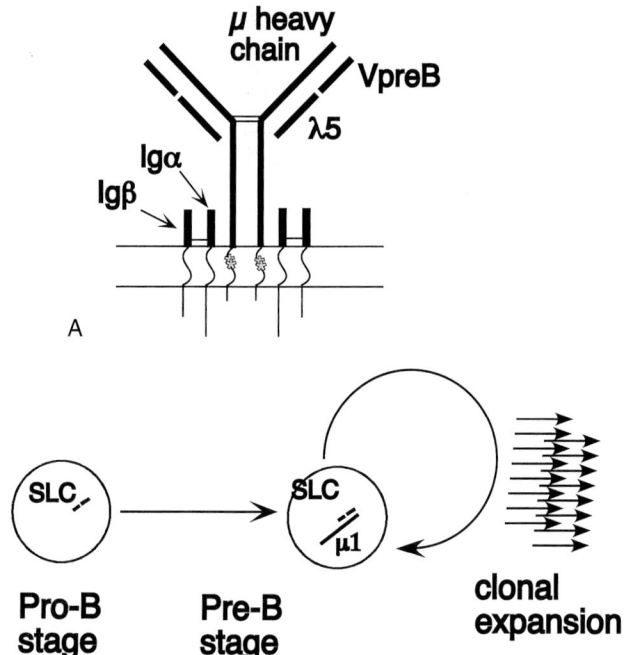

A

B

FIG. 10. A: Diagram of the pre-BCR, μ heavy chain with surrogate light chain ($\lambda 5$ and VpreB) in place of conventional light chain. As in the BCR, Ig-α and Ig-β serve to couple signals between the receptor and cytoplasmic components, such as BLNK and Syk. μ transmembrane residues (starred) are important in mediating interaction with Ig-α/Ig-β, as mutation of these diminishes BCR function. **B:** Clonal expansion mediated by pre-BCR assembly. Association of newly generated μ heavy chain with preexisting surrogate light-chain leads to a burst of proliferation at the pre-B stage.

little clonal expansion, so such cells will become under-represented at later stages of B-cell development relative to cells containing heavy chains that signal effectively. One explanation of the reason for this SLC assembly–mediated clonal expansion is that it serves a quality control function to test heavy-chain V regions for their potential to fold with real Ig light chain, a critical requirement if the cell is to express a complete BCR. An alternative (not necessarily mutually exclusive) explanation is that making pre–B-cell proliferation dependent on pre–BCR expression provides a simple mechanism for regulating the extent of clonal expansion, since an immediate consequence of pre–BCR signaling is to terminate SLC expression. Thereafter, SLC protein levels decay and are diluted by cell division, so that after several rounds of proliferation, pre–BCR levels will decrease to below the threshold required to provide the signal to maintain the cell in cycle. Fig. 11 illustrates a model for bone marrow B-cell development, showing the pre–BCR checkpoint.

One of the most striking examples of pre–BCR selection is seen with the D-proximal V_H gene, $V_H 81X$, where early precursors show biased over-utilization, due to preferential rearrangement of this V_H gene (11,219,220). $V_H 81X$ had also been identified as frequently rearranged in Abelson virus transformed pre–B cells (221), even though it was rarely seen in the mature B-cell compartment. The demonstration of the decrease in representation of cells with $V_H 81X$ rearrangements at the pre–B clonal expansion phase in bone marrow (222,223), together with the demonstration that heavy chains utilizing VH81X frequently fail to assemble functional pre-BCRs (215,216,224), explained this paradox. However, it is still curious that the most frequently rearranged V_H

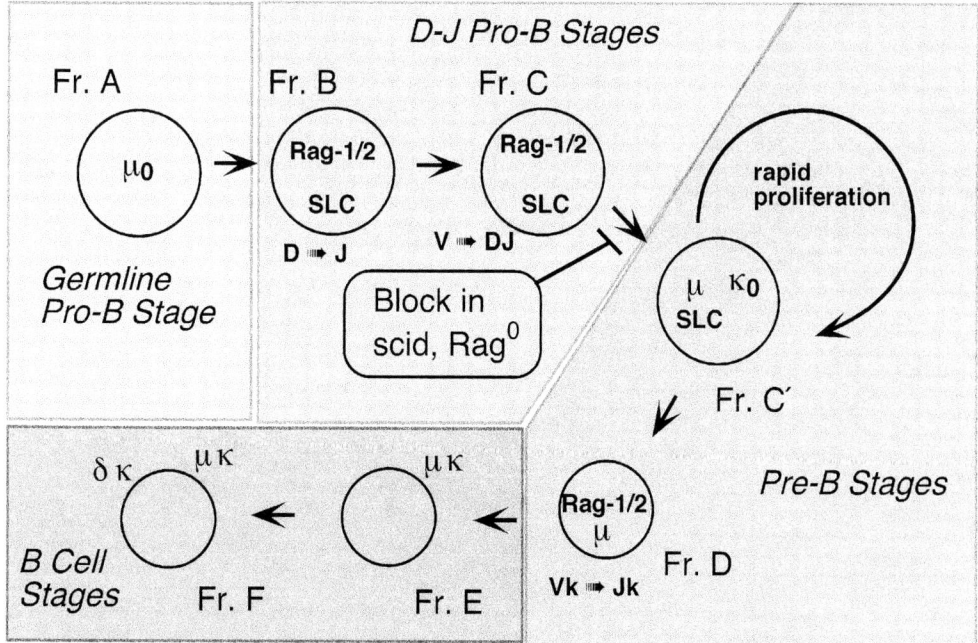

FIG. 11. Model for mouse bone-marrow B-cell development showing relationship of Ig rearrangement with progression and proliferation.

gene is so strongly selected *against* at the clonal expansion stage. A possible explanation may lie in comparisons of V_H utilization during fetal development. That is, in contrast with bone-marrow precursor cultures, the ratio of productive/nonproductive V_H81X does not decrease during cultures of fetal precursors (225,226). Furthermore, the proliferative burst that pre–BCR assembly provides to bone marrow pre–B cells may instead result in exit from cell cycle in fetal precursors (218), leading to selection of very different BCR repertoires during fetal and adult B-lymphopoiesis. The possible significance of this is discussed below in the section on B-1 B cells.

Light-Chain Rearrangement and Generation of Immature B Cells

Besides termination of TdT and SLC gene expression, pre–BCR signaling also results in the down-regulation of RAG1 and RAG2 expression and protein levels rapidly drop as cells enter the rapidly cycling stage. However, as pre–BCR levels decrease and cells exit from the cycle, the RAG genes are re-expressed at high levels. Sterile kappa transcripts become detectable during the cycling stage, likely reflecting chromatin remodeling to make the kappa light-chain locus accessible (209); thus, induction of RAG expression together with the rest of the recombinase machinery will initiate kappa light-chain V to J rearrangement. An interesting feature of the $V\kappa$ locus is that the approximately 100 genes are in both transcriptional orientations, and so these genes can rearrange either by deletion (generating an extrachromosomal excision circle) or by inversion (227). The absence of intervening D segments also means that it is possible for upstream V-kappa genes to rearrange to downstream J-kappa segments, "leapfrogging" the initial rearrangement, assuming it was to any $J\kappa$ other than $J\kappa5$. The successive association of different kappa chains with the same heavy chain in a B-cell is referred to as BCR "editing" and was originally observed in the context of autoreactivity, which maintains RAG expression even at the B-cell stage (228,229) (see following section on B-cell tolerance). Since assembly and expression of a complete BCR (i.e., not self-reactive) terminates RAG expression, an additional reason for light-chain editing in the bone marrow may be to replace an initial light chain that fails to assemble effectively with the particular heavy chain present in that pre–B cell. This is probably the explanation for multiple light-chain rearrangements detected in single early B-lineage cells (230).

Newly formed B cells can be distinguished from mature B cells on the basis of their inability to proliferate in response to BCR cross-linking; that is, they are functionally immature. This is also the stage where negative selection is reported in transgenic models of autoreactivity (231,232). Cells at this stage have a half-life of only a few days, compared to mature follicular B cells with a half-life measured in months. They can be distinguished by surface phenotype from other B cells based on expression of certain combinations of markers, such as IgM^+IgD^-, absence of CD23, and high-level expression

of CD24/HSA (233). Recently there are reports of single markers that are useful in distinguishing newly formed cells from any mature subset, such as the molecules recognized by monoclonal antibodies 493 (234) and AA4.1 (235). The AA4.1 target molecule has been cloned and identified as the mouse ortholog of a component of the human C1q receptor (236).

Cells similar to newly formed B cells can be generated to varying extent during stromal cell culture of B-cell precursors, although the more primitive cycling pre–B or pro–B cells are usually more abundant and tend to increase in frequency with prolonged culture. It is possible to induce differentiation of B cells in these cultures by withdrawing IL-7, which induces a wave of small pre–B and then newly formed B-cell generation. Such cells do not persist for more than a day, unless the cultures are established from Bcl-2 transgenic mice (99), suggesting that the short half-life of newly formed cells in these cultures, and possibly also *in vivo,* is due to their low level of anti-apoptotic mediators. Both Bcl-2 and Bcl-X_L mRNA are present at only very low levels in these cells, in contrast to other B-lineage stages where either one or the other predominates. Over-expression of Bcl-X_L from a transgene results in accumulation of a population of pro–B phenotype cells with nonfunctional rearrangements (237), implicating this protein in the process of pre–BCR selection of cells with functional rearrangements.

Peripheral Maturation Stages and Functional Subsets

Transitional B Cells

Newly formed immature B cells migrate to the spleen where they either die or undergo further maturation to mature B-cells. These maturing B cells can be subdivided based on differential expression of several surface proteins, including CD21, CD23, CD24/HSA, and AA4.1. These subdivisions have been referred to as "transitional B cells" (238). One recent subdivision based on CD21, CD23, AA4.1, and IgM level has shown progression from an $AA4.1^+CD21^-CD23^-$ T1 stage to an $AA4.1^+CD21^-CD23^+$ T2 stage, followed by down-regulation of IgM as a T3 stage, and finally loss of AA4.1 with up-regulation of CD21 to yield the mature follicular phenotype (235). As shown in Fig. 12, this approach also resolves two $AA4.1^-$ subsets that lack CD23, the B-1 subset with low CD21 and the MZ subset with very high CD21 (see below). The transitional stage cells are all short-lived as shown by bromodeoxyuridine incorporation (235,239). They are also not functionally competent, as shown by inability to proliferate after BCR cross-linking (233,240). Another well-characterized functional distinction is that B-cell tolerance, rather than an immune response, is induced by BCR cross-linking of immature B cells (241–243). More recent studies with transgenic models of self-reactivity have shown that these B cells can be deleted, undergo receptor editing, or rendered functionally unresponsive (anergic) by BCR signaling at the immature stage (228,231,244–248).

CD19+IgM+

AA4.1/CD23 Subsets

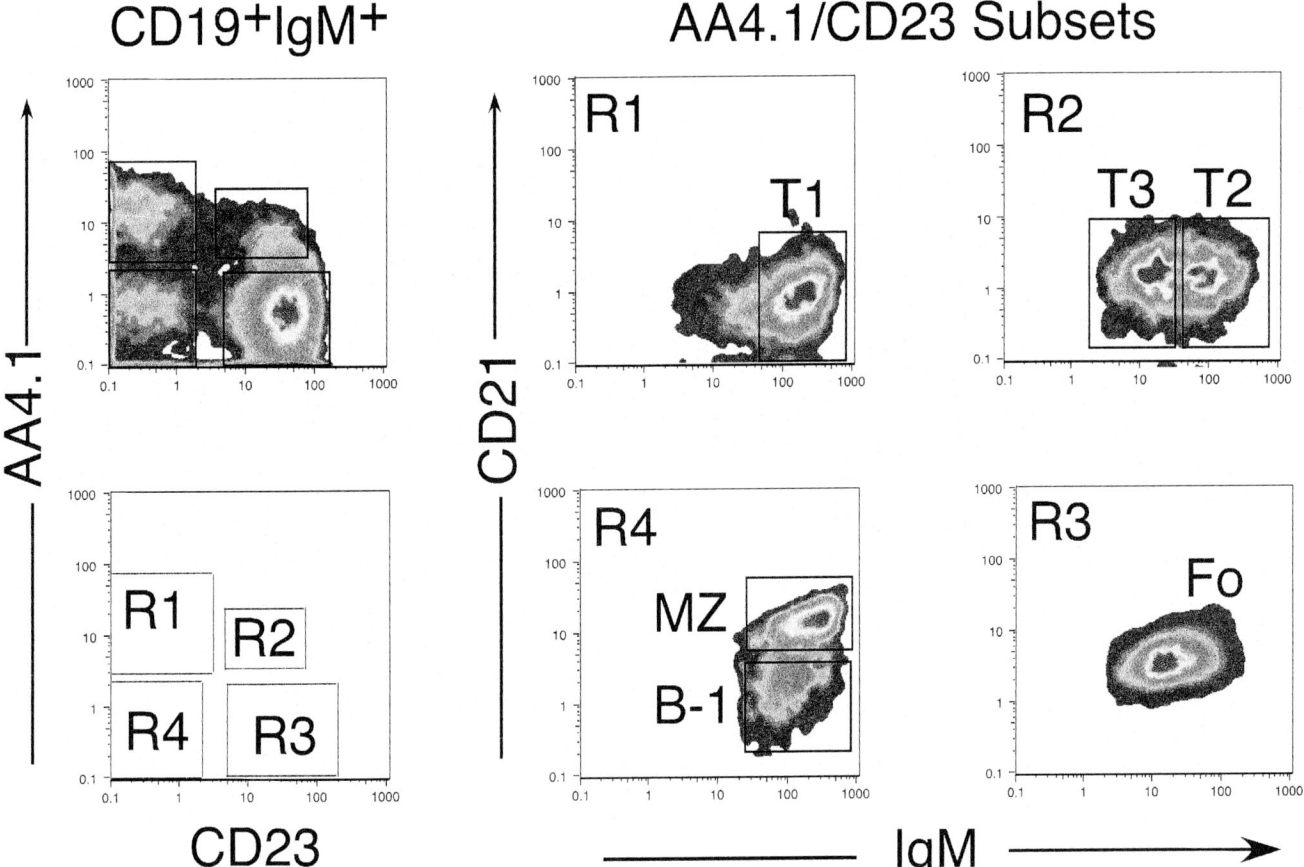

FIG. 12. Flow-cytometry approach for resolution of transitional (T1-T3) and mature (Fo, B-1, MZ) populations of B cells in mouse spleen. *Left panels* show the distribution of AA4.1 and CD23 on B cells (defined as CD19+IgM+). Cells in the boxed regions are then analyzed for correlated expression of CD21 and IgM, facilitating resolution of three AA4.1+ fractions (T1-T3), the follicular subset (AA4.1−CD23+CD21+), the marginal zone subset (AA4.1-CD23-CD21++) and the B-1 subset (AA4.1−CD23−CD21low).

It is not simply the inability to receive T-cell help due to differences in microenvironment or receptor expression that makes immature B cells incapable of responding as mature B cells. Cross-linking the BCR on purified populations of immature, but not mature, B cells has been shown to induce apoptosis, suggesting distinctions in the signaling pathways between these two stages (249,250). Studies with transgenic mice suggest that this apoptosis is not mediated through the Fas/Fas–ligand pathway, since central deletion is intact in Fas-mutant mice (251,252). Prior to induction of apoptosis, immature B cells have been shown to complete some of the early events associated with entry into cell cycle, while failing to complete this program (253). Distinct stages in maturation appear more or less capable of responding to BCR cross-linking by re-induction (or maintenance) of RAGs to facilitate receptor editing (232). Furthermore, it appears that immature B cells are more sensitive to smaller changes in intracellular free calcium, compared to mature B cells (254). It is possible that the capacity to up-regulate anti-apoptotic molecules, such as A1, may play a critical role in the inability of immature B cells to survive and complete a normal

response (255,256). The characterization of signaling pathways in different immature stages of developing B cells is ongoing and should eventually provide insights into the detailed mechanism for immature B-cell tolerance.

Analyses of various normally occurring or engineered mutant mice have provided approaches for investigation of the process of progressing from a newly formed B-cell to a mature follicular B-cell. B-cell populations and B-cell function have been studied for many years in CBA/N mice bearing the X-linked immunodeficiency (Xid) mutation. This mouse has a mutation in the Btk gene that produces a milder phenotype than the complete absence of peripheral B cells seen in humans. The Btk gene likely plays a role at several stages of B-cell development and activation, which complicates the analysis, but it appears clear that one major consequence is altered BCR signaling that has a profound effect on progression through the various transitional stages in the spleen. A likely consequence of diminished strength of BCR signaling is a compensatory requirement for higher-surface BCR expression that eventually produces at decreased frequency a type of "mature" B-cell that is still functionally handicapped

(257,258). Several groups have produced Xid mice on a nu/nu T-cell–less background that results in a more profound absence of mature B cells, suggesting a requirement for T cells or T-cell–produced factors in the maturation of Xid B cells (259,260). A more recent variation of this type of investigation is the production of Xid/CD40–deficient mice that show a similar deficit in mature B cells, suggesting a role for the CD40/CD40L interaction in the generation of mature B cells from transitional B cells, particularly when the BCR is handicapped by defective Btk (261).

Lyn is an Src-family protein kinase that is associated with the BCR and functions in signaling in mature B cells (262). Lyn-deficient mice exhibit defects in maturation of immature cells, suggesting a positive role for BCR/Lyn signaling at this stage, but these mice also develop a severe autoimmune condition, suggesting an additional negative regulatory role for Lyn in maintaining tolerance in mature B cells (263,264).

CD72 is a predominantly B-lineage restricted C-type lectin and ligating this molecule was recognized for many years (when it was known as Lyb2) as having functional consequences (265). Recent analyses of a CD72-null mouse have clarified its function in B-cell development and activation (266). CD72 has been shown to recruit SHP-1 to the BCR, supporting a negative regulatory role in BCR activation (267). Consistent with this model for CD72 function, null gene-targeted mice have been shown to produce B cells that are hyper-responsive (266). Interestingly, late stages of B-cell development are affected, with fewer mature B cells and relatively normal numbers of immature B cells in spleen (266). Thus, signaling that is too intense may also delay maturation of immature B cells.

Follicular B Cells

The major population of mature recirculating B cells in the spleen is located in the B-cell follicle region, hence the term "follicular B cells." Entry into this anatomical site appears to constitute a final stage in maturation for developing bone marrow B cells, as competition for this site is compromised in several transgenic models of B-cell tolerance (268–271). Cells in this compartment do not proliferate, but persist in the resting state for several months. A conditional knockout study, eliminating expression of the BCR (by deleting the V region), revealed that expression of the BCR is required for cell survival (197). It is not yet established whether this is due to "tonic signaling" (simple assembly of the BCR signaling complex) or instead reflects signaling by low-affinity binding to cross-reactive self-determinants, a kind of "positive selection."

The repertoire of the follicular B-cell pool appears to differ from the earlier immature splenic B-cell population, as assessed by sequence analysis of the light-chain repertoire in heavy-chain transgenic mice (272). The approach of fixing the heavy chain and then examining the light-chain repertoire simplifies the analysis and the results of this study were interpreted to indicate that BCR-mediated antigen selection is indeed operating. However, the resolution of the analysis probably could not have rigorously excluded populations known to show V-gene biases, such as B-1 or MZ B cells (see following sections), so further work will be required to provide convincing evidence of antigenic selection in the follicular B-cell pool.

B-Cell Migration and Maintenance

Newly formed B cells migrate from the bone marrow to the spleen, undergo further maturation in the red pulp, and eventually enter the follicle where they constitute the mature B-cell pool that recirculates. Their migration is dependent on chemokines/receptor interactions, notably the SLC(CCL21)/CCR7 interaction, as demonstrated by the inability of mature B cells to be retained normally in spleens of CCR7-null mice (273). The role of the CXCR5 receptor on B cells in homing to the lymphoid follicle due a gradient of the B-lymphocyte chemoattractant CXCL13 is also well known; moreover, CXCL13 can directly induce Ltα1β2 on the recruited cells (274). Finally, it is also possible that the SDF1(CXCL12)/CXCR4 interaction, critical for normal B-lymphopoiesis, may also be important at this later stage, although investigation of this issue is complicated by the early defect. This is an ongoing area of investigation and may eventually be clarified by developmentally regulated gene-targeting studies.

Recently, considerable interest has focused on the role of cytokine, a TNF family member—known variously as BAFF, BLyS, TALL-1, zTNF4, or THANK—in the process of peripheral B-cell maturation (275). BAFF is a TNF family member found to enhance survival of B cells or even produce autoimmunity in transgenic mice constitutively expressing it (276,277). Initially, two receptors defined for BAFF, BCMA, and TACI, provided a complex picture, as targeted inactivation of BCMA yielded no B-cell defect and deletion of TACI had increased B-cell numbers (suggesting that TACI might be a negative regulator). This puzzle was resolved by identification of a third receptor, BAFF-R/BR3 (278,279), which was mutated in a strain of mice known to lack most mature B cells, A/WySnJ (280). A second ligand, APRIL, can bind to BCMA and TACI, but not to BAFF/BR3, and this binding is proliferative rather than survival promoting (281). Thus, the critical interaction for maintenance of follicular B cells is BAFF/BLyS with its receptor. B-1 cells are not deficient in A/WySnJ (280), suggesting that their maintenance does not depend on this pathway, but instead is more BCR dependent.

B-Cell Turnover

It is estimated that 10 to 20 million B cells are produced in bone marrow of the mouse each day (282), yet it appears that only about 10% of this number reach the periphery (239). Thus, there is considerable loss at this bone-marrow–emigration stage/spleen-entry stage, possibly due to elimination of autoreactive cells (B-cell tolerance) or to homeostatic regulation. The latter possibility is supported by the observation that depletion of the mature B-cell population results in a relatively rapid recovery of this pool, suggesting that most of the immature B-cell population can enter the mature follicular subset in this situation (283).

Once functionally mature B cells are generated, it has been difficult to unambiguously determine their half-life, although accumulating data from several laboratories using bromodeoxyuridine labeling has led to the idea that follicular B cells have a relatively long half-life, on the order of months (239,284). A recent elegant study provided definitive confirmation of this by conditional elimination of RAG2 expression, which allowed termination of B-cell development in adult mice (285). This study showed that follicular B cells have a half-life of about 4.5 months. The same analysis showed that two other subsets of B cells—B-1 and MZ B cells—did not diminish over time, which is consistent with their well-known capacity for self-renewal and lifelong persistence.

Germinal Center B Cells

T-cell–dependent immune responses usually give rise to anatomically distinctive structures in spleen and lymph nodes that are referred to as germinal centers and contain large numbers of rapidly cycling B cells (286,287). These cells can be recognized in stained sections of spleen by binding of high levels of peanut agglutinin (PNA) and by the absence of IgD (288,289). Many of the B cells with this phenotype have down-regulated–BCL-2/up-regulated–Fas expression and, in the absence of strong BCR signaling, will likely die by apoptosis (290–293). The termination of IgD expression means that surface BCR expression decreases at least 10-fold; thus, limiting amounts of antigen will favor the cells with increased affinity for antigen, which are generated by a process termed somatic hypermutation. The molecular details of this mechanism are still unclear, but a major advance has been the recent discovery that activation-induced cytidine deaminase (AID), a putative RNA-editing enzyme that can induce class switch recombination in fibroblasts (294–296), is also a key player in the process of hypermutation (297,298). In fact, a third means for Ig gene diversification used in nonmammalian species, V-gene conversion, is also dependent on AID (299,300).

A potential means for repertoire diversification in the germinal center, distinct from somatic hypermutation, has been suggested by the finding that the RAG genes are induced in at least some GC B cells (301–304). Receptor editing is a potential consequence of this induction, but to date, it is unclear that there is any physiologic relevance for the induction of RAG in the periphery. Considering the important role that the pre-BCR and BCR play in regulating RAG expression in bone marrow development, it seems quite possible that the re-expression of RAG may be a consequence of hypermutation of the heavy or light chain (or both), which results in the generation of nonfunctional receptor genes. This could occur either from truncation by stop codons or by less severe alterations that result in an inability of Ig HL pairing. Consistent with this notion, it appears that much of the RAG expression by GC B cells is coincident with apoptotic cells in the GC (305). Recent RAG-reporter approaches have failed to indicate significant RAG re-induction in mature B cells (306,307). An alternative explanation for some peripheral RAG expression may be an influx of immature cells into the spleen, induced as a consequence of immunization (308).

The precise mechanism of selection for higher-affinity B cells generated by hypermutation of the BCR V regions remains to be fully understood, but regulation of pro- and anti-apoptotic genes likely plays a major role. B cells able to bind antigen with high affinity can present antigen to $CD4^+$ T cells that then signal the B cell through a CD40/CD40L interaction, resulting in the up-regulation of $Bcl-X_L$ (290–292). Most GC B cells have sharply down-regulated levels of Bcl-2 and up-regulated levels of Fas (292,293), and so in the absence of rescue by expression of the alternative anti-apoptotic mediator $Bcl-X_L$, cell death by apoptosis will be the fate of most B cells in the GC. Careful regulation of selection is critical to affinity maturation, and elimination of self-reactive cells that potentially could be generated during this process must also occur efficiently to avoid the potential of autoimmune disease. This is an active area of investigation and more players in this selection process are continuing to be identified (309).

Memory B Cells

Memory B cells were initially defined functionally as cells that could respond rapidly by production of high-affinity antibody when challenged in a host reconstituted with B cells and T cells from a primed animal (310–315). Subsequently, such cells have been purified based on their antigen-binding properties (316) and shown to consist primarily of isotype-switched (IgG^+) B cells that continue to express CD45R/B220 and have distinctively lower levels of cell-surface BCR (317). They arise during the T-cell–dependent immune response, probably only from follicular B cells, in the germinal center. They are very long-lived or self-regenerating, as cell transfer assays have shown that memory responses can be detected for long periods after the primary immunization (317,318).

It is not clear whether all B cells are capable of giving rise to memory B cells. Memory or "secondary" B cells were originally described as expressing distinctively low levels of CD24/HSA, recognized by the monoclonal antibody J11d (319). Some years later, fractionation of naïve spleen B-cell precursors into $J11d^{low}$ and $J11d^{high}$ subsets in a spleen-focus assay system showed that while rapid antibody secretion derived from $J11d^{high}$ cells, memory came largely from the $J11d^{low}$ subset (320). Subsequent experiments demonstrated that germinal centers (the site where most memory B cells are generated) were only produced in cell transfers of $J11d^{low}$ B cells and not with $J11d^{high}$ or $CD5^+$ B cells (321). Considering the rapid Ig secretory response of B-1 B cells and MZ B cells, both contained in the $CD24/HSA^{high}$ fraction, and the fact that most other $CD24/HSA^{high}$ cells are immature (transitional) B cells, likely to be highly susceptible to apoptosis, it seems quite reasonable that memory B cells would not be a major product of this fraction. Rather, the most likely candidate for the memory B-cell precursor is the follicular B-cell subset (Fo), which has a variable but lower expression of CD24/HSA. Whether there is heterogeneity for GC formation or memory B-cell generation within the Fo population remains to be determined.

Whether the maintenance of memory requires periodic restimulation by antigen has been a long-standing controversial issue. On the one hand, transfer of B cells and T cells into irradiated recipients usually required simultaneous challenge with antigen in order to elicit the full response and maintain B-cell memory in recipients (322). Antigenic fragments can persist for very extended periods on follicular dendritic cells (FDC), which are very potent antigen-presenting cells. Thus, in this model the memory B cells are periodically triggered to self-renew by interaction with antigen on FDC. However, on the other hand, memory B cells can be maintained in the apparent absence of T cells or FDC (323,324). Furthermore, analysis by bromodeoxyuridine labeling of memory B-cell populations showed that they were nondividing (318). This issue has recently been addressed in elegant experiments that used the inducible Cre recombinase system to switch the BCR on memory cells away from the immunizing antigen (325). Such antigen-negative memory cells still persisted for extended periods, clearly demonstrating that this was a physiological property of the cell type, independent of the presence of antigen.

B-1 B Cells

B-1 B cells, initially described as Ly-1/CD5$^+$ B cells, are distinguished from follicular B cells by phenotype, anatomical distribution, and function. The B-1 B–cell phenotype encompasses both CD5$^+$ and CD5$^-$ B cells that are IgM^{high}, IgD$^{low/-}$, CD23$^-$ and CD43$^+$. They constitute a large proportion of the B cells found in the peritoneal and pleural cavities (30% to 50% of B cells, around 10^6 cells), but are also found in spleen where they are present at numerically similar levels, but constitute a much lower proportion of the total B-cell pool (2% of B cells, around 10^6 cells). The B-1 B cells in the peritoneal cavity are also CD11b/Mac-1$^+$, unlike those in spleen. They appear early in ontogeny, representing 30% or more of the B cells in spleen of 1-week-old animals. They also have a distinctively higher frequency of λ light chain usage compared to follicular B cells (20% vs. 5%). Also, unlike follicular B cells, they maintain their population in adult animals largely by self-renewal (possibly dependent on periodic stimulation by self-antigen; see below), rather than by input from precursor cells, as shown in cell transfer studies (326).

Perhaps the most distinctive feature of CD5$^+$/B-1 B cells is their enrichment of certain self-reactive specificities, notably for branched carbohydrates, glycolipids, and glycoproteins, including phosphorylcholine, phosphatidylcholine (PtC), the Thy-1 glycoprotein, and bacterial cell-wall constituents (327–330). These antibodies, while autoantibodies, are not pathogenic, but rather referred to as "natural autoantibodies" whose existence has been recognized in serum for several decades (331–333). Their function is still under active investigation, but at least some natural autoantibodies are thought to function in clearance of senescent cells or proteins and to provide an initial immunity to common bacterial or viral pathogens, serving as a kind of "hard-wired" memory of the B-cell population (334–337).

Under physiologic conditions in normal mice most of the CD5$^+$ B cells in the B-1 population (so called "B-1a B cells") arise from precursors in fetal liver, as cell transfer studies showed many years ago that B cells with this phenotype were inefficiently generated from bone marrow precursors in adult mice, compared to fetal or neonatal precursors (338). This is very clearly shown by repopulation of SCID mice by pro–B stage cells isolated from fetal liver and adult bone marrow (Fig. 13). Part of the reason for this difference may be that novel BCRs are enriched by distinctive mechanisms of fetal B-lymphopoiesis, including recombination in the absence of TdT (thereby favoring rearrangement of certain D-J and V-D junctions possessing short regions of homology) (16) and distinctive pre–BCR selection (218,226,339). It is also possible, although not yet tested, that the threshold for elimination of self-reactive B cells at the newly formed stage may be less stringent during fetal development. Forced expression of transgenic BCRs cloned from CD5$^+$ B cells can give rise to CD5$^+$ B cells from bone marrow of adult animals, but the physiologic relevance of this remains to be carefully assessed. The development of B cells in bone marrow of such transgenic mice often appears handicapped, and the precise reason for this requires further study.

The development of B-1/CD5$^+$ B cells is thought to be more dependent on antigenic selection compared to follicular B cells. This idea was first suggested by the finding of particular specificities enriched in this population and strengthened by the observation of repeated occurrences of particular V_H/V_L pairs (340). Thus, for example, the anti-PtC specificity is predominantly encoded by $V_H11V_\kappa9$ and $V_H12V_\kappa4$, utilizing two V_H genes rarely found in conventional T-dependent immune responses (328,341). These cells appear to participate in T-independent responses, but in normal physiology may in fact provide an initial low-affinity "first wave" response to many pathogens that eventually will also elicit a T-dependent response (337,342).

Observations of their self-reactive bias, their capacity for self-renewal, and their restricted repertoire of distinctive BCRs are all consistent with an important role for BCR–antigen interaction in generation and maintenance of this population. This has been formally confirmed recently by studying mice bearing a BCR transgene specific for a glycosylation present only on the Thy-1 membrane protein (343). In these mice, transgene-encoded serum anti–Thy-1 autoantibody (329) was readily detected and there was a corresponding accumulation of a population of CD5$^+$ transgene BCR$^+$ B cells in the peritoneal cavity. Importantly, in Thy-1–null mice generated by gene targeting, neither serum

Fetal
Pro-B

Adult
Pro-B

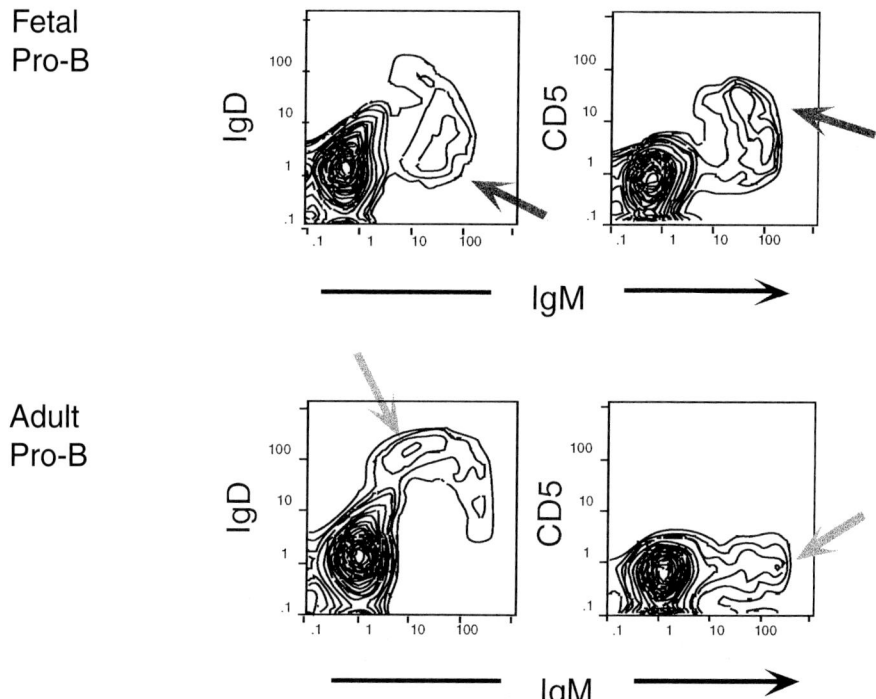

FIG. 13. Generation of B cells in SCID mice shows the distinctive phenotypes produced from fetal and adult pro–B cells. Similar numbers of Pro-B cells, isolated as in Fig. 5, Fr B/C, were injected intravenously into sublethally irradiated adult SCID mice, and then recipients were analyzed 3 weeks later for spleen-cell lymphocytes by staining as shown here.

autoantibody nor the B-cell population was found, demonstrating the critical role for antigen in selection of this B-cell population (344).

Consistent with the importance of antigen selection in the generation and/or maintenance of these cells, this population is often severely affected in mice bearing mutations that alter BCR signaling intensity. The loss of negative mediators such as PTP1C/SHP-1 in moth-eaten mice (345), of CD72 that recruits this phosphatase (345), and of the CD22 co-receptor (346,347), all result in an increased frequency of B-1/CD5+ B cells relative to follicular B cells. On the other hand, the loss of critical BCR signaling components or positive mediators in this pathway, such as an Ig-α tail mutant (348), Btk deficiency (in Xid or Btk-null mice) (349,350), CD19-null mice (351,352), CD21-null mice (353), CD45-null mice (342), and Vav-null mice (354) all negatively impact this B-cell population. In further conformation of this signal-dependent model, transgenic mice expressing different levels of human CD19 show increasing frequencies of B-1/CD5+ B cells. One novel finding is with IL-7$^{-/-}$ mice where it is reported that only B1 and MZ B cells are found (21).

Marginal Zone B Cells

MZ B cells are localized in a distinct anatomical region of the spleen that represents the major antigen-filtering and scavenging area (by specialized macrophages resident there). It appears that they are preselected to express a BCR repertoire similar to B-1 B cells, biased toward bacterial cell wall constituents (355) and senescent self-components (such as oxidized LDL) (356,357). Similar to B-1 B cells, they respond very rapidly to antigenic challenge, likely independently of T cells, but participating in the early phase of T-dependent responses (358,359).

There are similarities and differences in the cell-surface phenotype of MZ and B-1 B cells. Thus, they both are IgM^{+++}IgD$^{-/+}$, CD23$^-$, and CD9$^+$ (360). However, while B-1/CD5+ B cells express CD5 and CD43, MZ B cells do not, and MZ B cells express distinctively high levels of CD21, while B-1 cells have distinctively low levels (Fig. 12). Also, MZ B cells have high levels of CD1, while B-1 B cells do not (361). Certain mutant mice show similar effects on MZ and B-1 B cells, distinct from Fo B cells. For example, most of the mutations described for B-1 B cells that alter BCR signaling have similar consequences for MZ B cells (362), although cells phenotypically similar to MZ B cells are present in Xid/Btk–deficient mice, leading to some controversy in their origins (363). Both are decreased by a mutation in the Ig-α tail that weakens overall BCR signaling (364). They are also both decreased in the Aiolos transcription–factor null mouse (58). Interestingly, deletion of the Pyk-2 tyrosine kinase results in elimination of MZ B cells, while B-1 cells are still found (365).

MZ B-cell development can be studied in a heavy-chain transgenic mouse model system where large numbers of such cells are produced (355,366). In this V$_H$81X heavy-chain mouse, B cells with a specific light chain accumulate with a marginal zone phenotype. This MZ population is eliminated by deletion of CD19, Btk, or CD45, all genetic changes that weaken BCR signaling (362).

B-Cell Tolerance and Receptor Editing

The past decade has seen the development of several transgenic models for the study of B-cell tolerance. In two of these systems, high-affinity BCRs are expressed as IgM-IgD transgenes, one specific for the antigen hen egg–white lysozyme (HEL), and the other for a specific polymorphic determinant on MHC class I (228,244–246,367–369) (Table 2). The advantage of these systems is that they utilize antigens that can be regulated: Transgenic B cells can develop in either the presence or absence of antigen, and cell transfer experiments can be employed to alter the B-cell's antigenic milieu. These have been used initially to confirm ideas on B-cell tolerance that originated in work with nontransgenic B cells, namely that exposure to antigen is generally deleterious to developing B cells, resulting in their elimination or failure to mature (instead entering an "anergic" state). However, the resolution of these systems, coupled with advances in gene targeting and other molecular technologies have uncovered important new details regarding the way that self-reactive B cells develop (or

fail to develop). For example, studies in the anti–H-2 model uncovered an alternative to deletion in response to immature B-cell encounter with antigen—BCR editing to escape autoreactivity (228).

In the HEL system, differences have been uncovered in immature B-cell responses to soluble versus membrane-bound antigen, suggesting that differences in the extent of BCR cross-linking can influence cell fate (245). Furthermore, studies with this system on different mutant backgrounds that shift BCR signaling thresholds up or down have shown that such alterations can result in striking alterations in selection outcomes (370,371). More recently, work in this system has shown that one consequence of B-cell tolerance may be arrest of B-cell migration, so that follicular entry is inefficient (268,269). Presumably, failure to reach such follicular niches contributes to handicapping the autoreactive B cells, resulting in their relatively speedy elimination.

Another major line of investigation has focused on a more "physiologic" example of pathogenic autoreactivity, the anti-DNA antibodies produced in lpr (Fas-deficient) mice that are generally considered to model the human disease of systemic lupus erythematosus (SLE). Analysis of transgenic mice bearing a heavy-chain transgene known to be capable of generating anti-dsDNA reactivity with numerous light chains showed that only light chains with ssDNA activity were

TABLE 2. *Transgenic models of B-cell tolerance*

Ig transgene	Antigen	Background	Effect	Reference
3-83mk	MHC class I H-2Kk,b	H-2Kk	Deletion, receptor editing	228,246,369
3-83mk	" "	H2-Kd	Normal development	
3-83mk	" "	H-2Kk lpr autoimmune-prone	Deletion unaffected	252
anti-HEL md	HEL	sHEL-Tg	Anergy	244,367,368
anti-HEL md	" "	Wild-type	Normal development	
anti-HEL md	" "	mHEL-TG	Deletion	245
anti-HEL md	" "	HEL-Tg lpr autoimmune prone	Deletion unaffected	251
anti-HEL md	HEL	sHEL-Tg CD45 null	Self-antigen promoted development	371
anti-HEL md	HEL	sHEL-Tg motheaten	Deletion by lower-valency autoantigen	370
3H9 H-only	ssDNA with many light chains	BALB/c	No anti-DNA autoantibodies	247
3H9 H-only	" "	lpr autoimmune-prone	Anti-DNA autoantibodies	496
3H9 H/L	dsDNA	BALB/c	Deletion, editing	248
3H9 H/L	dsDNA	$J_H{}^-/J_K{}^-$	Deletion	231
3H9/λ	" "	Wild-type and lpr autoimmune-prone	Anergy	270,271
3H9-R/V$_K$4-R	dsDNA	BALB/c	Deletion, editing anergy	497
3H9-R/V$_K$8-R	ssDNA			
3H9-R/V$_K$4-R	dsDNA, ssDNA	RAG2$^-$	Deletion, activation	498
3H9-R/V$_K$8-R				
3H9/56R	dsDNA, ssDNA	BALB/c	Deletion, editing	499
3H9/56R76R				
Anti-erythrocyte	Red blood cell		Tg+ cells only in peritoneal cavity	375–377
V$_H$11, V$_H$12	PtC, BrMRBC	Wild-type	Increased number of B-1 B cells	500 501
6C10μ	ATA (glycosylation of Thy-1)	Wild-type Thy-1 null	ATA B cells ATA serum no ATA	344

tolerated in the periphery and even these did not contribute to the serum antibody pool (247). Follow-up work uncovered receptor editing in this model (248,372–374) and also showed that when such editing was blocked, the B cells were eliminated in the bone marrow at an immature stage (231). More recent work analyzing transgenic B cells expressing lambda light chain (or in kappa-null mice) where B cells have dsDNA binding has shown the failure of follicular entry previously described in the HEL system (270,271). Interestingly, similar analyses on an "autoreactive" (Fas-deficient) background have shown that this follicular exclusion is lost and production of pathogenic autoantibodies ensues, providing a powerful model for the further characterization of the development of autoimmunity due to breakdown of B-cell tolerance.

A different model of a pathogenic anti-erythrocyte autoantibody has shown another possible mechanism whereby self-reactive B cells may escape deletion or receptor editing, by sequestration from self-antigen (375,376). In this system, the transgenic B cells are largely absent from spleen, but instead survive in the peritoneal cavity, where exposure to the distinctive microenvironment may also contribute to the persistence of these cells. Eventual activation of the B cells by mitogen or antigen can lead to an autoimmune condition in these mice (377).

A common thread in all of the studies described above is the negative impact that the B-cell experiences upon interaction with self-antigen, an expected result for systems that model the regulation of pathogenic autoantibodies. However, a class of autoantibodies is produced in healthy individuals and these "natural autoantibodies" may play a role in early responses to certain classes of pathogens (334,335,337,378). Such a natural autoantibody has been used to construct a transgenic model system where the self-antigen can be regulated. Most natural self-antigens are common glycosylations or cell constituents such as PtC that cannot be eliminated, but a class of natural autoantibodies binds to thymocytes (antithymocyte autoantibody, ATA) and many of these recognize a glycolylation that is only present on the abundant thymocyte cell surface glycoprotein Thy-1 (344). Because Thy-1–null mice have already been generated (379), production of ATA transgenic mice enabled the study of the role of antigen in the generation of this natural autoantibody. Interestingly, both the production of serum ATA and accumulation of B cells with the appropriate light chain (by rearrangement of the endogenous kappa locus) for the ATA BCR required the presence of Thy-1 self-antigen (344). Thus, at least some B cells are selected for binding to self-antigen, although these may belong exclusively to specialized B-cell compartments, such as the B-1 B-cell subset.

Role of Complement, Serum Antibody, and CD5 in B-Cell Tolerance and Response

The importance of complement in the immune system has long been recognized, based on classic experiments showing that cobra toxin decreased responses (380–382). Over the past 10 years the importance of complement in immune responses, explaining the function of adjuvants, has become clearer (383). In the context of B-cell development, components of the complement system also play a role in modulating BCR responses and negative selection of B cells. At least in the HEL-Ig/sHEL system, altering the strength of the BCR signal, by CD45R or PTP1C/SHP1 inactivation, could either reduce or enhance B-cell deletion (371). Similar results could be obtained by altering the BCR-associated chain CD19 (384). Considering the role of complement as a co-receptor for modulating BCR signaling thresholds, the finding that HEL double-Tg mice that also are Cr2 (CD21/CD35) null develop peripheral B cells that are apparently not fully anergized, since they could still respond to antigen challenge, is not surprising (385). This could be due to an inefficient retention of antigen (sHEL) on stromal/dendritic cells and therefore weaker signaling by a monomeric soluble antigen to developing/transitional B cells in the bone marrow or spleen. Potentially, a major role for complement would be to localize self-antigens on bone marrow stromal and dendritic cells, facilitating tolerance at the newly formed B-cell stage. An implication of these findings is that complement deficiency could result in accumulation of functional autoreactive cells, possibly leading to autoimmunity.

Natural autoantibody, a major component of the serum, may have a role (together with complement) in maintaining tolerance to highly conserved self-antigens (383). It also appears that it plays a role in amplifying immune responses, as suggested by studies with a mutant mouse lacking the μ heavy-chain secretory exon (386). The deficit due to a lack of serum IgM was particularly severe in an acute peritonitis model, where some restoration of responsiveness could be obtained by injection of a monoclonal IgM antibody derived from CD5$^+$ B cells (386). Finally, in infection with influenza virus, it appears that early presence of natural autoantibody was equally as important as antibody induced during the course of infection in mediating viral clearance and survival (337). This work has led to the proposal of a two-phase description of immune responses: (a) early T-cell–independent phase dominated by natural autoantibody, which is likely critically dependent on innate immune recognition and activation of complement; and (b) T-cell dependent phase culminating in the germinal center reaction that prduces high-affinity antibody and memory B cells (387).

The presence of CD5 on many of the B-1 B cells has led to the question of whether it plays a direct role in maintaining such self-reactive B cells, particularly in light of its role in altering T-cell selection thresholds as demonstrated in the CD5-null mouse (388). Analysis of B-cell responses to BCR cross-linking in CD5-null mice suggested that the presence of CD5 makes the normal population less likely to respond by secreting IgM (389), effectively "raising the threshold" for their response, possibly by promoting interaction of the BCR with SHP-1 (390). Analysis of the effect of CD5 expression on tolerance in the HEL-Ig/sHEL system also suggested a modulating role, with absence of CD5 leading to a loss of B-cell tolerance and production of serum anti-HEL autoantibody (391).

B-CELL DEVELOPMENT IN HUMANS—SIMILARITIES AND DIFFERENCES WITH MICE

Fetal Development

As described for mouse, human B-cell development can be broadly divided into that taking place prior to birth and that operating after birth throughout life. The liver and spleen are major sites of fetal B-lymphopoiesis in humans and, as in mouse, the bone marrow is the predominant site in adults, with production continuing over most of an individual's lifespan, with some decrease in the aged. The fetal omentum has also been described as a site for B-cell development, similar to mouse (9,392). There is some indication that VH-gene usage is more restrictive in fetal development (393). TdT, absent from mouse fetal development, is similarly missing very early in human fetal development, but is expressed by the 8th or 9th week of gestation, based on detection of N-region addition (393). In general, there is more N-addition (and consequently longer CDR3 regions) in human antibodies compared to mouse at all stages of development, including the adult, although the significance of this is not known.

Bone Marrow Development

B-cell development can be detected in human bone marrow from 20 weeks of gestation and continues throughout life (394,395). Phenotypic subdivisions similar to those in the mouse have been described for developing bone marrow cells (396) (Fig. 14). Thus, CD19 identifies B-lineage cells at all stages, with the earliest stages also expressing CD34, a molecule found on multilineage progenitors (397). These CD19+CD34+ cells have been shown to express TdT, RAG1, and RAG2, the surrogate light-chain orthologs, and Ig-α/Ig-β (396). They contain D-J, but not productive V-D-J rearrangements. The next stage can be defined by loss of CD34, with a fraction that is still IgM− (pre–B cells) and another subset that is IgM+. The pre–B cells express heavy chain in their cytoplasm and have down-regulated expression of TdT (396). All of the IgM+ cells express a marker lost upon final maturation, CD10, so they are immature B cells.

Human early B-lineage cells have proven much more difficult to grow in culture than mouse cells, although conditions have now been defined that allow their expansion *in vitro*. One of the most surprising differences between mouse and human B-precursor growth has been much less dependence on IL-7, suggesting that a different cytokine may substitute in humans (398–400). The finding that lack of the cytokine common gamma chain (γc) in mouse blocks B-cell development, but spares T-cell development, while the reverse is the case in humans (124,401), demonstrates clear differences in cytokine dependence between mouse and human lymphopoiesis.

Human B precursors also express orthologs of λ5 and VpreB, although their organization and number differ from the mouse (402–404). Their expression occurs at a corresponding stage and analysis of the human EBF gene, showing that its targets are similar to those of mouse EBF, including Ig-α, Ig-β and 14.1 (the human ortholog of λ5) (405). Importantly, mutations in components of the pre-BCR lead to immunodeficiency diseases in humans, pointing out the similar and crucial role that pre–BCR signaling plays in human B-cell development (406–408).

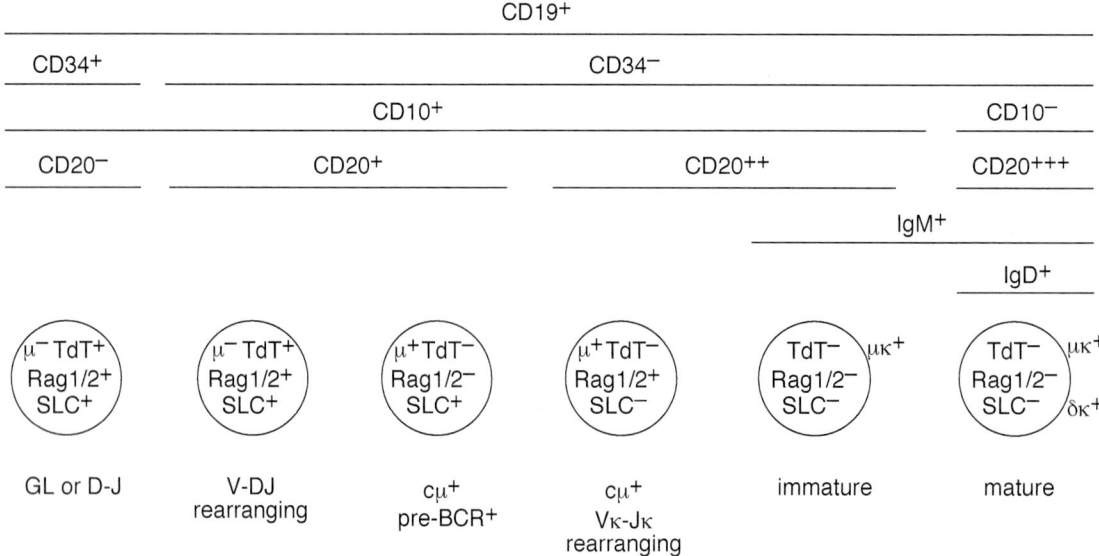

FIG. 14. Stages of developing B-lineage cells in human bone marrow can be delineated based on expression of combinations of cell surface proteins, similar to mouse.

Germinal Center Differentiation

As in mouse, germinal centers (GC) are anatomical structures in secondary lymphoid organs where T-dependent immune responses occur, selecting high-affinity clones during the process of somatic hypermutation and eventually generating memory B cells. The GC consists of B cells at a variety of differentiation states, from early-activated B cells through the plasmablast stage. Therefore, study of this process has benefited significantly from resolution of intermediate stages using multiparameter flow cytometry and carefully chosen cell-surface markers. In one study, this technique allowed definition of two IgD$^+$ stages, two GC stages, and a memory stage in tonsilar B cells (409). This work focused on the levels of somatic mutations accumulating as cells passed through this pathway, finding that it was first detected in the initial GC stage (centroblast). Subsequent work has shown that IgD$^+$ somatically mutated cells can be detected in peripheral blood, based on expression of CD27, suggesting that they are IgM+IgD+ memory B cells (409).

Recent work has found an interesting link between somatic hypermutation and certain B-cell lymphomas. Bcl-6 is a transcriptional repressor that is linked to both germinal center B cells and to B-lymphomas that likely derive from GC B cells (410,411). Bcl-6 expression is high in GC B cells and is required for formation of the germinal center (412). Strikingly, its 5′ regulatory region is mutated as a consequence of hypermutation in GC B cells, the first example of hypermutation targeted outside the Ig regions (410,411), and links this process to deregulated cell growth and lymphomagenesis. Subsequently, mutations have also been found, albeit at a lower level, in CD95/Fas, suggesting this as another potential cause for lymphomas of GC origin (413).

Abnormalities of Development

A key discovery in the past decade has been the finding that a well-known immunodeficiency, X-linked immunodeficiency (XLA), characterized by inability to respond to bacterial infections and a severe deficit in peripheral B cells (414), is due to mutations in Btk, Bruton's tyrosine kinase (415). Shortly after this finding, the mouse ortholog of Btk was shown to be the cause of murine Xid, an extensively studied mutation originally identified in CBA/N mice (416). Btk deficiency in humans is more severe than Xid, with little B-cell development past the early B-cell stage, in contrast with an absence of normal peripheral B-cell development in mouse and inability to respond to certain types of T-independent antigens (417). This difference is not simply due to specific differences in the mutations, as a complete null mutation in mouse is indistinguishable from Xid (350). Thus, human B-cell development, likely at the pre–BCR signaling stage, is much more dependent on Btk.

While XLA is by far the most common B-cell deficiency, amounting to over 80% of those identified, non–X-linked mutations have also been observed. These correspond to mutations in the pre–BCR signaling complex, and in most cases similar effects had been observed in the mouse. For example, deletions or mutations in the μ-constant regions accounted for another 5% (408). Examples have been found of mutations in the 14.1 gene, the human ortholog of the mouse surrogate light-chain λ5 protein (406) and also in Ig-α (407). In both of these cases, early B-lineage cells, identified as CD19$^+$CD34$^+$, were present in normal numbers in bone marrow, but CD19$^+$CD34$^-$ cμ$^+$ cells (pre–B cells) and all later stages were absent. Finally, a patient with a mutation in BLNK, an adaptor protein that links pre–BCR signaling from Syk to the rest of the signaling cascade, showed a similar phenotype (418).

Very few peripheral B cells are detected in any of these disorders, which suggests that pre–BCR signaling is more critical in human than in mouse, where mutations in λ5 and BLNK allow the generation of variable numbers of peripheral B cells. The reason for this difference is not yet understood. Interestingly, common variable immunodeficiency has been shown to result from mutations in the common gamma chain (124) or in the JAK3 gene (419), consistent with IL-7 playing a much less critical role in human pre–B-cell growth than in mouse. As had already been determined from culture studies (398,399), B-cell development is relatively intact, whereas T cells are ablated. The reverse is true for mouse (420,421).

New Insights into Treatment of B-Cell Malignancies

One of the principal reasons for studying the regulation of B-cell development is that defects in this process may result in lymphoma. Human B-lineage neoplasias can be viewed as transformed counterparts of normal B-cell developmental stages, such as pro–B, pre–B, immature B, mature B, or plasma cell, based on rearrangement status and surface phenotype (402). In some cases, transformed cells may even retain growth characteristics of the normal counterpart. This type of classification scheme, correlating features of neoplasias with their normal counterparts has been useful in diagnosis and prognosis of B-lineage neoplasias. For example, B-precursor acute lymphoblastic leukemia (ALL), the most common type of ALL in children (ALL accounts for 25% of childhood cancer), is a clonal expansion of a cell defined by surface phenotype and Ig rearrangement status as representing the pro–B stage (422–424). Recent analyses of B-precursor ALL suggests that they can be subdivided into a pro–B type, predominant in pediatric patients, and a pre–B type, more frequent in adults (425).

Whereas traditional chemotherapeutic agents typically target proliferating cells without specificity for malignant cells, the identification of molecular abnormalities that result in the abnormal survival and proliferation of leukemic cells may lead to the design of novel therapies that specifically target these cells. For example, the successful treatment of mice carrying human B-precursor leukemias with antisense strategies and tyrosine kinase inhibitors holds promise for efficacy in humans (426,427). The identification of novel translocations in B-precursor ALL also holds promise in understanding this disease at the molecular level (428–431).

Another therapeutic approach makes use of knowledge of the surface phenotype of the transformed cell, as in the recent development of anti-CD20 therapy for several types of B-lymphomas (432). CD20 is a 33-kDa phosphoprotein expressed highly on the surface of mature B cells (433–435). Antibodies to CD20, originally called B-1, were initially characterized by their stimulatory and inhibitory effects on human B cells, indicating the importance of CD20 in regulating B-cell proliferation and differentiation (436–438). Therapeutic anti-CD20, called Rituximab, is a chimeric antibody derived by fusing the V regions of a mouse antibody to the human IgG1 constant segment (439). The precise mechanism of depletion is not yet fully understood, but likely includes contributions from antibody-dependent cell-mediated cytotoxicity, complement mediated cytotoxicity, and direct antibody binding effects, including sensitization to apoptosis (432). As most of the cells in many indolent B-cell neoplasms, such as non-Hodgkin's lymphoma or chronic lymphocytic leukemia (CLL), are not predominantly in cycle, the problem may be more a failure to die appropriately, rather than a failure to regulate proliferation. A greater understanding of the growth and sensitivity to apoptosis of different types of lymphomas and leukemias may allow more specific targeting using this approach (440). For example, while CLL cells express relatively low levels of CD20, likely requiring higher doses of anti-CD20 for a response, a combination with another antibody, CD52, which recognizes a molecule that is highly expressed on CLL, has shown promise (441). Alternatively, treatment with anti-CD20 may render the cells generally more sensitive to apoptosis, so that use in combination with more conventional chemotherapeutic agents will be efficacious. These combination therapies are already in clinical trials.

Novel technologies may revolutionize our understanding of B-cell development and the relationship between normal and transformed cells. For example, recent gene-profiling analysis suggests that CLL can be subdivided into two types of disease, with different severity and different response to therapies (442). This analysis also challenges the earlier classification of the disease as a transformation of normal CD5$^+$ B cells, since there are more similarities with normal memory B cells. It is likely that advances in our understanding of the growth and differentiation of cells that represent transformed counterparts of normal developmental stages will suggest novel therapeutic approaches. In the case of CLL, the development of gene therapy has allowed introduction of a gene product, CD40, into patient leukemia cells that can then serve as stimulators for induction of anti-tumor responses (443).

ALTERNATIVE STRATEGIES FOR B-CELL DEVELOPMENT

The broad outlines, and even many of the details of B-cell development, are quite similar in mouse and man, but there are striking differences in other species. There is a notable common alternative approach that involves generation of Ig$^+$ cells during fetal/neonatal development with a relatively restricted repertoire that is then diversified by novel approaches (gene conversion or somatic hypermutation) in specialized lymphoid organs that are associated with the gut. In these species most development from Ig$^-$ precursors appears to cease by birth and the B-cell population is maintained by self-renewal of mature B cells. Here we consider the development and diversification of B cells in chicken and rabbit.

Chicken

B-cell development in the avian occurs in the bursa of Fabricius (444,445). In fact, the term "B" cell refers to "bursa-derived," reflecting the historical origins of research in lymphocyte development. In brief, removal of the bursa just after hatching eliminated the ability to mount an antibody response, demonstrating the importance of this organ in generating cells capable of antibody formation (444). In contrast with the bone marrow, the bursa, being associated with the gut (446), facilitates exposure of developing cells to external antigens and bacterial flora. B-cell development in chicken is usually divided into three stages: pre-bursal, bursal, and post-bursal (447).

During pre-bursal development, at day E5, early precursors can be identified in the para-aortic foci (448), likely corresponding with similar precursor stages localized in this anatomic site in mammals (2). B-lineage commitment, as indicated by D-J rearrangements is detected in the yolk sack at day E5/6, and V-gene rearrangement is found 3 days later (449). Unlike mammalian ordered development, light-chain rearrangement is detected at about the same time as heavy chain, and light chain can precede heavy chain (450). This means that there is no pre–B stage, per se, and also probably no requirement for surrogate light chain. Rearranging B-lineage precursors migrate into the bursal mesenchyme at about day E12, and thereafter these cells begin to proliferate in bursal epithelial buds. This proliferation selectively expands cells that have B-cell receptors. These receptors have very limited diversity, since the heavy chain is formed by rearrangement of a single VH, several Ds, and a single JH pairing with a light chain generated by rearrangement of a single VL with a single JL (451,452). As in mouse fetal development, there is no TdT-mediated N-region addition at the junctions (452).

This "pre-bursal" receptor is diversified by gene conversion by a set of V pseudo-genes during this proliferative phase. At about hatching, these cells become exposed to the contents of the bursal lumen that is connected to the gut lumen via the bursal duct, similar to the appendix. Thus, these proliferating B cells are exposed to the contents of the digestive tract and there is also reverse peristalsis at the end of the gut that transports external antigens into the bursal duct (446). At about this time, the level of apoptosis increases dramatically and it is possible that only 5% of the cells generated in the bursa eventually emerge (453). This death may be due to generation of nonfunctional receptors during the course of gene conversion or it may reflect antigenic selection.

At hatching, emigration of B cells from the bursa increases, but most of these cells constitute a population with a relatively short half-life, measured in days (454). The long-lived pool colonizes the peripheral lymphoid organs over several weeks as the bursa atrophies. By 3 weeks after hatching, bursectomy no longer results in agammaglobulinemia, indicating that the post-bursal phase has become established.

Rabbit

B-cell development in rabbit is similar to chicken, in that B cells initially are produced with limited BCR diversity (455–457) during fetal life, with little new production after birth (458,459). This repertoire is then expanded through gene conversion (455,460) and somatic hypermutation (460,461) in a specialized gut-associated organ, the appendix (462). However, unlike chicken, this diversification process is dependent on antigen availability (463–465).

Pre–B cells can be found in rabbit before birth in the liver, bone marrow, and omentum (458,466–468), but B-lymphopoiesis decreases at birth and is negligible in adult animals (459). Ig rearrangement during fetal and neonatal times is dominated by usage of the most D-proximal V_H gene paired with multiple V_L genes in the light chain (456,457,469–472). In contrast with chicken and mouse, there is significant N-addition (457,471). From 4 to 8 weeks after birth, there is a striking increase in the diversity of this primary repertoire that occurs during proliferation of B cells in the gut-associated lymphoid tissues (GALT) (459,460). V genes are diversified by both gene conversion (455) and also by somatic hypermutation (460,461). Importantly, surgical removal of GALT organs—appendix, saccutus rotundus, and the Peyer's patch—from neonatal rabbits led to unresponsiveness to many antigens, suggesting that this diversification was crucial for normal immune function (473). This finding has been confirmed by sequence analysis, demonstrating that removal of the GALT blocks diversification (462).

Considering the relatively late diversification in rabbit compared to the chicken, these gut areas will provide a milieu of microbial antigens and this appears to be a critical aspect of the diversification process. For example, surgery to prevent access of intestinal flora to the appendix blocked diversification in this organ (474,475); diversification could be restored by reversing the ligation (474). Furthermore, analysis of rabbits reared in germfree conditions revealed abnormal cellular development in the GALT (464) and a lack of responsiveness to certain antigens (463). The dependence of V-gene diversification on antigen has been directly demonstrated in animals where the sacchus rotundus and Peyer's patches were removed at birth and the appendix ligated. Testing the peripheral blood B-cell–V-gene repertoire showed an absence of diversification, in contrast to controls (465). Although the mechanism for this stimulation remains to be established,

possibilities include B-cell activation by a BCR superantigen (476–478) or through a B-cell Toll-like receptor (479).

Two B-Cell Developmental Pathways?

The similarities of chicken and rabbit B-cell development with that in other species such as sheep, swine, and cow suggests that the initial production of a limited BCR repertoire during fetal/neonatal life, diversification at a later time, and maintenance of the B-cell pool in adult life by self-renewal (rather than *de novo* generation from unrearranged precursors) is a major pattern in the design of the immune system (Fig. 15). This pattern contrasts with that described for mouse and man, where ordered heavy- and light-chain rearrangement, pre–BCR selection, and replacement of senescent B cells by newly generated B cells are major aspects of development. This raises the interesting question of whether there is an analogous B-cell development pathway in humans or mouse, perhaps as a vestige.

The idea of two pathways in bone marrow development was suggested previously, based on the observation that heavy- and light-chain ordering is not absolute: Light-chain rearrangements are detected in mice incapable of making heavy-chain rearrangements and can be detected in cells early in B-cell development (480). In one pathway, heavy chains rearrange first, and the pre-BCR is assembled and signals down-regulation of RAG1/2 expression (ending heavy-chain rearrangement), clonal expansion, and accessibility of the kappa locus. Cessation of proliferation is coincident with re-induction of RAG1/2 and light-chain rearrangement. Expression of a complete BCR signals final termination of RAG expression. In this model, pre-BCR and BCR mediate allelic exclusion by a feedback mechanism regulating RAG expression. Thus, most B cells have D-J or even V-D-J rearrangements on both alleles. In the alternative pathway, heavy and light chains rearrange stochastically and allelic exclusion is mediated by relative inaccessibility of the loci (and thereby low frequency of rearrangement). If this is the major pathway in chicken and rabbit, it is consistent with the observation that most chicken B cells have only one allele rearranged (452,481,482). Furthermore, the careful ordering of TdT expression, being down-regulated at the light-chain rearranging stage, is apparently not the case for rabbit, where a large percentage of light chains have N regions (472).

Most rabbit B cells express CD5 (483). In mouse, much of the CD5+ B-cell population is generated during fetal/neonatal development and persists in the adult through self-renewal (326). Furthermore, these cells express a relatively restricted BCR repertoire that is dependent on antigen selection (23). Finally, the pre–BCR selection phase of several heavy chains abundant in CD5 B cells appears to follow different rules than classical pre–BCR-mediated expansion (218). In fact, the process of development in mouse fetal liver may predominantly follow this alternative pathway (339). Thus, in mouse, fetal development, which culminates in production of B-1 B cells, may represent a type of alternative or

Human/Mouse Primary Pathway Bone Marrow B-Cell Development

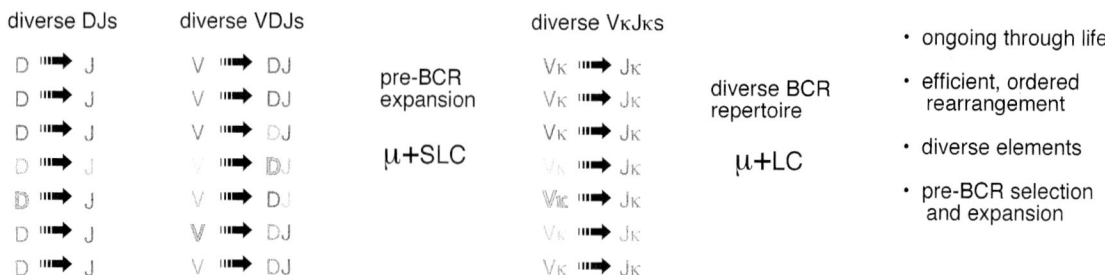

Chicken/Rabbit Alternate Pathway B-Cell Development

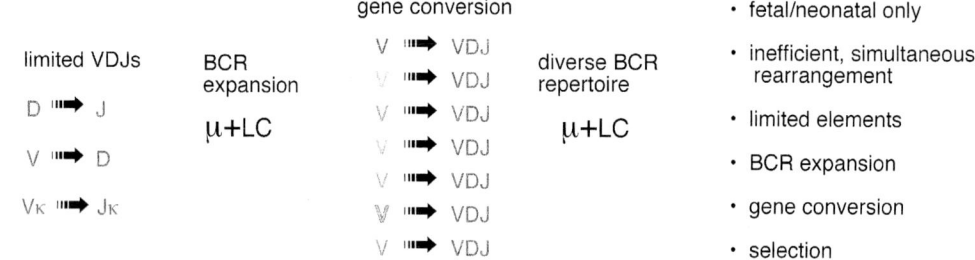

FIG. 15. Alternative strategies of repertoire diversification and B-cell development. In B-cell development in both mouse and human bone marrow, ordered rearrangement predominates, with a pre–BCR selection phase dividing heavy- and light-chain rearrangement. The eventual outcome is a population of newly formed B cells with a diverse set of BCRs that are produced throughout life. In the chicken and rabbit, Ig rearrangement appears less efficient (usually the other allele is germline) and much less diverse, with a single BCR for chicken. However, these cells proliferate and undergo gene conversion during fetal/neonatal life, followed by selection, eventually generating a set of B cells with a more diverse repertoire that persist for the life of the animal.

"primitive" B-cell development, as has been proposed previously (484). It is less clear whether a similar distinction exists in human B-cell development, as data are lacking. Nevertheless, one can envision a primordial pathway that randomly combines heavy and light chains and simply selects cells that express BCRs with weak reactivity to self or environmental antigens, as an alternative to an elaborate process fine tuned to generate more variation comprised of ordered rearrangement, pre–BCR selection, and BCR selection.

CONCLUDING REMARKS

There has been considerable progress over the past decade in understanding the mechanisms that regulate B-cell development, with important insights coming from application of the novel genetic approaches of transgenesis and gene targeting. In a sense, this has allowed progression from research with simple model systems using cell lines to analysis of "normal B cells" in whole animals. The use of such mutant mouse "reagents," together with much higher resolution of normal development made possible by multiparameter flow cytometry, has proven a powerful combination for unravel-

ing much of the complexity of this process. It is daunting to attempt to predict where new advances in the field will come, but undoubtedly the completion of the genome sequence for both mouse and human will provide impetus to large-scale gene profiles of B-cell development, as have already begun (485,486). A complementary approach to gene targeting based on such profiling will involve characterizing new mutant mice generated by chemical mutagenesis (487,488). Considering the recent unanticipated discoveries of AID in isotype switching and BAFF in peripheral B-cell development, it seems likely that the coming decade will provide many surprises. A goal will be to eventually understand how the interplay of the innate and adaptive immune systems generates protective responses, while avoiding autoimmune pathologies at the organism level.

ACKNOWLEDGMENTS

The work in my laboratory is supported by grants from the National Institutes of Health (CA06927, AI26782, and AI40946), and by an appropriation from the Commonwealth of Pennsylvania.

REFERENCES

1. Moore MA, Metcalf D. Ontogeny of the haemopoietic system: yolk sac origin of in vivo and in vitro colony forming cells in the developing mouse embryo. *Br J Haematol* 1970;18:279–296.

2. Godin IE, Garcia-Porrero JA, Coutinho A, et al. Para-aortic splanchnopleura from early mouse embryos contains B1a cell progenitors. *Nature* 1993;364:67–70.

3. Medvinsky AL, Samoylina NL, Muller AM, et al. An early pre-liver intraembryonic source of CFU-S in the developing mouse. *Nature* 1993;364:64–67.

4. Muller AM, Medvinsky A, Strouboulis J, et al. Development of hematopoietic stem cell activity in the mouse embryo. *Immunity* 1994;1:291–301.

5. Medvinsky A, Dzierzak E. Definitive hematopoiesis is autonomously initiated by the AGM region. *Cell* 1996;86:897–906.

6. Yoder MC, Hiatt K, Dutt P, et al. Characterization of definitive lymphohematopoietic stem cells in the day 9 murine yolk sac. *Immunity* 1997;7:335–344.

7. Owen JJ, Cooper MD, Raff MC. In vitro generation of B lymphocytes in mouse foetal liver, a mammalian 'bursa equivalent'. *Nature* 1974;249:361–363.

8. Strasser A, Rolink A, Melchers F. One synchronous wave of B cell development in mouse fetal liver changes at day 16 of gestation from dependence to independence of a stromal cell environment. *J Exp Med* 1989;170:1973–1986.

9. Solvason N, Lehuen A, Kearney JF. An embryonic source of Ly1 but not conventional B cells. *Int Immunol* 1991;3:543–550.

10. Gregoire KE, Goldschneider I, Barton RW, et al. Ontogeny of terminal deoxynucleotidyl transferase-positive cells in lymphohemopoietic tissues of rat and mouse. *J Immunol* 1979;123:1347–1352.

11. Li YS, Hayakawa K, Hardy RR. The regulated expression of B lineage associated genes during B cell differentiation in bone marrow and fetal liver. *J Exp Med* 1993;178:951–960.

12. Landau NR, Schatz DG, Rosa M, et al. Increased frequency of N-region insertion in a murine pre–B-cell line infected with a terminal deoxynucleotidyl transferase retroviral expression vector. *Mol Cell Biol* 1987;7:3237–3243.

13. Desiderio SV, Yancopoulos GD, Paskind M, et al. Insertion of N regions into heavy-chain genes is correlated with expression of terminal deoxytransferase in B cells. *Nature* 1984;311:752–755.

14. Gilfillan S, Dierich A, Lemeur M, et al. Mice lacking TdT: mature animals with an immature lymphocyte repertoire. *Science* 1993;261:1175–1178.

15. Feeney AJ. Lack of N regions in fetal and neonatal mouse immunoglobulin V-D-J junctional sequences. *J Exp Med* 1990;172:1377–1390.

16. Feeney AJ. Comparison of junctional diversity in the neonatal and adult immunoglobulin repertoires. *Int Rev Immunol* 1992;8:113–122.

17. Chang Y, Paige CJ, Wu GE. Enumeration and characterization of DJH structures in mouse fetal liver. *EMBO J* 1992;11:1891–1899.

18. Oltz EM, Yancopoulos GD, Morrow MA, et al. A novel regulatory myosin light chain gene distinguishes pre–B cell subsets and is IL-7 inducible. *EMBO J* 1992;11:2759–2767.

19. Hayakawa K, Tarlinton D, Hardy RR. Absence of MHC class II expression distinguishes fetal from adult B lymphopoiesis in mice. *J Immunol* 1994;152:4801–4807.

20. Lam KP, Stall AM. Major histocompatibility complex class II expression distinguishes two distinct B cell developmental pathways during ontogeny. *J Exp Med* 1994;180:507–516.

21. Carvalho TL, Mota-Santos T, Cumano A, et al. Arrested B lymphopoiesis and persistence of activated B cells in adult interleukin 7(-/)- mice. *J Exp Med* 2001;194:1141–1150.

22. Mebius RE, Miyamoto T, Christensen J, et al. The fetal liver counterpart of adult common lymphoid progenitors gives rise to all lymphoid lineages, CD45+CD4+CD3 cells, as well as macrophages. *J Immunol* 2001;166:6593–6601.

23. Hardy RR, Hayakawa K. B cell development pathways. *Annu Rev Immunol* 2001;19:595–621.

24. Stephan RP, Lill-Elghanian DA, Witte PL. Development of B cells in aged mice: decline in the ability of pro–B cells to respond to IL-7 but not to other growth factors. *J Immunol* 1997;158:1598–1609.

25. Stephan RP, Sanders VM, Witte PL. Stage-specific alterations in murine B lymphopoiesis with age. *Int Immunol* 1996;8:509–518.

26. Sherwood EM, Blomberg BB, Xu W, et al. Senescent BALB/c mice exhibit decreased expression of lambda5 surrogate light chains and reduced development within the pre–B cell compartment. *J Immunol* 1998;161:4472–4475.

27. Sherwood EM, Xu W, King AM, et al. The reduced expression of surrogate light chains in B cell precursors from senescent BALB/c mice is associated with decreased E2A proteins. *Mech Ageing Dev* 2000;118:45–59.

28. Ogawa M, Matsuzaki Y, Nishikawa S, et al. Expression and function of c-kit in hemopoietic progenitor cells. *J Exp Med* 1991;174:63–71.

29. Ikuta K, Weissman IL. Evidence that hematopoietic stem cells express mouse c-kit but do not depend on steel factor for their generation. *Proc Natl Acad Sci U S A* 1992;89:1502–1506.

30. Spangrude GJ, Heimfeld S, Weissman IL. Purification and characterization of mouse hematopoietic stem cells. *Science* 1988;241:58–62.

31. Morrison SJ, Weissman IL. The long-term repopulating subset of hematopoietic stem cells is deterministic and isolatable by phenotype. *Immunity* 1994;1:661–673.

32. Morrison SJ, Hemmati HD, Wandycz AM, et al. The purification and characterization of fetal liver hematopoietic stem cells. *Proc Natl Acad Sci U S A* 1995;92:10302–10306.

33. Kondo M, Weissman IL, Akashi K. Identification of clonogenic common lymphoid progenitors in mouse bone marrow. *Cell* 1997;91:661–672.

34. Akashi K, Traver D, Miyamoto T, et al. A clonogenic common myeloid progenitor that gives rise to all myeloid lineages. *Nature* 2000;404:193–197.

35. Traver D, Miyamoto T, Christensen J, et al. Fetal liver myelopoiesis occurs through distinct, prospectively isolatable progenitor subsets. *Blood* 2001;98:627–635.

36. Kondo M, Scherer DC, Miyamoto T, et al. Cell-fate conversion of lymphoid-committed progenitors by instructive actions of cytokines. *Nature* 2000;407:383–386.

37. Rolink A, Kudo A, Karasuyama H, et al. Long-term proliferating early pre B cell lines and clones with the potential to develop to surface Ig-positive, mitogen reactive B cells in vitro and in vivo. *EMBO J* 1991;10:327–336.

38. Krop I, de Fougerolles AR, Hardy RR, et al. Self-renewal of B-1 lymphocytes is dependent on CD19. *Eur J Immunol* 1996;26:238–242.

39. Li YS, Wasserman R, Hayakawa K, et al. Identification of the earliest B lineage stage in mouse bone marrow. *Immunity* 1996;5:527–535.

40. Rolink A, ten Boekel E, Melchers F, et al. A subpopulation of B220+ cells in murine bone marrow does not express CD19 and contains natural killer cell progenitors. *J Exp Med* 1996;183:187–194.

41. Tudor KS, Payne KJ, Yamashita Y, et al. Functional assessment of precursors from murine bone marrow suggests a sequence of early B lineage differentiation events. *Immunity* 2000;12:335–345.

42. Nakano H, Yanagita M, Gunn MD. CD11c(+)B220(+)Gr-1(+) cells in mouse lymph nodes and spleen display characteristics of plasmacytoid dendritic cells. *J Exp Med* 2001;194:1171–1178.

43. Nikolic T, Dingjan GM, Leenen PJ, et al. A subfraction of B220(+) cells in murine bone marrow and spleen does not belong to the B cell lineage but has dendritic cell characteristics. *Eur J Immunol* 2002;32:686–692.

44. Cumano A, Paige CJ, Iscove NN, et al. Bipotential precursors of B cells and macrophages in murine fetal liver. *Nature* 1992;356:612–615.

45. Nutt SL, Heavey B, Rolink AG, et al. Commitment to the B-lymphoid lineage depends on the transcription factor Pax5. *Nature* 1999;401:556–562.

46. Rolink AG, Nutt SL, Melchers F, et al. Long-term in vivo reconstitution of T-cell development by Pax5-deficient B-cell progenitors. *Nature* 1999;401:603–606.

47. Kozmik Z, Wang S, Dorfler P, et al. The promoter of the CD19 gene is a target for the B-cell–specific transcription factor BSAP. *Mol Cell Biol* 1992;12:2662–2672.

48. Allman D, Li J, Hardy RR. Commitment to the B lymphoid lineage occurs before DH-JH recombination. *J Exp Med* 1999;189:735–740.

49. Nutt SL, Urbanek P, Rolink A, et al. Essential functions of Pax5 (BSAP) in pro–B cell development: difference between fetal and adult B lymphopoiesis and reduced V-to-DJ recombination at the IgH locus. *Genes Dev* 1997;11:476–491.

50. Tsai FY, Keller G, Kuo FC, et al. An early haematopoietic defect in

mice lacking the transcription factor GATA-2. *Nature* 1994;371:221–226.

51. Okuda T, van Deursen J, Hiebert SW, et al. AML1, the target of multiple chromosomal translocations in human leukemia, is essential for normal fetal liver hematopoiesis. *Cell* 1996;84:321–330.

52. Niki M, Okada H, Takano H, et al. Hematopoiesis in the fetal liver is impaired by targeted mutagenesis of a gene encoding a non–DNA binding subunit of the transcription factor, polyomavirus enhancer binding protein 2/core binding factor. *Proc Natl Acad Sci U S A* 1997;94:5697–5702.

53. Wang Q, Stacy T, Binder M, et al. Disruption of the Cbfa2 gene causes necrosis and hemorrhaging in the central nervous system and blocks definitive hematopoiesis. *Proc Natl Acad Sci U S A* 1996;93:3444–3449.

54. Cai Z, de Bruijn M, Ma X, et al. Haploinsufficiency of AML1 affects the temporal and spatial generation of hematopoietic stem cells in the mouse embryo. *Immunity* 2000;13:423–431.

55. Georgopoulos K, Bigby M, Wang JH, et al. The Ikaros gene is required for the development of all lymphoid lineages. *Cell* 1994;79:143–156.

56. Molnar A, Georgopoulos K. The Ikaros gene encodes a family of functionally diverse zinc finger DNA-binding proteins. *Mol Cell Biol* 1994;14:8292–8303.

57. Wang JH, Nichogiannopoulou A, Wu L, et al. Selective defects in the development of the fetal and adult lymphoid system in mice with an Ikaros null mutation. *Immunity* 1996;5:537–549.

58. Wang JH, Avitahl N, Cariappa A, et al. Aiolos regulates B cell activation and maturation to effector state. *Immunity* 1998;9:543–553.

59. Scott EW, Simon MC, Anastasi J, et al. Requirement of transcription factor PU.1 in the development of multiple hematopoietic lineages. *Science* 1994;265:1573–1577.

60. McKercher SR, Torbett BE, Anderson KL, et al. Targeted disruption of the PU.1 gene results in multiple hematopoietic abnormalities. *EMBO J* 1996;15:5647–5658.

61. DeKoter RP, Singh H. Regulation of B lymphocyte and macrophage development by graded expression of PU.1. *Science* 2000;288:1439–1441.

62. Colucci F, Samson SI, DeKoter RP, et al. Differential requirement for the transcription factor PU.1 in the generation of natural killer cells versus B and T cells. *Blood* 2001;97:2625–2632.

63. DeKoter RP, Lee HJ, Singh H. PU.1 regulates expression of the interleukin-7 receptor in lymphoid progenitors. *Immunity* 2002;16:297–309.

64. Bain G, Maandag EC, Izon DJ, et al. E2A proteins are required for proper B cell development and initiation of immunoglobulin gene rearrangements. *Cell* 1994;79:885–892.

65. Bain G, Robanus Maandag EC, te Riele HP, et al. Both E12 and E47 allow commitment to the B cell lineage. *Immunity* 1997;6:145–154.

66. Romanow WJ, Langerak AW, Goebel P, et al. E2A and EBF act in synergy with the V(D)J recombinase to generate a diverse immunoglobulin repertoire in nonlymphoid cells. *Mol Cell* 2000;5:343–353.

67. Pui JC, Allman D, Xu L, et al. Notch1 expression in early lymphopoiesis influences B versus T lineage determination. *Immunity* 1999;11:299–308.

68. Ikawa T, Fujimoto S, Kawamoto H, et al. Commitment to natural killer cells requires the helix-loop-helix inhibitor Id2. *Proc Natl Acad Sci U S A* 2001;98:5164–5169.

69. Spits H, Couwenberg F, Bakker AQ, et al. Id2 and Id3 inhibit development of CD34(+) stem cells into predendritic cell (pre-DC)2 but not into pre-DC1. Evidence for a lymphoid origin of pre-DC2. *J Exp Med* 2000;192:1775–1784.

70. Yokota Y, Mansouri A, Mori S, et al. Development of peripheral lymphoid organs and natural killer cells depends on the helix-loop-helix inhibitor Id2. *Nature* 1999;397:702–706.

71. Koch U, Lacombe TA, Holland D, et al. Subversion of the T/B lineage decision in the thymus by lunatic fringe–mediated inhibition of Notch-1. *Immunity* 2001;15:225–236.

72. Izon DJ, Aster JC, He Y, et al. Deltex1 redirects lymphoid progenitors to the B cell lineage by antagonizing Notch1. *Immunity* 2002;16:231–243.

73. Lin H, Grosschedl R. Failure of B-cell differentiation in mice lacking the transcription factor EBF. *Nature* 1995;376:263–267.

74. O'Riordan M, Grosschedl R. Coordinate regulation of B cell differentiation by the transcription factors EBF and E2A. *Immunity* 1999;11:21–31.

75. Sigvardsson M, O'Riordan M, Grosschedl R. EBF and E47 collaborate to induce expression of the endogenous immunoglobulin surrogate light chain genes. *Immunity* 1997;7:25–36.

76. Kee BL, Murre C. Induction of early B cell factor (EBF) and multiple B lineage genes by the basic helix-loop-helix transcription factor E12. *J Exp Med* 1998;188:699–713.

77. Morrison AM, Nutt SL, Thevenin C, et al. Loss- and gain-of-function mutations reveal an important role of BSAP (Pax-5) at the start and end of B cell differentiation. *Semin Immunol* 1998;10:133–142.

78. Urbanek P, Wang ZQ, Fetka I, et al. Complete block of early B cell differentiation and altered patterning of the posterior midbrain in mice lacking Pax5/BSAP. *Cell* 1994;79:901–912.

79. Eastman Q, Grosschedl R. Regulation of LEF-1/TCF transcription factors by Wnt and other signals. *Curr Opin Cell Biol* 1999;11:233–240.

80. Reya T, O'Riordan M, Okamura R, et al. Wnt signaling regulates B lymphocyte proliferation through a LEF-1 dependent mechanism. *Immunity* 2000;13:15–24.

81. Lee G, Namen AE, Gillis S, et al. Normal B cell precursors responsive to recombinant murine IL-7 and inhibition of IL-7 activity by transforming growth factor-beta. *J Immunol* 1989;142:3875–3883.

82. Kee BL, Rivera RR, Murre C. Id3 inhibits B lymphocyte progenitor growth and survival in response to TGF-beta. *Nat Immunol* 2001;2:242–247.

83. Schilham MW, Oosterwegel MA, Moerer P, et al. Defects in cardiac outflow tract formation and pro–B-lymphocyte expansion in mice lacking Sox-4. *Nature* 1996;380:711–714.

84. Lenardo MJ, Baltimore D. NF-kappa B: a pleiotropic mediator of inducible and tissue-specific gene control. *Cell* 1989;58:227–229.

85. Horwitz BH, Scott ML, Cherry SR, et al. Failure of lymphopoiesis after adoptive transfer of NF-kappaB–deficient fetal liver cells. *Immunity* 1997;6:765–772.

86. Franzoso G, Carlson L, Xing L, et al. Requirement for NF-kappaB in osteoclast and B-cell development. *Genes Dev* 1997;11:3482–3496.

87. Corcoran LM, Karvelas M, Nossal GJ, et al. Oct-2, although not required for early B-cell development, is critical for later B-cell maturation and for postnatal survival. *Genes Dev* 1993;7:570–582.

88. Corcoran LM, Karvelas M. Oct-2 is required early in T cell-independent B cell activation for G1 progression and for proliferation. *Immunity* 1994;1:635–645.

89. Humbert PO, Corcoran LM. oct-2 gene disruption eliminates the peritoneal B-1 lymphocyte lineage and attenuates B-2 cell maturation and function. *J Immunol* 1997;159:5273–5284.

90. Kim U, Qin XF, Gong S, et al. The B-cell-specific transcription coactivator OCA-B/OBF-1/Bob-1 is essential for normal production of immunoglobulin isotypes. *Nature* 1996;383:542–547.

91. Schubart DB, Rolink A, Kosco-Vilbois MH, et al. B-cell-specific coactivator OBF-1/OCA-B/Bob1 required for immune response and germinal centre formation. *Nature* 1996;383:538–542.

92. Nielsen PJ, Georgiev O, Lorenz B, et al. B lymphocytes are impaired in mice lacking the transcriptional co-activator Bob1/OCA-B/OBF1. *Eur J Immunol* 1996;26:3214–3218.

93. Wolf I, Pevzner V, Kaiser E, et al. Downstream activation of a TATA-less promoter by Oct-2, Bob1, NF-kappaB directs expression of the homing receptor BLR1 to mature B cells. *J Biol Chem* 1998;273:28831–28836.

94. Schubart DB, Rolink A, Schubart K, et al. Cutting edge: lack of peripheral B cells and severe agammaglobulinemia in mice simultaneously lacking Bruton's tyrosine kinase and the B cell-specific transcriptional coactivator OBF-1. *J Immunol* 2000;164:18–22.

95. Hayashi S, Kunisada T, Ogawa M, et al. Stepwise progression of B lineage differentiation supported by interleukin 7 and other stromal cell molecules. *J Exp Med* 1990;171:1683–1695.

96. Era T, Ogawa M, Nishikawa S, et al. Differentiation of growth signal requirement of B lymphocyte precursor is directed by expression of immunoglobulin. *EMBO J* 1991;10:337–342.

97. Hardy RR, Carmack CE, Shinton SA, et al. Resolution and characterization of pro–B and pre–pro–B cell stages in normal mouse bone marrow. *J Exp Med* 1991;173:1213–1225.

98. Reichman-Fried M, Bosma MJ, Hardy RR. B-lineage cells in mutransgenic scid mice proliferate in response to IL-7 but fail to show evidence of immunoglobulin light chain gene rearrangement. *Int Immunol* 1993;5:303–310.

99. Rolink A, Grawunder U, Haasner D, et al. Immature surface Ig+ B cells can continue to rearrange kappa and lambda L chain gene loci. *J Exp Med* 1993;178:1263–1270.

100. Owen JJ, Raff MC, Cooper MD. Studies on the generation of B lymphocytes in the mouse embryo. *Eur J Immunol* 1976;5:468–473.

101. Owen JJ, Wright DE, Habu S, et al. Studies on the generation of B lymphocytes in fetal liver and bone marrow. *J Immunol* 1977;118:2067–2072.

102. Johnson P, Greenbaum L, Bottomly K, et al. Identification of the alternatively spliced exons of murine CD45 (T200) required for reactivity with B220 and other T200-restricted antibodies. *J Exp Med* 1989;169:1179–1184.

103. Johnson P, Maiti A, Ng DHW. CD45: A family of leukocyte-specific cell surface glycoproteins. In: Herzenberg LA, Weir DW, eds. *Weir's handbook of experimental immunology*. Cambridge, MA: Blackwell Science, 1997:62. 61–62.

104. Wang J, Walker H, Lin Q, et al. The mouse BP-1 gene: structure, chromosomal localization, regulation of expression by type I interferons and interleukin-7. *Genomics* 1996;33:167–176.

105. ten Boekel E, Melchers F, Rolink A. The status of Ig loci rearrangements in single cells from different stages of B cell development. *Int Immunol* 1995;7:1013–1019.

106. Whitlock CA, Witte ON. Long-term culture of B lymphocytes and their precursors from murine bone marrow. *Proc Natl Acad Sci U S A* 1982;79:3608–3612.

107. Whitlock CA, Robertson D, Witte ON. Murine B cell lymphopoiesis in long term culture. *J Immunol Methods* 1984;67:353–369.

108. Whitlock C, Denis K, Robertson D, et al. In vitro analysis of murine B-cell development. *Annu Rev Immunol* 1985;3:213–235.

109. Grawunder U, Melchers F, Rolink A. Interferon-gamma arrests proliferation and causes apoptosis in stromal cell/interleukin-7–dependent normal murine pre–B cell lines and clones in vitro, but does not induce differentiation to surface immunoglobulin-positive B cells. *Eur J Immunol* 1993;23:544–551.

110. Reininger L, Radaszkiewicz T, Kosco M, et al. Development of autoimmune disease in SCID mice populated with long-term "in vitro" proliferating (NZB × NZW)F1 pre–B cells. *J Exp Med* 1992;176:1343–1353.

111. Pietrangeli CE, Hayashi S, Kincade PW. Stromal cell lines which support lymphocyte growth: characterization, sensitivity to radiation and responsiveness to growth factors. *Eur J Immunol* 1988;18:863–872.

112. Miyake K, Underhill CB, Lesley J, et al. Hyaluronate can function as a cell adhesion molecule and CD44 participates in hyaluronate recognition. *J Exp Med* 1990;172:69–75.

113. Miyake K, Medina K, Ishihara K, et al. A VCAM-like adhesion molecule on murine bone marrow stromal cells mediates binding of lymphocyte precursors in culture. *J Cell Biol* 1991;114:557–565.

114. Miyake K, Weissman IL, Greenberger JS, et al. Evidence for a role of the integrin VLA-4 in lympho-hemopoiesis. *J Exp Med* 1991;173:599–607.

115. Lesley J, He Q, Miyake K, et al. Requirements for hyaluronic acid binding by CD44: a role for the cytoplasmic domain and activation by antibody. *J Exp Med* 1992;175:257–266.

116. Miyake K, Medina KL, Hayashi S, et al. Monoclonal antibodies to Pgp-1/CD44 block lympho-hemopoiesis in long-term bone marrow cultures. *J Exp Med* 1990;171:477–488.

117. Dorshkind K. IL-1 inhibits B cell differentiation in long term bone marrow cultures. *J Immunol* 1988;141:531–538.

118. Namen AE, Lupton S, Hjerrild K, et al. Stimulation of B-cell progenitors by cloned murine interleukin-7. *Nature* 1988;333:571–573.

119. Namen AE, Schmierer AE, March CJ, et al. B cell precursor growth-promoting activity. Purification and characterization of a growth factor active on lymphocyte precursors. *J Exp Med* 1988;167:988–1002.

120. Morrissey PJ, Conlon P, Charrier K, et al. Administration of IL-7 to normal mice stimulates B-lymphopoiesis and peripheral lymphadenopathy. *J Immunol* 1991;147:561–568.

121. Hirayama F, Shih JP, Awgulewitsch A, et al. Clonal proliferation of murine lymphohemopoietic progenitors in culture. *Proc Natl Acad Sci U S A* 1992;89:5907–5911.

122. Valenzona HO, Pointer R, Ceredig R, et al. Prelymphomatous B cell hyperplasia in the bone marrow of interleukin-7 transgenic mice: precursor B cell dynamics, microenvironmental organization and osteolysis. *Exp Hematol* 1996;24:1521–1529.

123. Park LS, Friend DJ, Schmierer AE, et al. Murine interleukin 7 (IL-7) receptor. Characterization on an IL-7–dependent cell line. *J Exp Med* 1990;171:1073–1089.

124. Noguchi M, Yi H, Rosenblatt HM, et al. Interleukin-2 receptor gamma chain mutation results in X-linked severe combined immunodeficiency in humans. *Cell* 1993;73:147–157.

125. Peschon JJ, Morrissey PJ, Grabstein KH, et al. Early lymphocyte expansion is severely impaired in interleukin 7 receptor–deficient mice. *J Exp Med* 1994;180:1955–1960.

126. Ray RJ, Furlonger C, Williams DE, et al. Characterization of thymic stromal-derived lymphopoietin (TSLP) in murine B cell development in vitro. *Eur J Immunol* 1996;26:10–16.

127. Levin SD, Koelling RM, Friend SL, et al. Thymic stromal lymphopoietin: a cytokine that promotes the development of IgM+ B cells in vitro and signals via a novel mechanism. *J Immunol* 1999;162:677–683.

128. Park LS, Martin U, Garka K, et al. Cloning of the murine thymic stromal lymphopoietin (TSLP) receptor: formation of a functional heteromeric complex requires interleukin 7 receptor. *J Exp Med* 2000;192:659–670.

129. Blagoev B, Nielsen MM, Angrist M, et al. Cloning of rat thymic stromal lymphopoietin receptor (TSLPR) and characterization of genomic structure of murine Tslpr gene. *Gene* 2002;284:161–168.

130. Isaksen DE, Baumann H, Trobridge PA, et al. Requirement for stat5 in thymic stromal lymphopoietin-mediated signal transduction. *J Immunol* 1999;163:5971–5977.

131. Migliaccio G, Migliaccio AR, Valinsky J, et al. Stem cell factor induces proliferation and differentiation of highly enriched murine hematopoietic cells. *Proc Natl Acad Sci U S A* 1991;88:7420–7424.

132. Metcalf D. Lineage commitment of hemopoietic progenitor cells in developing blast cell colonies: influence of colony-stimulating factors. *Proc Natl Acad Sci U S A* 1991;88:11310–11314.

133. Tsuji K, Lyman SD, Sudo T, et al. Enhancement of murine hematopoiesis by synergistic interactions between steel factor (ligand for c-kit), interleukin-11, other early acting factors in culture. *Blood* 1992;79:2855–2860.

134. Yasunaga M, Wang F, Kunisada T, et al. Cell cycle control of c-kit+IL-7R+ B precursor cells by two distinct signals derived from IL-7 receptor and c-kit in a fully defined medium. *J Exp Med* 1995;182:315–323.

135. Mackarehtschian K, Hardin JD, Moore KA, et al. Targeted disruption of the flk2/flt3 gene leads to deficiencies in primitive hematopoietic progenitors. *Immunity* 1995;3:147–161.

136. Jacobsen SE, Veiby OP, Myklebust J, et al. Ability of flt3 ligand to stimulate the in vitro growth of primitive murine hematopoietic progenitors is potently and directly inhibited by transforming growth factor–beta and tumor necrosis factor–alpha. *Blood* 1996;87:5016–5026.

137. Ray RJ, Paige CJ, Furlonger C, et al. Flt3 ligand supports the differentiation of early B cell progenitors in the presence of interleukin-11 and interleukin-7. *Eur J Immunol* 1996;26:1504–1510.

138. Veiby OP, Jacobsen FW, Cui L, et al. The flt3 ligand promotes the survival of primitive hemopoietic progenitor cells with myeloid as well as B lymphoid potential. Suppression of apoptosis and counteraction by TNF-alpha and TGF-beta. *J Immunol* 1996;157:2953–2960.

139. Veiby OP, Lyman SD, Jacobsen SE. Combined signaling through interleukin-7 receptors and flt3 but not c-kit potently and selectively promotes B-cell commitment and differentiation from uncommitted murine bone marrow progenitor cells. *Blood* 1996;88:1256–1265.

140. Billips LG, Petitte D, Dorshkind K, et al. Differential roles of stromal cells, interleukin-7, kit-ligand in the regulation of B lymphopoiesis. *Blood* 1992;79:1185–1192.

141. Collins LS, Dorshkind K. A stromal cell line from myeloid long-term bone marrow cultures can support myelopoiesis and B lymphopoiesis. *J Immunol* 1987;138:1082–1087.

142. Cumano A, Dorshkind K, Gillis S, et al. The influence of S17 stromal cells and interleukin 7 on B cell development. *Eur J Immunol* 1990;20:2183–2189.

143. Winkler TH, Melchers F, Rolink AG. Interleukin-3 and interleukin-7 are alternative growth factors for the same B-cell precursors in the mouse. *Blood* 1995;85:2045–2051.

144. Kee BL, Cumano A, Iscove NN, et al. Stromal cell independent growth of bipotent B cell—macrophage precursors from murine fetal liver. *Int Immunol* 1994;6:401–407.

145. Rolink AG, Winkler T, Melchers F, et al. Precursor B cell receptor-dependent B cell proliferation and differentiation does not require the bone marrow or fetal liver environment. *J Exp Med* 2000;191:23–32.

146. Faust EA, Saffran DC, Toksoz D, et al. Distinctive growth requirements and gene expression patterns distinguish progenitor B cells from pre–B cells. *J Exp Med* 1993;177:915–923.

147. Spanopoulou E, Roman CA, Corcoran LM, et al. Functional immunoglobulin transgenes guide ordered B-cell differentiation in Rag-1–deficient mice. *Genes Dev* 1994;8:1030–1042.

148. Gordon MY, Riley GP, Watt SM, et al. Compartmentalization of a haematopoietic growth factor (GM-CSF) by glycosaminoglycans in the bone marrow microenvironment. *Nature* 1987;326:403–405.

149. Borghesi LA, Yamashita Y, Kincade PW. Heparan sulfate proteoglycans mediate interleukin-7–dependent B lymphopoiesis. *Blood* 1999;93:140–148.

150. Kincade PW, Medina KL, Payne KJ, et al. Early B-lymphocyte precursors and their regulation by sex steroids. *Immunol Rev* 2000;175:128–137.

151. Igarashi H, Kouro T, Yokota T, et al. Age and stage dependency of estrogen receptor expression by lymphocyte precursors. *Proc Natl Acad Sci U S A* 2001;98:15131–15136.

152. Landreth KS, Narayanan R, Dorshkind K. Insulin-like growth factor–I regulates pro–B cell differentiation. *Blood* 1992;80:1207–1212.

153. Jardieu P, Clark R, Mortensen D, et al. In vivo administration of insulin-like growth factor-I stimulates primary B lymphopoiesis and enhances lymphocyte recovery after bone marrow transplantation. *J Immunol* 1994;152:4320–4327.

154. Zhang Y, Lu L, Furlonger C, et al. Hemokinin is a hematopoietic-specific tachykinin that regulates B lymphopoiesis. *Nat Immunol* 2000;1:392–397.

155. Montecino-Rodriguez E, Clark RG, Powell-Braxton L, et al. Primary B cell development is impaired in mice with defects of the pituitary/thyroid axis. *J Immunol* 1997;159:2712–2719.

156. Montecino-Rodriguez E, Clark R, Johnson A, et al. Defective B cell development in Snell dwarf (dw/dw) mice can be corrected by thyroxine treatment. *J Immunol* 1996;157:3334–3340.

157. Allman D, Karnell FG, Punt JA, et al. Separation of Notch1 promoted lineage commitment and expansion/transformation in developing T cells. *J Exp Med* 2001;194:99–106.

158. Izon DJ, Punt JA, Pear WS. Deciphering the role of Notch signaling in lymphopoiesis. *Curr Opin Immunol* 2002;14:192–199.

159. Wilson A, MacDonald HR, Radtke F. Notch 1-deficient common lymphoid precursors adopt a B cell fate in the thymus. *J Exp Med* 2001;194:1003–1012.

160. Jacobsen K, Osmond DG. Microenvironmental organization and stromal cell associations of B lymphocyte precursor cells in mouse bone marrow. *Eur J Immunol* 1990;20:2395–2404.

161. Bleul CC, Fuhlbrigge RC, Casasnovas JM, et al. A highly efficacious lymphocyte chemoattractant, stromal cell-derived factor 1 (SDF-1). *J Exp Med* 1996;184:1101–1109.

162. Nagasawa T, Kikutani H, Kishimoto T. Molecular cloning and structure of a pre–B-cell growth-stimulating factor. *Proc Natl Acad Sci U S A* 1994;91:2305–2309.

163. D'Apuzzo M, Rolink A, Loetscher M, et al. The chemokine SDF-1, stromal cell-derived factor 1, attracts early stage B cell precursors via the chemokine receptor CXCR4. *Eur J Immunol* 1997;27:1788–1793.

164. Nagasawa T, Tachibana K, Kishimoto T. A novel CXC chemokine PBSF/SDF-1 and its receptor CXCR4: their functions in development, hematopoiesis and HIV infection. *Semin Immunol* 1998;10:179–185.

165. Nagasawa T, Hirota S, Tachibana K, et al. Defects of B-cell lymphopoiesis and bone-marrow myelopoiesis in mice lacking the CXC chemokine PBSF/SDF-1. *Nature* 1996;382:635–638.

166. Ma Q, Jones D, Borghesani PR, et al. Impaired B-lymphopoiesis, myelopoiesis, derailed cerebellar neuron migration in CXCR4– and SDF-1–deficient mice. *Proc Natl Acad Sci U S A* 1998;95:9448–9453.

167. Zou YR, Kottmann AH, Kuroda M, et al. Function of the chemokine receptor CXCR4 in haematopoiesis and in cerebellar development. *Nature* 1998;393:595–599.

168. Ma Q, Jones D, Springer TA. The chemokine receptor CXCR4 is required for the retention of B lineage and granulocytic precursors within the bone marrow microenvironment. *Immunity* 1999;10:463–471.

169. Lennon GG, Perry RP. The temporal order of appearance of transcripts from unrearranged and rearranged Ig genes in murine fetal liver. *J Immunol* 1990;144:1983–1987.

170. Lennon GG, Perry RP. C mu-containing transcripts initiate heterogeneously within the IgH enhancer region and contain a novel 5′-nontranslatable exon. *Nature* 1985;318:475–478.

171. Nelson KJ, Haimovich J, Perry RP. Characterization of productive and sterile transcripts from the immunoglobulin heavy-chain locus: processing of micron and muS mRNA. *Mol Cell Biol* 1983;3:1317–1332.

172. Oettinger MA, Schatz DG, Gorka C, et al. RAG-1 and RAG-2, adjacent genes that synergistically activate V(D)J recombination. *Science* 1990;248:1517–1523.

173. Schatz DG, Oettinger MA, Baltimore D. The V(D)J recombination activating gene, RAG-1. *Cell* 1989;59:1035–1048.

174. Desiderio SV, Yancopoulos GD, Paskind M, et al. Insertion of N regions into heavy-chain genes is correlated with expression of terminal deoxytransferase in B cells. *Nature* 1984;311:752–755.

175. Ehlich A, Martin V, Muller W, et al. Analysis of the B-cell progenitor compartment at the level of single cells. *Curr Biol* 1994;4:573–583.

176. Kitamura D, Rajewsky K. Targeted disruption of mu chain membrane exon causes loss of heavy-chain allelic exclusion. *Nature* 1992; 356:154–156.

177. Bosma GC, Custer RP, Bosma MJ. A severe combined immunodeficiency mutation in the mouse. *Nature* 1983;301:527–530.

178. Hardy RR, Kemp JD, Hayakawa K. Analysis of lymphoid population in scid mice; detection of a potential B lymphocyte progenitor population present at normal levels in scid mice by three color flow cytometry with B220 and S7. *Curr Top Microbiol Immunol* 1989;152:19–25.

179. Blunt T, Finnie NJ, Taccioli GE, et al. Defective DNA-dependent protein kinase activity is linked to V(D)J recombination and DNA repair defects associated with the murine scid mutation. *Cell* 1995;80:813–823.

180. Peterson SR, Kurimasa A, Oshimura M, et al. Loss of the catalytic subunit of the DNA-dependent protein kinase in DNA double-strand-break-repair mutant mammalian cells. *Proc Natl Acad Sci U S A* 1995; 92:3171–3174.

181. Reichman-Fried M, Hardy RR, Bosma MJ. Development of B-lineage cells in the bone marrow of scid/scid mice following the introduction of functionally rearranged immunoglobulin transgenes. *Proc Natl Acad Sci U S A* 1990;87:2730–2734.

182. Kitamura D, Roes J, Kuhn R, et al. A B cell-deficient mouse by targeted disruption of the membrane exon of the immunoglobulin mu chain gene. *Nature* 1991;350:423–426.

183. Loffert D, Schaal S, Ehlich A, et al. Early B-cell development in the mouse: insights from mutations introduced by gene targeting. *Immunol Rev* 1994;137:135–153.

184. Karasuyama H, Kudo A, Melchers F. The proteins encoded by the VpreB and lambda 5 pre–B cell-specific genes can associate with each other and with mu heavy chain. *J Exp Med* 1990;172:969–972.

185. Sakaguchi N, Melchers F. Lambda 5, a new light-chain–related locus selectively expressed in pre–B lymphocytes. *Nature* 1986;324:579–582.

186. Kudo A, Melchers F. A second gene, VpreB in the lambda 5 locus of the mouse, which appears to be selectively expressed in pre–B lymphocytes. *EMBO J* 1987;6:2267–2272.

187. Kitamura D, Kudo A, Schaal S, et al. A critical role of lambda 5 protein in B cell development. *Cell* 1992;69:823–831.

188. Papavasiliou F, Jankovic M, Nussenzweig MC. Surrogate or conventional light chains are required for membrane immunoglobulin mu to activate the precursor B cell transition. *J Exp Med* 1996;184:2025–2030.

189. Sakaguchi N, Kashiwamura S, Kimoto M, et al. B lymphocyte lineage-restricted expression of mb-1, a gene with CD3-like structural properties. *EMBO J* 1988;7:3457–3464.

190. Hermanson GG, Eisenberg D, Kincade PW, et al. B29: a member of the immunoglobulin gene superfamily exclusively expressed on beta-lineage cells. *Proc Natl Acad Sci U S A* 1988;85:6890–6894.

191. Hombach J, Lottspeich F, Reth M. Identification of the genes encoding the IgM-alpha and Ig-beta components of the IgM antigen receptor complex by amino-terminal sequencing. *Eur J Immunol* 1990; 20:2795–2799.

192. Campbell KS, Hager EJ, Friedrich RJ, et al. IgM antigen receptor complex contains phosphoprotein products of B29 and mb-1 genes. *Proc Natl Acad Sci U S A* 1991;88:3982–3986.

193. Gong S, Nussenzweig MC. Regulation of an early developmental checkpoint in the B cell pathway by Ig beta. *Science* 1996;272:411–414.

194. Cheng AM, Rowley B, Pao W, et al. Syk tyrosine kinase required for mouse viability and B-cell development. *Nature* 1995;378:303–306.

195. Turner M, Mee PJ, Costello PS, et al. Perinatal lethality and blocked B-cell development in mice lacking the tyrosine kinase Syk. *Nature* 1995;378:298–302.

196. Wienands J, Larbolette O, Reth M. Evidence for a preformed transducer complex organized by the B cell antigen receptor. *Proc Natl Acad Sci U S A* 1996;93:7865–7870.

197. Lam KP, Kuhn R, Rajewsky K. In vivo ablation of surface immunoglobulin on mature B cells by inducible gene targeting results in rapid cell death. *Cell* 1997;90:1073–1083.

198. Hirabayashi Y, Lecerf JM, Dong Z, et al. Kinetic analysis of the interactions of recombinant human VpreB and Ig V domains. *J Immunol* 1995;155:1218–1228.

199. Wasserman R, Li YS, Hardy RR. Down-regulation of terminal deoxynucleotidyl transferase by Ig heavy chain in B lineage cells. *J Immunol* 1997;158:1133–1138.

200. Middendorp S, Dingjan GM, Hendriks RW. Impaired precursor B cell differentiation in Bruton's tyrosine kinase-deficient mice. *J Immunol* 2002;168:2695–2703.

201. Hayashi S, Witte PL, Kincade PW. The xid mutation affects hemopoiesis in long term cultures of murine bone marrow. *J Immunol* 1989;142:444–451.

202. Narendran A, Ramsden D, Cumano A, et al. B cell developmental defects in X-linked immunodeficiency. *Int Immunol* 1993;5:139–144.

203. Nisitani S, Satterthwaite AB, Akashi K, et al. Posttranscriptional regulation of Bruton's tyrosine kinase expression in antigen receptor–stimulated splenic B cells. *Proc Natl Acad Sci U S A* 2000;97:2737–2742.

204. Kurosaki T, Johnson SA, Pao L, et al. Role of the Syk autophosphorylation site and SH2 domains in B cell antigen receptor signaling. *J Exp Med* 1995;182:1815–1823.

205. Kurosaki T. Genetic analysis of B cell antigen receptor signaling. *Annu Rev Immunol* 1999;17:555–592.

206. Xu S, Tan JE, Wong EP, et al. B cell development and activation defects resulting in xid-like immunodeficiency in BLNK/SLP-65–deficient mice. *Int Immunol* 2000;12:397–404.

207. Xu S, Wong SC, Lam KP. Cutting edge: B cell linker protein is dispensable for the allelic exclusion of immunoglobulin heavy chain locus but required for the persistence of CD5+ B cells. *J Immunol* 2000;165:4153–4157.

208. Grawunder U, Leu TM, Schatz DG, et al. Down-regulation of RAG1 and RAG2 gene expression in preB cells after functional immunoglobulin heavy chain rearrangement. *Immunity* 1995;3:601–608.

209. Schlissel MS, Baltimore D. Activation of immunoglobulin kappa gene rearrangement correlates with induction of germline kappa gene transcription. *Cell* 1989;58:1001–1007.

210. Lin WC, Desiderio S. Regulation of V(D)J recombination activator protein RAG-2 by phosphorylation. *Science* 1993;260:953–959.

211. Li Z, Dordai DI, Lee J, et al. A conserved degradation signal regulates RAG-2 accumulation during cell division and links V(D)J recombination to the cell cycle. *Immunity* 1996;5:575–589.

212. Lee J, Desiderio S. Cyclin A/CDK2 regulates V(D)J recombination by coordinating RAG-2 accumulation and DNA repair. *Immunity* 1999;11:771–781.

213. Karasuyama H, Nakamura T, Nagata K, et al. The roles of preB cell receptor in early B cell development and its signal transduction. *Immunol Cell Biol* 1997;75:209–216.

214. Marshall AJ, Fleming HE, Wu GE, et al. Modulation of the IL-7 dose–response threshold during pro–B cell differentiation is dependent on pre–B cell receptor expression. *J Immunol* 1998;161:6038–6045.

215. Keyna U, Beck-Engeser GB, Jongstra J, et al. Surrogate light chain–dependent selection of Ig heavy chain V regions. *J Immunol* 1995;155:5536–5542.

216. Kline GH, Hartwell L, Beck-Engeser GB, et al. Pre–B cell receptor-mediated selection of pre–B cells synthesizing functional mu heavy chains. *J Immunol* 1998;161:1608–1618.

217. ten Boekel E, Melchers F, Rolink AG. Changes in the V(H) gene repertoire of developing precursor B lymphocytes in mouse bone marrow mediated by the pre–B cell receptor. *Immunity* 1997;7:357–368.

218. Wasserman R, Li YS, Shinton SA, et al. A novel mechanism for B cell repertoire maturation based on response by B cell precursors to pre–B receptor assembly. *J Exp Med* 1998;187:259–264.

219. Wu GE, Paige CJ. VH gene family utilization in colonies derived from B and pre–B cells detected by the RNA colony blot assay. *EMBO J* 1986;5:3475–3481.

220. Decker DJ, Boyle NE, Koziol JA, et al. The expression of the Ig H chain repertoire in developing bone marrow B lineage cells. *J Immunol* 1991;146:350–361.

221. Yancopoulos GD, Desiderio SV, Paskind M, et al. Preferential utilization of the most JH-proximal VH gene segments in pre–B-cell lines. *Nature* 1984;311:727–733.

222. Decker DJ, Boyle NE, Klinman NR. Predominance of nonproductive rearrangements of VH81X gene segments evidences a dependence of B cell clonal maturation on the structure of nascent H chains. *J Immunol* 1991;147:1406–1411.

223. Decker DJ, Kline GH, Hayden TA, et al. Heavy chain V gene–specific elimination of B cells during the pre–B cell to B cell transition. *J Immunol* 1995;154:4924–4935.

224. Keyna U, Applequist SE, Jongstra J, et al. Ig mu heavy chains with VH81X variable regions do not associate with lambda 5. *Ann N Y Acad Sci* 1995;764:39–42.

225. Marshall AJ, Wu GE, Paige GJ. Frequency of VH81x usage during B cell development: initial decline in usage is independent of Ig heavy chain cell surface expression. *J Immunol* 1996;156:2077–2084.

226. Marshall AJ, Paige CJ, Wu GE. V(H) repertoire maturation during B cell development in vitro: differential selection of Ig heavy chains by fetal and adult B cell progenitors. *J Immunol* 1997;158:4282–4291.

227. Shapiro MA, Weigert M. How immunoglobulin V kappa genes rearrange. *J Immunol* 1987;139:3834–3839.

228. Tiegs SL, Russell DM, Nemazee D. Receptor editing in self-reactive bone marrow B cells. *J Exp Med* 1993;177:1009–1020.

229. Lang J, Jackson M, Teyton L, et al. B cells are exquisitely sensitive to central tolerance and receptor editing induced by ultralow affinity, membrane-bound antigen. *J Exp Med* 1996;184:1685–1697.

230. Yamagami T, ten Boekel E, Andersson J, et al. Frequencies of multiple IgL chain gene rearrangements in single normal or kappaL chain-deficient B lineage cells. *Immunity* 1999;11:317–327.

231. Chen C, Nagy Z, Radic MZ, et al. The site and stage of anti-DNA B-cell deletion. *Nature* 1995;373:252–255.

232. Melamed D, Benschop RJ, Cambier JC, et al. Developmental regulation of B lymphocyte immune tolerance compartmentalizes clonal selection from receptor selection. *Cell* 1998;92:173–182.

233. Allman DM, Ferguson SE, Cancro MP. Peripheral B cell maturation. I. Immature peripheral B cells in adults are heat-stable antigenhi and exhibit unique signaling characteristics. *J Immunol* 1992;149:2533–2540.

234. Rolink AG, Andersson J, Melchers F. Characterization of immature B cells by a novel monoclonal antibody, by turnover and by mitogen reactivity. *Eur J Immunol* 1998;28:3738–3748.

235. Allman D, Lindsley RC, DeMuth W, et al. Resolution of three non-proliferative immature splenic B cell subsets reveals multiple selection points during peripheral B cell maturation. *J Immunol* 2001;167:6834–6840.

236. Petrenko O, Beavis A, Klaine M, et al. The molecular characterization of the fetal stem cell marker AA4. *Immunity* 1999;10:691–700.

237. Fang W, Mueller DL, Pennell CA, et al. Frequent aberrant immunoglobulin gene rearrangements in pro–B cells revealed by a bcl-xL transgene. *Immunity* 1996;4:291–299.

238. Carsetti R, Kohler G, Lamers MC. Transitional B cells are the target of negative selection in the B cell compartment. *J Exp Med* 1995;181:2129–2140.

239. Allman DM, Ferguson SE, Lentz VM, et al. Peripheral B cell maturation. II. Heat-stable antigen(hi) splenic B cells are an immature developmental intermediate in the production of long-lived marrow-derived B cells. *J Immunol* 1993;151:4431–4444.

240. Weiner HL, Moorhead JW, Claman HN. Anti-immunoglobulin stimulation of murine lymphocytes. I. Age dependency of the proliferative response. *J Immunol* 1976;116:1656–1661.

241. Nossal GJ, Pike BL, Battye FL. Mechanisms of clonal abortion tolerogenesis. II. Clonal behaviour of immature B cells following exposure to anti-mu chain antibody. *Immunology* 1979;37:203–215.

242. Metcalf ES, Klinman NR. In vitro tolerance induction of neonatal murine B cells. *J Exp Med* 1976;143:1327–1340.

243. Metcalf ES, Klinman NR. In vitro tolerance induction of bone marrow cells: a marker for B cell maturation. *J Immunol* 1977;118:2111–2116.

244. Goodnow CC, Crosbie J, Adelstein S, et al. Altered immunoglobulin expression and functional silencing of self-reactive B lymphocytes in transgenic mice. *Nature* 1988;334:676–682.

245. Hartley SB, Crosbie J, Brink R, et al. Elimination from peripheral lymphoid tissues of self-reactive B lymphocytes recognizing membrane-bound antigens. *Nature* 1991;353:765–769.

246. Nemazee DA, Burki K. Clonal deletion of B lymphocytes in a transgenic mouse bearing anti–MHC class I antibody genes. *Nature* 1989;337:562–566.

247. Erikson J, Radic MZ, Camper SA, et al. Expression of anti-DNA immunoglobulin transgenes in non-autoimmune mice. *Nature* 1991; 349:331–334.

248. Gay D, Saunders T, Camper S, et al. Receptor editing: an approach by autoreactive B cells to escape tolerance. *J Exp Med* 1993;177:999–1008.

249. Norvell A, Mandik L, Monroe JG. Engagement of the antigen-receptor on immature murine B lymphocytes results in death by apoptosis. *J Immunol* 1995;154:4404–4413.

250. Norvell A, Monroe JG. Acquisition of surface IgD fails to protect from tolerance-induction. Both surface IgM- and surface IgD-mediated signals induce apoptosis of immature murine B lymphocytes. *J Immunol* 1996;156:1328–1332.

251. Rathmell JC, Goodnow CC. Effects of the lpr mutation on elimination and inactivation of self-reactive B cells. *J Immunol* 1994;153:2831–2842.

252. Rubio CF, Kench J, Russell DM, et al. Analysis of central B cell tolerance in autoimmune-prone MRL/lpr mice bearing autoantibody transgenes. *J Immunol* 1996;157:65–71.

253. Carman JA, Wechsler-Reya RJ, Monroe JG. Immature stage B cells enter but do not progress beyond the early G1 phase of the cell cycle in response to antigen receptor signaling. *J Immunol* 1996;156:4562–4569.

254. Benschop RJ, Melamed D, Nemazee D, et al. Distinct signal thresholds for the unique antigen receptor–linked gene expression programs in mature and immature B cells. *J Exp Med* 1999;190:749–756.

255. Tomayko MM, Cancro MP. Long-lived B cells are distinguished by elevated expression of A1. *J Immunol* 1998;160:107–111.

256. Grumont RJ, Rourke IJ, Gerondakis S. Rel-dependent induction of A1 transcription is required to protect B cells from antigen receptor ligation–induced apoptosis. *Genes Dev* 1999;13:400–411.

257. Khan WN. Regulation of B lymphocyte development and activation by Bruton's tyrosine kinase. *Immunol Res* 2001;23:147–156.

258. Maas A, Hendriks RW. Role of Bruton's tyrosine kinase in B cell development. *Dev Immunol* 2001;8:171–181.

259. Mond JJ, Scher I, Cossman J, et al. Role of the thymus in directing the development of a subset of B lymphocytes. *J Exp Med* 1982;155:924–936.

260. Wortis HH, Burkly L, Hughes D, et al. Lack of mature B cells in nude mice with X-linked immune deficiency. *J Exp Med* 1982;155:903–913.

261. Oka Y, Rolink AG, Andersson J, et al. Profound reduction of mature B cell numbers, reactivities and serum Ig levels in mice which simultaneously carry the XID and CD40 deficiency genes. *Int Immunol* 1996;8:1675–1685.

262. Clark MR, Campbell KS, Kazlauskas A, et al. The B cell antigen receptor complex: association of Ig-alpha and Ig-beta with distinct cytoplasmic effectors. *Science* 1992;258:123–126.

263. Hibbs ML, Tarlinton DM, Armes J, et al. Multiple defects in the immune system of Lyn-deficient mice, culminating in autoimmune disease. *Cell* 1995;83:301–311.

264. Chan VW, Meng F, Soriano P, et al. Characterization of the B lymphocyte populations in Lyn-deficient mice and the role of Lyn in signal initiation and down-regulation. *Immunity* 1997;7:69–81.

265. Subbarao B, Mosier DE. Induction of B lymphocyte proliferation by monoclonal anti-Lyb 2 antibody. *J Immunol* 1983;130:2033–2037.

266. Pan C, Baumgarth N, Parnes JR. CD72-deficient mice reveal nonredundant roles of CD72 in B cell development and activation. *Immunity* 1999;11:495–506.

267. Adachi T, Flaswinkel H, Yakura H, et al. The B cell surface protein CD72 recruits the tyrosine phosphatase SHP-1 upon tyrosine phosphorylation. *J Immunol* 1998;160:4662–4665.

268. Cyster JG, Hartley SB, Goodnow CC. Competition for follicular niches excludes self-reactive cells from the recirculating B-cell repertoire. *Nature* 1994;371:389–395.

269. Cyster JG, Goodnow CC. Antigen-induced exclusion from follicles and anergy are separate and complementary processes that influence peripheral B cell fate. *Immunity* 1995;3:691–701.

270. Mandik-Nayak L, Bui A, Noorchashm H, et al. Regulation of anti-double-stranded DNA B cells in nonautoimmune mice: localization to the T-B interface of the splenic follicle. *J Exp Med* 1997;186:1257–1267.

271. Mandik-Nayak L, Seo SJ, Sokol C, et al. MRL-lpr/lpr mice exhibit a defect in maintaining developmental arrest and follicular exclusion of anti-double-stranded DNA B cells. *J Exp Med* 1999;189:1799–1814.

272. Levine MH, Haberman AM, Sant'Angelo DB, et al. A B-cell receptor–specific selection step governs immature to mature B cell differentiation. *Proc Natl Acad Sci U S A* 2000;97:2743–2748.

273. Forster R, Schubel A, Breitfeld D, et al. CCR7 coordinates the primary immune response by establishing functional microenvironments in secondary lymphoid organs. *Cell* 1999;99:23–33.

274. Ansel KM, Ngo VN, Hyman PL, et al. A chemokine-driven positive feedback loop organizes lymphoid follicles. *Nature* 2000;406:309–314.

275. Waldschmidt TJ, Noelle RJ. Immunology. Long live the mature B cell—a baffling mystery resolved. *Science* 2001;293:2012–2013.

276. Khare SD, Sarosi I, Xia XZ, et al. Severe B cell hyperplasia and autoimmune disease in TALL-1 transgenic mice. *Proc Natl Acad Sci U S A* 2000;97:3370–3375.

277. Khare SD, Hsu H. The role of TALL-1 and APRIL in immune regulation. *Trends Immunol* 2001;22:61–63.

278. Thompson JS, Bixler SA, Qian F, et al. BAFF-R, a newly identified TNF receptor that specifically interacts with BAFF. *Science* 2001;293:2108–2111.

279. Yan M, Brady JR, Chan B, et al. Identification of a novel receptor for B lymphocyte stimulator that is mutated in a mouse strain with severe B cell deficiency. *Curr Biol* 2001;11:1547–1552.

280. Lentz VM, Cancro MP, Nashold FE, et al. Bcmd governs recruitment of new B cells into the stable peripheral B cell pool in the A/WySnJ mouse. *J Immunol* 1996;157:598–606.

281. Yu G, Boone T, Delaney J, et al. APRIL and TALL-I and receptors BCMA and TACI: system for regulating humoral immunity. *Nat Immunol* 2000;1:252–256.

282. Opstelten D, Osmond DG. Pre-B cells in mouse bone marrow: immunofluorescence stathmokinetic studies of the proliferation of cytoplasmic mu-chain-bearing cells in normal mice. *J Immunol* 1983; 131:2635–2640.

283. Bazin H, Platteau B, Maclennan IC, et al. B-cell production and differentiation in adult rats. *Immunology* 1985;54:79–88.

284. Forster I, Rajewsky K. The bulk of the peripheral B-cell pool in mice is stable and not rapidly renewed from the bone marrow. *Proc Natl Acad Sci U S A* 1990;87:4781–4784.

285. Hao Z, Rajewsky K. Homeostasis of peripheral B cells in the absence of B cell influx from the bone marrow. *J Exp Med* 2001;194:1151–1164.

286. MacLennan IC. Germinal centers. *Annu Rev Immunol* 1994;12:117–139.

287. Przylepa J, Himes C, Kelsoe G. Lymphocyte development and selection in germinal centers. *Curr Top Microbiol Immunol* 1998;229:85–104.

288. Butcher EC, Rouse RV, Coffman RL, et al. Surface phenotype of Peyer's patch germinal center cells: implications for the role of germinal centers in B cell differentiation. *J Immunol* 1982;129:2698–2707.

289. Kraal G, Hardy RR, Gallatin WM, et al. Antigen-induced changes in B cell subsets in lymph nodes: analysis by dual fluorescence flow cytofluorometry. *Eur J Immunol* 1986;16:829–834.

290. Wang Z, Karras JG, Howard RG, et al. Induction of bcl-x by CD40 engagement rescues sIg-induced apoptosis in murine B cells. *J Immunol* 1995;155:3722–3725.

291. Tuscano JM, Druey KM, Riva A, et al. Bcl-x rather than Bcl-2 mediates CD40-dependent centrocyte survival in the germinal center. *Blood* 1996;88:1359–1364.

292. Zhang X, Li L, Choe J, et al. Up-regulation of Bcl-xL expression protects CD40-activated human B cells from Fas-mediated apoptosis. *Cell Immunol* 1996;173:149–154.

293. Takahashi Y, Ohta H, Takemori T. Fas is required for clonal selection in germinal centers and the subsequent establishment of the memory B cell repertoire. *Immunity* 2001;14:181–192.

294. Muramatsu M, Kinoshita K, Fagarasan S, et al. Class switch recombination and hypermutation require activation-induced cytidine deaminase (AID), a potential RNA editing enzyme. *Cell* 2000;102:553–563.

295. Fagarasan S, Kinoshita K, Muramatsu M, et al. In situ class switching

and differentiation to IgA-producing cells in the gut lamina propria. *Nature* 2001;413:639–643.

296. Okazaki IM, Kinoshita K, Muramatsu M, et al. The AID enzyme induces class switch recombination in fibroblasts. *Nature* 2002;416:340–345.

297. Martin A, Bardwell PD, Woo CJ, et al. Activation-induced cytidine deaminase turns on somatic hypermutation in hybridomas. *Nature* 2002;415:802–806.

298. Nagaoka H, Muramatsu M, Yamamura N, et al. Activation-induced deaminase (AID)-directed hypermutation in the immunoglobulin Smu region: implication of AID involvement in a common step of class switch recombination and somatic hypermutation. *J Exp Med* 2002;195:529–534.

299. Arakawa H, Hauschild J, Buerstedde JM. Requirement of the activation-induced deaminase (AID) gene for immunoglobulin gene conversion. *Science* 2002;295:1301–1306.

300. Harris RS, Sale JE, Petersen-Mahrt SK, et al. AID is essential for immunoglobulin V gene conversion in a cultured B cell line. *Curr Biol* 2002;12:435–438.

301. Han S, Zheng B, Schatz DG, et al. Neoteny in lymphocytes: Rag1 and Rag2 expression in germinal center B cells. *Science* 1996;274:2094–2097.

302. Hikida M, Mori M, Takai T, et al. Reexpression of RAG-1 and RAG-2 genes in activated mature mouse B cells. *Science* 1996;274:2092–2094.

303. Han S, Dillon SR, Zheng B, et al. V(D)J recombinase activity in a subset of germinal center B lymphocytes. *Science* 1997;278:301–305.

304. Papavasiliou F, Casellas R, Suh H, et al. V(D)J recombination in mature B cells: a mechanism for altering antibody responses. *Science* 1997;278:298–301.

305. Hikida M, Mori M, Kawabata T, et al. Characterization of B cells expressing recombination activating genes in germinal centers of immunized mouse lymph nodes. *J Immunol* 1997;158:2509–2512.

306. Yu W, Nagaoka H, Jankovic M, et al. Continued RAG expression in late stages of B cell development and no apparent re-induction after immunization. *Nature* 1999;400:682–687.

307. Gartner F, Alt FW, Monroe RJ, et al. Antigen-independent appearance of recombination activating gene (RAG)-positive bone marrow B cells in the spleens of immunized mice. *J Exp Med* 2000;192:1745–1754.

308. Nagaoka H, Gonzalez-Aseguinolaza G, Tsuji M, et al. Immunization and infection change the number of recombination activating gene (RAG)-expressing B cells in the periphery by altering immature lymphocyte production. *J Exp Med* 2000;191:2113–2120.

309. McHeyzer-Williams LJ, Driver DJ, McHeyzer-Williams MG. Germinal center reaction. *Curr Opin Hematol* 2001;8:52–59.

310. Herzenberg LA, Okumura K, Metzler CM. Regulation of immunoglobulin and antibody production by allotype suppressor T cells in mice. *Transplant Rev* 1975;27:57–83.

311. Jacobson EB, L'Age-Stehr J, Herzenberg LA. Immunological memory in mice. II. Cell interactions in the secondary immune response studies by means of immunoglobulin allotype markers. *J Exp Med* 1970;131:1109–1120.

312. L'Age-Stehr J, Herzenberg LA. Immunological memory in mice. I. Physical separation and partial characterization of memory cells for different immunoglobulin classes from each other and from antibody-producing cells. *J Exp Med* 1970;131:1093–1108.

313. Romano TJ, Mond JJ, Thorbecke GJ. Immunological memory function of the T and B cell types: distribution over mouse spleen and lymph nodes. *Eur J Immunol* 1975;5:211–215.

314. Okumura K, Metzler CM, Tsu TT, et al. Two stages of B-cell memory development with different T-cell requirements. *J Exp Med* 1976;144:345–357.

315. Herzenberg LA, Black SJ, Tokuhisa T. Memory B cells at successive stages of differentiation. Affinity maturation and the role of IgD receptors. *J Exp Med* 1980;151:1071–1087.

316. Yefenof E, Sanders VM, Snow EC, et al. Preparation and analysis of antigen-specific memory B cells. *J Immunol* 1985;135:3777–3784.

317. Hayakawa K, Ishii R, Yamasaki K, et al. Isolation of high-affinity memory B cells: phycoerythrin as a probe for antigen-binding cells. *Proc Natl Acad Sci U S A* 1987;84:1379–1383.

318. Schittek B, Rajewsky K. Maintenance of B-cell memory by long-lived cells generated from proliferating precursors. *Nature* 1990;346:749–751.

319. Bruce J, Symington FW, McKearn TJ, et al. A monoclonal antibody discriminating between subsets of T and B cells. *J Immunol* 1981;127:2496–2501.

320. Linton PL, Decker DJ, Klinman NR. Primary antibody-forming cells and secondary B cells are generated from separate precursor cell subpopulations. *Cell* 1989;59:1049–1059.

321. Linton PJ, Lo D, Lai L, et al. Among naïve precursor cell subpopulations only progenitors of memory B cells originate germinal centers. *Eur J Immunol* 1992;22:1293–1297.

322. Gray D, Skarvall H. B-cell memory is short-lived in the absence of antigen. *Nature* 1988;336:70–73.

323. Vieira P, Rajewsky K. Persistence of memory B cells in mice deprived of T cell help. *Int Immunol* 1990;2:487–494.

324. Karrer U, Lopez-Macias C, Oxenius A, et al. Antiviral B cell memory in the absence of mature follicular dendritic cell networks and classical germinal centers in TNFR1-/- mice. *J Immunol* 2000;164:768–778.

325. Maruyama M, Lam KP, Rajewsky K. Memory B-cell persistence is independent of persisting immunizing antigen. *Nature* 2000;407:636–642.

326. Hayakawa K, Hardy RR, Stall AM, et al. Immunoglobulin-bearing B cells reconstitute and maintain the murine Ly-1 B cell lineage. *Eur J Immunol* 1986;16:1313–1316.

327. Hayakawa K, Hardy RR, Honda M, et al. Ly-1 B cells: functionally distinct lymphocytes that secrete IgM autoantibodies. *Proc Natl Acad Sci U S A* 1984;81:2494–2498.

328. Hardy RR, Carmack CE, Shinton SA, et al. A single VH gene is utilized predominantly in anti-BrMRBC hybridomas derived from purified Ly-1 B cells. Definition of the VH11 family. *J Immunol* 1989;142:3643–3651.

329. Hayakawa K, Carmack CE, Hyman R, et al. Natural autoantibodies to thymocytes: origin, VH genes, fine specificities, the role of Thy-1 glycoprotein. *J Exp Med* 1990;172:869–878.

330. Masmoudi H, Mota-Santos T, Huetz F, et al. All T15 Id–positive antibodies (but not the majority of VHT15+ antibodies) are produced by peritoneal CD5+ B lymphocytes. *Int Immunol* 1990;2:515–520.

331. Boyden S. Autoimmunity and inflammation. *Nature* 1964;201:200–201.

332. Schlesinger M. Spontaneous occurrence of autoantibodies cytotoxic to thymus cells in the sera of mice of the 129 strain. *Nature* 1965;207:429–430.

333. Steele EJ, Cunningham AJ. High proportion of Ig-producing cells making autoantibody in normal mice. *Nature* 1978;274:483–484.

334. Ochsenbein AF, Fehr T, Lutz C, et al. Control of early viral and bacterial distribution and disease by natural antibodies. *Science* 1999;286:2156–2159.

335. Macpherson AJ, Gatto D, Sainsbury E, et al. A primitive T cell–independent mechanism of intestinal mucosal IgA responses to commensal bacteria. *Science* 2000;288:2222–2226.

336. Baumgarth N, Herman OC, Jager GC, et al. Innate and acquired humoral immunities to influenza virus are mediated by distinct arms of the immune system. *Proc Natl Acad Sci U S A* 1999;96:2250–2255.

337. Baumgarth N, Herman OC, Jager GC, et al. B-1 and B-2 cell-derived immunoglobulin M antibodies are nonredundant components of the protective response to influenza virus infection. *J Exp Med* 2000;192:271–280.

338. Hardy RR, Hayakawa K. A developmental switch in B lymphopoiesis. *Proc Natl Acad Sci U S A* 1991;88:11550–11554.

339. Hardy RR, Wasserman R, Li YS, et al. Response by B cell precursors to pre–B receptor assembly: differences between fetal liver and bone marrow. *Curr Top Microbiol Immunol* 2000;252:25–30.

340. Forster I, Rajewsky K. Expansion and functional activity of Ly-1+ B cells upon transfer of peritoneal cells into allotype-congenic, newborn mice. *Eur J Immunol* 1987;17:521–528.

341. Pennell CA, Sheehan KM, Brodeur PH, et al. Organization and expression of VH gene families preferentially expressed by Ly-1+ (CD5) B cells. *Eur J Immunol* 1989;19:2115–2121.

342. Martin F, Kearney JF. B-cell subsets and the mature preimmune repertoire. Marginal zone and B1 B cells as part of a "natural immune memory". *Immunol Rev* 2000;175:70–79.

343. Gui M, Wiest DL, Li J, et al. Peripheral CD4+ T cell maturation recognized by increased expression of Thy-1/CD90 bearing the 6C10 carbohydrate epitope. *J Immunol* 1999;163:4796–4804.

344. Hayakawa K, Asano M, Shinton SA, et al. Positive selection of natural autoreactive B cells. *Science* 1999;285:113–116.

345. Sidman CL, Shultz LD, Hardy RR, et al. Production of immunoglob-

ulin isotypes by Ly-1+ B cells in viable motheaten and normal mice. *Science* 1986;232:1423–1425.

346. O'Keefe TL, Williams GT, Davies SL, et al. Hyperresponsive B cells in CD22-deficient mice. *Science* 1996;274:798–801.

347. Sato S, Miller AS, Inaoki M, et al. CD22 is both a positive and negative regulator of B lymphocyte antigen receptor signal transduction: altered signaling in CD22-deficient mice. *Immunity* 1996;5:551–562.

348. Torres RM, Flaswinkel H, Reth M, et al. Aberrant B cell development and immune response in mice with a compromised BCR complex. *Science* 1996;272:1804–1808.

349. Hayakawa K, Hardy RR, Parks DR, et al. The "Ly-1 B" cell sub-population in normal immunodefective, autoimmune mice. *J Exp Med* 1983;157:202–218.

350. Khan WN, Alt FW, Gerstein RM, et al. Defective B cell development and function in Btk-deficient mice. *Immunity* 1995;3:283–299.

351. Engel P, Zhou LJ, Ord DC, et al. Abnormal B lymphocyte development, activation, differentiation in mice that lack or overexpress the CD19 signal transduction molecule. *Immunity* 1995;3:39–50.

352. Rickert RC, Rajewsky K, Roes J. Impairment of T-cell-dependent B-cell responses and B-1 cell development in CD19-deficient mice. *Nature* 1995;376:352–355.

353. Ahearn JM, Fischer MB, Croix D, et al. Disruption of the Cr2 locus results in a reduction in B-1a cells and in an impaired B cell response to T-dependent antigen. *Immunity* 1996;4:251–262.

354. Tarakhovsky A, Turner M, Schaal S, et al. Defective antigen receptor–mediated proliferation of B and T cells in the absence of Vav. *Nature* 1995;374:467–470.

355. Chen X, Martin F, Forbush KA, et al. Evidence for selection of a population of multi-reactive B cells into the splenic marginal zone. *Int Immunol* 1997;9:27–41.

356. Shaw PX, Horkko S, Chang MK, et al. Natural antibodies with the T15 idiotype may act in atherosclerosis, apoptotic clearance, protective immunity. *J Clin Invest* 2000;105:1731–1740.

357. Silverman GJ, Shaw PX, Luo L, et al. Neo-self antigens and the expansion of B-1 cells: lessons from atherosclerosis-prone mice. *Curr Top Microbiol Immunol* 2000;252:189–200.

358. Oliver AM, Martin F, Kearney JF. IgMhighCD21high lymphocytes enriched in the splenic marginal zone generate effector cells more rapidly than the bulk of follicular B cells. *J Immunol* 1999;162:7198–7207.

359. Martin F, Oliver AM, Kearney JF. Marginal zone and B1 B cells unite in the early response against T-independent blood-borne particulate antigens. *Immunity* 2001;14:617–629.

360. Martin F, Kearney JF. B1 cells: similarities and differences with other B cell subsets. *Curr Opin Immunol* 2001;13:195–201.

361. Amano M, Baumgarth N, Dick MD, et al. CD1 expression defines subsets of follicular and marginal zone B cells in the spleen: beta 2-microglobulin-dependent and independent forms. *J Immunol* 1998;161:1710–1717.

362. Martin F, Kearney JF. Positive selection from newly formed to marginal zone B cells depends on the rate of clonal production, CD19, btk. *Immunity* 2000;12:39–49.

363. Cariappa A, Tang M, Parng C, et al. The follicular versus marginal zone B lymphocyte cell fate decision is regulated by Aiolos, Btk, CD21. *Immunity* 2001;14:603–615.

364. Kraus M, Pao LI, Reichlin A, et al. Interference with immunoglobulin (Ig)alpha immunoreceptor tyrosine–based activation motif (ITAM) phosphorylation modulates or blocks B cell development, depending on the availability of an Igbeta cytoplasmic tail. *J Exp Med* 2001;194:455–469.

365. Guinamard R, Okigaki M, Schlessinger J, et al. Absence of marginal zone B cells in Pyk-2–deficient mice defines their role in the humoral response. *Nat Immunol* 2000;1:31–36.

366. Martin F, Chen X, Kearney JF. Development of VH81X transgene–bearing B cells in fetus and adult: sites for expansion and deletion in conventional and CD5/B1 cells. *Int Immunol* 1997;9:493–505.

367. Goodnow CC, Crosbie J, Jorgensen H, et al. Induction of self-tolerance in mature peripheral B lymphocytes. *Nature* 1989;342:385–391.

368. Goodnow CC, Adelstein S, Basten A. The need for central and peripheral tolerance in the B cell repertoire. *Science* 1990;248:1373–1379.

369. Russell DM, Dembic Z, Morahan G, et al. Peripheral deletion of self-reactive B cells. *Nature* 1991;354:308–311.

370. Cyster JG, Goodnow CC. PTP1C negatively regulates antigen receptor signaling in B lymphocytes and determines thresholds for negative selection. *Immunity* 1995;2:13–24.

371. Cyster JG, Healy JI, Kishihara K, et al. Regulation of B-lymphocyte negative and positive selection by tyrosine phosphatase CD45. *Nature* 1996;381:325–328.

372. Radic MZ, Erikson J, Litwin S, et al. B lymphocytes may escape tolerance by revising their antigen receptors. *J Exp Med* 1993;177:1165–1173.

373. Chen C, Radic MZ, Erikson J, et al. Deletion and editing of B cells that express antibodies to DNA. *J Immunol* 1994;152:1970–1982.

374. Prak EL, Trounstine M, Huszar D, et al. Light chain editing in kappa-deficient animals: a potential mechanism of B cell tolerance. *J Exp Med* 1994;180:1805–1815.

375. Murakami M, Tsubata T, Okamoto M, et al. Antigen-induced apoptotic death of Ly-1 B cells responsible for autoimmune disease in transgenic mice. *Nature* 1992;357:77–80.

376. Okamoto M, Murakami M, Shimizu A, et al. A transgenic model of autoimmune hemolytic anemia. *J Exp Med* 1992;175:71–79.

377. Murakami M, Tsubata T, Shinkura R, et al. Oral administration of lipopolysaccharides activates B-1 cells in the peritoneal cavity and lamina propria of the gut and induces autoimmune symptoms in an autoantibody transgenic mouse. *J Exp Med* 1994;180:111–121.

378. Fehr T, Rickert RC, Odermatt B, et al. Antiviral protection and germinal center formation, but impaired B cell memory in the absence of CD19. *J Exp Med* 1998;188:145–155.

379. Nosten-Bertrand M, Errington ML, Murphy KP, et al. Normal spatial learning despite regional inhibition of LTP in mice lacking Thy-1. *Nature* 1996;379:826–829.

380. Lay WH, Nussenzweig V. Receptors for complement of leukocytes. *J Exp Med* 1968;128:991–1009.

381. Pepys MB. Role of complement in induction of the allergic response. *Nat New Biol* 1972;237:157–159.

382. Pepys MB. Role of complement in the induction of immunological responses. *Transplant Rev* 1976;32:93–120.

383. Carroll MC. The role of complement in B cell activation and tolerance. *Adv Immunol* 2000;74:61–88.

384. Inaoki M, Sato S, Weintraub BC, et al. CD19-regulated signaling thresholds control peripheral tolerance and autoantibody production in B lymphocytes. *J Exp Med* 1997;186:1923–1931.

385. Prodeus AP, Goerg S, Shen LM, et al. A critical role for complement in maintenance of self-tolerance. *Immunity* 1998;9:721–731.

386. Boes M, Prodeus AP, Schmidt T, et al. A critical role of natural immunoglobulin M in immediate defense against systemic bacterial infection. *J Exp Med* 1998;188:2381–2386.

387. Baumgarth N. A two-phase model of B-cell activation. *Immunol Rev* 2000;176:171–180.

388. Tarakhovsky A, Kanner SB, Hombach J, et al. A role for CD5 in TCR-mediated signal transduction and thymocyte selection. *Science* 1995;269:535–537.

389. Bikah G, Carey J, Ciallella JR, et al. CD5-mediated negative regulation of antigen receptor-induced growth signals in B-1 B cells. *Science* 1996;274:1906–1909.

390. Bondada S, Bikah G, Robertson DA, et al. Role of CD5 in growth regulation of B-1 cells. *Curr Top Microbiol Immunol* 2000;252:141–149.

391. Hippen KL, Tze LE, Behrens TW. CD5 maintains tolerance in anergic B cells. *J Exp Med* 2000;191:883–890.

392. Solvason N, Kearney JF. The human fetal omentum: a site of B cell generation. *J Exp Med* 1992;175:397–404.

393. Pascual V, Verkruyse L, Casey ML, et al. Analysis of Ig H chain gene segment utilization in human fetal liver. Revisiting the "proximal utilization hypothesis". *J Immunol* 1993;151:4164–4172.

394. LeBien TW, Wormann B, Villablanca JG, et al. Multiparameter flow cytometric analysis of human fetal bone marrow B cells. *Leukemia* 1990;4:354–358.

395. Nunez C, Nishimoto N, Gartland GL, et al. B cells are generated throughout life in humans. *J Immunol* 1996;156:866–872.

396. Ghia P, ten Boekel E, Sanz E, et al. Ordering of human bone marrow B lymphocyte precursors by single-cell polymerase chain reaction analyses of the rearrangement status of the immunoglobulin H and L chain gene loci. *J Exp Med* 1996;184:2217–2229.

397. Simmons DL, Satterthwaite AB, Tenen DG, et al. Molecular cloning of a cDNA encoding CD34, a sialomucin of human hematopoietic stem cells. *J Immunol* 1992;148:267–271.

398. Dittel BN, LeBien TW. The growth response to IL-7 during normal human B cell ontogeny is restricted to B-lineage cells expressing CD34. *J Immunol* 1995;154:58–67.

399. Rawlings DJ, Quan SG, Kato RM, et al. Long-term culture system for selective growth of human B-cell progenitors. *Proc Natl Acad Sci U S A* 1995;92:1570–1574.

400. LeBien TW. Fates of human B-cell precursors. *Blood* 2000;96:9–23.

401. Gougeon ML, Drean G, Le Deist F, et al. Human severe combined immunodeficiency disease: phenotypic and functional characteristics of peripheral B lymphocytes. *J Immunol* 1990;145:2873–2879.

402. Bauer SR, Kubagawa H, Maclennan I, et al. VpreB gene expression in hematopoietic malignancies: a lineage- and stage-restricted marker for B-cell precursor leukemias. *Blood* 1991;78:1581–1588.

403. Bossy D, Milili M, Zucman J, et al. Organization and expression of the lambda-like genes that contribute to the mu-psi light chain complex in human pre–B cells. *Int Immunol* 1991;3:1081–1090.

404. Bauer SR, Kudo A, Melchers F. Structure and pre–B lymphocyte restricted expression of the VpreB in humans and conservation of its structure in other mammalian species. *EMBO J* 1988;7:111–116.

405. Gisler R, Jacobsen SE, Sigvardsson M. Cloning of human early B-cell factor and identification of target genes suggest a conserved role in B-cell development in man and mouse. *Blood* 2000;96:1457–1464.

406. Minegishi Y, Coustan-Smith E, Wang YH, et al. Mutations in the human lambda5/14. 1 gene result in B cell deficiency and agammaglobulinemia. *J Exp Med* 1998;187:71–77.

407. Minegishi Y, Coustan-Smith E, Rapalus L, et al. Mutations in Igalpha (CD79a) result in a complete block in B-cell development. *J Clin Invest* 1999;104:1115–1121.

408. Yel L, Minegishi Y, Coustan-Smith E, et al. Mutations in the mu heavy-chain gene in patients with agammaglobulinemia. *N Engl J Med* 1996;335:1486–1493.

409. Pascual V, Liu YJ, Magalski A, et al. Analysis of somatic mutation in five B cell subsets of human tonsil. *J Exp Med* 1994;180:329–339.

410. Pasqualucci L, Migliazza A, Fracchiolla N, et al. BCL-6 mutations in normal germinal center B cells: evidence of somatic hypermutation acting outside Ig loci. *Proc Natl Acad Sci U S A* 1998;95:11816–11821.

411. Staudt LM, Dent AL, Shaffer AL, et al. Regulation of lymphocyte cell fate decisions and lymphomagenesis by BCL-6. *Int Rev Immunol* 1999;18:381–403.

412. Dalla-Favera R, Ye BH, Lo Coco F, et al. BCL-6 and the molecular pathogenesis of B-cell lymphoma. *Cold Spring Harb Symp Quant Biol* 1994;59:117–123.

413. Muschen M, Re D, Jungnickel B, et al. Somatic mutation of the CD95 gene in human B cells as a side-effect of the germinal center reaction. *J Exp Med* 2000;192:1833–1840.

414. Conley ME, Parolini O, Rohrer J, et al. X-linked agammaglobulinemia: new approaches to old questions based on the identification of the defective gene. *Immunol Rev* 1994;138:5–21.

415. Tsukada S, Saffran DC, Rawlings DJ, et al. Deficient expression of a B cell cytoplasmic tyrosine kinase in human X-linked agammaglobulinemia. *Cell* 1993;72:279–290.

416. Rawlings DJ, Saffran DC, Tsukada S, et al. Mutation of unique region of Bruton's tyrosine kinase in immunodeficient XID mice. *Science* 1993;261:358–361.

417. Campana D, Farrant J, Inamdar N, et al. Phenotypic features and proliferative activity of B cell progenitors in X-linked agammaglobulinemia. *J Immunol* 1990;145:1675–1680.

418. Minegishi Y, Rohrer J, Coustan-Smith E, et al. An essential role for BLNK in human B cell development. *Science* 1999;286:1954–1957.

419. Macchi P, Villa A, Giliani S, et al. Mutations of Jak-3 gene in patients with autosomal severe combined immune deficiency (SCID). *Nature* 1995;377:65–68.

420. DiSanto JP, Muller W, Guy-Grand D, et al. Lymphoid development in mice with a targeted deletion of the interleukin 2 receptor gamma chain. *Proc Natl Acad Sci U S A* 1995;92:377–381.

421. Baird AM, Lucas JA, Berg LJ. A profound deficiency in thymic progenitor cells in mice lacking Jak3. *J Immunol* 2000;165:3680–3688.

422. Margolin JF, Poplack DG. Acute lymphoblastic leukemia. In: Pizzo PA, Poplack, DG, eds. *Principles and practice of pediatric oncology.* Philadelphia: Lippincott-Raven, 1997:409–462.

423. Cherepakhin V, Baird SM, Meisenholder GW, et al. Common clonal origin of chronic lymphocytic leukemia and high-grade lymphoma of Richter's syndrome. *Blood* 1993;82:3141–3147.

424. Felix CA, Poplack DG. Characterization of acute lymphoblastic leukemia of childhood by immunoglobulin and T-cell receptor gene patterns. *Leukemia* 1991;5:1015–1025.

425. Lemmers B, Arnoulet C, Fossat C, et al. Fine characterization of child-

426. Uckun FM, Evans WE, Forsyth CJ, et al. Biotherapy of B-cell precursor leukemia by targeting genistein to CD19-associated tyrosine kinases. *Science* 1995;267:886–891.

427. Meydan N, Grunberger T, Dadi H, et al. Inhibition of acute lymphoblastic leukaemia by a Jak–2 inhibitor. *Nature* 1996;379:645–648.

428. Bertrand FE, Vogtenhuber C, Shah N, et al. Pro-B-cell to pre–B-cell development in B-lineage acute lymphoblastic leukemia expressing the MLL/AF4 fusion protein. *Blood* 2001;98:3398–3405.

429. Brumpt C, Delabesse E, Beldjord K, et al. The incidence of clonal T-cell receptor rearrangements in B-cell precursor acute lymphoblastic leukemia varies with age and genotype. *Blood* 2000;96:2254–2261.

430. Pui CH. Acute lymphoblastic leukemia in children. *Curr Opin Oncol* 2000;12:3–12.

431. Domer PH, Fakharzadeh SS, Chen CS, et al. Acute mixed-lineage leukemia t(4;11)(q21;q23) generates an MLL-AF4 fusion product. *Proc Natl Acad Sci U S A* 1993;90:7884–7888.

432. Maloney DG, Smith B, Rose A. Rituximab: mechanism of action and resistance. *Semin Oncol* 2002;29:2–9.

433. Bhan AK, Nadler LM, Stashenko P, et al. Stages of B cell differentiation in human lymphoid tissue. *J Exp Med* 1981;154:737–749.

434. Nadler LM, Ritz J, Hardy R, et al. A unique cell surface antigen identifying lymphoid malignancies of B cell origin. *J Clin Invest* 1981;67:134–140.

435. Tedder TF, Streuli M, Schlossman SF, et al. Isolation and structure of a cDNA encoding the B1 (CD20) cell-surface antigen of human B lymphocytes. *Proc Natl Acad Sci U S A* 1988;85:208–212.

436. Golay JT, Clark EA, Beverley PC. The CD20 (Bp35) antigen is involved in activation of B cells from the G0 to the G1 phase of the cell cycle. *J Immunol* 1985;135:3795–3801.

437. Clark EA, Shu G, Ledbetter JA. Role of the Bp35 cell surface polypeptide in human B-cell activation. *Proc Natl Acad Sci U S A* 1985;82:1766–1770.

438. Ledbetter JA, Clark EA. Surface phenotype and function of tonsillar germinal center and mantle zone B cell subsets. *Hum Immunol* 1986;15:30–43.

439. Reff ME, Carner K, Chambers KS, et al. Depletion of B cells in vivo by a chimeric mouse human monoclonal antibody to CD20. *Blood* 1994;83:435–445.

440. Reed JC, Kitada S, Kim Y, et al. Modulating apoptosis pathways in low-grade B-cell malignancies using biological response modifiers. *Semin Oncol* 2002;29:10–24.

441. Nabhan C, Rosen ST. Conceptual aspects of combining rituximab and Campath-1H in the treatment of chronic lymphocytic leukemia. *Semin Oncol* 2002;29:75–80.

442. Rosenwald A, Alizadeh AA, Widhopf G, et al. Relation of gene expression phenotype to immunoglobulin mutation genotype in B cell chronic lymphocytic leukemia. *J Exp Med* 2001;194:1639–1647.

443. Wierda WG, Cantwell MJ, Woods SJ, et al. CD40-ligand (CD154) gene therapy for chronic lymphocytic leukemia. *Blood* 2000;96:2917–2924.

444. Glick G, Chang TS, Jaap RG. The bursa of Fabricius and antibody production. *Poult Sci* 1956;35:224–234.

445. Cooper MD, Raymond DA, Peterson RD, et al. The functions of the thymus system and the bursa system in the chicken. *J Exp Med* 1966;123:75–102.

446. Sorvari T, Sorvari R, Ruotsalainen P, et al. Uptake of environmental antigens by the bursa of Fabricius. *Nature* 1975;253:217–219.

447. McCormack WT, Tjoelker LW, Thompson CB. Avian B-cell development: generation of an immunoglobulin repertoire by gene conversion. *Annu Rev Immunol* 1991;9:219–241.

448. Dieterlen-Lievre F, Martin C. Diffuse intraembryonic hemopoiesis in normal and chimeric avian development. *Dev Biol* 1981;88:180–191.

449. Reynaud CA, Imhof BA, Anquez V, et al. Emergence of committed B lymphoid progenitors in the developing chicken embryo. *EMBO J* 1992;11:4349–4358.

450. Benatar T, Tkalec L, Ratcliffe MJ. Stochastic rearrangement of immunoglobulin variable-region genes in chicken B-cell development. *Proc Natl Acad Sci U S A* 1992;89:7615–7619.

451. Reynaud CA, Anquez V, Dahan A, et al. A single rearrangement event generates most of the chicken immunoglobulin light chain diversity. *Cell* 1985;40:283–291.

452. Reynaud CA, Dahan A, Anquez V, et al. Somatic hyperconversion

diversifies the single Vh gene of the chicken with a high incidence in the D region. *Cell* 1989;59:171–183.

453. Lassila O. Emigration of B cells from chicken bursa of Fabricius. *Eur J Immunol* 1989;19:955–958.

454. Paramithiotis E, Ratcliffe MJ. Bursa-dependent subpopulations of peripheral B lymphocytes in chicken blood. *Eur J Immunol* 1993;23:96–102.

455. Becker RS, Knight KL. Somatic diversification of immunoglobulin heavy chain VDJ genes: evidence for somatic gene conversion in rabbits. *Cell* 1990;63:987–997.

456. Raman C, Spieker-Polet H, Yam PC, et al. Preferential VH gene usage in rabbit Ig-secreting heterohybridomas. *J Immunol* 1994;152:3935–3945.

457. Tunyaplin C, Knight KL. Fetal VDJ gene repertoire in rabbit: evidence for preferential rearrangement of VH1. *Eur J Immunol* 1995;25:2583–2587.

458. McElroy PJ, Willcox N, Catty D. Early precursors of B lymphocytes. I. Rabbit/mouse species differences in the physical properties and surface phenotype of pre–B cells, in the maturation sequence of early B cells. *Eur J Immunol* 1981;11:76–85.

459. Crane MA, Kingzette M, Knight KL. Evidence for limited B-lymphopoiesis in adult rabbits. *J Exp Med* 1996;183:2119–2121.

460. Weinstein PD, Anderson AO, Mage RG. Rabbit IgH sequences in appendix germinal centers: VH diversification by gene conversion-like and hypermutation mechanisms. *Immunity* 1994;1:647–659.

461. Short JA, Sethupathi P, Zhai SK, et al. VDJ genes in VHa2 allotype-suppressed rabbits. Limited germline VH gene usage and accumulation of somatic mutations in D regions. *J Immunol* 1991;147:4014–4018.

462. Vajdy M, Sethupathi P, Knight KL. Dependence of antibody somatic diversification on gut-associated lymphoid tissue in rabbits. *J Immunol* 1998;160:2725–2729.

463. Tlaskalova-Hogenova H, Stepankova R. Development of antibody formation in germ-free and conventionally reared rabbits: the role of intestinal lymphoid tissue in antibody formation to E. coli antigens. *Folia Biol* 1980;26:81–93.

464. Stepankova R, Kovaru F, Kruml J. Lymphatic tissue of the intestinal tract of germfree and conventional rabbits. *Folia Microbiol* 1980;25:491–495.

465. Lanning D, Sethupathi P, Rhee KJ, et al. Intestinal microflora and diversification of the rabbit antibody repertoire. *J Immunol* 2000;165:2012–2019.

466. Hayward AR, Simons MA, Lawton AR, et al. Pre-B and B cells in rabbits. Ontogeny and allelic exclusion of kappa light chain genes. *J Exp Med* 1978;148:1367–1377.

467. Gathings WE, Mage RG, Cooper MD, et al. Immunofluorescence studies on the expression of VH a allotypes by pre–B and B cells of homozygous and heterozygous rabbits. *Eur J Immunol* 1981;11:200–206.

468. Solvason N, Chen X, Shu F, et al. The fetal omentum in mice and humans. A site enriched for precursors of CD5 B cells early in development. *Ann N Y Acad Sci* 1992;651:10–20.

469. Becker RS, Suter M, Knight KL. Restricted utilization of VH and DH genes in leukemic rabbit B cells. *Eur J Immunol* 1990;20:397–402.

470. Friedman ML, Tunyaplin C, Zhai SK, et al. Neonatal VH, D, JH gene usage in rabbit B lineage cells. *J Immunol* 1994;152:632–641.

471. Zhu X, Boonthum A, Zhai SK, et al. B lymphocyte selection and age-related changes in VH gene usage in mutant Alicia rabbits. *J Immunol* 1999;163:3313–3320.

472. Sehgal D, Johnson G, Wu TT, et al. Generation of the primary antibody repertoire in rabbits: expression of a diverse set of Igk-V genes may compensate for limited combinatorial diversity at the heavy chain locus. *Immunogenetics* 1999;50:31–42.

473. Cooper MD, Perey DY, Gabrielsen AE, et al. Production of an antibody deficiency syndrome in rabbits by neonatal removal of organized intestinal lymphoid tissues. *Int Arch Allergy Appl Immunol* 1998;33:65–88.

474. Perey DY, Good RA. Experimental arrest and induction of lymphoid development in intestinal lymphoepithelial tissues of rabbits. *Lab Invest* 1968;18:15–26.

475. Stramignoni A, Mollo F, Rua S, et al. Development of the lymphoid tissue in the rabbit appendix isolated from the intestinal tract. *J Pathol* 1969;99:265–269.

476. Berberian L, Goodglick L, Kipps TJ, et al. Immunoglobulin VH3 gene products: natural ligands for HIV gp120. *Science* 1993;261:1588–1591.

477. Pospisil R, Mage RG. B-cell superantigens may play a role in B-cell development and selection in the young rabbit appendix. *Cell Immunol* 1998;185:93–100.

478. Silverman GJ, Cary SP, Dwyer DC, et al. A B cell superantigen–induced persistent "hole" in the B-1 repertoire. *J Exp Med* 2000;192:87–98.

479. Chan VW, Mecklenbrauker I, Su I, et al. The molecular mechanism of B cell activation by toll-like receptor protein RP-105. *J Exp Med* 1998;188:93–101.

480. Ehlich A, Schaal S, Gu H, et al. Immunoglobulin heavy and light chain genes rearrange independently at early stages of B cell development. *Cell* 1993;72:695–704.

481. Reynaud CA, Anquez V, Grimal H, et al. A hyperconversion mechanism generates the chicken light chain preimmune repertoire. *Cell* 1987;48:379–388.

482. McCormack WT, Tjoelker LW, Barth CF, et al. Selection for B cells with productive IgL gene rearrangements occurs in the bursa of Fabricius during chicken embryonic development. *Genes Dev* 1989;3:838–847.

483. Raman C, Knight KL. CD5+ B cells predominate in peripheral tissues of rabbit. *J Immunol* 1992;149:3858–3864.

484. Herzenberg LA. Toward a layered immune system. *Cell* 1989;59:953–954.

485. Glynne R, Akkaraju S, Healy JI, et al. How self-tolerance and the immunosuppressive drug FK506 prevent B-cell mitogenesis. *Nature* 2000;403:672–676.

486. Hoffmann R, Seidl T, Neeb M, et al. Changes in gene expression profiles in developing B cells of murine bone marrow. *Genome Res* 2002;12:98–111.

487. Nelms KA, Goodnow CC. Genome-wide ENU mutagenesis to reveal immune regulators. *Immunity* 2001;15:409–418.

488. Loy AL, Goodnow CC. Novel approaches for identifying genes regulating lymphocyte development and function. *Curr Opin Immunol* 2002;14:260–265.

489. Lee G, Namen AE, Gillis S, et al. Recombinant interleukin-7 supports the growth of normal B lymphocyte precursors. *Curr Top Microbiol Immunol* 1988;141:16–18.

490. Hirayama F, Ogawa M. Cytokine regulation of early lymphohematopoietic development. *Stem Cells* 1996;14:369–375.

491. Baird AM, Gerstein RM, Berg LJ. The role of cytokine receptor signaling in lymphocyte development. *Curr Opin Immunol* 1999;11:157–166.

492. Funk PE, Kincade PW, Witte PL. Native associations of early hematopoietic stem cells and stromal cells isolated in bone marrow cell aggregates. *Blood* 1994;83:361–369.

493. Medina KL, Kincade PW. Pregnancy-related steroids are potential negative regulators of B lymphopoiesis. *Proc Natl Acad Sci U S A* 1994;91:5382–5386.

494. Smithson G, Couse JF, Lubahn DB, et al. The role of estrogen receptors and androgen receptors in sex steroid regulation of B lymphopoiesis. *J Immunol* 1998;161:27–34.

495. Foster MP, Montecino-Rodriguez E, Dorshkind K. Proliferation of bone marrow pro–B cells is dependent on stimulation by the pituitary/thyroid axis. *J Immunol* 1999;163:5883–5890.

496. Roark JH, Kuntz CL, Nguyen KA, et al. Breakdown of B cell tolerance in a mouse model of systemic lupus erythematosus. *J Exp Med* 1995;181:1157–1167.

497. Chen C, Prak EL, Weigert M. Editing disease-associated autoantibodies. *Immunity* 1997;6:97–105.

498. Xu H, Li H, Suri-Payer E, et al. Regulation of anti-DNA B cells in recombination-activating gene-deficient mice. *J Exp Med* 1998;188:1247–1254.

499. Li H, Jiang Y, Prak EL, et al. Editors and editing of anti-DNA receptors. *Immunity* 2001;15:947–957.

500. Chumley MJ, Dal Porto JM, Kawaguchi S, et al. A VH11V kappa 9 B cell antigen receptor drives generation of CD5+ B cells both in vivo and in vitro. *J Immunol* 2000;164:4586–4593.

501. Arnold LW, Pennell CA, McCray SK, et al. Development of B-1 cells: segregation of phosphatidyl choline-specific B cells to the B-1 population occurs after immunoglobulin gene expression. *J Exp Med* 1994;179:1585–1595.

CHAPTER 7

B-Cell Signaling Mechanisms and Activation

Michael McHeyzer-Williams

Overview
BCR Proximal Signaling Mechanisms
    The BCR Signaling Complex · Membrane Microdomains · Receptor Aggregation
Early Intracellular Activation Cascades
    SFK Recruitment and Activation · Syk Recruitment and Activation · A Role for Adaptor Molecules BLNK and BCAP · PI-3K Recruitment to Membrane · Btk Recruitment and Activation · PLC-γ2 Activation
Effector Signaling Pathways
    Mobilization of Intracellular Calcium Stores · Capacitative Calcium Entry · Calcium-Mediated Regulation of NF-ATc Activation · Regulation of NF-κB Activation · The PKC Pathway · PI-3K/Akt Signaling Pathway · Ras/MAPK Signaling Pathways
Surface-Expressed Modulators of BCR Signaling
    CD45 · CD22 · CD19 · FcγRIIb
Mature B-Cell Subsets
    B-1 B Cells · Marginal Zone B Cells
T-Cell–Independent B-Cell Responses
    Type 1 T–Independent B-Cell Responses · Type 2 T–Independent B-Cell Responses · Regulation of TI-2 B-Cell Responses
Helper T–Regulated B-Cell Responses
    Recruitment of Antigen-Specific T-Cell Help—Phase I · Delivery of T-Cell Help to Antigen–Prime B Cells—Phase II · The Germinal Center Reaction—Phase III · The B-Cell Memory Response—Phase IV
References

OVERVIEW

Humoral immunity provides immediate and long-term protection against a vast array of infectious agents as one vital component of the adaptive immune system. Expression of a B-cell receptor (BCR) signaling complex guides the development of immature B cells in the bone marrow and is required for the survival of mature B cells at homeostasis in the periphery. Infection disturbs homeostasis to signal and recruit antigen-specific B cells into the adaptive immune response.

In the first half of this chapter, I discuss BCR signaling mechanisms as the biochemical consequences of the initial encounter with antigen. Upon cross-linking with specific antigen, the BCR signaling complex translocates rapidly and aggregates in specialized membrane microdomains rich in signaling intermediates. These biophysical consequences of antigen-specific recognition are detected within seconds of antigen encounter and are discussed as the earliest BCR proximal signaling mechanisms. Surface BCR aggregation then initiates a rapid cascade of intracellular activation events recruiting kinases, adaptor molecules, and lipid-metabolizing

enzymes to the plasma membrane to amplify this initial BCR-mediated signal. These membrane-associated activities produce a number of secondary signaling intermediates that impact a multitude of downstream effector pathways. The separate effector pathways are described in detail highlighting their potential impact on cell fate through differential regulation of gene expression. A discussion of cell surface molecules able to modulate BCR signaling by either exerting their basal enzymatic activity or interpreting the form of antigen encountered by the B cells concludes the presentation of BCR signaling mechanisms.

In the second half of this chapter, the cellular impact of antigen-specific B-cell activation is discussed in detail. The activities of subspecialized B-cell compartments (B-1 and marginal zone MZ B cells) are presented and discussed in the context of their role in T-cell–independent B-cell responses. Emphasis is then placed on antigen-specific, helper T-cell–regulated B-cell immunity. This intriguing facet of adaptive immunity emerges as a series of interdependent Th-cell and B-cell development pathways that are highly focused on specific antigen clearance and long-term immune protection. The innate immune system is still required to recruit and shape the quality of the initial naïve Th- and B-cell response. Clonally expanded effector Th cells then deliver cognate help to antigen-activated B cells at the T/B borders of secondary lymphoid organs. Isotype switch recombination and plasma cell development constitute one option for specific B-cell development that proceeds within the T zones of these organs. The second major outcome of specific Th/B–cell interactions is the germinal center (GC) pathway to memory B-cell development. The quantity and quality of cognate cellular interaction (immune synapse) at each phase of development determines subsequent cell fate. A short discussion on the cellular organization of B-cell memory and the nature of antigen recall responses concludes the last section of the chapter.

BCR PROXIMAL SIGNALING MECHANISMS

Recognition of foreign antigens through the BCR complex is the central initiating event that leads to antigen-specific B-cell differentiation and the development of humoral immunity. The BCR signaling complex also plays a central role in B-cell development and the survival of mature B cells at homeostasis. Thus, it remains difficult to study the role of the BCR in isolation of its potential impact on the pre-immune status of the naïve B cell. Nevertheless, numerous analyses of BCR function in B-cell lines and genetically manipulated animal models provide insight into the steady-state organization of the BCR signaling complex and the earliest BCR proximal signaling mechanisms at the time of initial antigen encounter.

The BCR Signaling Complex

The BCR signaling complex consists of membrane immunoglobulin (mIg) to bind specific antigens and a heterodimer of Ig-α (CD79a) and Ig-β (CD79b) as its noncovalently associated signaling subunit (1–3) (Fig. 1). The membrane proximal heavy-chain constant region (CH) domain of mIg is required for stable association with Ig-α/β heterodimers. The 25-amino-acid transmembrane domain of mIg contains a series of polar residues on one side of a predicted α-helix that are conserved across all Ig isotype classes and for mIgM have been shown to bind Igα/β heterodimers (4). Using epitope-tagged Igα and the immunoprecipitation of the BCR complex from the J558L B-cell line, Schamel and Reth (5) demonstrated that each complex contained only one type of Igα (either tagged or untagged). These trends were further supported by biosynthetic labeling that quantified relative amounts of IgH, IgL, Igα, and Igβ. Thus, contrary to earlier expectations, there was a 1:1 stoichometry between mIg and Igα/Igβ. Using limiting detergent concentrations, further analyses indicate that co-expressed mIgM and mIgD form BCR oligomers that segregate in the cell membrane in an isotype-specific manner. These more complex structures may influence the lateral mobility of the BCR complex in

the cell membrane at homeostasis and impact the quality of initial antigen recognition events.

The Igα/Igβ molecules are disulphide-bonded, type I transmembrane proteins. They are the 34- and 40-kDa polypeptide products of the murine genes mb-1 and B29, respectively. Apart from glycosylation differences in Igα, all mIg classes associate with the same heterodimer (6,7). Each subunit expresses a single extracellular Ig domain, a transmembrane region with three polar amino acids (aa) and a cytoplasmic tail of 61aa for Igα and 48aa for Igβ. Both molecules display one immune-receptor tyrosine-based activation motif (ITAM) in their cytoplasmic tails that plays a critical role in BCR-mediated signal transduction (8). The ITAMs are characterized by six conserved amino acid residues (D/Ex$_7$D/Ex$_2$Yx$_2$L/Ix$_7$Yx$_2$L/I; single-letter code x = any aa) and are also found in the cytoplasmic domains of TCR signaling components, certain Fc receptors, and CD22. Cross-linking these receptors rapidly induces protein tyrosine kinase activation and intracellular calcium mobilization. Mutating either of the two conserved tyrosines abolishes this ITAM activity (3,9). Thus, the intracellular ITAMs of Igα/Ig$\beta$are one critical means for communicating a BCR recognition event to the signaling intermediates of a variety of intracellular pathways.

During B-cell development, the Igα/β heterodimer can be found on the surface of pro–B cells and is capable of signaling even in the absence of mIg (10). In pre–B cells, the presence of Igα/β is required for surface expression of rearranged Igμ heavy chains that associate with surrogate light chains (VpreB/λ5). Transgenic and gene ablation studies confirm the critical role of the Igα/β heterodimer in B-cell development (3). Animals deficient in Igβ display a complete block at the pro–B-cell stage, while those expressing truncated Igα lacking critical cytoplasmic domains, are compromised in B-cell development with a 100-fold decrease in mature B cells in the periphery (1–3). More recently, Lam et al. (11) used conditional gene ablation methods to delete mIg on mature B cells after normal development in the presence of expressed BCR. When mature naïve B cells lost mIg expression, they died rapidly by apoptosis with an associated up-regulation of CD95 (Fas). Thus, naïve B cells require mIg for their survival *in vivo* and presumably receive some basal signal through an intact BCR complex to maintain homeostasis.

Membrane Microdomains

The spatial organization of plasma membrane–associated receptors and their signaling intermediates serves to regulate cellular homeostasis. At physiological temperatures, cell membranes can be shown to contain segregated microdomains referred to as lipid rafts (12,13) (Fig. 1). These lipid rafts consist of dynamic assemblies of glycosphingolipids with saturated fatty acid chains that allow cholesterol to be more tightly packed than surrounding less-ordered phospholipid-rich regions of the plasma membrane (14). Operationally, lipid rafts are insoluble in nonionic detergents

EXTRACELLULAR

1. Membrane Microdomains
2. Partitioning of BCR complex
3. Raft Association of SFK
4. Cytoplasmic Syk
5. Cbp/Csk impact on SFK
6. Impact of CD22 & CD45

Phospholipid
Sphingolipid
Sat. Phospholipid
Cholesterol

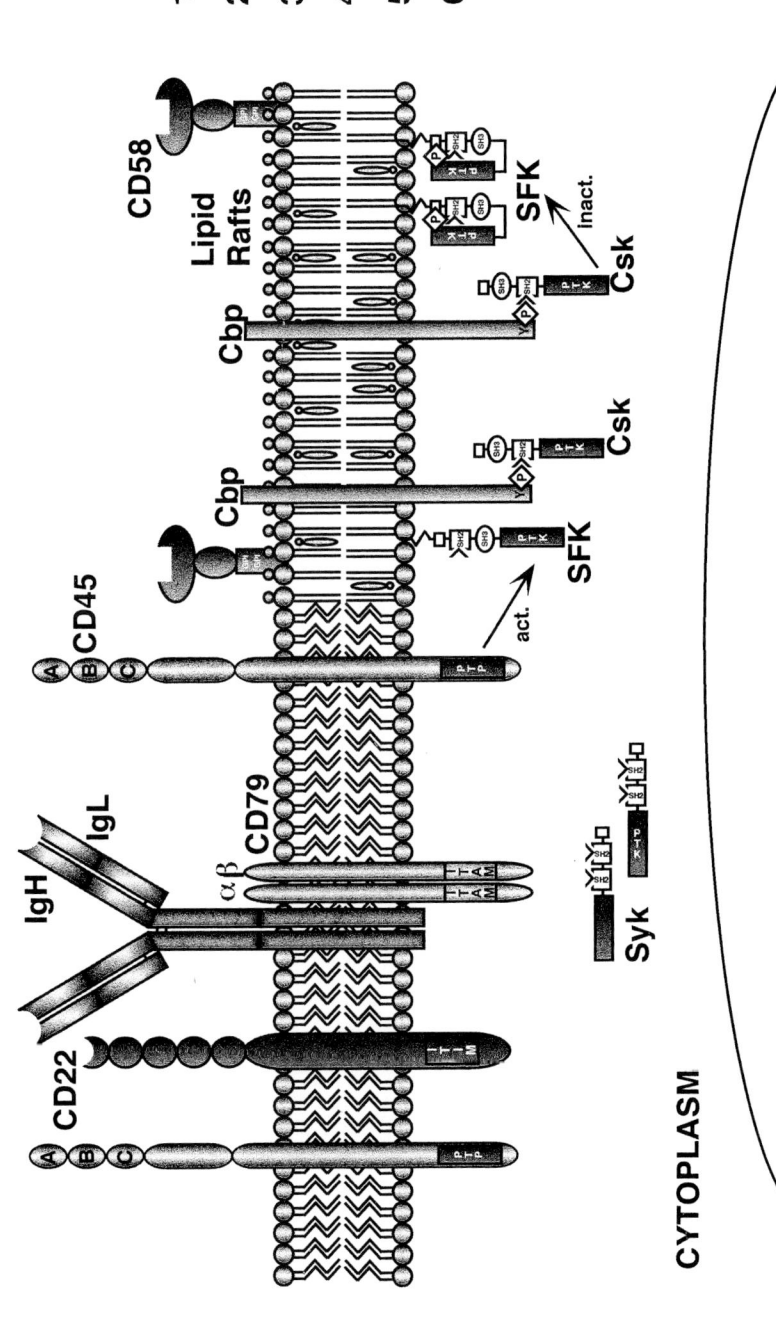

NUCLEUS

CYTOPLASM

FIG. 1. Dynamic equilibrium of BCR signaling at homeostasis. The BCR signaling complex consists of membrane immunoglobulin with heavy (IgH) and light (IgL) chain subunits noncovalently associated with a signaling subunit heterodimer of Igα (CD79a) and Igβ (CD79b). Prior to antigen engagement, the BCR complex is excluded from the cholesterol-rich membrane microdomains referred to as lipid rafts. The lipid rafts exclude most membrane proteins but concentrate proteins modified by saturated fatty acids, such as the adhesion molecule CD58 (LFA-3) and the Src family kinases (SFK). At homeostasis, the Syk/Zap 70 family kinase resides constitutively in the cytoplasm while the C-terminal Src kinase (Csk) is constitutively associated with a transmembrane adaptor protein, Csk binding protein (Cbp), which locates to lipid rafts. Csk serves to phosphorylate the inhibitory tyrosines of SFKs, an action antagonized by the phosphatase CD45 to maintain a basal level of activated SFKs in the lipid raft microdomains. The BCR signaling complex can be found in association with CD45 and another transmembrane tyrosine phosphatase, CD22, which are thought to exert positive and negative influences at homeostasis to dynamically maintain the naïve B cell in a signal-competent state.

at low temperatures, can be disrupted by the extraction of cholesterol from the membrane and can be detected by immunoblotting with cholera toxin B (CTB) subunits that bind GM1 gangliosides within rafts. These lipid rafts exclude most transmembrane proteins but concentrate proteins that are modified with saturated fatty acids. These include glycosylphosphatidylinositol-anchored proteins such as CD90 (Thy 1) and CD58 (LFA-3), doubly acylated proteins such as Src family kinases (SFK) and the Gα subunit of heterotrimeric G proteins, and palmitoylated proteins such as the linker of activated T cells (LAT) (15). Many of these molecules have been directly implicated in lymphocyte activation or as intermediates in antigen receptor–activated signaling events.

Receptor Aggregation

BCR ligation by multivalent antigen induces rapid translocation of the BCR signaling complex into lipid rafts (Fig. 2). Before activation, only 1% of BCR complexes pre-associate with these lipid rafts in mature B cells (16). Within seconds after cross-linking mIg, increased amounts of the BCR complex can be detected in GM1-ganglioside rich-membrane fractions (17). These BCR-containing lipid-raft fractions are also enriched for the activating Src family kinase (SFK) Lyn. Aggregating receptors on cell membranes is a powerful means to heighten ligand sensitivity and intensify the initial specific recognition event (10,18). In general, receptor aggregation allows ligand-activated receptors to induce ligand-independent activation of neighboring receptors. This type of signal amplification can also occur in B cells. Cross-linking mIgM in naïve B cells activates the co-expressed mIgD-associated Igα/Igβ heterodimers (19). Similarly, ligating epitope-tagged Igα with antibodies to the epitope tag, also activates untagged Igα in the same B cells (5). Stable translocation into lipid rafts is a selective property of only a few transmembrane proteins with the antigen receptor on T cells and FcϵRI on mast cells being two other notable examples (20). The exchange of transmembrane (TM) domains or mutations within the TM of these receptors reduces their translocation propensity (21).

Translocating the BCR signaling complex into lipid raft microdomains also acts to dissociate the potentially inhibiting effects of tyrosine phosphatase activity associated with CD22 and CD45 (22) (Fig. 2). These two transmembrane receptors remain excluded from the raft environment, altering the preexisting phosphatase/kinase balance associated with the BCR signaling complex at homeostasis.

In mature B cells, stable translocation into lipid rafts precedes BCR-induced tyrosine phosphorylation. This translocation event does not require SFK activation, Igα/Igβ phosphorylation or an intact cytoskeleton (12,13). Nevertheless, upon BCR ligation many intracellular signaling intermediates also rapidly re-locate to the cytoplasmic face of the plasma-membrane raft microenvironment. These include the partitioning of phosphatidylinositol 4,5-bis-phosphate (PIP$_2$) into

rafts suggesting that these sites may concentrate the action of lipid-metabolizing enzymes, phospholipase C (PLC) and phosphoinositide 3-kinase (PI-3K) (12,13). Interestingly, the rapid translocation into lipid rafts may be required for some aspects of BCR-mediated signal transduction such as mobilizing intracellular calcium (23), but appears dispensable for others, such as activating of protein kinase C (PKC) and mitogen-activated protein kinase (MAPK) signaling pathways (24). Nevertheless, the rapid relocation of BCR complexes into lipid rafts constitutes the earliest BCR proximal signal mechanism used by B cells in recognition of foreign antigen (Fig. 2).

EARLY INTRACELLULAR ACTIVATION CASCADES

BCR aggregation induces rapid intracellular tyrosine kinase recruitment and activation. Generally, the membrane-associated SFKs are the kinases most rapidly involved in the phosphorylation of Igα/Igβ ITAMs. The pITAMs then recruit the ZAP 70–related kinase, spleen tyrosine kinase (Syk), from the cytoplasm to further amplify the initial BCR-mediated signal. These early activation events propagate a cascade of kinase recruitment and activation through trans- and cross-phosphorylation that culminates in the assembly of nonenzymatic adaptor molecules into the growing signaling complex. Adaptors connect these early signaling activities with a multitude of downstream effector pathways. In the next section, two of these adaptor molecules (B-cell linker protein, BLNK, and B-cell cytoplasmic adaptor protein, BCAP) are considered with particular references to their impact on the formation of the calcium initiation complex. This complex comprises the membrane-associated lipid-metabolizing enzyme, PI-3K, the Tek family kinase, Bruton's tyrosine kinase (Btk), and activated PLC-γ2. Formation of this complex and the production of diacyl glycerol (DAG) and inositol (1,4,5) triphosphate (IP$_3$) signify the completion of the early intracellular activation cascades.

SFK Recruitment and Activation

Protein tyrosine phosphorylation accompanies receptor aggregation as one of the earliest detectable events following antigen-receptor oligomerization on mature B cells (1–3,25) (Fig. 2). This kinase activity is detected as early as 5 seconds and peaks within minutes after BCR engagement. The BCR complex itself has no intrinsic protein tyrosine kinase (PTK) activity and therefore, must recruit kinases in order to propagate downstream signaling events. Four SFKs—Lyn, Fyn, Blk, and Lck—are the earliest kinases activated upon BCR ligation (26). The SFKs are constitutively anchored to the inner leaflet of the plasma membrane via N-terminal myristylation of a common glycine residue at position 2 of the molecule. The SFKs Lyn and Fyn are also palmitylated on cysteine at position 3 or 5 from the N-terminal. These N-terminals preferentially enrich SFKs into lipid rafts and bring

EXTRACELLULAR

1. Ag ligates BCR
2. BCR translocates to Rafts
3. CD22/CD45 excluded
4. Cbp dephos. Csk dissoc.
5. Act. SFKs phos. ITAMs
6. pITAMs recruit Syk
7. Further trans/cross phos.

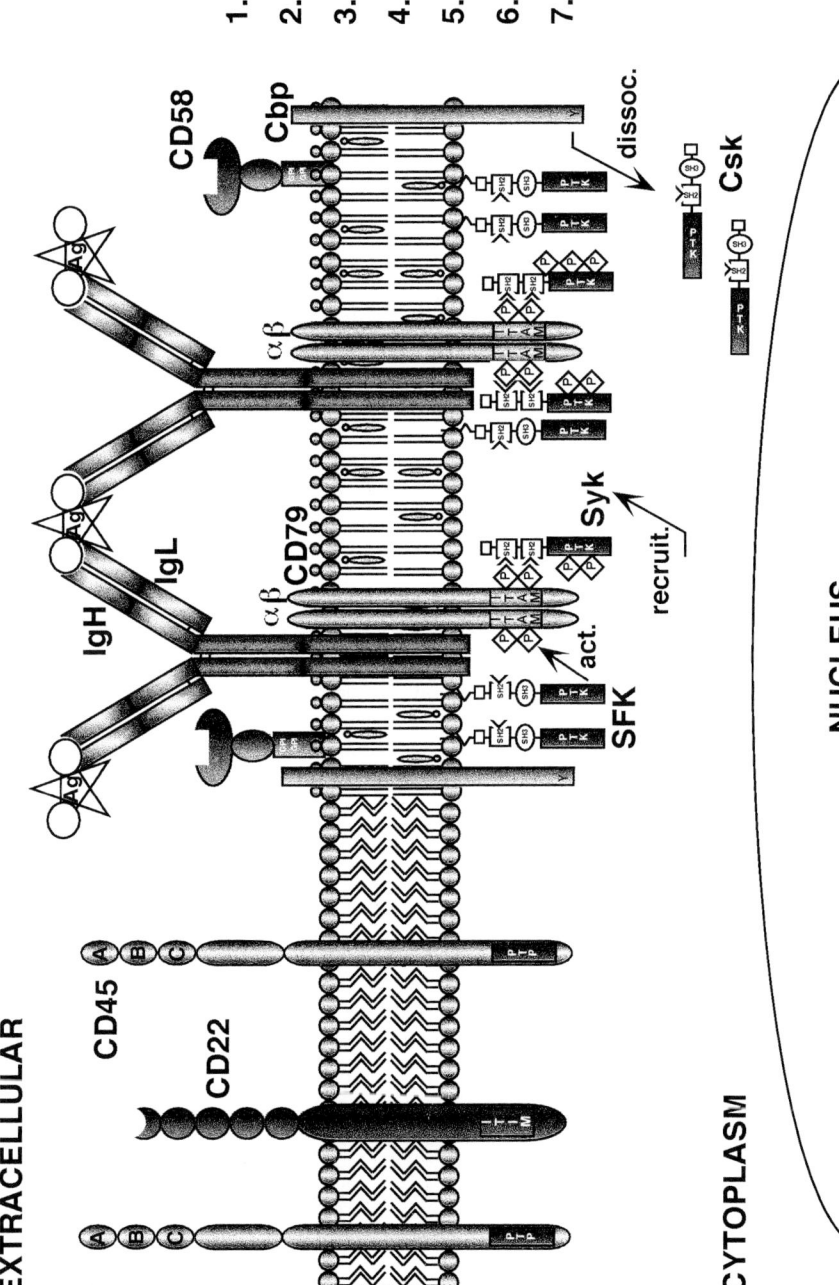

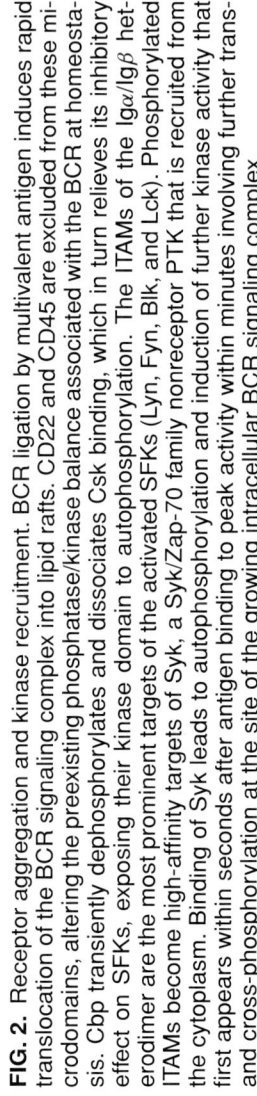

Phospholipid
Sphingolipid
Sat. Phospholipid
Cholesterol

NUCLEUS

CYTOPLASM

FIG. 2. Receptor aggregation and kinase recruitment. BCR ligation by multivalent antigen induces rapid translocation of the BCR signaling complex into lipid rafts. CD22 and CD45 are excluded from these microdomains, altering the preexisting phosphatase/kinase balance associated with the BCR at homeostasis. Cbp transiently dephosphorylates and dissociates Csk binding, which in turn relieves its inhibitory effect on SFKs, exposing their kinase domain to autophosphorylation. The ITAMs of the Igα/Igβ heterodimer are the most prominent targets of the activated SFKs (Lyn, Fyn, Blk, and Lck). Phosphorylated ITAMs become high-affinity targets of Syk, a Syk/Zap-70 family nonreceptor PTK that is recruited from the cytoplasm. Binding of Syk leads to autophosphorylation and induction of further kinase activity that first appears within seconds after antigen binding to peak activity within minutes involving further trans- and cross-phosphorylation at the site of the growing intracellular BCR signaling complex.

them into close proximity with translocated BCR complexes upon specific receptor engagement.

Upon BCR engagement, the most prominent targets for the initial kinase activity are the two tyrosines within the ITAM of Igα and to a lesser extent Igβ (1–3). There appear to be qualitative differences in SFK activity and target discrimination that indicate a hierarchy of action for these enzymes at the cellular level. Each SFK contains a unique N-terminal of ~30aa associated with protein interactions and a single Src homology domain 3 (SH3) that can bind proline-rich regions in many signaling intermediates. The next single SH2 domain in each kinase facilitates binding to phosphotyrosines and may target pITAMs of the Igα/Igβ heterodimer and help to amplify the initial signal. In B-cell lines, Fyn predominantly phosphorylates the N-terminal tyrosine of the Igα ITAM and then the C-terminal tyrosine, while Blk phosphorylates the C-terminal tyrosine, even if the N-terminal tyrosine has been mutated. Further, the expression of Lyn and Fyn alone is sufficient to phosphorylate Igα after BCR cross-linking (27). However, B cells from Lyn-deficient mice display exaggerated B-cell responsiveness revealing a negative regulatory role for this SFK *in vivo* (28). While Lyn is the most prominent SFK in naïve B cells, it is still not clear which of these molecules, or in what combination, are used at the time of initial antigen contact *in vivo*.

Syk Recruitment and Activation

Once the ITAMs of Igα/Igβ have been phosphorylated, they become high-affinity targets for the tandem SH2 domains of Syk, a Syk/Zap-70 family kinase (29). Syk is a nonreceptor PTK that resides constitutively in the cytoplasm. The binding of Syk to pITAMs recruits this kinase to the plasma membrane site of BCR aggregation (Fig. 2). Syk binding to pITAMs induces a conformational change similar to that seen on autophosphorylation that promotes phosphorylation of two adjacent tyrosines within the SH1 domain, inducing kinase activity (30). Alternatively, phosphorylation of Tyr519 also substantially increases Syk kinase activity, and mutation of this residue to Phe inhibits BCR signaling (31). The activated SFKs associated within the growing intracellular signaling complex have been implicated in this process with evidence in Lyn-deficient cell lines for greatly reduced Syk activity (32). Lyn and Syk can also be co-precipitated with the BCR complex from activated B cells lending support that the SH2 domains of SFKs may bind phosphorylated Syk. Therefore, the intracellular aspect of the BCR signaling complex contains activated SFKs, pITAMs, and activated Syk kinases that first appear within seconds of the initial recognition event, and then amplifies to peak activity within the first few minutes after BCR engagement.

It has been difficult to analyze the role of Syk in mature B cells *in vivo* because Syk-deficient mice display a significant developmental defect and accumulate B cells at the pro–B stage in the bone marrow (33). Even the expression of a transgenic BCR fails to promote the maturation of Syk-deficient B cells. However, binding of antigen to these immature Syk-deficient B cells does lead to phosphorylation of Igα/Igβ but this is insufficient to mobilize intracellular calcium.

A Role for Adaptor Molecules BLNK and BCAP

Adapter molecules represent another class of molecules that regulate antigen receptor–mediated signals (Fig. 3). These adaptor molecules possess no enzymatic or transcriptional activity, but express a variety of modular binding domains such as SH2, SH3, phosphotyrosine binding (PTB) and pleckstrin homology (PH) binding domains (34,35). The adaptor acts as protein scaffolding to couple signal-transducing complexes to a variety of intracellular effector mechanisms. While the list of adaptors and their potential binding partners is growing, there is general agreement that LAT and SLP-76 in T cells (15) and B-cell linker protein (BLNK; also known as SLP-65) in B cells (34,35) are central modulators of antigen-specific lymphocyte activation and critical to the initiation of sustained intracellular calcium responses.

BLNK is resident in the cytoplasm, contains an N-terminal region with five tyrosines in a YXXP context, a central portion containing several SH3-domain binding motifs, and a C-terminal SH2 domain (34,35). Upon BCR ligation, BLNK translocates to the membrane where it co-localizes with the PTK Syk (Fig. 3). Syk is required for tyrosine phosphorylation of BLNK, and phosphorylated BLNK is capable of binding the SH2 domains of PLC-γ2 (36). BLNK is also one of the major binding proteins for the SH2 domains of the Tek family kinase, Btk in B cells. Therefore, phosphorylated BLNK is thought to bring Btk into close proximity to PLC-γ2, allowing complete phosphorylation and full activation of this key lipid metabolizing enzyme. In support of this model, PLC-γ2 tyrosine phosphorylation and inositol-1,4,5-triphosphate (IP$_3$) production is absent in BLNK-deficient B cells (36,37). Furthermore, Syk-deficient B cells cannot phosphorylate PLC-γ2 or produce IP$_3$ (38). While Btk-deficient B cells display only a small decrease in PLC-γ2 phosphorylation, there is a complete loss of IP$_3$ production (39). Thus, BLNK recruits and facilitates the activation of Btk and PLC-γ2, two of the major constituents of the calcium initiation complex.

The third member of this membrane-associated calcium-initiation complex is PI-3K. While PI-3K is a constitutively active enzyme, it must be recruited to the membrane complex to exert and focus this metabolic activity. The B-cell cytoplasmic adaptor protein (BCAP) was identified through its binding to the p85 subunit of PI-3K based on the expectation that additional adaptor molecules exist to connect BCR signaling to PI-3K activation (40). BCAP contains 31 tyrosines that may be phosphorylated and four of these within the consensus binding motif for the SH2 domain of the p85 subunit of PI-3K. The rapid recruitment of this PI-3K subunit to the lipid rafts upon BCR engagement was dependent on the presence of BCAP (Fig. 3). In the DT-40 chicken B-cell line, both

EXTRACELLULAR

CYTOPLASM

NUCLEUS

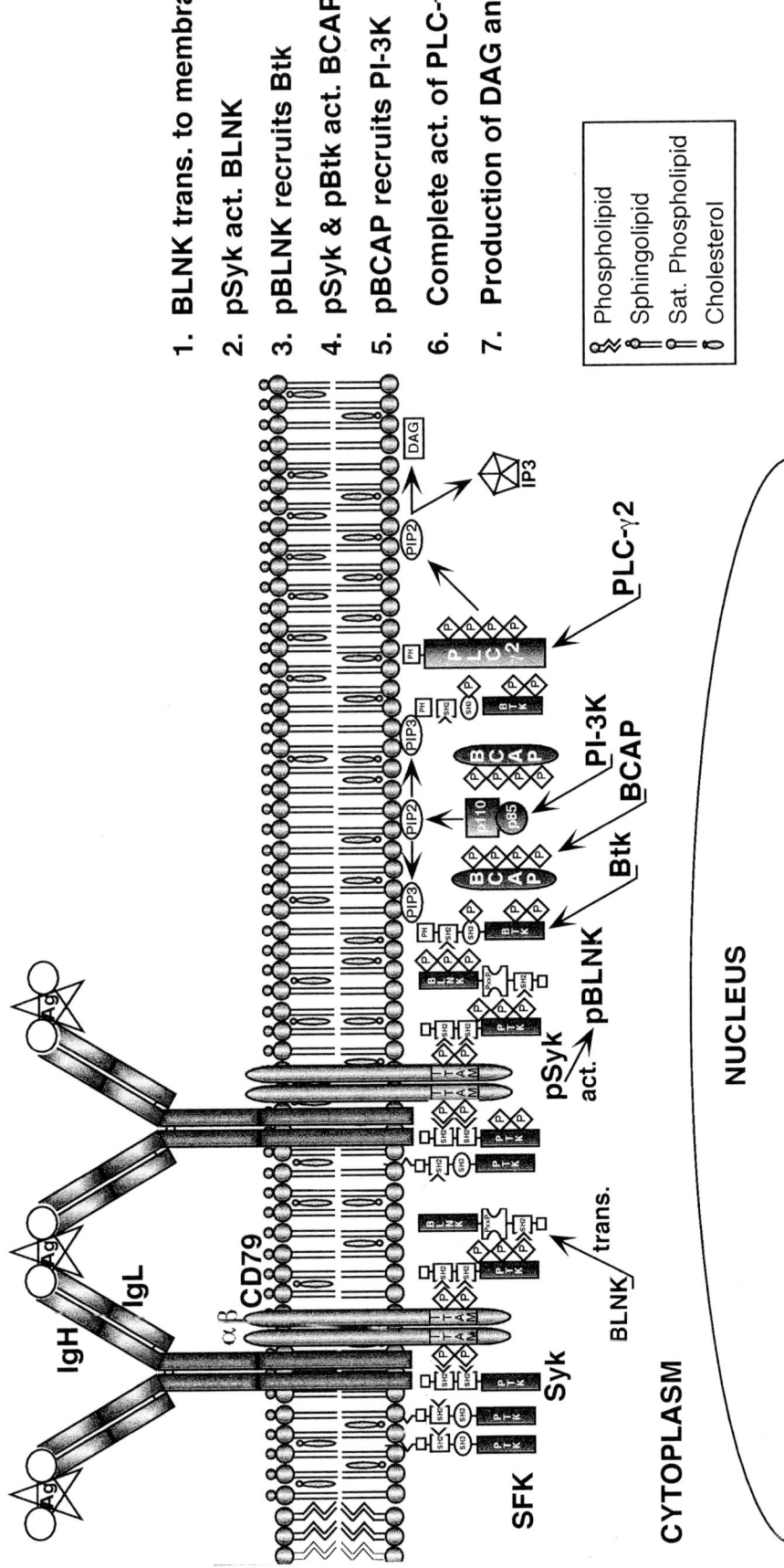

1. BLNK trans. to membrane
2. pSyk act. BLNK
3. pBLNK recruits Btk
4. pSyk & pBtk act. BCAP
5. pBCAP recruits PI-3K
6. Complete act. of PLC-γ2
7. Production of DAG and IP3

Phospholipid
Sphingolipid
Sat. Phospholipid
Cholesterol

FIG. 3. Adaptors and the formation of the calcium initiation complex. The adaptor protein B-cell linker protein (BLNK) is resident in the cytoplasm and translocates to the membrane upon BCR ligation, co-localizing with phosphorylated Syk (pSyk). pSyk phosphorylates BLNK, which allows subsequent binding PLC-γ2, relocating this critical lipid metabolizing enzyme to the membrane. pBLNK also binds the Tek family kinase Btk, bringing it to the membrane and into close proximity to SFKs, which facilitate its own full activation and close to PLC-γ2. pSyk and pBtk appear to help recruit and activate the B-cell cytoplasmic adaptor protein (BCAP), which in turn rapidly recruits another lipid-metabolizing enzyme, PI-3K, to the growing membrane complex. PI-3K phosphorylates PI(4,5)P₂ to produce focal accumulations of PI(3,4,5)P₃, which also serve to recruit enzymes such as Btk and PLC-γ2 via their pleckstrin homology (PH) domain to the membrane. Physical recruitment to the membrane together with pSyk and pBtk are required for full activation of PLC-γ2, which ultimately produces substantial quantities of DAG that accumulate at the plasma membrane and activates most protein kinase C (PKC) isoenzymes and IP₃ that diffuse into the cytoplasm to initiate mobilization of intracellular calcium.

Syk and Btk were shown to contribute to initiating and sustaining BCAP phosphorylation (40,41), while the SFK Lyn had an inhibitory effect, perhaps through the recruitment of tyrosine phosphatases (42). Mice deficient in BCAP have decreased numbers of mature B cells, reduced calcium responsiveness and proliferative responses *in vitro*. These data are consistent with the studies in cell lines (43). Thus, BCAP and PI-3K can be added to the list of molecules recruited rapidly into the intracellular signaling complex to regulate the impact of BCR-mediated signaling.

PI-3K Recruitment to Membrane

PI-3K plays an important role in PLC-γ2 activation, although both enzymes share a common membrane-associated lipid substrate. PI-3K phosphorylates the inositol group of the PLC-γ2 substrate PI(4,5)P$_2$ to produce PI(3,4,5)P$_3$. The subsequent focal accumulation of PI(3,4,5)P$_3$ recruits Btk to the membrane signaling complex by binding to its pleckstrin homology (PH) domain (44). This brings Btk into close apposition to PLC-γ2, which may itself bind to the membrane via its own PH domain. As discussed above, this direct membrane binding further encourages Btk activation by Syk and its subsequent activation of PLC-γ2. This molecular interdependence is again highlighted through the role of Syk and Btk in phosphorylating BCAP, the adaptor molecule that initially recruits PI-3K to the membrane complex (Fig. 3).

There are multiple forms of PI-3Ks but those associated with lymphocyte activation are the class 1 PI-3Ks (45). These comprise a heterodimer with one catalytic subunit and one regulatory subunit. The p110 catalytic subunit is constitutively active and exists in four isoforms (α, β, δ and γ). Hence, the key to regulating PI-3K activity is targeting catalysis to the plasma membrane through the regulatory subunit, which is encoded by three distinct genes, p85α, p85β, and p55 (45). The p85α subunit of PI-3K is the most abundant regulatory molecule and deletion of this isoform by gene targeting results in decreased B-cell development and diminished proliferative responses to BCR stimulation *in vitro*. However, genetic manipulation of PI-3K function is complicated and becomes difficult to interpret due to the multiple isoforms of both the catalytic and regulatory subunits. The PI-3K inhibitor wortmannin blocks BCR-induced PI(3,4,5)P$_3$ production, and has been useful in establishing the role of the latter in a range of cellular processes, such as cell cycle progression, cell motility, and adhesion. Wortmannin treatment also abrogates BCR-induced elevation of intracellular calcium, emphasizing the interplay among its activity, Btk activity, the complete activation of PLC-γ2, and the production of adequate levels of IP$_3$.

Btk Recruitment and Activation

BCR-mediated activation also leads to the rapid recruitment and activation of the Tek family kinase, Btk (Fig. 3). The Tek family of kinases share some structural homology with SFKs displaying similar SH2 and SH3 domains, but lack constitutive attachment to the plasma membrane with no N-terminal myristylation or palmitoylation sites (46). Complete activation of Teks requires localization to the membrane, phosphorylation of the activation loop by SFKs, and subsequent autophosphorylation of Tyr223 in the SH3 domain. Binding pBLNK through its SH2 domain and PI(3,4,5)P$_3$ through its PH domain brings Btk into close proximity to SFKs for activation and to its major substrate PLC-γ2. Lack of functional Btk causes severe B-cell immunodeficiencies that are characterized by decreased mature B-cell numbers and grossly impaired B-cell responsiveness (X-linked agammaglobulinemia, XLA in humans, and Xid in mice) (47,48). Mutations in the kinase, PH, SH2, and SH3 domains cause varying degrees of immunodeficiency. Ectopic expression of Btk can restore the blunted calcium responsiveness of the Xid B cells. Similarly, over-expression of Btk in B-cell lines augments intracellular calcium mobilzation. A negative regulator of Btk has also recently been described (49). This transinhibitor of Btk (IBtk) binds to the PH domain and can block downstream activities such as calcium responsiveness and NF-κB–driven transcription.

PLCc-γ2 Activation

Activated PLC-γ hydrolyzes the lipid substrate PI(4,5)P$_2$ to generate the secondary signaling activators DAG and IP$_3$. While DAG remains associated with the plasma membrane, IP$_3$ diffuses into the cytosol and binds to its receptors on the membrane of the endoplasmic reticuluum (ER) to initiate the release of Ca^{2+}. PLC-γ isoforms 1 and 2 uniquely contain two SH2 domains, an SH3 domain, and a PH domain. While PLC-γ1 is predominant in most cell types, including T cells, PLC-γ2 is the dominant isoform in B cells. Full activity of PLC-γ2 requires physical recruitment to the plasma membrane, direct phosphorylation of multiple tyrosines, and perhaps an SH2- and phosphorylation-mediated conformational change of the molecule (1).

In activated B cells, the C-terminal SH2 domain of PLC-γ2 can bind to a conserved phosphotyrosine residue between the SH2 and the kinase domain of activated Syk (50). As described above, PLC-γ2 can also bind to phosphorylated BLNK. Btk is capable of directly phosphorylating critical tyrosine residues required for activation; however, there is residual phosphorylation of PLC-γ2 in the absence of Btk that can be attributed to Syk activity. It is plausible that both Syk and Btk play a role in activating PLC-γ by phosphorylating different tyrosines, and this concerted action is facilitated through the SH2 docking site of BLNK. The PH domain can also directly recruit PLC-γ2 to the plasma membrane and contribute to the complete activation of this enzyme. Finally, to underscore the importance of PLC-γ2 to calcium responsiveness *in vivo*, IgM receptor–induced calcium flux and proliferation to B-cell mitogens are absent in PLC-γ2–deficient mice (51). The B-cell defects in PLC-γ2–deficient animals are similar to the Btk-deficient and BLNK-deficient animals arguing further that they lie within the same signal transduction pathway.

In summary, surface BCR aggregation nucleates an intracellular signaling complex at the inner leaflet of the plasma membrane through the rapid concerted action of activated SFKs, pITAMs, and activated Syk PTK. Recruitment and phosphorylation of the adaptors BLNK and BCAP encourage the lipid-metabolizing enzyme PI-3K and the Tek-family kinase Btk to join this complex and completely activate PLC-$\gamma 2$ (Fig. 3). Activated PLC-$\gamma 2$ ultimately produces substantial quantities of IP_3 that diffuses into the cytoplasm, binds IP_3 receptors, and initiates the mobilization of intracellular calcium stores.

EFFECTOR SIGNALING PATHWAYS

Sustained elevation of cytosolic Ca^{2+} regulates the activity of transcription factors such as NF-ATc and NF-κB with substantial impact on cell fate. This complex effector signaling pathway relies on IP_3-dependent mobilization of intracellular Ca^{2+} stores from the ER of activated B cells (Fig. 4). ER-store release of Ca^{2+} then triggers the influx of extracellular Ca^{2+} through Ca^{2+} release-activated Ca^{2+} (CRAC) channels by a poorly understood mechanism referred to as capacitive calcium entry (CCE). This elevated level of intracellular Ca^{2+} propagates Ca^{2+}/calmodulin–dependent activation of calcineurin and the nuclear translocation of NF-ATc, and together with PKC activation, the nuclear translocation of NF-κB. Three separate effector signaling pathways are presented in some detail in the last half of this section. The PKC activation pathway that has both positive and negative influences on BCR signaling activity. The PI-3K/Akt (PKB) activation pathway that has a significant impact on cell fate by regulating the pattern of gene expression and more directly promoting cell survival. Finally, the Ras/MAPK pathways are presented briefly as being associated with BCR-mediated cell proliferation, differentiation, and death. The details of these effector signaling pathways serve to highlight the diversity of intracellular regulatory mechanisms available to antigen-activated B cells and begin to outline how BCR-mediated signals are integrated at the cellular level.

Mobilization of Intracellular Calcium Stores

The complete activation of PLC-$\gamma 2$ converts the membrane component $PI(4,5)P_2$ into the two second messengers, DAG and IP_3. While DAG remains attached to the inner leaflet of the plasma membrane, IP_3 is water soluble and diffuses into the cytoplasm where it binds to IP_3Rs as the critical mediator of intracellular calcium mobilization (52,53) (Fig. 4). In B cells, the ER is the major intracellular store for calcium ions (Ca^{2+}). These stores are maintained dynamically through ATPase-dependent pumps associated with the ER membrane, referred to as the sarcoplasmic/endoplasmic reticulum Ca^{2+}-ATPase (SERCA) (54). There are also buffering proteins within the ER, such as calsequestrin, that help

to maintain the high intraluminal concentrations of Ca^{2+}. In naïve mature lymphocytes, the free cytoplasmic Ca^{2+} is maintained at around 100 nM prior to mobilization of intracellular stores. Within the first 5 to 15 seconds after antigen-receptor oligomerization, intracellular free calcium can reach levels of 400nM to in excess of 1000 nM, depending on the nature of the signal.

The IP_3R that mediates this release of intracellular Ca^{2+} stores is composed of a homotetramer of 310 kDa subunits, each capable of binding one IP_3 molecule at its positively charged Arg/Lys–rich N-terminal region (54). These receptors are inserted into the ER membrane and coexist in multiple isoforms with somewhat differing signaling patterns (55). IP_3R-1 is slowly inactivated by Ca^{2+}, while both IP_3R-2 and IP_3R-3 are resistant to Ca^{2+}. IP_3R-1 and IP_3R-2 mediate Ca^{2+} oscillations while IP_3R-3 mediates a single spike in intracellular Ca^{2+}. However, there appears to be a great deal of functional redundancy across these receptors as deletion of all three isoforms in DT40 chicken B cells was required to completely inhibit the BCR-mediated Ca^{2+} response (56). Chemicals such as thapsigargin have been useful in manipulating the ER stores of Ca^{2+}. These chemicals debilitate the SERCA pump and allow slow emptying of the ER stores that is independent of IP_3 production. The calcium ionophore, ionomycin, can also mediate ER store release of Ca^{2+} in the absence of antigen-receptor ligation, IP_3 production, or significant direct influx of extracellular calcium via the plasma membrane.

Capacitative Calcium Entry

Emptying the ER stores of Ca^{2+} triggers the influx of extracellular Ca^{2+} across the plasma membrane through specialized Ca^{2+} channels. The Ca^{2+} store release leads to an initial spike of cytoplasmic Ca^{2+}, while sustained elevation in the cytoplasm needed for subsequent impact on transcriptional activity, requires the influx of extracellular Ca^{2+}. As lymphocytes are nonexcitable cells, these channels represent a type of store-operated channel known as CRAC channels (53). The CRAC channels are highly selective for Ca^{2+}, and display an inwardly rectifying current-voltage relationship in patch–clamp studies of lymphocyte electrophysiology that can be blocked by Ni^{2+} and Cd^{2+} ions. While these functional analyses are sensitive and can identify CRAC channels and quantify the numbers of channels on the cell surface, cloning the genes associated with these activities has been more elusive. In B cells, CD20 has been proposed as a candidate CRAC channel; when transfected into T cells and nonlymphoid cells, it conferred Ca^{2+} conductance similar to what was seen in the B cells (57). CD20 belongs to the large family of MS4A genes with 20 closely related members, hence its requirement for Ca^{2+} flux in B cells has been difficult to confirm using gene-targeting experiments. More recently, a protein CaT1 whose gene was cloned from rat duodenum (58), when expressed in mammalian CHO cells, demonstrates cation selectivity and single channel currents in patch–clamp analysis that were

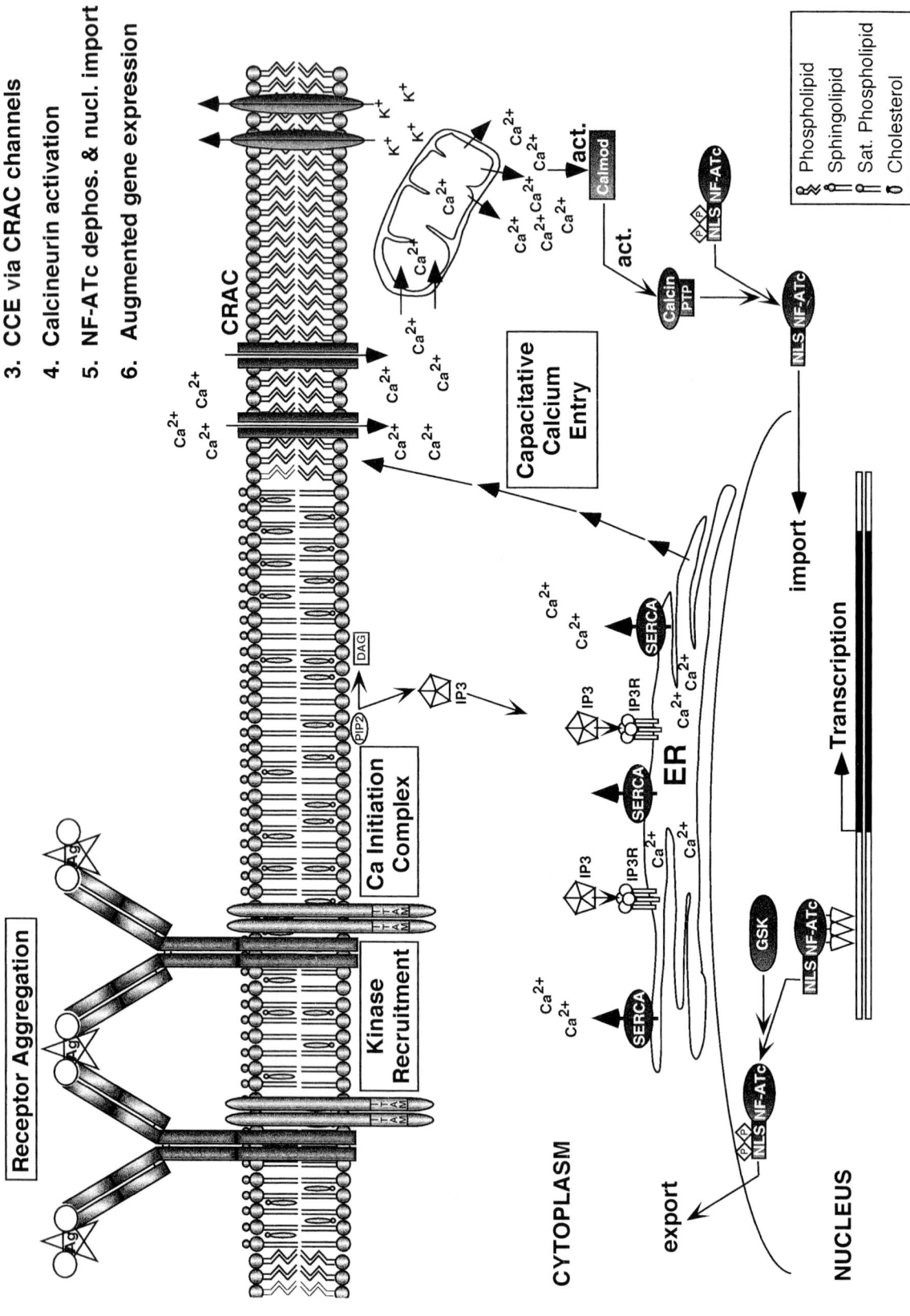

EXTRACELLULAR

Receptor Aggregation

Kinase Recruitment

Ca Initiation Complex

CRAC

1. IP3 binds IP3R on ER
2. Mobil. of ER Ca²⁺ stores
3. CCE via CRAC channels
4. Calcineurin activation
5. NF-ATc dephos. & nucl. import
6. Augmented gene expression

Capacitative Calcium Entry

CYTOPLASM

ER

SERCA

IP3R

IP3

PIP2

DAG

GSK

NLS NF-ATc

Calcin PTP

Calmod

act.

act.

import

export

Transcription

NUCLEUS

Phospholipid
Sphingolipid
Sat. Phospholipid
Cholesterol

indistinguishable from CRAC channels. This gene was also expressed in Jurkat T cells and is likely to at least represent a component of the CRAC channel in lymphocytes (59). Its relationship to CD20 is currently unclear.

The mechanism that facilitates the entry of Ca^{2+} through CRAC channels upon emptying of ER stores remains unknown, but the process is generally referred to as CCE (Fig. 4). It is possible that a soluble factor is released from the ER when Ca^{2+} stores are depleted and this calcium influx factor (CIF) would regulate opening of the CRAC channels. The initial evidence for such a factor was later found to induce store depletion itself, and hence acts upstream of CCE. Putney (60) suggests a physical interaction between the IP_3R and the CRAC channels upon store depletion that allows Ca^{2+} influx, referred to as the conformational coupling model. In Drosophila, there is evidence for such an association between IP_3R and store-operated transient-receptor potential (TRP) channels. However, TRPs do not behave exactly as CRAC channels in lymphocytes and require IP_3 itself for their activation (61). Further, receptor-independent CCE remains intact in B-cell lines that lack all IP_3R isoforms, arguing against a direct effect through IP_3 or an IP_3R regulating CCE in lymphocytes. Nevertheless, the contribution of CCE to sustained elevation of calcium is clearly demonstrated when intracellular stores are depleted either using receptor-mediated or receptor-independent means, in the absence of extracellular calcium (62). The magnitude and duration of the intracellular calcium response is greatly diminished under these conditions and can be used to demonstrate the basal Ca^{2+} level of the ER stores in these cells. Serafini et al. (63) have also isolated T-cell–mutant cell lines that are normal in primary Ca^{2+} mobilization but are defective in CCE. The level of defect in these lines may reside in the CRAC channels themselves or in the regulation of CCE.

Calcium-Mediated Regulation of NF-ATc Activation

Sustained high cytoplasmic Ca^{2+} levels are required for the activation of the transcription regulators, nuclear factor of activated T cells (NF-ATc), and nuclear factor κB (NF-κB).

The NF-AT family of transcription factors includes at least four calcium-regulated members that reside in the cytoplasm at homeostasis, with NF-ATc1 and NF-ATc2 being the major family members in lymphocytes (64). Without stimulation, NF-ATc proteins are all heavily phosphorylated on serine in a conserved serine-rich (SRR) and serine-proline rich (SP) region. Phosphorylation of serines in the SRR and SP regions are required to mask nuclear localization signals (NLS) and control basal cytoplasmic localization (65). Sustained and elevated intracellular Ca^{2+} targets the Ca^{2+}/calmodulin–dependent activation of the serine/threonine protein phosphatase, calcineurin. Activated calcineurin then targets NF-ATc dephosphorylation, exposing the NLS and promoting nuclear import (66) (Fig. 4). The immunosuppressive action of drugs such as cyclosporin and FK506 inhibit calcineurin activity and shift the distibution of NF-ATc toward cytoplasmic localization. Glycogen synthase kinase 3 (GSK-3) can oppose nuclear localization of NF-ATc by phosphorylating the serines within the SRR and SP regions and actively promoting nuclear export (67). GSK-3 is also constitutively active in resting lymphocytes and is inhibited by phosphorylation in response to antigen receptor–mediated activation. Lithium, an inhibitor of GSK-3 activity, increases the duration of NF-ATc residence in the nucleus. Hence, retention of NF-ATc in the nucleus requires both Ca^{2+}-dependent activation of nuclear import and the inhibition of nuclear export (Fig. 4).

The action of NF-ATc family members is also regulated at the transcriptional level. NF-ATc1 is induced upon antigen activation and NF-ATc1–deficient lymphocytes display impaired proliferative responses (68). In contrast, NF-ATc2 is repressed upon activation and animals deficient in NF-ATc2 display hyperactive peripheral lymphocytes, lymphoadenopathy, and susceptibility to apoptosis (69). Animals doubly deficient in NF-ATc1 and NF-ATc2 display hyperactivated T cells and B cells with exaggerated helper T-cell and plasma-cell differentiation (70). These studies emphasize the importance of NF-ATc in the balanced regulation of immune responses and highlights a level of interplay between family members *in vivo* that is still not clearly understood.

FIG. 4. Elevation of cytosolic calcium and alterations in gene expression. The complete activation of PLC-γ2 leads to the production of water-soluble IP_3, which diffuses into the cytoplasm where it binds IP_3R located in the membrane of the endoplasmic reticulum (ER). Binding to IP_3R mobilizes ER Ca^{2+} stores to the cytosol by altering a dynamic balance maintained through ATPase-dependent pumps within the membrane referred to as sarcoplasmic/ER Ca^{2+}-ATPase (SERCA). The depletion of ER Ca^{2+} triggers the influx of extracellular Ca^{2+} across the plasma membrane through Ca^{2+} release–activated Ca^{2+} (CRAC) channels by a poorly understood mechanism referred to as capacitative calcium entry (CCE). Sustained elevation of cytosolic calcium targets the Ca^{2+}/calmodulin–dependent activation of the serine/threonine protein phosphatase, calcineurin. Activated calcineurin dephosphorylates the transcription factor NF-ATc, exposing a nuclear localization signal (NLS) that promotes its nuclear import, allowing the modulation of gene expression for numerous gene products through binding to consensus sequences in many promoters. Glycogen synthase kinase-3 (GSK-3) that is resident in the nucleus can promote nuclear export of NF-ATc through phosphorylation and masking of the NLS, indicating a complex mechanism of nuclear retention for this transcription factor in B cells.

Regulation of NF-κB Activation

The elevation of intracellular Ca^{2+} and the activation of protein kinase C (PKC) act synergistically to promote nuclear translocation of NF-κB. NF-κB refers to a family of inducible dimeric transcription factors composed of members of the Rel family of DNA-binding proteins (71,72). At homeostasis, NLS sequences in NF-κB are masked by binding to a family of inhibitory proteins (IκBs) that localize NF-κB dimers to the cytoplasm (71). Activation of a multisubunit IκB kinase (IKK) regulates IκB phosphorylation, which in turn targets the inhibitory protein for ubiquitination and proteolytic degradation. Degradation of IκB reveals the NLS in NF-κB subunits and promotes its translocation to the nucleus. Once in the nucleus, NF-κB dimers are further regulated through phosphorylation of the Rel proteins that are required for full activation. Acute stimulation of B cells by antigen and phorbol ester (to activate PKC) leads to detectable NF-κB activation within 4 minutes as assayed by cytosolic degradation of IκBα and accumulation of Rel A in the nucleus (73). The Ca^{2+}/calmodulin–dependent activation of calcineurin and DAG-dependent activation of PKC converge to activate IKK under these stimuli. Calcineurin has been shown to synergize with PKC and either activate IKK or inactivate IκB. Interestingly, the amplitude and duration of the induced Ca^{2+} response in antigen-specific B cells differentially impact transcriptional regulators (73). While NF-κB and the c-Jun N-terminal kinase (JNK) are selectively activated by large transient Ca^{2+} response, NF-AT is efficiently activated by a low but sustained Ca^{2+} plateau.

Using a Ca^{2+} clamp technique to pulse store depleted Jurkat T cells, Dolmetsch et al. (74) also implicate the frequency of intracellular Ca^{2+} oscillations as a regulatory element in transcriptional activity. In these studies, oscillation with a periodicity of up to 400 seconds efficiently induced NF-AT translocation while maximal NF-κB activity was induced with a periodicity of as long as 1,800 seconds. Thus, modulators of signaling that affect the quantity and quality of the cytoplasmic Ca^{2+} response, such as PI-3K, Btk, and PLC-γ2 activation, can significantly impact the pattern of gene expression in antigen-activated B cells and may determine subsequent B-cell fate.

The PKC Pathway

The second product of $PI(4,5)P_2$ hydrolysis by PLC-γ2 is DAG that accumulates at the plasma membrane and activates most PKC isoenzymes (75). PKC refers to a ubiquitous group of at least 11 related serine/threonine kinases that are activated by calcium and/or the phospholipid, DAG. Phorbol myristate acetate (PMA) is a DAG analogue that can directly activate PKC isoforms and has been useful in elucidating the action of these isoenzymes. PKC rapidly relocates from the cytosol to the membrane-associated fraction of cells within seconds of direct activation. The isoforms expressed in B cells include α, β, δ, ζ, η, and θ, of which α, β, δ, and θ are regulated by DAG (3). PKCβ-deficient mice display reduced numbers of mature B cells and substantially impaired humoral responses. This is a B-cell phenotype similar to the X-linked immunodeficiency of Btk-deficient animals (76). BCR-mediated proliferation is also significantly reduced in the PKCβ-deficient mature B cells. These patterns indicate a positive role for PKCβ activity that appears to be downstream of Btk. In contrast, Kang et al. (77) report that the overall tyrosine phosphorylation of Btk is elevated in the PKCβ-deficient B cells. They demonstrate that PKCβ can uniquely interfere with Btk membrane recruitment through serine phosphorylation within the Btk Tek-homology (TH) domain. In this manner, PKCβ acts as a potent negative regulator of Btk-induced Ca^{2+} mobilization and thereby impacts the BCR signaling thresholds that ultimately modulate lymphocyte activity. Taken together, Kang et al. (77) suggest that exaggerated Btk signals may be as equally detrimental as deficient Btk, and that PKCβ may act to regulate its optimal balance at different stages of B-cell development *in vivo*.

At least one other PKC isoform has been implicated in regulating BCR-mediated activity. The atypical isoform PKCμ is activated upon BCR engagement and co-precipitates with the BCR complex, Syk and PLC-γ2. Activation of PKCμ appears to be Syk dependent as it does not occur in Syk-deficient, DT40 chicken B cells and can be rescued by constitutively activated Syk in these cells (78). Syk itself can then be phosphorylated on serine by activated PKCμ in a way that can inhibit its ability to activate PLC-γ2. While calcium does not influence PKCμ function *in vitro*, PKCμ does contain the tandem cysteine-rich, zinc-finger–like motifs that confer DAG binding. Hence, PKCμ also appears to function in a negative feedback loop that can regulate the extent of BCR-mediated signaling cascades.

PI-3K/Akt Signaling Pathway

Another serine/threonine kinase, Akt (also called protein kinase B; PKB) acts as a critical link between PI-3K activation and the cellular impact of BCR signaling (3,79,80). Activated PI-3K phosphorylates $PI(4,5)P_2$ to generate $PI(3,4,5)P_3$. The SH2 domain that contains inositol polyphosphate 5′-phosphatase (SHIP), helps to balance PI-3K activity by hydrolyzing $PI(3,4,5)P_3$ to generate $PI(3,4)P_2$ and may stimulate Akt in this manner (3). The $PI(3,4)P_2$ helps to activate Akt through binding to its PH domain. Binding to this membrane-associated lipid brings Akt into close proximity to a 3′-phosphoinositide-dependent protein kinase-1 (PDK1), a serine/threonine kinase that is activated by $PI(3,4,5)P_3$. Activated PDK1 can phosphorylate Akt on Thr308, which is a step required for complete activation of Akt (81). GSK-3 is one downstream target of activated Akt that loses its kinase activity upon serine phosphorylation leading to the enhanced nuclear retention of NF-ATc. Akt also inhibits the induction of apoptosis by inactivating pro-apoptotic proteins such as Bax, Bad, caspase 9, forkhead, and Nur 77, and by activating anti-apoptotic proteins such as NF-kB and cAmp response-element-binding protein (CREB) (82). Hence, the PI-3K/Akt pathway can indirectly regulate the pattern of gene expression but more directly promotes cell survival as one set of effector functions associated with antigen-specific BCR signaling.

Ras/MAPK Signaling Pathways

The Ras/MAPK signaling pathways have substantial impact on B-cell function and are implicated in the regulation of BCR-mediated cellular proliferation, differentiation, and death. The activation of Ras is determined by the nature of its bound guanine nucleotide. Ras is inactive when bound to guanosine diphosphate (GDP) and active when bound to guanosine triphosphate (GTP). Activation of PTKs promoted by BCR ligation leads to the accumulation of GTP-bound Ras at the intracellular site associated with receptor clustering (83). Inhibitors of PTK block the activation of Ras and part of this activation also appears dependent on PKC activation. Upon BCR ligation, the 46 kDa and 52 kDa isoforms of the PTB- and SH2-containing adaptor molecule, Shc translocates from the cytoplasm to the membrane (84). Shc, can bind the ITAMs of the Igα/Igβ *in vitro* and may directly associate with the BCR complex in this way (84). Activated Lyn and/or Syk phosphorylates Shc at Y^{239} and Y^{313} that act as the binding site for the SH2 domain of a second adaptor molecule, Grb2. Grb2 contains two SH3 domains that allow it to bind the proline-rich sequence of the Ras-guanine nucleotide exchange–factor SOS that positively regulates the activity of Ras.

The inositol phosphatase SHIP also associates with this multiprotein complex and Shc and Grb2 may help to localize it to the membrane complex to help balance the activation of Ras (85). Once tyrosine is phosphorylated, SHIP can compete with Grb2/SOS for binding to Shc, thereby inhibiting Ras activation. SHIP may inhibit Ras activity by hydrolyzing PI(3,4,5)P3 and preventing proper assembly of the signaling complex. The GTPase-activating protein, RasGAP, can also modulate Ras activity by enhancing the intrinsic GTPase activity of Ras and favoring the inactive GDP-bound form (86). RasGAP then associates through SH2 domains to another adaptor molecule, p62^dok. While the action of these inhibitors may balance BCR-mediated activation events, they strongly potentiate when FcγRIIb and the BCR are co–cross-linked (87). Under these conditions, tyrosine phosphorylation of p62^dok and binding to RasGAP are increased together with SHIP phosphorylation and binding to the PTB domain of p62^dok.

Accumulated RasGTP at the intracellular signaling complex promotes the activation of the best-characterized, mitogen-activated protein kinase (MAPK), the classical p42 and p44 isoforms of the extracellular signal-related kinases (ERK1 and ERK2) (3). In this cascade, RasGTP binds directly to Raf-1, the MAPK kinase kinase (MAPKKK) that in turn activates MEK-1 and MEK-2 (the MAPKK in this case) that phosphorylates ERK-1 and ERK-2. The phosphorylated ERKs form heterodimers, translocate into the nucleus and phosphorylates transcriptional regulators, including Fos, Jun, and Ets family members (3). PMA can induce ERK activation, implicating a role for PKC activation in this pathway.

The JNK MAPK kinase subfamily is activated by small GTP-binding proteins Rac-1 and Cdc 42 (88,89), and involves a cascade of MKK1, SEK1, and then JNK. Activated JNK translocates to the nucleus to target transcription factors c-Jun and ATF-1. JNK activation is sensitive to Ca^{2+} and can be inhibited by cyclosporine that blocks the activity of the Ca^{2+}/calmodulin–dependent serine phosphatase calcineurin. JNK remains inactive in the absence of IP_3R and the PKC isoform, PKCθ (90). Similarly, the third MAPK subfamily, p38 kinase, is also regulated by Rac-1 and Cdc42, however it only requires the activation of PKC and is not dependent on Ca^{2+} (88). The substrates in this pathway have not been as well characterized but activation of p38 has been correlated with BCR-induced apoptosis. BLNK-deficient B cells were unable to activate JNK and p38 following BCR ligation, indicating that this adaptor was needed for the initial activation of Rac-1 (36). Overall, these three MAPK pathways serve to highlight the diverse range of intracellular effector pathways that may be differentially triggered in B cells to influence B-cell fate.

SURFACE-EXPRESSED MODULATORS OF BCR SIGNALING

In this final section on BCR signaling mechanisms, the influence of four surface-expressed molecules and how they modulate BCR signaling will be discussed. CD45 is a transmembrane tyrosine phosphatase that has a positive regulatory impact on BCR signaling that exerts its influence at homeostasis to maintain the naïve B-cell in a signal-competent state. In contrast, CD22 has a negative regulatory impact on BCR signaling through its intracellular association with the tyrosine phosphatase, SHP-1. Finally, the form of antigen can influence the outcome of a BCR recognition event. Complement-decorated antigen co–cross-links complement receptors such as CD21 on naïve B cells and lead to substantial enhancement of the B-cell response. This enhancement is controlled by the recruitment of CD19 into the BCR signaling complex that acts like an adaptor molecule, efficiently recruiting signaling intermediates into the intracellular signaling cascade. If B cells encounter antigen as immune complexes, they co–cross-link the FcγRIIb into the BCR complex and recruit the inositol 5-phosphatase SHIP into the intracellular signaling complex. This phosphatase has a significant negative impact on the BCR signaling cascade. These details highlight the impact of microenvironmental context on the response to antigen and serve as a prelude to the range of complex interactions that can regulate the direction of B-cell differentiation *in vivo*.

CD45

Prior to contact with foreign antigen, naïve B cells dynamically maintain SFKs in a signal-competent state (Fig. 1). This homeostatic SFK activity is regulated through the action of C-terminal Src kinase (Csk) and the transmembrane protein tyrosine phosphatase (PTP), CD45 (91). Csk is a ubiquitously expressed cytoplasmic PTK with potent negative regulatory action through its propensity to phosphorylate the inhibitory carboxy-terminal tyrosine of SFKs. Once phosphorylated, this tyrosine provides an internal binding site for the SFKs' own SH2 domain and effectively closes the kinase domain and shuts off its activity (35,92). Csk is constitutively associated through its SH2 domain with a Csk-binding protein (Cbp) (93,94). Cbp is a transmembrane adaptor molecule that is itself constitutively tyrosine phosphorylated and locates to lipid rafts through palmitylation of its juxtamembrane cysteines. CD45 is thought to antagonize the action of Csk by dephosphorylating the inhibitory tyrosine of SFKs (95) (Fig. 1). Dephosphorylation of this site maintains the SFK in a primed state, capable of full activation. Consistent with this positive role, CD45–deficient B and T cells are hyper-phosphorylated at the inhibitory tyrosine in SFKs and fail to respond to antigen-receptor triggering (95). CD45-deficient animals also display a severe combined immunodeficiency.

Upon activation through the antigen receptor, Cbp transiently dephosphorylates and dissociates Csk binding (94). This relieves Csk phosphorylation of the inhibitory tyrosine in SFKs, thereby exposing the kinase domain to autophosphorylation. Interestingly, the antigen-receptor complex also rapidly translocates into lipid rafts that exclude CD45 (96), suggesting that continued local phosphatase activity may be detrimental to the development of the intracellular signaling complex at this point.

CD22

CD22 is expressed in the cytoplasm of pro–B cells and pre–B-cells and on the cell surface on mature recirculating B cells that co-express mIgM and mIgD. CD22 can be considered a cell surface adhesion receptor that recognizes N-glycolyl neuraminic acid residues on glycoprotein or glycolipid ligands expressed in the serum or on disparate hematopoeitic and nonhematopoeitic target cells (97,98). This adhesion molecule can be co-precipitated with the BCR in naïve B cells and becomes rapidly phosphorylated on tyrosine upon BCR engagement (99). The protein tyrosine phosphatase, SHP-1, rapidly associates with the activated CD22 at three of its six cytoplasmic tyrosines, each in the V/IxYxxL of the immune tyrosine-based inhibitory motif (ITIM) (100). The ITIMs act as a docking site for the SH2 domains of SHP-1.

In contrast to CD45, CD22 appears to have a negative impact on BCR signal transduction. B cells in CD22-deficient animals spontaneously down-modulate sIgM on peripheral B cells as well as exaggerated intracellular calcium responsiveness upon BCR cross-linking (101). These patterns are similar to the B-cell phenotype in SHP-1–deficient mice, further supporting CD22's role as a negative regulator (102) that may target the ITAMs of Igα/Igβ, Lyn, Syk, CD19, and PLCγ. While Lyn-deficient B cells can respond to BCR signals, they are unable to phosphorylate CD22 and recruit SHP-1, which leads to a hyperactivity of

B cells with delayed but exaggerated calcium responses (103). CD19/CD22 doubly deficient B cells were functionally similar to the CD19-deficient B cells, suggesting that CD19 activation of Lyn was also required to phosphorylate CD22 and subsequently recruit SHP-1 (103). Together these data argue for the negative and controlling role of CD22 in regulating the extent of the BCR-mediated cellular response that acts through and somewhat counter-regulates the action of CD19 *in vivo*.

CD19

CD19 and CD22 reciprocally regulate the BCR signaling complex. Both molecules associate with the sIgM at homeostasis and may control both the basal survival and the activation signals received by mature B cells through their BCR (103). CD19 is a 95 kDa transmembrane glycoprotein expressed on B cells from the pre–B-cell stage in the bone marrow and remains expressed throughout maturation (104). CD19 is associated noncovalently with CD21 (the complement receptor CR2); CD81 (TAPA-1); and Leu-13. Coligation of the BCR and CD19 using C3d-coupled antigen, greatly decreases the amount of antigen required for threshold cellular activation (1,000-fold less antigen) (105). Binding complement-tagged antigen co-translocates CD19/CD21 into lipid raft microdomains with prolonged residency compared to BCR cross-linking alone (106). The SFK Lyn is required for CD19 phosphorylation and CD19-deficient B cells have diminished levels of Lyn activity. Fujimoto et al. (107) demonstrate the initial phosphorylation of purified CD19 (at Y^{513}) by Lyn leads to the phosphorylation of a second tyrosine (Y^{482}) that serves to recruit a second Lyn molecule to CD19. This processive phosphorylation of CD19 and transphosphorylation of Lyn amplify both SFK and CD19 activity. CD19 also associates to some degree with the SFK Fyn and may impact the early phosphorylation of Igα/Igβ ITAMS. Upon co-ligation with the BCR, CD19 acts as a transmembrane adaptor protein with evidence for recruitment of PI-3K and Btk that impact the subsequent intracellular calcium response in activated B cells.

FcγRIIb

The other well-characterized surface modulator of BCR signal transduction is the Fc receptor for IgG on B cells, FcγRIIb (108). This single chain glycoprotein contains a ligand-binding extracellular domain and an ITIM motif in its cytopasmic domain. This FcR binds IgG with low affinity, interacting with immune complexes at physiological concentrations of antibody. The 13aa ITIM–containing motif is both necessary and sufficient to mediate the inhibition of BCR-mediated calcium mobilization and subsequent cellular proliferation. Upon co-ligation of the BCR and FcγRIIb, the tyrosine within the ITIM is phosphorylated, generating an SH2 recognition domain that recruits the inositol 5-phosphatase SHIP (109). SHIP mediates its inhibitory action by hydrolyzing the membrane inositol phosphate $PI(3,4,5)P_3$ to $PI(3,4)P_2$. This action reverses the accumulation of $PI(3,4,5)P_3$ at the plasma membrane interfering with the binding of PH-domain–containing molecules such as Btk and PLC-γ involved in calcium responsiveness. In support of this role, SHIP-deficient B cells are resistant to the negative effects of FcγRIIb co-ligation on calcium mobilization. Co-ligation of the FcγRIIb receptor also decreases CD19 phosphorylation and the recruitment of PI-3K to the membrane. As the appearance of IgG containing immune complexes is more associated with late primary B-cell responses or memory B-cell responses, the action of the FcγRIIb receptor is not likely to exert its effects on initial BCR-mediated activation of naïve B cells. Nevertheless, these molecules may play a role in the maintenance of peripheral B-cell tolerance and serve to control ongoing immunity and negatively regulate self-reactivity.

In summary, surface-expressed molecules can impact the basal survival signal received by naïve B cells and also play an important regulatory role at the time of antigen recognition when homeostasis is disturbed. As discussed, these molecules can have both positive and negative impacts on the extent of the BCR-mediated response. These molecules can be actively recruited based on the microenvironmental context of antigen presentation through ligation of their counter-receptors or exert their influence indirectly through dissociation of basal complexes. The form of the antigen itself can have a dramatic influence on the immune response that ensues by recruiting co-receptor molecules into the BCR signaling complex. In each case, these differential effects can impact the cell fate and influence the quality of the resultant humoral immune response generated and the efficacy of its long-term protection. In the remaining sections of this chapter, the cellular and molecular impact of these early signaling mechanisms are presented in their microenvironmental context as I consider B-cell activation and the progression of antigen-driven B-cell development.

MATURE B-CELL SUBSETS

All mature B cells are not the same and their developmental programs impact the quality of antigen responsiveness. B cells develop in the bone marrow (discussed in detail elsewhere in this volume) and exit this microenvironment as immature $mIgM^+mIgD^-$ B cells that appear in the spleen with a distinguishable transitional cell (T1 and T2) surface phenotype. The majority of these immature B cells have a short half-life in the spleen (2 to 3 days), while some get selected into the longer-lived recirculating B-cell compartment ($\sim$30-day half-life). These mature recirculating B cells are typically $mIgD^{++}mIgM^+$ and comprise more than 95% of naïve B cells found in peripheral lymph nodes (LN). These naïve B cells are referred to as conventional B cells or B-2 B cells, and are the precursors for Th-cell–dependent B-cell responses to most foreign protein antigens. The long-lived B cells in the spleen are more heterogeneous than the LN populations with

two other distinct subsets present, the B-1 B cells and the marginal zone (MZ) B cells.

B-1 B Cells

B-1 B cells represent a separate subset of mature B cells with distinct origins, cell surface phenotype, functional properties, and anatomical distribution. The B-1 subset was first identified based on its expression of CD5, phenotypic similarity to a set of B-cell lymphomas, and expansion within certain autoimmune-prone strains of mice (110,111). The origins of the B-1 B cells still remain a source of debate. Initially, they were shown to arise from precursors in the fetal liver and not from adult bone marrow. Transfer of B-1 B cells into an adoptive host demonstrated their capacity for self-renewal, a memory B-cell characteristic. However, V-region sequences analysis indicated the expression of germline V regions with no evidence for somatic hypermutation, and the expressed isotype was primarily IgM. The expressed V-region repertoire also indicated the use of a more restricted set of V regions than B-2 B cells. The junctions of these cells display fewer nontemplated nucleotide (N) junctional sequences typical of neonatal B cells with low terminal deoxynucleotidyl transferase (TdT) activity. Together these data gave rise to the notion that B-1 B cells represented the long-lived products of a separate lineage of B cells that emerged and stabilized during the neonatal period.

More recently, studies using various lines of BCR transgenic mice demonstrate that the mature phenotype of the B-cell population is dependent on the specificity of the expressed BCR (111–114). When the expressed BCR was selected from B-1 B cells, the mature BCR-transgenic B cells populated the B-1 B-cell compartment. Similarly, BCR selected from B-2 and MZ B cells gave rise to transgenic B cells of the same subset. These data more closely fit an induced-differentiation model in which the mature phenotype of the B-cell is a consequence of early antigen experience. In support of the induced-differentiation model, CD5 can be induced on B-2 B cells in vitro and B-1 B-cell development does appear to be dependent on efficient BCR signaling. Mutations in positive regulators of BCR signaling, such as CD19, BLNK, PI-3K, Vav, and Btk, result in decreased numbers of B-1 B cells (110,111,114). The converse is also true with an increase in B-1 B cells seen upon ablation of negative regulators of BCR signaling, such as CD22, Lyn, PD-1, and SHP-1 (110,111,114). In most of the latter models, there is an increase in B-1 B cells that express the phenotypic and functional attributes of B-1 B cells but lack CD5 (referred to as the B-1b B-cell subset).

The B-1 B-cell repertoire appears to be selected by self-antigen (115) and/or naturally occurring T-independent type 2 (TI-2) antigens with repetitive arrays of epitopes that can promote BCR cross-linking. Hayakawa et al. (116) demonstrated that B cells specific for a CD90-associated self-antigen only segregated and expanded into the B-1 compartment in the presence of that self-epitope. Nevertheless, it is still possible that the developmental status of the B-1 B-cell precursor predetermines the outcome of antigenic contact, such as up-regulation of CD5. If this is true, both hypotheses may still be correct and all B cells may not be created equal. This is a difficult question to address experimentally as the nature of the expressed BCR may itself influence the developmental programs available in the mature B cells.

Regardless of the controversy about their origins, B-1 B cells are clearly distinct in many ways from either MZ B cells or conventional B-2 B cells (110). Besides CD5 expression, low levels of sIgD, B220 (the B-cell isoform of CD45), CD21, CD23, and expression of CD11b, CD43, and high levels of sIgM distinguish the B-1 cells from their B-2 counterparts. Upon adoptive transfer in the absence of intentional immunization, the B-1 B cells are found to be the source of natural serum IgM antibodies and most of the IgG3. These IgM are polyreactive, weakly autoreactive and found to bind many common pathogen-associated carbohydrate antigens (110,111). These natural antibodies can be shown to play an important early role in the immune response to many bacteria and viruses but require complement fixation to influence antigen clearance. The B-1 B-cell compartment also gives rise to IgA plasma cells that are resident in the lamina propria and peyers patches of the gastrointestinal tract. The distribution of these cells may also relate to their antigen specificity, suggesting that their localization may best suit their ultimate function. While there are ~1% to 5% of B-1 B cells in the spleen and less than 1% in the peripheral lymph nodes, they comprise a substantial fraction of B cells among peritoneal exudate cells (PerC). Ansel et al. (117) recently demonstrated a critical role for the chemokine CXCL13 (B-lymphoid chemokine, BLC) in the development and localization of the B-1 B-cell compartment to the peritoneal and other body cavities (117).

Marginal Zone B Cells

MZ B cells are another distinct mature B-cell subset that segregate anatomically, and display unique cell-surface phenotype and immune response functions from their B-1 and B-2 B-cell counterparts. The splenic marginal zone is located at the juncture of white and red pulp and contains macrophage, dendritic cells, and MZ B cells. The MZ B-cell phenotype is closer to B-1 than B-2 B cells with low levels of B220 and high levels of sIgM. In contrast to B-1 B cells, MZ B cells do not express CD5 or CD11b and express high levels of the complement receptor CD21. The MZ B cells express higher basal and induced levels of B7-1 and B7-2. The specificity of the BCR impacts the propensity of B cells to develop into MZ B cells as discussed above (118). The generation of MZ B cells is markedly diminished in CD19-deficient mice, further supporting the notion of BCR-mediated subset selection in the periphery (118). Xid mice and Btk-deficient mice also have a decreased numbers of MZ B cells. In addition, MZ B cells fail to develop in Pyk-2 tyrosine kinase–deficient mice (119). Pyk is a PTK that regulates chemokine responsiveness,

which suggests that the defect in MZ B-cell development in the Pyk-deficient animals is due to impaired homing. The Pyk-deficient mice have severely diminished IgM and IgG3 responses to a TI-2 antigen, ficoll. MZ B cells also fail to develop in the absence of NF-γB p50 and Aiolos, a transcription factor of the Ikaros family that helps to regulate B-cell proliferation (120). While the assortment of B cells into distinctive cellular subsets and microenvironmental niches appears to be regulated by BCR specificity, it is not yet clear precisely how or why this discrimination occurs *in vivo*.

T-CELL–INDEPENDENT B-CELL RESPONSES

The initial antibody response to many infectious agents is largely based on the rapid T-cell–independent (TI) expansion of B cells and their subsequent differentiation into plasma cells. The B-1 and MZ B cells are largely responsible for these rapid TI humoral responses suggesting that some level of "natural memory" function resides in these B-cell subsets and may be predetermined in an evolutionarily conserved manner. T-cell–independent antigens can be separated into two broad categories, based on their ability to polyclonally activate B cells (TI-1) or require BCR recognition of multivalent epitope displays to induce B-cell differentiation in the absence of T-cell help (TI-2). TI-2 antigens can activate BCR signaling but require accessory signals to promote the development of antigen-specific plasma cells (regulation of TI-2 responses).

Type 1 T–Independent B-Cell Responses

Categorizing an antigen as TI-1 was originally based on the ability of the antigen to elicit an antibody response in immunocompromised mice with a defect in Btk function. This categorization indicated that some antigens stimulate B-cell clonal expansion regardless of effective BCR signal transduction. Many such polyclonal activators are compounds of bacterial cell walls, such as lipopolysaccharide (LPS); peptideoglycans (PGN);and lipoteichoic acid (LTA). A family of receptors with homology to the Toll receptor in Drosophila play an essential role in recognition of these pathogen-associated molecular patterns (PAMPs) (121,122). Mammalian Toll-like receptors (TLRs) are a family of highly conserved, germline-encoded transmembrane receptors that can directly activate the innate immune system and serve as a powerful mechanism to bridge the innate and adaptive immune responses (123,124). TLR expression on B cells allows for direct polyclonal activation. However, the more sensitive TLR-dependent responses of dendritic cells and macrophage and their ability to induce a plethora of accessory signals (125) still suggest a more indirect mechanism of activation for the B cells responding to these TI-1 polyclonal B-cell activators.

Type 2 T–Independent B-Cell Responses

The TI-2 antigens are typically repetitive polymers such as capsular polysaccharides in bacterial cell walls or the repetitive antigenic epitopes found in many viral particles. Studies using antigen coupled to polyacrylamide determined that a minimum of 12 to 16 haptens (small chemical antigens) per molecule are required to induce a strong TI-2 antibody response (126). The size of the epitope array indicates the aggregate BCR cluster required to initiate signal transduction at the cellular level. The backbone flexibility or the density of accessible epitope is also a factor in antigenicity. Even using a high ratio of hapten conjugated to protein molecules, the B-cell response still required T-cell help to induce antibody production. Dextran molecules have been used to conjugate anti-IgM and -IgD into potent TI-2 reagents that can stimulate phosphoinositde breakdown and intracellular Ca^{2+} responsiveness at much lower concentrations (many thousand-fold less) than the soluble antibody alone. Many TI-2 antigens can also fix complement and thereby co–cross-link the BCR complex and CD21/CD19 molecules. As discussed, involvement of CD19 in the BCR signaling cascade reduces the signaling threshold for activation of cellular responses.

While B-2 B cells can respond to TI stimuli *in vitro,* B-1 B cells and MZ B cells are the B-cell subsets predominantly recruited into TI-2 responses *in vivo* (114,127). IgA plasma cells in the gut are largely of B-1 B-cell origin and can be generated in the absence of T-cell help. Ochsenbein et al. (128) recently demonstrated that these IgA antibodies were specific for cell-wall antigens of commensal microorganisms. Furthermore, the generation of IgA plasma cells was induced by the presence of bacteria with specific binding not simply attributable to preexisting natural antibody. Thus, at the mucosal surfaces of the gut, a T-cell–independent mechanism of host defense is the preferred option for systemic immunity. The peritoneal cavity is enriched for B-1 B cells and intraperitoneal injection of TI-2 antigens is often cleared locally with little evidence of a response in the spleen. Alternatively, if the TI response is focused to the spleen using high doses of antigen or intravenous injection, both B-1 and MZ B cells are rapidly recruited (127). The MZ B cells are ideally located to sample blood-borne antigens and are rapidly drawn into the white pulp upon antigen exposure. Rapid clonal expansion of MZ and B-1 B cells is followed by the accumulation of plasma cells in the bridging channels and the red pulp of the spleen. Both B-1 and MZ B-cell clones can respond to the same TI challenges at levels commensurate with their respective precursor frequencies in the spleen prior to immunization (127). The ability to rapidly differentiate into plasma cells may be a direct consequence of the sensitivity to BCR-mediated signaling, the selection of distinct BCR repertoires and/or a developmental propensity to terminal differentiation in these specialized B-cell subsets.

Regulation of TI-2 B-Cell Responses

TI-2 antigens require accessory signals to drive B-cell proliferation and plasma cell differentiation. Many soluble antigens promote complement fixation and association with cells of the innate immune system. In this manner, the TI-2 antigens may be presented to B cells in the context of activated APCs producing a constellation of different accessory signals (128). The transmembrane activator and CAML interactor (TACI) is one candidate regulatory molecule in this process (128,129). TACI is a member of the tumor necrosis factor receptor (TNFR) family based on homology of its extracellular domain, and is expressed on mature B cells (130). TACI ligation can activate NF-κB, AP-1, and NF-AT transcription factors in mature B cells. Most pertinently, TACI-deficient mice display normal T-dependent B-cell responses, but responses to TI-2 antigens are completely abolished (131).

A ligand for TACI has been identified as the TNF homologue B lymphocyte stimulator (BlyS; also known as BAFF, TALL-1, THANK, or zTNF4) (132). BlyS is expressed on macrophage, monocytes, and dendritic cells, and is known to modulate B-cell development, survival, and activation. BlyS is most closely related to another TNF family member, a proliferation-inducing ligand, APRIL (133,134). Both BlyS and APRIL can bind to TACI and to another member of this family, BCMA (also constitutively expressed on mature B cells). Injection of BlyS or its continuous transgenic expression *in vivo* boosts the numbers of all mature B cells in the spleen, B-1, B-2, and MZ B cells, as well as the serum Ig levels. These animals also appear prone to autoimmune disease possibly through excess survival signals. Conversely, injection of soluble TACI-Ig blocks B-cell development at the transitional stage in the spleen, a phenotype similar to that in BlyS-deficient animals (135). Thus, TACI and BCMA expression on B cells appears to serve positively regulatory roles in the B-cell response to TI-2 antigens through their binding to BlyS and/or APRIL on antigen-presenting cells. The detailed itinerary of these overlapping sets of interactions is still a matter of great interest and importance to the regulation of TI-2 responses.

There are also molecular candidates for the negative regulation of TI-2 responses through the inhibition of BCR signaling events. These candidates include CD22, FcγRIIb, and CD5 (136,137). A more recent addition to this list is an ITIM-containing member of the Ig superfamily, PD-1. PD-1 is expressed on activated T and B cells; mice deficient for this molecule exhibit exaggerated IgG3 antibody responses to TI-2 antigens (138). The B cells from PD-1–deficient mice are also hyper-responsive to BCR stimulation *in vitro,* and the animals are prone to autoimmune disease. Co-ligation of PD-1 and BCR decreases tyrosine phosphorylation, Ca^{2+} responsiveness, and proliferation *in vitro.* Hence, this molecule may serve to counterbalance activating BCR-mediated signals presented by TI-2 antigens *in vivo.*

HELPER T-REGULATED B-CELL RESPONSES

While TI B-cell responses rapidly clear many infectious agents, the helper T-cell–regulated B-cell response produces affinity-matured B-cell immunity to most protein antigens. The T-dependent humoral response is the systemic outcome of a complex cascade of interdependent cellular and molecular interactions. The details of these events are presented across three broad phases of development that follow the initial exposure to antigen. Each phase of development relies on the successful cognate exchange of molecular information across intercellular immune synapses. Although these synaptic interactions have not been demonstrated *in vivo,* the terminology and conceptual framework help to focus our discussion of these still poorly understood molecular events.

Recruitment of Antigen-Specific T-Cell Help—Phase I

Phase I of this response begins with the initial local exposure to antigen and activation of the innate immune system (Fig. 5). Activated dendriditic cells (DC) as the most prominent antigen-presenting cells (APCs) for these responses migrate to the T zones of the draining LNs to recruit and activate naïve antigen-specific Th cells. Clonally expanded, antigen-activated, effector Th cells then migrate to the T/B borders

of secondary lymphoid organs and will regulate the development of antigen-primed B cells. The antigen-specific naïve B cells are recruited into the development pathway during this early phase of the response. Once activated, the B cells relocate to the T/B borders to increase the likelihood of cognate Th-cell contact. These naïve B cells recognize antigen and internalize, process, and present antigenic peptide/MHC on their cell surface in order to acquire cognate T-cell help.

Activation of Innate Immune System

Initial encounter with foreign protein antigen nonspecifically activates the uptake of antigen by the innate immune system (Fig. 5). Hence, adjuvants are used to aggravate the innate system at the site of antigen exposure. DC are the predominant APCs of the innate system involved in these early inflammatory responses. Immature DC reside in peripheral tissues and constitutively migrate to the draining LNs. These unactivated DC have no impact on naïve T cells, as they express only low

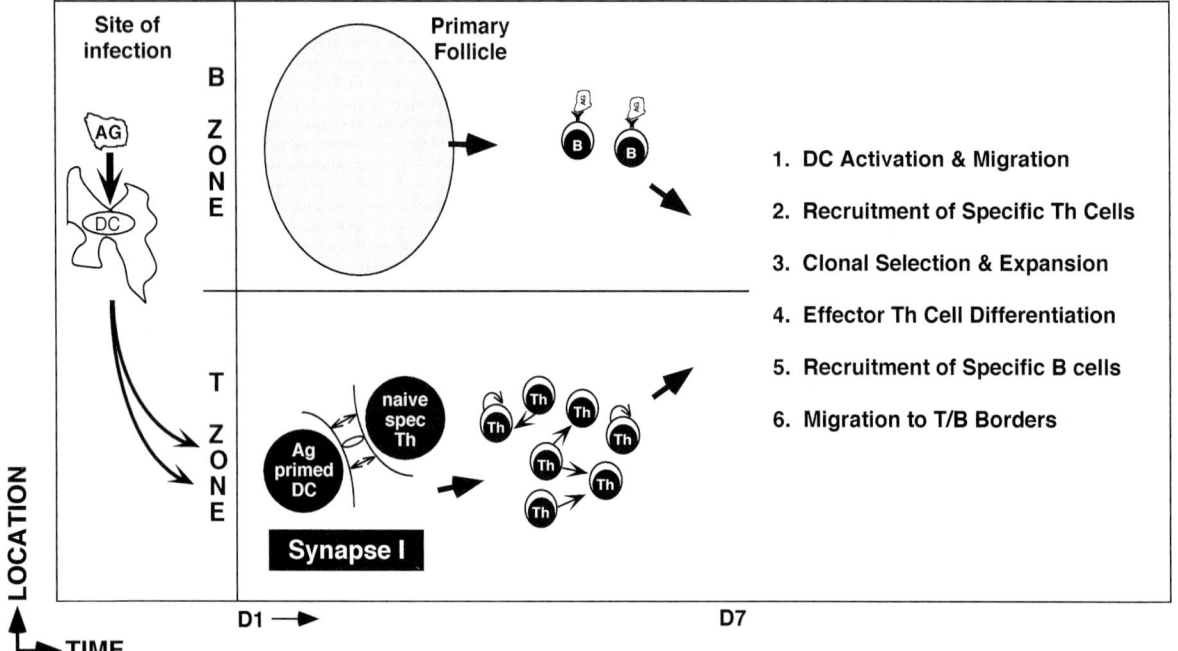

FIG. 5. Recruitment of antigen-specific T-cell help. Initial encounter with antigen (Ag) at the site if infection inflames local tissue and activates the resident dendritic cells (DC). Activated DC migrate to the T-cell zones of draining secondary lymphoid tissue. These DC up-regulate co-stimulatory molecules and process peptides from foreign proteins to present them in the context of MHC class II. In this manner, the activated DC remain in the T-cell zones to sample the naïve Th-cell compartment for those with TCR specific for the pMHC complex. Immune synapse I is formed between antigen-activated DC and naïve peptide-specific Th cells in the T-cell zones. Specific Th-cell clones with TCR of the best fit for pMHC are selected and preferentially expanded during this early phase of the adaptive immune response. Clonal expansion is followed by differentiation of effector Th cells that migrate toward the T-B borders of the lymphoid organs under the differential influence of chemokines and chemokine receptor expression. B cells can encounter antigen in soluble form and endocytose antigen and process and present peptides in a manner similar to DC. These antigen-activated B cells also migrate toward the T-B cell borders where they require cognate T-cell help to facilitate the development of the B-cell response to most protein antigens. The timescale is presented for the draining LN response to a model protein antigen such as pigeon cytochrome C (PCC) after base of tail injection in a nondepot adjuvant such as Ribi (an LPS derivative).

levels of co-stimulatory signals and little to no foreign peptide MHC (pMHC) complexes to initiate T-cell contact. In response to pathogens, DC produce bursts of inflammatory chemokines that recruit monocytes and promote their differentiation into DC under the influence of local cytokines such as type I interferons (IFN) (139). Activated DC up-regulate CCR7, a chemokine receptor that accelerates their migration to the T-cell zones in peripheral LNs (140) where CCR7-binding chemokines CCL19/ELC and CCL21/SLC are maintained at high concentration (141). Once in the T zones, these activated DC produce mainly CCR7 and CCR4 ligands to attract naïve Th cells and increase the ability to screen for TCR with the appropriate pMHC specificity.

There are multiple subsets of DC that mature along distinct pathways once activated in the periphery. Lymphoid DC are associated with thymic negative selection, but can be found in peripheral lymphoid tissue. In adaptive immunity, most attention is placed on the myeloid DC (MDC) and the plasmacytoid DC (PDC). MDC produce high levels of IL-12 under the influence of many bacteria and viruses. Freshly isolated PDC stimulated by virus produce high levels of type I IFNs and can prime T cells to produce IFN-γ and IL10 (142). DC mature differentially under the influence of inflammatory stimuli such as LPS, TNFα, IL-1, CD40L, and type I IFN. Recognition of PAMPs through differential expression of TLR2 (lipoprotein and PGN recognition), TLR4 (LPS responsiveness), and TLR9 (response to nonmethylated DNA) may also impact the balance of DC subset differentiation in response to infection. Finally, DC maturation involves up-regulation of co-stimulatory molecules CD80 (B7-1) and CD86 (B7-2) that serves to enhance first contact with antigen-specific naïve Th cells.

Immune Synapse I: Recruitment and Activation of Antigen-Specific T-Cell Help

Monks et al. (143) characterized the molecular organization of cognate interactions at the cellular interface between Th cells and antigen-presenting cells (APC) using high-resolution 3-D image analysis. Adhesion molecule interactions establish initial cell contact and then assort to the periphery of the supramolecular activation complex (pSMAC) that accumulates at the synaptic interface. TCR and pMHC interactions of sufficient strength concentrate to the center of this interface (cSMAC) together with signaling intermediates such as Zap70 and PKCθ. Grakoui et al. (144) and Bromley et al. (145) quantified the dynamics of formation for these immunological synapses using naïve T cells and labeled target proteins in lipid bilayers. In this system, TCR–pMHC interactions centralized at the membrane interface within 5 minutes of cell contact with the lipid bilayer. Some molecules, such as CD43, are excluded from the synapse, mainly due to the size of their extracellular domains. The actin cytoskeleton also plays a role in immune synapse formation by enabling the translocation of major co-stimulatory molecules to the cellular interface (146). As predicted from early bio-

chemical studies, the phosphorylated form of signaling intermediates are only transiently associated with the immune synapse, suggesting that sustained synapsis has a broader role to play in cellular differentiation (147). In support of this notion, stable intercellular synapsis for >2h was required for the progression of antigen-specific Th-cell differentiation.

Immune synapse formation can be considered one of the central checkpoints underlying the cognate regulation of developing immune responses in vivo. When activated DC first contact naïve antigen-specific Th cells in the T zones, the resultant immune synapse (synapse I) (Fig. 5) communicates the nature of the original antigenic insult to the adaptive immune system. Initial antigen-specific Th-cell development is heavily influenced by the DC expression pattern of cytokines (such as IL-12 and IL-6) and co-stimulatory molecules (such as CD80 and CD86) that reflect the initial inflammatory context of its activation. The strength and kinetics of the TCR–pMHC interaction can significantly impact Th-cell fate. Therefore, the available pre–immune TCR repertoire influences the outcome of this developing immune response. The antigen-primed Th cells can also deliver signals to the DC by way of cell contact (such as CD40L) and immediate early cytokine production such as TNF-α before dissociating the initial contact. Thus, immune synapsis encourages efficient local exchange of complex molecular information in an antigen-specific manner.

Clonal Selection, Expansion, and Effector Th-Cell Differentiation

Synapse I interactions result in extensive clonal expansion of the antigen-specific Th-cell compartment (Fig. 5). There are 100- to 500-fold increases in the numbers of antigen-responsive Th cells during the first week after initial antigen encounter (148). Selection for Th-cells with preferred TCR features can occur very rapidly between days 3 to 5 after priming. Early selection events are consolidated through preferential clonal expansion and appear to be driven by the kinetics of TCR–pMHC binding (149). Effector cell differentiation accompanies clonal expansion in the T zones (Fig. 5). Developmental programs initiated at synapse I are consolidated over this period of Th-cell expansion and differentiation. Autocrine and paracrine influences of cytokines may also play a major role in shaping the mix of Th-cell effector functions within the responsive population. Studies on cytokine production in vivo demonstrate a wide spectrum of effector Th-cell functions associated with the regulation of antigen-specific B-cell responses (150). Differential changes in cell-surface phenotype and alterations in T-cell physiology during this stage of development will impact the quality of T-cell help delivered to B cells. Over this first week after priming, clonally expanded effector Th cells migrate towards the T/B borders of the secondary lymphoid tissues. Ansel et al. (151) have demonstrated this to be due to the up-regulation of CXCR5 and response to CCL13/BLC in the B zones and a concomitant decrease in the response to the T-cell zone chemokines CCL19/ELC and CCL21/SLC. This combined pull-and-release mechanism allows the activated Th cells to enter the microenvironments in which they are most likely to encounter antigen-primed B cells (Fig. 5).

Recruitment and Activation of Naïve Antigen-Specific B Cells

To receive cognate T-cell help, antigen-specific B cells must have contacted their specific antigen, internalized, processed, and presented antigenic peptides in the context of MHC class II. The efficiency of antigen capture is a major determinant in the density of pMHC molecules presented on the cell surface. Early studies established that BCR-mediated processing is ~10^4-fold more sensitive that nonreceptor-mediated uptake through fluid pinocytosis. This is likely due to enhanced endocytosis as well as more efficient targeting to the intracellular class II peptide-loading compartment (152). Both antigen recognition and BCR signaling events appear to be involved as inhibitors of kinase activity block antigen processing. B cells do not efficiently present antigen that is in the form of immune complexes. Most likely, this leads to an aborted BCR signal in naïve B cells due to co-clustering of FcγRIIb and recruitment of SHP-1. Mutant sIgM that do not associate with the Igα/Igβ also lose much of their endocytic capacity and process antigen inefficiently. Addition of the cytoplasmic tail of Igβ is sufficient to restore normal processing in these cells. Further, BCR mutants containing a deletion in their cytoplasmic tail can constitutively associate with the lipid rafts but do not internalize antigen upon cross-linking (153). Hence, antigen recognition, BCR signaling, and endocytosis are required to accelerate appropriate antigen targeting, processing, and presentation of pMHC II (Fig. 5).

Antigen-activated B cells rapidly relocate to the T/B-cell interface of secondary lymphoid organs (Fig. 5). These earliest events in B-cell activation are difficult to access experimentally in normal nontransgenic animals due to the extremely low pre-immune precursor frequency for any known antigens. Adoptive transfer of BCR-transgenic B cells and TCR-transgenic Th cells has helped to overcome this limitation. Garside et al. (154) directly demonstrated these early B and Th-cell migration patterns and were able to visualize Th/B-cell conjugate formation that was antigen-specific. More recently, Reif et al. (155) demonstrated a chemokine-driven basis for the B-cell migration to these areas. B cells were shown to up-regulate the chemokine receptor CCR7 (specific for T-zone chemokines CCL19/ELC and CCL21/SLC) and this was sufficient to relocate activated B cells to the T/B borders. Curiously, the continued expression of CXCR5 (specific for B-zone chemokine CCL13/BLC) on the B cells seemed to create the right counterbalance for this migration event. Thus, at around days 5 to 7 after initial antigen priming, both the antigen-activated–effector Th cells and antigen-primed B cells are translocated to the same microenvironment to continue the regulation and development of the humoral immune response.

Delivery of T-Cell Help to Antigen-Primed B Cells—Phase II

The delivery of cognate T-cell help to the antigen-primed B cells requires the formation of Immune synapse II (Fig. 6). These interactions involve receptor-counter-receptor pairs of the TNFR and CD28/B7 families of molecules as well as the focal secretion of soluble factors that impact subsequent B-cell and Th-cell development. The cellular outcome for the B-cell bifurcates at this point with a GC pathway that proceeds in the B zone (discussed below) and a T-zone pathway that involves isotype switch recombination and the development of short-lived plasma cells.

Immune Synapse II

Immune synapse II forms between antigen-experienced and clonally expanded effector Th cells and antigen-primed B cells (Fig. 6). This intercellular contact is qualitatively and quantitatively distinct from the interaction between activated DC and naïve Th cells discussed in Phase I. While cytokines are sufficient to promote B-cell differentiation in bulk cell culture, it soon became apparent that inter-cellular contact is also a crucial factor that regulates B-cell fate in vivo. A signal through the pMHC expressed on these activated B cells could promote early biochemical changes, as well as cell cycle entry and plasma cell differentiation. However, the tumor necrosis family receptor (TNFR) family member, CD40, was one of the earliest co-stimulatory molecules identified as indispensable to effective Th-cell–regulated B-cell response (156). In the absence of this molecule, T-dependent immune responses generated IgM plasma cell formation without isotype switch recombination, germinal center formation, or affinity maturation (157). CD40 is constitutively expressed on B cells and its ligand, CD154 (CD40L), is expressed during the synapse I interactions of DC-induced Th-cell activation. At synapse II, there is an exchange of information through CD40–CD40L interactions with impact on both activated Th cells and antigen-primed B cells. In CD40-deficient animals, delivering a signal to the CD40L on the activated Th cells overcomes the defect in B-cell responsiveness (158,159). Hence, these specific molecular interactions significantly impact continued progression of lymphocyte development (Fig. 6).

Other TNF/TNFR family members play significant roles in shaping the fate of the B-cell response (160). OX40 (CD134) is expressed on activated Th cells, and its counter-receptor OX40-L (CD134L) is expressed on activated B cells. Mice deficient in CD134L have substantially reduced isotype switch recombination (161). Unlike the CD40-deficient animals, the CD134L-deficient mice can promote GC formation. Signals through CD134L on activated B cells can enhance the rate of IgG production in vitro by anti-CD40,

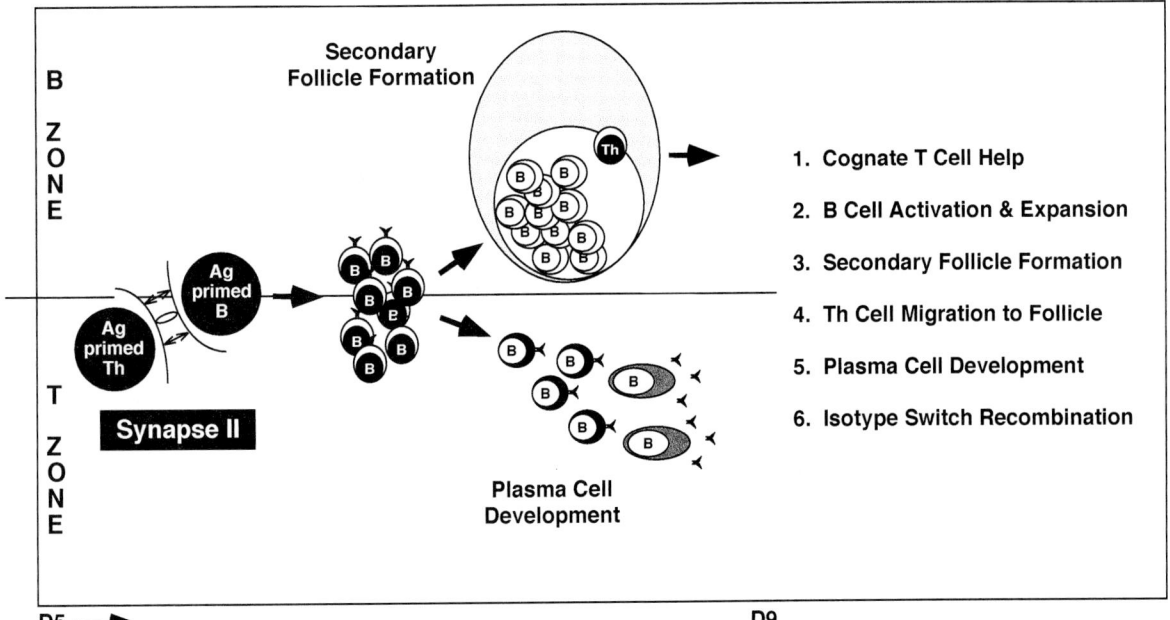

FIG. 6. Delivery of T-cell help to antigen-specific B cells. Immune synapse II forms between clonally expanded and differentiated antigen-specific Th cells and antigen-experienced B cells at the T-B cell borders of secondary lymphoid organs. The sets of co-receptor and co-stimulatory molecules potentially involved in this complex interaction are covered in detail in this chapter. The immediate impact of synapse II is rapid and substantial B-cell clonal expansion either within the B-cell zones or T-cell zones. The B-zone pathway leads to the formation of secondary follicles, the precursors of the germinal center reaction while the T-zone pathway involves the development of short-lived plasma cells and isotype switch recombination in the absence of somatic hypermutation. Some antigen-specific Th cells also remain in the T zones while the majority migrate to the secondary follicles to participate in the germinal center reaction.

IL-4, and IL-10–stimulated B cells suggesting a role in the regulation of antibody production distinct from CD40. Another TNFR family member, CD27, has been a useful marker of memory B cells in humans (162,163). The CD27 counter-receptor, CD70—a TNF family member expressed on T cells relatively late in activation—appears important in the regulation of plasma cell differentiation. CD27 is also expressed by many T cells and may serve to regulate the effect of CD70 on B cells as a decoy function. Two other sets of receptors in this family act as negative regulators of B-cell immunity. Signals through CD30 (TNFR family) or its ligand CD153 (TNF family) on activated B cells are reported to inhibit isotype switch and limit the extent of the B-cell response *in vivo* (164). However, the response to vesicular stomatitis virus in CD30-deficient animals appears to be normal and may suggest that there are redundant controlling mechanisms for the action of these molecules *in vivo* (165).

Finally, CD95 (Fas) (TNF family) and its ligand CD95L(TNFR family) have well-characterized effects on the B-cell response. Deficiencies in either member of this pair lead to marked lymphoproliferative defects together with autoimmune susceptibility. CD40 signals induce this molecule on activated B cells, increasing their susceptibility to apoptosis through CD95L expression on activated T cells (166). Thus, all these sets of molecules clearly have an

impact on the emerging B-cell response with substantial ability to regulate the quality of its outcome *in vivo*. However, the precise temporally and spatially defined events and how their molecular activities are distributed across antigen-specific–effector Th-cell and B-cell subsets remains to be thoroughly analyzed.

CD28 is another well-characterized T-cell co-stimulatory molecule primarily involved in sustained T-cell activation and appears critical for the initial DC-naïve Th interaction through the counter-receptors B7-1 (CD80) and B7-2 (CD86) (167). These counter-receptors are also up-regulated on antigen-primed B cells offering a means to increase stability of synapse II interactions or more directly enhance the TCR-pMHC interactions at this later stage of development *in vivo*. CTLA4 is another well-characterized member of this CD28/B7 family of molecules that has a dramatic impact on the decline of immune responses (168). In the absence of CTLA4, the animal develops a fatal lymphoproliferative disorder that is characterized by the presence of a huge number of infiltrating activated CD4 Th cells due to uncontrolled B7-1/B7-2 stimulation (169). Hence, a negative signal through CTLA4 appears important to reestablish homeostasis following antigen-driven clonal expansion.

Another more recently identified member of this CD28/B7 family is the inducible T-cell co-stimulator (ICOS)

(167,170). ICOS is homologous to CD28 with a distinct ligand-binding motif and cytoplasmic tail and no detectable B7-1 or B7-2 binding. ICOS is not expressed constitutively on Th cells but is rapidly up-regulated on TCR engagement. ICOS-L is expressed at low levels on resting B cells and is not strongly up-regulated upon activation with BCR or anti-CD40. Unlike CD28, interfering with ICOS/ICOS-L interactions with soluble ICOS-Ig has modest effects at the initiation of Th-cell responses *in vivo*, but appear to be more important in promoting sustained T-cell expansion. ICOS-deficient mice have clear defects in class switch recombination and cannot form GC to T-dependent antigen (171–173). CD40 stimulation can overcome these defects and suggest that ICOS interactions are upstream from CD40–CD40L interactions *in vivo*. These newly described sets of interactions clearly contribute to the ongoing development of effective B-cell immunity and display some level of temporal organization in a cascade of cellular activities and outcomes.

Isotype Switch Recombination

Antigen-specific B-cell development divides spatially and functionally at the end of immune synapse II (Fig. 6). One group of antigen-primed B cells clonally expands in the T zones and differentiates into short-lived plasma cells, while the second group returns to the B zones to initiate the GC reaction. Both pathways involve immunoglobulin class-switch recombination (CSR), while only the GC pathway undergoes somatic hypermutation and affinity-based maturation.

The switch of Ig isotype from IgM to IgG, IgE, or IgA is accompanied by CSR. CSR is regulated by Th-cell signals and is critical for the generation of functional diversity in the humoral immune response. CD40–CD154 (CD40L) are required for CSR, as the absence of these signals leads to elevated serum-IgM levels (hyperIgM syndrome) in the absence of IgG, IgE, and IgA (174). Soluble T-cell–derived factors are also implicated in this differentiation event. IL-4 drives the high-efficiency switch to IgG1 and IgE *in vitro* (175). However, IL-4–deficient animals display residual IgG1 production but absent IgE responses *in vivo* (176). TGF-β has been implicated in the regulation of IgA, while IFN-γ is thought to induce IgG2a switch and to counter-regulate the influence of IL-4.

CSR is an intrachromosonal deletional process between the switch (S) regions that reside 5' of each constant-region gene in B cells (except Cδ) (177). Signaling through CD40 and cytokine receptors induces germline transcription through the targeted S regions. The Sμ region and the targeted S region is then cleaved by a putative DNA-cleaving enzyme. The activation-induced deaminase (AID), a putative RNA-editing cytidine deaminase, is required and sufficient for the initiation of the CSR reaction in the activated locus (178); however, it is not yet clear if it does the cleaving or regulates the cleaving activity of a separate complex. AID-deficient animals (179) and humans (180) display no CSR or somatic hypermutation of the Ig genes. Repair and ligation through nonhomologous end joining completes the process and results in the looping-out and replacement of the Cμ heavy-chain constant-region gene (C$_H$) with other downstream C$_H$ genes. While isotype switch proceeds without somatic hypermutation in the T-zone pathway, the process within the GC reaction is thought to use the same molecular machinery.

Development of Short-lived Plasma Cells

The T-zone pathway to plasma cell differentiation induces the rapid production of germline-encoded antigen-specific antibody (Fig. 6). Within the first 3 to 5 days of a T-dependent response, small foci of B-cell blasts can be seen in the T zones (181). They expand and differentiate into plasma cells of multiple Ig isotypes that migrate via the bridging channel in the splenic marginal zones and lodge in the red pulp, and are found in the lymphatic sinus of the medullary cords in LN responses (182). In contrast to their GC counterparts, these T-zone B cells do not diversify their Ig receptors, and once differentiated into plasma cells, have short half-lives of 3 to 5 days. Plasma cells are terminally differentiated, post-mitotic, antibody-producing factories. They display a marked increase in IgH and IgL mRNA and prominent amounts of rough ER to accommodate translation and secretion of abundant Ig. They have reduced or lost numerous cell-surface molecules, including MHC II, B220, CD19, CD21, and CD22, with an increase in the proteoglycan syndecan-1 (CD138), often used as a distinguishing marker for plasma cells. Plasma cells decrease the expression of CXCR5 and CCR7, and up-regulate responsiveness to CXCL12/SDF-1, the CXCR4 ligand that is localized more to the red pulp and medullary cords (183).

Several transcription factors are also decreased or absent in plasma cells including B-cell lineage-specific activator (BSAP), the Pax-5 gene product and the class II transactivator (CIITA). Early B-cell factor (EBF), A-Myb, and BCL-6 that are also associated with B-cell development are down-regulated in plasma cells. In contrast, some transcription factors increase upon terminal differentiation. B-lymphocyte-induced maturation protein 1 (BLIMP-1) is induced upon cytokine-induced, plasma-cell differentiation of a murine B-cell lymphoma BCL-1 *in vitro* (184). This zinc-finger–containing transcriptional repressor has three identified targets. The repression of c-Myc may provide a mechanism for the cessation of cell cycle. The repression of CIITA may explain the decrease of MHC II expression and inability to receive further cognate T-cell signals, and Pax-5 repression may be required to release its control of XBP-1 transcription (185). While XBP-1–deficient mice are embryonic lethal, using the RAG complementation system, XBP-1–deficient B cells could develop normally *in vivo*, but were severely blocked in their ability to differentiate into plasma cells (186). XBP-1 is induced upon activation in splenic B cells and remains at high concentrations in plasma cells. IRF4 is another transcription factor up-regulated in plasma cells and IRF4-deficient animals cannot mount antibody responses

(187). Calame (185) proposes a complex regulatory cascade in antigen-activated B cells that integrates the action of XBP-1, BLIMP-1, and IRF4 to induce terminal differentiation and plasma cell commitment.

The Germinal Center Reaction—Phase III

The second broad cellular outcome of synapse II interactions is the GC reaction (Fig. 7). Antigen-primed B cells migrate to the B-zone follicular area after the delivery of cognate T-cell help and rapidly expand as sIgD⁻ B220⁺ B cells. This massive and rapid clonal expansion displaces mature resting B cells, creating regions within the B-cell follicular area now referred to as secondary follicles. At some point, the secondary follicle polarizes into the "dark zone" region of rapidly proliferating sIgM/D⁻ cells proximal to the T-cell areas, and a "light zone" region of nondividing cells that

express downstream sIg at the opposite pole (Fig. 7). The polarization of the secondary follicle signifies the beginning of the germinal center reaction. The dividing cells are referred to as centroblasts and the nondividing cells are centrocytes. Multiple specialized cell types participate in the GC reaction, giving rise to a cycle of activity that is focused on the development of high-affinity B-cell memory. Recruitment into the GC cycle involves massive clonal expansion and the random somatic diversification of the BCR. GC B cells expressing high-affinity variants are then selected for either re-entry into the GC cycle or export into the long-lived memory B-cell compartment.

Formation of Germinal Center Microenvironment

The formation of the GC reaction is generally thought to require T-cell help, as it is absent in athymic nude mice,

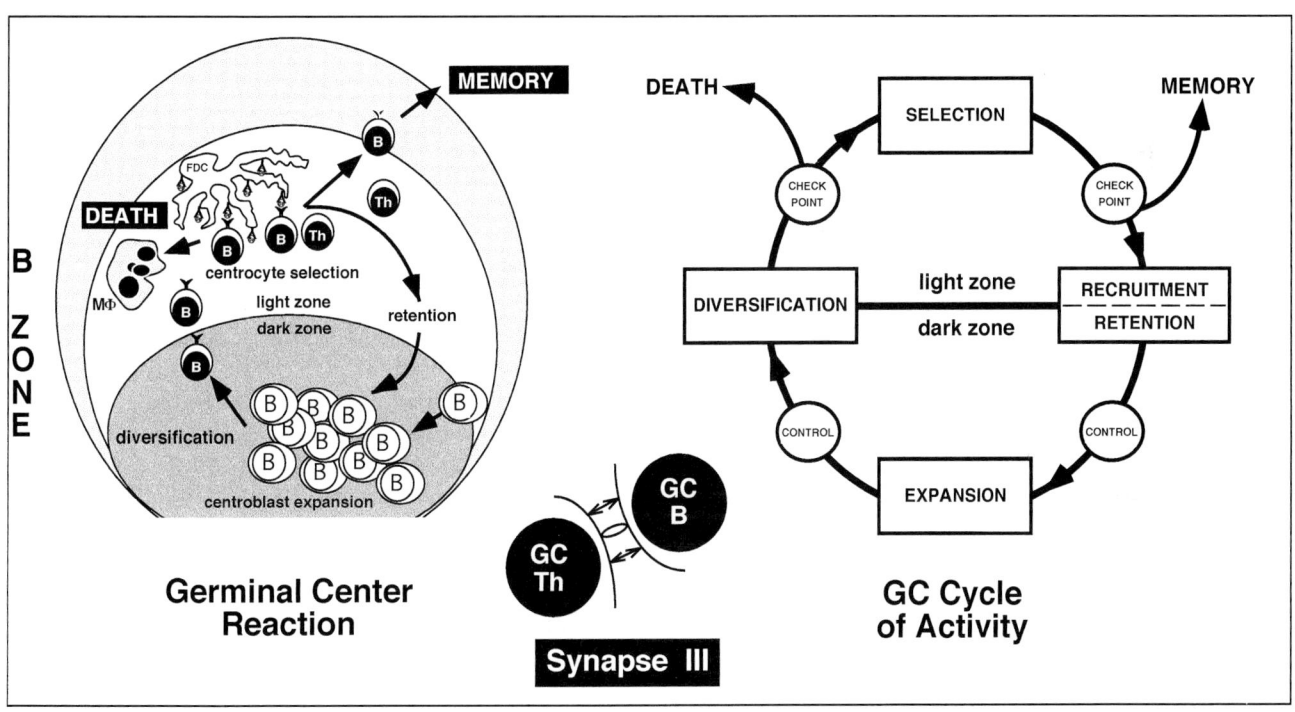

FIG. 7. Phase III: the germinal center reaction. Cells involved in the GC reaction and their location in the germinal center **(left),** and cycle of activity that accompanies these cellular events *in vivo* **(right).** The GC reaction officially begins when the secondary follicle polarizes into the dark zone of proliferating centroblasts and the light zone of centrocytes that have dropped out of the cell cycle and express variant Ig receptors. Antigen-specific B cells are initially recruitment into the GC pathway followed by massive clonal expansion and BCR diversification via somatic hypermutation. Cells expressing variant BCR then exit the cell cycle and migrate to light zones that are filled with follicular dendritic cells (FDC) displaying copious immune-complexed antigen and occasional antigen-specific Th cells. The majority of centrocytes die locally by apoptosis and are cleared rapidly by tingible body macrophage (Mφ). Some centrocytes with high-affinity variant BCR are selected to either re-enter the GC cycle of expansion, diversification, and selection or exit the GC reaction to enter the long-lived memory B-cell pool. This cell fate decision appears dependent on the quality of the BCR–antigen interaction and the nature of T-cell help delivered in a cognate manner by the resident antigen-specific GC Th cells (immune synapse III). The memory B-cell compartment exists in at least two major cellular fractions, the long-lived affinity-matured plasma cells and the affinity-matured memory-response precursors that are primed to respond rapidly to secondary antigen challenge.

CD40- and CD154 (CD40L)-deficient animals, and is diminished using reagents that block or deplete Th-cell function, such as anti-CD4, anti-CD40, and anti-CD28 (188–190). However, some T-independent antigens do induce a GC response and they can arise in T-deficient animals. In the latter case, the GC reaction appears with truncated kinetics and does not support somatic hypermutation (191). Using T-dependent antigens such as hapten–protein conjugates, there is evidence for the initiation of GC by 5 to 7 days after priming. Each GC develops as a discrete entity imposing the cycles of diversification and then selection upon an oligoclonal set of antigen-specific B cells. There is some evidence for secondary selection of the subset of antigen-specific B cells that enter the GC reaction compared with those in the T-zone pathway; however, these issues have not yet been carefully addressed. Upon committing to the GC pathway, clonal expansion that forms the secondary follicle proceeds with a B-cell doubling time of about 6 to 8 hours. This rapid doubling time continues in the GC dark zone over the course of the primary response GC reaction (~21 days) (182).

Somatic Hypermutation and BCR Diversification

Clonal expansion in the GC is associated with somatic diversification of the Ig receptor by a hypermutator mechanism (Fig. 7). Somatic hypermutation underpins affinity maturation in the B-cell compartment; however, the molecular mechanism that drives this process remains largely unresolved.

The B cells recruited into the GC reaction have already been selected based on the germline specificity of their rearranged V-region genes (Fig. 7). Upon expansion in the GC reaction, the B cells down-regulate this germline sIg and somatically diversify their variable-region genes. Single base substitutions, rare insertions, and deletions are introduced into a region spanning 1.5 to 2.0 kb downstream of the transcription initiation site (192). Activity peaks within the V(D)J region and decreases within the J-C intronic region of IgH and IgL V genes. The mutation rate approaches 10^{-3} per base pair per generation at six orders of magnitude higher than spontaneous mutation frequencies. Approximately one mutation is introduced with each cell division. Analysis of mutation in "passenger" Ig transgenes that are not under selection pressure indicates intrinsic sequence hot spots for the mutator mechanism (193). These analyses identify a motif referred to as RGYW (where R = A or G; Y = C or T; W = A or T), with AGC/T triplets for serine identified as preferred targets. Transitions are more frequent than transversions and A nucleotides in the coding strand are replaced more frequently than T nucleotides (referred to as strand bias). However, it is clear that mutation does not rely on the sequence of the target genes, but does require transcription of the target locus.

Double stranded DNA breaks (DSB) have been identified in the V(D)J regions of mutating B cells (194). Most of these DSB also occur preferentially at RGYW motifs and most often 5′ of the G and R residues. These DSB may represent the reaction intermediates of the hypermutation mechanism or entry points for an endonuclease to cleave DNA strands and initiate hypermutation. Mutations could be introduced into these lesions as mismatched nucleotides by an error-prone DNA polymerase during the repair process. Zan et al. (195) demonstrate a role for polymerase ζ (POLZ) in a human B-cell line that can hypermutate in vitro. POLZ effectively extends DNA past mismatch base insertions and is up-regulated in this B-cell line upon BCR engagement in the presence of T-cell help. Blocking its action impaired hypermutation frequency. Polymerase η (POLH) is also highly error prone, and while humans with defective enzyme appear to have normal frequency of hypermutation in their B cells, the pattern of mutation is significantly altered to less A/T and more G/C mutations (196). This suggests that multiple error-prone POLs may be involved in B cells. Polymerase ι (POLI) and μ (POLM) are two other highly error-prone polymerases that may play a role in hypermutation. However, after the introduction of mutations, there must be some means to subvert the mismatch repair mechanisms present in all cells. Curiously, mice deficient in nucleotide excision repair, mismatch repair, and base excision repair displayed normal levels of hypermutation, albeit with some differences in the overall patterns (197).

A most remarkable finding in this field by Muramatsu et al. (198) is a role for the activation-induced cytidine deaminase (AID) as a central component for both somatic hypermutation and CSR. Originally discovered through cDNA subtraction focused on novel genes in GC B cells (198), it was then found to be the defect associated with an autosomal recessive form of hyper-IgM syndrome (180). Mice deficient in AID were able to form the GC reaction but were unable to undergo CSR or somatic hypermutation (179). AID may function as a catalytic subunit of an RNA-editing enzyme complex as other members of this deaminase family and as such it may edit the RNA of a putative hypermutator and exert an indirect effect. Alternatively, it may function more directly as the enzyme that introduces nicks or single nucleotide gaps, as it can also deaminate deoxycytosines to uracil. If these lesions are not effectively repaired they have an increased spontaneous mutation rate causing G/C to A/T transitions. Although the precise role AID plays in hypermuation has yet to be resolved; it is clearly an early intermediate in two critical aspects of antigen-driven B-cell development—somatic hypermutation and CSR.

Antigen-Driven Selection and GC Th Cells—Immune Synapse III

Centroblast expansion and receptor diversification introduce different point mutations into the V-region genes of clonal progeny. GC microdissection, PCR amplification, and V-region sequence analysis directly identifies these clonally related genealogies in vivo (199,200). Noncycling centrocytes express the variant receptors and move into the light zones of the GC, a region rich in follicular dendritic cells (FDC) and scattered antigen-specific GC Th cells. FDC are nonphago-cytic stromal cells that are involved in the organization of primary follicles. These cells have been implicated in antigen-based GC selection events due to expression of FcγR and complement receptor-1 (CR-1) influencing their ability to trap native antigen as immune complexes. In contrast, animals lacking complement receptors, C3, or treatment with anti-CR1/2 displayed diminished or absent GCs and slower maturation of the humoral response (201). Using a BCR transgenic mouse model with B cells expressing only membrane-bound antibody that were unable to secrete (and thereby unable to form immune complexes; IC), Hannum et al. (202) demonstrated normal GC formation and affinity maturation. These data argue against the requirement for IC in GC selection events.

Antigen-specific Th cells are also enriched in the GC environment of an ongoing immune response (Fig. 7). These GC Th cells express low to negative levels of CD90 (Thy 1), unlike their non-GC counterparts, and are very sensitive to apoptosis induction via CD3 signaling (203). Anti-CD154 (CD40L) or anti-B7-2 antibody can disrupt ongoing GC reactions, presumably by interfering with cognate GC Th-cell–GC B-cell interactions. As the surface phenotype of the GC Th cells and the GC B cells are substantially different from their T-zone counterparts, it is reasonable to consider this distinct cognate cellular interchange as immune synapse III. The specialized function of the GC Th cells is not yet well understood, but these GC Th-B interactions serve to propagate B-cell memory and may help to interpret secondary antigen-selection events.

Most mutational events in the BCR are deleterious to antigen binding and result in loss of the variants by apoptosis in the GC reaction. In support of this idea, overexpression of anti-apoptotic molecules, Bcl-2 or Bcl-xL, results in the accumulation of low-affinity and/or autoreactive B cells as either long-lived plasma cells or memory B cells (204,205). CD95 (Fas) is also expressed in GC B cells and these cells are highly susceptible to CD95L-induced apoptosis. Mice with defective CD95 function (lpr mutation) display a lymphoproliferative disorder with accumulation of autoreactive B cells. There is evidence for an impact on clonal selection in the GC and subsequent entry into the memory B-cell compartment of these animals. GC B cells appear poised to undergo apoptosis expressing high levels of CD95, c-Myc, P^{53}, and Bax and low levels of bcl-2. Studies using human tonsillar GC B cells indicate preformed death-inducing signaling complex (DISC) that are held inactivated by c-FLIP (206). The c-FLIP is rapidly down-regulated *in vitro* in the absence of stimuli and can be prevented by CD40 ligation. Most studies support the susceptibility of GC B cells to apoptosis unless rescued by antigen and the appropriate T-cell help.

The B-Cell Memory Response—Phase IV

Exit from the GC reaction is one consequence of positive selection based on the increased affinity for antigen (Fig. 7).

These post–GC B cells exist long term as multiple cellular subsets that form the memory B-cell compartment. Stable maintenance of B-cell memory requires cell longevity that does not appear to need the continued expression of the affinity-matured BCR. These data argue that a continued antigen depot is not needed for memory B-cell survival. Finally, accelerated cellular expansion and rapid differentiation to high-affinity plasma cells is the hallmark of the memory B-cell response to antigen recall. This rapid cellular response is regulated by antigen-specific memory Th cells and constitutes Phase IV of the B-cell response that is controlled by the formation of immune synapse IV between memory Th cells and antigen-activated memory B cells (Fig. 8).

Memory B-Cell Subsets

Post–GC B cells can be considered to persist in two broad categories: long-lived plasma cells and memory response precursors. These long-lived plasma cells display evidence for somatic hypermutation, produce isotype-switched, high-affinity antibody, and preferentially home to the bone marrow with greatly extended half-lives compared to their T-zone/red-pulp plasma cell counterparts (207). Long-lived plasma cells do not appear to self-replenish but can survive in the absence of transferred antigen with half-lives ~140 days as estimated by Slifka et al. (208). Animals deficient in CXCR4 expression have increased antigen-specific plasma cells in the peripheral blood but a reduced cell number in the bone marrow. Plasma cells express high levels of the integrin α4β1, and animals deficient in its ligand VCAM1 are depleted of mature recirculating B cells in the bone marrow and display decreased T-dependent B-cell responses (209). Interestingly, CD22-deficient mice also have a decreased number of recirculating B cells in the bone marrow, and injecting normal mice with a soluble CD22-Fc to block interactions of CD22 with its ligands (α2,6-linked sialic acids on glycans) decreases the numbers of plasma cells in the bone marrow (210). Hence, there may be multiple mechanisms for regulating plasma-cell homing to the bone marrow that may represent signals for both homing and long-term survival in this specialized microenvironment.

Memory response precursors can be broadly defined as a residual population of antigen-experienced B cells that are not actively secreting antibody. Antigen experience preprograms these memory B cells to respond rapidly to secondary encounters with antigen under the regulation of memory Th cells. Accelerated clonal expansion and exaggerated plasma cell differentiation are the cardinal cellular characteristics of a memory response. Invariably, memory B cells will express isotype-switched and mutated BCR with evidence for affinity-based selection (211). Martin and Goodnow (212) recently demonstrated that the cytoplasmic tail of IgG was sufficient to increase the clonal burst potential of naïve B cells upon primary encounter with antigen. These data indicate one mechanism for quantitatively altering the memory B-cell response to antigen.

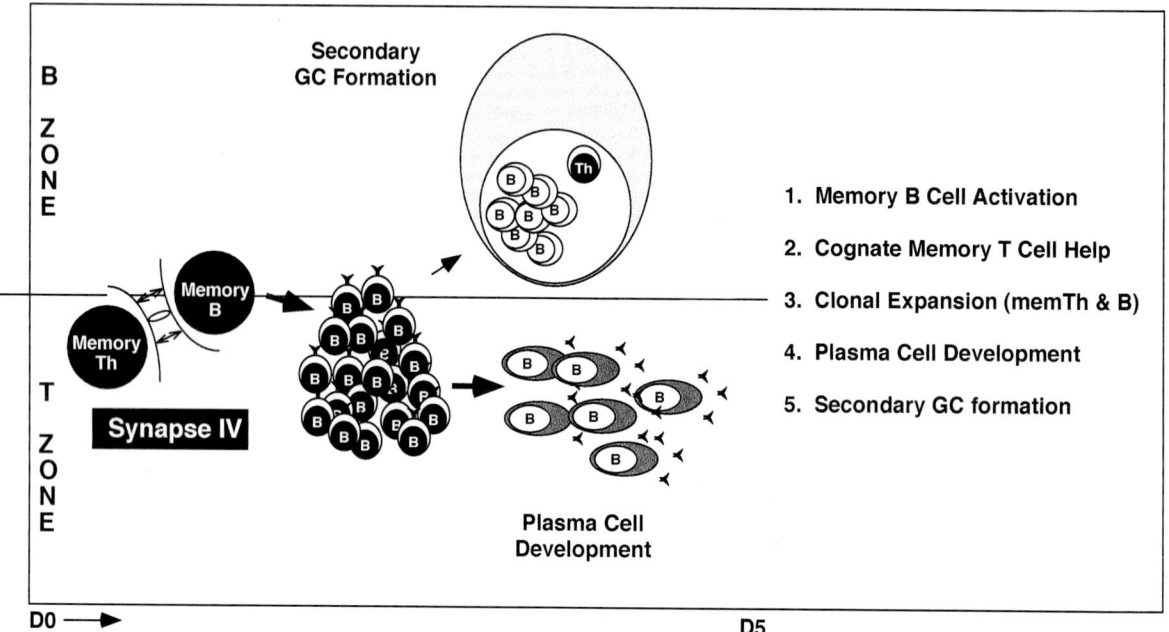

FIG. 8. Phase IV: memory response to antigen re-challenge. Memory B-cell responses to T-dependent antigens also require T-cell help. It is thought that the memory B cell acts as the main APC in these memory responses. Hence, immune synapse IV can be thought to occur between antigen-activated memory B cells and memory Th cells and most likely occurs in the T-cell zones of secondary lymphoid tissue. Massive and rapid clonal expansion ensues in both the memory B-cell and memory Th-cell compartments with substantial plasma cell production evident in the T zones of these organs. These plasma cells appear short-lived and secrete the affinity-matured range of BCR expressed by their memory cell precursors. There is also evidence of secondary-response germinal centers that may be seeded by memory response precursors or naïve B cells with a different spectrum of BCR.

Our group has recently identified multiple subsets of antigen-specific memory-response precursors based on the expression of cell-surface phenotype (mainly the expression of particular CD45 glycoform seen by mAb 6B2). The two main subsets (6B2$^+$ and 6B2$^-$) differ in localization (peripheral lymphoid tissue versus bone marrow, respectively), and proliferative and differentiative capacity upon adoptive transfer and antigen re-exposure (213,214). The cell-surface phenotype of these two main memory B-cell subsets also suggests they have overtly differing responses to BCR triggering with differences in co-receptor and complement-receptor expression (6B2$^+$CD19$^+$CD21$^+$CD22$^+$; 6B2$^-$CD19$^-$CD21$^+$CD11b$^+$CD22$^-$). Linton et al. (215) have identified multiple potentials for antigen responsiveness in the pre-immune compartment. They demonstrate subsets of naïve B cells that have a greater propensity to produce antibody-secreting cells (CD24 high) and others more likely to form memory-response precursors (CD24low). While the understanding of B-cell memory is still rudimentary, it is clear that its heterogeneous cellular organization indicates complex molecular regulation for both survival and response to recall.

Memory B-Cell Maintenance

The longevity of memory B cells appears independent of antigen. Initial transfer analyses by Gray and Skarvall (216)

suggested a constant source of antigen was required for long-term memory B-cell survival. Maruyama et al. (217) recently addressed this question in an elegant Cre-LoxP–mediated genetic manipulation of an animal model. Animals were engineered to express two Ig heavy-chain alleles with expected specificity to two separate antigens (the hapten, NP, and the protein phycoerythrin, PE with the heavy chain in the opposite orientation) and then immunized to NP. Once NP-specific memory B cells were produced after immunization, the BCR heavy chain was switched by Cre-mediated recombination to lose the NP specificity and express the PE heavy chain. These BCR-switched memory B cells survived for 15 weeks in the absence of any exposure to PE, thus indicating no requirement for specific antigen. The PE-specific response had been used previously by the same group to demonstrate that memory B cells survived for extended periods with very low cell turnover.

The Response to Antigen Recall—Immune Synapse IV

The role of memory Th cells in the regulation of memory B-cell responses has not been clearly addressed to date. Abrogation of CD4 Th cells using ablative anti-CD4 treatment clearly decreases subsequent memory B-cell responses *in vivo*. It is also apparent that all memory Th cells do not express similar functions, at least with respect to cytokine secretion

(150). The APC for the memory B-cell response are most likely antigen-specific memory B cells. These cells have high-affinity receptors for antigen, and memory responses can be triggered with very low doses of antigen in the absence of any adjuvant. In a similar manner to the APC impact on naïve Th cells in the primary response, the quality of the initial memory B-cell response to antigen recall could significantly impact the differentiation of memory T-cell help. Hence, the nature of cognate help in the induction of memory B-cell responses may again be qualitatively and quantitatively distinct from any previous synaptic interaction and can be considered immune synapse IV (Fig. 8). Synapse IV interactions will still be antigen specific and require pMHC expression by the memory B cells. However, the constellation of co-stimulatory/co-receptor molecules involved in this specialized molecular exchange has yet to be carefully investigated.

In summary, B-cell activation *in vivo* takes on multiple forms that depend on the nature of the antigen and the developmental program of the B cell recruited to respond. Some subsets of B cells appear to be specialized to respond to T-independent forms of antigen in a manner that suggests the presence of a natural, evolutionarily conserved B-cell memory. In contrast, the response to most protein antigens requires the activation of the innate immune system and the recruitment of antigen-specific Th cells. These T-dependent B-cell responses develop as elaborate cellular cascades of interdependent activity, critically regulated over time and spatially organized within specialized microenvironments. Cognate interactions of intercellular information exchange act as the key checkpoints to this complex process. The primary response can be divided into three broad phases of cellular development culminating in the development of high-affinity B-cell memory as the cellular product of the germinal center reaction. Long-term protection is served through the ability of these memory B cells to respond very rapidly to subclinical re-challenge with antigen under the regulation of memory Th cells and the heightened reactivity of this adaptive arm of the immune system.

REFERENCES

1. Reth M, Wienands J. Initiation and processing of signals from the B cell antigen receptor. *Annu Rev Immunol* 1997;15:453–479.
2. DeFranco AL. The complexity of signaling pathways activated by the BCR. *Curr Opin Immunol* 1997;9:296–308.
3. Kurosaki T. Genetic analysis of B cell antigen receptor signaling. *Annu Rev Immunol* 1999;17:555–592.
4. Shaw AC, Mitchell RN, Weaver YK, et al. Mutations of immunoglobulin transmembrane and cytoplasmic domains: effects on intracellular signaling and antigen presentation. *Cell* 1990;63:381–392.
5. Schamel WW, Reth M. Monomeric and oligomeric complexes of the B cell antigen receptor. *Immunity* 2000;13:5–14.
6. Campbell KS, Hager EJ, Cambier JC. Alpha-chains of IgM and IgD antigen receptor complexes are differentially N-glycosylated MB-1–related molecules. *J Immunol* 1991;147:1575–1580.
7. Venkitaraman AR, Williams GT, Dariavach P, et al. The B-cell antigen receptor of the five immunoglobulin classes. *Nature* 1991;352:777–781.
8. Reth M. Antigen receptor tail clue. *Nature* 1989;338:383–384.
9. Sanchez M, Misulovin Z, Burkhardt AL, et al. Signal transduction by immunoglobulin is mediated through Ig alpha and Ig beta. *J Exp Med* 1993;178:1049–1055.
10. Matsuuchi L, Gold MR. New views of BCR structure and organization. *Curr Opin Immunol* 2001;13:270–277.
11. Lam KP, Kuhn R, Rajewsky K. In vivo ablation of surface immunoglobulin on mature B cells by inducible gene targeting results in rapid cell death. *Cell* 1997;90:1073–1083.
12. Simons K, Toomre D. Lipid rafts and signal transduction. *Nat Rev Mol Cell Biol* 2000;1:31–39.
13. Pierce SK. Lipid rafts and B-cell activation. *Nature Rev Immunol* 2002;2:96–105.
14. Simons K, Ikonen E. Functional rafts in cell membranes. *Nature* 1997;387:569–572.
15. Zhang W, Trible RP, Samelson LE. LAT palmitoylation: its essential role in membrane microdomain targeting and tyrosine phosphorylation during T cell activation. *Immunity* 1998;9:239–246.
16. Guo B, Kato RM, Garcia-Lloret M, et al. Engagement of the human pre–B cell receptor generates a lipid raft- dependent calcium signaling complex. *Immunity* 2000;13:243–253.
17. Weintraub BC, Jun JE, Bishop AC, et al. Entry of B cell receptor into signaling domains is inhibited in tolerant B cells. *J Exp Med* 2000;191:1443–1448.
18. Bray D, Levin MD, Morton-Firth CJ. Receptor clustering as a cellular mechanism to control sensitivity. *Nature* 1998;393:85–88.
19. Gold MR, Matsuuchi L, Kelly RB, et al. Tyrosine phosphorylation of components of the B-cell antigen receptors following receptor crosslinking. *Proc Natl Acad Sci U S A* 1991;88:3436–3440.
20. Cherukuri A, Dykstra M, Pierce SK. Floating the raft hypothesis: lipid rafts play a role in immune cell activation. *Immunity* 2001;14:657–660.
21. Field KA, Holowka D, Baird B. Structural aspects of the association of FcepsilonRI with detergent-resistant membranes. *J Biol Chem* 1999;274:1753–1758.
22. Friedrichson T, Kurzchalia TV. Microdomains of GPI-anchored proteins in living cells revealed by crosslinking. *Nature* 1998;394:802–805.
23. Xavier R, Brennan T, Li Q, et al. Membrane compartmentation is required for efficient T cell activation. *Immunity* 1998;8:723–732.
24. Kabouridis PS, Janzen J, Magee AL, et al. Cholesterol depletion disrupts lipid rafts and modulates the activity of multiple signaling pathways in T lymphocytes. *Eur J Immunol* 2000;30:954–963.
25. Campbell MA, Sefton BM. Protein tyrosine phosphorylation is induced in murine B lymphocytes in response to stimulation with anti-immunoglobulin. *EMBO J* 1990;9:2125–2131.
26. Carter RH, Park DJ, Rhee SG, et al. Tyrosine phosphorylation of phospholipase C induced by membrane immunoglobulin in B lymphocytes. *Proc Natl Acad Sci U S A* 1991;88:2745–2749.
27. Flaswinkel H, Reth M. Dual role of the tyrosine activation motif of the Ig-alpha protein during signal transduction via the B cell antigen receptor. *EMBO J* 1994;13:83–89.
28. Wang J, Koizumi T, Watanabe T. Altered antigen receptor signaling and impaired Fas-mediated apoptosis of B cells in Lyn-deficient mice. *J Exp Med* 1996;184:831–838.
29. Chen T, Repetto B, Chizzonite R, et al. Interaction of phosphorylated FcepsilonRIgamma immunoglobulin receptor tyrosine activation motif-based peptides with dual and single SH2 domains of p72syk. Assessment of binding parameters and real time binding kinetics. *J Biol Chem* 1996;271:25308–25315.
30. Kimura T, Sakamoto H, Appella E, et al. Conformational changes induced in the protein tyrosine kinase p72syk by tyrosine phosphorylation or by binding of phosphorylated immunoreceptor tyrosine-based activation motif peptides. *Mol Cell Biol* 1996;16:1471–1478.
31. Kurosaki T, Johnson SA, Pao L, et al. Role of the Syk autophosphorylation site and SH2 domains in B cell antigen receptor signaling. *J Exp Med* 1995;182:1815–1823.
32. Weiss A, Littman DR. Signal transduction by lymphocyte antigen receptors. *Cell* 1994;76:263–274.
33. Turner M, Mee PJ, Costello PS, et al. Perinatal lethality and blocked B-cell development in mice lacking the tyrosine kinase Syk. *Nature* 1995;378:298–302.
34. Kurosaki T, Tsukada S. BLNK: connecting Syk and Btk to calcium signals. *Immunity* 2000;12:1–5.
35. Leo A, Schraven B. Adapters in lymphocyte signalling. *Curr Opin Immunol* 2001;13:307–316.

36. Ishiai M, Kurosaki M, Pappu R, et al. BLNK required for coupling Syk to PLC gamma 2 and Rac1-JNK in B cells. *Immunity* 1999;10:117–125.

37. Xu S, Tan JE, Wong EP, et al. B cell development and activation defects resulting in xid-like immunodeficiency in BLNK/SLP-65–deficient mice. *Int Immunol* 2000;12:397–404.

38. Takata M, Sabe H, Hata A, et al. Tyrosine kinases Lyn and Syk regulate B cell receptor-coupled Ca^{2+} mobilization through distinct pathways. *EMBO J* 1994;13:1341–1349.

39. Fluckiger AC, Li Z, Kato RM, et al. Btk/Tec kinases regulate sustained increases in intracellular Ca^{2+} following B-cell receptor activation. *EMBO J* 1998;17:1973–1985.

40. Okada T, Maeda A, Iwamatsu A, et al. BCAP: the tyrosine kinase substrate that connects B cell receptor to phosphoinositide 3-kinase activation. *Immunity* 2000;13:817–827.

41. Beitz LO, Fruman DA, Kurosaki T, et al. SYK is upstream of phosphoinositide 3-kinase in B cell receptor signaling. *J Biol Chem* 1999;274:32662–32666.

42. Tamir I, Dal Porto JM, Cambier JC. Cytoplasmic protein tyrosine phosphatases SHP-1 and SHP-2: regulators of B cell signal transduction. *Curr Opin Immunol* 2000;12:307–315.

43. Yamazaki T, Takeda K, Gotoh K, et al. Essential immunoregulatory role for BCAP in B cell development and function. *J Exp Med* 2002;195:535–545.

44. Takata M, Kurosaki T. A role for Bruton's tyrosine kinase in B cell antigen receptor-mediated activation of phospholipase C-gamma 2. *J Exp Med* 1996;184:31–40.

45. Ward SG, Cantrell DA. Phosphoinositide 3-kinases in T lymphocyte activation. *Curr Opin Immunol* 2001;13:332–338.

46. Tsukada S, Rawlings DJ, Witte ON. Role of Bruton's tyrosine kinase in immunodeficiency. *Curr Opin Immunol* 1994;6:623–630.

47. Thomas JD, Sideras P, Smith CI, et al. Colocalization of X-linked agammaglobulinemia and X-linked immunodeficiency genes. *Science* 1993;261:355–358.

48. Rawlings DJ, Saffran DC, Tsukada S, et al. Mutation of unique region of Bruton's tyrosine kinase in immunodeficient XID mice. *Science* 1993;261:358–361.

49. Liu W, Quinto I, Chen X, et al. Direct inhibition of Bruton's tyrosine kinase by IBtk, a Btk-binding protein. *Nat Immunol* 2001;2:939–946.

50. Law CL, Chandran KA, Sidorenko SP, et al. Phospholipase C-gamma1 interacts with conserved phosphotyrosyl residues in the linker region of Syk and is a substrate for Syk. *Mol Cell Biol* 1996;16:1305–1315.

51. Wang D, Feng J, Wen R, et al. Phospholipase Cgamma2 is essential in the functions of B cell and several Fc receptors. *Immunity* 2000;13:25–35.

52. Miyakawa T, Maeda A, Yamazawa T, et al. Encoding of Ca^{2+} signals by differential expression of IP3 receptor subtypes. *EMBO J* 1999;18:1303–1308.

53. Lewis RS. Calcium signaling mechanisms in T lymphocytes. *Annu Rev Immunol* 2001;19:497–521.

54. Clapham DE. Calcium signaling. *Cell* 1995;80:259–268.

55. Hagar RE, Burgstahler AD, Nathanson MH, et al. Type III InsP3 receptor channel stays open in the presence of increased calcium. *Nature* 1998;396:81–84.

56. Sugawara H, Kurosaki M, Takata M, et al. Genetic evidence for involvement of type 1, type 2 and type 3 inositol 1,4,5-trisphosphate receptors in signal transduction through the B-cell antigen receptor. *EMBO J* 1997;16:3078–3088.

57. Bubien JK, Zhou LJ, Bell PD, et al. Transfection of the CD20 cell surface molecule into ectopic cell types generates a Ca^{2+} conductance found constitutively in B lymphocytes. *J Cell Biol* 1993;121:1121–1132.

58. Peng JB, Chen XZ, Berger UV, et al. Molecular cloning and characterization of a channel-like transporter mediating intestinal calcium absorption. *J Biol Chem* 1999;274:22739–22746.

59. Yue L, Peng JB, Hediger MA, et al. CaT1 manifests the pore properties of the calcium-release-activated calcium channel. *Nature* 2001;410:705–709.

60. Putney JW. "Kissin' cousins": intimate plasma membrane–ER interactions underlie capacitative calcium entry. *Cell* 1999;99:5–8.

61. Ma HT, Patterson RL, van Rossum DB, et al. Requirement of the inositol trisphosphate receptor for activation of store-operated Ca^{2+} channels. *Science* 2000;287:1647–1651.

62. Bikah G, Pogue-Caley RR, McHeyzer-Williams LJ, et al. Regulating T helper cell immunity through antigen responsiveness and calcium entry. *Nat Immunol* 2000;1:402–412.

63. Serafini AT, Lewis RS, Clipstone NA, et al. Isolation of mutant T lymphocytes with defects in capacitative calcium entry. *Immunity* 1995;3:239–250.

64. Rao A, Luo C, Hogan PG. Transcription factors of the NFAT family: regulation and function. *Annu Rev Immunol* 1997;15:707–747.

65. Neilson J, Stankunas K, Crabtree GR. Monitoring the duration of antigen-receptor occupancy by calcineurin/glycogen-synthase-kinase-3 control of NF-AT nuclear shuttling. *Curr Opin Immunol* 2001;13:346–350.

66. Beals CR, Clipstone NA, Ho SN, et al. Nuclear localization of NF-ATc by a calcineurin-dependent, cyclosporin- sensitive intramolecular interaction. *Genes Dev* 1997;11:824–834.

67. Beals CR, Sheridan CM, Turck CW, et al. Nuclear export of NF-ATc enhanced by glycogen synthase kinase-3. *Science* 1997;275:1930–1934.

68. Ranger AM, Oukka M, Rengarajan J, et al. Inhibitory function of two NFAT family members in lymphoid homeostasis and Th2 development. *Immunity* 1998;9:627–635.

69. Hodge MR, Ranger AM, Charles de la Brousse F, et al. Hyperproliferation and dysregulation of IL-4 expression in NF-ATp–deficient mice. *Immunity* 1996;4:397–405.

70. Peng SL, Gerth AJ, Ranger AM, et al. NFATc1 and NFATc2 together control both T and B cell activation and differentiation. *Immunity* 2001;14:13–20.

71. Karin M, Ben-Neriah Y. Phosphorylation meets ubiquitination: the control of NF-[kappa]B activity. *Annu Rev Immunol* 2000;18:621–663.

72. Karin M, Lin A. NF-kappaB at the crossroads of life and death. *Nat Immunol* 2002;3:221–227.

73. Dolmetsch RE, Lewis RS, Goodnow CC, et al. Differential activation of transcription factors induced by Ca^{2+} response amplitude and duration. *Nature* 1997;386:855–858.

74. Dolmetsch RE, Xu K, Lewis RS. Calcium oscillations increase the efficiency and specificity of gene expression. *Nature* 1998;392:933–936.

75. Dorn GW 2nd, Mochly-Rosen D. Intracellular transport mechanisms of signal transducers. *Annu Rev Physiol* 2002;64:407–429.

76. Leitges M, Schmedt C, Guinamard R, et al. Immunodeficiency in protein kinase cbeta-deficient mice. *Science* 1996;273:788–791.

77. Kang SW, Wahl MI, Chu J, et al. PKCbeta modulates antigen receptor signaling via regulation of Btk membrane localization. *EMBO J* 2001;20:5692–5702.

78. Sidorenko SP, Law CL, Klaus SJ, et al. Protein kinase C mu (PKC mu) associates with the B cell antigen receptor complex and regulates lymphocyte signaling. *Immunity* 1996;5:353–363.

79. Fruman DA, Ferl GZ, An SS, et al. Phosphoinositide 3-kinase and Bruton's tyrosine kinase regulate overlapping sets of genes in B lymphocytes. *Proc Natl Acad Sci U S A* 2002;99:359–364.

80. Gold MR, Scheid MP, Santos L, et al. The B cell antigen receptor activates the Akt (protein kinase B)/glycogen synthase kinase-3 signaling pathway via phosphatidylinositol 3-kinase. *J Immunol* 1999;163:1894–1905.

81. Stokoe D, Stephens LR, Copeland T, et al. Dual role of phosphatidylinositol-3,4,5-trisphosphate in the activation of protein kinase B. *Science* 1997;277:567–570.

82. Tsuruta F, Masuyama N, Gotoh Y. The PI3K-Akt pathway suppresses Bax translocation to mitochondria. *J Biol Chem* 2002;12:12.

83. Graziadei L, Riabowol K, Bar-Sagi D. Co-capping of ras proteins with surface immunoglobulins in B lymphocytes. *Nature* 1990;347:396–400.

84. Harmer SL, DeFranco AL. The src homology domain 2-containing inositol phosphatase SHIP forms a ternary complex with Shc and Grb2 in antigen receptor-stimulated B lymphocytes. *J Biol Chem* 1999;274:12183–12191.

85. Tridandapani S, Kelley T, Cooney D, et al. Negative signaling in B cells: SHIP Grbs Shc. *Immunol Today* 1997;18:424–427.

86. Carpino N, Wisniewski D, Strife A, et al. p62(dok): a constitutively tyrosine-phosphorylated, GAP-associated protein in chronic myelogenous leukemia progenitor cells. *Cell* 1997;88:197–204.

87. Tamir I, Stolpa JC, Helgason CD, et al. The RasGAP-binding protein p62dok is a mediator of inhibitory FcgammaRIIB signals in B cells. *Immunity* 2000;12:347–358.

88. Hashimoto A, Okada H, Jiang A, et al. Involvement of guanosine triphosphatases and phospholipase C-gamma2 in extracellular signal-regulated kinase, c-Jun NH2-terminal kinase, and p38 mitogen-activated protein kinase activation by the B cell antigen receptor. *J Exp Med* 1998;188:1287–1295.

89. Jacinto E, Werlen G, Karin M. Cooperation between Syk and Rac1 leads to synergistic JNK activation in T lymphocytes. *Immunity* 1998;8:31–41.

90. Werlen G, Jacinto E, Xia Y, et al. Calcineurin preferentially synergizes with PKC-theta to activate JNK and IL-2 promoter in T lymphocytes. *EMBO J* 1998;17:3101–3111.

91. Latour S, Veillette A. Proximal protein tyrosine kinases in immunoreceptor signaling. *Curr Opin Immunol* 2001;13:299–306.

92. Cloutier JF, Veillette A. Cooperative inhibition of T-cell antigen receptor signaling by a complex between a kinase and a phosphatase. *J Exp Med* 1999;189:111–121.

93. Kawabuchi M, Satomi Y, Takao T, et al. Transmembrane phosphoprotein Cbp regulates the activities of Src-family tyrosine kinases. *Nature* 2000;404:999–1003.

94. Brdicka T, Pavlistova D, Leo A, et al. Phosphoprotein associated with glycosphingolipid-enriched microdomains (PAG), a novel ubiquitously expressed transmembrane adaptor protein, binds the protein tyrosine kinase csk and is involved in regulation of T cell activation. *J Exp Med* 2000;191:1591–1604.

95. Hermiston ML, Xu Z, Majeti R, et al. Reciprocal regulation of lymphocyte activation by tyrosine kinases and phosphatases. *J Clin Invest* 2002;109:9–14.

96. Batista FD, Iber D, Neuberger MS. B cells acquire antigen from target cells after synapse formation. *Nature* 2001;411:489–494.

97. Kelm S, Pelz A, Schauer R, et al. Sialoadhesin, myelin-associated glycoprotein and CD22 define a new family of sialic acid-dependent adhesion molecules of the immunoglobulin superfamily. *Curr Biol* 1994;4:965–972.

98. Engel P, Nojima Y, Rothstein D, et al. The same epitope on CD22 of B lymphocytes mediates the adhesion of erythrocytes, T and B lymphocytes, neutrophils, and monocytes. *J Immunol* 1993;150:4719–4732.

99. Tedder TF, Tuscano J, Sato S, et al. CD22, a B lymphocyte-specific adhesion molecule that regulates antigen receptor signaling. *Annu Rev Immunol* 1997;15:481–504.

100. Doody GM, Justement LB, Delibrias CC, et al. A role in B cell activation for CD22 and the protein tyrosine phosphatase SHP. *Science* 1995;269:242–244.

101. Sato S, Miller AS, Inaoki M, et al. CD22 is both a positive and negative regulator of B lymphocyte antigen receptor signal transduction: altered signaling in CD22-deficient mice. *Immunity* 1996;5:551–562.

102. Cyster JG, Goodnow CC. Protein tyrosine phosphatase 1C negatively regulates antigen receptor signaling in B lymphocytes and determines thresholds for negative selection. *Immunity* 1995;2:13–24.

103. Fujimoto M, Bradney AP, Poe JC, et al. Modulation of B lymphocyte antigen receptor signal transduction by a CD19/CD22 regulatory loop. *Immunity* 1999;11:191–200.

104. Tedder TF, Zhou LJ, Engel P. The CD19/CD21 signal transduction complex of B lymphocytes. *Immunol Today* 1994;15:437–442.

105. Dempsey PW, Allison ME, Akkaraju S, et al. C3d of complement as a molecular adjuvant: bridging innate and acquired immunity. *Science* 1996;271:348–350.

106. Cherukuri A, Cheng PC, Sohn HW, et al. The CD19/CD21 complex functions to prolong B cell antigen receptor signaling from lipid rafts. *Immunity* 2001;14:169–179.

107. Fujimoto M, Fujimoto Y, Poe JC, et al. CD19 regulates Src family protein tyrosine kinase activation in B lymphocytes through processive amplification. *Immunity* 2000;13:47–57.

108. Ravetch JV, Bolland S. IgG Fc receptors. *Annu Rev Immunol* 2001; 19:275–290.

109. D'Ambrosio D, Fong DC, Cambier JC. The SHIP phosphatase becomes associated with Fc gammaRIIB1 and is tyrosine phosphorylated during "negative" signaling. *Immunol Lett* 1996;54:77–82.

110. Hardy RR, Hayakawa K. B cell development pathways. *Annu Rev Immunol* 2001;19:595–621.

111. Berland R, Wortis HH. Origins and functions of B-1 cells with notes on the role of cd5. *Annu Rev Immunol* 2002;20:253–300.

112. Arnold LW, Pennell CA, McCray SK, et al. Development of B-1 cells: segregation of phosphatidyl choline-specific B cells to the B-1 population occurs after immunoglobulin gene expression. *J Exp Med* 1994;179:1585–1595.

113. Clarke SH, Arnold LW. B-1 cell development: evidence for an uncommitted immunoglobulin (Ig)M+ B cell precursor in B-1 cell differentiation. *J Exp Med* 1998;187:1325–1334.

114. Martin F, Kearney JF. B1 cells: similarities and differences with other B cell subsets. *Curr Opin Immunol* 2001;13:195–201.

115. Bendelac A, Bonneville M, Kearney JF. Autoreactivity by design: innate B and T lymphocytes. *Nature Rev Immunol* 2001;1:177–186.

116. Hayakawa K, Asano M, Shinton SA, et al. Positive selection of natural autoreactive B cells. *Science* 1999;285:113–116.

117. Ansel KM, Harris RB, Cyster JG. CXCL13 is required for B1 cell homing, natural antibody production, and body cavity immunity. *Immunity* 2002;16:67–76.

118. Martin F, Kearney JF. Positive selection from newly formed to marginal zone B cells depends on the rate of clonal production, CD19, and btk. *Immunity* 2000;12:39–49.

119. Guinamard R, Okigaki M, Schlessinger J, et al. Absence of marginal zone B cells in Pyk-2–deficient mice defines their role in the humoral response. *Nat Immunol* 2000;1:31–36.

120. Wang JH, Avitahl N, Cariappa A, et al. Aiolos regulates B cell activation and maturation to effector state. *Immunity* 1998;9:543–553.

121. Medzhitov R, Janeway CA Jr. Innate immunity: the virtues of a nonclonal system of recognition. *Cell* 1997;91:295–298.

122. Medzhitov R, Preston-Hurlburt P, Janeway CA Jr. A human homologue of the Drosophila Toll protein signals activation of adaptive immunity. *Nature* 1997;388:394–397.

123. Poltorak A, He X, Smirnova I, et al. Defective LPS signaling in C3H/HeJ and C57BL/10ScCr mice: mutations in Tlr4 gene. *Science* 1998;282:2085–2088.

124. Takeuchi O, Hoshino K, Kawai T, et al. Differential roles of TLR2 and TLR4 in recognition of gram-negative and gram-positive bacterial cell wall components. *Immunity* 1999;11:443–451.

125. Fearon DT, Locksley RM. The instructive role of innate immunity in the acquired immune response. *Science* 1996;272:50–53.

126. Dintzis HM, Dintzis RZ, Vogelstein B. Molecular determinants of immunogenicity: the immunon model of immune response. *Proc Natl Acad Sci U S A* 1976;73:3671–3675.

127. Martin F, Oliver AM, Kearney JF. Marginal zone and B1 B cells unite in the early response against T-independent blood-borne particulate antigens. *Immunity* 2001;14:617–629.

128. Ochsenbein AF, Fehr T, Lutz C, et al. Control of early viral and bacterial distribution and disease by natural antibodies. *Science* 1999;286:2156–2159.

129. von Bulow GU, Bram RJ. NF-AT activation induced by a CAML-interacting member of the tumor necrosis factor receptor superfamily. *Science* 1997;278:138–141.

130. Laabi Y, Egle A, Strasser A. TNF cytokine family: more BAFF-ling complexities. *Curr Biol* 2001;11:R1013–R1016.

131. von Bulow GU, van Deursen JM, Bram RJ. Regulation of the T-independent humoral response by TACI. *Immunity* 2001;14:573–582.

132. Gross JA, Johnston J, Mudri S, et al. TACI and BCMA are receptors for a TNF homologue implicated in B-cell autoimmune disease. *Nature* 2000;404:995–999.

133. Marsters SA, Yan M, Pitti RM, et al. Interaction of the TNF homologues BLyS and APRIL with the TNF receptor homologues BCMA and TACI. *Curr Biol* 2000;10:785–788.

134. Wu Y, Bressette D, Carrell JA, et al. Tumor necrosis factor (TNF) receptor superfamily member TACI is a high affinity receptor for TNF family members APRIL and BLyS. *J Biol Chem* 2000;275:35478–35485.

135. Gross JA, Dillon SR, Mudri S, et al. TACI-Ig neutralizes molecules critical for B cell development and autoimmune disease. impaired B cell maturation in mice lacking BLyS. *Immunity* 2001;15:289–302.

136. Fagarasan S, Honjo T. T-Independent immune response: new aspects of B cell biology. *Science* 2000;290:89–92.

137. Ravetch JV, Lanier LL. Immune inhibitory receptors. *Science* 2000; 290:84–89.

138. Nishimura H, Nose M, Hiai H, et al. Development of lupus-like autoimmune diseases by disruption of the PD-1 gene encoding an ITIM motif-carrying immunoreceptor. *Immunity* 1999;11:141–151.

139. Lanzavecchia A, Sallusto F. The instructive role of dendritic cells on

T cell responses: lineages, plasticity and kinetics. *Curr Opin Immunol* 2001;13:291–198.

140. Sallusto F, Mackay CR, Lanzavecchia A. The role of chemokine receptors in primary, effector, and memory immune responses. *Annu Rev Immunol* 2000;18:593–620.

141. Cyster JG. Chemokines and cell migration in secondary lymphoid organs. *Science* 1999;286:2098–2102.

142. Nakano H, Yanagita M, Gunn MD. CD11c(+)B220(+)Gr-1(+) cells in mouse lymph nodes and spleen display characteristics of plasmacytoid dendritic cells. *J Exp Med* 2001;194:1171–1178.

143. Monks CR, Freiberg BA, Kupfer H, et al. Three-dimensional segregation of supramolecular activation clusters in T cells. *Nature* 1998;395:82–86.

144. Grakoui A, Bromley SK, Sumen C, et al. The immunological synapse: a molecular machine controlling T cell activation. *Science* 1999;285:221–227.

145. Bromley SK, Iaboni A, Davis SJ, et al. The immunological synapse and CD28-CD80 interactions. *Nat Immunol* 2001;2:1159–1166.

146. Wulfing C, Davis MM. A receptor/cytoskeletal movement triggered by costimulation during T cell activation. *Science* 1998;282:2266–2269.

147. Lee KH, Holdorf AD, Dustin ML, et al. T cell receptor signaling precedes immunological synapse formation. *Science* 2002;295:1539–1542.

148. McHeyzer-Williams MG, Davis MM. Antigen-specific development of primary and memory T cells in vivo. *Science* 1995;268:106–111.

149. McHeyzer-Williams LJ, Panus JF, Mikszta JA, et al. Evolution of antigen-specific T cell receptors in vivo: preimmune and antigen-driven selection of preferred complementarity-determining region 3 (CDR3) motifs. *J Exp Med* 1999;189:1823–1838.

150. Panus JF, McHeyzer-Williams LJ, McHeyzer-Williams MG. Antigen-specific T helper cell function: differential cytokine expression in primary and memory responses. *J Exp Med* 2000;192:1301–1316.

151. Ansel KM, McHeyzer-Williams LJ, Ngo VN, et al. In vivo–activated CD4 T cells upregulate CXC chemokine receptor 5 and reprogram their response to lymphoid chemokines. *J Exp Med* 1999;190:1123–1134.

152. Watts C. Capture and processing of exogenous antigens for presentation on MHC molecules. *Annu Rev Immunol* 1997;15:821–850.

153. Cheng PC, Dykstra ML, Mitchell RN, et al. A role for lipid rafts in B cell antigen receptor signaling and antigen targeting. *J Exp Med* 1999;190:1549–1560.

154. Garside P, Ingulli E, Merica RR, et al. Visualization of specific B and T lymphocyte interactions in the lymph node. *Science* 1998;281:96–99.

155. Reif K, Ekland EH, Ohl L, et al. Balanced responsiveness to chemoattractants from adjacent zones determines B-cell position. *Nature* 2002;416:94–99.

156. Calderhead DM, Kosaka Y, Manning EM, et al. CD40-CD154 interactions in B-cell signaling. *Curr Top Microbiol Immunol* 2000;245:73–99.

157. Banchereau J, Bazan F, Blanchard D, et al. The CD40 antigen and its ligand. *Annu Rev Immunol* 1994;12:881–922.

158. Grewal IS, Xu J, Flavell RA. Impairment of antigen-specific T-cell priming in mice lacking CD40 ligand. *Nature* 1995;378:617–620.

159. van Essen D, Kikutani H, Gray D. CD40 ligand-transduced costimulation of T cells in the development of helper function. *Nature* 1995;378:620–623.

160. Bishop GA, Hostager BS. B lymphocyte activation by contact-mediated interactions with T lymphocytes. *Curr Opin Immunol* 2001;13:278–285.

161. Murata K, Ishii N, Takano H, et al. Impairment of antigen-presenting cell function in mice lacking expression of OX40 ligand. *J Exp Med* 2000;191:365–374.

162. Tangye SG, Liu YJ, Aversa G, et al. Identification of functional human splenic memory B cells by expression of CD148 and CD27. *J Exp Med* 1998;188:1691–1703.

163. Agematsu K, Hokibara S, Nagumo H, et al. CD27: a memory B-cell marker. *Immunol Today* 2000;21:204–206.

164. Cerutti A, Schaffer A, Shah S, et al. CD30 is a CD40-inducible molecule that negatively regulates CD40-mediated immunoglobulin class switching in non–antigen-selected human B cells. *Immunity* 1998;9:247–256.

165. Amakawa R, Hakem A, Kundig TM, et al. Impaired negative selection of T cells in Hodgkin's disease antigen CD30-deficient mice. *Cell* 1996;84:551–562.

166. Krammer PH. CD95's deadly mission in the immune system. *Nature* 2000;407:789–795.

167. Sharpe AH, Freeman GJ. The B7-CD28 superfamily. *Nature Rev Immunol* 2002;2:116–126.

168. Walunas TL, Lenschow DJ, Bakker CY, et al. CTLA-4 can function as a negative regulator of T cell activation. *Immunity* 1994;1:405–413.

169. Waterhouse P, Penninger JM, Timms E, et al. Lymphoproliferative disorders with early lethality in mice deficient in Ctla-4. *Science* 1995;270:985–988.

170. Coyle AJ, Lehar S, Lloyd C, et al. The CD28-related molecule ICOS is required for effective T cell-dependent immune responses. *Immunity* 2000;13:95–105.

171. McAdam AJ, Greenwald RJ, Levin MA, et al. ICOS is critical for CD40-mediated antibody class switching. *Nature* 2001;409:102–105.

172. Dong C, Juedes AE, Temann UA, et al. ICOS co-stimulatory receptor is essential for T-cell activation and function. *Nature* 2001;409:97–101.

173. Tafuri A, Shahinian A, Bladt F, et al. ICOS is essential for effective T-helper-cell responses. *Nature* 2001;409:105–109.

174. Armitage RJ, Fanslow WC, Strockbine L, et al. Molecular and biological characterization of a murine ligand for CD40. *Nature* 1992;357:80–82.

175. Coffman RL, Seymour BW, Lebman DA, et al. The role of helper T cell products in mouse B cell differentiation and isotype regulation. *Immunol Rev* 1988;102:5–28.

176. Kuhn R, Rajewsky K, Muller W. Generation and analysis of interleukin-4 deficient mice. *Science* 1991;254:707–710.

177. Honjo T, Kinoshita K, Muramatsu M. Molecular mechanism of class switch recombination: linkage with somatic hypermutation. *Annu Rev Immunol* 2002;20:165–196.

178. Okazaki I, Kinoshita K, Muramatsu M, et al. The AID enzyme induces class switch recombination in fibroblasts. *Nature* 2002;727:1–5.

179. Muramatsu M, Kinoshita K, Fagarasan S, et al. Class switch recombination and hypermutation require activation-induced cytidine deaminase (AID), a potential RNA editing enzyme. *Cell* 2000;102:553–563.

180. Revy P, Muto T, Levy Y, et al. Activation-induced cytidine deaminase (AID) deficiency causes the autosomal recessive form of the Hyper-IgM syndrome (HIGM2). *Cell* 2000;102:565–575.

181. Jacob J, Kassir R, Kelsoe G. In situ studies of the primary immune response to (4-hydroxy-3-nitrophenyl)acetyl. I. The architecture and dynamics of responding cell populations. *J Exp Med* 1991;173:1165–1175.

182. Liu YJ, Zhang J, Lane PJ, et al. Sites of specific B cell activation in primary and secondary responses to T cell-dependent and T cell-independent antigens. *Eur J Immunol* 1991;21:2951–2962.

183. Hargreaves DC, Hyman PL, Lu TT, et al. A coordinated change in chemokine responsiveness guides plasma cell movements. *J Exp Med* 2001;194:45–56.

184. Turner CA Jr, Mack DH, Davis MM. Blimp-1, a novel zinc finger-containing protein that can drive the maturation of B lymphocytes into immunoglobulin-secreting cells. *Cell* 1994;77:297–306.

185. Calame KL. Plasma cells: finding new light at the end of B cell development. *Nat Immunol* 2001;2:1103–1108.

186. Reimold AM, Iwakoshi NN, Manis J, et al. Plasma cell differentiation requires the transcription factor XBP-1. *Nature* 2001;412:300–307.

187. Mittrucker HW, Matsuyama T, Grossman A, et al. Requirement for the transcription factor LSIRF/IRF4 for mature B and T lymphocyte function. *Science* 1997;275:540–543.

188. Jacobson EB, Caporale LH, Thorbecke GJ. Effect of thymus cell injections on germinal center formation in lymphoid tissues of nude (thymusless) mice. *Cell Immunol* 1974;13:416–430.

189. Kawabe T, Naka T, Yoshida K, et al. The immune responses in CD40-deficient mice: impaired immunoglobulin class switching and germinal center formation. *Immunity* 1994;1:167–178.

190. Renshaw BR, Fanslow WC 3rd, Armitage RJ, et al. Humoral immune responses in CD40 ligand–deficient mice. *J Exp Med* 1994;180:1889–1900.

191. de Vinuesa CG, Cook MC, Ball J, et al. Germinal centers without T cells. *J Exp Med* 2000;191:485–494.

192. Neuberger MS, Milstein C. Somatic hypermutation. *Curr Opin Immunol* 1995;7:248–254.

193. Jolly CJ, Wagner SD, Rada C, et al. The targeting of somatic hypermutation. *Semin Immunol* 1996;8:159–168.

194. Bross L, Fukita Y, McBlane F, et al. DNA double-strand breaks in immunoglobulin genes undergoing somatic hypermutation. *Immunity* 2000;13:589–597.

195. Zan H, Komori A, Li Z, et al. The translesion DNA polymerase zeta plays a major role in Ig and bcl-6 somatic hypermutation. *Immunity* 2001;14:643–653.

196. Gearhart PJ, Wood RD. Emerging links between hypermutation of antibody genes and DNA polymerases. *Nature Rev Immunol* 2001;1:187–192.

197. Jacobs H, Bross L. Towards an understanding of somatic hypermutation. *Curr Opin Immunol* 2001;13:208–218.

198. Muramatsu M, Sankaranand VS, Anant S, et al. Specific expression of activation-induced cytidine deaminase (AID), a novel member of the RNA-editing deaminase family in germinal center B cells. *J Biol Chem* 1999;274:18470–18476.

199. Jacob J, Kelsoe G, Rajewsky K, et al. Intraclonal generation of antibody mutants in germinal centres. *Nature* 1991;354:389–392.

200. Berek C, Berger A, Apel M. Maturation of the immune response in germinal centers. *Cell* 1991;67:1121–1129.

201. Fearon DT, Carroll MC. Regulation of B lymphocyte responses to foreign and self-antigens by the CD19/CD21 complex. *Annu Rev Immunol* 2000;18:393–422.

202. Hannum LG, Haberman AM, Anderson SM, et al. Germinal center initiation, variable gene region hypermutation, and mutant B cell selection without detectable immune complexes on follicular dendritic cells. *J Exp Med* 2000;192:931–942.

203. Zheng B, Han S, Kelsoe G. T helper cells in murine germinal centers are antigen-specific emigrants that downregulate Thy-1. *J Exp Med* 1996;184:1083–1091.

204. Smith KG, Light A, O'Reilly LA, et al. bcl-2 transgene expression inhibits apoptosis in the germinal center and reveals differences in the selection of memory B cells and bone marrow antibody-forming cells. *J Exp Med* 2000;191:475–484.

205. Takahashi Y, Cerasoli DM, Dal Porto JM, et al. Relaxed negative selection in germinal centers and impaired affinity maturation in bcl-xL transgenic mice. *J Exp Med* 1999;190:399–410.

206. Hennino A, Berard M, Krammer PH, et al. FLICE-inhibitory protein is a key regulator of germinal center B cell apoptosis. *J Exp Med* 2001;193:447–458.

207. McHeyzer-Williams MG, Ahmed R. B cell memory and the long-lived plasma cell. *Curr Opin Immunol* 1999;11:172–179.

208. Slifka MK, Antia R, Whitmire JK, et al. Humoral immunity due to long-lived plasma cells. *Immunity* 1998;8:363–372.

209. Koni PA, Joshi SK, Temann UA, et al. Conditional vascular cell adhesion molecule 1 deletion in mice: impaired lymphocyte migration to bone marrow. *J Exp Med* 2001;193:741–754.

210. Nitschke L, Floyd H, Ferguson DJ, et al. Identification of CD22 ligands on bone marrow sinusoidal endothelium implicated in CD22-dependent homing of recirculating B cells. *J Exp Med* 1999;189:1513–1518.

211. McHeyzer-Williams MG, Nossal GJ, Lalor PA. Molecular characterization of single memory B cells. *Nature* 1991;350:502–505.

212. Martin SW, Goodnow CC. Burst-enhancing role of the IgG membrane tail as a molecular determinant of memory. *Nat Immunol* 2002;3:182–188.

213. McHeyzer-Williams LJ, Cool M, McHeyzer-Williams MG. Antigen-specific B cell memory: expression and replenishment of a novel b220(−) memory b cell compartment. *J Exp Med* 2000;191:1149–1166.

214. Driver DJ, McHeyzer-Williams LJ, Cool M, et al. Development and maintenance of a B220⁻ memory B cell compartment. *J Immunol* 2001;167:1393–1405.

215. Linton PL, Decker DJ, Klinman NR. Primary antibody-forming cells and secondary B cells are generated from separate precursor cell subpopulations. *Cell* 1989;59:1049–1059.

216. Gray D, Skarvall H. B-cell memory is short-lived in the absence of antigen. *Nature* 1988;336:70–73.

217. Maruyama M, Lam KP, Rajewsky K. Memory B-cell persistence is independent of persisting immunizing antigen. *Nature* 2000;407:636–642.

CHAPTER 8

T-Cell Antigen Receptors

Mark M. Davis and Yueh-Hsiu Chien

T-Cell Receptor Polypeptides
T-Cell Receptor Structure
   $\alpha\beta$ T-Cell Receptor Structure • $\gamma\delta$ T-Cell Receptor Structure
The CD3 Polypeptides
   Sequence and Structure of the CD3 Polypeptides • Intracellular Assembly and Degradation of the T-Cell Receptor–CD3 Complex • CD3 Structure
T-Cell Receptor Genes
   Organization of the T-Cell Receptor α/δ Locus • Organization of the T-Cell Receptor β Locus • Organization of the T-Cell Receptor γ Locus • Transcriptional Control of the T-Cell Receptor Genes • Chromosomal Locations of T-Cell Receptor Genes and Translocations Associated with Disease • Allelic Exclusion • Commitment to the $\alpha\beta$ Lineage versus the $\gamma\delta$ Lineage • Other Genetic Mechanisms
Biochemistry of $\alpha\beta$ T-Cell Receptor–Ligand Interactions
   Role of CD4 and CD8
Topology of T-Cell Receptor–Peptide/Major Histocompatibility Complex Interactions
   T-Cell Receptor Plasticity
$\alpha\beta$ T-Cell Receptor and Superantigens
A Second Type of Receptor: $\gamma\delta$-CD3
   Identification of $\gamma\delta$ T Cells • $\gamma\delta$ T Cells Contribute to Host Immune Defense Differently than $\alpha\beta$ T Cells • Antigen Recognition by $\gamma\delta$ T Cells Does Not Require Processing • Other Antigen Specificities of $\gamma\delta$ T Cells • Complementarity-Determining Region 3 Length Distribution Analysis shows $\gamma\delta$ T-Cell Receptors are more Immunoglobulin-like • Multivalence of the Ligands Is Required for Activation through the $\gamma\delta$ T-Cell Receptor
Complementary-Determining Region 3 Diversification: A General Strategy for T-Cell Receptors and Immunoglobulin Complementarity to Antigens?
Conclusions
Acknowledgments
References

The characteristics of T-lymphocyte recognition and the nature of T-cell antigen receptors (TCRs) has been a difficult and controversial area for immunologists. However, since 1983 there has been tremendous progress in identifying the molecules and genes that govern T cell recognition, and in more recent years, researchers have obtained the first concrete information on their biochemistry and structure. Although TCRs share many similarities, both structural and genetic, with B cell antigen receptors (immunoglobulins), they also possess a number of unique features related to their specific biological functions.

For classically defined helper and cytotoxic T cells, the most important of these differences was first suggested by the experiments of Zinkernagel and Doherty, who showed that viral antigen recognition by cytotoxic T cells was possible only with a certain major histocompatibility complex (MHC) haplotype on the infected cell (1,2). Evidence for this phenomenon of MHC restricted "recognition" was also demonstrated for helper T cells (3,4). It is now known that this type of T-cell recognition involves fragments of antigens (e.g., peptides) bound to specific MHC molecules (see Chapters 19 and 20). Because all antigens must eventually be degraded, this form of T-cell recognition is very complementary to that of B cells, in which pathogens can escape recognition by obscuring an antibody binding site or employing "decoy" molecules.

T-cell receptors occur as either of two distinct heterodimers, $\alpha\beta$ or $\gamma\delta$, both of which are expressed with the nonpolymorphic CD3 polypeptides γ, δ, ϵ, and ζ and, in some cases, the ribonucleic acid (RNA) splicing variant of ζ, η, or Fcϵ chains. The CD3 polypeptides, especially ζ and its variants, are critical for intracellular signaling (5). The $\alpha\beta$ TCR heterodimer–expressing cells predominate in most lymphoid compartments (90% to 95%) of humans and mice, and they are responsible for the classical helper or cytotoxic T cell

227

responses. In most cases, the $\alpha\beta$ TCR ligand is a peptide antigen bound to a class I or class II MHC molecule. T cells bearing $\gamma\delta$ TCR are less numerous than the $\alpha\beta$ type in most cellular compartments of humans and mice. However, they make up a substantial fraction of T lymphocytes in cows, sheep, and chickens (6). Studies of the structural characteristics and specificity of $\gamma\delta$ TCRs indicate that they are much more like immunoglobulins than like $\alpha\beta$ TCRs in their antigen recognition properties. In particular, they do not seem to require MHCs or other molecules to present antigens but instead appear to recognize antigens directly (7). Although it is not yet clear what role they play in the immune response, this is a very active area of current research, and many interesting leads are being pursued.

T-CELL RECEPTOR POLYPEPTIDES

The search for the molecules responsible for T-cell recognition first focused on deriving antisera or monoclonal antibodies specific for molecules on T-cell surfaces. Ultimately, a number of groups identified "clonotypic" sera (8) or monoclonal antibodies (9–13). A number of these antibodies were able to block antigen specific responses by the T cells they were raised against or, when coated on a surface, could activate the T cells for which they are specific. They were also able to immunoprecipitate 85,000- to 90,000—molecular weight (MW) disulfide-bonded heterodimers from different T cell clones or hybridomas consisting of two 40,000- to 50,000-MW glycosylated subunits referred to as α and β. Peptide mapping studies showed that there was a striking degree of polymorphism between heterodimers isolated from T cells of differing specificity, which thus suggests that these antigen recognition molecules may be akin to immunoglobulins (14,15).

Work in parallel to these serological studies exploited the small differences ($\sim$2%) observed between B- and T-cell gene expression (16) and isolated both a murine (17,18) and a human (19) T-cell specific gene that had antibody-like V, J, and C region sequences and could rearrange in T-lymphocytes (18). This molecule was identified as TCRβ by partial sequence analysis of immunoprecipitated materials (20). Subsequent subtractive cloning work rapidly identified two other candidate TCRs' complementary deoxyribonucleic acids (cDNAs) identified as TCRα (21,22) and TCRγ (23). It was quickly established that all antigen-specific helper or cytotoxic T-cell expressed TCR$\alpha\beta$ heterodimers. Where TCRγ fit in remained a puzzle until work by Brenner et al. (24) showed that it was expressed on a small (5% to 10%) subset of peripheral T cells together with another polypeptide, TCRδ. The nature of TCRδ remained unknown until it was discovered within the TCRα locus, between the Vα and Jα regions (25). Formal proof that the TCRα and TCRβ subunits were sufficient to transfer antigen/MHC recognition from one T cell to another came from gene transfection experiments (26,27), and equivalent experiments have also been performed with $\gamma\delta$ TCRs (28).

As shown in Fig. 1, all TCR polypeptides have a similar primary structure, with distinct variable (V) and diversity (D) regions in the case of TCRβ and TCRδ, and with joining (J), and constant (C) regions exactly analogous to their immunoglobulin counterparts. They also share many of the amino acid residues thought to be important for the characteristic variable and constant domains of immunoglobulins (29). The Cβ region is particularly homologous, sharing 40% of its amino acid sequence with CK and Cλ. The TCR polypeptides all contain a single C region domain (versus up to four for immunoglobulins) followed by a connecting peptide or hinge region, usually containing the cysteine for the disulfide linkage, which joins the two chains of the heterodimer [some human TCR$\gamma\delta$ isoforms lack this cysteine and consequently are not disulfide linked (30)]. N-linked glycosylation sites vary from two to four for each polypeptide, with no indications of O-linked sugar addition. C-terminals to the connecting peptide sequences are the hydrophobic transmembrane regions, which have no similarity to those of heavy immunoglobulin genes but instead have one or two positively charged residues that appear to be important for interaction with the CD3 molecules and T cell signaling, through interaction with the acidic residues found in all CD3 transmembrane regions. The newest member of the TCR polypeptide family is the pre–Tα chain, which serves as a chaperone for TCRβ in early thymocytes, which is similar to the role of λ5 in pre–B cells. It was first identified and cloned by Groettrup et al. (31) and Saint-Ruf et al. (32). It has an interesting structure that consists of a single immunoglobulin constant region–like domain followed by a cysteine-containing connecting peptide and a transmembrane region containing two charged residues: an arginine and a lysine spaced identically to those on the TCRα transmembrane region. The cysteine in the connecting peptide is presumably what allows heterodimer formation with TCRβ, and the similarity to TCRα in the transmembrane region is most likely to accommodate the CD3 polypeptides. In both mice and humans, the cytoplasmic tail is much longer than any of the TCR chains (37 and 120 amino acids, respectively), and the murine sequence contains two likely phosphorylation sites and sequences homologous to an SH3 domain–binding region. These are not present in the human sequence, however, and their functional significance is therefore questionable (32). Thus, the pre–Tα molecule could function as signaling intermediate independent of any of the CD3 polypeptides.

T-CELL RECEPTOR STRUCTURE

As just discussed, the sequences of TCR polypeptides show many similarities to immunoglobulins, and thus it has long been suggested that both heterodimers would be antibody-like in structure (18,19,33). These similarities include the number and spacing of specific cysteine residues within domains, which in antibodies form intrachain disulfide bonds. Also conserved are many of the interdomain and intradomain contact residues; in addition, secondary structure predictions

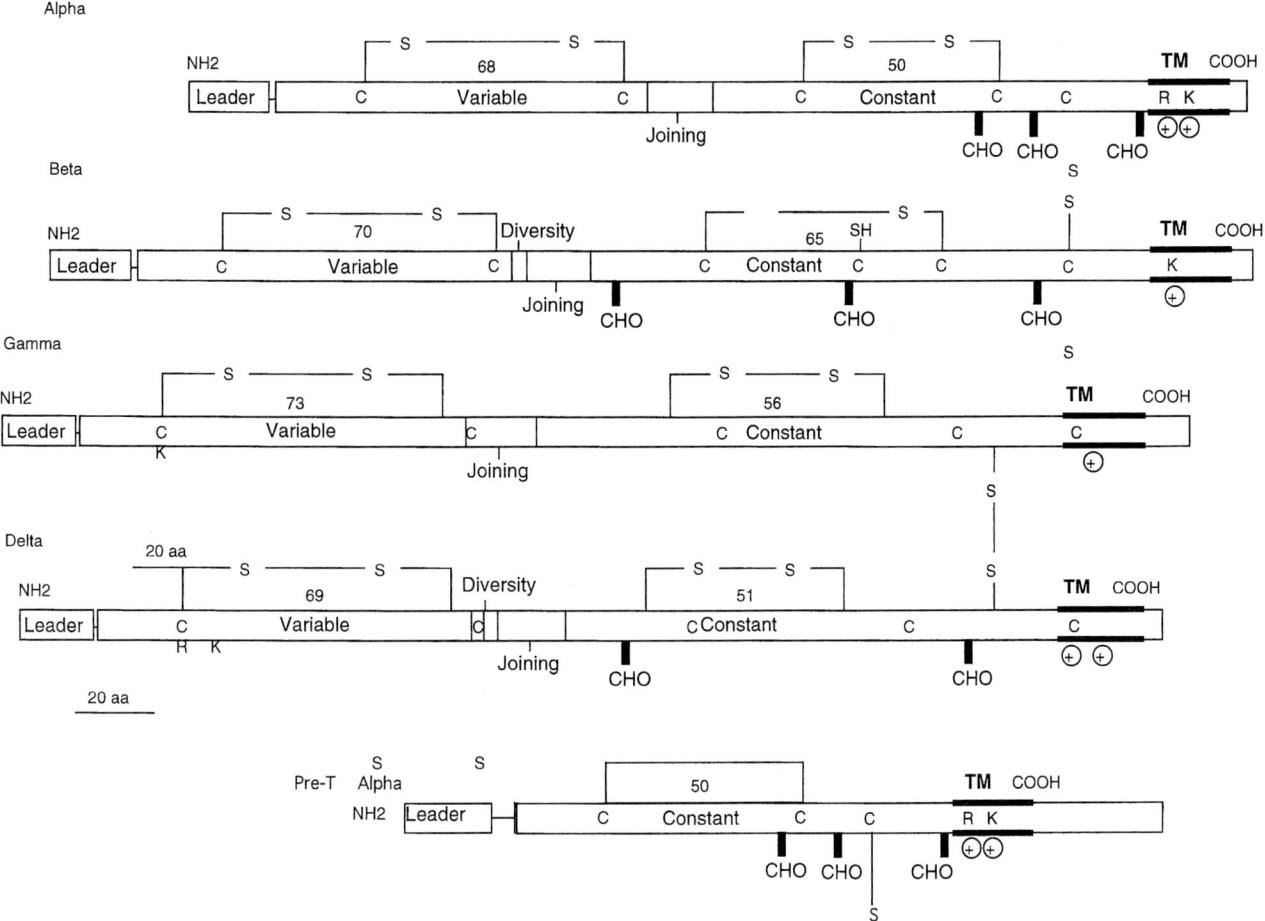

FIG. 1. Structural features of T-cell receptors and pre–T α polypeptides. Leader (L), variable (V), diversity (D), joining (J), and constant region (C) gene segments are indicated. TM and *bold horizontal lines* delineate the putative transmembrane regions; CHO indicates potential carbohydrate addition sites; C and S refer to cysteine residues that form interchain and intrachain disulfide bonds; R and K indicate the positively charged amino acids (arginine and lysine, respectively) that are found in the transmembrane regions.

are largely consistent with an immunoglobulin-like "β barrel" structure. This consists of three to four antiparallel β strands on one side of the "barrel" facing a similar number on the other side, with a disulfide bridge (usually) connecting the two β "sheets" (sets of β strands in the same plane) (Fig 2A). A diagrammatic representation of a typical V-region structure is shown in Fig. 2B. All immunoglobulin V- and C-region domains have this structure, with slight variations in the number of β strands in V-region domains (by convention, including V, D, and J sequences) in comparison with C-region domains.

αβ T-Cell Receptor Structure

Efforts to derive x-ray crystal structures of TCR heterodimers and fragments of heterodimers have encountered many technical hurdles. One reason is that it requires engineering the molecules into a soluble form. A second is that many of the TCRs are heavily glycosylated, and it was necessary to elim-

inate most or all of the carbohydrates on each chain to obtain high-quality crystals. An alternative is to express soluble TCRs in insect cells, which have compact N-linked sugars, or in *Escherichia coli,* which have none. The first successes in TCR crystallization come from the work of Bentley et al. (34), who solved the structure of a Vβ Cβ polypeptide, and Fields et al. (35), who then solved the structure of a Vα fragment. In general, these domains all are very immunoglobulin-like, with the classical β-barrel structure in evidence in all three domains. At each end of the barrel in each V-region domain, there are four loops between the β sheets, three of which form the complementarity-determining regions (CDRs) of immunoglobulins. The fourth loop, between the D and E strands, has been implicated in superantigen binding. The six CDR loops from the two variable domains form the antigen-binding surface of immunoglobulins and, as discussed later, TCRs as well. Whereas the Vβ domain depicted in Fig. 2A follows the canonical V domain β sheet structure, Vα differs significantly in that one of the

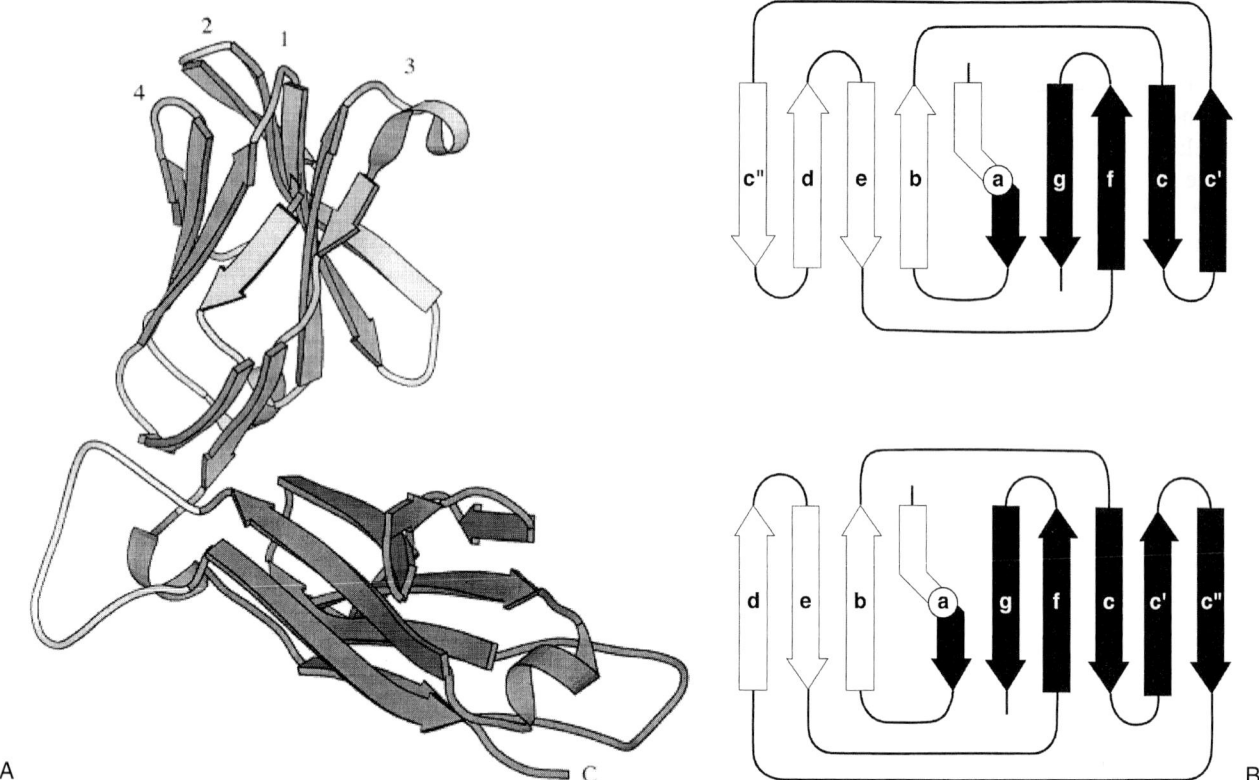

FIG. 2. T-cell receptors β and Vα. **A:** Ribbon diagram of the first T-cell receptor crystal structure (34), showing the antiparallel β sheets of a Vβ-Cβ polypeptide. The Vβ and Cβ domains show the classical eight and seven β-strand "barrels" characteristic of immunoglobulin V and C domains, respectively. Also shown are the positions of the complementarity-determining region loops 1, 2, and 3 at the end of Vβ and the fourth loop, which has been implicated in superantigen interactions. **B:** Schematic of the β strands in typical V region domain, which contrast with the alterations found in a Vα domain.

sheets has been translocated to the other half of the barrel (as schematized in Fig. 2B). This acts to remove a bulge in the side of the Vα domain, and it has been suggested that this would allow dimers of TCRs or perhaps higher order structures to assemble (35). Ultimately, Garcia et al. (36) were able to solve the structure of the Cα in the context of a complete heterodimer, and it has a remarkable variation of the classical immunoglobulin-like domain (Colorplate 1). Here there is only one half of the classical β-barrel—that is, one set (or "sheet") of β strands—whereas the rest of the somewhat truncated domain exhibits random coils. This type of structure is unprecedented in the immunoglobulin. The functional significance of such a variant structure in unknown, but it has been suggested that this incompletely formed immunoglobulin-like domain may be responsible for the observed lability of TCRα, and this may allow greater flexibility in the regulation of its expression. Another possible explanation is that this alteration may be designed to accommodate one or more of the CD3 molecules.

With regard to complete heterodimer structures, there are now data from four $\alpha\beta$ (36–40) and one $\gamma\delta$ heterodimer (41), and they largely resemble the crystallized fragment of an antibody (Fab). Although many features of these structures are shared with their antibody counterparts, several unusual features in the $\alpha\beta$ molecules may be significant. These include the following: (a) In one structure (36), four of seven N-linked sugars diffracted to high resolution, which indicates that they are not free to move very much and thus are likely to play a structural role, particularly in Cα:Cβ interactions. This correlates with mutagenesis data indicating that certain Cα sugars could not be eliminated without abolishing protein expression in mammalian cells (42) and the disordered state of a Cα domain in the structure of a TCR lacking glycosylation (37). (b) There is much more contact between Vβ and somewhat more between Vα and Cα than in the equivalent regions of antibodies. (c) The geometry of the interaction of Vα and Vβ more closely resembles that of the CH3 domains of antibodies than VH and VL domains. (d) Between the CDR3 loops of Vα and Vβ, there can be a pocket that, in at least one case (37)] accommodates a large side chain from the peptide bound to an MHC. Another key question is whether any conformational change occurs in the TCR upon ligand binding. Conformational changes in the TCR or in the CD3 polypeptides in particular may hold important clues as to the mechanism of signal transduction across the membrane after TCR engagement.

$\gamma\delta$ T-Cell Receptor Structure

The crystal structure of a $\gamma\delta$ TCR from a human T cell clone (41) that can be stimulated by small phosphate-containing compounds has been solved. Although both of its CDR3 loops are similar in length to those of $\alpha\beta$ TCRs whose structures have been determined, they protrude significantly from the rest of the putative binding surface and create a cleft between them. Portions of the CDR1γ, CDR1δ, and CDR2γ combine with the clefts between the CDR3 loops to form a pocket that may be the phosphoantigen binding site. This is because its structure is similar to those of pockets that are found in antibodies that bind phosphate-containing antigens, and it is surrounded by positively charged amino acid residues contributed by CDR2γ, CDR2δ, and CDR3γ, which is consistent with binding the negatively charged phosphate compounds (41).

A unique feature of this structure is the unusually small angle between the variable and constant regions of the $\gamma\delta$ TCR, in comparison with $\alpha\beta$ TCRs and antibodies. In addition, structural differences in Cγ and Cδ and the locations of the disulfide bond between them may indicate distinct recognition and signaling properties in comparison with $\alpha\beta$ TCRs.

THE CD3 POLYPEPTIDES

Immunoprecipitation of the TCR with anti-idiotypic antibodies after solubilization with the nonionic detergent noniodet P_{40} (NP$_{40}$) shows only the α- and β-chain heterodimer. However, the use of gentler detergents, such as digitonin or Triton-X100, reveals five other proteins [as reviewed by Terhorst et al. (5) and Klausner et al. (43)]. This is shown most clearly in a form of two-dimensional gel electrophoresis in which the first dimension is run without a reducing agent, whereas the second gel is run with one such agent (Fig. 3). The result is that most proteins can be graphed along a diagonal, whereas the subunits from disulfide-bonded multimeric proteins fall below the diagonal. Analysis of murine T cells by this technique shows the two TCR subunits (α, β) running at 40,000 MW together with CD3γ (20,000), CD3δ (25,000), CD3ϵ (20,000), and a fourth running below the diagonal at 16,000 MW (44) (ζ). The fact that the ϵ chain runs above the diagonal indicates that it migrates faster when disulfide bonds are intact than when they are broken. This in turn implies that there are intrachain disulfide bonds that hold the molecule in a compact configuration. The migration of the ζ chain is indicative of a disulfide-bonded homodimer; however, further studies have shown that the ζ chain can be part of a heterodimer in at least two forms. In murine T cells, the ζ chain can disulfide-bond with a minor variant called the η chain (45,46). This latter chain is an alternate splicing variant of the ζ-chain gene (47). This alternatively spliced species of the ζ chain is not found in significant quantities in human T cells (48). The second type of ζ chain containing heterodimer contains the γ chain associated with the FcϵRI (FcϵRIγ) and FcγRIII (CD16) receptors (49).

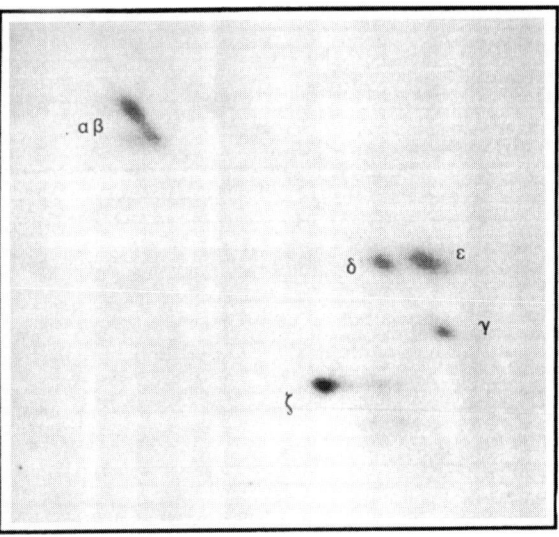

NR →

FIG. 3. T-cell receptor (TCR) $\alpha\beta$ CD3 complexes. Sodium dodecyl sulfate–polyacrylamide gel electrophoresis (SDS-PAGE) analysis of TCR-CD3 complexes studied with immunoprecipitation and the two-dimensional "diagonal" gel method of Goding et al. (291). T-cell hybridoma cells were surface labeled with iodine-125 and immunoprecipitated with an anti-TCR antibody. The first dimension was run on SDS-PAGE without reducing agents, and the second dimension included the reducing agents. Molecules that are not disulfide-linked multimers cluster along a diagonal, whereas those that are disulfide-linked multimers "fall off" the diagonal as their molecular weight decreases, as they dissociate into their component chains. Shown here are TCRα; TCRβ; and CD3 γ, δ, ϵ, and ζ chains, from Samelson et al. (44).

With regard to overall stoichiometry, current evidence suggests that there are two TCR heterodimers per CD3 cluster. This is based on a number of findings, particularly the work of Terhorst et al. (5) who showed that in a T-T hybridoma, a monoclonal antibody against one TCR$\alpha\beta$ pair could comodulate a second $\alpha\beta$ heterodimer. In addition, sucrose gradient centrifugation of TCR/CD3 showed a predicted molecular weight of 300 kD, more than 100 kD larger than expected from a minimal δ subunit complex (α, β, γ, δ, ϵ_2, ζ_2) (50). Another study suggesting that there are least two TCRs in a given CD3 complex is the Scatchard analysis, which indicated that the number of CD3ϵ molecules on a T-cell surface equals the number of $\alpha\beta$ TCRs (51–53). Finally, Fernandez-Miguel et al. (53a) showed that in T cells that have two transgenic TCRβ chains, antibodies to one Vβ can immunoprecipitate the other. It was also found that they are often close enough to allow fluorescence energy transfer, which means that the two TCRβ chains in a cluster are within 50 Å of each other (53a). Interestingly, it appears that the TCR complexes with CD3 have either CD3 γ or CD3δ but not both, and these two receptor types are expressed in different ratios in different cells. Furthermore, in cell types that express the FcϵRIγ chain, these two forms of the receptor can be further divided into those that contain the $\zeta\zeta$ homodimer and those

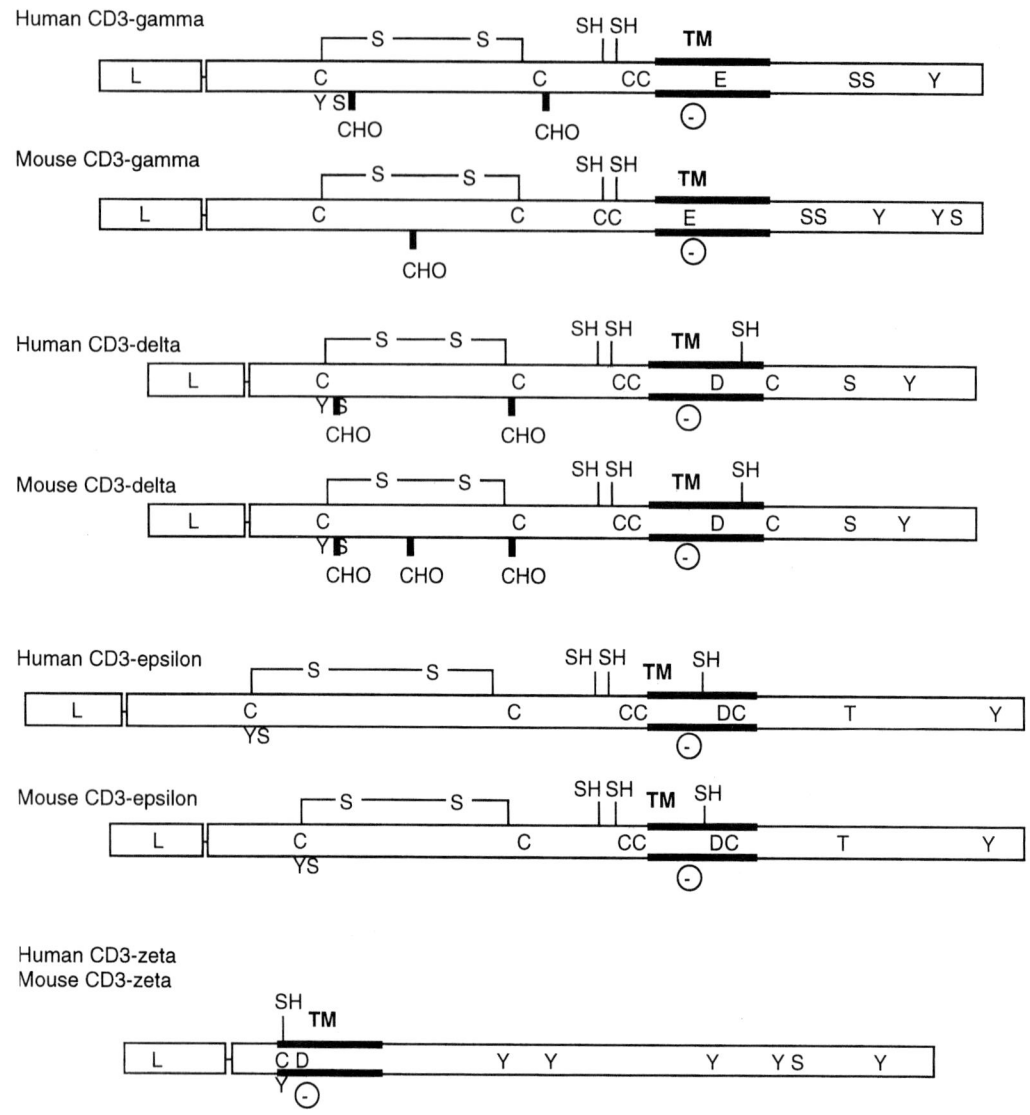

FIG. 4. Structural features of the CD3 molecules. As in Figure 1, transmembrane regions (TM) carbohydrate addition sites (CHO) and cysteine residues (C) are indicated. In addition, negatively charged transmembrane residues (D for aspartic acid and E for glutamic acid) as well putative phosphorylation sites are shown.

that have the $\zeta Fc\epsilon RI\gamma$ heterodimer (49). Thus, as shown in Fig. 4, much of the evidence to-date suggests a stoichiometry of the core cluster being $[\alpha\beta]_2[\gamma/\delta\epsilon]_2[\zeta\zeta]_4$, with a number of the variations involving FcϵR, as discussed previously. However, this has recently been disputed by Call and colleagues (53b), whose data support a single TCR heterodimer/CD3 complex.

Sequence and Structure of the CD3 Polypeptides

Figure 4 illustrates the principal structural features of the γ-, δ-, ϵ-, and ζ-chain polypeptides as derived from gene cloning and sequencing [as reviewed by Terhorst et al. (5) and Clevers et al. (54)]. The extracellular domains of the γ-, δ-, and ϵ-chains show a significant degree of similarity to one another. These domains retain the cysteines that have been shown to form intrachain disulfide bonds and each consists of a single immunoglobulin superfamily domain. The spacing of the cysteines in these domains indicates a compact immunoglobulin fold, similar to a constant region domain. All of the extracellular domains contain a pair of closely spaced cysteines just before the predicted membrane-spanning regions, and these are likely candidates for the formation of intermolecular disulfide bonds as described previously. The extracellular domain of the ζ chain consists of only nine amino acids and contains the only cysteine, which is responsible for the disulfide linkage of the $\zeta\zeta$ homodimer or the $\zeta Fc\epsilon RI\gamma$ heterodimer. In the transmembrane regions, it is particularly striking that all of the CD3 polypeptides have a conserved negatively charged amino acid, complementary to the positive charges seen in the TCR transmembrane regions and also necessary for proper assembly (55–57).

The intracellular domains of the γ, δ, ϵ, and ζ chains are the intracellular signaling "domains" of the TCR heterodimer. Each of these molecules contains an amino acid sequence motif that can mediate cellular activation (58). In T cells that are defective in ζ-chain expression, a small but significant amount of interleukin-2 production can be elicited through the use of either the superantigen SEA or an antibody specific for thy-1. However, the ζ chain is required for optimal stimulation by antigen, and the intracellular sequences responsible for this activation are contained within as few as 18 amino acids with the sequence X2YX2L/IX7YX2L/I. Both of the tyrosines in this sequence motif are absolutely required to mediate signal transduction, because mutation of either completely prevents the mobilization of free Ca^{2+} or cytolytic activity. This sequence occurs three times in the ζ chain and once in each of the CD3 γ, δ, ϵ, and $F_c\epsilon RI\gamma$ chains. There are also pairs of tyrosines present in the cytoplasmic domains of the γ, δ, ϵ, and ζ chains (Fig. 5). This sequence motif is also present in the mβ-1 and B29 chains associated with the (immunoglobulin) β-cell receptor and in the $F_c\epsilon RI\beta$ chain. The tyrosines in these cytoplasmic sequences are substrates for tyrosine phosphorylation, which is one of earliest steps in T cell signaling (58) and is thought to occur aberrantly in nonproductive T cell responses (e.g., antagonism, described later). Serine phosphorylation of the CD3γ also occurs upon antigen or mitogenic stimulation of T cells (59) and thus may play a role as well.

Intracellular Assembly and Degradation of the T-Cell Receptor–CD3 Complex

The assembly of newly formed TCRα- and TCRβ chains with the CD3 γ, δ, ϵ, and ζ chains and their intracellular fate have been studied in detail (5,43,60). Studies have focused on mutant hybridoma lines that fail to express TCR on their cell surface, and in transfection studies, cDNA has been used for the different chains in the receptor.

Experiments in a nonlymphoid cell system (61) have shown that TCRα can assemble with CD3δ and CD3ϵ but not with CD3γ and CD3ζ. In contrast, the TCRβ chain can assemble with any of the CD3 chains except the ζ chain. When the CD3ζ chain was transfected with α or β chain genes or with any of the three CD3 chains, no pairwise interaction occurred. Only when all six cDNAs were cotransfected was it shown that the ζ chain could be coprecipitated with the other chains (61). On the basis of these data, a model has been proposed to suggest that the TCRα chain pairs with CD3δ and CD3ϵ chains and that the TCRβ chain pairs with the CD3γ and CD3ϵ chains in the completed molecule. The CD3ζ chain is thought to join the TCR and other CD3 polypeptides in that last stage of assembly.

Pulse-chase experiments have shown that all six chains are assembled in the endoplasmic reticulum, transported to the Golgi apparatus, and then transferred to the plasma membrane. It also appears that the amount of ζ chain is rate limiting, as it is synthesized at only 10% the level of the other chains. This results in the vast majority of newly synthesized α, β or CD3 components being degraded within 4 hours of their synthesis. The remaining nondegraded chains are long-lived and form complete TCR/CD3 complexes with the limiting ζ chain (74). TCR/CD3 complexes lacking CD3ζ chains migrate through the endoplasmic reticulum and Golgi apparatus intact but then are transported to the lysosomes and degraded. Analysis using transfectants of individual chains or pairs of chains has shown that CD3γ and CD3δ chains contain endoplasmic reticulum retention signals. If these signals are removed, the chains are transported through the Golgi apparatus and rapidly degraded in the lysosomes. The immunological significance of this pre-Golgi degradation pathway is most evident in CD4$^+$CD8$^+$ thymocytes, in which, despite

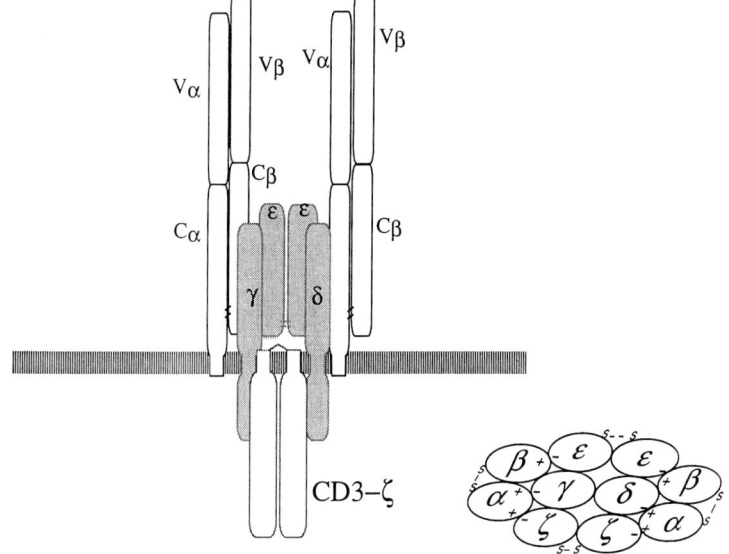

FIG. 5. A model of the T-cell receptor $\alpha\beta$–CD3 complex. Although the precise arrangement of T-cell receptor polypeptides and CD3 molecules in a given cluster is not known, the fragmentary data that exist have been schematized by Terhorst et al. (5) into this working model of the complex. This model is also consistent with the data of Fernandez-Miguel et al. (53a), but disputed by Call et al. (53b). From (5), with permission.

high levels of synthesis of both messenger RNA and protein for all the TCR, CD3, and ζ chains, surface expression is relatively low. The TCR chains in immature thymocytes seem to be selectively degraded (62). Thus, posttranslation regulation appears to be an important means of controlling the cell surface expression of TCR heterodimers.

CD3 Structure

It is very important, ultimately, to know the structure and dynamics of an entire TCR/CD3 complex. Although a number of TCR structures are now known, only recently have the first CD3 structures been solved (63). As expected, this CD3 $\epsilon\gamma$ heterodimer has immunoglobulin domains and yields some possible clues as to how it "fits" with a TCR heterodimer. It is hoped to be the harbinger of bigger pieces to this puzzle.

T-CELL RECEPTOR GENES

As shown in Fig. 6, TCR gene segments are organized similarly to segments of immunoglobulins, and the same recombination machinery is responsible for joining separate V and D segments to particular J and C segments. This was initially indicated by the fact that the characteristic seven- and nine-nucleotide conserved sequences adjacent to the V, D, and J regions with the 12- or 23-nucleotide spacing between them, first described for immunoglobulin genes, are also present in TCRs (64). The most conclusive evidence of this common rearrangement mechanism has been shown by the fact that both a naturally occurring recombination-deficient mouse strain [severe combined immune deficiency (65)] and mice engineered to lack recombinase activating genes (RAG) 1 (66) or 2 (67) are unable to rearrange either TCR or immunoglobulin gene segments properly. As with immunoglobulins, if the V region and J region gene segments are in the same transcriptional orientation, the intervening DNA is deleted during recombination. DNA circles of such material can be observed in the thymus (68,69), the principal site of TCR recombination (see later discussion). In the case of TCRβ and TCRδ, there is a single V region 3' to the C region in the opposite transcriptional orientation to J and

C regions. Thus, rearrangement of these gene segments occurs through an inversion. Variable points of joining are seen along the V, D, and J gene segments, as are random nucleotide addition (N regions) in postnatal TCRs. The addition of several nucleotides in an inverted repeat pattern, referred to a P element insertion, at the V-J junction of the TCRγ chains has also been observed (70).

Organization of the T-Cell Receptor α/δ Locus

In humans and in mice, there is a single α-chain C-region gene that is composed of four exons encoding (a) the constant region domain; (b) 16 amino acids, including the cysteine that forms the interchain disulfide bond; (c) the transmembrane and intracytoplasmic domains; and (d) the 3' untranslated region (Fig. 6). The entire α/δ locus in humans spans about 1.1 Mb (96) . The murine α/δ locus appears to be similar in size. There are 50 different J-region gene segments upstream of the C region in the murine locus. At least eight of the J-region gene elements are nonfunctional because of in-frame stop codons or rearrangement and splicing signals that are likely to be defective. A similar number of α-chain J regions are present in the human locus. This very large number of α-chain J regions, in comparison with the immunoglobulin loci, may indicate that the functional diversity contributed by the J segment of the TCR (which constitutes a major portion of the CDR3 loop) makes a special contribution to antigen recognition (see later discussion).

Both the murine and human Cδ, Jδ, and two Dδ gene segments are located between the Vα and Jα gene segments. In the murine system, there are two Jδ and two Dδ gene segments on the 5' side of Cδ, and the Cδ gene is approximately 75 kb upstream of the Cα gene but only approximately 8 kb upstream of the most 5' known Jα gene segments. The human organization is similar, with three Dα and two Jδ gene segments. Surprisingly, in both species, all of the D elements can be used in one rearranged gene rather than alternating, as is the case with TCRβ or heavy immunoglobulin; that is, Vδ, D_1, D_2, and Jδ rearrangements are frequently found in mice (71) and Vδ, D_1, D_2, D_3, and Jδ are frequently found in humans (72). This greatly increases the junctional or CDR3 diversity that is available, especially because of the potential

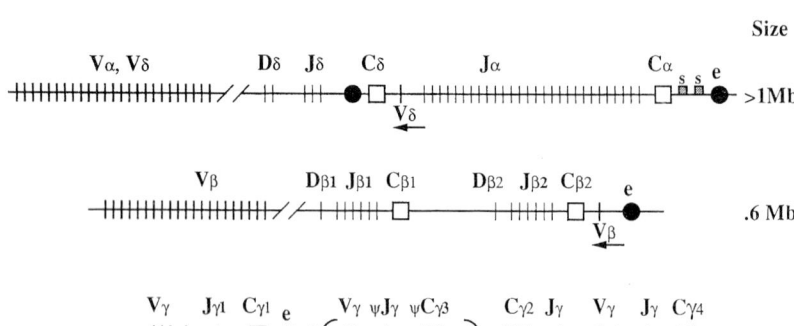

FIG. 6. T-cell receptor gene organization in mice and humans. Schematic of V, D, J, and C elements of the T-cell receptor genes. Transcriptional orientation is from left to right except where noted. The overall size of each locus is indicated on the right side. E, enhancers; S, silencer elements.

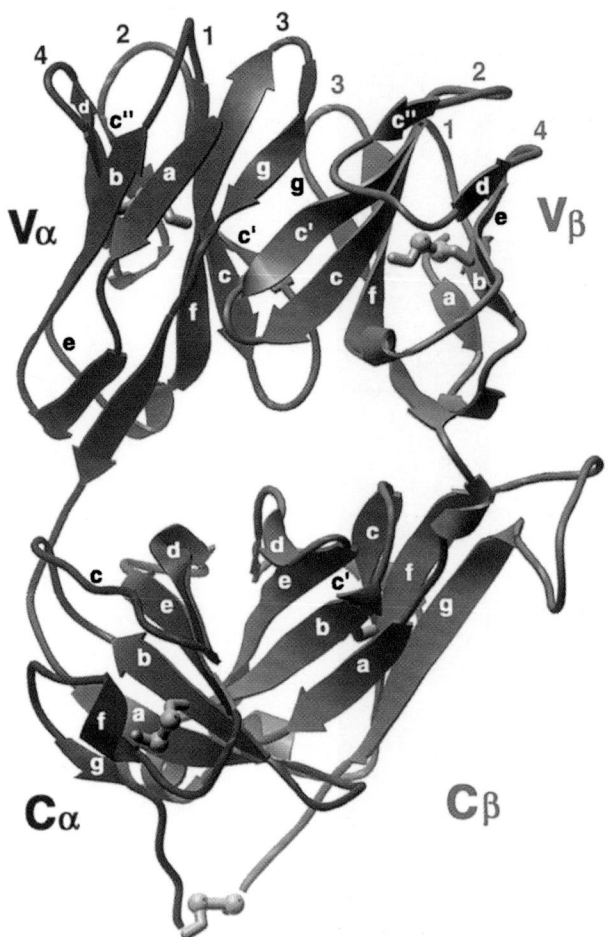

COLORPLATE 1. Complete T-cell receptor $\alpha\beta$ structure. A ribbon diagram of the first T-cell receptor $\alpha\beta$ heterodimer structure from Garcia et al. (36). In all domains, β strands are indicated by letters and the complementarity-determining regions 1, 2, 3, and 4 loops by numbers.

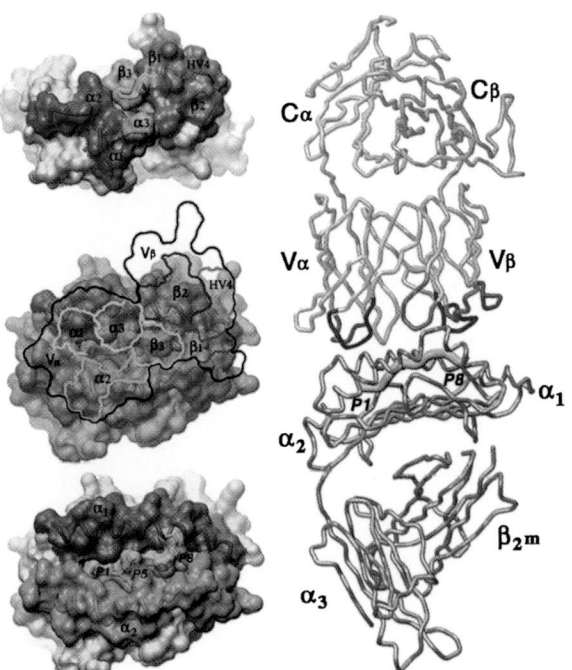

COLORPLATE 2. T-cell receptor (TCR)–peptide/major histocompatibility complex (MHC) crystal structure of a TCR-peptide/MHC complex. Peptide and complementary-determining regions are portrayed in different colors. From (36), with permission.

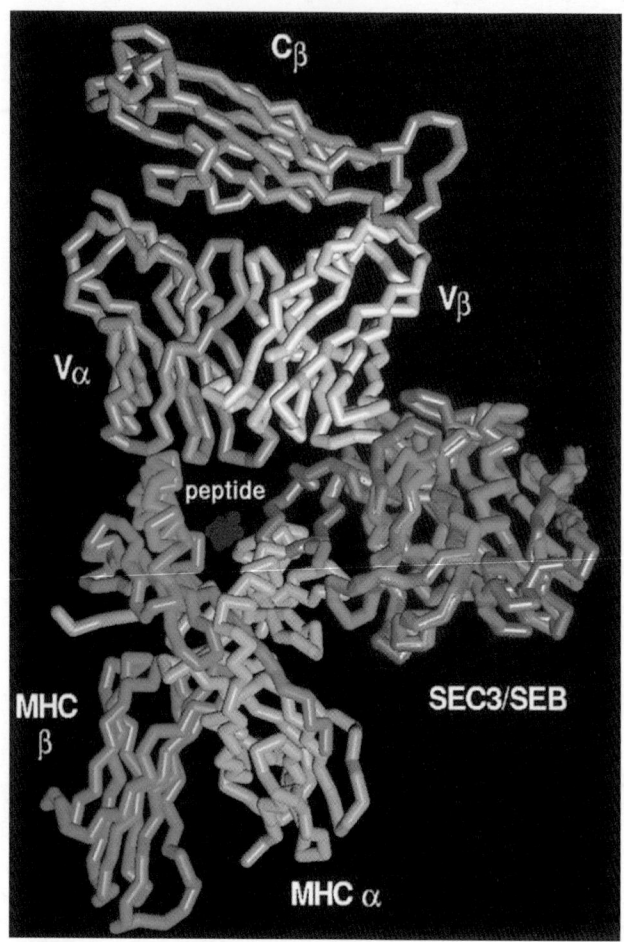

COLORPLATE 3. Crystal structure of a T-cell receptor (TCR) *β*/superantigen (SAg) complex. Fields et al. (208) crystallized TCR-SAg complexes and from the structure of the same superantigens with a class II major histocompatibility complex (MHC) molecule and were able to deduce the relative spatial arrangement of the three molecules. This model suggests that TCR does not contact the MHC very strongly, which is consistent with the relative peptide insensitivity of SAg activation.

for N-region addition in between each gene segment. This property makes TCRδ the most diverse of any of the antigens receptors known, with approximately 10^{12} to 10^{13} different amino acid sequences in a relatively small (10- to 15—amino acid) region (71).

The location of Dδ, Jδ, and Cδ genes between Vα and Jα gene segments raises the possibility that TCRδ and TCRα could share the same pool of V gene segments. There is some overlap in V gene usage; however, in the murine system, four of the commonly used Vδ genes (Vδ1, Vδ2, Vδ4, and Vδ5) are very different than known Vα sequences and they have not been found to associate with Cα (73). The other four Vδ gene families overlap with or are identical to Vα subfamilies (Vδ3, Vδ6, Vδ7, and Vδ8 with Vα6, Vα7, Vα4, and Vα11, respectively).

The mechanisms that account for the preferential usage of certain gene segments to produce δ versus α chain are not known. Although some Vδ genes are located closer to the Dδ and Jδ fragments than Vα genes (such as Vδ1), other Vδ genes (such as Vδ6) are rarely deleted by Vα-Jα rearrangements and thus seem likely to be located 5′ of many Vα gene segments.

One of the Vδ gene segments, Vδ5, is located approximately 2.5 kb to the 3′ of Cδ in the opposite transcriptional orientation and rearranges by inversion. Despite its close proximity to Dδ-Jδ gene segments, Vδ5 is not frequently found in fetal γδ T cells. Instead, the Vδ5→DJδ rearrangement predominates in adult γδ T cells.

An implicit characteristic of the α/δ gene locus is that a rearrangement of Vα to Jα deletes the entire D-J-C core of the δ-chain locus. In many αβ T cells, the α-chain locus is rearranged on both chromosomes, and thus no TCRδ could be made. In most cases, this results from Vα→Jα rearrangement, but evidence suggesting an intermediate step in the deletion of TCRδ has been reported (74). This involves rearrangements of an element termed TEA to a pseudo-Jα 3′ of Cδ. The rearrangement of TEA to this pseudo-Jα would eliminate the δ-chain locus in αβ T cells. Gene targeting of the TEA element has resulted in normal levels of αβ and γδ T cells, but usage of the most Jα genes was severely restricted (75), which suggests that its function has more to do with governing the accessibility of the most 5′ Jα genes for recombination.

Organization of the T-Cell Receptor β Locus

The entire human 685-kb β-chain gene locus was originally sequenced by Rowen et al. (76), and the organization is shown in Fig. 6. One interesting feature is the tandem nature of Jβ-Cβ in the TCRβ locus. This arrangement is preserved in all higher vertebrate species that have been characterized thus far (mouse, human, chicken, and frog). The two Cβ coding sequences are identical in the mouse and nearly so in humans and other species. Thus, it is unlikely that they represent two functionally distinct forms of Cβ. However, the Jβ clusters have relatively unique sequences, and this may thus be a mechanism for increasing the number of Jβ gene segments.

Together with the large number of Jα gene segments, there is far more combinatorial diversity (Jα × Jβ = 50 × 12 = 600) provided by J regions in αβ TCRs than in immunoglobulins.

Most of the V regions are located upstream of the J and C regions and in the same transcriptional orientation as the D and J gene element, and they rearrange to Dβ-Jβ genes through deletion. As in the case of Vδ5, a single Vβ gene, Vβ14, is located 3′ to C regions and in the opposite transcriptional orientation; thus, rearrangements involving Vβ14 occur through inversion.

In the NZW strain of mouse, there is a deletion in the β chain locus that spans from Cβ1 up to and including the Jβ2 cluster (77). In SJL, C57BR, and C57L mice, there is a large deletion (78) in the V-region locus from Vβ5 to Vβ9. These mice also express a V gene, Vβ17, which is not expressed in other strains of mice. Deletion of about half of the V genes (in SJL, C57BR, and C57L mice) does not seem to have any particular effect on the ability of these mice to mount immune responses whereas mice which have deleted the Jβ2 cluster show impaired responses (79).

Organization of the T-Cell Receptor γ Locus

The organization of the murine and human γ-chain loci are shown in Fig. 6. The human γ genes span about 150 kb (29) and are organized in a manner similar to that of the β chain locus with two Jγ-Cγ regions. An array of Vγ genes in which at least six of the V regions are pseudogenes (filled in) are located 5′ to these Jγ-Cγ clusters, and each of the V genes are potentially capable of rearranging to any of the five J regions. The sequences of the two human Cγ regions are very similar overall and differ significantly only in the second exon. In Cγ2, this exon is duplicated two or three times, and the cysteine that forms in the interchain disulfide bond is absent. Thus, Cγ2-bearing human T cells have an extra large γ chain (55,000 MW) that is not disulfide-bonded to its δ-chain partner.

The organization of the murine γ chain genes is very different from that of the human genes in that there are three separate rearranging loci that span about 205 kb (117). Of four murine Cγ genes, Cγ3 is apparently a pseudogene in BALB/c mice, and the Jγ3-Cγ3 region is deleted in several mouse strains, including C57 Bl/10. Cγ1 and Cγ2 are very similar in coding sequences. The major differences between these two genes is in the five–amino acid deletion in the Cγ2 gene, which is located in the C II exon at the amino acid terminal of the cysteine residue used for the disulfide formation with the δ chain. The Cγ4 gene differs significantly in sequences from the other Cγ genes (in 66% overall amino acid identity). In addition, the Cγ4 sequences contains a 17–amino acid insertion (in comparison with Cγ1) in the C II exon located at similar position as that of the five–amino acid deletion of the Cγ2 gene (G. Kershard and S. M. Hedrick, unpublished results).

Each of the Cγ genes is associated with a single Jγ gene segment. The sequences of Jγ1 and Jγ2 are identical at the amino acid level, whereas Jγ4 differs from Jγ1 and Jγ2 at 9 of 19 amino acid residues.

The murine Vγ genes usually rearrange to the Jγ-Cγ gene that is most proximal and in the same transcription orientation. Thus, Vγ1.1 rearranges to Jγ4; Vγ1.2 rearranges to Jγ2; and Vγ2, Vγ3, Vγ4, and Vγ5 rearrange to Jγ1. Interestingly, it appears that some Vγ genes are rearranged and expressed preferentially during γδ T cell ontogeny and in different adult tissues as well (80).

Transcriptional Control of the T-Cell Receptor Genes

Transcriptional regulation of the TCR genes has been studied extensively; enhancer sequences were first identified in the TCRβ locus, 3′ of Cβ2 (81,82) and subsequently for the other TCR loci as well [reviewed by Lefranc and Lefranc (29)], as indicated in Fig. 6. These TCR enhancers all share sequence similarities. Some of the transcriptional factors that bind to the TCR genes are also found to regulate immunoglobulin gene expressions. Work by Sleckman et al. (83) has shown that the TCRα enhancer (Eα) is not only important for normal rearrangement and expression for the α chain locus but is also required for a normal expression level of mature TCRδ transcripts. Also interesting is the work of Lauzurica and Krangel (84,85), who showed that a human TCRδ enhancer containing mini-locus in transgenic mice is able to rearrange equally well in αβ T cells as in αδ T cells but that an Eα-containing construct was active only in αβ-lineage T cells. Like immunoglobulin genes, promoter sequences are located 5′ to the V gene segments. Although D→Jβ rearrangement and transcription occur fairly often in B cells and in B-cell tumors (86), Vβ rearrangement and transcription appear highly specific to T cells. In addition to enhancers, there are also "silencer" sequences 3′ of Cα (87,88) and in the Cγ1 locus (89). It has been suggested that these "repressor sites" could turn off the expression of either of these genes, influencing T cell differentiation toward either the αβ or the γδ T-cell lineage.

Chromosomal Locations of T-Cell Receptor Genes and Translocations Associated with Disease

The chromosomal locations of the different TCR loci have been delineated in both mice and humans, and the results are summarized in Table 1. One significant factor in cancers of hematopoietic cells are chromosomal translocations, which result in the activation of genes that are normally turned off or in the inactivation of genes that are normally turned on. Thus, B or T lymphocyte neoplasia is frequently associated with interchromosomal or intrachromosomal rearrangements of immunoglobulin or TCR loci and, in some cases, both (90,91).

These translocations seemed to mediated by the V(D)J recombinase machinery, indicating the inherent danger and need for tight regulation of this pathway. Such rearrangements are particularly common in the α/δ locus, perhaps because this locus spans the longest developmental window

TABLE 1. *Chromosomal locations of T-cell receptor, immunoglobulin, and related loci in mouse and human*

	Mouse chromosome	Human chromosome
TCR-α	14	14(q11–q12)
TCR-δ	14	14(q11–q12)
IgH	12	14(qter)
TCR-β	6	7(q35)
CD4	6	12
CD8	6	2(p11)
Igκ	6	2(p12)
TCR-γ	13	7(p14)
CD3-γ	9	11(q23)
CD3-δ	9	11(q23)
CD3-ε	9	11(q23)
CD3-ζ	1	1
Thy-1	9	11(q23)
Igλ	16	22(q11.2)
MHC	17	6(p21)
Pre-Tα	17	6

Ig, immunoglobulin; IgH, heavy-chain immunoglobulin; MHC, major histocompatibility complex; TCR, T-cell receptor.

in terms of gene expression, with TCRδ being the first and TCRα the last gene to rearrange during T cell ontogeny (as discussed in more detail later). In addition, the α/δ locus is in excess of 1 Mb in size, and this provides a larger target for rearrangement than does either TCRβ or TCRγ. Interestingly, in humans, TCRαδ is on the same chromosome as the heavy immunoglobulin locus, and VH→Jα rearrangements (by inversion) have been observed in some human tumor material (92,93). The functional significance of this is not known.

Particularly frequent is the chromosome 8–14 translocation [t(8;14) (q24;q11)], which joins the α/δ locus to the c-myc gene, analogous to the C-myc→heavy immunoglobulin translocation in many murine myeloma tumors and in Burkitt's lymphomas in humans. In one cell line, a rearrangement occurs between the Jα-region coding sequences and in a region 3′ of c-myc (94). In both B- and T-cell malignancies, the translocation of c-myc into heavy immunoglobulin or TCRα/β appears to increase the expression of c-myc and may be a major factor in the unregulated cell growth that characterizes cancerous cells. Other putative proto-oncogenes that have been found translocated into the TCRα/β locus are the LIM domain–containing transcription factors Ttg-1 (95) and Ttg-2 (96,97), which are involved in neural development; the helix-loop-helix proteins Lyl-1 (98) and Scl (99), which are involved in early hematopoietic development; and the homeobox gene Hox 11 (100), which is normally active in the liver. How these particular translocations contribute to malignancy is unknown, but they presumably causes aberrations in gene expression that contribute to cell growth or escape from normal regulation. In patients infected with the human T-cell leukemia virus type I, there are large numbers of similar translocations, and it is thought that this virus itself is not directly leukemogenic but acts by causing aberrant rearrangements in the T cells that it infects, some of which become malignant.

Another disorder that exhibits frequent TCR and immunoglobulin locus translocations is ataxia telangiectasia, a autosomal recessive disorder characterized by ataxia, vascular telangiectasis, immunodeficiency, an increased incidence of neoplasia, and an increased sensitivity to ionizing radiation. Peripheral blood lymphocytes from patients with ataxia telangiectasia have an especially high frequency of translocations involving chromosomes 7 and 14 (101). These sites correspond to the TCRγ, TCRβ, and TCRα loci and to the immunoglobulin heavy-chain locus. Thus, it appears as though one of the characteristics of patients with ataxia telangiectasia is a relatively error-prone rearrangement process that indiscriminately recombines genes that have the TCR and immunoglobulin rearrangement signals (102).

Allelic Exclusion

In immunoglobulins, only one allele of the heavy chain locus and one of the light chain alleles are normally productively rearranged and expressed; this phenomenon is termed *allelic exclusion* (see Chapter 5). With regard to αβ TCR expression, current data indicate that, although TCRβ exhibits allelic exclusion (103), TCRα does not (104,105) and that some mature T cells express two functional TCRα chains. As the chances of forming an in-frame joint with any antigen receptor is only one in three, the probability that a T cell would have two productively rearranged TCRα genes is only 1/3 ×x 1/3 (1/9), or 11%. However, even when this happens, the two TCRα chains may not form heterodimers equally well with the single TCRβ that is expressed, and thus only one heterodimer may be expressed.

Data strongly suggest an important role for the pre-TCR heterodimer (e.g., pre-Tα:TCRβ) in blocking further TCRβ rearrangement and thus ensuring allelic exclusion at that locus (106,107). In particular, pre-Tα–deficient mice had a significant increase in the number of cells with two productive TCRβ rearrangements, in comparison with wild-type mice (106).

Commitment to the αβ Lineage versus the γδ Lineage

One important issue in T-cell development concerns the lineage relationship between αβ and γδ T cells: What governs the differentiation of the thymic stem cells to become either αβ or γδ T cells? Two models have been proposed. In one, which could be termed the *sequential rearrangement model* (24), the precursor cells first rearrange the γ- and δ-chain genes. The cells that fail to made a functional TCRγ or TCRδ would progress to the αβ lineage and attempt to rearrange the TCRβ- and TCRα-chain loci. According to the second model, referred to as the *separate lineage model,* T cells differentiate into two lineages before rearrangement. One line of evidence that supports the sequential rearrangement model is a study in which δ-chains were often found to be rearranged on chromosomes that undergo an α-chain rearrangement (108), but a subsequent more extensive investigation revealed most unrearranged sequences (109). Further

evidence in favor of the separate lineage model comes from transgenic mice bearing rearranged TCRγ- and TCRδ-chain genes. In these mice, although all of the precursor cells express functional γδ genes, there are normal numbers of αβ T cells in the thymus (110). This is the opposite of what would be expected if successful γδ TCR expression blocked the rearrangement of the α and β loci. In another study of early αβ precursor thymocytes, it was found that, in half the cells, TCRδ had not rearranged at all but the TEA transcript was being expressed (111), presumably just before Vα→Jα rearrangement. In mice that are defective in either αβ TCR or γδ TCR, there is no obvious effect on the development of the remaining lineage (112–114). Taken together, almost all of the data in the literature supports a separate lineage model and not sequential rearrangement.

Other Genetic Mechanisms

One important mechanism of antibody diversification that has not been reproducibly found in TCR genes is somatic hypermutation. In antibodies, this form of mutation typically raises the affinities of antigen-specific immunoglobulins several orders of magnitude, typically from the micromolar range (10^{-6} M) to the nanomolar range (10^{-9} M) for protein antigens. It is now known that most cell surface receptors that bind ligands on other cell surfaces, including TCRs, typically have affinities in the micromolar range but that they compensate for this relatively low affinity by engaging multiple receptors simultaneously (e.g., increasing the valency) and by functioning in a confined, largely two-dimensional volume (e.g., between two cells). Cells employing such receptors most probably require weak (but highly specific) interactions so that they can disengage quickly (115,116). The rapid "off" rate seen with TCRs has even been postulated to amplify the effects of small numbers of ligands (i.e. "the serial engagement model" described later).

There has also been no enduring evidence for a naturally secreted form of either an αβ or γδ TCR. Again, it can be argued that such a molecule would have no obvious use because it is too low in affinity to bind ligands efficiently. In the case of most TCRs, the concentration of protein would have to be very high to achieve an effect similar to soluble antibodies (in the milligram/milliliter range).

A third mechanism seen in antibodies but not TCRs is CH switching, which allows different immunoglobulin isotypes to maintain a given V region specificity and associate it with different C regions that have different properties in solution (such as complement fixation and basophil binding). Because there is no secreted form of the TCR, it is not obvious how this would be useful.

BIOCHEMISTRY OF αβ T-CELL RECEPTOR–LIGAND INTERACTIONS

Although it has long been established that T cells recognize a peptide in association with an MHC molecule, a formal biochemical demonstration that this was caused by TCR binding to a peptide/MHC complex took many years to establish. Part of the difficulty in obtaining measurements of this type has been the intrinsically membrane-bound nature of MHC and TCR molecules. Another major problem is that the affinities are relatively low, in the micromolar range, which is too unstable to measure by conventional means.

The problem of normally membrane-bound molecules can be circumvented by expressing soluble forms of TCR and MHC, which is also essential for structural studies (see previous discussion). For TCRs, there have been many successful strategies, including replacement of the transmembrane regions with signal sequences for glycolipid linkage (117), expression of chains without transmembrane regions in either insect or mammalian cells (36,118), or a combination of cysteine mutagenesis and *E. coli* expression (37). Unfortunately, no one method seems to work for all TCR heterodimers, although the combination of insect cell expression and leucine zippers at the C-terminal to stabilize heterodimer expression has been successful in many cases (119). The production of soluble forms of MHC molecule has a much longer history, starting with the enzymatic cleavage of detergent-solubilized native molecules (120), as well as some of the same methods employed for TCR such as glycophosphotidyl inositol linkage (121), *E. coli* expression and refolding (122,123), and insect cell expression of truncated (or leucine zippered) molecules (124). One interesting variant that seems necessary for the stable expression of some class II MHC molecules in insect cells has been the addition of a covalent peptide to the N-terminal of the β chain (125).

The first measurements of TCR affinities for peptide/MHC complexes were made by Matsui et al. (126) and Weber et al.

(127). Matsui et al. used a high concentration of soluble peptide/MHC to block the binding of a labeled anti-TCR Fab to T cells specific for those complexes, obtaining a binding constant (K_d) of approximately 50 μM for several different T cells and two different cytochrome peptide/IE^K complexes (as shown in Table 2). Weber et al. used a soluble TCR to inhibit the recognition of a flu peptide/IE^d complex by a T cell and obtained a K_d value of approximately 10 μM. Although these measurements were an important start in TCR biochemistry, they gave no direct information about the kinetics of TCR-ligand interactions. Fortunately, the development of surface plasmon resonance instruments, particularly the BIAcore^{TM} (Pharmacia Biosensor) with its remarkable sensitivity to weak macromolecular interactions (128), has allowed rapid progress in this area. In the BIAcore technique, one component is covalently cross-linked to a surface, and then buffer containing the ligand is passed in solution over it. The binding of even approximately 5% of the surface-bound material is sufficient to cause a detectable change in the resonance state of gold electrons on the surface. This method allows the direct measurement of association and dissociation rates—that is, kinetic parameters—and also has the advantage of being completely cell free. Figure 7 shows the type of resonance profile obtained contrasting the weak but specific binding of a particular peptide/MHC complex in solution to a bound TCR with the binding pattern of an antibody to the same TCR. The affinity of cytochrome c/IE^K/2B4 TCR measured with this instrument (129) matches well (Table 1) with previous results obtained from cell-based measurements. These and other data [reviewed by Davis et al. (116)] showed definitively that TCR and peptide-loaded MHC molecules

TABLE 2. *T-cell receptor–ligand binding*

T cell	Ligand	K_D (μM)	k_{on} (M^{-1}s^{-1})	k_{off} (s^{-1})	Method	Reference
T$_H$ cells						
5C.C7	MCC/E^k	50	—	—	anti-TCR comp.	Matsui et al. (126)
2B4	MCC/E^k	50	—	—	anti-TCR comp.	Matsui et al. (126)
2B4	MCC/E^k	30	—	—	anti-P/MHC comp.	Matsui et al. (129)
2B4	MCC/E^k	90	600	0.057	BIA1	Matsui et al. (129)
228.5	MCC 99E/E^k	50	—	—	anti-TCR comp.	Matsui et al. (126)
14.3.d	Flu H1N1/E^d	~10	—	—	sol. TCR	Weber et al. (127)
14.3.d	SEC1,2,3	5.4–18.2	>100,000	>0.1	BIA1	Malchiodi et al. (206)
HA1.7	HA/DR1	>25	—	—	BIA1	Seth et al. (281)
HA1.7	SEB	0.82	13,000	0.001	BIA1	Seth et al. (281)
T$_C$ cell						
2C	p2Ca/L^d	0.5	11,000	0.0055	anti-TCR comp.	Sykulev et al. (138)
2C	p2Ca/L^d	0.1	21,0000	0.026	BIA1	Corr et al. (282)
2C	QL9/L^d	0.065	53,000	0.003	Labeled MHC	Sykulev et al. (283)
4G3	pOV/L^b	0.65	22,000	0.02	Labeled MHC	Sykulev et al. (283)
42.12	OVA/K^b	6.5	3,135	0.02	BIA4	Alam et al. (140)
2C	p2Ca/L^d	3.3	8,300	0.027	BIA1	Garcia et al. (131)
HY	M80/D^b	23.4	6,200	0.145	BIA1	Garcia et al. (131)
HY	CD8 α/β + M80/D/^{b}	2.0	5,100	0.01	BIA1	Garcia et al. (131)
2C	CD8 α/β + p2Ca/L^d	0.32	1,2000	0.0038	BIA1	Garcia et al. (131)

Note: BIA1 = TCR amine coupled, BIA2 = TCR cysteine coupled, BIA3 = MHC–peptide amine coupled in competition experiment, and BIA4 = TCR coupled by using H57 antibody and MHC coupled via amine chemistry. comp. MHC, major histocompatibility complex; sol., soluble; TCR, T-cell receptor.

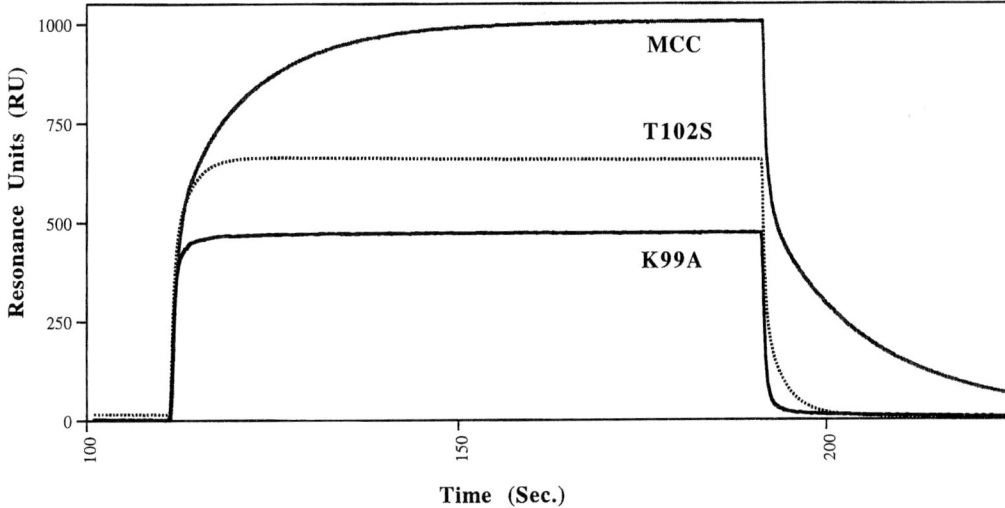

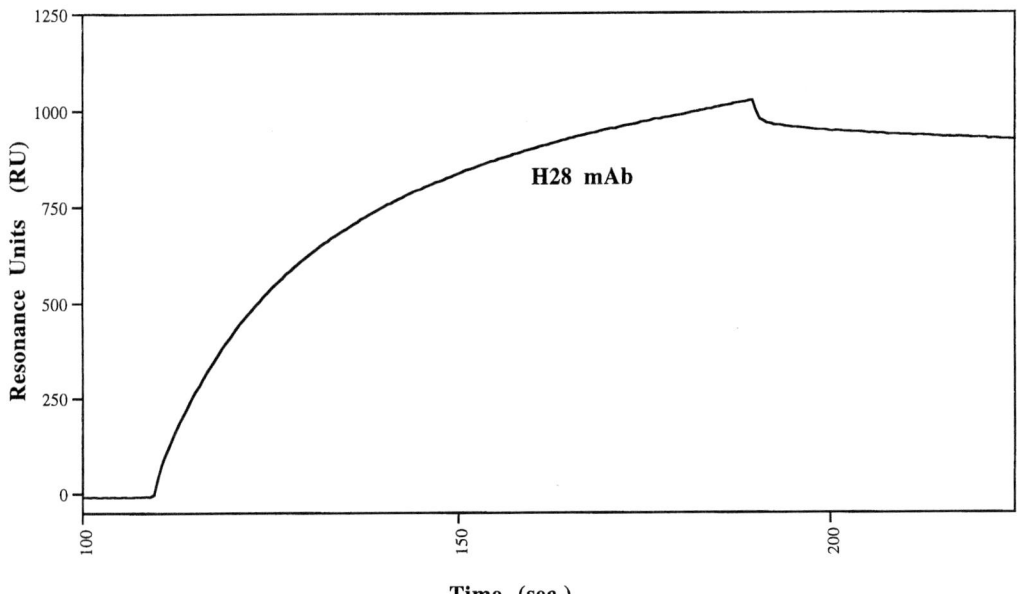

FIG. 7. T-cell receptor (TCR) binding to peptide/major histocompatibility complex (MHC). **Top:** A typical surface plasmon resonance analysis of the binding characteristics of a TCR specific for a cytochrome c peptide bound to the mouse class II MHC molecule, IE^K. Here the soluble TCR is fixed to a solid support and different peptide/MHCs are passed over it in solution. The most robust profile represents the original peptide MCC (residues 88 to 103) complexes to IE^K, a strong agonist, whereas T102s represents a weak agonist, K99A, a null peptide (see also Tables 1 and 2). These profiles are compared to the **bottom** trace in the figure, which shows an antibody specific for $C\alpha$ binding to the same TCR. Note the sharper initial phase, which is a measure of the association rate, and the very stable decay phase, which is a measure of the dissociation rate. The x-axis is the time in seconds, and the y-axis is in arbitrary resonance units. Figure courtesy of D. S. Lyons.

alone are able to interact and also that expression in a soluble form has not altered their ability to bind to each other. Because of its sensitivity and ease of use, the surface plasmon resonance technique has become the method of choice for measuring the kinetics of TCR binding to its ligands. As shown in Table 2, these measurements show that although the "on"

rates of TCRs binding to peptide/MHC molecules vary from very slow (1,000 M per second) to moderately fast (200,000 M per second), their "off" rates fall in a relatively narrow range (0.5 to 0.01 second^{-1}) or a $t_{1/2}$ of 12 to 30 seconds at 25°C. This is in the general range of other membrane-bound receptors that recognize membrane molecules on other cells

(114), but it has also been noted that most TCRs have very slow "on" rates (130), which seems to reflect a flexibility in the binding site that might help to foster cross-reactivity (see later discussion). In the case of the class I MHC-restricted TCR, 2C, this relatively fast "off" rate may be stabilized (10-fold) if soluble CD8 is introduced (131), but this result is controversial (132). CD8 stabilization of TCR binding has been seen by Renard et al. (133) in their unique cell-based TCR labeling assay; however, no enhancement of TCR binding has been seen with soluble CD4 (134). Although most of the BIAcore measurements cited earlier were performed at 25°C because of instrument limitations, the "off" rates are likely to be much faster (10 to 20 times) at 37°C (135).

To what extent can a T-cell response be predicted on the basis of the binding characteristic of its TCR to a ligand? One of the most intriguing discoveries concerning T-cell reactivity has been the phenomenon of altered peptide ligands. These are single–amino acid variants of antigenic peptides that change either the nature or the degree of the T-cell response (partial agonists) or prevent a response to a normally stimulating ligand (antagonists) (136,137). Discussions concerning the mechanism of these "altered peptide" responses have focused on whether they are caused by some conformational phenomenon involving TCRs or CD3 molecules or both or caused by affinity or kinetic characteristics. The data now available indicate that most, but not all, T-cell responses correlate very well with the binding characteristics of their T-cell receptors. In particular, Sykulev et al. (138) first noted that higher affinity peptide variants elicited more robust T-cell responses. Subsequently, Matsui et al. (129) found that in a series of three agonist peptides, increasing dissociation rates correlated with decreasing agonist activity. Lyons et al. (139) found that this correlation extended to antagonist peptides in the same antigen system (moth cytochrome c/E^k). They also showed that although an antagonist peptide might differ only slightly in affinity in comparison with the weakest agonist, its dissociation rate differed by 10-fold or more (see

Table 2). This data in a class II MHC-restricted system is largely supported by the studies of Alam et al. (140) in a class I MHC system, who also saw a drop-off in affinities and an increase in "off" rates (with one exception, as noted in Table 2) with antagonist versus agonist ligands. In the cell-based TCR labeling system of Luescher, a survey of related peptide ligands of varying potency also revealed a general, but not absolute, correlation between receptor occupancy and stimulatory ability (141). Thus, although there is a general trend toward weaker T-cell responses and faster "off" rates and lower affinities, this does not seem to be an absolute rule, and thus other factors may be important in some cases. Alternatively, Holler et al. (142) suggested that some or all of the discrepancies may derive from differences in peptide stability (in the MHC) between the relatively short (minutes) time scale of BIAcore analysis at 25°C, in comparison with the much longer (days) cellular assays at 37°C.

How might the relatively small differences in the binding characteristics of the ligands summarized in Tables 2 and 3 cause such different T-cell signaling outcomes as agonism or antagonism? As McKeithan (143) and Rabinowitz et al. (144) noted, any multistep system such as T-cell recognition has an inherent ability to amplify small differences in signals that are received on the cell surface to much larger differences at the end of the pathway—in this case, gene transcription in the nucleus. Thus, antagonism may occur at one threshold and an agonist response at another. Alternatively, an antagonist ligand may traverse the activation pathway just far enough to use up some critical substrate, as proposed by Lyons et al. (139). Yet another possibility that has also been suggested is that some antagonists may act even earlier, by blocking TCR clustering at the cell surface (145).

One controversy that bears on this data is the *serial engagement model* of Vallitutti et al. (146) and Viola and Lanzavecchia (147), which proposes that one way in which a small number of peptide/MHC complexes can initiate T-cell activation is by transiently binding many TCRs in a sequential

TABLE 3. *Weak agonist–antagonist binding*

T cell	Ligand	Type	K_D (μM)	k_{off}(S^{-1})	$t_{1/2}$	Method	Reference
2B4	MCC/E^k	Strong agonist	90	0.057	12	BIA1	Matsui et al. (129)
			40	0.063	11	BIA2	Lyons et al. (139)
2B4	PCC/E^k	Agonist	80	0.09	8.0	BIA1	Matsui et al. (129)
2B4	MCC 102S/E^k	Weak agonist	240	0.36	2.0	BIA2	Lyons et al. (139)
2B4	MCC 102N/E^k	Weak agonist	320	0.44	1.6	BIA2	Lyons et al. (139)
2B4	MCC 99R/E^k	Antagonist	500	4.8	0.15	BIA2	Lyons et al. (139)
			330	—	—	BIA3	
2B4	MCC 102G/E^k	Antagonist	1500	5.1	0.14	BIA2	Lyons et al. (139)
			900–1200	—	—	BIA3	
2B4	MCC 99Q/E^k	Weak antagonist	2100	—	—	BIA3	Lyons et al. (139)
42.12	OVA/K^b	Strong agonist	6.5	0.02	24.5	BIA4	Alam et al. (140)
42.12	OVA E1/K^b	Weak agonist	22.6	0.068	7.3	BIA4	Alam et al. (140)
42.12	V-OVA/K^b	Antagonist	29.8	0.039	12.9	BIA4	Alam et al. (140)
42.12	OVA R4/K^b	Antagonist	57.1	0.146	3.4	BIA4	Alam et al. (140)
42.12	OVA K4/K^b	Null	>360	>0.2	<2.5	BIA4	Alam et al. (140)

See Table 2 for explanation of BIAcore methods.

manner. Estimates based on TCR down-regulation have suggested that one peptide/MHC complex could bind to as many as 200 TCR molecules in succession (147). Although the dissociation rates reviewed here show that TCR binding is likely to be very transient, they do not in fact, support the statement that more interactions are better. This is because, in most cases, improvements in TCR-peptide/MHC stability within any one system result in a more robust T cell response. This has been shown most spectacularly in the work of Holler et al. (142), who selected a nanomolar-affinity TCR from a mutagenized library expressed in yeast. With an approximately 100-fold slower "off" rate than the original, this TCR should have been only poorly stimulatory, according to the serial engagement model. Instead, T cells bearing it were considerably more sensitive to antigen.

Role of CD4 and CD8

What is the role of CD4 and CD8 with regard to the T-cell response to agonist and antagonist peptides? In the case of a T helper cell response, the presence of CD4 greatly augments the amount of cytokine produced and, in some cases, determines whether there is a response at all [as reviewed by Janeway (148)]. Much of the effect of CD4 seems to come from the recruitment of Lck to the TCR/CD3 complexes. In addition, there is a significant positive effect even with CD4 molecules that are unable to bind Lck, and thus there appears to be an affect on TCR-ligand interaction as well. Nonetheless, although a weak binding of CD4 to class II MHC has been observed (134), there is no apparent cooperativity with regard to TCR binding to peptide/MHC, in contrast to the case of CD8 and class I–specific TCRs (see later discussion). Together with the low-resolution structure of CD4–class II MHC (149), the classical model of CD4 binding to the same MHC as a TCR that it is associated with (148) seems untenable. However, there is abundant evidence that CD4 molecules do associate with TCRs, especially on previously activated T cells (150). Thus, models in which CD4 cross-linking to class II MHC indirectly supports TCR binding to peptide/MHCs and potentiates signaling through the delivery of Lck seem more likely (see later discussion).

In addition, Irvine et al. (151), using a single-peptide labeling technique, showed an appreciable T-cell response to even one agonist peptide, resulting in a "stop" signal for the T cell and a small but detectable rise in intracellular calcium. Both of these effects are attenuated by antibody blockade of CD4, in such a way that many more (25 to 30) peptides are required in order to elicit a stop signal and a calcium flux. How could CD4 be facilitating the recognition of small numbers of peptides? Irvine et al. (151) proposed a "pseudodimer" model that suggests that a CD4 molecule associated with a TCR binding to an agonist peptide/MHC could bind laterally to an endogenous peptide/MHC that is also being bound by an adjacent TCR. This takes advantage of the apparent abundance of endogenous peptide/MHCs that can be bound by a given TCR (152) and uses two weak interactions (CD4→

class II MHC and TCR→endogenous peptide/MHC) to help create a dimeric "trigger" for activation.

CD8 also greatly augments the response of class I MHC-specific T cells (148) and binds to class I MHC in much the same manner as CD4 (153). Overall, it seems likely that each of these co-receptor molecules has two roles: to stabilize TCR–ligand interactions physically and to aid in signaling by recruiting Lck. Consistent with this are data showing that CD4 can convert an antagonist peptide into a weak agonist (154,155), although CD4 has no apparent effect on antagonism (156,157). These results indicate that CD4 acts to augment T cell responses, even of very weak ligands, but that antagonism per se exerts its effects before CD4 engagement.

TOPOLOGY OF T-CELL RECEPTOR–PEPTIDE/MAJOR HISTOCOMPATIBILITY COMPLEX INTERACTIONS

An analysis of TCR sequence diversity has shown that most amino acid variation resides in the region between the V- and J-region gene segments, which corresponds to the CDR3 regions of antibodies (158). This has led to models in which the CDR3 loops of $V\alpha$ and $V\beta$ make the principal contacts with the antigenic peptide bound to the MHC (158–160). Support for such a model has come from many studies that have shown that the CDR3 sequences of TCRs are important predictors of specificity [as reviewed by Davis and Bjorkman (158)] as well as the elegant mutagenesis studies of Engel and Hedrick (161), who showed that a single CDR3 point mutation could alter the specificity of a TCR, and Katayama et al. (162), who showed also that a CDR3 "transplant" could confer the specificity of the donor TCR onto the recipient. In addition, a novel approach to TCR-ligand interactions was developed by Jorgensen et al. (163,164), who made single–amino acid changes in an antigenic peptide at positions that affect T-cell recognition but not MHC binding. These variant peptides are then used to immunize mice that express either the α or β chain of a TCR that recognizes the original peptide, and the responding T cells are analyzed. Using these hemitransgenic mice allows the resulting T cells to keep half of the receptor constant while allowing considerable variation in the chain that pairs with it. The results from this study and from work in another system by Sant'Angelo et al. (165) are very similar in that every mutation at a TCR-sensitive residue triggered a change in the CD3 sequence of $V\alpha$, $V\beta$, or both and, in some cases, changed the $V\alpha$ or $V\beta$ gene segment as well (as summarized in Fig. 8). One of the more striking examples of a CDR3-peptide interaction occurred in the cytochrome c system, in which a Lys→Glu change in the central TCR determinant on the peptide triggered a Glu→Lys charge reversal in the $V\alpha$ CDR3 loop, which argues for a direct Lys→Glu contact between the two molecules (199).

Another interesting finding was the order of $V\alpha$→$V\beta$ preference going from the N-terminal to the C-terminal residues of the peptides. This led Jorgensen et al. (163,164) to propose a "linear" topology of TCR-peptide/MHC interaction in

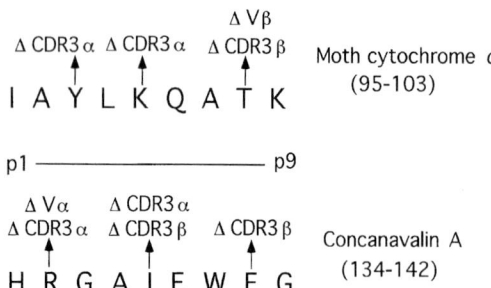

FIG. 8. Sensitivity of T-cell receptor (TCR) complementarity-determining region 3 (CDR3) sequences and Vα/Vβ usage to changes in the antigen peptide. This figure summarizes the data of Jorgensen et al. (163,164) and Sant'Angelo et al. (165), who immunized single-chain transgenic mice (TCRα or TCRβ) with antigenic peptides (MCC or CVA) altered at residues that influence T-cell recognition but not major histocompatibility complex binding. These data show that such changes invariably affect the CDR3 sequences of Vα or Vβ or both and that there appears to be a definite topology in which Vα governs the N-terminal region and Vβ seems more responsible for the c-terminal portion of the peptide.

which the CDR3 loops of Vα and Vβ line up directly over the peptide. Sant'Angelo et al. (165) proposed an orientation of the TCR in which the CDR3 loops are perpendicular to the peptide. This was based partially on intriguing data they found that suggested an interaction between the CDR1 of Vα and an N-terminal residue of the peptide. A third orientation was proposed by Sun et al. (166) on the basis of the analysis of a large number of class I MHC mutants and their effect on TCR reactivity. This produced a roughly diagonal footprint of TCRs over the MHC, in comparison with the two previous models. On the other hand, an extensive class II MHC mutagenesis study failed to reveal a consistent "footprint" of TCR interaction and furthermore revealed that the pattern of TCR sensitivity was remarkably labile and highly dependent on sequences in the TCR CDR3 region or the peptide (167).

This controversy has been largely resolved by the work of Garcia et al. (36) and Garboczi et al. (37), who, nearly simultaneously, solved the crystal structures of two different TCR-peptide/class I MHCs. These studies show a TCR binding surface much like an antibody fitting down between the two opposite "high points" of the class I MHC α helices, in a roughly diagonal configuration. In these structures, one of which is shown in Colorplate 2, the CDR3 loops are centrally located over the peptide, but the Vα CDR1 and the Vβ CDR1 are also in a position to contact the N-terminal and C-terminal peptide residues, respectively. Such a contact between Vα CDR1 and an N-terminal residue was seen in the structure of Garboczi et al., whereas that of Garcia et al. has insufficient resolution at this point. There are now many additional structures including two involving class II MHCs, all of which exhibit a similar orientation, albeit with an approximately

20° variation in orientation (168,169). This oriented recognition constitutes a major departure from antibody–antigen interactions and may reflect a need to accommodate other molecules into a particular configuration that is optimal for signaling.

T-Cell Receptor Plasticity

As αβ T-cell receptor heterodimers are first selected in the thymus for reactivity to self-peptides bound to MHC molecules (see Chapter 9), all foreign peptide–reactive TCRs could be considered to be inherently cross-reactive. Indeed, a number of T cells have reactivity to very different peptide sequences, as shown by Nanda et al. (170). It has also been argued by Mason (171) that the universe of peptides is so large that each T cell must, on average, be cross-reactive to approximately 10^6 different peptides (although many of the differences in peptide sequence in this calculation would not be accessible to the TCR, being buried in the MHC binding groove). A large-scale screen of a random nonamer-peptide library with different T cells does turn up a great many stimulatory peptides, most with nonaccessible residues, but some with significantly different sequences, so that, in some cases, peptides with completely different sequences can activate the same T cell (172). Analyses of a T-cell hybrid that could recognize either a lysine or a glutamic acid residue in the center of a cytochrome c peptide on a panel of MHC mutants revealed that a different MHC "footprint" was evident, depending on which peptide was recognized (167,173) (as shown in Fig. 9). This suggests a plasticity of TCR binding to particular peptide/MHC complexes. More direct evidence of TCR plasticity was obtained by Garcia et al. (174), who, in comparing the x-ray crystal structures of the same TCR bound to two different peptide/MHC ligands, found a large conformational change in the CDR3 loop and a smaller one in the CDR1α loop. An even larger conformational change (13 Å) has been found in the CDR3β residue of another TCR as it binds to a peptide/MHC complex (175). That each TCR may have many different conformations of its CDR3 loops is suggested by the two-dimensional nuclear magnetic resonance studies of Hare et al. (176) (Fig. 10), who found that the CDR3 regions of a TCR in solution were significantly more mobile than the rest of the structure. That this may be a general feature of most TCRs is supported by thermodynamic analyses of various TCRs binding to their peptide/MHC ligands, both class I and class II. This binding is invariably accompanied by a substantial loss of entropy (130,177) and, at least in some cases, an "induced fit" mechanism (178). This seems to be a situation in which an inherently flexible binding site achieves greater order upon binding. This mechanism is also employed by DNA recognition proteins; Boniface et al. (178) suggested that it might represent a common mechanism of "scanning" an array of very similar molecular structures (MHCs or DNA) rapidly for the few that "fit" properly. As mentioned

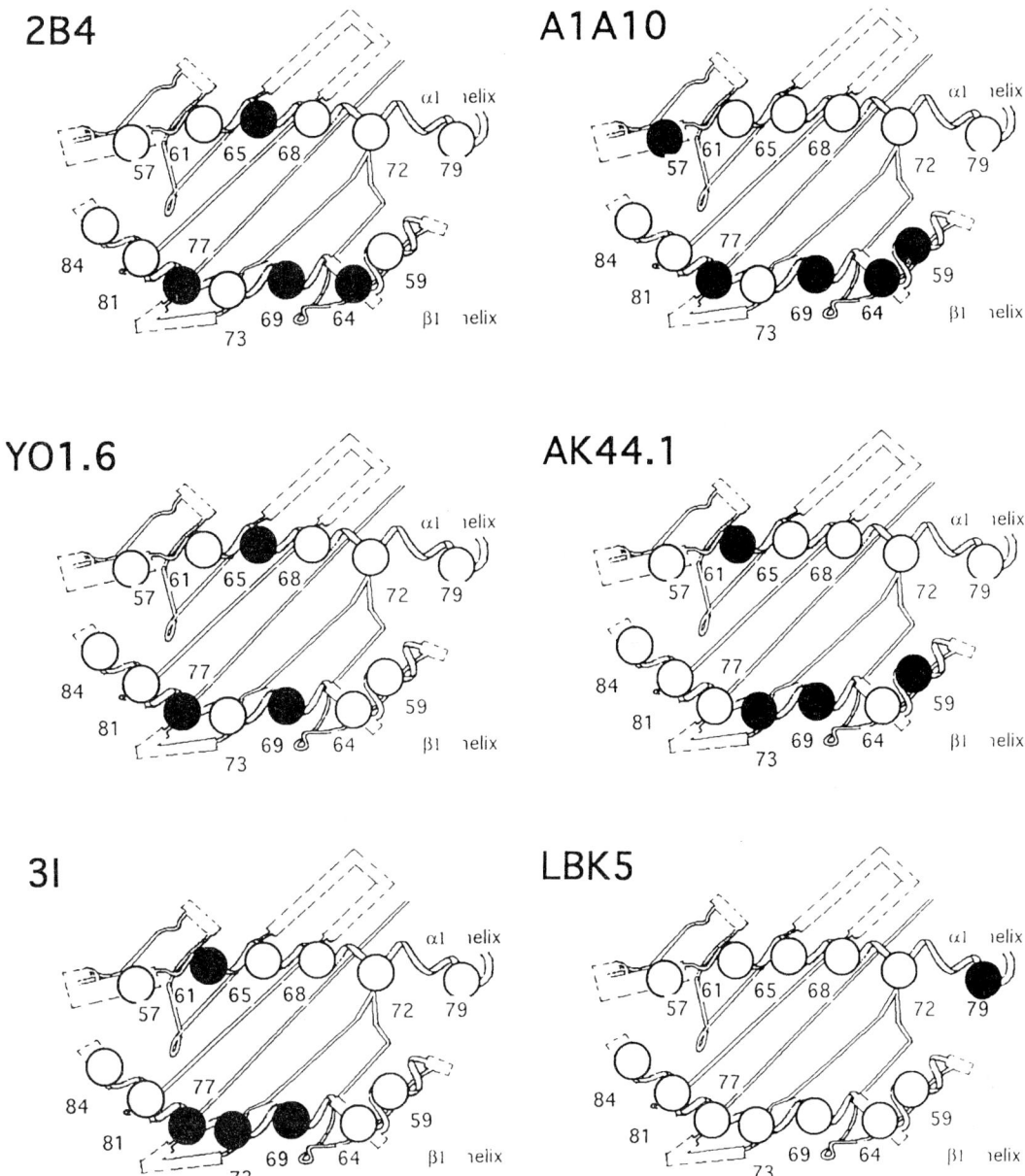

FIG. 9. A $\gamma\delta$ T-cell receptor does not recognize the same epitope as $\alpha\beta$ T-cell receptors. Shown here are the effects of a panel of mutation located on the α helices of the IE^K molecule on T-cell recognition. Inhibition of recognition is denoted by a *filled circle*. The one $\gamma\delta$ T cell is this survey, LBK5, does not recognize a part of the central peptide-binding groove. This is also consistent with its indifference to what peptides occupy this site (see text). From (244), with permission.

previously, the association rates are remarkably slow, in the range of 1,000 to 10,000 M per second (Table 2). This indicates either that a multistep process is occurring before stable binding can be achieved or that only a fraction of the TCRs in solution have the correct conformation. Just how such a scanning mechanism might work for TCRs has been shown by Wu and colleagues (179), who found that a cytochrome c/class II MHC-specific TCR derived most of its stability of binding, but very little of its initial activation energy, from antigenic peptide residues. In contrast, MHC

residues contributed by far the most to the initial binding but had relatively modest effects on stability. This indicates that "scanning" may be a process as shown in Fig. 11, first involving contact with (and orientation by) the α helices of the MHC and then a "fitting" process with and stabilization by peptide residues that involves a substantial loss of entropy. This model of TCR binding may help explain the striking efficiency and sensitivity of T-cell recognition with the MHC helices guiding the TCR into the correct orientation. It may also be the structural basis for cross-reactivity with

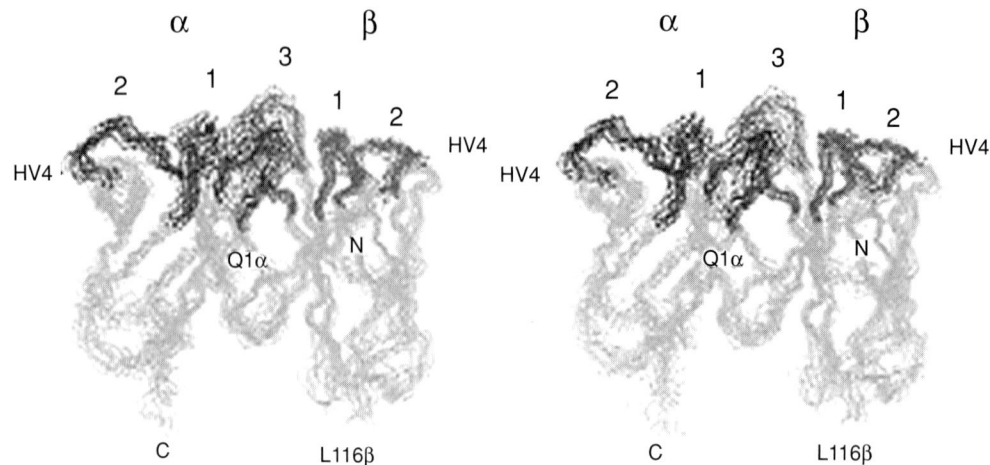

FIG. 10. T-cell receptor complementarity-determining region 3 (CDR3) loops are more mobile than other CDRs in the binding site. Two-dimensional nuclear magnetic resonance studies of a murine T-cell receptor by Reinherz and Wüthrich and colleagues (176) show greater mobility in the central CDR loop (CDR3α and CDR3β) than in the outer loops (CDR1 and CDR2 of TCRα and TCRβ).

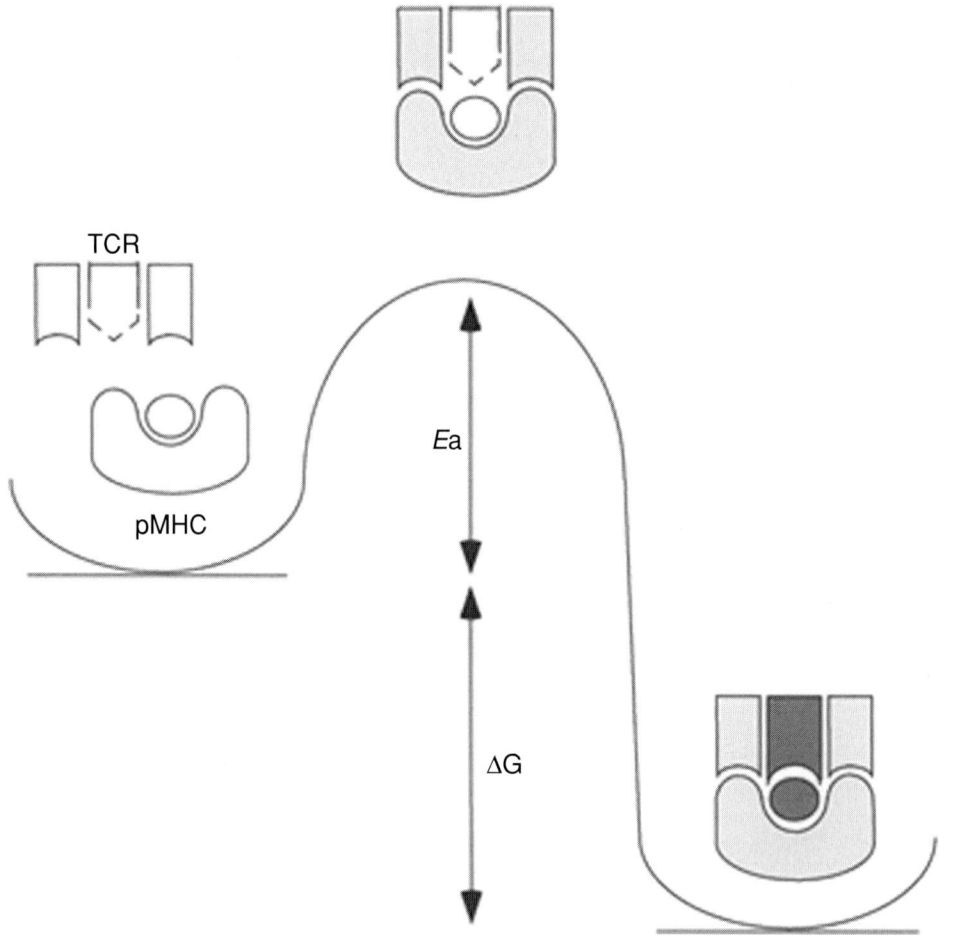

FIG. 11. As shown by Wu et al. (179), mutational analysis of T-cell receptor (TCR)–peptide/major histocompatibility complex (MHC) binding indicates that the TCR first contacts MHC residues (in the transition state), and the peptide has very little influence. Subsequently, however, the peptide residues contribute greatly to the stability of the complex. Thus, we have proposed that the transition state largely involves TCR-MHC contact followed by stabilization of mobile complementarity-determining region 3 residues into a stable state, usually involving significant conformational change and loss of entropy.

structurally very different peptides binding to the same MHC, inasmuch as the CDR3 regions of TCR could "fold" into the peptide in many possible configurations.

$\alpha\beta$ T-CELL RECEPTOR AND SUPERANTIGENS

One of the most interesting and unexpected discoveries to emerge from the study of $\alpha\beta$ T-cell reactivities is the that of superantigens. Whereas a particular antigenic peptide might be recognized by only 1 or fewer in 100,000 T cells in a naive organism, a given superantigen might stimulate 1% to 20% of the T cells (180–183). As discussed in more detailed later, the physical basis for this is that the superantigen binds to a Vβ domain of the TCR on T cells while simultaneously binding to a class II MHC molecule on an antigen-presenting cell (although not in the peptide-binding groove). This allows a single superantigen, such as SEA in Table 4, to stimulate virtually every murine T-cell–bearing Vβ 1, 3, 10, 11, 12, or 17 (~15% of all $\alpha\beta$ T cells), in most cases regardless of what Vα it is paired with or what CDR3 sequence is expressed. This is clearly a unique class of T-cell stimulatory molecule.

The first indication of a superantigen effect was the discovery of minor lymphocyte stimulating determinants by Festenstein (184) in the early 1970s. Many years later, Kappler et al. (185) characterized a mouse strain–specific deletion of T cells expressing a specific TCR Vβs that were attributable to these loci. It emerged that these effects were caused by endogenous retroviruses of the murine mammary tumor virus (MMTV) family (186–190). Different family members bind different TCR Vβ domains (as shown in Table 4) and stimulate T cells expressing them. Meanwhile, Janeway et al. (191) showed that *Staphylococcus* enterotoxins could polyclonally activate naive T cells in a Vβ-specific manner without a requirement for antigen processing. Many of these enterotoxins have been characterized extensively (180,182,183). Unlike the MMTV proteins, which are a type II membrane protein, the enterotoxins are secreted. Subsequently, proteins having similar properties have been isolated from other bacteria, such as *Yersinia pseudotuberculosis*

TABLE 4. Vβ specificity of exogenous and endogenous superantigens

Bacterial superantigen	Human Vβ specificity	Reference	Murine Vβ specificity	Reference
SEA	ND		1, 3, 10, 11, 12, 17	285, 286
SEB	3, 12, 14, 15, 17, 20	125,284	(3), 7, 8.1, 8.3, (11), (17)	285,287,288
SEC$_1$	12	284	7, 8.2, 8.3, 11	285
SEC$_2$	12, 13, 14, 15, 17, 20	125,284	8.2, 10	285
SEC$_3$	5, 12	284	(3), 7, 8.2	285
SED	5, 12	284	3, 7, (8.2), 8.3, 11, 17	285
SEE	5.1, 6.1–6.3, 8, 18	125,284	11, 15, 17	285
TSST-1	2	284	15, 16	285
ExFT	2	125	10, 11, 15	285
Strep M	2, 4, 8	194	ND	

Endogenous proviruses	Vβ specificity	Mls type[a]	Chromosome	Reference
Mtv-1	3	c, 4a	7	As reviewed in 181, 289
Mtv-2	14	NA	18	
Mtv-3	3, 17	c	11	
Mtv-6	3, 17	c, 3a	16	
Mtv-7	6, 7, 8.1, 9	a, 1a	1	
Mtv-8	11, 12	f, Dvbll.1	6	
Mtv-9	5, 11, 12	f, Etc-1,	12	
Mtv-11	11, 12	f, Dvbll.3	14	
Mtv-13	3	c, 2a	4	
Mtv-43	6, 7, 8.1, 9	Mls-like	ND	

Exogenous viruses	Vβ specificity	Mls type	Chromosome	Reference
MMTV-C3H	14, 15	NA		187,188
MMTV-SW	6, 7, 8.1, 9	Mls-like		290
Rabies			Suspected	197
EBV			Suspected	200
CMV			Suspected	198

Other pathogens	Vβ specificity	Name	Chromosome	Reference
Mycoplasma	h17, 6, 8.1, 8.3	MAM		195,196
Toxoplasma gondii			Suspected	201

Vβ in parentheses are reactive with commercial but not recombinant enterotoxins (180).
CMV, cytomegalovirus; EBV, Epstein-Barr virus; MMTV, mouse mammary tumor virus; NA, not applicable; ND, not determined.
[a]The nomenclature in use before the discovery that the phenotype resulted from endogenous retroviruses.

and *Y. enterocolitica* (192,193) and *Streptococcus* (194), and from *Mycoplasma* (195,196). There is also evidence of superantigen-like activities in other mammalian viruses such as rabies (197), cytomegalovirus (198), herpes virus (199), and Epstein-Barr virus (200) and also in *Toxoplasma gondii* (201). Because so many pathogenic or parasitic organisms possess these molecules, apparently by convergent evolution, there must be some selective advantage, but in most cases, there is no conclusive evidence as to what this might be. The one exception is the case of the MMTV superantigens, in which it has been shown that polyclonal T cell stimulation allows the virus to much more efficiently infect the B lymphocytes that are activated by the T cells (202,203). This may be a special case, however, and most authors writing on this subject have suggested that superantigens primarily serve to confuse and occupy the immune system while the pathogen escapes specific targeting and elimination. Large doses of superantigens have also been implicated in various "shock" syndromes, such as food poisoning or toxic shock (180), but this is probably not their everyday purpose, because it would violate the general rule that the host and parasite should coexist.

It has also been suggested that superantigens may be involved in triggering autoimmune diseases. The hypothesis is that a large number of some $V\beta$-bearing T cells are activated by a pathogenic superantigen and that subsequently self-reactive T cells within those activated cells are more easily stimulated by a particular tissue antigen. That this may occur in some cases is supported by the work of Stauffer et al. (204) on a human endogenous retrovirus which specifically stimulates $V\beta7$ T cells and is implicated in the initiation of type I diabetes. Another report implicates a superantigen in Crohn's disease, another autoimmune disorder (205).

Although the biochemistry of superantigen binding to TCR and MHC is similar to that of TCR peptide/MHC interactions (206), mutagenesis data and, in particular, x-ray structural data have shown that the topologies are both quite different and variable (207). In particular, it has been found that Mls-1a presentation to T cells is most affected by mutations on the "outside" surface of the $V\beta$ domain that do not affect peptide/MHC recognition (207). In contrast, CDR1 and CDR2 of regions of $V\beta$ chains are involved in bacterial superantigen reactivity.

An example of these data is shown in Colorplate 3, which shows how a model TCR-superantigen-MHC complex (derived from separate structures) would displace the TCR somewhat (but not entirely) away from the MHC binding groove (208), thus making the interaction largely insensitive to the TCR-peptide specificity. Other TCR-superantigen-MHC complexes have very different geometries (209–212).

Why do all the many independently derived superantigens interact with only the TCRβ-chain? One possibility is that the β-chain offers the only access to the TCR, perhaps because the CD4 molecules hinders access to the Vα side, as suggested by the antibody blocking studies of Rojo and Janeway (213).

A SECOND TYPE OF RECEPTOR: $\gamma\delta$-CD3

Identification of $\gamma\delta$ T Cells

Although $\alpha\beta$ T cells were originally defined on the basis of functional characteristics, such as providing T cell "help" or initiating cytotoxicity, $\gamma\delta$ TCR–bearing cells were not discovered through any cellular assay or by serological analysis but instead were identified through gene cloning. Thus, most work on these cells has been devoted to the understanding of what they recognize and how they function within the immune system. Although there has been substantial progress, these questions are still largely unresolved. We review here some of the salient characteristics of these enigmatic cells.

In the mouse, $\gamma\delta$ T cells first appear in the fetal thymus fully 2 days before $\alpha\beta$ T cells, but in later weeks, $\alpha\beta$ T cells quickly predominate. In both mouse and human adults, $\gamma\delta$ T cells represent only a small fraction (1% to 5%) of thymocytes (214,215) and lymphocytes in all of the secondary lymphoid organs. However, they are found in larger numbers in the mucus membranes of a variety of tissues such as the skin (216), small intestine (217), female reproductive tract (218), and lung (219).

One population of $\gamma\delta$ T cells that has been studied intensively are the CD4$^-$CD8$^-$ $\gamma\delta$T lymphocytes, which have a dendritic structure and are embedded in the epidermis (216,217). These cells have been termed *dendritic epidermal cells* (DECs). Curiously, 90% of these cells express a TCR with identical Vγ and Vδ sequences (217). It has been shown that most DECs arise during days 15 to 17 of fetal life (119). At this stage in development, there is a preference for V$\gamma3$ rearrangement, and little or no terminal deoxynucleotidyl transferase is expressed, and N-region diversity is consequently absent. In addition, the mechanism of gene rearrangement has been shown to be biased by nucleotide homologies between the end of the V region and the beginning of (in this case) the J region (221). Thus, there may be a limited repertoire of $\gamma\delta$ sequences at this stage, but the presence of so many identical ones so reproducibly indicates there is either some additional recombinational mechanism other than those cited or a strong selection for this particular outcome.

As to what these DEC cells "see," experiments have shown that they can respond to mouse keratinocytes or to an extract of keratinocytes added directly to the DECs (222). The nature of the determinant recognized is currently unknown. Other intraepithelial lymphocytes (IELs) show distinct receptor expression as well. The $\gamma\delta$ T cells found in the female reproductive epithelia and tongues of mice preferentially express V$\gamma4$ and V$\delta1$ (218). In the BALB/c strain of mice, most of the TCRδ sequences are the same (223), but others are diverse, and this phenomenon has not been seen in other strains.

Another population of $\gamma\delta$ T cells that has been studied extensively is resident in the epithelium of the small intestine (217). The gut IELs consist of a population of $\alpha\beta$ T cells and a population of $\gamma\delta$ T cells. They are phenotypically CD4$^-$CD8$^-$ or CD4$^-$CD8$^+$. Unlike CD8$^+$ $\alpha\beta$ T cells, the CD8 molecules on $\gamma\delta$ IELs contain α chains and no β chains (224,225). IEL$\gamma\delta$ TCRs use different Vγ and Vδ chains, and the CDR3 regions of both the γ and δ chains show significant diversity both in length and sequence, which suggests that they can "see" a wide variety of ligands.

How does this correlation between $\gamma\delta$ TCR expression and anatomically different epithelia reflect an immune function? Is it the result of a unique homing process, or does it reveal some aspect of ontogeny? No concrete answers to these questions are yet at hand.

$\gamma\delta$ T Cells Contribute to Host Immune Defense Differently than $\alpha\beta$ T Cells

Earlier studies showed that $\gamma\delta$ T cells can secrete a variety of lymphokines and mount cytolytic responses and therefore have the potential to function like $\alpha\beta$ T cells. Their preferential localization in the epithelium also suggested that they may be responsible for a first line of defense [reviewed by Allison and Havran (226)]. This hypothesis is supported by the increase of $\gamma\delta$ T lymphocytes occurring early in infections by some bacteria and a virulent Sendai virus strain, before $\alpha\beta$ T cell responses are observed (227,228). However, in other infection models, $\gamma\delta$ T cells accumulate within the inflammatory lesions late in the infection after the virus have been cleared [reviewed by Kaufmann (229)], which suggests that they may be responding to cells that are damaged or stressed by the infection. Consistent with this is the demonstration that some $\gamma\delta$ T cells can kill virus infected cells *in vitro* but that the recognition is not virus specific (230).

In addition, mice with deficiencies of $\alpha\beta$ or $\gamma\delta$ T cells have been used to dissect the role of these cells in the immune defense against intracellular pathogens (bacteria, protozoa, and viruses) (231–233). These T-cell deficiencies were induced by either the administration of a monoclonal antibody against $\alpha\beta$ or $\gamma\delta$ T lymphocytes or by disruption of a TCR gene through homologous recombination. It was found that the effect of a $\gamma\delta$ T cell deficiency differs, depending on the type of infection. In case of bacille Calmette-Guérin or *Salmonella* administration, $\alpha\beta$ but not $\gamma\delta$ T cells are essential in controlling the infection. In other cases, such as *Mycobacterium tuberculosis* and *Listeria monocytogenes,* $\gamma\delta$ T cells are able to compensate for the absence of $\alpha\beta$ T cells. Interestingly, in *L. monocytogenes* and *Hartmannella vermiformis* infections, a lack of $\gamma\delta$ T cells does not change the pathogen load but instead results in a different pathological process in the infected tissue (231–234). This has led to the suggestion that $\gamma\delta$ T cells may somehow regulate immune and nonimmune cells to maintain host tissue integrity (235). This possibility is supported by data showing that certain $\gamma\delta$ T cells can produce keratinocyte growth factor and chemokines (236), as well as regulate the development of epithelial cells (237) and influence $\alpha\beta$ T cell responses (238–241). It is also compatible with the analysis of $\gamma\delta$ T cell recognition requirements in that these cells can mediate cellular immune functions without a requirement for antigen processing and specialized antigen-presenting cells [reviewed by Hein and Mackay (6)]. There-

fore, they have the capacity to initiate immune responses by recognizing other lymphoid cells or damaged tissue cells directly. To gain insight into the scope of $\gamma\delta$ IEL responses, the gene expression profiles of $\gamma\delta$ IELs were surveyed with DNA microarrays (Affymetrix) (242) and the serial analysis of gene expression (243). These data suggest that $\gamma\delta$ IELs may modulate local immune responses and participate in the intestinal metabolism and physiology by using mechanisms not previously appreciated. More strikingly, the transcription profiles show that whereas lymph node CD8$^+$ $\alpha\beta$ T cells must be activated to become cytotoxic effectors, $\gamma\delta$ IELs are constitutively transcribing genes associated with activation and effector functions. In particular, even in uninfected animals, $\gamma\delta$ IELs constitutively express very high levels of granzyme A and B transcripts as well as natural killer cell–activating and inhibitory receptors. Thus, a cytolytic program could be readily turned on with little or no *de novo* transcription. An important implication is that the lytic activity of $\gamma\delta$ IELs may be induced without a requirement for TCR ligand recognition. This would allow $\gamma\delta$ IELs to deal with a broad range of pathological situations quickly, despite the diversity of the $\gamma\delta$ TCRs expressed by these cells. The expression of the T-cell receptor may give IELs an alternative route to induce cytotoxicity, such as by recognizing pathogens directly or by utilizing additional or different sets of effector programs, depending on the method of target recognition. Although all these experiments point to an unique role for $\gamma\delta$ T cell in the immune system, $\gamma\delta$ T cell specificity and their exact effector functions in any pathological situation remains undefined. It is interesting to note that the function of $\gamma\delta$ T cells has been studied mainly in mouse and human, but they are significantly more abundant in birds and artiodactyls (214,226). Thus, $\gamma\delta$ T cells in these species may encompass other functions as well.

Antigen Recognition by $\gamma\delta$ T Cells Does Not Require Processing

Since 1994, a number of studies have shown that $\gamma\delta$ T cells have profound differences in their antigen recognition requirements in comparison with $\alpha\beta$ T cells. Some $\gamma\delta$ T cells also seem to recognize an entirely different types of antigens. More specifically, these experiments suggest that the antigens recognized by many $\gamma\delta$ T cells do not have to be processed and presented and that they also do not have to be proteins [as reviewed by Hein and Mackay (6)].

Because most $\alpha\beta$ T cells recognize protein antigens processed inside the cell and presented by MHC molecules, it was originally assumed that $\gamma\delta$ T cells follow the same general pattern. Despite early work showing that classical MHC molecules are not involved in antigen recognition by $\gamma\delta$ T cells, it was assumed that nonclassical MHC molecules, heat shock proteins, or yet-unidentified surface proteins may play a similar role.

To date, the recognition requirements for $\gamma\delta$ T cells have been evaluated in three model systems that allow a precise interpretation of the results. They are the recognition of the mouse class II MHC molecules IE^K by the T cell clone LBK5 (244); the recognition of the murine nonclassical class I MHC molecules T10 and the closely related T22 molecule (94% identity) by the T cell clone G8 (244,245); and the recognition of a herpes simplex virus glycoprotein, gI, by the T cell clone TgI4.4 (246).

The IE^K encoded protein has been shown to bind peptides, whereas both biochemical (247) and structural studies (248) have shown that T10 and T22 do not. Furthermore, all three proteins have the potential to be degraded into peptides and "presented" for recognition. Strikingly, in all three cases, neither peptides bound to these proteins nor peptides derived from them are recognized by the $\gamma\delta$ T cell clones. Instead, protein antigens are recognized directly without any requirement for antigen processing. An example of these data is shown in Table 5, which shows the effect of temperature-sensitive endocytic compartment mutants on $\alpha\beta$ T cell recognition of a protein antigen versus the recognition of IE^K by LBK5 (244). Note that the endosomal mutants disrupt processing of cytochrome c but have no effect on $\gamma\delta$ T cell recognition. In addition, epitope mapping with mutant IE molecules shows that amino acid residues in the α helices of the IEα and IEβ chains that affect $\alpha\beta$ T cell recognition do not affect LBK5 stimulation (244).

Research on LBK5 recognition (250) has also shown a remarkable sensitivity to changes in N-linked glycosylation of the IE^K molecule. This is despite the fact that E. coli expressed (e.g., unglycosylated molecules) can be recognized. Because cells that are stressed, infected, or transformed often change the posttranslational modifications of their surface proteins, these findings suggest a way to regulate a $\gamma\delta$ T cell response by qualitative changes of self antigens.

T22 Tetramers Stain a Relatively Large Fraction of $\gamma\delta$ T Cells

Figure 12 shows the results of Crowley et al. (251), who used a T22 tetrameric straining reagent to show that a surprisingly large fraction (0.4% to 2.0%) of splenic $\gamma\delta$ T cells could be stained. More than 90% of these cells are CD4$^-$CD8$^-$, whereas the rest are either CD4 or CD8 single positive (about 3% to 4% each). A similar frequency of tetramer positive

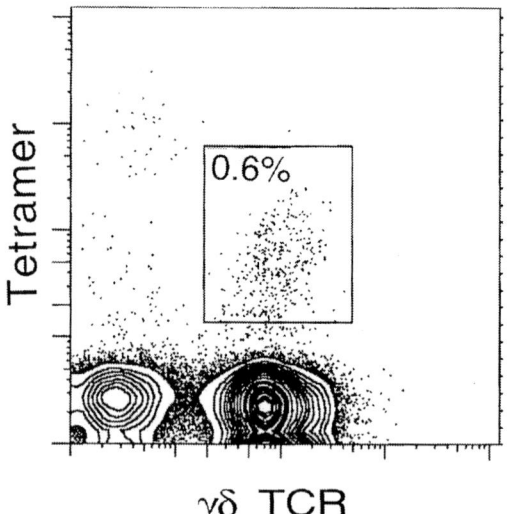

FIG. 12. T10/T22-specific $\gamma\delta$ T cells can be detected in normal mice through use of a tetrameric T22 staining reagent. As shown by Crowley et al. (247), a T22 tetrameric flow cytometry staining reagent, which was generated by similar methods as tetrameric peptide/MHC reagents, stained approximately 0.6% of splenic $\gamma\delta$ T cells in normal animals. More than 90% of these cells are CD4$^-$CD8$^-$; the rest are either CD4 or CD8 single positive (about 3% to 4% each). A similar frequency of tetramer-positive $\gamma\delta$ T cells was also found in the intestinal intraepithelial lymphocyte (IEL) population (data not shown).

$\gamma\delta$ T cells was also found in the intestinal IEL population. This represents a much higher frequency of this particular $\gamma\delta$ T cell specificity than is true of unimmunized $\alpha\beta$ T cells, which are in the range of 0.001 to 0.0001%. Also interesting is the finding that the T10 molecule is expressed at very low levels in the periphery (and T22 is not expressed at all) but is induced on activated cells (B and T lymphocytes, macrophages, and dendritic cells). This has led to the suggestion that T10/T22-specific $\gamma\delta$ T cells could regulate these cells during an immune response (251). Whether other $\gamma\delta$ T cell specificities occur in such large numbers is not known but seems very likely.

A human homologue of T10/T22, MICA/MICB, was found to stimulate human $\gamma\delta$ T cell lines derived from intestinal intraepithelial lymphocytes. Subsequent experiments

TABLE 5. *Effect of temperature-sensitive endocytic compartment mutants on $\alpha\beta$ T-cell recognition of antigen versus recognition of IE$_k$ by LBK-5*

	2B4 peptide ($\alpha\beta$)		2B4 protein ($\alpha\beta$)		A1A10 ($\alpha\beta$)		LBK5 ($\gamma\delta$)	
	34°C	39°C	34°C	39°C	34°C	39°C	34°C	39°C
IE^k-CHO	+++	++++	+++	++++	++	+++	++	+++
IE^k-G8.1 (end1)	+++	++++	++	0	+	0	++	+++
IE^k-25.2.2 (end2)	+++	++++	+++	+	+	0	++	+++
IE^k-G7.1 (end3)	+++	++++	++	0	+	0	++	+++

T-cell reactivity, from "0" (no T-cell activation) to "++++" strong activation.
From Schild H, Mavaddat N, Litzenberger C, et al. The nature of major histocompatibility complex recognition by $\gamma\delta$ T cells. *Cell* 1994;76:29.

demonstrated that MICA/MICB is a ligand for the natural killer cell activating receptor NKG2D (252). The reactivity of $\gamma\delta$ T cell line to MICA/MICB-expressing cells is inhibited by antibodies to NKG2D. It has been proposed that MICA/MICB may also act as a ligand for the $\gamma\delta$ TCR, because antibodies to the receptor also inhibit the reactivity.

$\gamma\delta$ T Cells Can Be Stimulated by Nonpeptide Antigens

$\gamma\delta$ T cells from healthy human peripheral blood and from patients with tuberculoid leprosy or rheumatoid arthritis respond to heat-killed mycobacteria. The major T-cell stimulatory components in the former are not the mycobacterial heat-shock proteins but instead have been identified to be phosphate-containing, nonpeptide molecules (253–258). Although the consensus is that phosphate is a necessary component, compounds identified from various laboratories with different mycobacteria-responsive clones appear to have distinctive structures (Table 6). These nonphosphate moieties include unusual carbohydrate and phosphate groups; a 5'-triphosphorylated thymidine or uridine substituted at its γ-phosphate group by a yet-uncharacterized low-molecular-weight structure; isopentenyl pyrophosphate and related prenyl pyrophosphate derivatives; synthetic alkenyl and prenyl derivatives of phosphate; and pyrophosphate and γ-monoethyl derivatives of nucleoside and deoxynucleoside triphosphates (253). Although the relative biological importance of these compounds remains to be determined, it is clear that a major class of stimulants are phosphate-containing nonpeptides. It is also clear that multiple phosphate-containing compounds are able to stimulate different clones with different efficacy.

An important finding is that all of these compounds can be found in both microbial and mammalian cells. Constant et al. (254) proposed that the mammalian TTP-X and UTP-X conjugate may be involved in a "salvage pathway" in DNA and RNA synthesis and thus could be involved in a metabolic pathway related to DNA or RNA synthesis such as cell proliferation. Such a molecule would fit with the "stress antigen" or "conserved primitive stimulus" expected for $\gamma\delta$ T cell ligands (226). Tanaka et al. (255,256) proposed that a link in the recognition of both microbial pathogens and hematopoietic tumor cells by these $\gamma\delta$ T cells is provided by the common

set of prenyl pyrophosphate intermediates, isopentenyl, and related prenyl pyrophosphate derivatives. These compounds are present in normal mammalian cells as precursors in lipid metabolism for the synthesis of farnesyl pyrophosphate. In mammalian cells, farnesyl addition has been proposed to be a critical modification for the membrane association of the ras protein and is required for transforming activity. The observation that this $\gamma\delta$ T-cell population accumulates in lesions caused by mycobacterial infections in humans (257,258) and is able to respond to virally and bacterially infected cells suggests that these $\gamma\delta$ cells respond to a class of antigens shared by a number of pathogens and transformed, damaged, or stressed cells.

Other Antigen Specificities of $\gamma\delta$ T Cells

Even the very earliest studies of $\gamma\delta$ T cell reactivities showed that classical MHC molecules are not the major ligands for these cells (214). Although some that can recognize either classical MHC or related molecules such as TL, Qa^d, or CD1 have been found, the frequency of such clones derived from a mixed lymphocyte reaction is low (about 1 in 100,000), which is much lower than the frequency of $\alpha\beta$ alloreactive generated in such reactions (1 in 10 to 100). In many cases, these $\gamma\delta$ T cells also show a broad cross-reactivity that is not seen for $\alpha\beta$ alloreactive T cells, which is consistent with the suggestion that there is a fundamental difference in their recognition properties.

There are also two reports indicating that the $\gamma\delta$ T-cell recognition may involve a "complexed antigen" on the cell surface: a $\gamma\delta$ T cell hybridoma that responded to synthetic copolymer Glu-Tyr (GT) in the presence of stimulator cells expressing the Qa-1b (but not the Qa-1a) molecule (259). Also, a human $\gamma\delta$ T cell clone from synovial fluid of a patient with early rheumatoid arthritis responding to a fragment C of tetanus toxin (260). The tetanus toxin response requires the presence of cells expressing a class II MHC molecule, DRw53, and can be inhibited by an anti-DRw53 antibody. In these two cases, it is not clear whether the Glu-Tyr copolymer and the tetanus toxin are "processed" and, if so, what kind of antigen processing is required. In addition to these specificities, $\gamma\delta$ T cells that are responsive to mycobacterial 60-kD heat-shock protein and peptide derived from it (261),

TABLE 6. *Nonpeptide mycobacterial antigens that stimulate human Vγ9Vδ2(Vγ2Vδ2) T cells*[a]

Name	Structure	Ref.
Phosphocarbohydrates	Unusual carbohydrates with terminal phosphorylation	Schoel et al. (253)
TUBag3	X-uridine 5'-triphosphate	J. J. Fournié, personal communication
TUBag4	X-thymidine 5'-triphosphate	Constant et al. (254)
Isopentenyl pyrophosphate	$CH_2=C(CH_3)CH_2CH_2=PP_i$	Tanaka et al. (255)

[a]All compounds have been isolated from myobacterial extracts and require some type of phosphorylation for stimulatory activity. The unknown structure "X," when phosphorylated, is the minimal active stimulatory component of the TUBag compounds. "X" is not a prenyl or alkenyl derivative (J. J. Fournié, personal communication).

staphylococcal enterotoxin A (262), and an immunoglobulin light chain–derived peptide in the context of the heat-shock protein have also been reported (263).

Complementarity-Determining Region 3 Length Distribution Analysis Shows $\gamma\delta$ T-Cell Receptors Are More Immunoglobulin-like

In an effort to find a molecular basis for these surprising differences in $\gamma\delta$ versus $\alpha\beta$ T cell recognition, Rock et al. (264) characterized the length distribution of CDR3 regions in three immune receptor chains: immunoglobulin, $\alpha\beta$ TCR, and $\gamma\delta$ TCR. Rock et al. found that the CDR3 lengths of both α and β TCR polypeptides are nearly identical and have very constrained length distributions. In contrast, CDR3 lengths of immunoglobulin heavy chains are long and variable, whereas those of light chains are much shorter and more constrained. As discussed previously, the CDR3 loops of $\alpha\beta$ TCRs are critical for recognizing antigenic peptides bound to MHC molecules. The constraints on α and β CDR3 length may reflect this functional requirement. Surprisingly, δ-chain CDR3 lengths are long and variable, but those of γ TCR chains are much shorter and constrained. In this regard, $\gamma\delta$ TCR and CDR3 length distributions are similar to those of immunoglobulins and distinct from those of $\alpha\beta$ TCR, as also indicated by the x-ray crystal structure of a $\gamma\delta$ TCR (41).

It has been observed that the frequency of $\gamma\delta$ T cell clones recognizing allogeneic MHC molecules in a mixed lymphocyte reaction is very low (in comparison with $\alpha\beta$ alloreactive clones) and that the majority of these clones show a high degree of cross-reactivity (only rarely seen with $\alpha\beta$ alloreactive clones) [reviewed by Hein and Mackay (6)]. These observations are consistent with the proposal that $\gamma\delta$ TCR recognition is more immunoglobulin-like, focusing on the common features shared by MHC molecules. It is noteworthy that the specificity of LBK5 (IE^B and IE^K but not IE^D) is the same as two previously described anti-IE antibodies (265,266).

Along these lines, human $\gamma\delta$ T cell clones from healthy donors that respond to mycobacteria extract have been found to express $V\gamma9$ and $V\delta2$ with diverse junctional (CDR3) sequences (267). This is reminiscent of the immunoglobulin receptor usage in naturally occurring murine B cells that recognize phosphorylcholine. There, it was found that only very restricted immunoglobulin heavy-chain (VH11, VH12, or Q52) and light-chain V gene segments are used, coupled with variable CDR3 junctional sequences (267a). In the latter case, the restricted usage of the V genes may be more significant, inasmuch as several hundred to a thousand VH gene segments are available to mount an immunoglobulin response.

The suggestion that $\gamma\delta$ TCR recognition is more immunoglobulin-like does not preclude the possibility that some $\gamma\delta$ T cells may recognize similar or identical ligands as $\alpha\beta$ T cells. It is clear, for example, that it is possible to make antibodies that are specific for different subtypes of MHC molecules or even particular peptide/MHC complexes (268–270).

As discussed earlier, by considering all elements that contribute to the variability of the junctional (CDR3) region, such as the numbers of D and J elements used, D-element reading frame, junctional diversity, and N-region nucleotide addition, it was calculated that the number of possible CDR3 sequences is the greatest for $\gamma\delta$ TCR, the least for immunoglobulin (irrespective of somatic mutation), and intermediate for $\alpha\beta$ TCR (158). This suggests that $\gamma\delta$ T cells have the potential to recognize a wide variety of different antigens.

Multivalence of the Ligands Is Required for Activation through the $\gamma\delta$ T-Cell Receptor

$\gamma\delta$ TCR, as with to $\alpha\beta$ TCR, needs to associate with CD3 molecules for cell surface expression. Therefore, signaling through the antigen receptor may utilize a multivalent form of the antigen so that the engaged receptors can be cross-linked. Cell surface molecules can be recognized as such, but soluble antigen must be rendered polyvalent. A demonstration of this requirement is that in the three cases of $\gamma\delta$ T cells recognizing cell surface molecules—IE^K, T10/T22, and HSV gI protein—a soluble form of the protein can be recognized only when bound to plastic plates: for example, presented in a multivalent form (244–246). Interestingly, the stimulation of mycobacterial extract reactive $\gamma\delta$ T-cell clones by small phosphate-containing compounds requires cell–cell contact, and all cell types are able to induce the recognition (271,272).

This apparent requirement for multivalent antigens would then suggest that soluble antigens—such as the phosphate-containing compounds—must be associated with certain cell surface molecules for their recognition. It is important to know whether the binding and display of soluble antigens is achieved by a variety of different molecules on the surface or by a limited set of molecules and whether they normally form part of the epitope recognized by the antigen receptors.

Although the recognition requirements just discussed are derived largely from observations with model systems, the identification of the *Mycobacterium* antigen clearly stems from a "physiologically relevant" event. It will be interesting to determine the generality of these rules in other systems, especially pathological ones. This should lead to a much better definition of the role or roles of $\gamma\delta$ T cells. This includes the identification of what $\gamma\delta$ T cells recognize and the consequence of such recognition in pathological situations.

The issue of $\gamma\delta$ T cell specificity is also important in understanding the development of these cells. Whereas some experiments with $\gamma\delta$ TCR transgenic mice have suggested that they are both positively and negatively selected much the same way as $\alpha\beta$ T cells, others have shown an entirely different mode of selection (273). Interestingly, the phosphate-containing compounds isolated from mycobacterial extracts can be found both in pathogens and in mammalian cells.

Thus, they are "self" as well as "nonself." However, $\gamma\delta$ T cells with this specificity seem not to have be eliminated from the normal repertoire.

COMPLEMENTARITY-DETERMINING REGION 3 DIVERSIFICATION: A GENERAL STRATEGY FOR T-CELL RECEPTORS AND IMMUNOGLOBULIN COMPLEMENTARITY TO ANTIGENS?

One interesting observation that emerges from a detailed analysis of the gene rearrangements that create both TCRs and immunoglobulins is how the diversity of the CDR3 loop region in one or both of the chains in a given TCR is so much greater than that available to the other CDRs. A schematic of this skewing of diversity is shown in Fig. 13 for human immunoglobulins and for $\alpha\beta$ and $\gamma\delta$ TCR heterodimers. In the case of $\alpha\beta$ TCRs, this concentration of diversity occurs in both Vα and Vβ CDR3 loops, and structural data (43,45) has confirmed that these loops sit largely over the center of the antigenic peptide (see previous section). Although this concentration of diversity in $\alpha\beta$ TCRs in the regions of principal contact with the many possible antigenic peptides seems reasonable, it is much harder to explain for immunoglobulin or $\gamma\delta$ TCRs. Clearly, there must be some chemical or structural "logic" behind this phenomenon. A clue as to what this might be comes from the elegant studies of Cunningham and Wells (274) and Clackson and Wells (275), who systematically mutated all of the amino acids (to alanine) at the interface of human growth hormone and its receptor, as determined by

x-ray crystallography. Interestingly, only a fourth of the approximately 30 mutations on either side had any effect on the binding affinity, even in cases in which the x-ray structural analysis showed that the amino acid side chains of most of the residues were "buried" in the other. These studies illustrate an important caveat to the interpretation of protein crystal structures: Although they are invaluable for identifying which amino acids could be important in a given interaction, they do not indicate which ones are the most important. This is presumably because the "fit" at that many positions is not "exact" enough to add significant binding energy to the interaction. In this context, Davis et al. (276) proposed a new model in which the principal antigen specificity of an immunoglobulin or TCR is derived from its most diverse CDR3 loops. In the case of antibodies, we imagine that most of the specific contacts (and hence the free energy) with antigen are made by the VH CDR3 and that the other CDRs provide "opportunistic" contacts that make, in general, only minor contributions to the energy of binding and specificity. Once antigen has been encountered and clonal selection activates a particular cell B, somatic mutation would then "improve" the binding of the CDR1 and CDR2 regions to convert the typically low-affinity antibodies to the higher affinity models, as observed by Berek and Milstein (277) and also by Patten et al. (278). As a test of this model, Xu and Davis (279) analyzed mice that had a severely limited immunoglobulin V-region repertoire, consisting of one VH and effectively two VL chains (Vλ1 and Vλ2). These mice are able to respond to a wide variety of protein and haptenic antigens, even

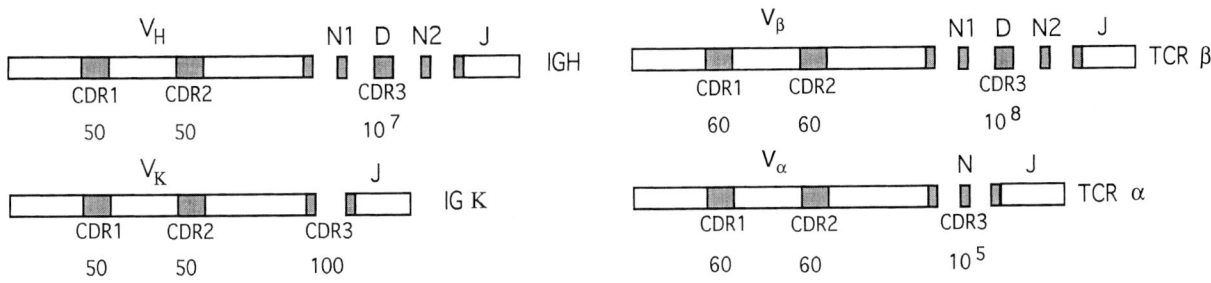

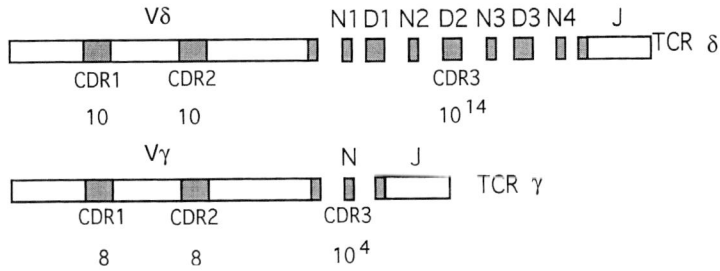

FIG. 13. Diversity "map" of immunoglobulins and T-cell receptors, showing the theoretical potential for sequence diversity in human antigen receptor molecules. N region addition is assumed to contribute 0 to 6 nucleotides to the junction of each gene segment, except for immunoglobulin K chains, in which this form of diversity is seldom utilized.

with this very limited complement of V regions. In several cases, hybridomas specific for very different antigens (e.g., ovalbumin vs. dinitrophenol) differ only in the V_H CDR3. A limited V-region repertoire also seemed no barrier to deriving high-affinity antibodies with somatic mutation, inasmuch as repeated immunizations produced immunoglobulin G monoclonal antibodies with very high affinities (10^{-9} to 10^{-10} M). The major immune deficit in these mice was their ability to produce antibodies to carbohydrates, which may require a special type of binding site or specific V region. Thus, although these experiments involved only one VH, the results are highly suggestive about the inherent malleability of VHV1 in general, at least with regard to protein and haptenic epitopes. With respect to $\alpha\beta$ TCRs, we expect that most of the energy of the interaction with a typical ligand resides in the CDR3-peptide contacts, and here again the CDR1 and CDR2 regions make less energetically important contacts. The case of $\gamma\delta$ TCRs would be more like an antibody only without the affinity improvements that are gained from somatic hypermutation. We have only an *ad hoc* explanation for the extremes of diversity seen in the TCRδ CDR3: It has to recognize both protein surfaces and small nonpeptidic molecules with a high degree of specificity. Perhaps the lack of somatic mutation forces it to provide more diversity in the initial repertoire.

CONCLUSIONS

Since TCR genes were first identified in the early 1980s, information about their genetics, biochemistry, structure, and function has accumulated to become almost a field unto itself. Despite this very real progress, many issues still remain unsolved: What do $\gamma\delta$ T cells normally "see," and what function do they serve? What do superantigens actually do during the course of a normal response, and how is this of benefit to the pathogen/parasite? What is the structural/chemical basis of TCR specificity? What sort of rearrangements or conformational charges occur in the TCR CD3 molecular ensemble upon ligand engagement? These and other questions should serve as a source of entertainment for many years to come.

ACKNOWLEDGMENTS

We are very grateful to Dr. Stephen Hedrick for allowing us to build so freely on his excellent previous chapters for this volume. This work was supported by grants from the National Institutes of Health (to Mark M. Davis and Yueh-Hsiu Chien) and from the Howard Hughes Medical Institute (to Mark M. Davis).

REFERENCES

1. Zinkernagel RM, Doherty PC. Immunological surveillance against altered self components by sensitized T lymphocytes in lymphocytic choriomeningitis. *Nature* 1974;251:547.
2. Zinkernagel R., Doherty P. H-2 compatibility requirement for T cell–mediated lysis of target cells infected with lymphocytic choriomeningitis virus: Different cytotoxic T cell specificities are associated with structures from H-3K or H-2D. *J Exp Med* 1975;141:1427.
3. Shevach EM, Rosenthal AS. Function of macrophages in antigen recognition by guinea pig T lymphocytes. II. Role of the macrophage in the regulation of genetic control of the immune response. *J Exp Med* 1973;138:1213.
4. Katz DH, Hamaoka T, Benacerraf B. Cell interactions between histoincompatible T and B lymphocytes. II. Failure of physiological cooperative interactions between T and B lymphocytes from allogeneic donor strains in humoral response to hapten-protein conjugates. *J Exp Med* 1973;137:1405.
5. Terhorst C, Spits H, Stall F, et al. T lymphocyte signal transduction. In Hames BD, Glover DM, eds. *Molecular immunology,* 2nd ed. Oxford, UK: IRL Press, 1996:132–188.
6. Hein WR, Mackay CR. Prominence of gamma delta T cells in the ruminant immune system. *Immunol Today* 1991;12:30.
7. Chien Y-H, Jores R, Crowley MP. Recognition by γ/δ T cells. *Annu Rev Immunol* 1996;14:511.
8. Infante AJ, Infante PD, Gillis S, et al. Definition of T cell idiotypes using anti-idiotype antisera produced by immunization with T cell clones. *J Exp Med* 1982;155:1100.
9. Allison JP, McIntyre BW, Bloch D. Tumor-specific antigen of murine T lymphoma defined with monoclonal antibody. *J Immunol* 1982;129:2293.
10. Meuer SC, Fitzgerald KA, Hussey RE, et al. Clonotypic structures involved in antigen specific human T cell function: relationship to the T3 molecular complex. *J Exp Med* 1983;157:705.
11. Haskins K, Kubo R, White J, et al. The major histocompatibility complex-restricted antigen receptor on T cells. I. Isolation with a monoclonal antibody. *J Exp Med* 1983;157:1149.
12. Kaye J, Procelli S, Tite J, et al. Both a monoclonal antibody and antisera specific for determinants unique to individual cloned helper T cell lines can substitute for antigen and antigen-presenting cells in the activation of T cells. *J Exp Med* 1983;158:836.
13. Samelson LE, Germain RN, Schwartz RH. Monoclonal antibodies against the antigen receptor on a cloned T cell hybrid. *Proc Natl Acad Sci U S A* 1983;80:6972.
14. MacIntyre BW, Allison JP. Biosynthesis and processing of murine T-cell antigen receptor. *Cell* 1984;38:654.
15. Kappler J, Kubo R, Haskins K, et al. The major histocompatibility complex–restricted antigen receptor on T cells in mouse and man. V. Identification of constant and variable peptides. *Cell* 1983;35:295.
16. Davis MM, Cohen DI, Nielsen EA, et al. The isolation of B and T cell–specific genes. In Vitteta E, ed. *UCLA symposia on molecular and cellular biology: B and T cell tumors,* vol. 24. New York: Academic Press, 1982:215.
17. Hedrick SM, Cohen DI, Nielsen EA, et al. Isolation of cDNA clones encoding T cell–specific membrane-associated proteins. *Nature* 1984;308:149.
18. Hedrick SM, Nielsen EA, Kavaler J, et al. Sequence relationships between putative T-cell receptor polypeptides and immunoglobulins. *Nature* 1984;308:153.
19. Yanagi Y, Yoshikai Y, Leggett K, et al. A human T cell–specific cDNA clone encodes a protein having extensive homology to immunoglobulin chains. *Nature* 1984;308:145.
20. Acuto O, Fabbi M, Smart J, et al. Purification and NH2-terminal amino acid sequencing of the beta subunit of a human T-cell antigen receptor. *Proc Natl Acad Sci U S A* 1984;81:3851.
21. Chien Y, Becker DM, Lindsten T, et al. A third type of murine T-cell receptor gene. *Nature* 1984;312:31.
22. Saito H, Kranz D, Takagaki Y, et al. A third rearranged and expressed gene in a clone of cytotoxic T lymphocytes. *Nature* 1984;312:36.
23. Saito H, Kranz DM, Takagaki Y, et al. Complete primary structure of a heterodimeric T-cell receptor deduced from cDNA sequences. *Nature* 1984;309:757.
24. Brenner MB, McLean J, Dialynas DP, et al. Identification of a putative second T-cell receptor. *Nature* 1986;322:145.
25. Chien YH, Iwashima M, Kaplan KB, et al. A new T-cell receptor gene located within the alpha locus and expressed early in T-cell differentiation. *Nature* 1987;327:677.

26. Dembic Z, Haas W, Weiss S, et al. Transfer of specificity by murine a and β T-cell receptor genes. *Nature* 1986;320:232.

27. Saito T, Weiss A, Miller J, et al. Specific antigen-Ia activation of transfected human T cells expressing murine Ti ab-human T3 receptor complexes. *Nature* 1987;325:125.

28. Havran WL, Chien YH, Allison JP Recognition of self antigens by skin-derived T cells with invariant gamma delta antigen receptors. *Science* 1991;252:1430.

29. Lefranc M-P, Lefranc G. *The T cell receptor: FactsBook.* London: Academic Press, 2001.

30. Brenner MB, McLean J, Scheft H, et al. Two forms of the T cell receptor gamma protein found on peripheral blood cytotoxic T lymphocytes. *Nature* 1987;325:689.

31. Groettrup M, Ungewiss K, Azogui O, et al. A novel disulfide-linked heterodimer on pre–T cells consists of the T cell receptor β chain and a 33 kDa glycoprotein. *Cell* 1993;75:283.

32. Saint-Ruf C, Ungewiss K, Groettrup M, et al. Analysis and expression of a cloned pre–T cell receptor gene. *Science* 1994;206:1208.

33. Novotny J, Tonegawa S, Saito H, et al. Secondary, tertiary, and quaternary structure of T-cell–specific immunoglobulin-like polypeptide chains. *Proc Natl Acad Sci U S A* 1986;83:742.

34. Bentley GA, Boulot G, Karjalainen K, et al. Crystal structure of the beta chain of a T cell antigen receptor. *Science* 1995;267:1984.

35. Fields BA, Ober B, Malchiodi EL, et al. Crystal structure of the V alpha domain of a T cell antigen receptor. *Science* 1995;270:1821–1824.

36. Garcia KC, Decagon M, Stanfield RL, et al. The structure of an αβ T-cell receptor at 2.5Å. *Science* 1996;274:209.

37. Garboczi DN, Ghosh P, Utz U, et al. Structure of the complex between human T-cell receptor, viral peptide and HLA-A2Å. *Nature* 1996;384:134.

38. Housset D, Mazza G, Gregoire C, et al. The three-dimensional structure of a T-cell antigen receptor V alpha V beta heterodimer reveals a novel arrangement of the V beta domain. *EMBO J* 1997;14:4205.

39. Reiser JB, Darnault C, Guimezanes A, et al. Crystal structure of a T cell receptor bound to an allogeneic MHC molecule. *Nat Immunol* 2002;1:291.

40. Hennecke J, Carfi A, Wiley DC. Structure of a covalently stabilized complex of a human αβ T-cell receptor, influenza HA peptide and MHC class II molecule, HLA-DR1. *EMBO J* 2000;19:5611.

41. Allison TJ, Winter CC, Fournie JJ, et al. Structure of a human gammadelta T-cell antigen receptor. *Nature* 2001; 411:820.

42. Strong RK, Penny DM, Feldman RM, et al. Engineering and expression of a secreted murine T cell receptor with reduced N-linked glycosylation. *J Immunol* 1994;153:4111.

43. Klausner RD, Lippincott-Schwartz J, Bonifacino JS. The T cell antigen receptor: insights into organelle biology. *Annu Rev Cell Biol* 1990;6:403.

44. Samelson LE, Harford HB, Klausner RD. Identification of the components of the murine T cell antigen receptor complex. *Cell* 1985;43:223.

45. Orloff DG, Frank SJ, Robey FA, et al. Biochemical characterization of the eta chain of the T-cell receptor. *J Biol Chem* 1989;264:14812.

46. Jin YJ, Clayton LK, Howard FD, et al. Molecular cloning of the CD3 eta subunit identifies a CD3 zeta–related product in thymus-derived cells. *Proc Natl Acad Sci U S A* 1990;87:3319.

47. Clayton LK, D'Adamio L, Howard FD, et al. CD3 eta and CD3 zeta are alternatively spliced products of a common genetic locus and are transcriptionally and/or post-transcriptionally regulated during T-cell development. *Proc Natl Acad Sci U S A* 1991;88:5202.

48. Rodewald HR, Arulanandam AR, Koyasu S, et al. The high affinity Fc epsilon receptor gamma subunit (Fc epsilon RI gamma) facilitates T cell receptor expression and antigen/major histocompatibility complex-driven signaling in the absence of CD3 zeta and CD3 eta. *J Biol Chem* 1991;266.15974.

49. Orloff DG, Ra C S, Frank SJ, et al. Family of disulphide-linked dimers containing the zeta and eta chains of the T-cell receptor and the gamma chain of Fc receptors. *Nature* 1990;347:189.

50. Koyasu S, D'Adamio L, Arulanandam AR, et al. T cell receptor complexes containing Fc epsilon RI gamma homodimers in lieu of CD3 zeta and CD3 eta components: a novel isoform expressed on large granular lymphocytes. *J Exp Med* 1992;175:203.

51. Exley M, Wileman T, Mueller B, et al. Evidence for multivalent structure of T cell antigen receptor complex. *Mol Immunol* 1995;32:829.

52. Blumberg RS, Ley S, Sancho J, et al. Structure of the T-cell receptor: Evidence for two CD3 epsilon subunits in the T-cell receptor–CD3 complex. *Proc Natl Acad Sci U S A* 1990;87:7220.

53. Jin YJ, Koyasu S, Moingeon P, et al. A fraction of CD3 epsilon subunits exists as disulfide-linked dimers in both human and murine T lymphocytes. *J Biol Chem* 1990;265:15850.

53a. Fernandez-Miguel G, Alarcón B, Iglesias A, et al. Multivalent structure of an αβ T cell receptor. *Science* 1999;96:1547.

53b. Call ME, Pyrdol J, Wiedmann M, et al. The organizing principal in the formation of the T cell receptor-CD3 complex. *Cell* 2002;111:967.

54. Clevers H, Alarcón B, Wileman T, et al. The T cell receptor/CD3 complex: a dynamic protein ensemble. *Annu Rev Immunol* 1988;6:629.

55. Cosson P, Lankford SP, Bonifacino JS, et al. Membrane protein association by potential intramembrane charge pairs. *Nature* 1991;351:414.

56. Hall C, Berkhout B, Alarcón B, et al. Requirements for cell surface expression of the human TCR/CD3 complex in non–T cells. *Int Immunol* 1991;3:359.

57. Alarcón B, Ley SC, Sanchez-Madrid F, et al. The CD3-gamma and CD3-delta subunits of the T cell antigen receptor can be expressed within distinct functional TCR/CD3 complexes. *EMBO J* 1991;10:903.

58. Klausner RD, Samelson LE. T cell antigen receptor activation pathways: the tyrosine kinase connection. *Cell* 1991;64:875.

59. Cantrell DA, Davies AA, Crumpton MJ. Activators of protein kinase C down-regulate and phosphorylate the T3/T–cell antigen receptor complex of human T lymphocytes. *Proc Natl Acad Sci U S A* 1985;82:8158.

60. Ashwell JD, Klausner RD. Genetic and mutational analysis of the T-cell antigen receptor. *Annu Rev Immunol,* 1990;8:139.

61. Minami Y, Weissman AM, Samelson LE, et al. Building a multichain receptor: synthesis, degradation and assembly of the T-cell antigen receptor. *Proc Natl Acad Sci U S A* 1987;84:2688.

62. Bonifacino JS, Suzuki CK, Klausner RD. A peptide sequence confers retention and degradation in the endoplasmic reticulum. *Science,* 1990;247:79.

63. Sun ZJ, Kim KS, Wagner G, et al. Mechanisms contributing to T cell receptor signaling and assembly revealed by the solution structure of an ectodomain fragment of the CD3εγ heterodimer. *Cell* 2001;105:913.

64. Chien Y, Gascoigne NRJ, Kavaler J, et al. Somatic recombination in a murine T-cell receptor gene. *Nature* 1984;309:322.

65. Bosma MJ. B and T cell leakiness in the SCID mouse mutant. *Immunodefic Rev* 1992;3:261.

66. Mombaerts P, Iacomini J, Johnson RS, et al. RAG-1–deficient mice have no mature B and T lymphocytes. *Cell* 1992;68:869.

67. Shinkai Y, Rathbun G, Lam KP, et al RAG-2–deficient mice lack mature lymphocytes owing to inability to initiate V(D)J rearrangement. *Cell* 1992;68:855.

68. Fujimoto S, Yamagishi H. Isolation of an excision product of T-cell receptor alpha-chain gene rearrangements. *Nature* 1987;327:242.

69. Okazaki K, Davis DD, Sakano HT. Cell receptor beta gene sequences in the circular DNA of thymocyte nuclei: direct evidence for intramolecular DNA deletion in V-D-J joining. *Cell* 1987;49:477.

70. Heilig JS, Tonegawa S. Diversity of murine gamma genes and expression in fetal and adult T lymphocytes. *Nature* 1986;322:836.

71. Elliott JF, Rock EP, Patten PA, et al. The adult T-cell receptor δ-chain is diverse and distinct from that of fetal thymocytes. *Nature* 1988;331:627.

72. Hata S, Satyanarayana K, Devlin P, et al. Extensive junctional diversity of rearranged human T cell receptor δ genes. *Science* 1988;250:1541.

73. Raulet DH. The structure, function, and molecular genetics of the γ/δ T cell receptor. *Annu Rev Immunol* 1989;7:175.

74. de Villartay JP, Lewis D, Hockett R, et al. Deletional rearrangement in the human T-cell receptor a chain locus *Proc Natl Acad Sci U S A* 1987;84:8608.

75. Villey I, Caillol D, Seiz F, et al. Defect in rearrangement of the most 5'TCR-Jα (TEA): implications for TCR α locus accessibility. *Immunity* 1996;5:331.

76. Rowen L, Koop BF, Hood L. The complete 685-kilobase DNA sequence of the human beta T cell receptor locus. *Science* 1996;272:1755.

77. Noonan DJ, Kofler R, Singer PA, et al. Delineation of a defect in

T cell receptor beta genes of NZW mice predisposed to autoimmunity. *J Exp Med* 1986;163:644.

78. Chou HS, Nelson CA, Godambe SA, et al. Germline organization of the murine T cell receptor beta-chain genes. *Science* 1987;238:545.

79. Woodland DL, Kotzin B, Palmer E. Functional consequences of a T cell receptor Dβ2 and Jβ2 gene segment deletion. *J Immunol* 1990;14:379.

80. Havran WL, Allison JP. Developmentally ordered appearance of thymocytes expressing different T cell antigen receptors. *Nature* 1988;335:443.

81. McDougall S, Peterson CL, Calame K. A transcriptional enhancer 3' of C β 2 in the T cell receptor β locus. *Science* 1988;241:205.

82. Krimpenfort P, de Jong R, Uematsu Y, et al. Transcription of T cell receptor β-chain genes is controlled by a down-stream regulatory element. *EMBO J* 1988;7:745.

83. Sleckman BP, Bardon CG, Ferrini R, et al. Function of the TCRα enhancer in αβ and γδ T cells. *Immunity* 1997;7:505.

84. Lauzurica P, Krangel MS. Temporal and lineage-specific control of T cell receptor alpha/delta gene rearrangement by T cell receptor alpha and delta enhancers. *J Exp Med* 1994;179:1913.

85. Lauzurica P, Krangel MS. Enhancer-dependent and -independent steps in the rearrangement of a human T cell receptor delta transgene. *J Exp Med* 1994;179:43.

86. Waldmann TA, Davis MM, Bongiovanni KF, et al. Rearrangements of genes for the antigen receptor on T cells as markers of lineage and clonality in human lymphoid neoplasms. *N Engl J Med* 1985;313:776.

87. Winoto A, Baltimore D. αβ lineage-specific expression of the T cell receptor α gene by nearby silencers. *Cell* 1989;59:649.

88. Diaz P, Cado D, Winoto A. A locus control region in the T cell receptor α/δ locus. *Immunity* 1994;1:207.

89. Ishida I, Verbeek S, Bonneville M, et al. T-cell receptor γδ and γ transgenic mice suggest a role of αγ transgenic mice suggest a role of a γ gene silencer in the generation of αβ T cells. *Proc Natl Acad Sci U S A* 1990;87:3067.

90. Korsmeyer SJ. Chromosomal translocations in lymphoid malignancies reveal novel proto-oncogenes. *Annu Rev Immunol* 1992;10:785.

91. Finger LR, Harvey RC, Moore RC, et al. A common mechanism of chromosomal translocation in T- and B-cell neoplasia. *Science* 1986;234:982.

92. Baer R, Chen K-C, Smith SD, et al. Fusion of an immunoglobulin variable gene and a T cell receptor constant gene in the chromosome 14 inversion associated with T cell tumors. *Cell* 1986;43:705.

93. Denny CT, Yoshikai YU, Mak TW, et al. A chromosome 14 inversion in a T cell lymphoma is caused by site-specific recombination between immunoglobulin and T cell receptor loci. *Nature* 1986;320:549.

94. Boehm T, Greenberg JM, Buluwela L, et al. An unusual structure of a putative T cell oncogene which allows production of similar proteins from distinct mRNAs. *EMBO J* 1990;9:857.

95. McGuire EA, Hockett RD, Pollock KM, et al. The t(11;14)(p15;q11) in a T cell acute lymphoblastic leukemia cell line activates multiple transcripts, including *Ttg-1*, a gene encoding a potential zinc finger protein. *Mol Cell Biol* 1989;9:2124.

96. Royer-Pokora B, Loos U, Ludwig W-D. *Ttg-2*, a new gene encoding a cysteine-rich protein with the LIM motif, is overexpressed in acute T-cell leukaemia with the t(11;14)(p13;q11). *Oncogene* 1991;6:1887.

97. Boehm T, Foroni L, Kaneko Y, et al. The rhombotin family of cysteine-rich LIM-domain oncogenes: distinct members are involved in T-cell translocations to human chromosomes 11p15 and 11p13. *Proc Natl Acad Sci U S A* 1991;88:4367.

98. Visvader J, Begley CG, Adams JM. Differential expression of the LYL, SCL and E2A helix-loop-helix genes within the hemopoietic system. *Oncogene* 1991;6:187.

99. Finger LR, Kagan J, Christopher G, et al. Involvement of the TCL5 gene on human chromosome 1 in T-cell leukemia and melanoma. *Proc Natl Acad Sci U S A* 1989;86:5039.

100. Hatano M, Roberts CWM, Minden M, et al. Deregulation of a homeobox gene *HOX11*, by the t(10;14) in T cell leukemia. *Science* 1991;253:79.

101. O'Conner RD, Brown MG, Francke U. Immunologic and karyotypic studies in ataxia-telangiectasia: specificity of break points on chromosomes 7 and 14 in lymphocytes from patients and relatives.In: Bridges BA, Harnden DG, eds. *Ataxia-telangiectasia—a cellular and molecular link between cancer, neuropathology and immune deficiency.* New York: John Wiley and Sons, 1982;259.

102. Lipkowitz S, Stern MH, Kirsch IR. Hybrid T cell receptor genes formed by interlocus recombination in normal and ataxia-telangiectasis lymphocytes. *J Exp Med* 1990;172:409.

103. Uematus Y, Ryser S, Dembic Z, et al. In transgenic mice the introduced functional T cell receptor beta gene prevents expression of endogenous beta genes. *Cell* 1988;52:831.

104. Padovan E, Casorati G, Dellabona P, et al. Expression of two T cell receptor alpha chains: dual receptor T cells. *Science* 1993;262:422.

105. Malissen M, Trucy J, Jouvin-Marche E, et al. Regulation of TCR alpha and beta gene allelic exclusion during T-cell development. *Immunol Today* 1992;13:315.

106. Aifantis I, Buer J, von Boehmer H, et al. Essential role of the pre–T cell receptor in allelic exclusion of the T cell receptor β locus. *Immunity* 1997;7:601.

107. O'Shea CC, Thornell AP, Rosewell IR, et al. Exit of the pre-TCR from the endoplasmic reticulum/cis-Golgi is necessary for signaling differentiation, proliferation, and allelic exclusion in immature thymocytes. *Immunity* 1997;7:591.

108. Takeshita S, Toda M, Yamagishi H. Excision products of T cell receptor gene support a progressive rearrangement model of the alpha/delta locus. *EMBO J* 1989;8:3261.

109. Winoto A, Baltimore D. Separate lineages of T cells expressing the alpha beta and gamma delta receptors. *Nature* 1989;338:430.

110. Dent AL, Matis LA, Hooshmand F, et al. Self-reactive gamma delta T cells are eliminated in the thymus. *Nature* 1990;343:714.

111. Wilson A, de Villartay J-P, MacDonald HR. T cell receptor δ gene rearrangement and T early α (TEA) expression in immature αβ lineage thymocytes: implications for αβ/γδ lineage commitment. *Immunity* 1996;4:37.

112. Mombaerts P, Clarke AR, Rudnicki MA, et al. Mutations in T-cell receptor genes α and β block thymocyte development at different stages. *Nature* 1992;360:225.

113. Philpott KL, Viney JL, Kay G, et al. Lymphoid development in mice congenitally lacking T cell receptor αβ-expressing cells. *Science* 1992;256:1448.

114. Itohara S, Mombaerts P, Lafaille J, et al. T cell receptor delta gene mutant mice: independent generation of alpha beta T cells and programmed rearrangements of gamma delta TCR genes. *Cell* 1993;72:337.

115. van der Merwe PA, Barclay AN. Transient intercellular adhesion: the importance of weak protein–protein interactions. *Trends Biochem Sci* 1994;19:354.

116. Davis MM, Boniface JJ, Reich Z, et al. Ligand recognition by αβ T cell receptors. *Annu Rev Immunol* 1998;16:523.

117. Lin AY, Devaux B, Green A., et al. Expression of T cell antigen receptor heterodimers in a lipid-linked form. *Science* 1990;249:677.

118. Gregoire C, Lin SY, Mazza G, et al. Covalent assembly of a soluble T cell receptor–peptide–major histocompatibility class I complex. *Proc Natl Acad Sci U S A,* 1996;14:7184.

119. Scott CA, Garcia, KC, Carbone FR, et al. Pairing for the production of functional soluble IA MHC class II molecules. *J Exp Med* 1996;183:2087.

120. Parham P, Alpert BN, Orr HT, et al. Carbohydrate moiety of HLA antigens. Antigenic properties and amino acid sequences around the site of glycosylation. *J Biol Chem* 1977;252:7555.

121. Wettstein DA, Boniface JJ, Reay PA, et al. Expression of a functional class II MHC heterodimer in a lipid-linked form with enhanced peptide/soluble MHC complex formation at low pH. *J Exp Med* 1991;174:219.

122. Garboczi DN, Hung DT, Wiley DC. HLA-A2–peptide complexes: refolding and crystallization of molecules expressed in *Escherichia coli* and complexed with single antigenic peptides. *Proc Natl Acad Sci U S A* 1992;89:3429.

123. Altman JD, Reay PA, Davis MM. Formation of functional class II MHC/peptide complexes from subunits produced in *E.coli*. *Proc Natl Acad Sci U S A* 1993;90:10330.

124. Jackson MR, Song ES, Yang Y, et al. Empty and peptide-containing conformers of class I major histocompatibility complex molecules expressed in *Drosophila melanogaster* cells. *Proc Natl Acad Sci U S A* 1992;89:12117.

125. Kozono H, White J, Clements J, et al. Production of soluble MHC

class II proteins with covalently bound single peptides. *Nature* 1994;369:151.

126. Matsui K, Boniface JJ, Reay PA, et al. Low affinity interaction of peptide–MHC complexes with T cell receptor. *Science* 1991; 254:1788.

127. Weber S, Traunecker A, Oliveri F, et al. Specific low-affinity recognition of major histocompatibility complex plus peptide by soluble T-cell receptor. *Nature* 1992;356:793.

128. Malmqvist M. Biospecific interaction analysis using biosensor technology. *Nature* 1993;361:186.

129. Matsui K, Boniface JJ, Steffner P, et al. Kinetics of T cell receptor binding to peptide-MHC complexes: correlation of the dissociation rate with T cell responsiveness. *Proc Natl Acad Sci U S A* 1994;91:12862.

130. Willcox BE, Gao GF, Wyer JR, et al. TCR binding to peptide-MHC stabilizes a flexible recognition interface. *Immunity* 1999;10:357.

131. Garcia K, Scott C, Brunmark A, et al. CD8 enhances formation of stable T-cell receptor/MHC class I molecule complexes. *Nature* 1996;384:577.

132. Wyer JR, Willcox BE, Gao GF, et al. T cell receptor and coreceptor CD8 alpha alpha bind peptide-MHC independently and with distinct kinetics. *Immunity* 1999;2:219.

133. Renard V, Romero P, Vivier E, et al. CD8 beta increases CD8 coreceptor function and participation in TCR-ligand binding. *J Exp Med* 1996;184:2439.

134. Xiong Y, Kern P, Chang H, et al. T cell receptor binding to a pMHCII ligand is kinetically distinct from and independent of CD4. *J Biol Chem* 2001;276:5659.

135. Boniface JJ, Reich Z, Lyons DS, et al. Thermodynamics of T cell receptor binding to peptide/MHC: evidence for a general mechanism of molecular scanning. *Proc Natl Acad Sci U S A* 1999;96:11446.

136. Kersh GJ, Allen PM. Essential flexibility in the T-cell recognition of antigen. *Nature* 1996;380:495.

137. Jameson SC, Bevan MJ. T cell receptor antagonists and partial agonists. *Immunity* 1995;2:1.

138. Sykulev Y, Brunmark A, Jackson M, et al. Kinetics and affinity of reactions between an antigen-specific T cell receptor and peptide–MHC complexes. *Immunity* 1994;1:15.

139. Lyons DS, Lieberman SA, Hampl J, et al. T cell receptor binding to antagonist peptide/MHC complexes exhibits lower affinities and faster dissociation rates than to agonist ligands. *Immunity* 1996;5:53.

140. Alam SM, Travers PJ, Wung JL, et al. T-cell–receptor affinity and thymocyte positive selection. *Nature* 1996;381:616.

141. Kessler BM, Bassanini P, Cerottini J-C, et al. Effects of epitope modification on T cell receptor–ligand binding and antigen recognition by seven H-2K^d-restricted cytotoxic T lymphocyte clones specific for a photoreactive peptide derivative. *J Exp Med* 1997;185:629.

142. Holler PD, Lim AR, Cho BK, et al. CD8$^-$ T cell transfectants that express a high affinity T cell receptor exhibit enhanced peptide-dependent activation. *J Exp Med* 2001;194:1043.

143. McKeithan K. Kinetic proofreading in T-cell receptor signal transduction. *Proc Natl Acad Sci U S A* 1995;92:5042.

144. Rabinowitz JD, Beeson C, Lyons DS, et al. Kinetic discrimination in T cell activation. *Proc Natl Acad Sci U S A* 1997;93:1401.

145. Reich Z, Boniface JJ, Lyons DS, et al. Ligand-specific oligomerization of T-cell receptor molecules. *Nature* 1997;387:617.

146. Valitutti S, Muller S, Cella M, et al. Serial triggering of many T-cell receptors by a few peptide–MHC complexes. *Nature* 1995;375:148.

147. Viola A, Lanzavecchia A. T cell activation determined by T cell receptor number and tunable thresholds. *Science* 1996;273:104.

148. Janeway CA Jr. The T cell receptor as a multicomponent signalling machine: CD4/CD8 coreceptors and CD45 in T cell activation. *Annu Rev Immunol* 1992;10:645.

149. Wang J-H, Meijers R, Xiong Y, et al. Crystal structure of the human CD4 N-terminal two-domain fragment complexed to a class II MHC molecule. *Proc Natl Acad Sci U S A* 2001;98:10799.

150. Krummel MF, Davis MM. Dynamics of the immunological synapse: finding, establishing and solidifying a connection. *Curr Opin Immunol* 2002;14:66.

151. Irvine DJ, Purbhoo MA, Krogsgaard M, et al. Direct observation of ligand recognition by T lymphocytes. *Nature* 2002;419:845.

152. Wülfing C, Sumen C, Sjaastad MD, et al. Costimulation and endogenous MHC ligands contribute to T cell recognition. *Nature Immunol* 2002;3:42.

153. Gao GF, Tormo J, Gerth UC, et al. Crystal structure of the complex between human CD8 alpha and HLA-A2. *Nature* 1997;387:630.

154. Mannie MD, Rosser JM, White GA. Autologous rat myelin basic protein is a partial agonist that is converted into a full antagonist upon blockade of CD4. Evidence for the integration of efficacious and nonefficacious signals during T cell antigen recognition. *J Immunol* 1995;154:2642.

155. Vidal K, Hsu BL, Williams CB, et al. Endogenous altered peptide ligands can affect peripheral T cell responses. *J Exp Med* 1996; 183:1311.

156. Hampl J, Chien Y, Davis MM. CD4 augments the response of a T cell to agonist but not to antagonist ligands. *Immunity* 1997;7:1.

157. Madrenas J, Chau, LA, Smith J, et al. The efficiency of CD4 recruitment to ligand-engaged TCR controls the agonist/ partial agonist properties of peptide–MHC molecule ligands. *J Exp Med* 1997;185:219.

158. Davis MM, Bjorkman PJ. T cell antigen receptor genes and T cell recognition. *Nature* 1988;334:395.

159. Chothia C, Boswell DR, Lesk AM. The outline structure of the T-cell alpha beta receptor. *EMBO J* 1988;7:3745.

160. Claverie JM, Prochinicka CA, Bouguelert L. Implications of a Fab-like structure for the T-cell receptor. *Immunol Today* 1989;10:10.

161. Engel I, Hedrick SM. Site-directed mutations in the VDJ junctional region of T cell receptor beta chain cause changes in antigenic peptide recognition. *Cell* 1988;54:473.

162. Katayama CD, Eidelman FJ, Duncan A, et al. Predicted complementarity determining regions of the T cell antigen receptor determine antigen specificity. *EMBO J* 1995;14:927.

163. Jorgensen JL, Esser U, Fazekas de St. Groth B, et al. Mapping T cell receptor/peptide contacts by variant peptide immunization of single-chain transgenics. *Nature* 1992;355:224.

164. Jorgensen JL, Reay PA, Ehrich EW, et al. Molecular components of T-cell recognition. *Annu Rev Immunol* 1992;10:835.

165. Sant'Angelo DB, Waterbury G, Preston-Hurlburt P, et al. The specificity and orientation of a TCR to its peptide-MHC class II ligands. *Immunity* 1996;4:367.

166. Sun R, Shepherd SE, Geier SS, et al. Evidence that the antigen receptors of cytotoxic T lymphocytes interact with a common recognition pattern on the H-2Kb molecule. *Immunity* 1995;3:573.

167. Ehrich EW, Devaux B, Rock EP, et al. T cell receptor interaction with peptide/MHC and superantigen/MHC ligands is dominated by antigen. *J Exp Med* 1993;178:713.

168. Hennecke J, Wiley DC. T cell receptor–MHC interactions up close. *Cell* 2001;104:1.

169. Reinherz EL, Tan K, Tang L, et al. The crystal structure of a T cell receptor in complex with peptide and MHC class II. *Science* 1999;286:1913.

170. Nanda NK, Arzoo KK, Geysen HM, et al. Recognition of multiple peptide cores by a single T cell receptor. *J Exp Med* 1995;182:531.

171. Mason D. A very high level of crossreactivity is an essential feature of the T-cell receptor. *Immunol Today* 1998;19:395.

172. Wilson DB, Pinilla C, Wilson DH, et al. Immunogenicity. I. Use of peptide libraries to identify epitopes that activate clonotypic CD4$^+$ T cells and induce T cell responses to native peptide ligands. *J Immunol* 1999;163:6424.

173. Chien Y, Davis MM. How $\alpha\beta$ T cell receptors "see" peptide/MHC complexes. *Immunol Today* 1993;14:597.

174. Garcia KC, Degano M, Pease LR, et al. Structural basis of plasticity in T cell receptor recognition of a self peptide–MHC antigen. *Science* 1998;279:1166.

175. Reiser JB, Gregoire C, Darnault C, et al. A T cell receptor CDR3beta loop undergoes conformational changes of unprecedented magnitude upon binding to a peptide/MHC class I complex. *Immunity* 2002;16:345.

176. Hare BJ, Wyss DF, Osburne MS, et al. Structure, specificity, and CDR mobility of a class II restricted single-chain T-cell receptor. *Nat Struct Biol* 1999;6:574.

177. Garcia KC, Radu CG, Ho J, et al. Kinetics and thermodynamics of T cell receptor–autoantigen interactions in murine experimental autoimmune encephalomyelitis. *Proc Natl Acad Sci U S A* 2001;8: 6818.

178. Boniface JJ, Reich Z, Lyons DS, et al. Thermodynamics of T cell receptor binding to peptide/MHC: evidence for a general mechanism of molecular scanning. *Proc Natl Acad Sci U S A* 1999;96: 11446.

179. Wu LC, Tuot DS, Lyons DS, et al. A two-step binding mechanism for T-cell receptor recognition of peptide MHC. *Nature* 2002:418:552.

180. Marrack P, Kappler J. The staphylococcal enterotoxins and their relatives. *Science* 1990;248:705.

181. McDonald KR, Acha-Orbea H. Superantigens of mouse mammary tumor virus. *Annu Rev Immunol* 1995;13:459.

182. Li H, Llera A, Malchiodi EL, et al. The structural basis of T cell activation by superantigens. *Annu Rev Immunol* 1999;17:435.

183. Sundberg EJ, Li Y, Mariuzza RA. So many ways of getting in the way: diversity in the molecular architecture of superantigen-dependent T-cell signaling complexes. *Curr Opin Immunol* 2002;14:36.

184. Festenstein H. Immunogenetic and biological aspects of *in vitro* lymphocyte allotransformation (MLR) in mouse. *Transplant Rev* 1973;15:62.

185. Kappler JW, Staerz U, White J, et al. T cell receptor Vb elements which recognize Mls-modified products of the major histocompatibility complex. *Nature* 1988;332:35.

186. Woodland DL, Happ MP, Gollob KJ, et al. An endogenous retrovirus mediating deletion of ab T cells. *Nature* 1991;349:529.

187. Marrack P, Kushnir E, Kappler J. A maternally inherited superantigen encoded by a mammary tumour virus. *Nature* 1991;349:524.

188. Choi Y, Kappler JW, Marrack P. A superantigen encoded in the open reading frame of the 3' long terminal repeat of mouse mammary tumour virus. *Nature* 1991;350:203.

189. Dyson PJ, Knight AM, Fairchild S, et al. Genes encoding ligands for deletion of Vb11 T cells cosegregate with mammary tumour virus genomes. *Nature* 1991;349:531.

190. Frankel WN, Rudy C, Coffin JM, et al. Linkage of *Mls* genes to endogenous mammary tumour viruses of inbred mice. *Nature* 1991;349:526.

191. Janeway CAJ, Yagi J, Conrad PJ, et al. T-cell responses to Mls and to bacterial proteins that mimic its behavior. *Immunol Rev* 1989;107:61.

192. Stuart PM, Woodward JG. *Yersinia enterocolitica* produces superantigenic activity. *J Immunol* 1992;148:225.

193. Abe J, Takeda T, Watanabe Y, et al. Evidence for superantigen production by *Yersinia pseudotuberculosis. J Immunol* 1993;151:4183.

194. Tomai M, Kotb M, Majumdar G, et al. Superantigenicity of streptococcal M protein. *J Exp Med* 1990;172:359.

195. Cole BC, Kartchner DR, Wells DJ. Stimulation of mouse lymphocytes by a mitogen derived from *Mycoplasma arthritidis*. VII. Responsiveness is associated with expression of a product(s) of the V beta 8 gene family present on the T cell receptor alpha/beta for antigen. *J Immunol* 1989;142:4131.

196. Friedman SM, Crow MK, Tumang JR, et al. Characterization of the human T cells reactive with the *Mycoplasma arthritidis*–derived superantigen (MAM): generation of a monoclonal antibody against Vb17, the T cell receptor gene product expressed by a large fraction of MAM-reactive human T cells. *J Exp Med* 1991;174:891.

197. Lafon M, Scott-Algara D, March PN, et al. Neonatal deletion and selective expansion of mouse T cells by exposure to rabies virus nucleocapsid superantigen. *J Exp Med* 1994;180:1207.

198. Dobrescu D, Ursea B, Pope M, et al. Enhanced HIV-1 replication in Vβ12 T cells due to human cytomegalovirus in monocytes: evidence for a putative herpesvirus superantigen. *Cell* 1995;82:753.

199. Yao Z, Maraskovsky E, Spriggs MK, et al. Herpesvirus saimiri open reading frame 14, a protein encoded by T lymphotropic herpesvirus binds to MHC class II molecules and stimulates T cell proliferation. *J Immunol* 1996;156:3260.

200. Sutkowski N, Conrad B, Thorley-Lawson DA, et al. Epstein-Barr virus transactivates the human endogenous retrovirus HERV-K18 that encodes a superantigen. *Immunity* 2001;15:57.

201. Denkers EY, Caspar P, Sher A. *Toxoplasma gondii* possesses a superantigen activity that selectively expands murine T cell receptor V beta 5–bearing CD8+ lymphocytes. *J Exp Med* 1994;180:985.

202. Held W, Waanders GA, Shakhov AN, et al. Superantigen-induced immune stimulation amplifies mouse mammary tumor virus infection and allows virus transmission. *Cell* 1993;74:529.

203. Golovkina TV, Chervonsky A, Dudley JP, et al. Transgenic mouse mammary tumor virus superantigen expression prevents viral infection. *Cell* 1992;69:637.

204. Stauffer Y, Marguerat S, Meylan F, et al. Interferon-induced endogenous superantigen: a model linking environment and autoimmunity. *Immunity* 2001;15:591.

205. Dalwadi H, Wei B, Kronenberg M, et al. The Crohn's disease–associated bacterial protein 12 is a novel enteric T cell superantigen. *Immunity* 2001;5:149.

206. Malchiodi EL, Eisenstein E, Fields BA, et al. Superantigen binding to a T cell receptor β chain of known three-dimensional structure. *J Exp Med* 1995;182:1.

207. Sundberg EJ, Li Y, Mariuzza RA. So many ways of getting in the way: diversity in the molecular architecture of superantigen-dependent T-cell signaling complexes. *Curr Opin Immunol* 2002;14:36.

208. Fields BA, Malchiodi EL, Li H, et al. Crystal structure of a T cell receptor beta-chain complexed with a superantigen. *Nature* 1996;384:188.

209. Arcus VL, Proft T, Sigrell JA, et al. Conservation and variation in superantigen structure and activity highlighted by the three-dimensional structures of two new superantigens from *Streptococcus pyogenes. J Mol Biol* 2000;299:157.

210. Li Y, Li H, Dimasi N, et al. Crystal structure of a superantigen bound to the high-affinity, zinc-dependent site on MHC class II. *Immunity* 2001;14:93.

211. Petersson K, Hakansson M, Nilsson H, et al. Crystal structure of a superantigen bound to MHC class II displays zinc and peptide dependence. *EMBO J* 2001;20:3306.

212. Li H, Llera A, Tsuchiya D, et al. Three-dimensional structure of the complex between a T cell receptor chain and the superantigen staphylococcal enterotoxin B. *Immunity* 1998;9:807.

213. Rojo JM, Janeway CAJ. The biologic activity of anti–T cell receptor V region monoclonal antibodies is determined by the epitope recognized. *J Immunol* 1988;140:1081.

214. Haas W, Pereira P, Tonegawa S. Gamma/delta cells. *Annu Rev Immunol* 1993;11:637.

215. Chien Y-H, Jores R, Crowley MP. Recognition by γ/δ T cells. *Annu Rev Immun* 1996;14:511.

216. Stingl G, Gunter KC, Tschachler E, et al. Thy-1+ dendritic epidermal cells belong to the T-cell lineage. *Proc Natl Acad Sci U S A* 1987; 84:2430.

217. Goodman T, Lefrancois L. Expression of the gamma-delta T-cell receptor on intestinal CD8+ intraepithelial lymphocytes. *Nature* 1988;333:855.

218. Itohara S, Farr AG, Lafaille JJ, et al. Homing of γδ thymocyte subset with homogeneous T-cell receptors to mucosal epithelia. *Nature* 1990;343:754.

219. Augustin A, Kubo RT, Sim GK. Resident pulmonary lymphocytes expressing the γ/δ T-cell receptor. *Nature* 1989;340:239.

220. Asarnow DM, Kuziel WA, Bonyhadi M, et al. Limited diversity of γδ antigen receptor genes of Thy-1+ dendritic epidermal cells. *Cell* 1988;55:837.

221. Feeney AJ. Predominance of VH-D-JH junctions occurring at sites of short sequence homology results in limited junctional diversity in neonatal antibodies. *J Immunol* 1992;149:222.

222. Havran WL, Chien YH, Allison JP. Recognition of self antigens by skin-derived T cells with invariant gamma delta antigen receptors. *Science* 1991;252:1430.

223. Sim G-K, Augustine A. Dominate expression of BID, an invariant undiversified T cell receptor δ chain. *Cell* 1990;61:397.

224. De Geus B, Van den Enden M, Coolen C, et al. Phenotype of intraepithelial lymphocytes in euthymic and athymic mice: implications for differentiation of cells bearing a CD3-associated γδ T cell receptor. *Eur J Immunol* 1990;20:291.

225. Cron RQ, Gajewski TF, Sharrow SO, et al. Phenotypic and functional analysis of murine CD3+, CD4−, CD8− TCR-gamma/delta–expressing peripheral T cells. *J Immunol* 1989;142:3754.

226. Allison JP, Havran WL. The immunobiology of T cells with invariant γδ antigen receptor. *Annu Rev Immunol* 1991;9:679.

227. Ohga S, Yoshikai Y, Takeda Y, et al. Sequential appearance of γδ- and αβ- bearing T cells in the peritoneal cavity during an i.p. infection with *Listeria monocytogenes. Eur J Immunol* 1990;20:533.

228. Ferrick D, Schrenzel M, Mulvania T, et al. Differential production of interferon-g and interleukin-4 in response to Th1- and Th2-stimulating pathogens by γδ T cells *in vivo. Nature* 1995;373:255.

229. Kaufmann S. Bacterial and protozoal infections in genetically disrupted mice. *Curr Opin Immun* 1994;6:518

230. Carding S, Allan W, Kyes S, et al. Late dominance of the inflammatory process in murine influenza by gamma/delta + T cells. *J Exp Med* 1990;172:1225.

231. Hiromatsu K, Yoshikai Y, Matsuzaki G, et al. A protective role of

γ/δ T cells in primary infection with *Listeria monocytogenes* in mice. *J Exp Med* 1992;175:49.

232. Roberts SJ, Smith AL, West AB, et al. T-cell alpha beta + and gamma delta + deficient mice display abnormal but distinct phenotypes toward a natural, widespread infection of the intestinal epithelium. *Proc Natl Acad Sci U S A* 1996;93:11774.

233. Mombaerts P, Arnoldi J, Russ F, et al. Different roles of αβ and γδ T cells in immunity against an intracellular bacterial pathogen. *Nature* 1993;365:53.

234. Kaufmann S, Ladel C. Role of T cell subsets in immunity against intracellular bacteria: Experimental infections of knock-out mice with *Listeria monocytogenes* and *Mycobacterium bovis* BCG. *Immunobiology* 1994;191:509.

235. Kaufmann, SHE. γ/δ and other unconventional T lymphocytes: what do they see and what do they do? *Proc Natl Acad Sci U S A* 1996;93:2272.

236. Witherden DA, Rieder SE, Boismenu R, et al. A role for epithelial gamma delta T cells in tissue repair. *Springer Semin Immunopathol* 2000;22:265.

237. Komano H, Fujiura Y, Kawaguchi M, et al. Homeostatic regulation of intestinal epithelia by intraepithelial γδ T cells. *Proc Natl Acad Sci U S A* 1995;92:6147.

238. Kaufmann S, Blum C, Yamamoto S. Crosstalk between alpha/beta T cells and gamma/delta T cells *in vivo*: activation of alpha/beta T-cell responses after gamma/delta T-cell modulation with the monoclonal antibody GL3. *Proc Natl Acad Sci U S A* 1993;90:9620.

239. McMenamin C, Pimm C, McKersey M, et al. Regulation of IgE responses to inhaled antigen in mice by antigen-specific gamma delta T cells. *Science* 1994;265:1869.

240. Wen L, Roberts S, Viney J, et al. Immunoglobulin synthesis and generalized autoimmunity in mice congenitally deficient in alpha beta(+) T cells. *Nature* 1994;369:654.

241. Viney J, Dianda L, Roberts J, et al. Lymphocyte proliferation in mice congenitally deficient in T-cell receptor alpha beta + cells. *Proc Natl Acad Sci U S A* 1994;91:11948.

242. Fahrer AM, Konigshofer Y, Kerr EM, et al. Attributes of gamma delta intraepithelial lymphocytes as suggested by their transcriptional profile. *Proc Natl Acad Sci U S A* 2001;98:10261.

243. Shires J, Theodoridis E, Hayday AC. Biological insights into TCRγδ + and TCRαβ+ intraepithelial lymphocytes provided by serial analysis of gene expression (SAGE). *Immunity* 2001;15:419.

244. Schild H, Mavaddat N, Litzenberger C, et al. The nature of major histocompatibility complex recognition by γδ T cells. *Cell* 1994;76:29.

245. Weintraub B, Jackson M, Hedrick S. Gamma delta T cells can recognize nonclassical MHC in the absence of conventional antigenic peptides. *J Immunol* 1994;153:3051.

246. Sciammas R, Johnson R, Sperling A, et al. Unique antigen recognition by a herpesvirus-specific TCR gamma delta cell. *J Immunol* 1994;152:5392.

247. Crowley MP, Reich Z, Mavaddat N, et al. The recognition of the nonclassical major histocompatibility complex (MHC) class I molecule, T10, by the gamma delta T cell, G8. *J Exp Med* 1997;185:1223.

248. Wingren C, Crowley MP, Degano M, et al. Crystal structure of a gamma delta T cell receptor ligand T22: a truncated MHC-like fold. *Science* 2000;287:310.

249. Van Kaer L, Wu M, Ichikawa Y, et al. Recognition of MHC TL gene products by gamma delta T cells. *Immunol Rev* 1991;120:89.

250. Hampl J, Schild H, Litzenberger C, et al. The specificity of a weak gamma delta TCR interaction can be modulated by the glycosylation of the ligand. *J Immunol* 1999;163:288.

251. Crowley MP, Fahrer AM, Baumgarth N, et al. A population of murine gamma delta T cells that recognize an inducible MHC class Ib molecule. *Science* 2000;287:314.

252. Bauer S, Groh V, Wu J, et al. Activation of NK cells and T cells by NKG2D, a receptor for stress-inducible MICA. *Science* 1999;285:727.

253. Schoel B, Sprenger S, Kaufmann S. Phosphate is essential for stimulation of V gamma 9V delta 2 T lymphocytes by mycobacterial low molecular weight ligand. *Eur J Immunol* 1994;24:1886.

254. Constant P, Davodeau F, Peyrat M, et al. Stimulation of human gamma delta T cells by nonpeptidic mycobacterial ligands. *Science* 1994;264:267.

255. Tanaka Y, Sano S, Nieves E, et al. Nonpeptide ligands for human gamma delta T cells. *Proc Natl Acad Sci U S A* 1994;91:8175.

256. Tanaka Y, Morita C, Tanaka Y, et al. Natural and synthetic nonpeptide antigens recognized by human gamma delta T cells. *Nature* 1995;375:155.

257. Janis EM, Kaufman SHE, Schwartz RH, et al. Activation of γδ T cells in the primary immune response to mycobacterium tuberculosis. *Science* 1989;244:713.

258. Modlin RL, Pirmez C, Hofman FM, et al. Lymphocytes bearing antigen-specific γδ T-cells receptors accumulate in human infectious disease lesions. *Nature* 1989;339:544.

259. Vidovic D, Roglic M, McKune K, et al. Qa-1 restricted recognition of foreign antigen by a gamma delta T-cell hybridoma. *Nature* 1989;340:646.

260. Holoshitz J, Vila LM, Keroack BJ, et al. Dual antigenic recognition by cloned human γ-δ T-cells. *J Clin Invest* 1992;89:308.

261. Born W, Hall L, Dallas A, et al. Recognition of a peptide antigen by heat shock reactive γδ T lymphocytes. *Science* 1990;249:67.

262. Loh EY, Wang M, Bartkowiak J, et al. Gene transfer studies of T-cell receptor-γ-δ recognition. Specificity for staphylococcal enterotoxin-A is conveyed by V-γ-9 alone. *J Immunol* 1994;152:3324.

263. Kim HT, Nelson EL, Clayberger C, et al. Gamma delta T cell recognition of tumor Ig peptide. *J Immunol* 1995;154:1614.

264. Rock E, Sibbald P, Davis M, et al. CDR3 length in antigen-specific immune receptors. *J Exp Med* 1994;179:323.

265. Lerner E, Matis L, Janeway CJ, et al. Monoclonal antibody against an Ir gene product? *J Exp Med* 1980;152:1085.

266. Ozato K, Mayer N, Sachs D. Hybridoma cell lines secreting monoclonal antibodies to mouse H-2 and Ia antigens. *J Immunol* 1980;124:533.

267. Fisch P, Malkovsky M, Kovats S, et al. Recognition by human Vγ9/Vδ2 T cells of a GroEL homolog on Daudi Burkitt's lymphoma cells. *Science* 1990;250:1269.

267a. Seidl K, Ph.D. diss. "Genetic Influences on development of B-1 cell repertoire". Stanford University, 1995.

268. Porgador A, Yewdell JW, Deng Y, et al. Localization, quantitation, and *in situ* detection of specific peptide-MHC class I complexes using a monoclonal antibody. *Immunity* 1997;6:715.

269. Dafaglio G, Nelson CA, Deck BM, et al. Characterization and quantitation of peptide-MHC complexes produced from hen egg lysozyme using a monoclonal antibody. *Immunity* 1997;6:727.

270. Reay PA, Matsui K, Haase K, et al. Determination of the relationship between T cell responsiveness and the number of MHC-peptide complexes using specific monoclonal antibodies. *J Immunol* 2000;164:5626.

271. Lang F, Peyrat M, Constant P, et al. Early activation of human Vγ9Vδ2 T cell broad cytotoxicity and TNF production by nonpeptidic mycobacterial ligands. *J Immunol* 1995;154:5986.

272. Morita CT, Beckman EM, Bukauri JF, et al. Direction presentation of nonpeptide prenyl pyrophosphate antigens to human γδ T cells. *Immunity* 1995;3:495.

273. Iwashima M, Green A, Bonyhadi M, et al. Expression of a fetal γδ T-cell receptor in adult mice triggers a non–MHC-linked form of selective depletion. *Int Immunol* 1991;3:385.

274. Cunningham BC, Wells JA. Comparison of a structural and a functional epitope. *J Mol Biol* 1993;234:554.

275. Clackson T, Wells JA. A hot spot of binding energy in a hormone-receptor interface. *Science* 1995;267:383.

276. Davis MM, Lyons DS, Altman JD, et al. T cell receptor biochemistry, repertoire selection and general features of TCR and Ig structure. In: *The molecular basis of cellular defence mechanisms.* Ciba Fdn, John Wiley and Sons 1997:94–104.

277. Berek C, Milstein C. The dynamic nature of the antibody repertoire. *Immunol Rev* 1988;105:5.

278. Patten PA, Gray NS, Yang PL, et al. The immunological evolution of catalysis. *Science* 1996;271:1078.

279. Xu JL, Davis MM. Diversity in the CDR3 region of VH is sufficient for most antibody specificities. *Immunity* 2000;13:37.

280. Taylor LD, Carmack CE, Huszar D, et al. Human immunoglobulin transgenes undergo rearrangement, somatic mutation and class switching in mice that lack endogenous IgM. *Int Immunol* 1994;6:579.

281. Seth A, Stern LJ, Ottenhoff THM, et al. Binary and ternary complexes between T-cell receptor, class II MHC and superantigen *in vitro.* *Nature* 1994;369:324.

282. Corr M, Slanetz A, Boyd L, et al. T cell receptor–MHC class I peptide interactions: affinity, kinetics, and specificity. *Science* 1994; 265:946.

283. Sykulev Y, Brunmark A, Tsomides TJ, et al. High-affinity reactions between antigen-specific T-cell receptors and peptides associated with allogeneic and syngeneic major histocompatibility complex class I proteins. *Proc Natl Acad Sci U S A* 1994;91:11487.

284. Stern LJ, Wiley DC. The human class II MHC protein HLA-DR1 assembles as empty alpha beta heterodimers in the absence of antigenic peptide. *Cell* 1992;68:465.

285. Callahan JE, Herman A, Kappler JW, et al. Stimulation of B10.BR T cells with superantigenic staphylococcal toxins. *J Immunol* 1990; 144:2473.

286. Takimoto H, Yoshikai Y, Kishihara K, et al. Stimulation of all T cells bearing V beta 1, V beta 3, V beta 11 and V beta 12 by staphylococcal enterotoxin A. *Eur J Immunol* 1990;20:617.

287. White J, Herman A, Pullen AM, et al. The V beta–specific superantigen staphylococcal enterotoxin B: stimulation of mature T cells and clonal deletion in neonatal mice. *Cell* 1989;56:27.

288. Yagi J, Baron J, Buxser S, et al. Bacterial proteins that mediate the association of a defined subset of T cell receptor: CD4 complexes with class II MHC. *J Immunol* 1990;144:892.

289. Herman A, Kappler JW, Marrack P, et al. Superantigens: mechanism of T-cell stimulation and role in immune responses. *Annu Rev Immunol* 1991;9:745.

290. Held W, Shakhov AN, Waanders G, et al. An exogenous mouse mammary tumor virus with properties of Mls-1a (Mtv-7). *J Exp Med* 1992;175:1623.

291. Goding JW, Harris AW. Subunit structure of cell surface proteins: disulfide bonding in antigen receptors, Ly-2/3 antigens, and transferrin receptors of murine T and B Lymphocytes. *Proc Natl Acad Sci U S A* 1981;78:4530.

CHAPTER 9

T-Cell Developmental Biology

Ellen V. Rothenberg, Mary A. Yui, and Janice C. Telfer

Overview of T-Cell Development
Key Molecules: Cell Stage Markers and T-Cell Receptor Genes · Narrative of T-Cell Development · Regulated Proliferation in T-Cell Development · Anatomical Path of T-Cell Development · Variations in Thymocyte Development in Ontogeny · Thymocyte Development in Species Other than Mouse · Plan of Chapter: Close-up Views of Key Events
Early Lineage Choices: Clues to Molecular Mechanisms
Developmental Potential of Earliest Intrathymic Precursors · Molecular Indices of T-Lineage Specification and Commitment · Genetic Requirements for T-Lineage Specification and Commitment
A Regulatory Upheaval: β Selection
Multiple Changes at the Transition from T-Cell Receptor–Independent to T-Cell Receptor–Dependent T-Cell Development · Triggering Requirements for β Selection · Constituent Events in the β Selection Cascade · Death Mechanisms and Other Checkpoint Controls · Significance of β Selection for Later T-Cell Differentiation
The Divergence of T-Cell Receptor $\alpha\beta$ and T-Cell Receptor $\gamma\delta$ Lineage Cells
Choices of Fate within the T-Cell Lineage: Differences between $\alpha\beta$ and $\gamma\delta$ T Cells · Generation of T-Cell Receptor $\gamma\delta$ Cells · Genetic Regulation of T-Cell Receptor $\alpha\beta$ versus T-Cell Receptor $\gamma\delta$ Cell Production · Models for the T-Cell Receptor $\alpha\beta$:T-Cell Receptor $\gamma\delta$ Lineage Choice
Positive and Negative Selection
The Double-Positive Thymocyte Stage · Time Windows for Positive and Negative Selection · Triggering and Results of Positive Selection · Strength of Signal versus Distinct Interaction Models for Positive and Negative Selection · Another Escape from Autoreactivity in the Thymic Cortex
CD4 Helper T-Cell versus CD8 Cytotoxic T-Cell Lineage Commitment
Major Histocompatibility Complex Restriction Regulates CD4 versus CD8 Lineage Differentiation · Models for CD4/CD8 Lineage Divergence · Molecules Implicated in the CD4/CD8 Lineage Choice · Maturation and Export of CD4 and CD8 Single-Positive Thymocytes · Relationships between Positive Selection, Negative Selection, and CD4/CD8 Lineage Choice
Frontiers for the Future: Mysteries and Alternatives in T-Cell Development
Alternative Pathway or Distinct Precursors: The Case of the NK T Cells · Variations on a Theme of Tolerance: Regulatory T Cells
Concluding Remarks
Acknowledgments
References

T-cell development is a composite of overlapping processes in the domains of developmental biology, immunology, and cell biology. It starts with purely hematopoietic developmental mechanisms leading to lymphoid commitment, T-lineage commitment, and later developmental choice points; then gradually, the basis for developmental choices becomes dominated by the immunology of T-cell receptor (TCR) repertoire selection. The underlying mechanisms by which these later choices are made can be understood only in terms of a richly complex cell biology of checkpoint enforcement, defining the two TCR-dependent fate-determination processes of β selection and positive/negative selection. Repertoire selection is crucial for establishing a functionally competent, mostly self-tolerant population of peripheral T cells, and it has attracted a great deal of interest in isolation from other aspects of T-cell development. In this chapter, we show how this cellular

process occurs, on the basis of mechanisms that emerge from a unique and fascinating developmental program. A recurrent theme is how the signals from various TCR complexes come to intertwine with underlying developmental mechanisms to control cell fate at a succession of distinct checkpoints and lineage choices.

To begin, this chapter introduces the broad map of T-cell developmental events. The subsequent sections focus in on the mechanisms involved at a few of its most interesting watersheds.

OVERVIEW OF T-CELL DEVELOPMENT

In mammals, most circulating T cells develop in the thymus. Bone marrow precursors in small numbers enter the thymus from the blood and undertake a course of proliferation, differentiation, and selection, which converts them into T cells in about 4 weeks (faster in fetal animals). The mature cells then emigrate from the thymus and take up their surveillance roles in the body. Precursors seed the thymus and differentiate into T cells continuously from midgestation throughout adult life. An additional site of development is in the intestinal epithelium, in which T cells that mostly remain associated with the gut epithelium appear to be generated. In either case, T cells distinguish themselves from most hematopoietic cell types by migrating away from the bone marrow in order to carry out their differentiation. It is in the thymus that most TCR gene rearrangement occurs and the cells first acquire their clonal recognition properties. The thymus not only promotes maturation but also rigorously screens each cohort of developing cells to eliminate those with either useless or dangerous TCRs, in a process called "repertoire selection."

Key Molecules: Cell Stage Markers and T-Cell Receptor Genes

At any one time after birth, the thymus contains cells in all stages of development, from the earliest precursors to cells that are virtually mature. Understanding of the process of T-cell differentiation has been possible because cells in different stages can be distinguished, and cells of each type can be isolated preparatively without being killed. At least seven developmental stages can be distinguished on the basis of their expression of useful surface molecules. These are introduced in Fig. 1. Key markers for subdividing the majority of thymocytes are TCR$\alpha\beta$, TCR$\gamma\delta$, and the co-receptors CD4 and CD8 (Fig. 1A). These help to identify cells in the later 2 weeks of intrathymic differentiation. The majority of thymocytes, approximately 80%, express both CD4 and CD8 and low levels of surface TCR$\alpha\beta$ complexes, a constellation of markers that is not seen in general on peripheral T cells (Fig. 1A). This distinctive population, called "double positive" (DP), is a key developmental intermediate that undergoes "TCR repertoire selection," the complex process that eliminates cells with either useless or autoreactive TCR specificities. The unique properties of DP cells make TCR repertoire selection possible. Minorities of the cells are CD4$^+$CD8$^-$ TCR$\alpha\beta^{high}$ or CD4$^-$CD8$^+$ TCR$\alpha\beta^{high}$, and these "single positive" (SP) thymocytes are the most mature cells.

Cells in the earlier 2 weeks of differentiation in the thymus lack any TCR expression as well as any expression of CD4 or CD8. Nevertheless, different stages can be distinguished in this "double negative" (DN) or "triple negative" (TN) population. In mice, they can be subdivided, on the basis of expression of the interleukin (IL)–2 receptor α-chain CD25 and the adhesion molecule CD44, into progressive developmental stages termed DN1, DN2, DN3, and DN4 (or TN1, TN2, and so forth) (Fig. 1B). Two other useful markers for these stages are the stem cell growth factor receptor c-kit (CD117), which is coexpressed with CD44, and the small phospholipid-linked heat-stable antigen (HSA, CD24) which is turned on with CD25 and remains on until the latest stages of thymocyte maturation. In the human system, different markers are useful for distinguishing corresponding stages, and they described later. An outline of the progression of mouse precursor cells through these stages is shown in Fig. 2 as a framework for this narrative.

TCR gene rearrangement plays a pivotal role in thymocyte fate. Ultimately, thymocytes can survive to maturity only if they successfully carry out combinations of gene rearrangements that will give them in-frame α and β chains or γ and δ chains, to be assembled into TCR$\alpha\beta$/CD3 or TCR$\gamma\delta$/CD3 complexes. The rules of the process are therefore worth reviewing. There are four TCR gene loci, each consisting of the constant region exons and multiple variable (V), joining (J), and sometimes diversity (D) segments of the TCRα, β, γ, and δ chain genes (see Chapter 8). The TCRβ and TCRδ loci have D segments as well as V and J segments to be rearranged, whereas the TCRα and TCRγ loci do not. Also, note that the TCRδ locus is embedded in the middle of the TCRα locus in such a way that any V-Jα rearrangement automatically deletes the TCRδ locus entirely, whether it had undergone rearrangement before or not. These features are important for the regulation of rearrangement and, as described later, for understanding the choice between becoming a TCR$\alpha\beta$- or a TCR$\gamma\delta$-lineage thymocyte. The rearrangement process is ordered, with D-Jβ rearrangements occurring before V-D-Jβ and V-Dδ rearrangements occurring before V-D-Jδ.

Narrative of T-Cell Development

Figure 2 traces the progress of cells through the best-known stages of T-cell development.

The cells that enter the thymus are capable of giving rise to all subsets of T cells plus natural killer (NK) cells and dendritic cells. As discussed later, they may be able to give rise to macrophages and B cells, too. These cells are initially c-kit$^+$, Thy-1^{low}, CD44^{high}, CD25$^-$, and CD24^{low}. At this stage, the TCR genes are not yet rearranged. These precursor cells form the key component of the subset called DN1 or TN1.

Once in the thymus, these cells undergo a major transition, losing much of their ability to give rise to anything but T cells, turning on the expression of multiple T-cell genes, and starting to proliferate. They begin to express Thy-1, CD25, and CD24, and CD44 and c-kit continue to be expressed on the cell surface, although at declining levels. The stage marked by this new phenotype is classified as DN2 (TN2) (Figs. 1B & 2). Proliferative expansion during this stage is considerable, approximately 6 to 10 rounds of division. This is the stage when TCR gene rearrangement begins. TCRγ, TCRδ, and TCRβ all appear to be similarly accessible to rearrangement during this initial period, but TCRα is not.

At the next stage, DN3, CD44, and c-kit are fully downregulated; most cell proliferation stops; and rearrangement of the TCRβ, γ, and δ genes occurs with maximum efficiency. The DN3 stage (Thy-1$^+$ c-kit$^-$ CD44$^-$ CD25$^+$ CD24$^+$ cells) is a landmark because, in both adult and fetal thymocytes,

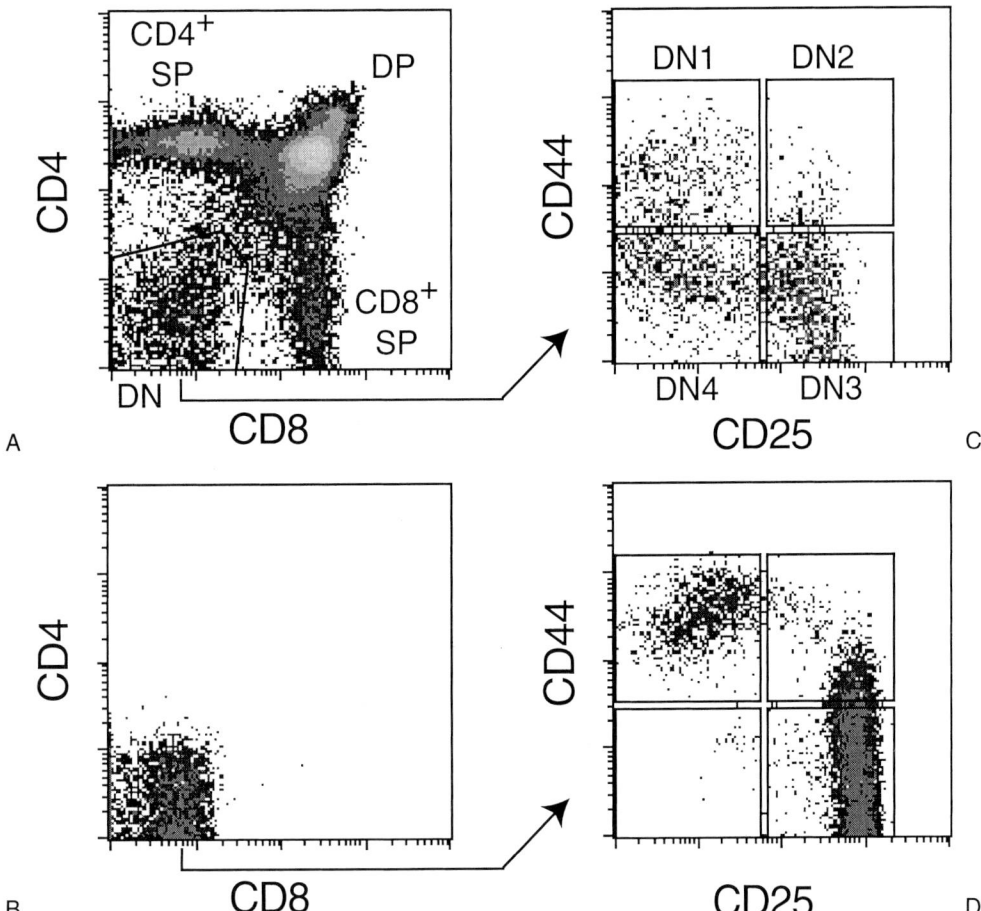

FIG. 1. Subsets of T-cell precursors: normal development versus. development without T-cell receptor (TCR) gene rearrangement. The major subsets of cells discussed in this chapter, as they appear in a typical flow cytometric analysis. Normal thymocytes are shown on the top (**A** and **C**), whereas thymocytes from recombination activating gene (RAG)–deficient mice, which cannot rearrange any TCR genes, are shown on the bottom (**B** and **D**). The cells are stained with fluorescent antibodies against CD4 and CD8 (**A** and **B**), and the double-negative (DN) cells are further stained with fluorescent antibodies against CD44 and CD25 (**C** and **D**). The axes represent increasing levels of these surface molecules on a 4-decade logarithmic scale: that is, a 10,000-fold range in fluorescent staining intensity. The main populations discussed in Fig. 2 are (DN, DP, CD4 SP, CD8 SP) (**A**), and the DN cells are subdivided into DN1, DN2, DN3, and DN4 (**C**). Comparison between the upper and lower panels shows that the recombinase-deficient thymocytes are developmentally arrested in the DN stages (**B**), with cells accumulating in the DN3 state and blocked from progressing forward to the DN4 state (**D**; cf. **C**). RAG-deficient thymocytes also accumulate only about 1/100 as many cells in the thymus as wild-type thymocytes ($\sim 4 \times 10^6$ vs. $\sim 3 \times 10^8$).

it is the first stage when the cells appear to have lost the ability to develop into anything but T cells. It is also the first stage when the protein products of rearranged TCR genes are detected in the cytoplasm. Beyond this stage, the proliferation and survival of the cells depend essentially on interactions mediated by TCR proteins. If they rearrange their TCR genes correctly, they can proceed, often with a burst of proliferation. If they fail, they die.

The exact path that the cells follow from this point depends on whether the cells succeed in making D-Jβ and V-D-Jβ rearrangements to form a productive TCRβ open-reading frame before they have completed productive rearrangements of both the γ and δ loci. In the first case, they develop into $\alpha\beta$ T cells; in the second case, they develop into $\gamma\delta$ T cells. The

$\gamma\delta$ cells mature with little additional proliferation and with few known changes to their surface phenotype other than down-regulation of CD25 and CD24. Cells that rearrange β, on the other hand, undergo a complex succession of events known as β selection. These cells proliferate in a rapid burst; down-regulate the DN2/DN3 marker CD25; turn on expression of CD4 and CD8; stop TCRβ, TCRγ, and TCRδ rearrangements; begin rearranging TCRα; and undergo profound functional transformations. Through this cascade of events, the cells are quickly transformed from DN3 to DP cells, through proliferating intermediates called DN4 and immature single positive (ISP) cells, usually CD8$^+$CD4$^-$CD3$^-$ (Fig. 2). DP cells are physiologically peculiar; these peculiarities make them uniquely poised for TCR-dependent

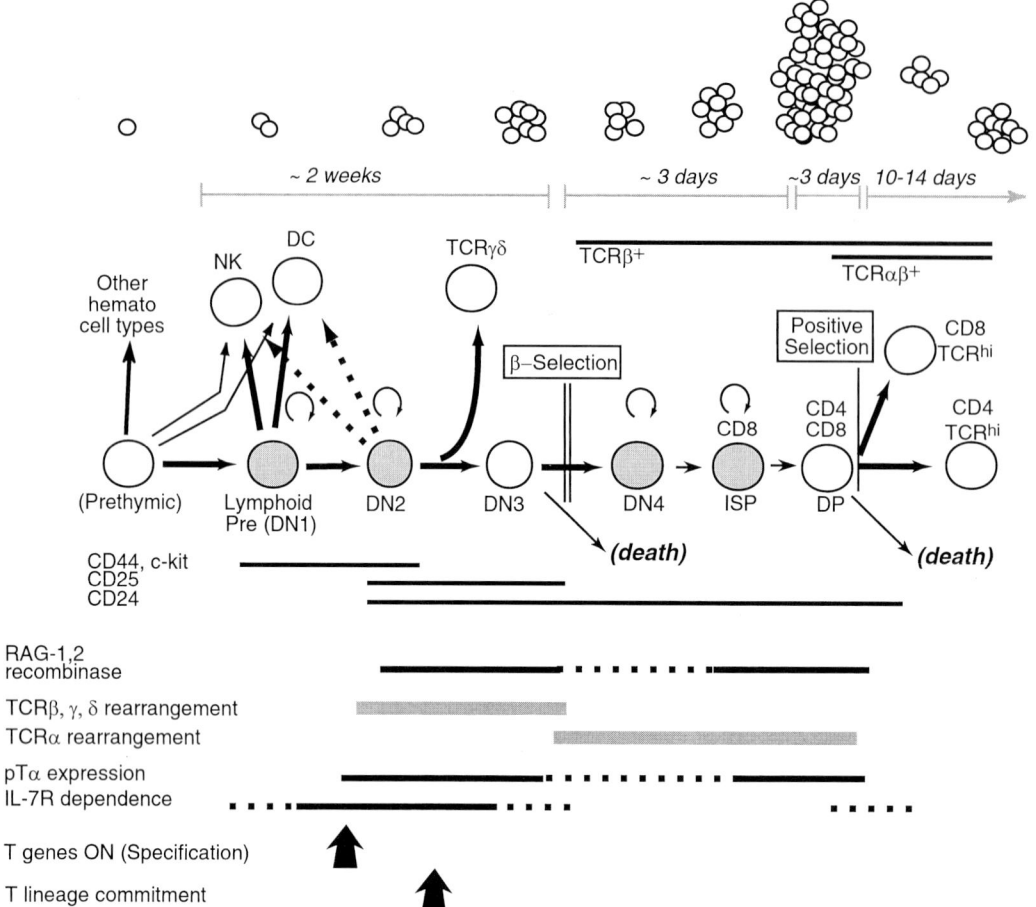

FIG. 2. Outline of events in T-cell development. Summary of the events occurring in normal mouse T-cell development, indicating the approximate time taken in each set of transitions, the developmental branch points, and key changes in gene expression and T-cell receptor (TCR) gene rearrangement status. Developmental branch points taken rarely are indicated by *broken-line arrows.* The two major checkpoints discussed in the chapter, β selection and positive selection, are indicated. The alternative to positive selection, death, includes both negative selection and death by "neglect," as discussed in the text. *Small curving arrows* over the double-negative 1 (DN1)→ DN2 and DN4→immature single positive (ISP) stages denote the extensive proliferation at these stages, also suggested by the cartoon at the top. Stages of development in which a majority of cells are seen to be in cycle are indicated by *gray filled circles.* Cells expressing rearranged TCRγ and TCRδ genes (TCR$\gamma\delta$) and cells expressing rearranged TCRβ genes either alone or together with rearranged TCRα genes are indicated above the main diagram. Below the main diagram, *bars* show the extents of expression of useful cell surface markers other than CD4, CD8, and the TCR complexes. Periods of recombinase expression, specific gene rearrangement, and key developmental events are also indicated by *horizontal bars. Broken bars* show reduced levels of expression. Common abbreviations of cell stages are given in the text. Hemato, hematopoietic; Lymphoid pre, lymphoid precursor.

repertoire selection. They are therefore key intermediates in the production of a self-tolerant T-cell population. As a rule, the DP cell fate is part of the $\alpha\beta$ program and not part of the $\gamma\delta$ program. Thus, although the choice of $\alpha\beta$ versus $\gamma\delta$ fate is based at least partly on the stochastic success or failure of rearrangements, it results in a real choice between developmental programs.

Cells that fail to complete any productive TCRβ or TCRγ and δ gene rearrangements die within a few days. In mutant mice that cannot make rearrangements at all, development cannot proceed beyond the DN3 stage (Fig. 1D), and death of

cells blocked at that point results in a thymus that is only about 1% of the normal cellularity. Besides the choice of TCR$\alpha\beta$ versus TCR$\gamma\delta$, the DN3 stage therefore represents a rigorous developmental checkpoint. The "β-selection checkpoint" is the first of two checkpoints at which survival is dependent on the TCR.

For cells taking the TCRβ^+ CD4$^+$CD8$^+$ path, rescue from death at the β-selection checkpoint is only a temporary, conditional reprieve. In these DP cells, TCRβ rearrangement must be followed by a successful TCRα gene rearrangement within about 3 days after the proliferative burst subsides, or else the cells die of "neglect." The selection for cells that have made an acceptable TCRαβ complex defines the second TCR-dependent checkpoint in T-cell development: "positive selection." The criteria for rearrangement success here are more stringent than for β selection. Any TCRβ gene rearrangement that generates a translatable protein coding sequence is adequate for β selection, but the TCRα rearrangement is evaluated both on the basis of a translatable protein coding sequence and on the basis of the recognition specificity that emerges from the new combination of TCRα chain with the previously fixed TCRβ chain. The cells must be able to interact with major histocompatibility complex (MHC) molecules in the microenvironment, but not too well, or else the cells die. The criterion is set so that individual CD4$^+$CD8$^+$ TCRβ$^+$ cells have less than a 5% chance of satisfying it. As a result, about 30% of this population dies each day in the young mouse thymus (over 90% die without maturing in the whole 3- to 4-day lifetime of each cell cohort) and must be replaced as a fresh cohort of CD4$^+$CD8$^+$ cells enters the selection pool.

DP cells are actually put through two tests. The first determines whether the newly expressed TCRαβ can make sufficiently strong interactions with MHC molecules to be useful, and the second assesses whether the interactions of this TCR with self-antigens in the thymus are weak enough to reduce the danger of autoimmunity. These thresholds are tested in two separable processes: positive selection and negative selection. Cells exceeding the minimum affinity threshold are positively selected, initiating a new cascade of phenotypic changes and enhancing the viability and functional responsiveness of the cells. Cells that exceed the maximum affinity threshold can be stripped of their receptors or negatively selected by induced apoptosis. Key changes that help trace progress through positive selection are the transient upregulation of the activation marker CD69, the stepwise increase in TCRαβ surface expression from low to intermediate to high, a parallel up-regulation of CD5 and MHC class I molecules, and ultimately the down-regulation of the immature cell marker CD24. Cells remain susceptible to negative selection for several days after the initiation of positive selection, however. They may even encounter the most potent negative selection stimuli in the period after positive selection. Only cells escaping both death by neglect and death by negative selection can complete their maturation and emigrate to the peripheral lymphoid system.

Positive selection also appears to drive a choice of maturation fates. It is in the emergence from the DP state that there occurs the first evidence of whether a cell will be a CD4$^+$ helper/regulatory cell or a CD8$^+$ killer cell. As described in detail later, detailed aspects of the TCR–ligand receptor interactions during this process guide or select cells to develop into one type of effector or the other. Cells with TCRs that recognize MHC class II molecules tend to develop as CD4$^+$ cells, whereas those with TCRs that recognize MHC class I molecules develop as CD8$^+$ cells. The basis of this profound differentiation choice is extremely interesting and appears to include subtle quantitative aspects of TCR/co-receptor interaction with MHC and the combination of TCR-generated signals with signals from other pathways.

Regulated Proliferation in T-Cell Development

Throughout T-cell development, phases of intense proliferation alternate with phases of little or no cycling. The differences in cell cycle activity are dramatic. As shown in Fig. 2, DN2 cells are cycling, DN3 cells halt, and then, after β selection, cells appear to go through six to eight rounds of division in about 3 days (1,2). After positive selection, in contrast, maturing cells appear to reside in the medulla for approximately 2 weeks without any significant proliferation. Each phase of proliferation tends to be driven by a different mechanism (3). The growth controllers used at various stages include many of the genes that are essential for progression through the T-cell developmental pathway, as discussed later.

In the first DN1 precursors, the initiation of cell division may be controlled by c-kit signaling. In the DN1-DN2 states, proliferation is mostly driven by signals from the interaction of IL-7, a cytokine secreted by the thymic stroma, with IL-7 receptor complexes, composed of IL-7Rα (CD127) and γc chains (CD132) (Fig. 2) (4–6). During β selection, population expansion is driven by signaling through the pre-TCR (TCRβ complex), which is discussed later in detail. The later events of positive selection and maturation do not involve significant proliferation; however, they completely depend on TCRαβ for survival signaling. These sequential requirements for survival have overlapping critical periods, so that the mutant phenotypes are slightly leaky but still have powerful quantitative effects (7). After export from the thymus, mature T-cell proliferation depends on TCRαβ triggering and signals through the IL-2, IL-4, or IL-7 receptors. The shift from one kind of proliferative stimulus to another is caused least in part by intrinsic developmental changes in the cells. It is an important factor contributing to the one-way polarity of developmental change.

The proliferative bursts are vital for setting up the large excess of precursors that makes it possible to use stringent selection at the checkpoints in T-cell development. The huge losses that occur in these selection processes seem shocking, except that the developmental program also provides for more than 10^5-fold clonal expansion from each precursor. Harsh selection against useless or autoreactive cells is a price the adaptive immune system must pay for its somatic generation of diversity in recognition structures. This suggests that the mechanisms used by lymphoid precursors to drive developmental proliferation are evolutionarily old and likely to have coevolved with the mechanisms generating clonal diversity.

The extents of proliferation at particular stages in T-cell development are somewhat flexible. Proliferation at β selection can compensate for poor precursor expansion in an earlier phase. Also, although positive selection per se does not involve proliferation, cells in the fetal and early postnatal thymus can undergo several cell cycles during the maturation period after positive selection. This presumably helps to supply T cells to the body quickly, during a period when peripheral T cells are rare. Later, in the adult thymus, maturation occurs with little if any proliferation. Development of T cells depends on proliferation but not in a way that rigidly links certain events to precise numbers of cell cycles.

Anatomical Path of T-Cell Development

The thymus is made up of lobes, each of which is divided into distinct zones with different stromal cells making up their microenvironments (8). The largest domain is the cortex, which is packed with DP thymocytes. The cortex surrounds an inner domain called the medulla, where the most advanced SP thymocytes are found. The outermost rim of the cortex (i.e., the subcapsular region) and the region defining the cortical/medullary junction are also specialized in some ways. The organization of the thymus is diagrammed schematically in Fig. 3.

From β selection onward, the pathway of thymocytes through the thymus is well known. Most of the proliferative expansion that follows β selection occurs in the subcapsular zone. As the cells are pushed away from the rim toward the inner cortex, they stop dividing. DP cells in the cortex continue to sink inward during their 3 days of postmitotic life, but they are not allowed to enter the medulla unless they pass positive selection. Those that do not succeed die in the cortex and are rapidly engulfed by resident macrophages.

The path taken from entry into the thymus until β selection has been less clear. Because of the enormous proliferative expansion during T-cell development, the number of cells in

the earliest stages, at any one time, is dwarfed by the number of cells in the later stages. All the DN stages together, representing approximately 2 weeks of developmental change, contribute only approximately 2% to 4% of a typical young adult thymus. The earliest precursors in the DN population have been estimated to be less than one one-hundredth of that frequency. Conceivably, a thymus that turns over approximately 5×10^7 cells per day may be resupplied with an input of only 50 to 100 cells per day. The low input numbers have made it hard to trace the path of precursors through intrathymic domains in their early development. Only since 2000 have DN1- and DN2-specific markers been used successfully to track the path of these thymic entrants specifically (9). This has revealed a more organized role for different subregions of the adult thymus than was previously suspected.

It now appears that blood-borne precursors enter the parenchyma of the postnatal thymus by exiting from the medium-sized blood vessels (postcapillary venules) at the cortical/medullary junction. These cells, in an early DN1 state, slowly make their way outward through the thymic cortex to the subcapsular zone, proliferating and differentiating through the DN2 and DN3 states over the next 2 weeks. Those cells becoming $\gamma\delta$ cells may not need to progress further than the midcortex. Those continuing on to become $\alpha\beta$ cells travel all the way to the periphery (Fig. 3). The β-selection checkpoint appears to be encountered mostly in the subcapsular zone. Numerous, rapidly proliferating blasts can be seen in the outer cortex; they represent the DN4, ISP, and early DP cells that have just passed this test. As they stop proliferating, DP thymocytes fall back into the cortex, being pushed progressively deeper by products of later cell divisions over the next 2 to 3 days. Those few that are positively selected, along with mature $\gamma\delta$ cells, migrate from the cortex to the medulla (Fig. 3) (9).

Maturation of the surviving cells occurs in the medulla over the following 2 weeks. The medullary epithelial cells are distinct from the cortical epithelial cells. It is not clear exactly how they influence final T-cell maturation, although evidence suggests that they may express a very wide range of self-antigens that may be valuable in negative selection (10). Dendritic cells, which are also specifically located in the medulla, present self-antigen to the newly SP cells in the most efficient way for the most stringent form of negative selection. It is only after surviving these encounters that the SP cells complete their maturation, changing their response physiology so that high-affinity interactions with antigen can lead to activation instead of paralysis or death.

The compartmentalization of functions in the thymus probably helps guide certain developmental transitions. As the cells change in intrinsic responsiveness to different proliferative signals, their migration may carry them from a zone rich in early stimuli (e.g., IL-7) to a zone that may be rich in later stimuli [possibly Wnt (11,12)]. Certain transitions from proliferation to G_1 arrest, such as from DN2 to DN3 or from β selection to a resting DP state, could result from migration

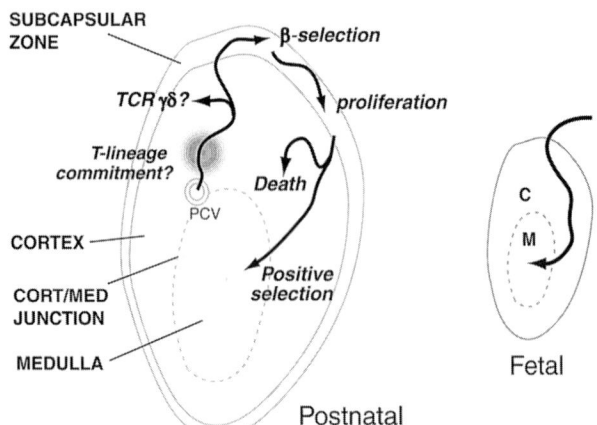

FIG. 3. Summary of migration pathways of thymocytes through the postnatal and fetal thymic microenvironments. The pathway of migration of adult thymocytes from the post-capillary venule (PCV) through the cortex, subcapsular zone, cortex and medulla is shown on the **left** (9). For comparison, the entry and migration through the fetal thymus is shown on the **right**.

of the cells into a zone where the most recent proliferative stimulus is no longer present. Also, the change in direction of migration of precursors through the cortex, from outbound to inbound, is likely to be a result of a change in the expression of adhesion molecules and chemokine receptors in the DN3 state or during β selection. There is evidence that could implicate particular integrins (e.g. $\alpha_4\beta_1$) in the outward migration of DN cells (13), and the roles of these important molecules are likely to become much clearer in the near future. At least one other adhesion molecule, CD44, is expressed very highly in the DN1 cells but then clearly turned off between the DN2 and DN3 state; this could be another participant in the early homing or guidance mechanisms or both. Later, at least one new chemokine receptor is turned on at β selection, and this may help attract DP cells back toward the interior (14–16). Migration between domains with different kinds of stromal cells allows a separation between positive and negative selection events in space and time. As discussed in a later section, this can clarify some otherwise confusing features of these processes.

Variations in Thymocyte Development in Ontogeny

The general outlines of thymocyte development are consistent between postnatal and fetal mice, but there are many differences, both subtle and overt. The mouse fetal thymic stroma develops from the outpocketing of third pharyngeal pouch endoderm, between 10 and 12.5 days of gestation (E10 to E12.5). It may undergo some inductive interaction with the overlying ectoderm and neural crest cells of the third branchial arch (17). The thymic epithelium, in any case, establishes a distinctive structure and gene expression pattern before any lymphoid precursors arrive (17,18). Seeding begins at about E12 as hematopoietic precursors migrate across the mesenchyme from the subclavian vessels to the tiny, nonvascularized epithelial rudiment (19,20). These cells are CD45$^+$, expressing certain lymphoid genes and marked by the presence of the lymphoid transcription factor Ikaros in the nucleus. The precursors collect around the thymus and then enter it directly from the outside; this is the one time that the future outer cortex is a point of entry (Fig. 3, right panel).

Lymphoid precursors proliferate exponentially in the fetal murine thymus, increasing from about 10^4 cells at E14.5 dpc to about 5×10^5 at E18. In contrast to the kinetics in the postnatal thymus, in the fetal thymus the first TCR$\alpha\beta$ DP cells are generated at about E16, the first SP CD4 cells about 2 days later, and CD8 cells a day after that, followed by birth at day 20; the first emigrants are exported to the periphery within 3 days after birth. Thus, the times in the DN state and in the medulla are each cut from approximately 14 days in the postnatal ("adult") thymus to less than 3 days in the fetal thymus.

The precursors that initially seed the fetal thymus are qualitatively different from any that enter it later. Radiation chimera experiments establish that they can generate the same types of T cells that are made from adult bone marrow–derived precursors, but they also have a capacity that adult precursors do not. The first thymic immigrants are uniquely capable of generating two classes of $\gamma\delta$ T cells that seed the skin, tongue, and reproductive organ epithelia in late fetal life but are not produced at all after birth (21). These "early-wave" $\gamma\delta$ cells use directed, predetermined V(D)J rearrangements without junctional diversification, so that their recognition specificities are completely invariant. They are, in fact, the first wave of TCR$^+$ thymocytes made in the mouse at all, maturing by E15.5 to E16.5, and they have a number of distinctive physiological properties, including growth factor requirements and transcription factor profiles (22). The precursors that make these cells may themselves be unusual in other ways as well. For example, it is not clear whether they ultimately originate in the intraembryonic hematopoietic tissues at all or from the molecularly unique precursor cells in the yolk sac (23).

At least one additional wave of precursors enters the thymus closer to the time of birth (24), and then further precursors can continue to enter throughout life. In the meantime, the properties of the major populations of hematopoietic precursors themselves continue to change, shifting from fetal liver to bone marrow and acquiring new molecular properties (23). Certain gene disruptions have sharply different effects on T-cell development in fetal, postnatal, and adult mice, because of intrinsic differences in the programming of different precursor cohorts (25–29) (detailed in the section on genetic requirements of T-lineage specification and commitment and in Fig. 5B later). It is intriguing that T-cell differentiation takes long enough, in relation to precursor cohort succession, so that considerable overlap could occur in young postnatal animals. Thus, we can even consider that in a 3- to 4-week-old weanling mouse, the bone marrow stem cells, intrathymic DN3 cells, and mature medullary SP thymocytes ready for export at that time could each represent progeny of distinct cohorts of progenitor cells, each with different genetic requirements, molecular expression properties, or both. Distinctions between results in fetal and adult systems are noted throughout this chapter.

Thymocyte Development in Species Other than Mouse

The overall organization of thymic lobes is conserved from mammals to cartilaginous fish. The overall roles of cortex and medulla for T-cell development seem to have been established early in vertebrate evolution. In chickens and *Xenopus*, there is also strong evidence for development of distinctive T-cell populations in the tadpole or embryo, unlike those made after hatching. Chicken thymocyte developmental studies have actually provided some of the first evidence for the distinctiveness of early-wave $\gamma\delta$ cells. However, markers are just becoming available to distinguish developmental stages in these animals (30,31), and much remains to be learned about homology or lack of homology of their T-cell developmental pathways with those in mice.

Thymocyte development has been studied in some detail in rats and humans as well as in mice. Comparison of features can indicate the most critical events in a developmental process, which tend to be conserved. One surprising finding is the relative lack of conservation of detailed patterns of surface marker expression, even over these short phylogenetic distances. The Thy-1 surface glycoprotein is not expressed in rat or human mature T cells, and CD25, which is distinctively up-regulated in murine DN2 and DN3 stages, is not up-regulated at a corresponding stage in human (32–34). Rat and human T cells can also express MHC class II molecules on activation, which is confined to non–T cells in mice, whereas CD2, which is T-cell specific in humans, is expressed by murine B and NK cells as well. The rat system has been more closely studied with reference to positive selection and its signaling requirements; some of the details of this process are different in rats than in mice (35). The timing of CD8 and CD4 expression relative to β selection is also slightly shifted from the mouse, which is, again, different from the human pattern (36). Homologous surface markers cannot always be assumed to mark homologous developmental stages in these three mammalian species.

Against this background of evolutionary variation, however, there are salient points of similarity, listed in Table 1. The human pathway starts with an uncommitted precursor (CD34$^+$CD38$^+$) that enters the thymus with a range of developmental potentials that is similar or identical to that of its mouse counterpart. The sequence of T-lineage commitment in relation to onset of T-cell gene expression and TCR gene rearrangement is similar to the timing in the murine system, as is the order of TCR gene rearrangement. The markers useful for distinguishing these stages are different, and CD4 and CD8 are turned on at a different time in relation to β selection. Nonetheless, the properties of DP thymocytes generated after β selection are grossly conserved, although they are generally more viable and responsive than their murine counterparts. As in the mouse, TCR^{high} SP thymocytes newly generated through positive selection remain functionally immature at first, which implies that maturation after positive selection is required (37,38). The cell surface markers that provide landmarks for this process are summarized in Table 1.

Plan of Chapter: Close-up Views of Key Events

This overview of intrathymic T-cell development gives a sense of the intricacy of the process, in terms of both the choices the cells must make and the constantly shifting interactions of the cells with their environment. The following sections of this chapter focus on five aspects of T-cell development in depth, in which underlying molecular mechanisms are beginning to be revealed. These areas offer insight into the ways T-cell precursors make the subtle and precise distinctions that are necessary to allow a complex hematopoietic developmental sequence to be governed by TCR specificity and self-tolerance.

EARLY LINEAGE CHOICES: CLUES TO MOLECULAR MECHANISMS

Developmental Potential of Earliest Intrathymic Precursors

The first question concerns when precursor cells are actually determined to become T cells at all. What is the relationship of this event to TCR gene rearrangement, to entry into the thymus, and to regulatory changes leading to expression of T-cell genes? Answers have emerged from experiments that define the functional properties of the least differentiated cells in the thymus.

The most primitive precursors in the thymus have been identified in two ways. One is on the basis of their time of appearance during gestation; that is, the first hematopoietic cells found in the thymus in the fetus. The other is in the adult thymus, through the use of multiple cell surface markers to purify subsets of cells that have immature characteristics (DN, c-kit$^+$) and then assays of their abilities to differentiate into T cells in adoptive transfer experiments. Adoptive transfer of cells to genetically distinct hosts has been the gold standard for proving developmental potential. Finely optimized fetal thymic organ cultures allow any T-lineage progeny to be studied on a smaller scale. In these assays, the most primitive of the precursors are identified as those that give the largest output of descendants per input cell, generate them over the longest time course, and give rise to other verified

TABLE 1. *T-cell development stage markers: a mouse–human comparison*

Stage	Mouse phenotype	Human phenotype
Intrathymic T/DC/NK precursor	CD44$^+$ c-kit$^+$ CD25$^-$	CD34$^+$ CD38^{lo}
Intrathymic T/NK precursor; TCRδ rearrangement	(Fetus only) NK1.1$^+$ CD122$^+$ CD44$^+$ c-kit$^+$ CD25$^-$	CD34$^+$ CD5$^+$ CD7$^+$
Committed T precursor	CD44$^-$ c-kit$^-$ CD25$^+$ CD24$^+$	CD34$^+$ CD5$^+$ CD7$^+$ CD1a$^+$
TCRβ, TCRγ, TCRδ rearrangement	CD44$^{+/-}$ c-kit$^{+/-}$ CD25$^+$ CD24$^+$	CD5$^+$ CD7$^+$ CD1a$^+$ CD4$^+$ CD8α^- CD8β^- (CD4 ISP)
β-selection	CD25$^+$ CD4$^-$ CD8$^-$ to CD25$^-$ CD4$^+$ CD8$^+$ (DN3 to DN4, ISP, DP)	CD8α^- to CD8α^+ (CD4 ISP to early DP)
TCRα rearrangement	CD4$^{+/-}$ CD8$\alpha\beta^+$ (ISP, DP)	CD1a$^+$ CD4$^+$ CD8$\alpha\beta^+$
Mature cells	TCR/CD3^{hi} and CD4$^+$ or CD8$\alpha\beta^+$	CD1a$^-$ TCR/CD3^{hi} and CD4$^+$ or CD8$\alpha\beta^+$

TCR, T-cell receptor; T/DC/NK, T cells/dendritic cells/natural killer cells.
Human data from Plum et al. (216) and Blom et al. (217).

T-lineage precursors as intermediates in the process. In the adult thymus, the most primitive precursors are found as a subpopulation within the DN1 class.

Adoptive transfer into irradiated mice or into fetal thymic organ cultures *in vitro* reveals that such cells actually have a range of developmental potentials, giving rise to non–T cells as well as T cells. This was shown first at the population level (39,40), and, more recently, it has been confirmed rigorously for single cells. In the murine fetal thymus and the postnatal human thymus, precursors are robust enough to be assayed in single-cell tests for multiple lineage precursor activity (41–43). These assays agree in showing that many early intrathymic precursors individually have the potential to give rise to dendritic cells, NK cells, and diverse classes of $\alpha\beta$ and $\gamma\delta$ T cells. In contrast, none of the intrathymic precursor populations have been reported to give rise to erythroid, megakaryocytic, or granulocytic cells. Thus, the precursors that enter the thymus are partially restricted in developmental potential but still uncommitted to the T-cell lineage.

Oligopotent, partially restricted cells may not be the only cells seeding the thymus. There is strong evidence that some cells can become committed to the T-cell lineage prethymically. This is indicated by the presence of partial TCR gene rearrangements and by the selective ability to generate T cells in adoptive transfer. Prethymic commitment of some cells to the T lineage is especially evident in the fetus (44,45). Some of these cells may be dedicated precursors of special, extrathymically developing lineages of T cells (46–49). Note that there is no known reason why T-lineage commitment could not occur both inside and outside the thymus; NK and mast cells are examples of other hematopoietic cell types that may undergo this step either in the bone marrow or in other sites. The mechanism that enables precursors to home to the thymus from the fetal liver or bone marrow is still poorly understood, but it presumably is a matter of altered expression of particular adhesion molecules and chemokine receptors. Conceivably, these alterations can occur at different times, in relation to other early T-lineage differentiation events, in fetal liver versus adult bone marrow precursor cells.

The most controversial question about early intrathymic precursors is whether they have B-cell as well as T-cell precursor activity. Because both B and T cells depend on the unique recombination activating gene (RAG) 1/RAG2–mediated receptor gene rearrangements and checkpoints in their development, it seems attractive to imagine that they are very closely related. In the adult, there are bone marrow common lymphoid precursors that can make colonies *in vitro* which differentiate selectively to B cells, NK cells, and T-cell precursors (50). Also, an evolutionarily conserved feature, across most jawed vertebrate classes, is the presence of at least some B cells as well as T cells in the thymus (51,52). The murine thymus itself includes a small number of B cells, as well as T cells, NK cells, and dendritic cells. Results of adoptive transfers and *in vitro* cultures of bulk cell populations have suggested that the B cells may arise from the same precursors that generate T cells (39,53,54). However, single-cell assays of precursors taken from the mouse

or human thymus have not confirmed a close B-/T-cell relationship (33,45); the cells that give rise to B cells are not the same as the T-cell precursors, at least not after they have arrived in the thymus. In assays of single cells from fetal liver, cells that show B- and T-cell precursor activity generally also show myeloid precursor activity (41,55,56).

One explanation seems to be provided by characteristics of the thymic microenvironment. Evidence suggests that many cells going to the thymus could differentiate efficiently into B cells in principle but that much of this activity is masked in the thymic environment by inhibitory signaling through the Notch-1 transmembrane receptor protein. Notch-1 signals are essential for T-cell development from the earliest detectable stages, and the thymic cortical microenvironment is evidently rich in Notch ligands. Notch ligand expression may be one of the conditions that makes the thymus (and some intestinal epithelial domains) uniquely permissive for T-cell development (57,58). This context is intensely suppressive of the development of B cells (58–60). Any of diverse strategies to inhibit Notch-1 activation allows production of thymic B cells at the expense of T cells (61–65). Thus, regardless of whether the cells populating the thymus have intrinsic B cell potential, this potential would normally be kept inoperative within the thymic cortex as long as the cells express Notch-1. The few B cells that do manage to reside in the thymus tend normally to be confined to the medulla; this may be a domain free of Notch ligands.

The cells gradually lose their developmental alternatives during the first T-lineage–differentiative transitions after precursor entry into the thymus. Single-cell analyses of fetal thymocytes show that many DN1 cells and a few DN2 cells can still differentiate into NK cells, and a large fraction of DN1-DN2 cells can give rise to dendritic cells (42,66–68). Under certain culture conditions, DN2 cells can even generate macrophages (69). The yield of these non–T cells is lower from DN2 thymocytes than from DN1 cells, and no B-cell potential is detected in the DN2 population. At the DN3 stage, the cells appear to have lost these residual alternatives and give rise only to T cells. The DN3 stage thus marks the completion of T-cell lineage commitment.

Molecular Indices of T-Lineage Specification and Commitment

Most genes associated with T-lineage development are already activated before commitment is complete. Some of these genes, such as CD3, Lck protein tyrosine kinase, and "sterile" transcripts from certain unrearranged $V\beta$ genes, are already expressed in DN1 cells (70–72). Most others are activated or up-regulated during the DN1→DN2 transition. Strikingly, cytokine and perforin genes used in responses of mature T cells are already expressed or inducible in the DN1 and DN2 cells. By the time the cells have reached the DN2 state, the cells are already expressing a full battery of T-lineage genes. We refer to these cells as "specified" for T-lineage differentiation. However, under appropriate conditions, as many as 50% to 75% of these cells (73) still remain capable of giving rise to dendritic cells *in vitro*. In the human system, committed dendritic cells continue to express the "T cell–specific" gene pTα (74). Thus, specification precedes commitment.

Expression of genes associated with a particular cell type before actual commitment is not an anomaly in hematopoietic development. For example, single-cell reverse-transcription polymerase chain reaction assays have shown that uncommitted erythromyeloid precursors and stem cells individually express a multilineage gene profile (75,76). In fact, using green fluorescent protein transgenes under the control of the Rag1 and pTα regulatory sequences, two groups have shown that both of these DN2-stage associated genes can be expressed at a low level even longer before commitment. They are both active in bone marrow precursors that are still pluripotent, and which shut off pTα when they differentiate into B cells and shut off Rag1 when they become NK cells (76a,76b). It is not surprising, therefore, that a population enriched for precursor activity within the DN1 subset expresses genes associated with non–T cell types as well as T cells, such as sterile transcripts of the immunoglobulin heavy chain, the macrophage colony–stimulating factor receptor, and the dendritic cell cytokine TARC (70, 70a). These non–T genes are not expressed in the DN2 and DN3 stages. This is consistent with the evidence from erythromyeloid systems that lineage commitment involves *repression of inappropriate genes,* in addition to *activation of lineage-specific genes.* Both the onset of T-lineage

gene expression and the shutting off of inappropriate genes are likely to be necessary for T-lineage differentiation. The regulatory genes that are necessary to guide T-cell development may contribute to either or both of these mechanisms.

Genetic Requirements for T-Lineage Specification and Commitment

T-cell development can be impaired by mutations of genes that act in specification of precursors, in survival and expansion in the DN2/DN3 states, in β selection, or in positive selection. None of the genes encoding TCR or pre-TCR components or the molecules that mediate TCR signaling cascades is needed before β selection. Instead, this early period depends on genes encoding growth factor receptors, their associated signaling components, several key transcription factors, and Notch-1. The developmental transitions dependent on the action of these genes are summarized in Fig. 4, and the effects of some of the knockout mutations on thymus size and cell number are illustrated in Fig. 5.

The growth factor receptors that are needed in the early stage are IL-7Rα/γc and c-kit (Fig. 4; cf. Fig. 2). Disruption of γc, IL-7, IL-7Rα, or c-kit alone causes a decline in the number of viable DN2 and DN3 cells, but a few cells escape to undergo essentially normal differentiation from β selection onward (3–6). Fig. 5A dramatically illustrates the importance of the IL-7/IL-7R pathway before β selection: If thymocytes

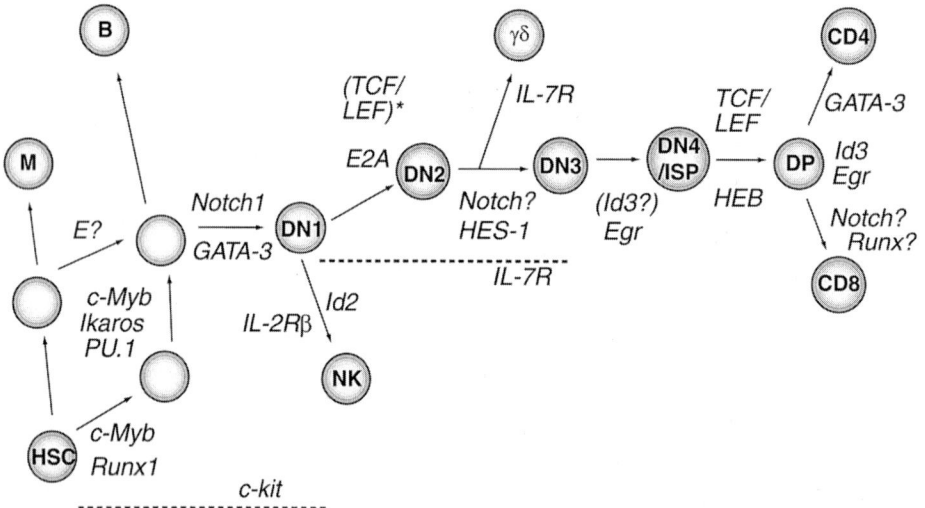

FIG. 4. Stage-specific requirements for transcription factor and growth factor receptor genes in development of T cells from hematopoietic stem cells. The stages of development at which the indicated genes work are shown, on the basis of the effects of loss or gain of function experiments. Cell types are indicated in *bold regular type* and genes are indicated in *italic type*. The genes shown in the figure are discussed extensively in the text. The roles of c-Myb and Runx1 are critical for establishment of definitive-type stem cells, making it difficult to assay any later effects. Ikaros and PU.1 also affect stem cells, at least in postnatal mice. It is not clear exactly which prethymic precursor types are affected by loss of function of these genes, and so two hypothetical pathways are shown, one involving a lymphoid/myeloid precursor, another less characterized. The T-cell factor (TCF) or lymphoid enhancer factor (LEF) is shown primarily acting at the transition from immature single positive (ISP) to double positive (DP), the first stage when these related factors appear to be needed in young mouse thymocytes; however, in older mice, the loss of TCF causes arrest at the transition from double negative (DN) 1 to DN2, indicated here by (TCF/LEF)*.HSC, hematopoietic stem cell; E?, possible role for some E protein, E2A, or HEB or a relative.

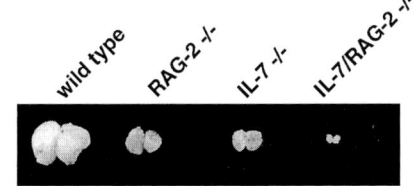

A

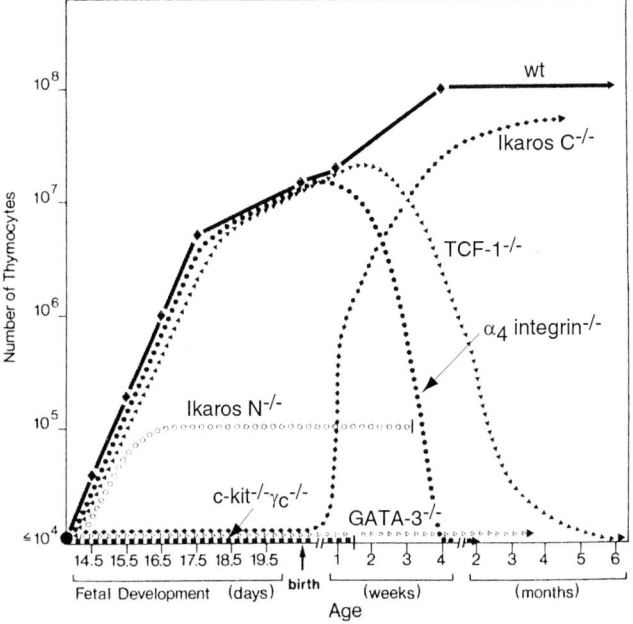

B

FIG. 5. Effects of mutations in growth factor and transcription factor genes on thymus population sizes. **A:** Evidence for a critical role of interleukin (IL)–7/IL-7R signaling in proliferation at a stage of T-cell development preceding β-selection. Thymus glands are shown from wild-type and the indicated mutant mice. The recombination activating gene 2 (RAG2)$^{-/-}$ mutation alone results in a 50- to 100-fold reduction in cell numbers because of a developmental block at β-selection. The IL-7$^{-/-}$ mutation alone has a similar impact on the size of the thymus. The multiplicative effect of the double mutation shows that IL-7 is needed for the proliferation that normally takes place in double negative (DN) cells in the RAG2$^{-/-}$ mouse thymus. From(5), with permission. **B:** Growth of cell numbers in the thymus from fetal life to adulthood in wild-type (wt) mice and mice with inactivating mutations in various genes. From (175), with permission. T-cell factor (TCF)–1 (TCF), GATA-3, and Ikaros are transcription factors discussed in the text. Ikaros-N$^{-/-}$ is a mutation that creates a dominant negative form; Ikaros-C$^{-/-}$ is a loss of function mutation (152). Double mutants lacking both c-kit and the common cytokine receptor chain γc do not generate any T-cell precursors, as discussed in the text. Mutants lacking α_4-integrin are defective in precursor migration, affecting T cell precursors after birth. The shifts in effects of some mutations between fetal life and postnatal life indicate the distinct molecular requirements for early and later T-cell development.

that cannot undergo β selection, such as RAG2$^{-/-}$ cells, attempt to differentiate in an IL-7–deficient environment, the thymus remains minute, much smaller than in the mutants of either the IL-7 or the RAG2 gene alone. Thus, the proliferation occurring at β selection may compensate for a shortage of precursors. The survival of any thymocytes to this point, in the absence of IL-7R signals, appears to be due to the ability of c-kit/stem cell factor interactions to sustain a few cells long enough for them to make a productive TCRβ gene rearrangement. Double mutation of both c-kit and the common γ subunit of the IL-7R prevents any detectable lymphoid precursors from appearing in the thymus (77). Growth factor receptors can be important to development both to provide survival/proliferation signals and, in some cases, to provide "instructive" signals to initiate a cell type–specific gene expression program. For T cell development in general, the roles of c-kit and the IL-7R complex can be explained entirely in terms of survival/proliferation. The only exception is that IL-7R receptor signaling may influence the direction of differentiation in the choice between TCR$\alpha\beta$ and TCR$\gamma\delta$ lineages, as discussed later.

The generation of precursors with the competence to become T cells depends on regulatory genes that include those coding for the transcription factors Ikaros, PU.1, c-Myb, and GATA3 (Figs. 4 and 5) (78–80). Ikaros, c-Myb, and GATA3 have all been shown to bind to specific target sites in T-cell differentiation genes [TCRα, TCRβ, TCRγ, TCRδ, CD3δ, and terminal deoxynucleotide transferase (TdT)], but mutation of any of these genes blocks thymocyte development long before any of these genes is required. PU.1 is not known to be required for any T-cell gene expression, but it may be used specifically in the precursors seeding the thymus in fetal life; loss of PU.1 eliminates all fetal T-cell development. The effects of PU.1 and Ikaros loss-of-function mutations (Ikaros C$^{-/-}$ in Fig. 5B) are quite leaky in postnatal T-cell development, in contrast to fetal T-cell development. This may simply be caused by transcription factor gene redundancy in the postnatal case, rather than true independence of these factors. Both the PU.1 and Ikaros genes are members of small families of related genes with overlapping expression in the postnatal thymus. Ikaros dominant-negative mutations that interfere with all family members result in complete ablation of T-cell development in the adult thymus as well as the fetal thymus. The genes regulated by Ikaros, PU.1, c-Myb, and GATA3 that are critical for early T-cell precursor function remain to be defined (78,79,81).

An additional set of transcription factors is required during the specification and expansion events in the DN2 and DN3 stage. Here, powerful quantitative effects result from loss-of-function mutations of the basic helix-loop-helix (bHLII) transcription factor E2A or the bHLH repressor Hes-1 (82,83). E2A gene products form heterodimers with related bHLH factors to help drive expression of the pTα and RAG1 genes (84–86), and this probably accounts for part of the E2A knockout effect. However, the effect of the E2A knockout is most severe in the DN2 and DN3 populations preceding β selection, before any of these target genes are needed. Thus, it is likely that additional target genes are involved. In the E2A mutants, T-lineage specification per se is not completely blocked; cells that manage to express some form of pre-TCR can undergo β selection and continue their development. The incomplete effect of E2A mutations may result from some overlap in function with the related bHLH factor HEB, which is expressed at high levels in T-cell development. It now appears that E2A carries out unique survival functions in lymphoid precursors, complementary to those mediated by IL-7R (87). These roles in survival of early precursors may explain some of the similarities between the severe early phenotypes of E2A knockouts and those of IL-7R component knockouts.

Hes-1 is a transcription factor that is directly induced by Notch signaling. It is therefore a potential component of the mechanism used by the Notch pathway to block B-cell development, enforce T-cell development of lymphoid precursors, or both (88). The mechanism that blocks progression through the DN2→DN3 stages in Hes-1 mutants also causes more severe effects on subsequent development than in E2A mutants, which is consistent with a direct effect on T-lineage specification. On the other hand, the block is somewhat leaky (83,89). It is possible that complementation by another Hes-related gene is responsible for the ability of a few cells to do without Hes-1, but it may also be that Hes-1 primarily provides a survival function. Mice with the Hes-1 mutation do not survive after birth, and their phenotype has been analyzed thus far only in the fetal thymus.

Figure 4 includes a number of factors that are most prominent at later stages, after T-lineage commitment. These include the bHLH transcription factor HEB, a relative of E2A, and the high-mobility group (HMG) box transcription factors T-cell factor 1 (TCF-1) and/or lymphoid enhancer factor (LEF), which have important roles in β selection. These are not absolutely required in earlier T-lineage specification events, but they probably participate to some extent; for example, HEB can provide a modest compensation for loss of E2A. As shown in Fig. 4, TCF-1 and LEF are not needed until after T-lineage commitment in fetal and young postnatal thymocytes, but the cohorts of precursors that populate the adult thymus need TCF-1 for earlier events, at the DN1-to-DN2 transition (25). Also shown in Fig. 4 is that transcription factors of the Egr family and an antagonist of bHLH positive regulators, Id3, have major roles later, in the TCR-dependent events of T-cell development, as discussed later.

Transcription factors are central players in establishing T-cell identity, for these molecules not only control the differentiation process but also enable the cell to maintain its characteristic pattern of gene expression once its differentiation is complete. The need for contributions from multiple factors is a normal consequence of the way this initial lineage choice works. It is probably a mistake to search for a gene that controls T-cell specification as such. Instead, these regulatory genes each appear to influence distinct developmental choices. The Notch pathway, acting through Hes-1 and other mediators, influences the ability to become a T cell versus a B cell but does not substantially affect the NK or dendritic cell developmental choices (90,91). In contrast, E2A and the genes of its family are crucial for the choice of either T- or B-cell development, as opposed to NK cell or myeloid/macrophage development (92). T-cell specification is likely to be defined by the combination of regulatory factors that permit lineage progression as they jointly eliminate all other developmental options (80).

Although none of them appear to be "master regulators" of T-cell identity, these genes are used throughout T-cell development. Notch family genes may participate in as many as three lineage choices within the T-cell pathway. E2A family and Id genes act in β selection and positive selection (93). GATA-3 influences not only the CD4/CD8 choice but also the postthymic differentiation of T_H1 and T_H2 effector subsets of helper T cells (94). Even Ikaros recurs in specific roles in later T-cell development. Thus, the interplay of these developmentally potent factors is a permanent feature of the T-cell regulatory apparatus, which may help to give mature T cells some of their richly nuanced repertoire of responses to their environment.

A REGULATORY UPHEAVAL: β-SELECTION

Multiple Changes at the Transition from T-Cell Receptor–Independent to T-Cell Receptor–Dependent T-Cell Development

The β-selection process is a watershed in T-cell development that marks the change from events dominated by hematopoietic-like mechanisms to events dominated by TCR interactions with the microenvironment. Understanding of the β-selection process advanced dramatically in just a few years, and several excellent reviews discuss this event in detail (95–98). As an immunological event, it has a significant impact on the eventual T-cell repertoire, but it is also fascinating as a complex, multistep cellular response triggered by a particularly well-studied signaling event. After 2 weeks of TCR-independent growth, β selection suddenly polarizes the fates of cells that have succeeded or failed at β-chain rearrangement: The successful ones are rewarded with proliferation and differentiation, and the failures are killed. It thus reflects the imposition of a novel criterion of viability, wresting the cells from their simple "hematopoietic" survival functions and making their futures TCR dependent. The proliferation it triggers sets up the large population of $TCR\beta^+$ cells that is needed to provide enough $TCR\beta$ diversity and cell numbers so that stringent positive/negative selection criteria can be applied later. This mitotic burst may also include some of the last cell cycles that T-cell precursors undergo, in adults, before they finish development and emerge to the periphery. β Selection is interesting, overall, in terms of the sweeping regulatory changes it brings about in cell physiology, the relationships among the intricate cascade of processes that it triggers, and its distinctive features in comparison with other TCR-dependent activation responses.

A summary of changes occurring in cells during β selection is presented in Fig. 6 and discussed in the next section. There

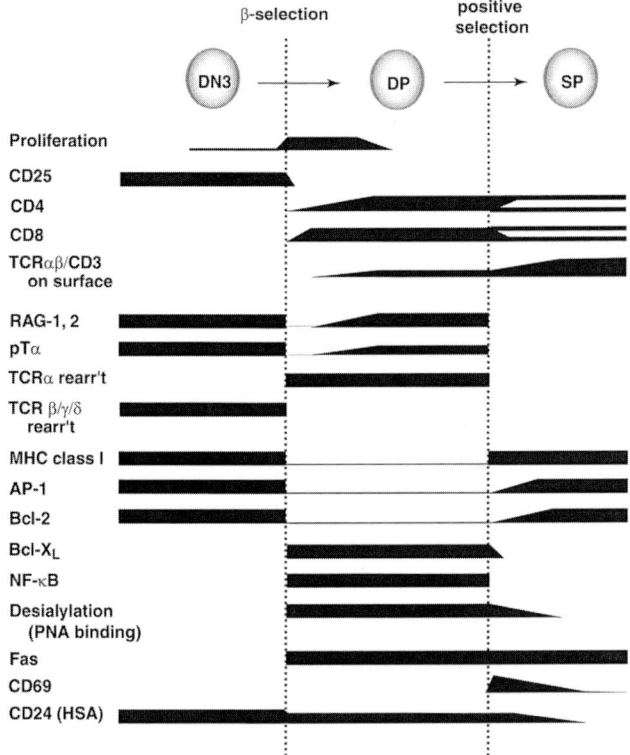

FIG. 6. Transformations of cell phenotype during β selection: comparison with later positive selection events. The changes in gene expression, rearrangement accessibility, and cell-surface phenotype at the transition from double negative (DN) 3 cells to double positive (DP) are compared with changes that occur later during positive selection. Changes in cell-surface phenotype where several distinct levels of marker expression are useful to distinguish among developmental states are distinguished by sloping or stepped forms, whereas others are simplified as all-or-none changes. For discussion, see text. Proliferation is shown as starting at a low level on the basis of the properties of DN3 cells that have not yet undergone productive T-cell receptor (TCR) β gene rearrangement (there is extensive proliferation in earlier DN subsets). Proliferation continues in mouse thymocytes through the DN4 and immature single positive (ISP) stages and into the beginning of the DP stage. CD4 and CD8 expression patterns are shown bifurcating at positive selection to represent the CD4/CD8 single positive (SP) lineage split. Recombination activating gene (RAG) 1 and RAG2 and pTα are transiently shut off during proliferation after β selection and then expressed again in DP thymocytes. AP-1 loss of function in DP thymocytes is a loss of inducibility of deoxyribonucleic acid (DNA) binding and transactivation activity, leading to broad defects in effector gene inducibility. NF-κB up-regulation is an elevated constitutive level of binding activity. The expression of surface glycoproteins deficient in sialic acid is detected by a sharp increase in binding to the lectin peanut agglutinin (PNA). Fas is a tumor necrosis factor (TNF) receptor family death receptor.

is, first, a powerful burst of proliferation, beginning before the cells change their DN3 phenotype (1). Cells responding to β selection were originally measured to have uncommonly fast cell cycles of only approximately 8 to 9 hours, with minimal G_1 and G_2 phases [reviewed by Rothenberg (99)]. This proliferation is apparently associated with a requirement

for new survival functions. There are also changes in cell surface phenotype, with gains of CD8 and CD4 expression and loss of CD25 expression (clearance of CD25 from the cell surface is aided by dilution as the cells proliferate; some CD25 persists in cases in which proliferation is partially blocked). Within the cell, TCRβ, TCRγ, and TCRδ genes become inaccessible to further rearrangement; and in a separable event, TCRα genes begin to be transcribed and become accessible for rearrangement for the first time.

The cells need new survival functions because they undergo rapid changes in their intrinsic survival potential and function that thrust them into a highly vulnerable state (100). This is associated with the loss of Bcl-2 expression, the onset of expression of the proapoptotic surface receptor Fas, and the replacement of Bcl-2 survival functions by Bcl-X$_L$ and NF-κB (101–104). In addition, changes in signaling physiology disable activation of normal AP-1 transcription factor, paralyzing cytokine gene expression and other functional responses that had been established previously in DN cells (105–108). At the same time, however, the cells paradoxically become more sensitive to interactions with cell-bound ligands and particularly hypersensitive to low-affinity TCR ligands (109–111), apparently because of an abrupt change in membrane glycoprotein processing (112,113). The suite of these processes results in DP thymocytes that are suspended in a state close to death and are easy to kill and yet are also uniquely capable of detecting encounters with low-avidity ligands for any TCR complexes they may form after TCRα gene rearrangement. These properties are exploited to the full, in the next 3 to 4 days, for the purposes of TCR repertoire selection.

Triggering Requirements for β Selection

β selection is triggered when a TCRβ gene rearrangement generates a sequence that can be translated into a β-chain protein. It was a mystery for a number of years how this response could occur so efficiently for diverse β chains, regardless of the binding specificities of their V regions. It now appears that this is the one case in which a TCR-like complex can undergo ligand-independent signaling. The β chain assembles into a pre-TCR complex with the surrogate α chain pTα and the CD3 components γ, δ, ϵ, and ζ_2, which are already being expressed in DN2 and DN3 cells (114–117), and thus enters the traffic to the plasma membrane. pTα, a key component of this complex, is an invariant transmembrane glycoprotein that is encoded by a nonrearranging immunoglobulin superfamily gene and expressed very specifically in DN and DP thymocytes (115,118). The TCRβ/pTα/CD3 complexes are segregated efficiently into cholesterol-rich lipid microdomains (lipid rafts) on the cell membrane (119). This is apparently possible because of distinctive features of the pTα transmembrane and submembrane regions, inasmuch as neither conventional TCR$\alpha\beta$ nor TCR$\gamma\delta$ complexes appear to partition to the rafts so effectively (119). Even at low levels of cell surface expression, the pre-TCR complexes cluster with each other in these rafts. The special organization or clustering of these rafts may depend on the Rho/Rac family of guanosine triphosphate (GTP)–binding proteins, which are also required for β selection (120). This clustering spontaneously triggers a potent signaling cascade that engages the kinase Lck, the adaptors SLP-76 and LAT, and the activation of protein kinase C, Ras, and MAP kinases to launch the complex β selection response. Figure 7 shows the mediators and pathways that have been implicated in this signaling response, in comparison with those triggered by the mature TCR in positive selection.

Substantial efforts have been made to find an extracellular ligand that may engage the pre-TCR. Some cross-linking stimulus was thought to be needed because, for years, one of the most effective ways known to induce a wave of β selection *in vivo* or *in vitro* has been to cross-link the sparse CD3ϵ-containing complexes on the surface of RAG-deficient thymocytes (121,122). However, it currently appears that in the normal case, no ligand is needed. Mutant forms of TCRβ and of pTα that completely lack extracellular immunoglobulin-like domains can mediate β selection in place of wild-type

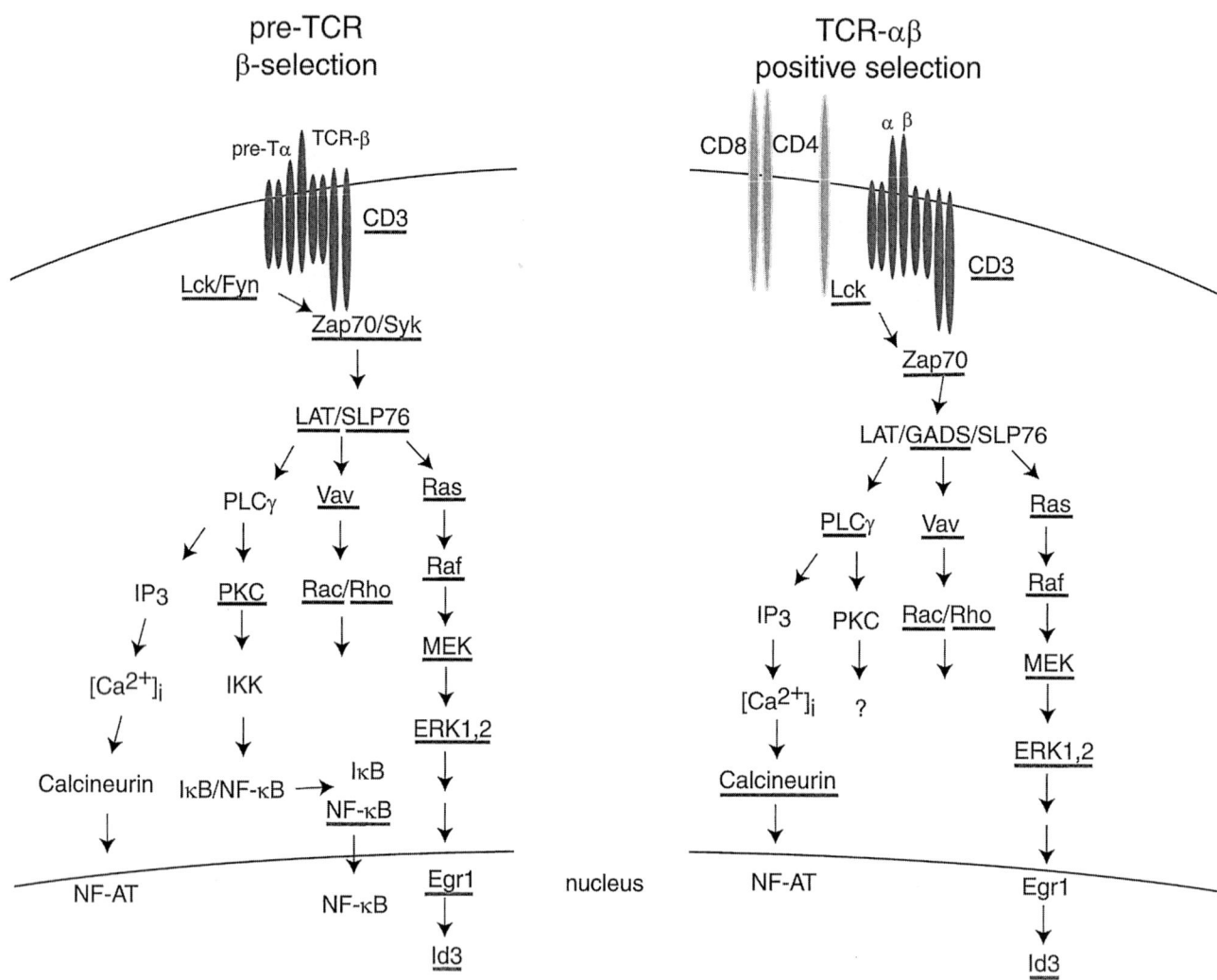

FIG. 7. Signaling cascades activated by pre–T-cell receptor (TCR) signaling during β selection: comparison with cascades activated by TCR$\alpha\beta$ complexes in positive selection. A simplified schematic is presented to show relationships discussed in the text. The figure focuses on mediators that are seen to be activated in β selection and positive selection. Those that appear to be essential for these transitions, on the basis of loss or gain of function experiments, are emphasized by *underlining*. There are certain to be other key mediators as well. Some differences are seen between the two activation processes. In β selection, there appears to be some redundancy in the roles for related kinases Lck and Fyn and for ZAP70 and Syk, whereas both Lck and ZAP70 are essential for positive selection. Lck cannot be brought to the pre-TCR by CD4 in β selection, at least not in mice, which do not express CD4 at this stage (in humans, however, CD4 is expressed before β selection), but it probably does depend on CD4 to bring it to TCR$\alpha\beta$ in positive selection. In spite of these differences, there is striking similarity between the two signaling cascades overall. In positive selection, several mediators that are essential in β selection are not underlined, only because the double positive (DP) thymocytes that are needed to undergo positive selection are not generated when these mediators are absent.

forms, at least when expressed as transgenes (123,124). Furthermore, pTα itself does not seem to mediate specific interactions with any distinctive set of signaling molecules, inasmuch as a form of pTα lacking most of its cytoplasmic domain is also capable of complementing a pTα deficiency. These structural perturbation results support the interpretation that assembly of the pTα::TCRβ::CD3 complex in lipid rafts itself is sufficient to trigger the signaling that leads to β selection.

The TCRα locus under normal conditions is neither rearranged nor transcribed appreciably until β selection. However, already-rearranged TCRα transgenes can be expressed early enough to enable the effects of TCRαβ complexes to be compared with the effects of pre-TCR (pTα:TCRβ) complexes at this transition. Up to a point, rearranged TCRα can replace pTα to mediate β selection. It certainly supports the differentiative changes induced during β selection, such as shutoff of CD25 expression and onset of CD4 and CD8 expression, together with a certain amount of proliferation. TCRαβ transgenic mice are capable of generating a DP population that is similar, in most respects, to the DP population in normal mice. Also, pTα$^{-/-}$ mutant mice do generate a small number of DP and SP cells in spite of their inability to make pre-TCR. Such cells appear to be generated through TCRαβ signaling, apparently because a few cells initiate TCRα rearrangement precociously. However, there is evidence that TCRαβ complexes are less effective than pre-TCR complexes in triggering the major proliferative expansion that normally occurs at β selection (125).

Constituent Events in the β Selection Cascade

Gene disruption and overexpression experiments show that the constituent events in β selection can be dissociated from one another. The whole process is therefore a short differentiation program rather than a single response to triggering. Components with distinct genetic requirements can be resolved in several ways: (a) early proliferation, with short-term protection from apoptosis (DN→ISP); (b) later proliferation (ISP→DP); (c) CD4, CD8, TCRα transcriptional activation (and CD25 down-regulation); (d) transient down-regulation of RAG1, RAG2, and pTα; (e) allelic exclusion (i.e., long-term shutoff of Vβ and Vγ rearrangement); and (f) antiapoptotic functions for ISP→DP cells. The roles of different genes in the process are shown vividly by the defects in or blockade of β selection when they are mutated, or by the ability to bypass the β-selection checkpoint when they are overexpressed.

The differentiation program from DN3 to DP can be triggered efficiently in the absence of pre-TCR expression by activated forms of signaling molecules that are normally mobilized by pre-TCR: activated Lck, activated Ras, or activated Raf (126–130). Any of these mediators allows cells to be generated with the CD4$^+$CD8$^+$CD25$^-$ phenotype of DP cells. Examples of these effects are shown in Fig. 8A and B. So far, only certain parts of the mechanism connecting the signaling events to the specific differentiation changes (events c and d)

are understood. The immediate-early response transcription factors of the Egr family are prominently activated during β selection, and these are probably responsible for inducing TCRα germline transcription and the shutoff of RAG1, RAG2, and pTα (131). However, the transcriptional mechanisms underlying CD4 and CD8 induction are still being studied (132,132a). Expression of CD4 and CD8 is controlled by complex positively and negatively acting factors, and those acting at β-selection appear to include some combination of Ikaros, bHLH factors, and Runx transcription factors as well as chromatin remodeling complexes (132b,132c,132d). None of these are known to be activated directly by pre-TCR signaling. Regulators of the other major changes resulting in DP cell properties are even less defined.

It is easy to explain the termination of the typical activities of DN2/DN3 thymocytes at this point by the shutoff of numerous regulatory genes (Fig. 6). The Ras signaling pathway can cause some of these changes itself, by activating the bHLH antagonist Id3, which is turned on by Egr-1 (133). When expressed any earlier, Id3 is a complete inhibitor of the entry of lymphoid precursors into the T lineage and a specific antagonist of the functions needed to prepare cells for β selection (134,135). Nothing could more emphasize how β selection terminates the immature stages of T-cell development than the activation of Id3 at this point.

Strangely, some of the obvious differentiative events (c and d) may not really depend on pre-TCR triggering at all. They may be events that the cells have been programmed to undergo during the DN3 stage but with a potent threat attached: that going forward from the DN3 state will lead to certain, rapid death unless a number of protective mechanisms are engaged. One look at the completeness of the block in RAG-deficient thymocytes (Fig. 1) might make this seem unlikely. However, that block to differentiation is dissipated substantially by a single genetic change: the mutational inactivation of the p53 tumor suppressor gene (136–138). This p53 gene product has many roles in cell biology, one of which is to impose G$_1$ arrest and another of which is to induce apoptosis under certain conditions, such as in case of deoxyribonucleic acid (DNA) damage. In pre-TCR–deficient thymocytes (e.g., RAG-knockout, pTα-knockout), the normal role of p53 appears to be mainly to punish differentiation with death, because if p53 function is removed, these cells develop efficiently into DP cells. In certain experimental situations, the death-dealing function of p53 at the β-selection checkpoint can also be counteracted by signals from the microenvironment (136,137,139,140).[1] Thus, although some uncertainty

---

[1] In a recombinase-deficient mutant thymus, cells become quiescent and arrest differentiation completely at the DN3 stage, but in adoptive transfer of recombinase-deficient cells to a wild-type thymus, some cells can pass through the DN4/ISP stages before dying in the DP state. The difference is likely to be the signals provided by the microenvironment. There is bidirectional communication between developing lymphocytes and the microenvironment at different stages (318), and the passage of a cohort of normal TCR$^+$ cells appears to cause the microenvironment to provide better mitogenic and signals to support "spontaneous" differentiation of DN3 cells. It is not known whether the level of checkpoint control that seems to be bypassed by stromal signals is the mechanism mediated by p53 or by TNF receptor/Fas$^+$ FADD.

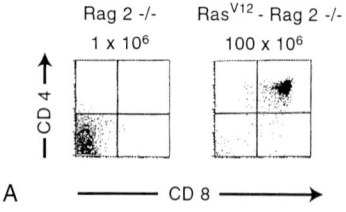

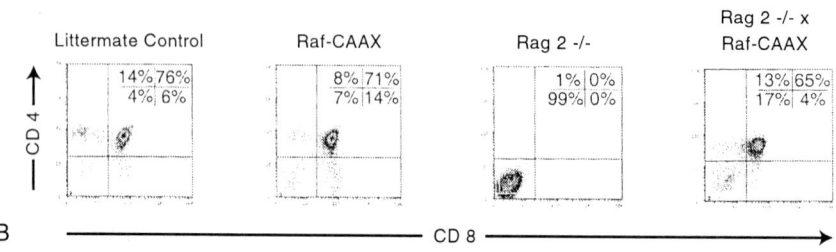

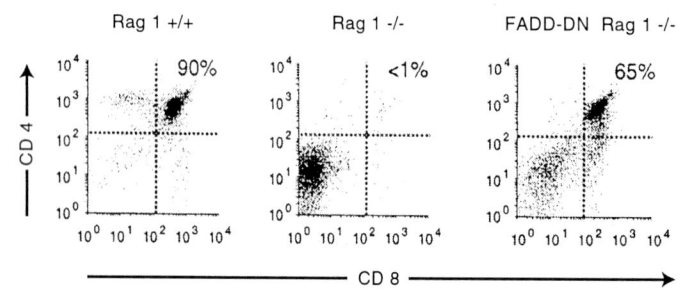

FIG. 8. Bypassing the β-selection checkpoint by Ras pathway activation or antagonism of FADD. **A:** The number and CD4/CD8 expression pattern of thymocytes from recombination activation gene (RAG) $2^{-/-}$ mice (**left**) are compared with those of thymocytes from RAG2$^{-/-}$ transgenic mice expressing a constitutively activated Ras transgene (Ras^{V12}) in the thymus. The elevated Ras activity causes a 100-fold expansion of cell numbers and a complete conversion from double negative (DN) to double positive (DP). The cells cannot progress further to CD4 or CD8 SP stages, because they still lack T-cell receptor (TCR) rearrangements and cannot be positively selected. From (130), with permission. **B:** A similar experiment is shown in which RAG2$^{-/-}$ mice were bred to express an activated Raf transgene (Raf-CAAX) in the thymus. Activated Raf alone has modest effects on normal thymocyte populations (compare Raf-CAAX, littermate control) but completely transforms the populations seen in RAG2$^{-/-}$ mice (compare RAG2$^{-/-}$, RAG2$^{-/-}$ with Raf-CAAX). From ref. (129), with permission. **C:** Not only activation of positive mediators but also competitive antagonism of a checkpoint enforcement function can allow the cells to break through β selection without a pre-TCR. Here a transgene encoding a dominant negative variant of FADD, which interferes with the normal functions of FADD, causes the appearance of DP and CD8 immature single positive (ISP) thymocytes when expressed in RAG1$^{-/-}$ thymocytes that would otherwise be blocked at the DN stage. The rescue is not complete (contrast wild-type control, **left**) but very pronounced in view of the fact that differentiation in this case occurs with little proliferation. From (147), with permission.

remains about how pre-TCR assembly causes differentiation, there is no question that it causes major shifts in susceptibility to apoptosis and proliferation.

Proliferation has to be induced and is not just a default, because when p53 is mutated, the differentiating cells remain limited in their ability to proliferate. What is needed to unleash this proliferation may include the removal of a specific brake: the antiproliferative adaptor molecule SOCS-1, which is highly expressed in DN3 cells and is abruptly shut off by pre-TCR triggering (141). Then, the roles of a succession of transcription factors distinguish early and late stages of β-selection-associated proliferation (events a and b). Early

proliferation (event a) appears to involve the Egr family transcription factors (131,142) and the HMG box transcription factor TCF-1 or LEF, or both (25,143). Later proliferation in the transition from ISP to DP (event b) can no longer be driven by Egr activation. Now, the cells depend acutely on TCF/LEF plus β-catenin (11,12). The discontinuity between the two phases may be caused by a switch in the need for bHLH transcription factors. In the first stage, proliferation is aided by the bHLH transcription factor antagonist Id3 (93). In the second phase, proliferation and differentiation depend on one of the molecules that Id3 should antagonize, the bHLH transcriptional activator HEB (144).

These stage-specific regulators work in collaboration with additional proliferative functions that may have broader roles. One is the proto-oncogene c-Myb, activated at β-selection by Pim-1 kinase (145). Yet another participant driving proliferation during β selection is a fascinating one in terms of checkpoint control: the bifunctional mediator FADD (146,147). FADD is an adaptor molecule transducing tumor necrosis factor (TNF) receptor family death signals, but it also seems to be vital for proliferation at β-selection. It is discussed further later.

The ability of pre-TCR/Lck complexes to initiate proliferation is probably mediated by the Ras pathway, inasmuch as this is sufficient to induce the mitogenic Egr (and Id3) family molecules. However, allelic exclusion (event e) has to be triggered through some mediator other than Ras, because activated Ras alone cannot close the TCRβ-chain genes to further rearrangement (129,130). Protein kinase C activity is also induced by pre-TCR signaling, upstream or parallel with Ras, and it has been suggested that that this is the mediator that is responsible for termination of TCRβ rearrangement (148).

Antiapoptotic functions (event f) need to be activated during β selection because of two kinds of threat: a general loss of survival support, which appears to be a default for DN3 cells, and a differentiation-linked susceptibility to apoptosis. Beyond the DN2/DN3 state, most thymocytes apparently lose their responsiveness to the IL-7R signaling that, until then, has supported most of their proliferation and kept them from death by inducing Bcl-2 gene expression. Furthermore, mitogenic stimulation itself can be risky. As noted previously, one of the molecules stimulating proliferation of DN3 cells, FADD, can also promote apoptosis. Two transcription factors, NF-κB/Rel (101) and activated TCF/LEF (11,12), appear to turn on the genes that protect cells from apoptosis. NF-κB appears to collaborate with TCF/LEF factors to turn on specific molecules that uncouple FADD from its apoptotic signaling cascade and restrict its effects to promoting growth (149). NF-κB and TCF/LEF factors activated by β-catenin can also help to turn on expression of Bcl-X$_L$ (Fig. 6), compensating in part for the shutoff of Bcl-2 (102,103,150).

Death Mechanisms and Other Checkpoint Controls

Under normal circumstances, DN3 thymocytes are probably prevented from spontaneous growth and differentiation by at least three mechanisms. Their ability to grow in response to IL-7R has been arrested by the high levels of the antiproliferative molecule SOCS-1 that they accumulate (141) and probably by a gradual down-regulation of IL-7Rα expression as well. They do not generally express substantial levels of p53, but through some mechanism not yet understood, any attempt they may make to differentiate is linked with p53 activation, which kills them. Furthermore, FADD plays a role. In addition to its role promoting growth, FADD function is needed to prevent differentiation to DP cells. When a dominant-negative FADD transgene is expressed in cells that cannot make pre-TCR, these cells break through the checkpoint and generate DP cells without TCR (Fig. 8C). FADD

is particularly interesting because it is not only expressed but also required to function when the cells receive their β-selection signal (147). It is expressed in concert with multiple receptors of the TNF receptor family that are linked with cell death, although the exact set of receptors expressed shifts from DN3 to DP stages (147). Thus, the pathway involving FADD has the opportunity to be triggered directly from the DN3 stage. There are complex relationships between p53 and the TNF receptor family death receptors, and this may account for their interconnected roles.

In addition to the death functions enforcing the checkpoint, there are a number of threshold-setting functions that appear to determine the magnitude of signal strength that will be needed to trigger β selection. One is Csk, the kinase that inhibits Src-family tyrosine kinases, such as Lck, by phosphorylating their C termini. Mutation of the csk gene allows Lck to be active constitutively, and the result is that cells without pre-TCR can spontaneously differentiate to DP cells (151).

Another gene product that appears to regulate stimulation thresholds turns out, surprisingly, to be the transcription factor Ikaros. Ikaros is a crucially important gene for all lymphocyte development (152), but it has been difficult to establish the nature of any target genes that it regulates positively; CD8 may be the first (132b). However, striking circumstantial evidence has associated Ikaros binding with the silencing of genes in the course of lymphoid development (153). Thus, it is noteworthy that Ikaros-mutant heterozygous mice show a dramatic breakthrough of pre-TCR–negative cells into the DP stage. Effects on the CD4 and CD8 genes themselves could be involved (132b), but this violation of the β-selection checkpoint, as in the case of Csk deficiency, is associated with a general T-cell hyper-reactivity (154). In the Ikaros+/− thymus, hyperreactivity is also a prelude to malignant transformation: These animals develop thymic lymphomas at a very high frequency. The gene dosage effect implies that Ikaros levels are tightly correlated with a precise regulator of activation.

Significance of β Selection for Later T-Cell Differentiation

As a developmental event, β-selection is momentous. The approximately 10^2-fold proliferation at β selection effectively erases the developmental alternatives for TCR$\alpha\beta$ cells, consummating not only T-lineage commitment but the separation of $\alpha\beta$ and $\gamma\delta$ cell fates. In adult mammals, this is the last significant proliferation that T-cell precursors undergo before being exported to the periphery. Thus, the form in which cells emerge from the various stages of β selection dictates the defaults for their responses to positive and negative selection signals.

Overall, β selection is a form of activation both in terms of specific gene expression and in terms of its use of stimulatory signaling cascades to trigger proliferation. However, transcriptional repression also seems to participate in differentiation or survival at this stage. The nuclear receptor co-repressor gene N-CoR turns out to be essential for β selection, because N-CoR$^{-/-}$ mutants are blocked at the DN stage (155). The target genes that may need to be repressed by N-CoR in the course of β selection have not yet been identified. However, several transcription factor messenger ribonucleic acids (RNAs) are abruptly silenced in T-lineage precursors during β selection (81,156), which suggests that this could represent a profound upheaval in gene-regulation potential as well as a major physiological change.

In certain ways, the immediate impact of β selection on the cells is the reverse of the impact of positive selection (see later discussion). In particular, the changes in Bcl-2, Bcl-X$_L$, NF-κB, and AP-1 activation, glycoprotein sialylation, and signaling thresholds will all be reversed when the cells are positively selected (Fig. 6). Nevertheless, many of the triggering functions used in β selection are the same as those used in positive selection (Fig. 7). Both involve triggering via Lck, SLP-76, LAT, Ras, Raf, Erk, and protein kinase C. Both involve Ca^{2+} fluxes and NF-AT transcription factor activation, at least as inferred from cyclosporine sensitivity (157–159), as well as induction of Egr family genes and Id3 (93,131,133,160). The signals may not be instructive but seem to act more as a toggle between alternative physiological states. The same threshold setting functions that limit activation in β selection are also used again to limit activation in positive selection.

Thus, the threshold-setting functions that act at β selection may turn out to be an important immunological legacy of the process. Of interest is whether the levels of threshold-setting function present in particular cells that undergo β selection, such as Csk and Ikaros, could be maintained through proliferation and into the DP population. If so, the positive/negative selection thresholds for individual DP cells could depend on the strength of the pre-TCR signals that triggered their β selection initially.

THE DIVERGENCE OF T-CELL RECEPTOR $\alpha\beta$ AND T-CELL RECEPTOR $\gamma\delta$ LINEAGE CELLS

Choices of Fate within the T-Cell Lineage: Differences between $\alpha\beta$ and $\gamma\delta$ T Cells

Cells committed to the T-cell lineage continue to make additional developmental choices as to what kind of T cell they will be. T cells that use TCR$\alpha\beta$ receptors differ in a number of respects from T cells that use TCR$\gamma\delta$ receptors. At later stages, CD4 SP and CD8 SP T cells exhibit divergent functional properties, and there is increasing evidence that another class of T cells, the NKT cells, represents yet a further discrete lineage. The intrathymic choice between TCR$\alpha\beta$ and TCR$\gamma\delta$ fate, like the choice between CD4$^+$ and CD8$^+$ fates, remains controversial because of two problems. The first problem is that the alternative fates are still relatively poorly defined in terms of multiple, independently measurable traits. As long as TCR$\gamma\delta$ complexes themselves (and failure to acquire CD4 and CD8) are the only clear markers for the $\gamma\delta$ cell fate, it is difficult to analyze the role of these complexes in bringing about this fate. The second problem is that the TCR structures on the cells making TCR$\gamma\delta$ versus TCR$\alpha\beta$ lineage choices are different in recognition specificity and other properties. Because of this, some of the behavioral differences between subsets could be caused by responses to differential TCR signaling, making it uncertain how much the cells may differ intrinsically.

There are two kinds of TCR$\gamma\delta$ cells that may be produced through distinct pathways. In mice and chickens, at least, the $\gamma\delta$ cells appearing first in ontogeny (before birth or hatching) display properties that distinguish them both from adult-type $\gamma\delta$ cells and from $\alpha\beta$ cells. For these early $\gamma\delta$ cells, a case can be made that a fundamentally different developmental program is used for these cells and that they arise from a cell type intrinsically different from TCR$\alpha\beta$ precursors. A summary of the properties of the early $\gamma\delta$, later $\gamma\delta$, and $\alpha\beta$ classes is presented in Table 2.

For adult-type TCR$\gamma\delta$ cells, the evidence that the precursors are intrinsically different from TCR$\alpha\beta$ precursors is shakier. In the periphery, TCR$\gamma\delta$ cells continue to carry out surveillance assignments that are different from those of TCR$\alpha\beta$ cells, although using many or all of the same effector functions as those used by $\alpha\beta$ cells. A general difference is that TCR$\gamma\delta$ cells in mice do not express CD4 or CD8β, in contrast to TCR$\alpha\beta$ cells. Because the cytoplasmic tails of CD4 and CD8 are the major known docking sites for Lck, their absence probably alters the way mature TCR$\gamma\delta$ cells can recruit Lck to lipid rafts with the TCR during antigen recognition. This could have multiple consequences for signaling and could contribute to the distinctive functions of TCR$\gamma\delta$ cells in the periphery. Developmentally, such

TABLE 2. *Properties of TCR$\alpha\beta$ and TCR$\gamma\delta$ cells: fetal versus postnatal*

Fetal-type TCR$\gamma\delta$ cells	Adult-type TCR$\gamma\delta$ cells	Adult-type TCR$\alpha\beta$ cells
Invariant TCR	Variable TCR	Variable TCR
Mucosal/skin targeting	No targeting (mice and humans)	No targeting
Low E2A requirement (Id expression tolerated)	High E2A requirement	High E2A requirement
Partially dependent on Jag2/Notch	Inhibited by Notch-1 signal	Enhanced by Notch-1 signal
No β-selection	No β-selection	β-selection required
No CD4, CD8	No CD4 or CD8	CD4 and CD8 induced, permanent CD4 or CD8 expression
IL-2Rβ/IL-15Rβ (CD122) dependent	Not IL-2Rβ/IL-15Rβ (CD122) dependent	Not IL-2Rβ/IL-15Rβ (CD122) dependent
IL-7Rα (CD127) dependent	IL-7Rα (CD127) dependent	Not IL-7Rα (CD127) dependent

IL, interleukin; TCR, T-cell receptor.

differences originate with the separation between TCRγδ and precursors of the TCRαβ cells in the thymus; this is because TCRγδ cells do not go through the full β-selection process.

Most prominently, TCRγδ cells are T cells that have succeeded in making both V-Jγ and V-D-Jγ gene rearrangements productively before they die or undergo complete β selection. The TCRγδ receptor is both their main distinguishing feature and their apparent cause of divergence from the TCRαβ path. In general, the rearrangements of TCRγ and nondeleted δ genes in TCRαβ cells are out of frame for protein translation (161,162) (see Chapter 8). On the other hand, there are some in-frame TCRβ rearrangements in γδ cells. These data can be interpreted to mean that cells keep "trying" to become TCRγδ cells by default; if they fail, they die unless they have been rescued by TCRβ rearrangement and β selection.

The first indication that the TCRαβ and TCRγδ differentiation programs can be separated from the use of these receptors came from analysis of TCRβ−/− mice. In these animals, DP thymocytes were generated in small numbers, even though β-selection as such could not take place (163). The DP thymocytes in this case used TCRγδ receptors and could be generated only if the TCRγ and δ genes were intact. However, DP thymocytes do not use TCRγδ receptors in normal mice. A careful analysis has shown that in several transgenic and knockout cases, TCRγδ receptors can apparently support development of cells with αβ-type characteristics when TCRαβ is unavailable, and vice versa (164,165). This is important evidence that cells are assigned to discrete differentiation programs that in some cases can be mismatched with the TCR class they express. In support of this view, researchers have identified several genes that can bias the lineage choice of developing cells to an αβ-like or γδ-like program independently of the TCR they express, as described in the following sections.

Generation of T-Cell Receptor γδ Cells

For adult-type γδ cells, separation from the TCRαβ pathway occurs after the DN2 stage (166,167). Successful rearrangement of both TCRγ and TCRδ genes rapidly downregulates CD25 expression and leads to generation of CD25− CD44low/int TCRγδ+ cells. These cells subsequently downregulate CD24 (HSA) as they complete their maturation. There are multiple points of contrast with the αβ pathway. First, there is little or no proliferation associated with TCRγδ development, in sharp contrast to β selection. Second, genes such as TCF-1 and HEB, which are required for completion of β selection, are dispensable for TCRγδ development (143,144). Third, the γδ program does not involve upregulation of CD4 or CD8β, and most γδ cells lack CD8α as well. TCRγδ cells use Lck for full maturation, but mutation of Lck has little effect on γδ cell numbers (168).

The lack of proliferation in TCRγδ cell development makes it easy to underestimate the percentage of intrathymic precursors taking this path. In steady state, TCRγδ+ cells constitute only 1% to 2% of thymocytes and circulating peripheral T cells in mice and humans, and so it is easy to regard them as a minor cell type. However, correcting for the approximately 100-fold expansion occurring in TCRαβ precursors at β selection, it can be argued that the absolute number of DN2 cells that will give rise to γδ cells is similar to the absolute number that will give rise to αβ cells.

What is the relationship between the αβ versus γδ lineage choice and β selection? The TCRγδ complex does not usually trigger β selection, but how its assembly differs functionally from those of the pre-TCR complex, on one hand, and the TCRαβ complex, on the other hand, is nonetheless an open question. Some evidence shows that TCRγδ is poorer than pre-TCR at spontaneous self-clustering in the pre–T cell membrane (119). This could explain its poorer activity in β selection. But the ability to generate TCRγδ DP cells under conditions in which there is no pre-TCR shows that these receptors can mediate certain aspects of β selection, at least the antiapoptotic ones. Also, the initial steps in β selection do not necessarily block the generation of γδ cells. Several groups have found TCRβ rearrangements that are apparently in frame in some TCRγδ thymocytes (162,169), and it has been argued that they are enriched above the level expected for random occurrence. Thus, there is a suggestion that some cells can undergo at least some β-selection–linked clonal expansion and still go on to differentiate into TCRγδ cells. These kinds of evidence tend to argue that there is an essential mechanism underlying TCRαβ and TCRγδ lineage divergence that is different from simple success or failure at triggering β selection.

Most precursors of γδ lineage cells separate from the αβ lineage earlier, before the β-selection checkpoint. As early as the DN2 stage, two populations can be distinguished on the basis of their levels of cell surface markers: one that can give rise to γδ cells as well as αβ cells, and one that is mostly or entirely restricted to the αβ lineage (170). The cells that retain γδ potential are the highest in IL-7Rα expression at the DN2 stage and low in pTα/pre-TCR surface expression at the DN3 stage (170,171). Both IL-7R and pTα/pre-TCR could participate in instructive signaling, but the very fact that their expression levels are heterogeneous provides evidence for additional, underlying regulatory differences that foreshadow the αβ/γδ lineage choice.

Genetic Regulation of T-Cell Receptor αβ versus T-Cell Receptor γδ Cell Production

Several genes appear to affect TCRαβ versus TCRγδ lineage choices or lineage-specific survival functions. Their roles appear to be distinct from those that alter the TCRαβ:TCRγδ ratio simply by enhancing or limiting the extent of proliferation at β selection. Some of these genes may primarily influence the choice between TCRαβ and TCRγδ fates in general, whereas others may actually affect the choice between adult-type and first-wave fetal-type T-cell development.

Particular growth factor receptor genes are disproportionately important for TCRγδ cell production. First-wave fetal TCRγδ thymocytes are greatly reduced by mutation or blockade of IL-2Rβ/IL-15Rβ (CD122), whereas other T-cell subsets are minimally affected (172,173) (Table 2). This correlates with the preferential expansion of these early cells in fetal thymic organ culture in response to moderate doses of IL-2 or IL-15 (174). Adult-type γδ thymocytes do not have this special response to IL-2 or IL-15, but they require IL-7/IL-7R interactions. More broadly, IL-7Rα (CD127) expression appears to be essential for all TCRγδ cell development, both fetal and adult type. The common cytokine receptor chain γc (CD132) is a component of both receptors and is essential for all TCRγδ cell development (175,176). This growth factor receptor dependence has two aspects. One is simply proliferative: Because TCRγδ cells cannot expand through β selection, the earlier IL-7–driven phases of their proliferation account for almost all the TCRγδ cells produced during differentiation. If IL-7–driven proliferation fails, there is no way to compensate by excess proliferation at a later stage (177). There is also evidence that something more instructive may be involved. IL-7R signaling directly facilitates rearrangement of the TCRγ genes (178). IL-7R signaling appears to increase transcription of the TCRγ genes before rearrangement, possibly via activation of the transcription factor Stat5 (179,180). There is evidence that Stat5 can open the TCRγ loci for rearrangement and preferentially target RAG1/RAG2 activity to these sites (181,182).

The transcription factor requirements for TCRγδ and TCRαβ lineage differentiation can also be distinguished. The difference between γδ and αβ cells may be regulated in part by the ratio of the E2A bHLH transcription factor to its antagonists of the Id family, especially Id2 and Id3. This regulatory influence emerges dramatically from experiments in which human lymphoid precursors were forced to express high levels of Id3. In early, uncommitted precursors, Id3 expression favors NK cell development and blocks T cell development altogether (135), but in T-lineage–committed precursors, the result is to block αβ cell development while promoting γδ cell generation (134). In mice, a related mechanism may be used naturally, especially to differentiate between fetal γδ cells and adult-type cells of both αβ and γδ types. The fetal thymus in general seems to tolerate levels of Id2 expression, in relation to E2A expression, that would be inhibitory to adult TCRαβ cell development (22). The reduced net E2A activity in the fetal thymus appears to help target TCRγδ rearrangement preferentially to the unique "first-wave" Vγ and Vδ gene segments, Vγ3(Vγ5), Vγ4(Vγ6), and Vδ1, while inhibiting adult-type gene rearrangements (22). Adult TCRαβ lineage cells in particular may also need higher levels of positively acting bHLH factors for multiple functions, beyond choosing the correct TCR to rearrange. For example, a dominant negative knock-in mutant form of HEB, which antagonizes both HEB and E2A activity, blocks the generation of DP cells even in the presence of a TCRαβ transgene, whereas TCRγδ cell development is spared (183).

Another regulator of the TCRαβ:TCRγδ ratio appears to be Notch-1. Notch-1$^{+/-}$ mice have normal thymocyte subsets, but in chimeras of Notch$^{+/-}$ and Notch$^{+/+}$ cells, a substantially increased percentage of Notch$^{+/-}$ thymocytes develop as TCRγδ cells. Thus, reduced Notch signaling, in relation to neighboring cells, favors the TCRγδ fate (184)[2]. Workers using a conditional knockout strategy to delete Notch-1 in DN2/DN3-stage thymocytes confirmed that committed T-lineage cells that have lost Notch-1 are specifically inhibited unless they develop as TCRγδ cells (184a). Although part of its effect may be on TCRβ gene rearrangement, Notch-1 signaling seems to act on the function that determines developmental path, irrespective of the TCR gene rearrangement in the cells. For example, although Notch-1 overexpression does not seem to increase the number of TCRαβ DP cells generated through β selection, it significantly enhances the ability of TCRγδ$^+$ cells to develop into DP cells (184). Other workers showed that Notch-1–activated transcription factors directly regulate pTα (185,186) and that high pTα expression is correlated with αβ lineage bias (171). Thus, in addition to its essential role in establishing T-lineage precursors, Notch-1 continues to influence their later developmental choices.

Models for the T-Cell Receptor αβ:T-Cell Receptor γδ Lineage Choice

Although TCRαβ:TCRγδ lineage divergence has not yet been solved, it is useful to compare a few ways of considering it, diagrammed in Fig. 9. The predominant view of the TCRαβ:TCRγδ choice is as a classic binary choice in which the cells reach a point in their development beyond which they can go forward only as an αβ cell in one path or as a γδ cell in the other (Fig. 9, options A1, A2). According to such a model, cells must actively determine whether to follow the developmental pathway involving β selection or the one or more distinct pathways that lead to fetal or adult types of γδ cells. The cells then have a problem to solve: how to coordinate their lineage choice accurately with the random success of their rearrangement of TCRβ or TCRγ and TCRδ genes. One way it could work is for the gene rearrangement to occur first and then for the pre-TCR and TCRγδ complexes to deliver different instructive signals for differentiation (119) (Fig. 9, option A1). Another way it can work is for the lineage choice to occur first and then the recombination accessibilities of TCRβ genes versus TCRγ and δ genes to become biased by some mechanism controlled by that developmental lineage choice. The latter case (Fig. 9, option A2) would explain why a bias may be detectable even before TCR gene rearrangement, with the surface density of IL-7Rα chains (170) used as a marker.

An additional model (Fig. 9B) is suggested by the numerous hints that αβ:γδ lineage divergence is asymmetrical. For example, IL-7Rα$^{low/-}$ or pTα^{high} DN2/DN3 cells can be

---

[2] Here an exception may be the "first wave" TCRγδ cells, since a large fraction of fetal γδ cell development depends on the Notch ligand Jagged-2 (319).

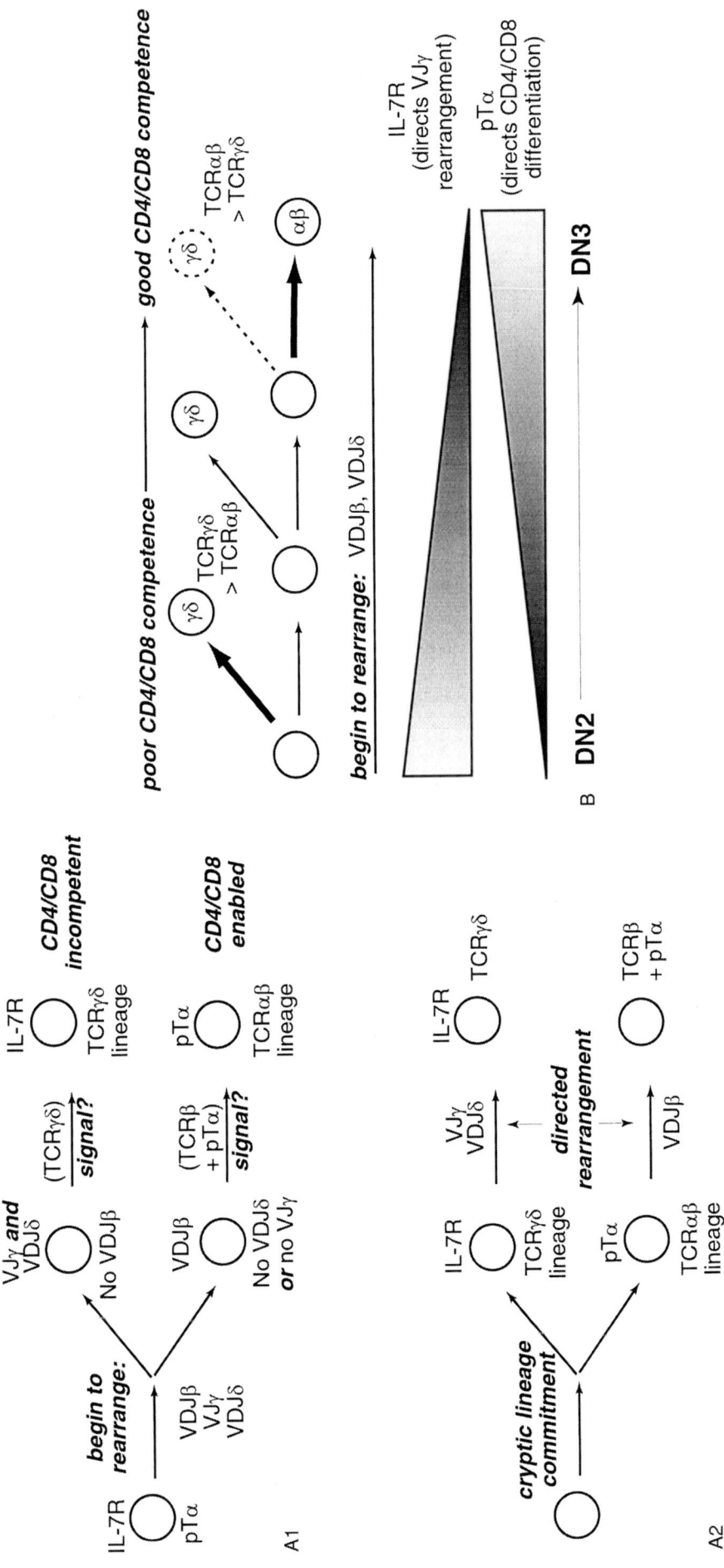

FIG. 9. Models for the divergence of T-cell receptor (TCR) $\alpha\beta$ and TCR$\gamma\delta$ lineages. The panels depict hypothetical choice points and their effects on the cells according to the models discussed in detail in the text. These changes are proposed to occur during the proliferation and differentiation events from the double negative (DN) 2 stage through the DN3 stage. **A:** The two versions of this model envision that the cells reach a discrete branch point at which they must decide whether to choose a TCR$\gamma\delta$ fate or a TCR$\alpha\beta$ fate; the only difference between these models is whether the choice involves a commitment to a developmental program or a successful gene rearrangement. In these models, the choice made instructively causes the cells to rearrange the appropriate genes or undergo the correct program thereafter. **B:** In this model, two stochastic processes are envisioned to overlap: a decreasing ability to make TCRγ gene rearrangements and an increasing ability to carry out the specific CD4/CD8 differentiation program associated with the TCR$\alpha\beta$ lineage. The *shaded wedges* represent decreasing and increasing expression of interleukin-7R and pTα, respectively. In this model, lineage commitment and TCR gene rearrangement could be matched stochastically without a unique choice point or an instructive process.

shown to have lost TCRγδ potential while retaining TCRαβ potential, but no comparable TCRγδ-committed precursor has been identified. IL-7Rα levels as a whole tend to fall and pTα levels tend to rise as cells differentiate from the DN2 to the DN3 state. The lack of proliferation in DN3 cells before β selection (1) could be a sign that the IL-7R signaling system has become completely disengaged, and thus unable to facilitate TCRγ rearrangement, by the time TCRβ rearrangement is maximal (166,187). There is also the asymmetry in gene rearrangement timing and effects in the two pathways. In principle, it should be easier to be β selected than to become a TCRγδ cell if the two pathways are in even competition and if success at TCRβ rearrangement were sufficient to make a cell undergo β selection. Instead, there are a substantial number of in-frame TCRβ rearrangements in TCRγδ cells. This suggests that some productive β-chain rearrangement can occur in precursors that cannot take advantage of it. This may be because they are precommitted to the TCRγδ lineage, but it could also be because they are not yet ready to undergo β selection.

Another type of option, then, may be envisioned as shown in Fig. 9B. The main point about such a model is that the cells never encounter any one, unique TCRαβ:TCRγδ choice point. Instead, they progress through a continuum of changes that make TCRγδ *rearrangement* less likely while making the cell better and better prepared for the TCRαβ/CD4/CD8 *differentiation* program. A separation in developmental time, and perhaps in thymic microenvironment, would coordinate the correct developmental program with the preferred TCR gene rearrangement.

IL-7R begins to be expressed by very primitive T-cell precursors and declines from the DN2 to the DN3 stage. This would bias generation of TCRγδ cells to earlier stages of the DN2/DN3 period. Meanwhile, pTα begins to be expressed at the DN1-to-DN2 transition and could accumulate in the DN2/DN3 stages over time. Furthermore, it is possible that additional regulation or signaling, or both, component changes that enhance the proliferative and differentiative capabilities that can be used at β selection could occur. Over time, the cells would thus become more likely to make vigorous β-selection responses and less likely to initiate TCRγ rearrangement. In the context of the slow migration of DN2/DN3 cells from the cortical/medullary border to the subcapsular zone of the thymus, this model would predict that most TCRγδ+ precursors would acquire their TCR in deeper parts of the cortex than the αβ lineage precursors.

The comparison between these models is useful in attempting to interpret the ways that molecules such as Notch-1 may work in this lineage choice. In the first kinds of models—A1 and A2 in Fig. 9—Notch-1 signaling could act synergistically with pre-TCR signaling to promote β selection (A1). Alternatively, it could act to enhance TCRβ rearrangement, in a discrete subset of precursors that will preferentially give rise to TCRαβ-lineage progeny (A2). In the second kind of model, Fig. 9B, Notch-1 signaling need only cause the cells to *delay* responding to early TCRγδ signals or to accelerate the clock

controlling their progress through the DN2-to-DN3 transition. Notch-1 activation is directly capable of turning on one gene that is critical for the αβ-lineage fate, pTα (185,186). However, precedents from erythromyeloid systems indicate that it may also control the timing of differentiation and selective responsiveness to growth factors in developing cells (188–191).

The roles of TCRαβ and TCRγδ cells in the periphery are increasingly revealed to be distinct. In the end, this divergence of T-cell lineages has great significance for the ability of the immune system to coordinate functions with the innate immune system and to focus the right kind of response for the nature of the threat. One of the great gaps in knowledge of the immune system is the sparse understanding of TCRγδ cells. Their development and their divergence from the αβ T-cell pathway is likely to become much clearer in the near future.

POSITIVE AND NEGATIVE SELECTION

Positive and negative selection became accessible to study as a result of the effects of expressing transgenes encoding pre-rearranged TCRα and TCRβ genes in developing T cells. Not only did these genes impose a predictable recognition specificity on the T cells, blocking most endogenous TCR gene rearrangement and diversity by allelic exclusion, but they also, dramatically, imposed a predictable developmental fate. Transgenes encoding a receptor that recognized some foreign peptide antigen in the context of the same MHC allelic forms expressed in the thymus could give thymocytes a greatly enhanced likelihood of survival (positive selection). Transgenes encoding a receptor that recognized both self-MHC and a self-peptide expressed in the thymus would cause the transgenic TCR+ cells to be eliminated (negative selection). Although details of the expression of the TCR transgenes are not normal (they are expressed at an earlier stage, typically, than normal TCR that depend on TCRα rearrangement), they have revealed the overwhelming importance of details of TCR signaling for thymocyte fate determination. This section describes the life/death decisions guided by TCR recognition events, and the next section examines the effect of TCR signaling on the choice of cells to be CD4 SP or CD8 SP.

The Double-Positive Thymocyte Stage

The CD4+ and CD8+ thymocytes produced through β selection are physiologically specialized for undergoing selection on the basis of TCR recognition. As already indicated in the discussion of the changes induced by β selection, these cells are a paradoxical combination of extreme sensitivity to TCR ligands and extreme functional paralysis. Unable to turn on any of the functional response genes of mature T cells in response to stimulation, they nevertheless do recognize TCR ligands with ultrasensitive dose–response relationships. Antigenic peptides presented on conventional antigen-presenting cells can trigger apoptosis of DP thymocytes with median effective dose values substantially lower ($\sim$10 fold) than those needed to trigger responses of mature T cells with the same TCR (109–111). This is especially surprising because the cell-surface density of TCR on DP thymocytes, even after productive TCRα rearrangement, is about 10-fold lower than on SP thymocytes. Operationally, this means that DP thymocytes can make responses to peptide/MHC complexes that are low-affinity ligands for their TCR, too low to be stimulatory for mature cells with the same TCR.

One important mechanism contributing to this ultrasensitivity is the distinctive glycosylation state of many DP thymocyte surface molecules. These are strikingly deficient in terminal sialylation, in comparison with surface glycoproteins of mature T cells and immature DN cells alike. These distinctive, developmentally regulated glycosylation properties of DP thymocytes were among the first characteristics of these cells to be noticed, in 1976 (192), long before their functional consequences were understood. Lack of sialylation not only gives DP thymocytes a highly specific reactivity with the lectin peanut agglutinin but also reduces electrostatic repulsion between DP thymocytes and other cells with a more typically strong negative surface charge. As a result, CD8 on DP thymocytes can bind MHC class I independently of class I haplotype or specific TCR recognition, under conditions in which CD8 on mature T cells cannot (112,113). On DP thymocytes, CD4 can also interact with class II MHC independently of TCR interactions (193), possibly also enabled by a lowered sialylation level. The DP cells themselves express neither class I nor class II MHC: the lack of class II is normal for murine T cells and the shutoff of class I MHC expression is another unique feature of the DP state (Fig. 6). Thus, both class I and class II binding by DP thymocyte CD8 and CD4 force the DP cells to interact with thymic epithelial cells even with low levels of TCR on their surfaces.

DP thymocytes have other features that bear on their eventual fates. Because of the regulatory changes that generate them during β selection, these cells are extremely sensitive to death induced by glucocorticoids, and, even without perturbation, they die quickly outside of the thymic microenvironment. These properties are especially pronounced in the mouse; human and rat DP thymocytes are somewhat more robust. The glucocorticoid sensitivity, exactly coincident with the peanut agglutinin–binding phenotype and the lack of class I MHC, is tightly developmentally regulated; it can be used as an efficient method to deplete DP cells specifically. Even mildly elevated physiological levels of glucocorticoids *in vivo* shrink the thymus dramatically through loss of DP cells.

The role of glucocorticoids in thymocyte homeostasis is complex. Adrenalectomy, which removes a major source of glucocorticoids, does result in an increase in DP cell numbers. However, low levels of glucocorticoids can antagonize DP thymocyte death in response to TCR cross-linking. This has been proposed as one of the mechanisms establishing the thresholds that distinguish positive from negative selec-

tion (194,195). On the other hand, a glucocorticoid receptor exon-disruption mutant has been generated, and the mutant mice show no perturbation of T-cell development (196,197). Thus, the role of glucocorticoids in selection is still under investigation. Nevertheless, it seems likely that glucocorticoid sensitivity is one of the physiological mechanisms limiting the life span of postmitotic DP cells that do not get selected, resulting in "death by neglect."

Time Windows for Positive and Negative Selection

Throughout the three-day period that is their average life span, DP thymocytes continue actively to carry on V-J rearrangement of the TCRα locus. This can begin early in the proliferation triggered by β selection (198), although in most cases it is likely to be aided by the increases in RAG activity that occur after proliferation stops (199) (Fig. 2). Individual cells can rearrange the α-chain genes on both chromosomes, not only once but many times, because the locus offers more than 50 possible Jα segments as well as Vα segments in a permissive topology. The first α rearrangements often involve Vα and Jα segments that are relatively close to each other, separated only by the δ locus. Subsequent rearrangements use more 5' Vα segments and more 3' Jα segments. There is no allelic exclusion of TCRα gene rearrangement; the process is terminated either by positive selection, which finally shuts off RAG expression, or by cell death (200–202).

Cells enter a thymic microenvironment in which they can be positively selected before they finish the proliferation that follows β selection. The critical aspect of the microenvironment in this domain is the possibility for intimate interaction with cortical epithelial cells. This specialized stromal cell type provides a rich source of MHC class I and class II surface complexes with a notable lack of co-stimulatory molecules for T cells. This is important because at the DP stage, co-stimulation causes not activation but negative selection (203,204). The cortical epithelial microenvironment is thus a uniquely forgiving testing ground for newly generated TCR recognition specificities.

Many cells are positively selected directly from a proliferating DP blast state (205,206). However, the cells remain rescuable even after they become small, postmitotic cells, perhaps as long as they survive, about 3 days after proliferation stops (207). The window of opportunity for positive selection is thus fairly extended. As a result, the same cell might audition for positive selection repeatedly, from its last cell cycle to 2 days later, with continuing TCRα gene rearrangements, so that each attempt tests a different TCR specificity.

The effect of this broad window is that there is no necessary size for the DP thymocyte pool. Under normal conditions, the pool contains about 3 days' accumulation of postmitotic, unselected cells. In disease, however, the DP thymocyte pool can be shrunk by stress-induced glucocorticoid elevation, and in mice with a transgenic TCR, input to the DP compartment can be significantly reduced by early positive selection. Meanwhile, the maximum fraction of cells eligible for positive selection, among cells with identical TCR, may be limited by competition for a finite number of "niches" (208,209). Thus, positive selection can be more efficient when the size of the DP cohort is smaller than the number of relevant peptide/MHC complexes on the whole cortical epithelium.

Negative selection has been found to affect thymocytes at two stages. It undoubtedly affects cells shortly after positive selection, aborting their differentiation into mature SP thymocytes or deleting newly made SP thymocytes that are not yet fully mature. At least for CD4 SP cells, negative selection is possible until the late stages after positive selection when the cells down-regulate CD24 (HSA) expression (210,211). By this time, the cells are in the medulla (Fig. 3). Most negative selection of CD4-lineage cells with class II MHC-restricted TCR can occur at this CD24$^+$ SP stage. In the cases of certain CD8 lineage cells, with class I MHC-restricted TCR, there is evidence that the cells can also be negatively selected before full differentiation into DP cells. Unlike class II MHC, class I MHC is expressed on many cells besides specialized thymic epithelial cells and dendritic cells, including the DN1 to DN3 cells themselves. Any of these could present antigen for negative selection of class I MHC-restricted cells, especially in TCR transgenics, in which TCR$\alpha\beta$ may be expressed before the DP stages. This shows that in principle, cells can become susceptible to negative selection during or immediately after β selection, depending on whether the target antigen and appropriate antigen-presenting cells are present as soon as TCRα is expressed.

Triggering and Results of Positive Selection

The signaling aspects of positive and negative selection have been studied intensively by many groups since 1995 and are discussed in depth in several excellent reviews (212–214). DP thymocytes are triggered to undergo positive selection when their TCR complexes and their CD4 or CD8 co-receptors engage a peptide/MHC complex presented by cortical epithelial cells. By far, the best TCR-ligand interactions for this purpose are of low affinity, for reasons to be described. As a result, a single peptide/MHC complex can positively select DP cells with any of numerous different TCR specificities, as long as they cross-react weakly with that complex (215). The heightened sensitivity of DP cells to weak TCR interactions means that the cross-reactivity with some peptide/MHC complex that allows a thymocyte to escape death may become undetectable, or detectable only as competitive antagonism, once the cell has matured into a peripheral T cell. However, mature T cells continue to recognize other peptides in association with the same class I or class II MHC molecule that mediated their positive selection. Thus, the MHC restriction of a population of mature T cells is generally determined by the MHC antigens that were expressed in the thymus where they differentiated.

The sequence of events set in train by positive selection begins with activation: the TCR/CD3/co-receptor engagement activates Lck, Ras, Vav, calcineurin, and protein kinase C

(Fig. 7). A major consequence of Ras pathway signaling here is the activation of the MAP kinase, ERK. These signaling mediators in turn must induce the transcription of Egr1 and Id3 (133,160,216), as in β selection, but this time there is little if any proliferation that results. Instead, CD69 is upregulated, and a dramatic transformation begins to unfold. The cells resume the Bcl-2 and class I MHC expression that they had lost at β selection and begin to recover the functional responsiveness (e.g., through AP-1 inducible effector genes) that had disappeared at that time (Fig. 6). Concomitantly, TCR complex expression at the cell surface is stabilized by more efficient assembly (217), and the cells immediately display higher steady-state levels of TCR/CD3. CD5 and TCR/CD3 expression increase in parallel. Glycoprotein processing is altered to a more "normal" pattern, so that new glycoproteins are once again fully sialylated. This restores electrostatic repulsion between DP and other cells and terminates the ability of CD4 and CD8 to interact with MHC independently of TCR. This is also the start of a 1- to 2-week maturation cascade that gradually leads to down-regulation of CD24 (HSA) on the cells as TCR/CD3 levels rise even higher, and CD69 expression finally subsides. These events appear to be common to all positively selected thymocytes.

Strength of Signal versus Distinct Interaction Models for Positive and Negative Selection

Positive and negative selection contribute to central tolerance because thymocytes with receptors that interact strongly with peptide/MHC complexes in the thymus are deleted, whereas those with receptors that interact weakly with thymic peptide/MHC complex are selected positively. A series of compelling studies from several groups in the early 1990s established these principles by using thymocytes with transgenic TCR of known specificity. Peptide/MHC complexes yielding high-affinity interactions with the TCR, which are good stimulators for mature T cells with that TCR, would induce death of thymocytes. Peptide/MHC complexes yielding low-affinity interactions, which could result in anergy or antagonism of mature T-cell responses, promoted positive selection and maturation of thymocytes. A simple bell-shaped dose–response function could thus be envisioned to govern thymocyte fate, as shown in Fig. 10 ("two-threshold model").

The striking features of this model are the sharp discontinuities in response at two points in a continuum of signal strength: separating nonselection from positive selection and separating positive selection from negative selection. If the cell had its fate determined in a single encounter, it would need extraordinarily precise computation of signal intensity levels. Small alterations in expression of signaling components, such as overexpression of a TCR complex or a downstream mediator in a transgenic mouse, might be expected to send the whole population into negative selection or nonselection catastrophes. However, the system is more robust than this. Moreover, it shows evidence of being tunable. In one model, in which thymocytes were made transgenic for

Two threshold model

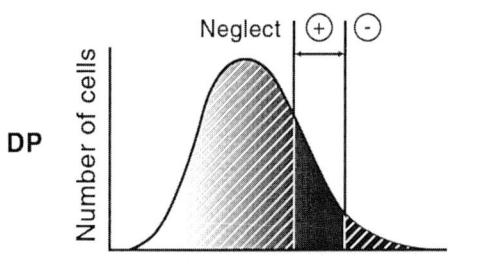

Sequential threshold model

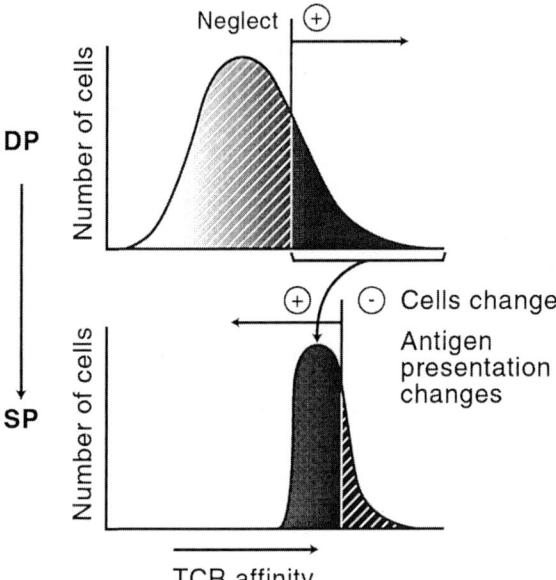

FIG. 10. Relation of T-cell receptor (TCR) affinity to thresholds for positive and negative selection. Two models are compared to indicate the range of TCR-ligand affinities that thymocytes must be able to distinguish in order to be directed correctly to positive selection (+), negative selection (−), or a failure of both (neglect). Histograms of the number of cells in hypothetical precursor populations with different levels of TCR affinity for major histocompatibility complex (MHC)/peptide ligands in the thymic microenvironment are shown. Most cells have receptors that interact too weakly to be positively selected (**left,** *stippled part of curves*). In the two-threshold model (**top**), double positive (DP) cells simultaneously determine whether to be positively selected (*nonstippled portion of curve*) and whether to be negatively selected (**right,** *stippled part of curve*). This choice must occur in the cortex, and it means that cells need to compare their TCR affinity with two reference values at once. In the sequential threshold model (**lower two panels**), DP cells in the cortex (**middle panel**) first need only compare their TCR affinity with a minimum threshold for positive selection. Those cells being positively selected (*bracket*) then differentiate toward the single positive (SP) state, enhancing their TCR expression level and migrating to the medulla, where they encounter highly active antigen-presenting cells (**lower panel**). They are then selected for TCR affinities below the threshold for negative selection. One reason the sequential threshold model is needed is that TCR surface expression increases 10-fold between the DP and SP stages, enabling SP cells to interact with ligands

a TCR with several possible ligands, positive selection could be promoted by several different peptide/MHC complexes with different affinities for the same TCR. However, the properties of the cells that matured were different, depending on the ligand that had selected them. In each case, the mature cells were anergic to the selecting ligand but responsive to stronger agonists (218,219). Thus, cellular properties distinct from the primary structure of the TCR ligands could contribute to positive selection thresholds. How could the sharp discontinuities in dose–response function be reconciled with this evidence for plasticity?

An important advance has been the demonstration that positive and negative selection involve qualitatively distinct signaling pathways. Through the use of transgenes with the Lck gene proximal promoter to direct thymocyte-specific expression of mutant signaling molecules, the Ras signaling pathway downstream of TCR signaling could be selectively manipulated. Such work showed that Ras and MEK signaling were critical for positive selection but unnecessary for negative selection (220). This result refuted the simple prediction that a stronger TCR-ligand interaction, as needed for negative selection, would necessarily be distinguished by activation of all the pathways used in positive selection plus additional ones.

More recently, mutation of specific TCR complex components has been found to disrupt positive selection but not negative selection. The results suggest that positive selection signals uniquely depend on a relay involving a domain of the TCRα chain itself and ultimately, ERK (221,222) [reviewed by Hogquist (214)]. Mutations of any of these components block positive selection without preventing negative selection. An implication is that particular substructures within the TCR complex engage a discrete set of downstream signaling components and that those needed for positive selection can be dissected from those used in other responses.

In subsequent work, negative selection has been found to depend on mediators of distinct signaling pathways [reviewed by Hogquist (214) and Mak et al. (223)], especially pathways triggered by signals from professional antigen-presenting cells that would be co-stimulatory for mature T cells (224). Interactions through certain TNF receptor family death receptors are especially potent ways of causing deletion (225,226). Both in the DP stage and in the HSA$^+$ SP stage, any of a variety of co-stimulatory ligand-receptor interactions can trigger negative selection. Within the thymocytes themselves, the GTPase Rac1, which helps activate the p38 stress kinase and enhances cytoskeletal reorganization, apparently

←
FIG. 10. (*continued*). with a higher avidity (affinity multiplied by number of interactions) than do DP cells with the same receptor. Cells with TCR that appeared to be innocuous in the DP stage could turn out to be autoreactive with their increased TCR levels in the SP stage, unless they were removed by a medullary negative selection mechanism.

promotes negative selection or even converts positive selection responses to death responses when chronically activated (227). Moreover, not all ways to kill immature thymocytes are reflections of the same negative selection process (228). In some cases, even IL-2/IL-2 receptor interaction can act as a cofactor for death (229). DP thymocytes die *in vivo* when animals are injected with anti-CD3 antibodies, at least in part because of TNFα release by mature T cells in the periphery, and this may mimic those forms of negative selection that are dependent on TNF receptor/Fas/CD40L family co-stimulation but not others.

Reflecting the importance of non–TCR-mediated inputs, positive and negative selection can often be mediated by distinct antigen-presenting cell types (230). This was not so clear in initial studies with class I MHC-restricted TCRαβ transgenes, which repeatedly tended to promote elimination of DP thymocytes within the cortex when the thymic microenvironment expressed a high-affinity MHC/peptide ligand. However, for cells with class II MHC-restricted TCR, which undergo positive selection to the CD4+ cell lineage, negative selection is triggered primarily in the thymic medulla. In fact, mice that are genetically manipulated to express class II MHC only in the cortex generate autoreactive CD4+ cells that cannot be eliminated and thus may end up causing autoimmune disease (231). The most effective antigen-presenting cells for negative selection are the hematopoietically derived dendritic cells (the same non-T population that can be derived from a common precursor with T cells). Dendritic cells not only express profuse class I and class II MHC but also display a wide variety of co-stimulatory molecules on their surfaces, from the immunoglobulin superfamily molecules CD80/CD86 to the TNF receptor family molecule CD40 and possibly ligands for CD5 as well. Positive and negative selection can thus take place sequentially; CD4+ cells positively selected in the cortex do not have an occasion to be negatively selected until they migrate to the medulla and encounter dendritic cells there.

This sequentiality is important because it relaxes some of the upper limit constraints on affinity that can be used for positive selection. Autoreactive CD4+ cells can afford to be positively selected, because under normal circumstances they can be negatively selected later (Fig. 10, sequential threshold model). This can be demonstrated in thymic organ culture reaggregates by using mixtures of genetically distinct cortical epithelial and dendritic cells with broader or narrower antigen-presentation capacities. In this system, it has been possible to generate mixed microenvironments in which at least 75% of the thymocytes positively selected in the cortex are subsequently destroyed in the thymic medulla (232). The medullary location is important, too, because, unlike the cortex, it is a site for expression or import of a large spectrum of genes used in peripheral somatic tissues (10). Thus, it provides a much better test panel of antigens than does the cortex to detect and eliminate self-reactivity. Sequentiality also frees positive selection to be mediated by TCR/co-receptor interactions with peptide/MHCs over a wider range of affinities

(Fig. 10, sequential threshold model). As discussed in the later section on CD4 helper T cell versus CD8 cytotoxic T cell lineage commitment, giving the cells a wider spectrum of affinities within which to be positively selected makes it easier to understand some of the aspects of the CD4/CD8 lineage choice.

Another Escape from Autoreactivity in the Thymic Cortex

Even if negative selection may normally be most efficient in the medulla, there can still be a penalty for extremely high-affinity interactions with self-MHC antigens in the cortex. Results of one study indicate one mechanism that is seen best by TCR genes in their native chromosomal context, not transgenes. High-avidity (i.e., affinity multiplied by density of interactions) interactions in the cortex do lead to disappearance of cells with the offending receptor, but not only because the cells are committed to negative selection. Instead, it appears that for many of them, such interactions so efficiently cause internalization of surface TCR that the cells never receive a sustained positive selection signal. Instead, they proceed as though their previous receptor gene rearrangement had yielded no TCRαβ complexes and continue with TCRα locus rearrangements, joining a Vα segment upstream of the previous one with a Jα segment downstream of the previous one, and so forth, until they receive a positive selection signal or reach the end of their DP cell life span (233). The ongoing rearrangement that leads to replacement of one TCR specificity by another is called *receptor editing*. Because of the large number of both V and J gene segments, this process can continue on both chromosomes to generate several rounds of receptor specificities. The result is that not only is the autoreactive TCR lost from the cell surface but also the TCRα gene rearrangement that created it is also commonly lost from the genome.

If this model is generally correct, then the first positive selection thresholds would thus be determined as the window between the minimum avidity required to trigger Ras activation and the maximum avidity that allows a significant number of TCR complexes to remain on the cell surface. Negative selection, occurring later in the medulla, offers a refinement in the context of a large spectrum of extrathymic self-peptides, but the cell biology of positive selection versus TCR internalization can provide an initial MHC affinity filter.

CD4 HELPER T-CELL VERSUS CD8 CYTOTOXIC T-CELL LINEAGE COMMITMENT

The most challenging aspect of positive selection is its apparent connection with a major developmental lineage decision, over and above the decision to live or die. Some of the positively selected cells become helper (CD4 SP) cells and others become killer (CD8 SP) cells. These subsets differ not only in recognition specificity, effector function, and co-receptor expression pattern but also in a whole host

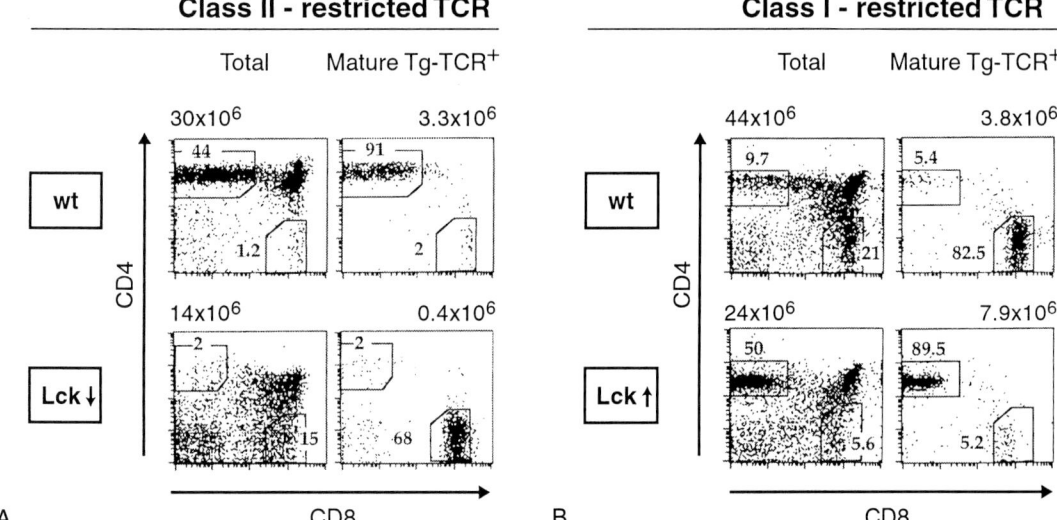

Class II - restricted TCR

Total   Mature Tg-TCR$^+$

Class I - restricted TCR

Total   Mature Tg-TCR$^+$

FIG. 11. CD4/CD8 lineage choice dictated by T-cell receptor (TCR) recognition specificity and by Lck activity levels. CD4/CD8 expression profiles of thymocytes from TCR-transgenic mice show the powerful effect of TCR specificity on CD4/CD8 lineage choice. In these analyses, thymocytes were stained to detect expression of CD4, CD8, and the specific transgenic TCR, and the right portion in each pair shows the CD4/CD8 pattern of the mature single positive (SP) cells expressing high levels of the transgenic TCR. The TCR-transgenic thymocytes are shown both in a normal genetic background (**upper panels**) and in genetic backgrounds which decrease or increase Lck activity in thymocytes (**lower panels**). **A:** Transgenic TCR$\alpha\beta$ that recognizes antigen in association with class II major histocompatibility complex (MHC) directs mature, TCR^{hi} development to the CD4 SP fate (**upper panels**). The bias is very strong in comparison to normal thymocytes (compare with Fig. 1, control samples in Fig. 8). In mice with this TCR transgene plus a transgene that reduces thymocyte Lck activity, however, the same transgenic TCR promotes development of CD8 SP cells (**lower panels**). **B:** Transgenic TCR$\alpha\beta$ that interacts with class I MHC overwhelmingly directs development of mature TCR^{hi} thymocytes to the CD8 SP fate (**upper panels**). However, when mice with this transgene are crossed with transgenic mice that express elevated levels of Lck in thymocytes, the double transgenics show transgenic TCR^{hi} thymocytes developing as CD4 SP cells (**lower panels**). Thus, the level of Lck activity appears to mediate the way the cell distinguishes between recognition of class I or class II MHC. From (251), with permission.

of characteristics regulating every aspect of cellular response from homeostatic mechanisms to growth factor responses. The challenge from a mechanistic point of view is how the apparently simple signal to live or die (or continue receptor editing) is intertwined with signals to undergo divergent pathways to maturation into richly different cell types, as described in detail in the later chapters of this book.

Major Histocompatibility Complex Restriction Regulates CD4 versus CD8 Lineage Differentiation

The problem of what determines the development of $\alpha\beta$ T cell lineage cells into either CD4$^+$ helper T cells or CD8$^+$ cytotoxic T cells has been intensely examined and passionately debated since 1990 but is still not settled (214,234–236). It is at the DP stage that the association among the CD4 or CD8 co-receptor, $\alpha\beta$ TCR specificity, and function appears to be established. When cells expressing an $\alpha\beta$ TCR that recognizes peptide in the context of the antigen-presentation molecule class I MHC are positively selected, they down-regulate the expression of CD4 and activate the gene program specific to a CD8 cytotoxic T cell. Conversely, cells express-

ing an $\alpha\beta$ TCR that recognizes peptide in the context of the antigen-presentation molecule class II MHC down-regulate the expression of CD8 and activate the gene program specific to a CD4 helper T cell. Examples are provided in virtually every thymus of animals with pre-rearranged TCR$\alpha\beta$ transgenes (Fig. 11A and B, wild type). Furthermore, CD8 SP cells are not generated in a thymus lacking class I MHC, and CD4 cells are not generated in a thymus lacking class II MHC.[3] It is not a coincidence that CD8 binds to class I MHC and CD4 binds to class II MHC—the simultaneous binding of class I by a class I–specific TCR and CD8 or class II by a class II–specific TCR and CD4 increases the affinity of the interaction and activates signaling pathways inside the T cell. Nevertheless, it is difficult to see how the cell perceives the difference in ligand binding to its TCR and co-receptor and then translates the signal into a choice of divergent differentiation programs.

There have been several problems in trying to solve the basis of this choice. First, the severe loss of cells from every DP

---

[3] The exception is one unconventional subset of CD4 SP cells that is actually selected by nonclassical class I MHC family molecules; this is the NK T-cell subset, discussed in the section on Frontiers for the Future.

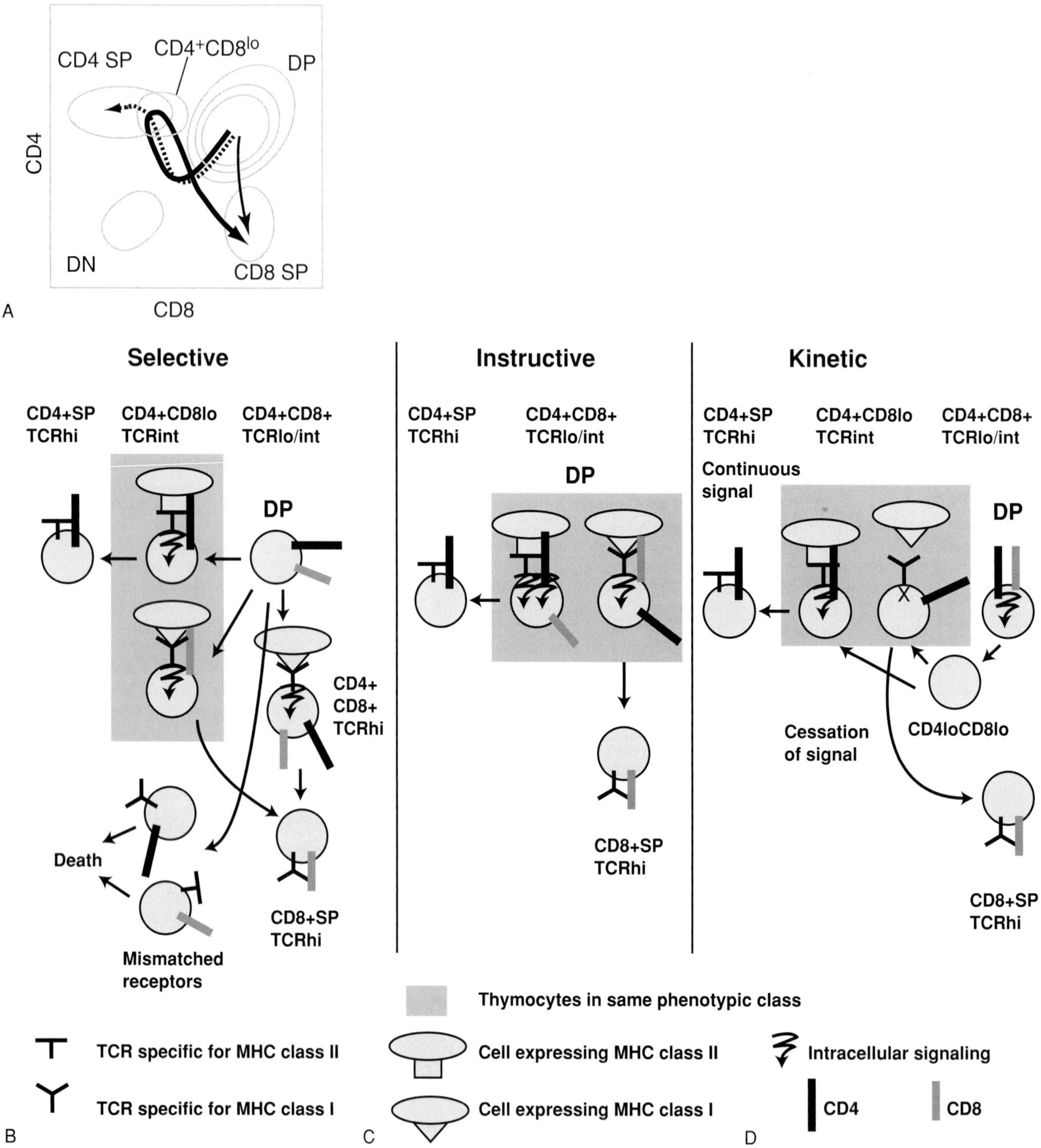

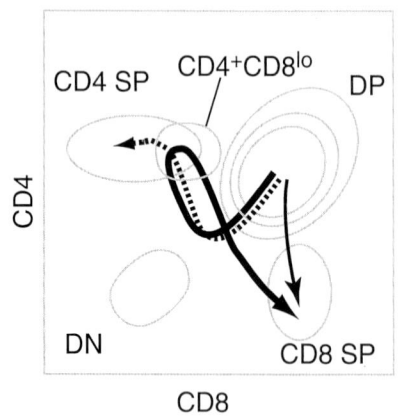

A

Selective

CD4+SP
TCRhi
CD4+CD8lo
TCRint
CD4+CD8+
TCRlo/int

DP

CD4+
CD8+
TCRhi

Death

Mismatched
receptors

CD8+SP
TCRhi

Instructive

CD4+SP
TCRhi
CD4+CD8+
TCRlo/int

DP

CD8+SP
TCRhi

Kinetic

CD4+SP
TCRhi
CD4+CD8lo
TCRint
CD4+CD8+
TCRlo/int

Continuous
signal

DP

Cessation
of signal

CD4loCD8lo

CD8+SP
TCRhi

Thymocytes in same phenotypic class

T   TCR specific for MHC class II

Y   TCR specific for MHC class I

Cell expressing MHC class II

Cell expressing MHC class I

Intracellular signaling

CD4   CD8

B   **C**   **D**

FIG. 12. Models of CD4/CD8 T cell lineage commitment. **A:** Schematic of changes in thymocyte phenotype during positive selection to the CD4 single positive (SP) or CD8 SP fate. The layout is that in which detailed interpretations of signaling and selection events are presented (**B** to **D**). An idealized flow cytometry plot is shown, with *arrows* denoting the path of differentiation taken by many CD8 SP precursors (*solid arrow*) and by CD4 SP precursors (*dotted arrow*). Both CD4 and CD8 expression are initially down-regulated, with transient recovery of CD4 expression, before the pathways of the two cell types are clearly seen to diverge. The following models depict the signaling events proposed to occur in each of the populations indicated. **B** to **D:** Symbols for cells that are proposed to be distinctly programmed but similar in surface phenotype are enclosed in *gray boxes*. **B:** Selective model. This model posits that before leaving the DP population, cells become programmed for different responses to positive selection

generation, which is common to most TCR-transgenic models as well as to normal mice, makes accounting impossible. Second, there is a critical shortage of markers that distinguish cells taking the CD4 path from those taking the CD8 path. As a result, much research is focused on the requirements for expression of the CD4 and CD8 molecules themselves. Because these vital co-receptors clearly participate in the process, however, there is an essential circularity in these analyses, which great ingenuity in experimental design has only partially succeeded in overcoming. Furthermore, the developmental expression of these molecules, even at the RNA level, is complex. There is strong evidence that the transit from DP to CD4 or CD8 SP involves not instant repression of the "wrong" co-receptor but rather a period of phenotypic instability going through CD4^{lo}CD8^{lo} and CD4^{+}CD8^{lo} intermediates to both end states (237–242) (Fig. 12A). With few markers capable of distinguishing between pre-CD4 and pre-CD8 intermediates at the earliest stages of their developmental divergence, studies have had to rely on measuring the output of mature CD4^{+} versus CD8^{+} cells. Full maturation is almost certain to rely on specialized survival signals for each committed lineage as well as the initial events that set the cells onto different pathways. Thus, much controversy has revolved around the respective roles of survival versus differentiation processes in the CD4/CD8 lineage choice.

Models for CD4/CD8 Lineage Divergence

Several models have been postulated to explain the correlation of TCR and co-receptor with mature T cell function (Fig. 12B, C, and D). A selective model postulates that CD4^{+}CD8^{+} thymocytes choose a CD4 SP helper versus CD8 SP killer lineage independently of their TCR recognition specificity. On the basis of this prior choice, they immediately begin down-regulating the unwanted co-receptor when positive selection begins. However, because sustained interactions are needed to complete maturation, the only thymocytes that survive are those that continue to express the co-receptor that binds to the same type of MHC molecule as the TCR (243,244). This model predicts that "mismatched" thymocytes would be generated—that is, that there would exist in the thymus transitional thymocytes expressing class I–specific TCR and CD4 or class II–specific TCR and CD8—but that such cells would be unable to finish their differentiation (Fig. 12B). Evidence for this is seen in a mouse model in which early commitment to the CD8 lineage can be traced by a silencing of a β-galactosidase gene "knocked into" the CD4 locus. In this mouse, 19% of cells apparently committed to the CD8 lineage express class II MHC-specific TCR, and 11% of cells apparently committed to the CD4 lineage express class I MHC-specific TCR (242). It is not clear whether these mismatched thymocytes die or whether they can reverse this early commitment, but they are not present in the mature T-cell population. The selective model also predicts that these mismatched cells could be rescued by constitutive expression of a co-receptor matching the specificity of the TCR. This has been shown in a mouse with a homozygous deletion of the CD4 silencer, which results in constitutive expression of CD4 in SP thymocytes and T cells and the development of CD8^{+}CD4^{+} class II MHC-restricted cytotoxic T cells (245). An argument against the selective model is that analysis of various TCR-transgenic mouse strains shows that the selection efficiency can be much higher than would be expected from the selective model (209).

The instructive model postulates that the lineage choice is made only in response to the positive selection signal, directed by a difference in signaling between TCR/CD4 recognition of class II MHC and TCR/CD8 recognition of class I MHC (Fig. 12C). This model is supported by evidence that signaling through the cytoplasmic tail of CD4 (246,247) and CD8 (248,249) leads to the development of CD4 SP and CD8 SP thymocytes, respectively. A difficulty with the instructive theory has been how to account for the differentiation between signals received from the CD4 and CD8 cytoplasmic tails, because both co-receptors associate with the same signaling molecules, most notably the Src family kinase p56^{Lck}

FIG. 12. (continued). signals. The co-receptors are programmed for down-regulation in a pattern that is independent of T-cell receptor (TCR), resulting in diverse combinations of CD4/CD8 phenotype and TCR specificity once positive selection begins. Cells that lose a co-receptor that is required to stabilize their TCR interactions with major histocompatibility complex (MHC) cannot continue to signal. Only cells capable of signaling, either through co-ligation of TCR and co-receptor by MHC or through ligation of a high-affinity TCR that is independent of co-receptor, will survive. C: Instructive model. This model is based on the idea that strong intracellular signals emanating from the co-ligation of a TCR specific for class II MHC and CD4 instruct the cells to silence CD8 and mature into a CD4^{+} helper T cell, whereas weaker intracellular signals emanating from the co-ligation of a TCR specific for class I MHC and CD8 lead to the silencing of CD4 transcription and the maturation of the thymocyte into a CD8^{+} cytotoxic T cell. This model does not predict the presence of thymocytes expressing inappropriate co-receptors for their TCR specificity unless signaling pathways are perturbed. D: Kinetic signaling model. This model holds that all thymocytes transit through an initial down-regulation of both co-receptors and then an up-regulation of CD4 to form a CD4^{+}CD8^{lo} population (A, broken arrow and heavy solid arrow). Cells expressing TCR specific for class I MHC cease signaling, because they lack sufficient CD8 to co-ligate class I MHC with the TCR. The cessation of signaling triggers the silencing of CD4 transcription and the maturation of these cells into CD8^{+} cytotoxic T cells. Thymocytes expressing a TCR specific for class II MHC continue to receive signals from the co-ligated TCR and CD4 and mature into CD4^{+} helper T cells.

(Lck). The two co-receptors do differ in the numbers of Lck molecules associated with their cytoplasmic tails: The cytoplasmic tail CD4 is associated with approximately 20 times more p56^{Lck} than is the cytoplasmic tail of CD8α (250). This difference is exacerbated by the fact that many DP thymocyte CD8α molecules are truncated so as not to bind any Lck at all. Increases in Lck activity promote the adoption of the CD4$^+$ lineage (251–253), whereas diminution of p56^{Lck} activity promotes the adoption of the CD8$^+$ lineage (251) (Fig. 11A and B, lower panels). The natural mixture of CD8α Lck-binding and nonbinding forms appears to promote CD8 SP cell development most efficiently, by stabilizing TCR-MHC interactions with the minimum of Lck recruitment (254).

An increased duration of signaling through the TCR is also associated with a commitment to the CD4$^+$ lineage (255). This is in agreement with results from a suspension culture system in which DP thymocytes can be directed into the CD4 SP or CD8 SP pathway with a combination of ionomycin (a calcium ionophore) and phorbol 12-myristate 13-acetate (PMA), depending on the length of time that the stimulation is applied. In this system, inducing DP thymocytes to commit to the CD4$^+$ lineage requires longer duration of treatment than the duration of treatment required to induce DP thymocytes to commit to the CD8$^+$ lineage (256). Some effects attributed to signal intensity may actually be signal duration effects. Even *in vivo,* in transgenic systems, Lck activity levels were most clearly seen to affect CD4/CD8 lineage choice when they were expressed in a sustained way over a period of days or from a promoter with increasing activity after the DP stage (252,257). This would associate the CD4$^+$ lineage choice again with a sustained elevation of Lck signaling, even after the positive selection process had begun.

Kinetic signaling models (Fig. 12D) define this difference in signal duration requirements for the CD4$^+$ and CD8$^+$ fates as being more important than the peak strengths of the signals. This class of model is supported by the observation that most DP thymocytes pass through an initial down-regulation of both co-receptors and then an up-regulation of CD4 to form a CD4$^+$CD8^{lo} population before the cells diverge to undergo differentiation to mature CD4 or CD8 SP states. During the CD4$^+$CD8^{lo} stage, interactions with class II MHC could continue, whereas interactions with class I MHC would naturally be weakened from loss of co-receptor contribution. The kinetic signaling models posit that continued signaling through TCR and CD4 leads to development into CD4 SP thymocytes; cessation of signaling triggers the down-regulation of CD4 and the up-regulation of CD8, leading to the development of CD8 SP thymocytes (258). After the basic lineage choice has been made, full maturation of CD8 SP cells appears to depend on non-TCR survival functions: either Notch family signaling (255) or IL-7R signaling (258). This kind of model can be integrated with signal strength or duration hypotheses, because thymocytes expressing class I MHC-restricted TCR in conjunction with a low level of class I MHC-ligated CD8 would naturally receive a lower strength signal than would thymocytes expressing class II MHC -restricted TCR in conjunction with high levels of class II MHC-ligated CD4.

A kinetic signaling model is supported by an experiment in which a hybrid molecule with a CD8α extracellular and transmembrane domain and a CD4 cytoplasmic tail is expressed in mice lacking class II MHC and CD8α (259). In this background, signals from the hybrid co-receptor promote the development of even more CD8 SP than of CD4 SP class I MHC-restricted thymocytes. In contrast, the instructive model predicts that the hybrid co-receptor would have preferentially promoted commitment to the CD4$^+$ lineage simply because of its CD4-promoting signal when the hybrid co-receptor co-ligated to class I MHC with a class I MHC-restricted TCR. Indeed, when class II MHC and endogenous CD8α are present, that is what is seen (247) but not when the occasion for CD4/class II MHC interaction is taken away. To understand how this works, recall that CD8 exists as a dimer (CD8$\alpha\beta$) and that the CD8β chain increases CD8α-associated Lck activity (248). Normally, both CD8α and CD8β are down-regulated in the CD4$^+$CD8^{lo} stage. The kinetic signaling model explains the increased numbers of CD8 SP thymocytes produced by the hybrid co-receptor by increased strength of signals during positive selection, increasing the number of cells entering the CD4$^+$CD8^{lo} compartment. Once the thymocytes enter the CD4$^+$CD8^{lo} compartment, however, endogenous CD8β is down-regulated, which decreases the signal resulting from class I MHC ligation of the hybrid co-receptor and results in direction of the thymocytes into the CD8 lineage.

Thus, the key issues that distinguish these models are (a) whether mismatched cells are generated at all, (b) whether the fates of such cells are to die or to be redirected into a different lineage, and (c) when the choice of fates is actually finalized. These properties of the three kinds of model are contrasted simply in Fig. 13. Data support the prediction that cells are generated initially that appear "mismatched," in conflict with the simplest version of an instructive model, but according to the kinetic signaling models, these cells simply have not yet finished receiving instructions about the types of cells they will be. Many, although perhaps not all (242), CD8 cells do appear to develop through a CD4$^+$CD8^{lo} intermediate, making the various kinetic signaling models plausible. However, there is still no direct proof that the developmental mechanisms needed for both CD4 and CD8 SP differentiation remain available to individual cells as late as the CD4$^+$CD8^{lo} stage. Thus, as in the cases of the earlier lineage choices, models based on selection and differential survival cannot yet be excluded. In any case, the challenge is to understand how these complex differences in intensity and duration of signaling can be translated into different developmental responses.

Molecules Implicated in the CD4/CD8 Lineage Choice

Signal intensity or duration does not necessarily mean an equal involvement of all the multiple branching pathways

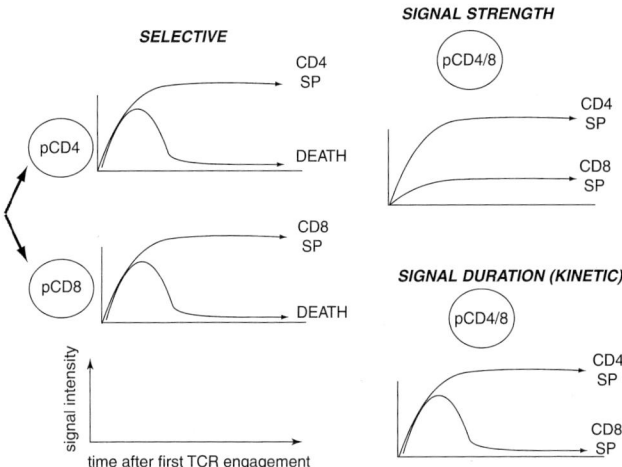

SELECTIVE

SIGNAL STRENGTH

SIGNAL DURATION (KINETIC)

FIG. 13. Developmental effects of intensity and time courses of T-cell receptor (TCR)/co-receptor signals in three models of CD4/CD8 lineage choice. Plots showing the intensity of predicted TCR/co-receptor signals over time and their effects on cell fate are compared in three models of CD4/CD8 lineage choice. **Left:** Selective model predicts initial divergence of pre-CD4 single positive (SP) and pre-CD8 SP cells, after which the only choice the cells need to make in response to TCR signals is to live or to die. Termination of signaling, the usual result of down-regulating the wrong co-receptor for the cell's TCR, leads to death in either lineage. **Upper right:** Signal strength model predicts that the intensity of TCR/co-receptor signaling instructs the cells whether to take a CD4 SP or a CD8 SP fate. It is assumed that the usable intensity range is limited by negative selection at the high end and by neglect at the low end. **Lower right:** Signal duration–based models such as the kinetic signaling model shown in Fig. 12D predict that transient signaling is a specific instructive signal for CD8 SP development, whereas sustained signaling is a specific instructive signal for CD4 SP development. In this kind of model, although TCR signaling itself may provide continuous survival functions for CD4 SP cells, additional kinds of survival functions are needed for CD8 SP cells (not shown).

activated by TCR ligation (Fig. 7). Mutant analyses show that the pathway most relevant to the signal duration/strength that will determine CD4 versus CD8 SP fate is the pathway involving Lck and ERK. Members of the Lck signaling cascade are essential for both but favor CD4 SP development over CD8 SP at high levels. Molecules other than TCR/co-receptor signaling components are also implicated in lineage-restricted roles, and this is an important step toward being able to resolve when the CD4 and CD8 gene expression programs actually diverge. To date, however, it is still debated whether the known molecules affect the choice itself or, rather, the efficiency of survival after the choice.

Lck activity levels have a powerful impact on the choice, as discussed (Fig. 11; compare upper and lower panels). From the DP stage onward, Lck is brought to the TCR signaling complex by CD4 or CD8, making the direction of CD4/CD8 lineage choice depend, by implication, on levels of co-receptor involvement in TCR triggering. Thus, the CD4/CD8 co-receptors have two separable roles in positive selection: They stabilize and initiate TCR complex signaling, and they do so either with a minimal amount of Lck—just enough to trigger ZAP70 and the rest of the TCR cascade—or with a "bonus" level of Lck, which CD4 can provide but CD8 cannot (244,247,254,259). For this to work, the cells must be able to distinguish between different levels of Lck signaling even in the context of equal levels of TCR complex/ZAP70 signaling. In this connection, it is interesting to note that the ratio of co-receptor–driven signaling to other TCR signaling may be expected to shift during the positive selection process in general, as TCR surface levels rise and the co-receptor-MHC interactions are weakened by increased surface sialylation (112,113). This shift would tend to amplify the effects of the CD8 down-regulation at the CD4⁺CD8^{lo} intermediate stage and enhance a signal duration or kinetic signaling mechanism.

One of the mediators that is preferentially activated by Lck is ERK. The involvement of the MAP kinase ERK in CD4 versus CD8 lineage commitment has been suggested by studies in which pharmacological inhibitors of ERK selectively block the development of CD4 SP thymocytes but not CD8 SP thymocytes (253,260,261). However, another study using ERK inhibitors shows a block in development of CD8 SP (262), as do genetic methods to reduce ERK activity, such as use of a dominant-negative MEK transgene (263) or a null mutation of ERK (264). One interpretation is that the disparate results may result from the inhibition of the activity of molecules other than ERK by the pharmaceutical inhibitors used. Alternatively, both lineages may require some ERK signaling, but a higher level or duration of ERK signaling may be critical for CD4 cell commitment or maturation, whereas a transient or low level of ERK signaling may be optimal for CD8 cell development.

In general, molecules that increase signaling (without promoting negative selection) favor CD4 cell production, whereas molecules that decrease signaling favor CD8 cell production. Thus, integrin-mediated enhancement of interactions is needed most urgently to make CD4 SP cells (265). A new DNA-binding protein that promotes CD8 cell development, TOX, appears to do so by reducing overall TCR signal strength (266). There is a role for Notch family molecules, to be discussed, and this too has been linked with effects on TCR signal strength (267). Even the threshold-setting functions of Ikaros for T-cell signaling, which were discussed previously in the context of β selection, could play a role again in the CD4/CD8 lineage choice: mice with Ikaros-deficient mutations generate a higher percentage of CD4 SP cells, as opposed to CD8 SP cells (154).

Genes that implement or stabilize the developmental effects of the positive selection signal to bring about CD4 SP or CD8 SP lineage differentiation have been harder to identify so far. Thus, there is a serious shortage of candidates for genes that actually define the long-term lineage identities of CD4 SP or CD8 SP cells.

One spontaneous mutation affects a gene that may prove to have a unique role in the development of the CD4 helper lineage. In the "helper-deficient" mutant mouse, class II MHC-restricted thymocytes are directed exclusively to the CD8 lineage, even in the absence of class I MHC ligation of the CD8 co-receptor. Positive selection signals in the helper-deficient mutant thymocytes appear to be normal (268). This suggests that although positive selection, mediated by signals through the TCR, and CD4 or CD8 lineage commitment occur at the same time, they are not the same process. Unfortunately, the gene mutated in this strain is not yet identified.

CD8 SP lineage cells apparently require more survival-promoting functions than CD4 SP cells (29). Either transgenic overexpression of Bcl-2 or stimulation of the IL-7R, which is expressed again after the DP stage (269), disproportionately enhances CD8 SP yields (258,270). Thus, some of the genes that enhance CD8 cell development could be doing so simply by providing survival functions. Among the most controversial of these effects is the impact of activation of Notch family genes.

Increased signaling by a constitutively activated cytoplasmic domain of the cell surface receptor Notch-1 has been shown to favor the development of CD8 SP thymocytes (271). The original report was highly important as the first demonstration that overexpression of a non-TCR gene could shift cells into the CD8 SP pathway even when their TCR had interacted with class II MHC. This effect has remained controversial, however, because expression of a larger piece of the intracellular domain of Notch-1, also constitutively activated, promotes the development of CD8 SP and, to a lesser degree, CD4 SP thymocytes (185). In vitro experiments diminishing Notch-1 activity in thymocytes that had already received co-receptor-TCR-MHC interaction signals have revealed that Notch-1 functioned only to promote the post-commitment maturation of CD8 SP thymocytes (255). In addition, a conditional deletion of Notch-1 shows no effect on CD4/CD8 lineage commitment if done after the earliest stages of thymocyte development (257).

One way the controversy may be resolved is that other Notch family members expressed in the thymus are able to substitute for Notch-1 in the CD4/CD8 lineage choice. Pharmaceutical inhibition of the enzymatic activation of all three Notch family members molecules in DP thymocytes does selectively decrease the number of CD8 SP thymocytes (64,65). These Notch inhibitor effects are dose and potency dependent, in such a way that greater inhibition of Notch impairs development of both CD4$^+$ SP and CD8$^+$ SP thymocytes and inhibition to a lesser degree impairs only the development of CD8$^+$ SP thymocytes.

The disparate effects seen in transgenic mice expressing activated Notch-1 can also be explained by dose and potency dependence. The activated Notch-1 domain that selectively promotes the development of CD8$^+$ SP thymocytes (271) is shorter and less potent than the activated Notch-1 domain that promotes the development of both CD4$^+$ SP and CD8$^+$ SP thymocytes (185). The expression of both of these constructs is driven by the Lck proximal promoter, which decreases in activity during the time that DP thymocytes commit to

either the CD4 or CD8 lineage. In contrast, expression of the full-length intracellular domain of Notch-1 from a constitutively active retroviral promoter inhibits development of both CD4 and CD8 SP thymocytes through attenuation of signals through the TCR(267). The lower effective dose of activated Notch-1 delivered from a proximal Lck promoter-driven transgene may promote development of CD8$^+$ SP thymocytes by lowering the strength or duration of the signal through the TCR, in keeping with the instructive models of T cell development, or by providing a lineage-specific survival function in committed CD8 precursors (255).

The physiological role that the Notch molecules really play in CD4 and CD8 cell lineage commitment still remains to be determined. Notch activity in DP thymocytes, at least as assessed by the expression of the downstream mediators Hes-1 and Deltex, is very low to undetectable (185). It may be that Notch-1 acts through other downstream mediators in DP thymocytes or that other Notch family members and a different set of downstream mediators play a more important role.

While the role of Notch family molecules and the transcription factors they control is being resolved, indications of other nuclear factors that appear to bias CD4/CD8 lineage choice have begun to appear. GATA-3 and Runx1 (AML1, CBFα2, or PEBP2αB), genes involved in T-cell development from the earliest stages (Fig. 4), also seem to be able to direct the output of positive selection to disproportionately CD4 SP or disproportionately CD8 SP pathways, respectively (272–274). These effects suggest a link to the functions that must coordinate CD4 and CD8 expression with effector function and other features of the mature CD4 and CD8 SP populations.

Maturation and Export of CD4 and CD8 Single-Positive Thymocytes

Commitment to the CD4$^+$ or CD8$^+$ lineage in thymocytes is characterized by the down-regulation of one co-receptor and the maintenance of expression of the other co-receptor, but it is important to remember that the commitment to the CD4$^+$ or CD8$^+$ lineage is also accompanied by a gene expression program specific to helper T cell functions (for CD4$^+$ class II MHC-restricted cells) or cytotoxic T cell functions (for CD8$^+$ class I MHC-restricted cells). The cells can begin expressing some of the effector genes associated with these distinctive pathways in vivo, long before their maturation is complete (158,251,275–277). In the long run, these sublineage-specific molecules that do not participate in antigen binding may provide the best indicators of the timing of the commitment of T-cell precursors to the CD4 and CD8 SP lineages.

As a general rule, in the rare cases in which the co-receptor is mismatched with the MHC restriction, the function of the cells is matched with the co-receptor, not with the specificity of the TCR (244,278,279). Genes integral to the function of CD8$^+$ cytotoxic T cells are expressed starting in the DP thymocytes, increasing only in cells that down-regulate CD4 mRNA (280). This suggests that down-regulation of the CD4 co-receptor and initiation of a program of cytotoxic gene expression occur simultaneously and are normally coordinated. However, CD4 down-regulation is not required for the establishment of a gene expression pattern specific to cytotoxic cells. Deletion of the CD4 silencer prevents the down-regulation of CD4 that normally occurs in the CD8 lineage, but the $CD4^+CD8^+$ cells that result develop as functional cytotoxic T cells (281). Conversely, helper and cytotoxic T cells can develop in the absence of CD4 or CD8, respectively.

In spite of the early flashes of effector gene expression, full functional maturation occurs over a substantially longer time than does the rescue of DP cells from death by neglect. The cells do not show full responsiveness to challenge with a TCR ligand and do not become resistant to apoptosis until the late stages of post–positive-selection processing, when the cells finally down-regulate CD24 (HSA) and CD69 and lose the markers that have distinguished them phenotypically from peripheral T cells. The process through which this occurs is still poorly understood. Perhaps what is needed is just time to reverse the numerous physiological adjustments that give DP thymocytes their unusual responses to stimulation. This could be a matter of waiting for key inhibitory molecules to decay physically. The process could also be more complex in itself, for example, if it involved a cascade of reciprocal cell–cell interactions with the medullary stroma. Finally, it remains possible that functional maturation includes a component of selection. Can helper or killer differentiation begin in a way that is mismatched with co-receptor or TCR specificity? If so, maturation could include rewarding (with survival) cells that happen to possess the right combinations of effector programming, co-receptor expression, and TCR specificity. In this case, effector maturation would be the actual conclusion of the CD4/CD8 lineage choice.

Finally, to detect the success of positive selection, the cells have to receive survival signals that make them permanently long-lived, a dramatic contrast from the DP thymocyte state. Sustained TCR/Lck signaling may provide much of this survival function for CD4 SP cells. For CD8 cells, the discontinuous or hit-and-run TCR/Lck signal may need to be supplemented by additional survival mechanisms. This would account for the enhanced importance of Bcl-2, IL-7R, and possibly Notch-family functions in CD8 SP lineage cells, as we have already noted, especially in the later period after CD8-lineage differentiation has begun. $CD4^+$ and $CD8^+$ mature cells continue to use different homeostatic maintenance and proliferation signals long after they leave the thymus, during their functions in the periphery; therefore, it is not surprising if a divergence is seen in these functions during maturation after positive selection.

The mature cells finally leave the thymus in a nonsynchronized manner, about 7 to 14 days after beginning positive selection (282,283). The emigration appears to depend on a G-protein–coupled chemokine receptor, possibly CCR7 (284,285). Very little is known yet about the signals that tell the cells when they are ready to leave. The developmental events that occur in the medulla, including the coordination of maturation and export, currently remain one of the important areas of mystery in T-cell development.

Relationships between Positive Selection, Negative Selection, and CD4/CD8 Lineage Choice

Positive selection, negative selection, and CD4/CD8 lineage choice all depend to some extent on quantitative aspects of signaling through the TCR. This leads to an obvious question of how the cells can interpret a particular TCR engagement to make the correct decision. If a cell with a class I MHC-restricted TCR has a particularly high affinity for intrathymic class I MHC/peptide complexes, how does that cell determine whether to be deleted or whether to be converted into a CD4 SP cell? The cells do appear to make the positive/negative selection decision independently of the CD4/CD8 decision. In transgenic TCR models, the deletion of self-reactive class I MHC-restricted cells occurs without any obvious redirection into the CD4 lineage (the CD4 SP cells that can be seen in such transgenic individuals generally do not use the transgenic TCR).

In principle, it may be possible to obtain four different outcomes from the single variable of signal strength, but the range of values directing negative selection, CD4 positive selection, and CD8 positive selection would each have to be tightly calibrated to distinguish them from one another as well as from death by neglect (Fig. 14A). Changes in TCR or co-receptor surface density, for example, would need to be held within sharply limited ranges. As far as can be determined, the system appears much more forgiving. Although TCR and co-receptor levels are finely regulated in normal development, transgenic manipulation can distort these levels quite substantially without altering the direction or predictability of CD4/CD8 lineage choice.

This, then, is an important attraction of the kinetic signaling/signal duration models: They add a second, independent parameter for the cells to use combinatorially with signal strength to compute the appropriate CD4/CD8 lineage choice (Fig. 14B). In a similar way, the importance of co-stimulatory interactions in many forms of negative selection gives the cells yet another independent parameter to help even further to distinguish the negative selection threshold from the CD4/CD8 differentiation threshold *in vivo* (Fig. 14C).

In CD4/CD8 lineage choice, there is a hint that in the repeated contacts the cells make with MHC/peptide ligands over the several days of positive selection, the balance of these pathways can change further. At least in the CD8 cell pathway, this would be caused by the increasing surface density of TCR complexes at the same time that glycosylation changes are reducing the ability of the CD8 to bind class I MHC on its own (see the section on positive and negative selection). A predicted effect would be that the signals delivered at the beginning of positive selection would be dominated more by the co-receptors and their signaling mediators, whereas the

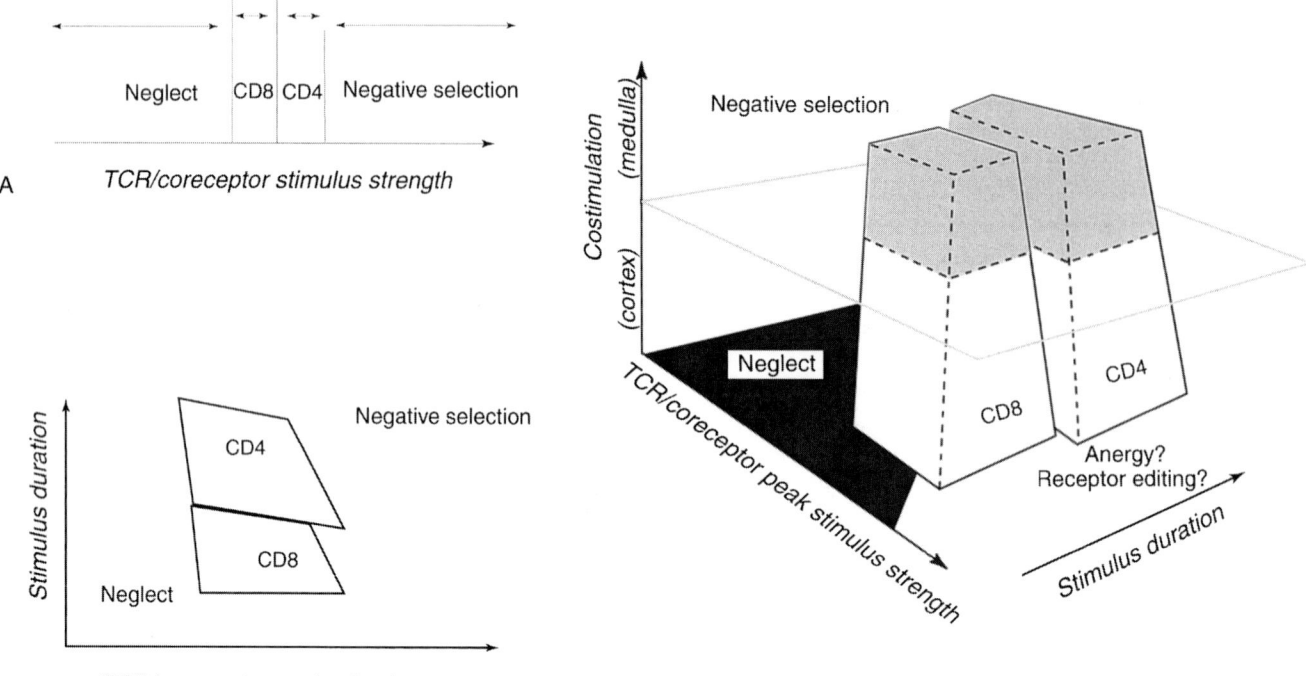

FIG. 14. Three schematic views of the signals that may determine thymocyte developmental fate during positive and negative selection. **A:** A simple stimulus strength model is depicted, in which the only parameter determining life, death, CD4 single positive (SP) cell fate, or CD8 SP cell fate is the intensity of signals through the T-cell receptor (TCR) and co-receptors. In this model, the cells compute TCR signaling intensity in the cortex and determine their fates immediately. **B:** A model in which stimulus strength and stimulus duration help the cell to distinguish between CD4 and CD8 cell fates and between these maturation pathways and death by neglect and by negative selection. Note the range of stimulus strengths (~TCR/co-receptor affinities) that can be used for positive selection in this model, wider than in the simple stimulus strength model (**A**) and the overlap in peak stimulus strength values (x-axis) that can give rise to either CD4 or CD8 cells. **C:** A model in which stimulus strength, stimulus duration, and the presence or absence of co-stimulation distinguish between CD4 and CD8 SP fates, neglect, and deletional and nondeletional forms of tolerance induction. This model is based on the idea that, for many cells, positive and negative selection choices can be encountered sequentially (also see Fig. 10, sequential threshold model). In this figure, high levels of co-stimulation that can lead to negative selection (*gray areas* on plots) are encountered only in the medulla, which cells are only allowed to enter if they have first been positively selected as CD4 SP or CD8 SP cells in the cortex.

signals delivered at the end of positive selection/maturation would be dominated more by the TCR. Thus, depending on when cells actually commit to a CD4 or CD8 SP fate, the composition of the "TCR signal" at the time of positive selection could shift substantially by the time that the maturing cells, now in the medulla, encounter their last negative selection threshold.

The need for survival functions after lineage commitment, which may be specialized for each lineage, offers a way to reconcile the more instructive models with key evidence for the selective model. Any experimental manipulation that removes the survival mechanism for CD4 or CD8 cells after lineage commitment would indeed lead to elimination of those cells and could be defined as a mismatch between programming and survival receptors. There is another implication as well. The asymmetrical survival requirements of CD4 and CD8 SP cells mean that failure of survival (i.e. negative selection) could be effected by different mechanisms, too. Thus,

the mechanism needed for negative selection may itself be an output of the CD4/CD8 lineage choice.

FRONTIERS FOR THE FUTURE: MYSTERIES AND ALTERNATIVES IN T-CELL DEVELOPMENT

There is some evidence that the main stream of thymocyte selection, branched and complex as it is, may not be the only pathway through which T cells mature. In the future, cells that take a somewhat different pathway may be recognized as extremely important for the regulation of the peripheral immune system and thus for human health. It is currently hard to be certain whether all T-lineage cells follow the same program or not. The more than 95% loss of each cohort of cortical thymocytes makes it difficult to track particular precursors from before β selection to maturation. One kind of evidence, however, suggests that there do exist substreams of T-cell development that are characterized by different surface marker expression patterns than are the majority of thymocytes. Some apparent intermediates in the transition from DN to DP to SP, for example, appear to preserve expression of the DN1/DN2 growth factor receptors c-kit and IL-7R all the way throughout β selection and positive selection (269,286). These c-kit$^+$ IL-7R$^+$ DP-like thymocytes appear to have better odds of maturing than do the mainstream c-kit$^-$ IL-7R$^-$ DP thymocytes. It is still unknown whether such cells develop into different kinds of T cells from the mainstream or whether they simply represent a lucky minority that have happened to undergo β selection early, before loss of key survival-enhancing functions.

One reason to consider that these cells could have a distinctive fate is that there are at least two unconventional minority subsets of TCR$\alpha\beta$ T cells that can be generated in the thymus, with functional properties clearly distinct from the majority. Both cell types appear to play important roles in the regulation of immune responses and the maintenance of peripheral self-tolerance. For this reason, the immunological functions and developmental history of these subsets are currently topics of great interest. Both lineages, it seems, could arise from variations in the mechanisms controlling positive or negative selection or both.

Alternative Pathway or Distinct Precursors: The Case of the NK T Cells

NK T cells are adult T cells that share characteristics with NK cells, most notably the expression of surface markers CD161 (NK1.1) and CD122 (IL-2Rβ); killer inhibitory receptors Ly49A, Ly49C/I, and Ly49G2; and cytolytic molecules perforin and granzyme (287–289). These cells appear to be important in controlling autoimmunity as well as immune responses to tumors and infectious diseases, perhaps because they produce very high levels of IL-4 and interferon-γ upon first encounter with antigen, unlike conventional T cells. They represent a kind of bridge from the adaptive to the innate immune system. More than 80% of the NK T cells in the thymus and liver express an invariant Vα14-Jα281; have a bias in Vβ usage to Vβ8, Vβ2, and Vβ7; and are specific for glycolipids bound by the nonclassical class I MHC relative CD1d. CD1d tetramers, which bind to the synthetic glycolipid α-galactosyl-ceramide (α-Gal-Cer), have been used successfully to identify these cells independently of NK1.1 (290,291). Most studies have shown that NK T cells do not appear until late in ontogeny, long after the first conventional $\alpha\beta$ T cells are seen. NK T cells binding the CD1d/glycolipid tetramers are not detectable in the fetal thymus at all and first appear 6 days after birth, increasing about 12- to 14-fold to 0.6% to 0.7% of thymocytes by 5 to 6 weeks of age (292). A striking thing about these cells is that they are mostly CD4$^+$ or DN, although they recognize a class I MHC-type ligand.

Beyond this CD1d-restricted NK1.1$^+$ majority, there are other cells classified as NK T cells that are highly heterogeneous with regard to expression of different surface markers, TCR repertoire, CD1d dependence, tissue localization, and even the NK1.1 expression that has typically been used to define the population. In addition, small populations of CD8$^+$NK1.1$^+$ and even TCR$\gamma\delta^+$NK1.1$^+$ cells have also been identified. This heterogeneity and the low abundance of these cells have made the study of NK T-cell function and development particularly difficult.

Most DN and CD4$^+$ NKT cells require a thymus for development, although some NK T cells may be generated extrathymically (293). NK T cells do not develop in neonatally thymectomized mice (294) or athymic nude mice (295), whereas they do develop in fetal thymic organ cultures (296). NK T cells probably represent a separate sublineage (or sublineages), inasmuch as they differ from conventional $\alpha\beta$ T cells in sensitivity to various mutations. Dominant-negative mutants of Ras and Mek do not appear to affect NK T-cell development (220), in sharp contrast to their effects on mainstream $\alpha\beta$ T cells, whereas NK T cells do not develop in mice with Fyn$^{-/-}$ (297,298) and transcription factor Ets1$^{-/-}$ (299), mutations that minimally affect $\alpha\beta$ T cells in general. NK T cells are also dependent on IL-15/IL-15R signals, like NK cells (300), and on lymphotoxin (LT)/LTβR (301). On the other hand, NK T cells require all the genetic functions needed by conventional $\alpha\beta$ T cells. They are also dependent on the presence of pTα (302), which suggests that they may go through β selection.

Positive selection of these cells is unusual; they are selected by interaction with a glycophospholipid antigen presented by a nonclassical class I MHC antigen, CD1d, and the interaction is with CD1d on hematopoietic cells, rather than epithelial cells. CD8 expression apparently makes these cells susceptible to negative selection and is thus generally excluded from the mature NK T-cell population. It may be that the unusual selection of these cells represents one case in which high-affinity class I MHC-restricted T cells are allowed to escape death by conversion to CD4 SP lineage after all. The combination of effector properties they wield, a mixture of T$_H$2 cytokines and NK cell–like cytolytic functions, makes it difficult to use these functions as criteria for deciding whether these cells are "naturally" unusual helper-lineage or unusual killer-lineage cells.

The developmental origins of NK T cells are controversial, and two models have been proposed [reviewed by Eberl et al. (303)]. According to the "precommitment model," NK T cells arise from a distinct committed precursor, before TCR rearrangement, which then rearranges a semi-invariant TCR for selection by CD1d molecules (304). In support of this model, ZAP70-deficient mice, which are blocked at β selection, were found to accumulate NK1.1$^+$ TCRβ^- thymocytes that had not undergone D-J or V-D-J rearrangements (305). When purified and stimulated with phorbol ester and ionomycin in neonatal thymic organ culture, NK1.1$^+$ TCRβ^+ cells were generated, some with Vα14-Jα281 rearrangements. In addition, NK1.1$^+$ cells have been detected in mice with CD3ζ- and/or p56^{Lck}-deficiencies, which are also blocked at β selection. These cells were found to have made V-D-J rearrangements in the TCRβ locus but express no surface TCRβ protein, which suggests that they may be blocked precommitted NK T cells (306). One problem with this model is that it provides no mechanism to explain why the Vα14-Jα281 rearrangement is so common in NK T cells. Although use of a recurrent rearrangement is reminiscent of the fetal-type TCR$\gamma\delta$ lineages, there is no evidence that Vα14-Jα281 rearrangement is directed in NK T cells (307). The second model is an instructive model in which NK T cells arise from the "mainstream" population of immature T cells with random TCR gene rearrangements that are positively selected by CD1d binding, rather than by conventional class I or II MHC, at the DP stage (287). The predominance of Vα14-Jα281 rearrangements would then be a result of selection for the few cells bearing TCRs with affinity for CD1d, which then diverts the cells to the NK T lineage. CD1d tetramer–binding NK T cells can develop from tetramer-nonbinding CD4$^+$CD8$^+$ TCRβ^- thymocytes sorted from 1-week-old mice, and they develop only when injected intrathymically into CD1d$^+$ recipients, which demonstrates that NK T cells can arise from DP cells and that they do require some kind of positive selection (292). Whether all NK T cells undergo this developmental pathway remains to be seen.

Variations on a Theme of Tolerance: Regulatory T Cells

Another subset of T cells that are potent suppressors of organ-specific autoimmunity have been identified and characterized (308,309). These CD4$^+$ $\alpha\beta$TCR cells express the activation surface marker CD25$^+$ (IL-2Rα), as do mature peripheral T cells that are anergic as a result of partial stimulation. They constitute approximately 5% of mature thymic CD4 SP cells (310). These cells also clearly require a thymus for their generation and appear to arise at the CD4 SP stage of development, during the time of negative selection and maturation, before export into the periphery (311,312). When isolated from the thymus, these cells are capable of suppressive activity similar to that found in peripheral CD4$^+$CD25$^+$ cells. These T regulatory cells require IL-2 for development or survival, or both (312).

There is some evidence that the affinity of the TCR to self peptide and MHC is of critical importance in the generation of CD4$^+$CD25$^+$ cells (309,313,314). Antigen presentation by thymic medullary epithelial cells has been shown to be capable of rendering T-cell populations tolerant even when it does not result in deletion (315). Thus, it is possible that tolerance induction by particular domains of the thymic stroma and distinctive profiles of TCR affinity translate into a distinct anergic and suppressive fate.

The characteristic T regulatory cell properties are established in these T cells by their expression of the transcription factor Foxp3 (Scurfin) (315a,315b,315c). This factor antagonizes conventional T-cell activation responses and not only distinguishes the T regulatory subset but also seems to be essential for its generation. Mutant mice with defects in this gene are subject to lethal autoimmunity as a result. Foxp3

expression alone may even be sufficient to convert conventional naïve T cells to T regulatory-like cells. An explanation for regulatory T cell development may thus emerge if specific cues from the thymic stroma can be linked to Foxp3 induction.

In view of the increasing importance of both NK T cells and regulatory T cells in systemic immune responses, filling in the picture of their development and selection is likely to become an active research frontier.

CONCLUDING REMARKS

We have focused in depth on several aspects of intrathymic T-cell development that are particularly significant in terms of developmental mechanisms or immunological impact. These are areas in which work since 1995 has offered new glimpses of understanding how a momentous developmental choice or transition will be made. But it is worth returning to the larger picture of T-cell development sketched in Fig. 2. In overview, it is striking how much functional diversity and lineage choice remain to cells after they have undergone T-lineage commitment. The cells take advantage of the intricate architecture of the thymus to migrate from one domain to another, using a core group of signaling molecules, carefully modulated interactions with environmental ligands, and a persistent set of transcription factors, to refine progressively what kind of T cell their initial T-lineage commitment will produce. Of course, the interactions that come to dominate the second half of T-cell development are TCR-mediated ones, but the responses they trigger depend on genes such as Notch, GATA-3, IL-7R, bHLH factors, Ikaros, and Lck kinase and its signaling partners, genes that have been used and reused from the earliest stages of T-cell development. T cells equip themselves with a well-stocked developmental toolkit that they use to generate the diverse regulatory functions that characterize our adaptive immune systems.

ACKNOWLEDGMENTS

The authors thank Tania Dugatkin for excellent help with the figures and the authors who kindly allowed their work to be reproduced for this chapter. We apologize to our many colleagues whose work and thoughtful interpretations we could not discuss adequately because of space limitations. Work in the authors' laboratory was supported by grants from the U.S. Public Health Service (AG13108 and CA92033), from the National Science Foundation (MCB-9983129), and from the National Aeronautics and Space Administration (NAG 2-1370), with initial support from a consortium of the Stowers Institute for Medical Research.

REFERENCES

1. Hoffman ES, Passoni L, Crompton T, et al. Productive T-cell receptor β-chain gene rearrangement: coincident regulation of cell cycle and clonality during development in vivo. *Genes Dev* 1996;10:948–962.

2. Penit C, Lucas B, Vasseur F. Cell expansion and growth arrest phases during the transition from precursor (CD4$^-$8$^-$) to immature (CD4$^+$8$^+$) thymocytes in normal and genetically modified mice. *J Immunol* 1995;154:5103–5113.

3. Di Santo JP, Rodewald H-R. *In vivo* roles of receptor tyrosine kinases and cytokine receptors in early thymocyte development. *Curr Opin Immunol* 1998;10:196–207.

4. Maraskovsky E, O'Reilly LA, Teepe M, et al. Bcl-2 can rescue T lymphocyte development in interleukin-7 receptor–deficient mice but not in mutant *RAG-1$^{-/-}$* mice. *Cell* 1997;89:1011–1019.

5. von Freeden-Jeffry U, Solvason N, Howard M, et al. The earliest T lineage-committed cells depend on IL-7 for Bcl-2 expression and normal cell cycle progression. *Immunity* 1997;7:147–154.

6. Candéias S, Muegge K, Durum SK. IL-7 receptor and VDJ recombination: trophic versus mechanistic actions. *Immunity* 1997;6:501–508.

7. Di Santo JP, Aifantis I, Rosmaraki E, et al. The common cytokine receptor γ chain and the pre–T cell receptor provide independent but critically overlapping signals in early α/β T cell development. *J Exp Med* 1999;189:563–573.

8. Anderson G, Moore NC, Owen JJ, et al. Cellular interactions in thymocyte development. *Annu Rev Immunol* 1996;14:73–99.

9. Lind EF, Prockop SE, Porritt HE, et al. Mapping precursor movement through the postnatal thymus reveals specific microenvironments supporting defined stages of early lymphoid development. *J Exp Med* 2001;194:127–134.

10. Derbinski J, Schulte A, Kyewski B, et al. Promiscuous gene expression in medullary thymic epithelial cells mirrors the peripheral self. *Nat Immunol* 2001;2:1032–1039.

11. Gounari F, Aifantis I, Khazaie K, et al. Somatic activation of β-catenin bypasses pre-TCR signaling and TCR selection in thymocyte development. *Nat Immunol* 2001;2:863–869.

12. Ioannidis V, Beermann F, Clevers H, et al. The β-catenin—TCF-1 pathway ensures CD4$^+$CD8$^+$ thymocyte survival. *Nat Immunol* 2001; 2:691–697.

13. Kitazawa H, Muegge K, Badolato R, et al. IL-7 activates $\alpha4\beta1$ integrin in murine thymocytes. *J Immunol* 1997;159:2259–2264.

14. Norment AM, Bogatzki LY, Gantner BN, et al. Murine CCR9, a chemokine receptor for thymus-expressed chemokine that is up-regulated following pre-TCR signaling. *J Immunol* 2000;164:639–648.

15. Uehara S, Song K, Farber JM, et al. Characterization of CCR9 expression and CCL25/thymus-expressed chemokine responsiveness during T cell development: CD3^{high}CD69$^+$ thymocytes and $\gamma\delta$TCR$^+$ thymocytes preferentially respond to CCL25. *J Immunol* 2002;168:134–142.

16. Wurbel MA, Malissen M, Guy-Grand D, et al. Mice lacking the CCR9 CC-chemokine receptor show a mild impairment of early T- and B-cell development and a reduction in T-cell receptor $\gamma\delta^+$ gut intraepithelial lymphocytes. *Blood* 2001;98:2626–2632.

17. Manley NR. Thymus organogenesis and molecular mechanisms of thymic epithelial cell differentiation. *Semin Immunol* 2000;12:421–428.

18. Manaia A, Lemarchandel V, Klaine M, et al. Lmo2 and GATA-3 associated expression in intraembryonic hemogenic sites. *Development* 2000;127:643–653.

19. Reya T, Yang-Snyder JA, Rothenberg EV, et al. Regulated expression and function of CD122 (interleukin-2/interleukin-15 R-β) during lymphoid development. *Blood* 1996;87:190–201.

20. Suniara RK, Jenkinson EJ, Owen JJ. Studies on the phenotype of migrant thymic stem cells. *Eur J Immunol* 1999;29:75–80.

21. Ikuta K, Kina T, NacNeil I, et al. A developmental switch in thymic lymphocyte maturation potential occurs at the level of hematopoietic stem cells. *Cell* 1990;62:863–874.

22. Bain G, Romanow WJ, Albers K, et al. Positive and negative regulation of V(D)J recombination by the E2A proteins. *J Exp Med* 1999; 189:289–300.

23. Dzierzak E, Medvinsky A, de Bruijn M. Qualitative and quantitative aspects of haematopoietic cell development in the mammalian embryo. *Immunol Today* 1998;19:228–236.

24. Jotereau F, Heuze F, Salomon-Vie V, et al. Cell kinetics in the fetal mouse thymus: precursor cell input, proliferation, and emigration. *J Immunol* 1987;138:1026–1030.

25. Verbeek S, Izon D, Hofhuis F, et al. An HMG-box–containing T-cell factor required for thymocyte differentiation. *Nature* 1995;374:70–74.

26. Wang J-H, Nichogiannopoulou A, Wu L, et al. Selective defects in the development of the fetal and adult lymphoid system in mice with an Ikaros null mutation. *Immunity* 1996;5:537–549.

27. McKercher SR, Torbett BE, Anderson KL, et al. Targeted disruption of the *PU.1* gene results in multiple hematopoietic abnormalities. *EMBO J* 1996;15:5647–5658.

28. Nakayama K, Nakayama K, Negishi I, et al. Disappearance of the lymphoid system in Bcl-2 homozygous mutant chimeric mice. *Science* 1993;261:1584–1588.

29. Veis DJ, Sorenson CM, Shutter JR, et al. Bcl-2-deficient mice demonstrate fulminant lymphoid apoptosis, polycystic kidneys, and hypopigmented hair. *Cell* 1993;75:229–240.

30. Ody C, Alais S, Corbel C, et al. Surface molecules involved in avian T-cell progenitor migration and differentiation. *Dev Immunol* 2000;7:267–277.

31. Chretien I, Marcuz A, Courtet M, et al. CTX, a *Xenopus* thymocyte receptor, defines a molecular family conserved throughout vertebrates. *Eur J Immunol* 1998;28:4094–4104.

32. Res P, Spits H. Developmental stages in the human thymus. *Semin Immunol* 1999;11:39–46.

33. Spits H, Blom B, Jaleco AC, et al. Early stages in the development of human T, natural killer and thymic dendritic cells. *Immunol Rev* 1998;165:75–86.

34. Plum J, De Smedt M, Verhasselt B, et al. Human T lymphopoiesis. *In vitro* and *in vivo* study models. *Ann N Y Acad Sci* 2000;917:724–731.

35. Mitnacht R, Bischof A, Torres-Nagel N, et al. Opposite CD4/CD8 lineage decisions of CD4$^+$8$^+$ mouse and rat thymocytes to equivalent triggering signals: correlation with thymic expression of a truncated CD8 alpha chain in mice but not rats. *J Immunol* 1998;160:700–707.

36. Hunig T. Cross-linking of the T cell antigen receptor interferes with the generation of CD4$^+$8$^+$ thymocytes from their immediate CD4$^-$8$^+$ precursors. *Eur J Immunol* 1988;18:2089–2092.

37. Yang SY, Denning SM, Mizuno S, et al. A novel activation pathway for mature thymocytes. Costimulation of CD2 (T,p50) and CD28 (T,p44) induces autocrine interleukin 2/interleukin 2 receptor–mediated cell proliferation. *J Exp Med* 1988;168:1457–1468.

38. Ramsdell F, Jenkins M, Dinh Q, et al. The majority of CD4$^+$8$^-$ thymocytes are functionally immature. *J Immunol* 1991;147:1779–1785.

39. Wu L, Antica M, Johnson GR, et al. Developmental potential of the earliest precursor cells from the adult mouse thymus. *J Exp Med* 1991;174:1617–1627.

40. Ardavin C, Wu L, Li CL, et al. Thymic dendritic cells and T cells develop simultaneously in the thymus from a common precursor population. *Nature* 1993;362:761–763.

41. Kawamoto H, Ohmura K, Katsura Y. Direct evidence for the commitment of hematopoietic stem cells to T, B, and myeloid lineages in murine fetal liver. *Int Immunol* 1997;9:1011–1019.

42. Res P, Martinez-Caceres E, Jaleco AC, et al. CD34$^+$CD38^{dim} cells in the human thymus can differentiate into T, natural killer, and dendritic cells but are distinct from pluripotent stem cells. *Blood* 1996;87:5196–5206.

43. Sanchez MJ, Muench MO, Roncarolo MG, et al. Identification of a common T/natural killer cell progenitor in human fetal thymus. *J Exp Med* 1994;180:569–576.

44. Rodewald HR, Kretzschmar K, Takeda S, et al. Identification of prothymocytes in murine fetal blood: T lineage commitment can precede thymus colonization. *EMBO J* 1994;13:4229–4240.

45. Kawamoto H, Ohmura K, Katsura Y. Cutting edge: presence of progenitors restricted to T, B, or myeloid lineage, but absence of multipotent stem cells, in the murine fetal thymus. *J Immunol* 1998;161:3799–3802.

46. Carding SR, Kyes S, Jenkinson EJ, et al. Developmentally regulated fetal thymic and extrathymic T-cell receptor $\gamma\delta$ gene expression. *Genes Dev* 1990;4:1304–1315.

47. Lefrancois L, Puddington L. Extrathymic intestinal T-cell development: virtual reality? *Immunol Today* 1995;16:16–21.

48. Bendelac A. Mouse NK1$^+$ T cells. *Curr Opin Immunol* 1995;7:367–374.

49. Dejbakhsh-Jones S, Garcia-Ojeda ME, Chatterjea-Matthes D, et al. Clonable progenitors committed to the T lymphocyte lineage in the

mouse bone marrow; use of an extrathymic pathway. *Proc Natl Acad Sci U S A* 2001;98:7455–7460.

50. Kondo M, Weissman IL, Akashi K. Identification of clonogenic common lymphoid progenitors in mouse bone marrow. *Cell* 1997;91:661–672.

51. Litman GW, Anderson MK, Rast JP. Evolution of antigen binding receptors. *Annu Rev Immunol* 1999;17:109–147.

52. Miracle AL, Anderson MK, Litman RT, et al. Complex expression patterns of lymphocyte-specific genes during the development of cartilaginous fish implicate unique lymphoid tissues in generating an immune repertoire. *Int Immunol* 2001;13:567–580.

53. Wu L, Li C-L, Shortman K. Thymic dendritic cell precursors: relationship to the T lymphocyte lineage and phenotype of the dendritic cell progeny. *J Exp Med* 1996;184:903–911.

54. Carlyle JR, Michie AM, Furlonger C, et al. Identification of a novel developmental stage marking lineage commitment of progenitor thymocytes. *J Exp Med* 1997;186:173–182.

55. Katsura Y, Kawamoto H. Stepwise lineage restriction of progenitors in lympho-myelopoiesis. *Int Rev Immunol* 2001;20:1–20.

56. Lacaud G, Carlsson L, Keller G. Identification of a fetal hematopoietic precursor with B cell, T cell, and macrophage potential. *Immunity* 1998;9:827–838.

57. Wilson A, Ferrero I, MacDonald HR, et al. Cutting edge: an essential role for Notch-1 in the development of both thymus-independent and -dependent T cells in the gut. *J Immunol* 2000;165:5397–5400.

58. Jaleco AC, Neves H, Hooijberg E, et al. Differential effects of Notch ligands Delta-1 and Jagged-1 in human lymphoid differentiation. *J Exp Med* 2001;194:991–1002.

59. Pui JC, Allman D, Xu L, et al. Notch1 expression in early lymphopoiesis influences B versus T lineage determination. *Immunity* 1999;11:299–308.

60. Varnum-Finney B, Xu L, Brashem-Stein C, et al. Pluripotent, cytokine-dependent, hematopoietic stem cells are immortalized by constitutive Notch1 signaling. *Nat Med* 2000;6:1278–1281.

61. Radtke F, Wilson A, Stark G, et al. Deficient T cell fate specification in mice with an induced inactivation of *Notch1*. *Immunity* 1999;10:547–558.

62. Koch U, Lacombe TA, Holland D, et al. Subversion of the T/B lineage decision in the thymus by lunatic fringe–mediated inhibition of Notch-1. *Immunity* 2001;15:225–236.

63. Wilson A, MacDonald HR, Radtke F. Notch 1-deficient common lymphoid precursors adopt a B cell fate in the thymus. *J Exp Med* 2001;194:1003–1012.

64. Doerfler P, Shearman MS, Perlmutter RM. Presenilin-dependent γ-secretase activity modulates thymocyte development. *Proc Natl Acad Sci U S A* 2001;98:9312–9317.

65. Hadland BK, Manley NR, Su D, et al. γ-secretase inhibitors repress thymocyte development. *Proc Natl Acad Sci U S A* 2001;98:7487–7491.

66. Ikawa T, Kawamoto H, Fujimoto S, et al. Commitment of common T/natural killer (NK) progenitors to unipotent T and NK progenitors in the murine fetal thymus revealed by a single progenitor assay. *J Exp Med* 1999;190:1617–1625.

67. Michie AM, Carlyle JR, Schmitt TM, et al. Clonal characterization of a bipotent T cell and NK cell progenitor in the mouse fetal thymus. *J Immunol* 2000;164:1730–1733.

68. Shortman K, Vremec D, Corcoran LM, et al. The linkage between T-cell and dendritic cell development in the mouse thymus. *Immunol Rev* 1998;165:39–46.

69. Lee C-K, Kim JK, Kim Y, et al. Generation of macrophages from early T progenitors *in vitro*. *J Immunol* 2001;166:5964–5969.

69a. Wang H, Rothenberg EV. Gene expression profiles distinguish multiple subsets of DN1 thymocytes. California Institute of Technology, 2000.

70. Wang H, Diamond RA, Rothenberg EV. Cross-lineage expression of Ig-β (B29) in thymocytes: positive and negative gene regulation to establish T-cell identity. *Proc Natl Acad Sci U S A* 1998;95:6831–6836.

71. Chen F, Rowen L, Hood L, et al. Differential transcriptional regulation of individual TCR V beta segments before gene rearrangement. *J Immunol* 2001;166:1771–1780.

72. Shimizu C, Kawamoto H, Yamashita M, et al. Progression of T cell lineage restriction in the earliest subpopulation of murine adult thymus

73. Lucas K, Vremec D, Wu L, et al. A linkage between dendritic cell and T-cell development in the mouse thymus: the capacity of sequential T-cell precursors to form dendritic cells in culture. *Dev Comp Immunol* 1998;22:339–349.

74. Res PCM, Couwenberg F, Vyth-Dreese FA, et al. Expression of a pTα mRNA in a committed dendritic cell precursor in the human thymus. *Blood* 1999;94:2647–2657.

75. Hu M, Krause D, Greaves M, et al. Multilineage gene expression precedes commitment in the hemopoietic system. *Genes Dev* 1997;11:774–785.

76. Delassus S, Titley I, Enver T. Functional and molecular analysis of hematopoietic progenitors derived from the aorta-gonad-mesonephros region of the mouse embryo. *Blood* 1999;94:1495–1503.

76a. Gounari F, Aifantis I, Martin C, Fehling HJ, Hoeflinger S, Leder P, von Boehmer H, Reizis B. Tracing lymphopoiesis with the aid of a pTα-controlled reporter gene. *Nat Immunol* 2002;3:489–96.

76b. Igarashi H, Gregory SC, Yokota T, Sakaguchi N, Kincade PW. Transcription from the RAG1 locus marks the earliest lymphocyte progenitors in bone marrow. *Immunity* 2002;17:117–30.

77. Rodewald H-R, Brocker T, Haller C. Developmental dissociation of thymic dendritic cell and thymocyte lineages revealed in growth factor receptor mutant mice. *Proc Natl Acad Sci U S A* 1999;96:15068–15073.

78. Kuo CT, Leiden JM. Transcriptional regulation of T lymphocyte development and function. *Annu Rev Immunol* 1999;17:149–187.

79. Staal FJ, Weerkamp F, Langerak AW, et al. Transcriptional control of T lymphocyte differentiation. *Stem Cells* 2001;19:165–179.

80. Rothenberg EV, Anderson MK. Elements of transcription factor network design for T-lineage specification. *Devel Biol* 2002;246:29–44.

81. Rothenberg EV, Telfer JC, Anderson MK. Transcriptional regulation of lymphocyte lineage commitment. *Bioessays* 1999;21:726–742.

82. Engel I, Murre C. The function of E- and Id proteins in lymphocyte development. *Nat Rev Immunol* 2002;1:193–199.

83. Tomita K, Hattori M, Nakamura E, et al. The bHLH gene *Hes1* is essential for expansion of early T cell precursors. *Genes Dev* 1999;13:1203–1210.

84. Reizis B, Leder P. The upstream enhancer is necessary and sufficient for the expression of the pre–T cell receptor α gene in immature T lymphocytes. *J Exp Med* 2001;194:979–990.

85. Kee BL, Murre C. Induction of early B cell factor (EBF) and multiple B lineage genes by the basic helix-loop-helix transcription factor E12. *J Exp Med* 1998;188:699–713.

86. Choi JK, Shen C-P, Radomska HS, et al. E47 activates the Ig-heavy chain and TdT loci in non–B cells. *EMBO J* 1996;15:5014–5021.

87. Kee BL, Bain G, Murre C. IL-7Rα and E47: independent pathways required for development of multipotent lymphoid progenitors. *EMBO J* 2002;21:103–113.

88. Osborne B, Miele L. Notch and the immune system. *Immunity* 1999;11:653–663.

89. Kaneta M, Osawa M, Sudo K, et al. A role for Pref-1 and HES-1 in thymocyte development. *J Immunol* 2000;164:256–264.

90. Radtke F, Ferrero I, Wilson A, et al. Notch1 deficiency dissociates the intrathymic development of dendritic cells and T cells. *J Exp Med* 2000;191:1085–1094.

91. Colucci F, Samson SI, DeKoter RP, et al. Differential requirement for the transcription factor PU.1 in the generation of natural killer cells versus B and T cells. *Blood* 2001;97:2625–2632.

92. Bain G, Murre C. The role of E-proteins in B- and T-lymphocyte development. *Semin Immunol* 1998;10:143–153.

93. Engel I, Johns C, Bain G, et al. Early thymocyte development is regulated by modulation of E2A protein activity. *J Exp Med* 2001;194:733–746.

94. Murphy KM, Ouyang W, Farrar JD, et al. Signaling and transcription in T helper development. *Annu Rev Immunol* 2000;18:451–494.

95. Kruisbeek AM, Haks MC, Carleton M, et al. Branching out to gain control: how the pre-TCR is linked to multiple functions. *Immunol Today* 2000;21:637–644.

96. von Boehmer H, Aifantis I, Feinberg J, et al. Pleiotropic changes controlled by the pre–T-cell receptor. *Curr Opin Immunol* 1999;11:135–142.

97. Levelt CN, Eichmann K. Receptors and signals in early thymic selection. *Immunity* 1995;3:667–672.
98. Borowski C, Martin C, Gounari F, et al. On the brink of becoming a T cell. *Curr Opin Immunol* 2002;14:200–206.
99. Rothenberg EV. The development of functionally responsive T cells. *Adv Immunol* 1992;51:85–214.
100. Rothenberg EV, Diamond RA, Chen D. Programming for recognition and programming for response: separate developmental subroutines in the murine thymus. *Thymus* 1994;22:215–244.
101. Voll RE, Jimi E, Phillips RJ, et al. NF-κB activation by the pre–T cell receptor serves as a selective survival signal in T lymphocyte development. *Immunity* 2000;13:677–689.
102. Gratiot-Deans J, Merino R, Nunez G, et al. Bcl-2 expression during T-cell development: Early loss and late return occur at specific stages of commitment to differentiation and survival. *Proc Natl Acad Sci U S A* 1994;91:10685–10689.
103. Linette GP, Grusby MJ, Hedrick SM, et al. Bcl-2 upregulated at the CD4⁺CD8⁺ stage during positive selection and promotes thymocyte differentiation at several control points. *Immunity* 1994;1:197–205.
104. Andjelic S, Drappa J, Lacy E, et al. The onset of Fas expression parallels the acquisition of CD8 and CD4 in fetal and adult alpha beta thymocytes. *Int Immunol* 1994;6:73–79.
105. Chen D, Rothenberg EV. Molecular basis for developmental changes in interleukin-2 gene inducibility. *Mol Cell Biol* 1993;13:228–237.
106. Rincon M, Flavell RA. Regulation of AP-1 and NFAT transcription factors during thymic selection of T cells. *Mol Cell Biol* 1996;16:1074–1084.
107. Sen J, Shinkai Y, Alt FW, et al. Nuclear factors that mediate intrathymic signals are developmentally regulated. *J Exp Med* 1994;180:2321–2327.
108. Chen F, Chen D, Rothenberg EV. Specific regulation of fos family transcription factors in thymocytes at two developmental checkpoints. *Int Immunol* 1999;11:677–688.
109. Davey GM, Schober SL, Endrizzi BT, et al. Preselection thymocytes are more sensitive to T cell receptor stimulation than mature T cells. *J Exp Med* 1998;188:1867–1874.
110. Lucas B, Stefanova I, Yasutomo K, et al. Divergent changes in the sensitivity of maturing T cells to structurally related ligands underlies formation of a useful T cell repertoire. *Immunity* 1999;10:367–376.
111. Vasquez NJ, Kane LP, Hedrick SM. Intracellular signals that mediate thymic negative selection. *Immunity* 1994;1:45–56.
112. Moody AM, Chui D, Reche PA, et al. Developmentally regulated glycosylation of the CD8αβ coreceptor stalk modulates ligand binding. *Cell* 2001;107:501–512.
113. Daniels MA, Devine L, Miller JD, et al. CD8 binding to MHC class I molecules is influenced by T cell maturation and glycosylation. *Immunity* 2001;15:1051–1061.
114. Wilson A, MacDonald HR. Expression of genes encoding the pre-TCR and CD3 complex during thymus development. *Int Immunol* 1995;7:1659–1664.
115. Bruno L, Rocha B, Rolink A, et al. Intra- and extra-thymic expression of the pre-T cell receptor α gene. *Eur J Immunol* 1995;25:1877–1882.
116. Malissen B, Malissen M. Functions of TCR and pre-TCR subunits: lessons from gene ablation. *Curr Opin Immunol* 1996;8:383–393.
117. Koyasu S, Clayton LK, Lerner A, et al. Pre-TCR signaling components trigger transcriptional activation of a rearranged TCR alpha gene locus and silencing of the pre-TCR alpha locus: implications for intrathymic differentiation. *Int Immunol* 1997;9:1475–1480.
118. Groettrup M, von Boehmer H. A role for a pre–T-cell receptor in T-cell development. *Immunol Today* 1993;14:610–614.
119. Saint-Ruf C, Panigada M, Azogui O, et al. Different initiation of pre-TCR and γδTCR signalling. *Nature* 2000;406:524–527.
120. Corre I, Gomez M, Vielkind S, et al. Analysis of thymocyte development reveals that the GTPase RhoA is a positive regulator of T cell receptor responses *in vivo*. *J Exp Med* 2001;194:903–914.
121. Chen J, Shinkai Y, Young F, et al. Probing immune functions in RAG-deficient mice. *Curr Opin Immunol* 1994;6:313–319.
122. Levelt CN, Ehrfeld A, Eichmann K. Regulation of thymocyte development through CD3. I. Timepoint of ligation of CD3ε determines clonal deletion or induction of developmental program. *J Exp Med* 1993;177:707–716.
123. Gibbons D, Douglas NC, Barber DF, et al. The biological activity of natural and mutant pTα alleles. *J Exp Med* 2001;194:695–703.
124. Irving BA, Alt FW, Killeen N. Thymocyte development in the absence of pre–T cell receptor extracellular immunoglobulin domains. *Science* 1998;280:905–908.
125. Lacorazza HD, Tucek-Szabo C, Vasovic LV, et al. Premature TCRαβ expression and signaling in early thymocytes impair thymocyte expansion and partially block their development. *J Immunol* 2001;166:3184–3193.
126. Mombaerts P, Anderson SJ, Perlmutter RM, et al. An activated *lck* transgene promotes thymocyte development in *RAG-1* mutant mice. *Immunity* 1994;1:261–267.
127. Swat W, Shinkai Y, Cheng H-L, et al. Activated Ras signals differentiation and expansion of CD4⁺8⁺ thymocytes. *Proc Natl Acad Sci U S A* 1996;93:4683–4687.
128. Fehling HJ, Iritani BM, Krotkova A, et al. Restoration of thymopoiesis in pTα−/− mice by anti-CD3ε antibody treatment or with transgenes encoding activated Lck or tailless pTα. *Immunity* 1997;6:703–714.
129. Iritani BM, Alberola-Ila J, Forbush KA, et al. Distinct signals mediate maturation and allelic exclusion in lymphocyte progenitors. *Immunity* 1999;10:713–722.
130. Gärtner F, Alt FW, Monroe R, et al. Immature thymocytes employ distinct signaling pathways for allelic exclusion versus differentiation and expansion. *Immunity* 1999;10:537–546.
131. Carleton M, Haks MC, Smeele SA, et al. Early growth response transcription factors are required for development of CD4⁻CD8⁻ thymocytes to the CD4⁺CD8⁺ stage. *J Immunol* 2002;168:1649–1658.
132. Ellmeier W, Sawada S, Littman DR. The regulation of CD4 and CD8 coreceptor gene expression during T cell development. *Annu Rev Immunol* 1999;17:523–554.
132a. Kioussis D, Ellmeier W. Chromatin and *CD4, CD8A* and *CD8B* gene expression during thymic differentiation. *Nat Rev Immunol* 2002;2:909–19.
132b. Harker N, Naito T, Cortes M, Hostert A, Hirschberg S, Tolaini M, Roderick K, Georgopoulos K, Kioussis D. The CD8α gene locus is regulated by the Ikaros family of proteins. *Mol Cell* 2002;10:1403–15.
132c. Taniuchi I, Osato M, Egawa T, Sunshine MJ, Bae S-C, Komori T, Ito Y, Littman DR. Differential requirements for Runx proteins in *CD4* repression and epigenetic silencing during T lymphocyte development. *Cell* 2002;111:621–33.
132d. Chi TH, Wan M, Zhao K, Taniuchi I, Chen L, Littman DR, Crabtree GR. Reciprocal regulation of CD4/CD8 expression by SWI/SNF-like BAF complexes. *Nature* 2002;418:195–9.
133. Bain G, Cravatt CB, Loomans C, et al. Regulation of the helix-loop-helix proteins, E2A and Id3, by the Ras-ERK MAPK cascade. *Nat Immunol* 2001;2:165–171.
134. Blom B, Heemskerk MHM, Verschuren MCM, et al. Disruption of αβ but not of γδ T cell development by overexpression of the helix-loop-helix protein Id3 in committed T cell progenitors. *EMBO J* 1999;18:2793–2802.
135. Heemskerk MHM, Blom B, Nolan G, et al. Inhibition of T cell and promotion of natural killer cell development by the dominant negative helix loop helix factor Id3. *J Exp Med* 1997;186:1597–1602.
136. Guidos CJ, Williams CJ, Grandal I, et al. V(D)J recombination activates a p53-dependent DNA damage checkpoint in *scid* lymphocyte precursors. *Genes Dev* 1996;10:2038–2054.
137. Jiang D, Lenardo MJ, Zúñiga-Pflücker JC. p53 prevents maturation to the CD4⁺CD8⁺ stage of thymocyte differentiation in the absence of T cell receptor rearrangement. *J Exp Med* 1996;183:1923–1928.
138. Haks MC, Krimpenfort P, van den Brakel JHN, et al. Pre-TCR signaling and inactivation of p53 induces crucial cell survival pathways in pre–T cells. *Immunity* 1999;11:91–101.
139. Petrie HT, Tourigny M, Burtrum DB, et al. Precursor thymocyte proliferation and differentiation are controlled by signals unrelated to the pre-TCR. *J Immunol* 2000;165:3094–3098.
140. Shores EW, Sharrow SO, Uppenkemp I, et al. T cell receptor–negative thymocytes from SCID mice can be induced to enter the CD4/CD8 differentiation pathway. *Eur J Immunol* 1990;20:69–77.
141. Trop S, De Sepulveda P, Zúñiga-Pflücker JC, et al. Overexpression of suppressor of cytokine signaling-1 impairs pre–T-cell receptor–induced proliferation but not differentiation of immature thymocytes. *Blood* 2001;97:2269–2277.

142. Miyazaki T. Two distinct steps during thymocyte maturation from CD4$^-$CD8$^-$ to CD4$^+$CD8$^+$ distinguished in the early growth response (Egr)-1 transgenic mice with a recombinase-activating gene-deficient background. *J Exp Med* 1997;186:877–885.

143. Okamura RM, Sigvardsson M, Galceran J, et al. Redundant regulation of T cell differentiation and TCRα gene expression by the transcription factors LEF-1 and TCF-1. *Immunity* 1998;8:11–20.

144. Barndt R, Dai MF, Zhang Y. A novel role for HEB downstream or parallel to the pre-TCR signaling pathway during αβ thymopoiesis. *J Immunol* 1999;163:3331–3343.

145. Pearson R, Weston K. c-Myb regulates the proliferation of immature thymocytes following β-selection. *EMBO J* 2000;19:6112–120.

146. Kabra NH, Kang C, Hsing LC, et al. T cell–specific FADD-deficient mice: FADD is required for early T cell development. *Proc Natl Acad Sci U S A* 2001;98:6307–6312.

147. Newton K, Harris AW, Strasser A. FADD/MORT1 regulates the pre-TCR checkpoint and can function as a tumour suppressor. *EMBO J* 2000;19:931–941.

148. Michie AM, Soh J-W, Hawley RG, et al. Allelic exclusion and differentiation by protein kinase C–mediated signals in immature thymocytes. *Proc Natl Acad Sci U S A* 2001;98:609–614.

149. Wu L, Strasser A. "Decisions, decisions...": β-catenin–mediated activation of TCF-1 and Lef-1 influences the fate of developing T cells. *Nat Immunol* 2001;2:823–824.

150. Chen C, Edelstein LC, Gelinas C. The Rel/NF-κB family directly activates expression of the apoptosis inhibitor Bcl-x$_L$. *Mol Cell Biol* 2000;20:2687–2695.

151. Schmedt C, Tarakhovsky A. Autonomous maturation of α/β T lineage cells in the absence of COOH-terminal Src kinase (Csk). *J Exp Med* 2001;193:815–826.

152. Georgopoulos K. Transcription factors required for lymphoid lineage commitment. *Curr Opin Immunol* 1997;9:222–227.

153. Brown KE, Guest SS, Smale ST, et al. Association of transcriptionally silent genes with Ikaros complexes at centromeric heterochromatin. *Cell* 1997;91:845–854.

154. Winandy S, Wu L, Wang J-H, et al. Pre–T cell receptor (TCR) and TCR-controlled checkpoints in T cell differentiation are set by Ikaros. *J Exp Med* 1999;190:1039–1048.

155. Jepsen K, Hermanson O, Onami TM, et al. Combinatorial roles of the nuclear receptor corepressor in transcription and development. *Cell* 2000;102:753–763.

156. Anderson MK, Hernandez-Hoyos G, Diamond RA, et al. Precise developmental regulation of Ets family transcription factors during specification and commitment to the T cell lineage. *Development* 1999;126:3131–3148.

157. Adachi S, Amasaki Y, Miyatake S, et al. Successive expression and activation of NFAT family members during thymocyte differentiation. *J Biol Chem* 2000;275:14708–14716.

158. Anderson G, Anderson KL, Conroy LA, et al. Intracellular signaling events during positive and negative selection of CD4$^+$CD8$^+$ thymocytes *in vitro*. *J Immunol* 1995;154:3636–3543.

159. Aifantis I, Gounari F, Scorrano L, et al. Constitutive pre-TCR signaling promotes differentiation through Ca^{2+} mobilization and activation of NF-κB and NFAT. *Nat Immunol* 2001;2:403–409.

160. Shao H, Kono DH, Chen LY, et al. Induction of the early growth response (Egr) family of transcription factors during thymic selection. *J Exp Med* 1997;185:731–744.

161. Dudley EC, Petrie HT, Shah LM, et al. T cell receptor β chain gene rearrangement and selection during thymocyte development in adult mice. *Immunity* 1994;1:83–93.

162. Burtrum DB, Kim S, Dudley EC, et al. TCR gene recombination and αβ-γδ lineage divergence: productive TCR-β rearrangement is neither exclusive nor preclusive of γδ cell development. *J Immunol* 1996;157:4293–4296.

163. Mombaerts P, Clarke AR, Rudnicki MA, et al. Mutations in T-cell antigen receptor genes α and β block thymocyte development at different stages. *Nature* 1992;360:225–231.

164. Terrence K, Pavlovich CP, Matechak EO, et al. Premature expression of T cell receptor (TCR)αβ suppresses TCRγδ gene rearrangement but permits development of γδ lineage T cells. *J Exp Med* 2000;192:537–548.

165. Bruno L, Fehling HJ, von Boehmer H. The αβ T cell receptor can replace the γδ receptor in the development of γδ lineage cells. *Immunity* 1996;5:343–352.

166. Capone M, Hockett RD Jr, Zlotnik A. Kinetics of T cell receptor β γ and δ rearrangements during adult thymic development: T cell receptor rearrangements are present in CD44$^+$CD25$^+$ pro-T thymocytes. *Proc Natl Acad Sci U S A* 1998;95:12522–12527.

167. Wilson A, Capone M, MacDonald HR. Unexpectedly late expression of intracellular CD3ε and TCR γδ proteins during adult thymus development. *Int Immunol* 1999;11:1641–1650.

168. Penninger J, Kishihara K, Molina T, et al. Requirement for tyrosine kinase p56^{lck} for thymic development of transgenic γδ T cells. *Science* 1993;260:358–361.

169. Wilson A, MacDonald HR. A limited role for β-selection during γδ T cell development. *J Immunol* 1998;161:5851–5854.

170. Kang J, Volkmann A, Raulet DH. Evidence that γδ versus αβ T cell fate determination is initiated independently of T cell receptor signaling. *J Exp Med* 2001;193:689–698.

171. Bruno L, Scheffold A, Radbruch A, et al. Threshold of pre–T-cell receptor surface expression is associated with αβ T-cell lineage commitment. *Curr Biol* 1999;9:559–568.

172. Tanaka R, Takeuchi Y, Shiohara T, et al. *In utero* treatment with monoclonal antibody to IL-2 receptor β-chain completely abrogates development of Thy-1$^+$ dendritic epidermal cells. *Int Immunol* 1992;4:487–491.

173. Ye S-K, Maki K, Lee H-C, et al. Differential roles of cytokine receptors in the development of epidermal γδ T cells. *J Immunol* 2001;167:1929–1934.

174. Leclercq G, Debacker V, De Smedt M, et al. Differential effects of interleukin-15 and interleukin-2 on differentiation of bipotential T/natural killer progenitor cells. *J Exp Med* 1996;184:325–336.

175. Rodewald H-R, Fehling HJ. Molecular and cellular events in early thymocyte development. *Adv Immunol* 1998;69:1–112.

176. Berg LJ, Kang J. Molecular determinants of TCR expression and selection. *Curr Opin Immunol* 2001;13:232–241.

177. Malissen M, Pereira P, Gerber DJ, et al. The common cytokine receptor γ chain controls survival of γ/δ T cells. *J Exp Med* 1997;186:1277–1285.

178. Durum SK, Candéias S, Nakajima H, et al. Interleukin 7 receptor control of T cell receptor γ gene rearrangement: role of receptor-associated chains and locus accessibility. *J Exp Med* 1998;188:2233–2241.

179. Kang J, Coles M, Raulet DH. Defective development of γ/δ T cells in interleukin 7 receptor–deficient mice is due to impaired expression of T cell receptor γ genes. *J Exp Med* 1999;190:973–982.

180. Lee H-C, Ye S-K, Honjo T, et al. Induction of germline transcription in the human TCRγ locus by STAT5. *J Immunol* 2001;167:320–326.

181. Ye S-K, Agata Y, Lee HC, et al. The IL-7 receptor controls the accessibility of the TCRγ locus by Stat5 and histone acetylation. *Immunity* 2001;15:813–823.

182. Huang J, Durum SK, Muegge K. Cutting edge: histone acetylation and recombination at the TCR gamma locus follows IL-7 induction. *J Immunol* 2001;167:6073–6077.

183. Barndt RJ, Dai M, Zhuang Y. Functions of E2A-HEB heterodimers in T-cell development revealed by a dominant negative mutation of HEB. *Mol Cell Biol* 2000;20:6677–6685.

184. Washburn T, Schweighoffer E, Gridley T, et al. Notch activity influences the αβ versus γδ T cell lineage decision. *Cell* 1997;88:833–843.

184a. Wolfer A, Wilson A, Nemir M, MacDonald HR, Radtke F. Inactivation of Notch1 impairs VDJβ rearrangement and allows pre-TCR-independent survival of early αβ lineage thymocytes. *Immunity* 2002;16:869–79.

185. Deftos ML, Huang E, Ojala EW, et al. Notch1 signaling promotes the maturation of CD4 and CD8 SP thymocytes. *Immunity* 2000;13:73–84.

186. Reizis B, Leder P. Direct induction of T lymphocyte–specific gene expression by the mammalian Notch signaling pathway. *Genes Dev* 2002;16:295–300.

187. Wilson A, Maréchal C, MacDonald HR. Biased Vβ usage in immature thymocytes is independent of DJβ proximity and pTα pairing. *J Immunol* 2001;166:51–57.

188. Bigas A, Martin DIK, Milner LA. Notch1 and Notch2 inhibit myeloid differentiation in response to different cytokines. *Mol Cell Biol* 1998;18:2324–2333.

189. Li L, Milner LA, Deng Y, et al. The human homolog of rat *Jagged1*

expressed by bone marrow stroma inhibits differentiation of 32D cells through interaction with Notch1. *Immunity* 1998;8:43–55.

190. Jones P, May G, Healy L, et al. Stromal expression of Jagged 1 promotes colony formation by fetal hematopoietic progenitor cells. *Blood* 1998;92:1505–1511.

191. Ohishi K, Varnum-Finney B, Serda RE, et al. The Notch ligand, Delta-1, inhibits the differentiation of monocytes into macrophages but permits their differentiation into dendritic cells. *Blood* 2001;98:1402–1407.

192. Reisner Y, Linker-Israeli M, Sharon N. Separation of mouse thymocytes into two subpopulations by the use of peanut agglutinin. *Cell Immunol* 1976;25:129–134.

193. Wiest DL, Yuan L, Jefferson J, et al. Regulation of T cell receptor expression in immature CD4$^+$CD8$^+$ thymocytes by p56^{Lck} tyrosine kinase: basis for differential signaling by CD4 and CD8 in immature thymocytes expressing both coreceptor molecules. *J Exp Med* 1993;178:1701–1712.

194. Ashwell JD, King LB, Vacchio MS. Cross-talk between the T cell antigen receptor and the glucocorticoid receptor regulates thymocyte development. *Stem Cells* 1996;14:490–500.

195. Vacchio MS, Lee JY, Ashwell JD. Thymus-derived glucocorticoids set the thresholds for thymocyte selection by inhibiting TCR-mediated thymocyte activation. *J Immunol* 1999;163:1327–1333.

196. Purton JF, Boyd RL, Cole TJ, et al. Intrathymic T cell development and selection proceeds normally in the absence of glucocorticoid receptor signaling. *Immunity* 2000;13:179–186.

197. Cole TJ, Myles K, Purton JF, et al. GRKO mice express an aberrant dexamethasone-binding glucocorticoid receptor, but are profoundly glucocorticoid resistant. *Mol Cell Endocrinol* 2001;173:193–202.

198. Yannoutsos N, Wilson P, Yu W, et al. The role of recombination activating gene (*RAG*) reinduction in thymocyte development *in vivo*. *J Exp Med* 2001;194:471–480.

199. Wilson A, Held W, MacDonald HR. Two waves of recombinase gene expression in developing thymocytes. *J Exp Med* 1994;179:1355–1360.

200. Thompson SD, Manzo AR, Pelkonen J, et al. Developmental T cell receptor gene rearrangements: relatedness of the α/β and the γ/δ T cell precursors. *Eur J Immunol* 1991;21:1939–1950.

201. Petrie HT, Livak F, Schatz DG, et al. Multiple rearrangements in T cell receptor α chain genes maximize the production of useful thymocytes. *J Exp Med* 1993;178:615–622.

202. Petrie HT, Livak F, Burtrum D, et al. T cell receptor gene recombination patterns and mechanisms: cell death, rescue, and T cell production. *J Exp Med* 1995;182:121–127.

203. Page DM. Cutting edge: thymic selection and autoreactivity are regulated by multiple coreceptors involved in T cell activation. *J Immunol* 1999;163:3577–3581.

204. Kishimoto H, Sprent J. Several different cell surface molecules control negative selection of medullary thymocytes. *J Exp Med* 1999;190:65–73.

205. Lucas B, Vasseur F, Penit C. Production, selection, and maturation of thymocytes with high surface density of TCR. *J Immunol* 1994;153:53–62.

206. Guidos CJ, Weissman IL, Adkins B. Intrathymic maturation of murine T lymphocytes from CD8$^+$ precursors. *Proc Natl Acad Sci U S A* 1989;86:7542–7546.

207. Lundberg K, Shortman K. Small cortical thymocytes are subject to positive selection. *J Exp Med* 1994;179:1475–1483.

208. Huesmann M, Scott B, Kisielow P, et al. Kinetics and efficacy of positive selection in the thymus of normal and T cell receptor transgenic mice. *Cell* 1991;66:533–540.

209. Itano A, Robey E. Highly efficient selection of CD4 and CD8 lineage thymocytes supports an instructive model of lineage commitment. *Immunity* 2000;12:383–389.

210. Kishimoto H, Sprent J. Negative selection in the thymus includes semimature T cells. *J Exp Med* 1997;185:263–271.

211. MacDonald HR, Lees RK. Programmed death of autoreactive thymocytes. *Nature* 1990;343:642–644.

212. Sebzda E, Mariathasan S, Ohteki T, et al. Selection of the T cell repertoire. *Annu Rev Immunol* 1999;17:829–874.

213. Sprent J, Kishimoto H. The thymus and central tolerance. *Philos Trans R Soc Lond B Biol Sci* 2001;356:609–616.

214. Hogquist KA. Signal strength in thymic selection and lineage commitment. *Curr Opin Immunol* 2001;13:225–231.

215. Ignatowicz L, Kappler J, Marrack P. The repertoire of T cells shaped by a single MHC/peptide ligand. *Cell* 1996;84:521–529.

216. Rivera RR, Johns CP, Quan J, et al. Thymocyte selection is regulated by the helix-loop-helix inhibitor protein, Id3. *Immunity* 2000;12:17–26.

217. Bonifacino JS, McCarthy SA, Maguire JE, et al. Novel post-translational regulation of TCR expression in CD4$^+$CD8$^+$ thymocytes influenced by CD4. *Nature* 1990;344:247–251.

218. Kawai K, Ohashi PS. Immunological function of a defined T-cell population tolerized to low-affinity self antigens. *Nature* 1995;374:68–69.

219. Sebzda E, Kundig TM, Thomson CT, et al. Mature T cell reactivity altered by peptide agonist that induces positive selection. *J Exp Med* 1996;183:1093–1104.

220. Alberola-Ila J, Hogquist KA, Swan KA, et al. Positive and negative selection invoke distinct signaling pathways. *J Exp Med* 1996;184:9–18.

221. Backstrom BT, Muller U, Hausmann B, et al. Positive selection through a motif in the alphabeta T cell receptor. *Science* 1998;281:835–838.

222. Werlen G, Hausmann B, Palmer E. A motif in the $\alpha\beta$ T-cell receptor controls positive selection by modulating ERK activity. *Nature* 2000;406:422–426.

223. Mak TW, Penninger JM, Ohashi PS. Knockout mice: a paradigm shift in modern immunology. *Nature Rev Immunol* 2001;1:11–19.

224. Li R, Page DM. Requirement for a complex array of costimulators in the negative selection of autoreactive thymocytes *in vivo*. *J Immunol* 2001;166:6050–6056.

225. Wang J, Chun T, Lo JC, et al. The critical role of LIGHT, a TNF family member, in T cell development. *J Immunol* 2001;167:5099–5105.

226. Wang ECY, Thern A, Denzel A, et al. DR3 regulates negative selection during thymocyte development. *Mol Cell Biol* 2001;21:3451–3461.

227. Gomez M, Kioussis D, Cantrell DA. The GTPase Rac-1 controls cell fate in the thymus by diverting thymocytes from positive to negative selection. *Immunity* 2001;15:703–713.

228. Page DM, Roberts EM, Peschon JJ, et al. TNF receptor-deficient mice reveal striking differences between several models of thymocyte negative selection. *J Immunol* 1998;160:120–133.

229. Bassiri H, Carding SR. A requirement for IL-2/IL-2 receptor signaling in intrathymic negative selection. *J Immunol* 2001;166:5945–5954.

230. Laufer TM, Glimcher LH, Lo D. Using thymus anatomy to dissect T cell repertoire selection. *Semin Immunol* 1999;11:65–70.

231. Laufer TM, DeKoning J, Markowitz JS, et al. Unopposed positive selection and autoreactivity in mice expressing class II MHC only on thymic cortex. *Nature* 1996;383:81–85.

232. Anderson G, Partington KM, Jenkinson EJ. Differential effects of peptide diversity and stromal cell type in positive and negative selection in the thymus. *J Immunol* 1998;161:6599–6603.

233. McGargill MA, Derbinski JM, Hogquist KA. Receptor editing in developing T cells. *Nat Immunol* 2000;1:336–341.

234. Basson MA, Zamoyska R. The CD4/CD8 lineage decision: integration of signalling pathways. *Immunol Today* 2000;21:509–514.

235. Singer A. New perspectives on a developmental dilemma: the kinetic signaling model and the importance of signal duration for the CD4/CD8 lineage decision. *Curr Opin Immunol* 2002;14:207–215.

236. Benoist C, Mathis D. T-lymphocyte differentiation and biology. In: Paul WE, ed. *Fundamental immunology*, 4th ed. Philadelphia: Lippincott-Raven Publishers, 1999:367–409.

237. Lucas B, Germain RN. Unexpectedly complex regulation of CD4/CD8 coreceptor expression supports a revised model for CD4$^+$CD8$^+$ thymocyte differentiation. *Immunity* 1996;5:461–477.

238. Lundberg K, Heath W, Köntgen F, et al. Intermediate steps in positive selection: differentiation of CD4$^-$8^{int} TCR^{int} thymocytes into CD4$^-$8$^+$ TCR^{hi} thymocytes. *J Exp Med* 1995;181:1643–1651.

239. Lucas B, Vasseur F, Penit C. Stochastic coreceptor shut-off is restricted to the CD4 lineage maturation pathway. *J Exp Med* 1995;181:1623–1633.

240. Kydd R, Lundberg K, Vremec D, et al. Intermediate steps in thymic positive selection. Generation of CD4$^-$8$^+$ T cells in culture from CD4$^+$8$^+$, CD4^{int}8$^+$, and CD4$^+$8^{int} thymocytes with up-regulated levels of TCR-CD3. *J Immunol* 1995;155:3806–3814.

241. Suzuki H, Punt JA, Granger LG, et al. Asymmetric signaling requirements for thymocyte commitment to the CD4$^+$ versus CD8$^+$ T cell

lineages: a new perspective on thymic commitment and selection. *Immunity* 1995;2:413–425.

242. Correia-Neves M, Mathis D, Benoist C. A molecular chart of thymocyte positive selection. *Eur J Immunol* 2001;31:2583–2592.

243. Chan SH, Cosgrove D, Waltzinger C, et al. Another view of the selective model of thymocyte selection. *Cell* 1993;73:225–236.

244. Davis CB, Killeen N, Casey Crooks ME, et al. Evidence for a stochastic mechanism in the differentiation of mature subsets of T lymphocytes. *Cell* 1993;73:237–247.

245. Leung RK, Thomson K, Gallimore A, et al. Deletion of the CD4 silencer element supports a stochastic mechanism of thymocyte lineage commitment. *Nat Immunol* 2001;2:1167–1173.

246. Itano A, Salmon P, Kioussis D, et al. The cytoplasmic domain of CD4 promotes the development of CD4 lineage T cells. *J Exp Med* 1996;183:731–741.

247. Seong RH, Chamberlain JW, Parnes JR. Signal for T-cell differentiation to a CD4 cell lineage is delivered by CD4 transmembrane region and/or cytoplasmic tail. *Nature* 1992;356:718–20.

248. Irie HY, Mong MS, Itano A, et al. The cytoplasmic domain of CD8 beta regulates Lck kinase activation and CD8 T cell development. *J Immunol* 1998;161:183–191.

249. Itano A, Cado D, Chan FK, et al. A role for the cytoplasmic tail of the βchain of CD8 in thymic selection. *Immunity* 1994;1:287–290.

250. Campbell KS, Buder A, Deuschle U. Interactions between the amino-terminal domain of p56[lck] and cytoplasmic domains of CD4 and CD8α in yeast. *Eur J Immunol* 1995;25:2408–2412.

251. Hernandez-Hoyos G, Sohn SJ, Rothenberg EV, et al. Lck activity controls CD4/CD8 T cell lineage commitment. *Immunity* 2000;12:313–322.

252. Legname G, Seddon B, Lovatt M, et al. Inducible expression of a p56[Lck] transgene reveals a central role for Lck in the differentiation of CD4 SP thymocytes. *Immunity* 2000;12:537–546.

253. Sharp LL, Hedrick SM. Commitment to the CD4 lineage mediated by extracellular signal-related kinase mitogen-activated protein kinase and lck signaling. *J Immunol* 1999;163:6598–6605.

254. Salmon P, Mong M, Kang X-J, et al. The role of CD8 α′ in the CD4 versus CD8 lineage choice. *J Immunol* 1999;163:5312–5318.

255. Yasutomo K, Doyle C, Miele L, et al. The duration of antigen receptor signalling determines CD4+ versus CD8+ T-cell lineage fate. *Nature* 2000;404:506–510.

256. Iwata M, Kuwata T, Mukai M, et al. Differential induction of helper and killer T cells from isolated CD4+CD8+ thymocytes in suspension culture. *Eur J Immunol* 1996;26:2081–2086.

257. Wolfer A, Bakker T, Wilson A, et al. Inactivation of Notch 1 in immature thymocytes does not perturb CD4 or CD8 T cell development. *Nat Immunol* 2001;2:235–241.

258. Brugnera E, Bhandoola A, Cibotti R, et al. Coreceptor reversal in the thymus: signaled CD4+8+ thymocytes initially terminate CD8 transcription even when differentiating into CD8+ T cells. *Immunity* 2000;13:59–71.

259. Bosselut R, Feigenbaum L, Sharrow SO, et al. Strength of signaling by CD4 and CD8 coreceptor tails determines the number but not the lineage direction of positively selected thymocytes. *Immunity* 2001;14:483–494.

260. Bommhardt U, Basson MA, Krummrei U, et al. Activation of the extracellular signal-related kinase/mitogen-activated protein kinase pathway discriminates CD4 versus CD8 lineage commitment in the thymus. *J Immunol* 1999;163:715–722.

261. Shao H, Wilkinson B, Lee B, et al. Slow accumulation of active mitogen–activated protein kinase during thymocyte differentiation regulates the temporal pattern of transcription factor gene expression. *J Immunol* 1999;163:603–610.

262. Mariathasan S, Ho SS, Zakarian A, Ohashi PS. Degree of ERK activation influences both positive and negative thymocyte selection. *Eur J Immunol* 2000;30:1060–1068.

263. Alberola-Ila J, Forbush KA, Seger R, et al. Selective requirement for MAP kinase activation in thymocyte differentiation. *Nature* 1995;373:620–623.

264. Pages G, Guerin S, Grall D, et al. Defective thymocyte maturation in p44 MAP kinase (Erk 1) knockout mice. *Science* 1999;286:1374–1377.

265. Schmeissner PJ, Xie H, Smilenov LB, et al. Integrin functions play a key role in the differentiation of thymocytes *in vivo. J Immunol* 2001;167:3715–3724.

266. Wilkinson B, Chen JY, Han P, et al. TOX: an HMG box protein implicated in the regulation of thymocyte selection. *Nat Immunol* 2002;3:272–280.

267. Izon DJ, Punt JA, Xu L, et al. Notch1 regulates maturation of CD4+ and CD8+ thymocytes by modulating TCR signal strength. *Immunity* 2001;14:253–264.

268. Keefe R, Dave V, Allman D, et al. Regulation of lineage commitment distinct from positive selection. *Science* 1999;286:1149–1153.

269. Akashi K, Kondo M, von Freeden-Jeffry U, et al. Bcl-2 rescues T lymphopoiesis in interleukin-7 receptor–deficient mice. *Cell* 1997;89:1033–1041.

270. Petrie HT, Strasser A, Harris AW, et al. CD4+8− and CD4−8+ mature thymocytes require different post-selection processing for final development. *J Immunol* 1993;151:1273–1279.

271. Robey E, Chang D, Itano A, et al. An activated form of Notch influences the choice between CD4 and CD8 T cell lineages. *Cell* 1996;87:483–492.

272. Nawijn MC, Ferreira R, Dingjan GM, et al. Enforced expression of GATA-3 during T cell development inhibits maturation of CD8 single-positive cells and induces thymic lymphoma in transgenic mice. *J Immunol* 2001;167:715–723.

273. Hayashi K, Abe N, Watanabe T, et al. Overexpression of AML1 transcription factor drives thymocytes into the CD8 single-positive lineage. *J Immunol* 2001;167:4957–4965.

274. Telfer JC, Laurent MN, Rothenberg EV. Runx1 expression influences both the αβ/γδ T cell and CD4/CD8 T cell lineage decisions. Submitted 2002.

275. Vandekerckhove BAE, Barcena A, Schols D, et al. *In vivo* cytokine expression in the thymus. CD3[high] human thymocytes are activated and already functionally differentiated into helper and cytotoxic cells. *J Immunol* 1994;152:1738–1743.

276. Vanhecke D, Verhasselt B, Debacker V, et al. Differentiation to T-helper cells in the thymus—gradual acquisition of T-helper cell–function by CD3+CD4+ cells. *J Immunol* 1995;155:4711–4718.

277. Wang H, Diamond RA, Yang-Snyder JA, et al. Precocious expression of T-cell functional response genes *in vivo* in primitive thymocytes before T-lineage commitment. *Int Immunol* 1998;10:1623–1635.

278. Corbella P, Moskophidis D, Spanopoulou E, et al. Functional commitment to helper T cell lineage precedes positive selection and is independent of T cell receptor MHC specificity. *Immunity* 1994;1:269–276.

279. Matechak EO, Killeen N, Hedrick SM, et al. MHC class II–specific T cells can develop in the CD8 lineage when CD4 is absent. *Immunity* 1996;4:337–347.

280. Bhandoola A, Kithiganahalli B, Granger L, et al. Programming for cytotoxic effector function occurs concomitantly with CD4 extinction during CD8+ T cell differentiation in the thymus. *Int Immunol* 2000;12:1035–1040.

281. Zou YR, Sunshine MJ, Taniuchi I, et al. Epigenetic silencing of CD4 in T cells committed to the cytotoxic lineage. *Nat Genet* 2001;29:332–336.

282. Tough DF, Sprent J. Thymic emigration—a reply. *Immunol Today* 1995;16:273–274.

283. Scollay R, Godfrey DI. Thymic emigration: conveyor belts or lucky dips? *Immunol Today* 1995;16:268–273.

284. Ueno T, Hara K, Willis MS, et al. Role for CCR7 ligands in the emigration of newly generated T lymphocytes from the neonatal thymus. *Immunity* 2002;16:205–218.

285. Chaffin KE, Perlmutter RM. A pertussis toxin–sensitive process controls thymocyte emigration. *Eur J Immunol* 1991;21:2565–2573.

286. Akashi K, Reya T, Dalma-Weiszhausz D, et al. Lymphoid precursors. *Curr Opin Immunol* 2000;12:144–150.

287. Bendelac A, Rivera MN, Park SH, et al. Mouse CD1-specific NK1 T cells: development, specificity, and function. *Annu Rev Immunol* 1997;15:535–562.

288. Godfrey DI, Hammond KJ, Poulton LD, et al. NKT cells: facts, functions and fallacies. *Immunol Today* 2000;21:573–583.

289. Wilson SB, Byrne MC. Gene expression in NKT cells: defining a functionally distinct CD1d-restricted T cell subset. *Curr Opin Immunol* 2001;13:555–561.

290. Benlagha K, Weiss A, Beavis A, et al. *In vivo* identification of glycolipid antigen–specific T cells using fluorescent CD1d tetramers. *J Exp Med* 2000;191:1895–1903.

291. Matsuda JL, Naidenko OV, Gapin L, et al. Tracking the response of natural killer T cells to a glycolipid antigen using CD1d tetramers. *J Exp Med* 2000;192:741–754.

292. Gapin L, Matsuda JL, Surh CD, et al. NKT cells derive from double-positive thymocytes that are positively selected by CD1d. *Nat Immunol* 2001;2:971–978.

293. MacDonald HR. NK1.1+ T cell receptor-α/β+ cells: new clues to their origin, specificity, and function. *J Exp Med* 1995;182:633–638.

294. Hammond K, Cain W, van Driel I, et al. Three day neonatal thymectomy selectively depletes NK1.1+ T cells. *Int Immunol* 1998;10:1491–1499.

295. Coles MC, Raulet DH. NK1.1+ T cells in the liver arise in the thymus and are selected by interactions with class I molecules on CD4+CD8+ cells. *J Immunol* 2000;164:2412–2418.

296. Bendelac A, Killeen N, Littman DR, et al. A subset of CD4+ thymocytes selected by MHC class I molecules. *Science* 1994;263:1774–1778.

297. Eberl G, Lowin-Kropf B, MacDonald HR. Cutting edge: NKT cell development is selectively impaired in Fyn-deficient mice. *J Immunol* 1999;163:4091–4094.

298. Gadue P, Morton N, Stein PL. The Src family tyrosine kinase Fyn regulates natural killer T cell development. *J Exp Med* 1999;190:1189–1196.

299. Walunas TL, Wang B, Wang CR, et al. Cutting edge: the Ets1 transcription factor is required for the development of NK T cells in mice. *J Immunol* 2000;164:2857–2860.

300. Ohteki T, Ho S, Suzuki H, et al. Role for IL-15/IL-15 receptor β-chain in natural killer 1.1+ T cell receptor-$\alpha\beta$+ cell development. *J Immunol* 1997;159:5931–5935.

301. Elewaut D, Brossay L, Santee SM, et al. Membrane lymphotoxin is required for the development of different subpopulations of NK T cells. *J Immunol* 2000;165:671–679.

302. Eberl G, Fehling HJ, von Boehmer H, et al. Absolute requirement for the pre–T cell receptor α chain during NK1.1+ TCR$\alpha\beta$ cell development. *Eur J Immunol* 1999;29:1966–1971.

303. MacDonald HR. Development and selection of NKT cells. *Curr Opin Immunol* 2002;14:250–254.

304. Sato H, Nakayama T, Tanaka Y, et al. Induction of differentiation of pre-NKT cells to mature Vα14 NKT cells by granulocyte/macrophage colony–stimulating factor. *Proc Natl Acad Sci U S A* 1999;96:7439–7444.

305. Iwabuchi K, Iwabuchi C, Tone S, et al. Defective development of NK1.1+ T-cell antigen receptor $\alpha\beta$+ cells in zeta-associated protein 70 null mice with an accumulation of NK1.1+ CD3− NK-like cells in the thymus. *Blood* 2001;97:1765–1775.

306. Baur N, Nerz G, Nil A, et al. Expression and selection of productively rearranged TCRβ VDJ genes are sequentially regulated by CD3 signaling in the development of NK1.1+ $\alpha\beta$ T cells. *Int Immunol* 2001;13:1031–1042.

307. Shimamura M, Ohteki T, Beutner U, et al. Lack of directed Vα14-Jα281 rearrangements in NK1+ T cells. *Eur J Immunol* 1997;27:1576–1579.

308. Sakaguchi S, Sakaguchi N, Asano M, et al. Immunologic self-tolerance maintained by activated T cells expressing IL-2 receptor alpha-chains (CD25). Breakdown of a single mechanism of self-tolerance causes various autoimmune diseases. *J Immunol* 1995;155:1151–1164.

309. Shevach EM. Regulatory T cells in autoimmmunity. *Annu Rev Immunol* 2000;18:423–449.

310. Itoh M, Takahashi T, Sakaguchi N, et al. Thymus and autoimmunity: production of CD25+CD4+ naturally anergic and suppressive T cells as a key function of the thymus in maintaining immunologic self-tolerance. *J Immunol* 1999;162:5317–5326.

311. Asano M, Toda M, Sakaguchi N, et al. Autoimmune disease as a consequence of developmental abnormality of a T cell subpopulation. *J Exp Med* 1996;184:387–396.

312. Papiernik M, de Moraes ML, Pontoux C, et al. Regulatory CD4 T cells: expression of IL-2Rα chain, resistance to clonal deletion and IL-2 dependency. *Int Immunol* 1998;10:371–378.

313. Jordan MS, Boesteanu A, Reed AJ, et al. Thymic selection of CD4+CD25+ regulatory T cells induced by an agonist self-peptide. *Nat Immunol* 2001;2:301–306.

314. Suto A, Nakajima H, Ikeda K, et al. CD4+CD25+ T-cell development is regulated by at least 2 distinct mechanisms. *Blood* 2002;99:555–560.

315. Ramsdell F, Lantz T, Fowlkes BJ. A nondeletional mechanism of thymic self tolerance. *Science* 1989;246:1038–1041.

315a. Hori S, Nomura T, Sakaguchi S. Control of regulatory T cell development by the transcription factor Foxp3. *Science* 2003;299:1057–61.

315b. Fontenot JD, Gavin MA, Rudensky AY. Foxp3 programs the development and function of CD4+CD25+ regulatory T cells. *Nat Immunol* 2003;4:330–6.

315c. Khattri R, Cox T, Yasayko SA, Ramsdell F. An essential role for Scurfin in CD4+CD25+ T regulatory cells. *Nat Immunol* 2003;4:337–42.

316. Plum J, De Smedt M, Verhasselt B, et al. In vitro intrathymic differentiation kinetics of human fetal liver CD34+CD38− progenitors reveals a phenotypically defined dendritic/T-NK precursor split. *J Immunol* 1999;162:60–68.

317. Blom B, Verschuren MC, Heemskerk MH, et al. TCR gene rearrangements and expression of the pre–T cell receptor complex during human T-cell differentiation. *Blood* 1999;93:3033–3043.

318. van Ewijk W, Wang B, Hollander G, et al. Thymic microenvironments, 3-D versus 2-D? *Semin Immunol* 1999;11:57–64.

319. Jiang R, Lan Y, Chapman HD, Shawber C, Norton CR, Serreze DV, Weinmaster G, Gridley T. Defects in limb, craniofacial, and thymic development in Jagged2 mutant mice. *Genes Dev* 1998;12:1046–57.

CHAPTER 10

Peripheral T-Lymphocyte Responses and Function

Marc K. Jenkins

Introduction
Naïve T Cells
  Generation · Recirculation · Survival
***In Vivo* Presentation of Peptide–MHC Ligands**
  Dendritic Cells · Presentation of Low-Affinity Self-Peptide–MHC Ligands · Presentation of High-Affinity Foreign Peptide–MHC Ligands
T-Cell Activation
  Signal Transduction · IL-2 Production and Proliferation · Effector Cells · Memory Cells
Summary
Acknowledgments
References

INTRODUCTION

A thymus-derived (T) lymphocyte becomes activated when its antigen receptor (TCR) binds to a major histocompatibility complex (MHC)–encoded protein containing a specific peptide on the surface of an antigen-presenting cell (APC) (1). The ensuing signal transduction and functional changes that occur in T cells have been studied extensively in culture systems and will be discussed in great detail in other chapters. The goal of this chapter is to provide the reader with a "big picture" of how T-cell activation occurs *in vivo* and how this activation results in immune memory.

Exposure of a normal host to virtually any foreign protein will activate a few naïve T cells that express TCRs with high affinity for peptide–MHC combinations produced from the antigen. Because of the vast diversity of the T-cell repertoire, the T cells expressing TCRs specific for a single foreign antigen are so rare that their activation cannot be detected after addition of a foreign antigen to an *in vitro* culture of blood or lymphoid tissue cells from a naïve host. On the other hand, *in vitro* culture with an antigen that the host has been exposed to in the past results in detectable signs of T-cell activation, such as proliferation, lymphokine production, and cell-mediated cytotoxicity (2). This *ex vivo* approach has been the mainstay for studying the ability of foreign antigens to induce T-cell activation *in vivo*. However, in addition to being too insensitive to detect the activation of naïve T cells in the polyclonal repertoire, cell culture approaches cannot reproduce the complex microenvironments in which T cells are activated

in vivo and are indirect measures of the products of activated T cells not direct measures of the T cells themselves.

These limitations have been remedied by new systems that allow direct *ex vivo* or *in situ* monitoring of antigen-specific T cells. One method relies on fluorochrome-labeled, homogenous, multimeric peptide–MHC I or II complexes (3–5). Peptide–MHC multimers bind to the T cells that express an appropriate TCR, allowing direct detection of antigen-specific T cells by flow cytometry or immunohistology. The strength of the peptide–MHC multimer approach is that it can theoretically measure all potentially responsive T cells in the normal repertoire. However, since the frequency of T cells specific for most peptide–MHC complexes in naïve individuals is below the limit of detection of flow cytometry (6–8), peptide–MHC multimers cannot currently be used to study the earliest events in T-cell activation that occur before proliferation.

One way to solve the clonal infrequency problem is adoptive transfer of T cells from TCR transgenic mice into syngeneic normal recipients (9). This maneuver produces a traceable naïve T-cell population of known peptide–MHC specificity, comprising ∼0.2% of cells in the secondary lymphoid organs of the recipient. The transferred cells can be distinguished from those of the recipient with antibodies specific for the transgenic TCR clonotype or an allelic marker such as Thy 1 or CD45. The earliest events in T-cell activation *in vivo* can be studied with this method because the antigen-specific T cells are abundant enough to be detected by flow cytometry or immunohistology before proliferation. A potential disadvantage is that even though only a small number of T cells are transferred, the resulting frequency of antigen-specific T cells is still higher than normal. This can create a situation in which the transferred T cells outcompete endogenous T cells of similar specificity under certain conditions (10–12). However, the kinetics and relative magnitude of proliferation and loss reported for transferred T cells after *in vivo* exposure to antigen are identical to those described for endogenous T cells tracked with peptide–MHC multimers (9). This chapter rests heavily on studies involving peptide–MHC multimers or TCR-transgenic T-cell adoptive transfer methods because they provide the most physiologically relevant information on the *in vivo* immune response.

NAÏVE T CELLS

Generation

As $\alpha\beta$ T cells develop in the thymus, TCR α and β gene segments are rearranged such that each clone eventually expresses a unique TCR (13). Developing thymocytes that produce a surface TCR express CD4 and CD8 co-receptors and undergo one of three fates, depending on the specificity and affinity of their TCRs for self-peptide–MHC ligands. Thymocytes that express TCRs with no affinity for self-peptide–MHC molecules die by a programmed cell death mechanism. Potentially harmful thymocytes that express TCRs with strong affinity for the self-peptide–MHC ligands expressed on cells in the thymus are eliminated via physical deletion (14), functional inactivation (15), or receptor editing (16). Only thymocytes that express TCRs with a low but significant affinity for self-peptide–MHC ligands on thymic stromal cells differentiate into mature T cells (17). Thymocytes expressing TCRs with a low affinity for self-peptide-class I MHC molecules (MHC I) become mature T cells that express CD8 but not CD4, whereas thymocytes expressing TCRs with a low affinity for self-peptide–class II MHC molecules (MHC II) mature into cells that express CD4 but not CD8. This process is termed "positive selection."

Recirculation

CD4 and CD8 T cells that survive positive selection leave the thymus and enter the secondary lymphoid organs. T cells that have not yet encountered a foreign peptide–MHC ligand for which their TCR has a high affinity are referred to as "naïve" T cells. These cells account for the majority of T cells in the secondary lymphoid organs in healthy young adults. Naïve T cells recirculate continuously through the secondary lymphoid organs, which include the spleen, lymph nodes, and mucosal lymphoid organs (e.g., the Peyer's patches of the intestines) (18,19). Secondary lymphoid organs are defined based on the presence of segregated T- and B-cell–rich regions and specialized blood vessels that facilitate the entry of naïve lymphocytes (20). Naïve T cells are found only in the T-cell–rich areas known as the paracortex in the lymph

nodes and mucosal lymphoid organs, and the periarteriolar lymphoid sheath (PALS) in the spleen (21,22). The predilection for lymph nodes is explained by the fact that naïve T cells express a unique set of receptors that bind ligands expressed on the specialized blood vessels of the lymph nodes and mucosal lymphoid organs known as high endothelial venules (HEV) (23). Naïve T cells use CD62L or $\alpha 4\beta 7$ integrin, CC chemokine receptor (CCR) 7, and LFA-1 (CD11a/CD18) for rolling, adhesion, and extravasation through the HEV in peripheral lymph nodes and mucosal lymphoid organs. HEV are the only blood vessels in the body that display all of the ligands for these receptors (23). Naïve T cells move from the blood into the spleen because blood is emptied from terminal branches of the central arteriole into marginal sinuses or directly into the red pulp (20). The T cells then move into the PALS by a poorly understood CD62L-independent, G protein–dependent mechanism (24). Naïve T cells are retained in the T-cell areas of the spleen for about 5 hours and the lymph nodes for about 1 day (18), in part via CCR7 signaling in response to CCL21 (SLC) and CCL19 (ELC) chemokines produced by stromal cells in the T-cell areas (20). Naïve T cells leave the lymph nodes via efferent lymphatic vessels that eventually merge into the blood stream via the thoracic duct, or the spleen via the splenic vein. Once in the blood, a naïve T-cell will quickly enter a new secondary lymphoid organ, repeating the processes described above. An exception to this scenario occurs for a short period after birth when naïve T cells recirculate through nonlymphoid tissues (25). This behavior may exist to induce tolerance in those naïve T cells that express TCRs specific for self-peptide–MHC combinations displayed only outside the thymus.

Survival

It is estimated that an individual naïve T-cell will on average circulate through the secondary lymphoid organs for several months (26,27). To have this normal lifespan, naïve CD4 T cells must be exposed to MHC II molecules and CD8 T cells to MHC I molecules (28,29). Thus, it is likely that T-cell survival is maintained by low-affinity TCR recognition of self-peptide–MHC complexes. This recognition results in a subset of the signals that emanate from the TCR when bound by a high-affinity ligand, including partial phosphorylation of the CD3-zeta chain (30). IL-7 is also required to maintain the survival of naïve T cells, as evidenced by the findings that IL-7 receptor–deficient naïve T cells have a short life span (31) and normal T cells survive poorly in IL-7–deficient recipients (32).

Although signals through the TCR and IL-7 receptor are required for the survival of naïve T cells, these signals do not cause the T cells to proliferate in hosts containing normal numbers of T cells. In contrast, naïve T cells proliferate when transferred into T-cell–deficient hosts (33–36). This "homeostatic" proliferation also depends on IL-7 (31,32) and low-affinity TCR recognition of self-peptide–MHC complexes—probably the self-peptide–MHC complex that caused the

T-cell to undergo positive selection in the thymus (34,35), but not IL-2 or the CD28 co-stimulatory receptor (37). Thus, the same signaling events that cause naïve T cells to survive in interphase in T-cell–sufficient hosts, cause these cells to proliferate in T-cell–deficient hosts, but using a program different from that engaged during the T-cell response to high-affinity TCR ligands. Survival and proliferation could both contribute to control of the number of naïve T cells in normal hosts. In young individuals, new naïve T cells are constantly produced by the thymus and exported to the secondary lymphoid organs to replace senescent naïve T cells. Since the secondary lymphoid organs would constantly be full under these conditions, the resident naïve T cells would survive in interphase. In contrast, in older individuals in whom thymic output is reduced or absent, and are thus susceptible to lymphopenia, senescent cells may be replaced by proliferation of remaining naïve T cells.

IN VIVO PRESENTATION OF PEPTIDE–MHC LIGANDS

As naïve T cells percolate through the T-cell areas of secondary lymphoid organs, they encounter a dense network of large, irregularly shaped dendritic cells that constitutively express the highest levels of MHC molecules of any cell in the body (38). Given their location in the T-cell areas, surface molecule repertoire, and potent capacity to stimulate naïve T cells in vitro (38), it is likely that dendritic cells play an important role in the presentation of low-affinity self-peptide–MHC ligands that maintains naïve T cells, as well as the initial presentation of high-affinity foreign peptide–MHC ligands that stimulates the proliferation and differentiation of naïve T cells.

Dendritic Cells

Dendritic cells exist in several subsets (39,40). In the mouse, the CD11c integrin appears to mark most large, MHC^{high} cells, although CD11c is also expressed on monocytes and a subset of antigen-experienced CD8 T cells (41). Three types of CD11c$^+$, MHC$^+$ dendritic cells are found in the spleen and lymph nodes (Fig. 1). One type expresses the myeloid marker CD11b and variably expresses CD4, but does not express CD8α or the CD205 integrin, and is often referred to as the "myeloid dendritic cell." These dendritic cells are found mainly in the red pulp or marginal zones of the spleen and the outer edges of the paracortex in the lymph nodes. A second type lacks CD11b and CD4 but expresses CD8α and CD205, and is often referred to as the "lymphoid dendritic cell." Lymphoid dendritic cells are located primarily in the PALS of the spleen and the central paracortex of the lymph nodes. Although the names imply derivation from separate lineages, recent work indicates that both myeloid and lymphoid dendritic cells can be derived from either common myeloid or lymphoid precursors (42,43). The common origin of these dendritic cells is supported by the recent finding that highly purified CD11b$^+$, CD205$^-$, CD8α^- myeloid dendritic cells give rise to CD11b$^-$, CD205$^+$, CD8α^+ lymphoid dendritic cells after adoptive transfer (44). Myeloid and lymphoid dendritic cells survive for about 10 days in the secondary lymphoid organs (45,46).

The third type of CD11c$^+$ dendritic cell in the spleen and lymph nodes lacks CD11b but expresses the B220 and Gr-1 molecules normally expressed by B cells and granulocytes, respectively (47). These cells have plasmacytoid morphology and are concentrated near the HEV (47) in the lymph nodes. The fact that the number of these dendritic cells is greatly reduced in the lymph nodes of CD62L-deficient mice (47) indicates that they enter the lymph nodes from the blood through the HEV. Plasmacytoid dendritic cells are potent producers of IFN-α, which plays a role in the generation of IFN-γ–producing memory T cells in humans (48).

The lymph nodes contain several additional dendritic populations (45,49,50) (Fig. 1B). All lymph nodes contain CD11c$^+$ cells that express CD11b and lack CD8α and are thus similar to myeloid dendritic cells, but also express CD205, albeit at a lower level than lymphoid dendritic cells. The absence of these cells in the spleen or Peyer's patches, which lack afferent lymphatic vessels, implies that these cells are migrants that move into the lymph node from interstitial tissue via afferent lymphatic vessels. These cells will be referred to as "interstitial dendritic cell migrants."

The superficial lymph nodes that drain the skin contain another population of dendritic cells that expresses high levels of CD205 and CD11b and intermediate levels of CD8α. These cells also express langerin (50), a protein that is expressed primarily by Langerhans cells (51). Therefore, it is very likely that CD11c$^+$, CD205$^+$, CD11b$^+$, CD8$\alpha^{intermediate}$ cells in the superficial lymph nodes are Langerhans cells that recently migrated from the skin. These Langerhans cell migrants are more long-lived than myeloid and lymphoid dendritic cells, as they survive for months in the secondary lymphoid organs (45).

The migration of dendritic cells from nonlymphoid organs to the lymph nodes, or red pulp of the spleen into the PALS, is driven by inflammatory stimuli such as LPS (52) or inflammatory cytokines including IL-1 and TNF-α (53,54). Dendritic cell migration from nonlymphoid organs into the secondary lymphoid organs is associated with a maturation process that results in changes in antigen processing and presentation potential (55). This maturation process can be mimicked by culturing immature nonlymphoid tissue–derived cells or their precursors in the presence of inflammatory cytokines (55). Immature dendritic cells efficiently engulf particles including apoptotic cells and extracellular fluid, and produce many peptide–MHC complexes from the ingested proteins, especially in the presence of inflammatory mediators such as TNF-α (56). Immature dendritic cells also display MHC II molecules that turn over rapidly (57). In contrast, mature dendritic cells that have been exposed to inflammatory cytokines for several days are inefficient at antigen uptake and processing and display stable MHC II molecules (57).

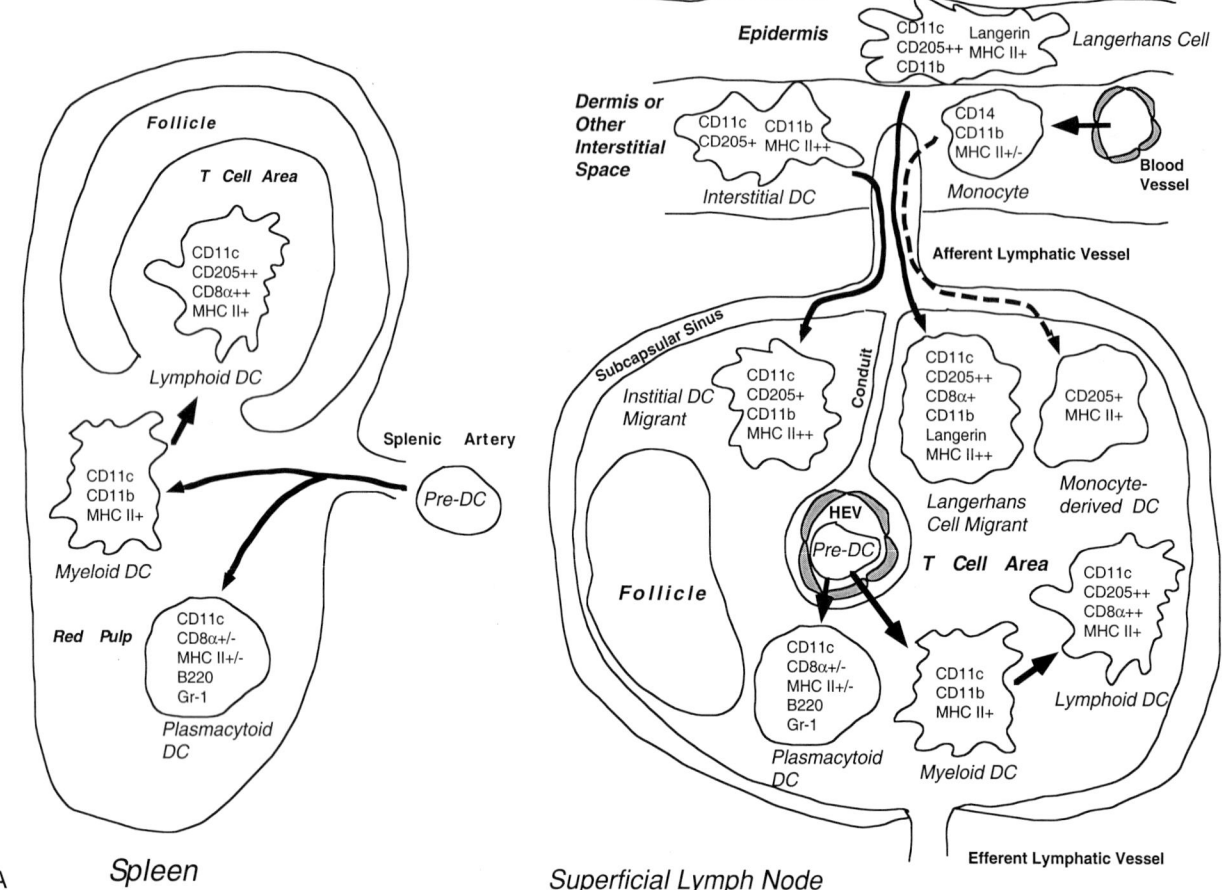

FIG. 1. A: Dendritic cell subsets of the spleen. **B:** Dendritic cell subsets of the lymph nodes. Molecules expressed by each dendritic subtype are shown. For certain molecules, the level of expression is indicated as high (++), intermediate (+), or low (+/−). *Arrows* indicate cellular movements. The *dashed arrow* indicates that the migration of monocytes and subsequent conversion to CD11c⁻ dendritic cells probably only operates in the presence of infection or tissue damage.

Together, these observations have led to the idea that *in vivo* antigen presentation to CD4 T cells depends heavily on immature dendritic cells that acquire antigens in nonlymphoid tissues, migrate to the secondary lymphoid organs, and in the process produce stable peptide–MHC II complexes. Inflammatory stimuli enhance this process, probably by increasing TNF-α and IL-1, and cause the migrated dendritic cells to increase expression of molecules in involved in co-stimulation (CD80, CD86, and CD40) (52).

**Presentation of Low-Affinity
Self-Peptide–MHC Ligands**

As mentioned above, naïve T cells must recognize low-affinity self-peptide–MHC ligands to have a normal life span. Dendritic cells probably play a role in this process because they are constantly in contact with T cells in the secondary lymphoid organs (58,59), and expression of MHC II molecules under the control of the dendritic cell-specific CD11c promoter is sufficient to maintain the survival of naïve CD4 T cells (58).

In the absence of infection or tissue damage, all dendritic cell populations in the secondary lymphoid organs exist in a resting state characterized by low expression of co-stimulatory molecules such as CD80 and CD86 (52). Recent discoveries indicate that this resting state is actively maintained by cytokines that are produced by phagocytes as they engulf senescent apoptotic cells. Engulfment of apoptotic cells is mediated by receptors that recognize unique molecules on apoptotic cells (60), for example, the phosphatidyl serine receptor (60,61), which trigger the production of TGF-β1, IL-10, and prostaglandins (62). These molecules are known to inhibit dendritic cell maturation and expression of co-stimulatory molecules (63). Together these results suggest a scenario, in which the dendritic cells that present self-peptide–MHC molecules to naïve T cells and maintain their survival are in a suppressed state brought about by anti-inflammatory cytokines produced by themselves or other phagocytes as they engulf senescent apoptotic cells, either in the lymphoid organs or in the nonlymphoid organs before migration. It is not clear which of the dendritic cell types found in the secondary lymphoid organs play this role.

Recent reports of autoimmune disease and immunopathology in mice with mutations that prevent disposal of apoptotic cells (64,65) suggest that the purpose of this inhibitory pathway is to prevent dendritic cells from activating self-reactive T cells *in the absence of inflammation.*

Presentation of High-Affinity Foreign Peptide–MHC Ligands

Unlike the presentation of low-affinity self-peptide–MHC ligands that maintains the survival of naïve T cells in interphase, the presentation of high-affinity foreign peptide–MHC ligands induces the specific T cells to produce lymphokines and proliferate. These more dramatic biological effects occur because the responding T cells express TCRs with high affinity for the foreign peptide–MHC ligands, and thus receive stronger or more durable signals through the TCR (66). In addition, foreign antigens naturally enter the body during infection or tissue damage and the accompanying inflammation improves the quantity, quality, and type of cells that present foreign peptide–MHC ligands to T cells (67,68). As detailed below (Table 1), the type of APC that presents foreign peptide–MHC ligands to naïve T cells is also influenced by the physical properties of the antigen and the site where it enters the body.

Particulate Antigens

The presentation of particulate antigens has been studied by tracking the fate of fluorescent microbeads (69). After subcutaneous injection, the beads are engulfed by monocytes that quickly enter the injection site from the blood, probably in response to inflammatory mediators made as a consequence of tissue damage resulting from the injection. Within 24 hours, cells containing more than one bead and expressing high amounts of MHC I and II molecules and the dendritic cell-specific molecules recognized by the MIDC-8 and 2A1 antibodies but low amounts of CD11c, appear in the draining lymph nodes. Monocytes that engulf particles and migrate *in vitro* across an artificial endothelial cell layer in

an abluminal-to-lumenal direction, also acquire these phenotypic characteristics (70). Together these results suggest that monocytes that enter tissue sites and engulf particles receive signals to differentiate into dendritic cells in the process of migrating from the tissue into the lumen of an afferent lymphatic vessel. These dendritic cells must appear in the lymph nodes transiently after tissue damage or change phenotype after migrating because CD11c[low], MHC[high] cells are rare in the secondary lymphoid organs under normal conditions. Although it is reasonable to assume that these cells would be capable of presenting peptide–MHC ligands to T cells after arriving in the T-cell areas, this remains to be determined. CD11c[high] cells containing one bead also appear in the draining lymph nodes after subcutaneous injection of fluorescent beads. It is therefore possible that these cells, which are probably interstitial dendritic cell migrants, could be the important APC for particulate antigens that enter the dermis. In either case, the bead-containing cells that appear in the lymph nodes after subcutaneous injection are most likely important for presentation of peptide–MHC II ligands to CD4 T cells because, as described next, a different dendritic cell type is responsible for presentation of peptide–MHC I ligands derived from particulate antigens.

Naïve CD8 T cells require signals through the TCR, CD28, and IL-12 receptor to proliferate maximally and differentiate into cytotoxic effector cells (71–73). Thus, although other cells express MHC I molecules in the T-cell areas, only dendritic cells express the ligands for these receptors and produce IL-12 (74), implying that dendritic cells play an important role as APC for naïve CD8 T cells. The TCR ligands for CD8 T cells are normally generated from endogenous proteins produced in the cytoplasm of the APC (75). This would be the case for particulate antigens, such as viruses that directly infect dendritic cells and replicate in the cytoplasm. However, if dendritic cells are necessary APC for naïve CD8 T cells, and peptide–MHC I complexes can only be produced from endogenous proteins, it is less clear how CD8 T-cell responses are initiated in cases where the antigen does not replicate directly within dendritic cells.

The answer to this question is provided by the existence of dendritic cells that violate the classical rules of antigen

TABLE 1. *Dendritic cell subsets that present peptide–MHC ligands* in vivo

Antigen	Entry route	Site of antigen presentation	Peptide–MHC produced	Dendritic cell subset
Particulate	Subcutaneous	Lymph node	II	CD11c[low], 2A1[+], MIDC-8[+], derived from monocytes at injection site
Reactive hapten	Skin surface	Draining lymph node	I and II	Langerhans cells and interstitial DC migrants
Soluble protein	Subcutaneous	Draining lymph node	II	Myeloid DC or interstitial DC migrants
Soluble protein LPS	Subcutaneous	Draining lymph node	II	Myeloid DC or interstitial DC migrants, lymphoid DC or Langerhans cells
Soluble protein	Intravenous	Spleen	II	Myeloid DC
Soluble protein LPS	Intravenous	Spleen	II	Myeloid DC, lymphoid DC
Soluble protein	Intravenous	Spleen	I	Lymphoid DC
Antigen-loaded splenocytes	Intravenous	Spleen	I	Lymphoid DC

processing and are capable of producing peptide–MHC I complexes from exogenous antigens. This capacity is sometimes called cross-presentation or cross-priming (76,77), and is particularly prominent for particulate antigens. Recent evidence indicates that the cross-priming APC is a CD11c$^+$, CD8α^+ dendritic cell. Intravenous injection of ovalbumin-pulsed, MHC I-deficient splenocytes into normal mice leads to the activation of ovalbumin peptide–MHC I-specific CD8 T cells (78). Because the injected cells are incapable of directly presenting ovalbumin peptide–MHC I complexes, cross-priming APC from the recipient must acquire ovalbumin from the injected cells and present ovalbumin peptide–MHC I complexes to the T cells. These cells are probably lymphoid dendritic cells because CD11c$^+$, CD8α^{high} but not CD11c$^+$, CD8α^- cells isolated from the spleens of injected mice stimulate ovalbumin peptide–MHC I-specific CD8 T cells in vitro. The simplest explanation for these results is that lymphoid dendritic cells are one of the few cell types in the body that deliver exogenous antigens into the cytosol and then the proteosome- and TAP-dependent MHC I processing pathway (79,80). This capacity of CD8α^+ dendritic cells is enhanced by CD4 T cells via a CD40-dependent mechanism (81,82). The facts that CD8α^+ dendritic cells are better IL-12 producers than CD8α^- dendritic cells (74) and that IL-12 enhances the proliferation of CD8 T cells (73) provide further evidence that CD8α^+ dendritic cells are important APC for CD8 T cells, at least when CD4 T cells are also present.

Skin-Surface Antigens

A rich literature suggests that Langerhans cells are involved in the presentation of antigens that enter the body through the epidermis (38,83,84). This contention is based largely on experiments done with reactive haptens that, when applied to the skin surface covalently attach to soluble proteins within the epidermis. Langerhans cells efficiently take up hapten-labeled proteins and could produce haptenated peptide– MHC I and II complexes via the exogenous antigen-processing pathway mentioned above (85–87). Alternatively, haptens could couple directly to self-peptide–MHC I or II molecules already on the surface of Langerhans cells (88). Chemically reactive haptens stimulate the production of inflammatory cytokines such as IL-1 and TNF-α within the epidermis (83,89). As mentioned above, these cytokines cause Langerhans cells to leave the epidermis (53,54), enter local afferent lymphatic vessels and migrate into the T-cell areas of the draining lymph nodes where they can be found about 24 hours after application of the hapten (45,83). Hapten-labeled interstitial dendritic cells from the dermis also arrive in the lymph nodes but only after 48 hours, probably because they are located further from the skin surface than Langerhans cells (45). Since inflammatory cytokines are also inducers of the maturation process, Langerhans cells or interstitial dendritic cells that migrate from inflamed skin express elevated levels of co-stimulatory molecules and are potent stimulators of CD4 and CD8 T cells (90–92). The finding that manipulations that reduce Langerhans cell density or function reduce the amount of T-cell priming induced by reactive haptens is evidence that migrating Langerhans cells present antigen to T cells in vivo (93).

Soluble Antigens

Along their length, mucosal surfaces have lymph node-like organs that abut the intestinal epithelium on the albumenal side (94). The best studied of these mucosal lymphoid organs are the Peyer's patches of the intestinal mucosa, although all mucosal surfaces probably have similar structures. The side of the mucosal lymphoid organ that attaches to the epithelium contains M cells that bring lumenal contents into the organ (94). Since mucosal lymphoid organs do not contain afferent lymphatic vessels, M cell sampling is the major mechanism whereby antigens enter these organs. Within the Peyer's patch, just beneath the M cells, lies the subepithelial dome, which is rich in CD11c$^+$, CD11b$^+$, CD8α^- dendritic cells (95). CD11c$^+$, CD11b$^-$, CD8α^+ dendritic cells are concentrated in the T-cell area, beneath the subepithelial dome. A third CD11c$^+$ population that lacks CD11b and CD8α, and found only in mucosal lymphoid organs, is located in the subepithelial dome and the T-cell area. The fact that CD11c$^+$, CD11b$^+$, CD8α^- dendritic cells are situated near the M cells where antigen enters the Peyer's patches suggests that these cells present peptide–MHC II ligands derived from antigens that enter through mucosal surfaces. This contention is further supported by the fact that CD11c$^+$, CD11b$^+$, CD8α^- dendritic cells migrate into the central T-cell areas in response to inflammation (95). The relationship between CD11c$^+$, CD11b$^+$, CD8α^- dendritic cells in mucosal lymphoid organs and those in other secondary lymphoid organs is unknown. However, since these cells express CD11b and lack CD8α and could not have migrated from nonlymphoid tissue via afferent lymphatic vessels, they are probably myeloid dendritic cells.

CD11c$^+$, CD11b$^+$, CD8α^- dendritic cells have also been implicated in the presentation of soluble antigens that enter lymph nodes from the mucosal surface of the trachea. Following instillation of labeled ovalbumin into the trachea, labeled CD11c$^+$, MHC^{high} cells appear in the lung-associated lymph nodes. When isolated, these dendritic cells stimulate ovalbumin-specific CD4 T cells in vitro (96). Since these cells express CD11b and CD205, but most lack CD8α, they are probably interstitial dendritic cell migrants. Manickasingham and Reis e Sousa (97) used a monoclonal antibody specific for a chicken lysozyme peptide–MHC II complex to show that CD8α^- dendritic cells also produce peptide–MHC II complexes derived from subcutaneously injected lysozyme. It is not clear from their studies whether the CD8α^- dendritic cells that produce peptide–MHC II ligands in this case are myeloid dendritic cells or interstitial dendritic cell migrants because CD205 and CD11b expression was not assessed. Manickasingham and Reis e Sousa (97) also showed that CD8α^+ dendritic cells produce lysozyme peptide–MHC II complexes if lysozyme is injected with lipopolysaccharide (LPS).

Although expression of CD8α indicates that these cells are lymphoid dendritic cells, they could have been Langerhans cell migrants if cells with intermediate levels of CD8α were included in the gate used to identify CD8+ cells. LPS-induced inflammation may cause CD8α+ lymphoid dendritic cells that acquire lysozyme within the T-cell areas to produce peptide–MHC II complexes from this material, or stimulate the migration of Langerhans cells from the subcutaneous injection site. B cells in the follicles also produce peptide–MHC II complexes from lysozyme within several hours of injection (98). However, these peptide–MHC II complexes are probably inaccessible to naïve CD4 T cells, which reside only in the T-cell areas (21,22).

The site where the dendritic cells in the aforementioned studies acquired antigen is not clear. They could have acquired antigen at the point of entry into the body before migrating to the lymph node, or they could have acquired lymph-borne antigen after arriving in the lymph node. Subcutaneously injected proteins are deposited in the extracellular fluid of the tissue at the injection site. This fluid, also know as lymph, is constantly siphoned from the tissues into blind-ended afferent lymphatic capillaries that are present in most organs. Thus, antigens that are injected into tissues would be drawn in the lymph into an afferent lymphatic vessel and then into the subcapsular sinus of a connected lymph node (99). Thin conduits connect the subcapsular sinus to perivenular spaces that surround the HEV that pass through the lymph node (100) (Fig. 1B). The conduits are composed of thin fibers of extracellular matrix proteins wrapped continuously on the outside with a coating composed of 90% reticular fibroblasts and 10% other cells, including dendritic cells (100). The lumen of each conduit is not completely filled with the fibers because soluble molecules pass from the subcapsular sinus through the conduits and into the perivenular space. Surprisingly, however, soluble molecules do not pass in large amounts from the subcapsular sinus or conduits into the T-cell–rich paracortex where naïve T cells reside (99). Thus, the resident dendritic cells that would have the best access to antigens present within the conduits would be those that coat the conduits and are exposed to high concentrations of antigen within the conduit lumen, or those that are near the conduits to take up the small amount of antigen that leaks out. CD11c+, CD11b+ dendritic cells are the best candidates because they are concentrated in the outer paracortex (101) where the conduit network is most dense (99). Expression of CD11b indicates that these cells are Langerhans cell migrants, interstitial dendritic cell migrants, or myeloid dendritic cells. If these cells produce peptide–MHC complexes from antigen that leaks from the conduits, then this implies that Langerhans cell migrants and interstitial dendritic cells migrants are still capable of antigen uptake and processing even after migrating.

If on the other hand, lymph-borne free antigen within the conduits is not accessible to APC in the lymph node, then the APC must acquire antigen before migrating to the lymph node. In this case, the CD11c+, CD8α− cells identified as APC in the studies of Vermaelen et al. (96) and

Manickasingham and Reis e Sousa (97) are probably interstitial dendritic cells that acquired the antigen in the tissue where it entered the body.

CD11b+, CD8α− dendritic cells are also involved in the splenic presentation of peptide–MHC II ligands derived from intravenously injected antigens. Pooley et al. (102) found that CD8α− dendritic cells isolated from the spleens of mice injected intravenously with ovalbumin were better CD4 T-cell stimulators than CD8α+ dendritic cells. These CD8α− dendritic cells are likely to be myeloid or plasmacytoid dendritic cells because these are the only CD8α− populations in the spleen. Since fluorescent-labeled ovalbumin was taken up by splenic CD8α+ dendritic cells in this case, Pooley et al. (102) attributed the failure of these cells to stimulate CD4 T cells to an inability to produce peptide–MHC II complexes from the internalized antigen. This finding is reminiscent of in vitro results in which immature dendritic cells took up antigen but did not produce peptide–MHC II complexes unless exposed to an inflammatory stimulus (56). However, this property does not explain the failure of CD8α+ dendritic cells to produce peptide–MHC II complexes from the internalized antigen, since addition of LPS to the injected ovalbumin did not correct the failure (102).

In contrast, another study that used a monoclonal antibody specific for a chicken lysozyme peptide–MHC II ligand showed that CD8α− and CD8α+ dendritic cells in the spleen participate in the presentation of peptide–MHC complexes derived from intravenously injected lysozyme (103). The number of CD8α− and CD8α+ dendritic cells displaying lysozyme peptide–MHC II complexes in the spleen is greatly enhanced in the presence of LPS-induced inflammation (103). Inflammation may stimulate the migration of dendritic cells from the red pulp into the T-cell areas as described by DeSmedt et al. (52).

As in the case of particulate antigens, CD11c+, CD8α+ dendritic cells in the spleen produce peptide–MHC I ligands from intravenously injected antigen (102), again suggesting that these cells are capable of producing peptide–MHC I ligands from exogenous material.

T-CELL ACTIVATION

Signal Transduction

In vitro experiments have shown that high-affinity TCR ligation activates protein tyrosine kinases such as Lck, which stimulate signaling cascades that elevate intracellular calcium, convert Ras into its active form, and activate the extracellular signal-regulated kinases (ERK1 and ERK2) and stress-activated protein kinases (Jun kinase and p38 mitogen-activated protein kinase) (104). These pathways culminate in the nuclear translocation and DNA binding of transcription factors that regulate lymphokine gene expression (105). Very little is known about early signaling events in naïve T cells in vivo because the assays used to measure most of these events rely on cell lines and in vitro culture methods. However, intracellular staining with antibodies that recognize the active forms of the c-Jun transcription factor and the p38 mitogen-activated protein kinase has been used to show that TCR signaling is initiated in antigen-specific naïve CD4 T cells in the spleen within minutes of intravenous injection of the relevant peptide (59). This rapid response is likely explained by the fact that the majority of naïve CD4 T cells are in contact with MHC II–expressing dendritic cells, at all times (59). Since the peptide used in this experiment does not require antigen processing (106), it would be able to immediately bind to MHC II molecules on dendritic cells, and activate the interacting antigen-specific T cells. Although these results show that *in vivo* TCR signaling commences very quickly after recognition of peptide–MHC complexes, this process would take longer in cases where the relevant APC must process the antigen and/or migrate into the T-cell areas from another location.

IL-2 Production and Proliferation

Naïve CD4 and CD8 T cells produce IL-2 *in vivo* within the first day after TCR ligation (107,108). *In vitro* experiments indicate that cell division by naïve, antigen-stimulated T cells is driven by autocrine production of IL-2 (109). Surprisingly, however, antigen-driven proliferation of naïve T cells is minimally dependent on IL-2 *in vivo* (107,110–113). Therefore, other signals or growth factors must be capable of driving T-cell proliferation *in vivo*, although IL-2 may contribute. As noted below, IL-2 plays an important role in the elimination of activated T cells. The dual function of IL-2 as both a T-cell growth factor early in the response and an inhibitory factor later, may make it difficult to reveal the growth factor activity of IL-2 in IL-2–deficient animals.

Naïve CD4 and CD8 T cells shown signs of DNA replication and cell division as early as 48 hours after exposure to antigen *in vivo* (21,108,114). These events are followed by an exponential increase in the number of antigen-specific T cells over the next several days. Depending on the stimulus, the number of antigen-specific T cells reaches its highest level in the relevant secondary lymphoid organs, 3 to 7 days after antigen enters the body (6,7,21,115–119) (Fig. 2). Recently it has been estimated that naïve mice contain about 200 CD8 T cells specific for a given peptide–MHC I complex (120). Since antigen-specific CD8 T cells specific for a single peptide–MHC I complex can increase to 10^7 cells at

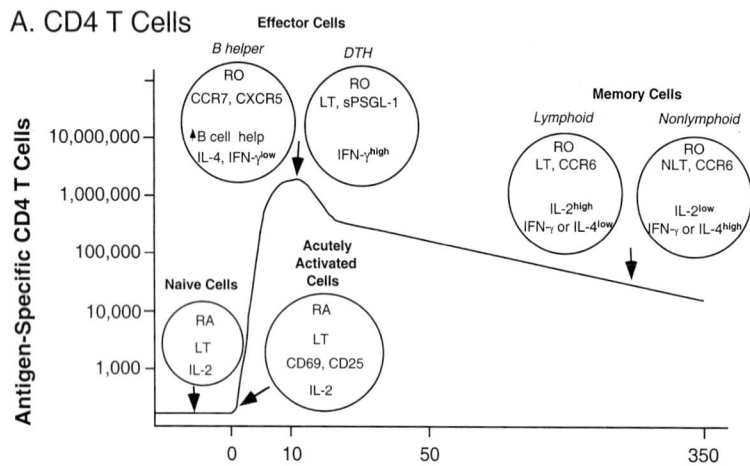

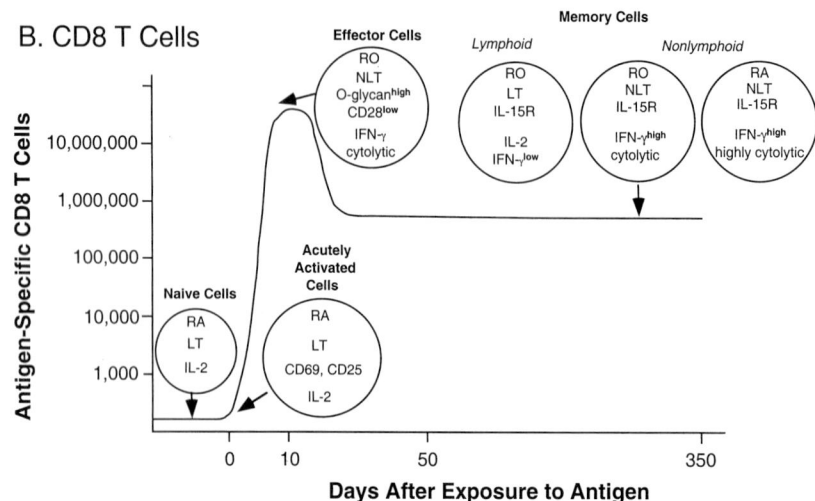

Days After Exposure to Antigen

FIG. 2. A: Kinetics, quantities, and phenotypes of antigen-specific CD4. **B:** Kinetics, quantities, and phenotypes of antigen-specific CD8. T cells during the primary immune response. RO and RA denote the CD45RO and CD45RA isoforms, respectively. LT denotes the set of molecules that are required for migration through HEV—CCR7, CD62L, and CD11a/CD18. NLT denotes the set of molecules involved in migration into nonlymphoid tissues, such as sPSGL-1, β1 and β7 integrins, and CCR5. Although a hypothetical situation is depicted, the number of cells shown is based on the work of Homann et al. (121), in which the number of CD4 or CD8 T cells specific for single peptide–MHC II or peptide–MHC I ligands was monitored during the course of a viral infection.

the peak of the primary response (121), it follows that CD8 T cells can expand 500,000-fold *in vivo*. Although naïve CD4 T cells are also capable of dramatic clonal expansion when stimulated appropriately, their burst size appears to be less than CD8 T cells (121).

Several factors influence the magnitude of *in vivo* T-cell proliferation. One is the size of the starting naïve population. The degree of proliferation is inversely correlated with the starting frequency of responding cells. In cases where the starting frequency is relatively high, for example after transfer of TCR transgenic T cells, the clonal burst size of this population is relatively low, probably as a result of competition between the T cells for peptide–MHC complexes (10,11).

In vivo T-cell proliferation is also regulated by co-stimulatory signals from APC. The proliferation of antigen-stimulated CD4 or CD8 T cells is reduced by two- to ten-fold in mice in which CD28 cannot interact with its ligands CD80 and CD86 (107,114,122,123). CD40 ligand deficiency has a similar effect on T-cell expansion (124–126), which may be related to the fact that CD40 signaling in APC induces CD80 and CD86 (127). Co-stimulatory signals regulate T-cell proliferation by enhancing growth factor production. Antigen-driven IL-2 production is greatly impaired when CD28 signaling is eliminated (107). Although it has been proposed that CD28 acts by promoting TCR aggregation in the synapse at the point of contact between the T-cell and APC (128), recent work indicates that CD28 is actually recruited into the synapse after it forms (129). CD28 then transduces signals that enhance lymphokine mRNA production and stability and promote T-cell survival by augmenting Bcl-XL production (130). Members of the TNF receptor family, such as OX40, CD27, and 4-1BB are induced on activated T cells several days into the primary response (131). These molecules bind ligands of the TNF family on the surface of APC and transduce signals that sustain the proliferation or survival of antigen-stimulated T cells (131,132).

Enhancement of co-stimulatory signals may underlie the observation that *in vivo* T-cell proliferation is also influenced by inflammation at the time of initial antigen presentation. The effect of inflammation is easily observed in the case of soluble antigens, where the magnitude of T-cell proliferation is several fold greater if antigen is administered with an adjuvant that induces inflammation or with inflammatory cytokines such as TNF-α, IL-1, or IL-12 (21,133–135). Adjuvant molecules are recognized by pattern recognition receptors (136), for example, Toll-like receptors (TLR) on cells of the innate immune system. The expansion of CD4 T cells in response to antigen plus complete Freund's adjuvant is deficient in mice that lack a functional TLR signaling pathway (137). The defect is probably related to the fact that TLR signaling stimulates tissue macrophages to produce TNF-α (138), which in turn stimulates dendritic cells to migrate from nonlymphoid tissues into the T-cell areas. TLR signaling causes APC to express higher levels of ligands for CD28 and produce inflammatory cytokines (139). Thus, adjuvants could enhance proliferation by driving more dendritic cells into the T-cell areas to present antigen, or by increasing the co-stimulatory capacity of the dendritic cells.

It is also likely that inflammatory cytokines stimulate proliferation by acting directly on the T cells. Support for this possibility comes from *in vitro* experiments that show that the proliferation of highly purified CD4 T or CD8 T cells in response to plastic surfaces coated with TCR and CD28 ligands is augmented by IL-1 or IL-12, respectively (73,140). These cytokines probably act by enhancing T-cell responsiveness to growth factors. For example, IL-1 has been shown to enhance IL-4–driven proliferation of CD4 Th2 clones (141).

Effector Cells

Antigen-specific T cells that are present at the time when the number of antigen-specific T cells reaches its peak express effector functions, and thus are sometimes to referred to as "effector cells" (142). Effector cells are blasts, express a different set of adhesion receptors, and possess different functional capabilities than naïve T cells. The functional properties that effector cells acquire are influenced by the presence of inflammatory cytokines and co-stimulatory ligands on APC present at the time of initial antigen presentation.

At least two types of antigen-specific effector CD4 T cells can be identified in the draining lymph nodes of mice injected subcutaneously with antigen and cholera toxin based on expression of CD62L and the functional, sialyated form of P-selectin ligand (sPSGL-1): CD62L$^+$, sPSGL-1$^+$ cells and CD62L-, sPSGL-1- cells (143) (Fig. 2A). The CD62L$^+$, sPSGL-1$^+$ cells are poor helpers of antibody production by B cells but are capable of IFN-γ production and cause delayed-type hypersensitivity (DTH) skin reactions when transferred into naïve recipients that are challenged with antigen. The DTH potential of these cells is explained by the fact that sPSGL-1 is critical for T-cell migration through CD62P-expressing blood vessels into inflamed skin (144). Once in the skin, IFN-γ production by CD62L$^+$, sPSGL-1$^+$ effector T cells likely causes some of the manifestations of the DTH reaction (145). Expression of sPSGL-1 on effector T cells is induced by exposure to IL-12 (146). The fact that IL-12 also controls acquisition of IFN-γ production capacity (147) probably underlies the finding that IFN-γ–producing effector cells are targeted preferentially to tissues like the skin that contains CD62P-expressing blood vessels (144).

Effector CD4 T cells capable of migrating into nonlymphoid tissues have been identified in several other types of immune responses. When antigen is initially presented in the mucosal lymphoid organs, the nonlymphoid trafficking population of effector CD4 T cells is induced to express the $\alpha4/\beta7$ integrin instead of sPSGL-1 (148), and would be expected to migrate to mucosal tissues instead of the skin. CD4 T cells capable of rapid IFN-γ production after challenge with antigen are found in the liver, lungs, thymus, salivary gland, and intestines of mice injected intravenously with antigen plus LPS (22). In addition, effector CD4 T cells capable of IL-4 production during *Leishmania* infection are found in the lungs (149). The fact that effector CD4 T cells produce IFN-γ after exposure to antigen plus cholera toxin or LPS, or IL-4 after to exposure to Leishmania, is probably related to differences in the early production of IL-12 or IL-4 by cells of the innate immune system. LPS stimulates IL-12 production, which favors the differentiation of IFN-γ–producing T cells, whereas Leishmania organisms stimulate IL-4 production, which favors the differentiation of IL-4–producing T cells (147). Together, these results suggest that antigenic stimulation within the secondary lymphoid organs produces a subset of IFN-γ- or IL-4–producing effector CD4 T cells that migrate into inflamed nonlymphoid organs and mediate immune reactions there. Such reactions lead to macrophage and granulocyte activation, which is an efficient means of eliminating microbes and parasites.

The CD62L$^-$, sPSGL-1$^-$ effector CD4 T cells found in the lymph nodes after injection of antigen and cholera toxin are efficient helpers of antibody production by B cells, do not cause DTH, and are poor IFN-γ producers (143). These may be the CD4 T cells that migrate into the B-cell–rich follicles during the primary response (21,117,143,150,151). Follicular migration is controlled by CXCR5, which is specific for the CXCL13 (BLC) chemokine produced by follicular stromal cells (20). CXCR5 expression is induced on T cells several days after in vivo exposure to antigen and adjuvant, but not antigen alone (152), probably because CXCR5 induction and follicular migration are dependent on signals through CD28 and OX40, the ligands for which are induced on dendritic cells by inflammation. Migration into follicles allows effector CD4 T cells to interact with and provide helper signals to antigen-specific B cells that display the relevant peptide–MHC complexes (125,153,154). Surprisingly, CD62L$^-$, sPSGL-1$^-$ effector CD4 T cells do not produce IL-4 (143), which is thought to be a critical component of T-cell–mediated promotion of antibody production (147). In addition, although the CD62L$^-$, sPSGL-1$^-$ effector CD4 T cells express CD40 ligand, another molecule that is critical for B-cell help, so do the CD62L$^+$, sPSGL-1$^+$ effector CD4 T cells that lack this activity (143). Therefore, the molecular basis for the potent B-cell helper function of CD62L$^-$, sPSGL-1$^-$ effector CD4 T cells is unclear. It is also not clear how the two different types of effector CD4 T cells are produced simultaneously in the same secondary lymphoid organs during the primary response.

Effector CD8 T cells also differ from their naïve precursors with respect to surface markers, function, and trafficking properties (Fig. 2B). Effector CD8 T cells that are generated during microbial infections express slightly lower levels of CD8 and more surface O-glycans than naïve cells (155), and in the human some effector CD8 T cells lose CD27 and CD28 but retain CD45RA (156). Unlike naïve cells, these effector CD8 T cells express perforin and granzymes, which are required for efficient cytolytic function (155). Expression of perforin and granzymes contributes to the defining feature of effector CD8 T cells, that is, the ability to directly kill target cells that display the appropriate peptide–MHC I

complexes. Interestingly, although large numbers of antigen-specific CD8 T cells accumulate in mice injected with a heat-killed microbe, these T cells do not acquire cytolytic function (157). Since the T cells undergo fewer cell divisions under these conditions, it is possible that CD8 T cells must divide many times before becoming effector cytolytic cells. Effector CD8 T cells gain the capacity to produce IFN-γ, but lose the capacity to produce IL-2, thus becoming dependent on IL-2 from CD4 T cells for further proliferation (158). The loss of CD28 function by effector CD8 T cells may contribute to the loss of IL-2 production capacity (159,160).

Effector CD8 T cells migrate out of the T-cell areas and into many nonlymphoid tissues, particularly inflamed sites of antigen deposition, such as the lungs during influenza infection (161,162) and the gut during vesicular stomatitis virus infection (163). In vitro experiments indicate that exposure to IL-2 is an important factor in the generation of nonlymphoid tissue-homing effector CD8 T cells (164). The migratory capacities of effector CD8 T cells correlate with loss of receptors involved in lymph node migration (CCR7 and CD62L) and acquisition of receptors such as $\alpha 4\beta 7$ integrin (165), which binds to MadCAM-1 expressed on blood vessels in mucosal organs. The migration of effector CD8 T cells with cytotoxic potential into nonlymphoid organs is an effective way of eliminating cells that display peptide–MHC I complexes from all parts of the body.

The number of effector T cells in the secondary lymphoid organs falls dramatically after the peak of proliferation (6,7,21,115–119) (Fig. 2). Some of this loss is due to the emigration of effector cells into nonlymphoid tissues as mentioned above (22). However, much of the loss must be due to cell death because apoptotic antigen-specific effector T cells can be identified in the secondary lymphoid organs (166), and because the total number of cells in the nonlymphoid organs declines shortly after its peak (22). The molecular basis for the death of effector T cells varies depending on the nature of the antigenic stimulus. The loss of effector CD8 T cells after the peak of proliferation in response to a single injection of antigen has been shown to be Fas-independent and Bcl-2 sensitive (167). This type of cell death has been observed in situations where cells are deprived of growth factors (168). This is a reasonable scenario because antigen-specific T cells stop making lymphokines at least 1 day before effector cells begin to disappear in hosts injected once with antigen (107). On the other hand, if antigen is presented chronically, TCR-mediated activation-induced cell death may occur (169). This type of apoptosis is dependent on Fas and is poorly inhibited by Bcl-2 (168). This scenario is plausible because chronic activation causes expression of Fas on T cells (170). In addition, a death pathway involving Fas could explain the role of IL-2 in activation-induced death of effector cells, because IL-2 prevents the activation of FLICE inhibitor protein, which normally inhibits Fas signaling (171). Yet another form of T-cell death has been described in studies of superantigen-induced T-cell activation. Superantigen-stimulated effector T cells die after peak proliferation by a mechanism that involves internal production of reactive oxygen species, but not Fas, TNF receptors, or caspases (172). Reactive oxygen species may damage mitochondrial membranes leading to metabolic dysfunction and apoptosis.

The death of effector T cells is regulated by inflammation. In the absence of inflammation, the loss of antigen-specific T cells from the secondary lymphoid and nonlymphoid organs after the peak of proliferation is nearly complete (22). In contrast, many more cells survive the loss phase in both types of organs after injection of antigen or superantigen plus adjuvants such as LPS or IL-1 (21,22,134,173). This sparing effect can be induced by injection of LPS 24 hours after superantigen injection (173), and equally well in normal and CD28-deficient mice (174). Because lymphokine production by antigen-stimulated T cells is CD28 dependent (107), it is unlikely that this is the target of this late adjuvant effect. It is possible that LPS promotes survival by protecting T cells from the toxic effects of reactive oxygen species by inducing the Bcl-3 survival protein (175).

Memory Cells

Although the vast majority of effector cells die after the peak of proliferation, a stable population of antigen-experienced T cells survives for long periods of time if the antigen was initially presented in an inflammatory context (142). These long-lived "memory" cells are capable of very rapid responses that can produce protective immunity to a later challenge with a microbe (176). Memory cells can be distinguished from effector cells in that most memory cells are not blasts, are not in the cell cycle, and many are not directly cytolytic or producing lymphokines (142). In many ways, memory cells can be thought of as effector cells that have returned to a basal activation state. Indeed, several lines of evidence suggest that effector cells are precursors of memory cells (177,178).

Memory CD8 T Cells

Antigen-specific memory CD8 T cells have been studied extensively in viral and bacterial infections. The number of naïve antigen-specific CD8 T cells in the secondary lymphoid organs increases manyfold during the first week after infection, falls dramatically as effector cells die, and achieves a stable level about 2 weeks after infection that is lower than the peak level but higher than the starting level (6,7,121) (Fig. 2B). The number of antigen-specific CD8 T cells then does not change for the life of the host, at least in the case of one viral infection in mice that have a life span of about 2 years (121,179).

Unlike naïve CD8 T cells, memory CD8 T cells do not depend on MHC I molecules for survival (180). Thus, memory CD8 T-cell survival cannot be explained by chronic TCR signaling as a result of recognition of peptide–MHC I complexes derived from persistent antigen. Whereas most memory CD8 T cells are not cycling, a small fraction of the memory CD8 T population is proliferating in an MHC I–independent fashion at all times (111,180). This proliferation must be balanced by death since the total number of antigen-specific memory CD8 T cells does not change over time. Several observations suggest that IL-15 plays a role in this process. The antigen-independent proliferation of memory CD8 T cells is accelerated by injection of IL-15 (181) and blocked by injection of antibodies that prevent IL-15 from binding to its receptor (111). In addition, memory CD8 T cells are diminished in IL-15–deficient mice (182). Since IL-15 is produced by non–T cells during the innate immune response, it is possible that memory CD8 T cells are maintained as a consequence of IL-15 produced in response to other infections (181,183).

Memory CD8 T cells are heterogeneous. Human memory CD8 T cells can be divided into at least three subsets with the following phenotypes: CD45RA$^-$, CCR7$^+$; CD45RA$^-$, CCR7$^-$; and CD45RA$^+$, CCR7$^-$ (156,184) (Fig. 2B). The CD45RA$^-$, CCR7$^+$ memory cells also express CD62L and therefore are expected to recirculate through secondary lymphoid organs including lymph nodes and mucosal lymphoid organs (184). CD45RA$^-$, CCR7$^+$ memory CD8 T cells lack perforin and thus would not be expected to be directly cytotoxic (184). Virus antigen-specific CD8 T cells with these features are present in the lymphoid organs of mice beginning several weeks after viral infection (163).

The two CCR7$^-$ subsets also lack CD62L (184) and therefore could not enter lymph nodes and mucosal lymphoid organs through HEV. On the other hand, subsets within these populations express high levels of β1 and β7 integrins, sPSGL-1, and CCR5 (184); these molecules facilitate migration into nonlymphoid tissues, especially in the presence of inflammation (185). Both of the CCR7$^-$ subsets contain perforin (184) and are thus likely to be cytotoxic. The CD45RA$^+$, CCR7$^-$ subset possesses especially high levels of perforin and the direct *ex vivo* cytotoxic function of these cells has been demonstrated (156,184). Both of the CCR7$^-$ subsets produce IFN-γ rapidly after *in vitro* stimulation (184). All things considered, the CCR7$^-$ subsets of memory CD8 T cells are very similar to effector CD8 T cells, and have in fact been referred to as effector memory cells (185). The finding of virus antigen-specific CD8 T cells with *ex vivo* cytotoxic function in the nonlymphoid organs of mice weeks after viral infection lends credence to the existence of these effector memory cells (163). It is possible that the subset of cycling memory CD8 T cells observed in murine studies are the effector memory cells.

Memory CD4 T Cells

The number of antigen-specific CD4 T cells in the body drops sharply several days after the peak accumulation of effector cells, to a level that is lower than the peak and greater than the starting level (21,116,117,121) (Fig. 2A). The antigen-specific CD4 T cells that are present at this time are not cycling blasts and thus can be considered memory cells. In one type of viral infection, the number of virus antigen-specific

CD4 T cells then continues to fall at a slow rate over the next year (121), indicating that memory CD4 T cells are not indefinitely maintained as are memory CD8 T cells (Fig. 2A). This possibility is supported by other evidence of instability, including the findings that memory CD4 T cells revert some surface markers to the naïve phenotype over time (186–188), and lose enhanced helper function in hosts that contain normal numbers of T cells (189). Memory in the CD4 compartment may wane because cells that die are not replaced by proliferation of other memory T cells from the same cohort as in the case of memory CD8 T cells. This possibility is supported by the finding that the IL-15 growth factor does not enhance the proliferation of memory CD4 T cells (181).

It should be noted that other experiments indicate that memory CD4 T cells are just as stable as memory CD8 T cells. For example, antigen-specific CD4 T cells that are stimulated *in vitro* with antigen and then transferred into T-cell–deficient hosts survive for months even in the absence of MHC II molecules (190,191). Similarly, antigen-specific CD4 T cells retain the CD44^{high} phenotype and the capacity to produce IFN-γ for months after exposure to antigen in hosts that lack T cells with other specificities (192). Although these experiments indicate that memory CD4 T cells can survive indefinitely in the absence of antigen, it is possible that persistence is related to the "space-filling" homeostatic proliferation that occurs in hosts that lack other T cells.

As in the case of CD8 T cells, the population of memory CD4 T cells that survives after the death of effector cells is heterogeneous. Humans have at least two populations of memory CD4 T cells in peripheral blood, both lacking CD45RA (and presumably expressing CD45RO); one expresses CCR7 and the other lacks CCR7 (184) (Fig. 2A). The CD45RA$^-$, CCR7$^+$ cells produce IL-2 rapidly when stimulated with anti-CD3 antibody *in vitro,* but do not produce IFN-γ or IL-4 (184). The cells in this population express high levels of CD62L and thus would be expected to circulate through secondary lymphoid organs including lymph nodes, although subsets express CCR4, CCR6, and CXCR3 and thus could migrate into certain sites of inflammation (184). The existence of such lymphoid tissue-seeking memory cells is supported by the presence of antigen-specific CD4 T cells capable of rapid IL-2 but not IFN-γ production in the lymph nodes of mice several months after exposure to antigen (22).

CD45RA$^-$, CCR7$^-$ memory CD4 T cells differ from CD45RA$^-$, CCR7$^+$ memory cells with respect to function and trafficking. CD45RA$^-$, CCR7$^-$ memory CD4 T cells produce IFN-γ, IL-4, and IL-5 rapidly when stimulated with anti-CD3 antibody *in vitro,* but are poor producers of IL-2 under these conditions (184). These cells express low or variable levels of CD62L and high levels of fPSGL-1, and/or β1 and β7 integrins (184). This expression pattern predicts that these cells would be excluded from lymph nodes but could enter nonlymphoid sites of inflammation. This possibility is supported by the fact that the nonlymphoid tissues, especially liver, lungs, and gut are major reservoirs of antigen-experienced CD4 T cells in mice after effector cells disappear

in a response induced by intravenous injection of antigen plus adjuvant (22). Like CD45RA$^-$, CCR7$^-$ human CD4 T cells, the murine memory CD4 T cells in nonlymphoid tissues are potent IFN-γ producers but produce IL-2 poorly (22). Because Mackay et al. (193) found that memory T cells are constantly coming out of tissues and into afferent lymphatic vessels, it is possible that memory CD4 T cells in nonlymphoid tissues are not fixed there but recirculate through the spleen and/or nonlymphoid tissues.

The relationship between the antigen-specific effector CD4 T cells that are present at the peak of the response and the memory cells that survive is unclear. The lymphoid tissue-seeking memory cells (22) are similar to the CD62L$^-$, sPSGL-1$^-$ effector CD4 T cells (143) with respect to poor IFN-γ and IL-4 production, and thus could be derived from these cells. If so, then the lymphoid tissue-seeking memory cells may be potent B cell helpers like their CD62L$^-$, sPSGL-1$^-$ effector precursors (143). However for this scenario to be correct, the CD62L$^-$, sPSGL-1$^-$ effector CD4 T cells must re-express CD62L to be able to recirculate through the lymph nodes as memory cells. The similar production of IFN-γ or IL-4 but not IL-2 by nonlymphoid–tissue seeking memory cells (22) and CD62L$^+$, sPSGL-1$^+$ effector CD4 T cells (143) suggests that the former derive from the latter. If this is correct, then the CD62L$^+$, sPSGL-1$^+$ effector CD4 T cells must lose CD62L as they become memory cells.

It is also possible that effector cells give rise to lymphoid tissue-seeking CD45RA$^-$, CCR7$^+$ central memory cells, which in turn give rise to nonlymphoid tissue-seeking CD45RA$^-$, CCR7$^-$ effector memory cells. This possibility is supported by the finding that human CD45RA$^-$, CCR7$^+$ memory cells lose CCR7 after 10 days of *in vitro* stimulation and acquire the capacity to produce IFN-γ (184). Confirmation of this linear relationship has been hampered by a lack of anti-mouse CCR7 antibodies. Thus, it has not been possible to analyze the CCR7 expression on a defined population of antigen-specific CD4 T cells at precise times and locations after a primary and secondary exposure to antigen.

SUMMARY

What follows is an attempt to unify the information presented above into a hypothetical sequence of events that occurs in the lives of antigen-specific CD4 and CD8 T cells from the time that they first encounter antigen as naïve cells until they become memory cells. Since this process is not completely understood, certain aspects of this sequence are speculative. Educated guesses have been made to marry analogous information from studies of mice and humans, assuming that T cells from these species behave similarly.

A naïve T cell spends its life of about 2 months, in a series of 1-day stops in the T-cell areas of different secondary lymphoid organs with intervening trips through the blood. While in the T-cell area, a naïve T cell receives survival signals through the IL-7 receptor as it binds to IL-7 made by stromal cells, and the TCR as it binds to the relevant selecting self-peptide–MHC ligand on the surface of an APC, probably a dendritic cell. In the absence of infection or tissue damage, these dendritic cells exist in a semisuppressed state characterized by low expression of co-stimulatory ligands, and caused by suppressive cytokines made by phagocytes as they engulf apoptotic senescent cells during normal homeostasis.

A naïve T cell is roused from its survival program when it encounters an APC bearing the foreign peptide–MHC ligand for which its TCR has a high affinity. This APC will be a resident dendritic cell that captured free antigen in the T-cell area as it flowed in from the afferent lymph or blood, or a dendritic cell that acquired the antigen in a nonlymphoid tissue and then migrated into the T-cell area, depending on the nature and entry point of the antigen. If the antigen is part of a microbe or is administered with an adjuvant, then signals from the innate immune system will directly or indirectly activate dendritic cells from their semisuppressed state, enhancing their rate of migration into the T-cell areas and increasing antigen processing, stabilization of peptide–MHC complexes on the cell surface, and expression of co-stimulatory ligands. Since dendritic cells are one of the few types in the body that are capable of producing both peptide–MHC I and peptide–MHC II ligands from exogenous antigens, they are uniquely suited for antigen presentation to naïve CD8 and CD4 T cells expressing the appropriate TCRs.

Naïve CD4 T cells produce IL-2 within several hours of encountering an activated dendritic cell expressing the appropriate peptide–MHC II complexes and increased levels of co-stimulatory ligands. IL-2, other unknown T-cell growth factors, and co-factors such as IL-1 then stimulate the CD4 T cells to proliferate extensively, eventually leading to the development of $CD62L^+$, $sPSGL$-1^+ and $CD62L^-$, $sPSGL^-1$-effector cells. The $CD62L^-$, $sPSGL^-$ effector cells gain expression of CXCR5, allowing them to sense the follicular chemokine CXCL13 and migrate into the follicles to provide helper signals to antigen-specific B cells. The $CD62L^+$, $sPSGL$-1^+ effector cells acquire the capacity to produce IFN-γ or IL-4, depending on the cytokines produced by innate immune cells, and then leave the secondary lymphoid organs through the efferent lymphatic vessels, enter the blood, and migrate into inflamed tissues where they produce IFN-γ or IL-4 in response to antigen presentation by tissue APC. The activating effects of these lymphokines and antibodies on the microbicidal activities of macrophages and granulocytes, lead to elimination of the antigen. At this point, most of the effector cells die by apoptosis. However, some of the effector cells return to a resting state and survive as memory cells. $CD62L^+$, $sPSGL$-1^+ effector cells give rise to $CCR7^-$ memory CD4 T cells that recirculate via the blood through the spleen, or the spleen and nonlymphoid tissues. This recirculation pattern would enable these memory cells to produce IFN-γ or IL-4 rapidly during secondary immune responses in nonlymphoid tissues where antigens enter the body. The $CD62L^-$, $sPSGL^-$ effector cells with B cell helper function may give rise to $CCR7^+$ memory CD4 T cells that re-express CD62L and recirculate via blood and efferent lymph through

spleen and lymph nodes like naïve cells. These memory cells may help memory B cells produce antibody in the lymphoid tissues during secondary immune responses, or they may proliferate to produce more effector cells. If antigen does not enter the body a second time, both populations of memory cells may disappear slowly over time because they do not proliferate to renew themselves.

Naïve CD8 T cells also produce IL-2 within several hours of encountering an activated dendritic cell expressing the appropriate peptide–MHC I ligands. IL-2, other unknown T-cell growth factors, and co-factors such as IL-12 then stimulate the CD8 T cells to proliferate extensively. Since CD8 T cells rapidly lose the ability to produce IL-2, their proliferation is aided by IL-2 produced by CD4 T cells. The proliferating CD8 T cells develop into perforin-expressing cytotoxic effector cells, many of which rapidly migrate into nonlymphoid tissues. These effector CD8 T cells then kill cells in nonlymphoid tissues that display the relevant peptide–MHC I complexes. As such cells are eliminated, most of the effector CD8 T cells die by apoptosis. However, some of the effector cells survive in nonlymphoid tissues for long periods of time as $CCR7^-$ memory cells and retain their cytotoxic potential. Other noncytotoxic $CCR7^+$ memory CD8 T cells survive in the lymphoid tissues. All memory CD8 T cells constitutively express the IL-15 receptor and use it to proliferate periodically in response to IL-15, which in turn is perhaps made in response to unrelated immune responses. This proliferation replaces memory cells that die and results in a constant number of memory CD8 cells for the life of the host, even in the absence of MHC I molecules. When exposed to antigen a second time, the memory CD8 T cells in nonlymphoid tissues rapidly kill cells displaying peptide–MHC I molecules, whereas the memory CD8 T cells in lymphoid organs cells proliferate extensively and rapidly acquire cytotoxic potential.

ACKNOWLEDGMENTS

I am grateful to Drs. Mathew Mescher, Daniel Mueller, Andre Itano, and Stephen Jameson for their helpful suggestions.

REFERENCES

1. Davis MM, Boniface JJ, Reich Z, et al. Ligand recognition by alpha beta T cell receptors. *Annu Rev Immunol* 1998;16:523.
2. Rothman AL, Yamada Y, Jameson J, et al. Assessment of human CD4+ and CD8+ T lymphocyte responses in experimental viral vaccine studies. *Dev Biol (Basel)* 1998;95:95.
3. Altman JD, Moss PAH, Goulder JR, et al. Phenotypic analysis of antigen-specific T lymphocytes. *Science* 1996;274:94.
4. Kozono H, White J, Clements J, et al. Production of soluble MHC class II proteins with covalently bound single peptides. *Nature* 1994; 369:151.
5. O'Herrin SM, Lebowitz MS, Bieler JG, et al. Analysis of the expression of peptide–major histocompatibility complexes using high affinity soluble divalent T cell receptors. *J Exp Med* 1997;186:1333.
6. Murali-Krishna K, Altman JD, Suresh M, et al. Counting antigen-specific CD8 T cells: a reevaluation of bystander activation during viral infection. *Immunity* 1998;8:177.

7. Busch DH, Pilip IM, Vijh S, et al. Coordinate regulation of complex T cell populations responding to bacterial infection. *Immunity* 1998;8:353.

8. Kotzin BL, Falta MT, Crawford F, et al. Use of soluble peptide-DR4 tetramers to detect synovial T cells specific for cartilage antigens in patients with rheumatoid arthritis. *Proc Natl Acad Sci U S A* 2000;97:291.

9. Jenkins MK, Khoruts A, Ingulli E, et al. *In vivo* activation of antigen-specific CD4 T cells. *Annu Rev Immunol* 2001;19:23.

10. Kedl RM, Rees WA, Hildeman DA, et al. T cells compete for access to antigen-bearing antigen-presenting cells. *J Exp Med* 2000;192:1105.

11. Smith AL, Wikstrom ME, Fazekas de St Groth B. Visualizing T cell competition for peptide/MHC complexes: a specific mechanism to minimize the effect of precursor frequency. *Immunity* 2000;13:783.

12. Laouar Y, Crispe IN. Functional flexibility in T cells: independent regulation of CD4+ T cell proliferation and effector function *in vivo*. *Immunity* 2000;13:291.

13. Davis MM. T cell receptor gene diversity and selection. *Annu Rev Biochem* 1990;59:475.

14. Kappler JW, Wade T, White J, et al. A T cell receptor Vb segment that imparts reactivity to a class II major histocompatibility complex product. *Cell* 1987;49:263.

15. Ramsdell F, Lantz T, Fowlkes BJ. A nondeletional mechanism of thymic self tolerance. *Science* 1989;246:1038.

16. McGargill MA, Derbinski JM, Hogquist KA. Receptor editing in developing T cells. *Nat Immunol* 2000;1:336.

17. Jameson SC, Hogquist KA, Bevan MJ. Positive selection of thymocytes. *Annu Rev Immunol* 1995;13:93.

18. Ford WL, Gowans JL. The traffic of lymphocytes. *Semin Hematol* 1969;6:67.

19. Mackay CR. Homing of naive, memory and effector lymphocytes. *Curr Opin Immunol* 1993;5:423.

20. Cyster JG. Chemokines and cell migration in secondary lymphoid organs. *Science* 1999;286:2098.

21. Kearney ER, Pape KA, Loh DY, et al. Visualization of peptide-specific T cell immunity and peripheral tolerance induction *in vivo*. *Immunity* 1994;1:327.

22. Reinhardt RL, Khoruts A, Merica R, et al. Visualizing the generation of memory CD4 T cells in the whole body. *Nature* 2001;410:101.

23. Campbell JJ, Butcher EC. Chemokines in tissue-specific and microenvironment-specific lymphocyte homing. *Curr Opin Immunol* 2000;12:336.

24. Cyster JG, Goodnow CC. Pertussis toxin inhibits migration of B and T lymphocytes into splenic white pulp cords. *J Exp Med* 1995;182:581.

25. Alferink J, Tafuri A, Vestweber D, et al. Control of neonatal tolerance to tissue antigens by peripheral T cell trafficking. *Science* 1998;282:1338.

26. Sprent J, Tough DF. Lymphocyte life-span and memory. *Science* 1994;265:1395.

27. Ferreira C, Barthlott T, Garcia S, et al. Differential survival of naive CD4 and CD8 T cells. *J Immunol* 2000;165:3689.

28. Rooke R, Waltzinger C, Benoist C, et al. Targeted complementation of MHC class II deficiency by intrathymic delivery of recombinant adenoviruses. *Immunity* 1997;7:123.

29. Tanchot C, Lemonnier FA, Perarnau B, et al. Differential requirements for survival and proliferation of CD8 memory T cells. *Science* 1997;276:2057–62.

30. Dorfman JR, Stefanova I, Yasutomo K, et al. CD4+ T cell survival is not directly linked to self–MHC-induced TCR signaling. *Nat Immunol* 2000;1:329.

31. Schluns KS, Kieper WC, Jameson SC, et al. Interleukin-7 mediates the homeostasis of naive and memory CD8 T cells *in vivo*. *Nat Immunol* 2000;1:426.

32. Tan JT, Dudl E, LeRoy E, et al. IL-7 is critical for homeostatic proliferation and survival of naive T cells. *Proc Natl Acad Sci U S A* 2001;98:8732.

33. Goldrath AW, Bevan MJ. Low-affinity ligands for the TCR drive proliferation of mature CD8+ T cells in lymphopenic hosts. *Immunity* 1999;11:183.

34. Bender J, Mitchell T, Kappler J, et al. CD4+ T cell division in irradiated mice requires peptides distinct from those responsible for thymic selection. *J Exp Med* 1999;190:367.

35. Ernst B, Lee DS, Chang JM, et al. The peptide ligands mediating positive selection in the thymus control T cell survival and homeostatic proliferation in the periphery. *Immunity* 1999;11:173.

36. Kieper WC, Jameson SC. Homeostatic expansion and phenotypic conversion of naive T cells in response to self peptide/MHC ligands. *Proc Natl Acad Sci U S A* 1999;96:13306.

37. Prlic M, Blazar BR, Khoruts A, et al. Homeostatic expansion occurs independently of costimulatory signals. *J Immunol* 2001;167:5664.

38. Banchereau J, Steinman RM. Dendritic cells and the control of immunity. *Nature* 1998;392:245.

39. Vremec D, Shortman K. Dendritic cell subtypes in mouse lymphoid organs: cross-correlation of surface markers, changes with incubation, and differences among thymus, spleen, and lymph nodes. *J Immunol* 1997;159:565.

40. Pulendran B, Lingappa J, Kennedy MK, et al. Developmental pathways of dendritic cells *in vivo*: distinct function, phenotype, and localization of dendritic cell subsets in FLT3 ligand–treated mice. *J Immunol* 1997;159:2222.

41. Huleatt JW, Lefrancois L. Antigen-driven induction of CD11c on intestinal intraepithelial lymphocytes and CD8+ T cells *in vivo*. *J Immunol* 1995;154:5684.

42. Traver D, Akashi K, Manz M, et al. Development of CD8alpha-positive dendritic cells from a common myeloid progenitor. *Science* 2000;290:2152.

43. Manz MG, Traver D, Miyamoto T, et al. Dendritic cell potentials of early lymphoid and myeloid progenitors. *Blood* 2001;97:3333.

44. del Hoyo GM, Martin P, Arias CF, et al. CD8alpha(+) dendritic cells originate from the CD8alpha(−) dendritic cell subset by a maturation process involving CD8alpha, DEC-205, and CD24 up-regulation. *Blood* 2002;99:999.

45. Ruedl C, Koebel P, Bachmann M, et al. Anatomical origin of dendritic cells determines their life span in peripheral lymph nodes. *J Immunol* 2000;165:4910.

46. Kamath AT, Pooley J, O'Keeffe MA, et al. The development, maturation, and turnover rate of mouse spleen dendritic cell populations. *J Immunol* 2000;165:6762.

47. Nakano H, Yanagita M, Gunn MD. CD11c(+)B220(+)GR-1(+) cells in mouse lymph nodes and spleen display characteristics of plasmacytoid dendritic cells. *J Exp Med* 2001;194:1171.

48. Rissoan MC, Soumelis V, Kadowaki N, et al. Reciprocal control of T helper cell and dendritic cell differentiation. *Science* 1999;283:1183.

49. Anjuere F, Martin P, Ferrero I, et al. Definition of dendritic cell subpopulations present in the spleen, Peyer's patches, lymph nodes, and skin of the mouse. *Blood* 1999;93:590.

50. Henri S, Vremec D, Kamath A, et al. The dendritic cell populations of mouse lymph nodes. *J Immunol* 2001;167:741.

51. Valladeau J, Ravel O, Dezutter-Dambuyant C, et al. Langerin, a novel C-type lectin specific to Langerhans cells, is an endocytic receptor that induces the formation of Birbeck granules. *Immunity* 2000;12:71.

52. DeSmedt T, Pajak B, Muraille E, et al. Regulation of dendritic cell numbers and maturation by lipopolysaccharide *in vivo*. *J Exp Med* 1996;184:1413.

53. Cumberbatch M, Kimber I. Dermal tumour necrosis factor-alpha induces dendritic cell migration to draining lymph nodes, and possibly provides one stimulus for Langerhans' cell migration. *Immunology* 1992;75:257.

54. Shornick LP, Bisarya AK, Chaplin DD. IL-1beta is essential for Langerhans cell activation and antigen delivery to the lymph nodes during contact sensitization: evidence for a dermal source of IL-1beta. *Cell Immunol* 2001;211:105.

55. Banchereau J, Briere F, Caux C, et al. Immunobiology of dendritic cells. *Annu Rev Immunol* 2000;18:767.

56. Turley SJ, Inaba K, Garrett WS, et al. Transport of peptide–MHC class II complexes in developing dendritic cells. *Science* 2000;288:522.

57. Cella M, Engering A, Pinet V, et al. Inflammatory stimuli induce accumulation of MHC class II complexes on dendritic cells. *Nature* 1997;388:782.

58. Brocker T. Survival of mature CD4 T lymphocytes is dependent on major histocompatibility complex class II–expressing dendritic cells. *J Exp Med* 1997;186:1223.

59. Zell T, Khoruts A, Ingulli E, et al. Single-cell analysis of signal transduction in CD4 T cells stimulated by antigen *in vivo*. *Proc Natl Acad Sci U S A* 2001;98:10805.

60. Savill J, Fadok V. Corpse clearance defines the meaning of cell death. *Nature* 2000;407:784.

61. Fadok VA, Bratton DL, Rose DM, et al. A receptor for phosphatidylserine-specific clearance of apoptotic cells. *Nature* 2000; 405:85.

62. Fadok VA, Bratton DL, Konowal A, et al. Macrophages that have ingested apoptotic cells *in vitro* inhibit proinflammatory cytokine production through autocrine/paracrine mechanisms involving TGF-beta, PGE2, and PAF. *J Clin Invest* 1998;101:890.

63. Yamaguchi Y, Tsumura H, Miwa M, et al. Contrasting effects of TGF-beta 1 and TNF-alpha on the development of dendritic cells from progenitors in mouse bone marrow. *Stem Cells* 1997;15:144.

64. Scott RS, McMahon EJ, Pop SM, et al. Phagocytosis and clearance of apoptotic cells is mediated by MER. *Nature* 2001;411:207.

65. Lu Q, Lemke G. Homeostatic regulation of the immune system by receptor tyrosine kinases of the Tyro 3 family. *Science* 2001;293:306.

66. Rosette C, Werlen G, Daniels MA, et al. The impact of duration versus extent of TCR occupancy on T cell activation: a revision of the kinetic proofreading model. *Immunity* 2001;15:59.

67. Janeway CA Jr. Approaching the asymptote? Evolution and revolution in immunology. *Cold Spring Harb Symp Quant Biol* 1989;54:1.

68. Matzinger P. Tolerance, danger, and the extended family. *Annu Rev Immunol* 1994;12:991.

69. Randolph GJ, Inaba K, Robbiani DF, et al. Differentiation of phagocytic monocytes into lymph node dendritic cells *in vivo*. *Immunity* 1999;11:753.

70. Randolph GJ, Beaulieu S, Lebecque S, et al. Differentiation of monocytes into dendritic cells in a model of transendothelial trafficking. *Science* 1998;282:480.

71. Whitmire JK, Ahmed R. Costimulation in antiviral immunity: differential requirements for CD4(+) and CD8(+) T cell responses. *Curr Opin Immunol* 2000;12:448.

72. Gajewski TF, Renauld JC, Van Pel A, et al. Costimulation with B7-1, IL-6, and IL-12 is sufficient for primary generation of murine antitumor cytolytic T lymphocytes *in vitro*. *J Immunol* 1995;154:5637.

73. Curtsinger JM, Schmidt CS, Mondino A, et al. Inflammatory cytokines provide a third signal for activation of naive CD4+ and CD8+ T cells. *J Immunol* 1999;162:3256.

74. Reis e Sousa C, Hieny S, Scharton-Kersten T, et al. *In vivo* microbial stimulation induces rapid CD40 ligand-independent production of interleukin 12 by dendritic cells and their redistribution to T cell areas. *J Exp Med* 1997;186:1819.

75. Pamer E, Cresswell P. Mechanisms of MHC class I-restricted antigen processing. *Annu Rev Immunol* 1998;16:323.

76. Bevan MJ. Cross-priming for a secondary cytotoxic response to minor H antigens with H-2 congenic cells which do not cross-react in the cytotoxic assay. *J Exp Med* 1976;143:1283.

77. Heath WR, Carbone FR. Cross-presentation, dendritic cells, tolerance and immunity. *Annu Rev Immunol* 2001;19:47.

78. den Haan JM, Lehar SM, Bevan MJ. CD8(+) but not CD8(-) dendritic cells cross-prime cytotoxic T cells *in vivo*. *J Exp Med* 2000;192: 1685.

79. Kovacsovics-Bankowski M, Rock KL. A phagosome-to-cytosol pathway for exogenous antigens presented on MHC class I molecules. *Science* 1995;267:243.

80. Brossart P, Bevan MJ. Presentation of exogenous protein antigens on major histocompatibility complex class I molecules by dendritic cells: pathway of presentation and regulation by cytokines. *Blood* 1997;90:1594.

81. Bennett SR, Carbone FR, Karamalis F, et al. Induction of a CD8+ cytotoxic T lymphocyte response by cross-priming requires cognate CD4+ T cell help. *J Exp Med* 1997;186:65.

82. Schoenberger SP, Toes RE, van der Voort EI, et al. T-cell help for cytotoxic T lymphocytes is mediated by CD40-CD40L interactions. *Nature* 1998;393:480.

83. Lappin MB, Kimber I, Norval M. The role of dendritic cells in cutaneous immunity. *Arch Dermatol Res* 1996;288:109.

84. Romani N, Ratzinger G, Pfaller K, et al. Migration of dendritic cells into lymphatics-the Langerhans cell example: routes, regulation, and relevance. *Int Rev Cytol* 2001;207:237.

85. Nalefski EA, Rao A. Nature of the ligand recognized by a hapten- and carrier-specific, MHC- restricted T cell receptor. *J Immunol* 1993; 150:3806.

86. Honda S, Zhang W, Kalergis AM, et al. Hapten addition to an MHC class I-binding peptide causes substantial adjustments of the TCR structure of the responding CD8(+) T cells. *J Immunol* 2001;167:4276.

87. Franco A, Yokoyama T, Huynh D, et al. Fine specificity and MHC restriction of trinitrophenyl-specific CTL. *J Immunol* 1999;162:3388.

88. Horton H, Weston SD, Hewitt CR. Allergy to antibiotics: T-cell recognition of amoxicillin is HLA-DR restricted and does not require antigen processing. *Allergy* 1998;53:83.

89. Flint MS, Dearman RJ, Kimber I, et al. Production and *in situ* localization of cutaneous tumour necrosis factor alpha (TNF-alpha) and interleukin 6 (IL-6) following skin sensitization. *Cytokine* 1998;10:213.

90. Nuriya S, Yagita H, Okumura K, et al. The differential role of CD86 and CD80 co-stimulatory molecules in the induction and the effector phases of contact hypersensitivity. *Int Immunol* 1996;8:917.

91. Jones DA, Morris AG, Kimber I. Assessment of the functional activity of antigen-bearing dendritic cells isolated from the lymph nodes of contact-sensitized mice. *Int Arch Allergy Appl Immunol* 1989;90:230.

92. De Creus A, Van Beneden K, Taghon T, et al. Langerhans cells that have matured *in vivo* in the absence of T cells are fully capable of inducing a helper CD4 as well as a cytotoxic CD8 response. *J Immunol* 2000;165:645.

93. Lynch DH, Gurish MF, Daynes RA. Relationship between epidermal Langerhans cell density ATPase activity and the induction of contact hypersensitivity. *J Immunol* 1981;126:1892.

94. Neutra MR, Mantis NJ, Kraehenbuhl JP. Collaboration of epithelial cells with organized mucosal lymphoid tissues. *Nat Immunol* 2001;2:1004.

95. Iwasaki A, Kelsall BL. Localization of distinct Peyer's patch dendritic cell subsets and their recruitment by chemokines macrophage inflammatory protein (MIP)-3alpha, MIP-3beta, and secondary lymphoid organ chemokine. *J Exp Med* 2000;191:1381.

96. Vermaelen KY, Carro-Muino I, Lambrecht BN, et al. Specific migratory dendritic cells rapidly transport antigen from the airways to the thoracic lymph nodes. *J Exp Med* 2001;193:51.

97. Manickasingham S, Reis e Sousa C. Microbial and T cell-derived stimuli regulate antigen presentation by dendritic cells *in vivo*. *J Immunol* 2000;165:5027.

98. Zhong G, Sousa CR, Germain RN. Antigen-unspecific B cells and lymphoid dendritic cells both show extensive surface expression of processed antigen-major histocompatibility complex class II complexes after soluble protein exposure *in vivo* or *in vitro*. *J Exp Med* 1997;186:673.

99. Gretz JE, Norbury CC, Anderson AO, et al. Lymph-borne chemokines and other low molecular weight molecules reach high endothelial venules via specialized conduits while a functional barrier limits access to the lymphocyte microenvironments in lymph node cortex. *J Exp Med* 2000;192:1425.

100. Ebnet K, Kaldjian EP, Anderson AO, et al. Orchestrated information transfer underlying leukocyte endothelial interactions. *Annu Rev Immunol* 1996;14:155.

101. Steinman RM, Pack M, Inaba K. Dendritic cells in the T-cell areas of lymphoid organs. *Immunol Rev* 1997;156:25.

102. Pooley JL, Heath WR, Shortman K. Intravenous soluble antigen is presented to CD4 T cells by CD8(−) dendritic cells, but cross-presented to CD8 T cells by CD8(+) dendritic cells. *J Immunol* 2001;166:5327.

103. Reis e Sousa C, Germain RN. Analysis of adjuvant function by direct visualization of antigen presentation *in vivo*: endotoxin promotes accumulation of antigen-bearing dendritic cells in the T cell areas of lymphoid tissue. *J Immunol* 1999;162:6552.

104. Kane LP, Lin J, Weiss A. Signal transduction by the TCR for antigen. *Curr Opin Immunol* 2000;12:242.

105. Crabtree GR. Generic signals and specific outcomes: signaling through Ca2+, calcineurin, and NF-AT. *Cell* 1999;96:611.

106. Sette A, Buus S, Colon S, et al. I-Ad-binding peptides derived from unrelated protein antigens share a common structural motif. *J Immunol* 1988;141:45.

107. Khoruts A, Mondino A, Pape KA, et al. A natural immunological adjuvant enhances T cell clonal expansion through a CD28-dependent, interleukin (IL)-2-independent mechanism. *J Exp Med* 1998;187:225.

108. Veiga-Fernandes H, Walter U, Bourgeois C, et al. Response of naive and memory CD8+ T cells to antigen stimulation *in vivo*. *Nat Immunol* 2000;1:47.

109. Schorle H, Holtschke T, Hunig T, et al. Development and function of T cells in mice rendered interleukin-2 deficient by gene targeting. *Nature* 1991;352:621.

110. Kneitz B, Herrmann T, Yonehara S, et al. Normal clonal expansion but impaired Fas-mediated cell death and anergy induction in interleukin-2-deficient mice. *Eur J Immunol* 1995;25:2572.

111. Ku CC, Murakami M, Sakamoto A, et al. Control of homeostasis of CD8+ memory T cells by opposing cytokines. *Science* 2000; 288:675.

112. Leung DT, Morefield S, Willerford DM. Regulation of lymphoid homeostasis by IL-2 receptor signals *in vivo*. *J Immunol* 2000;164: 3527.

113. Lantz O, Grandjean I, Matzinger P, et al. Gamma chain required for naive CD4+ T cell survival but not for antigen proliferation. *Nat Immunol* 2000;1:54.

114. Gudmundsdottir H, Wells AD, Turka LA. Dynamics and requirements of T cell clonal expansion *in vivo* at the single-cell level: effector function is linked to proliferative capacity. *J Immunol* 1999;162:5212.

115. Rocha B, von Boehmer H. Peripheral selection of the T cell repertoire. *Science* 1991;251:1225.

116. McHeyzer-Williams MG, Davis MM. Antigen-specific development of primary and memory T cells *in vivo*. *Science* 1995;268:106.

117. Gulbranson-Judge A, MacLennan I. Sequential antigen-specific growth of T cells in the T zones and follicles in response to pigeon cytochrome c. *Eur J Immunol* 1996;26:1830.

118. Luther SA, Gulbranson-Judge A, Acha-Orbea H, et al. Viral superantigen drives extrafollicular and follicular B cell differentiation leading to virus-specific antibody production. *J Exp Med* 1997;185: 551.

119. Zimmerman C, Brduscha-Riem K, Blaser C, et al. Visualization, characterization, and turnover of CD8+ memory T cells in virus-infected hosts. *J Exp Med* 1996;183:1367.

120. Blattman JN, Antia R, Sourdive DJ, et al. Estimating the precursor frequency of naive antigen-specific CD8 T cells. *J Exp Med* 2002; 195:657.

121. Homann D, Teyton L, Oldstone MB. Differential regulation of antiviral T-cell immunity results in stable CD8+ but declining CD4+ T-cell memory. *Nat Med* 2001;7:913.

122. Kearney ER, Walunas TL, Karr RW, et al. Antigen-dependent clonal expansion of a trace population of antigen-specific CD4+ T cells *in vivo* is dependent on CD28 costimulation and inhibited by CTLA-4. *J Immunol* 1995;155:1032.

123. Suresh M, Whitmire JK, Harrington LE, et al. Role of CD28-B7 interactions in generation and maintenance of CD8 T cell memory. *J Immunol* 2001;167:5565.

124. Grewal IS, Xu J, Flavell RA. Impairment of antigen-specific T-cell priming in mice lacking CD40 ligand. *Nature* 1995;378:617.

125. Garside P, Ingulli E, Merica RR, et al. Visualization of specific B and T lymphocyte interactions in the lymph node. *Science* 1998;281:96.

126. Buhlmann JE, Gonzalez M, Ginther B, et al. Sustained expansion of CD8+ T cells requires CD154 expression by Th cells in acute graft versus host disease. *J Immunol* 1999;162:4373.

127. Ranheim EA, Kipps TJ. Activated T cells induce expression of B7/BB1 on normal or leukemic B cells through a CD40-dependent signal. *J Exp Med* 1993;177:925.

128. Viola A, Schroeder S, Sakakibara Y, et al. T lymphocyte costimulation mediated by reorganization of membrane microdomains. *Science* 1999;283:680.

129. Bromley SK, Iaboni A, Davis SJ, et al. The immunological synapse and CD28-CD80 interactions. *Nat Immunol* 2001;2:1159.

130. Salomon B, Bluestone JA. Complexities of CD28/B7: CTLA-4 costimulatory pathways in autoimmunity and transplantation. *Annu Rev Immunol* 2001;19:225.

131. Watts TH, DeBenedette MA. T cell co-stimulatory molecules other than CD28. *Curr Opin Immunol* 1999;11:286.

132. Rogers PR, Song J, Gramaglia I, et al. Ox40 promotes bcl-xl and bcl-2 expression and is essential for long-term survival of CD4 T cells. *Immunity* 2001;15:445.

133. Schmidt CS, Mescher MF. Adjuvant effect of IL-12: conversion of peptide antigen administration from tolerizing to immunizing for CD8+ T cells *in vivo*. *J Immunol* 1999;163:2561.

134. Pape KA, Khoruts A, Mondino A, et al. Inflammatory cytokines enhance the *in vivo* clonal expansion and differentiation of antigen-activated CD4+ T cells. *J Immunol* 1997;159:591.

135. Sun S, Kishimoto H, Sprent J. DNA as an adjuvant: capacity of insect DNA and synthetic oligodeoxynucleotides to augment T cell responses to specific antigen. *J Exp Med* 1998;187:1145.

136. Medzhitov R, Janeway C Jr. Innate immune recognition: mechanisms and pathways. *Immunol Rev* 2000;173:89.

137. Schnare M, Barton GM, Holt AC, et al. Toll-like receptors control activation of adaptive immune responses. *Nat Immunol* 2001;2:947.

138. Jones BW, Means TK, Heldwein KA, et al. Different Toll-like receptor agonists induce distinct macrophage responses. *J Leukoc Biol* 2001;69:1036.

139. Kaisho T, Takeuchi O, Kawai T, et al. Endotoxin-induced maturation of MyD88-deficient dendritic cells. *J Immunol* 2001;166:5688.

140. Joseph SB, Miner KT, Croft M. Augmentation of naive, Th1 and Th2 effector CD4 responses by IL-6, IL-1 and TNF. *Eur J Immunol* 1998;28:277.

141. Lichtman AH, Chin J, Schmidt JA, et al. Role of interleukin 1 in the activation of T lymphocytes. *Proc Natl Acad Sci U S A* 1988;85:9699.

142. Dutton RW, Bradley LM, Swain SL. T cell memory. *Annu Rev Immunol* 1998;16:201.

143. Campbell DJ, Kim CH, Butcher EC. Separable effector T cell populations specialized for B cell help or tissue inflammation. *Nat Immunol* 2001;2:876.

144. Borges E, Tietz W, Steegmaier M, et al. P-selectin glycoprotein ligand-1 (PSGL-1) on T helper 1 but not on T helper 2 cells binds to P-selectin and supports migration into inflamed skin. *J Exp Med* 1997;185:573.

145. Fong TA, Mosmann TR. The role of IFN-gamma in delayed-type hypersensitivity mediated by Th1 clones. *J Immunol* 1989;143:2887.

146. Xie H, Lim YC, Luscinskas FW, et al. Acquisition of selectin binding and peripheral homing properties by CD4(+) and CD8(+) T cells. *J Exp Med* 1999;189:1765.

147. Murphy KM. T lymphocyte differentiation in the periphery. *Curr Opin Immunol* 1998;10:226.

148. Campbell DJ, Butcher EC. Rapid Acquisition of Tissue-specific Homing Phenotypes by CD4(+) T cells activated in cutaneous or mucosal lymphoid tissues. *J Exp Med* 2002;195:135.

149. Mohrs M, Shinkai K, Mohrs K, et al. Analysis of type 2 immunity *in vivo* with a bicistronic IL-4 reporter. *Immunity* 2001;15:303.

150. Fuller KA, Kanagawa O, Nahm MH. T cells within germinal centers are specific for the immunizing antigen. *J Immunol* 1993;151:4505.

151. Zheng B, Han S, Kelsoe G. T helper cells in murine germinal centers are antigen-specific emigrants that downregulate Thy-1. *J Exp Med* 1996;184:1083.

152. Ansel KM, McHeyzer-Williams LJ, Ngo VN, et al. *In vivo*-activated CD4 T cells upregulate CXC chemokine receptor 5 and reprogram their response to lymphoid chemokines. *J Exp Med* 1999;190:1123.

153. Cyster JG, Goodnow CC. Antigen-induced exclusion from follicles and anergy are separate and complementary processes that influence peripheral B cell fate. *Immunity* 1995;3:691.

154. Fulcher DA, Lyons AB, Korn SL, et al. The fate of self-reactive B cells depends primarily on the degree of antigen receptor engagement and availability of T cell help. *J Exp Med* 1996;183:2313.

155. Harrington LE, Galvan M, Baum LG, et al. Differentiating between memory and effector CD8 T cells by altered expression of cell surface O-glycans. *J Exp Med* 2000;191:1241.

156. Hamann D, Baars PA, Rep MH, et al. Phenotypic and functional separation of memory and effector human CD8+ T cells. *J Exp Med* 1997;186:1407.

157. Lauvau G, Vijh S, Kong P, et al. Priming of memory but not effector CD8 T cells by a killed bacterial vaccine. *Science* 2001;294:1735.

158. Matloubian M, Concepcion RJ, Ahmed R. CD4+ T cells are required to sustain CD8+ cytotoxic T-cell responses during chronic viral infection. *J Virol* 1994;68:8056.

159. Finch RJ, Fields PE, Greenberg PD. A transcriptional block in the IL-2 promoter at the -150 AP-1 site in effector CD8+ T cells. *J Immunol* 2001;166:6530.

160. Tham EL, Mescher MF. Signaling alterations in activation-induced nonresponsive CD8 T cells. *J Immunol* 2001;167:2040.

161. Flynn KJ, Belz GT, Altman JD, et al. Virus-specific CD8+ T cells in primary and secondary influenza pneumonia. *Immunity* 1998;8:683.

162. Hendriks J, Gravestein LA, Tesselaar K, et al. CD27 is required for generation and long-term maintenance of T cell immunity. *Nat Immunol* 2000;1:433.

163. Masopust D, Vezys V, Marzo AL, et al. Preferential localization of effector memory cells in nonlymphoid tissue. *Science* 2001;291:2413.

164. Weninger W, Crowley MA, Manjunath N, et al. Migratory properties of naive, effector, and memory CD8(+) T cells. *J Exp Med* 2001; 194:953.

165. Lefrancois L, Parker CM, Olson S, et al. The role of beta7 integrins in CD8 T cell trafficking during an antiviral immune response. *J Exp Med* 1999;189:1631.

166. Liblau RS, Tish R, Shokat K, et al. Intravenous injection of soluble antigen induces thymic and peripheral T cell apoptosis. *Proc Natl Acad Sci USA* 1996;93:3031.

167. Petschner F, Zimmerman C, Strasser A, et al. Constitutive expression of Bcl-xL or Bcl-2 prevents peptide antigen-induced T cell deletion but does not influence T cell homeostasis after a viral infection. *Eur J Immunol* 1998;28:560.

168. Lenardo M, Chan KM, Hornung F, et al. Mature T lymphocyte apoptosis—immune regulation in a dynamic and unpredictable antigenic environment. *Annu Rev Immunol* 1999;17:221.

169. Refaeli Y, Van Parijs L, Abbas AK. Genetic models of abnormal apoptosis in lymphocytes. *Immunol Rev* 1999;169:273.

170. Hiromatsu K, Aoki Y, Makino M, et al. Increased Fas antigen expression in murine retrovirus-induced immunodeficiency syndrome, MAIDS. *Eur J Immunol* 1994;24:2446.

171. Refaeli Y, Van Parijs L, London CA, et al. Biochemical mechanisms of IL-2-regulated Fas-mediated T cell apoptosis. *Immunity* 1998;8:615.

172. Hildeman DA, Mitchell T, Teague TK, et al. Reactive oxygen species regulate activation-induced T cell apoptosis. *Immunity* 1999;10:735.

173. Vella AT, McCormack JE, Linsley PS, et al. Lipopolysaccharide interferes with the induction of peripheral T cell death. *Immunity* 1995;2:261.

174. Vella AT, Mitchell T, Groth B, et al. CD28 engagement and proinflammatory cytokines contribute to T cell expansion and long-term survival *in vivo*. *J Immunol* 1997;158:4714.

175. Mitchell TC, Hildeman D, Kedl RM, et al. Immunological adjuvants promote activated T cell survival via induction of Bcl-3. *Nat Immunol* 2001;2:397.

176. Ahmed R, Gray D. Immunological memory and protective immunity: understanding their relation. *Science* 1996;272:54.

177. Opferman JT, Ober BT, Ashton-Rickardt PG. Linear differentiation of cytotoxic effectors into memory T lymphocytes. *Science* 1999;283:1745.

178. Jacob J, Baltimore D. Modelling T-cell memory by genetic marking of memory T cells *in vivo*. *Nature* 1999;399:593.

179. Jamieson BD, Ahmed R. T cell memory. Long-term persistence of virus-specific cytotoxic T cells. *J Exp Med* 1989;169:1993.

180. Murali-Krishna K, Lau LL, Sambhara S, et al. Persistence of memory CD8 T cells in MHC class I-deficient mice. *Science* 1999;286:1377.

181. Zhang X, Sun S, Hwang I, et al. Potent and selective stimulation of memory-phenotype CD8+ T cells *in vivo* by IL-15. *Immunity* 1998;8:591.

182. Kennedy MK, Glaccum M, Brown SN, et al. Reversible defects in natural killer and memory CD8 T cell lineages in interleukin 15-deficient mice. *J Exp Med* 2000;191:771.

183. Lodolce JP, Burkett PR, Boone DL, et al. T cell-independent interleukin 15Ralpha signals are required for bystander proliferation. *J Exp Med* 2001;194:1187.

184. Sallusto F, Lenig D, Forster R, et al. Two subsets of memory T lymphocytes with distinct homing potentials and effector functions. *Nature* 1999;401:708.

185. Sallusto F, Mackay CR, Lanzavecchia A. The role of chemokine receptors in primary, effector, and memory immune responses. *Annu Rev Immunol* 2000;18:593.

186. Bell EB, Sparshott SM. Interconversion of CD45R subsets of CD4 T cells *in vivo*. *Nature* 1990;348:163.

187. Tough DF, Sprent J. Turnover of naive- and memory-phenotype T cells. *J Exp Med* 1994;179:1127.

188. Merica R, Khoruts A, Pape KA, et al. Antigen-experienced CD4 T cells display a reduced capacity for clonal expansion *in vivo* that is imposed by factors present in the immune host. *J Immunol* 2000;164:4551.

189. Gray D, Matzinger P. T cell memory is short-lived in the absence of antigen. *J Exp Med* 1991;174:969.

190. Swain S. Generation and *in vivo* persistence of polarized Th1 and Th2 memory cells. *Immunity* 1994;1:543.

191. Swain SL, Hu H, Huston G. Class II-independent generation of CD4 memory T cells from effectors. *Science* 1999;286:1381.

192. Garcia S, DiSanto J, Stockinger B. Following the development of a CD4 T cell response *in vivo*: from activation to memory formation. *Immunity* 1999;11:163.

193. Mackay C, Marston W, Dudler L. Naive and memory T cells show distinct pathways of lymphocyte recirculation. *J Exp Med* 1990;171:801.

CHAPTER 11

T-Lymphocyte Activation

Arthur Weiss and Lawrence E. Samelson

Introduction
Experimental Models Used to Study T-Cell Activation
Responding T Cells and Antigen-Presenting Cells · Stimuli: Complex Antigens and Peptides · Stimuli: Superantigens · Stimuli: Lectins · Stimuli: Monoclonal Antibodies · Pharmacologic Agents
Requirements for the Initiation of T-Cell Activation
Primary Signal for T-Cell Activation: Requirement or Dependency for TCR Involvement · CD4 and CD8 Co-receptors Contribute to Primary Activation Signal · Accessory Molecules Increase Avidity of T-Cell–APC Interaction · Co-stimulatory Signal Is Required for T-Cell Activation
Signal Transduction by T-Cell Antigen Receptor
Complex Structure and Signal Transduction Function of TCR · TCR ITAMs and Cytoplasmic Protein-Tyrosine Kinases · Src PTKs Involved in TCR Signal Transduction · Function of SH2 Domains in Signal Transduction Pathways · Protein-Tyrosine Phosphatase (PTPase) CD45 Plays Critical Role in TCR Signal Transduction · Consequences of TCR-Mediated PTK Activation
Consequences of Early Signal Transduction Events
Early Biochemical Events · Cellular Responses · Gene Activation Events
Terminating T-Cell Responses
T-Cell Inactivation
Conclusion
References

INTRODUCTION

The immune system has evolved to provide a flexible and dynamic mechanism to respond specifically to a wide variety of antigens. In order for a response to occur following antigen challenge, antigen must not only be recognized by antigen-specific lymphocytes but such recognition must be translated into signal transduction events that are responsible for the initiation of cellular responses. T-lymphocytes, together with B-lymphocytes, represent the two antigen-specific components of the cellular immune system. The activation of resting T cells is critical to most immune responses and allows these cells to exert their regulatory or effector capabilities. During activation these relatively quiescent T cells in the G_0 stage of the cell cycle undergo complex changes resulting in cell differentiation and proliferation.

Since each T cell expresses T-cell antigen receptors (TCR) of a single antigen specificity, only a small subset of T cells is activated by any particular antigen (clonal selection). This results in the clonal expansion of antigen-reactive T cells that acquire differentiated functional capacities. However, the activation of T-lymphocytes is actually a consequence of multiple ligand–receptor interactions that occur at the interface of the T cell and an antigen-presenting cell (APC). In sum, these interactions initiate intracellular biochemical events within the T cells that culminate in cellular responses.

It is clear that a large number of different cell-surface molecules on the T-lymphocyte and the APC, only some of which are depicted in Fig. 1, may participate in the complex cell–cell interaction that occurs during antigen presentation. In view of the specificity of T-cell responses, antigen-induced T-lymphocyte activation must be directed by T-cell antigen receptors (TCR). The ligand for the TCR is a short peptide antigen fragment, derived by proteolysis from a larger molecule, which is bound to a syngeneic major histocompatibility complex (MHC) molecule (see Chapters 19 and 20). The antigen receptor is a multichain structure derived from at least six genes (Fig. 2). On most T cells, it contains at least one disulfide-linked α/β heterodimer responsible for antigen recognition (see Chapter 8). A small subset of T cells that recognize antigen with a γ/δ heterodimer, may preferentially play a role in immune responses in epithelial tissues. The α/β or γ/δ heterodimer is noncovalently associated with invariant chains derived from the ζ and CD3γ, δ, and ϵ genes that are responsible for coupling the receptor to intracellular signal-transduction components (1,2) (see below).

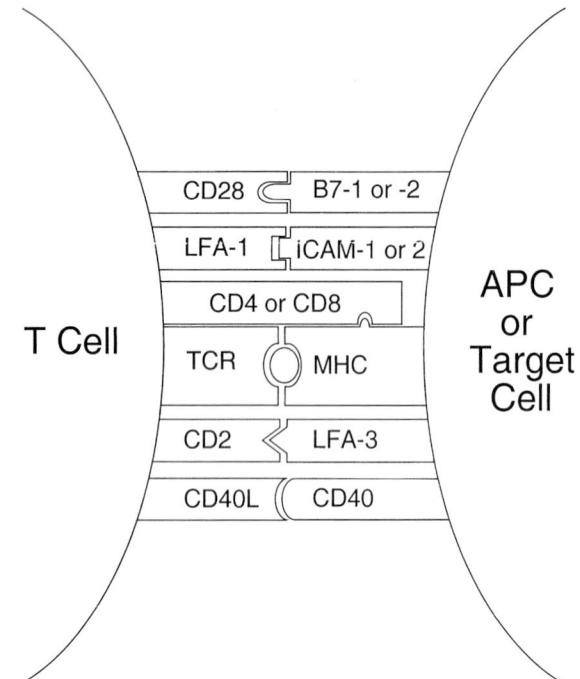

FIG. 1. Schematic representation of some of the ligand–receptor interactions that occur during the interaction of a T cell with an antigen-presenting cell (APC) or target cell.

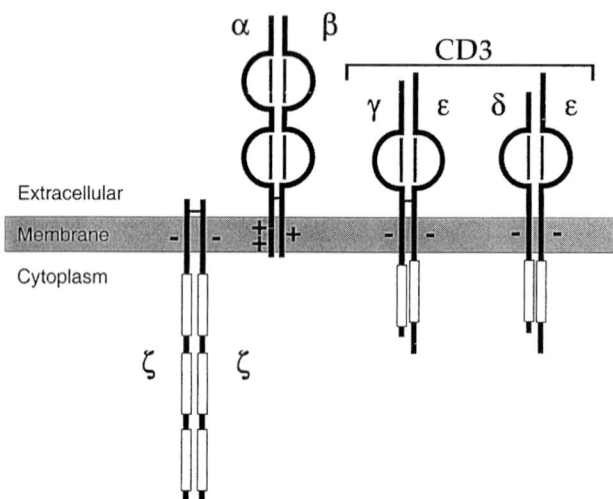

FIG. 2. The T-cell antigen receptor. Illustrated schematically is the antigen-binding subunit comprised of an $\alpha\beta$ heterodimer, and the associated invariant CD3 and ζ chains. Acidic ($-$) and basic ($+$) residues located within the plasma membrane are indicated. The open rectangular boxes indicate motifs (see Fig. 3) within the cytoplasmic domains that interact with cytoplasmic protein-tyrosine kinases.

Antigen-induced stimulation of the TCR delivers the primary signal in initiating activation. For naïve resting T cells, stimulation of the TCR alone is insufficient to induce proliferative responses by purified resting G_0 T cells, but may be sufficient to induce activation of more differentiated T-cell populations or to induce a state of unresponsiveness, termed "anergy" (reviewed in Schwartz [3]) (see also Chapter 29). Other cell-surface molecules expressed on T cells, by binding to their respective ligands, play a role in antigen-specific activation by functioning as accessory molecules in the initial antigen-specific events occurring between an APC and T cell. These accessory molecules may contribute to the initiation of cellular activation by (a) functioning as adhesion molecules, strengthening the interaction between the T cell and APC (e.g., LFA-1 and CD2); (b) modifying the transmembrane signal initiated via the antigen receptor (e.g., CD4 and CD8); and/or (c) initiating their own transmembrane signaling events, distinct from those of the TCR, which are necessary for cellular responses (e.g., CD28 and the interleukin-1 receptor). These latter signal transduction events are responsible for the requisite second signal, or co-stimulatory signal, required to activate resting T cells. A more detailed discussion of the structure and function of some of these accessory molecules is presented in Chapter 13.

The interaction of the TCR with its ligand, or the co-stimulatory receptor with its ligand, initiates cellular activation by inducing a series of rapid biochemical changes that have a number of important consequences. For example, activation of protein kinases results in phosphorylation of specific substrates. These phosphorylations can serve as binding sites for additional signaling molecules. This process of protein–protein interaction results in recruitment of a number of molecules, the creation of signaling complexes, and activation of signaling molecules. Among the latter are enzymes that induce formation of intracellular biochemical mediators called "second messengers." These second messengers as well as multiple activated enzymes can function to initiate or influence cellular response pathways. In resting T cells, such signals can alter a multitude of intracellular events. In differentiated effector T cells, such signals can initiate the activation of the cytolytic mechanism, a stimulus coupled-secretory response in which exocytosis of previously synthesized and packaged proteins involved in the cytolytic apparatus occurs.

During the process of T-cell activation, there are early responses occurring within minutes or hours after the initiation of signal transduction, while others may only occur days after the stimulating event. The early cellular responses may directly or indirectly be the result of TCR- or other receptor-mediated signal transduction. During the early phase of T-cell activation, T cells undergo enormous changes characterized by protein phosphorylation, membrane lipid and cytoskeletal changes, membrane reorganization, ion fluxes, cyclic nucleotide alterations, increased or decreased RNA synthesis of constitutive and newly activated gene products, and cell volume increases (blast transformation). The later cellular responses, such as proliferation, generally result from a complex cascade of gene activation events and the coordinated sequential influence of the products of these genes. For instance, stimulation of the TCR can drive a resting G_0 T cell into G_1, where it expresses lymphokine receptors, but further progression through the cell cycle requires the action of growth factors such as interleukin 2 (IL-2) or 4 (IL-4) to act on their respective receptors (4). The process of T-cell activation represents a contingent cascade of events in which each event is dependent on the expression of the previous components (5). Ultimately, activation of the resting T-lymphocyte may be manifested in a variety of ways but includes the expression of new cell-surface molecules, secretion of a host of lymphokines, cell proliferation, cellular differentiation, and even programmed cell death (apoptosis). All or only some of these events might be manifested by activated T cells and dominate a particular response.

EXPERIMENTAL MODELS USED TO STUDY T-CELL ACTIVATION

A great deal of interest has focused on the requirements for the induction of T-cell activation. This has primarily concerned the initial cellular and molecular interactions involved in the stimulation of resting previously unstimulated (naïve) T cells by antigen. However, several features of antigen-induced activation of T-lymphocytes have hampered such analyses. First, study of the interaction of the T cell with antigen, as it is presented on an APC, involves a cell–cell interaction. This interaction is extremely difficult to study due to the complexities of the stimulating ligand and the TCR. In addition, there are uncertainties regarding the diverse intermolecular ligand–receptor binding events involving other plasma membrane proteins that may occur during this cell–cell interaction (see Fig. 1). Second, the frequency of antigen-specific responding T cells for any given antigen is exceedingly low, representing tenths to hundredths of a percentage of unselected T cells. Third, the responding T-cell populations are heterogeneous, representing a mixture of subpopulations of T cells. Each T-cell subpopulation may have different requirements for activation or may respond in a different manner. Moreover, whether from tissues or blood, these T-cell populations are isolated mixed together with non–T cells that are difficult to completely remove. These non–T cells may play distinct roles in the initiation of the response. Fourth, the source of responding T cells influences the requirements for activation; freshly isolated naïve G_0 T cells have activation requirements that are more stringent than propagated T-cell lines, clones, or hybridomas. Fifth, the resulting response may not reflect the response to the initial stimulus, but instead may result from a response to products (for instance, lymphokines) of another responding cell population. Finally, these inherent ambiguities have been confounded by the various parameters used to assess T-cell activation experimentally. These parameters include: (a) early signal transduction events, such as protein-tyrosine phosphorylation or an increase in cytoplasmic free calcium ($[Ca^{2+}]_i$), that do not necessarily lead to a cellular response; (b) expression of new cell-surface activation antigens, including the α chain (CD25) of the interleukin-2 receptor (IL-2R), the transferrin receptor, class II MHC molecules on human T cells, and CD69, a molecule with as yet unknown function; (c) production of lymphokines, such as IL-2 or IL-4; (d) cell proliferation; and (e) cytolytic activity.

Responding T Cells and Antigen-Presenting Cells

In an effort to circumvent the inherent difficulties in studying the complex interactions that occur during antigen-induced T-cell activation, model systems have been developed to simplify the interacting cells as well as the stimulating ligands. T-cell populations that are used include T-cell clones, hybridomas, or leukemic lines. The major advantages of the use of such models are that they represent homogeneous clonal cell populations that can be obtained in large numbers and have well-characterized antigen receptors and responses. However, it is precisely these characteristics, as well as the immortality and other differentiated features, that may not permit extrapolation of all results to responses of resting naïve T cells. To avoid these problems, investigators have relied on purified fractionated preparations of T cells derived from more complex mixtures of cells. The major shortcomings of such studies, as discussed, are the difficulties in the isolation procedures and the compromises that are made in the purity of the cell populations obtained. The development of transgenic mice containing T cells that express TCRs of a single specificity has greatly facilitated such studies.

The most commonly used models of APCs have been B-cell lines or adherent cells isolated from peripheral-blood mononuclear cells or spleen cells. More emphasis is being placed on studies of dendritic cells, since these cells appear to be the most potent APCs (see Chapter 15). Differences in the abilities of these cell populations to present and/or process antigen is well documented (6). This should be considered in questions of how APCs participate in the processes that lead to T-cell activation. Additional differences in APC function relate to the ability of some, but not all, cells to provide a co-stimulatory signal (7,8). In addition, a variety of tumor lines and lymphoblasts have served as target cells to present antigen to cytolytically active T cells. The use of planar lipid membranes or lipid-coated beads that have been reconstituted with limited numbers of purified proteins to stimulate T-cell clones and hybridomas represents an attempt to further simplify the ligands on the APC as well as to eliminate the need for intact cell systems. Immobilization at high concentration of such molecules is probably required to achieve a sufficiently high avidity since the affinities in solution of the TCR to MHC bound peptide or accessory molecules with their ligands is so low, generally in the micromolar range (reviewed in Shaw et al. [9] and Dustin et al. [10]).

Through the use of gene transfer studies in cell lines or transgenic mice, as well as mice made deficient in expression of an ever-increasing number of molecules by homologous recombination, the role of surface molecules in T-cell activation is being explored. By expressing such molecules on the surface of a variety of functional T cells or APCs that do not normally express them, new cellular models to test the function of these molecules have been developed. T cells or APCs that develop in mice in which a particular gene has been inactivated or specifically replaced have provided important insights into the requirements for T-cell activation. Examining the function of expressed mutant or hybrid molecules in cells and mice underscores the power of current genetic analyses.

Stimuli: Complex Antigens and Peptides

Early studies of T-cell activation examined the responses of complex cell populations to complex cellular or soluble antigens. As efforts evolved to simplify the nature of the responding cell, so too have efforts to simplify the stimulating antigen. Alloantigens expressed on cells have received a great deal of attention since they represent a class of antigens for which the precursor frequency of antigen-responsive T cells is high enough to permit measurable responses following a primary antigen stimulus. Although allogeneic cells with many antigenic differences are often used, more recent studies have relied on cells expressing transfected cloned allogeneic molecules or the development of transgenic mice whose T cells express an allo-specific TCR. Further sophistication of this sort of analysis has included the use of transfected chimeric allogeneic molecules (11).

The study of responses to alloantigens has suffered from the necessity of using cells with the antigen expressed as an integral plasma-membrane molecule. In such analyses, the contribution of other cell-surface molecules or of processing of alloantigens to the activation events is largely undefined. Planar lipid membranes or lipid-coated beads have been reconstituted with purified preparations of MHC molecules to address such ambiguities (12,13). Soluble synthetic peptides derived from the primary sequence of alloantigens or other cellular proteins can be used as agonists or antagonists in sensitizing cells or purified MHC molecules (14). Such approaches with peptides have allowed the type of flexible manipulation of alloantigens that has existed for soluble antigens by permitting the use of MHC molecules containing homogeneous peptides.

The other major type of antigen stimulation that is widely used relies on well-defined soluble proteins presented by APCs. A major limitation in using such soluble antigens is the low frequency of antigen-responsive T cells in the spleen, lymph node, or blood, and the resultant difficulty in studying primary responses. However, the study of responses to soluble antigens has been greatly facilitated by the availability of homogeneous antigen-responsive T-cell clones, hybridomas, or T cells from TCR transgenic mice. Synthetic peptides prepared from the deduced sequence of more complex antigens

are now widely used. It has been possible to obtain near-pure populations of class I MHC molecule/peptide complexes by taking advantage of cells deficient in peptide transporters (15). Under these circumstances, synthetic peptides rescue the expression of unstable MHC molecules. The ability to load MHC molecules on APCs with uniform populations of peptides offers real advantages in studying the biochemical events involved in T-cell activation.

Stimuli: Superantigens

A rather unique group of bacterial and viral products, including bacterial enterotoxins, can activate large numbers of T cells and have been termed "superantigens". These superantigens stimulate T cells due to their abilities to interact with TCR Vβ framework regions outside the peptide–MHC–binding site (reviewed in Sundberg et al. [16]). As a consequence, 5% to 20% of T cells may be stimulated by some of these superantigens. The *in vivo* effects of such massive T-cell stimulation often results in disease, that is, toxic shock syndrome and food poisoning in humans. Unlike conventional peptide antigens that are bound to the antigen-binding groove in MHC molecules, superantigens interact with MHC molecules outside of the peptide-binding groove and do not require antigen processing. Although such superantigens may have dire consequences for the host *in vivo* as activators of large numbers of T cells, they have been quite useful for *in vitro* studies since their mode of T-cell stimulation seems similar, although perhaps not identical, to conventional antigens (17–19).

Stimuli: Lectins

A number of different reagents have been used to substitute for the stimulating antigen/MHC molecule. Many are polyclonal activators of T cells, thereby eliminating the difficulties encountered in studying small numbers of antigen-specific responding cells. Among these reagents are several lectins, plant-derived proteins that bind various carbohydrate groups (20). The lectins phytohemagglutinin (PHA), concanavalin A (Con A), and pokeweed mitogen (PWM) were among the first recognized polyclonal activators of T cells (21). Since they can induce the proliferative responses, they are among a class of reagents termed "mitogens." They bind to a number of glycoproteins expressed on the plasma membrane of a variety cells in addition to T cells. Con A and PHA are selective T-cell mitogens when compared to their effects on B cells, whereas PWM is a T- and B-cell mitogen (20). The relative mitogenic selectivity of lectins is not dependent on their binding specificity for particular cell populations but, rather, reflects the heterogeneity in the carbohydrate groups expressed on different glycoproteins of various cells. Their mitogenic effects for T cells are felt to depend on their ability to bind and cross-link relevant receptors involved in physiologic T-cell activation. Studies with PHA and Con A suggest that these lectins can bind to component chains of the TCR and that their ability to activate T cells is dependent on the expression and function of the TCR (22). However, it should be emphasized that their effects represent the summation of the effects of the binding of these lectins to a large number of distinct molecules, in addition to the TCR. Despite such heterogeneous interactions, stimulation of naïve T cells or resting T-cell clones with Con A still requires a co-stimulatory signal (23).

Stimuli: Monoclonal Antibodies

A major advance in the study of T-cell activation came from the use of monoclonal antibodies (mAbs) as specific probes to study the role of distinct T-cell surface molecules. These mAbs have been used as agonists or antagonists to mimic or interrupt the intermolecular interactions that occur between the T cell and APC or target cell. Among these are mAbs reactive with either the $\alpha\beta$ or the CD3 subunits of the TCR. These mAbs have been used to mimic the agonist effects of antigenic peptide–MHC or interrupt the binding of antigenic peptide–MHC to the TCR. Additional mAbs have been used to address whether other T-cell or APC surface molecules may participate in T-cell activation. A variation on this theme has come from the use of immunoglobulin fusion proteins linked to the extracellular domains of molecules expressed on the T cell or APC. This allows for a more physiologic interaction than may be obtained using mAbs. These approaches have led to the identification of a large number of T-cell and APC surface molecules that participate directly in initiating T-cell activation or may serve to modify the process of activation. Moreover, interruption of key protein–protein interactions involved in T-cell activation with such reagents has also been of considerable therapeutic use.

A degree of caution, however, must be exercised in the interpretation of studies that solely rely on mAbs or fusion proteins. It should be readily apparent that the binding of these reagents may not truly mimic the physiologic ligand-binding event with respect to epitope specificity, avidity, or valency. The non–antigen-binding portions of mAbs may influence the effects of the mAb used; notably, this has been well documented for anti–CD3 mAbs in which immobilization of these mAbs via the Fc receptor to adherent cells contained in cultures is critical for their mitogenic effects for T cells (24). The agonist or antagonist effects of mAbs may not completely mimic or interrupt the effects of the physiologic ligand but may have effects of their own. Confusion regarding the role of the physiologic receptor may thus arise; for instance, in the case of CD2, agonist as well as antagonist effects of mAbs reactive with this receptor have been observed depending on the experimental model and specific mAb used (25–27). In addition, the extensive cross-linking of all of the molecules reactive with a particular mAb is not a situation likely to be mimicked by physiologic ligands for such cell-surface molecules. Despite these cautionary notes, the use of mAbs has proven invaluable in approaching the problem of studying the complex intermolecular events that may occur between the T cell and APC during the initiation of T-cell activation.

Pharmacologic Agents

Pharmacologic agents that can mimic or inhibit some of the intracellular events associated with T-cell activation have been used as probes to address the importance of these events. Notably, the calcium ionophores A23187 and ionomycin, which increase cytoplasmic free calcium $[Ca^{2+}]_i$, and phorbol esters, which activate protein kinase C (PKC) and other proteins, can act synergistically to induce many of the gene activation events and proliferation responses observed during T-cell activation (28–30). The use of these reagents to mimic some of the events associated with ligands that bind to the TCR has been of considerable value in understanding the signal transduction function of the TCR (see below).

A large number of pharmacologic agents have been used as inhibitors of particular intracellular events or as agents that prevent certain cellular responses. Some of the more commonly used inhibitors are listed in Table 1. The targets of such inhibitors are diverse and often ill-defined. However, under some circumstances, these inhibitors are enormously helpful in assessing the contribution of a particular target in cellular responses. Notably, the inhibitors of protein-tyrosine kinases, genestein and herbimycin A, gave the first clues that protein-tyrosine kinases regulated the phosphatidylinositol pathway in T cells (31,32). Recently, a protein-tyrosine kinase inhibitor, STI-571, which specifically targets the Abl kinase has been developed. This agent, because it binds and inhibits Abl function, has an ameliorative effect on the course

TABLE 1. *Inhibitors used to study T-cell activation*

Inhibitor	Target
Neomycin	Phosphatidylinositol turnover
Lithium	Inositol phosphate phosphatase
H7	Protein kinase C
Sphingosine	Protein kinase C
Staurosporine	Protein kinase C
Genestein	Tyrosine kinase
Herbimycin A	Tyrosine kinase
Tyrphostin	Tyrosine kinase
Vanadate	Tyrosine phosphatase
Phenylarsine oxide	Tyrosine phosphatase
EDTA	Ca^{2+} and Mg^{2+}
EGTA	Ca^{2+}
Dimethylamiloride	Na^+/H^+ antiporter
Glucocorticoids	Glucocorticoid receptor; diverse effects
Cyclosporin A	Calcineurin
FK506	Calcineurin
Rapamycin	mTor
Wortmannin	Phosphatidylinositol 3-kinase
LY294002	Phosphatidylinositol 3-kinase

of chronic myelogenous leukemia (33). Additional agents of this sort of fine specificity may have a significant role in further dissecting biochemical pathways in lymphocytes as well as other cells.

Other inhibitors of T-cell activation have already found great utility in clinical medicine. Cyclosporin A, FK506, and Rapamycin have had a major role in tissue and organ transplantation treatment (see below and Chapter). Glucocorticoids have been used throughout medicine for treatment of inflammation and allergic responses. Many of these reagents have also led to important basic biological insights. For example *in vitro* studies exploring the mechanism of action of cyclosporin A and FK506 have led to the discovery of previously unrecognized molecular components of the TCR-regulated signal-transduction pathway. The use of inhibitors in the study of T-cell activation depends on their specificity and low toxicity. Unfortunately, in practice, few of these inhibitors have the required exquisite specificity and low toxicity. Nonetheless, through the use of several different pharmacologic inhibitors and agonists, much can be learned about the processes and events involved in T-cell activation.

Although each experimental model has its ambiguities and limitations, a great deal has been learned from such experimental approaches. These model systems provide the basis for much of the discussion in this and subsequent chapters on cell-surface molecules and events involved in T-cell activation.

REQUIREMENTS FOR THE INITIATION OF T-CELL ACTIVATION

Antigen-specific T-cell activation is initiated during an extraordinarily complex cell–cell interaction. Antigenic peptides bound to MHC molecules on APCs are recognized by T cells bearing antigen-specific TCRs. However, a large number of molecules, some of which are depicted in Fig. 1, also participate in the response. The TCR and other cell-surface molecules contribute to the initiation of T-cell activation by inducing signal transduction events and by contributing to the overall avidity of the T-cell–APC interaction. Considerable evidence has accumulated to suggest that at least one molecule, a co-stimulatory receptor, must initiate signal transduction events distinct from the TCR in order to initiate IL-2 secretion and induce a proliferative response in naïve T cells.

Primary Signal for T-Cell Activation: Requirement or Dependency for TCR Involvement

Clearly, the TCR is central to antigen activation of the T cell. Stimulation of the TCR delivers the primary signal required for the activation of resting T cells. The TCR has two functions in the antigen-induced activation of T cells. First, it must bind the specific peptide–MHC molecule complex on the surface of an APC. Second, this binding event must be converted into a transmembrane signal-transduction event in

which membrane and cytoplasmic signaling molecules that can regulate subsequent cellular responses are activated (see below for a detailed discussion of TCR signal transduction). It is clear from gene transfer studies that the TCR α/β heterodimer contains all of the information necessary for the recognition of the antigen peptide–MHC molecule. However, how peptide–MHC binding to the α/β heterodimer induces signal transduction by the associated CD3 and ζ chains of the TCR is not fully understood. This has become a growing area of interest as distinct or minimally altered peptides (altered peptide ligands; APL) bound to the same MHC molecule can induce distinct signal transduction events by the TCR (34–36). The analyses of the effects of the APLs on TCR signal transduction have been hampered by the complexity of the ligand (i.e., peptide–MHC molecule) and by the fact that this interaction occurs during a complex cell–cell interaction that involves many other molecules on the T cell and APC. Differences in signal transduction have been attributed to differences in the allosteric conformation of the TCR during peptide–MHC recognition, differences in the interaction of the TCR with accessory molecules, as well as to distinct on/off rates involved in these intermolecular interactions (10,37,38). The differences in signaling events induced by APLs are discussed below.

Efforts to study signal transduction by the TCR alone have also taken advantage of mAbs that react with distinct chains of the TCR. Monoclonal antibodies reactive with clone-specific variable or constant determinants of the α/β heterodimer as well as CD3 have been used as agonists to initiate T-cell activation (reviewed in Weiss and Imboden [39]). Under appropriate conditions, which usually require immobilization to a solid support or binding to an Fc receptor on adherent cells, these mAbs can induce resting T cells to secrete lymphokines (such as IL-2 and interferon-γ, IFN), to express a number of new cell-surface molecules (including the high affinity IL-2R and CD69), and to proliferate. Such mAbs also have been used to activate T-cell clones and tumor lines to produce lymphokines and to induce the cytolytic mechanism by differentiated cytolytic T-lymphocytes (CTL). Interestingly, mAbs reactive with the TCR α/β heterodimer differ in their ability to function as agonists (40,41). In addition, stimulation of the receptor with mAbs that selectively react either with α/β or CD3 components may differ in their functional effects (42). These observations together with studies of chimeric T-cell receptors (discussed below) suggest that structurally distinct domains and components of the TCR may have distinct signal transduction functions.

Monoclonal antibodies reactive with either CD3 or the α/β heterodimer can also function as antagonists to inhibit the antigen-specific interaction between T cells and APC or target cells. The ability of these mAbs to function as either agonists or antagonists in a particular experimental model probably depends on the conditions under which they are used. Immobilization of anti–TCR mAbs usually results in an agonist effect, but is not always necessary for an agonist effect. Such immobilization may prevent receptor internalization and enhance receptor cross-linking. Soluble anti–TCR mAbs have generally been used in experiments in which antagonist effects are observed.

The very low concentrations of peptide–MHC complexes or of mAbs required for activation suggests that occupancy of relatively few receptors, perhaps less than a few hundred, is sufficient to initiate T-cell activation (43–45). This is consistent with the relatively few relevant antigenic peptides that are likely to be associated with MHC molecules on the surface of an APC. An alternate possibility has emerged from recent studies that relates the relatively low affinity/short half-life of the TCR peptide–MHC interaction. Some experimental evidence suggests that relatively large numbers of TCRs may be serially engaged by the few specific peptide–MHC complexes on an APC, resulting in signal transduction by large numbers of TCRs that are engaged for relatively short periods of time before they are internalized (46). However, when mAbs are used, it is clear that engagement of only a few TCRs is sufficient to generate a signal that can result in T-cell activation.

In a similar manner, although less frequently, purified MHC molecules that have been pulsed with peptides have been used to stimulate T cells. Usually, any induced response requires multimerization or immobilization of these molecules to plastic surfaces, within lipid bilayers or on some other matrix (12). Successful activation with such purified molecules is usually only seen with hybridomas or some T-cell clones. Primary resting T cells, even if derived from TCR transgenic mice, have additional requirements for activation (47). The signal transduction events induced by such purified peptide–MHC complexes and anti–TCR mAbs are similar but may not be identical.

Superantigens such as staphylococcal enterotoxins or Mls antigens—molecules encoded by endogenous mouse-mammary tumor-virus genomes—have also been used to induce a primary signal via the TCR (reviewed in Herman et al. [48]). Responses to these superantigens are dependent on their interaction with class II MHC molecules on APCs and TCRs derived from appropriate $V\beta$ gene segments (as discussed above). Interestingly, stimulation with such antigens has variable outcomes. In some cases, polyclonal T-cell proliferative and lymphokine responses are observed. However, subsequent clonal deletion and anergy also occur in a process termed "activation-induced cell death" (AICD) (49). The reasons for the diversity in the responses is likely to depend on whether such superantigens are presented to T cells in the setting of an inflammatory response (50). This is not a special property of responses to superantigen, although it may be more easily recognized due to the large number of responsive T cells, as similar AICD of conventional antigen responsive T cells occurs in the absence of concomitant inflammation (51). There is some controversy regarding whether the signal transduction events observed with superantigens are identical to those induced by antigen or mAbs (17,19,52,53). Nevertheless, these bacterial and viral products have proven to be potent reagents in stimulating the TCR and valuable probes for the new insights they have provided.

Under appropriate conditions, stimulation of several other distinct cell-surface molecules is able to mimic this function of the TCR. Among those that have been most extensively studied, CD2, CD28, and, in the murine system, Thy-1 and Ly-6, can all induce signal transduction events similar to those initiated by the TCR (reviewed in Weiss and Imboden [39] and Bierer et al. [54]). With the exceptions of CD2 and CD28, the physiologic ligands of these other cell-surface molecules are as yet unidentified. Therefore, the physiologic significance of signal transduction events leading to T-cell activation via these molecules is not known. In general, in order for the non–TCR molecules to mediate such a primary activation signal, their extensive cross-linking, usually with mAbs, is required. Such a requirement is not likely to be met by physiologic ligands. Nor is it clear, when the ligand may be expressed fairly broadly, as is the case for CD2 ligands, how activation via these molecules would be regulated in a manner that is beneficial to the host. Some of these molecules may have other more important functions, including to increase the avidity of the T-cell–APC interaction or to mediate other distinct signal transduction events, as has been demonstrated for CD28 (8). Moreover, the dependency of these non–TCR molecules on the expression and functional competency of the TCR to initiate a primary activation signal suggests that the pathways by which these molecules induce a primary signal must converge with the TCR-regulated pathway (55). Thus, in some way, perhaps through a direct or indirect physical interaction that results from extensive cross-linking, the TCR appears to be responsible for some of the signal transduction events attributed to this group of molecules. This is consistent with the demonstration that the TCR ζ chain participates in and is required for CD2-mediated signaling events (56).

Engagement of the TCR by ligand is not sufficient for the full activation of T cells. However, before considering other signals required for T-cell activation, the requirements for activation via the TCR must be defined in terms of the parameters of activation examined and the cell population being stimulated. For instance, expression of CD25 (the α chain of the IL-2R) can be induced on naïve resting T cells in the absence of a demonstrable proliferative response by stimulating the TCR alone (57,58). In contrast, production of the lymphokine IL-2 by these cells is more stringently regulated and requires additional stimuli provided by co-stimulatory receptors (see below). Hence, a T-cell proliferative response is more likely to be limited by IL-2 production than by IL-2R expression.

Antigen or mAb-induced IL-2 production and proliferative responses by resting G0 T cells are dependent on several functions by the APC that influence the delivery of the primary signal. Some functions have been delineated by using anti–TCR mAbs. One function appears to involve the immobilization of the mAb via its Fc domain to Fc receptors on the APC (24,59). This function of the APC can be bypassed by stimulating the T cell with anti–TCR mAbs that have been bound to Sepharose beads or to a plastic culture dish. The immobilized mAb may be analogous to the cell-bound peptide–MHC complex when it is presented to a T cell. This suggests that the formation of a high local concentration or of a cross-linked array of TCRs by antigenic peptide–MHC molecules or mAbs may be important to initiate activation. Such multimerization of ligands will also serve to increase their effective valency and avidity. Alternatively, stimulation with immobilized rather than soluble ligands may serve to prevent TCR internalization and thus potentiate the duration and magnitude of the stimulus.

CD4 and CD8 Co-receptors Contribute to Primary Activation Signal

The CD4 and CD8 molecules are expressed on and define the two major subsets of mature α/β TCR-bearing T cells (see Chapter 13). They bind to nonpolymorphic regions of class II and class I MHC molecules, respectively. In general, CD4 cells are involved in T-helper cell function and participate in host responses to antigens that are processed via the endocytic pathway. In contrast, CD8 T cells give rise to cytolytic effector cells and recognize peptides that are derived from the endogenous biosynthetic pathway (60). The co-receptors function in concert with the TCR during antigen recognition to increase the sensitivity of TCR responsiveness to antigen and contribute to the primary activation stimulus delivered by the TCR.

CD4 and CD8 are integral membrane glycoproteins whose structures have been extensively studied (reviewed in Zamoyska [61]). The extracellular domain of CD4 consists of four immunoglobulin (Ig) domains joined in tandem. The two more membrane-distal or N-terminal domains interact with the β2 domain of class II MHC molecules, whereas the more membrane-proximal two Ig domains may play a role in homo-oligomerization. The two N-terminal Ig domains also are involved in the interaction with the envelope glycoprotein gp120 of the human immunodeficiency virus. CD8 on TCR-α/β–expressing T cells is a heterodimer of an α and a β chain, but can be expressed as an α/α homodimer on TCR-γ/δ–bearing T cells. The N-terminal Ig domain of the α chain binds to the α3 domain of class I MHC molecules. It is not clear whether the CD8β chain, which cannot be expressed independently of the CD8α chain, can bind Class I MHC molecules. The binding of CD4 and CD8 to MHC molecules is a relatively low-affinity interaction in the micromolar range. Interestingly, the interaction of CD8 with class I MHC molecules is regulated by the differential O-linked glycosylation of this molecule in thymocytes versus peripheral T cells (62). The ability of these co-receptors to interact with regions of the MHC molecule not involved with peptide recognition allows for the simultaneous binding of the TCR and co-receptor to a single peptide–MHC molecule. This can lead to the enhanced stability of the tetrameric complex (61). Hence, it is not surprising that many, although not all, functional interactions of TCRs with antigen are dependent on appropriate CD4 or CD8 co-receptor engagement.

The antigen responses that are co-receptor–independent frequently involve memory responses and may involve T cells with TCRs that have been selected for higher affinity.

Whereas the CD4 and CD8 co-receptors can contribute to the formation of a more stable interaction of the TCR with the peptide–MHC complex, they also communicate with intracellular signal transduction events through the interaction of their intracellular domains with the cytoplasmic protein-tyrosine kinase Lck. A more detailed discussion of the function of Lck in TCR signaling pathways follows below. Here, we focus on its role in co-receptor function.

Both co-receptors interact noncovalently with the N-terminal unique region of Lck via paired cysteine residues (reviewed in Basson and Zamoyska [63]). The interaction of Lck with CD4 is of higher affinity than with CD8. Some evidence suggests that the differences in the interaction of the co-receptors with Lck leads to distinct signal transduction events. This model may explain the distinct developmental outcomes that occur during positive selection in the thymus as well as the distinct functions of the resultant CD4 and CD8 subsets of mature T cells.

Co-ligation of the TCR with either co-receptor can markedly enhance signal transduction by the TCR (64). The contribution of Lck to CD4 and CD8 co-receptor function is important but not essential for effective TCR signaling function during development or at high antigen concentrations. The function of Lck in thymic development can be overcome, presumably by higher levels of co-receptor engagement (65). The role of Lck may be two-fold: A kinase-independent function of Lck has been identified that may be to deliver or strengthen the interaction of the co-receptor with the TCR-peptide–MHC complex (66). In fact, the strength of binding of CD4 or CD8 to MHC molecules may be regulated by TCR signal transduction events that influence the localization or interactions of Lck to cytoskeletal components (67) or to the stimulated TCR (68,69). This may lead to the formation and stabilization of the tetrameric complex. A second function is mediated by the kinase domain, which the co-receptor delivers to the stimulated TCR complex (63). In this case, the kinase domain of Lck may function by phosphorylating critical substrates (see below). These two functions probably act in concert, rather than independently, to increase the overall sensitivity of the TCR for antigen recognition.

Independent engagement of the co-receptors can lead to a signal that inhibits T-cell activation. Whereas the binding of CD4 and CD8 to MHC molecules has been demonstrated in cells that massively overexpress these molecules (70,71), stable, functionally important interactions probably occur normally only during simultaneous TCR recognition of peptide–MHC molecules. However, experimental ligation of CD4 with anti–CD4 mAbs primes T cells for apoptosis when the TCR is subsequently stimulated (72). *In vivo,* this may be relevant to interactions of the HIV envelope glycoprotein gp120 with CD4, where apoptosis results if the TCR is subsequently engaged (73). The mechanisms underlying these inhibitory events have not yet been determined.

In most primary immune responses, the involvement of CD4 or CD8 is required. Thus, in general, mAbs reactive with either CD4 or CD8 can block the responses of the appropriate subset of cells to antigens during primary but not secondary immune responses. However, the dependency of an individual T cell upon the involvement of CD4 or CD8 is highly clone dependent. In the case of CD4, its contribution to the antigen response depends not only on its extracellular domain that interacts with MHC class II molecules, but also on the sequences in its cytoplasmic domain that interact with Lck (74). This suggests critical roles for domains of these molecules that bind to MHC molecules and domains responsible for the redistribution of the Lck PTK. It is also clear from such studies that requirement for the interaction of CD4 or CD8 with an MHC molecule during antigen recognition requires that these molecules interact with the same MHC molecule that is presenting peptide to the TCR. This has at least two functions: First, it serves to increase the overall avidity of the antigen recognition complex. Second, it serves to deliver Lck into the close proximity to the TCR that is being stimulated by antigen, potentially allowing Lck to regulate this interaction.

Accessory Molecules Increase Avidity of T-Cell–APC Interaction

Several nonantigen-dependent molecular interactions have been identified that serve to increase the overall avidity of the interaction of T cells with APCs and may help to organize the complex intercellular interaction. These include the LFA-1 (CD11a/CD18) with ICAM-1 (CD54) or ICAM-2 (CD102); CD2 with LFA-3 (CD58) or CD59; and CD4 with MHC class II or CD8 with MHC class I (reviewed in Shaw and Dustin [9]). Whereas the TCR may dictate the specificity of the recognition event, these antigen-independent molecular interactions serve in a permissive manner to facilitate the interaction of the T-cell with the APC.

The affinity of the TCR for the specific peptide–MHC complex is relatively low, on the order of 10^{-5} M (75). For this reason, and because nonspecific cell conjugates have been observed between T cells and potential APCs, it has been proposed that the initial encounter of a T cell with a potential APC may not involve antigen-specific recognition (9,76). A nonspecific T-cell–APC conjugate may form initially and be mediated, in part, by the molecular interactions listed above. Such nonantigen-specific adhesion between a T cell and APC may permit the TCR to survey peptide–MHC molecules and, if engaged by sufficient specific complexes, to initiate signal transduction events. These signal transduction events not only can lead to the activation of biochemical pathways responsible for T-cell activation, but also increase the avidity of several of these accessory molecule pairs. Such a TCR-mediated increase in avidity has been observed for interactions of LFA-1 with ICAM-1 (77); CD2 with LFA-3 (78); and, CD8 with class I MHC molecules (67). This increase in avidity serves to further stabilize the interaction

between the T cell and APC and promotes the activation of the T cell by prolonging signal transduction. This TCR-mediated signaling appears to require a molecule now named ADAP (adhesion and degranulation promoting adapter protein) and previously named Fyb or SLAP-130. T cells from mice engineered to lack this protein fail to activate LFA-1 and other integrin receptors following TCR engagement (79). If the TCR does not encounter its specific peptide antigen during the initial interaction, signal transduction events that contribute to the increased avidity of the accessory molecules are not induced. This permits the disengagement of the T cell and APC from a low-avidity interaction and allows the T cell to move on to interactions with other potential APCs. Some of these accessory molecules undergo complex movement and sorting on the plasma membrane during the process of TCR interaction with the peptide MHC. This issue is discussed below. The functions of these accessory molecules are discussed in further detail in Chapter 13.

Co-stimulatory Signal Is Required for T-Cell Activation

As is clear, the molecules expressed in an APC provide many functions for the initiation of T-cell activation. In addition to peptide presentation and the adhesion functions, molecules on or secreted by the APC induce additional signal transduction events necessary for T-cell activation. This latter function is termed a co-stimulatory function or signal (3). The function of co-stimulation is to ensure that the antigenic peptide recognized is a non–self-peptide. This is accomplished by requiring that the resting T cell is only activated by peptide antigens presented by dedicated APCs such as dendritic cells, macrophages, or activated B cells. These dedicated APCs constitutively express or are induced by inflammatory stimuli to express ligands for co-stimulatory receptors on T cells.

The co-stimulatory function has been revealed primarily in studies involving the response of resting G_0 T cells or resting T-cell clones of the Th1 type that have been depleted of APCs contained in the adherent cell population. Purified resting T cells fail to produce IL-2 or proliferate in response to mitogenic lectins, immobilized anti–TCR mAbs, or antigen-pulsed fixed APCs (fixed APCs cannot provide a co-stimulatory signal), but they are induced to express IL-2 receptors and will proliferate if exogenous IL-2 is provided (57,58,80). In contrast, T-cell hybridomas and cytolytic T-cell clones will frequently produce IL-2 and/or proliferate in response to immobilized anti–TCR mAbs, antigen-pulsed fixed APCs alone, or even lipid membranes reconstituted with peptide–MHC molecules (12,13,81), whereas such stimulation of T-helper cell clones may fail to induce IL-2 production or proliferation and can induce an unresponsive state (3). This state of unresponsiveness will be discussed later in this chapter and in Chapter 29. The critical event necessary to avoid the anergic state is the response to IL-2 (82). In most cases this will reflect the production of IL-2 by the same T cell. The variable dependency of some T-cell clones and hybridomas on a co-stimulatory signal may reflect the state of differentiation of these cells. T-cell clones already express high-affinity IL-2 receptors, transferrin receptors, and, in the case of human clones, class II MHC molecules, characteristics not shared by resting naïve T cells. Thus, these observations suggest that the activation of resting naïve T cells and, in some cases, T-helper cell clones requires two independent signals for IL-2 production, proliferation, and differentiation. One signal is provided by the TCR. The other signal is provided by a soluble factor or by cell-surface molecules on the APC that interact with molecules on the T cell.

One molecule that functions as a co-stimulatory receptor on T cells is CD28 (reviewed in Foy et al. [83], Michel et al. [84], and Frauwirth and Thompson [85]). The function of CD28 is discussed in detail in Chapter 13. Briefly, CD28 is a disulfide-linked homodimer of 44 kD glycoprotein monomers. It is expressed on most T cells, but in the human approximately 50% of CD8 T cells do not express CD28. CD28 has two well-characterized ligands, B7-1 (CD80) and B7-2 (CD86), that are expressed on potent APCs, including activated B cells, activated macrophages and dendritic cells. Co-stimulatory function can be provided by anti–CD28 mAbs, soluble B7-immunoglobulin fusion proteins, or cells expressing B7 molecules. Interruption of the CD28–B7 interaction can block co-stimulatory function and prevent T-cell activation *in vitro* or *in vivo*, highlighting the importance of

this interaction. Moreover, mice made deficient in CD28 or both B7-1 and B7-2 have markedly impaired immune responses (85–87).

A critical event necessary for co-stimulatory function is the induction or up-regulation of B7 molecules on the surface of APCs, particularly when B cells function as APCs. This involves the sequential stimulation of the TCR on the interacting T cells and CD40 on the antigen-presenting B cell (83) (Fig. 3). During this interaction, stimulation of the TCR on a resting T cell results in the induced expression of gp39, the CD40 ligand (CD40L), a membrane-bound member of the tumor necrosis factor (TNF) family. This, in turn, allows for the stimulation of CD40 on the B cell, which induces up-regulation of B7-1 and B7-2 that can then stimulate CD28. Inflammatory mediators, such as lipopolysaccharide, have also been shown to up-regulate B7-1 and B7-2 expression, ensuring that co-stimulatory function will be provided at inflammation sites. This allows for the initial response of the innate immune system to recruit the adaptive immune system. Such a complex scheme has probably evolved to ensure that T cells are activated only under appropriate circumstances.

The mechanism by which CD28, which does not have intrinsic enzymatic activity, mediates signals responsible for co-stimulation remains elusive and controversial. CD28 engagement by B7 or with antibodies results in phosphorylation of tyrosine residues on its cytosolic tail. These events are

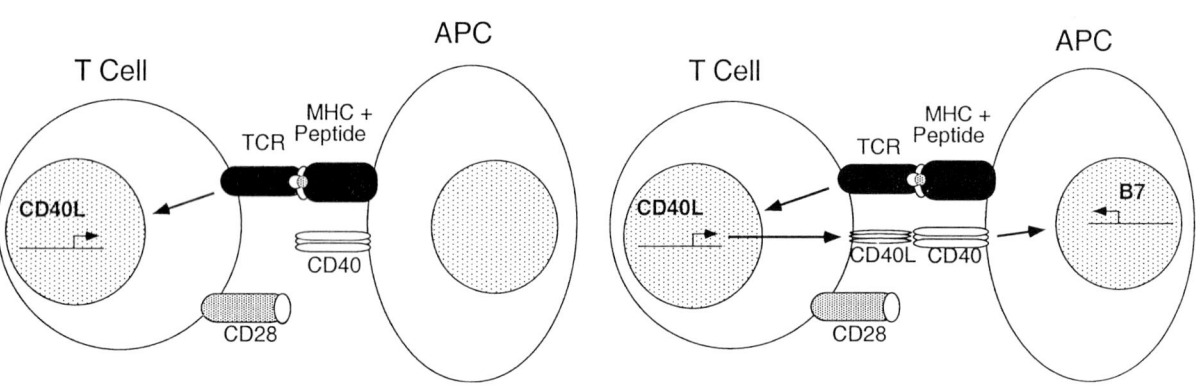

TCR stimulation induces CD40L

CD40 stimulation induces B7

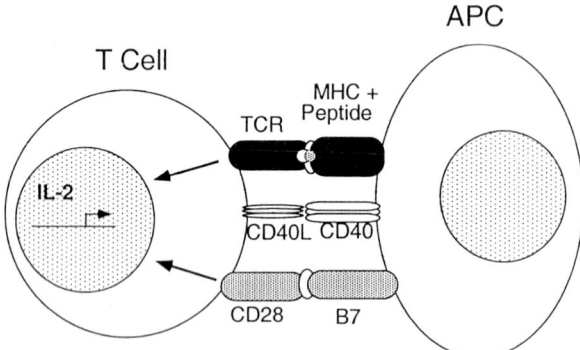

TCR + CD28 stimulation induces
IL-2 Gene Activation

FIG. 3. Interactions between a T cell and antigen-presenting cell (APC) that lead to IL-2 production. The sequential interactions of the TCR with peptide antigen/MHC complex lead to the induced expression of CD40L on the T cell that interacts with CD40 on the APC. This induces the expression of B7 molecules on the APC that can then stimulate CD28, the co-stimulatory receptor on the T cell. The two signals induced by the TCR and CD28 lead to IL-2 gene expression.

mediated by protein-tyrosine kinases of the Src family present in T cells. Phosphorylation events of this type and their complex consequences are critical to TCR-mediated activation as described extensively below. The phosphorylation of the CD28 tail creates binding sites for a number of important signaling molecules including Grb2 and the p85 regulatory subunit of PI-3 kinase. The latter enzyme can be activated by this recruitment. Investigators have also observed that CD28 engagement leads to activation of certain protein-tyrosine kinases such as Itk and Tec, as well as tyrosine phosphorylation of both Vav, an activator of Rho family G proteins and PLCγ. PLCγ is responsible for phosphoinositide breakdown, as well as production of diacylglycerol and inositol phosphates, the activators of protein kinase C and calcium, respectively. All of these actions can be detected following engagement of the TCR alone. Thus, there is a strong sense that the role of CD28 is to enhance or amplify TCR signaling (84,85). On the other hand, a number of functions associated with CD28 activation seem unique, and thus may serve to complement TCR-induced pathways. CD28 can promote TCR interactions with membrane microdomains called rafts, which are discussed below. CD28 is also coupled via PI3 kinase to the serine–threonine kinase Akt that regulates the function of NF-κB transcription factors and contributes to optimal activation of the IL-2 promoter. In this pathway, CD28 engagement targets the specific transcriptional element, CD28RE, which is a component of the IL-2 promoter. The relative importance of the various CD2γ pathways shared with the TCR or unique CD2γ, remains an active and vital area of research.

The signals responsible for IL-2 production have been studied most intensively, although CD28 regulates the production of several other T-cell–derived lymphokines (88,89). CD28 signals regulate the transcriptional activity of the IL-2 gene (discussed below) and its post-transcriptional regulation (reviewed in Powell et al. [90]). The cytoplasmic tail of CD28 is sufficient to mediate the signals required for co-stimulation of IL-2 gene transcription and production of the lymphokine (91), and residues critical for this function have been identified. The biochemical signals induced by CD28 stimulation that are responsible for its co-stimulatory function remain ill-defined. Several distinct events have been identified and will be described below and in Chapter 13.

Despite the importance of the interaction of CD28 with B7 molecules, blockade of the interactions or deficiency of the interaction in mice that do not express CD28 or B7 molecules does not always result in an anergic state. Indeed, CD28-deficient mice can mount a significant immune response to some pathogens (86,92). These results suggest that other molecules may provide similar, though perhaps not identical co-stimulatory functions. ICOS, for instance, is a CD28 homologue that is up-regulated following initial T-cell stimulation and binds a B7 family member. ICOS appears to play a preferential role in regulating Th2 cytokine production (93).

Of the other molecules on or secreted by the APCs, heat-stable antigen and interleukin-1 (IL-1) have received the greatest attention. The effects of IL-1 may be quite indirect.

For instance, IL-1 can up-regulate the expression of B7 (94). The intracellular events initiated by or modified by the binding of IL-1 to its receptor have not been well characterized. However, the cytoplasmic domain of IL-1 is homologous to the cytoplasmic domain of Drosophila Toll. Several mammalian Toll receptor homologues have been identified and are involved in the initiation of the innate immune response by functioning as pattern recognition receptors. They frequently recognize bacterial, fungal or viral products. Interestingly, stimulation of all these molecules activates NF-κB transcription factors via adaptor proteins such as MyD88 that ultimately activate IkB kinases (95–97). The activation of NF-κB plays a role in inducing the transcriptional activation of B7 and CD40 genes.

Other reagents and mAbs against other cell-surface molecules have produced second signals required for T-cell lymphokine production and proliferation. Some of these are likely to function indirectly to up-regulate B7 or CD40 genes. A second signal can also be provided by pharmacologic reagents, namely phorbol esters that activate protein kinase C isozymes (57,98). The mechanism by which phorbol esters provide a co-stimulatory signal is not clear since TCR stimulation should activate protein kinase C or Ras (see below). It seems likely that there are many ways to provide a second signal that can lead to T-cell activation. These signals may not necessarily be qualitatively equivalent and may not functionally activate the same T-cell populations.

SIGNAL TRANSDUCTION BY T-CELL ANTIGEN RECEPTOR

Complex Structure and Signal Transduction Function of TCR

The TCR contains an α/β or γ/δ heterodimer that is responsible for peptide antigen/MHC molecule recognition. These subunits are transported to the plasma membrane in an obligatory association with as many as six other invariant proteins derived from four genes, although the precise stoichiometry of the chains within the TCR complex is uncertain (1,2). Among the associated proteins are those comprising the CD3 complex. CD3 consists of three homologous noncovalently linked transmembrane proteins: γ, δ, and ε. The CD3 genes are closely linked and are presumed to have arisen via gene duplication (1). Within each TCR complex, there appear to be two copies of CD3ε that associate with either δ or γ to form dimers, but γ and δ cannot associate with each other. The crystal structure of the extracellular fragment of the CD3ε/γ heterodimer demonstrates a tight interface between the two chains (99). In addition, the TCR contains a disulfide-linked homodimer or heterodimer containing the ζ chain, which has little overall structural homology to the CD3 chains. The predominant form of the TCR contains ζ/ζ homodimers. On some CTL, ζ forms disulfide-linked dimers with the structurally homologous γ chain of the high-affinity IgE Fc receptor

(100). The function of such diversity in TCR structure is still not known, but it may allow for diversification of the signal transduction functions of the receptor.

The scant five residues in the cytoplasmic domains of the α and β chains do not contain sufficient information to couple to intracellular signal transduction machinery. Instead, the signal transduction function of the TCR complex is conveyed by the associated CD3 and ζ subunits. Initial clues to this function came from studies using mAbs reactive with extracellular domains of the CD3 complex that were able to mimic the effects of antigen by inducing many of the manifestations of T-cell activation (45). When the structural features of the CD3 and ζ chains are compared to the α and β chains, it is clear that although the cytoplasmic domains of the CD3 and ζ chains do not encode an intrinsic enzymatic activity, they are sufficiently large (40 to 113 residues) and more likely to interact with cytoplasmic signal transduction molecules.

Studies with chimeric molecules that included the cytoplasmic domain of ζ, CD3ϵ, or related molecules, provided evidence for this signal transduction function. Earlier studies had revealed that the regions surrounding and including the transmembrane domains of the TCR component contain the information necessary for the assembly of the TCR subunits (101,102). This permitted the development of a strategy in which the functions of the cytoplasmic domains of the individual chains of the TCR could be studied in isolation. Chimeric molecules were constructed in which the extracellular and, importantly, the transmembrane domains of CD4, CD8, CD16, or the IL-2 receptor α chain (which can be expressed independently of the TCR) were fused to the cytoplasmic domains of the TCR ζ, CD3ϵ, or IgE Fc–receptor γ chains (103–105). These chimeric molecules could be expressed independently of endogenous TCR chains in T-cell lines or clones or in basophil lines. Stimulation of these chimeras induced early signal transduction events and later manifestations of T-cell activation, such as lymphokine secretion and cytolytic activity associated with stimulation of the intact oligomeric TCR. Thus, the TCR ζ and CD3 chains can both couple the ligand-binding subunit of the TCR to intracellular signal transduction mechanisms. This is consistent with TCR reconstitution studies of a T-cell hybridoma that suggested that CD3 and ζ chains could function as independent signal transduction modules (106).

The apparent paradoxical redundancy of function of the CD3 and ζ subunits is explained by the recognition of a common sequence motif contained in the cytoplasmic domains of the non–ligand-binding subunits of many hematopoietic cell receptors involved in antigen recognition (107). Termed the "immunoreceptor tyrosine-based activation motif" (ITAM), this motif is (a) based on conservation of the consensus sequence $(D/E)XXYXXLX_{(6-8)}YXXL$; (b) triplicated within the cytoplasmic domain of the ζ chain; and (c) contained as a single copy in the cytoplasmic domains of each of the CD3 chains (Fig. 4). The ITAM is also contained in the β and γ chains of the IgE Fc receptor, the Igα and Igβ chains associated with the membrane immunoglobulin antigen

receptor on B cells, and DAP-12, which is associated with MHC recognition structures on natural killer (NK) cells (Fig. 4) (see Chapters 7, 12 and 22). The observations made with TCR chimeric receptors have been extended to other invariant chains of receptors associated with oligomeric receptors expressed on B cells (the B-cell antigen receptor); mast cells (the high-affinity IgE Fc receptor); and NK cells (the activating forms of the killer inhibitory receptors, KIR, or Ly49 molecules). Chimeric receptors containing only a single copy of most, but perhaps not all, ITAMs are sufficient to induce the early and late events associated with stimulation of the intact oligomeric TCR (105,108,109). The β chain of the IgE Fc receptor, which is the only ITAM with a six-residue spacer, appears to function as an amplifier rather than an independently functioning unit (110). Mutagenesis of the ITAM sequences has demonstrated the importance of the tyrosine and leucine residues in the ITAM signaling function. It is not surprising that ITAMs may have similar functions within distinct receptors since the exon–intron organization of the various ITAMs is conserved, suggesting a common evolutionary precursor (106).

The multiplicity of the ITAMs within the TCR is a striking feature of the receptor that is likely to have functional consequences. Although the precise stoichiometry of the chains comprising the TCR is not clear, if one assumes the most common model of receptor structure (Figs. 2 and 4), then a single TCR complex contains ten copies of this motif. The redundancy of this motif within the receptor allows a single TCR to interact with and activate multiple copies of the same signal transduction component. This can lead to amplification of signal transduction by a single ligand-binding event (109), thereby increasing the sensitivity of the TCR (111). Alternatively, the motifs contain sufficiently distinct sequences to allow them to interact with distinct intracellular signal-transduction molecules, which permits diversification of the signal transduction events. Thus, it is possible that selective involvement of ITAMs following TCR stimulation can lead to distinct cellular responses (35,112).

It is not surprising that viruses which target lymphocytes have acquired ITAM sequences that aid them in their pathogenic mechanisms. At least four viruses have ITAM-like sequences that can couple to intracellular signaling mechanisms in lymphocytes and have been shown to play important roles in pathology. The bovine-leukemia-virus envelope glycoproteins, gp130, contains an ITAM sequence. This virus, which transforms B cells in ruminants, depends on the ITAM sequence for infection and for high viral titers (113). The Epstein–Barr virus latent-membrane protein 2 (LMP2) plays an important role in maintaining viral latency in transformed B cells. The ITAM in LMP2 may activate B cells, but also contains a motif that facilitates ubiquitination and degradation of the Lyn kinase (114). An unusual isolate of the simian immunodeficiency virus (SIV) causes fulminant infection of resting T cells, in contrast to the chronic and latent infection observed with most SIV isolates. The highly unusual behavior of this virus has been mapped to two

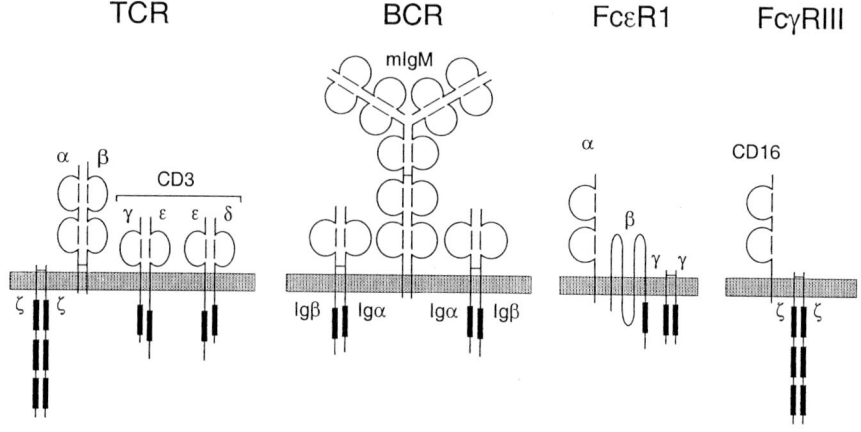

ITAMs
(Immunoreceptor Tyrosine-Based Activation Motif)

```
hζ1          N Q L Y N E L N L G R R E E - Y D V L
hζ2          E G L Y N E L Q K D K M A E A Y S E I
hζ3          D G L Y Q G L S T A T K D T - Y D A L

hCD3γ        D Q L Y Q P L K D R E D D Q - Y S H L
hCD3ε        N P D Y E P I R K G Q R D L - Y S G L
hCD3δ        D Q V Y Q P L R D R D D A Q - Y S H L

rIgE FcR γ   D A V Y T G L N T R N Q E T - Y E T L
rIgE FcR β   D R L Y E E L - H V Y S P I - Y S A L

mIg α        E N L Y E G L N L D D C S M - Y E D I
mIg β        D H T Y E G L N I D Q T A T - Y E D I

BLV gp30     D S D Y Q A L L P S A P E I - Y S H L
EBV LMP-2    H S D Y Q P L G T Q D Q S L - Y L G L
SIV Nef      G D L Y E R L L R A R G E T - Y G R L
HHV8 K1      L Q D Y Y S L H D L C T E D - Y T Q P

Consensus    D/E- - Y - - L - - - - - - - - Y - - L
```

FIG. 4. ITAMs in receptors involved in antigen recognition.

mutations in the viral Nef protein that create an ITAM sequence (115). Finally, the K1 gene product of the Kaposi's sarcoma herpes virus contains a functional ITAM-like sequence (116). This could play a role in facilitating the infection of B cells, thought to be an intermediate reservoir for the virus. Thus, these viral ITAM sequences appear to have taken advantage of the function of the ITAM present in the TCR or other antigen receptors in order to interact with intracellular signaling molecules involved in lymphocyte activation.

The CD3 chains may serve an additional regulatory function within the TCR. The human CD3γ and δ chains are phosphorylated on serine residues in response to events that lead to protein kinase C activation (see below) (117,118). This has been associated with diminished TCR signal transduction function. Thus, it may represent a feedback regulatory mechanism leading to receptor desensitization.

The mechanism by which the α/β chains transmit ligand occupancy to the CD3 and ζ subunits remains poorly understood. The ability to stimulate simple single- or double-chain chimeric receptors containing ζ or CD3ϵ cytoplasmic domains with mAbs is most consistent with a cross-linking or dimerization model. However, the complex structure of the receptor and the varying sensitivity of α/β and CD3 to stimulation by mAbs suggests that allosteric changes could play a role in receptor activation (42,119). The varying ability of peptide ligands with similar affinities to induce distinct signaling events also favors an allosteric model, although differences in kinetic parameters could also explain such differences (38). Finally, the CD3 and ζ chains may also serve a "docking" function to permit other cell-surface molecules, such as CD2, CD4, or CD8, to interact with the TCR in forming a properly assembled receptor complex. This latter function is consistent with observed stable or induced associations of the TCR with CD4 (38,120). Such a docking function is also consistent with the observed requirement for a functional TCR or ζ chain-containing chimera in CD2-mediated signal transduction (56).

TCR ITAMs and Cytoplasmic Protein-Tyrosine Kinases

Stimulation of the TCR by peptide antigen–MHC molecules or by agonist anti–TCR mAbs must induce intracellular biochemical events in order to initiate a cellular response. A number of intracellular biochemical changes occur during the first few seconds to minutes after stimulation of the TCR. These include protein phosphorylation, increases in cytoplasmic free calcium $[Ca^{2+}]_i$, pH changes, and changes in cyclic nucleotides. The primary sequences of the TCR component chains do not encode proteins with intrinsic enzymatic activity. Instead, the TCR ITAMs couple the TCR to intracellular enzymes.

The most rapid event associated with TCR stimulation is the induced phosphorylation of several proteins on tyrosine residues (121). Notably, among these phosphorylated substrates are the ITAMs of the TCR ζ and CD3 chains (122,123). Such tyrosine phosphorylation can be observed within seconds of TCR stimulation and persists for hours (103,121,124). Inhibitors of protein-tyrosine kinases (PTKs) can inhibit most if not all of the later events associated with TCR stimulation (31,32). Since the ITAMs contain all of the information necessary for TCR signal transduction function, it seemed likely that the ITAMs regulate the function of PTKs. Two families of cytoplasmic PTKs, the Src and Syk families, interact directly with TCR ITAMs in a sequential and highly coordinated manner (53). Members of these two families of PTKs have been shown to play critical roles in TCR signaling function. A third family of PTKs, the Tecs, although not directly interacting with the TCR, are intimately involved in TCR-mediated signaling (125).

Src PTKs Involved in TCR Signal Transduction

Lck and Fyn are the major Src family PTKs expressed in T cells. Both have been implicated in interactions with ITAMs and in TCR signal transduction. Prior to reviewing the specific role of each of these kinases, the overall common structural features (Fig. 5) and the functions of the domains of these PTKs will be discussed.

The Src kinases vary from approximately 50 to 60 kilodaltons (kDa) (126). At the N-terminus of each of these kinases, at position 2, is a glycine residue that is myristoylated. Some of the Src kinases, including Lck, are also palmitoylated at one or two cysteine residues contained within the first ten residues, and this modification may be dynamically regulated (127,128). The presence of these two lipid moieties is intimately involved in membrane localization of these PTKs, and, in particular, with localization to membrane microdomains called rafts. The function of raft localization is

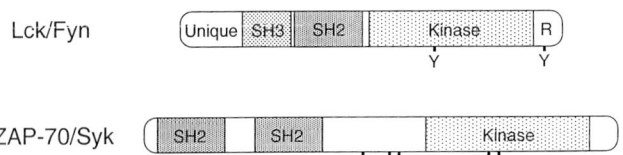

FIG. 5. Protein tyrosine kinases involved in TCR signal transduction. Shown are schematic representations of the Lck/Fyn and Syk/ZAP-70 PTKs. The unique, SH3, SH2, kinase, and regulatory domains are indicated. Also shown are the two sites of phosphorylation in Lck/Fyn and some of the sites in Syk/ZAP-70.

discussed below. Within the N-terminal, 40 to 70 residues are also the most distinguishing sequences among this family that probably play important roles in the unique functions and interactions of each of these kinases. The unique region is followed by the Src homology 3 (SH3) domain that consists of approximately 60 residues. The SH3 domain is involved in directing protein–protein interactions by binding in a sequence-specific context to residues contained in proline-rich regions. The SH3 domain is followed by a 100–amino-acid structural domain, the Src homology 2 (SH2) domain. The SH2 domain also is involved in protein–protein interactions by binding to phosphorylated tyrosine residues contained in a particular sequence-specific context.

The SH2 domain is followed by the catalytic domain, the kinase domain. The crystal structure of the activated Lck kinase domain has been solved and, like other kinase domains, it is a two-lobed structure consisting of approximately 250 residues (129). Like most kinases, the catalytic activity of the kinase is regulated by an activation loop. Within the activation loop of the Src family is a single tyrosine residue that regulates kinase activity. Phosphorylation of this tyrosine residue activates catalytic function by relocalization of the activation loop allowing for substrate access to the catalytic site.

At the C-terminal of the Src kinases is the regulatory domain. This short region contains the second well-characterized tyrosine phosphorylation site in Src kinases. Phosphorylation of this tyrosine results in the inactivation of the kinase. The crystal structures of two Src family kinases, Hck and Src, that are phosphorylated at this position have been solved and are remarkably similar (130,131). The structure reveals that in the inactive phosphorylated state, the kinase is in a closed conformation in which the C-terminal negative-regulatory-phosphorylated tyrosine interacts with the SH2 domain of the same molecule and that the SH3 domain interacts with a proline-containing spacer sequence between the SH2 and kinase domain. These interactions prevent the kinase domain from assuming an active conformation. Thus, activation of the kinase requires the dephosphorylation of the C-terminal tyrosine residue and phosphorylation of the tyrosine in the activation loop.

Fyn PTK

Several lines of evidence have implicated the Fyn PTK in TCR signal transduction. Fyn is a 59-kDa protein and is expressed ubiquitously but at particularly high levels in the brain and hematopoietic system. Two isoforms of Fyn exist that are differentially expressed in hematopoietic cells or the brain (132). The molecular basis for these two forms of Fyn is the tissue-specific alternative splicing of two homologous but nonidentical copies of exon 7 that encode a portion of the kinase domain. Overexpression of either of the two forms of Fyn in an antigen-specific T-cell hybridoma can have different functional consequences (133). Whereas both forms of Fyn-enhanced anti–TCR mAb increases in protein-tyrosine phosphorylation, only the Fyn isoform expressed in hematopoietic cells augmented antigen-induced IL-2 production. Thus, the two forms of Fyn may serve distinct functions, possibly by interacting with distinct intracellular signal transduction molecules.

The interaction of Fyn with the TCR has been difficult to study. Fyn can be co-immunoprecipitated with the TCR complex, albeit at low stoichiometry, if mild detergents are used to solubilize the complex (134). Fyn protein has also been reported to co-localize with the TCR when TCR capping is induced by anti–CD3 mAb, consistent either with a direct or indirect association (135). A specific association between Fyn and ζ, CD3γ or CD3ϵ fusion proteins could be detected in a sensitive heterologous expression system (136). This interaction mapped to the 10 most N-terminal residues of Fyn (which also encode the residues responsible for lipid modification and membrane localization) and sequences within ITAMs, although no single residue seemed critical in the interaction. Further investigation has shown that the dual fatty acylation (myristoylation and palmitoylation) of Fyn that occurs in the N-terminal region is responsible for localization of this PTK to membrane lipid rafts. In these microdomains Fyn can phosphorylate TCR ITAMS. These phosphorylated sites then serve to bind the Fyn SH2 domain, thus stabilizing the interaction of PTK and TCR (137). Thus, these biochemical and cellular studies suggest the possibility of an indirect as well as direct association of Fyn with the TCR.

The functional importance of the interaction of Fyn with the TCR has been addressed in a variety of biochemical and genetic approaches. Stimulation of the TCR induces an increase in Fyn PTK activity that is associated with an increase in tyrosine phosphorylation of Fyn-associated proteins (138). Expression of activated versions of both isoforms of Fyn in a T-cell hybridoma results in heightened TCR signal transduction (133). The activated version of Fyn here refers to a protein in which the C-terminal negative regulatory tyrosine has been mutated. Similar effects have been observed with other activated Src family members, so that this effect may not reveal a function specific to Fyn. An alternative approach has been used to express increased levels of normal Fyn as a transgene within the T-cell lineage. This resulted in heightened responses to TCR responsiveness, whereas mice expressing a kinase-deficient mutant of Fyn had diminished TCR signal transduction capability (139). Surprisingly, disruption of the *Fyn* gene by homologous recombination resulted in a relatively restricted deficiency in signal transduction function. Mature single positive thymocytes (CD4$^+$ or

CD8$^+$) had a rather striking impairment in TCR signal transduction, whereas double-positive (CD4$^+$CD8$^+$) and mature T-peripheral T cells had a more modest decrease in TCR signal transduction capacity (140,141). These experiments with the mice containing the disrupted Fyn gene suggest a potential role for Fyn in TCR signal transduction that is developmentally restricted to a specific stage in T-cell development. The loss of Fyn, however, did not appear to have untoward consequences on thymic development, suggesting the possibility of compensatory mechanisms involving other PTKs that may have redundant functions. Indeed, results discussed below suggest an important role for the Lck kinase.

Although redundancy among Src family members may be observed in developmental studies where selective pressures in the developing populations of cells are brought to bear, it is likely that each Src kinase may have specific functions as well, defined by specific substrates. A unique functional role for Fyn has been revealed in studies of the Pyk2 kinase, which is homologous to the focal adhesion kinase. Although the function for Pyk2 is not yet understood, its phosphorylation and catalytic activity are regulated by TCR signal transduction (142). However, in Fyn-deficient mice, Pyk2 is neither activated nor phosphorylated. These results suggest that Fyn is required to couple the TCR to Pyk2. Results in several studies suggest that Fyn has a specific role in binding to or phosphorylating ADAP (previously known as Fyb or SLAP-130), Cbl, and Vav. These substrate molecules are described further below.

Lck PTK

Lck, a 56-kD PTK of the Src family, plays a critical role in TCR signal transduction. It is expressed predominantly in T cells. Lck associates with CD4 and CD8 via interactions that involve cysteine residues present in the cytoplasmic domains of the co-receptors and within the unique N-terminal domain of Lck (143). Although not all Lck is associated with either CD4 or CD8, the stoichiometry is relatively high. This direct interaction of Lck with the co-receptors CD4 and CD8 positions it to play an important functional role in TCR signal transduction during antigen recognition.

The demonstrated role of CD4 and CD8 as co-receptors with the TCR during peptide–MHC interactions supports an important functional role for Lck during TCR signal transduction (60). Cross-linking of the TCR together with CD4, but not separately, with mAbs markedly enhances TCR-mediated signal transduction (64). This suggests a model in which the co-receptors CD4 and CD8 function not only to increase avidity of the TCR with the antigen peptide–MHC complex, but also to co-localize Lck with the signaling apparatus contained within the cytoplasmic domains of the TCR. This model has been supported by work involving a CD4-dependent antigen-specific T-cell hybridoma. Antigen-induced IL-2 production by this hybridoma was reconstituted by wild-type CD4, but not by mutants of CD4 that could not associate with Lck (74). Thus, Lck appears to play a critical role during CD4- and CD8-dependent TCR signal transduction.

A function for Lck in TCR-mediated signal transduction, independent of its association with CD4 or CD8, is suggested by a variety of observations. Some T-cell clones or hybridomas can respond to antigen in the absence of CD4 or CD8 expression. CD4 and CD8 participation in antigen recognition is generally less important in secondary immune responses. Expression of activated Lck within a class II MHC–restricted IL-2–secreting T-cell hybridoma that failed to express CD4 still markedly increased the sensitivity of this cell to antigen (144). At least an indirect interaction of Lck with the TCR is implied by experiments in which the expression of CD4 in a CD4-negative T-cell clone could inhibit the ability of anti–TCR mAbs from activating this cell through the TCR by apparently sequestering Lck away from the TCR (145). Moreover, Lck can be detected in immunoprecipitates of TCR components, although it is not clear whether the interaction is direct. The mechanism by which Lck might directly interact with TCR components has not been defined, although it is properly positioned at the plasma membrane and lipid rafts to interact with TCR components (146). Thus, Lck can contribute to TCR signal transduction through CD4/CD8-dependent and -independent mechanisms.

A critical role for Lck in TCR signal transduction is evident from genetic studies of mice and cell lines deficient in Lck function. TCR induction of protein-tyrosine phosphorylation as well as downstream events are markedly impaired in Lck-deficient T cells (147–150). Moreover, a critical role for Lck in thymic development, which likely involves its function within the pre-TCR and mature TCR signaling pathways, is well illustrated by the profound, but incomplete, arrest in thymic development in mice in which the Lck gene has been disrupted by homologous recombination (148). The major defect appears to occur at an early developmental checkpoint, the CD4⁻/CD8⁻ to CD4⁺/CD8⁺ transition, where the pre-TCR mediates a signal to indicate that the TCR β chain has been functionally rearranged and expressed on the cell surface (see Chapter 19). A complete block is observed at this developmental checkpoint in mice lacking both Lck and Fyn (151,152). Since no developmental defect is observed in the Fyn-deficient mice, these results suggest that Lck plays the major role in pre-TCR signaling function but that Fyn can partially compensate for its loss.

Cell lines deficient in Lck have proved useful in examining the function of the various Lck domains. In all these studies, Lck–deficient cell lines have been subjected to cDNA transfection to express either Lck with targeted mutations or wild-type, nonmutated Lck. Studies of this kind have demonstrated the importance of N-terminal Lck cysteine residues. These residues become acylated, targeting the PTK to rafts and ensuring proper signaling function. Expression of a mutation that blocks function of the Lck SH2 domain fails to restore TCR-mediated signaling. The mutation blocked interaction of Lck with the ZAP-70 PTK, which as discussed below, would have a deleterious effect on ZAP-70 function. Disruption of the Lck SH3 domain, assayed in the same manner, had a partial effect. In cells expressing this mutant form

of Lck, many signaling pathways were intact, but activation of MAPK (mitogen-activated protein kinase) serine kinase was significantly inhibited for unclear reasons (153–155).

The activation of Lck catalytic activity following TCR stimulation can be detected. In addition, a two-fold to four-fold increase in Lck kinase activity can also be detected following cross-linking of the CD4 molecule. Activation of the PTK activity is associated with phosphorylation of a tyrosine residue (Y394) within the activation loop of the kinase domain, a characteristic site of autophosphorylation of activated Src family members (155). This is presumed to allow access of the substrate to the catalytic site. It is noteworthy that although cross-linking of CD4 increases Lck catalytic activity, the characteristic increase in cellular tyrosine phosphoproteins associated with TCR stimulation is not observed (64). Therefore, Lck represents a critically important PTK involved in TCR signal transduction but it is not likely be the only PTK involved.

Syk Family PTKs Associate with Stimulated TCR

The Syk family of PTKs, consisting of only Syk and ZAP-70, plays an important role in TCR signal transduction (reviewed in Chu et al. [156]). ZAP-70 is expressed preferentially in T cells and NK cells. It was first identified as a 70-kDa TCR ζ-associated tyrosine phosphoprotein in immunoprecipitates isolated from TCR-stimulated cells. Syk is 72 kDa and is more broadly expressed within the hematopoietic lineage. However, within the T-cell lineage, it is expressed early in thymic ontogeny and is down-regulated in mature T cells, except for the γ/δ lineage, where it appears to be expressed in greater abundance (157,158). Both of these kinases have similar functions within signaling pathways mediated by receptors of cells of the hematopoietic lineages. They associate with doubly phosphorylated ITAMs and are inducibly phosphorylated following TCR stimulation (63).

The overall structure of ZAP-70 and Syk are similar. They each have two N-terminal SH2 domains and a more C-terminal catalytic domain (Fig. 5). It is now well recognized that the ZAP-70 SH2 domains bind in tandem to a single doubly phosphorylated ITAM with the relatively high affinity of 10 to 30 nM (159). This affinity is substantially higher than is seen with isolated SH2 domains that bind with micromolar affinities. The structure of the two ZAP-70 SH2 domains bound to a single doubly phosphorylated TCR ζ ITAM has been solved by x-ray crystallography (160). The phospho-ITAM has an extended structure and the more C-terminal SH2 (SH2C) domain has a typical structure and binds to the more N-terminal pYXXL sequences in the ITAM. In contrast, the N-terminal SH2 domain (SH2N) is atypical. It is an incomplete SH2 domain; the SH2N phosphotyrosine–binding pocket is only completed when it is brought into close apposition to SH2C. The close relationship between SH2N and SH2C when bound to the doubly phosphorylated ITAM emphasizes the importance of the critical spacing between the YXXL groups of the ITAM. Greater or fewer than the seven or eight residues would probably not permit appropriate binding to occur. The other interesting feature revealed from the structure is the formation of a coiled-coiled loop in interdomain A, which separates the SH2 domains. The function of interdomain A is not clear, although it may help to stabilize the bound structure. Based on studies of Syk, phosphorylation of this loop could regulate the binding of the SH2 domains to a phospho-ITAM (161). The structure of the Syk SH2 domains is similar but not identical (162). Both SH2 domains are structurally complete and there is some evidence that they exhibit more flexibility in their binding requirements.

Approximately 65 residues comprising interdomain B separate the ZAP-70 SH2 and kinase domains. This interdomain region has a regulatory function. Y292, within interdomain B, is an *in vivo* autophosphorylation site in ZAP-70 (218), and its phosphorylation inhibits ZAP-70 function (163–165). This phosphorylated site binds to the proto-oncogene product, Cbl, which is a negative regulator of a number of PTKs (166,167). The mechanism of Cbl action is discussed below. There are two other sites of phosphorylation within interdomain B in ZAP-70, Y315, and Y319. The homologous sites in Syk have been shown to be *in vitro* autophosphorylation sites (168). These sites serve a positive regulatory function by recruiting substrates to ZAP-70. Y315 is important for ZAP-70 function and for the phosphorylation of the proto-oncogene Vav (see below). Y319 has a significant effect on ZAP-70 function. When this site is mutated to phenylalanine, there is a marked inhibition of signaling events induced by this PTK. When phosphorylated, Y319 serves as a binding site for the SH2 domain of the Lck PTK (169). However, deletion of interdomain B has a net positive effect on ZAP-70 function, suggesting that the region has an overall negative regulatory function (165).

The catalytic domains of ZAP-70 and Syk are typical of PTK domains. TCR stimulation increases the catalytic activities of both of these kinases. Their catalytic activities are regulated by phosphorylation of residues contained within their putative activation loops. Phosphorylation of Y493 in the activation loop of ZAP-70 and of the homologous residue in Syk, Y519, increases kinase activity (170). In contrast, Y492 in ZAP-70 has a negative regulatory function (163,164,170). These two residues within the same activation loop may be sequentially phosphorylated in a dynamic feedback regulatory circuit (170). Interestingly, the intrinsic catalytic activity of Syk is greater than that of ZAP (171). Based on expression studies of mutant forms of ZAP-70 and Syk in cell lines and natural mutations of ZAP-70 in mice and a human patient (172,173), the catalytic activities of ZAP-70 and Syk are critical for their function.

The functional importance of ZAP-70 and Syk in T cells has been established from natural and experimental genetic models. A human severe combined immunodeficiency (SCID) syndrome characterized by defective TCR signal transduction and developmental abnormalities in the T-cell lineage results from ZAP-70 mutations (174–176). In these SCID patients, only mature CD4$^+$ T cells are detectable, but

these T cells have defective TCR signal transduction. In mice deficient in ZAP-70 protein or with a kinase-defective ZAP-70 protein (172,177), thymocyte development is blocked at the CD4$^+$ CD8$^+$ stage, a time when signal transduction by the mature TCR is required for positive selection. The ability to bypass the developmental checkpoint mediated by the pre-TCR may reflect compensation by the Syk kinase, which is expressed at higher levels earlier in thymocyte development (156). Differences between the phenotypes of humans and mice deficient in ZAP-70 remain unexplained, but could reflect differences in Syk expression (156,178). Mice made deficient in Syk expression by gene targeting best reveal the normal function of Syk in the T-cell lineage. In these mice, the predominant defect in T cells is the failure of epithelial T cells expressing the γ/δ TCR to develop (179). Cell lines deficient in Syk or ZAP-70 have proven useful to study these enzymes. Investigators have transfected them with DNA encoding mutated versions of these enzymes, and have achieved careful structure–function studies in this way. Collectively, all these approaches indicate that this family of kinases plays an important role in TCR signal transduction and that these kinases may be able to play some redundant and some unique functions.

Interaction of Src and Syk PTKs

The Src and Syk kinases interact with the TCR in a highly coordinated and sequential manner. In cell lines or T cells cultured *in vitro,* TCR ITAMs are inducibly phosphorylated following receptor stimulation. In *ex vivo* thymocytes or T cells, the TCR ζ ITAMs are constitutively phosphorylated, although CD3 ITAMs are inducibly phosphorylated (180). Both the inducible and constitutive phosphorylation of the ITAMs appear to be principally mediated by Lck (53,150). ZAP-70 or Syk bind to the doubly phosphorylated ITAMs. Once bound, they can be activated in the stimulated TCR complex by phosphorylation of their activation loops. Phosphorylation of Y493, the critical residue in the ZAP-70 activation loop, is thought to be mediated by Lck (53,170). In contrast, Syk may be able to autophosphorylate and activate its kinase activity on ITAM binding (181). Indeed, it appears that Syk may be less dependent on Src kinases in T cells for its activation. However, in *ex vivo* thymocytes and T cells, receptor stimulation is required for the inducible phosphorylation of ZAP-70 or Syk, which are constitutively associated with the TCR ζ chain (150). ITAM-bound Syk or ZAP-70 in the stimulated TCR complex forms a stable complex with Lck via the Lck SH2 domain (68,69). This likely leads to a further increase in PTK activity and substrate phosphorylation.

These studies suggest important interactions between Lck and Syk family PTKs that may occur during T-cell responses to antigen. One model that may account for the interaction of Lck and ZAP-70 is depicted in Fig. 6. During the recognition of peptide antigen bound to class II–MHC molecules, co-localization of the TCR and CD4 occurs. This recruits Lck into close proximity with the cytoplasmic domains of the

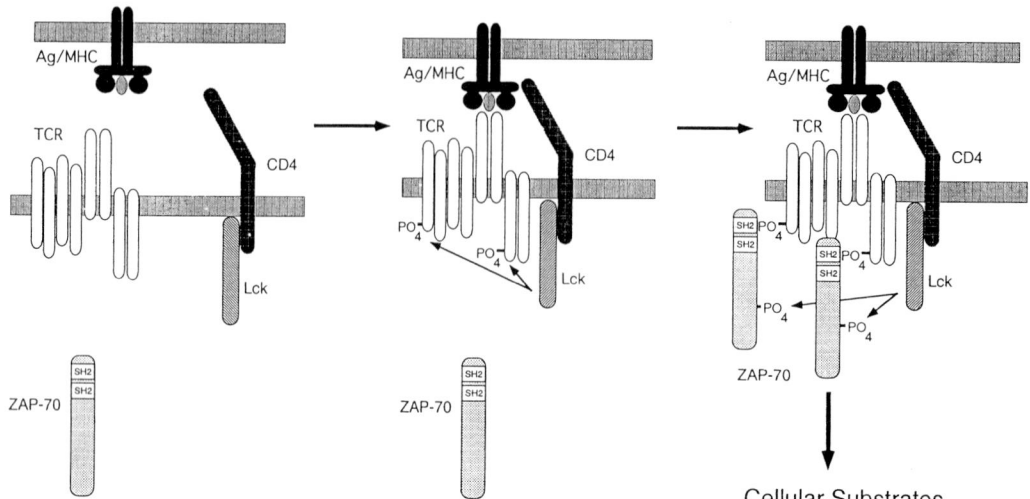

FIG. 6. A speculative model of the interaction of Lck and ZAP-70 during antigen recognition by a CD4$^+$ T cell. During TCR and CD4 engagement of an MHC class II molecule, Lck is brought into close proximity with the TCR cytoplasmic domain and phosphorylates CD3 and ζ chains. ZAP-70 is recruited to the tyrosine phosphorylated CD3 and ζ chains via its SH2 domains, which allows Lck to transphosphorylate and thereby activate ZAP-70.

TCR chains containing ITAMs. This could result in phosphorylation of tyrosine residues within the ITAMs. *In vivo,* it is likely that this only results in CD3 phosphorylation. Such tyrosine phosphorylation of ITAMs allows for the recruitment of ZAP-70 or Syk. Co-localization of ZAP-70 and/or Syk with Lck facilitates the interaction and transphosphorylation/ activation of these kinases. The ability of Lck to interact with activated ZAP-70 at phosphorylated Y319, discussed in the previous section, may ensure that additional ZAP-70 molecules are activated. A similar model may apply to the recognition of peptides bound to class I–MHC molecules by CD8$^+$ cells. However, this model does not account for the mechanism by which the TCR can induce signal transduction events independent of CD4 or CD8. In these situations, cytoplasmic or membrane-localized Lck that is not bound to CD4 or CD8 may be recruited to the TCR complex through oligomerization of the ITAMs. The net result of these interactions is the coordinated activation of these kinases leading to the tyrosine phosphorylation of downstream effector molecules and substrates that represent critical regulators in signaling pathways.

Function of SH2 Domains in Signal Transduction Pathways

The activation of the catalytic function of cytoplasmic PTKs by the TCR has several consequences. Certainly tyrosine phosphorylation of certain enzymes is well known to lead to their activation as discussed above in the section on T-cell PTKs. Over the past decade, an additional consequence of protein-tyrosine phosphorylation has been recognized and intensively studied. This is the use of tyrosine phosphorylation to facilitate protein–protein interactions. Considerable

progress has been made toward understanding how proteins in PTK or protein-tyrosine phosphatase (PTPase) signal transduction pathways interact since it has been recognized that sequences containing phosphotyrosine residues can bind to SH2 domains (reviewed in Pawson et al. [182]). SH2 domains are homologous sequences consisting of approximately 100 residues that are present in a variety of molecules that have been implicated in signal transduction pathways involving protein-tyrosine phosphorylation. Some of the proteins implicated in TCR signal transduction pathways that contain SH2 domains are listed in Table 2.

Isolated SH2 domains can independently interact with phosphoproteins or phosphopeptides with micromolar affinities. It has been possible to demonstrate specificity in these interactions that depends on the sequences that surround the phosphotyrosine residue (182,183). The structural basis for this specificity and for the interaction with phosphotyrosine is evident from the three-dimensional structure of SH2 domains. Each SH2 domain contains a binding pocket for phosphotyrosine, but sequences surrounding the binding pocket influence this interaction. Thus, the ability of this structural domain to recognize sequences surrounding phosphotyrosine can define the specificity of the interactions that occur among proteins in a signal transduction pathway.

SH2 domains may serve multiple functions. First, they can be responsible for recruiting signal transduction molecules to activated PTKs. Activated PTKs often contain sites of auto- or trans-phosphorylation that may represent the sites to which downstream signal transduction components bind via SH2 domains. For instance, the Vav SH2 domain binds to phospho-Y315 in ZAP-70 and this binding event facilitates the tyrosine phosphorylation and function of Vav (184). Second, they may protect tyrosine-phosphorylated sites from the

TABLE 2. *Proteins with Src homology-2 (SH2) domains that may be associated with T-cell activation*

Protein tyrosine kinases
  Fyn
  Lck
  Syk
  ZAP-70
  Csk
  Itk

Protein tyrosine phosphatases
  SHP-1
  SHP-2

Proteins with enzymatic functions
  Phospholipase C γ1 (PLC γ1)
  Phosphatidylinositol 3-kinase (PI 3-kinase), p85 subunit

Adaptors and regulators
  GTPase activating protein (GAP)
  SOS
  Vav
  Slp-76
  Shc
  Nck
  Grb2
  Crk

action of PTPases, thereby prolonging the effects of tyrosine phosphorylation (185). Third, they may permit the recruitment of kinases or phosphatases to potential substrates or sites of action. PTKs of the Src and Syk families all contain SH2 domains, as do at least some cytosolic tyrosine phosphatases (182). Fourth, SH2 domains may play important regulatory functions to enhance or inhibit enzymatic functions. For instance, the negative regulatory site of tyrosine phosphorylation in Src family PTKs interacts with the SH2 domain contained within these molecules to inhibit kinase activity (130,131). Thus, SH2 domains can play a variety of distinct roles by interacting with phosphotyrosine residues within proteins in a signal transduction pathway.

It is important to recognize that SH2 domains are not the only structural domains that bind phosphotyrosine and that other structural domains may contribute to protein–protein interactions within a signaling pathway. For instance, phosphotyrosine binding (PTB) domains bind to tyrosine-phosphorylated residues (186). The specificities of the PTB domain may be more limited. Many other modular domains that bind to residues other than phosphotyrosine contribute to the interactions observed in signaling pathways. These include the SH3, PH, WW, WD40, and PDZ domains. The SH2 domain is frequently found in tandem with one or more SH3 domains. As discussed above, SH3 domains bind to sequences rich in proline residues, so that no covalent post-translational modification is necessary for the interaction of SH3 domains with their targets. However, allosteric changes in the target sequence may be critical. The SH2 and SH3 domains of different molecules vary in sequence sufficiently to impart specificity in their binding events. The affinities of the SH2 and SH3 domains for their peptide ligands are only in the low micromolar range, and for SH2 domains this affinity is only 20-fold to 50-fold greater than for isolated phosphotyrosine. However, by using pairs or combinations of these protein modules, a much higher degree of specificity and affinity may be achieved in these protein–protein interactions (187).

Protein-Tyrosine Phosphatase (PTPase) CD45 Plays Critical Role in TCR Signal Transduction

Protein phosphorylation can be regulated by stimulating PTKs, but it can also be induced by inhibiting PTPases. Many PTPases are expressed in T cells (reviewed in Veillette et al. [188] and Mustelin et al. [189]). CD45 (leukocyte common antigen or T200), CD148, and PTPaseα (or LRP) are transmembrane tyrosine phosphatases. Many cytosolic PTPases (including T-cell phosphatase, PEP, SHP-1 and-2, and low-molecular-weight phosphatase) are expressed in T cells. Although all of these PTPases may contribute to TCR signal transduction, the role of CD45 in T cells is best understood.

CD45 represents a family of transmembrane PTPases consisting of various isoforms that are derived by the alternative splicing of exons 4 through 6 (190). All of the isoforms contain two tandem domains, of 300 amino acids each, that are homologous with other PTPases. Only the first domain has catalytic activity (191,192), but its activity depends on the second domain.

CD45 proteins are expressed at high levels on all cells of the hematopoietic lineage except mature erythrocytes. The individual CD45 isoforms, 180 to 220 kD, are expressed differentially in a tissue- and activation-specific manner. On T cells, these isoforms have been used to distinguish helper T-cell subsets (193) and resting or activated T cells (194). For instance, activated T cells express only the 180-kD isoform (CD45RO) in which the products of exons 4, 5, and 6 are excluded, but naïve T cells express higher molecular weight isoforms. The highly regulated expression of the various isoforms suggests that the extracellular domain has a specific function. This notion is supported by the ability of individual isoforms to differentially reconstitute CD45 function in an antigen-specific hybridoma (195). The ligands for the various isoforms, if they exist, have not been established. Both stimulatory and inhibitory effects of mAbs reactive with the various CD45 isoforms have been observed. Some investigators have suggested that CD45 isoforms differentially interact with other molecules such as CD4 on the same cell. Independent of ligand interactions, distinct roles have been proposed for CD45 isoforms, based on the size and charge differences of the isoforms, that influence the ability of T cells to interact with APCs (9). However, studies with a chimeric molecule in which the extracellular and transmembrane domains of the epidermal growth factor receptor were substituted for those of CD45 suggest that ligand-induced dimerization may inhibit CD45 function (196). These inhibitory effects have been attributed to the symmetrical interaction of a putative wedge-like structure in the juxtamembrane region of one monomer that blocks the catalytic site of the partner monomer during dimerization. Moreover, inactivation of this putative wedge leads to lymphoproliferation and autoimmunity, suggesting that inhibition of CD45 function by dimerization plays an important physiologic regulatory function (197). A function for CD45 has emerged from genetic studies in which mutant T-cell lines or mice, deficient in CD45 expression, have been isolated (reviewed in Hermiston et al. [198]). Loss of CD45 expression in most T-cell lines and clones is associated with selective loss in TCR signal transduction function, including the ability of the TCR to induce increases in tyrosine phosphoproteins. Similarly, developmental arrest and impairment in TCR function are found in mice made deficient in CD45 by gene targeting. The loss of this major membrane PTPase is not associated with a general increase in tyrosine phosphoproteins. Since the initial signal transduction event associated with TCR stimulation is activation of a PTK, CD45 appears to play a selective role in regulating the ability of the TCR to activate the PTK pathway.

Studies with CD45-deficient cells suggest that one target of this PTPase is the negative regulatory site of Lck and has led to the model of Lck regulation shown in Fig. 7. CD45 can dephosphorylate this site *in vitro*, resulting in the priming of Lck (199). This site in Lck, Y505, is hyperphosphorylated in CD45-deficient T-cell lines (200,201). The homologous site in Fyn is also affected, but to a lesser extent. The mechanism by which this site of phosphorylation inhibits kinase function was revealed when the structure of the inactive kinase was solved by x-ray crystallography (130,131). When phosphorylated at the C-terminal, the SH2 domain binds to this site in an intramolecular interaction and the SH3 domain contributes to the inactive conformation by binding to a proline helix encoded by sequences between the SH2 and kinase domains. As a result of these interactions, the kinase domain is kept in an inactive state. The tyrosine associated with negative regulation of kinase function is phosphorylated by a ubiquitous PTK, termed Csk, which shares

some homology with Src PTKs (188). Csk is recruited to the lipid rafts to inactivate Lck and other Src kinases via a protein called Cbp/PAG-85. Thus, CD45 opposes the action of Csk, serves to dephosphorylate the negative regulatory site in Lck (or other Src members) *in vivo,* and allows the kinase to become activated by transautophosphorylation of its activation-loop tyrosine, Y394, during TCR and co-receptor oligomerization. The Y505 hyperphosphorylated form of Lck in CD45-deficient cells would be blocked from participation in TCR signal transduction events. Thus, a complex and likely very dynamic relationship between Src PTKs and PTPases exists that influences the ability of the TCR to induce signal transduction events.

Lastly, CD45 has been reported to be a PTPase for various other substrates. These include the TCR ζ chain, Jak kinases that are involved in lymphokine receptor signaling and also the activation loop of various Src kinases (189).

Consequences of TCR-Mediated PTK Activation

TCR-mediated induction of PTK activity results in the tyrosine phosphorylation of a large number of cellular proteins, in addition to the component chains of the TCR and the Src and Syk family kinases. Some of the many proteins that are inducibly phosphorylated following TCR stimulation are listed in Table 3. Some of these substrate proteins—that is, LAT, Shc, and Slp-76—have no intrinsic enzymatic activity but instead function as adaptors, which mediate protein–protein interactions, thereby coupling the TCR to important intracellular pathways (202). Other substrates have well-characterized enzymatic activities, such as phospholipase C γ1 (PLCγ1), Itk, and mitogen-activated protein kinase (MAPK), that are influenced by tyrosine phosphorylation. Many others do not have a well-defined function in TCR signal transduction pathways.

Recent work on TCR signaling reveals that in addition to changes affecting phosphorylation or re-localization of

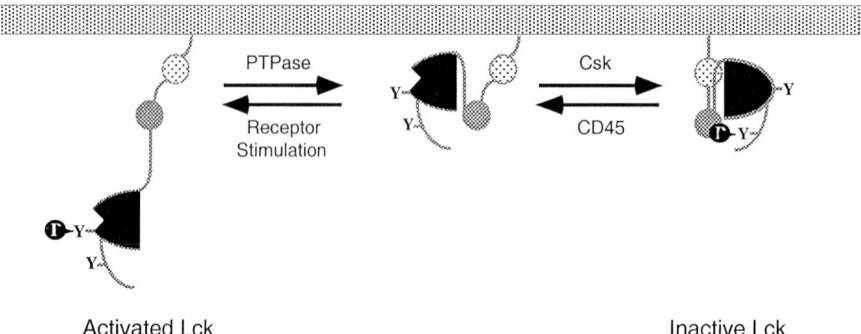

Activated Lck

Inactive Lck

FIG. 7. Dynamic regulation of Lck. A schematic representation of the regulation of the two phosphorylation sites of Lck. Csk phosphorylates Lck at the C-terminal negative regulatory site, driving the kinase into the "closed" inactive state. CD45 dephosphorylates this site, opening the kinase and allowing it to be activated by receptor stimulation. Receptor stimulation leads to the phosphorylation of the tyrosine in the activation loop, increasing kinase activity. An as-yet-unidentified PTPase dephosphorylates the activation loop, thereby decreasing kinase activity.

TABLE 3. *Some of the proteins that are tyrosine phosphorylated following TCR stimulation*

TCR subunits
  CD3 δ, ϵ, γ
  ζ

Protein tyrosine kinases
  Itk
  Lyn
  Lck
  MAPKs
  Pyk2
  Syk
  ZAP-70

Proteins with enzymatic function
  Phospholipase C γ1 (PLC γ1)
  Vav

Others
  ADAP
  Cbl
  Cbp
  CD5
  CD6
  Ezrin
  LAT
  Shc
  Slp-76
  Shc
  α Tubulin

individual proteins, activation of T cells results in major changes in macromolecular structures. Two important subjects discussed below include dynamic changes in the plasma membrane due to membrane lipid heterogeneity and the generation of large macromolecular arrays that form at the interface of the T cell and the APC.

Substrate Phosphorylation and Generation of Protein Signaling Complexes

A prominent PTK substrate observed after activation of the TCR is the adaptor molecule LAT (linker for activation of T cells), a protein of 36 to 38 kD (reviewed in Samelson [202] and Zhang and Samelson [203]). In early studies, this protein was detected in a complex with a number of other PTK substrates, including PLC-γ1 and the small linker molecule Grb2. LAT has a short extracellular sequence, a transmembrane domain and a long cytosolic component containing nine tyrosine residues conserved between mouse and human proteins. LAT contains two cysteine residues (C26 and C29) that are predicted to be near the inner leaflet of the plasma membrane. These cysteines are targets for post-translational palmitoylation, which is responsible for specific localization within the plasma membrane (see below).

LAT is rapidly phosphorylated on tyrosine residues following TCR engagement. Experiments in T cells indicate that ZAP-70 is the PTK most likely to be responsible for these events. The multiple phosphorylations on LAT provide binding sites for a number of critical signaling proteins. The significance of LAT as a site where these proteins interact is shown in studies comparing T-cell lines and mutant versions of these lines that lack LAT. The variants that lack LAT when activated by cross-linking the TCR show no activation of most of the distal signaling pathways described in subsequent sections. One exception is the activation of the Pak kinase, a kinase downstream of Rho GTPases, that likely plays a role in actin cytoskeleton remodeling (204). However, all signaling events are restored in cells in which LAT is replaced. These experiments show that LAT, as a proximal substrate of TCR-activated PTKs, is critical to subsequent signaling events.

The proteins that bind phosphorylated LAT fall in the same two categories described above for PTK substrates, enzymes and adaptor proteins. Some of these adaptor proteins are members of the Grb2 family, which consists of Grb2, Grap, and Gads (205). These molecules contain a central SH2 domain surrounded by two SH3 domains. The Gads protein, which is also known by a number of other names (e.g., Grpl, MONA, Grf40) contains an internal proline-rich region between the SH2 and the C-terminal SH3 domains. The SH2 domain of Grb2 family members bind to phosphorylated LAT at one or more of the three distal LAT tyrosines. Their SH3 domains bind a number of other signaling proteins. Thus, the interaction of LAT with Grb2 family members results in ways to recruit additional signaling molecules.

Grb2 is ubiquitously expressed and is known to bind many different proteins through its SH3 domains. In T cells, one such protein is Sos (son of sevenless), which is a well-characterized activator of the RasG protein. Cbl is another protein that binds Grb2. Both of these proteins can be detected in association with LAT. Their functions are discussed further below. Grap-associated proteins include Sos, dynamin, and Sam68. The role of Grap has not been extensively studied. Gads is only expressed in hematopoietic cells. Gads interacts with another critical adaptor molecule, SLP-76, and with the serine-threonine kinase HPK.

SLP-76 is another protein that was originally identified as a tyrosine kinase substrate (205). It is a 76-kD protein expressed exclusively in hematopoietic cells. SLP-76 is also an adaptor protein that binds multiple effector and linker molecules through three domains. The amino-terminal region contains multiple tyrosines that are phosphorylated following TCR activation. The central region contains multiple proline residues including those that bind the Gads SH3 domains. The carboxy-terminal end of the protein contains an SH2 domain. A cell line lacking SLP-76 also has major signaling defects that can be restored when the protein is restored. This cell line has been useful in studies designed to uncover the role of SLP-76 and its various domains.

Upon TCR engagement the amino terminal region of SLP-76 is phosphorylated on tyrosine residues by activated ZAP-70. These sites bind a number of other proteins that also contain SH2 domains. These include Vav, an activator of G proteins of the Rac family; Nck, which is also an adaptor molecule; and Itk, a member of the Tec PTK family. These various SLP-76–binding proteins are thought to be involved in a number of pathways involved in T-cell activation. SLP-76 binding to Itk potentially positions this PTK in close proximity to PLC-γ1, which is also bound to LAT and SLP-76. PLC-γ1, as discussed below, is an important regulator of phospholipids and calcium levels. Itk phosphorylation of this enzyme appears to have a positive regulatory effect. Vav and Nck are involved in biochemical pathways that regulate gene transcription and the cytoskeleton. The carboxy-terminal SH2 domain of SLP-76 binds a protein originally known as SLAP (SLP-76–associated phosphoprotein) or Fyb (Fyn-binding protein). By consensus it is now known as ADAP (adhesion and degranulation promoting adaptor protein). This molecule is involved in coupling TCR signals to adhesion molecules during T-cell activation (79,206).

This description gives a sense of the complexity of protein interactions that occur following TCR engagement. The central role of LAT, Grb2 family members, and SLP-76 should be apparent. The interactions that have been described, however, have been limited to these adaptor or linker molecules. Phosphorylated LAT and SLP-76 interact as well with the enzyme PLC-γ1. This protein is one of the best characterized of PTK substrates phosphorylated in response to TCR engagement.

The interaction of PLC-γ1 and a 36- to 38-kD protein was described prior to LAT isolation (202,203). This interaction was observed to depend on T-cell activation and on the two PLC-γ1 SH2 domains. The N-terminal SH2 domain appears to have higher affinity for phospho-LAT, but the C-terminal SH2 domain binds to LAT as well. The PLC-γ1 interaction with LAT depends primarily on tyrosine-132 in LAT (human sequence numbering). This residue is part of a consensus-binding sequence for PLC-γ1 SH2 domains. The conversion of this LAT tyrosine residue to phenylalanine has been tested, introducing this mutant form of the molecule into cells that lack LAT. In these experiments, the mutant form shows no PLC-γ1-LAT association and PLC-γ1 tyrosine phosphorylation is inhibited. A normal consequence of PLC-γ1 tyrosine phosphorylation is elevation of intracellular calcium, as discussed in the next section. This response was blocked in cells expressing only LAT with the mutation at residue 132. Simultaneous mutation of the three distal tyrosine residues of LAT also had a negative effect on PLC-γ1 activation. This effect either reflects a direct effect on PLC-γ1 binding and activation, or an indirect effect due to the loss of binding of another protein involved in regulating PLC-γ1 binding (202,203).

As noted above, the multidomain adaptor, SLP-76, is critical to T-cell activation; cell lines lacking this molecule fail to activate PLC-γ1 normally. An interaction of this adaptor with PLC-γ1 has been demonstrated. A region of the SLP-76 central domain, rich in prolines but distinct from the site of interaction with the Gads SH3 domains, interacts with the PLC-γ1 SH3 domain. As may be clear from the description of the various protein interactions with LAT and SLP-76, it is possible to define a complex of LAT-Gads-SLP-76 and PLC-γ1 held together by multiple sites of interaction.

Full PLC-γ1 phosphorylation and activation requires members of the Tec PTK family (125,207). Deletion of the Tec PTK (Itk), or deletion of two Tec PTKs (Itk and Txk/Rlk), results in defects in sustained calcium elevation following TCR activation. The Itk PTK can localize to the plasma membrane via its plextrin homology domain, a lipid-binding module. SH2 and SH3 domains of the Tec PTKs have been shown to interact in various assays with LAT, SLP-76, and PLC-γ1. Although the mode of interaction of these enzymes with signaling molecules contained in complexes is not yet entirely clear, such interactions would be likely to enhance substrate phosphorylation and thus PLC-γ1 activation.

Plasma Membrane Heterogeneity and Raft Model of T-Cell Activation

An added level of complexity in the current model of T-cell activation needs to be introduced now that the basic elements of TCR, PTKs, and proximal PTK substrates have been defined. TCR engagement, the recruitment and activation of PTKs, and the phosphorylation of substrates all occur at the plasma membrane. This structure had been assumed to be a homogeneous lipid bilayer, but this impression has been considerably revised. Instead, there is now considerable evidence that lipid heterogeneity exists within the membrane. In addition to glycerolipids, the membrane contains glycosphingolipids and cholesterol. These components self-associate and in so doing form microdomains that are distinct from diffuse glycerolipids. These domains have been named in many ways: GEMs (glycolipid-enriched microdomains); DIGs (detergent insoluble glycolipid-enriched membranes; DRMs (detergent-resistant membranes); or rafts (208,209). Some of these names refer to certain properties of the domains. In particular, this is the inability of nonionic detergents such as Triton X-100 to solubilize these domains from plasma membranes in the cold. These insoluble membrane components can be separated from solubilized material by sucrose gradient centrifugation.

These domains have been shown to have a significant impact on T-cell activation. They are enriched in a number of molecules relevant to TCR-mediated signaling, including the Src family PTKs, LAT, and the lipid substrates of PLC-γ1. The G protein Ras, which is described below, can be found in rafts, and some enzymes such as Itk are recruited to rafts upon cellular activation. Various signals determine whether proteins localize in rafts. One characteristic is that lipids can post-translationally modify several of these proteins. Thus, for example, most members of the Src family are modified by myristoylation and palmitoylation.

In addition to the fact that critical signaling molecules are in rafts, it has become clear that other signaling molecules are recruited to rafts with activation. In some studies, receptor engagement in T-cells increases the level of TCR localization in rafts. More easily demonstrated is the localization of LAT in rafts and the recruitment of signaling molecules to phosphorylated LAT following TCR engagement (202,203). Two

LAT cysteine residues (positions 26 and 29) adjacent to the putative transmembrane domain of the protein are palmitoylated. This modification, especially at Cys 26, is required for LAT localization to rafts and LAT tyrosine phosphorylation. Since LAT phosphorylation induces binding by a number of molecules, it is clear that those molecules, such as Grb2, PLC-γ1, and Cbl, are recruited to rafts in this fashion. The fraction of such LAT-binding proteins that shifts in this way is small, but this is presumably the fraction that is functionally active. In studies in which Cys 26 is mutated, there is no LAT tyrosine phosphorylation, no translocation of critical signaling molecules to the rafts, and no T-cell activation.

An unresolved issue is how the TCR and its associated PTKs, which may only loosely be associated with rafts, interact with LAT upon TCR engagement. Various possibilities have been suggested. Lck, which is located in rafts, and its SH2 domain, can bind a phosphorylated tyrosine residue in the activated ZAP-70 PTK (169). This intermolecular bridge may bring TCRs bearing activated ZAP-70 to rafts. The co-receptors CD4 and CD8 by virtue of their multiple interactions may also enhance TCR localization to rafts. Various adaptor molecules have been suggested as linkers between components. These are 3BP2, which can interact via its SH2 domain with both ZAP-70 and LAT, or Shb, which contains two separate phosphotyrosine-binding domains, one which binds TCR ζ chain on phosphorylated tyrosine residues, while the other binds phosphorylated LAT. A conclusion from another study supports the idea that TCR-LAT association is dependent on protein–protein interactions induced by TCR activation and tyrosine phosphorylation, and not on an interaction of the receptor with LAT via large lipid aggregations.

There is certainly strong evidence that membrane heterogeneity exists in model systems and in cells. There is much evidence that membrane microdomains are relevant for signaling in lymphocytes. Advances in this area will likely depend on the development of new techniques. To date many studies depend on a definition of rafts that simply reflects a failure of these structures to be solubilized in detergents. Methods that use advanced microscopic techniques to identify and track membrane heterogeneity in living cells and at physiologic conditions are much needed.

Generation of Immunologic Synapse: Supramolecular Array of Signaling Molecules Formed upon TCR Activation

Engagement of the TCR by peptide MHC complexes results in molecular rearrangements on a very large scale (210). These events have been recognized only recently, and their discovery relied on a number of technical advances. Investigators have enhanced standard immunofluorescent microscopic analysis of fixed cells with special computer software. Others have used high-resolution rapid microscopy of live cells to image signaling molecules containing fluorescent tags. These complementary approaches have provided novel insights into the molecular sorting that occurs following TCR

activation. In T cell clones that engaged and formed conjugates with peptide-loaded APCs a number of signaling molecules localized to the T-cell–APC contact site. Further investigation revealed that these various molecules were found in distinct zones at this site. The TCR and protein kinase Cθ were found to be co-localized at the center of the contact (211). Surrounding this central zone, the adhesion molecule LFA-1 and the cytoskeletal protein talin were found. These molecular assemblies have been named supramolecular activation clusters (SMACs) and the two zones are distinguished as the central SMAC (c-SMAC) and peripheral SMAC (p-SMAC) (210–212).

The dynamic nature of this molecular sorting was first revealed in an artificial antigen-presenting system to enable live cell imaging (212). Instead of APCs, lipids with fluorescently tagged, peptide-loaded MHC and ICAM-1 (the cellular ligand for LFA-1) molecules—both made with glycophosphatidyl tails—were applied to a glass surface. This technique ensured that the molecules that would engage two critical T-cell receptors, the TCR and ICAM-1, could freely move in the plane of the glass. Upon addition of T cells and in the first 30 seconds, an accumulation of ICAM-1 in the central contact area was observed. In this early period, the peptide–MHC complex appeared outside the central contact at points most closely apposed to the surface. Over the next 5 minutes, extensive rearrangement occurred, with the peptide–MHC complexes moving to the center and the ICAM-1 molecules moving to a ring around the central peptide–MHC molecules. This later distribution exactly mirrors what was seen in fixed cells in the previously mentioned study with T-cell clones, assuming, of course, that the peptide–MHC and ICAM-1 were engaged with TCR and LFA-1, respectively (211). Further investigation has identified other components of the c-SMAC, including Lck and CD28. Beyond the p-SMAC are found additional proteins, such as CD43, a large, heavily glycosylated membrane protein, anchored to cytoskeletal proteins such as ezrin and moesin. These molecular distributions are quite stable, lasting at least 1 hour.

As additional molecules are tagged and followed in the context of synapse formation, additional complexities of the process have been appreciated. The fate of CD45 is one example (213). In a number of studies, this large integral membrane tyrosine phosphatase has been observed to be excluded from the SMACs with CD43. However, careful imaging has shown that although much of the CD45 does migrate to periphery of the SMAC, some moves to a central region in the area of TCR–MHC contact. Additionally, some of this central CD45 actually localizes above the TCR and over the plane of contact. Additional experiments showed that CD45 in both peripheral, and to a lesser degree, central locations remain mobile and dynamic. The complex dynamics and localization of CD45 suggest that it may have a similarly complex function and interaction with multiple substrates over time and space.

The dynamics of CD4 have been studied in a similar system (214). In these experiments, chimeric proteins consisting of CD4 and TCR ζ coupled to the green fluorescent protein (GFP) were expressed in the T cells. These molecules could then be tracked with a rapid imaging system to simultaneously follow intracellular calcium levels using specific dyes. Both the TCR subunit and CD4 localized initially in a central area. Interestingly, the accumulation at the earliest time points were punctate, disperse clusters. This early picture corresponded in time with the onset of the initial calcium response. Over the next few minutes as the TCR coalesced and took on the distribution seen in the mature synapse, the CD4 molecule migrated from the central region and appeared as a peripheral ring. Co-localization with pSMAC molecules was not determined. The results with CD4 again indicate that localization varies over time and suggests also that molecular function may change over time as regulated by molecular localization.

The mechanisms underlying the molecular sorting involved in immunologic synapse formation are likely to be multiple and complex (215,216). One such factor is molecular size. There is considerable size heterogeneity of the molecules that sort into a synapse. The extracellular domains of the TCR and CD28 are about 7 nM; integrins are intermediate at about 20 nM; and CD43 and CD45, two very abundant, membrane glycoproteins, have extracellular domains that can be over 40 nM. It is notable that the final distribution of molecules in the synapse reflects this rank order of size: The TCR is in the cSMAC, LFA-1 in the pSMAC, and CD43 and the majority of CD45 are excluded from the SMAC entirely. To what extent sorting is driven by size segregation remains to be determined.

Active changes mediated by the cytoskeleton are certainly involved in molecular movement and synapse formation (215,216). The data supporting this conclusion are varied and extensive. The TCR is indirectly and directly coupled to elements of the cytoskeleton and to the process of cytoskeletal reorganization. The phosphorylation of LAT and recruitment of SLP-76 to phospho-LAT, as reviewed above, brings together a number of critical molecules that directly affect actin polymerization. The phosphorylated tyrosine residues bind the SH2 domain of Vav and Nck. Vav is a guanine-nucleotide-exchange factor (GEF) for the small G proteins Rac and Cdc42 (217). The importance for Vav in T-cell activation has been revealed in studies of mice in which the Vav gene is deleted. T cells from these mice demonstrate deficiencies in calcium flux, lymphokine production, and proliferation. Significantly, antibody-induced capping, a cytoskeleton-regulated event, was markedly inhibited in these cells. T cells that lack Vav show a defect in TCR and MHC accumulation at the point of cell contact (218). The Vav substrate Cdc42 has also been localized at this site (219,220).

SLP-76 binding to Nck can bring another critical cytoskeletal regulator, WASP (Wiskott Aldrich syndrome protein), to the site of activated TCRs. WASP recruitment might also be mediated by Grb2, another LAT-binding protein. WASP is a complex molecule that can be activated by binding Cdc42 and certain phospholipids. Activated WASP in turn binds the actin nucleation complex Arp2/3. This complex series of events results in actin polymerization mediated by Arp2/3. That all these molecules regulate cytoskeletal events upon TCR activation is suggested by the localization of WASP to the T-cell–APC contact, by the presence of cytoskeletal abnormalities in humans and mice lacking WASP, and by direct evidence that TCR engagement leads to actin polymerization (217,220).

An active role for the cytoskeleton and movement of molecules involved in synapse formation has been shown in studies of ICAM-1 (221). ICAM-1 on antigen-presenting B cells rapidly migrates to the T–B interface following engagement of the cells. This movement was shown to be dependent on the T-cell cytoskeleton in studies in which pretreatment with cytochalasin D blocked T-cell activation and decreased ICAM-1 redistribution. In a subsequent study, attaching beads with anti–ICAM-1 antibodies tracked ICAM-1 movement on T cells. Upon T–APC contact, the ICAM-1 molecules moved toward the interface. This movement could be blocked by addition of agents that poison myosin motors. These two experiments suggest that motors along actin filaments move these molecules. Alternatively, molecules could be directly attached to actin filaments and move as filaments that are dynamically modified. In this regard, it is notable that the TCR can be shown to bind actin via the TCR ζ chain.

Multiple studies have thus demonstrated that complex molecular sorting occurs at the interface of the T cell and APC following TCR engagement with stimulatory peptide–MHC molecules. The mechanisms behind these events are also complex and remain an area of active work. One last question is what the function of the synapse is for T cells. Clearly some signaling events such as tyrosine phosphorylation and calcium elevation begin before and while the molecular rearrangements occur. However, T-cell signaling needs to be sustained in order for optimal activation of transcriptional elements, and molecular organization may therefore be required. Synapse formation is also accompanied by reorientation of the microtubule-organizing center and the secretory apparatus behind the TCR. This allows for directed delivery of cytokines from the T cell to the APC or B cell, and in the case of cytotoxic T cells, it allows toxic cytolytic products to be delivered directly to the target. The synapse potentially will prevent dilution of critical products, and will prevent toxic material from inappropriate delivery outside the target.

Activation of Phosphatidylinositol Second-Messenger Pathway and Function of Second Messengers of Pathway

Classic biochemical pathways are activated by TCR engagement in the context of generation of protein complexes, redistribution of the membrane, and formation of the immune synapse. The consequences of the activation of PLC are the best studied of these events. Activation of PLCγ1 enzymes results in the generation of second messengers of the phosphatidylinositol (PI) pathway. The contribution of the PI pathway to T-cell activation has been well studied. Early studies with calcium ionophores and certain phorbol esters demonstrated that these reagents synergize in inducing lymphokine secretion, IL-2R expression, T-cell proliferation, and the activation of the cytolytic mechanism of CTL (reviewed in Weiss and Imboden [39]). Moreover, these reagents could induce lymphokine secretion in mutant cell lines that failed to express the TCR (28,222), suggesting that these pharmacologic reagents mimicked important signals downstream of the TCR. Since calcium ionophores induce an increase in cytoplasmic free calcium ($[Ca^{2+}]_i$) and agonist phorbol esters activate the serine/threonine kinase, PKC, this led to the notion that the TCR may function to initiate T-cell activation by a signal transduction mechanism that involves similar events.

The development of calcium sensitive fluorescent dyes (i.e., quin 2, indo 1, and fura 2) that can be used to monitor changes in $[Ca^{2+}]_i$ in small cells such as lymphocytes permitted the test of this hypothesis. These changes can be monitored in bulk populations within a spectrofluorimeter, within subsets of cells in a flow cytometer, or within individual cells with sensitive microscopic techniques. Indeed, increases in $[Ca^{2+}]_i$ from basal levels of approximately 100 nM to greater than 1.0 μM are induced within seconds to minutes and may be sustained for hours following stimulation of the TCR (28,222,223). Similarly, a rapid and sustained activation of PKC is observed following TCR stimulation (224). The agonist effects of calcium ionophores and phorbol esters suggest that the observed increase in $[Ca^{2+}]_i$ and activation of PKC induced by stimulation of the TCR are physiologically important intracellular events.

An increase in $[Ca^{2+}]_i$ and activation of PKC are characteristic events that result from a common receptor-mediated signal-transduction pathway, the phosphatidylinositol (PI) pathway. The key regulatory event in the PI pathway involves the hydrolysis of a relatively rare membrane phospholipid called phosphatidylinositol 4,5-bisphosphate (PIP2) (225). TCR stimulation activates the PI pathway through the tyrosine phosphorylation of PLC-γ1. Activation of this enzyme is associated with its cleavage of the phosphodiester linkage of PIP2, resulting in the formation of inositol 1,4,5-trisphosphate (1,4,5-IP3) and 1,2-diacylglycerol (DG) (Fig. 8). These molecules, in turn, function as intracellular "second messengers" to induce an increase in $[Ca^{2+}]_i$ and activation of PKC, respectively. Within seconds following stimulation of the TCR by antigen or anti–TCR mAb, a substantial increase in 1,4,5-IP3 and the immediate metabolite of DG, phosphatidic acid, are observed. Second-messenger generation has been shown to continue as long as occupancy of the receptor persists (22).

The role of 1,4,5-IP3 in increasing intracellular calcium has been studied intensively. This water-soluble sugar has specific intracellular receptors that regulate the mobilization of $[Ca^{2+}]_i$ from intracellular Ca^{2+} stores associated with the

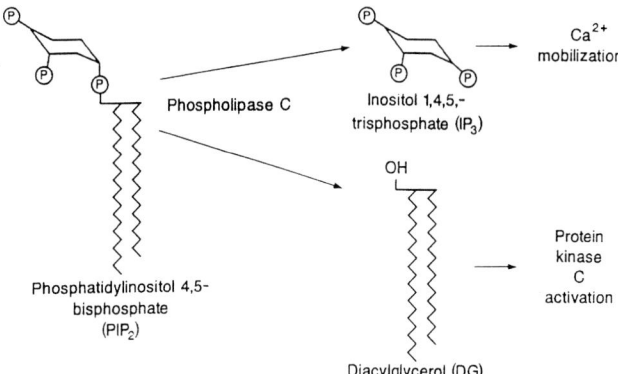

FIG. 8. The structure of phosphatidylinositol 4,5-bisphosphate (PIP₂) and the products of its hydrolysis by phospholipase C.

endoplasmic reticulum. The release of intracellular stores of Ca^{2+} by 1,4,5-IP3 can account for most of the initial increase in $[Ca^{2+}]_i$ that occurs during the first minute or two following TCR stimulation (226). However, at the cell population level, stimulation of the TCR induces increases in $[Ca^{2+}]_i$ that persist for several hours (22,227). At the level of individual cells, patch clamp and image analyses indicate that the sustained increase observed at the population level following TCR stimulation with various types of ligands reflects the summation of asynchronous oscillatory increases of $[Ca^{2+}]_i$ in individual cells (36,228). Both the sustained $[Ca^{2+}]_i$ increase and the persistence of oscillations require a transmembrane flux of calcium from outside the cell to the inside. The persistent response is necessary for certain cellular responses, notably the initiation of IL-2 gene transcription (22,227,229). The mechanism responsible for the regulation of the transmembrane flux of Ca^{2+} in T cells involves a non–voltage-gated Ca^{2+} channel that is regulated when intracellular stores are depleted. The molecular identity of this channel, referred to as iCRAC or SOCS, and its mechanism of regulation is still unclear (230). Once the intracellular stores are refilled from transmembrane fluxes of Ca^{2+}, the plasma membrane channel closes. This type of regulation of calcium currents is termed capacitative calcium entry. High levels of $[Ca^{2+}]_i$ appear to have a negative influence on transmembrane calcium currents. This negative feedback could account for the observed oscillations and function to keep $[Ca^{2+}]_i$ within the required relatively narrow physiologic range.

The potential contribution of inositol phosphates to events involved in cell activation is raised to an increased level of complexity by the various forms of inositol phospholipids, the large number of distinct inositol phosphate isomers, and the numerous enzymes that regulate these compounds (reviewed in Majerus et al. [231]). The possibility that each of these phospholipid or inositol phosphate isomers, as well as other forms not depicted, might regulate some intracellular event illustrates how receptors coupled to the PI pathway may exert effects on a number of intracellular events. For instance, IP4 has recently been shown to inhibit the function of IP3 phosphatase, thereby potentiating the action of IP3, and illustrating the manifold effects that one may anticipate from the various inositol isomers that can be generated (232).

One set of the inositol phosphate lipid metabolites deserves special mention, those formed by the action of phosphatidylinositol 3-kinase (PI3-kinase). This enzyme consists of two components, a p85 subunit that serves as an adaptor and regulatory subunit and a catalytic p110 subunit (233). This enzyme is activated through stimulation of a number of receptors, including the TCR, CD28, and IL-2R (234–236). Activation of PI3-kinase leads to the generation of several inositol phospholipids including PI 3-P, PI 3,4-P_2, and PI 3,4,5-P_3. The activity of PI3-kinase can be blocked by two inhibitors, wortmannin and LY294002. These inhibitors help to define the importance of PI3-kinase and its metabolites in receptor-mediated signaling events. These phospholipids and their inositol phosphate metabolites generated through the activation of PI3-kinase serve, in part, as localization signals. A number of critical enzymes bearing PH domains bind to PI-3 kinase metabolites located in the membrane and are thus recruited to receptor activation sites (237). Such enzymes include members of the Tec family of PTK, and the serine-threonine kinases, PDK1 and Akt, as well as PLC-γ1 itself. These and other enzymes, some described above, have been implicated in a number of important functions, including receptor endocytosis, cytoskeletal rearrangements, cell proliferation, and apoptosis (233).

The other hydrolysis product of PIP2 is DG. DG is also a potent "second messenger" that regulates a family of serine/threonine kinases consisting of the PKC isozymes (238). DG activates pkC isozymes by increasing the affinity of this kinase for phospholipid. Many of the isozymes are also Ca^{2+} dependent so that activation occurs through the synergistic actions of DG and Ca^{2+} at physiologic $[Ca^{2+}]_i$ levels. Activation of PKC isozymes has been observed in cells following TCR stimulation (224,239,240). Likewise, phorbol esters are also potent activators of PKC, explaining the ability of these reagents to synergize with calcium ionophores, together mimicking the effects of anti–TCR mAb.

PKC represents a family of closely related enzymes that share structural features and requirements for Ca^{2+}, phospholipid, and DG (238). All identified forms can be activated by agonist phorbol esters but differ in their calcium sensitivities. Many, but not all of the isozymes are expressed in T cells. Of those expressed, evidence is strongest for the importance of the pkC α, β, and θ isozymes (239,240). At least some T-cell responses, including IL-2 production, can occur in the absence of PKC β (241). Redundant function among some isozymes seems likely since expression of a constitutively active form of PKC β could induce IL-2 transcriptional activity in the presence of calcium ionophore stimulation only (242). It still remains possible, however, that distinct isozymes may have overlapping as well as distinct functions in T cells. A specific function for PKC θ is suggested by its specific local-

ization at the interface of the T cell and APC, as described above in the description of the immunologic synapse (211). This calcium-independent enzyme is the only PKC isozyme that relocalizes during an antigen-specific interaction. Recent evidence indicates that PKC θ interacts with Vav and the cytoskeleton (243).

The activation of PKC may be influenced in several ways (244). First, metabolism of DG to phosphatidic acid by DG kinase will serve to limit the availability of DG. Second, a calcium-activated protease, calpain, can cleave PKC *in vitro* into a cytosolic constitutively active 50-kD enzyme that is Ca^{2+} and phospholipid independent. Whether calpain activity contributes to the activation or modification of PKC in T cells is not known. Third, the nature of the stimulating ligand may influence the observed activation of PKC. Stimulation of T cells with immobilized anti–CD3 mAb induces more prolonged translocation of PKC activity to the plasma membrane than does the same mAb used in soluble form, probably the result of more sustained PIP2 turnover (224). Such sustained activation of PKC is important for subsequent T-cell proliferative responses (245). Thus, the activation and regulation of PKC may be more complex than first appreciated. One can expect that differences in the regulation of these intracellular events will impact on the cellular responses observed.

Consequences of Increases in [Ca²⁺]ᵢ and Activation of PKC

The synergistic effects of increases in $[Ca^{2+}]_i$ and activation of PKC must be explained by the impact of these intracellular events on subsequent signaling pathways. Although the details of the events leading from increases in $[Ca^{2+}]_i$ and activation of PKC to cellular responses are not known, considerable progress has been made. A model outlining these events leading from the TCR to the transcriptional activation of the IL-2 gene is depicted in Fig. 9. The increase in $[Ca^{2+}]_i$ influences calmodulin-dependent events, including the activation of calcineurin (PP2B) and Ca^{2+}/calmodulin–dependent kinase.

A critical role for calcineurin, the Ca^{2+}/calmodulin–dependent serine/threonine phosphatase, is now well established. Calcineurin is the molecular target for the immunosuppressives cyclosporin A (CsA) and FK506, drugs that have revolutionized clinical organ transplantation (reviewed in Schreiber and Crabtree [246]). CsA and FK506 form molecular complexes with their cellular receptors, cyclophilin and FKBP, respectively. It is these molecular complexes, not the isolated drugs, that inhibit the phosphatase function of calcineurin. Calcineurin is expressed ubiquitously, but is expressed at only low levels in T-lymphocytes. This probably accounts for the relative specificity of the immunosuppressive drugs in targeting T-cell function.

A critical function for calcineurin has been established in the regulation of IL-2 gene expression (5). One target

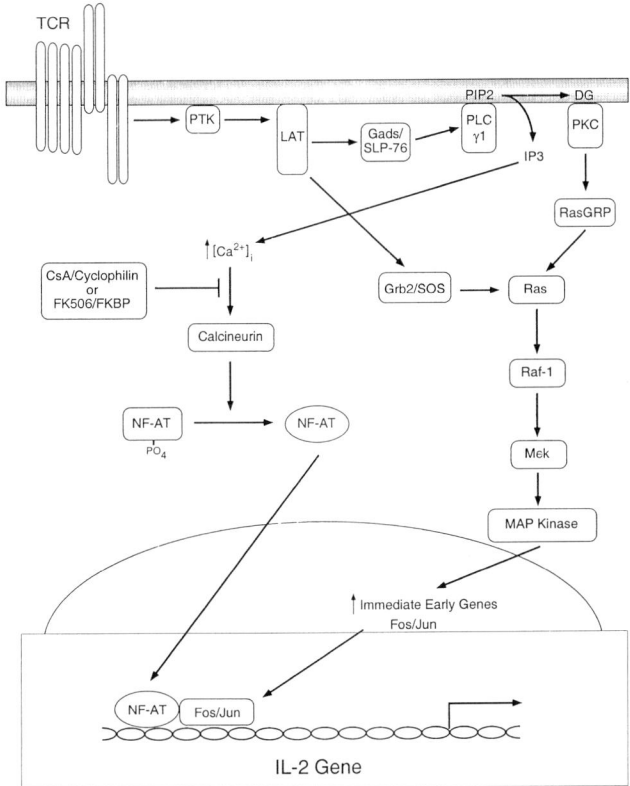

FIG. 9. Model of TCR-mediated signal transduction leading to lymphokine (IL-2) gene transcription. Note that the arrows between the protein components do not necessarily reflect direct interactions.

of calcineurin involves a protein(s) called nuclear factor of activated T cells, NF-AT, which is involved in the transcriptional regulation of many lymphokine genes including IL-2 (247,248). NF-AT constitutes a family of cytoplasmic phosphoproteins that translocate to the nucleus in response to calcium increases. This translocation is a critical regulatory event, since enforced nuclear localization of NF-AT activates its transcriptional function (229). Calcineurin phosphatase activity is critical for the activity of NF-AT transcriptional reporter constructs. Moreover, calcineurin can dephosphorylate NF-AT. This dephosphorylation reveals an NF-AT nuclear localization site that allows for its translocation. Thus, calcineurin activation resulting from an increase in $[Ca^{2+}]_i$ leads to the dephosphorylation and activation of a key transcriptional factor involved in lymphokine gene expression (see below).

Another enzyme that is responsive to increases in $[Ca^{2+}]_i$ is the multifunctional Ca^{2+}/calmodulin–dependent kinase (CAM-kinase). This kinase is activated following TCR stimulation. Activation of CAM-kinase alone appears to have a negative regulatory influence on IL-2 gene expression (249). This is consistent with the ability of calcium ionophores, when used alone, to induce anergy in T cells in some systems (23).

The relevant substrates of PKC are of considerable interest. A number of proteins are phosphorylated on serine or threonine residues as a result of PKC activation following treatment of T cells with phorbol esters or following TCR stimulation. Among these are the human CD3γ and δ chains (117); the murine CD3δ and CD3ϵ chains (250); CD4 (251); the transferrin receptor, the IL-2R; and HLA class I heavy chains (252). Some of these proteins are not direct substrates of PKC and the functional significance of these phosphorylations is not yet clear.

Activation of Ras Pathway

Stimulation of T cells with phorbol esters or with TCR ligands induces the rapid activation of the proto-oncogene Ras (253). Ras is a 21-kDa peripheral membrane protein and is one of many related proteins that can bind and hydrolyze guanine-nucleoside triphosphate (GTP). Ras is activated in the GTP-bound state and is inactive in the GDP-bound state. Its GTPase activity is regulated by interactions with guanine-nucleotide-exchange proteins, such as Sos, and GTPase-activating proteins (GAPs) (reviewed in Schlessinger [254]) (Fig. 10).

Activation of Ras by the TCR is the result of both PKC-dependent and PKC-independent mechanisms. How PKC activation leads to Ras activation remains unclear. Initial studies suggested that the activation of Ras in T cells following phorbol ester addition or TCR stimulation occurs as the result of inhibition of GAP activity (255). GAP is weakly tyrosine phosphorylated following TCR stimulation and associates with an induced 62-kDa tyrosine phosphoprotein called Dok (188). Dok, a negative regulatory adaptor protein, may serve to couple GAP proteins to stimulated complexes of proteins that contain Ras. An involvement of this complex in Ras regulation in T cells has been implicated in CD2- but not TCR-mediated signaling events (256). However, more recent studies have implicated the involvement of two guanine-nucleotide factors, Sos and RasGRP, as the means by which Ras function can be regulated in T cells. Several genetic and biochemical studies have implicated the

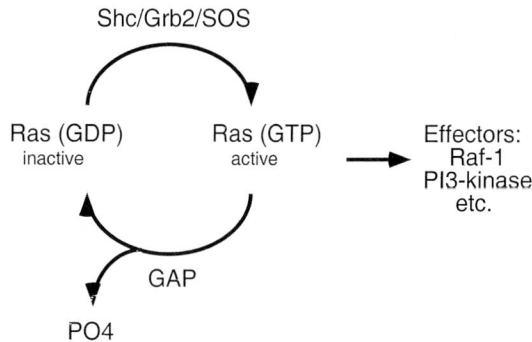

FIG. 10. Regulation of the Ras GTPase.

adaptor protein Grb2, which binds to the guanine-nucleotide-exchange protein Sos in Ras regulation (254). As previously discussed, Grb2 is an adaptor protein that is recruited to tyrosine phosphorylated LAT. Grb2 can also bind to another adaptor called Shc that appears to play an important, as yet undefined role, in linking the TCR to the MAPK pathway (257). One possibility may involve the recruitment of Shc to tyrosine-phosphorylated residues in the TCR ζ chain. The SH3 domains of Grb2 bind to proline-rich regions in Sos. Thus, TCR stimulation may activate Ras via the recruitment of a Grb2/Sos complex to tyrosine phosphorylated Shc bound to the TCR or to membrane-associated LAT. The membrane-associated Sos molecule can then activate Ras by inducing nucleotide exchange. More recently, a second Ras activator, RasGRP, has been identified and characterized in T cells (30). This guanine-nucleotide-exchange factor contains a carboxy-terminal domain that binds DG. This product of PLC-γ1 activation is thought to bring RasGRP to the plasma membrane in a manner analogous to its action on PKC. Membrane-bound RasGRP then activates Ras by inducing exchange of GTP for GDP. The relative importance of Sos and RasGRP is a current area of interest.

Ras has multiple downstream effectors, including Raf, PI3-kinase, and other GTP-binding proteins such as Rac and Cdc42 (258,259). The function of the Ras–Raf interaction is best characterized and has been shown to be important in TCR signaling function leading to IL-2 gene activation (240). Ras interacts directly with the serine/threonine kinase Raf-1. Raf-1 is activated in T cells following TCR stimulation or PKC activation with phorbol esters. Raf-1 can regulate the activation of a dual-specific tyrosine/serine/threonine kinase, MEK, which in turn activates MAPKs (253). In T cells, the activation of MAPKs has also been associated with PKC activation (260). This complex kinase cascade can function to regulate nuclear events involved in the growth and differentiation of a variety of cells.

The activation of Ras contributes to the transcriptional activation of the IL-2 gene (240). Expression of an activated form of Ras, which has reduced capacity to hydrolyze GTP, can substitute, in part, for phorbol esters in synergizing with calcium ionophores to induce transcription driven by the IL-2 upstream regulatory region or a multimer of the NF-AT site (261,262). Moreover, dominant-negative mutants of Ras or Raf inhibit TCR-induced IL-2 transcription (261,263). Among other things, activated Ras is involved in the induction of the MAPK pathway (264). The MAPKs that include Jnk, p38, and Erk kinases contribute to the regulation of a large number of transcriptional responses, including those that involve the AP-1 family of transcription factors. AP-1 proteins are heterodimers composed of Fos and Jun-related proteins and, among other things, form transcription factor complexes with NF-AT proteins (265). Expression of the Fos is highly dependent upon the activation of MAPKs. Thus, the integration of distinct branches of the TCR-induced signaling pathway, those mediating increases in $[Ca^{2+}]_i$, and those mediating activation of Ras, result in the activation of distinct transcriptional factors that coordinately regulate IL-2 gene expression (Fig. 9).

CONSEQUENCES OF EARLY SIGNAL TRANSDUCTION EVENTS

Early Biochemical Events

As a consequence of signal transduction events initiated by the TCR and presumably by other co-stimulatory and accessory receptors, a cascade of intracellular biochemical changes occur that contribute to the events that lead to a demonstrable cellular response. Among these early biochemical events are protein phosphorylation and activation of a variety of kinases (as discussed above), cytoplasmic alkalinization, fluxes in ions, and changes in levels of cyclic nucleotides. Such events are not confined to the T cell but have been widely observed in receptor-mediated activation of many cell types. They are likely to be important, through mechanisms that have yet to be elucidated, in regulating later cellular responses.

Changes in pH

One mechanism whereby intracellular functions may be influenced and could be envisioned to initiate a cellular response is by altering the cytoplasmic ionic milieu, specifically cytoplasmic pH. Changes in pH can have profound effects on the activities of enzymes. Cellular alkalinization is known to occur during receptor-initiated PIP2 hydrolysis in many cell types (266). An increase in pH has been demonstrated in T-cell lines and thymocytes following lectin stimulation or TCR stimulation by mAb (267,268). This appears to be the result of an increased activity of the plasma membrane Na^+/H^+ antiporter. Evidence suggests that this effect may be regulated by PIP2 hydrolysis since both dependency on extracellular calcium and the ability of PKC-activating phorbol esters to mimic the effect of lectins and TCR mAb have been reported (267,268).

Fluxes in Cyclic Nucleotides

Changes in the cyclic nucleotides, cyclic adenosine monophosphate (cAMP) and cyclic guanosine monophosphate (cGMP), regulate cellular functions in a variety of cell types. Changes in cyclic nucleotides in T-lymphocyte mitogenic responses received considerable attention in early work on T-cell activation. Following mitogenic lectin stimulation of T cells, both a rise followed by a fall in cAMP levels were thought to be important in T-cell proliferative responses (269). An increase in cAMP levels has been reported following stimulation of a T-cell line with anti–CD3 mAb (270). Inhibitory effects of high levels of cAMP on T-cell proliferative responses are well documented. High cAMP levels inhibit T-cell proliferative responses by blocking IL-2 production, but not by inhibiting the effects of IL-2 on its receptor (271). The mechanism for this inhibitory effect of cAMP on T-cell responses is somewhat controversial, although it is likely to involve the action of cAMP-dependent protein kinase. Inhibition of PIP2 hydrolysis by cAMP in T cells has been observed by some (272), but not all, investigators (273). Another target for cAMP-dependent kinase, PKA, is the Raf-1 kinase that can be inactivated by serine phosphorylation (274). Inhibition of any of these events would have an inhibitory effect. Since T cells express a variety of receptors that can induce an increase in cAMP, including β-adrenergic receptors, it is likely that immunologic and nonimmunologic mediators may influence T-cell function.

An increase in cGMP has also been observed following mitogenic lectin stimulation of T cells (275). The physiologic function of these cGMP increases has yet to be established.

Changes in Membrane Potential

Like other cells, T cells have an electrochemical gradient of ions across their plasma membranes. This gradient is established by the unequal distribution of ions on the two sides of the plasma membrane and is responsible for a resting negative electrical potential of approximately −70 mV. This negative resting potential influences the tendency of charged ions to cross the plasma membrane down their concentration gradients. However, the ability of ions such as Na^+, K^+, Cl^-, and Ca^{2+} to cross the plasma membrane is limited by the permeability of the plasma membrane to each of these ions. Events that result in changes in the membrane permeability of a particular ion, which can be receptor mediated, will change the membrane potential. In addition, rapid changes in membrane permeability, such as channel opening, will establish diffusion potential as long as the channel remains open and the ionic gradient persists. Thus, receptor-signal transduction may represent or influence changes in the plasma membrane permeability to certain ions. These changes in permeability may be manifested as changes in membrane potential.

Transient hyperpolarization (i.e., a more negative potential) followed later by depolarization (i.e., more positive potential) of T cells after lectin stimulation has been appreciated for many years. Using sensitive patch-clamping techniques, voltage-gated potassium channels have been shown to be important ion-gated channels in T cells (276). Heterogeneity of these potassium channels has been observed in murine T cells and thymocytes of various phenotypes. Three types of K^+ channels have been detected—n, n′, and l—although only n channels are present in human T cells. The functional significance of this heterogeneity is not clear. The gating properties of these channels change following the addition of T-cell mitogens, but it is not clear whether these channels can be regulated directly by T-cell surface molecules as a result of ligand–receptor interactions. Extracellular Ca^{2+} does not pass through these channels. The observed transient hyperpolarization response appears to be regulated by the increase in $[Ca^{2+}]_i$ (277). The mechanism explaining the later depolarization is not well understood. The relatively delayed changes in membrane potential depolarization observed in

T-cell mitogenic responses would suggest that these channels are regulated indirectly by membrane receptor–associated signal transduction. The importance of the activity of these channels has been suggested by the ability of K^+ channel blockers to inhibit T-cell proliferative responses (278,279). Blockade of K^+ channels with charybdotoxin appears to influence the extent of Ca^{2+} increase that is achieved following TCR stimulation. This does not appear to be an effect mediated on classic voltage-gated Ca^{2+} channels. Further work on understanding the functions of K+ channels is required.

Cellular Responses

Cytoskeletal Changes

The redistribution and reorientation of cytoskeletal elements in T cells have been studied during interactions between helper T-cell clones and APCs as well as cytolytic T-lymphocytes (CTL) and their targets (280). Many of the molecular sorting events that result in formation of the immunologic synapse are dependent on dynamic changes in the actin cytoskeleton, as discussed above. Additionally, a specific antigen-dependent reorientation of the microtubule-organizing center (MTOC) in the T-helper cell and CTL toward the cell with which either interacts occurs. This reorientation of the MTOC does not occur in the APC or target cell.

It is clear that TCR-mediated signaling is involved in the polarization of the cytoskeleton. A number of studies suggest that TCR ITAMs are required as are the TCR-regulated PTKs. The ITAM could serve as the focal point to orient the redirected cytoskeleton. The role of Src PTKs in cytoskeletal changes can be shown by studies with Src PTK inhibitors. Although the activation of Ras does not appear to be required for these events, other GTP-binding proteins, Cdc42 and Rac, have been implicated in the polarization of T cells (281). Since the guanine-nucleotide-exchange function (GEF) of Vav can regulate the activation of Cdc42 and Rac, and loss of Vav by gene ablations deleteriously affects antibody-induced clustering (capping) of surface molecules, it is likely that this GEF for Rho family GTPases could serve to reorient the T-cell cytoskeleton. It is also interesting that α-tubulin is tyrosine phosphorylated following TCR stimulation and that tyrosine-phosphorylated tubulin is found in the depolymerized fraction of cellular tubulin (282). This suggests the possibility that the tyrosine phosphorylation of tubulin might play a role in the polarization of the MTOC. Polarization of the cytoskeleton in T cells also depends on calcium (283). Myosin light-chain kinase, which can regulate cytoskeletal structure, is activated by elevations in $[Ca^{2+}]_i$, and myosin motors have been implicated in T-cell polarization using inhibitors (221). These observations suggest that complex mechanisms function to reorient the T-cell cytoskeleton to achieve properly oriented and localized T-cell responses.

An attractive notion for a functional consequence of this reorientation is the directional secretion of prepackaged or newly synthesized secretory products. In the case of the CTL, this could represent the focused secretion of cytolytic components (see below and Chapter 36) toward only the relevant antigen-bearing target cell. In the case of the helper T cell, newly synthesized lymphokines important in macrophage activation or B-cell differentiation/proliferation could be envisioned to be targeted toward the relevant APC. For the B cell that presents antigen to the T cell, this might serve to limit the effects of such lymphokines to antigen-specific B cells.

Activation of Cytolytic Mechanism

The initiation of the lytic process occurs during the complex cell–cell interaction between receptors on the CTL and ligands on the target cell. TCR-initiated signal transduction events contribute to the activation of the cytolytic mechanism. In keeping with this notion is the observation that in most instances extracellular Ca^{2+} is necessary for target cell lysis, but not for the binding of the CTL to its target (reviewed in Berke [284]). Moreover, calcium ionophores and phorbol esters synergize in inducing the lysis of bystander cells by CTL in an antigen-independent manner. Increases in $[Ca^{2+}]_i$ in CTL interacting with specific targets have been observed at the single cell level. Collectively, these observations strongly suggest that stimulation of the TCR on a CTL by target-cell antigens initiates transmembrane signaling events including PIP2 hydrolysis. The resultant increase in $[Ca^{2+}]_i$ and/or the activation of PKC leads to activation of a cytolytic mechanism.

Two cytolytic mechanisms are activated by TCR signaling events. These two mechanisms are discussed in detail in Chapter 36. Briefly, one mechanism involves the secretion of prepackaged cytolytic granules that contain perforin and serine esterase enzymes called granzymes (284). Perforin is a calcium-dependent pore-forming protein that contributes to the osmotic destruction of the target cell. Granzymes help to initiate the apoptotic pathway in target cells. Secretion of these granules can be induced by the reagents that mimic TCR-initiated PIP_2 hydrolysis, phorbol esters and calcium ionophores. The activation of this cytolytic mechanism by the TCR-induced signal transduction events involving PIP2 hydrolysis is consistent with the stimulus–secretion coupling mechanism that is observed in platelets, neutrophils, and mast cells that use similar receptor-mediated signal transduction mechanisms. In fact it has been possible to transfer perforin and granzymes into mast cell granules and induce these cells to kill sensitized target cells. In the case of the CTL, linking the reorientation of the cytoskeletal elements, particularly the MTOC, serves to focus the stimulus secretion of the cytolytic granules toward the relevant target and prevent non–antigen-specific bystander cell lysis (283). In contrast, the bystander lysis that is observed when calcium ionophores and phorbol esters are used to stimulate lysis is likely to represent a situation where cell-surface receptors play no role with resultant secretion of lytic granules in a nonfocused manner.

A second mechanism is used by CTL to induce target cell destruction. This involves the Fas system (see Chapters 24 and 36). Fas is a member of the TNF receptor family. Sequences in its cytoplasmic domain are responsible for interacting with proteins that can initiate the apoptotic pathway and destruction of the target cell. Only Fas-expressing target cells are sensitive to this cytolytic mechanism. In order for T cells to mediate destruction of target cells via the Fas system, they must be induced to express the Fas ligand (Apo-1), a member of the TNF family. Fas ligand expression is transcriptionally induced by TCR signal-transduction events and involves the activation of the NF-AT transcription factor. Thus, TCR signal-transduction events regulate two very distinct mechanisms that contribute to target cell destruction by CTLs.

Gene Activation Events

As a result of receptor-mediated signal transduction events in T cells, stimuli at the plasma membrane induce a set of specifically responsive genes to become transcriptionally active. These transcriptional events are responsible for the differentiation, proliferation, and survival of the stimulated T cells. Considerable progress has been made in our understanding of how cytoplasmic signal-transduction pathways lead to the activation of key transcription factors.

It has become increasingly clear that receptor-mediated signal transduction events leading to the proliferation and acquisition of differentiated functions by the T cell are not the result of a single wave of gene activation events. Instead, these are likely to result from a regulated cascade of sequential gene activation events that may be conditionally regulated. Hence, following initial signal transduction events that lead to the transcriptional activation of a certain set of genes, the products of this first wave of activated genes may contribute to the transcriptional activation of a second set of targeted genes, and so on. At some point, there is commitment to the final response (measured as differentiation or proliferation), although there is substantial evidence that T-cell responses are not quantal.

An appreciation of this type of cascade is readily apparent if one considers the activation of the IL-2 gene and its receptor, the IL-2R, which serve to regulate the proliferation and survival of T cells. Transcription of these genes begins during the first few hours of T-cell stimulation by antigen (reviewed in Crabtree and Clipstone [5] and Rao et al. [247]). The transcriptional activation of the IL-2 gene itself is dependent on protein synthesis and this reflects the requirement for the translation of the product(s) of a gene(s) needed for the initiation of IL-2 transcription. Once produced, the binding of IL-2 to its receptor initiates distinct signal transduction events, mediated by Jak kinases and STAT transcription factors, that result in a cascade of events involved in regulating cell growth. This is manifested many hours to days later as a proliferative response. For such a cascade of gene activation events to function, the activation of the initial set of responsive genes must be tightly regulated. Otherwise, uncontrolled proliferation or differentiation might ensue.

Early Gene Activation Events

The transcriptional activation of some genes is readily apparent in T cells within minutes of certain activating stimuli (5,247). This set of "immediate early activation genes" represents a relatively large number of newly transcribed genes, whose expression is not dependent on protein synthesis. Hence, the immediate early genes represent the first in a cascade of genes induced during T-cell activation. The ability of inhibitors of protein synthesis to prevent subsequent IL-2 gene transcriptional activation suggests that at least one of the products of these early activation genes influences IL-2 gene regulation (22,285). Thus, one or more members of this set of genes may contribute to the appearance of nuclear proteins that bind to or influence important regulatory sequences of the IL-2 gene (see below). Recent advances permit a more complete understanding of the regulation of these immediate early activation genes and their functions in the ensuing waves of gene activation that occur during T-cell responses.

Two proto-onocogenes, c-Myc and c-Fos, encode nuclear proteins that are immediate early genes involved in transcriptional regulation. They serve as useful models to study the set of immediate early activation genes. The long-sought function of c-Myc in cell growth remains ill-defined, but it can bind DNA, forms complexes with other nuclear proteins including Max, and can regulate transcription (286). In the case of c-Fos, it forms a dimer with another protein called c-Jun to form the transcriptional complex of AP-1 (265,287). Whereas the appearance of c-Myc and c-Fos mRNA is not restricted to T cells, these genes are among the first to become transcriptionally active following stimulation of the TCR on resting T cells. Transcripts for both c-Myc and c-Fos are readily detectable within 5 to 10 minutes of stimulation by PHA, or with mAbs reactive with the TCR or CD2 (288,289). In studies to examine the requirements for the transcriptional activation of c-Myc and c-Fos in T cells, an increase in $[Ca^{2+}]_i$, activation of PKC, or activation of Ras alone could induce their expression (290). However, synergy between these two events is evident from the combined effects of calcium ionophores and phorbol esters. Protein synthesis is not required for the transcriptional activation of either c-Myc or c-Fos in T cells, indicating that the transcription of these genes is directly regulated by the biochemical events that result from receptor-mediated signal transduction. MAPK family members, including Jun N-terminal kinase (Jnk) and Erk kinases, which are activated in T cells in response to antigen receptor signals together with phorbol esters or co-stimulatory signals, have been directly implicated in regulating c-Fos transcription by the phosphorylation of transcription factors such as Elk-1 that binds to the c-Fos promoter (287).

The products of such early activation genes, together with the effects of ongoing signal transduction events, initiate the next wave of gene activation. Indeed, several products of

early activation genes have been implicated in the regulation of IL-2 gene expression, including those comprising the AP-1 complex (291). Interestingly, persistent signal transduction is required for the transcriptional activation of the IL-2 gene even after the appearance of transcripts of the early activation genes. Although there are several possible explanations for this, the post-translational modification of products of the early activation genes may be required for their functions. Indeed, the post-translational phosphorylation of c-Fos and c-Jun by Jnk and an ill-defined c-Fos kinase are required for AP-1 transcriptional activity (287,292,293). Thus, a well-coordinated cascade of events involving signal transduction events and gene activation serves to regulate subsequent waves of gene activation that ultimately induce T-cell proliferative responses.

Activation of Lymphokine Genes

Many of the prominent manifestations of T-cell activation are mediated by one of the large number of T-cell–derived, secreted soluble proteins termed "lymphokines." These lymphokines exert a great diversity of effects on many cell types and tissues. In resting T cells, the production of lymphokines results from the transcriptional activation of the genes that encode them. Individual T cells produce different sets of lymphokines in response to similar stimuli. While distinct patterns of lymphokines may reflect the profiles of lymphokines secreted by the two major subsets of helper T cells (Th1 and Th2) (see Chapter 10), the molecular basis for the heterogeneity in expression of these inducible genes within distinct subsets is only partially understood. Differences in tissue-specific expression of regulatory factors certainly account for some of these differences in expression. For instance, persistence in the transcriptional factor GATA-3 is associated with the Th2 phenotype and T-bet is associated with the Th1 phenotype (reviewed in Ho and Glimcher [294]). Selective expression of the c-Maf transcription factor in the presence of NIP45—a recently identified NF-AT–binding protein—as well as NF-AT is also associated with the tissue-specific transcriptional activation of the IL-4 gene. The determinants involved in the tissue-specific expression of GATA-3 and c-Maf are not clear. IL-4 is a major determinant in Th2 subset commitment. Therefore, signaling pathways from the IL-4 receptor may influence the specific expression of c-Maf and/or GATA-3. Alternatively, interferon γ and IL-12 are the lymphokines that predominantly drive T cells to commit to the Th1 phenotype. These lymphokines could positively influence another set of transcriptional factors or negatively influence the expression of GATA-3 and/or c-Maf. Alternatively, there may be differences in the transmembrane signals generated by cell-surface receptors or cytoplasmic proteins expressed in different T-cell subsets or when T cells engage different receptors on distinct populations of APCs. Such events could contribute to the differences in the menu of lymphokine genes that becomes transcriptionally active. The varied manifestations of T-cell activation may reflect the summation of the effects of the products of the lymphokine genes that become transcriptionally active. A detailed discussion of the effects of the various lymphokines that are expressed during the course of T-cell activation is presented in Chaper 10.

Since substantial progress has been made in understanding the mechanisms involved in the transcriptional regulation of the IL-2 gene, the following discussion focuses on its regulation. It is likely that the general principles that hold for the regulation of the IL-2 gene will also apply to the transcriptional regulation of other lymphokine genes as well. As discussed above, signaling pathways emanating from the TCR that are regulated by protein-tyrosine phosphorylation are required for the transcriptional activation of the IL-2 gene.

Genomic DNA sequences involved in the regulation of the IL-2 gene were initially identified by their increased sensitivity to DNAase I digestion. More detailed analyses of the regulation of the IL-2 gene demonstrated that a 275–base-pair segment upstream from the transcription initiation site contains most of the sequences that regulate its transcriptional activation (5). This region is responsive to the synergistic actions of stimuli that increase $[Ca^{2+}]_i$ and induce the activation of PKC or Ras (261,295). From kinetic analyses and the ability of inhibitors of protein synthesis to block the transcriptional activation of IL-2, it is clear that products of immediate early genes are necessary for this activation (5). The involvement of c-Fos in many of the AP-1 sites offers at least a partial explanation for this requirement.

DNAse "footprint" analyses—assays with transcriptional reporter constructs—and electromobility shift analyses have demonstrated that there are several distinct nuclear protein-binding sites within this region that are responsive to TCR-derived and CD28-derived signal transduction events (5,296) (Fig. 11). The proteins that bind to this region contribute to the transcriptional activation, as well as to the suppression of transcription of the IL-2 gene. TCR signal transduction events that influence the binding and/or activity of at least six nuclear complexes are depicted in Fig. 11. All of these sites are required to coordinately respond to TCR-derived signal transduction events.

The NF-IL2A site binds Oct-1, a homeodomain transcription factor. The activity of this factor is regulated by a protein complex, termed OAP, which contains a Jun family member that associates with Oct-1 only after stimulation (291). The complex NF-IL2B site, which binds AP-1 or related proteins and the NF-AT transcription factor, appears to be a major

site of PKC and Jnk responsiveness (297,298). The failures to activate AP-1 proteins that bind to this site have also been implicated in anergic T cells (299). This is consistent with the impaired activation of MAPKs and Jnk proteins in anergic T cells (300,301), and the roles of MAPKs and Jnk in regulating AP-1 function. The NF-IL2C site has been reported to bind several distinct transcription factors including NF-κB and AP-3. However, the contribution of this site to the inducibility of the IL-2 gene has been questioned. The NF-IL2D site is another Oct-binding site. It has not been studied in detail.

At least two sites bind NF-AT transcription factors within the IL-2 regulatory region, the proximal NF-AT site adjacent to the NF-IL2B site and the NF-IL2E site (5,247,296). The DNA-binding and activation domain of the NF-AT family of proteins are homologous to the Rel family of transcription factors. The favored DNA binding site for NF-AT resembles Rel-binding sites. The NF-AT–binding sites in the IL-2 gene are actually composite transcriptional elements that bind proteins derived from one of the four NF-AT proteins in conjunction with AP-1 protein complexes. Binding of the entire protein complex is required for function. These NF-AT sites can be multimerized to create transcriptional reporter constructs that have been very useful in studying T-cell activation. The signals required for NF-AT translocation to the nucleus, where it can interact with a nuclear AP-1 complex that has been activated through the actions of MAPKs and Jnks, have been discussed above. However, it is clear that both NF-AT nuclear translocation, regulated by the calcium–calcineurin pathway (265), and nuclear export, regulated by Crm-1 and GSK3 (302), are under tight control. The delicate balance of signals that control NF-AT import and export from the nucleus will determine NF-AT–dependent responses.

Stimulation of CD28 can also regulate lymphokine gene transcription, if TCR-derived signals are also provided (89). As discussed above, the proximal signal transduction events regulated by CD28 that influence lymphokine gene expression are not clearly established, although they are CsA and FK506 insensitive. Some studies have implicated the involvement of the PI 3-kinase/Akt pathway while others have not. The ability of Akt to activate the NF-κB pathway via an indirect activating effect on the IkB kinases (IKKs) is particularly noteworthy since NF-κB family members have been implicated in co-stimulation. Moreover, heterologous expression of an activated allele of Akt can reconstitute CD28-deficient

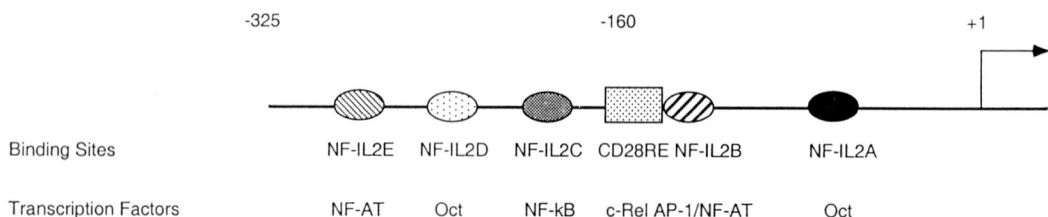

FIG. 11. IL-2 gene upstream (5′) regulatory regions with TCR-(ovals) and CD28-responsive elements (rectangle) indicated.

T cells (303). In the presence of TCR signals or calcium ionophore plus phorbol esters, CD28 stimulation induces nuclear factors that bind to a sequence element, the CD28RE, contained in multiple lymphokine genes, including IL-2, interferon γ, GM-CSF, and IL-3 (89). These sites are responsible for the effects of CD28 signals upon transcription of these genes and may, in part, be responsible for the co-stimulatory effects of CD28. The CD28RE has been reported to bind a number of the NF-κB Rel family transcription factors, particularly c-Rel, as well as NF-AT (304,305). The CD28RE site in the IL-2 gene is adjacent to the neighboring NF-IL2B site that binds AP-1. This site functions as a composite element to bind c-Rel and AP-1 (306,307). In this regard, it is noteworthy that T cells from c-Rel–deficient mice fail to produce IL-2 unless they are stimulated with calcium ionophore and phorbol ester (308). This site appears to be a signal integration locus where requirements for both TCR and CD28 signals are required for c-Rel and AP-1 activation.

Although transcriptional regulation represents a major mechanism for controlling lymphokine production, post-transcriptional regulation also represents an important regulatory mechanism. Most lymphokine transcripts, including IL-2, contain an AU-rich $3'$ untranslated sequence that confers instability to these mRNAs. Stimulation of T cells with phorbol esters or CD28 ligands has been reported to stabilize lymphokine mRNA (90,309). These observations on the transcriptional and post-transcriptional regulation of lymphokine genes suggest that complex regulatory mechanisms govern the expression of these important regulatory molecules.

Expression of New Cell Surface Molecules

A number of cell-surface molecules appear on the surface of the T cell during the events associated with their activation, differentiation, and proliferation. These include lymphokine receptors (i.e., CD25, the α chain of the IL-2R); nutrient receptors (i.e., the transferrin receptor and insulin receptor); class II MHC antigens on human T cells, but not on murine T cells; and, other cell-surface molecules, the functions of which are largely unknown (i.e., CD69 and 4F2). These proteins may subserve different roles in the growth, differentiation, and function of T cells following activation. The kinetics of the appearance of some of these proteins differ, with some appearing within minutes to hours after stimulation (i.e., CD25 and CD69) and others only appearing days (i.e., VLA-2) following T-cell activation. As the appearance of most of these proteins is transcriptionally regulated, different mechanisms of transcriptional regulation must be operative.

In addition to the appearance of new cell-surface molecules, new antigenic epitopes on existing cell-surface proteins indicate a different mechanism of functionally regulating certain receptors. For instance, concomitant with T-cell activation, a new antigenic epitope on the CD2 molecule (T11$_3$ epitope) is detected, probably the result of an allosteric change (26,54). Another mechanism responsible for the expression of new epitopes involves the regulated

alternative splicing of exons, as in the case of CD45. Activated T cells and some helper T-cell subsets express a distinct 180-kDa isoform of CD45, CD45RO, which lacks the products of exons 4, 5, and 6. This is in contrast to the 200- to 210-kDa CD45RA or CD45RB isoforms that include some of these exons and are expressed on resting T cells. This is the result of regulated alternative splicing of exons that encode a portion of the extracellular domain (190). It is tempting to speculate that such regulated splicing may affect the ligand-binding function of CD45 or its ability to homodimerize. Disruption of the splicing mechanism via single nucleotide polymorphism in exon 4, which interferes with an exonic splicing silencer site, has been associated with multiple sclerosis (310,311).

A detailed analysis of the regulation of all the cell-surface proteins induced during T-cell activation is beyond the scope of this chapter. However, a brief discussion of CD25, the α chain of the human IL-2R, a 55-kDa glycoprotein recognized by the anti–Tac mAb, is instructive (312). Expression of the IL-2R α chain is transcriptionally regulated. It is not expressed in most resting G0 T cells. The finding of at least three distinct sites of transcription initiation under different conditions that induce expression suggests that different modes of T-cell activation may influence distinct regulatory sequences flanking these sequences (313). Regulatory sequences responsive to certain stimuli involved in the activation of T cells have been identified in the upstream flanking regions of the IL-2R α chain gene. NF-κB appears to play a critical role in regulating the gene. The post-translational regulation of NF-κB function via IκB phosphorylation and degradation is the predominant means by which NF-κB is regulated (96). The recent identification of the IκB kinase that is responsible for the phosphorylation event that leads to IκB ubiquitination and degradation provides a link from cell-surface stimuli and the transcriptional regulation of IL-2R α chain (97).

The regulation of expression of the IL-2R α chain differs from the regulation of its ligand, IL-2 (312), as follows:

1. Reagents that activate PKC only are sufficient and more potent than those that increase $[Ca^{2+}]_i$ only to induce IL-2R α chain gene expression.
2. IL-2 itself up-regulates the expression of the IL-2R α chain via a transcriptional mechanism. This can, in part, account for the synergistic effects observed with reagents that increase $[Ca^{2+}]_i$ and activate PKC, that is, the resulting IL-2 up-regulates IL-2R α chain expression.
3. The induction of IL-2R α chain expression by PMA is not inhibitable by cyclosporin A, a potent inhibitor of IL-2 expression.
4. The expression of extremely high levels of IL-2R α chain expression on HTLV-1 transformed human T-cell lines in the absence of IL-2 production suggests another distinct mechanism of IL-2R α chain regulation (313).

Hence, the regulation of this lymphokine receptor chain is not as stringently regulated as the lymphokine itself. This allows for the recruitment of IL-2R expressing cells at sites of immune responses where other cells are producing IL-2, resulting in a paracrine effect. Since cells that have been previously activated continue to express low levels of IL-2R α chains, this would be a particularly attractive means by which the recruitment of memory T cells into an immune response might be facilitated. This paracrine effect is also the most widely accepted explanation for the synergy observed between CD4$^+$ IL-2 producing cells and CD8$^+$ CTL precursors that do not generally produce abundant quantities of IL-2. It is clear that the regulation of the IL-2R α chain during T-cell activation is complex. The regulation of the IL-2R α chain may have been raised to an increased level of complexity with the recognition that T cells that negatively regulate immune responses, Treg, constitutively express the IL-R α chain (314). It is likely that many other cell-surface receptors expressed during the activation of T cells have equally complex but distinct mechanisms of regulation.

TERMINATING T-CELL RESPONSES

An uncontrolled or unending T-cell response would be devastating to the host. Relatively little is known about how the levels of T-cell responses are regulated or how they are terminated. Exhaustion or elimination of a stimulating antigen may lead to termination of the input signal, but what determines when the response must end? Some regulatory mechanisms are known to exist. This is an area of research that is just evolving. However, it is useful to mention a few of the identified mechanisms that are likely to play important roles.

Of the signal transduction mechanisms that are induced during antigen recognition, most involve tyrosine or serine/threonine phosphorylation events. The PTKs and serine/threonine kinases exist in equilibrium with PTPases and serine/threonine phosphatases. The phosphatases themselves may be regulated through activation by phosphorylation or relocalization to substrates. PTPases with SH2 domains, such as SHP-1 and SHP-2, can be activated by their own tyrosine phosphorylation and can be targeted to relevant substrates via their SH2 domains (188). Mice deficient in SHP-1 have a lethal disease characterized by an overly active inflammatory system and have hyperresponsive Src kinase activities in their thymocytes.

A noteworthy example involves CTLA-4, which has been reported to interact with the SHP-2 PTPase (315). CTLA-4 is a transmembrane molecule that is homologous to CD28. It is up-regulated during T-cell activation. Mice deficient in CTLA-4 have a massive lymphoproliferative syndrome early in life, which appears to result from the unchecked polyclonal activation of T cells (316). Thus, CTLA-4 may serve in a negative feedback loop to autoregulate T-cell responses, once initiated, by recruiting the SHP-2 PTPase to the plasma membrane where it can act on relevant substrates associated with the TCR complex.

Csk, as mentioned above, is a PTK that has a critical role in negative regulation of Src family PTKs (188). This kinase

has a structure similar to Src PTKs, consisting of three major domains: SH3, SH2, and catalytic from amino to carboxy terminal. Initial studies demonstrated that it phosphorylates the negative carboxy-terminal regulatory sites in Src kinases, such as Lck (Tyr 505). Recent work indicates a more complex activity and regulation. Structure–function studies revealed that all three domains are critical to Csk function. The SH3 domain was shown to interact with a protein-tyrosine phosphatase known as PEP. This enzyme has as a target the activating tyrosine phosphorylation site on Src kinases, such as Lck Tyr 394. The effect of Lck interaction with the Csk-PEP complex would thus be inhibition by alteration of tyrosine phosphorylation at two sites potentially simultaneously.

Evaluation of the function of the Csk SH2 domain has led to further understanding of the complexity of Csk regulation. This domain binds the adaptor molecule known alternatively as PAG or Cbp when this molecule is phosphorylated. PAG/Cbp is a transmembrane protein sharing certain properties of the adaptor molecule LAT, which was described above. PAG/Cbp is also palmitoylated and a raft-resident protein. It is constitutively phosphorylated on tyrosine and a fraction of Csk is bound and thus found in rafts in resting T cells. This interaction is transiently lost with T-cell activation, but it is thought that re-phosphorylation of PAG/Cbp by Src kinase allows Csk to re-bind. This event would then bring Csk and PEP back to rafts allowing these enzymes to down-regulate the Src kinases that were activated by TCR engagement. This reasonable model requires much additional testing.

Down-regulation of receptors is a complex and important topic throughout cell biology and immunology in particular. Only recently have a number of investigators begun to probe the molecular mechanisms responsible for down-regulation of TCR and associated PTKs. One such mechanism is the targeted degradation of signaling molecules mediated by members of the Cbl family of ubiquitin ligases (166,167). These molecules have a complex yet conserved structure consisting of a phosphotyrosine-binding domain related to SH2 domains; a RING finger, which has E3 ubiquitin ligase activity; multiple sites of tyrosine phosphorylation and multiple proline-rich regions; and a leucine zipper-related sequence at the carboxy terminal. Extensive studies of the role of Cbl in cytokine receptor systems showed that Cbl can bind receptors, enzymes, and adaptor molecules using the Cbl phosphotyrosine–binding domain or via interaction with phosphorylated tyrosines or the multiple prolines. These interactions target Cbl to these proteins and allow the ubiquitin ligase RING domain access to the protein in question. The consequence is down-regulation of the target. In T cells, the consequence of overexpression of a Cbl protein with a mutated RING results in enhanced T-cell activation. In this setting, the mutant Cbl is serving as a dominant negative, presumably inhibiting the physiologic down-regulation of ZAP-70 mediated by Cbl. Cbl targets ZAP-70 using its SH2-related domain to bind to the PTK via a phosphorylated tyrosine (Y292) in the linker between the second SH2 and the kinase domain of ZAP-70. Other members of the Cbl family have different targets, and in particular, Cbl-b appears to bind and regulate the Vav molecule. Recent observations suggest that another molecule, SLAP, has a similar effect on T-cell activation as does Cbl. SLAP structure resembles Src kinases, but lacks a kinase domain. Overexpression studies with SLAP, like those with Cbl, suggest that these molecules negatively regulate TCR signal transduction. Mice deficient in SLAP have a thymic phenotype resembling c-Cbl–deficient mice, the main feature being an up-regulation of the TCR on CD4/CD8 double-positive thymocytes (317). This suggests that Cbl and SLAP play roles in controlling the levels of TCR expression.

Lymphokines are extremely potent biological mediators. Overproduction, such as occurs during food poisoning or toxic shock syndrome due to staphylococcal enterotoxins, can have devastating consequences on the host. Therefore, most lymphokines tend to be produced only transiently during an immune response. One mechanism to ensure their transient production is through the AU-rich $3'$ untranslated region present in most lymphokines (318). This AU-rich region confers instability on the mRNAs encoding lymphokines, ensuring only transient production of these potent mediators.

The final example of a mechanism that may contribute to the termination of T-cell activation during an immune response involves apoptosis. During the activation of antigen-responsive lymphocytes, the Fas ligand is up-regulated on responsive T cells (51). In fact, expression of the Fas ligand gene is regulated by the same TCR signals that regulate lymphokine responses (319). In the absence of appropriate inflammatory signals, the expansion of antigen-responsive T cells is followed by elimination of the activated T cells via apoptosis of Fas and Fas-ligand–expressing T cells (50). As yet ill-defined inflammatory cytokines or other signals of inflammation can prevent apoptosis of antigen-responsive T cells, thus perpetuating an immune response in an inflammatory setting. The failure of this system can have dire consequences as evidenced from the lymphoproliferative syndromes that result in humans with Fas mutations and in mice lacking functional Fas (lpr mice) or Fas ligand (gld mice) (320,321).

The termination and regulation of the immune response are as important as its initiation. The appropriate level of an immune response is critically important for the host. The regulatory systems involved in terminating the response are likely to be at least as complex as the systems that have evolved to initiate it.

T-CELL INACTIVATION

Stimulation of T cells, under certain *in vivo* conditions as well as certain *in vitro* culture conditions, with reagents that normally function as agonists can lead to a long-lived state in which they are unresponsive to subsequent TCR stimulation (80). This state of unresponsiveness has been termed "anergy." The unresponsive state has been induced in T-cell clones stimulated with mitogens, antigen, altered peptide ligands, anti–TCR mAb, and lymphokines. These experimental models may be relevant toward understanding certain forms of tolerance, particularly to peripheral (extrathymic) antigens, as well as in understanding how the outcomes of immune responses may differ as a result of different types of antigenic challenge.

Several factors appear to influence the ability of stimuli to induce unresponsiveness rather than activation of T-cell clones. A critical factor toward the induction of the unresponsive state is the nature of the responding cell. Unresponsiveness has only been induced in helper T-cell clones of the Th1 subtype (322,323). Under similar conditions, unresponsiveness could not be induced in cytolytic T-cell clones (324). Similar states of unresponsiveness have not been induced in T-cell hybridomas or leukemic lines. However, anergy has been induced by antigen injection in naïve mice (325).

The nature and the context of the stimulus are critical factors in the induction of unresponsiveness. Antigen presented on the surface of fixed APC or on planar lipid membranes reconstituted only with class II MHC molecules induces a long-lived state of unresponsiveness to subsequent antigenic challenge in antigen-specific murine helper T-cell clones, but not hybridomas, as measured by proliferative responses or IL-2 production (325,326). Inactivation is not complete and refers mainly to the proliferative response because suboptimal IFN-γ and IL-3 are produced in response to subsequent antigen challenge. Moreover, the proliferative response can be restored by exogenous IL-2 (23). The principle defect during the induction of the anergic state appears to be the reception of a TCR-derived signal, which involves a rise in $[Ca^{2+}]_i$, in the absence of a subsequent IL-2 stimulus (80,82).

The failure to produce IL-2 in most of these models is due to the failure of the T cell to receive a co-stimulatory signal. The preponderance of evidence suggests that the interaction of CD28 with either B7-1 or B7-2 is responsible for the co-stimulatory signal, as discussed above (reviewed in Foy et al. [83]). However, blockade of the CD28–B7 interaction only sometimes results in the induction of the anergic state. This suggests that there may be other co-stimulatory pathways that can lead to IL-2 production. Alternatively, under some circumstances of very potent TCR stimuli, it may be possible to induce IL-2 production in the absence of co-stimulation. This is consistent with the observations that CD28-deficient mice can still make some immune responses (84,92).

Altered peptide ligands can also induce an anergic state in the presence of appropriate co-stimulatory signals (34). In this setting, a subtle difference in the stimulatory peptide antigen or a mutation in the MHC molecule can result in marked alterations in the response of a particular T-cell clone. Biochemical analysis of these clones has consistently revealed a different pattern of TCR and PTK phosphorylation. As described above, TCR engagement with a fully stimulatory peptide–MHC combination normally leads to tyrosine phosphorylation of the TCR ζ chain. Close examination reveals two phosphotyrosine-containing bands on protein gels. These represent two phosphorylated forms of TCR ζ. One, known as p23, represents a fully phosphorylated TCR ζ chain, while the other, p21, is partially phosphorylated. Examination of the TCR following stimulation with altered antigens, in contrast, reveals only p21. The other main difference between stimulatory and altered antigens can be seen when the ZAP-70 associated with the TCR is examined. Optimal phosphorylation of ZAP-70 occurs only with stimulatory and not with altered antigen. Failure of full ZAP-70 activation presumably results in insufficient activation of distal pathways, and IL-2 production in this situation is also insufficient. In all these experimental systems, it is the failure to produce and respond to IL-2 that is the most important determinant of whether anergy is induced (82).

Establishing characterization of the unresponsive state has received considerable attention. Induction of the unresponsive state requires protein synthesis, suggesting that a newly synthesized protein may be required for the maintenance of the unresponsive state. Recent studies suggest a defect in Ras activation, with resulting defects in MAPK and Jnk activation following the stimulation of the TCR in anergized T cells (300,301). The failure to activate Ras and these kinases helps to explain previous results that demonstrated diminished AP-1 activity in an anergized T-cell clone (299). The failure to activate Ras may be explained via the activation of another GTPase called Rap-1, which antagonizes the activity of Ras by competing for binding with Ras GEFs. In anergic T cells, Rap-1 activity is elevated, perhaps through mechanisms that involve Fyn, Crk, and C3G, a GEF for Rap-1 (327). Further studies will be required to assess the general importance of this pathway.

CONCLUSION

The activation of T-lymphocytes is a complex process that results in cell growth and differentiation. Examples of the major events involved are presented in Table 4. T-cell activation is initiated by ligand–receptor interactions that occur at the interface of the T cell and APC or target cell. The TCR plays a prominent role in this interaction, but other molecules on the T cell and APC also contribute to the ultimate activation of the T cell. Stimulation of the TCR induces a highly ordered sequence of tyrosine phosphorylation events that are orchestrated by PTKs and are regulated by other PTKs and PTPases. These phosphorylation events lead to signaling pathways that activate a variety of enzymes and induce a multitude of protein interactions. Second messengers are produced and ion fluxes occur. Cascades of these signaling events determine the T-cell response. In some cases, effector functions are activated. In others, expression of a variety of genes is induced, which contributes to the clonal expansion and differentiation of appropriate antigen-specific T cells. In still others, where signaling events are inadequate, a state of unresponsiveness ensues. Future studies promise to unravel some of the complexities of the events that occur in signaling pathways that

TABLE 4. *Major events involved in T-cell activation*

Event	Example
Cell–cell interaction	T cell–APC CTL–target cell
Receptor–ligand binding	TCR–antigen/MHC
Transmembrane signal transduction	Activation of Lck
Generation of second messengers	1,4,5-IP$_3$ and DG
Second-messenger effects	Ca^{2+} mobilization Protein kinase C activation
Biochemical pathways	Phosphatidylinositol pathway Ras pathway
Cellular events	MTOC reorganization Secretion of cytolytic granules
Early gene activation	c-Myc, c-Fos
Intermediate gene activation	Lymphokines, lymphokine receptors, nutrient receptors
Late gene activation	Genes involved in cell proliferation 4F2, VLA-2

lead from the membrane to the nucleus. The activation of the T cell has proven to be a unique system to sample and explore the complex mechanisms regulating cell growth and differentiation.

REFERENCES

1. Clevers H, Alarcon B, Willeman T, et al. The T cell receptor/CD3 complex: a dynamic protein ensemble. *Annu Rev Immunol* 1988;6:629–662.
2. Weiss A. Molecular and genetic insights into T cell antigen receptor structure and function. *Annu Rev Genet* 1991;25:487–510.
3. Schwartz RH. Costimulation of T-lymphocytes: the role of CD28, CTLA-4, and B7/BB1 in interleukin-2 production and immunotherapy. *Cell* 1992;71:1065–1068.
4. Smith KA. Interleukin-2: inception, impact, and implications. *Science* 1988;240:1169–1176.
5. Crabtree GR, Clipstone NA. Signal transmission between the plasma membrane and nucleus of T-lymphocytes. *Annu Rev Biochem* 1994;63:1045–1083.
6. Marrack P, Kappler J. T cells can distinguish between allogeneic major histocompatibility complex products on different cell types. *Nature* 1988;332:840–843.
7. Linsley PS, Ledbetter JA. The role of the CD28 receptor during T cell responses to antigen. *Annu Rev Immunol* 1993;11:191–212.
8. Salomon B, Bluestone JA. Complexities of CD28/B7: CTLA-4 costimulatory pathways in autoimmunity and transplantation. *Annu Rev Immunol* 2001;19:225–252.
9. Shaw AS, Dustin ML. Making the T cell receptor go the distance: A topological view of T cell activation. *Immunity* 1997;6:361–369.
10. Dustin ML, Bromley SK, Davis MM, et al. Identification of self through two-dimensional chemistry and synapses. *Annu Rev Cell Biol* 2001;17:133–157.
11. Ronchese F, Schwartz RH, Germain RN. Functionally distinct subsites on a class II major histocompatibility complex molecule. *Nature* 1987;329:254–256.
12. Watts TH, Brian AA, Kappler JW, et al. Antigen presentation by supported planar membranes containing affinity-purified I-Ad. *Proc Natl Acad Sci U S A* 1984;81:7564–7568.
13. Goldstein SAN, Mescher MF. Cytotoxic T cell activation by class I protein on cell–size artificial membranes: antigen density and Lyt-2/3 function. *J Immunol* 1987;138:2034–2043.
14. Clayberger C, Parham P, Rothbard J, et al. HLA-A2 peptides can regulate cytolysis by human allogeneic T-lymphocytes. *Nature* 1987;330:763–765.

15. York I, Rock KL. Antigen processing and presentation by the class I major histocompatibility complex. *Annu Rev Immunol* 1996;14:369–396.

16. Sundberg EJ, Li Y, Mariuzza RA. So many ways of getting in the way: diversity in the molecular architecture of superantigen–dependent T-cell signaling complexes. *Curr Opin Immunol* 2002;14:36–44.

17. Fraser JD, Newton ME, Weiss A. CD28 and T cell antigen receptor signal transduction coordinately regulate interleukin 2 gene expression in response to superantigen stimulation. *J Exp Med* 1992;175:1131–1134.

18. Yamasaki S, Tachibana M, Shinohara N, et al. Lck-independent triggering of T-cell antigen receptor signal transduction by staphylococcal enterotoxin. *J Biol Chem* 1997;272:14787–14791.

19. Liu H, Lampe MA, Iregui MV, et al. Conventional antigen and superantigen may be coupled to distinct and cooperative T-cell activation pathways. *Proc Natl Acad Sci U S A* 1991;88:8705–8709.

20. Sharon N. Lectin receptors as lymphocyte surface markers. *Adv Immunol* 1983;34:213–298.

21. Kipatrick DC. Mechanisms and assessment of lectin-mediated mitogenesis. *Mol Biotechnol* 1999;11:55–65.

22. Weiss A, Shields R, Newton M, et al. Ligand–receptor interactions required for commitment to the activation of the interleukin 2 gene. *J Immunol* 1987;138:2169–2176.

23. Mueller DL, Jenkins MK, Schwartz RH. Clonal expansion vs functional inactivation: a costimulatory pathway determines the outcome of T cell antigen receptor occupancy. *Annu Rev Immunol* 1989;7:445–480.

24. Tax WJM, Hermes FFM, Willems RW, et al. Fc receptors for mouse IgG1 on human monocytes: polymorphism and its role in antibody-induced T cell proliferation. *J Immunol* 1984;133:1185–1189.

25. Palacios R, Martinez-Maza O. Is the E receptor on human T-lymphocytes a "negative signal receptor"? *J Immunol* 1982;129:2479–2485.

26. Meuer SC, Hussey RE, Fabbi M, et al. An alternative pathway of T-cell activation: a functional role of the 50 kd T11 sheep erythrocyte receptor protein. *Cell* 1984;36:897–906.

27. Yang SY, Chouaib S, Dupont B. A common pathway for T-lymphocyte activation involving both the CD3-Ti complex and CD2 erythrocyte receptor determinants. *J Immunol* 1986;137:1097–1100.

28. Weiss A, Imboden J, Shoback D, et al. Role of T3 surface molecules in human T-cell activation: T3-dependent activation results in an increase in cytoplasmic free calcium. *Proc Natl Acad Sci U S A* 1984;81:4169–4173.

29. Truneh A, Albert F, Golstein P, et al. Early steps of lymphocyte activation bypassed by synergy between calcium ionophores and phorbol ester. *Nature* 1985;313:318–320.

30. Ebinu JO, Stang SL, Teixeira C, et al. RasGRP links T-cell receptor signaling to Ras. *Blood* 2000;95:3199.

31. Mustelin T, Coggeshall KM, Isakov N, et al. T cell antigen receptor–mediated activation of phospholipase C requires tyrosine phosphorylation. *Science* 1990;247:1584–1587.

32. June CH, Fletcher MC, Ledbetter JA, et al. Inhibition of tyrosine phosphorylation prevents T cell receptor-mediated signal transduction. *Proc Natl Acad Sci U S A* 1990;87:7722–7726.

33. Mauro MJ, O'Dwyer M, Heinrich MC, et al. STI571: a paradigm of new agents for cancer therapeutics. *J Clin Oncol* 2002;20:325–334.

34. Sloan-Lancaster J, Evavold BE, Allen P. Induction of T-cell anergy by altered T-cell–receptor ligand on live antigen-presenting cells. *Nature* 1993;363:156–159.

35. Sloan-Lancaster J, Shaw AS, Rothbard JB, et al. Partial T cell signaling: altered phospho-zeta and lack of zap70 recruitment in APL-induced T cell anergy. *Cell* 1994;79:913–922.

36. Rabinowitz JD, Beeson C, Wulfing C, et al. Altered T cell receptor ligands trigger a subset of early T cell signals. *Immunity* 1996;5:125–135.

37. Lyons DS, Lieberman SA, Hampl J, et al. A TCR binds to antagonist ligands with lower affinities and faster dissociation rates than to agonists. *Immunity* 1996;5:53–61.

38. Madrenas J, Germain R. Variant TCR ligands: new insights into the molecular basis of antigen-dependent signal transduction and T cell activation. *Sem Immunol* 1996;8:83–101.

39. Weiss A, Imboden JB. *Cell* surface molecules and early events involved in human T-lymphocyte activation. *Adv Immunol* 1987;41:1–38.

40. Lanier LL, Ruitenberg JJ, Allison JP, et al. Distinct epitopes on the T cell antigen receptor of HPB-ALL tumor cells identified by monoclonal antibodies. *J Immunol* 1986;137:2286–2292.

41. Rojo JM, Janeway J, CA. The biological activity of anti–T cell receptor antibodies is determined by the epitope recognized. *J Immunol* 1988;140.

42. Finkel TH, Cambier JC, Kubo RT, et al. The thymus has two functionally distinct populations of immature ab+ T cells: one population is deleted by ligation of $\alpha\beta$TCR. *Cell* 1989;58:1047–1054.

43. Demotz S, Grey HM, Sette A. The minimal number of class II MHC–antigen complexes needed for T cell activation. *Science* 1990;249:1028–1030.

44. Harding CV, Unanue E. Quantitation of antigen-presenting cell MHC class II/peptide complexes necessary for T-cell stimulation. *Nature* 1990;346:574–576.

45. Van Wauwe JP, De Mey JR, Goosens JG. OKT3: a monoclonal anti-human T-lymphocyte antibody with potent mitogenic properties. *J Immunol* 1980;124:2708–2713.

46. Valitutti S, Muller S, Cella M, et al. Serial triggering of many T-cell receptors by a few peptide–MHC complexes. *Nature* 1995;375:148–151.

47. Sagerstrom CG, Kerr EM, Allison JP, et al. Activation and differentiation requirements of primary T cells *in vitro*. *Proc Natl Acad Sci U S A* 1993;90:8987–8991.

48. Herman A, Kappler JW, Marrack P, et al. Superantigens: mechanism of T-cell stimulation and role in immune responses. *Annu Rev Immunol* 1991;9:745–772.

49. Webb S, Morris C, Sprent J. Extrathymic tolerance of mature T cells: clonal elimination as a consequence of immunity. *Cell* 1990;63:1249–1256.

50. Vella AT, McCormack JE, Linsley PS, et al. Lipopolysaccharide interferes with the induction of peripheral T cell death. *Immunity* 1995;2:261–270.

51. van Parijs L, Abbas A. Role of Fas-mediated cell death in the regulation of immune responses. *Curr Opin Immunol* 1996;8:355–361.

52. O'Rourke AM, Mescher MF, Webb SR. Activation of polyphosphoinositide hydrolysis in T cells by H-2 alloantigen but not MLS determinants. *Science* 1990;249:171–174.

53. Iwashima M, Irving BA, van Oers NSC, et al. Sequential interactions of the TCR with two distinct cytoplasmic tyrosine kinases. *Science* 1994;263:1136–1139.

54. Bierer BE, Sleckman BP, Ratnofsky SE, et al. The biological roles of CD2, CD4, and CD8 in T-cell activation. *Immunol Rev* 1989;7:579–599.

55. Bockenstedt LK, Goldsmith MA, Dustin M, et al. The CD2 ligand LFA-3 activates T cells but depends on the expression and function of the antigen receptor. *J Immunol* 1988;141:1904–1911.

56. Howard FD, Moingeon P, Moebius U, et al. The CD3ζ cytoplasmic domain mediates CD2-induced T cell activation. *J Exp Med* 1992;176:139–145.

57. Hara T, Fu SM. Human cell activation: I. Monocyte-independent activation and proliferation induced by anti–T3 monoclonal antibodies in the presence of tumor promoter 12-o-tetradecanoyl phorbol-13-acetate. *J Exp Med* 1985;161:641–656.

58. Williams JM, Deloria D, Hansen JA, et al. The events of primary T cell activation can be staged by use of sepharose-bound anti–T3 (64.1) monoclonal antibody and purified interleukin 1. *J Immunol* 1985;135:2249–2255.

59. Ceuppens JL, Bloemmen FJ, Van Wauwe JP. T cell unresponsiveness to the mitogenic activity of OKT3 antibody results from a deficiency of monocyte Fcg receptors for murine IgG2α and inability to cross-link the T3-Ti complex. *J Immunol* 1985;135:3882–3886.

60. Janeway CA Jr. The T cell receptor as a multicomponent signalling machine: CD4/CD8 coreceptors and CD45 in T cell activation. *Annu Rev Immunol* 1992;10:645–674.

61. Zamoyska R. CD4 and CD8: modulators of T cell receptor recognition of antigen and of immune response? *Curr Opin Immunol* 1998;10:82–87.

62. Moody AM, Chui D, Reche PA, et al. Developmentally regulated glycosylation of the CD8alphabeta coreceptor stalk modulates ligand binding. *Cell* 2001;107:501–512.

63. Basson MA, Zamoyska R. The CD4/CD8 lineage decision: integration of signalling pathways. *Immunol Today* 2000;21:509–514.

64. Ledbetter JA, Gilliland LK, Schieven GA. The interaction of CD4 with

CD3/Ti regulates tyrosine phosphorylation of substrates during T cell activation. *Sem Immunol* 1990;2:99–106.

65. Killeen N, Littman DR. Helper T-cell development in the absence of CD4-p56^lck association. *Nature* 1993;364:729–732.

66. Xu H, Littman DR. A kinase-independent function of lck in potentiating antigen-specific T cell activation. *Cell* 1993;74:633–644.

67. O'Rourke AM, Mescher MF. Cytotoxic T-lymphocyte activation involves a cascade of signaling and adhesion events. *Nature* 1992; 358:253–255.

68. Thome M, Duplay P, Guttinger M, et al. Syk and ZAP-70 mediate recruitment of p56lck/CD4 to the activated T cell receptor/CD3/ζ complex. *J Exp Med* 1995;181:1997–2006.

69. Straus DB, Chan AC, Patai B, et al. SH2 domain function is essential for the role of the Lck tyrosine kinase in T cell receptor signal transduction. *J Biol Chem* 1996;271:9976–9981.

70. Doyle C, Strominger JL. Interaction between CD4 and class II MHC molecules mediates cell adhesion. *Nature* 1988;330:256–258.

71. Norment AM, Salter RD, Parham P, et al. Cell–cell adhesion mediated by CD8 and MHC class I molecules. *Nature* 1988;336:79–81.

72. Newell MK, Haughn LJ, Maroun CR, et al. Death of mature T cells by separate ligation of CD4 and the T-cell receptor for antigen. *Nature* 1990;347:286–289.

73. Banda NK, Bernier J, Kurahara DK, et al. Crosslinking CD4 by human immunodeficiency virus gp120 primes T cells for activation-induced apoptosis. *J Exp Med* 1992;176:1099–1106.

74. Glaichenhaus N, Shastri N, Littman DR, et al. Requirement for association of p56^lck with CD4 in antigen-specific signal transduction in T cells. *Cell* 1991;64:511–520.

75. Matsui K, Boniface JJ, Reay PA, et al. Low affinity interaction of peptide–MHC complexes with T cell receptors. *Science* 1991;254: 1788–1791.

76. Shimizu Y, van Seventer G, Horgan KJ, et al. Roles of adhesion molecules in T-cell recognition: Fundamental similarities between four integrins on resting human T cells (LFA-1, VLA-4, VLA-5, VLA-6) in expression, binding, and costimulation. *Immunol Rev* 1990;114:109–143.

77. Dustin ML, Springer TA. T-cell receptor cross-linking transiently stimulates adhesiveness through LFA-1. *Nature* 1989;341:619–624.

78. Hahn WC, Burakoff SJ, Bierer BE. Signal transduction pathways involved in T cell receptor-induced regulation of CD2 avidity for CD58. *J Immunol* 1993;150:2607–2619.

79. Peterson EJ, Woods ML, Dmowski SA, et al. Coupling of the TCR to integrin activation by SLAP-130/Fyb. *Science* 2001;293:2263–2265.

80. Schwartz RH. T cell clonal anergy. *Curr Opin Immunol* 1997;9: 351–357.

81. Shimonkevitz R, Kappler J, Marrack P, et al. Antigen recognition by H-2–restricted T cells. *J Exp Med* 1983;158:303–316.

82. Madrenas J, Schwartz RH, Germain RN. Interleukin 2 production, not the pattern of early T-cell antigen receptor-dependent tyrosine phosphorylation, controls anergy induction by both agonists and partial agonists. *Proc Natl Acad Sci U S A* 1996;93:9736–9741.

83. Foy TM, Aruffo A, Bajorath J, et al. Immune regulation by CD40 and its ligand GP39. *Annu Rev Immunol* 1996;14:591–617.

84. Michel F, Attal-Bonnefoy G, Mangino G, et al. CD28 as a molecular amplifier extending TCR ligation and signaling capabilities. *Immunity* 2001;15:935–945.

85. Frauwirth KA, Thompson CB. Activation and inhibition of lymphocytes by costimulation. *J Clin Invest* 2002;109:295–299.

86. Shahinian A, Pfeffer K, Lee KP, et al. Differential T cell costimulatory requirements in CD28-deficient mice. *Science* 1993;261:609–612.

87. Borriello F, Sethna MP, Boyd SD, et al. B7-1 and B7-2 have overlapping, critical roles in immunoglobulin class switching and germinal center formation. *Immunity* 1997;6:303–13.

88. Thompson CG, Lindstein T, Ledbetter JA, et al. CD28 activation pathway regulates the production of multiple T-cell–derived lymphokines/cytokines. *Proc Natl Acad Sci U S A* 1989;86:1333–1337.

89. Fraser JD, Weiss A. Regulation of T cell lymphokine transcription by the accessory molecule CD28. *Mol Cell Biol* 1992;12:4357–4363.

90. Powell JD, Ragheb JA, Kitagawa-Sakakida S, et al. Molecular regulation of interleukin-2 expression by CD28 co-stimulation and anergy. *Immunol Rev* 1998;165:287–300.

91. Stein PH, Fraser JD, Weiss A. The cytoplasmic domain of CD28 is both necessary and sufficient for costimulation of interleukin-2 secre-

tion and association with phosphatidylinositol 3'-kinase. *Mol Cell Biol* 1994;14:3392–3402.

92. Kundig TM, Shahinian A, Kawai K, et al. Duration of TCR stimulation determines costimulatory requirement of T cells. *Immunity* 1996;5:41–52.

93. Dong C, Juedes AE, Temann UA, et al. ICOS co-stimulatory receptor is essential for T-cell activation and function. *Nature* 2001;409:97–101.

94. Furue M, Chang CH, Tamaki K. Interleukin-1 but not tumour necrosis factor alpha synergistically upregulates the granulocyte–macrophage colony-stimulating factor-induced B7-1 expression of murine Langerhans cells. *Br J Dermatol* 1996;135:194–198.

95. Janeway CA, Medzhitov R. Innate immune recognition. *Annu Rev Immunol* 2002;20:197–216.

96. Baeuerle PA, Henkel T. Function and activation of NF-κB in the immune system. *Annu Rev Immunol* 1994;12:141–179.

97. DiDonato JA, Hayakawa M, Rothwarf DM, et al. A cytokine-responsive IkappaB kinase that activates the transcription factor NF-kappaB. *Nature* 1997;388:548–554.

98. Weiss A, Wiskocil R, Stobo JD. The role of T3 surface molecules in the activation of human T cells: a two stimulus requirement for IL-2 production reflects events occurring at a pre-translational level. *J Immunol* 1984;133:123–128.

99. Sun Z-Y J, Kim S, Wagner G, et al. Mechanisms contributing to T cell receptor signaling and assembly revealed by the solution structure of an ectodomain fragment of the CD3εγ heterodimer. *Cell* 2001;105:913–923.

100. Orloff DG, Ra C, Frank SJ, et al. Family of disulphide-linked dimers containing ζ and η chains of the T-cell receptor and the γ chain of Fc receptors. *Nature* 1990;347:189–191.

101. Manolios N, Letourneur F, Bonifacino JS, et al. Pairwise, cooperative and inhibitory interactions describe the assembly and probable structure of the T-cell antigen receptor. *EMBO J* 1991;10:1643–1651.

102. Tan L, Turner J, Weiss A. Regions of the T cell antigen receptor α and β chains that are responsible for interactions with CD3. *J Exp Med* 1991;173:1247–1256.

103. Irving B, Weiss A. The cytoplasmic domain of the T cell receptor ζ chain is sufficient to couple to receptor-associated signal transduction pathways. *Cell* 1991;64:891–901.

104. Romeo C, Seed B. Cellular immunity to HIV activated by CD4 fused to T cell or Fc receptor polypeptides. *Cell* 1991;64:1037–1046.

105. Letourneur F, Klausner RD. Activation of T cells by a tyrosine kinase activation domain in the cytoplasmic tail of CD3ε. *Science* 1992; 255:79–82.

106. Wegener A-MK, Letourneur F, Hoeveler A, et al. The T cell receptor/CD3 complex is composed of at least two autonomous transduction modules. *Cell* 1992;68:83–95.

107. Reth M. Antigen receptor tail clue. *Nature* 1989;338:383–384.

108. Romeo C, Amiot M, Seed B. Sequence requirements for induction of cytolysis by the T cell antigen/Fc receptor ζ chain. *Cell* 1992;68:889–897.

109. Irving BA, Chan AC, Weiss A. Functional characterization of a signal transducing motif present in the T cell receptor ζ chain. *J Exp Med* 1993;177:1093–1103.

110. Lin S, Cicala C, Scharenberg AM, et al. The FceR1β subunit functions as an amplifier of FceR1γ-mediated cell activation signals. *Cell* 1996;85:985–995.

111. Shores EW, Tran T, Grinberg A, et al. Role of the multiple T cell receptor (TCR)-ζ chain signaling motifs in selection of the T cell repertoire. *J Exp Med* 1997;185:893–900.

112. Combadière B, Freedman M, Chen L, et al. Qualitative and quantitative contributions of the T cell receptor zeta chain to mature T cell apoptosis. *J Exp Med* 1996;183:2109–2117.

113. Willems L, Gatot JS, Mammerickx M, et al. The YXXL signalling motifs of the bovine leukemia virus transmembrane protein are required for in vivo infection and maintenance of high viral loads. *J Virol* 1995;69:4137–4141.

114. Miller CL, Burkhardt AL, Lee JH, et al. Integral membrane protein 2 of Epstein–Barr virus regulates reactivation from latency through dominant negative effects on protein–tyrosine kinases. *Immunity* 1995;2:155–166.

115. Du Z, Lang SM, Sasseville VG, et al. Identification of a nef allele that causes lymphocyte activations and acute disease in macaque monkeys. *Cell* 1995;82:665–674.

116. Lagunoff M, Majeti R, Weiss A, et al. Deregulated signal transduction by the K1 gene product of Kaposi's sarcoma–associated herpesvirus. *Proc Natl Acad Sci U S A* 1999;96:5704–5709.

117. Cantrell DA, Davies AA, Crumpton MJ. Activators of protein kinase C down-regulate and phosphorylate the T3/T-cell antigen receptor complex of human T-lymphocytes. *Proc Natl Acad Sci U S A* 1985;82:8158–8162.

118. Dietrich J, Hou X, Wegener AM, et al. Molecular characterization of the di-leucine–based internalization motif of the T cell receptor. *J Biol Chem* 1996;271:11441–11448.

119. Goldsmith MA, Weiss A. Isolation and characterization of a T-lymphocyte somatic mutant with altered signal transduction by the antigen receptor. *Proc Natl Acad Sci U S A* 1987;84:6879–6883.

120. Dianzani U, Shaw A, Al-Ramadi BK, et al. Physical association of CD4 with the T cell receptor. *J Immunol* 1992;148:678–688.

121. Hsi ED, Siegel JN, Minami Y, et al. T cell activation induces rapid tyrosine phosphorylation of a limited number of cellular substrates. *J Biol Chem* 1989;264:10836–10842.

122. Baniyash M, Garcia-Morales P, Luong E, et al. The T cell antigen receptor ζ chain is tyrosine phosphorylated upon activation. *J Biol Chem* 1988;263:18225–18230.

123. Qian D, Griswold-Prenner I, Rosner MR, et al. Multiple components of the T cell antigen receptor complex become tyrosine-phosphorylated upon activation. *J Biol Chem* 1993;268:4488–4493.

124. June CH, Fletcher MC, Ledbetter JA, et al. Increases in tyrosine phosphorylation are detectable before phospholipase C activation after T cell receptor stimulation. *J Immunol* 1990;144:1591–1599.

125. Miller AT, Berg LJ. New insights into the regulation and functions of Tec family tyrosine kinases in the immune system. *Curr Opin Immunol* 2002;14:331–340.

126. Brown MT, Cooper JA. Regulation, substrates and functions of src. *Biochim Biophys Acta* 1996;1287:121–149.

127. Yurchak LK, Sefton BM. Palmitoylation of either Cys-3 or Cys-5 is required for the biological activity of the Lck tyrosine protein kinase. *Mol Cell Biol* 1995;15:6914–6922.

128. Shenoy-Scaria AM, Gauen LKT, Kwong J, et al. Palmitylation of an amino–terminal cysteine motif of protein tyrosine kinases p56[lck] and p59[fyn] mediates interactions with glycosyl-phosphatidylinositol–anchored protein. *Mol Cell Biol* 1993;13:6385–6392.

129. Yamaguchi H, Hendrickson WA. Structural basis for activation of human lymphocyte kinase Lck upon tyrosine phosphorylation. *Nature* 1996;384:484–489.

130. Sicheri F, Moarefi I, Kuriyan J. Crystal structure of the Src family tyrosine kinase Hck. *Nature* 1997;385:602–609.

131. Xu W, Harrison SG, Eck MJ. Three-dimensional structure of the tyrosine kinase c-Src. *Nature* 1997;385:595–602.

132. Cooke MP, Perlmutter RM. Expression of a novel form of the fyn proto-oncogene in hematopoietic cells. *New Biologist* 1989;1:66–74.

133. Davidson D, Chow LML, Fournel M, et al. Differential regulation of T cell antigen responsiveness by isoforms of the src-related tyrosine protein kinase p59[fyn]. *J Exp Med* 1992;175:1483–1492.

134. Samelson LE, Phillips AF, Luong ET, et al. Association of the fyn protein-tyrosine kinase with the T-cell antigen receptor. *Proc Natl Acad Sci U S A* 1990;87:4358–4362.

135. Gassmann M, Amrein KE, Flint NA, et al. Identification of a signaling complex involving CD2, ζ chain and p59[fyn] in T-lymphocytes. *Eur J Immunol* 1994;24:139–144.

136. Gauen LKT, Kong A-NT, Samelson LE, et al. p59[fyn] tyrosine kinase associates with multiple T-cell receptor subunits through its unique amino-terminal domain. *Mol Cell Biol* 1992;12:5438–5446.

137. van't Hof W, Resh MD. Dual fatty acylation of p59[fyn] is required for association with the T cell receptor ζ chain through phosphotyrosine–Src homology domain-2 interactions. *J Cell Biol* 1999;145:377–389.

138. Tsygankov AY, Spana C, Rowley RB, et al. Activation dependent tyrosine phosphorylation of Fyn-associated proteins in T-lymphocytes. *J Biol Chem* 1994;269:7792–7800.

139. Cooke MP, Abraham KM, Forbush KA, et al. Regulation of T cell receptor signaling by a src family protein–tyrosine kinase (p59[fyn]). *Cell* 1991;65:281–292.

140. Appleby MW, Gross JA, Cooke MP, et al. Defective T cell receptor signaling in mice lacking the thymic isoform of p59[fyn]. *Cell* 1992;70:751–763.

141. Stein PL, Lee H-M, Rich S, et al. pp59fyn mutant mice display differential signaling in thymocytes and peripheral T cells. *Cell* 1992;70:741–750.

142. Qian D, Lev S, van Oers NSC, et al. Tyrosine phosphorylation of Pyk2 is selectively regulated by Fyn during TCR signaling. *J Exp Med* 1997;185:1253–1259.

143. Veillette A, Bookman MA, Horak EM, et al. The CD4 and CD8 T cell surface antigens are associated with the internal membrane tyrosine–protein kinase p56[lck]. *Cell* 1988;55:301–308.

144. Abraham N, Miceli MC, Parnes JR, et al. Enhancement of T-cell responsiveness by the lymphocyte-specific tyrosine protein kinase p56[lck]. *Nature* 1991;350:62–66.

145. Haughn L, Gratton S, Caron L, et al. Association of tyrosine kinase p56lck with CD4 inhibits the induction of growth through the $\alpha\beta$ T-cell receptor. *Nature* 1992;358:328–331.

146. Ley SC, Marsh M, Bebbington CR, et al. Distinct intracellular localization of Lck and Fyn protein tyrosine kinases in human T-lymphocytes. *J Cell Biol* 1994;125:639–649.

147. Straus D, Weiss A. Genetic evidence for the involvement of the Lck tyrosine kinase in signal transduction throught the T cell antigen receptor. *Cell* 1992;70:585–593.

148. Molina TJ, Kishihara K, Siderovski DP, et al. Profound block in thymocyte development in mice lacking p56[lck]. *Nature* 1992;357:161–164.

149. Karnitz L, Sutor SL, Torigoe T, et al. Effects of p56[lck] on the growth and cytolytic effector function of an interleukin-2–dependent cytotoxic T-cell line. *Mol Cell Biol* 1992;12:4521–4530.

150. van Oers NSC, Killeen N, Weiss A. Lck regulates the tyrosine phosphorylation of the T cell receptor subunits and ZAP-70 in murine thymocytes. *J Exp Med* 1996;183:1053–1062.

151. van Oers NSC, Lowin-Kropf B, Finlay D, et al. $\alpha\beta$ T cell development is abolished in mice lacking both Lck and Fyn protein tyrosine kinases. *Immunity* 1996;5:429–436.

152. Groves T, Smiley P, Cooke MP, et al. Fyn can partially substitute for Lck in T-lymphocyte development. *Immunity* 1996;5:417–428.

153. Kabouridis PS, Magee AI, Ley SC. S-acylation of LCK protein tyrosine kinase is essential for its signalling function in T-lymphocytes. *EMBO J* 1997;16:4983–4998.

154. Strauss DB, Chan AC, Patai B, et al. SH2 domain function is essential for the role of the Lck tyrosine kinase in T cell receptor signal transduction. *J Biol Chem* 1996;271:9976–9981.

155. Xu H, Littman DR. The kinase-dependent function of Lck in T-cell activation requires an intact site for tyrosine autophosphorylation. *Ann N Y Acad Sci* 1995;766:99–116.

156. Chu DH, Morita CT, Weiss A. The Syk family of protein tyrosine kinases in T-cell activation and development. *Immunol Rev* 1998:165:167–180.

157. Chan AC, van Oers NSC, Tran A, et al. Differential expression of ZAP-70 and Syk protein tyrosine kinases, and the role of this family of protein tyrosine kinases in T cell antigen receptor signaling. *J Immunol* 1994;152:4758–4766.

158. Mallick-Wood CA, Pao W, Cheng AM, et al. Disruption of epithelial gd T cell repertoires by mutation of the Syk tyrosine kinase. *Proc Natl Acad Sci U S A* 1996;93:9704–9709.

159. Bu J-Y, Shaw AS, Chan AC. Analysis of the interaction of ZAP-70 and syk protein–tyrosine kinases with the T-cell antigen receptor by plasmon resonance. *Proc Natl Acad Sci U S A* 1995;92:5106–5110.

160. Hatada MH, Lu X, Laird ER, et al. Molecular basis for interaction of the protein tyrosine kinase ZAP-70 with the T-cell receptor. *Nature* 1995;377:32–38.

161. Keshvara LM, Isaacson C, Harrison ML, et al. Syk activation and dissociation from the B-cell antigen receptor is mediated by phosphorylation of tyrosine 130. *J Biol Chem* 1997;272:10377–10381.

162. Futterer K, Wong J, Grucza RA, et al. Structural basis for Syk tyrosine kinase ubiquity in signal transduction pathways revealed by the crystal structure of its regulatory SH2 domains bound to a dually phosphorylated ITAM peptide. *J Mol Biol* 1998;281:523–537.

163. Wange RL, Guitian R, Isakov N, et al. Activating and inhibitory mutations in adjacent tyrosines in the kinase domain of ZAP-70. *J Biol Chem* 1995;270:18730–18733.

164. Kong G, Dalton M, Wardenburg JB, et al. Distinct tyrosine phosphorylation sites in ZAP-70 mediate activation and negative regulation of antigen receptor function. *Mol Cell Biol* 1996;16:5026–5035.

165. Zhao Q, Weiss A. Enhancement of lymphocyte responsiveness by a gain-of-function mutation of ZAP-70. *Mol Cell Biol* 1996;16:6765–6774.

166. Thien CBF, Langdon WY. CBL: Many adaptations to regulate protein tyrosine kinases. *Mol Cell Biol* 2001;2:294–305.

167. Rao N, Dodge I, Band H. The Cbl family of ubiquin ligases: critical negative regulators of tyrosine kinase signaling in the immune system. *J Leukoc Biol* 2002;71:753–763.

168. Furlong MT, Mahrenholz AM, Kim KH, et al. Identification of the major sites of autophosphorylation of the murine protein-tyrosine kinase Syk. *Biochim Biophys Acta* 1997;1355:177–90.

169. Di Bartolo V, Mege D, Germain V, et al. Tyrosine 319, a newly identified phosphorylation site of ZAP-70, plays a critical role in T cell antigen receptor signaling. *J Biol Chem* 1999;274:6285–6294.

170. Chan AC, Dalton M, Johnson R, et al. Activation of ZAP-70 kinase activity by phosphorylation of tyrosine 493 is required for lymphocyte antigen receptor function. *EMBO J* 1995;14:2499–2508.

171. Latour S, Chow LML, Veillette A. Differential intrinisic enzymatic activity of Syk and Zap-70 protein-tyrosine kinases. *J Biol Chem* 1996;271:22782–22790.

172. Wiest DL, Ashe JM, Howcroft TK, et al. A spontaneously arising mutation in the DLAARN motif of murine ZAP-70 abrogates kinase activity and arrests thymocyte development. *Immunity* 1997;6:663–671.

173. Elder ME, Skodar-Smith S, Kadlecek TA, et al. Distinct T cell developmental consequences in humans and mice expressing identical mutations in the DLAARN motif of ZAP-70. *J Immunol* 2001;166:656–661.

174. Arpaia E, Shahar M, Dadi H, et al. Defective T cell receptor signaling and CD8+ thymic selection in humans lacking ZAP-70 kinase. *Cell* 1994;76:947–958.

175. Chan AC, Kadlecek TA, Elder ME, et al. ZAP-70 deficiency in an autosomal recessive form of severe combined immunodeficiency. *Science* 1994;264:1599–1601.

176. Elder ME, Lin D, Clever J, et al. Human severe combined immunodeficiency due to a defect in ZAP-70, a T-cell tyrosine kinase. *Science* 1994;264:1596–1599.

177. Negishi I, Motoyama N, Nakayama K-I, et al. Essential role for ZAP-70 in both positive and negative selection of thymocytes. *Nature* 1995;376:435–438.

178. Gelfand EW, Weinberg K, Mazer BD, et al. Absence of ZAP-70 prevents signaling through the antigen receptor on peripheral blood T cells but not thymocytes. *J Exp Med* 1995;182:1057–1066.

179. Harnett M. Syk deficiency—a knockout for B-cell development. *Immunol Today* 1996;17:4.

180. van Oers NSC, Tao W, Watts JD, et al. Constitutive tyrosine phosphorylation of the T cell receptor (TCR) ζ subunit: regulation of TCR-associated protein kinase activity by TCR ζ. *Mol Cell Biol* 1993;13:5771–5780.

181. Shiue L, Zoller MJ, Brugge JS. Syk is activated by phosphotyrosine-containing peptides representing the tyrosine-based activation motifs of the high affinity receptor for IgE. *J Biol Chem* 1995;270:10498–10502.

182. Pawson T, Gish GD, Nash P. SH2 domains, interaction modules and cellular wiring. *Trends Cell Biol* 2001;11:504–511.

183. Songyang Z, Shoelson SE, Chaudhuri M, et al. SH2 domains recognize specific phosphopeptide sequences. *Cell* 1993;72:767–778.

184. Wu J, Zhao Q, Kurosaki T, Weiss A. The Vav binding site (Y315) in ZAP-70 is critical for antigen receptor-mediated signal transduction. *J Exp Med* 1997;185:1877–1882.

185. Rotin D, Margolis B, Mohammadi M, et al. SH2 domains prevent tyrosine dephosphorylation of the EGF receptor, identification of Tyr992 as the high affinity binding site for SH2 domains of phospholipase Cγ. *EMBO J* 1992;11:559–567.

186. van der Geer P, Pawson T. The PTB domain: a new protein module implicated in signal transduction. *Trends Biochem Sci* 1995;20:277–80.

187. Ladbury JE, Arold S. Searching for specificity in SH domains. *Chem Biol* 2000;7:R3–R8.

188. Veillette A, Latour S, Davidson D. Negative regulation of immunoreceptor signaling. *Annu Rev Immunol* 2002;20:669–707.

189. Mustelin T, Feng GS, Bottini N, et al. Protein tyrosine phosphatases. *Front Biosci* 2002;7:d85–142.

190. Trowbridge IS, Thomas ML. CD45: an emerging role as a protein tyrosine phosphatase required for lymphocyte activation and development. *Annu Rev Immunol* 1994;12:85–116.

191. Johnson P, Ostergaard HL, Wasden C, et al. Mutational analysis of CD45: a leukocyte-specific protein tyrosine phosphatase. *J Biol Chem* 1992;12:8035–8041.

192. Desai DM, Sap J, Silvennoinen O, et al. The catalytic activity of the CD45 membrane proximal phosphatase domain is required for TCR signaling and regulation. *EMBO J* 1994;13:4002–4010.

193. Bottomly K, Luqman M, Greenbaum L, et al. A monoclonal antibody to murine CD45R distinguishes CD4 T cell populations that produce different cytokines. *Eur J Immunol* 1989;19:617–623.

194. Akbar AN, Terry L, Timms A, et al. Loss of CD45R and gain of UCHL1 reactivity is a feature of primed T cells. *J Immunol* 1988;140:2171–2178.

195. Novak TJ, Farber D, Leitenberg D, et al. Isoforms of the transmembrane tyrosine phosphatase CD45 differentially affect T cell recognition. *Immunity* 1994;1:109–119.

196. Desai DM, Sap J, Schlessinger J, et al. Ligand-mediated negative regulation of a chimeric transmembrane receptor tyrosine phosphatase. *Cell* 1993;73:541–554.

197. Majeti R, Xu Z, Parslow TG, et al. An inactivating point mutation in the inhibitory wedge of CD45 causes lymphoproliferation and autoimmunity. *Cell* 2000;103:1059–1070.

198. Hermiston ML, Xu Z, Majeti R, et al. Reciprocal regulation of lymphocyte activation by tyrosine kinases and phosphatases. *J Clin Invest* 2002;109:9–14.

199. Mustelin T, Coggeshall KM, Altman A. Rapid activation of the T-cell tyrosine protein kinase pp56^lck by the CD45 phosphotyrosine phosphatase. *Proc Natl Acad Sci U S A* 1989;86:6302–6306.

200. McFarland EDC, Hurley TR, Pingel JT, et al. Correlation between Src family member regulation by the protein-tyrosine-phosphatase CD45 and transmembrane signaling through the T-cell receptor. *Proc Natl Acad Sci U S A* 1993;90:1402–1406.

201. Sieh M, Bolen JB, Weiss A. CD45 specifically modulates binding of Lck to a phosphopeptide encompassing the negative regulatory tyrosine of Lck. *EMBO J* 1993;12:315–322.

202. Samelson LE. Signal transduction mediated by the T cell antigen receptor: the role of adapter proteins. *Annu Rev Immunol* 2002;20:371–394.

203. Zhang W, Samelson LE. The role of membrane-associated adaptors in T cell receptor signaling. *Sem Immunol* 2000;12:35–41.

204. Ku GM, Yablonsky D, Manser E, et al. A PAK1-PIX-PKL complex is activated by the T-cell receptor independent of Nck, Slp-76 and LAT. *EMBO J* 2002;20:457–465.

205. Myung PS, Boerthe NJ, Koretzky GA. Adapter proteins in lymphocyte antigen-receptor signaling. *Curr Opin Immunol* 2000;12:256–266.

206. Griffiths EK, Penninger JM. Communication between the TCR and integrins: role of the molecular adapter ADAP/Fyb/Slap. *Curr Opin Immunol* 2002;14:317–322.

207. Schaeffer EM, Schwartzberg PL. Tec family kinases in lymphocyte signaling and function: lymphocyte activation and effector functions. *Curr Opin Immunol* 2000;12:282–288.

208. Simons K, Ikonen E. Functional rafts in cell membranes. *Nature* 1997;387:569–572.

209. Brown DA, London E. Structure and function of sphingolipid- and cholesterol-rich membrane rafts. *J Biol Chem* 2000;275:17221–17224.

210. Bromley SK, Burack WR, Johnson KG, et al. The immunological synapse. *Annu Rev Immunol* 2001;19:375–396.

211. Monks CRF, Freiberg BA, Kupfer H, et al. Three-dimensional segregation of supramolecular activation clusters in T cells. *Nature* 395:82–86.

212. Grakoui A, Bromley SK, Sumen C, et al. The immunological synapse: a molecular machine controlling T cell activation. *Science* 1999;285:221–228.

213. Johnson KG, Bromley SK, Dustin ML, et al. A supramolecular basis for CD45 tyrosine phosphatase regulation in sustained T cell activation. *Proc Natl Acad Sci U S A* 2000;97:10138–10143.

214. Krummel MF, Sjaastad MD, Wilfing C, et al. Differential clustering of CD4 and CD3ζ during T cell recognition. *Science* 2000;289:1349–1352.

215. van der Merwe PA, Davis SJ, Shaw AS, et al. Cytoskeletal polarization and redistribution of cell-surface molecules during T cell antigen recognition. *Sem Immunol* 2000;12:5–21.

216. Dustin ML, Cooper JA. The immunological synapse and the actin cytoskeleton: molecular hardware for T cell signaling. *Nat Immunol* 2000;1:23–29.

217. Bustelo XR. Regulatory and signaling properties of the Vav famly. *Mol Cell Biol* 2000;20:1461–1477.
218. Wulfing C, Bauch A, Crabtree GR, et al. The vav exchange factor in actin-dependent receptor translocation to the lymphocyte-antigen–presenting cell interface. *Proc Natl Acad Sci U S A* 2000;97:10150–10155.
219. Krause M, Sechi AS, Konradt M, et al. Fyn-binding protein (Fyb)/SLP-76–associated protein (SLAP), Ena/vasodilator–stimulated phosphoprotein (VASP) proteins and the Arp2/3 complex link T cell receptor (TCR) signaling to the actin cytoskeleton. *J Cell Biol* 2000;149:181–194.
220. Cannon JL, Labno CM, Bosco G, et al. WASP recruitment to the T cell: APC contact site occurs independently of Cdc42 activation. *Immunity* 2001;15:249–259.
221. Wulfing C, Davis MM. A receptor/cytoskeletal movement triggered by costimulation during T cell activation. *Science* 1998;282:2266–2269.
222. Oettgen HC, Terhorst C, Cantley LC, et al. Stimulation of the T3-T cell receptor complex induces a membrane-potential–sensitive calcium influx. *Cell* 1985;40:583–590.
223. Rabinovitch PS, June CH, Grossman A, et al. Heterogeneity among T cells in intracellular free calcium responses after mitogen stimulation with PHA or anti-CD3, simultaneous use of indo-1 and immunofluorescence with flow cytometry. *J Immunol* 1986;137:952–961.
224. Manger B, Weiss A, Imboden J, et al. The role of protein kinase C in transmembrane signaling by the T cell receptor complex: effects of stimulation with soluble or immobilized T3 antibodies. *J Immunol* 1987;139:395–407.
225. Berridge MJ, Lipp P, Bootman ND. The calcium entry pas de deux. *Science* 2000;287:1604–1605.
226. Imboden JB, Stobo JD. Transmembrane signalling by the T cell antigen receptor: Perturbation of the T3-antigen receptor complex generates inositol phosphates and releases calcium ions from intracellular stores. *J Exp Med* 1985;161:446–456.
227. Goldsmith M, Weiss A. Early signal transduction by the antigen receptor without commitment to T cell activation. *Science* 1988;240:1029–1031.
228. Lewis RS. Calcium signaling mechanisms in T-lymphocytes. *Annu Rev Immunol* 2001;19:497–521.
229. Timmerman LA, Clipstone NA, Ho SN, et al. Rapid shuttling of NF-AT in discrimination of Ca^{2+} signals and immunosuppression. *Nature* 1996;383:837–840.
230. Putney JW, Bird GSJ. The signal for capacitative calcium entry. *Cell* 1993;75:199–201.
231. Majerus PW, Ross TS, Cunningham TW, et al. Recent insights in phosphatidylinositol signaling. *Cell* 1990;63:459–465.
232. Hermosura MC, Takeuchi H, Fleig A, et al. InsP4 facilitates store-operated calcium influx by inhibition of InsP3 5-phosphatase. *Nature* 2000;408:735–740.
233. Toker A, Cantley LC. Signaling through the lipid products of phosphatidylinositide-3-OH kinase. *Nature* 1997;387:673–676.
234. Ward SG, Westwick J, Hall ND, et al. Ligation of CD28 receptor by B7 induces formation of D-3 phosphoinositides in T-lymphocytes independently of T cell receptor/CD3 activation. *Eur J Immunol* 1993;23:2572–2577.
235. Ward SG, Reif K, Ley S, et al. Regulation of phosphoinositide kinases in T cells. *J Biol Chem* 1992;267:23862–23869.
236. Truitt KE, Mills GB, Turck CW, et al. SH2-dependent association of phosphatidylinositol 3′-kinase 85-kD regulatory subunit with the interleukin-2 receptor β chain. *J Biol Chem* 1994;269:5937–5943.
237. Hemmings BA. PH domains—a universal membrane adapter. *Science* 1997;275:1899.
238. Nishizuka Y. Protein kinase C and lipid signaling for sustained cellular responses. *FASEB J* 1995;9:484–496.
239. Genot EM, Parker PJ, Cantrell DA. Analysis of the role of protein kinase C-α, -ε, and -ζ in T cell activation. *J Biol Chem* 1995;270:9833–9839.
240. Cantrell D. T cell antigen receptor signal transduction pathways. *Annu Rev Immunol* 1996;14:259–274.
241. Koretzky GA, Wahi M, Newton ME, et al. Heterogeneity of protein kinase C isoenzyme gene expression in human T cell lines: Protein kinase C-β is not required for several T cell functions. *J Immunol* 1989;143:1692–1695.
242. Muramatsu M, Kaibuchi K, Arai K. A protein kinase C cDNA without

243. Isakov N, Altman A. Protein kinase Cθ in T cell activation. *Annu Rev Immunol* 2002;20:761–794.
244. Oancea E, Meyer T. Protein kinase C as a molecular machine for decoding calcium and diacylglycerol signals. *Cell* 1998;95:307–318.
245. Berry N, Ase K, Kishimoto A, et al. Activation of resting human T cells requires prolonged stimulation of protein kinase C. *Proc Natl Acad Sci U S A* 1990;87:2294–2298.
246. Schreiber SL, Crabtree GR. The mechanism of action of cyclosporin A and FK506. *Immunol Today* 1992;13:136–142.
247. Rao A, Luo C, Hogan PG. Transcription factors of the NFAT family: regulation and Function. *Annu Rev Immunol* 1997;15:707–747.
248. Stankunas K, Graef IA, Neilson JR, et al. Signaling through calcium, calcineurin, and NF-AT in lymphocyte activation and development. *Cold Spring Harb Symp Quant Biol* 1999;64:505–516.
249. Nghlem P, Ollick T, Gardner P, et al. Interleukin-2 transcriptional block by multifunctional Ca^{2+}/calmodulin kinase. *Nature* 1994;371:347–350.
250. Samelson LE, Harford JB, Klausner RD. Identification of the components of the murine T cell antigen receptor complex. *Cell* 1985;43:223–231.
251. Acres RB, Conlon PJ, Mochizuki DY, et al. Rapid phosphorylation and modulation of the T4 antigen on cloned helper T cells induced by phorbol myristate acetate or antigen. *J Biol Chem* 1986;261:16210–16214.
252. Shackelford DA, Trowbridge IS. Identification of lymphocyte integral membrane protein as substrates for protein kinase C. *J Biol Chem* 1986;261:8334–8341.
253. Genot E, Cantrell DA. Ras regulation and function in lymphcytes. *Curr Opin Immunol* 2000;12:289–294.
254. Schlessinger J. How receptor tyrosine kinases activate Ras. *Trends Biochem Sci* 1993;18:273–275.
255. Downward J, Graves JD, Warne PH, et al. Stimulation of p21^{ras} upon T-cell activation. *Nature* 1990;346:719–723.
256. Nemorin JG, Laporte P, Berube G, et al. p62dok negatively regulates CD2 signaling in Jurkat cells. *J Immunol* 2001;166:4408–4415.
257. Iwashima M, Takamatsu M, Yamagishi H, et al. Gentic evidence for Shc requirement in TCR-induced c-Rel nuclear translocation and IL-2 expression. *Proc Natl Acad Sci U S A* 2002;99:4544–4549.
258. McCormick F, Wittinghofer A. Interactions between Ras proteins and their effectors. *Curr Opin Biotechnol* 1996;7:449–456.
259. Rodriguez-Viciana P, Warne PH, et al. Role of phosphoinositide 3-OH kinase in cell transformation and control of the actin cytoskeleton by Ras. *Cell* 1997;89:457–67.
260. Nel AE, Hanekom C, Rheeder A, et al. Stimulation of map-2 kinase activity in T-lymphocytes by anti–CD3 or anti–Ti monoclonal antibody is partially dependent on protein kinase C. *J Immunol* 1990;144:2683–2689.
261. Rayter SI, Woodrow M, Lucas SC, et al. Downward J p21^{ras} mediates control of IL-2 gene promoter function in T cell activation. *EMBO J* 1992;11:4549–4556.
262. Woodrow MA, Rayter S, Downward J, et al. p21^{ras} function is important for T cell antigen receptor and protein kinase C regulation of nuclear factor of activated T cells. *J Immunol* 1993;150:3853–3861.
263. Owaki H, Varma R, Gillis B, et al. Raf-1 is required for T cell IL2 production. *EMBO J* 1993;12:4367–4373.
264. Dong C, Davis RJ, Flavell RA. MAP Kinases in the immune response. *Annu Rev Immunol* 2002;20:55–72.
265. Macian F, Lopez-Rodriguez C, Rao A. Partners in transcription: NFAT and AP-1. *Oncogene* 2001;20:2476–2489.
266. Grinstein S, Goetz-Smith JD, Stewart D, et al. Protein phosphorylation during activation of Na+/H2+ exchange by phorbol esters and by osmotic shrinking. *J Biol Chem* 1986;261:8009–8016.
267. Grinstein S, Goetz JD, Rothstein A. $^{22}Na^+$ fluxes in thymic lymphocytes: II. Amiloride sensitive Na+/H+ exchange pathway reversibility of transport and asymmetry of the modifier site. *J Gen Physiol* 1984;84:585–600.
268. Rosoff PM, Cantley LC. Stimulation of the T3-T cell receptor–associated Ca2+ influx enhances the activity of the Na+/H+ exchanger in a leukemic human T cell line. *J Biol Chem* 1985;260:14053–14059.
269. Wang T, Sheppard JR, Foker JE. The rise and fall of cAMP required for onset of lymphocyte DNA synthesis. *Science* 1978;201:155–157.

270. Ledbetter JA, Parsons M, Martin PJ, et al. Antibody binding to CD5 (Tp67) and Tp44 cell surface molecules: effects of cyclic nucleotides, cytoplasmic free calcium and cAMP-mediated suppression. *J Immunol* 1986;137:3299–3305.

271. Novogrodsky A, Patya M, Rubin AL, et al. Agents that increase cellular cAMP inhibit production of interleukin-2, but not its activity. *Biochem Biophys Res Commun* 1983;114:93–98.

272. Patel MD, Samelson LE, Klausner RD. Multiple kinases and signal transduction. *J Biol Chem* 1987;262:5831–5838.

273. Imboden JB, Shoback DM, Pattison G, et al. Cholera toxin inhibits the T-cell antigen receptor-mediated increases in inositol trisphosphate and cytoplasmic free calcium. *Proc Natl Acad Sci U S A* 1986;83:5673–5677.

274. Cook SJ, McCormick F. Inhibition of cAMP of Ras-dependent activation of raf. *Science* 1993;262:1069–1072.

275. Atkinson JP, Kelley JP, Weiss A, et al. Enhanced intracellular cGMP concentrations and lectin-induced lymphocyte transformation. *J Immunol* 1978;121:2282–2291.

276. DeCoursey TE, Chandy KG, Gupta S, et al. Voltage-gated K+ channel in human T-lymphocytes: a role in mitogenesis? *Nature* 1984;307:465–468.

277. Gray LS, Gnarra JR, Russell JH, et al. The role of K+ in the regulation of the increase in intracellular Ca²⁺ mediated by the T-lymphocyte antigen receptor. *Cell* 1987;50:119–127.

278. Chandy KG, DeCoursey TE, Cahalan MD, et al. Voltage-gated potassium channels are required for human T-lymphocyte activation. *J Exp Med* 1984;160:369–385.

279. Lin CS, Boltz RC, Blake JT, et al. Voltage-gated potassium channels regulate calcium-dependent pathways involved in human T-lymphocyte activation. *J Exp Med* 1993;177:637–645.

280. Morley SC, Bierer BE. The actin cytoskeleton, membrane lipid microdomains, and T cell signal transduction. *Adv Immunol* 2001;77:1–43.

281. Stowers L, Yelon D, Berg LJ, et al. Regulation of the polarization of T cells toward antigen-presenting cells by Ras-related GTPase CDC42. *Proc Natl Acad Sci U S A* 1995;92:5027–31.

282. Ley SC, Verbi W, Pappin DJC, et al. Tyrosine phosphorylation of a tubulin in human T-lymphocytes. *Eur J Immunol* 1994;24:99–106.

283. Kupfer A, Singer SJ, Dennert G. On the mechanism of unidirectional killing in mixtures of two cytotoxic lymphocytes. *J Exp Med* 1986;163:489–498.

284. Berke G. The binding and lysis of target cells by cytotoxic lymphocytes: molecular and cellular aspects. *Annu Rev Immunol* 1994;12:735–773.

285. Shaw J-P, Utz PJ, Durand DB, et al. Identification of a putative regulator or early T cell activation genes. *Science* 1988;241:202–205.

286. Grandori C, Cowley SM, James LP, et al. The Myc/Max/Mad network and the transcriptional control of cell behavior. *Annu Rev Cell Dev Biol* 2000;16:653–699.

287. Karin M, Liu Z, Zandi E. AP-1 function and regulation. *Curr Opin Cell Biol* 1997;9:240–246.

288. Reed JC, Alpers JD, Nowell PC, et al. Sequential expression of protooncogenes during lectin-stimulated mitogenesis of normal human lymphocytes. *Proc Natl Acad Sci U S A* 1986;83:3982–3986.

289. Ship MA, Reinherz E. Differential expression of nuclear protooncogenes in T cells triggered with mitogenic and nonmitogenic T3 and T11 activation signals. *J Immunol* 1987;139:2143–2148.

290. Grausz JD, Fradelizi D, Dautry F, et al. Modulation of c-fos and c-myc mRNA levels in normal human lymphocytes by calcium ionophore A23187 and phorbol ester. *Eur J Immunol* 1986;16:1217–1221.

291. Ullman KS, Northrup JP, Admon A, et al. Jun family members are controlled by a calcium-regulated, cyclosporin A–sensitive signaling pathway in activated T-lymphocytes. *Genes Dev* 1993;7:188–196.

292. Derijard B, Hibi M, Wu I-H, et al. JNK1: A protein kinase stimulated by UV light and Ha-Ras that binds and phosphorylates the c-Jun activation domain. *Cell* 1994;76:1025–1037.

293. Deng T, Karin M. c-Fos transcriptional activity stimulated by H-Ras–activated protein kinase distinct from JNK and ERK. *Nature* 1994;371:171–175.

294. Ho JC, Glimcher LH. Transcription: tantalizing times for T cells. *Cell* 2002;109:S109–S120.

295. Durand DB, Shaw J-P, Bush MR, et al. Characterization of antigen receptor response elements within the interleukin-2 enhancer. *Mol Cell Biol* 1988;8:1715–1724.

296. Serfling E, Avots A, Neumann M. The architecture of the interleukin-2 promoter: a reflection of T-lymphocyte activation. *Biochim Biophys Acta* 1995;1263:181–200.

297. Jain J, Valge-Archer VE, Sinskey AJ, et al. The AP-1 site at −150 bp, but not the NF-κB site, is likely to represent the major target of protein kinase C in the interleukin 2 promoter. *J Immunol* 1992;175:853–862.

298. Jain J, Valge-Archer VE, Rao A. Analysis of the AP-1 sites in the IL-2 promoter. *J Immunol* 1992;148:1240–1250.

299. Kang S-M, Beverly B, Tran A-C, et al. Transactivation by AP-1 is a molecular target of T cell clonal anergy. *Science* 1992;257:1134–1138.

300. Li W, Whaley CD, Mondino A, et al. Blocked signal transduction to the ERK and JNK protein kinases in anergic CD4+ T cells. *Science* 1996;271:1272–1276.

301. Fields PE, Gajewski TF, Fitch FW. Blocked Ras activation in anergic CD4+ T cells. *Science* 1996;271:1276.

302. Zhu J, McKeon F. NF-AT activation requires suppression of Crm1-dependent export by calcineurin. *Nature* 1999;398:256–260.

303. Kane LP, Andres PG, Howland KC, et al. Akt provides the CD28 costimulatory signal for up-regulation of IL-2 and IFN-gamma but not TH2 cytokines. *Nat Immunol* 2001;2:37–44.

304. Lai J-H, Horvath G, Subleski J, et al. RelA is a potent transcriptional activator of the CD28 response element within the interleukin 2 promoter. *Mol Cell Biol* 1995;15:4260–4271.

305. Ghosh P, Tan T-H, Rice NR, et al. The interleukin 2 CD28-responsive complex contains at least three members of the NFκB family: c-Rel, p50, and p65. *Proc Natl Acad Sci U S A* 1993;90:1696–1700.

306. Shapiro VS, Truitt KE, Imboden JB, et al. CD28 mediates transcriptional upregulation of the Interleukin-2 (IL-2) promoter through a composite element containing the CD28RE and NF-IL-2B AP-1 sites. *Mol Cell Biol* 1997;17:4051–4058.

307. McGuire KL, Iacobelli M. Involvement of Rel, Fos, and Jun proteins in binding activity to the IL-2 promoter CD28 response element/AP-1 sequence in human T cells. *J Immunol* 1997;159:1319–27.

308. Kontgen F, Grumont RJ, Strasser A, et al. Mice lacking the c-rel protooncogene exhibit defects in lymphocyte proliferation, humoral immunity, and interleukin-2 expression. *Genes Dev* 1995;9:1965–1977.

309. Chen CY, Del Gatto-Konczak F, Wu Z, et al. Stabilization of Interleukin-2 mRNA by the c-Jun NH2-terminal kinase pathway. *Science* 1998;280:1945–1949.

310. Jacobsen M, Schweer D, Ziegler A, et al. A point mutation in PTPRC is associated with the development of multiple sclerosis. *Nat Genet* 2000;26:495–499.

311. Lynch KW, Weiss A. A CD45 polymorphism associated with multiple sclerosis disrupts an exonic splicing silencer. *J Biol Chem* 2001;276:24341–24347.

312. Waldmann TA. The IL-2/IL-2 receptor system: a target for rational immune intervention. *Immunol Today* 1993;14:264–270.

313. Bohnlein E, Lowenthal JW, Siekevitz M, et al. The same inducible nuclear proteins regulates mitogen activation of both the interleukin-2 receptor–alpha gene and type 1 HIV. *Cell* 1988;53:827–836.

314. Shevach EM, McHugh RS, Piccirillo CA, et al. Control of T-cell activation by CD4+ CD25+ suppressor T cells. *Immunol Rev* 2001;182:58–67.

315. Marengere LEM, Waterhouse P, Duncan GS, et al. Regulation of T cell receptor signaling by tyrosine phosphatase SYP association with CTLA-4. *Science* 1996;272:1170–1173.

316. Waterhouse P, Penninger JM, Timms E, et al. Lymphoproliferative disorders with early lethality in mice deficient in Ctla-4. *Science* 1995;270:985–988.

317. Sosinowski T, Killeen N, Weiss A. The Src-like adaptor protein downregulates the T cell receptor on CD4+CD8+ thymocytes and regulates positive selection. *Immunity* 2001;15:457–466.

318. Shaw G, Kamen R. A conserved AU sequence from the 3′ untranslated region of GM–CSF mRNA mediates selective mRNA degradation. *Cell* 1986;46:659–667.

319. Latinis KM, Carr LL, Peterson EJ, et al. Regulation of CD95 (Fas) ligand expression by TCR-mediated signaling events. *J Immunol* 1997;158:4602–4611.

320. Fisher GH, Rosenberg FJ, Straus SE, et al. Dominant interfering Fas gene mutations impair apoptosis in a human autoimmune lymphoproliferative syndrome. *Cell* 1995;81:91.

321. Nagata S, Golstein P. The Fas death factor. *Science* 1995;267:1449–1456.

322. Wilde DB, Fitch FW. Antigen-reactive cloned helper T cells. I. Unresponsiveness to antigenic restimulation develops after stimulation of cloned helper T cells. *J Immunol* 1984;132:1632–1638.

323. Williams ME, Shea CM, Lichtman AH, et al. Antigen receptor-mediated anergy in resting T-lymphocytes and T cell clones: correlation with lymphokine secretion patterns. *J Immunol* 1992;149:1921–1926.

324. Nau GJ, Moldwin RL, Lancki DW, et al. Inhibition of IL 2–driven proliferation of murine T-lymphocyte clones by supraoptimal levels of immobilized anti–T cell receptor monoclonal antibody. *J Immunol* 1987;139:114–122.

325. Jenkins MK, Schwartz RH. Antigen presentation by chemically modified splenocytes induces antigen-specific T cell unresponsiveness *in vitro* and *in vivo*. *J Exp Med* 1987;165:302–319.

326. Quill H, Schwartz RH. Stimulation of normal inducer T cell clones with antigen presented by purified Ia molecules in planar lipid membranes: specific induction of a long-lived state of proliferative nonresponsiveness. *J Immunol* 1987;138:3704–3712.

327. Boussiotis VA, Freeman GJ, Berezovskaya A, et al. Maintenance of human T cell anergy: blocking of IL-2 gene transcription by activated Rap1. *Science* 1997;278:124–128.

CHAPTER 12

Natural Killer Cells

David H. Raulet

Overview
Discovery · Phenotype and Distribution
Target Cell Recognition by Natural Killer Cells
General Properties of Natural Killer Cell Receptors · The Missing Self Hypothesis · Major Histocompatibility Complex–Specific Inhibitory and Stimulatory Receptors · Stimulatory Receptors Specific for Non–Major Histocompatibility Complex Ligands · Integration of Stimulatory and Inhibitory Signaling
Natural Killer Cell Development and Differentiation
Natural Killer Cell Differentiation · Formation of the Repertoire and Self-Tolerance of Natural Killer Cells
Role of Natural Killer Cells in Disease and Pertinent Effector Functions
Natural Killer Cell Effector Functions · Viral Infections · Intracellular Microbes · Cancer
Natural Killer Cell Activation
Role of Natural Killer Cells in Mouse Cytomegalovirus Infection
Conclusion and Perspective
Acknowledgments
References

OVERVIEW

Discovery

Around 1970, it was first recognized that lymphocytes consist of several specialized cell types that are similar in appearance. These discoveries depended on a combination of approaches, including newly developed functional assays, mutant animals deficient in T cells, and antisera that stained specific lymphocyte subsets. It became clear that antibody-producing cells could be discriminated from thymus-derived cells. The latter cells were divisible into T-helper cells and cytotoxic T cells (CTLs). CTLs were generally specific for the cells that elicited the response, a characteristic of the adaptive immune response. Later, it became clear that CTLs recognize antigens in a major histocompatibility complex (MHC)–restricted manner.

Shortly after the discovery of B and T cells, a second set of cytotoxic lymphocytes was discovered in rodents that differed in several key ways from CTLs (1–3). These cells, called *natural killer* (NK) cells, lacked several cell surface markers of CTLs and other T cells. Whereas active CTLs typically arise only several days after immunization with foreign cells, pathogens, or tumor cells, NK cells were active even after isolation from unimmunized animals. Furthermore, NK cells lysed many different tumor cell lines. CTLs, in contrast,

are generally quite specific for a particular type of cell or pathogen. Because the newly discovered cytotoxic cells did not require specific immunization, they were termed "natural killer cells."

It has since become evident that NK cells represent a third class of lymphocytes distinct from B and T cells. The most striking distinction is that NK cells do not express a clonally distributed antigen receptor that is subject to somatic diversification. One clear indication of this is that NK cells do not rearrange B and T cell receptor genes (4), and, unlike B and T cells, arise normally in animals with deficiencies in genes that encode the V(D)J recombinase (5). As discussed in detail later, NK cells are now known to employ several types of stimulatory receptors specific for molecules associated with infected, transformed, or stressed cells. NK cells are also regulated by inhibitory receptors specific for class I MHC molecules. The distinctive specificity of the cells, along with their fast response and lack of a memory stage, is the basis for considering the cells part of the innate (as opposed to adaptive) immune system.

NK cells play several roles in immune responses. Once activated, NK cells are potent cytotoxic cells capable of lysing certain tumor cell lines, cells infected with various intracellular pathogens, and antibody-coated cells. Activated NK cells also produce cytokines, notably the inflammatory cytokines interferon-γ (IFN-γ) and tumor necrosis factor-α (TNF-α). These cytokines can directly induce antipathogen activity by macrophages and neutrophils and can also help to regulate the adaptive immune response to an antigen.

NK cells play a particularly important role in limiting the expansion of certain intracellular pathogens early in the infectious cycle, at a time when specific immunity has not yet fully developed. A role in attacking tumor cells is also suggested by *in vitro* and *in vivo* studies. Furthermore, NK cells can attack foreign cells, especially lymphohematopoietic cells such as bone marrow cells, and therefore can exert a barrier to bone marrow transplantation.

Phenotype and Distribution

Morphologically, many NK cells are large granular lymphocytes (LGLs). This structure is not a defining property of NK cells, however, because some NK cells are small and lack granules, and some other cells, such as CD8$^+$ T cells, can exhibit the LGL structure.

A list of markers expressed by NK cells is presented in Table 1. No single cell surface molecule is known to be obligatory for the function of NK cells, as is the case for T cells (the T-cell antigen receptor) or B cells (the B-cell antigen receptor). Indeed, although NK cells express distinctive cell surface markers, most are also expressed by some other cell type, usually one or another subset of T cells. For example,

CD56 is a good marker for NK cells in humans, but it is also expressed by a subset of T cells. Consequently, NK cells in humans are usually defined as cells that express CD56 but not the T-cell antigen receptor/CD3 complex (CD56$^+$CD3$^-$). Similarly, the NK1.1 and DX5 markers are widely used to identify NK cells in mice, but each is also expressed by a small percentage of T cells. Therefore, mouse NK cells are often defined as NK1.1$^+$CD3$^-$ or DX5$^+$CD3$^-$ cells. Studies demonstrate that essentially all NK cells are included in these phenotypically defined populations. It is less clear whether every cell defined in this way is an NK cell, although studies suggest that most are. In mice, NK cells also express cell surface asialoGM1, but many asialoGM1$^+$ cells are not NK cells. Nevertheless, injection of antibodies specific for asialoGM1 is often useful experimentally to deplete NK cells from mice.

NK cells are typically a minority population among lymphoid cell populations, constituting approximately 5% to 10% of peripheral blood lymphocytes in healthy humans and 3% of splenocytes in nonimmune mice. Similarly small percentages of NK cells are found among liver lymphocytes, bone marrow cells, and peritoneal lymphocytes. Even fewer NK cells are found in lymph nodes or other secondary lymphoid tissue, reflecting the absence of lymph node homing receptors on most of these cells. Although NK cells are less abundant overall than B and T cells, only a tiny fraction of B and T cells are specific for a given immunogen in a primary immune response. In contrast, most inductive stimuli

TABLE 1. *Cell surface markers of natural killer (NK) cells*

Marker	Molecule/function	Distribution
Relatively NK specific		
NK1.1	NKR-P1	~All NK cells, some T cells
DX5 (in rodents)	CD49b	~All NK cells, some T cells
CD16	Fc receptor	Most NK cells, some T cells
CD94 (KLRD1)	Pairs with NKG2A/C/E	~All NK cells (different levels), some T cells
NKG2A (KLRC1)	Inhibitory receptor	Subset of NK cells, some T cells
Ly49 (KLRA) (in rodents)	Inhibitory/stimulatory receptors	NK cells subsets, some T cells
KIR (in humans)	Inhibitory/stimulatory receptors	NK cells subsets, some T cells
NKp46	Stimulatory receptor	All NK cells (different levels)
NKp30	Stimulatory receptor	All NK cells (different levels)
NKp44	Stimulatory receptor	All NK cells (different levels)
Other		
NKG2D	Stimulatory/costimulatory receptor	~All NK cells, activated CD8$^+$ T cells, activated macrophages
CD2	Immune modulation	All NK cells, all T cells
CD5	Immune modulation	All NK cells, all T cells
CD11a	LFA-1α	NK and T cells, granulocytes, macrophages
CD11b	Mac-1α	NK cells, granulocytes, macrophages
CD11c	p150α	NK, T, and B cells; granulocytes; macrophages
CD18	β2 integrin	All leukocytes
CD45	B220	All leukocytes
CD56 (in humans)		NK cells, some T cells
CD57 (in humans)		NK cells, some T cells
2B4		All NK cells, some T cells
KLRG1 (MAFA)		NK subset, some T cells, possibly mast cells
gp49		NK cells, mast cells
IL-2/IL-15Rβ	Component of IL-2/IL15 receptor	NK cells, T cells

Fc, crystallizable fragment; IL, interleukin; LFA, leukocyte function–associated antigen; Mac, macrophage.

for NK cells activate a large fraction of the population. Therefore, most or all NK cells can be rapidly mobilized against a given challenge. After infection or the provision of certain NK cell stimuli, the percentage of NK cells may increase in an affected tissue or at the site of infection.

TARGET CELL RECOGNITION BY NATURAL KILLER CELLS

General Properties of Natural Killer Cell Receptors

Even clonal populations of NK cells lyse a wide variety of tumor cell lines. Molecules involved in target cell recognition by NK cells were sought for many years without success, in part because researchers expected the cells to express a unique type of stimulatory receptor akin to the T- and B-cell antigen receptors. However, it turned out that individual NK cells employ multiple stimulatory and inhibitory receptors. Since the early 1990s, a rapidly growing number of such receptors has been identified, and the number continues to grow. The receptors generally interact with counterreceptors (ligands) on the surface of other cells.

Because NK cells typically lyse tumor cells that vary in the class I MHC alleles that they express, or even lack class I MHC expression, they are often termed *MHC-unrestricted* to contrast their specificity with that of T cells. This label is misleading in the sense that it suggests the absence of MHC specificity. In fact, the first target cell–specific receptors to be identified on NK cells were specific for class I MHC molecules. Unlike the B- and T-cell receptors, however, many of the MHC-specific receptors expressed by NK cells are inhibitory in function. This accounts for a cardinal feature of NK cell recognition: the enhanced lysis of cells lacking class I MHC molecules (Fig. 1; see the later section on the missing self hypothesis).

Each of the inhibitory receptors is typically expressed by only a subset of NK cells, overlapping with subsets expressing other inhibitory MHC-specific receptors. The inhibitory receptors all contain one or more copies of a characteristic amino acid sequence motif in their cytoplasmic domains, called an *immunoreceptor tyrosine-based inhibitory motif* (ITIM), with the consensus sequence V/IxYxxL/V (Fig. 2) (6,7). Receptor engagement results in phosphorylation of the tyrosine residue in the ITIM, leading to the recruitment and activation of the protein tyrosine phosphatase SHP-1 (8). As discussed in more detail later, the activated phosphatase inhibits NK cell activation. Although the early discovery of inhibitory NK-specific receptors led to the notion that NK cell specificity is controlled primarily by inhibitory recognition, the discovery of several stimulatory receptors has revealed that stimulatory recognition plays an equally important role in that control. The balance of stimulatory and inhibitory recognition determines whether an NK cell will attack a given target cell (Fig. 1).

Stimulatory NK receptors lack an ITIM in their cytoplasmic domains and typically contain a basic amino acid

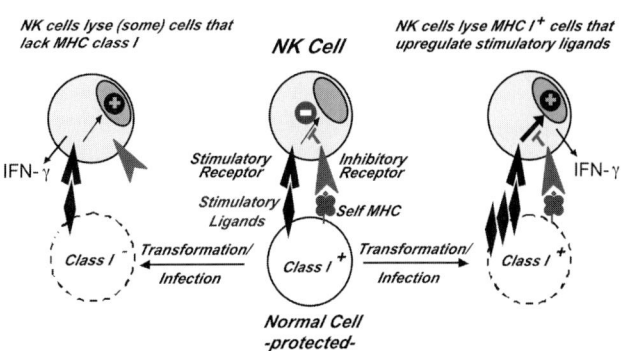

FIG. 1. Natural killer (NK) cells are regulated by the balance of signaling through stimulatory and inhibitory receptors. Each NK cell expresses inhibitory receptors specific for class I major histocompatibility complex (MHC) molecules and several types of stimulatory receptors specific for various ligands. Most normal cells express high levels of class I MHC molecules, which provide a strong inhibitory signal to the NK cell. Although some normal cell types (such as cells in the bone marrow) are believed to express ligands that stimulate NK cells, the inhibitory signal overrides stimulation, preventing NK cell activation. Infection or tumorigenesis of normal cells often leads to loss of class I MHC proteins (**left**) and/or up-regulation of ligands that stimulate NK cells (**right**). Either of these events may swing the balance of signaling in favor of NK cell activation, and both together have an even greater effect. The activated NK cells can secrete cytokines such as IFN-γ and lyse the susceptible target cell (indicated by disrupted membrane).

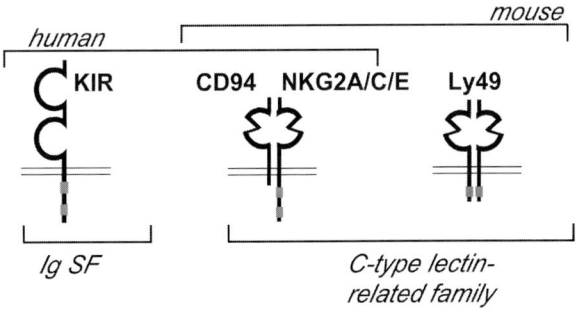

FIG. 2. Three types of class I major histocompatibility complex (MHC)–specific inhibitory receptors expressed by NK cells. The inhibitory receptors are divided into two structural classes: immunoglobulin superfamily [killer cell immunoglobulin-like receptor (KIR)] and lectin-like (Ly49 and CD94/NKG2A). Of the three receptor families, only CD94/NKG2A is clearly conserved in both mice and humans. KIR have not been well characterized in mice, and functional Ly49 receptors have not been found in humans. All three types of receptors impart inhibitory activity by virtue of immunoreceptor tyrosine-based inhibitory motifs (ITIM) located in their cytoplasmic tails, with the consensus sequence (I/V)xYxx(L/V).

residue within their transmembrane domains (9). T- and B-cell antigen receptors also contain charged amino acids in their transmembrane domains, which enable associations with other transmembrane proteins such as CD3 proteins or immunoglobulin (Ig) α and Igβ, which are responsible for transmitting the stimulatory signal. Most of the known stimulatory NK receptors associate with the signaling molecule variously called KARAP or DAP12, although others interact with FcεR1γ, CD3ζ, or KAP/DAP10 (Fig. 3) (9). These signaling molecules are transmembrane proteins with short extracellular domains and relatively long cytoplasmic domains that usually contain *immunoreceptor tyrosine-based activation motifs* (ITAMs). Engagement of the stimulatory receptor leads to tyrosine phosphorylation of the ITAMs on the associated signaling molecule and to the recruitment and activation of protein tyrosine kinases such as Syk (10).

The stimulatory receptors can be broadly divided by specificity into a group that recognizes class I MHC ligands and a group that does not. The non–MHC-specific receptors, which are not fully characterized, include some receptors that recognize cell surface ligands that are expressed poorly or not at all by normal cells but are up-regulated in transformed or infected cells. These receptors, some of which are expressed by all NK cells, are probably important for stimulating lysis of most tumor cells by NK cells (9,11). The stimulatory MHC-specific receptors, in contrast, are expressed by overlapping

subsets of NK cells (12). The existence of stimulatory MHC-specific receptors expressed by NK cells was not initially anticipated, inasmuch as they might be expected to negate the function of the MHC-specific inhibitory receptors. Some ideas as to the function of stimulatory MHC-specific NK cell receptors are discussed in a later section (Possible Functions of Stimulatory Major Histocompatibility Complex—Specific Natural Killer Cell Receptors).

Structurally, NK receptors can also be divided into two main groups, although each of these groups includes MHC-specific and non–MHC-specific members (Figs. 2 and 3). One group consists of dimeric type II transmembrane proteins similar in structure to C-type lectins (13), whereas the other group consists of type I transmembrane receptors of the immunoglobulin superfamily (IgSF) (6,14). The lectin-like receptors are encoded within the so-called NK cell gene complex (NKC) on human chromosome 12 and mouse chromosome 6 (Fig. 4). The NKC includes many other genes encoding lectinlike proteins that are involved in recognition by NK cells and other lymphocytes (13). Interestingly, several genes that influence disease susceptibility map in or near the NKC. In one case, a gene that controls susceptibility of mice to cytomegalovirus infection has been identified as one that encodes a specific NK receptor (Ly49H; see section on possible functions of stimulatory MHC-specific NK receptors). The immunoglobulin-like NK receptors are also encoded in a larger cluster of related genes: in this case, the leukocyte receptor complex (LRC), on human chromosome 19 and mouse chromosome 7 (Fig. 4) (15). The LRC includes a variety of other receptor genes expressed in immune cells that encode IgSF members.

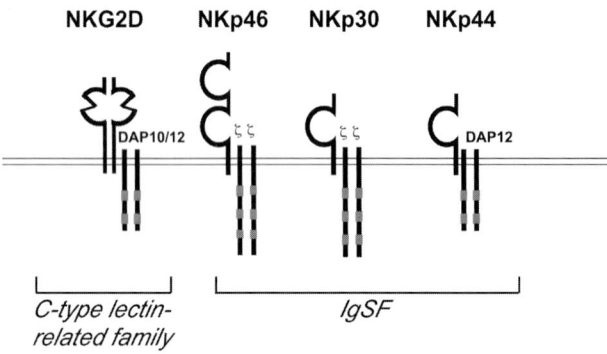

FIG. 3. Some of the stimulatory receptors employed by natural killer (NK) cells to recognize target cells. The four receptors shown participate in natural killing of tumor target cells. NKG2D is a lectin-like receptor, whereas the other three are immunoglobulin superfamily members. In mice and humans, NKG2D recognizes ligands that are induced in "distressed" cells (transformed, infected, or stressed). NKp46, NKp30, and NKp44 have been studied primarily in human NK cells, in which antibodies that block the receptors were shown to prevent lysis of various tumor target cell lines. The cellular ligands for NKp46, NKp30, and NKp44 have not been characterized. All four receptors provide stimulatory signals through noncovalent interactions with signaling adapter molecules such as DAP12, DAP10, and CD3ζ. These adapter proteins contain immunoreceptor tyrosine-based activation motifs (ITAMs) or other stimulatory sequences in their cytoplasmic domains.

The NK gene complex (NKC)-mouse and human

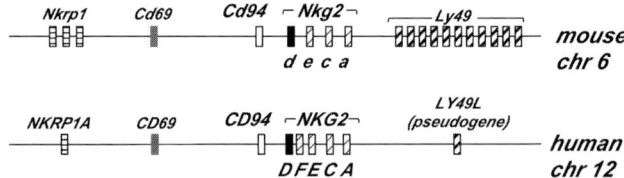

The human leukocyte receptor gene complex (LRC)

FIG. 4. Gene complexes encoding families of natural killer (NK) receptors. The NK cell gene complexes (NKCs) of mice and humans encode lectin-like inhibitory and stimulatory receptors expressed by NK cells and other leukocytes. The human leukocyte receptor complex (LRC) encodes immunoglobulin superfamily–type receptors expressed by NK cells and other leukocytes. The murine LRC is not well characterized. For simplicity, only some of the genes in each complex are depicted. The numbers of genes in each family are approximate and may vary in different strains or individuals.

The features of inhibitory and stimulatory recognition are described in the following section, beginning first with the early studies leading to the discovery of inhibitory recognition.

The Missing Self Hypothesis

The first real breakthrough in understanding NK cell recognition came from studies of the role of MHC molecules expressed by target cells. Mutations in tumor cell lines that reduced the expression of class I MHC molecules resulted in a greater sensitivity of the cells to attack by NK cells (16,17). The same mutations decreased the sensitivity of the tumor cells to cytotoxic T cells, which suggests that the principles of recognition by NK cells and CTLs are opposite in nature. Loss of class I MHC molecules occurs frequently in advanced tumors and in cells infected by viruses from several families (18,19). It was proposed that NK cells may help to counter this form of CTL evasion by specifically attacking cells that down-regulate class I MHC molecules (20).

Much earlier, studies of bone marrow transplantation had led to an unexpected discovery that could now be interpreted in a different light. The experiments showed that bone marrow grafts from an inbred mouse strain (call it strain A) were often rejected by a hybrid between strain A and a second strain, B, that expressed different MHC alleles (Table 2) (21,22). The hybrid mice are denoted $(A \times B)F_1$. The relevant genetic differences were mapped to the MHC. This pattern of rejection, "hybrid resistance," violated the accepted laws of transplantation. These "laws" were based on the fact that grafts of skin or various organs from strain A (or strain B) were uniformly accepted by $(A \times B)F_1$ mice. The hybrid was expected to express all the MHC molecules and other antigens of both parents, and therefore its T cells should have been immunologically tolerant of strain A cells. It later became clear that hybrid resistance is mediated by NK cells and not by T cells (23).

Although the recipients are often irradiated with gamma rays or x-rays before bone marrow transplantation, the NK cells can survive and function for several days, sufficient time to cause bone marrow graft rejection. Possible reasons why this form of rejection is limited primarily to bone marrow grafts are discussed in the later section on class I down-regulation and sensitivity of cells to NK cells.

The discoverers of hybrid resistance assumed that NK cells must be stimulated by recessively expressed foreign antigens present on bone marrow cells of the A strain but not on cells from the $(A \times B)F_1$ hybrid mice. Although the genes that cause hybrid resistance were known to be MHC-linked, class I and class II MHC molecules were not initially considered probable target antigens because they are expressed in a codominant manner and should therefore be found on cells from both types of mice.

The realization that recognition of class I MHC molecules could underlie hybrid resistance emerged when investigators contemplated the results of the tumor cell experiments just discussed. Those studies had shown that NK cells preferentially attack cells lacking class I MHC molecules, but a refined notion would be that NK cells attack cells lacking *self* class I MHC proteins. This would provide an explanation for why NK cells in $(A \times B)F_1$ mice attack strain A bone marrow cells. These bone marrow cells lack at least some of the class I molecules of the $(A \times B)F_1$ host. In this hypothesis, the relevant target molecules are self class I MHC proteins, but it is their *absence* from the target cell that provokes NK cells to attack. Consequently, the model is called the "missing self hypothesis" (20).

The missing self hypothesis received strong support from two types of experiments, both summarized in Table 2. In one, a transgene encoding a specific MHC molecule, D^d, was inserted into $H-2^b$ mice. "D" refers to the product of a specific class I gene (D), and the superscript "d" refers to the allelic form of that gene. H-2 is the mouse MHC, and the superscript

TABLE 2. *Genetics of bone marrow cell rejection mediated by natural killer cells*

Irradiated host[a]		Bone marrow graft donor[a]		
Strain	H-2 genotype	Strain	H-2 genotype	Outcome[b]
B6	$H-2^{b/b}$	B6	$H-2^{b/b}$	Accept
$(B6 \times B6-H-2^d)F_1$	$H-2^{b/d}$	B6	$H-2^{b/b}$	Reject
$(B6 \times B6-H-2^d)F_1$	$H-2^{b/d}$	$(B6 \times B6-H-2^d)F_1$	$H-2^{b/d}$	Accept
B6-(D^d transgenic)	$H-2^{b/b} + D^d$	B6	$H-2^{b/b}$	Reject
B6-(D^d transgenic)	$H-2^{b/b} + D^d$	B6-(D^d transgenic)	$H-2^{b/b} + D^d$	Accept
B6	$H-2^{b/b}$	$B6-\beta_2m^{-/-}$	No class I MHC	Reject
$B6-\beta_2m^{-/-}$	No class I MHC	$B6-\beta_2m^{-/-}$	No class I MHC	Accept

MHC, major histocompatibility complex.

[a]B6 refers to C57BL/6, an inbred $H-2^{b/b}$ mouse strain. $B6-H-2^d$ is a congenic strain that is identical to B6 except that it contains the segment of chromosome containing the $H-2^d$ MHC. D^d is a specific class I molecule encoded within the $H-2^d$ MHC; the D^d transgene was incorporated into B6 mice and is expressed by the same cells that normally express class Ia MHC genes. $B6-\beta_2m^{-/-}$ mice are B6 mice in which the gene for β_2-microglobulin is mutated by gene targeting; in the absence of β_2-microglobulin, class I proteins are not expressed at the cell surface.

[b]In all instances of bone marrow graft rejection in the table, natural killer cells are responsible for the rejection.

(*b* in this case) refers to a collection of specific alleles of all the various MHC genes. Thus, nontransgenic H-2^b mice express D^b but not D^d, whereas the transgenic mice express both molecules. Because D^d is expressed in the transgenic mice from the time of conception, it can be considered a self class I MHC protein. Confirming predictions arising from the hypothesis, the transgenic mice rejected bone marrow grafts from nontransgenic H-2^b mice, which lacked D^d but were otherwise identical to the transgenic mice (24). Thus, the specific absence of a single self class I gene is sufficient to render bone marrow cells susceptible to NK cells. In the second type of experiment, researchers examined bone marrow cells from mice that were genetically engineered to lack all class I MHC proteins. These cells were strongly rejected by otherwise identical but class I$^+$ mice (25). Both of these experiments demonstrated that absence of class I MHC proteins, especially self class I MHC molecules, is sufficient to render bone marrow cells sensitive to rejection by NK cells. Similar results were obtained in studies in which mitogen-activated T or B cells (lymphoblasts) from mice were used as target cells for NK cells *in vitro:* NK cells from wild-type mice could lyse target cells from class I–deficient mice (26), and NK cells from the D^d transgenic mice could lyse target cells from nontransgenic mice (27).

Two molecular mechanisms were initially proposed to account for missing self recognition (20). According to one model, NK cells express *stimulatory* receptors for *non-MHC* target molecules expressed by all normal cells. Class I MHC molecules expressed by the same target cell can associate with these target molecules, interfering with recognition of the target molecule by the NK cells. According to the second model (Fig. 1), NK cells express *inhibitory* receptors specific for *self class I MHC* molecules. Self class I MHC molecules on normal cells therefore inhibit NK cells, preventing cytotoxicity. The latter model was proved correct by the identification and characterization of three families of inhibitory class I MHC–specific receptors expressed by NK cells, as described in the following section.

Major Histocompatibility Complex–Specific Inhibitory and Stimulatory Receptors

The three major families of NK cell receptors specific for class I MHC proteins are designated KIR (killer cell immunoglobulin-like receptors), Ly49 receptors, and CD94/NKG2 receptors (Fig. 2). Each family is composed of several related isoforms. As their name implies, KIR are members of the immunoglobulin superfamily, whereas Ly49 and CD94/NKG2 receptors are structurally similar to C-type lectins. Ly49 genes were initially identified in mice (13). Although Ly49 genes may be functionally expressed in many species, including some primates (28), the human genome reportedly contains only a single nonfunctional Ly49 pseudogene (Fig. 4) (15). Conversely, KIR were discovered in humans and are found in various primates but have not been well studied in mice and other rodents (29). Despite their

dissimilar structures, KIR and Ly49 proteins function very similarly in NK cell recognition. CD94/NKG2 receptors are the only MHC-specific receptors that are known to be functionally expressed in both humans and rodents and presumably in most other animal species. Unlike KIR and Ly49 receptors, CD94/NKG2 receptors recognize classical class I MHC molecules in an indirect manner, as discussed later.

All three of these gene families were initially discovered as a result of the inhibitory function of some family members, each of which contain ITIMs in their cytoplasmic domains. Unexpectedly, each family also contains stimulatory isoforms, which are characterized by the presence of a charged amino acid residue in the transmembrane domain that enables the receptor to associate with the KARAP/DAP12 signaling molecule. Like the inhibitory isoforms, many if not all of the stimulatory isoforms recognize class I MHC molecules.

Ly49 Receptors

The first molecularly defined inhibitory receptors to be implicated in MHC recognition were the Ly49 family of proteins in mice. Ly49 proteins are homodimeric type II transmembrane proteins that are structurally similar to C-type lectins (Fig. 2). The fact that Ly49 receptors inhibit NK cells upon binding class I MHC molecules was demonstrated by exploiting monoclonal antibodies specific for one family member, Ly49A. Typical of inhibitory MHC-specific receptors, Ly49A is expressed by a subset of NK cells. It was shown that the sensitivity of a tumor cell line to lysis by purified Ly49A$^+$ NK cells depends on the allelic form of class I MHC molecules expressed by the tumor cells. The Ly49A$^+$ NK cells killed tumor cells from H-2^b mice but did not kill tumor cells from H-2^d mice (30). To test whether H-2^d class I MHC molecules were preventing cell lysis, susceptible H-2^b tumor cells were separately transfected with each of the three classical class I MHC molecules expressed in H-2^d mice (K^d, D^d, and L^d). Transfection with D^d protected the cells from Ly49A$^+$ NK cells, whereas K^d or L^d had no effect. The protection was prevented by adding antibodies specific for either D^d on the target cell or Ly49A on the NK cells. The results suggested that Ly49A is an inhibitory receptor that binds D^d. It was later confirmed that Ly49A binds D^d as well as some other class Ia MHC molecules.

Subsequent studies have identified MHC specificities for several other Ly49 receptors (31,32). These receptors interact with classical class I (also called class Ia) MHC molecules. Individual receptors typically bind to some class Ia allelic isoforms but not others, which accounts for the capacity of NK cells to differentiate between cells that express different MHC alleles. Binding of Ly49 receptors to class I MHC molecules is not highly specific for the peptide bound in the class I groove. Some interactions, such as Ly49A with D^d, occur with essentially any bound peptide (33). In other cases, such as Ly49I with K^d or Ly49C with K^b, the binding occurs with some bound peptides but not with others

(32,34). However, it appears that even in these cases, a relatively large number of peptides that are capable of binding to the class I molecule are compatible with receptor binding. This binding behavior contrasts markedly with T-cell antigen receptors, which are generally highly specific for the bound peptide.

Although C-type lectins bind carbohydrates, the structurally related Ly49 receptors bind quite well to unglycosylated class I MHC molecules (32,35). It remains possible that glycans linked to class I MHC molecules enhance the binding affinity. Ly49A binds to unglycosylated D^d molecules with a dissociation constant (K_D) of approximately 1 to 2×10^{-5} Molar (M) (36). Crystal structure analysis revealed two distinct Ly49A–D^d interfaces (37). One interface is at one end of the peptide-binding groove of D^d, near but not in contact with the N-terminus of the bound peptide. The other interface is in a cavity beneath the peptide-binding platform and involves contacts with all four domains of the class I MHC molecule (α_1, α_2, α_3, and β_2 microglobulin). It remains unclear whether one or both of these interactions occur in living cells. Some studies suggest that the latter site may be the major one involved in functional interactions between Ly49A on NK cells and D^d on target cells (38,39).

The majority of Ly49 proteins are inhibitory; the few that are stimulatory include Ly49D and Ly49H. Functional studies indicate that Ly49D is specific for several class I MHC molecules, including D^d (40,41). Accordingly, the reactivity of NK cells from C57BL/6 (H-2^b) mice with H-2^d–expressing cells is partly mediated by the Ly49D–D^d interaction. Furthermore, the receptor appears to cross-react in some cases with xenogeneic class I MHC molecules (42). Despite these functional results, direct binding of Ly49D to D^d or other class I MHC molecules has not been observed, which suggests that the interaction may be of low affinity.

Most of the approximately 10 *Ly49* genes in C57Bl/6 mice are encoded in a 500-kb region at one end of the murine NKC, although one relatively divergent *Ly49* gene (Ly49B) maps 700 kb to one side of this region (Fig. 4) (43). *Ly49* genes exhibit considerable genetic polymorphism in different mouse strains. In addition to considerable sequence diversity between alleles, specific *Ly49* genes appear to be completely absent in some strains of mice. Polymorphisms in *Ly49* genes can therefore contribute to disease susceptibility, as discussed later.

Killer Cell Immunoglobulin-like Receptors

The discovery of KIR and their role in NK cell recognition occurred in a manner similar to that of Ly49 receptors. After it was discovered that human NK cell clones can attack allogeneic cells (44), the genes encoding the target structures were mapped to the human MHC [the human leukocyte antigen (HLA)] (45). Monoclonal antibodies specific for the NK cell clones were prepared and shown to modulate target cell recognition (46). The monoclonal antibodies initially defined two types of KIR, often expressed by

different NK clones. It ultimately became clear that these receptors were inhibitory and recognized alternative allelic families of HLA-C molecules. Cloning of the receptor genes followed (47–49), and additional receptor family members were subsequently discovered, some of which react with other HLA molecules, including HLA-A and HLA-B alleles (12). Thus, KIR, like Ly49 receptors, generally recognize classical class I MHC molecules. Individual KIR typically interact with several class Ia MHC alleles. Originally labeled "killer cell inhibitory receptors," the receptor family was eventually renamed "killer cell immunoglobulin-like receptors."

As their name implies, KIR contain immunoglobulin-like ectodomains (Fig. 2). Most KIR contain two immunoglobulin domains, but some contain three. Most KIR are thought to be monomeric, but at least one is believed to form homodimers. Like Ly49 receptors, some KIR are inhibitory and contain cytoplasmic ITIMs, whereas others are stimulatory and carry charged residues in their transmembrane domains (12). Most of the known stimulatory KIR are specific for class I HLA-C molecules. The stimulatory isoforms contain a shorter cytoplasmic domain than the inhibitory isoforms. The nomenclature for KIR includes a designation of the number of immunoglobulin domains and whether the isoform has a long (L, inhibitory) or short (S, stimulatory) cytoplasmic tail. For example, KIR2DL1 contains two immunoglobulin domains and is a long (inhibitory) isoform.

The interaction of KIR with HLA-C molecules has been well studied. The binding affinity of inhibitory KIR with class I molecules is similar to that of Ly49, corresponding to a K_D of approximately 1 to 2×10^{-5} M (50). Stimulatory KIR appear to have a generally lower affinity for class I molecules (51). The crystal structure of a KIR with HLA-C reveals that two immunoglobulin domains of the receptor bind near one end of the class I groove, over the C-terminal portion of the bound peptide (52). This site is well separated from either of the two corresponding sites on murine class I molecules that have been shown to interact with Ly49A. The location of the binding site near the C-terminus of the bound peptide is in agreement with the finding that substitutions in the C-terminal amino acid residues of the peptide, especially at the seventh and eighth amino acid positions, leads to impaired recognition, which results in reduced inhibition (53). Thus, receptor binding is to some degree dependent on the sequence of the peptide. Nevertheless, because alterations in the other half of the peptide do not affect receptor binding, KIR binding to HLA-C is not nearly as specific for the MHC-bound peptide as is T-cell receptor binding. In this regard, KIR binding is similar to Ly49 binding.

Approximately 10 closely linked KIR genes span 160 kb of deoxyribonucleic acid (DNA) in the LRC (Fig. 4) (15). KIR genes exhibit substantial genetic polymorphism, both in sequence and in the presence or absence of specific KIR genes in the cluster (29). With the exception of genomic location, these and other features, too, are remarkably similar to those of Ly49 genes.

CD94/NKG2 Receptors

CD94/NKG2 receptors, like Ly49 receptors, are lectinlike type II transmembrane proteins (Fig. 2) (54–56). Among MHC-specific NK receptors, they are unique in their conservation between humans and rodents and in their heterodimeric structure. The CD94 chain can pair with NKG2A, NKG2B (a splice variant of the NKG2A gene), NKG2C, or NKG2E. These NKG2 proteins are highly related in amino acid sequence (90% or higher sequence identity). (In contrast, NKG2D represents a functionally distinct type of receptor that does not pair with CD94, as discussed later.) Depending on the NKG2 chain in the heterodimer, the resulting receptor is inhibitory or stimulatory. CD94/NKG2A is a major isoform that exhibits inhibitory activity, as a result of the presence of an ITIM in the NKG2A cytoplasmic domain. CD94/NKG2C and CD94/NKG2E are stimulatory isoforms as a result of charged residues in the NKG2C/E transmembrane domains that enable interactions with the KARAP/DAP12 signaling molecule (57).

All of the CD94/NKG2 isoforms recognize class Ia MHC molecules in an indirect and unique manner (Fig. 5). The actual ligand is a nonclassical class I (also called class Ib) molecule, known as HLA-E in humans (58,59) and Qa-1 in mice (55), complexed with a peptide derived from class Ia molecules. The nine–amino acid peptide is conserved in the

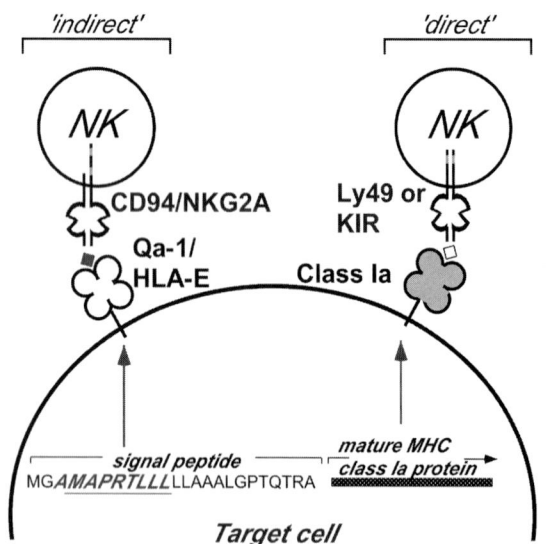

FIG. 5. Natural killer (NK) cells survey class Ia major histocompatibility complex (MHC) expression by target cells by using both a "direct" mechanism and an "indirect" mechanism. The direct mechanism employs Ly49 receptors (mouse) or killer cell immunoglobulin-like receptor (KIR) (human) to recognize the mature class Ia molecule itself. In the indirect mechanism, a nine–amino acid peptide sequence, which is well conserved in the signal peptide domain of many (but not all) class Ia molecules, is processed from the protein and presented to the outside of the cell in the peptide-binding groove of a nonclassical class I molecule called human leukocyte antigen E (HLA-E) in humans and Qa-1 in mice. The complex is specifically recognized by the CD94/NKG2A receptor.

cleaved signal sequences of a subset of class Ia molecules, including many HLA-A, HLA-B, and HLA-C molecules in humans and all known D and L molecules in mice (60,61). A similar peptide is present in the signal sequence of HLA-G, a nonclassical class I molecule expressed in trophoblast and placenta cells. Binding of CD94/NKG2 receptors is specific for the sequence of the bound peptide (62,63). Consequently, cells that fail to synthesize corresponding class Ia molecules fail to generate the complete ligand for CD94/NKG2 receptors. In the case of HLA-E, but not Qa-1, the absence of appropriate class Ia–derived peptides leads to destabilization of the molecule and low cell surface expression. Furthermore, because presentation of the class Ia peptide is dependent on the transporter associated with antigen processing (TAP) (64), cells lacking TAP also fail to generate effective ligands for CD94/NKG2 receptors. As a result, such cells fail to engage the inhibitory CD94/NKG2A isoform and may be susceptible to lysis by NK cells that express CD94/NKG2A. Thus, the CD94/NKG2A receptor system can be considered an indirect means of monitoring class Ia gene expression, in distinction with the direct mode of recognition employed by Ly49 receptors and KIR (Fig. 5).

Both the inhibitory and stimulatory CD94/NKG2 isoforms bind to the complex of class Ia leader peptide bound to HLA-E or Qa-1. CD94/NKG2A, the inhibitory isoform, binds to peptide-loaded HLA-E molecules with a K_D of approximately 10^{-5} M, similar to that of the other inhibitory MHC-specific NK receptors (65). The stimulatory CD94/NKG2C isoform binds with about fivefold lower affinity.

The *Cd94* and *Nkg2* genes are located together in a cluster within the NK gene complex, near the *Ly49* genes (Fig. 4) (56). Unlike *Ly49* and *KIR* genes, the *Cd94/Nkg2* genes are not highly polymorphic.

Leukocyte Immunoglobulin-like Receptors/Immunoglobulin-like Transcripts

A family of receptors called variously leukocyte immunoglobulin-like receptors (LIR) or immunoglobulin-like transcripts (ILT) is expressed in humans by B cells, monocytes, dendritic cells, granulocytes, and NK cells (66,67). The LIR/ILT genes are encoded in the LRC (Fig. 4), and the corresponding proteins include inhibitory and stimulatory isoforms. At least some of these proteins bind to classical class I MHC molecules. The available data suggest that LIR/ILT are expressed most prominently in cells of the myeloid lineages and only sporadically and weakly in NK cells. In some people, NK cells may not express these proteins at all. Therefore, although LIR/ILT may play a role in NK cell functions, it is likely that they play a greater role in myeloid lineage cells.

Lag-3 Receptors

Lag-3 is a protein related in structure to CD4. Lag-3 is expressed by activated T cells and NK cells. It appears to contribute to natural killing of at least some tumor target cells, as shown with NK cells from mice with a disrupted *Lag-3* gene, or by blocking Lag-3 on NK cells with an antiserum (68). The tumor cells whose lysis is most dependent on Lag-3 express class II MHC molecules, and there is some evidence that Lag-3 may bind class II molecules. In contrast, Lag-3 plays no detectable role in NK cell lysis of many other target cells, including class I MHC–deficient T-cell blasts or bone marrow cells. It remains to be established whether Lag-3 provides directly stimulatory, co-stimulatory or adhesion function in NK cell recognition.

Expression Patterns of Major Histocompatibility Complex–Specific Receptors

The well-characterized MHC-specific receptors (KIR, Ly49, and CD94/NKG2) share two key features:

1. *The different receptors all discriminate between allelic isoforms of class Ia MHC molecules.* In the case of CD94/NKG2 receptors, this occurs in an indirect manner as a consequence of the fact that some, but not all, class Ia proteins contain the critical HLA-E/Qa-1–binding peptide within their cleaved signal sequences.
2. *All of the receptors are expressed by NK cells in a characteristic variegated pattern* (69–71). This means that each receptor is expressed by a subset of NK cells but in an overlapping manner such that NK cells expressing almost any pair or trio of receptors can be easily detected. The number of different inhibitory receptors expressed by each NK cell varies, but the average is approximately four. The expression of each receptor occurs more or less randomly with regard to other receptors, as inferred from the fact that the frequency of NK cells expressing a given receptor combination can be estimated as the product of the frequencies of cells expressing each receptor (the "product rule") (69,71). As a consequence, many NK cells in a given host animal express inhibitory receptors specific for MHC molecules that are not present in that animal. Such receptors presumably have no function in that animal, although they may in its descendants. The apparent wastefulness is tolerated, possibly because it is inherent in the processes used to generate the repertoire.

The receptor repertoire is not completely random, as discussed in more detail later. Furthermore, the functional activity of NK cells expressing different receptor sets may vary. Each fully active NK cell is believed to express at least one inhibitory receptor specific for a *self* class Ia molecule. The self MHC-specific inhibitory receptor prevents the NK cell from attacking normal self cells (see the section on self tolerance).

These shared features account for a central property of NK cell recognition: the capacity of NK cells to attack cells that selectively lack expression of one or another, but not all, of the relatively small complement (<6, considering both parents) of class Ia MHC alleles that an individual possesses. The capacity of NK cells to attack cells with a selective loss of MHC molecules was presumably favored by natural selection because infected and transformed cells often exhibit selective down-regulation or loss of MHC expression (18,19). This characteristic of NK cell recognition also underlies the phenomenon of hybrid resistance discussed previously, in which *H-2* heterozygous mice can reject bone marrow grafts from an *H-2* homozygous parent but not from *H-2* heterozygous siblings. The same phenomenon is illustrated by the finding that NK cells from normal mice reject cells from otherwise identical mice that lack expression of a single class Ia gene as a result of gene targeting (72).

How does receptor variegation account for the lysis of cells with selective loss of class I MHC proteins? Because the inhibitory receptors are variegated in expression and can discriminate among MHC allelic forms, some NK cells express an inhibitory receptor specific for only one of the host's several class Ia molecules. When these NK cells encounter a potential target cell in which the corresponding class I molecule has been extinguished, no inhibition will occur. If the target cell can stimulate the NK cell, it will be lysed.

Stimulation can occur in at least two ways. If the target cell is infected or transformed, it may up-regulate non-MHC ligands that engage stimulatory receptors expressed by many or all NK cells (see the later section on NKG2D and its ligands). Alternatively, some of the NK cell stimulatory receptors, like the inhibitory receptors, are specific for class I MHC molecules and are variegated in expression. Because these receptors are expressed in an essentially random manner, NK cells with stimulatory receptors specific for one of the host's class I MHC molecules (H-2D, for example) often express an inhibitory receptor specific for a *different* host class I molecule (H-2K, for example). These NK cells may attack target cells in which the inhibitory ligand (H-2K in this example) is extinguished, even if the target cell fails to up-regulate other stimulatory ligands.

Class I Down-Regulation and Sensitivity of Cells to Natural Killer Cells

The loss of class I MHC molecules has been shown to be sufficient to render certain normal cell types sensitive to NK cells. Primary activated T cells or B cells from mice with targeted mutations in β_2-microglobulin, TAP, or K^b and D^b class I molecules are sensitive to NK cells from normal mice, and bone marrow cells from these mice are rejected *in vivo* by NK cells present in normal mice (25,26). Interestingly, however, primary fibroblasts from the same class I MHC–deficient mice are not NK sensitive (73). Furthermore, unlike bone marrow grafts, skin and organ grafts from class I MHC–deficient mice are not rejected by otherwise genetically identical class I$^+$ mice (73). The varying susceptibility of different cell types led to the suggestion that some normal cells (especially lymphohematopoietic cells) express non-MHC stimulatory ligands for NK cells, whereas many other cell types do not (74).

In the case of tumor cell lines, the loss of class I MHC expression is well correlated with enhanced susceptibility to NK cells *in vitro* and *in vivo*. MHC loss variants arise at a high rate in natural tumors (18), possibly because of the high rate of mutations that occur in tumors, coupled with selection against class I MHC expression by tumor-specific T cells. Class I MHC loss may result from alterations in expression of the class I genes themselves or in other molecules necessary to achieve normal levels of class I expression, such as β_2-microglobulin or TAP. Restoration of class I MHC expression typically protects the tumor cell from NK cell attack, both *in vitro* and *in vivo*. Nevertheless, some tumor cells that express high levels of class I MHC are sensitive to NK cells. It is likely that such tumor cells are highly stimulatory to NK cells, thus overwhelming the inhibitory signals delivered as a result of MHC recognition.

NK cells may play a significant role in tumor surveillance *in vivo*, as discussed in more detail later. Studies with tumor cell lines selected for class I MHC down-regulation suggest that MHC down-regulation can lead specifically to NK susceptibility *in vivo*. However, in the context of a naturally developing tumor, the relative roles of MHC down-regulation versus up-regulation of stimulatory ligands or other factors have not been clearly defined. Therefore, it remains to be proved that NK cells eliminate or impair the growth of endogenous tumors as a specific result of tumor cell class I MHC down-regulation.

Class I MHC loss also occurs in cells infected with many (but not all) types of viruses. Viruses have evolved a plethora of mechanisms for down-regulating class I MHC molecules, including inhibition of transcription, interference with peptide transport by TAP, targeting of newly synthesized class I MHC molecules for degradation, impairment of vesicular transport to the cell surface, and rapid turnover of class I MHC molecules from the cell surface (19). A given complex virus, such as cytomegalovirus, may employ several of these mechanisms to inhibit class I MHC expression. However, even a relatively simple virus, such as human immunodeficiency virus (HIV), has evolved two effective strategies. One viral protein (HIV-Vpu) destabilizes newly synthesized class I MHC molecules, and another protein (HIV-Nef) leads to the rapid internalization and degradation of cell surface class I molecules.

Because class I-down-regulation is expected to protect infected cells from T cell supervision, it makes sense that NK cells might be needed to provide compensatory protection. Indeed, it is generally proposed that the class I MHC–down-regulating activities of viruses served as the evolutionary selection pressure that gave rise to the capacity of NK cells to attack class I MHC–deficient cells. In accordance with this idea, the viruses in which NK cells play the most clearly defined protective role, such as cytomegalovirus and other herpesviruses, also tend to down-regulate class I MHC expression in infected cells.

Although this theory is attractive, there is little direct evidence that virus-induced loss of MHC expression in an infected cell is sufficient to induce NK sensitivity. The difficulty in addressing the question arises because viruses induce many changes in infected cells that may either enhance or inhibit NK sensitivity independently of any effects on class I MHC expression. For example, infection of cells with various herpesviruses results in both enhanced NK sensitivity and class I MHC down-regulation, but a direct connection between these events has not been demonstrated. Enhanced sensitivity of the cytomegalovirus-infected cells is also attributed to the induction of stimulatory ligands for NK cells, such as the MIC proteins (75) (see later section on NKG2D and its ligands), or to the up-regulation of adhesion molecules such as intercellular adhesion molecule 1 and leukocyte function–associated antigen 3 (76,77). Separating these and other events that occur in viral infection in order to dissect their roles is a challenge that remains for the future.

Interestingly, in some instances in which viruses cause class I MHC down-regulation, such as adenovirus type 12 infection of fibroblasts, the infected cells do not become sensitive to NK cells (78). Perhaps relevant to this finding are the findings of other studies indicating that class I MHC down-regulation is not sufficient to induce sensitivity of fibroblasts to NK cells (73,76). It is possible, therefore, that adenovirus type 12 fails to induce expression of NK-stimulatory ligands by fibroblasts. Alternatively, the virus may have evolved independent mechanisms to evade NK cells (78).

Viral Evasion of Natural Killer Cells through Inhibition

The existence of MHC-specific inhibitory receptors expressed by NK cells provides a potential mechanism for pathogens to evade the NK cell response. Indeed, certain viruses, such as cytomegaloviruses, encode class I MHC homologs that are expressed in infected cells and are proposed to function in immune evasion by serving as ligands for NK cell inhibitory receptors. Thus, a cytomegalovirus-infected cell might evade T-cell recognition by down-regulating class I MHC molecules but also evade NK cells by expressing a class I MHC homolog recognized by NK inhibitory receptors (but not T cells). For example, mouse cytomegalovirus (MCMV) encodes a class I MHC homolog called m144. An MCMV mutant in which the *m144* gene is deleted grows poorly in normal mice, in comparison to the vigorous replication of the wild-type virus. The poor growth of the mutant virus is reversed when NK cells are depleted from the mice (79). These findings suggest that *m144* normally inhibits NK cells. However, this conclusion has been difficult to confirm in studies with cell lines that have been transfected with *m144*. Such cell lines exhibit only a modest resistance to NK cells (80). Furthermore, although it might be proposed that *m144* binds to inhibitory Ly49 or CD94/NKG2A receptors, no correlation between expression of these receptors and inhibition has been observed to date, which raises the possibility that *m144* serves some other function for the virus.

Human cytomegalovirus (HCMV) also encodes a class I MHC homolog, called UL18. UL18 is unrelated to *m144*, which reflects the distance of the relation between MCMV and HCMV. There is some controversy over whether UL18 expression reduces (81) or enhances (76) sensitivity of cells to NK attack. Interestingly, UL18 was shown to bind to a member of the LIR family (67). As discussed above, most LIRs are inhibitory, and many also interact with classical class I HLA proteins. LIRs are expressed poorly by a small subset of NK cells, but B cells and monocytes exhibit much stronger LIR expression. It is therefore plausible that UL18 exerts its primary function *in vivo* through inhibition of one or both of the latter cell types. One possibility is that UL18 and, by extension, *m144* repress NK cell induction indirectly, by inhibiting production of NK cell–inducing cytokines by monocytes or dendritic cells. In summary, although class I MHC homologs exist in several viruses, they have not been clearly shown to inhibit NK cell function directly or to bind to the major inhibitory receptors employed by NK cells.

Another mechanism by which some pathogens may evade NK cell attack exploits the CD94/NKG2A inhibitory receptor. Some viruses encode membrane proteins containing within their signal sequences a peptide that exactly matches the nine–amino acid peptide in class Ia MHC molecules that binds to HLA-E or Qa-1 to create the ligand for CD94/NKG2A. An example is an HCMV protein of unknown function called UL40. Transfected cells expressing UL40 exhibit up-regulation of HLA-E and reduced sensitivity to lysis by NK cells, which supports the idea that the viral peptide provides protection to infected cells (82).

It has been proposed that some pathogens evade NK cells by down-regulating class I MHC molecules in a locus-selective manner. As one example, HIV-Nef expression leads to the selective down-regulation of HLA-A and HLA-B molecules, with little or no effect on HLA-C expression (83). Because most HIV-specific CTLs are restricted by HLA-A and HLA-B molecules, this tactic may enable the virus to evade CTL. At the same time, many of the inhibitory NK cell receptors in humans recognize HLA-C molecules, and so the sustained expression of HLA-C molecules by infected cells may help to protect them from attack by NK cells. It is notable that this proposed mechanism of evasion seems to conflict with the notion, discussed earlier, that NK cells are equipped to attack cells in which class I molecules are down-regulated selectively (see the earlier section on expression patterns of MHC-specific receptors). Indeed, because some of the inhibitory receptors are specific for HLA-A and HLA-B molecules, this mechanism of evasion is unlikely to be completely effective.

Possible Functions of Stimulatory Major Histocompatibility Complex–Specific Natural Killer Cell Receptors

The existence of stimulatory MHC-specific receptors expressed by NK cells was not initially anticipated, and their biological function is not well understood. One role, as proposed previously (in the section on expression patterns of MHC-specific receptors), may be to aid in attacking cells that selectively down-regulate class I MHC molecules. However, several other possibilities may be considered (70). One idea is that stimulatory MHC-specific receptors evolved to counter the evasion tactics that viruses employ to inhibit NK cells. If the stimulatory receptors bind to the class I "decoys" that some viruses encode, the balance of signaling could shift back in the direction of NK cell activation. Alternatively, stimulatory receptors may preferentially bind MHC molecules that have complexed with specific pathogen-derived peptides. Another possibility is suggested by the observation that stimulatory MHC-specific receptors are generally of lower affinity than are their inhibitory counterparts. In this scheme, stimulatory receptors are saturated only when class I MHC molecules on a target cell are overexpressed, as occurs in response to locally produced interferons at the site of infections. Saturation of the stimulatory receptors may overcome inhibitory signaling, leading to lysis of the class I–overexpressing cells. Finally, it is possible that some of the stimulatory receptors cross-react with non-MHC ligands associated with infection, such as pathogen-encoded molecules or host-encoded molecules whose expression is induced by infection.

Direct evidence demonstrates that at least one stimulatory receptor, called Ly49H, recognizes a virally encoded MHC "decoy." Although a member of the Ly49 family, Ly49H exhibits no known MHC reactivity. This receptor plays an important role in the NK cell response to MCMV. NK cells are known to play an important role in limiting cytomegalovirus replication early in the infectious cycle. The effectiveness of this response is under genetic control, in such a way that certain mouse strains, such as C57BL/6, are more resistant to the virus than others, such as DBA/2 or BALB/c. Genetic segregation studies demonstrated the existence of a key dominant gene, called *Cmv1ʳ*, that confers resistance to MCMV, especially affecting viral replication in the spleen (13). Genetic evidence suggests that *Cmv1ʳ* encodes Ly49H, and that virus-sensitive strains lack a functioning *Ly49h* gene (84–86). When virus-resistant C57BL/6 mice were injected with an antibody that blocks the Ly49H receptor, they became susceptible to the virus. In addition, virus infection leads to preferential accumulation of the subset of NK cells that express Ly49H. Apparently, MCMV infection leads to expression in target cells of a ligand that interacts with Ly49H, which triggers a strong NK cell response against the infected cells. The ligand was identified as a viral product called m157, which is structurally related to class I MHC proteins (87). Of significance is that the m157 protein also binds to certain inhibitory Ly49 receptors, which suggests that, in some circumstances, it can function as a "decoy" to aid the virus in evading NK cells. A plausible evolutionary scenario to explain these findings is that the inhibitory function of m157 evolved first as a viral adaptation to evade the immune system. Natural selection may then have given rise to Ly49H in the host as an evolutionary "countermeasure."

Stimulatory Receptors Specific for Non–Major Histocompatibility Complex Ligands

In this section, the growing list of stimulatory NK receptors specific for non-MHC ligands is described, along with receptors with unknown ligands that are thought to play a role in natural killing. An early finding was that nearly all NK cells express a CD16 or FcγRIII, a high affinity receptor for the Fc portion of antibodies. CD16 associates with the signaling molecule FcεR1γ. CD16 binds the Fc portion of several IgG isotypes, enabling NK cells to mediate potent antibody-dependent cellular cytotoxicity against antibody-coated cells (88). Natural killing of most susceptible target cells does not depend on antibodies, however. Consequently, a search has been undertaken for other stimulatory receptors responsible for recognition of tumor cells and infected cells. The search has unearthed several receptors and receptor families that participate in the stimulation of natural killing, including NKp46, NKp30, NKp44, NKR-P1, and NKG2D (Fig. 3). The first three are restricted in expression to NK cells, whereas NKR-P1 and NKG2D are expressed by certain other immune cells. Ligands have been definitively identified only in the case of one of these receptors, NKG2D, but none appear to bind conventional class I MHC molecules. Antibodies that block each receptor have been used to assess their role in target cell recognition by human NK cells. For some target cells, one receptor or the other plays a dominant role in NK cell activation, whereas other target cells appear to express ligands for several of the receptors (9,89). These findings accord with the idea that NK cells are equipped with several stimulatory receptors to detect various alterations in target cells.

NKG2D and Its Ligands

Certain stimulatory receptors expressed by all NK cells recognize "self" cell surface proteins that are induced in infected, transformed, or stressed target cells. The evolution of cellular genes that are up-regulated in distressed cells and serve to arouse an immune response represents a fascinating form of innate immunity. An example of a receptor for such proteins is NKG2D, a stimulatory homodimeric type II transmembrane receptor that is structurally similar to C-type lectins and well conserved in rodents and humans (Fig. 3) (54,90,91). Like other lectin-related NK receptor genes, the *Nkg2d* gene is located within the NKC on human chromosome 12 and mouse chromosome 6 (Fig. 4) (91). Despite its name, NKG2D differs dramatically in sequence from NKG2A, NKG2B, NKG2C, and NKG2E; does not form heterodimers with CD94; and exhibits a completely distinct ligand specificity. Thus, NKG2D is not considered a bona fide member of the NKG2 family.

NKG2D is constitutively expressed by essentially all NK cells, but it is also expressed by CD8+ T cells, γδ T cells, NK1.1+ T cells, activated macrophages, and possibly other cell types (92–94). NKG2D interacts with several families of

cell surface ligands, all of which are distantly related to class I MHC molecules. One family, consisting of two functional members, MICA and MICB, is encoded by genes within the human MHC (95). Although distantly related in sequence to class I MHC proteins and of a similar overall domain structure, MICA and MICB do not associate with the class I light chain β_2-microglobulin. Furthermore, the site corresponding to the peptide groove in class I molecules is closed off in MICA and MICB, preventing peptide binding (96). NKG2D interacts with the α-helical surface of MIC molecules in a manner similar to the T cell receptor interacting with MHC molecules (97). The K_D of the interaction is approximately 10^{-6} M, about 10-fold higher than most NK receptor–ligand interactions that have been characterized (97).

MICA is expressed by some intestinal epithelial cells in normal humans but not by other cells examined (95). Upon transformation, however, most tumors derived from epithelial cells strongly up-regulate MICA and MICB expression (98). Furthermore, infection of cells with cytomegalovirus and possibly other infectious agents induces expression of MICA or MICB or both (75). The up-regulation of MICA/MICB genes in infected or transformed cells probably results from the presence within their promoter regions of heat shock transcription elements (95). This class of transcription elements is activated by several forms of stress, including heat shock, infection, and transformation.

Surprisingly, no homologs of MICA and MICB have been identified in mice. However, mice have another family of ligands for NKG2D, retinoic acid early inducible–1 (Rae1), which is also up-regulated in tumor cells (93,94). The Rae1 proteins are encoded by the *Raet1* genes, a family of several highly homologous genes on chromosome 10, a different chromosome from that containing the mouse MHC (99). A related protein, H60, is also a ligand for NKG2D and is also encoded on chromosome 10 near the *Raet1* genes (93,94). H60 is not expressed in all mouse strains. Humans express a family of proteins related to Rae1 and H60, called ULBPs or human RAET1 proteins, which are encoded on chromosome 6 in a region syntenic to the *Raet1* and *H60* genes (100,101). Like MIC molecules, ULBPs are ligands for human NKG2D. Most Rae1 proteins and ULBPs are attached to the plasma membrane by a lipid linkage.

The Rae1, H60, and ULBP families exhibit only low sequence homology to each other but are encoded in syntenic chromosomal locations and have similar domain structures consisting of two N-terminal domains distantly related to the class 1 MHC α1 and α2 domains and a short third domain that is dissimilar to the class I α3 domain or to the corresponding region of MIC. Furthermore, all three of these protein families form a similar three-dimensional structure that is comparable with that of the α1 and α2 domains of MIC molecules or class I MHC molecules. As with MIC molecules, the site corresponding to the peptide-binding groove in class I MHC molecules is apparently inaccessible to peptides. NKG2D binds across the α-helical surfaces of Rae1 and ULBP molecules with an orientation similar to that of the

NKG2D-MIC complex, or the T-cell receptor–MHC complex. Thus, it appears that all of the ligand families, despite their dissimilar sequences, interact with a similar site on the NKG2D receptor. The affinity of murine NKG2D for Rae1 (K_D = approximately 0.5×10^{-6} M) is only slightly higher than that of human NKG2D for MICA, whereas its affinity for H60 is approximately fifty times higher (K_D = approximately 2×10^{-8} M) (102).

Few if any normal cells express Rae1 family members (99), but the genes are induced in many tumor cell lines of diverse origins, including carcinomas, lymphomas, and macrophage tumors (93). The signaling events leading to Rae1 up-regulation in tumor cells are not known. A possible clue is that expression of Rae1 is induced by retinoic acid in at least one cell line (99). In contrast to Rae1, H60 and ULBPs are expressed by at least some normal cells. Up-regulation may nevertheless occur in some tumor cells (93,94,103) or in infected cells.

Expression of NKG2D ligands by a target cell results in full stimulation of NK cells and activated macrophages (93,94,104). In contrast, target cell expression of NKG2D ligands is not sufficient to stimulate cytokine production or cytolysis by activated CD8$^+$ T cells (75,104). Instead, NKG2D ligands appear to provide a co-stimulatory signal to CTLs, which also receive a primary signal as a result of T-cell receptor triggering (75,104). The basis for this difference in signaling is not known. The receptor associates with signaling molecules, including one called DAP10, which has been found to have primarily co-stimulatory activity (105).

NKG2D ligand expression has a dramatic effect on tumor cell rejection *in vivo*. When NKG2D ligands such as Rae1 are introduced by transfection into tumor cells that lack them, the resulting cells are potently rejected by normal syngeneic mice when transferred subcutaneously (104,106). The rejection is mediated by NK cells and, in some cases, by CD8$^+$ T cells. Remarkably, the injected mice become immune to challenges with the same tumor cells lacking Rae1 or other NKG2D ligands (104). The immunity is mediated by CD8$^+$ T cells. The results indicate that Rae1 expression by tumor cells can result in the induction of a potent NK cell response as well as induction of protective memory CTLs.

NKp46, NKp30, and NKp44

Three stimulatory receptors expressed exclusively by NK cells—NKp46 (107), NKp30, (108) and NKp44 (109)—have also been shown to participate in target cell recognition by human NK cells (Fig. 3). All three are members of the IgSF. NKp46 contains two C2-type immunoglobulin-like domains in its extracellular portion, whereas NKp30 and NKp44 each contain a single V-type immunoglobulin-like domain (9). NKp46 is encoded within the LRC (15), whereas the NKp30 and NKp44 genes are located within the human MHC (110). A homolog of NKp46 has been identified in rodents (111).

All three receptors have charged residues within their transmembrane domains that allow interactions with signaling molecules, although the different receptors associate with different signaling molecules. NKp46 pairs with CD3ζ or FcεRIγ; NKp30 pairs with CD3ζ; and NKp44 pairs with KARAP/DAP12 (9). Engagement of each receptor leads to full NK cell activation.

NKp46 and NKp30 are expressed by NK cells freshly derived from a donor, but NKp44 expression is inducible by cytokines such as interleukin (IL)–2 (109). NKp44 induction may account for the fact that cytokine-activated NK cells attack certain tumor target cells that are resistant to freshly isolated NK cells.

Although most NK cells express NKp46 and NKp30, the percentage of NK cells expressing high levels of the two receptors (which are expressed coordinately) varies widely from individual to individual (9,108). The high or low expression level is maintained even as the cells are activated and expanded clonally in cell cultures. Cells within the two subsets express KIR and NKG2D receptors similarly, but CD94/NKG2A expression may be limited to the NKp46/NKp30-high subset. The genes or environmental factors that underlie this variable degree of receptor expression are unknown.

Results of blocking experiments with different combinations of antibodies specific for NKp46, NKp30, NKp44, and NKG2D suggest that different stimulatory receptors predominate in different NK-target cell combinations (108,112). Even tumor cells of the same type—for example, different melanoma cell lines—may stimulate through different receptors. One or more of these receptors may also participate in NK cell lysis of nontransformed mitogen-activated T cells or bone marrow cells; lysis of such cells can occur when MHC expression is impaired or blocked. The simultaneous blockade of all four receptors is effective in completely inhibiting lysis of most NK-sensitive target cells.

The ligands on tumor cells recognized by NKp46, NKp30, and NKp44 have not yet been identified, and so how the expression of such ligands is regulated is unknown. In addition to a role in tumor cell lysis, there is some evidence that NKp46 and possibly NKp44 participate in recognition of cells infected with influenza or parainfluenza viruses by binding to the viral hemagglutinin as it is expressed on the surface of infected cells (113).

NKR-P1

A set of lectinlike receptors called NKR-P1 proteins are encoded in the NKC (114,115). NKR-P1 receptors are expressed by all NK cells and a small fraction of T cells. Indeed, certain NKR-P1 family members encode the so-called NK1.1 antigen, which is used to define NK cells in some mouse strains. Some NKR-P1 isoforms are stimulatory, whereas others are inhibitory. Transfection studies provided evidence that stimulatory NKR-P1 isoforms may be involved in recognition of a subset of tumor cell lines (116). The putative ligands for NKR-P1 proteins have not been identified, but the available data suggest that they are not class I MHC proteins.

2B4

Another receptor implicated in NK cell activation is 2B4, a member of the CD2 family of receptors conserved in mice and humans (117–119). 2B4 is expressed by all NK cells, some T cells, and monocytes. The CD2 family are IgSF members that interact with each other in various combinations. The primary ligand for 2B4 is another CD2 family member called CD48, which is expressed by lymphocytes, monocytes, and endothelial cells (120). Engagement of 2B4 by CD48 appears to be insufficient for activation of NK cells, but it enhances the level of activation mediated by another NK cell receptor, such as NKp46 (121). Thus, 2B4 may function as a co-receptor or a co-stimulatory receptor in NK cell activation. The cytoplasmic domain of 2B4 interacts with several signaling molecules that may provide this co-receptor activity, including Src family protein tyrosine kinases, the linker for activated T cells (LAT), and the SLAM-associated protein (SAP) (9).

Integration of Stimulatory and Inhibitory Signaling

The outcome of an NK cell–target cell interaction is determined by the balance of stimulatory and inhibitory signaling (Fig. 1). Thus, even target cells that express high levels of inhibitory MHC molecules are susceptible to lysis by NK cells if they also express sufficient levels of a stimulatory ligand. For example, if a cell sufficiently up-regulates MICA/MICB or Rae1 expression as a result of infection or transformation, it becomes sensitive to NK cells, even if class I MHC expression remains high (89,92–94,104,106). If such cells also extinguish class I MHC expression, sensitivity to NK cells increases even further. On the other hand, some stimulatory interactions are insufficient to overcome normal levels of inhibitory signaling. For example, as discussed earlier (in the section on class I MHC down-regulation and sensitivity of cells to NK cells), certain normal cells such as bone marrow cells, T-cell blasts, and B-cell blasts appear to express stimulatory ligands for NK cells. These cells are nevertheless insensitive to NK cells because of the expression of normal levels of inhibitory class I MHC proteins. If class I MHC–mediated inhibition is prevented, these cell types become sensitive to lysis by NK cells. As one specific example, bone marrow cells that lack class I MHC molecules are sensitive to NK cells (25). Bone marrow cells from wild-type animals that express a foreign (allogeneic) MHC are also sensitive to NK cell attack, in part because some NK cells in the host do not express inhibitory receptors specific for the donor's MHC molecules (122,123). The failure of NK cells to attack many other allogeneic cell types, such as cells in a skin graft, may result from the failure of these cells to express the relevant stimulatory ligands for NK cell receptors. Validation of this proposition will require the identification of stimulatory ligands expressed by susceptible normal cell types.

As described previously, stimulatory receptors expressed by NK cells generally associate with signaling molecules that contain cytoplasmic ITAMs. Engagement of stimulatory receptors leads to rapid tyrosine phosphorylation of the ITAMs and recruitment and activation of protein tyrosine kinases of the syk/ZAP70 family (10). As in activation of other lymphocytes, these tyrosine kinases initiate a series of signaling pathways that lead to cytokine production and perforin release.

How do MHC-specific inhibitory receptors prevent NK cell activation? Although the detailed mechanism is unknown, important features of the process have been worked out. Engagement of inhibitory receptors results in rapid phosphorylation of the tyrosine residue in the cytoplasmic ITIM, presumably by Src family protein tyrosine kinase such as p56 Lck (124). The phosphorylated ITIM binds to the SH2 domain of a protein tyrosine phosphatase, principally SHP-1 but possibly also SHP-2 (8). Binding to the phosphorylated ITIM activates the phosphatase. The activated phosphatase is believed to dephosphorylate key substrates in the activation pathway, but these substrates have not been definitively identified (12). Studies demonstrate that inhibition is effective only when inhibitory receptors are clustered together on the cell surface with stimulatory receptors, which suggests that the phosphatase substrate is part of the proximal stimulatory apparatus (125). In accordance with this conclusion, inhibitory receptor engagement is known to prevent early events in the stimulatory signaling pathway, such as the flux of Ca^{2+} ions that occurs in NK cells shortly after stimulatory receptor engagement. The integration of stimulatory and inhibitory signals may reflect the balance between the competing phosphatase activity and kinase activity in the receptor clusters at the cell surface.

NATURAL KILLER CELL DEVELOPMENT AND DIFFERENTIATION

Natural Killer Cell Differentiation

NK cells, like other lymphocytes, are derived from pluripotent hematopoietic stem cells. Intermediate stages are thought to include a lymphocyte-restricted progenitor (restricted to T, B, and NK lineages), followed by a T/NK restricted intermediate (126–128). NK cell development but not T-cell development is impaired in mice treated with strontium 89 and other agents that disrupt the bone marrow, which suggests that critical phases of NK cell development occur primarily in the bone marrow (129,130). In contrast, although small numbers of NK cells do develop in the fetal thymus, NK cell development is not impaired in athymic mice, which lack conventional T cells. Thus, NK cell development does not require a maturation step in the thymus. Indeed, NK cell activity is often elevated in athymic mice in comparison with normal mice, perhaps because of compensatory mechanisms or a higher incidence of infections in such mice.

Analysis of mice with mutations in cytokine genes or their receptors has demonstrated that IL-15, a cytokine produced by bone marrow stromal cells, plays a central role in NK cell development or survival or both (131,132). Other cytokines

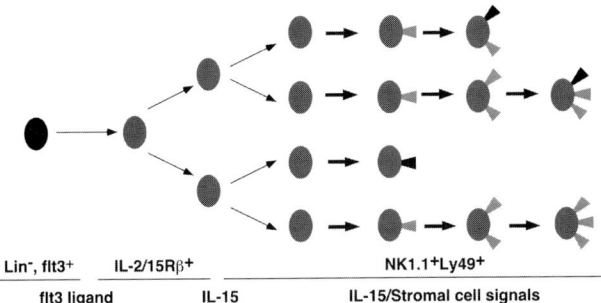

Lin⁻, flt3⁺   IL-2/15Rβ⁺   NK1.1⁺Ly49⁺
        flt3 ligand   IL-15   IL-15/Stromal cell signals

FIG. 6. A scheme of natural killer (NK) cell differentiation. NK cells are derived from an early lymphoid precursor cell type that lacks lineage markers (Lin⁻) and expresses flt3, the receptor for flt3 ligand. Exposure of the cell to flt3 ligand and other cytokines results in the expression of the receptor for interleukin (IL)–15. IL-15 from stromal cells induces NK cell differentiation, proliferation, or survival, or a combination of these, but is not sufficient to induce expression of most inhibitory NK cell receptors. Undefined stromal cell signals in conjunction with IL-15 stimulate expression Ly49 inhibitory receptors. The various Ly49 receptors are expressed more or less randomly in a given NK cell but are up-regulated over time in a cumulative manner. Initial expression of Ly49 receptors that do not interact with self class Ia major histocompatibility complex (MHC) molecules (lightly-shaded triangles) has no effect on subsequent expression of other Ly49 receptors. Expression of a Ly49 receptor that strongly interacts with self class I MHC molecules (black triangle) results in inhibition of new receptor expression. Some NK cells (such as the one depicted on the bottom row) may never succeed in expressing Ly49 receptors specific for self class I MHC proteins. Such cells exhibit a hyporesponsive functional phenotype.

are believed to be necessary at an earlier stage, in order to induce expression of IL-15 receptors on progenitor cells (Fig. 6) (133). Cell culture models of NK cell development suggest that stromal cells also supply additional undefined signals that enhance NK cell development and that cannot be replaced by any known cytokine (Fig. 6) (134,135).

As NK cells develop, they acquire various markers and receptors progressively. An early marker is the IL-2/IL-15 receptor β chain, expression of which is necessary for responsiveness to IL-15 and subsequent stages in development (133). Expression of at least some of the stimulatory receptors, such as NKG2D, appears to also be a relatively early event. In mice, expression of the NK1.1 antigen first occurs at a later stage, along with expression of many of the known inhibitory receptors (Fig. 6). Little is known about NK cell ontogeny in humans.

The transcription factor Ikaros is necessary for NK cell development, as well as for the development of other lymphohematopoietic cell types (136). Mutations in certain other transcription factors result in selectively defective NK cell development. Mutant mice lacking an interferon-inducible transcription factor called interferon regulatory factor–1 (IRF-1) fail to produce NK cells. The absence of NK cells is caused by the requirement of IRF-1 for transcription of IL-15 in bone marrow stromal cells (137). Mice with mutations of the Ets-1

or Id2 transcription factors also exhibit a selective defect in NK cell development, although the mechanistic basis of these defects is not known (138,139). Id proteins are helix-loop-helix transcription factors that inhibit the function of other helix-loop-helix transcription factors such as E-box binding (E) factors. The requirement for Id2 in NK cell development therefore suggests that specific E proteins may prevent NK cell development, perhaps by favoring another cell fate.

Formation of the Repertoire and Self-Tolerance of Natural Killer Cells

Inhibitory Receptor Expression during Natural Killer Cell Differentiation

Although a small set of functional NK cells can be detected in the murine fetal thymus and neonatal spleen, full NK cell functionality arises rather late, typically well after birth in mice (140). For unknown reasons, NK cells arising at different stages express different complements of inhibitory MHC-specific receptors. Most NK cells in newborn or fetal mice (141) or in the human fetal liver (142) express the CD94/NKG2A inhibitory receptor. In contrast, Ly49 receptors are generally not expressed in mice early in ontogeny (143,144). The fraction of NK cells expressing Ly49 receptors increases progressively during the first few weeks of life, whereas the percentage of cells expressing CD94/NKG2A receptors decreases. The pattern stabilizes after about 8 weeks, at which time nearly all NK cells express one or more Ly49 receptors and about 50% of the cells express CD94/NKG2A. Comparable information concerning KIR expression in human ontogeny is not yet available.

In cell differentiation studies *in vitro,* expression of CD94/NKG2 receptors is induced by IL-15 (142,145). In contrast, Ly49 gene expression requires undefined signals from stromal cells that cannot be replaced with any known cytokines (Fig. 6) (134,135). Cell differentiation experiments in mice indicate that individual developing NK cells "switch on" different Ly49 receptors over time in a cumulative manner (Fig. 6). Thus, the average number of Ly49 receptors expressed by each developing NK cell increases cumulatively as differentiation proceeds. The different genes are up-regulated in an ordered manner, although the exact order remains to be clarified (134,144,146). Once a Ly49 gene is expressed, its expression is stable even as the cell undergoes cell division (147).

Monoallelic Expression of Ly49 and NKG2A Genes

As discussed earlier, different inhibitory receptors (Ly49 family members and CD94/NKG2A) are expressed by overlapping subsets of NK cells. The mechanisms underlying the variegated expression pattern of these genes is of interest but still poorly understood. An interesting clue was the finding that each *Ly49* gene is usually transcribed from only one of the two alleles in each cell that expresses the gene (70,148), a pattern called *monoallelic gene expression*. The choice of allele is apparently random, so that each of the two alleles is expressed by equal numbers of cells in the same animal. A smaller subset of cells expresses both alleles. A similar pattern of expression occurs in the case of the NKG2A subunit of the CD94/NKG2A receptor, which suggests that the phenomenon may apply to all of the inhibitory NK receptor genes (149). Random monoallelic gene expression of this sort has been documented in only a few other autosomal genes, including olfactory receptor genes and some cytokine genes (150).

In the case of inhibitory NK cell receptors, it is likely that monoallelic expression is a consequence of a stochastic gene expression mechanism that equips each NK cell with a largely random combination of the possible receptors. Studies indicate that each *Ly49* allele is activated in only a fraction of cells and that expression of each allele occurs largely independently of expression of other *Ly49* alleles, including alleles of other *Ly49* genes and the opposing allele of the same *Ly49* gene (147,151). The result is variegated expression of each receptor and random expression of a different set of receptors in each cell.

T- and B-cell receptor genes are also expressed in a monoallelic manner. Allelic exclusion of T- and B-cell receptor genes serves to suppress the formation of cells expressing two receptors of different specificity. It appears unlikely that monoallelic expression of NK cell inhibitory receptors serves the same purpose, because the two alleles of a specific *Ly49* gene or *Nkg2a* gene usually encode receptors with the same specificity. Moreover, the mechanism of monoallelic expression is different in the two instances. T- and B-cell receptor genes are encoded by gene segments that must be assembled by somatic DNA recombination events, and the regulation of recombination is involved in imposing the monoallelic expression pattern. The *Ly49* and *Nkg2a* genes, in contrast, do not undergo rearrangement, and regulation occurs at the level of transcription.

As discussed previously, once an *Ly49* allele is expressed, expression is maintained even as the cell undergoes multiple rounds of cell division (147). The relatively stable expression pattern of these genes suggests that, although initiation of gene expression may be random, the expressed gene subsequently undergoes epigenetic modifications to maintain the gene in an active state.

Self-Tolerance

A key function of inhibitory NK receptors is to prevent the lysis of normal cells. However, because of the variegated expression of the receptors and the fact that they differ in specificity for MHC alleles, some NK cells in every animal are expected to lack inhibitory receptors specific for a given MHC molecule or set of MHC molecules. This largely explains the capacity of NK cells to attack foreign cells, as discussed previously. However, this line of reasoning also suggests that some NK cells that fail to express inhibitory receptors specific for *self* MHC molecules will arise. Nonetheless, it is known that NK cells exhibit self tolerance. What mechanisms prevent NK cell-mediated autoreactivity?

As one explanation for self-tolerance of NK cells, it has been proposed that all peripheral NK cells in fact do express at least one inhibitory receptor specific for self class I MHC molecules, presumably as the result of a selective or developmental process. Direct evidence for this model is sparse, however. To the contrary, there is some evidence that there exists a subset of mouse NK cells that lack inhibitory receptors specific for self MHC molecules (70). An alternative hypothesis to explain NK cell self-tolerance is that NK cells that lack receptors for self MHC molecules can arise in development, but such cells are functionally silenced. Such a mechanism is consistent with studies of gene targeted class I MHC–deficient mice. Despite the absence of class I MHC molecules in these mice, normal numbers of NK cells arise in development, but these NK cells are self-tolerant; that is, they do not attack class I MHC–deficient cells (25,26,152). Apparently, when developing NK cells are deprived of inhibitory receptor signaling, they fail to achieve full functionality and acquire a hyporesponsive phenotype. In a normal animal, therefore, a subset of NK cells that fails to express inhibitory receptors specific for self class I MHC molecules may also be functionally silenced (Fig. 6). According to this hypothesis, each fully functional NK cell expresses a self-MHC specific inhibitory receptor, but there exists a subset of hyporesponsive NK cells that lack such receptors.

The hyporesponsive state of NK cells in class I MHC–deficient mice bears similarities to the state of "anergy" described for B and T cells; that is, the NK cells from class I MHC–deficient mice are not completely devoid of functional activity. Instead, the cells are poorly responsive to stimulation through numerous NK cell–activating receptors (70). Presumably, the weak stimulation provided by neighboring MHC-deficient but otherwise normal cells is insufficient to activate the hyporesponsive cells, which accounts for the self-tolerance of the NK cells. It is not known whether the hyporesponsive state results from a deficit in signaling molecules or adhesion molecules or results from enhanced inhibition through unknown receptors specific for non-MHC ligands.

Results of bone marrow chimera experiments suggest that hyporesponsiveness occurs when developing NK cells are exposed to cells that lack appropriate MHC ligands, even when other cells that express such ligands are present in the animal (153,154). These findings suggest that the hyporesponsive state ensues when the differentiating NK cell receives unopposed stimulatory signals in some of its encounters, even if it encounters other cells that also provide inhibitory signaling. Although the hyporesponsive state must therefore persist for some time, it is not necessarily an irreversible phenotype. *In vitro*, for example, the hyporesponsive state can be reversed by culturing the cells in high doses of IL-2 (154). Whether this occurs *in vivo* is not known.

Major Histocompatibility Complex–Dependent Modulation of Cell Surface Ly49 Receptors

The shaping of the functional repertoire may also be influenced by MHC-dependent changes in inhibitory receptor expression levels. For example, the cell surface level of a given Ly49 receptor is generally significantly lower in mice that express an MHC ligand for that receptor (155). Each Ly49 receptor is affected independently, depending on its reactivity with available MHC molecules. The lowered cell surface level has been shown to correlate with a decreased sensitivity of the cell to inhibition through that receptor (156). These alterations may participate in fine-tuning the repertoire. For example, the level of a Ly49 receptor is expected to be higher in mice that express a weak MHC ligand for that receptor than in mice expressing a strong MHC ligand. The higher expression would presumably enhance the sensitivity of the NK cell to inhibition by the weak ligand. MHC-dependent alterations in cell surface receptor levels are not observed for either of the other MHC-specific inhibitory receptor families, KIR and CD94/NKG2A, which suggests that such fine-tuning is accomplished by other means for these receptors (71,149).

MHC-induced changes in the level of a Ly49 receptor on the cell surface is a post–messenger ribonucleic acid (RNA) event, which suggests that it may reflect receptor internalization after ligand engagement (157). In accordance with this possibility, the phenotype is not a stable property of the cell, as shown by cell transfer experiments (158).

A Developmental Process Prevents the Expression of "Too Many" Self–Major Histocompatibility Complex–Specific Receptors

The preceding discussion suggests that a selective process to equip all NK cells with at least one self MHC-specific inhibitory receptor is unlikely. However, MHC molecules of the host do influence the receptor repertoire in a different way. Several studies demonstrate that the frequency of NK cells expressing two or more receptors specific for self MHC molecules is limited by a developmental process (157,159). As discussed previously, during their development, NK cells "switch on" different Ly49 genes progressively in a cumulative manner. Once the cell acquires receptors specific for MHC molecules of the host, receptor engagement inhibits expression of new receptors by the cell (Fig. 6). One consequence of this process is that the NK cells in class I MHC–deficient mice express a greater average number of different Ly49 receptors per cell than do the NK cells in normal mice. Evidence for this feedback mechanism came from studies in which mice were provided a transgenically encoded Ly49 receptor expressed by all developing NK cells. In a host expressing the cognate class I MHC molecule, expression of endogenously encoded Ly49 receptors was reduced (134,157,160,161). In contrast, in mice lacking expression of class I MHC molecules, the transgene did not inhibit expression of endogenously encoded Ly49 receptors.

What is the adaptive value of such a process? The outcome is to constrain the number of different inhibitory receptors specific for self MHC that each NK cell expresses. As a result, the process prevents the development of NK cells that are overinhibited and therefore insensitive to modest reductions in class I MHC expression that may occur in infected or transformed cells. Furthermore, the process is expected to result in a greater percentage of NK cells that express inhibitory receptors for only one of the few self class I MHC molecules expressed by the animal. As discussed previously, such NK cells are of special use for attacking infected or transformed cells that selectively extinguish expression of some, but not all, of the host's class I MHC molecules.

ROLE OF NATURAL KILLER CELLS IN DISEASE AND PERTINENT EFFECTOR FUNCTIONS

Natural Killer Cell Effector Functions

The primary effector functions of NK cells are cytolysis and cytokine release. In several scenarios, a key biologically important function of these cells is production of proinflammatory cytokines, especially IFN-γ and TNF-α. IFN-γ is also produced by Th1 cells and CTLs, but in the early stages of many immune responses, the cytokine is produced principally by NK cells. IFN-γ, like other interferons, induces an antiviral state in uninfected cells, but it also has numerous activities distinct from those of the other interferons (162). Important among these is its capacity to activate macrophages. Activated macrophages are more effective in fusing phagosomes with lysozymes and produce potent antimicrobial substances such as oxygen radicals, nitric oxide, antimicrobial peptides, and proteases. Therefore, activated macrophages exhibit greatly enhanced capacity to destroy both intracellular and extracellular pathogens, including bacteria, parasites, and viruses. Activation of macrophages by IFN-γ is enhanced by TNF-α, which is also produced by stimulated NK cells.

Cytotoxicity by NK cells is another key effector function. NK cytotoxicity of most sensitive target cells *in vitro* is mediated through the production of cytotoxic granules containing perforin and granzymes, similar to CTL cytotoxicity (163). However, NK cells can also mediate cell lysis through several other mechanisms, including the Fas-Fas ligand pathway (164), the TNF-related apoptosis-inducing ligand (TRAIL) pathway (165), and membrane TNF-α pathway (166).

NK cells also have the potential to modulate adaptive immune responses in several ways. For example, in addition to activating macrophages as described previously, IFN-γ also induces expression of class II MHC by macrophages and certain other cells and higher levels of class I MHC expression on numerous cell types (162). Molecules involved in antigen processing, such as the TAP molecules, are also induced by IFN-γ. Induction of these molecules can lead to greatly enhanced T-cell responses to an antigen. Furthermore, IFN-γ is known to promote the differentiation of Th1 cells and to promote immunoglobulin class switching to IgG2a. Therefore, IFN-γ produced by NK cells early in an infection has the potential to influence the immune response in numerous ways. Following is a summary of some of the roles of NK cells in various infections and diseases, along with information regarding the effector systems involved.

Viral Infections

Depletion of NK cells renders mice more susceptible to infection with viruses in several families, among them herpesviruses [MCMV, herpes simplex virus 1 (HSV-1)], orthomyxoviruses (influenza virus), picornaviruses (Coxsackie virus), poxviruses (vaccinia virus, ectromelia virus), and a coronavirus (mouse hepatitis virus) (167) [reviewed by Biron et al. (168)]. In humans, an inverse correlation has been demonstrated between NK cell activity and susceptibility to infection with various viruses, including herpesviruses (HSV-1, Epstein-Barr virus, HCMV) and a papovavirus (papilloma virus) (168). In HIV-seropositive patients, low NK cell numbers correlate with more rapid progression toward the acquired immunodeficiency syndrome (168). Particularly informative was the study of a single patient with a specific deficiency in NK cells who acquired recurrent infections with various herpesviruses, including varicella-zoster virus (chicken pox), HCMV, and HSV (169). NK cells do not play a role in all viral infections, however. For example, NK cells play no demonstrable role in controlling infections of mice with lymphocytic choriomeningitis virus, despite the fact that the virus leads to strong early induction of NK cell cytotoxic activity (167).

Induction of NK cell effector functions generally occurs within a day or two after primary viral infection, long before the adaptive immune response develops (Fig. 7). Depletion of NK cells at this early time in mice can strongly impair control of the virus infection, leading in some cases to death (170). As the infection proceeds and the adaptive immune response develops, T cells generally play an increasingly important role in controlling the infection and are usually, if not always, necessary to actually eliminate the virus (Fig. 7). Furthermore, elimination of NK cells in the later stages of MCMV infection has been shown to have no effect on viral titers (170). Hence, in viral infections, NK cells are thought to play a central role primarily in the early stages of the response, in which they function to restrain viral replication until the adaptive immune response is sufficiently developed to control the infection.

IFN-γ produced by NK cells plays a key role in certain viral infections (168). In the case of MCMV, abundant IFN-γ is produced predominantly by NK cells early in the infection. Studies with neutralizing anti–IFN-γ antibodies or mutant mice with a disrupted IFN-γ receptor gene demonstrated that IFN-γ derived from NK cells is essential for controlling MCMV infection in the liver (171,172). In the absence of IFN-γ, there was a large increase of hepatic lesions and impaired control of viral replication in the liver (171). In

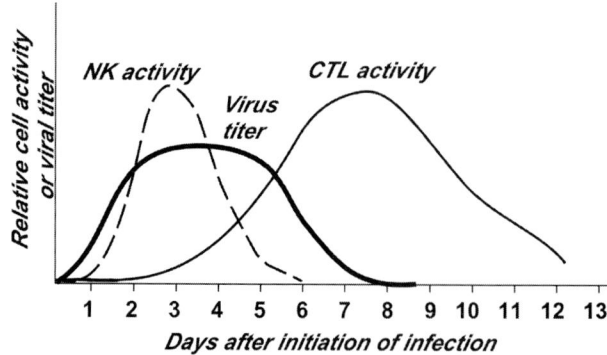

FIG. 7. Time course of effector cell induction in a "typical" primary viral infection. Natural killer (NK) cell activity is upregulated rapidly after infection. In the case of susceptible viruses, the activated NK cells can constrain viral replication in affected organs. Appreciable cytotoxic T-cell (CTL) activity is not detected until several days after onset of infection, in large part because the virus-specific CTLs are extremely rare in unprimed animals and must undergo considerable expansion to achieve an effective dose. CTLs are nevertheless necessary for clearance of most viruses. Viral titers usually do not decline until CTL activity reaches an appreciable level.

contrast, IFN-γ produced by NK cells is relatively unimportant in controlling MCMV replication in another site of infection, the spleen.

NK cell cytotoxicity against sensitive targets is also strongly up-regulated early in the course of MCMV infection. Studies of mice with a mutation in the perforin gene demonstrated that perforin-dependent cytotoxicity plays an important role in controlling MCMV replication in the spleen but little or no role in the liver (172,173). It therefore appears that both IFN-γ and cytotoxicity play important roles in controlling MCMV infection, albeit at different sites of infection. The differential role of cytotoxicity in the two organ sites may be related to the fact that different types of target cells are infected in the two sites: hepatocytes in the liver and lymphocytes in the spleen. In general, NK cells preferentially lyse lymphohematopoietic cells, in comparison with other cell types.

NK cytotoxicity through TRAIL has been implicated in control of another virus, encephalomyocarditis virus (EMCV). TRAIL expression by NK cells is up-regulated by IFN-α/IFN-β produced early in the infection. Blockade of TRAIL with antibodies impaired the early control of EMCV *in vivo,* and prevented the lysis of primary EMCV-infected fibroblasts *in vitro.*

Intracellular Microbes

NK cells also play a significant role in immunity against microbes that replicate intracellularly. Among those studied are bacteria [*Listeria monocytogenes* (174), *Mycobacteria avium* (175)] and parasites [*Leishmania major* (176), *Toxoplasma gondii* (177)]. In general, IFN-γ production by NK cells appears to play a significant role in controlling the early stages of these infections, before adaptive immune responses develop.

In the case of the intracellular bacterium *L. monocytogenes,* IFN-γ produced by NK cells in T cell–deficient mice leads to the induction of antimicrobial activity in infected macrophages and has been reported to limit a primary infection without eliminating the bacteria from the infected animal (174). Inhibitor studies suggest that nitric oxide production, induced in macrophages by IFN-γ, mediates a potent listericidal effect. NK cells are not essential for controlling the early stages of infection in at least some normal animals, however, because other cells also produce sufficient IFN-γ at these early stages (178). Although NK cells reportedly limit the early growth of *Listeria,* subsequent elimination of the bacteria requires the action of T cells.

In infections with intracellular parasites, NK cell activation of macrophages through the action of IFN-γ is also important. As in *Listeria* infections, NK cells appear to play a redundant role with T cells early in the course of infections with the intracellular parasite *T. gondii* (177). However, in the case of the protozoan intracellular parasite *L. major,* NK cells apparently play a significant nonredundant role. In a mouse strain that is genetically highly resistant to *L. major,* such as C3H/HeN mice, strong NK cell responses were observed in infected mice, and NK cell depletion resulted in reduced control of the parasites in the early stages of infection. The impaired immunity correlated with reduced IFN-γ production (176), in line with reports that early containment of *L. major* is abrogated in mice deficient in the capacity to produce nitric oxide (179). Mouse strains that generate a weaker NK cell response, such as C57BL/6 mice, tend to be less resistant to *L. major*; in these mice, IFN-γ produced by CD4$^+$ T cells plays a more important role in controlling the infection (180).

Cancer

The cancer immunosurveillance hypothesis, originally proposed by Burnet (181), postulated that the immune system destroys many nascent tumors. It is well established that various components of the immune system, including T cells, antibodies, and NK cells, can exert potent antitumor activity. In the case of NK cells, a hallmark activity is lysis of tumor cells *in vitro,* as discussed throughout this chapter. However, NK cells can also exert a potent barrier to tumor cell growth *in vivo,* as illustrated in many studies. For example, growth of certain subcutaneously transplanted tumor cell lines and metastasis of a malignant melanoma cell line are much more severe when NK cells are depleted in mice (16,182,183). Also, tumor cell lines expressing high levels of ligands for the NKG2D receptor are completely rejected by NK cells in syngeneic mice (104,106). Furthermore, the efficacy of several tumor vaccines depends on NK1.1$^+$ cells, which suggests that NK cells or NK1.1$^+$ T cells or both play a key role in these responses (184,185). Finally, the treatment of human cancer

patients with IL-2–activated autologous cell preparations that are highly enriched for NK cells (lymphokine-activated killer cells) has yielded some, albeit limited, clinical improvement and extended lifespan, especially in the case of patients with metastatic melanoma (186).

Despite the ability of various components of the immune system to reject tumors in the experimental models described previously, enthusiasm for the cancer immunosurveillance hypothesis waned when it was reported that certain immunodeficient mouse strains have no higher incidence of spontaneous tumors than do normal mice. However, reports have yielded contrasting results and have led to a resurgence of support for the hypothesis. One study demonstrated an increase in the incidence of spontaneous or carcinogen-induced tumors in mice lacking B and T cells because of a mutation in the recombination activating gene 2 (RAG2) component of the V(D)J recombinase (187). Equally striking were the reports of a higher incidence of tumors in mice harboring genetic deficiencies in molecules such as the IFN-γ receptor α chain or perforin (187–189). These molecules are made largely by T cells and NK cells, which suggests a critical role for one or both of these lymphocyte subsets in tumor surveillance. Although the published studies do not clearly discriminate the roles played by NK cells versus T cells, some of the evidence is consistent with a role for NK cells in antitumor immunity. In response to the carcinogen methylcholanthrene, for example, perforin-deficient mice developed sarcomas at a lower threshold dose than did normal mice, and the tumors appeared more rapidly at higher carcinogen doses (188). Depletion of CD8$^+$ T cells had no effect on the incidence or kinetics of sarcoma development, leaving NK cells or CD8$^-$ cytolytic T cells as likely effector cells. The tumors that developed in perforin-deficient mice expressed low levels of class I MHC molecules and were sensitive to NK cells but did not express class II MHC molecules necessary to stimulate CD4$^+$ T cells. Accordingly, it was proposed that NK cells provide significant protection from methylcholanthrene-induced sarcomas. In another study, the frequency of spontaneous disseminated lymphoma was much higher in perforin-deficient mice than in normal mice, but it was not determined whether perforin from T cells or NK cells was responsible for lymphoma surveillance in normal mice (189).

A role for TRAIL-induced killing by NK cells in tumor control has also been demonstrated. Blockade of TRAIL by antibodies led to a much higher rate of fibrosarcoma development in normal mice treated with limiting doses of the carcinogen methylcholanthrene. The protective effect of TRAIL was at least partly mediated by NK cells (190).

Mice deficient in IFN-γ or responsiveness to IFN-γ also exhibit higher rates of spontaneous and carcinogen-induced tumors (191). The protective effect of IFN-γ has been attributed in part to elevated expression of MHC molecules and other molecules involved in antigen processing and to the consequently enhanced T cell response, but other pathways may also be involved. For example, although RAG2 knockout mice developed spontaneous tumors at a higher rate than did normal mice, an even higher rate of tumor development was observed in mice deficient in both RAG2 and STAT1 (187). STAT1 is a transcription factor involved in signaling by the IFN-γ and IFN-α/IFN-β receptors. Furthermore, the double-deficient mice, unlike RAG2- or STAT1-deficient mice, developed mammary tumors at a high rate. These experiments suggest that tumor surveillance is mediated in part by IFN-dependent but T cell–independent mechanisms. The data are consistent with a role for NK cells in tumor surveillance, although this remains to be definitively tested.

NATURAL KILLER CELL ACTIVATION

It is commonly believed that NK cells are perpetually active and do not require prior stimulation ("priming"). It is true that the massive clonal expansion that often accompanies priming of B and T cells does not occur during NK cell activation. On the other hand, NK cells do require an activation step *in vivo* to achieve full effector status. For example, NK cells isolated directly from pathogen-free mice in a "clean" animal facility typically exhibit little if any activity against various NK-sensitive target cells. Preactivation of the cells *in vivo* or *in vitro* is necessary for the elaboration of full effector function. For experimental purposes, one commonly used NK cell activator *in vivo* is double-stranded RNA, typically in the form of polyinosine:polycytidylic acid [poly(I:C)] (see later discussion). *In vitro,* NK cells from unmanipulated animals are usually activated by culturing the cells in IL-2 or IL-15, which yields lymphokine-activated killer cells.

Under physiological circumstances, NK cell activation *in vivo* can probably occur by several pathways. In some cases, NK cell activation occurs as a consequence of direct interactions with other cells. As discussed previously, for example, infected, transformed, or stressed cells can up-regulate cell surface molecules that stimulate NK cells through stimulatory receptors such as NKG2D, NKp46, NKp30, or NKp44. In addition, dendritic cells (DCs) play an important role in activating NK cells (192) [reviewed by Zitvogel (193)]. The DCs must contact the NK cells in order to activate them, but the relevant NK cell receptors and ligands on the DC have not been identified. Freshly isolated DCs are relatively ineffective at stimulating NK cells *in vitro,* but "mature" DCs that have been exposed to inflammatory stimuli or appropriate cytokines are quite effective. This pathway provides one example in which inflammatory signals, such as microbial products that stimulate DCs, can indirectly activate NK cells. Reciprocally, studies indicate that NK cells, once activated, can stimulate DCs to mature. Therefore, stimuli that activate either cell type could lead to progressive activation of the other cell type. In cases of intense NK cell activation, the resulting positive-feedback loop may be dampened or terminated because activated NK cells can acquire the capacity to lyse immature DCs.

Cytokines also play a central role in the activation of NK cells. Sufficient levels of the appropriate cytokines may activate NK cells in the absence of NK receptor stimulation, but in some cases, cytokine signals act cooperatively with NK receptor signals. Among the cytokines that participate in activating NK cells are IFN-α/IFN-β, IL-12, IL-15, and IL-18. A key cytokine involved in NK cell function is IL-15. NK cells express functional IL-15 receptors, which are heterotrimeric molecules composed of the unique IL-15 receptor α chain, the shared IL-2/IL-15 receptor β chain, and the common γ chain shared by several interleukin receptors. IL-15, but not IL-2, is essential for NK cell development (see section on NK cell differentiation). Aside from its role in NK cell development, IL-15 is generally believed to be an important inducer of NK cell functional activity *in vivo* (Fig. 8). Physiologically relevant doses of IL-15 induce NK cell survival, proliferation, and cytotoxicity, and IL-15 and IL-12 synergize in the induction of IFN-γ production by NK cells (194,195). Although IL-2 can also stimulate NK cells, it is produced only by activated T cells, whereas NK cell activation *in vivo* is usually independent of T cells.

IL-15 is produced by stromal cells and activated monocytes, macrophages, and dendritic cells. The stimuli that regulate IL-15 production are incompletely characterized, but production by human monocytes can be stimulated by

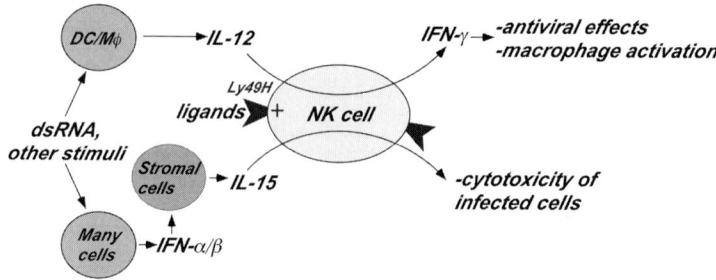

FIG. 8. The role of natural killer (NK) cells in mouse cytomegalovirus (MCMV) infections. Interferon (IFN)–γ, produced by NK cells in response to interleukin (IL)–12, plays a central role in control of viral replication in the liver. In contrast, for control of viral replication in the spleen, NK cytotoxicity induced by IFN-α/IFN-β is crucial. Both IL-12 and IFN-α/IFN-β are induced early in the infection in response to viral cues to the innate immune system, including double-stranded ribonucleic acid. IFN-α/IFN-β induces stromal cells to produce IL-15, which stimulates NK cell cytotoxicity. Signaling through cell surface receptors such as Ly49H is also crucial in mounting an effective NK cell response in both organs.

bacterial lipopolysaccharide, which suggests a role for Toll-like receptors in these cells. In bone marrow stromal cells, interferons probably play an important role in IL-15 production (Fig. 8). This conclusion is based on the finding that mutant mice lacking the transcription factor IRF-1 do not express IL-15 in bone marrow stromal cells and fail to produce NK cells. Furthermore, IRF-1 transactivates the IL-15 promoter in transfected cells (137).

IFN-α and IFN-β also play an important role in NK cell activation. These two interferon families exhibit similar biological activities and are induced in many cell types as a consequence of viral infection. IFN-α/IFN-β is induced in response to double-stranded RNA that arises in the life cycle of many viruses (Fig. 8). Double-stranded RNA can lead to cellular activation through intracellular pathways, including the double-stranded RNA–dependent protein kinase and RNA-dependent protein kinase (RNase L) (196). Alternatively, these cytokines are induced by the interaction of double-stranded RNA, including poly(I:C), with a membrane receptor called Toll-like receptor 3 that is expressed by macrophages and possibly other cells (197).

IFN-α/IFN-β clearly play a role in the induction of NK responses in certain viral infections. NK cell activation by IFN-α/IFN-β is probably caused partly by the induction of IL-15 secretion by stromal cells (Fig. 8) but may also result from direct effects on NK cells. In the case of MCMV, IFN-α/IFN-β are induced early in the infection, correlating with induction of NK cytotoxic activity. Furthermore, antibody neutralization of IFN-α/IFN-β impairs the induction of NK cytotoxicity (173). The capacity of NK cells to limit MCMV replication in the liver is also impaired by neutralization of IFN-α/IFN-β, though evidence suggests that this is not due to impaired NK cytotoxicity.

Interestingly, while IFN-α/IFN-β induce cytotoxic activity, they do not normally play a decisive role in induction of IFN-γ production by NK cells. In fact, relatively high but physiological doses of IFN-α/IFN-β can inhibit IFN-γ production by NK cells. For example, high systemic levels of IFN-α/IFN-β that are produced during infection with lymphocytic choriomeningitis virus, a virus unrelated to MCMV, appear to inhibit IFN-γ production by NK cells (198); this may be one reason why NK cells are unable to inhibit lymphocytic choriomeningitis virus replication (167).

IL-12, a cytokine produced by macrophages and DCs and originally called NK cell stimulatory factor, plays an important role in induction of IFN-γ production by NK cells (Fig. 8). Production of IL-12 by monocytes and DCs is induced by double-stranded RNA and other stimuli (197). In cell cultures, NK cells treated with IL-12 are induced to secrete IFN-γ. Several other cytokines, including IL-15, IL-2, and TNF-α, synergize with IL-12 in this response (199). In mice infected with MCMV, neutralization of IL-12 with specific antibodies impairs IFN-γ production by NK cells (200). Interestingly, IL-12 plays little role in induction of NK cell cytotoxicity in the MCMV response. However, because IFN-γ production is more important than cytotoxicity in controlling

MCMV infection in the liver, neutralization of IL-12 lowers the capacity of mice to limit MCMV replication in this organ and increases the incidence of hepatic lesions resulting from viral infection (200). Another cytokine, IL-18, appears to play a similar role to IL-12 in NK cell activation. This conclusion arises from the observation that NK cell activation is nearly abolished in knockout mice lacking both IL-12 and IL-18 but is only partially impaired in mice lacking one or the other of these cytokines (201).

ROLE OF NATURAL KILLER CELLS IN MOUSE CYTOMEGALOVIRUS INFECTION

The most detailed knowledge of the function of NK cells *in vivo* comes from studies of MCMV infection. Throughout this chapter, the NK cell response in MCMV infection has been discussed in different contexts. Because of the detailed knowledge of this infection, it is useful to summarize and elaborate on various aspects here in order to provide a comprehensive view of the NK cell response to a specific pathogen (Fig. 8).

In resistant strains of mice, NK cells are activated rapidly in response to primary MCMV infection, reaching a peak on the second to third days of infection. In the first week of infection, NK cells restrain but do not eliminate viral replication in both the liver and the spleen, two of the main sites of viral replication. Typical of other viral infections, the CD8$^+$ T-cell response develops rapidly in the first week and is ultimately necessary to clear the virus. The importance of NK cells in restraining virus replication in the early phases is illustrated by the fact that mice depleted of NK cells rapidly succumb to a relatively high infectious dose (170).

The NK cell response to MCMV in mice may be controlled in part by NKG2D or one of the other stimulatory NK cell receptors discussed previously. A precedent is the finding that the NKG2D ligands MICA and MICB are induced in human liver cells infected with HCMV, leading to activation of NK cells through NKG2D (75). However, direct homologs of MICA and MICB may not exist in mice, and it is not known whether MCMV induces expression of any of the known mouse NKG2D ligands such as Rae1 or H60. Furthermore, although MCMV and HCMV are members of the same virus family, they are not highly related, which raises the possibility that the immune responses to these viruses differ.

An important stimulatory receptor in the NK cell response to MCMV is Ly49H, the product of the *Cmv1^r* gene (85). The *Cmv* locus controls susceptibility to cytomegalovirus infection among inbred mouse strains. *Cmv1^s* is a null allele of *Ly49h*. The importance of the NK cell response through Ly49H is illustrated by the sensitivity of homozygous *Cmv1^s* mice to the lethal effects of MCMV infection (202).

Ly49H is expressed by approximately 50% of NK cells in normal mice. The Ly49H molecule pairs in the cell membrane with KARAP/DAP12, a signaling adapter molecule that contains ITAMs in its cytoplasmic domains. In *Cmv1^r* mice, Ly49H is presumably engaged by a ligand expressed as a consequence of MCMV infection. The ligand is a viral gene product called m157, which is expressed in infected cells. *Cmv1ˢ* (MCMV-susceptible) mice exhibit much higher viral titers than do *Cmv1ʳ* (MCMV-resistant) mice on the second to third days of infection, as do *Cmv1ʳ* mice that are injected with an antibody that blocks the Ly49H receptor (85). Thus, Ly49H plays a critical early role in controlling the infection. It is therefore somewhat surprising that both Ly49H⁺ and Ly49H⁻ NK cells are induced to proliferate and produce IFN-γ at these early stages (203). In view of this finding, it remains to be determined how Ly49H confers early resistance to the virus. It is likely that the Ly49H⁺ subset is preferentially stimulated, as revealed by a selective clonal expansion of these cells at later times during the infection (203).

Various organs are sites of MCMV infection, and the NK cell response differs in mechanism according to the affected organ. The liver and spleen have been studied in the greatest detail. NK cells play a central role in the early control of viral replication in both organs, as illustrated by cell-depletion experiments.

In the spleen, cytolysis of infected cells by NK cells plays a significant role in limiting viral replication, as illustrated by analysis of mice with a disrupted perforin gene (172). In contrast, perforin-dependent cytolysis by NK cells plays little or no role in controlling MCMV infection in the liver, perhaps because hepatocytes are generally less susceptible than lymphoid cells to cytolysis. Induction of actively cytotoxic NK cells from quiescent precursors is dependent on IFN-α/IFN-β, production of which is induced by viral infection (173). IL-15, itself regulated by IFN-α/IFN-β, probably also plays a role in the induction of cytotoxic activity, whereas IL-12 plays little or no role in this capacity during MCMV infection (200). It remains possible that IFN-α/IFN-β and IL-15 activate NK cells synergistically in conjunction with the stimulation of NK cell surface receptors by viral or cellular products that are up-regulated in infected cells. Ly49H engagement, however, is apparently not required for the induction of cytotoxic activity in NK cells (203). The Ly49H receptor may instead play a role in the effector phase of the response by triggering cytolysis of infected cells by previously activated NK cells.

IFN-γ production plays little role in controlling MCMV infection in the spleen, as illustrated by antibody neutralization studies or analyses of mice with a mutation in the IFN-γ receptor (171,172). Conversely, IFN-γ produced by NK cells is critical for limiting viral replication in the liver, where cytolysis plays no apparent role. IFN-γ production by NK cells in MCMV infection requires the action of IL-12, possibly in synergy with IL-15 or TNF-α or both. All three of these cytokines are produced by macrophages and DCs in response to double-stranded RNA and possibly other viral products. Stimulatory NK cell receptors may also play a role in IFN-γ production by NK cells, although Ly49H engagement does not appear to be required, at least in the initial phases of the response (203). IFN-α/IFN-β play no

demonstrable role in IFN-γ production by NK cells in this infection (198), although they appear to enhance the capacity of NK cells to control MCMV in the liver by an undefined mechanism.

IFN-γ produced by NK cells limits viral replication in the liver and reduces the incidence of hepatic lesions (171). Viral control by IFN-γ may involve induction of the antiviral state in hepatocytes, as well as stimulation of the synthesis of antimicrobial substances, such as nitric oxide, by macrophages (172). Although IFN-γ produced by NK cells outside of the liver could, in theory, act systemically in the liver, there is a clear requirement that the cells be focally concentrated in the liver for efficacy in that organ. NK cells are attracted to the liver by the action of the chemokine MIP-1α, which is produced there immediately after infection (204). In infected mice treated with neutralizing antibodies specific for MIP-1α or with a mutation in the MIP-1α gene, NK cells function normally in the spleen but fail to accumulate in the liver. As a consequence, these mice exhibit poor early control of MCMV replication in the liver. It is not yet established why NK cell penetration of the liver is required for control of MCMV. It may reflect a requirement for high local concentrations of IFN-γ in the liver, or it may indicate that contact with hepatocytes is necessary for the full elaboration of other necessary NK cell functions.

CONCLUSION AND PERSPECTIVE

It is fair to say that there has been an explosion in information concerning NK cells since the early 1990s, especially with regard to their receptors and specificity, the cytokine networks that regulate them, and their roles in certain diseases. Close scrutiny of the cells reveals that although they are appropriately considered effector cells of the innate immune system, they exhibit some features normally associated with adaptive immune cells such as B and T cells, especially with regard to the specificity of the cells at a population level. Furthermore, NK cells have evolved numerous interactions with cells of the adaptive immune system, as well as adaptations that appear to specifically back up or reinforce the adaptive immune response.

One feature of the NK cell compartment that is normally considered a hallmark of adaptive immunity is the existence of a repertoire of specificities (see the section on formation of the repertoire and self-tolerance of NK cells). As is the case for B and T cells, individual NK cells vary in specificity because of the selective expression of specific receptors. From a bank of 10 to 15 class I MHC–specific inhibitory receptor genes, a more or less random subset of a few receptors is expressed by each cell. Some of the stimulatory receptors are also expressed by subsets of NK cells. In fact, during MCMV infection, a subset of NK cells expressing a specific stimulatory receptor undergoes clonal expansion, another feature normally associated with adaptive immunity. Of course, the NK cell repertoire differs in key respects from that of B cells or T cells. Individual NK cells express more than one receptor, as opposed to the single specificity characteristic of most B and T cells, and many of the NK receptors are inhibitory rather than stimulatory. Moreover, the diversity of the repertoire is not as random or nearly as complex as that of B cells or T cells. Nevertheless, the distribution of different receptors to different cells means that NK cells, like B cells and T cells, exhibit clonally variable specificity for target cells.

The interactions between NK cells and the adaptive immune response are numerous. Induction of adaptive immunity may be enhanced or inhibited by NK cells, which can either stimulate DC maturation or kill DCs, depending on the specific circumstances (see the section on NK cell activation). Cytokines produced by NK cells, such as IFN-γ, may also, in some cases, influence the tenor of an adaptive immune response. Some of the receptors expressed by NK cells also suggest a close coevolution of these cells with the adaptive immune response. An obvious example is the Fc receptor, through which NK cells mediate antibody-dependent cellular cytotoxicity. A more striking set of examples is the MHC-specific inhibitory and stimulatory receptors (see the section on MHC-specific inhibitory and stimulatory receptors). It is generally believed that the inhibitory MHC-specific receptors are an evolutionary adaptation that enables NK cells to attack cells that down-regulate class I MHC molecules. Class Ia MHC molecules present antigens to T cells, and MHC downregulation is thought to occur in the context of evasion of T cell immunity. If these assumptions are correct, the implication is that the MHC-specific inhibitory receptor system arose in its present form after T cells appeared and has since coevolved with the T cell–MHC system.

The NK cell system is therefore particularly interesting in that it appears to blur some of the distinctions between adaptive and innate immunity. A possible lesson is that the labels *innate* and *adaptive* may apply more accurately to systems of molecules or receptors than to types of cells. It is likely that in the course of evolution, recognition systems were added or lost from a given cell type to diversify or restrict its functional potential, which makes it difficult to categorize the cell in the usual terms. In the case of NK cells, for example, it is possible that the recognition of ligands that are induced by infection or transformation are the most ancient functions. The MHC-specific receptors could have been "added" later to broaden the functional capabilities of the cells as the need arose. Some blurring between adaptive and innate functions has already been revealed for other immune cell types, and it appears likely that the distinctions will grow even hazier as the knowledge base grows.

ACKNOWLEDGMENTS

I thank the members of my laboratory since the late 1980s for providing stimulating discussions, innumerable ideas, and dedicated research in the field of NK cell biology and specificity. For providing excellent advice on the manuscript, I am particularly grateful to Drs. Christopher McMahon, Russell Vance, and Andreas Diefenbach.

REFERENCES

1. Herberman RB, Nunn ME, Lavrin DH, et al. Effect of antibody to theta antigen on cell-mediated immunity induced in syngeneic mice by murine sarcoma virus. *J Natl Cancer Inst* 1973;51:1509–1512.
2. Takasugi M, Mickey MR, Terasaki PI. Reactivity of lymphocytes from normal persons on cultured tumor cells. *Cancer Res* 1973;33:2898–2902.
3. Kiessling R, Klein E, Wigzell H. "Natural" killer cells in the mouse. I. Cytotoxic cells with specificity for mouse Moloney leukemia cells. Specificity and distribution according to genotype. *Eur J Immunol* 1975;5:112–117.
4. Ritz J, Campen TJ, Schmidt RE, et al. Analysis of T-cell receptor gene rearrangement and expression in human natural killer clones. *Science* 1985;228:1540–1543.
5. Dorshkind K, Pollack SB, Bosma MJ, et al. Natural killer (NK) cells are present in mice with severe combined immunodeficiency (SCID). *J Immunol* 1985;134:3798–3801.
6. Long EO, Burshtyn DN, Clark WP, et al. Killer cell inhibitory receptors: diversity, specificity and function. *Immunol Rev* 1997;155:135–144.
7. Vivier E, Daeron M. Immunoreceptor tyrosine-based inhibition motifs. *Immunol Today* 1997;18:286–291.
8. Burshtyn D, Scharenberg A, Wagtmann N, et al. Recruitment of tyrosine phosphatase HCP by the NK cell inhibitory receptor. *Immunity* 1996;4:77–85.
9. Moretta L, Bottino C, Vitale M, et al. Activating receptors and coreceptors involved in human natural killer cell–mediated cytolysis. *Annu Rev Immunol* 2001;19:197–223.
10. Brumbaugh KM, Binstadt BA, Billadeau DD, et al. Functional role for Syk tyrosine kinase in natural killer cell–mediated natural cytotoxicity. *J Exp Med* 1997;186:1965–1974.
11. Diefenbach A, Raulet DH. Strategies for target cell recognition by natural killer cells. *Immunol Rev* 2001;181:170–184.
12. Lanier LL. NK cell receptors. *Annu Rev Immunol* 1998;16:359–393.
13. Brown MG, Scalzo AA, Matsumoto K, et al. The natural killer gene complex: a genetic basis for understanding natural killer cell function and innate immunity. *Immunol Rev* 1997;155:53–65.
14. Moretta A, Bottino C, Vitale M, et al. Receptors for HLA class-I molecules in human natural killer cells. *Annu Rev Immunol* 1996;14:619–648.
15. Trowsdale J, Barten R, Haude A, et al. The genomic context of natural killer receptor extended gene families. *Immunol Rev* 2001;181:20–38.
16. Ljunggren H-G, Karre K. Host resistance directed selectively against H-2–deficient lymphoma variants. *J Exp Med* 1985;162:1745–1759.
17. Storkus WJ, Howell DN, Salter RD, et al. NK susceptibility varies inversely with target cell class I HLA antigen expression. *J Immunol* 1987;138:1657–1659.
18. Garrido F, Ruiz-Cabello F, Cabrera T, et al. Implications for immunosurveillance of altered HLA class I phenotypes in human tumours. *Immunol Today* 1997;18:89–95.
19. Tortorella D, Gewurz BE, Furman MH, et al. Viral subversion of the immune system. *Annu Rev Immunol* 2000;18:861–926.
20. Ljunggren HG, Karre K. In search of the "missing self": MHC molecules and NK cell recognition. *Immunol Today* 1990;11:237–244.
21. Cudkowicz G, Stimpfling JH. Induction of immunity and of unresponsiveness to parental marrow grafts in adult F1 hybrid mice. *Nature* 1964;204:450–453.
22. Bennett M. Biology and genetics of hybrid resistance. *Adv Immunol* 1987;41:333–445.
23. Murphy W, Kumar V, Bennett M. Rejection of bone marrow allografts by mice with severe combined immunodeficiency (SCID). *J Exp Med* 1987;165:1212–1217.
24. Ohlen C, Kling G, Höglund P, et al. Prevention of allogeneic bone

marrow graft rejection by H-2 transgene in donor mice. *Science* 1989;246:666–668.

25. Bix M, Liao N-S, Zijlstra M, et al. Rejection of class I MHC–deficient hemopoietic cells by irradiated MHC-matched mice. *Nature* 1991;349:329–331.

26. Liao N, Bix M, Zijlstra M, et al. MHC class I deficiency: susceptibility to natural killer (NK) cells and impaired NK activity. *Science* 1991;253:199–202.

27. Sentman CL, Olsson MY, Salcedo M, et al. H-2 allele–specific protection from NK cell lysis *in vitro* for lymphoblasts but not tumor targets. Protection mediated by alpha 1/alpha 2 domains. *J Immunol* 1994;153:5482–5490.

28. Takei F, McQueen KL, Maeda M, et al. Ly49 and CD94/NKG2: developmentally regulated expression and evolution. *Immunol Rev* 2001;181:90–103.

29. Valiante NM, Lienert K, Shilling HG, et al. Killer cell receptors: keeping pace with MHC class I evolution. *Immunol Rev* 1997;155:155–164.

30. Karlhofer FM, Ribaudo RK, Yokoyama WM. MHC class I alloantigen specificity of Ly-49+ IL-2 activated natural killer cells. *Nature* 1992;358:66–70.

31. Takei F, Brennan J, Mager DL. The Ly49 family: genes, proteins and recognition of class I MHC. *Immunol Rev* 1997;155:67–77.

32. Hanke T, Takizawa H, McMahon CW, et al. Direct assessment of MHC class I binding by seven Ly49 inhibitory NK cell receptors. *Immunity* 1999;11:67–77.

33. Correa I, Raulet DH. Binding of diverse peptides to MHC class I molecules inhibits target cell lysis by activated natural killer cells. *Immunity* 1995;2:61–71.

34. Franksson L, Sundback J, Achour A, et al. Peptide dependency and selectivity of the NK cell inhibitory receptor Ly-49C. *Eur J Immunol* 1999;29:2748–2758.

35. Matsumoto N, Ribaudo RK, Abastado JP, et al. The lectin like NK cell receptor Ly49A recognizes a carbohydrate independent epitope on its MHC ligand. *Immunity* 1998;8:245–254.

36. Natarajan K, Boyd LF, Schuck P, et al. Interaction of the NK cell inhibitory receptor Ly49A with H-2Dd: identification of a site distinct from the TCR site. *Immunity* 1999;11:591–601.

37. Tormo J, Natarajan K, Margulies DH, et al. Crystal structure of a lectin-like natural killer cell receptor bound to its MHC class I ligand. *Nature* 1999;402:623–631.

38. Matsumoto N, Mitsuki M, Tajima K, et al. The functional binding site for the C-type lectin-like natural killer cell receptor Ly49A spans three domains of its major histocompatibility complex class I ligand. *J Exp Med* 2001;193:147–157.

39. Nakamura MC, Hayashi S, Niemi EC, et al. Activating Ly-49D and inhibitory Ly-49A natural killer cell receptors demonstrate distinct requirements for interaction with H2-D(d). *J Exp Med* 2000;192:447–454.

40. Nakamura MC, Linnemeyer PA, Niemi EC, et al. Mouse Ly-49D recognizes H-2D(d) and activates natural killer cell cytotoxicity. *J Exp Med* 1999;189:493–500.

41. George TC, Mason LH, Ortaldo JR, et al. Positive recognition of MHC class I molecules by the Ly49D receptor of murine NK cells. *J Immunol* 1999;162:2035–2043.

42. Idris AH, Smith HR, Mason LH, et al. The natural killer gene complex genetic locus Chok encodes Ly-49D, a target recognition receptor that activates natural killing. *Proc Natl Acad Sci U S A* 1999;96:6330–6335.

43. Depatie C, Lee SH, Stafford A, et al. Sequence-ready BAC contig, physical, and transcriptional map of a 2-Mb region overlapping the mouse chromosome 6 host-resistance locus *Cmv1*. *Genomics* 2000;66:161–174.

44. Ciccone E, Viale O, Pende D, et al. Specific lysis of allogeneic cells after activation of CD3-lymphocytes in mixed lymphocyte culture. *J Exp Med* 1988;168:2403–2408.

45. Ciccone E, Colonna M, Viale O, et al. Susceptibility or resistance to lysis by alloreactive natural killer cells is governed by a gene in the human major histocompatibility complex between BF and HLA-B. *Proc Natl Acad Sci U S A* 1990;87:9794–9797.

46. Moretta A, Bottino C, Pende D, et al. Identification of four subsets of human CD3$^-$CD16$^+$ natural killer (NK) cells by the expression of clonally distributed functional surface molecules: correlation between subset assignment of NK clones and ability to mediate specific alloantigen recognition. *J Exp Med* 1990;172:1589–1598.

47. Wagtmann N, Biassoni R, Cantoni C, et al. Molecular clones of the p58 natural killer cell receptor reveal Ig-related molecules with diversity in both the extra- and intra-cellular domains. *Immunity* 1995;2:439–449.

48. Colonna M, Samaridis J. Cloning of immunoglobulin-superfamily members associated with HLA-C and HLA-B recognition by human natural killer cells. *Science* 1995;268:405–408.

49. D'Andrea A, Chang C, Bacon K, et al. Molecular cloning of NKB1: A natural killer cell receptor for HLA-B allotypes. *J Immunol* 1995;155:2306–2310.

50. Boyington JC, Brooks AG, Sun PD. Structure of killer cell immunoglobulin-like receptors and their recognition of the class I MHC molecules. *Immunol Rev* 2001;181:66–78.

51. Vales-Gomez M, Reyburn HT, Erskine RA, et al. Differential binding to HLA-C of p50-activating and p58-inhibitory natural killer cell receptors. *Proc Natl Acad Sci U S A* 1998;95:14326–14331.

52. Boyington JC, Motyka SA, Schuck P, et al. Crystal structure of an NK cell immunoglobulin-like receptor in complex with its class I MHC ligand. *Nature* 2000;405:537–543.

53. Peruzzi M, Parker KC, Long EO, et al. Peptide sequence requirements for the recognition of HLA-B*2705 by specific natural killer cells. *J Immunol* 1996;157:3350–3356.

54. Houchins JP, Yabe T, McSherry C, et al. DNA sequence analysis of NKG2, a family of related cDNA clones encoding type II integral membrane proteins on human natural killer cells. *J Exp Med* 1991;173:1017–1020.

55. Vance RE, Kraft JR, Altman JD, et al. Mouse CD94/NKG2A is a natural killer cell receptor for the nonclassical MHC class I molecule Qa-1b. *J Exp Med* 1998;188:1841–1848.

56. Vance RE, Jamieson AM, Raulet DH. Recognition of the class Ib molecule Qa-1(b) by putative activating receptors CD94/NKG2C and CD94/NKG2E on mouse natural killer cells. *J Exp Med* 1999;190:1801–1812.

57. Lanier LL, Corliss B, Wu J, et al. Association of DAP12 with activating CD94/NKG2C NK cell receptors. *Immunity* 1998;8:693–701.

58. Braud VM, Allan DSJ, O'Callaghan CA, et al. HLA-E binds to natural killer cell receptors CD94/NKG2A, B, and C. *Nature* 1998;391:795–799.

59. Lee N, Llano M, Carretero M, et al. HLA-E is a major ligand for the natural killer inhibitory receptor CD94/NKG2A. *Proc Natl Acad Sci U S A* 1998;95:5199–5204.

60. Braud V, Jones EY, McMichael A. The human major histocompatibility complex class Ib molecule HLA-E binds signal sequence-derived peptides with primary anchor residues at positions 2 and 9. *Eur J Immunol* 1997;27:1164–1169.

61. Kurepa Z, Forman J. Peptide binding to the class Ib molecule, Qa-1b. *J Immunol* 1997;158:3244–3251.

62. Llano M, Lee N, Navarro F, et al. HLA-E-bound peptides influence recognition by inhibitory and triggering CD94/NKG2 receptors: preferential response to an HLA-G–derived nonamer. *Eur J Immunol* 1998;28:2854–2863.

63. Kraft JR, Vance RE, Pohl J, et al. Analysis of Qa-1(b) peptide binding specificity and the capacity of CD94/NKG2A to discriminate between Qa-1–peptide complexes. *J Exp Med* 2000;192:613–624.

64. Aldrich CJ, DeCloux A, Woods AS, et al. Identification of a Tap-dependent leader peptide recognized by alloreactive T cells specific for a class Ib antigen. *Cell* 1994;79:649–658.

65. Valés-Gómez M, Reyburn HT, Erskine RA, et al. Kinetics and peptide dependency of the binding of the inhibitory NK receptor CD94/NKG2-A and the activating receptor CD94/NKG2-C to HLA-E. *EMBO J* 1999;18:4250–4260.

66. Samaridis J, Colonna M. Cloning of novel immunoglobulin superfamily receptors expressed on human myeloid and lymphoid cells: structural evidence for new stimulatory and inhibitory pathways. *Eur J Immunol* 1997;27:660–665.

67. Cosman D, Fanger N, Borges L, et al. A novel immunoglobulin superfamily receptor for cellular and viral MHC class I molecules. *Immunity* 1997;7:273–282.

68. Miyazaki T, Dierich A, Benoist C, et al. Independent modes of natural killing distinguished in mice lacking Lag3. *Science* 1996;272:405–408.

69. Raulet DH, Held W, Correa I, et al. Specificity, tolerance and developmental regulation of natural killer cells defined by expression of class I–specific Ly49 receptors. *Immunol Rev* 1997;155:41–52.

70. Raulet DH, Vance RE, McMahon CW. Regulation of the natural killer cell receptor repertoire. *Annu Rev Immunol* 2001;19:291–330.

71. Valiante N, Uhberg M, Shilling H, et al. Functionally and structurally distinct NK cell receptor repertoires in the peripheral blood of two human donors. *Immunity* 1997;7:739–751.

72. Grigoriadou K, Menard C, Perarnau B, et al. MHC class Ia molecules alone control NK-mediated bone marrow graft rejection. *Eur J Immunol* 1999;29:3683–3690.

73. Zijlstra M, Auchincloss HJ, Loring JM, et al. Skin graft rejection by beta 2-microglobulin–deficient mice. *J Exp Med* 1992;175:885–893.

74. Correa I, Corral L, Raulet DH. Multiple natural killer cell-activating signals are inhibited by major histocompatibility complex class I expression in target cells. *Eur J Immunol* 1994;24:1323–1331.

75. Groh V, Rhinehart R, Randolph-Habecker J, et al. Costimulation of CD8 $\alpha\beta$ T cells by NKG2D via engagement by MIC induced on virus-infected cells. *Nat Immunol* 2001;2:255–260.

76. Leong CC, Chapman TL, Bjorkman PJ, et al. Modulation of natural killer cell cytotoxicity in human cytomegalovirus infection: the role of endogenous class I major histocompatibility complex and a viral class I homolog. *J Exp Med* 1998;187:1681–1687.

77. Fletcher JM, Prentice HG, Grundy JE. Natural killer cell lysis of cytomegalovirus (CMV)–infected cells correlates with virally induced changes in cell surface lymphocyte function–associated antigen-3 (LFA-3) expression and not with the CMV-induced down-regulation of cell surface class I HLA. *J Immunol* 1998;161:2365–2374.

78. Raska K Jr, Gallimore PH. An inverse relation of the oncogenic potential of adenovirus-transformed cells and their sensitivity to killing by syngeneic natural killer cells. *Virology* 1982;123:8–18.

79. Farrell HE, Vally H, Lynch DM, et al. Inhibition of natural killer cells by a cytomegalovirus MHC class I homologue *in vivo*. *Nature* 1997;386:510–514.

80. Cretney E, Degli-Esposti MA, Densley EH, et al. m144, a murine cytomegalovirus (MCMV)–encoded major histocompatibility complex class I homologue, confers tumor resistance to natural killer cell–mediated rejection. *J Exp Med* 1999;190:435–444.

81. Reyburn HT, Mandelboim O, Vales-Gomez M, et al. The class I MHC homologue of human cytomegalovirus inhibits attack by natural killer cells. *Nature* 1997;386:514–517.

82. Tomasec P, Braud VM, Rickards C, et al. Surface expression of HLA-E, an inhibitor of natural killer cells, enhanced by human cytomegalovirus gpUL40. *Science* 2000;287:1031.

83. Cohen GB, Gandhi RT, Davis DM, et al. The selective downregulation of class I major histocompatibility complex proteins by HIV-1 protects HIV-infected cells from NK cells. *Immunity* 1999;10:661–671.

84. Lee SH, Girard S, Macina D, et al. Susceptibility to mouse cytomegalovirus is associated with deletion of an activating natural killer cell receptor of the C-type lectin superfamily. *Nat Genet* 2001;28:42–45.

85. Brown MG, Dokun AO, Heusel JW, et al. Vital involvement of a natural killer cell activation receptor in resistance to viral infection. *Science* 2001;292:934–937.

86. Daniels KA, Devora G, Lai WC, et al. Murine cytomegalovirus is regulated by a discrete subset of natural killer cells reactive with monoclonal antibody to Ly49H. *J Exp Med* 2001;194:29–44.

87. Arase H, Mocarski ES, Campbell AE, et al. Direct recognition of cytomegalovirus by activating and inhibitory NK cell receptors. *Science* 2002;296:1323–1326.

88. Hazenbos WL, Gessner JE, Hofhuis FM, et al. Impaired IgG-dependent anaphylaxis and Arthus reaction in Fc gamma RIII (CD16) deficient mice. *Immunity* 1996;5:181–188.

89. Pende D, Cantoni C, Rivera P, et al. Role of NKG2D in tumor cell lysis mediated by human NK cells: cooperation with natural cytotoxicity receptors and capability of recognizing tumors of nonepithelial origin. *Eur J Immunol* 2001;31:1076–1086.

90. Vance RE, Tanamachi DM, Hanke T, et al. Cloning of a mouse homolog of CD94 extends the family of C-type lectins on murine natural killer cells. *Eur J Immunol* 1997;27:3236–3241.

91. Ho EL, Heusel JW, Brown MG, et al. Murine Nkg2d and Cd94 are clustered within the natural killer complex and are expressed independently in natural killer cells. *Proc Natl Acad Sci U S A* 1998;95:6320–6325.

92. Bauer S, Groh V, Wu J, et al. Activation of NK cells and T cells by NKG2D, a receptor for stress-inducible MICA. *Science* 1999;285:727–729.

93. Diefenbach A, Jamieson AM, Liu SD, et al. Ligands for the murine NKG2D receptor: expression by tumor cells and activation of NK cells and macrophages. *Nat Immunol* 2000;1:119–126.

94. Cerwenka A, Bakker ABH, McClanahan T, et al. Retinoic acid early inducible genes define a ligand family for the activating NKG2D receptor in mice. *Immunity* 2000;12:721–727.

95. Groh V, Bahram S, Bauer S, et al. Cell stress-regulated human major histocompatibility complex class I gene expressed in gastrointestinal epithelium. *Proc Natl Acad Sci U S A* 1996;93:12445–12450.

96. Li P, Willie ST, Bauer S, et al. Crystal structure of the MHC class I homolog MIC-A, a gammadelta T cell ligand. *Immunity* 1999;10:577–584.

97. Li PW, Morris DL, Willcox BE, et al. Complex structure of the activating immunoreceptor NKG2D and its MHC class I–like ligand MICA. *Nat Immunol* 2001;2:443–451.

98. Groh V, Rhinehart R, Secrist H, et al. Broad tumor-associated expression and recognition by tumor-derived gamma delta T cells of MICA and MICB. *Proc Natl Acad Sci U S A* 1999;96:6879–6884.

99. Nomura M, Zou Z, Joh T, et al. Genomic structures and characterization of Rae1 family members encoding GPI-anchored cell surface proteins and expressed predominantly in embryonic mouse brain. *J Biochem* 1996;120:987–995.

100. Sutherland CL, Chalupny NJ, Cosman D. The UL16-binding proteins, a novel family of MHC class I–related ligands for NKG2D, activate natural killer cell functions. *Immunol Rev* 2001;181:185–192.

101. Radosavljevic M, Cuillerier B, Wilson MJ, et al. A cluster of ten novel MHC class I related genes on human chromosome 6q24.2–q25.3. *Genomics* 2002;79:114–123.

102. O'Callaghan CA, Cerwenka A, Willcox BE, et al. Molecular competition for NKG2D: H60 and RAE1 compete unequally for NKG2D with dominance of H60. *Immunity* 2001;15:201–211.

103. Sutherland CL, Chalupny NJ, Schooley K, et al. UL16-binding proteins, novel MHC class I–related proteins, bind to NKG2D and activate multiple signaling pathways in primary NK cells. *J Immunol* 2002;168:671–679.

104. Diefenbach A, Jensen ER, Jamieson AM, et al. Rae1 and H60 ligands of the NKG2D receptor stimulate tumour immunity. *Nature* 2001;413:165–171.

105. Wu J, Song Y, Bakker AB, et al. An activating immunoreceptor complex formed by NKG2D and DAP10. *Science* 1999;285:730–732.

106. Cerwenka A, Baron JL, Lanier LL. Ectopic expression of retinoic acid early inducible–1 gene (RAE-1) permits natural killer cell–mediated rejection of a MHC class I–bearing tumor *in vivo*. *Proc Natl Acad Sci U S A* 2001;98:11521–11526.

107. Sivori S, Vitale M, Morelli L, et al. p46, a novel natural killer cell–specific surface molecule that mediates cell activation. *J Exp Med* 1997;186:1129–1136.

108. Pende D, Parolini S, Pessino A, et al. Identification and molecular characterization of NKp30, a novel triggering receptor involved in natural cytotoxicity mediated by human natural killer cells. *J Exp Med* 1999;190:1505–1516.

109. Vitale M, Bottino C, Sivori S, et al. NKp44, a novel triggering surface molecule specifically expressed by activated natural killer cells, is involved in non–major histocompatibility complex–restricted tumor cell lysis. *J Exp Med* 1998;187:2065–2072.

110. Biassoni R, Cantoni C, Pende D, et al. Human natural killer cell receptors and co-receptors. *Immunol Rev* 2001;181:203–214.

111. Biassoni R, Pessino A, Bottino C, et al. The murine homologue of the human NKp46, a triggering receptor involved in the induction of natural cytotoxicity. *Eur J Immunol* 1999;29:1014–1020.

112. Moretta A, Biassoni R, Bottino C, et al. Natural cytotoxicity receptors that trigger human NK-cell–mediated cytolysis. *Immunol Today* 2000;21:228–234.

113. Mandelboim O, Lieberman N, Lev M, et al. Recognition of haemagglutinins on virus-infected cells by NKp46 activates lysis by human NK cells. *Nature* 2001;409:1055–1060.

114. Chambers WH, Vujanovic NL, DeLeo AB, et al. Monoclonal antibody to a triggering structure expressed on rat natural killer cells and adherent lymphokine–activated killer cells. *J Exp Med* 1989;169:1373–1389.

115. Yokoyama WM, Ryan JC, Hunter JJ, et al. cDNA cloning of mouse NKR-P1 and genetic linkage with Ly-49. Identification of a natural killer cell gene complex on mouse chromosome 6. *J Immunol* 1991;147:3229–3236.

116. Ryan J, Niemi E, Nakamura M, et al. NKR-P1A is a target-specific receptor that activates natural killer cell cytotoxicity. *J Exp Med* 1995;181:1911–1915.

117. Garni-Wagner BA, Purohit A, Mathew PA, et al. A novel function-associated molecule related to non–MHC-restricted cytotoxicity mediated by activated natural killer cells and T cells. *J Immunol* 1993;151:60–70.

118. Mathew PA, Garni-Wagner BA, Land K, et al. Cloning and characterization of the 2B4 gene encoding a molecule associated with non–MHC-restricted killing mediated by activated natural killer cells and T cells. *J Immunol* 1993;151:5328–5337.

119. Valiante NM, Trinchieri G. Identification of a novel signal transduction surface molecule on human cytotoxic lymphocytes. *J Exp Med* 1993;178:1397–1406.

120. Brown MH, Boles K, van der Merwe PA, et al. 2B4, the natural killer and T cell immunoglobulin superfamily surface protein, is a ligand for CD48. *J Exp Med* 1998;188:2083–2090.

121. Sivori S, Parolini S, Falco M, et al. 2B4 functions as a co-receptor in human NK cell activation. *Eur J Immunol* 2000;30:787–793.

122. George T, Yu YYL, Liu J, et al. Allorecognition by murine natural killer cells: lysis of T-lymphoblasts and rejection of bone marrow grafts. *Immunol Rev* 1997;155:29–40.

123. Hoglund P, Sundbäck J, Ollson-Alheim MY, et al. Host MHC class I gene control of NK cell specificity in the mouse. *Immunol Rev* 1997;155:11–28.

124. Binstadt BA, Brumbaugh KM, Leibson PJ. Signal transduction by human NK cell MHC–recognizing receptors. *Immunol Rev* 1997;155:197–203.

125. Eriksson M, Leitz G, Fällman E, et al. Inhibitory receptors alter natural killer cell interactions with target cells yet allow simultaneous killing of susceptible targets. *J Exp Med* 1999;190:1005–1012.

126. Kondo M, Weissman IL, Akashi K. Identification of clonogenic common lymphoid progenitors in mouse bone marrow. *Cell* 1997;91:661–672.

127. Rodewald HR, Moingeon P, Lucich JL, et al. A population of early fetal thymocytes expressing Fc gamma RII/III contains precursors of T lymphocytes and natural killer cells. *Cell* 1992;69:139–150.

128. Carlyle JR, Zúñiga-Pflücker JC. Requirement for the thymus in alpha beta T lymphocyte lineage commitment. *Immunity* 1998;9:187–197.

129. Kumar V, Ben-Ezra J, Bennett M, et al. Natural killer cells in mice treated with 89Sr: normal target-binding cell numbers but inability to kill even after interferon administration. *J Immunol* 1979;123:1832–1838.

130. Seaman WE, Gindhart TD, Greenspan JS, et al. Natural killer cells, bone, and the bone marrow: studies in estrogen-treated mice and in congenitally osteopetrotic (mi/mi) mice. *J Immunol* 1979;122:2541–2547.

131. Lodolce JP, Boone DL, Chai S, et al. IL-15 receptor maintains lymphoid homeostasis by supporting lymphocyte homing and proliferation. *Immunity* 1998;9:669–676.

132. Kennedy MK, Glaccum M, Brown SN, et al. Reversible defects in natural killer and memory CD8 T cell lineages in interleukin 15-deficient mice. *J Exp Med* 2000;191:771–780.

133. Williams NS, Moore TA, Schatzle JD, et al. Generation of lytic natural killer 1.1+, Ly-49− cells from multipotential murine bone marrow progenitors in a stroma-free culture: definition of cytokine requirements and developmental intermediates. *J Exp Med* 1997;186:1609–1614.

134. Roth C, Carlyle JR, Takizawa H, et al. Clonal acquisition of inhibitory Ly49 receptors on differentiating NK cell precursors is successively restricted and regulated by stromal cell class I MHC. *Immunity* 2000;13:143–153.

135. Williams NS, Klem J, Puzanov IJ, et al. Differentiation of NK1.1+, Ly49+ NK cells from flt3+ multipotent marrow progenitor cells. *J Immunol* 1999;163:2648–2656.

136. Wang JH, Nichogiannopoulou A, Wu L, et al. Selective defects in the development of the fetal and adult lymphoid system in mice with an Ikaros null mutation. *Immunity* 1996;5:537–549.

137. Ogasawara K, Hida S, Azimi N, et al. Requirement for IRF-1 in the microenvironment supporting development of natural killer cells. *Nature* 1998;391:700–703.

138. Barton K, Muthusamy N, Fischer C, et al. The Ets-1 transcription factor is required for the development of natural killer cells in mice. *Immunity* 1998;9:555–563.

139. Yokota Y, Mansouri A, Mori S, et al. Development of peripheral lymphoid organs and natural killer cells depends on the helix-loop-helix inhibitor Id2. *Nature* 1999;397:702–706.

140. Herberman RB, Nunn ME, Lavrin DH. Natural cytotoxic reactivity of mouse lymphoid cells against syngeneic and allogeneic tumors. I. Distribution of reactivity and specificity. *Int J. Cancer* 1975;16:216–229.

141. Sivakumar PV, Gunturi A, Salcedo M, et al. Cutting edge: expression of functional CD94/NKG2A inhibitory receptors on fetal NK1.1+Ly-49− cells: a possible mechanism of tolerance during NK cell development. *J Immunol* 1999;162:6976–6980.

142. Jaleco AC, Blom B, Res P, et al. Fetal liver contains committed NK progenitors, but is not a site for development of CD34+ cells into T cells. *J Immunol* 1997;159:694–702.

143. Sivakumar PV, Bennett M, Kumar V. Fetal and neonatal NK1.1+ Ly-49− cells can distinguish between major histocompatibility complex class I(hi) and class I(lo) target cells: evidence for a Ly-49–independent negative signaling receptor. *Eur J Immunol* 1997;27:3100–3104.

144. Dorfman JR, Raulet DH. Acquisition of Ly49 receptor expression by developing natural killer cells. *J Exp Med* 1998;187:609–618.

145. Mingari MC, Ponte M, Bertone S, et al. HLA class I–specific inhibitory receptors in human T lymphocytes: interleukin 15–induced expression of CD94/NKG2A in superantigen- or alloantigen-activated CD8+ T cells. *Proc Natl Acad Sci U S A* 1998;95:1172–1177.

146. Williams NS, Kubota A, Bennett M, et al. Clonal analysis of NK cell development from bone marrow progenitors in vitro: orderly acquisition of receptor gene expression. *Eur J Immunol* 2000;30:2074–2082.

147. Tanamachi DM, Hanke T, Takizawa H, et al. Expression of natural killer cell receptor alleles at different Ly49 loci occurs independently and is regulated by major histocompatibility complex class I molecules. *J Exp Med* 2001;193:307–315.

148. Held W, Roland J, Raulet DH. Allelic exclusion of Ly49 family genes encoding class I-MHC–specific receptors on NK cells. *Nature* 1995;376:355–358.

149. Vance RE, Jamieson AM, Cado D, et al. Implications of CD94 deficiency and monoallelic NKG2A expression for natural killer cell development and repertoire formation. *Proc Natl Acad Sci U S A* 2002;99:868–873.

150. Chess A. Expansion of the allelic exclusion principle? *Science* 1998;279:2067–2068.

151. Held W, Kunz B. An allele-specific, stochastic gene expression process controls the expression of multiple Ly49 family genes and generates a diverse, MHC-specific NK cell receptor repertoire. *Eur J Immunol* 1998;28:2407–2416.

152. Hoglund P, Ohlen C, Carbone E, et al. Recognition of β2-microglobulin–negative (β2m−) T-cell blasts by natural killer cells from normal but not from β2m− mice: nonresponsiveness controlled by β2m− bone marrow in chimeric mice. *Proc Natl Acad Sci U S A* 1991;88:10332–10336.

153. Wu M-F, Raulet DH. Class I–deficient hematopoietic cells and nonhematopoietic cells dominantly induce unresponsiveness of NK cells to class I–deficient bone marrow grafts. *J Immunol* 1997;158:1628–1633.

154. Johansson MH, Bieberich C, Jay G, et al. Natural killer cell tolerance in mice with mosaic expression of major histocompatibility complex class I transgene. *J Exp Med* 1997;186:353–364.

155. Karlhofer FM, Hunziker R, Reichlin A, et al. Host MHC class I molecules modulate in vivo expression of a NK cell receptor. *J Immunol* 1994;153:2407–2416.

156. Olsson-Alheim MY, Salcedo M, Ljunggren HG, et al. NK cell receptor calibration: effects of MHC class I induction on killing by Ly49Ahigh and Ly49Alow NK cells. *J Immunol* 1997;159:3189–3194.

157. Held W, Raulet DH. Ly49A transgenic mice provide evidence for a major histocompatibility complex–dependent education process in NK cell development. *J Exp Med* 1997;185:2079–2088.

158. Kase A, Johansson MH, Olsson-Alheim MY, et al. External and internal calibration of the MHC class I–specific receptor Ly49A on murine natural killer cells. *J Immunol* 1998;161:6133–6138.

159. Held W, Dorfman JR, Wu M-F, et al. Major histocompatibility complex class I–dependent skewing of the natural killer cell Ly49 receptor repertoire. *Eur J Immunol* 1996;26:2286–2292.

160. Fahlen L, Lendahl U, Sentman CL. MHC class I–Ly49 interactions shape the Ly49 repertoire on murine NK cells. *J Immunol* 2001;166:6585–6592.

161. Hanke T, Takizawa H, Raulet DH. MHC-dependent shaping of the inhibitory Ly49 receptor repertoire on NK cells: evidence for a regulated sequential model. *Eur J Immunol* 2001;31:3370–3379.

162. Boehm U, Klamp T, Groot M, et al. Cellular responses to interferon-gamma. *Annu Rev Immunol* 1997;15:749–795.

163. Kagi D, Ledermann B, Burki K, et al. Cytotoxicity mediated by T cells and natural killer cells is greatly impaired in perforin-deficient mice. *Nature* 1994;369:31–37.

164. Arase H, Arase N, Saito T. Fas-mediated cytotoxicity by freshly isolated natural killer cells. *J Exp Med* 1995;181:1235–1238.

165. Kayagaki N, Yamaguchi N, Nakayama M, et al. Expression and function of TNF-related apoptosis-inducing ligand on murine activated NK cells. *J Immunol* 1999;163:1906–1913.

166. Caron G, Delneste Y, Aubry JP, et al. Human NK cells constitutively express membrane TNF-alpha (mTNFalpha) and present mTNFalpha-dependent cytotoxic activity. *Eur J Immunol* 1999;29:3588–3595.

167. Bukowski JF, Woda BA, Habu S, et al. Natural killer cell depletion enhances virus synthesis and virus-induced hepatitis *in vivo. J Immunol* 1983;131:1531–1538.

168. Biron CA, Nguyen KB, Pien GC, et al. Natural killer cells in antiviral defense: function and regulation by innate cytokines. *Annu Rev Immunol* 1999;17:189–220.

169. Biron CA, Byron KS, Sullivan JL. Severe herpesvirus infections in an adolescent without natural killer cells. *N Engl J Med* 1989;320:1731–1735.

170. Bukowski JF, Woda BA, Welsh RM. Pathogenesis of murine cytomegalovirus infection in natural killer cell–depleted mice. *J Virol* 1984;52:119–128.

171. Orange JS, Wang B, Terhorst C, et al. Requirement for natural killer cell–produced interferon gamma in defense against murine cytomegalovirus infection and enhancement of this defense pathway by interleukin 12 administration. *J Exp Med* 1995;182:1045–1056.

172. Tay CH, Welsh RM. Distinct organ-dependent mechanisms for the control of murine cytomegalovirus infection by natural killer cells. *J Virol* 1997;71:267–275.

173. Orange JS, Biron CA. Characterization of early IL-12, IFN-alphabeta, and TNF effects on antiviral state and NK cell responses during murine cytomegalovirus infection. *J Immunol* 1996;156:4746–4756.

174. Unanue ER. Studies in listeriosis show the strong symbiosis between the innate cellular system and the T-cell response. *Immunol Rev* 1997;158:11–25.

175. Harshan KV, Gangadharam PR. *In vivo* depletion of natural killer cell activity leads to enhanced multiplication of *Mycobacterium avium* complex in mice. *Infect Immun* 1991;59:2818–2821.

176. Scharton TM, Scott P. Natural killer cells are a source of interferon gamma that drives differentiation of CD4$^+$ T cell subsets and induces early resistance to *Leishmania major* in mice. *J Exp Med* 1993;178:567–577.

177. Hunter CA, Subauste CS, Van Cleave VH, et al. Production of gamma interferon by natural killer cells from *Toxoplasma gondii*–infected SCID mice: regulation by interleukin-10, interleukin-12, and tumor necrosis factor alpha. *Infect Immun* 1994;62:2818–2824.

178. Andersson A, Dai WJ, Di Santo JP, et al. Early IFN-gamma production and innate immunity during *Listeria monocytogenes* infection in the absence of NK cells. *J Immunol* 1998;161:5600–5606.

179. Diefenbach A, Schindler H, Donhauser N, et al. Type 1 interferon (IFNalpha/beta) and type 2 nitric oxide synthase regulate the innate immune response to a protozoan parasite. *Immunity* 1998;8:77–87.

180. Wakil AE, Wang ZE, Ryan JC, et al. Interferon gamma derived from CD4(+) T cells is sufficient to mediate T helper cell type 1 development. *J Exp Med* 1998;188:1651–6.

181. Burnet FM. Immunological aspects of malignant disease. *Lancet* 1967;1:1171–1174.

182. Seaman W, Sleisenger M, Eriksson E, et al. Depletion of natural killer cells in mice by monoclonal antibody to NK-1.1. Reduction in host defense against malignancy without loss of cellular or humoral immunity. *J Immunol* 1987;138:4539–4544.

183. Kim S, Iizuka K, Aguila HL, et al. *In vivo* natural killer cell activi-

184. Levitsky HI, Lazenby A, Hayashi RJ, et al. *In vivo* priming of two distinct antitumor effector populations: the role of MHC class I expression. *J Exp Med* 1994;179:1215–1224.

185. van Elsas A, Hurwitz AA, Allison JP. Combination immunotherapy of B16 melanoma using anti-cytotoxic T lymphocyte-associated antigen 4 (CTLA-4) and granulocyte/macrophage colony–stimulating factor (GM-CSF)–producing vaccines induces rejection of subcutaneous and metastatic tumors accompanied by autoimmune depigmentation. *J Exp Med* 1999;190:355–366.

186. Rosenberg SA, Lotze MT, Yang JC, et al. Prospective randomized trial of high-dose interleukin-2 alone or in conjunction with lymphokine-activated killer cells for the treatment of patients with advanced cancer. *J Natl Cancer Inst* 1993;85:622–632.

187. Shankaran V, Ikeda H, Bruce AT, et al. IFN gamma and lymphocytes prevent primary tumour development and shape tumour immunogenicity. *Nature* 2001;410:1107–1111.

188. van den Broek M, Kagi D, Ossendorp F, et al. Decreased tumor surveillance in perforin-deficient mice. *J Exp Med* 1996;184:1781–1790.

189. Smyth MJ, Thia KYT, Street SEA, et al. Perforin-mediated cytotoxicity is critical for surveillance of spontaneous lymphoma. *J Exp Med* 2000;192:755–760.

190. Takeda K, Smyth MJ, Cretney E, et al. Critical role for tumor necrosis factor–related apoptosis-inducing ligand in immune surveillance against tumor development. *J Exp Med* 2002;195:161–169.

191. Kaplan DH, Shankaran V, Dighe AS, et al. Demonstration of an interferon gamma–dependent tumor surveillance system in immunocompetent mice. *Proc Natl Acad Sci U S A* 1998;95:7556–7561.

192. Fernandez NC, Lozier A, Flament C, et al. Dendritic cells directly trigger NK cell functions: cross-talk relevant in innate anti-tumor immune responses *in vivo. Nat Med* 1999;5:405–411.

193. Zitvogel L. Dendritic and natural killer cells cooperate in the control/switch of innate immunity. *J Exp Med* 2002;195:F9–F14.

194. Carson WE, Giri JG, Lindemann MJ, et al. Interleukin (IL) 15 is a novel cytokine that activates human natural killer cells via components of the IL-2 receptor. *J Exp Med* 1994;180:1395–1403.

195. Carson WE, Fehniger TA, Haldar S, et al. A potential role for interleukin-15 in the regulation of human natural killer cell survival. *J Clin Invest* 1997;99:937–943.

196. Jacobs BL, Langland JO. When two strands are better than one: the mediators and modulators of the cellular responses to double-stranded RNA. *Virology* 1996;219:339–349.

197. Alexopoulou L, Holt AC, Medzhitov R, et al. Recognition of double-stranded RNA and activation of NF-kappa B by Toll-like receptor 3. *Nature* 2001;413:732–738.

198. Nguyen KB, Cousens LP, Doughty LA, et al. Interferon alpha/beta–mediated inhibition and promotion of interferon gamma: STAT1 resolves a paradox. *Nat Immunol* 2000;1:70–76.

199. Trinchieri G. Interleukin-12—a proinflammatory cytokine with immunoregulatory functions that bridge innate resistance and antigen-specific adaptive immunity. *Annu Rev Immunol* 1995;13:251–276.

200. Orange JS, Biron CA. An absolute and restricted requirement for IL-12 in natural killer cell IFN-gamma production and antiviral defense. Studies of natural killer and T cell responses in contrasting viral infections. *J Immunol* 1996;156:1138–1142.

201. Takeda K, Tsutsui H, Yoshimoto T, et al. Defective NK cell activity and Th1 response in IL-18–deficient mice. *Immunity* 1998;8:383–390.

202. Scalzo AA, Fitzgerald NA, Simmons A, et al. *Cmv-1,* a genetic locus that controls murine cytomegalovirus replication in the spleen. *J Exp Med* 1990;171:1469–1483.

203. Dokun AO, Kim S, Smith HR, et al. Specific and nonspecific NK cell activation during virus infection. *Nat Immunol* 2001;2:951–956.

204. Salazar-Mather TP, Orange JS, Biron CA. Early murine cytomegalovirus (MCMV) infection induces liver natural killer (NK) cell inflammation and protection through macrophage inflammatory protein 1alpha (MIP-1alpha)–dependent pathways. *J Exp Med* 1998;187:1–14.

ties revealed by natural killer cell–deficient mice. *Proc Natl Acad Sci U S A* 2000;97:2731–2736.

CHAPTER 13

Accessory Molecules and Co-Stimulation

Arlene H. Sharpe, Yvette Latchman, and Rebecca J. Greenwald

General Aspects
The B7:CD28 Superfamily
  B7-1/B7-2:CD28/Cytotoxic T Lymphocyte–Associated Antigen 4 Pathway · The Inducible Co-Stimulator Ligand–Inducible Co-Stimulator Pathway · PD-Ligand/PD-1 Pathway · The CD40:CD154 Pathway · Other Tumor Necrosis Factor:Tumor Necrosis Factor Receptor Pathways with Co-Stimulatory Function
CD2 Superfamily
  CD2 and Its Ligands · CD150 (Signaling Lymphocyte-Activation Molecule, IPO-3) · CD244 (2B4) · CD84 · Signaling Lymphocyte-Activation Molecule–Associated Protein and Members of the CD2 Superfamily
Concluding Remarks
References

GENERAL ASPECTS

The "two-signal" concept of lymphocyte activation was originally proposed to explain how antigen recognition by mature peripheral B cells could result in either of two seemingly opposing outcomes: lymphocyte clonal expansion and antibody production or unresponsiveness (anergy). Bretscher and Cohn (1,2) developed this model to explain both discrimination of self from nonself and immunization versus tolerance induction for B-cell responses. Lafferty and Cunningham (3) extended this model to T cells. According to this model, T cells require two signals to become fully activated. The first signal, which gives specificity to the immune response, is provided by the interaction of antigenic peptide/major histocompatibility complex (MHC) with the T-cell receptor (TCR). The second, antigen-independent co-stimulatory signal, is delivered to T cells by antigen-presenting cells (APCs) to promote T-cell clonal expansion, cytokine secretion, and effector function. In the absence of the second signal, antigen-specific lymphocytes fail to respond effectively and are functionally inactivated and resistant to subsequent activation to the antigen (anergic). Thus, co-stimulation was postulated to have a critical role in determining T-cell activation versus anergy. Co-stimulation is of therapeutic interest because an understanding of these signals may provide methods for blocking undesired T-cell responses or stimulating immune responses. The two-signal model is useful but oversimplifies the contribution of the first and second signals in several ways. First, there is a quantitative influence of the strength of the TCR

signal on T-cell activation and differentiation (4). T-cell activation may occur under conditions of strong TCR stimulation without second signals. Second, there are both positive and negative second signals that can be delivered to T cells. Some negative second signals appear to be necessary for inducing T-cell tolerance, whereas positive second signals promote T-cell activation. Finally, although the two-signal hypothesis was proposed for naïve lymphocytes, the immune response is a dynamic process, and co-stimulatory signals can also be delivered to antigen-experienced effector and memory T cells.

There are now a large number of T-cell co-stimulatory molecules, with distinct and overlapping functions. Co-stimulation is provided by three major families—the B7:CD28 superfamily, a tumor necrosis factor:tumor necrosis factor receptor (TNF:TNFR) subfamily that lacks death domains, and the CD2 superfamily—as well as some integrins [CD44, CD43, and heat-stable antigen (HSA)]. In this section, we focus on the three major families, comparing their roles in regulating the activation of naïve and antigen-experienced T cells.

THE B7:CD28 SUPERFAMILY

The B7-1/B7-2:CD28/cytotoxic T lymphocyte–associated antigen 4 (CTLA-4) pathway is the best characterized T-cell co-stimulatory pathway and has a critical role in regulating T cell activation and tolerance [several reviews are available

(5–10)]. Additional B7 and CD28 family members have been identified, and two new pathways have been delineated: (a) one pathway involving inducible co-stimulator (ICOS) (11) that interacts with a ligand that we call ICOS ligand but is also known as B7h (12), GL50 (13), B7RP-1 (14), LICOS (15), and B7-H2 (16) and (b) a second pathway involving the PD-1 receptor (17) that interacts with two new B7 family members, PD-L1 (18) [B7-H1 (19)] and PD-L2 (20) [B7-DC (21)]. In addition, there is another B7 homolog, B7-H3 (22) (whose receptor remains to be identified), which suggests that there are still additional pathways within the B7:CD28 superfamily to be identified (Fig. 1).

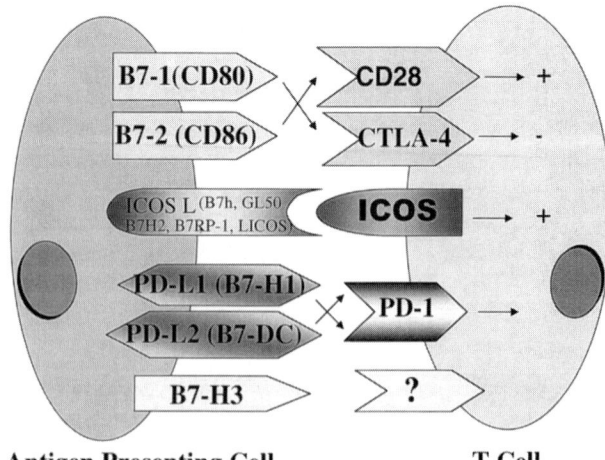

Antigen Presenting Cell   **T Cell**

FIG. 1. Summary of B7:CD28 superfamily. Receptors, ligands, and their interactions are shown. From Sharpe et al. Accessory molecules and co-stimulation.

B7-1/B7-2:CD28/Cytotoxic T Lymphocyte–Associated Antigen 4 Pathway

The B7:CD28/CTLA-4 pathway has a pivotal role in regulating T-cell activation and tolerance. The B7-1 (CD80) (23–25) and B7-2 (CD86) (26–28) co-stimulatory molecules provide a major signal for augmenting and sustaining T-cell responses through interaction with CD28 (29,30) but deliver inhibitory signals when they engage a second, higher affinity receptor on T cells, CTLA-4 (CD152) (31,32) (Table 1). The importance of this pathway *in vivo* has been illustrated by studies of pathway antagonists, which can enable long-term graft survival and suppress autoimmunity (7,33). CTLA-4 immunoglobulin (Ig), which blocks the interactions of B7-1 and B7-2 with both CD28 and CTLA-4, has entered phase I clinical trials (34,35).

TABLE 1. *Comparison of CD28 family of receptors*

Characteristic	CD28	CTLA-4	ICOS	PD-1
% Homology	100%	29%	24%	17%
Chromosome				
Human	2q33	2q33	2q33	2q37
Mouse	1C1 30.1cM	1C2, 30.1cM	1C2, 32cM	1D, 55cM
Structure				
Ligand-binding motif	MYPPPY	MYPPPY	FDPPPF	Unknown
Cytoplasmic domain	PI3k motif, PP2A	PI3K motif, PP2A, SHP2(?)	PI3K	ITIM motif, SHP2
Expression				
Cell type	T	T	T	T, B, M
Kinetics	Constitutive	Inducible	Inducible	Inducible
Function				
Naïve T cells				
Prolif/IL-2	Promotes	Inhibits	Promotes	Unknown*
Cell cycle	Promotes G_0/G_1 Reduce $p27^{kip1}$	Blocks G_1/S Increase $p27^{kip1}$	Unknown	Blocks G_1/S
T helper cell differentiation	Promotes	Inhibits (?)	Promotes	Unknown
Survival	Yes, bcl-xL	No	Unknown	No
Isotype class switch	Yes	No	Yes	Unknown
Effector T cells				
Proliferation	Promotes	Inhibits	Promotes	Inhibits
Cytokines	Indirect, related to expansion	Inhibits	Promotes	Inhibits
Survival	Promotes	No	Unknown	Unknown
Knockout phenotype	Viable	Early lethality	Viable	Late lethality; incomplete penetrance
Defects	Activation, differentiation, survival of naive T cells; Ig class switch	T cell proliferation, cell cycle progression	Differentiation, effector function, Ig class switch	B, myeloid cell proliferation, severe; T cell proliferation, mild

Ig, immunoglobulin; IL, interleukin.

CD28/CTLA-4 Structure and Expression

CD28 and CTLA-4 are type I transmembrane glycoproteins and Ig supergene family members with a single IgV-like extracellular domain. Both CD28 and CTLA-4 have a MYPPPY motif within the IgV-like domain that is required for binding B7-1 and B7-2 (36). CTLA-4 is the higher affinity receptor for B7-1 and B7-2 (37,38) with a 20- to 50-fold higher dissociation constant (K_d) than that of CD28. The cytoplasmic domain of CTLA-4 has only approximately 30% homology with the CD28 cytoplasmic domain but is 100% conserved across species, which suggests an important signaling function.

CD28 is constitutively expressed on the surface of T cells (39). CD28 is expressed on virtually all human CD4$^+$ T cells, 50% of human CD8$^+$ T cells, and all murine T cells. It is also expressed on some plasma cells and natural killer (NK) cells, but its function on these cell types remains uncertain. CD28 has a cysteine residue after the IgV-like domain, and this is involved in homodimerization.

In contrast to the constitutive expression of CD28, CTLA-4 is expressed after T cell activation and is rapidly up-regulated on CD4$^+$ and CD8$^+$ T cells with peak expression 24 to 48 hours after activation (40). Although CTLA-4 is expressed on the cell surface, the majority of CTLA-4 is in intracellular vesicles and is shuttled to the cell surface after antigen recognition. CTLA-4 can be expressed on the cell surface as both a monomer and a dimer, but it does not dimerize with CD28.

B7-1 and B7-2 Structure and Expression

B7-1 and B7-2 are type I transmembrane proteins with one IgV-like and one IgC-like extracellular domain, and short cytoplasmic tails (Table 2). Both bind CD28 with similar low affinities and CTLA-4 with similar 20- to 50-fold higher affinities. The fine specificity of the interaction of B7-1 and B7-2 with CTLA-4 is distinct. Mutation of a single amino acid in the MYPPPY motif of CTLA-4 destroys B7-2 binding but retains B7-1 binding. B7-1 has a slower "off" rate than B7-2 from both CD28 and CTLA-4 (38), which may account for distinct functional roles of these molecules in different types of in vivo immune responses.

B7-1 and B7-2 form back-to-back, noncovalent homodimers that interact with covalent homodimers of CD28 or CTLA-4 (41,42). Each CTLA-4 dimer can bind two independent B7 homodimers (42). The crystal structure of B7:CTLA-4 suggests that a linear zipper-like structure may form between B7 and CTLA-4 homodimers (42,43). Such a structure may promote the recruitment of inhibitory signaling molecules through interaction with either the cytoplasmic or extracellular domains in CTLA-4 and B7.

B7-1 and B7-2 have distinct expression patterns on APCs (44,45). B7-2 is constitutively expressed at low levels and is rapidly up-regulated on B cells, monocytes, and dendritic cells after their activation. B7-1 is generally absent on unstimulated APCs, and the kinetics of its up-regulation is slower than that of B7-2. The distinct temporal expression kinetics of B7-1 and B7-2 on APCs have suggested that B7-2 may be most important for initiating an immune response, and this has been confirmed by analyses of B7-1– and B7-2–deficient (−/−) mice. The expression of B7-1 and B7-2 on APCs can be up-regulated by CD40 ligation (46,47). Interleukin (IL)–4 and interferon (IFN)-γ stimulate B7-2 expression dramatically but have lesser effects on B7-1 (48). IL-10 blocks B7-1 and B7-2 up-regulation

TABLE 2. *Comparison of B7 family of co-stimulatory molecules*

Characteristic	B7-1 (CD80)	B7-2 (CD86)	ICOSL (B7h, B7-H2; B7RP-1)	PD-L1 (B7-H1)	PD-L2 (B7-DC)	B7-H3
% Homology	100%	23%	25%	22%	21%	24%
Chromosome						
Human	3q13	3q21	21q22	9p24	9p24	15q24
Mouse	16B, 32.8	16B, 26.9	10C1	19B	19B	9A
Expression						
Lymphoid	B, Mac, DC, T	B, Mac, DC, T	B, Mac, DC, T	B, Mac, DC, T	DC	Mac, DC
Nonlymphoid	Rare	Rare	Fibroblast Endothelial Others unknown	Endothelial Tumor cells Many tissues; high in heart, placenta	Tumor cells Many tissues; high in heart, placenta	Many tissues; absent in PBLs, bone marrow
Kinetics	I; later than B7-2	C and I	C and I	C and I	Unknown	I
Receptor	CD28 CTLA-4	CD28 CTLA-4	ICOS	PD-1	PD-1	Unknown
Knockout phenotype	Modest defects in T cell activation; overlap with B7-2	Some defects in T cell activation; overlap with B7-1	Unknown	Unknown	Unknown	Unknown

C, constitutive; DC, dendritic cell; I, inducible; Mac, macrophage.

on peritoneal macrophages, and granulocyte-macrophage colony-stimulating factor (GM-CSF) down-regulates B7-2 but not B7-1 on dendritic cells (48). B7-1 and B7-2 are also expressed on T cells, but the function of these B7 co-stimulators on T cells is not clear.

Functions

Roles in Regulating T Cell Proliferation and Survival

B7-1 and B7-2 provide important co-stimulatory signals for augmenting and sustaining a T-cell response through interaction with CD28 (48). CD28 transmits a signal that synergizes with the TCR signal to promote activation of naïve T cells (49). CD28 engagement usually does not have a physiological effect in the absence of TCR signaling. CD28 signaling regulates the threshold for T-cell activation and significantly decreases the number of TCR engagements needed for effective T-cell activation (4). CD28 co-stimulation results in enhanced T-cell proliferation, production of multiple cytokines (e.g., IL-2) and cytokine receptors (e.g., IL-2R), increased expression of proteins involved in cell cycle progression, and sustained CD40L expression (45,48). CD28 signals also induce bcl-x_L, which sustains T-cell survival (50), and have a critical role in regulating CD4$^+$ and CD8$^+$ T-cell differentiation (45,51). CD28 also optimizes responses of previously activated T cells, promoting IL-2 production and T-cell survival (45). B7:CD28 interactions also appear important for CD4$^+$CD25$^+$ regulatory T cell development or expansion, or both, inasmuch as CD28$^{-/-}$ and B7-1/B7-2$^{-/-}$ mice have markedly reduced numbers of these regulatory T cells (52). Some responses are CD28 independent, and it is not yet clear whether these responses are co-stimulation independent because of strong antigenic stimuli or redundancy in co-stimulatory pathways.

Although the co-stimulatory function of CD28 is well established, the function of CTLA-4 has been more controversial. Most data support a role for CTLA-4 as a negative regulator of T cell activation. The fatal lymphoproliferative disease that develops in CTLA-4$^{-/-}$ mice, as a result of uncontrolled B7-1/B7-2 co-stimulation, underscores the importance of CTLA-4 as a negative regulator of T cell responses (53,54). CTLA-4 blockade *in vitro* increases T-cell proliferation and cytokine production and *in vivo* augments antitumor immunity and exacerbates autoimmune responses (5,55–58). CTLA-4 inhibits TCR- and CD28-mediated signal transduction. CTLA-4 inhibits IL-2 synthesis and progression through the cell cycle and terminates T-cell responses (59,60). Some studies have suggested that CTLA-4 may exert inhibitory effects by regulating production of soluble inhibitory cytokines, such as transforming growth factor β, but this is controversial (61). Some studies suggest that CTLA-4 ligation may be needed for regulatory T-cell function and raise the possibility that the immune stimulatory consequences of CTLA-4 blockade may in part be caused by the inhibition of function of regulatory T cells (62,63).

Role in Regulating T Helper Cell Differentiation

B7-1/B7-2:CD28 interactions have important roles in T helper cell differentiation (45,48). *In vitro* and *in vivo* studies with monoclonal antibodies (mAbs) against B7-1 and B7-2 and *in vitro* studies with Chinese hamster ovary (CHO) cells transfected with B7-1 or B7-2 indicated that B7-1 and B7-2 may be distinct in their capacity to induce T-cell differentiation. When naïve TCR transgenic T cells were stimulated with APC lacking either or both B7 co-stimulators, both B7-1 and B7-2 were found to contribute to Th1 and Th2 cytokine production, which suggests that the different contributions of B7-1 and B7-2 may reflect their different levels and timing of expression. IL-4 production by naïve T cells is highly dependent on B7-1/B7-2 co-stimulation. Intense TCR stimulation alone is enough to induce some IL-2 dependent IFN-γ production in the absence of B7:CD28. Blockade of this pathway during the activation of a naïve T cell impairs T-cell proliferation and differentiation. Blockade of this pathway in previously activated T cells diminishes T-cell expansion but not effector cytokine production.

Role in Regulating Humoral Immune Responses

T helper cell–dependent antibody responses require reciprocal interactions between T and B cells that are dependent on antigen recognition and co-stimulatory signals. The B7:CD28 pathway provides co-stimulatory signals essential for cognate T cell–B cell interactions required for Ig class switching and germinal center (GC) formation. CD28$^{-/-}$ mice revealed a critical role for CD28 in GC formation (64). Potentially reactive B cells accumulate within lymphoid follicles of CD28$^{-/-}$ mice after antigenic stimulation but are not able to proliferate or undergo somatic mutation. B7-1/B7-2 antagonists given at the initiation of an immune response reduce or inhibit primary antibody responses, GC formation, and somatic hypermutation (65). Mice lacking both B7-1 and B7-2 fail to generate antigen-specific IgG1 and IgG2a responses and form GCs when immunized with adjuvant (66). B7-1$^{-/-}$ or B7-2$^{-/-}$ mice mount high-titer antigen-specific IgG responses when immunized with adjuvant, which indicates overlapping roles for B7-1 and B7-2 in Ig class switching. However, when B7-2$^{-/-}$ mice were immunized intravenously without adjuvant, there was a complete failure to switch antibody isotypes and form GCs, whereas B7-1$^{-/-}$ mice had responses comparable with those of wild-type mice. Together, these studies point to a dominant role for B7-2 in initiating T-cell responses and providing cognate help for B cells. The nature of the antigen stimulus also can influence the role of CD28 in Ig class switching. CD28$^{-/-}$ mice do not have impaired IgG production in response to infection with some parasites (67).

Role of CTLA-4 in Regulating Peripheral T-Cell Tolerance

CTLA-4 plays a critical role in regulating peripheral T-cell tolerance (60,68). Peripheral T-cell tolerance may be induced not because of the absence of B7-1/B7-2 mediated co-stimulation but as a consequence of CTLA-4:B7-1/B7-2 interactions (60,68). The outcome of an immune response involves a balance between CD28-mediated T-cell activation and CTLA-4–mediated inhibition. How signals through CD28 and CTLA-4 are coordinated is not clear. CTLA-4 may inhibit T-cell responses by outcompeting CD28 for binding to B7, by inducing immunosuppressive cytokines, or by directly antagonizing CD28-mediated signaling or TCR-mediated signaling or both. These mechanisms are not mutually exclusive.

Therapeutic Manipulation of the B7-1/B7-2: CD28/CTLA-4 Pathway

Because the B7-1/B7-2:CD28/CTLA-4 pathway delivers signals necessary for T-cell activation, there has been great interest in manipulating this pathway for therapy. Blockade could inhibit undesired T-cell responses occurring during autoimmunity, transplant rejection, or allergy, whereas stimulation through this pathway could promote T-cell responses for tumor and vaccine immunity.

Antitumor Immunity. Genetic modification of tumors to express B7-1 or B7-2 can enhance the host antitumor immune response (69,70). Administration of anti–CTLA-4 mAbs in animal models (57,58) can accelerate tumor rejection, presumably by enhancing T-cell activation. There is great interest in designing therapies that enhance the antitumor response by either stimulating expression of B7-1/B7-2 or blocking B7:CTLA-4 interactions.

Transplantation. The efficacy of co-stimulatory blockade in delaying graft rejection was first reported in a murine cardiac allograft model (71). Administration of CD28:B7 blockade prevents acute allograft rejection, induces donor-specific tolerance in several animal models, and prevents development and interrupts progression of chronic allograft rejection (33,72). Blockade of the B7:CD28/CTLA-4 pathway also has been a key strategy in prevention of graft-versus-host disease (GVHD) (73). GVHD occurs when transplanted T cells mount a vigorous immune response against host tissue alloantigens. GVHD is a major obstacle to the success of bone marrow transplantation. Treating recipients of mismatched donor bone marrow with CTLA-4Ig prevents the expansion and cytolytic activity of the donor T cells characteristic of acute GVHD, and this approach has been used in a clinical trial for bone marrow transplant recipients (35).

Autoimmunity. Blockade of the B7-1/B7-2:CD28 pathway has been effective in preventing the induction of autoimmune disease and the progression of established autoimmune disease in experimental animal models and in patients. The resistance of B7-1/B7-2$^{-/-}$ mice to experimental autoimmune encephalomyelitis (EAE) induction and to EAE after the adoptive transfer of encephalitogenic T cells demonstrated a key role for B7-1 and B7-2 not only during the induction phase but also during the effector phase of EAE (74). Results of studies indicate that EAE can develop in CD28$^{-/-}$ mice

if these mice are given a higher dose of myelin antigen or are immunized twice, which suggests that other pathways can be used for induction of autoimmunity in the absence of CD28 (75). Studies in models of collagen-induced arthritis, autoimmune thyroiditis, autoimmune uveitis, myasthenia gravis, and lupus implicate CD28 signals in the development of autoimmune disease. CD28 blockade may not completely prevent disease, but it alternatively may reduce severity and alter T-cell responsiveness. The distinct effects of anti-B7 antibodies or CTLA-4Ig in some models may result from differential blockade of positive (B7-CD28) and negative (B7-CTLA-4) signals within the B7-1/B7-2:CD28/CTLA-4 pathway, depending on the timing of administration (7). Results of studies suggest that CD28$^{-/-}$ and B7-1/B7-2$^{-/-}$ nonobese diabetic mice may be more susceptible to insulin-dependent diabetes mellitus because they lack CD4$^+$CD25$^+$ regulatory T cells (52).

In several models of autoimmunity, CTLA-4 has been shown to down-regulate T-cell responses during the course of an autoimmune disease. Treatment with blocking anti–CTLA-4 mAbs exacerbated EAE when given after adoptive transfer of primed T cells (5). Similar effects were observed in a TCR transgenic model of diabetes in which administration of anti–CTLA-4 mAbs accelerated the development of diabetes (76). The onset of diabetes was affected only when the anti–CTLA-4 mAb was given before the onset of insulitis. These results suggest a critical role for CTLA-4 at the initiation of the autoimmune response and at the down-regulation of the ongoing response.

CTLA-4Ig has been studied in patients in a phase I clinical trial for the treatment of the T cell–mediated autoimmune skin disease psoriasis vulgaris (34,77) and reduced clinical disease. These results are promising for the treatment of psoriasis vulgaris as well as other T cell–mediated autoimmune diseases.

Allergy. In a murine model of asthma, administration of CTLA-4Ig before antigen sensitization or before reexposure to antigen blocked asthma (78). Levels of IL-4, serum IgG1 and IgE, and pulmonary eosinophilia were markedly reduced. Although CTLA-4Ig treatment has been shown to be effective in some models of allergy, there is some evidence that Th2 cells may be more resistant to tolerance induction than are Th1 cells. An effective immunotherapy for allergy may require a strategy that prevents naïve, effector, and memory T cells from responding on subsequent exposure to the allergen.

Biochemical Basis for CD28 and CTLA-4 Function

Despite considerable investigation, the molecular mechanisms by which CD28 and CTLA-4 transduce signals are not well defined [reviewed by Alegre et al. (10), Rudd (79), and Slavik et al. (80)]. Whether CD28 increases TCR signaling or triggers TCR-independent signals has been controversial. Cyclosporine can inhibit TCR signals but partially blocks CD28 signals, which indicates that some events downstream of CD28 are TCR independent (10). CD28 ligation can enhance levels of Itk, a tec-related tyrosine kinase, in a TCR-independent manner. However, CD28 ligation also can amplify biochemical signals triggered by the TCR, including the activation of phosphatidylinositol 3-kinase (PI3K) and the Ras pathway. CD28 coaggregates with the TCR/CD3 complex when T cells bind to APCs displaying antigen. CD28 enhances the time that the TCR remains in membrane microdomains at the site of contact with APCs, the immunological synapse, and recruits lipid rafts to this site. The IL-2 transcription factor cJun is activated after CD28 engagement, but whether this transcription factor is required for CD28-mediated T cell co-stimulation is not established. Cross-linking of the TCR and CD28 results in the activation of the transcription factors nuclear factor of activated T cells (NF-AT), activator protein–1, and NFκB/rel. In contrast, stimulation of the TCR alone may be sufficient for the activation of NF-AT. Cbl-b may influence the CD28 dependence of T-cell activation by selectively suppressing TCR-mediated Vav activation (81).

CD28 has a 41–amino acid cytoplasmic domain containing four tyrosines, but it has no intrinsic catalytic activity. Lck, Fyn, and Itk can phosphorylate CD28. Protein phosphatase 2A binds to the conserved YMNM motif when Y170 is not phosphorylated, and it may serve a negative regulatory function and limit CD28 co-stimulation (82). When Y170 is phosphorylated, SH2-containing proteins, PI3K, and Grb2 are recruited. The role of the PI3K association with CD28 is not yet clear. Mutational analysis of CD28 has revealed that Y170 in mouse CD28 is critical for up-regulating bcl-x$_L$ expression but not for T-cell proliferation, IL-2 production, or B cell help (83).

CTLA-4 contains two tyrosine-containing motifs and lacks intrinsic enzymatic activity. Mutational analyses of CTLA-4 have indicated that mutations of Y201 within the YVKM motif and of Y218 do not prevent CTLA-4 inhibitory effects (84). The first tyrosine motif, YVKM, plays a pivotal role in the tightly controlled cellular localization of CTLA-4 and in the interaction with key signaling molecules (85). The nonphosphorylated YVKM can associate with the AP50 subunit of the clathrin-associated adapter complex AP-2, which is responsible for continuous translocation of CTLA-4 to and from the cell surface. Phosphorylation of CTLA-4 releases binding to AP-2 and results in increased cell surface expression. In a phosphorylated state, CTLA-4 can interact with PI3K, but the significance of this is not clear. Some studies suggest that the inhibitory activity of CTLA-4 is related to its ability to antagonize CD28-mediated activation by sequestering signaling molecules such as PI3K away from CD28. Another mechanism by which CTLA-4 may disrupt TCR-mediated signals is to dephosphorylate key signaling proteins. SHP-2 has been found to associate with the PI3K binding motif of CTLA-4, but whether this interaction is direct or indirect is not clear, because CTLA-4 does not have the motif that typically interacts with SHP-2 SH2 domains

(86). The functional significance of this interaction has not been demonstrated. Other studies indicate that CTLA-4 may bind to proteins of the TCR/CD3 complex and directly alter TCR signaling (87). There is evidence for an interaction of CTLA-4 with the CD3-ζ chain of the TCR complex intracellularly, which suggests that CTLA-4 interferes with very early TCR signaling events. Other studies have indicated that mutant CTLA-4 lacking the cytoplasmic tail could still suppress IL-2 production from T cells, which suggests that the more proximal regions of CTLA-4 may be involved in negative signaling (88). CTLA-4 cross-linking blocks activation of the mitogen-activated protein kinases JNK and ERK.

There is no evidence that B7-1 or B7-2 can function as signal transducers, and it appears likely that they serve only as ligands for the CD28/CTLA-4 signaling receptors.

The Inducible Co-Stimulator Ligand–Inducible Co-Stimulator Pathway

Structure and Expression of Inducible Co-Stimulator and Inducible Co-Stimulator Ligand

Although ICOS was first reported on activated human T cells, a previously characterized T-cell activation molecule called H4 was shown to be identical to ICOS (11,89). The rat ortholog of ICOS was cloned as activation inducible lymphocyte immunomodulatory molecule (90). Like CD28 and CTLA-4, ICOS is a glycosylated disulfide-linked homodimer. ICOS has an FDPPPF motif (11) instead of the MYPPPY motif and does not bind B7-1 or B7-2 (13,14,91) (Table 1). The ICOS cytoplasmic tail contains a YMFM motif that binds the p85 subunit of PI3K, analogous to the YMNM motif of CD28 (92). Whereas CD28 has a consensus SH3-kinase binding site PYAP that is crucial for T-cell proliferation and IL-2 production, ICOS lacks this PXXP site, which suggests a structural basis for distinct functions of these receptors.

In contrast to CD28, ICOS is not expressed constitutively on naïve T cells but is induced rapidly on T cells after TCR engagement (11,14,92,93). The inducible expression of ICOS shortly after T-cell activation suggests that ICOS may be particularly important in providing co-stimulatory signals to activated T cells. ICOS expression is influenced by both TCR and CD28 signals. TCR cross-linking induces ICOS cell surface expression by 12 hours after activation (92,93). CD28 co-stimulation enhances ICOS expression. ICOS up-regulation is markedly reduced in the absence of B7-1 and B7-2 (94,95), which suggests that some of the functions ascribed to CD28 may result in part from ICOS signaling. However, ICOS expression is not entirely dependent on CD28 signals, and this is functionally significant, as demonstrated by studies showing that T-cell responses in CD28$^{-/-}$ mice can be modulated with ICOS-Ig (96). ICOS is expressed on recently activated T cells and resting memory T cells, on both Th1 and Th2 cells during differentiation, but ICOS levels remain high on

Th2 cells and diminish on Th1 cells (92,95). ICOS expression also has been reported on rat B cells (90) but not on B cells from other species. ICOS is expressed in the human fetal and neonatal thymus (11) and in the thymic medulla and corticomedullary junction in mice (93), but studies in ICOS$^{-/-}$ mice do not indicate an essential role for ICOS in T-cell development (97–99).

ICOS ligand (ICOSL) is expressed on APCs and other cell types (12–14,16,94) (Table 2). ICOSL messenger ribonucleic acid (mRNA) is expressed constitutively in lymphoid and nonlymphoid tissues such as those of the kidney, liver, peritoneum, lung, and testes. ICOSL is expressed at low levels on resting B cells, on some macrophages and dendritic cells, and on a small subset of CD3$^+$ T cells (13). TNF-α and IFN-γ induce ICOSL mRNA expression in fibroblasts (12). IFN-γ induces ICOSL expression on B cells, monocytes, and some dendritic cells (14,94). B7-1 and B7-2 also can be up-regulated by IFN-γ, but the mechanisms appear to be distinct: B7-1/B7-2 induction by IFN-γ is NFκB dependent, whereas ICOSL induction is NFκB independent (94). Ig or CD40 cross-linking does not up-regulate ICOSL expression on human B cells, in contrast to B7-1 and B7-2 (94). ICOSL is expressed in the B-cell areas of lymph nodes in normal mice and in follicles in the spleen, Peyer's patches, and thymic medulla (14,93). The functional significance of ICOSL expression on nonlymphoid cells is not yet clear.

Functions of Inducible Co-Stimulator–Inducible Co-Stimulator Ligand Interactions

Role in Regulating T-Cell Proliferation and Differentiation

The effects of ICOS on naïve T-cell proliferation are modest in comparison with those of CD28 (11,14,16,92). ICOS-Ig does not inhibit T-cell proliferation of naïve DO.11.10 TCR transgenic T cells to peptide (95). Naïve ICOS$^{-/-}$ T cells exhibit modest defects in T-cell proliferation in most studies (95,99). ICOS co-stimulation can produce low levels of IL-2 that are necessary for initial proliferation but not sufficient for sustained proliferation (100). Thus, a major distinction between ICOS and CD28 is that CD28 has a unique role in the initial co-stimulation of IL-2 by naïve T cells and in sustained expansion of recently activated T cells.

Signals through ICOS appear to be more significant for regulating cytokine production by recently activated and effector T cells (11,92). Stimulatory anti-ICOS mAbs can enhance production of IL-4, IL-5, IL-10, IFN-γ, TNF-α, and GM-CSF. Blockade of ICOS during initial stimulation of naïve T cells enhances Th1 differentiation (95). Differentiated ICOS$^{-/-}$ T cells produce IFN-γ but fail to express IL-4 when restimulated (97–99). This defect in Th2 cytokine production reflects the crucial role for ICOS in regulating IL-4 and IL-13 production by effector T cells.

ICOS has an important role in regulating Th2 effector responses. In studies of allergic airway disease, Th2 effector function, but not Th2 differentiation, was prevented by ICOS blockade (101). ICOS blockade at the time of antigen priming had little effect on subsequent airway challenge in normal mice (92,102). Blockade of ICOS after priming significantly reduced lung inflammation after airway antigen challenge (102), whereas blockade of the B7:CD28 pathway after priming did not inhibit Th2 effector cytokine production. Thus, CD28 and ICOS have distinct functions in regulating Th2 responses: CD28 has a dominant role at the time of priming, whereas ICOS regulates effector Th2 responses.

ICOS also can regulate Th1 immune responses (103). When ICOS-Ig is given at the time of infection with *Nocardia brasiliensis,* both Th1 (IFN-γ) and Th2 (IL-4 and IL-5) cytokines are reduced (96). ICOS can also regulate CD8$^+$ T-cell responses (104). ICOSL can enhance IL-2 and IFN-γ production by CD8$^+$ T cells predominantly in recall responses, but CD8$^+$ lytic effector function does not appear to be ICOS dependent. ICOSL expression in an immunogenic, class I$^+$ MHC tumor enhanced tumor rejection in mice. Inhibition of the ICOS pathway does not diminish cytotoxic T-cell (CTL) responses to lymphocytic choriomeningitis virus (LCMV) or vesicular stomatitis virus infection in mice (96).

Role in Regulating Humoral Immune Responses

ICOS has an important role in T-cell:B-cell collaboration. Transgenic mice expressing a secreted form of ICOSL exhibit lymphoid hyperplasia and high serum IgG levels (14). ICOS$^{-/-}$ mice exhibit profound defects in Ig isotype class switching and GC formation after immunization with model protein antigens under most conditions (47,98,99). The defect in class switching and GC formation observed in ICOS$^{-/-}$ mice resembles that observed in B7-1/B7-2$^{-/-}$ mice (66). However, B7-1/B7-2$^{-/-}$ mice are unable to class switch or form GCs, irrespective of immunization route or adjuvant used, whereas ICOS$^{-/-}$ mice can class switch and form GCs under strong inflammatory conditions. This suggests that B7-1 and B7-2 can elicit class switching in the absence of ICOS. Therefore, ICOS and B7:CD28 interactions have overlapping and distinct critical roles in T:B collaboration.

Therapeutic Manipulation of the ICOS:ICOSL Pathway

Transplantation. In a Th1-mediated cardiac allograft rejection model, blockade or elimination of ICOS co-stimulation prolongs acute cardiac allograft survival and suppresses intragraft cytokine production, particularly IFN-γ and IL-10 (105). ICOS blockade also prevents transplant arteriosclerosis that develops when the CD40:CD40L pathway is blocked (105). B7:CD28 blockade similarly prevents graft arteriosclerosis (106). Thus, ICOS and CD28 similarly promote inflammation underlying graft arteriopathy.

Autoimmunity. Studies of EAE further demonstrate the influence of ICOS on Th1 responses and indicate that the outcome of ICOS blockade may be distinct when ICOS co-stimulation is blocked during T cell priming or effector phase of EAE (97,103,107). EAE is greatly exacerbated in ICOS$^{-/-}$ mice, with increased IFN-γ production, in comparison with wild-type mice (97). Similarly, ICOS blockade during induction of EAE worsens disease (107). ICOS blockade during priming leads to Th1 polarization of the response. The EAE resistance of mice lacking CD28 or both B7-1 and B7-2 (74) is in contrast with the exacerbated EAE that develops in ICOS$^{-/-}$ mice. These differences may reflect the predominant role of CD28 in stimulating T-cell clonal expansion. Elimination or blockade of CD28 or ICOS during priming skews Th cells to Th1, but because T-cell expansion is markedly impaired without CD28, the functional consequences of Th1 skewing are observed only when ICOS is blocked.

ICOS blockade during the effector phase of EAE can inhibit disease progression and ameliorate EAE (103,107), which suggests that ICOS co-stimulation has a key role in sustaining effector Th1 cells. When B7:CD28 interactions are blocked during the effector phase, EAE is transient and mild. Thus, B7:CD28 interactions are also critical for sustaining effector T cells (74). However, the effects of CD28 signaling are mainly on T-cell expansion, whereas ICOS mainly affects effector cytokine production.

Infection. Results of studies in murine models of virus and parasite infections have suggested synergies between ICOS and CD28. ICOS blockade in CD28$^{-/-}$ mice further reduced Th1/Th2 polarization in viral and parasitic infection models (96). ICOS-Ig abrogated IFN-γ production by virus-specific T cells from LCMV-infected CD28$^{-/-}$ mice. ICOS can regulate both CD28-dependent and CD28-independent CD4$^+$ subset responses. CTLA-4 can oppose T-cell activation by either CD28 or ICOS (100).

In summary, studies of ICOS pathway blockade suggest that this pathway may be an attractive target for blocking chronic inflammation. Because ICOS co-stimulation is important for IL-10 production (11), ICOS may be important for T-cell tolerance, when IL-10–producing T regulatory cells have a role in T-cell tolerance. Because CD28 and ICOS have both synergistic and overlapping effects (Table 1), combination therapy may be advantageous, particularly for inhibiting established immune responses.

PD-Ligand/PD-1 Pathway

Structure and Expression of PD-1 and Its Ligands

PD-1 has an extracellular domain with a single IgV domain lacking both the MYPPPY motif found in CD28/CTLA4 and the additional cysteine which allows these molecules to homodimerize (17,108) (Table 1). The PD-1 cytoplasmic domain has two tyrosines, one that constitutes an immunoreceptor tyrosine-based inhibitory motif. PD-1 only binds PD-L1 (B7-H1) and PD-L2 (B7-DC). The PD-1 ligands do not bind to any other CD28 family members (18–21).

PD-1 expression is much broader than that of CD28, CTLA-4 and ICOS. PD-1 is expressed in activated, but not resting CD4$^+$ and CD8$^+$ T cells, B cells, and myeloid cells. PD-1 mRNA is expressed in human CD4$^+$ and CD8$^+$ T cells activated by mitogen or anti-CD3(109). PD-1 protein expression is up-regulated by anti-IgM cross-linking but not by lipopolysaccharide. PD-1 is expressed in the thymus primarily on CD4$^-$CD8$^-$ (DN) T cells (109,110). $\gamma\delta$ DN thymocytes express high levels of PD-1 and NK T cells express low levels of PD-1 (110).

PD-L1 and PD-L2 are expressed in both lymphoid and non-lymphoid organs (18–20) (Table 2). Both are up-regulated after activation of lymphoid cells. IFN-γ stimulates their expression on monocytes, dendritic cells, and endothelial cells. Human and mouse T cells express PD-L1 but not PD-L2. Both PD-1 ligands are expressed in the heart and placenta at high levels, and in lung, spleen, lymph nodes, and thymus. Human pancreas, lung and liver, express PD-L2, but not PD-L1. Human fetal liver expresses PD-L1, but not PD-L2. PD-L1 and PD-L2 are also expressed in a variety of tumor cell lines.

Functions of PD-1: PD-L1/PD-L2 Interactions

The phenotype of PD-1$^{-/-}$ mice demonstrates a negative regulatory role for PD-1 *in vivo* (111–113). PD-1$^{-/-}$ mice develop splenomegaly with increased myeloid and B cells. PD-1$^{-/-}$ B cells respond more strongly to anti-IgM cross-linking, and PD-1$^{-/-}$ myeloid cells have an increased response to GM-CSF, whereas PD-1$^{-/-}$ T cell responses to anti-CD3 are unchanged (111). PD-1$^{-/-}$ mice on the C57Bl/6 background develop a late-onset, progressive arthritis and lupus-like glomerulonephritis (112). Introduction of the *lpr* (Fas gene) mutation into PD-1$^{-/-}$ mice accelerates disease. In contrast, PD-1$^{-/-}$ mice of the Balb/c background develop a dilated cardiomyopathy with an earlier onset (113). PD-1$^{-/-}$ recombination activating gene 2 (RAG2)$^{-/-}$ Balb/c mice do not develop the disease, which implicates T or B cells or both in this process. The expression of PD-L1 and PD-L2 at high levels in the heart (18–20) suggests a role for PD-1 ligands in preventing potentially self-reactive lymphocytes from causing tissue injury. PD-1$^{-/-}$ mice further show that PD-1 regulates CD8$^+$ T cells (110,112).

The functions of PD-L1 or PD-L2 in regulating T-cell responses are just becoming understood, and this is an area of some controversy. PD-L1 or PD-L2–Ig proteins coupled to beads together with anti-CD3 mAb inhibited T-cell proliferation and cytokine production by both resting and previously activated CD4$^+$ and CD8$^+$ T cells and even naïve T cells from umbilical cord blood (18). Inhibition was not seen when PD-1$^{-/-}$ T cells were incubated with anti-CD3 plus PD-L1–Ig, which indicates that the inhibitory signal was transduced by PD-1. Studies of CHO cells transfected with class II MHC and PD-L1 or PD-L2 in the presence or absence of B7-2 also support an inhibitory role for PD-1 (20). When previously activated TCR transgenic CD4$^+$ T cells were cultured with peptide and CHO cells expressing PD-L1 or PD-L2, T-cell proliferation and cytokine production were markedly reduced by CHO cells expressing PD-1 ligands. T-cell proliferation and cytokine production also were strongly reduced when the TCR transgenic T cells were cultured with CHO transfectants expressing B7-2 and PD-L1 or PD-L2 at low antigen concentrations. At high antigen concentrations, these transfectants reduced cytokine production but did not inhibit T-cell proliferation. The PD-1 ligands exert these effects by causing cell cycle arrest in G_0/G_1 but not cell death (20). These studies demonstrate overlapping functions of PD-L1 and PD-L2 and support a role for the PD-L:PD-1 pathway in down-regulating T-cell responses.

However, not all studies support a negative regulatory role for PD-L1 and PD-L2. In three studies, these B7 homologs stimulated T-cell proliferation (19,21,114). When resting T cells were stimulated with low levels of anti-CD3 and immobilized B7-H1–Ig (PD-L1–Ig), T-cell proliferation was modestly enhanced, IL-10 production was markedly increased, and IFN-γ and GM-CSF levels were modestly elevated, but there was little effect on IL-2 or IL-4 production. CD28$^{-/-}$ T cells were stimulated similarly to wild-type cells. Neither CTL generation nor lysis was stimulated. When resting CD4$^+$ T cells were incubated with immobilized anti-CD3 plus B7-DC–Ig (PD-L2–Ig), T-cell proliferation and IFN-γ production were strongly increased, but there was little effect on IL-2, IL-4, or IL-10 production. Little effect was observed on CD8 T-cell responses.

The reasons for the contradictory results of functional studies of the PD-1 ligand are not clear. Two major differences are the use of resting T cells in the majority of the studies that indicated a co-stimulatory function for PD-1 ligands and the use of previously activated T cells in studies that indicated an inhibitory function. It may be that, as with the B7-1/B7-2:CD28/CTLA-4 pathway, a second receptor for PD-1 ligands might exist with the capacity to deliver a stimulatory signal like CD28. However, PD-L1–Ig and anti-CD3 mAb do not stimulate PD-1$^{-/-}$ T cells; only a loss of inhibition is observed in PD-1$^{-/-}$ T cells, in comparison with wild-type T cells (18). Studies of blocking antibodies and knockout mice are needed to resolve these differences.

Biochemical Basis for PD-1 Function

The biochemical pathways by which PD-1 exerts its effects are beginning to be elucidated. PD-1 transduces a signal when cross-linked along with TCR or B-cell receptor but does not transduce a signal when cross-linked alone. Coligation of TCR and PD-1 on Jurkat cells stimulates rapid tyrosine phosphorylation and activation of SHP-2, which dephosphorylates signaling molecules in the membrane proximal TCR-signaling cascade (20). In a B lymphoma cell line model, coligation of the B-cell receptor with chimeric molecules, containing the extracellular domain of FcγRIIB fused to the PD-1 cytoplasmic domain, inhibited B-cell receptor–mediated growth retardation, Ca^{2+} mobilization, and tyrosine phosphorylation of Syk, PLCγ2, PI3K, Vav, and ERK1/ERK2 but

not Lyn or Dok (115). Both tyrosines in the PD-1 cytoplasmic domain were phosphorylated, which led to recruitment and activation of SHP-2 but not SHP-1 or SHIP. However, the more COOH-terminal tyrosine, and not the immunoreceptor tyrosine-based inhibitory motif tyrosine, has the major role in mediating the inhibitory signals of PD-1.

In summary, the phenotype of PD-1$^{-/-}$ mice implicates PD-1 in down-regulating immune responses and regulating tolerance of peripheral T or B cells or both. PD-L1 and PD-L2 expression in nonlymphoid tissues suggests that this pathway regulates inflammatory responses in peripheral tissues. Further studies are needed to elucidate PD-L1 and PD-L2 functions.

The CD40:CD154 Pathway

The CD40:CD154 pathway is required for effective T- and B-cell immune responses. The recognition of antigen by naïve CD4$^+$ T cells results in expression of CD154. Activated CD4$^+$ T cells express CD154 and bind to APCs expressing CD40. Engagement of CD40 provides critical signals for B-cell expansion, Ig production and isotype class switching, and memory cell development (Fig. 2). Cytokine secretion by the APCs stimulates T-cell differentiation and effector function. Thus, the CD40:CD154 pathway provides a critical initial step for the development of humoral and cell-mediated immunity.

CD40

CD40 is a 40- to 45-kD type I membrane protein and a member of the TNFR family (Table 3). CD40 is expressed on B cells, activated macrophages, follicular dendritic cells (FDCs), bone marrow–derived dendritic cells, thymic epithelium, and endothelial cells (116–120). CD40 on APCs binds

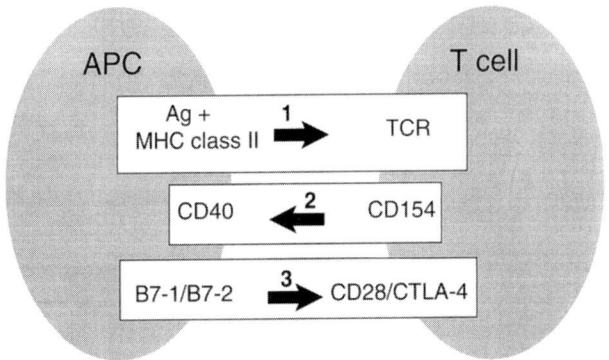

FIG. 2. Model of CD40:CD154 interactions. Stimulation of the T-cell receptor by recognition of antigen (Ag) in the context of class II major histocompatibility complex (MHC) molecules results in expression of CD154 on T cells. B7:CD28 interactions also promote CD154 expression. CD154 binds to CD40 on antigen-presenting cells (APCs) and enhances B7-1 and B7-2 expression. APCs produce cytokines that promote T-cell differentiation.

TABLE 3. *Expression and chromosome location of the TNF:TNFR superfamily*

Member	Family	Expression	Receptor/ligands	Chromosome location	
				Human	Murine
CD40	TNFR	B cells, dendritic cells, macrophages, FDCs, thymic epithelium, endothelial cells	CD154	20q13.12	2–97.0cM
CD154 (CD40L, gp39)	TNF	T cells, eosinophils, basophils, NK cells	CD40	Xq26	X–18.0cM
CD134 (OX40)	TNFR	T cells	CD134L	1p36	4–79.4cM
CD134L (OX40L)		Dendritic cells, B cells, vascular endothelial cells	CD134	1q25	1–84.9cM
4-1BB	TNFR	T cells, NK cells	4-1BBL	1p36	4–75.5cM
4-1BBL		B cells, dendritic cells, macrophages	4-1BB	19p13.3	17
CD70	TNF	T cells, B cells	CD27	19p13	17–20.0cM
CD27	TNFR	T cells, B cells, hematopoietic progenitor cells	CD70	12p13	6–60.35cM

FDC, follicular dendritic cell; NK, natural killer; TNF, tumor necrosis factor; TNFR, tumor necrosis factor receptor.

to CD154 on activated T cells. Triggering of CD40 on B cells results in B cell expansion, Ig production, isotype switching, GC formation, and memory cell development (121). Engagement of CD40 on dendritic cells and macrophages stimulates the production of IL-12, which is a potent inducer of Th1 differentiation. CD40 signals up-regulate cell surface molecules, including B7-1 and B7-2, CD23, intercellular adhesion molecule 1 (ICAM-1), and intracellular proteins such as NFκB and bcl-x_L (122–124). Thus, CD40 provides critical early activation signals to APCs that stimulate their activation and promote T cell differentiation.

CD154

CD154 (gp39, CD40L), the ligand for CD40 (125,126), is a 39-kD type II intramembrane protein and member of the TNF gene family. CD154 is expressed on activated CD4$^+$ T cells, some CD8$^+$ T cells, eosinophils, basophils, and NK cells (127–133). CD154 serves primarily as a ligand for CD40, and there is little evidence that engagement of CD40L delivers a signal to the T cell that directly promotes T-cell responses. On eosinophils, CD154 may be an important regulator of inflammation. Activated NK cells express CD154 and can lyse targets that express CD40.

Signaling through CD40

The CD40 cytoplasmic tail contains a binding site for TNFR-associated factors (TRAFs), which are involved in signal transduction pathways of TNFR superfamily members. TRAFs contain a conserved constant domain that binds to the cytoplasmic tails of TNFR family members and to other intracellular mediators. TRAF2 and TRAF3 have shown association with the CD40 cytoplasmic tail (134,135). After stimulation through CD40, TRAF3 binds the CD40 cytoplasmic tail in B cells (136). Binding of TRAF3 to CD40 is not required for Ig production (137). In fact, Ig production is blocked in B cells when TRAF3 is expressed at high

levels. Overexpression of a dominant-negative N-terminal–truncated TRAF3 in human B cells both interfered with CD40-mediated up-regulation of CD23 and B7-1 and rescued cells from Fas-mediated apoptosis (138). However, stimulation of TRAF3$^{-/-}$ B cells with anti-CD40L results in normal B cell proliferative responses and CD23 expression, which indicates that TRAF3 is not required for B-cell activation and cell survival (139). These studies suggest that expression of the TRAF3 constant domain at high levels disrupts the expression of other TRAF family members. Signaling through CD40 induces expression of TRAF2, which plays a role in NFκB-cell activation and B-cell differentiation (134). The signaling pathways between TRAFs that bind the CD40 cytoplasmic tail, other intracellular signaling molecules, and downstream transcription factors remains to be elucidated.

CD40:CD154 Interactions in the Germinal Center

The role of the CD40:CD154 pathway during *in vivo* immune response was established through the use of anti-CD154 mAbs and mice genetically deficient for CD40 and CD154. In CD40$^{-/-}$ and CD40L$^{-/-}$ mice, marked defects in B-cell responses, including Ig class switching and GC formation, were observed (140–144). The GC is the *in vivo* site of B-cell clonal expansion, affinity maturation, and memory development (145). FDCs form the framework for the GC reaction to occur and express CD40 and antigen complexes on their surface. Within the GCs, B cells express CD40 and interact with activated CD4$^+$ T cells that express high levels of CD154. The cognate interactions that occur between CD4$^+$ T cells, GC B cells, and FDCs are critical for the development of Ig-secreting B cells and memory cells. Blockade of CD154 immediately after priming with a thymus-dependent antigen prevented GC formation and reduced serum Ig to very low levels (65). However, delayed administration of anti-CD154 mAbs abrogated established GCs but had no effect on serum Ig production. These findings suggest that CD40:CD40L interactions are required for the initiation but not maintenance of B-cell differentiation for Ig production.

Genetic Defects in CD154: Hyper-Immunoglobulin M Syndrome

In humans, mutations in CD154 result in a rare immunodeficiency known as hyper-IgM syndrome. Patients with hyper-IgM syndrome have normal to high levels of polyclonal IgM; however, they exhibit low or absent levels of serum IgG, IgA, and IgE (146–150). Hyper-IgM can occur through either X-linked or autosomal modes of inheritance (151). This defect highlights the required role for CD40:CD154 interactions in Ig class switching. Although B cells from patients with hyper-IgM express CD40, defective CD154 protein expression prevents normal binding to CD40. In the absence of effective CD40:CD154 interactions, B-cell proliferative responses are impaired, which results in poor stimulation of T cells. In secondary lymphoid tissues of patients with hyper-IgM syndrome, lymphoid architecture is abnormal. FDCs are reduced in number and exhibit alterations in phenotypic markers. The defective expression and function of FDCs leads to defective GC formation (152).

Although hyper-IgM has been classified as a B-cell defect caused by the high levels of IgM and defective Ig class switching, circulating B-cell numbers in patients with hyper-IgM syndrome are often normal. Stimulation of hyper-IgM B cells with wild-type CD154 results in normal B-cell responses (150). Thus, defective B-cell responses are a consequence of abnormal expression of CD40L on T cells. Defects in T-cell responses also occur. T cells stimulated from patients with hyper-IgM demonstrate defects in IFN-γ and TNF-α [Jain 1999 #183]. In the absence of appropriate CD40:CD154 interactions, B7-1 and B7-2 are not up-regulated, and poor signaling through the B7:CD28/CTLA-4 pathway inhibits normal T-cell activation. Together, these defects in humoral and cell-mediated immunity increase the likelihood of recurrent infections in patients with hyper-IgM syndrome (153,154).

Role of the CD40:CD154 Pathway in Infection

The function of the CD40:CD154 pathway during the immune response to infectious pathogens has been investigated through the use of CD40$^{-/-}$ and CD154$^{-/-}$ mice. After infection with the intracellular parasites *Leishmania major* and *Leishmania amazonensis*, CD154$^{-/-}$ mice failed to mount a host protective immune response (155). On a genetically resistant background, wild-type mice resolve *Leishmania* infection by developing a Th1 immune response characterized by IFN-γ production by T cells and IL-12 production primarily by macrophages. IFN-γ activates nitric oxide pathways in macrophages, which kill phagocytosed *Leishmania* parasites. In *L. major*–infected CD154$^{-/-}$ mice, marked defects in IFN-γ production and IL-12 production were observed, and mice were unable to resolve the infection (156). Similar results

were observed in *L. amazonensis*–infected CD154$^{-/-}$ mice (157). Defects in IFN-γ, lymphotoxin–tumor necrosis factor, and nitric oxide production were detected, and CD154$^{-/-}$ mice developed progressive ulcerative lesions with high parasite numbers. Defects in serum Ig isotype class switching were also described after infection with *L. amazonensis*. Reduced parasite-specific IgG and IgE levels were observed in CD154$^{-/-}$ mice. In CD40$^{-/-}$ mice, the generation of the protective Th1 response and the activation of macrophages were also defective (158). These studies confirmed that mice deficient in CD40 or CD154 exhibited similar defects in humoral immune and cell-mediated responses to infection. Thus, CD40:CD154 interactions are critical for the development of the host protective immune response against an intracellular parasite.

The CD40:CD154 pathway is also critical for host immune responses against other infectious pathogens. Studies with anti-CD154 mAbs have demonstrated the requirement for CD40:CD154 interactions for resolution of *Pneumocystis carinii* (159,160). Interestingly, many patients with hyper-IgM syndrome have recurrent infections with *P. carinii*, which highlights the importance of the CD40:CD154 pathway in the host defense response against *P. carinii*.

The function of the CD40:CD154 pathway has been investigated during the immune response to several viral infections. CD40$^{-/-}$ and CD154$^{-/-}$ mice infected with LCMV or vesicular stomatitis virus exhibited profound deficits in the humoral immune response, memory B-cell development, and CD4$^+$ T-cell responses (161–163). In contrast, the CD8$^+$ CTL responses to LCMV were intact; however, memory CTL responses were impaired. Although the LCMV-specific CD8$^+$ response is potent in the CD154$^{-/-}$ mice, the ability to control infection is severely compromised (164). Thus, CD40:CD154 interactions are critical for resolving chronic viral infection, in addition to stimulating T- and B-cell responses.

Role of the CD40:CD154 Pathway in Autoimmunity

Blockade of CD154 has been one strategy for prevention or suppression of autoimmune disease. In systemic lupus erythematosus, early administration of anti-CD154 mAbs to genetically prone mice slowed progression of the disease (165). B cell activation and production of autoantibodies are required for disease progression. Because CD154 blockade diminishes the humoral immune response, the development of lupus was retarded. When the CD154 blockade was combined with CTLA-4Ig treatment, production of autoantibodies and renal disease were markedly suppressed, which suggests important synergies between the B7:CD28 and CD40:CD154 pathways. Similar results were observed in a model of myasthenia gravis. CD154$^{-/-}$ mice exhibited decreased levels of autoantibodies and amelioration of disease (166).

Blockade of the CD40:CD154 pathway also has been investigated in murine models of diabetes and multiple sclerosis. In a diabetes model, the onset of insulitis was blocked when anti-CD154 mAbs were administered to 3- to 4-week old nonobese diabetic mice, but delaying treatment beyond 9 weeks had no effect on disease (167). Thus, CD40:CD154 interactions are critical at the early stage of disease but not in the effector phase of disease. In EAE, the CD40:CD154 pathway is an important factor in disease progression within the central nervous system (168). In the absence of CD40 within the central nervous system, both inflammation in the central nervous system and disease severity are reduced even in the presence of normal peripheral T-cell responses. Thus, CD40:CD154 blockade at the onset of disease, coupled with therapies that target effector T-cell responses, may be an effective strategy for prevention of autoimmunity.

Blockade of the CD40:CD154 Pathway in Transplantation

Targeting the CD40:CD154 pathway with blocking anti-CD154 mAbs is one promising approach for prevention of transplant rejection (33). In a mouse cardiac allograft model, administration of Xanti-CD154 mAbs inhibited acute graft rejection (169). The survival of cardiac allografts and islet cell transplants were enhanced when donor cells were co-administered with anti-CD154 mAbs (170,171). It is unclear whether CD154 blockade alone will support long-term graft survival. In one study, blockade of CD154 prevented chronic rejection; however, in other model systems, graft rejection did occur (172–174). The finding that CD154 blockade alone may not be sufficient to promote healthy grafts have been supported by studies in CD154$^{-/-}$ mice. Although CD154$^{-/-}$ mice are able to support long-term graft survival, chronic allograft vasculopathy occurs over time (175). Thus, other co-stimulatory pathways may contribute to survival of allografts. Because of synergies between the B7:CD28 and CD40:CD154 pathways, combined blockade of both these pathways promotes graft survival in cardiac and skin transplant models. In primates, treatment with anti-CD154 mAbs and CTLA-4Ig prolonged renal and islet graft survival. Further studies are needed to understand the role of these pathways in order to optimize strategies for promoting long-term graft survival in animal models that may lead to clinical applications.

Other Tumor Necrosis Factor:Tumor Necrosis Factor Receptor Pathways with Co-Stimulatory Function

Within the TNF:TNFR superfamily, there are several pathways in addition to the CD40:CD154 pathway that are important for T-cell activation (176), and the receptors in these pathways lack the death domain that is present in other TNFRs. These pathways include the CD134 (OX40):CD134L, CD27:CD70, 4-1BB:4-1BBL, CD30:CD30L, RANK (OPG):RANKL, LIGHT:HVEM, and GITR:GITRL pathways. We focus on the functions of the CD134 (OX40):CD134L, CD27:CD70, and 4-1BB:4-1BBL pathways because their functions are the best understood.

CD134-CD134L Pathway

The TNFR family member CD134 (OX40) is not constitutively expressed but is up-regulated on CD4$^+$ and CD8$^+$ T cells at 24 to 48 hours after activation (177,178). CD134 expression is augmented by CD28 (179) but can occur independently of CD28 (180). The CD134 cytoplasmic domain associates with TRAF2 and TRAF5 (181). CD134 ligand (OX40L), a type II membrane protein with limited homology to TNF (182,183), is expressed on activated dendritic cells (184), B cells (185), and vascular endothelial cells (186) and also on human T-lymphocyte virus type 1–transformed T cells (182,183). CD134L is inducible on B cells and dendritic cells by CD40L (184).

The OX40:OX40L pathway appears to be particularly important for regulating the extent of CD4$^+$ T-cell expansion in the primary T cell response (187). CD134$^{-/-}$ T cells secrete IL-2 and proliferate normally during the initial period of activation but exhibit decreased survival over time and fail to sustain bcl-x$_L$ and bcl-2 production (188). CD134$^{-/-}$ mice generated lower frequencies of antigen-specific CD4$^+$ T cells late in the primary response *in vivo* and generated lower frequencies of surviving memory cells than did wild-type mice. Thus, this pathway is important for regulating primary T-cell expansion and T-cell memory.

CD134–CD134L interactions also regulate cytokine production. CD134 and CD134L$^{-/-}$ mice exhibit impaired Th1 and Th2 cytokine production (189–192). CD134$^{-/-}$ mice are severely impaired in their ability to generate a Th2 response to allergen induced airway disease (193). These mice also exhibit reduced lung inflammation and airway activity. CD134–CD134L blockade abrogated progressive leishmaniasis by suppressing the development of Th2 responses (180). Early studies suggested that CD134–CD134L interactions were required for B-cell activation and humoral immunity (185). However, studies of CD134 and CD134L$^{-/-}$ mice indicate that this pathway is not obligatory for GC formation or antibody responses to antigens or infectious agents (189–192). *In vivo* studies indicate that CD134–CD134L interactions are critical for autoimmune responses. Blocking this pathway ameliorated autoimmunity in models of EAE (194,195) and inflammatory bowel disease (196).

Although there is CD28-independent co-stimulation of T cells by CD134L (197), there are synergistic interactions between the CD28:B7 and CD134:CD134L pathways. Studies with fibroblast transfectants expressing B7-1 or CD134L or both demonstrated that CD134L and B7-1 together enhance T-cell proliferation and cytokine production, especially IL-2 (198). Anti-CD134 mAb protected CD28$^{-/-}$ mice immunized twice with myelin antigens from EAE (75). Thus, blockade of CD134 signals may enhance CD28 blockade, which may have therapeutic relevance.

CD27:CD70 Pathway

The TNF-R superfamily member CD27 is expressed on T cells, B cells, NK cells, and hematopoietic progenitor cells.

CD27 expression on T cells is constitutive but up-regulated after activation (199). The cytoplasmic domain of CD27 associates with Siva1, a proapoptotic protein and with TRAF2 and TRAF5 (200). Its ligand, CD70, is transiently induced on T and B cells after activation (199,201). TCR and co-stimulatory signals enhance CD70 expression. Proinflammatory cytokines, including IL-12 and TNF, also stimulate CD70 expression, but IL-4 and IL-10 reduce its expression.

The CD27:CD70 pathway appears to be particularly important for T-cell expansion and effector cell differentiation (200,202). CD27 ligation does not enhance IL-2 production and cell cycle progression, in contrast to CD28, but it does enhance TNF secretion (203), CTL generation, and prolong survival of anti-CD3–stimulated T cells (204). $CD27^{-/-}$ mice (204) exhibit impaired influenza virus–specific $CD4^+$ and $CD8^+$ T-cell expansion in primary and secondary responses. Effects of CD27 deficiency were most profound on T-cell memory, reflected by delayed response kinetics and markedly reduced $CD8^+$ virus-specific T-cell numbers.

CD70 on activated B cells can provide CD28-independent co-stimulatory signals to T cells. Transgenic mice constitutively expressing CD70 on B cells show that CD70 is a potent stimulus of T-cell expansion and effector cell differentiation (205). CD27:CD70 interactions also appear important in T cell–dependent B-cell differentiation after CD154:CD40–mediated expansion (206). Furthermore, CD27 signals can stimulate NK proliferation and IFN-γ production (202).

The function of this pathway in autoimmunity and tumor immunity has been evaluated in several studies. An anti-CD70 mAb prevented induction of EAE and suppressed TNF-α production (207). Co-expression of CD70 and B7-1 on tumor cells increased antitumor immune responses (208). In summary, the CD27:CD70 pathway appears most important for effector and memory T-cell generation, $CD8^+$, and NK cell functions.

4-1BB:4-1BBL Pathway

The TNFR family member 4-1BB (CD137) has a 30-kD monomeric form and a 55-kD homodimeric form (209). The cytoplasmic domain of 4-1BB interacts with TRAF1 and TRAF2 (181,210–212) but not TRAF3 and TRAF5. 4-1BB is expressed mainly on activated $CD4^+$ and $CD8^+$ T cells but also on NK cells. 4-1BB expression peaks 2 to 3 days after activation (213). 4-1BBL is expressed on activated B cells and macrophages (214) and mature dendritic cells (215). CD40 signals stimulate 4-1BBL expression (215).

4-1BB can stimulate high level IL-2 production by resting T cells in the absence of CD28 signals (215) and can stimulate primary and secondary responses of both $CD4^+$ and $CD8^+$ T cells. The role of 4-1BB on $CD4^+$ versus $CD8^+$ responses has been an area of some controversy; some studies suggest that 4-1BB has a preferential role in stimulating $CD8^+$ T cells, but others show significant effects of 4-1BB on $CD4^+$ T cells. In a comparison of $CD4^+$ and $CD8^+$ responses to 4-1BBL under similar conditions of antigenic stimulation

in which mixed lymphocyte reaction was used with purified $CD4^+$ or $CD8^+$ T cells from $CD28^{+/+}$ or $CD28^{-/-}$ mice, it was demonstrated that 4-1BBL can stimulate $CD4^+$ and $CD8^+$ proliferation and cytokine responses with similar efficacy (216). Similar roles for 4-1BB on $CD4^+$ and $CD8^+$ responses are also supported by studies of GVHD in which both $CD4^+$- and $CD8^+$-mediated GVHD were influenced by 4-1BB signals to a similar extent (217). 4-1BB does not appear to influence the synthesis of particular cytokines preferentially; rather, it influences overall levels of cytokines. 4-1BB promotes survival of both $CD4^+$ and $CD8^+$ T cells, as well as CTL responses (216). Thus, CD134 and 4-1BB appear to have similar roles in sustaining T-cell survival and enhancing effector T-cell function. However, there are some differences: Only 4-1BB, and not CD134, can stimulate IL-2 production in the absence of CD28. This may reflect differences in downstream signaling events triggered by CD134 and 4-1BB, differential expression of their ligands in vivo, or both.

Synergies between CD28 and 4-1BB have been demonstrated in vitro and in vivo. A number of studies support the idea that CD28 has a primary role in initial T-cell expansion, whereas 4-1BB:4-1BBL sustains T-cell responses (176,216,218). There is a delay in cell division in response to 4-1BB, in comparison with CD28 co-stimulation, and this may reflect constitutive expression of CD28 and inducible expression of 4-1BB (216). In primary mixed lymphocytic reactions, co-blockade with CTLA-4Ig plus 41BB-alkaline phosphatase conjugate completely abrogated the mixed lymphocytic reaction response (215). Similarly, $CD28^{-/-}$ T-cell killing of an allogeneic target was completely blocked by addition of 4-1BB-AP (215). Transfection of 4-1BBL and B7-1 or B7-2 into tumor cells enhanced antitumor responses (219), conferring long-lasting protection against subsequent challenge with parental tumor in vivo. $CD28/4-1BB^{-/-}$ mice exhibit prolonged skin graft survival (215). In summary, the 4-1BB:4-1BBL pathway appears to be most important during the later stages of an immune response and may sustain T cell activation after CD28.

CD2 SUPERFAMILY

Since 1990, the known number of molecules in the CD2 superfamily has grown from three to nine, and the functional significance of these molecules is still being elucidated. This family includes CD2, CD58, CD48, CD150, CD244, CD84, CD299, Ly–108, and BLAME. The prototype, CD2, is a member of the Ig superfamily, with IgV-like and IgC-like domains with intrachain disulfide bonds (220). The other family members have structural similarities, except CD299, which has a duplication of the IgV-IgC domains (221–233). All family members are type 1 transmembrane proteins, except for CD58 and CD48, which are glycosyl phosphatidyl inositol–linked proteins. CD58 also exists as a transmembrane protein with a short cytoplasmic domain (221). These genes are clustered at two locations on chromosome 1 (Table 4), with CD2 and CD58 at one locus and the rest of the

TABLE 4. *Structure, expression, and chromosome location of the CD2 superfamily*

Member	Structure	Expression	Receptor/ligands	Chromosome location	
				Human	Murine
CD2	Two Ig-like domains: IgV-IgC	T cells, NK cells, B cells (rodent)	CD58 (human), CD48 (human and rodents)	lp13	3–48.2cM
CD58	Two Ig-like domains: IgV-IgC GPI linked	Lymphocytes, myeloid cells, granulocytes, endothelial cells and fibroblasts	CD2	lp13	Not detected
CD48	Two Ig-like domains: IgV-IgC GPI linked	T cells, B cells, NK cells, dendritic cells	CD2, CD244	1q21–23	1–93.3cM
CD150 (SLAM)	Two Ig-like domains: IgV-IgC TxYxxV/A motif in cytoplasmic tail	Memory T cells, B cells, a subset of thymocytes. Upregulated on B cells, T cells, dendritic cells, NK cells	CD150	1q21.2–23	1–93.3cM
CD244 (2B4)	Two Ig-like domains: IgV-IgC TxYxxV/A motif in cytoplasmic tail	NK cells, $\gamma\delta$ T cells, a subset of CD8$^+$ T cells, monocytes, basophils	CD4	1q22	1–90.0cM
CD84	Two Ig-like domains: IgV-IgC TxYxxV/A motif in cytoplasmic tail	B cells, T cells, macrophages, platelets	CD84	1q24	1–93.3cM
CD299 (Ly-9)	Four Ig-like domains: IgV-IgC-IgV-IgC TxYxxV/A motif in cytoplasmic tail	T cells, B cells, thymocytes	Unknown	1q22	1–93.3cM
Ly-108	Two Ig-like domains: IgV-IgC	mRNA found in spleen, lymph nodes, B and T cell lines	Unknown	Unknown	1–89.5cM
BLAME	Two Ig-like domains: IgV-IgC	mRNA found in IFN-γ treated monocytes, bone marrow derived dendritic cells	Unknown	1q21	Unknown

GPI, glycoprotein I; IFN, interferon; Ig, immunoglobulin; mRNA, messenger ribonucleic acid; NK, natural killer.

family at another. In this section, we discuss the expression pattern and function of CD2 family members. The functions of CD299, Ly-108, and BLAME are not well characterized; therefore, these molecules are not discussed further.

CD2 and Its Ligands

Early studies identified CD2 as the receptor that bound sheep red blood cells in the isolation of human T cells (220). CD58 was recognized initially as the ligand for CD2 in humans with an affinity between 10 and 20 μM (234–236). Later, CD48 was reported also as a ligand for CD2 with a lower affinity (>100 μM) (237). However, the avidity of CD2 for CD58 is increased on TCR signaling through modifications in the cytoplasmic tail of CD2 (238). To date, a homolog for CD58 has not been found in rodents, and CD48 is the only ligand for CD2 (239,240). Murine and human CD48 also bind to CD244, another member of the CD2 superfamily, whereas no other ligands have been discovered for CD2 (241–243). Rodent CD48 has been shown to be a receptor for FimH-expressing *Escherichia coli* on macrophages and mast cells (244,245). Human CD48 also binds to heparin sulfate on epithelial cells (246).

CD2 is expressed on human and murine T cells, NK cells, and thymocytes (247). Murine CD2 is also expressed on B cells (248,249). In contrast to CD2, CD58 is more widely expressed on lymphocytes, myeloid cells, granulocytes, endothelial cells, and fibroblasts (250). Human CD48 (Blast-1) was originally discovered as an antigen expressed on B cells after transformation by Epstein-Barr virus (EBV) but is also found to be expressed on T cells, NK cells, and monocytes (250–253). Expression of murine CD48 is less broad than that of human CD58 and is restricted to lymphocytes, dendritic cells, and macrophages (239,254,255).

Function

The human CD2-CD58 receptor-ligand pair enhances T cell activation. Mitogenic anti-CD2 antibodies induce proliferation without the need for a TCR signal. Initial studies demonstrated the role for CD2 in T-cell activation by utilizing anti-CD2 mAb in combination with phorbol myristate acetate or anti-CD28 antibodies (256–259). In contrast, certain anti-CD2 mAbs have been shown to down-regulate immune responses by inducing apoptosis in activated T cells (260). Conjugate assays also demonstrated that CD2 can mediate adhesion to CD58-bearing target cells (261). The CD58:CD2 pathway can synergize with B7:CD28 pathway to enhance cell adhesion, T-cell activation and cytokine production (262). IL-1, IL-2, IL-4, IFN-γ, TNF-α, and IL-10 were enhanced when both the CD58:CD2 and B7:CD28 pathways were engaged, in comparison with B7-CD28 engagement alone (263–266). Co-engagement of the CD28 and CD2 pathways superinduced transcription factors such as activator protein–1 and NF-AT (267). CD58 co-stimulation of CD8$^+$ T cells induced higher levels of IFN-γ than did co-stimulation by the B7 family (268). Anti-CD2 antibodies also inhibited T cell–dependent B-cell activation, which indicates that CD2 and its ligands may play a role in humoral immunity (269). CD58:CD2 interactions also activate NK cells (256,270) and induce differentiation of a subset of T cells, which secretes elevated levels of IL-10 (271,272). Thus, this pathway may lead to the generation of a yet-undefined regulatory CD4$^+$ T cell population. In summary, data from human studies imply that the CD2:CD58 pathway is involved in cell adhesion, cytokine production, and the differentiation of cells, which regulate immune responses.

In murine studies, CD48:CD2 interactions have been addressed in *in vitro* and *in vivo* models. The expression of CD2 and CD48 on both APCs and T cells implies that the function of these molecules is important in APC–T-cell collaboration. Anti–murine CD2 suppressed phytohemagglutinin and anti-CD3 responses of CD4$^+$ T cells (239). Anti-CD48 antibodies inhibited the proliferation of T-cells *in vitro* (254). When DO11.10 TCR transgenic T cells were stimulated with CHO cells transfected with CD48 and class II-IA^d MHC, CD48 enhanced T-cell proliferation and IL-2 production (273). CD2 Fab$_2$ antibodies blocked this enhanced response. *In vivo*, anti-CD2 mAbs suppressed cell-mediated immunity and prolonged kidney allograft pancreatic islet cell allografts and xenograft survival (274–277). There was synergy between anti-CD2 and anti-CD48 antibodies in prolonging allograft survival (278). Anti-CD48 antibodies blocked hapten-induced contact sensitivity and CTL generation (279). The interpretation of *in vivo* studies with anti-CD48 antibodies needs to be revisited, because CD48 is now known also to be a ligand for CD244.

Initially, the CD2$^{-/-}$ mouse did not exhibit a detectable phenotype, although there was a suggestion that T cells from CD2$^{-/-}$ mice may be defective in proliferation and cytokine production (280,281). Infection of CD2$^{-/-}$ mice with LMCV showed normal antiviral responses (282). However, when CD2$^{-/-}$ mice were crossed with a T-cell transgenic specific for LCMV-derived peptide p33, there was 3- to 10-fold shift in the dose response to LMCV peptide in CD2$^{-/-}$ T cells *in vitro* and reduced expansion of the CD2$^{-/-}$ T cells *in vivo*, in comparison with the wild-type T cells (283). Further studies in another transgenic model have found that T cells of CD2$^{-/-}$ mice were less responsive to wild-type peptide and unresponsive to peptide agonists (284). This study also indicated a role for CD2 in thymic selection. CD48$^{-/-}$ mice show defects in CD4$^+$ T-cell activation and demonstrate a

role for CD48 on APCs as well as T cells (223). T cells in CD2$^{-/-}$CD28$^{-/-}$ mice showed decreased proliferation to concanavalin A, anti-CD3, and antigen, in comparison with CD2$^{-/-}$ or CD28$^{-/-}$ mice (285). This defect was more profound at lower antigen concentrations, which indicates a role for both pathways in modulating T-cell responses.

Although many studies have addressed the role of CD2 *in vivo* and *in vitro*, the molecular mechanism of CD2 function is still controversial. The cytoplasmic tail of CD2 is rich in proline and basic amino acids (220). The increased avidity of CD2 for CD58 on TCR signaling may enhance adhesion and may be one mechanism by which this pathway attenuates responses (238). Studies have demonstrated the association of Lck and Fyn with the cytoplasmic tail of CD2 (286,287), and an adaptor protein called CD2 binding protein (CD2BP1) in humans and PSTPIP in mice binds to the cytoplasmic tail of CD2 (288,289). Highly expressed in T cells and NK cells, CD2BP1 may be an adaptor protein that couples CD2 to a protein tyrosine phosphatase (288). A second protein, CD2BP2, binds to the proline-rich motif in the CD2 cytoplasmic tail. When CD2BP2 was overexpressed in Jurkat T cells, cross-linking of CD2 led to increased IL-2 production (290).

CD2 may have an important role in the immunological synapse (291). During formation of the immunological synapse, there are distinct clusters of molecules termed *supramolecular clusters* (SMACs) (291). Central SMACs contain the TCR/MHC complex and CD28, and outer SMACs contain ICAM and leukocyte function–associated antigen 1 (LFA-1). CD2 has been localized to the outer SMAC within the ICAM:LFA-1 ring, where larger molecules are excluded (291). Van der Merwe (292) postulated that the interaction of CD2 with its ligand may have two functions: (a) to optimize TCR engagement by placing the cell membranes at the correct distance for binding and (b) to maintain the integrity of the immunological synapse by "filtering out" molecules of the incorrect size after TCR triggering. Wild et al. (293) examined the effects of changing the dimensions of murine CD48 and measured the outcome by assessing T-cell activation. Wild-type or truncated CD48 enhanced T-cell activation, but an elongated CD48 inhibited T-cell activation. This study gave the first direct evidence that segregation of molecules of the same size into discrete contact zones was important in T-cell activation. Further studies have shown that the recruitment of murine CD48 to lipid raft resulted in enhanced ζ chain tyrosine phosphorylation and association with the actin cytoskeleton (294). Mutational studies have shown that binding of CD58 to CD2 is sufficient to translocate CD2 to lipid rafts (295). This process was independent of signaling through the cytoplasmic tail of CD2. Furthermore, co-stimulation of CD4$^+$ memory T cells by activated endothelial cells required the binding of CD58 to CD2 for the development of lipid rafts (296). The cytoplasmic tail of CD2 binds CD2-associated protein (CD2AP), which is essential for stabilizing contact between the APC and T cell (297). CD2AP$^{-/-}$ mice showed defects in T-cell activation;

however, these mice die of renal failure at 6 to 7 weeks because of the essential role of CD2AP2 in glomerular epithelial cell formation (298).

CD150 (Signaling Lymphocyte-Activation Molecule, IPO-3)

CD150, also known as signaling lymphocyte-activation molecule (SLAM) and IPO-3, was identified as an antigen expressed on human CD45RO$^+$ T cells, thymocytes, and B cells (224,299). It is up-regulated on activated human and murine B cells, T cells, dendritic cells, and NK cells (225,299–301). Both activated human T cells and B cells express three isoforms of CD150 (224,302), including membrane and soluble forms. The cytoplasmic tail of the membrane form of CD150 has three consensus sequence TxYxxV/A that are involved in recruitment of SH2-domain protein tyrosine phosphatases. The murine CD150 gene has membrane isoforms but no soluble form of CD150 (225). SAP (SLAM-associated protein) associates with the cytoplasmic tail of CD150 in T cells and NK cells (303). The consequences of the association of SAP with members of the CD2 superfamily are discussed later. In B cells and macrophages, another protein, EAT-2, has been shown to associate with the phosphorylated tail of CD150 (304). A ligand for CD150 has not been discovered; however, homophilic interaction between CD150 molecules has been described, but the interaction is of low affinity (305).

Function

Co–cross-linking of CD150 plus CD3-augmented T-cell cytokine production independent of CD28 (224). Cross-linking of CD3 plus CD150-enhanced production of IFN-γ by Th1 clones and redirected Th2 and Th0 clones to produce IFN-γ (224). Murine studies confirmed the enhancement of IFN-γ production by Th1 clones but did not find that IFN-γ was produced in Th2 clones (225). CD150 engagement seems to have little effect on IL-4 or IL-13 production (306). CD150 also enhances T-cell cytotoxicity (307). Together, these studies imply a role of CD150 in T-cell activation and effector functions. On APCs, soluble CD150 stimulated proliferation of human B cells induced by anti-IgM and augmented IgM, IgG, and IgA produced by anti-CD40–activated B cells (302). CD150 is up-regulated on dendritic cells in the presence of anti-CD40 or lipopolysaccharide (300). When dendritic cells were activated and subsequently stimulated with anti-CD150 mAbs, there was increased production of IL-12 and IL-8 but not IL-10, in comparison with control mAb. The homophilic interaction of CD150 or interaction with a yet-undefined ligand might be important in the APC and T-cell collaboration.

Human CD150 is the cellular receptor for measles virus, and the V region is essential for the measles virus binding (308,309). CD150 is down-regulated by infection of peripheral blood lymphocytes with measles virus. However, CD150 is not involved in the dominant negative signal, which leads to inhibition of proliferation induced by the virus (310).

CD244 (2B4)

Murine CD244 was originally cloned from a cytotoxic T-lymphocytic line 2 complementary deoxyribonucleic acid (cDNA) library (226, 311).

Murine CD244 exists as two isoforms, generated by alternative splicing, on the surface of activated NK cells: CD244L and CD244S (227). These are identical in the extracellular and transmembrane domains. Like CD150, the cytoplasmic tail of CD244L has four consensus tyrosine TxYxxV/A motifs, whereas CD244S has only two (227). Phosphorylated CD244L associates with SHP-2 but not SHP-1. Neither SHP-1 nor SHP-2 associates with CD244S, which indicates that SHP-2 binding involves one of the other two motifs in the cytoplasmic tail of CD244L (312). SAP and EAT-2 also are recruited to phosphorylated human and murine CD244. (301,304,313). Human CD244 has four consensus tyrosine motifs, similar to murine CD244L (314). To date, a shorter version of human CD244 has not been published. The promoter regions of murine and human CD244 have been cloned, and there is an indication that the activator protein–1 is involved in the transcription of the CD244 gene (315,316).

Human and murine CD244 are expressed on NK cells, $\gamma\delta$ T cells, and a subset of CD8$^+$ T cells (317–320). In human thymus, CD244 is expressed only on single positive CD8$^+$ thymocytes. CD244 is up-regulated on activated murine and human CD8$^+$ T cells (320–322). Both isoforms of murine CD244 are up-regulated on CD8$^+$ T cells after activation by IL-2 (322). Human CD244 is also expressed on CD14$^+$ monocytes and basophils (323) and binds CD48 (241–243). The affinity of human CD48 for CD244 is 8 μM, much higher than the interaction between CD48 and CD2 (242).

Function

Murine CD244 was originally thought to be an activating receptor on NK cells. The lytic activity of NK cells and non–MHC-restricted T cells was increased when CD244 was engaged on these cells (317). There was also an increase in IFN-γ production and granule release. The discovery of two isoforms of CD244 in the mouse led to evaluation of each isoform on NK cells (312). CD244L and CD244S were transfected into a rat NK cell line (RNK-16) and redirected cell lysis of P815 tumor cells lines was analyzed with an anti-CD244 antibody (312). CD244S was shown to be an activating receptor for NK cells, whereas CD244L was an inhibitory receptor. Engagement of human CD244 by various anti-CD244 antibodies or CD48 results in enhanced cytotoxicity and IFN-γ production (243,323). CD244 has been implicated as a co-receptor involved in natural cytotoxicity, and engagement of NK inhibitory receptors can interfere with the phosphorylation of CD244 (324,325). In humans, NK activation is dependent on the signals through activating receptors such as CD244 and signals through inhibitory receptors. Ligation of CD244 on epidermal $\gamma\delta$ T cells led to increased production of IFN-γ and IL-2 (319). However ligation of CD244 on human

CD8$^+$ T cells did not induce cytokine production, whereas anti-CD244 mAbs inhibited non–MHC-restricted cytolysis by IL-2 activated CD8$^+$ T cells (318,320,323). Anti-CD244 mAbs blocked the proliferation of the IL-2 activated but not naïve CD8$^+$ T cells. Anti-CD48 was also able to block the proliferation of IL-2–activated CD8$^+$ T cells, but there was no synergetic effect of adding both anti-CD244 and anti-CD48. These results demonstrate that the CD244/CD48 interaction serves as a T-cell co-stimulatory pathway (323). The function of CD244 on monocytes and basophils is still unknown.

CD84

CD84 was defined by three monoclonal antibodies in 1994 (228,229,326): SAP, SHP-2, and EAT-2, which associate with the phosphorylated tyrosine in the cytoplasmic tail of human CD84. (304,327).

Human CD84 is expressed as a highly glycolysated surface receptor. Expression is found on B cells, macrophages, T cells, and platelets (228). In the thymus, the highest expression of CD84 is found on CD4$^-$CD8$^-$ thymocytes with a slight decrease in expression when thymocytes mature to the single positive stage (228). In the periphery, CD45RO^{high} express elevated levels of CD84. mRNA for murine CD84 has been detected in bone marrow, lymph node thymus, spleen, and lung tissues, but surface expression of CD84 has not been confirmed in these tissues or on lymphoid cells (229).

CD84 binds to itself. Coligation of suboptimal doses of anti-CD3 and anti-CD84 leads to augmented IFN-γ production by human peripheral blood mononuclear cells, in comparison with anti-CD3 alone (328). CD84-Ig fusion protein immobilized by plastic in the presence of anti-CD3 also led to increased IFN-γ production by peripheral blood mononuclear cells.

Signaling Lymphocyte-Activation Molecule–Associated Protein and Members of the CD2 Superfamily

SAP, or SH2DIA, is a 128–amino acid molecule containing a single SH2 domain (301,329,330). SAP is expressed in human and murine T cells, NK cells, tonsillar B cells, and some B lymphoblastoid cell lines (301,331,332). The gene that encodes SAP is mutated or deleted in patients with X-linked lymphoproliferative (XLP) disease (333). Boys with this disease are unable to mount an effective immune response to EBV, and those exposed to EBV develop fatal mononucleosis (334). Children who survive can develop lymphoproliferative diseases such as Burkitt's lymphoma or dysgammaglobulinemia. The murine homolog of SAP is highly expressed in Th1 clones, in comparison with Th2 clones (331). SAP$^{-/-}$ mice exhibit increased T-cell activation and IFN-γ production when the mice are challenged with LCMV and *Toxoplasma gondii* but exhibit decreased responses to *L. major* (335,336), which suggests a role for SAP in limiting Th1 responses. During an EBV infection, XLP patients show increased IFN-γ production (337).

SAP has been shown to associate with four members of the CD2 family: CD150, CD244, CD84, and CD299. This association occurs with the phosphorylation of the TxYxxV/A motif in these molecules (301,303,313,327). It has been proposed that the association of SAP with phosphorylated CD150 in T cells, NK cells, and tonsillar B cells leads to the inhibition of SHP-2 binding (247,332), which may lead to positive signaling of the CD150 molecule. This is also thought to be the case in NK cells, in which SAP associates with CD244 (313). However, ligation of CD150 leads to SAP-dependent protein tyrosine phosphorylation of certain signaling molecules, including the Src-related tyrosine kinase FynT (338). These functions of SAP may not be mutually exclusive; SAP may bind to the cytoplasmic tail, preventing the binding of SHP-2 as well as causing conformational changes in the cytoplasmic tail to allow the binding of other signaling molecules. The link between SAP and XLP disease is not clear. Patients with XLP disease have a defect in NK cytotoxicity (339–341). Ligation of CD244 on NK cells from patients with XLP disease inhibited NK cytolysis. In the presence of EBV-transformed human leukocyte antigen–1 negative B-cell clones in which CD48 was highly expressed, NK killing was defective in patients with XLP disease (341). Because CD150, CD244, CD84, and CD299 are expressed on APCs, T cells, and NK cells, it will be intriguing to learn whether the defects exhibited by patients with XLP disease are caused by a lack of association with these molecules.

The CD2 superfamily is a newly emerging family of molecules that may contribute to enhancing responses of cells of the immune system. The role of CD2 in the immunological synapse and the involvement of the other family members in XLP disease have illuminated the importance of these molecules in APC–T-cell collaboration.

CONCLUDING REMARKS

A growing number of T-cell co-stimulatory pathways provide second signals that can regulate the activation, inhibition, and fine-tuning of T-cell responses. After TCR engagement, CD28 predominates and delivers critical stimulatory signals to naïve T cells that can prevent the development of anergy by promoting T-cell activation, differentiation, and survival. The effects of CD28 co-stimulation depend, in part, on the CD40:CD40L pathway, inasmuch as CD40 engagement results in APC activation, which up-regulates B7-1 and B7-2. Whereas CD28 has a primary role in initial T-cell activation, other co-stimulatory pathways sustain T cell activation after CD28. For example, ICOS regulates effector cytokine production, and CD134 and 4-1BB can sustain T-cell survival and effector functions. The expression ligands for some co-stimulatory receptors, such as ICOS and CD134, on non-APCs as wells as APCS, suggest a means for regulating effector T-cell responses in peripheral tissues. The CD2 family also is important for T cell and NK cell activation, but the relationships among CD2 family members and other co-stimulatory pathways is not yet clear. Signals through co-stimulatory pathways not only stimulate T-cell activation but also inhibit T-cell responses. CTLA-4 inhibits T-cell proliferation and IL-2 production and can promote the induction of anergy. PD-1 also can inhibit T-cell proliferation and cytokine production, and the expression of PD-1 ligands in a variety of tissues suggests a role for PD-1 in regulating T-cell responses and tolerance in the periphery. The critical role of co-stimulation in regulating T cell activation and tolerance has been demonstrated *in vivo* in models of autoimmunity, transplantation, and infectious diseases. Additional understanding of the functions of T-cell co-stimulatory pathways individually and their interplay may enable manipulation of co-stimulatory signals to promote T-cell activation or T-cell tolerance for therapeutic purposes.

REFERENCES

1. Bretscher P, Cohn M. A theory of self-nonself discrimination. *Science* 1970;169:1042–1049.
2. Bretscher PA. A two-step, two-signal model for the primary activation of precursor helper T cells. *Proc Natl Acad Sci U S A* 1999;96:185–190.
3. Lafferty KJ, Cunningham AJ. A new analysis of allogeneic interactions. *Aust J Exp Biol Med Sci* 1975;53:27–42.
4. Viola A, Lanzavecchia A. T cell activation determined by T cell receptor number and tunable thresholds. *Science* 1996;273:104–106.
5. Karandikar NJ, Vanderlugt CL, Bluestone JA, et al. Targeting the B7/CD28:CTLA-4 costimulatory system in CNS autoimmune disease. *J Neuroimmunol* 1998;89:10–18.
6. Oosterwegel MA, Greenwald RJ, Mandelbrot DA, et al. CTLA-4 and T cell activation. *Curr Opin Immunol* 1999;11:294–300.
7. Salomon B, Bluestone JA. Complexities of CD28/B7:CTLA-4 costimulatory pathways in autoimmunity and transplantation. *Annu Rev Immunol* 2001;19:225–252.
8. Chambers CA, Kuhns MS, Egen JG, et al. CTLA-4–mediated inhibition in regulation of T cell responses: mechanisms and manipulation in tumor immunotherapy. *Annu Rev Immunol* 2001;19:565–594.
9. Coyle AJ, Gutierrez-Ramos JC. The expanding B7 superfamily: increasing complexity in costimulatory signals regulating T cell function. *Nat Immunol* 2001;2:203–209.
10. Alegre M, Frauwirth K, Thompson C. T-cell regulation by CD28 and CTLA-4. *Nat Immunol Rev* 2001;1:220–228.
11. Hutloff A, Dittrich AM, Beier KC, et al. ICOS is an inducible T-cell co-stimulator structurally and functionally related to CD28. *Nature* 1999;397:263–266.
12. Swallow MM, Wallin JJ, Sha WC. B7h, a novel costimulatory homolog of B7.1 and B7.2, is induced by TNFalpha. *Immunity* 1999;11:423–432.
13. Ling V, Wu PW, Finnerty HF, et al. Cutting edge: identification of GL50, a novel B7-like protein that functionally binds to ICOS receptor. *J Immunol* 2000;164:1653–1657.
14. Yoshinaga SK, Whoriskey JS, Khare SD, et al. T-cell co-stimulation through B7RP-1 and ICOS. *Nature* 1999;402:827–832.
15. Brodie D, Collins AV, Iaboni A, et al. LICOS, a primordial costimulatory ligand? *Curr Biol* 2000;10:333–336.
16. Wang S, Zhu G, Chapoval AI, et al. Costimulation of T cells by B7-H2, a B7-like molecule that binds ICOS. *Blood* 2000;96:2808–2813.
17. Ishida Y, Agata Y, Shibahara K, et al. Induced expression of PD-1, a novel member of the immunoglobulin gene superfamily, upon programmed cell death. *EMBO J* 1992;11:3887–3895.
18. Freeman GJ, Long AJ, Iwai Y, et al. Engagement of the PD-1 immunoinhibitory receptor by a novel B7 family member leads to negative regulation of lymphocyte activation. *J Exp Med* 2000;192:1027–1034.
19. Dong H, Zhu G, Tamada K, et al. B7-H1, a third member of the B7 family, co-stimulates T-cell proliferation and interleukin-10 secretion. *Nat Med* 1999;5:1365–1369.
20. Latchman Y, Wood CR, Chernova T, et al. PD-L2 is a second ligand for PD-I and inhibits T cell activation. *Nat Immunol* 2001;2:261–268.
21. Tseng SY, Otsuji M, Gorski K, et al. B7-DC, a new dendritic cell molecule with potent costimulatory properties for T cells. *J Exp Med* 2001;193:839–846.
22. Chapoval AI, Ni J, Lau JS, et al. B7-H3: a costimulatory molecule for T cell activation and IFN-gamma production. *Nat Immunol* 2001;2:269–274.
23. Freeman GJ, Gray GS, Gimmi CD, et al. Structure, expression, and T cell costimulatory activity of the murine homologue of the human B lymphocyte activation antigen B7. *J Exp Med* 1991;174:625–631.
24. Freedman AS, Freeman G, Horowitz JC, et al. B7, a B-cell-restricted antigen that identifies preactivated B cells. *J Immunol* 1987;139:3260–3267.
25. Yokochi T, Holly RD, Clark EA. B lymphoblast antigen (BB-1) expressed on Epstein-Barr virus–activated B cell blasts, B lymphoblastoid cell lines, and Burkitt's lymphomas. *J Immunol* 1982;128:823–827.
26. Freeman GJ, Gribben JG, Boussiotis VA, et al. Cloning of B7-2: a CTLA-4 counter-receptor that costimulates human T cell proliferation. *Science* 1993;262:909–911.
27. Freeman GJ, Borriello F, Hodes RJ, et al. Murine B7-2, an alternative CTLA4 counter-receptor that costimulates T cell proliferation and interleukin 2 production. *J Exp Med* 1993;178:2185–2192.
28. Azuma M, Ito D, Yagita H, et al. B70 antigen is a second ligand for CTLA-4 and CD28. *Nature* 1993;366:76–79.
29. Aruffo A, Seed B. Molecular cloning of a CD28 cDNA by a high-efficiency COS cell expression system. *Proc Natl Acad Sci U S A* 1987;84:8573–8577.
30. Gross JA, St. John T, Allison JP. The murine homologue of the T lymphocyte antigen CD28. Molecular cloning and cell surface expression. *J Immunol* 1990;144:3201–3210.
31. Brunet JF, Denizot F, Luciani MF, et al. A new member of the immunoglobulin superfamily—CTLA-4. *Nature* 1987;328:267–270.
32. Linsley PS, Brady W, Urnes M, et al. CTLA-4 is a second receptor for the B cell activation antigen B7. *J Exp Med* 1991;174:561–569.
33. Salama AD, Remuzzi G, Harmon WE, et al. Challenges to achieving clinical transplantation tolerance. *J Clin Invest* 2001;108:943–948.
34. Abrams JR, Kelley SL, Hayes E, et al. Blockade of T lymphocyte costimulation with cytotoxic T lymphocyte-associated antigen 4–immunoglobulin (CTLA4Ig) reverses the cellular pathology of psoriatic plaques, including the activation of keratinocytes, dendritic cells, and endothelial cells. *J Exp Med* 2000;192:681–694.
35. Guinan EC, Boussiotis VA, Neuberg D, et al. Transplantation of anergic histoincompatible bone marrow allografts. *N Engl J Med* 1999;340:1704–1714.
36. Peach RJ, Bajorath J, Brady W, et al. Complementarity determining region 1 (CDR1)– and CDR3-analogous regions in CTLA-4 and CD28 determine the binding to B7-1. *J Exp Med* 1994;180:2049–2058.
37. Linsley PS, Greene JL, Tan P, et al. Coexpression and functional cooperation of CTLA-4 and CD28 on activated T lymphocytes. *J Exp Med* 1992;176:1595–1604.
38. Linsley PS, Greene JL, Brady W, et al. Human B7-1 (CD80) and B7-2 (CD86) bind with similar avidities but distinct kinetics to CD28 and CTLA-4 receptors. *Immunity* 1994;1:793–801.
39. Gross JA, Callas E, Allison JP. Identification and distribution of the costimulatory receptor CD28 in the mouse. *J Immunol* 1992;149:380–388.
40. Linsley PS, Bradshaw J, Greene J, et al. Intracellular trafficking of CTLA-4 and focal localization towards sites of TCR engagement. *Immunity* 1996;4:535–543.
41. Ikemizu S, Gilbert RJ, Fennelly JA, et al. Structure and dimerization of a soluble form of B7-1. *Immunity* 2000;12:51–60.
42. Schwartz JC, Zhang X, Fedorov AA, et al. Structural basis for costimulation by the human CTLA-4/B7-2 complex. *Nature* 2001;410:604–608.
43. Stamper CC, Zhang Y, Tobin JF, et al. Crystal structure of the B7-1/CTLA-4 complex that inhibits human immune responses. *Nature* 2001;410:608–611.
44. Hathcock KS, Laszlo G, Pucillo C, et al. Comparative analysis of B7-1 and B7-2 costimulatory ligands: expression and function. *J Exp Med* 1994;180:631–640.

45. McAdam AJ, Schweitzer AN, Sharpe AH. The role of B7 co-stimulation in activation and differentiation of CD4+ and CD8+ T cells. Immunol Rev 1998;165:231–247.
46. Ranheim EA, Kipps TJ. Activated T cells induce expression of B7/BB1 on normal or leukemic B cells through a CD40-dependent signal. J Exp Med 1993;177:925–935.
47. Roy M, Aruffo A, Ledbetter J, et al. Studies on the interdependence of gp39 and B7 expression and function during antigen-specific immune responses. Eur J Immunol 1995;25:596–603.
48. Lenschow DJ, Walunas TL, Bluestone JA. CD28/B7 system of T cell costimulation. Annu Rev Immunol 1996;14:233–258.
49. Lanzavecchia A, Lezzi G, Viola A. From TCR engagement to T cell activation: a kinetic view of T cell behavior. Cell 1999;96:1–4.
50. Boise LH, Minn AJ, Noel PJ, et al. CD28 costimulation can promote T cell survival by enhancing the expression of Bcl-X$_L$. Immunity 1995;3:87–98.
51. Rulifson IC, Sperling AI, Fields PE, et al. CD28 costimulation promotes the production of Th2 cytokines. J Immunol 1997;158:658–665.
52. Salomon B, Lenschow DJ, Rhee L, et al. B7/CD28 costimulation is essential for the homeostasis of the CD4+CD25+ immunoregulatory T cells that control autoimmune diabetes. Immunity 2000;12:431–440.
53. Tivol EA, Boyd SD, McKeon S, et al. CTLA-4Ig prevents lymphoproliferation and fatal multiorgan tissue destruction in CTLA-4–deficient mice. J Immunol 1997;158:5091–5094.
54. Waterhouse P, Penninger JM, Timms E, et al. Lymphoproliferative disorders with early lethality in mice deficient in Ctla-4. Science 1995;270:985–988.
55. Walunas TL, Bakker CY, Bluestone JA. CTLA-4 ligation blocks CD28-dependent T cell activation. J Exp Med 1996;183:2541–2550.
56. Krummel MF, Allison JP. CTLA-4 engagement inhibits IL-2 accumulation and cell cycle progression upon activation of resting T cells. J Exp Med 1996;183:2533–2540.
57. Leach DR, Krummel MF, Allison JP. Enhancement of antitumor immunity by CTLA-4 blockade. Science 1996;271:1734–1736.
58. van Elsas A, Sutmuller RP, Hurwitz AA, et al. Elucidating the autoimmune and antitumor effector mechanisms of a treatment based on cytotoxic T lymphocyte antigen–4 blockade in combination with a B16 melanoma vaccine: comparison of prophylaxis and therapy. J Exp Med 2001;194:481–489.
59. Brunner MC, Chambers CA, Chan FK, et al. CTLA-4–mediated inhibition of early events of T cell proliferation. J Immunol 1999;162:5813–5820.
60. Greenwald RJ, Boussiotis VA, Lorsbach RB, et al. CTLA-4 regulates induction of anergy in vivo. Immunity 2001;14:145–155.
61. Chen W, Jin W, Wahl SM. Engagement of cytotoxic T lymphocyte–associated antigen 4 (CTLA-4) induces transforming growth factor beta (TGF-beta) production by murine CD4(+) T cells. J Exp Med 1998;188:1849–1857.
62. Read S, Malmstrom V, Powrie F. Cytotoxic T lymphocyte–associated antigen 4 plays an essential role in the function of CD25(+)CD4(+) regulatory cells that control intestinal inflammation. J Exp Med 2000;192:295–302.
63. Takahashi T, Tagami T, Yamazaki S, et al. Immunologic self-tolerance maintained by CD25(+)CD4(+) regulatory T cells constitutively expressing cytotoxic T lymphocyte–associated antigen 4. J Exp Med 2000;192:303–310.
64. Ferguson SE, Han S, Kelsoe G, et al. CD28 is required for germinal center formation. J Immunol 1996;156:4576–4581.
65. Han S, Hathcock K, Zheng B, et al. Cellular interaction in germinal centers. Roles of CD40 ligand and B7-2 in established germinal centers. J Immunol 1995;155:556–567.
66. Borriello F, Sethna MP, Boyd SD, et al. B7-1 and B7-2 have overlapping, critical roles in immunoglobulin class switching and germinal center formation. Immunity 1997;6:303–313.
67. Gause WC, Lu P, Zhou XD, et al. H. polygyrus: B7-independence of the secondary type 2 response. Exp Parasitol 1996;84:264–273.
68. Perez VL, Van Parijs L, Biuckians A, et al. Induction of peripheral T cell tolerance in vivo requires CTLA-4 engagement. Immunity 1997;6:411–417.
69. Chen L, Ashe S, Brady WA, et al. Costimulation of antitumor immunity by the B7 counterreceptor for the T lymphocyte molecules CD28 and CTLA-4. Cell 1992;71:1093–1102.
70. Townsend SE, Allison JP. Tumor rejection after direct costimulation of CD8+ T cells by B7- transfected melanoma cells. Science 1993;259:368–370.
71. Turka LA, Linsley PS, Lin H, et al. T-cell activation by the CD28 ligand B7 is required for cardiac allograft rejection in vivo. Proc Natl Acad Sci U S A 1992;89:11102–11105.
72. Sayegh MH, Turka LA. The role of T-cell costimulatory activation pathways in transplant rejection. N Engl J Med 1998;338:1813–1821.
73. Blazar BR, Taylor PA, Linsley PS, et al. In vivo blockade of CD28/CTLA4: B7/BB1 interaction with CTLA4-Ig reduces lethal murine graft-versus-host disease across the major histocompatibility complex barrier in mice. Blood 1994;83:3815–3825.
74. Chang TT, Jabs C, Sobel RA, et al. Studies in B7-deficient mice reveal a critical role for B7 costimulation in both induction and effector phases of experimental autoimmune encephalomyelitis. J Exp Med 1999;190:733–740.
75. Chitnis T, Najafian N, Abdallah KA, et al. CD28-independent induction of experimental autoimmune encephalomyelitis. J Clin Invest 2001;107:575–583.
76. Luhder F, Hoglund P, Allison JP, et al. Cytotoxic T lymphocyte–associated antigen 4 (CTLA-4) regulates the unfolding of autoimmune diabetes. J Exp Med 1998;187:427–432.
77. Abrams JR, Lebwohl MG, Guzzo CA, et al. CTLA4Ig-mediated blockade of T-cell costimulation in patients with psoriasis vulgaris. J Clin Invest 1999;103:1243–1252.
78. Keane-Myers A, Gause WC, Linsley PS, et al. B7-CD28/CTLA-4 costimulatory pathways are required for the development of T helper cell 2–mediated allergic airway responses to inhaled antigens. J Immunol 1997;158:2042–2049.
79. Rudd CE. Upstream-downstream: CD28 cosignaling pathways and T cell function. Immunity 1996;4:527–534.
80. Slavik JM, Hutchcroft JE, Bierer BE. CD28/CTLA-4 and CD80/CD86 families: signaling and function. Immunol Res 1999;19:1–24.
81. Rudd CE, Schneider H. Lymphocyte signaling: Cbl sets the threshold for autoimmunity. Curr Biol 2000;10:R344–347.
82. Chuang E, Fisher TS, Morgan RW, et al. The CD28 and CTLA-4 receptors associate with the serine/threonine phosphatase PP2A. Immunity 2000;13:313–322.
83. Okkenhaug K, Wu L, Garza KM, et al. A point mutation in CD28 distinguishes proliferative signals from survival signals. Nat Immunol 2001;2:325–332.
84. Masteller EL, Chuang E, Mullen AC, et al. Structural analysis of CTLA-4 function in vivo. J Immunol 2000;164:5319–5327.
85. Bradshaw JD, Lu P, Leytze G, et al. Interaction of the cytoplasmic tail of CTLA-4 (CD152) with a clathrin-associated protein is negatively regulated by tyrosine phosphorylation. Biochemistry 1997;36:15975–15982.
86. Marengere LE, Waterhouse P, Duncan GS, et al. Regulation of T cell receptor signaling by tyrosine phosphatase SYP association with CTLA-4. Science 1996;272:1170–1173.
87. Lee KM, Chuang E, Griffin M, et al. Molecular basis of T cell inactivation by CTLA-4. Science 1998;282:2263–2266.
88. Nakaseko C, Miyatake S, Iida T, et al. Cytotoxic T lymphocyte antigen 4 (CTLA-4) engagement delivers an inhibitory signal through the membrane-proximal region in the absence of the tyrosine motif in the cytoplasmic tail. J Exp Med 1999;190:765–774.
89. Buonfiglio D, Bragardo M, Redoglia V, et al. The T cell activation molecule H4 and the CD28-like molecule ICOS are identical. Eur J Immunol 2000;30:3463–3467.
90. Tezuka K, Tsuji T, Hirano D, et al. Identification and characterization of rat AILIM/ICOS, a novel T-cell costimulatory molecule, related to the CD28/CTLA4 family. Biochem Biophys Res Commun 2000;276:335–345.
91. Beier KC, Hutloff A, Dittrich AM, et al. Induction, binding specificity and function of human ICOS. Eur J Immunol 2000;30:3707–3717.
92. Coyle AJ, Lehar S, Lloyd C, et al. The CD28-related molecule ICOS is required for effective T cell–dependent immune responses. Immunity 2000;13:95–105.
93. Mages HW, Hutloff A, Heuck C, et al. Molecular cloning and characterization of murine ICOS and identification of B7h as ICOS ligand. Eur J Immunol 2000;30:1040–1047.
94. Aicher A, Hayden-Ledbetter M, Brady WA, et al. Characterization of human inducible costimulator ligand expression and function. J Immunol 2000;164:4689–4696.

95. McAdam AJ, Chang TT, Lumelsky AE, et al. Mouse inducible cos-timulatory molecule (ICOS) expression is enhanced by CD28 cos-timulation and regulates differentiation of CD4$^+$ T cells. *J Immunol* 2000;165:5035–5040.

96. Kopf M, Coyle AJ, Schmitz N, et al. Inducible costimulator protein (ICOS) controls T helper cell subset polarization after virus and parasite infection. *J Exp Med* 2000;192:53–61.

97. Dong C, Juedes AE, Temann UA, et al. ICOS co-stimulatory receptor is essential for T-cell activation and function. *Nature* 2001;409:97–101.

98. McAdam AJ, Greenwald RJ, Levin MA, et al. ICOS is critical for CD40-mediated antibody class switching. *Nature* 2001;409:102–105.

99. Tafuri A, Shahinian A, Bladt F, et al. ICOS is essential for effective T-helper–cell responses. *Nature* 2001;409:105–109.

100. Riley JL, Blair PJ, Musser JT, et al. ICOS costimulation requires IL-2 and can be prevented by CTLA-4 engagement. *J Immunol* 2001;166:4943–4948.

101. Tesciuba AG, Subudhi S, Rother RP, et al. Inducible costimulator regulates Th2-mediated inflammation, but not Th2 differentiation, in a model of allergic airway disease. *J Immunol* 2001;167:1996–2003.

102. Gonzalo JA, Tian J, Delaney T, et al. ICOS is critical for T helper cell–mediated lung mucosal inflammatory responses. *Nat Immunol* 2001;2:597–604.

103. Sporici RA, Beswick RL, von Allmen C, et al. ICOS ligand co-stimulation is required for T-cell encephalitogenicity. *Clin Immunol* 2001;100:277–288.

104. Wallin JJ, Liang L, Bakardjiev A, et al. Enhancement of CD8$^+$ T cell responses by ICOS/B7h costimulation. *J Immunol* 2001;167:132–139.

105. Ozkaynak E, Gao W, Shemmeri N, et al. Importance of ICOS-B7RP-1 costimulation in acute and chronic allograft rejection. *Nat Immunol* 2001;2:591–596.

106. Furukawa Y, Mandelbrot DA, Libby P, et al. Association of B7-1 co-stimulation with the development of graft arterial disease. Studies using mice lacking B7-1, B7-2, or B7-1/B7-2. *Am J Pathol* 2000;157:473–484.

107. Rottman JB, Smith T, Tonra JR, et al. The costimulatory molecule ICOS plays an important role in the immunopathogenesis of EAE. *Nat Immunol* 2001;2:605–611.

108. Shinohara T, Taniwaki M, Ishida Y, et al. Structure and chromo-somal localization of the human PD-1 gene (PDCD1). *Genomics* 1994;23:704–706.

109. Agata Y, Kawasaki A, Nishimura H, et al. Expression of the PD-1 antigen on the surface of stimulated mouse T and B lymphocytes. *Int Immunol* 1996;8:765–772.

110. Nishimura H, Honjo T. PD-1: an inhibitory immunoreceptor involved in peripheral tolerance. *Trends Immunol* 2001;22:265–268.

111. Nishimura H, Minato N, Nakano T, et al. Immunological studies on PD-1 deficient mice: implication of PD-1 as a negative regulator for B cell responses. *Int Immunol* 1998;10:1563–1572.

112. Nishimura H, Nose M, Hiai H, et al. Development of lupus-like au-toimmune diseases by disruption of the PD-1 gene encoding an ITIM motif–carrying immunoreceptor. *Immunity* 1999;11:141–151.

113. Nishimura H, Okazaki T, Tanaka Y, et al. Autoimmune dilated car-diomyopathy in PD-1 receptor–deficient mice. *Science* 2001;291:319–322.

114. Tamura H, Dong H, Zhu G, et al. B7-H1 costimulation prefer-entially enhances CD28-independent T-helper cell function. *Blood* 2001;97:1809–1816.

115. Okazaki T, Maeda A, Nishimura H, et al. PD-1 immunoreceptor in-hibits B cell receptor–mediated signaling by recruiting src homology 2-domain–containing tyrosine phosphatase 2 to phosphotyrosine. *Proc Natl Acad Sci U S A* 2001;98:13866–13871.

116. Stamenkovic I, Clark EA, Seed B. A B-lymphocyte activation molecule related to the nerve growth factor receptor and induced by cytokines in carcinomas. *EMBO J* 1989;8:1403–1410.

117. Inaba K, Witmer-Pack M, Inaba M, et al. The tissue distribution of the B7-2 costimulator in mice: abundant expression on dendritic cells *in situ* and during maturation *in vitro. J Exp Med* 1994;180:1849–1860.

118. Alderson MR, Armitage RJ, Tough TW, et al. CD40 expression by human monocytes: regulation by cytokines and activation of monocytes by the ligand for CD40. *J Exp Med* 1993;178:669–674.

119. Galy AH, Spits H. CD40 is functionally expressed on human thymic epithelial cells. *J Immunol* 1992;149:775–782.

120. Karmann K, Hughes CC, Schechner J, et al. CD40 on human en-dothelial cells: inducibility by cytokines and functional regulation of adhesion molecule expression. *Proc Natl Acad Sci U S A* 1995;92:4342–4346.

121. Durie FH, Foy TM, Masters SR, et al. The role of CD40 in the regulation of humoral and cell-mediated immunity. *Immunol Today* 1994;15:406–411.

122. Ishida T, Kobayashi N, Tojo T, et al. CD40 signaling–mediated induc-tion of Bcl-X$_L$, Cdk4, and Cdk6. Implication of their cooperation in selective B cell growth. *J Immunol* 1995;155:5527–5535.

123. Kehry MR. CD40-mediated signaling in B cells. Balancing cell sur-vival, growth, and death. *J Immunol* 1996;156:2345–2348.

124. Gordon J. CD40 and its ligand: central players in B lymphocyte sur-vival, growth, and differentiation. *Blood Rev* 1995;9:53–56.

125. Armitage RJ, Fanslow WC, Strockbine L, et al. Molecular and biolog-ical characterization of a murine ligand for CD40. *Nature* 1992;357:80–82.

126. Hollenbaugh D, Grosmaire LS, Kullas CD, et al. The human T cell antigen gp39, a member of the TNF gene family, is a ligand for the CD40 receptor: expression of a soluble form of gp39 with B cell co-stimulatory activity. *EMBO J* 1992;11:4313–4321.

127. Roy M, Waldschmidt T, Aruffo A, et al. The regulation of the expres-sion of gp39, the CD40 ligand, on normal and cloned CD4$^+$ T cells. *J Immunol* 1993;151:2497–2510.

128. Armitage RJ, Tough TW, Macduff BM, et al. CD40 ligand is a T cell growth factor. *Eur J Immunol* 1993;23:2326–2331.

129. Fanslow WC, Clifford KN, Seaman M, et al. Recombinant CD40 ligand exerts potent biologic effects on T cells. *J Immunol* 1994;152:4262–4269.

130. Hermann P, Van-Kooten C, Gaillard C, et al. CD40 ligand-positive CD8$^+$ T cell clones allow B cell growth and differentiation. *Eur J Immunol* 1995;25:2972–2977.

131. Gauchat JF, Henchoz S, Fattah D, et al. CD40 ligand is functionally expressed on human eosinophils. *Eur J Immunol* 1995;25:863–865.

132. Sad S, Krishnan L, Bleackley RC, et al. Cytotoxicity and weak CD40 ligand expression of CD8$^+$ type 2 cytotoxic T cells restricts their po-tential B cell helper activity. *Eur J Immunol* 1997;27:914–922.

133. Carbone E, Ruggiero G, Terrazzano G, et al. A new mechanism of NK cell cytotoxicity activation: the CD40–CD40 ligand interaction. *J Exp Med* 1997;185:2053–2060.

134. Bradley JR, Pober JS. Tumor necrosis factor receptor–associated fac-tors (TRAFs). *Oncogene* 2001;20:6482–6491.

135. Hu HM, O'Rourke K, Boguski MS, et al. A novel RING finger pro-tein interacts with the cytoplasmic domain of CD40. *J Biol Chem* 1994;269:30069–30072.

136. Kuhne MR, Robbins M, Hambor JE, et al. Assembly and regula-tion of the CD40 receptor complex in human B cells. *J Exp Med* 1997;186:337–342.

137. Hostager BS, Bishop GA. Cutting edge: contrasting roles of TNF receptor–associated factor 2 (TRAF2) and TRAF3 in CD40-activated B lymphocyte differentiation. *J Immunol* 1999;162:6307–6311.

138. Cheng G, Cleary AM, Ye ZS, et al. Involvement of CRAF1, a relative of TRAF, in CD40 signaling. *Science* 1995;267:1494–1498.

139. Xu Y, Cheng G, Baltimore D. Targeted disruption of TRAF3 leads to postnatal lethality and defective T-dependent immune responses. *Immunity* 1996;5:407–415.

140. Foy TM, Shepherd DM, Durie FH, et al. *In vivo* CD40-gp39 in-teractions are essential for thymus-dependent humoral immunity. II. Prolonged suppression of the humoral immune response by an an-tibody to the ligand for CD40, gp39. *J Exp Med* 1993;178:1567–1575.

141. Xu J, Foy TM, Laman JD, et al. Mice deficient for the CD40 ligand. *Immunity* 1994;1:423–431.

142. Kawabe T, Naka T, Yoshida K, et al. The immune responses in CD40-deficient mice: impaired immunoglobulin class switching and germinal center formation. *Immunity* 1994;1:167–178.

143. Renshaw BR, Fanslow WC 3rd, Armitage RJ, et al. Humoral immune responses in CD40 ligand–deficient mice. *J Exp Med* 1994;180:1889–1900.

144. van Essen D, Kikutani H, Gray D. CD40 ligand–transduced co-stimulation of T cells in the development of helper function. *Nature* 1995;378:620–623.

145. Kelsoe G. Life and death in germinal centers (redux). *Immunity* 1996;4:107–111.
146. Padayachee M, Levinsky RJ, Kinnon C, et al. Mapping of the X linked form of hyper IgM syndrome (HIGM1). *J Med Genet* 1993;30:202–205.
147. Aruffo A, Farrington M, Hollenbaugh D, et al. The CD40 ligand, gp39, is defective in activated T cells from patients with X-linked hyper-IgM syndrome. *Cell* 1993;72:291–300.
148. Korthauer U, Graf D, Mages HW, et al. Defective expression of T-cell CD40 ligand causes X-linked immunodeficiency with hyper-IgM. *Nature* 1993;361:539–541.
149. DiSanto JP, Bonnefoy JY, Gauchat JF, et al. CD40 ligand mutations in X-linked immunodeficiency with hyper-IgM. *Nature* 1993;361:541–543.
150. Allen RC, Armitage RJ, Conley ME, et al. CD40 ligand gene defects responsible for X-linked hyper-IgM syndrome. *Science* 1993;259:990–993.
151. Callard RE, Smith SH, Herbert J, et al. CD40 ligand (CD40L) expression and B cell function in agammaglobulinemia with normal or elevated levels of IgM (HIM). Comparison of X-linked, autosomal recessive, and non–X-linked forms of the disease, and obligate carriers. *J Immunol* 1994;153:3295–3306.
152. Facchetti F, Appiani C, Salvi L, et al. Immunohistologic analysis of ineffective CD40–CD40 ligand interaction in lymphoid tissues from patients with X-linked immunodeficiency with hyper-IgM. Abortive germinal center cell reaction and severe depletion of follicular dendritic cells. *J Immunol* 1995;154:6624–6633.
153. Primary immunodeficiency diseases. Report of a WHO Scientific Group. *Clin Exp Immunol* 1995;99(Suppl 1):1–24.
154. Notarangelo LD, Duse M, Ugazio AG. Immunodeficiency with hyper-IgM (HIM). *Immunodefic Rev* 1992;3:101–121.
155. Noelle RJ. CD40 and its ligand in host defense. *Immunity* 1996;4:415–419.
156. Campbell KA, Ovendale PJ, Kennedy MK, et al. CD40 ligand is required for protective cell-mediated immunity to *Leishmania major*. *Immunity* 1996;4:283–289.
157. Soong L, Xu JC, Grewal IS, et al. Disruption of CD40–CD40 ligand interactions results in an enhanced susceptibility to *Leishmania amazonensis* infection. *Immunity* 1996;4:263–273.
158. Kamanaka M, Yu P, Yasui T, et al. Protective role of CD40 in *Leishmania major* infection at two distinct phases of cell-mediated immunity. *Immunity* 1996;4:275–281.
159. Wiley JA, Harmsen AG. CD40 ligand is required for resolution of *Pneumocystis carinii* pneumonia in mice. *J Immunol* 1995;155:3525–3529.
160. Garvy BA, Wiley JA, Gigliotti F, et al. Protection against *Pneumocystis carinii* pneumonia by antibodies generated from either T helper 1 or T helper 2 responses. *Infect Immun* 1997;65:5052–5056.
161. Borrow P, Tishon A, Lee S, et al. CD40L-deficient mice show deficits in antiviral immunity and have an impaired memory CD8$^+$ CTL response. *J Exp Med* 1996;183:2129–2142.
162. Oxenius A, Campbell KA, Maliszewski CR, et al. CD40–CD40 ligand interactions are critical in T-B cooperation but not for other anti-viral CD4$^+$ T cell functions. *J Exp Med* 1996;183:2209–2218.
163. Whitmire JK, Slifka MK, Grewal IS, et al. CD40 ligand–deficient mice generate a normal primary cytotoxic T-lymphocyte response but a defective humoral response to a viral infection. *J Virol* 1996;70:8375–8381.
164. Whitmire JK, Flavell RA, Grewal IS, et al. CD40–CD40 ligand co-stimulation is required for generating antiviral CD4 T cell responses but is dispensable for CD8 T cell responses. *J Immunol* 1999;163:3194–3201.
165. Daikh DI, Finck BK, Linsley PS, et al. Long-term inhibition of murine lupus by brief simultaneous blockade of the B7/CD28 and CD40/gp39 costimulation pathways. *J Immunol* 1997;159:3104–3108.
166. Shi FD, He B, Li H, et al. Differential requirements for CD28 and CD40 ligand in the induction of experimental autoimmune myasthenia gravis. *Eur J Immunol* 1998;28:3587–3593.
167. Balasa B, Krahl T, Patstone G, et al. CD40 ligand–CD40 interactions are necessary for the initiation of insulitis and diabetes in nonobese diabetic mice. *J Immunol* 1997;159:4620–4627.
168. Becher B, Durell BG, Miga AV, et al. The clinical course of experimental autoimmune encephalomyelitis and inflammation is controlled by the expression of CD40 within the central nervous system. *J Exp Med* 2001;193:967–974.
169. Larsen CP, Alexander DZ, Hollenbaugh D, et al. CD40-gp39 interactions play a critical role during allograft rejection. Suppression of allograft rejection by blockade of the CD40-gp39 pathway. *Transplantation* 1996;61:4–9.
170. Parker DC, Greiner DL, Phillips NE, et al. Survival of mouse pancreatic islet allografts in recipients treated with allogeneic small lymphocytes and antibody to CD40 ligand. *Proc Natl Acad Sci U S A* 1995;92:9560–9564.
171. Hancock WW, Sayegh MH, Zheng XG, et al. Costimulatory function and expression of CD40 ligand, CD80, and CD86 in vascularized murine cardiac allograft rejection. *Proc Natl Acad Sci U S A* 1996;93:13967–13972.
172. Hancock WW, Buelow R, Sayegh MH, et al. Antibody-induced transplant arteriosclerosis is prevented by graft expression of anti-oxidant and anti-apoptotic genes. *Nat Med* 1998;4:1392–1396.
173. Ensminger SM, Witzke O, Spriewald BM, et al. CD8$^+$ T cells contribute to the development of transplant arteriosclerosis despite CD154 blockade. *Transplantation* 2000;69:2609–2612.
174. Larsen CP, Elwood ET, Alexander DZ, et al. Long-term acceptance of skin and cardiac allografts after blocking CD40 and CD28 pathways. *Nature* 1996;381:434–438.
175. Shimizu K, Schonbeck U, Mach F, et al. Host CD40 ligand deficiency induces long-term allograft survival and donor-specific tolerance in mouse cardiac transplantation but does not prevent graft arteriosclerosis. *J Immunol* 2000;165:3506–3518.
176. Watts TH, DeBenedette MA. T cell co-stimulatory molecules other than CD28. *Curr Opin Immunol* 1999;11:286–293.
177. Baum PR, Gayle RB, 3rd, Ramsdell F, et al. Identification of OX40 ligand and and preliminary characterization of its activities on OX40 receptor. *Circ Shock* 1994;44:30–34.
178. Baum PR, Gayle RB 3rd, Ramsdell F, et al. Molecular characterization of murine and human OX40/OX40 ligand systems: identification of a human OX40 ligand as the HTLV-1–regulated protein gp34. *EMBO J* 1994;13:3992–4001.
179. Walker LS, Gulbranson-Judge A, Flynn S, et al. Co-stimulation and selection for T-cell help for germinal centres: the role of CD28 and OX40. *Immunol Today* 2000;21:333–337.
180. Akiba H, Miyahira Y, Atsuta M, et al. Critical contribution of OX40 ligand to T helper cell type 2 differentiation in experimental leishmaniasis. *J Exp Med* 2000;191:375–380.
181. Arch RH, Thompson CB. 4-1BB and OX40 are members of a tumor necrosis factor (TNF)–nerve growth factor receptor subfamily that bind TNF receptor–associated factors and activate nuclear factor kappaB. *Mol Cell Biol* 1998;18:558–565.
182. Akiba H, Atsuta M, Yagita H, et al. Identification of rat OX40 ligand by molecular cloning. *Biochem Biophys Res Commun* 1998;251:131–136.
183. Miura S, Ohtani K, Numata N, et al. Molecular cloning and characterization of a novel glycoprotein, gp34, that is specifically induced by the human T-cell leukemia virus type I transactivator p40tax. *Mol Cell Biol* 1991;11:1313–1325.
184. Ohshima Y, Tanaka Y, Tozawa H, et al. Expression and function of OX40 ligand on human dendritic cells. *J Immunol* 1997;159:3838–3848.
185. Stuber E, Neurath M, Calderhead D, et al. Cross-linking of OX40 ligand, a member of the TNF/NGF cytokine family, induces proliferation and differentiation in murine splenic B cells. *Immunity* 1995;2:507–521.
186. Imura A, Hori T, Imada K, et al. The human OX40/gp34 system directly mediates adhesion of activated T cells to vascular endothelial cells. *J Exp Med* 1996;183:2185–2195.
187. Gramaglia I, Jember A, Pippig SD, et al. The OX40 costimulatory receptor determines the development of CD4 memory by regulating primary clonal expansion. *J Immunol* 2000;165:3043–3050.
188. Rogers PR, Song J, Gramaglia I, et al. OX40 promotes Bcl-x$_L$ and Bcl-2 expression and is essential for long-term survival of CD4 T cells. *Immunity* 2001;15:445–455.
189. Chen AI, McAdam AJ, Buhlmann JE, et al. OX40-ligand has a critical costimulatory role in dendritic cell:T cell interactions. *Immunity* 1999;11:689–698.
190. Kopf M, Ruedl C, Schmitz N, et al. OX40-deficient mice are defective

in Th cell proliferation but are competent in generating B cell and CTL responses after virus infection. *Immunity* 1999;11:699–708.

191. Pippig SD, Pena-Rossi C, Long J, et al. Robust B cell immunity but impaired T cell proliferation in the absence of CD134 (OX40). *J Immunol* 1999;163:6520–6529.

192. Murata K, Ishii N, Takano H, et al. Impairment of antigen-presenting cell function in mice lacking expression of OX40 ligand. *J Exp Med* 2000;191:365–374.

193. Jember AG, Zuberi R, Liu FT, et al. Development of allergic inflammation in a murine model of asthma is dependent on the costimulatory receptor OX40. *J Exp Med* 2001;193:387–392.

194. Weinberg AD, Vella AT, Croft M. OX-40: life beyond the effector T cell stage. *Semin Immunol* 1998;10:471–480.

195. Nohara C, Akiba H, Nakajima A, et al. Amelioration of experimental autoimmune encephalomyelitis with anti-OX40 ligand monoclonal antibody: a critical role for OX40 ligand in migration, but not development, of pathogenic T cells. *J Immunol* 2001;166:2108–2115.

196. Higgins LM, McDonald SA, Whittle N, et al. Regulation of T cell activation *in vitro* and *in vivo* by targeting the OX40-OX40 ligand interaction: amelioration of ongoing inflammatory bowel disease with an OX40-IgG fusion protein, but not with an OX40 ligand–IgG fusion protein. *J Immunol* 1999;162:486–493.

197. Akiba H, Oshima H, Takeda K, et al. CD28-independent costimulation of T cells by OX40 ligand and CD70 on activated B cells. *J Immunol* 1999;162:7058–7066.

198. Gramaglia I, Weinberg AD, Lemon M, et al. OX-40 ligand: a potent costimulatory molecule for sustaining primary CD4 T cell responses. *J Immunol* 1998;161:6510–6517.

199. Lens SM, Tesselaar K, van Oers MH, et al. Control of lymphocyte function through CD27-CD70 interactions. *Semin Immunol* 1998;10:491–499.

200. Gravestein LA, Amsen D, Boes M, et al. The TNF receptor family member CD27 signals to Jun N-terminal kinase via Traf-2. *Eur J Immunol* 1998;28:2208–2216.

201. Tesselaar K, Gravestein LA, van Schijndel GM, et al. Characterization of murine CD70, the ligand of the TNF receptor family member CD27. *J Immunol* 1997;159:4959–4965.

202. Takeda K, Oshima H, Hayakawa Y, et al. CD27-mediated activation of murine NK cells. *J Immunol* 2000;164:1741–1745.

203. Hintzen RQ, Lens SM, Lammers K, et al. Engagement of CD27 with its ligand CD70 provides a second signal for T cell activation. *J Immunol* 1995;154:2612–2623.

204. Hendriks J, Gravestein LA, Tesselaar K, et al. CD27 is required for generation and long-term maintenance of T cell immunity. *Nat Immunol* 2000;1:433–440.

205. Arens R, Tesselaar K, Baars PA, et al. Constitutive CD27/CD70 interaction induces expansion of effector-type T cells and results in IFNgamma-mediated B cell depletion. *Immunity* 2001;15:801–812.

206. Jacquot S. CD27/CD70 interactions regulate T dependent B cell differentiation. *Immunol Res* 2000;21:23–30.

207. Nakajima A, Oshima H, Nohara C, et al. Involvement of CD70-CD27 interactions in the induction of experimental autoimmune encephalomyelitis. *J Neuroimmunol* 2000;109:188–196.

208. Braun-Falco M, Hallek M. Recombinant adeno-associated virus (rAAV) vector–mediated cotransduction of CD70 and CD80 into human malignant melanoma cells results in an additive T-cell response. *Arch Dermatol Res* 2001;293:12–17.

209. Pollok KE, Kim YJ, Zhou Z, et al. Inducible T cell antigen 4-1BB. Analysis of expression and function. *J Immunol* 1993;150:771–781.

210. Saoulli K, Lee SY, Cannons JL, et al. CD28-independent, TRAF2-dependent costimulation of resting T cells by 4-1BB ligand. *J Exp Med* 1998;187:1849–1862.

211. Cannons JL, Choi Y, Watts TH. Role of TNF receptor–associated factor 2 and p38 mitogen–activated protein kinase activation during 4-1BB–dependent immune response. *J Immunol* 2000;165:6193–6204.

212. Jang IK, Lee ZH, Kim YJ, et al. Human 4-1BB (CD137) signals are mediated by TRAF2 and activate nuclear factor–kappa B. *Biochem Biophys Res Commun* 1998;242:613–620.

213. Vinay DS, Kwon BS. Role of 4-1BB in immune responses. *Semin Immunol* 1998;10:481–489.

214. Pollok KE, Kim YJ, Hurtado J, et al. 4-1BB T-cell antigen binds to mature B cells and macrophages, and costimulates anti-mu–primed splenic B cells. *Eur J Immunol* 1994;24:367–374.

215. DeBenedette MA, Wen T, Bachmann MF, et al. Analysis of 4-1BB ligand (4-1BBL)–deficient mice and of mice lacking both 4-1BBL and CD28 reveals a role for 4-1BBL in skin allograft rejection and in the cytotoxic T cell response to influenza virus. *J Immunol* 1999;163:4833–4841.

216. Cannons JL, Lau P, Ghumman B, et al. 4-1BB ligand induces cell division, sustains survival, and enhances effector function of CD4 and CD8 T cells with similar efficacy. *J Immunol* 2001;167:1313–1324.

217. Blazar BR, Kwon BS, Panoskaltsis-Mortari A, et al. Ligation of 4-1BB (CDw137) regulates graft-versus-host disease, graft- versus-leukemia, and graft rejection in allogeneic bone marrow transplant recipients. *J Immunol* 2001;166:3174–3183.

218. Kim YJ, Kim SH, Mantel P, et al. Human 4-1BB regulates CD28 co-stimulation to promote Th1 cell responses. *Eur J Immunol* 1998;28:881–890.

219. Melero I, Johnston JV, Shufford WW, et al. NK1.1 cells express 4-1BB (CDw137) costimulatory molecule and are required for tumor immunity elicited by anti–4-1BB monoclonal antibodies. *Cell Immunol* 1998;190:167–172.

220. Seed B, Aruffo A. Molecular cloning of the CD2 antigen, the T-cell erythrocyte receptor, by a rapid immunoselection procedure. *Proc Natl Acad Sci U S A* 1987;84:3365–3369.

221. Wallner BP, Frey AZ, Tizard R, et al. Primary structure of lymphocyte function–associated antigen 3 (LFA-3). The ligand of the T lymphocyte CD2 glycoprotein. *J Exp Med* 1987;166:923–932.

222. Fisher RC, Thorley-Lawson DA. Characterization of the Epstein-Barr virus–inducible gene encoding the human leukocyte adhesion and activation antigen BLAST-1 (CD48). *Mol Cell Biol* 1991;11:1614–1623.

223. Gonzalez-Cabrero J, Wise CJ, Latchman Y, et al. CD48-deficient mice have a pronounced defect in CD4(+) T cell activation. *Proc Natl Acad Sci U S A* 1999;96:1019–1023.

224. Cocks BG, Chang CC, Carballido JM, et al. A novel receptor involved in T-cell activation. *Nature* 1995;376:260–263.

225. Castro AG, Hauser TM, Cocks BG, et al. Molecular and functional characterization of mouse signaling lymphocytic activation molecule (SLAM): differential expression and responsiveness in Th1 and Th2 cells. *J Immunol* 1999;163:5860–5870.

226. Mathew PA, Garni-Wagner BA, Land K, et al. Cloning and characterization of the 2B4 gene encoding a molecule associated with non–MHC-restricted killing mediated by activated natural killer cells and T cells. *J Immunol* 1993;151:5328–5337.

227. Stepp SE, Schatzle JD, Bennett M, et al. Gene structure of the murine NK cell receptor 2B4: presence of two alternatively spliced isoforms with distinct cytoplasmic domains. *Eur J Immunol* 1999;29:2392–2399.

228. de la Fuente MA, Pizcueta P, Nadal M, et al. CD84 leukocyte antigen is a new member of the Ig superfamily. *Blood* 1997;90:2398–2405.

229. de la Fuente MA, Tovar V, Pizcueta P, et al. Molecular cloning, characterization, and chromosomal localization of the mouse homologue of CD84, a member of the CD2 family of cell surface molecules. *Immunogenetics* 1999;49:249–255.

230. Tovar V, de la Fuente MA, Pizcueta P, et al. Gene structure of the mouse leukocyte cell surface molecule Ly9. *Immunogenetics* 2000;51:788–793.

231. Sandrin MS, Gumley TP, Henning MM, et al. Isolation and characterization of cDNA clones for mouse Ly-9. *J Immunol* 1992;149:1636–1641.

232. Peck SR, Ruley HE. Ly108: a new member of the mouse CD2 family of cell surface proteins. *Immunogenetics* 2000;52:63–72.

233. Kingsbury GA, Feeney LA, Nong Y, et al. Cloning, expression, and function of BLAME, a novel member of the CD2 family. *J Immunol* 2001;166:5675–5680.

234. Hunig T. The cell surface molecule recognized by the erythrocyte receptor of T lymphocytes. Identification and partial characterization using a monoclonal antibody. *J Exp Med* 1985;162:890–901.

235. Selvaraj P, Plunkett ML, Dustin M, et al. The T lymphocyte glycoprotein CD2 binds the cell surface ligand LFA-3. *Nature* 1987;326:400–403.

236. Davis SJ, van der Merwe PA. The structure and ligand interactions of CD2: implications for T-cell function. *Immunol Today* 1996;17:177–187.

237. Arulanandam AR, Moingeon P, Concino MF, et al. A soluble multimeric recombinant CD2 protein identifies CD48 as a low affinity ligand

for human CD2: divergence of CD2 ligands during the evolution of humans and mice. *J Exp Med* 1993;177:1439–1450.

238. Hahn WC, Bierer BE. Separable portions of the CD2 cytoplasmic domain involved in signaling and ligand avidity regulation. *J Exp Med* 1993;178:1831–1836.

239. Kato K, Koyanagi M, Okada H, et al. CD48 is a counter-receptor for mouse CD2 and is involved in T cell activation. *J Exp Med* 1992;176:1241–1249.

240. van der Merwe PA, McPherson DC, Brown MH, et al. The NH2-terminal domain of rat CD2 binds rat CD48 with a low affinity and binding does not require glycosylation of CD2. *Eur J Immunol* 1993;23:1373–1377.

241. Latchman Y, McKay PF, Reiser H. Identification of the 2B4 molecule as a counter-receptor for CD48. *J Immunol* 1998;161:5809–5812.

242. Brown MH, Boles K, van der Merwe PA, et al. 2B4, the natural killer and T cell immunoglobulin superfamily surface protein, is a ligand for CD48. *J Exp Med* 1998;188:2083–2090.

243. Kubin MZ, Parshley DL, Din W, et al. Molecular cloning and biological characterization of NK cell activation-inducing ligand, a counterstructure for CD48. *Eur J Immunol* 1999;29:3466–3477.

244. Baorto DM, Gao Z, Malaviya R, et al. Survival of FimH-expressing enterobacteria in macrophages relies on glycolipid traffic. *Nature* 1997;389:636–639.

245. Malaviya R, Abraham SN. Mast cell modulation of immune responses to bacteria. *Immunol Rev* 2001;179:16–24.

246. Ianelli CJ, DeLellis R, Thorley-Lawson DA. CD48 binds to heparan sulfate on the surface of epithelial cells. *J Biol Chem* 1998;273:23367–23375.

247. Tangye SG, Phillips JH, Lanier LL. The CD2-subset of the Ig superfamily of cell surface molecules: receptor–ligand pairs expressed by NK cells and other immune cells. *Semin Immunol* 2000;12:149–157.

248. Yagita H, Nakamura T, Karasuyama H, et al. Monoclonal antibodies specific for murine CD2 reveal its presence on B as well as T cells. *Proc Natl Acad Sci U S A* 1989;86:645–649.

249. Duplay P, Lancki D, Allison JP. Distribution and ontogeny of CD2 expression by murine T cells. *J Immunol* 1989;142:2998–3005.

250. Kishimoto T, Kikutani H, von dem Borne AEG, et al. *Leucocyte typing VI: white cell differentiation antigens.* New York: Garland Publishing Inc, 1997.

251. Thorley-Lawson DA, Schooley RT, Bhan AK, et al. Epstein-Barr virus superinduces a new human B cell differentiation antigen (B-LAST 1) expressed on transformed lymphoblasts. *Cell* 1982;30:415–425.

252. Yokoyama S, Staunton D, Fisher R, et al. Expression of the Blast-1 activation/adhesion molecule and its identification as CD48. *J Immunol* 1991;146:2192–2200.

253. Staunton DE, Fisher RC, LeBeau MM, et al. Blast-1 possesses a glycosyl-phosphatidylinositol (GPI) membrane anchor, is related to LFA-3 and OX-45, and maps to chromosome 1q21-23. *J Exp Med* 1989;169:1087–1099.

254. Reiser H. sgp-60, a signal-transducing glycoprotein concerned with T cell activation through the T cell receptor/CD3 complex. *J Immunol* 1990;145:2077–2086.

255. Ozawa H, Aiba S, Nakagawa S, et al. Murine epidermal Langerhans cells express CD48, which is a counter-receptor for mouse CD2. *Arch Dermatol Res* 1995;287:524–528.

256. Meuer SC, Hussey RE, Fabbi M, et al. An alternative pathway of T-cell activation: a functional role for the 50 kd T11 sheep erythrocyte receptor protein. *Cell* 1984;36:897–906.

257. Bernard A, Knowles RW, Naito A, et al. A unique epitope on the CD2 molecule defined by the monoclonal antibody 9-1: epitope-specific modulation of the E-rosette receptor and effects on T-cell functions. *Hum Immunol* 1986;17:388–405.

258. Van Lier RA, Brouwer M, De Groot ED, et al. T cell receptor/CD3 and CD28 use distinct intracellular signaling pathways. *Eur J Immunol* 1991;21:1775–1778.

259. Pierres A, Lopez M, Cerdan C, et al. Triggering CD 28 molecules synergize with CD 2 (T 11.1 and T 11.2)–mediated T cell activation. *Eur J Immunol* 1988;18:685–690.

260. Mollereau B, Deckert M, Deas O, et al. CD2-induced apoptosis in activated human peripheral T cells: a Fas-independent pathway that requires early protein tyrosine phosphorylation. *J Immunol* 1996;156:3184–3190.

261. Dustin ML, Sanders ME, Shaw S, et al. Purified lymphocyte function–

262. Parra E, Wingren AG, Hedlund G, et al. Costimulation of human CD4[+] T lymphocytes with B7 and lymphocyte function–associated antigen–3 results in distinct cell activation profiles. *J Immunol* 1994;153:2479–2487.

263. Cerdan C, Martin Y, Brailly H, et al. IL-1 alpha is produced by T lymphocytes activated via the CD2 plus CD28 pathways. *J Immunol* 1991;146:560–564.

264. Santis AG, Campanero MR, Alonso JL, et al. Regulation of tumor necrosis factor (TNF)–alpha synthesis and TNF receptors expression in T lymphocytes through the CD2 activation pathway. *Eur J Immunol* 1992;22:3155–3160.

265. Van der Pouw-Kraan T, Van Kooten C, Rensink I, et al. Interleukin (IL)–4 production by human T cells: differential regulation of IL-4 vs. IL-2 production. *Eur J Immunol* 1992;22:1237–1241.

266. Valentin H, Groux H, Gelin C, et al. Modulation of lymphokine release and cytolytic activities by activating peripheral blood lymphocytes via CD2. *J Immunol* 1990;144:875–882.

267. Parra E, Varga M, Hedlund G, et al. Costimulation by B7-1 and LFA-3 targets distinct nuclear factors that bind to the interleukin-2 promoter: B7-1 negatively regulates LFA-3–induced NF-AT DNA binding. *Mol Cell Biol* 1997;17:1314–1323.

268. Parra E, Wingren AG, Hedlund G, et al. The role of B7-1 and LFA-3 in costimulation of CD8[+] T cells. *J Immunol* 1997;158:637–642.

269. Sen J, Bossu P, Burakoff SJ, et al. T cell surface molecules regulating noncognate B lymphocyte activation. Role of CD2 and LFA-1. *J Immunol* 1992;148:1037–1042.

270. Siliciano RF, Pratt JC, Schmidt RE, et al. Activation of cytolytic T lymphocyte and natural killer cell function through the T11 sheep erythrocyte binding protein. *Nature* 1985;317:428–430.

271. Wakkach A, Cottrez F, Groux H. Differentiation of regulatory T cells 1 is induced by CD2 costimulation. *J Immunol* 2001;167:3107–3113.

272. Bullens DM, Rafiq K, Charitidou L, et al. Effects of co-stimulation by CD58 on human T cell cytokine production: a selective cytokine pattern with induction of high IL-10 production. *Int Immunol* 2001;13:181–191.

273. Latchman Y, Reiser H. Enhanced murine CD4[+] T cell responses induced by the CD2 ligand CD48. *Eur J Immunol* 1998;28:4325–4331.

274. Bromberg JS, Chavin KD, Altevogt P, et al. Anti-CD2 monoclonal antibodies alter cell-mediated immunity *in vivo. Transplantation* 1991;51:219–225.

275. Guckel B, Berek C, Lutz M, et al. Anti-CD2 antibodies induce T cell unresponsiveness *in vivo. J Exp Med* 1991;174:957–967.

276. Chavin KD, Lau HT, Bromberg JS. Prolongation of allograft and xenograft survival in mice by anti-CD2 monoclonal antibodies. *Transplantation* 1992;54:286–291.

277. Kapur S, Khanna A, Sharma VK, et al. CD2 antigen targeting reduces intragraft expression of mRNA-encoding granzyme B and IL-10 and induces tolerance. *Transplantation* 1996;62:249–255.

278. Qin L, Chavin KD, Lin J, et al. Anti-CD2 receptor and anti-CD2 ligand (CD48) antibodies synergize to prolong allograft survival. *J Exp Med* 1994;179:341–346.

279. Chavin KD, Qin L, Lin J, et al. Anti-CD48 (murine CD2 ligand) mAbs suppress cell mediated immunity *in vivo. Int Immunol* 1994;6:701–709.

280. Killeen N, Stuart SG, Littman DR. Development and function of T cells in mice with a disrupted CD2 gene. *EMBO J* 1992;11:4329–4336.

281. Teh SJ, Killeen N, Tarakhovsky A, et al. CD2 regulates the positive selection and function of antigen-specific CD4− CD8[+] T cells. *Blood* 1997;89:1308–1318.

282. Evans CF, Rall GF, Killeen N, et al. CD2-deficient mice generate virus-specific cytotoxic T lymphocytes upon infection with lymphocytic choriomeningitis virus. *J Immunol* 1993;151:6259–6264.

283. Bachmann MF, Barner M, Kopf M. CD2 sets quantitative thresholds in T cell activation. *J Exp Med* 1999;190:1383–1392.

284. Sasada T, Reinherz EL. A critical role for CD2 in both thymic selection events and mature T cell function. *J Immunol* 2001;166:2394–2403.

285. Green JM, Karpitskiy V, Kimzey SL, et al. Coordinate regulation of T cell activation by CD2 and CD28. *J Immunol* 2000;164:3591–3595.

286. Bell GM, Fargnoli J, Bolen JB, et al. The SH3 domain of p56lck binds to proline-rich sequences in the cytoplasmic domain of CD2. *J Exp Med* 1996;183:169–178.

287. Gassmann M, Amrein KE, Flint NA, et al. Identification of a signaling complex involving CD2, zeta chain and p59fyn in T lymphocytes. *Eur J Immunol* 1994;24:139–144.

288. Li J, Nishizawa K, An W, et al. A cdc15–like adaptor protein (CD2BP1) interacts with the CD2 cytoplasmic domain and regulates CD2-triggered adhesion. *EMBO J* 1998;17:7320–7336.

289. Bai Y, Ding Y, Spencer S, et al. Regulation of the association between PSTPIP and CD2 in murine T cells. *Exp Mol Pathol* 2001;71:115–124.

290. Nishizawa K, Freund C, Li J, et al. Identification of a proline-binding motif regulating CD2-triggered T lymphocyte activation. *Proc Natl Acad Sci U S A* 1998;95:14897–14902.

291. Bromley SK, Burack WR, Johnson KG, et al. The immunological synapse. *Annu Rev Immunol* 2001;19:375–396.

292. van der Merwe PA. A subtle role for CD2 in T cell antigen recognition. *J Exp Med* 1999;190:1371–1374.

293. Wild MK, Cambiaggi A, Brown MH, et al. Dependence of T cell antigen recognition on the dimensions of an accessory receptor-ligand complex. *J Exp Med* 1999;190:31–41.

294. Moran M, Miceli MC. Engagement of GPI-linked CD48 contributes to TCR signals and cytoskeletal reorganization: a role for lipid rafts in T cell activation. *Immunity* 1998;9:787–796.

295. Yang H, Reinherz EL. Dynamic recruitment of human CD2 into lipid rafts. Linkage to T cell signal transduction. *J Biol Chem* 2001;276:18775–18785.

296. Mestas J, Hughes CC. Endothelial cell costimulation of T cell activation through CD58–CD2 interactions involves lipid raft aggregation. *J Immunol* 2001;167:4378–4385.

297. Dustin ML, Olszowy MW, Holdorf AD, et al. A novel adaptor protein orchestrates receptor patterning and cytoskeletal polarity in T-cell contacts. *Cell* 1998;94:667–677.

298. Shih NY, Li J, Karpitskii V, et al. Congenital nephrotic syndrome in mice lacking CD2-associated protein. *Science* 1999;286:312–315.

299. Sidorenko SP, Clark EA. Characterization of a cell surface glycoprotein IPO-3, expressed on activated human B and T lymphocytes. *J Immunol* 1993;151:4614–4624.

300. Bleharski JR, Niazi KR, Sieling PA, et al. Signaling lymphocytic activation molecule is expressed on CD40 ligand–activated dendritic cells and directly augments production of inflammatory cytokines. *J Immunol* 2001;167:3174–3181.

301. Sayos J, Nguyen KB, Wu C, et al. Potential pathways for regulation of NK and T cell responses: differential X-linked lymphoproliferative syndrome gene product SAP interactions with SLAM and 2B4. *Int Immunol* 2000;12:1749–1757.

302. Punnonen J, Cocks BG, Carballido JM, et al. Soluble and membrane-bound forms of signaling lymphocytic activation molecule (SLAM) induce proliferation and Ig synthesis by activated human B lymphocytes. *J Exp Med* 1997;185:993–1004.

303. Sayos J, Wu C, Morra M, et al. The X-linked lymphoproliferative-disease gene product SAP regulates signals induced through the co-receptor SLAM. *Nature* 1998;395:462–469.

304. Morra M, Lu J, Poy F, et al. Structural basis for the interaction of the free SH2 domain EAT-2 with SLAM receptors in hematopoietic cells. *EMBO J* 2001;20:5840–5852.

305. Mavaddat N, Mason DW, Atkinson PD, et al. Signaling lymphocytic activation molecule (CDw150) is homophilic but self-associates with very low affinity. *J Biol Chem* 2000;275:28100–28109.

306. Isomaki P, Aversa G, Cocks BG, et al. Increased expression of signaling lymphocytic activation molecule in patients with rheumatoid arthritis and its role in the regulation of cytokine production in rheumatoid synovium. *J Immunol* 1997;159:2986–2993.

307. Henning G, Kraft MS, Derfuss T, et al. Signaling lymphocytic activation molecule (SLAM) regulates T cellular cytotoxicity. *Eur J Immunol* 2001;31:2741–2750.

308. Tatsuo H, Ono N, Tanaka K, et al. SLAM (CDw150) is a cellular receptor for measles virus. *Nature* 2000;406:893–897.

309. Ono N, Tatsuo H, Tanaka K, et al. V domain of human SLAM (CDw150) is essential for its function as a measles virus receptor. *J Virol* 2001;75:1594–1600.

310. Erlenhoefer C, Wurzer WJ, Loffler S, et al. CD150 (SLAM) is a receptor for measles virus but is not involved in viral contact-mediated proliferation inhibition. *J Virol* 2001;75:4499–4505.

311. Kubota K, Katoh H, Muguruma K, et al. Characterization of a surface membrane molecule expressed by natural killer cells in most inbred mouse strains: monoclonal antibody C9.1 identifies an allelic form of the 2B4 antigen. *Immunology* 1999;96:491–497.

312. Schatzle JD, Sheu S, Stepp SE, et al. Characterization of inhibitory and stimulatory forms of the murine natural killer cell receptor 2B4. *Proc Natl Acad Sci U S A* 1999;96:3870–3875.

313. Tangye SG, Lazetic S, Woollatt E, et al. Cutting edge: human 2B4, an activating NK cell receptor, recruits the protein tyrosine phosphatase SHP-2 and the adaptor signaling protein SAP. *J Immunol* 1999;162:6981–6985.

314. Boles KS, Nakajima H, Colonna M, et al. Molecular characterization of a novel human natural killer cell receptor homologous to mouse 2B4. *Tissue Antigens* 1999;54:27–34.

315. Chuang SS, Lee Y, Stepp SE, et al. Molecular cloning and characterization of the promoter region of murine natural killer cell receptor 2B4. *Biochim Biophys Acta* 1999;1447:244–250.

316. Chuang SS, Pham HT, Kumaresan PR, et al. A prominent role for activator protein–1 in the transcription of the human 2B4 (CD244) gene in NK cells. *J Immunol* 2001;166:6188–6195.

317. Garni-Wagner BA, Purohit A, Mathew PA, et al. A novel function-associated molecule related to non–MHC-restricted cytotoxicity mediated by activated natural killer cells and T cells. *J Immunol* 1993;151:60–70.

318. Valiante NM, Trinchieri G. Identification of a novel signal transduction surface molecule on human cytotoxic lymphocytes. *J Exp Med* 1993;178:1397–1406.

319. Schuhmachers G, Ariizumi K, Mathew PA, et al. Activation of murine epidermal gamma delta T cells through surface 2B4. *Eur J Immunol* 1995;25:1117–1120.

320. Peritt D, Sesok-Pizzini DA, Schretzenmair R, et al. C1.7 antigen expression on CD8$^+$ T cells is activation dependent: increased proportion of C1.7$^+$CD8$^+$ T cells in HIV-1–infected patients with progressing disease. *J Immunol* 1999;162:7563–7568.

321. Speiser DE, Colonna M, Ayyoub M, et al. The activatory receptor 2B4 is expressed *in vivo* by human CD8$^+$ effector alphabeta T cells. *J Immunol* 2001;167:6165–6170.

322. Kambayashi T, Assarsson E, Chambers BJ, et al. Cutting edge: regulation of CD8(+) T cell proliferation by 2B4/CD48 interactions. *J Immunol* 2001;167:6706–6710.

323. Nakajima H, Cella M, Langen H, et al. Activating interactions in human NK cell recognition: the role of 2B4-CD48. *Eur J Immunol* 1999;29:1676–1683.

324. Sivori S, Parolini S, Falco M, et al. 2B4 functions as a co-receptor in human NK cell activation. *Eur J Immunol* 2000;30:787–793.

325. Watzl C, Stebbins CC, Long EO. NK cell inhibitory receptors prevent tyrosine phosphorylation of the activation receptor 2B4 (CD244). *J Immunol* 2000;165:3545–3548.

326. Tedder TF, Wagner N, Engel P. B-cell section workshop. In: Schlossman SF, Boumsell L, Gilks W, et al., eds. *Leucocyte typing V: white cell differentiation antigens.* Oxford, UK: Oxford University Press, 1995:483–504.

327. Sayos J, Martin M, Chen A, et al. Cell surface receptors Ly-9 and CD84 recruit the X-linked lymphoproliferative disease gene product SAP. *Blood* 2001;97:3867–3874.

328. Martin M, Romero X, de la Fuente MA, et al. CD84 functions as a homophilic adhesion molecule and enhances IFN-gamma secretion: adhesion is mediated by Ig-like domain 1. *J Immunol* 2001;167:3668–3676.

329. Coffey AJ, Brooksbank RA, Brandau O, et al. Host response to EBV infection in X-linked lymphoproliferative disease results from mutations in an SH2-domain encoding gene. *Nat Genet* 1998;20:129–135.

330. Nichols KE, Harkin DP, Levitz S, et al. Inactivating mutations in an SH2 domain-encoding gene in X-linked lymphoproliferative syndrome. *Proc Natl Acad Sci U S A* 1998;95:13765–13770.

331. Wu C, Sayos J, Wang N, et al. Genomic organization and characterization of mouse SAP, the gene that is altered in X-linked lymphoproliferative disease. *Immunogenetics* 2000;51:805–815.

332. Shlapatska LM, Mikhalap SV, Berdova AG, et al. CD150 association with either the SH2-containing inositol phosphatase or the SH2-containing protein tyrosine phosphatase is regulated by the adaptor protein SH2D1A. *J Immunol* 2001;166:5480–5487.

333. Howie D, Sayos J, Terhorst C, et al. The gene defective in X-linked lymphoproliferative disease controls T cell dependent immune surveillance against Epstein-Barr virus. *Curr Opin Immunol* 2000;12:474–478.

334. Seemayer TA, Gross TG, Egeler RM, et al. X-linked lymphoproliferative disease: twenty-five years after the discovery. *Pediatr Res* 1995;38:471–478.

335. Wu C, Nguyen KB, Pien GC, et al. SAP controls T cell responses to virus and terminal differentiation of TH2 cells. *Nat Immunol* 2001;2:410–414.

336. Czar MJ, Kersh EN, Mijares LA, et al. Altered lymphocyte responses and cytokine production in mice deficient in the X-linked lymphoproliferative disease gene SH2D1A/DSHP/SAP. *Proc Natl Acad Sci U S A* 2001;98:7449–7454.

337. Morra M, Howie D, Grande MS, et al. X-linked lymphoproliferative disease: a progressive immunodeficiency. *Annu Rev Immunol* 2001;19:657–682.

338. Latour S, Gish G, Helgason CD, et al. Regulation of SLAM-mediated signal transduction by SAP, the X-linked lymphoproliferative gene product. *Nat Immunol* 2001;2:681–690.

339. Nakajima H, Cella M, Bouchon A, et al. Patients with X-linked lymphoproliferative disease have a defect in 2B4 receptor–mediated NK cell cytotoxicity. *Eur J Immunol* 2000;30:3309–3318.

340. Benoit L, Wang X, Pabst HF, et al. Defective NK cell activation in X-linked lymphoproliferative disease. *J Immunol* 2000;165:3549–3553.

341. Parolini S, Bottino C, Falco M, et al. X-linked lymphoproliferative disease. 2B4 molecules displaying inhibitory rather than activating function are responsible for the inability of natural killer cells to kill Epstein-Barr virus–infected cells. *J Exp Med* 2000;192:337–346.

CHAPTER 14

Lymphoid Tissues and Organs

David D. Chaplin

Introduction
Primary Lymphoid Organs
   Bone Marrow · Thymus
Secondary Lymphoid Tissues
   Overview of Secondary Lymphoid Organs · Lymph Nodes · Mucosal-Associated Lymphoid Tissues · Spleen Structure and Function · Signals Regulating Formation and Maintenance of Secondary Lymphoid Tissue Structure · Lymphocyte Recruitment to Secondary Lymphoid Tissues
Summary
References

INTRODUCTION

The mammalian adaptive immune system uses antigen-specific B cells and T cells to provide specific immunity against a constantly evolving universe of pathogenic microbes. Because each antigen-specific cell has the potential to proliferate and differentiate, this system has exceptional flexibility to react in a substantial way to new challenges and to provide focused and appropriate effector responses. Important in these effector responses is the formation of both B- and T-memory cells. While this type of antigen-specific immune system provides rich flexibility to the immune response, the implementation of the response presents a huge challenge. This challenge is the result of the need both to generate the repertoire of properly selected antigen-specific B and T cells, and to facilitate productive encounters between invading pathogens and the rare clonally defined B and T cells that can recognize each specific pathogen.

The primary lymphoid organs, in mammals the bone marrow and thymus, provide tissue microenvironments that support the development and initial maturation of antigen-specific lymphocytes and other hematopoietic cells. The secondary lymphoid organs provide sites where encounters between rare antigen-specific lymphocytes and their cognate antigens can occur efficiently, and where proper cellular interactions can occur to provide a well-regulated immune response. Over the past several years, substantial progress has been made in defining the molecular signals for the induction and maintenance of the normal primary and secondary lymphoid organs and in defining the ways in which these structures support normal immune responses. This chapter provides an overview of the structures of these key immune organs and reviews the factors that regulate their development and maintenance and that govern movement of antigen-specific and antigen-nonspecific cells into and within these tissues.

PRIMARY LYMPHOID ORGANS

Bone Marrow

Early Lymphocyte Maturation in the Bone Marrow—Hematopoietic Stem Cells

In the mouse, hematopoiesis begins in a poorly defined anterior region of the embryo, and then moves to the yolk sac where the expansion and differentiation of hematolymphoid precursors form blood islands (1). Hematopoietic stem cells (HSCs) detected in these blood islands represent a self-renewing population of precursor cells that sustain the formation of all required blood elements throughout the life of the individual. The formation of all hematopoietic lineages from HSCs is defined as definitive hematopoiesis. Investigations of the differentiation of HSC suggest that, in addition to giving rise to all hematopoietic lineages, these cells are also responsible for the formation of vascular endothelial cells and perhaps cells of other lineages (2). The observations that both hematopoietic and endothelial cells develop from common precursor cells *in vitro* and that early hematopoietic lineage cells share common surface markers (e.g., the vascular endothelial growth factor receptor 2, also designated Flk-1) (3,4) support this common ancestry of hematopoietic

419

cells and endothelial cells. These studies have suggested that there may be important functional interactions between these progeny of HSCs, with the microenvironment created by differentiation of HSCs to endothelial cells supporting the further development of HSCs to the classically defined hematopoietic lineages.

Shortly after the liver forms by differentiation from the definitive gut endoderm, HSCs take up residence in this richly vascular organ and hematopoiesis occurs here through most of normal gestation (5,6). Near the end of gestation, the major site of hematopoiesis moves to the developing spleen and then to the bone marrow (7). Under pathologic conditions, extramedullary hematopoiesis can re-emerge, with substantial hematopoiesis occurring particularly in the spleen (8).

Bone Marrow Structure and Function

Stem cells that are committed to the lymphoid lineages can be found in all of the major hematopoietic compartments, initially in the yolk sac, then in the fetal liver and spleen, and finally in the bone marrow (1). The bone marrow provides a microenvironment that is particularly supportive of the differentiation and maturation of B-lymphocytes (9) and natural killer (NK) cells (10). In mammals, the bone marrow appears to be the exclusive site for differentiation of B cells from stem cells. In contrast, B-cell differentiation in birds appears to occur predominantly in the bursa of Fabricius, an organ closely associated with the terminal portion of the gastrointestinal and genitourinary tracts (11). In sheep, important B-cell differentiation occurs in the Peyer's patches (12,13).

In adults, the bone marrow is the major hematopoietic organ, located within the central cavity of the major long bones as well as in the core of the spongy bones of the sternum, skull, and vertebral bodies. Although the marrow space grows as the developing organism grows, because it is surrounded by bone it cannot change its total size in response to acute changes in the need for different hematolymphoid cell types. The marrow contains a complex mixture of cells including the cells of the hematopoietic lineage, macrophages, connective tissue cells, stromal cells, and adipocytes (14). The biological role of bone marrow fat is not fully defined. It may provide a reservoir for key lipid soluble nutrients for hematopoietic cell development, including vitamins and membrane precursors. Adipocytes are increasingly appreciated as sources of cytokines and growth factors (15,16), and may therefore contribute in a regulatory fashion to the formation of hematopoietic cell lineages. Adipocytes also represent one of the cell lineages that can expand or contract in size to provide additional space for hematopoietic cell development. In human marrow, fat can fill 50% or more of the marrow space. In spite of the flexibility afforded by fat, there is a limited ability to manipulate the size of the marrow compartment. Consequently, it is not surprising that pathologic processes that ablate portions of the marrow space (e.g., myelofibrosis or hematologic malignancies) are associated with alterations in immune function (17).

The microanatomy of the bone marrow compartment has only been partially defined. It is likely that marrow compartments in cortical bone (characteristic of the long bones such as the femur) differ substantially in their organization from marrow compartments in trabecular bone (characteristic of spongy bone such as the sternum or vertebral bodies). Cells enter the marrow through terminal arterioles that penetrate the calcified portion of the bone, branch, and appear to empty into large venous sinusoids (Fig. 1). Venous drainage and transport of cells from the marrow space back into the circulation appears to occur by coalescence of sinusoid structures into large marrow venules and veins (18). The relationship of the hematopoietic compartment to the defined vessels remains poorly understood. It is likely, however, that hematopoiesis occurs primarily in an extravascular compartment and that regulated processes control the movement of nucleated cells into and out of the hematopoietic space (19). Supporting this is the observation that normal function of the chemokine receptor, CXCR4 (expressed on B-cell precursors, mature B and T cells and monocytes) is required for retention of B-lineage precursors within the bone marrow hematopoietic microenvironment (20).

The Microenvironment Created by Bone Marrow Stromal Cells

The selective differentiation and maturation of B-lymphocytes in the bone marrow suggests that this tissue provides a microenvironment particularly supportive of the differentiation of this lineage. This support most likely represents a combination of physical features of the tissue that facilitates localization of stem cell precursors and efflux of mature cells and the presence of stromal "feeder" cells that produce growth factors and hormones that are required for the differentiation process. The bone marrow also supports the differentiation of erythroid and myeloid lineages as well as early lymphoid precursors that populate the thymus for T-cell differentiation (21,22). It is, consequently, likely that different microenvironments may exist within the bone marrow, perhaps defined by different stromal elements, each adapted to providing an appropriate repertoire of factors suited to each of the major lineages that mature within this tissue.

Initial evidence of a specific microenvironment that supports functions required for development of hematopoietic lineages came from the studies of Lord et al. (23). These investigators observed that HSCs were localized close to the marrow/bone junction. A specialized cell layer designated the endosteum lines the inner surface of the bony compartment. The localization of stem cells near the endosteum suggests that this tissue compartment contains cellular elements that support stem cell functions including the initiation of their differentiation programs to produce the many cell lineages found in the marrow. Consistent with this, Hermans et al. (24) subsequently found clusters of developing pre–B cells located several cell layers internal to this endosteal compartment. This distribution of stem cells and developing

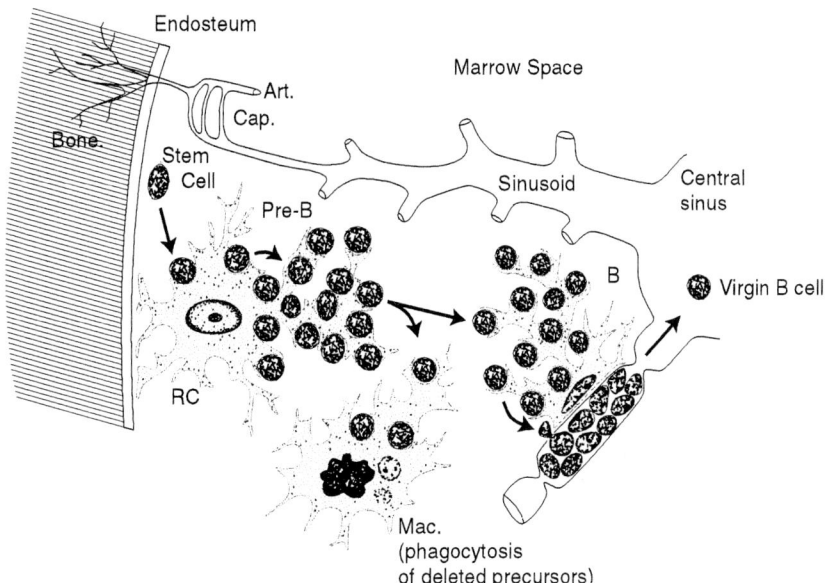

FIG. 1. Organization of the bone marrow and of B-cell development within this organ. Terminal bone marrow arterioles form capillary networks near the endosteum, marking the most peripheral portion of the marrow cavity. Hematopoietic stem cells appear to localize near the endosteum, probably nurtured by growth factors produced in high concentration in this area. Proliferation and differentiation of cells along the B-lineage pathway is dependent on reticular stromal cells (RC) that lie in the spaces surrounding venous sinusoids. B cells progress through pre–B-cell stages in association with these reticular stromal cells, undergoing progressive heavy-chain and light-chain rearrangement, ultimately resulting in the formation of virgin B cells that then enter the circulation. Generally, B-cell differentiation proceeds in a spatially organized fashion, with the most primitive B-cell precursors located near the endosteum and the differentiated virgin B cells emerging near the center of the marrow compartment. Once heavy-chain rearrangement is complete, a process of testing cells for successful Ig gene rearrangements is initiated and cells that fail to generate productive rearrangements are removed by apoptosis and cleared by phagocytosis by bone marrow macrophages. From Picker and Siegelman (17), with permission.

pre–B cells might represent differences in stromal cell types immediately subjacent to the endosteum and several cell layers more central in the marrow, or it might represent gradients of growth and differentiation factors produced from common endosteal stromal elements. More differentiated cells are found in a more central location in the marrow cavity, placing the most mature cells that are prepared for export from the marrow adjacent to the coalescing venous sinus. Thus, immature pro–B cells are detected close to the endosteal layer. Final maturation of B cells occurs in association with macrophage-like cells that infiltrate the central venous sinusoids (24,25).

Stromal Cell Cultures and Stromal Factors Supporting Lymphopoiesis

Evidence supporting the presence of different classes of stromal cells, each adapted to support of the differentiation of different hematopoietic lineages comes from *in vitro* culture systems that permit parts of the hematopoietic differentiation program to occur under well-defined conditions. Initial studies defined conditions under which mixed cultures of bone marrow stromal cells could support differentiation from stem cells along myelopoietic pathways (26) and along pathways

leading to formation of pre–B cells (27). These Dexter cultures and Whitlock-Witte cultures were subsequently adapted in order to isolate cloned stromal cell lines representing defined subsets that could support selectively the differentiation of HSCs to myeloid lineages (28) or pre–B lineages (29,30). These cloned stromal cell lines have permitted isolation of cells with HSC character that could generate long-term myeloid cultures and pre–B-cell cultures (31). The features of these stromal cell lines that permit them to support differentiation of myeloid and pre–B-cell lineages are not fully defined (32,33), but include the expression of specific cytokines, such as IL-3, IL-7, and IL-11, and growth factors, such as G-CSF, GM-CSF, c-kit, and IGF-1 (34–40), as well as the expression of adhesion molecules such as CD44, fibronectin, syndecan, and VLA-4 that support close interactions between the hematopoietic precursors and the stromal elements (41–45). The involvement of adhesion molecules initially suggested that contact between the stromal cell and the developing lymphocyte was particularly important. This hypothesis has been validated by experiments *in vitro* using cloned stromal lines and normal B progenitor cells (46,47). It is likely that the recent development of gene expression–profiling technology will permit the more complete delineation of stromal products that act to permit commitment of

HSC to specific cell lineages. More complex will be the identification of local signals that permit the self-renewal of HSC. These cells that represent less than 0.1% of total bone marrow cells persist through the life of the organism. In mice, adoptive transfer of as few as 10 of these cells is sufficient to reconstitute all hematopoietic lineages in a lethally irradiated recipient mouse for the life of the animal (23,48). Animals reconstituted in this way can themselves serve as donors of HSC to other lethally irradiated recipients, indicating that these stem cells can indeed self-renew. In fact, when as few as 20 to 30 HSC are adoptively transferred into a lethally irradiated recipient mouse, these cells expand to yield more than 10,000 new HSC (48).

Interestingly, when HSC are tested for their proliferative potential *in vitro,* they are found not to be in cell cycle and to be resistant to stimulation by a wide variety of growth factors including IL-1, IL-3, IL-4, IL-6, CSF-1, G-CSF, and GM-CSF (49). But, when these cells are injected *in vivo* into a lethally irradiated host, they can expand to yield a thousand-fold more hematopoietic stem cells and can differentiate to yield more than 10^{10} mature cells representing all arms of the hematopoietic spectrum. This underscores the key role of the normal bone marrow microenvironment in the proliferative and differentiative capacity of HSC.

Apoptosis in Normal Bone Marrow Function

Generation of rearranged heavy- and light-chain genes by a largely stochastic process results in the production of not only appropriately formed antibody molecules, but also nonfunctional immunoglobulin chains as well as potentially dangerous autoreactive chains. Removal of developing B cells with defective or autoreactive immunoglobulin chains is largely through an apoptotic mechanism (50–53). The molecular mechanisms regulating this central deletion of unwanted B cells are not well defined, but appear to involve the B-cell antigen receptor (54). Analysis of B-cell apoptosis *in situ* shows macrophages adjacent to the apoptotic cells (55–57). It is not yet clear, however, whether macrophages are involved as triggers of the apoptotic process, or if their presence is reactive, to facilitate removal of the apoptotic cells.

Stromal Cells Contributing to NK Cell Differentiation

An essential role of the bone marrow microenvironment has also been observed in the development of NK cells. Studies by Iizuka et al. (58) showed that numbers of NK cells are reduced in mice deficient in the membrane lymphotoxin-$\alpha_1\beta_2$ (LT$\alpha_1\beta_2$) heterotrimer (58). Interactions of this ligand with the LTβ receptor (LTβR) are required for the normal development of many aspects of the lymphoid tissue microenvironment (Fig. 6, see below), and deficiency of the ligand was found to be associated with deficient production of NK cells. Systemic blocking of LT$\alpha_1\beta_2$ in normal mice by treatment with a soluble LTβR-IgFcγ fusion protein from mid-gestation through the first 3 weeks after birth resulted in not only life-long deficiency of NK cells, but also inability to reconstitute NK-cell development by transplantation with normal bone-marrow precursor cells. Thus, signals mediated by the LT$\alpha_1\beta_2$ ligand are instructive for a microenvironment that is required for NK cell development.

Together, these studies leave us with a clear awareness of the complexity of the bone marrow microenvironment. In this compartment, diverse lineages of cells, including definitive HSCs, must survive, proliferate, and differentiate. Some of these processes are likely to be bone marrow autonomous, but others appear to be carefully regulated in response to needs defined in the peripheral tissues. Marrow stromal cells provide key signals allowing properly regulated growth and differentiation along the various bone marrow lineages. Additional studies to define further the characteristics of the stromal cell types that support each of the bone marrow hematopoietic lineages will be essential for our further understanding of how production of each of these lineages is regulated.

Thymus

Soon after the demonstration that neonatal thymectomy resulted in defective development of other lymphoid organs, impaired immune responses, and increased susceptibility to infection (59,60), the thymus was recognized as the site of maturation of antigen-specific T cells (61–63). To serve this function, the thymus must first be populated with precursor cells from the bone marrow. Once in the thymus, these cells proliferate and their progeny begin a complex differentiation pathway that results in selection of cells recognizing foreign antigens in the context of self–major histocompatibility complex (MHC) molecules, but tolerant to self-antigens (described in detail in Chapters 8 and 9). As is the case for B cells in the bone marrow, the initiation and progress of this developmental program are dependent on interactions between the developing T cells and stromal cells within the thymic microenvironment. For B-lymphocytes, the instructive actions of the bone marrow microenvironment appear to be limited to regulation of cell proliferation and to activation of an autonomous process of differentiation and maturation that includes activation of heavy- and light-chain immunoglobulin gene rearrangement. In contrast, for T-lymphocytes, differentiation and maturation in the thymus includes regulation of precursor cell proliferation; entry into the T-cell differentiation pathway; programmed activation of T-cell receptor α, β, γ, and δ gene rearrangement; positive selection for α/β T cells that are able to recognize antigens in the context of self-MHC; and negative selection of cells with dangerous reactivity against self-antigens (64). It is not unexpected, therefore, that the thymus contains additional classes of non-hematopoietic cells to support these additional processes.

Normal Anatomy of the Thymus

The thymus is a symmetric bi-lobed organ that sits in the anterior mediastinum, immediately over the pericardial surface and extending up into the base of the neck. The thymus forms relatively early in embryonic development, being detected in mice soon after mid-gestation, with initial phases of α/β T-cell development occurring by embryonic day 14. At birth, the thymus has attained its maximum relative weight, in association with the rapid production of T cells that occurs at this time. The organ continues to grow in size until 4 to 6 weeks of age (puberty in humans), and thereafter gradually involutes (65,66). In adults it appears to be almost entirely replaced by fatty and fibrous tissue and manifests production of only small numbers of mature T cells. In spite of its appearance, this involuted adult thymus appears to retain significant function. This is seen most clearly in pathologic conditions such as myasthenia gravis in which thymectomy can have a profoundly beneficial immunomodulatory role (67).

Each thymic lobe is subdivided by fibrous septae that extend centrally from the capsule to form discrete lobules each of which contains a distinct peripherally located cortex and a centrally located medulla (Fig. 2). The cortex contains a large population of small, immature thymocytes, specialized cortical epithelial cells, and scattered macrophages. These macrophages serve to remove cells undergoing apoptotic selection. The medulla contains nearly mature and mature T cells that are in close association with medullary epithelial cells, dendritic cells, and macrophages. The medulla also contains Hassall's corpuscles, made up of epithelial cells that also appear to contribute to removal of unwanted cells (68). The most peripheral part of each lobule consists of a thin subcapsular zone that appears to contain the most recent thymic immigrants and that may represent the site of activation of the T-cell differentiation pathway (69).

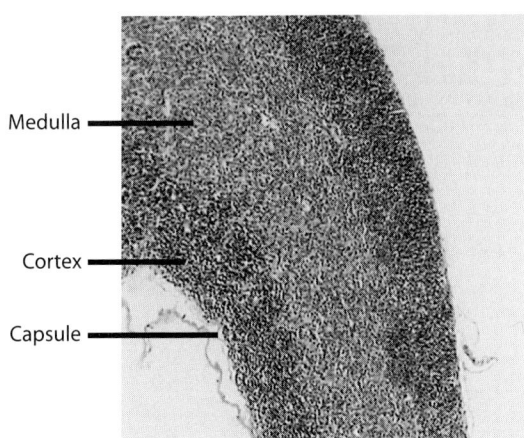

FIG. 2. Organization of thymic microarchitecture. Low-power view of a murine thymic lobe, showing the densely packed immature cells in the dark-staining thymic cortex and the less-densely cellular, lighter-staining thymic medulla. The most primitive thymocyte precursors are thought to lodge in peripheral portions of the thymus, in the subcapsular region. As the thymocytes mature, they move toward the center of the thymus, interacting with discrete subsets of epithelial cells in the cortex and the medulla. Positive selection is initiated near the cortico-medullary junction, and negative selection appears to occur predominantly in association with the medullary epithelial cells.

The interlobular septae serve as conduits for blood vessels, nerves, and efferent lymphatic vessels, and end near the cortico-medullary junction in an out-pouching that forms a compartment designated the perivascular space. This perivascular space appears to be a major site of nutrient and waste exchange between the circulation and each lobule compartment. Small branching vessels also leave this area to penetrate into the cortical and medullary compartments. The lymphatic vessels that arise in this area probably serve largely to maintain proper fluid homeostasis in the tissue and to remove from the thymus debris created during the negative selection of the developing thymocytes. It remains unclear to what extent appropriately selected, mature T cells use these lymphatics to leave the thymus and enter the circulation as opposed to entering directly via post-capillary venules near the cortico-medullary junction (70–72). Also unknown is the role of the nerves that course through the thymic lobular septae. They clearly control vascular tone in the thymus. Some nerves, however, extend into the cortex and medulla, terminating on or near epithelial structures in these areas (73). Organ transplantation experiments suggest that innervation may simulate lymphopoiesis with the thymus, indicating that the thymus may be a key site of regulation of the neuro-immune axis (74). The perivascular space also serves as a site for accumulation of B cells, plasma cells, myeloid cells, eosinophils, and mast cells (75). These generally are present as apparently unorganized collections of single cells, but can organize into follicles, particularly under pathologic conditions (76).

Embryologic Development of the Thymus

The thymus develops from endodermal and ectodermal components of the third pharyngeal pouch and the third branchial cleft, respectively (77). In mice, the thymus anlage is clearly detected by embryonic day 10. Studies in chickens, mice, and rats suggest that cells from several different sources must interact in a precisely timed sequence for the thymus to develop properly. An important early interaction occurs between neural crest immigrants and epithelial cells from the pharyngeal pouch to create an environment that will support the growth and development of the immature lymphoid cells. Surgical ablation of selected neural crest cells prevents normal thymus development (78,79). The developmental defect induced by ablation of these neural crest cells is similar to that seen in the human congenital immunodeficiency state designated DiGeorge syndrome (see Chapter 48) (80).

Additional interactions between the pharyngeal pouch epithelium and ectodermal cells from the branchial cleft subsequently permit expansion of the developing thymic epithelium (81). The "nude" mouse demonstrates clearly the requirement for an interaction between endodermal and ectodermal elements in order for normal thymus development. In this strain, the ectoderm of the third branchial cleft involutes after embryonic day 11.5, resulting in arrested development of the endodermal epithelium and failure of the tissue to support lymphocyte growth (82,83).

In addition to interactions between ectoderm, endoderm, and neural crest derivatives, normal thymic development requires signals generated by immigrant lymphoid cells. Circulating lymphoid cells localize in the thymus primordium between embryonic days 11 and 12. Interactions between these lymphoid cells and the developing thymic epithelium result in the formation of morphologically distinct cortical and medullary epithelium by embryonic day 13 (84). The ability of these lymphoid cells to signal development of the cortical epithelium is dependent on commitment to the T-cell lineage. Mice with a mutation that prevents the earliest phases of T-cell lineage commitment show failure of development of the thymic cortex (85). This defect can be corrected by transplantation into fetal but not adult mice of hematopoietic stem cells. Thus, developmentally restricted interactions between different cell lineages are essential for the development of the normal thymic microenvironment.

Genes controlling the developmental program that leads to formation of the normal thymus are just beginning to be identified. Because development of the thymus is dependent on cellular elements that are located in the third pharyngeal pouch, the third branchial cleft, and the neural crest, genes that are essential for normal development of these structures are expected to be required for thymus development as well. For example, normal function of the homeobox gene Hox-1.5 is required for development of parts of the hindbrain and spinal cord, including the neural crest (86). Targeted ablation of the Hox-1.5 locus results consequently in congenital absence of the thymus (87). This mutation also causes failure of parathyroid gland development, a consequence of the quite broad expression of the hox-1.5 gene in tissues giving rise to both of these structures. Compound mutations in both the Hoxa1 and Hoxb1 loci, two homeobox genes that are individually expressed in the first and second branchial arches in developing mice, also result in congenital athymia (88). Although neither the Hoxa1 nor the Hoxb1 gene is expressed in the critical third pharyngeal pouch or third branchial cleft, mutation of both loci induces sufficient distortion of structures adjacent to the second branchial arch that their ability to participate in normal developmental processes is impaired.

Recently, a set of four mammalian genes homologous to the *Drosophila eyes absent* (eya) gene have been isolated (89–93). These genes encode proteins with N-terminal transactivation domains and C-terminal domains that mediate protein–protein interaction. In mice, the eya1 gene product is widely expressed in sites of inductive tissue interaction during embryonic organogenesis. This gene is expressed at particularly high levels in the pharyngeal region around days 9 to 10 of mouse development (89). The eya1 gene is expressed in neural crest–derived pharyngeal arch mesenchyme, pharyngeal pouch endoderm, and branchial cleft ectoderm during the critical time that these three cell types interact during normal thymus development. Null mutation of eya1 results in congenital total absence of the thymus (94), underscoring the importance of these cellular interactions in thymus development.

The classical mutation affecting the development of the thymus was defined by the *nude* mouse. This spontaneous mutation affected both the formation of the thymus gland and the formation of normal hair follicles. Both of these tissues contain major ectodermal components. In the developing thymus, by embryonic day 12, ectoderm has extended over most of the endodermal portion. In nude mice, the proliferation of the ectoderm fails, leaving a cystic thymic rudiment that is unable to attract and support lymphocytes (83). The nude gene, initially localized to an approximately 1-megabase region of chromosome 11, was isolated using positional cloning and found to be a member of the winged-helix family of transcription factors. The isolated gene was named Whn (winged-helix nude, also designated FoxN1) and shown to be disrupted in both the mouse nude mutation and the rat rnuN nude mutation (95). Subsequent targeted disruption of the Whn gene recapitulated the phenotype of the nude mouse and proved definitively that the Whn gene determined the nude mutation (96). Recent studies have confirmed that the Whn gene encodes a sequence-specific DNA binding protein with characteristics of a regulatory transcription factor (97) and have identified the PD-L1 protein (programmed death ligand-1, also designated B7-H1) as a target of the Whn gene product (98). Whether PD-L1 is an essential mediator of the actions of Whn in development of normal thymic ectoderm, or whether its induction is an epiphenomenon of Whn activation, requires experimental examination. Interestingly, expression of Whn is regulated by Wnt glycoproteins that are themselves expressed by thymic epithelial cells and thymocytes (99). This, therefore, provides a mechanism for autocrine and paracrine regulation of Whn expression, underscoring the importance of lymphoid-cell/epithelial-cell interaction in the development of this tissue.

In addition to genes that have broad effects on lineages involved in thymus development, current studies are identifying genes that contribute to thymic development in a more thymus-specific fashion. For example, the RelB gene is required for the proper formation of medullary epithelial cells (distinguished by the expression of the UEA-1 surface marker) and of bone marrow–derived dendritic cells (distinguished by the expression of MIDC-8) (100–102). Targeted disruption of RelB results in nearly complete absence of medullary epithelial cells and interdigitating dendritic cells. Mice carrying this defect have peripheral T cells, indicating that some aspects of T-cell selection can occur without these thymic constituents, but manifest a severe inflammatory syndrome, suggesting that some aspect of proper regulation of T-cell function is imprinted in the thymic medulla (100,101).

A spontaneously arising mutation designated "alymphoplasia" (aly) also affects normal thymic development and function. This mutation causes a severe immunodeficiency expressed phenotypically as congenital absence of lymph nodes and Peyer's patches, disturbed structure of the spleen, and loss of a distinct cortical–medullary junction in the thymus (103). Alymphoplasia in mice is caused by a point mutation in the gene encoding the NFκB-inducing kinase (NIK)

(104,105). Adoptive transfer studies attribute at least part of the abnormal thymus phenotype in aly mice to abnormal medullary epithelial cells in this strain (106) and suggest that NIK provides essential signals for the normal development of this cell lineage.

A final spontaneous mutation affecting thymic epithelial cell function is seen in "undulated" mice. These mice, which were identified because of abnormalities in their vertebral skeleton, have a mutation in the Pax1 gene, a gene homologous to the Drosophila "paired box" family of transcriptional regulatory genes that control embryo segmentation (107). Pax1 is expressed by endodermal precursor cells of the thymus epithelium in the pharyngeal pouches, and remains expressed in thymic epithelial cells throughout ontogeny. In adult life, Pax1 is expressed by a small subset of cortical epithelial cells (108). Analysis of various alleles of the undulated mutant mice demonstrate that defective expression of Pax1 is associated with the formation of a small thymus and dramatically reduced numbers of thymic and peripheral T cells. Thus, this mutation expressed primarily in the thymic epithelial compartment results in dramatically impaired T-cell development.

Together, studies of mice mutant in either the organogenesis of the thymus or in the development of a normal thymic epithelium underscore the importance of cellular interactions in the formation of this complex organ. Any process that interrupts the temporally and spatially regulated program of these cellular interactions is likely to result in either total or partial failure of development of the organ.

Mature Architecture of the Thymus

Implicit in the above discussion of embryologic development of the thymus is the assertion that epithelial elements of the thymus are critical to its function. Although the cortical and medullary compartments of each thymic lobule differ in several of their constituent cellular elements, the epithelial component of each compartment is central to its biological function (109,110). Although the structure of the thymus changes steadily throughout the life of the organism, from its "mature" structure in the immediate postnatal period, through its initial period of growth peaking near puberty, to its gradual involution as the organism ages, the thymus contains several discrete epithelial compartments.

These discrete thymic epithelial compartments are defined both morphologically and functionally, and generally are positionally restricted (Fig. 3) (111). Beginning from the capsule and moving toward the center of the organ, at least three types of epithelial cells are encountered. First is the subcapsular–perivascular epithelium that lines the internal surface of the capsule and extends along the interlobular septae. This epithelial cell layer contributes to the structural integrity of the thymus, but unlike the cortical and medullary epithelium has no known functional interaction with the developing lymphoid cells. Because of its strategic location and its apparently complete envelopment of all the subcapsular

vascular structures, this epithelial layer has been thought to contribute importantly to the blood–thymus barrier. The possible existence of such a barrier was suggested by early studies showing exclusion of macromolecules from the thymic lymphoid compartment (75,112,113). A barrier layer was consistent with models in which T-cell development in the thymus was thought to occur in the absence of systemic antigens. While it remains likely that the thymic cortex is relatively protected from major fluctuations in circulating antigens, it is now clear that circulating macromolecules do cross from the thymic vasculature into the cortical and medullary lymphoid spaces (114–118). It remains possible that, although the subcapsular–perivascular epithelium may not represent an absolute barrier restricting access of circulating macromolecules, this epithelial layer modulates entry of systemic antigens in a way that is important for normal thymocyte development. Such transepithelial traffic of antigen is almost certainly supplemented by antigen-transport mechanisms in which phagocytic or dendritic cells may carry molecules from peripheral sites into the thymic cortex (119). Lastly, developing thymic lymphoid cells also appear to encounter "tissue-specific" self-antigens that are produced at low levels by cells located within the thymus (120–122).

Epithelial cells in the cortex manifest a dramatically different morphology compared to the subcapsular epithelial cells. The cortical epithelial cells have a more dendritic morphology, with their cellular processes in close contact with the developing cortical lymphoid cells (110,123). Immature thymocytes bind with substantial affinity to cortical epithelial cells in vitro (124). This together with the observation that thymic LFA-1 and epithelial ICAM-1 are major contributors to this interaction (125) suggests that direct contact between these two cell types is a necessary part of the cortical T-cell maturation process. Many studies have suggested that the existence of an additional epithelial cell type in the thymic cortex designated the thymic nurse cell because of its presumed role in fostering the maturation of developing thymocytes (126). These cells are defined by their association with large numbers of thymocytes (up to 200 lymphoid cells/epithelial cell). Nurse cells are thought to completely engulf the developing thymocytes into their cytoplasm, thus providing the immature lymphocytes with a protected environment in which to complete their initial differentiation program. It remains, however, controversial whether a lineage of nurse cells exists that is distinct from the well-characterized thymic cortical epithelium (127), and whether thymocytes truly reside in the cytoplasm of these cells. Considerable data exist to suggest that the apparent complete envelopment of thymocytes by the epithelial nurse cell is an artifact of the methods used for isolation of these large cell aggregates (123,128).

Epithelial cells in the thymic medulla appear morphologically distinct from the cortical epithelial cells (129). The density of lymphoid and epithelial cells in the medulla is reduced compared to the cortex. Although both cortical and medullary epithelial cells express high levels of class II MHC molecules, medullary epithelial cells show higher levels of

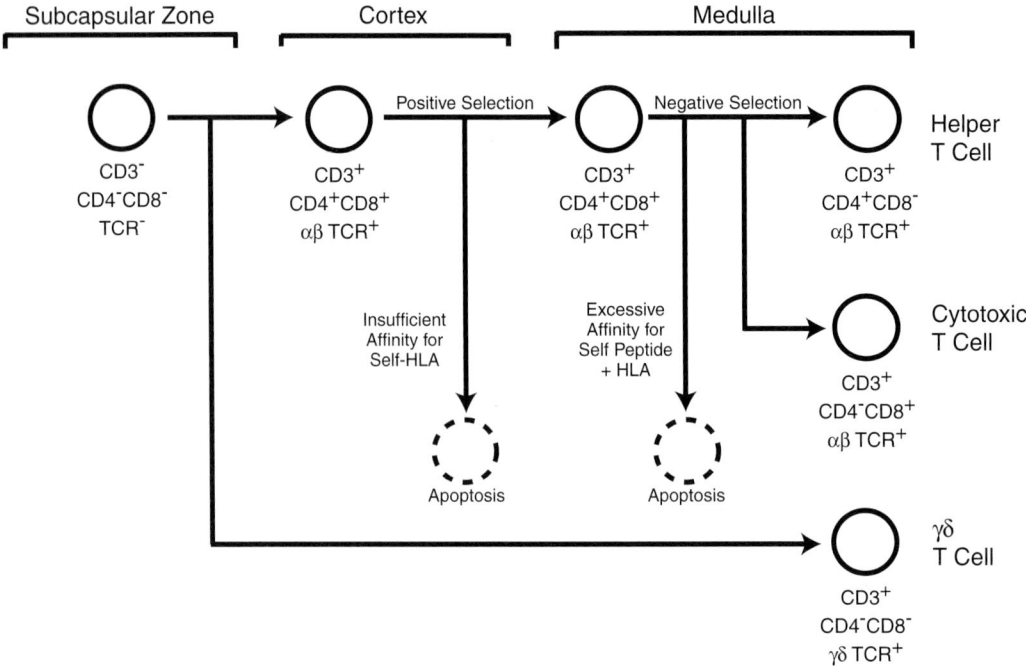

FIG. 3. Compartmentalization of T-cell development in the thymus. Discrete populations of epithelial cells are present in the thymic subcapsular zone, cortex, and medulla, with each epithelial population supporting the stages of thymic development that occur in each compartment. The subcapsular epithelial cells support the expansion of the thymocyte pool from a committed T-cell precursor population. T-cell receptor gene rearrangement is induced during the movement of cells from the subcapsular region to the cortex where double-positive cells are subjected to positive selection. Cells that fail positive selection are removed by apoptosis. Following positive selection, the developing thymocytes undergo negative selection on medullary epithelial cells that present a huge array of self-peptides. This is accompanied by transition to CD4+ or CD8+ single-positive cells. Again, failure of selection leads to death of the developing thymocyte by an apoptotic mechanism. A fraction of γ/δ T cells develop in the thymus, but the role of the defined thymic epithelial cell populations in differentiation of this lineage is not defined. Adapted from Chaplin (111), with permission.

class I molecules (130). Medullary epithelial cells also show high levels of HLA-DM (68), which suggests that these cells are particularly active in the loading of peptide antigens into class II molecules (Chapters 19 and 20). This may be consistent with the medulla as a site of negative selection of the developing thymocytes. The thymic medullary epithelium can be subdivided into two types based on surface expression of MHC molecules (131) and other cell-surface molecules including discrete forms of keratin (132). The functional significance of keratin expression in either cortical or thymic epithelial cells remains unknown. The medullary epithelial cells also can be separated into two subsets based on their expression of ligands for the *Ulex europeus* agglutinin (UEA-1). This lectin has specificity for a subset of fucosylated glycoproteins and identifies medullary epithelial cells with a dendritic morphology that form a reticular network throughout the medulla (133). The numbers of UEA-1+ cells gradually decrease as the animal ages, apparently paralleling the overall involution of the thymus with age. UEA-1⁻ epithelial cells have a less dendritic morphology and show fewer associations with the developing lymphoid cells. Some hypothesize that these represent spent epithelial cells that are in the

initial phases of involution prior to apoptosis. Finally, a third species of epithelial cells is identified in the medulla constituting the Hassall's corpuscles. These appear late in the first trimester of human fetal life as duct-like structures (134). By the time of birth, they have assumed their mature structure with concentrically organized, highly keratinized epithelial cells arranged in an onion-like fashion. They also express fucose-containing glycoproteins on their cell surfaces, but these show low reactivity with UEA-1 and high reactivity with the *Tetragonolobus purpureas* agglutinin (TPA). TPA+ cells remain prominent throughout life, apparently resistant to the involution of the thymus that occurs with aging. Although the functions of Hassall's corpuscles remain incompletely defined, they associate with fragments of dead cells. Thus, they are assumed to participate in the catabolism of either lymphoid or nonlymphoid cells that are removed during the process of negative selection.

Attempts to define the mechanisms by which thymic epithelial cells support the differentiation and maturation of T-lymphocytes have included studies of the secreted mediators they produce. These include cytokines such as IL-1 (135), IL-3 (136), IL-6 (137–139), and IL-7 (140–143),

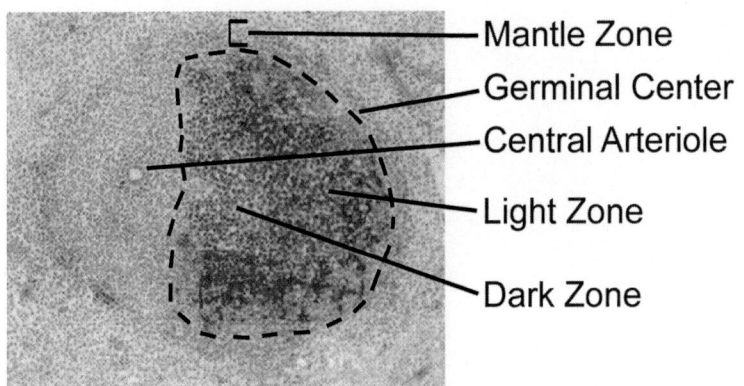

Mantle Zone
Germinal Center
Central Arteriole
Light Zone
Dark Zone

COLORPLATE 1. Architecture of a germinal center. This germinal center is within a splenic white pulp nodule. The center of the nodule is marked by the central arteriole. The germinal center is highlighted by a dashed line. Unactivated cells surround the germinal center constituting the mantle zone. The light zone of the germinal center represents rapidly proliferating, surface Ig$^-$ B cells, here stained brown with anti-B220 antibody. The light zone of cells undergoing selection for affinity maturation lie within a dense reticulum of follicular dendritic cells here stained blue with anti-CR2 antibody.

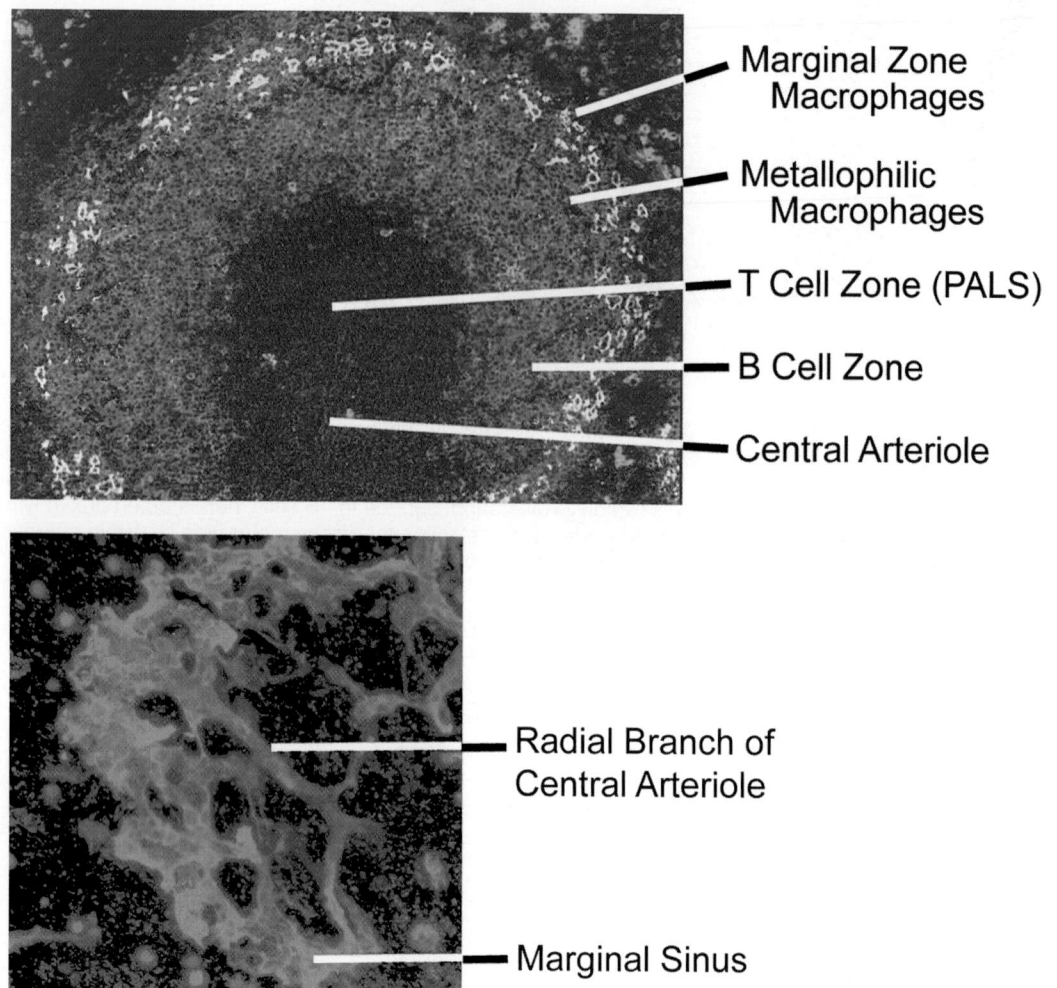

Marginal Zone
Macrophages

Metallophilic
Macrophages

T Cell Zone (PALS)

B Cell Zone

Central Arteriole

Radial Branch of
Central Arteriole

Marginal Sinus

COLORPLATE 2. Organization of the spleen white pulp. **Top panel:** Immunofluorescence stain of a white pulp unit in the mouse spleen. T cells (anti-CD4+anti-CD8, red) are localized around the central arteriole. B cells (anti-IgM, green) are localized in follicles around the T-cell area, and surrounded by a layer of metalophilic macrophages (labeled with monoclonal antibody MOMA-1, blue) and a more peripheral layer of marginal zone macrophages (labeled with monoclonal antibody ERTR-9, orange). The marginal sinus is located between the metalophilic macrophage and the marginal zone macrophage layers (not shown). From Martin and Kearney (314), with permission. **Bottom panel:** Structure of the marginal sinus in a thick (100 micrometer) frozen section of mice with targeted insertion of the Lac Z gene into the ephrin B2 locus (470). In the spleen, ephrin B2 expression is high in the central arteriole, in radial branches of the central arteriole and in the marginal sinus. Lac Z is visualized by staining with FITC-labeled anti–Lac Z antibody. Note the transition from discrete arteriolar vessels to a network of flattened vessels at the transition to the marginal sinus plexus. Lower panel courtesy of C. Zindl (University of Alabama at Birmingham, Birmingham, AL).

and chemokines such as interferon-inducible protein 10 (IP-10) (144), macrophage-derived chemokine (MDC) (145), monokine induced by interferon gamma (Mig) (144), EBI1-ligand chemokine (ELC) (145), secondary lymphoid tissue chemokine (SLC) (145), interferon-inducible T-cell alpha chemoattractant (I-TAC) (144), stromal-derived factor-1 (SDF-1) (146), and thymus-expressed chemokine (TECK) (147). Thymic epithelial cells also produce the peptide mediators leukemia inhibitory factor (LIF) (148), oncostatin M (148), M-CSF (148), stem cell factor (148), insulin-like growth factor 1 (149), thymosin-α1 (143), and thymic stromal lymphopoietin (TSLP) (150,151). Careful localization of the sites of production of these mediators has indicated different patterns of production by different subtypes of epithelial cells. For example, ELC, IP-10, Mig, and I-TAC are found selectively in medullary epithelial cells (144,145), whereas cells forming the Hassall's corpuscles are the producers of SDF-1 and MDC (145,152). It is likely that understanding the nature of the cells recruited by each of these chemokines to the central medullary zone and to the Hassall's corpuscles will provide clues to the biological roles of each of the compartments.

Nonlymphoid Bone Marrow–Derived Cells

In addition to its important vascular, nervous, epithelial, and lymphoid cell components, the thymus contains prominent populations of macrophages and dendritic cells. It is not known if these cells develop in situ in the thymus from partially differentiated precursors, or if they mature elsewhere and enter the thymus via the vascular channels that also supply the T-cell precursors.

As has been discussed in Chapters 8 and 9, the large population of α/β T cells acquire their antigen specificity and mature phenotype by processes involving assembly of functional T-cell receptor α- and β-chain genes, followed by selection of those cells whose receptors are competent to recognize antigen when presented bound to a class I or class II MHC molecule (positive selection) without reacting against self-antigens (negative selection) (Fig. 3). Because the assembly of individual V-, D-, and J-elements often results in T-cell receptor genes that are either unable to encode functional α or β chains, that have insufficient affinity for self-MHC molecules, or that have excessive self-reactivity, the vast majority of developing T cells are destroyed within the thymus. This removal of unwanted cells is accomplished primarily by induction of apoptosis of the lymphoid cell (153). It is not, therefore, surprising to find large numbers of macrophages in the thymic cortex and medulla. The cortical macrophages associate closely with developing lymphoid cells, with up to 80% of thymic macrophages forming rosettes with lymphoid cells (154). Up to 10% of these rosetted macrophages manifest internalized lymphoid cells that have been taken up because they have entered the apoptotic pathway. Macrophages are present also in the thymic medulla, although in smaller numbers, and less frequently containing detectable apoptotic

bodies. This may simply reflect the smaller number of lymphoid cells in this compartment, rather than a fundamentally different biological function of macrophages in the medulla. In addition to their role in apoptosis of unwanted lymphoid cells, cortical and medullary macrophages are known to express on their surfaces class II MHC molecules (154). They also express a spectrum of cytokines and growth factors (155). Consequently, although their direct participation in activation of thymocyte differentiation and maturation has not been proved, they have the potential to contribute both to activation of lymphoid cell development and to shaping the antigen specificity of the T-cell repertoire.

Thymic dendritic cells predominate in the medulla (156), where they contact both lymphoid and epithelial cells. These interdigitating dendritic cells bear high levels of class II MHC on their surfaces, express co-stimulatory molecules, and have potent ability to present antigen to mature T cells in vitro. It is likely, therefore, that they participate actively in the selection of the mature T-cell repertoire; however, the relative roles of these dendritic cells and of the medullary epithelial cells (also class II MHC$^+$) in this process have not been defined.

Relationship of Thymic Compartments to T-Lymphopoiesis

The preceding discussion has defined three physical compartments in each thymic lobule, beginning with the peripheral subcapsular zone, to the densely cellular cortex, and then the less dense medulla. Minimally differentiated T-cell precursors enter the mouse thymus at the cortico-medullary junction, probably from vessels branching at the termini of the interlobular septae (Fig. 3) (157). Because they are present in quite small numbers, it has been difficult to definitively characterize the phenotype of these earliest bone marrow–derived T-cell precursors, but it appears that they have committed to the T-lineage (158,159), having acquired expression of Thy-1 and low levels of CD4, although they retain all their T-cell receptor gene loci in the germline configuration (160,161). Once these cells enter from the circulation into the thymus near the cortico-medullary junction, they move to the subcapsular zone (162) where they appear to encounter stromal cells that propel them down the T-cell developmental pathway.

In the subcapsular zone, the developing cells complete their commitment to the T lineage, and begin the differentiative events that lead either to the α/β T-cell lineage or to the thymic γ/δ T-cell lineage. Because they show no expression of CD3, CD4, or CD8, these cells are referred to as triple negative (TN). The most immature TN cells are CD44^{hi}CD25$^-$ and can after adoptive transfer to irradiated recipients give rise to B cells, NK cells and dendritic cells in addition to cells of the T-cell lineage. They are not, therefore, irrevocably committed to the T-cell developmental pathway. Soon, however, they up-regulate CD25, proliferate rapidly, and then down-modulate CD44 expression to become CD44^{lo}CD25$^+$. It is in this compartment that the T-cell receptor β-chain gene begins to rearrange and a subset of cells commits to rearrangement of their γ-chain and δ-chain genes (163). A second population of γ/δ T cells develops outside the thymus. After successful β-chain gene rearrangement, the pre–TCR-α gene is expressed. The pre–TCRα-chain pairs with the rearranged β chain gene and the developing T cells again enter a rapidly proliferating phase. Pre-TCR$^+$ cells then move into the thymic cortex where expression of both CD4 and CD8 is induced (DP) and α-chain rearrangement is activated. Once the TCR α- and β-chains pair, the immature T cells can begin to undergo selection. In the cortex, cortical epithelial cells and cortical macrophages appear to mediate the process of positive selection, whereby cells that show insufficient affinity for self-MHC molecules are eliminated (164). In the course of this process, cells become either CD4 or CD8 single positive (SP) and move to the medulla where they are tested for excessive self-reactivity. This process appears to occur on medullary epithelial cells or the medullary interdigitating dendritic cells, and probably depends on the expression at low levels in this area of the vast majority of self-proteins (121,165).

Intriguing studies have indicated that medullary epithelial cells (and to a lesser extent subcapsular epithelial cells) express, in addition to classical MHC class I molecules, the class Ib molecule HLA-G (166). This molecule is of low polymorphism and prior to these studies had only been detected in the trophoblast cells of the placenta where it had been thought to contribute to maternal tolerance of the fetal allograft (see Chapters 19 and 28). In the thymus, HLA-G appears to be expressed both as a membrane protein in medullary epithelial cells and as a secreted product (167,168). It is likely that expression of HLA-G in this compartment provides the mechanisms for maternal lymphoid cells to acquire tolerance to this protein, thus permitting retention of the fetal allograft. Thus, selection in the thymus is not limited to cells encountering pathogen-based antigens, but includes preparation for the unique encounter with alloantigens that characterizes normal mammalian reproduction.

The entire process of maturation and selection in the thymus appears to require approximately 3 weeks, with fewer than 5% of the cells generated ultimately surviving the dual gauntlets of positive and negative selection. The final signals marking a lymphocyte as ready for export to the periphery have not yet been defined (169,170), nor has the exact location of cell exit from the thymus been identified (71,110). Most likely, emigrating cells leave from the corticomedullary junction via postcapillary venules or by entry into efferent lymphatic vessels.

SECONDARY LYMPHOID TISSUES

Overview of Secondary Lymphoid Organs

Once mature B- and T-lymphocytes are released from the bone marrow and thymus, they circulate in a resting state until they encounter the antigen that is specified by their antigen receptor. For B cells, this antigen is a conformational epitope generally displayed on the surface of a macromolecular antigen. For α/β T cells, the antigen is generally a linear peptide epitope that is displayed in association with a class I or class II MHC protein. While antigenic targets of B and T cells may include normal and abnormal self-molecules, it is generally thought that the primary targets of the adaptive immune system are pathogenic microbes. Most microbial pathogens enter the host at epithelial barriers including the skin and mucous membranes. These microbes begin to replicate rapidly after entering the rich culture medium of the mammalian host. This initiates a race between the microbe and the host, with the microbe trying to expand sufficiently to permit it to survive in spite of the host's immune response, and the host trying to activate its innate immune responses and to expand its repertoire of antigen-specific immune cells sufficiently to control the microbe. For some microbes, the innate response is largely able to contain the microbe, but for the majority of microbial challenges, a combination of innate responses and adaptive responses is required. In a naïve host, the total B-cell and T-cell repertoires each exceed 10^8 specificities (171–173). Thus, fewer than 1 in 10^8 B cells or T cells will carry a receptor specific for a given antigenic epitope on a pathogen. Consequently, a major challenge for the immune response is to facilitate the encounter of antigens from microbial pathogens with the rare, naïve pathogen-specific B and T cells soon after the pathogen has breached the protective epithelial barrier. The lymphoid vascular circulation and the secondary lymphoid tissues appear to have evolved to meet this challenge.

The secondary lymphoid tissues are the spleen, lymph nodes (LN), and organized lymphoid tissues associated with mucosal surfaces including the Peyer's patches (PP) (174,175), tonsils (176), bronchial-associated lymphoid tissues (BALT) (177,178), nasal-associated lymphoid tissues (NALT or adenoids) (179,180), and gut-associated lymphoid tissues (GALT) (181,182). Together, the tonsils and NALT constitute Waldeyer's ring (183,184), thought of as the guardian of the oropharynx. In addition to these easily identified lymphoid structures, there are other less well-defined clusters of lymphoid and other hematopoietic cells associated with the genitourinary (185–187), gastrointestinal (188,189), and respiratory tracts that contribute to host defense but whose formation and function may be governed by different rules than those determining the classical secondary lymphoid organs.

The secondary lymphoid tissues are situated at strategic sites where foreign antigens and pathogenic microbes may enter the body, either by penetrating the skin, by crossing a mucosal barrier, or by injection into the blood circulation by an arthropod vector. Although the individual types of secondary lymphoid tissues differ in their detailed structures, they each consist of a supporting stromal matrix that provides an organizing framework for T- and B-lymphocytes, antigen-transporting and antigen-presenting cells, and other regulatory cells (190,191). Each secondary lymphoid tissue also possesses a vascular supply that permits the delivery of both nutrients and naïve cells to the tissue, and removal of metabolic wastes and in some cases export of selected populations of cells.

Organizing lymphocytes and other cells of the immune system into the various lymphoid organs is thought to enhance the efficiency of the immune response by providing sites where antigens delivered from peripheral tissues either in soluble form or in association with MHC-bearing antigen-transporting and antigen-presenting cells can be concentrated, where rapidly circulating naïve and memory lymphocytes can interact with these antigen-loaded cells, and where activated cells can be either expanded or destroyed depending on the needs of the immune response. The enhanced efficiency that comes from gathering lymphoid and other immune cells into a specialized microenvironment can be appreciated by studies such as those of Kundig et al. (192) who showed that efficient T-cell sensitization to a fibrosarcoma cell line required immunization with 10^6 cells when the tumor cells were injected subcutaneously. In contrast, injection of as few as 500 cells directly into the spleen resulted in enduring T-cell sensitization. This type of experiment has suggested that both geographic localization of antigens to secondary lymphoid tissues and the maintenance of an appropriate quantity of antigen for an appropriate period of time are key variables that determine whether a properly regulated protective immune response occurs (193). Thus, the mechanisms by which secondary lymphoid organs concentrate antigens and retain them in association with the responding lymphoid cells are critical for immune homeostasis.

The signals that specify where and when secondary lymphoid tissues form are only beginning to be understood. It is likely that organized lymphoid tissues form near essentially any site where disruptive antigens can enter the organism. For example, organized lymphoid structures have even been found associated with salivary glands (194,195). Some of these tissues are present throughout the life of the organism, but some become visible only at selected times. In humans, the bronchial-associated lymphoid tissue (BALT), for example, is well developed and easily visible in childhood and adolescence, but involutes in early adult life becoming undetectable at a gross level (196). In adults, BALT is only observed in acute and chronic inflammatory states of the lung. Although it has not been tested directly, it is thought that the BALT seen in inflamed adult lungs is located at sites that constituted BALT in childhood, with the adult BALT representing re-population of a persistent childhood BALT remnant. Similarly, when normally nonpalpable lymph nodes become enlarged following their stimulation by a local infectious process or by infiltration with metastatic tumor cells, these nodes are thought to result from the influx of cells into structures that have been present continuously since infancy, rather than de novo formation of newly organized lymph node structures. In contrast, it is clear that new organized solitary lymphoid follicles can form in a variety of tissues under the influence of local inflammatory signals (197,198). Such ectopic lymphoid follicles have been seen in the inflamed, hyperplastic synovium of rheumatoid arthritis (199), in the parenchyma of the liver during chronic

viral hepatitis (200), and in inflamed thymus of subjects with myasthenia gravis (201). These ectopic structures appear to develop in response to chronic expression of certain lymphoid structure-inducing cytokines and chemokines, and are not associated with specialized stromal structures such as afferent and efferent lymphatics or an organ capsule. Additionally, they are characterized by organization as single lymphoid follicles (see below). The secondary lymphoid organs, in contrast, contain many follicles organized into a single structure. The induction of the inflammatory follicles can be modeled experimentally by ectopic transgenic expression of the cytokine lymphotoxin (198) or the chemokine CXCL13 (202). While these inflammatory signal–induced lymphoid structures can include many of the cellular constituents of lymph nodes, spleen, and other secondary lymphoid organs, it is assumed that if the inflammatory signal is extinguished, these ectopic organs will disappear without a trace. If a new inflammatory reaction were to arise, the location of any newly arising lymphoid follicles would be determined randomly, and not be influenced by the site of previous ectopic follicle formation.

While all secondary lymphoid tissues share some common features, the mechanisms that support recruitment of each of the key immune cell types to the tissue and that provide efficient delivery of antigens from the epithelial barrier are adapted to the particular epithelial surface that each tissue serves. I next describe the key anatomic features of each of the major secondary lymphoid tissues that render them well suited to facilitating immune responses against locally invading microbial antigens.

Lymph Nodes

Structure and Organization of Lymphatic Vessels and Lymph Nodes

The lymphatic system consists of the lymphatic vessels and lymph nodes. The lymphatic vessels serve at least three critical functions: (a) to return back into the circulation extracellular fluid that has leaked from the blood vasculature as a consequence of Starling forces (203); (b) to deliver both soluble antigens and antigen-transporting/antigen-presenting cells from the peripheral tissues to the lymph nodes (204–206); and (c) to carry water-insoluble nutrients from the gastrointestinal tract eventually into the circulation (207).

The most peripheral lymphatic vessels arise in the connective tissue of skin and mucosal tissues below the basement membrane that supports the epithelial layer. Their site of origin in solid organs has not been defined. The first ultrastructurally recognized lymphatic structures in the dermis and mucosal tissues are arranged in a capillary-like fashion thought to arise blindly in the interstitial spaces (208). These lymphatic capillaries are thought to be freely permeable to both interstitial fluid and particulate matter, including cells the size of lymphocytes and antigen-transporting cells. For example, radio-opaque dyes and India ink particles injected subcutaneously rapidly enter the lymphatic vessels and are

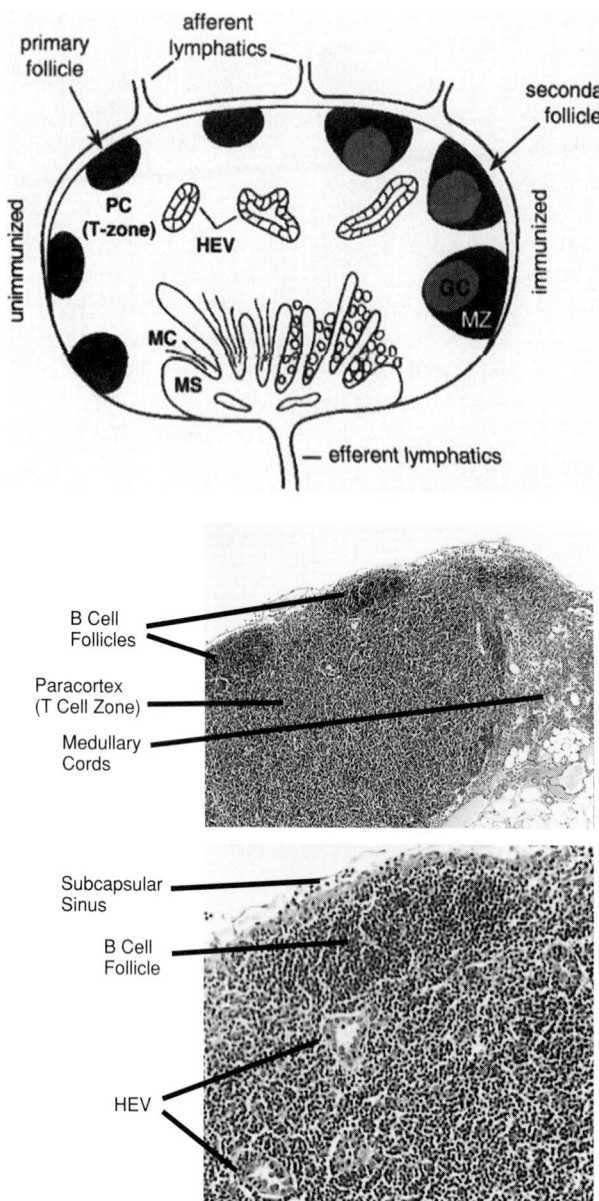

FIG. 4. The organization of peripheral lymph nodes. **Top panel:** Diagram of a peripheral lymph node highlighting the placement of afferent lymphatics on the convex surface of the node opposite the hilum. The efferent lymphatic vessel emerges from the hilum in close proximity to the lymphatic artery and vein (not shown). Primary and secondary follicles are located around the periphery of the node just below the subcapsular sinus. Secondary follicles are marked by the presence of germinal centers (GC) induced after activation of B cells with T-cell–dependent antigens. Surrounding the germinal center cells is a band of unactivated B cells designated the mantle zone (MZ). Between follicles is the paracortex (PC) consisting of T cells and MHC class II⁺ dendritic cells. Within the paracortex are the HEV where naïve cells are extracted from the circulation and recruited into the T-cell and B-cell compartments. Cells ready for return to the circulation move to the medullary cords (MC) and into the medullary sinus (MS) for delivery into the efferent lymphatic vessel. From Picker and Siegelman (17) with permission. **Middle panel:** Low-power view of the lymph node showing the densely staining primary

transported to the draining lymph nodes within a period from minutes to a few hours after their initial entry (209,210).

Ultrastructural evaluation of the terminal lymphatic capillaries suggests that they are supported and held in place by reticular anchoring filaments (211,212). These filaments keep the lymphatic channels open when extracellular fluid pressure increases, permitting bulk flow of fluid, particles, and cells into the vessels. Increases in extracellular fluid pressure are prominent at sites of tissue injury and inflammation, where they can result in an increased rate of delivery of subcutaneous antigen to the lymphoid tissue compartment.

The lymphatic capillaries are distributed widely, with the exception of the central nervous system (where the spinal fluid circulation appears to serve a similar function); the globe of the eye (where circulation of the aqueous humor supports a similar function); and the bone marrow (where venous sinusoids probably serve a similar function). The density of lymphatic capillaries is highest in the connective tissue of the dermis, and in the submucosa of the gastrointestinal, genitourinary, and respiratory tracts. These are sites where the largest quantities of antigens enter the body, and where substantial amounts of lymphatic fluid are generated. As the vessels move centrally from these peripheral tissues, the capillaries coalesce into larger afferent vessels that ultimately empty into a regional lymph node.

Formation of lymphatic vessels during embryonic development requires as an early signal expression of the homeobox gene Prox-1 (213). Prox-1 expression is observed at the site of formation of the earliest observed lymphatic sacs as buds off of developing venous structures, in mice at embryonic day 10.5 (E10.5). Over the next 5 days, the lymphatic sac endothelial cells acquire a distinctive endothelial phenotype, expressing VEGFR-3, CCL21 (secondary lymphoid tissue chemokine, SLC), and the CD44 homologue LYVE-1 (214,215), and by E15.5, the formation of the lymphatic vascular network appears complete.

The lymph nodes are small bean-shaped structures that are localized in clusters usually at sites of vascular junctions such as the popliteal, inguinal, and axillary regions, and near branches of the mesenteric artery and aorta. As will be described below, the lymph nodes arise as outpouchings of lymphatic vessels. Although there has been considerable progress in defining the molecular events that underlie the development of a normal lymph node, the nature of the signals that lead to the formation of lymph nodes at their characteristic locations remains to be defined.

The afferent lymphatic vessels enter the lymph node on its convex surface, penetrate the lymph node capsule, and empty into the subcapsular sinus (Fig. 4). It is typical for several afferent lymphatic vessels to enter a single lymph node. On the

FIG. 4. (*continued*). follicles in the subcapsular region. **Lower panel:** Higher-power view highlighting the HEV, showing circulating leukocytes adhering to the HEV luminal surface and transmigrating leukocytes in the HEV endothelial layer.

opposite side of the node, a nodal artery brings nutrients and naïve lymphoid cells into the tissue and a nodal vein returns blood and waste to the circulation. The insertion of these vessels into the node defines the lymph node hilum. The hilum also contains an efferent lymphatic vessel. This efferent lymphatic serves as a conduit for lymphatic fluid and lymphoid cells that are also returning to the circulation. The lymphatic vessels from different nodes join as they progress centrally, passing through additional more central lymph nodes and ultimately forming the large thoracic duct. The thoracic duct then empties into the superior vena cava, permitting the filtered lymph and recirculating lymphocytes to be diluted into the venous blood immediately before the blood enters the heart.

The lymph node itself is a complex structure with several distinct compartments. After the afferent lymphatic vessels penetrate the lymph node capsule, they empty into the subcapsular sinus. Immediately internal to this sinus is the lymph node cortex, consisting of the B-cell–enriched follicles and the intervening T-cell–enriched paracortex. The cortex overlies the lymph node medulla, which consists of alternating medullary sinuses and medullary cords. The medullary cords contain cells thought to be in transit out of the lymph node, including activated T and B cells and plasma cells that arise in the course of an ongoing immune response (216). The medullary sinuses coalesce as they approach the lymph node hilum and ultimately resolve to a single channel that becomes the efferent lymphatic vessel.

The paracortex contains a specialized vascular structure that mediates trafficking of naïve lymphocytes from the circulation into the lymph node. These vessels are postcapillary venules that stand out in this part of the node because they have a plump, cuboidal morphology. They bear important adhesion molecules on their luminal surface. The cuboidal morphology gives these vessels their designation as high endothelial venules (HEV). Circulating naïve lymphocytes interact with these HEV and transmigrate across the endothelial layer to enter the paracortex (Fig. 4). This is a highly efficient process with well over 50% of the naïve lymphocytes that enter the lymph node by its nodal artery leaving the circulation and entering the paracortical space. Interestingly, the normal structure of the HEV is dependent on ongoing delivery of antigens and perhaps other factors from the peripheral tissues. In germ-free mice, the HEV show a flattened endothelium with little evidence of ongoing lymphoid cell transmigration (217). When the microflora of germ-free mice is conventionalized (restored to normal microbial flora), the endothelial cells of the HEV rapidly acquire a cuboidal morphology, and large numbers of intramural lymphocytes are observed, indicating that cellular transmigration has been restored. Additionally, expression of adhesion molecules on the luminal surface of the HEV is induced following restoration of normal flora. Flattening of the HEV endothelium and loss of surface adhesion similar to that seen in germ-free mice has been observed following ligation of the afferent lymphatic vessels in several experimental animals, suggesting that ongoing delivery of factors from the peripheral tissue is critical for both the development and the maintenance of the HEV structure.

The selections of adhesion molecules that are expressed on the luminal surface of HEV vary in different lymphoid tissues. These molecules interact with ligands on circulating lymphocytes and mediate their specific extraction from the blood, so that selected subsets of lymphoid cells are recruited from the circulation in different lymphoid organs. In the peripheral lymph nodes, L-selectin (originally designated Mel-14) interacts with the sialylated oligosaccharides displayed on the peripheral node addressin (PNAd) molecules on the luminal surface of the HEV endothelial cells (218). In the mesenteric lymph node and other gut-associated lymphoid tissues, the integrin $\alpha 4\beta 7$ on naïve lymphocyte interacts with the mucosal addressin cell-adhesion molecule-1 (MAdCAM-1) on the HEV endothelial cells in those tissues to mediate emigration of the circulating cells into the lymphoid organ parenchyma (219,220). The selective expression of PNAd and MAdCAM-1 in the peripheral lymph nodes and gut-associated lymph nodes and lymphoid tissues determines distinct recirculation patterns of lymphoid cells particularly adapted to these tissue environments.

Unlike naïve lymphocytes, antigens from peripheral tissues enter the lymph node via the afferent lymphatics. These vessels empty into the subcapsular sinus, a narrow space immediately under the lymph node capsule. Lymph entering the subcapsular sinus consists of a mixture of extracellular fluid and cells that are migrating to the node from peripheral tissues. The cellular component consists primarily of antigen-carrying dendritic cells and macrophages, with only a few recirculating memory and effector lymphocytes. It is not surprising, therefore, that the subcapsular sinus contains few lymphocytes. When visualized using electron microscopy, the internal floor of the sinus that separates this compartment from the paracortex and follicles has a mosaic-like appearance without clear opening through which cells can pass (221).

Until recently, it had been assumed that the mosaic-like floor of the subcapsular sinus is characterized by loose intercellular junctions, permitting cells and lymphatic fluid to cross into the paracortex and follicles with little impediment. Thus, lymph-borne antigens that had been imported from peripheral tissues could simply move with bulk fluid flow from the subcapsular sinus through the paracortex and follicles into the lymph node medulla. Because of the dense packing of lymphoid and other cells in the paracortex and follicles, this model suggested that antigens carried in the lymph encountered a large number of lymphocytes as they were filtered by the node. Facilitating interactions of the lymph node lymphocytes and the filtered antigens was a scaffold designated the reticular network. The reticular network extended throughout the T-cell paracortex, and appeared excluded from the B-cell follicular area. Interestingly, at least a portion of the reticular network fibers appeared to radiate from the HEV to the subcapsular sinus (222), suggesting that it might represent a conduit between these two important structures. By electron microscopy, this network appeared to be composed of collagen-like fibers wrapped in fibroblast-like reticular cells (223). Lymphocytes were dispersed along the strands of this reticulum, appearing to use these fibers as a track along which to migrate. More detailed characterization of the protein composition of the fiber identified collagens I, III, and IV (224), elastin (225), fibronectin (226), laminin (227), tenascin (228), vitronectin (229), and heparan sulfate (230), suggesting that there were many potential ligands for lymphocyte–reticular fiber interaction. The structural features of the reticular network suggested that it was both a physical scaffold on which the lymph node was built, and a series of conduits that could facilitate the movement of both cells and fluid. A role in transport of cells and fluid was supported by direct visualization of rapid movement of tracer molecules along these conduits, from the subcapsular sinus to the HEV (231,232). The importance of these conduits for the function of lymph nodes is underscored by the observation that chemokines injected subcutaneously are rapidly delivered to the luminal surface of the HEV where they can have an important influence on the recruitment of circulating lymphocytes (233).

Recent studies by Gretz et al. (205,206) have added importantly to our understanding of how antigen moves within and through the lymph node. Using a variety of soluble, fluorescently tagged macromolecules, ranging in size from 300 to 2×10^6 daltons, they observed that after injection of these molecules subcutaneously in mice, all appeared rapidly (on the order of 2 to 10 minutes) in the subcapsular sinus (205,206). Unexpectedly, most of the molecules were excluded from the T-cell area of the cortical tissue. Low-molecular-weight dextrans ranging from 3,000 MW to 40,000 MW entered the T-cell zone, but were limited to close association with the reticular network. These low-molecular-weight molecules rapidly moved to and into the HEV. In contrast, high-MW dextrans (70,000 MW and larger) were excluded from the paracortex and largely remained in the subcapsular sinus. Thus, rather than permitting percolation of antigens from afferent lymph throughout its cellular compartments, the floor of the subcapsular sinus appears to present a barrier that restricts entry of soluble macromolecules into the lymphoid cell compartment. This suggests that delivery of moderate and large molecular weight antigens into the T-cell areas of the lymph node is regulated, with antigen-transporting and antigen-presenting cells playing an obligate role in this antigen entry (205). Requiring that soluble molecules must be taken up by antigen-presenting cells before they are transported to the T-cell areas of the lymph node offers a mechanism to protect the responding lymphocytes from toxicity or from unwanted activation by soluble microbial products.

In addition to the reticular network, the T-cell–rich paracortex contains substantial numbers of dendritic cells. As described in Chapter 15, different classes of dendritic cells predominate in the lymph node depending on the immune activation state of the organ. Many of these dendritic cells enter the lymph node via the afferent lymphatics after picking up antigens and receiving signals to mature in peripheral tissues (234,235). The extent to which dendritic cells can also enter the lymph node in an immature form by transmigrating across the HEV has not been defined; however, the detection of substantial numbers of immature dendritic cells in lymph nodes in the naïve, nonimmunized host suggests that entry of dendritic cells into the lymph node parenchyma directly from the blood circulation is an important pathway. In addition to stromal cells, T cells, and dendritic cells, the paracortex also contains small numbers of B-lymphocytes. Some of these represent naïve B cells that are in transit from the HEV to the B-cell follicles. Others are cells that have specifically entered the T-cell area in order to receive T-cell help for class switching, or that are on their way to the medullary sinusoids for circulation to other lymphoid organs or peripheral tissues (236).

B-Cell Follicles and Germinal Centers

In unimmunized hosts, lymph node B cells are organized into primary follicles that support the formation of germinal centers following immunization with a T-cell–dependent antigen (237). Primary follicles appear organized around a network of follicular dendritic cells. These cells represent a lineage distinct from the dendritic cells in the T-cell–rich paracortex. They are adapted to presentation of antigens in a conformation suitable for B-cell recognition, bearing abundant complement receptors (both complement receptor 1 and complement receptor 2), and immunoglobulin Fc receptors (particularly FcγRIIb) (238,239), and not expressing MHC class II proteins or T-cell co-stimulatory molecules. Follicular dendritic cells use their complement and Fc receptors to focus immune complexes of antigen and antibody-plus complement within the B-cell follicle in a fashion that supports the effective development of high-affinity, isotype-switched, and memory responses (238,240–243). Unlike class II MHC–expressing interdigitating dendritic cells, which are derived from bone marrow precursors, follicular dendritic cells appear not to be of the hematopoietic lineage (238). Under normal conditions, they cannot be transferred from one animal to another by bone marrow transplantation, suggesting that they may be of stromal origin (244). Interestingly, under conditions of transplantation of bone marrow cells or fetal liver cells into newborn mice less than 1 day postpartum, there can be engraftment with allofollicular dendritic cells (241). While this finding does not define the cell lineage from which follicular dendritic cells derive, it does demonstrate that follicular dendritic cells can develop *de novo* from precursor cells that are present in both bone marrow and fetal liver. This provides an assay that should permit better definition of the lineage from which these important cells derive and the factors that control differentiation of these cells from their precursors.

Primary follicles also contain macrophages that acquire the tingible body macrophage morphology after immunization, consistent with their having a role in the clearance of apoptotic cells as the B-cell immune response progresses (245,246). Additionally, B-cell follicles can contain a minority population of CD4$^+$ T cells. These T cells appear to be antigen-specific cells recruited to contribute to the germinal center reaction in response to specific antigen (236,247).

Morphologically and functionally, the B-cell zones of lymph nodes and other secondary lymphoid tissues can be subdivided into primary and secondary follicles. Primary follicles are quiescent, containing small, resting B cells that are distributed around a small cluster of loosely packed follicular dendritic cells, with few detectable T cells. Secondary follicles arise in response to immunization with a T-cell–dependent antigen (Colorplate 1). The secondary follicle is more intensely cellular, with a robust cluster of densely packed follicular dendritic cells, scattered CD4$^+$ T cells, activated B cells with enlarged cytoplasm, and tingible body macrophages. These reactive cells constitute the germinal center reaction and are usually surrounded by a ring of resting B cells similar in morphology to the primary follicle (237).

Germinal centers usually appear within 4 to 5 days after immunization and persist for 10 to 20 days (248–250). They reappear rapidly after a secondary immunization with the same antigen, but interestingly reach a smaller size with each successive antigen challenge (250). This suggests that a counter-regulatory activity may become increasingly prominent as the immune response matures.

Analysis of the cells that comprise the germinal center demonstrates this as a site for clonal expansion of antigen-specific B cells (251–253), somatic mutation of their immunoglobulin heavy- and light-chain genes (254), selection of cells with the highest affinity for antigen (254–257), and initiation of steps that lead B cells to differentiate either into plasma cells (256,257) or memory B cells (258–260). Cells constituting each of these germinal center subsets are located in specific compartments giving the germinal center its characteristic structural features. Rapidly proliferating B cells enter the germinal center from the T-cell zone where they have received T-cell help (253). Each germinal center represents an oligoclonal population, with on average one to three B-cell clones populating each center (249,252,261). The numbers of these proliferating B cells expand rapidly and acquire surface binding molecules for peanut agglutinin and the germinal center marker GL-7 (262–264). These rapidly expanding cells compress the surrounding nonreactive, uninvolved B cells into a band designated the mantle zone (265). After a brief period, the developing germinal center polarizes into a dark zone, proximal to the T-cell area, and a light zone, distal to the T-cell area. The dark zone contains rapidly proliferating, surface-immunoglobulin—negative-B cells designated centroblasts (266). Direct interactions between the centroblasts in the dark zone and germinal center follicular dendritic cells are limited to contacts with infrequent dendritic processes that infiltrate this zone. This may imply that surface immunoglobulin is necessary for maturing B cells to maintain substantial interactions with antigen-charged follicular dendritic cells. The light zone contains centrocytes, a

population of nondividing B cells that re-express their surface immunoglobulin. The light zone also contains a dense network of follicular dendritic cells. The light zone centrocytes express surface immunoglobulin molecules that have undergone somatic mutation (252,267,268). There is dramatic centrocyte apoptosis within this area, consistent with this area serving as the site for clonal selection of the somatically mutated cells (269,270). Some studies suggest the interesting likelihood that germinal center B cells may cycle from the centrocyte population back to the dark zone in order to undergo additional rounds of somatic mutation, then to the light zone again for selection (271,272). Such recycling would explain the observation that within a single germinal center, clonal lines of B cells exist that appear to have accumulated multiple somatic mutations of their immunoglobulin genes, each of which appears to contribute independently to the acquisition of higher affinity for the immunizing antigen (252,253,273).

The numbers of primary and secondary B-cell follicles in a lymph node are dependent on whether the cells in the node have been recently challenged by a T-cell–dependent antigen (274). Lymph nodes from a naïve animal may have only a few primary follicles. In contrast, lymph nodes from a recently immunized animal are enlarged, with an expanded cortex containing numerous secondary follicles (275). This response is clearly induced by local factors, since lymph nodes that drain tissues distant from the site of immunization do not show this hyperplastic response. Interestingly, if the lymph node receives its stimulus in the form of a potent T-cell–independent antigen such as dextran sulfate, profound disorganization of the follicular structure ensues, including elimination of macrophages from the subcapsular sinus and diffuse proliferation of B cells throughout the cortex (276). Thus, the primary follicles that exist to facilitate interactions between B- and T-lymphocytes appear to depend for maintenance of their integrity on a balance of T-cell and B-cell responses.

Mucosal-Associated Lymphoid Tissues

While the mucosal-associated lymphoid tissues (MALT) have structural features in common with lymph nodes, they manifest unique morphology and functions due to their role in focusing the immune response on a mucosal surface. Common functional characteristics of MALT include their support of the production of IgA-producing B cells and plasma cells as well as effector T cells adapted to support an IgA-specific response (277). Unlike lymph nodes, which are usually located at some distance from the tissues they sample, MALT is generally located immediately below the epithelium of the mucosal tissue, frequently displacing the epithelium characteristic of the specific mucosal site. Because antigen entry into MALT is largely, if not entirely, directly across the mucosal surface, MALT manifests no afferent lymphatic structures. Taking the place of afferent lymphatics are specialized epithelial cells. These specialized epithelia are specifically adapted to the individual mucosal tissue in which they are found.

Structural Features of Peyer's Patches

Nodules on the serosal surface of the small intestine were first described by the Swiss physician and anatomist, Johannes Conrad Peyer (1653–1712) in 1677 in his treatise entitled *Exercitatio anatomica—medica de glandulis intestinorum, earumque usu et affectionibus. Cui subjungitur anatome ventriculi galliinacei* (278). Peyer initially thought these structures represented glands, and it was not until the advent of microscopes and "modern" histologic techniques that it became apparent that these were lymphoid structures (Fig. 5). Although all mammals appear to have Peyer's patches, they vary considerably in distribution in different species. For example, in humans, there are on average approximately 30 Peyer's patches in the distal 200 cm of the ileum, with the majority in the distal 25 cm (279,280). In mice and rats, Peyer's patches are scattered along the length of the entire small intestine and number between 12 and 20 (281,282). In contrast, in pigs, sheep, and cattle, there are two discrete forms of Peyer's patches. Peyer's patches with structure typical of that seen in other species are scattered along the length of the jejunum. In addition, a large continuous patch is seen in the terminal 50 to 100 cm of the ileum (283–285). In spite of these differences in their number, size, and location, Peyer's patches in all of these species share the following features. Except when they cluster in the terminal ileum, Peyer's patches are located on the antimesenteric wall of the small intestine. They are covered on the luminal surface of the intestine by a specialized epithelial layer. These specialized epithelial cells are designated M cells because of their "microfold" luminal surface (Fig. 5). M cells have intercellular tight junctions and a polarized phenotype marking them as typical epithelial cells (286); however, they also possess specialized features that render them well adapted for their immune function. They serve as antigen-uptake cells from the intestine and can transport particles ranging in size from that of soluble proteins up to intact bacteria (174,287). This occurs by processes using clathrin-mediated endocytosis (288), pinocytosis (289), and phagocytosis (290). The M cells do not express the thick glycocalyx that coats the brush border of normal enterocytes (288). Absence of the glycocalyx facilitates rapid contact between luminal contents and the apical plasma membrane of the M cell. The basolateral surface of the M cell has a concave morphology, forming an invagination or "pocket" that is filled with B cells, T cells, and dendritic cells (288,291). This invagination brings the basolateral surface of the M cell into close proximity with the apical, luminal surface, perhaps facilitating transcytosis of luminal particles across this cell layer. Recent studies have shown uptake of many different pathogenic microbes across M cells. HIV can traffic from the gut into the Peyer's patch by M-cell transcytosis, and this transcytosis is receptor mediated (292). The development of an *in vitro* model for M-cell differentiation, in which co-culture of the intestinal epithelial cell line Caco-2 with

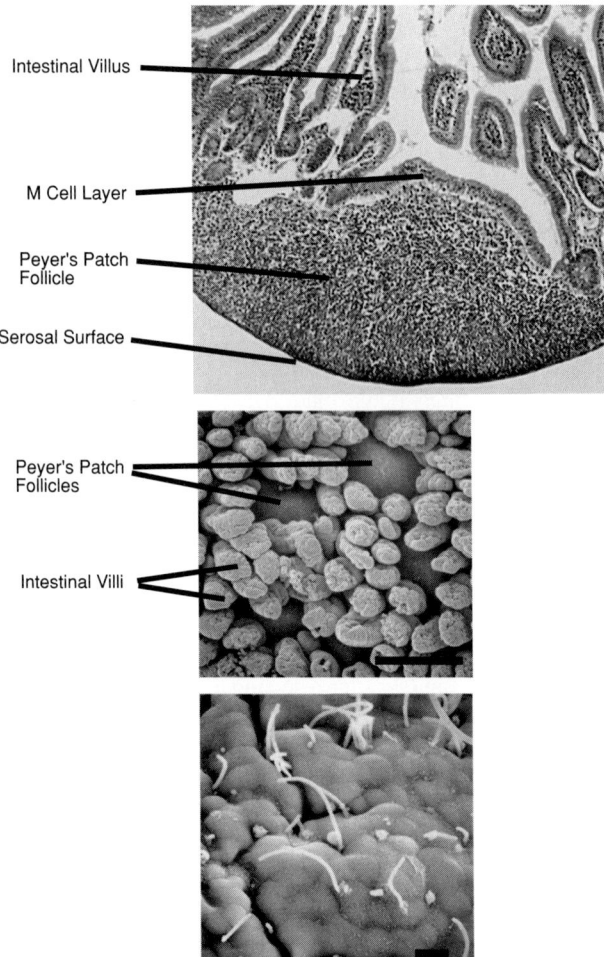

FIG. 5. Organization of the Peyer's patch. **Top panel:** The Peyer's patch is embedded in a region rich in small intestinal villi. The patch itself is overlaid by a dome of M cells that are adapted for transport of soluble and particulate antigens from the gut lumen into the lymphoid compartment of the patch. The lymphatic drainage of the Peyer's patch is difficult to visualize. Efferent lymphatic vessels appear to arise at the serosal surface of the patch. **Middle panel:** Scanning electron micrograph (60 X magnification) of a murine Peyer's patch showing the dome-like area of M-cell epithelium surrounded by small intestinal villi. The black bar represents 500 micrometers. **Bottom panel:** High-power scanning-electron-micrograph view (1200 X magnification) of the Peyer's patch surface showing resident enteric microbes interacting with the M-cell apical surface. The black bar represents 5 micrometers. Middle and lower panels courtesy of R. Newberry (Washington University, St. Louis, MO) and R. Lorenz (University of Alabama at Birmingham, Birmingham, AL).

mature B-lymphocytes results in transformation of the Caco-2 cells into cells with M-like morphology (293), now permits *in vitro* analysis of the transcytosis process, which should lead to rapid progress in understanding the biochemical processes underlying transepithelial transport. Such a model system has been used to demonstrate uptake of poliovirus by *in vitro* differentiated M cells (294). Specific antibodies augment pathogen uptake, and recent studies provide evidence for a novel IgA receptor on this cell type (295).

Like other secondary lymphoid tissues, Peyer's patches contain discrete B-cell and T-cell zones. Viewed from the luminal surface, the Peyer's patch is defined by a convex dome that is covered by M cells (Fig. 5). Immediately under the dome are several B-cell follicles separated by narrow wedges of parafollicular T-cell zone. Similar to follicles in the lymph node, the Peyer's patch B-cell follicles contain clusters of follicular dendritic cells, tingible body macrophages, and small numbers of CD4$^+$ T cells. The parafollicular T-cell zones contain dendritic cells, macrophages, and supporting stromal elements as well as robust HEV that support the delivery of B cells and T cells to this organ. A major adhesion molecule on the HEV luminal surface that supports lymphocyte recruitment to the Peyer's patch is MAdCAM-1 (219,220). In the absence of afferent lymphatics to this tissue, it is likely that immature dendritic cells also enter the Peyer's patch via the HEV, although the adhesion molecules that govern this recruitment are not well defined. Although the Peyer's patches do not have afferent lymphatics, they do have efferent lymphatics. These vessels emerge from lymphatic sinuses that arise on the serosal side of the patch and serve to carry mature lymphocytes, plasma cells, and antigen to the mesenteric lymph nodes and on to the thoracic duct for recirculation to other tissues (296).

B-cell follicles in Peyer's patches constitutively show features of secondary follicles, with most follicles showing activated B cells, occasional plasma cells, and staining with the germinal center-marker peanut agglutinin (263). This constitutive activity of Peyer's patch follicles may be a consequence of the constant delivery of dietary antigens and microbes of the intestinal microflora to this tissue. Interestingly, 70% of the B cells in Peyer's patch follicles express surface IgA, indicating that mechanisms controlling isotype switching to this Ig class are robustly active in this tissue. Switching to this isotype is probably determined by the secretory profile of Peyer's patch dendritic cells; however, whether this dendritic cell phenotype indicates that these cells are the product of a unique lineage, or is the result of differentiation in response to regulatory factors produced locally in the gut is not known. While Peyer's patches are a major site for the differentiation and maturation of IgA-producing B cells, they are not essential for the IgA response. Mice congenitally deficient in Peyer's patches remain competent to produce substantial numbers of lamina-propria IgA-secreting B cells (297). This Peyer's patch–independent production of mucosal IgA producing B cells is probably dependent on a coordinated immune response in the mesenteric lymph node that remains intact in these mice (297).

Respiratory Tract–Associated Lymphoid Tissues

Mucosal-associated lymphoid tissues are prominent in association with the epithelium of the respiratory tract. Like Peyer's patches, specific characteristics of the respiratory tract–associated lymphoid tissues vary among mammalian species. Bronchial-associated lymphoid tissue (BALT) is prominent in rabbits (298,299) where it is located at bifur-

cations of large- and medium-sized airways. This tissue is, however, not detected in the lungs of mice (300), and is only transiently expressed during childhood in humans (301). The BALT of rabbits has structural features similar to Peyer's patches in other species, with distinct B-cell follicles, follicular dendritic cells, and germinal centers, and intervening parafollicular T-cell zones. It is covered by a differentiated epithelium with morphologic features of M cells, although the extent to which these cells can import intact viruses and bacteria has not been defined.

In humans, the major airway-associated lymphoid tissues are the tonsils and adenoids (302,303). These tissues constitute Waldeyer's ring (303). Located at the openings to both the respiratory and the gastrointestinal tracts, the tonsils and adenoids represent the first defense against invading organisms for both these organ systems. These tissues include all of the typical features of mucosal-associated secondary lymphoid tissues with B-cell follicles, parafollicular T-cell zones, an M-cell–like epithelium, HEV, and an efferent lymphatic drainage system. Although they contain substantial numbers of IgA-producing B cells, IgG-producing B cells represent the largest cell population. Adhesion molecule expression on HEV includes peripheral node addressin and ICAM-1 and ICAM-2, but not MAdCAM-1 (304). In mice, the nasopharyngeal lymphoid tissue (NALT) is thought to be the functional equivalent of Waldeyer's ring. Comparisons of murine NALT to Peyer's patches has shown similarly organized B- and T-cell zones with an overlying M-cell–containing epithelium (305); however, T cells represent a higher proportion of total cells in the NALT (306,307). Intranasal immunization using cholera-toxin–B subunit as an adjuvant resulted in the induction of a strong IgA response in NALT cells, with large numbers of IgA-secreting B cells and plasma cells (307). IgA-producing antigen-specific memory cells could be detected in NALT for at least 8 months after the initial immunization, underscoring the significance of this tissue as an immune inductive site in the respiratory tract.

In summary, although there are structural and functional differences between different mucosal-associated lymphoid tissues, all of these secondary lymphoid tissues share the presence of B-cell follicles and adjacent T-cell zones; lymphatic drainage for dissemination of antigen-educated cells to other parts of the body; a specialized epithelium adapted to import a broad spectrum of antigens, including intact microbes, into the tissue; and regulatory cells that favor IgA and IgG humoral responses and immune memory. Because immune sensitization at these sites generally elicits strong IgA responses and enduring memory, considerable effort is now being applied to develop MALT-specific vaccination approaches.

Spleen Structure and Function

The spleen is the largest single secondary lymphoid organ in mammals, containing up to 25% of the body's mature lymphocytes (308). In humans, the spleen weighs 100 to 150 g (a little over 0.2% of the total body weight). It is separated into two major anatomic and functional compartments, the red pulp and the white pulp based on their appearances in a freshly cut surface of the tissue. The red pulp consists of a reticular network that contains stromal cells, macrophages, natural killer cells (309,310), variable numbers of plasma cells (311), and a large collection of aged or damaged red blood cells. The white pulp constitutes the organized lymphoid compartment (Colorplate 2). Like lymph nodes and mucosal-associated lymphoid tissues, the spleen white pulp contains organized B-cell follicles and T-cell zones adapted to supporting a regulated immune response. Unlike the lymph nodes and mucosal-associated lymphoid tissues, the spleen has only one way in. Both immune cells and antigens enter the spleen with the circulating blood via the splenic artery. In humans, the spleen receives approximately 5% of the total systemic blood flow (312,313).

The splenic artery branches within the tissue first to form trabecular arteries, and then central arterioles that penetrate each white pulp nodule. Surrounding each central arteriole is a T-cell–rich compartment designated the periarteriolar lymphoid sheath (PALS). This region is analogous to the paracortex of lymph nodes and contains, in addition to T cells, substantial numbers of interdigitating dendritic cells; however, the T-cell zone of the spleen contains no HEV structures. As the central arteriole courses through the PALS, it gives off smaller radial branches that ultimately empty into the marginal sinus. This sinus forms a vascular network around each white pulp nodule and defines a white pulp compartment, the marginal zone. The marginal zone contains a large collection of B-lymphocytes (314), including naïve, long-lived B cells, B-1 cells and memory B cells, a specialized layer of metalophilic macrophages (315), and a layer of marginal zone macrophages (316). The marginal sinus endothelium expresses on its surface MAdCAM-1 (317). By analogy to the MAdCAM-1–expressing HEV of the Peyer's patch and mesenteric lymph nodes, it has been assumed that the marginal sinus represented the site where naïve lymphoid cells and blood borne antigens leave the blood circulation to enter the white or the red pulp. Venous sinusoids are prominent in the red pulp, and it has been assumed that blood exited the circulation at the marginal sinus, percolated through the red pulp, and returned to the circulation via these red pulp venous sinusoids. Entry of cells into the white pulp was thought to be the consequence of chemoattractive activities released from the white pulp to capture cells as the moved from the marginal sinus towards the red pulp sinusoids. This model defined the blood flow through the spleen as an open circulation (318). Recent studies by Grayson et al. (319) using real-time, intravital confocal microscopy of the mouse spleen to visualize blood flow directly demonstrates that blood enters each white pulp nodule via the central arteriole, moves to the marginal sinus, and then moves back towards the PALS before appearing in the large draining vessels in the red pulp. Neither fluorescently conjugated high-molecular-weight dextran nor fluorescently labeled erythrocytes were dumped from the marginal sinus into the red pulp. This suggests that the splenic circulation is closed, and that lymphocytes that leave the circulation do so at a position central to the marginal sinus. Whether this happens by the lymphocytes crossing a vascular endothelium remains to be determined. Studies by Steiniger et al. suggest that the perifollicular zone of the human spleen contains a blood-filled space without a vascular lining, and that this compartment is the likely site of lymphocyte migration out of the circulation and into the white pulp. If so, this suggests that adhesion molecules play little role in regulating cellular movement into the white pulp of the spleen, but rather that this movement is controlled by chemoattractive molecules that draw cells from this blood-filled space into the organized lymphoid compartment. Indeed, this observation is consistent with the findings of others that blocking a broad range of adhesion molecules with neutralizing monoclonal antibodies had little impact on cell entry into the white pulp (317,320).

Between the PALS and the marginal zone are primary (quiescent) and secondary (reactive) B-cell follicles. These follicles have structure similar to those present in lymph nodes and mucosal lymphoid tissues, with a central cluster of follicular dendritic cells, macrophages, and a large population of B cells containing a few interspersed T cells. In the reactive secondary follicles observed after immunization with T-cell–dependent antigens, the follicular macrophages take on the tingible-body morphology, consistent with the substantial cellular apoptosis that accompanies B-cell selection in the germinal center (265,321).

Signals Regulating Formation and Maintenance of Secondary Lymphoid Tissue Structure

The anatomic features of the secondary lymphoid tissues are well defined; however, the signals that lead to the establishment and maintenance of these organized structures are only beginning to be understood. The observation that the overall structure of the various secondary lymphoid tissues is highly conserved suggests that the organized structure of these tissues is critical for their function; however, the relationship between the organized tissue structure and ability to generate a safe and effective immune response also is only beginning to be tested (193,209,322). Analysis of mice carrying spontaneous and targeted mutations in a growing number of genes is providing an increasingly sophisticated understanding of key signals that support the normal development of the secondary lymphoid tissues (323). Similarly, evaluation of the quality of the immune response in mice with congenital alterations in their secondary lymphoid tissues is affording an opportunity to investigate the relationship between normal lymphoid organ structure and normal immune function.

Spontaneous Mouse Mutations Affecting Spleen Development

Two spontaneous mouse mutations have been identified that manifest defects in spleen development. The first is the semidominant Dh (dominant hemimelia) mutation (324).

Heterozygous Dh/+ mice have skeletal abnormalities (particularly of the tibia in the hind limb, ribs, and vertebrae), a constellation of visceral defects including a small digestive tract and urogenital system, and nearly completely penetrant agenesis of the spleen (325,326). Homozygous mutant embryos show the same spectrum of skeletal and visceral defects but are more severely affected and usually die shortly after birth (324). The Dh gene maps to chromosome 1 and is closely linked, but not allelic, to the mouse En-1 gene (mouse homolog of the Drosophila *engrailed* locus) (327,328). In studies to investigate whether Dh/+ or Dh/Dh cells can contribute to the cellularity of the spleen, Suto et al. (325) formed chimeric embryo aggregates using morula cells from C3H/He and Dh/Dh or Dh/+ embryos. Cells derived from the Dh embryos were identified using a linked gene that encoded an allelic phenotypic marker. While most of the chimeric mice were asplenic, approximately 25% showed some splenic tissue. When spleen tissue was identified, it contained Dh cells and showed grossly normal histology (325). The absence of spleens in Dh/+ mice suggests that this defect is in a critical developmental decision point for formation of the spleen. But, the finding that cells carrying the Dh mutation are still able to localize within and contribute to the formation of the spleen in embryo chimeras demonstrates that Dh is not incompatible with spleen functions. Interestingly, Dh/+ mice show dramatically reduced numbers of mast cells in their popliteal lymph nodes compared to their wild-type littermates, suggesting the possibility either that mast cells may play a role in lymphoid organ development or that Dh contributes to mast-cell homing to lymphoid tissues (329).

Deliberate targeted mutations that lead to congenital asplenia have identified additional loci that are critical for the normal development of this organ. Homozygous knockout of the Hox11 gene, which encodes a homeobox-like DNA-binding protein, resulted in congenital asplenia (330,331). Targeted null mutations of this gene were created in order to define its function in the context of its identification at the sites of the t(10;14) translocation breakpoint in human T-cell acute lymphoblastic leukemia (332). Thus, the observation of asplenia in association with Hox11 deficiency was a serendipitous one, arising from experiments performed for reasons unrelated to studies of lymphoid organ development. The phenotypic abnormalities in Hox11$^{-/-}$ mice are focused on the spleen, with the only other detected alterations being an enlargement of the stomach and pancreas (333). Tracking of the expression of Hox11 in mouse embryos shows its expression early in several branchial arches and in motor neurons of several cranial nerves; however, deficiency of Hox11 resulted in no defect in these structures. This underscores the principle that expression of a gene in a developing tissue does not always indicate a critical role for the gene in that organ's development. Importantly, however, beginning at embryonic day 11.5, Hox11 expression was dramatically induced at a discrete site in the abdomen within mesodermal tissues that eventually develops into the spleen (333). Analysis of Hox11$^{-/-}$ embryos showed that at E11.5 spleen formation appears to begin normally, but that by E13.5 the developing splenic anlage has completely disappeared (331). In at least one study, the involution of the spleen anlage was associated with rapid cellular apoptosis, suggesting that the Hox11 gene product is required, not to initiate spleen development, but rather to sustain the survival of developing splenocytes as the tissue matures. However, subsequent studies using aggregation chimeras showed that at E13, Hox11$^{-/-}$ cells that initially were present in the developing spleen had moved out of the tissue and subsequently were excluded from the residual spleen anlage. Rather, they persisted as a disorganized cluster of cells between the stomach and the pancreas (334). This latter study suggested that loss by apoptosis was a characteristic of only a portion of the Hox11-dependent cells. The localization of Hox11-expressing cells near the pancreas suggested a possible relationship between spleen development and the development of the pancreas. This potential relationship is consistent with the observation that transgenic overexpression of the "sonic hedgehog" gene selectively in the pancreas leads to failure of development of both the pancreas and the spleen (335).

Asplenia has also been reported in mice homozygous for targeted mutations in Bapx1, the mouse homolog of Drosophila "bagpipes" (336,337). Bapx1$^{-/-}$ embryos show no evidence of spleen tissue at E14.5, and no evidence of Hox11 expression at E12, indicating that Bapx1 acts early in spleen formation, probably upstream of Hox11. Targeting of the Wilms tumor-suppressor gene WT1 also results in asplenia, but without suppression of Hox11 expression, defining this as a signaling pathway discrete from the Hox11/Bapx1 pathway in spleen development (338). Lastly, obliteration of capsulin, the basic helix-loop-helix transcription factor gene, also results in failure of the spleen anlage to develop beyond what is present at E12.5 (339). Expression of Hox11 and Bapx1 was not observed in the capsulin-deficient splenic anlage, suggesting that expression of capsulin is a prerequisite for subsequent expression of Hox11 and Bapx1. Together, these findings suggest that there is a critical event in spleen development that occurs either concomitantly with or shortly after the initial specification of the splenic anlage at day E12-E12.5, which requires expression of multiple transcription factors to sustain proper cell interactions in the developing tissue.

An additional spontaneous mouse mutation that has provided insight into lymphoid organ development is the aly/aly mutation (alymphoplasia). The impact of this mutation on thymus development was discussed earlier. This autosomal recessive single-gene mutation (103) leads to congenital absence of lymph nodes and Peyer's patches, structural abnormalities in the spleen and thymus, and an immunodeficiency affecting the T-cell (340), B-cell (341), and NK–T-cell (106) compartments. Unlike the Dh, Hox11, and Bapx1 mutations, aly/aly does not cause total asplenia. Rather, it results in the development of a substantially cellular spleen in which the normal internal compartmentalization has been lost. Although white pulp nodules develop, there is a prominent failure to form normal lymphoid follicles, including failure to develop the follicular dendritic cell network, to define the marginal zone, to establish marginal sinus expression of MAdCAM-1, and to induce normal segregation of the B-cell and T-cell zones (342,343). Nonlymphoid tissues appeared generally normal in structure in aly/aly mice, although changes in mammary gland structure have been described (344), and dramatic infiltration of the epididymis and vas deferens by eosinophils and macrophages has been observed (345). Changes in distribution of intraepithelial lymphocytes in the small intestine have also been seen (346). Whether these latter changes are a consequence of chronic infection secondary to the immunodeficiency caused by aly or are in some other way secondary to the primary lymphoid organ abnormalities has not been defined.

Using linkage analysis, Shinkura et al. (104) mapped the aly mutation to a 264-KB region of mouse chromosome 11. Using a reverse genetics approach, they determined that aly is a point mutation of the gene encoding the NFκB-inducing kinase (NIK) (104). NIK was discovered by virtue of its interaction with Traf2, a signal-transduction adaptor protein that interacts with TNF receptors I and II (347) and with the IκB-specific kinase α (IKKα) (348). The mutation in aly is located in the carboxy-terminal portion of the encoded protein, in a region predicted to be the subunit interaction domain that controls interactions of the NIK protein with IKKα, Traf 2, and Traf 5 (347,349). Thus, the aly allele is expected to retain kinase activity. Confirmation that NIK determines the aly phenotype came from subsequent studies by Yin et al. (105) who generated an independent targeted mutation in the NIK gene (eliminating the anticipated promoter and the majority of the first exon sequences) (105). NIK$^{-/-}$ mice showed a lymphoid tissue phenotype indistinguishable from the aly/aly strain. Interestingly, NIK$^{-/-}$ cells showed normal NFκB-mediated DNA-binding activity after activation using TNF, IL-1, and the lymphotoxin-α/β heterotrimer. Furthermore, ligation of the p55 or p75 TNF receptors in NIK$^{-/-}$ cells induced activation of gene transcription in an apparently normal fashion. Ligation of the lymphotoxin-β receptor (LTβR), however, resulted in abnormal transcription suggesting that the major critical functions of NIK may be mediated through this pathway.

The Role of Lymphotoxin in Lymphoid Organ Formation

The observation that NIK$^{-/-}$ mice show abnormal signaling via the LTβR is consistent with the existence of an important relationship between NIK and the LTβR. The LTβR is a member of the TNF receptor family. The prototypic ligands of the TNF family, TNFα (hereinafter designated TNF) and lymphotoxin (LT, also originally designated TNFβ) were first described as homotrimeric proteins (Fig. 6). TNF is synthesized as a type II transmembrane protein with a long N-terminal intracellular domain (350). Release of TNF from the cell that synthesizes it is the result of proteolytic cleavage by the cellular metaloproteinase designated the TNF-α

converting enzyme (TACE) (351,352). LT, in contrast, is synthesized with a signal peptide and is secreted from the cell via the typical vesicular transport pathway (353). Both TNF and LT exist in homotrimer forms in solution and bind with similar affinities to the two defined TNF cell-surface receptors (TNFR-I and TNFR-II) (354). LT also exists as a heterotrimer, with one copy of the originally defined LT protein (now designated LTα) associated with two copies of the lymphotoxin-β (LTβ) chain (355,356). The genes encoding TNF, LTα, and LTβ are encoded together in a small gene cluster located within the MHC (357,358). Like TNF, LTβ is a type II transmembrane protein, but unlike TNF, the LTβ chain is not a substrate for TACE. Thus, the LT$\alpha_1\beta_2$ protein appears to act as a cell-associated signaling protein throughout its life span. The LT$\alpha_1\beta_2$ heterotrimer (hereinafter referred to

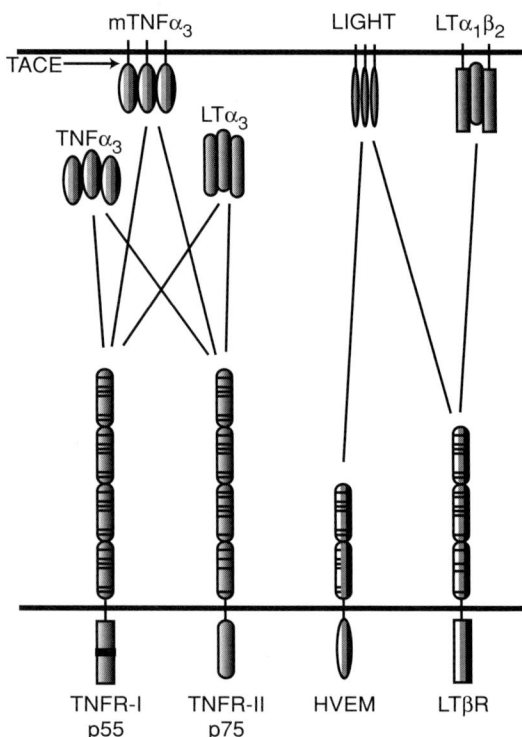

FIG. 6. The TNF/lymphotoxin family of ligands and receptors. The homotrimeric ligands, TNFα_3 and LTα_3 interact similarly with the two defined TNF receptors, TNFR-I (p55) and TNFR-II (p75). The LTα_3 homotrimer is synthesized as a conventionally secreted glycoprotein by a signal peptide–mediated mechanism. The TNFα_3 homotrimer is synthesized as a type II transmembrane protein that is released from the cell in soluble form by the action of the cellular protease TNFα converting enzyme (TACE). Ligation of TNFR-I can activate signaling via its intracellular "death domain" (black bar) to induce the apoptotic program in susceptible cells. LIGHT and the mLT heteromer (LT$\alpha_1\beta_2$) are type II transmembrane proteins that are not substrates for TACE. These trimers bind to the LTβR on lymphoid tissue stromal cells. LIGHT also binds the TNF receptor family member HVEM (Herpes simplex virus entry mediator). For the induction of normal lymphoid tissue development and organization, mLT appears to be the major physiologic ligand for the LTβR.

as membrane LT or mLT) has no measurable binding affinity for TNFR-I or TNFR-II. Rather, it activates the LTβR (359). Conversely, the homotrimer ligands, TNF and LTα_3, bind to TNFR-I and TNFR-II but have no measurable affinity for the LTβR. Whereas TNF is expressed at very high levels by activated mononuclear phagocytic cells, and can, following appropriate stimulation with inflammatory mediators, be expressed at lower levels on a broad variety of other cell types (ranging from endothelial cells to endocrine cells of the thyroid gland), mLT expression appears limited to activated CD4$^+$ Th1 cells, CD8$^+$ T cells, B cells, and NK cells. At the receptor level, expression of the TNF receptors TNFR-I and TNFR-II is nearly ubiquitous, whereas the LTβR is expressed with very limited tissue distribution, not on hematopoietic cell lineages, but rather on stromal cells within lymphoid tissues (360). Thus, the TNF/LT system functions as two distinct pathways. The homotrimeric ligands (TNF and LTα_3) act through TNFR-I and TNFR-II to form the first pathway, and the mLT heterotrimer acts through the LTβR to form the second pathway.

Gene-targeting experiments to discriminate the functions of LT and TNF have established that the mLT/LTβR pathway plays a critical role in the formation and maintenance of secondary lymphoid tissue structure (323). Initial studies targeting the LTα locus demonstrated that LTα deficiency resulted in a profound defect in formation of lymph nodes and complete absence of Peyer's patches (361,362). Deficiency of lymph nodes was not absolute, with 5% to 10% of LT$\alpha^{-/-}$ offspring retaining a small mesenteric lymph node (361,362). This suggests that the signals that induce mature lymph node formation are not identical for all nodes (363). The spleen, although it was present, showed grossly disturbed structure, with disturbances in essentially all aspects of normal spleen microarchitecture (244,361–365). The polarized organization of the white pulp nodules was lost with failure to form segregated T-cell and B-cell zones. There was loss of other aspects of B-cell follicle organization, including loss of follicular dendritic cells and the ability to form a germinal center, absence of a detectable MAdCAM-1$^+$ marginal sinus, absence of metalophilic macrophages, and loss of a defined marginal zone B-cell population (364–367). Interdigitating dendritic cells were also dramatically reduced (368). Similar findings were observed in LT$\beta^{-/-}$ and LTβR$^{-/-}$ mice, establishing that this phenotype defined a key role for the mLT/LTβR pathway in lymphoid organ development (369–371).

Complementary studies using blockade of mLT/LTβR signaling by systemic administration of a neutralizing LTβR-IgFc$_\gamma$ fusion protein (372,373) or by bone marrow transplantation of wild-type mice with mLT-deficient marrow (244,363,374,375) have demonstrated that some aspects of the mLT-dependent, organized lymphoid architecture are fixed, and some are plastic. Treatment with the LTβR-IgFc$_\gamma$ fusion protein has been particularly informative because this reagent, by virtue of its Igγ chain domain, efficiently crosses the placenta after administration to a pregnant mouse, thereby neutralizing mLT action in the developing embryos. Studies using this fusion protein showed that the mLT-dependent signals that support the formation of lymph nodes are delivered during the second half of murine gestation (372,373), with more central lymph nodes (mesenteric, para-aortic) specified first, and more peripheral (axillary, popliteal) specified later. Signals for development of Peyer's patches were given later still, near the last few days of mouse gestation and within the first day or two after birth. Development of Peyer's patches could, for example, be arrested by the action of an LTβR-IgFc$_\gamma$ transgene expressed under the control of a cytomegalovirus promoter that initiated expression only at the end of gestation (376). However, once the critical times for induction of the lymph nodes and Peyer's patches had passed, no nodes or Peyer's patches could form. Similarly, if mLT-expressing cells were removed from adult mice (either permanently by irradiation or temporarily by treatment with the LTβR-IgFc$_\gamma$ fusion protein), the lymph node and Peyer's patch tissues remain (374). This defines the development of lymph nodes and Peyer's patches as fixed characteristics.

Neutralization of mLT function in an adult animal, while it does not cause disappearance of lymph nodes or Peyer's patches, does cause loss of B-cell follicle organization in these tissues and a more extensive effacement of white pulp structure in the spleen (377). Within a few days after administration of the LTβR-IgFc$_\gamma$ fusion protein to an adult mouse, the follicular dendritic cell network disappears, MAdCAM-1 expression on the spleen marginal sinus endothelium is extinguished, and normal segregation of B-cell and T-cell zones is lost. Similarly, when an mLT-deficient mouse is reconstituted either by adoptive transfer of wild-type, mLT-producing splenocytes, or by transplantation with wild-type bone marrow (375), then a follicular dendritic cell network is induced, segregated B-cell and T-cell zones are formed, and the potential for antigen-dependent formation of germinal centers is restored. These observations define these aspects of lymphoid organ structure as plastic, dependent on ongoing mLT expression.

Analysis of additional mutant mouse strains complemented by studies using adoptive transfer of selective cell populations have defined the nature of the cell lineage that provides the lymphotoxin-dependent signal for the plastic lymphotoxin-dependent structures. Of the mature hematopoietic lineages, CD4$^+$ Th1 cells, CD8$^+$ T cells, activated B cells, and activated NK cells can express detectable surface lymphotoxin (323). Analysis of mouse strains deficient in α/β T cells or B cells has shown that B cells but not T cells are essential for the induction of the follicular dendritic cell network and for expression of MAdCAM-1 on the marginal sinus (378,379). Using adoptive transfer of B cells from either wild-type or LT$\alpha^{-/-}$ donors into RAG-1$^{-/-}$ recipients, it was shown that the B-cell signal for induction of the follicular dendritic cell network was mLT-dependent. This, therefore, defines a setting in which the B cell delivers a signal that supports the development of the lymphoid tissue structure that is itself required for the B cell to express its mature function. Subsequent studies have shown that the ability to deliver the mLT signal is acquired when the B cell enters the lymphoid tissue where it is stimulated by the locally produced chemokine CXCL13 (BLC) (380). Interestingly, while CXCL13 can be produced in modest amounts by currently uncharacterized lymphoid tissue stromal cells, it is robustly expressed by follicular dendritic cells themselves. This represents, therefore, a setting in which B cells provide an LT-dependent signal that induces and consolidates the follicular dendritic cell network. The follicular dendritic cells then produce CXCL13, which brings more B cells into the lymphoid organ and activates them for LT expression. In addition to directing the formation of the follicular dendritic cell network, B cells also provide both lymphotoxin-dependent and lymphotoxin-independent signals that lead to the recruitment of normal numbers of T cells to the spleen white pulp and normal segregation of the white pulp into discrete T zones containing interdigitating dendritic cells and B zones that are dendritic cell poor (381).

Other TNF/TNFR Family Members in Development of Secondary Lymphoid Tissues

Recent studies have demonstrated that there are additional members of the mLT/LTβR family. **LIGHT** (homologous to lymphotoxins, exhibits inducible expression, competes with HSV glycoprotein D for **HVEM**, a receptor expressed on **T** cells; also know as herpes simplex virus entry mediator-ligand, HVEM-L) (382) can interact with the LTβR as well as with the TNFR family members HVEM and DcR3 (Fas decoy receptor 3) (383,384). Knockout of the LIGHT gene, however, does not lead to disordered lymphoid organ development on its own. Rather, LIGHT$^{-/-}$ mice manifest depressed T-cell co-stimulation (385). However, a higher fraction of mice deficient for both LIGHT and LTβ show complete loss of mesenteric lymph nodes than do mice deficient in LTβ alone, demonstrating cooperation between LIGHT and LTβ for mesenteric lymph node formation.

Most closely related of the TNF/TNFR family members to mLT and the LTβR are TNF and the two TNF receptors TNFR-I and TNFR-II. Deficiency of TNFR-II (p75) resulted in no recognized abnormality in lymphoid tissue development or organization (364,386,387). Deficiency of either TNF or TNFR-I, in contrast, resulted in mice with reduced numbers of Peyer's patches and the Peyer's patches that did form were small in size (388,389). Lymph nodes, on the other hand, were retained in apparently normal numbers and a normal-sized spleen was present. Deficiency of either TNF or TNFR-I (p55), however, resulted in abnormal architecture of the spleen and peripheral lymph nodes, with a prominent loss of clustered follicular dendritic cells (364,386,387,390). Using gene targeting to modify the TNF locus so as to remove the TACE cleavage site so that only a membrane-anchored form of the cytokine was produced, Ruuls et al. (391) demon-

strated that this membrane form of TNF was sufficient to support normal secondary lymphoid tissue structures.

Unlike mLT-deficient and LTβR$^{-/-}$ mice that appeared to manifest a true lack of follicular dendritic-cell localization, the lack of a follicular dendritic-cell network in TNF$^{-/-}$ mice was a manifestation of defective follicular dendritic-cell localization. In the absence of TNF signals through TNFR-I, spleen follicular dendritic cells were found scattered in the marginal zone area (392). These abnormally positioned follicular dendritic cells could, however, be rescued by systemic treatment of TNF$^{-/-}$ with an activating monoclonal anti–TNFR-I antibody (393). Induction of signaling through TNFR-I was accompanied by up-regulation of CXCL13 (BLC) and down-regulation of CCL19 (ELC) and CCL21 (SLC), suggesting that normal clustering of follicular dendritic cells may be mediated by the action of specific chemokines.

Perhaps to be expected, when mice that lack follicular dendritic cells completely (LT$\alpha^{-/-}$ or LTβR$^{-/-}$ mice) were immunized with a T-cell–dependent antigen, there was a dramatic failure to develop high-affinity, somatically mutated antibody (371,375,394). Less expected was the finding that immunization of TNF$^{-/-}$ or TNFR-I$^{-/-}$ mice that retained follicular dendritic cells but in an unclustered configuration also manifested a failure of affinity maturation of the antibody response (387,395). This suggests either that clustering of follicular dendritic cells is integral to their normal function, or that the TNFR-I–mediated signal activates key follicular dendritic-cell functions that support affinity maturation in addition to those activities that drive cell clustering.

Other members of the TNF/TNFR family also contribute to the development of normal lymphoid organs. Mice deficient in either RANK (receptor-activating NFκB; also known as TRANCE-R) or its ligand osteoprotegrin ligand (OPGL) showed complete absence of peripheral lymph nodes, although the Peyer's patches and spleen were retained (396,397). Follicular dendritic cells appeared normal in number and distribution. These studies demonstrate that different signals control the formation of lymph nodes, Peyer's patches, and spleen.

Other Signals Controlling Formation of Secondary Lymphoid Tissues

Not surprisingly, deficiency of a number of intracellular signal transduction molecules that participate in signaling by key TNFR family members also are essential for normal secondary lymphoid tissue development. As already discussed, deficiency of NIK leads to extensive defects in secondary lymphoid tissue development, including absence of lymph nodes, Peyer's patches, and disorganized spleen (105). Targeting the genes encoding members of the NFκB/Rel family, including NFκB1, NFκB2, and Bcl-3 has led to defects of varying severity in Peyer's patch formation and in establishment of the follicular dendritic cell network in other lymphoid organs (398,399). This probably is a consequence of the participation by these transcription factors in the genetic programs initiated by signaling through TNFR family members. Similarly, mice deficient in the TNF receptor–associated factor 6 (Traf-6) showed dense absence of mesenteric and peripheral lymph nodes (400). Deficiency of the IL-2 receptor common gamma chain ($\gamma c^{-/-}$) (401,402) or of the signaling kinase JAK3 (403–405) also leads to loss of subsets of lymph nodes. Finally, targeted ablation of the gene encoding the retinoic acid receptor–related orphan receptor γ (ROR-γ) interrupts development of peripheral and mesenteric lymph nodes and Peyer's patches, while retaining development of spleen and nasal associated lymphoid tissue (406–408). The function of RORγ is not known. Its loss is associated with extinction of expression of the anti-apoptotic factor Bcl-xL in the thymus, leading to decreased survival of $CD4^+CD8^+$ thymocytes. There was also loss of a population of bone marrow–derived cells that normally express RORγ, distinguished by its surface expression of CD45 and CD4, but not CD3 (406). These cells, as discussed below, represent a major cell population present at the sites of development of many secondary lymphoid tissues and may be important organizers of the developmental program for these tissues (409). Interruption of any signal crucial for the development, function, or survival of such an organizing cell population would also be expected to result in disordered lymphoid organ development. Additionally, any genetic lesion that prevents appropriate localization of a key inducing cell population within the developing lymphoid organs may also lead to failure of normal establishment of that organ. Such a mechanism may underlie the defect in lymph node formation observed in mice deficient either in the receptor for the B-lymphocyte chemokine (BLR1, also designated CXCR5) or for the B-lymphocyte chemokine itself (BLC, also designated CXCL13) (380,410). Null mutations of either the CXCL13 chemokine or its receptor (CXCR5) result in reduced numbers of Peyer's patches and loss of selected populations of lymph nodes. Although major cellular targets of CXCL13 are the $CXCR5^+$ B cells, CXCR5 is also expressed in the $CD45^+CD4^+CD3^-$ cell population (411,412).

Cell Lineages That Signal for Normal Secondary Lymphoid Organ Structure

Analysis of the cells residing in early developing lymph nodes identified a distinctive population of $CD4^+$ cells that appeared hematopoietic in origin ($CD45^+$), but not of the T-cell lineage ($CD3^-$, T-cell receptor$^-$, Ig^-) (411). These cells were found to express surface LTα/β. They are thus excellent candidates to provide essential inductive signals for the formation of the lymphoid organs in which they are found. They also express the IL-7Rα chain and appear to require IL-7 signaling for their development (413). These cells are found in substantial numbers in developing embryonic lymph nodes (411,414), Peyer's patches (413,415,416), and nasal-associated lym-

phoid tissue (417), consistent with their playing an important role in development of these tissues. Furthermore, many of the mutant mouse strains that demonstrate abnormal secondary lymphoid tissue development show dramatic reductions or complete absence of these cells. Specifically, mice deficient in LTα (409), TRANCE (OPGL, RANKL) (418), or RORγ (406,407) show dramatically reduced numbers of $CD45^+CD4^+CD3^-$ cells in the mesenteric node rudiments that are present at birth, and at the sites where Peyer's patches would be expected to form. Additional recently described gene-targeted mouse strains also show altered numbers of $CD45^+CD4^+CD3^-$ cells in association with failure of secondary lymphoid tissue development. $Id2^{-/-}$ mice show complete lack of lymph nodes and Peyer's patches, but maintenance of normal spleen structure and spleen B-cell follicles (419). The failure of Peyer's patch development in $Id2^{-/-}$ mice was accompanied by complete absence of $CD45^+CD4^+CD3^-IL-7R\alpha^+$ cells in the developing small intestine. Id2 is an inhibitor of basic helix-loop-helix transcription factors. It is expressed in $CD45^+CD4^+CD3^-IL-7R\alpha^+$ cells where it may play an essential role in their differentiation from more primitive hematopoietic precursors or in their ability to express the phenotype required for Peyer's patch formation. Perhaps acting at an even more primitive level is the Ikaros gene, a member of the Kruppel family of zinc-finger DNA-binding proteins. $Ikaros^{-/-}$ mice lack all lymph nodes and Peyer's patches as well as the $CD45^+CD4^+CD3^-$ cell population (409,420,421).

Normal Steps in Secondary Lymphoid Organ Development

Elegant studies by Adachi et al. (415) have defined several landmarks in the normal development of mouse Peyer's patches. Using whole-mount *in situ* hybridization, this group has identified the clustering of characteristic cell populations at sites of Peyer's patch formation, defining three stages in Peyer's patch development. Around embryonic day 15.5, clusters of cells that are $VCAM-1^+ICAM-1^+$ are first seen on the antimesenteric surface of the developing small intestine. Whether these cells congregate in a stochastic fashion under the influence of natural signaling gradients within the tissue, or whether they are attracted by a currently unrecognized stromal element has not been defined. The $VCAM-1^+ICAM-1^+$ cells have been designated Peyer's patch organizing centers. Over the next 2 days, these organizing centers are infiltrated by a collection of $CD4^+CD3^-IL-7R\alpha^+$ cells of hematopoietic lineage (thought to be identical or equivalent to the $CD45^+CD4^+CD3^-$ cells observed in developing lymph nodes). Interestingly, it has just been shown that the VCAM-1/ICAM-1–expressing cells that constitute the organizing center express the chemokines CXCL13 (BLC) and CCL19 (ELC) (412). This may directly contribute to the recruitment of the mLT-expressing $CXCR5^+$ $CD45^+CD4^+CD3^-$ cell population. In the final stage beginning at E18.5, B- and T-lymphocytes begin to enter the tissue, accompanied by dendritic cells, and soon after birth by follicular dendritic cells. Interestingly, stages 1 and 2 of this process appeared to proceed normally in SCID mice, indicating that the initial steps of Peyer's patch specification are independent of B- and T-lineage cells. In contrast, aly/aly mice (deficient in the function of the signaling protein NIK) manifested no detectable clustering of VCAM-1$^+$ICAM-1$^+$ cells, suggesting either that these cells themselves are dependent on NIK function for their normal development, or that cells that provide the signals for their aggregation in the wall of the developing gut are dependent on NIK. While the structures that define stages one to three of Peyer's patch development appear robust and sufficient for Peyer's patch organ development, they remain labile as evidenced by their apparently complete regression in mice treated with the neutralizing LTβR–IgFcγ fusion protein during the first day after birth (372,373). Consequently, it may be appropriate to define a fourth stage of consolidation of Peyer's patch structure that takes place in mice in an mLT-dependent fashion during the first 7 to 10 days after birth. After this consolidation, the Peyer's patch structure is stable, even if mLT signals are removed.

Lymph node organogenesis has also been divided into discrete steps based on many different kinds of studies (418,422–425). Stage 1 represents the initiation at E10.5 in mice of the formation of lymphatic vessels, marked by the formation of endothelial buds from developing veins. Stage 2 marks the development of lymphatic vessels by endothelial sprouting from the lymphatic buds. Both stages 1 and 2 are dependent on normal function of Prox-1 (213). Stage 3 represents the formation of the true lymph node anlagen, with mesenchymal connective tissue cells protruding into the lumen of the growing lymph sacs. These invaginations contain reticular cells, fibroblasts, leukocytes, and vascular loops. These loops eventually develop into the afferent and efferent blood supply of the lymph node, including the high endothelial venules. Stage 4 is marked by influx of hematopoietic lineage cells and the formation of the subcapsular sinus. Stage 5 is the result of immigration of increasing numbers of B and T cells, and the formation of normal cellular compartmentalization within the node. The colonization of the developing lymph node anlagen with CD45$^+$CD4$^+$CD3$^-$ cells that are required for continued maturation of the node appears to occur during the latter half of stage 3. In the case of the developing lymph node, it is apparent that important localizing signals have been given to specify where the lymph node anlagen will emerge prior to the colonization with the CD45$^+$CD4$^+$CD3$^-$ cells. This is consistent with the observation that treatment of developing $LT\alpha^{-/-}$ embryos with an agonist monoclonal anti-LTβR antibody during mid-gestation to late gestation results in induction of morphologically normal lymph nodes at sites typical for normal lymph node formation (426). Again, as seen for Peyer's patches, the early forming lymph node anlagen is fragile and requires lymphotoxin-dependent signals in order for a stable organ to form. Thus, the mesenteric lymph node anlage are easily detected in newborn LT$\alpha^{-/-}$ or

TRANCE$^{-/-}$ mice (418). However, in the absence of mLT or TRANCE signals, this mesenteric node remnant disappears over the first 2 weeks after birth.

Lymphoid Organogenesis and Chronic Inflammation

Experiments to investigate the role of different intercellular mediators *in vivo* by transgenic ectopic expression in mice have identified unanticipated potential of some of these molecules to induce formation of organized lymphoid structures. The first such experiment was performed by Kratz et al. (198) and Picarella et al. (427) involved expression of lymphotoxin-α under the rat insulin promoter. This ectopic expression of LTα induced modest islet cell inflammation that did not progress to frank diabetes. Apparently, because the rat insulin promoter used was leaky in mice, inflammatory infiltrates were also seen in the kidneys and skin. Detailed histologic evaluation of the inflammatory infiltrates demonstrated that they contained B cells, both CD4$^+$ and CD8$^+$ T cells, plasma cells, dendritic cells, follicular dendritic cells, and vessels with high endothelial venule morphology and PNAd staining (198). These inflammatory foci had structural features typical of organized lymphoid tissues. Furthermore, following systemic immunization with sheep erythrocytes, they showed evidence of germinal center reactions, and contained B cells producing antisheep erythrocyte, isotype-switched antibodies. Thus, chronic expression of LTα in the islets led to formation of apparently functional lymphoid follicular structures. This process of inflammation-induced formation of lymphoid follicles has been termed lymphoid neogenesis (198).

The general importance of this phenomenon has been suggested by the finding of ectopic lymphoid nodules at sites of pathologic inflammation, including autoimmune thyroiditis (428,429), the salivary glands of patients with Sjogren's syndrome (430,431), the thymus in patients with myasthenia gravis (432,433), the synovial membranes of patients with rheumatoid arthritis (434–438), the gastric mucosa in subjects with chronic *Helicobacter pylori* stomach infections (439), chronic hepatitis C infection (200), and chronic arthritis due to *Borrelia burgdorferi* (440). In many of these conditions, local production of potentially pathologic antibodies has been demonstrated in these follicles, and there is potential that suppressing this local response could result in substantial clinical benefit.

Ectopic expression of other immunologic mediators has led to local formation of organized lymphoid structures. Expression of CXCL13 (BLC) under the control of the rat insulin promoter induced formation, in a lymphotoxin-dependent fashion, of organized lymphoid structures containing discrete B-cell and T-cell zones, high endothelial venules, follicular dendritic cells, stromal cells, and the chemokine CCL21 (SLC) (202). This indicated that the chemokine CXCL13 that normally serves to recruit B cells to sites of immune activation, but that also induces expression on their surface of the membrane lymphotoxin heterotrimer (380), is sufficient to initiate a series of events leading to formation of organized lymphoid tissue. Similarly, ectopic expression of CCL21 (SLC), again under the control of the rat insulin promoter, induced the formation of organized lymphoid nodules containing B cells, T cells, dendritic cells, and high endothelial venules (441,442). CXCL12 (SDF-1) and CCL19 (ELC) also could induce organized lymphoid tissue nodules, but these were smaller and included fewer T cells than the structures induced by CCL21 (442). Interestingly, the structures induced by CCL19 and CCL21 were ablated by treatment of the transgenic mice with the LTβR–IgFcγ fusion protein, indicating that their development was dependent on expression of mLT.

The relationship of these organized lymphoid structures to local expression of inflammatory cytokines and chemokines suggests that collections of interacting lymphoid cells may be a common feature of all chronic inflammatory processes. It also suggests the intriguing possibility that mammals have co-opted mechanisms used to elicit tissue inflammation for the purpose of inducing the development of lymphoid organs (443). Organized lymphoid tissue structures may be important in the expression of pathologic immunoglobulins at sites of chronic inflammation. This may be a central process in the expression of antibody-mediated autoimmune disorders (444).

Lymphocyte Recruitment to Secondary Lymphoid Tissues

When naïve lymphocytes are released from the bone marrow and thymus, they must traffic to secondary lymphoid tissues to ready themselves for an encounter with antigen. In order for the secondary lymphoid tissues to remain charged with cells representing a broad repertoire of antigen specificities, it is essential that their cellular composition be constantly renewed. This requires potent mechanisms for recruitment of cells from the circulation. After an immune encounter in the secondary lymphoid tissues, the mature, antigen-experienced effector cells must leave the tissue and traffic to peripheral tissue sites where they can appropriately express their effector functions. In order for these effector cells to provide effective immune surveillance, they appear to be constantly on patrol, continuously circulating from one potential site of antigen encounter to another. It is likely that most mature effector and memory lymphocytes are in constant motion, moving from efferent lymphatic vessels to the blood circulation, into peripheral tissues for antigen surveillance, to afferent lymphatics, to lymph node, and back to efferent lymphatics (445). Although it is difficult to calculate for all subsets of mature lymphocytes, evidence suggests that at least some subsets of cells may make one or two circuits from blood to tissue and back every day (446). It is likely that specific subsets of cells demonstrate selective recirculation patterns, based on the functions to which they are specifically adapted.

Naïve cells freshly exported from the bone marrow and thymus have very limited potential for localization in peripheral tissues, even under conditions of tissue inflammation. Rather, these cells home preferentially to secondary lymphoid tissues (447) where they can interact efficiently with newly encountered antigens. These naïve cells appear to move continuously from one secondary lymphoid tissue to another until they either encounter their specific antigen or are damaged and die (62,63,448). There is evidence that most lymphocytes can demonstrate tissue-specific trafficking by virtue of their recognition of organ-specific adhesion molecules on specialized postcapillary venules in each target tissue (449). For example, naïve lymphocytes harvested from the Peyer's patch largely recirculate to gut-associated lymphoid tissues by virtue of their expression of the integrin $\alpha4\beta7$ that interacts selectively with MAdCAM-1 expressed on the high endothelial venules of Peyer's patches, mesenteric lymph node, and other gut-associated lymphoid tissues (447,449). Alternatively, naïve cells from peripheral lymph nodes use L-selectin interacting with sialylated oligosaccharides on peripheral node addressin (PNAd) expressed on the high endothelial venules of peripheral nodes (218).

Data from many investigators support a multistep model for lymphocyte recruitment (450–452). The general features of this model have been confirmed by a combination of intravital microscopy and in vitro analysis of adhesion under conditions of physiologic flow (453–455). For entry of an $\alpha4\beta7^+$ L-selectin$^+$ naïve lymphocyte into the Peyer's patch, for example, the first recognizable event is an L-selectin–dependent initial attachment of the lymphocyte to MAdCAM-1 on the Peyer's patch high endothelial venule (455). This initial L-selectin–dependent contact proceeds to established rolling that depends on both L-selectin and $\alpha4\beta7$ interacting with MAdCAM-1 on the HEV. The requirement for interaction via both L-selectin and $\alpha4\beta7$ for rolling has been confirmed by gene-targeting experiments in which either L-selectin or the $\beta7$ integrin chain have been deleted (456,457). Rolling lymphocytes then arrest by the combined action of the integrins $\alpha4\beta7$ and LFA-1 in a process that requires signaling via a G-protein coupled receptor on the lymphocyte surface. The requirement for this G-protein coupled receptor activation is shown by the ability of pertussis toxin treatment of the lymphocytes to prevent firm adhesion completely (458).

Similar studies have defined a multistep process of lymphocyte recruitment into peripheral lymph nodes. Here, interactions between L-selectin and peripheral node addressin are required for attachment and rolling (218,459–462). Firm adhesion depended on a pertussis toxin–sensitive G-protein coupled receptor and LFA-1 (462–465).

The ligands for the G-protein coupled receptors that regulate the conversion from rolling to firm adhesion were initially assumed to be locally produced chemokines. While this may be true in many cases, studies by Baekkevold et al. (233) have demonstrated that the chemokine CCL21 (SLC) can be carried from a peripheral site such as the subcutaneous connective tissue to the draining lymph node and be presented to circulating lymphocytes on the luminal surface of the HEV. This expands the repertoire of chemokines that may control lymph node recruitment well beyond the molecules synthesized locally in the vascular endothelial cells and their surrounding tissue cells. Again, using intravital microscopy and a collection of mice targeted for mutations in chemokine receptors or bearing natural mutations in chemokine genes, it is now possible to test the role of specific chemokines in cell recruitment to individual secondary lymphoid tissues. Cells have been analyzed from chimeric mice deficient in CXCR4 (the receptor for CXCL12 (SDF-1) (20,466) and from CXCR5-deficient mice (410), as well as from the natural mutation **PLT** (**p**aucity of **l**ymph node **T** cells; mutant in CCL19 and the lymphoid tissue isoform of CCL21) (467,468). Results have demonstrated that homing of B cells to both Peyer's patches and peripheral lymph nodes is dependent on both SDF-1 signaling through CXCR4 and CCL21 signaling through CCR7 (469), with these chemokines mediating the transition of B cells from rolling to firm adhesions in the high endothelial venules. Furthermore, CXCL13 (BLC) acting through CXCR5 on the B cell contributes importantly to B-cell homing to Peyer's patches (469).

SUMMARY

Proper functioning of the immune response depends on complex functions of several specific tissue compartments. The primary lymphoid tissues include the bone marrow and thymus and represent sites where naïve B- and T-lymphocytes are produced. The secondary lymphoid tissues provide sites where these naïve cells can efficiently encounter antigen and cooperate with each other in the generation of a T-cell–dependent immune response. Our developing understanding of the molecular signals that support the formation and maintenance of the secondary lymphoid tissues give us an appreciation that these tissues are more plastic than originally recognized. Signaling molecules that modulate the plastic features of secondary lymphoid tissue structure and that alter cellular localization within these tissues may represent promising targets for immunomodulatory drug development.

REFERENCES

1. Orkin SH, Zon LI. Hematopoiesis and stem cells: plasticity versus developmental heterogeneity. *Nat Immunol* 2002;3:323–328.
2. Ogawa M, Fraser S, Fujimoto T, et al. Origin of hematopoietic progenitors during embryogenesis. *Int Rev Immunol* 2001;20:21–44.
3. Choi K, Kennedy M, Kazarov A, et al. A common precursor for hematopoietic and endothelial cells. *Development* 1998;125:725–732.
4. Schuh AC, Faloon P, Hu QL, et al. *In vitro* hematopoietic and endothelial potential of flk-1(−/−) embryonic stem cells and embryos. *Proc Natl Acad Sci U S A* 1999;96:2159–2164.
5. Medvinsky AL, Dzierzak EA. Development of the definitive hematopoietic hierarchy in the mouse. *Dev Comp Immunol* 1998;22:289–301.
6. Wolber F, Leonard E, Michael S, et al. Roles of spleen and liver in development of the murine hematopoietic system. *Exp Hematol* 2002;30:1010.
7. Tsai FY, Keller G, Kuo FC, et al. An early haematopoietic defect in mice lacking the transcription factor GATA-2. *Nature* 1994;371:221–226.
8. Freedman MH, Saunders EF. Hematopoiesis in the human spleen. *Am J Hematol* 1981;11:271–275.
9. Osmond DG, Nossal GJ. Differentiation of lymphocytes in mouse bone marrow. II. Kinetics of maturation and renewal of antiglobulin-binding cells studied by double labeling. *Cell Immunol* 1974;13:132–145.
10. Silvennoinen O, Renkonen R, Hurme M. Characterization of natural killer cells and their precursors in the murine bone marrow. *Cell Immunol* 1986;101:1–7.
11. Cooper MD, Raymond DA, Peterson RD, et al. The functions of the thymus system and the bursa system in the chicken. *J Exp Med* 1966;123:75–102.
12. Reynaud CA, Mackay CR, Muller RG, et al. Somatic generation of diversity in a mammalian primary lymphoid organ: the sheep ileal Peyer's patches. *Cell* 1991;64:995–1005.
13. Reynolds JD, Kennedy L, Peppard J, et al. Ileal Peyer's patch emigrants are predominantly B cells and travel to all lymphoid tissues in sheep. *Eur J Immunol* 1991;21:283–289.
14. Beutler E, Lichtman MA, Coller BS, et al. *Williams hematology.* 6th ed. New York: McGraw-Hill Professional, 2000.
15. Coppack SW. Pro-inflammatory cytokines and adipose tissue. *Proc Nutr Soc* 2001;60:349–356.
16. Gevers EF, Loveridge N, Robinson IC. Bone marrow adipocytes: a neglected target tissue for growth hormone. *Endocrinology* 2002; 143:4065–4073.
17. Picker LJ, Siegelman MH. Lymphoid tissues and organs. In: Paul WE, ed. *Fundamental immunology.* 4th ed. Philadelphia: Lippincott-Raven Publishers, 1999;479–531.
18. Weber MH, Sharp JC, Hassard TH, et al. Normal murine bone morphometry: a comparison of magnetic resonance microscopy with micro X-ray and histology. *Skeletal Radiol* 2002;31:282–291.
19. Dorshkind K. Regulation of hemopoiesis by bone marrow stromal cells and their products. *Annu Rev Immunol* 1990;8:111–137.
20. Ma Q, Jones D, Springer TA. The chemokine receptor CXCR4 is required for the retention of B lineage and granulocytic precursors within the bone marrow microenvironment. *Immunity* 1999;10:463–471.
21. Ford CE, Micklem HS, Evans EP, et al. The inflow of bone marrow cells to the thymus. Studies with part body–irradiated mice injected with chromosome-marked bone marrow and subjected to antigenic stimulation. *Ann NY Acad Sci* 1968;129:283–296.
22. Ezine S, Weissman IL, Rouse RV. Bone marrow cells give rise to distinct cell clones within the thymus. *Nature* 1984;309:629–631.
23. Lord BI, Testa NG, Hendry JH. The relative spatial distributions of CFUs and CFUc in the normal mouse femur. *Blood* 1975;46:65–72.
24. Hermans MH, Hartsuiker H, Opstelten D. An *in situ* study of B-lymphocytopoiesis in rat bone marrow. Topographic arrangement of terminal deoxynucleotidyl transferase–positive cells and pre-B cells. *J Immunol* 1989;142:67–73.
25. Jacobsen K, Osmond DG. Microenvironmental organization and stromal cell associations of B lymphocyte precursor cells in mouse bone marrow. *Eur J Immunol* 1990;20:2395–2404.
26. Dexter TM, Allen TD, Lajtaj LD, et al. *In vitro* analysis of self-renewal and commitment of hematopoietic stem cells. In: Clarkson B, Marks PA, Till JE, eds. *Differentiation of normal and neoplastic hematopoietic cells.* Cold Spring Harbor, NY: Cold Spring Harbor Laboratory Press, 1978;63–80.
27. Whitlock CA, Witte ON. Long-term culture of B lymphocytes and their precursors from murine bone marrow. *Proc Natl Acad Sci U S A* 1982;79:3608–3612.
28. Zipori D, Duksin D, Tamir M, et al. Cultured mouse marrow stromal cell lines. II. Distinct subtypes differing in morphology, collagen types, myelopoietic factors, and leukemic cell growth modulating activities. *J Cell Physiol* 1985;122:81–90.
29. Dorshkind K, Johnson A, Collins L, et al. Generation of purified stromal cell cultures that support lymphoid and myeloid precursors. *J Immunol Methods* 1986;89:37–47.
30. Whitlock CA, Tidmarsh GF, Muller-Sieburg C, et al. Bone marrow

stromal cell lines with lymphopoietic activity express high levels of a pre–B neoplasia-associated molecule. *Cell* 1987;48:1009–1021.

31. Weilbaecher K, Weissman I, Blume K, et al. Culture of phenotypically defined hematopoietic stem cells and other progenitors at limiting dilution on Dexter monolayers. *Blood* 1991;78:945–952.

32. Pietrangeli CE, Hayashi S, Kincade PW. Stromal cell lines which support lymphocyte growth: characterization, sensitivity to radiation and responsiveness to growth factors. *Eur J Immunol* 1988;18:863–872.

33. Kincade PW, Medina K, Pietrangeli CE, et al. Stromal cell lines which support lymphocyte growth. II. Characteristics of a suppressive subclone. *Adv Exp Med Biol* 1991;292:227–234.

34. Billips LG, Petitte D, Dorshkind K, et al. Differential roles of stromal cells, interleukin-7, and kit-ligand in the regulation of B lymphopoiesis. *Blood* 1992;79:1185–1192.

35. Landreth KS, Narayanan R, Dorshkind K. Insulin-like growth factor-I regulates pro-B cell differentiation. *Blood* 1992;80:1207–1212.

36. Namen AE, Lupton S, Hjerrild K, et al. Stimulation of B-cell progenitors by cloned murine interleukin-7. *Nature* 1988;333:571–573.

37. Ogawa M, Matsuzaki Y, Nishikawa S, et al. Expression and function of c-kit in hemopoietic progenitor cells. *J Exp Med* 1991;174:63–71.

38. Paul SR, Bennett F, Calvetti JA, et al. Molecular cloning of a cDNA encoding interleukin 11, a stromal cell-derived lymphopoietic and hematopoietic cytokine. *Proc Natl Acad Sci U S A* 1990;87:7512–7516.

39. Rolink A, Streb M, Nishikawa S, et al. The c-kit-encoded tyrosine kinase regulates the proliferation of early pre–B cells. *Eur J Immunol* 1991;21:2609–2612.

40. Sudo T, Ito M, Ogawa Y, et al. Interleukin 7 production and function in stromal cell–dependent B cell development. *J Exp Med* 1989;170:333–338.

41. Hahn BK, Piktel D, Gibson LF, et al. Hematopoiesis: the role of stromal integrin interactions in pro–B cell proliferation. *Hematol* 2000;5:153–160.

42. Bernardi P, Patel VP, Lodish HF. Lymphoid precursor cells adhere to two different sites on fibronectin. *J Cell Biol* 1987;105:489–498.

43. Miyake K, Underhill CB, Lesley J, et al. Hyaluronate can function as a cell adhesion molecule and CD44 participates in hyaluronate recognition. *J Exp Med* 1990;172:69–75.

44. Sanderson RD, Sneed TB, Young LA, et al. Adhesion of B lymphoid (MPC-11) cells to type I collagen is mediated by integral membrane proteoglycan, syndecan. *J Immunol* 1992;148:3902–3911.

45. Miyake K, Medina K, Ishihara K, et al. A VCAM-like adhesion molecule on murine bone marrow stromal cells mediates binding of lymphocyte precursors in culture. *J Cell Biol* 1991;114:557–565.

46. Miyake K, Medina KL, Hayashi S, et al. Monoclonal antibodies to Pgp-1/CD44 block lympho-hemopoiesis in long-term bone marrow cultures. *J Exp Med* 1990;171:477–488.

47. Miyake K, Weissman IL, Greenberger JS, et al. Evidence for a role of the integrin VLA-4 in lympho-hemopoiesis. *J Exp Med* 1991;173:599–607.

48. Spangrude GJ, Heimfeld S, Weissman IL. Purification and characterization of mouse hematopoietic stem cells. *Science* 1988;241:58–62.

49. Heimfeld S, Hudak S, Weissman I, et al. The *in vitro* response of phenotypically defined mouse stem cells and myeloerythroid progenitors to single or multiple growth factors. *Proc Natl Acad Sci U S A* 1991;88:9902–9906.

50. Deenen GJ, Van Balen I, Opstelten D. In rat B lymphocyte genesis sixty percent is lost from the bone marrow at the transition of nondividing pre–B cell to sIgM+ B lymphocyte, the stage of Ig light chain gene expression. *Eur J Immunol* 1990;20:557–564.

51. Motyka B, Reynolds JD. Apoptosis is associated with the extensive B cell death in the sheep ileal Peyer's patch and the chicken bursa of Fabricius: a possible role in B cell selection. *Eur J Immunol* 1991;21. 1951–1958.

52. Pabst R, Reynolds JD. Evidence of extensive lymphocyte death in sheep Peyer's patches. II. The number and fate of newly-formed lymphocytes that emigrate from Peyer's patches. *J Immunol* 1986;136:2011–2017.

53. Reynolds JD. Evidence of extensive lymphocyte death in sheep Peyer's patches. I. A comparison of lymphocyte production and export. *J Immunol* 1986;136:2005–2010.

54. Defrance T, Casamayor-Palleja M, Krammer PH. The life and death of a B cell. *Adv Cancer Res* 2002;86:195–225.

55. Osmond DG, Rico-Vargas S, Valenzona H, et al. Apoptosis and macrophage-mediated cell deletion in the regulation of B lymphopoiesis in mouse bone marrow. *Immunol Rev* 1994;142:209–230.

56. Lu L, Osmond DG. Apoptosis during B lymphopoiesis in mouse bone marrow. *J Immunol* 1997;158:5136–5145.

57. Lu L, Osmond DG. Apoptosis and its modulation during B lymphopoiesis in mouse bone marrow. *Immunol Rev* 2000;175:158–174.

58. Iizuka K, Chaplin DD, Wang Y, et al. Requirement for membrane lymphotoxin in natural killer cell development. *Proc Natl Acad Sci U S A* 1999;96:6336–6340.

59. Miller JFAP. Immunological function of the thymus. *Lancet* 1961; 2:748.

60. Miller JF. The discovery of thymus function and of thymus-derived lymphocytes. *Immunol Rev* 2002;185:7–14.

61. Miller JF, Osoba D. Current concepts of the immunological function of the thymus. *Physiol Rev* 1967;47:437–520.

62. Sprent J. Circulating T and B lymphocytes of the mouse. I. Migratory properties. *Cell Immunol* 1973;7:10–39.

63. Sprent J, Basten A. Circulating T and B lymphocytes of the mouse. II. Lifespan. *Cell Immunol* 1973;7:40–59.

64. Fowlkes BJ, Pardoll DM. Molecular and cellular events of T cell development. *Adv Immunol* 1989;44:207–264.

65. Muller-Hermelink HK, Steinmann G, Stein H. Structural and functional alterations of the aging human thymus. *Adv Exp Med Biol* 1982;149:303–312.

66. Steinmann GG. Changes in the human thymus during aging. *Curr Top Pathol* 1986;75:43–88.

67. Papatestas AE, Genkins G, Kornfeld P, et al. Effects of thymectomy in myasthenia gravis. *Ann Surg* 1987;206:79–88.

68. Douek DC, Altmann DM. T-cell apoptosis and differential human leucocyte antigen class II expression in human thymus. *Immunology* 2000;99:249–256.

69. Haynes BF, Hale LP. The human thymus. A chimeric organ comprised of central and peripheral lymphoid components. *Immunol Res* 1998;18:175–192.

70. Clark SL. The thymus in mice of strain 129/J studied with the electron microscope. *Am J Anat* 1961;112:1.

71. Kendall MD. The morphology of perivascular spaces in the thymus. *Thymus* 1989;13:157–164.

72. Kato S. Intralobular lymphatic vessels and their relationship to blood vessels in the mouse thymus. Light- and electron-microscopic study. *Cell Tissue Res* 1988;253:181–187.

73. Ghali WM, Abdel-Rahman S, Nagib M, et al. Intrinsic innervation and vasculature of pre- and post-natal human thymus. *Acta Anat (Basel)* 1980;108:115–123.

74. Singh U, Fatani J. Thymic lymphopoiesis and cholinergic innervation. *Thymus* 1988;11:3–13.

75. Bearman RM, Bensch KG, Levine GD. The normal human thymic vasculature: an ultrastructural study. *Anat Rec* 1975;183:485–497.

76. Malhotra V, Tatke M, Khanna SK, et al. Thymic histology in myasthenia gravis. *Indian J Chest Dis Allied Sci* 1992;34:117–121.

77. van Ewijk W. T-cell differentiation is influenced by thymic microenvironments. *Annu Rev Immunol* 1991;9:591–615.

78. Bockman DE, Kirby ML. Dependence of thymus development on derivatives of the neural crest. *Science* 1984;223:498–500.

79. Bockman DE, Kirby ML. Neural crest interactions in the development of the immune system. *J Immunol* 1985;135:766s–768s.

80. Hong R. The DiGeorge anomaly. *Clin Rev Allergy Immunol* 2001; 20:43–60.

81. Bockman DE. Development of the thymus. *Microsc Res Tech* 1997; 38:209–215.

82. Cordier AC, Heremans JF. Nude mouse embryo: ectodermal nature of the primordial thymic defect. *Scand J Immunol* 1975;4:193–196.

83. Cordier AC, Haumont SM. Development of thymus, parathyroids, and ultimo-branchial bodies in NMRI and nude mice. *Am J Anat* 1980; 157:227–263.

84. Boyd RL, Tucek CL, Godfrey DI, et al. The thymic microenvironment. *Immunol Today* 1993;14:445–459.

85. Hollander GA, Wang B, Nichogiannopoulou A, et al. Developmental control point in induction of thymic cortex regulated by a subpopulation of prothymocytes. *Nature* 1995;373:350–353.

86. Fainsod A, Awgulewitsch A, Ruddle FH. Expression of the murine homeo box gene Hox 1.5 during embryogenesis. *Dev Biol* 1987; 124:125–133.

87. Chisaka O, Capecchi MR. Regionally restricted developmental defects resulting from targeted disruption of the mouse homeobox gene hox-1.5. *Nature* 1991;350:473–479.

88. Rossel M, Capecchi MR. Mice mutant for both Hoxa1 and Hoxb1 show extensive remodeling of the hindbrain and defects in craniofacial development. *Development* 1999;126:5027–5040.

89. Xu PX, Woo I, Her H, et al. Mouse Eya homologues of the Drosophila eyes absent gene require Pax6 for expression in lens and nasal placode. *Development* 1997;124:219–231.

90. Abdelhak S, Kalatzis V, Heilig R, et al. A human homologue of the Drosophila eyes absent gene underlies branchio-oto-renal (BOR) syndrome and identifies a novel gene family. *Nat Genet* 1997;15:157–164.

91. Duncan MK, Kos L, Jenkins NA, et al. Eyes absent: a gene family found in several metazoan phyla. *Mamm Genome* 1997;8:479–485.

92. Zimmerman JE, Bui QT, Steingrimsson E, et al. Cloning and characterization of two vertebrate homologs of the Drosophila eyes absent gene. *Genome Res* 1997;7:128–141.

93. Borsani G, DeGrandi A, Ballabio A, et al. EYA4, a novel vertebrate gene related to Drosophila eyes absent. *Hum Mol Genet* 1999;8:11–23.

94. Xu PX, Zheng W, Laclef C, et al. Eya1 is required for the morphogenesis of mammalian thymus, parathyroid and thyroid. *Development* 2002;129:3033–3044.

95. Nehls M, Pfeifer D, Schorpp M, et al. New member of the winged-helix protein family disrupted in mouse and rat nude mutations. *Nature* 1994;372:103–107.

96. Nehls M, Kyewski B, Messerle M, et al. Two genetically separable steps in the differentiation of thymic epithelium. *Science* 1996;272:886–889.

97. Schlake T, Schorpp M, Nehls M, et al. The nude gene encodes a sequence-specific DNA binding protein with homologs in organisms that lack an anticipatory immune system. *Proc Natl Acad Sci U S A* 1997;94:3842–3847.

98. Bleul CC, Boehm T. Laser capture microdissection-based expression profiling identifies PD1–ligand as a target of the nude locus gene product. *Eur J Immunol* 2001;31:2497–2503.

99. Balciunaite G, Keller MP, Balciunaite E, et al. Wnt glycoproteins regulate the expression of FoxN1, the gene defective in nude mice. *Nat Immunol* 2002;3:1102–1108.

100. Weih F, Carrasco D, Durham SK, et al. Multiorgan inflammation and hematopoietic abnormalities in mice with a targeted disruption of RelB, a member of the NF-kappa B/Rel family. *Cell* 1995;80:331–340.

101. Burkly L, Hession C, Ogata L, et al. Expression of relB is required for the development of thymic medulla and dendritic cells. *Nature* 1995;373:531–536.

102. Carrasco D, Ryseck RP, Bravo R. Expression of relB transcripts during lymphoid organ development: specific expression in dendritic antigen-presenting cells. *Development* 1993;118:1221–1231.

103. Miyawaki S, Nakamura Y, Suzuka H, et al. A new mutation, aly, that induces a generalized lack of lymph nodes accompanied by immunodeficiency in mice. *Eur J Immunol* 1994;24:429–434.

104. Shinkura R, Kitada K, Matsuda F, et al. Alymphoplasia is caused by a point mutation in the mouse gene encoding NF-kappa B-inducing kinase. *Nat Genet* 1999;22:74–77.

105. Yin L, Wu L, Wesche H, et al. Defective lymphotoxin-beta receptor-induced NF-kappaB transcriptional activity in NIK-deficient mice. *Science* 2001;291:2162–2165.

106. Konishi J, Iwabuchi K, Iwabuchi C, et al. Thymic epithelial cells responsible for impaired generation of NK-T thymocytes in Alymphoplasia mutant mice. *Cell Immunol* 2000;206:26–35.

107. Balling R, Deutsch U, Gruss P. undulated, a mutation affecting the development of the mouse skeleton, has a point mutation in the paired box of Pax 1. *Cell* 1988;55:531–535.

108. Wallin J, Eibel H, Neubuser A, et al. Pax1 is expressed during development of the thymus epithelium and is required for normal T-cell maturation. *Development* 1996;122:23–30.

109. von Gaudecker B. Functional histology of the human thymus. *Anat Embryol* 1991;183:1–15.

110. Von Gaudecker B, Kendall MD, Ritter MA. Immuno-electron microscopy of the thymic epithelial microenvironment. *Microsc Res Tech* 1997;38:237–249.

111. Chaplin DD. Overview of the immune response. *J Allergy Clin Immunol* 2003;111:S442–459.

112. Toro I, Olah L. Studies on the blood–thymus barrier. *Acta Biol* 1967;18:135–150.

113. Raviola E, Karnovsky MJ. Evidence for a blood–thymus barrier using electron-opaque tracers. *J Exp Med* 1972;136:466–498.

114. Kouvalainen K, Gitlin D. Passage of antigens across the vascular barrier of the thymus. *Nature* 1967;214:592–593.

115. Hoffmann-Fezer G, Antica M, Schuh R, et al. Distribution of injected anti-Thy-1 monoclonal antibodies in mouse lymphatic organs: evidence for penetration of the cortical blood–thymus barrier, and for intravascular antibody-binding onto lymphocytes. *Hybridoma* 1989;8:517–527.

116. Henry L, Durrant TE, Anderson G. Pericapillary collagen in the human thymus: implications for the concept of the "blood–thymus" barrier. *J Anat* 1992;181 (Pt 1):39–46.

117. Roberts RL, Sandra A. Transport of transferrin across the blood–thymus barrier in young rats. *Tissue Cell* 1994;26:757–766.

118. Hess MW, Mueller C, Schaffner T, et al. Thymic lymphopoiesis: protected from, or influenced by, external stimulation? *Ann N Y Acad Sci* 1985;459:14–21.

119. Eggli P, Schaffner T, Gerber HA, et al. Accessibility of thymic cortical lymphocytes to particles translocated from the peritoneal cavity to parathymic lymph nodes. *Thymus* 1986;8:129–139.

120. Pugliese A, Brown D, Garza D, et al. Self-antigen–presenting cells expressing diabetes-associated autoantigens exist in both thymus and peripheral lymphoid organs. *J Clin Invest* 2001;107:555–564.

121. Derbinski J, Schulte A, Kyewski B, et al. Promiscuous gene expression in medullary thymic epithelial cells mirrors the peripheral self. *Nat Immunol* 2001;2:1032–1039.

122. Pugliese A, Diez J. Lymphoid organs contain diverse cells expressing self-molecules. *Nat Immunol* 2002;3:335–336; discussion 336.

123. Kyewski BA, Rouse RV, Kaplan HS. Thymocyte rosettes: multicellular complexes of lymphocytes and bone marrow-derived stromal cells in the mouse thymus. *Proc Natl Acad Sci U S A* 1982;79:5646–5650.

124. Munoz-Blay T, Nieburgs AC, Cohen S. Thymic epithelium *in vitro*. V. Binding of thymocytes to cultured thymic epithelial cells. *Cell Immunol* 1987;109:371–383.

125. Singer KH, Denning SM, Whichard LP, et al. Thymocyte LFA-1 and thymic epithelial cell ICAM-1 molecules mediate binding of activated human thymocytes to thymic epithelial cells. *J Immunol* 1990;144:2931–2939.

126. de Waal Malefijt R, Leene W, Roholl PJ, et al. T cell differentiation within thymic nurse cells. *Lab Invest* 1986;55:25–34.

127. van Vliet E, Melis M, van Ewijk W. Immunohistology of thymic nurse cells. *Cell Immunol* 1984;87:101–109.

128. Kyewski BA, Kaplan HS. Lymphoepithelial interactions in the mouse thymus: phenotypic and kinetic studies on thymic nurse cells. *J Immunol* 1982;128:2287–2294.

129. Van Vliet E, Jenkinson EJ, Kingston R, et al. Stromal cell types in the developing thymus of the normal and nude mouse embryo. *Eur J Immunol* 1985;15:675–681.

130. Rouse RV, Parham P, Grumet FC, et al. Expression of HLA antigens by human thymic epithelial cells. *Hum Immunol* 1982;5:21–34.

131. Surh CD, Gao EK, Kosaka H, et al. Two subsets of epithelial cells in the thymic medulla. *J Exp Med* 1992;176:495–505.

132. Farr AG, Braddy SC. Patterns of keratin expression in the murine thymus. *Anat Rec* 1989;224:374–378.

133. Farr AG, Anderson SK. Epithelial heterogeneity in the murine thymus: fucose-specific lectins bind medullary epithelial cells. *J Immunol* 1985;134:2971–2977.

134. Shier KJ. The thymus according to Schambacher: medullary ducts and reticular epithelium of thymus and thymomas. *Cancer* 1981;48:1183–1199.

135. Farr AG, Hosier S, Braddy SC, et al. Medullary epithelial cell lines from murine thymus constitutively secrete IL-1 and hematopoietic growth factors and express class II antigens in response to recombinant interferon-gamma. *Cell Immunol* 1989;119:427–444.

136. Dalloul AH, Arock M, Fourcade C, et al. Human thymic epithelial cells produce interleukin-3. *Blood* 1991;77:69–74.

137. Le PT, Lazorick S, Whichard LP, et al. Human thymic epithelial cells produce IL-6, granulocyte-monocyte-CSF, and leukemia inhibitory factor. *J Immunol* 1990;145:3310–3315.

138. Schluns KS, Cook JE, Le PT. TGF-beta differentially modulates epidermal growth factor-mediated increases in leukemia-inhibitory factor, IL-6, IL-1 alpha, and IL-1 beta in human thymic epithelial cells. *J Immunol* 1997;158:2704–2712.

139. Fiorini E, Marchisio PC, Scupoli MT, et al. Adhesion of immature and mature T cells induces in human thymic epithelial cells (TEC) activation of IL-6 gene trascription factors (NF-kappaB and NF-IL6) and IL-6 gene expression: role of alpha3beta1 and alpha6beta4 integrins. *Dev Immunol* 2000;7:195–208.

140. Chene L, Nugeyre MT, Guillemard E, et al. Thymocyte-thymic epithelial cell interaction leads to high-level replication of human immunodeficiency virus exclusively in mature CD4(+) CD8(−) CD3(+) thymocytes: a critical role for tumor necrosis factor and interleukin-7. *J Virol* 1999;73:7533–7542.

141. Erickson M, Morkowski S, Lehar S, et al. Regulation of thymic epithelium by keratinocyte growth factor. *Blood* 2002;100:3269–3278.

142. Hare KJ, Jenkinson EJ, Anderson G. An essential role for the IL-7 receptor during intrathymic expansion of the positively selected neonatal T cell repertoire. *J Immunol* 2000;165:2410–2414.

143. Knutsen AP, Freeman JJ, Mueller KR, et al. Thymosin-alpha1 stimulates maturation of CD34+ stem cells into CD3+4+ cells in an *in vitro* thymic epithelia organ coculture model. *Int J Immunopharmacol* 1999;21:15–26.

144. Romagnani P, Annunziato F, Lazzeri E, et al. Interferon-inducible protein 10, monokine induced by interferon gamma, and interferon-inducible T-cell alpha chemoattractant are produced by thymic epithelial cells and attract T-cell receptor (TCR) alphabeta+ CD8+ single-positive T cells, TCRgammadelta+ T cells, and natural killer-type cells in human thymus. *Blood* 2001;97:601–607.

145. Annunziato F, Romagnani P, Cosmi L, et al. Macrophage-derived chemokine and EBI1-ligand chemokine attract human thymocytes in different stage of development and are produced by distinct subsets of medullary epithelial cells: possible implications for negative selection. *J Immunol* 2000;165:238–246.

146. Zaitseva M, Kawamura T, Loomis R, et al. Stromal-derived factor 1 expression in the human thymus. *J Immunol* 2002;168:2609–2617.

147. Wurbel MA, Philippe JM, Nguyen C, et al. The chemokine TECK is expressed by thymic and intestinal epithelial cells and attracts double- and single-positive thymocytes expressing the TECK receptor CCR9. *Eur J Immunol* 2000;30:262–271.

148. Sempowski GD, Hale LP, Sundy JS, et al. Leukemia inhibitory factor, oncostatin M, IL-6, and stem cell factor mRNA expression in human thymus increases with age and is associated with thymic atrophy. *J Immunol* 2000;164:2180–2187.

149. de Mello Coelho V, Villa-Verde DM, Farias-de-Oliveira DA, et al. Functional insulin-like growth factor-1/insulin-like growth factor-1 receptor-mediated circuit in human and murine thymic epithelial cells. *Neuroendocrinology* 2002;75:139–150.

150. Sims JE, Williams DE, Morrissey PJ, et al. Molecular cloning and biological characterization of a novel murine lymphoid growth factor. *J Exp Med* 2000;192:671–680.

151. Reche PA, Soumelis V, Gorman DM, et al. Human thymic stromal lymphopoietin preferentially stimulates myeloid cells. *J Immunol* 2001;167:336–343.

152. Chantry D, Romagnani P, Raport CJ, et al. Macrophage-derived chemokine is localized to thymic medullary epithelial cells and is a chemoattractant for CD3(+), CD4(+), CD8(low) thymocytes. *Blood* 1999;94:1890–1898.

153. Murphy KM, Heimberger AB, Loh DY. Induction by antigen of intrathymic apoptosis of CD4+CD8+TCRlo thymocytes *in vivo*. *Science* 1990;250:1720–1723.

154. Epstein HD, Mitchell DS, Hunt JS, et al. Ia-positive macrophages bind and internalize viable lymphocytes in murine thymus. *Cell Immunol* 1985;95:15–34.

155. Ruco LP, Pisacane A, Pomponi D, et al. Macrophages and interdigitating reticulum cells in normal human thymus and thymomas: immunoreactivity for interleukin-1 alpha, interleukin-1 beta and tumour necrosis factor alpha. *Histopathology* 1990;17:291–299.

156. Kaiserling E, Stein H, Muller-Hermelink HK. Interdigitating reticulum cells in the human thymus. *Cell Tissue Res* 1974;155:47–55.

157. Ceredig R, Schreyer M. Immunohistochemical localization of host and donor-derived cells in the regenerating thymus of radiation bone marrow chimeras. *Thymus* 1984;6:15–26.

158. Bruno L, Res P, Dessing M, et al. Identification of a committed T cell precursor population in adult human peripheral blood. *J Exp Med* 1997;185:875–884.

159. Rodewald HR, Kretzschmar K, Takeda S, et al. Identification of pro-thymocytes in murine fetal blood: T lineage commitment can precede thymus colonization. *EMBO J* 1994;13:4229–4240.

160. Wu L, Scollay R, Egerton M, et al. CD4 expressed on earliest T-lineage precursor cells in the adult murine thymus. *Nature* 1991;349:71–74.

161. Sotzik F, Rosenberg Y, Boyd AW, et al. Assessment of CD4 expression by early T precursor cells and by dendritic cells in the human thymus. *J Immunol* 1994;152:3370–3377.

162. Penit C, Vasseur F. Sequential events in thymocyte differentiation and thymus regeneration revealed by a combination of bromodeoxyuridine DNA labeling and antimitotic drug treatment. *J Immunol* 1988;140:3315–3323.

163. Farr A, Hosier S, Nelson A, et al. Distribution of thymocytes expressing gamma delta receptors in the murine thymus during development. *J Immunol* 1990;144:492–498.

164. Surh CD, Sprent J. T-cell apoptosis detected *in situ* during positive and negative selection in the thymus. *Nature* 1994;372:100–103.

165. Klein L, Kyewski B. "Promiscuous" expression of tissue antigens in the thymus: a key to T-cell tolerance and autoimmunity? *J Mol Med* 2000;78:483–494.

166. Crisa L, McMaster MT, Ishii JK, et al. Identification of a thymic epithelial cell subset sharing expression of the class Ib HLA-G molecule with fetal trophoblasts. *J Exp Med* 1997;186:289–298.

167. Mallet V, Fournel S, Schmitt C, et al. Primary cultured human thymic epithelial cells express both membrane-bound and soluble HLA-G translated products. *J Reprod Immunol* 1999;43:225–234.

168. Lefebvre S, Adrian F, Moreau P, et al. Modulation of HLA-G expression in human thymic and amniotic epithelial cells. *Hum Immunol* 2000;61:1095–1101.

169. Scollay R, Godfrey DI. Thymic emigration: conveyor belts or lucky dips? *Immunol Today* 1995;16:268–273; discussion 273–264.

170. Gabor MJ, Scollay R, Godfrey DI. Thymic T cell export is not influenced by the peripheral T cell pool. *Eur J Immunol* 1997;27:2986–2993.

171. Rowen L, Koop BF, Hood L. The complete 685-kilobase DNA sequence of the human beta T cell receptor locus. *Science* 1996;272:1755–1762.

172. Hood L, Rowen L, Koop BF. Human and mouse T-cell receptor loci: genomics, evolution, diversity, and serendipity. *Ann N Y Acad Sci* 1995;758:390–412.

173. Fanning LJ, Connor AM, Wu GE. Development of the immunoglobulin repertoire. *Clin Immunol Immunopathol* 996;79:1–14.

174. Owen RL, Ermak TH. Structural specializations for antigen uptake and processing in the digestive tract. *Springer Semin Immunopathol* 1990;12:139–152.

175. Laissue JA, Chappuis BB, Muller C, et al. The intestinal immune system and its relation to disease. *Dig Dis* 1993;11:298–312.

176. Richtsmeier WJ, Shikhani AH. The physiology and immunology of the pharyngeal lymphoid tissue. *Otolaryngol Clin North Am* 1987;20:219–228.

177. Berman JS, Beer DJ, Theodore AC, et al. Lymphocyte recruitment to the lung. *Am Rev Respir Dis* 1990;142:238–257.

178. Berman JS. Lymphocytes in the lung: should we continue to exalt only BALT? *Am J Respir Cell Mol Biol* 1990;3:101–102.

179. Wu HY, Russell MW. Nasal lymphoid tissue, intranasal immunization, and compartmentalization of the common mucosal immune system. *Immunol Res* 1997;16:187–201.

180. Kuper CF, Koornstra PJ, Hameleers DM, et al. The role of nasopharyngeal lymphoid tissue. *Immunol Today* 1992;13:219–224.

181. Par A. Gastrointestinal tract as a part of immune defence. *Acta Physiol Hung* 2000;87:291–304.

182. Song F, Whitacre CC. The role of the gut lymphoid tissue in induction of oral tolerance. *Curr Opin Investig Drugs* 2001;2:1382–1386.

183. Goeringer GC, Vidic B. The embryogenesis and anatomy of Waldeyer's ring. *Otolaryngol Clin North Am* 1987;20:207–217.

184. Brook I. The clinical microbiology of Waldeyer's ring. *Otolaryngol Clin North Am* 1987;20:259–272.

185. Russell MW, Mestecky J. Humoral immune responses to microbial infections in the genital tract. *Microbes Infect* 2002;4:667–677.

186. Yeaman GR, Collins JE, Fanger MW, et al. CD8+ T cells in human uterine endometrial lymphoid aggregates: evidence for accumulation of cells by trafficking. *Immunology* 2001;102:434–440.

187. Yeaman GR, Guyre PM, Fanger MW, et al. Unique CD8+ T cell–rich lymphoid aggregates in human uterine endometrium. *J Leukoc Biol* 1997;61:427–435.

188. Ishikawa H, Saito H, Suzuki K, et al. New gut associated lymphoid tissue "cryptopatches" breed murine intestinal intraepithelial T cell precursors. *Immunol Res* 1999;20:243–250.

189. Suzuki K, Oida T, Hamada H, et al. Gut cryptopatches: direct evidence of extrathymic anatomical sites for intestinal T lymphopoiesis. *Immunity* 2000;13:691–702.

190. Goodnow CC. Chance encounters and organized rendezvous. *Immunol Rev* 1997;156:5–10.

191. Steinman RM, Pack M, Inaba K. Dendritic cells in the T-cell areas of lymphoid organs. *Immunol Rev* 1997;156:25–37.

192. Kundig TM, Bachmann MF, DiPaolo C, et al. Fibroblasts as efficient antigen-presenting cells in lymphoid organs. *Science* 1995;268:1343–1347.

193. Zinkernagel RM, Ehl S, Aichele P, et al. Antigen localisation regulates immune responses in a dose- and time-dependent fashion—a geographical view of immune reactivity. *Immunol Rev* 1997;156:199–209.

194. Nair PN, Schroeder HE. Duct-associated lymphoid tissue (DALT) of minor salivary glands and mucosal immunity. *Immunology* 1986;57:171–180.

195. Schroeder HE, Moreillon MC, Nair PN. Architecture of minor salivary gland duct/lymphoid follicle associations and possible antigen-recognition sites in the monkey *Macaca fascicularis*. *Arch Oral Biol* 1983;28:133–143.

196. Tschernig T, Pabst R. Bronchus-associated lymphoid tissue (BALT) is not present in the normal adult lung but in different diseases. *Pathobiology* 2000;68:1–8.

197. Drayton DL, Chan K, Lesslauer W, et al. Lymphocyte traffic in lymphoid organ neogenesis: differential roles of LTa and LTab. *Adv Exp Med Biol* 2002;512:43–48.

198. Kratz A, Campos-Neto A, Hanson MS, et al. Chronic inflammation caused by lymphotoxin is lymphoid neogenesis. *J Exp Med* 1996;183:1461–1472.

199. Magalhaes R, Stiehl P, Morawietz L, et al. Morphological and molecular pathology of the B cell response in synovitis of rheumatoid arthritis. *Virchows Arch* 2002;441:415–427.

200. Murakami J, Shimizu Y, Kashii Y, et al. Functional B-cell response in intrahepatic lymphoid follicles in chronic hepatitis C. *Hepatology* 1999;30:143–150.

201. Roxanis I, Micklem K, McConville J, et al. Thymic myoid cells and germinal center formation in myasthenia gravis; possible roles in pathogenesis. *J Neuroimmunol* 2002;125:185–197.

202. Luther SA, Lopez T, Bai W, et al. BLC expression in pancreatic islets causes B cell recruitment and lymphotoxin-dependent lymphoid neogenesis. *Immunity* 2000;12:471–481.

203. Taylor AE. Capillary fluid filtration. Starling forces and lymph flow. *Circ Res* 1981;49:557–575.

204. Romani N, Ratzinger G, Pfaller K, et al. Migration of dendritic cells into lymphatics—the Langerhans cell example: routes, regulation, and relevance. *Int Rev Cytol* 2001;207:237–270.

205. Gretz JE, Anderson AO, Shaw S. Cords, channels, corridors and conduits: critical architectural elements facilitating cell interactions in the lymph node cortex. *Immunol Rev* 1997;156:11–24.

206. Gretz JE, Norbury CC, Anderson AO, et al. Lymph-borne chemokines and other low molecular weight molecules reach high endothelial venules via specialized conduits while a functional barrier limits access to the lymphocyte microenvironments in lymph node cortex. *J Exp Med* 2000;192:1425–1440.

207. Ohtani O, Ohtsuka A. Three-dimensional organization of lymphatics and their relationship to blood vessels in rabbit small intestine. A scanning electron microscopic study of corrosion casts. *Arch Histol Jpn* 1985;48:255–268.

208. Casley-Smith JR. The fine structure and functioning of tissue channels and lymphatics. *Lymphology* 1980;13:177–183.

209. Rennert PD, Hochman PS, Flavell RA, et al. Essential role of lymph nodes in contact hypersensitivity revealed in lymphotoxin-alpha-deficient mice. *J Exp Med* 2001;193:1227–1238.

210. Sainte-Marie G, Peng FS. Depopulation of lymphocyte migration sites in the lymph node by irradiation and colloidal carbon. *Rev Can Biol Exp* 1983;42:285–293.

211. Leak LV, Burke JF. Electron microscopic study of lymphatic capillaries in the removal of connective tissue fluids and particulate substances. *Lymphology* 1968;1:39–52.

212. Leak LV, Burke JF. Fine structure of the lymphatic capillary and the adjoining connective tissue area. *Am J Anat* 1966;118:785–809.

213. Wigle JT, Oliver G. Prox1 function is required for the development of the murine lymphatic system. *Cell* 1999;98:769–778.

214. Kaipainen A, Korhonen J, Mustonen T, et al. Expression of the fms-like tyrosine kinase 4 gene becomes restricted to lymphatic endothelium during development. *Proc Natl Acad Sci U S A* 1995;92:3566–3570.

215. Banerji S, Ni J, Wang SX, et al. LYVE-1, a new homologue of the CD44 glycoprotein, is a lymph-specific receptor for hyaluronan. *J Cell Biol* 1999;144:789–801.

216. Straus W. Staining patterns for the anti-horseradish peroxidase antibody reaction in proplasma cells developing in the medulla of rat popliteal lymph nodes during the secondary response. *J Histochem Cytochem* 1981;29:525–530.

217. Manolios N, Geczy CL, Schrieber L. High endothelial venule morphology and function are inducible in germ-free mice: a possible role for interferon-gamma. *Cell Immunol* 1988;117:136–151.

218. Gallatin WM, Weissman IL, Butcher EC. A cell-surface molecule involved in organ-specific homing of lymphocytes. *Nature* 1983;304:30–34.

219. Berlin C, Berg EL, Briskin MJ, et al. Alpha 4 beta 7 integrin mediates lymphocyte binding to the mucosal vascular addressin MAdCAM-1. *Cell* 1993;74:185.

220. Hamann A, Andrew DP, Jablonski-Westrich D, et al. Role of alpha 4–integrins in lymphocyte homing to mucosal tissues *in vivo*. *J Immunol* 1994;152:3282–3293.

221. Racz P, Tenner-Racz K, Myrvik QN, et al. The "mosaic" structure of the sinuses in the hilar lymph node complex of the lungs in rabbits undergoing a pulmonary cell-mediated reaction: an electron microscopic study. *J Reticuloendothel Soc* 1978;24:527–545.

222. Clark SLJ. The reticulum of lymph nodes in mice studied with the electron microscope. *Am J Anat* 1962;110:217–257.

223. Moe RE. Fine structure of the reticulum and sinuses of the lymph node. *Am J Anat* 1963;112:311–335.

224. Konomi H, Sano J, Nagai Y. Immunohistochemical localization of type I, III and IV (basement membrane) collagens in the liver. *Acta Pathol Jpn* 1981;31:973–978.

225. Miyata K, Takaya K. Elastic fibers associated with collagenous fibrils surrounded by reticular cells in lymph nodes of the rat as revealed by electron microscopy after orcein staining. *Cell Tissue Res* 1981;220:445–448.

226. Stenman S, Vaheri A. Distribution of a major connective tissue protein, fibronectin, in normal human tissues. *J Exp Med* 1978;147:1054–1064.

227. Karttunen T, Alavaikko M, Apaja-Sarkkinen M, et al. Distribution of basement membrane laminin and type IV collagen in human reactive lymph nodes. *Histopathology* 1986;10:841–849.

228. Ocklind G, Talts J, Fassler R, et al. Expression of tenascin in developing and adult mouse lymphoid organs. *J Histochem Cytochem* 1993;41:1163–1169.

229. Gloghini A, Carbone A. Dendritic reticulum cell-related immunostaining in follicular and diffuse B-cell lymphomas. *Virchows Arch A Pathol Anat Histopathol* 1990;416:197–204.

230. Kramer RH, Rosen SD, McDonald KA. Basement-membrane components associated with the extracellular matrix of the lymph node. *Cell Tissue Res* 1988;252:367–375.

231. Sainte-Marie G, Peng FS. Diffusion of a lymph-carried antigen in the fiber network of the lymph node of the rat. *Cell Tissue Res* 1986;245:481–486.

232. Anderson AO, Anderson ND. Studies on the structure and permeability of the microvasculature in normal rat lymph nodes. *Am J Pathol* 1975;80:387–418.

233. Baekkevold ES, Yamanaka T, Palframan RT, et al. The CCR7 ligand elc (CCL19) is transcytosed in high endothelial venules and mediates T cell recruitment. *J Exp Med* 2001;193:1105–1112.

234. Caux C, Ait-Yahia S, Chemin K, et al. Dendritic cell biology and regulation of dendritic cell trafficking by chemokines. *Springer Semin Immunopathol* 2000;22:345–369.

235. Caux C, Vanbervliet B, Massacrier C, et al. Regulation of dendritic cell recruitment by chemokines. *Transplantation* 2002;73:S7–11.

236. Garside P, Ingulli E, Merica RR, et al. Visualization of specific B and

T lymphocyte interactions in the lymph node. *Science* 1998;281:96–99.

237. Kelsoe G. The germinal center reaction. *Immunol Today* 1995;16:324–326.

238. Tew JG, Wu J, Fakher M, et al. Follicular dendritic cells: beyond the necessity of T-cell help. *Trends Immunol* 2001;22:361–367.

239. Qin D, Wu J, Vora KA, et al. Fc gamma receptor IIB on follicular dendritic cells regulates the B cell recall response. *J Immunol* 2000;164:6268–6275.

240. Burton GF, Conrad DH, Szakal AK, et al. Follicular dendritic cells and B cell costimulation. *J Immunol* 1993;150:31–38.

241. Kapasi ZF, Qin D, Kerr WG, et al. Follicular dendritic cell (FDC) precursors in primary lymphoid tissues. *J Immunol* 1998;160:1078–1084.

242. Liu Y-J, Xu J, de Bouteiller O, et al. Follicular dendritic cells specifically express the long CR2/CD21 isoform. *J Exp Med* 1997;185:165–170.

243. Tew JG, Wu JH, Qin DH, et al. Follicular dendritic cells and presentation of antigen and costimulatory signals to B cells. *Immunol Rev* 1997;156:39–52.

244. Matsumoto M, Fu Y-X, Molina H, et al. Distinct roles of lymphotoxin-α and the type I tumor necrosis factor (TNF) receptor in the establishment of follicular dendritic cells from non-bone marrow-derived cells. *J Exp Med* 1997;186:1997–2004.

245. Smith JP, Kosco MH, Tew JG, et al. Thy-1 positive tingible body macrophages (TBM) in mouse lymph nodes. *Anat Rec* 1988;222:380–390.

246. Smith JP, Burton GF, Tew JG, et al. Tingible body macrophages in regulation of germinal center reactions. *Dev Immunol* 1998;6:285–294.

247. Zheng B, Han S, Kelsoe G. T helper cells in murine germinal centers are antigen-specific emigrants that downregulate Thy-1. *J Exp Med* 1996;184:1083–1091.

248. MacLennan IC, Oldfield S, Liu YJ, et al. Regulation of B-cell populations. *Curr Top Pathol* 1989;79:37–57.

249. Liu YJ, Zhang J, Lane PJ, et al. Sites of specific B cell activation in primary and secondary responses to T cell–dependent and T cell–independent antigens. *Eur J Immunol* 1991;21:2951–2962.

250. Hollowood K, Macartney J. Cell kinetics of the germinal center reaction—a stathmokinetic study. *Eur J Immunol* 1992;22:261–266.

251. Nieuwenhuis P, Kroese FG, Opstelten D, et al. *De novo* germinal center formation. *Immunol Rev* 1992;126:77–98.

252. Jacob J, Kelsoe G, Rajewsky K, et al. Intraclonal generation of antibody mutants in germinal centres. *Nature* 1991;354:389–392.

253. Jacob J, Kelsoe G. *In situ* studies of the primary immune response to (4-hydroxy-3-nitrophenyl)acetyl. II. A common clonal origin for periarteriolar lymphoid sheath-associated foci and germinal centers. *J Exp Med* 1992;176:679–687.

254. Rajewsky K. Clonal selection and learning in the antibody system. *Nature* 1996;381:751–758.

255. Liu YJ, Joshua DE, Williams GT, et al. Mechanism of antigen-driven selection in germinal centres. *Nature* 1989;342:929–931.

256. Ziegner M, Steinhauser G, Berek C. Development of antibody diversity in single germinal centers: selective expansion of high-affinity variants. *Eur J Immunol* 1994;24:2393–2400.

257. Berek C, Berger A, Apel M. Maturation of the immune response in germinal centers. *Cell* 1991;67:1121–1129.

258. Coico RF, Bhogal BS, Thorbecke GJ. Relationship of germinal centers in lymphoid tissue to immunologic memory. VI. Transfer of B cell memory with lymph node cells fractionated according to their receptors for peanut agglutinin. *J Immunol* 1983;131:2254–2257.

259. MacLennan IC. Germinal centers. *Annu Rev Immunol* 1994;12:117–139.

260. Ahmed R, Gray D. Immunological memory and protective immunity: understanding their relation. *Science* 1996;272:54–60.

261. Jacob J, Kassir R, Kelsoe G. *In situ* studies of the primary immune response to (4-hydroxy-3-nitrophenyl)acetyl. I. The architecture and dynamics of responding cell populations. *J Exp Med* 1991;173:1165–1175.

262. Han S, Zheng B, Schatz DG, et al. Neoteny in lymphocytes: Rag1 and Rag2 expression in germinal center B cells. *Science* 1996;274:2094–2097.

263. Butcher EC, Reichert RA, Coffman RL, et al. Surface phenotype and migratory capability of Peyer's patch germinal center cells. *Adv Exp Med Biol* 1982;149:765–772.

264. Reichert RA, Gallatin WM, Weissman IL, et al. Germinal center B cells lack homing receptors necessary for normal lymphocyte recirculation. *J Exp Med* 1983;157:813–827.

265. Kelsoe G. Life and death in germinal centers (redux). *Immunity* 1996;4:107–111.

266. Pascual V, Liu YJ, Magalski A, et al. Analysis of somatic mutation in five B cell subsets of human tonsil. *J Exp Med* 1994;180:329–339.

267. McHeyzer-Williams MG, McLean MJ, Nossal GJ, et al. The dynamics of T cell–dependent B cell responses *in vivo*. *Immunol Cell Biol* 1992;70:119–127.

268. McHeyzer-Williams MG, McLean MJ, Lalor PA, et al. Antigen-driven B cell differentiation *in vivo*. *J Exp Med* 1993;178:295–307.

269. Kimoto H, Nagaoka H, Adachi Y, et al. Accumulation of somatic hypermutation and antigen-driven selection in rapidly cycling surface Ig+ germinal center (GC) B cells which occupy GC at a high frequency during the primary anti-hapten response in mice. *Eur J Immunol* 1997;27:268–279.

270. Hennino A, Berard M, Krammer PH, et al. FLICE-inhibitory protein is a key regulator of germinal center B cell apoptosis. *J Exp Med* 2001;193:447–458.

271. Han S, Zheng B, Dal Porto J, et al. *In situ* studies of the primary immune response to (4-hydroxy-3-nitrophenyl)acetyl. IV. Affinity-dependent, antigen-driven B cell apoptosis in germinal centers as a mechanism for maintaining self-tolerance. *J Exp Med* 1995;182:1635–1644.

272. Kepler TB, Perelson AS. Cyclic re-entry of germinal center B cells and the efficiency of affinity maturation. *Immunol Today* 1993;14:412–415.

273. Jacob J, Przylepa J, Miller C, et al. *In situ* studies of the primary immune response to (4-hydroxy-3-nitrophenyl)acetyl. III. The kinetics of V region mutation and selection in germinal center B cells. *J Exp Med* 1993;178:1293–1307.

274. Wu X, Jiang N, Fang YF, et al. Impaired affinity maturation in Cr2−/− mice is rescued by adjuvants without improvement in germinal center development. *J Immunol* 2000;165:3119–3127.

275. Rife U. Antigenically-induced changes in lymph nodes during the primary antibody response. *Int Arch Allergy Appl Immunol* 1969;36:538–545.

276. Horie K, Hoshi H, Hamano K, et al. Morphological changes in the mouse popliteal lymph node after local injection of dextran sulfate. *Tohoku J Exp Med* 1994;172:175–193.

277. Kiyono H, Bienenstock J, McGhee JR, et al. The mucosal immune system: features of inductive and effector sites to consider in mucosal immunization and vaccine development. *Reg Immunol* 1992;4:54–62.

278. Peyer JC. *Exercitatio anatomico-medica de usu et affectionibus. Cui subjungitur anatome ventriculi galliinacei.* Scafusae, Switzerland: Onophrius et Waldkeirch, 1677.

279. Cornes JS. Peyer's patches in the human gut. *Proc R Soc Med* 1965;58:716.

280. Van Kruiningen HJ, West AB, Freda BJ, et al. Distribution of Peyer's patches in the distal ileum. *Inflamm Bowel Dis* 2002;8:180–185.

281. Friedberg SH, Weissman IL. Lymphoid tissue architecture. II. Ontogeny of peripheral T and B cells in mice: evidence against Peyer's patches as the site of generation of B cells. *J Immunol* 1974;113:1477–1492.

282. Sminia T, Janse EM, Plesch BE. Ontogeny of Peyer's patches of the rat. *Anat Rec* 1983;207:309–316.

283. Binns RM, Licence ST. Patterns of migration of labelled blood lymphocyte subpopulations: evidence for two types of Peyer's patch in the young pig. *Adv Exp Med Biol* 1985;186:661–668.

284. Makala LH, Kamada T, Nishikawa Y, et al. Ontogeny of pig discrete Peyer's patches: distribution and morphometric analysis. *Pathobiology* 2000;68:275–282.

285. Reynolds J, Pabst R, Bordmann G. Evidence for the existence of two distinct types of Peyer's patches in sheep. *Adv Exp Med Biol* 1985;186:101–109.

286. Neutra MR, Mantis NJ, Krachenbuhl JP. Collaboration of epithelial cells with organized mucosal lymphoid tissues. *Nat Immunol* 2001;2:1004–1009.

287. Owen RL, Cray WC, Jr., Ermak TH, et al. Bacterial characteristics and follicle surface structure: their roles in Peyer's patch uptake and transport of *Vibrio cholerae*. *Adv Exp Med Biol* 1988;237:705–715.

288. Frey A, Giannasca KT, Weltzin R, et al. Role of the glycocalyx in regulating access of microparticles to apical plasma membranes of

intestinal epithelial cells: implications for microbial attachment and oral vaccine targeting. *J Exp Med* 1996;184:1045–1059.

289. Owen RL. Uptake and transport of intestinal macromolecules and microorganisms by M cells in Peyer's patches—a personal and historical perspective. *Semin Immunol* 1999;11:157–163.

290. Jones BD, Ghori N, Falkow S. *Salmonella typhimurium* initiates murine infection by penetrating and destroying the specialized epithelial M cells of the Peyer's patches. *J Exp Med* 1994;180: 15–23.

291. Iwasaki A, Kelsall BL. Unique functions of CD11b+, CD8 alpha+, and double-negative Peyer's patch dendritic cells. *J Immunol* 2001; 166:4884–4890.

292. Fotopoulos G, Harari A, Michetti P, et al. Transepithelial transport of HIV-1 by M cells is receptor-mediated. *Proc Natl Acad Sci U S A* 2002;99:9410–9414.

293. Kerneis S, Bogdanova A, Kraehenbuhl JP, et al. Conversion by Peyer's patch lymphocytes of human enterocytes into M cells that transport bacteria. *Science* 1997;277:949–952.

294. Ouzilou L, Caliot E, Pelletier I, et al. Poliovirus transcytosis through M-like cells. *J Gen Virol* 2002;83:2177–2182.

295. Mantis NJ, Cheung MC, Chintalacharuvu KR, et al. Selective adherence of IgA to murine Peyer's patch M cells: evidence for a novel IgA receptor. *J Immunol* 2002;169:1844–1851.

296. Pellas TC, Weiss L. Migration pathways of recirculating murine B cells and CD4+ and CD8+ T lymphocytes. *Am J Anat* 1990;187: 355–373.

297. Yamamoto M, Rennert P, McGhee JR, et al. Alternate mucosal immune system: organized Peyer's patches are not required for IgA responses in the gastrointestinal tract. *J Immunol* 2000;164:5184–5191.

298. Myrvik QN, Racz P, Racz KT. Ultrastructural studies on bronchial-associated lymphoid tissue (BALT) and lymphoepithelium in pulmonary cell–mediated reactions in the rabbit. *Adv Exp Med Biol* 1979;121B:145–153.

299. Gehrke I, Pabst R. The epithelium overlying rabbit bronchus-associated lymphoid tissue does not express the secretory component of immunoglobulin A. *Cell Tissue Res* 1990;259:397–399.

300. Kolopp-Sarda MN, Bene MC, Massin N, et al. Immunohistological analysis of macrophages, B-cells, and T-cells in the mouse lung. *Anat Rec* 1994;239:150–157.

301. Pabst R. Is BALT a major component of the human lung immune system? *Immunol Today* 1992;13:119–122.

302. van Kempen MJ, Rijkers GT, Van Cauwenberge PB. The immune response in adenoids and tonsils. *Int Arch Allergy Immunol* 2000;122: 8–19.

303. Hellings P, Jorissen M, Ceuppens JL. The Waldeyer's ring. *Acta Otorhinolaryngol Belg* 2000;54:237–241.

304. Baekkevold ES, Jahnsen FL, Johansen FE, et al. Culture characterization of differentiated high endothelial venule cells from human tonsils. *Lab Invest* 1999;79:327–336.

305. van der Ven I, Sminia T. The development and structure of mouse nasal-associated lymphoid tissue: an immuno- and enzyme-histochemical study. *Reg Immunol* 1993;5:69–75.

306. Heritage PL, Underdown BJ, Arsenault AL, et al. Comparison of murine nasal-associated lymphoid tissue and Peyer's patches. *Am J Respir Crit Care Med* 1997;156:1256–1262.

307. Wu HY, Nikolova EB, Beagley KW, et al. Induction of antibody-secreting cells and T-helper and memory cells in murine nasal lymphoid tissue. *Immunology* 1996;88:493–500.

308. Brown AR. Immunological functions of splenic B lymphocytes. *Crit Rev Immunol* 1992;11:395–417.

309. Salazar-Mather TP, Ishikawa R, Biron CA. NK cell trafficking and cytokine expression in splenic compartments after IFN induction and viral infection. *J Immunol* 1996;157:3054–3064.

310. Dokun AO, Chu DT, Yang L, et al. Analysis of *in situ* NK cell responses during viral infection. *J Immunol* 2001;167:5286–5293.

311. Manz RA, Arce S, Cassese G, et al. Humoral immunity and long-lived plasma cells. *Curr Opin Immunol* 2002;14:517–521.

312. Koyama K. Hemodynamics of the spleen in Banti's syndrome. *Tohoku J Exp Med* 1967;93:199–217.

313. Yamauchi H. Estimation of blood flow in the Banti spleen on anatomical basis. *Tohoku J Exp Med* 1968;95:63–77.

314. Martin F, Kearney JF. B-cell subsets and the mature preimmune repertoire. Marginal zone and B1 B cells as part of a "natural immune memory." *Immunol Rev* 2000;175:70–79.

315. Kraal G, Janse M. Marginal metallophilic cells of the mouse spleen identified by a monoclonal antibody. *Immunology* 1986;58:665–669.

316. Geijtenbeek TB, Groot PC, Nolte MA, et al. Marginal zone macrophages express a murine homologue of DC-SIGN that captures blood-borne antigens *in vivo*. *Blood* 2002;100:2908–2916.

317. Kraal G, Schornagel K, Streeter PR, et al. Expression of the mucosal vascular addressin, MAdCAM-1, on sinus-lining cells in the spleen. *Am J Pathol* 1995;147:763–771.

318. Steiniger B, Barth P, Hellinger A. The perifollicular and marginal zones of the human splenic white pulp: do fibroblasts guide lymphocyte immigration? *Am J Pathol* 2001;159:501–512.

319. Grayson MH, Chaplin DD, Karl IE, et al. Confocal fluorescent intravital microscopy of the murine spleen. *J Immunol Methods* 2001;256:55–63.

320. Lu TT, Cyster JG. Integrin-mediated long-term B cell retention in the splenic marginal zone. *Science* 2002;297:409–412.

321. Kelsoe G. The germinal center: a crucible for lymphocyte selection. *Semin Immunol* 1996;8:179–184.

322. Karrer Y, Althage A, Odermatt B, et al. On the key role of secondary lymphoid organs in antiviral immune responses studied in alymphoplastic (aly/aly) and spleenless (hox11(−/−)) mutant mice. *J Exp Med* 1997;185:2157–2170.

323. Fu Y-X, Chaplin DD. Development and maturation of secondary lymphoid tissues. *Annu Rev Immunol* 1999;17:399–433.

324. Searle AG. The genetics and morphology of two "luxoid" mutants in the house mouse. *Genet Res* 1964;5:171–197.

325. Suto J, Wakayama T, Imamura K, et al. Incomplete development of the spleen and the deformity in the chimeras between asplenic mutant (dominant hemimelia) and normal mice. *Teratology* 1995;52:71–77.

326. Suto J, Wakayama T, Imamura K, et al. Skeletal malformations caused by the Dh (dominant hemimelia) gene in mice. *Exp Anim* 1996;45:95–98.

327. Martin GR, Richman M, Reinsch S, et al. Mapping of the two mouse engrailed-like genes: close linkage of En-1 to dominant hemimelia (Dh) on chromosome 1 and of En-2 to hemimelic extra-toes (Hx) on chromosome 5. *Genomics* 1990;6:302–308.

328. Higgins M, Hill RE, West JD. Dominant hemimelia and En-1 on mouse chromosome 1 are not allelic. *Genet Res* 1992;60:53–60.

329. Wlodarski K, Morrison K, Michowski D. The effect of dominant hemimelia (Dh) genes on the number of mast cells in lymph nodes. *Folia Biol (Praha)* 1982;28:254–258.

330. Roberts CW, Shutter JR, Korsmeyer SJ. Hox11 controls the genesis of the spleen. *Nature* 1994;368:747–749.

331. Dear TN, Colledge WH, Carlton MB, et al. The Hox11 gene is essential for cell survival during spleen development. *Development* 1995;121:2909–2915.

332. Hatano M, Roberts CW, Minden M, et al. Deregulation of a homeobox gene, HOX11, by the t(10;14) in T cell leukemia. *Science* 1991;253:79–82.

333. Roberts CW, Sonder AM, Lumsden A, et al. Development expression of Hox11 and specification of splenic cell fate. *Am J Pathol* 1995;146:1089–1101.

334. Kanzler B, Dear TN. Hox11 acts cell autonomously in spleen development and its absence results in altered cell fate of mesenchymal spleen precursors. *Dev Biol* 2001;234:231–243.

335. Apelqvist A, Ahlgren U, Edlund H. Sonic hedgehog directs specialised mesoderm differentiation in the intestine and pancreas. *Curr Biol* 1997;7:801–804.

336. Lettice LA, Purdie LA, Carlson GJ, et al. The mouse bagpipe gene controls development of axial skeleton, skull, and spleen. *Proc Natl Acad Sci U S A* 1999;96:9695–9700.

337. Tribioli C, Lufkin T. The murine Bapx1 homeobox gene plays a critical role in embryonic development of the axial skeleton and spleen. *Development* 1999;126:5699–5711.

338. Herzer U, Crocoll A, Barton D, et al. The Wilms tumor suppressor gene wt1 is required for development of the spleen. *Curr Biol* 1999;9:837–840.

339. Lu J, Chang P, Richardson JA, et al. The basic helix-loop-helix transcription factor capsulin controls spleen organogenesis. *Proc Natl Acad Sci U S A* 2000;97:9525–9530.

340. Matsumoto M, Yamada T, Yoshinaga SK, et al. Essential role of NF-kappa B–inducing kinase in T cell activation through the TCR/CD3 pathway. *J Immunol* 2002;169:1151–1158.

341. Karrer U, Althage A, Odermatt B, et al. Immunodeficiency of alymphoplasia mice (aly/aly) *in vivo:* structural defect of secondary lymphoid organs and functional B cell defect. *Eur J Immunol* 2000;30:2799–2807.

342. Yasumizu R, Miyawaki S, Koba M, et al. Pathology of ALY mice: congenital immunodeficiency with lymph node and Peyer's patch defects. *Immunobiology* 2000;202:213–225.

343. Koike R, Nishimura T, Yasumizu R, et al. The splenic marginal zone is absent in alymphoplastic aly mutant mice. *Eur J Immunol* 1996;26:669–675.

344. Nishimura T, Koike R, Miyasaka M. Mammary glands of Aly mice: developmental changes and lactation-related expression of specific proteins, alpha-casein, GLyCAM-1 and MAdCAM-1. *Am J Reprod Immunol* 2000;43:351–358.

345. Itoh M, Miyamoto K, Ooga T, et al. Spontaneous accumulation of eosinophils and macrophages throughout the stroma of the epididymis and vas deferens in alymphoplasia (aly) mutant mice: I. A histological study. *Am J Reprod Immunol* 1999;42:246–253.

346. Suzuki H, Jeong KI, Doi K. Regional variations in the distribution of small intestinal intraepithelial lymphocytes in alymphoplasia (aly/aly) mice and heterozygous (aly/+) mice. *Immunol Invest* 2001;30:303–312.

347. Malinin NL, Boldin MP, Kovalenko AV, et al. MAP3K-related kinase involved in NF-kappaB induction by TNF, CD95 and IL-1. *Nature* 1997;385:540–544.

348. Woronicz JD, Gao X, Cao Z, et al. IkappaB kinase-beta: NF-kappaB activation and complex formation with IkappaB kinase-alpha and NIK. *Science* 1997;278:866–869.

349. Lin X, Mu Y, Cunningham ET, Jr., et al. Molecular determinants of NF-kappaB–inducing kinase action. *Mol Cell Biol* 1998;18:5899–5907.

350. Kriegler M, Perez C, DeFay K, et al. A novel form of TNF/cachectin is a cell surface cytotoxic transmembrane protein: ramifications for the complex physiology of TNF. *Cell* 1988;53:45–53.

351. Black RA, Rauch CT, Kozlosky CJ, et al. A metalloproteinase disintegrin that releases tumour-necrosis factor-alpha from cells. *Nature (London)* 1997;385:729–733.

352. Moss ML, Jin S-LC, Milla ME, et al. Cloning of a disintegrin metalloproteinase that processes precursor tumour-necrosis factor-alpha. *Nature (London)* 1997;385:733–736.

353. Gray PW, Aggarwal BB, Benton CV, et al. Cloning and expression of cDNA for human lymphotoxin, a lymphokine with tumour necrosis activity. *Nature* 1984;312:721–724.

354. Ruddle NH. Tumor necrosis factor (TNF-α) and lymphotoxin (TNF-β). *Curr Opin Immunol* 1992;4:327–332.

355. Browning JL, Androlewicz MJ, Ware CF. Lymphotoxin and an associated 33-kDa glycoprotein are expressed on the surface of an activated human T cell hybridoma. *J Immunol* 1991;147:1230–1237.

356. Browning JL, Ngam-ek A, Lawton P, et al. Lymphotoxin β, a novel member of the TNF family that forms a heteromeric complex with lymphotoxin on the cell surface. *Cell* 1993;72:847–856.

357. Lawton P, Nelson J, Tizard R, et al. Characterization of the mouse lymphotoxin-beta gene. *J Immunol* 1995;154:239–246.

358. Pokholok DK, Maroulakou IG, Kuprash DV, et al. Cloning and expression analysis of the murine lymphotoxin beta gene. *Proc Natl Acad Sci U S A* 1995;92:674–678.

359. Crowe PD, VanArsdale TL, Walter BN, et al. A lymphotoxin-β-specific receptor. *Science* 1994;264:707–710.

360. Ware CF, VanArsdale TL, Crowe PD, et al. The ligands and receptors of the lymphotoxin system. *Curr Top Microbiol Immunol* 1995;198:175–218.

361. De Togni P, Goellner J, Ruddle NH, et al. Abnormal development of peripheral lymphoid organs in mice deficient in lymphotoxin. *Science* 1994;264:703–707.

362. Banks TA, Rouse BT, Kerley MK, et al. Lymphotoxin α–deficient mice. Effects on secondary lymphoid organ development and humoral immune responsiveness. *J Immunol* 1995;155:1685–1693.

363. Fu Y-X, Huang G, Matsumoto M, et al. Independent signals regulate development of primary and secondary follicle structure in spleen and mesenteric lymph node. *Proc Natl Acad Sci U S A* 1997;94:5739–5743.

364. Matsumoto M, Mariathasan S, Nahm MH, et al. Role of lymphotoxin and type I TNF receptor in the formation of germinal centers. *Science* 1996;271:1289–1291.

365. Matsumoto M, Lo SF, Carruthers CJ, et al. Affinity maturation without germinal centers in lymphotoxin-α (LTα) deficient mice. *Nature* 1996;382:462–466.

366. Amiot F, Bellkaid Y, Lebastard M, et al. Abnormal organisation of the splenic marginal zone and the correlated leukocytosis in lymphotoxin-alpha and tumor necrosis factor alpha double deficient mice. *Eur Cytokine Netw* 1996;7:733–739.

367. Korner H, Winkler TH, Sedgwick JD, et al. Recirculating and marginal zone B cell populations can be established and maintained independently of primary and secondary follicles. *Immunol Cell Biol* 2001;79:54–61.

368. Wu Q, Wang Y, Wang J, et al. The requirement of membrane lymphotoxin for the presence of dendritic cells in lymphoid tissues. *J Exp Med* 1999;190:629–638.

369. Alimzhanov MB, Kuprash DV, Kosco-Vilbois MH, et al. Abnormal development of secondary lymphoid tissues in lymphotoxin-β–deficient mice. *Proc Natl Acad Sci U S A* 1997;94:9302–9307.

370. Koni PA, Sacca R, Lawton P, et al. Distinct roles in lymphoid organogenesis for lymphotoxins alpha and beta revealed in lymphotoxin beta–deficient mice. *Immunity* 1997;6:491–500.

371. Futterer A, Mink K, Luz A, et al. The lymphotoxin β receptor controls organogenesis and affinity maturation in peripheral lymphoid tissues. *Immunity* 1998;9:59–70.

372. Rennert PD, Browning JL, Mebius R, et al. Surface lymphotoxin α/β complex is required for the development of peripheral lymphoid organs. *J Exp Med* 1996;184:1999–2006.

373. Rennert PD, Browning JL, Hochman PS. Selective disruption of lymphotoxin ligands reveals a novel set of mucosal lymph nodes and unique effects on lymph node cellular organization. *Int Immunol* 1997;9:1627–1639.

374. Mariathasan S, Matsumoto M, Baranyay F, et al. Absence of lymph nodes in lymphotoxin-α (LTα)–deficient mice is due to abnormal organ development, not defective lymphocyte migration. *J Inflamm* 1995;45:72–78.

375. Fu Y-X, Molina H, Matsumoto M, et al. Lymphotoxin-α supports development of splenic follicular structure that is required for IgG responses. *J Exp Med* 1997;185:2111–2120.

376. Ettinger R, Browning JL, Michie SA, et al. Disrupted splenic architecture, but normal lymph node development in mice expressing soluble lymphotoxin-beta receptor–IgG1 Fc chimeric fusion protein. *Proc Natl Acad Sci U S A* 1996;93:13102–13107.

377. Mackay F, Browning JL. Turning off follicular dendritic cells. *Nature* 1998;395:26–27.

378. Fu Y-X, Huang G, Wang Y, et al. B lymphocytes induce the formation of follicular dendritic cell clusters in a lymphotoxin-α dependent fashion. *J Exp Med* 1998;187:1009–1018.

379. Gonzalez M, Mackay F, Browning JL, et al. The sequential role of lymphotoxin and B cells in the development of splenic follicles. *J Exp Med* 1998;187:997–1007.

380. Ansel KM, Ngo VN, Hyman PL, et al. A chemokine-driven positive feedback loop organizes lymphoid follicles. *Nature* 2000;406:309–314.

381. Ngo VN, Cornall RJ, Cyster JG. Splenic T zone development is B cell dependent. *J Exp Med* 2001;194:1649–1660.

382. Mauri DN, Ebner R, Montgomery RI, et al. LIGHT, a new member of the TNF superfamily, and lymphotoxin α are ligands for herpesvirus entry mediator. *Immunity* 1998;8:21–30.

383. Pitti RM, Marsters SA, Lawrence DA, et al. Genomic amplification of a decoy receptor for Fas ligand in lung and colon cancer. *Nature* 1998;396:699–703.

384. Hsu TL, Chang YC, Chen SJ, et al. Modulation of dendritic cell differentiation and maturation by decoy receptor 3. *J Immunol* 2002;168:4846–4853.

385. Scheu S, Alferink J, Potzel T, et al. Targeted disruption of LIGHT causes defects in costimulatory T cell activation and reveals cooperation with lymphotoxin beta in mesenteric lymph node genesis. *J Exp Med* 2002;195:1613–1624.

386. Le Hir M, Bluethmann H, Kosco-Vilbois MH, et al. Tumor necrosis factor receptor-1 signaling is required for differentiation of follicular dendritic cells, germinal center formation, and full antibody responses. *J Inflamm* 1995;47:76–80.

387. Le Hir M, Bluethmann H, Kosco-Vilbois MH, et al. Differentiation of follicular dendritic cells and full antibody responses require

tumor necrosis factor receptor-1 signaling. *J Exp Med* 1996;183:2367–2372.

388. Neumann B, Luz A, Pfeffer K, et al. Defective Peyer's patch organogenesis in mice lacking the 55-kD receptor for tumor necrosis factor. *J Exp Med* 1996;184:259–264.

389. Pasparakis M, Alexopoulou L, Grell M, et al. Peyer's patch organogenesis is intact yet formation of B lymphocyte follicles is defective in peripheral lymphoid organs of mice deficient for tumor necrosis factor and its 55-kDa receptor. *Proc Natl Acad Sci U S A* 1997;94:6319–6323.

390. Pasparakis M, Alexopoulou L, Episkopou V, et al. Immune and inflammatory responses in TNF alpha-deficient mice: a critical requirement for TNF alpha in the formation of primary B cell follicles, follicular dendritic cell networks and germinal centers, and in the maturation of the humoral immune response. *J Exp Med* 1996;184:1397–1411.

391. Ruuls SR, Hoek RM, Ngo VN, et al. Membrane-bound TNF supports secondary lymphoid organ structure but is subservient to secreted TNF in driving autoimmune inflammation. *Immunity* 2001;15:533–543.

392. Pasparakis M, Kousteni S, Peschon J, et al. Tumor necrosis factor and the p55TNF receptor are required for optimal development of the marginal sinus and for migration of follicular dendritic cell precursors into splenic follicles. *Cell Immunol* 2000;201:33–41.

393. Mandik-Nayak L, Huang G, Sheehan KC, et al. Signaling through TNF receptor p55 in TNF-alpha–deficient mice alters the CXCL13/CCL19/CCL21 ratio in the spleen and induces maturation and migration of anergic B cells into the B cell follicle. *J Immunol* 2001;167:1920–1928.

394. Eugster HP, Muller M, Karrer U, et al. Multiple immune abnormalities in tumor necrosis factor and lymphotoxin-alpha double–deficient mice. *Int Immunol* 1996;8:23–36.

395. Wang Y, Huang G, Wang J, et al. Antigen persistence is required for somatic mutation and affinity maturation of immunoglobulin. *Eur J Immunol* 2000;30:2226–2234.

396. Dougall WC, Glaccum M, Charrier K, et al. RANK is essential for osteoclast and lymph node development. *Genes Dev* 1999;13:2412–2424.

397. Kong YY, Yoshida H, Sarosi I, et al. OPGL is a key regulator of osteoclastogenesis, lymphocyte development and lymph-node organogenesis. *Nature* 1999;397:315–323.

398. Franzoso G, Carlson L, Poljak L, et al. Mice deficient in nuclear factor (NF)-kappa B/p52 present with defects in humoral responses, germinal center reactions, and splenic microarchitecture. *J Exp Med* 1998;187:147–159.

399. Paxian S, Merkle H, Riemann M, et al. Abnormal organogenesis of Peyer's patches in mice deficient for NF-kappaB1, NF-kappaB2, and Bcl-3. *Gastroenterology* 2002;122:1853–1868.

400. Naito A, Azuma S, Tanaka S, et al. Severe osteopetrosis, defective interleukin-1 signalling and lymph node organogenesis in TRAF6-deficient mice. *Genes Cells* 1999;4:353–362.

401. Cao X, Shores EW, Hu-Li J, et al. Defective lymphoid development in mice lacking expression of the common cytokine receptor γ chain. *Immunity* 1995;2:223–238.

402. Leonard WJ, Shores EW, Love PE. Role of the common cytokine receptor gamma chain in cytokine signaling and lymphoid development. *Immunol Rev* 1995;148:97–114.

403. Nosaka T, van Deursen JM, Tripp RA, et al. Defective lymphoid development in mice lacking Jak3. *Science* 1995;270:800–802.

404. Park SY, Saijo K, Takahashi T, et al. Developmental defects of lymphoid cells in Jak3 kinase–deficient mice. *Immunity* 1995;3:771–782.

405. Thomis DC, Gurniak CB, Tivol E, et al. Defects in B lymphocyte maturation and T lymphocyte activation in mice lacking Jak3. *Science* 1995;270:794–797.

406. Sun Z, Unutmaz D, Zou YR, et al. Requirement for RORgamma in thymocyte survival and lymphoid organ development. *Science* 2000;288:2369–2373.

407. Kurebayashi S, Ueda E, Sakaue M, et al. Retinoid-related orphan receptor gamma (RORgamma) is essential for lymphoid organogenesis and controls apoptosis during thymopoiesis. *Proc Natl Acad Sci U S A* 2000;97:10132–10137.

408. Harmsen A, Kusser K, Hartson L, et al. Cutting edge: organogenesis of nasal-associated lymphoid tissue (NALT) occurs independently of lymphotoxin-alpha (LT alpha) and retinoic acid receptor–related orphan receptor-gamma, but the organization of NALT is LT alpha dependent. *J Immunol* 2002;168:986–990.

409. Cupedo T, Kraal G, Mebius RE. The role of CD45+CD4+CD3– cells in lymphoid organ development. *Immunol Rev* 2002;189:41–50.

410. Forster R, Mattis AE, Kremmer E, et al. A putative chemokine receptor, BLR1, directs B cell migration to defined lymphoid organs and specific anatomic compartments of the spleen. *Cell* 1996;87:1037–1047.

411. Mebius RE, Rennert P, Weissman IL. Developing lymph nodes collect CD4$^+$CD3$^-$ LTβ^+ cells that can differentiate to APC, NK cells, and follicular cells but not T or B cells. *Immunity* 1997;7:493–504.

412. Honda K, Nakano H, Yoshida H, et al. Molecular basis for hematopoietic/mesenchymal interaction during initiation of Peyer's patch organogenesis. *J Exp Med* 2001;193:621–630.

413. Adachi S, Yoshida H, Honda K, et al. Essential role of IL-7 receptor alpha in the formation of Peyer's patch anlage. *Int Immunol* 1998;10:1–6.

414. Mebius R, Akashi K. Precursors to neonatal lymph nodes: LT beta+CD45+CD4+CD3– cells are found in fetal liver. *Curr Top Microbiol Immunol* 2000;251:197–201.

415. Adachi S, Yoshida H, Kataoka H, et al. Three distinctive steps in Peyer's patch formation of murine embryo. *Int Immunol* 1997;9:507–514.

416. Yoshida H, Honda K, Shinkura R, et al. IL-7 receptor alpha+ CD3(−) cells in the embryonic intestine induces the organizing center of Peyer's patches. *Int Immunol* 1999;11:643–655.

417. Fukuyama S, Hiroi T, Yokota Y, et al. Initiation of NALT organogenesis is independent of the IL-7R, LTbetaR, and NIK signaling pathways but requires the Id2 gene and CD3(−)CD4(+)CD45(+) cells. *Immunity* 2002;17:31–40.

418. Kim D, Mebius RE, MacMicking JD, et al. Regulation of peripheral lymph node genesis by the tumor necrosis factor family member TRANCE. *J Exp Med* 2000;192:1467–1478.

419. Yokota Y, Mansouri A, Mori S, et al. Development of peripheral lymphoid organs and natural killer cells depends on the helix-loop-helix inhibitor Id2. *Nature* 1999;397:702–706.

420. Georgopoulos K, Bigby M, Wang JH, et al. The Ikaros gene is required for the development of all lymphoid lineages. *Cell* 1994;79:143–156.

421. Wang JH, Nichogiannopoulou A, Wu L, et al. Selective defects in the development of the fetal and adult lymphoid system in mice with an Ikaros null mutation. *Immunity* 1996;5:537–549.

422. Sabin FR. On the origin of the lymphatic system from the veins and the development of the lymph hearts and thoracic ducts in the pig. *Am J Anat* 1902;1:367–389.

423. Sabin FR. The lymphatic system in human embryos, with a consideration of the morphology of the system as a whole. *Am J Anat* 1909;9:43–91.

424. Eikelenboom P, Nassy JJ, Post J, et al. The histogenesis of lymph nodes in rat and rabbit. *Anat Rec* 1978;190:201–215.

425. Bailey RP, Weiss L. Ontogeny of human fetal lymph nodes. *Am J Anat* 1975;142:15–27.

426. Rennert PD, James D, Mackay F, et al. Lymph node genesis is induced by signaling through the lymphotoxin beta receptor. *Immunity* 1998;9:71–79.

427. Picarella DE, Kratz A, Li CB, et al. Insulitis in transgenic mice expressing tumor necrosis factor beta (lymphotoxin) in the pancreas. *Proc Natl Acad Sci U S A* 1992;89:10036–10040.

428. Armengol MP, Juan M, Lucas-Martin A, et al. Thyroid autoimmune disease: demonstration of thyroid antigen-specific B cells and recombination-activating gene expression in chemokine-containing active intrathyroidal germinal centers. *Am J Pathol* 2001;159:861–873.

429. Knecht H, Saremaslani P, Hedinger C. Immunohistological findings in Hashimoto's thyroiditis, focal lymphocytic thyroiditis and thyroiditis de Quervain. Comparative study. *Virchows Arch A Pathol Anat Histol* 1981;393:215–231.

430. Harris NL. Lymphoid proliferations of the salivary glands. *Am J Clin Pathol* 1999;111:S94–103.

431. Aziz KE, McCluskey PJ, Wakefield D. Characterisation of follicular dendritic cells in labial salivary glands of patients with primary Sjogren syndrome: comparison with tonsillar lymphoid follicles. *Ann Rheum Dis* 1997;56:140–143.

432. Shiono H, Fujii Y, Okumura M, et al. Failure to down-regulate Bcl-2 protein in thymic germinal center B cells in myasthenia gravis. *Eur J Immunol* 1997;27:805–809.

433. Murai H, Hara H, Hatae T, et al. Expression of CD23 in the germinal center of thymus from myasthenia gravis patients. *J Neuroimmunol* 1997;76:61–69.

434. Krenn V, Souto-Carneiro MM, Kim HJ, et al. Histopathology and molecular pathology of synovial B-lymphocytes in rheumatoid arthritis. *Histol Histopathol* 2000;15:791–798.

435. Berek C, Kim HJ. B-cell activation and development within chronically inflamed synovium in rheumatoid and reactive arthritis. *Semin Immunol* 1997;9:261–268.

436. Kim HJ, Berek C. B cells in rheumatoid arthritis. *Arthritis Res* 2000;2:126–131.

437. Weyand CM, Klimiuk PA, Goronzy JJ. Heterogeneity of rheumatoid arthritis: from phenotypes to genotypes. *Springer Semin Immunopathol* 1998;20:5–22.

438. Takemura S, Braun A, Crowson C, et al. Lymphoid neogenesis in rheumatoid synovitis. *J Immunol* 2001;167:1072–1080.

439. Eidt S, Stolte M. Prevalence of lymphoid follicles and aggregates in Helicobacter pylori gastritis in antral and body mucosa. *J Clin Pathol* 1993;46:832–835.

440. Steere AC, Duray PH, Butcher EC. Spirochetal antigens and lymphoid cell surface markers in Lyme synovitis. Comparison with rheumatoid synovium and tonsillar lymphoid tissue. *Arthritis Rheum* 1988;31: 487–495.

441. Fan L, Reilly CR, Luo Y, et al. Cutting edge: ectopic expression of the chemokine TCA4/SLC is sufficient to trigger lymphoid neogenesis. *J Immunol* 2000;164:3955–3959.

442. Luther SA, Bidgol A, Hargreaves DC, et al. Differing activities of homeostatic chemokines CCL19, CCL21, and CXCL12 in lymphocyte and dendritic cell recruitment and lymphoid neogenesis. *J Immunol* 2002;169:424–433.

443. Nishikawa SI, Hashi H, Honda K, et al. Inflammation, a prototype for organogenesis of the lymphopoietic/hematopoietic system. *Curr Opin Immunol* 2000;12:342–345.

444. Weyand CM, Kurtin PJ, Goronzy JJ. Ectopic lymphoid organogenesis: a fast track for autoimmunity. *Am J Pathol* 2001;159:787–793.

445. Gowans JL, Knight EJ. The route of recirculation of lymphocytes in the rat. *Proc R Soc Lond B Biol* 1964;159:257–282.

446. Smith ME, Ford WL. The recirculating lymphocyte pool of the rat: a systematic description of the migratory behaviour of recirculating lymphocytes. *Immunology* 1983;49:83–94.

447. Butcher EC, Picker LJ. Lymphocyte homing and homeostasis. *Science* 1996;272:60–66.

448. Sprent J, Schaefer M, Hurd M, et al. Mature murine B and T cells transferred to SCID mice can survive indefinitely and many maintain a virgin phenotype. *J Exp Med* 1991;174:717–728.

449. Butcher EC, Scollay RG, Weissman IL. Organ specificity of lymphocyte migration: mediation by highly selective lymphocyte interaction with organ-specific determinants on high endothelial venules. *Eur J Immunol* 1980;10:556–561.

450. Butcher EC. Leukocyte-endothelial cell recognition: three (or more) steps to specificity and diversity. *Cell* 1991;67:1033–1036.

451. Shimizu Y, Newman W, Tanaka Y, et al. Lymphocyte interactions with endothelial cells. *Immunol Today* 1992;13:106–112.

452. Springer TA. Traffic signals for lymphocyte recirculation and leukocyte emigration: the multistep paradigm. *Cell* 1994;76:301–314.

453. von Andrian UH, Chambers JD, McEvoy LM, et al. Two-step model of leukocyte-endothelial cell interaction in inflammation: distinct roles for LECAM-1 and the leukocyte beta 2 integrins *in vivo*. *Proc Natl Acad Sci U S A* 1991;88:7538–7542.

454. Lawrence MB, Berg EL, Butcher EC, et al. Rolling of lymphocytes and neutrophils on peripheral node addressin and subsequent arrest on ICAM-1 in shear flow. *Eur J Immunol* 1995;25:1025–1031.

455. Bargatze RF, Jutila MA, Butcher EC. Distinct roles of L-selectin and integrins alpha 4 beta 7 and LFA-1 in lymphocyte homing to Peyer's patch-HEV *in situ:* the multistep model confirmed and refined. *Immunity* 1995;3:99–108.

456. Arbones ML, Ord DC, Ley K, et al. Lymphocyte homing and leukocyte rolling and migration are impaired in L-selectin–deficient mice. *Immunity* 1994;1:247–260.

457. Wagner N, Lohler J, Kunkel EJ, et al. Critical role for beta7 integrins in formation of the gut-associated lymphoid tissue. *Nature* 1996; 382:366–370.

458. Bargatze RF, Butcher EC. Rapid G protein-regulated activation event involved in lymphocyte binding to high endothelial venules. *J Exp Med* 1993;178:367–372.

459. Streeter PR, Rouse BT, Butcher EC. Immunohistologic and functional characterization of a vascular addressin involved in lymphocyte homing into peripheral lymph nodes. *J Cell Biol* 1988;107:1853–1862.

460. Streeter PR, Berg EL, Rouse BT, et al. A tissue-specific endothelial cell molecule involved in lymphocyte homing. *Nature* 1988;331:41–46.

461. Xu J, Grewal IS, Geba GP, et al. Impaired primary T cell responses in L-selectin–deficient mice. *J Exp Med* 1996;183:589–598.

462. Warnock RA, Askari S, Butcher EC, et al. Molecular mechanisms of lymphocyte homing to peripheral lymph nodes. *J Exp Med* 1998; 187:205–216.

463. Hamann A, Jablonski-Westrich D, Duijvestijn A, et al. Evidence for an accessory role of LFA-1 in lymphocyte-high endothelium interaction during homing. *J Immunol* 1988;140:693–699.

464. Schmits R, Kundig TM, Baker DM, et al. LFA-1–deficient mice show normal CTL responses to virus but fail to reject immunogenic tumor. *J Exp Med* 1996;183:1415–1426.

465. Spangrude GJ, Braaten BA, Daynes RA. Molecular mechanisms of lymphocyte extravasation. I. Studies of two selective inhibitors of lymphocyte recirculation. *J Immunol* 1984;132:354–362.

466. Ma Q, Jones D, Borghesani PR, et al. Impaired B-lymphopoiesis, myelopoiesis, and derailed cerebellar neuron migration in CXCR4- and SDF-1–deficient mice. *Proc Natl Acad Sci U S A* 1998;95:9448–9453.

467. Gunn MD, Kyuwa S, Tam C, et al. Mice lacking expression of secondary lymphoid organ chemokine have defects in lymphocyte homing and dendritic cell localization. *J Exp Med* 1999;189:451–460.

468. Luther SA, Tang HL, Hyman PL, et al. Coexpression of the chemokines ELC and SLC by T zone stromal cells and deletion of the ELC gene in the plt/plt mouse. *Proc Natl Acad Sci U S A* 2000;97:12694–12699.

469. Okada T, Ngo VN, Ekland EH, et al. Chemokine requirements for B cell entry to lymph nodes and Peyer's patches. *J Exp Med* 2002;196: 65–75.

470. Wang HU, Chen ZF, Anderson DJ. Molecular distinction and angiogenic interaction between embryonic arteries and veins revealed by ephrin-B2 and its receptor Eph-B4. *Cell* 1998;93:741–753.

CHAPTER 15

Dendritic Cells

Muriel Moser

Discovery and Definition
Distribution of Dendritic Cells *In Vivo*: a Multimember Family
Langerhans Cells · Interstitial Dendritic Cells · Veiled Cells · Dendritic Cell Precursors · Monocyte-Derived Dendritic Cells · Plasmacytoid-Derived Dendritic Cells
Hallmarks of Cells from the Dendritic Family
Co-Stimulation and Adhesion · The Process of Maturation · Antigen Uptake · Antigen Processing · Migratory Properties · Cytokine Release
Dendritic Cells and T-Cell–Mediated Immunity
Immunostimulatory Properties *In Vitro* · Adoptive Transfer · Dendritic Cells as Physiological Adjuvant · T-Cell/Dendritic Cell Synapses · Antigen-Independent Clustering · Adjuvants · Immune Escape
Dendritic Cells and the Polarization of the Immune Response
Role of Antigen-Presenting Cells · Polarizing Dendritic Cell–Derived Cytokines · Mechanisms of Dendritic Cell Polarization
Dendritic Cells and T-Cell Tolerance
Central Tolerance · Peripheral Tolerance
Dendritic Cells and B-Cell Activation
Dendritic Cells and Natural Killer Cells
Dendritic Cells and Natural Killer T Cells
Dendritic Cell–Based Immunotherapy for Cancer
Conclusions
Acknowledgments
References

DISCOVERY AND DEFINITION

In the 1960s, several research groups demonstrated that a population of adherent cells was required for the induction of B- and T-cell responses *in vitro* and *in vivo*. Most immunologists believed at that time that macrophages were the critical "accessory" cells, on the basis of their adherent properties (1).

In 1973, during the course of observations of murine splenic cells that adhere to glass and plastic surfaces, Steinman and Cohn (2) noticed large stellate cells whose cytoplasm was arranged in pseudopods of varying length and form. These authors reported that these cells, named *dendritic cells* (DCs) because of their branch-like projections (from δενδρεον, tree), undergo characteristic movements, do not exhibit the endocytic capacities of macrophages, and adhere to glass. The function of DCs was elucidated 5 years later when it was reported that these cells were the most potent stimulators of the primary mixed leukocyte reaction in mice, which led to the suggestion that DCs instead of macrophages could be the accessory cells required in the generation of many immune responses (3). This hypothesis was amply demonstrated in the following years.

The dendritic family includes many members located throughout the body that share phenotypic and functional properties:

- Dendritic morphology (at least at some stage) and low buoyant density
- Elevated expression of major histocompatibility complex (MHC) molecules (class I and class II) and intermediate to high expression of co-stimulatory molecules
- Motility
- Specialization of function over time: that is, a shift from an antigen-capturing mode to a T-cell sensitizing mode

The hallmark of the DC family is the conversion of these cells from immature sentinels to mature immunostimulatory cells, a phenomenon called *maturation*.

455

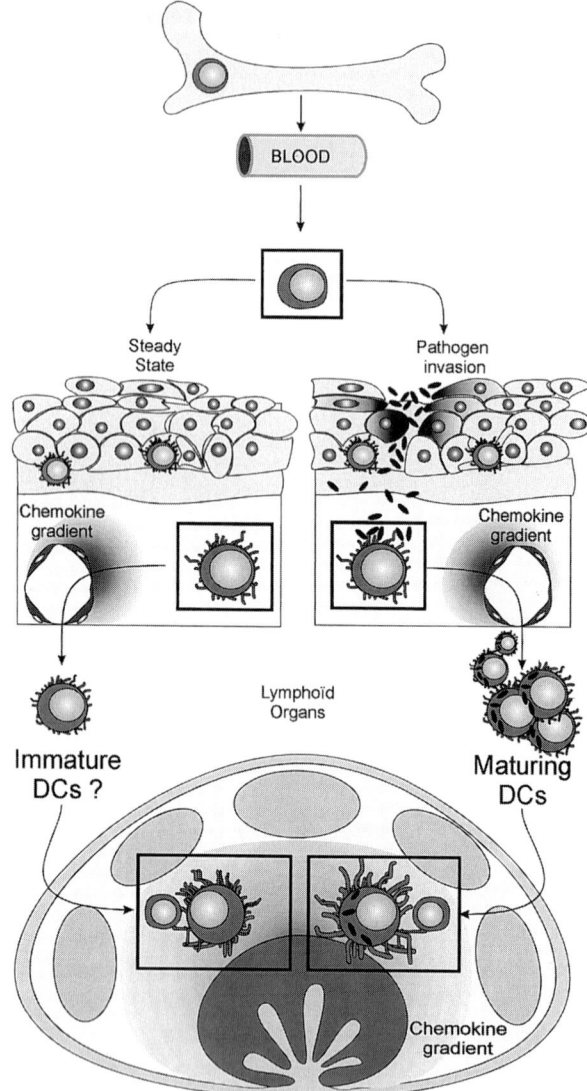

FIG. 1. Developmental stages of dendritic cells (DCs) *in vivo*. The generation of DC precursors in the bone marrow, the recruitment of immature DCs in peripheral tissues, and the migration of DCs into the lymphoid organs are illustrated. The maturation of DCs into potent antigen-presenting cells in case of infection or inflammation and their migration have been amply documented (**right**), but there is also evidence that in the "steady state"—that is, in the absence of a "danger signal"—these immature DCs may migrate into the lymphoid organs while remaining at the immature stage (**left**). The phenotype of the DC migrating in baseline conditions is still unclear. The movement of maturing DCs and the "constitutive" migration of immature DCs have been shown to depend on chemokine gradients.

Figure 1 illustrates the development of DCs *in vivo* at the precursor, immature, and mature stages. The right column corresponds to the induction of DC maturation by a "danger signal" (pathogen invasion), and their subsequent migration to lymphoid organs. The left column describes the movement of (presumably immature) DCs at the steady state. These pathways are described in the following chapters.

DISTRIBUTION OF DENDRITIC CELLS *IN VIVO*: A MULTIMEMBER FAMILY

CD34$^+$ hematopoietic stem cells differentiate into common myeloid progenitors (CMP) and common lymphoid progenitors (CLP) in the bone marrow (Fig. 2). The CMP give rise to two types of *immature DCs* (CD11c$^+$CD14$^+$ and CD11c$^+$CD14$^-$ in humans, undefined in mice) that become interstitial DCs and Langerhans cells when homing to epithelia or other tissues, respectively. The CMP also give rise to two types of *DC precursors,* monocytes and plasmacytoid cells, which play a role in innate and adaptive immunity and undergo differentiation and maturation in the presence of cytokines or microbial products (Fig. 2) (4). In contrast to monocytes, DCs can also arise from a CLP *in vivo,* as clearly demonstrated in the mouse (5). In particular, splenic DCs of CD8α$^+$ and CD8α$^-$ phenotypes can be generated from CMP or CLP *in vivo.* Although human DCs can be generated *in vitro* from lymphoid-committed precursors, the physiological differentiation from CLP *in vivo* is still a matter of speculation (6). There is some evidence that human plasmacytoid–derived DCs may be related to lymphoid lineage, inasmuch as they express messenger ribonucleic acid (mRNA) specific for lymphocytes as pre-Tα, immunoglobulin (Ig) λ–like 14.1, and Spi-B (7).

The four main DC populations differ by their phenotype (Table 1) and function (see the following sections).

Langerhans Cells

Cells with a dendritic structure were visualized in the skin by Paul Langerhans in 1868. They were described as cells displaying long processes and were considered to belong to the nervous system. The nature of these so-called Langerhans cells remained obscure until they were shown to be derived from bone marrow and to express class II MHC and were identified as the active cells in epidermis for presenting antigen to T cells (8–10). The relationship of these epidermal Langerhans cells to DCs was suggested by the observations that murine epidermal Langerhans cells mature into potent immunostimulatory DCs *in vitro* (11).

Ultrastructurally, Langerhans cells are characterized by a unique pentalamellar cytoplasmic organelle: the Birbeck granule. Valladeau et al. (12) identified a type II Ca^{2+}-dependent lectin displaying mannose-binding specificity, exclusively expressed by Langerhans cells. This lectin was called *langerin* and is constitutively associated with Birbeck granules. Although the role of Birbeck granules remains enigmatic, they are attractive candidate receptors for nonconventional antigen routing in Langerhans cells. Because the lectin domain of langerin recognizes mannose, antigens bearing this sugar, which is common on microorganisms, may be internalized into Birbeck granules after their binding to langerin. In addition, Langerhans cells express E-cadherin,

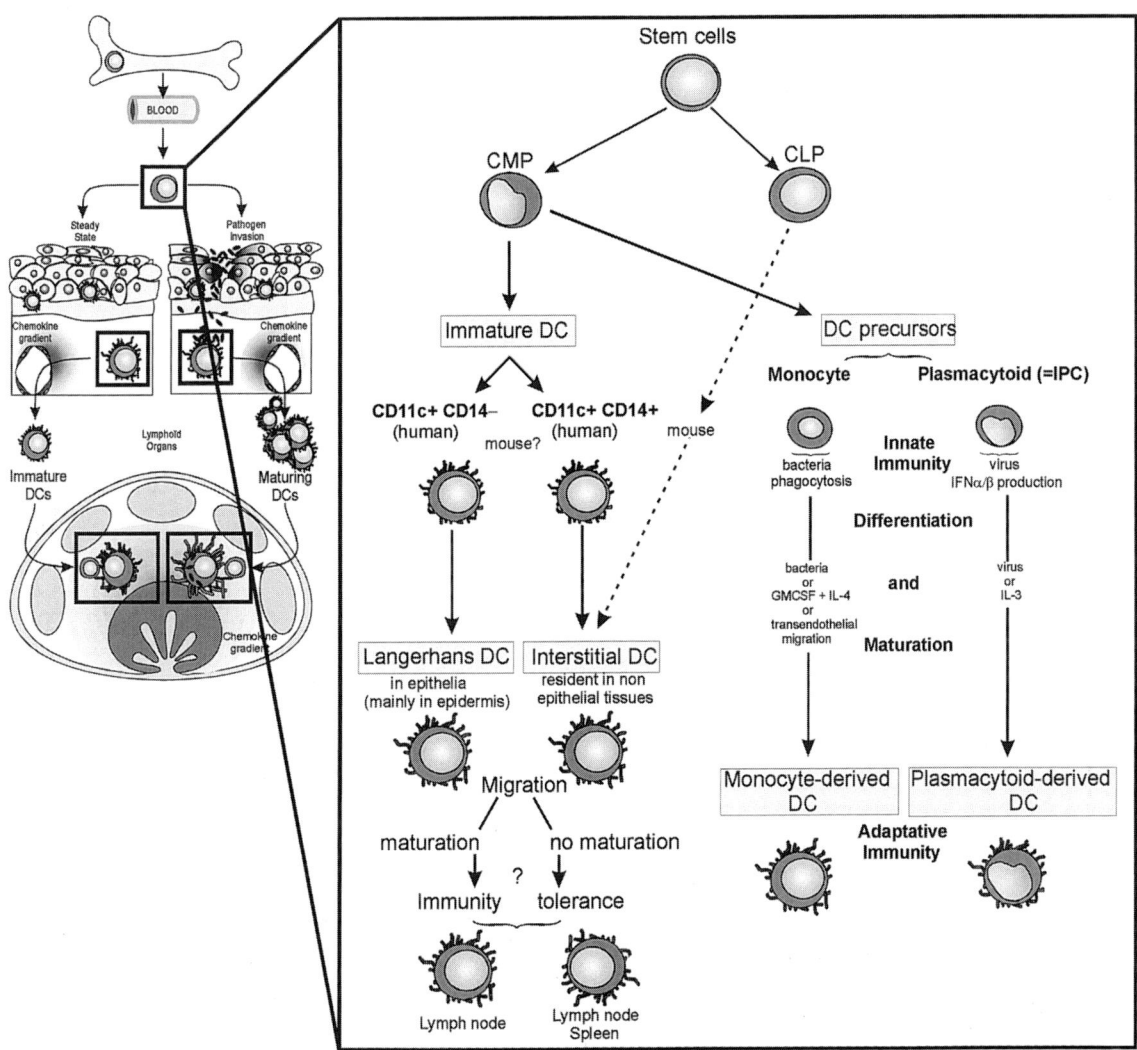

FIG. 2. Dendritic cell (DC) development and diversification in mice and humans. Common myeloid progenitors (CMP) and common lymphoid progenitors (CLP) are generated in the bone marrow. The CMP give rise to two types of immature DCs and two types of DC precursors: monocytes and plasmacytoid cells. *Immature DCs* migrate to epithelia or other tissues, where they become Langerhans cells or interstitial DCs, respectively. These tissue-resident DCs may further migrate at the immature or the mature state to lymphoid organs, where they may perform different functions. *DC precursors* are monocytes and plasmacytoid cells that may differentiate into mature DCs in the presence of indicated stimuli and play a role in innate and adaptive immunity.

which permits, through homotypic interactions, the residence of Langerhans cells in epidermis.

Interstitial Dendritic Cells

DCs are found as immature cells in virtually all organs (except the brain) within the interstitial spaces that are drained by afferent lymphatic vessels. DCs have been isolated from the heart, kidney, dermis, liver, and other organs.

DCs are found in mucosal surfaces, such as those of the lung and intestine. In the lung, the network of airway DCs is particularly well developed to capture inhaled antigens (13). Its location above the basement membrane of the airway epithelium ensures accessibility to inhaled antigens. There

is some evidence that these DCs are maintained in an immature state by an inhibitory mechanism that may involve macrophages (14,15). In the intestine, DCs from Peyer's patches have been characterized and are known to contain three populations that differ by their phenotype and function (16,17).

In the mouse, all splenic DCs express similar amounts of CD11c, class II MHC, and co-stimulatory molecules CD80, CD86, and CD40, but they can be subdivided into three subtypes on the basis of their expression of CD4 and the CD8α homodimer: CD8α^-CD4$^-$, CD8α^-CD4$^+$, and CD8α^+CD4$^-$ (18). The subsets also differ by their localization: the majority of DCs in the marginal zone are CD8α^-, whereas most DCs in the T-cell areas express the CD8α

TABLE 1. *Dendritic cell lineages and their phenotypes in mouse and humans*

Characteristic	Mouse	Human
Common phenotype	MHC classes I and II$^{lo/high}$, CD80$^{lo/high}$, CD86$^{lo/high}$, CD40$^{lo/high}$, [for review, see references (6,216)]	MHC classes I and II$^{lo/high}$, CD80$^{lo/high}$, CD86$^{lo/high}$, CD40$^{lo/high}$
Langerhans cells	CD11c$^+$, Birbeck granules$^+$, E-cadherin$^+$, Langerin$^+$, DEC205$^+$, CD11b$^+$, CD4$^+$ (subset), CD8α^-, 33D1$^-$ (subset)	CD11c$^+$, CD11b$^+$, CD13$^+$, CD33$^+$, CD4$^+$, CD1a$^+$, Birbeck granules$^+$, Langerin$^+$, DC-LAMP$^+$, IL-3R$^{+/-}$
Interstitial dendritic cells	CD11c$^+$, Birbeck granules$^-$, E-cadherin$^-$, Langerin$^-$, DEC205$^+$ (subset), CD11b$^+$ (subset), CD8α^+ (subset)	CD11c$^+$, CD11b$^+$, CD13$^+$, CD33$^+$, CD4$^+$, CD1a$^-$, Birbeck granule$^-$, DC-LAMP$^+$, IL-3R$^-$
Monocyte-derived dendritic cells		
Cytokines *in vitro*	CD11c$^+$, CD54$^+$, DEC-205$^+$, CD4$^+$ (26)	CD11c$^+$, CD11b$^+$, CD1$^+$, CD13$^+$, CD33$^+$, CD44$^+$, ICAM-1$^+$, CD14$^-$ (24)
Transendothelial migration *in vitro*		CD14$^-$, CD32$^-$, CD64$^-$, CD11b$^-$, CD83$^{+/-}$, CD1a$^-$ (25)
Transendothelial migration *in vivo*	CD11c^{lo}, MIDC8$^+$, 2A1$^+$, DEC-205$^+$ (subset), B220$^-$, CD8α^- (27)	
Plasmacytoid-derived dendritic cells	CD11c^{lo}, CD8α^+ (fraction), CD11b$^-$, Ly6C/Gr1$^+$, B220$^+$, CD54$^+$, DEC205^{lo} (29,30)	CD11c$^-$, IL-3R$^+$, CD11b$^-$, CD4$^+$, CD1a$^-$, CD13$^-$, CD33$^-$, DC-Lamp$^+$ (23)

MHC, major histocompatibility complex.

homodimer. The three splenic DC subtypes seem to behave as rapidly turning-over products of three independent developmental lineages (19). The DC populations in lymph nodes appear to be even more complex. In addition to the three populations present in the spleen, two DC subtypes that may be dermal and epidermal derived DCs (20) have been described. The mouse thymus (18) has been shown to contain two DC types that differ at the level of CD8α expression.

The DCs localized in the T-cell areas of lymphoid organs are called *interdigitating cells,* because they extend numerous processes between the T cells.

Veiled Cells

Typical DCs are found in afferent lymphatic vessels and are called veiled cells because of their sheetlike appearance. Early studies underscored the crucial role of the afferent lymphatics during cell-mediated immunity: priming to skin transplants were shown to be blocked by lymphatic ablation (21). In contrast, efferent lymphatic vessels seem to lack DCs, which suggests that they do not leave the lymph nodes. Indeed, there is evidence that mature DCs undergo apoptosis in the lymphoid organ (22).

Dendritic Cell Precursors

Stem cells also give rise to two types of DC precursors: monocytes [also called pre-DC1s after their functional properties (23)] and plasmacytoid cells (also named pre-DC2s), which do not have dendrites and do not display the phenotype and function of DCs but seem to serve as effector cells in antimicrobial innate immunity. Monocytes and plasmacytoid cells have the capacity to differentiate in culture into DCs. The monocyte- and plasmacytoid-derived DCs display distinct functional properties and, in particular, differentially regulate the development of T helper 1 and 2 (Th1 and Th2) cells *in vitro* (detailed later).

Monocyte-Derived Dendritic Cells

Human monocytes have been shown to differentiate into DCs in culture with granulocyte-macrophage colony-stimulating factor (GM-CSF) and interleukin (IL)–4 (24), as well as in an *in vitro* model of transendothelial migration that involves a layer of endothelial cells over a collagen matrix. Monocytes migrate across the endothelial barrier onto collagen matrix, mimicking entry of monocytes into tissues, and become tissue macrophages. Of note, some transmigrate back across the endothelial barrier, mimicking transit from tissues to lymph, and become DCs. The process is markedly enhanced if particulate material is phagocytosed in the collagen matrix (25). Murine monocytes have been shown to differentiate into DCs when cultured in the presence of GM-CSF and IL-4 (26). Furthermore, Randolph et al. investigated the differentiation and trafficking *in vivo* of inflammatory monocytes that phagocytosed subcutaneously injected fluorescent microspheres. They found that most of the monocytes became macrophages in the subcutaneous tissue but that 25% of latex$^+$ cells migrated to the T-cell area of draining lymph nodes, where they expressed DC-restricted markers and high levels of co-stimulatory molecules (27). The various pathways of differentiation of DCs from monocytes *in vitro* and *in vivo* are illustrated in Table 1.

Plasmacytoid-Derived Dendritic Cells

CD4⁺CD11c⁻ DC precursors (pre-DC2s) with plasmacytoid structures have been identified in human blood and are
identical to natural interferon (IFN) α/β–producing cells,
which secrete high amounts of IFN-α/β in response to
viruses. These plasmacytoid cells give rise to DC2s *in vitro*
in the presence of IL-3 or during viral infection. IFN-α/β and
tumor necrosis factor (TNF-) α produced by virus-activated
pre-DC2s act as an autocrine survival factor and a DC differentiation factor, respectively (28). These cells appear therefore to play a role in innate immune responses as IFN-α
producers and in adaptive immune responses as antigen-
presenting cells (APCs).

The equivalent murine type of type I IFN-producing cells
(mIPCs) has been described only as recently as 2001 and consists of a population of immature DCs Ly6C/Gr-1⁺, B220⁺,
CD11cˡᵒ, and CD4⁺ (29,30), showing a homogeneous plasmacytoid structure—that is, a round shape, a smooth surface,
and an eccentric nucleus. Upon activation, these cells display
a more irregular shape, up-regulate their immunostimulatory
properties, and produce IFN-α, IL-12, or both, depending on
the stimulus.

HALLMARKS OF CELLS FROM THE DENDRITIC FAMILY

Among the populations of APCs, which include DCs,
B-lymphocytes, and macrophages, DCs display some unique
properties aimed at sensitizing T-lymphocytes specific for
dangerous antigens encountered earlier in periphery. Indeed,
pathogens often invade peripheral tissues, whereas the immune response is initiated in lymphoid structures in which
T- and B-lymphocytes reside (31). DCs appear to form a
physical link between the periphery and the secondary lymphoid organs: they act as sentinels for "dangerous" antigens
in the peripheral tissues and then migrate to the areas where
T cells are located to transmit information about the nature of
the pathogen and the infected tissues. To efficiently perform
these different tasks, DCs have a specialization of function
over time and location. During the process of maturation, often associated with their migration from the periphery to the
lymphoid organs, DCs shift from an antigen-capturing mode
to a T cell–sensitizing mode. The maturation process is induced by microbial products and inflammatory chemokines,
thereby favoring the sensitization of T-lymphocytes specific for non–self-infectious antigens (Fig. 3). The following

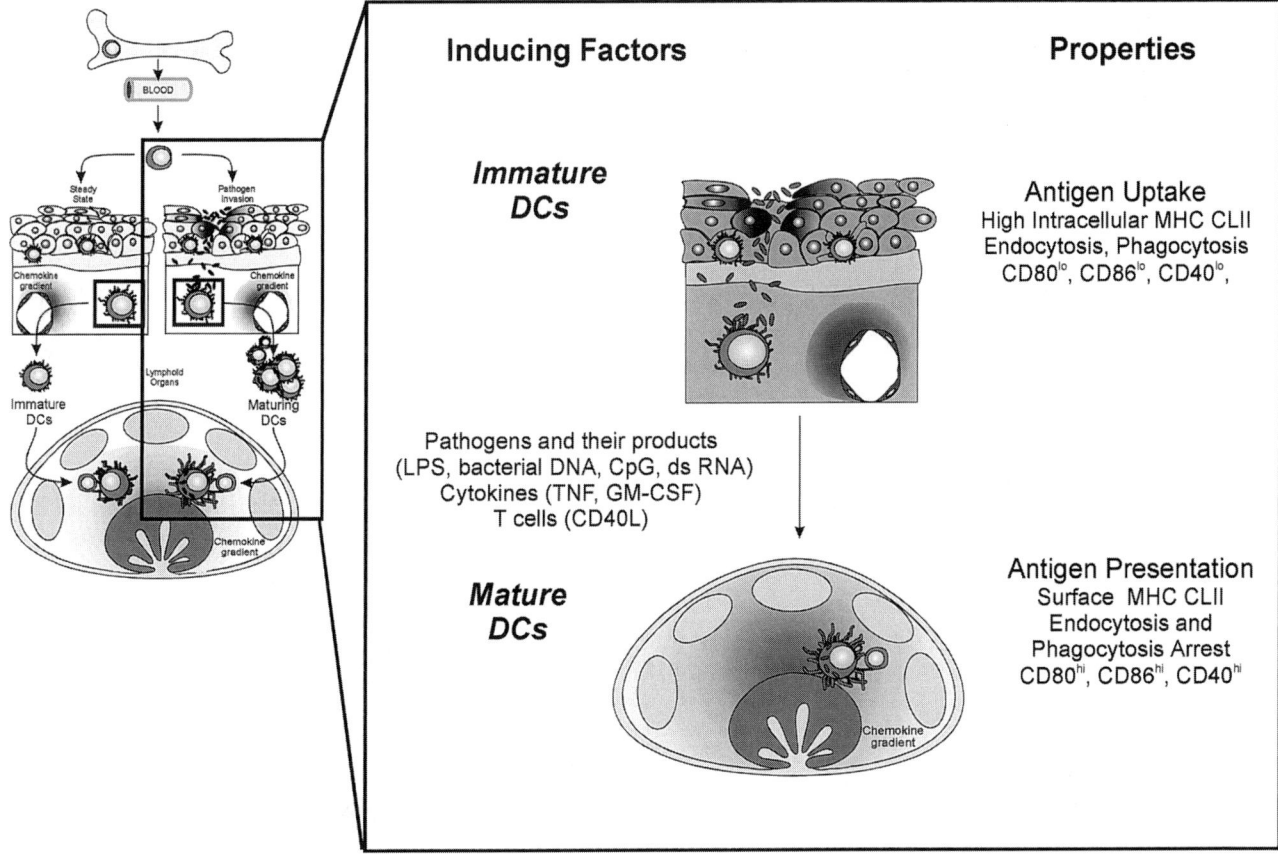

FIG. 3. The phenomenon of maturation. In the presence of inflammatory cytokines, microbial products or
antigen-activated T-lymphocytes, dendritic cells undergo a phenomenon of maturation: that is, they shift
from an antigen-capturing mode to a T cell–sensitizing mode. The phenotypic and functional changes
are associated with their migration into the T-cell area of lymphoid organs.

sections review the properties of DCs that confer on them the capability to focus the adaptive immune response on pathogens, avoiding autoimmunity.

Co-Stimulation and Adhesion

To recognize antigen, T cells need to establish contact with APCs by forming an immunological synapse, in which T-cell receptors (TCRs) and co-stimulatory molecules are congregated in a central area surrounded by a ring of adhesion molecules. The zone contains multiple copies of molecular couples, such as the TCR and peptide/MHC, leukocyte function–associated antigen 1 (LFA-1) and intercellular adhesion molecule 1 (ICAM-1), CD2 and CD48, and CD28 and ligands (Fig. 4).

The B7 family has been shown to contain six members, which positively or negatively regulate the expansion or function of T cells, or both [for review, see Coyle and Gutierrez-Ramos (32)]. The CD80 and CD86 molecules, the first CD28 ligands, have been shown to promote clonal expansion of resting T cells through CD28 and to inhibit T-cell expansion through interactions with CTLA-4. The biological role of CD80 may be to generate stable signaling complexes with CTLA-4 to terminate T-cell activation. The expression of CD80 and CD86 is strongly up-regulated during DC maturation (33,34). B7RP-1 has been shown to be expressed by human but not murine DCs. Its expression is down-regulated during activation, and its counterreceptor is inducible co-stimulator (ICOS). Evidence is emerging that B7RP-1

delivers a critical signal that favors Th2 production. PD-L1 (or B7-H1) and PD-L2 interact with programmed death 1 (PD-1) on T cells and function similarly in their ability to oppose T-cell activation and attenuate cytokine production. The most newly discovered member, B7-H3, is expressed at high levels on immature DCs and seems to regulate IFN-γ production by T cells.

Of note, the CD86 co-stimulatory molecule is not only abundant on DCs but also associates with antigen-presenting MHC products in stable patches on the DC surface. The polyvalent configuration may facilitate the activation of quiescent T cells (35).

Other molecules expressed by DCs seem to be involved in co-stimulation. CD24 (heat-stable antigen, HSA) is a protein of 30- to 60-kD molecular mass with size heterogeneity resulting from variable cell type–specific glycosylation. HSA is expressed by freshly isolated Langerhans cells and, in contrast to CD80 and CD86, is down-regulated during maturation in culture. Data suggesting that HSA is required for activation of Th1 but not Th2 have been reported (36).

Several molecules belonging to the TNF superfamily appear to function as co-stimulatory molecules and include 4-1BB, OX40, and LIGHT (37).

Early studies indicated that DCs and T cells tend to form clusters in an antigen-independent manner (38). In addition to co-stimulatory molecules, adhesion molecules and their corresponding ligands—LFA-3/CD2 and LFA-1/ICAM-1, -2 or -3—are probably involved in these DC–T-cell interactions. Geijtenbeek et al. (39) developed an adhesion assay

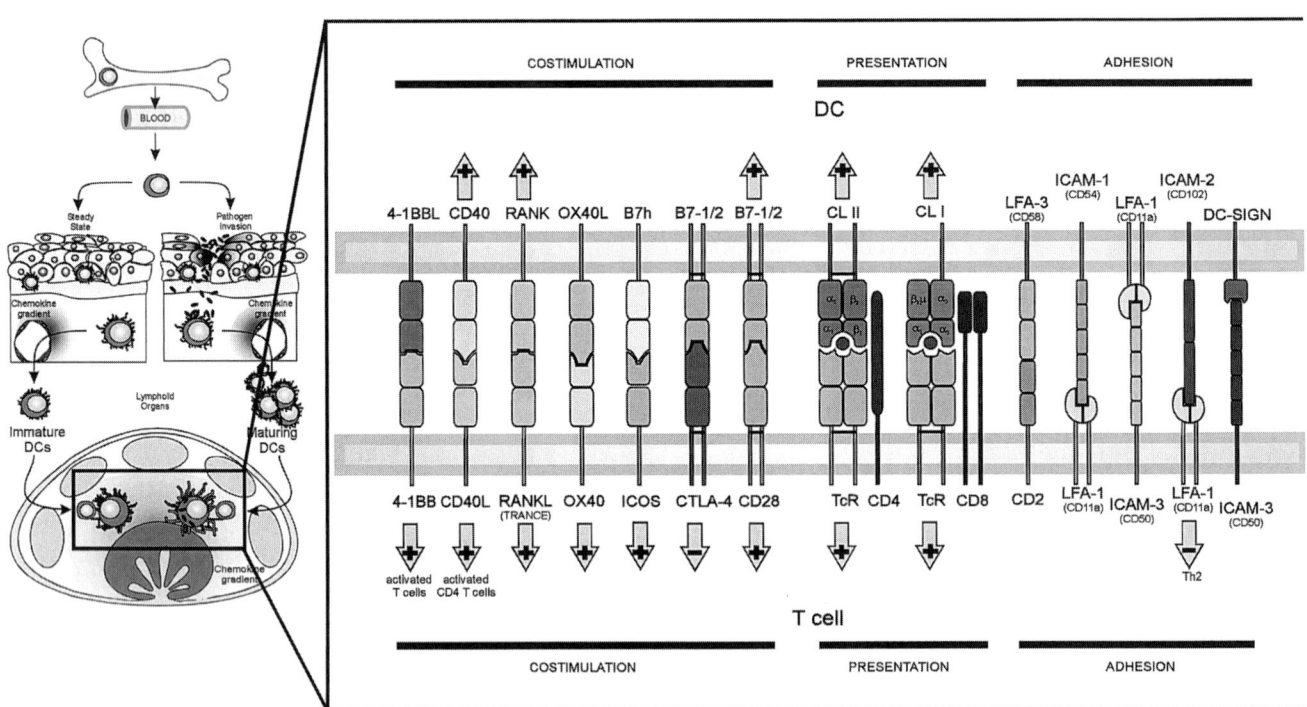

FIG. 4. Molecules involved in the T-cell/dendritic cell synapse. The interaction between dendritic cells and T-lymphocytes involves several ligand/receptor pairs that include MHC molecules, adhesion and co-stimulatory molecules.

to address the role of ICAM-3 and identified a novel DC-specific adhesion receptor. They showed that both DCs and monocytes bind to fluorescent beads coated with ICAM-3-Fc. ICAM-3 binding by monocytes is mediated mainly by LFA-1, whereas binding of ICAM-3 by DCs is completely independent of LFA-1 but dependent on a novel molecule, DC-SIGN. DC-SIGN is a type II membrane protein with an external mannose-binding, C-type lectin domain. It was named DC-SIGN because it is a *DC-s*pecific, ICAM-3–grabbing *n*onintegrin. The interaction of DC-SIGN with ICAM-3 establishes the initial contact of the DC with the resting T cells, appears restricted to DCs, and is essential for T-cell activation. In addition, DC-SIGN has been shown to be a special kind of viral receptor, promoting binding and transmission of human immunodeficiency virus type I to T cells, rather than viral entry into the DCs (40).

The Process of Maturation

The relationship of Langerhans cells to DCs isolated from lymphoid organs was provided in 1985 by Schuler and Steinman (11). The authors showed that fresh Langerhans cells are weak stimulators of T-cell proliferation but undergo a progressive increase in stimulatory capacity *in vitro*. The development of enhanced stimulatory activity during culture was called *maturation* (Fig. 3) and could not be ascribed only to an increase in the level of class II MHC molecules. The authors suggested that functioning DCs, present in lymphoid organs, may be derived from less mature precursors located in nonlymphoid tissues. By comparing the efficacy of fresh and cultured DCs to present a protein to T-cell clones, Romani et al. (41) showed that the capacity of DC populations to present proteins varies inversely with stimulating activity in the mixed leukocyte reaction (MLR). Freshly isolated Langerhans cells are very active in presenting proteins, whereas spleen DCs and cultured epidermal Langerhans cells present native protein weakly. These observations suggested that DCs in nonlymphoid tissues such as skin act as sentinels for presenting antigens *in situ*, whereas DCs in lymphoid organs have the capacity to sensitize naïve T cells.

Therefore, cells of the dendritic family have a specialization of function over time, as they shift from an antigen-capturing mode to a T cell–sensitizing mode during a process called *maturation* (Fig. 3). DC maturation induces multiple alterations in the function and intracellular transport of class II MHC molecules, leading to the redistribution of class II MHC from intracellular compartments to the plasma membrane (see later discussion). Expression of ligands for the CTLA-4/CD28 molecules was shown to be up-regulated on epidermal Langerhans cells (34) and splenic DCs (33,42) during their functional maturation *in vitro*. The process of maturation also occurs *in vivo*: Systemic administration of endotoxin [lipopolysaccharide (LPS)] induces the migration of most splenic DCs from the marginal zone between the red and white pulp to the T-cell area in the white pulp (43,44). This movement parallels a maturation process, as assessed

by down-regulation of processing capacity and up-regulation of immunostimulatory properties (44).

Maturation can be mediated by inflammatory cytokines (TNF-α, IL-1), T cells (through CD40/CD40L interaction), microbial constituents (LPS, CpG oligonucleotides), and stress (necrosis, transplantation). DC maturation has been shown to involve signaling cascades initiated by the Toll/interleukin-1 receptor homology domains of Toll-like receptor (TLR) family that can lead to activation of nuclear factor κB (NFκB) and mitogen-activated protein kinase (MAPK). TLR4 is the mammalian homolog of *Drosophila* Toll, which is involved in dorsoventral patterning and in host defense against fungal infection. To date, more than 10 members have been reported to belong to the TLR family in mammals and seem involved in recognizing pathogen-associated molecular patterns [for review, see Kaisho and Akira (45)]. Recent findings in myeloid differentiation factor 88 (MyD88)–knockout and Toll-like receptor (TLR)–knockout mice have shown that TLR4 activates two pathways: one that is MyD88 dependent and crucial for cytokine production and another that is MyD88 independent and induces phenotypic and functional maturation of DCs (45). In contrast, TLR9-mediated DC maturation and cytokine release are dependent on MyD88.

An interesting question is whether DCs stimulated through TLR ligands differentiate exclusively to "type 1" DCs, as suggested by LPS and CpG, and whether "type 2" DCs are less mature cells (see following discussion).

Antigen Uptake

At the immature stage, DCs exhibit potent endocytic activity. To sample their environment in peripheral tissues, they constitutively macropinocytose extracellular fluid and concentrate the macrosolutes in the endocytic compartment. The fluid volume taken up per hour by a single DC has been estimated to be 1,000 to 1,500 μm^3, a volume that is close to that of the cell itself (46). The large volume of fluid that is continuously taken up through macropinocytosis must be eliminated by the DCs to maintain their volume. Two mechanisms that may be involved in the volume regulatory system have been described: the amiloride-sensitive epithelial sodium channel that increases the transport of ions (46) and aquaporins that facilitate the flow of water in accordance with the salt gradient. Two members of the aquaporin family, aquaporins 3 and 7, are highly expressed in immature DCs and are down-regulated upon maturation. Blocking aquaporins inhibits uptake and concentration of macrosolutes taken up by fluid phase endocytosis but does not affect receptor-mediated endocytosis through the mannose receptor, which suggests that aquaporins are essential elements of macropinocytosis by DCs (47).

In addition, DCs express various receptors mediating endocytosis and phagocytosis of antigens, pathogens, and dying cells: crystallized fragment (Fc) receptors for IgE and IgG, which internalize immune complexes receptors for heat shock proteins; receptors, such as CD36 and avb5, which bind and phagocytose apoptotic bodies; and C-type lectins, such as macrophage mannose receptor and DEC-205 (48), which contain 8 and 10 contiguous C-type lectin domains, respectively (49). Whereas most receptors, including the macrophage mannose receptor, internalize and recycle through early endosomes, the DEC-205 cytosolic domain mediates a unique recycling pathway through late endosomes or lysosomes, rich in antigen-presenting class II MHC products, and greatly enhances antigen presentation relative to the mannose receptor tail (50).

The antigen uptake is down-modulated during the process of maturation (46). Most receptors are expressed at lower levels on mature DCs, except DEC-205 in the mouse, which is expressed at higher levels. In addition, endocytosis and macropinocytosis are down-regulated. Garrett et al. (51) found that endocytic down-regulation reflects a decrease in endocytic activity controlled by Rho family guanosine triphosphatase Cdc42. Blocking Cdc42 function in immature DCs abrogates endocytosis, whereas injection of active Cdc42 in mature DCs reactivates endocytosis (51), which suggests that the regulation of endocytosis during maturation is at least partly controlled by the levels of active Cdc42. Another report, however, demonstrates that the Rho-family guanosine triphosphatases Cdc42 and Rac are required for constitutive macropinocytosis by DCs but do not control its regulation (52).

Whether distinct DC subpopulations present distinct pathogens is still unclear. The differential expression of TCRs on the human DC subsets could form the basis of a selective response to different pathogens. TCRs are highly conserved from *Drosophila* to humans and recognize molecular patterns specific to microbial pathogens. The pDC1 and pDC2 have been shown to express different sets of pattern-recognition receptors and show corresponding differences in reactivity to different microbial products. Monocytes (pDC1) express TLR1, TLR2, TLR4, TLR5, and TLR8 and respond to peptidoglycan, lipoteichoic acid, and LPS, whereas pDC2 express TLR7 and TLR9 and respond to CpG oligonucleotides. The CD11c interstitial DCs express TLR3 and are reactive to double-strand deoxyribonucleic acid (DNA) (53). In addition, C-type lectins appear differentially expressed on DCs, depending on the subset, activation state, and tissue localization (49).

In the mouse, Pulendran et al. (54) reported observations suggesting that LPS from different bacteria that signal through distinct TLR, may differentially activate DCs. In favor of this notion, CD8α^- and CD8α^+ DCs have been shown to respond to distinct microbial stimuli (55).

Antigen Processing

Class II Major Histocompatibility Complex–Restricted Presentation

Stimulation of naïve T- and B-lymphocytes is likely to occur in primary lymphoid organs, which are organized to favor cellular interactions. Because DCs are posted as sentinels in peripheral organs, an initial step of the immune response most probably requires the migration of DCs to the zone where lymphocytes reside. Of importance is that DCs have the unique capability to present antigens encountered earlier in periphery after they have migrated to lymphoid organs (Fig. 5). This property, a form of "antigenic memory," results from (a) a shift in class II MHC half-life in mature versus immature DCs, (b) the sequestration of class II MHC/peptide combinations intracellularly in immature DCs, and (c) a blockade of the peptide-loading step in immature DCs. Each of these is discussed as follows.

A Shift in Class II Half-Life in Mature versus Immature Dendritic Cells

Class II MHC molecules of immature DCs are expressed at low levels at the plasma membrane but are abundant in endocytic compartments. In contrast, mature DCs express high levels of class II MHC loaded with peptides at the surface. The mechanisms that control class II MHC expression in DCs are still unclear, but they are known to involve the modulation of cathepsin S activity and the rate of endocytosis. According to the first model, cathepsin S activity is inhibited by the presence of protease inhibitor cystatin C in the class II MHC compartments of immature DCs, thereby preventing the full degradation of the invariant chain. The complexes formed by the class II MHC and partly degraded invariant chain would be transported to lysosomes and degraded. In mature DCs, cystatin C would be down-regulated, thereby enabling cathepsin S to fully degrade the invariant chain and class II MHC to bind antigenic peptides and shuttle to the cell surface. These findings suggest that the ratio of cystatin C to cathepsin S in developing DCs would determine the fate of newly synthesized class II MHC molecules (56). However, the similar regulation of class II MHC expression for cathepsin S–independent class II MHC allotypes and in cathepsin S–deficient mice (57) argues against this hypothesis. The second model suggests that class II MHC expression is regulated in murine (57) and human (58) DCs by controlling the rate of endocytosis and subsequent degradation of peptide-loaded class II MHCs. In immature DCs, class II MHC molecules are rapidly internalized and recycled, turning over with a half-life of about 10 hours, whereas in mature DCs, there is a rapid and transient boost of class II MHC synthesis, and the half-life of class II MHC molecules increases over 100 hours. Indeed, in immature DCs, biotinylated Fab fragments of an anti-DR antibody bound to surface class II molecules are rapidly internalized and recycled back to the cell surface, whereas the pool of recycling class II molecules progressively disappears after maturation (58). Thus, delivery of class II MHC/peptide combinations to the cell surface would proceed similarly in immature and mature DCs, but immature DCs would reendocytose and degrade the complexes much faster than the mature DCs.

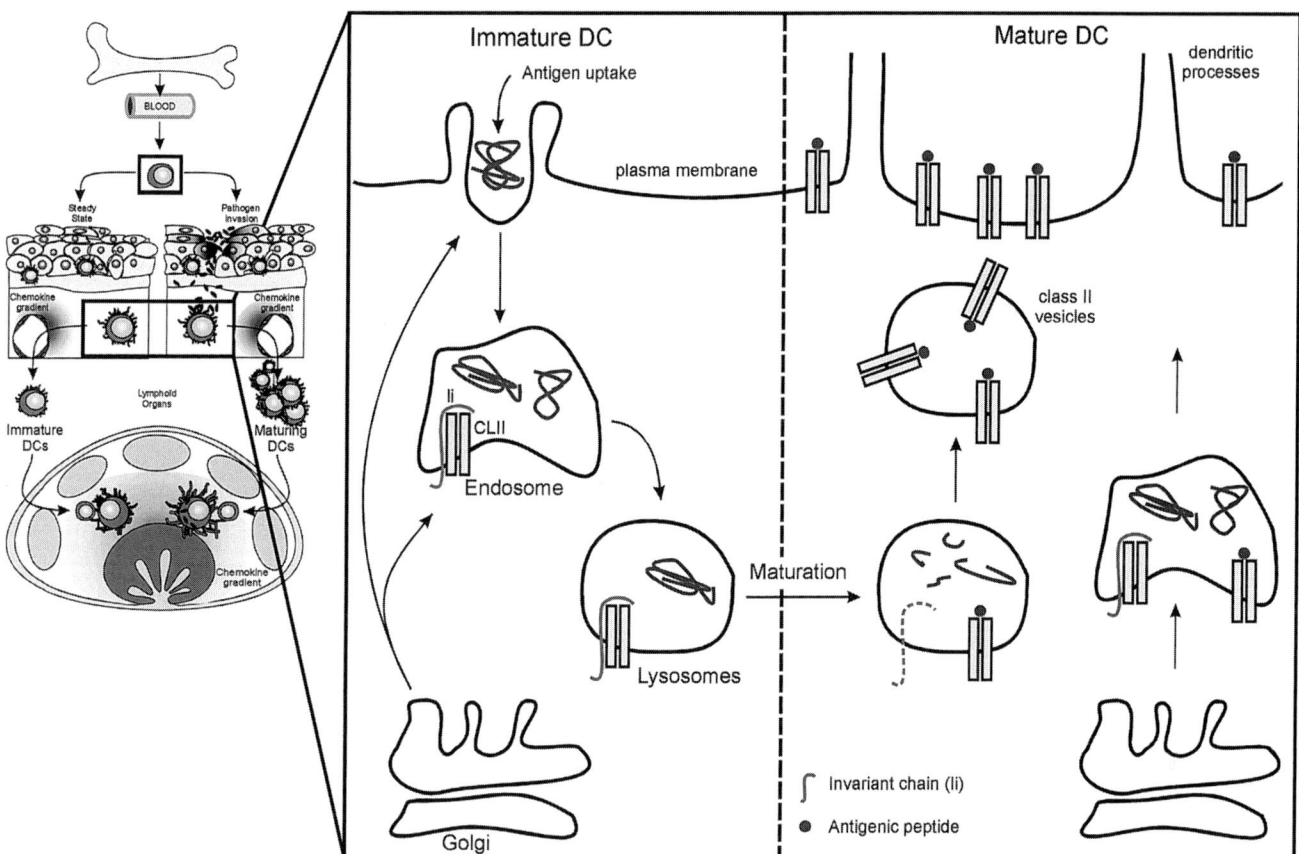

FIG. 5. Antigen handling and class II major histocompatibility complex (MHC) expression in immature and mature dendritic cells (DCs). The maturation of DCs is associated with a redistribution of class II MHC molecules from intracellular compartments to the plasma membrane. In immature DCs (**left**), class II MHC molecules are associated mainly with invariant chain and are sequestered intracellularly in lysosomes. Indeed, the activity of cathepsin S (which has a major role in the cleavage of the class II MHC–associated invariant chain) remains low, thereby slowing the processing of the invariant chain, which contains a lysosomal targeting signal in its cytoplasmic domain. Although the majority of new class II MHC molecules are targeted directly to endosomes and lysosomes upon exit from the trans-Golgi network, some class II MHC molecules also seem to reach lysosomes after endocytosis from the plasma membrane. Maturation (**right**) has been shown to enhance the peptide loading of class II MHC molecules that have accumulated in lysosomes before maturation. The peptide/MHC combinations are then transported to the class II MHC vesicles and reach the cell surface as small clusters, partly associated with CD86 (not shown). In addition, the activity of cathepsin S is enhanced, allowing a greater fraction of new class II MHC molecules to avoid lysosomes and reach the cell surface after antigen loading in endosomes. Redrawn from Mellman and Steinman (217), with permission.

The Sequestration of Class II/Peptide Combinations Intracellularly in Immature Dendritic Cells

There is evidence that immature DCs exhibit a phenotype in which most class II MHC molecules are intracellular and localized to lysosomes. Upon maturation, these cells progressively differentiate into cells in which intracellular class II MHC molecules are found in peripheral nonlysosomal vesicles and then into mature DCs that express almost all of their class II MHC molecules on the plasma membrane (35,59). Of note, although early DCs do not present antigen immediately after uptake, they efficiently present previously internalized antigen after maturation. By delaying antigen presen-

tation, DCs retain the memory of antigens encountered in the periphery.

Blockade of the Peptide-Loading Step in Immature Dendritic Cells

There is evidence that DCs also regulate the intracellular formation of immunogenic class II MCH/peptide combinations. Indeed, although a protein antigen has been shown to colocalize with class II MHC products in late endosomes and lysosomes, class II MHCs do not form unless the DCs are exposed to maturation agents. These observations suggest an arrest to antigen presentation at the peptide-loading step at the immature stage (60).

Of importance is that the down-regulation of antigen processing may help avoid induction of autoimmune reactions. Indeed, by turning off endocytosis, a mature DC arriving in the lymph node with pathogenic peptides would be unable to pick up self antigens and would present only epitopes generated at sites of infection. Of note, adjacent DCs in the T-cell area in the steady state may present self antigens and contribute to peripheral tolerance (see later discussion).

An unusual extracellular presentation pathway has been described in immature DCs. At the cell surface, these cells express empty or peptide-receptive class II MHC molecules, as well as H-2M or HLA-DM. Immature DCs may therefore use alternative pathways for loading of class II MHC molecules, in addition to the endosomal pathway (61).

Class I Major Histocompatibility Complex–Restricted Presentation

In most cells, class I MHC molecules associate exclusively with peptides derived from endogenous cytosolic proteins, such as virus-encoded proteins or tumor antigens. In contrast, peptides derived from internalized exogenous antigens associate not with class I MHC molecules but, instead, with class II MHC molecules. The class I MHC–restricted presentation of endogenous but not exogenous antigens should prevent cytotoxic T-cell (CTL) lysis of noninfected neighboring cells that have phagocytosed infected cells.

The class I MHC–restricted presentation of antigens in DCs is similar to that seen in other cells, except for three features:

1. There is a marked increase in class I MHC synthesis during maturation, and half-life is increased (62).
2. Several proteasome subunits characteristics of the immunoproteasome are induced during maturation (63).
3. DCs appear very efficient in presenting exogenous internalized antigens in the context of class I MHC molecules, a processed referred to as cross-presentation. Albert et al. (64) demonstrated that human DCs have the capability to efficiently present antigens derived from apoptotic, influenza-infected cells and to stimulate class I MHC–restricted CD8$^+$ cytotoxic T-lymphocytes. Regnault et al. (65) showed that Fcγ receptors induce the maturation of DCs and mediate efficient internalization of immune complexes. This process requires proteasomal degradation and is dependent on functional peptide transporters associated with antigen processing (TAP) 1 and 2. Glycoprotein 96–associated antigens can be cross-presented on class I MHC by DCs (66) as well as foreign proteins expressed by bacteria (62). There is evidence that internalized antigens may access the cytosol for processing by the proteasome and loading in the endoplasmic reticulum. DCs have developed a unique membrane transport pathway for the export of exogenous antigens from endocytic compartments to the cytosol. Endosome-to-cytosol transport is restricted to DCs and allows internalized antigens to gain access to the cytosolic antigen-processing machinery and to the conventional class I MHC antigen-presentation pathway (67).

Of importance is that the cross-presentation can lead to the generation of cytotoxic responses to viruses that do not infect DCs themselves. This pathway may also account for the *in vivo* phenomenon of cross-priming, whereby antigens derived from tumor cells or transplants are presented by host APCs.

A potentially critical role of cross-presentation could be to allow DCs in the steady state to present self antigens on class I MHC and thereby to induce tolerance (see later discussion). This process would be essential to prevent the induction of autoimmunity when DCs capture dying infected cells (68).

Migratory Properties

The trafficking events that bring together T cells, B-lymphocytes, and DCs involve chemokines, which are small basic proteins that engage seven transmembrane receptors on responsive cells and promote chemotaxis (69).

Chemokines and their receptors regulate the movement and interaction of APCs such as DCs and T cells. CC chemokine receptor (CCR) 2 has been shown to be required for Langerhans cell migration to the lymph nodes and is also an important determinant of splenic DC migration, especially in the localization of CD8α^+ cells (see later discussion) (70). Two other chemokines have been suggested to serve a homing function in the T-cell compartment: the secondary lymphoid tissue chemokine (SLC)/6Ckine and the Epstein-Barr virus–induced molecule 1 ligand chemokine (ELC)/macrophage inflammatory protein (MIP)–3β. SLC and ELC are structurally related chemokines, and both bind the receptor CCR7. Immature DCs express CCR6 and respond to MIP-3α, whereas maturing DCs down-regulate expression of CCR6, up-regulate expression of CCR7, and chemotactically respond to ELC/MIP-3β (71). SLC appears to be needed for efficient passage of DCs from lymphatic vessels into the T-cell zone of lymph nodes (72). Interaction of CXCR4 on DCs with stromal cell factor might also contribute to the localization of DCs into the T-cell area.

The tight regulation of chemokine receptors allows DCs to be recruited to inflammatory sites and to leave these sites after antigen capture to reach secondary lymphoid organs. Mature DCs have been shown to produce ELC/MIP-3β, an observation that correlates with their unique capacity to organize the structure of T-cell areas within the lymph nodes by attracting antigen-carrying DCs as well as naïve T cells (73).

There is evidence that C-type lectin receptors regulate the migration of DCs (49). In particular, DC-SIGN appears to support tethering and rolling of DC-SIGN–positive cells on the vascular ligand ICAM-2 under shear flow, which suggests a potential role in emigration from blood (74).

Migration In Situ

The capability of DCs to transport antigen has been illustrated in several models *in situ*. Larsen et al. (75) showed that, when mouse skin is transplanted, the DCs enlarge, express higher levels of class II MHC, and begin to migrate. Xia et al. (76) showed that primary sensitization of naïve T cells after an airway challenge occurs predominantly within local lymph nodes and not in the lung or bronchial associated lymphoid tissues and that antigen presentation by DCs shifts from lung to lymph node during the response to inhaled antigen. Antigen transport from the airway mucosa to the thoracic lymph nodes was studied by intratracheal instillation of fluorescein isothiocyanate (FITC)–conjugated macromolecules (ovalbumin). After instillation, FITC$^+$ cells with stellate structure were found in the T-cell area of thoracic lymph nodes. The FITC signal was detected only in migratory airway-derived lymph node DCs, which display a mature phenotype and present ovalbumin to TCR transgenic T cells specific for an ovalbumin peptide (77). In the intestine, Huang et al. (78) identified a DC subset that constitutively endocytoses and transports apoptotic epithelial cells to T-cell areas of mesenteric lymph nodes *in vivo*.

Cytokine Release

Interleukin-12

In 1995, Macatonia et al. (79) demonstrated that murine splenic DCs produce IL-12 and direct the development of Th1 cells *in vitro*. Similar observations were reported by Koch et al. (80), who further showed that ligation of either CD40 or class II MHC molecules independently triggered IL-12 production in splenic DCs and that IL-12 production was down-regulated by IL-4 and IL-10. More recently, Biedermann et al. (81) found, however, that IL-4, when present during the initial activation of bone marrow-derived DCs, could instruct these cells to produce bioactive IL-12.

Although previous *in vitro* studies had suggested that the macrophage was a major source of the IL-12 produced on microbial stimulation, DCs but not macrophages were shown to be the initial cells to synthesize IL-12 in the spleens of mice exposed *in vivo* to an extract of *Toxoplasma gondii* or to LPS (43). The major producers of IL-12 are CD8α^+ DCs in response to bacterial or intracellular parasite infection (43, 84), whereas plasmacytoid DCs can produce IL-12 in response to various viruses, to CpG oligodeoxynucleotides, and *in vivo* to mouse cytomegalovirus (MCMV) (30). Iwasaki and Kelsall (16,17) demonstrated that CD11b$^-$CD8α^+ Peyer's patch DCs but not CD11b$^+$CD8α^- or double negative subset produce IL-12 p70 on stimulation *in vitro*.

Although the CD8α^+ DC subset seems to have the greatest capacity for IL-12 production, different stimuli can change the balance. *Escherichia coli* LPS induces IL-12 p70 in the CD8α^+ DC subset, presumably through TLR4, whereas *Porphyromonas gingivalis* LPS does not. Both LPSs activate the two DC subsets to up-regulate co-stimulatory molecules and produce IL-6 and TNF-α (54). Of note, all three splenic populations respond with increased IL-12 p70 production *in vitro* when IL-4 is present during stimulation, whereas only CD8α^+ DCs produce IL-12 in the absence of IL-4 (82) [for review, see Maldonado-López and Moser (83)]. Both subsets have the capacity to produce IL-12 after *in vivo* priming with *Toxoplasma* extracts (84). CD8α^- DCs from IL-10–deficient animals have an increased capacity to produce IL-12, in comparison with DCs from wild-type animals, which suggests that IL-12 release is tightly controlled in this subset (85).

In humans, Langerhans cells, particularly after maturation, have been shown to release functional IL-12 heterodimer *in vitro* (86). Rissoan et al. (23) reported that CD40L activation up-regulates the expression of mRNA for IL-12 p40 in human monocyte-derived but not plasmacytoid-derived DCs *in vitro*.

IL-12 exerts a powerful positive regulatory influence on the development of Th1 helper T-cell immune responses and is a potent inducer of IFN-γ production and cytotoxic differentiation and function, which suggests that DCs could dictate the class selection of the subsequent adaptive response (see later discussion).

The release of heterodimeric IL-12 p70, which is potentially harmful, appears tightly regulated *in vivo*. The production of IL-12 has been shown to depend on two signals: initial APC activation by a microbial stimulus and an amplifying signal through DC-T interaction (55). Negative regulatory mechanisms have been described: IL-10 has been shown to down-regulate the production of IL-12 by murine splenic DCs (85); IL-12 production by DCs is rapid and intense but relatively short-lived (84,87). This paralysis of DC IL-12 production is likely to prevent infection-induced immunopathology (84).

IL-12 is a disulfide-like 70-kD heterodimer composed of 35-kD (p35) and 40-kD (p40) subunits, each of which is encoded by a distinct gene. Although the regulation of IL-12 expression may be largely focused on p40 in other cell types, one report demonstrated that the regulation of IL-12 p70 expression at the transcriptional level by Rel/NFκB is controlled through both the p35 and p40 genes in CD8α^+ DCs (88).

Interferon-α

In the mouse, a population of plasmacytoid cells has been shown to produce IFN-α when cultured with inactivated influenza virus. These cells were detected in low numbers in the spleen, bone marrow, thymus, lymph nodes, blood, lungs, and liver. *In vivo* activated CD8α^+Ly6G/C$^+$CD11b$^-$ DCs appear to be the major producers of IFN-α/β during MCMV but not LCMV infection, and they probably derive from plasmacytoid CD11c$^+$CD8α^-Ly6G/C$^+$CD11b$^-$ immature APCs (30,89). Interestingly, IFN-α/β appear to regulate DC cytokine production by enhancing their own expression while inhibiting IL-12 synthesis during MCMV infection (89). Another report demonstrates that among the splenic DCs, only the CD4$^-$CD8$^+$ DCs produced IFN-α in culture when stimulated by a combination of CpG and polyinosine:polycytidylic acid poly(I:C)(82). The relationship between both IFN-α–producing populations requires further studies, especially because a proportion of plasmacytoid APCs has been shown to express CD8α (30). In humans, plasmacytoid-derived DCs release IFN-α during viral infection or inflammation (28,90).

Interleukin-2

The analysis of genes that are differentially expressed upon maturation induced by exposure to gram-negative bacteria revealed that IL-2 mRNA was transiently up-regulated at early time (4 to 6 hours) points after bacterial encounter (91). The same authors showed that DC-derived IL-2 mediates T-cell activation, inasmuch as the ability of IL-2$^{-/-}$ DCs to induce proliferation of allogeneic CD4$^+$ and CD8$^+$ T cells was severely impaired. The production of IL-2 by DCs may explain the unique ability of these cells to prime T-lymphocytes. In addition, DCs have been shown to produce IL-6 (92), IL-10, and IFN-γ (93,94). Mature DCs, predominantly of CD8α phenotype, appear to constitutively produce small amounts of IL-12, which induces the secretion of IFN-γ, leading to up-regulation of IL-12 production. Liver-derived DC progenitors (95) and freshly isolated Peyer's patch DCs (17) have the capacity to produce IL-10.

DENDRITIC CELLS AND T-CELL–MEDIATED IMMUNITY

Immunostimulatory Properties *In Vitro*

The first evidence that DCs have a potent capacity to activate T cells was provided in 1978 by Steinman and Witmer (3), who showed that these cells are at least 100 times more effective as mixed leukocyte reaction stimulators than are other splenic cells. Selective removal of DCs dramatically reduced stimulation of the primary mixed leukocyte reaction, whereas populations enriched in DCs were potent stimulators (96). DCs have been shown to activate both CD4$^+$ and CD8$^+$ T-lymphocytes in various models (97–99). Although DCs have the capacity to directly sensitize CD8$^+$ T cells, differentiation of CD8$^+$ T cells into killer cells requires help from CD4$^+$ T-lymphocytes. The classical model suggests that T helper and T killer cells recognize their specific antigens simultaneously on the same APC and that cytokines (such as IL-2) produced by the activated T helper cells facilitate the differentiation of the killer cell. The three-cell interaction seems unlikely, inasmuch as all cell types are rare and migratory. According to an alternative theory, proposed by P. Matzinger and demonstrated by three independent groups (100–102), the interaction could occur in two steps: the helper cell can first engage and condition the DC, which then becomes empowered to stimulate a killer cell.

Adoptive Transfer

DCs were further shown to be powerful stimulators of immune responses *in vivo* after adoptive transfer. Injection of epidermal Langerhans cells (103) or splenic DCs (104), coupled to trinitrophenyl, was shown to activate effector T cells in mice, in contradiction to other coupled cells. In a model of rat kidney allograft, Lechler and Batchelor (105) found that injection of small numbers of donor strain DCs triggers an acute rejection response, which suggests that intrarenal DCs provide the major stimulus of a kidney allograft. The *in vivo* priming capacity of DCs has been documented in several CD4$^+$ (92,106) and CD8$^+$ T-cell responses in rodents and in humans (see later section on tumor immunity). In addition, adoptive transfer of syngeneic DCs, pulsed extracorporeally with an antigen, induces a primary humoral response characterized by the secretion of IgG1 and IgG2a antibodies (107).

Whether the very same DCs that have captured antigen migrate to the T-cell areas in lymphoid organs and directly sensitize T-lymphocytes is still a matter of speculation. Direct priming by injected antigen-pulsed DCs has been suggested by studies showing that, in F1 recipient mice, parental DCs prime only T cells restricted to the MHC of the injected DCs (106,108). In addition, migratory DCs (which may be apoptotic) can be processed, distributing their peptides widely and efficiently to other DCs to form MHC/peptide combinations (109). Surprisingly, a protein from phagocytosed cells can be presented 1,000 to 10,000 times better than preprocessed peptide. DCs that have captured the antigen may also transfer their antigen through the release of antigen-bearing vesicles (exosomes) (110).

In favor of an indirect priming, Knight et al. (111) provided evidence for a transfer of antigen between DCs in the stimulation of primary T cell proliferation. Collectively, these observations suggest that different DCs may pick up the antigen and process or present it in the lymph nodes.

Dendritic Cells as Physiological Adjuvant

Several observations suggest that DCs play a major role in the initiation of immune responses in physiological situations *in situ*. DCs are the major cell type transporting the antigen in an immunogenic form for T cells. Rat intestinal DCs have been shown to acquire antigen administered orally, can stimulate sensitized T cells *in vitro,* and can prime popliteal lymph node CD4$^+$ T cells *in vivo* after footpad injection (108). DCs but not B cells present antigenic complexes to class II MHC–restricted T cells after administration of protein in adjuvants (112). Pulmonary DCs are able to present a soluble antigen shortly after it is introduced into the airways (76). In spleens of mice injected with protein antigens, DCs are the main cell type that carries the protein in a form that is immunogenic for T cells (113). DCs have been shown to migrate rapidly out of mouse cardiac allografts into the recipient's spleens, where they home to the peripheral white pulp and associate predominantly with CD4$^+$ T lymphocytes. This movement probably represents the initiation of the graft rejection (114). The essential role of DCs in the activation of T cells *in vivo* has been demonstrated in a model of asthma. Lambrecht et al. (115) used conditional depletion of airway DCs by treatment of thymidine kinase–transgenic mice with the antiviral drug ganciclovir to deplete DCs during the second exposure to ovalbumin. The depletion of DCs before challenge with inhaled antigen results in a decrease in the number of bronchoalveolar CD4 and CD8 T-lymphocytes and B-lymphocytes and prevents the Th2 cytokine–associated eosinophilic airway inflammation (115).

DCs are presented as nature's adjuvant as they function to initiate immune responses *in vivo*. In line with this hypothesis, DCs are activated by endogenous signals received from cells that are stressed, virally infected, or killed necrotically (116).

T-Cell/Dendritic Cell Synapses

The concept of synapse proposes a central contact zone between APCs and T cells and is characterized by the large-scale segregation of cell surface molecules into concentric zones. Synapse formation has been shown to follow and depend on T-cell antigen receptor signaling and may fulfill several roles: It participates in sustained TCR signaling, facilitates co-stimulation, polarizes the T-cell secretory apparatus towards the APC, and may play a role in the late signaling. The zone contains multiple copies of molecular couples: the TCR and peptide/MHC molecules and the adhesion and co-stimulatory molecules (Fig. 4).

Observations made *in vitro* have suggested that a large number of productive interactions (5,000 to 20,000) are needed for T-cell activation. According to the serial triggering model, proposed by Valitutti et al. (117), the threshold could be reached by serial engagement of a limited number of MHC molecules loaded by the cognate peptide on each APC (117). The immunological synapse appears dynamic, as, when offered another APC displaying ligands in greater quantities, T cells that have been activated by encounter with a first APC can form a new synapse within minutes (118). The time of commitment of naïve CD4$^+$ cells varies from 6 hours (high antigen and co-stimulatory APCs) to more than 30 hours (low antigen or absence of co-stimulation). In contrast, primed CD4$^+$ cells respond rapidly, within 0.5 to 2 hours. (119). Some results suggest that CD8$^+$ T cells might achieve commitment more rapidly than CD4$^+$ T cells (120). Indeed, naïve CTLs become committed after as little as 2 hours of exposure to APCs, and their subsequent division and differentiation can occur without the need for further antigenic stimulation, whether priming is *in vitro* or *in vivo*.

An elegant study explored the *in vivo* significance of the number of molecules engaged and the duration of engagement in transgenic mice expressing TCRs in a quantitatively and temporally controlled manner (121). Very few surface TCR molecules were found to be needed for T cells to respond to immunization *in vivo* (100 or less). These results would be compatible with models in which TCR:MHC/peptide combinations form on a one-to-one basis and persist for a long time, rather than forming serial engagements. Whether *in vivo* T-cell differentiation requires stimulation by a single DC or by continuously recruited DCs is still a matter of speculation.

Zell et al. (122) analyzed signaling events in individual CD4 T cells after antigen recognition *in vivo*. Phosphorylation of c-jun and p38 MAPK was detected within minutes in virtually all antigen-specific CD4 T cells in secondary lymphoid organs after injection of peptide antigen into the bloodstream. The rapidity of signaling correlates with the finding that about 60% to 70% of the naïve DO11.10 T cells are constantly interacting with class II$^+$ MHC CD11c$^+$ (presumably DCs) in the T-cell zones of lymphoid organs. Contrary to predictions from *in vitro* experiments, the rate and magnitude of c-jun phosphorylation appears independent of CD28 signals. Collectively, these observations highlight the efficiency of T cell sensitization under physiological conditions *in vivo*, in comparison with *in vitro* models.

Antigen-Independent Clustering

Studies have shown that DCs may signal T cells in the absence of exogenous antigen. In the mouse, Revy et al. (123) showed that, in the absence of antigen and even of MHC molecules, T-cell/DC synapses are formed and lead to several T-cell responses: a local increase in tyrosine phosphorylation, induction of small Ca^{2+} currents, weak proliferation, and long-term survival. Kondo et al. (124) showed that DCs mediate a signal that correlates with increased *in vitro* survival of human T cells and results in antigen-independent cytokine gene expression. Thus, in the absence of antigen, DCs generated from peripheral blood monocytes by cytokine stimulation induced increased amounts of IL-12Rβ2 chain and IFN-γ mRNA, which suggests a new role for DCs in shaping the cytokine milieu.

These observations are reminiscent of earlier studies showing that mouse (124a) and rat (125) DCs could physically cluster with T cells in the absence of antigen.

Adjuvants

The induction of immune response *in vivo* is typically performed with antigens administered in external adjuvants. The presence of adjuvants has been shown to increase the level of antibodies and the duration of the immune response, to modify the Th1/Th2 balance, and to induce an anamnestic response. The mechanism by which adjuvants coinitiate an immune response is still poorly understood. Their role could be to provide a signal of "danger" that is necessary to turn on the immune system and could be detected by DCs (116). In favor of this hypothesis, it was shown that the adjuvant monophosphoryl lipid A provokes the migration and maturation of DCs *in vivo* (126). LeBon et al. (127) demonstrated that type I interferons, the major ones of which are IFN-α and IFN-β, potently enhance humoral immunity and can promote isotype switching by stimulating DCs *in vivo*. Adjuvants such as poly(I:C) or complete Freund's adjuvant (containing heat-killed mycobacteria) may act through the induction of endogenous type I IFN production and the subsequent stimulation of DCs by type I IFN (127).

Immune Escape

Viruses and parasites have developed various means to evade the immune response. MCMV infects and productively replicates in DCs and strongly impairs their endocytic and stimulatory capacities (128). Of note, infected DCs appear incapable of transducing the "danger" signals required to induce antiviral immune responses. DCs appear to be the major target of measles virus proteins, which is related to the profound defect in lymphocyte priming. The capacity of DCs to stimulate T cells was shown to be impaired after measles virus infection *in vitro,* and their production of IL-12 was down-regulated *in vitro* and *in vivo* (129). Schistosomes have been shown to inhibit Langerhans cell migration *in vivo*, probably through the production of prostaglandin D2 (130).

DENDRITIC CELLS AND THE POLARIZATION OF THE IMMUNE RESPONSE

There is evidence that the onset of an immune response may not be sufficient to eliminate all pathogens but that the character of the response (the Th1/Th2 balance) determines its efficiency. Of importance is that an inadequate immune response may even be deleterious and result in tissue damage, allergic reactions, or disease exacerbation. Th1 cells, by their production of IFN-γ and lymphotoxin, are responsible for the eradication of intracellular pathogens, but they may also cause organ-specific autoimmune diseases if dysregulated. Th2 cells, by their production of IL-4 and IL-5, can activate mast cells and eosinophils and induce humoral immune responses, but they can also provoke atopy and allergic inflammation. The identification of the factors that affect T helper subset development is therefore a prerequisite for the development of effective vaccination strategies.

Role of Antigen-Presenting Cells

Several observations suggest that APCs may govern the development of T helper cell populations:

1. The development of Th1 versus Th2 cells seems to be determined early on, at the stage of antigen presentation. Indeed, T cell proliferation and up-regulation of mRNA for interferon-γ in response to Swiss-type murine mammary tumor virus and IL-4 in response to haptenated protein has been shown to start on the third day after immunization (131).
2. Antigen-presenting-cells release cytokines (IL-12, IFN-γ, IL-10), which play a central role in Th1/Th2 differentiation.
3. The strength of interaction mediated through the TCR and MHC/peptide combination or the dose of antigen appears to affect lineage commitment (132). The number of TCR molecules engaged has also been correlated with the outcome [for review, see Lanzavecchia et al. (133)].
4. Membrane-bound co-stimulators, as CD80 or CD86, may influence Th development *in vitro* and *in vivo*.

In favor of this notion, it was shown that the nature of the cell presenting the antigen *in vitro* and *in vivo* (92) strongly influences the development of Th1 versus Th2 cells.

Polarizing Dendritic Cell–Derived Cytokines

IL-12 plays a major role in immunity to intracellular pathogens by governing the development of IFN-γ–dependent host resistance [for review, see O'Garra (134)]. IL-12 receptor–deficient patients display severe mycobacterial and *Salmonella* infections, which indicates an essential role of IL-12 and type 1 cytokine pathway in resistance to infections by intracellular bacteria (135).

DCs appear to be the initial cells to synthesize IL-12 in the spleens of mice exposed to microbial stimulants. The production of IL-12 in mice exposed to an extract of *T. gondii* or to LPS occurs very rapidly, is independent of signals from T-lymphocytes, and is associated with DC redistribution to the T-cell areas, which suggests that DCs function simultaneously as APCs and as initiators of the Th1 response (43). It was subsequently shown that CD40 ligation induces a significant increase in IL-12 p35 and IL-12 p70 heterodimer production (55). Thus, production of high levels of bioactive IL-12 appears to be dependent on two signals: a microbial priming signal and a T cell–derived signal.

There is strong evidence that the Th1-prone capacity of murine DCs is strictly dependent on its IL-12 production, although the role of IL-23 [a combination of p19 and the p40 subunit of IL-12 (136)] and IL-18 (137) has not been clearly assessed *in vivo*. The crucial role of IL-12 in Th1 priming by DCs has been demonstrated by experiments with mice genetically deficient in IL-12 (138). In parallel with the loss of IL-12 production, human DCs appear to switch from a Th1- to a Th2-inducing mode (87). An important determinant of Th1 development in CD4$^+$ T cells is STAT4 activation by IL-12 (139), although a STAT4-independent pathway has been reported. Among the transcription factors selectively expressed in Th1 cells, T-bet seems to play a crucial role, and its overexpression by retroviruses in T cells increases the frequency with which Th1 and Th2 cells that produce IFN-γ develop (140).

There is no evidence so far that indicates that DCs produce a Th2-prone cytokine. In contrast to IL-12, IL-4 has been shown to skew the development of naïve T cells toward an IL-4–producing Th2 phenotype (141). Activated CD4$^+$ T cells themselves may provide the IL-4 required for Th2 differentiation. The contribution of DCs to Th2 development does not appear to require APC-derived IL-4, inasmuch as injection of DCs from wild-type or IL-4–deficient mice induces similar Th2-type responses in wild-type recipients (85). Also, in humans, activated plasmacytoid-derived DCs do not seem to produce detectable amounts of IL-4, and blocking IL-4 at the beginning of culture does not prevent generation of IL-4–producing cells (23). This view is, however, still controversial (142,143). The co-stimulatory molecule CD86 has been shown to be required for Th2 development *in vitro* and *in vivo* (92, 144), whereas CD80 is a more neutral co-stimulatory molecule. Of note, CD28 signaling alone appears to induce the pro-Th2 transcription factor GATA-3 and the presence of IL-12 has been shown to repress Th2 development *in vivo*. Indeed, CD8α^+ DCs from IL-12–deficient mice prime for Th2, whereas the same subset from wild-type animals primes for Th1 (138). It is therefore conceivable that Th2 is a default pathway—that is, that type 2 T cells would develop spontaneously in the absence of IL-12. The hypothesis that Th2 is a default pathway suggests that IL-12 has a greater opportunity to drive naïve T cells to polarize to Th1 than Th2-prone stimuli such as IL-4. In favor of this notion, TCR ligation has been shown to transiently desensitize IL-4R by inhibiting STAT6 phosphorylation (145). The mechanism by which IL-12 would prevent Th2 priming is still unclear, but it involves inhibition of GATA-3 expression by IL-12 signaling through STAT4, indirect inhibition through IFN-γ production, or both. The requirements for Th2 induction may therefore be less stringent and may require only priming and relief from Th1 induction.

Neutralization of IL-4 has been shown to prevent the differentiation of Th2 responses, and IL-4 acts as antagonist of Th1-induced inflammatory responses. However, it has been clearly demonstrated that, paradoxically, IL-4 may promote Th1 development and induce IL-12 production by DCs. These contradictory observations were resolved by a report showing that IL-4 has opposite effects on DC development versus T-cell differentiation. When present during the initial activation of DCs by infectious agents, IL-4 instructs DCs to produce IL-12 (146–148) and favor Th1 development, but when present later, during the period of T-cell priming, IL-4 includes Th2 differentiation (81). These opposing effects correlate with resistance/sensitivity to *Leishmania major in vivo* (81).

Unlike murine T cells, human T cells respond to type I interferons by inducing Th1 development. The basis of selective Th1 induction by IFN-α in human T cells appears to be a difference in IFN-α signaling between the mice and humans (149). In particular, IFN-α has been shown to activate STAT4 in human but not mouse T cells. Of note, it has been reported that the COOH-terminal region of human

and murine STAT2, which acts as an adapter for STAT4, are widely divergent, because of the insertion of a minisatellite region in mouse exon 23 (which encodes this region).

Mechanisms of Dendritic Cell Polarization

Kalinski et al. (150) suggested that migrating DCs not only provide an antigen-specific signal 1 and a co-stimulatory signal 2 but also carry an additional signal 3, contributing to the initial commitment of naïve T helper cells into Th1 or Th2 subsets. This would allow the efficient induction of T helper cells with adequate cytokine profiles during early infections without requirement for a direct contact between antigen-specific T cells and the pathogens (150).

Reports in the literature are consistent with three models through which DCs may control T cell polarization: (a) subclasses of DCs; (b) the nature of the stimuli that activate DCs; and (c) the kinetics of DC activation.

Dendritic Cell Subclasses

In the mouse, three *in vivo* studies have demonstrated that DC subsets differed in the cytokine profiles that they induce in T cells. In one study (151), TCR transgenic T cells from DO11.10/SCID mice were adoptively transferred into Balb/c recipients. CD11c$^+$CD11b$^{dull/-}$ (mainly CD8α^+) or CD11c$^+$CD11b^{bright}CD8α^- cells were loaded with ovalbumin peptide *in vitro* and injected into the footpads of transferred animals. Both DC subpopulations induced antigen-specific proliferation *in vivo* and *in vitro* upon restimulation with the antigen. Assessment of cytokine production revealed that both subsets induced IFN-γ and IL-2 production but that the CD11c$^+$CD11b^{bright}CD8α^- subset induced much greater levels of IL-10 and IL-4 production. The differences in the cytokine profiles of T cells correlated with class-specific differences in the antibody profiles. In the second study (138), antigen-pulsed CD8α^+ and CD8α^- DCs were injected into the footpads of syngeneic recipients. Administration of CD8α^- DCs induced a Th2-type response, whereas injection of CD8α^+ DCs led to Th1 differentiation. Similar experiments with mice genetically deficient in IL-12 underscored the crucial role of IL-12 in Th1 development by CD8α^+ DCs. In a third study, CD11b$^+$CD8α^- DCs from murine Peyer's patch have been shown to prime naïve T cells to secrete high levels of IL-4 and IL-10 *in vitro,* whereas the CD11b$^-$CD8α^+ and double negative subsets from the same tissue primed for IFN-γ production. (16).

In humans, monocyte-derived DCs were found to induce Th1 differentiation, whereas DCs derived from plasmacytoid cells favor Th2 development of allogeneic T cells (23). Subsequent work has demonstrated, however, that the T-cell stimulatory function of DC2s was regulated by the environment: Virus-induced plasmacytoid DC2s stimulate naïve T cells to produce IFN-γ and IL-10, whereas IL-3 induced DC2s stimulate naïve T cells to produce Th2-type cytokines (IL-4, IL-5, and IL-10) (28). Cella et al. (90) reported that blood plasmacytoid DCs represent the principal source of type I interferon during inflammation and participate in antiviral Th1-type responses.

There is evidence that DC subsets express distinct pattern-recognition and presentation receptors. Human monocyte-derived pre-DC1s express TLR2 and TLR4 and rapidly produce large amounts of proinflammatory cytokines such as TNF-α, IL-6, and IL-12 in response to TLR2 and TLR4 ligands such as glycoproteins from mycobacteria and gram-positive bacteria. In contrast, plasmacytoid-derived DCs express TLR7 and TLR9 and produce type 1 IFN in response to TLR9 ligand and bacterial DNA rich in unmethylated CpG motifs.

Nature of the Stimuli

Vieira et al. (152) showed that the Th1- and Th2-inducing function of human monocyte-derived DCs is not an intrinsic attribute but depends on environmental instruction. DCs that matured in the presence of IFN-γ induce Th1 responses, whereas DCs that matured in the presence of prostaglandin E$_2$ induce Th2 responses. Similarly, the presence of IL-10 during maturation has been shown to lead to the development of DCs with Th2-driving function, whereas incubation of DC subsets with IFN-γ favors the priming of Th1 cells to the detriment of Th2 cell development (85,150,153). This provides evidence for the adaptation of DC function to the conditions that they encounter in the pathogen-invaded tissue.

The antigen itself has been shown to regulate DC function. DCs have the capacity to discriminate between yeasts and hyphae of the fungus *Candida albicans* and release distinct cytokines (142). Using oligonucleotides microarrays, Huang et al. (154) measured gene expression profiles of DCs in response to *E. coli, C. albicans,* and influenza virus. The data show that a common set of 166 genes, as well as particular subsets of genes, is regulated by each pathogen, which demonstrates that DCs discriminate between diverse pathogens and elicit tailored pathogen-specific immune responses (154).

Kinetics of Dendritic Cell Activation

In addition to the nature of the maturation stimulus, the kinetics of activation may influence the capacity of DCs to induce different types of T-cell responses. Recent *in vitro* observations suggest that, indeed, DCs produce IL-12 during a narrow time window and afterwards become refractory to further stimulation. The exhaustion of cytokine production has been shown to affect the T-cell polarizing process: DCs taken at early times after induction of maturation (active DCs) prime strong Th1 responses, whereas the same cells taken at later times ("exhausted" DCs) preferentially prime Th2 and nonpolarized cells (87). These observations, although made *in vitro,* suggest a dynamic regulation of the generation of effector and memory cells during the immune response.

Two subsets of memory T-lymphocytes with distinct homing potentials and effector functions have been described (155). Expression of CCR7, a chemokine receptor that controls homing to secondary lymphoid organs, divides memory T cells into CCR7$^-$ effector memory cells, which migrate to inflamed tissues and display immediate effector function, and CCR7$^+$ central memory cells, which home in the lymph nodes and lack immediate effector function. Both subsets may persist for years, and the central memory cells give rise to effector memory upon secondary stimulation.

It has been proposed that the nature of DCs bearing antigen and co-stimulatory molecules, as well as the amount and duration of TCR triggering, determines whether effector memory or central memory cells are generated. A short TCR stimulation may expand nonpolarized T cells that home to lymph nodes and respond promptly to antigenic stimulation. In contrast, a prolonged stimulation in the presence of polarizing cytokines may drive differentiation of Th1 or Th2 effector cells that home to inflamed peripheral tissues.

DENDRITIC CELLS AND T-CELL TOLERANCE

Central Tolerance

The normal development of T cells in the thymus requires both positive and negative selection. During positive selection, thymocytes mature only if their TCRs react with some specificity to host MHC and host peptides. Laufer et al. (156) used the keratin promoter to reexpress a class II MHC antigen in class II–negative mice and showed that autoimmunity develops in transgenic mice in which class II MHC products are expressed only by epithelial cells and not by bone marrow-derived APCs. Autoreactive cells that constitute up to 5% of the peripheral CD4 T cells were generated.

During negative selection, developing T cells reacting strongly to self-peptide/self MHC combinations are eliminated. Brocker et al. (157) demonstrated that thymic DCs are sufficient to mediate negative selection *in vivo*. Using a CD11c promoter, they targeted the expression of an MHC class II I-E transgene to DCs and showed that tolerance to I-E was induced. These observations demonstrate that thymocyte development is a sequential process: Positive selection occurs on thymic cortical epithelium independently of negative selection, which is mediated by thymic DCs.

Of note, a report demonstrates that the level of class I MHC protein is 10-fold higher on thymic DCs than on thymic epithelial cells and that an increase in the level of a particular cognate peptide/MHC ligand may be sufficient to result in negative rather than positive selection. This finding suggests a role for the quantitative differences in the level of MHC expression in thymic selection (158).

Peripheral Tolerance

Many proteins, however, may not have access to the thymus during development, and a significant proportion of self-reactive T cells have been shown to escape negative selection, which suggests that a mechanism must be able to silence autoreactive T cells in the periphery. Bouneaud et al. (159) studied a peptide-specific T-cell repertoire in the presence and absence of the deleting ligand. The authors used mice transgenic for the TCR-β chain of an anti-HY T-cell clone and compared the preimmune repertoire reactive to the male-specific peptide in male and female animals. Interestingly, their results showed that a large proportion of CD8$^+$ T cells specific for the male-specific peptide persist in male animals, as detected by MHC/peptide tetramer staining and functional assays. Of note, male T cells (specific to the male peptide) that escape clonal deletion do not react with the endogenous male peptide, as predicted by the observation that the threshold of antigenic stimulation is lower for negative selection that for activation of mature cells, but those cells are still capable of functional reactivity with self peptides when facing high doses of antigen.

There is evidence that, besides their immunostimulatory functions, DCs may also maintain and regulate T-cell tolerance in the periphery. This control function may be exerted by certain maturation stages, specialized subsets, or cells influenced by immunomodulatory agents such as IL-10.

Immature Dendritic Cells

In the periphery, immature DCs are specialized for antigen capture but display weak stimulatory properties for naïve CD4$^+$ and CD8$^+$ T cells. Some results suggest that immature DCs retain antigen in endosomal compartments and do not display antigenic peptide/MHC combinations at levels detectable by microscopy until they receive a maturation stimulus. This would imply that immature DCs could not present peptides derived from self proteins. However, several observations (57,58) show that immature DCs express MHC/peptide combinations, albeit at low levels. On the basis of in vitro studies showing that TCR engagement in the absence of co-stimulation may lead to anergy of T-cell clones (160), it was postulated that immature DCs may induce a state of unresponsiveness in antigen-specific T-lymphocytes. This hypothesis would be in agreement with several observations: (a) Both immature and mature DCs are constantly acquiring peptide cargo, although immature DCs clearly display lower levels of antigen/MHC combinations; (b) immature DCs are in close contact with T-lymphocytes in lymphoid organs; and (c) immature DCs present self antigens (161).

Hawiger et al. (162) examined the function of murine DCs in the steady state, using as antigen delivery system a monoclonal antibody to a DC-restricted endocytic receptor DEC-205. Targeting the antigen on DCs resulted in transient antigen-specific T-cell activation, followed by T-cell deletion and unresponsiveness. T cells initially activated by DCs in these conditions could not be reactivated when the mice were challenged with the same antigen in complete Freund's adjuvant. In contrast, coinjection of the DC-targeted antigen and anti-CD40 agonistic antibody resulted in prolonged

T-cell activation and immunity. These observations suggest that, in the steady state, the primary function of DCs may be to maintain peripheral tolerance. Consistently, an initial burst of CD8$^+$ T-cell proliferation followed by deletion was observed when antigen was expressed as transgene in pancreatic β cells, in kidney proximal tubular cells, and in the testes of male mice. The antigen was shown to be presented not by pancreatic β cells but by bone marrow–derived APCs in the draining lymph nodes (163). Similar results were obtained by Morgan et al. (164), who further demonstrated a direct correlation between the amounts of antigen expressed in the periphery and the rate of tolerance of specific CD8$^+$ T cells. Another study showed that administration of immature DCs may prolong cardiac allograft survival in nonimmunosuppressed recipients (165). Collectively, these observations support the hypothesis that activation of T cells in a noninflammatory environment, presumably by immature DCs, could be part of a normal mechanism of peripheral tolerance.

In humans, Dhodapkar et al. (166) analyzed the immune response induced after injection of immature DCs pulsed with influenza matrix peptide and keyhole limpet hemocyanin (KLH) in two healthy subjects. A decline in matrix peptide–specific IFN-γ–producing T cells was observed, whereas such cells were detected in both subjects before immunization as expected, because most adults have been exposed to the influenza virus. Of note, the decline in IFN-γ production was associated with the appearance of IL-10–producing cells specific for the same antigen. KLH priming was much greater when mature DCs were used and KLH-specific, IFN-γ-secreting cells were detected. In vitro studies (167) have shown that repetitive stimulation with immature human DCs induced nonproliferating, IL-10–producing CD4$^+$ T cells. These T cells, in coculture experiments, have been shown to inhibit the antigen-driven proliferation of Th1 cells in a contact- and dose-dependent but antigen-nonspecific manner.

The Existence of Specialized Subsets of Dendritic Cells

The existence of these cells, which would display tolerogenic properties, is still a matter of speculation. Initial in vitro studies by Suss and Shortman (168) demonstrated that splenic CD8α^- DCs induced a vigorous proliferative response in CD4$^+$ T cells, whereas CD8α^+ DCs induced a lesser response that was associated with T-cell apoptosis. This programmed cell death was shown to be caused by interaction of Fas on T cells with FasL on CD8α^+ DCs. Similarly, CD8α^+ DCs regulated the response of naïve CD8 T cells by limiting their IL-2 production (169). These findings led to the appealing hypothesis that FasL$^+$ CD8α^+ DCs could be involved in the tolerance of peripheral T-lymphocytes, whereas the classical CD8α^- DCs would induce immunity. This notion was consistent with the reduced phagocytic capacity of CD8α^+ DCs, their poor migratory properties (170), their localization in T-cell zones of lymphoid organs, and the high levels of self peptide/MHC combinations expressed by DCs in the T-cell areas (161). This hypothesis was in line with the tolerogenic properties of thymic DCs. The tolerogenic capacity of CD8α^+ DCs was demonstrated *in vivo* in one report, but the negative regulatory effect appears restricted to tumor/self peptide P815AB and was not observed with other antigens (171). The potential role of CD8α^+ DCs in peripheral tolerance was challenged by numerous reports showing that these DCs are the major producers of IL-12 and induce the development of IFN-γ–producing T cells *in vivo* (see earlier discussion).

Interleukin-10

IL-10 has been shown to suppress multiple activities of the immune response. The immunosuppressive properties of IL-10 on DCs are caused by a reduction in the up-regulation of expression of class II MHC, co-stimulatory, and adhesion molecules, as well as an inhibition of the production of inflammatory cytokines (IL-1, IL-6, TNF-α, and IL-12). Of note, IL-10 modulates the function of immature DCs but has little effect on mature DCs [for review, see Jonuleit et al. (172)]. In the mouse, splenic DCs that have undergone maturation *in vitro* in the presence of IL-10 have an impaired capability to induce Th1-type response *in vivo,* leading to the development of Th2 cells only (153). Human DCs generated from peripheral progenitors and exposed to IL-10 for the last 2 days of culture were shown to induce a state of antigen-specific anergy in T cells (173). The tolerogenic properties of these IL-10–treated DCs correlate with a reduced expression of class II MHC molecules, CD58 and CD86 co-stimulatory molecules, and the DC-specific antigen CD83. The role of IL-10–producing DCs has been illustrated in the lung (174). Pulmonary DCs from mice exposed to respiratory antigen transiently produce IL-10 and induce antigen unresponsiveness in recipient mice. Although they are phenotypically mature, these DCs stimulate the development of CD4$^+$ T regulatory cells that also produce high amounts of IL-10. Upon transfer, these pulmonary DCs induce antigen unresponsiveness in recipient mice.

A number of CD4$^+$ T-cell subpopulations capable of inhibiting the response of other T cells have been described and include naturally occurring CD4$^+$CD25$^+$ T cells, which inhibit Th cells through cell contact; Tr1 cells, which secrete IL-10 and TGF-β; and Th3 cells, which produce TGF-β [for review, see Waldmann and Cobbold (175) and Maloy and Powrie (176)].

In accordance with tolerogenic properties of DCs, several reports suggest a major flux of tissue antigens through DCs migrating to the lymph nodes. Huang et al. (78) identified in rats a DC subset (OX41$^-$) that constitutively transports apoptotic bodies derived from the intestinal epithelium to T-cell areas of mesenteric lymph nodes *in vivo*. OX41$^-$ DCs are weak APCs despite expressing high levels of B7 molecules and may play a role in inducing and maintaining self-tolerance. In addition, rat intestinal lymph contains another subset of OX41$^+$ DCs that are strong APCs but may not reach the

T-cell area in the absence of inflammation. Specific migratory DCs rapidly transport antigen from the airways to the thoracic lymph nodes in baseline conditions (Fig. 6) (77). These observations suggest that DCs internalize potential self-antigens from tissues and from noninfectious environmental proteins. It is important to note that exposure of DCs to primary tissue cells or apoptotic cells do not induce their maturation (177). These observations led to the hypothesis (178) that immature DCs phagocytose tissue cells undergoing normal cell turnover by apoptosis, leading to unresponsiveness of self-reactive T cells in the draining lymph node.

In addition to the induction of anergy/hyporesponsiveness in T-lymphocytes, APCs may regulate the Th1/Th2 balance. The study of autoimmune models suggests that mature DCs, expressing high levels of CD80 and CD86, may induce a shift toward Th2 responses and may therefore be effective in preventing autoimmune diseases dominated by Th1 responses [for comment, see Morel and Feili-Hariri (179)].

DENDRITIC CELLS AND B-CELL ACTIVATION

Several observations have underscored the role of DCs in the induction of humoral responses. Inaba et al. (180,181) demonstrated that DCs were required for the development of T cell–dependent antibody responses by murine and human lymphocytes *in vitro*. Injection of syngeneic DCs, which have been pulsed *in vitro* with soluble protein antigen, induced a strong antibody response in mice that were boosted with soluble antigen (107). Antigen-specific antibodies of isotypes similar to the immunoglobulin classes produced after immunization with the same antigen in complete Freund's adjuvant were detected in treated animals. In particular, IgG1 and IgG2a antibodies were produced, which suggests that Th1 and Th2 cells are activated and a memory response was induced.

The classical view of DC function in antibody formation was that these cells activate CD4$^+$ T helper cells, which in turn interact directly with B cells to provide help. However, more recent findings have suggested a role for direct DC–B cell interaction. CD40-activated DCs have been shown to enhance both the proliferation and IgM secretion of CD40-activated B-lymphocytes (182) and to switch naïve IgD$^+$ cells to become IgA secretors in the presence of IL-10 (183). Of note, it has been found that DCs themselves produce IL-2 (91), which may contribute to the ability of DCs to activate B cells, because exogenous IL-2 is required for the up-regulation of IgM secretion by resting naïve B cells cultured with CD40-activated DCs.

Furthermore, Grouard et al. (184) identified a population of DCs capable of stimulating T cells in germinal center. This population of germinal center DCs is distinct from the follicular DCs, which retain immune complexes and promote the activation and selection of high-affinity B cells. Germinal center DCs express CD11c and CD4 and represent 0.5% to 1% of all germinal center cells in human tonsils, spleen, and lymph nodes. Germinal center DCs display much stronger

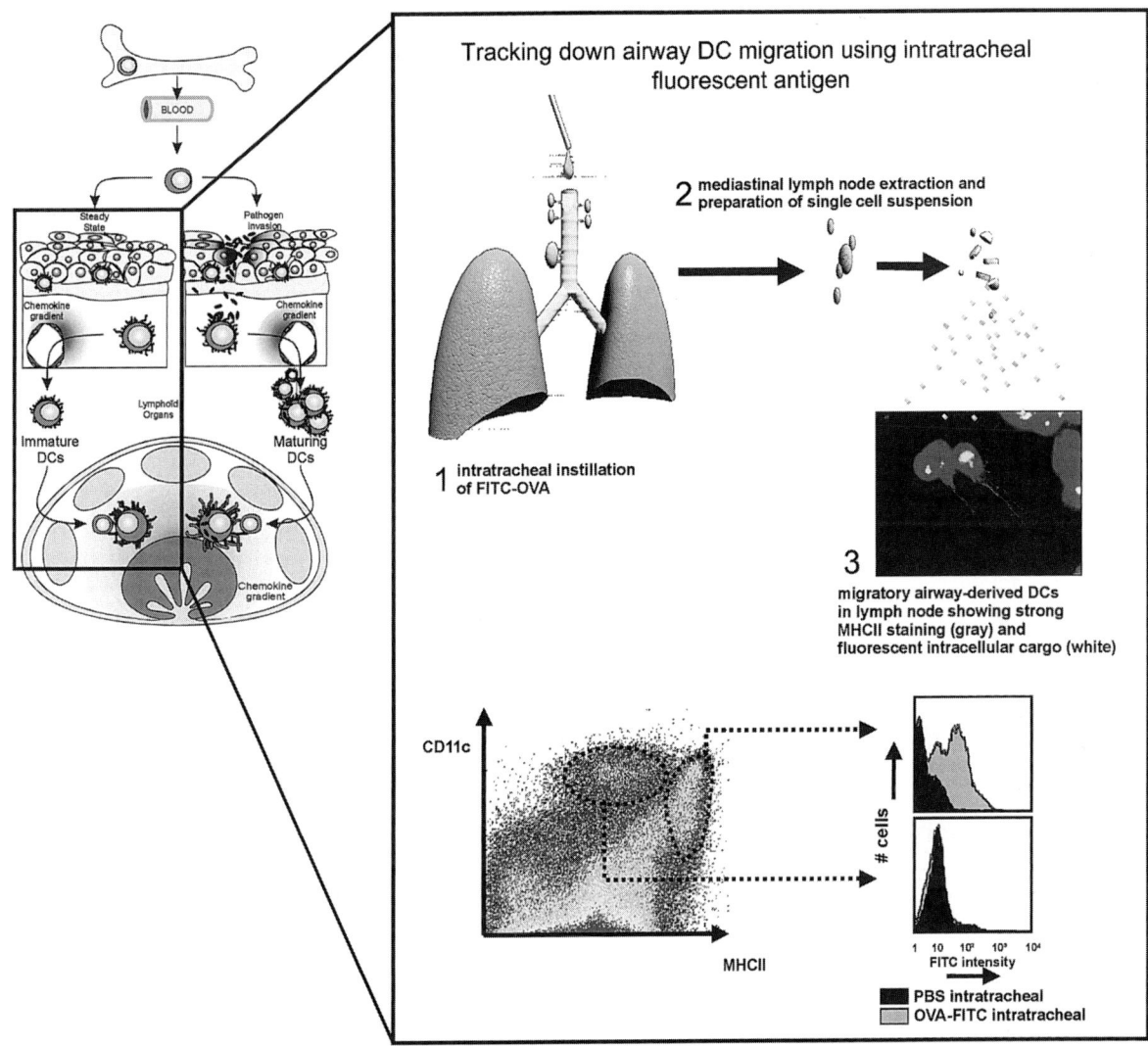

Tracking down airway DC migration using intratracheal fluorescent antigen

2 mediastinal lymph node extraction and preparation of single cell suspension

1 intratracheal installation of FITC-OVA

3 migratory airway-derived DCs in lymph node showing strong MHCII staining (gray) and fluorescent intracellular cargo (white)

PBS intratracheal
OVA-FITC intratracheal

FIG. 6. Steady-state flux of DCs. After instillation of fluorescein isothiocyanate (FITC)–conjugated oval-bumin in the airway, FITC+ cells with dendritic structure are detected in the T-cell area of thoracic lymph nodes. The FITC signal is detected in CD11c+ class II^{high} MHC cells representing migratory airway-derived lymph node DCs. Redrawn from Vermaelen et al. (77) by copyright permission of the Rockefeller University Press.

T-cell stimulatory function than do germinal center B cells and were found in close association with memory T cells *in situ,* which suggests that they may maintain the germinal center reaction by sustaining the activation state of germinal center memory T cells.

DENDRITIC CELLS AND NATURAL KILLER CELLS

In addition to their major role in the induction or adaptative immune responses, DCs appear to activate the innate arm of antitumor immunity; that is, natural killer (NK) and NK T effector cells.

NK cells participate in the innate response against trans-formed cells *in vivo* (185). Murine DCs have been shown to enhance proliferation, cytotoxicity properties, and IFN-γ

production by NK cells *in vitro* (186). Moreover, in mice with class I MHC–negative tumors, DCs promote NK-dependent antitumor effects *in vivo*. The activation depends on direct DC–NK cell contact and on secreted factors that include IL-12, IL-18, and possibly IL-15. In addition, IL-2 released by DCs (91) could play a role in the activation of NK functions by DCs.

Gerosa et al. (1987) analyzed the interaction between human peripheral blood NK cells and monocyte-derived DCs. Fresh NK cells were activated, and their cytolytic activity was strongly augmented by contact with mature DCs. Reciprocally, fresh NK cells culture with immature DCs strongly enhance DC maturation and IL-12 production (187).

Direct killing of DCs by NK cells has also been demonstrated. Murine bone marrow–derived DCs can be lysed by NK1.1+ cells *in vitro* (188), and mouse splenic DCs can be targeted *in vitro* by stimulated NK cells (189). Activated human NK cells and NK cell lines have been shown to lyse both autologous DCs derived from peripheral blood monocytes and Langerhans cells derived from $CD34^+$ stem cells (190).

DENDRITIC CELLS AND NATURAL KILLER T CELLS

NK T cells are $TCR\alpha/\beta^+$ $CD4^+$ or $CD4^-CD8^-$ T cells that display distinctive phenotypic and functional properties (191–193). They can be distinguished from conventional T cells by their expression of the NK cell locus-encoded C-type lectin molecule NK1.1. Another hallmark of murine NK T cells is their restricted TCR repertoire: the great majority express an invariant TCR-α chain structure. Both mouse and human NK T cells rapidly secrete cytokines associated with both Th1 (IFN-γ) and Th2 (IL-4) responses upon TCR engagement or stimulation with the synthetic CD1d ligand, the α-galactosylceramide. NK T cells are relevant in innate antitumor immunosurveillance. Studies have revealed that murine DCs at an immature stage were unable to induce NK T cells triggering because of an H-2 class I–mediated constitutive inhibitory pathway. Of note, mature DCs have been shown to overcome the inhibition through B7/CD28 interaction, thereby promoting CD1d-dependent IFN-γ production by NK T cells *in vitro* (193a). The cytokine profiles of human NK T cells appear regulated by the type of DCs: addition of plasmacytoid DC2 enhances the development of neonatal NK T cells into $IL-4^+$ $IFN-\gamma^-$ NKT2 cells, whereas addition of monocyte-derived DC1 cells induces polarization toward IFN-γ–producing NKT1 cells (194).

Collectively, these observations suggest that DCs are involved in the interaction between innate and adaptive immune responses. Innate immunity may control the development of adaptive immunity. The interactions of DCs with NK cells or NK T cells or both may result in release of antigens (as apoptotic or necrotic bodies) and production of cytokines (such as IFN-γ or IL-4) that may direct the polarization of T helper cells.

DENDRITIC CELL–BASED IMMUNOTHERAPY FOR CANCER

The first experimental evidence that lack of immunogenicity could be caused by the tumor's inability to activate the immune system rather than the absence of tumor antigens was provided by Boon and Kellerman in 1977 (195). This observation was confirmed in various tumor models and paved the way for a vaccination therapy of cancer.

As a complement to other less specific therapies, the immunotherapy may be highly beneficial to tumor patients because it would ideally induce an antigen-specific, widespread, long-term protection. DCs are currently under active clinical investigation, mostly for their immunostimulatory properties in cancer.

A large body of literature involves animal models showing that DCs loaded with tumor-associated antigens are able to induce a protective immune response, even to established tumors. In mice, successful protection against a B-cell lymphoma was achieved by immunization with idiotype-pulsed splenic DCs (196). Naïve mice injected with bone marrow–derived DCs pulsed with tumor-associated, class I–restricted peptides were protected against a subsequent lethal tumor challenge and against preestablished C3 sarcoma cells or 3LL lung carcinoma cells (197).

In addition, immunity has been induced against unidentified antigens by injecting DCs pulsed with tumor cell membranes, RNA from tumors, peptides eluted from class I MHC molecules, or DC/tumor cell hybrids. The fusion of DCs with tumor cells has been shown to generate hybrid cells that display the functional properties of DCs and present one or more tumor antigens. Administration of hybrid cells prevents the growth of preimplanted tumor cells in various models, induces long-lasting tumor resistance *in vivo* (198–200), and can reverse unresponsiveness to a tumor-associated antigen (201). Another strategy is to expand DCs *in vivo* through administration of Fms-like tyrosine kinase 3 (FLT-3) ligand, which results in mobilization of DC precursors from the bone marrow and induction of antitumor immunity. FLT-3 ligand and CD40L synergize in the generation of immune response against two poorly immunogenic tumors, leading to complete rejection in a high proportion of mice and long-lasting protection (202).

Although animal studies provided the proof of principle for antigen-pulsed DC vaccination against cancer, this approach is still in an early stage in humans.

The use of DCs as adjuvants for immunotherapy of cancer has been possible because of the discovery that DCs might be generated from peripheral monocytes or CD34 bone marrow precursors, in the presence of certain cytokines such as GM-CSF, IL-4, and TNF-α (24).

DCs loaded with tumor antigens have been used in a number of trials in humans [for review, see Fong and Engelman (203) and Gunzer and Grabbe (204)]. It was initially demonstrated that DCs can be used to vaccinate B-cell lymphoma patients with the induction of antigen-specific T cells, and clinical responses were achieved in two of four patients (205). DCs were further used to treat melanoma, prostate cancer, and bladder cancer [for review, see Nestle (206)]. Nestle et al. (207) injected the DC preparation directly under ultrasound control in a normal inguinal lymph node (207). KLH was added as a CD4 helper antigen and immunological tracer molecule. DC vaccination induced delayed-type hypersensitivity reactivity toward KLH in all 16 patients and toward peptide-pulsed DCs in 11 patients. Objective clinical responses were obtained in five patients.

In another trial (208), injection of mature monocyte-derived DCs, pulsed with a MAGE-3 peptide and a recall antigen, was shown to enhance circulating MAGE-3–specific cytotoxic effectors in patients with melanoma and to lead to regression of individual metastases in 6 of 11 patients. Antigen-specific immune response was induced after intradermal injection but decreased after intravenous injection (208).

In another study, Banchereau et al. (209) used DCs derived from CD34$^+$ cells that consist of two phenotypically and functionally distinct populations: Langerhans cells and the interstitial/dermal DCs (similar to those derived from blood monocytes). Patients with metastatic melanoma received subcutaneous injections of CD34 progenitor–derived autologous DCs, pulsed with peptides derived from four melanoma antigens, as well as control antigens (influenza matrix peptide and KLH). DCs induced an immune response to control antigens in most patients, who also responded to at least one melanoma antigen.

A critical aspect of immunotherapy is the identification of immunologic markers that will permit prediction of clinical efficacy. Interestingly, the development of T-cell response to multiple tumor antigens was associated with a favorable early clinical outcome (209). Four patients who had metastatic MAGE-3$^+$ bladder cancer with measurable lesions were treated with autologous DCs prepared from peripheral blood mononuclear cells with one MAGE-3 epitope peptide; three showed significant reductions in the size of lymph node metastases, liver metastasis, or both (210). In one clinical trial, DCs expanded in patients after FLT-3 ligand treatment were used. These FLT-3 ligand–mobilized DCs were loaded with altered peptide derived from carcinoembryonic antigen and injected intravenously into patients with recurrent or metastatic colon cancer or non–small-cell lung cancer. Clinical response was observed in 5 of 12 patients and correlated with the expansion of CD8$^+$ T cells that recognized both the native and altered epitopes and displayed cytotoxic function (211).

Fusions were generated with primary human breast carcinoma cells and autologous DCs (212) and with human ovarian carcinoma cells with autologous or allogeneic DCs (213). The fusion cells retain the functional potency of DCs and activate CTL responses against autologous breast tumor cells *in vitro*.

Although promising, DC vaccination is in an early stage, and several parameters that may be critical for the immunological and clinical outcome need to be defined: the DC type, antigen loading, site of injection, DC dosage, and frequency of injections. Labeling studies with radioactive tracers have demonstrated significant differences in the distribution of DCs administered by different routes. Subcutaneous injection was shown to be ineffective in causing DC migration to regional lymphatic vessels, intravenous administration resulted in DC migration in the spleen, and intradermal administration led to regional transit in some patients (214). Another study (215) compared the efficacy of DC vaccines given by intravenous, intradermic, and intralymphatic routes. Patients with metastatic prostate cancer received two monthly injections of *ex vivo*–enriched DCs. The results indicated that DCs can

prime CD4 T-cell responses when administered by any of the studied routes but that the cytokine profile differs with route of administration: intradermic and intralymphatic injections induce Th1 immunity, whereas intravenous administration is associated with higher frequency and titer of antigen-specific antibodies.

CONCLUSIONS

DCs perform several tasks with high efficiency. They present the antigenic sample at the time of danger through evolutionary conserved pattern-recognition systems and sensitize lymphocytes specific for these dangerous antigens. They also seem to play an active role in central and peripheral tolerance by silencing autoreactive T cells generated by the stochastic recombination of the T-cell variable pattern-recognition receptors. There is indeed evidence that DCs constitutively present self antigens and that tolerogenic DCs that directly or indirectly prevent the activation of T cells specific to self may exist.

The immune system is confronted with the difficult task of combining the detection of potential pathogens in the periphery with the ability of adequately instruct cells of the adaptive immune system often located in lymphoid organs distant from the infection site. In general, when distant cells of a multicellular organism must communicate with one another, they secrete chemicals (hormones) that travel in the bloodstream to reach their target cells (endocrine communication). The immune system has developed a unique form of cell–cell communication, implying the migration of DCs carrying the biological information gathered at the site of infection (signals 1, 2, and 3) to the lymphoid organ, where they establish immunological synapses with lymphoid cells, exchanging information through locally secreted (paracrine communication) or membrane-bound molecules. This unique form of cell communication (which may be referred to as *motocrine communication*), combines long-distance communication between the peripheries of the lymphoid organs, with the confidentiality and specificity of a short-range synapse.

ACKNOWLEDGMENTS

I am grateful to Ralph Steinman for careful review and excellent suggestions; Oberdan Leo for interesting discussions; and Roberto Maldonado-López, Guillaume Oldenhove, and Karim Vermaelen for drawing the figures.

REFERENCES

1. Mosier D. A requirement for two cell types for antibody formation *in vitro*. *Science* 1967;158:1573–1575.
2. Steinman RM, Cohn ZA. Identification of a novel cell type in peripheral lymphoid organs of mice. I. Morphology, quantitation, tissue distribution. *J Exp Med* 1973;137:1142–1162.
3. Steinman RM, Witmer MD. Lymphoid dendritic cells are potent

stimulators of the primary mixed leukocyte reaction in mice. *Proc Natl Acad Sci U S A* 1978;75:5132–5136.

4. Liu YJ. Dendritic cell subsets and lineages, and their functions in innate and adaptive immunity. *Cell* 2001;106:259–262.

5. Manz MG, Traver D, Miyamoto T, et al. Dendritic cell potentials of early lymphoid and myeloid progenitors. *Blood* 2001;97:3333–3341.

6. Ardavin C, Martinez del Hoyo G, Martin P, et al. Origin and differentiation of dendritic cells. *Trends Immunol* 2001;22:691–700.

7. Bendriss-Vermare N, Barthelemy C, Durand I, et al. Human thymus contains IFN-alpha–producing CD11c(−), myeloid CD11c(+), and mature interdigitating dendritic cells. *J Clin Invest* 2001;107:835–844.

8. Katz SI, Tamaki K, Sachs DH. Epidermal Langerhans cells are derived from cells originating in bone marrow. *Nature* 1979;282:324–326.

9. Klareskog L, Tjernlund U, Forsum U, et al. Epidermal Langerhans cells express Ia antigens. *Nature* 1977;268:248–250.

10. Rowden G, Lewis MG, Sullivan AK. Ia antigen expression on human epidermal Langerhans cells. *Nature* 1977;268:247–248.

11. Schuler G, Steinman RM. Murine epidermal Langerhans cells mature into potent immunostimulatory dendritic cells *in vitro*. *J Exp Med* 1985;161:526–546.

12. Valladeau J, Ravel O, Dezutter-Dambuyant C, et al. Langerin, a novel C-type lectin specific to Langerhans cells, is an endocytic receptor that induces the formation of Birbeck granules. *Immunity* 2000;12:71–81.

13. Schon-Hegrad MA, Oliver J, McMenamin PG, et al. Studies on the density, distribution, and surface phenotype of intraepithelial class II major histocompatibility complex antigen (Ia)–bearing dendritic cells (DC) in the conducting airways. *J Exp Med* 1991;173:1345–1356.

14. Pavli P, Woodhams CE, Doe WF, et al. Isolation and characterization of antigen-presenting dendritic cells from the mouse intestinal lamina propria. *Immunology* 1990;70:40–47.

15. Holt PG, Oliver J, Bilyk N, et al. Downregulation of the antigen presenting cell function(s) of pulmonary dendritic cells *in vivo* by resident alveolar macrophages. *J Exp Med* 1993;177:397–407.

16. Iwasaki A, Kelsall BL. Unique functions of CD11b[+], CD8 alpha[+], and double-negative Peyer's patch dendritic cells. *J Immunol* 2001;166:4884–4890.

17. Iwasaki A, Kelsall BL. Freshly isolated Peyer's patch, but not spleen, dendritic cells produce interleukin 10 and induce the differentiation of T helper type 2 cells. *J Exp Med* 1999;190:229–239.

18. Vremec D, Pooley J, Hochrein H, et al. CD4 and CD8 expression by dendritic cell subtypes in mouse thymus and spleen. *J Immunol* 2000;164:2978–2986.

19. Kamath AT, Pooley J, O'Keeffe MA, et al. The development, maturation, and turnover rate of mouse spleen dendritic cell populations. *J Immunol* 2000;165:6762–6770.

20. Henri S, Vremec D, Kamath A, et al. The dendritic cell populations of mouse lymph nodes. *J Immunol* 2001;167:741–748.

21. Barker CF, Billingham RE. The role of afferent lymphatics in the rejection of skin homografts. *J Exp Med* 1968;128:197–221.

22. De Smedt T, Pajak B, Klaus GG, et al. Antigen-specific T lymphocytes regulate lipopolysaccharide-induced apoptosis of dendritic cells *in vivo*. *J Immunol* 1998;161:4476–4479.

23. Rissoan MC, Soumelis V, Kadowaki N, et al. Reciprocal control of T helper cell and dendritic cell differentiation. *Science* 1999;283:1183–1186.

24. Sallusto F, Lanzavecchia A. Efficient presentation of soluble antigen by cultured human dendritic cells is maintained by granulocyte/macrophage colony-stimulating factor plus interleukin 4 and downregulated by tumor necrosis factor alpha. *J Exp Med* 1994;179:1109–1118.

25. Randolph GJ, Beaulieu S, Lebecque S, et al. Differentiation of monocytes into dendritic cells in a model of transendothelial trafficking. *Science* 1998;282:480–483.

26. Schreurs MW, Eggert AA, de Boer AJ, et al. Generation and functional characterization of mouse monocyte-derived dendritic cells. *Eur J Immunol* 1999;29:2835–2841.

27. Randolph GJ, Inaba K, Robbiani DF, et al. Differentiation of phagocytic monocytes into lymph node dendritic cells *in vivo*. *Immunity* 1999;11:753–761.

28. Kadowaki N, Antonenko S, Lau JY, et al. Natural interferon alpha/beta–producing cells link innate and adaptive immunity. *J Exp Med* 2000;192:219–226.

29. Nakano H, Yanagita M, and Gunn MD. Cd11c(+)b220(+)gr-1(+) cells in mouse lymph nodes and spleen display characteristics of plasmacytoid dendritic cells. *J Exp Med* 2001;194:1171–1178.

30. Asselin-Paturel C, Boonstra A, Dalod M, et al. Mouse type I IFN-producing cells are immature APCs with plasmacytoid morphology. *Nat Immunol* 2001;2:1144–1150.

31. Zinkernagel RM, Ehl S, Aichele P, et al. Antigen localisation regulates immune responses in a dose- and time-dependent fashion: a geographical view of immune reactivity. *Immunol Rev* 1997;156:199–209.

32. Coyle AJ, Gutierrez-Ramos JC. The expanding B7 superfamily: increasing complexity in costimulatory signals regulating T cell function. *Nat Immunol* 2001;2:203–209.

33. Inaba K, Witmer-Pack M, Inaba M, et al. The tissue distribution of the B7-2 costimulator in mice: abundant expression on dendritic cells *in situ* and during maturation *in vitro*. *J Exp Med* 1994;180:1849–1860.

34. Larsen CP, Ritchie SC, Pearson TC, et al. Functional expression of the costimulatory molecule, B7/BB1, on murine dendritic cell populations. *J Exp Med* 1992;176:1215–1220.

35. Turley SJ, Inaba K, Garrett WS, et al. Transport of peptide-MHC class II complexes in developing dendritic cells. *Science* 2000;288:522–527.

36. Enk AH, Katz SI. Heat-stable antigen is an important costimulatory molecule on epidermal Langerhans' cells. *J Immunol* 1994;152:3264–3270.

37. Tamada K, Shimozaki K, Chapoval AI, et al. LIGHT, a TNF-like molecule, costimulates T cell proliferation and is required for dendritic cell–mediated allogeneic T cell response. *J Immunol* 2000;164:4105–4110.

38. Steinman RM, Cohn ZA. Identification of a novel cell type in peripheral lymphoid organs of mice. II. Functional properties *in vitro*. *J Exp Med* 1974;139:380–397.

39. Geijtenbeek TB, Torensma R, van Vliet SJ, et al. Identification of DC-SIGN, a novel dendritic cell-specific ICAM-3 receptor that supports primary immune responses. *Cell* 2000;100:575–585.

40. Geijtenbeek TB, Kwon DS, Torensma R, et al. DC-SIGN, a dendritic cell–specific HIV-1–binding protein that enhances trans-infection of T cells. *Cell* 2000;100:587–597.

41. Romani N, Koide S, Crowley M, et al. Presentation of exogenous protein antigens by dendritic cells to T cell clones. Intact protein is presented best by immature, epidermal Langerhans cells. *J Exp Med* 1989;169:1169–1178.

42. Moser M, De Smedt T, Sornasse T, et al. Glucocorticoids downregulate dendritic cell function *in vitro* and *in vivo*. *Eur J Immunol* 1995;25:2818–2824.

43. Reis e Sousa C, Hieny S, Scharton-Kersten T, et al. *In vivo* microbial stimulation induces rapid CD40 ligand–independent production of interleukin 12 by dendritic cells and their redistribution to T cell areas. *J Exp Med* 1997;186:1819–1829.

44. De Smedt T, Pajak B, Muraille E, et al. Regulation of dendritic cell numbers and maturation by lipopolysaccharide *in vivo*. *J Exp Med* 1996;184:1413–1424.

45. Kaisho T, Akira S. Dendritic-cell function in Toll-like receptor–and MyD88-knockout mice. *Trends Immunol* 2001;22:78–83.

46. Sallusto F, Cella M, Danieli C, et al. Dendritic cells use macropinocytosis and the mannose receptor to concentrate macromolecules in the major histocompatibility complex class II compartment: downregulation by cytokines and bacterial products. *J Exp Med* 1995;182:389–400.

47. de Baey A, Lanzavecchia A. The role of aquaporins in dendritic cell macropinocytosis. *J Exp Med* 2000;191:743–748.

48. Jiang W, Swiggard WJ, Heufler C, et al. The receptor DEC-205 expressed by dendritic cells and thymic epithelial cells is involved in antigen processing. *Nature* 1995;375:151–155.

49. Figdor CG, van Kooyk Y, Adema GJ. C-type lectin receptors on dendritic cells and Langerhans cells. *Nat Rev* 2002;21:77–84.

50. Mahnke K, Guo M, Lee S, et al. The dendritic cell receptor for endocytosis, DEC-205, can recycle and enhance antigen presentation via major histocompatibility complex class II–positive lysosomal compartments. *J Cell Biol* 2000;151:673–684.

51. Garrett WS, Chen LM, Kroschewski R, et al. Developmental control of endocytosis in dendritic cells by Cdc42. *Cell* 2000;102:325–334.

52. West MA, Prescott AR, Eskelinen EL, et al. Rac is required for constitutive macropinocytosis by dendritic cells but does not control its downregulation. *Curr Biol* 2000;10:839–848.

53. Kadowaki N, Ho S, Antonenko S, et al. Subsets of human dendritic cell precursors express different Toll-like receptors and respond to different microbial antigens. *J Exp Med* 2001;194:863–869.

54. Pulendran B, Kumar P, Cutler CW, et al. Lipopolysaccharides from distinct pathogens induce different classes of immune responses *in vivo*. *J Immunol* 2001;167:5067–5076.

55. Schulz O, Edwards DA, Schito M, et al. CD40 triggering of heterodimeric IL-12 p70 production by dendritic cells *in vivo* requires a microbial priming signal. *Immunity* 2000;13:453–462.

56. Pierre P, Mellman I. Developmental regulation of invariant chain proteolysis controls MHC class II trafficking in mouse dendritic cells. *Cell* 1998;93:1135–1145.

57. Villadangos JA, Cardoso M, Steptoe RJ, et al. MHC class II expression is regulated in dendritic cells independently of invariant chain degradation. *Immunity* 2001;14:739–749.

58. Cella M, Engering A, Pinet V, et al. Inflammatory stimuli induce accumulation of MHC class II complexes on dendritic cells. *Nature* 1997;388:782–787.

59. Pierre P, Turley SJ, Gatti E, et al. Developmental regulation of MHC class II transport in mouse dendritic cells. *Nature* 1997;388:787–792.

60. Inaba K, Turley S, Iyoda T, et al. The formation of immunogenic major histocompatibility complex class II–peptide ligands in lysosomal compartments of dendritic cells is regulated by inflammatory stimuli. *J Exp Med* 2000;191:927–936.

61. Santambrogio L, Sato AK, Carven GJ, et al. Extracellular antigen processing and presentation by immature dendritic cells. *Proc Natl Acad Sci U S A* 1999;96:15056–15061.

62. Rescigno M, Citterio S, Thery C, et al. Bacteria-induced neobiosynthesis, stabilization, and surface expression of functional class I molecules in mouse dendritic cells. *Proc Natl Acad Sci U S A* 1998;95:5229–5234.

63. Morel S, Levy F, Burlet-Schiltz O, et al. Processing of some antigens by the standard proteasome but not by the immunoproteasome results in poor presentation by dendritic cells. *Immunity* 2000;12:107–117.

64. Albert ML, Sauter B, Bhardwaj N. Dendritic cells acquire antigen from apoptotic cells and induce class I–restricted CTLs. *Nature* 1998;392:86–89.

65. Regnault A, Lankar D, Lacabanne V, et al. Fcgamma receptor–mediated induction of dendritic cell maturation and major histocompatibility complex class I–restricted antigen presentation after immune complex internalization. *J Exp Med* 1999;189:371–380.

66. Singh-Jasuja H, Toes RE, Spee P, et al. Cross-presentation of glycoprotein 96–associated antigens on major histocompatibility complex class I molecules requires receptor-mediated endocytosis. *J Exp Med* 2000;191:1965–1974.

67. Rodriguez A, Regnault A, Kleijmeer M, et al. Selective transport of internalized antigens to the cytosol for MHC class I presentation in dendritic cells. *Nat Cell Biol* 1999;1:362–368.

68. Steinman L. Absence of "original antigenic sin" in autoimmunity provides an unforeseen platform for immune therapy. *J Exp Med* 1999;189:1021–1024.

69. Baggiolini M. Chemokines and leukocyte traffic. *Nature* 1998;392:565–568.

70. Sato N, Ahuja SK, Quinones M, et al. CC chemokine receptor (CCR)2 is required for Langerhans cell migration and localization of T helper cell type 1 (Th1)–inducing dendritic cells. Absence of CCR2 shifts the *Leishmania major*–resistant phenotype to a susceptible state dominated by Th2 cytokines, B cell outgrowth, and sustained neutrophilic inflammation. *J Exp Med* 2000;192:205–218.

71. Dieu MC, Vanbervliet B, Vicari A, et al. Selective recruitment of immature and mature dendritic cells by distinct chemokines expressed in different anatomic sites. *J Exp Med* 1998;188:373–386.

72. Gunn MD, Kyuwa S, Tam C, et al. Mice lacking expression of secondary lymphoid organ chemokine have defects in lymphocyte homing and dendritic cell localization. *J Exp Med* 1999;189:451–460.

73. Sallusto F, Schaerli P, Loetscher P, et al. Rapid and coordinated switch in chemokine receptor expression during dendritic cell maturation. *Eur J Immunol* 1998;28:2760–2769.

74. Geijtenbeek TB, Krooshoop DJ, Bleijs DA, et al. DC-SIGN–ICAM-2 interaction mediates dendritic cell trafficking. *Nat Immunol* 2000;1:353–357.

75. Larsen CP, Steinman RM, Witmer-Pack M, et al. Migration and maturation of Langerhans cells in skin transplants and explants. *J Exp Med* 1990;172:1483–1493.

76. Xia W, Pinto CE, Kradin RL. The antigen-presenting activities of Ia+ dendritic cells shift dynamically from lung to lymph node after an airway challenge with soluble antigen. *J Exp Med* 1995;181:1275–1283.

77. Vermaelen KY, Carro-Muino I, Lambrecht BN, et al. Specific migratory dendritic cells rapidly transport antigen from the airways to the thoracic lymph nodes. *J Exp Med* 2001;193:51–60.

78. Huang FP, Platt N, Wykes M, et al. A discrete subpopulation of dendritic cells transports apoptotic intestinal epithelial cells to T cell areas of mesenteric lymph nodes. *J Exp Med* 2000;191:435–444.

79. Macatonia SE, Hosken NA, Litton M, et al. Dendritic cells produce IL-12 and direct the development of Th1 cells from naïve CD4+ T cells. *J Immunol* 1995;154:5071–5079.

80. Koch F, Stanzl U, Jennewein P, et al. High level IL-12 production by murine dendritic cells: upregulation via MHC class II and CD40 molecules and downregulation by IL-4 and IL-10. *J Exp Med* 1996;184:741–746.

81. Biedermann T, Zimmermann S, Himmelrich H, et al. IL-4 instructs TH1 responses and resistance to *Leishmania major* in susceptible BALB/c mice. *Nat Immunol* 2001;2:1054–1060.

82. Hochrein H, Shortman K, Vremec D, et al. Differential production of IL-12, IFN-alpha, and IFN-gamma by mouse dendritic cell subsets. *J Immunol* 2001;166:5448–5455.

83. Maldonado-López R, Moser M. Dendritic cell subsets and the regulation of Th1/Th2 responses. *Semin Immunol* 2001;13:275–282.

84. Reis e Sousa C, Yap G, Schulz O, et al. Paralysis of dendritic cell IL-12 production by microbial products prevents infection-induced immunopathology. *Immunity* 1999;11:637–647.

85. Maldonado-Lopez R, Maliszewski C, Urbain J, et al. Cytokines regulate the capacity of cd8alpha(+) and cd8alpha(−) dendritic cells to prime Th1/Th2 cells *in vivo*. *J Immunol* 2001;167:4345–4350.

86. Kang K, Kubin M, Cooper KD, et al. IL-12 synthesis by human Langerhans cells. *J Immunol* 1996;156:1402–1407.

87. Langenkamp A, Messi M, Lanzavecchia A, et al. Kinetics of dendritic cell activation: impact on priming of TH1, TH2 and nonpolarized T cells. *Nat Immunol* 2000;1:311–316.

88. Grumont R, Hochrein H, O'Keeffe M, et al. c-Rel regulates interleukin 12 p70 expression in CD8(+) dendritic cells by specifically inducing p35 gene transcription. *J Exp Med* 2001;194:1021–1032.

89. Dalod M, Salazar-Mather TP, Malmgaard L, et al. IFN-α/β and IL-12 responses to viral infections: pathways regulating dendritic cell cytokine expression *in vivo*. *J Exp Med* 2002;195:517–528.

90. Cella M, Facchetti F, Lanzavecchia A, et al. Plasmacytoid dendritic cells activated by influenza virus and CD40L drive a potent TH1 polarization. *Nat Immunol* 2000;1:305–310.

91. Granucci F, Vizzardelli C, Pavelka N, et al. Inducible IL-2 production by dendritic cells revealed by global gene expression analysis. *Nat Immunol* 2001;2:882–888.

92. De Becker G, Moulin V, Tielemans F, et al. Regulation of T helper cell differentiation *in vivo* by soluble and membrane proteins provided by antigen-presenting cells. *Eur J Immunol* 1998;28:3161–3171.

93. Ohteki T, Fukao T, Suzue K, et al. Interleukin 12–dependent interferon gamma production by CD8alpha+ lymphoid dendritic cells. *J Exp Med* 1999;189:1981–1986.

94. Fukao T, Matsuda S, Koyasu S. Synergistic effects of IL-4 and IL-18 on IL-12–dependent IFN-gamma production by dendritic cells. *J Immunol* 2000;164:64–71.

95. Khanna A, Morelli AE, Zhong C, et al. Effects of liver-derived dendritic cell progenitors on Th1- and Th2-like cytokine responses *in vitro* and *in vivo*. *J Immunol* 2000;164:1346–1354.

96. Steinman RM, Gutchinov B, Witmer MD, et al. Dendritic cells are the principal stimulators of the primary mixed leukocyte reaction in mice. *J Exp Med* 1983;157:613–627.

97. Nussenzweig MC, Steinman RM, Gutchinov B, et al. Dendritic cells are accessory cells for the development of anti-trinitrophenyl cytotoxic T lymphocytes. *J Exp Med* 1980;152:1070–1084.

98. Macatonia SE, Taylor PM, Knight SC, et al. Primary stimulation by dendritic cells induces antiviral proliferative and cytotoxic T cell responses *in vitro*. *J Exp Med* 1989;169:1255–1264.

99. Inaba K, Young JW, Steinman RM. Direct activation of CD8$^+$ cytotoxic T lymphocytes by dendritic cells. *J Exp Med* 1987;166:182–194.

100. Ridge JP, Di Rosa F, Matzinger P. A conditioned dendritic cell can be a temporal bridge between a CD4$^+$ T-helper and a T-killer cell. *Nature* 1998;393:474–478.

101. Schoenberger SP, Toes RE, van der Voort EI, et al. T-cell help for cytotoxic T lymphocytes is mediated by CD40–CD40L interactions. *Nature* 1998;393:480–483.

102. Bennett SR, Carbone FR, Karamalis F, et al. Help for cytotoxic T-cell responses is mediated by CD40 signalling. *Nature* 1998;393:478–480.

103. Ptak W, Rozycka D, Askenase PW, et al. Role of antigen-presenting cells in the development and persistence of contact hypersensitivity. *J Exp Med* 1980;151:362–375.

104. Britz JS, Askenase PW, Ptak W, et al. Specialized antigen-presenting cells. Splenic dendritic cells and peritoneal-exudate cells induced by mycobacteria activate effector T cells that are resistant to suppression. *J Exp Med* 1982;155:1344–1356.

105. Lechler RI, Batchelor JR. Restoration of immunogenicity to passenger cell-depleted kidney allografts by the addition of donor strain dendritic cells. *J Exp Med* 1982;155:31–41.

106. Inaba K, Metlay JP, Crowley MT, et al. Dendritic cells pulsed with protein antigens *in vitro* can prime antigen-specific, MHC-restricted T cells *in situ*. *J Exp Med* 1990;172:631–640.

107. Sornasse T, Flamand V, De Becker G, et al. Antigen-pulsed dendritic cells can efficiently induce an antibody response *in vivo*. *J Exp Med* 1992;175:15–21.

108. Liu LM, MacPherson GG. Antigen acquisition by dendritic cells: intestinal dendritic cells acquire antigen administered orally and can prime naïve T cells *in vivo*. *J Exp Med* 1993;177:1299–1307.

109. Inaba K, Turley S, Yamaide F, et al. Efficient presentation of phagocytosed cellular fragments on the major histocompatibility complex class II products of dendritic cells. *J Exp Med* 1998;188:2163–2173.

110. Thery C, Regnault A, Garin J, et al. Molecular characterization of dendritic cell-derived exosomes. Selective accumulation of the heat shock protein hsc73. *J Cell Biol* 1999;147:599–610.

111. Knight SC, Iqball S, Roberts MS, et al. Transfer of antigen between dendritic cells in the stimulation of primary T cell proliferation. *Eur J Immunol* 1998;28:1636–1644.

112. Guery JC, Ria F, Adorini L. Dendritic cells but not B cells present antigenic complexes to class II–restricted T cells after administration of protein in adjuvant. *J Exp Med* 1996;183:751–757.

113. Crowley M, Inaba K, Steinman RM. Dendritic cells are the principal cells in mouse spleen bearing immunogenic fragments of foreign proteins. *J Exp Med* 1990;172:383–386.

114. Larsen CP, Morris PJ, Austyn JM. Migration of dendritic leukocytes from cardiac allografts into host spleens. A novel pathway for initiation of rejection. *J Exp Med* 1990;171:307–314.

115. Lambrecht BN, Salomon B, Klatzmann D, et al. Dendritic cells are required for the development of chronic eosinophilic airway inflammation in response to inhaled antigen in sensitized mice. *J Immunol* 1998;160:4090–4097.

116. Gallucci S, Lolkema M, Matzinger P. Natural adjuvants: endogenous activators of dendritic cells. *Nat Med* 1999;5:1249–1255.

117. Valitutti S, Muller S, Cella M, et al. Serial triggering of many T-cell receptors by a few peptide-MHC complexes. *Nature* 1995;375:148–151.

118. Valitutti S, Muller S, Dessing M, et al. Signal extinction and T cell repolarization in T helper cell–antigen-presenting cell conjugates. *Eur J Immunol* 1996;26:2012–2016.

119. Iezzi G, Karjalainen K, Lanzavecchia A. The duration of antigenic stimulation determines the fate of naïve and effector T cells. *Immunity* 1998;8:89–95.

120. van Stipdonk MJ, Lemmens EE, Schoenberger SP. Naïve CTLs require a single brief period of antigenic stimulation for clonal expansion and differentiation. *Nat Immunol* 2001;2:423–429.

121. Labrecque N, Whitfield LS, Obst R, et al. How much TCR does a T cell need? *Immunity* 2001;15:71–82.

122. Zell T, Khoruts A, Ingulli E, et al. Single-cell analysis of signal transduction in CD4 T cells stimulated by antigen *in vivo*. *Proc Natl Acad Sci U S A* 2001;98:10805–10810.

123. Revy P, Sospedra M, Barbour B, et al. Functional antigen-independent synapses formed between T cells and dendritic cells. *Nat Immunol* 2001;2:925–931.

124. Kondo T, Cortese I, Markovic-Plese S, et al. Dendritic cells signal T cells in the absence of exogenous antigen. *Nat Immunol* 2001;2:932–938.

124a. Inaba K, Steinman RM. Accessory cell-T lymphocyte interactions. Antigen-dependent and -independent clustering. *J Exp Med* 1986;163:247–261.

125. Green J, Jotte R. Interactions between T helper cells and dendritic cells during the rat mixed lymphocyte reaction. *J Exp Med* 1985;162:1546–1560.

126. De Becker G, Moulin V, Pajak B, et al. The adjuvant monophosphoryl lipid A increases the function of antigen-presenting cells. *Int Immunol* 2000;12:807–815.

127. Le Bon A, Schiavoni G, D'Agostino G, et al. Type I interferons potently enhance humoral immunity and can promote isotype switching by stimulating dendritic cells *in vivo*. *Immunity* 2001;14:461–470.

128. Andrews DM, Andoniou CE, Granucci F, et al. Infection of dendritic cells by murine cytomegalovirus induces functional paralysis. *Nat Immunol* 2001;2:1077–1084.

129. Marie JC, Kehren J, Trescol-Biemont MC, et al. Mechanism of measles virus–induced suppression of inflammatory immune responses. *Immunity* 2001;14:69–79.

130. Angeli V, Faveeuw C, Roye O, et al. Role of the parasite-derived prostaglandin D2 in the inhibition of epidermal Langerhans cell migration during schistosomiasis infection. *J Exp Med* 2001;193:1135–1147.

131. Toellner KM, Luther SA, Sze DM, et al. T helper 1 (Th1) and Th2 characteristics start to develop during T cell priming and are associated with an immediate ability to induce immunoglobulin class switching. *J Exp Med* 1998;187:1193–1204.

132. Constant SL, Bottomly K. Induction of Th1 and Th2 CD4$^+$ T cell responses: the alternative approaches. *Annu Rev Immunol* 1997;15:297–322.

133. Lanzavecchia A, Iezzi G, Viola A. From TCR engagement to T cell activation: a kinetic view of T cell behavior. *Cell* 1999;96:1–4.

134. O'Garra A. Cytokines induce the development of functionally heterogeneous T helper cell subsets. *Immunity* 1998;8:275–283.

135. de Jong R, Altare F, Haagen IA, et al. Severe mycobacterial and *Salmonella* infections in interleukin-12 receptor–deficient patients. *Science* 1998;280:1435–1438.

136. Oppmann B, Lesley R, Blom B, et al. Novel p19 protein engages IL-12p40 to form a cytokine, IL-23, with biological activities similar as well as distinct from IL-12. *Immunity* 2000;13:715–725.

137. Stoll S, Jonuleit H, Schmitt E, et al. Production of functional IL-18 by different subtypes of murine and human dendritic cells (DC): DC-derived IL-18 enhances IL-12-dependent Th1 development. *Eur J Immunol* 1998;28:3231–3239.

138. Maldonado-Lopez R, De Smedt T, Michel P, et al. CD8alpha$^+$ and CD8alpha$^-$ subclasses of dendritic cells direct the development of distinct T helper cells *in vivo*. *J Exp Med* 1999;189:587–592.

139. Jacobson NG, Szabo SJ, Weber-Nordt RM, et al. Interleukin 12 signaling in T helper type 1 (Th1) cells involves tyrosine phosphorylation of signal transducer and activator of transcription (Stat)3 and Stat4. *J Exp Med* 1995;181:1755–1762.

140. Szabo SJ, Kim ST, Costa GL, et al. A novel transcription factor, T-bet, directs Th1 lineage commitment. *Cell* 2000;100:655–669.

141. Paul WE, Seder RA. Lymphocyte responses and cytokines. *Cell* 1994;76:241–251.

142. d'Ostiani CF, Del Sero G, Bacci A, et al. Dendritic cells discriminate between yeasts and hyphae of the fungus *Candida albicans*. Implications for initiation of T helper cell immunity *in vitro* and *in vivo*. *J Exp Med* 2000;191:1661–1674.

143. Kelleher P, Maroof A, Knight SC. Retrovirally induced switch from production of IL-12 to IL-4 in dendritic cells. *Eur J Immunol* 1999;29:2309–2318.

144. Freeman GJ, Boussiotis VA, Anumanthan A, et al. B7-1 and B7-2 do not deliver identical costimulatory signals, since B7-2 but not B7-1

preferentially costimulates the initial production of IL-4. *Immunity* 1995;2:523–532.

145. Zhu J, Huang H, Guo L, et al. Transient inhibition of interleukin 4 signaling by T cell receptor ligation. *J Exp Med* 2000;192:1125–1134.

146. Ebner S, Ratzinger G, Krosbacher B, et al. Production of IL-12 by human monocyte-derived dendritic cells is optimal when the stimulus is given at the onset of maturation, and is further enhanced by IL-4. *J Immunol* 2001;166:633–641.

147. Hochrein H, O'Keeffe M, Luft T, et al. Interleukin (IL)–4 is a major regulatory cytokine governing bioactive IL-12 production by mouse and human dendritic cells. *J Exp Med* 2000;192:823–833.

148. Kalinski P, Smits HH, Schuitemaker JH, et al. IL-4 is a mediator of IL-12p70 induction by human Th2 cells: reversal of polarized Th2 phenotype by dendritic cells. *J Immunol* 2000;165:1877–1881.

149. Farrar JD, Smith JD, Murphy TL, et al. Selective loss of type I interferon–induced STAT4 activation caused by a minisatellite insertion in mouse Stat2. *Nat Immunol* 2000;1:65–69.

150. Kalinski P, Hilkens CM, Wierenga EA, et al. T-cell priming by type-1 and type-2 polarized dendritic cells: the concept of a third signal. *Immunol Today* 1999;20:561–567.

151. Pulendran B, Smith JL, Caspary G, et al. Distinct dendritic cell subsets differentially regulate the class of immune response *in vivo. Proc Natl Acad Sci U S A* 1999;96:1036–1041.

152. Vieira PL, de Jong EC, Wierenga EA, et al. Development of Th1-inducing capacity in myeloid dendritic cells requires environmental instruction. *J Immunol* 2000;164:4507–4512.

153. De Smedt T, Van Mechelen M, De Becker G, et al. Effect of interleukin-10 on dendritic cell maturation and function. *Eur J Immunol* 1997;27:1229–1235.

154. Huang Q, Liu do N, Majewski P, et al. The plasticity of dendritic cell responses to pathogens and their components. *Science* 2001;294:870–875.

155. Sallusto F, Lenig D, Forster R, et al. Two subsets of memory T lymphocytes with distinct homing potentials and effector functions. *Nature* 1999;401:708–712.

156. Laufer TM, DeKoning J, Markowitz JS, et al. Unopposed positive selection and autoreactivity in mice expressing class II MHC only on thymic cortex. *Nature* 1996;383:81–85.

157. Brocker T, Riedinger M, Karjalainen K. Targeted expression of major histocompatibility complex (MHC) class II molecules demonstrates that dendritic cells can induce negative but not positive selection of thymocytes *in vivo. J Exp Med* 1997;185:541–550.

158. Delaney JR, Sykulev Y, Eisen HN, et al. Differences in the level of expression of class I major histocompatibility complex proteins on thymic epithelial and dendritic cells influence the decision of immature thymocytes between positive and negative selection. *Proc Natl Acad Sci U S A* 1998;95:5235–5240.

159. Bouneaud C, Kourilsky P, Bousso P. Impact of negative selection on the T cell repertoire reactive to a self-peptide: a large fraction of T cell clones escapes clonal deletion. *Immunity* 2000;13:829–840.

160. Schwartz RH. Models of T cell anergy: is there a common molecular mechanism? *J Exp Med* 1996;184:1–8.

161. Inaba K, Pack M, Inaba M, et al. High levels of a major histocompatibility complex II–self peptide complex on dendritic cells from the T cell areas of lymph nodes. *J Exp Med* 1997;186:665–672.

162. Hawiger D, Inaba K, Dorsett Y, et al. Dendritic cells induce peripheral T cell unresponsiveness under steady state conditions *in vivo. J Exp Med* 2001;194:769–779.

163. Kurts C, Kosaka H, Carbone FR, et al. Class I–restricted cross-presentation of exogenous self-antigens leads to deletion of autoreactive CD8(+) T cells. *J Exp Med* 1997;186:239–245.

164. Morgan DJ, Kreuwel HT, Sherman LA. Antigen concentration and precursor frequency determine the rate of CD8+ T cell tolerance to peripherally expressed antigens. *J Immunol* 1999;163:723–727.

165. Lutz MB, Suri RM, Niimi M, et al. Immature dendritic cells generated with low doses of GM-CSF in the absence of IL-4 are maturation resistant and prolong allograft survival *in vivo. Eur J Immunol* 2000;30:1813–1822.

166. Dhodapkar MV, Steinman RM, Krasovsky J, et al. Antigen-specific inhibition of effector T cell function in humans after injection of immature dendritic cells. *J Exp Med* 2001;193:233–238.

167. Jonuleit H, Schmitt E, Schuler G, et al. Induction of interleukin 10-producing, nonproliferating CD4(+) T cells with regulatory properties by repetitive stimulation with allogeneic immature human dendritic cells. *J Exp Med* 2000;192:1213–1222.

168. Suss G, Shortman K. A subclass of dendritic cells kills CD4 T cells via Fas/Fas-ligand–induced apoptosis. *J Exp Med* 1996;183:1789–1796.

169. Kronin V, Winkel K, Suss G, et al. A subclass of dendritic cells regulates the response of naïve CD8 T cells by limiting their IL-2 production. *J Immunol* 1996;157:3819–3827.

170. Fazekas de St Groth B. The evolution of self-tolerance: a new cell arises to meet the challenge of self-reactivity. *Immunol Today* 1998;19:448–454.

171. Grohmann U, Bianchi R, Ayroldi E, et al. A tumor-associated and self antigen peptide presented by dendritic cells may induce T cell anergy *in vivo*, but IL-12 can prevent or revert the anergic state. *J Immunol* 1997;158:3593–3602.

172. Jonuleit H, Schmitt E, Steinbrink K, et al. Dendritic cells as a tool to induce anergic and regulatory T cells. *Trends Immunol* 2001;22:394–400.

173. Steinbrink K, Wolfl M, Jonuleit H, et al. Induction of tolerance by IL-10–treated dendritic cells. *J Immunol* 1997;159:4772–4780.

174. Akbari O, DeKruyff RH, Umetsu DT. Pulmonary dendritic cells producing IL-10 mediate tolerance induced by respiratory exposure to antigen. *Nat Immunol* 2001;2:725–731.

175. Waldmann H, Cobbold S. Regulating the immune response to transplants. a role for CD4+ regulatory cells? *Immunity* 2001;14:399–406.

176. Maloy KJ, Powrie F. Regulatory T cells in the control of immune pathology. *Nat Immunol* 2001;2:816–822.

177. Sauter B, Albert ML, Francisco L, et al. Consequences of cell death: exposure to necrotic tumor cells, but not primary tissue cells or apoptotic cells, induces the maturation of immunostimulatory dendritic cells. *J Exp Med* 2000;191:423–434.

178. Steinman RM, Turley S, Mellman I, et al. The induction of tolerance by dendritic cells that have captured apoptotic cells. *J Exp Med* 2000;191:411–416.

179. Morel PA, Feili-Hariri M. How do dendritic cells prevent autoimmunity? *Trends Immunol* 2001;22:546–547.

180. Inaba K, Steinman RM, Van Voorhis WC, et al. Dendritic cells are critical accessory cells for thymus-dependent antibody responses in mouse and in man. *Proc Natl Acad Sci U S A* 1983;80:6041–6045.

181. Inaba K, Witmer MD, Steinman RM. Clustering of dendritic cells, helper T lymphocytes, and histocompatible B cells during primary antibody responses *in vitro. J Exp Med* 1984;160:858–876.

182. Dubois B, Vanbervliet B, Fayette J, et al. Dendritic cells enhance growth and differentiation of CD40-activated B lymphocytes. *J Exp Med* 1997;185:941–951.

183. Fayette J, Dubois B, Vandenabeele S, et al. Human dendritic cells skew isotype switching of CD40-activated naïve B cells towards IgA1 and IgA2. *J Exp Med* 1997;185:1909–1918.

184. Grouard G, Durand I, Filgueira L, et al. Dendritic cells capable of stimulating T cells in germinal centres. *Nature* 1996;384:364–367.

185. Trinchieri G. Biology of natural killer cells. *Adv Immunol* 1989;47:187–376.

186. Fernandez NC, Lozier A, Flament C, et al. Dendritic cells directly trigger NK cell functions: cross-talk relevant in innate anti-tumor immune responses *in vivo. Nat Med* 1999;5:405–411.

187. Gerosa F, Baldani-Guerra B, Nisii C, et al. Reciprocal activating interaction between natural killer cells and dendritic cells. *J Exp Med* 2002;195:327–333.

188. Chambers BJ, Salcedo M, Ljunggren HG. Triggering of natural killer cells by the costimulatory molecule CD80 (B7-1). *Immunity* 1996;5:311–317.

189. Geldhof AB, Moser M, Lespagnard L, et al. Interleukin-12–activated natural killer cells recognize B7 costimulatory molecules on tumor cells and autologous dendritic cells. *Blood* 1998;91:196–206.

190. Wilson JL, Heffler LC, Charo J, et al. Targeting of human dendritic cells by autologous NK cells. *J Immunol* 1999;163:6365–6370.

191. MacDonald HR. NK1.1+ T cell receptor-alpha/beta+ cells: new clues to their origin, specificity, and function. *J Exp Med* 1995;182:633–638.

192. Kawano T, Cui J, Koezuka Y, et al. CD1d-restricted and TCR-mediated activation of Valpha14 NKT cells by glycosylceramides. *Science* 1997;278:1626–1629.

193. Spada FM, Koezuka Y, Porcelli SA. CD1d-restricted recognition of synthetic glycolipid antigens by human natural killer T cells. *J Exp Med* 1998;188:1529–1534.

193a. Ikarashi Y, Mikami R, Bendelac A, et al. Dendritic cell maturation overrules H-2-mediated natural killer T (NKT) cell inhibition: critical role for B7 in CD1d-dependent NKT cell interferon gamma production. *J Exp Med* 2001;194:1179–1186.

194. Kadowaki N, Antonenko S, Ho S, et al. Distinct cytokine profiles of neonatal natural killer T cells after expansion with subsets of dendritic cells. *J Exp Med* 2001;193:1221–1226.

195. Boon T, Kellermann O. Rejection by syngeneic mice of cell variants obtained by mutagenesis of a malignant teratocarcinoma cell line. *Proc Natl Acad Sci U S A* 1977;74:272–275.

196. Flamand V, Sornasse T, Thielemans K, et al. Murine dendritic cells pulsed *in vitro* with tumor antigen induce tumor resistance *in vivo*. *Eur J Immunol* 1994;24:605–610.

197. Mayordomo JI, Zorina T, Storkus WJ, et al. Bone marrow–derived dendritic cells pulsed with synthetic tumour peptides elicit protective and therapeutic antitumour immunity. *Nat Med* 1995;1:1297–1302.

198. Gong J, Chen D, Kashiwaba M, et al. Induction of antitumor activity by immunization with fusions of dendritic and carcinoma cells. *Nat Med* 1997;3:558–561.

199. Wang J, Saffold S, Cao X, et al. Eliciting T cell immunity against poorly immunogenic tumors by immunization with dendritic cell–tumor fusion vaccines. *J Immunol* 1998;161:5516–5524.

200. Lespagnard L, Mettens P, Verheyden AM, et al. Dendritic cells fused with mastocytoma cells elicit therapeutic antitumor immunity. *Int J Cancer* 1998;76:250–258.

201. Gong J, Chen D, Kashiwaba M, et al. Reversal of tolerance to human MUC1 antigen in MUC1 transgenic mice immunized with fusions of dendritic and carcinoma cells. *Proc Natl Acad Sci U S A* 1998;95:6279–6283.

202. Borges L, Miller RE, Jones J, et al. Synergistic action of fms-like tyrosine kinase 3 ligand and CD40 ligand in the induction of dendritic cells and generation of antitumor immunity *in vivo*. *J Immunol* 1999;163:1289–1297.

203. Fong L, Engleman EG. Dendritic cells in cancer immunotherapy. *Annu Rev Immunol* 2000;18:245–273.

204. Gunzer M, Grabbe S. Dendritic cells in cancer immunotherapy. *Crit Rev Immunol* 2001;21:133–145.

205. Hsu FJ, Benike C, Fagnoni F, et al. Vaccination of patients with B-cell lymphoma using autologous antigen-pulsed dendritic cells. *Nat Med* 1996;2:52–58.

206. Nestle FO. Dendritic cell vaccination for cancer therapy. *Oncogene* 2000;19:6673–6679.

207. Nestle FO, Alijagic S, Gilliet M, et al. Vaccination of melanoma patients with peptide- or tumor lysate–pulsed dendritic cells. *Nat Med* 1998;4:328–332.

208. Thurner B, Haendle I, Roder C, et al. Vaccination with Mage-3A1 peptide–pulsed mature, monocyte-derived dendritic cells expands specific cytotoxic T cells and induces regression of some metastases in advanced stage IV melanoma. *J Exp Med* 1999;190:1669–1678.

209. Banchereau J, Palucka AK, Dhodapkar M, et al. Immune and clinical responses in patients with metastatic melanoma to CD34(+) progenitor–derived dendritic cell vaccine. *Cancer Res* 2001;61:6451–6458.

210. Nishiyama T, Tachibana M, Horiguchi Y, et al. Immunotherapy of bladder cancer using autologous dendritic cells pulsed with human lymphocyte antigen-A24-specific MAGE-3 peptide. *Clin Cancer Res* 2001;7:23–31.

211. Fong L, Hou Y, Rivas A, et al. Altered peptide ligand vaccination with Flt3 ligand expanded dendritic cells for tumor immunotherapy. *Proc Natl Acad Sci U S A* 2001;98:8809–8814.

212. Gong J, Avigan D, Chen D, et al. Activation of antitumor cytotoxic T lymphocytes by fusions of human dendritic cells and breast carcinoma cells. *Proc Natl Acad Sci U S A* 2000;97:2715–2718.

213. Gong J, Nikrui N, Chen D, et al. Fusions of human ovarian carcinoma cells with autologous or allogeneic dendritic cells induce antitumor immunity. *J Immunol* 2000;165:1705–1711.

214. Morse MA, Coleman RE, Akabani G, et al. Migration of human dendritic cells after injection in patients with metastatic malignancies. *Cancer Res* 1999;59:56–58.

215. Fong L, Brockstedt D, Benike C, et al. Dendritic cells injected via different routes induce immunity in cancer patients. *J Immunol* 2001;166:4254–4259.

216. Pulendran B, Banchereau J, Maraskovsky E, et al. Modulating the immune response with dendritic cells and their growth factors. *Trends Immunol* 2001;22:41–47.

217. Mellman I, Steinman RM. Dendritic cells: specialized and regulated antigen processing machines. *Cell* 2001;106:255–258.

CHAPTER 16

Macrophages and the Immune Response

Siamon Gordon

Introduction
Some Landmarks in the Study of Macrophages
Properties of Macrophages and Their Relation to Immune Functions
    Overview · Growth and Differentiation: Life History and Turnover · Tissue Distribution and Phenotypic Heterogeneity of Resident Macrophages in Lymphoid and Nonlymphoid Organs · Enhanced Recruitment of Monocytes by Inflammatory and Immune Stimuli: Activation *In Vivo* · Phagocytic Recognition and Intracellular Infection · Gene expression and secretion · Modulation of Macrophage Activation *In Vitro*
Conclusions and Some Remaining Issues
Acknowledgments
References

INTRODUCTION

Macrophages (Mϕ) represent a family of mononuclear leukocytes that are widely distributed throughout the body, within and outside lympho-hemopoietic organs. They vary considerably in life span and phenotype, depending on their origin and local microenvironment. Mature Mϕ are highly phagocytic, relatively long-lived cells, and adaptable in their biosynthetic responses to antigens and microbial stimuli. The functions of Mϕ within tissues are homeostatic, regulating the local and systemic milieu through diverse plasma membrane receptors and varied secretory products. They react to as well as generate signals that influence growth, differentiation, and death of other cells, recognizing and engulfing senescent and abnormal cells. These activities contribute substantially to recognition and defense functions against invading microorganisms, foreign particulates, and other immunogens. Innate immune functions of Mϕ complement their contributions to acquired humoral and cellular immunity, in which they regulate activation of T- and B-lymphocytes; this is achieved in part through their specialized derivatives, dendritic cells (DC) of myeloid origin. With or without DC, Mϕ process and present antigen, and produce chemokines and cytokines (e.g., IL-1, IL-6, IL-12, IL-18, TNFα, and IL-10), and phagocytose apoptotic and necrotic cells. Acting directly or under the influence of other immune cells, Mϕ capture extra- and intra-cellular pathogens, and eliminate invaders and deliver them to appropriate subcompartments of lymphoid organs. As key regulators of the specific as well as natural immune response, Mϕ boost as well as limit induction and effector mechanisms of the specific immune response by positive and negative feedback.

The properties and roles of DC are described in detail elsewhere in this volume. Here we focus on other members of the Mϕ lineage, consider their interrelationship and outline specialized properties that underlie their roles in the execution and regulation of immune responses. The following works deal with the history and broad aspects of Mϕ immunobiology: Metchnikoff (1), Karnovsky and Bolis (2), Tauber and Chernyak (3), Van Furth (4), Gordon (5–7), and Burke and Lewis (8).

SOME LANDMARKS IN THE STUDY OF MACROPHAGES

Our understanding of Mϕ developed in parallel with the growth of immunology as an experimental science. Metchnikoff, a comparative developmental zoologist, is widely credited for his recognition of phagocytosis as a fundamental host defense mechanism of primitive, as well as highly developed multicellular organisms (1–3). He clearly stated the link between capture of infectious microorganisms by the spleen and subsequent appearance of reactive substances (antibodies) in the blood, although mistakenly ascribing their production to the phagocytes themselves. The importance of systemic clearance of particles by Mϕ, especially Kupffer cells in liver and other endothelial cells, was memorialized in the term "reticulo-endothelial system" (RES). Although rejected by influential investigators in the field in favor of the term "mononuclear phagocyte system" (MPS), the understanding that sinus-lining Mφ in liver and elsewhere share common properties with selected endothelial cells is worth preserving (4). Earlier studies by Florey and his students, including Gowans, established that circulating monocytes give rise to tissue Mφ. Van Furth and colleagues investigated the life history of Mφ by kinetic labeling methods; subsequently, the development of membrane antigen markers facilitated a more precise definition of specialized Mφ subpopulations in tissues such as brain (9). The appearance and potential importance of Mφ during development also became evident as a result of sensitive immunocytochemical methods. Morphologic and functional studies by Humphrey and many others drew attention to striking diversity among Mφ-like cells in secondary lymphoid organs, especially within the marginal zone of the spleen, where complex particulates and polysaccharides are captured from the circulation (10).

The era of modern cell biology impinged on Mφ studies following the studies of Cohn and Hirsch and colleagues (11). Their work touched on many aspects of cell structure and function, including phagocytosis (the zipper mechanism of Silverstein), fluid and receptor-mediated endocytosis, secretion, and antimicrobial resistance. Isolation and *in vitro* culture systems became available for cells from mouse and human, especially after the identification of specific growth and differentiation factors such as CSF-1 (M-CSF) (12). It is perhaps fitting that the earliest known natural knockout (KO) affecting macrophages, a natural mutation in the op gene in the osteopetrotic mouse, should involve CSF-1 (13). Cell lines retaining some, but not all features of mature Mφ, have been useful for many biochemical and cellular studies (5). Macrophages and dendritic cells can be readily derived from embryonic stem cells by growth in appropriate culture conditions.

The role of Mφ as antigen-processing cells able to initiate adaptive immune responses had false trails—"immunogenic RNA" was thought to be involved at one time. It also encompassed early genetic strategies: Mφ of mice selected for high anti-sheep erythrocyte antibody responses by Biozzi and colleagues displayed enhanced degradative properties; adherent cells from defined guinea pig strains were shown to play an important role in Ia (MHC) restricted anti-insulin responses. For many years, the antigen-presenting cell (APC) functions of adherent cells were highly controversial as promoted by Unanue, who concentrated on intracellular processing by Mφ and Steinman, who discovered the specialized role of "dendritic cells" in antigen presentation to naïve T-lymphocytes. The importance of Mφ as effector cells in immunity to intracellular pathogens such as *Mycobacterium tuberculosis* was recognized early by Lurie and Dannenberg. Mackaness made use of Listeria monocytogenes and BCG infection in experimental models and developed the concept of Mφ activation as an antigen-dependent, but immunologically nonspecific, enhancement of antimicrobial resistance. The subsequent delineation of T-lymphocyte subsets and characterization of

interferon gamma (14) as the major lymphokine involved in macrophage activation, including MHC II induction, merged with increasing knowledge of the role of reactive oxygen, and later, nitrogen metabolites as cytotoxic agents (15). The role of virus-infected Mφ as MHC I–restricted targets for antigen-specific CD8$^+$ killer cells was part of the initial characterization of this phenomenon by Zinkernagel and Doherty. D'Arcy Hart was an early investigator of the intracellular interactions between Mφ and invaders of the vacuolar system, especially mycobacteria, which survive within Mφ by evading host resistance mechanisms. Mouse breeding studies by several groups defined a common genetic locus involved in resistance to BCG, Leishmania, and Salmonella organisms. The host phenotype was shown to depend on expression in Mφ and, many years later, the gene (termed N-ramp for natural resistance–associated membrane protein) was identified by positional cloning by Skamene, Gross, and their colleagues (16). Positional cloning by Beutler and associates led to the identification of the gene responsible for lipopolysaccharide (LPS) resistance in particular mouse strains. Together with studies by Hoffman and colleagues on the Toll pathway in *Drosophila,* this work resulted in an explosion of interest in the identification of Toll-like receptors (TLR) and their role in innate immunity to infection (17).

This brief survey concludes with the identification of Mφ as key target cells for infection, dissemination, and persistence of HIV (18), and tropic for macrophages by virtue of their expression of CD4, chemokine co-receptors, and DC-SIGN, a C-type lectin also expressed by DC (19). Although Mφ had been implicated by earlier workers such as Mims as important in antiviral resistance generally, their role in this regard was neglected before the emergence of HIV as a major pathogen.

Many molecules have been identified as important in Mφ functions in immunity and serve as valuable markers to study their properties in mouse and human. These include Fc (20) and complement (21) receptors, important in opsonic phagocytosis; killing and immunoregulation; nonopsonic lectin receptors, such as the mannose receptor (MR) (22) and β glucan receptor (BGR) (23); and secretory products such as lysozyme (24), neutral proteinases, TNFα (25), chemokines, and many other cytokines. A range of membrane antigens (Ag) expressed by human and rodent mononuclear phagocytes has been characterized and reagents made available for further study of Mφ in normal and diseased states (9). Recently, the role of DNA-binding transcription factors including members of the NFκB and Ets (PU.1) families has received increased attention in the study of differential gene expression by Mφ (26,27). Gene inactivation has confirmed the important role of many of these molecules within the intact host, although little use has yet been made of cell-specific or conditional KO animals to uncover the role of Mφ in immunologic processes. Naturally occurring inborn errors in man such as the leukocyte adhesion–deficiency syndrome and chronic granulomatous disease have contributed to the analysis of important leukocyte functions, including those of Mϕ, in host resistance to infection. Mutations to a monocyte-expressed gene (NOD2), initially thought to be involved in LPS signaling and NFκB activation, have been implicated in a subset of individuals with an enhanced susceptibility to Crohn's disease (28). The validity of murine KO models for human genetic deficiencies has been confirmed for key molecules involved in Mϕ activation, such as IFNγ and IL-12. Others will undoubtedly follow.

PROPERTIES OF MACROPHAGES AND THEIR RELATION TO IMMUNE FUNCTIONS

Overview

Mϕ participate in the production, mobilization, activation, and regulation of all immune effector cells. They interact reciprocally with other cells while their own properties are modified to perform specialized immunologic functions. As a result of cell-surface, auto- and paracrine interactions, Mϕ display marked heterogeneity in phenotype (9,29), a source of interest and considerable confusion to the investigator. Increasing knowledge of cellular and molecular properties of Mϕ bears strongly on our understanding of their role in the immune response. I review these briefly below, with emphasis on functional significance, and draw attention to unresolved and controversial issues.

Growth and Differentiation: Life History and Turnover

In contrast with T- and B-lymphocytes, monocytes from blood give rise to terminally differentiated Mϕ that cannot recirculate or re-initiate DNA replication except in a limited way; DC may represent specialized migratory derivatives of mononuclear cells. Unlike other myeloid granulocytic cells, Mϕ can be long-lived and retain the ability to synthesize RNA and protein to a marked extent, even when in a relatively quiescent state, as "resident" cells. These are distributed throughout the tissues of the body and constitute a possible alarm-response system, but also mediate poorly understood trophic functions. Following inflammatory and immune stimuli, many more monocytes can be recruited to local sites and give rise to "elicited" or "immunologically activated" Mϕ with altered surface, secretory, and cytotoxic properties. The origins of Mϕ from precursors are well known, from yolk sac (and possibly earlier para-aortic progenitors), migrating to fetal liver, and then spleen and bone marrow, before and after birth (30). In the fetus, mature Mϕ proliferate actively during tissue remodeling in developing organs. In the normal adult, tissue Mϕ do not self-renew extensively except in specialized microenvironments such as the lung or pituitary; after injury there can be considerable further replication at local sites of inflammation. Growth and differentiation are tightly regulated by specific growth factors (e.g., IL-3, CSF-1, GM-CSF, IL-4, IL-13) and inhibitors (e.g., IFN-α/β,

TGF β, LIF) that vary considerably in their potency and selectivity. These processes are modulated by interactions with adjacent stromal and other cells—for example, through c-kit/ligand and Flt-3/ligand interactions. The growth response of the target cell to an extrinsic stimulus decreases progressively and markedly (from 10^8 or more to 10^0) during differentiation from stem cell to committed precursor to monoblast, monocyte, and Mϕ, yet even the most terminally differentiated Mϕ such as microglial cells can be "reactivated" to a limited extent by local stimuli (31). Elicited/activated Mϕ respond more vigorously than resident Mϕ to growth stimuli in vivo and in vitro, but the molecular basis for their enhanced proliferation is unknown.

Although the general picture of blood monocyte to tissue Mϕ differentiation has been clear for some time, as a result of parabiosis, adoptive transfer and irradiation-reconstitution experiments, there are still major unsolved issues. Are all "monocytes" equivalent or is there heterogeneity in the circulating mononuclear cell pool corresponding with the ultimate tissue localization of their progeny? Our present understanding of DC and osteoclast differentiation is compatible with a relatively simple model (Fig. 1) in which major Mϕ populations in tissues can be characterized by selected Ag markers such as F4/80 (Emr1, a member of a new family of EGF-TM7 molecules) (32) and macrosialin (CD68), a pan-Mϕ endosomal glycoprotein related to the lysosome-associated membrane protein (LAMP) family (33). The DC of myeloid origin can be viewed as products of Langerhans-type cells in nonlymphoid organs such as skin and airway epithelium, which undergo further differentiation and migrate to secondary lymphoid organs in response to an antigenic stimulus. Circulating precursors of DC and recirculating progeny are also normally present in the mononuclear fraction of blood in small numbers and may be already "marked" for distribution to peripheral sites as Langerhans cells. Monocytes that have crossed the endothelium may be induced to "reverse migrate" into circulation by selected stimuli in tissues (34).

Circulating mononuclear precursors for osteoclasts are less defined and differentiate into mononucleate cells in bone and cartilage, where they fuse to form multinucleate bone-resorbing osteoclasts. Local stromal cells, growth factors such as CSF-1, steroids (vitamin D metabolites) and hormones (e.g., calcitonin for which osteoclasts express receptors), all contribute to local maturation. Recently, it has been found that osteoprotegerin, a naturally occurring secreted protein with homology to members of the TNF receptor family, interacts with TRANCE, a TNF-related protein, to regulate osteoclast differentiation and activation in vitro and in vivo.

Ag markers such as CD34 on progenitors and CD14 and CD16 on monocytes, and the use of multichannel FACS analysis make it possible to isolate leukocyte subpopulations and study their progeny and differential responses. The mononuclear fraction of blood may contain precursors of other tissue

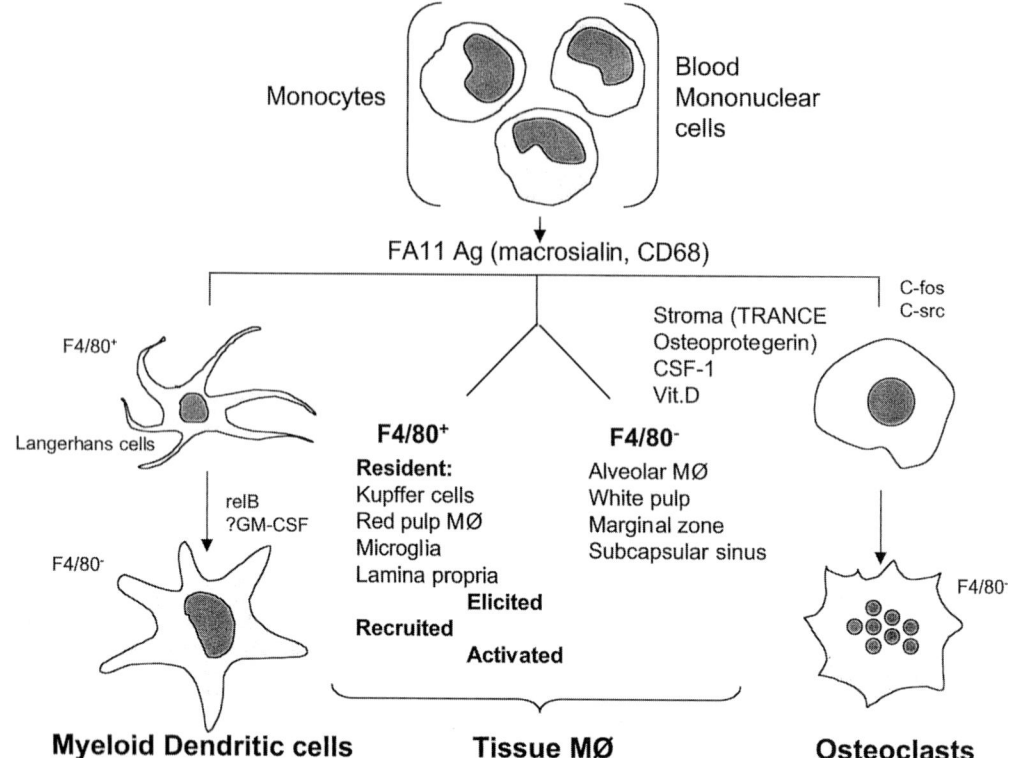

FIG. 1. Differentiation of mononuclear phagocytes, based on antigen markers FA-11 (macrosialin, murine CD68) and F4/80.

cells, including "fibrocytes," thought to be hemopoietic yet able to synthesize matrix proteins such as collagen, and some endothelial cells. Perhaps the mysterious follicular dendritic cells (FDC), with mixed hemopoietic and mesenchymal properties, fall into this category.

The large-scale production of immature and mature DC-like cells from bulk monocytes in cytokine-supplemented culture systems (IL-4, GM-CSF, TNFα), has revolutionized the study of these specialized APC (35). Individually, the same cytokines give rise to Mφ-like cells, and early during in vitro differentiation, the cellular phenotype is reversible. Later, when mature DC with high MHC II, APC function and other characteristic markers are formed, differentiation is irreversible. This process is independent of cell division, although earlier progenitors in bone marrow and G-CSF–mobilized blood mononuclear cells can be stimulated to multiply, as well as differentiate, in vitro. These examples of terminal differentiation observed with DC and osteoclasts may extend to other specialized, more obvious Mφ-like cells. Mature Mφ can be derived by growth and differentiation in steroid-supplemented media in Dexter-type long-term bone marrow cultures that contain stromal fibroblasts and hemopoietic elements. These Mφ express adhesion molecules responsible for divalent cation–dependent cluster formation with erythroblasts (EbR) (36). This receptor, possibly related to V-CAM, cannot be induced on terminally differentiated peritoneal Mφ if these are placed in the same culture system. This contrasts sharply with the ready adaptation

of many tissue Mφ to conventional cell culture conditions, when the cells often adopt a common, standard phenotype. Irreversible stages of Mφ differentiation may therefore occur in specialized microenvironments in vitro or in vivo.

Little is known about determinants of Mφ longevity and turnover. Growth factors such as CSF-1 enhance Mφ survival and prevent induction of an apoptotic program. The expression of Fas-L and Fas on Mφ has been less studied than on lymphocytes; they and other members of the TNF and its receptor family may play a major role in determining Mφ survival, especially in induced populations, where cell turnover is markedly enhanced. Tissue Mφ vary greatly in their life span, from days to months. Apart from inflammatory and microbial stimuli, local and systemic environmental factors such as salt loading and hormones, including oestrogen, are known to influence Mφ turnover.

Tissue Distribution and Phenotypic Heterogeneity of Resident Macrophages in Lymphoid and Nonlymphoid Organs

The use of the F4/80 plasma membrane Ag made it possible to detect mature Mφ in developing and adult murine tissues and define their anatomic relationship to other cells in endothelium, epithelium, and connective tissue, as well as the nervous system (9,37). Subsequently, other membrane Ag (38)—macrosialin (33) and sialoadhesin (Sn) (39,40)—were identified as useful markers for Mφ in situ (Table 1).

TABLE 1. *Differentiation antigens used to study murine macrophage heterogeneity*

Ab	Ag	Structure	Ligands	Cellular expression	Function	Comment
F4/80	F4/80 (EMR1)	EGF-TM7	?	Mature Mφ Absent T areas	?	Useful marker development, CNS
FA-11	Macrosialin (CD68)	Mucin-Lamp	OX-LDL	Pan-Mφ, DC	Late endosomal	Glycoforms regulated by inflammation and phagocytosis
5C6	CR3 (CD11b, CD18)	β2 integrin	iC3b, ICAM	Monocytes, microglia, PMN, NK cells	Phagocytosis Adhesion	Important in inflammatory recruitment, PMN apoptosis
2F8	SR-A (I,II)	Collagenous, type II glycoprotein Isoforms differ Cysteine-rich domain	Polyanions -LTA,LPS -modified proteins -β amyloid	Mφ Sinusoidal Endothelium	Adhesion Endocytosis Phagocytosis of apoptotic cells and bacteria	Protects host against LPS-induced shock Promotes atherosclerosis
SER-4 3D6	Sn (Siglec-1)	Ig superfamily	Sialyl glycoconjugates, e.g., CD43	Subsets tissue Mφ	Lectin	Strongly expressed marginal zone metallophils in spleen and subcapsular sinus of lymph nodes

Mφ subpopulations in different tissues display considerable heterogeneity in expressing these and selected receptor antigens (CR3 [41] and SR-A [42]), drawing attention to mechanisms of homing, emigration and local adaptation to particular microenvironments. From the viewpoint of immune responses, a few aspects deserve comment.

Fetal Liver and Bone Marrow

Mature Mφ form an integral part of the hemopoietic microenvironment and play a key role in the production, differentiation, and destruction of all hemopoietic cells. The fetal liver is a major site of definitive erythropoiesis from midgestation. The bone marrow becomes active in the production of hemopoietic cells from shortly before birth and Mφ are a prominent component of the hemopoietic stroma throughout adult life. Mature "stromal" Mφ in fetal liver and adult bone marrow express nonphagocytic adhesion molecules such as Sn, an Ig-superfamily sialic acid–binding lectin (39,40) (Table 1), and the EbR referred to above (36), which is also involved in adhesion of developing myeloid and possibly lymphoid cells (Fig. 2). VLA-4 has been implicated as a ligand for EbR. Ligands for Sn include CD43 on developing granulocytes and on lymphocyte subpopulations. Sn clusters at sites of contact between stromal Mφ and myeloid, but not erythroid cells. Chemokines are able to induce polarized expression of adhesion molecules such as ICAMs and CD43 in leukocytes, but the significance of altered ligand distribution for interactions between Mφ and bound hemopoietic cells is unknown. Adhesion of immature cells to stromal Mφ may play a role in regulating their intermediate stages of development before release into the blood stream, whereas fibroblasts in the stroma associate with earlier progenitors, as well as with Mφ. Discarded nuclei of mammalian erythroid cells are rapidly engulfed by stromal Mφ, but the receptors involved in their binding and phagocytosis are unknown. Mφ also phagocytose apoptotic hemopoietic cells generated in bone marrow, including large numbers of myeloid and B cells. We still know little about the plasma membrane molecules and cytokine signals operating within this complex milieu, but it is clear that stromal Mφ constitute a neglected constituent within the hemopoietic microenvironment.

Thymus

Apart from their remarkable capacity to remove apoptotic thymocytes, the possible role of Mφ in positive and negative selection of thymocytes has been almost totally overlooked; more attention has been given to local DC, which may share markers with lymphoid, rather than myeloid cells. Mature Mφ with specialized properties are present in cortex and medulla. Clusters of viable thymocytes and Mφ can be isolated from the thymus of young animals by collagenase digestion and adherence to a substratum (Fig. 2). The nonphagocytic adhesion receptors responsible for cluster formation are more highly expressed by thymic than other Mφ, but their nature is unknown (N. Platt, remain unpublished from this laboratory). These Mφ also express MHC class II Ag and other

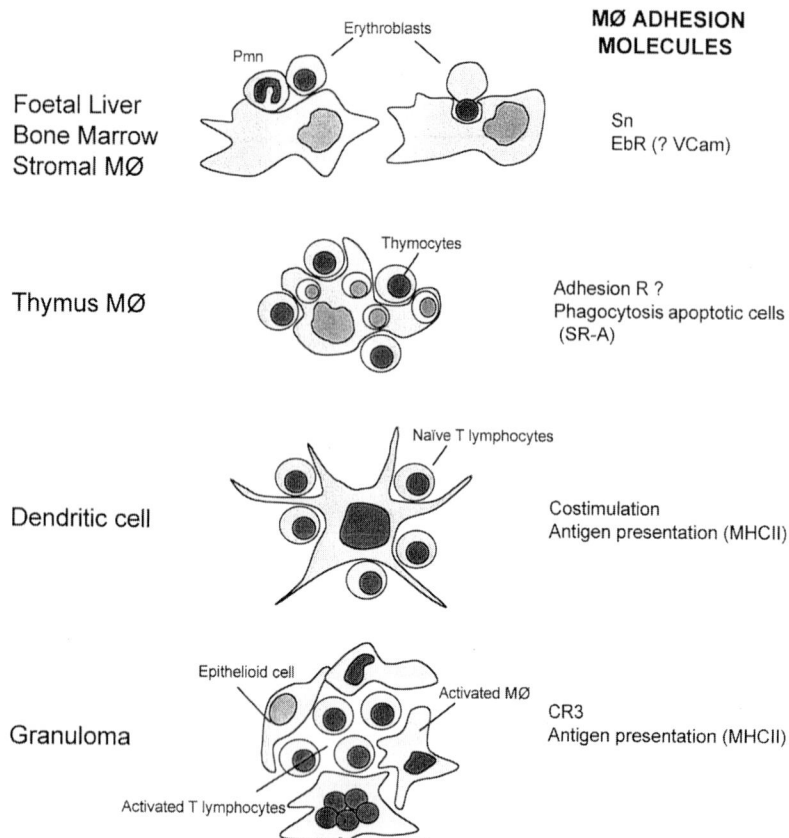

MØ ADHESION MOLECULES

Foetal Liver
Bone Marrow
Stromal MØ

Sn
EbR (? VCam)

Thymus MØ

Adhesion R ?
Phagocytosis apoptotic cells
(SR-A)

Dendritic cell

Costimulation
Antigen presentation (MHCII)

Granuloma

CR3
Antigen presentation (MHCII)

FIG. 2. Associations of tissue macrophages with other haemopoietic cells to illustrate variations on a common theme.

receptors such as the class A scavenger receptor (SR-A) (see below), which contributes to phagocytosis of apoptotic thymocytes (43). Other markers such as the F4/80 Ag are poorly expressed *in situ,* but can be readily detected after cell isolation. A striking difference between thymic and several other tissue MØ subpopulations is their independence of CSF-1; the CSF-1–deficient op/op mouse lacks osteoclasts and some MØ populations, including monocytes, peritoneal cells, and Kupffer cells, but contains normal numbers of thymic MØ, as well as DC and selected MØ in other sites. Factors involved in constitutive recruitment of thymic MØ are unknown; following death of thymocytes induced by ionizing radiation or glucocorticoids, intensely phagocytic MØ appear in large numbers; it is not known what proportion arises locally and by recruitment.

Spleen

From the viewpoint of the MØ, the spleen is perhaps the most complex organ in the body. It contributes to hemopoiesis, which persists postnatally in some species or can be induced by increased demand, and to the turnover of all blood elements at the end of their natural life span. In addition, the spleen filters a substantial proportion of total cardiac output, captures particulate and other antigenic materials from the blood stream, and plays an important role in natural and acquired humoral and cellular immunity. The organ is rich in

subpopulations of MØ that differ in microanatomical localization, phenotype, life history, and functions (Fig. 3). MØ are central to antigen capture, degradation, transport, and presentation to T- and B-lymphocytes, and contribute substantially to antimicrobial resistance. Since other hemopoietic and secondary lymphoid organs can replace many of these functions after maturation of the immune system, the unique properties of the spleen have been mainly recognized in the immature host and in immune responses to complex polysaccharides. Splenectomy in the adult renders the host susceptible to infection by pathogenic bacteria such as pneumococci that contain saccharide-rich capsular antigens; the marginal zone of the spleen in particular may play an essential role in this aspect of host resistance (10).

The properties of MØ in the unstimulated mature mouse spleen are very different according to their localization in red or white pulp, and the marginal zone. MØ are intimately associated with the specialized vasculature. Species differences in splenic anatomy are well recognized, but MØ display broadly common features in man and rodent, where studied. Subpopulations of MØ, DC, and cells with mixed phenotypes, have been characterized by *in situ* analysis with Ag markers, toxic liposome–depletion studies, various immunization and infection protocols, and, recently, cytokine and receptor-gene KO models in the mouse (44). The results raise questions about the dynamics and molecular basis of cell production, recruitment, differentiation, emigration, and death within each

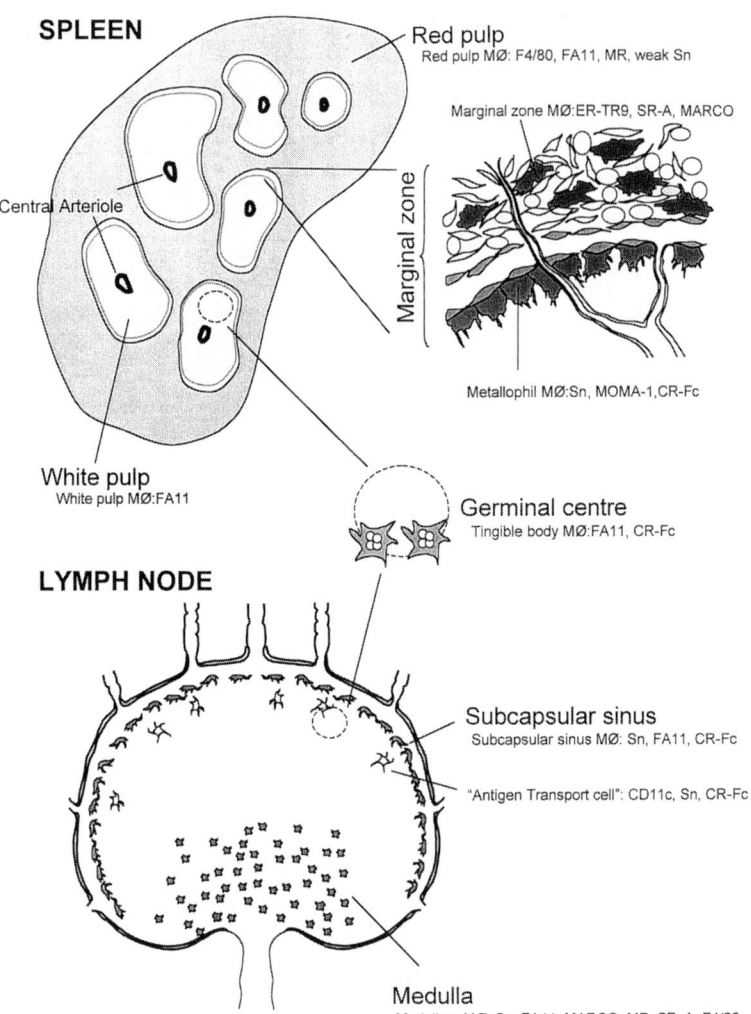

SPLEEN

Red pulp
Red pulp MØ: F4/80, FA11, MR, weak Sn

Marginal zone MØ:ER-TR9, SR-A, MARCO

Central Arteriole

Metallophil MØ:Sn, MOMA-1,CR-Fc

White pulp
White pulp MØ:FA11

Germinal centre
Tingible body MØ:FA11, CR-Fc

LYMPH NODE

Subcapsular sinus
Subcapsular sinus MØ: Sn, FA11, CR-Fc

"Antigen Transport cell": CD11c, Sn, CR-Fc

Medulla
Medullary MØ: Sn, FA11, MARCO, MR, SR-A, F4/80

FIG. 3. Microheterogeneity of macrophages in spleen, and resting and antigen-stimulated lymph nodes. (See text for markers.)

distinct splenic compartment. Cell isolation methods are still primitive in correlating *in vitro* properties with those of MØ subpopulations *in vivo,* and provide an important challenge for the future. Detailed aspects of splenic architecture, DC origin and function, and of T- and B-lymphocyte induction and differentiation, are described elsewhere in this volume. I shall highlight some features of MØ in the normal and immunoreactive organ.

Marginal Zone Macrophages

The spleen marginal zone consists of a complex mixture of resident cells (reticular and other fibroblasts, endothelium), MØ, DC, and lymphoid cells, including subpopulations of B-lymphocytes (10). It constitutes an important interface with the circulation, which delivers cells, particulates, or soluble molecules directly into the marginal sinus or via the red pulp. Resident MØ are present as specialized metallophilic cells in the inner marginal zone and other MØ are found in the outer zone; the latter may be more phagocytic. Sn is very strongly expressed by the marginal metallophils, compared with only weak expression in red pulp, and its virtual

absence in the white pulp. Sn$^+$ cells appear in this zone 2 to 4 weeks postnatally in the mouse as the white pulp forms. Liposomes containing clodronate, a cytotoxic drug, can be delivered systemically and deplete Sn$^+$ cells and other MØ; regeneration of different MØ subpopulations in spleen occurs at different times and this procedure has been used to correlate their reappearance with distinct immunologic functions. Marginal zone MØ lack F4/80, but express the type 3 complement receptor (CR$_3$), which is absent on red pulp MØ. Marginal zone MØ express other phagocytic receptors, such as SR-A, which is more widely present on tissue MØ, as well as MARCO, a distinct collagenous scavenger receptor that is almost exclusively present on these MØ in the normal mouse. The structures and possible role of these pattern-recognition receptors in uptake of microbes will be discussed below. Recent studies have shown that a MØ lectin, the MR, may be involved in transfer of mannosylated ligands to the site of an immune response in the white pulp (22). The MR contains a highly conserved cysteine-rich domain, not involved in mannosyl recognition, that reacts strongly with ligands on marginal metallophilic MØ (45), sulphated glycoforms of Sn and CD45 among others. This has been demonstrated with a chimeric probe of the cysteine-rich domain of the MR and human Fc (CR-Fc) and by immunochemical analysis of tissue sections and affinity chromatography of spleen ligands (46). After immunization this probe additionally labels undefined cells in the FDC network of germinal centers, as well as tingible body Mφ. It is possible that marginal zone Mφ can be induced to migrate into white pulp as described after LPS injection; alternatively, they may shed complexes of soluble MR-glycoprotein ligand, for transfer to other CR-Fc⁺ cells, which may be resident or newly recruited mononuclear cells. Finally, the marginal metallophilic Mφ population depends on CSF-1 for its appearance (44), and on members of the TNF receptor family, as shown with op/op and experimentally produced KO mice (47).

White Pulp Macrophages

The F4/80 Ag is strikingly absent on murine white pulp Mφ which do express FA-11, (macrosialin), the murine homolog of CD68. Actively phagocytic Mφ express this intracellular glycoprotein in abundance, compared with DC. After uptake of a foreign particle—for example, sheep erythrocytes, or an infectious agent (e.g., BCG, *Plasmodium yoelii*)—white pulp Mφ become more prominent, although it is not known whether there is migration of cells into the white pulp or transfer of phagocytosed material and reactivation of previous resident Mφ. Tingible body Mφ appear to be involved in uptake and digestion of apoptotic B-lymphocytes.

Red Pulp Macrophages

Red pulp macrophages express F4/80 Ag and MR (48) strongly, and in the mouse include stromal-type Mφ involved in hemopoiesis. Extensive phagocytosis of senescent erythrocytes results in accumulation of bile pigments and ferritin. The role of various phagocytic receptors in clearance of host cells and pathogens by red pulp Mφ requires further study.

There is no evidence that Mφ, other than interdigitating DC, associate directly with CD4⁺ T-lymphocytes in the normal spleen. Following infection by BCG, for example, or by other microorganisms such as Salmonella, there is massive recruitment and local production of Mφ, many of which associate with T-lymphocytes. Newly formed granulomata often appear first in the marginal zone (focal accumulations of activated Mφ and activated T cells). As infections spread into the white and red pulp the granulomata become confluent and less localized, obscuring and/or disrupting the underlying architecture of the spleen. The possible role of activated Mφ in T-cell apoptosis and clearance in spleen has not been defined.

Lymph Nodes

F4/80 Ag is relatively poorly expressed in lymph node, but many macrosialin (CD68) ⁺cells are present (Fig. 3). The subcapsular sinus is analogous to the marginal zone and

contains strongly Sn⁺ cells; this is the site where afferent lymph enters, containing antigen and migrating DC derived from Langerhans cells. The medulla contains Sn⁺, CD68⁺ Mφ, which also express high levels of SR-A. As in the spleen marginal zone, subcapsular sinus Mφ are strongly labeled by the CR-Fc probe. Following primary or secondary immunization, the staining pattern moves deeper into the cortex and eventually becomes concentrated in germinal centers. The kinetics of this process strongly suggest a transport process by Mφ-related cells resembling antigen transport cells described previously. CR-Fc⁺ cells can be isolated by digestion of lymph nodes and form clusters with CR-Fc⁻ lymphocytes. Adoptive transfer has shown that FACS-isolated CR-Fc⁺ cells resemble DC in their ability to home to T-cell areas and to present antigen to naïve T and B cells (49). Overall, there is considerable heterogeneity in the population of migratory APC involved in antigen capture, transport, and delivery to T and B cells, and it may turn out that specialized tissue Mφ as well as myeloid-type DC can migrate in response to immunologic stimuli, especially of a particulate nature.

Peyer's Patch

While less studied, the Mφ in Peyer's patch resemble the CD68⁺ F4/80⁻ cells described in spleen and white pulp, and in other T-cell–rich areas. They are well placed to interact with gut-derived antigens and pathogens taken up via specialized epithelial M cells in the dome, and deliver antigens to afferent lymphatics, as myeloid DC. These cells are distinct from abundant F4/80⁺ cells in the lamina propria found all the way down the gastrointestinal tract and may play a role in the induction of mucosal immunity.

Nonlymphoid Organs

Regional F4/80⁺ and CD68⁺ Mφ are well described in liver (Kupffer cells), dermis, in neuro-endocrine and reproductive organs, and in serosal cavities where they are able to react to systemic and local stimuli. In the lung, alveolar Mφ are strongly CD68⁺ but only weakly F4/80⁺, and are distinct from interstitial Mφ and intra-epithelial DC (50). Additionally, resident Mφ are found throughout connective tissue and within the interstitium of organs, including heart, kidney, and pancreas. These cells vary greatly depending on their local microenvironment; for example, in the central nervous system microglia within the neuropil differ strikingly from Mφ in the meninges or choroid plexus. Perivascular Mφ in the brain can be distinguished from resident microglia by their expression of endocytic receptors, such as the SR-A and MR, and of MHC I and II antigens. Microglia are highly ramified, terminally differentiated cells of monocytic origin and many Mφ markers are down-regulated; their phenotype is influenced by the blood–brain barrier, normally absent in circumventricular organs, and disrupted by inflammatory stimuli. Microglia can be reactivated by local LPS and neurocytotoxins, and are then difficult to distinguish from newly recruited monocytes that acquire microglial features once they enter the parenchyma of the brain (51). Resting microglia are unusual among many tissue Mφ in that they constitutively express high levels of CR3 and respond to CR3 ligands, such as mAb, by induced DNA synthesis and apoptosis (31). Natural ligands for CR3 in the central nervous system are not defined.

Enhanced Recruitment of Monocytes by Inflammatory and Immune Stimuli: Activation *In Vivo*

In response to local tissue and vascular changes, partly induced by resident Mφ during (re)activation by inflammatory and immunologic stimuli, monocytes are recruited from marrow pools and blood in increased numbers; they diapedese and differentiate into Mφ with altered effector functions as they enter the tissues. These Mφ are classified as "elicited" when cells are generated in the absence of γ interferon, and as "immunologically activated" after exposure to γ interferon. Enhanced recruitment can also involve that of other myeloid or lymphoid cells; selectivity of the cellular response depends on the nature of the evoking stimulus (immunogenic or not), the chemokines produced, and the receptors expressed by different leukocytes. Mφ as well as other cells produce a range of different chemokines and express multiple-7 transmembrane, G-protein–coupled chemokine receptors. The chemokines can also act in the marrow compartment, especially if anchored to matrix and glycosaminoglycans, and may display other growth regulatory functions. Locally bound or soluble chemokines induce the surface expression and activity of adhesion molecules on circulating white cells, as well as directing their migration through and beyond endothelium. Feedback mechanisms from periphery to central stores and within the marrow stroma may depend on cytokines and growth factors such as MIP1α and GM-CSF, which inhibit or enhance monocyte production, respectively. The adhesion molecules involved in recruitment of monocytes, originally defined by studies in humans with inborn errors and by use of inhibitory antibodies in experimental animal models, overlap with those of PMN and lymphocytes and include L-selectin, β_2 integrins, especially CR3, CD31, an Ig superfamily molecule, and CD99 (52). Additional monocyte adhesion molecules for activated endothelium include CD44, VCAM, β_1 integrins, and newly described receptors. The mechanisms of constitutive entry of monocytes into developing and adult tissues, in the absence of an inflammatory stimulus, are unknown.

The migration and differentiation of newly recruited monocytes once they have left the circulation are poorly understood. They are able to enter all tissues, undergoing alterations in membrane molecules and secretory potential under the influence of cytokines and surface interactions with endothelial cells, leukocytes, and other local cells. Phenotypic changes mentioned below have been characterized by a range of *in vitro* and *in vivo* studies. Well-studied examples include murine peritoneal Mφ, resident, elicited by thioglycollate broth or biogel polyacrylamide beads, and immunologi-

cally activated by BCG infection. The latter provides a useful model of granuloma formation in solid organs, but does not fully mimic the human counterpart associated with *M. tuberculosis* infection. Granuloma Mφ vary in their turnover and immune effector functions and display considerable heterogeneity; lesions contain recently recruited monocytes, mature epithelioid Mφ (described as secretory cells), and Langerhans giant cells. Interactions with T-lymphocytes, other myeloid cells, DC, and fibroblasts, as well as microorganisms, yield a dynamic assembly of cells as the granuloma evolves, heals, and resolves (Fig. 2). Apoptosis and necrosis of Mφ and other cells contribute to the balance of continued recruitment and local proliferation. The emigration of Mφ rather than DC from sites of inflammation is less evident, although it has become clear that elicited Mφ within the peritoneal cavity, for example, migrate actively to draining lymph nodes.

Gene KO models have confirmed the role of molecules previously implicated in recruitment, activation, and granuloma formation. These include the adhesion molecules listed above; their ligands such as ICAM 1; and key cytokines such as γ interferon, IL-12, and TNFα, as well as their receptors. Antimicrobial resistance and Mφ cytotoxicity resulting from production of reactive oxygen and nitrogen metabolites, are now accessible to study in KO of the phagocyte oxidase and iNOS. Knockouts of membrane molecules of immunologic interest expressed by Mφ and other cells include MHC class II and I, CD4 and CD40L, other accessory molecules such as B7-1 and B7-2, and the Mφ-restricted, intracellular molecule N-ramp.

The use of KO and/or antibodies (53) or soluble receptors has brought insight into essential, nonredundant contributions of molecules that regulate Mφ activation, immunopathology syndromes such as septic shock, and autoimmunity. Examples include myeloid antigens such as TREM-1, receptor–ligand pairs involving OX2 and suppressors of cytokine signaling (SOCS) proteins. TNFα is essential for host resistance to infection (54), and contributes to immunopathology. Highly effective anti-TNFα therapy for chronic inflammatory diseases such as rheumatoid arthritis (55) can result in reactivation of latent tuberculosis.

The potential for Th1- and Th2-type regulation of Mφ demonstrated *in vitro,* and discussed below, can result in highly complex, often co-existent, heterogeneity of Mφ phenotype *in situ* (Fig. 4). While almost all granuloma Mφ express lysozyme, only minor subpopulations express cytokines such as IL-1β, IL-6, and TNFα. Pro- and anti-inflammatory cytokines, IL-12, IL-18, IL-10, and TGFβ, produced by Mφ themselves and other cells, modulate the phenotype of Mφ *in vivo.*

Apart from the local interactions outlined, Mφ regulate systemic host reactions to immune and infectious stimuli by producing circulating cytokines such as IL-6, and arachidonate- and other lipid-derived metabolites. These act on neural and endocrine centers, crossing the blood–brain barrier, or are generated locally by reactive microglia and Mφ. Glucocorticosteroids are powerful immunomodulators

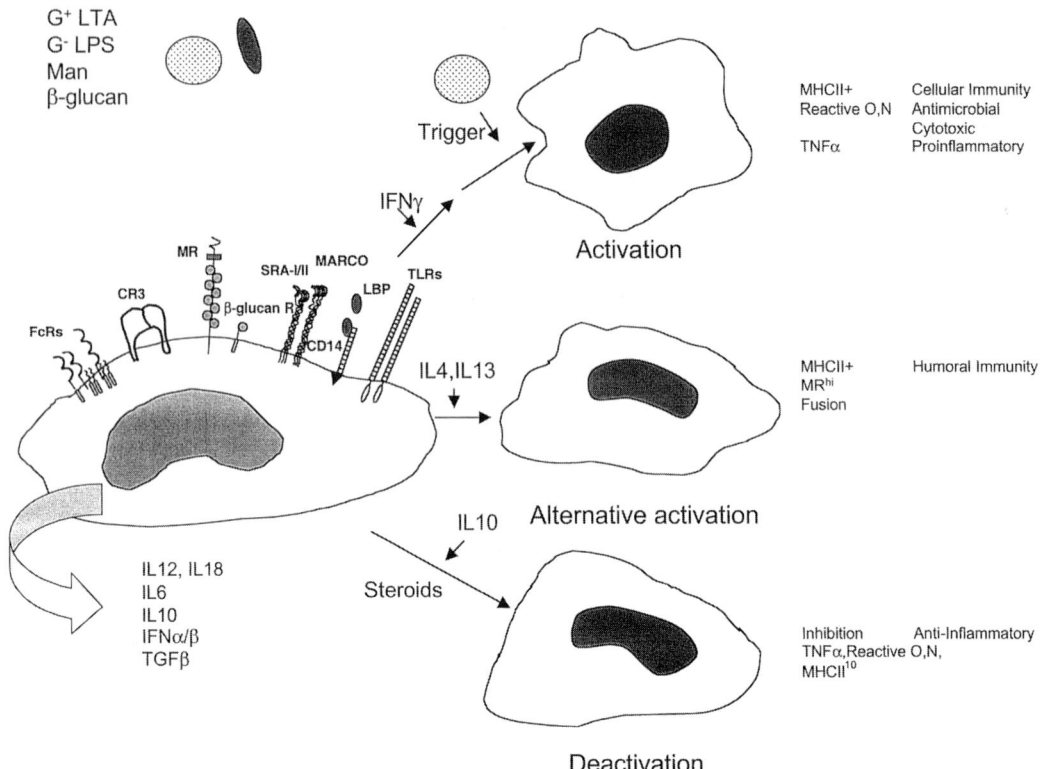

G+ LTA
G- LPS
Man
β-glucan

Trigger

IFNγ

Activation

MHCII+   Cellular Immunity
Reactive O,N   Antimicrobial
              Cytotoxic
TNFα   Proinflammatory

FcRs
CR3
MR
SRA-I/II
MARCO
β-glucan R
CD14
LBP
TLRs

IL4,IL13

Alternative activation

MHCII+   Humoral Immunity
MRhi
Fusion

IL12, IL18
IL6
IL10
IFNα/β
TGFβ

IL10

Steroids

Deactivation

Inhibition   Anti-Inflammatory
TNFα,Reactive O,N,
MHCII10

FIG. 4. Macrophage activation. Role of microbial stimuli and cytokines.

and form part of a regulatory network that may involve Mφ, through circulating mediators such as MIF (migration inhibition factor). Mφ also contain potent enzymes involved in steroid biosynthesis and catabolism.

While the immunologic relevance of Mφ-induced responses may seem evident, many aspects remain unclear. For example, do Mφ actively destroy activated T-lymphocytes, thus contributing to regulation of immune responses and peripheral tolerance, or are Mφ only passive removers of dying cells? Do Mφ contribute to recruitment, differentiation, and death of DC at sites of inflammation before their migration to secondary lymphoid organs? Do adjuvant-stimulated Mφ interact with B-lymphocytes, directing their migration into germinal centers? Are interactions of activated Mφ with antibody and complement, through different Fc and complement receptors, implicated in fine-tuning humoral responses? Are activated Mφ themselves cytocidal for infected host cells and to what extent do they in turn provide targets for attack by NK cells and CTL? Study of a range of experimental models and disease processes *in vivo* should yield new insights, as well as extending and confirming mechanisms already defined *in vitro*.

Phagocytic Recognition and Intracellular Infection

The initiation and localization of an immune response depend on recognition by Mφ and other cells of particulate agents or soluble proteins that are foreign or modified self.

Phagocytic and endocytic recognition by Mφ and DC depends on opsonic (mainly antibody, complement) and nonopsonic pattern-recognition receptors that interact with a range of related ligands (56–58). Innate and acquired responses are thus interlinked. Different FcR are involved in uptake and destruction of targets as well as in negative regulation of effector functions. Complement receptors are also heterogeneous; CR3 interacts with C_3-derived ligands formed by activation of the classical, alternate, or lectin pathways, and mediate phagocytosis, cell migration, and cell activation. Other ligands include I-CAM. CR3 functions are modulated by fibronectin, via integrins, other adhesion molecules, and inflammatory stimuli. FcR ligation and cross-linking activates tyrosine kinases such as Syk that are essential for phagocytosis (58). CR3 signaling is less defined and may not trigger a respiratory burst or arachidonate release, unlike FcR, thus favoring pathogen entry. Antibody-mediated uptake targets an organism or soluble antigen to a different, degradative compartment, and usually results in its neutralization and destruction, although enhancement of infection can also occur in Mφ. For example, flavivirus infection in the presence of specific antibody can result in the dengue hemorrhagic shock syndrome. Immune complexes, with or without complement, localize antigens to FDC and other FcR+ CR+ cells. Mφ themselves are able to produce all components of the complement cascade in significant amounts at local sites, which may be less accessible to circulating proteins made by hepatocytes.

TABLE 2. *Toll-like receptors and their ligands*

Receptor	Ligands
TLR2/6 or unknown	Peptidoglycan (gram-positive), LPS (leptospira, P gingivalis)
	Bacterial lipoprotein, lipoarabinomannan, zymosan, GPI anchor (T. cruzi)
TLR3	Double-stranded RNA
TLR4	LPS (gram-negative), taxol (plant), F protein (respiratory syncytial virus), heat-shock protein 60 (host), fibronectin fragments
TLR5	Flagellin
TLR9	CpG DNA

Nonopsonic receptors reacting directly with ligands on microorganisms include CR3, lectins, especially the MR (22) and β glucan receptor (23), the scavenger receptors (59) SR-A and MARCO, and a newly defined family of TLR (17) (Fig. 4, Table 2). MR are present on Mφ, DC, and sinusoidal endothelium. They mediate phagocytosis and endocytosis, including macropinocytosis, and structurally resemble another multilectin, Dec 205, present on DC as well as tissue Mφ and epithelial cells in thymus; carbohydrate recognition by the latter has not been demonstrated. The MR has eight C-type lectin domains, homologous to the mannose-binding protein (MBP), a circulating hepatocyte-derived acute-phase reactant. MBP contains a single lectin domain per polypeptide, which oligomerizes like other collectins to achieve multivalent interactions and activate complement via associated serine proteases. MR expression on Mφ is selectively down- and up-regulated by IFNγ and IL-4/13, respectively (60). The possible role of the cysteine-rich domain in transport of immunogenic glycopeptides within secondary lymphoid organs has been noted. The β glucan receptor, previously reported as dectin 1, is related to C-type lectins, and is responsible for phagocytic recognition of nonopsonized zymosan and for Mφ activation.

The SR-A mediates endocytosis of modified proteins, such as acetylated lipoproteins, and selected polyanions, such as LPS and lipoteichoic acid. In addition, it can serve as an adhesion molecule (42), and contributes to phagocytic clearance of apoptotic thymocytes (43) and gram-negative as well as gram-positive bacteria (59). The newly described phosphatidylserine receptor has been implicated in the recognition of novel lipid ligands expressed on the surface of apoptotic cells (61). CD36 (thrombospondin receptor) (62), vitronectin receptors, and CD44 have also been implicated in the uptake of senescent PMN by Mφ. A role for Mφ SR-A in immune induction has not been demonstrated, but studies in SR-A KO mice have revealed an important inhibitory role in limiting TNFα production by immunologically activated Mφ (63). Wild-type, BCG-primed mice produce granulomata rich in SR-A⁺ Mφ; SR-A KO mice restrict growth of this organism and form normal granulomata containing activated MHC II⁺ Mφ; upon additional challenge with LPS, the KO mice die

approximately ten-fold more readily than wild-type animals. TNFα levels in the circulation rise markedly, because of unopposed triggering via CD14, a receptor for the LPS-binding protein, and contribute to septic shock, since blocking anti-TNF mAb protects these mice (64).

The family of TLR consists of homo- or hetero-dimeric transmembrane molecules related to the IL-1 receptor, which are involved in innate immunity to microbial constituents, and activation of Mφ responses (Table 2) (17,65–67). Downstream signaling depends on association with other soluble and membrane molecules, as well as with intracellular proteins. MyD88, for example, has been implicated in many, but not all TLR-induced signaling resulting in transcription factor regulation, cell activation, or apoptosis.

Naturally occurring microbial ligands for these nonopsonic receptors are still poorly defined; individual receptors mediate microbial binding and uptake of microorganisms, although each contributes only part of total binding. Particle uptake involves the cytoskeleton, bulk membrane flow, and remodeling, as well as multiple plasma membrane receptors (68). Phagosome formation and maturation resemble endocytic uptake, initiating Mφ vesicle trafficking and recirculation, fusion with lysosomes, acidification, ion fluxes, and digestion. GTP-binding proteins and complex signaling cascades play an important role in these dynamic events. A key issue that needs to be resolved is how cell and receptor functions are modulated so that microbial phagocytosis or invasion induce inflammatory responses, unlike the uptake of apoptotic cells (69). The MHC II biosynthesis and subcellular localization and proteolytic processing of peptide antigens in vacuolar and cytosolic compartments of APC are discussed elsewhere in this volume. Cytokines, especially IL-4/13, IL-10, and IFNγ, influence endocytosis via MR-dependent and MR-independent pathways, and selectively alter vesicle dynamics.

Pathogens vary in utilizing Mφ plasma membrane molecules for entry and modify the composition of the resultant phagosome membrane. Mycobacteria, for example, employ a range of mechanisms to evade killing by Mφ, including delayed maturation of phagosomes and inhibition of fusion with lysosomes and acidification. Listeria monocytogenes escape into the cytosol by disruption of the phagosome membrane, whereas Leishmania multiplies in phagolysosomes. Humoral (antibody, complement) and cellular (γ interferon) mechanisms overcome parasitization of Mφ by diversion to lysosomes, or induce killing via O/N-dependent and other mechanisms.

Clearance of proteinase–inhibitor complexes (e.g., by CD91) and of haptoglobin–hemoglobin complexes by the Mφ receptor CD163 are essential homeostatic functions of tissue Mφ, limiting potentially injurious extracellular molecules (70).

Major unsolved questions remain concerning phagocytosis, intracellular infection, and immune responses. How do particulate antigens and microbial agents induce T-cell responses? What are the relative contributions to this process of Mφ and DC, highly and minimally efficient phagocytes, respectively? What determines the balance between total antigen degradation and loading of MHC molecules? What interactions take place between intracellular pathogens and host Mφ, especially in regard to nutritional requirements of the organism? What is the role of pathogen-derived secretory products in the vacuolar milieu, in recruitment of organelles such as endoplasmic reticulum and mitochondria and in effects on host cell biosynthesis? What are the intracellular killing mechanisms and how can organisms survive, or become latent, within Mφ? Finally, what receptor-mediated signals induce the secretion of Mφ molecules such as IL-12 that direct the resultant specific immune response?

Gene Expression and Secretion

Knowledge of Mφ gene expression and protein synthesis is growing rapidly from the application of gene array and proteomic technologies (71). Following surface and endocytic stimulation, the mature Mφ is able to secrete a very large range of high- and low-molecular-weight products. These include enzymes involved in antimicrobial resistance (lysozyme), neutral proteinases, and arachidonate metabolites that contribute to inflammation and tissue repair, cytokines such as IL-1 and TNFα that modulate the activities of other leukocytes and endothelium, and reactive oxygen and nitrogen intermediates implicated in host defense (72). Pro-inflammatory cytokines account for part of the effects of immune adjuvants in promoting, broadening, and sustaining humoral responses. The ability to release these products depends on the prior history of the Mφ, whether resident, recruited, or activated (primed); its encounters with microbial wall products, including LPS; and exposure to cytokines and other immunomodulatory molecules in its immediate environment. Ligation of specific receptors induces various signaling pathways and is able to alter gene expression in the Mφ selectively. Transcription factors such as the NFκB and PU.1 families contribute to Mφ-restricted or activation-dependent changes in gene expression (27). Product expression depends further on translational regulation, post-translational modification such as proteolytic processing, and co-expression of inhibitors such as IL-10. mRNA turnover varies greatly for different products, due to the presence or absence of specific 3′ instability sequences. Many Mφ products are labile and act close to the cell surface; overproduction results in tissue catabolism and systemic effects associated with widespread infection or chronic inflammation, often as a result of an immunologically driven disease process.

While most bioactivities have been defined *in vitro,* there is evidence that expression of Mφ secretory activities may be quite different *in situ;* lysozyme production is characteristic of all Mφ in culture, but is down-regulated on most resident cells *in vivo* and depends on induction by immune or phagocytic stimuli (24). 5′ promoter sequences of human lysozyme (73) and CD68 (74) transgenes have been used to target tissue- and Mφ-activation–specific expression of a reporter molecule *in vivo.* The promoters of these and other Mφ-restricted molecules may, in due course, make it possible to direct Mφ biosynthetic activities precisely to boost or inhibit immune responses.

Modulation of Macrophage Activation *In Vitro*

Our understanding of Mφ activation derives from studies of induction of MHC II antigen, of effector functions such as proteinase, TNFα, ROI and RNI release, of expression of membrane receptors such as MR and of resistance to infectious agents, such as Mycobacteria, Listeria, Candida, and HIV. Generalizations can be made, but it must be remembered that organisms vary considerably in their ability to evade or survive Mφ-restriction mechanisms, and interact with Mφ in individual ways. Various inhibitory cell-surface molecules (e.g., killer inhibitory receptors) are known to regulate Mφ activation through poorly defined interactions with other activating plasma-membrane receptors.

Fig. 4 illustrates various pathways of Mφ activation that result from microbial, cellular, and cytokine interactions. Knowledge is based mainly on *in vitro* experiments, and *in vivo* challenge of selected animal models. Analysis of the actions of individual cytokines (IFNγ, IL-10, IL-4/13) on defined Mφ targets (murine peritoneal Mφ and human monocyte-derived Mφ) reveals three characteristic and distinctive *in vitro* phenotypes across a spectrum of activation. IFNγ and its own production and amplification via IL-12 or IL-18 play a central role in MHC II induction, enhanced antimicrobial resistance, and pro-inflammatory cytokine production, which are characteristic of Th1-type responses. Conversely, IL-10 suppresses markers of activation, while inducing selective expression of other Mφ genes. A comparable link between Mφ/APC and the induction of Th2-type responses has proved elusive to identify. IL4/IL-13 have closely overlapping functions and induce an alternative activation phenotype in Mφ consistent with increased APC function and humoral responses (75). It is important to distinguish modulation of Mφ immunologic properties by IL4/13 from marked deactivation and inhibition of pro-inflammatory and cytotoxic functions by IL-10. The interplay of cytokines derived from Mφ themselves, from activated T- and B-lymphocytes, and from other cells (NK, endothelial cells) results in reciprocal positive or negative interactions and time-dependent changes in activating and inhibitory signals. Some predictions from *in vitro* studies can be extended to the intact host. For example, IFNγ and IL-12 deficiency results in inability to restrict opportunistic organisms in murine models and in man, and iNOS is important for resistance to a range of infectious agents. IL-10 deficiency, on the other hand, results in overactive Th1-dependent inflammation (e.g., in the gut). IL-4 deficiency by itself has little effect on Mφ phenotype *in vivo,* since IL-13 mimics many of its actions. These cytokines share a common receptor subunit and it will be interesting to study further Mφ from KO mice that lack the ability to respond to both IL-4 and IL-13.

The above analysis is oversimplified. Combinations of cytokines *in vitro* have different effects on Mφ than the sum of the parts. For example, the combination of IL-4 and GM-CSF induces differentiation of human monocytes into immature DC, while each alone induces cells with distinctive Mφ properties. Furthermore, a particular "Th2-type" cytokine such as IL-10 can display radically different effects on antimicrobial (iNOS dependent) killing, which is markedly suppressed, and anti-HIV activities of Mφ, which are enhanced. While IFNγ and IL-4 may have opposing actions on MR expression and phagocytosis of yeasts, in combination they synergize to markedly enhance uptake. Other combinations of cytokines, such as αβ IFN and IFNγ, can antagonize each other, presumably by competition for signaling pathways. Although extrapolations with predictive value can be made in some situations, a great deal remains to be learned about Mφ behavior in complex immune environments *in vivo*.

CONCLUSIONS AND SOME REMAINING ISSUES

Mφ influence and respond to all other cells involved in immunity during both afferent and efferent limbs. Many of the molecules that mediate particular functions are now defined, but their role within the Mφ and in intercellular interactions is often poorly understood. Mφ developed during the evolution of multicellular organisms before immunologically specific, clonotypic responses of B- and T-lymphocytes emerged. Mφ themselves diversified in parallel with T-helper lymphocytes, generating DC as specialized APC for naïve T-lymphocytes, and yielding a range of effector cell phenotypes in response to diverse activated T cells, both CD4+ and CD8+. Mφ and their derivatives cluster with differentiating hemopoietic cells in fetal liver and bone marrow, developing thymocytes, naïve CD4+ T-lymphocytes and antigen during immune induction, and activated T cells and microbial pathogens in granuloma formation (Fig. 2). In addition, they associate with antigen-stimulated B-lymphocytes during cell expansion, diversification, and apoptosis. A major challenge will be to define the role of specific and accessory surface molecules by which Mφ discriminate between live and dying cells, and to uncover the intrinsic and extrinsic factors that control Mφ activities within these diverse immune-cell interactions.

Our understanding of the multiple roles of Mφ and DC in immunoregulation is also evolving, as we better appreciate their specializations and adaptations. The following central issues in the immunobiology of Mφ remain obscure and interesting for further investigation:

Mφ display broad functions in homeostasis, beyond host defense and immunity, which may be special instances of a more general role in preserving host integrity, comparable to that of the CNS and endocrine systems. Their dispersion, plasticity, and responsiveness raise obvious questions for the biologist. In particular, what are their roles in development and in trophic interactions within different organs?

The Mφ lies at the heart of the classic immunologic question of recognition of altered or non-self, especially of particulates. What are the actual ligands recognized by the diverse range of plasma membrane receptors capable of direct discrimination and what determines whether uptake of a target is immunologically silent or productive? How can this information be harnessed to vaccine development?

Once activated, Mφ change their ability to recognize and destroy targets, directly or in concert with antibody, complement and other less-defined opsonins. Can Mφ directly kill virus-infected and other immunologically activated cells? If so, do they use MHC matching, even in a limited way, and do they contribute to tolerance and, by implication, autoimmunity by failure to perform a suppressive function?

A special case in which Mφ are present in large numbers at a site of "failure" to respond immunologically, is the fetoplacental unit. CSF-1 is produced locally at high levels. Does this deactivate Mφ or make them switch to perform a trophic role? Do tumors that are rich in Mφ adopt a similar strategy? Catabolism of tryptophan by Mφ enzymes has been put forward as another mechanism to prevent local destruction of an allogeneic fetus (75).

Although Mφ express a large number of genes involved in household functions, and share expression of others with a limited range of cell types, they also express highly restricted molecules, responsible for unique functions. Can these be harnessed for Mφ-specific gene targeting at selected microanatomic sites to deliver functionally precise signals at predetermined times? Techniques are becoming available for at least part of this fantasy, and should provide new insights into the multiple roles of the Mφ in immunity.

ACKNOWLEDGMENTS

I thank the members of my laboratory for discussions, Dr. Luisa Martinez-Pomares for illustrations, and Christine Holt for preparing the manuscript. Research in my laboratory is supported by grants from the Medical Research Council of the United Kingdom, the Wellcome Trust, Arthritis and Rheumatism Research Council, and the British Heart Foundation.

REFERENCES

1. Metchnikoff E. *Immunity in infective disease.* Cambridge: Cambridge University Press, 1905. Binnie FG, translator.
2. Karnovsky MC, Bolis L, eds. *Phagocytosis: past and future.* New York: Academic Press, 1982.
3. Tauber AI, Chernyak L. *Metchnikoff and the origins of immunology: from metaphor to theory.* New York: Oxford University Press, 1991.
4. Van Furth R, ed. *Mononuclear phagocytes: biology of monocytes and macrophages.* Dordrect, The Netherlands: Kluwer, 1992.
5. Gordon S, ed. Section 26. The myeloid system. In: Herzenberg LA, Weir DM, Herzenberg LA, et al., eds. *Weir's handbook of experimental immunology,* 5th ed., vol. 4. Cambridge, MA: Blackwell Scientific Publications, 1997:153–175.
6. Gordon S, ed. *Phagocytosis—the host.* Vol. 5 of *Advances in cell and molecular biology of membranes and organelles.* Stamford, CT: JAI Press, 1999.
7. Gordon S, ed. *Microbial invasion.* Vol. 6 of *Advances in cell and*

molecular biology of membranes and organelles. Stamford, CT: JAI Press, 1999.

8. Burke B, Lewis CE, eds. *The macrophage,* 2nd ed. New York: Oxford University Press, 2002:138–209.

9. Gordon S, Lawson L, Rabinowitz S, et al. Antigen markers of macrophage differentiation in murine tissues. In: Russell S, Gordon S, eds. *Macrophage biology and activation.* Berlin: Springer-Verlag, 1992;8:1–37.

10. Kraal G. Cells in the marginal zone of the spleen. *Int Rev Cytol* 1992; 132:31–74.

11. Steinman RM, Moberg CL. Zanvil Alexander Cohn 1926–1993. An appreciation of the physician-scientist. The macrophage in cell biology and resistance to infectious disease. *J Exp Med* 1994;179:1–30.

12. Gordon S. My favourite cell: the macrophage. *Bioessays* 1995;17:977–986.

13. Wiktor-Jedrzejczak W, Gordon S. Cytokine regulation of the Mø system using the colony stimulating factor-1 deficient op/op mouse. *Physiol Rev* 1996;76:927–947.

14. Dalton DK, Pitts-Meek S, Keshav S, et al. Multiple defects of immune cell function in mice with disrupted interferon-γ genes. *Science* 1993;259:1739–1742.

15. MacMicking J, Xie Q-W, Nathan C. Nitric oxide and macrophage function. *Annu Rev Immunol* 1997;15:323–350.

16. Gruenheid S, Pinner E, Desjardins M, et al. Natural resistance to infection with intracellular pathogens: the Nramp1 protein is recruited to the membrane of the phagosome. *J Exp Med* 1997;185:717–730.

17. Akira S, Takeda K, Kaisho T. Toll-like receptors: critical proteins linking innate and acquired immunity. *Nat Immunol* 2001;2:675–680.

18. Zink W, Ryan L, Gendelman HE. Macrophage–virus interactions. 1:38–209.

19. Geijtenbeek TB, Engering A, Van Kooyk Y. DC-SIGN, a C-type lectin on dendritic cells that unveils many aspects of dendritic cell biology. *J Leuk Biol* 2002;7:923–931.

20. Ravetch JV, Bolland S. IgG Fc receptors. *Annu Rev Immunol* 2001; 19:275–290.

21. Barrington R, Zhang M, Fischer M, et al. The role of complement in inflammation and adaptive immunity. *Immunol Rev* 2001;180:5–15.

22. Martinez-Pomares L, Gordon S. The Mannose receptor and its role in antigen presentation. *Immunologist* 1999;7:119–123.

23. Brown GD, Gordon S. A new receptor for β-glucans. *Nature* 2001; 413:36–37.

24. Keshav S, Chung L-P, Milon G, et al. Lysozyme is an inducible marker of macrophage activation in murine tissues as demonstrated by *in situ* hybridization. *J Exp Med* 1991;174:1049–1058.

25. Kindler V, Sappino A-P, Grau GE, et al. The inducing role of tumor necrosis factor in the development of bactericidal granulomas during BCG infection. *Cell* 1989;56:731–740.

26. Anderson KL, Smith KA, Conners K, et al. Myeloid development is selectively disrupted in PU.1 null mice. *Blood* 1998;91:3702–3710.

27. Clarke S, Gordon S. Myeloid-specific gene expression. *Rev J Leuk Biol* 1998;63:153–168.

28. Ahmad T, Armuzzi A, Bunce M, et al. The molecular classification of the clinical manifestation of Crohn's disease. *Gastroenterology* 2002;122:854–866.

29. Gordon S. Mononuclear phagocytes in immune defense. In: Roitt I, Brostoff B, Male D, eds. *Immunology,* 6th ed. Edinburgh: Mosby, 2001:147–162.

30. Morris L, Graham CF, Gordon S. Macrophages in haemopoietic and other tissues of the developing mouse detected by monoclonal antibody F4/80. *Development* 1991;112:517–526.

31. Reid DM, Perry VH, Andersson P-B, et al. Mitosis and apoptosis of microglia *in vivo* induced by an anti-CR3 monoclonal antibody which crossed the blood–brain barrier. *Neuroscience* 1994;56:529–533.

32. Stacey M, Lin H-H, Gordon S, McKnight AJ. LNB-TM7, a novel group of seven-transmembrane proteins related to family-B G-protein–coupled receptors. Trends Biochem *Sci* 2000;25:284–289.

33. Holness CL, da Silva RP, Fawcett J, et al. Macrosialin, a mouse macrophage restricted glycoprotein, is a member of the lamp/lgp family. *J Biol Chem* 1993;268:9661–9666.

34. Randolph GJ, Inaba K, Robbiani DF, et al. Differentiation of phagocytic monocytes into lymph node dendritic cells *in vivo. Immunity* 1999;11:753–761.

35. Shortman K, Liu Y-J. Mouse and human dendritic cell subtypes. *Nat Immunol* 2002;2:151–161.

36. Morris L, Crocker PR, Gordon S. Murine foetal liver macrophages bind developing erythroblasts by a divalent cation-dependent haemagglutinin. *J Cell Biol* 1988;106:649–656.

37. Perry VH, Andersson P-B, Gordon S. Macrophages and inflammation in the central nervous system. *Trends Neurosci* 1993;16:268–273.

38. McKnight AJ, Gordon S. Membrane molecules as differentiation antigens of murine macrophages. *Adv Immunol* 1998;68:271–314.

39. Crocker PR, Mucklow S, Bouckson V, et al. Sialoadhesin, a macrophage-specific adhesion molecule for haemopoietic cells with 17 immunoglobulin-like domains. *EMBO J* 1994;13:4490–4503.

40. Crocker PR, Hartnell A, Munday J, et al. The potential role of sialoadhesin as a macrophage recognition molecule in health and disease. *Glycoconj J* 1997;14:601–609.

41. Rosen H, Gordon S. Monoclonal antibody to the murine type 3 complement receptor inhibits adhesion of myelomonocytic cells in vitro and inflammatory cell recruitment *in vivo. J Exp Med* 1987;166:1685–1701.

42. Fraser IP, Hughes DA, Gordon S. Divalent cation–independent macrophage adhesion inhibited by monoclonal antibody to murine scavenger receptor. *Nature* 1993;364:343–346.

43. Platt N, Suzuki H, Kurihara Y, et al. Role for the Class A macrophage scavenger receptor in the phagocytosis of apoptotic thymocytes. *Proc Natl Acad Sci U S A* 1996;93:12456–12460.

44. Witmer-Pack MD, Hughes D, Schuler G, et al. Identification of macrophages and dendritic cells in the osteopetrotic [op/op] mouse. *J Cell Sci* 1993;104:1021–1029.

45. Martinez-Pomares L, Kosco-Vilbois M, Darley E, et al. Fc chimeric protein containing the cysteine-rich domain of the murine mannose receptor binds to macrophages from splenic marginal zone and lymph node subcapsular sinus, to germinal centres. *J Exp Med* 1996;184:1927–1937.

46. Martinez-Pomares L, Crocker PR, da Silva R, et al. Cell-specific glycoforms of sialoadhesin and CD45 are counter receptors for the cysteine-rich domain of the mannose receptor. *J Biol Chem* 1999;274:35211–35218.

47. Yu P, Wang Y, Chin RK, et al. B cells control the migration of a subset of dendritic cells into B cell follicles via CXC chemokine ligand 13 in a lymphotoxin-dependent fashion. *J Immunol* 2002;168:5117–5123.

48. Linehan SA, Martinez-Pomares L, Stahl PD, et al. Mannose receptor and its putative ligands in normal murine lymphoid and non-lymphoid organs. *In situ* expression of mannose receptor by selected macrophages, endothelial cells, perivascular microglia and mesangial cells, but not dendritic cells. *J Exp Med* 1999;189:1961–1972.

49. Berney C, Herren S, Power CA, et al. A member of the dendritic cell family that enters B cell follicles and stimulates primary antibody responses identified by a mannose receptor fusion protein. *J Exp Med* 1999;190:851–860.

50. Gordon S, Hughes DA. Macrophages and their origins: heterogeneity in relation to tissue microenvironment. In: Lipscomb M, Russell S, eds. *Lung macrophages and dendritic cells in health and disease.* New York: Marcel Dekker, 1997:3–31.

51. Andersson P-B, Perry VH, Gordon S. The acute inflammatory response to lipopolysaccharide in CNS parenchyma differs from that in other body tissues. *Neuroscience* 1992;48:169–186.

52. Schenkel AR, Mamdouh Z, Chen X, et al. CD99 plays a major role in the migration of monocytes through endothelial junctions. *Nat Immunol* 2002;3:143–150.

53. Hutchings P, Rosen H, O'Reilly L, et al. Transfer of diabetes in mice prevented by blockade of adhesion-promoting receptor on macrophages. *Nature* 1990;348:639–642.

54. Havell EA. Production of tumor necrosis factor during murine listeriosis. *J Immunol* 1987;139:4225–4231.

55. Feldman M, Nagase H, Saklatvala J, et al., eds. The scientific basis of rheumatology. *Arthritis Res* 2002;4[Suppl 3].

56. Janeway CA Jr. Approaching the asymphote? Evolution and revolution in immunology. *Cold Spring Harb Symp Quant Biol* 1989;54:1–13.

57. Innate recognition systems (Forum in Immunology). *Microbes Infect* 2000;2.

58. Crowley MT, Costello PS, Fitzer-Attas CJ, et al. A critical role for Syk in signal transduction and phagocytosis mediated by Fcγ receptors on macrophages. *J Exp Med* 1997;186:1027–1039.

59. Peiser L, Mukhopadhyay S, Gordon S. Scavenger receptors in innate immunity. *Curr Opin Immunol* 2002;14:123–128.

60. Stein M, Keshav S, Harris N, et al. IL-4 potently enhances murine macrophage mannose receptor activity; a marker of alternative immune macrophage activation. *J Exp Med* 1992;176:287–293.

61. Henson PM, Bratton DL, Fadok VA. Apoptotic cell removal. *Curr Biol* 2001;11:795–805.
62. Ren Y, Silverstein RL, Allen J, et al. CD36 gene transfer confers capacity for phagocytosis of cells undergoing apoptosis. *J Exp Med* 1995;181:1857–1862.
63. Haworth R, Platt N, Keshav S, et al. The macrophage scavenger receptor type A (SR-A) is expressed by activated macrophages and protects the host against lethal endotoxic shock. *J Exp Med* 1997;186:1431–1439.
64. Haziot A, Ferrero E, Kontgen F, et al. Resistance to endotoxin shock and reduced dissemination of gram-negative bacteria in CD14-deficient mice. *Immunity* 1996;4:407–414.
65. Underhill DM, Ozinsky A, Hajjar AM, et al. The Toll-like receptor 2 is recruited to macrophage phagosomes and discriminates between pathogens. *Nature* 1999;401:811–815.
66. Ozinsky A, Underhill DM, Fontenot JD, et al. The repertoire for pattern recognition of pathogens by the innate immune system is defined by co-operation between toll-like receptors. *Proc Natl Acad Sci U S A* 2000;97:13766–13771.
67. Schnare M, Barton GM, Holt AC, et al. Toll-like receptors control activation of adaptive immune responses. *Nat Immunol* 2001;2:947–950.
68. Aderem A, Underhill DM. Mechanisms of phagocytosis in macrophages. *Annu Rev Immunol* 1999;17:593–623.
69. Freire-de-Lima CG, Nascimento DO, Soares MB, et al. Uptake of apoptotic cells drives the growth of a pathogenic trypanosome in macrophages. *Nature* 2000;403:199–203.
70. Kristiansen M, Graverson JH, Jacobsen C, et al. Identification of the haemoglobin scavenger receptor. *Nature* 2001;409:198–201.
71. Ehrt S, Schnappinger D, Bekiranov S, et al. Reprogramming of the macrophage transcriptome in response to interferon-γ and *Mycobacterium tuberculosis:* signaling roles of nitric oxide synthase-2 and phagocyte oxidase. *J Exp Med* 2001;194:1123–1139.
72. Shiloh MU, MacMicking JD, Nicholson S, et al. Phenotype of mice and macrophages deficient in both phagocyte oxidase and inducible nitric oxide synthase. *Immunity* 1999;10:29–38.
73. Clarke S, Greaves DR, Chung L-P, et al. The human lysozyme promoter directs reporter gene expression to activated myelomonocytic cells in transgenic mice. *Proc Natl Acad Sci U S A* 1996;93:1434–1438.
74. Lang R, Rutschman RL, Greaves DR, et al. Autocrine deactivation of macrophages in transgenic mice constitutively overexpressing IL-10 under control of the human CD68 promotor. *J Immunol* 2002;168:3402–3411.
75. Gordon S. Alternative activation of macrophages. *Native Reviews* 2003;3:23–35.
76. Mellor AL, Sivakumar J, Chandler P, et al. Prevention of T cell–driven complement activation and inflammation by tryptophan catabolism during pregnancy. *Nat Immunol* 2001;2:64–68.

CHAPTER 17

The Innate Immune System

Ruslan Medzhitov

Introduction
Innate Immune Recognition
  Strategies of Innate Immune Recognition: "Microbial Non-self" and "Missing Self" · Targets of Innate Immune Recognition
The Receptors of the Innate Immune System
  Toll-like Receptors · Phagocytic Receptors · Secreted Pattern-Recognition Molecules · Intracellular Recognition Systems
The Cells of the Innate Immune System
  Macrophages · Neutrophils · Mast Cells · Eosinophils · Dendritic Cells · Surface Epithelium
The Effector Mechanisms of the Innate Immune System
  Lysozyme · Chitinases · Phospholipase A2 · BPI · Defensins · Cathelicidins · Serprocedins · Lactoferrin, NRAMP, and Calprotectin · Phagocyte Oxidase, Myeloperoxidase, and Nitric Oxide Synthase · The Antiviral Effector Mechanisms of the Innate Immune System
Control of Adaptive Immunity by the Innate Immune System
Conclusions
Acknowledgments
References

INTRODUCTION

Host defense against microbial infection is mediated by a variety of mechanisms that fall into two categories: innate and adaptive (or acquired). The adaptive immune system is found only in jawed vertebrates and apparently developed as a result of the acquisition of the RAG genes by common ancestors of the vertebrate lineage (1). Accordingly, the adaptive immune system exists only in the context of vertebrate physiology and relies on the function of the RAG genes for somatic recombination of gene segments that encode antigen receptors. Clonal distribution and selection of antigen receptors from a randomly generated and highly diverse repertoire of specificities are the two unifying principles of the adaptive immune system. Innate immunity, on the other hand, is evolutionarily ancient and a universal form of host defense found in all multicellular organisms studied. Innate immunity is not a function of a single defined physiologic system; rather, it is a product of multiple and diverse defense mechanisms. Some of these mechanisms appeared early in evolution and are present in all studied species of plant and animal kingdoms. The other mechanisms are unique to different lineages of metazoans, demonstrating the significant diversity of molecular mechanisms and pathways involved in host defense.

INNATE IMMUNE RECOGNITION

Strategies of Innate Immune Recognition: "Microbial Non-self" and "Missing Self"

The innate immune system uses at least two distinct strategies of immune recognition: recognition of "microbial non-self" and recognition of "missing self." The first strategy is based on the recognition of molecular structures that are unique to microorganisms and that are not produced by the host (2,3). Recognition of these microbial products directly leads to the activation of immune responses. The second strategy is based on the recognition of molecular structures expressed only on normal, uninfected cells of the host (4). These structures function as molecular "flags" of normal (i.e., healthy) self because they are not produced by microorganisms and their expression is lost on infected and transformed cells. These flags are recognized by inhibitory receptors (e.g., on natural killer [NK] cells), or by proteins that inhibit activation of innate immune effector mechanisms (e.g., factor H of complement). Recognition of missing self plays an important role in the function of NK cells and complement and is discussed in the context of NK and complement biology in Chapters 12 and 33, respectively.

Targets of Innate Immune Recognition

The strategy of innate immune recognition is based on the detection of conserved molecular structures produced by microbial pathogens, but not by the host organism (2). There are multiple differences between the metabolic pathways of prokaryotic and eukaryotic cells, as well as of protozoan pathogens and multicellular hosts. Some of the pathways that are unique to microbial metabolism have essential physiologic functions, and therefore are found in all microorganisms of a given class. The products of these metabolic pathways, as well as some individual gene products, are referred to as pathogen-associated molecular patterns (PAMPs) and represent targets of innate immune recognition. The receptors of the innate immune system that evolved to recognize PAMPs are called pattern-recognition receptors (PRRs) (2,5).

The best-known examples of PAMPs include lipopolysaccharide (LPS) of gram-negative bacteria; lipoteichoic acids (LTA) of gram-positive bacteria; peptidoglycan; lipoproteins generated by palmitylation of the N-terminal cysteines of many bacterial cell wall proteins; lipoarabinomannan of mycobacteria; double-stranded RNA (dsRNA), which is produced by most viruses during the infection cycle; and β-glucans and mannans found in fungal cell walls. All these structures are produced by different classes of microbial pathogens, but importantly, not by the host organisms. Therefore, they function as "molecular signatures" of microbial metabolism, and their recognition by the innate immune system signals the presence of infection.

PAMPs derived from different species of pathogens may differ from one another in the details of their chemical structure, but they always share a common molecular pattern. For example, the lipid A region of LPS is highly conserved across a wide range of gram-negative bacteria and is responsible for the proinflammatory activity of LPS, whereas the core region and the O side chain can be variable even among closely related strains and are not recognized by the innate immune system.

Although different PAMPs are not structurally related to each other, they all share several features that reflect the evolutionary strategy of innate immune recognition (2,5). First, all PAMPs are produced by microbes, but not by the host organism. This is the basis of self/non-self discrimination, a key aspect of innate immune recognition that enables innate and adaptive immune responses to be mounted only against microbial cells and antigens. Second, PAMPs are invariant among pathogens of a given class. This allows a limited number of germline-encoded PRRs to detect any microbial infection. For example, recognition of the conserved lipid-A portion of LPS allows a single PRR to detect the presence of almost any gram-negative bacterial infection. Third, PAMPs often perform physiologic functions that are essential for microbial survival, which means that loss or mutational change of PAMPs would be lethal or at least highly disadvantageous for the microorganism. Therefore, microbial pathogens are

limited in their ability to either mutate or lose expression of PAMPs in order to avoid recognition by the innate immune system.

It is important to note that while PAMPs are unique to microorganisms, they are not unique to pathogens. Indeed, all the known PAMPs are produced by both pathogenic and nonpathogenic (e.g., commensal) microorganisms. For example, LPS derived from commensal gram-negative bacteria is as potent in inducing host macrophages as LPS derived from pathogenic species of bacteria. This means that the receptors of the innate immune system cannot distinguish between pathogens and nonpathogenic microbes. This distinction, however, clearly has to be made by the innate immune system, because all multicellular organisms live in constant contact with commensal microflora. Failure to tolerate or ignore PAMPs derived from commensal microbes would have disastrous consequences to the host. The mechanisms that allow the innate immune system to distinguish between pathogens and commensals are not well understood. Presumably, anti-inflammatory cytokines (such as IL-10 and TGF-β) and compartmentalization (confinement of the commensals to the apical side of the surface epithelia) play an important role in preventing the inappropriate triggering of innate immune responses.

THE RECEPTORS OF THE INNATE IMMUNE SYSTEM

The innate immune system detects infection using a variety of PRRs that recognize PAMPs and trigger various effector responses (6). Several classes of PRRs that evolved to perform these functions differ in expression profile, localization (cell surface, cytosolic, secreted into serum and tissue fluids), and function. All PRRs can be broadly categorized into three functional classes (Fig. 1):

1. PRRs that signal the presence of infection. These can be expressed on the cell surface or intracellularly. In either case, recognition of PAMPs by these receptors leads to the activation of "pro-inflammatory" signaling pathways, typically NFκB, Jun N-terminal kinase (JNK), and p38 MAP kinase. Activation of these evolutionarily conserved signaling pathways by PRRs leads to the induction of numerous genes. There are three categories of gene products induced by PRRs: (a) proteins and peptides that have direct antimicrobial effector functions (e.g., antimicrobial peptides and lysozyme); (b) inflammatory cytokines and chemokines (e.g., TNF-α, Il-1, Il-8) that induce multiple physiologic reactions aimed at optimizing conditions to combat the infection); and (c) gene products that control activation of the adaptive immune response (e.g., MHC, CD80/CD86). The best-known receptors of this class are the family of Toll-like receptors (TLRs). Some intracellular PRRs also belong to this category (Fig. 1A and B).
2. Phagocytic (or endocytic) PRRs (Fig. 1C). These receptors are expressed on the surface of macrophages, neutrophils

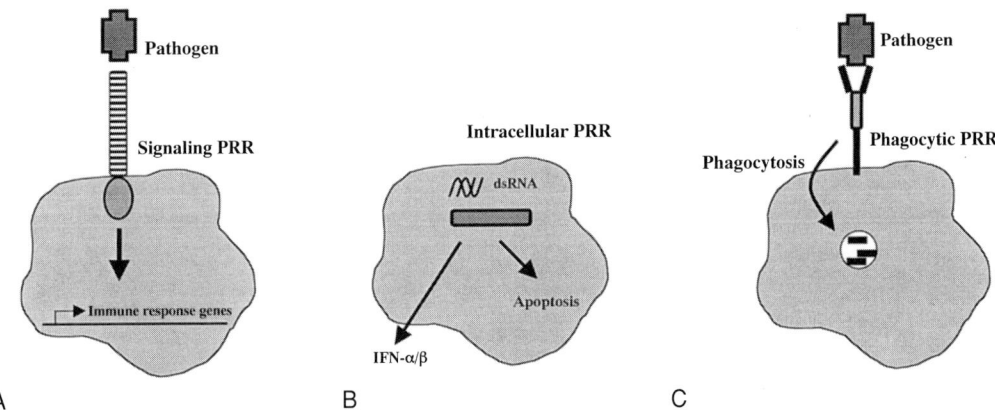

A

B

C

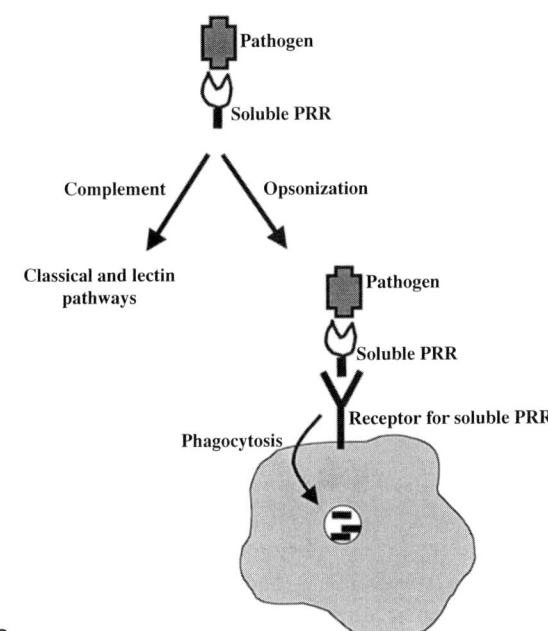

D

FIG. 1. Functional classes of pattern recognition receptors. **A:** Signaling PRRs recognize pathogens and pathogen-derived products and initiate signaling pathways that induce inflammatory responses. In specialized professional antigen-presenting cells, PRR-triggered signaling pathways also induce the expression of accessory molecules necessary for the induction of adaptive immune responses. **B:** Intracellular PRRs. These receptors recognize intracellular pathogens and pathogen-derived products (e.g., viral dsRNA) and induce production of IFN-α/β, which in turn induces an antiviral state in the infected cell as well as in neighboring cells. In some cases, recognition of an intracellular pathogen can induce apoptosis of the infected cell, thus preventing the pathogen from spreading to other cells of the host. **C:** Phagocytic PRRs bind to pathogens directly, without the aid of opsonins. Binding is followed by phagocytosis and delivery of pathogens or pathogen-derived products into lysosomal compartments. In specialized professional antigen-presenting cells, pathogen-derived proteins are degraded and presented on the cell surface on MHC molecules for recognition by T cells. **D:** Secreted PRRs, upon binding to pathogen cell walls, activate complement and function as opsonins. Both the classical and the lectin pathways of complement can be induced, depending on the PRR. Opsonization is followed by phagocytosis, which is mediated by a receptor expressed on phagocytes that binds to the PRR complexed with the pathogen.

and dendritic cells. As the name implies, these PRRs recognize PAMPs on pathogen surfaces and mediate their uptake into the phagocytes. Phagocytosed microorganisms are delivered into lysosomal compartments where they are killed by several effector mechanisms available in phagocytes. In dendritic cells and macrophages, phagocytosis is followed by processing of pathogen-derived proteins and their presentation by MHC molecules for recognition by T cells. PRRs of this class include the macrophage mannose receptor (MR) and MARCO (macrophage receptor with collagenous structure).

3. Secreted PRRs (Fig. 1D). PRRs of this class perform three types of functions: They activate complement, opsonize microbial cells to facilitate their phagocytosis, and, in the case of some PRRs, function as accessory proteins for PAMP recognition by transmembrane receptors, such as TLRs. Some PRRs are secreted by macrophages and epithelial cells into tissue fluids. Most, however, are secreted into the serum by the liver; many of these are acute-phase reactants, as their production is increased dramat-

ically during the acute-phase response. Examples of secreted PRRs are the mannan-binding lectin (MBL) and peptidoglycan-recognition proteins (PGRPs).

Toll-like Receptors

The Toll-like receptors play a unique and essential role in innate immune recognition. TLRs comprise a family of type I transmembrane receptors that are characterized by leucine-rich repeats (LRRs) in the extracellular portion and an intracellular TIR (Toll/IL-1 receptor) domain, which is homologous to the intracellular domain of IL-1 receptor family members (7,8). LRRs are found in many functionally distinct proteins where they appear to be involved in protein interactions and ligand recognition (9). The TIR domain is a conserved signaling module, found in a number of cytoplasmic proteins in animals and plants in addition to Tolls and IL-1 receptors. Interestingly, most, if not all, TIR domain-containing proteins in animals and plants are involved in host defense pathways.

There are at least ten TLRs in mammalian species (10–14), all of which appear to function as receptors of the innate immune system. TLRs differ from one another in their expression pattern, their ligand specificities, the signaling pathways they utilize, and the cellular responses they induce. Although not all TLR ligands are known at the moment, the ones that are known are PAMPs derived from all the major classes of pathogens—bacterial, viral, and protozoan (Fig. 2). It is not yet known if any of the TLRs can recognize molecular products associated with multicellular parasites. The PAMPs that are known to signal through TLRs are structurally quite diverse, and, importantly, lack any common chemical features. The exact mechanism of PAMP recognition by TLRs is not yet known, but the available information suggests that TLRs directly recognize their ligands and therefore may function as *bona fide* PRRs (15–17). It is interesting in this regard that at least some of the TLRs can recognize more than one ligand, and again, these ligands can be structurally unrelated to each other. Another important feature of TLR function is that at least some TLRs use accessory proteins for ligand recognition.

TLR4

Human TLR4 is expressed on many cell types, most predominantly in the cells of the immune system, including macrophages, dendritic cells, neutrophils, mast cells, and B cells (10). TLR4 is also expressed on various nonhematopoietic cell types, including endothelial cells, fibroblasts, surface epithelial cells, and muscle cells. TLR4 is the signal-transducing receptor for LPS. This was discovered by positional cloning of the Lps gene in the LPS-unresponsive C3H/HeJ mouse strain (18,19) and was confirmed in Tlr4 knockout mice (20). In C3H/HeJ mice, TLR4 fails to signal in response to LPS due to a point mutation in the TIR domain that results in the substitution of proline for histidine at position 712 (18–20).

Analysis of C3H/HeJ mice and TLR4 knockout mice demonstrated that TLR4 is absolutely crucial for LPS recog-

nition and responsiveness by macrophages, dendritic cells, and B cells. *In vivo* responses to LPS (such as endotoxic shock) are also completely abrogated in TLR4-deficient mice (20).

The mechanism of LPS recognition by TLR4 is quite complex and requires several accessory proteins. LPS first binds to LBP (LPS-binding protein), a serum protein that binds LPS monomers and transfers them to CD14 (21). CD14 is a GPI-linked protein expressed on the surface of macrophages and some subpopulations of dendritic cells. CD14 also exists as a soluble protein in the serum. Both forms of CD14 bind LPS with high affinity (21). The mechanism of CD14 function is unknown, but appears to be important for LPS recognition, as demonstrated by the profound defect in LPS responsiveness in CD14-deficient mice (22). The ectodomain of TLR4 is associated with another accessory protein called MD-2. MD-2 is a small protein that lacks a transmembrane domain but is expressed on the cell surface in a complex with TLR4 (23). The function of MD-2 is not known except that it is required for LPS recognition by TLR4 (24). Several experimental approaches have indicated that TLR4 and MD-2 make a direct contact with LPS (15–17), although much remains to be learned about the composition of the TLR4 complex and the mechanism of LPS recognition.

The issue of LPS recognition is complicated even further by the discovery of another cell-surface receptor that appears to cooperate with TLR4 in LPS recognition in B cells. This protein, called RP105 (25), is expressed almost exclusively on B cells and has an ectodomain closely related to that of TLR4. Similar to TLR4, RP105 is associated through its ectodomain with an accessory protein called MD-1, which is a homolog of MD-2 (26,27). Unlike TLR4, however, RP105 lacks a TIR domain, and instead has a short cytoplasmic tail that contains the tyrosine phosphorylation motif, YXXI (25). Cross-linking of RP105 leads to B-cell proliferation and up-regulation of CD80/CD86 co-stimulatory molecules, similar to the effect of LPS stimulation (27). RP105 is also known to induce activation of Src-family tyrosine kinases, including Lyn (28). Deletion of the RP105 gene results in reduced

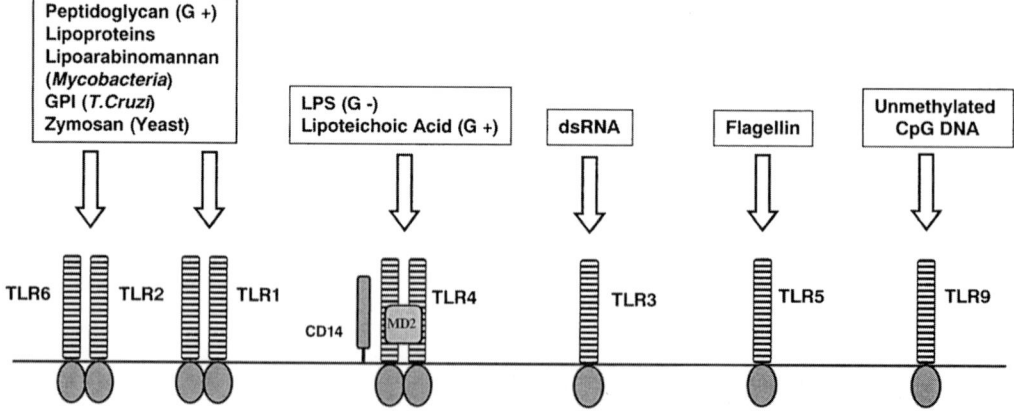

FIG. 2. Microbial products recognized by TLRs.

responsiveness of B cells to LPS stimulation, although the defect is not nearly as complete as the defect seen in TLR4-deficient B cells (29). Thus, RP105 appears to cooperate with TLR4 in LPS recognition in B cells, but the mechanism of this cooperation remains unknown.

In addition to LPS, TLR4 is involved in recognition of several other ligands. Lipoteichoic acid (LTA), a component of gram-positive bacterial cell walls, was shown in one study to signal through TLR4 (30), although in another study LTA was demonstrated to signal through TLR2 (31). The reason for this discrepancy is not yet clear. It is likely that the LTA preparation used in one of the studies was contaminated with another TLR ligand. A heat-sensitive factor associated with the cell walls of *Mycobacterium tuberculosis* was also shown to signal through TLR4, but the chemical nature of the ligand is not yet known (32). TLR4, as well as TLR2, has also been implicated in recognition of the heat-shock protein 60 (Hsp60) (33,34). Because these studies employed recombinant Hsp60 expressed in bacteria, it is difficult to rule out the possibility of contamination by some unknown bacterial product that signals through TLR4 and/or TLR2. Hsp60 is a molecular chaperone highly conserved from bacteria to humans. Host-derived Hsp60 is normally not available for recognition, but presumably can be released from cells dying by necrosis. Necrotic cells are known to induce inflammatory responses, which could be mediated in part by Hsp60, and these responses could be mediated by TLRs. However, the inflammatory response induced by necrotic cells may be primarily, if not exclusively, involved in wound healing and tissue remodeling, rather than in immune responses (35).

TLR4 along with CD14 was also shown to mediate responsiveness to the fusion (F) protein of respiratory syncytial virus (RSV) (36). However, it is not clear yet whether TLR4 recognizes some feature of the F protein that is shared with other viral fusion proteins. In other words, it is not clear if TLR4 evolved to recognize the F protein, or if the F protein evolved to bind to TLR4 and trigger its activation because it provides some unknown benefit to RSV.

TLR2, TLR1, and TLR6

TLR2 is involved in recognition of a surprisingly broad range of microbial products. These include peptidoglycan from gram-positive bacteria (30,31), bacterial lipoproteins (37–39), mycoplasma lipoprotein (39,40), mycobacterial lipoarabinomannan (32,41), a phenol-soluble modulin from *Staphylococcus epidermidis* (42), zymosan of yeast cell walls (43), and glycosylphosphotidylinositol from *Trypanosoma cruzi* (44). TLR2 was also shown to mediate recognition of two kinds of atypical LPS, one derived from *Leptospira interrogans* (45) and the other from *Porphyromonas gingivitis* (46). In addition, according to some studies, TLR2 is also responsible for the recognition of LTA (31) (see above). In terms of their structure, most of these ligands are completely distinct from each other. In fact, the only thing common to them is that they are all PAMPs. It is puzzling, then, how all these

different microbial products can signal through the same receptor. Although the answer to this question is unknown at the moment, there are at least two factors that can help explain the broad range of ligands recognized by TLR2. One is the use of accessory proteins. Indeed, recognition of some TLR2 ligands (e.g., peptidoglycan) requires CD14 (21). It is quite possible that recognition of at least some other TLR2 ligands may be assisted by additional accessory proteins. Different accessory proteins could conceivably recognize structurally distinct PAMPs and then bind to and trigger TLR2. The second factor that contributes to the diversity of TLR2 ligands is the cooperation of TLR2 with other TLRs, in particular TLR1 and TLR6, such that the TLR2/TLR1 heterodimer recognizes one set of ligands, whereas the TLR2/TLR6 heterodimer recognizes a different set of ligands (40,47). These observations were made using mice with targeted deletions in either the TLR2 or TLR6 genes: While both triacylated (tripalmitylated) bacterial lipopeptides and MALP-2 (mycoplasmal macrophage-activating lipopeptide 2kD) failed to signal in TLR2 knockout cells, only MALP-2 (but not tripalmitylated bacterial lipopeptides) required TLR6 for cellular responsiveness (40). Therefore, TLR2 cooperates with TLR6 for the recognition of MALP-2, and with another TLR for the recognition of bacterial lipopeptides (40). *In vitro* studies, which showed that TLR2 can heterodimerize and signal cooperatively with TLR1 and TLR6 (47), are also consistent with these observations. Interestingly, the only relevant difference between the two ligands is that bacterial lipopeptides have a third palmityl chain attached to the amino group of their N-terminal cysteine, while MALP-2 does not.

It is not yet known if any of the other TLRs can heterodimerize for ligand recognition and signaling, but *in vitro* studies suggest that at least TLR4 and TLR5 may function as homodimers (47).

TLR2 is expressed constitutively on macrophages, dendritic cells, and B cells, and can be induced in some other cell types, including epithelial cells. TLR1 and TLR6, on the other hand, are expressed almost ubiquitously (48). In human dendritic cells, expression of TLR2 and TLR4 is restricted to monocyte-derived dendritic cells. Accordingly, this subtype of dendritic cells, but not plasmocytoid dendritic cells that do not express TLR2 and TLR4, respond to TLR2 and TLR4 ligands (LPS and peptidoglycan, respectively) by producing IL-12 (49–51).

TLR3

TLR3 functions as a cell-surface receptor for dsRNA (52). dsRNA is a molecular pattern associated with viral infections, as most viruses produce dsRNA at some point of their infection cycle. dsRNA and its synthetic analog, poly(IC), have long been known to activate inflammatory responses. As discussed in the next sections, dsRNA is recognized by at least two intracellular recognition systems that mediate antiviral responses in infected cells. Protein kinase R (PKR), in particular, has been characterized extensively as an intracellular receptor for dsRNA (53). However, mice and cells deficient in PKR can still respond to dsRNA and poly(IC), suggesting that another receptor may mediate these responses (54). This receptor appears to be TLR3, as TLR3 can mediate responses to poly(IC), and TLR3 knockout mice and cells are deficient in their responsiveness to poly(IC) and viral dsRNA (52). These findings strongly suggest that TLR3 is involved in viral recognition, although the contribution of TLR3 to antiviral immunity remains to be demonstrated.

TLR3 is expressed on dendritic cells, macrophages, and surface epithelial cells, including intestinal epithelium. Interestingly, expression of TLR3 in human dendritic cells is restricted to plasmocytoid dendritic cells (49–51). This subtype of dendritic cells produces large amounts of type I interferons in response to dsRNA, further implicating TLR3 in antiviral defense.

TLR5

TLR5 is the receptor for flagellin, the protein that polymerizes to form bacterial flagella (55). An interesting aspect of this TLR ligand is that, unlike most other PAMPs, flagellin does not undergo any posttranslational modifications that would distinguish it from cellular proteins. However, flagellin is extremely conserved at its amino- and carboxyl-termini, which presumably explains why it was selected as a ligand for innate immune recognition.

TLR5 is expressed on epithelial cells as well as on macrophages and dendritic cells. Interestingly, expression of TLR5 on intestinal epithelium is polarized such that TLR5 is expressed only on the basolateral side of the cell (56). It is likely that other TLRs that are expressed on surface epithelium are also expressed exclusively on the basolateral surface. Since pathogenic but not commensal microbes cross the epithelial barrier, confining TLRs to the basolateral side would enable the host to recognize and be activated by pathogenic but not commensal microbes.

TLR9

DNA that contains unmethylated CpG dinucleotides has long been known for its immunostimulatory properties (57,58). Oligonucleotides that contain unmethylated CpG motifs strongly induce B-cell proliferation and cytokine production by dendritic cells and murine macrophages (57,58). Permutation of a single nucleotide or methylation of the CpG motif results in a complete loss of activity (57,58). The stimulatory property of CpG DNA is due to its ability to trigger TLR9 (59). TLR9 knockout mice are completely unresponsive to CpG DNA, demonstrating that all the known effects of CpG DNA are mediated by this TLR (59).

CpG DNA is an unusual PAMP. Cytosine methylation exists in mammalian but not bacterial cells, and most (but not all) CpG in the mammalian genome is methylated. Therefore, unmethylated CpG DNA may signal the presence of microbial infection. Unmethylated CpG motifs, however, are not

strictly restricted to bacteria. Moreover, it is hard to envision how bacterial DNA can become accessible for recognition during infection. DNA can be released from dying cells, or from phagocytosed cells. Interestingly in this regard, signaling by CpG DNA requires its internalization into late endosomal/lysosomal compartments (58,60). Viral DNA may also be available in these compartments, and it is possible that TLR9 is involved in viral recognition as well.

Optimal responsiveness to CpG DNA by mouse versus human cells requires a slightly different sequence motif flanking the CpG dinucleotide (57). Interestingly, the CpG motifs that preferentially stimulate mouse cells also induce a much stronger activation of transfected mouse TLR9, and correspondingly, the CpG motif that elicits optimal responsiveness in human cells preferentially activates transfected human TLR9. This observation suggests that TLR9 itself can distinguish between the two CpG motifs, and therefore that it presumably recognizes CpG DNA directly (61).

Expression of TLR9 in humans is restricted to B cells and plasmocytoid dendritic cells. In the mouse, TLR9 is also expressed in macrophages. Expression of TLR9 in type I interferon producing plasmocytoid dendritic cells (49–51) further suggests that TLR9 may be involved in antiviral host defense. The precise physiologic function of TLR9 in innate immunity remains to be elucidated using TLR9-deficient mice.

TLR Signaling Pathways

Activation of TLRs by microbial products leads to the induction of numerous genes that function in inflammatory and immune responses. These include inflammatory cytokines, (e.g., TNF-α, IL-1, IL-6 and IL-12), chemokines (e.g., the neutrophil chemoattractant IL-8), antimicrobial effector molecules (e.g., inducible nitric oxide synthase and antimicrobial peptides), and MHC and co-stimulatory molecules (7,8,10).

Stimulation of TLRs activates the NFκB pathway as well as three MAP kinase-signaling pathways, JNK, p38, and ERK (7,8,10). The functions of several components of the TLR signaling pathways have been elucidated through biochemical and/or gene knockout approaches. These complications include the adaptor proteins MyD88 and Tollip, the serine/threonine protein kinase IRAK (IL-1 receptor–associated kinase), the ubiquitin ligase TRAF6 (TNF receptor–associated factor 6), the MAP kinase kinase kinase (MAP3K) TAK1, and the IκB kinases IKKα and IKKβ. All these components function in both TLR and IL-1 receptor–signaling pathways (7,8) (Fig. 3).

Ligation of TLRs induces receptor dimerization (or higher-order oligomerization) and/or a conformational change that triggers downstream signaling events. Activated TLRs recruit the adaptor proteins MyD88 and Tollip (62–65). MyD88 consists of an N-terminal death domain and a C-terminal TIR domain. The TIR domain of MyD88 interacts with the TIR domain of the TLRs, while the death domain interacts with the death domain of IRAK (62–65). MyD88 therefore functions

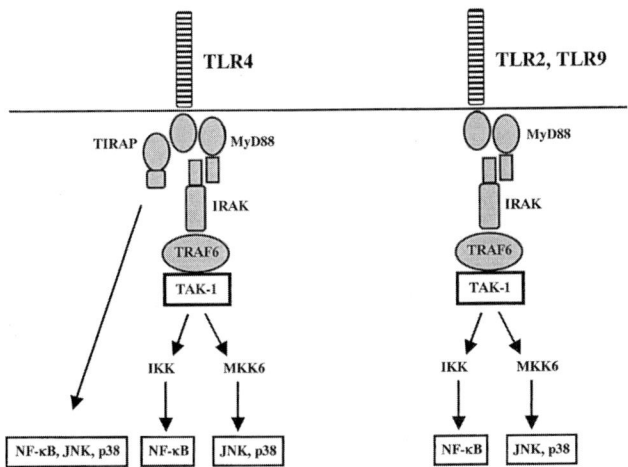

FIG. 3. TLR signaling pathways. All mammalian TLRs signal through the adaptor protein MyD88, the protein kinase IRAK, and the ubiquitin E3 ligase TRAF6. Activation of TRAF6 leads to the induction of NFκB and MAP kinase signaling via the protein kinase TAK-1. TLR4, in addition to engaging a MyD88-dependent pathway, also activates a second adaptor protein, TIRAP. The MyD88-independent signaling pathway downstream of TLR4 also activates NFκB and MAP kinases JNK and p38, although most of the components of this pathway are currently unknown.

to recruit IRAK to activated receptors, and, as demonstrated by gene-targeting studies, has a crucial role in signaling downstream of the IL-1R and TLRs (66,67). Tollip is also associated with IRAK and has been shown to recruit IRAK to the receptor complex; how its function differs from that of MyD88 is therefore not yet clear (65). Notably, Tollip lacks a TIR domain, but has a C2 domain, which in other proteins mediates binding to membrane lipids. In addition to IRAK, two closely related kinases, IRAK2 and IRAKM, have also been identified and reported to function in the TLR and IL-1R signaling pathways (63,68). The existence of multiple IRAKs, at least some of which may have similar or redundant functions, may explain why mice deficient in IRAK1 (unlike those lacking MyD88) have only a mild defect in TLR signaling (69).

Recruitment of IRAK to the receptors results in IRAK autophosphorylation and dissociation from the receptor complex. Once IRAK is phosphorylated, it interacts with and activates TRAF6 (70,71). TRAF6 is a member of the TRAF family of RING-finger E3 ubiquitin ligases (72). Other members of the TRAF family mediate signal transduction by receptors of the TNF receptor superfamily (73). Activation of TRAF6 is thought to be triggered by oligomerization induced by interaction with phosphorylated IRAK. Once activated, TRAF6 functions in concert with the noncanonical E2 ubiquitin–conjugating enzymes, Ubc13 and Uev1A, to conjugate polyubiquitin chains onto itself (and perhaps other as yet unidentified targets) (72). Unlike the polyubiquitin chains that target substrates for degradation by the 26S proteasome, which are linked through K48 of ubiquitin, TRAF6 catalyzes conjugation of noncanonical K63-linked polyubiquitin chains (72). In *in vitro* reconstitution systems, this ubiquitination event

is necessary and sufficient for subsequent activation of the IKK complex by the kinase TAK1 (74). As TAK1 does not seem to be a target of ubiquitination, how autoubiqutination of TRAF6 activates TAK1 is not yet clear. Nevertheless, TRAF6-activated TAK1 phosphorylates IKKβ, which leads to activation of the NFκB pathway (see below) (74). In addition, TRAF6-activated TAK1 also phosphorylates the MAP kinase kinase MKK6, which in turn phosphorylates the MAPK JNK. Therefore, activation of TAK1 by a TRAF6-catalyzed ubiquitination reaction leads to activation of both the NFκB and AP-1 pathways (74). In addition to TAK1, other kinases (such as the MAP3K NIK) reportedly can also activate the IKK complex in *in vitro* systems. Gene-targeting studies, however, do not support a crucial role for these kinases in TLR- (or IL-1R-) mediated IKK activation; it remains to be seen whether TAK1-deficient mice will have a defect in this regard.

The NFκB family of transcription factors plays a crucial role in innate immunity. In flies as well as mammals, most inducible host defense genes are critically regulated, at least in part, by the NFκB pathway (75,76). NFκB is usually composed of a heterodimer of two Rel/NFκB family transactivators (most commonly p50 and p65) bound to an inhibitory subunit called IκB (inhibitor of κB). In unstimulated cells, IκB masks the nuclear localization signal on NFκB and thus blocks its nuclear translocation. Upon stimulation by TLR ligands and IL-1 (as well as other signals), IκB is rapidly phosphorylated and degraded by the 26S proteasome. Freed of its cytosolic anchor, NFκB can then translocate to the nucleus, where it turns on expression of target genes (75,76).

Phosphorylation-dependent degradation of IκB, a pivotal checkpoint in activating NFκB, is controlled by the IKK (IκB kinase) complex (77). The IKK complex consists of two kinases, IKK-α and IKK-β and a third noncatalytic subunit, IKK-γ. Mutagenesis studies have established serines 32 and 36 of IκB as the targets of IKK-β phosphorylation (77). Phosphorylation at these sites enables recognition of IκB by the F-box/WD protein, β-TrCP, the receptor subunit of a multisubunit SCF ubiquitin ligase complex that subsequently ubiquitinates IκB, thereby targeting IκB for degradation (75,76).

While all TLRs (as well as the IL-1R) can induce the signaling pathway described above, it is clear that some, if not all of them, must also activate additional pathways. The first evidence of differential signaling by TLRs came with an analysis of cells derived from MyD88-deficient mice. MyD88-deficient macrophages failed to produce any inflammatory cytokines in response to LPS stimulation, but surprisingly retained the ability to activate NFκB and MAP kinases (67). As TLR4 is required for all cellular responses to LPS, these observations suggested the existence of a MyD88-independent pathway that can induce NFκB and MAP kinases. Intriguingly, some TLRs do not elicit any cellular responses in the absence of MyD88. TLR ligands can therefore be divided into two categories with respect to the signaling pathways they induce: CpG and MALP-2 (which signal through TLR9 and TLR2, respectively) require MyD88 for all responses analyzed (39,78), while LPS and poly(IC) (which signal through TLR4 and TLR3, respectively) require MyD88 for cytokine production but can activate NFκB and MAP kinases in the absence of MyD88 (52,67). Moreover, TLR3 and TLR4 can induce DC maturation through a MyD88-independent pathway (52,79). IL-1R also has an absolute requirement for MyD88 to signal (66). Therefore, TLR2, TLR9, and the IL-1R appear to signal only through the MyD88-dependent pathway, while TLR4 and TLR3 can signal as well through a MyD88-independent pathway.

A novel TIR domain-containing protein that might trigger the MyD88-independent pathway downstream of TLR4 is TIRAP (for TIR domain–containing adaptor protein, also known as Mal, for MyD88-like adaptor) (80,81). This adaptor, which contains a C-terminal TIR domain, was implicated in MyD88-independent signaling because a dominant negative form of TIRAP inhibits TLR4- but not TLR9- nor IL-1R-induced NFκB activation (80) (Fig. 3). Another protein that may also have a role in triggering MyD88-independent responses is the interferon-regulated kinase, PKR (also discussed below). PKR is activated by LPS, poly(IC), and CpG in wild-type macrophages, and by LPS and poly(IC) but not by CpG in their MyD88-deficient counterparts (80). PKR associates with TIRAP, suggesting that TIRAP may regulate activation of PKR in the MyD88-independent pathway downstream of TLR4 (80).

Targets of the MyD88-independent signaling pathway have been identified by a subtractive hybridization study comparing wild-type and MyD88-deficient macrophages stimulated with the TLR4 ligand LPS (82). These genes encode the chemokine IP-10, and the interferon-induced genes GARG16 and IRG1. The TLR2 ligand MALP-2, which induces IL-12 and TNF-α as do ligands for other TLRs, does not induce IP-10 expression (82). IP-10 is therefore an example of a gene that is up-regulated by a subset of TLRs. Identification of other such genes and responses regulated differentially by different TLRs will be important in understanding how TLR-mediated recognition is translated into appropriate immune responses.

Phagocytic Receptors

Scavenger Receptors

Scavenger receptors (SRs) are cell-surface glycoproteins that are defined by their ability to bind to modified low-density lipoprotein (LDL) (83). There are six classes of structurally unrelated SRs (84). The class A SRs include the macrophage SR (SR-A), the founding member of the SR family, and MARCO (macrophage receptor with collagenous structure). Both SR-A and MARCO are type II transmembrane glycoproteins that contain a collagenous region and a so-called scavenger receptor cysteine-rich (SRCR) domain. The SR-A isoforms generated by alternative splicing are referred to as SR-AI and SR-AII. SR-AII is the shorter isoform that lacks the C-terminal SRCR domain. Both SR-A and MARCO are

homotrimeric proteins. SR-A also contains an α-helical—coiled coil region that is absent in MARCO.

SR-A is expressed in most macrophage subtypes, as well as in endothelial cells. This receptor has an unusually broad ligand specificity and has been reported to bind, in addition to oxidized and acetylated LDL, a variety of microbial ligands, including gram-negative and gram-positive bacteria, LPS, LTA, and poly(IC) (83). Interestingly, SR-AI and SR-AII have almost identical ligand-binding specificities, suggesting that the SRCR domain is not required for ligand binding. Indeed, binding of the polyanionic ligands has been shown to be mediated by the collagenous domain (83).

The role of SR-A in host defense is demonstrated by the increased susceptibility of SR-A–deficient mice to *Listeria monocytogenes,* herpes simplex virus, and malaria infection (85). SR-A–deficient mice are also more susceptible to endotoxic shock than wild-type mice, suggesting that SR-A may be involved in the clearance of LPS from the circulation (86).

MARCO is expressed predominantly in the macrophages of the marginal zone of the spleen, but its expression can be induced in other macrophage subsets by LPS and inflammatory cytokines (87,88). MARCO binds gram-positive and gram-negative bacteria but not yeast zymosan (87,88), and mediates phagocytosis of bound bacteria (88,89). Unlike SR-A, MARCO binds its ligands through the SRCR domain (90). A definitive demonstration of the role of MARCO in host defense will have to await the generation of MARCO-deficient mice.

Macrophage Mannose Receptor

The macrophage mannose receptor (MR) is a 175-kD type I transmembrane protein expressed primarily in macrophages (91). The MR contains cysteine-rich and fibronectin–type 2 domains at the N-terminus followed by eight carbohydrate recognition domains (CRD) of the C-type lectin family (91,92). Individual CRDs of the MR appear to have different carbohydrate specificities with CRD4 being primarily responsible for mannose specificity (93). Although the MR has been implicated in the recognition of microbial carbohydrates, it can also recognize oligo-mannoses found in host-derived, high-mannose asparagine-linked carbohydrates. Indeed, in addition to microbial ligands, the MR has been shown to endocytose several host-derived, high-mannose glycoproteins (94).

Although the MR appears to be a multiligand receptor and may have several physiologic roles, the main function of MR is thought to be in phagocytosis of microorganisms (91,94). Indeed, the MR has been implicated in the phagocytosis of a variety of pathogens. Many of these studies are based on the inhibition of MR-mediated phagocytosis by soluble carbohydrate ligands, such as mannan. As microorganisms contain multiple carbohydrate ligands that presumably engage several receptors on the host cell, some of these analyses are inconclusive and will need to be confirmed using MR-deficient macrophages. A combination of inhibition and transfection studies demonstrated that MR is involved in phagocytosis of bacterial (*M. tuberculosis, Pseudomonas aeruginosa, Klebsiella pneumoniae*), fungal (*Saccharomyces cerevisiae, Candida albicans*) and protozoan pathogens (*Pneumocystis carinii*) (91,94). Upon recognition of microbial ligands, the MR presumably delivers them to the late endosome/lysosome. Thus, the MR was shown to deliver mycobacterial lipoglycan lipoarabinomannan (LAM) into the late endosomal compartment where LAM binds to CD1b for subsequent presentation to T cells (95).

While the MR clearly can mediate phagocytosis of microorganisms, the outcome of MR-mediated phagocytosis is not well defined and appears to depend on several factors, including the activation and differentiation status of the macrophage. At least some carbohydrate structures recognized by the MR on microorganisms (e.g., α-linked branched oligo-mannoses) are similar to mammalian high-mannose oligosaccharides. However, these structures may be present as a particulate ligand (in the context of a microbial cell), or as a soluble ligand (in host glycoproteins). As the mechanism of uptake differs for particulate and soluble ligands, the effect of MR ligation may be distinct depending on the origin of the carbohydrate that is bound. The most important factor influencing the outcome of MR ligation by microbial versus host-derived ligand, however, is the co-ligation of the microbial cell by other cell-surface receptors, in particular the TLRs. Some of the results implicating the MR in inducing cytokine production may be due to the co-engagement of TLRs by complex microbial structures, such as yeast cell walls.

The MR is structurally related to DEC205, a member of the C-type lectin family expressed preferentially on dendritic cells (96). Although the binding of DEC205 to microbial cell walls has not yet been demonstrated, this protein is very likely to function as a PRR, given the high degree of similarity between the CRD domain structures of the MR and DEC205. Moreover, DEC205 has been shown to direct bound material into antigen-processing compartments in dendritic cells (96), supporting the notion that it may function as a phagocytic PRR.

β-Glucan Receptor

Dectin-1 is a type II transmembrane receptor that contains one CRD at the C-terminal portion of the protein and an ITAM motif in the N-terminal, cytoplasmic region (97). The CRD of dectin-1 belongs to the C-type lectin-like subfamily of the CTL domain. Unlike the classical CTL domain, the C-type lectin-like domain lacks amino acid residues required for calcium binding and therefore binds its ligands in a calcium-independent manner. Dectin-1 was first identified as a dendritic cell-specific lectin, but was later found to be expressed on macrophages as well (98). An expression-cloning approach led to the identification of dectin-1 as a β-glucan receptor (98). Dectin-1 is specific for β-1,3–linked and β-1,6–linked glucans, which are PAMPs found in fungal and other microbial cell walls. The signaling capabilities of dectin-1

are not yet established, but the presence of the ITAM motif suggests that this receptor may signal through Src-family tyrosine kinases. Dectin-1 binds and phagocytoses β-glucan–rich zymosan and therefore functions as a phagocytic PRR on macrophages and dendritic cells (98).

Secreted Pattern-Recognition Molecules

Secreted pattern-recognition receptors (or pattern-recognition molecules, PRMs), similar to PRRs expressed on the cell surface, are specific to microbial PAMPs, but their physiologic roles in host defense are different. The two main functions of secreted PRMs are activation of complement and opsonization of microbial cells for phagocytosis. In addition, some secreted PRMs have direct bactericidal effects on bound bacteria.

Soluble PRMs are produced and secreted into the circulation mainly by the liver (primarily by hepatocytes), and to a lesser degree by several other cell types, including phagocytes. The serum concentration of these PRMs increases dramatically during the acute-phase response, a systemic inflammatory response induced by inflammatory cytokines such as IL-6, IL-1, and TNF-α. Secreted PRMs therefore are sometimes referred to as acute-phase proteins.

Depending on their domain composition secreted PRMs fall into four major structural classes: collectins, pentraxins, lipid transferases and peptidoglycan recognition proteins (PGRPs). The function of each of these classes will be discussed next.

Collectins

Collectins comprise a group of structurally related PRMs characterized by the presence of a carbohydrate recognition domain of the C-type lectin family at the C-terminus, and a collagenous domain at the N-terminus (99). The CRD domains of the collectins are engaged in ligand recognition, whereas the collagenous portions are responsible for the effector functions, such as activation of the complement cascade. All collectins form multimers in solution, which permits higher avidity interactions with their cognate ligands (100). Multimerization is also responsible for orienting the CRD domains such that they match the spatial arrangement of their carbohydrate ligands on the microbial surface, thereby allowing the collectins to distinguish microbial carbohydrates from mannose residues on self-glycoproteins (101).

Mannose binding lectin (MBL) is the best-characterized member of the collectin family. MBL binds to terminal mannose and fucose residues in a calcium-dependent manner and has been reported to recognize a broad range of pathogens, including gram-positive (*Staphylococcus aureus, Streptococcus pneumonia*) and gram-negative (*P. aeruginosa, K. pneumonia, Escherichia coli, Salmonella enteritidus*) bacteria; mycobacteria (*M. tuberculosis*); yeast (*Cryptococcus neoformans, C. albicans, S. cerevisiae*); viruses (influenza A, HSV, HIV); and protozoan pathogens (*T. cruzi, P. carinii*) (102).

The main function of MBL is to activate the lectin pathway of complement. MBL is associated with two serine proteases, MASP-1 and MASP-2 (MBL-associated serine proteases). Upon binding to microbial cells, MBL induces a conformational change in the associated MASPs that leads to MASP activation, similar to the activation of C1r and C1s by antibody-bound C1q. Activated MASPs then cleave C2 and C4 complement components, thus initiating the complement cascade. In addition to the triggering of the lectin pathway of complement, MBL can function as an opsonin. MBL bound to pathogen cell walls promotes phagocytosis by interacting with C1qRp, a receptor for C1q and MBL expressed on phagocytes (102).

Surfactant proteins A and D (SP-A and SP-D) are collectins expressed in the lung and secreted by airway epithelial cells into the alveolar fluid. Both SP-A and SP-D interact with a variety of pathogens, including gram-positive and gram-negative bacteria, fungi, and several viruses (103). Similar to MBL, SP-A and SP-D recognize terminal mannose, fucose and N-acetyl glucosamine residues expressed on microbial surfaces. SP-A and SP-D proteins function as opsonins and bind to several macrophage receptors that mediate the phagocytosis of the bound microorganism (100). SP-A, similar to MBL and C1q, binds C1qRp expressed on macrophages. SP-D binds to Gp340 (also known as hensin), a receptor expressed in macrophages and epithelial cells (103). It is not yet clear if Gp340 plays any role in phagocytosis (103).

SP-A–deficient mice show increased susceptibility to infection with a number of bacterial, fungal and viral pathogens, for example, *Group B streptococci, S. aureus, P. aeroginosa, K. pneumoniae, P. carinii,* and respiratory syncytial virus (RSV) (103). SP-D–deficient mice are also compromised in their resistance to several pathogens; however, this defect is difficult to interpret because deletion of SP-D leads to abnormalities of alveolar macrophages and surfactant homeostasis (103).

C-Reactive Protein and Serum Amyloid A

C-reactive protein (CRP) and serum amyloid A (SAM) are two structurally related proteins that belong to the pentraxin family (104). Both CRP and SAP are acute-phase proteins that bind to bacterial surfaces, in part through recognition of phosphorylcholine (105). These PRRs function as opsonins and can activate the classical pathway of complement by binding to and activating C1q (104,106).

LBP and BPI

LPS-binding protein (LBP) and bactericidal permeability increasing protein (BPI) are members of a lipid transferase family that also includes cholesteryl ester transfer protein (CETP) and phospholipid transfer protein (PLTP). All four proteins are related to each other in primary structure, which suggests a common origin; however, unlike LBP and BPI, CETP and PLTP do not play any role in host defense, but rather function as lipid carriers in the serum. Both LBP and BPI are components of the acute-phase response, although BPI can also be produced by activated phagocytes. Given that BPI functions as a bactericidal protein, it will be discussed later, along with other effector mechanisms of innate immunity.

LBP functions as a transfer protein for LPS and various host-derived lipids. In this sense, LBP is not a true pattern-recognition receptor. However, LBP does play a role in LPS recognition by monomerizing LPS from aggregates or micelles and transferring it onto CD14, the high-affinity LPS receptor (21,107). LBP can also function as an opsonin—LBP bound to LPS or gram-negative bacteria was shown to bind to CD14 expressed on the macrophage plasma membrane (107). This binding can subsequently lead to endocytosis of the bound bacteria and/or LPS. The physiologic significance and mechanism of LBP-mediated phagocytosis are currently unknown. The function of LBP in LPS recognition may be redundant as LBP-deficient mice exhibit normal responsiveness to LPS injection *in vivo* (21).

PGRPs

PGRPs comprise a family of recently discovered PRRs that function as receptors for peptidoglycan in evolutionarily distant organisms, including insects and mammals (108–110). All PGRPs contain a highly conserved peptidoglycan-binding domain. Some PGRPs have putative transmembrane regions and presumably function as cell surface receptors, whereas other PGRPs are secreted proteins (109,110). There are four known PGRPs in humans, but more are likely to exist. Human PGRPs are differentially expressed, with one gene predominantly expressed in the liver, one in neutrophils, and one in the esophagus (110). The function of mammalian PGRPs is unknown, but one mammalian PGRP was shown to inhibit bacterial growth, suggesting that at least some PGRPs may function as bactericidal effector molecules (111). Surprisingly, one PGRP that has been analyzed so far inhibited phagocytosis of gram-positive bacteria by macrophages (111). This PGRP also blocked peptidoglycan-induced cytokine production and oxidative burst in macrophages. These effects were presumably due to competition for peptidoglycan binding between PGRP and PGN-binding cell-surface receptors such as TLR2.

Since PGRPs were shown to trigger a serine protease cascade in insects in response to bacterial infection, it is likely that at least some mammalian PGRPs may have a similar role—for example, in inducing the complement cascade—to the way in which the lectin pathway is activated by MBL upon microbial recognition (21,107).

Intracellular Recognition Systems

Although most of the initial recognition of microbial infection occurs outside the host cell, many pathogens, and in particular viruses, gain access to intracellular compartments such as the cytosol. Several intracellular recognition systems have evolved to detect pathogens in the cytosol of infected cells. In addition to the typical outcomes of innate immune recognition—induction of microbicidal effector mechanisms and production of cytokines that activate effector cells—intracellular immune recognition often leads to apoptosis of the infected cell. This is true for both innate and adaptive immune systems (compare NK and CD8 T-cell functions). Apoptosis of the infected cell can be cell autonomous, or it can be triggered by specialized effectors, the NK cells.

The two best-characterized intracellular recognition systems are the protein kinase R (PKR) and oligoadenylate synthase (OAS) systems, both of which play a role in antiviral host defense. The NOD family of intracellular signaling proteins resembles the proteins that trigger host defense reactions in plants and is likely to function in innate immune recognition and/or signaling, although its precise function remains to be elucidated.

PKR

PKR is a serine/threonine protein kinase that contains three double-stranded RNA (dsRNA) binding domains at the N-terminal part of the protein and a C-terminal kinase domain. PKR can be activated by dsRNA and thus functions as an intracellular sensor of viral infection, as dsRNA of the length that is sufficient to activate PKR is produced by many viruses, but not by host cells. PKR is expressed ubiquitously, and its expression can be further induced by interferons. Activation of PKR by viral dsRNA has several consequences. First, it leads to the induction of inflammatory signaling pathways, such as NFκB, MAP kinases, STATs, and IRFs (112). Activation of these pathways leads to the production of inflammatory cytokines and type I interferons. Interferons α/β, in turn, activate NK cells and induce antiviral genes in neighboring cells that are likely to get infected by the same virus. Second, activated PKR phosphorylates the translation initiation factor eIF-2α on Ser 51, which results in a block of cellular and viral protein synthesis (53). Finally, activation of PKR leads to the induction of apoptosis in infected cells, thus preventing the further spread of the virus (Fig. 4).

2'-5'-Oligoadenylate Synthase and RNaseL

2'-5'-Oligoadenylate synthases (OAS) are a family of IFN-inducible enzymes that synthesize an unusual polymer—2'5' oligoadenylate (113,114). Activation of OAS requires dsRNA and therefore is triggered by viral infection. 2'5' Oligoadenylate produced by activated OAS then induces dimerization and activation of a dormant endonuclease, RNaseL. Once activated, RNaseL degrades viral and cellular RNA, including ribosomal RNA, which leads to a block of mRNA translation and to apoptosis (113,114) (Fig. 5). There are at least three genes encoding OAS proteins, and one of them can induce apoptosis through an additional pathway—by binding the antiapoptotic proteins Bcl2 and BclX$_L$ via the

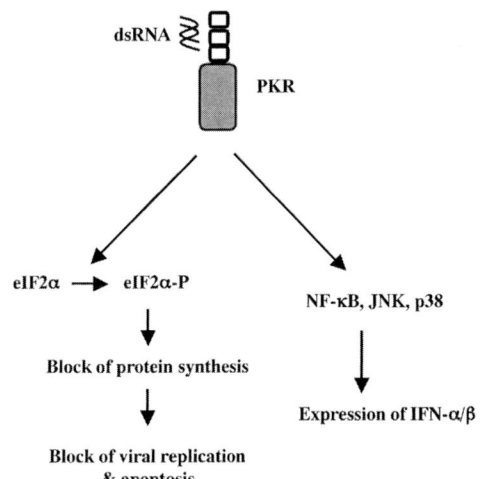

FIG. 4. Recognition of viral infection by PKR. PKR is activated upon binding to viral dsRNA. Activated PKR phosphorylates the translation initiation factor eIF2α, which results in an inhibition of translation. This block of cellular and viral protein synthesis limits viral replication and can lead to apoptosis of the infected cell. In addition, activation of PKR leads to the induction of NFκB and MAP kinase signaling pathways that turn on the expression of IFN-α/β genes.

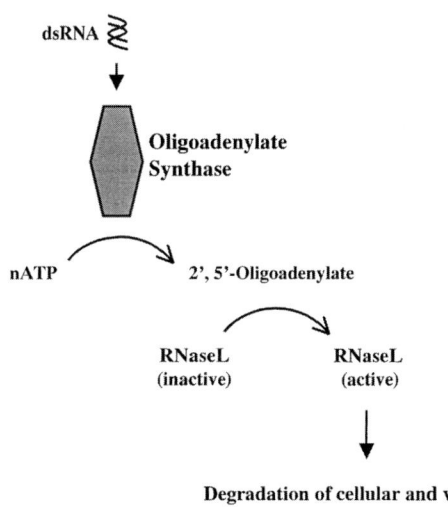

FIG. 5. Recognition of viral infection by oligoadenylate synthase (OAS). OAS is activated by viral dsRNA and generates 2',5'-oligoadenylate, which functions as a second messenger to activate a dormant ribonuclease, RNaseL. Once activated by 2'5'-oligoadenylate, RNaseL degrades cellular and viral RNA, which results in an inhibition of viral replication. Activated RNase L can also trigger pathways that lead to apoptosis of the infected cell. Some OAS proteins can induce apoptosis more directly by additional pathways that involve the sequestration of the antiapoptotic members of the Bcl 2 family.

C-terminal BH3 domain of the OAS. Sequestration of Bcl2 and BclX$_L$ then results in apoptosis of virally infected cells. Interestingly, the dsRNA-binding specificity of OAS evolved independently of that of PKR, as the dsRNA-binding domains in OAS and PKR are not related to each other. The importance of the OAS/RNaseL system in antiviral defense is demonstrated by the increased susceptibility of RNaseL-deficient mice to ECMV infection (114).

The NOD Family

The NOD family of intracellular proteins is characterized by a nucleotide-binding domain (NBD) followed by a leucine-rich repeat (LRR) region (115–118). In addition, some members of the family contain one or two CARD (caspase activation and recruitment domain) domains at the N-terminus, while others have a pyrin domain, a domain structurally related to the CARD domain (119). Although the function of NOD proteins is not known, there are three reasons to believe that these proteins play important roles in the innate immune system. First, NODs are structurally similar to a family of resistance gene products that confer protection against phytopathogens in plants. Second, some NOD proteins, including NOD1, NOD2, and NOD10—all of which contain CARD domains—activate NFκB and MAP-kinase signaling pathways (115–118), which are the same pathways activated by proinflammatory stimuli such as PAMPs. Finally, three proteins of the NOD family have been implicated in the pathogenesis of several inflammatory diseases—Crohn's disease (NOD2) (120,121), Mediterranean fever (pyrin) (122), and cold fever (cryopyrin) (123).

In plants, the products of R genes interact with pathogens and induce the hypersensitive response (HR), the plant equivalent of the inflammatory response in animals (124). The LRR region is thought to function in ligand recognition, the NBD domain in oligomerization, and the N-terminal domain in inducing downstream signaling events (124). The N-terminal CARD domains of several mammalian NOD proteins interact with and activate the serine/threonine protein kinase RIP2, which in turn induces the NFκB and MAP-kinase signaling pathways (115–117). The signals that activate NODs and the outcomes of this activation are presently unknown. It is widely speculated, however, that similar to the plant R-gene products, NOD proteins may function as intracellular receptors for pathogens.

THE CELLS OF THE INNATE IMMUNE SYSTEM

Unlike antigen receptors of the adaptive immune system, which are expressed exclusively on lymphocytes, the receptors of the innate immune system are expressed on many cell types. In fact, some of these receptors, most notably the intracellular receptors involved in the detection of viral infections, are expressed in almost every cell type. In this sense, innate host defense is not a function of a few specialized cell types. However, several cell types do have specialized functions related to innate immunity, although some of these cell types have other functions unrelated to immunity as well. Among these cells are macrophages, neutrophils, NK cells, mast cells, basophils, eosinophils, and surface epithelial cells. These cells are specialized to function at different stages of infection and to deal with different types of pathogens.

Macrophages

Macrophages have the most central and essential functions in the innate immune system, and have multiple roles in host defense. Mature, resident macrophages differentiate from circulating monocytes and occupy peripheral tissues and organs where they are most likely to encounter pathogens during the early stages of infection. Upon encounter with infectious agents, macrophages can employ a broad array of antimicrobial effector mechanisms, including phagocytosis of the pathogen and the induction of microbicidal effector systems, such as reactive oxygen and nitrogen intermediates and antimicrobial proteins and peptides. In addition, interaction of macrophages with pathogens leads to the induction of a plethora of inflammatory mediators, such as TNF-α, IL-1, and IL-6, and chemokines, such as KC-1 (and IL-8 in humans). TNF-α and IL-1 induce a local inflammatory response, and at higher concentrations, these cytokines (along with IL-6) induce the acute-phase response by triggering the expression of acute-phase genes in the liver. IL-8, a neutrophil chemoattractant produced by resident macrophages, recruits neutrophils to the site of infection. Production of antimicrobial effector genes, cytokines, and chemokines is mediated primarily by TLRs, whereas phagocytosis is mediated by multiple phagocytic PRRs. Many of the effector functions of macrophages are strongly augmented by IFN-γ, which comes from either NK cells or Th1 cells. IFN-γ also induces the antigen-presenting functions of macrophages by turning on the expression of a battery of genes involved in antigen processing and presentation.

In addition to their roles in host defense, macrophages have multiple "housekeeping functions," the most appreciated of which is their function as the body's scavengers. Macrophages phagocytose apoptotic cells, cell debris, oxidized lipoproteins, and other by-products of the normal physiology of multicellular organisms. Kuppfer cells (liver macrophages) remove from circulation senescent cells and desialated glycoproteins through phagocytosis mediated by asialoglycoprotein receptors (101). Similarly, macrophages located in the red pulp of the spleen phagocytose and remove from circulation senescent erythrocytes. Thus, in addition to the recognition of microbial non-self by PRRs, macrophages are equipped with a separate set of receptors for the recognition of "altered self" (desialated self-glycoproteins and phosphotidylserine exposed on apoptotic cells) and missing self (e.g., the lack of expression of CD47 on senescent erythrocytes) (125–127).

It is important to note that, unlike the phagocytosis of pathogens, which is mediated by PRRs and is followed by the induction of inflammatory mediators, phagocytosis of apoptotic and senescent cells is immunologically "silent" in that it does not lead to the induction of inflammatory responses. In fact, recognition and phagocytosis of apoptotic cells result in the production of the anti-inflammatory cytokine TGF-β (128). This phagocytosis pathway is mediated by the recently characterized macrophage receptor specific for phosphatidylserine (129). Thus, functionally distinct receptors expressed on macrophages determine the functional outcome of phagocytosis mediated by these versatile cells.

Neutrophils

Neutrophils are short-lived cells (average life span is about 24 to 48 hours) equipped with numerous antimicrobial effector mechanisms. Unlike resident macrophages, mast cells, and immature dendritic cells, neutrophils do not reside in peripheral tissues prior to infection. Rather, neutrophils are recruited from the circulation to the site of infection by cytokines and chemokines produced by resident macrophages and mast cells that have encountered pathogens. Recruited neutrophils accumulate at the site of infection and phagocytose and kill pathogens using several microbicidal mechanisms. In addition to reactive oxygen and nitrogen intermediates, neutrophils employ a number of antimicrobial proteins and peptides that are stored in neutrophil granules. Neutrophils contain several types of granules, including primary (or azurophil) granules, and secondary (or specific) granules that are specialized for the storage and secretion of antimicrobial products. Neutrophils are capable of both extracellular and intracellular killing of microorganisms, depending on the type of granules used. The content of primary granules is predominantly secreted into the extracellular space, whereas antimicrobial peptides of the secondary granules are predominantly released into the phagolysosome for the intracellular killing of pathogens.

Mast Cells

Although mast cells are best known as effectors of allergic responses, they are also an important component of innate immunity. Mature mast cells reside in connective and mucosal tissues where they encounter and phagocytose infecting microorganisms and produce inflammatory mediators that play an important role in leukocyte recruitment (130–132). The role of mast cells in innate host defense has been addressed using Kit^w/Kit^{w-v} mice, which carry an inactivating mutation in the c-kit gene and are essentially mast cell-deficient. Experiments carried out in these mice demonstrated that mast cells play an essential role in antibacterial defense in a model of acute septic peritonitis (133,134). Moreover, the protective role of mast cells is mediated mainly by the rapid production of TNF-α and leucotriene B4, which in turn are

responsible for neutrophil recruitment to the site of infection (131,133,134). The dramatic effect of mast cell deficiency revealed in the acute septic peritonitis experiments performed on Kit^w/Kit^{w-v} mice reflects the unique ability of mast cells to store preformed TNF-α that can be quickly secreted upon interaction with pathogens (135). Mast cells also produce lipid mediators of inflammation and a vast array of cytokines, including the "type II cytokines" IL-4, IL-5, and IL-13 (131,132).

Eosinophils

Mature eosinophils are found mainly in tissues, primarily in the respiratory, intestinal, and genitourinary tracts. Eosinophils, similar to mast cells, are rich in granules and produce a variety of cytokines and lipid mediators. In addition, eosinophil granules contain several cationic effector proteins that have potent toxic effects against parasitic worms (136). Unlike neutrophils and macrophages, eosinophils are poor phagocytes, and consequently release the content of their granules into the extracellular space. The production of various cationic antiparasitic proteins (which include major basic protein, eosinophil cationic protein, and eosiniphil-derived neurotoxic protein), as well as the fact that eosinophilia is induced in several model parasitic infections, implicate this cell type as an effector involved in host defense against parasite infections.

Dendritic Cells

Immature dendritic cells reside in peripheral tissues and are highly active in macropinocytosis and receptor-mediated endocytosis (137). DCs express a number of PRRs, including phagocytic receptors and TLRs. DCs are best known for their role in the initiation of adaptive immune responses, but these cells can also contribute to direct antimicrobial responses as well (137). Thus, stimulation of DCs with microbial products leads to the induction of several antimicrobial effector responses, such as nitric oxide production. The role of DCs in the initiation of the adaptive immune responses is discussed later in this chapter. The biology of DCs is described in more detail in Chapter 15.

Surface Epithelium

The epithelial cells that line the mucosal surfaces of the intestinal, respiratory, and genitourinary tracts provide an important physical barrier that separates the host from the environment. Mucins, which are highly glycosylated glycoproteins expressed on the surface of these cells, help to prevent pathogen attachment and invasion. In addition to providing physical separation of the host from the microbial environment, surface epithelial cells produce antimicrobial effectors, such as β-defensins and lysozyme, and secrete a number of cytokines and chemokines that contribute to the local inflammatory response and to the recruitment of leukocytes to the site of pathogen entry (138).

THE EFFECTOR MECHANISMS OF THE INNATE IMMUNE SYSTEM

The innate immune system possesses a wide variety of antimicrobial effector mechanisms that differ in inducibility, site of expression, mechanism of action, and activity against different pathogen classes. The major categories of antimicrobial effectors are as follows:

1. Enzymes that hydrolyze components of microbial cell walls (lysozyme, chitinases, phospholipase A2)
2. Antimicrobial proteins and peptides that disrupt the integrity of microbial cell walls (BPI, defensins, cathelicidins, complement, eosinophil cationic protein)
3. Microbicidal serine proteases (serprocidins)
4. Proteins that sequester iron and zinc (lactoferrin, NRAMP, calprotectin)
5. Enzymes that generate toxic oxygen and nitrogen derivatives (phagocyte oxidase, nitric oxide synthase, myeloperoxidase)

The major sites of expression of antimicrobial effectors are granulocytes (especially neutrophils), macrophages, and surface epithelium. It is worth pointing out that the antimicrobial activities of most of these effectors were demonstrated *in vitro;* physiologic roles in *in vivo* host defense have only been demonstrated for a few of these gene products.

Lysozyme

Lysozyme (also known as muramidase) and its antimicrobial properties were first described by Alexander Fleming in 1921. Lysozyme is a 14-kD enzyme that degrades the peptidoglycan of some gram-positive bacteria by cleaving the β 1,4-glycosidic linkage between N-acetylmuramic acid and N-acetylglucosamine. Disruption of the peptidoglycan layer leads to the osmotic lysis of the bacteria. Some gram-positive pathogens with highly cross-linked peptidoglycans are resistant to the action of lysozyme, and gram-negative bacteria as well are generally protected from lysozyme by their outer membrane. Lysozyme is highly concentrated in secretions such as tears and saliva. In humans, there is a single lysozyme gene that is expressed in neutrophils and macrophages. In the mouse there are two lysozymes: lysozyme M, which is expressed in macrophages, and lysozyme P, which is expressed by Paneth cells of the small intestine.

Chitinases

Chitinases comprise a family of enzymes that degrade chitin, a structural polysaccharide that forms the cell wall of fungi and the exoskeleton of insects. Chitinases are secreted by activated macrophages and presumably play a role in antifungal defense, although direct evidence for this function is lacking

(139). Several members of the chitinase family are enzymatically inactive due to amino acid substitutions in their catalytic sites. Some of them are expressed in human neutrophils, but their physiologic role is not known.

Phospholipase A2

Phospholipase A2 (PLA2) belongs to a family of disulfide-rich enzymes that share similar structures and catalytic mechanisms, but differ in substrate preferences and disulfide arrangements. Group II PLA2 is a 14-kD enzyme that hydrolyses the ester bonds at the 2-acyl position in the phospholipids of bacterial membranes. PLA2 is found in primary granules of neutrophils (and therefore is secreted upon degranulation), Paneth cells, and epithelial secretions (e.g., in tear fluid), and is produced by the liver as an acute-phase protein. The bactericidal activity of PLA2 is strongly potentiated by other antimicrobial products of neutrophils and by complement (141). PLA2 is particularly efficient against gram-positive bacteria (142). Killing of gram-negative bacteria is potentiated by antimicrobial effectors that disrupt the outer membrane, such as BPI. The important role of PLA2 in innate host defense is demonstrated by the finding that PLA2-deficient mice are more susceptible to infection with *S. aureus* than their wild-type controls (143,144).

BPI

Bactericidal permeability-increasing protein (BPI) is a cationic 55-kD protein that has several effector activities against gram-negative bacteria, but is inactive against gram-positive bacteria (145). BPI is structurally related to the acute-phase reactant LBP and, similar to LBP, BPI binds to the conserved lipid-A portion of LPS. BPI exerts its bactericidal activity by disrupting the integrity of the outer and inner membranes of gram-negative bacteria, thereby increasing their permeability and susceptibility to the action of other antimicrobial proteins such as PLA2. BPI can also function as an opsonin by binding to gram-negative bacteria and facilitating their uptake by neutrophils. Unlike LBP, which functions by potentiating LPS recognition by CD14/TLR4, BPI neutralizes free LPS and inhibits LPS signaling (145).

BPI is expressed predominantly in neutrophils, where it is found in large quantities in the primary granules and is secreted into inflammatory fluids upon neutrophil activation (145).

Defensins

Defensins are small (3 to 4 kD) cationic peptides with a broad spectrum of antimicrobial activities. Defensins are active against gram-positive and gram-negative bacteria, fungi, parasites, and some enveloped viruses (136,146). Defensins kill microorganisms by forming multimeric voltage–dependent pores in their membranes. The selective toxicity of defensins toward microbial cells can be explained in part by the differences in phospholipid composition between microbial and mammalian cell membranes and by the presence of choles-terol in mammalian but not bacterial membranes (147).

Defensins are characterized by a common structural feature—a hydrophobic β sheet stabilized by three disul-fide bonds. Depending on the pattern of disulfide bond for-mation between the six conserved cysteines, vertebrate de-fensins fall into two classes—α-defensins and β-defensins (136,146,147). The α-defensins are generally presynthesized and stored in granules of neutrophils (in humans but not in mice) and Paneth cells of the small intestine. The β-defensins, in contrast, are produced by epithelial cells and in most cases are not stored in cytoplasmic granules (136,146,147). The secretion of β-defensins is controlled primarily at the level of gene transcription and is inducible by microbial products (through TLRs) and by inflammatory cytokines (136,146,147).

Like all known antimicrobial peptides, defensins are syn-thesized as inactive precursors that contain a prodomain (which includes a leader sequence) and an acidic region that neutralizes and inactivates the cationic mature peptide. Pro-cessing of defensins results in the generation of active pep-tides. In neutrophils, active (processed) defensins are stored in the granules, whereas the epithelial defensins are secreted as propeptides and are processed in the lumen of the crypt (136,146,147). For mouse α-defensins the lumenal process-ing enzyme has been shown to be the matrix metalloprotease matrilysin (148). Matrilysin-deficient mice do not contain active α-defensins in their intestinal crypts and consequently are susceptible to intestinal infection (148).

Cathelicidins

Cathelicidins comprise a family of antimicrobial peptides that contain a conserved N-terminal prodomain called cathelin, and a C-terminal peptide that becomes active after cleavage from the cathelin domain. The C-terminal peptide is highly divergent between different cathelicidins within and between mammalian species (149,150). In the single human member of the cathelicidin family, the C-terminal peptide is 37 amino acids long and lacks cysteines but can form an amphipathic α helix that allows it to interact with microbial membranes. Cathelicidins are active against gram-positive and gram-negative bacteria and fungi and can act synergistically with other antimicrobial proteins (149,150). Cathelicidins are pro-duced in neutrophils and stored as inactive proproteins in the secondary granules. Activation of cathelicidins occurs when the neutrophil protease elastase cleaves off the cathelin domain. Interestingly, elastase is stored in the primary gran-ules of neutrophils and gains access to cathelicidin precursors only when the primary and secondary granules fuse with the phagosomes of activated neutrophils (136,149).

Serprocedins

Serprocedins comprise a family of 25- to 35-kD cationic serine proteases with antimicrobial activity and include neutrophil elastase, proteinase 3, cathepsin G, and azuro-cidin/CAP37 (136,151). Unlike other members of the family, azurocidin/CAP37 is catalytically inactive. Serprocedins are localized in the primary granules of neutrophils and are struc-turally related to the granzymes of NK cells and CD8 T cells. Serprocedins exert their antimicrobial activity either by di-rect perturbation of microbial membranes, or by proteolysis (136,151). Neutrophil elastase, as discussed above, converts cathelicidin precursors into active bactericidal peptides. Mice deficient for neutrophil elastase are more susceptible to gram-negative and fungal infections (152).

Lactoferrin, NRAMP, and Calprotectin

The antimicrobial activities of lactoferrin, NRAMP, and cal-protectin are due to their ability to sequester iron and zinc, which are essential for microbial metabolism and replication.

Lactoferrin is an 80-kD iron-chelating protein of the tras-ferrin family that contains two iron-binding sites. Lactoferrin is found in the secondary granules of neutrophils, in epithe-lial secretions such as breast milk, in the intestinal epithe-lium of infants, and in airway fluids. Lactoferrin has two mechanisms of antimicrobial activity: bacteriostatic and mi-crobicidal. The bacteriostatic effect is due to iron sequestra-tion (153). Pathogens depend on iron provided by the host and iron deprivation is an efficient strategy to block micro-bial metabolism, as iron is critically required for both oxida-tive and anaerobic pathways of ATP generation. In addition, lactoferrin can be processed by limited proteolysis to yield a cationic microbicidal peptide called lactoferricin (154). The bactericidal effect of lactoferricin is not dependent on iron sequestration and is thought to be due to a perturbation of microbial membranes (154).

NRAMP (natural resistance–associated macrophage pro-tein) is a 65-kD integral membrane protein that functions as an ion pump in the phagocytic vacuoles of macrophages and neutrophils (155). NRAMP is thought to function by pumping out iron from phagocytic vacuoles that harbor mycobacteria and other such bacteria that can persist in these vacuoles. In-deed, the gene encoding NRAMP is mutated in mouse strains that are highly susceptible to mycobacterial infections (155). NRAMP is inducible by IFN-γ.

Calprotectin, a member of the S-100 family of calcium-binding proteins, is composed of 8- and 14-kD subunits and is found in large amounts in the cytoplasm of neutrophils. The antimicrobial activity of this protein resides in its histidine-rich regions, which chelate and sequester zinc ions (156).

Phagocyte Oxidase, Myeloperoxidase, and Nitric Oxide Synthase

Phagocytes (granulocytes and macrophages) are equipped with an enzymatic machinery that generates highly toxic reactive oxygen and nitrogen intermediates that have po-tent antimicrobial activities (157). The induction of these antimicrobial effector responses is tightly regulated and is triggered upon interaction of phagocytes with pathogens (157,158).

Phagocyte oxidase (also known as NADPH oxidase) is responsible for the mitochondria-independent respiratory burst induced in phagocytes during the phagocytosis of microorganisms. NADPH oxidase is a multicomponent enzymatic complex that consists of three cytosolic subunits ($p40^{phox}$, $p47^{phox}$, and $p67^{phox}$) and a membrane-associated flavocytochrome complex ($p22^{phox}$ and $p91^{phox}$). Assembly of the subunits into a functional NADPH complex is induced by phagocyte activation through a Rac GTPase–dependent pathway. Once the complex is assembled, it produces superoxide anions (a primary product) and hydrogen peroxide (a secondary product), which are released into phagocytic vacuoles or outside the cell where they exert their direct and potent microbicidal effect. Mice deficient for various components of the NADPH complex are susceptible to multiple microbial infections (157,158).

Superoxide and hydrogen peroxide, in addition to their own antimicrobial activity, can also be used as substrates for another neutrophil enzyme called myeloperoxidase (157,158). Myeloperoxidase is stored in the primary granules of neutrophils and is also expressed in monocytes. Using the products of the NADPH oxidase as substrates, myeloperoxidase generates hypochlorous acid and chloramines as well as other reactive oxygen intermediates, all of which have potent microbicidal activities. Myeloperoxidase-deficient mice are highly susceptible to infection with *Candida albicans* (157,158).

Inducible nitric oxide synthase (iNOS) is expressed in neutrophils and macrophages and generates large amounts of nitric oxide (NO). NO is toxic to bacteria, although the exact mechanism(s) of its toxicity is not yet known (159). iNOS is inducible by IFN-γ and TLR ligands such as LPS (in mouse but not in human macrophages) (159). The role of iNOS and NO in the innate immune resistance to infection has been demonstrated in mice deficient for this enzyme. iNOS knockout mice are more susceptible than their wild-type counterparts to infection with multiple bacterial, viral, and protozoan pathogens (158,159). Interestingly, mice deficient for both NADPH oxidase and iNOS are severely immunocompromised and are highly susceptible not only to infection with pathogens, but also to commensal microorganisms (160).

The Antiviral Effector Mechanisms of the Innate Immune System

NK cells, which play a major role in the innate antiviral host defense, are discussed in depth in Chapter 12. Therefore, the discussion here is focused on cell-autonomous effector mechanisms that appear to be unique to antiviral defense. These mechanisms include the induction of apoptosis in virally infected cells and the inhibition of the viral life cycle by IFN-α/β-inducible gene products. Apoptosis of infected cells is an efficient way to prevent viral spread and can be induced either by cell-autonomous mechanisms (e.g., through PKR and OAS pathways, as discussed earlier in this chapter), or with the help of NK or CD8 T cells.

The best-characterized IFN-inducible gene products with intrinsic antiviral activity are members of the Mx protein family (161). The Mx protein and the closely related GBP (guanylate-binding protein) are members of the dynamin family of GTPases. The antiviral function of Mx proteins was discovered by the demonstration that the mouse Mx-1 gene confers resistance to influenza virus infection in A2G mice, whereas most other mouse strains carry a defective allele of Mx-1 and consequently are highly susceptible to influenza infection (161). Mx-1 appears to block transcription of the viral genome by inhibiting the influenza-virus polymerase complex (162–164). The second mouse Mx protein, Mx-2, is also mutated in most inbred strains of mice, except in the feral mouse strains NJL and SPR. In these mice, IFN-inducible Mx-2 protein confers resistance to VSV infection. Unlike the Mx-1 protein, which functions in the nucleus, the Mx-2 protein is cytoplasmic (165).

In human cells, there are two IFN-inducible Mx proteins, Mx-A and Mx-B. Mx-A is a cytoplasmic protein that inhibits replication of several viruses, including influenza, measles virus and VSV. Transgenic expression of the Mx-A protein in mice deficient for the IFN-α receptor protects these mice from lethal viral infections and demonstrates that Mx-A has intrinsic antiviral activity independently of other IFN-inducible genes (162,166).

GBP proteins are structurally related to Mx proteins, and likewise are inducible by IFN-α/β and confer resistance to some viral infections (167).

Not all the mechanisms of the antiviral function of Mx and GBP are known. Cytoplasmic Mx and GBP proteins may interfere with viral infection by blocking viral assembly, as suggested by the similarity of these proteins to other members of the dynamin family that play a role in vesicular trafficking and fusion.

CONTROL OF ADAPTIVE IMMUNITY BY THE INNATE IMMUNE SYSTEM

In addition to directly activating antimicrobial effector responses, innate immune recognition leads to the induction of three types of signals that control the activation of adaptive immunity (2). First, recognition of microbial infection leads to the induction of a local inflammatory response, which is mediated primarily through TLRs expressed on resident macrophages and endothelial cells. Second, recognition of PAMPs by TLRs and other PRRs expressed on dendritic cells induces dendritic cell maturation and an increase in the cell-surface expression of MHC class II and co-stimulatory molecules (CD80 and CD86) (Fig. 6). Finally, innate immune recognition triggers the induction of effector cytokines that

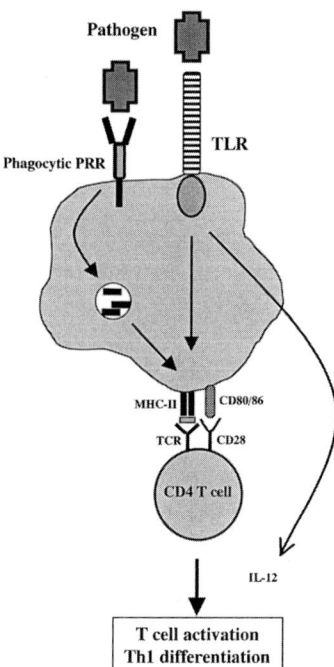

FIG. 6. Innate immune recognition and control of adaptive immune responses. Recognition of pathogens or PAMPs by PRRs expressed on dendritic cells leads to dendritic cell maturation and activation of naïve T cells. Phagocytic PRRs internalize pathogens into antigen-processing compartments, where pathogen-derived proteins are processed into antigenic peptides that are subsequently presented by MHC class II molecules on the cell surface. Therefore, expression of MHC-II/peptide complexes, induction of co-stimulatory molecules (CD80/CD86) and production of inflammatory cytokines (e.g., IL-12) are all induced by TLRs upon stimulation by microbial ligands. TLR-induced IL-12 directs T-cell differentiation into Th1 effector cells. The receptors involved in the recognition and initiation of Th2 responses are currently unknown.

critically control the type of effector responses mounted by the adaptive immune system.

Innate immune recognition is required for the activation of adaptive immune responses in part because the innate immune system can determine the origin of the antigen (2,3,5). Adaptive immune recognition relies on two types of antigen receptors—the T-cell receptor (TCR) and the B-cell receptor (BCR). The specificities of these receptors are generated by random processes such as gene rearrangement, and therefore are not predetermined to recognize pathogen-derived antigens. Both T and B cells undergo a process of negative selection that deletes lymphocytes specific for certain self-antigens. However, central tolerance does not eliminate all self-reactive lymphocytes. Those autoreactive lymphocytes that do mature and reach the peripheral lymphoid compartments are normally kept in an inactive state due to peripheral tolerance. The basis of peripheral tolerance lies in the dependence of T-lymphocytes on two signals for

activation: One signal is the antigen itself and the other is the co-stimulatory molecules of the B7 family (CD80/CD86). According to a theory proposed by Janeway (2,3), PRRs of the innate immune system control the expression of co-stimulatory molecules on antigen-presenting cells, and therefore make the activation of the adaptive immune responses dependent on the recognition of microbial infection by the innate immune system.

TLRs play a particularly important role in the control of adaptive immune responses. The specificity of TLRs to PAMPs allows them to distinguish self from non-self and to signal the presence of infection. Recognition of microbial products by TLRs expressed on DCs induces DC maturation (7,8). Immature DCs are located in peripheral tissues where they are likely to encounter invading pathogens (137). Interaction of DCs with pathogens leads to the activation of TLRs and the phagocytosis of pathogens by phagocytic PRRs, such as DEC205 and the mannose receptor. Once activated through TLRs, DCs begin to express high levels of MHC class II and co-stimulatory molecules, and migrate to the T-cell zone in the draining lymph nodes where they present pathogen-derived antigens to T-lymphocytes (7,8,137). In addition, TLRs induce expression by DCs of cytokines, including IL-12, which control T-cell differentiation into Th1 effector cells (168).

The role of TLRs in the control of adaptive immune responses has been demonstrated using MyD88 knockout mice. These mice have a profound defect in T-cell proliferation, IFN-γ production, and the generation of antigen-specific IgG2a responses to model antigens administered in complete Freund's adjuvant (CFA) (169). These results demonstrate the crucial role of Toll-mediated recognition in the initiation of Th1 immune responses. Th2 responses, on the other hand, are not diminished under the same experimental conditions, suggesting that the Toll pathway may only be required for Th1 but not Th2 adaptive immune responses (169). It is likely therefore, that Th2 responses are controlled by some other PRRs that perhaps recognize molecular patterns associated with "type 2" pathogens, such as helminthes. Additionally, that MyD88-deficient mice suffer a complete block of Th1 responses to antigen administered with CFA demonstrates that CFA and other similar adjuvants function by triggering TLRs on antigen-presenting cells.

CONCLUSIONS

Innate immunity is an evolutionarily ancient and universal system of host defense. Innate immunity is a function of multiple cell types, receptors, signaling systems, and effector mechanisms. Innate immune recognition is directed at conserved molecular patterns unique to microorganisms, which allows the innate immune system to distinguish self from microbial non-self. Recognition of infectious microorganisms by the innate immune system leads to the induction of antimicrobial effector mechanisms and thus provides the first line of host defense. In addition, the innate immune system plays an essential role in the initiation of adaptive immune responses and in the control of the effector responses of the adaptive immune system.

ACKNOWLEDGMENTS

This work is supported by the Howard Hughes Medical Institute and by the National Institutes of Health through grants AI44220-01 and AI46688-01.

REFERENCES

1. Agrawal A, Eastman QM, Schatz DG. Transposition mediated by RAG1 and RAG2 and its implications for the evolution of the immune system. *Nature* 1998;394:744.
2. Janeway CA Jr. Approaching the asymptote? Evolution and revolution in immunology. *Cold Spring Harb Symp Quant Biol* 1989;54:1.
3. Janeway CA Jr. The immune system evolved to discriminate infectious nonself from noninfectious self. *Immunol Today* 1992;13:11.
4. Karre K. How to recognize a foreign submarine. *Immunol Rev* 1997; 155:5.
5. Medzhitov R, Janeway CA Jr. Innate immunity: the virtues of a non-clonal system of recognition. *Cell* 1997;91:295.
6. Medzhitov R, Janeway CA Jr. Innate immunity: impact on the adaptive immune response. *Curr Opin Immunol* 1997;9:4.
7. Medzhitov R. Toll-like receptors and innate immunity. *Nature Reviews Immunology* 2001;1:135.
8. Akira S, Takeda K, Kaisho T. Toll-like receptors: critical proteins linking innate and acquired immunity. *Nat Immunol* 2001;2:675.
9. Kobe B, Deisenhofer J. Proteins with leucine-rich repeats. *Curr Opin Struct Biol* 1995;5:409.
10. Medzhitov R, Preston-Hurlburt P, Janeway CA Jr. A human homologue of the *Drosophila* Toll protein signals activation of adaptive immunity. *Nature* 1997;388:394.
11. Rock FL, Hardiman G, Timans JC, et al. A family of human receptors structurally related to *Drosophila* Toll. *Proc Natl Acad Sci U S A* 1998;95: 588.
12. Takeuchi O, Kawai T, Sanjo H, et al. TLR6: a novel member of an expanding Toll-like receptor family. *Gene* 1999;231:59.
13. Chuang TH, Ulevitch RJ. Cloning and characterization of a sub-family of human Toll-like receptors: hTLR7, hTLR8 and hTLR9. *Eur Cytokine Netw* 2000;11:372.
14. Chuang T, Ulevitch RJ. Identification of hTLR10: a novel human Toll-like receptor preferentially expressed in immune cells. *Biochim Biophys Acta* 2001;1518:157.
15. da Silva Correia J, Soldau K, Christen U, et al. Lipopolysaccharide is in close proximity to each of the proteins in its membrane receptor complex. Transfer from cd14 to tlr4 and md-2. *J Biol Chem* 2001;276:21129.
16. Poltorak A, Ricciardi-Castagnoli P, Citterio S, et al. Physical contact between lipopolysaccharide and Toll-like receptor 4 revealed by genetic complementation. *Proc Natl Acad Sci U S A* 2000;97: 2163.
17. Lien E, Means TK, Heine H, et al. Toll-like receptor 4 imparts ligand-specific recognition of bacterial lipopolysaccharide. *J Clin Invest* 2000;105:497.
18. Poltorak A, He X, Smirnova I, et al. Defective LPS signaling in C3H/HeJ and C57BL/10ScCr mice: mutations in Tlr4 gene. *Science* 1998;282:2085.
19. Qureshi ST, Lariviere L, Leveque G, et al. Endotoxin-tolerant mice have mutations in Toll-like receptor 4 (Tlr4). *J Exp Med* 1999;189: 615.
20. Hoshino K, Takeuchi O, Kawai T, et al. Cutting edge: Toll-like receptor 4 (TLR4)-deficient mice are hyporesponsive to lipopolysaccharide: evidence for TLR4 as the Lps gene product. *J Immunol* 1999;162: 3749.
21. Wright SD. Innate recognition of microbial lipids. In: Gallin JI, Snyderman R,eds. *Inflammation: basic principles and clinical correlates,* 3rd ed. Philadelphia: Lippincott Williams & Wilkins, 1999: 525.
22. Haziot A, Ferrero E, Kontgen F, et al. Resistance to endotoxin shock and reduced dissemination of gram-negative bacteria in CD14-deficient mice. *Immunity* 1996;4:407.
23. Shimazu R, Akashi S, Ogata H, et al. MD-2, a molecule that confers lipopolysaccharide responsiveness on Toll-like receptor 4. *J Exp Med* 1999;189:1777.
24. Schromm AB, Lien E, Henneke P, et al. Molecular genetic analysis of an endotoxin nonresponder mutant cell line. A point mutation in a conserved region of md-2 abolishes endotoxin-induced signaling. *J Exp Med* 2001;194:79.
25. Miyake K, Yamashita Y, Ogata M, et al. RP105, a novel B cell surface molecule implicated in B cell activation, is a member of the leucine-rich repeat protein family. *J Immunol* 1995;154:3333.
26. Miyake K, Shimazu R, Kondo J, et al. Mouse MD-1, a molecule that is physically associated with RP105 and positively regulates its expression. *J Immunol* 1998;161:1348.
27. Miura Y, Shimazu R, Miyake K, et al. RP105 is associated with MD-1 and transmits an activation signal in human B cells. *Blood* 1998;92:2815.
28. Chan VW, Mecklenbrauker I, Su I, et al. The molecular mechanism of B cell activation by Toll-like receptor protein RP-105. *J Exp Med* 1998;188:93.
29. Ogata H, Su I, Miyake K, et al. The Toll-like receptor protein RP105 regulates lipopolysaccharide signaling in B cells. *J Exp Med* 2000;192:23.
30. Takeuchi O, Hoshino K, Kawai T, et al. Differential roles of TLR2 and TLR4 in recognition of gram-negative and gram-positive bacterial cel wall components. *Immunity* 1999;11:443.
31. Schwandner R, Dziarski R, Wesche H, et al. Peptidoglycan- and lipoteichoic acid-induced cell activation is mediated by Toll-like receptor 2. *J Biol Chem* 1999;274:17406.
32. Means TK, Wang S, Lien E, et al. Human Toll-like receptors mediate cellular activation by Mycobacterium tuberculosis. *J Immunol* 1999; 163:3920.
33. Ohashi K, Burkart V, Flohe S, et al. Cutting edge: heat shock protein 60 is a putative endogenous ligand of the Toll-like receptor-4 complex. *J Immunol* 2000;164:558.
34. Vabulas RM, Ahmad-Nejad P, da Costa C, et al. Endocytosed heat shock protein 60s use TLR2 and TLR4 to activate the Toll/interleukin-1 receptor signaling pathway in innate immune cells. *J Biol Chem* 2001;11:11.
35. Li M, Carpio DF, Zheng Y, et al. An essential role of the NF-kappa B/Toll-like receptor pathway in induction of inflammatory and tissue-repair gene expression by necrotic cells. *J Immunol* 2001;166: 7128.
36. Kurt-Jones EA, Popova L, Kwinn L, et al. Pattern recognition receptors TLR4 and CD14 mediate response to respiratory syncytial virus. *Nat Immunol* 2000;1:398.
37. Aliprantis AO, Yang RB, Mark MR, et al. Cell activation and apoptosis by bacterial lipoproteins through Toll-like receptor-2. *Science* 1999;285:736.
38. Brightbill HD, Libraty DH, Krutzik SR, et al. Host defense mechanisms triggered by microbial lipoproteins through Toll-like receptors. *Science* 1999;285:732.
39. Takeuchi O, Kaufmann A, Grote A, et al. Cutting edge: preferentially the R-stereoisomer of the mycoplasmal lipopeptide macrophage-activating lipopeptide-2 activates immune cells through a Toll-like receptor 2- and MyD88-dependent signaling pathway. *J Immunol* 2000; 164:554.
40. Takeuchi O, Kawai T, Muhlradt PF, et al. Discrimination of bacterial lipoproteins by Toll-like receptor 6. *Int Immunol* 2001;13:933.
41. Means TK, Lien E, Yoshimura A, et al. The CD14 ligands lipoarabinomannan and lipopolysaccharide differ in their requirement for Toll-like receptors. *J Immunol* 1999;163:6748.
42. Hajjar AM, O'Mahony DS, Ozinsky A, et al. Cutting edge: functional interactions between Toll-like receptor (TLR) 2 and TLR1 or TLR6 in response to phenol-soluble modulin. *J Immunol* 2001;166:15.
43. Underhill D, Ozinsky A, Hajjar A, et al. The Toll-like receptor 2 is recruited to macrophage phagosomes and discriminates between pathogens. *Nature* 1999;401:811.

44. Campos MA, Almeida IC, Takeuchi O, et al. Activation of Toll-like receptor-2 by glycosylphosphatidylinositol anchors from a protozoan parasite. *J Immunol* 2001;167:416.

45. Werts C, Tapping RI, Mathison JC, et al. Leptospiral lipopolysaccharide activates cells through a TLR2-dependent mechanism. *Nat Immunol* 2001;2:346.

46. Hirschfeld M, Weis JJ, Toshchakov V, et al. Signaling by Toll-like receptor 2 and 4 agonists results in differential gene expression in murine macrophages. *Infect Immun* 2001;69:1477.

47. Ozinsky A, Underhill DM, Fontenot JD, et al. The repertoire for pattern recognition of pathogens by the innate immune system is defined by cooperation between Toll-like receptors. *Proc Natl Acad Sci U S A* 2000;97:13766.

48. Muzio M, Bosisio D, Polentarutti N, et al. Differential expression and regulation of Toll-like receptors (TLR) in human leukocytes: selective expression of TLR3 in dendritic cells. *J Immunol* 2000;164:5998.

49. Jarrossay D, Napolitani G, Colonna M, et al. Specialization and complementarity in microbial molecule recognition by human myeloid and plasmacytoid dendritic cells. *Eur J Immunol* 2001;31:3388.

50. Krug A, Towarowski A, Britsch S, et al. Toll-like receptor expression reveals CpG DNA as a unique microbial stimulus for plasmacytoid dendritic cells which synergizes with CD40 ligand to induce high amounts of IL-12. *Eur J Immunol* 2001;31:3026.

51. Kadowaki N, Ho S, Antonenko S, et al. Subsets of human dendritic cell precursors express different Toll-like receptors and respond to different microbial antigens. *J Exp Med* 2001194:863.

52. Alexopoulou L, Holt AC, Medzhitov R, et al. Recognition of double-stranded RNA and activation of NF-kappaB by Toll-like receptor 3. *Nature* 2001;413:732.

53. Williams BR. PKR: a sentinel kinase for cellular stress. *Oncogene* 1999;18:6112.

54. Chu WM, Ostertag D, Li ZW, et al. JNK2 and IKKbeta are required for activating the innate response to viral infection. *Immunity* 1999;11:721.

55. Hayashi F, Smith KD, Ozinsky A, et al. The innate immune response to bacterial flagellin is mediated by Toll-like receptor 5. *Nature* 2001;410:1099.

56. Gewirtz AT, Navas TA, Lyons S, et al. Cutting edge: bacterial flagellin activates basolaterally expressed tlr5 to induce epithelial proinflammatory gene expression. *J Immunol* 2001;167:1882.

57. Krieg AM. The role of CpG motifs in innate immunity. *Curr Opin Immunol* 2000;12:35.

58. Krieg AM, Yi AK, Matson S, et al. CpG motifs in bacterial DNA trigger direct B-cell activation. *Nature* 1995;374:546.

59. Hemmi H, Takeuchi O, Kawai T, et al. A Toll-like receptor recognizes bacterial DNA. *Nature* 2000;408:740.

60. Hacker H, Mischak H, Miethke T, et al. CpG-DNA-specific activation of antigen-presenting cells requires stress kinase activity and is preceded by non-specific endocytosis and endosomal maturation. *Embo J* 1998;17:6230.

61. Bauer S, Kirschning CJ, Hacker H, et al. Human TLR9 confers responsiveness to bacterial DNA via species-specific CpG motif recognition. *Proc Natl Acad Sci U S A* 2001;98:9237.

62. Medzhitov R, Preston-Hurlburt P, Kopp E, et al. MyD88 is an adaptor protein in the hToll/IL-1 receptor family signaling pathways. *Mol Cell* 1998;2:253.

63. Muzio M, Ni J, Feng P, et al. IRAK (Pelle) family member IRAK-2 and MyD88 as proximal mediators of IL-1 signaling. *Science* 1997;278:1612.

64. Muzio M, Natoli G, Saccani S, et al. The human Toll signaling pathway: divergence of nuclear factor kappaB and JNK/SAPK activation upstream of tumor necrosis factor receptor-associated factor 6 (TRAF6). *J Exp Med* 1998;187:2097.

65. Burns K, Clatworthy J, Martin L, et al. Tollip, a new component of the IL-1RI pathway, links IRAK to the IL-1 receptor. *Nat Cell Biol* 2000;2:346.

66. Adachi O, Kawai T, Takeda K, et al. Targeted disruption of the MyD88 gene results in loss of IL-1- and IL-18-mediated function. *Immunity* 1998;9:143.

67. Kawai T, Adachi O, Ogawa T, et al. Unresponsiveness of MyD88-deficient mice to endotoxin. *Immunity* 1999;11:115.

68. Wesche H, Gao X, Li X, et al. IRAK-M is a novel member of the Pelle/interleukin-1 receptor-associated kinase (IRAK) family. *J Biol Chem* 1999;274:19403.

69. Thomas JA, Allen JL, Tsen M, et al. Impaired cytokine signaling in mice lacking the IL-1 receptor-associated kinase. *J Immunol* 1999;163:978.

70. Cao Z, Xiong J, Takeuchi M, et al. TRAF6 is a signal transducer for interleukin-1. *Nature* 1996;383:443.

71. Cao Z, Henzel WJ, Gao X. IRAK: a kinase associated with the interleukin-1 receptor. *Science* 1996;271:1128.

72. Deng L, Wang C, Spencer E, et al. Activation of the IkappaB kinase complex by TRAF6 requires a dimeric ubiquitin-conjugating enzyme complex and a unique polyubiquitin chain. *Cell* 2000;103:351.

73. Arch RH, Gedrich RW, Thompson CB. Tumor necrosis factor receptor-associated factors (TRAFs)—a family of adapter proteins that regulates life and death. *Genes Dev* 1998;12:2821.

74. Wang C, Deng L, Hong M, et al. TAK1 is a ubiquitin-dependent kinase of MKK and IKK. *Nature* 2001;412:346.

75. Silverman N, Maniatis T. NF-kappaB signaling pathways in mammalian and insect innate immunity. *Genes Dev* 2001;15:2321.

76. Ghosh S, May MJ, Kopp EB. NF-kappa B and Rel proteins: evolutionarily conserved mediators of immune responses. *Annu Rev Immunol* 1998;16:225.

77. Karin M, Delhase M. The I kappa B kinase (IKK) and NF-kappa B: key elements of proinflammatory signalling. *Semin Immunol* 2000;12:85.

78. Schnare M, Holt AC, Takeda K, et al. Recognition of CpG DNA is mediated by signaling pathways dependent on the adaptor protein MyD88. *Curr Biol* 2000;10:1139.

79. Kaisho T, Takeuchi O, Kawai T, et al. Endotoxin-induced maturation of myd88-deficient dendritic cells. *J Immunol* 2001;166:5688.

80. Horng T, Barton GM, Medzhitov R. TIRAP: an adapter molecule in the Toll signaling pathway. *Nat Immunol* 2001;2:835.

81. Fitzgerald KA, Palsson-McDermott EM, Bowie AG, et al. Mal (MyD88-adapter-like) is required for Toll-like receptor-4 signal transduction. *Nature* 2001;413:78.

82. Kawai T, Takeuchi O, Fujita T, et al. Lipopolysaccharide stimulates the MyD88-independent pathway and results in activation of IFN-regulatory factor 3 and the expression of a subset of lipopolysaccharide-inducible genes. *J Immunol* 2001;167:5887.

83. Krieger M, Herz J. Structures and functions of multiligand lipoprotein receptors: macrophage scavenger receptors and LDL receptor-related protein (LRP). *Annu Rev Biochem* 1994;63:601.

84. Pearson AM. Scavenger receptors in innate immunity. *Curr Opin Immunol* 1996;8:20.

85. Suzuki H, Kurihara Y, Takeya M, et al. A role for macrophage scavenger receptors in atherosclerosis and susceptibility to infection. *Nature* 1997;386:292.

86. Haworth R, Platt N, Keshav S, et al. The macrophage scavenger receptor type A is expressed by activated macrophages and protects the host against lethal endotoxic shock. *J Exp Med* 1997;186:1431.

87. van der Laan LJ, Kangas M, Dopp EA, et al. Macrophage scavenger receptor MARCO: in vitro and in vivo regulation and involvement in the anti-bacterial host defense. *Immunol Lett* 1997;57:203.

88. Kraal G, van der Laan LJ, Elomaa O, et al. The macrophage receptor MARCO. *Microbes Infect* 2000;2:313.

89. Palecanda A, Paulauskis J, Al-Mutairi E, et al. Role of the scavenger receptor MARCO in alveolar macrophage binding of unopsonized environmental particles. *J Exp Med* 1999;189:1497.

90. Elomaa O, Sankala M, Pikkarainen T, et al. Structure of the human macrophage MARCO receptor and characterization of its bacteria-binding region. *J Biol Chem* 1998;273:4530.

91. Fraser IP, Koziel H, Ezekowitz RA. The serum mannose–binding protein and the macrophage mannose receptor are pattern recognition molecules that link innate and adaptive immunity. *Semin Immunol* 1998;10:363.

92. Taylor ME, Conary JR, Lennartz MR, et al. Primary structure of the mannose receptor contains multiple motifs resembling carbohydrate-recognition domains. *J Biol Chem* 1990;265:12156.

93. Taylor ME, Bezouska K, Drickamer K. Contribution to ligand binding by multiple carbohydrate-recognition domains in the macrophage mannose receptor. *J Biol Chem* 1992;267:1719.

94. Linehan SA, Martinez-Pomares L, Gordon S. Macrophage lectins in host defence. *Microbes Infect* 2000;2:279.

95. Prigozy TI, Sieling PA, Clemens D, et al. The mannose receptor delivers lipoglycan antigens to endosomes for presentation to T cells by CD1b molecules. *Immunity* 1997;6:187.

96. Jiang W, Swiggard WJ, Heufler C, et al. The receptor DEC-205 expressed by dendritic cells and thymic epithelial cells is involved in antigen processing. *Nature* 1995;375:151.

97. Ariizumi K, Shen GL, Shikano S, et al. Identification of a novel, dendritic cell-associated molecule, dectin-1, by subtractive cDNA cloning. *J Biol Chem* 2000;275:20157.

98. Brown GD, Gordon S. A new receptor for beta-glucans. *Nature* 2001; 413:36.

99. Holmskov U, Malhotra R, Sim RB, et al. Collectins: collagenous C-type lectins of the innate immune defense system. *Immunol Today* 1994;15:67.

100. Clark HW, Reid KB, Sim RB. Collectins and innate immunity in the lung. *Microbes Infect* 2000;2:273.

101. Weis WI, Drickamer K. Structural basis of lectin-carbohydrate recognition. *Annu Rev Biochem* 1996;65:441.

102. Fraser I, Ezekowitz RAB. Receptors for microbial products: carbohydrates. In: Gallin JI, Snyderman R,eds. *Inflammation: basic principles and clinical correlates,* 3rd. ed. Philadelphia: Lippincott Williams & Wilkins, 1999:515.

103. Crouch E, Wright JR. Surfactant proteins A and D and pulmonary host defense. *Annu Rev Physiol* 2001;63:521.

104. Gewurz H, Mold C, Siegel J, et al. 1982. C-reactive protein and the acute phase response. *Adv Intern Med* 1982;27:345.

105. Schwalbe RA, Dahlback B, Coe JE, et al. Pentraxin family of proteins interact specifically with phosphorylcholine and/or phosphorylethanolamine. *Biochemistry* 1992;31:4907.

106. Agrawal A, Shrive AK, Greenhough TJ, et al. Topology and structure of the C1q-binding site on C-reactive protein. *J Immunol* 2001; 166:3998.

107. Ulevitch RJ, Tobias PS. Receptor-dependent mechanisms of cell stimulation by bacterial endotoxin. *Annu Rev Immunol* 1995;13:437.

108. Kang D, Liu G, Lundstrom A, et al. A peptidoglycan recognition protein in innate immunity conserved from insects to humans. *Proc Natl Acad Sci U S A* 1998;95:10078.

109. Werner T, Liu G, Kang D, et al. A family of peptidoglycan recognition proteins in the fruit fly *Drosophila* melanogaster. *Proc Natl Acad Sci U S A* 2000;97:13772.

110. Liu C, Xu Z, Gupta D, et al. Peptidoglycan recognition proteins: a novel family of four human innate immunity pattern recognition molecules. *J Biol Chem* 2001;276:34686.

111. Liu C, Gelius E, Liu G, et al. Mammalian peptidoglycan recognition protein binds peptidoglycan with high affinity, is expressed in neutrophils, inhibits bacterial growth. *J Biol Chem* 2000;275:24490.

112. Clemens MJ, Elia A. The double-stranded RNA-dependent protein kinase PKR: structure and function. *J Interferon Cytokine Res* 1997;17:503.

113. Kumar M, Carmichael GG. Antisense RNA: function and fate of duplex RNA in cells of higher eukaryotes. *Microbiol Mol Biol Rev* 1998;62:1415.

114. Samuel CE. Antiviral actions of interferons. *Clin Microbiol Rev* 2001; 14:778.

115. Bertin J, Nir WJ, Fischer CM, et al. Human CARD4 protein is a novel CED-4/Apaf-1 cell death family member that activates NF-kappaB. *J Biol Chem* 1999;274:12955.

116. Inohara N, Koseki T, del Peso L, et al. Nod1, an Apaf-1-like activator of caspase-9 and nuclear factor-kappaB. *J Biol Chem* 1999;274: 14560.

117. Ogura Y, Inohara N, Benito A, et al. Nod2, a Nod1/Apaf-1 family member that is restricted to monocytes and activates NF-kappaB. *J Biol Chem* 2001;276:4812.

118. Wang L, Guo Y, Huang WJ, et al. Card10 is a novel caspase recruitment domain/membrane-associated guanylate kinase family member that interacts with BCL10 and activates NF-kappa B. *J Biol Chem* 2001;276:21405.

119. Kastner DL, O'Shea JJ. A fever gene comes in from the cold. *Nat Genet* 2001;29:241.

120. Cho JH. The Nod2 gene in Crohn's disease: implications for future research into the genetics and immunology of Crohn's disease. *Inflamm Bowel Dis* 2001;7:271.

121. Hampe J, Cuthbert A, Croucher PJ, et al. Association between insertion mutation in NOD2 gene and Crohn's disease in German and British populations. *Lancet* 2001;357:1925.

122. Consortium TFF. A candidate gene for familial Mediterranean fever. *Nat Genet* 1997;17:25.

123. Hoffman HM, Mueller JL, Broide DH, et al. Mutation of a new gene encoding a putative pyrin-like protein causes familial cold autoinflammatory syndrome and Muckle-Wells syndrome. *Nat Genet* 2001;29:301.

124. Hammond-Kosack K, Jones J. Plant disease resistance genes. *Annu Rev Plant Physiol Plant Mol Biol* 1997;48:575.

125. Fadok VA, Voelker DR, Campbell PA, et al. Exposure of phosphatidylserine on the surface of apoptotic lymphocytes triggers specific recognition and removal by macrophages. *J Immunol* 1992;148: 2207.

126. Fadok VA, de Cathelineau A, Daleke DL, et al. Loss of phospholipid asymmetry and surface exposure of phosphatidylserine is required for phagocytosis of apoptotic cells by macrophages and fibroblasts. *J Biol Chem* 2001;276:1071.

127. Oldenborg PA, Zhelezsnyak A, Fang YF, et al. Role of CD47 as a marker of self on red blood cells. *Science* 2000;288:2051.

128. Henson PM, Bratton DL, Fadok VA. Apoptotic cell removal. *Curr Biol* 2001;11:R795.

129. Fadok VA, Bratton DL, Rose DM, et al. A receptor for phosphatidylserine-specific clearance of apoptotic cells. *Nature* 2000; 405:85.

130. Zhang Y, Ramos BF, Jakschik BA. Neutrophil recruitment by tumor necrosis factor from mast cells in immune complex peritonitis. *Science* 1992;258:1957.

131. Ramos BF, Zhang Y, Qureshi R, et al. Mast cells are critical for the production of leukotrienes responsible for neutrophil recruitment in immune complex-induced peritonitis in mice. *J Immunol* 1991;147:1636.

132. Galli SJ. Mast cells and basophils. *Curr Opin Hematol* 2000;7:32.

133. Echtenacher B, Mannel DN, Hultner L. Critical protective role of mast cells in a model of acute septic peritonitis. *Nature* 1996;381:75.

134. Malaviya R, Ikeda T, Ross E, et al. Mast cell modulation of neutrophil influx and bacterial clearance at sites of infection through TNF-alpha. *Nature* 1996;381:77.

135. Gordon JR, Galli SJ. Mast cells as a source of both preformed and immunologically inducible TNF-alpha/cachectin. *Nature* 1990; 346:274.

136. Levy O. Antimicrobial proteins and peptides of blood: templates for novel antimicrobial agents. *Blood* 2000;96:2664.

137. Banchereau J, Steinman RM. Dendritic cells and the control of immunity. *Nature* 1998;392:245.

138. Kagnoff MF, Eckmann L. Epithelial cells as sensors for microbial infection. *J Clin Invest* 1997;100:6.

139. Boot RG, Renkema GH, Strijland A, et al. Cloning of a cDNA encoding chitotriosidase, a human chitinase produced by macrophages. *J Biol Chem* 1995;270:26252.

140. Renkema GH, Boot RG, Au FL, et al. Chitotriosidase, a chitinase, the 39-kDa human cartilage glycoprotein, a chitin-binding lectin, are homologues of family 18 glycosyl hydrolases secreted by human macrophages. *Eur J Biochem* 1998;251:504.

141. Wright GC, Weiss J, Kim JS, et al. Bacterial phospholipid hydrolysis enhances the destruction of Escherichia coli ingested by rabbit neutrophils. Role of cellular and extracellular phospholipases. *J Clin Invest* 1990;85:1925.

142. Qu XD, Lehrer RI. Secretory phospholipase A2 is the principal bactericide for staphylococci and other gram-positive bacteria in human tears. *Infect Immun* 1998;66:2791.

143. Laine VJ, Grass DS, Nevalainen TJ. Resistance of transgenic mice expressing human group II phospholipase A2 to Escherichia coli infection. *Infect Immun* 2000;68:87.

144. Laine VJ, Grass DS, Nevalainen TJ. Protection by group II phospholipase A2 against Staphylococcus aureus. *J Immunol* 1999;162:7402.

145. Elsbach P, Weiss J. Role of the bactericidal/permeability-increasing protein in host defence. *Curr Opin Immunol* 1998;10:45.

146. Martin E, Ganz T, Lehrer RI. Defensins and other endogenous peptide antibiotics of vertebrates. *J Leukoc Biol* 1995;58:128.

147. Boman HG. Peptide antibiotics and their role in innate immunity. *Annu Rev Immunol* 1995;13:61.

148. Wilson CL, Ouellette AJ, Satchell DP, et al. Regulation of intestinal alpha-defensin activation by the metalloproteinase matrilysin in innate host defense. *Science* 1999;286:113.

149. Zanetti M, Gennaro R, Romeo D. The cathelicidin family of antimicrobial peptide precursors: a component of the oxygen-independent defense mechanisms of neutrophils. *Ann N Y Acad Sci* 1997;832: 147.

150. Zanetti M, Gennaro R, Romeo D. Cathelicidins: a novel protein family with a common proregion and a variable C-terminal antimicrobial domain. *FEBS Lett* 1995;374:1.
151. Gabay JE, Almeida RP. Antibiotic peptides and serine protease homologs in human polymorphonuclear leukocytes: defensins and azurocidin. *Curr Opin Immunol* 1993;5:97.
152. Belaaouaj A, McCarthy R, Baumann M, et al. Mice lacking neutrophil elastase reveal impaired host defense against gram negative bacterial sepsis. *Nat Med* 1998;4:615.
153. Jurado RL. Iron, infections, anemia of inflammation. *Clin Infect Dis* 1997;25:888.
154. Hoek KS, Milne JM, Grieve PA, et al. Antibacterial activity in bovine lactoferrin–derived peptides. *Antimicrob Agents Chemother* 1997;41:54.
155. Vidal SM, Malo D, Vogan K, et al. Natural resistance to infection with intracellular parasites: isolation of a candidate for Bcg. *Cell* 1993;73:469.
156. Loomans HJ, Hahn BL, Li QQ, et al. Histidine-based zinc-binding sequences and the antimicrobial activity of calprotectin. *J Infect Dis* 1998;177:812.
157. Klebanoff SJ. Oxygen metabolites from phagocytes. In: Gallin JI, Snyderman R, eds. *Inflammation: basic principles and clinical correlates,* 3rd ed. Philadelphia: Lippincott Williams & Wilkins, 1999:721.
158. Bogdan C, Rollinghoff M, Diefenbach A. Reactive oxygen and reactive nitrogen intermediates in innate and specific immunity. *Curr Opin Immunol* 2000;12:64.
159. MacMicking J, Xie QW, Nathan C. Nitric oxide and macrophage function. *Annu Rev Immunol* 1997;15:323.
160. Shiloh MU, MacMicking JD, Nicholson S, et al. Phenotype of mice and macrophages deficient in both phagocyte oxidase and inducible nitric oxide synthase. *Immunity* 1999;10:29.
161. Arnheiter H, Skuntz S, Noteborn M, et al. Transgenic mice with intracellular immunity to influenza virus. *Cell* 1990;62:51.
162. Pavlovic J, Arzet HA, Hefti HP, et al. Enhanced virus resistance of transgenic mice expressing the human MxA protein. *J Virol* 1995;69:4506.
163. Pavlovic J, Staeheli P. The antiviral potentials of Mx proteins. *J Interferon Res* 1991;11:215.
164. Pavlovic J, Schroder A, Blank A, et al. Mx proteins: GTPases involved in the interferon-induced antiviral state. *Ciba Found Symp* 1993;176:233.
165. Landolfo S, Gribaudo G, Angeretti A, et al. Mechanisms of viral inhibition by interferons. *Pharmacol Ther* 1995;65:415.
166. Hefti HP, Frese M, Landis H, et al. Human MxA protein protects mice lacking a functional alpha/beta interferon system against La crosse virus and other lethal viral infections. *J Virol* 1999;73:6984.
167. Anderson SL, Carton JM, Lou J, et al. Interferon-induced guanylate binding protein-1 (GBP-1) mediates an antiviral effect against vesicular stomatitis virus and encephalomyocarditis virus. *Virology* 1999;256:8.
168. Abbas AK, Murphy KM, Sher A. Functional diversity of helper T lymphocytes. *Nature* 1996;383:787.
169. Schnare M, Barton GM, Holt AC, et al. Toll-like receptors control activation of adaptive immune responses. *Nat Immunol* 2001;2:947.

CHAPTER 18

Evolution of the Immune System

Martin F. Flajnik, Kristina Miller, and Louis Du Pasquier

Introduction
Components of Adaptive Immune System
  T-cell receptors · Immunoglobulins · Major Histocompatibility Complex · Lymphoid Tissues and Cells of Jawed Vertebrates · Rearrangement and Diversification of TCR and Ig Genes During Lymphocyte Differentiation · Adaptive Immune Responses · Cytokines and Chemokines · Evolution of Hematopoiesis
Evolution of Innate Immunity
  Invertebrate Cells · Recognition · Signaling · Allorecognition
Origins of Adaptive Immunity
  MHC Origins · Origins of Rearranging Receptors
Conclusions
Acknowledgments
Publications Worth Noting
References

INTRODUCTION

All living organisms have the capacity to defend themselves against invasion by pathogens. The number of mechanisms that have evolved for immune protection is remarkable and we are headed toward at least a chronicling of most of the molecules used for defense in some vertebrates and invertebrates; obviously a gestalt *understanding* of the interplay of these molecules and mechanisms will occupy us for the rest of our natural lives. Furthermore, there will certainly be novel mechanisms that we never anticipated: For example, the recently discovered phenomenon by which the genome adaptively "responds" to foreign nucleic acid (RNA silencing) was a surprise to most comparative immunologists (R1).

Innate defense mechanisms are found in all living things, while adaptive immunity grounded on somatically generated immunoglobulin (Ig), T-cell receptors (TCR), and the major histocompatibility complex (MHC) is only present in jawed vertebrates (Figs. 1 and 2). Because of clonal selection, positive and negative selection in the thymus, MHC-regulated initiation of all adaptive responses, and so on, the major elements of the adaptive immune system are locked in a co-evolving Ig-TCR-MHC unit. This system was superimposed onto an innate system inherited from primitive invertebrates, from which some innate molecules were co-opted for the initial phase of the adaptive response and others for effector mechanisms at the completion of adaptive responses. In

jawed vertebrates (gnathostomes), we observe fine-tuning or adaptations (or degeneration) in each taxon and generally not a regular progression from fish to mammals as is seen, for example, in evolution of the telencephalon (forebrain) in the nervous system or in heart specialization. Given that all basic adaptive immune system features are present in cartilaginous fish and none were lost, we see only variation on the theme (differential usage) rather than progressive installation of new elements (Fig. 2 displays the vertebrate tree). As we shall see, there are only a few cases of increasing complexity in the adaptive system superimposed on the vertebrate phylogenetic tree, but many examples of contractions/expansions of existing gene families; thus, on average "more (or less) of the same" rather than "more and more new features" is the rule. We watch a bush growing from a short stem rather than a tall tree, and thus deducing the primitive traits is not easy. The quality of immune responses, however, is not the same between cold-blooded and warm-blooded vertebrates or even among all mammalian species.

Figure 1 displays the extant animal phyla ranging from the single-celled protozoa to the advanced protostome and deuterostome lineages. It is often suggested or assumed that molecules or mechanisms found in living protostomes, like the well-studied *Drosophila*, are ancestral to similar molecules/mechanisms in mouse and human. While this may be true in some cases, one should instead recognize that *Drosophila* and mouse/human have taken just as long

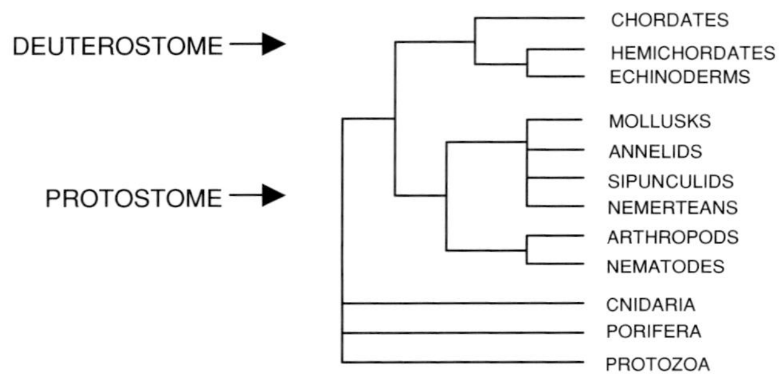

FIG. 1. Immune system elements throughout the animal kingdom.

	METAZOA												
	PORIFERA	CNIDARIA	BILATERIA										
			PROTOSTOMATA						DEUTEROSTOMATA				
			LOPHOTROCHOZOANS				ECDYSOZOANS			CHORDATA			
												VERTEBRATA	
			NEMERTEANS	SIPUNCULIDA	ANNELIDS	MOLLUSKS	NEMATODES	ARTHROPODS	ECHINODERMS	UROCHORD.	CEPH. CHORD.	AGNATHA	GNATHOSTOMATA
	sponges	*sea anemones*	*ribbon worms*	*sip. worms*	*earthworms*	*snails*	*C. elegans*	*insects and crust.*	*sea urchins*	*tunicates*	*amphioxus*	*hagfish*	*shark - man*
RECOGNITION													
-Allorecognition	+	+		+	+				+	+		+	+
-Pathogens	+	+		+	+	+		+	+	+		+	+
CELLS													
-Macrophages	+	+	+	+	+	+	+	+	+	+	+	+	+
-Mesodermal origin			+	+	+	+		+	+	+		+	+
-Hematopoiec transx. fac.		+						+	+	+		+	+
-Specific clonal expansion													+
-(memory)	-	?	?		?				?			?	+
SURFACE RECEPTORS													
-Igsf V domains	+	+				+	+	+	+	+			+
C2 domains	+	+				+	+	+		+			+
C1 domains													
-Lectins	+	+			+	+	+	+	+	+		+	+
-Scavenger receptors							+	+	+				+
-Peptidoglycan receptors								+					+
-Toll (-like)							+	+			+		+
SIGNALLING													
-NFKB	-					+	-	+		+			+
-SYK		+					-	+					+
-JAK-STAT								+					+
EFFECTOR MECHANISMS													
-Anti-Mic peptides	+	+			+	+		+	+	+		+	+
-Complement family								+	+	+		+	+
-Thioester a2m like	+							+	+	+		+	+
-C3 and Bf like	+								+	+		+	+
-Melanization (PPO)	+	?			+	+		+	+	+		?	?
-Clotting								+					+
STRATEGY FOR DIVERSITY													
-Multigene family						+		+	+			+	+
-Alternate splicing									+				+
-Somatic rearrangement												-	+
-Somatic mutation													+

DEUTEROSTOME →

PROTOSTOME →

CHORDATES
HEMICHORDATES
ECHINODERMS
MOLLUSKS
ANNELIDS
SIPUNCULIDS
NEMERTEANS
ARTHROPODS
NEMATODES
CNIDARIA
PORIFERA
PROTOZOA

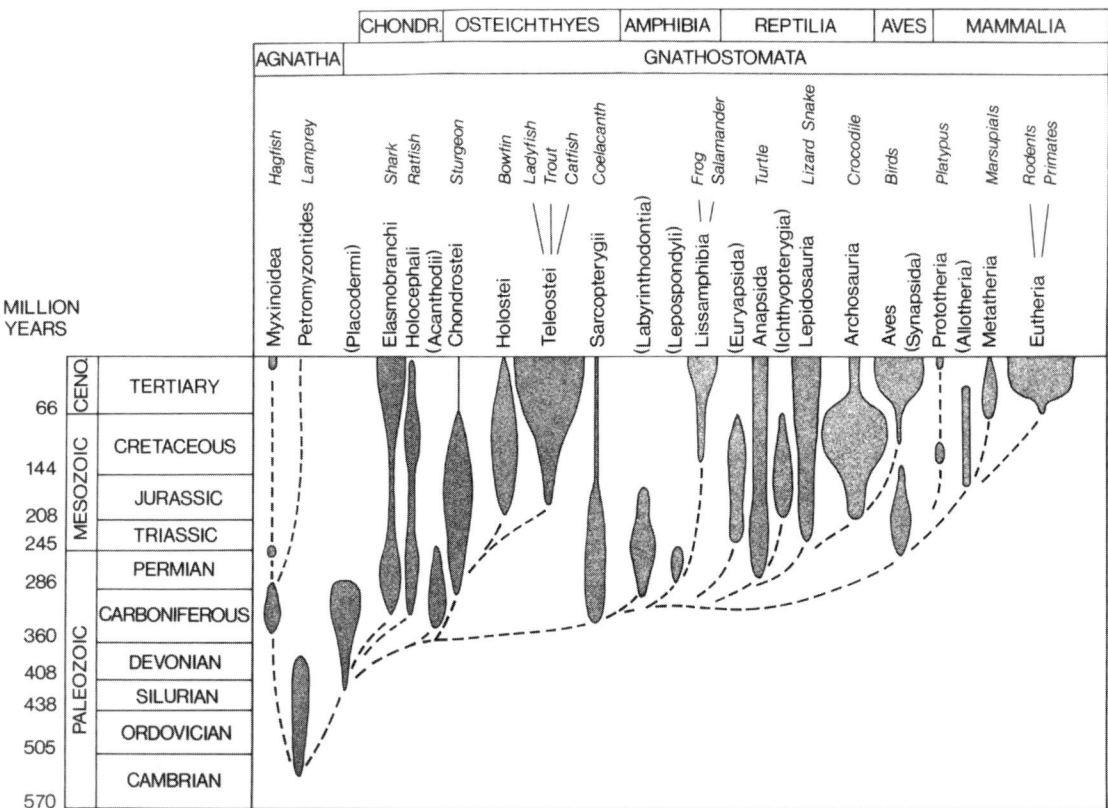

FIG. 2. The vertebrate phylogenetic tree. The size of the shaded areas indicates the number of extant species.

(over 600 million years) to evolve from a common ancestral triploblastic coelomate (an animal with three germ layers and a mesoderm-lined body cavity, features shared by protostomes and deuterostomes), and clearly *Drosophila* is not our ancestor; that is, the manner by which flies and mouse/human utilize certain families of defense molecules may be quite different and both may be nothing like the common ancestor. Thus, knowing how model invertebrates and vertebrates perform certain immune tasks is always an important first step, but we only understand what is primordial or derived when we have examined similar immune mechanisms/molecules in species from a range of animal phyla. We touch upon all defense molecule families listed in Fig. 1 and emphasize which ones have been conserved evolutionarily (clearly the minority), and those that have evolved rapidly.

In previous editions of *Fundamental Immunology,* we began our analysis with immune responses of the invertebrates, concentrating on allorecognition phenomena, most of which are still undefined at the molecular level. (We ask readers to refer to an earlier edition for a detailed discussion of the subject.) In this edition, we begin with the elements of the adaptive immune system, found only in the jawed vertebrates, then review the burgeoning (and surprisingly young) field of innate immunity in animals and plants, and conclude with speculations on origins of adaptive immunity. As predicted over 10 years ago by Zasloff (2), it is informative from both intellectual and applied viewpoints to understand how *all*

living things defend themselves; few would argue against the premise that studies of *Drosophila* humoral immunity has fueled great interest in innate immunity, both for its own sake and in the way it regulates adaptive immunity (R3). In this edition we also have expanded the section on MHC population genetics/polymorphism to complement the comparative, structural features.[*]

COMPONENTS OF ADAPTIVE IMMUNE SYSTEM

T-Cell Receptors

Ig, TCR, and MHC class I and class II are all composed of immunoglobulin superfamily (Igsf) domains (Fig. 3). The membrane-proximal domains of each Ig/TCR/MHC chain are Igsf C1-set domains, a type thus far restricted to the jawed vertebrates (see below). The N-terminal domains of Ig and TCR proteins are V-set domains encoded by genes generated via rearrangement of two or three gene segments during ontogeny (Figs. 4 to 6). The membrane-distal domains of MHC are a special case (see below). In all vertebrates studied to

---

[*] Because of space restrictions, we have limited references to recent review articles, the most classic papers in the field, and some recent articles that have modified our view of comparative immunology. References denoting reviews are marked with a capital R followed by the respective number, e.g. R1. We have compiled a supplementary list of references that is available on the CD-ROM.

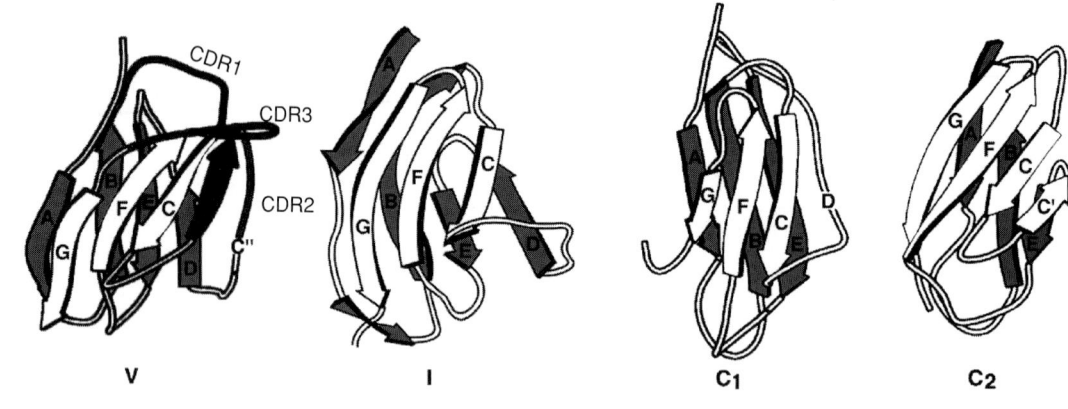

V   **I**   **C₁**   **C₂**

Dimer interface; C, C', C'', F, G   **Dimer interface; A, B, D, E**

FIG. 3. Different types of immunoglobulin superfamily domains. The sheets are composed of ABDE and C(C′C″)FG in all domains. The CDR of V domains are shown in black. Note that dimers of V and C domains interact through different sheets. Modified from Du Pasquier (7), with permission.

```
Alpha                          extracellular constant
D                PSVY L     S   S    CLATDFSP N             K SAV        SYS V     K        consensus
PKRDEELK----------PSVYVLRPPPASPDDRQAPAACLATDYFPNKYDLTMTMDGTSKTSSNNSAQVSIKDRSYSLLSFINGSTPQS  ray
EEKRE------------PSIYKLP--------SDEQEYCLATRFTVHNTTNGTWPTNEY-KEDAV-RFEGEGY--YSRLLR-NIKD---   catfish
REKHD------------PSYYSLK--------SRNTTACLAIDFSAHNATT---HLELFNKTEAT-RMNGDSY--YSQVAL-GGEN---   trout
DATEDECRIGINNIPDSPPSVYLLKPASES--EGHGRLCCLTDFSPVNKVKVFRNDTEEGKREATLVQSQMKW-SYGIVEW-STKQNDT   axolotl
DIT------------PSPSVYRLTSEDD-----KDLEMCLITDYSPEKLDLS----SVDSKTETVVEVATSENKHEASYLS-TYWAKKD   chicken
D------------IQNPDPAVYQLR---DS--KSSDKSVCLFTDFDSQTNVSQSKDSDVYITDKTVLDMRSMDFKSNSAVAW-SNK---S  human

        C      I   D   G   C       FETDE LNFLSLSVLGLRILFLK I FN LMTLRLW S    consensus
81 EITCELEPNTPNIAETDV----GQMSCIPLEETD---EDGEYMRGISLTVFGMRMLFVKGVIFNILMSVRVWTS  ray
62 ---CPE----------------NETMCDSSKSEDGGFKSDAKTNFLGLSIFWLRVVLFLKTIVFNILMTLKVWMS  catfish
60 ---CTEV--------------GGSEKCEANWY----FDTDAKINFLSLTILGLRILFLKTIVFNVLITLRLWMS  trout
87 QFQCNAKYKD-TMYTAQEIKGGVQIACPVMAVNES-FETDEQLNTLSLTVLGLKIIFLKSIGFNLLMTLRLWTN  axolotl
68 EMQCGAKHEGFGILKGDDPEAGASTVCITGMSLL--FKTDENLNMLTFSQLGLKIIFMKAVIFNVLITMLMWKKNQ  chicken
70 DFACANAFNN-SIIPEDTFFPSPESSCDVKLVEKS-FETDTNLNFQNLSVIGFRILLLKVAGFNLLMTLRLWSS  human

             constant                    transmembrane    cytoplasmic

Beta                          extracellular constant
        P V  F PS  EI     K KATLVCLA  F PDHV  W VN          TD           YS SSRLR    A  W   consensus
LDPKFKLRPPQVTILQPSDREI----KNKGKATVVCLITDFYPDNIKIRWIFDDVVQDKDSDNIHTDASSQSEDEGMTFSISSRFRLD-ARDY  ray
GEND-TIRPAKVTVFEPSPEEI----REKKKATVVCLVSDFYPDNIKIHWLVDGKEKDANDTNIHTDLNAILSKENTSYSISSRLRFD-ALDW  shark
-DPDMKLQAPTVTVLNVSEKEVCT----KENVTLVCVAKGFYPDHVKVYWTVDEVNRTIDVSTDEAAVQG----SDKYYTISSRLNIDYKTEW  catfish
-DPNIKVTEPTVKVLAPSAKK-CEDRNKKKKKTLVCVATRFYPDHVTVFWQVNNVNRTEGAGTDNRALWD----KDGLYSITSRLRVP-ANEW  trout
-EEGLSVTQPSVVLFDPSPQEI----KKKGKATLVCLATNFYPDHVTLRWSVNDQVTTTGVKTDDSPIRG----SDRMYSLSSRLRLT-KMDW  axolotl
EKGQEEKNVANVAIFRPNPKE----QTDHGYLSIVCLASGFFPEHVQLQWKVNKKERDGS--------QGKAIKTGDTYSISSRLSLT-KNEY  xenopus
-GKNSEIIEPDVVIFSPSKQEI----QEKKKATLVCLASGFFPDHLNLVWKVNGVKRTEGVGTD-----EISTSNGSTYSLTSRLRIS-AQEW  chicken
--DLRNVTPPKVSLFEPSKAEI----ANKQKATLVCLARGFFPDHVELSWWVNGKEVHSGVSTDPQAYKE----SNYSYCLSSRLRVS-ATFW  mouse
-EDLNKVFPPEVAVFEPSEAEI----SHTQKATLVCLATGFFPDHVELSWWVNGKEVHSGVSTDPQPLKEQPALNDSRYCLSSRLRVS-ATFW  human

     P N   C VF                    I     G   CG          Y  L  KS  YG  V              K   consensus
95 KTEK-IVCEVDHYRNGSTPQ-----TEQGTHYIKKET-----CGLSKEAKIQTMETAKLTYLILICKSILYGIIVSVLACKAKTSYNKRFV  ray
94 RSKN-VECRVDLYTNESVPT-----TSSSTLAVKAEM-----CGISKEAKIQSMATAKLTYLILICKSIFYTIFISTIAWKTKTSYSKRFD  shark
91 TR-GKTFTCIVNFFNGTG-IN--------YKDSITGPKLTIDEDNYET--YVRSVKTTMLRYGMFVAKSIAYGIFIMYIVRR-QGFMSK  catfish
94 HKPENRFTCIVSFYDGTDNIR--------VNDTISGDLQGQSGGEITTDYYVKSTQTAKLAYSIFIAKSTFYGLVVMVMIWKFQGSSEKQI  trout
91 MNPHNTFRCSVYF-------------DPENITVSRETKGREGCGVTEDSFRSSAKIGRFAYLLLVSKSAAYGLFVT--ISMCRV-K---L  axolotl
88 YNPDNTFECSAGL----------RGRTDVKTESIR----GEKSCGVSPDELKRIVNNGVYSYILILCKTALYGLIVTAIVLRKKAIANAY  xenopus
90 FNPLNRFECIANFF------------KNGTQQSIQKIIYGDTGCITFKENYQRSATAGKFVYIMLIFKSILYGIFVMGMMLWY----KKMY  chicken
90 HNPRNHFRCQVQFHGLSEEDKWPEGSPKPVTQNISAEAWGRADCGITSASYHQGVLSATIYEILLGKATLYAVLVSGLVLMAMV-KKKNS  mouse
95 QNPRNHFRCQVQFYGLSENDEWTQDRAKPVTQIVSAEAWGRADCGFTSVSYQQGVLSATILYEILLGKATLYAVLVSALVLMAMV-KRKDF  human

   solvent exposed insertion        hinge           transmembrane    cytoplasmic
```

FIG. 4. Alignment of TCR α- and β-chain constant domains. Note the absence of the "solvent-exposed region" in all nonmammalian vertebrates and the low degree of identity among the sequences.

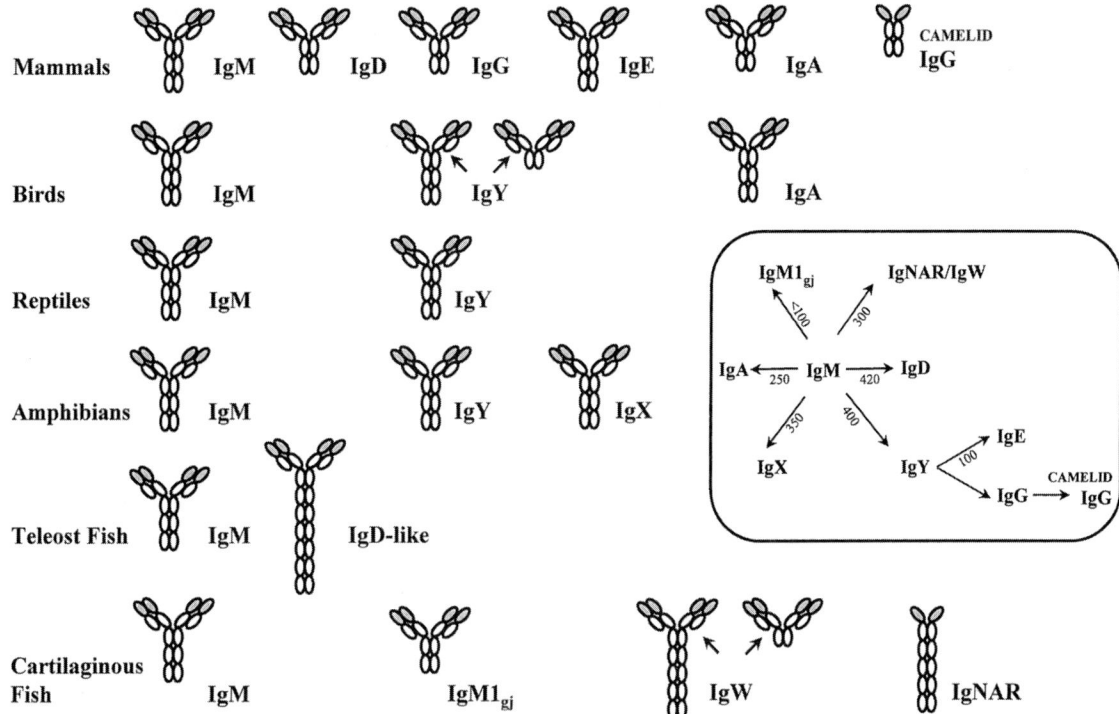

FIG. 5. Immunoglobulin heavy-chain isotypes in the jawed vertebrates. Note that based on amino acid sequences there are no detectable hinge regions in the majority of nonmammalian vertebrate isotypes (18), despite the "Y" shape shown in the figures. Note also that IgM is predominantly multimeric in all vertebrate groups except cartilaginious fish, in which it is found in multimeric and monomeric forms.

date, TCR are membrane bound and never secreted, while almost all Ig proteins have transmembrane and secreted forms.

α/β Constant Domains

Genes encoding the two types of TCR, α/β (which accounts for all known MHC-restricted regulatory and effector functions) and γ/δ (which recognizes antigens in an Ig-like manner and may play immunoregulatory roles during certain infections), existed in the earliest jawed vertebrates (R4,R5). cDNA sequences from species in the oldest vertebrate class (cartilaginous fish) revealed genes homologous to all four mammalian TCR chains (6). Although many Igsf members exist in the invertebrates (Fig. 1), thus far no Ig/TCR sequences (i.e., Igsf genes generated by somatic rearrangements) have been isolated from jawless vertebrates or invertebrates, a theme that will be repeated throughout the chapter. While TCR genes have been cloned from representatives of most vertebrate classes, few biochemical data are available, except in birds where α/β and γ/δ TCR have been identified with monoclonal antibodies (mAbs). In amphibians, the *Xenopus* α/β TCR was co-immunoprecipitated with cross-reactive antibodies raised against human CD3 chains (see below). A comparison of all TCR α- and β-chain C regions is presented in Fig. 4. α chains from diverse vertebrates are poorly conserved and the structure of the Cα Igsf domain itself is problematic: Only strands A, B, C, E, and F can be identified, although strands E and F are shorter than those of

mammals and strand D is absent (7). The lack of conservation in this extracellular domain as well as deletions found in bird and teleost fish TCR (especially in the connecting peptide) suggest that the co-receptor may be structurally distinct from mammalian CD3 complex components. Even within a class the sequence divergence is great: Catfish Cα has only 44% and 29% amino acid identity to trout and pufferfish Cα, respectively. Pre-Tα, which associates with TCR β chains during thymocyte development, has been identified only in mammals (R7). Interestingly, the pre–Tα gene is near to MHC in mouse/human, and phylogenetic studies should be performed to determine whether this linkage group is ancient (see below).

The transmembrane (TM) region and cytoplasmic tail of Cα are the most conserved parts of the molecules. Cα and Cβ TM segments in all species have the so-called CART motif, in which conserved amino acids form an interacting surface with the CD3 complex (R8). Besides CART, the opposite TM face with residues Ile-Lys-Leu may be conserved for interactions with other CD3 components. The cytoplasmic region is remarkably conserved among teleosts, birds, and mammals. TCR β genes have been sequenced in four species of cartilaginous and bony fish and two species of amphibians (axolotl and *Xenopus*). In addition to the typical Igsf domain features, there are several conserved regions among vertebrate TCRβ chains, especially at positions 81 to 86, which might be involved in TCR dimerization. There are also remarkable differences: The solvent-exposed segment

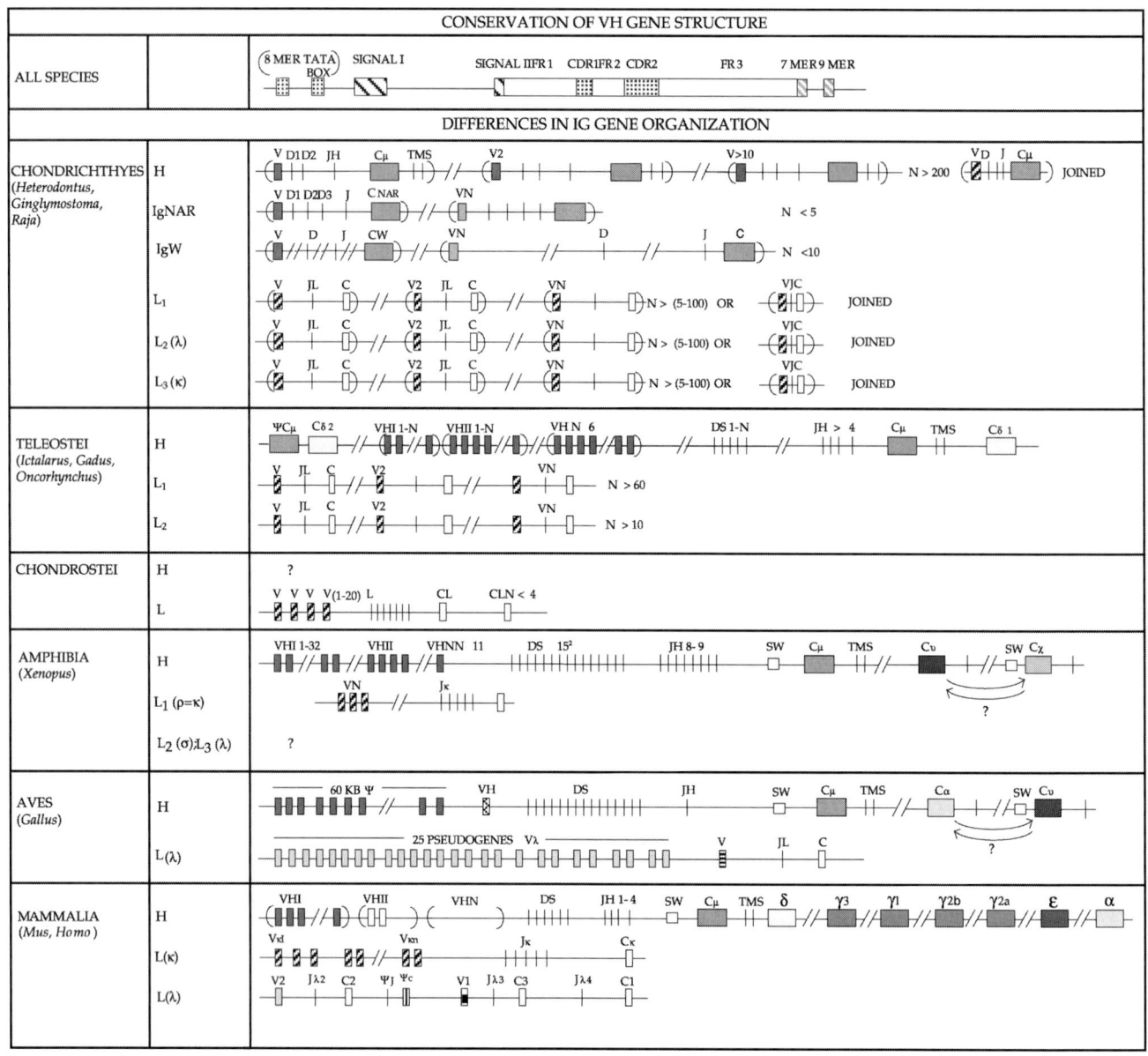

FIG. 6. Immunoglobulin gene organization in the various vertebrates. FR, framework; 7mer and 9mer, heptamer and nonamer; TM, transmembrane segment.

98 to 120 in mammals is absent in all nonmammalian vertebrates. This loop has recently been shown in mouse TCR to be important in negative selection events in the thymus (R9); perhaps the absence of this region in nonmammalian vertebrates results in subtle differences in tolerance induction as compared to mouse/human. The number of $C\beta$ genes varies in different species: Horned shark has more TCR $C\beta$ genes than the skate, but its genome size is largest of any elasmobranch thus far studied. Unlike all other vertebrates, the axolotl has four $C\beta$ genes as well as four $DJC\beta$ clusters that rearrange to the same collection of $V\beta$. Only one $C\beta$ gene has been detected in chicken and in *Xenopus laevis*, even though it is a pseudotetraploid species (see below).

Like $C\alpha$, $C\beta$ sequences are not well conserved in evolution; for example, the *X. laevis* $C\beta$ gene does not crosshybridize with *X. tropicalis* genomic DNA, and catfish $C\beta$ has only 41% to 42% identity with other teleost $C\beta$ and 26% identity with horned shark $C\beta$. Two different catfish $C\beta$ cDNA sequences were identified, suggesting the existence of either two loci or allotypes, as is found in mammals. Indeed, very recently Kamper and McKinney (10) showed that the damselfish $C\beta$ is encoded by two polymorphic genes, and this feature seems to extend to other teleosts. As the polymorphic sites are believed to interact with the associated CD3-signaling molecules, the authors suggested that signals might be transduced to T cells in different ways depending on the particular expressed $C\beta$ allele.

α/β Variable Domains

Because T-cell recognition is MHC restricted, TCR V regions may have been evolutionary selected for different properties as compared to Ig; indeed, TCR V regions are much less similar to each other than are Ig V regions. Furthermore, TCR Vs, unlike IgV$_H$, have conserved CDR3 lengths, suggesting that there is a restricted size for recognition of MHC-peptide complexes (11). Four Vα families were identified among only six skate cDNA clones, and six Vα families were identified in trout and three in channel catfish. In the axolotl, five Vα and at least 14 Jα segments were identified and 32 different trout Jα have been sequenced. Thus, α loci in all vertebrates examined have many J segments, and consistent with the mammalian paradigm, the absence of D and the large numbers of J segments favors the potential for receptor editing during thymic positive selection (R4). A large number of Vβ gene families are another evolutionarily conserved feature. At least seven TCR Vβ families were isolated from horned sharks; four to six in skate; at least four in trout (one with limited amino acid–sequence similarity to the human Vβ 20 family), and 19 in *Xenopus*. In axolotls, Vβ are classified into nine categories each with 75% or more nucleotide identity; since only 35 genes were cloned there are probably more families, and several are related to mammalian Vβ genes (human Vβ13 and Vβ20). N regions were present in ~40% and 73% of V-D-J junctions in 2.5-month-old larvae and 10- to 25-month-old animals, respectively. In axolotl, ~30% of the β chains cDNAs were defectively rearranged. Many of the axolotl TCRβ CDR3 are the same in animals of different origins (see discussion below).

Little is known about the architecture of the TCR loci besides what has been inferred above (R4,R5). Recent identification of the *Fugu* α/δ locus suggests an organization similar to mouse/human, but with more rearrangement by inversion (12). (Interestingly, it is similar to the Ig L-chain loci in teleosts, as discussed below.) Based on Southern blot analyses, each catfish locus appears to be arranged in a translocon (as opposed to multicluster) organization with multiple V elements and a single or few copies of C-region DNA. Pulsed-field gel analysis suggested that the horned shark α and δ TCR loci are closely linked (6). The D segment GGGACAGGGG (Dβ of mammals and chicken) is encountered in all vertebrate classes, alone or in conjunction with other Dβ. These segments usually encode glycines, suggesting a selection for flexibility in TCR CDR3 (11). There are 10 trout Jβ and at least 11 in *Xenopus*.

γ/δ TCR

cDNA sequences from the skate have significant identity with prototypic mammalian γ and δ TCR genes with extensive V-region diversity, putative D segments in δ, and varying degrees of junctional diversity. In amphibians, axolotl Cδ TM regions shows most conservation to mammalian TCRβ. Some of the six Vα can associate with Cδ and no specific Vδ has been detected, strongly suggesting that like mammals, the axolotl δ locus lies within the α locus (13). Two Jδ were found, but interestingly no D to date. Vδ diversity was diminished in thymectomized animals and TCR δ chains are expressed by cells in lymphoid organs, skin, and intestine. Chicken γ/δ

T cells were identified long ago (R4,14). Expression is found in thymus, spleen, and a γ/δ T-cell line, but not in B cells or α/β T-cell lines. Three V subfamilies, three J gene segments, and one C gene were identified at the TCR γ locus. All Vγ subfamilies participate in rearrangement during the first wave of thymocyte development, and the γ repertoire diversifies from embryonic day 10 onwards with random V-J recombination, nuclease activity, and P- and N-nucleotide addition. Chicken TCRδ genes were deleted on both alleles in some α/β T-cell lines, suggesting that, like in mammals the δ locus is located between Vα and Cα. Vα and Vδ gene segments rearrange to one, both, or neither of the two Dδ segments and either of the two Jδ segments.

Mouse and human γ/δ TCR repertoires are much less diverse than that of α/β. In ruminants and chickens (so-called "GALT species"—see below) the two repertoires are quite diverse and there seems to be ligand-mediated selection of γ/δ cells during ontogeny. In sheep, where γ/δ TCR diversity is thymus dependent and follows a developmentally regulated progression, no invariant γ/δ TCRs are found. The degree of γ/δ expression is correlated with the evolution of the TCR V families in warm-blooded vertebrates. Indeed, mammals/chickens can be classified into "γ/δ low" (humans and mice, in which γ/δ T cells constitute limited portion of the T-cell population) and "γ/δ high" (chicken, sheep, cattle, and rabbits, in which such γ/δ cells comprise up to 60% of T cells). TCR V genes form subgroups in phylogenetic analyses, and humans and mice have representative loci in most subgroups whereas the other species appear to have lost some (15). Thus, γ/δ-low species have a high degree of TCR-V gene diversity, while γ/δ-high species have limited diversity. Interestingly, this pattern is similar to that found for IgV$_H$ genes (see below).

CD3 Complex

CD3 chains (γ, δ, ϵ), which associate noncovalently with both types of TCR, are each composed of single extracellular C2-set Igsf domains and they transduce signals via ITAM motifs in their cytoplasmic tails (R7,R8,R9). CD3 genes or proteins have been isolated from birds, amphibians, and teleost fish. In *Xenopus,* one CD3 gene is encoded by five exons, a structure resembling the mammalian CD3 δ gene rather than the seven-exon CD3 γ gene. As there was no evidence for a γ-like related gene, the one clone probably represents an ancestral form of mammalian CD3 δ and γ genes. Similarly, a chicken cDNA clone encoding a CD3 chain was difficult to assign to δ or γ, and phylogenetic analysis suggests that this gene is also derived from an ancestral form. Motifs in the CD3 ϵ cytoplasmic domain important for signal transduction in mammals are highly conserved in chickens and flounder, and all CD3 chains analyzed to date have conserved features (R8,16).

As an example of this conservation, immunohistology of *Xenopus* tissues with an antiserum raised to the cytoplasmic part of the human CD3-chain stained T cells and perhaps NK cells, confirmed by double-staining with a

CD8-specific mAb. The antiserum immunoprecipitated a putative *Xenopus* TCR/CD3 complex since an associated 75-kDa α/β heterodimer was reduced into two chains of predicted size. Two CD3-like proteins that comigrated at approximately 19 kDa were noncovalently associated with the TCR heterodimer; removal of N-linked glycans yielded CD3 proteins of 19 kDa and 16.5 kDa, probably the *Xenopus* CD3ϵ and CD3γ/δ proteins, respectively. These properties of the *Xenopus* TCR/CD3 complex support a stepwise evolutionary model of the CD3 protein family (17).

Immunoglobulins

A typical Ig molecule is composed of four polypeptide chains (two heavy [H] and two light [L]) joined into a macromolecular complex via several disulfide bonds. Each chain is composed of a linear combination of Igsf domains, much like the TCR (Fig. 5) (see Chapter 3), and almost all molecules studied to date can be expressed in secreted or transmembrane forms.

Ig Heavy-Chain Isotypes

No Ig-like molecule has been isolated from hagfish or lampreys, despite the capacity of these animals to make humoral "responses" to antigens (see below). Like all other building blocks of the adaptive immune system, Ig is present in all jawed vertebrates (Figs. 1 and 5). Sequences of IgH-chain C-region genes, however, are not well conserved in evolution and insertions and deletions in loop segments occur more often in C than in V domains. As a consequence, relationships among non-μ isotypes (and even μ isotypes among divergent taxa) are difficult to establish (R18). Despite these obstacles, recent work has allowed us to infer a working evolutionary tree among all of the isotypes (Fig. 5). Cartilaginous fish have evolved "dead-end" isotypes that seem specific only to this vertebrate class, while evolutionary relationships can be detected for most of the unique isotypes in nonmammalian vertebrates and mouse/human.

IgM

The secretory μ H chain is found in all vertebrates and consists of one V and four C1 domains, and is heavily glycosylated. H chains associate with each other and with L chains through disulfide bridges in most species, and IgM subunits form pentamers or hexamers in all vertebrate classes except teleost fish where tetramers are clearly found (R19). The μ C_H4 domain is most evolutionarily conserved, especially in its C-terminal region. There are several μ-specific residues in each of the four C_H domains among vertebrates (see Chapter 3) suggesting a continuous line of evolution, which is supported by phylogenetic analyses (R18). Like TCR TM regions described above, μ TM regions are also well conserved among sharks, mammals, and amphibians, but the process

by which the Ig TM mRNA is assembled varies in different species. In all vertebrate classes except teleosts, the μ TM region is encoded by separate exons that are spliced to a site on μ mRNA located $\sim$30 bp from the end of the C_H4-encoding exon. In contrast, splicing of teleost fish μ mRNA takes place at the end of C_H3 exon (R20). In holostean fish (gar and sturgeon), cryptic splice donor sites are found in the C_H4 sequence that could lead to conventional splicing, but in the bowfin there is another cryptic splice donor site in C_H3. Some modifications apparently related to the particular environment were noticed in the Antarctic fish *Trematomus bernacchii*. There are two remarkable insertions, one at the V_H–C_H1 boundary and another at the C_H2–C_H3 boundary; the latter insertion results in a very long CH2–CH3 hinge region. These unusual features (also unique glycosylation sites) may permit flexibility of this IgM at very low temperatures (21).

IgM_{1gj}

Nurse shark *Ginglymostoma cirratum* expresses an IgM subclass in neonates (22) (Fig. 5). The V_H gene underwent V-D-J rearrangement in germ cells ("germline-joined" or "gj"; see below). Expression of H_{1gj} is detected in primary and secondary lymphoid tissues early in life, but in adults only in the primary lymphoid tissue, the epigonal organ (see below). H_{1gj} associates covalently with L chains and is most similar in sequence to IgM H chains, but like mammalian IgG, it has three rather than the typical four IgM constant domains (Fig. 5); deletion of the ancestral IgM second domain thus defines both IgG and IgM_{1gj}. Because sharks are in the oldest vertebrate class known to possess antibodies, unique or specialized antibodies expressed early in ontogeny in sharks and other vertebrates were likely present at the inception of the adaptive immune system. IgM_{1gj} may aid in removal of catabolic products as was proposed by Grabar (23) in theorizing on the original function of antibodies.

IgNAR

A dimer found in the serum of nurse sharks and so far restricted to cartilaginous fish, IgNAR (Ig new antigen receptor) is composed of two H chains, each containing a V domain generated by rearrangement and five constant C1 domains (Fig. 5). IgNAR was originally found in sera, but TM forms exist as cDNA and cell-surface staining is detected with specific mAbs (24,R25). The single V resembles a fraction of camel/llama (camelid) IgG that binds to antigen in a monovalent fashion with a single V region (26). In phylogenetic trees, NAR V domains cluster with TCR and L-chain V domains rather with that V_H. A molecule with similar characteristics has also been reported in ratfish, although it was independently derived from IgM like the camelid molecule emerged from *bona fide* IgG (26,27). IgNAR V-region genes accumulate a high frequency of somatic mutations (see below).

IgR/IgNARC/IgW/IgX

Originally discovered as a second Ig class in the skate *Raja kenojei* named IgR, this non-μ isotype was later cloned from another skate species and designated IgX (R18,R25). (Do not confuse with *Xenopus* IgX; see discussion below.) The IgX H-chain C region consists of two Ig domains and an unusual cysteine-rich C-terminal segment (Fig. 5). Later, cDNAs encoding long forms of IgX were detected in sandbar shark (called IgW) and nurse sharks (called IgNARC because of the C-domain similarities to IgNAR). These long forms are composed of an amino-terminal V domain followed by six C1-type constant domains and a C-terminal tail typical of secreted IgM and IgA. The two amino-terminal C domains are orthologous to skate IgX and the last four domains are homologous to IgNAR (28). The long form was subsequently found in skates and the short form in sharks, suggesting that all elasmobranchs have both forms of IgW, presumably generated via alternative splicing (Fig. 5). H chains predicted from cDNA sequences are likely to associate with L chains, a characteristic that was verified biochemically. In skate, the V and C segments are in a cluster-type organization like IgM, and Southern blotting also suggests a cluster organization for shark IgW (Fig. 6). Like the teleost TM form of IgM, IgW TM segments are alternatively spliced onto the CH4-domain mRNA, thus encoding an H chain of the same size as the typical vertebrate IgM TM form.

IgD Homologues

Previously found only in primates and rodents, IgD was thought to be a recently evolved Ig. However, a novel Ig first discovered in channel catfish and later in other teleosts (salmonids and gadids) is homologous, in part, to δ H chains (R18,29) (Fig. 5). Like mammalian δ genes, the teleost gene is immediately downstream of the μ gene. The TM form of the mature protein is "chimeric," containing a V domain, C_H1 of μ, and seven C domains encoded by the δ homolog. In catfish, two different genes encode the secretory and TM forms of the molecule, a phenomenon unique to vertebrate Ig genes (note that a complete cDNA of secretory IgD has not been identified yet). The IgD TM form is co-expressed with μ in some but not all B cells. Larger but apparently less flexible than mouse/human IgD (no hinge region in fish IgD), fish and mammalian IgD may not be analogous. Phylogenetic trees indicate a relationship between teleost and mammalian IgD primarily because of the similarity between fish $\delta5$ and human $\delta2$ domains (the corresponding domain in mouse IgD was deleted). The teleost $\delta1$ and $\delta6$ sequences are most similar to domains of other non-IgM isotypes, including those of cartilaginous fish. Specific differences in cod IgD such as deletion of some δ domains, a tandem duplication, and translocations of part of the locus, developed after divergence of the catfish and salmon lineages (R18).

Other Isotypes Related to IgG, IgE, IgA, and the Switch

Other isotypes consist of four C domains in nonmammalian vertebrates, including *Xenopus* IgY and IgX, non-μ isotypes of *Rana*, IgY of axolotl, and IgA and IgY of birds (Fig. 5) (R18). In *Xenopus*, IgY is thymus dependent; IgM and IgX are not, although thymectomy impacts specific IgM antibody production (i.e., antigen-specific IgM can be produced but there is neither an increase in affinity after immunization nor elicitation of plaque-forming cells). IgM and IgX plasma cells are abundant in the gut, while IgY is expressed primarily in spleen (30). Axolotl IgM is present in the serum early during development, and represents the bulk of specific antibody synthesis after antigenic challenge. In contrast to *Xenopus* IgY, the axolotl ortholog appears late in development and is relatively insensitive to immunization. From 1 to 7 months post-hatching, axolotl IgY is present in the gut epithelium associated with a secretory component. IgY progressively disappears from the gut and is undetectable in the serum of 9-month-old animals. Thus, axolotl IgY, like *Xenopus* IgX, may be analogous to mammalian IgA (31). *Xenopus* IgX and IgY are not homologous to any mammalian non-μ Ig isotype and are most similar to IgM. The TM and cytoplasmic domains of *Xenopus* TM IgY, however, share residues with avian IgY and mammalian IgG and IgE, suggesting that mammalian/avian isotypes share a common ancestry with amphibian IgY (32). This similarity is especially interesting since a recent mouse study suggested that the IgG cytoplasmic tail is the central molecular element promoting rapid memory responses (33).

Although cartilaginous and teleost fish have multiple Ig isotypes, the class switch appears first in evolution in amphibians (R18,34). The *Xenopus* switch μ (Sμ) region (5 kb) (Fig. 6) contains 23 repeats approximately 150 bp long, consisting of shorter internal repeats and palindromes, such as AGCT (like in mammals). In IgX-expressing cells, the μ gene has been deleted and Sμ and Sχ are joined. Both S boxes are AT-rich (not G-rich as in mammals), but Sχ is not homologous to Sμ and contains TGCA palindromes. Recombination usually occurs at microsites where single-stranded DNA folding programs predict a transition from a stem to a loop structure. This structural feature, also conserved in mammalian switch junctions, implicates such microsites for targeting of the recombination breakpoint. Thus, the capacity of S regions to recombine is regulated by DNA secondary structure rather than base composition, with the repetitive occurrence of palindromes being most essential; this hypothesis was confirmed recently in elegant transfection experiments in mammals (35).

A single gene can encode different Ig forms, such as for duck IgY, cartilaginous fish IgW, and camel IgG loci (Fig. 5). It has been suggested that the avian IgY short and long forms could be the functional equivalents of both IgE and IgG, respectively (36); the same may be true of the cartilaginous fish IgW short and long forms with two and six C domains, respectively (Fig. 5).

V_H Regions

A rearranged V_H gene consists of a leader (encoded by a split exon) followed by four framework regions and three CDRs (Fig. 6). Canonical V_H CDR1 nucleotide sequences are conserved in all jawed vertebrates, perhaps as targets for somatic hypermutation (37). A major germline difference is the lack of conserved octamers and TATA box in the 5' region of shark Vs (Fig. 6). In all species, functional V genes are assembled by rearrangement and joining of germline V, D, and J elements. Cartilaginous fish H chains are encoded by large numbers of clusters (>100 in horned shark) (4,38). For IgNAR there are only four V regions/haploid genome and only a few IgW V genes are detected in nurse sharks (but a large number in skates) (R25). In teleosts, seven V_H families have been characterized in the catfish, each containing up to seven to ten genes (most with open reading frames), and in the trout, 11 V_H families were identified. *Xenopus* has at least 11 V families, three of which (V_{H1-3}) contain 20 to 30 members and ~10% to 30% pseudogenes; the other families are smaller (1 to 8 genes), so the total number of functional V_H elements is ~90 to 100. Reptiles have very large pools of V_H segments: The turtle *Pseudemys scripta* has four families, with ~700 V_H/haploid genome (10% to 20% pseudogenes), and at least 125 genes homologous to the mouse V_H S107 gene were detected in another turtle species, *Chelydra serpentine* (39). Importantly, the V_H complexity does not seem to limit diversity of the antibody repertoire in any ectothermic vertebrate studied to date. There are actually fewer functional human V_H(44 functional, 79 pseudogenes that fall into seven families) than in many ectotherms. Dynamic reorganization of the H-chain V regions seems to have occurred at least eight times between 133 and 10 million years ago (R40). Perhaps species that utilize somatic mutation/selection "optimally" rely less on germline diversity and therefore fewer functional genes are required. Only ~10% of *Xenopus* V_H are pseudogenes in the three families (V_{H1-3}) that have been exhaustively studied; thus, *Xenopus* with fewer lymphocytes has a greater number of functional V_H genes than humans.

D Segments

D segments are always present in one of the two loci encoding an Ig/TCR heterodimer (IgH and TCR β,δ), and it is not known what pressure maintains this asymmetry (R5). Cartilaginous fish have one or two D genes/H-chain cluster and there are only minor variations among the clusters (Fig. 6). In teleosts, amphibians, and reptiles where the organization of the H-chain locus is similar to humans, the number of Ds deduced from cDNAs ranges from 10 to 16. Two germline D segments have been identified in *Xenopus,* and their recombination signal sequences (RSS) follow the rules defined in mammals. In birds, there are 15 very similar D_H.

There seem to be several reasons why D segments have been preserved throughout evolution. Incorporation of D segments augments CDR3 diversity and size, obviously directly influencing the combining site. Three different Ds contribute to IgNAR CDR3, and besides generating great diversity, CDR3 length and amino acid composition fulfill special tertiary structure requirements: D-encoded cysteine residues bond with cysteine(s) in the body of the V domain, thereby stabilizing a loop involved in the antigen binding of this unusual monomeric receptor (R25). A similar situation has been reached by convergence in the monomeric variant of camel IgG (R25,26). Anther potential function for Ds is in the rearrangement itself. As mentioned, in Ig or TCR heterodimers only one chain has D-encoded regions, and if D were maintained solely to promote diversity, it is likely that both chains of one receptor would have acquired Ds in some species. The receptor chain locus containing D segments rearranges first in two of the three antigen-receptor types (IgH and TCRβ), suggesting that a molecular constraint is linked to the rearrangement mechanism. In fact, after V-D-J rearrangement further rearrangement is difficult, since all Ds are deleted and remaining unrearranged V and J segments have incompatible RSS spacers. Thus, after rearrangement, IgH and TCRβ loci are "locked" in pre–B/pre–T cells, followed by a proliferative phase prior to rearrangement of the IgL or TCRα locus in immature lymphocyte progeny. In summary, D may have been selected to generate diversity in the various receptors by allowing N-region addition at the joins, and this may have been the driving force for D evolution if a monomeric receptor like NAR was primordial. If the original antigen receptor was a dimer, then the selective pressure for evolving a D was perhaps to "lock the locus," or to promote haplotype exclusion (R41).

J Segments

J segments encode the G strand (FR 4) of an Igsf domain, which contains a highly conserved diglycine bulge that is vital for the structure of the dimeric receptor (Figs. 3 and 7) (see below). In cartilaginous fish there is one J segment in each gene cluster and it thus promotes diversity only through junctional diversity achieved during rearrangement. In teleosts, for example, channel catfish, nine J_H segments are tightly clustered within 2.2 kb. Strong sequence homologies, as well as unified length of repeat sequences, indicate that segments J_H3 to J_H7 arose by unequal crossing over (42). Each J_H segment is potentially functional and CDR3 junctional diversity is prominent in cDNA clones. The characteristic structure and organization of J_H segments in higher vertebrates thus evolved early in vertebrate phylogeny. In *Xenopus,* depending on the species there are eight or nine J_H segments (one pseudogene). Some J_H spacers contain pseudo nonamers that allow direct joining to V segments. In the turtle *Pseudemys,* at least 16 J_H were found, each with unique RSS. Birds have only one J_H.

V_H Evolution

Diversity of the immune repertoire depends on the variety of V segments inherited in the germline and on the further diversification by rearrangement (CDR3 only) and somatic

A   B   C   C'   C"   D   E   F   G

```
           A                    B              C            C'             C"        D                      E                          F              G
LAMBDA   ----LTQ-PRSVSGSP- GQSDTISCTGTSSDVGGYN ---F-VSW- YQQHPGKAPKLM --IY- --DAT- KRPSGVPIRPSGSKSGNT --- ASLTISGLQAEDRADYYCCSYAGD --- YTPGVVPGGGTKLTVLV-
KAPPA    -EIVLTQSPSFLSAFV- GDRITITCR-ASQGISS ----Y-LAW- YQQKPGKAPKLL --IY- --DAS- TLQRGVPSRFSGRRSGTD- FTLTISSLQPEDVGTYYCQKYKS ---- VP-LTFGGGTKLEIKRAA
H HUM    -QTQLVQ-SGAEVRKP- GASVRVSCK-ASGYTFIDS ---V-IHW- IRQAPGEGLEWVGNINFNSGGT- NYAPRPQGRVMTRDASFS- TAYMDLRSLRSDDSAVFYCAKSDPF- WSSYTLDVWGQGTTVTVS-
HFTCRβ   --VLIQQTPASISHSP- GSPVRIECI-YIRATASS ----V-FNW- YRWHLDREPRNH- FYS-YPAGT- ITPSGEVTGFTARRPNNSH- FYLESSLQVNQSAVYCAWNQDR--- NAGEAYFGDGTKLVVLG-
NAR      --ARVDQTPQTITKEI- GESLTINCV-LRNSACALS --- T-TYW- YRKKSASTNEES--IS- ----KGG-- RVETVNSGSKS-FSLRNDLITVEDSGTYRCMVLRCA-- SWILDDVYGGGTVTVNP-
IgW      ---LNQ-TESVVKKL- GESHKITCH-ESEFGLSG ----YGIHW- VRQATGKGLEWLTAIL-TSGAK- YYAPAIQDRFEISKDSDT-- VYLKVTNLTVDDTAIYCARGYHSGHATPYYLDYWDGTFLEVTS-
A33      ---ISVETPQDVLRASQGKSVTLPCT-YHTSTSSREQ --L-IQW- DELLLTHTERVV-IWPFSNKNY- IHGELYKNRVSISNNAEQS-DASITDLQLTNADNGTYECSVSLMS--- DLEGNTKSRVRLLVL-
BUTY     APFDVIGPPEPILAVV- GEDAELPCR-LSPNASAEHL --E-LRW- FRKKVSPAVLVH-RDGRE-QEA- EQMPEYRGRATLVQDGLAKGRVALRIRGVRVSDDGEYTCF---- FREDGSYEEALV-
HS1C7    -ALWVSQPPEIRTLE- GSSAFLPCSFNASQGRLAIG ---S-VTW- FRDEVVPGKEVR--NG- ----T- PEFRGRLAPLASSRFLHDH- QAELHIRDVRGHDASIYCRVEVLG--- LGVGTGNGTRLV-
RAGE     --GAVVG-AQNITARI- GEPLVLKCK-GAPKKPPQ ----R-LEW- KLNTGRTEAWK-VLS- ----PQGGG-- PWDSVARVLPN--GSLFLPAVGIQDEGIFRCRANNRN--- GKETKSNYRVRVYQI-
BG       -QITVVAPSLRVTAIV- GQDVVLRCH-LSPCKDVRNS --D-IRW- IQQRSRLVHHY-RNG- ---VDL- GQMEEVKGRTELLRDGLSDGNLDRITAVTSSDSGSYSCAVQ---- ESSQQGKILLTVL-
CTX      --VQVTIQNPIINVTSGQNATLYCT-YILNNQNKNN --Y-ILNNQNKNN-IFQAKSQNQETV- PPYQN-GQS- LSGPSYKNRVTAANSPGN-- ATITSNNQSQDTGIYTCEVLNLP-- ESSQGKILLTV-
ZFCTX1   -VLLKSTNSKPWVNEF- ESIELSCM-IESITTTKP --R-IEW- KKIKNGDPSYVY- FD-- ---NI- VLDGIIQPNFNNGRFSIVN-PSSLQISESIKTDTGSYTCLVTLPN-- DQKSFDEILISLTV-
CTXCION1 ---NGAASPLPIEVTL- GNPITLACS-YQPENGNAQD --ARLEW- LYSTNMDGTSTS--GQ- ---NI- VLDGIIQPNFNNGRFSIVN-PSSLQISESIKTDTGSYTCLVTLPN-- DTPSKGSGTYNLTVNV-
AMA      --VISQISKDVVASV- GDSVEPNCT-VEEVGQLS ----VSWAKRPSESDTNSVV-LSMRNILSL- PDKRYNVTVTEGPKTGSAI- YTFRIQNIEVSDMGPYECQVLVS--- ATEKVTKKLSLQ-
FREP4*2  -RLSFYANVEKFNEVI- QPLKLTCTFQISKNDSDNDSQVLFMS-IYHETKRVIASISKYQPVATSLYPSVTKVQGHIYHSNESKDS-YIQVTWTHPKLSESGKYFCLAHAWN--- STSQNSV-
PREP2    SWLNFTGNSETIRELI- QPLKLTCTFQISKNDSDNDSQVLFMS-IYHETKRVIASISKYQPVATSLYPSVTKVQGHIYHSNESKDS-YIQVTWTHPKLSESGKYFCLAHAWN--- STSQNSV-
GEODIA   LIVEVDSSGLVVREG- SEVIVLTCE-VYGYPRDSS --P-PNN- ---SPGRNLESG-RFN---- IT-PRYTGTLSNGSVSSSDKVA-LSQLTIFNITVADEGEYKCS--------- VDGESASFRVDL-
```

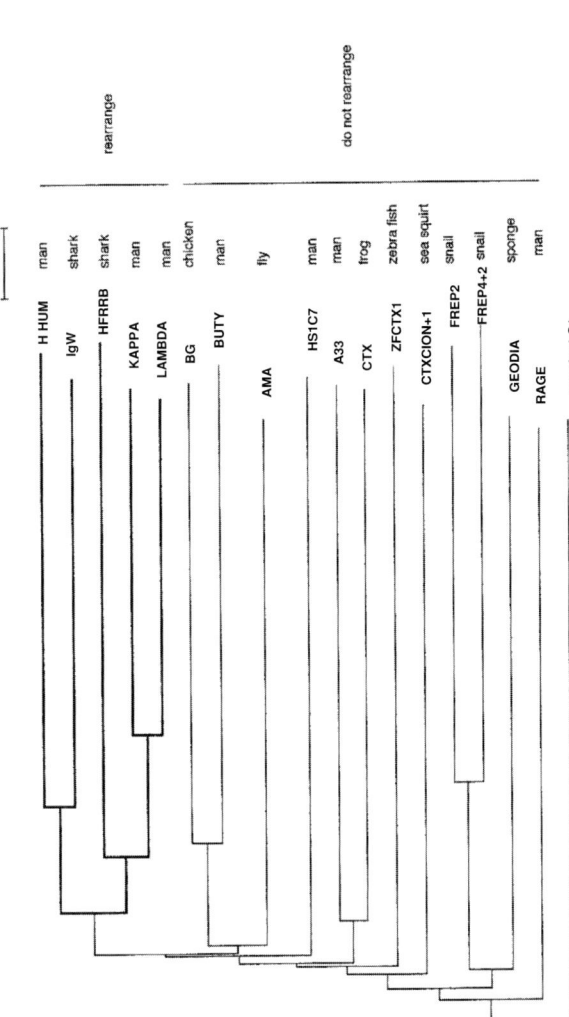

rearrange

do not rearrange

0.05

H HUM — man
IgW — shark
HFRRB — shark
KAPPA — man
LAMBDA — man
BG — chicken
BUTY — man
AMA — fly
HS1C7 — man
A33 — man
CTX — frog
ZFCTX1 — zebra fish
CTXCION+1 — sea squirt
FREP2 — snail
FREP4+2 — snail
GEODIA — sponge
RAGE — man
constant C1

FIG. 7. Evolution of variable domains. The shaded areas indicate regions of high conservation among members of all domains or of only one type (rearranging or nonrearranging). Modified from Du Pasquier (7), with permission. H hum: IgM human; hfrb: shark TCRβ; kappa: human LK; BG: chicken MHC-linked; Buty: butrophilin; Ama: amalgam; HS1C7: NKD30; A33: CTX member chr.1; CTX: cortical thymocyte *Xenopus*; ZFCTX: zebrafish CTX homologue; CTXciona: *Ciona* CTX homologue; FREP: fibrinogen-related protein biomphalaria; *Geodia*: V/I set domain with tyrosine kinase; RAGE: receptor for advanced glycosylation end product.

hypermutation (all CDR). Early in life the repertoire depends chiefly on the inheritable genes as one finds little N-region diversity and somatic mutation (for exceptions, see below). A central question is how antibody-germline V genes diversify CDR during evolution while they are subject to homogenizing forces operating in most multigene families. Perhaps environmental antigens have played a major role in shaping the germline repertoire, and have selected some V_H/V_L germline sequences used by neonates. V_H families arose prior to the mammalian radiation and have been conserved for hundreds of millions of years (R40). Conserved regions defining families are found on solvent-exposed faces of the V_H, at some distance from the antibody-combining site. Phylogenetic analyses show clustering of V_H into groups A, B, C, D, and E (Fig. 8). Almost all cartilaginous fish V_H belong to the monophyletic group E; bony-fish V_H genes cluster into all groups (one group [D] unique only to them). By contrast, group C includes bony fish sequences as well as V_H from all other classes except cartilaginous fish. Another phylogenetic analysis classifies mammalian V_H genes in three "clans" (I, II, and III) that have coexisted in the genome for more than 400 million years (43). Only in cartilaginous fish does it appear that V_H-gene families have been subjected to concerted evolution that homogenized member genes (except for the IgM_{1gj} V region described above) (22). It has been debated whether Ig V genes could be under direct positive selection or not because these genes hypermutate somatically. However, several features (e.g., codon bias) and discovery of high replacement/silent ratios in germline gene CDR codons indeed argue for positive selection during evolution.

In summary, much of the V_H germline repertoire has been conserved over extremely long periods of vertebrate

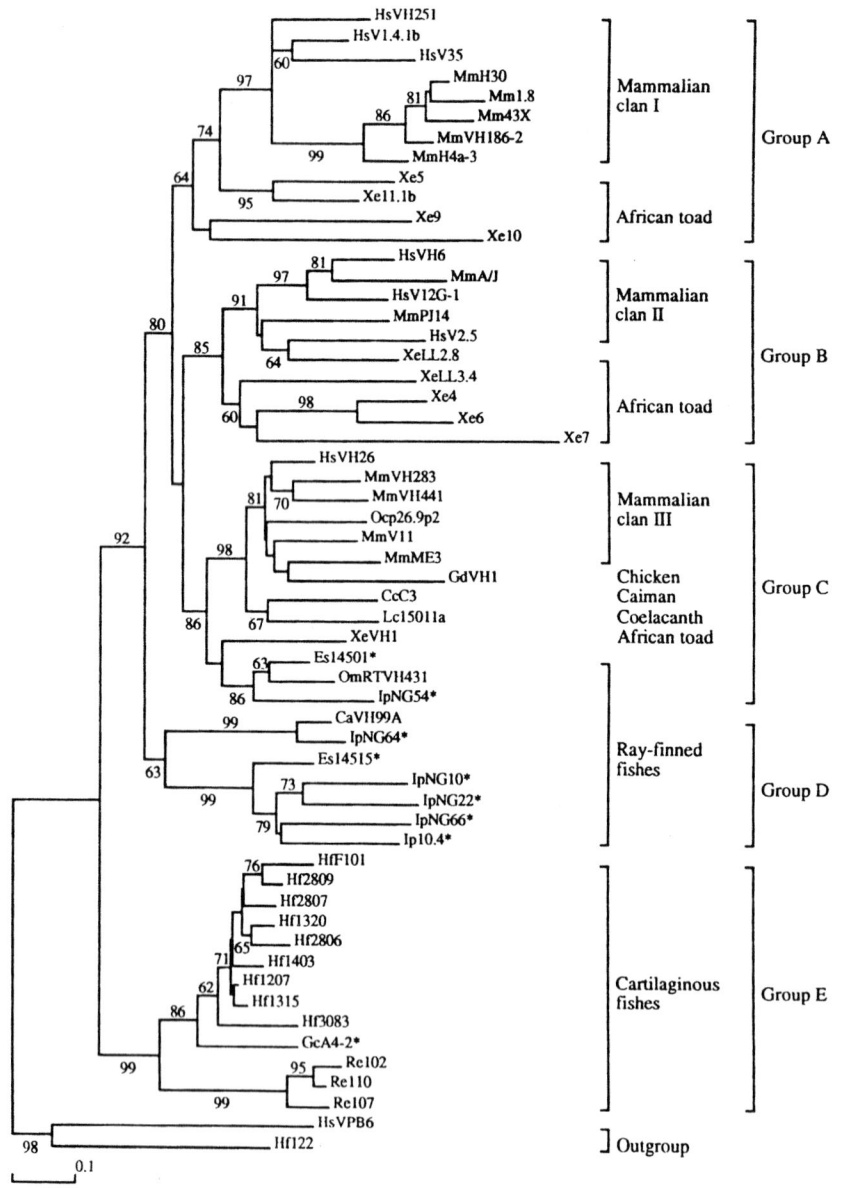

FIG. 8. Phylogenetic tree of 56 VH and two VL (outgroup) sequences. The number on each interior branch is the confidence probability. Modified from Ota et al. (40), with permission.

evolution. The birds and some mammalian species that rely on gut-associated lymphoid tissue (GALT) to generate Ig diversity, are exceptions with a reduced germline repertoire (at least expressed repertoire), but as will be seen below, gene conversion and somatic hypermutation compensate for this situation in formation of the primary repertoire. Even in the cartilaginous fish where there is a single V_H family, there is nevertheless heterogeneity in CDR1 and CDR2 sequences that must boost diversity in the expressed repertoire (R44).

Ig Light Chains

L chains can be classified phylogenetically not only by their sequence similarity, but also by the orientation of their V and J RSS, which differ for mammalian λ and κ. There is much debate regarding the affiliations of L chains in various vertebrates, but as sequences have accumulated, a picture starts to emerge (Fig. 6). Contrary to what was believed, the κ and λ L chains emerged early in vertebrate evolution, probably in an ancestor of the cartilaginous fish (R18,R25).

Elasmobranchs have three L-chain isotypes (type I, II, and III), and the combined data suggest that they are present in all elasmobranchs (45). Type I seems to be the ancestral group and resembles the unusual *Xenopus* σ L chain (see below). Type II L chains are arguably more like λ of birds, *Xenopus,* and mammals, and have been cloned from sharks and skates. The type III is clearly κ-like, at least in the V region (and RSS orientation). As mentioned, the λ-κ dichotomy therefore arose at the origins of adaptive immunity, and intermediates explaining L-chain history are lacking. These relationships to L chains of higher vertebrates are noted for the cartilaginous fish V domains, as the C domains form their own elasmobranch supercluster; this suggests that there were (are) different selection pressures on the V and C domains that resulted in their independent evolution. Different elasmobranch species express the L-chain isotypes preferentially, for example, type III in nurse sharks, type I in horned sharks, and type II in sandbar sharks. This pattern of expression may be due to expansions/contractions of the different isotype genes in various elasmobranch lineages (R46). Multiple L-chain isotypes (molecular weight, 22 to 26 kDa) are also found in teleosts. In some species, mAbs were produced that distinguish L-chain classes, such as the F and G L chains of the catfish. CodL1, catfish F and G, trout type L1, and the sturgeon (chondrostean) L chains appear to be κ homologs, and a second trout isotype (L2) seems most related to the cartilaginous fish type I and *Xenopus* σ (R18,R46).

MAb studies suggested the existence of three *Xenopus* L-chain isotypes of 25, 27, and 29 kDa with heterogeneous 2D gel patterns and preferential association of some L-chain isotypes with IgY H chains. Indeed, three *Xenopus* L-chain genes have been isolated: ρ (κ-like), σ, and λ (R46). Only one C gene is present in the ρ locus, and it encodes the most abundant L chain. The V and J RSS are of the κ type and the five identified J segments are nearly identical. The locus is deleted, like mammalian κ, when the other isotype genes are rearranged. Southern hybridizations with genomic DNA from different animals showed V_L sequences to be both diverse and polymorphic. The third *X. laevis* L-chain isotype predicted from biochemical studies is related to mammalian λ genes and consists of six distinct V_L families. In the σ locus, the J segment has an unusual replacement of the diglycine bulge by two serines. The Rana major L-chain type has an unusual intrachain disulfide bridge that seemingly precludes covalent association of its H and L chains.

Two L-chain types were identified in reptiles. Chickens and turkeys only express one L chain (λ) with a single functional V and J gene (Fig. 6), and the manner by which diversity is generated is likely responsible for this unusual evolutionarily derived arrangement (see below). Nonproductive rearrangements are not detected on the unexpressed L-chain allele, and thus there is a strong pressure to generate functional joints (see below). Such a system probably rendered a second (or third) L-chain locus superfluous (R18). Within mammals (marsupial *Monodelphis domestica*), the Vλ repertoire is comprised of at least three diverse families related to distinct placental families, suggesting the divergence of these genes before the separation of metatherians and eutherians more than 100 million years ago (R47). Opossum λJC sequences are phylogenetically clustered, as if these gene duplications were recent and the complexity of the λ locus seems greater than that found at the H-chain locus.

Thus, all vertebrate groups except the birds have two or three L-chain isotypes, but we are still at a loss to understand the significance of possessing multiple isotypes since there is scant evidence that L chains have any effector functions (R46). It has been suggested that different isotypes may provide distinct CDR conformations in association with H chains, or there may be L-chain/H-chain preferences that provide some advantage that is not obvious (R18,45).

J Chain

The joining (J) chain is a small polypeptide, expressed by mucosal and glandular plasma cells, which regulates polymer formation of IgA and IgM. J-chain incorporation into dimeric IgA and pentameric IgM endows these antibodies with the ability to be transported across epithelial cell barriers (48). J chain facilitates creation of the binding site for poly Ig receptor (spIgR, secretory component (SC) in the Ig polymers), not only by regulating the polymeric structure but apparently also by interacting directly with the receptor. Therefore, both the J chain and the pIgR/SC are key proteins in secretory immunity. Mouse IgM is synthesized as hexamers in the absence of J chain and as pentamers in its presence. Since some *Xenopus* EM studies suggested the existence of Ig hexamers, it was of interest to examine J-chain conservation over evolutionary time. J-chain cDNAs have been reported in the amphibians *Rana* and *Xenopus* (49), and in chickens (55% to 71% sequence identity to mammalian J chains). The existence of *Xenopus* J chain suggests that, unlike mouse IgM, *Xenopus* IgM forms hexamers with J chain; alternatively the previous EM studies identified IgX as the hexameric isotype (the χ chain has a stop codon before the Cys of C_{H4} domain and thus cannot make a covalent attachment to J chain). The highest level of J-chain expression was detected in frog and bird intestine, correlating well with a role for J chain in mucosal immunity (although obviously not for IgX secretion). There was a claim for J chain's presence in many protostomic invertebrates since a homolog was cloned in earthworms (50), but no J-chain sequences have appeared in the invertebrate databases (e.g., *Caenorhabditis elegans, Drosophila*).

Gene Organization

Chondrichthyan Germline-Joined Genes

In all vertebrate species, functional Ig genes are assembled by rearranging DNA segments scattered on the chromosome. However, in cartilaginous fish some V genes are the products of V(D)J rearrangement in eggs/sperm (R51). Are germline-rearranged genes relics of archaic genes before the "RAG transposon" invasion (see below), or are they the result of rearrangements in germ cells? Type I L-chain genes are all germline joined in skates but split in horned sharks, and the piecemeal germline joins (e.g., V-D, V-D-D, V-D-D-J) found in many horned shark H-chain gene clusters strongly suggest that the germline joining is a derived feature (R5,38). Definitive proof came from a study of a germline-joined nurse shark type III L-chain gene, shown by phylogenetic analysis to have been joined within the last 10 million years (52). When there is a *mixture* of joined and conventional genes, the split genes are expressed in adults, while the joined genes are expressed at significant levels only early in ontogeny. When *all* of the genes in a particular family are joined (e.g., skate type I L-chain genes and type II L chains in all elasmobranchs), they continue to be expressed into adult life at high levels. In mammals what may appear like germline-rearranged V genes are in most cases processed pseudogenes (e.g., pseudo Vκ on chromosome 22 in human or in mouse). However, it is possible that the surrogate L-chain gene VpreB is the product of a germline-joining event in the line leading to mammals (52).

Organization of Rearranging Genes

As mentioned, shark IgH-chain genes are structured into perhaps hundreds of clusters, each consisting of V, D, J, and C elements; all evidence from studies in horned shark, nurse shark, skate, and sandbar shark (and holocephalan ratfish) suggests that V, D, and J genes rearrange only within one cluster (5,25,38). While there is extensive N-region diversity and sometimes usage of two D segments (three Ds in IgNAR), and there are V_H subfamilies having substantial CDR1/2 heterogeneity (R44), diversity of the primary repertoire is lower than in other vertebrates since there is no rearrangement between clusters. Little is known about control of Ig expression in cartilaginous fish, but the presence of a TCR-like promoter instead of conserved octamer in V_H gene promoters

is worth study. The special constitution of the shark H- and L-chain loci suggests an exclusion mechanism similar to that of mouse TCR γ loci, also in clusters. Recent evidence suggests that only one V_H transcript is expressed in each lymphocyte, consistent with isotypic exclusion, despite the many clusters. Bony fish (teleosts and chondrosteans like the sturgeon), frogs, reptiles, and mammals have very similar architectures of their H-chain locus—the so-called translocon configuration (R18) (Fig. 6). As described above, multiple families of V_H genes, each consisting of many apparently functional elements (1 to 30 per family), are separated from a smaller number of genomic D and J elements. The possibility of combinatorial rearrangement enables more diversification than is possible with the cartilaginous fish clusters for a given number of segments. In birds the organization is similar but all V genes except those most 3' to the D elements are pseudogenes (see below).

L-chain gene organization is more variable. In elasmobranchs, the organization is the same (i.e., in clusters) as the H-chain locus without the D segments. The prototypic horned shark, type I L chain has a cluster organization in which V, J, and C segments are closely linked. In bony fish, L-chain genes have the shark cluster-type organization, but in the majority of their clusters V and J gene segments rearrange by inversion (R18,53,54), in contrast to cartilaginous fish (Fig. 6). Interestingly, sturgeon L-chain genes are in the translocon configuration, arguing that the cluster organizations in bony and cartilaginous fish L-chain genes arose independently. In *Xenopus* there are multiple Vκ(ρ) presumably derived from one family, 5J, and a single C-gene segment. In cartilaginous fish and birds, there has been co-evolution of Ig gene architecture for H and L loci, but the teleosts have shown that this is not a rule.

Major Histocompatibility Complex

T cells distinguish self from non-self through the presentation of small peptides bound to MHC class I and class II molecules, that is, MHC restriction. The genetic restriction of T-cell–APC collaboration, processing of antigen by professional APCs, and T-cell education in the thymus described in mice hold true for most vertebrate classes (R55). No MHC-regulated T-cell responses have been documented in cartilaginous fish, but the identification of polymorphic class I and II and rearranging TCR genes (see above) strongly suggest that functional analyses will reveal MHC restriction of adaptive responses. Similarly, urodele amphibians are notorious for their poor immune responses (see below), and biochemical and recent molecular evidence suggests that class II polymorphism is low in the axolotl. In addition, like the cod, axolotls have very high numbers of expressed class I loci, which might play into their dismal adaptive immunity.

Class I/II Structure

The three-dimensional organizations of class I and class II are remarkably similar (R56) (alignment in Fig. 9), although

PBR

	S1	S2	S3	S4	H1	H2	H2
	-----	-----	-----	-----	-----	-----	-----

```
                                                              Y-7                                                  Y-59                          Y/R-84
HLA-A2a-1   --GSHSMRYFFTSVSRPGRGEPRFIAVGYVDDTQFVRFDSDAASGRMEPRAPWIEQEGPEYWDGETRKVKAHSQTHRVDLGTLRGYYNQSEA
DR1a-1      IKEEHVIIQAEFYLNPD----QSGEFMFDFDGDEIFHVDM------AKKETVWRLEEFGRFASFEAQGALANIAVDKANLEIMTKRSNYTPITN
                                                              F S-53    N-62    N-69 ===
```

PBR

	S1	S2	S3	S4	H1	H2	H3
	-----	-----	-----	-----	-----	-----	-----

```
              101#                                                    T KW-146,7        164#       Y-171
HLA-A2a-2   ----GSHTVQRMYGCDVGSDWRFLRGYHQYAYDGKDYIALKEDLRSWTAADMAAQITKHKWEAA-HVAEQLRAYLEGTCVEWLRRYLENGKETLQRT
DR1b-1      GDTRPRFLWQLKFECHFFNGTERVRLLERCIYNQEESVRFDSDVGEYRAVTELGRPDAEYWNSQKDLLEQRRAAVDTYCRHNYGVGESFTVQRR
              15# ===                                                W-61                          79# HN-81,2
```

C-1 Igsf

	S1(A)	S2(B)	S3(C)	S4(D)	S5(E)	S6(F)	S7(G)
	-----	-----	-----	-----	-----	-----	-----

```
            P         L C    FYP    W  NG                                      P              P   Y C V H        P
HLA-A2a-3   --DAPKTHM--THHAVSDHEATLRCWALSFYPAEITLTWQRDGEDQTQDTELVETRPAGDGTFQKWAAVVVPSGQEQRYTCHVQHEGLPKPLTLRW----
DR1a-2      --VPPEVTVLTNSPVELREPNVLICFIDKFTPPVVNVTWLRNGKPVTTGVSETVFLPREDHLFRKFHYLPFLPSTEDVYDCRVEHWGLDEPLTKHW----
DR1b-2      --VHPKVTVYPSKTQPLQHHNLLVCSVSGFYPGSIEVRWFRNGQEEKTGVVSTGLIHNGDWTFQTLVMLETVPRSGEVTCQVEHPSVSPLTVEW----
b2m         IQRTPKIQVYSRHPAENGKSNFLNCYVSGFHPSDIEVDLLKNGERIEK-VEHSDLSFSKDWSFYLLYYTEFTPTEKDEYACRVNHVTLSQPKIVKWDRDM
```

TM/CYT

```
            TRANSMEMBRANE        CYTOPLASMIC
HLA-A2      IVGIIAGLVLFGAVITGAVVAAV  MWRRKSSDRKGGSYSQAASSDSAQGSDVSLTACKV
DR1a        NVVCALGLTVGLVGIIIGTIFII   KGVRKSNAAERRGP
DR1b        MLSGVGGFVLGLLFLGAGLFI     YFRNQKGHSGIQPRGFLS
CON. PIECE  EPSSQPTIP
            EFDAPSPLPETTE
            RARSESASQSK
```

FIG. 9. Amino acid residues conserved in classical class I and class II molecules in all vertebrates. Displayed are sequences of HLA-A2 and DR1 for which crystal structures exist for the extracellular domains (210,211). Bold residues indicate that they are found in the majority of classical class I/II sequences from members of all vertebrate classes (or all but one class). Residues above the alignments for class I PBR a-1 and a-2 (Y-7, Y-59, Y/R-84, T-123, K-146, W-147, Y-171; note that Y-84 is invariant in mammals but is R in all other vertebrates) and below the alignments in class II PBR a-1 and b-1 (Fa-53, Sa-55, Na-62, Na-69, Wb-61, Hb-78, Nb-82) are invariant residues that bind to main-chain atoms of acquired peptides. For the Igsf C1 domains, residues above the alignment are conserved in all C1-set domains (212) and are found in at least four sequences. Double-underlined residues are conserved glycosylation sites. Strands (S) and helices (H) for the PBR and strands (S) for the Igsf domains are displayed (see Fig. 15). See Kaufman et al. (56).

recent evidence from crystal structures of class I/II suggests that minor differences in the α1 helix force TCR to dock either diagonally (class I) or orthogonally (class II or class I) onto the peptide-binding region (PBR) (R57). The two membrane-distal domains of both molecules form a PBR composed of two antiparallel α helices resting on a floor of eight β strands, and the two membrane-proximal domains are Igsf C1. Although sequence identity among class I and class II genes in vertebrates is low (like most other immune genes), the four extracellular domain organization and other conserved features are likely to be found in the ancestral class I/II gene (Fig. 9). An intrachain disulfide bridge exists within the class I

PBR α2 and class IIβ1 domains, but not the class I/II PBR α1 domains, and phylogenetic trees show that these respective domains are most similar (58,59). Bony fish class II α1 domains, like class II DMα molecules that are as old as the *bona fide* class II genes (see Fig. 12) do have a disulfide bridge. The exon/intron structure of class I and class II extracellular domains is also well conserved, but some teleosts have acquired an intron in the exon encoding the Igsf β2 domain. Other conserved features of class I genes (Fig. 9) include a glycosylation site on the loop between the α1 and α2 domains (shared with class II β chains), a Tyr and one to three Ser in the cytoplasmic regions that can be phosphorylated in

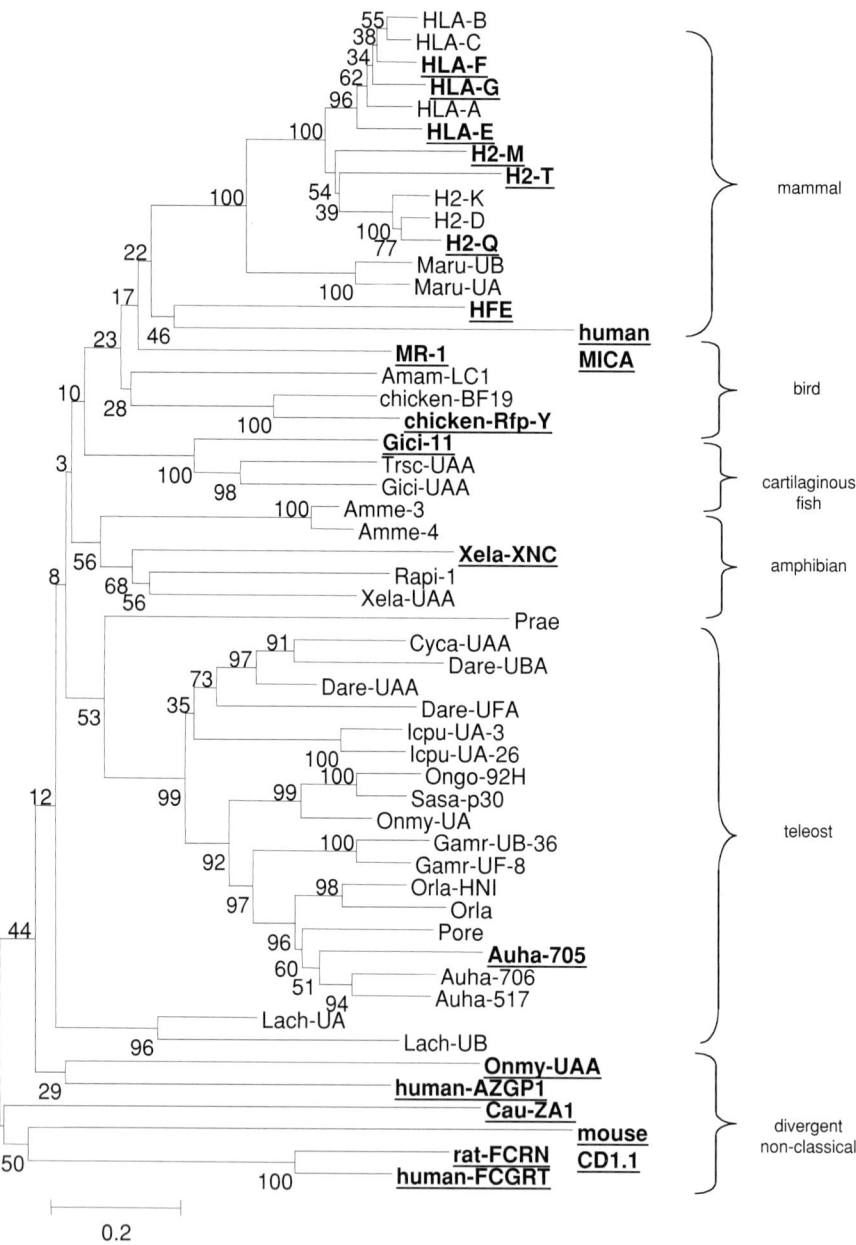

FIG. 10. Phylogenetic tree of classical and nonclassical class I molecules from all vertebrates. The nonclassical proteins are underlined and bolded. Note that there are two types of nonclassical class I: one type recently derived within a taxon, and another type that is ancient, emerging at about the same time class I split from class II.

mammals, as well as several stabilizing ionic bonds. Class II with its two TM regions differs from class I with only one; conserved residues in the class II α and β TM/cytoplasmic regions facilitate dimerization (Fig. 9). In summary, because sequence similarity is very low among MHC genes in different taxa, these conserved features are important for function and maintenance of structure.

β2m was the second Igsf molecule (C1 type) ever to be identified, originally found at high levels in the urine of patients with kidney disease. It associates with most class I molecules (see below). Besides mammals, β2m genes have been cloned from several teleost fish and two avian species. The β2m gene is outside the MHC and is a single-copy gene in all species except cod and trout, in which it has undergone multiple duplications, such as in Shum et al. (60).

Classical and Nonclassical Class I and Class II

Class Ia (classical) and class Ib (nonclassical) genes are found in all of the major groups of jawed vertebrates (R61). Class Ia genes are defined by their ubiquitous expression, their presence in the MHC proper, and by high polymorphism (56). In addition, class Ia proteins almost always have eight conserved residues at both ends of the PBR that interact with main-chain atoms of bound peptides and constrain their size to eight or nine residues (Fig. 9); this feature often distinguishes class Ia from class Ib (see below). Thus, tight binding of peptides, a likely source of conformational changes in class I allowing transport through the ER and cell-surface expression, is an evolutionarily conserved trait.

The class Ia/Ib distinction holds in most taxa: One to three polymorphic class Ia genes are expressed ubiquitously in most species while other minimally polymorphic or monomorphic class Ib genes can be expressed in a tissue-specific fashion. The class Ib genes can be split into two major groups: one set that is most related to the class Ia genes within a taxon (Fig. 10) and thus recently derived, and one group that is ancient and emerged near the origin of the adaptive immune system (R61). In the first set are class Ib genes found in chicken (Rfpy) and *Xenopus* (XNC) in gene clusters on the same chromosome as the MHC proper but far enough away to segregate independently from MHC (62,63). One *Xenopus* class Ib gene is expressed specifically in the lung and thus likely has a specialized function, and chicken Rfpy is associated with resistance to pathogens. Thus, class Ib genes that arise in each taxon seem to have true class I–like functions, but perhaps have become specialized (sometimes the distinction between class Ia and class Ib is blurry; see below). The second set of older class Ib genes that predates divergence of taxa can have very different functions (R61). For example, the neonatal Fc receptor (FCRN or FCGRT) is involved in binding and transport of IgG molecules across epithelia as well as protecting them from degradation, and zinc α2 glycoprotein (AZGP1) is believed to function in zinc transport. Furthermore, molecules have recently been discovered in mouse/human that are composed only of a PBR without Igsf domains; these unusual class I molecules do not bind

peptides but rather are important for regulation of NK- and T-cell function during infection. The paradigm for these SOS responses is the MIC class Ib molecule, which does have an Igsf domain but clearly does not bind peptides (R64). Some teleost class Ib genes that fall outside the major cluster of fish class I genes may fit into this category (R65). Finally, molecules like CD1 bind nonpeptidic antigens for presentation to innate-like NK T cells. The phylogenetic analysis predicts that CD1 and FcRN are old class I genes, which may be present today in all vertebrates; the age revealed by the phylogenetic tree also correlates well with the hypothesis that ancient duplication events predating the emergence of jawed vertebrates resulted in the appearance of CD1, FcRN, and MHC-linked class I genes (Fig. 11). Was the original function of class I linked to antigen presentation (peptidic or otherwise), induction of an SOS response, or to housekeeping functions? Currently we do not have the answer since class Ia and class Ib molecules are just as ancient. The discovery of class I–like genes in animals derived from ancestors predating adaptive immunity (if such genes exist) will help resolve this question.

Class II molecules also have nearly invariant residues that bind to main-chain atoms of peptides, but these are in the center of the groove (Fig. 9). Thus, tight binding to main-chain peptide atoms occurs in the center of the class II PBR, and peptides are free to protrude from both ends (R56). The only nonclassical class II molecules so far identified are the previously mentioned DM molecules that lack these residues. DM molecules so far have been cloned only from mammalian and avian species, but they are likely to be present in all species with canonical class II molecules (Fig. 12).

Polymorphism of MHC Genes

High levels of polymorphism and genetic diversity are characteristic of most classical MHC genes. MHC variation among taxa has been classically derived via mutation, gene conversion, and recombination. However, it is the retention of ancient allelic lineages through selection that accounts for the high levels of diversity observed within species (R66). The repertoire of antigens recognized by MHC alleles is determined by the amino acids in the PBR, such that different MHC alleles recognize different sets of peptide derivatives. Although even minor alterations of the anchor residues in the PBR can drastically change the peptide-binding capacity of an MHC molecule, in general, MHC alleles that differ by only a few amino acids can overlap considerably in their peptide-binding repertoires while highly divergent alleles bind unique sets of peptides (R67,R68). The differential binding capacities of MHC alleles form the basis of two models of balancing selection proposed to account for the extreme diversity observed at MHC. Overdominance, or heterozygote advantage, assumes that heterozygous individuals are capable of binding a wider array of pathogenic peptides than homozygous individuals; hence they should be selectively favored (69). Alternately, negative frequency-dependent selection is based on the premise that a co-evolutionary arms race between host

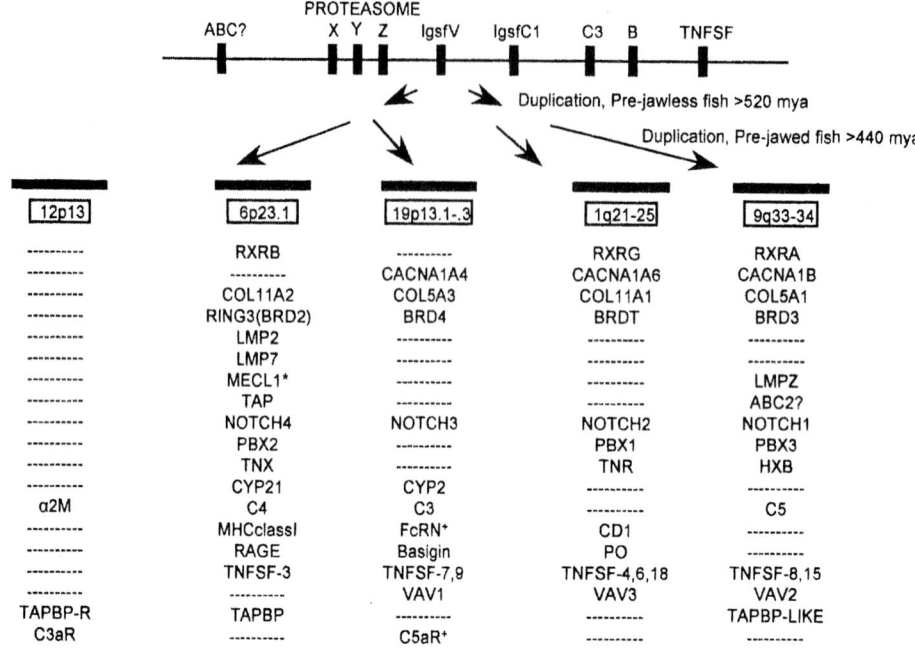

FIG. 11. Gene duplication model of MHC evolution. The MHC paralogous regions identified by Kasahara et al. (88) are displayed, with some of the genes found in the syntenic groups that are described in the text. For a more detailed view of these regions, see Flajnik and Kasahara (R55). Modified from Flajnik and Kasahara (R55), with permission.

MHC and pathogens exists, resulting in the development of escape mechanisms by pathogens to common MHC alleles and according an advantage to rare alleles. Although numerous individual studies exist providing support for one or the other of these selective mechanisms, from a population genetics standpoint, they give very similar theoretical results and are difficult to distinguish (70).

Studies of MHC gene population dynamics generally support the influence of balancing (diversifying) selection maintaining diversity of MHC genes, although deviations from theoretical expectations exist. At the molecular level, pathogen-driven selection should operate primarily on the codons of the PBR that determine the peptide-binding repertoire. For almost all classical MHC class I and II genes studied to date, excesses in nonsynonymous mutation of the PBR codons are observed (69,71). Within populations, both types of balancing selection should result in the evening of allele frequencies relative to neutral distributions, because rare alleles are increased in frequency by their presence in heterozygous individuals. Allele frequencies more even than expected under neutrality have been shown in a variety of species and populations. However, in many species the evening of allele frequencies does not lead to the maintenance of equal frequencies, indicating that not all heterozygotes have equal fitness and/or allele frequencies are influenced by additional selective forces or genetic drift (72). Balancing selection may also affect the distribution of genetic variability at MHC loci among populations (73). Theoretical models show that balancing selection should counteract the effects of genetic drift driving the differentiation among populations. Immigrant alleles will be selected for as a result of their exclusive oc-

currence in heterozygous individuals; hence, higher effective migration rates are expected for loci under balancing selection. This leads to a reduction, relative to neutral variation, in genetic divergence among proximate populations experiencing similar selective regimes. For the few studies with comparable population data for neutral loci and MHC loci, this expectation is not generally supported. Some studies show similar levels and patterns of differentiation among proximate populations, suggesting a greater role of drift relative to selection maintaining the observed variation at MHC. Many of the recent studies on teleosts fish show higher levels of interpopulation differentiation at MHC loci than at neutral microsatellite loci, and in some cases, different patterns of differentiation at MHC loci (71).

Two recent studies suggest that heterogeneity in the levels of balancing selection exists among MHC loci and among populations at a single MHC locus (71,74). In humans, intensities of selection for HLA-B are 2.5 to 4 times the levels observed for HLA-A, while levels of selection among populations vary by as much as half an order of magnitude (74). Moreover, the levels of selection among populations among loci are not consistent. Similarly, selection intensities at HLA-DRB1 are generally higher than those observed at HLA-DQA1, but variation among populations for both loci is relatively low. Variation in selection intensities at MHC loci also exists among salmonid populations (71). Examination of MHC class II–allele frequencies in sockeye salmon populations indicated that balancing selection had led to an overall evening of allele frequencies in some populations and an evening of frequencies of allelic lineages in an even greater number of populations. The study indicated

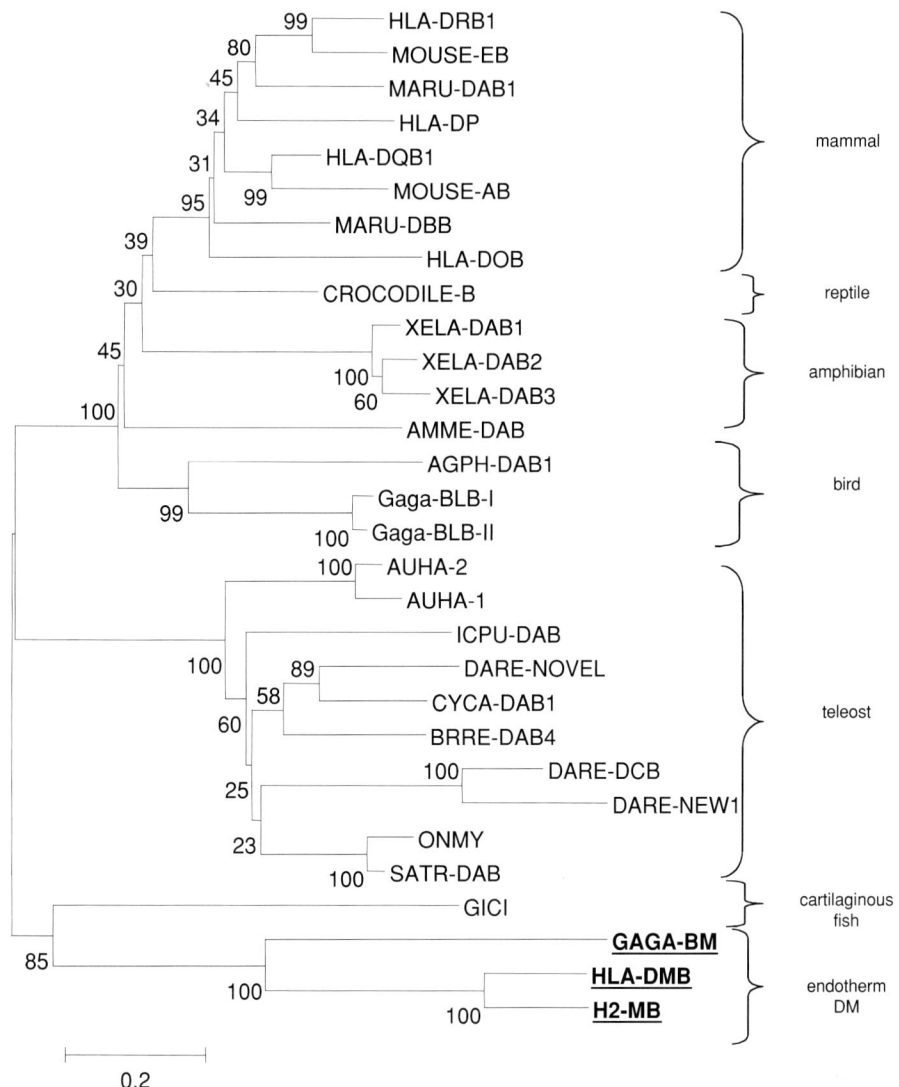

FIG. 12. Phylogenetic tree of class II beta (B) from various species and DM molecules of chickens, humans, and mice. Note that DM branches off near the root of the tree, suggesting that it arose early in the evolution of the adaptive immune system.

that in certain geographic regions divergent allele advantage, whereby heterozygotes containing highly differentiated alleles are selectively favored, led to balancing selection. However, some populations that possessed high levels of variation at neutral loci were depauperate of MHC variation, reflecting a lack of selection or directional selection at the MHC locus. Near fixation of different allelic lineages among MHC-depauperate populations that were connected by gene flow to each other and to populations rich in MHC allelic diversity was observed. This suggested that spatial and/or temporal variability in pathogen-driven directional selection as well as heterozygotes with unequal fitness levels can contribute to the maintenance and distribution of MHC variation.

Disease Associations

Due to the crucial role of MHC genes in immunity, it is often assumed that selection maintaining MHC diversity is pathogen-driven. Direct evidence of increased fitness of heterozygous individuals under pathogen challenge has been documented in only two studies. The first showed that maximum HLA heterozygosity of class I loci delays the onset of AIDS in patients infected with HIV, while the second documented a lowered response to hepatitis B vaccine in homozygous versus heterozygous individuals. Indirect evidence of pathogen-driven selection is also somewhat limited and is usually in the form of MHC haplotype associations with susceptibility or resistance to specific pathogens. Examples of disease associations documented in humans include malaria, HIV, tuberculosis, hepatitis B, leprosy, and Epstein-Barr virus; in mice, *Streptococcus pyogenes*, *Plasmodium chabauidi*, and *Trichuris muris;* and in chickens, Marek's disease, Rouse sarcoma virus, fowl cholera, *Staphylococcus aureas*, and *Eimeria tenella* (R75). Most associations are weakened by their limitation to specific populations or ethnic groups, suggesting the additional influence of background genes. The overall difficulty in documenting disease associations may be a consequence of very weak selective forces exerted by individual pathogens due to the overall redundancy both in the MHC (most mammalian species express multiple polymorphic MHC class I and class II genes) and in the numbers of peptide epitopes produced by pathogens for MHC recognition. The strongest associations of MHC haplotypes with infectious disease resistance tend to be with small viral pathogens with limited numbers of epitopes, and a greater strength and number of disease associations are found in chickens that contain a "minimal essential MHC" (single dominantly expressed class I and II genes) (R76). These observations suggest that MHC redundancies make it difficult for individual pathogens to escape recognition and confer a strong selective force on MHC diversity. In addition, most of the selection documented from single pathogens is directional, that is, certain haplotypes are associated with susceptibility or resistance, and therefore selection is not diversity generating. Under these circumstances, the generation of MHC diversity through pathogen-driven selection requires cumulative effects of selection exerted by multiple pathogens, each responsible for small haplotype-specific differences in survival and/or reproduction (R77).

Mating Preferences

Balancing selection on MHC genes may also be influenced by reproductive mechanisms, such as maternal–fetal compatibility and mate choice. Studies on humans have shown decreased survival of homozygous fetuses, lower fertility in couples sharing HLA-DR alleles, and a correlation in couples between unexplained recurrent abortions and the sharing of MHC antigens. In mice, survival of homozygous fetuses is negatively influenced by the viral infection status of the pregnant female. Also in mice, the "Bruce effect," whereby up to 90% of pregnant females block implantation when exposed to an unfamiliar male or his odor, is strongest when new males are from different MHC congenic strains from the parental male than when they are from the same strain. These findings suggest that in viviparous species, abortional selection can contribute to the maintenance of MHC diversity.

Substantial evidence of MHC-based disassortative mating exists in mice. Early studies on congenic mice that differed only in their MHC genes showed that males and females choose mates that are dissimilar to their familial MHC haplotypes, a finding that was later confirmed in studies on semi-wild mice and humans. The mechanism of MHC-based mate recognition lies in the lymphatic system, where MHC haplotype–specific odors are emitted. Mice for which the hematopoietic system is destroyed and replaced with cells of an MHC dissimilar congenic donor acquire the MHC distinctive odor of the donor. Direct evidence that MHC haplotypes contribute to odor came from a recent study by Montag et al. (78), where they measured, using a novel device termed the "e-nose," differences in odors of urine and serum between

mice differing only in their MHC genes. There are a number of hypotheses to explain how MHC genes affect odor, the most plausible of which may be one proposed by Penn and Potts (R79), which suggests that commensal microflora in microbe-harboring glands volatize metabolites of peptides carried by MHC molecules. Hence, individual odor is determined by unique sets of peptides recognized by the PBR of MHC alleles. In addition, MHC molecules may influence odor by controlling the commensal microbial flora within the glands, as originally proposed by Howard and supported by a recent study comparing the bacterial cellular fatty acid profiles of fecal microfloras in mice differing only in their MHC genes (80).

By selectively choosing mates with different MHCs, disassortative mating can generate diversity not only of MHC genes, but could potentially promote genome-wide diversity. Whether MHC-based mate recognition evolved to avoid inbreeding, in a manner similar to the plant histocompatibility genes or the tunicate S locus genes (see below), or to produce MHC heterozygous offspring that are more resistant to multiple pathogens, or both, is currently under much debate (74,R79). Certainly, the finding in both mice and humans that mating preferences are based on familial rather than self-MHC haplotypes suggests the role of MHC in inbreeding avoidance. However, familial imprinting would be limited to social species with prolonged parental care. Alternately, a recent study in mice (81) and two recent studies in fish (82,83) demonstrated a preference for partners that maximized the complexity of progeny MHC genotypes, but did not necessarily maximize genome-wide diversity. In the threespine stickleback, a species in which MHC class II is polygenic, with variable numbers of loci present in individual haplotypes, mate choice by female sticklebacks was based on the number of alleles over all loci carried by the males (82). Females did not necessarily avoid males with similar MHC haplotypes or choose males with the maximum number of alleles, but chose mates that would input an apparently "optimal" level of MHC diversity to the offspring. Thus, females possessing high numbers of alleles may be less selective in mate choice than females with low numbers of class II alleles. In salmon, which contain only a single MHC class II gene, and in mice, females apparently maximized the complexity of MHC in their offspring by choosing males with the most functionally divergent MHC alleles (81,83). This finding supports the suggestion that balancing selection based on divergent allele advantage governs the level of MHC allelic diversity in many sockeye salmon (71) and human (68) populations.

Selection on Locus Complexity

Diversifying selection on MHC genes is not likely controlled by any one factor alone, but is gained through a combination of selective forces, including pathogen-driven selection, mate choice, maternal–fetal interactions, and possibly other as yet undefined mechanisms. Perhaps the strength and contribution of each of these forces varies among species and over time and space within species. Certainly, although MHC diversity is generally high relative to other coding loci in all of the vertebrate species studied to date, variation in the absolute amount of diversity exists both among species and among populations. Species vary not only in the number of expressed MHC genes, but also in the numbers and divergence of alleles found within genes. For instance, salmon are likely capable of binding a wide repertoire of peptides by the maintenance of highly divergent allelic lineages, with up to 40% divergence in PBR-encoding exons, possibly gained by convergence of multiple ancient loci into a single ubiquitously expressed classical class I locus. Alternately, many neoteleost species, such as cod, pufferfish, and cichlids, maintain diversity through the presence of multiple MHC class I and II genes (84). As with the recurring theme of this chapter, there is no progression of MHC gene complexity among classes of organisms. And although selection favors MHC diversity, there appears to be an optimal level of diversity tolerated, possibly controlled by the potential of negative selection on T cells producing holes in the T-cell repertoire into which pathogens can escape recognition (R85). In fact, most species contain only one to three classical class I and class II MHC genes, which vary among them in levels of diversity and expression. In polyploid species of *Xenopus* ranging from 2n to 12n, the number of expressed class I and class II genes is kept stable through diploidization (one class Ia gene and two or three class II genes/haploid genome), while most other genes are maintained for ten of millions of years (86). The silencing of MHC genes is neither immediate nor compulsory for survival because laboratory-bred polyploids express multiple MHCs, and presumably reflects the pressure to limit expression of polymorphic class Ia/class II. Furthermore, in species that carry greater numbers of expressed genes, the number of encoded genes present in individuals is limited through haplotype variation. Exceptions to this "rule" might be found in the cod where up to 42 recently duplicated MHC genes were isolated from the cDNA of an individual fish (84), or in the axolotl (R87), which also has a very large number of MHC-linked expressed class I genes. However, even in these examples, many genes may be in the process of degeneration from class Ia to class Ib genes, as measured by the conservation of PBR codons.

MHC Gene Organization

Because class I and class II proteins are structurally similar, it is no surprise that their genes are linked, a primordial trait subsequently lost only in bony fish. But why are structurally unrelated class I–processing genes, including the immune proteasome components LMP2 and LMP7 and the TAP genes, also found in the MHC (Fig. 13)? There are two possible scenarios: primordial linkage of ancestral processing and presenting genes in the MHC or later recruitment of either the processing/presenting genes into a primordial MHC. Based on the presence of similar clusters of MHC genes on paralogous chromosomal regions in humans and mice, Kasahara et al. (88) proposed that ancestors of class I, class II, proteasome, transporter, and class III genes were already linked before the emergence of the adaptive immune system (Fig. 11) (see below). Genome-wide duplications around the time of the origin of vertebrates, as proposed by Ohno (89), may have provided the raw material from which the immune system genes were assembled (see discussion below). As for all other adaptive immune genes described so far, neither class I/II nor immune proteasome/TAP have been isolated from hagfish nor lampreys, and all of these genes as well as CD1 and FcRN could have emerged as a consequence of the duplications. Because class I genes are found on two or three of the clusters (Fig. 11), class I–like molecules may have predated class II in evolution. Indeed, NK-like recognition of a class I molecule encoded in an ancestral linkage group may have been at the origin of the adaptive immune system (We discuss this topic further in the last section.)

In birds, bony fish, and amphibians, unlike mammals, the LMP and TAP genes are closely linked to class I genes, not to class II, in a true "class I region" (Fig. 13). This result is most striking in bony fish (*Fugu,* zebrafish, medaka, trout) because class I/LMP/TAP/TAPBP and class II are found on different chromosomes (R90). The class III region, historically defined by the innate immune genes such as factor B and C4 are also present in the *Xenopus* and elasmobranch MHC, showing that association of class I/II with such genes is ancient. If Kasahara's interpretation is correct—that is, MHC syntenic groups found on different mammalian chromosomes resulted from ancient block duplications—it is expected that the physical association of ancestral class I, II, and III genes predated the emergence of jawed vertebrates, and such syntenies in ectothermic vertebrates are not surprising. Indeed, linkage studies in nonvertebrates *Amphioxus* and sea urchin do support an ancient linkage of class I, II, and III genes (91) (see below). Taken together, the data suggest that lack of synteny of class I, class II, and class III genes in teleosts is a derived characteristic. Independent assortment of class I and class II may allow these genes to evolve at different rates: In trout, class Ia alleles form ancient, slowly evolving lineages, whereas class II genes evolve at similar rates as mammalian MHC alleles (92).

The chicken MHC, the B complex, is on a microchromosome, and intron sizes and intergenic distances are both quite small so that the entire complex is only 92 kb as compared to over 4,000 kb in humans (93) (Fig. 13). Class Ia (BF), class IIβ (BL and DM), and TAP genes are in the MHC, but there is no evidence for immune proteasome genes, and almost all class III genes have been deleted except for C4. Although most class III genes will likely be found on other chromosomes, LMP2/7 seems to be absent from the genome; indeed, peptides bound to chicken class I molecules sometimes have C-terminal glutamic acid or aspartic acid, which are rare after proteolysis by mammalian proteasomes containing LMP2 and LMP7. To explain the correlation of diseases with particular haplotypes, Kaufman et al. (R76) proposed that the

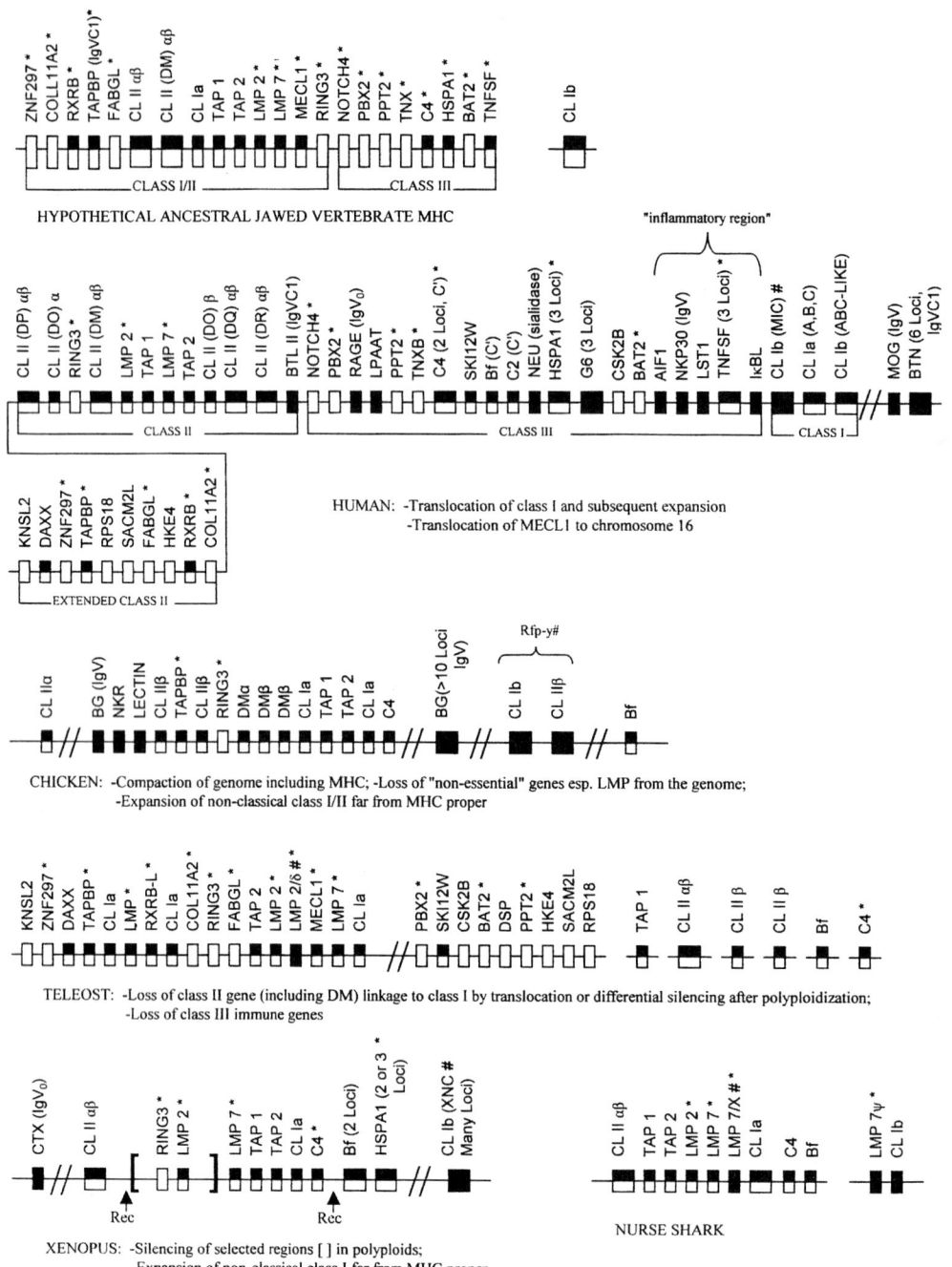

FIG. 13. MHC gene evolution. *White* indicates that the gene is found in at least one other species besides human; *black* designates a gene with known or inferred immune function; *asterisk* designates an old gene found on at least two paralogous regions in humans or at least one other species besides human; *pound sign* indicates a species-specific characteristic; *large box* indicates at least two genes in that region; *double slash* indicates linkage far away on the same chromosome; *space between lines* indicates that the genes are on different linkage groups. The teleost MHC is a composite of the zebrafish, *Fugu*, medakafish maps. Modified from Flajnik and Kasahara (55), with permission.

chicken has a minimal essential MHC composed of only those genes absolutely required to remain in the complex (see above).

In summary, in all nonmammalian species studied, classical class I genes map closely to the TAP and LMP genes, suggesting that the processing, transport, and presenting genes were in an original "class I region" (R55). The tight linkage of the functionally, but not structurally, related genes strongly suggests that such genes co-evolve within particular MHC haplotypes. Although teleosts underwent an explosive adaptive radiation 100 million years ago, there are deep lineages of class Ia genes in many species, also found for *Xenopus* and cartilaginous fish class Ia genes. In mammals, the class I region is not closely linked to LMP/TAP and is very unstable, with rapid duplications/deletions expected in a multigene complex; the same class I instability extends to the non-MHC–linked class Ib genes in *Xenopus* species. It will be interesting to determine whether the neoteleost species that have high numbers of class I genes are linked to the processing/transport genes, or are in another region of the genome as in sharks, frogs, and chickens.

Class I/II Expression

In *Xenopus* species, immunocompetent larvae express high levels of class II on APCs such as B cells, but express only very low levels of class Ia molecules on hematopoietic cells until metamorphosis (R94). Expression of the immune proteasome element LMP7 and all identified class Ib isotypes is also very low. Larval skin and gut, organs with epithelia in contact with the environment, appear to coexpress class I (transcripts) and class II. Such expression may provide immune protection during larval life; perhaps expression of class Ia is limited to organs that undergo massive destruction and remodeling at metamorphosis. Class II molecules also change their distribution after metamorphosis and are highly expressed by unstimulated T cells. Axolotl class II molecules are also regulated differentially during ontogeny, expressed in young animals on B cells and then expanding to all hematopoietic cells, including erythrocytes, later in life. Changes in MHC expression are not correlated with cryptic metamorphosis in axolotls, but class II expression by erythrocytes is correlated to the switch from larval to adult globins (95). Unlike *Xenopus*, class I transcripts isolated so far are expressed early in ontogeny, from hatching onward. Carp class I and class II transcripts are detected in embryos 1 day after fertilization and reach a plateau at day 14. However, the suspected class Ia protein does not appear until week 13, whereas β2m can be detected several weeks earlier. It was suggested that another class I molecule is expressed during early development of the carp hematopoietic system, perhaps one of the unusual nonclassical molecules that groups outside the teleost cluster (R65) (Fig. 10).

Lymphoid Tissues and Cells of Jawed Vertebrates

In addition to the molecules and functions characteristic of adaptive immunity, primary (lymphocyte-generating) and secondary (immune response-generating) lymphoid tissues also define the specific immune system (R96,R97). The thymus is present in all jawed vertebrates, but not in the jawless fish, further solidifying the lack of (at least) conventional T cells outside the gnathostomes. All animals have hematopoietic cell-generating tissues, and outside of the so-called GALT species (15), B cells develop in such bone marrow equivalents in all jawed vertebrates. With the advent of clonal selection, the accumulation and segregation of T and B cells in specialized organs for antigen presentation became necessary and indeed the spleen as such an organ is found in all jawed vertebrates, but not in agnathans or invertebrates.

Cartilaginous Fish

Like all other major adaptive immune system components, cartilaginous fish are the first in evolution to possess a thymus originating from pharyngeal pouches (Fig. 14). As in mammals, it has a distinct cortex/medulla structure, and terminal deoxyribonucleotidyl transferase [TdT] expression was detected in thymocytes with cross-reactive antisera (98) and more recently by northern blotting (22). GALT is also important in elasmobranchs, but lymphoid tissue in the spiral valve (intestine) does not have typical secondary lymphoid tissue structure; the spleen is the only tissue with compartmentalization of cells into discrete T-cell and B-cell zones. The Leydig and epigonal organs (associated with the gonads) are lymphopoietic and erythropoietic, producing mainly granulocytes and lymphocytes and there is high RAG expression in these tissues (see below). Lymphocytes form nodules in the epigonal organ, likely to be indicative of differentiative events. Macrophage–lymphocyte clusters in dogfish brain may be established only after specific stimulation, perhaps preventing foreign materials from entering the parenchyme.

During dogfish development, the liver is the first tissue to contain Ig+ cells at 2 months, followed by the interstitial kidney at 3 months. The thymus, spleen, and Leydig organ appear at 4 months, and the epigonal and GALT are the last tissues to differentiate (99). The hematopoietic/lymphoid nature of the kidney and thymus disappears after hatching, whereas the other lymphomyeloid tissues persist through adult life. At hatching when embryos are exposed to waterborne antigens, structural development of the lymphomyeloid tissues is well advanced. In the nurse shark, neonatal spleen white pulp consists entirely of class II–negative B cells; by 5 months after birth, T-cell zones containing class II dendritic-like cells appear adjacent to the B-cell zones. Both the B-cell and T-cell zones are vascularized, and no detectable marginal zone separates red pulp from white pulp.

Bony Fish

The teleost thymus gland originates from the pharyngeal pouches and can be uni-, bi-, or tri-lobed, depending on the species. It is the first organ to become lymphoid, and its structure may differ from species to species. The cortex/medulla architecture is not as precise in other vertebrate species, but the duality of the compartment is apparent, at least in trout and the sea bass (R97). The spleen contains the basic elements seen in other vertebrates—blood vessels, red pulp, and white pulp—but the distinction between red and white pulp is less obvious (the white pulp being poorly developed). In spleen the ellipsoids, which are actually terminal capillaries, have a thin endothelial layer surrounded by fibrous reticulum and an accumulation of cells, mainly macrophages. Lymphocyte accumulations are often seen in their vicinity, especially during immune responses, which have been suggested to be primitive germinal centers, but they are not homologous. Red pulp is rich in melanomacrophage centers, which are groups of pigment-containing cells at bifurcations of large blood

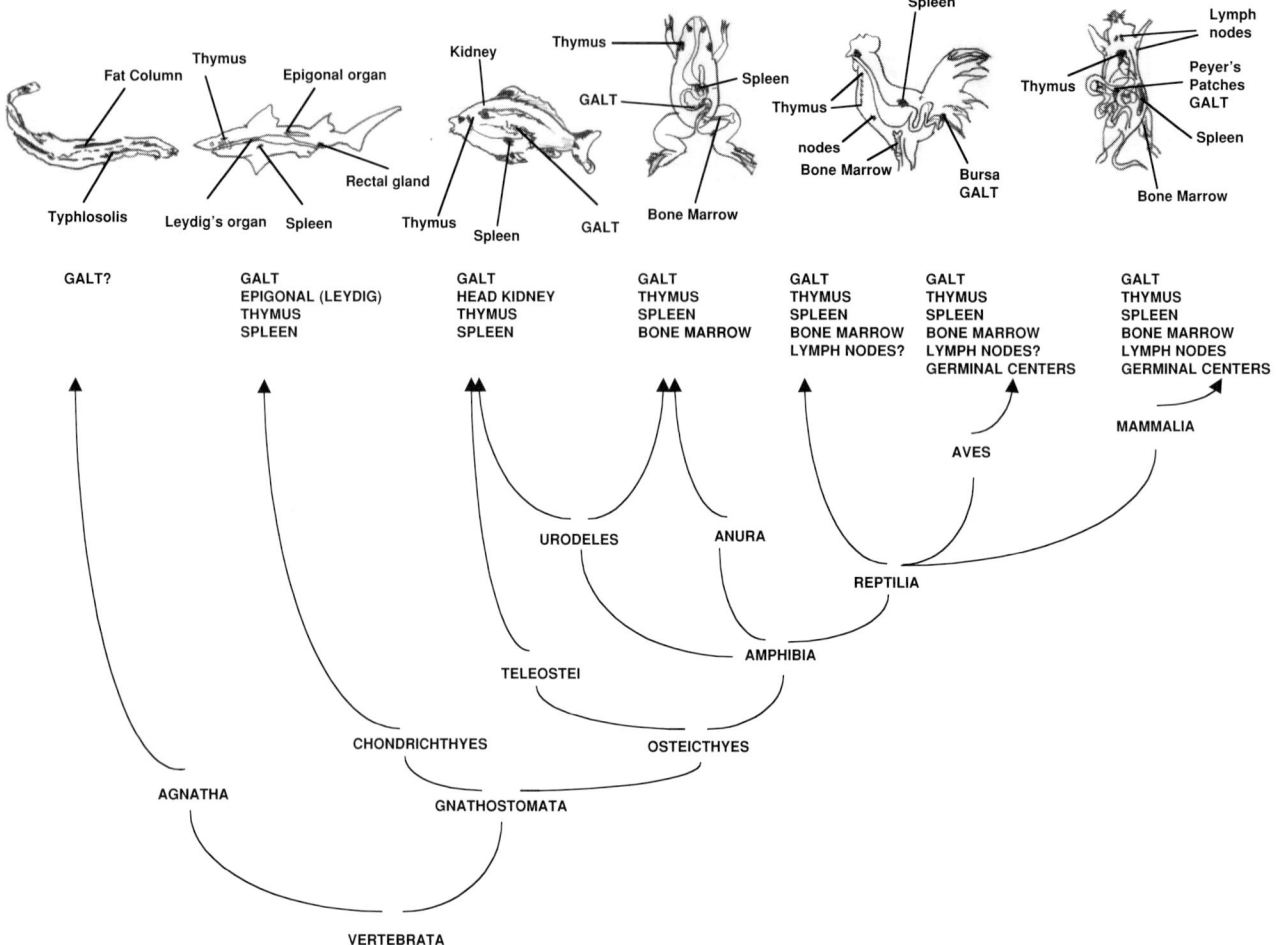

FIG. 14. Evolution of lymphoid tissues in all vertebrate classes.

vessels that may regulate immune responses. The other main lymphoid organ is head kidney, believed to function as mammalian bone marrow (100).

Lymphocyte heterogeneity resembling that of mammals exists in the trout. Thymus cells respond exclusively to T mitogens (e.g., ConA), head kidney lymphocytes respond exclusively to B mitogens (LPS), and spleen cells respond to both. PBL can be activated in MLR in the trout, carp, and catfish. In sea bass, functional T cells monitored with mAbs appear among thymocytes 30 days after hatching. Similar cells appear on day 45 in the gut mucosa, spleen, and kidneys. B cells are detected by day 80. Thymectomy of young mouth breeders (*Tilapia*) impairs allograft and antibody responses. During immune responses, plaque-forming cells are detected in the thymus, similar to studies in mammals after intrathymic immunization. Antibody-forming cells can be found in the spleen or head kidney of many species. Only T cells (surface Ig⁻) respond in MLR, whereas T cells, B cells, and macrophages stimulate responses, which suggests that all lymphocytes express MHC class II molecules and display other features required for T-cell activation. In addition, some mAbs react with a distinct mucosal T-cell population and could identify the homolog of γ/δ T cells,

abundant in various mammalian epithelia. For antibody production *in vitro* to thymus-dependent hapten-carrier immunogens, macrophages (or some APC), T cells, and B cells are necessary, whereas for thymus-independent antigens, only macrophages (APC) and B cells are required. These experiments provide the strongest evidence for T cells, B cells, and accessory cells in this vertebrate class.

Amphibians

In anurans the thymus develops from the dorsal epithelium of the visceral pouches (the number of the pouches involved varies with species) and is the first tissue to become lymphopoietic. It is colonized from days 6 or 7 onward by precursors derived from lateral plate and ventral mesoderm through the head mesenchyme. Precursors proliferate *in situ* as the epithelium begins to express MHC class II molecules but not classical class I molecules. By day 8, thymic cortex/medulla architecture resembles that of other vertebrates. Amphibians possess a spleen with red and white pulp, GALT with no organized secondary lymphoid tissue, and many nodules (but no lymph nodes), with lymphopoietic activity in the kidney, liver, mesentery, and gills. The general morphology of lymphoid organs varies greatly according to species and changes with the season. In *Xenopus* splenic white pulp is delineated by a boundary layer, and the central arteriole of the white pulp follicle terminates in the red pulp perifollicle area, a T-dependent zone. As described above for fish, anuran spleens lack true germinal centers. In *Bufo calamita*, colloidal carbon particles injected via the lymph sac are trapped by free macrophages in the red pulp, which then move through the marginal zone to the white pulp. Giant, ramified, non-phagocytic cells found in both white and red pulp have been proposed to be dendritic cells. *Xenopus* bone marrow does not appear to be a major lymphoid organ from histologic observation, but high RAG expression in this tissue suggests lymphopoietic activity. The maintenance of RAG expression throughout adult life suggests that lymphocytes are continually produced.

Thymectomy decreases or abolishes allograft rejection capacity, MLR and PHA responsiveness, IgY antibody synthesis, and all antibody responses that increase in affinity to classic thymus-dependent antigens (R101). MLR reactivity matures before the ability to mount IgY responses in primary responses. Thymectomy at age 7 days delays allograft rejection and abrogates specific IgY responses, whereas later in life it only abrogates antibody responses. Thymectomy performed later greatly affects the pool of peripheral T cells, as monitored with mAbs specific for XTLA.1, CD5, and CD8. Early thymectomy results in the complete absence of T cells, but lymphocytes with T-cell markers, perhaps corresponding to NK T cells, can still be detected. In *Xenopus,* thymocytes induce weak GVH reactions, whereas splenic T cells are good helpers and strong GVH inducers. The thymus contains some IgM-producing B cells and memory cells poised to switch to IgY synthesis, and *in vitro* responses are down-regulated by naïve thymus cells. Nitrosomethylurea (NMU) eliminates T cells and thereby abrogates alloreactivity, but rejection of xenografts is not abolished and thus may be controlled by thymus-independent mechanisms. *Xenopus* B cells respond *in vitro* to low doses of LPS not by proliferation, but rather by Ig synthesis, and also respond to PMA. Old reports of B-cell proliferation can be attributed to contaminants in LPS preparations.

NK cells were detected in *Xenopus* by *in vitro* ^{51}Cr assays. Splenocyte effectors from early thymectomized frogs spontaneously lyse allogeneic thymus tumor cell lines that lack MHC antigen expression (R101,102). This activity is increased after the injection of tumor cells or after treating the splenocytes *in vitro* with mitogens, suggesting lymphokine activation of the killers. Spontaneous killers also were identified in *Rana* species. Few lineage-restricted surface glycoproteins have been characterized in amphibians. Nevertheless, the following homologs have been identified by mAbs and, in some cases, gene isolation: CD5, CD8, CD45, XTLA.1, and CTX.

Urodele embryos initially produce five pairs of thymic buds, the first two of which disappear. This results in a three-lobe thymus in *Ambystoma*, but in *Pleurodeles* and *Triturus* it forms one lobe. No cortex or medulla can be distinguished,

and the thymus generally resembles the cortex of a mammalian/anuran thymus (R97). There are at least three types of stromal epithelial cells. There is no lymphopoietic activity in axolotl bone marrow, and hematopoeisis takes place in the spleen and in the peripheral layer of the liver (Fig. 14). The spleen is not clearly divided into white and red pulp.

Axolotl lymphocytes proliferate *in vitro* with diverse mitogenic agents. In larval or adult axolotls, a population of B cells is specifically stimulated by LPS and can synthesize and secrete both IgM and IgY. T-cell responses to mitogens or allogeneic determinants are allegedly poor, but adult (older than 10 months) splenocytes and thymocytes respond well to PHA when the medium is supplemented with 0.25% bovine serum albumin, rather than 1% fetal bovine serum. T cells are activated in these experiments, as shown by cell depletion with mAbs *in vitro,* and *in vivo* by thymectomy. Axolotl lymphocytes, like mammalian lymphocytes, proliferate *in vitro* when stimulated by staphylococcal enterotoxins A and B (SEA and SEB superantigens).

Reptiles

In all reptiles studied, the thymic cortex and medulla are clearly separated. The spleen has well-defined white and red pulp regions, but T- and B-cell zones have not been delineated with precision. In *Chrysemys scripta,* white pulp is composed of two lymphoid compartments: Lymphoid tissue surrounds both central arterioles and thick layers of reticular tissue called ellipsoids (R97). Even after paratyphoid vaccine injection, splenic germinal centers are not formed, as in fish and amphibians. Splenic red pulp is composed of a system of venous sinuses and cords. In *Python reticulatus,* dendritic cells involved in immune complex trapping have been identified and may be related to mammalian follicular dendritic cells. GALT develops later than spleen during development and it appears to be a secondary lymphoid organ (but does not seem to contain the equivalent of the bursa of Fabricius). Lymph node–like structures, especially in snakes (*Elaphe*) and lizards (*Gehyra*) have been reported.

Reptiles, the evolutionary precursors of both birds and mammals, are a pivotal group, but unfortunately the functional heterogeneity of reptile lymphocytes is poorly documented. There seems to be T/B-cell heterogeneity because an antithymocyte antiserum altered some T-cell–dependent functions in the viviparous lizard *Chalcides ocellatus.* Embryonic thymocytes responded in MLR at all stages, but ConA responsiveness increased gradually during successive stages and declined at birth. In the alligator (*Alligator mississippiensis*), like in mammals after glass-wool filtration, nonadherent PBL responded to PHA and not to LPS, whereas adherent cells were stimulated by LPS.

Birds

The thymus, which develops in chickens from the third and fourth pharyngeal pouches, consists of two sets of seven lobes each with definitive cortex/medulla. The thymus becomes lymphoid around day 11 of incubation. Splenic architecture is less differentiated than in mammals. It is not lymphopoietic during embryogenesis, as RAG-positive cells are found mainly in yolk sac and blood. Birds are the first vertebrate group where follicular germinal centers and T-dependent areas comprising the periarteriolar lymphatic sheath (PALS) are encountered. Plasma cells are located in the red pulp. γ/δ TCR$^+$ T-lymphocytes are chiefly concentrated in sinusoids, whereas α/β T cells fill the PALS. Lymph nodes seem to be present in water and shore birds but not in chickens and related birds.

The bursa of Fabricius is a primary lymphoid organ unique to birds in which B cells are produced (103). It arises at day 5 of development and involutes 4 weeks later (see B-cell differentiation). T–B heterogeneity is obviously well defined in birds (indeed, the "B" in B-cell stands for bursa.) The effects of thymectomy—T- and B-cell collaboration and generation of MHC-restricted helper and killer cells—are very similar to mammals, the other class of warm-blooded vertebrates.

In summary, the organization of the lymphoid tissues is perhaps the only element of the immune system that shows increasing complexity that can be superimposed on the vertebrate phylogenetic tree. The absence of primary and secondary lymphoid tissues (thymus and spleen) is correlated with the absence of a rearranging receptor family in jawless vertebrates. While all jawed vertebrates have a true secondary lymphoid tissue (spleen), ectotherms lack lymph nodes and organized GALT. In addition, while ectotherms clearly have B-cell zones resembling follicles, germinal centers with follicular dendritic cells are not formed after immunization, and clearly this was a major advance in the evolution of the vertebrate immune system (see below).

Rearrangement and Diversification of TCR and Ig Genes During Lymphocyte Differentiation

All vertebrate species rearrange their antigen-receptor genes (except the case mentioned above for some cartilaginous-fish germline-joined genes). Besides rearrangement, with combinatorial joining of gene segments and imprecision of the joins, there are two other sources of diversity to generate the repertoires: the TdT enzyme that modifies boundaries of rearranging gene segments, and somatic mutations, found exclusively in B cells usually introduced during immune responses. However, progression of rearrangement during B- and T-cell development and diversification follow different rules in different vertebrates (R5,15). It is conceivable that species hatching early with just a few lymphocytes are under pressures to develop a rapid response and may not use the same mechanisms as species protected by the mother's uterine environment. It is also possible that immune systems of species with small progenies are under stronger pressures than species that have many offspring, and this might be reflected in the manner that diversity is generated. Studies of B- and T-cell differentiation have been performed in many vertebrates. RAG and TdT genes have been cloned in representatives of many classes, probes that allow us to follow

lymphocyte generation. Reagents have become available that permit an accurate monitoring of T-cell appearance in the lymphoid organs of ectotherms (cross-reactive anti-CD3 sera or TCR probes), as well as mAbs and gene probes specific for Ig H/L chains that allow examination of B cells. As a rule, the thymus is the first organ to become lymphoid during development. Another emerging rule is that development of the thymus-dependent MHC-restricted T-cell repertoire is similar in all species, and this is reflected in the evolution of TCR gene organization described above. In contrast (R4,R5), B-cell repertoire generation differs drastically among different species, even within the same class of vertebrates (R40,R104).

Cartilaginous Fish

In the skate *Raja eglanteria,* Ig and TCR expression is sharply up-regulated relatively late in development (8 weeks). At this age, TCR and TdT expression is limited to the thymus; later, TCR gene expression appears in peripheral sites in hatchlings and adults. IgM expression is first detected in the spleen of young skates but IgX is expressed first in gonad, liver, Leydig organ, and thymus (105). In adults, Leydig organ and spleen are sites of the highest IgM and IgX expression. In nurse sharks, 19S IgM appears in the serum before 7S IgM and IgNAR, and this profile is reflected in the lack of IgNAR$^+$ cells in the spleen until 2 months after birth. RAG and TdT expression in the thymus and epigonal organ of the nurse shark suggests that lymphopoiesis is ongoing in adult life (22). In contrast to most other vertebrates, N-region diversity is detected in skate and nurse shark IgM and IgNAR CDR3 from the earliest stages analyzed, suggesting that a full-blown diverse repertoire is important for young elasmobranchs (105). As mentioned above, a subset of Ig genes is prearranged in the germline of chondrichthyans, and many of those germline-joined genes are transcribed in the embryo and hatchling, but not in the adult. This pattern fits with the expression of the nurse shark IgM$_{1gj}$ with its germline-joined V region (22), and suggests that some germline-joined genes "take advantage" of their early transcriptional edge and thus some clusters can be selected for specialized tasks in early development. With the hundreds of gene clusters, it is not known how "clusteric exclusion" is achieved at the molecular level (and why the germline-joined gene expression is extinguished in adult life), but as mentioned above preliminary experiments suggest that only one H-chain cluster is expressed in each lymphocyte.

The architecture of cartilaginous fish Ig loci allows greatest diversity only in CDR3 since the CDR2 and CDR1 are always encoded in the germline and V segments do not combine with (D),J segments from other clusters. Yet the number of possible CDR3 is essentially limitless and the number of germline clusters is also high (and usually three rearrangement events take place since two D segments are in each cluster). Thus, as described previously the potential diversity is greater than the number of lymphocytes.

Bony Fish

In the sea bass *Dicentrarchus labrax,* a mAb detects differentiating T cells (perhaps pre-T cells) as well as mature T cells as evidenced by the presence of TCR mRNA in the sorted populations (106). Cells seem to migrate from surrounding mesenchyme and subsequently mature in the thymus, like in all vertebrates studied so far. T cells appear earlier in ontogeny (between 5 and 12 days after hatching) than cytoplasmic Ig$^+$ pre–B cells, which are detected only at 52 days post-hatching. Adult levels of T and B cells are reached between 137 and 145 days after hatching, quite a long time compared to young amphibians. In all teleosts examined, the thymus is the primary organ for T-lymphocyte generation and head kidney the primary organ for B-cell development.

RAG1 of the trout *Oncorhynchus mykiss* differs from mammalian RAG1 genes by the presence of an intron of 666 bp. Compared with other RAG1 sequences, trout RAG1 has a minimum of 78% similarity for the complete sequence and 89% similarity in the conserved region (aa 417 to 1042). RAG1 transcripts are detected chiefly in thymus, pronephros, mesonephros, spleen, and intestine starting at day 20 after fertilization (R96). Trout TdT is highly expressed within the thymus and to a lesser extent in the pronephros beginning at 20 days post-fertilization, which correlates with the appearance of theses two tissues (100). Because the H-chain cluster is in the translocon configuration and there are many V$_H$ families, it is assumed that diversity is generated in the mouse/human mode. However, a study of L-chain diversity could be interesting since the genes are encoded in clusters with many loci that rearrange by inversion; thus, this system might allow for high levels of receptor editing.

Amphibians

Amphibians show major differences in the timing of rearrangement and in usage of TdT. Whereas precursor lymphocytes in axolotls start to rearrange at 6 weeks (3 weeks later than teleosts) until ~1 year later, in the anuran *Xenopus* RAG expression is detected at hatching on day 2 after fertilization. In 6-week-old axolotl larvae, RAG1 mRNAs were first detected in the thymus until its involution after 12 months of age (R107). The first appearance of RAG1 gene products is well correlated with the appearance of the rearranged T-cell and B-cell receptor mRNAs, 40 to 60 days after fertilization. RAG1 transcripts were present in the spleen and liver of young larvae, but neither in the liver after 4.5 months nor in the spleen after 8 months. Other investigators reported RAG1 transcription as early as the neurula stages of development, and in addition to the thymus expression was detected in spleen, brain, and eyes of adults.

About 40% of TCRβ V-D-J junctions in 2.5-month-old *Ambystoma* larvae have N nucleotides, compared to about 73% in 10- to 25-month-old animals. These V-D-J junctions had ~30% defective rearrangements at all stages of development, which could be due to the slow rate of cell division

in the axolotl lymphoid organs, and the large genome in this urodele (108). As mentioned above, many axolotl CDRβ3 sequences, deduced from in frame V-D-J rearrangements, are the same in animals of different origins. In contrast, in *Xenopus* rearrangement starts on day 5 after fertilization for the V$_H$ locus, and within 9 days all V$_H$ families are used. V$_H$1 rearranges first, followed by V$_H$3; by day 9 or 10 V$_H$ 2, 6, 9, and 10 begin being rearranged, and then V$_H$ 5, 7, 8, and 11 on day 13. For VL, the κ locus is the first to rearrange on day 7 (2 days after V$_H$), a situation similar to that found in mammals. During this early phase, B cells are present in the liver, where their number increases to ~500 cells. Later in larval life, rearrangement stops and then resumes at metamorphosis as suggested by the low incidence of pre–B cells and by the re-expression of RAG during the second histogenesis of the lymphoid system. RAG is expressed in adult bone marrow, as examined by northern blotting and by isolation of DNA excision circles, landmarks of ongoing rearrangements. T cells show a similar type of RAG expression/cell renewal during ontogeny as the B cells, and the larval and adult Vβ T-cell repertoires differ significantly. Even early in development, tadpoles express a highly variable TCR β repertoire despite the small number of lymphocytes present at these early stages (8,000 to 10,000 splenic T cells); little redundancy in TCR cDNA recovered from young larvae implies that clone sizes must be extremely small, unlike the axolotl situation described above.

In *Xenopus* no lymphoid organ except the thymus is detectable until day 12 when the spleen appears and with it the ability to respond to antigen. For B cells until this time no selection occurs as suggested by the random ratio of productive/nonproductive V-D-J rearrangements (2:1). After day 12 this ratio becomes 1:1; that is, the rearrangements have been selected. cDNA sequences on day 10 to 12 (when the number of B cells increases from 80 to 500) are not redundant as if each sequence was represented by one cell (R107). RAG expression together with the detection of DNA rearrangement circles in the bone marrow suggests that rearrangement is ongoing throughout life and is not restricted to an early period like in birds. Tadpole rearrangements are characterized by a lack of N-region diversity, like in mammals but not axolotls or shark/skate (see above), and thus very short CDR3. During ontogeny, TdT appears at significant levels in thymus of tadpoles at metamorphic climax but little expression is detected at earlier stages, which correlates well with the paucity of N-region addition in larval IgH-chain sequences (107,109). Studies of the ontogeny of the *Xenopus* immune system have revealed a less efficient tadpole immune response (skin graft rejection and Ig heterogeneity and affinity); the absence of TdT expression during tadpole life fits well with the findings of lower larval Ig (and TCR) diversity (see below).

Birds

During the embryonic period, chicken stem cells found in yolk sac and blood rearrange their IgH and Ig light (L)V genes simultaneously over a very restricted period of time, and very few cells colonize each bursal follicle (about 10^4 follicles). Three weeks after hatching, these cells have differentiated in the bursa and then seed the secondary lymphoid tissues after which time B cells are no longer be generated from multipotent stem cells; thus, only $\sim 2 \times 10^4$ productive Ig rearrangements occur in the life of the chicken (110). When an antiserum to chicken IgM is administered *in ovo* to block this early bursal immigration, there are no stem cells arising later in development that can colonize the bursa, and these chickens lack B cells for their entire lives (111). Although the general Ig locus architecture is similar to that of frogs and mammals, only one rearrangement is possible as there is only one functional V_L or V_H on each allele. Diversity is created during bursal ontogeny by a hyperconversion mechanism in which a pool of pseudogenes (25 ψL and approximately 80 ψH) (Fig. 6) act as donors and the unique rearranged gene acts as an acceptor (Fig. 4) during a proliferative phase in bursal follicles (112,113). For H chains, the situation is more complex as there are multiple D elements. During ontogeny selection of productive rearrangements parallels the selection of a single D reading frame, suggesting that the many D segments favor D-D joins to provide junctions that are diversified by gene conversion; the hyperconversion mechanism can also modify Ds because most donor pseudogenes are fused V-D segments. The gene conversion process requires the enzyme activation-induced deaminase (AID), which is also required for somatic hypermutation and class switch (114).

Since diversification by gene conversion occurs after Ig rearrangement and cellular entry into bursal follicles, and there is only a single germline V_H and V_L expressed on all developing B cells, it was tempting to implicate a bursal ligand binding to cell-surface IgM to initiate and sustain cellular proliferation and gene conversion. However, surface expression of IgM devoid of V regions permitted the typical B-cell developmental progression, demonstrating that such receptor–ligand interactions are not required (115). Thus, currently we know little of how cells enter the bursa, which signals induce them to proliferate/convert, and how cells arrest their development and seed the periphery.

Mammals

Perhaps surprisingly, mechanisms leading to the generation of repertoire diversity vary among mammalian species (15,R40,R104). At the rabbit H locus, as in the chicken, a single V_H is expressed in most peripheral B cells. During development B cells that have rearranged this particular V in the bone marrow (and other sites) migrate to the appendix where this rearranged gene is diversified by gene conversion using upstream donor V segments (116). In ruminants, the ileal Peyer's patches (IPP) are the bursa-like primary B-cell-generating tissue (117). Although bursa, appendix, and sheep IPPs show morphologic similarities, the mechanisms generating diversity are different: conversion in the chicken and

hypermutation in sheep, and both in the rabbit. As data accumulate, categories can be made depending upon the mode of B-cell development: Rabbits, cattle, swine and chickens, unlike fish, amphibians, reptiles and primates/rodents, use a single V_H family, of which only a few members (sometimes only one) are functional. This so-called "GALT group" uses gene conversion or hypermutation in hindgut follicles early in life (rather than bone marrow throughout life) to diversify their antibody repertoire. The "GALT group" also appears to lack IgD; thus IgD might serve some purpose in repertoire development in some groups of mammals and not in others (R118). It would be interesting to study the generation of diversity in teleost fish, where an IgD homolog has been found (see above), yet in which the gene organization is of the translocon type with many V_H families.

In conclusion, the potential repertoire of Ig- and TCR-combining sites is enormous in all jawed vertebrates. The potential antigen-receptor repertoire in all species for both T and B cells is far greater than could ever be expressed in an animal because of cell number limitations. Not all species or all gene families use combinatorial joining for repertoire building, but all species assemble V, (D), and J gene segments to generate their functional Ig genes during B-cell ontogeny, and the imprecision of this assembly creates great somatic diversity. Thus, from this survey in various species one could not predict that there would be major differences in immune responses in representatives of different vertebrate classes, and yet in the next section we shall see that mouse/human antibody responses are superior to those in many taxa.

Adaptive Immune Responses

The quality of T-cell and B-cell responses depends on the heterogeneity and the diversity of the antigen-receptor repertoires and on the ability to select cells in secondary lymphoid tissues. As described, because of the indefinite and huge number of potential Ig/TCR V region sequences, potential diversity exceeds the number of available lymphocytes. Yet, while potential repertoires are diverse in all vertebrate classes, and polymorphic MHC class I and II and TCR genes have been isolated from all classes, antibody diversity in non-mammalian vertebrates is low. The expressed repertoire has been studied by indirect methods based on structural studies, affinity measurements during the maturation of the immune response, enumeration of antigen-binding Igs by isoelectrofocusing (IEF), and idiotypic analysis. Sequences of Ig and TCR genes expressed over the course of a response help to estimate diversity at another level, allowing studies of V genes diversified by gene conversion and/or somatic mutation during a response in a precise way. In the following survey we describe studies of specific antibody synthesis, T-cell responsiveness (T–B collaboration, MHC restriction). NK and NK–T cells will be considered in this section as well. Because of space limitations, we focus on ectothermic vertebrates and to a certain extent on birds.

Agnatha

Hagfish and lampreys were reported to mount humoral responses to sheep red blood cells (SRBC), keyhole limpet hemocyanin (KLH), bacteriophage, *Brucella,* and human RBC. For antigroup A streptococcal antigens, hagfish "antibodies" recognize predominantly rhamnose, while mammals recognize N-acetylglucosamine. These "antibodies" were actually the complement component C3 (119). The alternative complement pathway was known in cyclostomes from earlier studies (see below), and now most investigators believe that hagfish/lamprey have no rearranging Ig/TCR genes. They do, however, possess cells resembling lymphocytes and plasma cells, but the quest for RAG or VC1 gene segments has been a failure. The report of specific memory in allograft rejection is difficult to reconcile with absence of the rearranging machinery and the possibility to generate specific lymphocyte clones, but it is possible that some sort of adaptive immunity exists in these animals (120).

Cartilaginous Fish

Natural antibodies binding many antigens have been detected at surprisingly high levels in chondrichthyans and in some teleosts (R121). After immunization (for instance, with 2-furyloxazolone- *Brucella,* or p-azobenzenearsonate), the horned shark mounts a low-affinity 19S IgM antibody response, which varies little among individuals and does not increase in affinity after prolonged immunization (R25,122). Variation of L chains isolated from individuals is limited, with the major bands having identical isoelectric points. Nurse sharks immunized to heat-killed streptococcal A–variant vaccine produced antibodies that among six outbred individuals had very different L-chain gel electrophoresis patterns. However, L-chain diversity does not increase with time after immunization.

The relative homogeneity and large number of V genes hindered somatic mutation studies until a single unique reference horned shark IgM V_H gene was found (123). Mutations in this gene were slightly more frequent than those in *Xenopus* (see below). Mutation rates could not be calculated and no correlation with an immune response was attempted. The mutations were predominantly found at GC bases and the frequency was rather low. Nevertheless, this work proved that somatic mutation preceded diversity obtained by combinatorial association of gene segments in evolution. In contrast to mutations in the IgM V_H genes, unusual patterns of somatic mutation were detected in nurse shark type II germline-joined L chains. Half of the mutations (338 of 631) occur in tandem without the GC bias seen in *Xenopus* or shark H-chain V genes (124). Tandem mutations and point mutations take place simultaneously and are unlikely to be generated by gene conversion since there are no repeated patterns or potential donor genes. The germline-joined L-chain genes can only diversify through somatic hypermutation, perhaps like the hypothetical prototype V region gene prior to RAG-

mediated rearrangement; that is, somatic hypermutation may have preceded gene rearrangement as the primordial somatic diversification mechanism (see below). The small number of IgNAR genes made it possible to analyze somatic mutation, but as in all shark mutation studies, random cDNAs were examined (24,125). The mutation frequency is about 10 times that of *Xenopus* and horned shark IgM, and even higher than in most studies in mammals. It is difficult to establish a pattern for the mutations due to their high frequency and because they are often contiguous, like in the L-chain gene study described above; however, mutations were not targeted to GC bases and analysis of synonymous sites suggested that the mechanism is similar to human/mouse. Mutations appeared to be under positive selection in IgNAR secretory but not TM clones, strongly suggesting that mutations do not generate the primary repertoire like in sheep but arise only after antigenic stimulation (125).

The role of T cells in shark immune responses has not been studied in detail. No thymectomy experiments have been performed and T cells have not been monitored during an immune response. Shark MLR and graft rejection have been attempted—MLR with little success (probably for technical reasons) and grafts with the demonstration of a chronic type of rejection for which the genetics has not been analyzed. However, from the MHC and TCR studies it is clear that all of the molecular components are available for proper antigen presentation in sharks and skates, and recent studies of splenic architecture suggestive of T-cell zones containing class II$^+$ dendritic cells argue for a prominent T-cell regulatory role in adaptive immunity.

Bony Fish

There are high levels of low-affinity natural antibody (up to 11% of total Ig) to nitrophenylacetate (NP) in some bony fish (R121). Natural antibodies in catfish have been correlated with resistance to virus infection or furonculosis. As a rule and like in cartilaginous fish, little affinity maturation has been detected in fish although some changes in fine specificities were noticed in the trout with a sensitive ELISA-based test (126). B-cell and Ig heterogeneity was demonstrated in carp using mAbs, and DNP-specific antibody-secreting cells were identified with the ELISPOT assay in pronephros and spleen cell suspensions after immunization. The number of IEF antigen-specific bands per individual is small (up to 23), and there is little variation from one outbred individual to another. In sea bass, extremely low variability was reported in CDR1, and no variability in CDR2 or CDR3 in DNP-specific L chains, suggesting expression of dominant monospecific antibodies.

The mild increase in trout antibody affinity (similar to that found in *Xenopus*) is attributed to selection of either minor preexisting B-cell populations or somatic mutants (126). In partially inbred self-fertilized or gynogenetic trout, variability of specific responses is even more restricted. Affinity measured by equilibrium dialysis was of the order of

2.0 × 10⁻⁶ M for TNP-specific antibodies. The percentage of L chains of the catfish "F" and "G" types can vary greatly in the course of a response (2 weeks vs. 3 months). A large literature deals with vaccination attempts in teleost fish, due to their economic importance. The availability of catfish B-cell, macrophage, and T-cell lines have been instrumental in analyses of antibody production (R127). There are puzzling differences in responses from different teleost groups, much like differences between urodeles and anurans (amphibians). Cod, for example, do not respond well to specific antigen and have very high levels of "natural antibodies."

Like the cartilaginous fish, isolation of TCR genes and the existence of a polymorphic class I and class II molecules suggest that antigen presentation is operative teleosts, but unlike sharks functional experiments examining mammalian-like T–APC interactions have been performed. TCR mRNAs are selectively expressed, and specific TCR rearrangements have been detected in catfish clonal cell lines that produce factor(s) with leukocyte growth-promoting activity (R127). Modifications of the trout T-cell repertoire during an acute viral infection have also been followed. In nonintentionally immunized trout, adaptation of the spectratyping technique for TCRβ CDR3 length revealed a polyclonal naïve T-cell repertoire (128). After an acute infection with viral hemorrhagic septicemia virus (VHSV), CDR3 size profiles were skewed for several Vβ/Jβ combinations, corresponding to T-cell clonal expansions. Both "public" and "private" T-cell expansions were detected in the infected, genetically identical individuals. The "public" response resulted in expansion of Vβ4/Jβ1–positive T cells that appeared first in the primary response and were boosted during the secondary response. Thus, like B cells, careful investigations reveal much more heterogeneity in T-cell responses than previously theorized.

We have seen that species living in extreme cold develop (adaptive?) structural differences in their Igs. At the level of global immune response temperature exerts a great influence in ectothermic vertebrates in general, low temperature generally being immunosuppressive. Lowering the water temperature from 23°C to 11°C over a 24-hour period suppresses both B- and T-cell functions of catfish for 3 to 5 weeks as assessed by *in vitro* responses (129). Virgin T cells are most sensitive to this cold-induced suppression, a property shared with mammals when tested appropriately. Fish have developed ways to adapt to the lack of fluidity of their B-cell membranes by altering the composition of fatty acid by using more oleic acid at low temperatures. After appropriate *in vivo* acclimation, catfish T cells are better able to cap cell-surface molecules at low assay temperatures than are B cells, suggesting that capping is not the low temperature–sensitive step involved in T-cell immunosuppression in catfish.

Evidence that fish possess cytotoxic cells was derived from allograft rejections and graft versus host reaction (GVR) studies. *In vitro* studies have now shown that leukocytes from immunized fish specifically kill a variety of target cells (allogeneic erythrocytes and lymphocytes, hapten-coupled autologous cells); fish cytotoxic T-lymphocyte (CTL) of the αβ (and perhaps γδ) lineages as well as NK cells were found.

Naïve catfish leukocytes spontaneously kill allogeneic cells and virally infected autologous cells without sensitization, and allogeneic cytotoxic responses were greatly enhanced by *in vitro* alloantigen stimulation (130). Cloned cytotoxic cells contain granules and likely induce apoptosis in sensitive targets via a putative perforin/granzyme or by Fas/FasL–like interactions. An Fc receptor for IgM (FcμR) was detected on some catfish NK-like cells that appears to "arm" these cells with surface IgM. All catfish cytotoxic cell lines express a signal-transduction molecule with homology to the Fcγ chain of mammals. This chain with an ITAM motif is an accessory molecule for the activating receptor NKP46 on mammalian NK cells. Importantly, these cytotoxic cells do not express a marker for catfish nonspecific cytotoxic cells (NCC). NCC have been found in other fish species, including trout, carp, damselfish, and tilapia, and they spontaneously kill a variety of xenogeneic targets, including certain fish parasites and traditional mammalian NK cell targets. Unlike mammalian NK cells, NCCs are small agranular lymphocytes found in lymphoid tissues (pronephros and spleen), but rarely in blood. Recently, the gene for catfish NCCRP-1 was sequenced, and found to be a novel type III membrane protein with no sequence homology to any known mammalian leukocyte receptor (R131).

Amphibians

Differences in immune system features between urodele (axolotl) and anuran (*Xenopus*) amphibians, already discussed for MHC and Ig complexity, are also seen in immune responses. Rarely is such divergence seen within one vertebrate class (although the two groups diverged over 250 million years ago!). Urodeles express a very restricted antibody repertoire in response to specific antigen that peaks at 40 days post-immunization, and is entirely of the IgM class, even though the serum also contains IgY (132). They do not respond well to thymus-dependent antigens, which may be due to lack of T-cell help, yet their expressed TCR diversity looks normal (R4). Perhaps the huge number of expressed class I molecules (like that seen in the cod) is a hindrance. A population of axolotl B cells proliferates specifically in response to LPS and also secretes both IgM and IgY. Moreover, a distinct lymphocyte subpopulation proliferates significantly in response to the T-cell mitogens Con A. T cells from young axolotls (before 10 months) do not have this functional ability. As mentioned above, axolotl T cells also can be stimulated with to SEA/SEB known from mammalian studies to be superantigens.

Anuran larvae can respond specifically (with only 10⁶ lymphocytes) to many antigens, with a modest affinity maturation of the IgM anti-DNP response. In adults the number of different anti-DNP antibodies does not exceed 40, versus 500 in mammals (133). In secondary responses, the peak of the response is about ten-fold higher and is reached in 2 weeks; there are no major changes in affinity over this initial rise. Anti–DNP Abs, or even nonimmune Ig pools, yield easily interpretable sequences for the first 16 N-terminal residues of both H- and L-chain V regions. However, this simple view was challenged when a great heterogeneity of cDNA sequences could be detected in animals after immunization. Isogenic *Xenopus* produce homogenous antibodies to DNP, xenogenic RBC, or phosphorylcholine with identical or similar IEF spectrotypes and idiotypes, while outbred individuals differ. Both IEF spectrotypes and idiotypes are inheritable, which suggests that diversity is a reflection of the germline repertoire without a major contribution from somatic mutations. Thus, somatic mutations were followed during the course of an antigen-specific immune response at the peak of the modest affinity maturation in larvae and adults (134). The V_H genes, like their mammalian homologs, contain sequence motifs (A/G G C/T A/T) reported to target hypermutation. Of the 32 members of the V_H1 family involved in the anti-DNP response, expression of only five was detected, indicating that immunization was being monitored. Few mutations were detected (average: 1.6 mutations per gene; range: 1 to 5), and there was not a strong preference for mutations in CDR1 and CDR2 and virtually none in CDR3. Like in the shark IgM study noted above (but not IgNAR or type II L chains), the mutations were targeted to GC bases, and such a pattern has been suggested to be the first phase of the somatic hypermutation phase in mouse/human (R135); perhaps *Xenopus* has lost the second phase of the process that results in an evening of mutation frequency for all bases. While the mutation frequency was lower than in mammalian B cells, the rates were only four- to seven-fold less in *Xenopus*. Thus, there is no shortage of variants, and the reasons for the low heterogeneity and poor affinity maturation may be due to less- than-optimal selection of the mutants. Indeed, because of a relatively low ratio of replacement to silent mutations in the CDRs, it was argued that there is no effective mechanism for selecting mutants, which in turn might be related to the absence of germinal centers in *Xenopus*. In summary, the data from hypermutation, cDNA heterogeneity, and spectrotype dominance suggests that in the absence of refined modes of selection in late-developing clones, B cells producing somatic mutants may be out-competed by antibodies generated earlier in the response.

Essential T-cell functions in anurans were shown with *in vitro* assays for T–B collaboration and MHC restriction, demonstrating the similarity of the role of MHC in *Xenopus* and mammals. Regulatory T cells have been shown indirectly in hematopoietic/thymic chimeras for control of CTL generation and in antibody responses (R136). Ig synthesis can be enhanced following thymectomy in axolotl or *Xenopus,* again implying a role for thymic-dependent regulatory cells. As described previously, the class switch first occurs in amphibians, and thymectomy early in life totally prevents IgY, but not IgX synthesis; thus, T cells are absolutely required for the switch and also for high-affinity IgM responses. Switching can also be induced in tadpoles, although one must hyperimmunize animals for this response, due to a paucity of T cells in larvae. The switch is also very much temperature-dependent, and as described above for channel catfish, ectotherm T cells are quite temperature sensitive.

Recently, similar to studies in mammals, the chaperone gp96 has been shown to shuttle peptides into target cells to make such cells targets for MHC-restricted CTL lysis. Immunization of frogs with gp96 from a thymic tumor results in the elicitation of CTL that display antitumor activity. Heroic experiments with gp96 vaccination have also shown that CTL activity against minor histocompatibility antigens is MHC restricted (137). As mentioned above, NK cells have been characterized in *Xenopus* with mAbs that recognize non–B/T cells (R101,102). Those cells kill MHC class I–negative target tumor cells but not class I$^+$ lymphocytes, and after thymectomy these cells are enriched in the spleen. More recently, CD8$^+$ cells expressing TCR were isolated with the same mAb, suggesting the existence of amphibian NK-T cells. Expression of the mAb epitope on cells is induced by PMA/ionomycin, and is also detected in CTL when MHC-dependent cytotoxicity is reduced.

Reptiles

Lack of an increase in affinity and homogeneity of IEF spectrotypes suggest low antibody heterogeneity in reptiles. In the turtle *Pseudemys scripta* a number of genomic VH sequences, representing possibly four families, were isolated, as was a genomic Cμ, all shown to be encoded at a single locus. In Northern hybridizations, the Cμ4 probe detected two transcripts; of the four VH groups, only one was expressed, and multiple bands indicated the presence of at least two non-μ transcripts. Among 32 unique V-D-J rearrangements from one animal, there were 22 sequence variants in FR 4, suggesting either a large number of J segments or somatic modification (39). The latter interpretation is supported by point mutations found in framework 3 and CDR3. For T cells there are no data on T-effector function, but studies on the behavior of T-cell populations change due to seasonal and hormonal variations. Thymocytes from the turtle *Mauremys caspica* proliferate in response to PHA and ConA, and can kill tumor target cells by both ADCC-mediated and NK-mediated cytotoxicity. Proliferative responses to PHA and Con A were higher for both sexes in spring and for females in winter than in the other seasons.

Birds and Mammals

Sequence data and L-chains patterns on 2-D gel electrophoresis showed less antibody heterogeneity in chicken than in mouse. The poor increase in affinity of chicken anti-DNP and antifluorescein antibodies again indicates lower heterogeneity. Few changes occur after immunization, even if one waits 1 year after several injections. Perhaps similar to the trout study described above, a restricted population of high-affinity antibodies was found only after immunization in Freund's complete adjuvant. Hyperconversion and somatic mutation in Ig genes have been found in splenic germinal center B cells after immunization (138). The relatively poor affinity maturation of the chicken response may be due to a balance between gene conversion and somatic mutation. Indeed, modifications of V genes with large segments of DNA is not an optimal strategy for fine-tuning antibody responses. In the rabbit there is also conversion/mutation by B cells in germinal centers after immunization. Within mammals large variations are found in marsupials with no obvious secondary response, to mouse with 1,000-fold increases in affinity, but the basis for the relatively poor responses has not been established.

In conclusion, although all vertebrates have a very large potential for generating diverse antibodies after immunization, only some mammals studied to date make the most of this potential. Perhaps pressures on the immune system of cold-blooded vertebrates have been less intense due to a stronger innate immunity and architecture of their lymphoid system is not optimal for selecting somatic mutants, or the great rises in affinity detected in antihapten responses are not physiologically relevant. An immune system using somatic diversification at its "best" is well adapted to species where the value of single individuals is important (i.e., species with small progenies). Has that been the condition for the creation and selection of somatic rearrangement and of the optimal usage of somatic mutations? If this explanation provides a rationale for the utilization of somatic mechanisms in generating a repertoire and improving it, it does not tell us why it works so well in certain species and not in others. Perhaps the key is the organization of secondary lymphoid organs. Likely a combination of factors—for example, endothermy, secondary lymphoid tissues, mutation versus conversion, the hypermutation mechanism itself, rates of proliferation (pathogen and lymphocyte), and so on—are at work in the regulation of antibody responses.

Cytokines and Chemokines

Many cytokines/chemokines and their receptors, like most molecules of the immune system, evolve rapidly. It has not been easy to isolate their genes and proteins by degenerate PCR/cross-hybridization/cross-reactive antibodies, although with the rapid analyses of ESTs and genes from sequencing projects in many species this situation is rapidly changing. The largest number of cytokine genes has been isolated from birds (mainly chickens) and teleosts (especially rainbow trout and flounder, but also carp and sea bass), with amphibians and reptiles trailing far behind. A comprehensive list of teleost (R139) and chicken (R140) cytokines identified to date has recently been published; here we provide the highlights, especially when some functional analyses have been performed.

Inflammatory Cytokines IL-1, IL-8, and TNF

IL-1, IL-6, TNFα, and IL-8 are the prototypic cytokines associated with inflammatory responses, which are defined by induction of vasodilation and vascular permeability, and up-regulation of innate immune system molecules that have direct functions or that co-stimulate/attract T and B cells. Some of these activities can be assayed in supernatants from LPS-stimulated phagocytes by determining whether thymocytes

are stimulated to proliferate when one also adds suboptimal concentrations of T-cell mitogens. It is perhaps reasonable to imagine that such cytokines, which act both at a distance as well as in a cognate fashion, might be found in the invertebrates. Indeed, IL-1–like activities have been described for echinoderm coelomocytes (either IL-1–like production by such cells, or the ability of the cells to respond to mammalian IL-1), but unfortunately no molecular data revealing the structures of the active invertebrate cytokine/cytokine receptor have been reported (R141). A molecule from earthworms capable of activating the prophenoloxidase defense pathway cross-reacted with a mAb directed to mammalian TNFα. However, this molecule had no homology to TNFα upon sequencing, but its activity is nonetheless quite interesting (142). Thus, we still await identification of invertebrate cytokines related to those in jawed vertebrates, which will likely come from the sequencing projects in prochordates and echinoderms. Furthermore, only one cyto(chemo)kine, with homology to IL-8, has been identified in agnathans (lamprey).

IL-1 activity, as measured by the thymocyte co-stimulation assay, has been detected in teleosts, amphibians, and chickens, and it has been cloned from several teleost species (e.g., rainbow trout and flounder). IL-1β up-regulation has been detected after treatment of macrophages with LPS, consistent with its inflammatory function in mammals. In addition, injection of gram-negative bacteria into trout induced IL-1β expression in many tissues. Identity with the mammalian IL-1β gene ranges from 32% to 40% (identity between mammalian IL-1α and IL-1β is about 25%). The first cytokine gene, IL-1β, from a cartilaginous fish recently was identified, and it shares all of the properties expected from studies in teleosts (143). TNFα homologs have also been cloned from trout and flounder (but surprisingly not yet from birds), and its expression in leukocytes is up-regulated within 4 hours after treatment with LPS, IL-1β, and PMA. Both chicken IL-1β and the IL-1R were identified and have been expressed as recombinant proteins. The IL-1R homology to mammalian orthologs is quite high (61% identity) but the highest similarity is found in the cytoplasmic domains. In addition, there are four blocks of high similarity to the cytoplasmic tail of Toll/TLR proteins, and IL-1R and TLR use similar signal transduction cascades (see below). IL-8 has been identified in the jawless lamprey (144) and in various gnathostomes such as trout, flounder, and perhaps chicken; a chicken CXC chemokine called K60 clusters with IL-8 in phylogenetic trees, and is up-regulated in macrophages stimulated with LPS, IL-1β, and IFN. Interestingly, Marek's disease virus expresses an IL-8 homolog (v-IL-8), which may be involved in inducing immune deviation.

Interleukin 2

Co-stimulation assays of thymocytes, as described for IL-1, and perpetuation of T-cell lines with stimulated T-cell supernatants are performed to detect IL-2 or T-cell growth factor activities. Unlike IL-1, IL-2–like factors generally stimulate cells only from the same species, and it is a "cognate" cytokine, meant for release only between closely opposed cells. From teleost fish to mammals, stimulated T-cell supernatants co-stimulate thymocyte proliferation or can maintain the growth of T-cell blasts (R140,145). The chicken IL-2 protein is only 24% identical to human IL-2 and only 70% identical to a near cousin, the turkey. Initially, it was difficult to determine whether the bird molecule was actually IL-2, its relative IL-15, or perhaps a precursor that predated their divergence. However, recent EST analysis suggests that both chicken genes exist. A candidate IL-2R in chicken was identified by a mAb recognizing a 50-kDa molecule only on stimulated T cells (thus and IL-2Rα homolog). This mAb blocks co-stimulation by IL-2–like molecules in chicken T-cell supernatants and also reduces the capacity of T-cell blasts to absorb IL-2–like activity from supernatants. It has yet to be determined whether candidate cDNA clones for IL-2Rα encode the molecule recognized by the mAb. Common γ chain (γC) is the signaling subunit of the IL-2, IL-4, IL-7, IL-9, IL-15, and IL-21 receptors; absence of this chain in mammals leads to major defects in lymphocyte development ("boy in the bubble"). A γC homolog was cloned in rainbow trout with unusually high identity (44% to 46%) to mouse/human genes (146). IL-1β, but not LPS, up-regulated the trout gene in macrophage cultures and a fibroblast cell line. Identification of this protein subunit should allow isolation of several fish cytokine receptors.

In summary, similar phenomena described in mammals for IL-2 and IL-2R expression seem to exist in all jawed vertebrates. Future studies will lead not only to an understanding of IL-2 evolution at the structural level, but also insight into the seasonal changes in T-cell stimulation in reptiles, the differential capacity of larval and adult amphibian T cells to produce or respond to T-cell growth factors, and hyperstimulation of T cells in the mutant obese chicken strain.

Interferons

Type I IFN is expressed in leukocytes (IFN-α) and virus-infected fibroblasts (IFN-β) and induces inhibition of viral replication in neighboring cells, as well as molecules of the innate immune system such as iNOS and IRF-1. In contrast, type II IFN (IFN-γ or immune IFN) is synthesized by activated T cells, activates macrophages, and up-regulates class I, class II, immune proteasome subunits, and TAP, and a large number of other genes (R55).

IFN has not been detected in the invertebrates, and in general cellular immunity in the invertebrates has lagged behind the explosion of data on humoral immunity (see below). However, an IFN consensus response element (GAAANN) is found in the promoter of the antibacterial diptericin gene in *Drosophila;* this sequence binds to a 45-kDa protein that cross-reacts with an antiserum specific for mouse IFN regulatory factor I (IRF1), which seems to be specifically expressed in immune tissues such as fat bodies and leukocytes (147). Antiviral activity is detected in supernatants from virally infected fish fibroblasts, epithelial cell lines, and leukocytes.

All of the biochemical properties of mammalian type I IFN (e.g., acid stable, temperature resistant) are present in these fish supernatants, and the putative IFN reduces viral cytopathic effects in homologous cell lines infected with virus, but no cDNA or genomic clones have been identified yet. *In vivo* passive transfer of serum from virally infected fish protects naïve fish from acute viral pathogenesis (R148). Similar activities have been detected in tortoises. In chickens there are up to ten closely related, intronless type I–IFN genes (140). Sequence identity to human type I IFN ranges from 25% to 80% with the apparent functional gene having highest similarity.

Type II IFN, like IL-2, has been difficult to isolate from lower vertebrates. In trout, a macrophage-activating factor (MAF) was identified in ConA-stimulated purified T cells. It induces macrophage phagocytosis, spreading, respiratory burst, and nitric oxide production. Chicken type II IFN, as a T-cell product with potent macrophage activation properties, has been cloned. Whether MAF is identical to type II IFN is unclear, but it is very likely since an antiserum raised to recombinant IFN blocks macrophage activation. The gene is 35% identical to human type II IFN and only 15% identical to chicken type I IFN. Recombinant chicken IFN stimulates nitric oxide production and class II expression by macrophages.

Transforming Growth Factor β

TGF forms a large family with pleiotropic effects in many developmental systems. For the immune system, TGFβ isoforms are best known for their capacity to suppress adaptive immune responses across species barriers, although they can also stimulate lymphocytes under certain conditions (149). TGF-β inhibits macrophage activation in trout and growth of T-cell lines in *Xenopus* species. Trout TGF-β, most similar to mammalian TGF-β1 and TGF-β5 (62% to 66% identity), is expressed in lymphoid tissues and brain, but not in the liver. Two forms of TGF-β were isolated in *Xenopus* species, both of which act on embryonic ectoderm to induce mesoderm. Recombinant *Xenopus* TGF-β, like the mammalian form, also can inhibit IL-2–like dependent growth of splenic lymphoblasts. Four TGFβ isoforms were isolated from chickens, but no functional work has been done with their products. However, recombinant human TGF-β1 inhibits chicken T-cell proliferation (also in trout) and seemingly supports the maturation of suppressor cells.

The isolation of nonmammalian cytokines and cytokine receptor genes has lagged behind molecular characterization of antigen receptors and MHC. Nevertheless, cytokine assay systems in many species and certain disease states, especially in fish and birds, suggest that the majority of vital mammalian cytokines and chemokines will be found in other vertebrates, and soon we will know the structures of all cytokine/chemokine genes in several ectothermic vertebrates. Teleost fish have led the way in analyses of innate responses to viruses, and the general pathways from cell-surface receptor to targets of transcriptional up-regulation will most likely be understood quite soon. We think it will be quite interesting to uncover which cytokines are ancestral to the major branches described here, once genome projects have revealed cytokine families in prochordates and echinoderms; indeed, will molecules related to the pro-inflammatory cytokines and type I interferons be most ancient as anticipated? Furthermore, with the explosion of knowledge concerning chemokines and their receptors, and their roles not only in immune responses but also in lymphoid organ formation, we anxiously await their identification in deuterostomes from ancestors predating the jawed vertebrates. Since chemokine receptors are members of the ancient family of seven transmembrane G-protein coupled receptors, it will be exciting to unravel their phylogenetic relationships to such molecules in animals without adaptive immunity.

Evolution of Hematopoiesis

Antigen-receptor genes rearrange and are expressed in the lymphoid lineage. What is the origin of pathways leading to the emergence of lymphocytes and are they conserved? In vertebrates the lymphocyte development is characterized by ventrolateral mesoderm induction, hematopoietic stem-cell specification, and cell lineage differentiation. Some of the key regulatory steps in this process have been uncovered by studies in mouse, chicken, zebrafish, and *Xenopus*. Evolutionary conservation of several pathways in vertebrates and invertebrates point to fundamental roles of various transcription factors such as FlK-1, Lmo-2, SCl, GATA, FOG (friend of GATA), molecules with the runt domain, PEBP2αA/CBFA1, Ets/Erg, AML, Ikaros, and so on in the control of hematopoiesis (R150). Indeed, homologs of transcription factors involved in vertebrate hematopoiesis even have been discovered in protostomes such as *Drosophila* and *C. elegans*. For instance a cDNA encoding the homolog of mammalian PEBP2α was discovered in *C. elegans* where no functional data are available (PEBP2αA/CBFA1 and PEBP2αB/CBFA2 function in vertebrate osteogenesis and hematopoiesis). The *C. elegans* PEBP2α homolog contains a region that is highly homologous to *Drosophila* runt and lozenge (Lz) and to members of the same family in vertebrates (see below). The hematopoietic functions of several transcription factor homologs have been investigated in *Drosophila* and some conservation in the genetics and principles of blood cell development have been discovered, despite the huge physiologic and phylogenetic differences between fly and vertebrate blood cells (151). In some cases, the conservation extends to the cascade of events leading to the generation of a certain cell type; for example, the two primary classes of hematopoietic cells in *Drosophila* are plasmatocytes/macrophages and crystal cells, and both can be involved in the immune responses of the animals. The *Drosophila* GATA protein Srp (Serpent) is required for the expression of both Lz and Gcm (glial cells missing), themselves required later to specify crystal cells (Gcm) or plasmatocytes and macrophages (Lz). Given the similarities of Srp

and Lz to mammalian GATA and AML1, there seems to be conservation of the pathway (152). In addition, there appears to be two waves of hematopoiesis in flies, much like during embryogenesis in vertebrates: Embryonic hematopoiesis takes place in head mesoderm, whereas larval and then adult hematopoiesis occurs in the larval lymph gland, perhaps the analog of mammalian bone marrow. In addition, embryonic crystal cells do not persist to late larval stages. These observations suggest that, as in the vertebrate system, a second wave of hematopoiesis produces *Drosophila* larval and adult hemocytes. Thus, conservation of the pathway resulting in the macrophage/granulocyte lineages is visible in protostomes, as are some innate immune mechanisms expressed in these cells (see below). In deuterostomes—for example, the sea urchin *Strongylocentrotus purpuratus*—several transcription factors have been cloned although few functional studies have been performed. In addition, a sea urchin runt domain–containing protein has been detected and is expressed in coelomocytes where it is up-regulated upon bacterial challenge (also urchin NFκB), and a GATA factor equally related to GATA1 and GATA3 was cloned and shown to be expressed in coelomocytes (R153).

In summary, transcription factors of the family PAX 2/5/8, GATA 1,2,3, Ets/Erg, and runt domain–containing factors have been cloned in several invertebrates. One plausible model to explain the genesis of true lymphocytes in vertebrates is that closely related members of transcription factor families are the result of relatively late divergence in lineage pathways followed by specialization of duplicated genes. These duplications could be those that apparently occurred during the history of chordates (see MHC Origins section below). Within deuterostomes, the generation of true GATA 2 and 3 probably occurred after echinoderms diverged from the chordate branch and the GATA, Ets, EBF, Pax5-dependent pathways of T/B–cell differentiation are thus specific to vertebrates (R150). Studies in prochordates and cyclostomes should now reveal when the duplications took place. It is already known that lampreys express a member of the purine box 1 (PU.1)/spleen focus-forming virus integration–B (Spi-B) gene family that is critically and specifically involved in jawed vertebrate lymphocyte differentiation (154). Expression has been detected in the gut, which may be related to the fundamental nature of "GALT" as a lymphoid cell-producing organ. In jawed vertebrates, the possibility of screening for lineage-specific mutations and the availability of transgenics in teleost fish (*Danio rerio*) and amphibians (*Xenopus*) should help in understanding lineage-specific gene expression, as well as provide information on the evolution of lymphocyte lineage-determination pathways.

In vertebrates, the generation of T-, B-, and NK-lymphocyte lineages from pluripotent hematopoietic stem cells depends on the early and tissue-specific expression of Ikaros (and related loci), which by means of alternative splicing produces a variety of zinc finger DNA–binding transcription factors. The orthologs of Ikaros, *Aiolos*, *Helios*, and *Eos* have been identified in the chondrichthyan *Raja eglanteria* where two of the four Ikaros family members are expressed in their specialized hematopoietic tissues (epigonal and Leydig organs; see discussion above) like in mammals (155). An Ikaros-related gene has been identified in the lamprey *Petromyzon marinus*, in which neither Ig nor TCRs have been identified. In teleost fish and amphibians Ikaros cDNA from trout and *Xenopus* show roughly 75% amino acid conservation with mammalian Ikaros. In mice and humans, Ikaros produces six alternatively spliced isoforms, but in trout there are two additional novel splice variants expressed early in ontogeny. In trout and zebrafish, as in mammals, Ikaros is a single-copy gene, but in *X. laevis,* Ikaros has been duplicated, most likely a result of polyploidization. The conservation of Ikaros structure and expression reinforces its role as a master switch of hematopoiesis (R156).

RAG and TdT: Lymphocyte Markers

Most models propose that the generation of somatically rearranging receptors occurred abruptly in evolution via the generation of the RAG machinery made of two lymphocyte-specific proteins, RAG1 and RAG2 (see below). Unique to gnathostomes, RAG genes have so far been isolated in all classes of jawed vertebrates excluding reptiles, and have been quite conserved. In every case examined, RAG1 and RAG2 genes are closely linked and in opposite transcriptional orientation. Some regions of RAG1 and RAG2 are similar to bacterial recombinases or to molecules involved in DNA repair (e.g., RAD16), or the regulation of gene expression (such as Rpt-1r). Similarities to prokaryotic proteins and the gene structure suggest that vertebrates acquired the RAG machinery by horizontal transfer and transposition from bacteria; thus, unlike the transcription factors described above, RAG-related genes are unlikely to be found in any invertebrate (R156). Indeed, RAG genetic organization has some transposon characteristics: The RSS are reminiscent of sequences involved in targeting excision of transposons (see below).

Another source of somatic antigen-receptor diversity shared by all gnathostomes characterized to date is a unique DNA polymerase, terminal deoxynucleotidyl transferase (TdT), which diversifies CDR3 during Ig and TCR gene rearrangement through the addition of nucleotides in a template-independent fashion. Furthermore, as detailed above, its expression serves as an unambiguous developmental marker for the sites of lymphopoiesis. TdT has been highly conserved in both sequence (>70% aa similarity, >50 aa identity) and overall structure during vertebrate evolution. An amino-acid alignment of all known TdT sequences reveals that some, but not all, structural motifs believed to be critical for TdT activity are particularly well conserved in chicken, mouse, human, cattle, and trout (100). TdT protein alignments, and the crystal structure for rat β-polymerase, support the hypothesis that both evolved from a common ancestral DNA repair gene. In addition, four protein kinase C–phosphorylation sites are conserved, and hence may be involved in TdT regulation.

Thus, unlike RAG, TdT has evolved by gradual evolution from a polymerase family and was recruited for immune system function.

EVOLUTION OF INNATE IMMUNITY

Of the over 1 million described species of animals (Fig. 1) ~95% are invertebrates representing 33 phyla, some with one species (Placozoa, Cycliophora) and others with over 1 million (Arthropoda). Since they have major differences in body plans, development, size, habitat, and so on, wildly different types of immune systems in diverse species should be expected. Early studies of invertebrate immunology reached no consensus of how immunity should be examined, but because vertebrate immunity was often defined through transplantation reactions, attempts to reveal specific memory by allograft rejection as detailed below was often used. After (mostly failed) attempts to demonstrate memory of such responses in the invertebrates, and after extensive molecular studies, a consensus was reached that an invertebrate adaptive immune system involving somatic generation of antigen receptors and their clonal expression was highly unlikely. Of course, invertebrates may have adaptive systems of different kinds, but without the fine specificity acquired with gene rearrangement/somatic mutation. In contrast, we expect that some characteristics that evolved early in animal evolution will be maintained in the vertebrate lineage. Phagocytosis has long been cited as one example of such conservation, together with several proteins of the acute-phase response and complement cascades (R157). All invertebrate immune responses studied to date are of the innate or nonadaptive type. In innate responses in which memory to a particular antigen does not exist, selection is at the level of species polymorphism and diversity. However, the term "innate" sometimes is too rigid and masks the possibility of other somatic alterations of invertebrate immune system molecules, such as alternate splicing. We classify the invertebrate responses into different phases: (a) cells involved in the responses; (b) recognition molecules; and (c) signaling in the systemic responses to fungi, bacteria, and eukaryotic cells (parasites). We make comparisons to the vertebrates throughout.

Invertebrate Cells

The cell types involved, besides direct interaction with the external layer of cells on the skin, or external teguments, are specialized cells of mesodermal origin devoted to defense. This is true for all coelomates where effector cells have been identified such as sipunculids, annelids, mollusks, arthropods, and all deuterostomes (Fig. 1). The cells can be circulating or sessile, and often are found associated with the gut. In the splanchnopleura of *Drosophila,* there are three cell types: plasmacyte, crystal cells, and lamellocytes. As described above, an understanding of lineage determination is at its beginning stages, but mutations in *Toll* and *cactus* cause abnormal differentiation and hyperproliferation. The conserved JAK/STAT pathway is also involved in the control of hematopoiesis, a further analogy with mammals (R158). Several morphologically distinct hemocyte types in insects cooperate in immune responses: They attach to invading organisms and isolate them, trapping larger organisms in nodules or forming large multicellular capsules around them. Indirect evidence for the role of hemocytes in immune responses can be derived by contrasting properties of such cells in healthy and parasitized animals—that is, modifications in adherence and opsonic activity. In sipunculids, cells resembling NK cells with their granules were seen. Since that report, numerous examples of cells with activities and morphologies similar to CTL or NK cells have been described in invertebrate taxa, such as echinoderms, annelids, and mollusks. As usual (and we cannot state this too strongly), caution regarding analogy versus homology must be exercised when describing these similarities.

Recognition

Initiation of an immune reaction can theoretically involve either the recognition of non-self, altered self, or the absence of self (R3). Non-self recognition can take place with receptors (PRR, pattern-recognition receptors or pattern-recognition molecules) for the so-called pathogen associated molecular patterns (PAMP), which are defined as evolutionarily conserved epitopes expressed by molecules of pathogens but not host cells. The second mode, altered self, is typified by molecules that are induced in self-cells during infections and recognized by conserved defense molecules, similar to the

SOS systems mentioned above (R64). A third mechanism, "Am I still myself," depends on recognition of self-tags and their changes in expression, such as NK recognition of self-MHC molecules through KIR and C-type lectins. These latter two mechanisms have not been described in the invertebrates for immune defense against pathogens, but it would not be surprising if they were revealed in the future. However, NK-like recognition phenomena are found in allorecognition reactions in some invertebrates (and in plants by one well-understood mechanism, as discussed below), which are governed by polymorphic systems that have yet to be analyzed at the molecular level.

Whether the invader is related to an animal host (cells from individuals of the same species or cells from a parasitoid) or are very distant from the host (fungi and bacteria), there are different principles of recognition. Yet PAMP determinants have been identified on very different organisms (sugars such as β1,3 glucan of fungi, LPS and peptidoglycans of bacteria, and phosphoglycan of some parasites) and they can trigger the same cascade of events (R3,R157). The foreign ligand can be bound by a molecule in solution that initiates an effector proteolytic cascade (e.g., clotting or the complement cascade). On the other hand, a proteolytic cascade can be initiated and result in the production of a self-ligand that interacts with a cell-surface receptor. In this way, there need not be a great diversity of cell-surface receptors, an advantage in the absence of clonal selection. The indirect membrane triggering may delay responses but it is economical, and might explain why *Drosophila* Toll receptors do not bind directly to a range of PAMPs, as in mammals (Fig. 15) (see below).

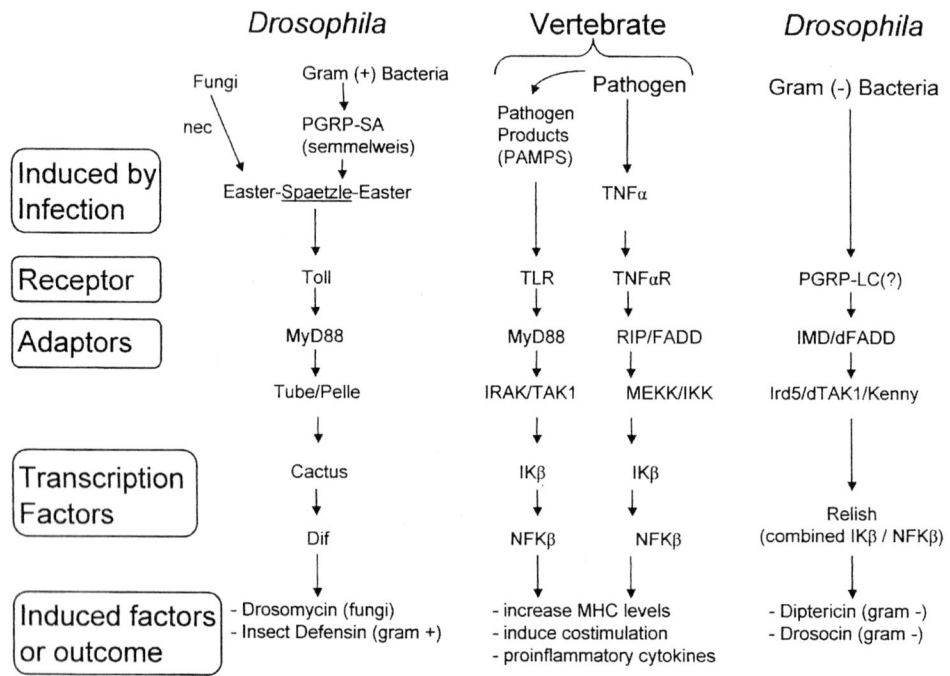

FIG. 15. Evolution of the Toll/TLR pathways in flies and vertebrates. (Only mammals have been analyzed thus far.)

First Line: Defense Molecules, Complement, and Gene Up-regulation

The accumulation of cDNA subtractive libraries following immunizations with pathogens in many animal phyla has shown that species challenged by pathogens respond by enhanced production of many different molecules. This immune response dubbed "nonspecific" by disdainful vertebrate immunologists can be quite complex, diverse, and specific. There are many types of responses and doubtless many more defense mechanisms will be uncovered.

An immediate innate response in annelids results in production of fetidin, a peroxidase-containing protein that is produced by coelomocytes in large amounts following physical challenge. Fetidin, which shows both polymorphism and polylocism, induces the production of massive amounts of lysine in the peritoneal fluid that kills all but self-cells (159). Crustacean (shrimp and crayfish) tissue extracts have activity against DNA viruses and nonenveloped RNA virus, and act during the virus-attachment phase (160). Whether the molecule(s) actually evolved for immune defense is not known, but if not, there should be antiviral activity since there can be 10 billion viral particles/liter of seawater and viral infections are common in Crustaceans (e.g., blue crabs can be infected by rotavirus, enterovirus, Newcastle disease virus, and polioviruses).

Diverse gene families (some with known structures, like the Toll and SRCR discussed below, and others with no recognizable mammalian homologs) are up-regulated in sea urchins. Many other proteins in several invertebrate phyla are involved in cell attachment, hemolysis, nodulation, encapsulation, and agglutination, whether related to an adhesion molecule like Igsf members (hemolin, MDM, FREPs) or not (limunectin, croquemort). Peroxidase-containing molecules tend to form a new group even if the activities of the molecules are quite different from earthworm fetidin described above. Often, and it almost becomes a rule with pathways and molecules involved in defense, they can be involved in development or regeneration. Sometimes the concentration of a defense peptide will increase without gene up-regulation: Crustaceans have an array of molecules with antifungal or antibacterial activities, and in one case shrimp use a respiratory pigment to cleave a peptide from the C-terminal region of hemocyanin, which increases in relative concentration after infection, and adds another function to the already multifunctional crustacean respiratory pigment (161). Finally, defense molecules can differ in body fluid concentration depending on the species examined: The well-conserved complement component C3 is found at very high levels in vertebrate serum, but appears to be absent in quiescent sea urchins until the animals are challenged by injury or infection (see below).

Ig Superfamily

Most invertebrate Ig-like defense molecules have been uncovered in mollusks, arthropods, and echinoderms. Mollusk FREPS (see origins of rearranging receptors section and Figs. 1 and 7 for further information) are proteins found in the hemolymph with an Igsf moiety (one or two V-like domains) and a fibrinogen domain; the level to which they can be induced is not known but they bind to schistosomes, common parasites of mollusks (162). The diversity is remarkable in that there are many polymorphic genes and alternate mRNA splicing within these genes. It is not known which region(s) is the "working end" of FREPS, but the fibrinogen domain can be associated with one of the molecules' extremities as if it could be an effector domain associated with an Igsf recognition domain. A huge diversity is seen within and among individuals that could be explained by somatic variation of some kind (see below).

Pentraxins

Acute-phase proteins like C-reactive protein (CRP) and serum amyloid P (SAP) are induced up to 100- to 1,000-fold within minutes after infection in many vertebrates (but not mice). CRP is highly conserved since homologs exist in many invertebrate taxa (Fig. 1). Vertebrate CRP and SAP are composed of five identical subunits and CRP is the prototype for the small family of pentraxin proteins (R141). CRP was discovered and named in 1930 as a Ca^{++}-dependent immunoprecipitin that bound to the C-polysaccharide of streptococcal capsules and cell walls; however, its binding specificity is confined to the phosphocholine (PC) group (SAP has a higher affinity for phosphoethanolamine, and its physiologic function may be to clear cellular debris following cell death). Conserved biological activities of CRP are consistent with its role as an effector of innate host resistance, since it shares with IgG and mannose-binding lectin (MBL) (see discussion below) the abilities to activate complement and enhance phagocytosis. Several horseshoe crab (*Limulus*) CRPs have been identified (R163), but although the binding specificities seem similar to the vertebrate version, their structures are different from the pentagonal rings seen in the vertebrates.

Lectins

We are only now starting to appreciate the diverse roles lectins play, not only in defense, but also in the homeostasis of immune systems (R164). Lectins can also be acute-phase proteins that recognize pathogen-specific carbohydrates. These molecules are conserved in many phyla, even though their structure and the number of binding sites can vary. Most lectins isolated from marine invertebrates are calcium-dependent lectins (C-type lectins) and form the most abundant family. A common lectin in all phyla is the galactoside-binding lectin family (galectins), which has several protein architectures and is involved in many physiologic processes besides defense (R141,R164). They can be found either in the plasma or on the hemocyte surface, and can be induced upon infection. Lectins can be involved in direct effector functions such as lysis or agglutination, in triggering of proteolytic cascades (e.g., see complement), or in opsonization.

Defensins

Each phylum, including Vertebrata, produces a variety of molecules with intrinsic antimicrobial activity. Some families can be conserved but usually they diverge rapidly and orthologous relationships are not apparent (R165). (Numerous reviews are available at *http://www.bbcm.univ.trieste.it/~tossi/pag4.htm#uno.*) The best-studied group of antimicrobials are the defensins, which are amphipathic cationic proteins; their positively charged surface allows them to associate with negatively charged membranes (more common in pathogens), and a hydrophobic surface that allows them to disrupt the membranes (either by disordering lipids or actually forming pores). Most of the molecules are proteins, but an antimicrobial lipid called squalamine, which also is modeled to have hydrophobic and positively charged surfaces, is found at very high levels in dogfish body fluids (166). Defensins can either be constitutively expressed, such as in respiratory epithelia in mammals, or inducible (e.g., see below for *Drosophila*). Certain responses that seem systemic like the production of *Drosophila* defensins can also take place locally in the damaged tissues themselves; otherwise, a systemic response is initiated in organs distant from the site of infection such as the fat body in *Drosophila* where induction of bactericidal peptides takes place.

Defensins are the focus of great attention in commercially bred species such as oysters, mussels, and crustaceans, and it is hoped that they will be applied to medicine whether they are derived from invertebrates or from vertebrates. Although they diverge rapidly, two members of the insect defensin family of antibacterial peptides have been found in mollusks, indicating that mollusk and arthropod defensins have a common ancestry, but the presence of two extra cysteines and of one modified amino acid in the mollusk protein suggest that it is a previously unknown member of that family (167). Located most of the time in different subtypes of circulating hemocytes, defensins and mytilins can be expressed in the same cell, and even in the same granule.

Scavenger receptors. The initial phase of an innate immune response (especially in the absence of adaptive immunity) might require a vast diversity of receptors. Within 6 hours after bacterial injection, sea urchin coelomocytes up-regulate a variety of genes including a very diverse family of scavenger receptors cysteine-rich (SRCR). An outstanding number of ~1,200 genes are present, but each individual may express different groups of SRCR genes at different levels (with differential splicing!). To assume that they are all involved in defense is premature, since SRCR genes can be both up- and down-regulated after infection with bacteria (168). In mammals, the scavenger-receptor family as a whole is also poorly defined but is involved in endocytosis, phagocytosis, and adhesion, and some members acts as PRR that bind to LPS or other bacterial components. One mammalian SRCR (gp340) is secreted into the saliva where it binds streptococci and heli-

cobacter. Molecules with scavenger domains and serine protease domains have been cloned in insects and are produced by hemocytes; in *Anopheles* such a protein, sp22d, does not bind to bacteria but rather to chitin and is only slightly up-regulated after bacterial injection (169).

Proteolytic Cascades

Proteolytic cascades are initiated immediately following interaction of foreign material bound by preformed proteins in solution, and this principle is conserved throughout evolution. Indeed, the proteolytic cascade upstream of production of the Toll ligand spaetzle (see below) resembles the complement or clotting cascades. The prophenoloxidase cascade of arthropods leading to melanization and the genesis of antibacterial products is another example in which peptidoglycans on microbial surfaces initiate the cascade resulting in the degranulation of hemocytes.

The best-studied immune proteolytic cascade that is (perhaps) surprisingly well conserved in the animal kingdom is complement (Fig. 16). In contrast to the other defense molecules that we have discussed, orthologous complement genes can be detected in all of the deuterostomes without a great deal of expansion/contraction of the gene family (R170,R171). The three major functions of complement in jawed vertebrates are: (a) coating of pathogens to promote uptake by phagocytes (opsonization); (b) initiation of inflammatory responses by stimulating smooth muscle contraction, vasodilation, and chemoattraction of leukocytes; and (c) lysis of pathogens via membrane disruption (Fig. 16) (see Chapter 34). The focal point of complement is C3, which lies at the intersection of the alternative, classical, and lectin pathways of complement activation. It is the only known immune recognition molecule (besides its homolog C4) that makes a covalent bond with biologic surfaces. C3 has a nonspecific recognition function and it interacts with many other proteins, including proteases, opsonic receptors, complement activators, and inhibitors. In the alternative pathway, C3 apparently exposes its thioester bond in solution, and in the presence of host cell surfaces lacking regulatory proteins that stop C3 in its tracks (by cleaving it into iC3b), it associates with the protease factor B (B). After binding to C3, B becomes susceptible to cleavage by the spontaneously active factor D, resulting in formation of the active protease Bb that in combination with the covalently attached C3 cleaves many molecules of C3 in an amplification step (Fig. 16). Another nonadaptive recognition system, the lectin pathway, starts with the mannose-binding lectin (MBL), which is a PRR of the collectin family that binds mannose residues on the surface of pathogens and can act as an opsonin (172). MBL is analogous to C1q with its high-avidity binding to surfaces by multiple interaction sites through globular C-terminal domains, but apparently it is not homologous to C1q. Like C1q, which associates with the serine proteases C1r and C1s, the MASP proteases (MBL-associated serine proteases) physically interact with MBL and not only activate the classical pathway of complement by splitting of C4 and C2 (the same function as C1s; MASP2

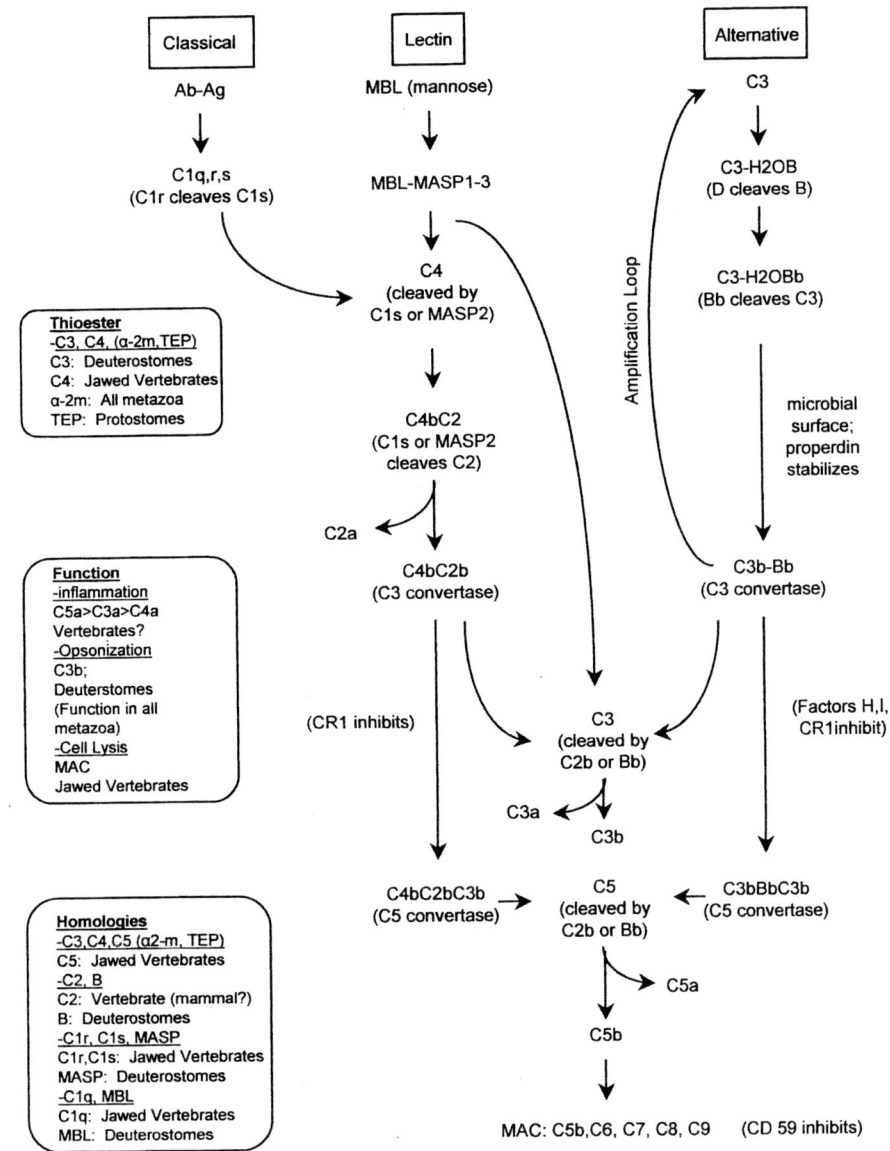

FIG. 16. The three major pathways of complement activation and the presence of various features of complement in the metazoa.

appears to be the active protease), but also can activate the alternative pathway in ways that are not understood and thus completely bypass the classical pathway (Fig. 16). Indeed, MASP-1 and -2 are homologs of C1r and C1s. Both C1q and MBL can be involved in promoting the uptake of apoptotic bodies by pahagocytes via receptors that remain elusive. Finally, the classical pathway, which is dependent on antibody molecules bound to a surface, results in the same potential effector outcomes described above for the alternative pathway. Novel molecules initiating this pathway are C1q, C1r, C1s, C4, and C2, as well as specific negative regulatory proteins.

C3 and MBL are vital players in the immediate innate immune response in vertebrates, and both have been described in nonvertebrate deuterostomes (R170). Thus far, the best-studied invertebrate systems for investigation of C3 evolution are the sea urchin and the ascidians *Halocynthia* and *Ciona*, in which C3 and B molecules and genes have been analyzed

in some detail. In contrast to the very high levels of C3 found in the plasma of jawed vertebrates, sea urchin C3 is not expressed at high levels but is induced in response to infection in coelomocytes (173). The C3 opsonic function clearly has been identified, but so far initiation of inflammatory or lytic responses (if they exist) has not been obvious. Receptors involved in the opsonization in echinoderms have not been identified, but in the ascidian gene fragments related to the C3 integrin–receptor CR3 were identified, and antisera raised to one of the receptors inhibited C3-dependent opsonization (174).

Hagfish and lamprey C3-like genes were thought to be ancestral C3/C4 genes because the sequence predicts two processing sites (leading to a three-chain molecule), like C4, but a C3-like properdin-binding site is clearly present. However, like C3 in other animals the hagfish protein is composed of only two chains of 115 and 72 kDa, and sea urchin and ascidian C3 sequences predict only two chains (one prote-olytic processing site). The lamprey, but not sea urchin or ascidian C3, has a recognizable C3a fragment known from mammals to be involved in inflammation, so complement's role in inflammation may be a vertebrate invention. Thioester-containing proteins (TEPs) were isolated from *Drosophila* and the mosquito *Anopheles* (175). While the molecules function in a C3-like fashion in mosquitoes (opsonization), phylogenetic analysis does not show them to be more related to C3 or α2-macroglobulin. Nevertheless, regardless of the lack of orthology, it is likely that the capacity for defense molecules to make covalent bonds with pathogens and then induce uptake by phagocytic cells is an ancient function pre-dating the protostome/deuterostome ancestor. In jawed verte-brates, both teleost and cartilaginous fish can have more than one C3 gene, suggesting that the innate system might com-pensate in animals that do not optimally exploit their adaptive immune system. Changes in the amino-acid composition of the C3-binding site are found that may somehow regulate the types of surfaces bound by the different isotypes (R170).

Like Ig/TCR/MHC, the classical pathway appears first in cartilaginous fish. However, since MBL can activate the clas-sical pathway in mammals it is possible that some portion of this pathway exists in prejawed vertebrates. Nevertheless, C4 and C2 genes have not been detected to date in jawless fish or invertebrates. Furthermore a *bona fide* C2 homolog has not been identified in nonmammalian vertebrates, al-though duplicate B genes were isolated from cartilaginous fish, teleost fish, and amphibians, and thus may function both in the classical and alternative pathways (176). The lytic pathway, with the formation of the membrane attack com-plex (MAC) initiated by the cleavage of C5 into C5a and C5b, also has not been described in taxa older than cartilagi-nous fish. Thus, opsonization and perhaps the induction of inflammatory responses were the primordial functions of the lectin/complement pathways. However, one should remain open-minded, as a cDNA clone for CD59, a molecule that inhibits MAC formation in self-cells, was identified from a hagfish library (177), and an *Amphioxus* EST with homol-ogy to C6 was isolated recently (178). We are still in for surprises.

C3, C4, C5, and α2m are members of the same small fam-ily. The protease inhibitor α2m, clearly present in inverte-brates (protostomes and deuterostomes) and vertebrates, is thought to be the oldest, but this must be viewed with cau-tion (R179). Along with its ubiquitous ability to bind to and inactivate proteases of all known specificities through a "bait region," it has been shown to be opsonic as well in some sit-uations. Given that α2m, C3, and C4 have internal thioester sites, this feature is primordial; C5 subsequently lost the site. The first divergence probably occurred between α2m and C3, with C5 and then C4 emerging later in the jawed verte-brates (180). Consistent with the vertebrate polyploidization scheme is the fact that C3, C4, and C5 genes are located on three of the four previously described paralogous clusters in mammals (Fig. 12), and this is also fits with the absence of classical (no antibody) and lytic (no MAC) pathways in phyla

older than cartilaginous fish (R170). α2m is encoded at the border of the NK complex in mice and human, and there are some tantalizing similarities between these regions and the other MHC paralogues (see below). The C3a and C5a recep-tors that promote the inflammatory responses upon comple-ment activation have so far only been identified in mammals; they are G-protein coupled receptors whose genes are also found on the Kasahara paralogues (C3aR, Chr 12p13; C5aR, Chr 19q13) (Fig. 11).

Phagocytosis

To obtain phagocytosis at the site of microorganism inva-sion implies recruitment of cells via chemoattraction (R157). In vertebrates this can be done by several categories of molecules such as chemokines like IL-8 or the complement fragments C3a and C5a. As mentioned above, a C3a fragment as we know from mammals is not found in nonvertebrates, but perhaps C3 is cleaved in different ways in the invertebrates. C3b, MBL, and many other lectins can function as opsonins, and further studies of invertebrate defense molecules will cer-tainly add to this list. Ingestion follows phagocytosis, and then killing occurs by an oxidative mechanism with the production of reactive oxygen radicals and nitric oxide. These mecha-nisms are conserved in phylogeny, for instance, in lamelli-branch mollusks where it has been demonstrated after incu-bation of hemocytes with PMA, or during phagocytosis of yeast in gastropods, in which nitric oxide is involved in the killing of schistosome sporocysts. Unique to mammals and presumably all jawed vertebrates, the activation of phago-cytes also leads to up-regulation of the antigen-processing machinery, co-stimulatory molecules, and pro-inflammatory cytokines that can enhance adaptive immunity (Fig. 14).

Signaling

Three pathways of innate immunity triggering have con-served elements in the plant and animal kingdoms (Fig. 15): the Toll/TLR–like receptor pathway, the TNFα/IMD recep-tor pathway, and the intracellular Nod pathway. Although Toll receptors have been found in all triploblastic coelomates, most of the work and the elucidation of pathways has been accomplished in *Drosophila* because of the well-known ad-vantages of the model; Toll was originally discovered for its role in fly embryonic development (181). In *C. elegans,* the homologs do not seem to be involved in defense. In mol-lusks (oyster), a component of the signalosome leading to NFκB activation has been cloned, which possesses the char-acteristic organization of mammalian IKK proteins; when transfected into human cell lines, oyster IKK activated the expression of NFκB-controlled reporter gene. The diversity of peptides that can be produced via the Toll/IMD pathways is substantial, and is classified in several categories depending upon the type of pathogen that is recognized (e.g., gram posi-tive, drosocin; gram negative, diptericin; fungal, drosomycin) with different effector functions (R182). *Drosophila* antimi-crobial molecules, originally discovered by Hans Boman and colleagues in 1981 (183), heralded the molecular analyses of innate immunity in invertebrates. It seems amazing that an animal living just a few days has these sophisticated mechanisms. Perhaps it illustrates the danger of trusting only an innate immune system: This may be sufficient with ten peptides and four major pathways in *Drosophila*, but in long-lived vertebrates a combinatorial system may have been required. Long-lived invertebrates would be interesting to study in detail for novel adaptive and innate mechanisms.

Toll and IMD Pathways

Invertebrate toll receptors are homologous to the Toll-like receptors (TLR) of mammals (see Chapter 17 and Fig. 15) in the sense that they are integral membrane proteins with an external leucine-rich repeat-binding region (R157,R182). *Drosophila* Toll is activated after it binds spaetzle, the product of a proteolytic cascade activated in solution after the interaction of molecules produced by fungi or gram-positive bacteria with soluble PRR. The TIR cytoplasmic domain of the Toll receptor then interacts with MyD88 (itself having a TIR domain) followed by Tube and Pelle, leading to activation of the homologous NFκB system (Cactus or Diff) that then induces transcription of various defense peptides. This is remarkably similar to the cascade of events following activation of mammalian Toll-like receptors (TLR), where after their interaction with PAMPs at the cell surface, a cascade is induced through TLR including MyD88, IRAK, TRAF, and TAK1, to NFκB via the IKK signalosome (Fig. 13). Thus, infection-induced Toll activation in *Drosophila* and TLR-dependent activation in mammals reveal a common ancestry in primitive coelomates, in which defense genes under the control of a common signaling pathway lead to activation of Rel family transactivators. However, in *Drosophila* the recognition events take place in solution via the PRR, followed by zymogen cascades ending in the proteolysis that produces spaetzle that binds Toll; in mammals each of nine different TLR apparently recognize (with or without co-receptors?) different microbial epitopes directly, like a family of germline-encoded receptors. The phylogenetic history of different Toll receptors in the different phyla also suggests independent emergence of the two groups of families, probably due to their different specializations (184).

Because *Drosophila* Toll/vertebrate TLR are similar in some respects to the mammalian IL1R, and the cascade leading to NFκB activation is also similar in flies and vertebrates, Toll/TLR bridges the immune systems of protostomes and vertebrates and has raised much interest in evolutionary biology. There is less conservation of pathways than of elements when one compares the pathways implicating Toll/TIR in plants and animals. To date the only similarity in plants and animals is the TIR domain (R157), which binds to a cytosolic molecule similar to MyD88; the closest plant analog is Pto, which is actually downsteam in the activation cascade (pto requires binding to the pathogen product as well as interaction with an NB-LRR without TIR domain called Prf). It may or may not be linked to an NFκB cascade. The diversity of the

plant molecules is enormous, since the defense system was originally found for plant resistance (R) genes in which there is a one-to-one relationship between molecules produced by pathogens and the plant receptors (185).

The IMD pathway is employed for *Drosophila* responses to gram-negative bacteria (Fig. 15). After interaction with a newly characterized cell-surface receptor (the pattern-recognition receptor PGRP-LC), in a cascade similar to the mammalian TNFαR signaling pathway, *Drosophila* Tak1, an IKK signalosome, and a Relish-mediated (instead of Diff) NFκB step, results in transcription of antibacterial peptides like diptericin. The *Drosophila* intracellular pathway is like the mammalian TNFα receptor cascade, which also progresses via a death domain Mekk3, the signalosome, and NFκB resulting in cytokine production. In both cases, a link to pathways leading to programmed cell death is possible; overexpression of *Drosophila* IMD leads to apoptosis. When the activation of either the fly Toll or IMD pathway is considered, they are analogous to a mammalian cytokine/cytokine receptor system (e.g., TNFα) in which a soluble self-molecule activates cells via a surface receptor (illustrated in Fig. 15).

NOD proteins (intracellular nucleotide binding plus leucine-rich repeat proteins [NB-LRR]) are in a third category of recognition molecules involved in innate immunity in animals and plants (R3,R157). They have an N-terminal CARD domain, followed by a nucleotide-binding domain (NBD) and leucine-rich repeat (LRR). As described above for plants, NOD binds its ligand intracellularly, and the CARD domain associates with a kinase (RIP2) that activates the NFκB/MAP kinase cascade. In mammals, NOD2 mutants lead to the potential for Crohn's Disease, a chronic inflammatory bowel disease.

The diversity of external recognition systems is not matched by an equivalent diversity of intracellular signaling pathways. There are a few signaling cascades and those are connected to the receptors, giving the impression of conservation of the innate immunity pathways. But these pathways are also used in development (for developmental pathways spaetzle binds Toll, but it is proteolytically generated by a different set of enzymes), and which is primordial is an open question. It is a common exploitation of a well-designed and probed tool, like the Vostok rocket of the Soviet Union. The NFκB conservation is clearly one example, although it does not exist in all species. *C. elegans* lacks it but do all members of its phylum?

Recognition of Parasites and Parasitoids

Because most attention has been focused on Toll pathways, virtually nothing is known about how invertebrates recognize eukaryotic invaders. For example, endoparasitoids within insects are more closely related to their hosts than are fungi or bacteria, and the host may use "hidden self"–recognition molecules to attack foreign material coming through the open circulatory system (R186). Is this a connection to mechanisms involved in allorecognition or vice versa? Still, the melanization pathways are induced. With distantly related individuals the same Toll cascade can be triggered by different organisms provided that they have certain surface carbohydrates. Insects resist parasitoids by encapsulation and, like in plants, the ability to encapsulate depends on one major gene for each parasite, except that the two genes discovered to influence encapsulation of *Leptopilina* and *Asobara* are not members of a cluster like the R genes of plants (R187). No correlation was found between the humoral response of the fly and its cellular immunity against the parasite.

Allorecognition

When one thinks of the pressures to develop an immune system, the necessity to prevent invasion by microorganisms and parasites first comes to mind. There are other pressures. In some ancient categories of invertebrates (many marine metazoa such as Porifera and Cnidaria) or in the more recent Tunicates, the possibility of fusion or contamination with cells from other members of one's own species may have exerted a strong pressure to develop mechanisms to resist such invasions (R188). This pressure seems to have disappeared within vertebrates, but in metazoan phylogeny it might have been a key factor to build up "immune systems" of which remnants may have survived long enough to participate in the elaboration of modern systems. There is an almost universal occurrence of allorecognition followed by "rejection"; in most cases the genetics and mechanisms of rejection are unknown. Certainly these mechanisms are at work in sponges, Cnidarians, Bryozoans, Echinoderms, and Ascidians. Less sure are studies of Nemerteans, where in the absence of allorecognition, xenorecognition has been studied and shown to involve effector cells of mesoderm origin, or in arthropods where possibilities of transplantation exist across genera. As mentioned above, for some time the hypothesis of the conservation of a specific adaptive immune system across the animal kingdom encouraged experiments on allograft rejection in invertebrates. It is no wonder that in the golden age of transplantation studies in mammals, when the adaptive immunity aspects of graft rejection were being discovered, that one thought similar phenomena would be encountered in the invertebrates (R189). Now that this hypothesis has been abandoned because of the paucity of evidence for specific memory, there are nevertheless interesting phenomena. In all living organisms from plants to vertebrates, highly polymorphic loci are associated with mechanisms of recognition. Perhaps the vertebrate MHC and the self-incompatibility (S locus) in flowering plants (see below) are the best-known examples at the molecular level of extreme allelic polymorphism maintained by frequency-dependent selection.

We do not know whether allorecognition mechanisms in the great range of invertebrates might be molecularly related, but at least in distantly related phyla they are almost certainly due to convergence. The situation is clearly different from the vertebrate MHC, but the analogy between histocompatibility loci in invertebrates and vertebrates remains intellectually challenging. In no case does the phenomenon outside of vertebrates lead to an adaptive response with specific memory. Doubt remains in some cases (190), and given the surprisingly diverse families of receptors and the surprising individual variations in local cellular or systemic responses it is likely that new mechanisms will be uncovered. The polymorphism of the recognized structure is always enormous, compatible with a self-recognition rather than a non–self-recognition model (with caveats, as discussed below). Many hypotheses have been put forward to explain the polymorphism. This type of "immune system" could be selected to maintain heterosis and linked to mate selection; other mechanisms will then be used against pathogens.

What is puzzling is that there are only one or few loci per species that achieve this great level of polymorphism. In other words, functionally speaking these animals utilize a major histocompatibility locus or complex, much more so than the jawed vertebrates! Yet certainly the effector mechanisms or even the substrates of the polymorphism are not the same when the surface molecules have been identified. There is an evolutionary strategy in common. In all cases, revealing the different recognition mechanisms will be important to understand co-evolution of the polymorphism and its effector mechanism. Unfortunately, molecular mechanisms have not been simple to dissect for the histocompatibility reactions in the prochordate *Botryllus* (R188), or cnidarians *Hydra* and *Hydractinia* (191) genetic models that have been studied for a many years (see below). Similarly in corals effector phenomena (now understandable as induced-apoptosis) take place following recognition but the nature of the highly polymorphic determinant (dozens of alleles) remains unknown (190). The apoptotic events and the first genes to be up-regulated during the response are now being examined.

Species-specific cell recognition in sponges is mediated by supramolecular proteoglycan-like complexes called "aggregation factors." A surprising characteristic of sponges, considering their phylogenetic position, is that they possess such a sophisticated histocompatibility system. Grafting between two different individuals (allograft) is almost invariably incompatible in the many species investigated, exhibiting a variety of transitive qualitatively and quantitatively different responses, which can only be explained by the existence of a highly polymorphic gene system (192). Individual variability of protein and glycan components in the aggregation factor of the red beard sponge, *Microciona prolifera,* matches the elevated sponge alloincompatibility, suggesting an involvement of the cell adhesion system in sponge allogeneic reactions and, therefore, an evolutionary relationship between cell adhesion and histocompatibility systems. Cell adhesion molecules are often members of the Ig superfamily and a bridge with molecules used in the vertebrate immune system is possible (192). Indeed, there are such polymorphic molecules on the surface of sponge cells but the relationship to allorecognition events (if one exists) is not established. Similar events may take place in sponges like *Geodia.* Interestingly, in this sponge polymorphic Igsf I- and V-set domains have been identified but their functions are not known (193).

One of the most informative models is the diploblastic cnidarian *Hydractinia,* where the genetics of histocompatibility are well understood. Using animals inbred for fusibility, Mokady and Buss (191) employed a standard back-cross/intercross analysis, which revealed that allorecognition is controlled by a single co-dominant Mendelian locus (ARL, allorecognition locus) such that colonies fuse when they share one or two alleles; such rules of histocompatibility are also found in the prochordates (see below). This model should allow the identification of the locus responsible for the incompatibility reaction. The effector phase involves the growth of hyperplastic stolons and the use of nematocysts, which should be amenable to functional and biochemical approaches (191).

In deuterostomes, the model originally developed by Oka and Watanabe (194) in the tunicate *Botryllus,* a colonial ascidian, is also quite interesting. In this polymorphic system, it was originally believed that recognition of polymorphic self-markers turned off a destructive response between colonies, as described above for NK-cell recognition (R3,R64). However, there may be weak reactions to allo; thus the situation is not so simple. What attracted extra attention was the discovery that the locus controlling histocompatibility was linked to or was the same locus as that controlling fertilization by preventing self-fertilization; in this case the sperm must be genetically disparate from the egg. This fertilization reaction has been studied recently in a solitary ascidian, with the suggestion that some features of the process may be related to MHC evolution (195). The great complexity of self–non-self recognition alleles involved in fertilization, and the involvement of an Hsp70 and the proteasome in processing self-sterility factors, suggested to the authors that the reproductive mechanisms might be evolutionarily related to the vertebrate immune system. We are waiting for the smoke to clear.

The prevention of self-fertilization has also evolved several times in the plant kingdom. In one case, the molecular mechanism for the phenomenon has been elucidated in study of the highly polymorphic self-recognition (S) locus of crucifers (R196). Genes encoding transmembrane-receptor Ser/Thr kinases called SRK (S-locus receptor protein kinase) are expressed in the stigma and closely linked to genes for soluble SCR (S-locus cysteine-rich) proteins expressed by pollen. Both genes are highly polymorphic, and if a self-SCR is recognized by an SRK, pollen tube growth and hence self-fertilization is inhibited. SRKs are members of a plant gene family that have been recruited for this purpose, and the SCRs have structural similarities to the amphipathic defensins described above; thus, perhaps molecules involved in microbial pattern recognition were co-opted for this new purpose. Here, two very different linked genes must co-evolve, in ways not understood, within each haplotype to ensure mutual binding of the self-gene products. Thus, while similar mechanisms at the genetic and population levels described above (e.g., balancing selection, ancient allelic lineages, co-evolution of linked genes, etc.) are operational for S locus,

MHC, and other recognition systems, clearly pressures can co-opt wildly different types of gene families for involvement in the recognition events. Working out molecular details of many allorecognition systems may shed new light on the sometimes unexpected relationships between apparently unrelated fields of research such as mating preference, kin recognition, olfactory receptors, and MHC.

ORIGINS OF ADAPTIVE IMMUNITY

The immune system of vertebrates is unique because the antigen-specific receptor expressed by lymphocytes, which initiates cascades leading to activation of the adaptive immune system, is not the product of a complete germline-inherited gene. Rather, receptors are generated somatically during lymphocyte ontogeny from gene segments scattered at a particular locus. As described above, the receptors are members of the immunoglobulin superfamily (Igsf) composed of variable (V) and constant (C) domains, with the C domains being of the rare "C1" type, which is shared by MHC class II and class I molecules (R7).

There are many specific questions, such as the following: (a) Did MHC class I or class II come first? (b) What is the origin of the MHC PBR? (c) Was the MHC involved with innate immunity before the emergence of adaptive immunity? (d) Did somatic rearrangement or somatic mutation come first to diversify antigen receptors? (e) Which of the extant antigen receptors, α/β TCR, γ/δ TCR, or IgH/L (if any) resembles the primordial receptor? The answers to these questions will always remain speculative, but deductions can be made based upon the wealth of genetic data accrued over the past few years. We base many of our arguments on the large-scale duplications that were noticed for MHC by Kasahara in 1996 (88) (Fig. 12). There is great controversy as to whether the paralogous regions arose via the Ohno-esque genome-wide duplications (197), but the remarkable syntenies of paucicopy genes on the paralogous regions, and the recent finding that an animal that predated the duplications (*Amphioxus*) has only single copy genes in the same syntenic group orthologous to the four mammalian copies (91), makes it incontrovertible that at least *en bloc* duplications were involved. Further analysis of this region in *Amphioxus* and other deuterostomes will begin to answer at least the first three questions above. Genetic analyses in protostome lineages have not been very informative, but we must have a second look once we piece together data from the deuterostomes.

MHC Origins

Class I and class II molecules have been found only on the jawed vertebrates. Based on phylogenetic analyses (58,R59) and thermodynamic arguments (198), most investigators believe that class II preceded class I in evolution. However, as stated above, class I is much more plastic than class II, as there are many different types of class I molecules, including some that do not even bind to peptides. Since class I genes are on two or three MHC paralogues, and they can have functions outside the immune system, this is evidence that the primordial "PBR" may not have even bound to anything. If this is true, and since class I and class II do bind peptides, it would suggest class I arose first. Again, genome scans of jawless fish and deuterostomes should be informative on this point.

From the paralogue data, genes encoding the complement components C3 and B, TNFSF members, the signaling molecule Vav, and proteasome subunits among other genes should have been present in the proto-MHC before emergence of the adaptive immune system (Fig. 12). Some of these genes were found in the *Amphioxus* "MHC" linkage groups (91), and C3 and B genes are linked in the sea urchin (R153). A fifth paralogous region on human Chr 12p13 contains the α2-macroglobulin gene (recall the C3/4/5 homolog), a tapasin homolog, the C3a receptor, and this "complex" is linked to the natural-killer cell complex (NKC). Taken together, the data suggest that the proto MHC included vital nonhomologous genes of the innate immune system, which perhaps were linked to allow coordinate regulation of expression. After the *en bloc* duplications, Abi et al. (R199) have suggested that "functional restraints upon the complex were relaxed," and hence the duplicated members could evolve new functions, including features indispensable to the adaptive system. If indeed innate immunity genes were already linked to allow up-regulation at times of infection, it is no surprise that the adaptive immune system piggybacked on such a gene complex. A final point: Why did the duplicate genes survive rather well over hundreds of millions of years? Cis duplicates have been shown to degenerate rapidly over evolutionary time (200). Evidence suggests that duplicates arising from polyploidy (and by inference, large *en bloc* duplications) survive better than cis duplicates, most likely because they cannot be inactivated by unequal crossovers; the ability of the genes to survive over very long periods, perhaps combined with strong selection pressures, would allow for subspecialization (201).

Origins of Rearranging Receptors

Rearranging Machinery

Somatic rearrangement is dependent on RAG1 and RAG2 enzymes, found only in jawed vertebrates and with no close relatives in other deuterostomes; all putative homologs among DNA-associated enzymes in other animal phyla are only distantly related to RAG. It seems that a "horizontal" acquisition of a RAG-laden transposon occurred at some point during the history of the vertebrates (R156,202). The structure of the receptor gene itself, in the region where rearrangements occur, suggests the introduction of a transposon. Recombination signal sequences (RSS) flanking the rearranging gene segments (e.g., V and J for L chains) are reminiscent of LTRs in a transposon. The lack of introns in most RAG genes is another sign of prokaryotic origins. In principle, RAG activity is confined

to lymphocytes but the existence of germline rearrangements of shark Ig genes suggests that RAG can remain an active force, modifying the genome in some vertebrates. As the enzyme itself is not so informative for phylogenetic analysis of origins of the adaptive immune system (197), one must turn to the history of the substrate, that is, the VC Igsf domains (see below). Introduction of RAG genes from a unicellular organism would be a unique example of a modification of the primordial immune system by horizontal transfer. In this case, microorganisms that interacted with ancestral vertebrates would not simply select the variation coming from the inside of the species on which it exerts its pressure, but it would introduce a new source of variation in the immune system. One must think of the cellular lineage in which somatic rearrangement was introduced. Such a dangerous innovation could not be tolerated under conditions where it would be ubiquitously expressed since it might jeopardize the whole genome. Most likely the introduction into a gene was expressed in a lymphoid cell lineage where a mistake would not threaten the whole individual (perhaps one that already was part of an adaptive immune system governed by somatic hypermutation; see below). Another scenario postulates that RAG was inactive until specific factors coevolved to permit lymphocyte-specific expression. The discovery that neighboring RAG1 and RAG2 genes are controlled by a single switch in a small piece of DNA next to one end of the RAG2 gene may explain why, over the 450 million years since the genes first appeared, they have remained closely linked. What was important is that the original transposon became under the control of regulatory regions active in only one cell type. Perhaps there were several "attempts" at transposition in evolution resulting in catastrophes or in other activities such as translocation or deletions. An ideal candidate would be a locus control region regulating expression of activating receptors with VC1 domains in NK-like cells, perhaps in the proto MHC. The MHC paralogous region described above near the NKC on Chr 12p13 and could be derived from the ancestral gene complex. In the same way as RAG1/2 genes remain linked because of regulatory elements close to RAG2, an NK cell–specific region under the control of a regulatory region might have controlled expression of a set of genes.

Rearrangement or Somatic Hypermutation First?

Since all antigen-receptor genes use somatic rearrangement of V genes to generate diversity in CDR3 regions as well as to promote combinatorial diversity, there is no doubt that this mechanism is at the heart of adaptive immunity (202). Indeed, as described, most investigators believe that the introduction of the tranposable element into a V gene was *the* driving force in the abrupt appearance of vertebrate adaptive immunity. However, it cannot be overemphasized that somatic hypermutation is also at the origins of the immune system (203); furthermore, all evidence to date suggests a gradual evolution of the hypermutation machinery rather than the "hopeful monster" generated by the famous RAG transposon (135,204). Thus, diversity generated via mutation may have existed in an adaptive immune system prior to rearrangement, and V-gene rearrangement was superimposed onto this already existing system. Perhaps it is no accident that the one gene discovered so far to be indispensable for somatic hypermutation, AID (activation-induced deaminase), is encoded smack-dab in the aforementioned Chr 12p13 region (204). If mutation indeed preceded rearrangement, we may find examples of it today in extant prochordates and invertebrates.

Which Antigen Receptor First?

Phylogenetic analyses have suggested that a γ/δ TCR-like ancestor may have predated α/β TCR and Ig H/L. This would suggest that direct antigen recognition, perhaps by a cell-surface receptor, arose first in evolution followed by a secreted molecule and an MHC-restricted one (205). Glusman et al. (206) argue that phylogenetic analyses over such large evolutionary distances obscure true relationships among the antigen-receptor genes (e.g., the relationships of the molecules in the phylogenetic trees have to impose multiple loss/gain of D segments in the various antigen-receptor families), and suggest a model based on genomic organization. They propose an alternative phylogeny in which an ancestral chromosomal region with linked genes encoding both chains of an ancestral antigen-receptor heterodimer, one having D segments and one not. One en bloc duplication gave rise to the Ig and TCR divergence, and a second to the α/β and γ/δ TCR gene complexes. The α and δ loci are still closely linked in all vertebrates analyzed (human Chr 14), and a pericentric inversion is suggested to have separated the TCR β and γ loci (linked on human Chr 7). This model predicts that D segments only emerged once, and also explains the existence of inverted V elements in the TCR β and δ loci. This model does not predict which antigen receptor is oldest, but does provide a simple view of receptor evolution, consistent with the Kasahara model (88,R199).

For the origin of the rearranging receptors, Igsf lineages have to be traced back through phylogeny since receptors generated by somatic rearrangement do not exist outside the jawed vertebrates. In a quest for molecules related to ancestors, without focusing on genes expressed in the immune systems of various phyla (i.e., structure is more important than function in this case), the most homologous sequences and gene architectures in the various metazoan phyla must be scrutinized.

V and C1 Domains

C1 domains are found in the antigen receptors, MHC class I and class II, and very few other molecules (Figs. 3 and 17). This Igsf domain is thus far restricted to gnathostomes, as if C1 domains arose concurrently with the adaptive immune system and co-evolved with it. What was the value of the C1

domain and why is it found almost exclusively in adaptive immune system-related molecules? All of these molecules interact with co-receptors such as CD3 (TCR), Igα and β chains (Ig on B cells), CD4, and CD8 (with MHC on opposing cells), and it is conceivable that in sections of Igsf domain in which C1 differs from the C2, there is a specific region favoring interaction with other molecules (R7,R207).

Possible features of V domain ancestors of the dimeric antigen receptor of vertebrates are depicted in Figs. 3 and 7. The G strand of Ig/TCR V domains is encoded by the J gene segment, separated from the V region–encoded A to F strands, and rearrangement is necessary in order to assemble a complete V gene. The primary structure of each Ig/TCR chain bears hallmarks of the dimeric nature of the receptor in which they participate. A diglycine bulge (Gly-X-Gly), present in all V domains, is thought either to be a beneficial adaptation, or to promote dimer formation by inducing a twist in the G strand that results in V domain pairing that appropriately orients the CDR. Monitoring this feature, therefore, might reveal genes that had the ability to form dimers similar to that of modern antigen-specific receptors. In V genes that do not somatically rearrange, the G stand is an integral part of the V exon. In other remotely related Igsf genes, introns have invaded the V domain exon creating a variety of V gene families. Many examples of such events can be found in the history of the Ig superfamily, such as in the genes encoding CD4 and CTX, for instance.

As described, no Ig/TCR genes have been isolated from hagfish or lampreys. Were Ig and TCR "invented" in a class of vertebrates now extinct (e.g., the placoderms, which are more primitive than cartilaginous fish but more advanced than agnathans) (Fig. 2)? Do cyclostomes have any features of a typical vertebrate immune system? It is not known whether agnathans have C1 domains, although from the study of the mammalian MHC paralogous regions, relatively recent jawed vertebrate ancestor should have had such domains. The discovery of the three tapasin paralogues, all with C1 domains, suggests an origin prior to the full establishment of the vertebrate genome (Fig. 12).

V and VC1 Segments in Evolution

V domains, either alone (e.g., NAR) or in association with another V domain (e.g., Ig H/L), recognize the antigenic epitope, and are therefore the most important elements for recognition. For this reason, they will be the first to be traced back in metazoan evolution by asking whether V domains exist in invertebrates. Domains with the typical V fold, whether belonging to the true V-set or the I-set, have been found from sponges to insects (although not necessarily involved in immune reactions; the first ones were discovered by nonimmunologists among molecules involved in nervous system differentiation in invertebrates, such as amalgam, lachesin, and fascicilin). Invertebrates also use Igsf members in immunity, although so far they are not V domains, but more I- or C2-set (e.g., MDM and hemolin). However, the mollusk

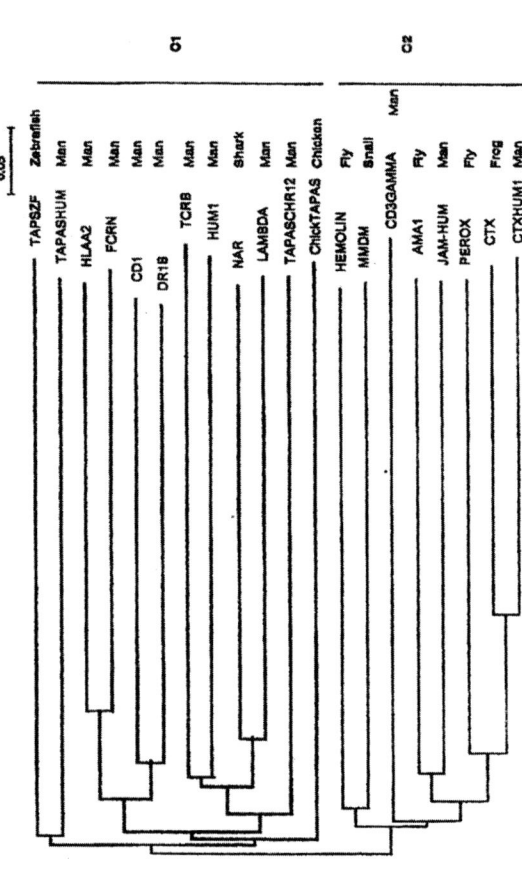

FIG. 17. Evolution of constant Igsf domains. *Shaded areas* indicate regions of high conservation among members of all domains or of only one type (C1 or C2). Modified from Du Pasquier (7), with permission. TAPZF: zebrafish tapasin; Tapashum: human tapasin; HLAA2: MHC class I human; FCRN: neonatal FC receptor; HUM1: Human IgM C1 domain; NAR: novel antigen receptor; TAPASCHR12: human tapasin homologue chr 12; ChickTAPAS: chicken tapasin; Ama1: amalgam first C domain; JAM-HUM: junction adhesion molecule human; PEROX: peroxidasin; CTXHUM1: human CTX homologue C1 domain; CTX: cortical thymocyte *Xenopus*.

FREPS (fibrinogen-related proteins) have a V domain at their distal end, associated with a fibrinogen-like domain. As described, they are involved in antiparasitic reactions and form a multigenic family with polymorphism (162).

Besides searching for VC1-encoding genes in nonvertebrates, surveying the human genome for such genes has proved fruitful (Fig. 12). Indeed, nonrearranging V-containing molecules, either V alone, VC1, or C1 alone, have been found in the human genome. Interestingly, many of them are encountered in the MHC class III region (human chromosome 6p21) or its paralogues (Fig. 12). Two MHC-linked gene segments stand out: a single V, NKP30, and a gene containing a VC1 core, tapasin, involved in antigen processing. NKP30, made of a single Ig domain of the V type, is an NK cell–activating receptor and it may offer a link to cell types encountered (analog or homolog?) in invertebrates. It could be a relative of an ancient receptor whose history is linked to the emergence of MHC class II and class I. In order to resemble an ancestor, the NKP30 V domain need only be associated with a C1 domain. In fact, a C1 single domain gene, pre–TCRα, is also encountered in this region of the genome. Besides Ig and TCR, tapasin is one of the rare cases, if not the only other case, of a gene segment with a VC1 structure existing on several paralogous linkage groups (6, 9q33, 19q13). In other words, while this gene is related to the rearranging receptor structure, it is undoubtedly very old, and probably predated the ancient block (genome-wide) duplications. It could have acted as a donor of C1 to a V domain-containing gene in the MHC class III region, which then could have been the first substrate of the rearrangement. Another set of molecules, the SIRPs, with a distal VC1 segment and the poliovirus receptor (VC1C2) could represent another group linked to the history of the Ig and TCR. TREM1 and TREM2, two related receptors on monocytes/neutrophils involved in inflammatory responses, are composed of single Igsf V domains whose genes are MHC linked. MOG and P0, two single V domains involved in the synthesis of myelin sheath, are encoded in the MHC paralogous region on chromosome 1. Chicken BG, which is related to MOG but probably having a different function, is encoded in the chicken MHC. Butyrophilin, CD83, and tapasin all have V domains, and butyrophilin also has a C1-type domain. More distant relatives with VC2-based architectures are also found in MHC (RAGE, CTX, lectin-related genes), and some of these genes related to the rearranging receptor ancestors, are found on several paralogues (whether the MHC paralogues or other) suggesting that the V-C1 core was generated early in vertebrate evolution subsequent to the emergence of the chordate superphylum (7,207). Among all these molecules, butyrophilin is perhaps not on the direct track to antigen-specific receptors. Its C domain, although proven to be C1 through its crystalline structure, is more like a C2 at the primary sequence level, and belongs to the CD80/86 family, rather than the TCR.

In teleost fish, Litman et al. (R208) have examined a very large family of genes (NITR, novel immune-type receptors), each having a V domain, C2 domain, and cytoplasmic tail often containing ITIMs. The V genes show greatest similarity to Ig/TCR V genes and NITRs may be related to the Igsf genes found in the mammalian LRC. Tracing this gene family back and forwards in evolution may lead us to an understanding of the original NKC/LRC/MHC, as well as identifying candidate genes related to the ancestral gene invaded by the RAG transposon.

Many invertebrate molecules not involved in immune responses are present as a distal V domain associated with one or more C2-type domains (Figs. 7 and 17). In the vertebrates, many molecules, such as CD2 and CTX, have retained this feature. Some members resemble "primitive" antigen receptors and several of them map to the MHC or its paralogous regions. Many form dimers and are expressed in lymphocytes, where they form a family of adhesion molecules. A recent crystal structure analysis of a CTX-related molecule (JAM or junctional adhesion molecule) revealed a unique form of dimerization, suggesting that the diversity of ligand binding and domain interactions used by different Igsf domain is extensive (209). Two JAM molecules form a U-shaped dimer with highly complementary interactions between the N-terminal domains. Two salt bridges are formed in a complementary manner by a novel dimerization motif, R (V, I, L) E. The RAGE gene (receptor for advanced glycosylation end products) has a rather "generic" receptor function since it recognizes aged cells exposing particular carbohydrate motifs.

In summary, there is no shortage of antigen receptor–related Igsf molecules in the metazoa and it is conceptually entertaining to imagine the MHC/NKC region as the ancestral backbone containing genes encoding all of the key molecules in the vertebrate adaptive immune system. Linkage studies and extension of the Igsf to prochordate species like *Amphioxus* should provide useful information on all of these problems of origins.

CONCLUSIONS

Many innate immune system features have persisted in animals that have evolved adaptive immunity. For example, cell-autonomous immunity is found in somatic cells of jawed vertebrates that produce type I interferons, and even some cells like keratinocytes that are capable of synthesizing inflammatory cytokines and antimicrobial peptides. In addition, systemic immunity (exemplified by the complement component C3 described above) is another innate feature that seems to be well conserved. Generally, however, such innate mechanisms were not able to sustain populations of long-lived organisms over evolutionary time, and somatic diversification mechanisms such as rearrangement and hypermutation evolved to protect *individuals* by sacrificing infected self cells via a highly discriminatory adaptive system (R3). However, perhaps we should not be surprised, when more information is obtained from invertebrate immune systems, that somatic mechanisms (RNA splicing, hypermutation, gene conversion) may have arisen by convergent evolution, especially in long-lived species.

In the next 10 years we expect to gain much more information concerning the molecules important for innate immune responses in the invertebrates. *Drosophila* has been the prototypic model to date, but studies of other insects (like *Anopheles*) (213) and representatives of other protostome classes will reveal which aspects of immunity are universal and those that are specific to particular groups of organisms. Further molecular studies in hagfish and lamprey and in non-vertebrate deuterostomes will perhaps permit a better understanding of the events leading to emergence of the adaptive immune system.

ACKNOWLEDGMENTS

MFF is supported by National Institutes of Health Grants AI28077 and RR6603. KM is supported by the Department of Fisheries and Oceans Strategic Science Fund in Newfoundland. We are grateful to Rebecca Lohr for production of the figures.

PUBLICATIONS WORTH NOTING

While this manuscript was in press, there have been several interesting publications worth noting.

In our review we state that IgW and IgNAR are "dead end" Ig isotypes, found only in the cartilaginous fish (Fig. 5). Ota et al (*Proc. Natl. Acad. Sci.* 2003, 100:2501–2506) now have shown that the lungfish (Osteichthyes) also has an IgW homologue, which has seven rather than the six C domains in the shark/skate version. This result suggests that the common ancestor of all jawed vertebrates had both IgM- and IgW-like molecules.

Concerning the problem of whether jawless fish have any molecules related to adaptive immunity, the Cooper group (Mayer et al *Proc. Natl. Acad. Sci.* 2002, 99:14350–14355 and Uinuk-Ool et al *Proc. Natl. Acad. Sci.* 2002, 99:14356–14361) isolated lymphocyte-like cells (based upon their size) from the lamprey and did not detect MHC, Ig, or TCR sequences in a random sequencing of genes expressed by these cells (typical EST project). However, these authors did find some homologous genes that are expressed rather exclusively in lymphocytes of jawed vertebrates, further suggesting that jawless fish indeed have lymphocytes. In this same vein, the urochordate Ciona intestinalis genome sequencing project (*Science* 2002, 298:2157–2167) also failed to reveal any Ig/MHC/TCR genes; nor were there immunoproteasome genes (LMP2, LMP7, or MECL-1), suggesting again that these genes all arose in a proximal vertebrate ancestor.

The tunicate *Botryllus* was shown to have a homologue of CD94, a C-type lectin expressed predominantly in vertebrate NK cells (Khalturin et al *Proc. Natl. Acad. Sci.* 2003, 100:622–627.) Based upon expression and polymorphism of

this gene, the authors suggest that it may be involved in allorecognition, but this hypothesis should be viewed with caution.

Bengten et al (*J. Immunol.* 2002, 169:2488–2497) surprisingly showed that the transmembrane and secretory forms of catfish IgD (Fig. 5) are encoded by different genes in the catfish. Transmembrane/secretory forms of Ig isotypes in all other vertebrates studied to date are derived by alternative splicing of a single gene.

In the chapter, we described work in sheep that suggested that the primary Ig repertoire is generated chiefly via somatic hypermutation. New work by Jenne et al (*J. Immunol.* 2003, 170:3739–3750) has shown that there are many more germline V genes than previously believed, suggesting that combinatorial (V-(D)-J) mechanisms plays an important role in primary repertoire generation.

REFERENCES

1. Plasterk RH. RNA silencing: the genome's immune system. *Science* 2002;296:1263–1265.
2. Jacob L, Zasloff M. Potential therapeutic applications of magainins and other antimicrobial agents of animal origin. *Ciba Found Symp* 1994;186:197–216.
3. Janeway CA Jr, Medzhitov R. Innate immune recognition. *Annu Rev Immunol* 2002;20:197–216.
4. Charlemagne J, Fellah JS, De Guerra A, et al. T-cell receptors in ectothermic vertebrates. *Immunol Rev* 1998;166:87–102.
5. Litman GW, Anderson MK, Rast JP. Evolution of antigen-binding receptors. *Annu Rev Immunol* 1999;17:109–147.
6. Rast JP, Anderson MK, Strong SJ, et al. Alpha, beta, gamma, and delta T cell antigen receptor genes arose early in vertebrate phylogeny. *Immunity* 1997;6:1–11.
7. Du Pasquier L. Relationships among the genes encoding MHC molecules and the specific antigen receptors. *Curr Top Microbiol Immunol* 2000;248:53–65.
8. Goebel TWF, Bollinger L. Evolution of the T cell receptor signal transduction units. *Curr Topics Microbiol Immunol* 2000;248:303–320.
9. Wang J, Reinherz E. Structural basis of cell–cell interactions in the immune system. *Curr Opin Struct Biol* 2000;10:656–661.
10. Kamper SM, McKinney EC. Polymorphism and evolution in the constant region of the T-cell receptor beta chain in an advanced teleost fish. *Immunogenetics* 2002;53:1047–1054.
11. Rock EP, Sibbald PR, Davis MM, et al. CDR3 length in antigen-specific immune receptors. *J Exp Med* 1994;179:323–328.
12. Fischer C, Bouneau L, Ozouf-Costaz C, et al. Conservation of the T-cell receptor α/δ linkage in the teleost fish *Tetradon nigroviridis*. *Genomics* 2002;79:241–248.
13. Fellah JS, Andre S, Kerfourn F, et al. Structure, diversity, and expression of the TCR-delta chains in the Mexican axolotl. *Eur J Immunol* 2002;32:1349–1358.
14. Sowder JT, Chen CL, Ager LL, et al. A large subpopulation of avian T cells express a homologue of the mammalian T gamma/delta receptor. *J Exp Med* 1988;67:315–322.
15. Su C, Jakobsen I, Gu X, et al. Diversity and evolution of T-cell receptor variable region genes in mammals and birds. *Immunogenetics* 1999;50:301–308.
16. Park CI, Hirono I, Enomoto J, et al. Cloning of Japanese flounder *Paralichthys olivaceus* CD3 cDNA and gene, and analysis of expression. *Immunogenetics* 2001;53:130–135.
17. Goebel TW, Meier EL, Du Pasquier L. Biochemical analysis of the *Xenopus laevis* TCR/CD3 complex supports the "stepwise evolution" model. *Eur J Immunol* 2000;30:2775–2781.
18. Bengten E, Wilson M, Miller N, et al. Immunoglobulin isotypes: structure, function, and genetics. *Curr Top Microbiol Immunol* 2000;248:189–219.

19. Kaattari S, Evans D, Klemer J. Varied forms of teleost IgM: an alternate to isotypic diversity? *Immunol Rev* 1998;166:133–142.
20. Ross DA, Wilson MR, Miller NW, et al. Evolutionary variation of immunoglobulin mu heavy chain RNA processing pathways: origins, effects, and implications. *Immunol Rev* 1998;166:143–151.
21. Coscia MR, Morea V, Tramontano A, et al. Analysis of a cDNA sequence encoding the immunoglobulin heavy chain of the Antarctic teleost *Trematomus bernacchii*. *Fish Shellfish Immunol* 2000;10:343–357.
22. Rumfelt LL, Avila D, Diaz M, et al. A shark antibody heavy chain encoded by a nonsomatically rearranged VDJ is preferentially expressed in early development and is convergent with mammalian IgG. *Proc Natl Acad Sci U S A* 2001;98:1775–1780.
23. Grabar P. Hypothesis. Auto-antibodies and immunological theories: an analytical review. *Clin Immunol Immunopathol* 1975;4:453–466.
24. Greenberg AS, Avila D, Hughes M, et al. A new antigen receptor gene family that undergoes rearrangement and extensive somatic diversification in sharks. *Nature* 1995;374:168–173.
25. Flajnik MF, Rumfelt LL. The immune system of cartilaginous fish. *Curr Top Microbiol Immunol* 2000;248:249–270.
26. Nguyen VK, Su C, Muyldermans S, et al. Heavy chain antibodies in *Camelidae*: a case of evolutionary innovation. *Immunogenetics* 2002;54:39–47.
27. Rast JP, Amemiya CT, Litman RT, et al. Distinct patterns of IgH structure and organization in a divergent lineage of chondrichthyan fishes. *Immunogenetics* 1998;47: 234–245.
28. Anderson MK, Strong SJ, Litman RT, et al. A long form of the skate IgX gene exhibits a striking resemblance to the new shark IgW and IgNARC genes. *Immunogenetics* 1999;49:56–67.
29. Wilson M, Bengten E, Miller NW, et al. A novel chimeric Ig heavy chain from a teleost fish shares similarities with IgD. *Proc Natl Acad Sci U S A* 1997;46:192–198.
30. Mussmann R, Du Pasquier L, Hsu E. Is *Xenopus* IgX and analog of IgA? *Eur J Immunol* 1996;26:2823–2830.
31. Fellah JS, Iscaki S, Vaerman JP, et al. Transient expression of IgY and secretory component-like protein in the gut of the axolotl *Ambystoma mexicanum*. *Dev Immunol* 1992;2:181–190.
32. Mussman R, Wilson M, Marcuz A, et al. Membrane exon sequences of the three *Xenopus* Ig classes explain the evolutionary origin of mammalian isotypes. *Eur J Immunol* 1996;26:409–414.
33. Martin SW, Goodnow CC. Burst-enhancing role of the IgG membrane tail as a molecular determinant of memory. *Nat Immunol* 2002;3:182–188.
34. Mussmann R, Courtet M, Schwager J, et al. Microsites for immunoglobulin switch recombination breakpoints from *Xenopus* to mammals. *Eur J Immunol* 1997;27:2610–2619.
35. Tashiro J, Kinoshita K, Honjo T. Palindromic but not G-rich sequences are targets of class switch recombination. *Int Immunol* 2001;13:495–505.
36. Magor KE, Higgins DA, Middleton DL, et al. One gene encodes the heavy chains for three different forms of IgY in the duck. *J Immunol* 1995;153:5549–5555.
37. Hsu E. Mutation, selection, and memory in B lymphocytes in exothermic vertebrates. *Immunol Rev* 1998;162:25–36.
38. Hinds KR, Litman GW. Major reorganization of immunoglobulin VH segmental elements during vertebrate evolution. *Nature* 1986;320:546–549.
39. Turchin A, Hsu E. The generation of antibody diversity in the turtle. *J Immunol* 1996;156:3797–3805.
40. Ota T, Sitnikova T, Nei M. Evolution of vertebrate immunoglobulin variable segments. *Curr Top Microbiol Immunol* 2000;248:221–245.
41. Cohn M, Langman RE. The protecton: the unit of humoral immunity selected by evolution. *Immunol Rev* 1990;115:11–147.
42. Ventura-Holman T, Lobb CJ. Structural organization of the immunoglobulin heavy chain locus in the channel catfish: the IgH locus represents a composite of two gene clusters. *J Immunol* 2002;38:557–564.
43. Kirkham PM, Mortari F, Newton JA, et al. Immunoglobulin VH clan and family identity predicts variable domain structure and may influence antigen binding. *EMBO J* 1992;11:603–609.
44. Shen SX, Bernstein RM, Schluter SF, et al. Heavy chain variable

regions in carcharhine sharks: development of a comprehensive model for the evolution of VH domains among the gnathostomes. *Immunol Cell Biol* 1996;74:357–364.
45. Rast JP, Anderson MK, Ota T, et al. Immunoglobulin light chain class multiplicity and alternative organizational forms in early vertebrate phylogeny. *Immunogenetics* 1994;40:83–89.
46. Lee SS, Greenberg AS, Hsu E. Evolution and somatic diversification of immunoglobulin light chains. *Curr Top Microbiol Immunol* 2000;248:285–300.
47. Miller RD, Belov K. Immunoglobulin genetics of marsupials. *Dev Comp Immunol* 2000;24:485–490.
48. Johansen FE, Braathen R, Brandtzaeg P. The J chain is essential for polymeric Ig receptor-mediated epithelial transport of IgA. *J Immunol* 2001;167:5185–5192.
49. Hohman VS, Stewart SE, Willett CE, et al. Sequence and expression pattern of J chain in the amphibian, *Xenopus laevis*. *Mol Immunol* 1997;34:995–1002.
50. Takahashi T, Iwase T, Tahibana T, et al. The joining (J) chain is present in invertebrates that do not express immunoglobulins. *Proc Natl Acad Sci U S A* 1996;93:1886–1891.
51. Yoder JA, Litman GW. Immune-type diversity in the absence of somatic rearrangement. *Curr Top Microbiol Immunol* 2000;248:271–282.
52. Lee SS, Fitch D, Flajnik MF, et al. Rearrangement of immunoglobulin genes in shark germ cells. *J Exp Med* 2000;191:1637–1648.
53. Daggfeldt A, Bengten E, Pilstrom L. A cluster type organization of the loci of the immunoglobulin light chain in Atlantic cod and rainbow trout indicated by nucleotide sequences of cDNAs and hybridization analysis. *Immunogenetics* 1993;38:199–209.
54. Ghaffari SH, Lobb CJ. Structure and genomic organization of a second class of immunoglobulin light chain genes in the channel catfish. *J Immunol* 1997;159:250–258.
55. Flajnik MF, Kasahara M. Comparative genomics of the MHC: glimpses into the evolution of the adaptive immune system. *Immunity* 2001;15:351–362.
56. Kaufman J, Salomonsen J, Flajnik MF. Evolutionary conservation of MHC class I and class II molecules—different yet the same. *Semin Immunol* 1994;6:411–424.
57. Wang J, Reinherz E. Structural basis of T cell recognition of peptides bound to MHC molecules. *Mol Immunol* 2002;38:1039–1049.
58. Hughes AL, Nei M. Evolutionary relationships of the classes of major histocompatibility complex genes. *Immunogenetics* 1993;37:337–346.
59. Klein J, O'hUigin C. Composite origin of major histocompatibility complex genes. *Curr Opin Genet Dev* 1993;3:923–930.
60. Shum BP, Azumi K, Zhang S, et al. Unexpected beta2-microglobulin diversity in individual rainbow trout. *Proc Natl Acad Sci U S A* 1996;93:2779–2784.
61. Hughes AL, Yeager M, Ten Elshof AE, et al. A new taxonomy of mammalian MHC class I molecules. *Immunol Today* 1999;20:22–26.
62. Miller MM, Goto RM, Taylor RL, et al. Assignment of Rfp-Y to the chicken MHC/NOR microchromosome and evidence for high frequency recombination associated with the nucleolar organizer region. *Proc Natl Acad Sci U S A* 1996;93:3958–3862.
63. Courtet M, Flajnik MF, Du Pasquier L. Major histocompatibility complex and immunoglobulin loci visualized by *in situ* hybridization on *Xenopus* chromosomes. *Dev Comp Immunol* 2001;25:149–157.
64. Cerwenka A, Lanier LL. Ligands for natural killer cell receptors: redundancy or specificity. *Immunol Rev* 2001;181:158–169.
65. Dixon B, Stet RJ. The relationship between major histocompatibility complex receptors and innate immunity in teleost fish. *Dev Comp Immunol* 2001;25:683–699.
66. Klein J. Origin of major histocompatibility complex polymorphism: the trans-species hypothesis. *Hum Immunol* 1087;19:155–162.
67. Wakeland EK, Boehme S, She JX, et al. Ancestral polymorphisms of MHC class II genes: divergent allele advantage. *Immunol Rev* 1990;9:115–122.
68. Sidney J, Grey HM, Kubo RT, et al. Practical, biochemical and evolutionary implications of the discovery of HLA class I supermotifs. *Immunol Today* 1996;17:261–266.
69. Hughes AL. Maintenance of MHC polymorphism. *Nature* 1992;335:402–403.
70. Takahata N, Nei M. Allelic genealogy under overdominant and frequency-dependent selection and polymorphism of major histocompatibility complex loci. *Genetics* 1990;124:967–978.

71. Miller KM, Kaukinen KH, Beacham TD, et al. Geographic heterogeneity in natural selection on an MHC locus in sockeye salmon. *Genetica* 2001;111:237–257.

72. Salamon H, Klitz W, Esteal S, et al. Evolution of HLA class II molecules: allelic and amino acid site variability across populations. *Genetics* 1999;152:393–400.

73. Schierup MH, Vekemans X, Charlesworth D. The effect of subdivision on variation at multi-allelic loci under balancing selection. *Genet Res Camb* 2000;76:51–62.

74. Slatkin M, Muirhead CA. A method for estimating the intensity of overdominant selection from the distribution of allele frequencies. *Genetics* 2000;156:2119–2126.

75. Apanius V, Penn D, Slev P, et al. The nature of selection on the major histocompatibility complex. *Crit Rev Immunol* 1997;17:179–224.

76. Kaufman J, Völk H, Wallny HJ. A "minimal essential Mhc" and an "unrecognized Mhc": two extremes in selection for polymorphism. *Immunol Rev* 1995;143:63–88.

77. Potts WK, Slev PR. Pathogen-based models favoring MHC genetic diversity. *Immunol Rev* 1995;143:181–197.

78. Montag S, Frank M, Ulmer H, et al. "Electronic nose" detects major histocomplatibility complex-dependent prerenal and postrenal odor components. *Proc Natl Acad Sci U S A* 2001;98:9249–9254.

79. Penn D, Potts WK. How do major histocompatibility complex genes influence odor and mating preference? *Adv Immunol* 1998;69:411–435.

80. Toivanen P, Vaahtovuo J, Eerola E. Influence of major histocompatibility complex on bacterial composition of fecal flora. *Infect Immun* 2001;69:2372–2377.

81. Carroll LS, Penn DJ, Potts WK. Discrimination of MHC-derived odors by untrained mice is consistent with divergence in peptide-binding region residues. *Proc Natl Acad Sci U S A* 2002;99:2187–2192.

82. Reusch TB, Haberli MA, Aeschlimann PB, et al. Female sticklebacks count alleles in a strategy of sexual selection explaining MHC polymorphism. *Nature* 2001;414:300–302.

83. Landry C, D Garant D, Duchesne P, et al. 'Good genes as heterozygosity': the major histocompatibility complex and mate choice in Atlantic salmon (*Salmo salar*). *Proc R Soc Lond B* 2001;268:1279–1285.

84. Miller KM, Kaukinen KH, Schulze AD. Expansion and contraction of major histocompatibility complex genes: a teleostean example. *Immunogenetics* 2002;53:941–963.

85. Takahata N. MHC diversity and selection. *Immunol Rev* 1995;143:225–247.

86. Du Pasquier L, Miggiano V, Kobel HR, et al. The genetic control of histocompatibility reactions in natural and laboratory-made polyploidy individuals in the clawed toad *Xenopus*. *Immunogenetics* 1977;5:129–141.

87. Sammut B, Du Pasquier L, Ducoroy P, et al. Axolotl MHC architecture and polymorphism. *Immunol Rev* 1998;166:259–277.

88. Kasahara M, Hayashi M, Tanaka K, et al. Chromosomal localization of the proteasome Z subunit gene reveals an ancient chromosomal duplication involving the major histocompatibility complex. *Proc Natl Acad Sci U S A* 1996;156:4245–4253.

89. Ohno S. Gene duplication and the uniqueness of vertebrate genomes circa 1970–1999. *Semin Cell Dev Biol* 1999;10:517–522.

90. Klein J, Sato A. Birth of the major histocompatibility complex. *Scand J Immunol* 1998;47:199–209.

91. Abi-Rached L, Gilles A, Shiina T, et al. Evidence of *en bloc* duplication in vertebrate genomes. *Nat Genet* 2002;1:100–105.

92. Shum BP, Guethlein L, Flodin LR, et al. Modes of salmonid MHC class I and class II evolution differ from the mammalian paradigm. *J Immunol* 2001;166:3297–3308.

93. Kaufman J, Milne S, Goebel TW, et al. The chicken B locus is a minimal essential major histocompatibility complex. *Nature* 1999;401:923–925.

94. Rollins-Smith LA. Metamorphosis and the amphibian immune system. *Immunol Rev* 1998;166:221–230.

95. Voelk H, Charlemagne J, Tournefier A, et al. Wide tissue distribution of axolotl class II molecules occurs independently of thyroxin. *Immunogenetics* 1998;47:339–349.

96. Hansen JD, Zapata AG. Lymphocyte development in fish and amphibians. *Immunol Rev* 1998;166:199–220.

97. Zapata A, Amemiya CT. Phylogeny of lower vertebrates and their immunological structures. *Curr Top Microbiol Immunol* 2000;248:67–107.

98. Luer CA, Walsh CJ, Bodine AB, et al. The elasmobranch thymus: anatomical, histological, and preliminary functional characterization. *J Exp Zool* 1995;273:342–354.

99. Lloyd-Evans P. Development of the lymphomyeloid system in the dogfish, *Scyliorhinus canicula*. *Dev Comp Immunol* 1993;17:501–514.

100. Hansen JD. Characterization of rainbow trout terminal deoxynucleotidyl transferase structure and expression. TdT and RAG1 co-expression defines the trout primary lymphoid tissues. *Immunogenetics* 1997;46:367–375.

101. Horton JD, Horton TL, Dzialo R, et al. T-cell and natural killer cell development in thymectomized *Xenopus*. *Immunol Rev* 1998;166:245–258.

102. Horton TL, Ritchie P, Watson MD, et al. Natural cytotoxicity towards allogeneic tumour targets in *Xenopus* mediated by diverse splenocyte populations. *Dev Comp Immunol* 1998;22:217–230.

103. Cooper MD, Raymond DA, Petersen RD, et al. The functions of the thymus system and the bursa system in the chicken. *J Exp Med* 1966;123:75–102.

104. Weill JC, Reynaud CA. Rearrangement/hypermutation/conversion: when, where, and why? *Immunol Today* 1996;17:92–97.

105. Miracle AL, Anderson MK, Litman RT, et al. Complex expression patterns of lymphocyte-specific genes during the development of cartilaginous fish implicate unique lymphoid tissues in generating the immune repertoire. *Intl Immunol* 2001;13:567–580.

106. Romano N, Abelli L, Mastrolia L, et al. Immunocytochemical detection and cytomorphology of lymphocyte subpopulations in a teleost fish *Dicentrarchus labrax*. *Cell Tissue Res* 1997;289:163–171.

107. Du Pasquier L, Robert J, Courtet M, et al. B-cell development in the amphibian *Xenopus*. *Immunol Rev* 2000;175:201–213.

108. De Guerra A, Charlemagne J. Genomic organization of the TCR beta chain diversity and joining segments in the rainbow trout: presence of many repeated sequences. *Mol Immunol* 1997;34:653–662.

109. Lee A, Hsu E. Isolation and characterization of the *Xenopus* terminal deoxynucleotidyl transferase. *J Immunol* 1994;152:4500–4507.

110. Weill JC, Reynaud CA, Lassila O, et al. Rearrangement of chicken immunoglobulin genes is not an ongoing process in the embryonic bursa of Fabricius. *Proc Natl Acad Sci U S A* 1986;83:3336–3340.

111. Ratcliffe MJ, Ivanyi J. Allotype suppression in the chicken. IV. Deletion of B cells and lack of suppressor cells during chronic suppression. *Eur J Immunol* 1981;11:306–310.

112. Reynaud CA, Anquez V, Grimal H, et al. A hyperconversion mechanism generates the chicken light chain preimmune repertoire. *Cell* 1987;48:379–388.

113. Thompson CB, Neiman PE. Somatic diversification of the chicken immunoglobulin light chain gene is limited to the rearranged variable gene segment. *Cell* 1987;48:369–378.

114. Arakawa H, Hauschild J, Buerstedde JM. Requirement of the activation-induced deaminase (AID) gene for immunoglobulin gene conversion. *Science* 2002;295:1301–1306.

115. Sayegh CE, Drury G, Ratcliffe MJ. Efficient antibody diversification *in vivo* in the absence of selection for V(D)J-encoded determinants. *EMBO J* 1999;18:6319–6328.

116. Becker RS, Knight KL. Somatic diversification of immunoglobulin heavy chain VDJ genes: evidence for somatic gene conversion in rabbits. *Cell* 1990;63:987–997.

117. Reynaud CA, Garcia C, Hein WR, et al. Hypermutation generating the sheep immunoglobulin repertoire is an antigen-independent process. *Cell* 1995;80:115–125.

118. Butler JE. Immunoglobulin gene organization and the mechanism of repertoire development. *Scand J Immunol* 1997;45:455–462.

119. Hanley PJ, Hook JW, Raftos DA, et al. Hagfish humoral defense protein exhibits structural and functional homology with mammalian complement components. *Proc Natl Acad Sci U S A* 1992;89:7910–7914.

120. Klein J, Sato A, Mayer WE. Jaws and AIS. In: Kasahara M, ed. *Major histocompatibility complex: evolution, structure, and function*. Tokyo: Springer, 2000:3–26.

121. Flajnik MF, Rumfelt LL. Early and natural antibodies in non-mammalian vertebrates. *Curr Top Microbiol Immunol* 2000;252:233–240.

122. Makela O, Litman GW. Lack of heterogeneity in antihapten antibodies of a phylogenetically primitive shark. *Nature* 1980;255:6532–6534.

123. Hinds-Frey KR, Nishikata H, Litman RT, et al. Somatic variation precedes extensive diversification of germline sequences and combinatorial joining in the evolution of immunoglobulin heavy chain diversity. *J Exp Med* 1993;178:815–824.

124. Lee SS, Tranchina D, Ohta Y, et al. Hypermutation in immunoglobulin light chain genes results in contiguous substitutions. *Immunity* 2002;16:571–582.

125. Diaz M, Greenberg AS, Flajnik MF. Somatic hypermutation of the new antigen receptor gene (NAR) in the nurse shark does not generate the repertoire: possible role in antigen-driven reactions in the absence of germinal centers. *Proc Natl Acad Sci U S A* 1998;95:14343–14348.

126. Kaattari SL, Zhang HL, Khor IW, et al. Affinity maturation in trout: clonal dominance of high affinity antibodies late in the immune response. *Dev Comp Immunol* 2002;26:191–200.

127. Clem LW, Bly JE, Wilson M, et al. Fish immunology: the utility of immortalized lymphoid cells—a minireview. *Vet Immunol Immunopathol* 1996;54:137–1144.

128. Boudinot P, Boubekeur S, Benmansour A. Rhabdovirus infection induces public and private T cell responses in teleost fish. *J Immunol* 2001;167:6202–6209.

129. Bly JE, Clem LW. Temperature-mediated processes in teleost immunity: *in vitro* immunosuppression induced by channel catfish peripheral blood cells. *Vet Immunol Immunopathol* 1991;28:365–377.

130. Shen L, Stuge TB, Zhou H, et al. Channel catfish cytotoxic cells: a mini-review. *Dev Comp Immunol* 2002;26:141–149.

131. Jaso-Friedmann L, Leary JH 3rd, Evans DL. The non-specific cytotoxic cell receptor (NCCRP–1): molecular organization and signaling properties. *Dev Comp Immunol* 2001;25:701–711.

132. Charlemagne J. Antibody diversity in amphibians. Noninbred axolotls use the same unique heavy chain and a limited number of light chains for their anti–2,4-dinitrophenyl antibody responses. *Eur J Immunol* 1987;17:421–424.

133. Wabl MR, Du Pasquier L. Antibody patterns in genetically identical frogs. *Nature* 1976;264:642–644.

134. Wilson M, Hsu E, Marcuz A, et al. What limits affinity maturation of antibodies in *Xenopus*—the rate of mutation or the ability to select mutants? *EMBO J* 1992;11:4337–4347.

135. Neuberger MS, Lanoue A, Ehrenstein MR, et al. Antibody diversification and selection in the mature B cell compartment. *Cold Spring Harb Symp Quant Biol* 1999;64:211–216.

136. Du Pasquier L, Schwager J, Flajnik MF. The immune system of *Xenopus*. *Annu Rev Immunol* 1989;7:251–275.

137. Robert J, Gantress J, Rau L, et al. Minor histocompatibility complex-specific MHC-restricted CD8 T cell responses elicited by heat shock proteins. *J Immunol* 2002;168:1697–1703.

138. Arakawa H, Furusawa S, Ekino S, et al. Immunoglobulin gene hyperconversion ongoing in chicken splenic germinal centers. *EMBO J* 1996;15:2540–2546.

139. Secombes CJ, Bird S, Hong S, et al. Phylogeny of vertebrate cytokines. *Adv Exp Med Biol* 2001;484:89–94.

140. Staehli P, Puehler F, Schneider K, et al. Cytokines of birds: conserved functions—a largely different look. *J Interferon Cytokine Res* 2001;21:993–1010.

141. Magor BG, Magor KE. Evolution of effectors and receptors of innate immunity. *Dev Comp Immunol* 2001;25:651–682.

142. Beschin A, Bilej M, Brys L, et al. Convergent evolution of cytokines. *Nature* 1999;400:627–628.

143. Bird S, Wang T, Zou J, et al. The first cytokine sequence within cartilaginous fish: IL–1β in the small spotted catshark (*Scyliorhinus canicula*). *J Immunol* 2002;168:3329–3340.

144. Najakshin AM, Mechetina LV, Alabyev BY, et al. Identification of an IL–8 homologue in lamprey (*Lampetra fluviatillis*): early evolutionary divergence of chemokines. *Eur J Immunol* 1999;29:375–382.

145. Haynes F, Cohen L. Further characterization of an interleukin–2-like cytokine produced by *Xenopus* laevis T lymphocytes. *Dev Immunol* 1993;3:231–238.

146. Wang T, Secombes CJ. Cloning and expression of a putative common cytokine receptor γ chain (γC) gene in rainbow trout (*Oncorhynchus mykiss*). *Fish Shellfish Immunol* 2001;11:233–244.

147. Georgel P, Kappler C, Langley E, et al. *Drosophila* immunity. A sequence homologous to mammalian interferon consensus response element enhances the activity of the diptericin promoter. *Nucleic Acids Res* 1995;23:1140–1145.

148. Ellis AE. Innate host defense mechanisms of fish against viruses and bacteria. *Dev Comp Immunol* 2001;25:827–839.

149. Gorelik L, Flavell RA. Transforming growth factor-β in T-cell biology. *Nature Rev Immunol* 2002;2:46–53.

150. Anderson MK, Rothenberg EV. Transcription factor expression in lymphocyte development: clues to the evolutionary origins of lymphoid cell lineages? *Curr Top Microbiol Immunol* 2000;248:137–155.

151. Fossett N, Schulz RA. Functional characterization of hematopoietic factors in *Drosophila* and vertebrates. *Differentiation* 2001;69:83–90.

152. Lebetsky T, Chang T, Hartenstein V, et al. Specification of *Drosophila* hematopoietic lineage by conserved transcription factors. *Science* 2000;288:146–149.

153. Rast JP, Pancer Z, Davidson EH. New approaches towards an understanding of deuterostome immunity. *Curr Top Microbiol Immunol* 2000;248:3–16.

154. Shintani S, Terzic J, Sato A, et al. Do lampreys have lymphocytes? The Spi evidence. *Proc Natl Acad Sci U S A* 2000;97:7417–7422.

155. Anderson MK, Sun X, Miracle AL, et al. Evolution of hematopoiesis: three members of the PU.1 transcription factor family in a cartilaginous fish *Raja eglanteria*. *Proc Natl Acad Sci U S A* 2001;98:553–558.

156. Hansen JD, McBlane JF. Recombination-activating genes, transposition, and the lymphoid-specific combinatorial immune system: a common evolutionary connection. *Curr Top Microbiol Immunol* 2000;248:111–135.

157. Kimbrell DA, Beutler B. The evolution and genetics of innate immunity. *Nat Rev Genet* 2001;2:256–267.

158. Luo H, Dearholf CR. The JAK/STAT pathway and *Drosophila* development. *Bioessays* 2001;23:1138–1147.

159. Milochau A, Lasségues M, Valembois P. Purification, characterization and activities of two hemolytic and antibacterial proteins from coelomic fluid of the annelid *Eisenia fetida andrei*. *Biochim Biophys Acta* 1997;1337:123–132.

160. Pan J, Kurosky A, Xu B, et al. Broad antiviral activity in tissues of crustaceans. *Antiviral Res* 2000;48:39–47.

161. Destoumieux-Garzon D, Saulnier D, Garnier J, et al. Crustacean immunity. Antifungal peptides are generated from the C-terminus of shrimp hemocyanin in response to microbial challenge. *J Biol Chem* 2001;276:47070–47077.

162. Zhang SM, Leonard PM, Adema CM, et al. Parasite-responsive IgSF members in the snail *Biomphalaria glabrata* : characterization of novel genes with tandemly arranged Igsf domains and a fibrinogen domain. *Immunogenetics* 2001;53:684–694.

163. Iwanaga S. The molecular basis of innate immunity in the horseshoe crab. *Curr Opin Immunol* 2002;14:87–95.

164. Vasta GR, Quesenberry M, Ahmed H, et al. C-type lectins and galectins mediate innate and adaptive immune functions: their roles in the complement activation pathway. *Dev Comp Immunol* 1999;23:401–420.

165. Zasloff M. Antimicrobial peptides of multicellular organisms. *Nature* 2002;415:389–395.

166. Moore KS, Wehrli S, Roder H, et al. Squalamine: an aminosterol antibiotic from the shark. *Proc Natl Acad Sci U S A* 1993;90:1354–1358.

167. Mitta G, Vandenbulcke F, Noel T, et al. Differential distribution and defence involvement of antimicrobial peptides in mussel. *J Cell Sci* 2000;113:2759–2769.

168. Pancer Z. Dynamic expression of multiple scavenger receptor cysteine-rich genes in coelomocytes of the purple sea urchin. *Proc Natl Acad Sci U S A* 2000;97:13156–13161.

169. Gorman MJ, Andreeva OV, Paskewitz SM. Sp22D: a multidomain serine protease with a putative role in insect immunity. *Gene* 2000;251:9–17.

170. Nonaka M. Evolution of the complement system. *Curr Opin Immunol* 2001;13:69–73.

171. Smith LC, Clow LA, Terwilliger DP. The ancestral complement system in sea urchins. *Immunol Rev* 2001;180:16–34.

172. Gadjeva M, Thiel S, Jensenius JC. The mannan-binding –lectin pathway of the innate immune response. *Curr Opin Immunol* 2001;13: 74–78.

173. Clow LA, Gross PS, Shih CS, et al. Expression of C3, the sea urchin complement component, in response to lipopolysaccharide. *Immunogenetics* 2000;51:1034–1044.

174. Miyazawa S, Azumi K, Nonaka M. Cloning and characterization of integrin alpha subunits from the solitary ascidian *Halocynthia roretzi*. *J Immunol* 2001;166:1710–1715.

175. Levashina EA, Moita LF, Blandin S, et al. Conserved role of a complement-like protein in phagocytosis revealed by dsRNA knockout in cultured cells of the mosquito, *Anopheles gambiae*. *Cell* 2001; 104:709–718.

176. Sunyer JO, Zarkadis I, Sarrias MR, et al. Cloning, structure, and function of two rainbow trout Bf molecules. *J Immunol* 1998;161:4106–4114.

177. Dos Remedios NJ, Ramsland PA, Hook JW, et al. Identification of a homologue of CD59 in a cyclostome: implications for the evolutionary development of the complement system. *Dev Comp Immunol* 1999;23:1–14.

178. Suzuki MM, Satoh N, Nonaka M. C6-like and C3-like molecules from a cephalochordate, amphioxus, suggest a cytolytic complement system in invertebrates. *J Mol Evol* 2002;54:671–679.

179. Dodds AW, Law SKA. The phylogeny and evolution of the thioester bond-containing proteins C3, C4, and α_2-macroglobulin. *Immunol Rev* 1998;166:15–26.

180. Hughes AL. Phylogeny of the C3/C4/C5 complement-component gene family indicates that C5 diverged first. *Mol Biol Evol* 1994;11:417–425.

181. St Johnston D, Nusslein-Volhard C. The origin of pattern and polarity in the *Drosphila* embryo. *Cell* 1992;68:201–219.

182. Hoffmann JA, Reichhart J-M. *Drosophila* innate immunity: an evolutionary perspective. *Nature Immunol* 2002;3:121–126.

183. Steiner H, Hultmark D, Engstrom A, et al. Sequence and specificity of two antibacterial proteins involved in insect immunity. *Nature* 1981;292:246–248.

184. Friedman R, Hughes AL. Molecular evolution of the NF-κB system. *Immunogenetics* 2002;53:964–974.

185. Dangl JL, Jones JDG. Plant pathogens and integrated defence responses to infection. *Nature* 2001;411:826–833.

186. Schmidt O, Theopold U, Strand M. Innate immunity and its evasion and suppression by hymenopteran parasitoids. *Bioessays* 2001;23:344–351.

187. Caton Y, Nappi AJ. Immunogenetic aspects of the cellular immune response against parasitoids. *Immunogenetics* 2001;52:157–164.

188. Magor BG, De Tomaso A, Rinkevich B, et al. Allorecognition in colonial tunicates: protection against predatory cell lineages? *Immunol Rev* 1999;167:69–79.

189. Burnet FM. Evolution of the immune process in vertebrates. *Nature* 1968;218:426–430.

190. Theodor JL. Distinction between "self" and "not-self" in lower vertebrates. *Nature* 1970;227:690–692.

191. Mokady O, Buss LW. Transmission genetics of allorecognition in *Hydractinia symbiolongicarpus* (Cnidaria: Hydrozoa). *Genetics* 1996; 143:823–827.

192. Fernandez-Busquets X, Burger MM. Cell adhesion and histocompatibility in sponges. *Microsc Res Tech* 1999;44:203–218.

193. Blumbach B, Diehl-Seifert B, Seack J, et al. Cloning and expression of new receptors belonging to the immunoglobulin superfamily from the marine sponge *Geodia cydonium*. *Immunogenetics* 1999;49:751–763.

194. Oka H, Watanabe H. Colony specificity in compound ascidians as tested by fusion experiments (a preliminary report). *Proc Jpn Acad Sci* 1957;33:657–658.

195. Marino R, De Santis R, Giuliano P, et al. Follicle cell proteasome activity and acid extract from the egg vitelline coat prompt the onset of self-sterility in *Ciona intestinalis* oocytes. *Proc Natl Acad Sci U S A* 1999;96:9633–9636.

196. Nasrallah JB. Recognition and rejection of self in plant reproduction. *Science* 2002;296:305–308.

197. Hughes AL. Genomic catastrophism and the origin of vertebrate immunity. *Arch Immunol Ther Exp* 1999;47:347–353.

198. Kaufman J. Vertebrates and the evolution of the major histocompatibility complex (MHC) class I and class II molecules. *Verh Dtsch Zool Ges* 1989;81:131–144.

199. Abi Rached L, McDermott MF, Pontarotti P. The MHC Big Bang. *Immunol Rev* 1999;167:33–45.

200. Lynch M, O'Hely M, Walsh B, et al. The probability of preservation of a newly arisen gene duplicate. *Genetics* 2001;159:1789–1804.

201. Hughes ML, Hughes AL. Evolution of duplicate genes in a tetraploid animal, *Xenopus laevis*. *Mol Biol Evol* 1993;10:1360–1369.

202. Agrawal A, Eastman QM, Schatz DG. Transposition mediated by RAG1 and RAG2 and its implication for the evolution of the immune system. *Nature* 1998;394:744–751.

203. Du Pasquier L, Wilson M, Greenberg AS, et al. Somatic mutation in ectothermic vertebrates: musings on selection and origins. *Curr Top Microbiol Immunol* 1998;229:199–216.

204. Honjo T, Kinoshita K, Muramatsu M. Molecular mechanism of class switch recombination: linkage with somatic mutation. *Annu Rev Immunol* 2002;20:165–196.

205. Richards MH, Nelson JL. The evolution of vertebrate receptors: a phylogenetic approach. *Mol Biol Evol* 2000;17:146–155.

206. Glusman G, Rowen L, Lee I, et al. Comparative genomics of the human and mouse T cell receptor loci. *Immunity* 2001;15:337–349.

207. Du Pasquier L, Chretien I. CTX, a new lymphocyte receptor in *Xenopus,* and the early evolution of Ig domains. *Res Immunol* 1996;147:218–226.

208. Litman GW, Hawke NA, Yoder JA. Novel immune-type receptor genes. *Immunol Rev* 2001;181:250–259.

209. Kostrewa D, Brockhaus M, D'Arcy A, et al. X-ray structure of junctional adhesion molecule: structural basis for homophilic adhesion via a novel dimerization motif. *EMBO J* 2001;20:4391–4398.

210. Bjorkman PJ, Saper MA, Samraoui B, et al. Structure of the human class I histocompatibility antigen, HLA-A2. *Nature* 1987;329:506–512.

211. Brown JH, Jardetzky TS, Gorga JC, et al. Three-dimensional structure of the human class II histocompatibility antigen HLA-DR1. *Nature* 1993;364:33–39.

212. Williams AF, Barclay AN. The immunoglobulin superfamily domains for cell surface recognition. *Annu Rev Immunol* 1988;6:381–405.

213. Christophides GK, Zdobnov E, Barillas-Mury C, et al. Immunity-related genes and gene families in *Anopheles gambiae*. *Science* 2002;298:159–165.

The Major Histocompatibility Complex and Its Encoded Proteins

David H. Margulies and James McCluskey

A Note on Nomenclature
The Immunological Function of Major Histocompatibility Complex Molecules
The Major Histocompatibility Complex
Major Histocompatibility Complex Genetic Maps · Major Histocompatibility Complex Polymorphism · Major Histocompatibility Complex Evolutionary Mechanisms · The Major Histocompatibility Complex and Transplantation · The Major Histocompatibility Complex and Clinical Transplantation · Family Studies in Histocompatibility Testing · Functional Tests of Human Leukocyte Antigen Compatibility · The Major Histocompatibility Complex and Disease · Mutations at the *H-2* Locus · Expression of Major Histocompatibility Complex Molecules
Structure of Major Histocompatibility Complex Molecules
Amino Acid Sequences: Primary Structure · Identification of Peptides Bound by Major Histocompatibility Complex Molecules · High Resolution Crystallographic Structures
Molecular Interactions of Major Histocompatibility Complex Molecules
Physical Assays · Multivalent Major Histocompatibility Complex/Peptide Complexes
Summary
Acknowledgments
References

The molecular center of the immune system consists of major histocompatibility complex (MHC) molecules: the cell surface receptors that govern, by interaction with membrane-expressed molecules on crucial cells of the innate and adaptive immune systems, the initiation, perpetuation, and regulation of cellular activation in response to infection and neoplasia. The MHC molecules are not static surface receptors that merely bind another set of receptors to indicate their presence and number. They are structurally and conformationally dynamic: they modulate their structure by incorporating peptides derived from ingested foreign molecules or dysregulated proteins expressed in the same cell, and they sense the presence of proteins from viruses and other cellular pathogens that affect the nature or efficiency of the MHC molecules' cell surface expression. In addition to providing the functional focal point for molecular recognition in the immune system, molecules encoded by the *Mhc* represent a microcosm of complex molecular biology. Members of the family of *Mhc*-encoded molecules interact extensively with a number of other molecules, during both their biosynthesis and intracellular trafficking. These interactions regulate the quality and rate of their appearance in specialized intracel-lular compartments as well as their arrival at the cell surface. When poised at the cell surface as ligands for specific molecules on T cells and natural killer (NK) cells, they control the response of these immunoeffectors. Understanding the MHC molecules in detail therefore provides a springboard for comprehending the layers of complex regulation to which the immune system is servant. The genetics of the *Mhc* offers a groundwork for understanding immunological selection and also reveals living footprints of molecular genetic evolution. Since the publication of the previous edition of this chapter, advances in the study of the *Mhc* as a genetic region, as well as in the understanding of its encoded molecules in structural and functional terms, have enabled a comprehensive understanding of this focal point of immune recognition. More facets of MHC function have been discovered, as the role of these molecules in sensing viral infection and in activating cells of the innate immune system has become better understood. Although an earlier view was that the *Mhc*-encoded molecules were uniquely involved in recognition by T cells, it is now overwhelmingly clear that MHC molecules interact with receptors on NK cells as well. As the strict definitions of MHC molecules based purely on the location of their encoding genetic loci have given way to looser groupings based on similarities of the protein structures or on functional relationships, we now appreciate that a larger family of genes, molecules, and functions should be included in this chapter. Our efforts are to preserve some sense of the historical development of this exciting field of study but also to focus on paradigmatic genetic, structural, and functional features that unify this extensive gene/protein family. Finally, the *Mhc* provides a genetic link from immune responsiveness to autoimmune disease—those well-known strong associations of particular *Mhc* genes to particular human diseases—and we outline the molecular basis for such associations.

The *Mhc* is a set of linked genes, located on chromosome 6 of the human, chromosome 17 of the mouse, chromosome 20 of the rat, and cluster I of the chicken that was first identified by its effects on tumor or skin transplantation and control of immune responsiveness (1–3). More recently, partly because of evolutionary interest and partly because of the importance of *Mhc* loci in species that serve as models for human disease, particularly human immunodeficiency virus, extensive information has been gathered on the MHC genes of several primate species (4). The *Mhc* also plays a role in resistance to infection. Early observations indicated an *Mhc*-linked control of immune responsiveness (5–9) and have culminated in a molecular understanding of the critical details of genetically encoded cellular recognition in the immune system. The control of transplantation and the immune response is the phenotypic consequence of the function of molecules encoded in the *Mhc*. Therefore, researchers gain a deeper understanding of the *Mhc* as they explore it in molecular and cellular terms. MHC molecules are cell surface receptors that bind antigen fragments and display them to various cells of the immune system: T cells that bear $\alpha\beta$ receptors (10–12), NK cells (13–15), and T cells that express $\gamma\delta$ receptors (16). Molecules structurally similar to class I MHC (MHC-I) molecules, but encoded beyond the strict genetic bounds of the *Mhc* and in some cases lacking the full complement of MHC-I domains, are now known to be expressed on particular subsets of somatic cells, some tumors, and cells of the placenta. In addition, a certain population of T cells, known as NK T cells, that express both NK cell receptors and a restricted set of T-cell receptors, are activated by the class Ib MHC (MHC-Ib) molecule CD1d (17–20). Thus, there has been a transition in knowledge from that of mysterious genetic entities, with ill-defined mechanism but distinct immunological function and genetic location, to a biochemical understanding of specific molecules with known structure, biosynthetic pathway, biophysical parameters of interaction, and temporal expression that convey specific signals between and within cells and that map precisely to defined regions of the chromosome. The study of the *Mhc* has accordingly also made a transition, from that of genetics and cellular immunology to detailed molecular mechanisms.

Major improvements in knowledge resulted from many complementary developments: the widespread availability of inbred and recombinant mouse strains; an increasing library of well-characterized monoclonal antibodies that detect cell surface markers with specificity and potency; genomic and complementary deoxyribonucleic acid (cDNA) clones for *Mhc*-encoded proteins derived from many different species; high-resolution linkage maps and complete sequences based on whole genome sequencing methods; methods for the controlled expression of *Mhc* genes in transfectant cell lines and transgenic mice; knockout and conditional knockout animals with directed and conditional mutations of relevant genetic loci; expression systems for producing large amounts of homogeneous, soluble analogues of MHC molecules and their protein ligands; and high resolution x-ray crystallographic structures of MHC molecules and their complexes with important associated proteins such as co-receptors, superantigens, and T-cell and NK cell receptors. In addition, the availability of computer-accessible databases for obtaining current information on the nucleotide and amino acid sequence, as well as the three-dimensional structures of many of these factors, make the study of the *Mhc* particularly exciting, challenging, and rewarding.

The focus of this chapter is the *Mhc,* and our primary goal is to outline the general principles of molecular organization and function both of the genetic regions that encode MHC molecules as well as of the functional cell surface molecules themselves. Human disease associations, molecular typing of MHC molecules and *Mhc* genes, and relevant functional polymorphisms complete our explication of these markers of immunological function.

A NOTE ON NOMENCLATURE

One of the most confusing topics for students of the *Mhc* has been its nomenclature. Like language, nomenclature evolves, and attempts at standardization are inevitably incompletely successful. With new discoveries, additional complexities are recognized, and a need for greater precision undermines the simpler systems of the past. Current usage differs from species to species, journal to journal, and writer to writer, although there are standards of which the informed scientist should be aware. For the mouse *Mhc,* these are available in several publications: *Genetic Variants and Strains of the Laboratory Mouse* (21), now in its third edition, and the Jackson Laboratory home page (http://www.informatics.jax.org/mgihome/nomen/). For the human *Mhc,* there is a standard World Health Organization (WHO) nomenclature that is periodically evaluated and revised (22). By convention, genes or genetic loci are indicated by designations in italics and the encoded protein product or phenotypic descriptions are shown in a standard font. For the genes of the human *Mhc,* this convention is often overlooked, whereas for those of the mouse and other species, it is frequently followed. The mouse *Mhc* is referred to as *H-2* because it was the second genetic locus involved in control of expression of erythrocyte antigens to be identified by Gorer (23,24). The *Mhc* is now known to consist of many loci, and the extended genetic region is referred to as the complex; thus the general term used for all species is the *Mhc* or *MHC*. (With the use of databases and computerized maps, the tendency is to eliminate the use of the hyphen; thus *H-2* is evolving to *H2*.) The *Mhc* in the rat is known as *RT1*, the human locus is known as human leukocyte antigen (*HLA*), and other common usages include *DLA* for the dog, *GPLA* for the guinea pig, *SLA* for the swine, and *RLA* for the rabbit. For other species, in accordance with a suggestion by Klein et al. (25), the taxonomic name forms the basis for the designation, contributing the first two letters of the genus and the first two of the species to name the locus. Thus, *Patr* is used for the chimpanzee (*Pan troglodytes*), *Gogo* for the gorilla (*Gorilla gorilla*), *Mamu* for the rhesus macaque (*Macaca mulatta*), and *Papa* for the bonobo (*Pan paniscus*).

Because the first genes of the *Mhc* to be identified were those that encoded cell surface molecules that could be detected by antibodies or by transplantation responses, these are the ones that are referred to as *Mhc* genes. More than 400 genes that map to the human or mouse *Mhc* are now known, and although technically they are all *"Mhc"* genes, the "MHC" molecules refer specifically to the MHC-I or class II MHC (MHC-II) molecules that are related in structure and function. Other *Mhc*-encoded molecules with distinct structure and function are referred to by their more specific names.

Particular *Mhc* genes are designated by one or more letters for the locus (e.g., *H-2K*, *H-2D*, *H-2L*, and *H-2IA* in the mouse; *HLA-A*, *HLA-B*, *HLA-C*, *HLA-E*, *HLA-F*, *HLA-G*, *HLA-H*, *HLA-J*, *HLA-K*, *HLA-L*, *HLA-DR*, *HLA-DQ*, *HLA-DO*, and *HLA-DP* in the human). *HLA-H*, *HLA-J*, *HLA-K*, and *HLA-L* are pseudogenes. *HLA-DRA*, *HLA-DQA1*, *HLA-DMA*, *HLA-DQA1*, *HLA-DQA2*, *HLA-DPA1*, and *HLA-DPA2* encode the α chains, and *HLA-DRB1* through *HLA-DRB9* (including pseudogenes), *HLA-DQB1* through *HLA-DQB3*, and *HLA-DOB*, *HLA-DMB*, *HLA-DPB1*, and *HLADPB2* encode the respective β chains. Allelic genes (and their expressed cell surface protein products) have been denoted in the mouse by the addition of a superscript (e.g., *H-2K^b* and *H-2K^d* are distinct alleles at the same locus) and in the human by the addition of a number or a letter and a number (*HLA-A2* and *HLA-A3* are alleles, as are *HLA-B8* and *HLA-B27*). Precise designation of human genes is by a nomenclature that includes a four-digit or longer number that follows the locus (e.g., *HLA-A*0101* and *HLA-DRB1*0101*; see Table 1 for clarification of the nomenclature of the HLA alleles). Clarity in understanding the human designations requires a conversion table to align the older nomenclature, which is based on serological findings, with the more recent one, which is based on DNA typing (Tables 2 and 3).

For the *Mhc* class II genes, the designation in the human is *HLA-D* (including *HLA-DM*, *HLA-DO*, *HLA-DP*, *HLA-DQ*, and *HLA-DR*); in the mouse, *H-2IAa*, *H-2IAb*, *H-2IEa*, and *H-2IEb* are used and frequently shortened to *IAa*, *IAb*, *IEa*, and *IEb*, respectively. *a* and *b* refer to the *a* or α (alpha) and *b* or β (beta) chain–encoding genes, respectively. Some authors prefer *H2-Aa*, *H2-Ab*, *H2-Ea*, and *H2-Eb*. Current usage

TABLE 1. *Nomenclature of human leukocyte antigen (HLA) loci and alleles*

Nomenclature	Definition
HLA	The HLA region and prefix for an HLA gene
HLA-DRB1	A particular HLA locus (i.e., DRB1)
HLA-DRB1*13	A group of alleles that encode the DR13 antigen defined serologically by microlymphocytotoxicity or by mixed lymphocyte reactivity
HLA-DRB1*1301	A specific HLA allele
HLA-DRB1*1301N	A null allele (i.e., nonexpressed)
HLA-DRB1*13012	An allele that differs by a synonymous mutation (i.e., identical amino acid encoded by a different codon)
HLA-DRB1*1301102	An allele that contains a mutation outside the coding region
HLA-DRB1*1301102N	A null allele that contains a mutation outside the coding region

Adapted from IMGT Website http://www.ebi.ac.uk/imgt/hla/.

tends to include the Roman letter for the gene designation and the Greek letter for the encoded protein chain. The MHC-II molecules are often referred to as IA or IE with a superscript denoting the haplotype (i.e., IA^b, IA^d, or IE^d). Several murine MHC-II–like genes, originally named *H-2Ma*, *H-2Mb1*, and *H-2Mb2*, which are homologues of the human *HLA-DMA* and *HLA-DMB* genes, are now called *H2-DMA*, *H2-DMB1*, and *H2-DMB2* in an effort to emphasize their structural and functional similarity to the human *HLA-DMA* and *HLA-DMB* genes, as well as to distinguish them from the *H-2M* genes that lie most distal on chromosome 17 (26). Another complication that demands the precise use of gene and encoded protein names is that the number of genes in a particular homologous genetic region can differ between strains or between individuals. In the mouse, whereas some strains have only a single gene at the D locus (e.g., *H-2D^b*), other strains may have as many as five genes in the homologous region (*H-2D^d*, *H-2D2^d*, *H-2D3^d*, *H-2D4^d*, and *H-L^d*) (27).

An important description commonly used is "haplotype," which refers to the linkage of particular alleles at distinct loci that occur as a group on a parental chromosome (28). The concept of haplotype is important in typing the *HLA* loci in the human, where the linked *Mhc* genes of one chromosome of one parent generally segregate as a linkage group to the children. Individual haplotypes of the *Mhc* in the mouse are referred to by a superscript lowercase letter as *H-2^b*, *H-2^d*, or *H-2^k*. Thus, the *H-2^k* haplotype refers to the full set of linked genes, *H-2K^k*, *H-2IA^k*, *H-2IE^k*, and *H-2D^k* and extends to the genes of the Q and T regions as well (29,30). (Some haplotype designations, such as *H-2^a*, refer to natural recombinants and thus include some of the linked genes from one haplotype and some from another). The realization that the similar *H-2* haplotypes represented by different mouse strains have

TABLE 2. *Listing of class I human leukocyte antigen (HLA) alleles*

HLA-A		HLA-B		HLA-C	
Serology	Alleles	Serology	Alleles	Serology	Alleles
A1	A*0101-0109	B7	B*07021-0731	Cw1	Cw*0102-0106
A2	A*0201-0258	B8	B*0801-0815	Cw2	Cw*02021-0205
A3	A*0301-0309	B13	B*1301-1310	Cw3	Cw*03021-0315
A11	A*1101-1110	B14	B*1401-14062	Cw4	Cw*0401101-0409
A23(9)	A*2301-2308	B15	B*1501101-1573	Cw5	Cw*0501-0505
A24(9)	A*2402-2433	B18	B*1801-1818	Cw6	Cw*0602-0607
A25(10)	A*2501-2504	B27	B*2701-2725	Cw7	Cw*07011-0716
A26(10)	A*2601-2618	B35	B*35011-3541	Cw8	Cw*08011-0809
A29(19)	A*2901-2905	B37	B*3701-3705	—	Cw*12021-1208
A30(19)	A*3001-3012	B38(16)	B*3801-3808	—	Cw*1301
A31(19)	A*3101-3108	B39(16)	B*39011-3926	—	Cw*14021-1405
A32(19)	A*3201-3207	B40	B*40011-4044	—	Cw*15021-1511
A33(19)	A*3301-3306	B41	B*4101-4106	—	Cw*1601-16041
A34(10)	A*3401-3404	B42	B*4201-4204	—	Cw*1701-1703
A36	A*3601-3603	B44(12)	B*44021011-4432	—	Cw*1801-1802
A43	A*4301	B45(12)	B*4501-4506	—	
A66	A*6601-6604	B46	B*4601-4602	—	
A68(28)	A*6801-6822	B47	B*4701101-4704		
A69(28)	A*6901	B48	B*4801-4807		
A74(19)	A*7401-7408	B49(21)	B*4901-4903		
—	A*8001	B50(21)	B*5001-5004		
		B51(5)	B*51011-5129		
		B52(5)	B*52011-5203		
		B53	B*5301-5309		
		B54(22)	B*5401-5402		
		B55(22)	B*5501-5512		
		B56(22)	B*5601-5608		
		B57(17)	B*57011-5709		
		B58(17)	B*5801-5806		
		B59	B*5901		
		B67	B*67011-6702		
		B73	B*7301		
		B78	B*7801-7805		
		—	B*7901		
		—	B*8101		
		—	B*8201-8202		
		—	B*8301		

HLA-E	HLA-F	HLA-G
* E*0101-0104	— F*0101	— G*01011-0106

This list summarizes the designations of the human class I major histocompatibility complex HLA gene products as they have been known based on serology, and they have been assigned by nucleotide (and thus inferred amino acid) sequences. Current serological designations are given in the "serology" columns, with older (broader) serological assignments listed in parentheses. Serological assignments are usually based on reactivity with alloantisera in a microlymphocytotoxicity assay. Some of the most recently identified HLA polymorphisms and products of nonclassical loci (e.g., HLA-E and HLA-G) have no historical serological designation. Note that the serologically defined HLA-B15 antigen comprises 83 allelic members (B*1501101-1573) and HLA A2 comprises 56 members (A*0201-0258) as of July 2002. The table is based on a listing of alleles maintained by Dr. Steve Marsh on behalf of the World Health Organisation Nomenclature Committee for Factors of the HLA System. All new and confirmatory sequences are generally submitted directly to the committee via the IMGT/HLA Database through the sequence submission tool provided. The IMGT/HLA Database may be accessed via the World Wide Web at *http://www.ebi.ac.uk/imgt/hla*.

significant differences, particularly in the number and allelic identity of *MHC-Ib* genes, has supported a proposal to refine the nomenclature. Table 4 is a summary of the haplotypes of common mouse strains.

In parallel with the genetic nomenclature system, investigators have developed a system that focuses on the expressed proteins rather than just on the genes and, by its use, emphasizes both structural and functional differences. The main distinction of MHC molecules is between the MHC-I and MHC-II molecules. [Class III MHC molecules (MHC-III) have also been included in a group originally characterized as serum molecules involved in the complement system

TABLE 3. *Listing of class II human leukocyte antigen (HLA) alleles*

HLA-DR

Serology	Alleles
α chain	
DRA	
—	DRA*0101-01022
β chain	
DRB1	
DR1	DRB1*0101-0108
DR15(2)	DRB1*15011-1513
DR16(2)	DRB1*16011-08
DR3	DRB1*03011-0322
DR4	DRB1*04011-0444
DR11(5)	DRB1*11011-1143
DR12(5)	DRB1*12011-1208
DR13(6)	DRB1*13011-1351
DR14(6)	DRB1*14011-1443
DR7	DRB1*07011-0706
DR8	DRB1*08011-0824
DR9	DRB1*09012-0902
DR10	DRB1*10011-10012
DRB3	
DR52	DRB3*01011-0110
	DRB3*0201-0217
	DRB3*03011-0303
DRB4	
DR53	DRB4*01011-0106
—	DRB4*0201N
—	DRB4*0301N
DRB5	
DR51	DRB5*01011-0110N
	DRB5*0202-0205
DRB6	
—	DRB6*0101
—	DRB6*0201-0202
DRB7	DRB7*01011-01012
DRB8	DRB8*0101
DRB9	DRB9*0101

HLA-DO

Serology	Alleles
α chain	
DOA1	
—	DQA1*01011-0106
—	DQA1*0201
—	DQA1*03011-0303
—	DQA1*0401
—	DQA1*05011-0505
—	DQA1*06011-06012
β chain	
DOB1	
DQ5(1)	DQB1*05011-0504
DQ6(1)	DQB1*06011-0620
DQ2	DQB1*0201-0203
DQ3(7,8,9)	DQB1*03011-0313
DQ4	DQB1*0401-0402

HLA-DP

Serology	Alleles
α chain	
DPA1	
—	DPA1*01031-0108
—	DPA1*02011-0203
—	DPA1*0301-0302
—	DPA1*0301-0302
β chain	
DPB1	
DPw1	DPB1*01011-01012
DPw2	DPB1*02012-0202
DPw3	DPB1*03011-03012
DPw4	DPB1*0401-0402
DPw5	DPB1*0501
DPw6	DPB1*0601
—	DPB1*0801
—	DPB1*0901
	DPB1*1001
	DPB1*11011-11012
	DPB1*1301-4101
	DPB1-4401-9201

HLA-DM and HLA-DO

Serology	Alleles
α chain	
DMA	DMA*0101-0104
DOA	DOA*01011-01015
β chain	
DMB	DMB*0101-0106
DOB	DOB*0101101-0104102

The table is based on a listing of alleles maintained by Dr. Dr. Steve Marsh on behalf of the World Health Organisation Nomenclature Committee for Factors of the HLA System, as of July 2002. All new and confirmatory sequences are generally submitted directly to the committee via the IMGT/HLA Database through the sequence submission tool provided. The IMGT/HLA Database may be accessed via the World Wide Web at *http://www.ebi.ac.uk/imgt/hla*. Note that the serological assignments of HLA class II.

TABLE 4. *Commonly used mouse strains: H-2 haplotypes*

Strain	Haplotype	H-2 complex							
		K	Ab	Aa	Eb	Ea	D	Oa1	Tla
Common strains									
129/J	bc	b	b	b	b	—	b	b	f
AKR/J	k	k	k	k	k	k	k	b	b
ASW/Sn	s	s	s	s	s	—	s	b	b
BALB/c	d	d	d	d	d	d	d	b	c
C3H/Hej	k	k	k	k	k	k	k	b	b
CBA/J	k	k	k	k	k	k	k	b	b
C57BL/6	b	b	b	b	b	—	b	b	b
C57BL/10	b	b	b	b	b	—	b	b	b
C57BR	k	k	k	k	k	k	k	a	a
DBA/2J	d	d	d	d	d	d	d	b	c
NOD/LtJ	g7	d	g7	d	—	—	b		
NON/LtJ	nb1	b	nb1	Unknown	k	k	b		
NZB/BINJ	d2	d	d	d	d	d	d	a	a
NZW/LacJ	z	u	u	u	u	u	z		
P/J	p	p	p	p	p	p	p	a	e
PL/J	u	u	u	u	u	u	d		
RIII	r	r	r	r	r	r	r	c(r)	b
SJL	s2	s	s	s	s	—	s	a	a
Congenic strains									
B10.BR	k2	k	k	k	k	k	k		
B10.D2	d	d	d	d	d	d	d		
B10.S	s	s	s	s	s	—	s		
BALB.B	b	b	b	b	b	—	b		
BALB.K	k	k	k	k	k	k	k		
C3H.SW	b	b	b	b	b	—	b		
Recombinant strains									
A	a	k	k	k	k	k	d		
A.TL	t1	s	k	k	k	k	d		
B10.A	a	k	k	k	k	k	d		
B10.A(1R)	h1	k	k	k	k	k	b		
B10.A(2R)	h2	k	k	k	k	k	b		
B10.A(3R)	l3	b	b	b	b/k	k	d		
B10.A(4R)	h4	k	k	k	k/b	—	b		
B10.A(5R)	l5	b	b	b	b/k	k	d		
B10.T(6R)	y2	q	q	q	q	—	d		
B10.S(7R)	t2	s	s	s	s	—	d		
B10.S(8R)	as1	k	k	k	k/s	—	s		
B10.S(9R)	t4	s	s	s	s/k	k	d		
B10.HTT	t3	s	s	s	sd/k	k	d		

Dashes indicate abnormal gene expression, although precise mechanism may differ in different strains (446). Blanks indicate insufficient data for characterization. Additional strains may be identified at *http://jaxmice.jax.org/html/jaxnotes/jaxn433c.shtml*.

Adapted from Kruisbeek (444) and Undahl (445), with permission.

(C4/C2/Bf) but now also include products of the genetically linked loci mapping between the class I and class II regions of the *Mhc*.] All MHC-I molecules consist of a heavy chain (also called an α chain) that is noncovalently assembled with a monomorphic (genetically invariant, or almost so) light chain known as β_2-microglobulin (β_2m), encoded by the *B2m* gene. All MHC-I molecules are subclassified into the MHC class Ia (MHC-Ia) and MHC-Ib groups, distinctions based on amino acid sequence differences as well as on gene location (31,32). MHC-II molecules are heterodimeric, consisting of noncovalently assembled α and β chains. The bulk of the serologically defined differences in HLA-DR molecules reside in the β chain. The heterodimers usually consist of the assem-

bled products of the linked genes encoding the two chains. In the mouse, the products of the *IAa* (also known as *IAα*) and *IAb* (or *IAβ*) genes assemble to form the IA heterodimer; similarly, the products of the *IEa* (*IEα*) and *IEb* (*IEβ*) genes assemble to form IE. IA and IE are often referred to as "isotypes." The allelic forms are usually referred to as *IA^b*, *IA^d*, or *IA^k*. Under some circumstances, mixed heterodimers that can be of immunological importance are observed (33–38). Thus, to refer to a mixed heterodimer consisting of the α chain of IE^d and the β chain of IA^d, the more precise but cumbersome description IAβ^dEα^d (IAb^{d}Ea^d) must be used. In the human, particularly in referring to MHC-II molecules, the distinctions between molecules identified by antibodies and those identified by DNA sequence typing must be made (Tables 2 and 3).

THE IMMUNOLOGICAL FUNCTION OF MAJOR HISTOCOMPATIBILITY COMPLEX MOLECULES

MHC molecules are a molecular reflection of the health status of either the cell that synthesizes them (for MHC-I molecules) or the local environment in which the cell resides (for MHC-II). The structure of the MHC molecule reflects the amino acid sequences of the two polypeptide chains [α and β for MHC-II and heavy (or α) and β_2m for MHC-I] that form the core of the complex and also the sequence of the variable bound peptide that forms an integral part of the trimer. The MHC molecule, governed by the sequence of the encoding structural genes for *Mhc-I* heavy chain and the *Mhc-II* α and β chains, as well as other genes involved in antigen processing and presentation that map to the *Mhc,* must satisfy at least two distinct recognition functions: (a) the binding of peptides or, in some cases, nonpeptidic molecules, and (b) the interaction with either T or NK cells through their respective receptors. The T-cell receptor (TCR) may augment its interaction with the MHC molecule by virtue of interaction of a T cell expressed co-receptor (CD8 for MHC-I and CD4 for MHC-II). [There is evidence that some NK receptors, when expressed on T cells, may also serve as co-receptors (39).] The binding of peptides by an MHC-I or MHC-II molecule is the initial selective event that permits the cell expressing the MHC molecule [the antigen-presenting cell (APC) or, when this cell is to be the recipient of a cytolytic signal, the target cell] to sample fragments derived either from its own proteins (for MHC-I–restricted antigen presentation) or from proteins ingested from the immediate extracellular environment (for the case of MHC-II).

In particular, cell surface MHC-I glycoproteins gather from the cell's biosynthetic pathway fragments of proteins derived from infecting viruses, intracellular parasites, or self molecules, expressed either normally or in a dysregulated manner as a result of tumorigenesis, and then display these molecular fragments, in complex with the mature MHC-I molecule, at the cell surface (12,40–43). Here, the cell-bound MHC-I/β_2m/peptide complex on the APC is exposed to the extracellular milieu and is available for interaction with T cells or NK cells. The T cell bearing an $\alpha\beta$ receptor recognizes the particular MHC/peptide complex by virtue of a specific physical binding interaction. Each T cell is representative of a clonal population and bears a unique TCR encoded by somatically rearranged TCR genetic elements. T cells bearing $\alpha\beta$ receptors undergo a complex selective process in the thymus, and only a small proportion of T cells that enter the thymus ultimately reach peripheral lymphoid organs, such as lymph nodes and the spleen. A particular TCR can bind only a very limited selection of MHC/peptide complexes. The recognition by T cells is known as *MHC-restricted* in that only a limited set of MHC molecules can bind a particular TCR and is also termed *antigen-specific*

in that a particular T cell "sees" a particular peptide. For any given T-cell clone, single amino acid substitutions of either the MHC or the peptide may severely diminish, or even obliterate, the functional interaction of the TCR with the MHC/peptide complex. The MHC-I system draws its spectrum of peptides from proteins in the cytosol that are (a) degraded by the multiproteolytic proteasome complex to peptides that are transported from the cytosol to the endoplasmic reticulum with the aid of the intrinsic membrane peptide transporter, the transporter associated with antigen processing (TAP), (b) then trimmed at their amino terminus, and (c) cooperatively folded as an intrinsic component of the newly synthesized MHC-I molecule (44).

MHC-II molecules, in contrast to MHC-I, are expressed on a more limited set of somatic cells—B cells, macrophages, dendritic cells, and activated but not resting T cells in the human—and have a somewhat more specific function in peptide selection and presentation. In general, they bind peptides derived from the degradation of proteins ingested by the APC, and they sort their MHC-II molecules into endosomal cellular compartments in which the degraded peptides are generated and catalytically transferred to the binding site of the MHC-II. The MHC-II antigen presentation pathway is based on the initial assembly of the MHC-II $\alpha\beta$ heterodimer with a dual-function molecule, the invariant chain (Ii), which serves as a chaperone to direct the $\alpha\beta$ heterodimer to an endosomal, acidic protein-processing location, where it encounters antigenic peptides and which also serves to protect the antigen binding site of the MHC-II molecule so that it will be preferentially loaded with antigenic peptides in this endosomal/lysosomal location (45–48). The loading of the MHC-II molecule with antigenic peptide, a process dependent on the release of the class II associated invariant chain peptide (CLIP), in part dependent on the MHC-II–like molecule, HLA-DM in the human, (49,50), then leads to the cell surface expression of MHC-II/peptide complexes. The MHC-II–recognizing T cells then secrete lymphokines and may also be induced to proliferate or to undergo programmed cell death. Such MHC-restricted lymphokine production that facilitates and augments the recruitment of additional inflammatory cells as well as APCs and antibody-producing cells is a contemporary explanation for what was historically referred to as "T-cell help."

Distinct from TCRs that recognize MHC molecules, a number of NK cell receptors, both activating and inhibitory, bind MHC-I molecules, and several NK receptors interact with MHC-I–like molecules (51). In general, the NK/MHC-I interaction, in comparison with the TCR/MHC interaction, shows considerably less peptide specificity, although the interaction is peptide dependent and, in some cases, may exhibit clear-cut peptide preferences (13,52–54). The functional purpose of the MHC-I or MHC-I–like molecule in NK cell recognition appears to be more subtle than that in T-cell recognition. The NK cell is tuned to a balance of inhibitory and activating signals conveyed to it through MHC interaction, and, in its resting state, the inhibitory signals predominate.

MHC-I is a sensor of the biosynthetic and metabolic state of the cell in which it is synthesized: When dysregulated by tumorigenesis or viral infection, the altered level of MHC-I can be detected by the NK cell. This ability of the NK cell to sense altered levels of MHC-I on target cells is the basis of the "missing self hypothesis," which holds that NK cells detect and lyse cells defective in MHC-I expression as a result of the loss of the inhibitory signal that results from engagement of NK receptors by MHC-I (55–57). The prototype NK receptor is the mouse NK inhibitory receptor, Ly49A, a C-type lectin-like molecule that delivers an inhibitory signal to the cell expressing it as a result of its interaction with normally expressed MHC-I molecule, H-2D^d (58). Distinct clones of NK cells differ in the combinatorial expression of different NK receptors that have different MHC preferences. Thus, in the

mouse, each distinct NK clone may express a different combination of NK inhibitory receptors such as Ly49A, Ly49C, Ly49G2, and Ly49I (59). Because each inhibitory molecule may exhibit slight differences in its MHC-I or peptide preference and specificity, this kind of combinatorial expression of NK activity offers a breadth of specificity toward different potential target cells.

MHC-I and MHC-II molecules, because of differences in the cellular compartments that they traverse from their biosynthesis to their maturation, reveal strong preferences for the origin of the proteins that they sample for antigen presentation (60,61). The MHC-I antigen presentation pathway is most easily thought of as an "inside-out" pathway by which protein fragments of molecules synthesized by the cell are delivered to and bound by the MHC-I molecule

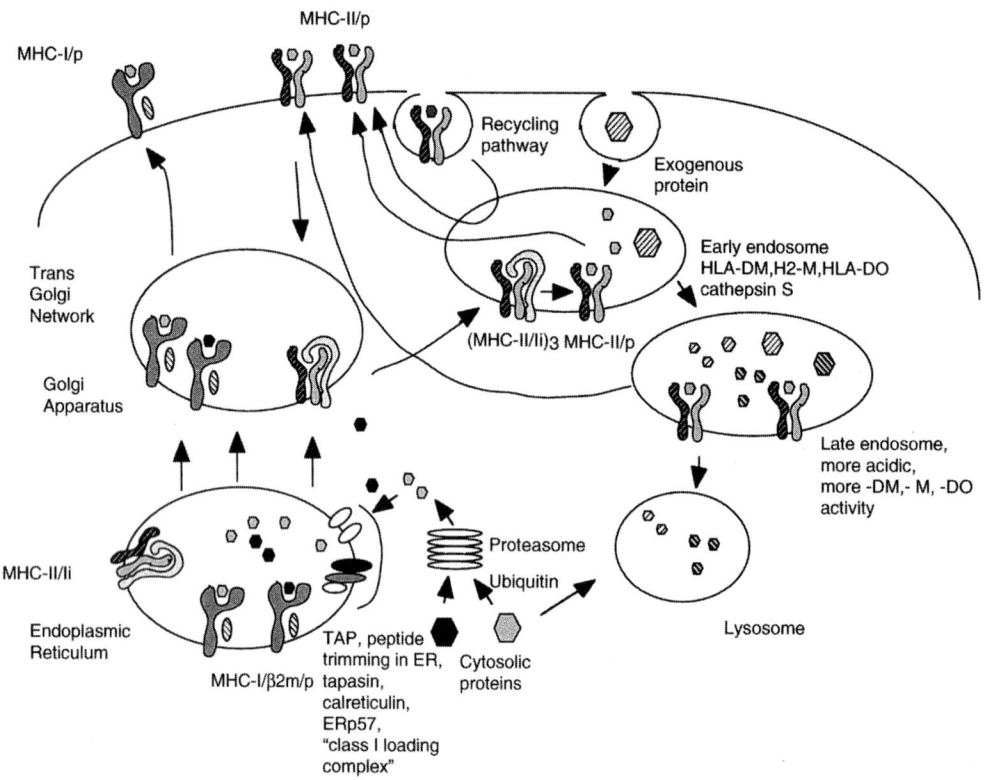

FIG. 1. Antigen processing and presentation. The major pathways of processing and presentation are shown. Cytosolic proteins (*shaded hexagons*) are degraded in proteasomes, sometimes after ubiquitination, to peptide fragments that are then transported into the endoplasmic reticulum by transporter associated with antigen processing (TAP) where they assemble with class I major histocompatibility complex (MHC)/β_2-microglobulin complexes. Proteolytic trimming of these peptides occurs following entry into the endoplasmic reticulum (450,451). For some MHC/peptide complexes, tapasin plays a crucial role in peptide loading. The thiol oxidoreductase ERp57 contributes to peptide loading and binding by facilitating the formation of a crucial disulfide bond between the class I MHC $\alpha2$ helix and the β strand floor of the peptide binding groove. From the endoplasmic reticulum, MHC/peptide complexes pass through the Golgi apparatus and trans-Golgi network, undergoing a variety of steps of carbohydrate addition and maturation, before emerging at the cell surface. Exogenous proteins (striped hexagons) enter the endosomal pathway through endocytosis, and in early or late endosomes or lysosomes, they are progressively degraded to peptides. In early and late endosomes, class II MHC/invariant chain complexes (those that have been trafficked there from the endoplasmic reticulum) are converted to class II MHC/corticotropin-like intermediate peptide (CLIP) complexes that are loaded with peptides with the catalytic aid of human leukocyte antigen–DM. These class II MHC/peptide complexes then go to the plasma membrane. This figure is adapted from those described elsewhere (62,265).

during its biosynthesis. In contrast, the MHC-II antigen presentation pathway is best visualized as an "outside-in" one in which ingested proteins are degraded by enzymes in the endosomal/lysosomal system and are delivered to MHC-II molecules in that degradative compartment (12,43,62,63). Careful analysis of peptides delivered to the class II pathway reveals that under some conditions, peptides generated in the cytoplasm can also be presented through the MHC-II pathway (64,65). [Cellular compartments for MHC-II peptide loading have been called MIIC, but it has been argued that this is an imprecise term that has limited utility (66).] The processes of antigen processing and presentation are schematically illustrated in Fig. 1 and are described in more detail elsewhere in this book. The biochemical steps involved in the production of antigen fragments from large molecules are collectively known as *antigen processing,* whereas those that concern the binding of antigen fragments by MHC molecules and their display at the cell surface are known as *antigen presentation.*

The understanding of the complexities of antigen processing and presentation continues to improve. The importance of MHC-I loading of proteasome components in controlling the specificity of the degradation of proteins in the cytoplasm has been recognized (42). Contributions made by the chaperone tapasin (67), by ubiquitination (42,68), and by amino terminal trimming of peptides in the endoplasmic reticulum (69) and the role of disulfide interchange as controlled by the resident endoplasmic reticulum protein Erp57 in peptide loading during MHC-I assembly (70) have also been recognized. MHC-II peptide loading is controlled in part by the multifunctional chaperone/groove protector, Ii, as well as the important catalytic machinery of the endosomes, molecules known as HLA-DM and HLA-DO in the human and H-2M and H-2O in the mouse (67) (Fig. 1).

In addition to showing preference for distinct pathways of antigen presentation, the MHC-I and MHC-II molecules also show preferential restriction to T cells of the CD8- or CD4-bearing subsets. This is related to the observation that CD8 binds to the nonpolymorphic $\alpha 3$ domain of MHC-I molecules (71–74), whereas CD4 interacts with membrane proximal domains of MHC-II (75–79). The CD8 and CD4 molecules serve as "co-receptors" on the surface of the T-lymphocyte, providing both adhesion (avidity increase) and specific activating signals that modulate the avidity of the T cell in a time dependent manner (80,81). The precise location of the site of interaction of the CD8$\alpha\alpha$ homodimer with MHC-I has been observed crystallographically for both human and murine molecules (82,83). In addition, the two amino terminal immunoglobulin-like domains of human CD4 complexed with a murine MHC-II molecule, I-A^k, have been visualized crystallographically (79). The numerous interactions of MHC molecules with other cellular components and with the wide variety of peptides and of various immunological receptors reflect the robust potential of the MHC structure as a molecular sensor and as a master regulator of immune responses. These molecular interactions then read out in different cell

trafficking and signaling functions. Table 5 summarizes some of these interactions, emphasizing the similarities and differences between MHC-I and MHC-II molecules.

THE MAJOR HISTOCOMPATIBILITY COMPLEX

Major Histocompatibility Complex Genetic Maps

The MHC is an extended region of the genome that spans approximately 4 million base pairs (Mb) on the short arm of human chromosome 6 in the region of 6p21.3. One analysis (84) suggested that the extended *Mhc* covers as much as 8 Mb. Although *Mhc* genes were among the first to be mapped in this region, it is now clear that a large proportion of genes with function unrelated to immune recognition also reside in this region. The interested reader is referred to the continually updated maps and linkages available at various websites, including *http://www.ebi.ac.uk/imgt/hla* and the MHC haplotype project at *http://www.sanger.ac.uk/HGP/Chr6/.*

Figure 2 shows a schematic map of some of the major genes of the human (85), mouse, and rat *Mhc,* which includes those that encode MHC-I and MHC-II proteins. These comparative maps are not drawn to scale and do not show every gene identified in the region. Three markers, Ke2, Bat1, and Mog, serve to define the gross colinearity of the MHC of the three species (86), although there are clearly major differences between strains and even detectable differences between individuals within a species as well. Bat1 and Mog define the boundaries of the MHC-I regions in all three species. The mapping and sequence information now available for the human is more extensive than that available for the mouse and the rat, although data on these are accumulating rapidly. A database of the human *Mhc* is available (*http://www.hgmp.mrc.ac.uk*) (87). The homology of the MHC region of mouse chromosome 17 to that region on human chromosome 6 can be found at *http://www.ncbi.nlm.nih.gov/Homology/,* and extensive maps of syntenic regions of the human and mouse are available there and in the recent publication of the physical map of the mouse genome (88). Large stretches of the rat MHC-I (89,90) and MHC-II (91) regions have been linked.

The human MHC map reveals clusters of genes grouped approximately into an *Mhc-II* region covering about 1,000 kb, an *Mhc-III* region of about 1,000 kb, and an *Mhc-I* region spanning 2,000 kb (Fig. 2). *HLA-DP* genes (*DPA,* which encodes the α chain, and *DPB,* which encodes the β chain) are proximal to the centromere on the short arm of the chromosome and are linked to the genes encoding the related HLA-DM molecule (*DMB* and *DMA*). Between these and the *DQ* genes lie the genes for low-molecular-weight proteins (*LMP*) (92–95)] and *TAP* (96–101). *LMP* and *TAP* genes encode molecules that are involved in peptide generation in the cytosol and peptide transport across the endoplasmic reticulum membrane, respectively. The current view of the LMPs is that they are subunits of the multicatalytic proteolytic proteasome complex that regulate the specificity of cleavage of proteins

TABLE 5. *Comparison of class I and class II MHC molecules*

Characteristic	MHC-Ia and -Ib	Class II MHC
Genetics	Multiple heavy-chain loci; many linked to the MHC Light-chain β_2-microglobulin is genetically unlinked	Several heavy- and light-chain loci, α and β chain genes linked to each other
Polymorphism	Highly polymorphic heavy chain; few alleles of β_2-microglobulin	β chain most polymorphic α chain shows some allelic diversity
Tissue specific expression	MHC Ia: ubiquitous MHC-Ib: on various cell subsets	MHC-II on B cells, macrophages, dendritic cells, Langerhans cells (in the mouse); in human, also found on T cells and many activated cell types
Molecular structure	Heavy chain/light chain form heterodimer; obligate cell surface molecule; heavy chain has three extracellular domains: $\alpha 1$, $\alpha 2$, and $\alpha 3$; $\alpha 1/\alpha 2$ form peptide binding site; α_3 and β_2-m are immunoglobulin-like Only heavy chain is membrane bound, β_2-microglobulin is noncovalently assembled (some MHC-Ib, like MICA, not β_2-microglobulin associated)	α and β chains form heterodimer of four domains; $\alpha 1/\beta 1$ form peptide binding site; $\alpha 2$ and $\beta 2$ are Ig-like Both chains are membrane bound Association of nascent MHC-II with invariant chain
Site of peptide acquisition	In endoplasmic reticulum during biosynthesis Role of Erp57 oxidoreductase in peptide loading; at cell surface when exposed to exogenous peptides	In endosome or lysosome where degraded products of ingested proteins are encountered

Nature of peptides bound	MHC-Ia
	    Preference for octamers to decamers; although longer peptides can be bound
	    "Motif" residues for particular class I MHC molecules
	MHC-Ib
	    CD1 capable of binding lipid antigens
	    MICA, RAE1, HL-60, FcRn, no Peptide binding cleft
		Longer peptides are acceptable

Rules for peptide binding	Defined termini; anchor residues crucial	Core motif of nine residues may be extended variably At either N or C terminal; anchors more subtle Role for backbone interactions
T-cell recognition	Primarily CD8$^+$	Primarily CD4$^+$
NK cell recognition	Interaction with both NK-activating and NK-inhibitory receptors	No known binding by NK receptors
Associated molecules	β_2-microglobulin TAP Tapasin Calnexin	Ii-invariant chain H-2M (HLA-DM)

FcRn, crystallized fragment receptor n; HLA, human leukocyte antigen; MHC, major histocompatibility complex; MHC-Ia, class Ia MHC; MHC-Ib, class Ib MHC; MICA, MHC-I related chain, A; NK, natural killer; RAE1, retinoic acid early inducible–1; TAP, transporter associated with antigen processing.

and thus modulate the repertoire of peptides available for MHC-I–restricted antigen presentation (102–105). The *TAP* genes encode a two-chain intrinsic membrane protein that resides in the endoplasmic reticulum of all cells and functions as an adenosine triphosphate–dependent transporter that pumps peptides generated in the cytosol into the lumen of the endoplasmic reticulum (106,107). The selective transport of cytoplasmically generated peptides by different TAP proteins in the rat demonstrates that the spectrum of MHC/peptide complexes expressed at the cell surface can be significantly altered by differences in the antigen presentation pathway (108–110). Such evidence suggesting that different peptide repertoires are related to different allelic forms of LMPs or of TAP has raised the possibility that genetic variation of LMPs or TAP may be related to autoimmune or malignant disease (111–113). However, the potential relationship between LMP2 expression and autoimmune diabetes in nonobese diabetic mice has provoked considerable discussion (114,115).

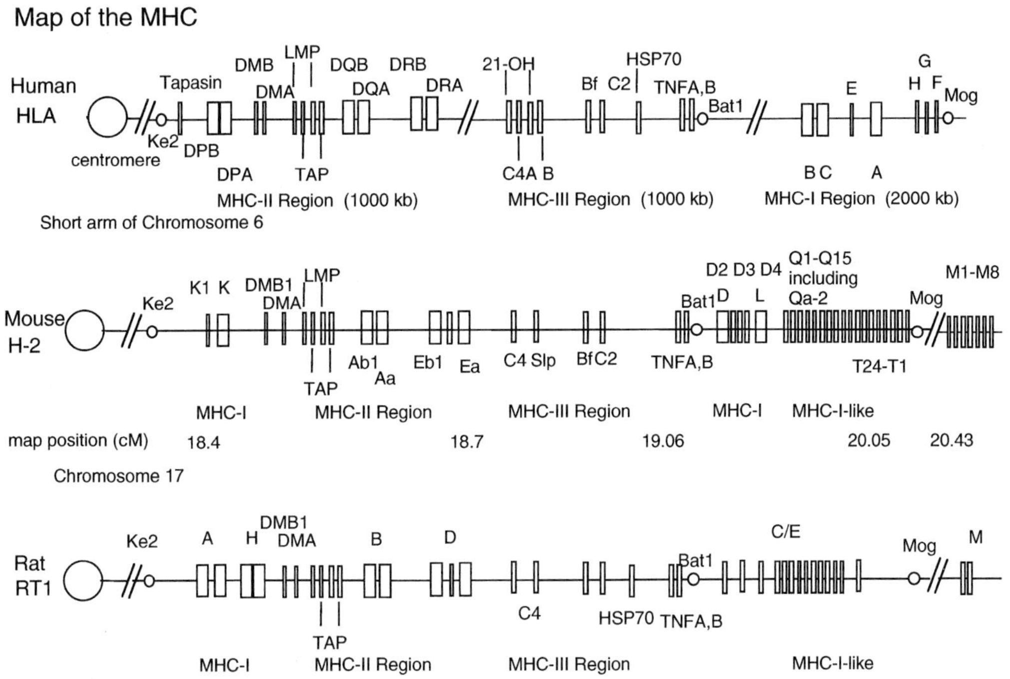

Map of the MHC

FIG. 2. Genetic maps of the major histocompatibility complex (*Mhc*). Comparative map of the human, mouse, and rat MHC. This schematic map is not complete or drawn to scale; it is derived from maps available elsewhere (86,87,89–91,149,158,452). The centromere and major genes are indicated.

The major *Mhc-II* genes of the human are *HLA-DRA* and *HLA-DRB,* which encode the chains that form the HLA-DR molecule, a major antigen presentation element. Genetic mapping of the human DRB region now indicates that several alternative arrangements of different DRB pseudogenes and functional genes account for the varied serotypes and genotypes observed among individuals (Fig. 3). Because these are carried as sets of genes in linkage disequilibrium, they are frequently referred to as *haplotypes.* The *Mhc-III* region is important in immunological terms for several reasons: The structural genes for several complement components map here, as do the structural genes for 21-hydroxylase (CYP21A2) (116,117), an enzyme critical in the biosynthesis of glucocorticoids, a deficiency of which can lead to congenital adrenal hyperplasia. Also linked in the *Mhc-III* region are the structural genes for tumor necrosis factors α and β (TNF-α and TNF-β), which are lymphokines made by activated T cells (118–120). TNF-β is also known as lymphotoxin α.

The more distal region of the *Mhc* encodes other MHC molecules; in the human, the cluster of the major *Mhc-I* genes lies here, spanning 2 Mb and including the genes encoding HLA-B, HLA C, HLA-E, and HLA-A, as well as HLA-H, HLA-G, and HLA-F. In humans, HLA-A, HLA-B, and HLA-C are the major MHC-I molecules. (A summary of the serological and genetic identification of these is in Table 2). Serological identification of HLA-C molecules has been difficult and imprecise; however, HLA-C molecules interact directly with NK receptors of the killer cell immunoglobulin-like

receptor (KIR) KIR2D family. Direct binding studies have analyzed the kinetics of the interaction of the KIR2 receptors (121–123), and three-dimensional structures of KIR2DL2 in complex with HLA-Cw3 and of KIR2DL1 in complex with HLA-Cw4 have been published (124,125). The precise functions of HLA-E, HLA-F, and HLA-G are not yet clear. HLA-E and its murine analog Qa-1 bind the hydrophobic leader peptides derived from some MHC-I molecules, forming a complex that is recognized by the C-type lectin-like NK receptor CD94/NKG2 (126–130). This implies an important function for HLA-E because these molecules are expressed on placental trophoblast cells and would be expected to bind the inhibitory NK receptor CD94/NKG2A, preventing NK-mediated rejection of the fetus (131,132). HLA-E has been shown to serve as a recognition element for some T cells as well, and so it seems capable of a more classical as well as a unique functional role (129,133,134). Some evidence now also supports an antigen presentation function of HLA-F and HLA-G (135,136) and the tissue-restricted expression of HLA-G. It has also been observed that a soluble form leads to apoptosis of CD8+ T cells, which suggests that this molecule may be involved in the mother's immunological tolerance of the fetus (137). *HLA-H* (138) is a pseudogene mapping to this region. This should not be confused with the more distantly related *HLA-HFE,* an *Mhc-Ib* gene erroneously called *HLA-H* by some authors (139,140), that controls hereditary hemochromatosis by virtue of its role in iron metabolism that results from its interaction with the transferrin receptor (141–146).

MHC Class II Region (~1 Megabase)

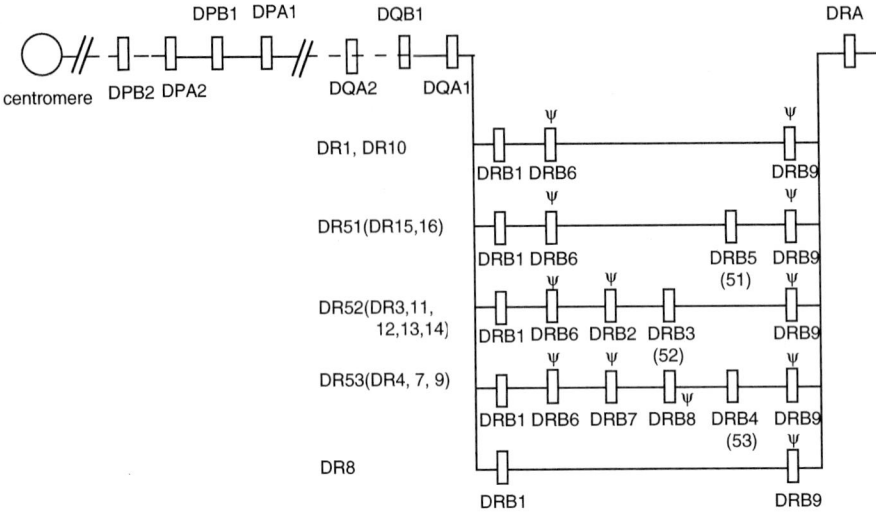

FIG. 3. Genetic basis of the structural variation in human leukocyte antigen (HLA) class II haplotypes. All HLA class II haplotypes contain DPA1, DPB1, DQA1, DQB1, DRA, and DRB1 loci; however, there is variation in the number of additional DRB loci found on different haplotypes. The DRB9 pseudogene (labeled with a ψ) is common to all haplotypes; however, a DRB3 locus product is also expressed on haplotypes containing any of the serological DRB1 specificities DR3, DR5 (11,12), or DR6 (13,14). The DRB3 β chain forms a cell surface heterodimer with the DRA α chain and creates the serological specificity DR52. These haplotypes also contain DRB6 and DRB2 loci that are pseudogenes. The DRB5 locus is found on most haplotypes containing the serological DRB1 specificity DR2, but this gene product is also occasionally expressed on other DRB1 haplotypes (164).

Comparison of the mouse, rat, and human *Mhc* maps reveals several interesting differences (147–150). The *Mhc* genes proximal to the centromere of the mouse and rat belong to the *Mhc-I* family, rather than to the *Mhc-II* family, as they do in the human. This mapping has suggested that an intrachromosomal recombination event that occurred in some common rodent ancestor displaced some of the *Mhc-I* genes from a more distal location to the proximal site (151). Inspection of the current human, mouse, and rat maps clearly indicates similarities in the relative locations and organization of *Mhc-II*, *Mhc-III*, and the distal *Mhc-I* genes (149). The major rat MHC-I molecule is RT1.A. Various genetic expansions and contractions are obvious as well. In particular, the mouse Q and T regions have expanded the pool of *Mhc-I* genes, which are relatively few in the human and the rat. Early studies of congenic mouse strains mapped multiple genes to the Q and T regions (152–154), and more recent evidence suggests significant differences in the number of genes of this region in different strains. The mouse has some MHC-Ib genes that seem to be relatively unique in function. In particular, the *H-2M3* gene (not to be confused with the *Mhc-II H-2Ma* and *H-2Mb* genes, which encode the homologues of the human HLA-DMA and HLA-DMB proteins), which maps distal to the Q and T regions, encodes a protein that exhibits a preference for binding peptides that have *N*-formyl amino terminal modifications, an antigen presenta-

tion function that may be geared to bacterial, protozoal, and mitochondrial antigens (155–157). Rat homologues of the mouse *H-2M3* and *H-2M2* genes have been identified (158).

Major Histocompatibility Complex Polymorphism

The *Mhc's* function in immune responsiveness is also reflected in its genetic polymorphism. Polymorphism is the presence at any given time of a larger-than-expected number of genetic variants in a population. As populations change and evolve, genetic variants are expected to arise, but because of constraints on the function of some genetic markers, relatively few of these genetic variants are able to persist. The generally accepted convention is that a genetic locus that exhibits more than 1% of the alleles as variant at any one time is *polymorphic*. A polymorphic locus or gene, therefore, is one that has a high frequency (not number) of genetic variants (1). A genetic locus that is relatively invariant is often referred to as *monomorphic*, even if more than one allele is recognized. *HLA* genes exhibit a high degree of polymorphism, and a number of different mechanisms may contribute to the generation and maintenance of polymorphism. Among these are the suggested selective advantage of a pool of antigen-presenting elements that might allow the binding and presentation of antigenic peptides derived from a wide variety of environmental pathogens. Limited polymorphism would make the entire population susceptible to a chance infectious agent to which all individuals would be unable to respond, whereas widespread polymorphism would be expected to allow the APCs of at least a proportion of the population to bind and present antigens derived from invading pathogens effectively (159,160). Such a view was originally based on HLA molecules as presenting elements for pathogen-derived peptide fragments to T cells and their antigen-specific TCRs; more recent studies suggest an additional role for MHC-I–related resistance to viral infection through an NK cell–mediated recognition (161,162).

The human *Mhc-I* and *Mhc-II* genes are clearly polymorphic; more than 50 alleles at each of the *HLA-A, HLA-B,* and *HLA-DRB* loci have been identified (163,164) (Tables 2 and 3). In experimental animals, it is more difficult to demonstrate polymorphism in terms of population genetics, although typing of wild mice has confirmed the impression gained from the analysis of inbred strains and mutants derived from them (165). The polymorphism of *Mhc-I* and *Mhc-II* genes, so evident in human and mouse, has also been documented in analyses of cichlid fishes, animals that diverged at least several hundred million years ago from the line leading to mammals (166–168).

Major Histocompatibility Complex Evolutionary Mechanisms

As both an extended genetic region and a group of genes with many belonging to the immunoglobulin supergene family (169,170), the *Mhc* has served as a prototype for elucidating and understanding mechanisms that contribute to the evolution of a multigene family and that add to the polymorphism that is such a dominant characteristic of the classical MHC molecules (150). The analysis of mutations in the mouse, mostly those of *Mhc-I* genes, has led to the understanding of the mechanisms that give rise to polymorphism. The mutations have been identified in mice by screening large numbers of animals by skin grafting of siblings. Both induced and spontaneous mutations affecting skin graft acceptance or rejection have been identified, and many of these have been mapped to the *Mhc*. Gross recombinational events have been documented (171,172), as have more subtle mutations, many of which are multiple amino acid substitutions in a relatively small part of the protein that seem to derive from nonreciprocal crossing-over events. Such a nonreciprocal recombinational event that occurs over short sequences is known as *gene conversion* because of its similarity to a phenomenon that occurs in yeast (171–178).

The mechanism of gene conversion in mice is now better understood because nucleotide sequence analysis and oligonucleotide-specific hybridization have been used not only to characterize the mutations that have occurred but also to identify the *Mhc* genes that have been the donors of the mutant sequences. Although the precise enzymatic details are not clear, it is now understood that gene conversion is a genetic event that allows the copying or transposition of short

sequences from a donor gene to a recipient. Some of the polymorphisms of *Mhc* genes that have been identified clearly reflect point mutations (164). The most important *H-2* mutants and the identified donor genes are summarized in Table 4. Structural studies have shown that the profound immunological effects of mutations of the *H-2* genes *H-2K*^{bm1} and *H-2K*^{bm8} result from minimal detectable structural changes that may affect thermostability (179). In addition to such mouse mutants, a number of somatic cell variants and mutants, some resulting from major deletions or regulational defects and others clearly from point mutants of structural genes, have been described (180). The characterization of three mutants of the *H2K*^{b} gene, mutants that have a complex set of several mutations over a more extended region of DNA, suggests that no single donor gene can be identified for these mutants. An effort to identify the donor gene for the *H2K*^{bm3}, *H2K*^{bm23}, and *H2D*^{bm23} mutations led to the conclusion that these complex mutations must have arisen by the contribution of at least two different donor genes acting either in sequence or in synergy (180).

The Major Histocompatibility Complex and Transplantation

Although the early description of the genes of the *Mhc* was based on identification of loci involved in tumor and allograft rejection (the rejection of grafts from genetically disparate donors of the same species), and although these genes clearly play a role in such complex phenomena, a contemporary understanding of the function of *Mhc* genes in immunology requires little understanding of the rules of transplantation. The early history of transplantation is chronicled extensively in several books (1,3) and reflects a developing interest in tumor immunology and congenic mouse strains. The most extensively studied species for tumor, tissue, and organ transplantation has been the mouse, and so a brief description of some relevant principles is in order. Comprehensive manuals and reviews are available (181). Propagation of a mouse strain by repeated matings of brothers and sisters leads to the establishment of an inbred strain, a group of animals that are genetically identical at all loci. More complete descriptions of the process by which brother–sister mating leads to homozygosity at all loci are given elsewhere (1,3). The probability of fixation of all loci (P_{fix}) as a function of the number of generations, n, is given by $P_{fix} = 1 - (7/8)^{n-1}$. Thus, after five generations of brother–sister matings, the probability of all loci being identical is 0.414; after 10 generations, 0.7; after 15 generations, 0.85; and after 20 generations, 0.91.

"Congenic" mouse strains, also known as "congenic-resistant" mouse strains, are those derived by first crossing two inbred strains that differ in a histocompatibility phenotype (such as resistance to a transplantable tumor or ability to reject a skin graft) and then successively backcrossing to one parental strain; in this way, the resistance phenotype is preserved. After at least 10 backcross generations (N10), $(1/2)^9 = 0.002$ of the genes of the selected strain should be present, the new strain is propagated by brother–sister mating. From such breeding schemes, a number of strains critical to genetic studies of the *Mhc* have been derived. Several relevant inbred mouse strains, congenic-resistant strains, are listed in Table 4 along with their *H-2* designations.

The availability of numerous polymerase chain reaction–based genetic markers throughout the mouse genome allows the direct identification of the progeny that have a greater proportion of the desired background at each generation. Selective backcrossing, taking advantage of the genotype of a large number of such genetic markers distributed widely throughout the genome, a process known as "speed congenics," can hasten the process of establishing a homogeneous background for a particular mutant or knock-in trait (182,183). Because strains obtained by brother–sister matings may reveal genetic drift as spontaneous mutations accumulate in the strain, it is crucial to keep track of the stock from which the animals were derived and the number of generations that they have been propagated without backcrossing to founder stock. This has been of particular concern because various lines of embryonic stem cells derived from different lines of strain 129 have been used for genetic manipulation (gene knockout experiments) (184) and there are clearly differences in histocompatibility (185).

The early rules of transplantation were determined by observation of the ability of either transplantable tumors or allografts (usually from skin) to survive in a particular inbred mouse strain host. The graft rejection phenomenon is an extremely sensitive and specific bioassay that permits the detection of genetic differences as small as a single amino acid in an MHC protein. It has been particularly valuable in assessing spontaneous and induced mutants (see previous discussion) and remains the absolute experimental discriminator of histocompatibility.

In addition to the *Mhc* genes, there exist the genes that encode minor histocompatibility antigens. In the mouse, these were originally identified as genetic loci responsible for graft rejection after extended periods of time. More recently, several minor histocompatibility loci have been identified as those that encode polymorphic proteins that give rise to peptides presented by MHC molecules (186–189), and the complexities of transplantation tolerance are now understood not only in terms of *Mhc* genes but also in terms of numerous proteins that may give rise to variant peptides for T-cell recognition.

The Major Histocompatibility Complex and Clinical Transplantation

Processed foreign antigen complexed to class I or class II HLA molecules is recognized by a specific clonally distributed TCR for antigen on the surface of T-lymphocytes. The T cell bearing an $\alpha\beta$ receptor is capable of recognizing the structure of the HLA molecule itself coordinately with the exposed parts of the peptide antigen. Co-recognition of HLA and peptide antigen means that T-cell antigen receptors are highly specific and genetically restricted to recognizing HLA molecules of the individual from which they were derived. Thus, a killer (cytotoxic) T cell raised against an influenza virus peptide in an individual expressing HLA-A2 does not confer any influenza immunity when passively transferred to an individual expressing HLA-A1. This concept is known as *MHC-restriction* and was first described by Zinkernagel and Doherty (8) for recognition of viral antigens, by Shevach and Rosenthal (7) for recognition of alloantigens, and by Shearer et al. (6) for recognition of altered self ligands. Given that T cells are MHC restricted, it is difficult to understand why they should ever recognize a foreign HLA type. However, in practice they do, and it is generally believed that they do so with alarmingly high frequency. Estimates of between 1/10 to 1/1,000 activated clonally distinct T cells are capable of responding to any random allogeneic HLA molecule (190–193). In view of the number of T cells in the human lymphoid system, this represents a striking tendency for T cells that are normally restricted to recognizing self HLA molecules complexed to foreign peptides to cross-react on allogeneic HLA molecules. This cross-reaction can arise from direct recognition of the allogeneic HLA/peptide complex, which usually depends on the peptide antigen as well as on the allogeneic HLA molecule. Alternatively, allorecognition by T cells can occur indirectly (194,195). In this case, peptides derived from the allogeneic HLA molecules are presented as nominal antigen after processing by the host cells bearing self HLA molecules. In the normal course of events, T-cell alloreactivity is an *in vitro* curiosity, although it is still not entirely clear why the fetal "allograft" does not stimulate the maternal immune system. However, the clinical transplantation of organs and hematopoietic stem cells across HLA incompatibility barriers produces graft rejection or graft-versus-host disease (GVHD) because of T cell alloreactivity. Fully allogeneic transplants theoretically expose the recipient immune system to up to 12 non-self HLA alleles expressed by the allograft. Moreover, the "self-peptides" constitutively presented by allogeneic HLA molecules are likely to be quite distinct from those presented by syngeneic HLA molecules because the polymorphisms of the peptide antigen-binding cleft of the MHC-I molecule that distinguish HLA alleles alter the spectrum of selected peptides. Allogeneic HLA/peptide complexes probably stimulate powerful T-cell responses because of the high density of unusual determinants and the diversity of new peptide ligands presented by the allogeneic HLA/peptide complexes. (Because there are so many genes encoding a host of proteins, superficially lacking immunological function, that are linked to the different HLA haplotypes—see previous section on MHC genetic maps—it is likely that polymorphisms in these molecules contribute significantly to the alloresponse.) Accordingly, many studies have demonstrated an incremental improvement in long-term graft survival with progressively higher levels of HLA matching at HLA-B and HLA-DR loci. For this reason, HLA matching is required, or desirable, in many forms of transplantation. The degree of HLA matching usually required for

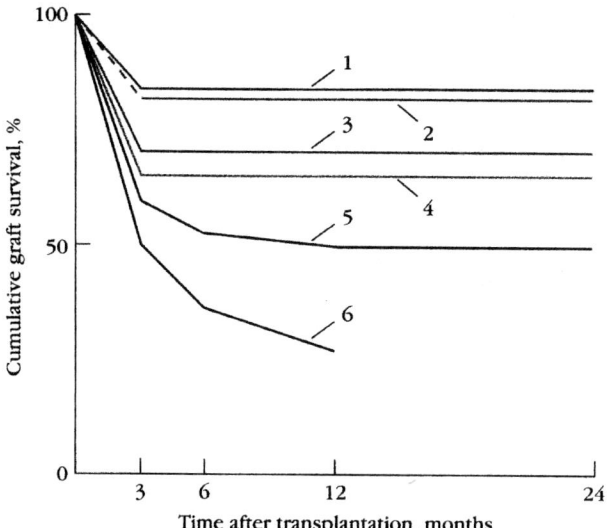

	HLA mismatches (no.)	
Curve no.	Class I	Class II
1	0	0
2	1 or 2	0
3	3 or 4	0
4	0	1 or 2
5	1 or 2	1 or 2
6	3 or 4	1 or 2

FIG. 4. Renal graft survival improves with fewer human leukocyte antigen (HLA) mismatches. Cumulative data for graft survival are plotted as a function of time. Curves 1, 2, and 3 represent the groups with no class II HLA mismatches and four or fewer class I HLA mismatches, whereas curve 4 shows the graft survival of those with fewer than two class II mismatches and no class I mismatch. The worst survivals are clearly those with both HLA class I and class II mismatches.

renal transplantation is shown in Fig. 4, and that required for bone marrow transplantation is shown in Table 6.

In addition to the allogeneic cellular response, the antibody response to HLA molecules and ABO blood groups can also cause rejection of certain grafts, especially when these antibodies are preformed and therefore present at the time of organ transplantation. Antibodies to ABO blood group antigens react with these determinants on vascular endothelium, and therefore ABO-incompatible solid organs can be rapidly rejected by humoral mechanisms. In patients who have undergone transfusion or previous transplantation or in multiparous women, exposure to allogeneic HLA molecules can also result in the production of anti–class I HLA antibodies. These preformed antibodies can lead to acute and hyperacute rejection of grafts expressing the particular HLA molecules recognized by these antibodies. Therefore, for solid organ transplants, not only are individuals matched as closely as possible for their HLA types to avert cellular rejection but it is also necessary to ensure ABO compatibility and to exclude preformed antidonor HLA antibodies in the host.

Paradoxically, some patients who have received multiple blood transfusions before transplantation appear to develop some form of T cell tolerance to allogeneic donor HLA alleles, and renal graft survival is actually enhanced in these individuals. This is known as the *"transfusion effect,"* and in some centers, pretransplantation transfusion and even donor-specific transfusions are routinely carried out. Transfusion of potential renal transplant recipients, however, carries the risk of inducing undesirable anti-HLA antibodies in the patient.

Testing for anti-HLA antibodies is known as the *crossmatch.* In practice, many laboratories crossmatch only for anti–class I HLA antibodies. Crossmatch compatibility to exclude anti–class I HLA antibodies is essential in renal transplantation and is widely practiced in heart-lung transplantation. Crossmatching for liver transplantation is practiced at only some centers, and the evidence that a positive crossmatch predicts allogeneic liver graft rejection has not convinced everyone of its importance in routine matching. Patients awaiting renal transplantation are usually monitored regularly for anti–class I HLA antibodies because the level and specificity of these antibodies can change with time. This monitoring involves regular crossmatching of the patient's serum against a panel of randomly selected cells bearing different HLA types. The percentage of positively reacting cells is known as

TABLE 6. *MHC matching versus success of bone marrow transplantation*

MHC compatibility survival	Risk of graft rejection (%)	Risk of graft-versus-host disease (%)	
		Acute	3-year
Share two haplotypes (HLA-identical sibling)	2	40	50
Share one haplotype plus			
Phenotypically identical	7	40	50
1 HLA mismatch	9	70	50
>2 HLA mismatches	21	80	15
Share zero haplotypes			
Unrelated			
"Matched"	3	80	35
"Mismatched"	5	95	35

HLA, human leukocyte antigen; MHC, major histocompatibility complex.
From Christiansen and Witt (447), with permission.

the *panel reactivity*. When performing a crossmatch between a patient's serum and donor cells, many centers test the current as well as "historical peak" serum from the patient. The historical peak is defined as the patient serum sample giving the highest panel reactivity throughout the monitoring period and is thought to be a sensitive reflection of previous HLA sensitization.

The role of antibody crossmatching in hematopoietic stem cell transplantation is unclear, and most centers do not take the class I or class II crossmatch into account when identifying a bone marrow transplant donor. On the other hand, some large centers place some importance on a positive crossmatch as a predictor of bone marrow rejection, and it is therefore advisable to crossmatch bone marrow donor–recipient pairs when there is a high risk of rejection (e.g. aplastic anemia). Crossmatching is also used to detect anti-HLA antibodies that cause refractoriness to platelet transfusion with random platelets.

Family Studies in Histocompatibility Testing

The linkage of HLA loci on chromosome 6 means that individuals usually inherit a set of nonrecombined HLA alleles encoded at linked HLA loci from each parent. This set of genes (the haplotype) is often identifiable in family studies in which all the alleles that are present on one chromosome cosegregate. In identifying donors for hematopoietic stem cell transplantation, testing of family members is essential for accurately determining haplotypes (196,197). This is

because sharing of HLA antigens from different haplotypes is quite common in families, and so subtype mismatches are easily overlooked because of mistaken haplo-identity of siblings or other family members. Because unrecognized HLA mismatching is poorly tolerated in hematopoietic stem cell transplantation, very careful matching is required to avoid GVHD (198–200). An example of haplotyping in a family study is shown in Fig. 5.

The role of HLA-DP in allogeneic stem cell transplantation is still unclear, and so testing for this locus is not routine clinically except when several donors are available and a rational choice of the best donor has to be made (201,202). Typically, an HLA typing laboratory would test for HLA-A, HLA-B, HLA-DRB1, HLA-DRB3, HLA-B4, HLA-B5, and HLA-DQ loci (203). In the family study shown in Fig. 5, the mother and father are mismatched at both haplotypes. Among the children, John and Andrew are haploidentical (and therefore phenotypically identical). Jane and Jim share a single haplotype, as do Tom and Jim. Jane's paternal haplotype is a recombinant involving a crossover event between HLA-A and -B. Recombination is observed between HLA-A and HLA-B and between HLA-B and HLA-DR in about 1% of meiotic events. The implications of this family study are that Andrew and John would be ideal bone marrow donors for each other but none of the other siblings would be suitable as a donor for these brothers. Even though there is sharing of a single haplotype between Tom and both Andrew and John, the complete mismatch in the second haplotype would make Tom unsuitable as a donor for hematopoietic stem cell

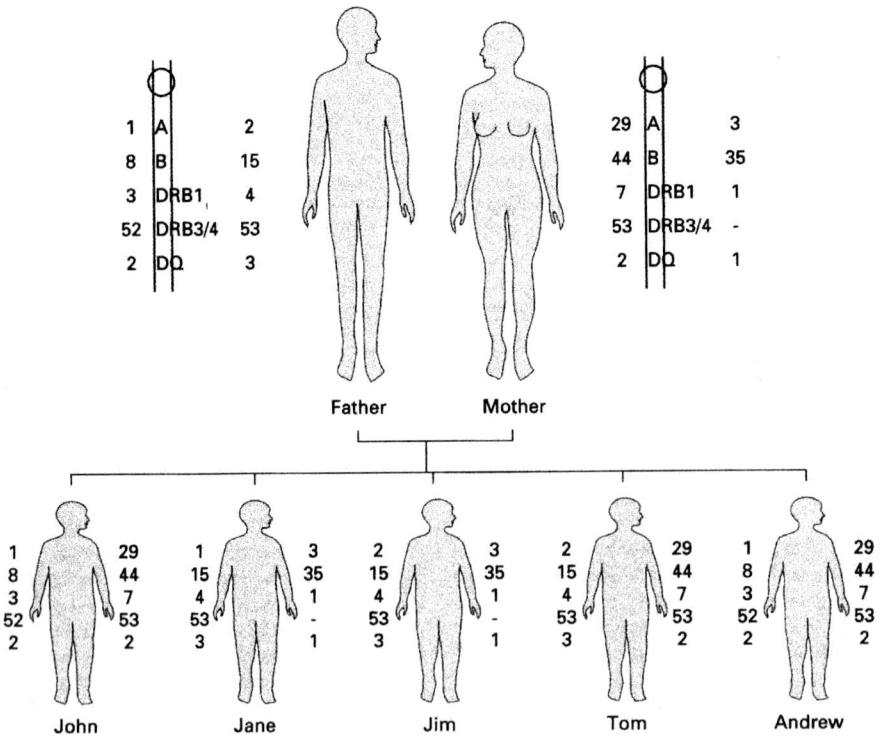

FIG. 5. Segregation of human leukocyte antigen haplotypes in a family. From McCluskey (453), with permission.

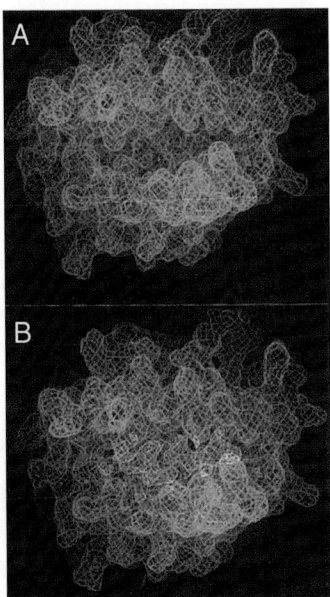

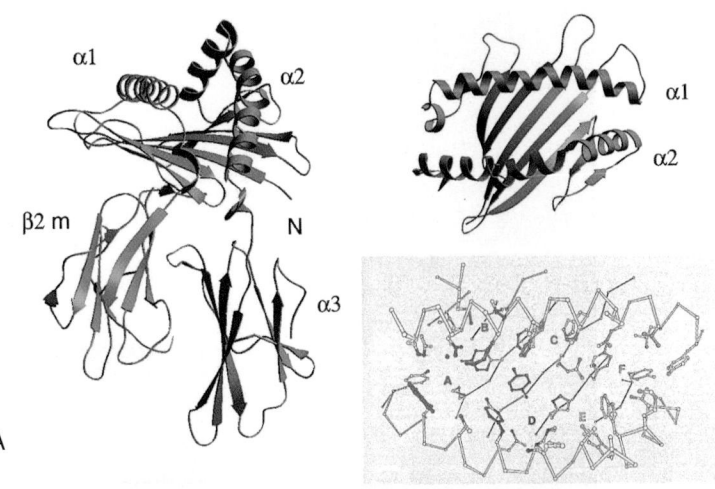

A

C

COLORPLATE 1. Electron density in the cleft of human leukocyte antigen (HLA)–A*0201. **A:** A surface representation of the HLA-A2 structure is shown in *blue.* **B:** The electron density not accounted for by the amino acid sequence of the protein is in *red.* From Bjorkman et al. (321), with permission.

COLORPLATE 2. Color ribbon representation of human leukocyte antigen (HLA)–A*0201. **A:** side view. **B:** top view. **C:** top view with positions of pockets A through F indicated. Panels A and B were made with SETOR (456), based on the protein data bank [PDB, ref. (455)] coordinates of 3HLA (349). Panel C is from Saper et al. (349), with permission.

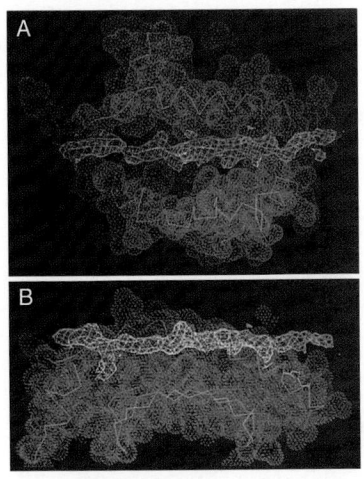

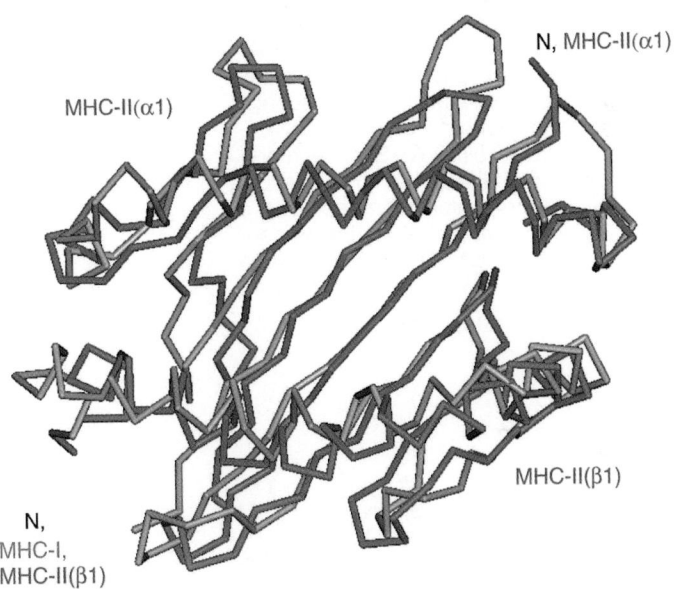

COLORPLATE 3. The location of the electron density in the cleft of human leukocyte antigen (HLA)–DR1. **A:** A classical top view of the class II major histocompatibility complex (MHC)–binding cleft with the α1 helix above and the β1 helix below. **B:** The orthogonal view of the same site from the side. The β1 helix is proximal to the viewer. The class II MHC surface is in *blue,* and the bound peptide electron density in *red.* From Brown et al. (362), with permission.

COLORPLATE 4. Superposition of the α-carbon backbones of a class I major histocompatibility complex (MHC) [PDB (455), 3HLA (349)] molecule and a class II MHC [1DLH (364)] molecule. The backbone tracings were displayed and superposed with QUANTA 97 (Molecular Simulations, Inc). Class I MHC is shown in *blue* and class II MHC in *red.* Amino termini are labeled *N.*

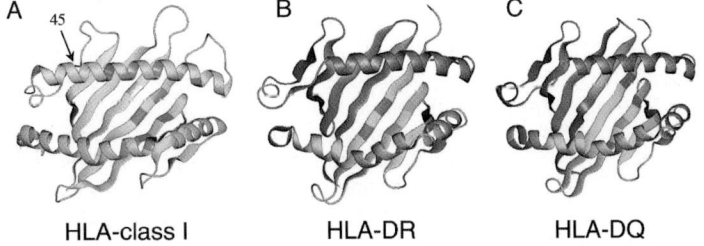

COLORPLATE 5. Location of polymorphic amino acid residues in MHC-I and MHC-II molecules. Variability plots were calculated as described in legend to Figure 9 and level of variability illustrated on ribbon diagrams [generated in QUANTA 2000 (Accelrys) of 3HLA (349)(HLA-class I), 1DLH (364) (HLA-DR), and 1JK8 (457)(HLA-DQ)] where greatest variability is *red,* intermediate is *green* and least is *blue.*

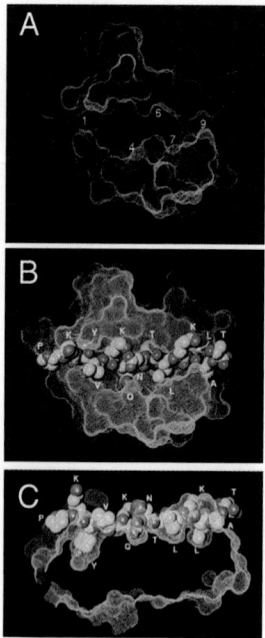

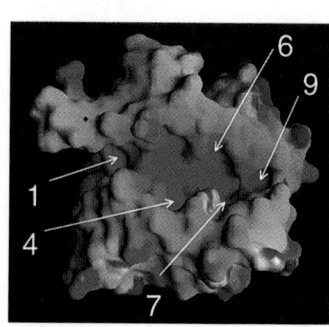

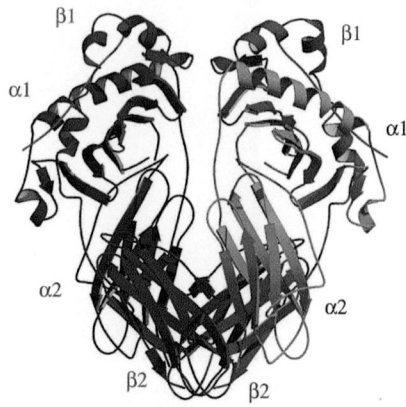

COLORPLATE 6. Location of pockets in human leukocyte antigen (HLA)–DR1 based on the cocrystal of HLA-DR1 with a peptide derived from the influenza hemagglutinin. The surface representation of the α1 and β1 domains is in *blue*. **A:** Surface representation of HLA-DR1 without peptide. **B:** Same representation, including a space-filling model of the bound peptide, PKYVKQNTLKLAT. **C:** A side view of part B. From Stern et al. (364), with permission.

COLORPLATE 7. Numbering of the major binding pockets of human leukocyte antigen (HLA)–DR1, according to Stern et al. (364). The structure of HLA-DR1, PDB (455) file 1DLH (364), was displayed with GRASP (458).

COLORPLATE 8. Ribbon diagram of the structure of human leukocyte antigen (HLA)–DR1 showing the dimer of dimers and the individual domains of the protein. α Chains are in *blue* and *yellow,* β chains are in *red* and *green,* and peptide is in *red*. The illustration was generated from 1DLH (364) in MOLSCRIPT (459) and rendered in RASTER3D (460).

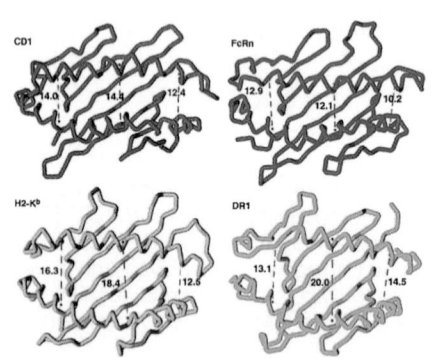

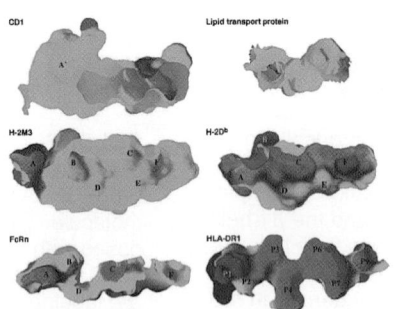

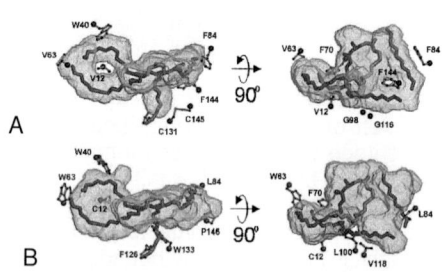

COLORPLATE 9. Comparison of the α-carbon backbone tracings and size of the potential peptide-binding cleft of class I major histocompatibility complex (MHC) molecule H-2K^b, class II MHC human leukocyte antigen (HLA)–DR1, and class Ib MHC molecules CD1d and FcRn. From Zeng et al. (378), with permission.

COLORPLATE 10. Shape, size, and charge of the binding groove of CD1d in comparison with those of several other major histocompatibility complex (MHC) molecules and with a lipid transport protein. Surface representation of the ligand binding cleft is displayed with acidic regions in *red,* basic regions in *blue,* and hydrophobic regions in *green*. From Zeng et al. (378), with permission.

COLORPLATE 11. Structural differences between the binding grooves of CD1b and CD1d. **A:** Orthogonal views for CD1b. **B:<** Orthogonal views for CD1d. The hydrophobic groove and key side chains for CD1b and CD1d are in *blue* and *green*, respectively. Position of alkyl chains and detergent visualized in CD1b are colored with regard to the binding channels they occupy: A′ in *red*, C′ in *yellow*, F′ in *pink*, and T′ in *violet*. From Gadola et al. (379), with permission.

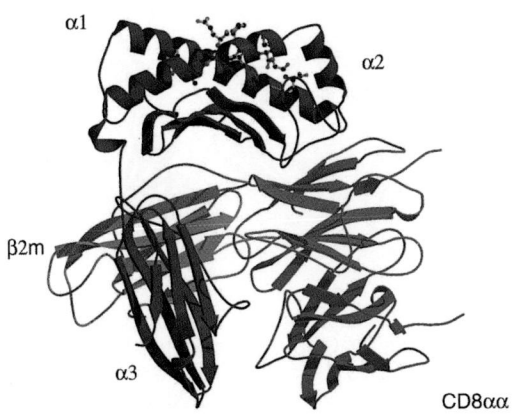

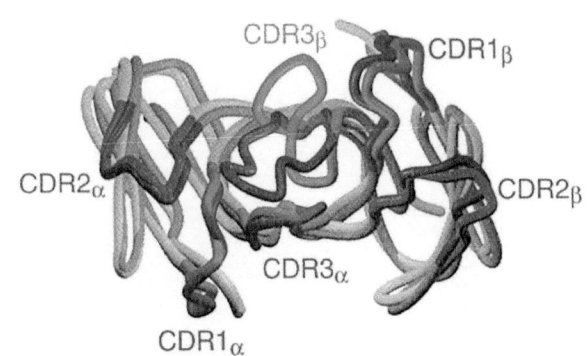

COLORPLATE 12. Structure of the FcRn complexed with Fc. Ribbon diagram of the FcRn (*purple*), β_2-microglobulin (*green*) interacting with the Fc (*magenta* and *brown*) heterodimer consisting of the wild type (wt) and nonbinding (nb) engineered chain. For comparison, the homodimer of the nbFc is shown on the right. [These are PDB (455) files, 1I1A and 1I1C (398) respectively.] From Martin et al. (398) with permission.

COLORPLATE 13. Structure of a class I major histocompatibility complex (MHC)/peptide/T-cell receptor (TCR) complex. H-2K^b bound to the peptide dEV8 (EQYKFYSV) in complex with the 2C TCR is shown. The TCR α and β chains (*magenta* and *light blue*) as well as H-2K^b (*green*) and peptide (*yellow*) are shown. Complementarity determining regions (CDRs) of the TCR, colored in contrasting colors, and labeled 1, 2, and 3 are also indicated. From Garcia et al. (402), with permission.

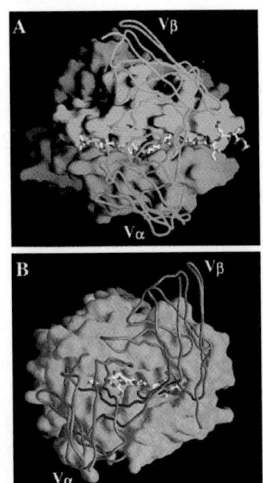

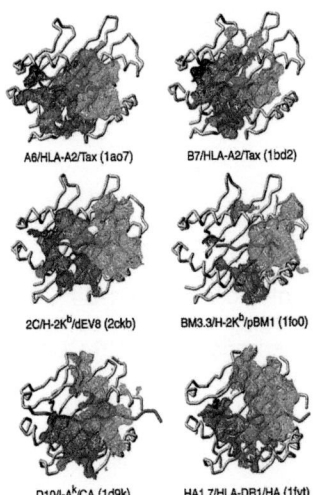

COLORPLATE 14. Footprints of CDRs of six different major histocompatibility complex (MHC)/peptide/T-cell receptor (TCR) complexes. The surfaces imprinted by different CDRs are color-coded: CDR1α in *dark blue*, CDR2α in *magenta*, CDR3α in *green*, CDR1β in *cyan*, CDR2β in *pink*, and CDR3β in *yellow*. From Rudolph et al. (461), with permission.

COLORPLATE 15. Different docking modes of T-cell receptor (TCR) Vα and Vβ in different major histocompatibility complex (MHC)/peptide/TCR complexes. **A:** Docking of scD10 TCR on IA^k/CA structure; the IA α chain is shown in *light green*, the β chain in *orange*, the Vα chain in *green*, and the Vβ chain in *light blue*. **B:** Docking of 2C TCR on H-2K^b/dEV8 structure; H-2K^b is shown in *orange* and Vα and Vβ in *magenta*. From Reinherz et al. (374), with permission.

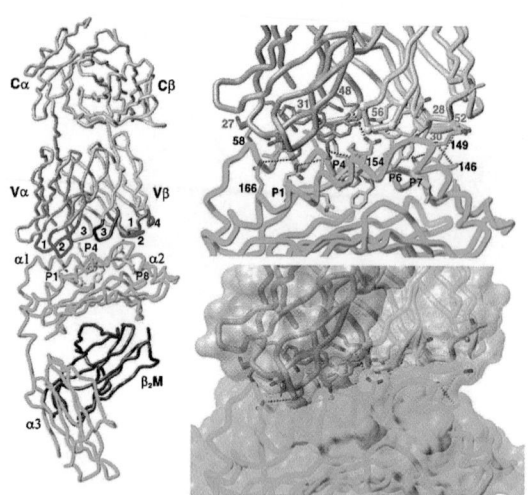

COLORPLATE 16. CDR3 plasticity. Backbone tracings of the KB5-C20 T-cell receptor (TCR) CDR loops free or bound to the major histocompatibility complex (MHC)/peptide complex are superposed. The unliganded forms are in lighter colors. From Reiser et al. (403), with permission.

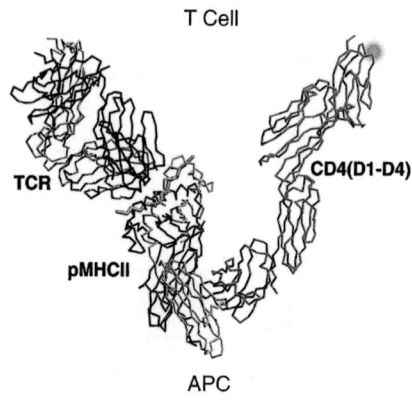

COLORPLATE 18. Model of T-cell receptor (TCR)/class II major histocompatibility complex (MHC)/peptide complex interacting with CD4. Superposition of class II MHC/CD4 D1D2 structure with that of a complete D1-D4 CD4 structure results in this model, which suggests how class II MHC may contribute to multimerization of a TCR/CD4 complex. From Wang et al. (79), with permission.

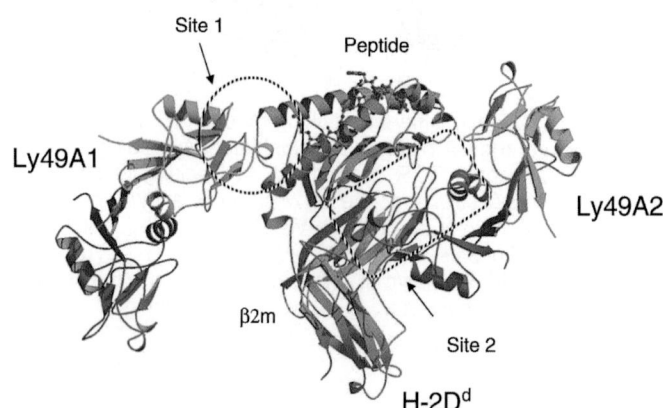

COLORPLATE 20. H-2D^d interactions with the C-type lectin-like receptor, Ly49A. The crystallographic determination of two distinct sites of H-2D^d interacting with the Ly49A homodimer is shown. Extensive mutagenesis and binding studies suggest that the functional site of interaction is site 2. From Natarajan et al. (13), with permission.

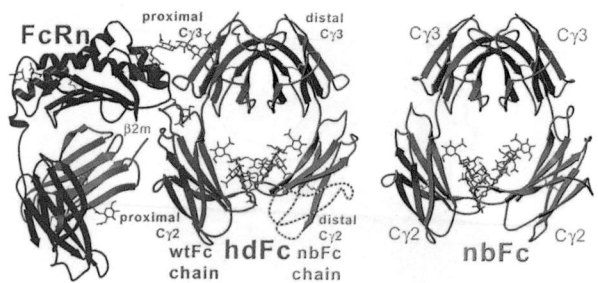

COLORPLATE 17. Class I major histocompatibility complex (MHC) binding site for CD8$\alpha\alpha$ homodimer lies beneath the peptide binding groove. Human leukocyte antigen (HLA)–A2 heavy chain is shown in *red*, β_2-microglobulin is shown in *orange*, and peptides (ball-and-stick) are shown in complex with the CD8$\alpha\alpha$ homodimer (*red* and *blue*). MOLSCRIPT (459) illustration is based on the PDB (455) file 1AKJ (83).

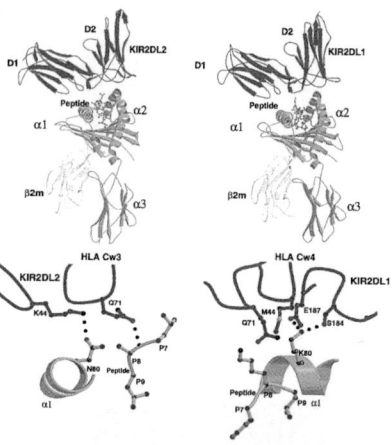

COLORPLATE 19. Interactions of killer cell immunoglobulin-like receptor, two-domain (KIR2D) molecules with their human leukocyte antigen (HLA)–Cw ligands. KIR2DL2 (**A, C**) and KIR2DL1 (**B, D**) are shown (*magenta*) in complex with their respective HLA-Cw3 and HLA-Cw4 ligands. From Natarajan et al. (13), with permission.

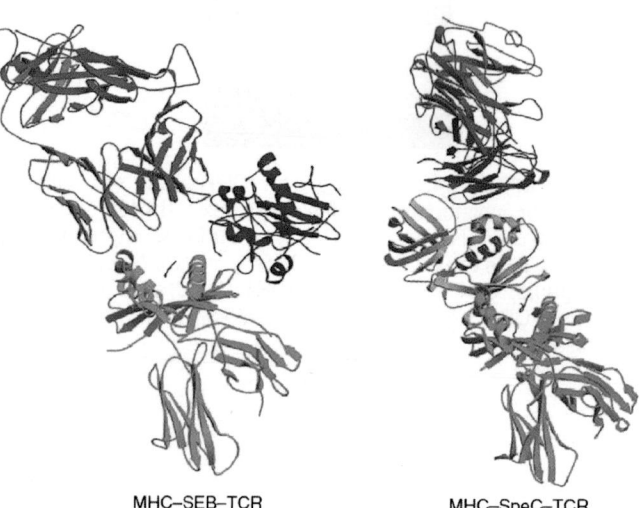

MHC–SEB–TCR   MHC–SpeC–TCR

COLORPLATE 21. Different superantigens. Staphylococcal enterotoxin B (SEB) (**A**) and SpeC (**B**) interact differently with T-cell receptor and class II major histocompatibility complex. From Sundberg et al. (462), with permission.

transplantation, which requires very close matching of HLA. On the other hand, haplotype mismatching is common in renal transplantation, in which perfect HLA matching is not absolutely required or routinely achievable (because of the narrow time frame for acquisition of acceptable cadaver donor grafts). However, for renal and other solid organ transplantation, ABO blood group compatibility is essential because these determinants are expressed on vascular endothelium, where recognition by isohemagglutinins leads to rapid vascular coagulation and organ failure.

When a matched sibling donor does not exist for a patient requiring allogeneic hematopoietic stem cell transplantation (70% cases), searching of the extended family or unrelated bone marrow registries is indicated. The National Marrow Donor Panel (NMDP: *http://www.marrow.org/*) has more than 1 million potential donors suitable for unrelated-donor stem cell transplantation, and marrow from these donors is used in the United States and worldwide. Bone marrow donor registries also exist in Europe, Australia, Hong Kong, and Japan, and these registries often provide donor marrow for patients in other parts of the world. Mobilization of stem cells in the blood after administration of hematopoietic growth factors is now widely used to avoid the need for marrow collections from donors.

Umbilical cord blood banks have also been established around the world (204). However, cord blood donation of stem cells is often unsuitable for adult transplantation because of limitations in the volume of cord blood collections. Cord blood registries offer the advantages of finding donors faster than adult unrelated registries (205) and, theoretically, providing banked stem cells from ethnic minority groups that are not well represented in bone marrow registries (206). Cord blood transplants induce GVHD less often than do bone marrow or peripheral blood stem cell transplants, but posttransplantation engraftment is slower (207).

Functional Tests of Human Leukocyte Antigen Compatibility

Testing for HLA identity at all HLA loci is a daunting task for most laboratories because of the very large number of alleles present in the population.

Moreover, in renal transplantation some mismatches appear to be well tolerated and are associated with long-term graft survival, whereas other mismatches of similar genetic disparity are poorly tolerated and are associated with early rejection (208). Reliable methods for predicting these "taboo" mismatches are not readily available. Similarly, high-resolution HLA typing does not predict all GVHD in selection of suitable unrelated donors for hematopoietic stem cell transplantation (199,209). Therefore, there has been a great deal of interest in developing functional or *in vitro* cellular tests of overall donor–recipient compatibility. Unfortunately, none of the tests so far developed provides convincing predictability of impending graft rejection or, more important, GVHD. Among the tests historically used for assessing func-

tional compatibility are the mixed lymphocyte reactivity (MLR), or mixed lymphocyte culture, test and the allogeneic T helper or cytotoxic T-cell (CTL) precursor studies. The MLR test involves measuring T-cell proliferation of host T cells in response to donor lymphocytes and vice versa. In a one-way MLR test, the stimulating lymphocytes are irradiated to prevent their proliferation, whereas in the two-way MLR test, both stimulator and responder cells are allowed to proliferate. The proliferation of responding T cells is normalized as a percentage of the maximal response achieved by the same T cells when stimulated by the lectin phytohemagglutinin or by a pool of histoincompatible (i.e., HLA-nonidentical) stimulator cells, usually derived from three or more unrelated individuals. This percentage is known as the relative response. In MLR studies, it is necessary to include controls to show that all responder cells can respond and that all stimulator cells can stimulate across an appropriate barrier such as third-party donor cells. Relative responses can vary widely, and individual laboratories use their own cutoff values defining negative (i.e., nonreactive) and positive (reactive) MLR results (209). Interpretation and reproducibility of the MLR is problematic, and enthusiasm for this test as a predictor of GVHD or HLA incompatibility is now limited (209). Unfortunately, known HLA mismatches can be present in a negative MLR result, and a positive MLR result can be obtained between phenotypically HLA-identical individuals. Because the MLR is biased toward measuring class II HLA discrepancies, many laboratories have abandoned this test and implemented high-resolution polymerase chain reaction–based class II HLA typing instead.

Allogeneic CTL or helper T-cell precursor frequencies are measured at specialized bone marrow transplantation centers, but this test is not universally accepted as being predictive of GVHD (210,211). The test is very labor intensive and requires a skilled technician for its reproducibility. Precursor frequencies are estimated by limit dilution analysis of donor versus host lymphocytes (i.e., T cells expected to cause GVHD). High precursor frequencies (up to 1 in 104 cells) are thought to be associated with a greater risk of acute GVHD (212). It is possible that precursor studies detect major and minor incompatibilities, and so, theoretically, they might give a broad measure of the transplantation barrier, but technical improvements are required before this test is widely adopted in clinical practice (213).

The Major Histocompatibility Complex and Disease

In addition to the control of transplant acceptance or rejection and immune responsiveness, the *Mhc* in the human plays an important role in the etiology of a number of diseases, many of which are autoimmune in nature (214,215). Several of the human diseases are associated with the *Mhc-III* genes, because some of the structural genes for enzymes involved in the adrenal steroid biosynthetic pathway [i.e., 21-hydroxylase (CYP21A2)] map to this region. More than 40 diseases have well-established genetic linkages to the

TABLE 7. *Human leukocyte antigen (HLA) disease associations*

Disease	Antigen	Race	Frequency[a] Patients	Frequency[a] Controls
Narcolepsy	HLA-DR2	White	1.0	0.22
		Asian	1.0	0.34
Ankylosing spondylitis	HLA-B27	White	0.89	0.09
		Asian	0.81	0.01
		Black	0.58	0.04
Reiter's disease	HLA-B27	White	0.47	0.10
Insulin-dependent	HLA-B8	White	0.40	0.21
diabetes	HLA-B15	White	0.22	0.14
mellitus	HLA-DR3	White	0.52	0.22
	HLA-DR4	White	0.74	0.24
	HLA-DR2	White	0.04	0.29
	HLA-DRB1*0301	White	0.54	0.27
	HLA-DRB1*0401	White	0.59	0.25
	HLA-DQA1*0301	White	0.85	0.35
	HLA-DQB1*0302	White	0.81	0.23
Rheumatoid arthritis	HLA-DR4	White	0.68	0.25
		Asian	0.66	0.39
		Black	0.44	0.10
Hodgkin's disease	HLA-A1	White	0.40	0.32
	HLA-DRB1*1104[b]	White	0.058	0.013
Hemochromatosis	HLA-A3	White	0.76	0.28
Psoriasis	HLA-Cw6	White	0.87	0.33
Celiac disease	HLA-DR3	White	0.79	0.26
Multiple sclerosis	HLA-DR2	White	0.59	0.26

[a]The frequencies given are the total genotypic frequencies of all individuals with at least one copy of the designated allele. Both homozygous and heterozygous individuals are included.

[b]In this case, the frequencies are based on allele frequencies, not genotype frequencies.

From Thomson (215), with permission.

Mhc (215,216), and the most important are summarized in Table 7. The precise mechanisms underlying the association of most of these diseases with the particular *Mhc* haplotypes are unknown, but several models have been proposed, including the cross-reactivity of antimicrobial antibodies with particular MHC molecules (217) and the molecular mimicry of viral antigens that might induce T-cell responses to self antigens (218–224). The very high incidence of some diseases associated with certain *HLA* genes assists in the diagnosis, as does the counseling of patients and their families. Several of these diseases are of particular note. Because virtually 100% of patients with narcolepsy have *HLA-DQB1*0602* (associated with *HLA-DR2*) (225,226), HLA typing can be used as a test of disease exclusion. Thus, a diagnosis of narcolepsy can be excluded with reasonable certainty if the patient does not have HLA-DQB1*0602. On the other hand, the presence of HLA-DQB1*0602 is of little predictive value in diagnosis of narcolepsy because this HLA type is relatively common in many populations and is frequently present in the absence of disease.

Ankylosing spondylitis is so strongly associated with the *Mhc-I* allele *HLA-B27* and the presence of some bacterial pathogens that it is a popular hypothesis that the disease is caused by the stimulation of particular T cells by HLA-B27 presented bacterial antigens that cross-react on self tissues. These T cells are then thought to initiate an inflammatory cascade. Despite the strong association of HLA with spondyloarthropathy, critical evaluation of the literature brings a postinfectious etiology into question, and certainly more studies are indicated (227).

Hereditary hemochromatosis is one of the commonest genetic disorders in white populations (with a prevalence of 1 in 300 to 1 in 400), and the gene controlling this condition (HFE) is MHC-linked mapping approximately 3 Mb telomeric to the HLA-A locus (143). The HFE protein is a MHC-I–like molecule, the structure of which has been solved (228,229). The HFE protein assembles with β_2m and is expressed in the intestinal mucosa and placenta, where it plays a role in regulating iron uptake and transport (230,231). Mice homozygous for an induced defect of β_2m and those with targeted inactivation of the *HFE* gene suffer from iron overload and hemochromatosis (232,232a,232b,232c), although there are also mutations at loci other than β_2m or *HFE* that also lead to the same disease phenotype (233). HFE regulates the affinity of the transferrin receptor for transferrin, altering the efficiency of iron transport. The most common molecular defect associated with hereditary hemochromatosis involves a point mutation that results in a Cys282Tyr substitution in the α3 domain of this MHC-I–like molecule (143). This mutation accounts for more than 80% of cases of hereditary hemochromatosis (234). The disruption of the disulfide bond in the α3 domain at this site prevents efficient assembly with

β_2m, and therefore the HFE protein is not expressed properly, which results in a failure to down-regulate the affinity of the transferrin receptor for its ligand, transferrin. This presumably leads to increased iron uptake by cells, and the resulting iron overload damages tissues. A second common *HFE* mutation, 187G, results in a His63Asp substitution and a very slight increase in susceptibility to developing hereditary hemochromatosis, depending on the genotype of the individual. Incomplete penetrance of even the high risk Cys282Tyr *HFE* genotypes can be partly explained by natural iron deficiency from limited dietary intake and menstrual losses in women.

As summarized in Table 7 and discussed previously, a number of autoimmune diseases are associated with particular alleles of class II HLA loci, especially with DR and DQ (235). These diseases include type 1 diabetes mellitus, rheumatoid arthritis, thyrogastric autoimmunity, multiple sclerosis, systemic lupus erythematosus, and Sjögren's syndrome. Rheumatoid arthritis is strongly associated with HLA-DR4 subtypes that share a common sequence motif within the DRβ chain (236), which suggests preferential antigen presentation of self epitopes by these molecules. The relative risk of severe rheumatoid arthritis is increased in DR4 homozygotes, particularly compound heterozygotes with high-risk alleles (237,238), which indicates a gene dose effect in susceptibility to autoimmune inflammation.

The number of different class I and class II *HLA* alleles that are associated with insulin-dependent diabetes mellitus clearly indicates that this relatively common disease has a complex etiology. However, the identification of a novel *Mhc-II* haplotype in the mutant nonobese diabetic mouse (239–243) and the recognition that particular TCRs can mediate disease (244) suggest that a cross-reactive response to a common self or environmental antigen may play an important role in the etiology of this disease as well. In human type 1 diabetes, the incidence of disease is significantly increased in white persons with HLA-DR3–HLA-DQ2 and HLA-DR4–HLA-DQ8 haplotypes (245,246). These haplotypes impart a synergistically increased relative risk when they occur as a heterozygous combination in comparison with the risk of disease conferred by either haplotype alone (235,245,246). This raises the possibility that trans-complementation of HLA-DQ gene products produce new molecules involved in antigen presentation (247).

Mutations at the *H-2* Locus

Mutations at the *H-2* locus have been identified in animals screened by skin grafting in extensive experiments carried out over a 25-year period (248,249). By grafting tail skin of siblings to and from each other, spontaneous or induced mutant animals that displayed a "gain," a "loss," or a "gain-plus-loss" transplantation phenotype were identified. "Gain" mutants are those that express a new transplantation antigen, and thus their skin is rejected by their nonmutant siblings; "loss" mutants have lost a transplantation antigen, and thus

they recognize the skin of their siblings as foreign and reject that graft. "Gain-plus-loss" mutations produce effects in both directions: Affected animals reject the skin of their siblings, and their skin is rejected by their siblings as well. In a classic series of experiments over an extended time, Melvold, Kohn, and their colleagues (248,249) screened a large number of mouse progeny. Both homozygous inbred and F1 animals were examined, and a total of 25 *H-2* mutations were identified at *K, D, L,* and *Ab* loci, and an additional 80 mutations of non–*H-2* histocompatibility genes were found. Although earlier studies suggested that all *H-2* genes might be hypermutable, a more complete retrospective evaluation of the available data suggests that, with the exception only of the *H-2K*^{b} gene, the spontaneous mutation rate for *H-2* genes was comparable with that for non–*H-2* genes. The characterization of these mutant animals, first based on peptide maps and amino acid sequences of the H-2 proteins (250–253) and later based on the nucleotide sequences of the cloned cDNAs or genes (175,176), provided some of the basic biochemical information on which later studies of structure and function and mechanism of gene evolution were based. The amino acid substitutions that have been identified among the more commonly used H-2K^b mutant strains are summarized in Table 8.

TABLE 8. *Sequence changes of some of the common H-2 ^{b} haplotype mutants*

Mutant	Altered amino acid	Donor gene
K^{bm1}	E152A	Q10
	R155Y	
	L156Y	
K^{bm3}	D77S	
	A89K	
K^{bm4}	K173E	
	N174L	
K^{bm5}	F116Y	
K^{bm16}	F116Y	
K^{bm6}	F116Y	Q4
	C121R	
K^{bm7}	F116Y	
	C121R	
K^{bm9}	F116Y	Q4
	C121R	
K^{bm8}	F22Y	
	I23M	
	E24S	
K^{bm10}	T163A	K1
	V165M	
	W167S	
	K173E	
	N174L	
K^{bm11}	D77S	D ^{b}
	T80N	
D^{bm28}	Q97W	
	S99Y	
H-2^{dm1}	D^d L^d recombinant	
H-2^{dm2}	L^d deletion	

Amino acid substitutions and donor gene designations are summarized by Nathenson et al. (176) and Klein (1).

X-ray structure determination of the H-2K^{bm1} and H-2K^{bm8} mutants suggests explanations for the differences in T-cell recognition that result from what might appear to be subtle amino acid substitutions (179).

Expression of Major Histocompatibility Complex Molecules

MHC molecules, synthesized in the endoplasmic reticulum and destined for cell surface expression, are controlled at many steps before their final disposition as receptors available for interaction with either T cells or NK cells. The MHC-I molecules should be viewed as trimers, consisting of the polymorphic heavy chain, the light chain β_2m, and the assembled self peptide. Because there are numerous steps in the biosynthesis of the MHC-I molecule, regulatory controls can be exerted at almost every step. In addition, reflecting

the continuous struggle between the immune system of the vertebrate organism and rapidly adaptable infectious agents, a number of steps in biosynthesis and expression are inhibited by virus-encoded proteins.

The first level of control of MHC-I expression (Fig. 6) is genetic: that is, the genes for a particular chain must be present for the trimer to be expressed. This is, of course, most relevant for β_2m, which is the obligate light chain for the complex. Induced β_2m-defective animals ($B2m^{0/0}$) (254,255) lack normal levels of MHC-I expression, although for some molecules, detectable amounts are present.

The next level of MHC-I expression control is transcriptional, and interferon-γ–dependent regulation is particularly important (256). For the most part, class Ia MHC (MHC-Ia) molecules are ubiquitously expressed, and their expression is dependent on a complex trans-regulatory process that coordinately controls the transcription of both MHC-I molecules

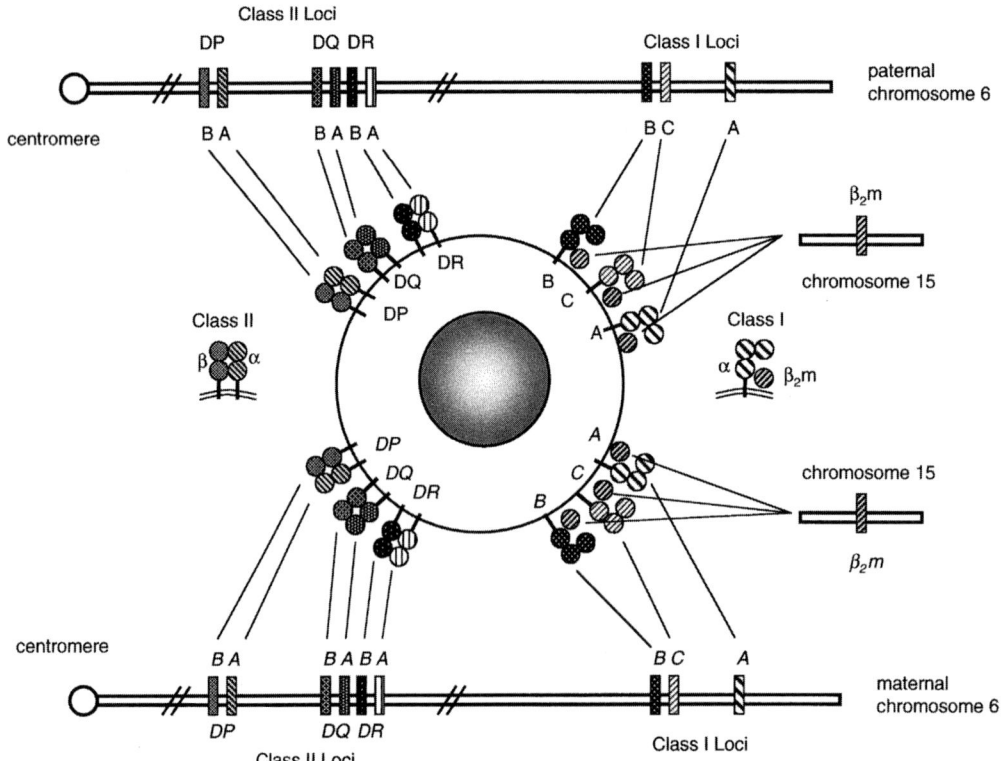

FIG. 6. Codominant expression of human leukocyte antigen (HLA) gene products encoded by the major histocompatibility complex. The *HLA-A, HLA-B,* and *HLA-C* class I loci, and the linked *HLA-DR, HLA-DQ,* and *HLA-DP* class II loci are located on the short arm of chromosome 6 (6p21), and the class I light chain locus *β2M* is encoded on chromosome 15. HLA genes and their respective proteins are shaded to reflect the different loci encoding these proteins and the inheritance of different alleles from the two parental chromosomes. The separate HLA class II α and β chain loci are also shown. The products of both maternal and paternal chromosomes are codominantly expressed on the surface of antigen presenting cells, resulting in expression up to six distinct class I allotypes. The number of expressed class II gene products can be even higher, because some haplotypes have extra DRB loci that produce additional β chains capable of assembling with DRα. In addition, pairing of certain DQα molecules from the DQA locus encoded on one chromosome, with DQβ chains derived from the other chromosome, can result in expression of new DQ *cis-trans* isotypes. The HLA class I and class II loci are separated by the class III region of the major histocompatibility complex (not shown). HLA class II molecules are only constitutively expressed on B cells, macrophages, and dendritic cells, whereas class I molecules are found on nearly all nucleated cell types.

and β_2m (257–259). The basis of the more limited tissue-specific expression of MHC-Ib molecules is of interest because of the potential importance in the role of some of the MHC-Ib molecules in tolerance to the placenta. HLA-E and HLA-G, expressed on placenta, and HLA-F, another MHC-Ib molecule with limited tissue-specific expression, have been examined in considerable detail (260–264). The rest of the MHC-I biosynthetic pathway is dependent on proper generation of cytosolic peptides by the proteasome and delivery to the endoplasmic reticulum by TAP, appropriate core glycosylation in the endoplasmic reticulum, transport through the Golgi apparatus, and arrival at the plasma membrane (265). A number of persistent viruses have evolved mechanisms for subverting this pathway of expression (266). The herpes simplex virus encodes a protein, infected cell peptide 47 (ICP47) (267–269), that blocks the activity of TAP (270). Several proteins encoded by the human cytomegalovirus, unique short region proteins 2 and 11 (US2 and US11), cause rapid protein degradation of MHC-I molecules (271). Another human cytomegalovirus protein, unique long region protein 18 (UL18), which has sequence similarity to MHC-I molecules, may affect normal MHC-I function by limiting β_2m availability. The biological effect may be related to functional inhibition of NK recognition of virus-infected cells (272–275). In addition to the human cytomegalovirus, murine cytomegalovirus (276) and adenovirus 2 (277,278) also have genes that function in blocking the transfer of folded assembled MHC-I molecules from the endoplasmic reticulum to the Golgi apparatus.

MHC-II molecules are also susceptible to regulation at multiple steps. The clear-cut tissue dependence of MHC-II expression—MHC-II molecules are generally found on cells that have specific antigen-presentation functions, such as macrophages, dendritic cells, Langerhans cells, thymic epithelial cells, and B cells, and can also be detected on activated T cells of the human and rat—suggests that transcriptional regulation plays an important role. Extensive studies of the promoter activities of *Mhc-II* genes have defined a number of specific transcriptional regulatory sequences (279), and one transcriptional activator, MHC-II transcriptional activator, clearly plays a major role (257,279–281). Considerations of differential expression of MHC-II molecules in different tissues, MHC-II deficiency diseases known as "bare lymphocyte syndromes" (281–286), and current views of the role of the balance of Th1 and Th2 T-lymphocyte subsets lead to a provocative hypothesis that suggests that the contribution of MHC-II differential expression and the resulting balance of Th1- and Th2-derived lymphokines are critical in the control of autoimmune disease (287–289).

A unique aspect of MHC-II regulation is the combination of both the need to protect its peptide binding site from loading of self peptides in the endoplasmic reticulum and the requirement to traffic to an acidic endosomal compartment where antigenic peptides, the products of proteolytic digestion of exogenous proteins, can be obtained. These two functions are provided by the MHC-II membrane protein invariant chain, Ii (45,290–292), that forms a nine-subunit complex

(consisting of three Ii and three $\alpha\beta$ MHC-II heterodimers). The region of Ii that protects the MHC-II peptide-binding groove, CLIP, is progressively trimmed from Ii and is ultimately released from the MHC-II by the action of HLA-DM and/or HLA-DO in the endosome to allow exchange for peptides generated there. The important role of Ii in regulating MHC-II expression has been emphasized by the behavior of mice with induced mutations that lack normal Ii (293–295), which exhibit a profound defect in MHC-II function and expression.

STRUCTURE OF MAJOR HISTOCOMPATIBILITY COMPLEX MOLECULES

> "There is nothing that living things do that cannot be understood from the point of view that they are made of atoms acting according to the laws of physics."—Richard Feynman (296)

So central are *Mhc* genes and their encoded molecules to both the regulation and the effector function of the immune system that it has been apparent almost since their discovery that an understanding of their structure and structural interactions would be fundamental to a comprehension of their physiological effects. The first hints of structural relationships of MHC molecules came from the understanding of serological differences, first with alloantiserum and then with monoclonal antibodies, among the expressed protein products of different *Mhc* alleles. Subsequently, analysis of the biochemistry of the H-2 and HLA molecules, initially by comparisons using peptide mapping techniques, followed by amino acid sequence determination of MHC-I and MHC-II chains. Amino acid sequence comparisons suggested a domain structure for the MHC-I molecules. With the identification first of cDNA and then of genomic clones of the genes encoding MHC molecules, it became routine to determine the encoded protein sequences of a large number of molecules. Databases of these sequences are maintained and enable determination of relationships of different genes on the basis of multiple alignment. Expression of recombinant clones encoding MHC molecules in several expression systems—mammalian cells, insect cells, and bacteria—then permitted the accumulation and purification of molecules for functional, binding, and, ultimately, x-ray structural studies. High-resolution three-dimensional structures of more than 100 different MHC/peptide, MHC/peptide/TCR, MHC/peptide/co-receptor, and MHC/peptide/NK receptor complexes are now available and allow an atomic understanding of the function of these molecules. The details of these structures also pose a number of questions that may be addressed only by additional functional experiments in whole animals complemented by biophysical methods applied *in vitro*. The molecular biological, functional, and structural studies have led to the development of the use of MHC multimers as extremely powerful tools for imaging specific T cells and NK cells. This section of this chapter summarizes these developments with explanation of function by structure, to reveal some of the current quandaries that continue to confound the understanding of the function of the *Mhc*.

Amino Acid Sequences: Primary Structure

Before the cloning of *Mhc* genes, the biochemical purification and amino acid sequence determination of the human MHC-I molecules HLA-A2 and HLA-B7 and of the mouse molecule H-2K^b (297,298) indicated that the MHC molecules showed similarities to immunoglobulins in their membrane proximal regions. Early goals were to identify the differences between allelic gene products as well as the differences between MHC proteins encoded at different loci. With the cloning of cDNAs and genomic clones for MHC-I molecules (173,299–301) and then for MHC-II molecules (302–304), the encoded amino acid sequences of a large number of MHC molecules of a number of species quickly became available. The comparison of gene and cDNA structures gave an indication of the exon/intron organization of the genes and explained the evolution of the MHC molecules as having been derived from primordial single-domain structures of a unit size of a single immunoglobulin domain (such as the light chain β_2m) that duplicated to form the basic unit of the MHC-II chain (two extracellular domains) and the MHC-I chain (three extracellular domains) (150). This gene/exon organization is illustrated in Fig. 7. Thus, the canonical MHC-I molecule has a heavy chain that is an intrinsic type I integral membrane protein with amino terminal domains called $\alpha1$, $\alpha2$, and $\alpha3$; is embedded in the cell membrane by a hydrophobic transmembrane domain; and extends into the cytoplasm of the cell with a carboxy-terminal tail. The light chain of the MHC-I molecule, β_2m, is a single-domain molecule. [Indeed, several alleles of β_2m have been identified in both inbred strains and wild mouse populations (305,306), although it should not be considered polymorphic.] The MHC-II molecule consists of two chains, an α chain and a β chain, inserted in the membrane. These chains consist of two major extracellular domains—for the α chain, $\alpha1$ and $\alpha2$, and for the β chain, $\beta1$ and $\beta2$—each linked to a transmembrane domain and cytoplasmic sequences. Thus, both MHC-I and MHC-II molecules are noncovalently assembled heterodimers consisting of four extracellular domains: The two membrane proximal domains ($\alpha3$ and β_2m for MHC-I and $\alpha2$ and $\beta2$ for MHC-II) of each molecule are immunoglobulin-like, whereas the two amino terminal domains ($\alpha1$ and $\alpha2$ of MHC-I and $\alpha1$ and $\beta1$ of MHC-II) are not. The $\alpha1$ domains of both MHC-I and MHC-II lack the intradomain disulfide bond characteristic of the other extracellular domains. The cytoplasmic domain of MHC-I molecules can be regulated by splicing and differential phosphorylation or other modification and is likely to play a role in cell surface stability and cycling between the cell surface and other intracellular compartments (307–311). However, analysis of directed mutants of MHC-I in some systems indicates that the cytoplasmic domain is

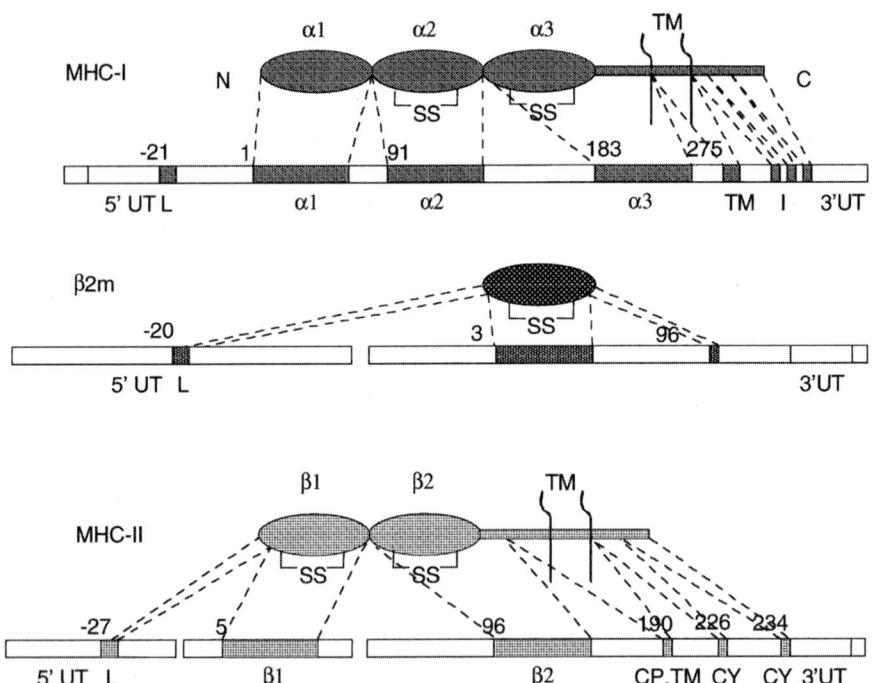

FIG. 7. Intron–exon organization of major histocompatibility complex (MHC) and β_2-microglobulin–expressing genes. Examples of class I MHC heavy chain, β_2-microglobulin, and a class II MHC β chain are shown with their domains corresponding to the canonical gene structure. The proteins are shown above and the genes below; 5′- and 3′-untranslated (UT) regions are indicated. Disulfide bonds in the heavy chain $\alpha2$ and $\alpha3$ domains, β_2-microglobulin, and the class II MHC $\beta1$ and $\beta2$ domains are shown. (The $\alpha1$ domain of the class II MHC α chain lacks a disulfide). Adapted from Margulies and McCluskey (454), with permission.

not required for cytoskeletal association or surface recycling (312). The MHC-II transmembrane and cytoplasmic domains have clear effects on the level of cell surface expression, the efficiency of antigen presentation, and the rate of lateral diffusion of the molecules in the cell membrane (313,314). Amino acid sequence alignments of MHC-I and MHC-II proteins, particularly of the human molecules, are available in a number of databases, such as *http://www.ebi.ac.uk/imgt/hla/*.

With the realization that MHC molecules were encoded by genes with modular exon structure, a number of laboratories began to explore the structure/function relationship of MHC molecules by generating various recombinants of the encoding genes *in vitro* and analyzing the expressed proteins after transfection into suitable cell types. These early studies allowed the mapping of serological epitopes (315,316), which are sites for recognition by monoclonal antibodies, and the mapping of various *Mhc*-restricted responses such as the recognition by either allospecific or antigen-specific cytolytic T-lymphocytes (317–319). The general results of these kinds of experiments were that the membrane distal domains of the MHC molecules—the $\alpha 1$ and $\alpha 2$ domains of the MHC-I molecules—acted together to form a functional element for the recognition by T cells. A clearer understanding of the significance of these finding was obtained with the determination of the three-dimensional structure of the MHC-I molecule HLA-A2 as purified after papain cleavage from tissue culture cells (320,321).

Figure 7 shows the canonical relationship between the gene that encodes an MHC-I or MHC-II molecule and the encoded protein. For the *Mhc-I* genes, there is a single transcriptional unit (exon) that encodes 5′ untranslated region, as well as the signal peptide that denotes that the protein is destined for the lumen of the endoplasmic reticulum. This exon is spliced to the coding block for the first extracellular domain of the encoded protein, an exon of about 270 nucleotides, encoding the first domain (the $\alpha 1$ domain), which is about 90 amino acids in length. The third exon encodes the second extracellular domain ($\alpha 2$ domain), and the fourth exon encodes the third extracellular domain ($\alpha 3$). The transmembrane exon of the *Mhc-I* gene encodes the transmembrane domain of the protein, and the remainder of the gene encodes several small exons that can be alternatively spliced, that can serve as phosphorylation sites, and that may play a role in the cycling of the molecule to the cell surface.

Similarly, the *Mhc-II* genes exhibit an exon/domain correspondence, although for the MHC-II molecules there are two extracellular domains ($\alpha 1$ and $\alpha 2$ for the α chain and $\beta 1$ and $\beta 2$ for the β chain, respectively) for each polypeptide chain, and both chains have transmembrane regions.

Identification of Peptides Bound by Major Histocompatibility Complex Molecules

Many different lines of evidence coalesced over a period of a few years to prove that MHC molecules function by binding peptides. From functional experiments, MHC-II–restricted T-cell responses to protein antigens were shown to be dependent on peptide fragments (322). The first direct evidence of MHC/peptide interactions came from the demonstrations that purified MHC-II proteins could bind synthetic peptides in a specific, saturable, and stable manner (323,324) with measurable affinity and remarkably slow dissociation rate (324). For MHC-I molecules, the results were at first less clear, but the realization that some cell lines defective in MHC-I surface expression could be induced to express higher levels of surface MHC-I molecules by exposure to the appropriate peptides (325,326) led the way for direct measurement of MHC-I peptide binding (327).

Several laboratories were successful in developing methods for the partial purification and identification of the peptides that copurified with MHC molecules. One approach for identifying the peptide derived from a virus that was bound by the MHC-I molecule H-2K^b involved recovering MHC molecules from infected cells, fractionating the bound peptides chromatographically, identifying a peak of functional biological activity in a CTL assay, and determining the amino acid sequence of the recovered peptide by radiochemical techniques (328). Another method that was useful for identifying both virus-derived peptides and the "motif" of self peptides by particular MHC-I molecules involved first the isolation of a large amount of detergent solubilized MHC-I with appropriate antibodies, the elution of the bound peptides, their partial purification as pools by reverse-phase high-pressure liquid chromatography, and the determination of the amino acid sequence of the bound peptides by classic Edman degradation of the peptide pools (329–331). The unpredictable and surprising results obtained from these studies of MHC-I–derived peptides were that specific amino acid residues were favored at particular positions of the sequence, depending on the MHC-I molecule from which the peptides were obtained, and that the length of the bound peptides was well defined and short, ranging from 8 to 10 amino acids. From such experiments, a number of peptide "motifs" of peptides bound to particular MHC-I molecules and allelic products were identified. Often, specific amino acids were identified at particular Edman degradation steps, which indicated a common, highly preferred residue at the same spacing from the amino terminal of the peptide. Thus, the peptide "motif" could be determined even from heterogeneous pools of peptides eluted from particular MHC-I molecules. Further refinements in methodology included the application of mass spectrometry to the identification of individual peptides and their sequencing (332,333). Alternative approaches for identifying peptide motifs include the use of soluble analogues of MHC-I molecules to ease the purification (334,335) or the use of peptide display libraries to identify the peptides that can bind the MHC (336,337). A summary of MHC-I peptide motifs is given in Table 9. An online database that is regularly maintained is at *http://syfpeithi.bmi-heidelberg.com/* (338). An algorithm that allows the prediction of candidates for MHC-I–restricted peptides on the basis of the amino acid sequence of the protein of interest is available (*http://www-bimas.dcrt.nih.gov/molbio/hla_bind/index.html*) (339). The distinction between "motif" residues of an MHC-restricted

TABLE 9. *Peptide-binding motifs for some class I MHC molecules* [a]

Molecule	Position								
	1	2	3	4	5	6	7	8	9
HLA-A1	—	(TS)	DE	—	—	—	(L)	—	Y
HLA-A*0201	—	LM	—	—	—	(V)	—	—	VL
HLA-A*0301	—	IL	—	—	—	—	—	—	KY
HLA-A*1101	—	VIFY	MLFYIA	—	—	—	LIYVF	—	KR
HLA-A3	—	LVM	FY	—	—	IMFVL	ILMF	—	KYE
HLA-B*07	—	P	(R)	—	—	—	—	—	LF
HLA-B*0801	—	—	K	—	—	—	—	—	—
HLA-B*2702	—	R	—	—	—	—	—	—	FYILW
HLA-B*2705	—	R	—	—	—	—	—	—	LFYRHK
HLA-B*3501	—	P	—	—	—	—	—	—	YFKLI
HLA-B*5301	—	P	—	—	—	—	—	—	WFL
H-2Kb	—	—	(Y)	—	FY	—	—	LMIV	—
H-2Kd	—	YF	—	—	—	—	—	—	ILV
H-2Kk	—	E	—	—	—	—	—	—	IV
H-2Db	—	—	—	—	N	—	—	—	MIL
H-2Dd	—	G	P	—	(RK)	—	—	—	LIF
H-2Ld	—	PS	—	—	—	—	—	—	FLM
Qa-2	—	(MLQ)	(NI)	—	(VI)	(KMI)	H	—	LIF
H-2M3	N-formyl-met	—	—	—	—	—	—	—	—
RT1.A1	—	(ASV)	FY	—	—	—	—	—	YFLM

MHC, major histocompatibility complex.

[a]Peptide-binding motifs for the indicated class I MHC molecules are shown in the single amino acid code. "Position" refers to the amino acid position of the peptide from the amino terminus. Only the most common residues are shown. Assignments in parenthesis are less common that the others. These motifs are taken from the more extensive summary of *http://syfpeithi.bmi-heidelberg.com/* and from the extensive description of Biddison and Martin (448).

peptide and "anchor" residues is an important one. *Motif* refers to the amino acid residues that are identified on the basis of the sequences of self or antigenic peptides that have been demonstrated to bind or copurify with a particular MHC molecule. *Anchor* implies a biophysical function of the particular amino acid residue as specifically interacting with a particular part of the MHC molecule itself. The designation of a residue as an anchor residue may be inferred by analysis of binding to peptide variants in the context of the parental peptide. Alternatively, anchors can be defined from knowledge of the x-ray structure of the peptide complexed to the MHC-I molecule.

The identification of MHC-II–bound self or antigenic peptides by biochemical methods similar to those employed for MHC-I molecules has proved more difficult, because the MHC-II molecules do not have the rigorous requirement for a defined amino terminal or the restricted length that MHC-I molecules need. Whereas MHC-I molecules bind peptides with a particular motif residue at a specific position as defined by the amino terminal, resulting in the ability to identify the dominant residue at a particular step in the Edman degradation even amidst a pool of peptides, MHC-II molecules bind peptides with "ragged ends," and little information is obtained from the sequencing of pools of peptides (340–343). Identification of MHC-II peptide binding motifs by bacteriophage display is also possible (344). In accord with the view that MHC-II molecules present peptides derived from an "outside-in" pathway, many of the peptides that copurify

with MHC-II molecules represent molecules derived from the extracellular milieu of the medium in which the cells were grown. Analysis of MHC-II/peptide complexes with cloned T cells and monoclonal antibodies with MHC/peptide specificity reveals that—partly because of the ability of MHC-II molecules to accommodate peptides with extensions at their amino and carboxy terminals and partly because of the smaller role that anchor residues seem to play in peptide binding by MHC-II molecules—occasionally even a unique peptide can bind a particular MHC-II molecule in more than one frame (345–347). As a result of structural studies (summarized later) and compilation of peptide sequences of the peptides bound by particular MHC-II molecules, the general conclusion is that all MHC-II molecules have four binding pockets, spaced at positions, P1, P4, P6, and P9 (or i, i +3, i+5, and i+9). Careful alignment of identified peptides permits the motifs summarized in Table 10.

High-Resolution Crystallographic Structures

Class I Major Histocompatibility Complex Molecules

The most graphic description of the relationship of form and function of the MHC molecule was first made by Bjorkman et al. (320,321), who determined the three-dimensional structure of the human MHC-I molecule HLA-A2 by x-ray crystallography. The extracellular, soluble portion of the membrane-associated molecule was cleaved from the surface of tissue

THE MAJOR HISTOCOMPATIBILITY COMPLEX AND ITS ENCODED PROTEINS / 595

TABLE 10. *Peptide-binding motifs for some class II MHC molecules* [a]

Molecule	i (P1)	i+1	i+2	i+3 (P4)	i+4	i+5 (P6)	i+6	i+7	i+8 (P9)	i+9
						Position [b]				
DRB1*0101	YVLFIAMW	—	—	LAIVMNQ	—	AGSTCP	—	—	LAIVMFY	—
DRB1*0301(DR17)	LIFMV	—	—	D	—	KRHEQN	—	—	YLF	—
DRB1*0401(DR4Dw4)	FYWILVM	—	—	PWILVADE	—	NSTQHR	many	—	many	—
DRB1*0405(DR4Dw15)	FYWVILM	—	—	VILMDE	—	NSTQKD	—	—	DEQ	—
DQA1*0501/B1*0301(DQ7)	WYAVM	—	—	A	—	ANTS	—	—	QN	—
IA^b(H2-A^b)[c]	—	—	—	—	—	—	—	—	—	—
IA^d(H2-A^d)	STYE (+)	—	—	VLIA	—	AV	—	—	—	—
IA^{g}7(H2-A^{g7})	KHSAV	—	—	L	—	VA	—	—	DSE	—
IA^s(H2-A^s)[c]	—	—	—	—	—	—	—	—	—	—
IE^b(H2-E^b)[d]	WFYILV	—	—	LIFSA	—	QNASTHRE	—	—	KR	—
IE^d(H2-E^d)	WFYILV	—	—	KRIV	—	ILVG	—	—	KR	—
IE^{g}7(H2-E^{g7})	ILVFWM	—	—	DESMV	—	QNASTED (+)	—	—	RKMF	—
IEK(H2-E^k)	ILVFYW	—	—	ILVFSA	—	QNASTHRE	—	—	KRG	—

MHC, major histocompatibility complex.

[a]Class II MHC, peptide-binding motifs. These are drawn from the more extensive summary of Biddison and Martin (448) and from *http://syfpeithi.bmi-heidelberg.com/*.

[b]As indicated, the peptide positions are relative; i is the amino acid residue that is thought to be situated in pocket P1, i+1, P2, and so forth.

[c]No motif assigned because of great variation in alignment possibilities.

[d]Motif assigned based on structural similarity to IE^D and IE^K (449).

culture cells by papain cleavage and further purified. At the time, there was no clear appreciation either of the role of peptide in the assembly of the molecule or of the nature of the recognition of the MHC molecule by TCRs or, for that matter, NK receptors. The most important insights in the interpretation of the electron density map derived were that part of the density, and thus part of the structure, was attributable to a heterogeneous collection of peptides bound tightly by the molecule and that this density could not be modeled on the basis of the known amino acid sequence of HLA-A2. This is illustrated in Colorplate 1. The molecular surface representation is shown in panel A (in blue), revealing the top of the MHC-I molecule exposed to the solvent without the additional density of the bound peptide. Panel B illustrates the same surface representation along with the peptide-assigned density in red.

This first MHC-I structure clarified several important aspects of the mechanism by which the MHC-I molecule carries out its peptide-binding function. The amino terminal domains (α1 and α2) of the MHC-I heavy chain form the binding site for peptide. This consists of a floor of eight strands of antiparallel β-pleated sheet that support two α helices, one contributed from the α1 domain and one from the α2 domain, aligned in an antiparallel orientation. The membrane proximal α3 domain has a fold similar to that of immunoglobulin domains and pairs asymmetrically with the other immunoglobulin domain of the molecule contributed by β_2m. The nature of recognition by T cells was suggested by a comparison of the location of the amino acid residues that had been characterized as being strong elements in T-cell recognition, residues that distinguished closely related allelic gene products, and residues that had been identified as responsible for the transplant rejection of the mutants of the *H-2K^b*

series (321). Amino acid residues of the MHC-I molecule responsible for T-cell recognition were most clearly classified into one of two categories, or an overlapping set: the residues that were "on the top of the molecule," exposed to solvent and available for direct interaction with the TCR, and those whose side chains pointed into the peptide-binding groove and might be considered crucial in the peptide-binding specificity of the particular MHC molecule. The original publications, which were based on a structure determined to a resolution of 3.5 Å, focused mainly on the structural outline of the molecule. The positions and numbering of the α-carbon atoms of the α1/α2 domain peptide binding unit are shown in Fig. 8. Ribbon diagrams of HLA-A2 as seen from the side (Colorplate 2A) and from the top (Colorplate 2B) indicate how the entire structure of the molecule is designed: The peptide-binding site is supported by the β-sheet floor, and the floor in turn is supported by the two immunoglobulin-like domains.

The comparison of this structure and higher resolution refinement of it to that of the closely related human MHC-I molecule HLA-Aw68 (now known as HLA-A68 or, more accurately, HLA-A*68011) (Table 2), suggested that surface depressions in the groove of the MHC-I molecule, now known as pockets A through F, would be available for interactions with some of the side chains of the bound peptide (348,349). The amino acid side chains that contribute to these six pockets are illustrated in Colorplate 2C. These MHC-I structures were determined of molecules purified from tissue culture cells and containing a heterogeneous spectrum of self peptides. Concurrently with the structural studies, a number of laboratories developed methods for identifying the motifs of peptides bound by particular MHC-I molecules (see previous discussion of MHC-bound peptides). Concomitant with the determination of the x-ray structure of the human

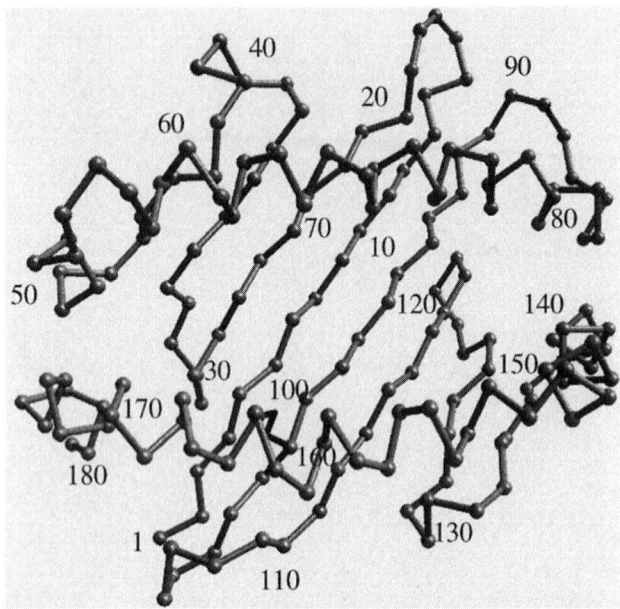

FIG. 8. α-Carbon backbone illustration of the peptide binding α1α2 domain unit of human leukocyte antigen (HLA)–A2. A top view of the HLA-A2 crystal structure (349) PBD ID: 3HLA (protein data bank [PDB (455); *http://www.rcsb.org/pdb/*]) was generated by means of the graphics program SETOR (456).

MHC-I molecule HLA-B*2705 (350), the motif of the peptides that were recovered from this molecule was determined, enabling the more precise modeling of the bound peptide in the cleft of the MHC-I (351). For HLA-B27, this was of particular interest because the bound peptides had a strong overrepresentation of arginine at position 2 of the bound peptide, and scrutiny of the HLA-B27 structure suggested that the amino acid residues lining the B pocket, particularly the acidic glutamic acid at position 45 as well as cysteine 67, were complementary to the long, positively charged arginine side chain of the peptide amino acid at position 2 (350). These structural studies supported a view of MHC-I/peptide binding in which the side chain of the carboxy terminal residue of the bound peptide sits deep in the F pocket. In addition, the amino terminal amino group forms strong hydrogen bonds with the hydroxyl groups of conserved amino acids tyrosine 59 and tyrosine 171. A hydrogen bond from the amino group of conserved tryptophan 147 to the backbone carbonyl oxygen of the penultimate peptide amino acid (usually position 8) also seems important, as do charge interactions and hydrogen bonds of the free carboxy group at the carboxy terminal of the peptide with tyrosine 84, threonine 143, and lysine 146.

Other structures of MHC-I molecules were determined of complexes produced with homogeneous peptide, assembled either *in vitro* from bacterially expressed proteins with synthetic peptide (352), or exploiting MHC proteins expressed in insect cells (353, 354). The structures of the H-2K^b molecule

complexed with synthetic peptides derived from Sendai virus, vesicular stomatitis virus, or chicken ovalbumin revealed that the same MHC molecule can bind peptides of different sequence and structure by virtue of their conserved motifs. Although small conformational changes of the MHC are detectable on binding the different peptides, the main distinction in the recognition of different peptides bound by the same MHC molecule concerns the location, context, size, and charge of amino acid side chains of the peptide displayed when bound by the MHC molecule.

The most consistent rule learned from the first x-ray structures and complemented by peptide recovery and early binding studies was that MHC-I–bound peptides were required to embed the side chain of their carboxy terminal amino acid into the F pocket. However, with further studies, it became clear that MHC-I molecules could bind longer peptides that extended beyond the residue anchored in the F pocket (355), a view that was confirmed by a crystallographic structure (356). An additional variation on the theme of MHC-I binding peptides that is based on particular anchor residues includes the demonstration that glycopeptides, anchored at their terminals in the MHC-I molecule with the carbohydrate moiety extending into solvent, are available for TCR interaction (357–359). This provides a structural basis for T-cell recognition of carbohydrate moieties on glycopeptides. An extreme example of a 13-residue peptide bound to its MHC-I presenting element, the rat MHC-I molecule RT1-Aa, was crystallized and shown to produce a peptide/MHC complex with a large central bulge. Two different complexes consisting of the same MHC and peptide reveal significantly different conformations in this central bulge region (360).

Class II Major Histocompatibility Complex Structures

Before any MHC-II structure was available, an initial model was based on the alignment of amino acid sequences and the available MHC-I three-dimensional structure (361). This model made several valid predictions that were borne out by the subsequent structure determination of HLA-DR1 (362). The MHC-II molecule clearly showed structural similarity to MHC-I and formed its binding groove by the juxtaposition of the α1 and β1 domains. The position of the electron density representing the heterogeneous peptide that copurified with the HLA-DR1 was identified. Colorplate 3 shows the electron density of the copurifying peptides superimposed on the van der Waals surface of the HLA-DR1 structure. In comparison to the MHC-I structure (Colorplate 1), the peptides bound to the MHC-II molecule extend through the binding groove, rather than being anchored in it by both ends.

A comparison of the α-carbon backbone of the peptide-binding region of the MHC-I structure with that of the MHC-II structure is shown in Colorplate 4. The structures are remarkably similar whether the binding domain is built from the α1 and α2 domains from the same chain (for MHC-I) or from the α1 and β1 domains that derive from two chains (for

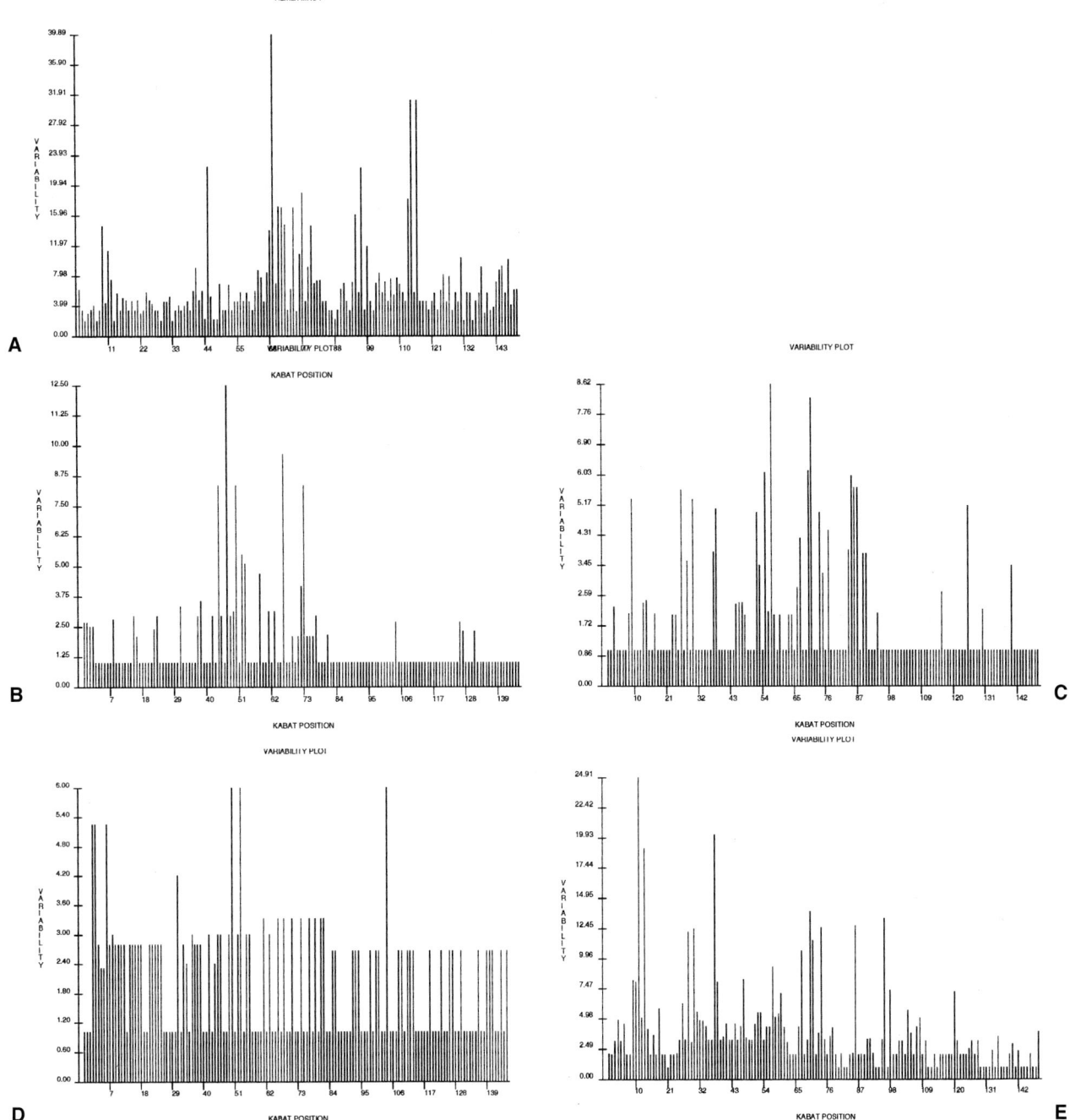

FIG. 9. Kabat-Wu variability plots. Human class I major histocompatibility complex (MHC) **(A)**, human leukocyte antigen (HLA)–DQA **(B)**, HLA-DQB **(C)**, HLA-DRA **(D)**, and HLA-DRB **(E)** were generated from calculations made according to Wu and Kabat (363), as implemented at *http://immuno.bme.nwu.edu/variability.html.*

MHC-II). The location of polymorphic residues can be determined by variability plots (Fig. 9) on the basis of multiple sequence alignments, as originally suggested by Wu and Kabat (363). Comparative ribbon diagrams (Colorplate 5), in which the location of the amino acid residues that are polymorphic for the human MHC-I and MHC-II chains are indicated, show that the bulk of the polymorphism derives

from amino acid variability in regions that line the peptide-binding groove. This suggests that MHC polymorphism is necessary to allow the MHC molecules—and, as a result, the organism and its species—to respond to a changing antigenic environment.

As with MHC-I, a further understanding of the details of the interactions of peptides with the MHC-II molecule came from crystallographic studies of molecules prepared with homogeneous peptide: in the first case, HLA-DR1 complexed with an antigenic peptide derived from the hemagglutinin of influenza virus (364). Colorplate 6 shows a top view (panel A) of the electron density associated with the HLA-DR1 protein without visualizing the bound peptide. With a space-filling model of the peptide position superposed, panels B and C show top and side views, respectively. On the basis of this structure, a set of pockets was initially designated, numbered for the peptide position that is bound. For the influenza peptide studied in this example, the major interactions were from peptide positions 1, 4, 6, 7, and 9, which are indicated in Colorplate 6A and in Colorplate 7. The deep P1 pocket accommodates the tyrosine (the third position of the peptide PKYVKQNTLKLAT) and the pockets indicated by 4, 6, 7, and 9 fit the Q, T, L, and L residues, respectively. The MHC-II is similar in its mode of binding to MHC-I but reveals important differences: the lack of need for free amino and carboxy terminals of the peptide, the binding of the peptide in a relatively extended conformation (like that of a type II polyproline helix), and a number of hydrogen bonds between conserved amino acids that line the binding cleft main chain atoms of the peptide.

Among the most provocative observations from the first MHC-II structures was that the molecule was visualized as a dimer of dimers, and this moved a number of investigators to consider the possibility that activation of the T cell through its receptor might require the dimerization or multimerization of the TCR, an event thought to be dependent on the propensity of the MHC/peptide complex to self-dimerize. The simple elegance of this dimer of dimers is illustrated in Colorplate 8. Several arguments support the dimerization hypothesis: the finding of a dimer of dimers in the crystals of HLA-DR that formed in several different space groups (362,364), the observation that a TCR Vα domain formed tight dimers and in its crystals formed dimers of the dimers (365), the demonstration of the ability to immunoprecipitate MHC-II dimers from B cells (366), the apparent requirement for purified MHC-I dimers for stimulation of a T cell in an *in vitro* system (367), and the finding that MHC-II/peptide/TCR complexes could form higher order multimers in solution as detected by quasi-elastic light scattering (368). However, a number of strong counterarguments draw this hypothesis into question. MHC-II molecules other than HLA-DR1 that have been crystallized do not seem to form the same kind of dimer of dimers in their crystals (369,370). None of the MHC-I molecules that have been examined by x-ray crystallography shows dimers in the same orientation as the MHC-II ones reported. A different Vα domain fails to dimerize even at high concentration (371). The reported x-ray structures of TCR/MHC/peptide complexes (372–375) fail to show dimerization. Therefore, despite its simple elegance, it is likely that additional experimentation is necessary to understand the topological requirements for T-cell activation through the αβ TCR.

Additions to the library of MHC-II structures include the I-A^{g7} molecule, a unique MHC-II molecule that provides one link in the model of susceptibility to insulin-dependent diabetes in the mouse (376,377). Although the structure fails to provide direct evidence to explain the linkage to diabetes, it suggests that the novelty in peptide repertoire bound by this MHC-II molecule reflects unique features of the wider peptide-binding groove.

Class Ib Major Histocompatibility Complex Molecules

H2-M3

To this point, our description of MHC-I molecules has focused on the classical molecules, represented by HLA-A, HLA-B, and HLA-C in the human and by H-2K, H-2D, and H-2L in the mouse. Several MHC-Ib molecules, for which three-dimensional structures have been determined, are of particular interest: the CD1 molecules (378,379), H2-M3 (380,381), MICA (382,383), nFcR (384), and Rae1 (385). H2-M3 is of particular note because of its ability to bind and present peptide antigens that contain amino terminal *N*-formyl groups. H2-M3 was originally identified as the MHC-Ib molecule that presents an endogenous peptide derived from the mitochondrially encoded protein ND1 that has been called maternally transmitted factor (MTF) (157,386). Thus, it was of interest to understand in structural terms how this molecule binds such *N*-formylated peptides (381,387). The crystal structure of H2-M3 complexed with an *N*-formylated nonamer peptide, fMYFINILTL, revealed that the structure of the A pocket—highly conserved among MHC-Ia molecules, which have tyrosine 7, tyrosine 59, tyrosine 159, tryptophan 167, and tyrosine 171—is quite different, so that it can accommodate the *N*-formyl group in the A pocket. In particular, H2-M3 has hydrophobic residues, leucine at 167 and phenylalanine at 171, and because of the side chain orientation of leucine 167, the A pocket is dramatically reduced in size, causing the amino terminal nitrogen of the *N*-formylated peptide to be positioned where the peptide position 2 amino nitrogen would lie in a MHC-Ia molecule. Thus, the unique peptide selectivity of H2-M3 is explained in structural terms.

CD1

Another MHC-Ib molecule of great interest is CD1, representative of a class of MHC-I molecules that map outside of the MHC, have limited tissue specific expression, and seem capable of interaction with both αβ and γδ T cells (388). In the human, there are two clearly distinct groups of CD1 molecules: one consisting of CD1a, CD1b, CD1c, and CD1e and another consisting of CD1d alone (389). CD1a, CD1b, and CD1c are capable of binding and presenting various nonpeptidic mycobacterial cell wall components such as mycolic acid–containing lipids and lipoarabinomannan lipoglycans (390,391). A minor subset of αβ-bearing T cells, believed to be an independent lineage, and defined by the expression of the NK1.1 marker, is restricted to CD1 recognition

(17). The crystal structure of murine CD1d1, which corresponds to human CD1d, has been determined (378), revealing a classic MHC-I structure with a basic α-carbon fold and β_2m association quite similar to that of the MHC-Ia molecules. Remarkably, this molecule was purified without the addition of either exogenous lipid or peptidic antigen, but the crystallographic structure revealed some poorly defined electron density in the binding cleft region. In accordance with its apparent biological function of binding hydrophobic lipid–containing molecules, its binding groove is somewhat narrower and deeper than that of either MHC-Ia molecules or MHC-II molecules. The backbone configuration of the $\alpha 1\alpha 2$ domain structure of CD1 is shown in Colorplate 9, where it is compared with the homologous region of H-2K^b, HLA-DR1, and another MHC-Ib molecule, the FcRn, a neonatal crystallized fragment (Fc) receptor. To get a three-dimensional understanding of the shape and charge distribution of the peptide-binding grooves of several examples of MHC-Ia, MHC-Ib, and MHC-II molecules, Zeng et al. (378) displayed a surface representation of the binding regions with electrostatic potentials mapped to that surface (Colorplate 10). Despite the narrowness of the entrance to the groove resulting from the distance between the α helices, the CD1 binding groove, because of its depth, has the largest volume. The depth of the groove results from the merging of pockets to form what have been termed the A$'$ and F$'$ pockets in place of the MHC-Ia A through F pockets (Colorplate 2C). The A$'$ pocket is about the size of the binding site of a nonspecific lipid-binding protein. For comparison, the groove of H-2M3, with a small charged A pocket and deep B and F pockets, is shown. An example of an MHC-Ia molecule, H-2D^b (392), shows how different charge distribution occurs in molecules of this group, and the depiction of HLA-DR1 reveals the depth of side chain pockets there. The very narrow groove of FcRn (see next section) appears to lack sufficient space to accommodate a conventional peptide antigen.

In an effort to understand more precisely how CD1 molecules bind lipid antigens, Gadola et al. (379) crystallized human CD1b complexed with either phosphatidylinositol (PI) or ganglioside GM2 (GM2) and determined their x-ray structures. The structures were essentially identical for the CD1b heavy chain and β_2m in the two complexes and revealed a network of four hydrophobic channels at the core of the $\alpha 1\alpha 2$ domain, which accommodate four hydrocarbon chains of length from 11 to 22 carbon atoms. These channels are called A$'$, C$'$, and F$'$ for the three analogous to the A, C, and F pockets of the MHC-Ia molecules, and a fourth, termed T$'$, is a distinct tunnel. An illustration of the binding groove with the bound alkyl chains is shown in Colorplate 11, which shows orthogonal views of the binding pocket of CD1b (panel A) in comparison with the pocket of CD1d with the hydrocarbon chains superposed (panel B). These features illustrate quite elegantly how the binding site of a classical MHC-I molecule may have evolved from (or to) the binding site of molecules such as CD1 to provide antigen selectivity

for a distinct set of molecules that would be common to a set of important mycobacterial pathogens.

FcRn

Another example of an MHC-Ib molecule, noteworthy because it serves as an example of a novel function of MHC molecules, is the neonatal Fc receptor. Originally described in the rat as a molecule of the intestinal epithelium that is involved in the transport of colostral immunoglobulin from the lumen to the bloodstream (393,394), homologues in the mouse and human have also been described (395–397), and the structure of the rat molecule has been determined crystallographically (384). As suggested by the amino acid sequence similarity of the FcRn to MHC-I proteins, the three-dimensional structure revealed considerable similarity to MHC-Ia molecules (384). Specifically, $\alpha 1$ and $\alpha 2$ domains have topology similar to that of the MHC-I molecule, although, as discussed previously, what would be the peptide-binding groove in the MHC-Ia molecules is closed tightly and lacks space sufficient for a ligand. Initially, the structure of the complex was determined only at low resolution (6.5 Å), but, more recently, a variant, engineered Fc has been used to obtain higher quality crystals (398). The most provocative feature of the structure of the FcRn/Fc complex is that the MHC-I–like FcRn interacts with the Fc through contacts from the $\alpha 2$ and β_2m domains to interact with the Fc C$_\gamma$2–C$_\gamma$3 interface. In comparison with the structure of the unliganded Fc, the complex reveals both conformational changes in the Fc and the presence of several titratable groups in the interface that must play a role in the pH-dependent binding and release of immunoglobulin molecules from the FcRn. This is illustrated in Colorplate 12. The FcRn has taken the MHC-I fold and diverted its function to an interaction with the Fc of the immunoglobulin. Amino acids at what would classically be considered the "right side" of the peptide-binding groove make contact with the Fc interface that lies between C$_\gamma$2 and C$_\gamma$3 domains. The FcRn serves as an excellent example of similar structures in the immune system being diverted for alternative purposes. The importance of the FcRn has been underscored by the observations of differences in the serum half-life of immunoglobulin in animals that, as a result of an induced deletion of β_2m, lack the normal expression FcRn as well and seem to metabolize serum immunoglobulin aberrantly (399).

Complexes of Major Histocompatibility Complex Molecules with Ligands

Our structure/function survey is completed by brief descriptions of the interactions of MHC-I and MHC-II molecules with $\alpha\beta$ TCRs and with the T cell co-receptors CD8 and CD4 and the interactions of MHC-I molecules with NK receptors. A brief description of interactions of MHC-II molecules with superantigen follows. Each of these structural studies complements a host of biological experiments that have led to an appreciation of the importance of understanding the structural basis of these immune reactions.

Major Histocompatibility Complex–T-Cell Receptor Interactions

Perhaps the most exciting of the recent structural observations have been the solution of x-ray structures of MHC molecules complexed with both specific peptides and TCR. This has been accomplished in several systems (372–374,400,401). The first examples were of MHC-I–restricted TCR, one from the mouse (373) and one from the human (372). The mouse MHC-I molecule H-2K^b was analyzed in complex with a self peptide, dEV8, and a TCR known as 2C (373,402), and the human HLA-A2 complexed with the Tax peptide was studied with its cognate TCR derived from a cytolytic cell known as A6 (372). Both of these structures offered a consistent first glimpse at the orientation of the TCR on the MHC/peptide complex, but additional structures, particularly those involving a murine MHC-II–restricted TCR, suggest that more molecular variations may exist. As a canonical example of the MHC/peptide/TCR complex, we include an illustration of the H-2K^b/dEV8/2CTCR complex (402) (Colorplate 13). The footprints of both the human and mouse TCRs as mapped onto their respective MHC/peptide complexes are illustrated in Colorplate 14. This illustration shows that the complementarity-determining regions (CDRs) of the TCR sit symmetrically on the MHC/peptide complexes. For the 2C/H-2K^b/dEV8 complex (Colorplate 14A), the region contacted by the CDRs of the Vα domain of the TCR lie to the left, and that contacted by the CDRs of the Vβ domain lie to the right. The regions contacted by CDR3, labeled α3 (for that contacted by CDR3 of Vα) and β3, are at the center of the bound peptide, whereas the regions contacted by CDR1 and CDR2 of both Vα and Vβ lie peripherally. The footprint of the A6 TCR on the HLA-A2/Tax peptide complex (Colorplate 14B) is somewhat different in that, although the contacts from the CDRs of the Vα domain are similar to those in the other MHC/TCR complex, the contacts of the Vβ domain are almost exclusively from the CDR3. This may in part result from the relatively long CDR3β of this particular TCR.

With the publication of additional MHC/peptide/TCR structures, several additional points have been made: (a) There is considerable variability in the orientation of the TCR Vα and Vβ domains with regard to the MHC/peptide complex. Although the first MHC-II/peptide/TCR structure discovered suggested that an orthogonal disposition—in which Vβ makes the most contacts with the MHC-II α1 domain, and the Vα interacts predominantly with the β1 domain—might be the preference for MHC-II/TCR interactions (374), additional MHC-II/peptide/TCR structures (375,400) suggest that this disposition is not indicative of MHC-I in comparison with MHC-II but rather reveals the wide variety of possibilities. (The two most extreme examples are illustrated in Colorplate 15.) (b) Considerable plasticity in the conformation of the CDR loops of the TCR, particularly long CDR3 loops, is observed in the comparison of TCR free or bound to their cognate MHC/peptide ligands (402,403). A striking example of this is illustrated by the structure of the KB5-C20 TCR alone in comparison with its complex with H-2K^b/peptide (Colorplate 16).

Major Histocompatibility Complex–Co-Receptor Interactions

The major co-receptors for recognition by $\alpha\beta$ TCRs are CD8, which interacts with MHC-I molecules, and CD4, which interacts with MHC-II. Co-receptor function probably plays a role in signaling the T cell in addition to or distinct from any contribution that the co-receptor MHC interaction may provide in increasing apparent avidity between the MHC/peptide and the TCR complexes. CD8, the co-receptor on MHC-I–restricted $\alpha\beta$ T cells, exists as a cell surface homodimer of two α chains or a heterodimer of α and β chains and plays an important role both in the activation of mature peripheral T cells and in the thymic development of MHC-I–restricted lymphocytes (404,405). The three-dimensional structures of human and mouse MHC-I/CD8 $\alpha\alpha$ complexes have been reported (82,83). These structures have localized the binding site of the CD8 immunoglobulin-like $\alpha\alpha$ homodimer to a region beneath the peptide-binding platform of the MHC, focusing an antibody-like combining site on an exposed loop of the MHC-I α3 domain. This interaction is illustrated in Colorplate 17, which shows the flexible loop of residues 223 to 229 clamped into the CD8 combining site.

The T-cell co-receptor associated with cells restricted to MHC-II antigens, CD4, has also been the subject of detailed structural studies, in part because of its role as a receptor for attachment and entry of the human immunodeficiency virus (406). The x-ray structure determination of the complete extracellular portion of the molecule (domains D1 through D4) indicates that there is segmental flexibility between domains D2 and D3, and both crystallographic and biochemical data suggest that dimerization of cell surface CD4 occurs (407). These results have been interpreted as supporting a role for CD4-mediated MHC-II–dependent dimerization in facilitating TCR dimerization and signaling. The geometry that facilitates the CD4/MHC-II/TCR interaction has been suggested by a crystal structure of an MHC-II/CD4 D1D2 complex and the superposition modeling of this with both a TCR/MHC structure and the full structure of the D1-D4 homodimer (79) (Colorplate 18).

Major Histocompatibility Complex–Natural Killer Cell Interactions

A cellular system that parallels T cells in recognition of cells altered by oncogenesis or pathogens is that of the innate immune system. The crucial cells that perform this recognition function are NK cells, and their NK receptors interact with classical MHC-I molecules either on their targets or their structural relatives. Since the mid-1990s, not only has appreciation of the complexity of NK/MHC recognition increased but also researchers have learned some of the structural and functional details by which different NK receptors identify potentially harmful cells (13,51). In addition to their expression on NK cells, some of the NK receptors are now known to be expressed on subsets of T cells and other hematopoietic cells. The NK receptors in general belong to two major functional categories: activating receptors and inhibitory receptors. In general, each of these classes of NK receptors also belongs to two structural groups: the immunoglobulin-like receptors and the C-type lectinlike receptors. Because of their functional interactions with MHC-I and MHC-I–like molecules, and because several different systems have evolved to recognize MHC-I molecules differently, it is worthwhile to examine the structures of several MHC-I/NK receptor complexes.

In the human, the major NK receptors are known as KIRs. These molecules are of the immunoglobulin superfamily and are distinguished by the number of their extracellular domains (classified as KIR2D or KIR3D for those with two or three extracellular domains, respectively), their amino acid sequence, and length of their transmembrane and cytoplasmic domains. The short KIRs (e.g., KIR3DS and KIR2DS molecules) are considered activating because they have the potential to interact with the DAP12 (KARAP12) signal-transducing molecule, and the long KIRs (e.g., KIR3DL and KIR2DL) are inhibitory because they have cytoplasmic domains that contain immunoreceptor tyrosine-based inhibitory motifs ITIMs.

The KIR2DL1 and KIR2DL2 molecules have been studied extensively. They interact with the human MHC-I molecules HLA-Cw4 and HLA-Cw3, respectively, and show some preferences for MHC-I molecules complexed with particular peptides. Among the polymorphic amino acid residues that distinguish HLA-Cw3 and HLA-Cw4 are Asn80 of HLA-Cw3 and Lys80 of HLA-Cw4. Thus, it was of interest when the structures of KIR2DL2/HLA-Cw3 (124) and KIR2DL1/HLA-Cw4 (125) complexes were reported. These structures are illustrated in Colorplate 19. The important conclusions from these structures are that the recognition of the MHC-I is through amino acid residues of the elbow bend joining the two immunoglobulin-like domains of the KIR and that residues that vary among different KIRs determine the molecular specificity of the interaction with the particular allelic product of HLA-C. In addition, the interaction of the KIR with the HLA-C is also modulated by the particular bound peptide, which explains the results of binding/peptide specificity studies.

The mouse exploits a set of NK receptors of a different structural family to provide the same function. In particular, the predominant and best studied mouse NK receptors are those of the Ly49 family, of which Ly49A is the best studied. Functional experiments had demonstrated that Ly49A interacts with the MHC-I molecule H-2D^d and also that for appropriate interaction, the H-2D^d needs to be complexed with a peptide. In contrast to human NK recognition, however, surveys of H-2D^d-binding peptides reveal little if any peptide preference or specificity. This would explain the function of the NK inhibitory receptor in that they are, at baseline, chronically stimulated by normal MHC-I on somatic cells, turning off the NK cell. When MHC-I is dysregulated by tumorigenesis or by pathogenic infection, the lower level of surface MHC-I diminishes the KIR-mediated signal, and the NK cell is activated. The structure of the mouse Ly49A inhibitory receptor in complex with its MHC-I ligand, H-2D^d (Colorplate 20), reveals several crucial features of the interaction: (a) The Ly49A C-type lectinlike molecule is a homodimer; (b) the Ly49A molecule makes no direct contact with residues of the MHC-bound peptide; and (c) in the x-ray structure, there are two potential sites for Ly49A interaction with the MHC molecule–site 1 at the end of the $\alpha 1$ and $\alpha 2$ helices and site 2, an extensive region making contact with the floor of the peptide binding groove, at the $\alpha 3$ domain of the MHC-I molecule and the β_2m domain as well. The ambiguity suggested by the x-ray structure has been resolved by extensive mutagenesis studies that are consistent with the view that site 2 is the functionally significant recognition site (408,409). Several other NK receptors have been studied structurally. These include the Ly49I inhibitory receptor, which interacts functionally with H-2K^b, which in turn has been crystallized without a ligand, revealing a basic fold similar to that of Ly49A but with a somewhat different dimeric arrangement (410). Both human and mouse NKG2D C-type lectinlike activation receptors have been examined by crystallography as well. The human NKG2D molecule forms a complex with an MHC-I–like molecule, MICA, which is expressed on epithelial cells and a wide variety of epithelial tumors (382). The murine NKG2D molecule has been crystallized in complex both with RAE-1β (385), a distantly related MHC-I–like molecule that lacks the $\alpha 3$ and β_2m domains of the classical MHC-I molecules, and with another MHC-I–like $\alpha 1\alpha 2$ domain molecule, ULBP3 (411). The general lesson learned from the studies of NKG2D interactions are that (a) this C-type lectinlike receptor, unlike Ly49A, binds to MHC-like molecules spanning the $\alpha 1$ and $\alpha 2$ domains of the MHC-I–like ligands and (b) NKG2D has considerable plasticity in its ability to interact with several different molecules while maintaining the same general docking orientation (412).

Class II Major Histocompatibility Complex Superantigen

Superantigens are molecules, frequently toxic products of bacteria, that bind MHC molecules on the cell surface and are then presented to a large subset of T cells, usually defined by the expression of a particular family of TCR V regions (413). Most of the known superantigens bind MHC-II molecules, although one, the agglutinin from *Urtica dioica*, the stinging nettle, can be bound by both MHC-I and MHC-II molecules and presented to T cells of the Vβ8.3 family (414). Its structure in complex with carbohydrate ligand has been reported (415,416). MHC-II interactions with superantigens, such as those derived from pathogenic bacteria, are the first step in the presentation of the multivalent array of the APC-bound superantigen to T cells bearing receptors of the family or class that can bind the superantigen (413). A number of structural studies examining the interaction of superantigen both with their MHC-II ligands and with TCR have been reported (417). Structural analysis of crystals derived from staphylococcal enterotoxin B (SEB) complexed with HLA-DR1 (418) and from toxic shock syndrome toxin–1 (TSST-1) complexed with HLA-DR1 (419) revealed that the two toxins bind to an overlapping site, primarily on the MHC-II α chain, and indicated that the SEB site would not be expected to be influenced by the specific peptide bound by the MHC, but the TSST-1 site would. The view that superantigens exert their biological effects by interaction with conserved regions of the MHC-II molecule as well as well conserved regions of the TCR has been challenged by the determination of two structures: that of *Staphylococcus aureus* enterotoxin H complexed with HLA-DR1 (420) and that of streptococcal pyrogenic toxin C in complex with HLA-DR2a (421). Both of these studies indicate that these superantigens can interact with the MHC-II β chain through a zinc-dependent site that includes superantigen contacts to bound peptide. From models for the complete complex of MHC-II/SEB/TCR and MHC-II/*Streptococcus pyogenes* exotoxin C SpeC/TCR based on these structures, a sense of the biological variety available for superantigen presentation to TCR was developed. These models are shown in Colorplate 21.

MOLECULAR INTERACTIONS OF MAJOR HISTOCOMPATIBILITY COMPLEX MOLECULES

Physical Assays

Whereas the crystal structures provide a vivid static illustration of the interactions of MHC molecules with their peptide, FcRn, CD8, CD4, superantigen, NK receptor, and TCR ligands, the dynamic aspects of these binding steps can be approached by a variety of biophysical methods (422). It is important to note that affinities and kinetics of interaction of MHC/peptide complexes for TCR have been determined by several methods in a variety of systems (423–430). In addition, MHC interactions with NK receptors (121,122,431,432) have been quantified by similar techniques. Although there are clear differences in the affinity and kinetics of binding of different TCR and NK receptors for their respective cognate MHC/peptide complexes, the generally consistent findings are that the affinities are low to moderate (i.e., $K_d = 5 \times 10^{-5}$ to 10^{-7} M) and are characterized by relatively rapid dissociation rates (i.e., $k_d = 10^{-1}$ to 10^{-3} sec^{-1}).

Multivalent Major Histocompatibility Complex/Peptide Complexes

A major development since the mid-1990s has been the engineering and application of multivalent MHC/peptide complexes for the identification, quantification, purification, and functional modulation of T cells with particular MHC or MHC/peptide specificity. Two general approaches have been exploited: one based on the enzymatic biotinylation of soluble MHC/peptide molecules generated in bacterial expression systems that are then multimerized by binding of the biotinylated molecules to the tetravalent streptavidin (433) and another based on the engineering of dimeric MHC/immunoglobulin fusion proteins (434). These reagents can be used in flow cytometric assays that permit the direct enumeration of MHC/peptide–specific T cells taken directly *ex vivo*. In either of these methods, multivalent MHC/peptide complexes are generated, and the relatively weak intrinsic affinity of the MHC/peptide complex for its cognate TCR is effectively magnified by the gain in avidity obtained by the increase in valency. For MHC-I molecules, the technology has been so reliable in producing multivalent (tetrameric) molecules loaded homogeneously with synthetic peptides that a wide variety of specific peptide/MHC-I multimers are available either from a resource facility sponsored by the National Institute of Allergy and Infectious Diseases (*http://www.niaid.nih.gov/reposit/tetramer/index.html*) or from commercial suppliers that offer either the tetramer or the immunoglobulin multimer. The MHC-I peptide multimers have also been exploited for identification of specific populations of NK cells and for assignment of various NK receptor specificities (126,435–437). For some MHC-II molecules, similar success has been achieved in the production of such multimers, using insect cell or mammalian cell expression systems for molecules produced by either the tetramer or immunoglobulin chimera strategy (438–442). Despite many reports of successful application of these MHC-II multimers for identification of specific MHC-II/peptide–directed T cells, the current technology seems less predictable than for MHC-I molecules. Further methodological improvements are no doubt needed (443).

SUMMARY

We have surveyed the *Mhc* as a genetic region and a source for molecules crucial to immune regulation and immunological disease. These genes reflect the panoply of mechanisms involved in the evolution of complex systems and encode cell surface proteins that interact through a complex orchestration with small molecules, including peptides and glycolipids, as well as with receptors on T cells and NK cells. The MHC-I molecules provide the immune system with a window for viewing the biological health of the cell in which they are expressed, and MHC-II molecules function as scavengers to taste and display the remnants of the cellular environment. Viruses and bacterial pathogens contribute enormously to the genetic dance—they modulate and compete in the control of MHC expression—and the host, by adjusting its T cell and NK cell repertoire on the time scale of both the individual organism and the species, resists the push to extinction. Through the concerted action of its MHC molecules, TCR,

NK receptors, and antibodies, as well as a host of other regulatory molecules, the immune system dynamically, resourcefully, creatively provides, an organ system vital not only to the survival of the individual but also to the success of the species. As the molecular functions of the MHC are better understood, the rational approaches to manipulating the immune system in the prevention, diagnosis, and treatment of immunological and infectious diseases should be better understood as well.

ACKNOWLEDGMENTS

We first accept responsibility for all errors of fact and citation throughout this review. We ask our colleagues to forgive our shortcomings in the proper crediting of their work, in terms of either priority or importance. We thank the members of our laboratories, particularly Sophie Candon and Kannan Natarajan, for their comments and criticism, and we thank our families for their encouragement and forbearance.

REFERENCES

1. Klein J. *Natural history of the major histocompatibility complex.* New York: Wiley-Interscience, 1986.
2. Kaufman J, Milne S, Gobel TW, et al. The chicken B locus is a minimal essential major histocompatibility complex. *Nature* 1999;401:923–925.
3. Snell GD, Dausset J, Nathenson S. *Histocompatibility.* New York: Academic Press, 1976:401.
4. Adams EJ, Parham P. Species-specific evolution of MHC class I genes in the higher primates. *Immunol Rev* 2001;183:41–64.
5. Benacerraf B, McDevitt HO. Histocompatibility-linked immune response genes. *Science* 1972;175:273–279.
6. Shearer GM, Rehn TG, Garbarino CA. Cell-mediated lympholysis of trinitrophenyl-modified autologous lymphocytes. Effector cell specificity to modified cell surface components controlled by H-2K and H-2D serological regions of the murine major histocompatibility complex. *J Exp Med* 1975;141:1384–1364.
7. Shevach EM, Rosenthal AS. Function of macrophages in antigen recognition by guinea pig T lymphocytes. II. Role of the macrophage in the regulation of genetic control of the immune response. *J Exp Med* 1973;138:1213–1229.
8. Zinkernagel RM, Doherty PC. Restriction of *in vitro* T cell–mediated cytotoxicity in lymphocytic choriomeningitis within a syngeneic or semiallogeneic system. *Nature* 1974;248:701–702.
9. Zinkernagel RM, Doherty PC. The discovery of MHC restriction. *Immunol Today* 1997;18:14–17.
10. Luz JG, Huang M, Garcia KC, et al. Structural comparison of allogeneic and syngeneic T cell receptor–peptide–major histocompatibility complex complexes: a buried alloreactive mutation subtly alters peptide presentation substantially increasing V(beta) interactions. *J Exp Med* 2002;195:1175–1186.
11. Germain RN. MHC-dependent antigen processing and peptide presentation: providing ligands for T lymphocyte activation. *Cell* 1994;76:287–299.
12. York IA, Rock KL. Antigen processing and presentation by the class I major histocompatibility complex. *Annu Rev Immunol* 1996;14:369–396.
13. Natarajan K, Dimasi N, Wang J, et al. Structure and function of natural killer cell receptors: multiple molecular solutions to self, nonself discrimination. *Annu Rev Immunol* 2002;20:853–885.
14. Yokoyama WM, Daniels BF, Seaman WE, et al. A family of murine NK cell receptors specific for target cell MHC class I molecules. *Semin Immunol* 1995;7:89–101.
15. Hoglund P, Sundback J, Olsson-Alheim MY, et al. Host MHC class I gene control of NK-cell specificity in the mouse. *Immunol Rev* 1997;155:11–28.
16. Chien YH, Hampl J. Antigen-recognition properties of murine gamma delta T cells. *Springer Semin Immunopathol* 2000;22:239–250.
17. Bendelac A, Rivera MN, Park SH, et al. Mouse CD1-specific NK1 T cells: development, specificity, and function. *Annu Rev Immunol* 1997;15:535–562.
18. Elewaut D, Kronenberg M. Molecular biology of NK T cell specificity and development. *Semin Immunol* 2000;12:561–568.
19. Porcelli SA, Brenner MB. Antigen presentation: mixing oil and water. *Curr Biol* 1997;7:R508–R511.
20. Gapin L, Matsuda JL, Surh CD, et al. NKT cells derive from double-positive thymocytes that are positively selected by CD1d. *Nat Immunol* 2001;2:971–978.
21. Lyon MF, Rastan S, Brown SDM, eds. *Genetic variants and strains of the laboratory mouse,* 3rd ed. Oxford, UK: Oxford University Press, 1996.
22. Marsh SG. Nomenclature for factors of the HLA system, update March 2002. *Eur J Immunogenet* 2002;29:279–280.
23. Gorer PA. Studies in antibody response of mice to tumour inoculation. *Br J Cancer* 1950;4:372–379.
24. Gorer P. The detection of antigenic differences in mouse erythrocyte by the employment of immune sera. *Br J Exp Pathol* 1936;17:42–50.
25. Klein J, Bontrop RE, Dawkins RL, et al. Nomenclature for the major histocompatibility complexes of different species: a proposal. *Immunogenetics* 1990;31:217–219.
26. Rodgers JR, Levitt JM, Cresswell P, et al. A nomenclature solution to mouse MHC confusion. *J Immunol* 1999;162:6294.
27. Duran LW, Horton RM, Birschbach CW, et al. Structural relationships among the H-2 D-regions of murine MHC haplotypes. *J Immunol* 1989;142:288–296.
28. Ceppellini R. *Histocompatibility testing, 1967.* Copenhagen: Munksgaard, 1967:149.
29. Yoshino M, Xiao H, Jones EP, et al. Genomic evolution of the distal Mhc class I region on mouse Chr 17. *Hereditas* 1997;127:141–148.
30. Yoshino M, Xiao H, Jones EP, et al. BAC/YAC contigs from the H2-M region of mouse Chr 17 define gene order as Znf173-Tctex5-mog-D17Tu42-M3-M2. *Immunogenetics* 1998;47:371–380.
31. Fischer Lindahl K. Peptide antigen presentation by non-classical MHC class I molecules. *Semin Immunol* 1993;5:117–126.
32. Stroynowski I, Lindahl KF. Antigen presentation by non-classical class I molecules. *Curr Opin Immunol* 1994;6:38–44.
33. Natarajan K, Burstyn D, Zauderer M. Major histocompatibility complex determinants select T-cell receptor alpha chain variable region dominance in a peptide-specific response. *Proc Natl Acad Sci U S A* 1992;89:8874–8878.
34. Moore JC, Zauderer M, Natarajana K, et al. Peptide binding to mixed isotype Abeta(d)Ealpha(d) class II histocompatibility molecules. *Mol Immunol* 1997;34:145–155.
35. Germain RN, Quill H. Unexpected expression of a unique mixed-isotype class II MHC molecule by transfected L-cells. *Nature* 1986;320:72–75.
36. Malissen B, Shastri N, Pierres M, et al. Cotransfer of the Ed alpha and Ad beta genes into L cells results in the surface expression of a functional mixed-isotype Ia molecule. *Proc Natl Acad Sci U S A* 1986;83:3958–3962.
37. Spencer JS, Kubo RT. Mixed isotype class II antigen expression. A novel class II molecule is expressed on a murine B cell lymphoma. *J Exp Med* 1989;169:625–640.
38. Mineta T, Seki K, Matsunaga M, et al. Existence of mixed isotype A beta E alpha class II molecules in Ed alpha gene-introduced C57BL/6 transgenic mice. *Immunology* 1990;69:385–390.
39. Jamieson AM, Diefenbach A, McMahon CW, et al. The role of the NKG2D immunoreceptor in immune cell activation and natural killing. *Immunity* 2002;17:19–29.
40. Germain RN, Margulies DH. The biochemistry and cell biology of antigen processing and presentation. *Annu Rev Immunol* 1993;11:403–450.
41. Yewdell JW, Bennink JR. Cell biology of antigen processing and presentation to major histocompatibility complex class I molecule–restricted T lymphocytes. *Adv Immunol* 1992;52:1–123.
42. Androlewicz MJ. Peptide generation in the major histocompatibility complex class I antigen processing and presentation pathway. *Curr Opin Hematol* 2001;8:12–16.

43. Watts C, Powis S. Pathways of antigen processing and presentation. *Rev Immunogenet* 1999;1:60–74.
44. Heemels MT, Ploegh H. Generation, translocation, and presentation of MHC class I–restricted peptides. *Annu Rev Biochem* 1995;64:463–491.
45. Cresswell P. Invariant chain structure and MHC class II function. *Cell* 1996;84:505–507.
46. Amigorena S, Webster P, Drake J, et al. Invariant chain cleavage and peptide loading in major histocompatibility complex class II vesicles. *J Exp Med* 1995;181:1729–1741.
47. Thery C, Amigorena S. The cell biology of antigen presentation in dendritic cells. *Curr Opin Immunol* 2001;13:45–51.
48. Newcomb JR, Carboy-Newcomb C, Cresswell P. Trimeric interactions of the invariant chain and its association with major histocompatibility complex class II alpha beta dimers. *J Biol Chem* 1996;271:24249–24256.
49. Denzin LK, Hammond C, Cresswell P. HLA-DM interactions with intermediates in HLA-DR maturation and a role for HLA-DM in stabilizing empty HLA-DR molecules. *J Exp Med* 1996;184:2153–2165.
50. Pierre P, Denzin LK, Hammond C, et al. HLA-DM is localized to conventional and unconventional MHC class II-containing endocytic compartments. *Immunity* 1996;4:229–239.
51. Lanier LL. NK cell receptors. *Annu Rev Immunol* 1998;16:359–393.
52. Correa I, Raulet DH. Binding of diverse peptides to MHC class I molecules inhibits target cell lysis by activated natural killer cells. *Immunity* 1995;2:61–71.
53. Malnati MS, Peruzzi M, Parker KC, et al. Peptide specificity in the recognition of MHC class I by natural killer cell clones. *Science* 1995;267:1016–1018.
54. Orihuela M, Margulies DH, Yokoyama WM. The natural killer cell receptor Ly-49A recognizes a peptide-induced conformational determinant on its major histocompatibility complex class I ligand. *Proc Natl Acad Sci U S A* 1996;93:11792–11797.
55. Karre K. How to recognize a foreign submarine. *Immunol Rev* 1997;155:5–9.
56. Karre K. NK cells, MHC class I molecules and the missing self. *Scand J Immunol* 2002;55:221–228.
57. Ljunggren HG, Karre K. In search of the "missing self": MHC molecules and NK cell recognition. *Immunol Today* 1990;11:237–244.
58. Karlhofer FM, Ribaudo RK, Yokoyama WM. MHC class I alloantigen specificity of Ly-49+ IL-2–activated natural killer cells. *Nature* 1992;358:66–70.
59. Dorfman JR, Raulet DH. Acquisition of Ly49 receptor expression by developing natural killer cells. *J Exp Med* 1998;187:609–618.
60. Yewdell JW, Bennink JR. The binary logic of antigen processing and presentation to T cells. *Cell* 1990;62:203–206.
61. Germain RN. Immunology. The ins and outs of antigen processing and presentation. *Nature* 1986;322:687–689.
62. Brodsky FM, Guagliardi LE. The cell biology of antigen processing and presentation. *Annu Rev Immunol* 1991;9:707–744.
63. Harding CV. Class II antigen processing: analysis of compartments and functions. *Crit Rev Immunol* 1996;16:13–29.
64. Dongre AR, Kovats S, deRoos P, et al. *In vivo* MHC class II presentation of cytosolic proteins revealed by rapid automated tandem mass spectrometry and functional analyses. *Eur J Immunol* 2001;31:1485–1494.
65. Mukherjee P, Dani A, Bhatia S, et al. Efficient presentation of both cytosolic and endogenous transmembrane protein antigens on MHC class II is dependent on cytoplasmic proteolysis. *J Immunol* 2001;167:2632–2641.
66. Neefjes J. CIIV, MIIC and other compartments for MHC class II loading. *Eur J Immunol* 1999;29:1421–1425.
67. Brocke P, Garbi N, Momburg F, et al. HLA-DM, HLA-DO and tapasin: functional similarities and differences. *Curr Opin Immunol* 2002;14:22–29.
68. Sijts A, Zaiss D, Kloetzel PM. The role of the ubiquitin-proteasome pathway in MHC class I antigen processing: implications for vaccine design. *Curr Mol Med* 2001;1:665–676.
69. Shastri N, Schwab S, Serwold T. Producing nature's gene-chips: the generation of peptides for display by MHC class I molecules. *Annu Rev Immunol* 2002;20:463–493.
70. Dick TP, Bangia N, Peaper DR, et al. Disulfide bond isomeriza-
71. Salter RD, Benjamin RJ, Wesley PK, et al. A binding site for the T-cell co-receptor CD8 on the alpha 3 domain of HLA-A2. *Nature* 1990;345:41–46.
72. Connolly JM, Potter TA, Wormstall EM, et al. The Lyt-2 molecule recognizes residues in the class I alpha 3 domain in allogeneic cytotoxic T cell responses. *J Exp Med* 1988;168:325–341.
73. Norment AM, Salter RD, Parham P, et al. Cell–cell adhesion mediated by CD8 and MHC class I molecules. *Nature* 1988;336:79–81.
74. Salter RD, Norment AM, Chen BP, et al. Polymorphism in the alpha 3 domain of HLA-A molecules affects binding to CD8. *Nature* 1989;338:345–347.
75. Doyle C, Shin J, Dunbrack RL Jr, et al. Mutational analysis of the structure and function of the CD4 protein. *Immunol Rev* 1989;109:17–37.
76. Doyle C, Strominger JL. Interaction between CD4 and class II MHC molecules mediates cell adhesion. *Nature* 1987;330:256–259.
77. Konig R. Interactions between MHC molecules and co-receptors of the TCR. *Curr Opin Immunol* 2002;14:75–83.
78. Konig R, Fleury S, Germain RN. The structural basis of CD4-MHC class II interactions: coreceptor contributions to T cell receptor antigen recognition and oligomerization-dependent signal transduction. *Curr Top Microbiol Immunol* 1996;205:19–46.
79. Wang JH, Meijers R, Xiong Y, et al. Crystal structure of the human CD4 N-terminal two-domain fragment complexed to a class II MHC molecule. *Proc Natl Acad Sci U S A* 2001;98:10799–10804.
80. Luescher IF, Vivier E, Layer A, et al. CD8 modulation of T-cell antigen receptor–ligand interactions on living cytotoxic T lymphocytes. *Nature* 1995;373:353–356.
81. Arcaro A, Gregoire C, Bakker TR, et al. CD8beta endows CD8 with efficient coreceptor function by coupling T cell receptor/CD3 to raft-associated CD8/p56(lck) complexes. *J Exp Med* 2001;194:1485–1495.
82. Kern PS, Teng MK, Smolyar A, et al. Structural basis of CD8 coreceptor function revealed by crystallographic analysis of a murine CD8alphaalpha ectodomain fragment in complex with H-2Kb. *Immunity* 1998;9:519–530.
83. Gao GF, Tormo J, Gerth UC, et al. Crystal structure of the complex between human CD8alpha(alpha) and HLA-A2. *Nature* 1997;387:630–634.
84. Rhodes D, Trowsdale J. Genetics and molecular genetics of the MHC. *http://www-immuno.path.cam.ac.uk/~immuno/mhc/mhc.html*. Cambridge University, 1998.
85. Campbell RD, Trowsdale J. MHC—centre fold poster. *Immunol Today* 1997;18.
86. Rolstad B, Vaage JT, Naper C, et al. Positive and negative MHC class I recognition by rat NK cells. *Immunol Rev* 1997;155:91–104.
87. Newell WR, Trowsdale J, Beck S. MHCDB: database of the human MHC (release 2). *Immunogenetics* 1996;45:6–8.
88. Gregory SG, Sekhon M, Schein J, et al. A physical map of the mouse genome. *Nature* 2002;418:743–750.
89. Ioannidu S, Walter L, Dressel R, et al. Physical map and expression profile of genes of the telomeric class I gene region of the rat MHC. *J Immunol* 2001;166:3957–3965.
90. Walter L, Gunther E. Physical mapping and evolution of the centromeric class I gene–containing region of the rat MHC. *Immunogenetics* 2000;51:829–837.
91. Walter L, Hurt P, Himmelbauer H, et al. Physical mapping of the major histocompatibility complex class II and class III regions of the rat. *Immunogenetics* 2002;54:268–275.
92. Monaco JJ, McDevitt HO. H-2–linked low–molecular weight polypeptide antigens assemble into an unusual macromolecular complex. *Nature* 1984;309:797–799.
93. Martinez CK, Monaco JJ. Post-translational processing of a major histocompatibility complex-encoded proteasome subunit, LMP-2. *Mol Immunol* 1993;30:1177–1183.
94. Monaco JJ, McDevitt HO. The LMP antigens: a stable MHC-controlled multisubunit protein complex. *Hum Immunol* 1986;15:416–426.
95. van Endert PM, Lopez MT, Patel SD, et al. Genomic polymorphism, recombination, and linkage disequilibrium in human major histocompatibility complex–encoded antigen-processing genes. *Proc Natl Acad Sci U S A* 1992;89:11594–11597.

96. Suh WK, Mitchell EK, Yang Y, et al. MHC class I molecules form ternary complexes with calnexin and TAP and undergo peptide-regulated interaction with TAP via their extracellular domains. *J Exp Med* 1996;184:337–348.

97. Spies T, Cerundolo V, Colonna M, et al. Presentation of viral antigen by MHC class I molecules is dependent on a putative peptide transporter heterodimer. *Nature* 1992;355:644–646.

98. Powis SJ. Major histocompatibility complex class I molecules interact with both subunits of the transporter associated with antigen processing, TAP1 and TAP2. *Eur J Immunol* 1997;27:2744–2747.

99. Hill A, Ploegh H. Getting the inside out: the transporter associated with antigen processing (TAP) and the presentation of viral antigen. *Proc Natl Acad Sci U S A* 1995;92:341–343.

100. Alberts P, Daumke O, Deverson EV, et al. Distinct functional properties of the TAP subunits coordinate the nucleotide-dependent transport cycle. *Curr Biol* 2001;11:242–251.

101. Yang Y, Sempe P, Peterson PA. Molecular mechanisms of class I major histocompatibility complex antigen processing and presentation. *Immunol Res* 1996;15:208–233.

102. Nandi D, Jiang H, Monaco JJ. Identification of MECL-1 (LMP-10) as the third IFN-gamma–inducible proteasome subunit. *J Immunol* 1996;156:2361–2364.

103. Driscoll J, Brown MG, Finley D, et al. MHC-linked LMP gene products specifically alter peptidase activities of the proteasome. *Nature* 1993;365:262–264.

104. Kuckelkorn U, Frentzel S, Kraft R, et al. Incorporation of major histocompatibility complex–encoded subunits LMP2 and LMP7 changes the quality of the 20S proteasome polypeptide processing products independent of interferon-gamma. *Eur J Immunol* 1995;25:2605–2611.

105. Ehring B, Meyer TH, Eckerskorn C, et al. Effects of major-histocompatibility-complex–encoded subunits on the peptidase and proteolytic activities of human 20S proteasomes. Cleavage of proteins and antigenic peptides. *Eur J Biochem* 1996;235:404–415.

106. Elliott T, Willis A, Cerundolo V, et al. Processing of major histocompatibility class I–restricted antigens in the endoplasmic reticulum. *J Exp Med* 1995;181:1481–1491.

107. Velarde G, Ford RC, Rosenberg MF, et al. Three-dimensional structure of transporter associated with antigen processing (TAP) obtained by single particle image analysis. *J Biol Chem* 2001;276:46054–46063.

108. Powis SJ, Young LL, Joly E, et al. The rat cim effect: TAP allele–dependent changes in a class I MHC anchor motif and evidence against C-terminal trimming of peptides in the ER. *Immunity* 1996;4:159–165.

109. Livingstone AM, Powis SJ, Diamond AG, et al. A trans-acting major histocompatibility complex-linked gene whose alleles determine gain and loss changes in the antigenic structure of a classical class I molecule. *J Exp Med* 1989;170:777–795.

110. Livingstone AM, Powis SJ, Gunther E, et al. Cim: an MHC class II–linked allelism affecting the antigenicity of a classical class I molecule for T lymphocytes. *Immunogenetics* 1991;34:157–163.

111. Hayashi T, Faustman D. A role for NF-kappaB and the proteasome in autoimmunity. *Arch Immunol Ther Exp (Warsz)* 2000;48:353–365.

112. Yan G, Fu Y, Faustman DL. Reduced expression of Tap1 and Lmp2 antigen-processing genes in the nonobese diabetic (NOD) mouse due to a mutation in their shared bidirectional promoter. *J Immunol* 1997;159:3068–3080.

113. Fu Y, Yan G, Shi L, et al. Antigen processing and autoimmunity. Evaluation of mRNA abundance and function of HLA-linked genes. *Ann N Y Acad Sci* 1998;842:138–155.

114. Kessler BM, Lennon-Dumenil AM, Shinohara ML, et al. LMP2 expression and proteasome activity in NOD mice. *Nat Med* 2000;6:1064; discussion, 1065–1066.

115. Runnels HA, Watkins WA, Monaco JJ. LMP2 expression and proteasome activity in NOD mice. *Nat Med* 2000;6:1064–1065; discussion, 1065–1066.

116. White PC, Chaplin DD, Weis JH, et al. Two steroid 21-hydroxylase genes are located in the murine S region. *Nature* 1984;312:465–467.

117. White PC, New MI, Dupont B. HLA-linked congenital adrenal hyperplasia results from a defective gene encoding a cytochrome P-450 specific for steroid 21-hydroxylation. *Proc Natl Acad Sci U S A* 1984;81:7505–7509.

118. Lawton P, Nelson J, Tizard R, et al. Characterization of the mouse lymphotoxin-beta gene. *J Immunol* 1995;154:239–246.

119. Browning JL, Ngam-ek A, Lawton P, et al. Lymphotoxin beta, a novel member of the TNF family that forms a heteromeric complex with lymphotoxin on the cell surface. *Cell* 1993;72:847–856.

120. Iraqi F, Teale A. Polymorphisms in the Tnfa gene of different inbred mouse strains. *Immunogenetics* 1999;49:242–245.

121. Vales-Gomez M, Reyburn HT, Mandelboim M, et al. Kinetics of interaction of HLA-C ligands with natural killer cell inhibitory receptors. *Immunity* 1998;9:337–344.

122. Vales-Gomez M, Reyburn HT, Erskine RA, et al. Differential binding to HLA-C of p50-activating and p58-inhibitory natural killer cell receptors. *Proc Natl Acad Sci U S A* 1998;95:14326–14331.

123. Fan QR, Garboczi DN, Winter CC, et al. Direct binding of a soluble natural killer cell inhibitory receptor to a soluble human leukocyte antigen–Cw4 class I major histocompatibility complex molecule. *Proc Natl Acad Sci U S A* 1996;93:7178–7183.

124. Boyington JC, Motyka SA, Schuck P, et al. Crystal structure of an NK cell immunoglobulin-like receptor in complex with its class I MHC ligand. *Nature* 2000;405:537–543.

125. Fan QR, Long EO, Wiley DC. Crystal structure of the human natural killer cell inhibitory receptor KIR2DL1-HLA-Cw4 complex. *Nat Immunol* 2001;2:452–460.

126. Braud VM, Allan DS, O'Callaghan CA, et al. HLA-E binds to natural killer cell receptors CD94/NKG2A, B and C. *Nature* 1998;391:795–799.

127. Braud V, Jones EY, McMichael A. The human major histocompatibility complex class Ib molecule HLA-E binds signal sequence-derived peptides with primary anchor residues at positions 2 and 9. *Eur J Immunol* 1997;27:1164–1169.

128. Aldrich CJ, DeCloux A, Woods AS, et al. Identification of a Tap-dependent leader peptide recognized by alloreactive T cells specific for a class Ib antigen. *Cell* 1994;79:649–658.

129. Soloski MJ, DeCloux A, Aldrich CJ, et al. Structural and functional characteristics of the class IB molecule, Qa-1. *Immunol Rev* 1995;147:67–89.

130. Kurepa Z, Hasemann CA, Forman J. Qa-1b binds conserved class I leader peptides derived from several mammalian species. *J Exp Med* 1998;188:973–978.

131. Loke YW, King A. Immunology of implantation. *Baillieres Best Pract Res Clin Obstet Gynaecol* 2000;14:827–837.

132. King A, Hiby SE, Gardner L, et al. Recognition of trophoblast HLA class I molecules by decidual NK cell receptors—a review. *Placenta* 2000;21(Suppl A):S81–S85.

133. Lowen LC, Aldrich CJ, Forman J. Analysis of T cell receptors specific for recognition of class IB antigens. *J Immunol* 1993;151:6155–6165.

134. Garcia P, Llano M, de Heredia AB, et al. Human T cell receptor–mediated recognition of HLA-E. *Eur J Immunol* 2002;32:936–944.

135. Le Bouteiller P, Solier C, Proll J, et al. Placental HLA-G protein expression *in vivo*: where and what for? *Hum Reprod Update* 1999;5:223–233.

136. Le Bouteiller P, Lenfant F. Antigen-presenting function(s) of the nonclassical HLA-E, -F and -G class I molecules: the beginning of a story. *Res Immunol* 1996;147:301–313.

137. Fournel S, Aguerre-Girr M, Huc X, et al. Cutting edge: soluble HLA-G1 triggers CD95/CD95 ligand-mediated apoptosis in activated CD8+ cells by interacting with CD8. *J Immunol* 2000;164:6100–6104.

138. Chorney MJ, Sawada I, Gillespie GA, et al. Transcription analysis, physical mapping, and molecular characterization of a nonclassical human leukocyte antigen class I gene. *Mol Cell Biol* 1990;10:243–253.

139. Bodmer JG, Parham P, Albert ED, et al. Putting a hold on "HLA-H." The WHO Nomenclature Committee for Factors of the HLA System. *Nat Genet* 1997;15:234–235.

140. Mercier B, Mura C, Ferec C. Putting a hold on "HLA-H." *Nat Genet* 1997;15:234.

141. Gerhard GS, Ten Elshof AE, Chorney MJ. Hereditary haemochromatosis as an immunological disease. *Br J Haematol* 1998;100:247–255.

142. Gerhard GS, Levin KA, Price Goldstein J, et al. *Vibrio vulnificus* septicemia in a patient with the hemochromatosis HFE C282Y mutation. *Arch Pathol Lab Med* 2001;125:1107–1109.

143. Feder JN, Gnirke A, Thomas W, et al. A novel MHC class I–like gene

is mutated in patients with hereditary haemochromatosis. *Nat Genet* 1996;13:399–408.

144. Mura C, Le Gac G, Raguenes O, et al. Relation between HFE mutations and mild iron-overload expression. *Mol Genet Metab* 2000; 69:295–301.

145. Hanson EH, Imperatore G, Burke W. HFE gene and hereditary hemochromatosis: a HuGE review. Human genome epidemiology. *Am J Epidemiol* 2001;154:193–206.

146. Fleming RE, Sly WS. Mechanisms of iron accumulation in hereditary hemochromatosis. *Annu Rev Physiol* 2002;64:663–680.

147. Klein J, Figueroa F. Evolution of the major histocompatibility complex. *Crit Rev Immunol* 1986;6:295–386.

148. Vincek V, Nizetic D, Golubic M, et al. Evolutionary expansion of Mhc class I loci in the mole-rat, *Spalax ehrenbergi. Mol Biol Evol* 1987;4:483–491.

149. Gunther E, Walter L. The major histocompatibility complex of the rat (*Rattus norvegicus*). *Immunogenetics* 2001;53:520–542.

150. Lawlor DA, Zemmour J, Ennis PD, et al. Evolution of class-I MHC genes and proteins: from natural selection to thymic selection. *Annu Rev Immunol* 1990;8:23–63.

151. Bodmer WF. HLA structure and function: a contemporary view. *Tissue Antigens* 1981;17:9–20.

152. Steinmetz M, Minard K, Horvath S, et al. A molecular map of the immune response region from the major histocompatibility complex of the mouse. *Nature* 1982;300:35–42.

153. Margulies DH, Evans GA, Flaherty L, et al. H-2-like genes in the Tla region of mouse chromosome 17. *Nature* 1982;295:168–170.

154. Pease LR, Nathenson SG, Leinwand LA. Mapping class I gene sequences in the major histocompatibility complex. *Nature* 1982; 298:382–385.

155. Shawar SM, Vyas JM, Rodgers JR, et al. Antigen presentation by major histocompatibility complex class I-B molecules. *Annu Rev Immunol* 1994;12:839–880.

156. Kurlander RJ, Shawar SM, Brown ML, et al. Specialized role for a murine class I-b MHC molecule in prokaryotic host defenses. *Science* 1992;257:678–679.

157. Lindahl KF, Byers DE, Dabhi VM, et al. H2-M3, a full-service class Ib histocompatibility antigen. *Annu Rev Immunol* 1997;15:851–879.

158. Gunther E, Walter L. Comparative genomic aspects of rat, mouse and human MHC class I gene regions. *Cytogenet Cell Genet* 2000;91:107–112.

159. Moore CB, John M, James IR, et al. Evidence of HIV-1 adaptation to HLA-restricted immune responses at a population level. *Science* 2002;296:1439–1443.

160. Gilbert SC, Plebanski M, Gupta S, et al. Association of malaria parasite population structure, HLA, and immunological antagonism. *Science* 1998;279:1173–1177.

161. Michael NL. Host genetics and HIV removing the mask. *Nat Med* 2002;8:783–785.

162. Martin MP, Gao X, Lee JH, et al. Epistatic interaction between KIR3DS1 and HLA-B delays the progression to AIDS. *Nat Genet* 2002;31:429–434.

163. Parham P, Ohta T. Population biology of antigen presentation by MHC class I molecules. *Science* 1996;272:67–74.

164. Marsh SG, Parham P, Barber LD. *The HLA FactsBook.* FactsBook Series. San Diego, CA: Academic Press. 2000:398.

165. Figueroa F, Tichy H, McKenzie I, et al. Polymorphism of lymphocyte antigens-encoding loci in wild mice. *Curr Top Microbiol Immunol* 1986;127:229–235.

166. Sultmann H, Mayer WE, Figueroa F, et al. Zebrafish Mhc class II alpha chain-encoding genes: polymorphism, expression, and function. *Immunogenetics* 1993;38:408–420.

167. Sato A, Klein D, Sultmann H, et al. Class I mhc genes of cichlid fishes: identification, expression, and polymorphism. *Immunogenetics* 1997;46:63–72.

168. Murray BW, Shintani S, Sultmann H, et al. Major histocompatibility complex class II A genes in cichlid fishes: identification, expression, linkage relationships, and haplotype variation. *Immunogenetics* 2000;51:576–586.

169. Williams AF. Immunoglobulin-related domains for cell surface recognition. *Nature* 1985;314:579–580.

170. Hood L, Steinmetz M, Malissen B. Genes of the major histocompatibility complex of the mouse. *Annu Rev Immunol* 1983;1:529–568.

171. Sun YH, Goodenow RS, Hood L. Molecular basis of the dm1 mutation

in the major histocompatibility complex of the mouse: a D/L hybrid gene. *J Exp Med* 1985;162:1588–1602.

172. Burnside SS, Hunt P, Ozato K, Sears DW. A molecular hybrid of the H-2Dd and H-2Ld genes expressed in the dm1 mutant. *Proc Natl Acad Sci U S A* 1984;81:5204–5208.

173. Evans GA, Margulies DH, Camerini-Otero RD, et al. Structure and expression of a mouse major histocompatibility antigen gene, H-2Ld. *Proc Natl Acad Sci U S A* 1982;79:1994–1998.

174. Schulze DH, Pease LR, Geier SS, et al. Comparison of the cloned H-2Kbm1 variant gene with the H-2Kb gene shows a cluster of seven nucleotide differences. *Proc Natl Acad Sci U S A* 1983;80:2007–2011.

175. Geliebter J, Zeff RA, Schulze DH, et al. Interaction between Kb and Q4 gene sequences generates the Kbm6 mutation. *Mol Cell Biol* 1986;6:645–652.

176. Nathenson SG, Geliebter J, Pfaffenbach GM, et al. Murine major histocompatibility complex class-I mutants: molecular analysis and structure-function implications. *Annu Rev Immunol* 1986;4:471–502.

177. Nathenson SG, Kesari K, Sheil JM, et al. Use of mutants to analyze regions on the H-2Kb molecule for interaction with immune receptors. *Cold Spring Harb Symp Quant Biol* 1989;54(Pt 1):521–528.

178. Hasenkrug KJ, Nathenson SG. Nucleic acid sequences of the H-2Ks and H-2Ksm1 genes. *Immunogenetics* 1991;34:60–61.

179. Rudolph MG, Speir JA, Brunmark A, et al. The crystal structures of K(bm1) and K(bm8) reveal that subtle changes in the peptide environment impact thermostability and alloreactivity. *Immunity* 2001;14:231–242.

180. Witte T, Smolyar A, Spoerl R, et al. Major histocompatibility complex recognition by immune receptors: differences among T cell receptor versus antibody interactions with the VSV8/H-2Kb complex. *Eur J Immunol* 1997;27:227–233.

181. Silver LM. *Mouse genetics: concepts and applications.* New York: Oxford University Press, 1995:362.

182. Wakeland E, Morel L, Achey K, et al. Speed congenics: a classic technique in the fast lane (relatively speaking). *Immunol Today* 1997;18:472–477.

183. Visscher PM. Speed congenics: accelerated genome recovery using genetic markers. *Genet Res* 1999;74:81–85.

184. Simpson EM, Linder CC, Sargent EE, et al. Genetic variation among 129 substrains and its importance for targeted mutagenesis in mice. *Nat Genet* 1997;16:19–27.

185. Sechler JM, Yip JC, Rosenberg AS. Genetic variation among 129 substrains: practical consequences. *J Immunol* 1997;159:5766–5768.

186. Simpson E, Roopenian D, Goulmy E. Much ado about minor histocompatibility antigens. *Immunol Today* 1998;19:108–112.

187. Simpson E, Scott D, James E, et al. Minor H antigens: genes and peptides. *Transpl Immunol* 2002;10:115–123.

188. Mendoza LM, Villaflor G, Eden P, et al. Distinguishing self from nonself: immunogenicity of the murine H47 locus is determined by a single amino acid substitution in an unusual peptide. *J Immunol* 2001;166:4438–4445.

189. Malarkannan S, Shih PP, Eden PA, et al. The molecular and functional characterization of a dominant minor H antigen, H60. *J Immunol* 1998;161:3501–3509.

190. Lindahl KF, Wilson DB. Histocompatibility antigen–activated cytotoxic T lymphocytes. I. Estimates of the absolute frequency of killer cells generated *in vitro. J Exp Med* 1977;145:500–507.

191. Lindahl KF, Wilson DB. Histocompatibility antigen–activated cytotoxic T lymphocytes. II. Estimates of the frequency and specificity of precursors. *J Exp Med* 1977;145:508–522.

192. Matzinger P, Bevan MJ. Hypothesis: why do so many lymphocytes respond to major histocompatibility antigens? *Cell Immunol* 1977;29:1–5.

193. Maryanski JL, MacDonald HR, Cerottini JC. Limiting dilution analysis of alloantigen-reactive T lymphocytes. IV. High frequency of cytolytic T lymphocyte precursor cells in MLC blasts separated by velocity sedimentation. *J Immunol* 1980;124:42–47.

194. Dalchau R, Fangmann J, Fabre JW. Allorecognition of isolated, denatured chains of class I and class II major histocompatibility complex molecules. Evidence for an important role for indirect allorecognition in transplantation. *Eur J Immunol* 1992;22:669–677.

195. Auchincloss H Jr, Sultan H. Antigen processing and presentation in transplantation. *Curr Opin Immunol* 1996;8:681–687.

196. Tiercy JM. Molecular basis of HLA polymorphism: implications in clinical transplantation. *Transpl Immunol* 2002;9:173–180.

197. Hansen JA, Yamamoto K, Petersdorf E, et al. The role of HLA matching in hematopoietic cell transplantation. *Rev Immunogenet* 1999;1:359–373.

198. Mickelson EM, Petersdorf E, Anasetti C, et al. HLA matching in hematopoietic cell transplantation. *Hum Immunol* 2000;61:92–100.

199. Hansen JA, Petersdorf E, Martin PJ, et al. Impact of HLA matching on hematopoietic cell transplants from unrelated donors. *Vox Sang* 2000;78:269–271.

200. Petersdorf E, Anasetti C, Martin PJ, et al. Genomics of unrelated-donor hematopoietic cell transplantation. *Curr Opin Immunol* 2001; 13:582–589.

201. Varney MD, Lester S, McCluskey J, et al. Matching for HLA DPA1 and DPB1 alleles in unrelated bone marrow transplantation. *Hum Immunol* 1999;60:532–538.

202. Petersdorf EW, Gooley T, Malkki M, et al. The biological significance of HLA-DP gene variation in haematopoietic cell transplantation. *Br J Haematol* 2001;112:988–994.

203. Rubinstein P. HLA matching for bone marrow transplantation—how much is enough? *N Engl J Med* 2001;345:1842–1844.

204. Hakenberg P, Kogler G, Wernet P. NETCORD: a cord blood allocation network. *Bone Marrow Transplant* 1998;22(Suppl 1):S17–S18.

205. Barker JN, Krepski TP, DeFor TE, et al. Searching for unrelated donor hematopoietic stem cells: availability and speed of umbilical cord blood versus bone marrow. *Biol Blood Marrow Transplant* 2002;8:257–260.

206. Gluckman E, Rocha V, Chastang C. Peripheral stem cells in bone marrow transplantation. Cord blood stem cell transplantation. *Baillieres Best Pract Res Clin Haematol* 1999;12:279–292.

207. Gluckman E, Rocha V, Chevret S. Results of unrelated umbilical cord blood hematopoietic stem cell transplant. *Transfus Clin Biol* 2001;8:146–154.

208. Doxiadis, II, Smits JM, Schreuder GM, et al. Association between specific HLA combinations and probability of kidney allograft loss: the taboo concept. *Lancet* 1996;348:850–853.

209. Mickelson EM, Longton G, Anasetti C, et al. Evaluation of the mixed lymphocyte culture (MLC) assay as a method for selecting unrelated donors for marrow transplantation. *Tissue Antigens* 1996;47:27–36.

210. Pei J, Martin PJ, Longton G, et al. Evaluation of pretransplant donor anti-recipient cytotoxic and helper T lymphocyte responses as correlates of acute graft-vs.-host disease and survival after unrelated marrow transplantation. *Biol Blood Marrow Transplant* 1997;3:142–149.

211. Wang XN, Taylor PR, Skinner R, et al. T-cell frequency analysis does not predict the incidence of graft-versus-host disease in HLA-matched sibling bone marrow transplantation. *Transplantation* 2000;70:488–493.

212. Kaminski E, Hows J, Man S, et al. Prediction of graft versus host disease by frequency analysis of cytotoxic T cells after unrelated donor bone marrow transplantation. *Transplantation* 1989;48:608–613.

213. Oudshoorn M, Doxiadis, II, van den Berg-Loonen PM, et al. Functional versus structural matching: can the CTLp test be replaced by HLA allele typing? *Hum Immunol* 2002;63:176–184.

214. Nepom GT, Erlich H. MHC class-II molecules and autoimmunity. *Annu Rev Immunol* 1991;9:493–525.

215. Thomson G. HLA disease associations: models for the study of complex human genetic disorders. *Crit Rev Clin Lab Sci* 1995;32:183–219.

216. Tiwari JL, Terasaki PI. *HLA and disease associations.* New York: Springer-Verlag, 1985.

217. Baines M, Ebringer A. HLA and disease. *Mol Aspects Med* 1992; 13:263–378.

218. von Herrath MG, Oldstone MB. Virus-induced autoimmune disease. *Curr Opin Immunol* 1996;8:878–885.

219. Oldstone MB. Molecular mimicry and autoimmune disease. *Cell* 1987;50:819–820.

220. Oldstone MD. Virus-induced autoimmunity: molecular mimicry as a route to autoimmune disease. *J Autoimmun* 1989;2(Suppl):187–194.

221. Oldstone MB. Viruses and autoimmune diseases. *Scand J Immunol* 1997;46:320–325.

222. Wucherpfennig KW. Structural basis of molecular mimicry. *J Autoimmun* 2001;16:293–302.

223. Wucherpfennig KW, Yu B, Bhol K, et al. Structural basis for major histocompatibility complex (MHC)–linked susceptibility to autoimmunity: charged residues of a single MHC binding pocket confer selective presentation of self-peptides in pemphigus vulgaris. *Proc Natl Acad Sci U S A* 1995;92:11935–11939.

224. Wucherpfennig KW, Strominger JL. Molecular mimicry in T cell–mediated autoimmunity: viral peptides activate human T cell clones specific for myelin basic protein. *Cell* 1995;80:695–705.

225. Mignot E, Tafti M, Dement WC, et al. Narcolepsy and immunity. *Adv Neuroimmunol* 1995;5:23–37.

226. Ellis MC, Hetisimer AH, Ruddy DA, et al. HLA class II haplotype and sequence analysis support a role for DQ in narcolepsy. *Immunogenetics* 1997;46:410–417.

227. Ringrose JH. HLA-B27 associated spondyloarthropathy, an autoimmune disease based on crossreactivity between bacteria and HLA-B27? *Ann Rheum Dis* 1999;58:598–610.

228. Lebron JA, Bennett MJ, Vaughn DE, et al. Crystal structure of the hemochromatosis protein HFE and characterization of its interaction with transferrin receptor. *Cell* 1998;93:111–123.

229. Bennett MJ, Lebron JA, Bjorkman PJ. Crystal structure of the hereditary haemochromatosis protein HFE complexed with transferrin receptor. *Nature* 2000;403:46–53.

230. Trinder D, Olynyk JK, Sly WS, et al. Iron uptake from plasma transferrin by the duodenum is impaired in the Hfe knockout mouse. *Proc Natl Acad Sci U S A* 2002;99:5622–5626.

231. Waheed A, Grubb JH, Zhou XY, et al. Regulation of transferrin-mediated iron uptake by HFE, the protein defective in hereditary hemochromatosis. *Proc Natl Acad Sci U S A* 2002;99:3117–3122.

232. Zhou XY, Tomatsu S, Fleming RE, et al. HFE gene knockout produces mouse model of hereditary hemochromatosis. *Proc Natl Acad Sci U S A* 1998;95:2492–2497.

232a. Santos M, Clevers HC, Marx JJ. Mutations of the hereditary hemochromatosis candidate gene HLA-H in porphyria cutanea tarda. *N Engl J Med,* 1997;336(18):1327–1328.

232b. Santos M, Schilham MW, Rademakers LH, et al. Defective iron homeostasis in beta 2-microglobulin knockout mice recapitulates hereditary hemochromatosis in man. *J Exp Med* 1996;184:1975–1985.

232c. Rothenberg BE, Voland JR. Beta2 knockout mice develop parenchymal iron overload: a putative role for class I genes of the major histocompatibility complex in iron metabolism. *Proc Natl Acad Sci U S A* 1996;93:1529–1534.

233. Fleming RE, Ahmann JR, Migas MC, et al. Targeted mutagenesis of the murine transferrin receptor-2 gene produces hemochromatosis. *Proc Natl Acad Sci U S A* 2002;99:10653–10658.

234. A simple genetic test identifies 90% of UK patients with haemochromatosis. The UK Haemochromatosis Consortium. *Gut* 1997;41:841–844.

235. Lechler R, Warren A. *Handbook of HLA and disease,* 2nd ed. London: Academic Press, 1998.

236. Wordsworth P. Rheumatoid arthritis. *Curr Opin Immunol* 1992;4: 766–769.

237. Wordsworth P, Pile KD, Buckely JD, et al. HLA heterozygosity contributes to susceptibility to rheumatoid arthritis. *Am J Hum Genet* 1992;51:585–591.

238. Hall FC, Weeks DE, Camilleri JP, et al. Influence of the HLA-DRB1 locus on susceptibility and severity in rheumatoid arthritis. *Qjm* 1996;89:821–829.

239. Hattori M, Buse JB, Jackson RA, et al. The NOD mouse: recessive diabetogenic gene in the major histocompatibility complex. *Science* 1986;231:733–735.

240. Acha-Orbea H, McDevitt HO. The first external domain of the nonobese diabetic mouse class II I-A beta chain is unique. *Proc Natl Acad Sci U S A* 1987;84:2435–2439.

241. Atkinson MA, Leiter EH. The NOD mouse model of type 1 diabetes: as good as it gets? *Nat Med* 1999;5:601–604.

242. Wicker LS, Miller BJ, Fischer PA, et al. Genetic control of diabetes and insulitis in the nonobese diabetic mouse. Pedigree analysis of a diabetic H-2nod/b heterozygote. *J Immunol* 1989;142:781–784.

243. Quartey-Papafio R, Lund T, Chandler P, et al. Aspartate at position 57 of nonobese diabetic I-Ag7 beta-chain diminishes the spontaneous incidence of insulin-dependent diabetes mellitus. *J Immunol* 1995;154:5567–5575.

244. Tisch R, McDevitt H. Insulin-dependent diabetes mellitus. *Cell* 1996;85:291–297.

245. Undlien DE, Thorsby E. HLA associations in type 1 diabetes: merging genetics and immunology. *Trends Immunol* 2001;22:467–469.

246. Undlien DE, Lie BA, Thorsby E. HLA complex genes in type 1 diabetes and other autoimmune diseases. Which genes are involved? *Trends Genet* 2001;17:93–100.

247. Morton NE, Green A, Dunsworth T, et al. Heterozygous expression of insulin-dependent diabetes mellitus (IDDM) determinants in the HLA system. *Am J Hum Genet* 1983;35:201–213.

248. Kohn HI, Melvold RW. Spontaneous histocompatibility mutations detected by dermal grafts: significant changes in rate over a 10-year period in the mouse H-system. *Mutat Res* 1974;24:163–169.

249. Melvold RW, Wang K, Kohn HI. Histocompatibility gene mutation rates in the mouse: a 25-year review. *Immunogenetics* 1997;47:44–54.

250. Yamaga KM, Pfaffenbach GM, Pease LR, et al. Biochemical studies of H-2K antigens from a group of related mutants. I. Identification of a shared mutation in B6-H-2bm5 and B6-H-2bm16. *Immunogenetics* 1983;17:19–29.

251. Pease LR, Ewenstein BM, McGovern D, et al. Biochemical studies on the H-2K mutant B6.C-H-2bm10. *Immunogenetics* 1983;17:7–17.

252. Ewenstein BM, Uehara H, Nisizawa T, et al. Biochemical studies on the H-2K antigens of the MHC mutants bm3 and bm11. *Immunogenetics* 1980;11:383–395.

253. Yamaga KM, Pfaffenbach GM, Pease LR, et al. Biochemical studies of H-2K antigens from a group of related mutants. II. Identification of a shared mutation in B6-H-2bm6, B6.C-H-2bm7, and B6.C-H-2bm9. *Immunogenetics* 1983;17:31–41.

254. Zijlstra M, Li E, Sajjadi F, et al. Germ-line transmission of a disrupted beta 2-microglobulin gene produced by homologous recombination in embryonic stem cells. *Nature* 1989;342:435–438.

255. Koller BH, Smithies O. Inactivating the beta 2-microglobulin locus in mouse embryonic stem cells by homologous recombination. *Proc Natl Acad Sci U S A* 1989;86:8932–8935.

256. Boehm U, Klamp T, Groot M, et al. Cellular responses to interferon-gamma. *Annu Rev Immunol* 1997;15:749–795.

257. Gobin SJ, van Zutphen M, Westerheide SD, et al. The MHC-specific enhanceosome and its role in MHC class I and beta(2)-microglobulin gene transactivation. *J Immunol* 2001;167:5175–5184.

258. Gobin SJ, van den Elsen PJ. Locus-specific regulation of HLA-A and HLA-B expression is not determined by nucleotide variation in the X2 box promoter element. *Blood* 2001;97:1518–1521.

259. van den Elsen PJ, Gobin SJ. The common regulatory pathway of MHC class I and class II transactivation. *Microbes Infect* 1999;1:887–892.

260. Wainwright SD, Biro PA, Holmes CH. HLA-F is a predominantly empty, intracellular, TAP-associated MHC class Ib protein with a restricted expression pattern. *J Immunol* 2000;164:319–328.

261. Houlihan JM, Biro PA, Harper HM, et al. The human amnion is a site of MHC class Ib expression: evidence for the expression of HLA-E and HLA-G. *J Immunol* 1995;154:5665–5674.

262. Le Bouteiller P, Rodriguez AM, Mallet V, et al. Placental expression of HLA class I genes. *Am J Reprod Immunol* 1996;35:216–225.

263. McMaster MT, Librach CL, Zhou Y, et al. Human placental HLA-G expression is restricted to differentiated cytotrophoblasts. *J Immunol* 1995;154:3771–3778.

264. Gobin SJ, van den Elsen PJ. Transcriptional regulation of the MHC class Ib genes HLA-E, HLA-F, and HLA-G. *Hum Immunol* 2000;61:1102–1107.

265. Wiertz EJ, Mukherjee S, Ploegh HL. Viruses use stealth technology to escape from the host immune system. *Mol Med Today* 1997;3:116–123.

266. Fruh K, Ahn K, Peterson PA. Inhibition of MHC class I antigen presentation by viral proteins. *J Mol Med* 1997;75:18–27.

267. Easterfield AJ, Austen BM, Westwood OM. Inhibition of antigen transport by expression of infected cell peptide 47 (ICP47) prevents cell surface expression of HLA in choriocarcinoma cell lines. *J Reprod Immunol* 2001;50:19–40.

268. Berger C, Xuereb S, Johnson DC, et al. Expression of herpes simplex virus ICP47 and human cytomegalovirus US11 prevents recognition of transgene products by CD8(+) cytotoxic T lymphocytes. *J Virol* 2000;74:4465–4473.

269. Furukawa L, Brevetti LS, Brady SE, et al. Adenoviral-mediated gene transfer of ICP47 inhibits major histocompatibility complex class I expression on vascular cells *in vitro*. *J Vasc Surg* 2000;31:558–566.

270. Jugovic P, Hill AM, Tomazin R, et al. Inhibition of major histocompatibility complex class I antigen presentation in pig and primate cells by herpes simplex virus type 1 and 2 ICP47. *J Virol* 1998;72:5076–5084.

271. Rehm A, Engelsberg A, Tortorella D, et al. Human cytomegalovirus gene products US2 and US11 differ in their ability to attack major histocompatibility class I heavy chains in dendritic cells. *J Virol* 2002;76:5043–5050.

272. Vitale M, Castriconi R, Parolini S, et al. The leukocyte Ig-like receptor (LIR)–1 for the cytomegalovirus UL18 protein displays a broad specificity for different HLA class I alleles: analysis of LIR-1 + NK cell clones. *Int Immunol* 1999;11:29–35.

273. Reyburn HT, Mandelboim O, Vales-Gomez M, et al. The class I MHC homologue of human cytomegalovirus inhibits attack by natural killer cells. *Nature* 1997;386:514–517.

274. Odeberg J, Cerboni C, Browne H, et al. Human cytomegalovirus (HCMV)–infected endothelial cells and macrophages are less susceptible to natural killer lysis independent of the downregulation of classical HLA class I molecules or expression of the HCMV class I homologue, UL18. *Scand J Immunol* 2002;55:149–161.

275. Park B, Oh H, Lee S, et al. The MHC class I homolog of human cytomegalovirus is resistant to down-regulation mediated by the unique short region protein (US)2, US3, US6, and US11 gene products. *J Immunol* 2002;168:3464–3469.

276. Koszinowski UH, Reddehase MJ, Del Val M. Principles of cytomegalovirus antigen presentation *in vitro* and *in vivo*. *Semin Immunol* 1992;4:71–79.

277. Burgert HG, Kvist S. An adenovirus type 2 glycoprotein blocks cell surface expression of human histocompatibility class I antigens. *Cell* 1985;41:987–997.

278. Burgert HG, Kvist S. The E3/19K protein of adenovirus type 2 binds to the domains of histocompatibility antigens required for CTL recognition. *EMBO J* 1987;6:2019–2026.

279. Boss JM. Regulation of transcription of MHC class II genes. *Curr Opin Immunol* 1997;9:107–113.

280. Fontes JD, Kanazawa S, Nekrep N, et al. The class II transactivator CIITA is a transcriptional integrator. *Microbes Infect* 1999;1:863–869.

281. Jabrane-Ferrat N, Nekrep N, Tosi G, et al. Major histocompatibility complex class II transcriptional platform: assembly of nuclear factor Y and regulatory factor X (RFX) on DNA requires RFX5 dimers. *Mol Cell Biol* 2002;22:5616–5625.

282. Rohn WM, Lee YJ, Benveniste EN. Regulation of class II MHC expression. *Crit Rev Immunol* 1996;16:311–330.

283. Reith W, Mach B. The bare lymphocyte syndrome and the regulation of MHC expression. *Annu Rev Immunol* 2001;19:331–373.

284. Abdulkadir SA, Ono SJ. How are class II MHC genes turned on and off? *FASEB J* 1995;9:1429–1435.

285. Hume CR, Shookster LA, Collins N, et al. Bare lymphocyte syndrome: altered HLA class II expression in B cell lines derived from two patients. *Hum Immunol* 1989;25:1–11.

286. Mach B. MHC class II regulation—lessons from a disease. *N Engl J Med* 1995;332:120–122.

287. Mitchison NA, Schuhbauer D, Muller B. Natural and induced regulation of Th1/Th2 balance. *Springer Semin Immunopathol* 1999;21:199–210.

288. Mitchison NA, Roes J. Patterned variation in murine MHC promoters. *Proc Natl Acad Sci U S A* 2002;99:10561–10566.

289. Guardiola J, Maffei A, Lauster R, et al. Functional significance of polymorphism among MHC class II gene promoters. *Tissue Antigens* 1996;48:615–625.

290. Stumptner-Cuvelette P, Benaroch P. Multiple roles of the invariant chain in MHC class II function. *Biochim Biophys Acta* 2002;1542:1–13.

291. Roche PA, Marks MS, Cresswell P. Formation of a nine-subunit complex by HLA class II glycoproteins and the invariant chain. *Nature* 1991;354:392–394.

292. Roche PA, Cresswell P. Invariant chain association with HLA-DR molecules inhibits immunogenic peptide binding. *Nature* 1990;345:615–618.

293. Bikoff EK, Huang LY, Episkopou V, et al. Defective major histocompatibility complex class II assembly, transport, peptide acquisition, and CD4+ T cell selection in mice lacking invariant chain expression. *J Exp Med* 1993;177:1699–1712.

294. Viville S, Neefjes J, Lotteau V, et al. Mice lacking the MHC class II–associated invariant chain. *Cell* 1993;72:635–648.

295. Bonnerot C, Marks MS, Cosson P, et al. Association with BiP and aggregation of class II MHC molecules synthesized in the absence of invariant chain. *EMBO J* 1994;13:934–944.

296. Feynman RP, Leighton RB, Sands ML, eds. *The Feynman lectures on physics*. Reading, MA: Addison-Wesley, 1963:5.

297. Orr HT, Lopez de Castro JA, Parham P, et al. Comparison of amino acid sequences of two human histocompatibility antigens, HLA-A2 and HLA-B7: location of putative alloantigenic sites. *Proc Natl Acad Sci U S A* 1979;76:4395–4399.

298. Coligan JE, Kindt TJ, Uehara H, et al. Primary structure of a murine transplantation antigen. *Nature* 1981;291:35–39.

299. Steinmetz M, Frelinger JG, Fisher D, et al. Three cDNA clones encoding mouse transplantation antigens: homology to immunoglobulin genes. *Cell* 1981;24:125–134.

300. Sood AK, Pereira D, Weissman SM. Isolation and partial nucleotide sequence of a cDNA clone for human histocompatibility antigen HLA-B by use of an oligodeoxynucleotide primer. *Proc Natl Acad Sci U S A* 1981;78:616–620.

301. Ploegh HL, Orr HT, Strominger JL. Molecular cloning of a human histocompatibility antigen cDNA fragment. *Proc Natl Acad Sci U S A* 1980;77:6081–6085.

302. Choi E, McIntyre K, Germain RN, et al. Murine I-A beta chain polymorphism: nucleotide sequences of three allelic I-A beta genes. *Science* 1983;221:283–286.

303. Hood L, Steinmetz M, Goodenow R, et al. Genes of the major histocompatibility complex. *Cold Spring Harb Symp Quant Biol* 1983;47 Pt 2:1051–1065.

304. Mathis DJ, Benoist CO, Williams VE 2nd, et al. The murine E alpha immune response gene. *Cell* 1983;32:745–754.

305. Robinson PJ, Steinmetz M, Moriwaki K, et al. Beta-2 microglobulin types in mice of wild origin. *Immunogenetics* 1984;20:655–665.

306. Michaelson J. Genetic polymorphism of beta 2-microglobulin (B2m) maps to the H-3 region of chromosome 2. *Immunogenetics* 1981;13:167–171.

307. Lew AM, Margulies DH, Maloy WL, et al. Alternative protein products with different carboxyl termini from a single class I gene, H-2Kb. *Proc Natl Acad Sci U S A* 1986;83:6084–6088.

308. Lew AM, McCluskey J, Maloy WL, et al. Multiple class I molecules generated from single genes by alternative splicing of pre-mRNAs. *Immunol Res* 1987;6:117–132.

309. Handy DE, McCluskey J, Lew AM, et al. Signals controlling alternative splicing of major histocompatibility complex H-2 class I pre-mRNA. *Immunogenetics* 1988;28:81–90.

310. Vega MA, Strominger JL. Constitutive endocytosis of HLA class I antigens requires a specific portion of the intracytoplasmic tail that shares structural features with other endocytosed molecules. *Proc Natl Acad Sci U S A* 1989;86:2688–2692.

311. Balomenos D, Poretz RD. An acidic modification of the cytoplasmic domain contributes to the charge heterogeneity of the MHC class I antigens. *Immunogenetics* 1998;47:381–389.

312. Gur H, Geppert TD, Lipsky PE. Structural analysis of class I MHC molecules: the cytoplasmic domain is not required for cytoskeletal association, aggregation and internalization. *Mol Immunol* 1997;34:125–132.

313. St-Pierre Y, Nabavi N, Ghogawala Z, et al. A functional role for signal transduction via the cytoplasmic domains of MHC class II proteins. *J Immunol* 1989;143:808–812.

314. Nabavi N, Freeman GJ, Gault A, et al. Signalling through the MHC class II cytoplasmic domain is required for antigen presentation and induces B7 expression. *Nature* 1992;360:266–268.

315. Evans GA, Margulies DH, Shykind B, et al. Exon shuffling: mapping polymorphic determinants on hybrid mouse transplantation antigens. *Nature* 1982;300:755–757.

316. Bluestone JA, Foo M, Allen H, et al. Allospecific cytolytic T lymphocytes recognize conformational determinants on hybrid mouse transplantation antigens. *J Exp Med* 1985;162:268–281.

317. Ozato K, Evans GA, Shykind B, et al. Hybrid H-2 histocompatibility gene products assign domains recognized by alloreactive T cells. *Proc Natl Acad Sci U S A* 1983;80:2040–2043.

318. Ozato K, Evans GA, Margulies DH, et al. The use of hybrid H-2 genes for localizing the positions of polymorphic determinants recognized by antibodies and by cytotoxic T cells. *Transplant Proc* 1983;15:2074–2076.

319. Reiss CS, Evans GA, Margulies DH, et al. Allospecific and virus-specific cytolytic T lymphocytes are restricted to the N or C1 domain of H-2 antigens expressed on L cells after DNA-mediated gene transfer. *Proc Natl Acad Sci U S A* 1983;80:2709–2712.

320. Bjorkman PJ, Saper MA, Samraoui B, et al. The foreign antigen binding site and T cell recognition regions of class I histocompatibility antigens. *Nature* 1987;329:512–518.

321. Bjorkman PJ, Saper MA, Samraoui B, et al. Structure of the human class I histocompatibility antigen, HLA-A2. *Nature* 1987;329:506–512.

322. Schwartz RH. Immune response (Ir) genes of the murine major histocompatibility complex. *Adv Immunol* 1986;38:31–201.

323. Babbitt BP, Allen PM, Matsueda G, et al. Binding of immunogenic peptides to Ia histocompatibility molecules. *Nature* 1985;317:359–361.

324. Buus S, Sette A, Colon SM, et al. Isolation and characterization of antigen-Ia complexes involved in T cell recognition. *Cell* 1986;47:1071–1077.

325. Townsend A, Ohlen C, Foster L, et al. A mutant cell in which association of class I heavy and light chains is induced by viral peptides. *Cold Spring Harb Symp Quant Biol* 1989;54(Pt 1):299–308.

326. Townsend A, Ohlen C, Bastin J, et al. Association of class I major histocompatibility heavy and light chains induced by viral peptides. *Nature* 1989;340:443–448.

327. Boyd LF, Kozlowski S, Margulies DH. Solution binding of an antigenic peptide to a major histocompatibility complex class I molecule and the role of beta 2-microglobulin. *Proc Natl Acad Sci U S A* 1992;89:2242–2246.

328. Van Bleek GM, Nathenson SG. Isolation of an endogenously processed immunodominant viral peptide from the class I H-2Kb molecule. *Nature* 1990;348:213–216.

329. Rotzschke O, Falk K, Deres K, et al. Isolation and analysis of naturally processed viral peptides as recognized by cytotoxic T cells. *Nature* 1990;348:252–254.

330. Rotzschke O, Falk K, Wallny HJ, et al. Characterization of naturally occurring minor histocompatibility peptides including H-4 and H-Y. *Science* 1990;249:283–287.

331. Rammensee HG, Falk K, Rotzschke O. Peptides naturally presented by MHC class I molecules. *Annu Rev Immunol* 1993;11:213–244.

332. Arnott D, Shabanowitz J, Hunt DF. Mass spectrometry of proteins and peptides: sensitive and accurate mass measurement and sequence analysis. *Clin Chem* 1993;39:2005–2010.

333. Hunt DF, Henderson RA, Shabanowitz J, et al. Characterization of peptides bound to the class I MHC molecule HLA-A2.1 by mass spectrometry. *Science* 1992;255:1261–1263.

334. Corr M, Boyd LF, Frankel SR, et al. Endogenous peptides of a soluble major histocompatibility complex class I molecule, H-2Lds: sequence motif, quantitative binding, and molecular modeling of the complex. *J Exp Med* 1992;176:1681–1692.

335. Corr M, Boyd LF, Padlan EA, et al. H-2Dd exploits a four residue peptide binding motif. *J Exp Med* 1993;178:1877–1892.

336. Gavin MA, Dere B, Grandea AG 3rd, et al. Major histocompatibility complex class I allele–specific peptide libraries: identification of peptides that mimic an H-Y T cell epitope. *Eur J Immunol* 1994;24:2124–2133.

337. Gavin MA, Bevan MJ. Major histocompatibility complex allele–specific peptide libraries and identification of T-cell mimotopes. *Methods Mol Biol* 1998;87:235–248.

338. Rammensee H, Bachmann J, Emmerich NP, et al. SYFPEITHI: database for MHC ligands and peptide motifs. *Immunogenetics* 1999;50:213–219.

339. Parker KC, Bednarek MA, Coligan JE. Scheme for ranking potential HLA-A2 binding peptides based on independent binding of individual peptide side-chains. *J Immunol* 1994;152:163–175.

340. Rudensky A, Preston-Hurlburt P, Hong SC, et al. Sequence analysis of peptides bound to MHC class II molecules. *Nature* 1991;353:622–627.

341. Chicz RM, Urban RG, Lane WS, et al. Predominant naturally processed peptides bound to HLA-DR1 are derived from MHC-related molecules and are heterogeneous in size. *Nature* 1992;358:764–768.

342. Janeway CA Jr, Mamula MJ, Rudensky A. Rules for peptide presentation by MHC class II molecules. *Int Rev Immunol* 1993;10:301–311.

343. Urban RG, Chicz RM, Vignali DA, et al. The dichotomy of peptide

presentation by class I and class II MHC proteins. *Chem Immunol* 1993;57:197–234.

344. Hammer J, Takacs B, Sinigaglia F. Identification of a motif for HLA-DR1 binding peptides using M13 display libraries. *J Exp Med* 1992;176:1007–1013.

345. Carrasco-Marin E, Petzold S, Unanue ER. Two structural states of complexes of peptide and class II major histocompatibility complex revealed by photoaffinity-labeled peptides. *J Biol Chem* 1999;274:31333–31340.

346. Gugasyan R, Velazquez C, Vidavsky I, et al. Independent selection by I-Ak molecules of two epitopes found in tandem in an extended polypeptide antigen. *J Immunol* 2000;165:3206–3213.

347. Cease KB, Berkower I, York-Jolley J, et al. T cell clones specific for an amphipathic alpha-helical region of sperm whale myoglobin show differing fine specificities for synthetic peptides. A multiview/single structure interpretation of immunodominance. *J Exp Med* 1986;164:1779–1784.

348. Garrett TP, Saper MA, Bjorkman PJ, et al. Specificity pockets for the side chains of peptide antigens in HLA-Aw68. *Nature* 1989;342:692–696.

349. Saper MA, Bjorkman PJ, Wiley DC. Refined structure of the human histocompatibility antigen HLA-A2 at 2.6 A resolution. *J Mol Biol* 1991;219:277–319.

350. Madden DR, Gorga JC, Strominger JL, et al. The three-dimensional structure of HLA-B27 at 2.1 A resolution suggests a general mechanism for tight peptide binding to MHC. *Cell* 1992;70:1035–1048.

351. Jardetzky TS, Lane WS, Robinson RA, et al. Identification of self peptides bound to purified HLA-B27. *Nature* 1991;353:326–329.

352. Zhang W, Young AC, Imarai M, et al. Crystal structure of the major histocompatibility complex class I H-2Kb molecule containing a single viral peptide: implications for peptide binding and T-cell receptor recognition. *Proc Natl Acad Sci U S A* 1992;89:8403–8407.

353. Fremont DH, Matsumura M, Stura EA, et al. Crystal structures of two viral peptides in complex with murine MHC class I H-2Kb. *Science* 1992;257:919–927.

354. Fremont DH, Stura EA, Matsumura M, et al. Crystal structure of an H-2Kb–ovalbumin peptide complex reveals the interplay of primary and secondary anchor positions in the major histocompatibility complex binding groove. *Proc Natl Acad Sci U S A* 1995;92:2479–2483.

355. Joyce S, Kuzushima K, Kepecs G, et al. Characterization of an incompletely assembled major histocompatibility class I molecule (H-2Kb) associated with unusually long peptides: implications for antigen processing and presentation. *Proc Natl Acad Sci U S A* 1994;91:4145–4149.

356. Collins EJ, Garboczi DN, Wiley DC. Three-dimensional structure of a peptide extending from one end of a class I MHC binding site. *Nature* 1994;371:626–629.

357. Kastrup IB, Stevanovic S, Arsequell G, et al. Lectin purified human class I MHC-derived peptides: evidence for presentation of glycopeptides *in vivo*. *Tissue Antigens* 2000;56:129–135.

358. Speir JA, Abdel-Motal UM, Jondal M, et al. Crystal structure of an MHC class I presented glycopeptide that generates carbohydrate-specific CTL. *Immunity* 1999;10:51–61.

359. Glithero A, Tormo J, Haurum JS, et al. Crystal structures of two H-2Db/glycopeptide complexes suggest a molecular basis for CTL cross-reactivity. *Immunity* 1999;10:63–74.

360. Speir JA, Stevens J, Joly E, et al. Two different, highly exposed, bulged structures for an unusually long peptide bound to rat MHC class I RT1-Aa. *Immunity* 2001;14:81–92.

361. Brown JH, Jardetzky T, Saper MA, et al. A hypothetical model of the foreign antigen binding site of class II histocompatibility molecules. *Nature* 1988;332:845–850.

362. Brown JH, Jardetzky TS, Gorga JC, et al. Three-dimensional structure of the human class II histocompatibility antigen HLA-DR1. *Nature* 1993;364:33–39.

363. Wu TT, Kabat EA. An analysis of the sequences of the variable regions of Bence Jones proteins and myeloma light chains and their implications for antibody complementarity. *J Exp Med* 1970;132:211–250.

364. Stern LJ, Brown JH, Jardetzky TS, et al. Crystal structure of the human class II MHC protein HLA-DR1 complexed with an influenza virus peptide. *Nature* 1994;368:215–221.

365. Fields BA, Ober B, Malchiodi EL, et al. Crystal structure of the V alpha domain of a T cell antigen receptor. *Science* 1995;270:1821–1824.

366. Schafer PH, Malapati S, Hanfelt KK, et al. The assembly and stability of MHC class II-(alpha beta)2 superdimers. *J Immunol* 1998;161:2307–2316.

367. Abastado JP, Lone YC, Casrouge A, et al. Dimerization of soluble major histocompatibility complex–peptide complexes is sufficient for activation of T cell hybridoma and induction of unresponsiveness. *J Exp Med* 1995;182:439–447.

368. Reich Z, Boniface JJ, Lyons DS, et al. Ligand-specific oligomerization of T-cell receptor molecules. *Nature* 1997;387:617–620.

369. Fremont DH, Hendrickson WA, Marrack P, et al. Structures of an MHC class II molecule with covalently bound single peptides. *Science* 1996;272:1001–1004.

370. Fremont DH, Dai S, Chiang H, et al. Structural basis of cytochrome c presentation by IE(k). *J Exp Med* 2002;195:1043–1052.

371. Plaksin D, Chacko S, McPhie P, et al. A T cell receptor V alpha domain expressed in bacteria: does it dimerize in solution? *J Exp Med* 1996;184:1251–1258.

372. Garboczi DN, Ghosh P, Utz U, et al. Structure of the complex between human T-cell receptor, viral peptide and HLA-A2. *Nature* 1996;384:134–141.

373. Garcia KC, Degano M, Stanfield RL, et al. An alphabeta T cell receptor structure at 2.5 A and its orientation in the TCR-MHC complex. *Science* 1996;274:209–219.

374. Reinherz EL, Tan K, Tang L, et al. The crystal structure of a T cell receptor in complex with peptide and MHC class II. *Science* 1999;286:1913–1921.

375. Hennecke J, Carfi A, Wiley DC. Structure of a covalently stabilized complex of a human alphabeta T-cell receptor, influenza HA peptide and MHC class II molecule, HLA-DR1. *EMBO J* 2000;19:5611–5624.

376. Corper AL, Stratmann T, Apostolopoulos V, et al. A structural framework for deciphering the link between I-Ag7 and autoimmune diabetes. *Science* 2000;288:505–511.

377. Latek RR, Suri A, Petzold SJ, et al. Structural basis of peptide binding and presentation by the type I diabetes–associated MHC class II molecule of NOD mice. *Immunity* 2000;12:699–710.

378. Zeng Z, Castano AR, Segelke BW, et al. Crystal structure of mouse CD1: an MHC-like fold with a large hydrophobic binding groove. *Science* 1997;277:339–345.

379. Gadola SD, Zaccai NR, Harlos K, et al. Structure of human CD1b with bound ligands at 2.3 A, a maze for alkyl chains. *Nat Immunol* 2002;3:721–726.

380. Wang CR, Esser L, Smagula CS, et al. Identification, expression, and crystallization of the protease-resistant conserved domain of synapsin I. *Protein Sci* 1997;6:2264–2267.

381. Wang CR, Lindahl KF, Deisenhofer J. Crystal structure of the MHC class Ib molecule H2-M3. *Res Immunol* 1996;147:313–321.

382. Li P, Morris DL, Willcox BE, et al. Complex structure of the activating immunoreceptor NKG2D and its MHC class I–like ligand MICA. *Nat Immunol* 2001;2:443–451.

383. Li P, Willie ST, Bauer S, et al. Crystal structure of the MHC class I homolog MIC-A, a gammadelta T cell ligand. *Immunity* 1999;10:577–584.

384. Burmeister WP, Gastinel LN, Simister NE, et al. Crystal structure at 2.2 A resolution of the MHC-related neonatal Fc receptor. *Nature* 1994;372:336–343.

385. Li P, McDermott G, Strong RK. Crystal structures of RAE-1beta and its complex with the activating immunoreceptor NKG2D. *Immunity* 2002;16:77–86.

386. Loveland B, Wang CR, Yonekawa H, et al. Maternally transmitted histocompatibility antigen of mice: a hydrophobic peptide of a mitochondrially encoded protein. *Cell* 1990;60:971–980.

387. Wang CR, Castano AR, Peterson PA, et al. Nonclassical binding of formylated peptide in crystal structure of the MHC class Ib molecule H2-M3. *Cell* 1995;82:655–664.

388. Moody DB, Besra GS, Wilson IA, et al. The molecular basis of CD1-mediated presentation of lipid antigens. *Immunol Rev* 1999;172:285–296.

389. Calabi F, Jarvis JM, Martin L, et al. Two classes of CD1 genes. *Eur J Immunol* 1989;19:285–292.

390. Shamshiev A, Donda A, Carena I, et al. Self glycolipids as T-cell autoantigens. *Eur J Immunol* 1999;29:1667–1675.

391. Rosat JP, Grant EP, Beckman EM, et al. CD1-restricted microbial lipid antigen–specific recognition found in the CD8+ alpha beta T cell pool. *J Immunol* 1999;162:366–371.

392. Young AC, Zhang W, Sacchettini JC, et al. The three-dimensional structure of H-2Db at 2.4 A resolution: implications for antigen-determinant selection. *Cell* 1994;76:39–50.

393. Simister NE, Rees AR. Isolation and characterization of an Fc receptor from neonatal rat small intestine. *Eur J Immunol* 1985;15:733–738.

394. Simister NE, Mostov KE. Cloning and expression of the neonatal rat intestinal Fc receptor, a major histocompatibility complex class I antigen homolog. *Cold Spring Harb Symp Quant Biol* 1989;54(Pt 1): 571–580.

395. Ahouse JJ, Hagerman CL, Mittal P, et al. Mouse MHC class I–like Fc receptor encoded outside the MHC. *J Immunol* 1993;151:6076–6088.

396. Story CM, Mikulska JE, Simister NE. A major histocompatibility complex class I–like Fc receptor cloned from human placenta: possible role in transfer of immunoglobulin G from mother to fetus. *J Exp Med* 1994;180:2377–2381.

397. Simister NE. IgG Fc receptors that resemble class I major histocompatibility complex antigens. *Biochem Soc Trans* 1993;21:973–976.

398. Martin WL, West AP Jr, Gan L, et al. Crystal structure at 2.8 A of an FcRn/heterodimeric Fc complex: mechanism of pH-dependent binding. *Mol Cell* 2001;7:867–877.

399. Israel EJ, Wilsker DF, Hayes KC, et al. Increased clearance of IgG in mice that lack beta 2-microglobulin: possible protective role of FcRn. *Immunology* 1996;89:573–578.

400. Hennecke J, Wiley DC. Structure of a complex of the human alpha/beta T cell receptor (TCR) HA1.7, influenza hemagglutinin peptide, and major histocompatibility complex class II molecule, HLA-DR4 (DRA*0101 and DRB1*0401): insight into TCR cross-restriction and alloreactivity. *J Exp Med* 2002;195:571–581.

401. Reiser JB, Darnault C, Guimezanes A, et al. Crystal structure of a T cell receptor bound to an allogeneic MHC molecule. *Nat Immunol* 2000;1:291–297.

402. Garcia KC, Degano M, Pease LR, et al. Structural basis of plasticity in T cell receptor recognition of a self peptide-MHC antigen. *Science* 1998;279:1166–1172.

403. Reiser JB, Gregoire C, Darnault C, et al. A T cell receptor CDR3beta loop undergoes conformational changes of unprecedented magnitude upon binding to a peptide/MHC class I complex. *Immunity* 2002;16:345–354.

404. Devine L, Kavathas PB. Molecular analysis of protein interactions mediating the function of the cell surface protein CD8. *Immunol Res* 1999;19:201–210.

405. Gao GF, Jakobsen BK. Molecular interactions of coreceptor CD8 and MHC class I: the molecular basis for functional coordination with the T-cell receptor. *Immunol Today* 2000;21:630–636.

406. Maddon PJ, Dalgleish AG, McDougal JS, et al. The T4 gene encodes the AIDS virus receptor and is expressed in the immune system and the brain. *Cell* 1986;47:333–348.

407. Wu H, Kwong PD, Hendrickson WA. Dimeric association and segmental variability in the structure of human CD4. *Nature* 1997; 387:527–530.

408. Matsumoto N, Yokoyama WM, Kojima S, et al. The NK cell MHC class I receptor Ly49A detects mutations on H-2Dd inside and outside of the peptide binding groove. *J Immunol* 2001;166:4422–4428.

409. Wang J, Whitman MC, Natarajan K, et al. Binding of the natural killer cell inhibitory receptor Ly49A to its major histocompatibility complex class I ligand. Crucial contacts include both H-2Dd AND beta 2-microglobulin. *J Biol Chem* 2002;277:1433–1442.

410. Dimasi N, Sawicki MW, Reineck LA, et al. Crystal structure of the Ly49I natural killer cell receptor reveals variability in dimerization mode within the Ly49 family. *J Mol Biol* 2002;320:573–585.

411. Radaev S, Rostro B, Brooks AG, et al. Conformational plasticity revealed by the cocrystal structure of NKG2D and its class I MHC–like ligand ULBP3. *Immunity* 2001;15:1039–1049.

412. Strong RK. Asymmetric ligand recognition by the activating natural killer cell receptor NKG2D, a symmetric homodimer. *Mol Immunol* 2002;38:1029–1037.

413. Herman A, Kappler JW, Marrack P, et al. Superantigens: mechanism of T-cell stimulation and role in immune responses. *Annu Rev Immunol* 1991;9:745–772.

414. Rovira P, Buckle M, Abastado JP, et al. Major histocompatibility class I molecules present *Urtica dioica* agglutinin, a superantigen of vegetal origin, to T lymphocytes. *Eur J Immunol* 1999;29:1571–1580.

415. Harata K, Muraki M. Crystal structures of *Urtica dioica* agglutinin and its complex with tri-*N*-acetylchitotriose. *J Mol Biol* 2000;297: 673–681.

416. Saul FA, Rovira P, Boulot G, et al. Crystal structure of *Urtica dioica* agglutinin, a superantigen presented by MHC molecules of class I and class II. *Structure Fold Des* 2000;8:593–603.

417. Papageorgiou AC, Acharya KR. Microbial superantigens: from structure to function. *Trends Microbiol* 2000;8:369–375.

418. Jardetzky TS, Brown JH, Gorga JC, et al. Three-dimensional structure of a human class II histocompatibility molecule complexed with superantigen. *Nature* 1994;368:711–718.

419. Fields BA, Malchiodi EL, Li H, et al. Crystal structure of a T-cell receptor beta-chain complexed with a superantigen. *Nature* 1996; 384:188–192.

420. Petersson K, Hakansson M, Nilsson H, et al. Crystal structure of a superantigen bound to MHC class II displays zinc and peptide dependence. *EMBO J* 2001;20:3306–3312.

421. Li Y, Li H, Dimasi N, et al. Crystal structure of a superantigen bound to the high-affinity, zinc-dependent site on MHC class II. *Immunity* 2001;14:93–104.

422. Fremont DH, Rees WA, Kozono H. Biophysical studies of T-cell receptors and their ligands. *Curr Opin Immunol* 1996;8:93–100.

423. Matsui K, Boniface JJ, Reay PA, et al. Low affinity interaction of peptide-MHC complexes with T cell receptors. *Science* 1991;254:1788–1791.

424. Matsui K, Boniface JJ, Steffner P, et al. Kinetics of T-cell receptor binding to peptide/I-Ek complexes: correlation of the dissociation rate with T-cell responsiveness. *Proc Natl Acad Sci U S A* 1994;91:12862–12866.

425. Khilko SN, Jelonek MT, Corr M, et al. Measuring interactions of MHC class I molecules using surface plasmon resonance. *J Immunol Methods* 1995;183:77–94.

426. Corr M, Slanetz AE, Boyd LF, et al. T cell receptor–MHC class I peptide interactions: affinity, kinetics, and specificity. *Science* 1994; 265:946–949.

427. Sykulev Y, Brunmark A, Jackson M, et al. Kinetics and affinity of reactions between an antigen-specific T cell receptor and peptide-MHC complexes. *Immunity* 1994;1:15–22.

428. Alam SM, Travers PJ, Wung JL, et al. T-cell-receptor affinity and thymocyte positive selection. *Nature* 1996;381:616–620.

429. Alam SM, Davies GM, Lin CM, et al. Qualitative and quantitative differences in T cell receptor binding of agonist and antagonist ligands. *Immunity* 1999;10:227–237.

430. Willcox BE, Gao GF, Wyer JR, et al. TCR binding to peptide-MHC stabilizes a flexible recognition interface. *Immunity* 1999;10:357–365.

431. Natarajan K, Boyd LF, Schuck P, et al. Interaction of the NK cell inhibitory receptor Ly49A with H-2Dd: identification of a site distinct from the TCR site. *Immunity* 1999;11:591–601.

432. Vales-Gomez M, Reyburn HT, Erskine RA, et al. Kinetics and peptide dependency of the binding of the inhibitory NK receptor CD94/NKG2-A and the activating receptor CD94/NKG2-C to HLA-E. *EMBO J* 1999;18:4250–4260.

433. Altman JD, Moss PA, Goulder PJ, et al. Phenotypic analysis of antigen-specific T lymphocytes. *Science* 1996;274:94–96.

434. O'Herrin SM, Lebowitz MS, Bieler JG, et al. Analysis of the expression of peptide–major histocompatibility complexes using high affinity soluble divalent T cell receptors. *J Exp Med* 1997;186:1333–1345.

435. Hanke T, Takizawa H, McMahon CW, et al. Direct assessment of MHC class I binding by seven Ly49 inhibitory NK cell receptors. *Immunity* 1999;11:67–77.

436. Mehta IK, Smith HR, Wang J, et al. A "chimeric" C57l-derived Ly49 inhibitory receptor resembling the Ly49D activation receptor. *Cell Immunol* 2001;209:29–41.

437. Mehta IK, Wang J, Roland J, et al. Ly49A allelic variation and MHC class I specificity. *Immunogenetics* 2001;53:572–583.

438. Cameron T, Norris P, Patel A, et al. Labeling antigen-specific CD4(+) T cells with class II MHC oligomers. *J Immunol Methods* 2002;268:51.

439. Hugues S, Malherbe L, Filippi C, et al. Generation and use of alternative multimers of peptide/MHC complexes. *J Immunol Methods* 2002;268:83.

440. Malherbe L, Filippi C, Julia V, et al. Selective activation and expansion of high-affinity CD4+ T cells in resistant mice upon infection with *Leishmania major*. *Immunity* 2000;13:771–782.

441. Lebowitz MS, O'Herrin SM, Hamad AR, et al. Soluble, high-affinity dimers of T-cell receptors and class II major histocompatibility complexes: biochemical probes for analysis and modulation of immune responses. *Cell Immunol* 1999;192:175–184.
442. Crawford F, Kozono H, White J, et al. Detection of antigen-specific T cells with multivalent soluble class II MHC covalent peptide complexes. *Immunity* 1998;8:675–682.
443. Hackett CJ, Sharma OK. Frontiers in peptide-MHC class II multimer technology. *Nat Immunol* 2002;3:887–889.
444. Kruisbeek A. Commonly used mouse strains. In: Bierer B, Coligan JE, Margulies DH, et al., eds. *Current protocols in immunology.* New York: John Wiley & Sons, 2002:Appendix 1C.
445. Lindahl KF. On naming *H2* haplotypes: functional significance of MHC class Ib alleles. *Immunogenet* 1997;46:53–62.
446. Mathis DJ, Benoist C, Williams VE 2nd, et al. Several mechanisms can account for defective E alpha gene expression in different mouse haplotypes. *Proc Natl Acad Sci U S A* 1983;80:273–277.
447. Christiansen FT, Witt CS. Allogeneic bone marrow transplantation. In: Bradley J, McCluskey J, eds. *Clinical immunology.* Oxford, UK: Oxford University Press, 1997:445.
448. Biddison WE, Martin R. Appendix 1I: peptide binding motifs for MHC class I and class II molecules. In: Bierer B, Coligan JE, Margulies DH, et al, eds. *Current protocols in immunology.* New York: John Wiley & Sons, 2002.
449. Schild H, Gruneberg U, Pougialis G, et al. Natural ligand motifs of H-2E molecules are allele specific and illustrate homology to HLA-DR molecules. *Int Immunol* 1995;7:1957–1965.
450. Brouwenstijn N, Serwold T, Shastri N. MHC class I molecules can direct proteolytic cleavage of antigenic precursors in the endoplasmic reticulum. *Immunity* 2001;15:95–104.
451. Fruci D, Niedermann G, Butler RH, et al. Efficient MHC class I–independent amino-terminal trimming of epitope precursor peptides in the endoplasmic reticulum. *Immunity* 2001;15:467–476.
452. Gruen JR, Weissman SM. Evolving views of the major histocompatibility complex. *Blood* 1997;90:4252–4265.
453. McCluskey J. The human leucocyte antigens and clinical medicine. In: Bradley J, McCluskey J, eds. *Clinical immunology.* Oxford, UK: Oxford University Press, 1997:415–427.
454. Margulies DH, McCluskey J. Exon shuffling: new genes from old. *Surv Immunol Res* 1985;4:146–159.
455. Berman HM, Westbrook J, Feng Z, et al. The protein data bank. *Nucleic Acids Res* 2000;28:235–242.
456. Evans SV. SETOR: hardware-lighted three-dimensional solid model representations of macromolecules. *J Mol Graph* 1993;11:134–138, 127–128.
457. Lee KH, Wucherpfennig KW, Wiley DC. Structure of a human insulin peptide-HLA-DQ8 complex and susceptibility to type 1 diabetes. *Nat Immunol* 2001;2:501–507.
458. Nicholls A, Sharp KA, Honig B. Protein folding and association: insights from the interfacial and thermodynamic properties of hydrocarbons. *Proteins* 1991;11:281–296.
459. Kraulis PJ, Domaille PJ, Campbell-Burk SL, et al. Solution structure and dynamics of ras p21.GDP determined by heteronuclear three- and four-dimensional NMR spectroscopy. *Biochemistry* 1994;33:3515–3531.
460. Merritt EA, Bacon DJ. Raster3D: photorealistic molecular graphics. *Methods Enzymol* 1997;277:505–524.
461. Rudolph MG, Luz JG, Wilson IA. Structural and thermodynamic correlates of T cell signaling. *Annu Rev Biophys Biomol Struct* 2002;31:121–149.
462. Sundberg EJ, Li Y, Mariuzza RA. So many ways of getting in the way: diversity in the molecular architecture of superantigen-dependent T-cell signaling complexes. *Curr Opin Immunol* 2002;14:36–44.

CHAPTER 20

The Biochemistry and Cell Biology of Antigen Processing

Peter Cresswell

Antigen Recognition by T-Cell Receptors
Class I Major Histocompatibility Complex–Restricted Antigen Presentation
  Peptide Generation · Peptide Transport into the Endoplasmic Reticulum · Assembly of Class I Major Histocompatibility Complex/Peptide Complexes · The Source of Class I Major Histocompatibility Complex–Associated Peptides · Release of Class I Major Histocompatibility Complex Molecules from the Endoplasmic Reticulum · Class I Major Histocompatibility Complex–Restricted Presentation of Extracellular Proteins
Class II Major Histocompatibility Complex–Restricted Antigen Presentation
  Class II Assembly of Major Histocompatibility Complex Molecules in the Endoplasmic Reticulum · Endocytic Processing of the Invariant Chain · Class II Peptide Loading of Major Histocompatibility Complex Molecules · Delivery of Class II Major Histocompatibility Complex Molecules to the Cell Surface · Endocytosis of Proteins and Peptide Generation by Antigen-Presenting Cells
Concluding Remarks
Acknowledgments
References

ANTIGEN RECOGNITION BY T-CELL RECEPTORS

Unlike antibodies, which can recognize almost any kind of chemical structure, the structurally similar receptors on T-lymphocytes exclusively recognize class I or class II major histocompatibility complex (MHC) molecules or their homologues, such as CD1 molecules. The antigen recognized by T-lymphocytes during an immune response is actually a complex between the MHC molecule and a peptide derived from a foreign protein: for example, one derived from a bacterium or virus. The integration of the peptide into a polymorphic binding groove, structurally defined by two antiparallel α helices overlaying an eight strand β sheet (see Chapter 19), generates a variable surface that interacts with the T-cell receptor in a defined orientation. Recognition of such complexes is described as "MHC-restricted antigen presentation," meaning that the receptor of a particular T cell is restricted to the recognition of a specific peptide in association with a single class I or class II MHC allele.

MHC molecules are integral membrane glycoproteins that acquire their associated peptides by complex mechanisms that are interwoven with their pathways of biosynthesis and intracellular transport. This is a constitutive process, and in the absence of infection, MHC molecules are associated with peptides derived from autologous proteins. The peptide generation and loading mechanisms are collectively referred to as antigen processing and are very different for the two classes of MHC molecules. Class I MHC molecules bind to short peptides of 8 to 10 amino acids in the endoplasmic reticulum (ER). These peptides are generated by proteolysis of proteins in the cytosol of the cell. Class II MHC molecules bind peptides of 13 to 24 amino acids that are almost exclusively derived from extracellular proteins, lysosomal proteins, or the luminal regions of integral membrane proteins. These peptides are generated by proteolysis in the endocytic pathway, which terminates in lysosomes. The successful cell surface expression of both classes of MHC molecules with their associated peptides relies on the same quality control mechanisms that govern the proper folding and surface expression of other membrane glycoproteins, although, in each case, specific adaptations to these conventional processes that facilitate peptide binding have evolved.

CLASS I MAJOR HISTOCOMPATIBILITY COMPLEX–RESTRICTED ANTIGEN PRESENTATION

Peptide Generation

The initial step in class I MHC–restricted antigen processing is the generation of peptides from proteins in the cytosol. The

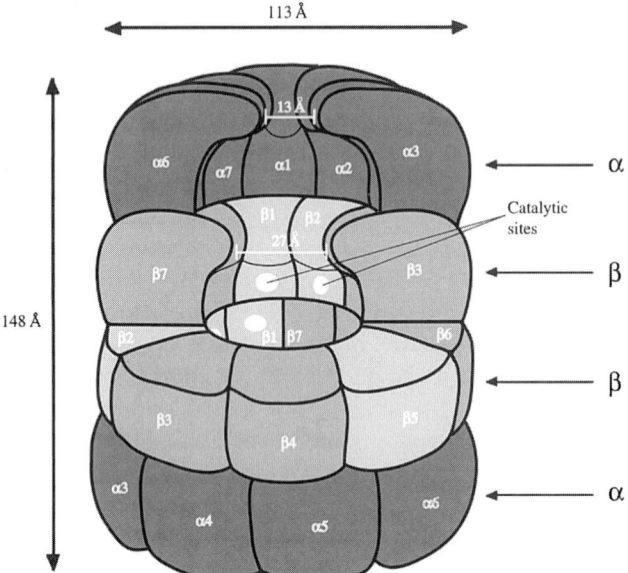

113 Å

13 Å

α6 α7 α1 α2 α3

β1 β2

21 Å

β7   β3

Catalytic
sites

148 Å

β2 β1 β7   β6

β3   β5

β4

α3

α4 α5   α6

α

β

β

α

FIG. 1. Schematic diagram of the structure of the 20S proteasome. Four heptameric rings of α subunits and β subunits make up the complete structure. The upper pair of rings are cut away to reveal the interior of the barrel-shaped structure. The proteolytically active β subunits (β1, β2, and β5) are shown in the lightest shade, and the active sites are indicated. Access of proteins to the interior is regulated by additional multisubunit components (19S and PA28) that bind to the ends of the proteasome, as described in the text and reviewed by Kloetzel (11).

dominant responsible protease is the proteasome. Much of the evidence for this comes from the use of specific inhibitors of proteasomal degradation (1,2). The proteasome is a complex multisubunit protease responsible for the turnover of the majority of cytosolic and nuclear proteins (3). The core of the proteasome is a cylindrical structure, the 20S proteasome, formed from four stacked rings of seven subunits each (4) (Fig. 1). The two inner rings are formed from the β subunits, three of which—β1, β2, and β5—are catalytically active, and thus there are six active sites per proteasome. The two outer rings consist of α subunits. The β subunits are synthesized as N-terminally extended precursors and undergo cleavage upon incorporation into the proteasome, which reveals an N-terminal threonine residue, an essential feature of the active site (5,6). The active sites are situated in a central chamber in the interior of the cylinder, and proteins must enter the cylinder for degradation to occur.

Access to the interior of the proteasome is regulated by an additional complex of proteins, which associates with the 20S core. This set of proteins is known as the 19S regulator. The combination of the 20S and two 19S complexes constitutes the 26S proteasome. The 19S regulator contains subunits with adenosine triphosphatase activities that unfold proteins, allowing them to penetrate the interior of the 20S catalytic core, and a subunit that recognizes ubiquitin, a small protein that is enzymatically added as an oligomeric chain to lysine

residues of cytosolic proteins to mark them for degradation (7–9). Three enzymes operating in sequence are responsible for ubiquitin addition: E1 activates the ubiquitin, E2 transfers the ubiquitin to E3, and E3 transfers the ubiquitin to the target protein. Regulated degradation of a number of cytosolic and nuclear proteins, including cyclins (which regulate the cell cycle) and a variety of transcription factors, is accomplished by their ubiquitination by a specific E3 enzyme, followed by proteasomal degradation (10).

A number of specific modifications are constitutively present in proteasomes in antigen-presenting cells (APCs) and are induced in a variety of normal cells upon treatment with γ-interferon (11). First, the three enzymatically active β subunits (β1, β2, and β5) are replaced by novel inducible active subunits, β1i, β2i, and β5i, which were originally called LMP2, MECL-1, and LMP7, respectively (12). Such modified proteasomes, frequently called *immunoproteasomes,* must be freshly assembled from newly synthesized subunits, and so the replacement process is slow upon γ-interferon treatment. The β1i (LMP2) and β5i (LMP7) subunits are encoded in the MHC (12–14); this, when discovered, immediately led to the suggestion that they might be involved with antigen processing. Considerable data have suggested that incorporation of the γ-interferon–inducible subunits into the proteasome changes its cleavage specificity (15–17). This results in the generation of more peptides that terminate in hydrophobic or basic residues, which, depending on the allele, are the preferred C-terminal residues of class I MHC–associated peptides. Support for the immunological importance of the inducible β subunits comes from studies of knockout mice. Mice lacking the β1i subunit have fewer CD8 cells and diminished cytotoxic T-cell responses than do wild-type mice when they are infected with influenza virus (18). β5i Knockout mice have reduced levels of cell surface expression of class I MHC molecules, which is often diagnostic of poor peptide binding (see later discussion), and their cells are poorly recognized by certain class I MHC–restricted T cells (19).

A second modification occurring upon γ-interferon treatment involves the induction of a novel regulator of the proteasome, which replaces the 19S regulator. This is proteasome activator 28 (PA28), also called the 11S regulator, and consists of a heptameric ring containing two subunits, PA28α and PA28β (20). No adenosine triphosphatase activity is associated with the 11S regulator, but it does enhance the peptidase activity of 20S proteasomes (21,22). Biochemical studies with purified components and oligopeptide or protein substrates have shown that the cleavage patterns of the substrates can be modified by association of the proteasome with the 11S regulator. One study indicated that a coordinated double cleavage by such modified proteasomes might preferentially generate class I MHC–restricted epitopes from larger precursors (23). Overexpression of the PA28 α subunit in cell lines was found to enhance presentation of certain viral epitopes (24). Again, knockout mice have provided evidence for an important role of the 11S regulator in antigen processing,

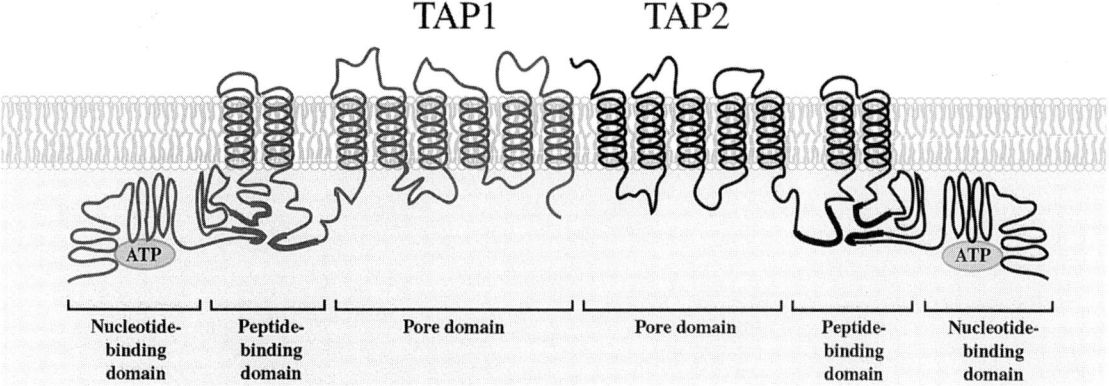

FIG. 2. Schematic diagram of transporter associated with antigen processing (TAP), which translocates peptides from the cytosol into the endoplasmic reticulum. The predicted organization of the TAP1 and TAP2 transmembrane segments is based on the work of Vos et al. (197). The peptide-binding regions, defined by Nijenhuis et al. (31), who used photoactivatable peptide derivatives, are indicated as thicker lines. The linear structure shown is predicted to form a pore in the endoplasmic reticulum membrane through which associated peptides are translocated upon adenosine triphosphate hydrolysis (198).

although there are conflicts in the literature over what the precise role may be. According to one report, PA28β knock-out mice express neither PA28β nor PA28α, which suggests that they necessarily function as a hetero-oligomer, and antiviral CD8[+] cytotoxic T-lymphocyte responses in these mice were seriously impaired (25). The incorporation of the γ-interferon–inducible β subunits into the proteasomes of these mice was inhibited, which suggests an as yet unexplained connection between the 11S regulator and assembly of the immunoproteasome. In another study, however, mice lacking both PA28 subunits assembled immunoproteasomes normally (26). Their cells showed reduced adenosine triphosphate (ATP)–dependent proteolytic activity, which implies an interaction between the PA28 and 19S regulatory complexes, perhaps corresponding to "hybrid proteasomes," with 20S cores associated with a PA28 complex at one end and a 19S complex at the other. Responses to two antigens, ovalbumin and influenza virus, were unimpaired, whereas the response to a third, a melanoma tumor antigen, was almost eliminated.

Peptides destined for class I MHC binding that are generated by proteasomal degradation already have the appropriate C-terminal amino acid residue. They may, however, be extended at the N-terminal (27). N-terminal trimming of such peptides can occur in the cytosol, and one enzyme capable of this reaction, leucine aminopeptidase, is inducible by γ-interferon, which argues perhaps for a specific role in antigen processing (28). Additional N-terminal trimming may occur in the ER, as described in the next section.

Peptide Transport into the Endoplasmic Reticulum

Class I MHC assembly and peptide binding occur in the ER, and peptides generated in the cytosol must be therefore be translocated across the ER membrane. This is achieved by a specific transporter, the transporter associated with antigen processing (TAP), which is composed of two MHC-encoded subunits, TAP1 and TAP2 (29) (Fig. 2). TAP is a member of a large family of related molecules, known as ATP binding cassette (ABC) transporters, that use ATP hydrolysis to move a variety of small molecules across membranes (30). All of the family members have a similar structure consisting of two hydrophobic domains, each with multiple transmembrane segments, and two hydrophilic domains with characteristic sequences, including the so-called Walker A and B motifs, which define sites for ATP binding and hydrolysis. Most ABC transporters contain all four of these domains in a single polypeptide, but in the case of TAP, each subunit includes a single hydrophobic N-terminal domain and a hydrophilic C-terminal domain. TAP molecules are located in the ER membrane, and the C-terminal ATP hydrolytic domains protrude into the cytosol.

Experiments using photoactivatable peptide derivatives, which can form covalent bonds upon exposure to ultraviolet light, have defined a TAP peptide-binding site. It is composed of elements of the transmembrane segments of both TAP1 and TAP2, particularly those adjacent to the hydrophilic C-terminal domain (31). Peptides ranging in length from 8 to 13 or more amino acids can bind and be transported. Binding and transport are quite independent of amino acid sequence, which suggests that interactions between TAP and the polyamide backbone of the peptide are mainly responsible for binding. Certain residues at some positions—for example, proline at position 2—inhibit peptide translocation. Peptides with basic or hydrophobic residues at the C-terminal are transported more efficiently than peptides with C-terminal acidic residues, and, as pointed out earlier, such peptides are preferentially produced by immunoproteasomes and also bind preferentially to class I MHC molecules (32–35). Peptide binding to TAP appears to be ATP independent in that it is unaffected by ATP depletion, although mutational analysis of the Walker A and B motifs of the TAP1 and TAP2 subunits indicates that ATP hydrolysis by TAP2 is critical for both binding and transport. ATP hydrolysis by TAP1 is not absolutely required for translocation of peptides into the ER but may be required for the transporter to return to a peptide-receptive and transport-competent conformation after one round of translocation (36–39).

Peptides associated with class I MHC molecules are short, generally between 8 and 10 residues in length. Peptides that are longer than this must be trimmed to fit into the binding groove. As described previously, at least one enzyme can mediate amino-terminal trimming in the cytosol, but considerable evidence suggests that further trimming occurs in the ER after translocation by TAP. Although the enzymes responsible have not been defined, there is biochemical evidence for such an activity (40,41). Certain alleles preferentially bind peptides with a proline residue in the second position. As described previously, such peptides are poor TAP substrates, and the implication is that amino-terminal trimming must occur after larger precursors are transported into the ER. N-terminally extended precursors can be found in association with class I MHC molecules when cells are incubated with certain inhibitors of aminopeptidases, such as leucinethiol (42). This is consistent with an early hypothesis that suggested that the class I MHC molecule may serve as a template for trimming, binding peptides initially by the C-terminal and completing the binding process only when the N-terminal is appropriately cleaved.

Assembly of Class I Major Histocompatibility Complex/Peptide Complexes

Many experiments since the mid-1990s have shown that the association of TAP-translocated peptides with class I MHC molecules is not a simple bimolecular ligand–receptor interaction. Rather, it is a complex process that has much in common with the assembly of many multisubunit glycoproteins in the ER, with roles for a variety of chaperones that facilitate the process. The assembly process is schematically presented in Fig. 3.

Class I MHC heavy chains are cotranslationally glycosylated and associate rapidly with the transmembrane chaperone calnexin soon after their introduction into the ER (43). The interaction with calnexin is not essential, and the soluble Hsp70 homologue Bip has also been reported to associate with free heavy chains (44–46). The association of the heavy chain with β_2-microglobulin coincides with dissociation of calnexin and the association of the class I MHC molecule with the soluble chaperone calreticulin (47). Both calnexin and calreticulin are "housekeeping" molecules that bind to the asparagine (N)-linked glycans of newly synthesized glycoproteins when they are in the monoglucosylated form (48). This is generated by the removal by the enzyme glucosidase I of two of the three glucose residues present on the glycan when it is initially transferred to the asparagine acceptor residue of the protein from a dolichol phosphate precursor. Calnexin and calreticulin participate in a quality control cycle in which removal of the third glucose residue by glucosidase

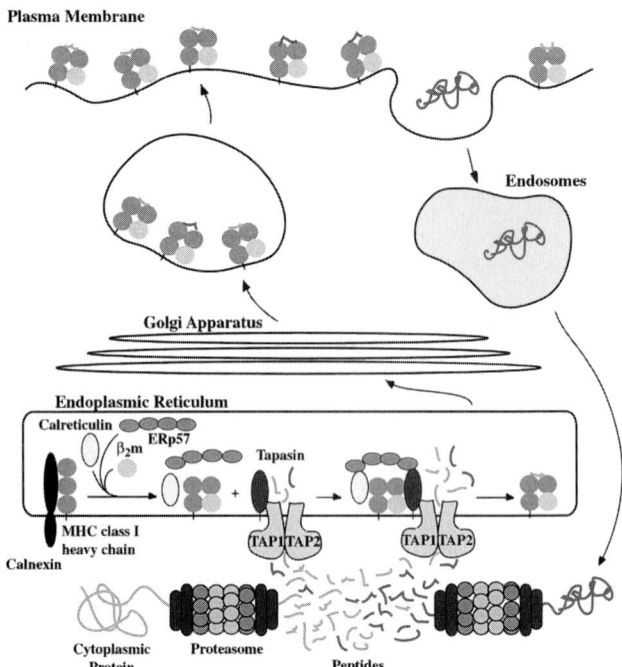

FIG. 3. The class I major histocompatibility complex (MHC) assembly pathway. Peptides generated in the cytosol by proteases (depicted as 20S proteasomes with associated 19S regulatory complexes) are transported into the endoplasmic reticulum by the transporter associated with antigen processing (TAP). Class I MHC–β_2-microglobulin dimers, assembled with the help of calnexin, associate with TAP through tapasin. ERp57 and calreticulin complete the loading complex. Successful association of a peptide with the class I MHC–β_2-microglobulin dimer causes its release from the loading complex, allowing transit through the Golgi apparatus to the plasma membrane. Also indicated is the ill-understood cross-priming pathway, in which protein antigens internalized by dendritic cells are introduced into the cytosol for processing via the class I pathway.

II induces dissociation of the chaperone. If the glycoprotein is appropriately folded, it escapes further interaction. However, if it remains misfolded, the glycan is reglucosylated by the enzyme uridine diphosphate-glucose glycoprotein glucosyl transferase, which can discriminate between native and nonnative protein structures (49). Upon reglucosylation, calnexin or calreticulin can rebind, allowing another attempt at folding. The differential binding of the free heavy chain to calnexin and the heavy chain–β_2-microglobulin dimer to calreticulin presumably reflects additional protein–protein interactions between the chaperone and the substrate.

The association of class I MHC molecules with calreticulin cannot be temporally separated from their interaction with another "housekeeping" molecule, ERp57, and with an ER resident transmembrane glycoprotein, tapasin (47,50–53). Tapasin is apparently dedicated to assisting class I MHC assembly and, like the TAP subunits, is encoded by a gene in the MHC (54). Tapasin, calreticulin, ERp57, and the class I MHC heavy chain–β_2-microglobulin dimer are all incorporated into a large assembly, often called the class I loading complex, which also includes the TAP1/TAP2 heterodimer (55) (Fig. 3). Various interactions between the components of the loading complex have been defined. The association of tapasin with TAP is independent of class I interaction and is lost if the transmembrane domain is removed to create a soluble tapasin molecule (56). The N-linked glycan of the class I MHC heavy chain is required for association of class I MHC with the complex (57). The glycan of class I MHC, but not that of tapasin, is largely in the monoglucosylated form in the loading complex, which implies that this glycan is involved in the calreticulin interaction. In addition, there is a labile disulfide bond linking ERp57 to tapasin that can be stabilized by treatment of cells with the sulfhydryl-reactive, membrane-impermeable reagent N-ethyl maleimide before purification of the loading complex (58).

Precisely how formation of the loading complex facilitates the assembly of class I MHC/peptide complexes is still unclear, but the evidence that it does is unequivocal. Mutant human cell lines or knockout mice lacking TAP fail to transport peptides into the ER, and, therefore, no peptides are associated with class I MHC molecules, with the exception of a few peptides derived from signal sequences of certain proteins translocated into the ER (59). TAP-negative cells express very low levels of surface class I MHC molecules because the majority of them fail to leave the ER. The class I MHC molecules that do escape to the cell surface are unstable (60–62). Class I MHC cell surface expression in tapasin-negative human cell lines or in knockout mice lacking tapasin is also low, although the level of expression depends on the individual allele, and in no such case is it as low as it is in the absence of TAP (53,63–65). The class I MHC molecules expressed are less stable than in wild-type cells, and the profile of associated peptides is different (66,67). This has been interpreted to suggest that tapasin has a "peptide editing" function, which normally ensures that only class I MHC molecules associated with high-affinity peptides are permitted to leave the ER. There are currently no calreticulin- or ERp57-negative human cell lines. Calreticulin knockout mice die in utero, but class I MHC assembly and transport is impaired in embryonic fibroblasts derived from them, which indicates that calreticulin is required for proper class I MHC peptide loading (68).

ERp57 is a homologue of the enzyme protein disulfide isomerase and shares with it the ability to promote proper disulfide bond formation in newly synthesized proteins in the ER. It functions in concert with calnexin and calreticulin and is believed to be specifically involved in disulfide bond formation in newly synthesized glycoproteins (69,70). Its role in the loading complex, performed in concert with tapasin, appears to be to maintain in an oxidized state the class I MHC heavy chain disulfide bond that anchors the $\alpha2$ domain α helix to the floor of the peptide-binding groove (see Chapter 19). Mutation of the cysteine residue at position 95 in human tapasin, which binds ERp57 to the loading complex by a disulfide bond, results in the accumulation of partially reduced class I MHC molecules in the loading complex. Unstable class I MHC molecules, presumably with a cohort of low-affinity peptides, accumulate on the surface of cells that express this mutant form of tapasin (58).

The Source of Class I Major Histocompatibility Complex–Associated Peptides

As described previously, the peptides associated with class I MHC molecules are derived from the cytosol (71). There is evidence that the majority of them derive from newly synthesized proteins. It has been shown, with the use of TAP proteins tagged with green fluorescent protein combined with real-time immunofluorescence microscopy, that the lateral mobility of TAP in the ER membrane is decreased when it is not actively transporting peptides. Mobility is reduced, for example, when peptide generation is blocked by the proteasome inhibitor lactacystin. The lateral mobility of TAP is also rapidly reduced in the presence of the protein synthesis inhibitor cycloheximide, which suggests that proteins that have just been synthesized are the predominant peptide source (72). It has been hypothesized that defective proteins, perhaps posttranslationally modified or prematurely terminated and released from cytoplasmic ribosomes, are the major source of class I MHC–associated peptides (73). The acronym DRiP, for "defective ribosomal products," has been suggested for these highly unstable and transient species, which may constitute as many as 30% of total translated proteins (74). The value of such a source for a rapid immune response lies in the speed with which foreign peptides derived from viral proteins synthesized in infected cells could bind and be presented by class I MHC molecules on the cell surface. The intrinsic stability and turnover rates of the mature viral proteins would be unimportant.

Certain epitopes recognized by CD8-positive T cells and associated with class I MHC molecules are derived from the luminal regions of membrane proteins: for example, influenza virus hemagglutinin. Such peptides could be generated from DRiPs that fail to translocate into the ER. Alternatively, they could be generated from a subset of the glycoproteins that are retrotranslocated into the cytosol from the ER and subsequently degraded by the proteasome. This process is the major pathway for the degradation of misfolded proteins, including class I MHC molecules themselves, that fail to be transported from the ER to the Golgi apparatus (75). The channel used appears to be the translocon, or Sec61 complex, normally responsible for the introduction into the ER through signal sequences of secreted proteins synthesized on membrane-associated ribosomes, but in this case operating in reverse (76,77). The same pathway may also be used to remove TAP translocated peptides from the ER if they fail to associate with class I MHC molecules (78).

Release of Class I Major Histocompatibility Complex Molecules from the Endoplasmic Reticulum

Tapasin, calreticulin, ERp57, and TAP are all retained in the ER: tapasin, by a cytoplasmic tail retention signal;

calreticulin and ERp57, by C-terminal so-called KDEL (lysine, aspartic acid, glutamic acid, leucine, or a close homologue) sequences; and TAP, by an unknown mechanism. They are all long-lived proteins and can participate in multiple rounds of class I MHC assembly and peptide loading. After class I MHC/peptide complexes are successfully assembled, they dissociate from the loading complex and, like other proteins destined for export, move to specialized exit sites in the ER, from which they are transported to the Golgi apparatus and ultimately to the plasma membrane (79). In transit, their carbohydrate side chains mature into complex (N)-linked glycans, in common with other membrane glycoproteins. Once expressed on the plasma membranes, class I MHC/peptide complexes are very stable, with half lives of 6 to 7 hours (80,81), a testament to the efficiency of the ER processes that promote their formation regardless of the allele and its preferred peptide binding motif.

Class I Major Histocompatibility Complex–Restricted Presentation of Extracellular Proteins

Although the general rule is that the peptides associated with class I MHC molecules are derived from cytoplasmic proteins, animals immunized with soluble or cell-associated antigenic proteins can make class I MHC–restricted T-cell responses to them. This was first observed in allogeneic responses to certain minor histocompatibility antigens, and the process is often called *cross-priming* (82). There is evidence that the ability to process external antigens and present them in a class I MHC–restricted manner is, in the main, a specific function of dendritic cells (83).

The precise mechanism of cross-priming is unclear, but endocytosis of the protein antigens or phagocytosis of apoptotic or necrotic cells by dendritic cells is certainly the first step. Two possible scenarios have been suggested to follow this. Proteolysis may occur in the endocytic pathway, and the peptides generated then bind to class I MHC molecules that recycle between the endosome and the plasma membrane. Alternatively, proteins internalized by dendritic cells, or large fragments of proteins generated in the endocytic pathway, may enter the cytosol by an as yet unidentified mechanism. These proteins or fragments would then be processed and peptides transported into the ER by the same mechanisms normally used to generate class I MHC/peptide complexes. Logically, it seems more likely that the latter hypothesis is the correct one. Priming of CD8 T cells to a particular epitope by dendritic cells—for example, during an antiviral response— is useful only if the same epitope is generated in normal cells when they are virally infected. If it is not, the virally infected cells would not be recognized by the CD8-positive T cells that are induced. That the proteases and exopeptidases in the endocytic pathway would generate the same peptides as those in the cytosol and ER seems highly unlikely.

Current evidence tends to suggest that an endosome to cytosol pathway exists for macromolecules in dendritic cells. Fluorescent protein and dextran derivatives have been observed to enter the cytosol after endocytosis by dendritic cells (84). Cross-priming is also often inhibited by proteasomal inhibitors, which implies that cytosolic degradation is required. Finally, TAP knockout mice appear to be incapable of cross-priming (85), and tapasin knockout mice are also deficient (65). It has been shown that in Langerhans cells, class I MHC molecules are mobilized from late endocytic compartments to the cell surface when the cells mature (86). However, it remains unclear where in the cell these class I MHC molecules acquire their peptides, although the ER, after TAP-mediated translocation, is perhaps the most likely site.

The generation of $CD8^+$ T-cell responses to cell-associated antigens may involve a variety of stress-induced proteins in the antigenic cells. These include glycoprotein 96 (gp96; also called GRP94), an ER stress protein or chaperone which, if isolated from a tumor or a virus-infected cell, can induce cytosolic class I MHC–restricted T cells when used to immunize mice (87). Considerable evidence suggests that this is a result of the association of gp96 with antigenic peptides derived from the tumor or virus. It has been suggested that a receptor on dendritic cells binds gp96/peptide complexes, facilitating their endocytosis (88). The receptor was previously defined as the α_2-macroglobulin receptor. Presumably, endocytosis of the gp96/peptide complex followed by its introduction into the cytosol allows the peptide, or a processed version of it, to be introduced into the ER by TAP, where it can bind to assembling class I MHC molecules. Other chaperones, including Hsp70 and calreticulin, share the property of facilitating the introduction of cell-associated antigens into the class I processing pathway (87,89).

CLASS II MAJOR HISTOCOMPATIBILITY COMPLEX–RESTRICTED ANTIGEN PRESENTATION

Class II Assembly of Major Histocompatibility Complex Molecules in the Endoplasmic Reticulum

Unlike class I MHC molecules, class II MHC molecules bind peptides in the endocytic pathway. This means that the initial assembly in the ER of the class II MHC heterodimer is independent of peptide association. The peptide-binding site, formed by the membrane distal domains of the α chain and β chain, is an open-ended groove with a propensity to bind to long peptides and unfolded segments of proteins. This is prevented in the ER because newly synthesized class II MHC molecules associate with a third glycoprotein, called the *invariant chain*. The invariant chain contains a segment, class II MHC–associated invariant chain peptide (CLIP), that protects the peptide-binding groove until the class II MHC/invariant chain complex enters the endocytic pathway.

The invariant chain is a type II transmembrane glycoprotein. Although there is no allelic polymorphism, there is alternative splicing, which gives rise to two forms called p33 and p41, based on their molecular weights (Fig. 4A) (90–92). In general, p33 is the most abundant form of the invariant

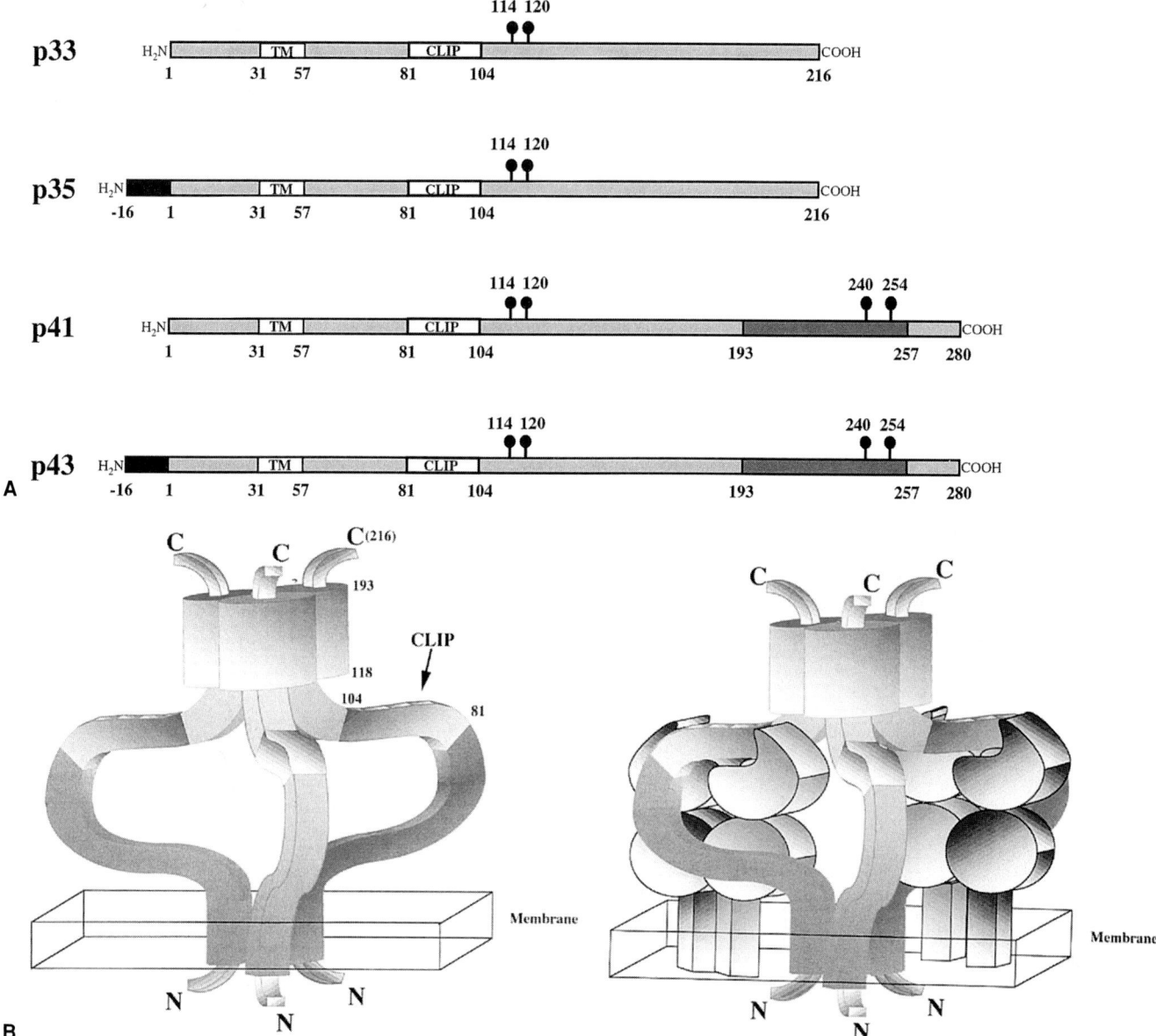

FIG. 4. A: Four forms of human invariant chain are generated by a combination of alternative splicing and alternative initiation of translation. The N-terminal segment shared by p35 and p43 contains a strong endoplasmic reticulum retention signal. The additional domain shared by p41 and p43 is an inhibitor of the lysosomal protease cathepsin L. The transmembrane domain (TM) and the region associated with the class II binding groove [class II MHC–associated invariant chain peptide (CLIP)] are also indicated. **B:** Models of the invariant trimer (*left*) and the trimer with associated class II αβ dimers (*right*). For simplicity, only two αβ dimers are indicated on the right rather than three. From Cresswell P. Invariant chain structure and MHC class II function. *Cell* 1996;84:505–507, with permission).

chain present in APCs. The additional segment in p41 is homologous to similar domains in thyroglobulin and functions as a protease inhibitor, specifically for cathepsin L (93,94), a property that is reviewed later. In humans, but not in mice, additional variation arises as a result of alternative initiation of translation. This causes an N-terminal extension of 16 amino acids and means that in humans there are four forms of the invariant chain; p35 and p43 are the extended forms of p33 and p41, respectively. The N-terminal extension contains a

strong ER retention sequence (95–97). A small fraction of the invariant chain, in both humans and mice, is modified by the addition of a chondroitin sulfate side chain, at serine residue 201 of the p33 form (98,99). Adding further complexity, the invariant chain forms noncovalently associated trimers, which may be homotrimers or mixed trimers, containing one or two subunits of any of the four forms (Fig. 4B) (100–102). Trimer formation is independent of class II MHC association.

Class II MHC/invariant chain complexes are nonameric, with three $\alpha\beta$ dimers associated with an invariant chain trimer (Fig. 4B) (103). Calnexin is an important chaperone involved in class II MHC assembly. Partial complexes containing one or two $\alpha\beta$ dimers associated with an invariant chain trimer are retained in the ER in association with calnexin (104). Export of free invariant chain trimers from the ER is slow, and virtually nonexistent if the trimer contains one or more p35 or p43 subunits (101). The C-terminal segment of the invariant chain forms a compact, cylindrical trimeric structure (105). The N-terminal region, including the transmembrane domain, also contributes to trimerization of the intact invariant chain (106,107). The region from the membrane-spanning domain through the CLIP sequence is disordered in solution, according to nuclear magnetic resonance analysis of soluble recombinant invariant chain (108). Thus, it seems likely that the CLIP region itself associates with the peptide-binding groove of the class II MHC molecule as a linear sequence, in a manner similar to a class II MHC–bound peptide (see Chapter 19). This is borne out by the crystallographic structure of the complex of DR3 with CLIP peptide, which is similar to that of other class II MHC/peptide complexes (109). When assembly of the class II MHC–invariant chain nonamer is complete, interactions with chaperones cease, ER retention

signals in p35 and p43 are overridden, and the complex leaves the ER.

Endocytic Processing of the Invariant Chain

Shared by all forms of the invariant chain are two so-called dileucine motifs in the N-terminal cytoplasmic domain (110). These interact with cytoplasmic adaptor proteins at the trans-Golgi network or at the plasma membrane to direct class II MHC/invariant chain complexes into the endocytic pathway (95,96,111–113). The complexes are exposed to progressively more acidic and proteolytically active environments as they move through the endocytic pathway. As a consequence, the invariant chain is degraded (Fig. 5). Ultimately, the class II MHC molecules arrive in deep endocytic compartments that share many characteristics with lysosomes, including the presence of mature hydrolytic enzymes. These compartments were called class II MHC compartments (MIICs) by their original discoverers, who defined them as membrane-rich, multivesicular or multilaminar compartments enriched for intracellular class II MHC molecules (114) (Fig. 6). Available evidence suggests that the multivesicular vesicles mature into the multilaminar MIICs and that these compartments are part of the conventional endocytic

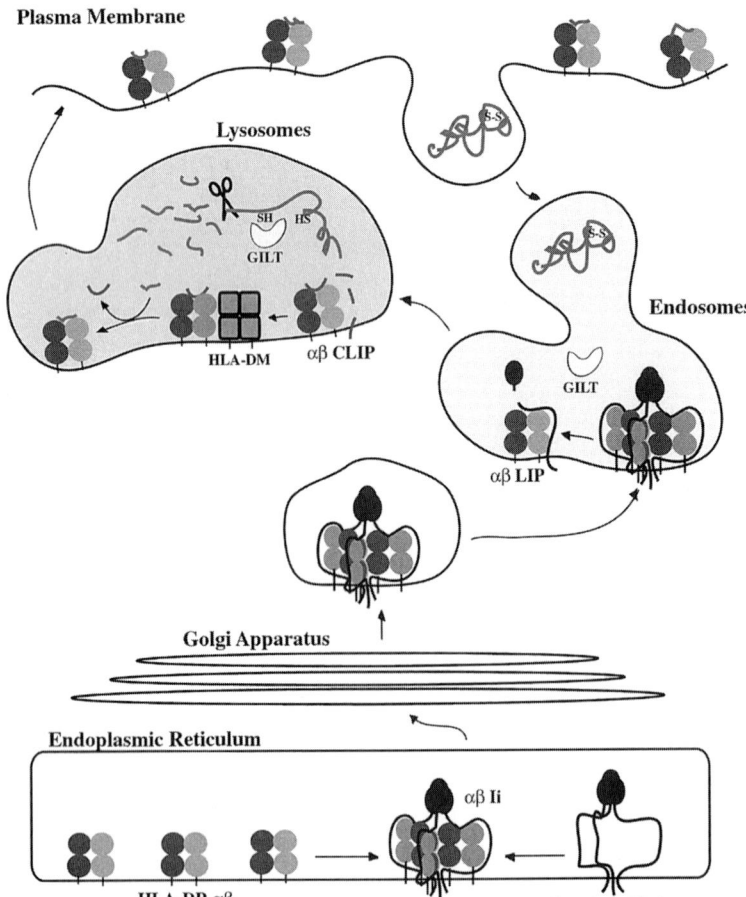

FIG. 5. Assembly and transport of class II major histocompatibility complex (MHC)–invariant chain complexes. Nonameric $\alpha\beta$–invariant chain complexes are assembled in the endoplasmic reticulum, transported through the Golgi apparatus, and diverted into the endocytic pathway. Here, invariant chain is progressively degraded until only class II MHC–associated invariant chain peptide (CLIP) remains associated with the binding groove. CLIP is exchanged for endocytically generated peptides before expression of class II MHC/peptide complexes on the cell surface.

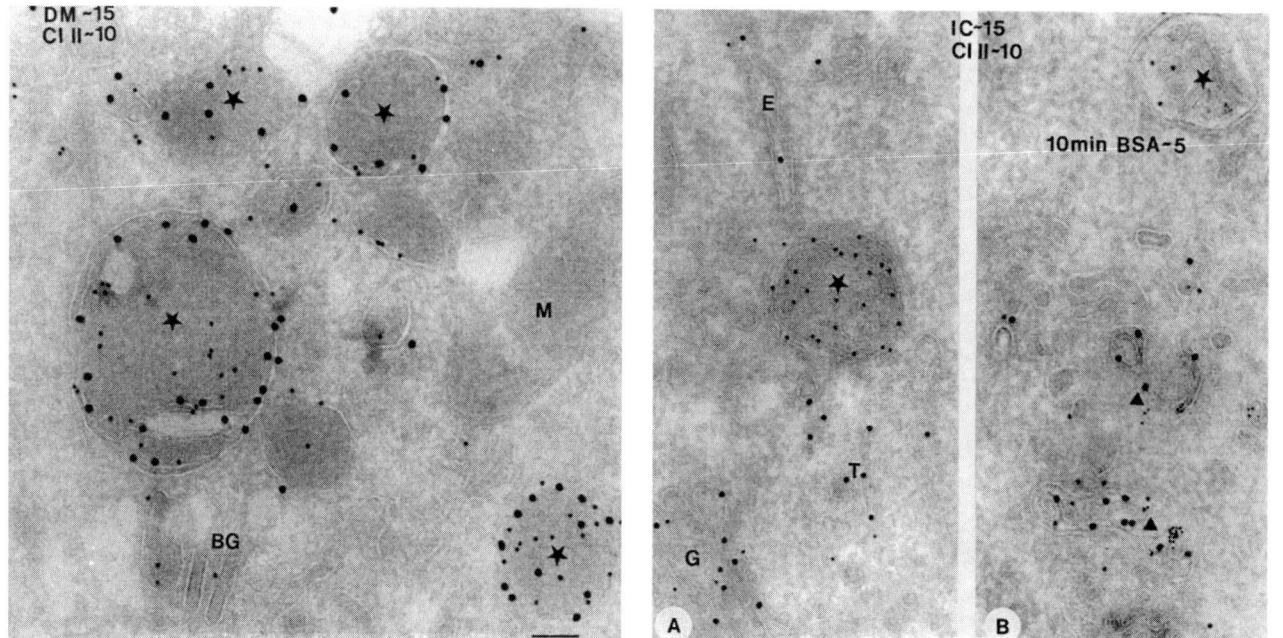

FIG. 6. A: Ultrathin cryosection of a human skin Langerhans cell, immunogold-labeled for human leukocyte antigen (HLA)–DM with 15-nm gold (DM-15) and for class II with 10-nm gold (CII-10). Several class II major histocompatibility complex (MHC) compartments (MIICs) (*asterisks*) are labeled for class II, as well as for DM (primarily at the periphery). MIICs in Langerhans cells typically have electron-dense contents. BG, Birbeck granules; M, mitochondrion. Bar represents 100 nm. **B:** Ultrathin cryosections of human B cells double-immunogold–labeled with antibodies against the C terminal domain of the invariant chain with 15-nm gold (IC-15) and class II with 10-nm gold (CII-10) (*a*). Labeling for invariant chain can be seen in the Golgi complex (G), the trans-Golgi network (T), and in the rough endoplasmic reticulum, whereas class II is primarily located in a multilaminar MIIC (*asterisk*). Note that the use of a C-terminal–specific anti–invariant chain antibody limits detection of proteolytically cleaved material in late endosomal/lysosomal organelles. Before being processed for immuno–electron microscopy, the cell had endocytosed 5-nm gold particles derivatized with bovine serum albumin (BSA) for 10 minutes (*b*). The endocytosed BSA-gold particles are present in irregularly shaped multivesicular compartments, so-called early MIICs (*triangles*) that are strongly labeled for invariant-chain C terminus. The MIIC (*asterisk*) is labeled only for class II. Bar represents 200 nm. Images courtesy of Monique Kleijmeer and Hans J. Geuze, Laboratory of Cell Biology, Medical School, Utrecht University, the Netherlands.

pathway (115). It is in these compartments that the majority of class II MHC molecules acquire their complement of peptides, most of which are derived from endocytosed proteins.

Degradation of the invariant chain has been studied by observing the effect of various protease inhibitors on the process. It was initially observed that incubation of human B-cell lines with leupeptin, which inhibits a number of lysosomal cysteine proteases, causes the intracellular accumulation of class II MHC molecules associated with a glycosylated N-terminal fragment of the invariant chain of approximately 25 kD (116). Additional studies showed that inhibitors of acid proteases further inhibit invariant chain degradation (117). More recently, it has been found that a specific lysosomal protease, cathepsin S, is critically involved in the final stages of invariant chain degradation (118). An inhibitor of cathepsin S, N-morpholinourea-leucine-homophenylalanine-vinylsulfone-phenyl (LHVS),

when added to APCs, causes the accumulation of a small, nonglycosylated, N-terminal invariant chain fragment of approximately 10 kD. These findings have given rise to a model (Fig. 5) in which the invariant chain is progressively degraded until only CLIP remains associated with the peptide-binding groove of the class II MHC molecule, with cathepsin S responsible for cleavage at the N-terminal end of CLIP. For reasons that are ill understood, in murine thymic epithelium, cathepsin L, rather than cathepsin S, appears to be involved in the final step in the generation of class II MHC/CLIP complexes. Because of this, cathepsin L knockout mice exhibit partial deficiency in thymic selection of CD4 T cells (119), and cathepsin S knockout mice are deficient in generating some, but not all, complexes of class II MHC molecules with antigenic peptides in peripheral APCs (120). Biochemical analysis suggests that invariant chain degradation is delayed in APCs from cathepsin S knockout mice rather than being completely

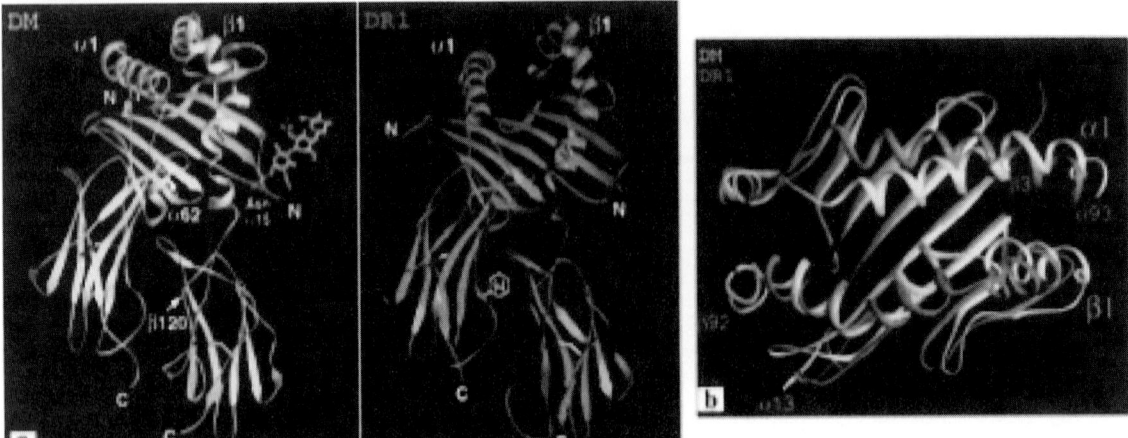

FIG. 7. Comparison of the structures of human leukocyte antigen (HLA)–DM and HLA-DR. **A:** DM and DR1. **B:** Superimposition of the α1 and β1 domain structure of DM and DR1. The two structures are very similar except that the two α helices that flank the peptide-binding groove in the DR molecule are closer together in the DM $\alpha\beta$ dimer, which indicates that DM is not a peptide-binding molecule. From Mosyak et al. (127), with permission.

inhibited. Nevertheless, this enzyme is important, and its co-induction with class II MHC subunits and invariant chain by γ-interferon in non-APCs argues for a specific role in class II MHC–restricted antigen processing.

Class II Peptide Loading of Major Histocompatibility Complex Molecules

The ultimate product of invariant chain degradation is the class II MHC/CLIP complex, which structurally resembles other class II MHC/peptide complexes (109). To generate class II MHC $\alpha\beta$ dimers associated with peptides from foreign or endogenous proteins, CLIP must be removed. Some class II alleles, such as human leukocyte antigen (HLA)–DR52 in humans and I-A^k in mice, have low affinity for CLIP (121). However, other alleles, such as HLA-DR1 and I-A^b, have a high affinity, and it is difficult to understand how CLIP could be efficiently released from these alleles. A major breakthrough in understanding class II MHC peptide loading came from the observation that certain human B-cell lines, mutagenized and selected for the loss of reactivity with a particular monoclonal antibody reactive with HLA-DR3, were incapable of class II MHC–restricted antigen processing (122). The loss of reactivity with the antibody correlated with the almost exclusive expression on these cells of HLA-DR3/CLIP complexes (123,124). On the basis of these observations, it was suggested that a specific gene product catalyzes the exchange of CLIP for other endosomally generated peptides. The protein was eventually identified and is called HLA-DM in humans and H2-M, or, more recently, H2-DM in mice (125). Mice lacking functional DM have major defects in processing antigens for presentation to class II MHC molecules, and H2^b DM knockout mice express I-A^b/CLIP complexes on their APCs.

DM is a heterodimer of two transmembrane glycoproteins, each of which is encoded by an MHC-linked gene. It is, in fact, a close homologue of class II MHC molecules, with a virtually identical structure (126,127) (Fig. 7). The major feature unique to DM is that the groove between the α and β subunit α helices, which is the peptide-binding site in conventional class II MHC molecules, is closed. There is a tyrosine-containing endocytic motif in the cytoplasmic tail of the DM β subunit that effectively restricts DM to late endocytic compartments (Fig. 6A) (128,129). In APCs, DM is almost exclusively localized to MIICs, although it can be detected in earlier endocytic compartments and even to some extent on the cell surface (130–132). Figure 8 shows a schematic view of the peptide exchange reaction catalyzed in MIICs by DM. Evidence suggests that DM transiently associates with class II MHC/CLIP complexes in the plane of the membrane (133,134). The interaction results in a conformational alteration of the peptide-binding groove such that the affinity of the class II MHC molecule for CLIP is reduced. Although the precise mechanism is not well understood, there is suggestive evidence that the DM–class II MHC interaction disturbs the hydrogen bonding pattern underlying the class II MHC interaction with the peptide backbone of CLIP, perhaps particularly those hydrogen bonds interacting with N-terminal residues (135). The dissociation reaction can be performed in solution with purified DM and DR/CLIP complexes, is optimal at an acidic pH, and follows classical Michaelis-Menten kinetics (136–139). When such *in vitro* reactions are carried out in the presence of specific class II MHC–binding peptides, they replace CLIP in the peptide-binding groove, which suggests that this is what happens *in vivo*.

Considerable evidence suggests that the dissociation of CLIP, followed by association with a replacement peptide, is not the end of the DM-mediated reaction. DM catalyzes the dissociation of any class II MHC–associated peptide.

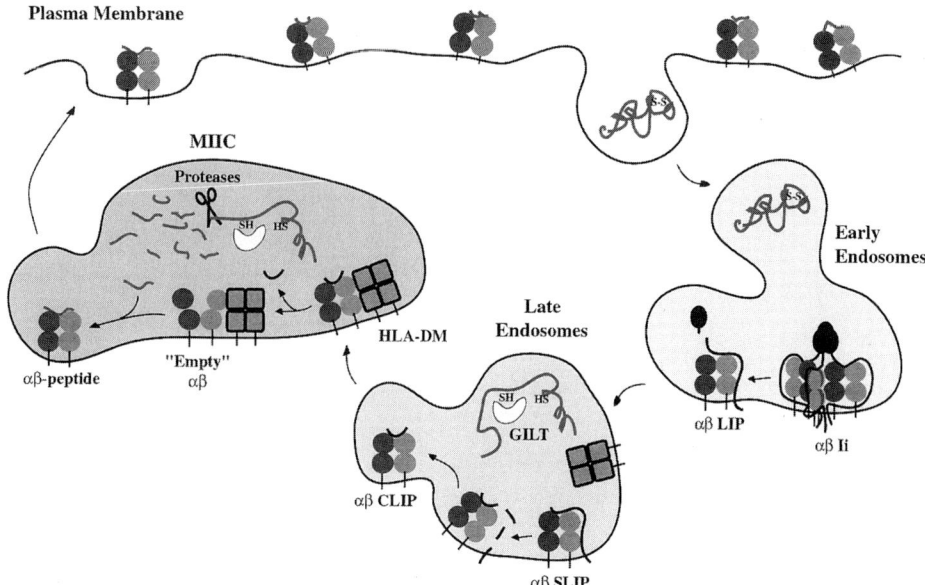

FIG. 8. Processing of antigens in the class II major histocompatibility complex (MHC) pathway. Entry of class II MHC–invariant chain nonamers into the endocytic pathway results in progressive invariant chain degradation. Proteins entering the endocytic pathway are unfolded by a combination of denaturation, resulting from acidification, and reduction of their disulfide bonds, mediated by γ-interferon–inducible lysosomal thiol reductase (GILT). In class II MHC compartments (MIICs), the interaction of class II MHC/CLIP complexes with DM reduces their affinity for CLIP, causing CLIP dissociation. Peptides with the appropriate sequence generated from the unfolded protein bind to the "empty" class II MHC molecules. Reiteration of this process, called peptide editing, generates class II MHC molecules associated with high-affinity peptides, which are then expressed on the cell surface.

The lower the affinity of a particular peptide for a class II MHC molecule, the higher the dissociation rate induced by DM (140,141). Because of this, it has been suggested that DM "edits" the peptide repertoire associated with class II MHC molecules in the endocytic pathway in a reiterative process involving successive dissociation–association reactions. This serves to maximize peptide affinities before the class II MHC/peptide complexes are expressed on the plasma membrane, ensuring their stability. Like class I MHC/peptide complexes, class II MHC/peptide complexes are very stable on the cell surface, with half-lives of 24 hours or more (81,142).

There is an additional homologue of class II MHC molecules encoded in the MHC, called HLA-DO in humans and H2-O in mice. DO is also composed of two transmembrane α and β subunits. Whereas classical class II MHC molecules and DM are expressed in all APCs, DO seems to be restricted to thymic epithelium and B cells (143). A peculiarity of the DO heterodimer is that it is dependent on DM for release from the ER (144). In fact, DM and DO associate with each other in the ER, and the DM/DO complex accumulates in MIICs, like DM. The precise role of DO remains somewhat obscure. Unlike DM molecules, DM/DO complexes poorly catalyze class II MHC peptide exchange *in vitro,* and overexpression of DO in DM-positive cell lines causes class II MHC–CLIP accumulation on the cell surface,

as is observed in DM-negative cells (145,146). These data argue that DO is an inhibitor of DM. It remains unclear why DM function should be regulated this way in only B cells and thymic epithelium. One suggestion, based on some *in vitro* experimental evidence, is that the efficiency of inhibition of DM function by DO is affected by pH, so that, at the low pH (4.5 to 5.0) characteristic of lysosomes and MIICs, the inhibitory effect is reduced (147,148). Immuno–electron microscopic analysis suggests that DO is more concentrated in earlier endocytic compartments in relation to DM, which is consistent with the idea that DO may actually dissociate in later compartments, releasing active DM (149). Thus, one possibility is that antigens internalized by binding to surface immunoglobulin, delivered to MIICs and preferentially presented by B cells (see later discussion), may be made more available for class II MHC binding than are antigens internalized by fluid-phase endocytosis. B cells from mice lacking the DO α subunit, and therefore any functional DO heterodimers, do indeed induce CD4 T cell responses to antigens internalized by fluid-phase endocytosis that are enhanced in relation to responses induced by wild-type, DO-positive B cells (148).

There are a substantial number of reports in the literature that peptides can also bind to class II MHC molecules that are recycling between the endocytic pathway and the plasma membrane (150–152). The phenomenon is essentially a process of peptide exchange and is restricted to early endosomes rather than to the MIICs (153,154). Peptide exchange even in early endosomes is catalyzed by HLA-DM (155). Class II MHC does not appear to recycle in all cell types (156). In situations in which class II MHC recycling does occur, it appears to be dependent on an endocytic signal in the cytoplasmic tail of the class II MHC β subunit (157). The contribution of the recycling pathway to the overall level of class II MHC–restricted antigen processing that occurs *in vivo* is unclear.

Delivery of Class II Major Histocompatibility Complex Molecules to the Cell Surface

The precise mechanism by which class II MHC/peptide complexes leave the endocytic pathway and are delivered to the plasma membrane remains poorly understood. Transport of membrane glycoproteins between intracellular compartments generally involves their segregation into limited regions of the source membrane (exit sites), incorporation into small transport vesicles, and fusion of these vesicles with the target membrane. Various accessory molecules, including the small guanosine triphosphatases known as rab proteins, are involved in these processes (158). There is evidence from two cell types, one being normal dendritic cells and the other a class II MHC–positive melanoma cell line, that a different mechanism may be at work in the transport from MIIC to plasma membrane for class II MHC molecules.

In resting dendritic cells, surface expression of class II MHC molecules is low, while the level of intracellular class II is high (159,160). One reason for this is that cathepsin S activity in these cells is also low, perhaps held in check by expression of the lysosomal protease inhibitor cystatin C (160,161). This limits invariant chain degradation, reduces generation of class II MHC $\alpha\beta$ dimers, and prolongs the retention of class II MHC molecules in MIICs. When the dendritic cells receive a maturation signal, such as exposure to lipopolysaccharide (see Chapter 15), cathepsin S activity is enhanced, and there is a radical change in the distribution of class II MHC molecules (Fig. 8). First, they move from MIICs to more peripheral vesicles that lack lysosomal markers and then to the cell surface. The peripheral vesicles, or class II vesicles (162), are much larger than the transport vesicles commonly associated with vesicular trafficking—between the ER and the *cis*-Golgi apparatus, for example—but their proximity to the plasma membrane has been taken to imply that they may directly fuse with the plasma membrane. Such fusion events have been observed in a melanoma cell line expressing class II MHC molecules, actually DR molecules, in which the β subunit has a green fluorescent protein tag attached to the cytoplasmic tail (163). It is not clear, however, whether the frequency of such fusion events is sufficient to completely account for the delivery of peptide-loaded class II MHC molecules from the endocytic pathway to the cell surface.

Endocytosis of Proteins and Peptide Generation by Antigen-Presenting Cells

The sources of peptides associated with class II MHC molecules are limited to proteins that enter endocytic compartments. There are occasional peptides derived from cytoplasmic proteins (164,165) that may be directly introduced from the cytosol by a direct pathway defined by Agarraberes et al. (166,167) that involves their association with cytosolic Hsc70, and perhaps other cytoplasmic chaperones. Some come from lysosomal enzymes, and many from plasma membrane proteins, including class I and class II MHC molecules themselves, which are internalized and degraded (165). Perhaps the most important sources, however, are soluble proteins internalized by APCs. Immature, or resting, dendritic cells, in particular, indulge in large-scale fluid-phase endocytosis (168), efficiently internalizing their extracellular liquid environment and concentrating its protein components in the endocytic pathway. Excess water is eliminated from the cells by specific transporters called aquaporins (169). Maturation shuts down fluid-phase endocytosis in dendritic cells as class II MHC/peptide complex formation and surface expression of class II MHC increases (168).

Pathogen-derived proteins can be specifically internalized by binding to endocytic receptors, such as the mannose receptor (170,171). In the case of B cells, as alluded to earlier, the membrane immunoglobulin can function as an antigen-specific receptor, internalizing bound antigen with such high efficiency that antigen-specific B cells can present cognate antigen more than 1,000 times as efficiently as can nonspecific B cells (172). Specific signaling by the immunoreceptor tyrosine-based activation motifs of the B-cell receptor associated immunoglobulin α and β chains may be partially responsible for the increased processing efficiency (173,174). Signal-dependent reorganization and fusion of B-cell MIICs has been observed when B cells are activated through the B-cell receptor. Various endocytic receptors on dendritic cells, such as DEC-205, may also play a specific role in antigen internalization (175). Dendritic cells also bind apoptotic cells through the $\alpha_V\beta_3$ integrin (176) or perhaps by the phosphatidyl serine receptor (177). This facilitates internalization and subsequent generation of both class I and class II MHCs containing peptides derived from the internalized cells (178–180).

Some of the least understood aspects of class II MHC–restricted antigen processing are the precise mechanisms governing the degradation of protein antigens after their endocytosis. It has been known for many years that inhibitors of lysosomal acidification, such as chloroquine, inhibit antigen processing (181). It is generally accepted that this is because lysosomal proteases, necessary for degrading protein antigens, have acidic pH optima. A further potential reason is that these proteases are also involved in the degradation of invariant chain, which is necessary for generating peptide-receptive class II MHC molecules in MIICs (182). Protease inhibitors, such as leupeptin, can also function at the level of protein antigen degradation and invariant chain processing.

MIICs are modified lysosomes, and lysosomes generally degrade proteins to their constituent amino acids. Thus, it seems likely that the degradative processes are modified in MIICs in such a way as to maximize the generation of large peptides that associate with class II MHC molecules. The demonstration that the additional domain present in the p41 and p43 forms of the invariant chain has protease inhibitory activity suggests that this might temper the proteolytic activity of MIICs (93,94,183). The p41 form actually downregulates the degradation rate of p33 when they are coexpressed (94,102), and results of experiments with transfected cell lines as APCs suggest that cells expressing p41 are superior to those expressing p33 in presenting antigens to T cells (184). However, these results have not been supported by experiments in which normal cells derived from mice expressing only the p41 form were used as APCs (185). Also, the p41-specific domain appears to preferentially inhibit cathepsin L, which is only one of a multitude of lysosomal cathepsins. There is evidence that the p41-specific domain is critical for the normal maturation of cathepsin L, a finding difficult to correlate specifically with a role in antigen processing (186).

Perhaps the most likely component of MIICs to modify protein antigen degradation is the class II MHC molecule itself. As discussed earlier and detailed in Chapter 19, the class II MHC binding groove is open ended, which means that peptides can, and do, protrude from the ends. In fact, variable trimming of the ends of class II MHC–associated peptides is the rule rather than the exception (165). A quite old idea in the field is that the binding of class II MHC molecules to the epitopes of internalized proteins may occur before significant degradation has occurred and that the cleavages on either side of the binding groove may happen after binding. There are examples of intact proteins or large protein fragments associating with class II MHC molecules in the endocytic pathway of MIICs, which is consistent with this idea (187–189).

The three-dimensional structures of many protein antigens are stabilized by intrachain and interchain disulfide bonds, and reduction of such bonds before adding antigens to APCs can enhance the presentation of such antigens to CD4 T cells (190–192). This may be because reduction facilitates protein unfolding and the exposure of epitopes normally buried in the three-dimensional structure, allowing binding of the epitope to class II MHC $\alpha\beta$ dimers before antigen degradation. There is evidence that such a process can occur physiologically. An enzyme, γ-interferon–inducible lysosomal thiol reductase (GILT), which localizes to MIICs and catalyzes the reduction of protein disulfide bonds at low pH (188,193,194), appears to facilitate this process *in vivo*. As the name implies, GILT is inducible in non-APCs by γ-interferon but is constitutively expressed in APCs. Mice that lack GILT show a reduction in their ability to respond to protein antigens containing multiple disulfide bonds (195). In fact, the response to some epitopes is completely eliminated.

Further modifications of lysosomes that facilitate antigen-processing functions in MIICs are likely to be revealed in the future. The current view is that proteolytic processing can be mediated by any one of a number of cathepsins, depending on the antigen. In the case of one antigen, tetanus toxin, a particular asparagine-specific protease, asparaginyl endopeptidase, is essential (196). Whether this enzyme is critical for additional protein antigens is unknown.

CONCLUDING REMARKS

Progress in understanding antigen processing at the molecular level has been remarkable since the phenomenon was uncovered in the early 1980s. However, a number of questions remain. For example, it is unclear exactly how the various components of the class I MHC loading complex—that is, tapasin, calreticulin, and ERp57—facilitate peptide binding after TAP-mediated peptide transport. The peptidases in the ER responsible for the N-terminal trimming of peptides before class I binding remain to be identified. For class II MHC, a major problem remains in uncovering the precise role of DO. Is it simply a pH-regulated modulator of DM function in B cells, or does it have a more specific function? What other modifications of lysosomes are made in the MIICs of APCs that facilitate antigen processing? Are there other molecules besides GILT that regulate the processing of protein antigens to peptides?

Currently perhaps the most intensive areas of study in the field of antigen processing concern the mechanisms governing the functions of dendritic cells. In the case of class I MHC, the mechanisms governing cross-presentation of external protein antigens to CD8$^+$ T cells remain poorly understood. In the case of class II MHC, the molecular mechanisms regulating peptide binding to class II MHC molecules and their subsequent redistribution during maturation are under intense investigation. Are there similar maturation-dependent modifications of the class I MHC loading pathway? These areas are likely to occupy investigators working in the field for some time to come.

ACKNOWLEDGMENTS

I thank Nancy Dometios for preparation of the manuscript and Anne Ackerman for valuable assistance in preparing the figures. This work was supported by the Howard Hughes Medical Institute and by National Institutes of Health grant R37 AI23081.

REFERENCES

1. Rock KL, Gramm C, Rothstein L, et al. Inhibitors of the proteasome block the degradation of most cell proteins and the generation of peptides presented by MHC class I molecules. *Cell* 1994;78:761–771.
2. Fenteany G, Standaert RF, Lane WS, et al. Inhibition of proteasome activities and subunit-specific amino-terminal threonine modification by lactacystin. *Science* 1995;268:726–731.

3. Coux O, Tanaka K, Goldberg AL. Structure and functions of the 20S and 26S proteasomes. *Annu Rev Biochem* 1996;65:801–847.

4. Groll M, Ditzel L, Lowe J, et al. Structure of 20S proteasome from yeast at 2.4 A resolution. *Nature* 1997;386:463–471.

5. Chen P, Hochstrasser M. Autocatalytic subunit processing couples active site formation in the 20S proteasome to completion of assembly. *Cell* 1996;86:961–972.

6. Schmidtke G, Kraft R, Kostka S, et al. Analysis of mammalian 20S proteasome biogenesis: the maturation of beta-subunits is an ordered two-step mechanism involving autocatalysis. *EMBO J* 1996;15:6887–6898.

7. Glickman MH, Rubin DM, Coux O, et al. A subcomplex of the proteasome regulatory particle required for ubiquitin-conjugate degradation and related to the COP9-signalosome and eIF3. *Cell* 1998;94:615–623.

8. Deveraux O, Ustrell V, Pickart C, et al. A 26S protease subunit that binds ubiquitin conjugates. *J Biol Chem* 1994;269:7059–7061.

9. Braun BC, Glickman M, Kraft R, et al. The base of the proteasome regulatory particle exhibits chaperone-like activity. *Nat Cell Biol* 1999;1:221–226.

10. Hochstrasser M. Ubiquitin-dependent protein degradation. *Annu Rev Genet* 1997;30:405–439.

11. Kloetzel PM. Antigen processing by the proteasome. *Nat Rev Mol Cell Biol* 2001;2:179–187.

12. Ortiz-Navarrete V, Seelig A, Gernold M, et al. Subunit of the "20S" proteasome (multicatalytic proteinase) encoded by the major histocompatibility complex. *Nature* 1991;353:662–664.

13. Martinez CK, Monaco JJ. Homology of proteasome subunits to a major histocompatibility complex-linked LMP gene. *Nature* 1991;353:664–667.

14. Glynne R, Powis SH, Beck S, et al. A proteasome-related gene between the two ABC transporter loci in the class II region of the human MHC. *Nature* 1991;353:357–360.

15. Gaczynska M, Rock KL, Goldberg AL. Gamma-interferon and expression of MHC genes regulate peptide hydrolysis by proteasomes. *Nature* 1993;365:264–267.

16. Driscoll J, Brown MG, Finley D, et al. MHC-linked LMP gene products specifically alter peptidase activities of the proteasome. *Nature* reticulum 1993;365:262–264.

17. Boes B, Hengel H, Ruppert T, et al. Interferon gamma stimulation modulates the proteolytic activity and cleavage site preference of 20S mouse proteasomes. *J Exp Med* 1994;179:901–909.

18. Van Kaer L, Ashton-Rickardt PG, Eichelberger M, et al. Altered peptidase and viral-specific T cell response in LMP2 mutant mice. *Immunity* 1994;1:533–541.

19. Fehling H, Swat W, Laplace C, et al. MHC class I expression in mice lacking the proteasome subunit LMP7. *Science* 1994;265:1234–1237.

20. Knowlton JR, Johnston SC, Whitby FG, et al. Structure of the proteasome activator REGalpha (PA28alpha). *Nature* 1997;390:639–643.

21. Ma CP, Slaughter CA, DeMartino GN. Identification, purification, and characterization of a protein activator (PA28) of the 20 S proteasome (macropain). *J Biol Chem* 1992;267:10515–10523.

22. Dubiel W, Pratt G, Ferrell K, et al. Purification of an 11S regulator of the multicatalytic protease. *J Biol Chem* 1992;267:22369–22377.

23. Dick TP, Ruppert T, Groettrup M, et al. Coordinated dual cleavages induced by the proteasome regulator PA28 lead to dominant MHC ligands. *Cell* 1996;86:253–262.

24. Groettrup M, Soza A, Eggers M, et al. A role for the proteasome regulator PA28a in antigen presentation. *Nature* 1996;381:166–168.

25. Preckel T, Fung-Leung WP, Cai Z, et al. Impaired immunoproteasome assembly and immune responses in PA28−/− mice. *Science* 1999;286:2162–2165.

26. Murata S, Udono H, Tanahashi N, et al. Immunoproteasome assembly and antigen presentation in mice lacking both PA28alpha and PA28beta. *EMBO J* 2001;20:5898–5907.

27. Cascio P, Hilton C, Kisselev AF, et al. 26S Proteasomes and immunoproteasomes produce mainly N-extended versions of an antigenic peptide. *EMBO J* 2001;20:2357–2366.

28. Beninga J, Rock KL, Goldberg AL. Interferon-gamma can stimulate post-proteasomal trimming of the N-terminus of an antigenic peptide by inducing leucine aminopeptidase. *J Biol Chem* 1998;273:18734–18742.

29. Karttunen JT, Trowsdale J, Lehner PJ. Antigen presentation: TAP dances with ATP. *Curr Biol* 1999;9:R820–R824.

30. Holland IB, Blight MA. ABC-ATPases, adaptable energy generators fuelling transmembrane movement of a variety of molecules in organisms from bacteria to humans. *J Mol Biol* 1999;293:381–399.

31. Nijenhuis M, Schmitt S, Armandola EA, et al. Identification of a contact region for peptide on the TAP1 chain of the transporter associated with antigen processing. *J Immunol* 1996;156:2186–2195.

32. Androlewicz MJ, Cresswell P. Human transporters associated with antigen processing possess a promiscuous peptide-binding site. *Immunity* 1994;1:7–14.

33. Neefjes J, Gottfried E, Roelse J, et al. Analysis of the fine specificity of rat, mouse and human TAP peptide transporters. *Eur J Immunol* 1995;25:1133–1136.

34. Van Endert PM, Riganelli D, Greco G, et al. The peptide-binding motif for the human transporter associated with antigen processing. *J Exp Med* 1995;182:1883–1895.

35. Uebel S, Kraas W, Kienle S, et al. Recognition principle of the TAP transporter disclosed by combinatorial peptide libraries. *Proc Natl Acad Sci U S A* 1997;94:8976–8981.

36. Knittler MR, Alberts P, Deverson EV, et al. Nucleotide binding by TAP mediates association with peptide and release of assembled MHC class I molecules. *Curr Biol* 1999;9:999–1008.

37. Lapinski PE, Neubig RR, Raghavan M. Walker A lysine mutations of TAP1 and TAP2 interfere with peptide translocation but not peptide binding. *J Biol Chem* 2001;276:7526–7533.

38. Alberts P, Daumke O, Deverson EV, et al. Distinct functional properties of the TAP subunits coordinate the nucleotide-dependent transport cycle. *Curr Biol* 2001;11:242–251.

39. Karttunen JT, Lehner PJ, Gupta SS, et al. Distinct functions and cooperative interaction of the subunits of the transporter associated with antigen processing (TAP). *Proc Natl Acad Sci U S A* 2001;98:7431–7436.

40. Fruci D, Niedermann G, Butler RH, et al. Efficient MHC class I–independent amino-terminal trimming of epitope precursor peptides in the endoplasmic reticulum. *Immunity* 2001;15:467–476.

41. Brouwenstijn N, Serwold T, Shastri N. MHC class I molecules can direct proteolytic cleavage of antigenic precursors in the endoplasmic reticulum. *Immunity* 2001;15:95–104.

42. Serwold T, Gaw S, Shastri N. ER aminopeptidases generate a unique pool of peptides for MHC class I molecules. *Nat Immunol* 2001;2:644–651.

43. Degen E, Cohen-Doyle MF, Williams DB. Efficient dissociation of the p88 chaperone from major histocompatibility complex class I molecules requires both β_2-microglobulin and peptide. *J Exp Med* 1992;175:1653–1661.

44. Scott JE, Dawson JR. MHC class I expression and transport in a calnexin-deficient cell line. *J Immunol* 1995;155:143–148.

45. Sadasivan BK, Cariappa A, Waneck GL, et al. Assembly, peptide loading, and transport of MHC class I molecules in a calnexin-negative cell line. *Cold Spring Harb Symp Quant Biol* 1995;55:267–275.

46. Noessner E, Parham P. Species-specific differences in chaperone interaction of human and mouse histocompatibility complex class I molecules. *J Exp Med* 1995;181:327–337.

47. Sadasivan B, Lehner PJ, Ortmann B, et al. Roles for calreticulin and a novel glycoprotein, tapasin, in the interaction of MHC class I molecules with TAP. *Immunity* 1996;5:103–114.

48. Hammond C, Helenius C. Quality control in the secretory pathway. *Curr Opin Cell Biol* 1995;7:523–529.

49. Sousa MC, Ferrero-Garcia MA, Parodi AJ. Recognition of the oligosaccharide and protein moieties of glycoproteins by the UDP-Glc:glycoprotein glucosyltransferase. *Biochemistry* 1992;31:97–105.

50. Hughes EA, Cresswell P. The thiol oxidoreductase ERp57 is a component of the MHC class I peptide-loading complex. *Curr Biol* 1998;8:709–712.

51. Lindquist JA, Jensen ON, Mann M, et al. ER-60, a chaperone with thiol-dependent reductase activity involved in MHC class I assembly. *EMBO J* 1998;17:2186–2195.

52. Morrice NA, Powis SJ. A role for the thiol-dependent reductase ERp57 in the assembly of MHC class I molecules. *Curr Biol* 1998;8:713–716.

53. Ortmann B, Copeman J, Lehner PJ, et al. A critical role for tapasin in the assembly and function of multimeric MHC class I–TAP complexes. *Science* 1997;277:1306–1309.

54. Herberg JA, Sgouros J, Jones T, et al. Genomic analysis of the tapasin gene, located close to the TAP loci in the MHC. *Eur J Immunol* 1998;28:459–467.
55. Cresswell P, Bangia N, Dick T, et al. The nature of the MHC class I peptide loading complex. *Immunol Rev* 1999;172:21–28.
56. Lehner PJ, Surman MJ, Cresswell P. Soluble tapasin restores MHC class I expression and function in the tapasin negative cell line .220. *Immunity* 1998;8:221–231.
57. Harris MR, Lybarger L, Yu YY, et al. Association of ERp57 with mouse MHC class I molecules is tapasin dependent and mimics that of calreticulin and not calnexin. *J Immunol* 2001;166:6686–6692.
58. Dick T, Bangia N, Peaper D, et al. Disulfide bond isomerization and the assembly of MHC class I–peptide complexes. *Immunity* 2002;16:87–98.
59. Wei ML, Cresswell P. HLA-A2 molecules in an antigen-processing mutant cell contain signal sequence-derived peptides. *Nature* 1992;356:443–446.
60. Spies T, De Mars R. Restored expression of major histocompatibility class I molecules by gene transfer of a putative peptide transporter. *Nature* 1991;351:323–324.
61. Ljunggren H-G, Stam NJ, Ohlen C, et al. Empty MHC class I molecules come out in the cold. *Nature* 1990;346:476–480.
62. Van Kaer L, Ashton-Rickardt PG, Ploegh HL, et al. TAP1 mutant mice are deficient in antigen presentation, surface class I molecules, and CD4⁻8⁺ T cells. *Cell* 1992;71:1205–1214.
63. Grandea IAG, Androlewicz MJ, Athwal RS, et al. Dependence of peptide binding by MHC class I molecules on their interaction with TAP. *Science* 1995;270:105–108.
64. Grandea AG 3rd, Golovina TN, Hamilton SE, et al. Impaired assembly yet normal trafficking of MHC class I molecules in tapasin mutant mice. *Immunity* 2000;13:213–222.
65. Garbi N, Tan P, Diehl AD, et al. Impaired immune responses and altered peptide repertoire in tapasin-deficient mice. *Nat Immunol* 2000;1:234–238.
66. Peh CA, Burrows SR, Barnden M, et al. HLA-B27–restricted antigen presentation in the absence of tapasin reveals polymorphism in mechanisms of HLA class I peptide loading. *Immunity* 1998;8:531–542.
67. Purcell AW, Gorman JJ, Garcia-Peydro M, et al. Quantitative and qualitative influences of tapasin on the class I peptide repertoire. *J Immunol* 2001;166:1016–1027.
68. Gao B, Adhikari R, Howarth M, et al. Assembly and antigen-presenting function of MHC class I molecules in cells lacking the ER chaperone calreticulin. *Immunity* 2002;16:99–109.
69. Oliver JD, Roderick HL, Llewellyn DH, et al. ERp57 functions as a subunit of specific complexes formed with the ER lectins calreticulin and calnexin. *Mol Biol Cell* 1999;10:2573–2582.
70. Helenius A, Aebi M. Intracellular functions of N-linked glycans. *Science* 2001;291:2364–2369.
71. Hunt DF, Michel H, Dickinson TA, et al. Peptides presented to the immune system by the murine class II major histocompatibility complex molecule I-Ad. *Science* 1992;256:1817–1820.
72. Reits EA, Vos JC, Gromme M, et al. The major substrates for TAP *in vivo* are derived from newly synthesized proteins. *Nature* 2000;404:774–778.
73. Yewdell JW, Anton LC, Bennink JR. Defective ribosomal products (DRiPs): a major source of antigenic peptides for MHC class I molecules? *J Immunol* 1996;157:1823–1826.
74. Schubert U, Anton LC, Gibbs J, et al. Rapid degradation of a large fraction of newly synthesized proteins by proteasomes. *Nature* 2000;404:770–774.
75. Wiertz EJHJ, Tortorella D, Bogyo M, et al. Sec61-mediated transfer of a membrane protein from the endoplasmic reticulum to the proteasome for destruction. *Nature* 1996;384:432–438.
76. Pilon M, Schekman R, Romisch K. Sec61p mediates export of a misfolded secretory protein from the endoplasmic reticulum to the cytosol for degradation. *EMBO J* 1997;16:4540–4548.
77. Ye Y, Meyer HH, Rapoport TA. The AAA ATPase Cdc48/p97 and its partners transport proteins from the ER into the cytosol. *Nature* 2001;414:652–656.
78. Koopmann JO, Albring J, Huter E, et al. Export of antigenic peptides from the endoplasmic reticulum intersects with retrograde protein translocation through the Sec61p channel. *Immunity* 2000;13:117–127.
79. Spiliotis ET, Manley H, Osorio M, et al. Selective export of MHC class I molecules from the ER after their dissociation from TAP. *Immunity* 2000;13:841–851.
80. Smith JD, Lie WR, Gorka J, et al. Disparate interaction of peptide ligand with nascent versus mature class I major histocompatibility complex molecules: comparisons of peptide binding to alternative forms of Ld in cell lysates and the cell surface. *J Exp Med* 1992;175:191–202.
81. Davis JE, Cresswell P. Lack of detectable endocytosis of B lymphocyte MHC class II antigens using an antibody-independent technique. *J Immunol* 1990;144:990–997.
82. Bevan MJ. Cross-priming for a secondary cytotoxic response to minor H antigens with H-2 congenic cells which do not cross-react in the cytotoxicity assay. *J Exp Med* 1976;143:1283–1288.
83. Heath WR, Carbone FR. Cross-presentation, dendritic cells, tolerance and immunity. *Annu Rev Immunol* 2001;19:47–64.
84. Rodriguez A, Regnault A, Kleijmeer M, et al. Selective transport of internalized antigens to the cytosol for MHC class I presentation in dendritic cells. *Nat Cell Biol* 1999;1:362–368.
85. Huang AY, Bruce AT, Pardoll DM, et al. In vivo cross-priming of MHC class I–restricted antigens requires the TAP transporter. *Immunity* 1996;4:349–355.
86. MacAry PA, Lindsay M, Scott MA, et al. Mobilization of MHC class I molecules from late endosomes to the cell surface following activation of CD34-derived human Langerhans cells. *Proc Natl Acad Sci U S A* 2001;98:3982–3987.
87. Li Z, Menoret A, Srivastava P. Roles of heat-shock proteins in antigen presentation and cross-presentation. *Curr Opin Immunol* 2002;14:45–51.
88. Basu S, Binder RJ, Ramalingam T, et al. CD91 is a common receptor for heat shock proteins gp96, hsp90, hsp70, and calreticulin. *Immunity* 2001;14:303–313.
89. Suto R, Srivastava PK. A mechanism for the specific immunogenicity of heat shock protein–chaperoned peptides. *Science* 1995;269:1585–1588.
90. Strubin M, Berte C, Mach B. Alternative splicing and alternative initiation of translation explain the four forms of the Ia antigen-associated invariant chain. *EMBO J* 1986;5:3483–3488.
91. O'Sullivan DM, Noonan D, Quaranta V. Four Ia invariant chain forms derive from a single gene by alternate splicing and alternate initiation of transcription/translation. *J Exp Med* 1987;166:444–460.
92. Koch N, Lauer W, Habicht J, et al. Primary structure of the gene for the murine Ia antigen–associated invariant chains (Ii). An alternatively spliced exon encodes a cysteine-rich domain highly homologous to a repetitive sequence of thyroglobulin. *EMBO J* 1987;6:1677–1683.
93. Bevec T, Stoka V, Pungercic G, et al. Major histocompatibility complex class II–associated p41 invariant chain fragment is a strong inhibitor of lysosomal cathepsin L. *J Exp Med* 1996;183:1331.
94. Guncar G, Pungercic G, Klemencic I, et al. Crystal structure of MHC class II–associated p41 Ii fragment bound to cathepsin L reveals the structural basis for differentiation between cathepsins L and S. *EMBO J* 1999;18:793–803.
95. Bakke O, Dobberstein B. MHC class II–associated invariant chain contains a sorting signal for endosomal compartments. *Cell* 1990;63:707–716.
96. Lotteau V, Teyton L, Peleraux A, et al. Intracellular transport of class II MHC molecules directed by invariant chain. *Nature* 1990;348:600–605.
97. Schutze MP, Peterson PA, Jackson MR. An N-terminal double-arginine motif maintains type II membrane proteins in the endoplasmic reticulum. *EMBO J* 1994;13:1696–1705.
98. Sant AJ, Cullen SE, Giacoletto KS, et al. Invariant chain is the core protein of the Ia-associated chondroitin sulfate proteoglycan. *J Exp Med* 1985;162:1916–1934.
99. Miller J, Hatch JA, Simonis S, et al. Identification of the glycosaminoglycan attachment site of mouse invariant chain proteoglycan core protein by site-directed mutagenesis. *Proc Natl Acad Sci U S A* 1989;85:1359–1363.
100. Marks MS, Blum JS, Cresswell P. Invariant chain trimers are sequestered in the rough endoplasmic reticulum in the absence of association with HLA class II antigens. *J Cell Biol* 1990;111:839–855.
101. Lamb CA, Cresswell P. Assembly and transport properties of invariant chain trimers and HLA-DR–invariant chain complexes. *J Immunol* 1992;148:3478–3482.

102. Arunachalam B, Lamb CA, Cresswell P. Transport properties of free and MHC class II–associated oligomers containing different isoforms of human invariant chain. *Int Immunol* 1993;6:439–451.

103. Roche PA, Cresswell P. Invariant chain association with HLA-DR molecules inhibits immunogenic peptide binding. *Nature* 1990; 345:615–618.

104. Anderson KS, Cresswell P. A role for calnexin (IP90) in the assembly of class II MHC molecules. *EMBO J* 1994;13:675–682.

105. Jasanoff A, Wagner G, Wiley DC. Structure of a trimeric domain of the MHC class II–associated chaperonin and targeting protein Ii. *EMBO J* 1998;17:6812–6818.

106. Newcomb JR, Carboy-Newcomb C, Cresswell P. Trimeric interactions of the invariant chain and its association with major histocompatibility complex class II ab dimers. *J Biol Chem* 1996;271: 24249–24256.

107. Ashman JB, Miller J. A role for the transmembrane domain in the trimerization of the MHC class II–associated invariant chain. *J Immunol* 1999;163:2704–2712.

108. Jasanoff A, Park SJ, Wiley DC. Direct observation of disordered regions in the major histocompatibility complex class II–associated invariant chain. *Proc Natl Acad Sci U S A* 1995;92:9900–9904.

109. Ghosh P, Amaya M, Mellins E, et al. The structure of an intermediate in class II MHC maturation: CLIP bound to HLA-DR3. *Nature* 1995;378:457–462.

110. Pond L, Kuhn LA, Teyton L, et al. A role for acidic residues in di-leucine motif-based targeting to the endocytic pathway. *J Biol Chem* 1995;270:19989–19997.

111. Romagnoli P, Layet C, Yewdell J, et al. Relationship between invariant chain expression and major histocompatibility complex class II transport into early and late endocytic compartments. *J Exp Med* 1993;177:583–596.

112. Roche PA, Teletski CL, Stang E, et al. Cell surface HLA-DR–invariant chain complexes are targeted to endosomes by rapid internalization. *Proc Natl Acad Sci U S A* 1993;90:8581–8585.

113. Hofmann MW, Honing S, Rodionov D, et al. The leucine-based sorting motifs in the cytoplasmic domain of the invariant chain are recognized by the clathrin adaptors AP1 and AP2 and their medium chains. *J Biol Chem* 1999;274:36153–36158.

114. Peters PJ, Neefjes JJ, Oorschot V, et al. Segregation of MHC class II molecules from MHC class I molecules in the Golgi complex for transport to lysosomal compartments. *Nature* 1991;349:669–676.

115. Kleijmeer MJ, Morkowski S, Griffith JM, et al. Major histocompatibility complex class II compartments (MIICs) in human and mouse B lymphoblasts represent conventional endocytic compartments. *J Cell Biol* 1997;139:639–649.

116. Blum JS, Cresswell P. A role for proteases in the processing and transport of class II HLA antigens. *Proc Natl Acad Sci U S A* 1988;85:3975–3979.

117. Maric MA, Taylor MD, Blum JS. Endosomal aspartic proteinases are required for invariant-chain processing. *Proc Natl Acad Sci U S A* 1994;91:2171–2175.

118. Riese RJ, Wolf PR, Bromme D, et al. Essential role for cathepsin S in MHC class II–associated invariant chain processing and peptide loading. *Immunity* 1996;4:357–366.

119. Nakagawa T, Roth W, Wong P, et al. Cathepsin L: critical role in Ii degradation and CD4 T cell selection in the thymus. *Science* 1998;280:450–453.

120. Shi GP, Villadangos JA, Dranoff G, et al. Cathepsin S required for normal MHC class II peptide loading and germinal center development. *Immunity* 1999;10:197–206.

121. Sette A, Southwood S, Miller J, et al. Binding of major histocompatibility complex class II to the invariant chain–derived peptide, CLIP, is regulated by allelic polymorphism in class II. *J Exp Med* 1995;181:677–683.

122. Mellins E, Smith L, Arp B, et al. Defective processing and presentation of exogenous antigens in mutants with normal HLA class II genes. *Nature* 1990;343:71–74.

123. Riberdy JM, Newcomb JR, Surman MJ, et al. HLA-DR molecules from an antigen-processing mutant cell line are associated with invariant chain peptides. *Nature* 1992;360:474–477.

124. Sette A, Ceman S, Kubo RT, et al. Invariant chain peptides in most HLA-DR molecules of an antigen-processing mutant. *Science* 1992; 258:1801–1804.

125. Morris P, Shaman J, Attaya M, et al. An essential role for HLA-DM in antigen presentation by class II major histocompatibility molecules. *Nature* 1994;368:551–554.

126. Fremont DH, Hendrickson WA, Marrack P, et al. Structures of an MHC class II molecule with covalently bound single peptides. *Science* 1996;272:1001–1004.

127. Mosyak L, Zaller DM, Wiley DC. The structure of HLA-DM, the peptide exchange catalyst that loads antigen onto class II MHC molecules during antigen presentation. *Immunity* 1998;9:377–383.

128. Marks MS, Roche PA, van Donselaar E, et al. A lysosomal targeting signal in the cytoplasmic tail of the beta chain directs HLA-DM to MHC class II compartments. *J Cell Biol* 1995;131:351–369.

129. Copier J, Kleijmeer MJ, Ponnambalam S, et al. Targeting signal and subcellular compartments involved in the intracellular trafficking of HLA-DMB. *J Immunol* 1996;157:1017–1027.

130. Sanderson F, Kleijmeer MJ, Kelly A, et al. Accumulation of HLA-DM, a regulator of antigen presentation, in MHC class II compartments. *Science* 1994;266:1566–1569.

131. Pierre P, Denzin LK, Hammond C, et al. HLA-DM is localized to conventional and unconventional MHC class II–containing endocytic compartments. *Immunity* 1996;4:229–239.

132. Santambrogio L, Sato AK, Carven GJ, et al. Extracellular antigen processing and presentation by immature dendritic cells. *Proc Natl Acad Sci U S A* 1999;96:15056–15061.

133. Mellins E, Cameron P, Amaya M, et al. A mutant human histocompatibility leukocyte antigen DR molecule associated with invariant chain peptides. *J Exp Med* 1994;179:541–549.

134. Weber DA, Dao CT, Jun J, et al. Transmembrane domain–mediated colocalization of HLA-DM and HLA-DR is required for optimal HLA-DM catalytic activity. *J Immunol* 2001;167:5167–5174.

135. Sant AJ, Beeson C, McFarland B, et al. Individual hydrogen bonds play a critical role in MHC class II:peptide interactions: implications for the dynamic aspects of class II trafficking and DM-mediated peptide exchange. *Immunol Rev* 1999;172:239–253.

136. Denzin LK, Cresswell P. HLA-DM induces CLIP dissociation from MHC class II ab dimers and facilitates peptide loading. *Cell* 1995;82:155–165.

137. Sherman MA, Weber DA, Jensen PE. DM enhances peptide binding to class II MHC by release of invariant chain–derived peptides. *Immunity* 1995;3:197–205.

138. Sloan VS, Cameron P, Porter G, et al. Mediation by HLA-DM of dissociation of peptides from HLA-DR. *Nature* 1995;375:802–806.

139. Vogt AB, Kropshofer H, Moldenhauer G, et al. Kinetic analysis of peptide loading onto HLA-DR molecules mediated by HLA-DM. *Proc Natl Acad Sci U S A* 1996;93:9724–9729.

140. Kropshofer H, Vogt AB, Moldenhauer G, et al. Editing of the HLA-DR–peptide repertoire by HLA-DM. *EMBO J* 1996;15:6144–6154.

141. Weber DA, Evavold BD, Jensen PE. Enhanced dissociation of HLA-DR–bound peptides in the presence of HLA-DM. *Science* 1996;274:618–620.

142. Lanzavecchia A, Reid PA, Watts C. Irreversible association of peptides with class II MHC molecules in living cells. *Nature* 1992;357:249–252.

143. Karlsson L, Surh CD, Sprent J, et al. A novel class II MHC molecule with unusual tissue distribution. *Nature* 1991;351:485–488.

144. Liljedahl M, Kuwana T, Fung-Leung WP, et al. HLA-DO is a lysosomal resident which requires association with HLA-DM for efficient intracellular transport. *EMBO J* 1996;15:4817–4824.

145. Denzin LK, Sant'Angelo DB, Hammond C, et al. Negative regulation by HLA-DO of MHC class II–restricted antigen processing. *Science* 1997;278:106–109.

146. van Ham SM, Tjin EPM, Lillemeier BF, et al. HLA-DO is a negative modulator of HLA-DM–mediated MHC class II peptide loading. *Curr Biol* 1997;7:950–957.

147. van Ham M, van Lith M, Lillemeier B, et al. Modulation of the major histocompatibility complex class II–associated peptide repertoire by human histocompatibility leukocyte antigen (HLA)–DO. *J Exp Med* 2000;191:1127–1136.

148. Liljedahl M, Winvist O, Surh CD, et al. Altered antigen presentation in mice lacking H2-O. *Immunity* 1998;8:233–243.

149. Mommaas AM, Mulder AA, Jordens R, et al. Human epidermal Langerhans cells lack functional mannose receptors and a fully developed endosomal/lysosomal compartment for loading of HLA class II molecules. *Eur J Immunol* 1999;29:571–580.

150. Harding RM. More on the X files. *Proc Natl Acad Sci U S A* 1999; 96:2582–2584.

151. Adorini L, Appella E, Doria G, et al. Competition for antigen presentation in living cells involves exchange of peptides bound by class II MHC molecules. *Nature* 1989;342:800–803.

152. Pinet V, Vergelli M, Martin R, et al. Antigen presentation mediated by recycling of surface HLA-DR molecules. *Nature* 1995;375:603–606.

153. Reid PA, Watts C. Cycling of cell-surface MHC glycoproteins through primaquine-sensitive intracellular compartments. *Nature* 1990;346:655–657.

154. Griffin JP, Chu R, Harding CV. Early endosomes and a late endocytic compartment generate different peptide–class II MHC complexes via distinct processing mechanisms. *J Immunol* 1997;158:1523–1532.

155. Pathak SS, Lich JD, Blum JS. Cutting edge: editing of recycling class II:peptide complexes by HLA-DM. *J Immunol* 2001;167:632–635.

156. Simonsen A, Momburg F, Drexler J, et al. Intracellular distribution of the MHC class II molecules and the associated invariant chain (Ii) in different cell lines. *Int Immunol* 1993;5:903–917.

157. Zhong G, Sousa CR, Germain RN. Antigen-unspecific B cells and lymphoid dendritic cells both show extensive surface expression of processed antigen–major histocompatibility complex class II complexes after soluble protein exposure *in vivo* or *in vitro*. *J Exp Med* 1997;186:673–682.

158. Der CJ, Balch WE. GTPase traffic control. *Nature* 2000;405:749, 751–742.

159. Cella M, Engering A, Pinet V, et al. Inflammatory stimuli induce accumulation of MHC class II complexes on dendritic cells. *Nature* 1997;388:782–787.

160. Pierre P, Mellman I. Developmental regulation of invariant chain proteolysis controls MHC class II trafficking in mouse dendritic cells. *Cell* 1998;93:1135–1145.

161. Villadangos JA, Cardoso M, Steptoe RJ, et al. MHC class II expression is regulated in dendritic cells independently of invariant chain degradation. *Immunity* 2001;14:739–749.

162. Turley SJ, Inaba K, Garrett WS, et al. Transport of peptide–MHC class II complexes in developing dendritic cells. *Science* 2000;288:522–527.

163. Wubbolts R, Fernandez-Borja M, Oomen L, et al. Direct vesicular transport of MHC class II molecules from lysosomal structures to the cell surface. *J Cell Biol* 1996;135:611–622.

164. Nuchtern JG, Biddison WE, Klausner RD. Class II MHC molecules can use the endogenous pathway of antigen presentation. *Nature* 1990; 343:74–76.

165. Chicz RM, Urban RG, Groga JC, et al. Specificity and promiscuity among naturally processed peptides bound to HLA-DR alleles. *J Exp Med* 1993;178:27–47.

166. Agarraberes F, Terlecky S, Dice J. An intralysosomal hsp70 is required for a selective pathway of lysosomal protein degradation. *J Cell Biol* 1997;137:825–834.

167. Agarraberes FA, Dice JF. A molecular chaperone complex at the lysosomal membrane is required for protein translocation. *J Cell Sci* 2001;114:2491–2499.

168. Sallusto F, Cella M, Danieli C, et al. Dendritic cells use macropinocytosis and the mannose receptor to concentrate macromolecules in the major histocompatibility complex class II compartment: downregulation by cytokines and bacterial products. *J Exp Med* 1995;182:389–400.

169. de Baey A, Lanzavecchia A. The role of aquaporins in dendritic cell macropinocytosis. *J Exp Med* 2000;191:743–748.

170. Tan MC, Mommaas AM, Drijfhout JW, et al. Mannose receptor–mediated uptake of antigens strongly enhances HLA class II–restricted antigen presentation by cultured dendritic cells. *Eur J Immunol* 1997;27:2426–2435.

171. Engering AJ, Cella M, Fluitsma D, et al. The mannose receptor functions as a high capacity and broad specificity antigen receptor in human dendritic cells. *Eur J Immunol* 1997;27:2417–2425.

172. Lanzavecchia A. Antigen-specific interaction between T and B cells. *Nature* 1985;314:537–539.

173. Siemasko K, Eisfelder BJ, Williamson E, et al. Signals from the B lymphocyte antigen receptor regulate MHC class II containing late endosomes. *J Immunol* 1998;160:5203–5208.

174. Siemasko K, Eisfelder BJ, Stebbins C, et al. Igα and Igβ are required for efficient trafficking to late endosomes and to enhance antigen presentation. *J Immunol* 1999;162:6518–6525.

175. Mahnke K, Guo M, Lee S, et al. The dendritic cell receptor for endocy-

tosis, DEC-205, can recycle and enhance antigen presentation via major histocompatibility complex class II–positive lysosomal compartments. *J Cell Biol* 2000;151:673–684.

176. Rubartelli A, Poggi A, Zocchi MR. The selective engulfment of apoptotic bodies by dendritic cells is mediated by the alpha(v)beta3 integrin and requires intracellular and extracellular calcium. *Eur J Immunol* 1997;27:1893–1900.

177. Henson PM, Bratton DL, Fadok VA. The phosphatidylserine receptor: a crucial molecular switch? *Nat Rev Mol Cell Biol* 2001;2:627–633.

178. Albert ML, Sauter B, Bhardwaj N. Dendritic cells acquire antigen from apoptotic cells and induce class I–restricted CTLs. *Nature* 1998;392:86–89.

179. Inaba K, Turley S, Yamaide F, et al. Efficient presentation of phagocytosed cellular fragments on the major histocompatibility complex class II products of dendritic cells. *J Exp Med* 1998;188:2163–2173.

180. Inaba K, Turley S, Iyoda T, et al. The formation of immunogenic major histocompatibility complex class II–peptide ligands in lysosomal compartments of dendritic cells is regulated by inflammatory stimuli. *J Exp Med* 2000;191:927–936.

181. Ziegler HK, Unanue ER. Decrease in macrophage antigen catabolism caused by ammonia and chloroquine is associated with inhibition of antigen presentation to T cells. *Proc Natl Acad Sci U S A* 1982;79:175–178.

182. Nowell J, Quaranta V. Chloroquine affects biosynthesis of Ia molecules by inhibiting dissociation of invariant (gamma) chains from alpha-beta dimers in B cells. *J Exp Med* 1985;162:1371–1376.

183. Fineschi B, Sakaguchi K, Appela E, et al. The proteolytic environment involved in MHC class II–restricted antigen presentation can be modulated by the p41 form of invariant chain. *J Immunol* 1996;157: 3211.

184. Peterson M, Miller J. Invariant chain influences the immunological recognition of MHC class II molecules. *Nature* 1990;345:172–174.

185. Takaesu NT, Lower JA, Yelon D, et al. *In vivo* functions mediated by the p41 isoform of the MHC class II–associated invariant chain. *J Immunol* 1997;158:187–199.

186. Lennon-Dumenil AM, Roberts RA, Valentijn K, et al. The p41 isoform of invariant chain is a chaperone for cathepsin L. *EMBO J* 2001; 20:4055–4064.

187. Davidson H, Reid PA, Lanzavecchia A, et al. Processed antigen binds to newly synthesized MHC class II molecules in antigen-specific B-lymphocytes. *Cell* 1991;67:105–116.

188. Arunachalam B, Pan M, Cresswell P. Intracellular formation and cell surface expression of a complex of an intact lysosomal protein and MHC class II molecules. *J Immunol* 1998;160:5797–5806.

189. Castellino F, Zappacosta F, Coligan JE, et al. Large protein fragments as substrates for endocytic antigen capture by MHC class II molecules. *J Immunol* 1998;161:4048–4057.

190. Collins DS, Unanue ER, Harding CV. Reduction of disulfide bonds within lysosome is a key step in antigen processing. *J Immunol* 1991;147:4054–4059.

191. Jensen PE. Acidification and disulfide reduction can be sufficient to allow intact proteins to bind class II MHC. *J Immunol* 1993;150:3347–3356.

192. Jensen PE. Antigen unfolding and disulfide reduction in antigen presenting cells. *Semin Immunol* 1995;7:347–353.

193. Arunachalam B, Phan UT, Geuze HJ, et al. Enzymatic reduction of disulfide bonds in lysosomes: characterization of a gamma-interferon–inducible lysosomal thiol reductase (GILT). *Proc Natl Acad Sci U S A* 2000;97:745–750.

194. Phan UT, Arunachalam B, Cresswell P. Gamma-interferon–inducible lysosomal thiol reductase (GILT): maturation, activity and mechanism of action. *J Biol Chem* 2001;275:25907–25914.

195. Maric M, Arunachalam B, Phan UT, et al. Defective antigen processing in GILT-free mice. *Science* 2001;294:1361–1365.

196. Manoury B, Hewitt EW, Morrice N, et al. An asparaginyl endopeptidase processes a microbial antigen for class II MHC presentation. *Nature* 1998;396:695–699.

197. Vos JC, Spee P, Momburg F, et al. Membrane topology and dimerization of the two subunits of the transporter associated with antigen processing reveal a three-domain structure. *J Immunol* 1999;163:6679–6685.

198. Reits EAJ, Griekspoor AC, Neefjes J. How does TAP pump peptides? Insights from DNA repair and traffic adenosine triphosphatases. *Immunol Today* 2000;21:598–600.

CHAPTER 21

Immunogenicity and Antigen Structure

Jay A. Berzofsky and Ira J. Berkower

The Nature of Antigenic Determinants Recognized by Antibodies
    Haptens · Carbohydrate Antigens · Immunogenicity of Polysaccharides · Protein and Polypeptide Antigenic Determinants
Antigenic Determinants Recognized by T Cells
    Mapping Antigenic Structures · Sequential Steps that Focus the T-Cell Response on Immunodominant Determinants · Prediction of T-Cell Epitopes
Relationship between Helper T-Cell Epitopes and B-Cell Epitopes on a Complex Protein Antigen
References

THE NATURE OF ANTIGENIC DETERMINANTS RECOGNIZED BY ANTIBODIES

Haptens

In the antigen–antibody binding reaction, the antibody-binding site is often unable to accommodate the entire antigen. The part of the antigen that is the target of antibody binding is called an antigenic determinant, and there may be one or more antigenic determinants per molecule. In order to study antibody specificity, antibodies against single antigenic determinants must be considered. Small functional groups that correspond to a single antigenic determinant are called *haptens*. For example, these may be organic compounds, such as trinitrophenyl or benzene arsonate; a monosaccharide or oligosaccharide, such as glucose or lactose; or an oligopeptide, such as pentalysine. Although these haptens can bind to antibody, immunization with them usually does not provoke an antibody response [for exceptions, see Goodman (1)]. Immunogenicity often can be achieved by covalently attaching haptens to a larger molecule, called the *carrier*. The carrier is immunogenic in its own right, and immunization with the hapten–carrier conjugate elicits an antibody response to both hapten and carrier. However, the antibodies specific for hapten can be studied by equilibrium dialysis with pure hapten (without carrier), by immunoprecipitation with hapten coupled to a different (and non–cross-reacting) carrier, or by inhibition of precipitation with free hapten.

This technique, pioneered by Landsteiner (2), helped elucidate the exquisite specificity of antibodies for antigenic determinants. For instance, the relative binding affinity of antibodies prepared against succinic acid–serum protein conjugates shows marked specificity for the maleic acid analogue, which is in the *cis*-configuration, in comparison with the fumaric acid (*trans*) form (3). Presumably, the immunogenic form of succinic acid corresponds to the *cis* form (3). This ability of antibodies to distinguish *cis* from *trans* configurations was reemphasized in later studies measuring relative affinities of antibodies to maleic and fumaric acid conjugates (4) (Table 1, section A). Section B of Table 1 shows the specificity of antibodies prepared against *p*-azobenzene arsonate coupled to bovine gamma globulin (5). Because the hapten is coupled through the *p*-azo group to aromatic amino acids of the carrier, haptens containing bulky substitutions in the *para* position would most resemble the immunizing antigen. In fact, *p*-methyl–substituted benzene arsonate has a higher binding affinity than unsubstituted benzene arsonate. However, methyl substitution elsewhere in the benzene ring reduces affinity, presumably because of interference with the way hapten fits into the antibody-binding site. Thus, methyl substitutions can have positive or negative effects on binding energy, depending on where the substitution occurs. Section C of Table 1 shows the specificity of antilactose antibodies for lactose versus cellobiose (6). These disaccharides differ only by the orientation of the hydroxyl attached to C4 of the first sugar either above or below the hexose ring. The three examples in this table, as well as many others (1), show the marked specificity of antibodies for *cis–trans, ortho–meta–para,* and stereoisomeric forms of the antigenic determinant.

Comparative binding studies of haptens have been able to demonstrate antibody specificity despite the marked heterogeneity of antibodies. Unlike the antibodies against a multideterminant antigen, the population of antibodies specific for

TABLE 1. *Exquisite specificity of antihapten antibodies*

Hapten	Structure	K_{rel} of antibody specific for	
A.		Maleic (cis)	Fumaric (trans)
Maleanilate		1.0	<0.01
Fumaranilate		<0.01	1.0
B.		Parasubstituted benzene arsonate	
Benzene arsonate		1.0	
o-Methyl benzene arsonate		0.2	
m-Methyl benzene arsonate		0.8	
p-Methyl benzene arsonate		1.9	
C.		Lactose	
Lactose	β gal (1→4) glu	1.00	
Cellobiose	β glu (1→4) glu	0.0025	

Part A from (4); part B from (5); and part C ref. (6), with permission.

a single hapten determinant is a relatively restricted population, because of the shared structural constraints necessary for hapten to fit within the antibody-combining site. However, the specificity of an antiserum depends on the collective specificities of the entire population of antibodies, which are determined by the structures of the various antibody-binding sites. In the cross-reactions of hapten analogues, some haptens bind all antibodies, but with reduced K_A. Other hapten analogues reach a plateau of binding, inasmuch as they fit some antibody-combining sites quite well but not others (see discussion of cross-reactivity in Chapter 4). Antibodies raised in different animals may show different cross-reactivities with related haptens. Even within a single animal, antibody affinity and specificity are known to increase over time after immunization under certain conditions (7). Thus, any statements about the cross-reactivity of two haptens reflect both structural differences between the haptens that affect antigen–antibody fit and the diversity of antibody-binding sites that are present in a given antiserum.

Carbohydrate Antigens

The antigenic determinants of a number of biologically important substances consist of carbohydrates. These often occur as glycolipids or glycoproteins. Examples of the former include bacterial cell wall antigens and the major blood group antigens, whereas the latter group includes "minor" blood group antigens such as Lewis antigen. In addition, the capsular polysaccharides of bacteria are important for virulence and are often targeted by protective antibodies. A number of spontaneously arising myeloma proteins have been found to show carbohydrate specificity, which possibly reflects the fact that carbohydrates are common environmental antigens. Before hybridoma technology, these carbohydrate specific myeloma proteins provided an important model for studying the reaction of antigen with a monoclonal antibody.

Empirically, the predominant antigenic determinants of polysaccharides often consist of short oligosaccharides (one to five sugars long) at the nonreducing end of the polymer chain (8). This situation is analogous to a hapten consisting of several sugar residues linked to a large nonantigenic polysaccharide backbone. The remainder of the polysaccharide is important for immunogenicity, just as the carrier molecule is important for haptens. In addition, branch points in the polysaccharide structure allow for multiple antigenic determinants to be attached to the same macromolecule. This is important for immunoprecipitation by lattice formation, as discussed in Chapter 4. Several examples illustrating structural studies of oligosaccharide antigens are given later.

The technique used most widely to analyze the antigenic determinants of polysaccharides is called *hapten inhibition* (8). In this method, the precipitation reaction between antigen and antibody is inhibited by adding short oligosaccharides. These oligosaccharides are large enough to bind with the same affinity and specificity as the polysaccharide, but because they are monomeric, no precipitate forms. As more inhibitor is added, fewer antibody-combining sites remain available for precipitation. By using antiserum specific for a single antigenic determinant, it is often possible to block precipitation completely with a short oligosaccharide corresponding to the nonreducing end of the polysaccharide chain. Besides showing the "immunodominance" of the nonreducing end of the chain, this result also shows that the structure of the antigenic determinant of polysaccharides depends on the sequence of carbohydrates and their linkage, rather than on their conformation. For inhibition by hapten to be complete, the antigen–antibody system studied must be made specific for a single antigenic determinant. For optimal sensitivity, the equivalence point of antigen and antibody should be used.

We illustrate the types of carbohydrate antigens encountered by examining three classic examples in more detail: the *Salmonella* O antigens, the blood group antigens, and dextrans that bind to myeloma proteins.

Immunochemistry of Salmonella O Antigens

The antigenic diversity among numerous *Salmonella* species resides in the structural differences of the lipopolysaccharide (LPS) component of the outer membrane (9). These molecules are the main target for anti-*Salmonella* antibodies. The polysaccharide moiety contains the antigenic determinant, whereas the lipid moiety is responsible for endotoxin

Lipopolysaccharide Structure

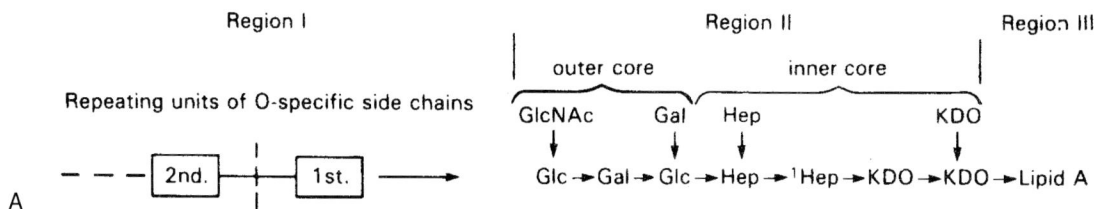

Oligosaccharide Antigens (Region I)

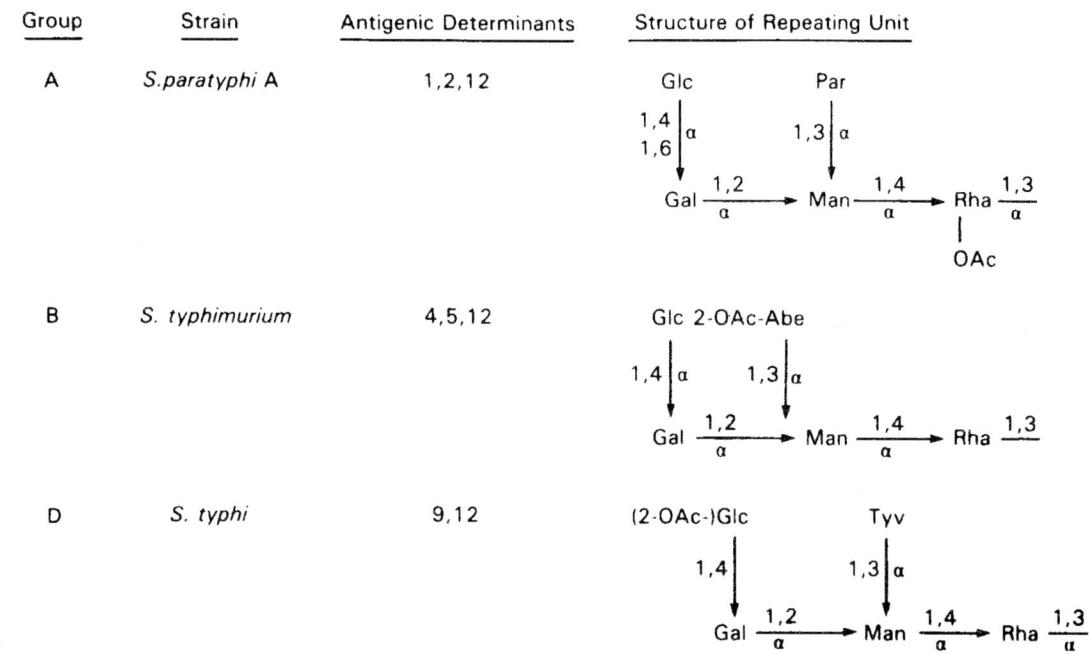

FIG. 1. Structure of *Salmonella* lipopolysaccharide. Region I contains the unique O-antigen determinants, which consist of repeating units of oligosaccharides. These are attached to lipid moiety through the core polysaccharide. Three examples of oligosaccharide units are shown (9). (A: Adapted from Kabat (8), with permission; B: based on Jann and Westphal (9).)

effects. The chemical structure of LPS can be divided into three regions (Fig. 1). Region I contains the antigenic O–specific polysaccharide, usually made up of repeated oligosaccharide units, which vary widely among different strains. Region II contains an oligosaccharide "common core" shared among many different strains. Failure to synthesize region II oligosaccharide or to couple completed region I polysaccharide to the growing region II core results in R (rough) mutants, which have "rough" colony structure and lack the O antigen. Region III is the lipid part, called lipid A, which is shared among all *Salmonella* species and serves to anchor LPS on the outer membrane. Early immunological attempts to classify the O antigens of different *Salmonella* species revealed a large number of cross-reactions between different strains. These were detected by researchers who prepared antiserum to one strain of *Salmonella* and used it to agglutinate bacteria of a second strain. Each cross-reacting

determinant was assigned a number, and each strain was characterized by a series of O antigen determinants (in aggregate, the "serotype" of the strain), on the basis of its pattern of cross-reactivity. Each strain was classified within a group, on the basis of sharing a strong O determinant. For example, group A strains share determinant 2, whereas group B strains share determinant 4 (Table 2). However, within a group, each strain possesses additional O determinants, which serve to differentiate it from other members of that group. Thus, determinant 2 coexists with determinants 1 and 12 on *Salmonella paratyphi* A. This problem of cross-reactivity based on sharing of a subset of antigenic determinants is commonly encountered in complex antigen–antibody systems. The problem may be simplified by making antibodies monospecific for individual antigenic determinants. To do this, either antibodies are absorbed to remove irrelevant specificities or cross-reactive strains that share only a single determinant

TABLE 2. Salmonella *Q antigen serotyping*

Salmonella strain	Serogroup	O antigenic determinants
S. paratyphi A	A	1, 2, 12
S. paratyphi B	B	1, 4, 5, 12
S. typhi	D	9, 12

Antiserum	Absorbed	Tested on	Single determinant measured
Anti–*S. typhi*		*S. paratyphi* B	12
Anti–*S. typhi*	*S. paratyphi* A	*S. typhi*	9

Reprinted with permission (8).

with the immunizing strain are chosen. The reaction of each determinant with its specific antibody can be thought of as an antigen–antibody system. Thus, for the strains shown in Table 2, antiserum to *Salmonella typhi* (containing anti-9 and anti-12 antibodies) may be absorbed with *S. paratyphi* A to remove anti-12, leaving a reagent specific for antigen 9 (Table 2). Alternatively, the unabsorbed antiserum may be used to study the system antigen 12–anti-12 by allowing it to agglutinate *S. paratyphi* B, which shares only antigen 12 with the immunogen. Because the other determinants on *S. paratyphi* B were absent from the immunizing strain, the antiserum contains no antibodies to them.

Once the antigen–antibody reaction is made specific for a single determinant, a variety of oligosaccharides can be added to test for hapten inhibition. Because the O antigens contain repeating oligosaccharide units, it is often possible to obtain model oligosaccharides by mild chemical or enzymatic degradation of the LPS itself. When the most inhibitory oligosaccharide is found, its chemical structure is determined. Alternatively, a variety of synthetic monosaccharides, disaccharides, trisaccharides, and oligosaccharides are tested for hapten inhibition of precipitation. For example, as shown in Table 3, antigen 1–anti-1 antibody precipitation is inhibited by methyl-α-D-glucoside. Therefore, various disaccharides incorporating this structure were tested, of which α-D-Glu(1→6)D-Gal was the most inhibitory. Then various trisaccharides incorporating this sequence were tested. The results indicate the sequence and size of the determinant recognized by anti-1 antibodies to be a disaccharide with the structure just described. The test sequences can be guessed by analyzing the oligosaccharide breakdown products of the LPS, which include tetramers of D-Glu-D-Gal-D-Man-L-

Rham. The results in Table 3 also suggest that the difference between determinants 1 and 19 is the length of oligosaccharide recognized by antibodies specific for each determinant. This hypothesis is supported by the observation that determinant 1 is found in some strains with, and in other strains without, determinant 19, whereas determinant 19 is always found with determinant 1. As shown in Table 3, determinant 19 requires the full tetrasaccharide for maximal hapten inhibition, including the sequence coding for determinant 1. Besides identifying the antigenic structures, these results indicate that there is variation in the size of different antigenic determinants of polysaccharides.

Blood Group Antigens

The major blood group antigens A and B were originally detected by the ability of serum from persons lacking either determinant to agglutinate red blood cells bearing them [for reviews, see Kabat (8), Springer (10), Marcus (11), and Watkins (12)]. In addition, persons with serogroup O have an H antigenic determinant that is distinct from A or B types, and persons in all three groups may have additional determinants such as the Lewis (Le) antigens. Although the ABH and Le antigenic determinants are found on a carbohydrate moiety, the carbohydrate may occur in a variety of biochemical forms. On cell surfaces, they are either glycolipids that are synthesized within the cell (AB and H antigens) or glycoproteins taken up from serum (Le antigens). In mucinous secretions, such as saliva, they occur as glycoproteins. Milk, ovarian cyst fluid, and gastric mucosa contain soluble oligosaccharides that express blood group reactivity. In addition, these antigens occur frequently in other species, including about

TABLE 3. *Analysis of* Salmonella *O-antigen structure by hapten inhibition*

Maximum inhibition by hapten (%)	Antigen system	
	1.anti-1	19.anti-19
D-Glu	—	0
Me-α-D-Glu	35	10
α-D-Glu(1 → 6)-D-Gal	80	25
Glu.Gal.Man	80	70
Glu.Gal.Man.L-Rham	>70	>70
Deduced structure	α-D-Glu(1→6)-D-Gal	D-Glu-D-Gal-D-Man-L-Rham

Reprinted with permission (8).

half of the bacteria in the normal flora of the gut (10). This widespread occurrence may account for the ubiquitous anti-AB reactivity of human sera, even in people never previously exposed to human blood group substances through transfusion or pregnancy.

The immunochemistry of these antigens was simplified greatly by the use of oligosaccharides in hapten inhibition studies. Group A oligosaccharides, for example, would inhibit the agglutination of group A red blood cells by anti-A antibodies. They could also inhibit the immunoprecipitation of group A–bearing glycoproteins by anti-A antibodies. Because the oligosaccharides are monomeric, their reaction with antibody does not form a precipitate but does block an antibody-combining site.

The inhibitory oligosaccharides from cyst fluid were purified and found to contain D-galactose, L-fucose, N-acetyl galactosamine, and N-acetylglucosamine. The most inhibitory oligosaccharides for each antigen are indicated in Fig. 2. As shown in the figure, the ABH and Le antigens all share a common oligosaccharide core sequence, and the antigens appear to differ from each other by the sequential addition of individual sugars at the end or at branch points. Besides hapten inhibition, other biochemical data support this relationship among the different determinants. Enzymatic digestion of A, B, or H antigens yields a common core oligosaccharide from each. This product cross-reacts with antiserum specific for pneumococcal polysaccharide type XIV, which contains structural elements shared with blood group determinants, as shown at the bottom of Fig. 2. In addition, this structure, known as precursor substance, has been isolated from ovarian cyst fluid.

Starting from precursor substance, the H determinant results from the addition of L-fucose to galactose, whereas Lewis a (Le^a) determinant results from the addition of L-fucose to N-acetylglucosamine, and Lewis b (Le^b) determinant results from the addition of L-fucose to both sugars. Addition of N-acetylgalactosamine to H substance produces the A determinant, whereas addition of galactose produces the B determinant, in each case blocking reactivity of the H determinant.

The genetics of ABH and Le antigens is explained by this sequential addition of sugars through glycosyltransferases. The allelic nature of the AB antigens is explained by the addition of N-acetylgalactosamine, galactose, or nothing to the H antigen. The rare inherited trait of inability to synthesize the H determinants from precursor substance (Bombay phenotype) also blocks the expression of A and B antigens, because the A and B transferases lack an acceptor substrate. However, the appearance of the Le^a on red blood cells is independent of H antigen synthesis. Its structure, shown in Fig. 2, can be derived directly from precursor substance without going through an H antigen intermediate. In different individuals, the appearance of Le^a antigen on red blood cells is correlated with its presence in saliva, because the Le^a antigen is not an intrinsic membrane component but must be absorbed from serum glycoproteins, which, in turn, depend on secre-

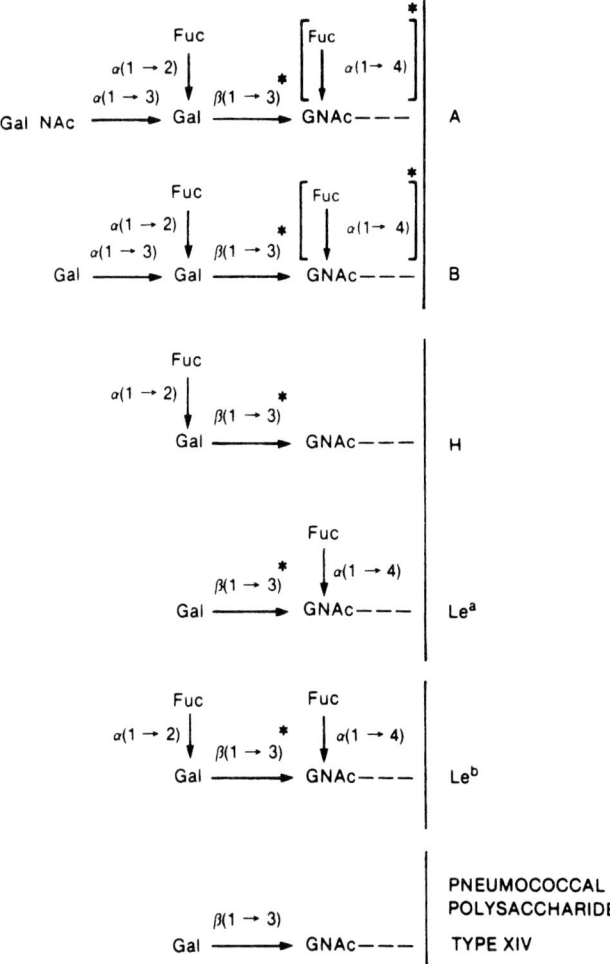

FIG. 2. Oligosaccharide chain specificity. Structure of the ABH and Lewis (Le) blood group antigens, as determined by hapten inhibition studies (8,11). There are two variants of each of these determinants. In type 1, the Gal-GNAc linkage is $\beta(1\rightarrow3)$, whereas in type 2, the Gal–GNAc linkage is $\beta(1\rightarrow4)$. In addition, there is heterogeneity in the A and B antigens with respect to the presence of the Le fucose attached to the GNAc. In the molecules that contain the extra fucose, when the Gal-GNAc linkage is $\beta(1\rightarrow3)$ (type 1), the fucose must be linked $\alpha(1\rightarrow4)$, whereas the type 2 molecules, with the $\beta(1\rightarrow4)$ Gal-GNAc linkage, contain $\alpha(1\rightarrow3)$-linked fucose. The *asterisks* indicate the sites of this variability in linkage.

tion. In addition to the independent synthetic pathway, the secretion of Le^a antigen is also independent of the secretory process for ABH antigens. Therefore, salivary nonsecretors of ABH antigens (20% of persons) may nonetheless secrete Le^a antigen if they have the fucosyl transferase encoded by the Le gene. In contrast, salivary secretion of ABH is required for red blood cells to express Le^b.

Dextran-Binding Myeloma Proteins

Because polysaccharides are common environmental antigens, it is not surprising that randomly induced myeloma proteins were frequently found to have carbohydrate specificities. Careful studies of these monoclonal antibodies support the clonal expansion model of antibody diversity: Heterogeneous antisera behave as the sum of many individual clones of antibody with regard to affinity and specificity. In the case of the immunoglobulin Aκ myeloma proteins W3129 and W3434, both antibodies were found to be specific for dextrans containing α-glu$(1\rightarrow6)$glu bonds (12). Hapten inhibition with a series of monosaccharides or oligosaccharides of increasing chain length indicated that the percentages of binding energy derived from the reaction with one, two, three, and four glucoses were 75%, 95%, 95% to 98%, and 100%, respectively. This suggests that most binding energy between antidextran antibodies and dextran is derived from the terminal monosaccharide and that oligosaccharides of chain length four to six commonly fill the antibody-combining site. Human antidextran antisera behaved similarly, with tetrasaccharides contributing 95% of the binding energy. These experiments provided the first measure of the size of an antigenic determinant: four to six residues (13,14). In addition, as was observed for antisera, binding affinity of myeloma proteins was highly sensitive to modifications of the terminal sugar and highly specific for $\alpha(1\rightarrow6)$ versus $\alpha(1\rightarrow3)$ glycosidic bonds. However, modification of the third or fourth sugar of an oligosaccharide had relatively less effect on hapten inhibition of either myeloma protein or polyclonal antisera reacting with dextran.

Studies with additional dextran-binding myeloma proteins (15) revealed that not all antipolysaccharide monoclonal antibodies are specific for the nonreducing end, as exemplified by myeloma protein QUPC 52. Competitive inhibition with monosaccharides and oligosaccharides revealed that less than 5% of binding energy derived from monosaccharides or disaccharides, 72% from trisaccharides, 88% from tetrasaccharides, and 100% from hexasaccharides, in marked contrast to other myeloma proteins. A second distinctive property of QUPC 52 was its ability to precipitate unbranched dextran of chain length 200. Because the unbranched dextran has only one nonreducing end, and because the myeloma protein has only one specificity, lattice formation resulting from cross-linking between the nonreducing ends is impossible, and precipitation must be explained by binding some other determinant. Therefore, QUPC 52 appears to be specific for internal oligosaccharide units of 3 to 7 chain length. W3129 is specific for end determinants and does not precipitate unbranched dextran chains. Antibodies precipitating linear dextran were also detected in six antidextran human sera, which comprise 48% to 90% of the total antibodies to branched-chain dextran. Thus, antidextrans can be divided into those specific for terminal oligosaccharides and those specific for internal oligosaccharides; monoclonal examples of both types are available, and both types are present in human immune serum. Cisar et al. (15) speculated as to the different topology of the binding sites of W3129 or QUPC 52 necessary for terminal or internal oligosaccharide specificity. Both terminal and internal oligosaccharides have nearly identical chemical structures, differing at a single C—OH or glycoside bond. Perhaps the terminal oligosaccharide specificity of W3129 results from the shape of the antibody-combining site: a cavity into which only the end can fit—whereas the internal oligosaccharide-binding site of QUPC 52 could be a surface groove in the antibody, which would allow the rest of the polymer to protrude at both ends. A more definitive answer depends on x-ray crystallographic studies of the combining sites of monoclonal antibodies with precisely defined specificity, performed with antigen occupying the binding site.

With the advent of hybridoma technology, it became possible to produce monoclonal antibodies of any desired specificity. Immunizing mice with nearly linear dextran (the preferred antigen of QUPC 52), followed by fusion and screening (with linear dextran) for dextran-binding antibodies, yielded 12 hybridomas (16), all with specificity similar to that of QUPC 52. Oligosaccharide inhibition of all 12 monoclonal antibodies showed considerable increments in affinity up to hexasaccharides, with little affinity for disaccharides and only 49% to 77% of binding energy derived from trisaccharides (17). Second, all 12 monoclonal antibodies had internal $\alpha(1\rightarrow6)$ dextran specificity, inasmuch as they all could precipitate linear dextran. Third, 9 of 11 BALB/c monoclonal antibodies shared cross-reactive idiotype with QUPC 52, whereas none shared idiotype with W3129 (18). These data support the hypothesis that different antibodies with similar specificity and similar groove-type sites may be derived from the same family of germline VH genes bearing the QUPC 52 idiotype (18).

The large number of environmental carbohydrate antigens and the high degree of specificity of antibodies elicited in response to each carbohydrate antigen suggest that a tremendous diversity of antibody molecules must be available, from which some antibodies can be selected for every possible antigenic structure. In studies of a series of 17 monoclonal anti-$\alpha(1\rightarrow6)$ dextran hybridomas (19,20), researchers have investigated whether the binding sites of closely related antibodies were derived from a small number of variable region genes, for both heavy and light chains, or whether antibodies of the same specificity could derive from variable region genes with highly divergent sequences. Each monoclonal antibody had a groove-type site that could hold six or seven sugar residues (with one exception), on the basis of inhibition of immunoprecipitation by different-length oligosaccharides. Thus, unlike monoclonal antibodies to haptenated proteins, the precise epitope could be well characterized and was generally quite similar among the entire series.

Studies of the Vκ sequences revealed that only three Vκ groups were used in these hybridomas. Use of each Vκ group correlated with the particular antigen used to immunize the animals, whether linear dextran or short oligosaccharides; 10 of the monoclonal antibodies from mice immunized the same way all used the same Vκ.

In contrast, the 17 VH chains were derived from at least five different germline genes from three different VH gene families (21). The two most frequently used germline VH genes were found in seven and five monoclonal antibodies, respectively, with minor variations explainable by somatic mutations. The remarkable finding is that very different VH chains (about 50% homologous) can combine with the same Vκ sequence to produce antibody-binding sites with nearly the same size, shape, antigen specificity, and affinity. Even when different VH sequences combine with different Vκ sequences, they can produce antibodies with very similar properties. Dextran binding depends on the antigen's fitting into the groove and interacting favorably with the residues forming the sides and bottom of the groove. The results indicate that divergent variable region sequences, both in and out of the complementarity-determining regions, can be folded to form similar binding site contours, which result in similar immunochemical characteristics. Similar results have been reported in other antigen–antibody systems, such as phenyloxazolone (22).

More detailed genetic studies were carried out with 34 groove-type monoclonal anti-α(1→6) dextran-binding hybridomas (23), of which 10 used heavy chain VH19.1.2 and 11 used VH9.14.7. Starting with different VH genes, these two families of monoclonal antibodies provide an experiment of nature concerning the ability of each VH gene to combine with different light chain Vκ and Jκ genes, as well as heavy chain D and JH genes to produce a groove-shaped binding site of a given specificity. In every one of these 21 monoclonal antibodies, the same light chain Vκ-OX1 gene was used, but the VH19 family used a single Jκ sequence exclusively (Jκ2), whereas the VH9 family included all four of the active Jκ segments (Jκ1, Jκ2, Jκ4, and Jκ5). Similarly, the heavy chain JH sequences of the VH19 family were all of a single type (JH3), whereas those of the VH9 family included three types (JH1, JH2, and JH3). A single D region was used by both families (DFL16.1), but the junctional sequences between VH–D and D–JH were different: The VH19 used minimal substitutions, and the VH9 allowed more variability in junctional sequences, depending on the size of the JH with which it was joining. Although the amino acid sequences of these two VH genes are 73% identical, they use markedly different strategies to arrive at the same groove-type binding site with nearly identical size and specificity. The results suggest that the two heavy chain variable regions, perhaps because of their conformation, may place different structural constraints on which mini-gene components can successfully contribute to forming a particular site. Two different strategies for generating the same antibody specificity are apparent, even though identical Vκ and D mini-genes were used by both families. For the VH19 family, the α(1→6) dextran specificity depended on holding both J sequences and the D junctions constant. For the VH9 family, a wide variety of JH, Jκ, and VH–D and D–JH sequences were used to generate the groove-type site. These two blueprints for constructing a binding site may also reflect distinct cellular pathways for generating antibody diversity.

Immunogenicity of Polysaccharides

Capsular polysaccharides are the main target of protective antibodies against bacterial infection. In adults, the chain length of the polysaccharide is an important determinant of immunogenicity, and the polysaccharides induce a T cell–independent response that cannot be boosted on repeat exposure. In young children, who most need immunity to pathogens such as *Haemophilus influenzae* type b and *Streptococcus pneumoniae* of multiple serotypes, the T cell–independent response to these polysaccharides is weak, regardless of chain length. To immunize children, the polysaccharides were coupled to a protein carrier to create a new T cell–dependent antigen, which gained immunogenicity from T-cell help and boosted antibody titers with each successive dose. This strategy has produced highly successful conjugate vaccines against *H. influenzae* type b (24), resulting in a markedly reduced incidence of meningitis caused by this agent in immunized children (25,26) and evidence of herd immunity even among unimmunized children. The same strategy has produced an effective vaccine against invasive disease (27) and otitis media (28) caused by the most prevalent serotypes of *S. pneumoniae*.

Protein and Polypeptide Antigenic Determinants

Like the proteins themselves, the antigen determinants of proteins consist of amino acid residues in a particular three-dimensional array. The residues that make contact with complementary residues in the antibody-combining site are called *contact residues.* To make contact, of course, these residues must be exposed on the surface of the protein, not buried in the hydrophobic core. Because the complementarity-determining residues in the hypervariable regions of antibodies have been found to span as much as 30 to 40 Å × 15 to 20 Å × 10 Å (D. R. Davies, personal communication 1983), these contact residues that constitute the antigenic determinant may cover a significant area of protein surface, as now measured in a few cases by x-ray crystallography of antibody–protein antigen complexes (29–32). The size of the combining sites has also been estimated by using simple synthetic oligopeptides of increasing length, such as oligolysine. In this case, a series of elegant studies (33–35) suggested that the maximum length of chain that a combining site could accommodate was six to eight residues, corresponding closely to that found earlier for oligosaccharides (13,14), discussed previously.

Several types of interactions contribute to the binding energy. Many of the amino acid residues exposed to solvent on the surface of a protein antigen are hydrophilic. These are likely to interact with antibody contact residues through polar interactions. For instance, an anionic glutamic acid carboxyl group may bind to a complementary cationic lysine amino group on the antibody, or vice versa, or a glutamine amide side chain may form a hydrogen bond with the antibody. However, hydrophobic interactions can also play a major role. Proteins cannot exist in aqueous solution as stable monomers with too many hydrophobic residues on their surface. The hydrophobic residues that are on the surface can contribute to binding to antibody for exactly the same reason. When a hydrophobic residue in a protein antigenic determinant or, similarly, in a carbohydrate determinant (8) interacts with a corresponding hydrophobic residue in the antibody-combining site, the water molecules previously in contact with each of them are excluded. The result is a significant stabilization of the interaction. These aspects of the chemistry of antigen–antibody binding were thoroughly reviewed by Getzoff et al.(36).

Mapping Epitopes: Conformation Versus Sequence

The other component that defines a protein antigenic determinant, besides the amino acid residues involved, is the way these residues are arrayed in three dimensions. Because the residues are on the surface of a protein, this component can also be thought of as the topography of the antigenic determinant. Sela (37) divided protein antigenic determinants into two categories, sequential and conformational, depending on whether the primary sequence or the three-dimensional conformation appeared to contribute the most to binding. On the other hand, because the antibody-combining site has a preferred topography in the native antibody, it seems a priori that some conformations of a particular polypeptide sequence would produce a better fit than others and therefore would be energetically favored in binding. Thus, conformation or topography must always play some role in the structure of an antigenic determinant.

Moreover, by looking at the surface of a protein in a space-filling model, it is not possible to ascertain the direction of the backbone or the positions of the helices (contrast Figs. 3 and 4) (38–42). It is hard to recognize whether two residues that are side by side on the surface are adjacent on the polypeptide backbone or whether they come from different parts of the sequence and are brought together by the folding

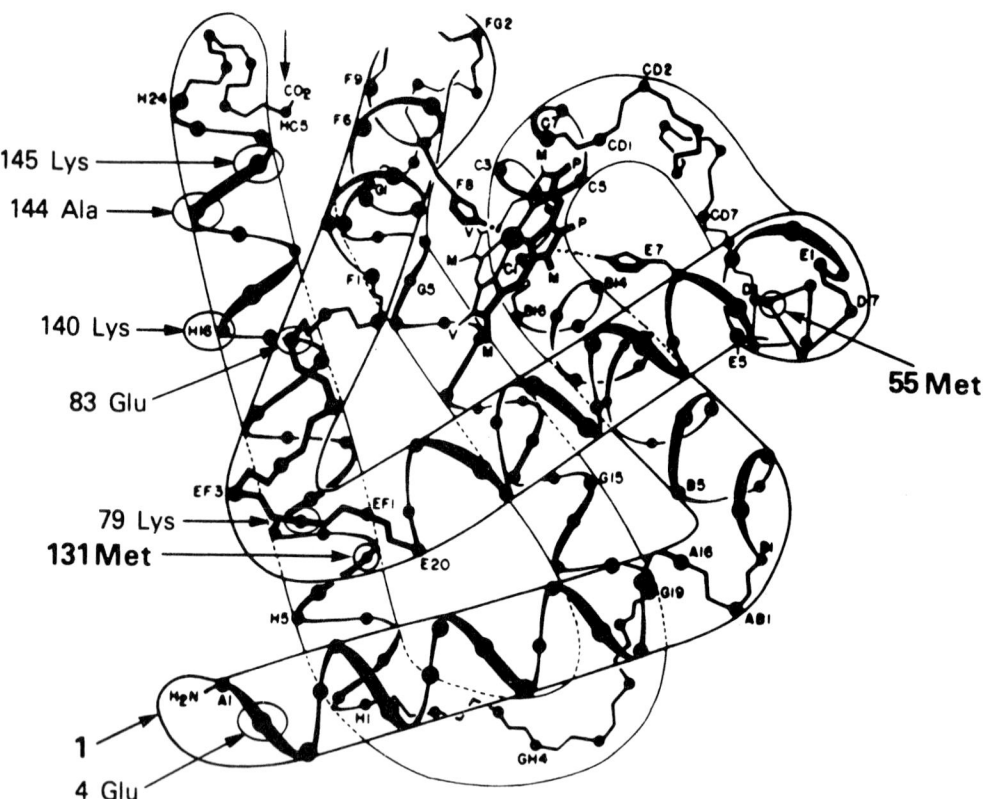

FIG. 3. Artist's representation of the polypeptide backbone of sperm whale myoglobin in its native three-dimensional conformation. The α helices are labeled A through H from the amino terminal to the carboxy terminal. Side chains are omitted, except for the two histidine rings (F8 and E7) involved with the heme iron. Methionines at positions 55 and 131 are the sites of cleavage by cyanogen bromide (CNBr), allowing myoglobin to be cleaved into three fragments. Most of the helicity and other features of the native conformation are lost when the molecule is cleaved. A less drastic change in conformation is produced by removal of the heme to form apomyoglobin, because the heme interacts with several helices and stabilizes their positions in relation to one another. The other labeled residues (4 Glu, 79 Lys, 83 Glu, 140 Lys, 144 Ala, and 145 Lys) are residues that have been found to be involved in antigenic determinants recognized by monoclonal antibodies (38). Note that cleavage by CNBr separates Lys 79 from Glu 4 and separates Glu 83 from Ala 144 and Lys 145. The "sequential" determinant of Koketsu and Atassi (39) (residues 15 to 22) is located at the elbow, lower right, from the end of the A helix to the beginning of the B helix. (Adapted from Dickerson (40), with permission.)

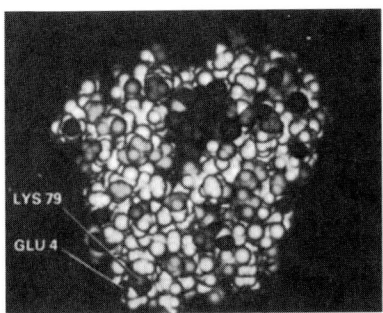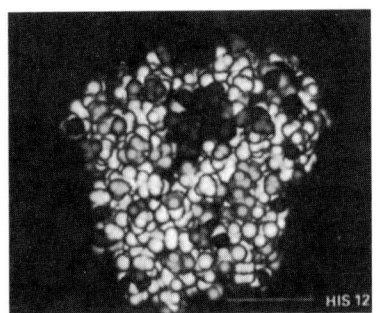

FIG. 4. Stereoscopic views of a computer-generated space-filling molecular model of sperm whale myoglobin, based on Takano's (41) x-ray diffraction coordinates. This orientation, which corresponds to that in Fig. 3, is arbitrarily designated the "front view." The computer method was described by Feldmann et al. (42). The heme and aromatic carbons are shaded darkest, followed by carboxyl oxygens, then other oxygen molecules, then primary amino groups, then other nitrogens, and finally side chains of aliphatic residues. The backbone and the side chains of nonaliphatic residues, except for the functional groups, are shown in white. Note that the direction of the helices is not apparent on the surface, in contrast to the backbone drawing in Fig. 3. The residues Glu 4, Lys 79, and His 12 are believed to be part of a topographic antigenic determinant recognized by a monoclonal antibody to myoglobin (38). This stereo pair can be viewed in three dimensions with an inexpensive stereoviewer such as the "stereoscopes" sold by Abrams Instrument Corp., Lansing, MI, or Hubbard Scientific Co., Northbrook, IL. Adapted from Berzofsky et al. (38), with permission.

of the molecule. If a protein maintains its native conformation when an antibody binds, then it must similarly be hard for the antibody to discriminate between residues that are covalently connected directly and those connected only through a great deal of intervening polypeptide. Thus, the probability that an antigenic determinant on a native globular protein consists of only a consecutive sequence of amino acids in the primary structure is likely to be rather small. Even if most of the determinant were a continuous sequence, other nearby residues would probably play a role as well. Only if the protein were cleaved into fragments before the antibodies were made would there be any reason to favor connected sequences.

This concept was analyzed and confirmed quantitatively by Barlow et al. (43), who examined the atoms lying within spheres of different radii from a given surface atom on a protein. As the radius increases, the probability that all the atoms within the sphere are from the same continuous segment of protein sequence decreases rapidly. Correspondingly, the fraction of surface atoms that would be located at the center of a sphere containing only residues from the same continuous segment falls dramatically as the radius of the sphere increases. For instance, for lysozyme, with a radius of 8 Å, fewer than 10% of the surface residues would lie in such a "continuous patch" of surface. These residues are primarily in regions that protrude from the surface. With a radius of 10 Å, almost none of the surface residues fall in the center of a continuous patch. Thus, for a contact area of about 20 Å × 25 Å, as found for a lysozyme–antibody complex studied by x-ray crystallography, none of the antigenic sites could be completely continuous segmental sites (see later discussion and Fig. 5).

Antigenic sites consisting of amino acid residues that are widely separated in the primary protein sequence but brought together on the surface of the protein by the way it folds in its native conformation have been called *assembled topographic* sites (44,45) because they are assembled from different parts of the sequence and exist only in the surface topography of the native molecule. In contrast, the sites that consist of only a single continuous segment of protein sequence have been called *segmental* antigenic sites (44,45).

In contrast to T-cell recognition of "processed" fragments retaining only primary and secondary structures, there is overwhelming evidence that most antibodies are made against the native conformation when the native protein is used as immunogen. For instance, antibodies to native staphylococcal nuclease were found to have about a 5,000-fold higher affinity for the native protein than for the corresponding polypeptide on which they were isolated (by binding to the peptide attached to Sepharose) (46). An even more dramatic example is that demonstrated by Crumpton (47) for antibodies to native myoglobin or to apomyoglobin. Antibodies to native ferric myoglobin produced a brown precipitate with myoglobin but did not bind well to apomyoglobin, which, without the heme, has a slightly altered conformation. On the other hand, antibodies to the apomyoglobin, when mixed with native (brown) myoglobin, produced a white precipitate. These antibodies so strongly favored the conformation of apomyoglobin, from which the heme was excluded, that they trapped the molecules that vibrated toward that conformation and pulled the equilibrium state over to the apo form. It could almost be said, figuratively, that the antibodies squeezed the heme out of the myoglobin. Thermodynamically, it is clear that the conformational preference of the antibody for the apo versus native forms, in terms of free energy, had to be greater than the free energy of binding of the heme to myoglobin. Thus, in general, antibodies that are very specific for the conformation of the protein used as immunogen are made.

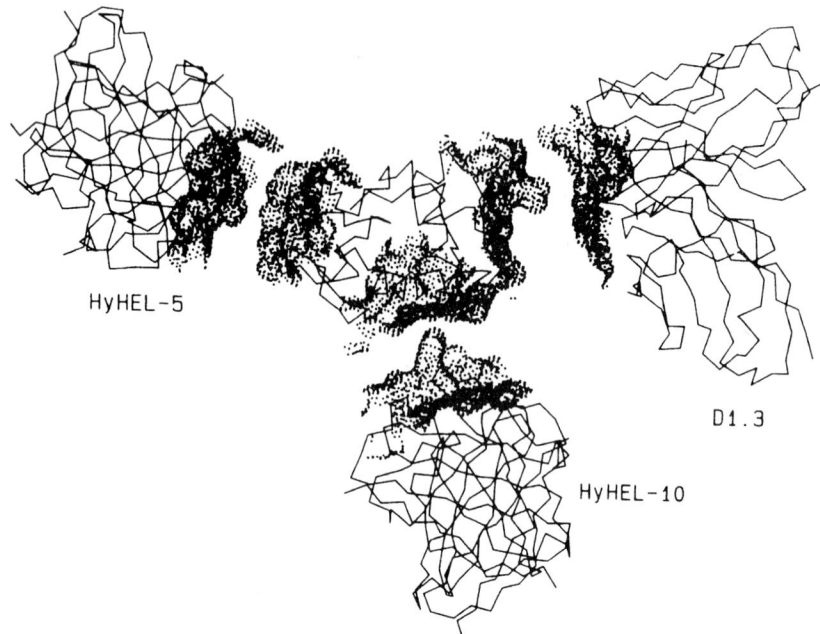

HyHEL-5

D1.3

HyHEL-10

FIG. 5. Assembled topographic sites of lysozyme illustrated by the footprints of three nonoverlapping monoclonal antibodies. Shown are the α carbon backbones of lysozyme in the center and the Fv portions of three antilysozyme monoclonal antibodies D1.3, HyHEL-5, and HyHEL-10. The footprints of the antibodies on lysozyme and lysozyme on the antibodies—that is, their interacting surfaces—are shown by a dotted representation. Note that the three antibodies each contact more than one continuous loop of lysozyme and thus define assembled topographic sites. From Davies and Padlan (32), with permission.

Synthetic peptides corresponding to segments of the protein antigen sequence can be used to identify the structures bound by antibodies specific for segmental antigenic sites. To identify assembled topographic sites, more complex approaches have been necessary. The earliest was the use of natural variants of the protein antigen with known amino acid substitutions, in which such evolutionary variants exist (44). Thus, substitution of different amino acids in proteins in the native conformation can be examined. The use of this method, which is illustrated later, is limited to the study of the function of amino acids that vary among homologous proteins: that is, those that are polymorphic. Its use may now be extended to other residues by use of site-directed mutagenesis. A second method is to use the antibody that binds to the native protein to protect the antigenic site from modification (48) or proteolytic degradation (49). A related but less sensitive approach makes use of competition with other antibodies (50–52). A third approach, taking advantage of the capability of producing thousands of peptides on a solid-phase surface for direct binding assays (53), is to study binding of a monoclonal antibody to every possible combination of six amino acids (53). If the assembled topographic site can be mimicked by a combination of six amino acids not corresponding to any continuous segment of the protein sequence but structurally resembling a part of the surface, then a "mimotope" defining the specificity of that antibody can be produced (53).

Myoglobin also serves as a good model protein antigen for studying the range of variation of antigenic determinants from those that are more sequential in nature to those that do not even exist without the native conformation of the protein (Fig. 3). A good example of the first, more segmental type of determinant is that consisting of residues 15 to 22 in the amino-terminal portion of the molecule. Crumpton and Wilkinson (54) first discovered that the chymotryptic

cleavage fragment consisting of residues 15 to 29 had antigenic activity for antibodies raised to either native or apomyoglobin. Two other groups (39, 55) then found that synthetic peptides corresponding to the shorter sequence 15 to 22 bind antibodies made to native sperm whale myoglobin, even though the synthetic peptides were only seven to eight residues long. Peptides of this length do not spend much time (in solution) in a conformation corresponding to that of the native protein. On the other hand, these synthetic peptides had a several hundred–fold lower affinity for the antibodies than did the native protein. Thus, even if most of the determinant was included in the consecutive sequence 15 to 22, the antibodies were still much more specific for the native conformation of this sequence than for the random conformation peptide. Moreover, there was no evidence to exclude the participation of other residues, nearby on the surface of myoglobin but not in this sequence, in the antigenic determinant (56–59).[1]

A good example of the importance of secondary structure is the case of the loop peptide (residues 64 to 80) of hen egg-white lysozyme (60). This loop in the protein sequence is created by the disulfide linkage between cysteine residues 64 and 80 and has been shown to be a major antigenic determinant for antibodies to lysozyme (60). The isolated peptide 60 to 83, containing the loop, binds antibodies with high

---

[1] This is the only segmental antigenic determinant of myoglobin that has clearly been confirmed by more than one independent group of investigators. Crumpton and Wilkinson (54) did measure antigenic activity for a chymotryptic fragment, 147-153, that overlaps one of the other reported sequential determinants (56). However, two of the other reported sequential determinants (56), corresponding to residues 56 to 62 and 94 to 100, have not been reproducible when tested with other antisera, even raised in the same species (57). For related studies, see Hurrell et al. (58) and East et al. (59).

affinity, but opening of the loop by cleavage of the disulfide bond destroys most of the antigenic activity for antilysozyme antibodies (60).

At the other end of the range of conformational requirements are the determinants involving residues far apart in the primary sequences that are brought close together on the surface of the native molecule by its folding in three dimensions. Myoglobin also provides a good example of these determinants, called *assembled topographic determinants* (44,45). Of six monoclonal antibodies to sperm whale myoglobin studied by Berzofsky et al. (38,61), none bound to any of the three cyanogen bromide cleavage fragments of myoglobin that together span the whole sequence of the molecule. Therefore, these monoclonal antibodies (all with affinities between 2×10^8 and 2×10^9 M^{-1}) were all highly specific for the native conformation. These were studied by comparing the relative affinities for a series of native myoglobins from different species with the known amino acid sequences of these myoglobins. With the myoglobins available, this approach allowed the definition of some of the residues involved in binding to three of these antibodies. The striking result was that two of these three monoclonal antibodies were found to recognize topographic determinants, as defined previously. One recognized a determinant that included Glu 4 and Lys 79, which are on the A helix and the E–F corner of the myoglobin molecule but come within about 2 Åof each other to form a salt bridge in the native molecule (Fig. 4). The other antibody recognized a determinant involving Glu 83 in the E–F corner and Ala 144 and Lys 145 on the H helix of the myoglobin molecule (Fig. 3). Again, these are far apart in the primary sequence but are brought within 12 Åof each other by the folding of the molecule in its native conformation. Similar examples have been reported for monoclonal antibodies to human myoglobin (62) and to lysozyme (32,50). Other examples of such conformation-dependent antigenic determinants have been suggested with the use of conventional antisera to such proteins as insulin (63), hemoglobin (64), tobacco mosaic virus protein (65), and cytochrome c (66). Moreover, the crystallographic structures of lysozyme–antibody (29,31,32) and neuraminidase–antibody (30) complexes show clearly that, in both cases, the epitope bound is an assembled topographic site. In the case of the three monoclonal antibodies binding to nonoverlapping sites of lysozyme (Fig. 5), it is clear that the footprints of all three antibody-combining sites cover more than one loop of polypeptide chain and thus each encompasses an assembled topographic site (32). This result beautifully illustrates the concept that the majority of antibody combining sites must interact with more than a continuous loop of polypeptide chain and thus must define assembled topographic sites (43). Another important example is represented by neutralizing antibodies to the human immunodeficiency virus (HIV) envelope protein that similarly bind assembled topographic sites (67,68) (see also the end of this section).

How frequent are antibodies specific for topographic determinants in comparison with those that bind consecutive

sequences when conventional antisera are examined? This question was studied by Lando et al. (69), who passed goat, sheep, and rabbit antisera to sperm whale myoglobin over columns of myoglobin fragments, together spanning the whole sequence. After removal of all antibodies binding to the fragments, there remained 30% to 40% of the antibodies that still bound to the native myoglobin molecule with high affinity but did not bind to any of the fragments in solution by radioimmunoassay. Thus, in four of four antimyoglobin sera tested, 60% to 70% of the antibodies could bind peptides and 30% to 40% could bind only native-conformation intact protein.

On the basis of studies such as these, it has been suggested that much of the surface of a protein molecule may be antigenic (44,70) but that the surface can be divided up into antigenic domains (38,58,59,62). Each of these domains consists of many overlapping determinants recognized by different antibodies.

An additional interesting point is that in three published crystal structures of protein antigen–antibody complexes, the contact surfaces were broad, with local complementary pairs of concave and convex regions in both directions (29–32). Thus, the concept of an antigen's binding in the groove or pocket of an antibody may be oversimplified, and antibodies may sometimes bind by extending into pockets on an antigen.

Further information on the subjects discussed in this section is available in the reviews by Sela (37), Crumpton (47), Reichlin (71), Kabat (72), Benjamin et al. (44), Berzofsky (45), Getzoff et al. (36), and Davies and Padlan (32).

Conformational Equilibria of Protein and Peptide Antigenic Determinants

There are several possible mechanisms to explain why an antibody specific for a native protein binds a peptide fragment in random conformation with lower affinity. Of course, the peptide may not contain all the contact residues of the antigenic determinant, so that the binding energy would be lower. However, for cases in which all the residues in the determinant are present in the peptide, several mechanisms still remain. First, the affinity may be lower because the topography of the residues in the peptide may not produce as complementary a fit in the antibody-combining site as the native conformation would. Second, the apparent affinity may be reduced because only a small fraction of the peptide molecules is in a native-like conformation at any time, assuming that the antibody binds only to the native conformation. The concentration of peptide molecules in native conformation is lower than the total peptide concentration by a factor that corresponds to the conformational equilibrium constant of the peptide; therefore, the apparent affinity is also lower by this factor. This model is analogous to an allosteric model. A third, intermediate hypothesis suggests that initial binding of the peptide in a nonnative conformation occurs with submaximal complementarity and is followed by an intramolecular conformational change in the peptide to achieve energy minimization by assuming a native-like conformation. This third hypothesis corresponds to an induced-fit model. The loss of affinity results from the energy required to change the conformation of the peptide, which in turn corresponds to the conformational equilibrium constant in the second hypothesis. To some extent, these models could be distinguished kinetically, because the first hypothesis predicts a faster "on" rate and a faster "off" rate than does the second hypothesis (73).

Although not the only way to explain the data, the second hypothesis is useful because it provides a method for estimating the conformational equilibria of proteins and peptides (46,74). The method assumes the second hypothesis, which can be expressed as follows:

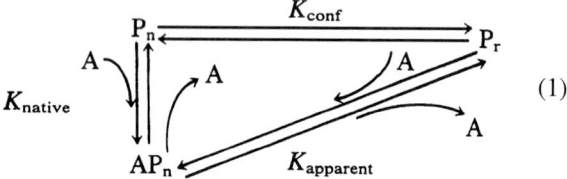

$$(1)$$

where A is antibody, P_n is native peptide, and P_r is random conformation peptide, so that

$$K_{apparent} = K_{conf} K_{native} \qquad (2)$$

Thus, the ratio of the apparent association constant for peptide to the measured association constant for the native molecule should yield the conformational equilibrium constant of the peptide. Note the implicit assumption that the total peptide concentration can be approximated by $[P_r]$. This is generally true, because most peptide fragments of proteins demonstrate little native conformation; that is, $K_{conf} = [P_n]/[P_r]$ is much less than 1. Also note that if the first hypothesis (or third) occurs to some extent, this method will overestimate K_{conf}. On the other hand, if the affinity for the peptide is lower because it lacks some of the contact residues of the determinant, this method will underestimate K_{conf} (by assuming that all the affinity difference results from conformation). To some extent, the two errors may partially cancel out. When this method was used to determine the K_{conf} for a peptide staphylococcal nuclease, a value of 2×10^{-4} was obtained (46). Similarly, when antibodies raised to a peptide fragment were used, it was possible to estimate the fraction of time that the native nuclease spends in nonnative conformations (74). In this case, the K_{conf} was found to be about 3,000-fold in favor of the native conformation.

Antipeptide Antibodies that Bind to Native Proteins at a Specific Site

In light of the conformational differences between native proteins and peptides and the observed K_{conf} effects shown by antibodies to native proteins when tested on the corresponding peptides, it was somewhat surprising to find that antibodies to synthetic peptides show extensive cross-reactions with native proteins (75,76). These two types of cross-reactions can be thought of as working in opposite directions: The binding

of antiprotein antibodies to the peptide is inefficient, whereas the binding of antipeptide antibodies to the protein is quite efficient and commonly observed. This finding is quite useful, because automated solid-phase peptide synthesis has become readily available. This has been particularly useful in three areas: exploitation of protein sequences deduced by recombinant deoxyribonucleic acid (DNA) methods, preparation of site-specific antibodies, and the attempt to focus the immune response on a single protein site that is biologically important but may not be particularly immunogenic. This section focuses on the explanation of the cross-reaction, uses of the cross-reaction, and the potential limitations with regard to immunogenicity.

The basic assumption is that antibodies raised against peptides in an unfolded structure bind the corresponding site on proteins folded into the native structure (76). This is not immediately obvious, because antibody binding to antigen is the direct result of the antigen's fitting into the binding site. Affinity is the direct consequence of "goodness of fit" between antibody and antigen, whereas antibody specificity results from the inability of other antigens to occupy the same site. How, then, can the antipeptide antibodies overcome the effect of K_{conf} and still bind native proteins with good affinity and specificity? The whole process depends on the antibody-binding site's forming a three-dimensional space and the antigen's filling it in an energetically favorable way.

Because the peptides are randomly folded, they rarely occupy the native conformation, so they are not likely to elicit antibodies against a conformation that they do not maintain. If the antibodies are specific for a denatured structure, then, as in the case of the myoglobin molecules that were denatured to apomyoglobin by antibody binding (47), the cross-reaction may depend on the native protein's ability to assume different conformational states. If the native protein is quite rigid, then the possibility of its assuming a random conformation is quite small, but if it is a flexible three-dimensional spring, then local unfolding and refolding may occur all the time. Local unfolding of protein segments may permit the immunological cross-reaction with antipeptide antibodies, because a flexible segment could assume many of the same conformations as the randomly folded peptide (76).

In contrast, the proteins' ability to crystallize (a feature that allows the study of their structure by x-ray crystallography) has long been taken as evidence of protein rigidity (77). In addition, the existence of discrete functional states of allosteric enzymes (78) provides additional evidence of stable structural states of a protein. Finally, the fact that antibodies can distinguish native from denatured forms of intact proteins is well known for proteins such as myoglobin (47).

However, protein crystals are a somewhat artificial situation, inasmuch as the formation of the crystal lattice imposes order on the components, each of which occupies a local energy minimum at the expense of considerable loss of randomness (entropy). Thus, the crystal structure may have artificial rigidity that exceeds the actual rigidity of protein molecules in solution. On the contrary, some of the considerable difficulty in crystallizing proteins may be attributed to disorder within the native conformation. Second, allosterism may be explained by two distinct conformations that are discrete without being particularly rigid. Finally, the ability to generate antiprotein antibodies that are conformation specific does not rule out the existence of antipeptide antibodies that are not. All antibodies are probably specific for some conformation of the antigen, but this need not be the crystallographic native conformation in order to achieve a significant affinity for those proteins or protein segments that have a "loose" native conformation.

Antipeptide antibodies have proved to be very powerful reagents when combined with recombinant DNA methods of gene sequencing (76,79). From the DNA sequence, the protein sequence is predicted. A synthetic peptide is constructed, coupled to a suitable carrier molecule, and used to immunize animals. The resulting polyclonal antibodies can be detected with a peptide-coated enzyme-linked immunosorbent assay plate (see Chapter 4). They are used to immunoprecipitate the native protein from a sulfur 35–labeled cell lysate and thus confirm expression of the gene product in these cells. The antipeptide antibodies can also be used to isolate the previously unidentified gene product of a new gene. The site-specific antibodies are also useful in detecting posttranslational processing, because they bind all precursors and products that contain the site. In addition, because the antibodies bind only to the site corresponding to the peptide, they are useful in probing structure–function relationships. They can be used to block the binding of a substrate to an enzyme or the binding of a virus to its cellular receptor.

Immunogenicity of Proteins and Peptides

Up to this point, the ability of antibodies to react with proteins or peptides as antigens has been discussed. However, *immunogenicity* refers to the ability of these compounds to elicit antibodies after immunization. Several factors limit the immunogenicity of different regions of proteins, and these have been divided into those that are intrinsic to protein structure itself and those extrinsic to the antigen that are related to the responder and vary from one animal or species to another (45). In addition, we consider the special case of peptide immunogenicity as it applies to vaccine development. The features of protein structure that have been suggested to explain the results include surface accessibility of the site, hydrophilicity, flexibility, and proximity to a site recognized by helper T cells.

When the x-ray crystallographic structure and antigenic structure are known for the same protein, it is not surprising to find that a series of monoclonal antibodies binding to a molecule such as influenza neuraminidase interact with an overlapping pattern of sites at the exposed head of the protein (80). The stalk of neuraminidase is not immunogenic, apparently because it is almost entirely covered by carbohydrate.

Beyond such things as carbohydrate, which may sterically interfere with antibody binding to protein, accessibility on the

surface is clearly a *sine qua non* for an antigenic determinant to be bound by an antibody specific for the native conformation, without any requirement for unfolding of the structure (45). Several measures of such accessibility have been suggested. All these require knowledge of the x-ray crystallographic three-dimensional structure. Some have measured accessibility to solvent by rolling a sphere with the radius of a water molecule over the surface of a protein (81,82). Other authors have suggested that accessibility to water is not the best measure of accessibility to antibody and have demonstrated a better correlation by rolling a sphere with the radius of an antibody-combining domain (83). Another approach to predicting antigenic sites on the basis of accessibility is to examine the degree of protrusion from the surface of the protein (84). This was done by modeling the body of the protein as an ellipsoid and examining which amino acid residues remained outside ellipsoids of increasing dimensions. The most protruding residues were found to be part of antigenic sites bound by antibodies, but usually these sites had been identified by using short synthetic peptides and so were segmental in nature. As noted previously, for an antigenic site to be contained completely within a single continuous segment of protein sequence, the site is likely to have to protrude from the surface, because otherwise residues from other parts of the sequence would fall within the area contacting the antibody (43).

Because the three-dimensional structure of most proteins is not known, other ways of predicting surface exposure have been proposed for most antigens. For example, hydrophilic sites tend to be found on the water-exposed surface of proteins. Thus, hydrophilicity has been proposed as a second indication of immunogenicity (85–87). This model has been used to analyze 12 proteins with known antigenic sites: The most hydrophilic site of each protein was indeed one of the antigenic sites. However, among the limitations are the facts that a significant fraction of surface residues can be nonpolar (81,82) and that several important examples of hydrophobic and aromatic amino acids involved in the antigenic sites are known (37,65,88,89). Specificity of antibody binding probably depends on the complementarity of surfaces for hydrogen bonding and polar bonding as well as van der Waals contacts (90), and hydrophobic interactions and the exclusion of water from the interacting surfaces of proteins may contribute a large but nonspecific component to the energy of binding (90).

A third factor suggested to play a role in immunogenicity of protein epitopes is mobility. Measurement of mobility in the native protein is largely dependent on the availability of a high-resolution crystal structure, and so its applicability is limited to only a small subset of proteins. Furthermore, it has been studied only for antibodies specific for segmental antigenic sites; therefore, it may not apply to the large fraction of antibodies to assembled topographic sites. Studies of mobility have taken two directions. The case of antipeptide antibodies, in which antibodies made to peptides corresponding to more mobile segments of the native protein were more likely to bind to the native protein, has already been discussed (76,91). This is not considered just a consequence of the fact that more mobile segments are likely to be those on the surface and therefore more exposed, because in the case of myohemerythrin (which was used as a model), two regions of the native protein that were equally exposed but less mobile did not bind nearly as well to the corresponding antipeptide antibodies (92). However, as is clear from the earlier discussion, this result applies to antibodies made against short peptides and therefore is not directly relevant to immunogenicity of parts of the native protein. Rather, it concerns the cross-reactivity of antipeptide antibodies with the native protein and is therefore of considerable practical importance for the purposes outlined in the section on antipeptide antibodies.

Studies in the other direction—that is, of antibodies raised against native proteins—are by definition more relevant to the question of immunogenicity of parts of the native protein. Westhof et al. (93) used a series of hexapeptides to determine the specificity of antibodies raised against native tobacco mosaic virus protein and found that six of the seven peptides that bound antibodies to native protein corresponded to peaks of high mobility in the native protein. The correlation was better than could be accounted for just by accessibility, because three peptides that corresponded to exposed regions of only average mobility did not bind antibodies to the native protein. However, when longer peptides—on the order of 20 amino acid residues—were used as probes, it was found that antibodies that bound to less mobile regions of the protein were present in the same antisera (94); they simply had not been detected with the short hexapeptides with less conformational stability. Thus, it was not that the more mobile regions were necessarily more immunogenic but rather that antibodies to these were more easily detected with short peptides as probes. A similar good correlation of antigenic sites with mobile regions of the native protein in the case of myoglobin (93) may also be attributed to the fact that seven of the nine sites were defined with short peptides of six to eight residues (56). Again, this result becomes a statement about cross-reactivity between peptides and native protein rather than about the immunogenicity of the native protein. For reviews, see Van Regenmortel (95) and Getzoff et al. (36).

To address the role of mobility in immunogenicity, an attempt was made to quantitate the relative fraction of antibodies specific for different sites on the antigen myohemerythrin (96). The premise was that, although the entire surface of the protein may be immunogenic, certain regions may elicit significantly more antibodies than others and therefore may be considered immunodominant or at least more immunogenic. Because this study was done with short synthetic peptides from 6 to 14 residues long on the basis of the protein sequence, it was limited to the subset of antibodies specific for segmental antigenic sites. Among these, it was clear that the most immunogenic sites were in regions of the surface that were most mobile, convex in shape, and often of negative electrostatic potential. The role of these parameters has been reviewed (36).

These results have important practical and theoretical implications. First, to use peptides to fractionate antiprotein antisera by affinity chromatography, peptides corresponding to more mobile segments of the native protein should be chosen when possible. If the crystal structure is not known, it may be possible to use peptides from amino or carboxy terminals or from exon–intron boundaries, because these are more likely to be mobile (91). Second, these results may explain how a large but finite repertoire of antibody-producing B cells can respond to any antigen in nature or even artificial antigens never encountered in nature. Protein segments that are more flexible may be able to bind by induced fit in an antibody-combining site that is not perfectly complementary to the average native structure (36,45). Indeed, there is evidence from the crystal structure of antigen–antibody complexes (97–99) that mobility in the antibody-combining site as well as in the antigen may allow both reactants to adopt more complementary conformations on binding to each other: that is, a two-way induced fit. An example comes from the study of antibodies to myohemerythrin (98), in which the data suggested that initial binding of exposed side chains of the antigen to the antibody promoted local displacements that allowed exposure and binding of other, previously buried residues that served as contact residues. The only way this could occur would be for such residues to become exposed during the course of an induced-fit conformational change in the antigen (36,98). In a second very clear example of induced fit, the contribution of antibody mobility to peptide binding was demonstrated for a monoclonal antibody to peptide 75-110 of influenza hemagglutinin, which was crystallized with or without peptide in the binding site and analyzed by x-ray crystallography for evidence of an induced fit (99). Despite flexibility of the peptide, the antibody-binding site probably could not accommodate the peptide without a conformational change in the third complementarity-determining region of the heavy chain, in which an asparagine residue of the antibody was rotated out of the way to allow a tyrosine residue of the peptide to fit in the binding pocket of the antibody (99).

With regard to host-limited factors, immunogenicity is certainly limited by self-tolerance. Thus, the repertoire of potential antigenic sites on mammalian protein antigens such as myoglobin or cytochrome c can be thought of as greatly simplified by the sharing of numerous amino acids with the endogenous host protein. For mouse, guanaco, or horse cytochrome c injected into rabbits, each of the differences between the immunogen and rabbit cytochrome c is seen as an immunogenic site on a background of immunologically silent residues (44,66,100). In another example, rabbit and dog antibodies to beef myoglobin bound almost equally well to beef or sheep myoglobin (101). However, sheep antibodies bound beef but not sheep myoglobin, even though these two myoglobins differ by just six amino acids. Thus, the sheep immune system was able to screen out the clones that would be autoreactive with sheep myoglobin.

Immune response (Ir) genes of the host also play an important role in regulating the ability of an individual to make antibodies to a specific antigen (102). These antigen-specific immunoregulatory genes are among the major histocompatibility complex (MHC) genes that code for transplantation antigens. Structural mutations, gene transfer experiments, and biochemical studies (102) all indicate that Ir genes are actually the structural genes for MHC antigens. The mechanism of action of the MHC antigens works through their effect on helper T cells (described later). There appear to be constraints on B cells in which a T cell of a given specificity can help (103,104), a process called T–B reciprocity (105). Thus, if Ir genes control helper T-cell specificity, they will in turn limit which B cells are activated and thus which antibodies are made.

The immunogenicity of peptide antigens is also limited by intrinsic and extrinsic factors. With less structure to go on, each small peptide must presumably contain some nonself structural feature in order to overcome self-tolerance. In addition, the same peptide must contain antigenic sites that can be recognized by helper T cells as well as by B cells. When no T cell site is present, three approaches may be helpful: graft on a T-cell site, couple the peptide to a carrier protein, or overcome T-cell nonresponsiveness to the available structure with various immunologic agents, such as interleukin 2.

An example of a biologically relevant but poorly immunogenic peptide is the asparagine–alanine–asparagine–proline (NANP) repeat unit of the circumsporozoite (CS) protein of malaria sporozoites. A monoclonal antibody to the repeat unit of the CS protein can protect against murine malaria (106). Thus, it would be desirable to make a malaria vaccine of the repeat unit of *Plasmodium falciparum* $(NANP)_n$. However, only mice of one MHC type (H-2^b) of all mouse strains tested were able to respond to $(NANP)_n$ (107,108). One approach to overcome this limitation is to couple $(NANP)_n$ to a site recognizable by T cells, perhaps a carrier protein such as tetanus toxoid (109). In human trials, this conjugate was weakly immunogenic and only partially protective. Moreover, as helper T cells produced by this approach are specific for the unrelated carrier, a secondary or memory response would not be expected to be elicited by the pathogen itself.

Another choice might be to identify a T cell site on the CS protein itself and couple the two synthetic peptides together to make one complete immunogen. The result with one such site, called Th2R, was to increase the range of responding mouse MHC types by one, to include H-2^k as well as H-2^b (110). This approach has the potential advantage of inducing a state of immunity that could be boosted by natural exposure to the sporozoite antigen. Because both CS-specific T and B cells are elicited by the vaccine, natural exposure to the antigen could help maintain the level of immunity during the entire period of exposure.

Another strategy to improve the immunogenicity of peptide vaccines is to stimulate the T- and B-cell responses artificially by adding interleukin (IL)–2 to the vaccine. Results with myoglobin indicate that genetic nonresponsiveness can be overcome by appropriate doses of IL-2 (111). The same effect was found for peptides derived from malaria proteins

(112) (K. Akaji, D. T. Liu, and I. J. Berkower, unpublished results).

One of the most important possible uses of peptide antigens is as synthetic vaccines. However, even though it is possible to elicit with synthetic peptides anti-influenza antibodies to nearly every part of the influenza hemagglutinin (75), antibodies that neutralize viral infectivity have not been elicited by immunization with synthetic peptides. This may reflect the fact that antibody binding by itself often does not result in virus inactivation. Viral inactivation occurs only when antibody interferes with one of the steps in the life cycle of the virus, including binding to its cell surface receptor, internalization, and virus uncoating within the cell. Apparently, antibodies can bind to most of the exposed surface of the virus without affecting these functions. Only antibodies that bind to certain "neutralizing" sites can inactivate the virus. In addition, as in the case of the VP1 coat protein of poliovirus, certain neutralizing sites are found only on the native protein and not on the heat-denatured protein (113). Thus, not only the site but also the conformation that is bound by the antibodies may be important for the antibody to inactivate the virus. These sites may often be assembled topographic sites not mimicked by peptide segments of the sequence. Perhaps binding of an antibody to such an assembled site can alter the relative positions of the component subsites so as to induce an allosteric neutralizing effect. Alternatively, antibodies to such an assembled site may prevent a conformational change necessary for activity of the viral protein.

One method of mapping neutralizing sites is based on the use of neutralizing monoclonal antibodies. The virus is grown in the presence of neutralizing concentrations of the monoclonal antibody, and virus mutants are selected for the ability to overcome antibody inhibition. These are sequenced, revealing the mutation that permits "escape" by altering the antigenic site for that antibody. This method has been used to map the neutralizing sites of influenza hemagglutinin (114) as well as poliovirus capsid protein VP1 (115). The influenza-escaping mutations are clustered to form an assembled topographic site, with mutations distant from each other in the primary sequence of hemagglutinin but brought together by the three-dimensional folding of the native protein. At first, it was thought that neutralization was the result of steric hindrance of the hemagglutinin-binding site for the cell surface receptor of the virus (116). However, similar work with poliovirus revealed that neutralizing antibodies that bind to assembled topographic sites may inactivate the virus at less than stoichiometric amounts, when at least half of the sites are unbound by antibody (117). The neutralizing antibodies all cause a conformational change in the virus, which is reflected in a change in the isoelectric point of the particles from pH 7 to pH 4 (115,118). Antibodies that bind without neutralizing do not cause this shift. Thus, an alternative explanation for the mechanism of antibody-mediated neutralization is the triggering of the virus to self-destruct.

Perhaps the reason that neutralizing sites are clustered near receptor-binding sites is that occupation of such sites by antibody mimics events normally caused by binding to the cellular receptor, causing the virus to prematurely trigger its cell entry mechanisms. However, in order to transmit a physiological signal, the antibody may need to bind viral capsid proteins in the native conformation (especially assembled topographic sites), which antipeptide antibodies may fail to do. Antibodies of this specificity are similar to the viral receptors on the cell surface, some of which have been cloned and expressed without their transmembrane sequences as soluble proteins. The soluble recombinant receptors for poliovirus (119) and HIV-1 (120–122) exhibit high-affinity binding to the virus and potent neutralizing activity in vitro. The HIV-1 receptor, CD4, has been combined with the human immunoglobulin heavy chain in a hybrid protein, CD4–Ig (123), which spontaneously assembles into dimers and resembles a monoclonal antibody, in which the binding site is the same as the receptor-binding site for HIV-1. In these recombinant constructs, high-affinity binding depends on the native conformation of the viral envelope glycoprotein 120 (gp120).

For HIV-1, two types of neutralizing antibodies have been identified. The first type binds a continuous or segmental determinant, such as the "V3 loop" sequence between amino acids 296 and 331 of gp120 (124–126). Antipeptide antibodies against this site can neutralize the virus (124). However, because this site is located in a highly variable region of the envelope, these antibodies tend to neutralize a narrow range of viral variants with nearly the same sequence as the immunogen. The second type of neutralizing antibody binds conserved sites on the native structure of gp120, allowing them to neutralize a broad spectrum of HIV-1 isolates. These antibodies are commonly found in the sera of infected patients (127), and a panel of neutralizing monoclonal antibodies derived from these subjects has been analyzed.

These monoclonal antibodies can be divided into three types. One group, possibly the most common ones in human polyclonal sera, bind at or near the CD4 receptor–binding site of gp120 (128–132). A second type of monoclonal antibody, 2G12, binds a conformational site on gp120 that also depends on glycosylation but has no direct effect on CD4 binding (133). A third type, quite rare in human sera, is represented by monoclonal antibody 2F5 (134) and binds a conserved site on the transmembrane protein gp41. Although this site is contained on a linear peptide, ELDKWA, antibodies like 2F5 cannot be elicited by immunizing with the peptide, which again suggests the conformational aspect of this site (135,136).

These monoclonal antibodies neutralize fresh isolates, as well as laboratory-adapted strains, and they neutralize viruses tropic for T cells or macrophages (137), regardless of the use of CXCR4 or CCR5 as second receptor. These monoclonal antibodies, which target different sites, act synergistically. A cocktail combining all three types of monoclonal antibodies can protect monkeys against intravenous or vaginal challenge with a simian immunodeficiency virus/HIV hybrid, which indicates the potential for antibodies alone to prevent HIV infection (138,139). Because each of the three conserved neutralizing determinants depends on the native conformation of the protein (140), a prospective gp120 vaccine (or gp160 vaccine) would need to be in the native conformation to be able to elicit these antibodies.

ANTIGENIC DETERMINANTS RECOGNIZED BY T CELLS

Mapping Antigenic Structures

Studies of T-cell specificity for antigen were motivated by the fact that the immune response to protein antigens is regulated at the T-cell level. A hapten, not immunogenic by itself, will elicit antibodies only when coupled to a protein that elicits a T-cell response in that animal. This ability of the protein component of the conjugate to confer immunogenicity on the hapten has been termed the carrier effect. Recognition of the carrier by specific helper T cells induces the B cells to make antibodies. Thus, the factors contributing to a good T-cell response appear to control the B-cell response as well.

"Nonresponder" animals display an antigen-specific failure to respond to a protein antigen, both for T cells and for antibody responses. The "high responder" phenotype for each antigen is a genetically inheritable, usually dominant trait. Among inbred strains of mice, the genes controlling the immune response were found to be tightly linked to the MHC genes (102,141). MHC-linked immune responsiveness has been shown to depend on the T-cell recognition of antigen bound within a groove of MHC antigens of the antigen-presenting cell (APC) (discussed later; see also Chapters 18 and 19). The recognition of antigen in association with MHC molecules of the B cell is necessary for carrier specific T cells to expand and provide helper signals to B cells.

In contrast to the range of antigens recognized by antibodies, the repertoire recognized by helper and cytotoxic T cells appears to be limited largely to protein and peptide antigens, although exceptions, such as the small molecule tyrosine–azobenzene arsonate (142), exist. Once the antigenic determinants on proteins recognized by T cells are identified, it may be possible to better understand immunogenicity and perhaps even to manipulate the antibody response to biologically relevant antigens by altering the helper T-cell response to the antigen.

Polyclonal T-Cell Response

Significant progress in understanding T-cell specificity was made possible by focusing on T-cell proliferation in vitro, mimicking the clonal expansion of antigen-specific clones in vivo. The proliferative response depends on only two cells: the antigen-specific T cell and an APC, usually a macrophage, dendritic cell, or B cell. The growth of T cells in culture is measured as the incorporation of [^{3}H] thymidine into newly formed DNA. Under appropriate conditions, thymidine incorporation increases with antigen concentration. This assay permits the substitution of different APCs and is highly useful in defining the MHC and antigen-processing requirements of the APCs.

Using primarily this assay, researchers have taken several different approaches to mapping T cell epitopes. First, T cells immunized to one protein have been tested for a proliferative response *in vitro* to the identical protein or to a series of naturally occurring variants. By comparing the sequences of stimulatory and nonstimulatory variants, it was possible to identify potential epitopes recognized by T cells. For example, the T-cell response to myoglobin was analyzed by immunizing mice with sperm whale myoglobin and testing the resulting T cells for proliferation in response to a series of myglobins from different species with known amino acid substitutions. The T cells responded to about half of the 12 myoglobin variants tested (143). Conversely, when mice were immunized to horse myoglobin, the reciprocal pattern was observed. The response to the cross-stimulatory myoglobins was as strong as the response to the myoglobin used to immunize the mice. This suggested that a few shared amino acid residues formed an immunodominant epitope that was essential for T-cell activation and that most substitutions had no effect on the dominant epitope. A comparison of the amino acid residues that were conserved in the stimulatory myoglobins with those that were substituted in the nonstimulatory myoglobins revealed that substitutions at a single residue could explain the pattern observed. All myoglobins that cross-stimulated sperm whale–immune T cells had Glu at position 109, whereas all those that cross-stimulated horse-immune T cells had Asp at position 109. No member of one group could stimulate T cells from donors immunized with a myoglobin of the other group. This suggested that an immunodominant epitope recognized by T cells was centered on position 109, regardless of which amino acid was substituted. Usually, this approach has led to correct localization of the antigenic site in the protein (143–145), but the possibility of long-range effects on antigen processing must be kept in mind (see the section on antigen processing). Also, this approach is limited in that it can focus on the correct region of the molecule but cannot define the boundaries of the site or identify all the critical residues because it is limited to testing positions at which amino acid substitutions occur in natural variants. Site-directed mutagenesis may therefore expand the capabilities of this approach.

A second approach is to use short peptide segments of the protein sequence, taking advantage of the fact that T cells specific for soluble protein antigens appear to recognize only segmental antigenic sites, not assembled topographic ones (102,146–150). These may be produced by chemical or enzymatic cleavage of the natural protein (148–156), solid-phase peptide synthesis (155,157–160), or recombinant DNA expression of cloned genes or gene fragments (161). In the case of class I MHC molecule–restricted cytotoxic T cells, viral gene deletion mutants expressing only part of the gene product have also been used (162–164).

In the case of myoglobin-specific T cells, mapping of an epitope to residue Glu 109 was confirmed by use of a synthetic peptide 102-118, which stimulated the T cells (159,165). The T cells elicited by a myoglobin with either Glu or Asp at position 109 could readily distinguish between synthetic peptides containing Glu or Asp at this position. Similar results were obtained with cytochrome c, for which the predominant site recognized by T cells was localized with sequence variants to the region around residue 100 at the carboxyl end of cytochrome (144). Furthermore, the response to cytochrome c peptide 81-104 was as great as the response to the whole molecule. This indicated that a 24–amino acid peptide contained an entire antigenic site recognized by T cells. The T cells could distinguish between synthetic peptides with Lys or Gln at position 99, although both were immunogenic with the same MHC molecule (166–168). This residue determined T-cell memory and specificity and so presumably was interacting with the T-cell receptor. A similar conclusion could be drawn for residue 109 of myoglobin. However, this type of analysis must be used with caution. When multiple substitutions at position 109 were examined for T-cell recognition and MHC binding, residue 109 was found to affect both functions (169). The ultimate use of synthetic peptides to analyze the segmental sites of a protein that are recognized by T cells was to synthesize a complete set of peptides, each staggered by just one amino acid from the previous peptide, corresponding to the entire sequence of hen egg lysozyme peptide HEL (170). Around each immunodominant site, a cluster of several stimulatory peptides was found. The minimum "core" sequence consisted of just the residues shared by all antigenic peptides within a cluster, whereas the full extent of sequences spanning all stimulatory peptides within the same cluster defined the "determinant envelope." These two ways of defining an antigenic site differ, and one interpretation is that each core sequence corresponds to an MHC binding site, whereas the determinant envelope includes the many ways for T cells to recognize the same peptide bound to the MHC.

In each case, the polyclonal T cell response could be mapped to a single predominant antigenic site. These results are consistent with the idea that each protein antigen has a limited number of immunodominant sites (possibly one) recognized by T cells in association with MHC molecules of the high responder type. If none of the antigenic sites could associate with MHC molecules on the APCs, then the strain would be a low responder, and the antigen would have little or no immunogenicity.

Monoclonal T Cells

Further progress in mapping T-cell sites depended on the analysis of cloned T-cell lines. These were either antigen specific T-cell lines made by the method of Kimoto and Fathman (171) or T-cell hybridomas made by the method of Kappler et al. (172). In the former method, T cells are stimulated to proliferate in response to antigen and APCs, rested, and then restimulated. After stimulation, the blasts can be cloned by limiting dilution and grown from a single cell in the presence of IL-2. In the second method, enriched populations of antigen-specific T cells are fused with a drug-sensitive T-cell tumor, and the fused cells are selected for their ability to grow in the presence of the drug. Then the antigen specificity of each fused cell line must be determined. The key to determining this in a tumor line is that antigen-specific stimulation of a T-cell hybridoma results in release of IL-2 even though proliferation is constitutive. T cells produced by either method are useful in defining epitopes, measuring their MHC associations, and studying antigen-processing requirements.

Monoclonal T cells may be useful in identifying which of the many proteins from a pathogen are important for T-cell responses. For instance, Young and Lamb (173) developed a way to screen proteins separated by sodium dodecyl sulfate (SDS)–polyacrylamide gel electrophoresis and blotted onto nitrocellulose for stimulation of T-cell clones and have used this to identify antigens of *Mycobacterium tuberculosis* (174). Mustafa et al. (175) even used T-cell clones to screen recombinant DNA expression libraries to identify relevant antigens of *Mycobacterium leprae*. Use of T cells to map epitopes has been important in defining tumor antigens (176–181).

These findings can be generalized to characterize a large number of epitopes recognized by T cells from a number of protein antigens (Table 4) (182–197). In each case, the entire site is contained on a short peptide. Class I MHC–restricted antigens also follow this rule (198), even when the protein antigen is normally expressed on the surface of infected cells. This applies to viral glycoproteins, such as influenza hemagglutinin, that are recognized by cytolytic T cells after antigen processing (199) (see later section on antigen processing).

Sequential Steps that Focus the T-Cell Response on Immunodominant Determinants

In contrast to antibodies that bind all over the surface of a native protein (44) (see section on protein and polypeptide antigenic determinants), it has been observed that T cells elicited by immunization with the native protein tend to be focused on one or a few immunodominant sites (200–202). This is true whether they were elicited with model mammalian or avian proteins such as cytochrome c (149), myoglobin (148,150), lysozyme (152,185,203,204), insulin (157,189), and ovalbumin (153) or with bacterial, viral, and parasitic proteins from pathogens, such as influenza hemagglutinin (187) or nucleoprotein (198), staphylococcal nuclease (205), or malarial CS protein (110,206). Because the latter category of proteins shares no obvious homology to mammalian proteins, the immunodominance of a few sites cannot be attributed simply to tolerance for the rest of the protein because of homologous host proteins. Moreover, immunodominance is not simply the preemption of the response by a single clone of predominant T cells, because it has been observed that immunodominant sites tend to be the focus for a polyclonal response of a number of distinct T-cell clones that recognize overlapping subsites within the antigenic site or that have

TABLE 4. *Examples of immunodominant T-cell epitopes recognized in association with class II MHC molecules*

Protein	T-cell antigenic sites (reference)	Amphipathic segments
Sperm whale myoglobin	69–78 (148)	64–78
	102–118 (159)	99–117
	132–145 (155)	128–145
Pigeon cytochrome c	93–104 (158)	92–103
Beef cytochrome c	11–25 (192)	9–29
	66–80 (193)	58–78
Influenza	109–119 (186)	97–120
Hemagglutinin	130–140 (187)	—
A/PR/8/34	302–313 (187,188)	291–314
Pork insulin	B 5–16 (157)	4–16
	A 4–14 (189)	1–21
Chicken lysozyme	46–61 (185)	—
	74–86 (184)	72–86
	81–96 (175)	86–102
	109–119 (145)	—
Chicken ovalbumin	323–339 (153)	329–346
Foot and mouth virus VP1	141–160 (191)	148–165
Hepatitis B virus		
Pre-S	120–132 (190)	121–135
Major surface antigen	38–52 (194)	36–49
	95–109 (194)	—
	140–154 (194)	—
λ Repressor protein CI	12–26 (195)	8–25
Rabies virus–spike glycoprotein precursor	32–44 (196)	29–46

MHC, major histocompatibility complex.
Adapted with permission (188).

different sensitivities to substitutions of amino acids within the site (152,153,158,159,170,184,185,207).

Immunodominant antigenic sites appear to be qualitatively different from other sites. For example, in the case of myoglobin, when the number of clones responding to different epitopes after immunization with native protein was quantitated by limiting dilution, it was observed that the bulk of the response to the whole protein in association with the high-responder class II MHC molecules was focused on a single site within residues 102 to 118 (165) (Fig. 6). When T cells in the high × low responder F1 hybrid restricted to each MHC haplotype were compared, there was little difference in the responses to nondominant epitopes, and all the overall difference in magnitude of response restricted by the high versus low responder MHCs could be attributed to the high response to the immunodominant determinant in the former and the complete absence of this response in the latter (Fig. 6). Similar results were found for two different high-responder and two different low-responder MHC haplotypes (165). Why did the response to the other sites not compensate

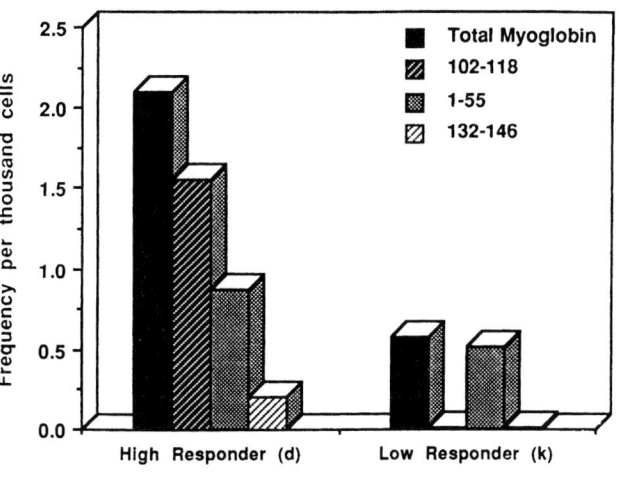

FIG. 6. Frequency of high- and low-responder major histocompatibility complex (MHC)–restricted T cells in F1 hybrid. High responsiveness may be accounted for by the response to a single immunodominant epitope. Lymph node T cells from [low-responder (H-2^k) × high-responder (H-2^b)]F1 hybrid mice immunized with whole myoglobin were plated at different limiting dilutions in microtiter wells with either high-responder or low-responder presenting cells and myoglobin as antigen. The cells growing in each well were tested for responsiveness to whole myoglobin and to various peptide epitopes of myoglobin. The frequency of T cells of each specificity and MHC restriction was calculated from Poisson statistics and is plotted on the ordinate. Most of the difference in T-cell frequency between high- and low-responder restriction types (*solid bars*) can be accounted for by the presence of T cells responding to the immunodominant site at residues 102 to 118, accounting for more than two thirds of the high-responder myoglobin–specific T cells, in contrast to the absence of such T cells restricted to the low-responder MHC type. Based on the data from Kojima et al. (165).

for the lack of response to the immunodominant site in the low responders? The greater frequency of T cells specific for the immunodominant site may in part be attributed to the large number of ways this site can be recognized by different T-cell clones, as mentioned previously, but this only pushes the problem back one level. Why is an immunodominant site the focus for so many different T-cell clones? Because the answer cannot depend on any particular T cell, it must depend on other factors, primarily involved in the steps in antigen processing and presentation by MHC molecules.

It has also been observed that some peptides may be immunogenic themselves, but the T-cell response they elicit is specific only for the peptide and does not cross-react with the native protein, and T cells specific for the native protein do not recognize this site (208–210). These peptides are called *cryptic determinants* (210). The reasons for these differences may involve the way the native protein is processed to produce fragments distinct from but including or overlapping the synthetic peptides used in experiments, and also the competition among sites within the protein for binding to the same MHC molecules, as discussed further in a later section. To understand these factors that determine dominance or crypticity, it is necessary to understand the steps through which an antigen must go before it can stimulate a T-cell response.

In contrast to B cells, T-cell recognition of antigen depends on the function of another cell, the APC (211). Antigen must pass through a number of intracellular compartments and survive processing and transport steps before it can be effectively presented to T cells. After antigen synthesis in the cell (as in a virally infected cell) or antigen uptake through phagocytosis, pinocytosis, or, in some cases, receptor-mediated endocytosis, the subsequent steps include (a) partial degradation ("processing") into discrete antigenic fragments that can be recognized by T cells, (b) transport of these fragments into a cellular compartment in which MHC binding can occur, (c) MHC binding and assembly of a stable peptide/MHC complex, and (d) recognition of that peptide/MHC complex by the expressed T-cell repertoire. At each step, a potential antigenic determinant runs the risk of being lost from the process—for example, by excessive degradation or failure to meet the binding requirements needed for transport to the next step. Only the peptides that surmount the four selective hurdles prove to be antigenic for T cells. Each step is now considered in detail, for its contribution to the strength and specificity of the T-cell response to protein antigens.

Antigen Processing

Influence of Antigen Processing on the Expressed T-Cell Repertoire

Several lines of evidence indicate that antigen processing plays a critical role in determining which potential antigenic sites are recognized and therefore what part of the potential T-cell repertoire is expressed upon immunization with a protein antigen. Because the T cell recognizes not the native antigen but only the products of antigen processing, it is not unreasonable that the nature of these products would at least partly determine which potential epitopes could be recognized by T cells.

One line of evidence that processing plays a major role in T-cell repertoire expression came from comparisons that were made of the immunogenicity of peptide versus native molecule in the cases of myoglobin (208) and lysozyme (209). In the case of myoglobin, a site of equine myoglobin (residues 102 to 118) that did not elicit a response when H-2^k mice were immunized with native myoglobin was nevertheless found to be immunogenic when the mice were immunized with the peptide (208). Thus, the low responsiveness to this site in mice immunized with the native myoglobin did not result from either of the classical mechanisms of Ir gene defects: namely, a hole in the T-cell repertoire or a failure of the site to interact with MHC molecules of that strain. However, the peptide-immune T cells responded only poorly to native equine myoglobin *in vitro*. Thus, the peptide and the native molecule did not cross-react well in either direction. The problem was not simply a failure to process the native molecule to produce this epitope, because (H-2^k × H-2^s)F1-presenting cells could present this epitope to H-2^s T cells when given native myoglobin but could not present it to H-2^k T cells. Also, because the same results applied to individual T-cell clones, the failure to respond to the native molecule was apparently not caused by suppressor cells induced by the native molecule. Similar observations were made for the response to the peptide 74-96 of hen lysozyme in B10.A mice (209). The peptide, not the native molecule, induced T cells specific for this site, and these T cells did not cross-react with the native molecule. With the previously discussed alternative mechanisms excluded, the conclusion is that an appropriate peptide was produced, but it differed from the synthetic peptide in such a way that a hindering site outside the minimal antigenic site interfered with presentation by presenting cells of certain MHC types. Further evidence consistent with this mechanism came from the work of Shastri et al. (212), who found that different epitopes within the 74-to-96 region of lysozyme were immunodominant in H-2^b mice when different forms of the immunogen were used.

Another line of evidence came from fine specificity studies of individual T-cell clones. Shastri et al. (213) observed that H-2^b T-cell clones specific for hen lysozymes were about 100-fold more sensitive to ring-necked pheasant lysozyme than to hen lysozyme. Nevertheless, they were equally sensitive to the cyanogen bromide cleavage fragments containing the antigenic sites from both lysozymes. Thus, regions outside the minimal antigenic site removable by cyanogen bromide cleavage presumably interfered with processing, presentation, or recognition of the corresponding site in hen lysozyme. Similarly, it was observed that a T-cell clone specific for sperm whale myoglobin, not equine myoglobin, responded equally well to the minimal epitope synthetic peptides from the two species (208). In this case, too, residues outside the actual site must be distinguishing equine from

sperm whale myoglobin. Experiments using F1-presenting cells that can clearly produce this epitope for presentation to other T cells proved that the problem was not a failure to produce the appropriate fragment from hen lysozyme (209) or equine myoglobin (208). Thus, these cases provide evidence that a structure outside the minimal site can hinder presentation in association with a particular MHC molecule.

Such a hindering structure was elegantly identified in a study by Grewal et al. (214), who compared hen egg lysozyme peptides presented by strains C57BL/6 and C3H.SW that share H-2^b but differ in non-MHC genes. After immunization with whole lysozyme, a strong T-cell response to peptide 46-61 was seen in C3H.SW mice but not at all in C57BL/6 mice. Because the F1 hybrids of these two strains responded, the lack of response in one strain was not caused by a hole in the T-cell repertoire produced by self-tolerance. It was found that peptide 46-60 bound directly to the IA^b class II MHC molecule, whereas peptide 46-61 did not, which indicates that the C-terminal Arg at position 61 hindered binding. Evidently, a non-MHC–linked difference in antigen processing allowed this Arg to be cleaved off the peptide 46-61 in C3H.SW mice, in which the peptide was dominant, but not in C57BL/6 mice, in which the peptide was cryptic.

Even a small peptide that does not need processing may nevertheless be processed, and that processing may affect its interaction with MHC molecules. Fox et al. (215) found that substitution of a tyrosine for isoleucine at position 95 of cytochrome c peptide 93-103 enhanced presentation with Eβ^b but diminished presentation with Eβ^k when live APCs were used but not when the APCs were fixed and could not process antigen. Therefore, the tyrosine residue was not directly interacting with the different MHC molecule but was affecting the way the peptide was processed, which in turn affected MHC interaction.

In addition to the mechanisms suggested previously, Gammon et al. (209) and Sercarz et al. (216) proposed the possibility of competition between different MHC-binding structures ("antigen-restriction-topes," or "agretopes") within the same processed fragment. If a partially unfolded fragment first binds to MHC by one such site already exposed, further processing may stop, and other potential binding sites for MHC may never become accessible for binding. Such competition could also occur between different MHC molecules on the same presenting cell (209). For instance, BALB/c mice, expressing both A^d and E^d, produce a response to hen lysozyme specific for 108 to 120, not for 13 to 35 (209), and this response is restricted to E^d. However, B10.GD mice that express only A^d respond well to 13 to 35 when immunized with lysozyme. BALB/c mice clearly express an A^d molecule, and so the failure to present this 13 to 35 epitope may result from competition from E^d, which may preempt presentation by binding the 108 to 120 site with higher affinity and preventing the 13 to 35 site from binding to A^d. Competition between different peptides binding to the same MHC molecule could also occur.

All these results together indicate that antigen processing not only facilitates interaction of the antigenic site with the MHC molecule or the T-cell receptor, or both, but also influences the specificity of these interactions and, in turn, the specificity of the elicited T-cell repertoire. The molecular mechanisms behind such effects are just now being elucidated, as described in the next sections.

Processing of Antigen for T Cells Restricted to Class II Major Histocompatibility Complex Molecules

It has long been known that T-cell responses such as delayed hypersensitivity *in vivo* or T-cell proliferation *in vitro* to exogenous proteins can be stimulated not only by the native protein but also by denatured protein (146) and fragments of native protein (189). Indeed, this feature, along with the requirement for recognition in association with class II MHC molecules, distinguishes T- from B-cell responses. In a number of cases, the site recognized by cloned T cells has been pinpointed to a discrete synthetic peptide corresponding to a segment of the primary sequence of the protein. Examples include insulin (157,189), cytochrome c (158), lysozyme (152,184), and myoglobin (148,155,159). In each case, the stimulatory peptide must contain all the information required

for antigen presentation and T-cell stimulation. The lack of conformational specificity does not indicate a lack of T-cell receptor specificity. Rather, it results from antigen processing into peptide fragments that destroys conformational differences before binding the T-cell receptor. One way to accomplish this is through antigen processing, which involves the partial degradation of a protein antigen into peptide fragments (see Fig. 7).

Evidence of processing came from the fact that a single protein antigen could stimulate T cells to different epitopes, each specific for a different MHC antigen. For example, when a series of myoglobin-specific T-cell clones were tested for both antigen specificity and MHC restriction, six clones were found to be specific for a site centering on amino acid Glu 109, and all six recognized the antigen in association with IA^d. Nine additional T-cell clones were specific for a second epitope centered on Lys 140 and were restricted to a different MHC antigen, IE^d. Thus, the antigen behaved as if it was split up into distinct epitopes, each with its own ability to bind MHC (182).

That T cells recognize processed antigen was demonstrated by the fact that inhibitors of processing can block antigen presentation. Early experiments by Ziegler and Unanue (217) showed that processing depends on intracellular degradative

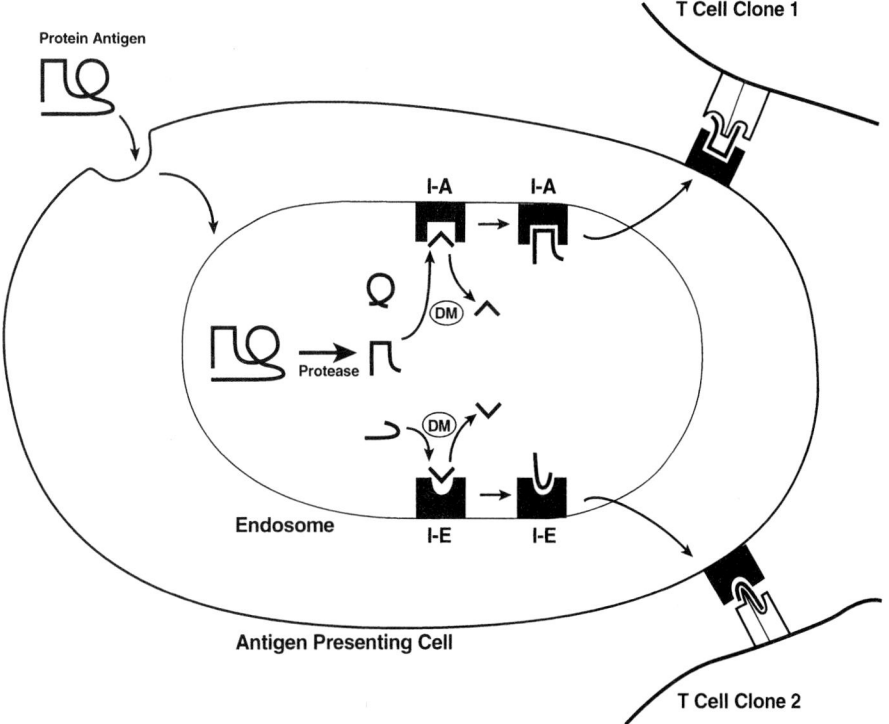

FIG. 7. Steps in antigen presentation by class II major histocompatibility complex (MHC) molecules. Soluble antigen enters the presenting cell by phagocytosis, pinocytosis, or receptor-mediated endocytosis. It is partially degraded to peptide fragments by acid-dependent proteases in endosomes. Antigenic peptides associate with class II MHC molecules (IA or IE in the mouse) to form an antigenic complex that is transported to the cell surface. Before a class II MHC molecule can bind the peptide, it must release the class II-associated invariant chain peptide (CLIP) fragment of invariant chain from the binding groove, which is catalyzed by human leukocyte antigen–DM. Binding of T cell receptors to the peptide/MHC complex triggers T-cell proliferation, resulting in clonal expansion of antigen-specific T cells.

endosomes, because drugs such as chloroquine and NH_4Cl, which raise endosomal pH and inhibit acid-dependent proteases, could block the process. However, prior degradation of proteins into peptide fragments allows them to trigger T cells even in the presence of these inhibitors of processing (218). For example, T-cell clone 14.5 recognizes the Lys 140 site of myoglobin equally well on the antigenic peptide (residues 132 to 153) as on the native protein (Fig. 8). The difference between these two forms of antigen is brought out by inhibition of processing. Leupeptin, for example, inhibits lysosomal proteases and blocks the T-cell responses to native myoglobin but not to peptide 132 to 153. Thus, native myoglobin cannot stimulate T cells without further processing, whereas the peptide requires little or no additional processing (219).

Why is antigen processing necessary? For class II MHC molecules, experiments suggest that antigen processing may uncover functional sites that are buried in the native protein structure. For example, a form of intact myoglobin that has

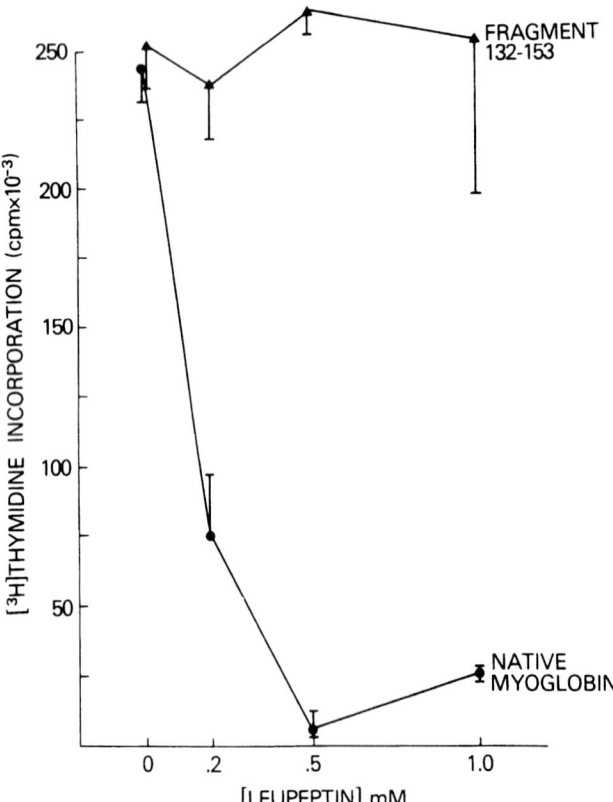

FIG. 8. Inhibition of antigen presentation by the protease inhibitor leupeptin: differential effect on presentation of the same epitope of native myoglobin or peptide 132 to 153 to the same monoclonal T-cell population. Splenic antigen-presenting cells, were incubated with leupeptin at the concentration indicated for 15 minutes before and during exposure to 2-μM native myoglobin or 1-μM peptide fragment, washed, irradiated, and cultured with T cells of clone 14.5 specific for this epitope; thymidine incorporation was measured after 4 days of culture. See Streicher et al. (219).

been partially unfolded through chemical modification can behave like a myoglobin peptide and can be presented by APC even in the presence of enough protease inhibitor or chloroquine to completely block the presentation of native myoglobin (219). Denatured lysozyme could also be presented without processing to one T-cell clone (154). This result suggests that the requirement for processing may simply be a steric requirement—that is, to uncover the two sites needed to form the trimolecular complex between antigen and MHC and between antigen and T-cell receptor. Thus, unfolding may be sufficient without proteolysis, and proteolysis may simply accomplish an unfolding analogous to Alexander's approach to the Gordian knot.

The importance of antigen unfolding for T-cell recognition and the ability of unfolding to bypass the need for antigen processing apply to a range of polypeptide sizes from small peptides to extremely large proteins. At one extreme, Lee et al. (220) found that even fibrinogen, of Mr 340,000, does not need to be processed if the epitope recognized is on the carboxy-terminal portion of the α chain, which is naturally unfolded in the native molecule. At the other extreme, even a small peptide of only 18 amino acid residues, apamin, requires processing unless the two disulfide bonds that hold it in the native conformation are cleaved artificially to allow unfolding (221). Therefore, large size does not mandate processing, and small size does not necessarily obviate the need for processing, at least for class II MHC presentation. The common feature throughout the size range seems to be the need for unfolding. This evidence, taken together with the earlier data on unfolding of myoglobin and lysozyme, strongly supports the conclusion that unfolding, rather than size reduction, is the primary goal of antigen processing and that either antigen presentation by MHC molecules or T-cell receptor recognition frequently requires exposure of residues not normally exposed on the surface of the native protein. This conclusion is supported by studies of peptides eluted from class II MHC molecules, and the crystal structures of class II MHC/peptide complexes, which show that longer peptides can bind with both ends extending beyond the two ends of the MHC groove (222–224) (see later section on antigen interaction with MHC molecules).

Besides proteolysis, unfolding may require the reduction of disulfide bonds between or within protein antigens. A γ-interferon–inducible lysosomal thiol reductase (GILT) is expressed in APCs and localizes to the late endosomal and lysosomal compartments where MHC class II peptide loading occurs (225). Unlike thioredoxin, this enzyme works at the acid pH of endosomes and uses Cys but not glutathione as a reducing agent. APCs from GILT knockout mice were tested for the ability to present hen egg lysozyme to HEL-specific T-cell lines (226). For two epitopes, the T-cell response was insensitive to the GILT defect, even though they involved a disulfide bond in the native protein. However, for one epitope, located between disulfide bonds, the T-cell response was completely inhibited when the APCs lacked GILT. In this case, reduction of disulfide bonds was an essential step for antigen presentation, presumably needed to generate free peptides for class II MHC binding.

Processing of Antigen for T Cells Restricted to Class I Major Histocompatibility Complex Molecules

In contrast to class II MHC–restricted T cells, it was widely assumed that class I MHC–restricted T cells, such as cytolytic T cells (CTLs) specific for virus-infected cells, responded mainly to unprocessed viral glycoproteins expressed on the surface of infected cells. However, in the mid-1980s, evidence that CTL also recognized processed antigens began to appear. For example, influenza nucleoprotein (NP) was found to be a major target antigen for influenza-specific CTLs, even though NP remains in the nucleus of infected cells and none is detectable on the cell surface (227). Further support came from the finding that target cells that take up synthetic NP peptide 366-379 were lysed by NP-specific CTLs (198). This constitutes evidence that antigen presented in association with class I MHC molecules requires processing into antigenic fragments. Also, the demonstration that synthetic peptides could sensitize targets for CTLs introduced a powerful tool for mapping and studying CTL epitopes.

Even for hemagglutinin, surface expression of native antigen was found not to be required for antigenicity, which implies that the processed antigen stimulates a T-cell response. Target cells expressing leader-negative hemagglutinin, which is not transported to the cell surface but remains in the cytosol, were lysed equally well as those with surface hemagglutinin (199). Similar conclusions were drawn from anchor-negative mutants (228). Indeed, studies of HIV-1 pg160 genes with or without a leader sequence suggest that removal of the leader sequence can increase the amount of protein that is retained in the cytosol and is available for processing and presentation through the class I MHC processing pathway (229). The explanation may be that the signal peptide results in cotranslational translocation of the growing peptide chain into the endoplasmic reticulum, whereas proteins without a signal peptide are synthesized in full and remain in the cytosol, where they are accessible to the processing machinery of the class I MHC pathway (see later discussion). This cytosolic protein processing machinery consists primarily of the 26S proteasomes (230,231). The specificity of such proteasomes to cleave at certain positions in a protein sequence thus provides the first hurdle that a potential epitope must surmount to be presented by class I MHC molecules, to be cut out correctly but not destroyed by the proteasome.

In the standard proteasome, 14 distinct subunits assemble to form a high-molecular-weight complex of about 580 kDa with five distinct protease activities, located at distinct sites. The proteasome is a barrel-shaped structure, with the protease activities arrayed on the inner surface, and unfolded proteins are believed to enter the barrel at one end, leaving as peptides at the other end. The different proteases cut preferentially after aromatic or branched-chain amino acids (chymotryptic-like activity), branched-chain amino acids (primarily aliphatic), basic amino acids (trypsin-like activity), acidic residues (glutamate preferring), or small neutral amino acid residues (232,233). Protease activity is increased against misfolded proteins, such as senescent proteins or viral proteins produced during infection, and proteins synthesized with artificial amino acids are particularly susceptible to degradation by proteasomes. The products of protease digestion are peptides, including nonamers, of just the right size for MHC binding. The chymotryptic and trypsin-like activities may be particularly important for antigenic peptides, because many peptides that naturally bind MHC end in hydrophobic or basic residues (234).

The proteasome is the major processing machinery of the nonendosomal processing pathway. This is shown by the effect of proteasome inhibitors on class I MHC assembly and antigen presentation and by the effect of low-molecular-weight protein (LMP)–2 and LMP-7 mutations on antigen processing. A family of proteasome inhibitors described (232,233,235) as consisting of short peptides, three to four amino acids in length, ending in an aldehyde, such as Ac-Leu Leu norLeu-al and carbobenzoxy-Leu Leu norVal-al (233), or nonpeptides such as lactacystin (236). Although the peptides appear to be directed primarily at the chymotrypsin-like protease activity, as false substrates, they actually inhibit all three types of protease activity.

By inhibiting antigen processing, these inhibitors induce a phenotype of reduced expression of class I MHC and inability to present antigen to class I MHC–restricted CTL (233). The class I MHC heavy chains remain in the endoplasmic reticulum, as shown by failure to become resistant to endoglycosidase H (237), which occurs in the Golgi apparatus. They are also unable to form stable complexes with β_2-microglobulin, because of a lack of peptides. These effects are specific for the protease function, because the inhibitors do not block presentation of synthetic peptides, which also rescue class I MHC expression, and because inhibition is reversible when inhibitor is removed. These results suggest that proteasomes are the primary supplier of antigenic peptides for class I MHC, inasmuch as other pathways are unable to compensate. However, it is possible that the inhibitors could block other potential processing enzymes as well. One alternative processing pathway is provided by signal peptidase. As signal peptides are cleaved from proteins entering the endoplasmic reticulum, these hydrophobic peptides can bind class I MHC (238). Particularly for MHC molecules such as human leukocyte antigen (HLA)–A2, which prefer hydrophobic sequences, this peptidase can be an important source of antigenic peptides that are independent of proteasomes and transporter associated with antigen processing types 1 and 2 (TAP1 and TAP2) transport (see the following section), because they are formed inside the endoplasmic reticulum.

Interestingly, the MHC itself encodes, near the class II MHC region, three proteins, known as LMP-2, LMP-7, and multicatalytic endopeptidase complex–like 1, (MECL-1), that contribute to the proteasome structure. The LMP-2,

MECL-1, and LMP-7 subunits are up-regulated by interferon-γ and substitute for the subunits β1, β2, and β5, respectively, forming what has been dubbed an *immunoproteasome,* present in professional APCs. All complexes with LMPs contain proteasome proteins, but only 5% to 10% of proteasomes contain LMP-2 and LMP-7.

These MHC-encoded subunits of the immunoproteasome shift the preference of proteasomes for cleaving after certain sequences, resulting in the production of different peptide fragments (239–241). Proteasomes lacking LMP-2 through mutation or gene knockout have the same affinity but decreased cleavage rate for sequences ending in hydrophobic or basic amino acids. The effect is specific for these proteolytic sites, because the activity against of sequences containing acidic amino acids is actually increased (240). Despite the shift in specific peptides released, the overall level of class I MHC expression was reduced only slightly in LMP-7 knockouts (241) and not at all in the LMP-2 knockouts. However, presentation of specific epitopes of the male H-Y antigen or of influenza nucleoprotein was reduced by threefold to fivefold in these knockouts. Toes et al. (242) quantitatively compared the cleavage fragments produced by standard proteasomes and immunoproteasomes and defined the prevalence of different amino acids on each side of the cleavage site. In accordance with the earlier studies, there was a strong preference for both to cleave after leucine and also, to a lesser extent, after other hydrophobic residues, both aliphatic and aromatic. However, the immunoproteasomes have a stronger tendency to cleave after such hydrophobic residues and a much reduced cleavage frequency after acidic residues Asp and Glu than do standard or constitutive proteasomes. This shift in specificity is concordant with the observation that class I MHC molecules tend to bind peptides with C-terminal hydrophobic or basic residues, not acidic ones. Thus, the immunoproteasomes in professional APCs may be more effective at generating antigenic peptides that can be presented by MHC molecules (239,242). Immunoproteasomes were shown to be essential for production of a hepatitis B virus core antigenic epitope (243), and to increase production of epitopes from adenovirus (244) and lymphocytic choriomeningitis virus (245). On the other hand, some epitopes are generated more effectively by the constitutive proteasome than by the immunoproteasome (246). When the repertoires of seven defined class I MHC–restricted epitopes were compared in an elegant quantitative study in LMP-2–deficient and wild-type C57BL/6 mice, it was found that responses to the two epitopes that are immunodominant in wild-type mice were greatly reduced in the LMP-2–deficient mice, which lack immunoproteasomes, and two normally subdominant epitopes became dominant (247). However, from adoptive transfer experiments in both directions, it was found that the reduced response to one normally dominant epitope was caused by decreased production without immunoproteasomes but the reduced response to the other was caused by an altered T-cell repertoire in the LMP-2–deficient mice, presumably as a result of alterations in the peptides presented in the thymus. Furthermore, the increased response to one of the subdominant determinants was related to increased production of this peptide by the constitutive proteasomes in comparison with the immunoproteasomes. Thus, the immunoproteasome specificity plays a significant role in determining the repertoire of epitopes presented and in selecting those that are immunodominant, as well as regulating the CD8$^+$ T-cell repertoire generated in the thymus.

Another protein associated with proteasomes is PA28, which assembles into 11S structures (248). Like LMP-2 and LMP-7 (239), PA28 is inducible by interferon-γ, and its induction causes a shift in proteasome function that may lead to the production of different antigenic peptides. For example, synthetic substrates were designed to test the ability of proteasomes to generate authentic MHC binding peptides. These substrates contained the MHC binding ligand flanked by the natural sequence as found in the original protein.

To generate the MHC binding ligand, the proteasome would have to cleave the substrate twice (249). By itself, the 20S proteasome was able to produce singly cleaved fragments, but with added PA28, doubly cut peptides were generated preferentially. Thus, PA28 favored the production of antigenic peptides, possibly by keeping the peptide in the proteasome until processing was complete. Alternatively, PA28 may coordinate the proteolytic activity of two adjacent sites to generate doubly cut peptides of just the right length (octamers to nonamers) to fit in the MHC groove. The distance between these nearby sites would determine the size of the peptides produced. PA28 has been shown to increase generation of a dominant lymphocytic choriomeningitis virus epitope independently of the presence of the other interferon-γ–inducible components LMP-2, LMP-7, and MECL-1 (250).

The specificity of this proteasomal processing system determines the first step in winnowing the number of protein segments that can become CTL epitopes, by selectively producing some peptide fragments in abundance and destroying others. Thus, it is probably not just coincidental that the C-terminal residues produced by proteasomal cleavage often serve as anchor residues for binding class I MHC molecules or that the lengths of peptides produced are optimal for class I MHC binding (239,251). A better understanding of the specificity of proteasomes will contribute to the new methods for predicting dominant CD8$^+$ T-cell epitopes (202).

Transport into a Cellular Compartment where Major Histocompatibility Complex Binding Can Occur

The second hurdle that a potential epitope must surmount is to be transported into the cellular compartment for loading onto MHC molecules. These compartments are different for class I and class II MHC molecules, as noted earlier.

Transport Pathways Leading to Class I Major Histocompatibility Complex Presentation

The second hurdle for peptide presentation by class I MHC molecules is to get from the cytosol, where the peptides are produced, to the endoplasmic reticulum, where the newly synthesized class I MHC molecules are assembled and loaded with peptide. The discovery of a specific active transporter suggested that specificity of transport could further restrict the repertoire of peptides available to load onto class I MHC molecules. Genetic analysis of mutant cell lines that failed to load endogenous peptides onto class I MHC molecules revealed homozygous deletions of part of the class II MHC region near the DR locus. Molecular cloning of DNA from this region revealed at least 12 genes, of which two, TAP1 and TAP2, showed a typical sequence for adenosine triphosphate binding cassette transporter proteins (252–254). Their function is to transport processed peptides from the cytosol to the endoplasmic reticulum. Once in this compartment, peptides are handed off by TAP to newly formed class I MHC molecules and stabilize a trimolecular complex with β_2-microglobulin. This complex is then transported to the cell surface, where antigen presentation occurs. Without the peptide transporters, empty dimers of class I MHC with β_2-microglobulin form, but these are unstable. Excess free peptide would rescue class I MHC by stabilizing the few short-lived empty complexes that reach the surface, as shown by Townsend et al. (255) and Schumacher et al. (256). Thus, MHC-linked genes coding for proteolysis, peptide transport, and presentation at the cell surface have been identified. In effect, the MHC now appears to encode a complex system of multiple elements devoted to the rapid display of foreign protein determinants on the surface of an infected cell. By continuously sampling the output of the protein synthesizing machinery, this system permits rapid identification and destruction of infected cells by CTL before infectious virus can be released.

In an infected cell, as soon as viral proteins are made, peptide fragments generated by the proteasome become available to the TAP1 and TAP2 transporter proteins (Fig. 9). These transport the peptide fragments into the endoplasmic reticulum for association with newly formed class I MHC molecules, which would carry them to the cell surface for antigen presentation, all within 30 minutes. Indeed, the finding of a physical association between TAP and the nascent class I MHC heavy chain/β_2-microglobulin complex suggests that the peptide may be directly handed off from TAP to the new MHC molecule without being free in solution (257,258). If TAP transport is highly selective, then some cytosolic peptides may fail to enter the endoplasmic reticulum for presentation with class I MHC, but if it is promiscuous, then some peptides that were better off not presented, such as those leading to autoimmunity, may be transported.

The idea that other proteins may control accessibility of class I MHC binding sites for peptides originally came from the observation that two rat strains with the same MHC type (RT1.A^a) were nevertheless not histocompatible, and CTL could recognize the difference between them (259). The difference, called a class I modification (cim) effect, occurred because different peptides were binding the same MHC in the two strains (260,261). The rat has two alleles for a peptide transporter supplying peptides to the MHC. TAP2A has peptide specificity matching that of RT1.A^a and delivers a broad set of peptides for MHC binding. The other transporter allele,

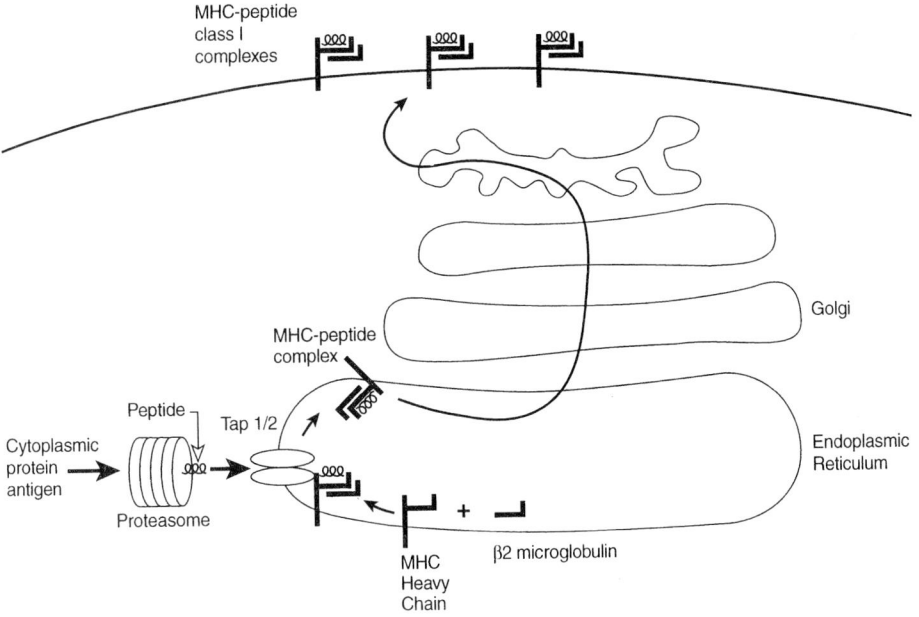

FIG. 9. Cytoplasmic antigen processing pathway leading to class I major histocompatibility complex (MHC) presentation. Cytoplasmic antigen is degraded to fragments in the proteasome, which are transported into the endoplasmic reticulum by the transporter associated with antigen processing (TAP). Peptide supplied by TAP forms a stable complex with class I MHC heavy chains and β_2-microglobulin, and the complex is transported through the Golgi apparatus, where it achieves mature glycosylation, and out to the cell surface for presentation to class I MHC–restricted T cells.

TAP2B, supplies a different set of peptides that are discordant with RT1.A^a, and so fewer types of peptides are bound. Although RT1.A^a would prefer to bind peptides with Arg at position 9, it has to settle for peptides with hydrophobic terminals as provided by TAP2B (262), thereby accounting for the apparent histocompatibility difference. Thus, the specificity of TAP transport was shown to provide a selective step in narrowing the potential repertoire of CTL epitopes.

To measure TAP specificity in other species, a transportable peptide bearing an N-terminal glycosylation site was added to cells made permeable by treatment with streptolysin. If the peptide was transported by TAP, it would enter the endoplasmic reticulum and *cis*-Golgi apparatus, where it would be glycosylated (263–265). The extent of glycosylation served as a measure of TAP function. When competitor peptides were added as well, TAP-mediated transport of the reporter peptide decreased, which indicated saturation of peptide-binding sites. In this way, a series of related peptides could be tested for the ability to compete for TAP binding and transport in order to identify the requirements for TAP binding and transport.

TAP binding and transport depended strongly on peptide length (265,266). Mouse TAP was shown to have a strong preference for peptides of nine residues or longer (266). For human TAP, peptides shorter than seven amino acids long were not transported, regardless of sequence (265). Almost all peptides 8 to 11 amino acids long were transported, with some variation in binding affinities, depending on sequence. Peptides 14 to 21 amino acids in length were transported selectively, whereas those longer than 24 amino acids were almost never transported intact. Thus, human TAP transport selected against peptides less than 7 or more than 24 amino acids in length, regardless of sequence.

Although TAP can and must transport a wide variety of peptides, it may nonetheless have preferences for which peptides are transported most efficiently and which MHC types are provided with the peptides they need. For example, a self-peptide that naturally binds HLA-B27 was modified slightly to produce an N-terminal glycosylation site, resulting in the sequence RRYQNSTEL (265). When the glycosylation of this peptide was used to measure transport, saturation of TAP by homologous peptides occurred with a 50% inhibitory concentration of less than 1 μM. Other peptides with unrelated sequences also inhibited, often with equally high affinity. Not only did natural HLA-binding peptides compete but so did peptide variants lacking the MHC binding motif at positions 2 and 9 (see later discussion). Clearly, peptides binding different MHC types were transported by the same TAP protein, and even peptides that bound mouse MHC were transported by human TAP. In another example, in which rat TAP proteins were used, peptides with Pro at position 2, 6, or 9 were found to be poor competitors for transport of a reference peptide (264).

In another approach, in which a baculovirus system overexpressing TAP proteins in microsomes was used, the affinity of TAP binding was determined for a wide variety of synthetic peptides, allowing mapping of the important residues (267,268). Binding, rather than transport, appears to be the major step determining TAP peptide selectivity (269). Indeed, artificial neural networks have been developed to predict peptide binding to human TAP (270). With this scheme, it was found that peptides eluted from three different human class I MHC molecules had higher predicted affinities for TAP than did a control set of peptides with equal binding to those class I MHC molecules, which supported the hypothesis that TAP specificity contributes to the selection of the subset of peptides able to bind a class I MHC molecule that actually bind *in vivo* (270). Unlike class I MHC, there were no anchor positions at which a specific amino acid was required. However, there were several positions where substituting the wrong amino acid caused a marked reduction in TAP binding. In a typical class I MHC–binding nonamer, the strongest substitution effects were observed at position 9 (P9), followed by substitutions at P2 and P3, followed by P1. At the carboxy-terminal P9 position, the preferred residues were Tyr and Phe (as well as Arg and Lys), whereas Glu was worst, causing a 3-log reduction in binding. Similarly, substituting Pro at P2 caused a 1.5- to 2-log reduction in binding, in comparison with preferred residues Arg, Val, and Ile. TAP preferences such as these would selectively transport some peptides more than others from cytoplasm to the endoplasmic reticulum. Use of combinatorial peptide libraries independently confirmed that the critical residues influencing TAP transport were the first three N-terminal residues and the last C-terminal residue (271).

Interestingly, these preferred residues are many of the same ones forming the class I MHC binding motifs (P2 and P9). However, because the MHC binding motifs differ from each other, it is not possible for TAP preferences to match them all. For example, the TAP preference for Arg at P2 and for Phe, Tyr, Leu, Arg, or Lys at P9 overlaps with the binding motif of HLA-B27 and may favor the transport of peptide ligands for this MHC type. Remarkably, the variant B*2709, which does not prefer Tyr or Phe at P9, is not associated with autoimmune disease as in the more common form of HLA-B27. In contrast, HLA-B7 requires a Pro at P2, which greatly decreases TAP binding. Similarly, some peptides binding HLA-A2 have hydrophobic residues unfavorable for TAP binding, which suggests suboptimal compatibility between TAP and the most common class I HLA allele. Measurements with a series of naturally presented peptides from HLA-A2 and HLA-B27 indicated a mean 300-fold higher affinity of TAP for the HLA-B27 peptides than for those from HLA-A2, and some of the HLA-A2 peptides did not bind TAP at all (270). How are these low-affinity peptides delivered to MHC? One suggestion is that peptide ligands for HLA-A2 and HLA-B7 may be transported as a larger precursor peptide containing the correct amino acids, which are then trimmed off to fit the MHC groove. A series of studies support this mechanism, showing that longer peptide precursors are trimmed at the N-terminal by aminopeptidases in the endoplasmic reticulum to form HLA-A2–binding peptides (272) and that peptides with a Pro at position 2, needed to bind to certain MHC molecules but poorly transported, are produced from longer precursors, which are transported, by N-terminal trimming in the endoplasmic reticulum by aminopeptidases (273). In fact, the inability of the aminopeptidase to cleave beyond a residue preceding a Pro naturally leads to trimming of peptides to produce ones with a Pro at position 2. Alternatively, some of these peptides may derive from signal peptides and enter the endoplasmic reticulum in a TAP-independent manner. The significance of selective peptide transport may be to limit immunity to self-peptides. If the match between HLA-B27 and TAP specificity is too good, it may contribute to the increased incidence of autoimmune disease associated with HLA- B27 (267). An effect of human TAP specificity in loading of peptides in viral infection has confirmed the biological significance of TAP specificity (274). TAP binding specificity also limited the repertoire of alloantigenic peptides presented by HLA-B27 (275).

The importance of TAP proteins to antiviral immunity is shown by the fact that certain herpesviruses have targeted TAP1 function as a way to interfere with antigen presentation to CD8$^+$ CTL. A herpes simplex virus (HSV) type 1 immediate early viral protein called ICP47 binds to TAP and inhibits its function, causing reduced expression of new class I MHC molecules on the cell surface and inability to present viral or other antigens with class I MHC molecules (276–278). As a way to evade immune surveillance, this strategy could contribute to viral persistence in chronic infection and viral activation in recurrent disease, as frequently occurs with HSV-1 and HSV-2. These findings also raise the possibility of making a live attenuated ICP47-defective HSV vaccine that would be more immunogenic than natural infection.

Transport Pathways Leading to Class II Major Histocompatibility Complex Presentation

Unlike the class I MHC pathway, which delivers peptides to MHC, the class II MHC pathway transports MHC molecules to the endosomal compartment, where antigenic peptides are produced. During transport, the peptide-binding groove must be kept free of endogenous peptides. The cell uses one protein, called invariant chain [and its processed fragment, class II-associated chain peptide (CLIP)], to block the binding site until needed and another protein, HLA-DM, to facilitate release of CLIP peptides and their exchange for antigenic peptides as they become available.

Class II MHC molecules assemble in the endoplasmic reticulum, where α and β chains form a complex with invariant chain (279–281). Invariant chain binds MHC and blocks the peptide-binding groove, so that endogenous peptides transported into the endoplasmic reticulum, for example by TAP, cannot bind (280,282–287). The complex of α, β, and invariant chains, consisting of nine polypeptide chains in all (288), is transported via the Golgi apparatus and directed by signals on invariant chain into endosome/lysosome–like vesicles called *class II MHC compartments*. The compart-

ments contain acid-activated proteases capable of digesting foreign proteins into antigenic peptides. In addition, they degrade invariant chain to CLIP, which corresponds to amino acids 80 to 103. As long as CLIP remains in the binding groove, antigenic peptides cannot bind, and so the rate of CLIP release limits the capacity of MHC to take up antigenic peptides.

Peptide loading can be measured by its effect on MHC structure. When a class II MHC molecule binds a peptide, it changes conformation, and certain monoclonal antibodies are specific for the peptide-bound conformation (289). Also, the α-β complex becomes more stable after peptide binding, which can be detected by running the MHC on an SDS gel without boiling. The peptide-bound form runs on gels as a large α-β dimer, whereas MHC without peptides (but still bound to CLIP) is unstable under these conditions and falls apart to yield α and β chain monomers on SDS gels (290).

Mutant cell lines have been generated with a deletion between HLA-DP and HLA-DQ genes on chromosome 6 (289,291–293). These cells express normal levels of class II MHC structural proteins, HLA-DQ, and HLA-DR but fail to present protein antigens (293). Some of their class II MHC proteins appear on the cell surface, but more are retained in the class II MHC compartments. Biochemically, they still contain CLIP peptides (294), rather than peptide antigens, and they have not achieved the conformation (289) or SDS stability of peptide-binding class II MHCs (295). The defect was discovered to result from loss of either of the two chains of a class II molecule, HLA-DM, and the phenotype can be corrected by adding back the missing gene (296). In the presence of normal HLA-DM, MHC releases CLIP and binds antigenic peptides for presentation to T cells.

The importance of HLA-DM function for T-cell help *in vivo* was studied in H2-DM knockout mice (297). These mice have reduced numbers of T cells, their class II MHC molecules reach the cell surface bearing high levels of CLIP peptide, and their B cells are unable to present certain antigens, such as ovalbumin, to T cells. When H2-DM knockout mice were immunized with 4-hydroxy 5-nitrophenyl acetyl ovalbumin, specific immunoglobulin G antibodies were reduced 20-fold, in comparison to the wild type. Germinal center formation and class switching were greatly reduced, and affinity maturation was not observed. The phenotype was more pronounced for some MHC types, such as IA^b, than for others, such as IA^k. Because of tighter binding of CLIP peptides, these MHC types may be more dependent on H2-DM to maintain empty class II MHC molecules in a peptide-receptive state.

In vitro studies with purified class II MHC molecules and biotin-labeled peptides have shown that HLA-DM can accelerate loading of exogenous peptides into HLA-DR binding sites (298,299). For example, loading of myelin basic protein fragment 90-102 was accomplished in 9 minutes with HLA-DM, as opposed to 60 minutes without it (Table 5). Other peptides were also loaded at the same rate, which

TABLE 5. *Effect of HLA-DM on peptide on rates and off rates for binding to HLA-DR1*

Peptide	HLA-DM	Half-life for binding	Half-life for release
CLIP (80–103)	−	60 min	11 hr
	+	9 min	0.3 hr
MBP (90–102)	−	62 min	86 hr
	+	9 min	1 hr
HA (307–319)	−	67 min	144 hr
	+	10 min	144 hr

The on (association) and off (dissociation) rates of biotinylated peptide from purified soluble HLA-DR1 were measured by fluorescence assay, in the presence or absence of HLA-DM. The on rates of all three peptides are increased similarly in the presence of HLA-DM and probably reflect the rate-limiting dissociation of the bound CLIP fragment of the invariant chain. In contrast, once the peptides are bound, the off rates differ as a result of differences in affinity. Thus, HLA-DM catalyzes release of more weakly binding peptides and allows stable binding of higher affinity peptides. In effect, this is an editing function of HLA-DM.

CLIP, class II-associated invariant chain peptide; HA, hemagglutinin; HLA, human leukocyte antigen; MBP, myelin basic protein.

Adapted from the data of Sloan et al. (298).

suggests that the rate-limiting step was the same for each: removal of CLIP peptides to expose the peptide binding sites on HLA-DR. The kinetic effect was optimal between pH 4.5 and pH 5.8, which is typical of the endosomal/lysosomal compartment in which HLA-DM operates. HLA-DM did not affect the affinity, as measured by half maximal binding, but it had a marked effect on the kinetics of binding.

Conversely, when biotinylated peptides were allowed to saturate HLA-DR binding sites overnight and then free peptides were removed, the "off rate" could be measured over time (298, 299). As shown in Table 5, the "off" rate for different peptides could be compared in the absence or presence of HLA-DM. The half-life for CLIP peptides was reduced from 11 hours to 20 minutes by the addition of HLA-DM. This could explain the enhanced loading of all other peptides, inasmuch as they must wait for CLIP to come off. In the case of antigenic peptides, myelin basic protein 90-112 was released 80-fold faster in the presence of DM than in its absence. However, another peptide, influenza hemagglutinin 307-319, was not affected at all. The differential effect on these antigenic peptides suggests that HLA-DM can serve a potential role in editing which peptides stay on MHC long enough to be presented and which are removed (298). By releasing myelin basic protein preferentially and not the hemagglutinin peptide, HLA-DM would favor the stable MHC binding and presentation of hemagglutinin peptides over myelin basic protein peptides. The affinity of each peptide is determined by the fit between peptide and MHC groove, not by HLA-DM. However, HLA-DM can amplify the impact of the difference in affinity (i.e., signal-to-noise ratio), by facilitating release of low-affinity peptides and allowing the high-affinity ones to remain. This editing function could have an

important effect on which peptides get presented and elicit a T-cell response and which do not. HLA-DM could contribute to immunodominance of a peptide-binding MHC with high affinity, by releasing its lower affinity competitors. Alternatively, HLA-DM could contribute to self-tolerance by releasing self-peptides of low affinity before they could stimulate self-reactive T cells.

Major Histocompatibility Complex Binding and Assembly of a Stable Major Histocompatibility Complex/Peptide Complex

Antigen Interaction with Major Histocompatibility Complex Molecules

Perhaps the most selective step a potential antigenic site must pass is to bind with sufficiently high affinity to an appropriate MHC molecule.

The response of T cells to antigens on APCs or target cells provided a number of hints that antigen interacts directly with MHC molecules of the APCs. First, inheritable genes coding for immune responsiveness to a specific antigen are tightly linked to the inheritance of genes for MHC-encoded cell surface molecules (102, 141). Second, it became apparent that T-cell recognition of antigen is the step at which MHC restriction occurs (102,149,189,300). For example, in vitro T-cell responses to small protein and polypeptide antigens were found to parallel in vivo responses controlled by Ir genes, and T cells were exquisitely sensitive to differences in MHC antigens of the APC in all their antigen recognition functions. This observation in vitro made it possible to separate the MHC of the T cell from that of the APC. The T-cell response to antigenic determinants on each chain of insulin depended on the MHC antigens of the APC. This was particularly apparent when T cells from an (A × B)F1 animal responded to antigen presented by APCs of either the A or B parental MHC type (189,301). Neither parental APC stimulated an allogeneic response from (A × B)F1 T cells, and the response to antigen was now limited by the MHC of the APC. This ability of the APC to limit what could be presented to the T cells was termed *determinant selection* (189,301). It became obvious that even in a single (A × B)F1 animal, there exist distinct sets of antigen specific T cells that respond to each antigenic determinant only in association with type A or type B MHC (302).

Experiments on the fine specificity of antigen-specific T-cell clones suggested that the MHC of the APC could influence the T-cell response in more subtle ways than just allowing or inhibiting it. Determinant selection implied that a given processed peptide should contain both a site for MHC interaction and a distinct functional site for T-cell receptor binding. Thus, a protein with multiple determinants could be processed into different peptides, each with a different MHC restriction, which is consistent with the independent Ir gene control of the response to each antigenic determinant on the same protein (151). For example, T-cell clones specific for myoglobin responded to different antigenic determinants on different peptide fragments of myoglobin (182): Those specific for one of the epitopes were always restricted to IA, whereas those specific for the other were always restricted to IE. The simplest interpretation was that each antigenic peptide contained an MHC association site for interacting with IA or IE. At the level of Ir genes, mouse strains lacking a functional IE molecule could respond to one of the sites only, and those with neither IA nor IE molecules capable of binding to any myoglobin peptide would be low responders to myoglobin.

Evidence for a discrete MHC association site on peptide antigens came from studies with pigeon cytochrome c. The murine T-cell response to pigeon cytochrome c and its carboxy-terminal peptide (81–104) depends on the IE molecules of the APCs (149). However, distinct structural sites on the synthetic peptide antigen appear to constitute two functional sites: an epitope site for binding to the T-cell receptor and an agretope site for interacting with the MHC molecule of the APC (149,166–168). Amino acid substitutions for Lys at position 99 on the peptide destroyed the ability to stimulate T-cell clones specific for the peptide, whereas the difference between Ala and a deletion at position 103 determined T-cell stimulation in association with some MHC antigens but not others, independent of the T-cell fine specificity. In addition, immunizing with the peptides substituted at position 99 elicited new T-cell clones that responded to the substituted peptide but not to the original and showed the same pattern of genetic restriction, correlated with the residue at position 103, as the clones specific for the original peptide. These results implied that the substitutions at position 99 had not affected the MHC association site but independently altered the epitope site that interacts directly with the T-cell receptor. In contrast, position 103 was a probable subsite for MHC interaction, without altering the T-cell receptor binding site.

It remained to be shown that MHC molecules without any other cell surface protein were sufficient for presentation of processed peptide antigens. This was demonstrated by Watts et al. (303), who showed that glass slides coated with lipid containing purified IA molecules could present an ovalbumin peptide to an ovalbumin-specific T-cell hybridoma. This result meant that no other special steps were required other than antigen processing and MHC association. Likewise, Walden et al. (304) specifically stimulated T-cell hybridomas with liposomes containing nothing but antigen and MHC molecules. Norcross et al. (305) transformed mouse L cells with the genes for the IA α and β chains and converted the fibroblasts (which do not express their own class II MHC molecules) into IA-expressing cells. These cells were able to present several antigens to IA-restricted T-cell clones and hybridomas (305), and similar IE transfectants presented to IE-restricted T cells (182). Thus, whatever processing enzymes are required are already present in fibroblasts, and the only additional requirement for antigen-presenting function is the expression of IA or IE antigens.

The planar membrane technique has been applied to determine the minimum number of MHC–antigen complexes per APC necessary to induce T-cell activation (306). After pulsing the presenting cells with antigen, the cells were studied for antigen-presenting activity, and some of the cells were lysed to produce a purified fraction containing MHC charged with antigenic peptides. These MHC/peptide complexes were used to reconstitute planar membranes, and their potency was compared to a reference MHC preparation pulsed with a high peptide concentration in vitro and presumed to be fully loaded. In this way, the relative peptide occupancy of MHC binding sites corresponding to any level of antigen presentation could be determined. For B cells and macrophages, the threshold of antigen loading necessary for triggering T cells was 0.2% of IE^d molecules occupied by peptide, corresponding to about 200 MHC/peptide complexes per presenting cell. For artificial presenting cells, such as L cells transfected with IE^d, the threshold was 23 times greater, or 4.6% of MHC occupied by peptide. Similarly, when MHC/peptide binding was measured directly, using radiolabeled peptide to determine the minimum level of MHC/peptide complexes required for T-cell triggering, B cells were capable of presenting antigen with as few as 200 to 300 MHC/peptide complexes per cell (307). A similar number of peptide/class I MHC molecule complexes was reported to be required on a cell for recognition by $CD8^+$ CTLs (308). These results explain how newly generated peptide antigens can bind enough MHC molecules to stimulate a T-cell response, even in the presence of competing cellular antigens, because a low level of MHC occupancy is sufficient. In addition, this threshold of presentation may explain how multivalent protein antigens, such as viral particles, with 100 to 200 protein copies each, can be over 10^3-fold more immunogenic than the same weight of protein monomers (309–311). Studies on the number of T-cell receptors needed for triggering, based on titrating peptide and recombinant soluble class I MHC molecules on plastic, suggested that interaction of three to five T-cell receptors with peptide/MHC complexes was sufficient, which was consistent with several T cells interacting with one APC (312,313). Biochemical evidence for the direct association between processed peptide and MHC molecules was demonstrated by competition between peptides for antigen presentation (195,314–317) and then more directly by equilibrium dialysis (318), molecular sieve chromatography (319), and affinity labeling (320). Equilibrium dialysis was performed by incubating detergent-solubilized class II MHC molecules with fluoresceinated or radioactive antigenic peptides, followed by dialysis against a large volume of buffer. Peptide can pass in or out of the dialysis bag, but the class II MHC molecules are trapped inside. In the absence of binding by class II MHC molecules, the labeled peptide would distribute itself equally between the inside and outside of the dialysis chamber. However, when the appropriate class II MHC molecules were added to the chamber, extra peptide molecules were retained inside it because of formation of a complex with class II MHC. In this way, direct binding of antigen and MHC was shown, and an affinity constant was determined (318,319).

A second approach was to form the antigen/MHC complex over 48 hours, followed by rapid passage over a Sephadex G50 sizing column. The bound peptide came off the column early, because it is the size of class II MHC molecules (about 58 kDa), whereas free peptide was usually included in the column and eluted later, because it is only approximately 2 kDa (319). Peptide bound to specific and saturable sites on MHC. Competitive binding showed that different peptide antigens with the same MHC restriction bind to the same site on the class II MHC molecule (321,322). For example, Table 6 shows the results with peptide antigens that are known to be presented with IA or IE antigens of the d or k haplotype. Ovalbumin peptide 323-339, which is presented with IA^d, also binds well to purified IA^d, whereas nonradioactive peptide competes for the peptide-binding sites of the IA^d molecule. Similarly, the other IA^d-restricted peptide, myoglobin 106-118, competes with ovalbumin peptide 323-339 for the same site. However, myoglobin 132-153, which is not restricted to IA^d, does not compete for it but does compete for its own restriction element, IE^d. Similarly, pigeon cytochrome c competes best for its restriction element IE^k rather than IA^k or IE^d, which do not present cytochrome. Conversely, recombinant $E\beta$ genes have been used to map separate sites on a class II MHC molecule for binding to peptide antigen and to the T-cell receptor (323).

Through the use of these two biochemical methods, it has been possible to explain major losses of peptide antigenicity resulting from amino acid substitutions in terms of their adverse effect on epitope or agretope function. For example, the response of each of two ovalbumin-specific T-cell clones was mapped to peptide 325-335 by using a nested set of synthetic peptides. Five substitutions were made for each amino acid in the peptide, and each of the resulting 55 different peptides was tested for the ability to stimulate the clone (324). Presumably, the peptides that failed to stimulate could be defective at an epitope or an agretope functional site. In fact, only two amino acids (Val 327 and Ala 332) were essential for MHC interaction, and changes at either of these resulted in a loss of antigenicity for the clone. Seven other amino acids were critical for T-cell stimulation but did not affect MHC binding; thus, these must have been part of the functional epitope. Interestingly, certain substitutions for His 328, Ala 330, and Glu 333 had effects on MHC binding,

whereas others had effects on T-cell stimulation without affecting MHC binding. These amino acids might participate in both agretope and epitope functional sites, or, alternatively, the substitutions may affect the conformation of the peptide as it binds, thus indirectly affecting T-cell recognition (325) (see later discussion). The fact that substitutions at 9 of 11 amino acids could be tolerated without affecting MHC binding is consistent with the determinant selection hypothesis in that multiple antigenic peptides are capable of interacting with the same antigen binding site on the MHC molecule.

Similarly, through the use of a T-cell clone specific for peptide 52-61 of hen egg lysozyme, substitutions at each amino acid were analyzed for the ability to bind to IA^k and stimulate the clone (326). Substitutions at 4 of 11 amino acid residues had no effect, whereas substitutions at three positions resulted in reduced binding to IA^k. Substitutions at the remaining three positions resulted in decreased T-cell stimulation without affecting MHC association. The epitope was very sensitive to substitutions, even conservative ones such as changing Leu 56 to Ile, norLeu, or Val. The results in both of these studies confirmed by competitive binding that the MHC molecule contains a single saturable site for peptide binding. This site must be capable of binding a broad range of antigenic peptides. In binding the MHC groove, antigenic peptides assume the extended conformation that exposes the epitope for recognition by the T-cell receptor.

Although a full set of general principles explaining the specificity of antigen presentation and T cell recognition has not yet emerged, studies such as these, combined with complementary structural studies characterizing the antigen-interacting portions of MHC molecules (185,223,224,323, 327–334) (see Chapter 19) and of T-cell receptors (335–341) (see Chapter 8) will ultimately lead to an understanding of these principles.

One observation that came out of this type of structure–function study was that a single peptide can bind to a class II MHC molecule in more than one way and thus can be recognized by different T cells in different orientations or conformations (325,342). The same conclusion can be reached from an entirely different type of study, in which mutations are introduced into the MHC molecule. Mutations in the floor of the peptide-binding groove, which cannot directly interact with the T-cell receptor, can differentially affect recognition of a peptide by one clone and not another (343–345). In a particularly thoroughly studied case, it was clear that

TABLE 6. *Correlation between MHC restriction and binding to MHC molecules*

Competitor peptide		Ova + A^d	Myo + E^d	HEL + A^k	Cyto + E^k
Ova	323–339	++++	−	++	+
Myo	106–118	++++	−	++	+/−
Myo	132–153	−	++++	−	++
HEL	46–61	+	+	++++	+
Cytochrome c	88–104	++	+/−	++	++++

MHC, major histocompatibility complex.
Data from Buus et al. (322).

the quantitative level of peptide binding was not affected by the mutation; rather, the change in the floor of the groove imposed an altered conformation on the peptide that differentially affected recognition by different T cells (345). If indeed the T-cell receptor cannot detect the mutation in the MHC molecule except indirectly by its effect on the peptide conformation, then it must be concluded that different T cells have preferences for different conformations of the same peptide bound to (what appears to the T cell as) the same MHC molecule.

Another general observation to come from this type of study is that substitution of amino acids often affects presentation by MHC and recognition by T cells through introduction of dominant negative interactions or interfering groups, whereas only a few residues are actually essential for peptide binding (346). Both for class II MHC binding (346–349) and for class I MHC binding (350), most residues can be replaced with Ala or sometimes Pro without losing MHC binding, as long as a few critical residues are retained. Of course, T-cell recognition may require retention of other residues. If many of the amino acid side chains are not necessary for binding to the MHC molecule, then side chains of noncritical amino acids may be expected to occasionally interfere with binding, either directly or through an effect on conformation. That is exactly what was observed for a helper epitope from the HIV-1 envelope protein when a heteroclitic peptide—that is, one that stimulated the T cells at much lower concentrations than did the wild-type peptide—was obtained by replacing a negatively charged Glu with Ala or with Gln, which has the same size but no charge (346). An Asp, negatively charged but smaller, behaved like the Glu. Thus, this residue was not necessary for binding to the class II MHC molecule, but a negatively charged side chain interfered with binding to the MHC molecule as measured by competition studies. Information about residues that interfere with binding has allowed the refinement of sequence motifs for peptides binding to MHC molecules to permit more reliable prediction of binding (351) (see later discussion).

This observation also provides a novel approach to make more potent vaccines by "epitope enhancement," the process of modifying the internal sequence of epitopes to make them more potent—for example, by increasing affinity for an MHC molecule or T cell receptor—or able to induce more broadly cross-reactive T cells specific for multiple strains of a virus (352–355). Proof of principle that this approach can make more potent peptide vaccines has been obtained (355). The modified "enhanced" helper T-cell epitope from the HIV-1 envelope protein described previously (346), with Ala substituted for Glu, was shown to be immunogenic at 10- to 100-fold lower doses for in vivo immunization than the wild-type HIV-1 peptide to induce a T-cell proliferative response specific for the wild-type peptide. Furthermore, when a peptide vaccine construct with this helper epitope coupled to a CTL epitope (356,357) was modified with the same Glu-to-Ala substitution, it was more potent at inducing CD8[+] CTL specific for the CTL epitope than was the original

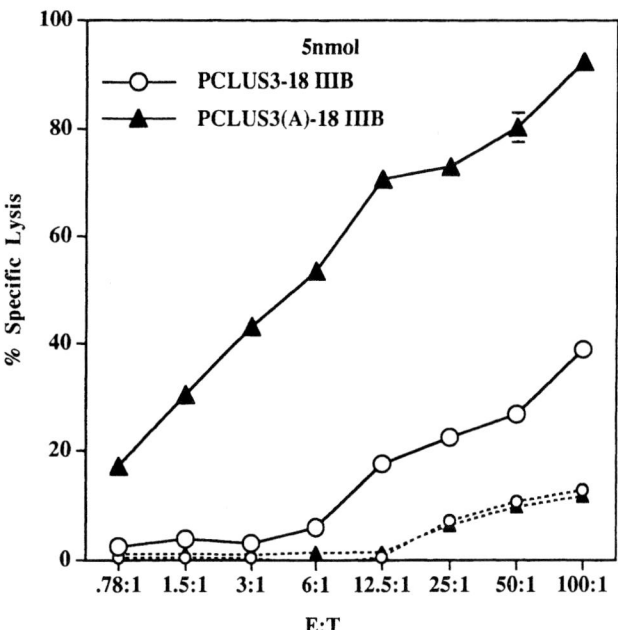

FIG. 10. Enhancement of immunogenicity of a peptide vaccine for induction of class I major histocompatibility complex (MHC)–restricted cytotoxic T-lymphocytes by modification of the class II MHC–binding portion to increase CD4[+] T-cell help. Peptide vaccine PCLUS3-18 IIIB contains a class II MHC–binding helper region, consisting of a cluster of overlapping determinants from the human immunodeficiency virus (HIV)–1 envelope protein, glycoprotein 160 (gp160), and a class I MHC–binding cytotoxic T cell (CTL) eptitope, P18 IIIB. Modification of the helper epitope to remove an adverse negative charge by replacement of a Glu with an Ala residue was shown to increase binding to the class II MHC molecule (346). Here, introduction of the same modification of the helper epitope, to produce PCLUS3(A)-18IIIB, is shown to greatly increase immunogenicity in vivo for induction of CTL to the class I MHC–binding P18IIIB portion. Immunization of A.AL mice with 5 nmol of either vaccine construct subcutaneously in Montanide ISA 51 adjuvant, and stimulation of resulting spleen cells with P18IIIB for 1 week in culture, resulted in 33-fold more lytic units for lysing targets coated with P18IIIB when mice were immunized with the modified second-generation vaccine than when they were immunized with the original construct with the natural sequence. Thus, class II MHC–restricted CD4[+] T-cell help has a major impact on induction of class I MHC–restricted CTL, and this process of "epitope enhancement" can be used to make vaccines more potent than the natural viral antigens. Targets: BALB/c 3T3 fibroblasts with P18IIIB (*solid lines*) or no peptide (*dashed lines*). (Modified from Ahlers et al. (355), with permission.)

vaccine construct, even though the CTL epitope was unchanged (Fig. 10) (355). The increased potency of the vaccine construct was shown to result from improved class II MHC–restricted help by genetic mapping, through the use of congenic strains of mice expressing the same class I MHC molecule to present the CTL epitope and the same background genes but differing in class II MHC molecules (355). Thus, class II MHC–restricted help makes an enormous difference in induction of class I MHC–restricted CTL, and epitope enhancement can allow construction of more potent vaccines, providing greater protection against viral infection (358). Furthermore, the improved help was found to be qualitatively, not just quantitatively, different, skewed more toward Th1 cytokines (358). The mechanism was found to involve greater induction of CD40 ligand on the helper T cells, resulting in greater IL-12 production by the antigen-presenting dendritic cells, which in turn polarized the helper cells toward the Th1 phenotype (358). The dendritic cells conditioned with the helper T cells and the higher affinity peptide and then purified were also more effective at activating CD8+ CTL precursors in the absence of helper cells, supporting a mechanism of help mediated through activation of dendritic cells (359–361). This study showed also that such help was mediated primarily through up-regulation of IL-12 production and CD80 and CD86 expression on the dendritic cell (358). Understanding this mechanism of epitope enhancement may contribute to the design of improved vaccines.

Similar epitope enhancement has been carried out for class I MHC–binding viral or tumor peptides as well (362–364) and, in one case, has been found to result in greater clinical efficacy of a melanoma vaccine used for human immunotherapy (365). These results emphasize the importance of affinity for MHC molecules in vaccine efficacy (366) and suggest that rational design of vaccines with higher affinity epitopes may produce more effective second-generation vaccines (367,368). To that end, the discovery of sequence motifs predicting MHC molecule binding and the development of bioinformatics strategies to predict peptide affinity have proved a great impetus to the field (369).

In the case of class I MHC molecules, results defining sequence-binding motifs generalize the conclusion that only a few critical "anchor" residues determine the specificity of binding to the MHC molecule (Table 7) (234,350,370–374). These motifs were defined (a) by a detailed study of one peptide/MHC system (372), (b) by sequencing the mixture of natural peptides eluted from a class I MHC molecule and finding that at certain positions in the sequence the same residue was shared by most of the peptides (370), and (c) by separating and sequencing individual natural peptides eluted from a class I MHC molecule and finding a conserved residue at certain positions (371). These two studies also yielded the important observation that the natural peptides eluted from class I MHC molecules were all about the same length, eight

TABLE 7. *Examples of motifs for peptides binding to class I and II MHC molecules*

MHC molecule	Residue number								
	1	2	3	4	5	6	7	8	9
Class I									
H-2K^d		Y							I, L, V
H-2D^b					N				M, I
H-2K^b					F, Y			L, M	
H-2L^d		P			(hydrophilic K, R)				M, L, F
H-2D^d		G	P		K, R				L
H-2K^k		E						I	
HLA-A2.1		L, M							V
HLA-A3		L	(F)						Y, K
HLA-B27	K, R, G	R	I, Y, F, W						K, R
Class II									
DRB1*0101	Y, V, L, F, I, A			L, A		A, G			L, A
DRB1*0301	L, I, F, M, V			D		K, R, E, Q			Y, L, F
DRB1*0401 (DR4Dw4)	F, Y, W		no	R, K		N, S, T, Q, Aliphatic	Polar Charged		Polar Aliphatic K
DRB1*0402 (DR4Dw10)	V, I, L, M		no	D, E		N, Q, S, T, K	R, K, H, N, Q, P		Polar Aliphatic H
DRB1*1501 (DR2b)	L, V, I			F, Y, I			I, L, V, M, F		
DQA1*0501 DQB1*0301	F, Y, I, M, L, V				V, L, I, M, Y		Y, F, M, L, V, I		

MHC, major histocompatibility complex.
Data from references 234, 350, and 370–374.

or nine residues, and this was confirmed for a much larger collection of peptides eluted from HLA-A2 and analyzed by tandem mass spectrometry (373). This finding was consistent with other studies demonstrating that a minimal nonapeptide was many orders of magnitude more potent than longer peptides in presentation by class I MHC molecules to T cells (375,376). This conservation of length was critical to the success of the approach of sequencing mixtures of peptides eluted from a class I MHC molecule (370), because such a method requires that the conserved anchor residues all be at the same distance from the N-terminal. The fact that Falk et al. (370) could find a single amino acid at certain positions, such as a Tyr at position 2 in peptides eluted from K^d, implies not only that most or all of the peptides bound to K^d had a Tyr that could be aligned but also that the peptides were already aligned as bound to the MHC molecule, each one having just one residue N-terminal to the Tyr. This result implies that the position of the N-terminal residue is fixed in the MHC molecule. It is this fact that has made the identification of motifs for binding to class I MHC molecules much more straightforward than finding motifs for binding class II MHC molecules.

This conclusion has been not only confirmed but also explained by the x-ray crystallographic data on class I MHC/peptide complexes (330–332). It appears that both the N-terminal α amino group and the C-terminal carboxyl group are fixed in pockets at either end of the MHC groove, independent of which amino acids are occupying those positions, and that the rest of the peptide spans these fixed points in a more or less extended conformation. The minimum length that can span the distance between these pockets is 8 residues, but 9 or 10 residues can be accommodated with a slight bulge or β turn in the middle of the peptide, which explains the narrow restriction on length. Between these ends, one or two pockets in the groove can accommodate the side chain of an amino acid, usually either at position 2 binding in the B pocket or at position 5 binding in the C pocket, depending on the particular MHC molecule. In addition, the side chain of the C-terminal residue serves as an anchor in the F pocket at the end of the groove. These residues that fit into pockets correspond exactly to the "anchor" residues, at position 2 or 5 and position 8, 9, or 10, defined by the sequence motifs, and appear to be the primary determinants of specificity for peptide binding, inasmuch as the rest of the interactions are largely with peptide backbone atoms, including the α amino and carboxyl groups, and therefore do not contribute to sequence specificity. This finding can explain both the breadth of peptides that can bind to a single MHC molecule, because most of the binding involves only backbone atoms common to all peptides, and the exquisite specificity of binding, determined by the anchor residues, that accounts for the Ir gene control of responsiveness.

In contrast, when natural self-peptides were eluted from class II MHC molecules (222,377), the lengths were much more variable, ranging from 13 to 18 residues, and several variants of the same peptide were found with different lengths

of extra sequence at one end or the other ("ragged ends"). This finding suggested that both ends of the peptide-binding groove of class II MHC molecules are open, in contrast to class I, so that additional lengths of peptide can hang out either side, and trimming does not have to be precise. However, a corollary is that the peptides eluted from class II MHC molecules would not be aligned in a motif starting from the exact amino-terminal residue, and that was indeed what was found. Although a moderately conserved motif was found in some of the peptides eluted from the murine class II MHC molecule IA^d, which is consistent with the motif defined on the basis of known antigenic peptides binding to IA^d (378), the motif was neither so clearly defined nor so highly conserved as in the class I case, and aligning of sequences was necessary to identify a core motif of about nine amino acid residues (377). Subsequently, a number of motifs for peptides binding to human class II MHC molecules have been defined (234,379–384). Unlike peptides eluted from class I MHC grooves, these class II MHC binding peptides may locate the core binding motif at various distances from the amino or carboxy end of the peptide.

The crystal structure of a peptide bound to a human class II MHC molecule, DR1, revealed that, indeed, the ends of the groove are open and the peptide can extend beyond the groove in either direction (224,385). In addition, the more broadly defined class II MHC motifs in Table 7 can be explained by less stringent requirements for amino acid side chains to interact with binding pockets in class II. In general, the class II MHC binding pockets are shallower than those of class I, and a selected peptide derives less binding energy from each pocket. In fact, the pockets form fewer H bonds with the peptide side chains, and more H bonds are directed at the peptide backbone, allowing a variety of different peptides to bind. Rather than requiring a specific amino acid at each position, the shallow binding pockets of MHC class II tend to exclude peptides on the basis of unfavorable interactions, such as side chains too large to fit the binding pocket. Even one amino acid side chain that binds strongly to an MHC pocket is sufficient to anchor the peptide to MHC class II and set the frame for the interaction of the rest of the peptide with the MHC groove.

For example, binding of three peptides to the class II MHC molecules IA in mice or HLA-DQ in humans are shown in Fig. 11. The first residue of the peptide motif is designated P1, the next is P2, and so on. The α helical walls and β sheet floor of the class II MHC groove (Chapter 19) are peeled away to reveal the peptide backbone and side chains in relation to MHC binding pockets. For the ovalbumin peptide Ova$_{323-329}$ binding to IA^d, residues P1, P4, and P9 all point down into the binding pockets (386). The best fit is between Val 327 and the P4 pocket, which creates mainly hydrophobic interactions with MHC and serves as the anchor residue. Residues P5 (His 328) and P8 (His 331) project upward for binding to the T-cell receptor. The shallow P4 pocket can tolerate only small hydrophobic side chains, such as Val, and that dictates which peptides can bind in it. The other MHC pockets, P1

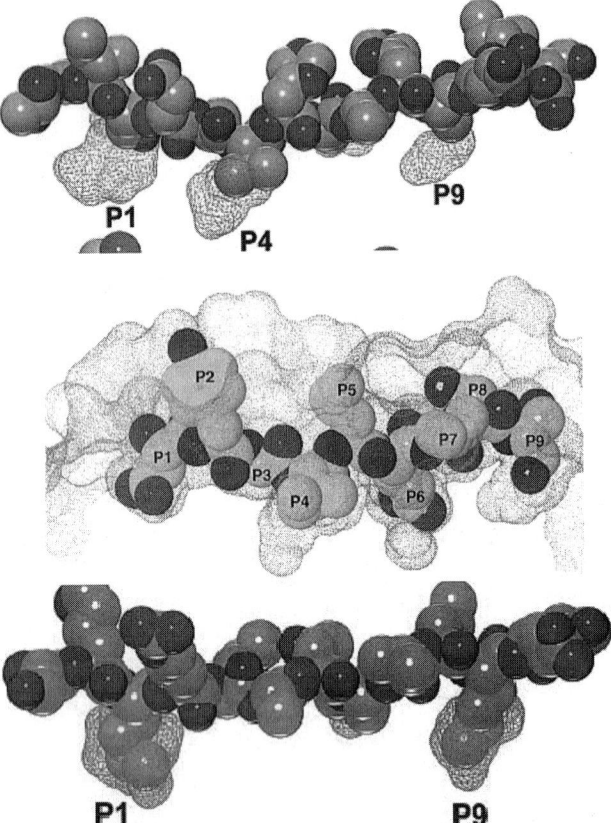

FIG. 11. Interaction of peptides with the binding groove of major histocompatibility complex (MHC) class II, as determined by x-ray crystallography. Anchor residue side chains (solid) fill binding pockets (stripped) to a greater or lesser extent, supplemented by H-bonds to the peptide backbone. Examples include IA^d with ovalbumin peptide 323-334 (**top**) (386), IA^k with hen egg lysozyme 52-60 (**middle**) (387), and human leukocyte antigen–DR3 with class II-associated invariant chain peptide (**bottom**) (388).

and P9, accommodate many different residues, so they have little effect on which peptides can be presented by IA^d.

For hen egg lysozyme peptide HEL$_{50-62}$ binding to IA^k, interactions with MHC are observed for P1, P4, P6, and P9 (387). The P1 interaction is very different from IA^d, inasmuch as the P1 pocket is a perfect fit for Asp and has an arginine at the end of the tunnel to neutralize charge. This structure explains why nearly all peptides presented by IA^k must have Asp at this position. In contrast, the P4 and P9 pockets are partially filled and tolerate a number of different side chains at these positions. The P6 pocket requires a Glu or Gln, even though the MHC residues deep in the pocket are acidic. It is presumed that one of the Glu residues must be protonated to allow Glu binding at this position. This arrangement of the peptide leaves P2, P5, and P8 exposed to solvent in the crystal structure and to the T-cell receptor during antigen presentation.

For the CLIP peptide binding to HLA-DR3, deep pockets at P1 and P9 are more fully occupied by the peptide side chains (388). pH-Dependent binding is important, because

CLIP must be stable at neutral pH and unstable at acid pH in the presence of HLA-DM in order to perform its function.

On the basis of affinity for MHC, these interactions explain the peptide-binding motifs for class II MHC that select which peptides can be presented to T cells. In addition, these interactions orient the peptide in the MHC groove and determine which residues are accessible for recognition by the T-cell receptor.

T-Cell Receptor Recognition

The last hurdle that a potential antigenic determinant must surmount is recognition by a T-cell receptor within the repertoire of the individual responding. This repertoire may be limited by the availability of combinations of V, D, and J genes in the genome that can combine to form an appropriate receptor, in view of the lack of somatic hypermutation in T-cell receptors in contrast to antibodies (337,389), and then by self-tolerance, as mediated by thymic or peripheral negative selection, or by limits on the repertoire that is positively selected in the thymus on existing self-peptide/MHC complexes. The available repertoire may also be influenced by prior exposure to cross-reactive antigens. In general, however, it has been hard to find holes in the repertoire (390). Furthermore, when T-cell receptor repertoires of mice and humans were compared for peptides presented by HLA-A2.1, they seemed to be capable of recognizing the same spectrum of peptides (391). Eleven peptides from hepatitis C virus proteins, each of which had a motif for binding to HLA-A2.1, were tested for recognition by CTL from HLA-A2.1 transgenic mice and human HLA-A2.1-positive patients infected with hepatitis C virus. The same four peptides that were recognized by the T cells from the mice were the ones recognized by the human T cells, whereas the others were not recognized well by either murine or human T cells. The selection of which peptides were recognized seemed to be determined by binding to the HLA-A2.1 molecule, rather than by the availability of T cells. Thus, despite the differences in T-cell receptor genes in mice and humans, the repertoires are plastic enough that if a peptide passes the other three hurdles of processing, transport, and binding to MHC molecules, T cells can be elicited to respond to it in either species (391).

On the other hand, there exists evidence that MHC binding is not the whole story. Schaeffer et al. (392) examined 14 overlapping peptides covering the sequence of staphylococcal nuclease with different class II MHC molecules, constituting 54 different peptide-MHC combinations. Clearly, MHC binding plays a major role because 12 of 13 immunogenic peptides were high or intermediate binders to MHC molecules, whereas only 1 of 37 poor binders were immunogenic. Of high-affinity binders, all five peptides were immunogenic. However, for intermediate affinity MHC-binding peptides, only 7 of 12 were immunogenic. Thus, MHC binding alone is not sufficient to ensure immunogenicity. The T-cell repertoire was one factor suggested that might limit the spectrum of immunogenic peptides.

Indeed, examples for selection at the level of the T-cell receptor repertoire exist. A particularly elegant example described by Moudgil et al. (393) is one in which a peptide (46-61) of mouse lysozyme presented by IA^k is recognized by T cells from CBA/J and B10.A mice, which express IA^k and IE^k, but not by T cells from B10.A(4R) mice, which express only IA^k, even though the APC from B10.A(4R) mice can present the peptide to T cells from the other strains. T cells from the B10.A(4R) mice can respond to peptide 46-61 variants in which the C-terminal Arg is replaced by Ala, Leu, Phe, Asn, or Lys, which indicates that the C-terminal Arg is hindering recognition but not binding by IA^k and, in this case, is not processing because the B10.A(4R) APC can present the peptide. It appears that the hindrance interferes with recognition by T-cell receptors available in B10.A(4R) mice but not T-cell receptors available in B10.A, CBA/J, or [B10.A(4R) × CBA/J]F1 mice. Because the B10.A mice are congenic with the B10.A(4R) mice, the difference is not one of non–MHC-linked genes such as T-cell receptor structural genes or non-MHC self-antigens producing self-tolerance. Furthermore, because the F1 mice respond, the difference is not due to a hole in the repertoire produced by a self-antigen of the B10.A(4R) mice. It was concluded that the CBA/J and B10.A mice contain an additional repertoire, positively selected on IE^k or possibly an H-2D/L class I molecule in which these strains differ, that can recognize peptide 46-61 despite the hindering Arg at the C-terminal. An alternative related explanation is that strains that express IE^k or D^k or D^d/L^d have an additional repertoire of T-cell receptors positively selected on IA^k-presenting self-peptides from processing of these other MHC molecules in the thymus. This example illustrates a case in point that subtle differences in T-cell receptor, presumably caused in this case by positive selection, can lead to responsiveness or nonresponsiveness to a determinant that has already passed all of the three earlier hurdles (processing, transport, and MHC binding). Another elegant example of T-cell repertoire limitations on immunodominance comes from a study of mice deficient in LMP-2 and therefore unable to make immunoproteasomes. Whereas loss of immunodominance of one influenza epitope was shown to result from decreased production by constitutive proteasomes, reduced response to another normally immunodominant influenza epitope was found by T-cell adoptive transfer studies to result from an alteration in the T-cell repertoire, presumably because of altered processing of self-peptides in the thymus (247).

As more is understood about the molecular basis of T-cell receptor recognition, with crystallographic data now available (340,341,394), it becomes possible to apply epitope enhancement in a rational way to the affinity of the peptide/MHC complex for the T-cell receptor, as was described for the peptide affinity for MHC molecules previously. Sequence modifications in the peptide that increase the affinity for the T-cell receptor were shown to be more effective at expanding *in vivo* the T cells specific for tumor antigens (395–397). Most of these modifications were found empirically,

but a systematic study of substitutions throughout a number of peptides revealed a pattern in which peptides with conservative substitutions at positions 3, 5, or 7 were most likely to yield increased T-cell receptor affinity, which narrows the candidate list of peptides that require empirical screening (398). This strategy provides a second type of epitope enhancement, derived from basic immunological principles, to produce more effective vaccines.

Epitope Mapping

Precise mapping of antigenic sites recognized by T cells was made possible by the fact that T cells would respond to peptide fragments of the antigen when they contain a complete antigenic determinant. A series of overlapping peptides can be used to walk along the protein sequence and find the antigenic site. Then, by truncating the peptide at either end, the minimum antigenic peptide can be determined. For example, in the case of myoglobin, a critical amino acid residue, such as Glu 109 or Lys 140, was found by comparing the sequences of stimulatory and nonstimulatory myoglobin variants and large cyanogen bromide cleavage fragments (183), and then a series of truncated peptides containing the critical residue was synthesized with different overlapping lengths at either end (155,159). Because solid-phase peptide synthesis starts from a fixed carboxyl end and proceeds toward the amino end, it can be stopped at various positions to produce a nested series of peptides that vary in length at the amino end. Each peptide is then tested in the proliferation assay. In this way, it was found that two of the Glu 109–specific T-cell clones responded to synthetic peptides 102-118 and 106-118 but not to peptide 109-118 (159). One clone responded to peptide 108-118, whereas the other did not. Thus, the amino end of the peptide recognized by one clone was Ser 108, whereas the other clone required Phe 106, Ile 107, or both. Similar fine specificity differences have been observed with T-cell clones specific for the peptides 52-61 and 74-96 of hen egg lysozyme (152,184,185), the peptide 323-339 of chicken ovalbumin (153), and the peptide 81-104 of pigeon cytochrome c (158): The epitopes recognized by several T-cell clones overlap but are distinct. In addition, nine T-cell clones recognized a second T-cell determinant in myoglobin located around Lys 140, and each one responded to the cyanogen bromide cleavage fragment 132-153 (182). Further studies with a nested series of synthetic peptides (peptide 135-146 vs. 136-146 vs. 137-146 and so forth) showed that the stimulatory sequence is contained in peptide 136-146, and additional studies with peptides trimmed at the carboxyl end with carboxypeptidases B and A showed that Lys 145 is necessary, but Tyr 146 is not, although it contributes to antigenic potency (155). What these studies and others demonstrated about epitopes recognized by T cells is that they are segmental determinants, contained on synthetic peptides consisting of no more than about 12 to 17 amino acid residues for class II MHC or 8 to 10 residues for class I MHC. Within this size, they must contain all the information necessary to survive processing within the APC, associate with the MHC antigen, and bind to the T-cell receptor.

Mapping by Amino Acid Substitution and Effects of Altered Peptide Ligands

Once an antigenic peptide is identified, the next step is to map key amino acid residues by making a series of variant peptides, each of which differs from the native sequence by a single amino acid substitution, as described previously in the section on MHC binding. One approach, an alanine scan, substitutes Ala for the natural amino acid at each position in the peptide or uses Ser or Gly to replace naturally occurring Ala. Ala is used because the side chain is only a methyl group, and so it replaces whatever functional side chain is present with the smallest one other than that of Gly, which is not used because of its effects on conformation. By this means, the investigator can determine whether the loss of the naturally occurring side chain affects function, without the introduction of a new side chain that might itself affect function. In general, each peptide has several amino acids where Ala substitution destroys antigenicity. Some of these correspond to contact residues for the T-cell receptor, whereas others are contact residues for MHC. In many cases, the MHC binding residues can be determined by testing the substituted peptides in a competitive MHC binding assay (discussed previously). The amino acid substitutions that knock out T-cell proliferation but not MHC binding are presumed to be in the epitope recognized by the T-cell receptor directly, and these can be studied with additional substitutions. For example, this technique was used to compare the residues interacting with the MHC molecule or T-cell receptor when the same HIV-1 V3 loop peptide P18 (residues 308 to 322) was presented by three different MHC molecules: a human class I molecule, a murine class I molecule, and a murine class II molecule (Fig. 12) (399,400). Interestingly, there was a striking concordance of function of several of the residues as presented by all three MHC molecules (Fig. 12). For example, Pro and Phe interacted with the MHC in all three cases, and the same Val interacted with the T-cell receptor in all three cases. Also, the same Arg in the middle of the peptide interacted with both the murine class I and the murine class II molecules, and the C-terminal Ile was an anchor residue for both human and murine class I molecules (399,400).

In the case of autoimmune T cells, these techniques have been used to study the number and variety of epitopes recognized by self-reactive T cells. In the nonobese diabetic mouse, the B chain of insulin is a major target of T cells recovered from pancreatic islet cells (401). Alanine scanning of B chain peptide 9-23 revealed two patterns of T-cell recognition for the same peptide. Some T cells recognize peptide 9-16; others respond to peptide 13-23. Each epitope appears to have distinct sites for MHC and T-cell receptor binding, even though they come from the same peptide chain. Similarly, in systemic lupus erythematosus, human T cells specific for the Sm antigen are narrowly restricted to a few epitopes that are found on

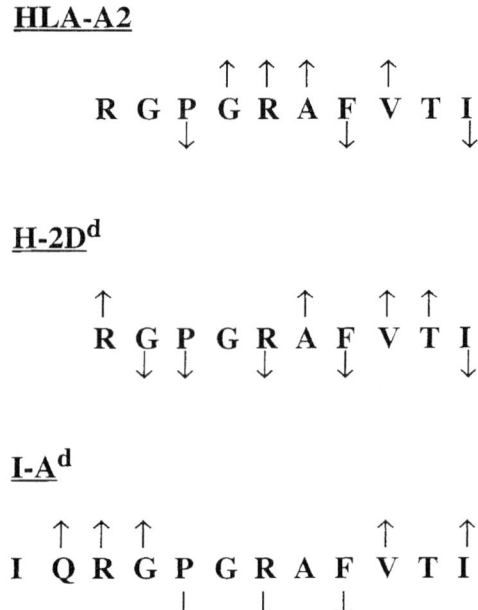

FIG. 12. Comparison of the major histocompatibility complex (MHC)–interacting ("agretopic") and T-cell receptor interacting ("epitopic") residues of the same HIV-1 envelope V3 loop peptide as it is presented by human class I, murine class I, and murine class II MHC molecules to CD8+ cytotoxic T cell (CTL) and CD4+ helper T cells. Shown is the sequence of the optimal binding portion of peptide P18 IIIB from the human immunodeficiency virus (HIV)–1 envelope protein V3 loop for each MHC molecule, in single-letter amino acid code. *Arrows pointing up* indicate residues determined to interact with the T-cell receptor, and *arrows pointing down* indicate residues determined to interact with the MHC molecule. Mapping of residue function for binding to the human class I MHC molecule HLA-A2.1 was described by Alexander-Miller et al. (400), and binding to the murine class I MHC molecule H-2Dd and the murine class II MHC molecule IAd was described Takeshita et al. (399). Note the common use of the Pro and Phe for binding all three MHC molecules and the use of the key Val residue for binding all the T-cell receptors. Also, both the murine MHC molecules use the central Arg residue as a contact residue, whereas both class I MHC molecules use the C-terminal Ile residue as an anchor residue. Thus, there is a surprising degree of concordance.

a small group of proteins (402). On the Sm-B antigen, three epitopes were recognized. On Sm-D antigen, there were two. In each case, alanine scans showed that the same epitopes were recognized by distinct T-cell clones. These results are consistent with the hypotheses that the autoimmune response to insulin or to Sm antigen may be induced by abnormal exposure of a very few cryptic epitopes, or they may depend on selective loss of tolerance for a limited number of epitopes shared by a small subset of self-proteins.

T-cell receptors may distinguish different chemical classes of amino acid side chains. An example of structural differences between amino acid side chains recognized by the T-cell receptor comes from an analysis of non–cross-reactive CTLs that distinguish homologous peptides from the V3 loop of different strains of HIV-1 envelope protein. The residue at position 8 in the minimal determinant was identified as a key "epitopic" T-cell receptor contact residue both in strain IIIB, which has a Val at this position, and in strain MN, which has a Tyr at this position (399,403,404). CTLs specific for strain IIIB do not recognize the MN sequence but do recognize peptides identical to MN except for the substitution of any aliphatic amino acid at that position, such as Val, Leu, or Ile (354). In contrast, CTLs specific for the MN strain do not recognize the IIIB sequence but do recognize the IIIB peptide if the Val at this position is replaced by a Tyr (403). Moreover, they recognize any MN variant in which the Tyr is replaced by another aromatic amino acid, such as Phe, Trp, or His (354). Thus, the two non–cross-reactive T-cell receptors recognize similar peptides but discriminate strongly between peptides with amino acids with aliphatic versus aromatic side chains. On the other hand, they do not distinguish strongly among different aliphatic residues or among different aromatic residues. Interestingly, however, in each category, the least active is the bulkiest member of the category, Ile and Trp, respectively, which suggests that these residues must fit into a pocket of limited size in the T-cell receptor.

The interaction of peptide ligand with T-cell receptor can be studied by introducing single substitutions of conservative amino acids at these contact residues, such as Glu for Asp, Ser for Thr, or Gln for Asn. The T-cell receptor readily distinguishes among peptides with these minor differences at a single residue, and the results have been revealing. Depending on affinity for the T-cell receptor, closely related (altered) peptides can elicit very different responses in T cells. Thus, although a substituted peptide may be very weak or nonstimulatory by itself, it may nonetheless act as a partial agonist or even a strong antagonist of an ongoing T-cell response. Antagonistic peptides can be demonstrated by pulsing APCs with native peptide antigen first, so that competition for binding to MHC molecules is not measured, followed by pulsing with a 10-fold or greater excess of the antagonist, before adding T cells. In the case of influenza hemagglutinin peptide 307-319 presented with HLA-DR1, peptide analogues such as Gln substituted for Asn 313 inhibited the proliferation of a human T-cell clone, even though they did not stimulate the clone. Anergy was not induced, and the antagonist peptide had to be present throughout the culture to inhibit the response (405,406). Thus, lack of antagonist activity is another feature of the interaction between peptide (in complex with MHC molecule) and T-cell receptor that is required for the peptide to be a stimulatory antigenic determinant.

Partial agonists were first demonstrated with the use of T-cell clones specific for an allelic form of murine hemoglobin. These T cells were from CE/J mice, which express the Hb^s allele of mouse hemoglobin, after immunization with the Hb^d allele. The minimum antigenic peptide corresponds to amino acids 67 to 76 of the Hb^d sequence and differs from Hb^s at positions 72, 73, and 76 (407). Peptides substituted at each residue from amino acids 69 to 76 were tested for T-cell proliferation and cytokine release. Some substitutions, such as Gln for Asn at position 72, blocked T-cell

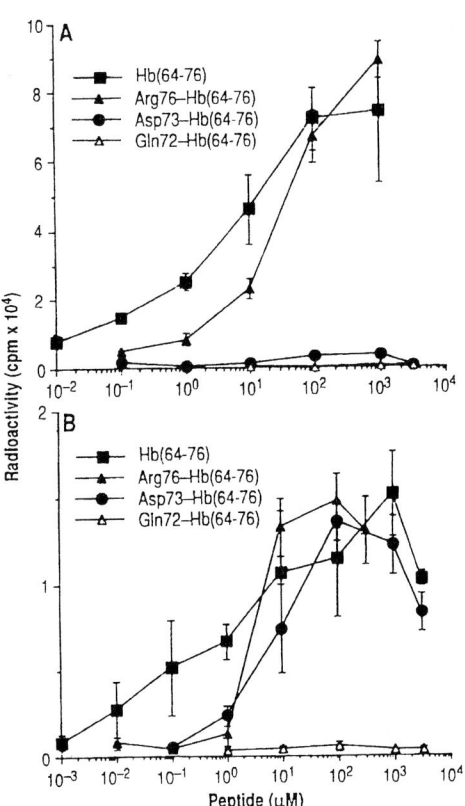

FIG. 13. Differential effect of altered peptide ligands on the response to peptide 64-76 from hemoglobin. **A:** Proliferative response of a T-cell line incubated with antigen-presenting cells and the natural hemoglobin (64-76) peptide or with peptides substituted at positions 72, 73, and 76. **B:** Interleukin-4 release by the T-cell line under the same conditions. The peptide substituted with Asp for Glu at position 73 is unable to induce T-cell proliferation, but it can still induce production of interleukin-4, and so it is a partial agonist. In contrast, substitution of Gln for Asn at position 72 knocks out both responses equally. Modified from Evavold and Allen (408), with permission.

stimulation completely in both assays. Other substituted peptides, such as Asp for Glu at position 73, lost T-cell proliferation but still stimulated IL-4 release, and these are considered partial agonists (Fig. 13) (408). Lack of stimulation was not caused by failure to bind MHC, inasmuch as both substituted peptides gave reasonable binding in a competitive binding assay (409). Similar alteration of cytokine profile by altering the peptide ligand can be seen in other systems (406,410,411).

For one of the hemoglobin 64-76–specific T-cell clones, PL.17, substitutions at amino acid 70, 72, 73, or 76 reduced antigenic potency by 1,000-fold or more, even though conservative amino acids were substituted. Although substitution of Ser for Ala 70 prevented T-cell stimulation in both assays, there was clearly some response to this peptide, inasmuch as it induced expression of the IL-2 receptor (412). In addition, once T cells were exposed to the Ser 70 peptide, they became unresponsive to subsequent exposure to the natural Hb^d peptide. This phenomenon closely resembled T-cell anergy and persisted for a week or more. The Ser 70 substitution alters a contact residue of the peptide for the T-cell receptor of clone PL.17 and affects its affinity. Other T-cell clones, however, can respond to this peptide presented on the same MHC molecule (IE^K). Other *Hb^d* peptides substituted at this position, such as Met and Gly 70, also induced anergy but not proliferation, whereas nonconservative substitutions such as Phe, Asn, Asp, and His 70 induced neither (413).

Another well-studied example is influenza hemagglutinin peptide 306-318 as presented on human HLA-DR1. On the basis of the known crystal structure of the peptide/MHC complex (223), amino acid substitutions could be targeted to contact residues for the T-cell receptor, at positions 307, 309, 310, 312, 315, and 318 (414). At each position, nonconservative substitutions often rendered the peptide inactive, whereas conservative substitutions at several sites yielded either full antigenicity or progressively lower stimulatory activity, down to 1,000-fold less than native peptide while retaining the ability to induce anergy. For example, substituting His or Gly for Lys 307 yielded 1,000-fold reduced stimulation of T-cell proliferation but full ability to induce tolerance. Similarly, substituting His for Lys 315 produced complete loss of stimulation but nearly full anergy-inducing activity. As before, induction of the IL-2 receptor (CD25) was a sign of T-cell activation by these altered peptide ligands, even when they did not induce proliferation. Unlike these peptides, the antagonists do not induce interleukin receptors or secretion, and they do not cause long-lasting tolerance. Overall, researchers have identified a number of altered peptide ligands that, in appropriate complexes with MHC molecules, induce anergy or act as antagonists of the T-cell receptor and block activation by agonist ligands by delivering an abortive signal (406).

Several methods have been found to anergize T cells to a specific antigen for up to a week, and all have the common theme of delivering a partial signal through the T-cell receptor, which results in tolerance rather than stimulation. The first method was to expose the T cells to peptide plus APCs treated with the carbodiimide cross-linker ECDI (415). This treatment may prevent accessory molecules on the presenting cell from interacting with the T-cell receptor complex or co-stimulatory signals from contributing to T-cell activation. The second method was to present peptide on presenting cells with mutated IE molecules (416,417). The third method was to use altered peptide ligands that act as T-cell receptor antagonists as described previously (406,413,414). The final method was to block CD4 function with a monoclonal antibody, which would delay the recruitment of CD4 to the engaged T-cell receptor (418). Because generation of a complete stimulatory signal requires the interaction of the T-cell receptor and accessory molecules, modifications that affect either component can block signaling. An altered peptide ligand, with decreased affinity for the T-cell receptor, may form an unstable complex, which cannot stay together long enough to recruit accessory molecules and generate a complete signal (418,419). Altered peptide ligands with low affinity for the T-cell receptor can also act as partial agonists that can compete with optimal agonists and reduce T-cell stimula-

tion through a similar mechanism (short dwell time of peptide/MHC complex on the T-cell receptor) (169).

Abnormal T-cell receptor signaling can be demonstrated by following the activity of protein kinases. Normal signaling produces phosphorylation of T-cell receptor subunits, such as ζ chain, as well as phosphorylation and activation of receptor-associated tyrosine kinases, such as ZAP70. These kinases generate the downstream signal needed for T-cell activation. However, in each case studied, partial antigen signaling resulted in ζ chain phosphorylation without phosphorylation or activation of ZAP70 (413,417,418), and so downstream activation did not occur. This abnormal pattern occurred regardless of the method of anergy induction.

Partial signaling may be important for T-cell survival during negative selection in the thymus or in maintaining peripheral tolerance. By responding to self-antigens as if they were altered ligands presented in the thymus, T cells can use anergy induction as a successful strategy for avoiding clonal deletion. Similarly, peripheral tolerance may be an important mechanism for preventing autoimmune disease. Immunotherapy with altered peptide ligands can be envisioned as a way to block an ongoing response or induce tolerance to a specific antigen, such as the synovium in arthritis, or foreign MHC antigens in allograft rejection. However, a potential pitfall is that different T cells recognize the same peptide differently, and so a peptide that is seen as an altered peptide ligand by some T-cell clones may be seen as a complete antigen by others. In addition, the choice of peptide would vary with MHC type. To be effective, an altered peptide ligand should antagonize or anergize polyclonal T cells and should work with each patient's MHC type.

A similar mechanism may be invoked to explain the generally weak immunogenicity of tumor antigens. According to this hypothesis, the only T cells capable of responding to self-antigens on tumors may have low-affinity receptors for them. In effect, the natural sequence is the altered ligand that induces tolerance. In some cases, this anergy can be overcome with modified peptides that have greater affinity for the T-cell receptor and induce a full stimulatory signal, resulting in an effective immune response to the tumor antigens (395), as described previously in the section on epitope enhancement.

Prediction of T-Cell Epitopes

The fact that T cells recognize processed fragments of antigens presented by MHC molecules leads to the ironic situation that T-cell recognition of antigen, which is more complex than antibody recognition because of the ternary complex needed among T-cell receptor, antigen, and MHC molecule, may actually be focused on simpler structures of the antigen than those seen by most antibodies specific for native protein antigens. In contrast to the assembled topographic antigenic sites seen by many antibodies (44,45), T cells specific for processed antigens are limited to recognizing short segments of continuous sequence (147,203). Therefore, the tertiary structure of the protein plays little if any role in the structure of the epitope recognized by T cells, except as it may influence processing. However, the structure of the T-cell antigenic site itself must be limited to primary (sequence) and secondary structure, the latter depending only on local rather than long-range interactions. This limitation greatly simplifies the problem of identifying structural properties important to T-cell recognition, because it is possible to deal with sequence information, which can be obtained from DNA without having a purified protein, and with the secondary structure implicit therein without having to obtain an x-ray crystallographic three-dimensional structure of the native protein, a much more difficult task.

Because the key feature necessary for a peptide to be recognized by T cells is its ability to bind to an MHC molecule, most approaches for predicting T-cell epitopes are based on predictions of binding to MHC molecules. These approaches, which have been reviewed (369,420), can be divided into those that focus on specific individual MHC molecules one at a time, such as motif-based methods, and those that concern general structural properties of peptide sequences. We discuss first the methods based on general properties and then those directed to individual MHC molecules.

The first structural feature of amino acid sequences found associated with T-cell epitopes that remains in use today is helical amphipathicity (197,421–424), which is statistically significant independent of the tendency to form a helix per se (422). Because the x-ray crystallographic structures of both class I (330–332,425) and class II MHC molecules (223,388) have consistently shown peptides to be bound in extended, not α helical conformation, helicity per se has been abandoned as an associated structural feature of T-cell epitopes. However, as discussed later, there are other explanations of amphipathic structures that do not require the peptide to be bound to the MHC molecule as an α helix. Amphipathicity is the property of having hydrophobic and hydrophilic regions separated in space. It was observed that the immunodominant T-cell epitopes myoglobin and cytochrome c corresponded to amphipathic helices (155,159,426). To see whether this observation was true of immunodominant T-cell antigenic sites in other proteins as well, DeLisi and Berzofsky (421) developed an algorithm to search for segments of protein sequence that could fold as amphipathic helices. The approach was based on the idea that the hydrophobicity of the amino acids in the sequence must oscillate around an amphipathic helix. For the hydrophobic residues to line up on one side and the hydrophilic residues on the other, the periodicity of this oscillation must be approximately the same as the structural periodicity of the helix, about 100 degrees per turn (360 degrees/3.6 residues per turn) (Fig. 14).

A microcomputer program implementing this analysis was published (424). Subsequently, Margalit et al. (197) optimized the original approach (421), correctly identifying 18 of the 23 immunodominant helper T-cell antigenic sites from the 12 proteins in an expanded database ($p < 0.001$) (197) (Table 4). Indeed, when the database was expanded to

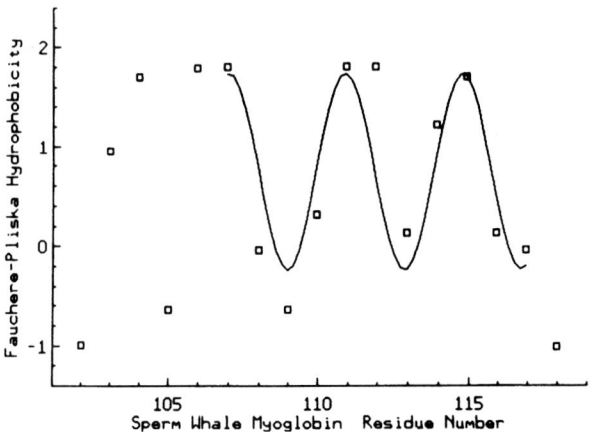

FIG. 14. Plot of hydrophobicity of each amino acid in sperm whale myoglobin 102-118, according to the scale of Fauchère and Pliska (488), as a function of amino acid sequence, showing least-squares fit of a sinusoidal function to the sequence of hydrophobicities from 107 to 117. From Berzofsky (150), with permission.

twice and then four times its original size, the correlation remained highly significant, and the fraction of sites predicted remained relatively stable (34 of 48 sites = 71%, $p < 0.003$; 61 of 92 sites = 66%, $p < 0.001$) (427,428). A similar correlation was found for 65% of peptides presented by class I MHC molecules (428). A primary sequence pattern found in a substantial number of T-cell epitopes by Rothbard and Taylor (429) was consistent with one turn of an amphipathic helix. Another approach, the "strip-of-the-helix" algorithm, that searches for helices with a hydrophobic strip down one face, found a correlation between amphipathic helices and determinants presented by both class II and class I MHC molecules (423,430).

Newer data suggest at least two explanations, not mutually exclusive, for this correlation in the absence of helical structure found in the peptides bound to MHC molecules (431). First, crystal structures of peptides bound to class II MHC molecules have revealed that the peptides are bound in an extended conformation, but with a −130-degree twist like that of a type II polyproline helix (223,388). The first such structure discovered, that of an influenza peptide bound to HLA-DR1 (223), was actually quite amphipathic because of this twist. Although the −130-degree twist is distinct from that of an α helix, it gives a periodicity similar enough to be detected. Second, it was observed that spacing of the anchor residues in the motifs for peptides binding to class I and II MHC molecules was consistent with the spacing of turns of an α helix: for example, at positions 2 and 9 (seven residues apart as in two turns of a helix) or at positions 5 and 9 (spaced like one turn of a helix) (431). Because the anchor residues are most often hydrophobic, this pattern resulted in an amphipathic periodicity pattern like that of an amphipathic α helix for just the anchor residues alone, seen in the majority of motifs (431). Thus, if the other residues have a random pattern, the anchor residue spacing alone, which is enforced by the spacing of the pockets in the MHC molecules that bind these anchor residues, produces the amphipathic helical signal, even though the peptide is bound in an extended conformation. This amphipathic helical periodicity has held up as a correlate for peptides defined as T-cell epitopes (431) and has continued to be a useful predictive tool for identifying potential epitopes, successful in a number of studies, when it is not desirable to focus on individual MHC alleles or to find regions of high epitope density.

Other approaches to predicting T-cell epitopes are generally based on sequences found to bind to specific MHC molecules (369,420). The simplest approach is to apply standard sequence search algorithms to known protein sequences to locate motifs for peptides binding to particular MHC molecules, using collections of motifs identified in the literature (234). This approach showed early success for epitopes in proteins from *Listeria monocytogenes* (432) and malaria (433), but it also became apparent that only about 30% of sequences bearing motifs actually bound to the corresponding MHC molecules (432,434,435). This discrepancy may relate to adverse interactions created by nonanchor residues (346,351,436) and could be overcome to some extent by generating extended motifs, taking into account the role of each residue in the sequence (351,436).

To determine whether regions of proteins with high densities of motifs for binding multiple MHC molecules could be located, Meister et al. (437) developed the algorithm, Epimer, which determined the density of motifs per length of sequence. A surprising result was that the motifs were not uniformly distributed, but clustered. This clustering may reflect the facts that many motifs are related and that the same anchor residues are shared by several motifs, perhaps because MHC molecules are also related and their variable segments that define some of the binding pockets are sometimes exchanged by gene conversion events (438). This hypothesis has been confirmed and extended by studies showing that each anchor pocket can be grouped into families of MHC molecules sharing similar pockets and, therefore, anchor residues; however, the families for the B, C, and F pockets do not coincide, and so there is a reassortment between pockets (439,440). These observations allow prediction of motifs for additional MHC molecules. In the case of HIV, the densities of motifs for class I MHC binding were anomalous at both the low and high ends of the spectrum (441). Clustering at the high end may result from anchor sharing and showed no correlation with conserved or variable regions of the sequence. However, at the low end, long stretches with low motif density occurred preferentially in variable regions, which suggests that the virus was mutating to escape the CTL immune system (441). This clustering may be useful in vaccine development, because identification of sequences containing overlapping motifs for multiple MHC molecules may define promiscuously presented peptides that would elicit responses in a broad segment of the population (437).

Another type of MHC allele–specific approach is the use of matrices defining the positive or negative contribution of each amino acid possible at each position in the sequence toward binding to an MHC molecule. A positive or negative value is assigned to each of the 20 possible amino acids that can occur at each position in a peptide sequence, and these are summed to give the estimated potential of that peptide for binding. The values in the matrix are derived either from experimental binding studies with peptide panels with single positions substituted with each possible amino acid (384,442–444) or from comparisons of peptides known to bind in a compilation of the literature, if the number known is sufficiently large (420,445). Davenport et al. (446,447) also developed a motif method based on Edman degradation sequencing of pooled peptides eluted from MHC molecules. All of these methods have had some success in predicting peptides binding to particular MHC molecules (420); however, they all require the assumption that each position in a peptide must be acting independently of its neighbors, which is a reasonable first approximation, but exceptions are known (448). The more experimental data that go into generating the matrix, the more reliable the predictions are. Therefore, the predictive success may be greater for some of the more common HLA molecules for which more data exist. This matrix approach has been used for both class I and class II MHC molecules.

A potentially very useful observation is the finding that HLA class I molecules can be grouped into families (HLA supertypes) that share similar binding motifs (383,442,449,450). The broader motifs that encompass several MHC molecules have been called *supermotifs*. For example, HLA-A*0301, HLA-A*1101, HLA-A*3101, HLA-A*3401, HLA-A*6601, HLA-A*6801, and HLA-A*7401 all belong to the HLA-A3 superfamily (449). A peptide that carries this supermotif should be active in a broader range of individuals than one that is presented by a single HLA molecule. Moreover, because several HLA supertypes have been defined, it should be possible to design a vaccine effective in a large fraction of the population with only a limited number of well-selected antigenic determinants (451).

Another approach for predicting peptides that bind to MHC molecules is based on free energy calculations of peptides docked into the groove of a known MHC structure, for which the crystallographic coordinates are known, or on structural modeling of the MHC molecule by homologous extension from another MHC molecule, when the crystal structure is not known, followed by peptide docking calculations (452,453). It is important to use free energy rather than energy, because the latter alone cannot find the most stable orientation of a side chain and cannot correctly rank-order different side chains at the same position. This approach correctly predicts the structure of several known peptide/MHC complexes when starting with the crystal structure of a different complex, in each case to within a 1.2- to 1.6-Å all-atom root mean square deviation (453). Using this structural modeling can allow extending motifs to nonanchor positions for cases in which only anchor residue motifs are known, and can allow one to predict new motifs for MHC molecules whose motifs have not yet been determined.

Yet another approach to predicting MHC binding sequences is to use a technique called *threading* that has been developed for predicting peptide secondary structure, based on threading a sequence through a series of known secondary structures and calculating the energies of each structure. Altuvia et al. (454) showed that threading could be applied to peptides in the groove of MHC molecules, because when several peptides that bind to the same MHC molecule are compared crystallographically, the conformations of the peptides are fairly similar, as, for example, in several peptides crystallized bound to HLA-A2.1 (425). In testing the threading approach, Altuvia et al. (454) showed that known antigenic peptides are highly ranked among all peptides in a given protein sequence, and the rank order of peptides in competitive binding studies could be correctly predicted. The advantage of this approach is that it is independent of known binding motifs and can identify peptides that bind despite lack of the common motif for the MHC molecule in question. It can also be used to rank a set of peptides all containing a known motif.

Finally, artificial neural networks can be trained on a set of peptides that bind to a given MHC molecule to recognize patterns present in binding peptides (455). When the predictions of the artificial neural network are tested, the results can be used to further train the network to improve the predictive capability in an iterative manner.

As all these methods are further developed and refined, they will allow accurate prediction of peptides that will bind to different MHC molecules and thus allow the design of vaccines without empirical binding studies until the end of the process. Furthermore, localization of clusters of adjacent or overlapping binding sequences in a short segment of protein sequence can also be useful for selecting sequences that will be broadly recognized.

RELATIONSHIP BETWEEN HELPER T-CELL EPITOPES AND B-CELL EPITOPES ON A COMPLEX PROTEIN ANTIGEN

As discussed, the factors that determine the location of antigenic sites for T cells and for B cells, with the possible exception of self-tolerance, are largely different. Indeed, if B cells (with their surface antibody) bind sites that tend to be especially exposed or protruding—sites that are also more accessible and susceptible to proteolytic enzymes—then there is reason to think that T cells may have a lower probability of being able to recognize these same sites, which may be more likely to be destroyed during processing. Certainly, assembled topographic sites are destroyed during processing. On the other hand, there are examples in which T cells and antibodies seem to recognize the same, or very closely overlapping, sites on a protein (38,155,182,456–458), although fine specificity analysis usually indicates that the antibody and T-cell fine specificities are not identical. The question dealt with here is whether there are any functional or regula-

tory factors in T cell–B cell cooperation that would produce a relationship between helper T-cell specificity and B-cell specificity for the same protein antigen.

Early evidence that helper T cells might influence the specificity of the antibodies produced came from a number of studies showing that Ir genes, which appeared to act through effects of T-cell help, could influence the specificity of antibodies produced to a given antigen (151,459–466). It was hard to imagine how MHC-encoded Ir genes could determine which epitopes of a protein elicit antibodies, when such antibodies are generally not MHC restricted. One explanation suggested was that the Ir genes first select which helper T cells are activated, and these in turn influence which B cells, specific for particular epitopes, can be activated (105). Because, for cognate help, the B cell has to present the antigen in association with an MHC molecule to the helper T cell, the Ir gene control of antibody specificity must operate at least partly at this step by selecting which helper T cell can be activated by and help a given B cell. Conversely, if the helper T cell selects a subset of B cells to be activated on the basis of their antibody specificity, then there is a reciprocal interaction between T and B cells that influences each other's specificity. Therefore, this hypothesis was called *T–B reciprocity* (105). Steric constraints on the epitopes that could be used by helper T cells to help a B cell specific for another particular epitope of the same protein were also proposed by Sercarz et al. (467).

The concept was first tested by limiting the fine specificity of helper T cells to one or a few epitopes and then determining the effect on the specificities of antibodies produced in response to the whole molecule. This was accomplished by inducing T-cell tolerance to certain epitopes (468) and by using T cells from animals immune to peptide fragments of the protein (103,469,470). In each case, the limitation on the helper T-cell specificity repertoire influenced the repertoire of antibodies produced.

One purpose of the B-cell surface immunoglobulin is to take up the specific antigen with high affinity, which is then internalized by receptor-mediated endocytosis and processed like any other antigen (471–478). Therefore, it was proposed that the surface immunoglobulin, which acts as the receptor to mediate endocytosis, sterically influences the rate at which different parts of the antigen are processed, because what the B cell is processing is not free antigen but a monoclonal antibody–antigen immune complex (105). This concept presupposes that many antibody–antigen complexes are stable near pH 6 in the endosome and that what matters is the kinetics of production of large fragments, rather than the products of complete digestion, when both the antigen and the antibody may be degraded to single amino acids. Such protection from proteolysis of antigen epitopes by bound antibody can be demonstrated at least *in vitro* (49). More recently, the effect of antigen-specific B-cell surface immunoglobulin on the fragments produced by proteolytic processing of antigen was elegantly demonstrated by Davidson and Watts (479). They showed that the pattern of fragmentation of tetanus toxoid, as measured by SDS–polyacrylamide gel electrophoresis, produced during processing by B lymphoblastoid clones specific for tetanus toxoid, varied among B-cell clones, depending on their specificity for different epitopes within the antigen. Binding to the antibody may also influence which fragments are shuttled to the surface and which are shunted into true lysosomes for total degradation. Thus, different B cells bearing different surface immunoglobulin would preferentially process the antigen differently to put more of some potential fragments than others on their surface, in contrast to nonspecific presenting cells that would process the antigen indifferently. By this mechanism, it was proposed that B-cell specificity leads to selective antigen presentation to helper T cells and therefore to selective help from T cells specific for some epitopes more than from T cells specific for others (105)

To test this hypothesis, Ozaki and Berzofsky (104) made populations of B cells effectively monoclonal for purposes of antigen presentation by coating polyclonal B cells with a conjugate of monoclonal antimyoglobin coupled to anti–immunoglobulin M antibodies. B cells coated with one such conjugate presented myoglobin less well to one myoglobin-specific T-cell clone than to others. B cells coated with other conjugates presented myoglobin to this clone equally well as to other clones. Therefore, the limitation on myoglobin presentation by this B cell to this T-cell clone depended on the specificity of both the monoclonal antibody coating the B cell and the receptor of the T-cell clone. It happened in this case that both the monoclonal antibody and the T-cell clone were specific for the same or closely overlapping epitopes. Therefore, it appears that the site bound by the B-cell surface immunoglobulin is less well presented to T cells. This finding is also consistent with results of a study of chimeric proteins in which one or more copies of an ovalbumin helper T-cell determinant were inserted in different positions (480). Although the position of the ovalbumin determinants did not affect the antibody response to one epitope, the position did matter for antibody production to an epitope of the chimeric protein derived from insulin-like growth factor I. An ovalbumin determinant inserted distal to this epitope was much more effective in providing help than was one inserted adjacent to the same epitope, when both constructs were used as immunogens, even though both constructs elicited similar levels of ovalbumin-specific T-cell proliferation in the presence of nonspecific presenting cells *in vitro,* as a control for nonspecific effects of flanking residues on processing and presentation of the helper T-cell determinants. However, circumstantial evidence from the Ir gene studies mentioned previously suggests that T cells may preferentially help B cells that bind with some degree of proximity to the T-cell epitope, inasmuch as there was a correlation between T cell and antibody specificity for large fragments of protein antigens under Ir gene control (102,105,151,462,463,466). Therefore, antibodies may have both positive and negative selective effects on processing. Further studies on presentation of β-galactosidase–monoclonal antibody complexes by nonspe-

cific APCs suggest similar conclusions (481,482). Presumably, the conjugates are taken up via crystallized fragment (Fc) receptors on the presenting cells and processed differentially according to the site bound by the antibody, so that they are presented differentially to different T cell clones. Thus, non–B-presenting cells can be made to mimic specific B-presenting cells. This also suggests that circulating antibody may have a role in the selection of which T cells are activated in a subsequent exposure to antigen.

The issue of whether bound antibody enhanced or suppressed presentation of specific determinants to T cells was explored further by Watts and Lanzavecchia (483) and Simitsek et al. (484). They first found that a particular tetanus toxoid–specific Epstein-Barr virus–transformed human B-cell clone 11.3 failed to present the tetanus toxoid epitope 1174-1189 to specific T cells, whereas it presented another epitope as well as did other B cells, and another B-cell clone presented the 1174-1189 epitope well. Moreover, the free 11.3 antibody also inhibited presentation of this epitope to T cells at the same time that it enhanced presentation of other epitopes by Fc receptor–facilitated uptake (483). They subsequently found that the same 11.3 B cell and antibody actually enhanced presentation of another epitope of tetanus toxoid, 1273-1284, by about 10-fold, even though both epitopes were within the footprint of the antibody, as determined by protection from proteolytic digestion (484). The enhancement could be mediated also by free antibody as well as antibody fragments thereof, indicating that the mechanism did not involve Fc receptor–facilitated uptake. Furthermore, the 11.3 antibody had no effect on presentation of another determinant in the same tetanus toxoid C fragment, 947-967, that was not within the footprint of the antibody, and another antibody to the C fragment did not enhance presentation of 1273-1284. The authors concluded that the same antibody or surface immunoglobulin can protect two determinants from proteolysis but sterically hinder the binding of one to class II MHC molecules while facilitating the binding of the other (484). The facilitation may involve protection from degradation. This antibody-mediated enhancement of presentation of selected epitopes to helper T cells can greatly lower the threshold for induction of a T-cell response and may thereby elicit responses to otherwise subdominant epitopes. It can also contribute to epitope spreading: for example, in autoimmune disease, in which an initial response to one dominant determinant leads to a subsequent response to other subdominant determinants, perhaps by helping for antibody production, which in turn facilitates presentation of the other determinants.

Taken together, these results support the concept of T–B reciprocity in which helper T cells and B cells each influence the specificity of the other's expressed repertoire (105). This mechanism may also provide an explanation for some of the cases in which Ir genes have been found to control antibody idiotype (485,486). These relationships probably play a significant role in regulating the fine specificity of immune response of both arms of the immune system. Therefore, they will also be of importance in the design of synthetic or recombinant fragment vaccines that incorporate both T and B cell epitopes to elicit an antibody response.

REFERENCES

1. Goodman JW. Antigenic determinants and antibody combining sites. In: Sela M, ed. *The antigens.* New York: Academic Press, 1975:127–187.
2. Landsteiner K. *The specificity of serological reactions,* Cambridge, MA: Harvard University Press, 1945.
3. Landsteiner K, Van der Scheer J. Serological studies on azoproteins antigens containing azo components with aliphatic side chains. *J Exp Med* 1934;59:751–768.
4. Pressman D, Grossberg AL. *The structural basis of antibody specificity,* New York: Benjamin, 1968.
5. Pressman D, Siegel M, Hall LAR. The closeness of fit of antibenzoate antibodies about haptens and the orientation of the haptens in combination. *J Am Chem Soc* 1954;76:6336–6341.
6. Karush F. The interaction of purified anti-lactoside antibody with haptens. *J Am Chem Soc* 1957;79:3380–3384.
7. Eisen HN, Siskind GW. Variations in affinities of antibodies during the immune response. *Biochemistry* 1964;3:996–1008.
8. Kabat EA. *Structural concepts in immunology and immunochemistry,* 2nd ed. New York: Holt, Rinehart & Winston, 1976.
9. Jann K, Westphal O. Microbial polysaccharides. In: Sela M, ed. *The antigens.* New York: Academic Press, 1975:1–125.
10. Springer GF. Blood group and Forssman antigenic determinants shared between microbes and mammalian cells. In: Kallos P, Waksman BH, eds. *Progress in allergy.* Basel: Karger, 1971:9–77.
11. Marcus DM. The ABO and Lewis blood-group system. Immunochemistry, genetics, and relation to human disease. *N Engl J Med* 1969;280:994–1006.
12. Watkins WM. Biochemistry and genetics of the ABO, Lewis, and P blood group systems. *Adv Hum Genet* 1980;10:1–136.
13. Kabat EA. The upper limit for the size of the human antidextran combining site. *J Immunol* 1960;84:82–85.
14. Kabat EA. The nature of an antigenic determinant. *J Immunol* 1966;97:1–11.
15. Cisar J, Kabat EA, Dorner MM, et al. Binding properties of immunoglobulin combining sites specific for terminal or nonterminal antigenic determinants in dextran. *J Exp Med* 1975;142:435–459.
16. Sharon J, Kabat EA, Morrison SL. Studies on mouse hybridomas secreting IgM or IgA antibodies to α(1→6)-linked dextran. *Mol Immunol* 1981;18:831–846.
17. Sharon J, Kabat EA, Liao J, et al. Immunochemical characterization of binding sites of hybridoma antibodies specific for α(1→6) linked dextran. *Mol Immunol* 1982;19:375–388.
18. Sharon J, D'Hoostelaere L, Potter M, et al. A cross-reactive idiotype, QUPC 52 IdX, present on most but not all anti-α(1→6) dextran-specific IgM and IgA hydriboma antibodies with combining sites of different sizes. *J Immunol* 1982;128:498–500.
19. Sikder SK, Akolkar PN, Kaladas PM, et al. Sequences of variable regions of hybridoma antibodies to α(1→6) dextran in BALB/c and C57BL/6 mice. *J Immunol* 1985;135:4215–4221.
20. Akolkar PN, Sikder SK, Bhattacharya SB, et al. Different VL and VH germline genes are used to produce similar combining sites with specificity for α(1→6) dextrans. *J Immunol* 1987;138:4472–4479.
21. Brodeur PM, Riblet R. The immunoglobulin heavy chain variable region (Igh-v) locus in the mouse I. One-hundred Igh-v genes comprise seven families of homologous genes. *Eur J Immunol* 1984;14:922–930.
22. Griffiths GM, Berek C, Kaartinen M, et al. Somatic mutation and the maturation of immune response to 2-phenxyloxazolone. *Nature* 1984;14:271–275.
23. Wang D, Chen H-T, Liao J, et al. Two families of monoclonal antibodies to α(1-6)dextran, VH19.1.2. and VH9.14.7, show distinct patterns of JK and JH minigene usage and amino acid substitutions in CDR3. *J Immunol* 1990;145:3002–3010.
24. Schneerson R, Barrera O, Sutton A, et al. Preparation, characterization, and immunogenicity of *Haemophilus influenzae* type b polysaccharide–protein conjugates. *J Exp Med* 1980;152:361–376.
25. Robbins JB, Schneerson R, Anderson P, et al. The 1996 Albert Lasker Medical Research Awards. Prevention of systemic infections, especially meningitis, caused by *Haemophilus influenzae* type b. Impact on public health and implications for other polysaccharide-based vaccines. *JAMA* 1996;276:1181–1185.
26. Murphy TV, White KE, Pastor P, et al. Declining incidence of *Haemophilus influenzae* type b disease since introduction of vaccination. *JAMA* 1993;269:246–248.
27. Black S, Shinefield H, Fireman B, et al. Efficacy, safety and immunogenicity of heptavalent pneumococcal conjugate vaccine in children. Northern California Kaiser Permanente Vaccine Study Center Group. *Pediatr Infect Dis J* 2000;19:187–195.
28. Eskola J, Kilpi T, Palmu A, et al. Efficacy of a pneumococcal conjugate vaccine against acute otitis media. *N Engl J Med* 2001;344:403–409.
29. Amit AG, Mariuzza RA, Phillips SEV, et al. Three-dimensional structure of an antigen–antibody complex at 2.8 Åresolution. *Science* 1986;233:747–758.
30. Colman PM, Laver WG, Varghese JN, et al. Three-dimensional structure of a complex of antibody with influenza virus neuraminidase. *Nature* 1987;326:358–363.
31. Sheriff S, Silverton EW, Padlan EA, et al. Three-dimensional structure of an antibody–antigen complex. *Proc Natl Acad Sci U S A* 1987;84:8075–8079.
32. Davies DR, Padlan EA. Antibody–antigen complexes. *Annu Rev Biochem* 1990;59:439–473.
33. Schlossman SF, Yaron A, Ben-Efraim S, et al. Immunogenicity of a series of αN-DNP-L-lysines. *Biochemistry* 1965;4:1638–1645.
34. Schlossman SF, Levine H. Desensitization to delayed hypersensitivity reactions. With special reference to the requirement for an immunogenic molecule. *J Immunol* 1967;99:111–114.
35. Van Vunakis H, Kaplan J, Lehrer H, et al. Immunogenicity of polylysine and polyornithine when complexed to phosphorylated bovine serum albumin. *Immunochemistry* 1966;3:393–402.
36. Getzoff ED, Tainer JA, Lerner RA, et al. The chemistry and mechanisms of antibody binding to protein antigens. *Adv Immunol* 1988;43:1–98.
37. Sela M. Antigenicity: some molecular aspects. *Science* 1969;166:1365–1374.
38. Berzofsky JA, Buckenmeyer GK, Hicks G, et al. Topographic antigenic determinants recognized by monoclonal antibodies to sperm whale myoglobin. *J Biol Chem* 1982;257:3189–3198.
39. Koketsu J, Atassi MZ. Immunochemistry of sperm-whale myoglobin-XVI: accurate delineation of the single region in sequence 1–55 by immunochemical studies of synthetic peptides. Some conclusions concerning antigenic structures of proteins. *Immunochemistry* 1974;11:1–8.
40. Dickerson RE. X-ray analysis and protein structure. In: Neurath H, ed. *The proteins.* New York: Academic Press, 1964:603–778.
41. Takano T. Structure of myoglobin refined at 2.0 Åresolution. I. Crystallographic refinement of metmyoglobin from sperm whale. *J Mol Biol* 1977;110:537–568.
42. Feldmann RJ, Bing DH, Furie BC, et al. Interactive computer surface graphics approach to the study of the active site of bovine trypsin. *Proc Natl Acad Sci U S A* 1978;75:5409–5412.
43. Barlow DJ, Edwards MS, Thornton JM. Continuous and discontinuous protein antigenic determinants. *Nature* 1986;322:747–748.
44. Benjamin DC, Berzofsky JA, East IJ, et al. The antigenic structure of proteins: a reappraisal. *Annu Rev Immunol* 1984;2:67–101.
45. Berzofsky JA. Intrinsic and extrinsic factors in protein antigenic structure. *Science* 1985;229:932–940.
46. Sachs DH, Schechter AN, Eastlake A, et al. An immunological approach to the conformational equilibria of polypeptides. *Proc Natl Acad Sci U S A* 1972;69:3790–3794.
47. Crumpton MJ. Protein antigen: the molecular bases of antigenicity and immunogenicity. In: Sela M, ed. *The antigens.* New York: Academic Press, 1974:1–79.
48. Burnens A, Demotz S, Corradin G, et al. Epitope mapping by chemical modification of free and antibody-bound protein antigen. *Science* 1987;235:780–783.
49. Jemmerson R, Paterson Y. Mapping epitopes on a protein antigen by the proteolysis of antigen–antibody complexes. *Science* 1986;232:1001–1004.
50. Smith-Gill SJ, Wilson AC, Potter M, et al. Mapping the antigenic

epitope for a monoclonal antibody against lysozyme. *J Immunol* 1982; 128:314–322.

51. Kohno Y, Berkower I, Minna J, et al. Idiotypes of anti-myoglobin antibodies: shared idiotypes among monoclonal antibodies to distinct determinants of sperm whale myoglobin. *J Immunol* 1982;128:1742–1748.

52. Streicher HZ, Cuttitta F, Buckenmeyer GK, et al. Mapping the idiotopes of a monoclonal anti-idiotypic antibodies: detection of a common idiotope. *J Immunol* 1986;136:1007–1014.

53. Geysen HM, Rodda SJ, Mason TJ, et al. Strategies for epitope analysis using peptide synthesis. *J Immunol Methods* 1987;102:259–274.

54. Crumpton MJ, Wilkinson JM. The immunological activity of some of the chymotryptic peptides of sperm-whale myoglobin. *Biochem J* 1965;94:545–556.

55. Smith JA, Hurrell JGR, Leach SJ. A novel method for delineating antigenic determinants: peptide synthesis and radioimmunoassay using the same solid support. *Immunochemistry* 1977;14:565–568.

56. Atassi MZ. Antigenic structure of myoglobin: the complete immunochemical anatomy of a protein and conclusions relating to antigenic structures of proteins. *Immunochemistry* 1975;12:423–438.

57. Berzofsky JA, Buckenmeyer GK, Hicks G, et al. Topographic antigenic determinants detected by monoclonal antibodies to myoglobin. In: Celada F, Sercarz E, Shumaker V, eds. *Protein conformation as immunological signal.* New York: Plenum Press, 1983:165–180.

58. Hurrell JGR, Smith JA, Todd PE, et al. Cross-reactivity between mammalian myoglobins: linear vs. spatial antigenic determinants. *Immunochemistry* 1977;14:283–288.

59. East IJ, Todd PE, Leach SJ. On topographic antigenic determinants in myoglobins. *Mol Immunol* 1980;17:519–525.

60. Maron E, Shiozawa C, Arnon R, et al. Chemical and immunological characterization of a unique antigenic region in lysozyme. *Biochemistry* 1971;10:763–771.

61. Berzofsky JA, Hicks G, Fedorko J, et al. Properties of monoclonal antibodies specific for determinants of a protein antigen, myoglobin. *J Biol Chem* 1980;255:11188–11191.

62. East IJ, Hurrell JGR, Todd PE, et al. Antigenic specificity of monoclonal antibodies to human myoglobin. *J Biol Chem* 1982;257:3199–3202.

63. Arquilla ER, Bromer WW, Mercola D. Immunology conformation and biological activity of insulin. *Diabetes* 1969;18:193–205.

64. Lau HKF, Reichlin M, Noble RW. Preparation of antibodies that bind to HbF but not to the isolated α and γ subunits. *Fed Proc* 1975;34:975.

65. Benjamini E, Shimizu M, Yound JD, et al. Immunochemical studies on the tobacco mosaic virus protein. VII. The binding of octanoylated peptides of the tobacco mosaic virus protein with antibodies to the whole protein. *Biochemistry* 1968;7:1261–1264.

66. Urbanski GJ, Margoliash E. Topographic determinants on cytochrome c: I. The complete antigenic structures of rabbit, mouse, and guanaco cytochromes c in rabbits and mice. *J Immunol* 1977;118:1170–1180.

67. Kwong PD, Wyatt R, Robinson J, et al. Structure of an HIV gp120 envelope glycoprotein in complex with the CD4 receptor and a neutralizing human antibody. *Nature* 1998;393:648–659.

68. Wyatt R, Kwong PD, Desjardins E, et al. The antigenic structure of the HIV gp120 envelope glycoprotein. *Nature* 1998;393:705–711.

69. Lando G, Berzofsky JA, Reichlin M. Antigenic structure of sperm whale myoglobin: I. Partition of specificities between antibodies reactive with peptides and native protein. *J Immunol* 1982;129:206–211.

70. White TJ, Ibrahimi IM, Wilson AC. Evolutionary substitutions and the antigenic structure of globular proteins. *Nature* 1978;274:92–94.

71. Reichlin M. Amino acid substitution and the antigenicity of globular proteins. *Adv Immunol* 1975;20:71–123.

72. Kabat EA. The structural basis of antibody complementarity. *Adv Protein Chem* 1978;32:1–76.

73. Berzofsky JA, Schechter AN. The concepts of crossreactivity and specificity in immunology. *Mol Immunol* 1981;18:751–763.

74. Furie B, Schechter AN, Sachs DH, et al. An immunological approach to the conformational equilibria of staphylococcal nuclease. *J Mol Biol* 1975;92:497–506.

75. Green N, Alexander H, Wilson A, et al. Immunogenic structure of the influenza virus hemagglutinin. *Cell* 1982;28:477–487.

76. Lerner R. Antibodies of predetermined specificity in biology and medicine. *Adv Immunol* 1984;36:1–44.

77. Perutz MF. Hemoglobin structure and respiratory transport. *Sci Am* 1978;239:92–125.

78. Monod J, Wyman J, Changeux J-P. On the nature of allosteric transitions: a plausible model. *J Mol Biol* 1965;12:88–118.

79. Papkoff J, Lai MH-T, Hunter T, et al. Analysis of transforming gene products from Moloney murine sarcoma virus. *Cell* 1981;27:109–119.

80. Colman PM, Varghese JN, Laver WG. Structure of the catalytic and antigenic sites in influenza virus neuraminidase. *Nature* 1983;303:41–44.

81. Lee B, Richards FM. The interpretation of protein structures: estimation of static accessibility. *J Mol Biol* 1971;55:379–400.

82. Connolly ML. Solvent-accessible surfaces of proteins and nucleic acids. *Science* 1983;221:709–713.

83. Novotny J, Handschumacher M, Haber E, et al. Antigenic determinants in proteins coincide with surface regions accessible to large probes (antibody domains). *Proc Natl Acad Sci U S A* 1986;83:226–230.

84. Thornton JM, Edwards MS, Taylor WR, et al. Location of "continuous" antigenic determinants in protruding regions of proteins. *EMBO J* 1986;5:409–413.

85. Hopp TP, Woods KR. Prediction of protein antigenic determinants from amino acid sequences. *Proc Natl Acad Sci U S A* 1981;78:3824–3828.

86. Fraga S. Theoretical prediction of protein antigenic determinants from amino acid sequences. *Can J Chem* 1982;60:2606–2610.

87. Hopp TP. Protein surface analysis: methods for identifying antigenic determinants and other interaction sites. *J Immunol Methods* 1986; 88:1–18.

88. Leach SJ. How antigenic are antigenic peptides? *Biopolymers* 1983; 22:425–440.

89. Todd PEE, East IJ, Leach SJ. The immunogenicity and antigenicity of proteins. *Trends Biochem Sci* 1982;7:212–216.

90. Chothia C, Janin J. Principles of protein-protein recognition. *Nature* 1975;256:705–708.

91. Tainer JA, Getzoff ED, Paterson Y, et al. The atomic mobility component of protein antigenicity. *Annu Rev Immunol* 1985;3:501–535.

92. Tainer JA, Getzoff ED, Alexander H, et al. The reactivity of antipeptide antibodies is a function of the atomic mobility of sites in a protein. *Nature* 1984;312:127–133.

93. Westhof E, Altschuh D, Moras D, et al. Correlation between segmental mobility and the location of antigenic determinants in proteins. *Nature* 1984;311:123–126.

94. Al Moudallal Z, Briand JP, Van Regenmortel MHV. A major part of the polypeptide chain of tobacco masaic virus protein is antigenic. *EMBO J* 1985;4:1231–1235.

95. Van Regenmortel MHV. Antigenic cross-reactivity between proteins and peptides: new insights and applications. *Trends Biochem Sci* 1987;12:237–240.

96. Geysen HM, Tainer JA, Rodda SJ, et al. Chemistry of antibody binding to a protein. *Science* 1987;235:1184–1190.

97. Edmundson AB, Ely KR, Herron JN. A search for site-filling ligands in the Meg Bence-Jones dimer: crystal binding studies of fluorescent compounds. *Mol Immunol* 1984;21:561–576.

98. Getzoff ED, Geysen HM, Rodda SJ, et al. Mechanisms of antibody binding to a protein. *Science* 1987;235:1191–1196.

99. Rini JM, Schulze-Gahmen U, Wilson IA. Structure evidence for induced fit as a mechanism for antibody-antigen recognition. *Science* 1992;255:959–965.

100. Jemmerson R, Margoliash E. Topographic antigenic determinants on cytochrome c. Immunoadsorbent separation of rabbit antibody populations directed against horse cytochrome c. *J Biol Chem* 1979; 254:12706–12716.

101. Cooper HM, East IJ, Todd PEE, et al. Antibody response to myoglobins: effect of host species. *Mol Immunol* 1984;21:479–487.

102. Berzofsky JA. Ir genes: antigen-specific genetic regulation of the immune response. In: Sela M, ed. *The antigens.* New York: Academic Press, 1987:1–146.

103. Manca F, Kunkl A, Fenoglio D, et al. Constraints in T–B cooperation related to epitope topology on *E.coli* β-galactosidase. I. The fine specificity of T cells dictates the fine specificity of antibodies directed to conformation-dependent determinants. *Eur J Immunol* 1985;15:345–350.

104. Ozaki S, Berzofsky JA. Antibody conjugates mimic specific B cell

presentation of antigen: relationship between T and B cell specificity. *J Immunol* 1987;138:4133–4142.

105. Berzofsky JA. T-B reciprocity: An Ia-restricted epitope-specific circuit regulating T cell–B cell interaction and antibody specificity. *Surv Immunol Res* 1983;2:223–229.

106. Potocnjak P, Yoshida N, Nussenzweig RS, et al. Monovalent fragments (Fab) of monoclonal antibodies to a sporozoite surface antigen (Pb44) protect mice against malarial infection. *J Exp Med* 1980;151:1504.

107. Good MF, Berzofsky JA, Maloy WL, et al. Genetic control of the immune response in mice to a *Plasmodium falciparum* sporozoite vaccine: widespread non-responsiveness to a single malaria T epitope in highly repetitive vaccine. *J Exp Med* 1986;164:655–660.

108. Del Giudice G, Cooper JA, Merino J, et al. The antibody response in mice to carrier-free synthetic polymers of *Plasmodium falciparum* circumsporozoite repetitive epitope is I-Ab–restricted: possible implications for malaria vaccines. *J Immunol* 1986;137:2952–2955.

109. Herrington DA, Clyde DF, Losonsky G, et al. Safety and immunogenicity in man of a synthetic peptide malaria vaccine against *Plasmodium falciparum* sporozoites. *Nature* 1987;328:257–259.

110. Good MF, Maloy WL, Lunde MN, et al. Construction of a synthetic immunogen: use of a new T-helper epitope on malaria circumsporozoite protein. *Science* 1987;235:1059–1062.

111. Kawamura H, Rosenberg SA, Berzofsky JA. Immunization with antigen and interleukin-2 *in vivo* overcomes Ir genetic low responsiveness. *J Exp Med* 1985;162:381–386.

112. Good MF, Pombo D, Lunde MN, et al. Recombinant human interleukin-2 (IL-2) overcomes genetic nonresponsiveness to malaria sporozoite peptides. Correlation of effect with biological activity of IL-2. *J Immunol* 1988;141:972–977.

113. Le Bouvier GL. The D→C change in poliovirus particles. *Br J Exp Pathol* 1959;40:605–620.

114. Gerhard W, Yewdell JW, Frankel ME, et al. Antigenic structure of influenza virus hemagglutinin defined by hybridoma antibodies. *Nature* 1981;290:713–717.

115. Emini EA, Kao S-Y, Lewis AJ, et al. Functional basis of poliovirus neutralization determined with mono-specific neutralizing antibodies. *J Virol* 1983;46:466–474.

116. Wiley DC, Wilson EA, Skehel JJ. Structural identification of the antibody-binding sites of Hong Kong influenza haemagglutinin and their involvement in antigenic variation. *Nature* 1981;289:373–378.

117. Icenogle J, Shiwen H, Duke G, et al. Neutralization of poliovirus by a monoclonal antibody: kinetics and stoichiometry. *Virology* 1983;127:412–425.

118. Mandel B. Interaction of viruses with neutralizing antibodies. In: Fraenkel-Conrat H, Wagner RR, eds. *Comprehensive virology 15: viral–host interactions.* New York: Plenum Press, 1979:37–121.

119. Kaplan G, Freistadt MS, Racaniello VR. Neutralization of poliovirus by cell receptors expressed in insect cells. *J Virol* 1990;64:4697–4702.

120. Smith DH, Byrn RA, Marsters SA, et al. Blocking of HIV-1 infectivity by a soluble, secreted form of the CD4 antigen. *Science* 1987;238:1704–1707.

121. Fisher RA, Bertonis JM, Meier W, et al. HIV infection is blocked *in vitro* by recombinant soluble CD4. *Nature* 1988;331:76–78.

122. Hussey RE, Richardson NE, Kowalski M, et al. A soluble CD4 protein selectively inhibits HIV replication and syncytium formation. *Nature* 1988;331:78–81.

123. Capon DJ, Chamow SM, Mordenti J, et al. Designing CD4 immunoadhesins for AIDS therapy. *Nature* 1989;337:525–531.

124. Palker TJ, Clark ME, Langlois AJ, et al. Type-specific neutralization of the human immunodeficiency virus with antibodies to env-encoded synthetic peptides. *Proc Natl Acad Sci U S A* 1988;85:1932–1936.

125. Rusche JR, Javaherian K, McDanal C, et al. Antibodies that inhibit fusion of HIV infected cells bind a 24 amino acid sequence of the viral envelope, gp120. *Proc Natl Acad Sci U S A* 1988;85:3198–3202.

126. Goudsmit J, Debouck C, Meloen RH, et al. Human immunodeficiency virus type 1 neutralization epitope with conserved architecture elicits early type-specific antibodies in experimentally infected chimpanzees. *Proc Natl Acad Sci U S A* 1988;85:4478–4482.

127. Berkower I, Smith GE, Giri C, et al. Human immunodeficiency virus–1: predominance of a group-specific neutralizing epitope that persists despite genetic variation. *J Exp Med* 1989;170:1681–1695.

128. Kang C-Y, Nara P, Chamat S, et al. Evidence for non–V3-specific neutralizing antibodies that interfere with gp120/CD4 binding in

human immunodeficiency virus 1–infected humans. *Proc Natl Acad Sci U S A* 1991;88:6171–6175.

129. Berkower I, Murphy D, Smith CC, et al. A predominant group-specific neutralizing epitope of human immunodeficiency virus type 1 maps to residues 342 to 511 of the envelope glycoprotein gp120. *J Virol* 1991;65:5983–5990.

130. Thali M, Olshevsky U, Furman C, et al. Characterization of a discontinuous human immunodeficiency virus type 1 gp120 epitope recognized by a broadly reactive neutralizing human monoclonal antibody. *J Virol* 1991;65:6188–6193.

131. Tilley SA, Honnen WJ, Racho ME, et al. A human monoclonal antibody against the CD4-binding site of HIV1 gp120 exhibits potent, broadly neutralizing activity. *Res Virol* 1991;142:247–259.

132. Kessler JA 2nd, McKenna PM, Emini EA, et al. Recombinant human monoclonal antibody IgG1b12 neutralizes diverse human immunodeficiency virus type 1 primary isolates. *AIDS Res Hum Retroviruses* 1997;13:575–582.

133. Trkola A, Purtscher M, Muster T, et al. Human monoclonal antibody 2G12 defines a distinctive neutralization epitope on the gp120 glycoprotein of human immunodeficiency virus type 1. *J Virol* 1996; 70:1100–1108.

134. Muster T, Steindl F, Purtscher M, et al. A conserved neutralizing epitope on gp41 of human immunodeficiency virus type 1. *J Virol* 1993;67:6642–6647.

135. Eckhart L, Raffelsberger W, Ferko B, et al. Immunogenic presentation of a conserved gp41 epitope of human immunodeficiency virus type 1 on recombinant surface antigen of hepatitis B virus. *J Gen Virol* 1996;77:2001–2008.

136. Burton DR. A vaccine for HIV type 1: the antibody perspective. *Proc Natl Acad Sci U S A* 1997;94:10018–10023.

137. Trkola A, Ketas T, Kewalramani VN, et al. Neutralization sensitivity of human immunodeficiency virus type 1 primary isolates to antibodies and CD4-based reagents is independent of coreceptor usage. *J Virol* 1998;72:1876–1885.

138. Baba TW, Liska V, Hofmann-Lehmann R, et al. Human neutralizing monoclonal antibodies of the IgG1 subtype protect against mucosal simian-human immunodeficiency virus infection. *Nat Med* 2000;6:200–206.

139. Mascola JR, Stiegler G, VanCott TC, et al. Protection of macaques against vaginal transmission of a pathogenic HIV-1/SIV chimeric virus by passive infusion of neutralizing antibodies. *Nat Med* 2000;6:207–210.

140. Steimer KS, Scandella CJ, Skiles PV, et al. Neutralization of divergent HIV-1 isolates by conformation-dependent human antibodies to Gp120. *Science* 1991;254:105–108.

141. Benacerraf B, McDevitt HO. Histocompatibility-linked immune response genes. *Science* 1972;175:273–279.

142. Godfrey WL, Lewis GK, Goodman JW. The anatomy of an antigen molecule: functional subregions of L-tyrosine-*p*-azobenzenearsonate. *Mol Immunol* 1984;21:969–978.

143. Berkower I, Buckenmeyer GK, Gurd FRN, et al. A possible immunodominant epitope recognized by murine T lymphocytes immune to different myoglobins. *Proc Natl Acad Sci U S A* 1982;79:4723–4727.

144. Solinger AM, Ultee ME, Margoliash E, et al. The T-lymphocyte response to cytochrome c. I. Demonstration of a T-cell heteroclitic proliferative response and identification of a topographic antigenic determinant on pigeon cytochrome c whose immune recognition requires two complementing major histocompatibility complex–linked immune response genes. *J Exp Med* 1979;150:830–848.

145. Katz ME, Maizels RM, Wicker L, et al. Immunological focusing by the mouse major histocompatibility complex: mouse strains confronted with distantly related lysozymes confine their attention to very few epitopes. *Eur J Immunol* 1982;12:535–540.

146. Gell PGH, Benacerraf B. Studies on hypersensitivity. II. Delayed hypersensitivity to denatured proteins in guinea pigs. *Immunology* 1959; 2:64–70.

147. Berzofsky JA. The nature and role of antigen processing in T cell activation. In: Cruse JM, Lewis RE Jr, eds. *The year in immunology 1984–1985.* Basel: Karger, 1985:18–24.

148. Livingstone A, Fathman CG. The structure of T cell epitopes. *Annu Rev Immunol* 1987;5:477–501.

149. Schwartz RH. T-lymphocyte recognition of antigen in association with gene products of the major histocompatibility complex. *Annu Rev Immunol* 1985;3:237–261.

150. Berzofsky JA, Cease KB, Cornette JL, et al. Protein antigenic structures recognized by T cells: potential applications to vaccine design. *Immunol Rev* 1987;98:9–52.

151. Berzofsky JA, Richman LK, Killion DJ. Distinct H-2–linked Ir genes control both antibody and T cell responses to different determinants on the same antigen, myoglobin. *Proc Natl Acad Sci U S A* 1979;76:4046–4050.

152. Manca F, Clarke JA, Miller A, et al. A limited region within hen egg-white lysozyme serves as the focus for a diversity of T cell clones. *J Immunol* 1984;133:2075–2078.

153. Shimonkevitz R, Colon S, Kappler JW, et al. Antigen recognition by H-2–restricted T cells. II. A tryptic ovalbumin peptide that substitutes for processed antigen. *J Immunol* 1984;133:2067–2074.

154. Allen PM, Unanue ER. Differential requirements for antigen processing by macrophages for lysozyme-specific T cell hybridomas. *J Immunol* 1984;132:1077–1079.

155. Berkower I, Buckenmeyer GK, Berzofsky JA. Molecular mapping of a histocompatibility-restricted immunodominant T cell epitope with synthetic and natural peptides: implications for antigenic structure. *J Immunol* 1986;136:2498–2503.

156. Kurokohchi K, Akatsuka T, Pendleton CD, et al. Use of recombinant protein to identify a motif-negative human CTL epitope presented by HLA-A2 in the hepatitis C virus NS3 region. *J Virol* 1996;70:232–240.

157. Thomas JW, Danho W, Bullesbach E, et al. Immune response gene control of determinant selection. III. Polypeptide fragments of insulin are differentially recognized by T but not by B cells in insulin immune guinea pigs. *J Immunol* 1981;126:1095–1100.

158. Schwartz RH, Fox BS, Fraga E, et al. The T lymphocyte response to cytochrome c. V. Determination of the minimal peptide size required for stimulation of T cell clones and assessment of the contribution of each residue beyond this size to antigenic potency. *J Immunol* 1985;135:2598–2608.

159. Cease KB, Berkower I, York-Jolley J, et al. T cell clones specific for an amphipathic alpha helical region of sperm whale myoglobin show differing fine specificities for synthetic peptides: a multiview/single structure interpretation of immunodominance. *J Exp Med* 1986;164:1779–1784.

160. Kurata A, Palker TJ, Streilein RD, et al. Immunodominant sites of human T-cell lymphotropic virus type 1 envelope protein for murine helper T cells. *J Immunol* 1989;143:2024–2030.

161. Lamb JR, Ivanyi J, Rees ADM, et al. Mapping of T cell epitopes using recombinant antigens and synthetic peptides. *EMBO J* 1987;6:1245–1249.

162. Townsend ARM, Gotch FM, Davey J. Cytotoxic T cells recognize fragments of the influenza nucleoprotein. *Cell* 1985;42:457–467.

163. Walker BD, Flexner C, Birch-Limberger K, et al. Long-term culture and fine specificity of human cytotoxic T lymphocyte clones reactive with human immunodeficiency virus type 1. *Proc Natl Acad Sci U S A* 1989;86:9514–9518.

164. Hosmalin A, Clerici M, Houghten R, et al. An epitope in HIV-1 reverse transcriptase recognized by both mouse and human CTL. *Proc Natl Acad Sci U S A* 1990;87:2344–2348.

165. Kojima M, Cease KB, Buckenmeyer GK, et al. Limiting dilution comparsion of the repertoires of high and low responder MHC-restricted T cells. *J Exp Med* 1988;167:1100–1113.

166. Heber-Katz E, Hansburg D, Schwartz RH. The Ia molecule of the antigen-presenting cell plays a critical role in immune response gene regulation of T cell activation. *J Mol Cell Immunol* 1983;1:3–14.

167. Matis LA, Longo DL, Hedrick SM, et al. Clonal analysis of the major histocompatibility complex restriction and the fine specificity of antigen recognition in the T cell proliferative response to cytochrome c. *J Immunol* 1983;130:1527–1535.

168. Hansburg D, Heber-Katz E, Fairwell T, et al. Major histocompatibility complex–controlled antigen presenting cell-expressed specificity of T cell antigen recognition. *J Exp Med* 1983;158:25–39.

169. England RE, Kullberg MC, Cornette JL, et al. Molecular analysis of a heteroclitic T-cell response to the immunodominant epitope of sperm whale myoglobin: implications for peptide partial agonists. *J Immunol* 1995;155:4295–4306.

170. Gammon G, Geysen HM, Apple RJ, et al. T cell determinant structure: cores and determinant envelopes in three mouse major histocompatibility complex haplotypes. *J Exp Med* 1991;173:609–617.

171. Kimoto M, Fathman CG. Antigen-reactive T cell clones. I. Transcomplementing hybrid I-A–region gene products function effectively in antigen presentation. *J Exp Med* 1980;152:759–770.

172. Kappler JW, Skidmore B, White J, et al. Antigen-inducible H-2–restricted interleukin-2–producing T cell hybridomas. Lack of independent antigen and H-2 recognition. *J Exp Med* 1981;153:1198–1214.

173. Young DB, Lamb JR. T lymphocytes respond to solid-phase antigen: a novel approach to the molecular analysis of cellular immunity. *Immunology* 1986;59:167–171.

174. Lamb JR, Young DB. A novel approach to the identification of T-cell epitopes in *Mycobacterium tuberculosis* using human T-lymphocyte clones. *Immunology* 1987;60:1–5.

175. Mustafa AS, Gill HK, Nerland A, et al. Human T-cell clones recognize a major *M. leprae* protein antigen expressed in *E. coli*. *Nature* 1986;319:63–66.

176. De Plaen E, Lurquin C, Van Pel A, et al. Immunogenic (tum−) variants of mouse tumor P815: cloning of the gene of tum− antigen P91A and identification of the tum− mutation. *Proc Natl Acad Sci U S A* 1988;85:2274–2278.

177. Van der Bruggen P, Traversari C, Chomez P, et al. A gene encoding an antigen recognized by cytolytic T lymphocytes on a human melanoma. *Science* 1991;254:1643–1647.

178. Guilloux Y, Lucas S, Brichard VG, et al. A peptide recognized by human cytolytic T lymphocytes on HLA-A2 melanomas is encoded by an intron sequence of the *N*-acetylglucosaminyltransferase B gene. *J Exp Med* 1996;183:1173–1183.

179. Kawakami Y, Eliyahu S, Delgado CH, et al. Cloning of the gene coding for a shared human melanoma antigen recognized by autologous T cells infiltrating into tumor. *Proc Natl Acad Sci U S A* 1994;91:3515–3519.

180. Robbins PF, El-Gamil M, Li YF, et al. A mutated β-catenin gene encodes a melanoma-specific antigen recognized by tumor infiltrating lymphocytes. *J Exp Med* 1996;183:1185–1192.

181. Wang R-F, Parkhurst MR, Kawakami Y, et al. Utilization of an alternative open reading frame of a normal gene in generating a novel human cancer antigen. *J Exp Med* 1996;183:1131–1140.

182. Berkower I, Kawamura H, Matis LA, et al. T cell clones to two major T cell epitopes of myoglobin: effect of I-A/I-E restriction on epitope dominance. *J Immunol* 1985;135:2628–2634.

183. Berkower I, Matis LA, Buckenmeyer GK, et al. Identification of distinct predominant epitopes recognized by myoglobin-specific T cells under control of different Ir genes and characterization of representative T-cell clones. *J Immunol* 1984;132:1370–1378.

184. Shastri N, Oki A, Miller A, et al. Distinct recognition phenotypes exist for T cell clones specific for small peptide regions of proteins. Implications for the mechanisms underlying major histocompatibility complex–restricted antigen recognition and clonal deletion models of immune response gene defects. *J Exp Med* 1985;162:332–345.

185. Allen PM, McKean DJ, Beck BN, et al. Direct evidence that a class II molecule and a simple globular protein generate multiple determinants. *J Exp Med* 1985;162:1264–1274.

186. Hackett CJ, Dietzschold B, Gerhard W, et al. Influenza virus site recognized by a murine helper T cell specific for H1 strains. *J Exp Med* 1983;158:294–302.

187. Hurwitz JL, Heber-Katz E, Hackett CJ, et al. Characterization of the murine TH response to influenza virus hemagglutinin: evidence for three major specificities. *J Immunol* 1984;133:3371–3377.

188. Lamb JR, Eckels DD, Lake P, et al. Human T cell clones recognize chemically synthesized peptides of influenza hemagglutinin. *Nature* 1982;300:66–69.

189. Rosenthal AS. Determinant selection and macrophage function in genetic control of the immune response. *Immunol Rev* 1978;40:136–152.

190. Milich DR, McLachlan A, Chisari FV, et al. Nonoverlapping T and B cell determinants on an hepatitis B surface antigen pre-S(2) region synthetic peptide. *J Exp Med* 1986;164:532–547.

191. Francis MJ, Fry CM, Rowlands DJ, et al. Immunological priming with synthetic peptides of foot and mouth disease virus. *J Gen Virol* 1985;66:2347–2352.

192. Corradin GP, Juillerat MA, Vita C, et al. Fine specificity of a BALB/c T cell clone directed against beef apo cytochrome c. *J Mol Immunol* 1983;20:763–768.

193. Corradin GP, Wallace CJA, Proudfoot AEI, et al. Murine T cell response specific for cytochrome c. In: Sercarz EE, Berzofsky JA, eds. *The

immunogenicity of protein antigens: repertoire and regulation. Boca Raton, FL: CRC Press, 1987:43–48.

194. Milich DR, Peterson DL, Leroux-Roels GG, et al. Genetic regulation of the immune response to hepatitis B surface antigen (HBsAg). VI. Fine specificity. *J Immunol* 1985;134:4203–4211.

195. Guillet J-G, Lai M-Z, Briner TJ, et al. Interaction of peptide antigens and class II major histocompatibility complex antigens. *Nature* 1986;324:260–262.

196. Macfarlan RI, Dietzschold B, Wiktor TJ, et al. T cell responses to cleaved rabies virus glycoprotein and to synthetic peptides. *J Immunol* 1984;133:2748–2752.

197. Margalit H, Spouge JL, Cornette JL, et al. Prediction of immunodominant helper T-cell antigenic sites from the primary sequence. *J Immunol* 1987;138:2213–2229.

198. Townsend ARM, Rothbard J, Gotch FM, et al. The epitopes of influenza nucleoprotein recognized by cytotoxic T lymphocytes can be defined with short synthetic peptides. *Cell* 1986;44:959–968.

199. Townsend AR, Bastin J, Gould K, et al. Cytotoxic T lymphocytes recognize influenza haemagglutinin that lacks a signal sequence. *Nature* 1986;324:575–577.

200. Berzofsky JA. Structural features of protein antigenic sites recognized by helper T cells: what makes a site immunodominant? In: Cruse JM, Lewis RE Jr, eds. *The year in immunology 1985–1986.* Basel: Karger, 1986:28–38.

201. Berzofsky JA. Immunodominance in T lymphocyte recognition. *Immunol Letters* 1988;18:83–92.

202. Yewdell JW, Bennink JR. Immunodominance in major histocompatibility complex class I–restricted T lymphocyte responses. *Annu Rev Immunol* 1999;17:51–88.

203. Allen PM. Antigen processing at the molecular level. *Immunol Today* 1987;8:270–273.

204. Goodman JW, Sercarz EE. The complexity of structures involved in T-cell activation. *Annu Rev Immunol* 1983;1:465–498.

205. Finnegan A, Smith MA, Smith JA, et al. The T cell repertoire for recognition of a phylogenetically distant protein antigen: peptide specificity and MHC restriction of staphylococcal nuclease specific T cell clones. *J Exp Med* 1986;164:897–910.

206. Good MF, Pombo D, Quakyi IA, et al. Human T cell recognition of the circumsporozoite protein of *Plasmodium falciparum.* Immunodominant T cell domains map to the polymorphic regions of the molecule. *Proc Natl Acad Sci U S A* 1988;85:1199–1203.

207. Nanda NK, Arzoo KK, Geysen HM, et al. Recognition of multiple peptide cores by a single T cell receptor. *J Exp Med* 1995;182:531–539.

208. Brett SJ, Cease KB, Berzofsky JA. Influences of antigen processing on the expression of the T cell repertoire: evidence for MHC-specific hindering structures on the products of processing. *J Exp Med* 1988;168:357–373.

209. Gammon G, Shastri N, Cogswell J, et al. The choice of T-cell epitopes utilized on a protein antigen depends on multiple factors distant from as well as at the determinant site. *Immunol Rev* 1987;98:53–73.

210. Sercarz EE, Lehmann PV, Ametani A, et al. Dominance and crypticity of T cell antigenic determinants. *Annu Rev Immunol* 1993;11:729–766.

211. Unanue ER. Antigen-presenting function of the macrophage. *Annu Rev Immunol* 1984;2:395–428.

212. Shastri N, Gammon G, Horvath S, et al. The choice between two distinct T cell determinants within a 23 amino acid region of lysozyme depends upon structure of the immunogen. *J Immunol* 1986;137:911–915.

213. Shastri N, Miller A, Sercarz EE. Amino acid residues distinct from the determinant region can profoundly affect activation of T cell clones by related antigens. *J Immunol* 1986;136:371–376.

214. Grewal IS, Moudgil KD, Sercarz EE. Hindrance of binding to class II major histocompatibility complex molecules by a single amino acid residue contiguous to a determinant leads to crypticity of the determinant as well as lack of response to the protein antigen. *Proc Natl Acad Sci U S A* 1995;92:1779–1783.

215. Fox BS, Carbone FR, Germain RN, et al. Processing of a minimal antigenic peptide alters its interaction with MHC molecules. *Nature* 1988;331:538–540.

216. Sercarz E, Wilbur S, Sadegh-Nasseri S, et al. The molecular context of a determinant influences its dominant expression in a T cell response hierarchy through "fine processing." In: Cinader B, Miller RG, eds.

Progress in immunology VI. New York: Academic Press, 1986:227–237.

217. Ziegler HK, Unanue ER. Decrease in macrophage antigen catabolism caused by ammonia and chloroquine is associated with inhibition of antigen presentation to T cells. *Proc Natl Acad Sci U S A* 1982;79:175–178.

218. Shimonkevitz R, Kappler J, Marrack P, et al. Antigen recognition by H-2 restricted T cells. I. Cell free antigen processing. *J Exp Med* 1983; 158:303–316.

219. Streicher HZ, Berkower IJ, Busch M, et al. Antigen conformation determines processing requirements for T-cell activation. *Proc Natl Acad Sci U S A* 1984;81:6831–6835.

220. Lee P, Matsueda GR, Allen PM. T cell recognition of fibrinogen. A determinant on the A α-chain does not require processing. *J Immunol* 1988;140:1063–1068.

221. Régnier-Vigouroux A, Ayeb ME, Defendini M-L, et al. Processing by accessory cells for presentation to murine T cells of apamin, a disulfide-bonded 18 amino acid peptide. *J Immunol* 1988;140:1069–1075.

222. Rudensky AY, Preston-Hurlburt P, Hong S-C, et al. Sequence analysis of peptides bound to MHC class II molecules. *Nature* 1991;353:622–627.

223. Stern LJ, Brown JH, Jardetzky TS, et al. Crystal structure of the human class II MHC protein HLA-DR1 complexed with an influenza virus peptide. *Nature* 1994;368:215–221.

224. Stern LJ, Wiley DC. Antigenic peptide binding by class I and class II histocompatibility proteins. *Structure* 1994;2:245–251.

225. Arunachalam B, Phan UT, Geuze HJ, et al. Enzymatic reduction of disulfide bonds in lysosomes: characterization of a gamma-interferon–inducible lysosomal thiol reductase (GILT). *Proc Natl Acad Sci U S A* 2000;97:745–750.

226. Maric M, Arunachalam B, Phan UT, et al. Defective antigen processing in GILT-free mice. *Science* 2001;294:1361–1365.

227. Townsend ARM, Skehel JJ. The influenza A virus nucleoprotein gene controls the induction of both subtype specific and crossreactive cytotoxic T cells. *J Exp Med* 1984;160:552–563.

228. Braciale TJ, Braciale VL, Winkler M, et al. On the role of the transmembrane anchor sequence of influenza hemagglutinin in target cell recognition by class I MHC–restricted hemagglutinin-specific cytolytic T lymphocytes. *J Exp Med* 1987;166:678–692.

229. Tobery T, Siliciano RF. Targeting of HIV-1 antigens for rapid intracellular degradation enhances cytotoxic T lymphocytes (CTL) recognition and the induction of *de novo* CTL responses *in vivo* after immunization. *J Exp Med* 1997;185:909–920.

230. York IA, Goldberg AL, Mo XY, et al. Proteolysis and class I major histocompatibility complex antigen presentation. *Immunol Rev* 1999;172:49–66.

231. Yewdell JW, Bennink JR. Cut and trim: generating MHC class I peptide ligands. *Curr Opin Immunol* 2001;13:13–18.

232. Vinitsky A, Antón LC, Snyder HL, et al. The generation of MHC class I–associated peptides is only partially inhibited by proteasome inhibitors: involvement of nonproteasomal cytosolic proteases in antigen processing? *J Immunol* 1997;159:554–564.

233. Rock KL, Gramm C, Rothstein L, et al. Inhibitors of the proteasome block the degradation of most cell proteins and the generation of peptides presented on MHC class I molecules. *Cell* 1994;78:761–771.

234. Rammensee H-G, Friede T, Stevanović S. MHC ligands and peptide motifs: first listing. *Immunogenetics* 1995;41:178–228.

235. Vinitsky A, Cardozo C, Sepp-Lorenzino L, et al. Inhibition of the proteolytic activity of the multicatalytic proteinase complex (proteasome) by substrate-related peptidyl aldehydes. *J Biol Chem* 1994;269:29860–29866.

236. Fenteany G, Standaert RF, Lane WS, et al. Inhibition of proteasome activities and subunit-specific amino-terminal threonine modification by lactacystin. *Science* 1995;268:726–731.

237. Hughes EA, Ortmann B, Surman M, et al. The protease inhibitor, N-acetyl-L-leucyl-L-leucyl-L norleucinal, decreases the pool of major histocompatibility complex class I–binding peptides and inhibits peptide trimming in the endoplasmic reticulum. *J Exp Med* 1996;183:1569–1578.

238. Henderson RA, Michel H, Sakaguchi K, et al. HLA-A2.1-associated peptides from a mutant cell line: a second pathway of antigen presentation. *Science* 1992;255:1264–1266.

239. Gaczynska M, Rock KL, Goldberg AL. γ-Interferon and expression

of MHC genes regulate peptide hydrolysis by proteasomes. *Nature* 1993;365:264–267.

240. Van Kaer L, Ashton-Rickardt PG, Eichelberger M, et al. Altered peptidase and viral-specific T cell response in LMP2 mutant mice. *Immunity* 1994;1:533–541.

241. Fehling HJ, Swat W, Laplace C, et al. MHC class I expression in mice lacking the proteasome subunit LMP-7. *Science* 1994;265:1234–1237.

242. Toes RE, Nussbaum AK, Degermann S, et al. Discrete cleavage motifs of constitutive and immunoproteasomes revealed by quantitative analysis of cleavage products. *J Exp Med* 2001;194:1–12.

243. Sijts AJ, Ruppert T, Rehermann B, et al. Efficient generation of a hepatitis B virus cytotoxic T lymphocyte epitope requires the structural features of immunoproteasomes. *J Exp Med* 2000;191:503–514.

244. Sijts AJ, Standera S, Toes RE, et al. MHC class I antigen processing of an adenovirus CTL epitope is linked to the levels of immunoproteasomes in infected cells. *J Immunol* 2000;164:4500–4506.

245. Schwarz K, van Den Broek M, Kostka S, et al. Overexpression of the proteasome subunits LMP2, LMP7, and MECL-1, but not PA28 alpha/beta, enhances the presentation of an immunodominant lymphocytic choriomeningitis virus T cell epitope. *J Immunol* 2000;165:768–778.

246. Morel S, Levy F, Burlet-Schiltz O, et al. Processing of some antigens by the standard proteasome but not by the immunoproteasome results in poor presentation by dendritic cells. *Immunity* 2000;12:107–117.

247. Chen W, Norbury CC, Cho Y, et al. Immunoproteasomes shape immunodominance hierarchies of antiviral CD8(+) T cells at the levels of T cell repertoire and presentation of viral antigens. *J Exp Med* 2001;193:1319–1326.

248. Dubiel W, Pratt G, Ferrell K, et al. Purification of an 11 S regulator of the multicatalytic protease. *J Biol Chem* 1992;267:22369–22377.

249. Dick TP, Ruppert T, Groettrup M, et al. Coordinated dual cleavages induced by the proteasome regulator PA28 lead to dominant MHC ligands. *Cell* 1996;86:253–262.

250. van Hall T, Sijts A, Camps M, et al. Differential influence on cytotoxic T lymphocyte epitope presentation by controlled expression of either proteasome immunosubunits or PA28. *J Exp Med* 2000;192:483–494.

251. Goldberg AL, Rock KL. Proteolysis, proteasomes and antigen presentation. *Nature* 1992;357:375–379.

252. Monaco JJ, Cho S, Attaya M. Transport protein genes in the murine MHC: possible implications for antigen processing. *Science* 1990;250:1723–1726.

253. Deverson EV, Gow IR, Coadwell WJ, et al. MHC class II region encoding proteins related to the multidrug resistance family of transmembrane transporters. *Nature* 1990;348:738–741.

254. Trowsdale J, Hanson I, Mockridge I, et al. Sequences encoded in the class II region of the MHC related to the "ABC" superfamily of transporters. *Nature* 1990;348:741–743.

255. Townsend A, Öhlén C, Bastin J, et al. Association of class I major histocompatibility heavy and light chains induced by viral peptides. *Nature* 1989;340:443–448.

256. Schumacher TNM, Heemels M-T, Neefjes JJ, et al. Direct binding of peptide to empty MHC class I molecules on intact cells and *in vitro*. *Cell* 1990;62:563–567.

257. Ortmann B, Androlewicz MJ, Cresswell P. MHC class I/β_2-microglobulin complexes associate with TAP transporters before peptide binding. *Nature* 1994;368:864–867.

258. Suh W-K, Cohen-Doyle MF, Fruh K, et al. Interaction of MHC class I molecules with the transporter associated with antigen processing. *Science* 1994;264:1322–1326.

259. Livingstone AM, Powis SJ, Diamond AG, et al. A trans-acting major histocompatibility complex–linked gene whose alleles determine gain and loss changes in the antigenic structure of a classical class I molecule. *J Exp Med* 1989;170:777–795.

260. Livingstone AM, Powis SJ, Günther E, et al. Cim: An MHC class II–linked allelism affecting the antigenicity of a classical class I molecule for T lymphocytes. *Immunogenetics* 1991;34:157–163.

261. Powis SJ, Deverson EV, Coadwell WJ, et al. Effect of polymorphism of an MHC-linked transporter on the peptides assembled in a class I molecule. *Nature* 1992;357:211–215.

262. Powis SJ, Young LL, Joly E, et al. The rat cim effect: TAP allele–dependent changes in a class I MHC anchor motif and evidence against C-terminal trimming of peptides in the ER. *Immunity* 1996;4:159–165.

263. Neefjes JJ, Momburg F, Hämmerling GJ. Selective and ATP-dependent translocation of peptides by the MHC-encoded transporter. *Science* 1993;261:769–771.

264. Neefjes JJ, Gottfried E, Roelse J, et al. Analysis of the fine specificity of rat, mouse and human TAP peptide transporters. *Eur J Immunol* 1995;25:1133–1136.

265. Androlewicz MJ, Cresswell P. Human transporters associated with antigen processing possess a promiscuous peptide-binding site. *Immunity* 1994;1:7–14.

266. Schumacher TNM, Kantesaria DV, Heemels M-T, et al. Peptide length and sequence specificity of the mouse TAP1/TAP2 translocator. *J Exp Med* 1994;179:533–540.

267. van Endert PM, Riganelli D, Greco G, et al. The peptide-binding motif for the human transporter associated with antigen processing. *J Exp Med* 1995;182:1883–1895.

268. van Endert PM. Peptide selection for presentation by HLA class I: a role for the human transporter associated with antigen processing? *Immunol Res* 1996;15:265–279.

269. Gubler B, Daniel S, Armandola EA, et al. Substrate selection by transporters associated with antigen processing occurs during peptide binding to TAP. *Mol Immunol* 1998;35:427–433.

270. Daniel S, Brusic V, Caillat-Zucman S, et al. Relationship between peptide selectivities of human transporters associated with antigen processing and HLA class I molecules. *J Immunol* 1998;161:617–624.

271. Uebel S, Kraas W, Kienle S, et al. Recognition principle of the TAP transporter disclosed by combinatorial peptide libraries. *Proc Natl Acad Sci U S A* 1997;94:8976–8981.

272. Fruci D, Niedermann G, Butler RH, et al. Efficient MHC class I–independent amino-terminal trimming of epitope precursor peptides in the endoplasmic reticulum. *Immunity* 2001;15:467–476.

273. Serwold T, Gaw S, Shastri N. ER aminopeptidases generate a unique pool of peptides for MHC class I molecules. *Nat Immunol* 2001;2:644–651.

274. Lauvau G, Kakimi K, Niedermann G, et al. Human transporters associated with antigen processing (TAPs) select epitope precursor peptides for processing in the endoplasmic reticulum and presentation to T cells. *J Exp Med* 1999;190:1227–1240.

275. Paradela A, Alvarez I, Garcia-Peydro M, et al. Limited diversity of peptides related to an alloreactive T cell epitope in the HLA-B27–bound peptide repertoire results from restrictions at multiple steps along the processing-loading pathway. *J Immunol* 2000;164:329–337.

276. York IA, Roop C, Andrews DW, et al. A cytosolic herpes simplex virus protein inhibits antigen presentation to CD8$^+$ T lymphocytes. *Cell* 1994;77:525–535.

277. Früh K, Ahn K, Djaballah H, et al. A viral inhibitor of peptide transporters for antigen presentation. *Nature* 1995;375:415–418.

278. Hill A, Jugovic P, York I, et al. Herpes simplex virus turns off the TAP to evade host immunity. *Nature* 1995;375:411–415.

279. Stockinger B, Pessara U, Lin RH, et al. A role of Ia-associated invariant chains in antigen processing and presentation. *Cell* 1989;56:683–689.

280. Brodsky FM, Guagliardi LE. The cell biology of antigen processing and presentation. *Annu Rev Immunol* 1991;9:707–744.

281. Germain RN, Margulies DH. The biochemistry and cell biology of antigen processing and presentation. *Annu Rev Immunol* 1993;11:403–450.

282. Elliot WL, Stille CJ, Thomas LJ, et al. An hypothesis on the binding of an amphipathic, a helical sequence in Ii to the desetope of class II antigens. *J Immunol* 1987;138:2949–2952.

283. Roche PA, Cresswell P. Invariant chain association with HLA-DR molecules inhibits immunogenic peptide binding. *Nature* 1990;345:615–618.

284. Teyton L, O'Sullivan D, Dickson PW, et al. Invariant chain distinguishes betweeen the exogenous and endogenous antigen presentation pathways. *Nature* 1990;348:39–44.

285. Roche PA, Cresswell P. Proteolysis of the class II–associated invariant chain generates a peptide binding site in intracellular HLA-DR molecules. *Proc Natl Acad Sci U S A* 1991;88:3150–3154.

286. Bodmer H, Viville S, Benoist C, et al. Diversity of endogenous epitopes bound to MHC class II molecules limited by invariant chain. *Science* 1994;263:1284–1286.

287. Long EO, LaVaute T, Pinet V, et al. Invariant chain prevents the HLA-DR–restricted presentation of a cytosolic peptide. *J Immunol* 1994;153:1487–1494.

288. Roche PA, Marks MS, Cresswell P. Formation of a nine-subunit

complex by HLA class II glycoproteins and the invariant chain. *Nature* 1991;354:392–394.

289. Fling SP, Arp B, Pious D. HLA-DMA and -DMB genes are both required for MHC class II/peptide complex formation in antigen-presenting cells. *Nature* 1994;368:554–558.

290. Sadegh-Nasseri S, Stern LJ, Wiley DC, et al. MHC class II function preserved by low-affinity peptide interactions preceding stable binding. *Nature* 1994;370:647–650.

291. Mellins E, Kempin S, Smith L, et al. A gene required for class II–restricted antigen presentation maps to the major histocompatibility complex. *J Exp Med* 1991;174:1607–1615.

292. Riberdy JM, Newcomb JR, Surman MJ, et al. HLA-DR molecules from an antigen-processing mutant cell line are associated with invariant chain peptides. *Nature* 1992;360:474–477.

293. Morris P, Shaman J, Attaya M, et al. An essential role for HLA-DM in antigen presentation by class II major histocompatibility molecules. *Nature* 1994;368:551–554.

294. Sette A, Ceman S, Kubo RT, et al. Invariant chain of peptides in most HLA-DR molecules of an antigen-processing mutant. *Science* 1992;258:1801–1804.

295. Denzin LK, Cresswell P. HLA-DM induces CLIP dissociation from MHC class II $\alpha\beta$ dimers and facilitates peptide loading. *Cell* 1995; 82:155–165.

296. Denzin LK, Robbins NF, Carboy-Newcome C, et al. Assembly and intracellular transport of HLA-DM and correction of the class II antigen-processing defect in T2 cells. *Immunity* 1994;1:595–606.

297. Alfonso C, Han JO, Williams GS, et al. The impact of H2-DM on humoral immune responses. *J Immunol* 2001;167:6348–6355.

298. Sloan VS, Cameron P, Porter G, et al. Mediation by HLA-DM of dissociation of peptides from HLA-DR. *Nature* 1995;375:802–806.

299. Sherman MA, Weber DA, Jensen PE. DM enhances peptide binding to class II MHC by release of invariant chain–derived peptide. *Immunity* 1995;3:197–205.

300. Benacerraf B. A hypothesis to relate the specificity of T lymphocytes and the activity of I region–specific Ir genes in macrophages and B lymphocytes. *J Immunol* 1978;120:1809–1812.

301. Rosenthal AS, Barcinski MA, Blake JT. Determinant selection is a macrophage dependent immune response gene function. *Nature* 1977;267:156–158.

302. Paul WE, Shevach EM, Pickeral S, et al. Independent populations of primed F1 guinea pig T-lymphocytes respond to antigen-pulsed parental peritoneal exudate cells. *J Exp Med* 1977;145:618–630.

303. Watts TH, Brian AA, Kappler JW, et al. Antigen presentation by supported planar membranes containing affinity-purified I-A^d. *Proc Natl Acad Sci U S A* 1984;81:7564–7568.

304. Walden P, Nagy ZA, Klein J. Induction of regulatory T-lymphocyte responses by liposomes carrying major histocompatibility complex molecules and foreign antigen. *Nature* 1985;315:327–329.

305. Norcross MA, Bentley DM, Margulies DH, et al. Membrane Ia expression and antigen-presenting accessory cell function of L cells transfected with class II major histocompatibility genes. *J Exp Med* 1984;160:1316–1337.

306. Demotz S, Grey HM, Sette A. The minimal number of class II MHC–antigen complexes needed for T cell activation. *Science* 1990;249:1028–1030.

307. Harding CV, Unanue ER. Quantitation of antigen-presenting cell MHC class II/peptide complexes necessary for T-cell stimulation. *Nature* 1990;346:574–576.

308. Christinck ER, Luscher MA, Barber BH, et al. Peptide binding to class I MHC on living cells and quantitation of complexes required for CTL lysis. *Nature* 1991;352:67–70.

309. Cabral GA, Marciano-Cabral F, Funk GA, et al. Cellular and humoral immunity in guinea pigs to two major polypeptides derived from hepatitis B surface antigen. *J Gen Virol* 1978;38:339–350.

310. Kirnbauer R, Booy F, Cheng N, et al. Papillomavirus L1 major capsid protein self-assembles into virus-like particles that are highly immunogenic. *Proc Natl Acad Sci U S A* 1992;89:12180–12184.

311. Stoute JA, Slaoui M, Heppner G, et al. A preliminary evaluation of a recombinant circumsporozoite protein vaccine against *Plasmodium falciparum* malaria. *N Engl J Med* 1997;336:86–91.

312. Takeshita T, Kozlowski S, England RD, et al. Role of conserved regions of class I MHC molecules in the activation of CD8$^+$ CTL by peptide and purified cell-free class I molecules. *Int Immunol* 1993;5:1129–1138.

313. Brower RC, England R, Takeshita T, et al. Minimal requirements for peptide mediated activation of CD8$^+$ CTL. *Mol Immunol* 1994;31:1285–1293.

314. Werdelin O. Chemically related antigens compete for presentation by accessory cells to T cells. *J Immunol* 1982;129:1883–1891.

315. Rock KL, Benacerraf B. Inhibition of antigen-specific T lymphocyte activation by structurally related Ir gene–controlled polymers. Evidence of specific competition for accessory cell antigen presentation. *J Exp Med* 1983;157:1618–1634.

316. Rock KL, Benacerraf B. Inhibition of antigen-specific T lymphocyte activation by structurally related Ir gene–controlled polymers. II. Competitive inhibition of I-E. *J Exp Med* 1984;160:1864–1879.

317. Guillet J-G, Lai M-Z, Briner TJ, et al. Immunological self, nonself discrimination. *Science* 1987;235:865–870.

318. Babbitt BP, Allen PM, Matsueda G, et al. The binding of immunogenic peptides to Ia histocompatibility molecules. *Nature* 1985;317:359–361.

319. Buus S, Sette A, Colon SM, et al. Isolation and characterization of antigen-Ia complexes involved in T cell recognition. *Cell* 1986; 47:1071–1077.

320. Phillips ML, Yip CC, Shevach EM, et al. Photoaffinity labeling demonstrates binding between Ia molecules and nominal antigen on antigen-presenting cells. *Proc Natl Acad Sci U S A* 1986;83:5634–5638.

321. Babbitt BP, Matsueda G, Haber E, et al. Antigenic competition at the level of peptide-Ia binding. *Proc Natl Acad Sci U S A* 1986;83:4509–4513.

322. Buus S, Sette A, Colon SM, et al. The relation between major histocompatibility complex (MHC) restriction and the capacity of Ia to bind immunogenic peptides. *Science* 1987;235:1353–1358.

323. Ronchese F, Schwartz RH, Germain RN. Functionally distinct subsites on a class II major histocompatibility complex molecule. *Nature* 1987;329:254–256.

324. Sette A, Buus S, Colon S, et al. Structural characteristics of an antigen required for its interaction with Ia and recognition by T cells. *Nature* 1987;328:395–399.

325. Kurata A, Berzofsky JA. Analysis of peptide residues interacting with MHC molecule or T-cell receptor: can a peptide bind in more than one way to the same MHC molecule? *J Immunol* 1990;144:4526–4535.

326. Allen PM, Matsueda GR, Evans RJ, et al. Identification of the T-cell and Ia contact residues of a T-cell antigenic epitope. *Nature* 1987;327:713–717.

327. Brown JH, Jardetzky T, Saper MA, et al. A hypothetical model of the foreign antigen binding site of class II histocompatibility molecules. *Nature* 1988;332:845–850.

328. Bjorkman PJ, Saper MA, Samraoui B, et al. Structure of the human class I histocompatibility antigen HLA-A2. *Nature* 1987;329:506–512.

329. Bjorkman PJ, Saper MA, Samraoui B, et al. The foreign antigen binding site and T cell recognition regions of class I histocompatibility antigens. *Nature* 1987;329:512–518.

330. Madden DR, Gorga JC, Strominger JL, et al. The structure of HLA-B27 reveals nonamer self-peptides bound in an extended conformation. *Nature* 1991;353:321–325.

331. Matsumura M, Fremont DH, Peterson PA, et al. Emerging principles for the recognition of peptide antigens by MHC class I molecules. *Science* 1992;257:927–934.

332. Fremont DH, Matsumura M, Stura EA, et al. Crystal structures of two viral peptides in complex with murine MHC class I H-2K^b. *Science* 1992;257:919–927.

333. Germain RN, Ashwell JD, Lechler RI, et al. "Exon-shuffling" maps control of antibody- and T-cell-recognition sites to the NH2-terminal domain of the class II major histocompatibility polypeptide A beta. *Proc Natl Acad Sci U S A* 1985;82:2940–2944.

334. Glimcher LH. T cells recognize multiple determinants on a single class II molecule, some of which depend on tertiary conformation. In: Sercarz EE, Berzofsky JA, eds. *Immunogenicity of protein antigens: repertoires and regulation.* Boca Raton, FL: CRC Press, 1987:131–138.

335. Haskins K, Kappler J, Marrack P. The major histocompatibility complex–restricted antigen receptor on T cells. *Annu Rev Immunol* 1984;2:51–66.

336. Meuer SC, Acuto O, Hercend T, et al. The human T-cell receptor. *Annu Rev Immunol* 1984;2:23–50.

337. Davis MM. Molecular genetics of the T cell-receptor beta chain. *Annu Rev Immunol* 1985;3:537–560.

338. Kronenberg M, Siu G, Hood LE, et al. The molecular genetics of the T-cell antigen receptor and T-cell antigen recognition. *Annu Rev Immunol* 1986;4:529–591.

339. Vasmatzis G, Cornette J, Sezerman U, et al. TcR recognition of the MHC-peptide dimer: structural properties of a ternary complex. *J Mol Biol* 1996;261:72–89.

340. Garcia KC, Degano M, Stanfield RL, et al. An $\alpha\beta$ T cell receptor structure at 2.5Å and its orientation in the TCR-MHC complex. *Science* 1996;274:209–219.

341. Garboczi DN, Ghosh P, Utz U, et al. Structure of the complex between human T-cell receptor, viral peptide and HLA-A2. *Nature* 1996;384:134–141.

342. Bhayani H, Paterson Y. Analysis of peptide binding patterns in different major histocompatibility complex/T cell receptor complexes using pigeon cytochrome c–specific T cell hybridomas. Evidence that a single peptide binds major histocompatibility complex in different conformations. *J Exp Med* 1989;170:1609–1625.

343. Brett SJ, McKean D, York-Jolley J, et al. Antigen presentation to specific T cells by Ia molecules selectively altered by site-directed mutagenesis. *Int Immunol* 1989;1:130–140.

344. McMichael AJ, Gotch FM, Santos-Aguado J, et al. Effect of mutations and variations of HLA-A2 on recognition of a virus peptide epitope by cytotoxic T lymphocytes. *Proc Natl Acad Sci U S A* 1988;85:9194–9198.

345. Racioppi L, Ronchese F, Schwartz RH, et al. The molecular basis of class II MHC allelic control of T cell responses. *J Immunol* 1991;147:3718–3727.

346. Boehncke W-H, Takeshita T, Pendleton CD, et al. The importance of dominant negative effects of amino acids side chain substitution in peptide—MHC molecule interactions and T cell recognition. *J Immunol* 1993;150:331–341.

347. Rothbard JB, Busch R, Howland K, et al. Structural analysis of a peptide—HLA class II complex: identification of critical interactions for its formation and recognition by T cell receptor. *Int Immunol* 1989;1:479–486.

348. Jardetzky TS, Gorga JC, Busch R, et al. Peptide binding to HLA-DR1: a peptide with most residues substituted to alanine retains MHC binding. *EMBO J* 1990;9:1797–1803.

349. Rothbard JB, Busch R, Bal V, et al. Reversal of HLA restriction by a point mutation in an antigenic peptide. *Int Immunol* 1989;1:487–495.

350. Maryanski JL, Verdini AS, Weber PC, et al. Competitor analogs for defined T cell antigens: peptides incorporating a putative binding motif and polyproline or polyglycine spacers. *Cell* 1990;60:63–72.

351. Ruppert J, Sidney J, Celis E, et al. Prominent role of secondary anchor residues in peptide binding to HLA-A2.1 molecules. *Cell* 1993;74:929–937.

352. Berzofsky JA. Epitope selection and design of synthetic vaccines: molecular approaches to enhancing immunogenicity and crossreactivity of engineered vaccines. *Ann N Y Acad Sci* 1993;690:256–264.

353. Berzofsky JA. Designing peptide vaccines to broaden recognition and enhance potency. *Ann N Y Acad Sci* 1995;754:161–168.

354. Takahashi H, Nakagawa Y, Pendleton CD, et al. Induction of broadly cross-reactive cytotoxic T cells recognizing an HIV-1 envelope determinant. *Science* 1992;255:333–336.

355. Ahlers JD, Takeshita T, Pendleton CD, et al. Enhanced immunogenicity of HIV-1 vaccine construct by modification of the native peptide sequence. *Proc Natl Acad Sci U S A* 1997;94:10856–10861.

356. Shirai M, Pendleton CD, Ahlers J, et al. Helper-CTL determinant linkage required for priming of anti-HIV CD8$^+$ CTL *in vivo* with peptide vaccine constructs. *J Immunol* 1994;152:549–556.

357. Ahlers JD, Dunlop N, Alling DW, et al. Cytokine-in-adjuvant steering of the immune response phenotype to HIV-1 vaccine constructs: GM-CSF and TNF α synergize with IL-12 to enhance induction of CTL. *J Immunol* 1997;158:3947–3958.

358. Ahlers JD, Belyakov IM, Thomas EK, et al. High affinity T-helper epitope induces complementary helper and APC polarization, increased CTL and protection against viral infection. *J Clin Invest* 2001;108:1677–1685.

359. Ridge JP, Di Rosa F, Matzinger P. A conditioned dendritic cell can be a temporal bridge between a CD4$^+$ T-helper and a T-killer cell. *Nature* 1998;393:474–478.

360. Bennett SRM, Carbone FR, Karamalis F, et al. Help for cytotoxic-T-cell responses is mediated by CD40 signalling. *Nature* 1998;393:478–480.

361. Schoenberger SP, Toes REM, van der Voort EIH, et al. T-cell help for cytotoxic T lymphocytes is mediated by CD40–CD40L interactions. *Nature* 1998;393:480–483.

362. Pogue RR, Eron J, Frelinger JA, et al. Amino-terminal alteration of the HLA-A*0201-restricted human immunodeficiency virus pol peptide increases complex stability and *in vitro* immunogenicity. *Proc Natl Acad Sci U S A* 1995;92:8166–8170.

363. Parkhurst MR, Salgaller ML, Southwood S, et al. Improved induction of melanoma-reactive CTL with peptides from the melanoma antigen gp100 modified at HLA-A*0201-binding residues. *J Immunol* 1996;157:2539–2548.

364. Sarobe P, Pendleton CD, Akatsuka T, et al. Enhanced *in vitro* potency and *in vivo* immunogenicity of a CTL epitope from hepatitis C virus core protein following amino acid replacement at secondary HLA-A2.1 binding positions. *J Clin Invest* 1998;102:1239–1248.

365. Rosenberg SA, Yang JC, Schwartzentruber DJ, et al. Immunologic and therapeutic evaluation of a synthetic peptide vaccine for the treatment of patients with metastatic melanoma. *Nat Med* 1998;4:321–327.

366. Sette A, Vitiello A, Reherman B, et al. The relationship between class I binding affinity and immunogenicity of potential cytotoxic T cell epitopes. *J Immunol* 1994;153:5586–5592.

367. Berzofsky JA, Ahlers JD, Derby MA, et al. Approaches to improve engineered vaccines for human immunodeficiency virus (HIV) and other viruses that cause chronic infections. *Immunol Rev* 1999;170:151–172.

368. Berzofsky JA, Ahlers JD, Belyakov IM. Strategies for designing and optimizing new generation vaccines. *Nat Rev Immunol* 2001;1:209–219.

369. DeGroot AS, Meister GE, Cornette JL, et al. Computer prediction of T-cell epitopes. In: Levine MM, Woodrow GC, Kaper JB, et al., eds. *New generation vaccines*. New York: Marcel Dekker, 1997:127–138.

370. Falk K, Rötzschke O, Stevanovic S, et al. Allele-specific motifs revealed by sequencing of self-peptides eluted from MHC molecules. *Nature* 1991;351:290–296.

371. Jardetzky TS, Lane WS, Robinson RA, et al. Identification of self peptides bound to purified HLA-B27. *Nature* 1991;353:326–329.

372. Romero P, Corradin G, Luescher IF, et al. H-2K^d–restricted antigenic peptides share a simple binding motif. *J Exp Med* 1991;174:603–612.

373. Hunt DF, Henderson RA, Shabanowitz J, et al. Characterization of peptides bound to the class I MHC molecule HLA-A2.1 by mass spectrometry. *Science* 1992;255:1261–1263.

374. Corr M, Boyd LF, Padlan EA, et al. H-2D^d exploits a four residue peptide binding motif. *J Exp Med* 1993;178:1877–1892.

375. Schumacher TNM, De Bruijn MLH, Vernie LN, et al. Peptide selection by MHC class I molecules. *Nature* 1991;350:703–706.

376. Tsomides TJ, Walker BD, Eisen HN. An optimal viral peptide recognized by CD8$^+$ T cells binds very tightly to the restricting class I major histocompatibility complex protein on intact cells but not to the purified class I protein. *Proc Natl Acad Sci U S A* 1991;88:11276–11280.

377. Hunt DF, Michel H, Dickinson TA, et al. Peptides presented to the immune system by the murine class II major histocompatibility complex molecule I-A^d. *Science* 1992;256:1817–1820.

378. Sette A, Buus S, Appella E, et al. Prediction of major histocompatibility complex binding regions of protein antigens by sequence pattern analysis. *Proc Natl Acad Sci U S A* 1989;86:3296–3300.

379. Chicz RM, Urban RG, Gorga JC, et al. Specificity and promiscuity among naturally processed peptides bound to HLA-DR alleles. *J Exp Med* 1993;178:27–47.

380. Chicz RM, Urban RG, Lane WS, et al. Predominant naturally processed peptides bound to HLA-DR1 are derived from MHC-related molecules and are heterogeneous in size. *Nature* 1992;358:764–768.

381. Hammer J, Takacs B, Sinigaglia F. Identification of a motif for HLA-DR1 binding peptides using M13 display libraries. *J Exp Med* 1992;176:1007–1013.

382. Hammer J, Valsasnini P, Tolba K, et al. Promiscuous and allele-specific anchors in HLA-DR-binding peptides. *Cell* 1993;74:197–203.

383. Sinigaglia F, Hammer J. Motifs and supermotifs for MHC class II binding peptides. *J Exp Med* 1995;181:449–451.

384. Marshall KW, Wilson KJ, Liang J, et al. Prediction of peptide affinity to HLA DRB1*0401. *J Immunol* 1995;154:5927–5933.

385. Jardetzky TS, Brown JH, Gorga JC. Three-dimensional structure of a human class II histocompatibility molecule complexed with superantigen. *Nature* 1994;368:714–717.

386. Scott CA, Peterson PA, Teyton L, et al. Crystal structures of two I-A(d)–peptide complexes reveal that high affinity can be achieved without large anchor residues. *Immunity* 1998;8:319–329.

387. Fremont DH, Monnaie D, Nelson CA, et al. Crystal structure of I-A(k) in complex with a dominant epitope of lysozyme. *Immunity* 1998;8:305–317.

388. Ghosh P, Amaya M, Mellins E, et al. The structure of an intermediate in class II MHC maturation: CLIP bound to HLA-DR3. *Nature* 1995;378:457–462.

389. Davis MM, Bjorkman PJ. T-cell antigen receptor genes and T-cell recognition. *Nature* 1988;334:395–402.

390. Ogasawara K, Maloy WL, Schwartz RH. Failure to find holes in the T cell repertoire. *Nature* 1987;325:450–452.

391. Shirai M, Arichi T, Nishioka M, et al. CTL responses of HLA-A2.1-transgenic mice specific for hepatitis C viral peptides predict epitopes for CTL of humans carrying HLA-A2.1. *J Immunol* 1995;154:2733–2742.

392. Schaeffer EB, Sette A, Johnson DL, et al. Relative contribution of "determinant selection" and "holes in the T-cell repertoire" to T-cell responses. *Proc Natl Acad Sci U S A* 1989;86:4649–4653.

393. Moudgil KD, Grewal IS, Jensen PE, et al. Unresponsiveness to a self-peptide of mouse lysozyme owing to hindrance of T cell receptor–major histocompatibility complex/peptide interaction caused by flanking epitopic residues. *J Exp Med* 1996;183:535–546.

394. Ding YH, Smith KJ, Garboczi DN, et al. Two human T cell receptors bind in a similar diagonal mode to the HLA-A2/Tax peptide complex using different TCR amino acids. *Immunity* 1998;8:403–411.

395. Slansky JE, Rattis FM, Boyd LF, et al. Enhanced antigen-specific antitumor immunity with altered peptide ligands that stabilize the MHC-peptide-TCR complex. *Immunity* 2000;13:529–538.

396. Zaremba S, Barzaga E, Zhu M, et al. Identification of an enhancer agonist cytotoxic T lymphocyte peptide from human carcinoembryonic antigen. *Cancer Res* 1997;57:4570–4577.

397. Fong L, Hou Y, Rivas A, et al. Altered peptide ligand vaccination with Flt3 ligand expanded dendritic cells for tumor immunotherapy. *Proc Natl Acad Sci U S A* 2001;98:8809–8814.

398. Tangri S, Ishioka GY, Huang X, et al. Structural features of peptide analogs of human histocompatibility leukocyte antigen class I epitopes that are more potent and immunogenic than wild-type peptide. *J Exp Med* 2001;194:833–846.

399. Takeshita T, Takahashi H, Kozlowski S, et al. Molecular analysis of the same HIV peptide functionally binding to both a class I and a class II MHC molecule. *J Immunol* 1995;154:1973–1986.

400. Alexander-Miller MA, Parker KC, Tsukui T, et al. Molecular analysis of presentation by HLA-A2.1 of a promiscuously binding V3 loop peptide from the HIV-1 envelope protein to human CTL. *Int Immunol* 1996;8:641–649.

401. Abiru N, Wegmann D, Kawasaki E, et al. Dual overlapping peptides recognized by insulin peptide B:9-23 T cell receptor AV13S3 T cell clones of the NOD mouse. *J Autoimmun* 2000;14:231–237.

402. Talken BL, Schafermeyer KR, Bailey CW, et al. T cell epitope mapping of the Smith antigen reveals that highly conserved Smith antigen motifs are the dominant target of T cell immunity in systemic lupus erythematosus. *J Immunol* 2001;167:562–568.

403. Takahashi H, Merli S, Putney SD, et al. A single amino acid interchange yields reciprocal CTL specificities for HIV gp160. *Science* 1989;246:118–121.

404. Takahashi H, Houghten R, Putney SD, et al. Structural requirements for class-I MHC molecule–mediated antigen presentation and cytotoxic T-cell recognition of an immunodominant determinant of the HIV envelope protein. *J Exp Med* 1989;170:2023–2035.

405. De Magistris MT, Alexander J, Coggeshall M, et al. Antigen analog–major histocompatibility complexes act as antagonists of the T cell receptor. *Cell* 1992;68:625–634.

406. Sette A, Alexander J, Ruppert J, et al. Antigen analogs/MHC complexes as specific T cell receptor antagonists. *Annu Rev Immunol* 1994; 12:413–431.

407. Lorenz RG, Allen PM. Direct evidence for functional self-protein/Ia-molecule complexes *in vivo*. *Proc Natl Acad Sci U S A* 1988;85: 5220–5223.

408. Evavold BD, Allen PM. Separation of IL-4 production from Th cell proliferation by an altered T cell receptor ligand. *Science* 1991; 252:1308–1310.

409. Evavold BD, Williams SG, Hsu BL, et al. Complete dissection of the Hb(64-76) determinant using Th1, Th2 clones and T cell hybridomas. *J Immunol* 1992;148:347–353.

410. Pfeiffer C, Stein J, Southwood S, et al. Altered peptide ligands can control CD4 T lymphocyte differentiation *in vivo*. *J Exp Med* 1995;181:1569–1574.

411. Chaturvedi P, Yu Q, Southwood S, et al. Peptide analogs with different affinities for MHC alter the cytokine profile of T helper cells. *Int Immunol* 1996;8:745–755.

412. Sloan-Lancaster J, Evavold BD, Allen PM. Induction of T-cell anergy by altered T-cell-receptor ligand on live antigen-presenting cells. *Nature* 1993;363:156–159.

413. Sloan-Lancaster J, Shaw AS, Rothbard JB, et al. Partial T cell signaling: altered phospho-ζ and lack of Zap70 recruitment in APL-induced T cell anergy. *Cell* 1994;79:913–922.

414. Tsitoura DC, Holter W, Cerwenka A, et al. Induction of anergy in human T helper 0 cells by stimulation with altered T cell antigen receptor ligands. *J Immunol* 1996;156:2801–2808.

415. Mueller DL, Jenkins MK, Schwartz RH. Clonal expansion versus functional clonal inactivation: a costimulatory signalling pathway determines the outcome of T cell antigen receptor occupancy. *Annu Rev Immunol* 1989;7:445–480.

416. Racioppi L, Ronchese F, Matis LA, et al. Peptide–major histocompatibility complex class II complexes with mixed agonist/antagonist properties provide evidence for ligand-related differences in T cell receptor–dependent intracellular signaling. *J Exp Med* 1993;177:1047–1060.

417. Madrenas J, Wange RL, Wang JL, et al. ζ Phosphorylation without ZAP-70 activation induced by TCR antagonists or partial agonists. *Science* 1995;267:515–518.

418. Madrenas J, Chau LA, Smith J, et al. The efficiency of CD4 recruitment to ligand-engaged TCR controls the agonist/partial agonist properties of peptide–MHC molecule ligands. *J Exp Med* 1997;185:219–229.

419. McKeithan TW. Kinetic proofreading in T-cell receptor signal transduction. *Proc Nat Acad Sci U S A* 1995;92:5042–5046.

420. DeGroot AS, Jesdale BM, Berzofsky JA. Prediction and determination of MHC ligands and T cell epitopes. In: Kaufmann SHE, Kabelitz D, eds. *Immunology of infection*. London: Academic Press, 1998:79–108.

421. DeLisi C, Berzofsky JA. T cell antigenic sites tend to be amphipathic structures. *Proc Natl Acad Sci U S A* 1985;82:7048–7052.

422. Spouge JL, Guy HR, Cornette JL, et al. Strong conformational propensities enhance T-cell antigenicity. *J Immunol* 1987;138:204–212.

423. Stille CJ, Thomas LJ, Reyes VE, et al. Hydrophobic strip-of-helix algorithm for selection of T cell-presented peptides. *Mol Immunol* 1987;24:1021–1027.

424. Sette A, Doria G, Adorini L. A microcomputer program for hydrophilicity and amphipathicity analysis of protein antigens. *Mol Immunol* 1986;23:807–810.

425. Madden DR, Garboczi DN, Wiley DC. The antigenic identity of peptide–MHC complexes: a comparison of the conformations of five viral peptides presented by HLA-A2. *Cell* 1993;75:693–708.

426. Carbone FR, Fox BS, Schwartz RH, et al. The use of hydrophobic α-helix–defined peptides in delineating the T cell determinant for pigeon cytochrome c. *J Immunol* 1987;138:1838–1844.

427. Cornette JL, Margalit H, DeLisi C, et al. Concepts and methods in the identification of T cell epitopes and their use in the construction of synthetic vaccines. *Methods Enzymol* 1989;178:611–634.

428. Cornette JL, Margalit H, DeLisi C, et al. The amphipathic helix as a structural feature involved in T-cell recognition. In: Epand RM, ed. *The amphipathic helix*. Boca Raton: CRC Press, 1993:333–346.

429. Rothbard JB, Taylor WR. A sequence pattern common to T cell epitopes. *EMBO J* 1988;7:93–100.

430. Reyes VE, Chin LT, Humphreys RE. Selection of class I MHC restricted peptides with the strip-of-helix hydrophobicity algorithm. *Mol Immunol* 1988;25:867–871.

431. Cornette JL, Margalit H, Berzofsky JA, et al. Periodic variation in side-chain polarities of T-cell antigenic peptides correlates with their structure and activity. *Proc Natl Acad Sci U S A* 1995;92:8368–8372.

432. Pamer EG, Harty JT, Bevan MJ. Precise prediction of a dominant class I MHC–restricted epitope of *Listeria monocytogenes*. *Nature* 1991;353:852–855.

433. Hill AVS, Elvin J, Willis AC, et al. Molecular analysis of the association of HLA-B53 and resistance to severe malaria. *Nature* 1992;360:434–439.

434. Lipford GB, Hoffman M, Wagner H, et al. Primary *in vivo* responses to ovalbumin: probing the predictive value of the Kb binding motif. *J Immunol* 1993;150:1212–1222.

435. Nijman HW, Houbiers JGA, Vierboom MPM, et al. Identification of peptide sequences that potentially trigger HLA-A2.1-restricted cytotoxic T lymphocytes. *Eur J Immunol* 1993;23:1215–1219.

436. Altuvia Y, Berzofsky JA, Rosenfeld R, et al. Sequence features that correlate with MHC restriction. *Mol Immunol* 1994;31:1–19.

437. Meister GE, Roberts CGP, Berzofsky JA, et al. Two novel T cell epitope prediction algorithms based on MHC-binding motifs; comparison of predicted and published epitopes from *Mycobacterium tuberculosis* and HIV protein sequences. *Vaccine* 1995;13:581–591.

438. Kaufman JF, Auffray C, Korman AJ, et al. The class II molecules of the human and murine major histocompatibility complex. *Cell* 1984;36:1–13.

439. Zhang C, Anderson A, DeLisi C. Structural principles that govern the peptide-binding motifs of class I MHC molecules. *J Mol Biol* 1998;281:929–947.

440. Sturniolo T, Bono E, Ding J, et al. Generation of tissue-specific and promiscuous HLA ligand databases using DNA microarrays and virtual HLA class II matrices. *Nat Biotechnol* 1999;17:555–561.

441. Zhang C, Cornette JL, Berzofsky JA, et al. The organization of human leukocyte antigen class I epitopes in HIV genome products: implications for HIV evolution and vaccine design. *Vaccine* 1997;15:1291–1302.

442. Hammer J, Bono E, Gallazzi F, et al. Precise prediction of major histocompatibility complex class II–peptide interaction based on peptide side chain scanning. *J Exp Med* 1994;180:2353–2358.

443. Parker KC, Bednarek MA, Coligan JE. Scheme for ranking potential HLA-A2 binding peptides based on independent binding of individual peptide side-chains. *J Immunol* 1994;152:163–175.

444. Fleckenstein B, Kalbacher H, Muller CP, et al. New ligands binding to the human leukocyte antigen class II molecule DRB1*0101 based on the activity pattern of an undecapeptide library. *Eur J Biochem* 1996;240:71–77.

445. Jesdale BM, Mullen L, Meisell J, et al. EpiMatrix and Epimer, tools for HIV research. In: *Vaccines '97*. Cold Spring Harbor, NY: Cold Spring Harbor Laboratory Press, 1997:0.

446. Davenport MP, Ho Shon IAP, Hill AVS. An empirical method for the prediction of T-cell epitopes. *Immunogenetics* 1995;42:392–397.

447. Davenport MP, Godkin A, Friede T, et al. A distinctive peptide binding motif for HLA-DRB1*0407, an HLA-DR4 subtype not associated with rheumatoid arthritis. *Immunogenetics* 1997;45:229–232.

448. Leggatt GR, Hosmalin A, Pendleton CD, et al. The importance of pairwise interactions between peptide residues in the delineation of T cell receptor specificity. *J Immunol* 1998;161:4728–4735.

449. Sidney J, Grey HM, Southwood S, et al. Definition of an HLA-A3–like supermotif demonstrates the overlapping peptide-binding repertoires of common HLA molecules. *Hum Immunol* 1996;45:79–93.

450. Kropshofer H, Max H, Halder T, et al. Self-peptides from four HLA-DR alleles share hydrophobic anchor residues near the NH2-terminal including proline as a stop signal for trimming. *J Immunol* 1993;151:4732–4742.

451. Sette A, Sidney J. Nine major HLA class I supertypes account for the vast preponderance of HLA-A and -B polymorphism. *Immunogenetics* 1999;50:201–212.

452. Vajda S, Weng Z, Rosenfeld R, et al. Effect of conformational flexibility and solvation on receptor-ligand binding free energies. *Biochemestry* 1994;33:13977–13988.

453. Sezerman U, Vajda S, DeLisi C. Free energy mapping of class I MHC molecules and structural determination of bound peptides. *Protein Sci* 1996;5:1272–1281.

454. Altuvia Y, Schueler O, Margalit H. Ranking potential binding peptides to MHC molecules by a computational threading approach. *J Mol Biol* 1995;249:244–250.

455. Brusic V, Rudy G, Harrison LC. Prediction of MHC binding peptides using artificial neural networks. In: Stonier RJ, Yu XH, eds. *Complex systems: mechanism of adaptation*. Amsterdam: IOS Press, 1994:253–260.

456. Takahashi H, Cohen J, Hosmalin A, et al. An immunodominant epitope of the HIV gp160 envelope glycoprotein recognized by class I MHC

457. Langton BC, Mackewicz CE, Wan AM, et al. Structural features of an antigen required for cellular interactions and for T-cell activation in an MHC-restricted response. *J Immunol* 1988;141:447–456.

458. Thomas DB, Skehel JJ, Mills KHG, et al. A single amino acid substitution in influenza haemagglutinin abrogates recognition by a monoclonal antibody and a spectrum of subtype-specific L3T4+ T cell clones. *Eur J Immunol* 1987;17:133–136.

459. Mozes E, McDevitt HO, Jaton J-C, et al. The nature of the antigenic determinant in genetic control of antibody response. *J Exp Med* 1969;130:493–504.

460. Mozes E, McDevitt HO, Jaton J-C, et al. The genetic control of antibody specificity. *J Exp Med* 1969;130:1263–1278.

461. Bluestein HG, Green I, Maurer PH, et al. Specific immune response genes of the guinea pig. V: influence of the GA and GT immune response genes on the specificity of cellular and humoral immune responses to a terpolymer of L-glutamic acid, L-alanine, and L-tyrosine. *J Exp Med* 1972;135:98–109.

462. Berzofsky JA, Schechter AN, Shearer GM, et al. Genetic control of the immune response to staphyloccal nuclease III. Time course and correlation between the response to native nuclease and the response to its polypeptide fragments. *J Exp Med* 1977;145:111–112.

463. Berzofsky JA, Schechter AN, Shearer GM, et al. Genetic control of the immune response to staphylococcal nuclease IV. H-2–linked control of the relative proportions of antibodies produced to different determinants of native nuclease. *J Exp Med* 1977;145:123–145.

464. Campos-Neto A, Levine H, Schlossman SJ. T cell regulation of specific B cell responses. *J Immunol* 1978;121:2235–2240.

465. Campos-Neto A, Levine H, Schlossman SJ. Immune response gene control of antibody specificity. *Cell Immunol* 1982;69:128–137.

466. Kohno Y, Berzofsky JA. Genetic control of the immune response to myoglobin. V. Antibody production *in vitro* is macrophage and T cell-dependent and is under control of two determinant-specific Ir genes. *J Immunol* 1982;128:2458–2464.

467. Sercarz E, Cecka JM, Kipp D, et al. The steering function of T cells in expression of the antibody repertoire directed against multideterminant protein antigen. *Ann Immunol Inst Pasteur* 1977;128:599.

468. Cecka JM, Stratton JA, Miller A, et al. Structural aspects of immune recognition of lysozymes. III: T cell specificity restriction and its consequences for antibody specificity. *Eur J Immunol* 1976;6:639–646.

469. Ferguson TA, Peters T Jr, Reed R, et al. Immunoregulatory properties of antigenic fragments from bovine serum albumin. *Cell Immunol* 1983;78:1–12.

470. Kawamura H, Berkower I, Glover C, et al. Helper T cell epitope specificity regulates B cell (antibody) specificity. *J Cell Biochem* 1984;8A:211.

471. Chesnut RW, Colon SM, Grey HM. Antigen presentation by normal B cells, B cell tumors and macrophages: functional biochemical comparison. *J Immunol* 1982;128:1764–1768.

472. Chesnut RW, Colon SM, Grey HM. Requirements for the processing of antigen by antigen-presenting cells. I: Functional comparison of B cell tumors and macrophages. *J Immunol* 1982;129:2382–2388.

473. Lanzavecchia A. Antigen-specific interaction between T cells and B cells. *Nature* 1985;314:537–539.

474. Chesnut RW, Grey HM. Studies on the capacity of B cells to serve as antigen-presenting cells. *J Immunol* 1981;126:1075–1079.

475. Malynn BA, Wortis HH. Role of antigen-specific B cells in the induction of SRBC-specific T cell proliferation. *J Immunol* 1984;132:2253–2258.

476. Rock KL, Benacerraf B, Abbas AK. Antigen presentation by hapten-specific B lymphocytes. I. Role of surface immunoglobulin receptors. *J Exp Med* 1984;160:1102–1113.

477. Tony H-P, Parker DC. Major histocompatibility complex–restricted polyclonal B cell responses resulting form helper T cell recognition of antiimmunoglobulin presented by small B lymphocytes. *J Exp Med* 1985;161:223–241.

478. Kawamura H, Berzofsky JA. Enhancement of antigenic potency *in vitro* and immunogenicity *in vivo* by coupling the antigen to anti-immunoglobulin. *J Immunol* 1986;136:58–65.

479. Davidson HW, Watts C. Epitope-directed processing of specific antigen by B lymphocytes. *J Cell Biol* 1989;109:85–92.

480. Löwenadler B, Lycke N, Svanholm C, et al. T and B cell responses to

chimeric proteins containing heterologous T helper epitopes inserted at different positions. *Mol Immunol* 1992;29:1185–1190.

481. Manca F, Fenoglio D, Kunkl A, et al. Differential activation of T cell clones stimulated by macrophages exposed to antigen complexed with monoclonal antibodies. A possible influence of paratope specificity on the mode of antigen processing. *J Immunol* 1988;140:2893–2898.

482. Manca F, Fenoglio D, Li Pira G, et al. Effect of antigen/antibody ratio on macrophage uptake, processing, and presentation to T cells of antigen complexed with polyclonal antibodies. *J Exp Med* 1991;173:37–48.

483. Watts C, Lanzavecchia A. Suppressive effect of antibody on processing of T cell epitopes. *J Exp Med* 1993;178:1459–1463.

484. Simitsek PD, Campbell DG, Lanzavecchia A, et al. Modulation of antigen processing by bound antibodies can boost or suppress class II major histocompatibility complex presentation of different T cell determinants. *J Exp Med* 1995;181:1957–1963.

485. Bekoff MC, Levine H, Schlossman SF. T cell and Ir gene regulation of expression of a cross-reactive idiotype. *J Immunol* 1982;129:1173–1180.

486. Kawamura H, Kohno Y, Busch M, et al. A major anti-myoglobin idiotype: Influence of H-2—linked Ir genes on idiotype expression. *J Exp Med* 1984;160:659–678.

487. Germain RN. The ins and outs of antigen processing and presentation. *Nature* 1986;322:687–689.

488. Fauchère JL, Pliska V. Hydrophobic parameters p of amino-acid side chains from the partitioning of *N*-acetyl—amino-acid amides. *Eur J Med Chem* 1983;18:369–374.

CHAPTER 22

Fc Receptors

Jeffrey V. Ravetch

Historical Background
Structure and Expression
   Molecular Genetics · Protein Heterogeneity · Expression · Three-Dimensional Structure
In Vitro **Activity**
   Binding Properties · Effector Cell Activation · B-Lymphocyte Suppression
Signaling
   Immunoreceptor Tyrosine-Based Activation Motif Pathways · Immunoreceptor Tyrosine-Based Inhibitory Motif Pathways
In Vivo **Functions**
   Fcγ Receptors in the Afferent Response · Fcγ Receptors in the Efferent Response
Disease Associations
   Autoimmunity and Tolerance · Inflammation
Summary and Conclusions
Acknowledgments
References

HISTORICAL BACKGROUND

Cellular receptors for immunoglobulins were anticipated by the description of cytophilic antibodies of the immunoglobulin (Ig) G class, identified by Boyden and Sorkin in 1960 (1). These antibodies conferred upon normal cells, like macrophages, the capacity to specifically absorb antigen. Using sheep red blood cells (RBCs) as the antigen resulted in rosette formation between the cytophilic anti–sheep RBC antibodies and macrophages and provided a convenient means of visualization of the binding of cytophilic antibodies with normal cells. Subsequent studies by Berken and Benacerraf (2) suggested that the crystallized fragment (Fc) of the cytophilic antibody interacted with a cell surface receptor on macrophages. Similar studies on B-lymphocytes extended the generality of these receptors and led to the term *Fc receptor* (FcR) to denote the surface molecules on lymphoid and myeloid cells that are capable of interacting with the Fc of immunoglobulin molecules (3). Studies on IgE, IgM, and IgA demonstrated the existence of distinct receptors for those isotypes as well on various immune cell types. Detailed biochemical characterization of Fc receptors was inaugurated by the studies of Kulczycki et al. (4) on the high-affinity IgE FcR of mast cells, revealing a hetero-oligomeric $\alpha\beta\gamma_2$ subunit structure. A distinction between FcRs for the IgE and IgG isotypes emerged with the observation of the very high (10^{10} M^{-1}) binding affinity of IgE for its receptor in comparison with the low binding (10^6 M^{-1}) of IgG1 to its receptor. This distinction led to the realization that the functional IgG1 ligand was exclusively in the form of an immune complex, whereas IgE binding occurred through monomer interaction with its receptor. This difference in binding affinity had significant functional implications for the structures of these receptors and mechanisms by which each isotype activated its target cell. Determination of the structure of these receptors was facilitated by their molecular cloning, beginning with the IgG FcRs (5,6), followed by the IgE FcR (7). Two distinct types of IgG receptors, differing in their transmembrane and cytoplasmic sequences, were identified, which thus offered a molecular explanation for the apparent contradictory activation and inhibitory activities attributed to IgG FcRs. The primary structure of the subunits of the high-affinity IgE FcR revealed homology in the ligand binding α subunit to its IgG counterparts. However, the extent of similarity between these receptors became apparent with the observation that the γ chain subunit was common to both IgG and IgE FcRs, providing both assembly and signaling functions to these activation receptors (8,9). This common structure suggested a functional link between immune complex diseases and allergic reactions, a prediction that was confirmed through mouse knockout studies of IgG FcRs (10,11). The FcRs, through their dependence on the immunoreceptor tyrosine-based activation motif (ITAM) pathway of cellular activation, belonged to the family of immunoreceptors that included the antigen receptors on B cells and T cells. Three-dimensional crystal structures have been solved for the low-affinity IgG FcRs (12,13) and the high-affinity IgE FcR (14), alone and in complex with their immunoglobulin ligands (15,16), further establishing the close structural link between these immunoglobulin receptors.

The functional roles of IgG FcRs were suggested by the distribution of these receptors on both lymphoid and myeloid cells (17). On myeloid cells, they were presumed to mediate effector cell activation, resulting in phagocytosis, antibody-dependent cellular cytotoxicity (ADCC) and release of inflammatory mediators. However, the well-known ability of the classical pathway of complement to generate activated fragments in response to immune complexes capable of inducing inflammatory responses by myeloid cells complicated the interpretation of the physiological role of IgG FcRs. Thus, the contribution of IgG FcRs to the mechanism of immune complex–mediated inflammation, as distinct from the role of complement, remained uncertain. Insight into this distinction was gained through the generation of mouse strains specifically deficient in either FcRs (10,18,19) or components of the classical complement pathway (20). Studies on immune complex–mediated inflammatory responses in these animals, such as the Arthus reaction, led to the realization that IgG FcRs and not the classical pathway of complement activation were the functional mediators of inflammatory responses triggered by immune complexes (21,22). The situation for IgE was less confounding, and the identification and characterization of a high-affinity receptor for this isotype on mast cells offered a plausible explanation for many of the inflammatory features of allergic reactions (23), validated later by mouse knockouts of this receptor. IgG immune complexes had also been observed to mediate suppression of B-cell responses; thus, the presence of an IgG FcR activity on B cells provided a possible, but uncharacterized, mechanism for this inhibitory activity. Molecular characterization of this inhibitory activity for the B-cell FcR, FcRIIB, resulted in the first detailed description of an inhibitory motif, now termed the immunoreceptor tyrosine-based inhibitory motif (ITIM) (24,25), and the signaling pathway by which it abrogates ITAM-triggered activation. The ITIM mechanism is now recognized as ubiquitous, and has resulted in the recognition of a large family of inhibitory receptors on immune cells that function to maintain proper thresholds for activation and abrogate activation responses to terminate an immune reaction (26).

FcRs are now recognized as central mediators of antibody-triggered responses, coupling the innate and adaptive immune responses in effector cell activation (27). In addition to these specialized roles, the IgG FcRs have served as an example of the emerging class of balanced immunoreceptors, in which activation and inhibition are tightly coupled in response to ligand binding. Perturbations in either arm of the response

have been shown to lead to pathological consequences and have been taken as a paradigm of how these systems are likely to work for those paired immunoreceptors with unknown ligand-binding functions. The newly described roles for FcRs in maintaining peripheral tolerance, shaping the antibody repertoire, regulating antigen-presenting cell (APC) maturation, and promoting mast cell survival indicate the diversity of functions that these receptors possess and their central role in modulating both afferent and efferent responses in the immune response.

This chapter focuses primarily on the IgG and IgE FcRs, for which substantial data on their structure, function, regulation, and role in a variety of physiological and pathological conditions are now available. The similarity in structure and signaling between those receptors and other members of this family, such as the IgA FcR, is also discussed. Other immunoglobulin receptors with specialized functions in the transport of immunoglobulins, such as the FcRn (28) and the poly-Ig FcR (29), will be discussed elsewhere in this volume.

STRUCTURE AND EXPRESSION

Molecular Genetics

Two general classes of FcRs are now recognized: the activation receptors, characterized by the presence of a cytoplasmic ITAM sequence associated with the receptor, and the inhibitory receptor, characterized by the presence of an ITIM sequence. These two classes of receptors function in concert and are usually found coexpressed on the cell surface. Because activation and inhibitory receptors bind immunoglobulin with comparable affinity and specificity, coengagement of both signaling pathways is thus the rule, setting thresholds for and ultimately determining the physiological outcome of effector cell responses.

Subunit Composition

FcRs are typically type I integral membrane glycoproteins consisting of, at the least, a ligand recognition α subunit that confers isotype specificity for the receptor. α subunits for IgG, IgE and IgA have been described [reviewed by Ravetch and Kinet (17,23) and Daëron (30)]. These subunits typically consist of two extracellular domains of the immunoglobulin V type superfamily: a single transmembrane domain and a relatively short intracytoplasmic domain. In activation FcRs, a signaling subunit of the γ family is often found, resulting in an $\alpha\gamma_2$ complex. The inhibitory FcRIIB molecule, in contrast, is expressed as a single-chain receptor. The α subunits have apparent molecular weights of between 40 and 75 kDa and share significant amino acid sequence homology in their extracellular domains. Alternatively spliced forms of FcγRIIB modify the intracytoplasmic domain of this molecule. For example, the B2 form lacks sequences that inhibit internalization and thus demonstrates enhanced internalization of immune complexes, in comparison with RIIB1. However, all the splice variants contain the ITIM motif, a necessary and sufficient domain for mediating inhibitory signaling. The conservation of this sequence in mice and humans, its presence in all splice variants, and the hyperresponsive phenotypes generated in mice deficient in this receptor all support inhibition as the central function of RIIB. The specific structures of the α subunits are shown in Fig. 1. The notable exceptions to the general structure just outlined are seen for the high-affinity FcγRIα subunit, which has three extracellular domains; the activation FcγRIIAα subunit, which does not require additional subunits for assembly or signaling; and the (GPI)–linked FcγRIIIB, which attaches to the cell surface through a glycosyl-phosphatidylinositol linkage, rather than through a transmembrane domain.

The γ subunit is found associated with activation IgG, IgE, and IgA FcRs, as well as with non-FcR molecules, such as paired immunoglobulin-like receptor A (PIR-A) and natural killer (NK) cell cytotoxicity receptors (31–33). It is required for assembly of the α subunits of these receptors by protecting these subunits from degradation in the endoplasmic reticulum. The γ chain is found as a disulfide linked homodimer, with a short extracellular domain containing the cysteine involved in dimerization, a transmembrane domain, and an intracytoplasmic domain containing the ITAM. An aspartic acid residue found in the transmembrane domain is often associated with a basic amino acid residue in the transmembrane domain of the α subunit. The γ subunit belongs to a gene family that includes the T-cell receptor–associated ζ chain and the NK receptor DAP-10– and DAP-12–associated molecules (34). FcγRIIIA can associate with the ζ chain, resulting in the $\alpha\zeta_2$ complex found in human NK cells.

A third subunit is found associated with the activation FcRs FcϵRI and FcγRIII, the β subunit. This 33-kDa subunit has four transmembrane-spanning domains and amino and carboxy intracytoplasmic domains, belonging to the CD20 family of tetraspan molecules (23). An ITAM sequence is found in the intracytoplasmic carboxy domain. In mast cells and basophils, the β chain assembles into an $\alpha\beta\gamma_2$ complex with the α chain belonging to either FcγRIII or FcϵRI. Its presence is required for assembly of FcϵRI in rodents. In humans,

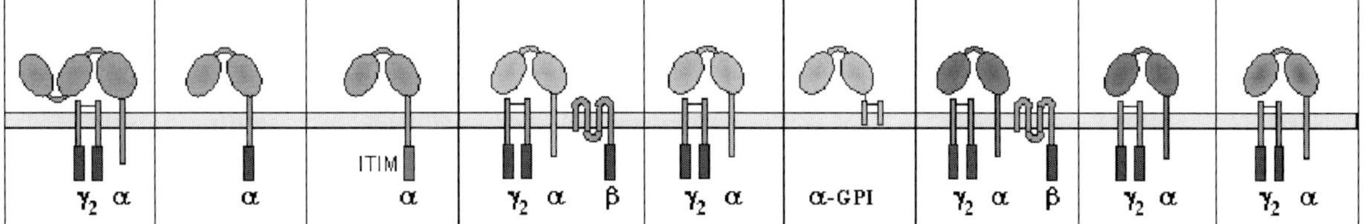

	FcγRI CD64	FcγRIIA CD32	FcγRIIB CD32	FcγRIIIA CD16		FcγRIIIB CD16	FcεRI		FcαRI CD89
Structure									
Subunit composition	γ₂ α	α	ITIM α	γ₂ α β	γ₂ α	α-GPI	γ₂ α β	γ₂ α	γ₂ α
Ka	10^8 M^{-1}	2×10^6 M^{-1}	2×10^6 M^{-1}	5×10^5 M^{-1}	5×10^5 M^{-1}	2×10^5 M^{-1}	10^{10} M^{-1}	10^{10} M^{-1}	5×10^7 M^{-1}
Binding Specificity	1. IgG1=IgG3 2. IgG4 3. IgG2	1. IgG1 2. IgG2=IgG3 3. IgG4	1. IgG1 2. IgG2=IgG3 3. IgG4	1. IgG1=IgG3	1. IgG1=IgG3	1. IgG1=IgG3	IgE	IgE	IgA₁=IgA₂
Expression	Macrophages Neutrophils Eosinophils Dendritic Cells	Macrophages Neutrophils Mast cells Eosinophils Platelets Dendritic Cells	Macrophages Neutrophils Mast cells Eosinophils Dendritic Cells FDC B cells	Mast cells Basophils	Macrophages Mast cells Basophils NK cells Dendritic Cells	Neutrophils	Mast cells Basophils	Mast cells Basophils Eosinophils Platelets Dendritic Cells	Macrophages Neutrophils Eosinophils
Class Function	Activation -Inducible by inflammatory cytokines -Enhance effector responses at inflammatory sites -IC capturing by DC	Activation -Effector cell activation by IC's, cytotoxic Ab	Inhibition -Set threshold for effector cell activation by Fc -B cell repression -Maintain tolerance	Activation -Dominant pathway for effector activation by IgG -In vivo ADCC -Arthus reaction -IC capture by DC		Decoy -Sink for IC -Focus IC to PMN -Synergize with FcγRIIA	Activation -Degranulation -Allergic reactions (Type I)	Activation -Degranulation -Allergy -Antigen caption by DC	Activation -IgA binding -IgA activation of effector cells

FIG. 1. Summary of FcR structures, expression patterns and *in vivo* functions. The immunoreceptor tyrosine-based activation motif (ITAM) signaling motif is indicated by the green rectangle; the immunoreceptor tyrosine-based inhibitor motif (ITIM) is indicated as a red rectangle. Alleles of FcRIIA and FcRIIIB and their binding properties are discussed in the text.

however, $\alpha\gamma_2$ complexes of FcεRI are found in monocytes, Langerhans cells, and dendritic cells, in addition to the $\alpha\beta\gamma_2$ complexes found in mast cells and basophils. The ITAM motif found in the β subunit is not an autonomous activation sequence but functions as a signaling amplifier of the ITAM found in the γ subunits (35).

Gene Organization, Linkage and Polymorphisms

All α subunits share a common gene organization, which indicates that the evolution of this family of receptors resulted from gene duplication from a common ancestor (36). Sequence divergence then resulted in the acquisition of distinctive specificities for these related sequences. Most of the genes belonging to the FcR family are found on the long arm of chromosome 1, including the γ chain and the α chains of FcγRI, FcγRII, FcγRIII, and FcεRI (37,38). This region is syntenic with a comparable region on mouse chromosome 1; however, FcγRIα is found on mouse chromosome 3. In humans, the α subunit of the IgA receptor is found on chromosome 19, and the β subunit is on chromosome 11. The FcγRII–FcγRIII locus on chromosome 1 is further linked to a variety of lupus susceptibility genes found in that region, including the *Sle1* cluster (39). A locus linked to atopy has been identified at 11q12–13 and further delineated polymorphisms of the β chain (I181V and V183L) that are associated with a heightened risk of atopy. However, a direct functional association of these polymorphisms with the known biological activities of the β chain has not been found (40).

Polymorphisms in the α chains of the FcγRs have been described, most notably in FcγRIIA and FcγRIII; these polymorphisms result in differences in binding affinity to specific IgG subclasses (41). For example, a histidine at position 131 in FcγRIIA results in higher affinity binding to IgG2 and IgG3 than does an arginine at that position. Similarly, FcγRIIIA with valine at position 158 of the α chain has a higher binding affinity for IgG1 and 3 than does the polymorphic form with phenylalanine at that position. This polymorphism translates into a more robust ADCC response for the val/val haplotype *in vitro* and has been positively correlated with the degree of an *in vivo* response to a B cell–depleting, anti-CD20 antibody (42). Four amino acids are polymorphic for FcγRIIIB at positions 18, 47, 64, and 88, which contributes to the neutrophil antigen polymorphisms for this receptor. Several studies have attempted to link specific FcR polymorphisms to autoimmune diseases, specifically to systemic lupus erythematosus. Although linkage to this region of chromosome 1 is well established in a variety of autoimmune diseases, the specific allelic associations that have been reported are not conclusive or consistent throughout these studies. Rather, these linkages are more likely to be indicative of linkage disequilibrium with other genes in this locus, such as the inhibitory FcγRIIB gene, for which functional evidence of a contribution to autoimmunity has been established in a variety of murine models.

Species Comparisons

Detailed comparisons between FcRs in mice and humans have revealed several notable differences in both structure and expression of these molecules. Whereas IgG and IgE FcRs are conserved in these species, IgA FcRs are not. To date, a murine homolog for the IgA FcR has not been identified. In general, the murine IgG FcRs are less complex than their human counterparts (36). For example, FcγRI is encoded by a single gene in the mouse, in comparison with three genes in the human (38). Mice have only a single FcγRII gene, the inhibitory FcγRIIB molecule. Two additional genes, FcγRIIA and C, are found in the human, which is notable because of their unusual single-chain activation structure (43). An analogous situation is found for FcγRIII. A single gene, FcγRIIIA, is found in the mouse, whereas two genes, FcγRIIIA and FcγRIIIB, are encoded in the human (44). As mentioned previously, FcγRIIIB is unique among FcRs in being expressed as a GPI-anchored protein. Its expression is limited to human neutrophils, in comparison with FcγRIIIA, which is expressed widely on cells of the myeloid lineage, such as macrophages, NK cells, mast cells, and dendritic cells. The genes for the IgE FcR are conserved in mice and humans. The difference that is observed relates to the requirement for the β chain to achieve surface expression in mice, precluding the expression of the $\alpha\gamma_2$ complex (23). In humans, this form of the receptor is widely expressed on monocytes, Langerhans cells, and dendritic cells and is likely to be found on mast cells and basophils as well. This difference in FcεRI subunit composition is likely to result in functional differences as well. Although these specific interspecies differences are important, the fundamental organization of the FcR system, with activation and inhibitory signaling through a shared ligand specificity coupled to opposing signaling pathways, is well conserved. Thus, conclusions regarding the function of this system in immunity by the analysis of murine models are relevant to an understanding of the role of these receptors to human immunity as well.

Expression

FcRs are expressed widely on cells of the myeloid lineage, including monocytes, macrophages, dendritic cells, mast cells, basophils, neutrophils, eosinophils, and NK cells (17,30). In addition, B cells and follicular dendritic cells (FDCs) express the inhibitory FcRIIB receptor, whereas T cells are generally negative for FcR expression. The specific expression pattern for each receptor varies, and these patterns are summarized in Fig. 1. Because FcRs represent a balanced system of activation and inhibition, the general rule of coexpression of FcRs of these classes is maintained. B cells use the B-cell antigen receptor as the activation co-receptor for FcRIIB, whereas NK cells appear to utilize NK inhibitory receptors to modulate FcγRIIIA activation. The decoy FcγR, FcγRIIIB, is expressed exclusively on human neutrophils, on which it functions to concentrate and focus immune complexes without directly triggering cell activation, perhaps also playing role in neutrophil recruitment (45). The FcγRIIA–FcγRIIB pair functions on neutrophils to modulate immune complex activation. FcεRI can be modulated by FcγRIIB, as demonstrated both *in vitro* and *in vivo*; mice deficient in FcγRIIB display enhanced IgE-triggered anaphylaxis (46) by virtue of the ability of IgE to bind with high affinity to FcεRI and with low affinity for FcγRIIB. Other mast cell inhibitory receptors, such as glycoprotein 49B1, modulate mast cell sensitivity to IgE: Mice deficient in this molecule display enhanced anaphylactic responses to IgE stimulation (47). Expression of the common γ chain is broad: It has been found on all myeloid and lymphoid cells examined to date. In contrast, the β chain appears to be quite restricted in its expression: It has been found only on mast cells and basophils.

Regulation of FcR expression can occur at several levels. In general, cytokines involved in activation of inflammatory responses induce expression of activation FcγRs, whereas inhibitory cytokines down regulate these activation receptors. Transcriptional regulation of α chain levels has been documented for a variety of cytokines, including interferon-γ, IL-4, and transforming growth factor β (48,49). Induction of FcγRI, FcγRIIA, and FcγRIIIA α and γ chains in myeloid cells occurs upon interferon-γ treatment: IL-4 generally inhibits expression of these activation receptors but induces expression of the inhibitory FcγRIIB. The situation in B cells is likely to be more complex, whereby regulation of FcγRIIB is critical for the process of affinity maturation and maintenance of peripheral tolerance. Germinal center B cells down-regulate FcγRIIB, perhaps in response to IL-4 production by T cells. Regulation of FcR expression has also been documented to occur upon binding of ligand. IgE regulates the expression of FcεRI by stabilizing the intracellular pool of receptor upon receptor engagement (50). Thus, high IgE levels result in the induction of surface expression of FcεRI. However, this same mechanism of regulation is not seen for FcγRs: Mice deficient in IgG have FcγR levels comparable with those of wild-type animals. Competition for limiting subunits also contributes to regulation of receptor expression. In mast cells, it appears that the level of γ chain is limiting. Competition between α chains for the limiting concentration of γ chain has been documented in mouse knockouts, whereby levels of one receptor increase if the α chain of the other receptor is reduced (51). This type of reciprocal regulation is likely to be significant in the cross-regulation of FcRs by different isotypes of immunoglobulin.

Three-Dimensional Structure

The crystal structures of FcγRIIA, FcγRIIB, FcγRIIIA, and FcεRI have been solved, along with the cocrystals of FcγRIIIA–IgG1 Fc and FcεRI–IgE Fc (52) (Fig. 2). These

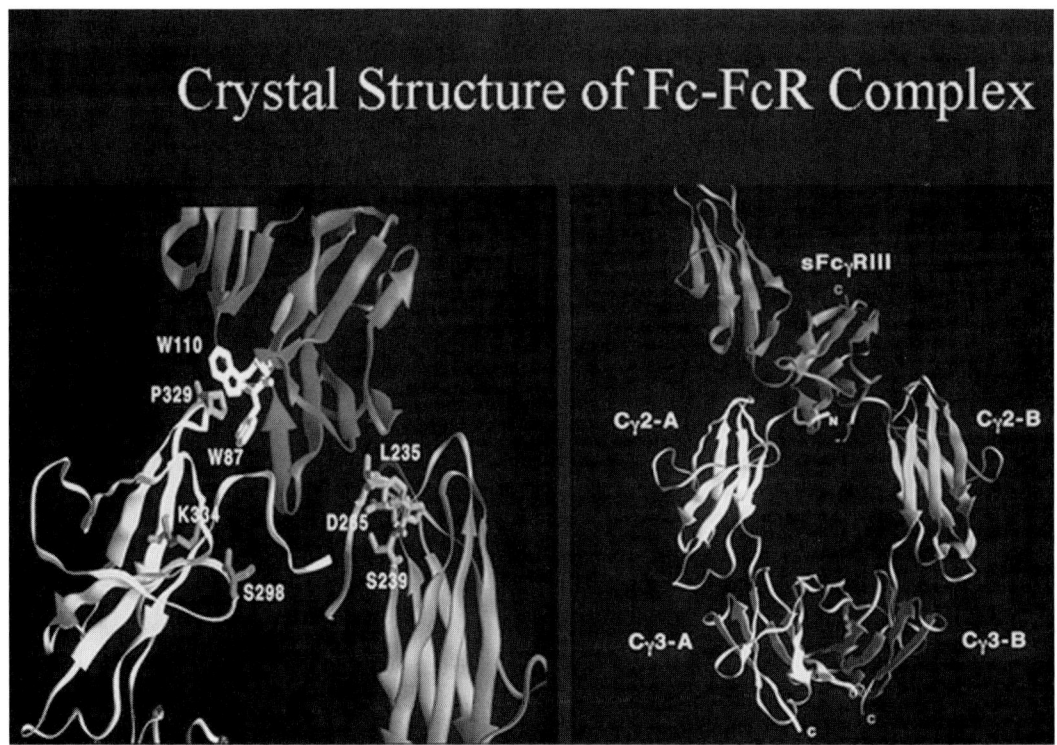

FIG. 2. Ribbon diagram of crystallizable fragment (Fc) receptor III–immunoglobulin G1 (IgG1) Fc structure. The carbohydrate moiety has been removed from the IgG1 Fc fragment in this visualization, although it is present in the crystal structure. The extracellular domains of Fc receptor III are shown, together with the Fc fragment of IgG1. Some of the contact residues are shown for the binding interface. See text for details. Adapted from Sondermann et al. (15), with permission.

studies demonstrate that the receptors have a common structure in which the two extracellular immunoglobulin domains fold in a strongly bent overall structure, arranged into a heart-shaped domain structure. A 1:1 stoichiometry between the receptor and ligand is observed, with the receptor inserted into the cleft formed by the two chains of the Fc fragment ($C\gamma2$ or $C\epsilon3$). The binding region of the FcR to Fc fragments consists mainly of rather flexible loops that rearrange upon complex formation. Only domain 2 and the linker region connecting domains 1 and 2 interact in the complex with different regions of both chains of the Fc. Conserved tryptophans located on the FcRs interact with proline to form a "proline sandwich." A solvent-exposed hydrophobic residue at position 155 is conserved among all FcRs and represents a binding site for the important IgG1 residue Leu 235 (not found in IgE). Specificity is generated among the receptor–ligand pairs in a variable region connecting the two extracellular domains that is in contact with the lower hinge region of the Fc fragment (residues 234 to 238), a region not conserved among the IgGs and IgE. The binding region of FcRs to their immunoglobulin ligands does not overlap with other Fc binding molecules such as protein A, protein G, and FcRn.

The structure of the FcR bound to their ligand reveal that the antigen-binding fragment (Fab) arms are quite sharply bent and may adopt a perpendicular orientation toward the Fc. This arrangement would give the Fab arms maximal flexibility to bind antigen when the Fc fragment is oriented parallel to the membrane of the FcR-expressing cell. The asymmetrical interaction of the two Fc chains with a single FcR prevents a single antibody molecule from triggering dimerization of receptors and initiating signaling. Instead, dimerization is initiated by the interaction of antigen with the Fab arms, thus linking adaptive responses to effector cell triggering.

IN VITRO ACTIVITY

Binding Properties

As outlined in Fig. 1, immunoglobulin binding to FcRs falls into either high- or low-affinity binding classes. The high-affinity binding class is typified by $Fc\epsilon RI$, with a binding affinity of 10^{10} M^{-1} for IgE, which ensures a monomeric interaction between IgE and its receptor. $Fc\gamma RI$ binds with relatively high affinity for IgG1 and IgG3 (human) and IgG2a (mouse) with an affinity constant of 10^{8} M^{-1}. In contrast to these high-affinity FcRs, the low-affinity receptors, such as $Fc\gamma RIIA$, $Fc\gamma RIIB$, $Fc\gamma RIIIA$, $Fc\gamma RIIIB$, and $Fc\alpha RI$, bind with affinities ranging from 5×10^{5} M^{-1} ($Fc\gamma RIII$) to 5×10^{7} M^{-1} ($Fc\alpha RI$). This low-affinity binding ensures that these receptors interact with immune complexes and not monomeric ligands. As described later, this dependence on high-avidity and low-affinity interactions ensures that these receptors are activated only by physiologically relevant immune complexes and not by circulating monomeric immunoglobulin, thus avoiding inappropriate activation of

effector responses. In general, low-affinity $Fc\gamma Rs$ bind IgG1 and IgG3 preferentially; binding to IgG2 and IgG4 is observed at even lower affinities. As mentioned previously, polymorphisms in $Fc\gamma RIIA$ and $Fc\gamma RIIIA$ affect binding to IgG2 and IgG1, respectively, which may have significance *in vivo* in predicting responses to specific cytotoxic antibodies. Binding has been observed between aglycosyl FcRs and immunoglobulin, with Ka values similar to that observed for the glycosylated forms. Subunit interactions have also been reported to influence affinity for ligand, as demonstrated for the common γ chain associating with $Fc\gamma RIIIA$ (53). Its affinity for IgG1 is higher than the GPI-anchored form of this receptor, $Fc\gamma RIIIB$.

The crystal structures of IgG1-$Fc\gamma RIIIA$ and IgE-$Fc\epsilon RI$ reveal similarities in the binding properties of these two complexes. Of significance is the 1:1 stoichiometry of the complexes, which ensures that a single receptor binds to a single immunoglobulin molecule (15,16). This property in turn ensures that activation occurs upon cross-linking of receptor complexes by multivalent ligands. Two binding sites on the receptor interact asymmetrically with two sites on the Fc molecule. The FcR inserts into the cleft formed by the two chains of the Fc molecule, burying a binding surface of 895 Å for each binding site. Alterations in the Fc structure that reduce the cleft, such as deglycosylation of IgG, inhibit FcR binding. Four distinct regions have been defined in the Fc domains involved in FcR interactions. For IgE, this includes residues 334 to 336, 362 to 365, 393 to 396, and 424. The homologous regions for IgG are residues 234 to 239, 265 to 269, 297 to 299, and 327 to 332. Interactions of these residues occur with the carboxy-terminal domain 2 of the respective FcRs. In view of the similarities of these complexes and the homologies among the receptors and their ligands, an obvious question that arises concerns the molecular basis for specificity. Attempts to resolve that question have relied on mutagenesis studies of the ligands and domain exchanges between receptors. For example, exchange of the FG loop in domain 2 of $Fc\epsilon$ to $Fc\gamma$ receptors confers detectable IgE binding; similarly, variation in this loop in $Fc\gamma Rs$ may provide interactions that determine IgG specificity for these receptors. Mutagenesis of IgG1 revealed that a common set of residues is involved in binding to all $Fc\gamma Rs$, but $Fc\gamma RII$ and $Fc\gamma RIII$ also utilize distinct residues (54). Several IgG1 residues not found at the IgG–FcR interface by crystallographic determination had a profound effect on binding, which indicates the greater complexity of these interactions in solution.

The implications of these structural studies are that the Fc domain of IgG may be selectively mutated to direct its binding to specific $Fc\gamma Rs$. Fc mutants that selectively engage activation FcRs (IIIA and IIA) while minimally interacting with inhibitory and decoy FcRs (IIB and IIIB) would confer optimal cytotoxic potential for tumoricidal applications. Indications that such Fc engineering is possible are suggested by IgG mutants with selective binding to FcRIII or FcRII.

Effector Cell Activation

The critical step in triggering effector cell response by FcRs is mediated by the cross-linking of these receptors by immunoglobulin. This can occur either by interactions of low-affinity, high-avidity IgG immune complexes or of IgG opsonized cells with activation FcγRs or by the cross-linking of monomeric IgG or IgE bound to FcγRI or FcεR, respectively, by multivalent antigens binding to the Fab of the antibody. Cross-linking of ITAM-bearing FcRs results in common cellular responses, determined by the cell type, rather than the FcR. Thus, for example, FcεRI or FcγRIII cross-linking of mast cells results in degranulation of these cells, whereas cross-linking of macrophage expressed FcαRI or FcγRIII by opsonized cells triggers phagocytosis. These functions underlie the functional similarity of activation FcRs in which cross-linking mediates cellular responses by ITAM-mediated tyrosine kinase cascades. In addition to degranulation and phagocytosis, activation FcR cross-linking has been demonstrated to induce ADCC, the oxidative burst, and the release of cytokines and other inflammatory cell mediators. A sustained calcium influx is associated with these functions, as are transcription of genes associated with the activated state.

Cellular activation initiated by ITAM-bearing activation FcRs can be enhanced by coengagement with integrin and complement receptors. Although the ability of these receptors to mediate phagocytosis, for example, are modest, synergistic interactions with FcRs result in sustained activation and enhancement. Synergistic interactions between activation FcRs and toll receptors, mannose receptors, and other pattern-recognition molecules have also been reported *in vitro* and suggest that interplay between the innate and adaptive effector mechanisms of an immune response are involved in mediating efficient protection from microbial pathogens.

In contrast to the activation of effector cell responses triggered by cross-linking of ITAM-bearing FcRs *in vitro*, cross-linking of an ITIM-bearing inhibitory receptor to an ITAM-bearing receptor results in the arrest of these effector responses. Homoaggregation of FcRIIB by its cross-linking on effector cells by immune complexes does not result in cellular responses; rather, it is the coengagement of ITAM- and ITIM-bearing receptors that results in the functional generation of an inhibitory signal. *In vitro*, it is possible to ligate any ITAM-bearing receptor to any ITIM-bearing receptor with a resulting inhibitory response. This activity is used functionally to define putative ITIMs and has proved to be a useful device in dissecting the signaling pathways induced by ITAM-ITIM coligation.

B-Lymphocyte Suppression

B-cell stimulation through the B-cell antigen receptor can be arrested by the coligation of FcγRIIB to the B-cell receptor (BCR). This occurs naturally when immune complexes, retained on FDCs in the germinal center, interact with both the BCR and FcγRIIB during the affinity maturation of an antibody response. *In vitro* suppression of B-cell activation has been demonstrated by coligation of BCR and FcγRIIB, resulting in arrest of calcium influx and proliferative responses triggered by the BCR (24,55), the result of recruitment of the SH2-containing inositol 5′-phosphatase (SHIP)–1 (56). Calcium release from the endoplasmic reticulum is not affected, and there is thus an initial rise in intracellular calcium; however, this calcium flux is not sustained, because SHIP recruitment blocks calcium influx by uncoupling of the capacitance channel. A third activity has been defined for FcγRIIB that is independent of the ITIM sequence. Homoaggregation of FcγRIIB by immune complexes triggers apoptosis in B cells, as demonstrated in the DT40 B-cell line and in murine splenocyte preparations (57). This activity is retained in ITIM mutants and is dependent on the transmembrane sequence of FcγRIIB. This pathway has been proposed to provide a mechanism for negative selection of somatically mutated B cells that have reduced affinity for BCR. The loss of FcγRIIB on B cells results in the loss of peripheral tolerance, which may be explained by the loss of this censoring pathway in the germinal center reaction.

SIGNALING

Immunoreceptor Tyrosine-Based Activation Motif Pathways

The general features of signal transduction through ITAM receptors are conserved among all members of this family, including T-cell receptors, BCRs, and various FcRs. The 19–amino acid–conserved ITAM is necessary and sufficient to generate an activation response, as demonstrated by the analysis of chimeric receptors. With a single exception, FcRs associate with accessory subunits that contain these signaling motifs. As described previously, the common γ chain contains an ITAM and is associated with FcεRI, FcγRI, FcγRIII, and FcαRI. In addition, both FcεRI and FcγRIII may associate with the β subunit in mast cells. The ITAM found in the β chain does not function as an autonomous activation cassette, as has been found for most other ITAMs. Rather, it functions to amplify the activation response generated by the γ chain ITAM by increasing the local concentration of Lyn available for activation upon aggregation of the receptor (35). FcγRIIA contains an ITAM in the cytoplasmic domain of its ligand recognition α subunit and is thus able to activate in the absence of any associated subunit.

Upon sustained receptor aggregation Src family kinases that may be associated with the receptor in an inactive form become activated and rapidly tyrosine-phosphorylate the ITAM sequences, creating SH2 sites for the docking and subsequent activation of Syk kinases. Ligands that become rapidly dissociated from the receptors result in nonproductive signaling complexes that fail to couple to downstream events and behave as antagonistic ligands (58). The specific Src kinase involved for each FcR depends on the receptor and cell type in which it is studied. Thus, Lyn is associated with the

FcεRI pathway in mast cells, Lck is associated with FcγRIIIA in NK cells, and both of these kinases as well as Hck are associated with FcγRI and FcγRIIA in macrophages. After activation of the Src kinase, tyrosine phosphorylation of the ITAM motif rapidly ensues, leading to the recruitment and activation of Syk kinases. This two-step process is absolutely necessary to transduce the aggregation signal to a sustainable intracellular response. Once activated, Syk kinases lead to the phosphorylation or recruitment of a variety of intracellular substrates, including PI3K, Btk and other Tec family kinases, phospholipase C-γ (PLCγ), and adaptor proteins such as SLP-76 and BLNK. The Ras pathway is also activated through Sos bound to Grb2 that is recruited upon phosphorylation of Shc. Ras phosphorylates Raf, which in turn leads to MEK kinase and MAP kinase activation. A summary of these intracellular pathways is shown in Fig. 3. A crucial step in this sequential activation cascade occurs with the activation of PI3K by Syk. By generating phosphatidyl inositol polyphosphates, such as PIP₃, PI3K leads to the recruitment of pleckstrin homology (PH) domain–expressing proteins such as Btk and PLCγ, which in turn leads to the generation of inositol triphosphate (IP3) and diacylglycerol (DAG), intermediates crucial to the mobilization of intracellular calcium and activation of protein kinase C (PKC), respectively.

Immunoreceptor Tyrosine-Based Inhibitory Motif Pathways

The inhibitory motif, embedded in the cytoplasmic domain of the single-chain FcγRIIB molecule, was defined as a 13–amino acid sequence AENTITYSLLKHP, shown to be both necessary and sufficient to mediate the inhibition of BCR-generated calcium mobilization and cellular proliferation (24,25). Significantly, phosphorylation of the tyrosine of

this motif was shown to occur upon BCR coligation and was required for its inhibitory activity. This modification generated an SH2 recognition domain that is the binding site for the inhibitory signaling molecule SHIP (56,59). In addition to its expression on B cells, where it is the only IgG FcR, FcγRIIB is widely expressed on macrophages, neutrophils, mast cells, dendritic cells, and FDCs, absent only from T and NK cells. Studies on FcγRIIB provided the impetus to identify similar sequences in other surface molecules that mediated cellular inhibition and resulted in the description of the ITIM, a general feature of inhibitory receptors.

FcγRIIB displays three separable inhibitory activities, of which two are dependent on the ITIM and one is independent of this motif. Coengagement of FcγRIIB to an ITAM-containing receptor leads to tyrosine phosphorylation of the ITIM by the Lyn kinase, recruitment of SHIP, and the inhibition of ITAM-triggered calcium mobilization and cellular proliferation (56,60,61). These two activities result from different signaling pathways; calcium inhibition requires the phosphatase activity of SHIP to hydrolyze PIP₃ and the ensuing dissociation of PH domain—containing proteins such as Btk and PLCγ (62) (Fig. 4). The net effect is to block calcium influx and prevent sustained calcium signaling. Calcium-dependent processes such as degranulation, phagocytosis, ADCC, cytokine release, and proinflammatory activation are all blocked. Arrest of proliferation in B cells is also dependent on the ITIM pathway, through the activation of the adaptor protein Dok and subsequent inactivation of MAP kinases (63,64). The role of SHIP in this process has not been fully defined, inasmuch as it can affect proliferation in several ways. SHIP, through its catalytic phosphatase domain, can prevent activation of the PH domain survival factor Akt by hydrolysis of PIP₃ (65,66). SHIP also contains PTB domains that could act to recruit Dok to the membrane and provide access to the Lyn kinase that is involved in its activation. Dok-deficient

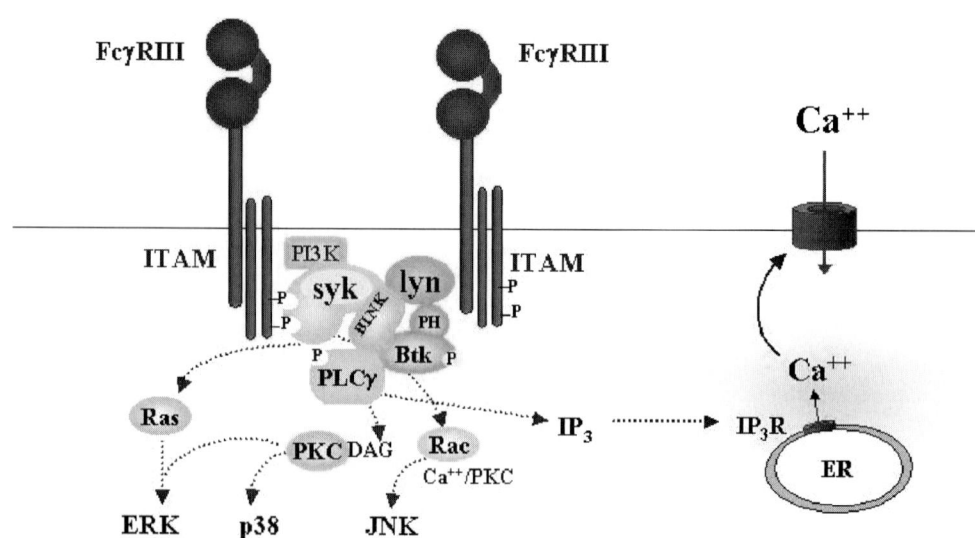

FIG. 3. Signaling by activation FcRs. FcRIII signaling in natural killer cells is shown as an example of the activation class of FcRs. Cross-linking by an immune complex initiates the signaling cascade. The specific Src family kinase varies, depending on the cell type.

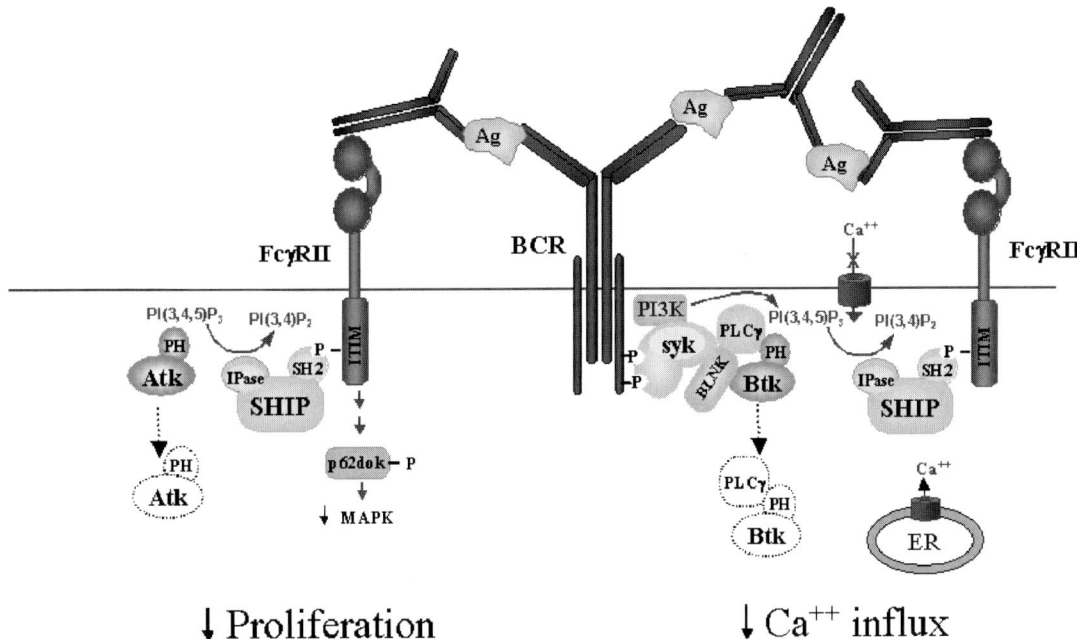

FIG. 4. Signaling pathways triggered by B-cell receptor–FcR IIB coligation. Cellular activation is inhibited by the recruitment of the SH2-containing inositol 5′-phosphatase (SHIP) to the FcR-phosphorylated immunoreceptor tyrosine-based inhibitor motif (ITIM).

B cells are unable to mediate FcγRIIB–triggered arrest of BCR-induced proliferation, while retaining their ability to inhibit a calcium influx, which demonstrates the dissociation of these two ITIM-dependent pathways.

The third inhibitory activity displayed by FcγRIIB is independent of the ITIM sequence and is displayed upon homoaggregation of the receptor. Under these conditions of FcγRIIB clustering, a proapoptotic signal is generated through the transmembrane sequence (Fig. 5). This proapoptotic signal is blocked by recruitment of SHIP, which occurs upon coligation of FcγRIIB to the BCR, because of the Btk requirement for this apoptotic pathway (57). This novel activity has been reported only in B cells and has been proposed

to act as a means of maintaining peripheral tolerance for B cells that have undergone somatic hypermutation. Support for this model comes from the *in vivo* studies of FcγRIIB-deficient mice in induced and spontaneous models of autoimmunity.

IN VIVO FUNCTIONS

Fcγ Receptors in the Afferent Response

The ability of IgG immune complexes to influence the afferent response has been known since the 1950s and can be either enhancing or suppressive, depending on the precise

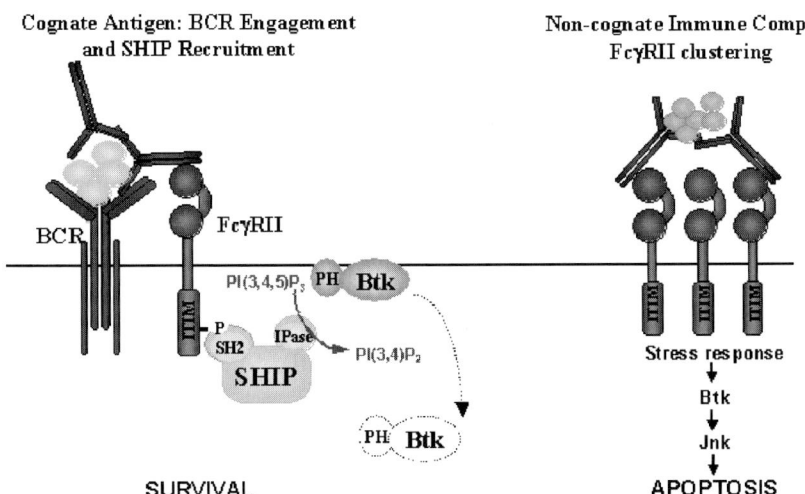

FIG. 5. A model for the role of FcR IIB in affinity maturation of germinal center B cells. Higher affinity B-cell receptors rescue somatically hypermutated B cells from FcRIIB-triggered apoptosis and negative selection by coligation to FcRIIB, leading to the recruitment of SH2-containing inositol 5′-phosphatase (SHIP) and release of the plekstrin homology (PH) domain–containing protein Btk.

combination of antibody and antigen and the mode of administration (67). Investigators have attempted to define the molecular mechanisms behind these activities with the availability of defined mouse strains with mutations in activation or inhibitory FcRs. Direct effects on B cells stem from the ability of the inhibitory FcγRIIB molecule to influence the state of B-cell activation and survival by providing a means of discriminating between the rare somatically hypermutated germinal center B cells that have high-affinity cognate antigen binding and the predominant population with low-affinity and potentially cross-reactive specificities. Because antigen is retained in the form of immune complexes on FDCs, it can interact with B cells either through FcγRIIB alone, resulting in apoptosis, or by coengaging FcγRIIB with BCR, favoring survival, as summarized in Fig. 5. Support for this model comes from the B-cell autonomous loss of peripheral tolerance in FcγRIIB knockout mice on the C57Bl/6 background (68). Those animals develop anti-DNA and antichromatin antibodies and die of a fatal, autoimmune glomerulonephritis at 8 months of age. The phenotype is strain dependent and is not seen in BALB/c or 129 strains of mice. FcγRIIB thus acts as a genetic susceptibility factor for autoimmune disease, under the control of epistatic modifiers to suppress the emergence of autoreactivity and maintain peripheral tolerance. Further support for this conclusion is provided by the observations that autoimmune disease–prone strains of mice, such as New Zealand black (NZB), BXSB, SB/Le, MRL, and nonobese diabetic (NOD), have reduced surface expression of FcγRIIB attributed to DNA polymorphisms in the promoter region of the gene encoding this receptor (69,70). This reduced expression of FcγRIIB is thus suggested to contribute to the increased susceptibility of these animals to the development of autoantibodies and autoimmune disease.

If FcγRIIB indeed functions *in vivo* to maintain peripheral tolerance, then its loss should allow for the emergence of autoantibodies when otherwise resistant animals are challenged with potentially cross-reactive antigens. This hypothesis has been validated in models of collagen-induced arthritis and Goodpasture's syndrome. FcγRIIB-deficient mice, with the nonpermissive H-2^b haplotype, develop arthritis when immunized with bovine type II collagen (71). The loss of FcγRIIB thus bypasses the requirement for the specific H-2^q and H-2^r alleles previously demonstrated to be necessary in this model by allowing FcγRIIB-deficient autoreactive B cell clones to expand and produce pathogenic autoantibodies. When the permissive DBA/1 strain (H-2^q) is made deficient in FcγRIIB, autoantibody development is augmented and disease is greatly enhanced. In a similar manner, immunization of H-2^b mice deficient in FcγRIIB with bovine type IV collagen results in cross-reactive autoantibodies to murine type IV collagen, with dramatic pathogenic effects (72). These mice develop hemorrhagic lung disease and glomerulonephritis with a "ribbon deposition" pattern of immune complexes in the glomeruli. These characteristics are indicative of Goodpasture's syndrome, a human disease not previously modeled in an animal species.

Expression of the inhibitory FcγRIIB on B cells thus provides a mechanism for the suppressive effects of immune complexes on antibody production, particularly during the germinal center reaction when immune complexes retained on FDCs interact with somatically hypermutated B cells. The enhancing property of immune complexes on the afferent response is likely to arise from the expression of FcRs on APCs, such as dendritic cells (73–75). Dendritic cells express all three classes of IgG FcRs as well as FcεRI. Although *in vitro* studies have suggested that triggering of activation FcRs can induce dendritic cell maturation, the *in vivo* significance of this pathway has not been established (76). The ability of FcRs, particularly FcγRI, to internalize immune complexes could provide a mechanism for enhanced presentation and augmented antibody responses, whereas the presence of the inhibitory FcγRIIB molecule appears to reduce the enhancing effect. Mice deficient in FcγRIIB display enhanced antibody responses to soluble antibody–antigen complexes, in some cases dramatically so, which is likely to result from enhanced presentation (77,78). In addition, *in vitro* studies suggest that internalization through specific FcRs on APCs may influence the epitopes presented and T-cell response generated as a result. At present, a growing body of data suggests that FcRs are indeed involved in enhancement of the afferent response, by influencing antigen presentation and cognate T-cell interactions. It is also possible that FcRs function on APCs in the establishment of tolerance by influencing the differentiation of dendritic cells and their capacity to induce either anergy or T-cell activation. Defining the precise role of each FcR expressed on APCs will require conditional knockouts of these molecules on specific dendritic cell populations to resolve the contribution of these systems to the generation of an appropriate antibody response.

Fcγ Receptors in the Efferent Response

The first FcR knockout to be described was for the common activation subunit, the γ chain, which resulted in the loss of surface assembly and signaling of FcγRI and FcγRIII as well as FcεRI (10). Mice deficient in the common γ chain were systematically studied in diverse models of inflammation and found to be unable to mediate IgG-triggered inflammatory responses, which was attributed to the loss of the low-affinity activation receptor FcγRIII; the FcγRI played a minimal role in the *in vivo* inflammatory response triggered by IgG (21,79–81). The results were further confirmed by comparisons of mice deficient in either FcγRI or FcγRIII (19,82). The loss of FcεRI ablated IgE-mediated anaphylaxis; this was demonstrated independently by gene disruption in the α subunit of that receptor (11). Subsequent studies on mice deficient in the inhibitory FcγRIIB molecule established the opposing action of this receptor, in which mice deficient in that receptor displayed enhanced B-cell responses, autoimmunity, and augmented IgG-mediated inflammation (18,81,83). The general finding, which is discussed in detail later, illustrates that IgGs initiate their effector responses *in vivo* through coengagement of activating and inhibitory FcRs. The physiological response is thus the net of the opposing activation and inhibitory signaling pathways that each receptor triggers and is determined by the level of expression of each receptor and the selective avidity of the IgG ligand. The absence of a murine homolog for FcαRI has precluded similar studies for that receptor. Studies on mice bearing a human transgene of FcαRI suggest that this receptor is involved in IgA nephropathy (Berger's disease) (84).

Type I: Immediate Hypersensitivity

Both cutaneous and systemic models of passive anaphylaxis, induced by IgE, were studied in FcRγ chain–deficient mice and were found to be absent, a finding fully consistent with the observations obtained in FcεRI-deficient mice and confirming the role of the high-affinity IgE receptor in mediating IgE-induced anaphylactic responses (10,11,35,85). FcγRIIB-deficient mice, challenged in this model, displayed an unexpected enhancement of IgE-mediated anaphylaxis, which suggests a physiological interaction between this inhibitory receptor and FcεRI (46). The molecular basis for this modulation of FcεRI signaling by FcγRIIB has not been determined, although previous studies have indicated that IgE can bind with low affinity to FcγRII/FcγIII, which suggests that there exists a mechanism for coengagement of these receptors. Deletion of the mast cell inhibitory receptor glycoprotein 49B1 also results in enhanced IgE-induced anaphylaxis (47). In addition to FcεRI, mast cells also express the IgG FcRIIB and FcRIII. Passive systemic anaphylaxis induced by IgG was attenuated in FcRγ chain–deficient and FcγRIII-deficient mice, which indicates the capacity of IgG and FcγRIII to mediate mast cell activation in vivo. FcγRIIB-deficient mice displayed enhanced IgG-induced anaphylaxis. Active anaphylaxis, induced by immunization with antigen in alum, was enhanced in FcεRI-, FcγRIIB-, and glycoprotein 49B1–deficient mice and attenuated in FcRγ- and FcγRIII-deficient mice. All these animals displayed antigen-specific antibodies for IgE and IgGs, which indicates that the active anaphylaxis seen was attributed primarily to IgG antibodies. The reason for the enhancement of anaphylactic responses in FcεRI-deficient animals resulted from the increased expression of FcγRIII on mast cells in these mice, normally limited by competition of α chains for the available pool of the common γ chain (51). In the absence of FcεRI α chain, FcRγ chain is available to associate with FcγRIII α chain and assemble on the cell surface as a functional signaling receptor. These studies indicated the importance of the γ chain in regulating the level of surface expression of FcεRI and FcγRIII. Because γ chain is also associated with other members of the activation/inhibition paired receptors expressed on mast cells, such as PIR-A/PIR-B, the intracellular competition between these diverse α subunits and the common γ chain determines the level of surface expression of individual receptors and thus their ability to respond to specific biological stimuli. The absolute level of surface expression of FcRs on mast cells is clearly of therapeutic significance in both IgE- and IgG-mediated inflammatory responses; modulation of γ chain expression could thus represent a new therapeutic avenue for intervention in diseases such as anaphylaxis and asthma.

Type II Inflammation: Cytotoxic Immunoglobulin G

Cytotoxic IgGs are found in a variety of autoimmune disorders and have been developed for therapeutic indications in the treatment of infectious and neoplastic diseases. The mechanisms by which these antibodies trigger cytotoxicity in vivo have been investigated in FcR knockout mice. Anti-RBC antibodies trigger erythrophagocytosis of IgG-opsonized RBCs in an FcR-dependent manner; γ chain-deficient mice were protected from the pathogenic effect of these antibodies, whereas complement C3–deficient mice were indistinguishable from wild-type animals in their ability to clear the targeted RBCs (86,87). FcγRIII plays the exclusive role in this process for mouse IgG1 and IgG2b isotypes of antibodies; murine IgG3 antibodies were not pathogenic, which is consistent with the minimal engagement of IgG3 by FcRs. Murine IgG2a anti-RBC antibodies utilize primarily the FcγRIII receptor pathway despite the singular ability of murine IgG2a antibodies to bind as monomers to FcγRI. These and other studies suggest that the role of the high-affinity FcγRI in IgG-mediated inflammation is likely to be restricted to augmenting the effector response (determined by FcγRIII) in situations that involve high concentrations of murine IgG2a or human IgG1 antibodies that are found at localized inflammatory sites where FcγRI expression is induced on recruited macrophages.

Experimental models of immune thrombocytopenic purpura (ITP) in which murine IgG1 antiplatelet antibodies trigger thrombocytopenia, yielded results similar to those of the anti-RBC studies cited previously; FcRγ- or FcγRIII-deficient mice were protected from the pathogenic activity of these antibodies, whereas FcγRI- or C3-deficient mice were fully susceptible to antibody-induced thrombocytopenia. FcγRIIB-deficient mice were indistinguishable from wild-type animals in their ability to mediate either anti-RBC or antiplatelet clearance, which indicates that the specific effector cells involved in clearance were not expressing significant levels of this inhibitory receptor constitutively. In a passive protection model of Cryptococcus neoformans–induced disease, passive immunization with mouse IgG1, IgG2a, and IgG2b antibodies resulted in protection in wild-type animals but not in FcRγ chain–deficient animals; murine IgG3 antibodies enhanced disease in wild-type and FcR-deficient strains, which again indicates that a distinct pathway, not requiring known FcγRs, is involved in murine IgG3 antibody–mediated internalization of this pathogen (88).

IgG antibodies raised to murine glomerular basement membrane preparations induce acute glomerulonephritis in wild-type but not FcRγ- or FcγRIII-deficient animals (89,90). FcγRIIB-deficient animals displayed enhanced disease in this model, which indicates that the effector cells involved were constitutively expressing significant levels of FcγRIIB. Similar results were obtained when DBA/1 animals were immunized with bovine type II collagen to induce arthritis. Deficiency of FcRγ chain protected these mice from the pathogenic effects of the anticollagen antibodies that were generated (91). As mentioned previously, deficiency of FcγRIIB in the DBA/1 collagen-induced arthritis model resulted in enhanced disease, through increased autoantibody production and elevated effector responses.

A dramatic example of the importance of these pathways in determining the *in vivo* activity of cytotoxic antibodies was obtained in models of antitumor antibody response. In a syngenic murine model of metastatic melanoma, a murine IgG2a antimelanocyte antibody was able to reduce tumor metastasis in wild-type animals but was ineffective in FcRγ-deficient mice (92) (Fig. 6). In the absence of FcγRIIB, the activity of the antibody was enhanced 50-fold, which indicates that the *in vivo* cytotoxic activity of the antibody was the net of activation and inhibitory receptor engagement (83). Identical results were obtained in xenograft models in nude mice,

with human breast carcinoma or lymphoma lines and either murine IgG1 or humanized IgG1 antibodies [trastuzumab (Herceptin) and rituximab (Rituxan)]. A point mutation that eliminated FcR binding of the anti-Her2/neu antibody 4D5 abolished the *in vivo* cytotoxic activity of the antibody against a human xenograft but did not affect the *in vitro* growth inhibitory activity; this again illustrates the difference between *in vivo* and *in vitro* mechanisms. The conclusions that can be drawn from these studies support a dominant role for FcγRIII in mediating cytotoxicity by IgG antibodies. FcγRIIB restricts the effector response in situations in which the effector cell expresses this inhibitory molecule.

Type III Responses: Immune Complex–Mediated Inflammation

The classic example of this reaction, the Arthus reaction, has been studied in a variety of FcR- and complement-deficient animals. The initial studies were performed by using the cutaneous reverse passive Arthus reaction, in which antibody was injected intradermally and antigen was given intravenously. An inflammatory response, characterized by edema, hemorrhage, and neutrophil infiltration, developed within 2 hours. This reaction was elicited in a variety of complement- and FcR-deficient animals. The results from several independent studies confirmed the initial observations: that IgG immune complexes triggered cutaneous inflammatory reactions even in the absence of complement but displayed an absolute requirement for FcγRIII activation. FcγRIIB modulated the magnitude of the response, with enhanced Arthus reactions observed in FcγRIIB-deficient strains. The effector cell in the cutaneous reaction was determined to be the mast cell, as demonstrated by the use of mast cell–deficient strains and by mast cell reconstitution studies. The generality of this result was demonstrated in similar reactions performed in the lung, illustrating the FcR dependence and relative complement independence of this response. Thus, all studies have demonstrated an absolute dependence on FcR expression in the Arthus reaction. One model for immune complex–induced arthritis, the KRN/NOD model, has been shown to depend on both FcRIII and C3 but not on components of the classical pathway, such as C1q and C4; transfer of serum to animals deleted for FcRIII or C3 prevented the development of disease (93,94). The difference between the Arthus reaction induced in the KRN/NOD model and provoked in the reverse passive reaction has not been determined but may be related to the solubility, stability, or membrane association of the immune complex formed in each reaction. Deficiency in the late components of complement, such as C5a or its receptor, have also been reported to result in a partial reduction in the magnitude of the response in immune complex–induced lung inflammation (95) and a result in a complete block in the KRN/NOD arthritis model. These studies have led to a revision of the hypotheses about the mechanism of immune complex–mediated inflammation, typified by the Arthus reaction, in which there is an absolute requirement for FcγRIII in initiating mast cell

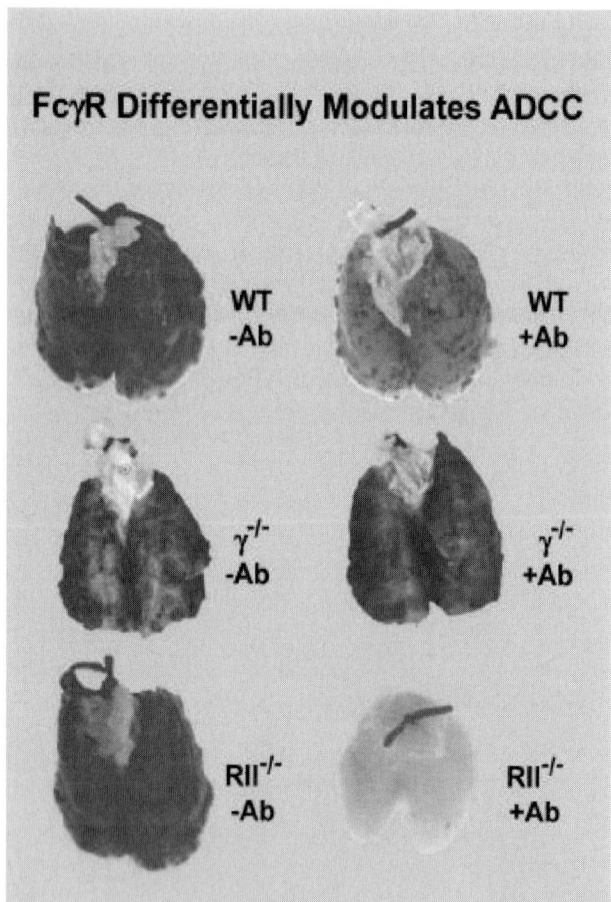

FIG. 6. Passive protection from pulmonary metastasis is modulated by FcR expression. Mice were injected intravenously with B16 melanoma cells on day 0 and with monoclonal antibody TA99 on alternate days. Lungs were harvested on day 14. Adapted from Clynes et al. (83), with permission.

activation by immune complexes. $Fc\gamma RIII$ activation is, in turn, modulated by the inhibitory receptor $Fc\gamma RIIB$. The ratio of these two molecules determines the concentration threshold for immune complex activation and the magnitude of the effector response that can be obtained. The classical pathway of complement activation is not required; however, C3 activation, through the alternative pathway, may be required under some circumstances, perhaps because of its ability to stabilize the immune complex and interact with the macrophage. Late components of complement, such as C5a, are generated as a result of FcRIII activation, along with other inflammatory mediators (vasoactive amines, chemokines, and cytokines). These mediators lead to the hallmarks of this reaction: edema, hemorrhage, and neutrophil infiltration at the site of immune complex deposition.

The significance of the FcR pathway in initiating immune complex inflammation in autoimmune disease was further established by investigating a spontaneous murine model of lupus, the B/W F1 mouse. The Arthus reaction results predicted the absolute requirement of activation $Fc\gamma R$ in initiating inflammation and tissue damage in immune complex diseases such as lupus. The $FcR\gamma$ chain deletion was backcrossed onto the NZB and New Zealand white strains for eight generations, and the intercrossed progeny were segregated into B/W $FcR\gamma^{-/-}$ and $FcR\gamma^{+/-}$. Anti-DNA antibodies and circulating immune complexes developed in all animals; immune complex and complement C3 deposition was similarly observed in all animals. However, mice deficient in the common γ chain showed no evidence of glomerulonephritis and had normal life expectancy, despite comparable levels of circulating immune complexes and glomerular deposition of these complexes along with complement C3. Mice heterozygous for the γ chain mutation were indistinguishable from B/W F1 animals with wild-type γ chains in developing glomerulonephritis and displaying reduced viability (80). This spontaneous model supports the conclusions stated previously about the absolute requirement for FcRIII in the activation of inflammatory disease by immune complexes: In the absence of this receptor, deposited immune complexes and C3 are not sufficient to trigger effector cell activation, which indicates that it is possible to uncouple pathogenic immune complexes from inflammatory disease by removing FcRIII engagement. These results further indicate that intervention in the effector stage of immune complex diseases, such as lupus, would be accomplished by blocking $Fc\gamma RIII$ activation to prevent initiation of effector cell responses.

DISEASE ASSOCIATIONS

Autoimmunity and Tolerance

In view of their functional capacity to link autoantibodies to effector cells, FcRs have naturally been considered to have a pathogenic role in the development of autoimmune diseases. Several studies have attempted to correlate specific polymorphisms in FcRIIA, FcRIIIA, or FcRIIIB with incidence or severity of lupus or rheumatoid arthritis (96). In view of the heterogeneity of these diseases, it is perhaps not surprising that inconsistent results have been obtained. Alleles that increase the ability of FcRIIA to bind IgG2 or FcRIIIA to bind IgG1 might be expected to correlate with disease severity in some populations. Indeed, these types of associations have been reported in some studies but not in others. These variable results have often been explained as an indication that other genes may be in linkage disequilibrium with the FcR alleles under investigation. This is a plausible explanation when viewed in light of the autoimmunity susceptibility genes mapping in or near the region of the FcR genes, chromosome 1q21–24 (97). This region of chromosome 1 has been implicated in a variety of human and murine linkage studies. For example, the Sle1 alleles derived from NZB flank the FcRIIB gene and form a linkage group with the ability to break tolerance to nuclear antigens, resulting in production of antichromatin antibodies. FcRIIB interacts with Sle1, as demonstrated by the construction of hybrids between these two loci. As heterozygotes, neither gene is capable of driving autoantibody production. However, the double heterozygote of Sle1 and RIIB develops antichromatin antibodies with a high degree of penetrance (97a). These data further support the hypothesis put forward that FcRIIB functions in the maintenance of peripheral tolerance by eliminating B cells expressing potentially cross-reactive BCRs from the germinal center. Other epistatic interactions between FcRIIB and lupus susceptibility genes have been demonstrated in the murine lupus model of B6.RIIB. Crossing the *yaa* gene to this strain accelerates the development of disease; 50% survival is decreased from 8 months to 4 months, with 100% fatality by 8 months. This increase in severity correlates with a change in the specificity of the autoantibodies, from diffuse antinuclear antibodies to antibodies that stain with a punctate, nucleolar pattern on antinuclear antibody staining. Together, these studies point to FcRIIB as a susceptibility factor in the development of autoimmunity with the ability to interact with other susceptibility factors to modify both the afferent and efferent limbs of the autoimmune response. Future studies aimed at demonstrating an association between RIIB expression on lymphoid and myeloid cells and the incidence and severity of autoimmune disease are necessary to extend this model to human disease.

Inflammation

Antibody-mediated inflammatory diseases have been clearly demonstrated to involve the coupling of pathogenic autoantibodies or immune complexes to cellular FcRs. Therapeutics targeted to disrupt these interactions are in development, beginning with a monoclonal antibody to human IgE that functions to reduce IgE binding to its high-affinity receptor and thereby prevent allergic and anaphylactic reactions (98). Because IgE is required for the survival of mast cells as well as in the regulation of $Fc\epsilon RI$ expression, reduction in IgE has synergistic effects on the ligand, receptor, and effector cell.

The success of this approach will undoubtedly lead to other approaches that target the receptor or its signaling pathway. Blocking FcγRIII is expected to mimic the phenotype of FcRIII-deficient animals in models of IgG-induced disease. Early attempts to use this approach in ITP were promising but limited by the cross-reactivity to receptors on neutrophils, which led to neutropenia and the development of immune response to the murine antibody (99). Development of second-generation anti-FcRIII antibodies with greater specificity and reduced toxicity now appears to be a viable approach for the treatment of autoimmune diseases.

An alternative approach to limiting the activation of FcRs is to utilize the endogenous inhibitory pathway to abrogate IgE or IgG activation of their cognate receptors through coligation to FcγRIIB. This mechanism has been proposed to explain the ability to induce desensitization for the treatment of allergic diseases (30). Inducing production of IgG antibodies to an allergen may facilitate cross-linking of FcγRIIB to FcϵRI. The ability to exploit the inhibitory pathway to reduce the activity of activation FcγRs has been demonstrated to account for some of the anti-inflammatory activity associated with high-dose intravenous gamma globulin (IVIG) (100). The use of IVIG for the treatment of ITP and other autoimmune diseases is well established, although the mechanism of action has been elusive. With a murine model of ITP, it has been demonstrated that protection by IVIG is dependent on the presence of FcRIIB; deletion of FcRIIB or blocking FcRIIB by a monoclonal antibody eliminates the ability of IVIG to protect the animal against the thrombocytopenia induced by a pathogenic antiplatelet antibody. IVIG was demonstrated to lead to the *in vivo* induction of FcRIIB on splenic macrophages, which would raise the threshold required for platelet clearance by FcRIII on these cells. These results suggest that inducing expression of FcRIIB is a clinically feasible approach and would be effective at modulating pathogenic autoantibodies from activation effector cell responses through FcRIII.

Studies on the FcαRI receptor have demonstrated a role for this molecule in the pathogenesis of IgA nephropathy, in which circulating macromolecular complexes are deposited in the mesangium, resulting in hematuria and eventually leading to renal failure. Soluble FcαRI is found in the circulating IgA complexes, which suggests a role for the receptor in the formation of these pathogenic complexes. A transgenic mouse expressing FcαRI spontaneously develops IgA nephropathy resulting from the interaction of polymeric mouse IgA and the human FcαRI receptor to release soluble receptor–IgA complexes, which leads to deposition in the mesangium and the sequelae of IgA neuropathy.

SUMMARY AND CONCLUSIONS

Receptors for the Fc of immunoglobulins provide an essential link between the humoral and adaptive response, translating the specificity of antibody diversity into cellular responses. These receptors mediate their biological responses through the coupling of Fc recognition to ITAM/ITIM-based signaling motifs. A diverse array of biological responses depends on the FcR system, influencing both the afferent and efferent limbs of the immune response. Detailed biochemical, structural, and molecular biological data have provided a detailed understanding of how these receptors are regulated, are assembled, bind their ligand, and transduce specific cellular signals. FcRs play a significant role *in vivo* in maintaining peripheral tolerance by deleting autoreactive B cells that potentially arise during somatic hypermutation in germinal centers, in augmenting T-cell responses by enhancing antigen presentation and maturation by dendritic cells, and in mediating the coupling of antigen recognition to effector cell activation. They are the primary pathways by which pathogenic IgG and IgE antibodies trigger inflammatory responses *in vivo*. Allergic reactions, cytotoxic IgG responses, and immune complex–mediated inflammation are all critically dependent on FcR cross-linking and have resulted in a fundamental revision of such classic immunological responses as the Arthus reaction. Blocking of these receptors uncouples the pathogenic potential of autoantibodies and represents an important new therapeutic target for the development of anti-inflammatory therapeutic agents. Central to the correct functioning of these responses is the balance that is maintained through the pairing of activation and inhibitory receptors that coengage the IgG ligand; perturbations in either component result in pathological responses. The study of FcRs defined the ubiquitous inhibitory motif, the ITIM, and has provided a paradigm for how these pathways modulate ITAM-based activation responses. Studies in mice deficient in individual FcRs have provided the necessary insights for defining comparable activities in human autoimmune diseases and suggest ways in which manipulation of the IgG–FcR interaction may lead to new classes of therapeutics for the treatment of these diseases. Modulation of the inhibitory response, a novel activity associated with IVIG to account for some of its anti-inflammatory activity *in vivo*, represents a novel approach to the regulation of immunoglobulin-mediated inflammation and suggests that therapeutic agents based on those pathways are likely to be effective. Conversely, engineering of therapeutic antibodies targeted to eliminate infectious or neoplastic disease will probably benefit from optimization of their Fc domains for interaction with specific FcRs.

ACKNOWLEDGMENTS

I thank the members of my laboratory at The Rockefeller University for helpful comments and suggestions and for assistance in preparing the figures shown in this chapter. I am grateful to Drs. Henry Metzger, Victor Nuzzenzweig, and Baruj Benacerraf for their insights into the historical background of FcRs. Ms. Cynthia Ritter provided, as always, invaluable assistance in the preparation of the manuscript. My laboratory of Molecular Genetics and Immunology at the

Rockefeller University is supported by the National Institutes of Health, the Alliance for Lupus Research, and Theresa and Eugene Lang.

REFERENCES

1. Boyden SV, Sorkin E. The adsorption of antigen by spleen cells previously treated with antiserum *in vivo*. *Immunology* 1960;3:272.
2. Berken A, Benacerraf B. Properties of antibodies cytophilic for macrophages. *J Exp Med* 1966;123:119.
3. Paraskevas F, Lee ST, Orr KB, et al. A receptor for Fc on mouse B-lymphocytes. *J Immunol* 1972;108;1319.
4. Kulczycki A Jr, Isersky C, Metzger H. The interaction of IgE with rat basophilic leukemia cells. I. Evidence for specific binding of IgE. *J Exp Med* 1974;139:600.
5. Ravetch JV, Luster AD, Weinshank R, et al. Structural heterogeneity and functional domains of murine immunoglobulin G Fc receptors. *Science* 1986;234:718.
6. Lewis VA, Koch T, Plutner H, et al. A complementary DNA clone for a macrophage-lymphocyte Fc receptor. *Nature* 1986;324:372.
7. Kinet JP, Metzger H, Hakimi J, et al. A cDNA presumptively coding for the alpha subunit of the receptor with high affinity for immunoglobulin E. *Biochemistry* 1987;26:4605.
8. Ra C, Jouvin MH, Blank U, et al. A macrophage Fcγ receptor and the mast cell receptor for IgE share an identical subunit. *Nature* 1989;341:752.
9. Kurosaki T, Ravetch JV. A single amino acid in the glycosyl phosphatidylinositol attachment domain determines the membrane topology of FcγRIII. *Nature* 1989;342:805.
10. Takai T, Li M, Sylvestre D, et al. FcR γ chain deletion results in pleiotrophic effector cell defects. *Cell* 1994;76:519.
11. Dombrowicz D, Flamand V, Brigman KK, et al. Abolition of anaphylaxis by targeted disruption of the high affinity immunoglobulin E receptor alpha chain gene. *Cell* 1993;75:969.
12. Sondermann P, Huber R, Jacob U. Crystal structure of the soluble form of the human Fcγ-receptor IIb: a new member of the immunoglobulin superfamily at 1.7 Åresolution. *EMBO J* 1999;18:1095.
13. Maxwell KF, Powell MS, Hulett MD, et al. Crystal structure of the human leukocyte Fc receptor, FcγRIIa. *Nat Struct Biol* 1999;6:437.
14. Garman SC, Kinet JP, Jardetzky TS. Crystal structure of the human high-affinity IgE receptor. *Cell* 1998;95:951.
15. Sondermann P, Huber R, Oosthuizen V, et al. The 32-A crystal structure of the human IgG1 Fc fragment–Fc gammaRIII complex. *Nature* 2000;406:267.
16. Garman SC, Wurzburg BA, Tarchevskaya SS, et al. Structure of the Fc fragment of human IgE bound to its high-affinity receptor Fc epsilonRI alpha. *Nature* 2000;406:259.
17. Ravetch JV, Kinet JP. Fc receptors. *Annu Rev Immunol* 1991;9:457.
18. Takai T, Ono M, Hikida M, et al. Augmented humoral and anaphylactic responses in Fc-gamma-RII–deficient mice. *Nature* 1996;379:346.
19. Hazenbos WL, Gessner JE, Hofhuis FM, et al. Impaired IgG-dependent anaphylaxis and Arthus reaction in FcgRIII (CD16) deficient mice. *Immunity* 1996;5:181.
20. Carroll MC. The role of complement and complement receptors in induction and regulation of immunity. *Annu Rev Immunol* 1998;16:545.
21. Sylvestre DL, Ravetch JV. Fc receptors initiate the Arthus reaction: redefining the inflammatory cascade. *Science* 1994;265:1095.
22. Ravetch JV, Clynes RA. Divergent roles for Fc receptors and complement *in vivo*. *Annu Rev Immunol* 1998;16:421.
23. Kinet JP. The high-affinity IgE receptor (FcεRI): from physiology to pathology. *Annu Rev Immunol* 1999;17:931.
24. Muta T, Kurosaki T, Misulovin Z, et al. A 13–amino-acid motif in the cytoplasmic domain of FcγRIIB modulates B-cell receptor signalling. *Nature* 1994;369:340.
25. Amigorena S, Bonnerot C, Drake JR, et al. Cytoplasmic domain heterogeneity and functions of IgG Fc receptors in B lymphocytes. *Science* 1992;256:1808.
26. Ravetch JV, Lanier LL. Immune inhibitory receptors. *Science* 2000;290:84.
27. Ravetch JV, Bolland S. IgG Fc receptors. *Annu Rev Immunol* 2001;19:275.
28. Ghetie V, Ward ES. Multiple roles for the major histocompatibility complex class I–related receptor FcRn. *Annu Rev Immunol* 2000;18:739.
29. Mostov KE. Transepithelial transport of immunoglobulins. *Annu Rev Immunol* 1994;12:63.
30. Daëron, M. Fc receptor biology. *Annu Rev Immunol* 1997;15:203.
31. Kubagawa H, Chen CC, Ho LH, et al. Biochemical nature and cellular distribution of the paired immunoglobulin-like receptors, PIR-A and PIR-B. *J Exp Med* 1999;189:309.
32. Maeda A, Kurosaki M, Kurosaki T. Paired immunoglobulin-like receptor (PIR)–A is involved in activating mast cells through its association with Fc receptor γ chain. *J Exp Med* 1998;188:991.
33. Moretta A, Bottino C, Vitale M, et al. Activating receptors and coreceptors involved in human natural killer cell–mediated cytolysis. *Annu Rev Immunol* 2001;19:197.
34. Lanier LL. Face off—the interplay between activating and inhibitory immune receptors. *Curr Opin Immunol* 2001;13:326.
35. Dombrowicz D, Lin S, Flamand V, et al. Allergy-associated FcRβ is a molecular amplifier of IgE- and IgG-mediated *in vivo* responses. *Immunity* 1998;8:517.
36. Qiu WQ, de Bruin D, Brownstein BH, et al. Organization of the human and mouse low-affinity FcγR genes: duplication and recombination. *Science* 1990;248:732.
37. Su Y, Brooks DG, Li L, et al. Myelin protein zero gene mutated in Charcot-Marie-Tooth type 1B patients. *Proc Natl Acad Sci U S A* 1993;90:10856.
38. Maresco DL, Chang E, Theil KS, et al. The three genes of the human FCGR1 gene family encoding Fc gamma RI flank the centromere of chromosome 1 at 1p12 and 1q21. *Cytogenet Cell Genet* 1996;73:157.
39. Morel L, Blenman KR, Croker BP, et al. The major murine systemic lupus erythematosus susceptibility locus, Sle1, is a cluster of functionally related genes. *Proc Natl Acad Sci U S A* 2001;98:1787.
40. Sandford AJ, Moffatt MF, Daniels SE, et al. A genetic map of chromosome 11q, including the atopy locus. *Eur J Hum Genet* 1995;3:188.
41. van der Pol W, van de Winkel JG. IgG receptor polymorphisms: risk factors for disease. *Immunogenetics* 1998;48:222.
42. Houghton AN, Scheinberg DA. Monoclonal antibody therapies—a "constant" threat to cancer. *Nat Med* 2000;6:373.
43. Brooks DG, Qiu WQ, Luster AD, et al. Structure and expression of human IgG FcRII(CD32). Functional heterogeneity is encoded by the alternatively spliced products of multiple genes. *J Exp Med* 1989;170:1369.
44. Ravetch JV, Perussia B. Alternative membrane forms of Fc gamma RIII(CD16) on human natural killer cells and neutrophils.Cell type–specific expression of two genes that differ in single nucleotide substitutions. *J Exp Med* 1989;170:481.
45. Coxon A, Cullere X, Knight S, et al. Fc gamma RIII mediates neutrophil recruitment to immune complexes. A mechanism for neutrophil accumulation in immune-mediated inflammation. *Immunity* 2001;14:693.
46. Ujike A, Ishikawa Y, Ono M, et al. Modulation of immunoglobulin (Ig)E–mediated systemic anaphylaxis by low-affinity Fc receptors for IgG. *J Exp Med* 1999;189:1573.
47. Daheshia M, Friend DS, Grusby MJ, et al. Increased severity of local and systemic anaphylactic reactions in gp49B1-deficient mice. *J Exp Med* 2001;194:227.
48. de Andrés B, Mueller AL, Verbeek S, et al. A regulatory role for Fcγ receptors CD16 and CD32 in the development of murine B cells. *Blood* 1998;92:2823.
49. Pricop L, Redecha P, Teillaud JL, et al. Differential modulation of stimulatory and inhibitory Fc gamma receptors on human monocytes by Th1 and Th2 cytokines. *J Immunol* 2001;166:531.
50. Yamaguchi M, Lantz CS, Oettgen HC, et al. IgE enhances mouse mast cell Fc(epsilon)RI expression *in vitro* and *in vivo*: evidence for a novel amplification mechanism in IgE-dependent reactions. *J Exp Med* 1997;185:663.
51. Dombrowicz D, Flamand V, Miyajima I, et al. Absence of FcεRI α chain results in upregulation of FcγRIII-dependent mast cell degranulation and anaphylaxis. *J Clin Invest* 1997;99:915.
52. Sondermann P, Kaiser J, Jacob U. Molecular basis for immune complex recognition: a comparison of Fc-receptor structures. *J Mol Biol* 2001;309:737.
53. Miller KL, Duchemin AM, Anderson CL. A novel role for the Fc

receptor gamma subunit: enhancement of Fc gamma R ligand affinity. *J Exp Med* 1996;183:2227.

54. Shields RL, Namenuk AK, Hong K, et al. High resolution mapping of the binding site on human IgG1 for Fc gamma RI, Fc gamma RII, Fc gamma RIII, and FcRn and design of IgG1 variants with improved binding to the Fc gamma R. *J Biol Chem* 2001;276:6591.

55. Choquet D, Partiseti M, Amigorena S, et al. Cross-linking of IgG receptors inhibits membrane immunoglobulin-stimulated calcium influx in B lymphocytes. *J Cell Biol* 1993;121:355.

56. Ono M, Bolland S, Tempst P, et al. Role of the inositol phosphatase SHIP in negative regulation of the immune system by the receptor Fc(gamma)RIIB. *Nature* 1996;383:263.

57. Pearse RN, Kawabe T, Bolland S, et al. SHIP recruitment attenuates FcγRIIB-induced B cell apoptosis. *Immunity* 1999;10:753.

58. Torigoe C, Inman JK, Metzger H. An unusual mechanism for ligand antagonism. *Science* 1998;281:568.

59. Tridandapani S, Pradhan M, LaDine JR, et al. Protein interactions of Src homology 2 (SH2) domain–containing inositol phosphatase (SHIP): association with Shc displaces SHIP from FcγRIIb in B cells. *J Immunol* 1999;162:1408.

60. Daëron M, Latour S, Malbec O, et al. The same tyrosine-based inhibition motif, in the intracytoplasmic domain of Fc gamma RIIB, regulates negatively BCR-, TCR-, and FcR-dependent cell activation. *Immunity* 1995;3:635.

61. Malbec O, Fong DC, Turner M, et al. Fcε receptor I-associated Lyn-dependent phosphorylation of Fcγ receptor IIB during negative regulation of mast cell activation. *J Immunol* 1998;160:1647.

62. Bolland S, Pearse RN, Kurosaki T, et al. SHIP modulates immune receptor responses by regulating membrane association of Btk. *Immunity* 1998;8:509.

63. Tamir I, Stolpa JC, Helgason CD, et al. The RasGAP-binding protein p62dok is a mediator of inhibitory FcγRIIB signals in B cells. *Immunity* 2000;12:347.

64. Yamanashi Y, Tamura T, Kanamori T, et al. Role of the rasGAP-associated docking protein p62(dok) in negative regulation of B cell receptor–mediated signaling. *Genes Dev* 2000;14:11.

65. Aman MJ, Lamkin TD, Okada H, et al. The inositol phosphatase SHIP inhibits Akt/PKB activation in B cells. *J Biol Chem* 1998;273:33922.

66. Liu Q, Sasaki T, Kozieradzki I, et al. SHIP is a negative regulator of growth factor receptor–mediated PKB/Akt activation and myeloid cell survival. *Genes Dev* 1999;13:786.

67. Heyman B. Regulation of antibody responses via antibodies, complement, and Fc receptors. *Annu Rev Immunol 18:709* 2000;18:709.

68. Bolland S, Ravetch JV. Spontaneous autoimmune disease in Fc(gamma)RIIB–deficient mice results from strain-specific epistasis. *Immunity* 2000;13:277.

69. Jiang Y, Hirose S, Abe M, et al. Polymorphisms in IgG Fc receptor IIB regulatory regions associated with autoimmune susceptibility. *Immunogenetics* 2000;51:429.

70. Pritchard NR, Cutler AJ, Uribe S, et al. Autoimmune-prone mice share a promoter haplotype associated with reduced expression and function of the Fc receptor FcgammaRII. *Curr Biol* 2000;10:227.

71. Yuasa T, Kubo S, Yoshino T, et al. Deletion of fcγ receptor IIB renders H-2(b) mice susceptible to collagen-induced arthritis. *J Exp Med* 1999;189:187.

72. Nakamura A, Yuasa T, Ujike A, et al. Fcγ receptor IIB–deficient mice develop Goodpasture's syndrome upon immunization with type IV collagen: a novel murine model for autoimmune glomerular basement membrane disease. *J Exp Med* 2000;191:899.

73. Banchereau J, Steinman RM. Dendritic cells and the control of immunity. *Nature* 1998;392:245.

74. Amigorena S, Bonnerot C. Fc receptors for IgG and antigen presentation on MHC class I and class II molecules. *Semin Immunol* 1999;11:385.

75. Hamano Y, Arase H, Saisho H, et al. Immune complex and Fc receptor–mediated augmentation of antigen presentation for *in vivo* Th cell responses. *J Immunol* 2000;164:6113.

76. Regnault A, Lankar D, Lacabanne V, et al. Fcγ receptor–mediated induction of dendritic cell maturation and major histocompatibility complex class I–restricted antigen presentation after immune complex internalization. *J Exp Med* 1999;189:371.

77. Wernersson S, Karlsson MCI, Dahlström J, et al. IgG-mediated enhancement of Ab responses is low in FcRγ chain deficient mice and increased in FcγRII deficient mice. *J Immunol* 1999;163:618.

78. Baiu DC, Prechl J, Tchorbanov A, et al. Modulation of the humoral immune response by antibody-mediated antigen targeting to complement receptors and Fc receptors. *J Immunol* 1999;162:3125.

79. Clynes R, Ravetch JV. Cytotoxic antibodies trigger inflammation through Fc receptors. *Immunity* 1995;3:21.

80. Clynes R, Dumitru C, Ravetch RV. Uncoupling of immune complex formation and kidney damage in autoimmune glomerulonephritis. *Science* 1998;279:1052.

81. Clynes R, Maizes JS, Guinamard R, et al. Modulation of immune complex-induced inflammation *in vivo* by the coordinate expression of activation and inhibitory Fc receptors. *J Exp Med* 1999;189:179.

82. Hazenbos WL, Heijnen IA, Meyer D, et al. Murine IgG1 complexes trigger immune effector functions predominantly via FcγRIII (CD16). *J Immunol* 1998;161:3026.

83. Clynes RA, Towers TL, Presta LG, et al. Inhibitory Fc receptors modulate *in vivo* cytoxicity against tumor targets. *Nat Med* 2000;6:443.

84. Launay P, Grossetete B, Arcos-Fajardo M, et al. Fcalpha receptor (CD89) mediates the development of immunoglobulin A (IgA) nephropathy (Berger's disease). Evidence for pathogenic soluble receptor–Iga complexes in patients and CD89 transgenic mice. *J Exp Med* 2000;191:1999.

85. Miyajima I, Dombrowicz D, Martin TR, et al. Systemic anaphylaxis in the mouse can be mediated largely through IgG1 and FcγRIII. *J Clin Invest* 1997;99:901.

86. Sylvestre D, Clynes R, Ma M, Warren H, et al. Immunoglobulin G–mediated inflammatory responses develop normally in complement-deficient mice. *J Exp Med* 1996;184:2385.

87. Fossati-Jimack L, Ioan-Facsinay A, Reininger L, et al. Markedly different pathogenicity of four immunoglobulin G isotype-switch variants of an antierythrocyte autoantibody is based on their capacity to interact *in vivo* with the low-affinity Fcγ receptor III. *J Exp Med* 2000;191:1293.

88. Yuan R, Clynes R, Oh J, et al. Antibody-mediated modulation of *Cryptococcus neoformans* infection is dependent on distinct Fc receptor functions and IgG subclasses. *J Exp Med* 1998;187:641.

89. Suzuki Y, Shirato I, Okumura K, et al. Distinct contribution of Fc receptors and angiotensin II–dependent pathways in anti-GBM glomerulonephritis. *Kidney Int* 1998;54:1166.

90. Park SY, Ueda S, Ohno H, et al. Resistance of Fc receptor–deficient mice to fatal glomerulonephritis. *J Clin Invest* 1998;102:1229.

91. Kleinau S, Martinsson P, Heyman B. Induction and suppression of collagen-induced arthritis is dependent on distinct fcγ receptors. *J Exp Med* 2000;191:1611.

92. Clynes R, Takechi Y, Moroi Y, et al. Fc receptors are required in passive and active immunity to melanoma. *Proc Natl Acad Sci U S A* 1998;95:652.

93. Korganow AS, Ji H, Mangialaio S, et al. From systemic T cell self-reactivity to organ-specific autoimmune disease via immunoglobulins. *Immunity* 1999;10:451.

94. Matsumoto I, Staub A, Benoist C, et al. Arthritis provoked by linked T and B cell recognition of a glycolytic enzyme. *Science* 1999;286:1732.

95. Baumann U, Köhl J, Tschernig T, et al. A codominant role of FcγRI/III and C5aR in the reverse Arthus reaction. *J Immunol* 2000;164:1065.

96. Dijstelbloem HM, van de Winkel JG, Kallenberg CG. Inflammation in autoimmunity: receptors for IgG revisited. *Trends Immunol* 2001;22:510.

97. Wakeland EK, Liu K, Graham RR, et al. Delineating the genetic basis of systemic lupus erythematosus. *Immunity* 2001;15:397.

97a. Bolland S, Yim Y-S, Tus K, et al. Genetic modifiers of systemic lupus erythematosus in FcγRIIB(−/−) mice. *J Exp Med* 2002;195:1167.

98. Heusser C, Jardieu P. Therapeutic potential of anti-IgE antibodies. *Curr Opin Immunol* 1997;9:805.

99. Bussel JB. Fc receptor blockade and immune thrombocytopenic purpura. *Semin Hematol* 2000;37:261.

100. Samuelsson A, Towers TL, Ravetch JV. Anti-inflammatory activity of IVIG mediated through the inhibitory Fc receptor. *Science* 2001;291:484.

CHAPTER 23

Type I Cytokines and Interferons and Their Receptors

Warren J. Leonard

Overview and Issues of Nomenclature
Type I Cytokines and Their Receptors
  Type I Cytokines: Structural Considerations · Receptors for Type I Cytokines · Type I Cytokine Receptors Are Homodimers, Heterodimers, or Higher Order Receptor Oligomers
Type I Cytokine Receptor Families and Their Relations
  Cytokines that Share the Common Cytokine Receptor γ Chain (Interleukins-2, -4, -7, -9, -15, and -21) · Cytokine Receptors that Share the Common β Chain, β_c (IL-3, IL-5, and GM-CSF) · Cytokine Receptors that Share gp130 (IL-6, IL-11, Oncostatin M, Ciliary Neurotropic Factor, Leukemia Inhibitory Factor, Cardiotrophin-1, and NNT/BSF-3) · Significance of the Sharing of Receptor Chains · Other Receptors with Similarities to gp130 (G-CSF Receptor, Obesity Receptor, and IL-12R) · Other Examples of Shared Receptor Molecules · An Example of Multiple Affinities of Binding for a Single Cytokine: Three Classes of IL-2 Receptors · Erythropoietin, Thrombopoietin, and Stem Cell Factor
Cytokine Pleiotropy, Cytokine Redundancy, Cytokine Receptor Pleiotropy, and Cytokine Receptor Redundancy
Soluble Receptors
Interferons (Type II Cytokines) and Their Receptors
  Interleukin-10, a Type II Cytokine, and Related Cytokines IL-19, IL-20, IL-22, IL-24, IL-26, IL-28, and IL-29
Species Specificity of Cytokines
Signaling through Interferon and Cytokine Receptors
Overview of Janus Kinases and STATs
  Jaks · Importance of Janus Kinases in Signaling · Jak3 Mutations Result in an Autosomal Recessive Form of Severe Combined Immunodeficiency that Is Indistinguishable from X-Linked Severe Combined Immunodeficiency Disease
Activation of Janus Kinases and the Janus Kinase–STAT Paradigm
STAT Proteins Are Substrates for Janus Kinases that at Least in Part Help Determine Specificity
  Docking of STATs on Receptors or Other Molecules, Tyrosine Phosphorylation of STATs, and STAT Dimerization · STAT Nuclear Translocation, DNA Binding, and Tetramerization · Optimal Binding Sites for STATs · Transcription Activation by STATs · Specificity of STATs · STATs Are Evolutionarily Old · What Are the Functions of STATs? · Do Other Proteins Bind to γ-Interferon–Activated Sequence Motifs?
Other Latent Transcription Factors as Examples of Cytoplasmic-to-Nuclear Signaling (NFκB, NF-AT, and SMADs)
Other Substrates for Janus Kinases
Other Signaling Molecules Important for Cytokines
  Other Tyrosine Kinases besides Janus Kinases · Insulin Receptor Substrate Proteins · Phosphatidylinositol 3-Kinase · The Ras/Mitogen-Activated Protein Kinase Pathway
Down-modulation of Cytokine Signals
The CIS/SOCS/JAB/SSI Family of Inhibitory Adapter Proteins
PIAS Proteins
Th1/Th2 Cells: The T Helper Paradigm
Diseases of Cytokine Receptors and Related Molecules
  Range of Cytokine-Related Causes of Severe Combined Immunodeficiency Disease · Defects in the Ability to Clear Mycobacterial Infections · Mutations in the WSX-1/TCCR Type I Receptor · Other Diseases Associated with Cytokine Receptors
Concluding Comments
References

OVERVIEW AND ISSUES OF NOMENCLATURE

Cytokines are proteins that are secreted by cells and exert actions either on the cytokine-producing cell (autocrine actions) or on other target cells (paracrine actions). Cytokines exert these effects by interacting with and transducing signals through specific cell surface receptors. From this operational type of definition, it is clear that the distinction among cytokines, growth factors, and hormones is often imprecise. In general, cytokines and growth factors can be thought of quite similarly, except that molecules involved in host defense that act on white blood cells (leukocytes) are generally called *cytokines,* whereas those that act on other somatic cell types are more typically described as *growth factors.* However, there is a major difference between hormones and the majority of cytokines: Cytokines generally act locally. For example, in the interaction between a T cell and an antigen-presenting cell, cytokines are produced and usually exert potent actions only locally, and have rather limited half-lives in the circulation. In contrast, following their release, hormones are generally disseminated by the bloodstream throughout the body, acting on a wide range of distal target organs. However, certain cytokines can act at longer distances as well, which makes the distinction between hormones and cytokines less absolute.

In the immune system, terms such as *lymphokines* and *monokines* were originally used to identify the cellular source for the cytokine (1). Thus, interleukin-1 (IL-1), which was first recognized to be made by monocytes, was a monokine, whereas IL-2, which was first described as a T-cell growth factor, was a lymphokine. A major limitation of this nomenclature became evident when it was recognized that many of these lymphokines and monokines were in fact produced by a wide spectrum of cell types; this recognition resulted in the adoption of the term *cytokine,* first coined by Stanley Cohen in 1974 (2,3). The term, in effect, refers to a factor made by a cell ("cyto") that acts on target cells. The range of actions of cytokines is diverse, including the abilities to induce growth, differentiation, cytolytic activity, apoptosis, and chemotaxis. The term *interleukin* refers to cytokines that are produced by one leukocyte and act on another leukocyte (4). In many cases, however, some interleukins (e.g., IL-1 and IL-6) are additionally produced by other cell types and/or can additionally act on other cell types, and IL-7 is produced by stromal cells rather than by typical leukocytes. A number of cytokines have more distinctive names, such as thymic stromal lymphopoietin (TSLP); however, such names are also not always descriptive, inasmuch as one of the major sources of human TSLP is epithelial cells and a site for its action is on dendritic cells (discussed later).

Among the many different cytokines, the "type I" cytokines share a similar four–α helical bundle structure, as detailed later, and their receptors correspondingly share characteristic features that have led to their description as the cytokine receptor superfamily, or type I cytokine receptors (5–8). Although many of the interleukins are type I cytokines, not all are molecules of this class. For example, of the "proin-flammatory cytokines" IL-1, tumor necrosis factor α (TNF-α), and IL-6, IL-6 is a type I cytokine, whereas IL-1 and TNF-α are not (IL-1 and TNF-α are discussed in Chapters 24 and 25). One interleukin, IL-8, is a chemokine (see Chapter 26). Moreover, as discussed later, IL-10, IL-19, IL-20, IL-22, IL-24, IL-26, IL-28, and IL-29 are more similar to interferons and are denoted type II cytokines. Thus, the term *interleukin* refers to a relationship to leukocytes, whereas the characterization of a cytokine as type I or type II has implications regarding the three-dimensional structure of the cytokine and evolutionary considerations for both the cytokines and their receptors that are important for ligand binding and the mechanisms of signal transduction. In reality, however, the fact that a molecule is an "interleukin" generally provides little more information than its being a type I or type II cytokine of immunological interest, although actions of interleukins are certainly not limited to the immune system. For example, IL-6 can exert actions related to the heart.

In addition to molecules that primarily are of immunological interest, other extremely important proteins, including growth hormone, prolactin, erythropoietin, thrombopoietin, and leptin are also type I cytokines, and their receptors are type I cytokine receptors. As detailed later, these nonimmunological type I cytokines share important signal transduction pathways with type I cytokines of immunological interest. Thus, the grouping in this chapter emphasizes evolution and signaling pathways, rather than common functions. Hence, although IL-6 exerts many actions that overlap those of IL-1 and TNF-α, these latter molecules are discussed elsewhere because the signaling pathways they use are very different from those used by type I cytokines and their receptors. This, however, raises the important concept that similar end functions can be mediated via more than one type of signaling pathway.

The field of interferon (IFN) research started earlier but then developed in parallel to the cytokine field. IFNs were first recognized as antiviral agents and, as such, have been of great excitement both for basic science and for potential clinical uses. Over time, it has become clear that the type I cytokines and IFNs share a number of features, so that they are addressed together in one chapter in this book. It is also noteworthy that the International Interferon Society changed its name to the International Society of Interferon and Cytokine Research and that the International Cytokine Society focuses on the IFNs as well as on cytokines; together, these developments emphasize the importance of the common themes of IFNs and cytokines that are the subject of part of this chapter.

TYPE I CYTOKINES AND THEIR RECEPTORS

Type I Cytokines: Structural Considerations

Despite the existence of extremely limited amino acid sequence similarities between different type I cytokines, it is striking that all type I cytokines whose structures have been solved (by nuclear magnetic resonance or x-ray crystallographic methods) are known to have similar three-dimensional structures (5–8). Moreover, type I cytokines whose structures have not yet been solved also appear, on the basis of modeling and comparison to the solved structures, to have similar three-dimensional structures (5–8). Type I cytokines are appropriately described as four–α helical bundle cytokines, because they exhibit characteristic three-dimensional structures containing four α helices (Fig. 1). In their structures, the first two and last two α helices are each connected by long-overhand loops. This results an "up-up-down-down" topological structure, because the first two helices (A and B) can be oriented in an "up"-orientation and the last two helices (C and D) can be oriented in a "down"-orientation, as viewed from the NH$_2$- to COOH-terminal direction. As shown in Fig. 1, the N- and C-terminals of the cytokines are positioned on the same part of the molecule.

Type I cytokines can be grouped as either short-chain and long-chain four–α helical bundle cytokines, according to their sizes (8). The short-chain cytokines include IL-2, IL-3, IL-4, IL-5, granulocyte-macrophage colony-stimulating factor (GM-CSF), IL-7, IL-9, IL-13, IL-15, macrophage colony-stimulating factor (M-CSF), stem cell factor (SCF), and TSLP; the long-chain cytokines include growth hormone, prolactin, erythropoietin, thrombopoietin, leptin, IL-6, IL-11, leukemia inhibitory factor (LIF), oncostatin M (OSM), ciliary neurotrophic factor (CNTF), cardiotrophin-1 (CT-1), novel neurotrophin 1/B cell–stimulating factor 3 (NNT-1/BSF-3), and granulocyte colony-stimulating factor (G-CSF) (Table 1) (8,9). In addition to a difference in the length of the helices, which typically are approximately 15 amino acids long for

TABLE 1. *Four helical-bundle cytokines*

Short-chain cytokines	Long-chain cytokines
IL-2	IL-6
IL-4	IL-11
IL-7	Oncostatin M
IL-9	Leukemia inhibitory factor
IL-13	Ciliary neurotrophic factor
IL-15	Cardiotropin-1
IL-21	NNT-1/BSF-3
TSLP	
IL-3	Growth hormone
IL-5[a]	Prolactin
GM-CSF	Erythropoietin
	Thrombopoietin
M-CSF[ab]	Leptin
SCF[b]	G-CSF

[a]Dimers.

[b]Different from the other four helical bundle cytokines in that the M-CSF and SCF receptors (CSF-1R and c-kit, respectively) have intrinsic tyrosine kinase activity and are not type I cytokine receptors.

BSF-3, B-lymphocyte–stimulating factor 3; G-CSF, granulocyte colony-stimulating factor; GM-CSF, granulocyte-macrophage colony-stimulating factor; IL, interleukin; M-CSF, macrophage colony-stimulating factor; NNT-1, novel neurotrophin 1; SCF, stem cell factor; TSLP, thymic stromal lymphopoietin.

the short-chain helical cytokines and 25 amino acids long for the long-chain helical cytokines, there are differences in the angles between the pairs of helices, and the AB loop is "under" the CD loop in the short cytokines but "over" the CD loop in the long cytokines (Fig. 1) (7,8,10). Short-chain, but not long-chain, cytokines have β structures in the AB and CD loops. The groupings according to short-chain and long-chain cytokines have evolutionary considerations and also correlate with grouping of receptor chains for these two subfamilies of type I cytokines. An analysis of short-chain cytokines has revealed that 61 residues constitute the family framework, including most of the 31 residues that contribute to the buried inner core. The similarities and differences in the structures of IL-2, IL-4, and GM-CSF have been carefully analyzed (6). Among these cytokines, there is considerable variation in the intrachain disulfide bonds that stabilize the structures. For example, IL-4 has three intrachain disulfide bonds, GM-CSF has two, and IL-2 has only one. In IL-4, the first disulfide bond (between Cys 24 and Cys 65) connects loop AB to BC, the second disulfide bond (between Cys 46 and Cys 99) connects helix B and loop CD, and the third disulfide bond (between Cys 3 and Cys 127) connects the residue preceding helix B with helix D. In GM-CSF, the N-terminal of helix B and the N-terminal of β strand CD are connected by one disulfide bond, whereas the other disulfide bond connects the C-terminal of helix C and a strand that follows helix D. In IL-2, a single essential disulfide bond between Cys 58 and Cys 105 connects helix B to strand CD. Thus, each cytokine has evolved distinct disulfide bonds to stabilize its structure, although it is typical that helix B is

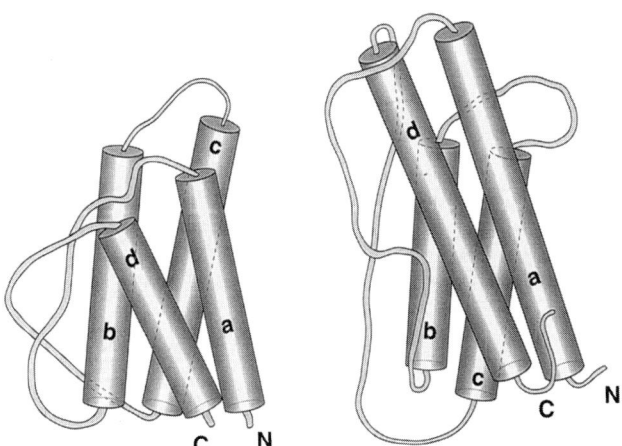

FIG. 1. Four–α helical bundle cytokines. Schematic drawing showing typical short-chain and long-chain four–helical bundle cytokines. Although both of these exhibit an "up-up-down-down" topology to their four α helices, note that in the short-chain cytokines, the AB loop is behind the CD loop, whereas in the long-chain cytokines, the situation is reversed. See text. The figure was provided by Dr. Alex Wlodawer, National Cancer Institute.

connected to the CD loop. The structures formed by helices A and D are more rigorously conserved than those formed by helices B and C, primarily because of the interhelical angles; helix D and the connecting region are the most highly conserved elements among the three cytokines (6). This is of particular interest, because the regions of type I cytokines that are most important for cytokine–cytokine receptor interactions (according to analogy to the growth hormone receptor structure; see later discussion) include helices A and D and residues in the AB and CD loops, whereas helices B and C do not form direct contacts (6).

Certain variations on these typical structures can occur. For example, IL-5 is unusual in that it is a dimer, positioned in such a way so that the ends containing the N- and C-terminals are juxtaposed (11). Helix D is "exchanged" between the two covalently attached molecules, so that helix D of each molecule actually forms part of the four-helix bundle of the other monomer (11). M-CSF is also a helical cytokine dimer, but no exchange of helix D occurs (10). The IFNs achieve related albeit somewhat different structures and also are known as type II cytokines (8). IFN-β has an extra helix that is positioned in place of the CD strand (12). IFN-γ is a dimer, each molecule of which consists of six helices (13), as can be seen in Fig. 2. Two of these helices are interchanged, including one from each four-helix bundle (10,13). IL-10, which is closely related to IFN-γ, has a similar structure (14), and it can be predicted that more recently identified IL-10–like molecules, such as IL-19, IL-20, IL-22, IL-24, IL-26, IL-28, and IL-29, presumably have similar structures. It is interesting that the majority of helical cytokines have four exons, with helix A in exon 1, helices B and C in exon 3, and helix D in exon 4 (7). A related organization is found for IFN-γ as well as for the long-chain helical cytokines, growth hormone, and G-CSF. However, there are a number of exceptions: For example, IL-15 is divided into nine exons and IFN-β has only one exon, being devoid of introns. Thus, there are general "rules," but each of these has exceptions.

Receptors for Type I Cytokines

The first published report suggesting that type I cytokine receptors had shared features came from a comparison of the sequences of the erythropoietin receptor and the IL-2 receptor β chain (15), but an analysis of a larger number of type I cytokine receptors provided a much clearer view of this superfamily (16). Type I cytokine receptors are generally type I membrane-spanning glycoproteins (N-terminal extracellular, C-terminal intracellular), the only exceptions being proteins such as the CNTF receptor α chain (see later discussion) that lack a cytoplasmic domain and instead have a glycosylphosphatidylinositol (GPI) anchor; however, the orientation of this protein is otherwise similar to that of a type I membrane protein. In their extracellular domains, a number of conserved similarities have been noted (Table 2). These include four conserved cysteine residues that were predicted to be involved in intrachain disulfide bonding and a tryptophan

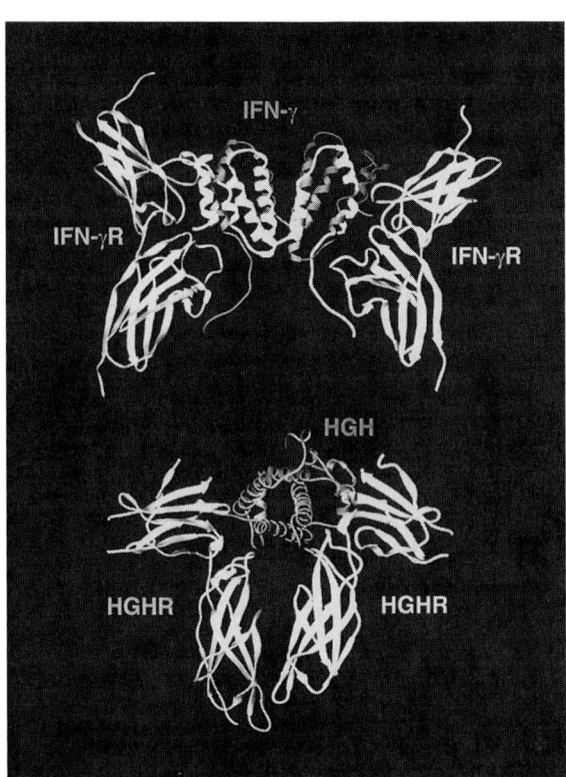

FIG. 2. Structure of the growth hormone and interferon (IFN) γ receptors. Shown are ribbon diagrams of the structures of the IFN-γ receptor (above) and growth hormone receptor (below) as examples of type II and type I cytokine receptors. In the IFN-γ receptor, only IFNGR-1 complexed to the IFN-γ dimer is shown, inasmuch as the full structure with IFNGR-2 is not yet known. For growth hormone, both growth hormone receptor monomers are shown. See text for discussion of the structures. The growth hormone/growth hormone receptor structure is from de Vos et al. (23), and the IFN-γ-IFNGR-1 structure is from Walter et al. (242). The figure was provided by Dr. Alex Wlodawer, National Cancer Institute.

residue, located two amino acids C-terminal to the second conserved cysteine. In addition, a membrane proximal region WSXWS (Trp-Ser-X-Trp-Ser) motif is generally conserved, although, again, exceptions exist: For example, in the growth hormone receptor, the motif is a substantially different YGEFS (Tyr-Gly-Glu-Phe-Ser) sequence, and in the IL-23 receptor, it is a more similar WQPWS (Trp-Gln-Pro-Trp-Ser) motif.

TABLE 2. *Features common to type I cytokine receptors*

Extracellular domain
Four conserved cysteine residues, involved in intrachain disulfide bonds
WSXWS motif
Fibronectin type III modules

Cytoplasmic domain
Box 1/box 2 regions: the box 1 region is a proline-rich region that is involved in the interaction of Janus family tyrosine kinases

Interestingly, an analysis of a number of the receptors reveals that the two sets of cysteines are typically encoded in two adjacent exons, and the exon containing the WSXWS motif is typically just 5' to the exon encoding the transmembrane domain. Although serines can be encoded by six different codons (i.e., sixfold degeneracy in codon usage), the codons used to encode the serines in WSXWS motif are far more limited, with two of the six possible codons (AGC and AGT) dominating. These data are consistent with a common ancestral precursor. Although complementary deoxyribonucleic acids (cDNAs) encoding many of the known cytokine receptors were identified on the basis of expression cloning with a defined ligand, the limited degeneracy of the WSXWS motif facilitated the cDNA cloning of several type I cytokine receptor members by the use of polymerase chain reaction, leading to the first identification of IL-11R (17,18), IL-13Rα (19), and an OSM receptor (20). With the advances in sequencing the human genome, receptors have also been identified on the basis of computer predictions of open reading frames that appeared to encode type I receptors (e.g., IL-21 receptor) (21) and have allowed computer-based homology searches when homology was too low for cloning by hybridization (e.g., identifying the human TSLP receptor on the basis of the sequences of the murine TSLP receptor) (22). Another shared feature of type I cytokine receptors is the presence of fibronectin type III domains. In some cases, such as the common cytokine receptor β chain, β_c, which is shared by the IL-3, IL-5, and GM-CSF receptors (see later discussion), the extracellular domain is extended, with a duplication of the domains containing the four conserved cysteines and the WSXWS motif.

Overall, the different receptor molecules, like the cytokines, have extremely limited sequence identity. Nevertheless, they appear to form similar structures, according to the known structures for the growth hormone, prolactin, erythropoietin, and IL-4 receptors (23–26) and the modeling of other cytokine receptor molecules on the basis of the known structures. Thus, the available data indicate closely related three-dimensional structures for the different type I cytokines and closely related structures for type I cytokine receptors, despite the widely divergent sequences. Of importance, however, is that the only type I cytokine receptors whose structures have been completely solved correspond to long-chain type I cytokines. A partial structure is available for the IL-4 receptor, containing IL-4 and IL-4Rα but not either of the essential second possible chains (γ_c or IL-13Rα1, which are part of the type I and type II IL-4 receptors, respectively). The cytokines and their receptors have presumably coevolved, whereby the differences in amino acid sequences between different cytokines allow for their distinctive interactions with their cognate receptor chains. At times, however, as illustrated later, despite amino acid differences, there are a number of sets of cytokines that are capable of interacting with shared receptor chains, allowing a number of the different cytokines and their receptors to be grouped into subfamilies (8).

In addition to the similarities just noted in the extracellular domains, there are sequence similarities that are conserved in the cytoplasmic domain of cytokine receptors. In particular, a membrane proximal area known as the Box 1/Box 2 regions are conserved (Table 2), with a proline-rich Box 1 region being the most conserved (27). This is discussed in greater detail later.

Type I Cytokine Receptors Are Homodimers, Heterodimers, or Higher Order Receptor Oligomers

The first cytokine receptor structure to be solved was that for growth hormone (Fig. 2) (23). Before the x-ray crystallographic analysis, it was believed that growth hormone bound to its receptor with a stoichiometry of 1:1. Remarkably, however, the x-ray crystal structure solution was necessary to establish that a single growth hormone molecule interacted with a dimer of the growth hormone receptor, in which each receptor monomer contributes a total of seven β strands. Perhaps the most striking finding was that totally different parts of the growth hormone molecule interacted with the same general region of each growth hormone receptor monomer. The three-dimensional x-ray crystal structure for the growth hormone/growth hormone receptor complex is shown in Fig. 2. Solving the structure also clarified the basis for the assembly of the growth hormone receptor complex (23). Kinetically, growth hormone is believed to interact first with one receptor monomer via a relatively large and high-affinity interaction surface (site I), spanning approximately 1,230 Å^2. A second receptor monomer then interacts with the growth hormone/growth hormone receptor complex via two contact points: one on growth hormone (spanning approximately 900 Å^2) (site II) and the other on the first receptor monomer (spanning approximately 500 Å^2) (site III), located much more proximal to the cell membrane. Thus, a total of three extracellular interactions are responsible for the formation and stabilization of the growth hormone/growth hormone receptor complex (23). Intuitively, critical mutations in site I should prevent growth hormone from binding to its receptor, whereas mutations in site II would potentially prevent dimerization and signal transduction, providing a rational method for the design of antagonists.

The growth hormone/growth hormone receptor structure revealed that the growth hormone receptor extracellular domain is composed of two fibronectin type III modules, each of which is approximately 100 amino acids long and contains seven β strands, resulting in the formation of an immunoglobulin-like structure. The contact surface between ligand and receptor occurs in the hinge region that separates these two fibronectin type III modules. Analysis of a growth hormone/prolactin receptor complex revealed the anticipated similar structure for the prolactin receptor (24).

The growth hormone/growth hormone receptor structure was obviously of great importance in the growth hormone field. In addition, however, the structure has been of great importance by serving as a paradigm for the structures of all type I cytokine receptors. Because the growth hormone receptor forms a homodimer, it immediately served as a model for other homodimers, such as the erythropoietin receptor, whose structure has also been solved (25). Interestingly, the structure of the erythropoietin receptor complex was solved by using a small protein mimetic (20–amino acid–long peptide) of erythropoietin that was identified through the use of random phage display peptide libraries and affinity selective methods (28). These studies on erythropoietin provided direct evidence that a small molecule not only mimicked erythropoietin action, but also could induce dimerization of the erythropoietin receptor, thus forming a structure similar to that of the growth hormone receptor. The greatest difference, however, is that the "site III" stem region interaction surface in the erythropoietin receptor is much smaller than that in the growth hormone receptor, comprising only 75 $\mathring{A}^2$ (25).

In addition to the similarities between the structures for the growth hormone (23) and erythropoietin (25) receptors and presumably with other homodimeric receptors, it is immediately evident that the same type of structure could be achieved by heterodimeric receptors, as demonstrated by the growth hormone–growth hormone receptor/prolactin receptor structure (24), in which one of the growth hormone receptor monomers is replaced by the prolactin receptor monomer. Thus, the growth hormone/growth hormone receptor system can be viewed as a specialized system in which two parts of growth hormone interact with the same receptor chain. It is reasonable to hypothesize that cytokine-receptor systems with a homodimeric receptor evolutionarily might be older than those with heterodimeric receptors and that the coordination of two different receptor chains in heterodimeric receptors might reflect added levels of specialization that have evolved. Because type I cytokines and their receptors are members of superfamilies, if there were a single original primordial type I cytokine receptor molecule from which all the others have been derived, it is reasonable to hypothesize that the original type I cytokine/receptor system might have involved a receptor that formed homodimers. In this regard, it is interesting that growth hormone and erythropoietin, whose actions are vital for growth and erythropoiesis, bind to receptors that are homodimers, whereas the heterodimeric structures that typify the immune system are perhaps more "specialized" functions that arose later in evolution.

Interestingly, all type I cytokines known to interact with homodimers (growth hormone, prolactin, erythropoietin, and G-CSF) are long-chain helical cytokines, although other long-chain helical cytokines [e.g., the cytokines whose receptors contain glycoprotein 130 (gp130); see later discussion] interact with heteromeric receptors. The short-chain cytokines that signal through homodimers are SCF and M-CSF, but in these cases, the receptors (c-kit and CSF-1 receptor, respectively) are different from type I cytokine receptors in that they contain intrinsic tyrosine kinase domains. Thus, SCF and M-CSF are not typical type I cytokines, and all other short-chain cytokines signal through heterodimers or more complex receptor structures (e.g., IL-2 and IL-15 signal through high-affinity receptors that have three components).

By analogy to the structure of the growth hormone receptor, for cytokines whose receptors are heterodimers, it is easy to envision that heterodimeric receptors would occur with cytokines in which site II on the cytokine had evolved to a point at which it interacted with a different receptor molecule than did site I, resulting in formation of a heterodimer rather than a homodimer. This latter situation is the case for many cytokines, including all short-chain type I cytokines except for SCF and M-CSF. Overall, there are a number of distinct groups of cytokines, and each group shares at least one common receptor component. This phenomenon is true for certain sets of both short-chain and long-chain four–α helical bundle cytokines, and, depending on the set of cytokines, the shared chain interacts with either site I or site II.

TYPE I CYTOKINE RECEPTOR FAMILIES AND THEIR RELATIONS

Cytokines that Share the Common Cytokine Receptor γ Chain (Interleukins-2, -4, -7, -9, -15, and -21)

The receptors for six different immunologically important cytokines—IL-2, IL-4, IL-7, IL-9, IL-15, and IL-21—share the common cytokine receptor γ chain, γ_c (CD132) (29–37) [reviewed by Leonard (38,39)]. These cytokines are all short-chain four–helical bundle cytokines; basic features of these cytokines are summarized in Table 3. The properties of these cytokines and their unique receptor chains are summarized, followed by a discussion of the discovery that they share a common receptor component and the implications thereof.

Mature IL-2 is a 133–amino acid–long peptide that is produced solely by activated T-lymphocytes and is the major T-cell growth factor, in keeping with its original discovery as a T-cell growth factor (40). IL-2 has other important actions as well, however, including its ability to exert effects on a number of other lineages; most notably, it can increase immunoglobulin synthesis and J chain transcription in B cells (41,42), potently augment the cytolytic activity of natural killer (NK) cells (43–45), and induce the cytolytic activity of lymphokine-activated killer cells. In addition, IL-2 plays an important role related to the elimination of autoreactive cells in a process known as antigen-induced (or activation-induced) cell death (AICD) (46,47) (Table 3). This is discussed further in Chapter 27.

IL-2 is particularly important historically, because it is the first type I cytokine that was cloned (48) and the first type I cytokine for which a receptor component was cloned (49,50). Many general principles were derived from this cytokine, including its being the first cytokine that was demonstrated to act in a growth factor–like manner through specific high-affinity receptors, which is analogous to the growth factors being studied by endocrinologists and biochemists (47,51).

Although not produced by resting T cells, production of IL-2 is rapidly and potently induced after antigen encounter

TABLE 3. *Features of cytokines whose receptors share γ_C*

Cytokine	Major source	Size[a]	Actions	Chromosomal location (human/mouse)	Genomic organization
IL-2	Activated T cells (preferentially from Th1 cells)	Human: 153 aa/20 aa Mouse: 169 aa/20 aa 15.5 kD	T cell growth factor B-cell growth, Ig production, J chain expression Induces LAK activity Induces tumor infiltrating lymphocyte activity Augments NK activity Critical role in antigen-induced cell death (AICD) Stimulates macrophage/monocytes Antitumor effects	4q26–27/3	4 exons
IL-4	Activated T cells (Th2 cells) CD4+NK1.1+ natural T cells	Human: 153 aa/24 aa Mouse: 140 aa/20 aa 18 kD	B-cell proliferation Ig class switch: IgG1, IgE production Augments MHC II, Fcε receptors, IL-4Rα and IL-2Rβ expression Th2 cell differentiation Antitumor effects	5q31.1/11	4 exons
IL-7	Stromal cells	Human: 177 aa/25 aa Mouse: 154 aa/25 aa 17–25 kD	Thymocyte growth T-cell growth Pre–B cell growth in mice but not humans Survival and growth of peripheral T cells	8q12–13/3	6 exons
IL-9	Activated helper T cells	Human: 144 aa/18 aa Mouse: 144 aa/18 aa 14 kD	T helper clones Erythroid progenitors B cells Mast cells Fetal thymocytes	5q31–35/13	5 exons
IL-15	Monocytes and many cells outside the immune system[b]	Human: 162 aa/48 aa Mouse: 162 aa/48 aa 14–15 kD	Mast cell growth NK cell development and activity T-cell proliferation, memory T-cell homeostasis	4q31/8	9 exons
IL-21	Activated CD4+ T cells	Human: 162 aa/31 aa Mouse: 146 aa/24 aa ~15kD	Comitogen for T-cell proliferation Inhibits B-cell proliferation to anti-IgM and IL-4 Augments B-cell proliferation to anti-CD40 Conflicting reports related to NK cells	4q26–27	5 exons

Fcε, crystallized ε fragment; Ig, immunoglobulin; IL, interleukin; LAK, lymphocyte-activated killer; MHC, major histocompatibiity complex; NK, natural killer; Th2, T helper cell 2.

[a]The number of amino acids (aa) refers to the length of the open reading frame/length of signal peptide. The number of amino acids in the mature protein is therefore the difference between these numbers. Note that for IL-15, residues 1–29 have been identified as a signal peptide and 30–48 as a propeptide.

[b]More IL-15 mRNA is produced in skeletal muscle, kidney, placenta, and lung than in thymus or spleen. It is important to note, however, that IL-15 mRNA is widely expressed without concomitant production of IL-15 protein so that the source of biologically meaningful IL-15 may be more limited.

with resting T cells. As a result, transcription and synthesis of IL-2 are often used as key indicators of successful T-cell receptor activation. Although the antigen determines the specificity of the T-cell immune response, the interaction of IL-2 with high-affinity IL-2 receptors helps regulate the magnitude and duration of the response, on the basis of the amount of IL-2 produced, the levels of high affinity receptors expressed, and the duration of IL-2 production and receptor expression. IL-2 can act in either an autocrine or paracrine manner, depending on whether the producing cell is also the responding cell or whether the responding cell is a nonproducing cell. IL-2, as noted previously, is also important for the process of AICD (46). The gene encoding IL-2 is located on chromosome 4 (52), and, like many other helical cytokines, its gene consists of four exons (7).

IL-2 binds to three classes of receptors. These are formed by different combinations of three chains: IL-2Rα (49,50,53), IL-2Rβ (54–57), and a protein initially called IL-2Rγ (29) but now known as the common cytokine receptor γ chain, γ_c (31,39). The different classes of IL-2 receptors are discussed later.

Like IL-2, IL-4 is produced primarily by activated CD4$^+$ T cells (58,59). IL-4 is also produced by CD4$^+$NK1.1$^+$ "natural" T cells (60), and by mast cells and basophils [reviewed by Nelms et al. (59)]. IL-4 is the major B-cell growth factor and is vital for immunoglobulin class switch, enhancing the production and secretion of immunoglobulins (Ig) G1 and E (59). IL-4 induces expression of class II major histocompatibility complex molecules on B cells and increases cell surface expression of crystallized fragment ϵ receptor I (FcϵRI) (the receptor for IgE) on B cells. In addition to its actions on B cells, IL-4 can also act as a T-cell growth factor, inducing proliferation in both human and murine T cells, and the differentiation of T helper 2 (Th2) cells (discussed later). When combined with phorbol myristate acetate (PMA), IL-4 is also a potent comitogen for thymocytes. Of importance is that IL-4 can inhibit certain responses of cells to IL-2 [reviewed by Paul (61)]. Moreover, IL-4 can exert actions on macrophages, hematopoietic precursor cells, stromal cells, and fibroblasts (58). Human IL-4 is 129 amino acids long, and its gene is located on human chromosome 5 (5q31.1–31.2) and mouse chromosome 11 (58,62), in the same region as IL-3, IL-5, IL-13, and GM-CSF. Its receptor on T cells and other hematopoietic cells consists of the 140-kDa IL-4Rα protein (59,63–65) and γ_c (30,32). This form of receptor is known as the type I IL-4 receptor. Expression of IL-4Rα tends to be quite low, and cells that potently respond to IL-4 often express only a few hundred receptors per cell. As discussed later, in addition to the type I IL-4 receptor, an alternative form of the receptor, containing IL-4Rα and IL-13Rα (now denoted IL-13Rα1), although not expressed on T cells, is expressed on a number of other cell types and can transduce IL-4 signals into these cells.

IL-7 is not a lymphokine (i.e., it is not produced by lymphocytes) but instead is produced by stromal cells (66,67).

Its major role is to enhance thymocyte growth, survival, and differentiation (68–72), as well as low-affinity peptide-induced proliferation and thus homeostatic proliferation of naïve and CD8$^+$ memory T cells (72–74). IL-7 has some activity for the growth of mature T cells (72,75,76). It also is vital for the growth of murine pre–B cells (66,70,71,76), but from studies of humans with defective IL-7 signaling [patients with X-linked severe combined immunodeficiency disease (SCID), Janus kinase 3 (Jak3)–deficient SCID, and IL-7Rα-deficient SCID; see later discussion], it is now clear that human B cells can develop in the absence of IL-7 responsiveness. This demonstrates that in humans, IL-7 is not as vital for the growth of human pre–B cells as for that of thymocytes (39,77). IL-7 is 152 amino acids long (67), and its gene is located on human chromosome 8q12–13 (78) and on murine chromosome 3. The functional IL-7 receptor contains the 75-kDa IL-7Rα (79) and γ_c (31,33). According to chemical cross-linking experiments and Scatchard analyses, there is a suggestion, however, that the receptor may contain a third component as well (31), although such a protein has not yet been identified.

IL-9 was originally described as a murine T-cell growth factor (80). Human and murine forms of IL-9 are 126 amino acids long (80,81). IL-9 is produced by activated T cells and supports the growth of T helper clones but not cytolytic clones (82). In contrast to IL-2, its production is much more delayed, which suggests its involvement in later, perhaps secondary signals. In the mouse, IL-9 has also been reported to exert effects on erythroid progenitors, B cells (including B1 cells), mast cells, and fetal thymocytes. With regard to mast cells, IL-9 has been shown to be identical to mast cell growth–enhancing activity, a factor present in conditioned medium derived from splenocytes (83). IL-9 can also synergize with IL-3 for maximal proliferation of these cells. The action of IL-9 on thymocytes *in vitro* is interesting in view of the development of thymomas in IL-9 transgenic mice, coupled to the observation that IL-9 is a major antiapoptotic factor for thymic lymphomas (84). Nevertheless, IL-9 knockout mice do not have a defect in T-cell development (85). Instead, they exhibit a defect in pulmonary goblet cell hyperplasia and mastocytosis after challenge with *Schistosoma mansoni* eggs, a synchronous pulmonary granuloma formation model; however, there was no defect in eosinophilia or granuloma formation (85). Interestingly, mice in which transgenic IL-9 is expressed in the lung exhibit airway inflammation and bronchial hyperresponsiveness; nevertheless, in the IL-9$^{-/-}$ mice, there was normal eosinophilia and airway hyperreactivity in an ovalbumin-mediated allergen (ovalbumin)–induced inflammatory model (86–88). Thus, although IL-9 clearly can contribute to allergic/pulmonary responses, it appears that there are compensatory cytokines that substitute for IL-9 in at least certain settings. Whereas murine IL-9 is active on human cells, human IL-9 is not biologically active on murine cells (the situation opposite that for IL-2). Human IL-9 is located on chromosome 5 in the 5q31–35 region (89), which is also the location for the genes encoding IL-3, IL-4, IL-5, IL-13, and GM-CSF. In contrast, murine IL-9 is "isolated" on chromosome 13, whereas IL-3, IL-4, IL-5, IL-13, and GM-CSF are clustered on chromosome 11. IL-9 binds to the 64-kDa IL-9Rα–binding protein, which is similar in size to γ_c (90), and the functional IL-9 receptor, which binds IL-9 with a dissociation constant (K_d) of 100 pM, consists of IL-9Rα plus γ_c (34,35).

IL-15 was identified as a novel T-cell growth factor that was also unexpectedly expressed in the supernatants of a human T-lymphocyte virus type I (HTLV-I)–transformed T-cell line (91,92). Although IL-15 messenger ribonucleic acid (mRNA) is produced by a range of nonlymphocytic cell types, it is quite difficult to detect IL-15 protein production (93). IL-15 is located at human chromosome 4q31 and at murine chromosome 8. Thus, a clear understanding of the cellular sources of actual production is important and still requires further investigation. IL-15 receptors are widely expressed, but IL-15 appears to be most important for NK cell development (94–96) and the development of CD8 memory T-cell development (95,96). Interestingly, the receptor for IL-15 on T cells contains IL-2Rβ (36,93,97), γ_c (36), and one unique protein, IL-15Rα. IL-15Rα shares a number of structural similarities with IL-2Rα, including the presence of so-called sushi domains (98), and the *IL2RA* and *IL15RA* genes are closely positioned on human chromosome 10p14 (99). An alternative form of receptor for IL-15, denoted IL-15RX has been detected on mast cells (100), with apparently distinctive signaling features, but cDNAs have not been identified. If more than one type of IL-15 receptor does exist, then it is possible that distinct types of IL-15 signals may be induced in distinct cell lineages. In contrast to IL-2, which is both a growth factor and a mediator of AICD, the role of IL-15 appears to be more focused on growth (101).

IL-21 is the most recently identified member of the IL-2 family of cytokines. The IL-21 binding protein (IL-21R) was identified as an open reading frame as part of a genomic DNA sequencing project (21) and independently as a novel expressed sequence tag (102). IL-21 was then cloned by an expression approach, on the basis of its ability to bind IL-21R (102). At least *in vitro*, IL-21 can bind to and has been reported to have effects on T, B, and NK cells. It augments T-cell proliferation as a comitogen (102), augments B-cell proliferation when combined with anti-CD40, and inhibits proliferation in response to anti-IgM plus IL-4 (102). On NK cells, it has been reported to cooperate with IL-15 and Flt-3 ligand to increase development (102) but oppose the actions of IL-15 (103). A clear understanding of the biological role for this cytokine is still emerging. The receptor for IL-21 consists of IL-21R plus γ_c (37) [reviewed by Leonard (39)]. IL-21R is most related to IL-2Rβ, and, like IL-2Rβ, its expression is induced after cellular stimulation with anti-CD3 or phytohemagglutinin; in addition, its expression is augmented in T cells after transformation with HTLV-I (21). Both human and murine IL-21 can act on cells of one another's species,

although a rigorous comparison of the relative potency on cells of the homologous versus heterologous species has not been reported. IL-21 is on chromosome 4q26–27, whereas its receptor is on chromosome 16p11.

Thus, IL-2, IL-4, IL-7, IL-9, IL-15, and IL-21 collectively exhibit overlapping roles related to T cells, NK cells, B cells, and mast cells and together are expected to play vital roles for normal development or function, or both, of these cellular lineages. The fact that these six cytokines share γ_c is therefore of particular interest, and a historical review of the basis for the discovery that IL-2, IL-4, IL-7, IL-9, IL-15, and IL-21 share a common chain is instructive.

X-Linked Severe Combined Immunodeficiency Disease Results from Mutations in γ_c

The γ chain was originally identified as a third component of the IL-2 receptor (29), after it became clear that IL-2 receptor α and β chains alone were not sufficient to transduce an IL-2 signal. The hypothesis that the γ chain was a shared component of receptors in addition to the IL-2 receptor was motivated from a comparison of the clinical phenotypes in humans that result from defective expression of IL-2 versus γ_c. In 1993, it was reported that the γ chain was located on the X chromosome and that it was the gene that was mutated in X-linked severe combined immunodeficiency (XSCID; the disease is formally designated as SCIDX1) (104) (see also Chapter 49). XSCID is characterized by profoundly diminished numbers of T cells and NK cells (38,39,105–107) (Table 4). Although the B cells are normal in number, they are nonfunctional, apparently because of a lack of T-cell help as well as an intrinsic B-cell defect that is not typically corrected solely by the addition of T cells (38,107,108). In contrast to the profound decrease in the number of T cells in patients with XSCID, IL-2–deficient humans (109,110) and mice (111) were found to have normal numbers of T cells [the phenotypes of mice deficient in type I and type II cytokines, their receptor, Janus kinases (Jaks), and signal transducer and activator of transcription (STAT) proteins are summarized later in Table 14]. This observation seemed to greatly minimize

TABLE 4. *Features of XSCID*

1. Absence or profoundly diminished numbers of T cells and mitogen responses
2. Absence of NK cells
3. Normal numbers of B cells but defective B cell responses
4. IgM can be normal, but immunoglobulins of other classes are greatly diminished
5. Female XSCID carriers exhibit nonrandom X-inactivation patterns in their T cells and NK cells; the X-inactivation pattern is random in surface IgM–positive B cells but nonrandom in more terminally differentiated B cells

IgM, immunoglobulin M; NK, natural killer; XSCID, X-linked severe combined immunodeficiency disease.

the possibility that a component of the IL-2 receptor would be defective in XSCID; therefore, the finding that the γ chain was mutated in XSCID was all the more unexpected. Thus, the conundrum was why a defect in a component of a receptor would be more severe than a defect in the corresponding cytokine. This led to the hypothesis that the γ chain was part of other immunologically important cytokine receptors as well (104). In this model, the defects in XSCID would be explained by the combination of defects resulting from simultaneous inactivation of multiple signaling pathways, rather than from a selective defect in IL-2 signaling (38,104). The initial two cytokines for which it was hypothesized that the γ chain might play a role were IL-4 and IL-7. The reasons for this were as follows [reviewed by Leonard (38)]: (a) IL-7 was known to be the major thymocyte growth factor, so that defective IL-7 signaling could potentially explain the basis for defective T-cell development. (b) Defective IL-4 and IL-7 signaling might explain the defects in B-cell function in XSCID. In XSCID, B-cell function was often known not to improve after successful bone marrow transplantation with T-cell engraftment, which suggested that there may be an intrinsic B-cell defect that persisted even when T-cell help was provided. Moreover, the γ chain appeared to be required for terminal B-cell differentiation, according to random X chromosome inactivation patterns in immature surface IgM$^+$ B cells from XSCID female carriers but nonrandom X-inactivation patterns in their more mature surface IgM B cells (i.e., only those B cells containing the active X chromosome with wild-type γ_c could mature) [reviewed by Noguchi et al. (104)]. Because both IL-4 and IL-7 were known to be important for B-cell function, defective IL-4 and IL-7 signaling could help explain these defects. (c) At the time of the studies, only a single chain had been identified for both the IL-4 and IL-7 receptors; therefore, it was reasonable that a second type I cytokine receptor chain might form part of their receptors. (d) Like IL-2, both IL-4 and IL-7 could exert actions as T-cell growth factors; thus, it was possible that the sharing of a common chain might partially account for shared actions. (e) In at least some situations, IL-2 and IL-4 were known to have opposing actions. If IL-2 and IL-4 competed for the recruitment of a shared receptor component present in limited amounts, this could help to explain how they might have opposing actions (discussed later). A series of experiments, including chemical cross-linking, Scatchard analyses on cells reconstituted with IL-4Rα with or without γ_c or with IL-7Rα with or without γ_c, and functional analyses, led to the establishment that the γ chain was also an essential functional component of both the IL-4 and IL-7 receptors on T cells (30–33). In view of its multifactorial role, the γ chain was renamed as the common cytokine receptor γ chain, γ_c (31,32). IL-9, another T-cell growth factor, was subsequently shown to also use γ_c, whereas the receptor on T cells for IL-15, a cytokine quite similar to IL-2, shares both IL-2Rβ and γ_c [reviewed by Leonard (39)] and differs only in that it has a different α chain. IL-15 appears even more dependent on IL-15Rα than is IL-2 on IL-2Rα for binding, inasmuch as

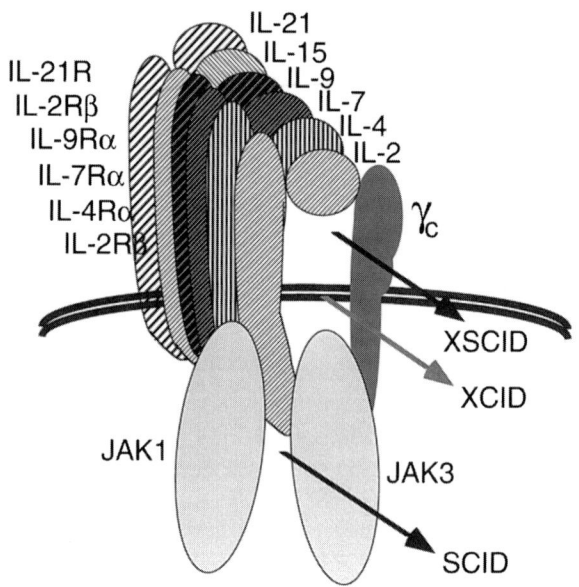

FIG. 3. Schematic of the receptors for interleukin (IL)–2, IL-4, IL-7, IL-9, IL-15, and IL-21, showing interactions with Janus kinases 1 and 3 (Jak1 and Jak3). The illustration shows that IL-2, IL-4, IL-7, IL-9, IL-15, and IL-21 all share γ_c. IL-2Rα and IL-15Rα are not shown. Whereas the distinctive chains associate with Jak1, γ_c associates with Jak3. Mutations in γ_c cause X-linked severe combined immunodeficiency disease or more moderate forms of X-linked immunodeficiency. Mutations in Jak3 cause an autosomal recessive form of severe combined immunodeficiency disease (see text).

the IL-15/IL-2Rβ/γ_c complex appears to be less stable than the IL-2/IL-2Rβ/γ_c complex (112). Most recently, IL-21 was also shown to share γ_c, so that at least six cytokines share γ_c (39) (Fig. 3).

In view of the sharing of γ_c by six different cytokine receptors, XSCID is clearly a disease of defective cytokine signaling, and it is reasonable to try to explain the major deficiencies in XSCID in terms of the disrupted signaling pathways. T-cell development is dramatically diminished not only in IL-7–deficient (71) and IL-7Rα–deficient mice (70) but also in *IL7R*-deficient humans with T$^-$B$^+$NK$^+$ SCID (113,114); however, T-cell development is normal in mice deficient in IL-2 (111), IL-4 (115,116), in both IL-2 and IL-4 (117), in IL-9 (85), in IL-15 (96), or in IL-15Rα (95). On the basis of these observations, it seems likely that most if not all of the defect in T-cell development in patients with XSCID results from defective IL-7 signaling [reviewed by Leonard (39)]. It is nevertheless possible that other γ_c-dependent cytokines might contribute, in view of, for example, the responsiveness of thymocytes to IL-9 and the fact that IL-15 is a T-cell growth factor and important for the development of CD8$^+$ memory T cells. As noted previously, IL-21 receptors are expressed on T cells, B cells, and NK cells and thus theoretically may contribute to T-cell or NK-cell development as well. Additional work is necessary to determine whether this is the case.

In addition to profoundly diminished numbers of T-cells, humans with XSCID lack NK cells. As discussed previously, NK-cell development is defective in IL-15– and IL-15Rα– deficient mice, which indicates that defective IL-15 signaling is responsible for the defective NK cell development in XS-CID [reviewed by Leonard (39)].

In contrast to the greatly diminished number of T cells and absence of NK cells in XSCID patients, the B-cell numbers are normal. This is in marked contrast to the greatly diminished numbers of B cells in γ_c-deficient mice (118,119) and in mice deficient in either IL-7 or IL-7Rα, and it strongly suggests that IL-7 is not required for pre–B cell development in humans. Indeed, as noted previously, *IL7R*-deficient SCID patients have a $T^-B^+NK^+$ form of SCID (114). Although B cells develop, they are nonfunctional. This results in part from a lack of T-cell help (in view of the near absence of T cells in XSCID), but various data have suggested an intrinsic B-cell defect as well (39). Indeed, defective γ_c-dependent signaling (and, in particular, defective signaling by cytokines that act on B cells, such as IL-4 and IL-21) may explain the intrinsic B-cell defect in XSCID (119a), and these cytokines may be required for the transition from random to nonrandom X chromosome inactivation patterns in surface IgM$^+$ versus IgM$^-$ B cells from XSCID female carriers.

Rationale for the Sharing of γ_c

Why should there have been evolutionary pressure to maintain the sharing of γ_c, in view of the obvious increased risk that sharing a receptor component has when mutations arise? There are at least two types of models (38,120). First, because IL-2, IL-4, IL-7, IL-9, IL-15, and IL-21 can each act as T-cell growth factors, at least *in vitro,* it is possible that γ_c might couple to one or more signal-transducing molecules that would promote this function. The second type of model, which is diametrically different, suggests that the sharing of γ_c is a means by which each cytokine can modulate the signals of the other cytokines whose receptors contain γ_c. To understand this model, it is important to emphasize that cytokine receptors individually are targeted to the cell surface and that the formation or stability of different receptor complexes is dependent on the ligand. This was suggested previously in the discussion of the growth hormone receptor, wherein the second receptor monomer recognizes the combined surface of growth hormone and the first growth hormone receptor monomer (23). Moreover, there are direct data for the IL-2 receptor, in which γ_c was originally detected as a receptor component that could be coprecipitated with IL-2Rβ in the presence but not in the absence of IL-2 (121), and dimerization of IL-2Rβ and γ_c is known to be required for efficient signaling (122,123). Thus, receptor heterodimerization at a minimum is stabilized by the cytokine and physiologically may be absolutely dependent on the presence of the cytokine. However, BIAcore optical biosensor experiments have indicated that, under the proper experimental conditions, dimers between IL-2Rα and IL-2Rβ (only the

latter of which is a type I cytokine receptor) can form in the absence of IL-2 (124,125). In the absence of stable preformed cytokine receptor complexes between γ_c and the other receptor chains, γ_c might differentially associate with the different γ_c-dependent cytokine receptors, depending on which cytokine was present. This model allows for the possibility that γ_c is differentially recruited to different receptors according to the relative amount of a cytokine or its relative binding efficiency. In a situation in which γ_c is limiting, a cytokine then not only might induce its own action but also could simultaneously inhibit the action of another cytokine that was less efficient at recruiting γ_c to its cognate receptor complex.

An analysis of mice deficient in IL-2 (111), IL-2Rα (126), IL-2Rβ (127), and γ_c (118,119) provides the rather interesting observation that, although the mice lacking γ_c have defective signaling in six different cytokine pathways, mice deficient in IL-2, IL-2Rα, and IL-2Rβ appear to be less healthy than the γ_c-knockout mice when maintained under specific pathogen-free conditions, although a direct comparison of all of the mice with the same genetic background in the same animal facility has not yet been performed. Although all of the mice have activated T cells, the development of autoimmunity is apparently less severe in γ_c-deficient mice. This suggests that the signals induced by IL-2 may normally be counterbalanced by signals from other γ_c-dependent cytokines and that when γ_c itself is mutated or deleted, there is something of a normalization of the balance of signals. These and other data suggest that γ_c plays a major role in regulating lymphoid homeostasis (128).

Cytokine Receptors that Share the Common β Chain, β_c (IL-3, IL-5, GM-CSF)

The hematopoietic cytokines, IL-3, IL-5, and GM-CSF (Table 5) are all synthesized by T cells and exert effects on cells of hematopoietic lineage (129–131). These cytokines are vital for proliferation as well as differentiation of myeloid precursor cells. Of these three cytokines, IL-3 is the most pluripotent (130) and historically was also called multi–colony-stimulating factor (multi-CSF), which reflects the large number of lineages on which it can act. It can act to promote proliferation, survival, and development of multipotent hematopoietic progenitor cells and of cells that have become dedicated to a range of different lineages, including granulocyte, macrophage, eosinophil, mast cell, megakaryocyte, and erythroid lineages. IL-3 also can exert end-function effects, such as enhancing phagocytosis and cytotoxicity. GM-CSF is mainly restricted to the granulocyte and monocyte/macrophage lineages, but its actions are nevertheless quite broad (129). It is both a growth and survival factor. In addition, it can expand the number of antigen-presenting cells, such as dendritic cells, and thereby may greatly expand the ability of the host to respond to antigen. Whereas IL-3 and GM-CSF can act on eosinophils, they act at much earlier stages than does IL-5, presumably expanding the number of eosinophil-committed precursor cells. IL-5 stimulates

TABLE 5. *Features of cytokines whose receptors share β_C*

Cytokine	Major source	Size[a]	Cellular targets	Chromosomal location (human/mouse)	Genomic organization
IL-3	T cells	Human: 152/19 aa Mouse: 166/26 aa 22–34 kD	Multiple lineages	5q31.1/11	5 exons
IL-5	T cells	Human: 139/22 aa Mouse: 133/21 aa 45 kD dimer	Eosinophils B cells (?)	5q31.1/11	4 exons
GM-CSF	T cells	Human: 144/17 aa Mouse: 141/17 aa 23 kD	Granulocytes Macrophages	5q31.1/11	4 exons

GM-CSF, granulocyte-macrophage colony-stimulating factor; IL, interleukin.
[a]The number of amino acids (aa) refers to the length of the open reading frame/length of signal peptide.

the eosinophilic lineage and eosinophil release from the bone marrow, is essential for expanding eosinophils after helminth infections (132,133), and can mediate the killing of *S. mansoni*. IL-5 can also induce immunoglobulin production in B cells activated by contact with activated T helper cells in murine systems, and IL-5 and IL-5Rα knockout mice have diminished numbers of CD5+ B1 cells and thymocytes until approximately 6 weeks of age (132,133).

On cells that express receptors for more than one of these cytokines, such as eosinophilic progenitors that express receptors for IL-3, IL-5, and GM-CSF, or on murine pre–B cells, which express receptors for IL-3 and IL-5, the signals induced are indistinguishable (130,131). Thus, we can conclude that the differential lineage specificities of these cytokines are determined by the cellular distribution of their receptors rather than by fundamental differences in the signals that are induced by each cytokine. These observations are explained by studies demonstrating that each of these three cytokines has its own unique 60- to 80-kDa α chain (i.e., IL-3Rα, IL-5Rα, and GM-CSFRα) (134–139) but that they share a common 120- to 130-kDa β chain, β_c (140,141) [reviewed by Geijsen et al. (131) and Miyajima et al. (142)]. The α chains are the principal binding proteins for the cytokines, whereas the shared β_c subunit can augment binding affinity but does not exhibit binding activity in the absence of the proper α chain. The α chains have relatively short cytoplasmic domains (approximately 55 amino acids each for IL-3Rα, IL-5Rα, and GM-CSFRα) and are not believed to play major roles in signaling function, whereas β_c, with its cytoplasmic domain of 432 amino acids, is the primary determinant of the signal. As a result, there is a relative compartmentalization of binding and signaling function for these cytokines, although the cytoplasmic domains of the GM-CSFRα and IL-5Rα chains (and by analogy, perhaps the IL-3Rα chains) as well as that of β_c appear to be capable of at least modulating the growth signals in transfected cells (131,143–145). In any case, the sharing of β_c helps explain why the signals induced by IL-3, IL-5, and GM-CSF are similar on cells that can respond to more than one of these cytokines. The situation for the β_c family of cytokines is therefore quite different from that of the receptors for IL-2, IL-4, IL-7,

IL-9, IL-15, and IL-21 wherein the chains with the largest cytoplasmic domains (IL-2Rβ, IL-4Rα, IL-7Rα, IL-9Rα, and IL-21R) not only contribute most to signaling specificity but also are the proteins principally involved in binding the ligands. (Note that in the case of IL-2 and IL-15, the IL-2Rα and IL-15Rα chains importantly cooperate with IL-2Rβ for this function.) The shared chain, γ_c, serves a vital accessory function that, when disrupted, causes XSCID, but it plays little role in cytokine binding and does not provide an obvious basis for signaling specificity (see later discussion).

One of the surprising features of the hematopoietic cytokines is that, despite their potent *in vitro* effects as well as some *in vivo* effects, there appears to be considerable redundancy of function, so that knockout mice that lack the ability to respond to GM-CSF, IL-3, and IL-5 (mice that lack β_c as well as a murine IL-3–specific β_c–like protein, discussed later) exhibit relatively normal hematopoiesis. These observations do not minimize the potency of these particular cytokines; instead, they underscore a substantial redundancy for a particularly important set of functions (130,131,146). It is noteworthy that β_c-deficient mice exhibit defective host responses to infectious challenge, which suggests that these hematopoietic cytokines play a vital role in promoting immune function.

Cytokine Receptors that Share gp130 (IL-6, IL-11, Oncostatin M, Ciliary Neurotropic Factor, Leukemia Inhibitory Factor, Cardiotrophin-1, and NNT/BSF-3)

Seven cytokines are now known to utilize gp130 as a signal-transducing molecule (17,147–155). Some of the properties of these cytokines are summarized in Table 6. This family is sometimes referred to as the IL-6 family of cytokines and includes IL-6, IL-11, OSM, LIF, CNTF, CT-1, and NNT/BSF-3. This group of cytokines comprises molecules with a diverse range of actions, ranging beyond the hematopoietic and immune systems to also include the central nervous system and cardiovascular systems, and thus they are even more "multifunctional" than the γ_c and β_c families of

TABLE 6. *Cytokines whose receptors share gp130*

Cytokine	Chromosomal location (human/mouse)
IL-6	7p21/5
IL-11	19q13.3–13.4/7
LIF	22q12.1–12.2/11
OSM	22q12.1–12.2/11
CNTF	11q12.2/19
CT-1	16p11.1–11.2/7
NNT-1/BSF-3	11q13/?

Overlapping actions of several gp130 cytokines	IL-6	IL-11	LIF	OSM	CNTF	CT-1
Growth of myeloma cells	+	−	+	+	+	?
Maintenance of embryonic stem cell pluripotency	−	−	+	+	+	+
Induction of hepatic acute phase proteins	+	+	+	+	+	+
Induction of cardiac hypertrophy	−	+	+	+	+/−	+
Induction of osteoclast formation	−	+	+	+	?	?
Enhanced neuronal survival/differentiaion	+	+	+	+	+	+
Inhibit adipogenesis	?	+	+	?	?	?

Most of the data in the lower part of table are derived from reference 152.

Note that NNT-1 can support survival of chicken embryonic and sympathetic neurons, can induce amyloid A, and, analogous to IL-6, can induce B-cell hyperplasia.

BSF-3, B-lymphocyte–stimulating factor 3; CNTF, ciliary neurotrophic factor; CT-1, cardiotropin-1; gp, glycoprotein; IL, interleukin; LIF, leukemia inhibitory factor; NNT-1, novel neutrophin 1; OSM, oncostatin M.

cytokines, which appear to exert actions largely restricted to the lymphoid and hematopoietic systems.

IL-6 was the first member of this family to be recognized. It was originally identified and then cloned as a B-cell differentiation factor that stimulated terminal differentiation/maturation of B cells into antibody-producing plasma cells (156). However, IL-6 also can exert effects for T-cell growth and differentiation (and thus is a thymocyte "comitogen"); induce myeloid differentiation into macrophages; induce acute-phase protein synthesis of hepatocytes; and exert actions on keratinocytes, mesangial cells, hematopoietic stem cells, the development of osteoclasts, and neural differentiation of PC12 cells [reviewed by Taga and Kishimoto (152)]. IL-6 binds to an 80-kDa IL-6–binding protein, denoted IL-6Rα, which has a comparatively short (82–amino acid–long) cytoplasmic domain (157). This IL-6/IL-6Rα complex then interacts with and recruits the 130-kDa signal-transducing molecule, gp130, which together with IL-6Rα can form a functional IL-6 receptor (152). Gp130 is the molecule that is the common component of the receptors for the family of cytokines being discussed in this section. Of interest from a structural perspective is that gp130 contains a total of six fibronectin type III modules, with the four conserved cysteine residues and the WSXWS motif located in the second and third of these modules, starting from the N-terminal. These regions are topologically positioned a greater distance external to the cell membrane than is the case for the other type I cytokine receptors discussed previously.

Remarkably, the IL-6 system illustrates a novel twist on the properties of their principal binding proteins: The cytoplasmic domain of IL-6Rα is superfluous for signaling; a soluble form of the IL-6Rα extracellular domain is sufficient for ligand binding and coordination with gp130. Thus, in the presence of soluble IL-6Rα and IL-6, many cell types that express gp130 but not IL-6Rα are capable of signaling. It was observed that IL-6 signaling requires the dimerization of gp130 (158,159). In fact, subsequent data revealed that IL-6 signals through a complex containing two molecules each of IL-6, IL-6Rα, and gp130 (a dimer of a trimer) (160), providing a possible paradigm for the stoichiometry of subunits for other members of the IL-6 family of cytokines.

IL-11 was originally identified as a factor produced by a stromal cell line in response to stimulation with IL-1 [reviewed by Du and Williams (161) and Goldman (162)]. It was noted to exert a number of effects on hematopoiesis, particularly in combination with IL-3 and SCF. Because IL-11 exhibited "IL-6–like activities," a cDNA was isolated on the basis of the presence of IL-6–like activity in the presence of antibodies to IL-6 (163). Other actions of IL-11 include the ability to stimulate the proliferation of lymphoid and hematopoietic progenitor cells, stimulate megakaryocytic progenitors and megakaryocyte maturation, and stimulate erythroid progenitors (an action not shared by IL-6). Like IL-6, IL-11 can induce acute-phase proteins and augment antigen-specific B-cell responses, but it does not stimulate human myeloma cells (161–164). Subsequently, adipogenesis inhibitory factor was cloned and found to be identical to IL-11 (165); this finding revealed another action of IL-11. IL-11 is also produced in the lung eosinophils and various structural cells in the lung and is expressed in patients with modest to severe asthma (166). IL-11 signals through a receptor complex containing both IL-11Rα and gp130 (17). Interestingly, IL-11Rα mRNA can be alternatively spliced to yield a form lacking the cytoplasmic domain, and, like IL-6Rα, a soluble form of IL-11Rα can coordinate with IL-11 to signal in cells expressing gp130 (167). Studies on the stoichiometry of the IL-11 receptor complex failed to reveal dimerization of gp130 to itself or LIFRβ. Thus, assuming that it forms a hexameric receptor complex, only five of the members—two molecules of IL-11 and IL-11Rα and one of gp130—are known, which suggests that another component may still be found (168). IL-11 is located at human chromosome 19q13.3—13.4 and murine chromosome 7.

LIF is another multifunctional cytokine originally cloned on the basis of the activity associated with its name (169). LIF can suppress the differentiation of pluripotent embryonic stem cells, inhibit adipogenesis, and induce monocyte differentiation of the M1 murine leukemia cell line, thus mimicking a number of the actions of IL-6 [reviewed by Hilton and Gough (170)]. In addition, it exerts a number of actions in the central nervous system and was shown to be identical to cholinergic neural differentiation factor (171), which can induce acetylcholine synthesis while simultaneously suppressing catecholamine production, thereby inducing cholinergic function while suppressing noradrenergic function (171). LIF has been shown to be essential for embryo implantations (172). LIF binds to a receptor (LIFRβ) that is structurally related to gp130 (173), but the functional LIF receptor requires the heterodimerization of LIFRβ and gp130 as well (148).

CNTF was discovered on the basis of its ability to promote neuronal survival (174,175). CNTF signals through a receptor comprising LIFRβ and gp130 but additionally requires a specific binding protein (176,177), now denoted CNTFRα. Interestingly, the CNTFRα chain lacks transmembrane and cytoplasmic domains and instead is a GPI-linked receptor molecule. CNTFRα appears to provide a receptor-cytokine surface with which gp130 and LIFRβ can interact. Thus, CNTF is like IL-6 in that each requires initial binding to a receptor component (CNTFRα or IL-6Rα) that does not require its own cytoplasmic domain for signaling. Whereas IL-6 signaling involves homodimerization of gp130, CNTF signaling involves the heterodimerization of LIFRβ and gp130. In fact, the functional CNTF receptor appears to be a hexameric structure containing two molecules of CNTF, two of CNTFRα, and one each of gp130 and LIFRβ (178). The receptor is expressed largely within the nervous system and in skeletal muscle, accounting for largely restricted actions of CNTF (176).

OSM was originally identified on the basis of its ability to inhibit the growth of A375 human melanoma cells (179), and cloning confirmed its actions as a growth regulator (180). OSM is a potent growth factor for Kaposi's sarcoma in patients with acquired immunodeficiency syndrome (AIDS) (181,182). OSM can bind directly to gp130 and signals through a receptor combination of gp130 and LIFRβ (148), but it also has an alternative receptor comprising a specific OSM receptor subunit (OSMRβ) and gp130 (20). These are now known as the type I and type II OSM receptors, respectively. OSM is known to enhance the development of both endothelial cells and hematopoietic cells, possibly by

increasing hemangioblasts, a common precursor for endothelial and hematopoietic cells (153).

(CT-1 was initially isolated on the basis of its actions on cardiac muscle cells (183). However, it is now clear that it is a multifunctional cytokine with hematopoietic, neuronal, and developmental effects, in addition to its effects on cardiac development and hypertrophy (184,185). The basis for these multifunctional actions became clear when it was found that, like OSM and LIF, CT-1 can also signal through a heterodimer of LIFRβ and gp130 (151). Interestingly, the CT-1 receptor on motor neurons may involve a third receptor component, possibly GPI-linked (186,187).

NNT-1/BSF-3, like CNTF, can also support the survival of chicken embryonic sympathetic and motor neurons (155). Interestingly, in mice, NNT-1/BSF-3 can augment the effects of IL-1 and IL-6 and is a B-cell stimulating factor. The NNT-1 receptor contains LIFRβ and gp130 (155). NNT-1 is also known as cardiotrophin-like cytokine (CLC) and forms a complex with a soluble receptor protein known as cytokine-like factor 1 (CLF-1). Together, this complex is a second ligand for CNTFR (188).

Thus, seven cytokines (IL-6, IL-11, LIF, CNTF, OSM, CT-1, NNT-1/BSF-3) all have receptors that are dependent on gp130 [reviewed by Ozaki and Leonard (189)]. These can be divided into two sets of cytokines: those known not to require LIFRβ (namely, IL-6 and IL-11) and those that use both gp130 and LIFRβ (LIF, CT-1, OSM, CNTF, and NNT-1/BSF-3) (Table 7). As noted previously, OSM has two forms of receptors, each of which contains gp130 but only one of which contains LIFRβ. When cytokines share essentially the same receptor, two cytokines might exert identical

TABLE 7. *Composition of receptors for the interleukin-6 family of cytokines*

Cytokines whose receptors do not contain LIFRβ	
Cytokine	*Receptor components*
IL-6	IL-6Rα + gp130
IL-11	IL-11Rα + gp130
OSM	OSMRβ + gp130
Cytokines whose receptors contain LIFRβ	
Cytokine	*Receptor components*
LIF	LIFRβ + gp130
OSM	LIFRβ + gp130
CNTF	CNTFRα + LIFRβ + gp130
CT-1	LIFRβ + gp130 + ?CT-1Rα
NNT-1/BSF-3/CLC + CLF-1	CNTFRα + LIFRβ + gp130

Note that there is evidence for CT1Rα, but it has not been cloned. It is conceivable but unproven that OSMRα and LIFRα proteins might also exist. Note that the share of CNTFRα by CNTF and the dimeric NNT-1/BSF-3/CLC–CLF-1 ligand helps to explain why the phenotype in CNTF⁻/⁻ mice is less severe than that found in CNTFRα⁻/⁻ mice.

BSF-3, B-lymphocyte–stimulating factor 3; CLC, cardiotrophin-like cytokine; CLF-1, cytokine-like factor 1; CNTF, ciliary neurotrophic factor; CT-1, cardiotropin-1; IL, interleukin; LIF, leukemia inhibitory factor; NNT-1, novel neurotrophin 1; OSM, oncostatin M.

actions on cells that can respond to both cytokines. It is clear that the presence of IL-6Rα, IL-11Rα, and CNTFRα (either on the cell surface or as a soluble receptor form, discussed later) determines whether a cell can respond to IL-6, IL-11, and CNTF. This raises the interesting question as to whether functional homologs of IL-6Rα, IL-11Rα, and CNTFRα also exist for LIF, OSM, CT-1, and NNT-1/BSF-3. As noted previously, this may well be the case for CT-1. There is added complexity, at least for OSM, in that it can also signal through the OSMRβ/gp130 heterodimer in a manner apparently independent of LIFRβ.

Significance of the Sharing of Receptor Chains

Interestingly, γ_c, β_c, and gp130 all contribute to signaling, but none of these shared cytokine receptor proteins has primary binding activity for any known cytokine. Instead, they each increase binding affinity in the context of the primary binding protein for each cytokine. Consequently, the capacity of a cell to respond to a given cytokine is determined by the unique binding chain, but signaling pathways can be shared.

Other Receptors with Similarities to gp130 (G-CSF Receptor, Obesity Receptor, and IL-12R)

As noted previously, LIFRβ, and OSMRβ bear some similarities to gp130 (20). In addition, the G-CSF receptor, the leptin receptor [also denoted obesity receptor (OB-R)], and the IL-12 receptor resemble gp130. The amino acid identity among these different receptors, compared pairwise, ranges from 18% to 32%; LIFRβ and OSMRβ are the most similar.

Leptin

Leptin is the product of the obesity (*ob*) gene, an adipose tissue–derived signaling factor that plays a role in body weight homeostasis (190,191). The leptin receptor, OB-R, was cloned and found to be most closely related to the gp130 signal transducer, G-CSF receptor, and LIFRβ (192). Interestingly, this receptor is encoded by the "diabetes gene," which is mutated in *db/db* mice (193).

IL-12 and IL-23

IL-12 is produced primarily by phagocytic cells in response to bacterial and intracellular parasites, such as *Toxoplasma gondii*, but it is also produced by other antigen-presenting cells, such as B cells (194). IL-12 potently induces the production of IFN-γ by NK cells and T cells and is also a growth factor for preactivated but not resting NK and T cells. IL-12 was originally discovered as NK cell stimulatory factor (195). IL-12 is a unique inducer of T helper 1 (Th1) cell differentiation (see later discussion). IL-12 can also induce the production of IL-2, IL-3, GM-CSF, IL-9, TNF-α, and M-CSF, although inducing IFN-γ is probably its most im-

portant recognized action (194). As is discussed later in the section on immunodeficiency diseases, IL-12 is essential for the proper clearing of mycobacterial infections.

IL-12 can be thought of as having vital roles in both innate immunity and later immune responses. It is rapidly produced by NK cells and then T cells in response to antigens or foreign pathogens. This rapid response facilitates the activation of first-line defense against infections. In addition, however, IL-12 is also required for the subsequent differentiation of specialized T-cell populations, including the priming of Th1 cells for optimal production of IFN-γ and IL-2 (discussed later). IL-12 also has the ability to act synergistically with hematopoietic growth factors, such as IL-3 and SCF, to support the proliferation and survival of hematopoietic stem cells (194). Structurally, IL-12 is a covalent dimer of 35- and 40-kDa peptides (194); thus, successful production of IL-12 requires that a cell be able to transcribe both the *p35* and *p40* genes (196). Interestingly, whereas *p35* bears sequence similarity to IL-6 and G-CSF, *p40* is homologous to the extracellular domains of IL-6Rα, CNTFRα, and G-CSF receptor and bears some of the features typical of type I receptors, including four conserved cysteines, a conserved tryptophan, and a WSEWAS motif, which has obvious similarity to the typical WSXWS motif [reviewed by Trinchieri (194)]. Moreover, because both IL-12 receptor (IL-12Rβ1 and IL-12Rβ2) chains bear some similarity to gp130 (195–197), *p40* can be considered a functional homolog of the soluble p80 IL-6Rα chain. Thus, for this cytokine, part of the "receptor" has become part of the cytokine. Interestingly, all the cells that produce IL-12 synthesize a much greater amount of *p40* than *p35*, which suggests that the careful control of signaling is at the level of the "primordial" *p35* cytokine part of IL-12. The *p40* gene is on human chromosome 5q31–33, whereas *p35* is on 3p12–13.2 (194).

IL-23 is a more recently recognized cytokine that is similar to IL-12 in that *p40* is part of the cytokine (199). However, rather than representing a *p35–p40* heterodimer, IL-23 is a dimer of a *p40* and *p19,* a more recently recognized gene product. IL-23 signals through a receptor containing IL-12Rβ1 but not IL-12Rβ2 (200). Instead, another receptor chain, denoted IL-23R, is the second component of the IL-23 receptor (201); both IL-12Rβ2 and IL-23R are located on chromosome 1 with 150 kb of each other (201). Both IL-12 and IL-23 activate Jak2 and tyrosine kinase 2 (Tyk2). Although IL-12 and IL-23 can activate STAT1, STAT3, STAT4, and STAT5, STAT4 is clearly the dominant STAT protein activated by IL-12, and the complexes induced by IL-23 are somewhat different (201). Interestingly, in comparison with human IL-23R, murine IL-23R contains a 20–amino acid duplicated region that spans the WQPWS motif.

IL-27

Another IL-6–related cytokine has been reported (202). This cytokine is denoted IL-27 and represents a dimer of the p28 protein and Epstein Barr virus–induced gene 3 (EBI3) that can induce proliferation of naïve CD4$^+$ T cells. IL-27, IL-12, IL-23, and CLC/CLF-1 are four cytokines that represent dimers, including a type I cytokine and a soluble receptor-like protein. IL-27 signals through the WSX-1/ T-cell cytokine receptor (TCCR) (202) (discussed later in the section on diseases of cytokine receptors and related molecules).

Other Examples of Shared Receptor Molecules

IL-7 and Thymic Stromal Lymphopoietin Share IL-7R

In addition to IL-7, a second stromal factor, TSLP, that shares at least some actions with IL-7 (203,204) and whose receptor is a heterodimer of TSLP receptor and IL-7Rα (205,206) has been identified. Interestingly, TSLP receptor is 24% identical to γ_c, and it is thus the cytokine receptor most like γ_c in available databases (205). Human TSLP and murine TSLP share only 43% amino acid identity, and human and murine TSLP receptors share only 39% amino acid identity (22). These percentages are extremely low for human and murine ortholog cytokine receptors; for example, human and murine γ_c are 70% identical (207). In addition to their wide sequence divergence, murine TLSP and human TSLP appear to differ functionally. So far, the known major actions of murine TSLP are as a B-cell differentiation factor that is important for the development of IgM$^+$ immature B-cells from pre–B cells and as a weak thymic comitogen. In contrast, human TSLP appears not to exert effects on these lineages but instead to be important for dendritic cell activation related to Th2 allergic responses, an action not known to be shared by murine TSLP (208) [reviewed by Leonard (209)]. This underscores a basic important principle: that there can be different effects of cytokines in different species. As a result, it is vital to evaluate effects in human systems *in vitro* and, when possible, *in vivo* to confirm the relevance of murine findings to human physiology and pathophysiology.

Two Types of IL-4 Receptors, One of which Also Responds to IL-13

As detailed previously, on T cells, IL-4 acts through a receptor comprising IL-4Rα and γ_c (now known as the type I IL-4 receptor) (30,32). However, it has been demonstrated that IL-4 can also signal through receptors on non–T cells (type II IL-4 receptors) that do not express γ_c (or Jak3, which is the Janus family tyrosine kinase that couples to γ_c; see later discussion) (210). Other studies suggested that IL-13, another T-cell derived cytokine that is very similar to IL-4 in action, could induce signals identical to those of IL-4 on non–T cells that respond to IL-4 but had no effect in T cells, because these cells do not bind IL-13 (211). The shared actions of IL-4 and IL-13 include the abilities to (a) decrease expression of inflammatory cytokines, (b) induce class II major histocompatibility complex expression, (c) induce CD23 expres-

sion and IgE production by B cells, (d) inhibit IL-2–induced proliferation of chronic lymphocytic leukemia cells of B-cell origin, and (e) co-stimulate with anti-CD40 antibodies.

In addition to the shared biological actions on non–T cells, a variety of data indicated that IL-4Rα was a component of both the IL-4 and IL-13 receptors (210–213) but that IL-4Rα could bind only IL-4. Specifically, antibodies to IL-4Rα inhibited both IL-4 and IL-13–induced proliferation, whereas soluble IL-4Rα could inhibit only IL-4–induced proliferation, which is consistent with its serving a major role for binding IL-4 but not IL-13. It was also shown that IL-13 as well as IL-4 could induce phosphorylation of IL-4Rα, which again suggests that it was a component of the IL-13 receptor. It was therefore hypothesized (210) and subsequently confirmed (19,214) that the type II IL-4 receptor consists of IL-4Rα plus IL-13Rα1 and that both IL-4 and IL-13 induce indistinguishable signals on cells expressing these receptors. Interestingly, IL-4 binds primarily to IL-4Rα and IL-13 binds primarily to IL-13Rα1. This situation may be analogous to the situation for LIF, CT-1, and OSM, all of which can act through receptors containing LIFRβ and gp130 but differ in their abilities to directly interact with each of these receptor proteins. An additional IL-13 binding protein that has much higher binding affinity for IL-13 than does IL-13Rα1 was identified (215). This protein, now denoted IL-13Rα2, appears to be nonfunctional in terms of signaling and perhaps functions as a "decoy" receptor.

IL-13 may be vital in the treatment of asthma, inasmuch as blocking IL-13 can inhibit pathophysiological changes of asthma (216,217). The phenotype of IL-13 knockout mice has revealed an important role for IL-13 in Th2 cell development and the ability to expel helminths (218).

An Example of Multiple Affinities of Binding for a Single Cytokine: Three Classes of IL-2 Receptors

Although cytokines typically signal through a single class of high-affinity cell surface receptor, more complex situations can exist. One particularly well-studied system in which there are three distinct classes of receptor is the IL-2 system. The high-affinity IL-2 receptor, which contains IL-2Rα, IL-2Rβ, and γ_c, was discussed previously. The IL-2 system provides the very interesting illustration of a system with three classes of affinities of receptors (Table 8). In addition to the high-affinity receptor ($K_d = 10^{-11}$ M), there are both low-affinity receptors (for IL-2Rα alone, $K_d = 10^{-8}$ M) and intermediate-affinity receptors (for IL-2Rβ plus γ_c, $K_d = 10^{-9}$ M) [reviewed by Lin and Leonard (47,51)]. Low- and high-affinity receptors are expressed on activated lymphocytes, whereas intermediate-affinity receptors are found on resting lymphocytes, particularly on NK cells. Both intermediate- and high-affinity receptors can signal, which thus suggests that IL-2Rβ and γ_c are necessary and sufficient for signaling, in keeping with the theme of dimerization indicated previously. Because the intermediate-affinity

TABLE 8. *Classes of interleukin-2 receptors*

Affinity	K_d	Where expressed	Composition	Functional
Low	10^{-8} M	Activated cells	IL-2Rα	No
Intermediate	10^{-9} M	Resting cells	IL-2Rβ and γ_C	Yes
High	10^{-11} M	Activated cells	IL-2Rα, IL-2Rβ, and γ_C	Yes

IL, interleukin; M, molar; R, receptor.

form is functional, what then is the rationale for having a high-affinity IL-2 receptor that also contains IL-2Rα? This is a particularly relevant question in view of the fact that IL-2Rα has an extremely short cytoplasmic domain that does not appear to play a role in signaling. The importance of IL-2Rα is clearly demonstrated by the severely abnormal phenotype of IL-2Rα-deficient mice, which exhibit autoimmunity, inflammatory bowel disease, and premature death (126), and by the recognition that IL-2Rα mutations can cause an autoimmune syndrome in humans as well (219). One of the clues to the importance of IL-2Rα comes from the kinetics of association of IL-2 with each chain. Although the IL-2Rα appears to lack a direct signaling function, it has a very fast "on" rate for IL-2 binding (220). Thus, the combination of this rapid "on" rate with the slow "off" rate from IL-2Rβ/γ_c dimers results in high-affinity binding that is vital for responding to the very low concentrations of IL-2 that are physiologically present *in vivo*. Moreover, as T cells express approximately 10 times as many low-affinity as high-affinity receptors, IL-2Rα may serve as an efficient means of recruitment and concentration of IL-2 on the cell surface, allowing more efficient formation of IL-2/IL-2Rβ/γ_c signaling complexes.

As mentioned previously, IL-2Rα is not a type I cytokine receptor. In the mid-1980s, it was noted to have homology to the recognition domain of complement factor B (221). However, the IL-15 receptor α chain was subsequently shown to have a similar structure (98); both IL-2Rα and IL-15Rα have sushi domains. The fact that both IL-2 and IL-15 have related α chains is consistent with the close relationship between IL-2 and IL-15 and the fact that the receptors for both IL-2 and IL-15 contain both IL-2Rβ and γ_c.

Of importance is that, as IL-2Rα cannot transduce a signal by itself, the detection of IL-2Rα on the cell surface does not necessarily reflect IL-2 responsiveness. Because IL-2Rα was discovered before IL-2Rβ and γ_c, many early reports in the literature evaluated IL-2 receptor expression based on IL-2Rα expression without studying IL-2Rβ or γ_c. Thus, for example, the presence of IL-2Rα on a subpopulation of double-negative thymocytes is a useful phenotypic marker corresponding to a stage of development, but it does not reflect IL-2 responsiveness. Each of the components of the IL-2 receptor is located on a different chromosome: In humans, IL-2Rα is located on chromosome 10p14–15 (222); IL-2Rβ is located at chromosome 22q (223,224), and γ_c is located at Xq13.1 (104); the murine homologs are located at chromosomes 2, 15, and X, respectively.

Erythropoietin, Thrombopoietin, and Stem Cell Factor

Erythropoietin is vital for erythropoiesis and thrombopoietin for thrombopoiesis. These cytokines each bind to receptors that are homodimers (25,225). Interestingly, erythropoietin signaling may depend in part on the functional cooperation of the erythropoietin receptor and c-kit, the receptor for SCF (226). This latter receptor has intrinsic tyrosine kinase activity and is not a type I cytokine receptor.

CYTOKINE PLEIOTROPY, CYTOKINE REDUNDANCY, CYTOKINE RECEPTOR PLEIOTROPY, AND CYTOKINE RECEPTOR REDUNDANCY

It is well recognized that many cytokines exhibit the phenomena of cytokine "pleiotropy" and "redundancy" (189). Cytokine pleiotropy is the ability of a cytokine to exert many different types of responses, often on different cell types, whereas cytokine redundancy refers to the fact that many different cytokines can induce similar signals. One set of cytokines that exhibit cytokine pleiotropy is the family of cytokines whose receptors contain γ_c. For example, IL-2 can induce T-cell growth, augment B-cell immunoglobulin synthesis, increase the cytolytic activity of lymphokine-activated killer and NK cells, and play an essential role in mediating AICD; IL-4 can induce B-cell growth and immunoglobulin class switch; and IL-7 plays a major role in thymocyte development but also can stimulate mature T cells and, at least in the mouse, can act as a pre–B cell growth factor. The gp130 set of cytokines also exhibit broad actions. For example, IL-6 exerts effects ranging from that of a co-mitogen for thymocyte activation to that of a mediator of the acute-phase response in liver cells. With regard to cytokine redundancy, it has already been highlighted that IL-2, IL-4, IL-7, IL-9, IL-15, and IL-21, whose receptors contain γ_c, can act as T-cell growth factors and that IL-3 has actions that overlap with those of IL-5 and GM-CSF.

The recognition that cytokines not only have overlapping actions but also share receptor components led to the concepts of "cytokine receptor pleiotropy" and "cytokine receptor redundancy" [reviewed by Ozaki and Leonard (189)]. The first of these terms can be defined by the ability of a single cytokine receptor subunit to function in more than one receptor. Thus, examples include the sharing of γ_c, β_c, and gp130, as summarized previously, as well as the sharing of IL-2Rβ by IL-2 and IL-15 receptors and the sharing of IL-4Rα and

IL-13Rα in type II IL-4 receptors and IL-13 receptors. Another way of viewing receptor pleiotropy is to regard certain receptor chains as useful "modules." In other words, just as domains of proteins, such as src homology domains 2 and 3 (SH2 and SH3), are used by many different proteins, shared receptor chains can be thought of as an analogous situation in which entire receptor chains is a module that functions in more than one context.

The final concept, cytokine receptor subunit redundancy, is the one with fewest examples. There is one well-documented example in mice but none in humans. IL-3 signals through IL-3Rα plus either β_c or an alternative unique IL-3Rβ [also known as β_{IL-3} (227)], which shares 91% amino acid identity with β_c and appears to be a completely functionally redundant protein for IL-3 signaling, but β_{IL-3} cannot substitute for β_c in the context of IL-5 or GM-CSF signaling (142). Other potential examples exist. For example, in type I and type II IL-4 receptors, IL-4Rα coordinates with either γ_c or IL-13Rα, respectively, and there are two types of OSM receptors, both of which contain gp130 but one of which contains a specific OSM receptor, and the other contains LIFRβ. What remains unknown, however, is whether the signals mediated by these different types of receptors are truly identical so that there is redundancy, or whether there are distinctive features to the signals that IL-4, OSM, and IL-15 induce through the different receptors.

In addition to the examples related to type I cytokines just mentioned, the IL-10 subfamily of type II cytokines is interesting in that IL-10Rβ, IL-20Rα, IL-20Rβ, and IL-22Rα are each shared components, collectively affecting signaling in response to IL-10, IL-19, IL-20, IL-22, and IL-24 [reviewed by Ozaki and Leonard (189) and in later-mentioned references related to the IL-10 family of cytokines]. Specifically, IL-10 signals through a receptor containing IL-10Rα and IL-10Rβ, IL-19 signals through a receptor containing IL-20Rα and IL-20Rβ, IL-20 signals through receptors containing IL-20Rβ and either IL-20Rα or IL-22Rα, IL-22 signals through receptors containing IL-10Rβ and IL-22Rα, and IL-24 signals through receptors containing IL-20Rβ plus either IL-20Rα or IL-22Rα.

SOLUBLE RECEPTORS

Soluble forms of many cytokine receptors have been identified, including those for IL-1, IL-2, IL-4, IL-5, IL-6, IL-7, GM-CSF, type I and type II IFNs, and TNF (228,229). As is clear from this list of cytokines, soluble receptors are not restricted to receptors that are type I cytokine receptors, and in the case of IL-2, the principal soluble receptor protein is IL-2Rα, which is not a type I cytokine receptor. Soluble receptors can be created by alternative splicing that truncates the protein N-terminal to the transmembrane domain, resulting in a secreted protein rather than a membrane-anchored membrane in the case of IL-4Rα, IL-5Rα, IL-6Rα, IL-7Rα, IFN-αR β chain (IFNAR-2), and GM-CSFRα. Alternatively, they can be created by proteolytic cleavage of the membrane

TABLE 9. *Soluble cytokine receptors*

Generated by alternative splicing
sIL-4Rα
sIL-5Rα
sIL-6Rα
sIL-7Rα
sGM-CSFRα
sIFNAR2

Generated by proteolytic cleavage of mature receptor
sIL-2Rα
sTNFR

GM-CSF, granulocyte-macrophage colony-stimulating factor; IFN, interferon; IL, interleukin; R, receptor; s, soluble; TNF, tumor necrosis factor.

receptor, as is found for the receptors for IL-2Rα and TNFRI and TNFRII [reviewed by Fernandez-Botran et al. (229)] (Table 9). Although it is theoretically possible that a distinct gene might encode the soluble forms of a receptor, no such examples have been reported. In the cases in which proteolytic cleavage occurs, the identity of the proteases has not been identified. The major questions related to these soluble receptors are as follows: (a) Do they have physiological or pathophysiological functions? (b) How do their affinities compare to the corresponding cell surface receptor? (c) Do they have diagnostic, prognostic, and therapeutic applications?

Unfortunately, there is little information available on the *in vivo* role of soluble receptors. In general, in *in vitro* studies, soluble receptors can compete with their corresponding cell surface receptors, thereby serving negative regulatory roles. However, soluble IL-6Rα exerts an agonistic role, because, as summarized previously, IL-6 signaling occurs equally well through gp130 when the soluble rather than transmembrane form of IL-6Rα interacts with IL-6. Nevertheless, a mutated form of IL-6Rα that cannot interact with gp130 but still binds IL-6 can effectively inhibit (230). In the case of IL-2Rα, there is no reported physiological function for soluble IL-2Rα, because the affinity of the released receptor is, as expected, similar to that of the low-affinity receptor ($K_d = 10^{-8}$ M), which makes it unlikely to effectively compete with the high-affinity cell surface receptor ($K_d = 10^{-11}$ M). However, this and other soluble receptors could serve as cytokine carrier proteins and potentially could increase stability of a cytokine by protecting it from proteolysis (229). Nevertheless, there are potential diagnostic and prognostic uses for measuring the numbers of these shed IL-2 receptors (Table 10).

INTERFERONS (TYPE II CYTOKINES) AND THEIR RECEPTORS

IFNs represent an evolutionarily conserved family (Table 11) of cytokines that, as noted previously, are related to the type I cytokines. IFNs were discovered in 1957 on the basis of their antiviral activity (231). Because of the existence of both type I and type II IFNs (232–237), the nomenclature of IFNs is reviewed first. Type I IFNs include IFN-α (originally known as

TABLE 10. *Soluble interleukin-2 receptors in human disease*

Malignancies
Hematological
  Adult T-cell leukemia
  Hairy cell leukemia
  Acute lymphocytic leukemia
  Chronic lymphocytic leukemia (B cell)
  Acute myelogenous leukemia
  Chronic myelogenous leukemia, especially in blast crisis
  Malignant lymphomas
    Hodgkin's disease
    Non-Hodgkin's lymphomas
Nonhematological
  Adenocarcinoma of lung, breast, pancreas
  Small cell bronchogenic carcinoma
  Ovarian, cervical, and endometrial cancers
  Nasopharyngeal carcinoma
  Melanoma
Infections
HIV
Tuberculosis
Rubeola
Infectious mononucleosis
Other diseases
End-stage renal disease
Rheumatoid arthritis
Systemic lupus erythematosus
Scleroderma
Sarcoidosis
After transplantation
After IL-2 administration

HIV, human immunodeficiency virus; IL, interleukin.

[a]In adults, the mean soluble IL-2Rα levels are 280 ± 161 units/mL (levels tend to be higher in pediatric populations). The situations in which the levels exceed 5,000 units/mL are adult T-cell leukemia, hairy cell leukemia, chronic myelogenous leukemia, and after IL-2 administration. The situations in which levels are between 1,000 and 5,000 units/mL include acute myelogenous leukemia, chronic lymphocytic leukemia, nonHodgkin's lymphomas, acquired immunodeficiency syndrome associated with Kaposi's sarcoma, tuberculosis, rubeola, and end-stage renal disease.

Data are from references 228 and 229.

TABLE 11. *Type II cytokines*

Type of cytokine	Number of genes	Chromosomal location (human/mouse)
Type I interferons		
IFN-α	Many genes	9p22/4
IFN-β	Single gene	9p21/4
IFN-ω	Single gene	9p21/4
IFN-τ	Many genes	
Type II interferon		
IFN-γ	Single gene	12q14/10
IL-10 family cytokines		
IL-10	Single gene	1q31–32/1
IL-19	Single gene	1q32/—
IL-20	Single gene	1q32/1
IL-22	Single gene	12q15/—
IL-24	Single gene	1q32/—
IL-26	Single gene	12q15/—
IL-28	Single gene	
IL-29	Single gene	

IFN, interferon; IL, interleukin.

leukocyte IFN), IFN-β (originally known as fibroblast IFN), and IFN-ω. IFN-ω is closely related to the IFN-αs and was formerly designated as an IFN-α. There are a large number of IFN-αs. In contrast, the other type I IFNs, IFN-β and IFN-ω, are each encoded by single human and murine genes near the IFN-α cluster, and there are multiple pseudogenes most closely related to IFN-α and IFN-ω. The type I IFNs are clustered on human chromosome 9 and murine chromosome 4. Type II IFN is IFN-γ, which is encoded by a single gene on human chromosome 12 and murine chromosome 10. In addition, another IFN, denoted IFN-δ, has been reported (238).

The grouping of IFN-α and IFN-β together as type I IFNs is logical not only because of the similar amino acid sequences and structures of these IFNs but also because they share the same receptor and induce essentially the same signals [reviewed by Stark et al. (233) and Langer et al.

(239)]. Although DNA array analysis does show some differences in the genes induced by IFN-α and IFN-β, the basis for these differences are unclear (240). These signals include antiproliferative and antiviral activities and also the ability to stimulate cytolytic activity in lymphocytes, NK cells, and macrophages. In contrast, IFN-γ has a distinct receptor. Type I and type II IFN receptors share a degree of similarity to each other sufficient to form a family (241). The structure of the IFN-γ receptor (242) is shown in Fig. 2. IFN receptors are referred to as type II cytokine receptors to reflect the substantial differences between these receptors and the type I cytokine receptors (8). Because both type I and type II IFNs bind to type II cytokine receptors, IFNs are occasionally referred to as type II cytokines but more generally are referred to as IFNs, which helps to minimize confusion of nomenclature. On the basis of the similarity of the IL-10 receptor to the IFN-γ receptors (8), IL-10 was designated as a type II cytokine, and, indeed, when its x-ray crystal was determined, IL-10 was found to be topologically related to IFN-γ (14). As noted previously, a series of IL-10–related cytokines has been identified, including IL-19, IL-20, IL-22, IL-24, IL-26, IL-28, and IL-29, and these are also designated as type II cytokines. Among type II cytokines, IFN-γ has helices similar to those of the type I short-chain helical cytokines, but its short helices that occupy the AB and CD loops exhibit the long-chain cytokine-like AB-over-CD topology. IL-10 and IFN-αβ have long-chain structures (8). Thus, the short-chain and long-chain theme of type I cytokines also extends to the IFNs and the IL-10 family of type II cytokines.

Type I IFNs signal through a receptor containing a receptor known as the type I IFN receptor (232,233). This receptor consists of at least two chains (243–246). In contrast to the chains' being denoted as α and β chains, which is analogous to the nomenclature for type I cytokine receptors, the Interferon Nomenclature Committee proposed that the chains be denoted as IFNAR-1 (previously also denoted IFN-αR1,

IFNAR1, and IFN-Rα) and IFNAR-2 [previously also known as IFN-α/β receptor (IFN-α/βR), IFN-αR2, IFNAR2, and IFN-Rβ] (238). Accordingly, this nomenclature is used in this chapter.

Interestingly, IFNAR-2 has both short and long forms as well as a soluble form (247). The long form has a much larger cytoplasmic domain and serves a more important role in signal transduction. Whereas IFNAR-1 cannot bind IFN-α, IFNAR-2 binds with low affinity, and the combination of both chains results in high-affinity binding (247) and function. As detailed later, IFNAR-1 binds the Tyk2, whereas IFNAR-2 binds Jak1. In addition to these cellular receptors, it is interesting that vaccinia virus and other orthopoxviruses encode a soluble form of type I IFN receptor that is related to the IL-1 receptors and that is capable of binding IFN-α, IFN-β, and IFN-ω (248,249). This form of IFN receptor is therefore not a member of the type II cytokine family but, rather, is a member of immunoglobulin superfamily. Usually IFN-αs are species specific, so that the human IFN-αs do not typically bind to the murine receptor. However, IFN-α8 is unusual in that it is one of the few or perhaps the only human type I IFN that can bind to the murine receptor. IFNAR-1 confers species specificity of binding.

IFN-γ was cloned in 1982 (250) [see Farrar and Schreiber (232), Stark et al. (233), and Bach et al. (251)]. IFN-γ is encoded by four exons on chromosome 12. IFN-γ forms a homodimer with an apparent molecular weight of 34 kDa. Little of the monomeric form can be detected, and it is not biologically active. As noted previously, each IFN-γ monomer has six α helices, four of which resemble the short-chain helical cytokines, and there is no β sheet structure. The subunits interact in an antiparallel manner. In contrast to IFN-α, which is produced by many different cells, IFN-γ is produced only by NK cells, CD8$^+$ T cells, and the Th1 subclass of CD4$^+$ T cells [reviewed by Farrar and Schreiber (232); see later discussion]. IFN-γ exerts its effects through specific receptors that are expressed on all cells except for erythrocytes. Interestingly, even platelets express IFN-γ receptors, which raises the possibility that they can serve a function in transporting IFN-γ in the circulation (232). The functional human receptor consists of two chains (252): IFNGR-1, also denoted IFN-γR1 or IFN-γRα (238,253), a 90-kDa protein whose gene is located on human chromosome 6q16–22 and murine chromosome 10 (251), and IFNGR-2, also denoted as IFN-γRβ (254,255), located on human chromosome 21q22.1 and murine chromosome 16 (251). IFNGR-1 is required for ligand binding, whereas IFNGR-2 plays a role in signaling. Jak1 associates with the Leu-Pro-Lys-Ser sequence in the membrane proximal region of the cytoplasmic domain of IFNGR-1 (256), whereas Jak2 binds to IFNGR-2 (257). Interestingly, as noted previously, IFN-γ itself is a homodimer. Thus, binding of IFN-γ induces the homodimerization of IFNGR-1, which then allows the recruitment of IFNGR-2, and the functional IFN-γ receptor is believed to contain two molecules each of IFNGR-1 and IFNGR-2. Normal IFN-γ production is dependent on IL-12,

and defective IFN-γ signaling is associated with failure to appropriate clear mycobacterial infections (discussed later).

Interleukin-10, a Type II Cytokine, and Related Cytokines IL-19, IL-20, IL-22, IL-24, IL-26, IL-28, and IL-29

IL-10 is a cytokine that is produced by activated T cells, B cells, monocytes, and keratinocytes (258). The IL-10 gene is divided into five exons and is located on chromosome 1 in both mice and humans (258). IL-10 has an open reading frame of 178 amino acids, including the signal peptide, and the mature protein is 18 kDa. Human IL-10 receptor maps to 11q23.3. It can inhibit the production of a number of cytokines, including IL-2, IL-3, IFN-γ, GM-CSF, and TNF and belongs to the category of a Th2 cytokine (258) (see below). IL-10 inhibits monocyte-dependent T-cell proliferation, in part by markedly decreasing synthesis of a variety of cytokines. Nevertheless, in addition to these indirect effects on T cells, IL-10 appears to exert direct stimulatory effects on thymocytes and T cells in vitro. Interestingly, the BCRF1 protein that is encoded by Epstein Barr virus is very similar to IL-10 and shares many of its biological properties as a macrophage "deactivating" factor and as a co-stimulator of proliferation of B cells (258,259). The EBV IL-10 homolog is a selective agonist, although its binding to the IL-10 receptor is somewhat impaired (259). IL-10 is a major inhibitor of Th1 functions (258). Although it was suggested that IL-10 might also favor Th2 development, it is clear that IL-4 is the major mediator of Th2 cell development. It is clear that IL-10 plays a major role in limiting and terminating inflammatory responses (258).

As noted previously, the IL-10 receptor is most closely related to IFN receptors, which makes it a type II rather than type I cytokine receptor (260,261). This corresponds to the close structural relationship of IL-10 to IFN-γ. An IL-10Rα chain was initially isolated. The previously recognized "orphan" IFN receptor family member denoted CRF2-4 that is located on chromosome 21 within 35 kb of IFNGR-2 (262,263) is now known to be the IL-10Rβ chain (258).

A series of IL-10-related cytokines have been been identified, including IL-19, IL-20, IL-22, IL-24, IL-26, IL-28, and IL-29 (264–269,269a,269b). Data on biological roles of some of these proteins is limited. IL-19 was discovered as a gene that was induced in lipopolysaccharide-stimulated monocytes. IL-20 was found in epidermal cells, with overexpression resulting in aberrant epidermal differentiation; it was suggested to have a role in psoriasis. IL-22 was found as an IL-9–induced cytokine that can in turn induce acute-phase reactant production by hepatocytes. IL-24 was originally discovered as melanoma differentiation–associated antigen 7, and IL-26 was originally discovered as AK155. Interestingly, IL-10, IL-19, IL-20, and IL-24 co-localize at human chromosome 1q32 whereas IL-22 and IL-26 are at 12q15 [see Fickenschur et al. (270) for a review]. IL-28 and IL-29 share IL-10Rβ and additionally use IL-28Rα (269a, 269b).

SPECIES SPECIFICITY OF CYTOKINES

There are no general rules for the species specificity of human and murine cytokines and how the cytokines and their receptor chains have coevolved. As examples of each situation, human IL-2 can stimulate both human and murine cells, whereas murine IL-2 exhibits little action on human cells (41). Conversely, human IL-12 does not work on murine cells, whereas murine IL-12 is biologically active on both murine and human cells (194). This selective property of IL-12 is dependent on the species origin of p35. Finally, IL-4 exhibits rather strict specificity so that human and murine IL-4 induce responses only on human and murine cells, respectively (58,62). In addition to these examples, varying degrees of relative species specificity have been demonstrated, depending on the cytokine; in other words, at times a cytokine from one species will work on another species but with attenuated potency. Thus, virtually any combination of species specificities has been observed.

SIGNALING THROUGH INTERFERON AND CYTOKINE RECEPTORS

Our understanding of signaling through IFN and cytokine receptors has increased tremendously over the past decade. Multiple signaling pathways/molecules have been observed for various cytokines. Collectively, these include the Jak-STAT pathway, the Ras–mitogen-activated protein (MAP) kinase pathway, Src and ZAP70 and related proteins, phosphatidyl inositol 3-kinase (PI3K), insulin receptor substrates 1 and 2 (IRS-1 and IRS-2), and phosphatases. Each of these pathways is discussed in turn, with an initial focus on Janus kinases and STAT proteins.

OVERVIEW OF JANUS KINASES AND STATS

The Jak-STAT pathway (39,233,271–273) is particularly exciting in that it serves as a rapid mechanism by which signals can be transduced from the membrane to the nucleus. Jaks are also known as Janus family tyrosine kinases. STAT proteins are substrates for Jaks. There is now a tremendous amount of

information on Jaks and STATs that demonstrate their importance related to development, differentiation, proliferation, cellular transformation, and tumorigenesis.

Janus Kinases

The Jaks are 116 to 140 kDa and comprise approximately 1,150 amino acids (233,272). The seven regions of conserved sequences in Jaks, denoted JH1 to JH7, are depicted in Fig. 4. One of the hallmark features of these kinases is that, in addition to the presence of a catalytic tyrosine kinase domain (JH1), there is also a pseudo-kinase region (JH2), respectively. The name *Janus kinase* reflects the two faces of the mythological Roman god, with one face representing the true kinase and the other the pseudo-kinase. Although the JH nomenclature has been used historically, it has obvious limitations in that, except for the JH1 catalytic domain and JH2 pseudo-kinase domain, it remains unclear whether the other JH regions correspond to discrete domains. Moreover, sequence analysis suggests that Jaks may have an SH2 domain, which spans approximately two of the JH domains. So far, the three-dimensional structures have not been solved for any of the Jaks.

There are four mammalian Jaks: Jak1 (274), Jak2 (275), Jak3 (276,277), and Tyk2 (278). Interestingly, none of the Jaks was cloned on the basis of purification or function. Instead, all the Jaks were identified as parts of studies intended to identify new kinases (272). At least one Jak is activated by every IFN and cytokine, and some cytokines activate two or three Jaks (233,271–273). Table 12 lists a number of features of each Jak, whereas Table 13 summarizes the Jaks that are activated by a variety of cytokines.

Because Jak1, Jak2, and Tyk2 are ubiquitously expressed, each cell type expresses either three or all four Jaks. The Jaks that are activated within the cells are those that can physically bind to the receptor chains. Jaks physically bind to the membrane proximal Box 1/Box 2 regions of the cytoplasmic domains (277–282), and the N-terminal region of the Jaks is required for this function (283–285). The Box 1 regions are proline-rich (27), which suggests that Jaks may have SH3-like

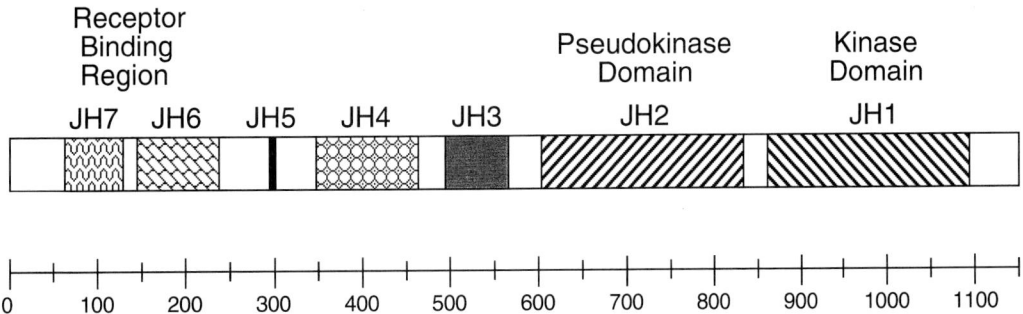

FIG. 4. Schematic of Janus kinases. Shown are the locations of the seven JH domains. JH1 is the catalytic domain. JH2 is the pseudo-kinase domain, the presence of which prompted the naming of this family as Janus family tyrosine kinases. As noted in the text, the JH nomenclature has limitations and in fact masks the presence of an SH2 domain that spans parts of the JH4 and JH3 domains. Also shown is the conserved tyrosine (Y1007 in Jak2) whose phosphorylation is required for maximal catalytic activity.

TABLE 12. *Features of Janus family kinases*

Kinase	Inducible vs. constitutive	Size	Chromosomal location (human/mouse)
Jak1	Constitutive	135 kD	1p31.3/4
Jak2	Constitutive	130 kD	9p23–24/19
Jak3	Inducible	116 kD	19p13/8
Tyk2	Constitutive	140 kD	19p13.2/—

Jak, Janus kinase; Tyk, tyrosine kinase.

domains in their N-terminal regions to mediate these interactions. Because each receptor is a homodimer, heterodimer, or higher order oligomer, it is reasonable to assume that at least two Jak molecules (either two molecules of one Jak or one molecule each of two different Jaks) will be activated, inasmuch as one Jak is associated with each receptor chain. In accord with their ubiquitous expression, Jak1, Jak2, and Tyk2 are activated by a variety of different sets of cytokines (Tables 12 and 13). For example, Jak1 is activated not only by

TABLE 13. *Cytokines and the Jaks they activate*

Cytokine	Jak kinases activated
IFN-α/β	Jak1, Tyk2
IFN-γ	Jak1, Jak2
Growth hormone	Jak2
Prolactin	Jak2
Erythopoietin	Jak2
Thrombopoietin	Jak2
IL-10	Jak1, Tyk2
IL-12	Jak2, Tyk2
G-CSF	Jak1, Jak2
γ_C family	
IL-2, IL-4,[a] IL-7, IL-9, IL-15,[b] IL-21	Jak1, Jak3
β_C family	
IL-3, IL-5, GM-CSF	Jak2, ?Jak1
gp130 family	
IL-6, IL-11, CNTF, LIF, OSM, CT-1	Jak1, Jak2, Tyk2
TSLP	No Jak appears to activated by murine TSLP

For murine TSLP, so far, no Jak has been identified that is activated; instead, it has been suggested that murine TSLP may activate a Tec family kinase (482).

CNTF, ciliary neurotrophic factor; CT-1, cardiotropin-1; G-CSF, granulocyte colony-stimulating factor; GM-CSF, granulocyte-macrophage colony-stimulating factor; IFN, interferon; IL, interleukin; Jak, Janus kinase; LIF, leukemia inhibitory factor; OSM, oncostatin M; TSLP, thymic stromal lymphopoietin; Tyk, tyrosine kinase.

[a]Note that IL-4 activates Jak1 and Jak3 when it acts through the type I IL-4 receptor (IL-4Rα and γ_C, found for example on T cells). However, Jak3 is not activated when IL-4 signals through the type II IL-4 receptors (IL-4Rα and IL-13Rα1, a form of receptor that is expressed on a number of non–T cells, including fibroblasts).

[b]Note that IL-15 activates Jak1 and Jak3 when it acts through the type I IL-15 receptor (IL-15Rα and IL-2Rβ and γ_C, found for example on T cells). However, Jak2 is instead activated when IL-15 signals through the type II IL-15 receptor (denoted IL-15RX) found, for example, on mast cells.

type I and type II IFNs but also by the γ_C family of cytokines (e.g., IL-2, IL-4, IL-7, IL-9, IL-15, and IL-21), and Jak2 is activated not only by IFN-γ but also by growth hormone, erythropoietin, prolactin, and the hematopoietic cytokines IL-3, IL-5, and GM-CSF (271,272). Tyk2 is somewhat more restricted in that it is activated by IFN-$\alpha\beta$ and IL-12/IL-23; the significance of its activation by gp130 family cytokines is less clear. Interestingly, Jak1, Jak2, and Tyk2 are all recruited by each of the cytokines that share gp130 as a signal transducing molecule; this raises the question as to whether in this context three Jaks are required or whether any one or two are sufficient. At least for IL-6, Jak1 is absolutely vital (286,287), whereas the importance of Jak2 and Tyk2 is less clear.

Jak3 is different from the other Jaks in that it is much more inducible. Moreover, Jak3 is activated by only the cytokines whose receptors contain γ_C [reviewed by Sprang and Bazan (8) and Leonard (39)]. It is interesting that each cytokine whose receptor contains γ_C activates not only Jak3 but also Jak1. The basis for the activation of both Jak1 and Jak3 by IL-2, IL-4, IL-7, IL-9, IL-15, and IL-21 is that Jak1 associates with each of the unique signaling chains (IL-2Rβ, IL-4Rα, IL-7Rα, IL-9Rα, and IL-21R), whereas Jak3 associates with γ_C (38,39). Although this could be coincidental, these observations raise the possibility that Jak1 is the Jak that can most efficiently cooperate functionally with Jak3. In view of the wide range of cytokines that activate any particular Jak and because in some cases multiple cytokines can activate the same set of Jaks, it is clear that the Jaks by themselves do not determine signaling specificity. For example, IL-2, IL-4, IL-7, IL-9, IL-15, and IL-21 all activate Jak1 and Jak3 but induce a range of signals. Moreover, Jak2 is the only Jak that is activated by growth hormone and erythropoietin, cytokines with little in common in terms of function. Interestingly, Jak2 is the Jak that interacts with all cytokine receptors that form homodimers. Because homodimeric receptors are probably the oldest cytokine receptors in evolution, Jak2 might be the "first" Jak from which others evolved.

Importance of Janus Kinases in Signaling

In addition to the activation of Jaks by multiples cytokines and IFNs, various other data indicate their importance for signaling. One of the vital series of experiments that led to the establishment of the critical role of Jaks in IFN signaling involved a group of mutant cell lines that were defective for IFN signaling but wherein signaling could be rescued by genetic complementation [reviewed by Stark et al. (233)]. Defective signaling in response to IFN-α and IFN-β was found in a mutant cell line (U1 cells) lacking Tyk2; defective signaling in response to IFN-α, IFN-β, and IFN-γ was found in a mutant cell line lacking Jak1 (U4 cells); and defective IFN-γ signaling was found in cells lacking Jak2 (γ1 cells) (233). Various other data have indicated the importance of Jaks for other cytokine pathways. First, a dominant negative Jak2 inhibits signaling by erythropoietin and growth hormone (288,289), whereas a dominant negative Jak3 inhibits signaling in response to IL-2 (290), and, as noted previously, Jak1 is vital for IL-6 signaling. Second, humans (291,292) and mice (293–295) deficient in Jak3 exhibit developmental and signaling defects consistent with defective signaling. Third, in *Drosophila*, the *hopscotch* gene encodes a Jak wherein loss-of-function alleles result in lethality and decreased proliferation, whereas a gain-of-function allele, *hopscotch*$^{Tumorous-lethal}$, results in melanotic tumors and hypertrophy of the hematopoietic organs (296–297). Fourth, in zebrafish, Jak1 is vital for normal cell migration and anterior specification (298). Fifth, as discussed later, Jaks are constitutively activated in many cell lines infected with a number of viruses, including HTLV-I, v-Abl, spleen focus forming virus, and with v-Src (299–302). Sixth, a Jak2 inhibitor inhibited the growth of acute lymphoblastic leukemia cells *in vitro* (303). These data together demonstrate the vital role of Jaks in cytokine signaling. Depending on the function of the particular cytokine (e.g., development, differentiation, or proliferation), the particular Jaks may therefore be involved in a variety of processes, and when dysregulated, in at least certain settings, they appear to contribute to cellular transformation.

Janus Kinase 3 Mutations Result in an Autosomal Recessive Form of Severe Combined Immunodeficiency that is indistinguishable from X-Linked Severe Combined Immunodeficiency

As mentioned previously, mutations in γ_c result in XS-CID in humans. A very large number of different mutations have been observed in XSCID (these are summarized on the World Wide Web; see *http://www.nhgri.nih.gov/DIR/LGT/SCID/IL2RGbase.html*). As might be expected, in cases in which it has been examined, amino acid substitutions in the extracellular domain result in defective cytokine binding [reviewed by Kimura et al. (35)]. In contrast, mutations or truncations in the γ_c cytoplasmic domain result in defective signaling. Analysis of an interesting family in which a number of boys and men exhibit a moderate form of X-linked combined immunodeficiency (XCID) revealed that this disease also resulted from a mutation in γ_c (34). The mutation (Leu 271→Gln) was found to result in a decrease, but not total loss, of Jak3 association, in contrast to the loss of Jak3 interaction seen with mutations in the γ_c cytoplasmic domain that cause XSCID. The severity of the immunodeficiency therefore appeared to inversely correlate with the degree of Jak3 activation. Thus, XSCID is truly a disease of defective cytokine signaling (38,39). Moreover, it was predicted that Jak3 was required for T-cell and NK-cell development and that mutations in Jak3 might result in a clinical phenotype indistinguishable from that in XSCID (34). Indeed, this is indeed the case in humans (291,292). As would be hypothesized, a number of distinct mutations in Jak3 were found (272). Presumably, any mutation that interferes with its interaction with γ_c, with its catalytic activity, or with recruitment of substrates could result in clinical disease.

TABLE 14. *Cytokines and the STATs they activate*

Cytokine	STATs activated
IFN-α/β	STAT1, STAT2
IFN-γ	STAT1
Growth hormone	STAT5a, STAT5b
Prolactin	STAT5a, STAT5b
Erythopoietin	STAT5a, STAT5b
Thrombopoietin	STAT5a, STAT5b
IL-10	STAT3
IL-12	STAT4, STAT3
G-CSF	STAT3
γ_c family	
IL-2, IL-7, IL-9, IL-15, IL-21	STAT5a, STAT5b, STAT3, STAT1
IL-4	STAT6
IL-13	STAT6
TSLP	STAT5a, STAT5b
β_c family	
IL-3, IL-5, GM-CSF	STAT5a, STAT5b
gp130 family	
IL-6, IL-11, CNTF, LIF, OSM, CT-1	STAT3
Leptin	STAT3

Note that for IL-2, IL-7, IL-9, and IL-15, STAT5a and STAT5b appear to be the major STATs that are activated, although STAT3 in particular and STAT1 can also be activated. For IL-21, at least in certain cell types, STAT1 may be more potently activated (37).

CNTF, ciliary neurotrophic factor; CT-1, cardiotropin-1; G-CSF, granulocyte colony-stimulating factor; GM-CSF, granulocyte-macrophage colony-stimulating factor; IFN, interferon; IL, interleukin; LIF, leukemia inhibitory factor; OSM, oncostatin M; STAT, signal transducer and activator of transcription; TSLP, thymic stromal lymphopoietin.

In an analogy to the similarity of XSCID and SCID associated with Jak3 deficiency, mice deficient in either γ_c or Jak3 also have very similar phenotypes (118,119,293–295). These *in vivo* data underscore the vital role of Jak3 in mediating γ_c-dependent functions and suggest that Jak3 would be essential for most if not all γ_c functions. Some *in vitro* data indicate that γ_c may do more than recruit Jak3 (290,304), but the recruitment of Jak3 is clearly essential, and the defects in T-cell and NK-cell development associated with γ_c or Jak3 deficiency are indistinguishable. Theoretically, it is possible that Jak3 might interact with one or more other important cytokine receptor chains that have not yet been identified. However, because Jak3 deficiency is not clinically or phenotypically worse than γ_c deficiency in humans and mice, it seems likely that Jak3 associates only with γ_c. One report has suggested that Jak3 is associated with CD40 (305), which raises the possibility of a role for Jak3 is a system distinct from cytokine receptors, although a functional role for Jak3 in CD40 signaling has not yet been established and this finding has been questioned (306). The phenotypes of mice lacking each of the four Jaks are summarized as part of Table 14.

ACTIVATION OF JANUS KINASES AND THE JANUS KINASE–STAT PARADIGM

Although the vital roles of Jaks in cytokine signaling have been discussed, little regarding how they are activated, how they are regulated, and how they phosphorylate substrates has been mentioned. The paradigm of Jak-STAT activation is included in Fig. 5, which also shows activation of other pathways, such as the Ras-MAP kinase and PI3K/Akt/p70 S6 kinase pathways. After IFN or cytokine engagement, dimerization or higher order oligomerization of receptor complexes is induced. This in turn allows the juxtapositioning of Jaks, allowing their potential transphosphorylation and activation. In receptors with only two chains, the direct transphosphorylation of one Jak by the other seems likely to occur. In more complex receptors, additional subtleties may exist. For example, for the IFN-γ system, because the receptor is a heterotetramer with two α (IFNGR-1) chains (each of which binds Jak1) and two β (IFNGR-2) chains (each of which binds Jak2), it is not clear whether Jak1 and Jak2 transactivate each other or whether one of the Jaks plays a dominant role. In fact, one study suggested that Jak2 may play the dominant role and that it is responsible for phosphorylating both itself

and Jak1, thereby increasing the catalytic activities of both kinases (307). Jak1 in turn phosphorylates IFNGR-1, allowing the recruitment of STAT1. In this model, it is additionally suggested that Jak2 phosphorylates STAT1 (307). Interestingly, a kinase-dead mutant of Jak1 was able to mediate the induction of certain IFN-γ-induced genes, which indicates a potential "structural" role for Jak1, but catalytically active Jak1 was essential for the establishment of the antiviral state (307), which emphasizes the essential role of both Jak1 and Jak2 catalytic activities for normal IFN-γ function.

In the preceding discussion, it is assumed that transphosphorylation of Jaks is a mechanism for the amplification of catalytic activity. Unless other kinases are involved, however, implicit in this idea is that the Jaks themselves must exhibit some basal activity that is amplified to a higher level by autophosphorylation or transphosphorylation. Consistent with activation of Jaks by phosphorylation, mutagenesis of a critical tyrosine in Tyk2 (308) or Jak2 (309) (e.g., tyrosine

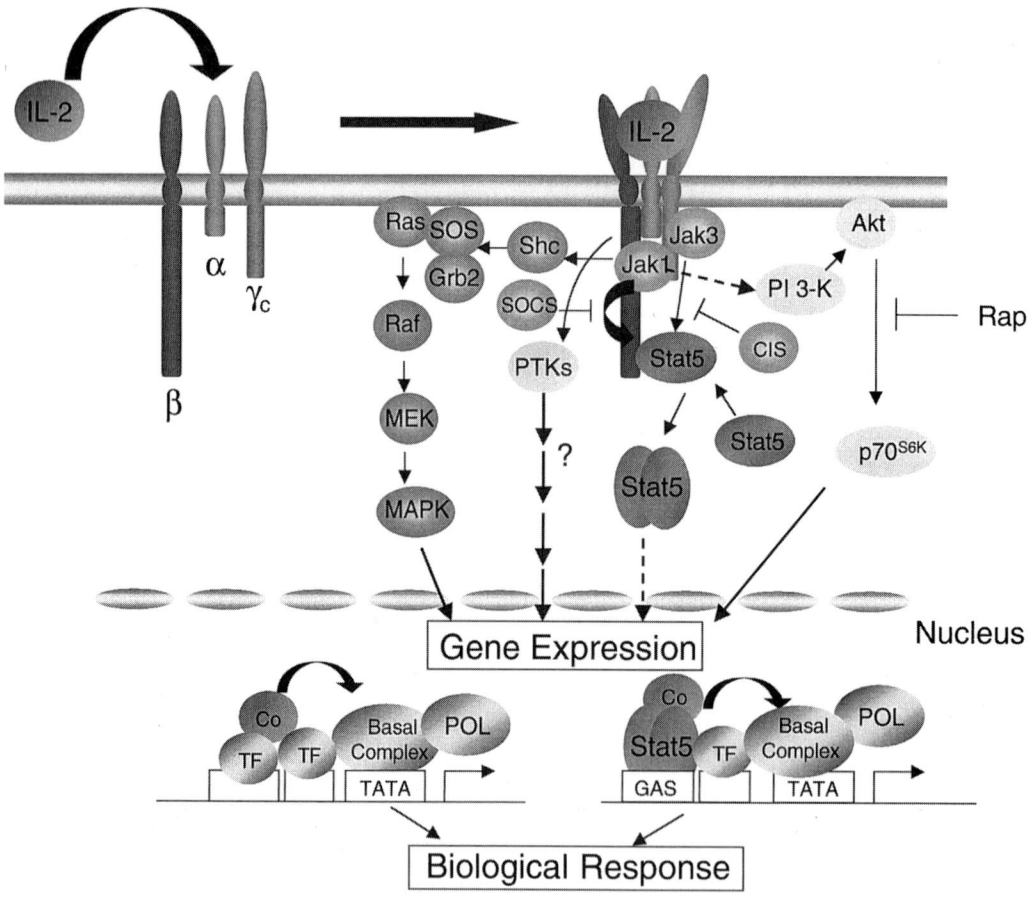

FIG. 5. Schematic of cytokine signaling showing multiple signaling pathways activated by IL-2. Shown is the association of Janus kinases 1 and 3 (Jak1 and Jak3) with different chains of the receptor. Activation of Jaks results in tyrosine phosphorylation of interleukin-2 receptor β (IL-2Rβ). This allows the docking of signal transducer and activator of transcription (STAT) 5 proteins through their SH2 domain. The STATs themselves are tyrosine-phosphorylated, dimerize, and translocate to the nucleus, where they modulate expression of target genes. The schematic also indicates that another phosphotyrosine mediates recruitment of Shc, which then can couple to the Ras/Raf/MEK/mitogen-activated protein (MAP) kinase pathway. Also shown is the important phosphatidylinositol 3-kinase pathway. These and other pathways are activated by many type I cytokines.

1007 in the case of Jak2) in the activation loop of the kinase domain inhibits activity. It is conceivable that phosphorylation of other tyrosines on the Jaks may create appropriate motifs for the recruitment of additional signaling molecules, but mutation of other tyrosines has not so far had obviously deleterious functional effects (310).

The function of the pseudo-kinase domain remains unclear. No other metazoan protein tyrosine kinases contain such a domain. The JH2 lacks the third glycine in the critical Gly-X-Gly-X-X-Gly motif, is missing an aspartic acid that serves as the proton acceptor that is typically conserved in the catalytic loop of both tyrosine and serine kinases, and is missing the conserved phenylalanine in the Asp-Phe-Glu motif that binds ATP [reviewed by Leonard and O'Shea (272)]. The absence of the critical amino acids previously summarized presumably explains the lack of catalytic function of the JH2 domain (274). Despite the lack of catalytic activity of the JH2 domain, there are increasing data in support of vital functions for this region. Although the kinase domain alone can act as an active kinase, it is interesting that a mutation in the Jak JH2 domain can hyperactivate the *Drosophila* (*hopTum-l*/D-STAT) Jak-STAT pathway and that the corresponding Glu695-to-Lys mutation in murine Jak2 also resulted in increased autophosphorylation of Jak2 and phosphorylation of STAT5 in transfected cells (311). Moreover, the JH2 domain may play an important role in mediating the interaction of Jaks with STAT proteins (312).

Because Jaks are associated with cytokine receptors and activated by cytokines, it is important to achieve an understanding of the range of cytokine signals that are mediated by these kinases. These include important roles in development (as demonstrated by the lack of T-cell and NK cell development associated with Jak3 deficiency, a defect at least partially caused by defective signaling in response to IL-7 and IL-15), in signaling in response to cytokines that are mitogenic growth factors (e.g., IL-2, IL-3), and in the antiviral response (IFNs). The analysis of the role of Jak1 in zebrafish was interesting not only in that it showed a role for Jak1 in early vertebrate development but also because it was demonstrated that during early development Jak1 kinase was exclusively of maternal origin (298). These developmental roles for Jak1 in zebrafish are consistent with the importance of a Jak in early *Drosophila* development as well (313).

Although the significance is unknown, splice variants have been found for Jak3 (314). One Jak, Jak2, is involved in a chromosomal translocation to create the Tel-Jak2 fusion protein that is causally related to leukemia (315).

STAT PROTEINS ARE SUBSTRATES FOR JANUS KINASES THAT AT LEAST IN PART HELP DETERMINE SPECIFICITY

Because the Janus family kinases cannot by themselves determine specificity (as demonstrated by the facts that different cytokines with different actions activate the same Jaks), a reasonable hypothesis was that the same Jaks might have

different substrates, depending on the receptor. The best characterized substrates for Jaks are STATs (271–273). Among the mutant cell lines with defects in IFN signaling, in addition to the ones with defects in Jaks noted previously, others were defective in STAT proteins. These data were among the first to prove a vital role for STAT proteins in signaling in response to IFNs.

STAT proteins are latent transcription factors that initially exist in the cytosol and then are translocated to the nucleus. STATs were first discovered on the basis of the identification of factors that were capable of binding to the promoters of IFN-inducible genes. There are seven mammalian STAT proteins: STAT1 (316), STAT2 (317), STAT3 (318,319), STAT4 (320,321), STAT5a (322–326), STAT5b (324–327), and STAT6 (328). Table 15 summarizes the cytokines that activate each of the STATs. Although the STATs conserve a reasonable level of homology, STAT5a and STAT5b are unusually closely related: They are 91% identical at the amino acid level (324–327). Although these proteins might be thought to have redundant functions, it is interesting that murine and human STAT5a are more related than are STAT5a and STAT5b within the same species. The same is true for murine and human STAT5b. Together, these data suggest that there has been evolutionary pressure to maintain the difference between STAT5a and STAT5b and that these two proteins, at least in part, have important distinctive actions and may selectively activate different target genes. Indeed, STAT5a and STAT5b knockout mice exhibit a number of major differences in their phenotypes (329–332).

As active STAT proteins exist as dimers, the ability of at least some STATs to form heterodimers [e.g., STAT1 with STAT2 or STAT3; reviewed by Horvath and Darnell (273)] increases the number of different complexes that can form. In addition, further complexity can be generated by the ability of at least some of the STATs to exist in alternatively spliced forms (327,333). Some of these forms are inactive, and if alternative splicing of certain forms were regulated, it would allow for negative regulation.

A schematic of STAT proteins is shown in Fig. 6. The STATs can be divided into two basic groups: those that are longer (STAT2 and STAT6, approximately 850 amino acids) and those that are shorter (STAT1, STAT3, STAT4, STAT5a, and STAT5b, between 750 and 800 amino acids). Interestingly, the chromosomal locations of the STATs suggest three different clusters. Both murine STAT2 and STAT6 are located on chromosome 10; STAT1 and STAT4 are located on chromosome 1; and STAT3, STAT5a, and STAT5b are located on chromosome 11 (334). Correspondingly, human STAT5a and STAT5b are closely positioned on chromosome 17q (327).

In order for STATs to be "activated" and to be able to function as transcriptional activators, a number of cellular events must occur. They must be able to bind to phosphorylated tyrosines, to be tyrosine-phosphorylated, to dimerize, to translocate from the cytosol to the nucleus, to bind to target DNA sequences, and to activate gene expression. A number of conserved structural features common to all STATs help to

TABLE 15. *Phenotypes of mice deficient in type I and type II cytokines, their receptors, Jaks, and STATs*

Type I cytokines and their receptors

γc family

IL-2 (111,483–484)	Normal thymic and peripheral T-cell development. Decreased polyclonal T-cell responses *in vitro* but more normal *in vivo* responses to pathogenic challenges. Autoimmunity with marked changes in levels of serum immunoglobulin isotypes. Ulcerative colitis–like inflammatory bowel disease.
IL-4 (115,116)	Defective Th2 cytokine responses and class switch; defective IgG1 and IgE production.
IL-2/IL-4 (117)	Some features of both IL-2 and IL-4 knockout mice. No gross abnormalities of T-cell development.
IL-7 (71)	Greatly diminished thymic and peripheral T-cell development and B-lymphopoiesis, resulting in profound lymphopenia.
IL-9 (85,87)	No T-cell defect. Defect in pulmonary goblet cell hyperplasia and mastocytosis after challenge with *Schistosoma mansoni* eggs. No defect in eosinophil or granuloma formation.
IL-15 (96)	Defective NK cell development. Defect in CD8 memory T-cell homeostasis.
IL-2Rα (126)	Normal initial lymphoid development but massive enlargement of peripheral lymphoid organs, polyclonal T- and B-cell expansions, and activated T cells, with impaired activation-induced cell death. Autoimmunity with increasing age, including hemolytic anemia and inflammatory bowel disease.
IL-2Rβ (127)	Severe autoimmunity, including autoimmune hemolytic anemia. Death within approximately 3 months. Deregulated T-cell activation. Dysregulated B-cell differentiation and altered immunoglobulin profile.
γc (118,119)	Greatly diminished thymic development, but double negative, double positive, and single positive cells all represented. Age-dependent accumulation of peripheral CD4$^+$ T cells with an activated memory phenotype. Greatly diminished numbers of conventional B cells, although B1 cells are present. No NK cells or γδ cells. Absent gut-associated lymphoid tissue, including Peyer's patches.
IL-4Rα (485)	As in IL-4$^{-/-}$ mice, defective Th2 cytokine responses and class switch; defective IgG1 and IgE production. In addition, inability to expel *Nippostrongylus brasiliensis*, presumably because of defective IL-13 signaling.
IL-7Rα (70)	Greatly diminished thymic and peripheral T-cell development and B-lymphopoiesis, resulting in profound lymphopenia.
IL-15α (95)	Defective NK-cell development. Defect in CD8 memory T-cell homeostasis.
IL-13 (218)	Defective Th2 cell development and defective ability to expel helminths.

βc family

IL-5 (486)	Decreased basal level of eosinophils and defective induction of eosinophils after infectious challenge. Developmental defect in CD5$^+$ B1 cells. Normal antibody and cytotoxic T cell responses.
GM-CSF (487,488)	Normal basal hematopoiesis. Unexpected abnormalities of the lung; abnormal pulmonary homeostasis.
βIL-3 (489)	No defects (because of redundant function of βc).
βc (146,489)	Defective responses to IL-5 and GM-CSF, but normal responses to IL-3 (because of redundant function of βIL-3). Diminished eosinophils: both basal levels and in responses to infectious challenge. Unexpected abnormalities of the lung, characterized by pulmonary proteinosis and reduced phagocytosis by alveolar macrophages. In other words, the defects are a combination of those found in the IL-5– and GM-CSF–deficient mice.
IL-3Rβ and IL-3Rβc double knockout (489)	Same phenotype as in βc-deficient mice, except inability to respond to IL-3.

gp130 family

IL-6 (490)	Impaired acute-phase responses after infection or tissue damage. Decreased numbers of hematopoietic progenitor cells.
gp130 (491,492)	Embryonic lethality. Extreme hypoplastic development of the myocardium; although the ventricular wall is very thin, traveculation within the ventricle chamber is normal. Hematological abnormalities characterized by greatly reduced CFU-Gm and BFU-E. Markedly diminished size of thymus and numbers of thymocytes. Reduced numbers of primordial germ cells in embryonic gonads. Diminished size of placenta.
LIF (493–495)	Decreased hematopoietic progenitor cells. Normal sympathetic neurons but deficient neurotransmitter switch *in vitro*. Defective blastocyst implantation.
LIFRβ (496,497)	Postnatal lethality. Normal hematopoietic and germ cell compartments, but multiple neurological, skeletal, placental, and metabolic defects. The greater severity than found in LIF-deficient mice reflects the fact that LIFRβ is shared by several cytokines, including CNTF, LIF, OSM, and CT1.
CNTF (498)	Progressive atrophy and loss of motor neurons.
CNTFRα (499)	Severe motor neuron deficiency resulting in perinatal mortality. The more severe phenotype than in CNTF-deficient mice was an unexpected discovery and suggests that another cytokine may utilize CNTFRα.
IL-11Rα (500)	Blastocysts can implant but decidualization cannot occur, which is associated with failure of pregnancy. Fetal lethal phenotype.

IL-12 family

IL-12 p40 (501)	Impaired but not completely lacking in their ability to produce IFN-γ and to mount a Th1 response *in vivo*. Elevated secretion of IL-4; normal production of IL-2 and IL-10. Substantially decreased CTL responses.
IL-12Rβ1 (502)	Defective IL-12 signaling. IL-2 but not IL-12 could augment NK activity. Defective IFN-γ production in response to ConA or anti-CD3. Severe defect in Th1 differentiation.

726

Epo, Tpo, G-CSF, and M-CSF family

Epo (503)	Embryonic lethality. Complete block of fetal liver erythropoiesis, resulting in severe anemia, yet normal development of BFU-E and CFU-E progenitor cells.
EpoR (504)	Same as as Epo-deficient mice.
TpoR (505)	Decreased numbers of megakaryocytes and platelets, but other hematopoietic cells are present in normal numbers.
G-CSF (506)	Neutropenia and impaired neutrophil mobility. Diminished numbers of granulocytes and macrophage precursors.
M-CSF (507,508)	Osteopetrosis, absence of teeth. Females are infertile, which suggests an unexpected role for M-CSF.
M-CSF and GM-CSF (5C8)	A combination of defects of both M-CSF and GM-CSF, with osteopetrosis and alveolar proteinosis. Early death from pneumonia.

Type II cytokines and their receptors

IFNAR-1 (509–511)	Normal development. Defective immune defense against most viral infections tested, including lymphocytic choriomeningitis virus, Semliki forest virus, Theiler's virus, and vesicular stomatitis virus. Normal resistance to *Listeria monocytogenes*, *Leishmania major*, *Mycobacterium bovis*, and *Mycobacterium avium*.
IFN-γ (512–514)	Normal lymphoid development. Impaired resistance to *Listeria monocytogenes*, *Leishmania major*, *Mycobacterium bovis*, and *Mycobacterium avium*. Ability to mount curative responses to a number of viruses. CD4$^+$ effector cells default of the Th2 pathway after infection with *Leishmania*. Infection with *Toxoplasmosis gondii* is fatal.
IFNGR-1 (510,511,515)	Normal lymphoid development. Impaired resistance to *Listeria monocytogenes*, *Leishmania major*, *Mycobacterium bovis*, and *Mycobacterium avium*. Ability to mount curative responses to a number of viruses.
IL-10 (258,516)	Normal lymphocyte development and antibody responses. Chronic entercolitis, anemia, and growth retardation. Augmented inflammatory responses.

STATs and Jaks

STAT1 (369,370)	Defective responses to both type I and type II IFNs. Defective response to certain viruses and bacterial antigens.
STAT2 (371)	Defective signaling in response to type I IFNs; interestingly, the defect in not as severe in STAT2-deficient macrophages as it is in STAT2-deficient fibroblasts.
STAT3 (372–375)	Embryonic lethality. Embryos implant but cannot grow. The fact that this phenotype is even more severe than that seen with gp130 suggests a role for STAT3 through a gp130-independent cytokine. By Cre-lox methodology, STAT3 was also selectively targeted in T cells, which exhibit defective IL-2-induced proliferation that correlates with a defect in IL-2-induced IL-2Rα expression; as expected, T cells also exhibit defective signaling in response to IL-6. STAT3-deficient neutrophils and macrophages show defective IL-10 signaling. STAT3 is also essential for normal involution of the mammary epithelium, for wound healing, and for normal hair cycle processes.
STAT4 (376,377)	Defective Th1 development. Essentially the same phenotype as in IL-12–deficient mice, including defective IL-12–mediated boosting of NK cell cytolytic activity.
STAT5a (329,381)	Defective lobuloalveolar development in the mammary gland, a syndrome resulting from defective prolactin signaling. Defective IL-2–induced IL-2Rα expression and associated defects in IL-2–induced T-cell proliferation. Defective superantigen-induced expansion of Vβ8 T cells. Defective antigen-induced recruitment of eosinophils into the lung as well as defective antigen-induced IgG1 production.
STAT5b (330,382)	Defective growth analogous to Laron dwarfism, a disease of defective growth hormone signaling. Defective IL-2–induced IL-2Rα expression. More severe defects in IL-2–induced T-cell proliferation and NK cell proliferation. Defective antigen-induced recruitment of eosinophils into the lung as well as defective antigen-induced IgG1 production. Defective NK cytolytic activity.
STAT5a/STAT5b (331,332,383)	Defective signaling in response to prolactin and growth hormone. Absence of NK cell development. Major defect in T-cell proliferation and TCR signaling. Anemia.
STAT6 (378–380)	Defective Th2 development, essentially the same phenotype as in IL-4–deficient mice. Defective B-cell proliferation.
Jak1 (287)	Perinatal lethality, with defective signaling by gp130-dependent cytokines (IL-6, IL-11, CNTF, OSM, LIF, CT-1, and NNT-1/BSF-3). Defective signaling by γc-dependent cytokines (IL-2, IL-4, IL-7, IL-9, IL-15, IL-21; of these, IL-2 and IL-7 were formally evaluated).
Jak2 (517,518)	Fetal lethality with profound anemia caused by defective signaling in response to erythropoietin.
Jak3 (293–295)	Phenotype is very similar and possibly identical to that of γc-deficient mice. Defective signaling in response to γc-dependent cytokines (IL-2, IL-4, IL-7, IL-9, IL-15, IL-21). Greatly diminished T cells in thymus and spleen, but then age-dependent peripheral expansion of CD4$^+$ T cells. Unlike humans with JAK3 mutations, Jak3-deficient mice have greatly diminished B-cell numbers as well.
Tyk2 (519–521)	Mice lacking Tyk2 exhibit diminished signaling in response to IFN-α/IFN-β and IL-12, but it is not abrogated. Primarily STAT3 activation is diminished, even though STAT1/STAT2 and STAT4, respectively, are the STAT proteins that are primarily activated by IFN-α, IFN-β, and IL-12. In addition, there are diminished responses to IFN-γ and IL-18.

BFU-E, burst-forming unit–erythrocyte; BSF-3, B-lymphocyte–stimulating factor 3; CFU-E, colony-forming unit–erythrocyte; CFU-GM, colony-forming unit–granulocyte-macrophage; CFU-S, colony-forming unit–spleen; CNTF, ciliary neurotrophic factor; CTL, cytotoxic T cell; Epo, erythropoietin; G-CSF, granulocyte colony-stimulating factor; GM-CSF, granulocyte-macrophage colony-stimulating factor; gp, glycoprotein; IFN, interferon; Ig, immunoglobulin; IL, interleukin; Jak, Janus kinase; LIF, leukemia inhibitory factor; M-CSF, macrophage colony-stimulating factor; NK, natural killer; NNT-1, novel neurotrophin 1; OSM, oncostatin M; STAT, signal transducer and activator of transcription; TCR, T-cell receptor; Th, T helper (cell); Tpo, thrombopoietin; Tyk, tyrosine kinase.

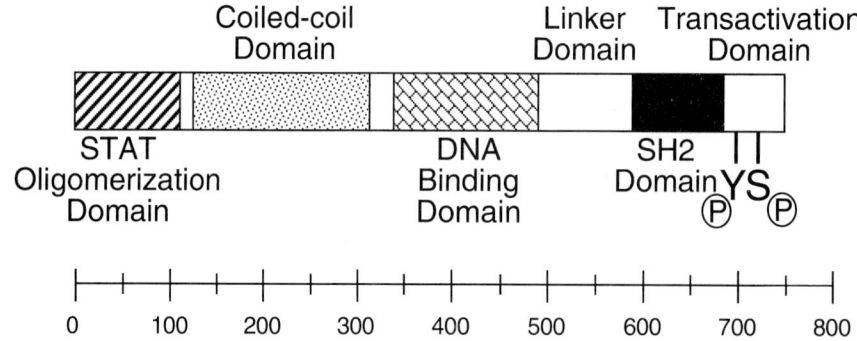

FIG. 6. Architecture of a typical signal transducer and activator of transcription (STAT) protein. Shown are the locations of the following important regions: (1) The N-terminal region has been shown to mediate the interaction of STAT dimers bound to adjacent γ-interferon–activated sequence (GAS) sites (known to be important for STAT1, but presumably true for all STATs), (2) the DNA–binding domain, (3) the SH2 domain that mediates STAT docking on receptors and STAT homodimerization/heterodimerization after tyrosine phosphorylation, and (4) the location of the conserved tyrosine whose phosphorylation allows the SH2-mediated dimerization. At least in STAT1 and STAT3, serine 727, which is C-terminal to the conserved tyrosine, is an important site for phosphorylation. In the case of STAT1, p48 interacts downstream of the STAT dimerization domain. CBP/p300 interacts with two sites: at both the N-terminal and the C-terminal. Although it has been suggested that the region between the DNA-binding domains and the SH2 domain is an SH3 domain, this remains unproven, and no interactions with proline-rich regions have been reported; as a result, this region is not labeled as an SH3 domain. Note that this structure is typical of that for STAT1, STAT3, STAT4, STAT5a, and STAT5b. The main features are conserved in STAT2 and STAT6, but these are approximately 50 to 100 amino acids longer.

explain these functions. These include an SH2 domain, a conserved tyrosine residue, a DNA binding domain, a C-terminal transactivation domain, and an N-terminal STAT tetramerization region. Other regions as well contribute important functions. These special features of STATs are discussed as follows.

Docking of STATs on Receptors or Other Molecules, Tyrosine Phosphorylation of STATs, and STAT Dimerization

Each STAT protein has an SH2 domain that plays two important roles: (a) for receptor docking, as, for example, has been shown for STAT1 docking on IFNGR-1 (335), STAT2 docking on IFNAR-1 (336), STAT3 docking on gp130 (337), STAT5 docking on IL-2Rβ and IL-7Rα (210,338), and STAT6 docking on IL-4Rα (339), and (b) for STAT dimerization, wherein dimerization is mediated by the SH2 of one STAT protein interacting with the conserved phosphorylated tyrosine of another STAT protein. In the case of the IFN-α receptor, no STAT1 docking site on IFNAR-1 or IFNAR-2 has been identified, and it is believed that STAT1 may interact with STAT2 after STAT2 is itself tyrosine phosphorylated (272). It is also possible that STATs can dock on Jaks, given the ability to directly coprecipitate Jaks and STATs (299,312). After docking has occurred, a conserved tyrosine (e.g., tyrosine 701 in STAT1, tyrosine 694 in STAT5a) can be phosphorylated. This phosphorylation is required for the SH2-domain–mediated dimerization of STATs, and the phosphorylation probably occurs while the STAT is docked on the receptor in physical proximity to receptor-associated Jaks.

After STAT protein phosphorylation, the STAT protein dissociates from the receptor, and its dimerization with itself or another STAT is then favored over its reassociation with the cytokine receptor chain. One reason for favoring STAT dimerization over receptor reassociation is that STAT dimerization involves two phosphotyrosine–SH2 interactions (a bivalent interaction), whereas docking on a receptor involves only one (a monovalent interaction). Thus, efficient activation of STATs requires the presence in STATs of a conserved SH2 domain and a critical tyrosine.

It is interesting that whereas IFNGR-1 (335) and IL-7Rα (210) each have only a single STAT docking site (for STAT1 and STAT5, respectively), a number of receptor molecules, including IL-2Rβ (210,338), IL-4Rα (339), gp130 (337), erythropoietin receptor (340), and IL-10Rα (341), have more than one docking site for their respective STATs. The presence of more than one site provides functional redundancy but also potentially could allow the simultaneous activation of two STATs, providing a high local concentration of phosphorylated STATs that facilitates their dimerization.

STAT Nuclear Translocation, DNA Binding, and Tetramerization

After dimerization, the STATs translocate into the nucleus, where they can bind DNA. The mechanism for nuclear translocation has been poorly understood because of the absence of an obvious nuclear localization signal (342). However, it has been shown that tyrosine phosphorylated STAT1 dimers can directly interact with importin-α5, allowing internalization. This suggests that there indeed is a nuclear localization signal that is normally masked, and mutation of Leu407 does not interfere with tyrosine phosphorylation, dimerization, or DNA binding, but it does prevent nuclear localization (342). After its dephosphorylation, nuclear STAT1 is exported to the cytosol by a process that is dependent on the chromosome region maintenance 1 export reporter (343). Thus, both import and export of STAT1 appear to be regulated processes. Whether these considerations generalize to other STAT proteins is unknown and requires additional investigation.

Whereas the majority of STAT dimers directly bind DNA, in the case of IFN-α/β, STAT1-STAT2 heterodimers are formed, and these bind DNA in conjunction with a 48-kDa DNA binding protein; the STAT1-STAT2-p48 complex is known as ISGF3 [reviewed by Horvath and Darnell (273)]. In the case of other STAT dimers, accessory proteins are not required for DNA binding. The motif recognized by ISGF3 complexes is an AGTTTNCNTTTCC motif, known as an for IFN-stimulated response element (ISRE), whereas the other STAT complexes tend to bind more semi-palindromic motifs TTCNmGAA [γ-IFN–activated sequence (GAS) motifs], which reflects their original discovery in the context of IFN-γ (233,271,272). Some variation is allowed in these GAS motifs, as discussed later.

DNA binding is mediated by a DNA-binding domain (339). A series of chimeric STATs were used to delineate a region of approximately 180 amino acids, with two conserved subdomains, as conferring DNA binding specificity. Although many of the STATs can bind to the same motifs, their relative efficiencies can vary considerably, which indicates the fine specificities conferred by the different DNA binding domains. For example, whereas STAT1 homodimers favor a TTCN3GAA motif, STAT6 prefers a TTCN4GAA motif (339). These differences between the different STATs in terms of their DNA binding specificity provide part of the basis to explain why different STATs modulate the expression of nonidentical sets of target genes. The structures of STAT1 and STAT3β bound to DNA have been solved (344,345). The structure of STAT1 (Fig. 7) almost resembles that of a vertebral column, wherein the DNA represents the spinal cord. The N-terminal and coiled-coil domains are spatially the farthest from the DNA, whereas the DNA-binding domain, the linker, and the SH2 domain surround the DNA; the stability is apparently provided by the SH2–phosphotyrosine interaction between the STAT monomers and each STAT monomer–DNA interaction with the DNA, presumably through a "half GAS site" (346).

N-terminal regions can mediate cooperative DNA binding of STAT proteins when multiple STAT binding sites are in close proximity (347,348). Such situations have been shown for the IFN-γ gene, in which multiple STAT binding sites are present (347); this also occurs, for example, in the well-studied IL-2 receptor α chain gene, in which two IL-2 response elements have been described (one in the 5′ regulatory region and one in the first intron), each of which has more than one GAS motif that are closely juxtaposed and are known to

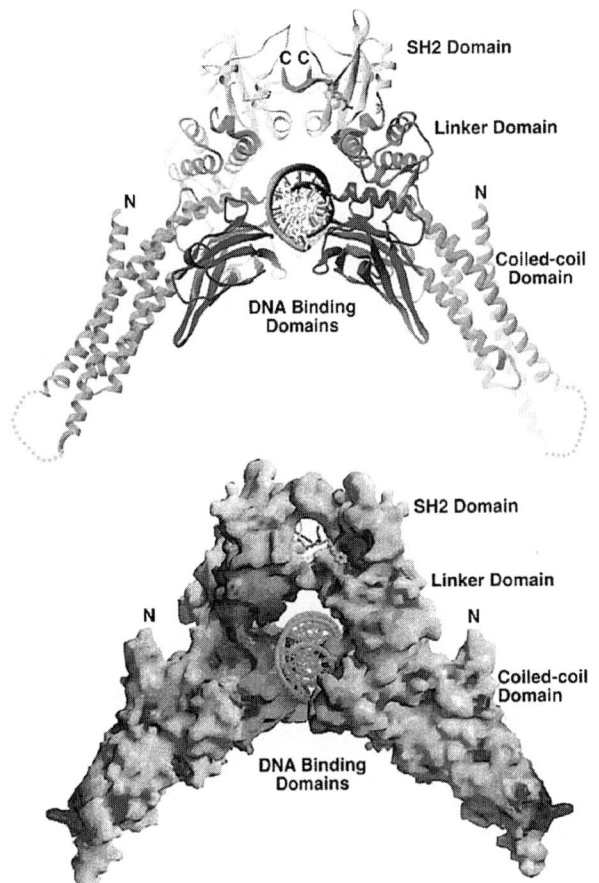

FIG. 7. Three-dimensional structure of a STAT1 bound to deoxyribonucleic acid (DNA). Reproduced from Chen et al. (344), with permission of Dr. Kuriyan and Cell Press.

functionally cooperate for IL-2–induced IL-2Rα transcription (349–352). The N-terminal domains (N-domains) allow formation of STAT tetramers and potentially higher order STAT oligomers (346–348,352a,352b).

Historically, STAT proteins were the first transcription factors that were recognized to be targets for tyrosine phosphorylation. Previously, tyrosine phosphorylation was associated primarily with membrane proximal events. A key feature of STATs is that the tyrosine phosphorylation is in fact associated with a membrane proximal event, but this phosphorylation then allows the rapid dimerization that facilitates nuclear localization and DNA binding. STATs can interact directly with Jaks, as was first shown for STAT5 and Jak3 (299), which provides added support for the idea that STATs are indeed phosphorylated by Jaks and also suggesting that STATs may at times dock on Jaks rather than on receptors.

In addition to the classical tyrosine phosphorylation–mediated dimerization and nuclear translocation, it is now clear that STAT proteins can exist in the nucleus even without being tyrosine phosphorylated (353,354) and, at least in the case of STAT1, are capable of modulating the expression of at least certain genes. It is reasonable to assume that this type of situation will apply to other STAT proteins as well.

Optimal Binding Sites for STATs

Optimal binding motifs for a number of STAT proteins have been determined. For STAT1, STAT3, and STAT4, a TTCC-SGGAA motif was defined (273,347); STAT5a and STAT5b optimally bind a TTCYNRGAA motif; and STAT6 binds a TTCNTNGGAA motif (in which S is C or G, Y is C or T and R is G or A) (346). An unexpected finding was that purified STAT5a expressed in a baculoviral expression system efficiently binds either as a dimer or tetramer, whereas similarly prepared STAT5b binds primarily as a dimer. This suggests a greater efficiency for homotetramerization of STAT5a than for STAT5b (346). Interestingly, whereas dimeric STAT protein binding strongly preferred canonical motifs, the range of sequences recognized by STAT5a tetramers was quite broad, so that very often tetrameric binding was found to occur not in two canonical motifs but rather in the setting of two imperfect motifs or with one canonical motif that appeared to be separated from a "half GAS motif" that comprises, for example, the "TTC" or "GAA." The optimal inter–GAS motif spacing appears to be 5 to 7, although some naturally occurring sites, such as that in the PRRIII element of the IL-2Rα gene, have a spacing of 11 (346). The presence of suboptimal GAS motifs spaced at appropriate distances to allow tetrameric binding has been suggested to allow greater specificity through cooperative binding of STAT oligomers. It is indeed interesting that a number of STAT-regulated genes, such as bcl-x and Pim-1, have such half GAS motifs located at appropriate distances from the GAS motifs that had been recognized, which suggests that tetrameric binding is involved in the regulation of these genes.

Transcriptional Activation by STATs

An area of considerable interest is how STAT proteins trigger the initiation of transcription. In addition to tyrosine phosphorylation, some STATs can be phosphorylated on serine. For example, for STAT1 and STAT3, it has been shown that serine phosphorylation is required for full activity (355,356), whereas STAT2 is not serine-phosphorylated (273). The phosphorylation site in STAT1 and STAT3 (Ser 727) is located in the C-terminal region of the protein, within the C-terminal transactivation domain (357,358). Interestingly, the region of Ser 727 resembles a MAP kinase recognition site, and one study has indicated that MAP kinase activity is required for IFN-α/β–induced gene expression (359). Ser 727 is important for the interaction of STAT1 with MCM5, a member of the minichromosome maintenance family of proteins; this interaction presumably is important for maximal transcriptional activation (360). Interestingly, STAT5a and STAT5b are also targets for serine phosphorylation, but the motif is different from that found in STAT1 and STAT3, and it is unclear that this phosphorylation is important for transcriptional activation.

STAT1 has also been shown to be a target for arginine methylation (361), a posttranslational modification that is essential for transcriptional activation. Inhibition of this methylation results in impaired gene induction and antiproliferative responses to IFN-α/β.

In addition to this regulated modification of the STAT proteins, considerable interest has focused on the ability of STATs to interact with other factors. As noted previously, STAT1-STAT2 heterodimers bind DNA only in the context of a DNA binding protein. The STAT1-STAT2-p48 complex is known as ISGF3 (273), and it is now clear that the region between amino acids 150 and 250 of STAT1 is required for the interaction with p48 (273). STAT1 has been reported to interact with and synergize with Sp1 for transcriptional activation in the intercellular adhesion molecule 1 gene (362). An alternatively spliced shorter form of STAT3, denoted STAT3β, was found to associate with c-Jun in a yeast two-hybrid analysis and that this interaction enhanced transcriptional activity of a reporter construct (363). Moreover, both STAT1 and STAT2 have been shown to interact with the potent transcriptional activators CBP/p300 (364–366), and these co-activators have been shown to interact with other STAT proteins as well. In the case of STAT1, this interaction appears to be mediated by interactions involving both the N-terminal and C-terminal regions of STAT1 and the CREB and E1A binding regions of CBP, respectively (365). STAT5a has been shown to associate with the glucocorticoid receptor (367). In addition, the well-defined IL-2 response element in the IL-2Rα gene requires not only STAT5 binding but also the binding of Elf-1, an Ets family transcription factor, to a nearby site (349). Thus, active STAT complexes appear to involve the coordination of STAT proteins with other factors. The co-repressor silencing mediator for retinoic acid receptor and thyroid hormone receptor (SMRT) was identified as a potential STAT5-binding partner. SMRT binds to both STAT5a and STAT5b and potentially plays a negative regulatory role related to the action of STAT5 proteins (368).

Specificity of STATs

In the analysis of STAT protein activation in response to different cytokines, it was observed that, in an analogy to the Jaks, the same STATs were induced by multiple cytokines. The degree of specificity conferred by the different STATs was therefore unclear. There are now published reports on at least the phenotypes of mice lacking expression of each of the seven STAT proteins. STAT1 knockout mice exhibit defects that are very selective for the actions of type I and type II IFNs, which suggests that STAT1 is vital only for the actions of IFNs, even though a variety of other cytokines have been reported to activate STAT1 (369,370). Although it is possible that STAT1 plays an important but redundant role for at least some of these other cytokines, the phenotype of STAT1-deficient mice indicates a need for caution in the interpretation of in vitro experiments that employ very high concentrations of cytokines and cell lines expressing very large numbers of receptors, because it is possible that these experiments may not always yield physiologically relevant patterns of STAT activation. STAT2-deficient mice exhibit defects consistent with selective inactivation of IFN-α/β signaling (371). STAT3-deficient mice die *in utero,* and lethality is evident early in embryogenesis (372). Interestingly, the embryos implant, but they exhibit defective development and growth. With Cre-loxP methods, STAT3 has also been selectively deleted within specific lineages. Mice that lack STAT3 in T cells (373) have normal lymphoid development but exhibit a defect in IL-2–induced IL-2Rα expression, which is somewhat analogous to what is seen in STAT5a and STAT5b-deficient mice (see later discussion). Neutrophils and macrophages lacking STAT3 exhibit defective signaling to IL-10, and it is known that STAT3 is important for the normal involution of the mammary epithelium, for wound healing, and for normal hair growth cycle (374,375). STAT4-deficient mice exhibit a phenotype indistinguishable from that of IL-12–deficient mice (i.e., defective Th1 development), a finding consistent with the observation that STAT4 is activated only by IL-12 (376,377). Analogously, STAT6-deficient mice exhibit a phenotype indistinguishable from that of IL-4–deficient mice (i.e., defective Th2 development) (378–380), in keeping with the observation that STAT6 is activated only by IL-4 and the closely related cytokine, IL-13. Interestingly, mice lacking STAT5a exhibit a defect in prolactin-mediated effects, including defective lobuloalveolar proliferation (381), whereas mice lacking STAT5b have defective growth similar to that found in Laron dwarfism (382). Thus, although STAT5a and STAT5b appear to always be coordinately induced, it is clear that these similar STATs cannot substitute for each other and have distinctive actions. In addition to these defects, both STAT5a-deficient and STAT5b-deficient mice have defects in T-cell development and signaling (329,330). STAT5a-deficient mice have diminished numbers of splenocytes and exhibit a defect in IL-2–induced IL-2Rα expression (329). STAT5b-deficient mice have similar defects but also have diminished numbers of thymocytes (330). The most dramatic finding is that these mice have a major defect in the proliferation of freshly isolated splenocytes (330). In accordance with the observation that the NK population of cells has the greatest degree of proliferation among fresh splenocytes, NK cytolytic activity is also decreased in these animals. As expected, STAT5a/STAT5b double-knockout mice have a more severe phenotype, characterized by a greater defect in T-cell proliferation as well as no development of NK cells (331). Presumably, this latter phenotype is related to defective IL-15–dependent STAT5 activation. Another dramatic defect seen in double-knockout mice is the severe anemia that develops in the STAT5a/STAT5b double-knockout mice (383).

STATs Are Evolutionarily Old

Just as *Drosophila* has a Jak, there is a *Drosophila* STAT, denoted as either DSTAT or STAT92E (384,385). The existence of Jaks and STAT proteins in lower organisms suggest that the system is evolutionarily old, and these other systems may help to elucidate some of the subtleties of this sys-

tem. In addition, a STAT has been identified in *Dictyostelium* that recognizes the sequence TTGA (386). This STAT has highest sequence similarity to STAT5b and can bind mammalian ISREs (386). Interestingly, *Saccharomyces cerevisiae* do not appear to have STATs, inasmuch as no DNA sequence encoding SH2 domains have been identified in the entire *S. cerevisiae* genome.

What Are the Functions of STATs?

Because STAT proteins translocate to the nucleus and bind DNA, it is self-evident that they can bind to the regulatory regions of the target genes and influence transcription. Although STAT proteins are generally assumed to be activators of transcription, at least in the case of the *c-Myc* gene, STAT1 has been shown to also be capable of functioning as a transcriptional repressor (387). Presumably, STAT proteins can negatively regulate the expression of other genes as well.

STAT proteins were originally discovered on the basis of the study of IFN-inducible genes as part of studies intended to understand the cellular differentiation events that lead to development of the antiviral state. However, it is quite evident that, rather than being solely differentiation factors, STAT proteins can contribute to mitogenic/proliferative responses that typify hematopoietic and immunological cytokines, such as IL-3, IL-5, GM-CSF, IL-2, IL-4, and IL-7, and also can be important as survival factors. Indeed, a variety of observations indicate roles in proliferation partially reviewed by Leonard and O'Shea (272): As noted previously, a number of *in vitro* systems have demonstrated that viruses or viral oncogenes are associated with activated Jak-STAT pathways, which suggests a role for STATs in cellular transformation. Second, there is diminished proliferation in a number of the STAT knockout mice that have been analyzed. For example, STAT4-deficient cells exhibit diminished proliferation to IL-12 (376,377), whereas STAT6-deficient mice exhibit diminished proliferation in response to IL-4 (378,379), and STAT5-deficient mice have diminished T-cell proliferation in response to IL-2 (329,330). However, it is not clear that the effect of STAT proteins on proliferation is always through a direct mechanism. For example, STAT6-deficient mice exhibit decreased IL-4Rα expression, which suggests that the effect on proliferation may be indirect. Similarly, mutation of the key tyrosines in IL-2Rβ that results in decreased proliferation also results in decreased IL-2Rα expression (388). Thus, although there are strong data suggesting a role for a number of STATs in proliferation, in at least some cases, the effect may be indirect, resulting from regulating the level of receptor components. STAT5a and STAT5b appear to regulate bcl-xL induction, indicating their ability to affect cell survival (383). Finally, it is interesting that STAT1 has been linked to cell growth arrest and induction of the CDK inhibitor p21$^{\text{WAF1/CIP1}}$ (389) and that activation of STAT1 occurs in thanatophoric dysplasia type II dwarfism as the result of a mutant fibroblast growth factor receptor (FGFR3) (390). In this chondrodysplasia, the mutant FGFR3 induces nuclear translocation of STAT1, expression of p21$^{WAF1/CIP1}$, and growth arrest, which suggests a possible relationship to the disease. Thus, different STATs may potentially mediate either growth expansion or growth arrest. Moreover, STATs may potentially play other types of roles as well. For example, STAT3 has been reported to serve as an adapter to couple PI3K to the IFNAR-1 component of type I IFN receptors (391). A more complete understanding of the actions of the different STAT proteins should in part be achieved when investigators have collectively compiled a complete list of the genes that are regulated by each STAT. Progress in this area has been made for a number of cytokines but particularly for the IFNs (240). Of importance, however, is that not all cytokine signals are dependent on STATs, as has been well demonstrated—for example, in the case of IFNs, in which there are STAT1-independent IFN signals (392).

Do Other Proteins Bind to γ-Interferon–Activated Sequence Motifs?

Although additional STAT proteins have not been identified, one non-STAT protein that binds to GAS motifs has been discovered. The bcl-6 gene is frequently found to be mutated or to have undergone translocations in diffuse large cell (B-cell) lymphomas. Interestingly, Bcl-6 binds to GAS motifs capable of binding STAT6 and specifically can inhibit IL-4 action (393). These data suggest that dysregulated IL-4/IL-13 signaling may contribute to the development of these lymphomas. Furthermore, mice lacking expression of Bcl-6 exhibit defective germinal center formation, which suggests that formation of germinal centers is dependent on Bcl-6-regulated (presumably negative) control of certain STAT-responsive genes (393).

OTHER LATENT TRANSCRIPTION FACTORS AS EXAMPLES OF CYTOPLASMIC-TO-NUCLEAR SIGNALING (NFκB, NF-AT, AND SMADS)

One of the exciting features of STAT proteins is that they exist in an inactive form in the cytosol and then are rapidly translocated to the nucleus. The rapid activation within minutes of signals from cell membrane to nuclear DNA binding makes the STAT acronym seem very appropriate, in view of the urgency associated with physician's "STAT" emergency orders in clinical medicine. The rapid activation of STAT proteins is somewhat analogous to several other systems (394). In the case of NFκB, there is rapid nuclear translocation, but this uses a completely different mechanism from STATs. In contrast to STAT proteins, for which the tyrosine phosphorylation of the STATs is an initiator of nuclear translocation, for NFκB it is the serine phosphorylation and/or ubiquitination of IκB that results in its dissociation and/or destruction, allowing the release and translocation of NFκB (395–397). A third example of cytosolic-to-nuclear translocation occurs with nuclear factor of activated T-cell (NF-AT) family proteins (398,399), which are vital for regulating transcription

of a number of cytokines, including IL-2, IL-4, and GM-CSF. In this case, NF-AT is translocated to the nucleus, where it associates with AP-1 family proteins to form a functional complex. The activation of calcineurin and the dephosphorylation of NF-AT allow its nuclear translocation. A fourth example of cytosolic-to-nuclear translocation occurs with the Sma- and Mad-related proteins (SMAD) that mediate transforming growth factor β signaling. In this case, the phosphorylation is on serine, and the kinase is intrinsic to the receptor, but there are a number of basic parallel features in terms of the rapid activation of latent transcription factors after binding of a growth factor. Thus, multiple different types of mechanisms, each involving phosphorylation or dephosphorylation, have evolved to allow nuclear-to-cytoplasmic translocation of latent transcription factors (400).

OTHER SUBSTRATES FOR JANUS KINASES

As Jaks are potent cytosolic tyrosine kinases, it is immediately evident that the activation of STATs may not be the sole function of Jaks. Various data indicate that Jaks have the ability to phosphorylate tyrosine on receptors where STAT proteins dock, as well as the ability to phosphorylate STATs. There are also in vitro data that indicate that Jaks can phosphorylate tyrosines on receptor chains other than those that are docking sites for STATs. For example, in overexpression experiments in COS cells, Jak1 appears to phosphorylate IL-2Rβ not only on tyrosines 392 and 510, which are needed for docking STAT proteins, but also on tyrosine 338, which is the docking site for Shc (338). Simultaneous mutation of all three of these tyrosines abrogates proliferation, which suggests that the molecules that dock on these tyrosines couple to vital pathways. Thus, Jaks may facilitate the recruitment of additional substrates to the receptors; in addition, it is well known that Jaks can phosphorylate themselves (autophosphorylate) or transphosphorylate other Jaks. Because Jaks contain a number of conserved tyrosine residues, it is possible that some of these are phosphorylated and serve as docking sites for important signaling molecules. Multiple other molecules, including the signal-transducing adapter molecule (401) and the p85 subunit of PI3K, are potentially phosphorylated by Jaks (402).

OTHER SIGNALING MOLECULES IMPORTANT FOR CYTOKINES

Other Tyrosine Kinases besides Janus Kinases

In addition to their activation of Jaks, a number of cytokines can activate Src family kinases. For example, IL-2 can activate p56 Lck (403,404) in T cells and p59 Fyn and p53/p56 Lyn in B-cell lines (405,406). The activation of some of these kinases has been reported to be mediated by association with the A region of IL-2Rβ. Another tyrosine kinase, Syk, has been reported to associate with the S region of IL-2Rβ (407). However, the significance of these interactions is less clear than that for Jaks. First, cells lacking Lck can vigorously proliferate in response to IL-2 (408,409). Second, when the A region is deleted, proliferation still occurs, albeit at a lower level than seen with wild-type IL-2Rβ (410). However, Y338, which is required for the recruitment of Shc, is in the A region and is required for normal proliferation (338). Thus, it is possible that the decrease in proliferation associated with deletion of the A region is related more to the loss of Y338 than to the loss of association of Lck. Moreover, in IL-2R$\beta^{-/-}$ mice reconstituted with an IL-2Rβ A-region mutant, proliferation is increased rather than diminished (411). Additional investigation is necessary to clarify the role of activation of Src family kinases by IL-2 and for other cytokines as well. The significance of the Syk interaction also remains unclear. Because both Syk and Jak1 associate with the S region of IL-2Rβ, mutations that delete the S region simultaneous prevent both associations, making it impossible if the effect is caused solely by a loss of one of these. The fact that Syk-deficient mice exhibit normal IL-2 proliferation (412) further suggests that Syk may not play an important role in IL-2–induced proliferation. Analogously, the G-CSF receptor forms a complex with Lyn and Syk (413), but, again, Syk-deficient mice do not exhibit a defect in G-CSF signaling (412). With regard to other kinases, β_c has been reported to interact with Src family kinases (414). Gp130 has been reported to associate with a number of other kinases, including Btk, Tec, and Fes (415–417), and IL-4Rα has been shown to interact with Fes (418). Overall, outside of the essential role of Jaks, relatively little is known about the significance of other tyrosine kinases in cytokine signaling. It is possible that they play important roles that have been difficult to evaluate, perhaps in part because of the existence of redundant pathways.

Insulin Receptor Substrate Proteins

IRS-1 was originally noted to be a tyrosine-phosphorylated substrate of the insulin receptor (419). Interestingly, both insulin and IL-4 could induce tyrosine phosphorylation of an IRS-1–like molecule in hematopoietic cells, and 32D myeloid progenitor cells lack IRS-1 and could signal in response to insulin or IL-4 only when they were transfected with IRS-1 (420). Both the insulin receptor and IL-4Rα proteins contain NPXY sequences that are important for IRS-1 or IRS-2 binding; in IL-4Rα, this is contained within a sequence called the I4R motif (421).

Other cytokines have subsequently been shown to activate IRS-1 or IRS-2 or both. For example, growth hormone can induce phosphorylation of IRS-1 (422) and IRS-2 (423), IFN-γ and LIF induce phosphorylation of IRS-2 (423), and the γ_c-dependent cytokines, IL-2, IL-7, and IL-15, can induce tyrosine phosphorylation of IRS-1 and IRS-2 in T cells (424). The significance of these findings remain unclear, because 32D cells (which constitutively express γ_c) can proliferative vigorously in response to IL-2 when they are transfected with only IL-2Rβ (408), whereas, as noted previously, in these same cells, IL-4 responsiveness requires coexpression of both IL-4Rα and IRS-1. Thus, IRS proteins appear to have differential importance for different cytokines. Because IRS proteins have a large number of phosphotyrosine docking sites, particularly for the p85 subunit of PI3K, they presumably serve to recruit important accessory molecules, and perhaps these differ in importance for mediating proliferation in response to different cytokines.

Phosphatidylinositol 3-Kinase

PI3K is a lipid kinase that consists of an 85-kDa regulatory subunit and a 110-kDa catalytic subunit (425). PI3K phosphorylation and activation can be induced by a number of cytokines (426–429), and the use of inhibitors, such as wortmannin or LY294002, has demonstrated its importance in signaling for at least certain cytokines. IRS-1 has multiple docking sites for PI3K (YXXM motifs), and thus for some cytokines, such as IL-4, the association of IRS-1 might be the mechanism by which PI3K can be recruited.

The Ras/Mitogen-Activated Protein Kinase Pathway

Another major signaling pathway for a number of cytokines is the Ras/MAP kinase pathway (430). This pathway presumably is used by cytokines whose receptors recruit the Shc adaptor molecule, which in turn mediates the recruitment of Grb2 and Sos, eventually leading to the activation of Ras. In turn, Ras couples to the MAP kinase pathway through a well-established signaling cascade. Certain cytokines, such as IL-2, appear to use this pathway, whereas others, such as IL-4, do not. Thus, like other pathways, this pathway is differentially important, depending on the cytokine that is being used.

DOWN-MODULATION OF CYTOKINE SIGNALS

Much of the preceding discussion has centered on the mechanisms by which cytokines induce signals. However, the mechanisms by which cytokine signals can be terminated are also extremely important. There are multiple levels at which negative regulation can occur. In broad mechanistic terms, these include (a) a balance among the production (transcriptional and translational control) of the cytokine, its receptor, or downstream signaling molecules and the degradation of these same molecules and (b) regulation of the activation state of the receptor and downstream signaling molecules.

Transcriptional control of cytokine production is a widely used mechanism. Many T cell–derived cytokines such as IL-2, IL-3, and IL-4 are produced only by activated T cells, and their production is lost with the loss of activation. IL-15 provides an example in which translation of the protein is carefully regulated, in part by the existence of multiple upstream ATGs (93). Most cytokine receptor chains are constitutive, but some, such as IL-21R and IL-2Rβ, are regulated in part by signals that act through the T-cell receptor. The most regulated receptor chain may be the IL-2 receptor

α chain, whose expression is absent on resting lymphocytes but strongly induced after stimulation with antigens, mitogens, and certain cytokines; however, the transcriptional/translational control of most cytokine receptors has been poorly studied.

Because phosphorylation events are vital for the creation of phosphotyrosine docking sites, dephosphorylation is an obvious mechanism of control. Indeed, two tyrosine phosphatases, Shp-1 (formerly also known as SHP, HCP, SH-PTP1, and PTP1C) and Shp-2 (formerly also known as Syp and PTP1D) have been shown to play roles related to cytokine signaling (431,432). The most well-studied example is Shp-1, mutations of which cause the motheaten (*me*) and viable motheaten (*me*v) phenotypes in mice (433,434). The viable motheaten mouse has a less severe phenotype that is associated with increased numbers of erythroid progenitor cells and hyperresponsiveness to erythropoietin (Epo) (435), which suggests that Shp-1 might normally diminish responsiveness to Epo. Indeed, it was demonstrated that Shp-1 binds directly to the Epo receptor when Y429 is phosphorylated (436). This tyrosine is located in a "negative" regulatory region of the Epo receptor and, when it is mutated, Epo-responsive cells can grow in lower concentrations of Epo. After Shp-1 binding to Y429, dephosphorylation and inactivation of Jak2 is facilitated (436). Thus, the negative regulation of Epo signaling appears to be at the level of a receptor-dependent inactivation of a Jak. Shp-1 has also been shown to interact with β_c and to mediate diminished IL-3–induced signaling (437) and to be able to associate with both Tyk-2 (438) and Jak2 (439).

Shp-2 has generally been thought to be more of an "activating" phosphatase; it is therefore interesting that it has also been shown that it can interact with Jak1, Jak2, and Tyk2 (440). In addition to the presumed dephosphorylation of Jaks by phosphatases, STAT proteins appear to be regulated at the level of tyrosine dephosphorylation (441). Finally, another type of phosphatase, the lipid phosphatases, known as Sh2-containing inositol 5′-phosphatase (SHIP) and SHIP2, can act as negative regulators of cytokine signals (442).

In addition to dephosphorylation, another mode of negative regulation is by degradation. In addition to the degradation of receptor molecules, STAT1 is regulated by the ubiquitin-proteasome pathway (443). Finally, it is possible that regulation also can occur at the level of alternative splicing. In this regard, alternatively spliced versions of some of the STATs (273,327,333) have been reported.

THE CIS/SOCS/JAB/SSI FAMILY OF INHIBITORY ADAPTER PROTEINS

In the 1990s, an interesting class of proteins that modulate the actions of cytokines was discovered. The prototype molecule was discovered in 1995 and was named CIS, for cytokine-inducible, SH2-containing protein (444). CIS was observed to be rapidly induced by a variety of cytokines, including IL-2, IL-3, GM-CSF, and erythropoietin; to physically associate with both the β_c and erythropoietin receptors; and to

be a negative regulator of cytokine action (444,445). Subsequently, researchers identified a related protein, variably denoted SOCS-1 (suppressor of cytokine signal 1), JAB (Jak-binding protein), and SSI-1 (STAT-induced STAT inhibitor 1), that could negatively regulate the activity of other cytokines, including IL-6 (446–448) and IL-2. Interestingly, this protein could associate with Jak family kinases, whereas this function has not been reported for CIS. A total of eight CIS/SOCS/JAB/SSI family members that collectively regulate signals in response to multiple cytokines have been identified (449,450). These proteins are now most typically denoted as SOCS proteins. They share an SH2 domain and a region known as a SOCS box. Additional SOCS box–containing proteins lack SH2 domains. The knowledge of the range of actions mediated by these proteins is still evolving, primarily on the basis of multiple-knockout mice that have been created. Mice with knockouts for each of the SOCS proteins are being prepared, alone and in combination. Interestingly, the analysis of SOCS1$^{-/-}$ mice revealed an essential role for this protein in thymocyte differentiation, and that these mice die at a very young age as the result of augmented responsiveness to IFN-γ. SOCS3$^{-/-}$ mice reveal an important role for this protein in erythropoiesis in the fetal liver [reviewed by Kovanen and Leonard (451)].

PIAS PROTEINS

Protein inhibitor of activated STAT (PIAS) proteins are other negative regulators of cytokine actions (452–456); PIAS-1 is an inhibitor of STAT1 binding activity, and PIAS-3 is a similar inhibitor of STAT3 binding activity. Two other members, PIASx (which has both α and β splice variants) and PIASy, have also been described, and the interactions are not restricted to the context of STAT inhibition. For example, PIASy is a nuclear matrix–associated small ubiquitin-related modifier (SUMO) E3 ligase (a ubiquitin-related protein) that can repress the activity of the Wnt-responsive transcription factor LEF1 (455). PIASy coexpression results in the covalent modification of LEF1 by SUMO. Thus, as a class, PIAS proteins have more than one type of action, and it is interesting to consider whether STAT proteins might be targets for SUMO-based modification.

TH1/TH2 CELLS: THE T HELPER PARADIGM

Th1 and Th2 cells were originally described on the basis of the patterns of cytokine production by murine T cells (457), but the paradigm was extended to human cells as well (458–462). Th1 cells secrete IL-2, IFN-γ, and lymphotoxin, whereas Th2 cells produce IL-4, IL-5, IL-6, IL-9, IL-10, and IL-13. The cytokines produced by Th1 and Th2 cells are sometimes referred to as type 1 and type 2 cytokines (for Th1 and Th2 cytokines); unfortunately, this results in potential confusion, because IL-4 is a type I (four–α helical bundle) cytokine that is functionally a type 2 cytokine (in that it is produced by Th2 cells).

In humans, the Th1 and Th2 patterns are similar, but not all the cytokines are as tightly restricted (458–462). IFN-γ is the cytokine most reliably produced by Th1 cells, whereas IL-4, IL-5, and IL-9 are produced by Th2 cells. In both species, certain cytokines, including IL-3 and GM-CSF, are produced by both Th1 and Th2 cells. The Th1/Th2 division of T helper cells has proved useful in correlating the function of Th1 cells with cell-mediated immunity (inflammatory responses, delayed-type hypersensitivity, and cytotoxicity) and that of Th2 cells with humoral immunity. Of the Th2 cytokines, IL-4 is particularly important in driving IgE responses. Because the division of Th1 and Th2 cells is not always perfect, when cells produce both Th1 and Th2 cytokines, they are called Th0 cells, whereas Th3 cells produce high levels of transforming growth factor β.

A number of murine and human physiological and disease states correspond to Th1 or Th2 responses/patterns [reviewed in detail by Mosmann and Sad (458), Abbas et al. (459), Lucey et al. (460), and Romagnani (462)]. In general, among infectious diseases, resistance to intracellular bacteria, fungi, and protozoa is linked to mounting a successful Th1 response. Th1 responses can also be linked to pathological conditions, such as arthritis, colitis, and other inflammatory states. Effective protection against extracellular pathogens, such as helminths, requires a Th2 response, and the enhanced humoral immunity may result in successful neutralization of pathogens by the production of specific antibodies. In humans, Th1 and Th2 cytokines each have dominant roles in the different types of lesions found in leprosy: Th1 cytokines dominate in tuberculoid lesions, and Th2 cytokines dominate in lepromatous lesions. In HIV, a simple Th1/Th2 pattern does not exist. The situation has been complicated by the fact that IL-4 expression is relatively transient, whereas IL-10 expression is more sustained. This has led to the thought that IL-10 and IL-12 may be the most important cytokines controlling disease progression in AIDS (460). Interestingly, Th0 and Th2 cells seem to be more susceptible to HIV than are Th1 cells, which potentially explains why the virus can persist even in the absence of Th1 cells. Overall, human diseases that are characterized primarily by Th1 responses include Hashimoto's thyroiditis, Graves' ophthalmopathy, multiple sclerosis, type 1 diabetes mellitus, Crohn's disease, rheumatoid arthritis, lyme arthritis, reactive arthritis, acute allograft rejection, unexplained recurrent abortions, *Helicobacter pylori*–induced peptide ulcer, and sarcoidosis. In contrast, diseases characterized primarily by Th2 responses include Omenn syndrome, vernal conjunctivitis, atopic disorders, progressive systemic sclerosis, cryptogenic fibrosing alveolitis, chronic periodontitis, progression to AIDS in HIV infection, and tumor progression (462).

It is believed that Th1 and Th2 cells are derived from a common precursor (Thp cells). IL-12 is the major driving force to induce Th1 differentiation, whereas IL-4 induces Th2 differentiation. In accordance with these findings, as discussed earlier, STAT4-deficient mice are defective in IL-12 signaling and exhibit a defect in Th1 development. Lineage commitment to Th1 and Th2 is now better understood in terms of transcription factors, whereby T-bet and ERM are transcription factors influencing Th1 commitment and c-Maf and GATA-3 are specific for Th2 cells [reviewed by Okamura and Rao (463) and Ho and Glimcher (464)]. The process by which the differentiated T helper cells produce cytokines is one in which the genetic loci need to become competent for efficient transcription. This process can be thought of as involving an initiation phase, dependent on STAT proteins; a commitment phase, mediated by factors such as T-bet and GATA3; and a final stabilization phase, in which transcription is maintained without further stimulation (465). Part of this process involves chromatin remodeling, a process that involves histone-modifying enzymes as well as specific transcription factors. Such a process allows coordinated transcription—for example, of the IL-4/IL-13 locus (465).

In addition to the major differences between Th1 and Th2 cells in the production of IFN-γ, it was observed that T helper subsets differed markedly in their abilities to respond to IFN-γ, whereby the proliferation of Th2 clones was inhibited and that of Th1 clones was not (466). Interestingly, the unresponsiveness of Th1 clones resulted from the absence of IFNGR-2, whereas Th2 cells express IFNGR-2 (467,468). Thus, Th1 cells produce IFN-γ and can thereby inhibit the proliferation of Th2 cells. As noted previously, IL-12 is the major inducer of Th1 cells. It is therefore interesting that Th2 cells do not respond to IL-12, and it is now clear that this extinction of IL-12 signaling results from their loss of expression of the IL-12Rβ2 subunit of the IL-12 receptor (469). Apparently, IL-4 inhibits IL-12Rβ2 expression, whereas IFN-γ overcomes this inhibition (469). The ability of mice to survive infections is critically linked to the T helper patterns of cytokines. For example, the ability to survive toxoplasmosis is strictly depend on IFN-γ/IL-12 production (a Th1 pattern) (461).

DISEASES OF CYTOKINE RECEPTORS AND RELATED MOLECULES

Range of Cytokine-Related Causes of Severe Combined Immunodeficiency Disease

As detailed previously, mutations in the common cytokine receptor γ chain, γ_c, causes a profound immunodeficiency known as XSCID, a T$^-$B$^+$NK$^-$ SCID. This indicates that XSCID is a disease of defective cytokine signaling and suggests that defects in molecules in downstream signaling pathways might also result in clinical disease. Indeed, it was directly confirmed that mutations in Jak3 also resulted in T$^-$B$^+$NK$^-$ SCID. Because γ_c-dependent cytokines activate primarily STAT5a and STAT5b as signaling molecules downstream of the Jaks, it remains an open question as to whether mutations in these STAT proteins also cause human disease. Although it might have been assumed that mutations in either STAT5a or STAT5b alone might not cause a phenotype because of their similarity and potential redundancy, mice lacking either STAT5a or STAT5b alone do have distinctive phenotypes. For example, STAT5a-deficient female mice exhibit a prolactin-related deficiency (381), whereas STAT5b-deficient mice have defective growth and a syndrome similar to that found in Laron dwarfism (382). Moreover, both STAT5a and STAT5b-deficient mice exhibit defects in T-cell proliferation and NK cytolytic activity. Mice lacking both STAT5a and STAT5b have an even more profound defect, with more defective T-cell proliferation and a lack of NK cell development (331). Because STAT5a and STAT5b are tandem genes on human chromosome 17, it seems likely that if both genes were simultaneously inactivated—for example, by a deletion of the STAT5a/STAT5b region of chromosome 17—that a SCID phenotype would be observed.

It can be predicted that human immunodeficiencies might also result from mutations in some of the cytokines whose receptors contain γ_c or from mutations in other components of the receptors for these cytokines. Indeed, as noted previously, patients with IL-2 deficiency exhibit a SCID-like syndrome, characterized by inadequate function of their T cells, and an unusual immunodeficiency has been found to result from a mutation in IL-2Rα (219). One patient with defective IL-2Rβ expression also had an immunodeficiency syndrome characterized by autoimmunity (470), somewhat analogous to the situation in IL-2Rβ-deficient mice. Because mutations in IL-7Rα in humans cause T$^-$B$^+$NK$^+$ SCID (113), mutations in IL-7 might be predicted to cause a similar syndrome. The one major difference might be that IL-7–deficient humans might not be capable of receiving a successful bone marrow transplant if stromal IL-7 is required for the graft. In any case, such patients have not yet been identified. In view of the defective NK cell development and CD8$^+$ memory T-cell development in IL-15– and IL-15Rα–deficient mice, it is likely that these types of defects would also occur in humans lacking either of these proteins. However, such individuals have not yet been identified. Although IL-9 transgenic mice develop lymphomas (81), IL-9–deficient mice exhibit defects related to mast cells and mucus production rather than lymphoid defects. Thus, defects related to the IL-9 system seem unlikely as causes of SCID. At least for the moment, defects in expression of IL-2, IL-2Rα, IL-2Rβ, IL-7Rα, γ_c, and Jak3 are the only cytokine-related mutations that have been found to cause SCID. More time is necessary to determine whether mutations in other cytokines, cytokine receptors, Jaks, or STATs can also cause SCID.

Defects in the Ability to Clear Mycobacterial Infections

A number of immunodeficiencies in which affected individuals cannot properly clear mycobacterial infections have been characterized. These have also turned out to be diseases of defective cytokine signaling. Mutations have been found in the components of either IL-12 itself or in the IFN or IL-12/IL-23 receptors, specifically in either the gene encoding the p40 subunit of IL-12 (which, as noted previously, is also a com-

ponent of IL-23) (471), in IL-12Rβ1 (which, as noted previously, is a component of both the IL-12 and IL-23 receptors) (472), or in either the IFNGR1 or IFNGR2 components of IFN-γ receptors (473,474). The critical role of IL-12 for Th1 cell–mediated differentiation and production of IFN-γ provides the explanation for finding similar clinical syndromes in humans lacking the p40, IL-12Rβ1, IFNGR1, or IFNGR2. Moreover, one patient with a mutation in the STAT1 gene was also identified with a similar clinical syndrome (475), which indicates that, as anticipated, STAT1 is a critical mediator of the IFN-γ signal. Interestingly, this patient had a mutation on only one STAT1 allele, but the mutation was a dominant negative mutation that selectively inhibits the formation of STAT1 dimers (hence abrogating IFN-γ signaling) but yet had at most only a modest effect on the ability to form ISGF3, which thus left signaling in response to IFN-α/β relatively intact.

Mutations in the WSX-1/TCCR Type I Receptor

The type I cytokine receptor denoted TCCR or WSX-1 is related to IL-12β2, and its mutations result in defective T-cell responses and diminished IFN-γ production (476,477). Interestingly, TCCR/WSX-1 is an essential component of the receptor for IL-27 (202).

Other Diseases Associated with Cytokine Receptors

A number of other diseases that related to cytokine receptors have been reported. First, mutations in the growth hormone receptor have been found in a form of dwarfism (Laron dwarfism) in which target cells cannot respond to growth hormone (478); interestingly, some aspects of STAT5b deficiency are related to this syndrome. Second, a single patient with a form of congenital neutropenia (Kostmann's syndrome) has been found to have a mutation in one of his G-CSF receptor alleles (479). Third, a kindred of patients with familial erythrocytosis has truncation in the erythropoietin receptor, which results in hypersensitivity to erythropoietin (480). Finally, it is interesting that the thrombopoietin receptor (c-Mpl) was first identified as an orphan cytokine receptor when a viral oncogene, v-Mpl, was originally identified as the oncogene of the myeloproliferative leukemia virus (481).

CONCLUDING COMMENTS

Type I cytokines and IFNs are involved in the regulation of an enormous number of immunological and nonimmunological processes. There has been a progressive transition from viewing these as discrete molecules with special actions to viewing them as sets of molecules that can be grouped according to shared receptor components and common signaling pathways. Signaling is one area in which the understanding has greatly expanded; the pathways that are activated are similar for many cytokines, even when the biological functions that they induce are dramatically different. Although some of the differences can be explained by "compartmentalization" according to which cells produce the cytokine and which cells express receptors that allow them to respond to the cytokine, a tremendous amount still needs to be learned about how distinctive signals are triggered and about the sets of genes that are induced by each cytokine. This knowledge will provide vital information important to the quest to completely understand the mechanisms by which type I cytokines and IFNs can effect their actions. At the same time, the generation of mice with knockouts for most cytokines and their receptors, as well as many signaling molecules, has provided *in vivo* clues as to vital functions served by these cytokines. Caution is clearly needed, however, in generalizing from these findings to human biology, in view of some apparently major differences in roles served, such as the fact that IL-7 plays an essential role in both humans and mice for T-cell development, whereas IL-7 is also essential for B-cell development in mice but not in humans. The identification of so many humans disorders associated with cytokines and cytokine receptors has tremendously helped to teach more about human biology as well.

REFERENCES

1. Dumonde DC, Wolstencroft RA, Panayi GS, et al. Lymphokines: non-antibody mediators of cellular immunity generated by lymphocyte action. *Nature* 1969;224:38.
2. Cohen S, Bigazzi PE, Yoshida T. Commentary. Similarities of T cell function in cell-mediated immunity and antibody production. *Cell Immunol* 1974;12:150.
3. Waksman BH, Oppenheim JJ. The contribution of the cytokine concept to immunology, In: Gallagher RB, Gilder J, Nossal FJV, et al., eds. *Immunology, the making of a modern science.* New York: Academic Press, 1995:33.
4. Oppenheim JJ, Gery I. From lymphodrek to interleukin 1 (IL-1). *Immunol Today* 1993;14:232.
5. Bazan JF. Neurotropic cytokines in the hematopoietic fold. *Neuron* 1991;7:1.
6. Wlodawer A, Pavlovsky A, Gustchina A: Hematopoietic cytokines: similarities and differences in the structures, with implications for receptor binding. *Protein Sci* 1993;2:1373.
7. Rozwarski DA, Gronenborn AM, Clore GM, et al. Structural comparisons among the short-chain helical cytokines. *Structure* 1994;2:159.
8. Sprang SR, Bazan JF. Cytokine structural taxonomy and mechanisms of receptor engagement. *Curr Opin Struct Biol* 1993;3:815.
9. Zhang F, Basinski MB, Beals JM, et al. Crystal structure of the obese protein leptin-E100. *Nature* 1997;387:206.
10. Davies DR, Wlodawer A. Cytokines and their receptor complexes. *FASEB J* 1995;9:50.
11. Milburn MV, Hassell AM, Lambert MH, et al. A novel dimer configuration revealed by the crystal structure at 2.4 Å resolution of human interleukin-5. *Nature* 1993;363:172.
12. Senda T, Shimazu T, Matsuda S, et al. Three-dimensional crystal structure of recombinant murine interferon-β. *EMBO J* 1992;11:3193.
13. Ealick SE, Cook WJ, Vijay-Kumar S, et al. Three-dimensional structure of recombinant human interferon-γ. *Science* 1991;252:698.
14. Zdanov A, Schalk-Hihi C, Gustchina A, et al. Crystal structure of interleukin-10 reveals the functional dimer with an unexpected topological similarity to interferon γ. *Structure* 1995;3:591.
15. D'Andrea AD, Fasman GD, Lodish HF. Erythropoietin receptor and interleukin-2 receptor β chain: a new receptor family. *Cell* 1989;58:1023.
16. Bazan JF. Structural design and molecular evolution of a cytokine receptor superfamily. *Proc Natl Acad Sci U S A* 1990;87:6934.
17. Hilton DJ, Hilton AA, Raicevic A, et al. Cloning of a murine IL-11 receptor α-chain: requirement for gp130 for high affinity binding and signal transduction. *EMBO J* 1994;13:4765.
18. Cherel M, Sorel M, Lebeau B, et al. Molecular cloning of two isoforms of a receptor for the human hematopoietic cytokine interleukin-11. *Blood* 1995;86:2534.
19. Hilton DJ, Zhang, J-G, Metcalf D, et al. Cloning and characterization of a binding subunit of the interleukin 13 receptor that is also a component of the interleukin 4 receptor. *Proc Natl Acad Sci U S A* 1996;93:497.
20. Mosley B, De Imus C, Friend D, et al. Dual oncostatin M (OSM) receptors: cloning and characterization of an alternative signaling subunit conferring OSM-specific receptor activation. *J Biol Chem* 1996;271:32635.
21. Ozaki K, Kristine K, Michalovich D, et al. Cloning of a type I cytokine receptor most related to the IL-2 receptor beta chain. *Proc Natl Acad Sci U S A* 2000;97:11439.
22. Reche PA, Soumelis V, Gorman DM, et al. Human thymic stromal lymphopoietin preferentially stimulates myeloid cells. *J Immunol* 2001;167:336.
23. de Vos AM, Ultsch M, Kossiakoff AA: Human growth hormone and extracellular domain of its receptor: crystal structure of the complex. *Science* 1992;255:306.
24. Somers W, Ultsch M, De Vos AM, et al. The X-ray structure of a growth hormone-prolactin receptor complex. *Nature* 1994;372:478.
25. Livnah O, Stura EA, Johnson DL, et al. Functional mimicry of a protein hormone by a peptide agonist: the EPO receptor complex at 2.8 Å. *Science* 1996;273:464.
26. Hage T, Sebald W, Reinemer P. Crystal structure of the interleukin-4/receptor alpha chain complex reveals a mosaic binding interface. *Cell* 1999;97:271.
27. Murakami M, Narazali M, Hibi M, et al. Critical cytoplasmic region of the interleukin 6 signal transducer gp130 is conserved in the cytokine receptor family. *Proc Natl Acad Sci U S A* 1991;88:11349.
28. Wrighton NC, Farrell FX, Chang R, et al. Small peptides as potent mimetics of the protein hormone erythropoietin. *Science* 1996;273:458.
29. Takeshita T, Asao H, Ohtani K, et al. Cloning of the γ chain of the human IL-2 receptor. *Science* 1992;257:379.
30. Kondo M, Takeshita T, Ishii N, et al. Sharing of the interleukin-2 (IL-2) γ chain between receptors for IL-2 and IL-4. *Science* 1993;262:1874.
31. Noguchi M, Nakamura Y, Russell SM, et al. Interleukin-2 receptor γ chain: a functional component of the interleukin-7 receptor. *Science* 1993;262:1877.
32. Russell SM, Keegan AD, Harada N, et al. Interleukin-2 receptor γ chain: a functional component of the interleukin-4 receptor. *Science* 1993;262:1880.
33. Kondo M, Takeshita T, Higuchi M, et al. Functional participation of the IL-2 receptor γ chain in IL-7 receptor complexes. *Science* 1994;263:1453.
34. Russell SM, Johnston JA, Noguchi M, et al. Interaction of IL-2Rβ and γ_c chains with Jak1 and Jak3: implications for XSCID and XCID. *Science* 1994;266:1042.
35. Kimura M, Ishii N, Nakamura M, et al. Sharing of the IL-2 receptor γ chain with the functional IL-9 receptor complex. *Int Immunol* 1995;7:115.
36. Giri JG, Ahdieh M, Eisenman J, et al. Utilization of the β and γ chains of the IL-2 receptor by the novel cytokine IL-15. *EMBO J* 1994;13:2822.
37. Asao H, Okuyama C, Kumaki S, et al. The common gamma-chain is an indispensable subunit of the IL-21 receptor complex. *J Immunol* 2001;167:1.
38. Leonard WJ. The molecular basis of X-linked combined immunodeficiency: defective cytokine receptor signaling. *Annu Rev Med* 1996;47:229.
39. Leonard WJ. Cytokines and immunodeficiency diseases. *Nat Rev Immunol* 2001;1:200.
40. Morgan DA, Ruscetti FW, Gallo R. Selective *in vitro* growth of T lymphocytes from normal human bone marrows. *Science* 1976;193:1007.
41. Waldmann, T. A. The multi-subunit interleukin-2 receptor. *Annu Rev Biochem* 1989;58:875.

93. Waldmann TA, Tagaya Y. The multifaceted regulation of interleukin-15 expression and the role of this cytokine in NK cell differentiation and host response to intracellular pathogens. *Annu Rev Immunol* 1999;17:19.

94. Carson WE, Giri JG, Lindemann MJ, et al. Interleukin (IL) 15 is a novel cytokine that activates human natural killer cells via components of the IL-2 receptor. *J Exp Med* 1994;180:1395.

95. Lodolce JP, Boone DL, Chai S, et al. IL-15 receptor maintains lymphoid homeostasis by supporting lymphocyte homing and proliferation. *Immunity* 1998;9:669.

96. Kennedy MK, Glaccum M, Brown SN, et al. Reversible defects in natural killer and memory CD8 T cell lineages in interleukin 15–deficient mice. *J Exp Med* 2000;191:771.

97. Bamford RN, Grant AJ, Burton JD, et al. The interleukin (IL) 2 β chain is shared by IL-2, and a cytokine, provisionally designated IL-T, that stimulates T-cell proliferation and the induction of lymphokine-activated killer cells. *Proc Natl Acad Sci U S A* 1994;91:4940.

98. Giri JG, Kumaki S, Ahdieh M, et al. Identification and cloning of a novel IL-15 binding protein that is structurally related to the α chain of the IL-2 receptor. *EMBO J* 1995;14:3654.

99. Anderson DM, Kumaki S, Ahdieh M, et al. Functional characterization of the human interleukin-15 receptor α chain and close linkage of IL15RA and IL2RA genes. *J Biol Chem* 1995;270:29862.

100. Tagaya T, Burton JD, Miyamoto Y, et al. Identification of a novel receptor signal transduction pathway for IL-15/T in mast cells. *EMBO J* 1995;15:4928.

101. Waldmann TA, Dubois S, Tagaya Y. Contrasting roles of IL-2 and IL-15 in the life and death of lymphocytes: implications for immunotherapy. *Immunity* 2001;14:105.

102. Parrish-Novak J, Dillon SR, Nelson A, et al. Interleukin 21 and its receptor are involved in NK cell expansion and regulation of lymphocyte function. *Nature* 2000;408:57.

103. Kasaian MT, Whitters MJ, Carter LL, et al. IL-21 limits NK cell responses and promotes antigen-specific T cell activation: a mediator of the transition from innate to adaptive immunity. *Immunity* 2002;16:559.

104. Noguchi M, Yi H, Rosenblatt HM, et al. Interleukin-2 receptor γ chain mutation results in X-linked severe combined immunodeficiency in humans. *Cell* 1993;73:147.

105. Conley ME. Molecular approaches to analysis of X-linked immunodeficiencies. *Annu Rev Immunol* 1992;10:215.

106. Fischer A, Cavazzana-Calvo M, de Saint Basile G, et al. Naturally occurring primary deficiencies of the immune system. *Annu Rev Immunol* 1997;15:93.

107. Buckley RH. Primary immunodeficiency diseases due to defects in lymphocytes. *N Engl J Med* 2000;343:1313.

108. Haddad E, Le Deist F, Aucouturier P, et al. Long-term chimerism and B-cell function after bone marrow transplantation in patients with severe combined immunodeficiency with B cells: a single-center study of 22 patients. *Blood* 1999;94:2923.

109. Weinberg K, Parkman R. Severe combined immunodeficiency due to a specific defect in the production of interleukin-2. *N Engl J Med* 1990;322:1718.

110. Chatila T, Castigli E, Pahwa R, et al. Primary combined immunodeficiency resulting from defective transcription of multiple T-cell lymphokine genes. *Proc Natl Acad Sci U S A* 1990;87:10033.

111. Schorle H, Holtschke T, Hunig T, et al. Development and function of T cells in mice rendered interleukin-2 deficient by gene targeting. *Nature* 1991;352:621.

112. de Jong JL, Farner NL, Widmer MB, et al. Interaction of IL-15 with the shared IL-2 receptor β and γ_c subunits. The IL-15/β/γ_c receptor–ligand complex is less stable than the IL-2/β/γ_c receptor–ligand complex. *J Immunol* 1996;156:1339.

113. Puel A, Ziegler SF, Buckley RH, et al. Defective IL7R gene expression in $T^-B^+NK^+$ severe combined immunodeficiency. *Nat Genet* 1998;20:394.

114. Puel A, Leonard WJ. Mutations in the gene for the IL-7 receptor result in $T(-)B(+)NK(+)$ severe combined immunodeficiency disease. *Curr Opin Immunol* 2000;12:468.

115. Kuhn R, Rajewsky K, Muller W. Generation and analysis of interleukin-4 deficient mice. *Science* 1991;254:707.

116. Kopf M, Le Gros G, Bachmann M, et al. Disruption of the murine IL-4 gene blocks Th2 cytokine responses. *Nature* 1993;362:245.

117. Sadlack B, Kuhn R, Schorle H, et al. Development and proliferation of lymphocytes in mice deficient for both interleukins-2 and -4. *Eur J Immunol* 1994;24:281.

118. DiSanto JP, Muller W, Guy-Grand D, et al. Lymphoid development in mice with a targeted deletion of the interleukin 2 receptor γ chain. *Proc Natl Acad Sci U S A* 1995;92:377.

119. Cao X, Shores EW, Hu-Li J, et al. Defective lymphoid development in mice lacking expression of the common cytokine receptor γ chain. *Immunity* 1995;2:223.

119a. Ozaki K, Spolski R, Feng CG, et al. A critical role for IL-21 in regulating immunoglobulin production. *Science* 2002;298:1630.

120. Leonard WJ. Dysfunctional cytokine receptor signaling in severe combined immunodeficiency. *J Investig Med* 1996;44:303.

121. Takeshita T, Asao H, Suzuki J, et al. An associated molecule, p64, with high-affinity interleukin 2 receptor. *Int Immunol* 1990;2:477.

122. Nakamura Y, Russell SM, Mess SA, et al. Heterodimerization of the interleukin-2 receptor β and γ cytoplasmic domains is required for signaling. *Nature* 1994;369:330.

123. Nelson B, Lord JD, Greenberg PD. Cytoplasmic domains of the interleukin-2 receptor β and γ chains mediate the signal for T-cell proliferation. *Nature* 1994;369:333.

124. Balasubramanian S, Chernov-Rogan T, Davis AM, et al. Ligand binding kinetics of IL-2 and IL-15 to heteromers formed by extracellular domains of the three IL-2 receptor subunits. *Int Immunol* 1995;7:1839.

125. Myszka DG, Arulanantham PR, Sana T, et al. Kinetic analysis of ligand binding to interleukin-2 receptor complexes created on an optical biosensor surface. *Protein Sci* 1996;5:2468.

126. Willerford DM, Chen J, Ferry JA, et al. Interleukin-2 receptor a chain regulates the size and content of the peripheral lymphoid compartment. *Immunity* 1995;3:521.

127. Suzuki H, Kundig TM, Furlonger C, et al. Deregulated T cell activation and autoimmunity in mice lacking interleukin-2 receptor β. *Science* 1995;268:1472.

128. Nakajima H, Shores EW, Noguchi M, et al. The common cytokine receptor γ chain plays an essential role in regulating lymphoid homeostasis. *J Exp Med* 1997;185:189.

129. Metcalf D. *The hematopoietic colony stimulating factors.* Amsterdam: Elsevier, 1984.

130. Hara T, Miyajima A. Functional and signal transduction mediated by the interleukin 3 receptor system in hematopoiesis. *Stem Cells* 1996;14:605.

131. Geijsen N, Koenderman L, Coffer PJ. Specificity in cytokine signal transduction: lessons learned from the IL-3/IL-5/GM-CSF receptor family. *Cytokine Growth Factor Rev* 2001;12:19.

132. Kopf M, Brombacher F, Hodgkin PD, et al. IL-5–deficient mice have a developmental defect in CD5$^+$ B-1 cells and lack eosinophilia but have normal antibody and cytotoxic T cell responses. *Immunity* 1996;4:15.

133. Yoshida T, Ikuta K, Sugaya H, et al. Defective B-1 cell development and impaired immunity against *Angiostrongylus cantonensis* in IL-5R alpha-deficient mice. *Immunity* 1996;4:483.

134. Kitamura T, Sato N, Arai K, et al. Expression cloning of the human IL-3 receptor cDNA reveals a shared β subunit for the human IL-3 and GM-CSF receptors. *Cell* 1991;66:1165.

135. Hara T, Miyajima T. Two distinct functional high affinity receptors for mouse IL-3. *EMBO J* 1992;10:1875.

136. Takaki S, Tominaga A, Hitoshi Y, et al. Molecular cloning and expression of the murine interleukin-5 receptor. *EMBO J* 1990;9:4367.

137. Tavernier J, Devos R, Cornelis S, et al. A human high affinity interleukin-5 receptor (IL-5R) is composed of an IL-5-specific α chain and a β chain shared with the receptor for GM-CSF. *Cell* 1991;66:1174.

138. Gearing DP, King JA, Gough NM, et al. Expression cloning of a receptor for human granulocyte-macrophage colony stimulating factor. *EMBO J* 1989;8:3667.

139. Park LS, Martin U, Sorensen R, et al. Cloning of the low-affinity murine granulocyte-macrophage colony stimulating factor receptor and reconstitution of a high-affinity receptor complex. *Proc Natl Acad Sci U S A* 1992;89:4295.

140. Gorman DM, Itoh N, Kitamura T, et al. Cloning and expression of a gene encoding an interleukin 3 receptor-like protein: identification of another member of the cytokine receptor gene family. *Proc Natl Acad Sci U S A* 1990;87:5459.

141. Hayashida K, Kitamura T, Gorman DM, et al. Molecular cloning of a second subunit of the receptor for human granulocyte-macrophage colony-stimulating factor (GM-CSF): reconstitution of a high affinity GM-CSF receptor. *Proc Natl Acad Sci U S A* 1990;87:9655.

142. Miyajima A, Kitamura T, Harada N, et al. Cytokine receptors and signal transduction. *Annu Rev Immunol* 1992;10:295.

143. Sakamaki K, Miyajima I, Kitamura T, et al. Critical cytoplasmic domains of the common β subunit of the human GM-CSF, IL-3 and IL-5 receptors for growth signal transduction and tyrosine phosphorylation. *EMBO J* 1992;11:3541.

144. Cornelis S, Fache I, Van der Heyden J, et al. Characterization of critical residues in the cytoplasmic domain of the human interleukin-5 receptor α chain required for growth signal transduction. *Eur J Immunol* 1995;25:1857.

145. Kouro T, Kikuchi Y, Kanazawa H, et al. Critical proline residues of the cytoplasmic domain of the IL-5 receptor α chain and its function in IL-5-mediated activation of Jak kinase and Stat5. *Int Immunol* 1996;8:237.

146. Nishinakamura R, Miyajima A, Mee PJ, et al. Hematopoiesis in mice lacking the entire granulocyte-macrophage colony-stimulating factor/interleukin-3/interleukin-5 functions. *Blood* 1996;88:2458.

147. Hibi M, Murakami M, Saito M, et al. Molecular cloning and expression of an IL-6 signal transducer, gp130. *Cell* 1990;63:1149.

148. Gearing DP, Comeau MR, Friend DJ, et al. The IL-6 signal transducer, gp130: an oncostatin M receptor and affinity converter for the LIF receptor. *Science* 1992;255:1434.

149. Taga T, Narazaki M, Yasukawa K, et al. Functional inhibition of hematopoietic and neurotrophic cytokines by blocking the interleukin 6 signal transducer gp130. *Proc Natl Acad Sci U S A* 1992;89:10998.

150. Yin T, Taga T, Tsang ML, et al. Involvement of IL-6 signal transducer gp130 in IL-11-mediated signal transduction. *J Immunol* 1993;151:2555.

151. Pennica D, Shaw KJ, Swanson TA, et al. Cardiotrophin-1. Biological activities and binding to the leukemia inhibitory factor receptor/gp130 signaling complex. *J Biol Chem* 1995;270:10915.

152. Taga T, Kishimoto T. Gp130 and the interleukin-6 family of cytokines. *Annu Rev Immunol* 1997;15:797.

153. Miyajima A, Kinoshita T, Tanaka M, et al. Role of Oncostatin M in hematopoiesis and liver development. *Cytokine Growth Factor Rev* 2000;11:177.

154. Bravo J, Heath JK. Receptor recognition by gp130 cytokines. *EMBO J* 2000;19:2399.

155. Senaldi G, Varnum BC, Sarmiento U, et al. Novel neurotrophin-1/B cell-stimulating factor-3: a cytokine of the IL-6 family. *Proc Natl Acad Sci U S A* 1999;96:11458.

156. Hirano T, Yasukawa K, Harada H, et al. Complementary DNA for a novel human interleukin (BSF-2) that induces B lymphocytes to produce immunoglobulin. *Nature* 1986;324:73.

157. Yamasaki K, Taga T, Hirata Y, et al. Cloning and expression of the human interleukin-6 (BSF-2/IFNβ2) receptor. *Science* 1988;241:825.

158. Murakami M, Hibib M, Nakagawa N, et al. IL-6–induced homodimerization of gp130 and associated activation of a tyrosine kinase. *Science* 1993;260:1808.

159. Panonessa G, Graziani R, Serio AD, et al. Two distinct and independent sites on IL-6 trigger gp130 dimer formation and signalling. *EMBO J* 1995;14:1942.

160. Ward LD, Howlett GJ, Discolo, et al. High affinity interleukin-6 receptor is a hexameric complex consisting of two molecules each of interleukin-6, interleukin-6 receptor, and gp-130. *J Biol Chem* 1994;269:23286.

161. Du XX, Williams DA. Interleukin-11: a multifunctional growth factor derived from the hematopoietic microenvironment. *Blood* 1994;83:2023.

162. Goldman SJ. Preclinical biology of interleukin 11: a multifunctional hematopoietic cytokine with potent thrombopoietic activity. *Stem Cells* 1995;13:462.

163. Paul SR, Bennett F, Calvetti JA, et al. Molecular cloning of a cDNA encoding interleukin 11, a stromal derived lymphopoietic and hematopoietic cytokine. *Proc Natl Acad Sci U S A* 1990;87:7512.

164. Kobayashi S, Teramura M, Oshimi K, et al. Interleukin-11. *Leuk Lymphoma* 1994;15:45.

165. Kawashima I, Ohsumi J, Mita-Honjo K, et al. Molecular cloning of cDNA encoding adipogenesis inhibitory factor and identity with interleukin-11. *FEBS Lett* 1991;283:199.

166. Zheng T, Zhu Z, Wang J, et al. IL-11: insights in asthma from overexpression transgenic modeling. *J Allergy Clin Immunol* 2001;108:489.

167. Baumann H, Wang Y, Morella KK, et al. Complex of the soluble IL-11 receptor and IL-11 acts as IL-6-type cytokine in hepatic and nonhepatic cells. *J Immunol* 1996;157:284.

168. Neddermann P, Graziani R, Ciliberto G, et al. Functional expression of soluble human interleukin-11 (IL-11) receptor α and stoichiometry of in vitro IL-11 receptor complexes with gp130. *J Biol Chem* 1996;271:30986.

169. Gearing DP, Gough NM, King JA, et al. Molecular cloning and expression of cDNA encoding a murine myeloid leukaemia inhibitory factor (LIF). *EMBO J* 1987;6:3995.

170. Hilton DJ, Gough NM. Leukemia inhibitor factor: a biological perspective. *J Cell Biochem* 1991;46:21.

171. Yamamori T, Kukada K, Abersold R, et al. The cholinergic neuronal differentiation factor from heart cells is identical to leukemia inhibitory factor. *Science* 1989;246:1412.

172. Piccinni MP, Scaletti C, Vultaggio A, et al. Defective production of LIF, M-CSF and Th2-type cytokines by T cells at fetomaternal interface is associated with pregnancy loss. *J Reprod Immunol* 2001;52:35.

173. Gearing DP, Thut CJ, VandenBos T, et al. Leukemia inhibitory factor receptor is structurally related to the IL-6 signal transducer, gp130. *EMBO J* 1991;10:2839.

174. Lin L-FH, Mismer D, Lile JD, et al. Purification, cloning, and expression of ciliary neurotrophic factor (CNTF). *Science* 1989;246:1023.

175. Stockli KA, Lottspeich F, Sendtner M, et al. Molecular cloning, expression and regional distribution of rat ciliary neurotrophic factor. *Nature* 1989;342:920.

176. Davis S, Aldrich TH, Valenzuela DM, et al. The receptor for ciliary neurotrophic factor. *Science* 1991;253:59.

177. Davis S, Aldrich TH, Stahl N, et al. LIFRβ and gp130 as heterodimerizing signal transducers of the tripartite CNTF receptor. *Science* 1993;260:1805.

178. De Serio A, Graziani R, Laufer R, et al. *In vitro* binding of ciliary neurotrophic factor to its receptors: evidence for the formation of an IL-6-type hexameric complex. *J Mol Biol* 1995;254:795.

179. Zarling JM, Shoyab M, Marquardt H, et al. Oncostatin M: a growth regulator produced by differentiated histiocytic lymphoma cells. *Proc Natl Acad Sci U S A* 1986;83:9739.

180. Malik N, Kalestad JC, Gunderson NL, et al. Molecular cloning, sequence analysis, and functional expression of a novel growth regulator, oncostatin M. *Mol Cell Biol* 1989;9:2847.

181. Nair BC, DeVico AL, Nakamura S, et al. Identification of a major growth factor for AIDS–Kaposi's sarcoma cells as oncostatin M. *Science* 1992;255:1430.

182. Miles SA, Martinez-Maza O, Rezai A, et al. Oncostatin M as a potent mitogen for AIDS–Kaposi's sarcoma derived cells. *Science* 1992;255:1432.

183. Pennica D, King KL, Shaw KL, et al. Expression cloning of cardiotrophin-1, a cytokine that induces cardiac myocyte hypertrophy. *Proc Natl Acad Sci U S A* 1995;92:1142.

184. Pennica D, Wood WI, Chien KR. Cardiotrophin-1: a multifunctional cytokine that signals via LIF receptor-gp130 dependent pathways. *Cytokine Growth Factor Rev* 1996;1:81.

185. Latchman DS. Cardiotrophin-1: a novel cytokine and its effects in the heart and other tissues. *Pharmacol Ther* 2000;85:29.

186. Pennica D, Arce V, Swanson TA, et al. Cardiotrophin-1, a cytokine present in embryonic muscle, supports long-term survival of spinal motoneurons. *Neuron* 1996;17:63.

187. Robledo O, Fourcin M, Chevalier S, et al. Signaling of the cardiotrophin-1 receptor. Evidence for a third receptor component. *J Biol Chem* 1997;272:4855.

188. Elson GC, Lelievre E, Guillet C, et al. CLF associates with CLC to form a functional heteromeric ligand for the CNTF receptor complex. *Nat Neurosci* 2000;3:867.

189. Ozaki K, Leonard WJ. Cytokine and cytokine receptor pleiotropy and redundancy. *J Biol Chem* 2002;277:29355.

190. Zhang Y, Proenca R, Maffei M, et al. Positional cloning of the mouse obese gene and its human homologue [Published erratum in *Nature* 1995;374:479]. *Nature* 1994;372:425.

191. Friedman JM, Halaas JL. Leptin and the regulation of body weight in mammals. *Nature* 1998;395:763.

192. Tartaglia LA, Dembski M, Weng X, et al. Identification and expression cloning of a leptin receptor, OB-R. *Cell* 1995;83:1263.

193. Chen H, Charlat O, Tartaglia LA, et al. Evidence that the diabetes gene encodes the leptin receptor: identification of a mutation in the leptin receptor gene in db/db mice. *Cell* 1996;84:491.

194. Trinchieri G. Interleukin-12: a proinflammatory cytokine with immunoregulatory functions that bridge innate resistance and antigen-specific adaptive immunity. *Annu Rev Immunol* 1995;13:251.

195. Kobayashi M, Fitz L, Ryan M, et al. Identification and purification of natural killer cell stimulatory factor (NKSF), a cytokine with multiple biologic effect on human lymphocytes. *J Exp Med* 1989;170:827.

196. Gubler U, Chua AO, Schoenhaut DS, et al. Coexpression of two distinct genes is required to generate secreted bioactive cytotoxic lymphocyte maturation factor. *Proc Natl Acad Sci U S A* 1991;88:4143.

197. Chua AO, Wilkinson VL, Presky DH, et al. Cloning and characterization of a mouse IL-12 receptor–β component. *J Immunol* 1995;155:4286.

198. Presky DH, Yang H, Minetti LJ, et al. A functional interleukin 12 receptor complex is composed of two β-type cytokine receptor subunits. *Proc Natl Acad Sci U S A* 1996;93:14002.

199. Gubler U, Presky DH. Molecular biology of interleukin-12 receptors. *Ann N Y Acad Sci* 1996;795:36.

200. Oppmann B, Lesley R, Blom B et al. Novel p19 protein engages IL-12p40 to form a cytokine, IL-23, with biological activities similar as well as distinct from IL-12. *Immunity* 200013:715.

201. Parham C, Chirica M, Timans J, et al. A receptor for the heterodimeric cytokine IL-23 is composed of IL-12Rβ1 and a novel cytokine receptor subunit, IL-23R. *J Immunol* 2002;168:5699.

202. Pflanz S, Timans JC, Cheung J, et al. IL-27, a heterodimeric cytokine composed of EBI3 and p28 protein, induces proliferation of naïve CD4$^+$ T cells. *Immunity* 2002;16:779.

203. Friend SL, Hosier S, Nelson A, et al. A thymic stromal cell line supports *in vitro* development of surface IgM$^+$ B cells and produces a novel growth factor affecting B and T lineage cells. *Exp Hematol* 1994;22:321.

204. Sims JE, Williams DE, Morrissey PJ, et al. Molecular cloning and biological characterization of a novel murine lymphoid growth factor. *J Exp Med* 2000;192:671.

205. Pandey A, Ozaki K, Baumann H, et al. Cloning of a receptor subunit required for signaling by thymic stromal lymphopoietin. *Nat Immunol* 2000;1:59.

206. Park LS, Martin U, Garka K, et al. Cloning of the murine thymic stromal lymphopoietin (TSLP) receptor: formation of a functional heteromeric complex requires interleukin 7 receptor. *J Exp Med* 2000;192:659.

207. Cao X, Kozak CA, Liu YJ, et al. Protein characterization of cDNAs encoding the murine interleukin 2 receptor (IL-2R) gamma chain: chromosomal mapping and tissue specificity of IL-2R gamma chain expression. *Proc Natl Acad Sci U S A* 1993;90:8464.

208. Soumelis V, Reche PA, Kanzler H, et al. Human epithelial cells trigger dendritic cell mediated allergic inflammation by producing TSLP. *Nat Immunol* 2002;3:673.

209. Leonard WJ. TSLP: finally in the limelight. *Nat Immunol* 2002;3:605.

210. Lin J-X, Migone T-S, Tsang M, et al. The role of shared receptor motifs and common Stat proteins in the generation of cytokine pleiotropy and redundancy by IL-2, IL-4, IL-7, IL-13, and IL-15. *Immunity* 1995;2:331.

211. Zurawski G, de Vries JE. Interleukin 13, an interleukin 4-like cytokine that acts on monocytes and B cells, but not on T cells. *Immunol Today* 1994;15:19.

212. Smerz-Bertling C, Duschl A. Both interleukin 4 and interleukin 13 induce tyrosine phosphorylation of the 140-kDa subunit of the interleukin 4 receptor. *J Biol Chem* 1994;270:966.

213. Zurawski SM, Chomarat P, Djossou O, et al. The primary binding subunit of the human interleukin-4 receptor is also a component of the interleukin-13 receptor. *J Biol Chem* 1995;270:13869.

214. Aman MF, Tayebi N, Obiri NI, et al. cDNA cloning and characterization of the human interleukin-13 receptor α chain. *J Biol Chem* 1996;271:29265.

215. Caput D, Laurent P, Kaghad M, et al. Cloning and characterization of a specific interleukin (IL)-13 binding protein structurally related to the IL-5 receptor α chain. *J Biol Chem* 1996;271:16921.

216. Grunig G, Warnock M, Wakil AE, et al. Requirement for IL-13 independently of IL-4 in experimental asthma. *Science* 1998;282:2261.

217. Wills-Karp M, Luyimbazi J, Xu X, et al. Interleukin-13: central mediator of allergic asthma. *Science* 1998;282:2258.

218. McKenzie GJ, Emson CL, Bell SE, et al. Impaired development of Th2 cells in IL-13–deficient mice *Immunity* 1998;9:423.

219. Sharfe N, Dadi HK, Shahar M, et al. Human immune disorder arising from mutation of the α chain of the interleukin-2 receptor. *Proc Natl Acad Sci U S A* 1997;94:3168.

220. Smith KA. The interleukin 2 receptor. *Annu Rev Cell Biol* 1989;5:397.

221. Leonard WJ, Depper JM, Kanehisa M, et al. Structure of the human interleukin-2 receptor gene. *Science* 1985;230:633.

222. Leonard WJ, Donlon TA, Lebo RV, et al. The gene encoding the human interleukin-2 receptor is located on chromosome 10. *Science* 1985;228:1547.

223. Gnarra JR, Otani H, Wang MG, et al. Human interleukin 2 receptor β chain gene: chromosomal localization and identification of 5' regulatory sequences. *Proc Natl Acad Sci U S A* 1990;87:3440.

224. Shibuya H, Yoneyama M, Nakamura Y, et al. The human interleukin-2 receptor β chain gene: genomic organization, promoter analysis and chromosomal assignment. *Nucl Acids Res* 1990;18:3697.

225. Watowich SS, Wu H, Socolovsky M, et al. Cytokine receptor signal transduction and the control of hematopoietic cell development. *Annu Rev Cell Dev Biol* 1996;12:91.

226. Wu H, Klingmuller U, Besmer P, et al. Interaction of the erythropoietin and stem-cell-factor receptors. *Nature* 1995;377:242.

227. Itoh N, Yonehara S, Schreurs J, et al. Cloning of an interleukin-3 receptor gene: a member of a distinct receptor gene family. *Science* 1990;247:324.

228. Kurman CC, Rubin LA, Nelson DL. Soluble products of immune activation: soluble interleukin-2 receptor (sIL-2R, Tac protein). In: Rose NR, deMacario EC, Fahey JL, et al., eds. *Manual of clinical laboratory immunology*. Washington, DC: American Society for Microbiology, 1992:256.

229. Fernandez-Botran R, Chilton PM, Ma Y. Soluble cytokine receptors: their roles in immunoregulation, disease, and therapy. *Adv Immunol* 1996;63:269.

230. Salvati AL, Lahm A, Paonessa G, et al. Interleukin-6 (IL-6) antagonism by soluble IL-6 receptor α mutated in the predicted gp130-binding interface. *J Biol Chem* 1995;270:12242.

231. Isaacs A, Lindermann J. Virus interference. I. The interferon. *Proc R Soc Lond (Biol)* 1957;147:258.

232. Farrar MA, Schreiber RD. The molecular cell biology of interferon-γ and its receptor. *Annu Rev Immunol* 1993;11:571.

233. Stark GR, Kerr IM, Williams BR, et al. How cells respond to interferons. *Annu Rev Biochem* 1998;67:227.

234. DeMaeyer E, Demaeyer-Guignard J. Type I interferons. *Int Rev Immunol* 1998;17:53.

235. Roberts RM, Liu L, Alexenko A. New and atypical families of type I interferons in mammals: comparative functions, structures, and evolutionary relationships. *Prog Nucleic Acid Res Mol Biol* 1997;56:287.

236. Hayes MP, Zoon KC. Production and action of interferons: new insights into molecular mechanisms of gene regulation and expression. *Prog Drug Res* 1994;43:239.

237. Roberts RM, Liu L, Guo Q, et al. The evolution of the type I interferons. *J Interferon Cytokine Res* 1998;18:805.

238. Nomenclature for interferon receptors and interferon δ. *Int Soc Interferon Cytokine Res Newslett* 1997;4:1.

239. Langer J, Garotta G, Pestka S. Interferon receptors. *Biotherapy* 1996;8:163.

240. de Veer MJ, Holko M, Frevel M, et al. Functional classification of interferon-stimulated genes identified using microarrays. *J Leukoc Biol* 2001;69:912.

241. Bazan JF. Shared architecture of hormone binding domains in type I and type II interferon receptors. *Cell* 1990;61:753.

242. Walter MR, Windsor WT, Nagabhushan TL, et al. Crystal structure of a complex between interferon-γ and its soluble high-affinity receptor. *Nature* 1995;376:230.

243. Uze G, Lutfalla G, Gresser I. Genetic transfer of a functional human interferon receptor into mouse cells: cloning and expression of its cDNA. *Cell* 1990;60:225.

244. Novick D, Cohen B, Rubinstein M. The human interferon α/β receptor: characterization and molecular cloning. *Cell* 1994;77:391.

245. Domanski P, Witte M, Kellum M, et al. Cloning and expression of a long form of the β subunit of the interferon α receptor that is required for interferon signaling. *J Biol Chem* 1995;270:21606.

246. Lutfalla G, Holland SJ, Cinato E, et al. Mutant U5A cells are complemented by an interferon $\alpha\beta$ receptor subunit generated by alternative processing of a new member of a cytokine receptor gene cluster. *EMBO J* 1995;14:5100.

247. Domanski P, Colamonici OS. The type-1 interferon receptor: the long and short of it. *Cytokine Growth Factor Rev* 1996;7:143.

248. Symons JA, Alcami A, Smith GL. Vaccinia virus encodes a soluble type I interferon receptor of novel structure and broad species-specificity. *Cell* 1995;81:551.

249. Spriggs MK. Poxvirus-encoded soluble cytokine receptors. *Virus Res* 1994;33:1.

250. Gray PW, Leung DW, Pennica D, et al. Expression of human immune interferon cDNA in *E. coli* and monkey cells. *Nature* 1982;295:503.

251. Bach EA, Aguet M, Schreiber RD. The IFNγ receptor: a paradigm for cytokine receptor signaling. *Annu Rev Immunol* 1997;15:563.

252. Marsters SA, Pennica D, Bach E, et al. Interferon γ signals via a high-affinity multisubunit receptor complex that contains two types of polypeptide chain. *Proc Natl Acad Sci U S A* 1995;92:5401.

253. Aguet M, Dembic Z, Merlin G. Molecular cloning and expression of the human interferon-γ receptor. *Cell* 1988;55:273.

254. Soh J, Donnelly RJ, Kotenko S, et al. Identification and sequence of an accessory factor required for activation of the human interferon γ receptor. *Cell* 1994;76:793.

255. Hemmi S, Bohni R, Stark G, et al. A novel member of the interferon receptor family complements functionality of the murine interferon γ receptor in human cells. *Cell* 1994;76:803.

256. Kaplan DH, Greenlund AC, Tanner JW, et al. Identification of an interferon-gamma receptor α chain sequence required for JAK-1 binding. *J Biol Chem* 1996;271:9.

257. Sakatsume M, Igarashi K, Winestock KD, et al. The Jak kinases differentially associate with the α and β (accessory factor) chains of the interferon γ receptor to form a functional receptor unit capable of activating STAT transcription factors. *J Biol Chem* 1995;270:17528.

258. Moore KW, de Waal Malefyt R, Coffman RL, et al. Interleukin-10 and the interleukin-10 receptor. *Annu Rev Immunol* 2001;19:683.

259. Ying L, de Waal Malefyt R, Briere F, et al. The EBV IL-10 homologue is a selective agonist with impaired binding to the IL-10 receptor. *J Immunol* 1997;158:604.

260. Ho AS, Liu Y, Khan TA, et al. A receptor for interleukin 10 is related to interferon receptors. *Proc Natl Acad Sci U S A* 1993;90:11267.

261. Liu Y, Wei SH, Ho AS, et al. Expression cloning and characterization of a human IL-10 receptor. *J Immunol* 1994;152:1821.

262. Lutfalla G, Gardiner K, Uze G. A new member of the cytokine receptor gene family maps on chromosome 21 at less than 35 kb from IFNAR. *Genomics* 1993;16:366.

263. Fibbs VC, Pennica D. CRF2-4: isolation of cDNA clones encoding the human and mouse proteins. *Gene* 1997;186:97.

264. Dumoutier L, Leemans C, Lejeune D, et al. STAT activation by IL-19, IL-20 and mda-7 through IL-20 receptor complexes of two types. *J Immunol* 2001;167:3545.

265. Wang M, Tan Z, Zhang R, et al. Interleukin 24 (MDA-7/MOB-5) signals through two heterodimeric receptors, IL-22R1/IL-20R2 and IL-20R1/IL-20R2. *J Biol Chem* 2002;277:7341.

266. Gallagher G, Dickensheets H, Eskdale J, et al. Cloning, expression and initial characterization of interleukin-19 (IL-19), a novel homologue of human interleukin-10 (IL-10). *Genes Immun* 2000;1:442.

267. Blumberg H, Conklin D, Xu WF, et al. Interleukin 20: discovery, receptor identification, and role in epidermal function. *Cell* 2001;104:9.

268. Xie MH, Aggarwal S, Ho WH, et al. Interleukin (IL)–22, a novel human cytokine that signals through the interferon receptor-related proteins CRF2-4 and IL-22R. *J Biol Chem* 2000;275:31335.

269. Jiang H, Lin JJ, Su ZZ, et al. Subtraction hybridization identifies a novel melanoma differentiation associated gene, mda-7, modulated during human melanoma differentiation, growth and progression. *Oncogene* 1995;11:2477.

269a. Sheppard P, Kindsvogel W, Xu W, et al. IL-28, IL-29 and their class II cytokine receptor IL-28R. *Nature Immunol* 2003;4:63.

269b. Kotenko SV, Gallagher G, Baurin VV, et al. IFN-λs mediate antiviral protection through a distinct class II cytokine receptor complex. *Nature Immunol* 2003;4:69.

270. Fickenscher H, Hor S, Kupers H, et al. The interleukin-10 family of cytokines. *Trends Immunol* 2002;23:89.

271. Darnell JE Jr, Kerr IM, Stark GR. Jak-STAT pathways and transcriptional activation in response to IFNs and other extracellular signaling proteins. *Science* 1994;264:1415.

272. Leonard WJ, O'Shea JJ. Jaks and STATS: biological implications. *Annu Rev Immunol* 1998;16:293.

273. Horvath CM, Darnell JE. The state of the STATs: recent developments in the study of signal transduction to the nucleus. *Curr Opin Cell Biol* 1997;9:233.

274. Wilks AF, Harpur AG, Kurban RR, et al. Two novel protein-tyrosine kinases, each with a second phosphotransferase-related catalytic domain, define a new class of protein kinase. *Mol Cell Biol* 1991;11:2057.

275. Harpur AG, Andres AC, Ziemiecki A, et al. JAK2, a third member of the JAK family of protein tyrosine kinases. *Oncogene* 1992;7:1347.

276. Johnston JA, Kawamura M, Kirken RA, et al. Phosphorylation and activation of the Jak-3 Janus kinase in response to interleukin-2. *Nature* 1994;370:151.

277. Witthuhn BA, Silvennoinen O, Miura O, et al. Involvement of the Jak-3 Janus kinase in signalling by interleukins 2 and 4 in lymphoid and myeloid cells. *Nature* 1994;370:153.

278. Krolewski JJ, Lee R, Eddy R, et al. Identification and chromosomal mapping of new human tyrosine kinase genes. *Oncogene* 1990;5:277.

279. Witthuhn BA, Quelle FW, Silvennoinen O, et al. JAK2 associates with the erythropoietin receptor and is tyrosine phosphorylated and activated following stimulation with erythropoietin. *Cell* 1993;74:227.

280. DaSilva L, Howard OMZ, Rui H, et al. Growth signaling and Jak2 association mediated by membrane-proximal cytoplasmic regions of the prolactin receptor. *J Biol Chem* 1994;269:18267.

281. Gurney AL, Wong SC, Henzel WJ, et al. Distinct regions of c-mpl cytoplasmic domain are coupled to the JAK-STAT signal transduction pathway and Shc phsophorylation. *Proc Natl Acad Sci U S A* 1995;92:5292.

282. Tanner JW, Chen W, Young RL, et al. The conserved Box 1 motif of cytokine receptors is required for association with Jak kinases. *J Biol Chem* 1995;270:6523.

283. Zhao, Y, Wagner F, Frank SJ, et al. The amino-terminal portion of the Jak2 protein kinase is necessary for binding and phosphorylation of the granulocyte-macrophage colony-stimulating factor receptor β_c. *J Biol Chem* 1995;270:13814.

284. Kohlhuber F, Rogers NC, Watling D, et al. A JAK1/JAK2 chimera can sustain alpha and gamma interferon responses. *Mol Cell Biol* 1997;17:695.

285. Chen M, Cheng A, Chen Y-Q, et al. The amino terminus of JAK3 is necessary and sufficient for binding to the common γ chain and confers the ability to transmit interleukin 2–mediated signals. *Proc Natl Acad Sci U S A* 1997;94:6910.

286. Guschin D, Rogers N, Briscoe J, et al. A major role for the protein tyrosine kinase JAK1 in the JAK/STAT signal transduction pathway in response to interleukin-6. *EMBO J* 1995;14:1421.

287. Rodig SJ, Meraz MA, White JM, et al. Disruption of the Jak1 gene demonstrates obligatory and nonredundant roles of the Jaks in cytokine-induced biologic responses. *Cell* 1998;93:373.

288. Zhuang H, Patil SV, He T-C, et al. Inhibition of erythropoietin-induced mitogenesis by a kinase-deficient form of Jak2. *J Biol Chem* 1994;269:21411.

289. Frank SJ, Yi W, Zhao Y, et al. Regions of the JAK2 tyrosine kinase required for coupling to the growth hormone receptor. *J Biol Chem* 1995;270:14776.

290. Kawahara A, Minami Y, Ihle JN, et al. Critical role of the interleukin 2 (IL-2) receptor γ-chain–associated Jak3 in the IL-2 induced c-fos and c-myc but not bcl-2 induction. *Proc Natl Acad Sci U S A* 1995;92:8724.

291. Macchi P, Villa A, Gillani S, et al. Mutations of Jak-3 gene in patients with autosomal severe combined immune deficiency (SCID). *Nature* 1995;377:65.

292. Russell SM, Tayebi N, Nakajima H, et al. Mutation of Jak3 in a patient with SCID: Essential role of Jak3 in lymphoid development. *Science* 1995;270:797.

293. Thomis DC, Gurniak CB, Tivol E, et al. Defects in B lymphocyte maturation and T lymphocyte activation in mice lacking Jak3. *Science* 1995;270:794.

294. Nosaka T, van Deursen JMA, Tripp RA, et al. Defective lymphoid development in mice lacking Jak3. *Science* 1995;270:800.

295. Park SY, Saijo K, Takahashi T, et al. Developmental defects of lymphoid cells in Jak3 kinase–deficient mice. *Immunity* 1995;3:771.

296. Luo H, Hanratty WP, Dearolf CR. An amino acid substitution in the *Drosophila hopTum-l* Jak kinase causes leukemia-like hematopoietic defects. *EMBO J* 1995;14:1412.

297. Harrison DA, Binari R, Nahreini TS, et al. Activation of a *Drosophila* Janus kinase (JAK) causes hematopoietic neoplasia and developmental defects. *EMBO J* 1995;14:2857.

298. Conway G, Margoliath A, Wong-Madden S, et al. Jak1 kinase is required for cell migrations and anterior specification in zebrafish embryos. *Proc Natl Acad Sci U S A* 1997;94:3082.

299. Migone T-S, Lin J-X, Cereseto A, et al. Constitutively activated Jak-Stat pathway in T cells transformed with HTLV-I. *Science* 1995;269:79.

300. Danial NN, Pernis A, Rothman PB. Jak-STAT signaling induced by the v-abl oncogene. *Science* 1995;269:1875.

301. Ohashi T, Masuda M, Ruscetti SK. Induction of sequence-specific DNA-binding factors by erythropoietin and the spleen focus-forming virus. *Blood* 1995;84:1454.

302. Yu CL, Meyer DJ, Campbell GS, et al. Enhanced DNA-binding activity of a Stat3-related protein in cells transformed by the Src oncoprotein. *Science* 1995;269:81.

303. Meydan N, Grunberger T, Dadi H, et al. Inhibition of acute lymphoblastic leukaemia by a Jak-2 inhibitor. *Nature* 1996;379:645.

304. Nelson BH, McIntosh BC, Rosencrans LL, et al. Requirement for an initial signal from the membrane-proximal region of the interleukin 2 receptor γ_c chain for Janus kinase activation leading to T cell proliferation. *Proc Natl Acad Sci U S A* 1997;94:1878.

305. Hanissian SH, Geha RS. Jak3 is associated with CD40 and is critical for CD40 induction of gene expression in B cells. *Immunity* 1997;6:379.

306. Jabara HH, Buckley RH, Roberts JL, et al. Role of JAK3 in CD40-mediated signaling. *Blood* 1998;92:2435.

307. Briscoe J, Rogers NC, Witthuhn BA, et al. Kinase-negative mutants of JAK1 can sustain interferon-γ inducible gene expression but not an antiviral state. *EMBO J* 1996;15:799.

308. Gauzzi MC, Velazaquez L, McKendry R, et al. Interferon-α–dependent activation of Tyk2 requires phosphorylation of positive regulatory tyrosines by another kinase. *J Biol Chem* 1996;271:20494.

309. Feng J, Witthuhn BA, Matsuda T, et al. Activation of Jak2 catalytic activity requires phosphorylation of Y1007 in the kinase activation loop. *Mol Cell Biol* 1997;17:2497.

310. Kohlhuber F, Rogers NC, Watling D, et al. A JAK1/JAK2 chimera can sustain alpha and gamma interferon responses. *Mol Cell Biol* 1997;17:695.

311. Luo H, Rose P, Barber D, et al. Mutation in the Jak kinase JH2 domain hyperactivates *Drosophila* and mammalian Jak-Stat pathways. *Mol Cell Biol* 1997;17:1562.

312. Fujitani Y, Hibi M, Fukada T, et al. An alternative pathway for STAT activation that is mediated by the direct interaction between JAK and STAT. *Oncogene* 1997;14:751.

313. Binari R, Perrimon N. Stripe-specific regulation of pair-rule genes by hopscotch, a putative Jak family tyrosine kinase in *Drosophila*. *Genes Dev* 1994;8:300.

314. Lai KS, Jin Y, Graham DK, et al. A kinase-deficient splice variant of the human JAK3 is expressed in hematopoietic and epithelial cancer cells. *J Biol Chem* 1995;270:25028.

315. Lacronique V, Boureux A, Valle VD, et al. A TEL-JAK2 fusion protein with constitutive kinase activity in human leukemia. *Science* 1997;278:1309.

316. Fu XY. A transcription factor with SH2 and SH3 domains is directly activated by an intereferon alpha-induced cytoplasmic protein tyrosine kinase(s). *Cell* 1992;70:323.

317. Fu XY, Schindler C, Improta T, et al. The proteins of ISGF-3, the interferon alpha–induced transcriptional activator, define a gene family involved in signal transduction. *Proc Natl Acad Sci U S A* 1992;89:7840.

318. Zhong Z, Wen Z, Darnell JE Jr. Stat3: a STAT family member activated by tyrosine phosphorylation in response to epidermal growth factor and interleukin-6. *Science* 1994;264:95.

319. Akira S, Nishio Y, Inoue M, et al. Molecular cloning of APRF, a novel IFN-stimulated gene factor 3 p91-related transcription factor involved in the gp130-mediated signaling pathway. *Cell* 1994;77:63.

320. Zhong Z, Wen Z, Darnell JE Jr. Stat3 and Stat4: members of the family of signal transducers and activators of transcription. *Proc Natl Acad Sci U S A* 1994;91:4806.

321. Yamamoto K, Quelle FW, Thierfelder WE, et al. Stat4, a novel gamma interferon activation site–binding protein expressed in early myeloid differentiation. *Mol Cell Biol* 1994;14:4342.

322. Wakao H, Gouilleux F, Groner B. Mammary gland factor (MGF) is a novel member of the cytokine regulated transcription factor gene family and confers the prolactin response. *EMBO J* 1994;13:2182.

323. Hou J, Schindler U, Henzel WJ, et al. Identification and purification of human Stat proteins activated in response to interleukin-2. *Immunity* 1995;2:321.

324. Mui AL, Wakao H, O'Farrell A, et al. Interleukin-3, granulocyte-macrophage colony stimulating factor and interleukin-5 signal through two STAT5 homologs. *EMBO J* 1995;14:1166.

325. Azam M, Erdjument-Bromage H, Kreider BL, et al. Interleukin-3 signals through multiple isoforms of Stat5. *EMBO J* 1995;14:1402.

326. Liu X, Robinston GW, Gouilleux F, et al. Cloning and expression of Stat5 and an additional homolgue (Stat5b) involved in prolactin signal transduction in mouse mammary tissue. *Proc Natl Acad Sci U S A* 1995;92:8831.

327. Lin J-X, Mietz J, Modi WS, et al. Cloning of human Stat5B: reconstitution of interleukin-2–induced Stat5A and Stat5B DNA binding activity in COS-7 cells. *J Biol Chem* 1996;271:10738.

328. Hou J, Schindler U, Henzel WJ, et al. An interleukin-4 induced transcription factor: IL-4 Stat. *Science* 1994;265:1701.

329. Nakajima H, Liu XW, Wynshaw-Boris A, et al. An indirect effect of Stat5a in IL-2–induced proliferation: a critical role for Stat5a in IL-2–mediated IL-2 receptor α chain induction. *Immunity* 1997;7:691.

330. Imada K, Bloom ET, Nakajima H, et al. Stat5b is essential for natural killer cell-mediated proliferation and cytolytic activity. *J Exp Med* 1998;188:2067.

331. Teglund S, McKay C, Schuetz E, et al. Stat5a and Stat5b proteins have essential and nonessential, or redundant, roles in cytokine responses. *Cell* 1998;93:841.

332. Moriggl R, Topham DJ, Teglund S, et al. Stat5 is required for IL-2–induced cell cycle progression of peripheral T cells. *Immunity* 1999;10:249.

333. Wang D, Stravopodis D, Teglund S, et al. Naturally occurring dominant negative variants of Stat5. *Mol Cell Biol* 1996;16:6141.

334. Copeland NG, Gilbert DJ, Schindler C, et al. Distribution of the mammalian Stat gene family in mouse chromosomes. *Genomics* 1995;29:225.

335. Greenlund AC, Farrar MA, Viviano BL, et al. Ligand induced IFNγ receptor phosphorylation couples the receptor to its signal transduction system (p91). *EMBO J* 1994;13:1591.

336. Yan H, Krishnan K, Greenlund AC, et al. Phosphorylated interferon-alpha receptor 1 subunit (IFNaR1) acts as a docking site for the latent form of the 113 kDa STAT2 protein. *EMBO J* 1996;15:1064.

337. Stahl N, Farruggella TJ, Boulton TG, et al. Choice of STATs and other substrates specified by modular tyrosine-based motifs in cytokine receptors. *Science* 1995;267:1349.

338. Friedmann MC, Migone T-S, Russell SM, et al. Different interleukin 2 receptor β-chain tyrosines couple to at least two signaling pathways and synergistically mediate interleukin 2–induced proliferation. *Proc Natl Acad Sci U S A* 1996;93:2077.

339. Schindler U, Wu P, Rother M, et al. Components of a Stat recognition code: evidence for two layers of molecular selectivity. *Immunity* 1995;2:686.

340. Klingmuller U, Bergelson S, Hsiao JG, et al. Multiple tyrosine residues in the cytosolic domain of the erythropoietin receptor promote activation of STAT5. *Proc Natl Acad Sci U S A* 1996;93:8324.

341. Weber-Nordt RM, Riley JK, Greenlund AC, et al. Stat3 recruitment by two distinct ligand-induced, tyrosine-phosphorylated docking sites in the interleukin-10 receptor intracellular domain. *J Biol Chem* 1996;271:27954.

342. McBride KM, Banninger G, McDonald C, et al. Regulated nuclear import of the STAT1 transcription factor by direct binding of importin-alpha. *EMBO J* 2002;21:1754.

343. McBride KM, McDonald C, Reich NC. Nuclear export signal located within the DNA-binding domain of the STAT1 transcription factor. *EMBO J* 2000;19:6196.

344. Chen X, Vinkemeier U, Zhao Y, et al. Crystal structure of a tyrosine phosphorylated STAT-1 dimer bound to DNA. *Cell* 1998;93:827.

345. Becker S, Groner B, Muller CW. Three-dimensional structure of the Stat3beta homodimer bound to DNA. *Nature* 1998;394:145.

346. Soldaini E, John S, Moro S, et al. DNA binding site selection of dimeric and tetrameric Stat5 proteins reveals a large repertoire of divergent tetrameric Stat5a binding sites. *Mol Cell Biol* 2000;20:389.

347. Xu X, Sun Y-L, Hoey T. Cooperative DNA binding and sequence-selective recognition conferred by the STAT amino-terminal domain. *Science* 1996;273:794.

348. Vinkemeier U, Cohen SL, Moarefi I, et al. DNA binding of *in vitro* activated Stat1 alpha, Stat1 beta and truncated Stat1: interaction between NH$_2$-terminal domains stabilizes binding of two dimers to tandem DNA sites. *EMBO J* 1996;15:5616.

349. Sperisen P, Wang SM, Soldaini E, et al. Mouse interleukin-2 receptor alpha gene expression. Interleukin-1 and interleukin-2 control transcription via distinct cis-acting elements. *J Biol Chem* 1995;270:10743.

350. John S, Robbins CM, Leonard WJ. An IL-2 response element in the human IL-2 receptor alpha chain promoter is a composite element that binds Stat5, Elf-1, HMG-I(Y), and a GATA family protein. *EMBO J* 1996;15:5627.

351. Lecine P, Algarte M, Rameil P, et al. Elf-1 and Stat5 bind to a critical element in a new enhancer of the human interleukin-2 receptor α gene. *Mol Cell Biol* 1996;16:6829.

352. Kim HP, Kelly J, & Leonard WJ. The basis for IL-2–induced IL-2 receptor alpha chain gene regulation: importance of two widely separated IL-2 response elements. *Immunity* 2001;15:159.

352a. Vinkemeier U, Moarefi I, Darnell JE Jr, Kuriyan J. Structure of the amino-terminal protein interaction site of Stat4. *Science* 1998;279:1048.

352b. John S, Vinkemeier U, Soldaini E, Darnell JE Jr, Leonard WJ. The significance of tetramerization in promoter recruitment by Stat5. *Mol Cell Biol* 1999;19:1910.

353. Chatterjee-Kishore M, Wright KL, Ting JP, et al. How Stat1 mediates constitutive gene expression: a complex of unphosphorylated Stat1 and IRF1 supports transcription of the LMP2 gene. *EMBO J* 2000;19:4111.

354. Meyer T, Begitt A, Lodige I, et al. Constitutive and IFN-gamma–induced nuclear import of STAT1 proceed through independent pathways. *EMBO J* 2002;21:344.

355. Zhang X, Blenis J, Li HC, et al. Requirement of serine phosphorylation for formation of STAT-promoter complexes. *Science* 1995;267:1990.

356. Wen Z, Zhong Z, Darnell JE Jr. Maximal activation of transcription by Stat1 and Stat3 requires both tyrosine and serine phosphorylation. *Cell* 1995;82:241.

357. Horvath CM, Darnell JE Jr. The antiviral state induced by alpha interferon and gamma interferon requires transcriptionally active Stat1 protein. *J Virol* 1996;70:647.

358. Morrigl R, Berchtold S, Friedrich K, et al. Comparison of the transactivation domains of Stat5 and Stat6 in lymphoid cells and mammary epithelial cells. *Mol Cell Biol* 1997;17:3663.

359. David M, Petricon E III, Benjamin C, et al. Requirement for MAP kinase (ERK2) activity in interferon alpha and interferon beta stimulated gene expression through Stat proteins. *Science* 1995;269:1721.

360. Zhang JJ, Zhao Y, Chait BT, et al. Ser727-dependent recruitment of MCM5 by Stat1alpha in IFN-gamma–induced transcriptional activation. *EMBO J* 1998;17:6963.

361. Mowen KA, Tang J, Zhu W, et al. Arginine methylation of STAT1 modulates IFNalpha/beta-induced transcription. *Cell* 2001;104:731.

362. Look DC, Pelletier MR, Tidwell RM, et al. Stat1 depends on transcriptional synergy with Sp1. *J Biol Chem* 1995;270:30264.

363. Schaefer TS, Sanders LK, Nathans D. Cooperative transcriptional activity of Jun and Stat3 beta, a short form of Stat3. *Proc Natl Acad Sci U S A* 1995;92:9097.

364. Bhattacharya S, Eckner R, Grossman S, et al. Cooperation of Stat2 and p300/CBP in signalling induced by interferon-α. *Nature* 1996;383:344.

365. Zhang JJ, Vinkemeier U, Gu W, et al. Two contact regions between Stat1 and CBP/p300 in interferon gamma signaling. *Proc Natl Acad Sci U S A* 1996;93:15092.

366. Horvai AE, Xu L, Korzus E, et al. Nuclear integration of JAK/STAT and Ras/AP-1 signaling by CBP and p300. *Proc Natl Acad Sci U S A* 1997;94:1074.

367. Stocklin E, Wissler M, Gouilleux F, et al. Functional interactions between Stat5 and the glucocorticoid receptor. *Nature* 1996;383:726.

368. Nakajima H, Brindle PK, Handa M, et al. Functional interaction of STAT5 and nuclear receptor co-repressor SMRT: implications in negative regulation of STAT5-dependent transcription. *EMBO J* 2001;20:6836.

369. Meraz MA, White JM, Sheehan KC, et al. Targeted disruption of the Stat1 gene in mice reveals unexpected physiologic specificity in the JAK-STAT signaling pathway. *Cell* 1996;84:431.

370. Durbin JE, Hackenmiller R, Simon MC, et al. Targeted disruption of the mouse Stat1 gene results in compromised immunity to viral disease. *Cell* 1996;84:443.

371. Park C, Li S, Cha E, et al. Immune response in Stat2 knockout mice. *Immunity* 2000;13:795.

372. Takeda K, Noguchi K, Shi W, et al. Targeted disruption of the mouse Stat3 gene leads to early embryonic lethality. *Proc Natl Acad Sci U S A* 1997;94:3801.

373. Akaishi H, Takeda K, Kaisho T, et al. Defective IL-2–mediated IL-2 receptor alpha chain expression in Stat3-deficient T lymphocytes. *Int Immunol* 1998;10:1747.

374. Akira, S. Roles of STAT3 defined by tissue-specific gene targeting. *Oncogene* 2000;19:2607.

375. Chapman RS, Lourenco PC, Tonner E, et al. Suppression of epithelial apoptosis and delayed mammary gland involution in mice with a conditional knockout of Stat3. *Genes Dev* 1999;13:2604.

376. Thierfelder WE, van Deursen J, Yamamoto K, et al. Requirement for Stat4 in interleukin-12–mediated responses of natural killer cells. *Nature* 1996;382:171.

377. Kaplan MH, Sun Y-L, Hoey T, et al. Impaired IL-12 responses and enhanced development of Th2 cells in Stat4-deficient mice. *Nature* 1996;382:174.

378. Kaplan MH, Schindler U, Smiley ST, et al. Stat6 is required for mediating responses to IL-4 and for the development of Th2 cells. *Immunity* 1996;4:313.

379. Takeda K, Tanaka T, Shi W, et al. Essential role of Stat6 in IL-4 signalling. *Nature* 1996;380:627.

380. Shimoda K, van Deursen J, Sangster MY, et al. Lack of IL-4–induced Th2 response and IgE class switching in mice with disrupted *Stat6* gene. *Nature* 1996;380:630.

381. Liu X, Robinson GW, Wagner K-U, et al. Stat5a is mandatory for adult mammary gland development and lactogenesis. *Genes Dev* 1997;11:179.

382. Udy GB, Towers RP, Snell RG, et al. Requirement of STAT5b for sexual dimorphism of body growth rates and liver gene expression. *Proc Natl Acad Sci U S A* 1997;94:7239.

383. Socolovsky M, Fallon AE, Wang S, et al. Fetal anemia and apoptosis of red cell progenitors in Stat5a−/−5b−/− mice: a direct role for Stat5 in Bcl-X(L) induction. *Cell* 1999;98:181.

384. Hou XS, Melnick MB, Perrimon N. Marelle acts downstream of the *Drosophila* HOP/JAK kinase and encodes a protein similar to the mammalian STATs. *Cell* 1996;84:411.

385. Yan R, Small S, Desplan C, et al. Identification of a Stat gene that functions in *Drosophila* development. *Cell* 1996;84:421.

386. Kawata T, Shevchenko A, Fukuzawa M, et al. SH2 signaling in a lower eukaryote: a STAT protein that regulates stalk cell differentiation in *Dictyostelium*. *Cell* 1997;89:909.

387. Ramana CV, Grammatikakis N, Chernov M, et al. Regulation of c-myc expression by IFN-gamma through Stat1-dependent and -independent pathways. *EMBO J* 2000;19:263.

388. Ascherman DP, Migone T-S, Friedmann M, et al. Interleukin-2 (IL-2)–mediated induction of the IL-2 receptor α chain gene: critical role of two functionally redundant tyrosine residues in the IL-2 receptor β chain cytoplasmic domain and suggestion that these residues mediate more than Stat5 activation. *J Biol Chem* 1997;272:8704.

389. Chin YE, Kitagawa M, Su WC, et al. Cell growth arrest and induction of cyclin-dependent kinase inhibitor p21$^{WAF1/CIP1}$ mediated by STAT1. *Science* 1996;272:719.

390. Su W-C S, Kitagawa M, Xue N, et al. Activation of Stat1 by mutant fibroblast growth-factor receptor in thanatrophoric dysplasia type II dwarfism. *Nature* 1997;386:288.

391. Pfeffer LM, Mullersman JE, Pfeffer SR, et al. STAT3 as an adapter

to couple phosphatidylinositol 3-kinase to the IFNAR1 chain of the type I interferon receptor. *Science* 1997;276:1418.

392. Ramana CV, Gil MP, Schreiber RD, et al. Stat1-dependent and -independent pathways in IFN-gamma–dependent signaling. *Trends Immunol* 2002;23:96.

393. Dent AL, Shaffer AL, Yu X, et al. Control of inflammation, cytokine expression and germinal center formation by BCL-6. *Science* 1997;276:589.

394. Brivanlou AH, Darnell JE Jr. Signal transduction and the control of gene expression. *Science* 2002;295:813.

395. Baldwin AS Jr. The NF-κB and IκB proteins: new discoveries and insights. *Annu Rev Immunol* 1996;14:649.

396. Lee FS, Hagler J, Chen ZJ, et al. Activation of the IkappaB alpha kinase complex by MEKK1, a kinase of the JNK pathway. *Cell* 1997; 88:213.

397. Karin M. How NF-kappaB is activated: the role of the IkappaB kinase (IKK) complex. *Oncogene* 1999;18:6867.

398. Macian F, Lopez-Rodriguez C, Rao A. Partners in transcription: NFAT and AP-1. *Oncogene* 2001;20:2476.

399. Crabtree GR, Olson EN. NFAT signaling: choreographing the social lives of cells. *Cell* 2002;109(Suppl):S67.

400. Wotton D, Massague J. Smad transcriptional corepressors in TGF beta family signaling. *Curr Top Microbiol Immunol* 2001;254:145.

401. Takeshita T, Arita T, Higuchi M, et al. STAM, signal transducing adaptor molecule, is associated with Janus kinases and involved in signaling for cell growth and c-myc induction. *Immunity* 1997;6: 449.

402. Migone T-S, Rodig S, Cacalano NA, et al. Functional cooperation of the interleukin-2 receptor beta chain and Jak1 in phosphatidylinositol 3-kinase recruitment and phosphorylation. *Mol Cell Biol* 1998;18: 6416.

403. Horak ID, Gress RE, Lucas PJ, et al. T-lymphocyte interleukin 2–dependent tyrosine protein kinase signal transduction involves the activation of p56lck. *Proc Natl Acad Sci U S A* 1991;88:1996.

404. Hatakeyama M, Kono T, Kobayashi N, et al. Interaction of the IL-2 receptor with the src-family kinase p56lck: identification of novel intermolecular association. *Science* 1991;252:1523.

405. Torigo T, Saragovi HU, Reed JC. Interleukin-2 regulates the activity of the lyn protein tyrosine kinase in a B-cell line. *Proc Natl Acad Sci U S A* 1992;89:2674.

406. Kobayashi N, Kono T, Hatakeyama M, et al. Functional coupling of the src-family protein tyrosine kinases p59fyn and p53/56lyn with the interleukin 2 receptor: implications for redundancy and pleiotropism in cytokine signal transduction. *Proc Natl Acad Sci U S A* 1993;90: 4201.

407. Minami Y, Nakagawa Y, Kawahara A, et al. Protein tyrosine kinase Syk is associated with and activated by the IL-2 receptor: possible link with the c-myc induction pathway. *Immunity* 1995;2:89.

408. Otani H, Siegel JP, Erdos M, et al. Interleukin (IL)–2 and IL-3 induce distinct but overlapping responses in murine IL-3 dependent 32D cells transduced with human IL-2 receptor β chain: involvement of tyrosine kinases other than p56lck. *Proc Natl Acad Sci U S A* 1992;89: 2789.

409. Karnitz L, Sutor SL, Torigoe T, et al. Effects of p56lck deficiency on the growth and cytolytic effector function of an interleukin-2–dependent cytotoxic T-cell line. *Mol Cell Biol* 1992;12:4521.

410. Hatakeyama M, Mori H, Doi T, et al. A restricted cytoplasmic region of IL-2 receptor β chain is essential for growth signal transduction but not for ligand binding and internalization. *Cell* 1989;59:837.

411. Fujii H, Ogasawara K, Otsuka A, et al. Functional dissection of the cytoplasmic subregions of the IL-2 receptor betac chain in primary lymphocyte populations. *EMBO J* 1998;17:6551.

412. Turner M, Mee PJ, Costello PS, et al. Perinatal lethality and blocked B-cell development in mice lacking the tyrosine kinase Syk. *Nature* 1995;378:298.

413. Corey SJ, Burkhardt AL, Bolen JB, et al. Granulocyte colony-stimulating factor receptor signaling involves the formation of a three-component complex with lyn and syk protein tyrosine kinases. *Proc Natl Acad Sci U S A* 1994;91:4683.

414. Rao P, Mufson RA. A membrane proximal domain of the human interleukin-3 receptor βc subunit that signals DNA synthesis in NIH 3T3 cells specifically binds a complex of src and Janus family tyrosine kinases and phosphatidylinositol 3-kinase. *J Biol Chem* 1995; 270:6886.

415. Ernst M, Gearing DP, Dunn AR. Functional and biochemical association of Hck with the LIF/IL-6 receptor signal transducing subunit gp130 in embryonic stem cells. *EMBO J* 1994;13:1574.

416. Matsuda T, Fukada T, Takahashi-Tezuka M, et al. Activation of Fes tyrosine kinase by gp130, an interleukin-6 family cytokine signal transducer, and their association. *J Biol Chem* 1995;270:11037.

417. Matsuda T, Takahashi-Tezuka M, Fukada T, et al. Association and activation of Btk and Tec tyrosine kinases by gp130, a signal transducer of the interleukin-6 family of cytokines. *Blood* 1995;85:627.

418. Izuhara K, Feldman RA, Greer P, et al. Interaction of the c-fes proto-oncogene product with the interleukin-4 receptor. *J Biol Chem* 1994;269:18623.

419. Burks DJ, White MF. IRS proteins and beta-cell function. *Diabetes* 2001;50(Suppl 1):S140.

420. Wang L-M, Myers MG Jr, Sun S-J, et al. IRS-1: essential for insulin- and IL-4–stimulated mitogenesis in hematopoietic cells. *Science* 1993;261:1591.

421. Keegan AD, Nelms K, White M, et al. An IL-4 receptor region containing an insulin receptor motif is important for IL-4 mediated IRS-1 phosphorylation and cell growth. *Cell* 1994;76:811.

422. Ridderstrale M, Degerman E, Tornqvist H. Growth hormone stimulates the tyrosine phosphorylation of the insulin receptor substrate-1 and its association with phosphatidylinositol 3-kinase in primary adipocytes. *J Biol Chem* 1995;270:3471.

423. Argetsinger LS, Norstedt G, Billestrup N, et al. Growth hormone, interferon-gamma, and leukemia inhibitory factor utilize insulin receptor substrate-2 in intracellular signaling. *J Biol Chem* 1996;271: 29415.

424. Johnston JA, Wang LM, Hanson EP, et al. Interleukins 2, 4, 7, and 15 stimulate tyrosine phosphorylation of insulin receptor substrates 1 and 2 in T cells. Potential role of JAK kinases. *J Biol Chem* 1995; 270:28527.

425. Fruman DA, Meyers RE, Cantley LC. Phosphoinositide kinases. *Annu Rev Biochem* 1998;67:481.

426. Truitt KE, Mills GB, Turck CW, et al. SH2-dependent association of phosphatidylinositol 3-kinase 85-kDa regulatory subunit with the interleukin-2 receptor β chain. *J Biol Chem* 1994;269:5937.

427. Damen JE, Cutler RL, Jiao H, et al. Phosphorylation of tyrosine 503 in the erythropoietin receptor (EpR) is essential for binding of the p85 subunit of phosphatidylinositol (PI) 3-kinase and for EpR-associated PI 3-kinase activity. *J Biol Chem* 1995;270:23402.

428. Jucker M, Feldman RA. Identification of a new adapter protein that may link the common β subunit of the receptor for granulocyte/macrophage colony stimulating factor, interleukin-3 (IL-3), and IL-5 to phosphatidylinositol 3-kinase. *J Biol Chem* 1995;270:27817.

429. Karnitz LM, Burns LA, Sutor SL, et al. Interleukin-2 triggers a novel phosphatidylinositol 3-kinase–dependent MEK activation pathway. *Mol Cell Biol* 1995;15:3049.

430. Dong C, Davis RJ, Flavell RA. MAP kinases in the immune response. *Annu Rev Immunol.* 2002;20:55.

431. Neel BG, Tonks NK. Protein tyrosine phosphatases in signal transduction. *Curr Opin Cell Biol* 1997;9:193.

432. Li L, Dixon JE. Form, function, and regulation of protein tyrosine phosphatases and their involvement in human diseases. *Semin Immunol* 2000;12:75.

433. Tsui HW, Siminovitch KA, de Souza L, et al. Motheaten and viable motheaten mice have mutations in the haematopoietic cell phosphatase gene. *Nat Genet* 1993;4:124.

434. Shultz LD, Schweitzer PA, Rajan TV, et al. Mutations at the murine motheaten locus are within the hematopoietic cell protein-tyrosine phosphatase (Hcph) gene. *Cell* 1993;73:1445.

435. van Zant G, Schultz L. Hematologic abnormalities of the immunodeficient mouse mutant, viable motheaten (meV). *Exp Hematol* 1989; 17:81.

436. Klingmuller U, Lorenz U, Cantley LC, et al. Specific recruitment of SH-PTP1 to the erythropoietin receptor causes inactivation of JAK2 and termination of proliferative signals. *Cell* 1995;80:729.

437. Yi T, Mui AL, Krystal G, et al. Hematopoietic cell phosphatase associates with the interleukin-3 (IL-3) receptor β chain and down-regulates IL-3 induced tyrosine phosphorylation and mitogenesis. *Mol Cell Biol* 1993;13:7577.

438. Yetter A, Uddin S, Krolewski JJ, et al. Association of the interferon-dependent tyrosine kinase Tyk-2 with the hematopoietic cell phosphatase. *J Biol Chem* 1995;270:18179.

439. Jiao H, Berrada K, Yang W, et al. Direct association with and dephosphorylation of Jak2 kinase by the SH2-domain-containing protein tyrosine phosphatase SHP-1. *Mol Cell Biol* 1996;16:6985.

440. Yin T, Shen R, Feng GS, et al. Molecular characterization of specific interactions between SHP-2 phosphatase and JAK tyrosine kinases. *J Biol Chem* 1997;272:1032.

441. Haspel RL, Salditt-Georgieff M, Darnell JE Jr. The rapid inactivation of nuclear tyrosine phosphorylated Stat1 depends upon a protein tyrosine phosphatase. *EMBO J* 1996;15:6262.

442. Krystal G. Lipid phosphatases in the immune system. *Semin Immunol* 2000;12:397.

443. Kim TK, Maniatis T. Regulation of interferon-γ-activated STAT1 by the ubiquitin-proteasome pathway. *Science* 1996;273:1717.

444. Yoshimura A, Ohkubo T, Kiguchi T, et al. A novel cytokine-inducible gene CIS encodes an SH2-containing protein that binds to tyrosine-phosphorylated interleukin 3 and erythropoietin receptors. *EMBO J* 1995;14:2816.

445. Matsumoto A, Masuhara M, Mitsui K, et al. CIS, a cytokine inducible SH2 protein, is a target of the JAK-STAT5 pathway and modulates STAT5 activation. *Blood* 1997;89:3148.

446. Starr R, Willson TA, Viney EM, et al. A family of cytokine-inducible inhibitors of signalling. *Nature* 1997;387:917.

447. Endo TA, Masuhara M, Yokouchi M, et al. A new protein containing an SH2 domain that inhibits JAK kinases. *Nature* 1997;387:921.

448. Naka T, Narazaki M, Hirata M, et al. Structure and function of a new STAT-induced STAT inhibitor. *Nature* 1997;387:924.

449. Yasukawa H, Sasaki A, Yoshimura A. Negative regulation of cytokine signaling pathways. *Annu Rev Immunol* 2000;18:143.

450. Krebs DL, Hilton DJ. SOCS proteins: negative regulators of cytokine signaling. *Stem Cells* 2001;19:378.

451. Kovanen PE, Leonard WJ. Inhibitors keep cytokines in check. *Curr Biol* 1999;9:R899.

452. Chung CD, Liao J, Liu B, et al. Specific inhibition of Stat3 signal transduction by PIAS3. *Science* 1997;278:1803.

453. Liu B, Liao J, Rao X, et al. Inhibition of Stat1-mediated gene activation by PIAS1. *Proc Natl Acad Sci U S A* 1998;95:10626.

454. Kile BT, Nicola NA, Alexander WS. Negative regulators of cytokine signaling. *Int J Hematol* 2001;73:292.

455. Sachdev S, Bruhn L, Sieber H, et al. PIASy, a nuclear matrix-associated SUMO E3 ligase, represses LEF1 activity by sequestration into nuclear bodies. *Genes Dev* 2001;15:3088.

456. Jackson PK. A new RING for SUMO: wrestling transcriptional responses into nuclear bodies with PIAS family E3 SUMO ligases. *Genes Dev* 2001;15:3053.

457. Mosmann TR, Cherwinski H, Bond MW, et al. Two types of murine helper T cell clones. 1. Definition according to profiles of lymphokine activities and secreted proteins. *J Immunol* 1986;136:2348.

458. Mosmann TR, Sad S. The expanding universe of T-cell subsets: Th1, Th2 and more. *Immunol Today* 1996;17:138.

459. Abbas AK, Murphy KM, Sher A. Functional diversity of helper T lymphocytes. *Nature* 1996;383:787.

460. Lucey DR, Clerici M, Shearer GM. Type 1 and type 2 cytokine dysregulation in human infectious, neoplastic, and inflammatory diseasee. *Clin Microbiol Rev* 1996;9:532.

461. Jankovic D, Sher A, Yap G. Th1/Th2 effector choice in parasitic infection: decision making by committee. *Curr Opin Immunol* 2001;13:403.

462. Romagnani S. TH1/TH2 interleukins. In: Oppenheim J, Feldman M, eds. *Cytokine reference*, vol 1. New York Academic Press, 2001:99.

463. Okamura H, Rao A. Transcriptional regulation in lymphocytes. *Curr Opin Cell Biol* 2001;13:239.

464. Ho IC, Glimcher LH. Transcription: tantalizing times for T cells. *Cell* 2002;109(Suppl):S109.

465. Avni O, Rao A. T cell differentiation: a mechanistic view. *Curr Opin Immunol* 2000;12:654.

466. Gajewski TF, Fitch FW. Anti-proliferative effect of IFN-γ in immune regulation. I. IFN-γ inhibits the proliferation of Th2 but not Th1 murine helper T lymphocyte clones. *J Immunol* 1988;140:4245.

467. Pernis A, Gupta S, Gollob KJ, et al. Lack of interferon γ receptor β chain and the prevention of interferon γ signaling in TH1 cells. *Science* 1995;269:245.

468. Bach EA, Szabo SJ, Dighe AS, et al. Ligand-induced autoregulation of IFN-γ receptor β chain expression in T helper cell subsets. *Science* 1995;270:1215.

469. Szabo SJ, Dighe AS, Gubler U, et al. Regulation of the interleukin (IL)–12Rβ2 subunit expression in developing T helper 1 (Th1) and Th2 cells. *J Exp Med* 1997;185:817.

470. Gilmour KC, Fujii H, Cranston T, et al. Defective expression of the interleukin-2/interleukin-15 receptor β subunit leads to a natural killer cell–deficient form of severe combined immunodeficiency. *Blood* 2001;98:877.

471. Altare F, Lammas D, Revy P, et al. Inherited interleukin 12 deficiency in a child with bacille Calmette-Guérin and *Salmonella enteritidis* disseminated infection. *J Clin Invest* 1998;102:2035.

472. Altare F, Durandy A, Lammas D, et al. Impairment of mycobacterial immunity in human interleukin-12 receptor deficiency. *Science* 1998;280:1432.

473. Jouanguy E, Lamhamedi-Cherradi S, Altare F, et al. Partial interferon-gamma receptor 1 deficiency in a child with tuberculoid bacillus Calmette-Guérin infection and a sibling with clinical tuberculosis. *J Clin Invest* 1997;100:2658.

474. Doffinger R, Jouanguy E, Dupuis S, et al. Partial interferon-gamma receptor signaling chain deficiency in a patient with bacille Calmette-Guérin and *Mycobacterium abscessus* infection. *J Infect Dis* 2000;181:379.

475. Dupuis S, Dargemont C, Fieschi C, et al. Impairment of mycobacterial but not viral immunity by a germline human STAT1 mutation. *Science* 2001;293:300.

476. Chen Q, Ghilardi N, Wang H, et al. Development of Th1-type immune responses requires the type I cytokine receptor TCCR. *Nature* 2000;407:916.

477. Yoshida H, Hamano S, Senaldi G, et al. WSX-1 is required for the initiation of Th1 responses and resistance to L. major infection. *Immunity* 2001;15:569.

478. Amselem S, Duquesnoy P, Attree O, et al. Laron dwarfism and mutations of the growth hormone receptor gene. *N Engl J Med* 1989;321:989.

479. Dong F, Hoefsloot LH, Schelen AM, et al. Identification of a nonsense mutation in the granulocyte–colony-stimulating factor receptor in severe congenital neutropenia. *Proc Natl Acad Sci U S A* 1994;91:4480.

480. de la Chapelle A, Traskelin AL, Juvonen E. Truncated erythropoietin receptor causes dominantly inherited benign human erythrocytosis. *Proc Natl Acad Sci U S A* 1993;90:4495.

481. Souyri M, Vigon I, Penciolelli J-F, et al. A putative truncated cytokine receptor gene transduced by the myeloproliferative leukemia virus immortalizes hematopoietic progenitors. *Cell* 1990;63:1137.

482. Isaksen DE, Baumann H, Trobridge PA, et al. Requirement for Stat5 in thymic stromal lymphopoietin-mediated signal transduction. *J Immunol* 1999;163:5971.

483. Kundig TM, Schorle H, Bachmann MF, et al. Immune responses in interleukin-2–deficient mice. *Science* 1993;262:1059.

484. Sadlack B, Merz H, Schorle H, et al. Ulcerative colitis–like disease in mice with a disrupted interleukin-2 gene. *Cell* 1993;75:253.

485. Noben-Trauth N, Shultz LD, Brombacher F, et al. An IL-4–independent pathway for CD4+ T cell IL-4 productionis revealed in IL-4 receptor–deficient mice. *Proc Natl Acad Sci U S A* 1997;94:10838.

486. Kopf M, Brombacher F, Hodgkin PD, et al. IL-5-deficient mice have a developmental defect in CD5+ B-1 cells and lack eosinophilia but have normal antibody and cytotoxic T cell responses. *Immunity* 1996;4:15.

487. Dranoff G, Crawford AD, Sadelain M, et al. Involvement of granulocyte-macrophage colony-stimulating factor in pulmonary homeostasis. *Science* 1994;264:713.

488. Stanley E, Lieschke GJ, Grail D, et al. Granulocyte/macrophage colony-stimulating factor–deficient mice show no major perturbation of hematopoiesis but develop a characteristic pulmonary pathology. *Proc Natl Acad Sci U S A* 1994;91:5592.

489. Nishinakamura R, Nakayama N, Hirabayashi Y, et al. Mice deficient for the IL-3/GM-CSF/IL-5 βc receptor exhibit lung pathology and impaired immune response while βIL-3 receptor–deficient mice are normal. *Immunity* 1995;2:211.

490. Kopf M, Baumann H, Freer G, et al. Impaired immune and actue-phase responses in interleukin-6–deficient mice. *Nature* 1994;368:339.

491. Yoshida K, Taga T, Saito M, et al. Targeted disruption of gp130, a common signal transducer for the interleukin 6 family of cytokines,

leads to myocardial and hematological disorders. *Proc Natl Acad Sci U S A* 1996;93:407.

492. Akira S, Yosha K, Tanaka T, et al. Targeted disruption of the IL-6 related genes: gp130 and NF-IL6. *Immunol Rev* 1995;148:221.

493. Stewart CL, Kaspar P, Brunet LJ, et al. Blastocyst implantation depends on maternal expression of leukaemia inhibitory factor. *Nature* 1992:359:76.

494. Escary JL, Perreau J, Dum'enil D, et al. Leukaemia inhibitory factor is necessary for maintenance of hematopoietic stem cells and thymocyte stimulation. *Nature* 1993:363:361.

495. Rao MS, Sun Y, Escary JL, et al. Leukaemia inhibitory factor mediates an injury response but not a target-directed developmental transmitter switch in sympathetic neurons. *Neuron* 1993;11:1175.

496. Ware CB, Horowitz MC, Renshaw BR, et al. Target disruption of the low-affinity leukemia inhibitory factor receptor gene causes placental, skeletal, neural and metabolic defects and results in perinatal death. *Development* 1995;121:1283.

497. Li M, Sendtner M, Smith A. Essential function of LIF receptor in motor neurons. *Nature* 1995;378:724.

498. Masu Y, Wolf E, Holtmann B, et al. Disruption of the CNTF gene results in motor neuron degeneration. *Nature* 1993;365:27.

499. DeChiara TM, Bejsada R, Poueymirou WT, et al. Mice lacking the CNTF receptor, unlike mice lacking CNTF, exhibit profound motor neuron deficits at birth. *Cell* 1995;83:313.

500. Robb L, Li R, Hartley L, et al. Infertility in female mice lacking the receptor for interleukin 11 is due to a defective uterine response to implantation. *Nat Med* 1998;4:303.

501. Magram J, Connaughton SE, Warrier RR, et al. IL-12–deficient mice are defective in interferon-γ production and type 1 cytokine responses. *Immunity* 1996;4:471.

502. Wu C, Ferrante J, Gateley MK, et al. Characterization of IL-12 receptor β1 chain (IL-12Rβ1)–deficient mice. *J Immunol* 1997;159:1658.

503. Wu H, Liu X, Jaenisch R, et al. Generation of committed erythroid BFU-E and CFU-E progenitors does not require erythropoietin or the erythropoietin receptor. *Cell* 1995;83:59.

504. Lin CS, Lim SK, D'Agati V, et al. Differential effects of an erythropoietin receptor gene disruption on primitive and definitive erythropoiesis. *Genes Dev* 1996;10:154.

505. Gurney AL, Carver-Moore K, de Sauvage FJ, et al. Thrombocytopenia in c-mpl deficient mice. *Science* 1994;265:1445.

506. Lieschke GJ, Grail D, Hodgson G, et al. Mice lacking granulocyte colony-stimulating factor have chronic neutropenia, granulocyte and macrophage progenitor cell deficiency, and impaired neutrophil mobilization. *Blood* 1994;84:1737.

507. Yoshida H, Yayashi S-I, Kunisada T, et al. The murine mutation osteopetrosis is in the coding region of the macrophage colony stimulating factor gene. *Nature* 1990;345:442.

508. Metcalf D. The granulocyte-macrophage regulators: reappraisal by gene inactivation. *Exp Hematol* 1995;23:569.

509. Muller U, Steinhoff U, Reis LF, et al. Functional role of type I and type II interferons in antiviral defense. *Science* 1994;264:1918.

510. van den Broek MF, Muller U, Huang S, et al. Immune defence in mice lacking type I and/or type II interferon receptors. *Immunol Rev* 1995;148:5.

511. van den Broek MF, Muller U, Huang S, et al. Antiviral defense in mice lacking both alpha/beta and gamma interferon receptors. *J Virol* 1995;69:4792.

512. Dalton DK, Pitts-Meek S, Keshav S, et al. Multiple defects of immune cell function in mice with disrupted interferon-γ genes. *Science* 1993;259:1739.

513. Wang ZE, Reiner SL, Zheng S, et al. CD4+ effector cells default to the Th2 pathway in interferon γ–deficient mice infected with *Leishmania major. J Exp Med* 1994;179:1367.

514. Scharton-Kersten, TM, Wynn TA, Denkers EY, et al. In the absence of endogenous IFN-g, mice develop unimpaired IL-12 responses to *Toxoplasma gondii* while failing to control acute infection. *J Immunol* 1996;157:4045.

515. Huang S, Hendriks W, Althage A, et al. Immune response in mice that lack the interferon γ receptor. *Science* 1993;259:1742.

516. Kuhn R, Lohler J, Rennick D, et al. Interleukin-10–deficient mice develop chronic enterocolitis. *Cell* 1993;75:263.

517. Parganas E, Wang D, Stravopodis D, et al. Jak2 is essential for signaling through a variety of cytokine receptors. *Cell* 1998;93:385.

518. Neubauer H, Cumano A, Müller M, et al. Jak2 deficiency defines an essential developmental checkpoint in definitive hematopoiesis. *Cell* 1998;93:397.

519. Karaghiosoff M, Neubauer H, Lassnig C, et al. Partial impairment of cytokine responses in Tyk2-deficient mice. *Immunity* 2000;13:549.

520. Shimoda K, Kato K, Aoki K, et al. Tyk2 plays a restricted role in IFN alpha signaling, although it is required for IL-12–mediated T cell function. *Immunity* 2000;13:561.

521. Shimoda K, Tsutsui H, Aoki K, et al. Partial impairment of interleukin-12 (IL-12) and IL-18 signaling in Tyk2-deficient mice. *Blood* 2002;99:2094.

CHAPTER 24

The Tumor Necrosis Factor Superfamily and Its Receptors

Lyle L. Moldawer

Introduction
Structure–Function Relationships in the TNF Superfamily
Structure–Function Relationships in the TNF Receptor Superfamily
Regulation of TNF-α Expression
Biological Functions of TNF-α
TNF-α Signaling Through Its Two Receptors
Lymphotoxin, Not Just Another TNF
LIGHT or HVEM Ligand
Fas and Fas Ligand
RANK Ligand, RANK, and Osteoprotegerin
TNF-Related Apoptosis-Inducing Ligand (TRAIL)
    TRAIL Receptors · TRAIL as a Cancer Chemotherapeutic
TWEAK
T-Lymphocyte Co-stimulatory Molecules: CD27, CD30, 4-1BB, and OX40
    CD27 · CD30 · 4-1BB · OX40 and OX40 Ligand
BLyS and APRIL: B-Lymphocyte Co-stimulators
Ectodysplasin and EDAR
Conclusions
References

INTRODUCTION

The TNF superfamily is comprised of at least 19 genes encoding 20 type II (i.e., intracellular N-terminus, extracellular C-terminus) transmembrane proteins (Table 1). Included are several well-known members, such as TNF-α (formerly termed cachectin), TNF-β (lymphotoxin-α, LT-α), Fas ligand (FasL), and CD40 ligand (CD40L), as well as an increasing number of newly described mediators, including APRIL (a proliferation-inducing ligand), TRAIL (TNF-related apoptosis inducing ligand), TWEAK (TNF-like and weak inducer of apoptosis), BLyS (B-lymphocyte stimulator), LIGHT (homologous to lymphotoxins, exhibits inducible expression, and competes with HSV glycoprotein D for herpesvirus entry mediator [HVEM], a receptor expressed by T-lymphocytes), CD27 ligand, CD30 ligand, OX40 ligand, 4-1BB ligand, ED1, and RANK ligand (receptor activator of NFκB ligand), among others. In 1998, a unified nomenclature similar to that

accepted for the chemokine family was adopted, composed of the term TNFSF for TNF superfamily or TNFRSF for TNF receptor superfamily and a number (1).

The biological activities of TNF-α and lymphotoxin were first described in the 1960s and 1970s with the identification of macrophage- and lymphocyte-derived products that produced hemorrhagic necrosis of solid tumors (2–4). The physical structure of the two proteins has been known for approximately 20 years, having been cloned and sequenced in the mid-1980s by several laboratories nearly simultaneously (5–7). Within a few years of its sequence and cloning, the principal biological activities of TNF-α had been identified and reproduced using purified or recombinant protein, including its ability to cause hemorrhagic necrosis of tumors, tissue injury, and shock through its pro-inflammatory properties on the vascular endothelium; to induce apoptosis in some cancerous or transformed cell lines, and in lymphocyte and epithelial cell populations; and to alter intermediate substrate

TABLE 1. *Members of the tumor necrosis factor (TNF) superfamily and their known receptors*

TNF superfamily		TNF receptor superfamily	
Systematic name	Functional names	Systematic name	Functional names
TNFSF1	LT, LTα, TNF-β	TNFRSF1A	TNF-RI, CD120α
		TNFRSF1B	TNF-RII, CD120β
TNFSF2	TNF-α, DIF	TNFRSF1A	TNF-RI, CD120α
		TNFRSF1B	TNF-RII, CD120β
TNFSF3	LTβ, TNF-γ, p33	TNFRSF3	LTβR, TNF-RIII, TNF-Rrp, TNF-γR, CD18
TNFSF4	OX40L, gp34, TXGP1	TNFRSF4	OX40, ACT35, TXGP1L
TNFSF5	CD40L, CD154, TRAP, gp39, IMD3, HIGM1	TNFRSF5	CD40, p50
TNFSF6	FasL, Apo 1L	TNFRSF6	Fas, Apo 1, CD95, APT1
		TNFRSF6B	DcR3
TNFSF7	CD27L, CD70	TNFRSF7	CD27, Tp55, S152
TNFSF8	CD30L	TNFRSF8	CD30, Ki-1, D1S166E
TNFSF9	4-1BBL, CD137L	TNFRSF9	4-1BB, CD137, ILA
TNFSF10	TRAIL, Apo 2L, TL2	TNFRSF10A	TRAIL-R1, DR4, Apo 2
		TNFRSF10B	TRAIL-R2, DR5, KILLER, TRICK-2
		TNFRSF10C	TRAIL-R3, DcR1, TRID, LIT
		TNFRSF10D	TRAIL-R4, DcR2, TRUNDD
TNFSF11	RANKL, OPGL, ODF	TNFRSF11A	RANK
		TNFRSF11B	OPG, OCIF, TR1
TNFSF12	TWEAK, DR3L, Apo 3L	TNFRSF12	TRAMP, DR3, WSL-1, LARD, TR3, Apo 3
TNFSF13	APRIL	TNFRSF13	TACI, BCMA
TNFSF13B	BAFF, BLyS, TALL-1, THANK	—	TACI, BCMA, BAFF-R
TNFSF14	LIGHT, LTγ, HVEML	TNFRSF14	LIGHT-R, HVEM, HVEA, ATAR, TR2
TNFSF15	TL1, VEGI	TNFRSF15	—
TNFSF16	—	TNFRSF16	NGF-R, p75NTR
TNFSF17	—	TNFRSF17	BCMA
TNFSF18	AITRL, TL6, GITRL	TNFRSF18	AITR, GITR
TNFSF19	—	TNFRSF19	TAJ, TROY

TNFRSF, tumor necrosis factor receptor superfamily; TNFSF, tumor necrosis factor superfamily.
Note that ED1 and EDAR have not been assigned names according to the new nomenclature.
Adapted from http://www.gene.ucl.ac.uk/users/hester/tnftop.html, the Centre for Human Genetics, University College, London, United Kingdom.

and energy metabolism and induce cachexia (for review, see Beutler and Cerami [8]).

However, it took another 10 to 15 years to fully realize that TNF-α and lymphotoxin were only two members of an ever-increasing family of proteins with both structural and functional homology. Large-scale sequencing of many similar expressed sequence tags identified related ligands in the same "superfamily." Their biological functions have often overlapped with TNF-α and lymphotoxin; but not unexpectedly, their activities have also demonstrated considerable diversity. In addition, the roles of many of these TNF superfamily ligands are not so much as orchestrators of the acquired or innate immune responses, but rather critical parts in development and organogenesis. (For review, see Wallach et al. [9], Mackay and Kalled [10], Zhou et al. [11], Griffith and Lynch [12], Idriss and Naismith [13], Schluter and Deckert [14], Sedgwick et al. [15], and Locksley et al. [16].) Not surprisingly, the receptors for these ligands of the TNF superfamily also comprise a related gene superfamily with common and distinct structure and signal transduction pathways (Table 1 and Fig. 1).

All of the diverse functions of the TNF superfamily ligands are still not fully known, and their roles in normal growth and development, as well as in disease pathogenesis have only been partially established. However, there is general recognition that ligands of the TNF superfamily regulate and control the inflammatory and immune response. Nevertheless, the range of activities that these ligands have on specific components of the immune response has only begun to be appreciated, and in many ways, their diversity is quite remarkable. For example, during development and organogenesis, ligands such as TNF-α, lymphotoxin-α, RANK ligand, and LT-α/β provide critical signals for the development of secondary lymphoid organs (17). Knockout mice lacking the genes for these proteins show abnormal lymph node development. The development and maturation of several key lymphocyte and myeloid cell populations are also dependent on the organized and timed release of several TNF superfamily ligands, including BLyS, CD40 ligand, 4-1BB ligand, OX40 ligand, CD27 ligand, CD30 ligand, and RANK ligand. Equally important, several ligands of the superfamily, including TNF-α, FasL, and TRAIL, provide the cytotoxic activity of effector cells and are responsible for the removal and re-establishment of homeostasis of leukocyte populations via activation induced cell death (10). Several members of this family—most notably TNF-α, TWEAK, and FasL—also

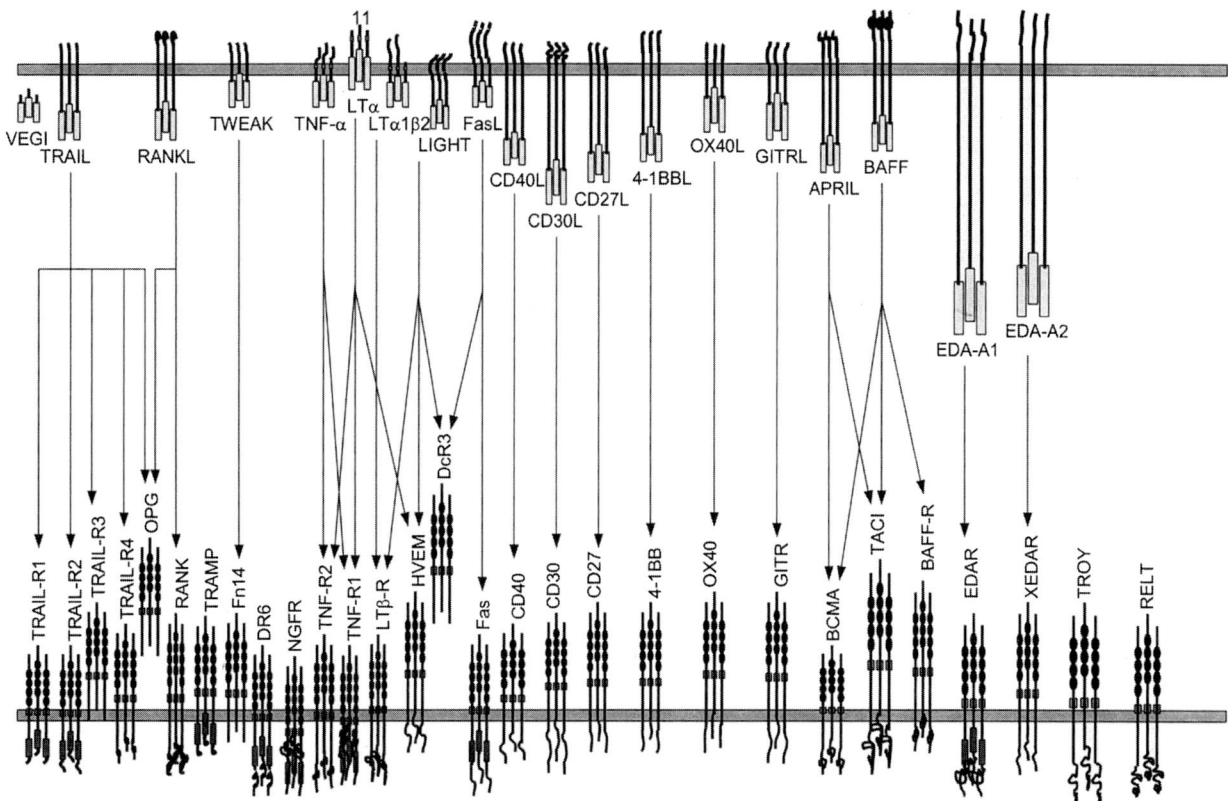

FIG. 1. Interrelationships among members of the TNF superfamily and the TNF receptors. Members of the TNF superfamily with the exception of APRIL/BLyS and lymphotoxin-α/β2 are homotrimers, while lymphotoxin-α/β2 is a heterotrimer comprised of a single lymphotoxin-α chain and two lymphotoxin-β chains. Adapted from Bodmer et al. (20), with permission.

appear to play critical roles in the communication between immune and parenchymal or endothelial cells, which is particularly important for induction of the acute-phase response and maintenance of vascular hemostasis (reviewed below). These proteins provide the fundamental communication between immune and somatic tissues. Other TNF superfamily ligands regulate the differentiation and development of epithelial structures (ED1) and bone-resorbing osteoclasts (RANK ligand and TNF-α).

Most notably, TNF superfamily ligands and their receptors are associated with several disorders that are secondary to either genetic defects or acquired processes. Two chronic inflammatory diseases in particular, rheumatoid arthritis and inflammatory bowel disease, have been shown to be caused by exaggerated and inappropriate local production of TNF-α, and two FDA-approved TNF inhibitors (Embrel™ and Remicaid™) have now been approved for rheumatoid arthritis (18). However, inappropriate production of TNF-α has also been implicated in the pathogenesis of a number of other chronic and acute inflammatory diseases, such as septic shock, meningococcemia, adult-respiratory distress syndrome, otitis media, hepatitis B and C infection, Reyes' syndrome, and cerebral malaria, among others (reviewed in Ksontini et al. [19]). Several hereditary diseases of the immune system are also associated with mutations in the ligands

or receptors of the TNF superfamily, including hyper IgM syndrome (CD40L), type I autoimmune lymphoproliferative syndrome (FasL/FAS), and the TNF receptor I–associated periodic fever syndrome (Table 2). Mutations in either the ED1 ligand or EDAR lead to devastating defects in skin, hair, and teeth development associated with ectodermal dysplasia syndrome. Because our knowledge of the functions of other ligands of the TNF superfamily is considerably less than for TNF-α and FasL, it is likely that other relationships between ligands of the TNF superfamily and diseases will be discovered in the future.

STRUCTURE–FUNCTION RELATIONSHIPS IN THE TNF SUPERFAMILY

The most identifiable single structural characteristic of individual ligands of the TNF superfamily is their propensity to trimerize. All members of the TNF superfamily with the exception of APRIL/BLyS and lymphotoxin-α/β2 are homotrimers, while lymphotoxin-α/β2 is a heterotrimer comprised of a single lymphotoxin-α chain and two lymphotoxin-β chains (Fig. 2). APRIL and BLyS also can apparently form heterotrimers, comprised of one or two of the respective members. The key to homotrimerization of the other species is a generally conserved 150-amino-acid–long C-terminal

TABLE 2. *Major classification of TNF ligands, their receptors, and their association with autoimmune diseases and infections*

Ligands	Receptor	Function	Disease
TNF-α	TNF-RI, TNF-RII	Inflammation	Rheumatoid arthritis, SLE, inflammatory bowel disease, multiple sclerosis, type I diabetes
LTα	TNF-RI, TNF-RII	Inflammation	Rheumatoid arthritis, SLE, inflammatory bowel disease, multiple sclerosis, type I diabetes
LTα/β	LTβ-R	Lymph node, spleen organization	Rheumatoid arthritis, SLE, inflammatory bowel disease, multiple sclerosis, type I diabetes
LIGHT	LTβ-R, HVEM	T-cell activation, thymocyte survival	Diabetes, rheumatoid arthritis
Fas ligand	FAS	Apoptosis, PMN recruitment	SLE, EAE, multiple sclerosis, thyroid disease, autoimmune hepatitis
TRAIL	TRAIL-R1, TRAIL-R2, TRAIL-R3, TRAIL-R4, OPG	Induces tumor cell death, blocks T-cell proliferation	Autoimmune thyroid disease, multiple sclerosis
RANK ligand	RANK, OPG	Osteoclast formation, dendritic cell maturation	Rheumatoid arthritis
CD30 ligand	CD30	T-cell co-stimulation	Rheumatoid arthritis, autoimmune thyroiditis, SLE, primary biliary cirrhosis
4-1BB ligand	4-1BB	T-cell co-stimulation	Rheumatoid arthritis, SLE
OX40 ligand	OX40	T-cell co-stimulation	Rheumatoid arthritis, multiple sclerosis, inflammatory bowel disease

EAE, experimental autoimmune encephalomyelitis; HVEM, herpesvirus entry mediator; LT, lymphotoxin; OPG, osteoprotegerin; PMN, polymorphonuclear neutrophil; RANK, receptor-activator of NFκB; SLE, systemic lupus erythematosus; TNF, tumor necrosis factor; TRAIL, TNF-related apoptosis-inducing ligand.

domain that has recently been coined the "TNF-homology domain" or THD (20). It is this trimeric domain that is responsible for ligand binding to its receptor, and it contains a conserved region of aromatic and hydrophobic residues. Although the THDs among TNF superfamily members do vary somewhat at their primary amino acid structure, they share a near identical tertiary folding to create β-pleated sheets that adopt a "jelly-roll"–like complex (21,22). Trimeric THDs are approximately 60 angstroms in height comprised of bell-shaped, truncated pyramids with loops of variable size extending from a compact core of conserved β-sheets (20). The trimer is assembled in such a manner that each subunit is tightly packed against the inner sheet of its neighbor, creating a very stable hydrophobic interface (20–22). It is at these three grooves that the TNF-superfamily ligand interacts with its cellular or soluble receptor and provides its specificity of binding.

Similarities in this topology between the THD and the globular gC1q domain of the C1q family suggest a distant evolutionary link between the two families (23). C1q, for example, is comprised of 18 chains, six heterotrimeric gC1q domains held together by a bundle of collagen domains. C1q is involved in the recognition of immune complexes and initiation of the classical complement pathway (24). It is enticing to suggest that these two families of immune regulatory proteins may have arisen from a common ancestral gene.

STRUCTURE–FUNCTION RELATIONSHIPS IN THE TNF RECEPTOR SUPERFAMILY

Like the TNF-α ligand superfamily, the TNF receptor family comprises a large number (at least 29) of primarily type I (extracellular N-terminus, intracellular C-terminus) transmembrane proteins (Table 1, Fig. 1). (For review, see Idriss and Naismith [13] and Locksley et al. [16].) There are, however,

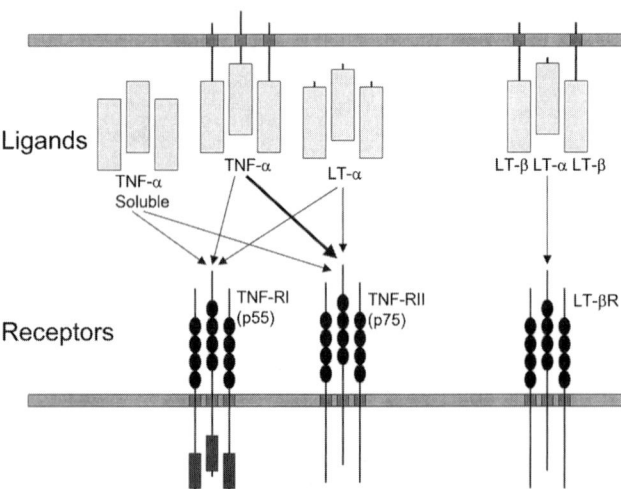

FIG. 2. TNF-α and lymphotoxin ligands and their receptors. TNF-α exists exclusively as a homotrimer, and binds to both the TNF-RI and TNFR-II receptors. Lymphotoxin is comprised of an α and a β chain. Homotrimeric lymphotoxin-α binds to similar receptors as TNF-α, whereas lymphotoxin heteromers comprised of α and β chains bind to a unique Ltβ-R.

some notable exceptions including BCMA, TACI, BAFFR, and ZEDAR, which are type III proteins (lacking a signal peptide), and OPG and DcR3, which are essentially secreted as soluble proteins. Many of the membrane-associated receptors can be further processed by proteolytic cleavage to soluble receptors (such as CD27, CD30, CD40, TNF-RI, and TNF-RII) while soluble forms of others can be generated by alternative splicing (Fas and 4-1BB). Several of these secreted or soluble receptors are biologically active, and can either serve as receptor antagonists for their corresponding ligands (as seen for OPG and the TNF-RI, under certain circumstances) or serve as ligand passers (as may be the case for TNF-RII). Most of the TNF superfamily receptors show high specificity for specific ligands with the exception of the NGF receptor, which will also bind with low affinity to several neurotrophins, including BDNF and NGF.

All members of the TNF receptor superfamily share extracellular domains characterized by cysteine-rich domains (CRDs) that typically contain six cysteine residues with three disulfide bonds. The number of CRDs, however, can vary from one to four, with the notable exception of CD30 where there are six CRDs in the human but not the mouse (20,25). The CRDs also vary in their primary amino acid sequence, numbers of modules and their distance from the three disulfide bridges, all of which determine their specificity for their respective ligand. The presence of these CRDs confers onto the receptor an elongated shape and often contains the "pre-ligand association domain" (PLAD), which is required for self-association and oligomerization of the receptors (25).

REGULATION OF TNF-α EXPRESSION

Human TNF-α is translated as a 233–amino acid, 26-kDa pro-protein that lacks a classic signal peptide. Newly synthesized pro-TNF-α is first displayed on the plasma membrane and is then cleaved in the extracellular domain to release the mature monomer through the actions of matrix metalloproteases (Fig. 3) (26). The primary enzyme responsible for the processing of cell-associated to secreted TNF-α is TNF-α converting enzyme (TACE) (27). TACE is an adamalysin, a member of a class of membrane-associated enzymes that contain both disintegrin and matrix metaloprotease domains. This class of enzymes appears to play a critical role in the processing of several membrane-associated proteins, including TNF-α, FasL, the TNF receptors, and the EGF receptor. At the present time, the primary substrates for TACE and other matrix metalloproteases are not completely known. The functions of TACE, however, are not limited solely to the processing of TNF-α, since ablation of the TACE gene is developmentally lethal in the mouse (28), whereas TNF-α gene ablation results in normal development, growth, and reproduction (29).

Membrane-associated TNF-α is biologically active and is thought to mediate the cytotoxic and inflammatory effects of TNF-α through cell-to-cell contact (30,31). After proteolytic cleavage, the pro-protein is converted to the 157–amino acid,

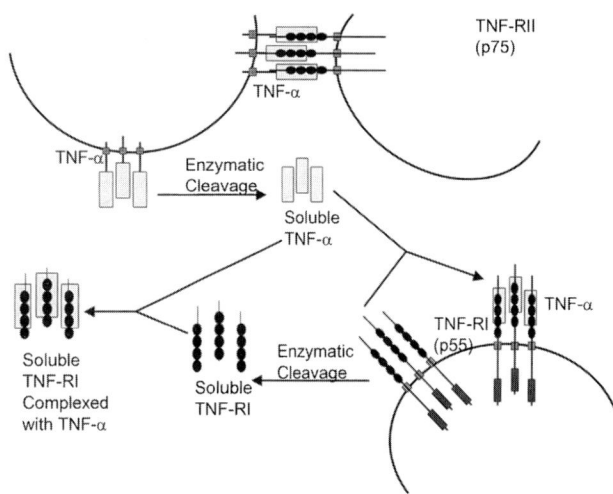

FIG. 3. Processing of cell-associated TNF-α and its receptors. TNF-α is first presented as a cell-associated molecule that can signal in a juxtacrine fashion. However, both TNF-α and its cellular receptors can be cleaved from the cell surface by proteases, and the soluble TNF-α can still serve as a ligand. The cleaved or shed receptors, however, can still bind the ligand, and depending upon their relative concentrations, can serve as either inhibitors or "ligand passers."

17.3-kDa secreted protein, which circulates as a homotrimer. The C-terminus of each subunit is embedded in the base of the trimer, and the N-terminus is relatively free of the base structure. Thus, the N-terminus does not participate in trimer interactions, and is not crucial for the biological activities of TNF-α. Results from mutational analysis have shown that each TNF-α trimer has three receptor interaction sites located in grooves between the subunits near the base of the trimer structure (13).

TNF-α is produced by numerous cell types that include immune cells (B cells and T cells, basophils, eosinophils, dendritic cells, NK cells, neutrophils, and mast cells); nonimmune cells (astrocytes, fibroblasts, glial cells, granulosa cells, keratinocytes, neurons, osteoblasts, retinal pigment epithelial cells, smooth muscle cells, and spermatogenic cells); and many kinds of tumor cells (32). However, monocytes and tissue macrophages are the primary cell sources for TNF-α synthesis. TNF-α synthesis is stimulated by a wide variety of agents. In macrophages, TNF-α synthesis is induced by biologic, chemical, and physical stimuli that include viruses, bacterial and parasitic products, tumor cells, complement, cytokines (IL-1, IL-2, IFN-g, GM-CSF, M-CSF, and TNF-α itself), ischemia, trauma, and irradiation. In other cell types, other stimuli are effective: LPS in monocytes, engagement of the T-cell receptor in T-lymphocytes, cross-linking of surface immunoglobulin in B-lymphocytes, ultraviolet light in fibroblasts, and phorbol esters and viral infections in many other cell types (32).

Biosynthesis of TNF-α is tightly controlled at several levels to ensure the silence of the TNF-α gene in the absence of exogenous stimulation, or in tissues that are not destined to synthesize the protein. Therefore, TNF-α is produced only in barely detectable quantities in quiescent cells, but is one of the major factors secreted by activated macrophages (33). The gene for TNF-α is one of the "immediate early" genes induced by a variety of stimuli. Early studies suggest that in blood monocytes and tissue macrophages, levels of TNF-α mRNA increase 5- to 50-fold after exposure to an inciting agent (34). Furthermore, the efficiency of mRNA translation can increase over 100-fold. Both the human and mouse TNF-α promoter region have been shown to contain multiple sites capable of binding NFκB. A particular site at -655 in the mouse promoter is of particular interest because it is conserved in all mammalian species (35). However, there have been some curious contradictory results between the human and murine systems regarding the quantitative importance of NFκB to TNF-α gene expression. In the human system, there is some controversy over whether NFκB-binding sites are required for transcriptional regulation of TNF-α (36–38), although in murine systems, LPS induction of TNF-α gene transcription is dependent on NFκB signaling (35,39).

Levels of TNF-α mRNA increase sharply within 15 to 30 minutes with no requirement for *de novo* protein synthesis. However, TNF-α production is also regulated post-transcriptionally. The 3' region of TNF-α mRNA includes a series of AU sequences that confer instability to the TNF-α message (mRNA) and determine its translational efficiency (40). These sequences are common in mRNA for several pro-inflammatory cytokines (41), and the presence of these sequences ensures that TNF-α mRNA cannot be translated, but is rapidly degraded by cytosolic RNAases without some de-repression. These AU-rich elements are known to be recognition sequences for several RNA-binding proteins, of which only a few have been characterized to date (e.g., AU, HU, TIA, TTP, and Tpl2) (42–44). Some of these proteins appear to be involved in determining TNF-α mRNA stability, while others are involved in translational silencing. The presence of these 3' AU-rich elements was responsible for both the suppression of TNF-α mRNA expression in the unstimulated state, as well as the derepression that occurs following stimulation of macrophages with bacterial endotoxin. The varying capabilities of different tissues to express TNF-α appears to depend as much upon its transcriptional regulation as well as the ability to derepress these translational signals in the AU-rich 3' untranslated region (40). These findings also explain how activated complement, IL-1, and TNF-α itself may induce TNF-α mRNA expression (45,46), but not translation, since these stimuli are not efficient at derepressing the translational blockade that exists in resting macrophages.

Many of the downstream mediators induced by TNF-α also serve to down-regulate TNF-α expression both transcriptionally and post-transcriptionally. For example, induction of corticosteroids and prostanoids by TNF-α down-regulates expression, as does the induction of anti-inflammatory cytokines such as IL-10 (47). Corticosteroids also appear to suppress the translation of the TNF-α mRNA (47,48). The net result of this feedback loop is an integrated effort to restrict the duration and magnitude of TNF-α expression once induced. This becomes particularly important in chronic inflammatory diseases in which TNF-α production becomes inappropriately sustained, as occurs in the arthritic synovium. Under these conditions, increased endogenous production of prostaglandins, corticosteroids, and IL-10 is generally ineffective at preventing sustained TNF-α expression. In fact, the use of NSAIDs in rheumatoid arthritis patients may actually increase TNF-α production (49,50).

BIOLOGICAL FUNCTIONS OF TNF-α

TNF-α was characterized simultaneously in the 1980s as a factor that produced tumor necrosis *in vivo* and exhibited anti-tumor activity by inducing cell apoptosis. It has subsequently been recognized that TNF-α (a) modulates growth, differentiation, and metabolism in a variety of cell types; (b) produces cachexia *in vivo* by stimulating lipolysis and inhibiting lipoprotein lipase activity in adipocytes and by stimulating hepatic lipogenesis; (c) initiates apoptosis in malignant or transformed cells, virally-infected cells, T-lymphocytes, and epithelial cells; and (d) produces inflammation (reviewed in Ksontini et al. [19] and Dinarello and Moldawer [51]).

Like IL-1, TNF-α is a powerful inducer of the inflammatory response and is a central regulator of the innate immune response. Inflammatory responses to TNF-α are mediated both directly and through stimulation of the expression of IL-1 and more distal pro-inflammatory cytokines. Secondary mediators that are known to be induced by systemically administered TNF-α include the cytokines (IL-1, IL-2, IL-4, IL-6, IL-10, IL-12, IL-18, and IFN-γ), transforming growth factor-β (TGF-β), LIF, and migration inhibitory factor (MIF); hormones (cortisol, epinephrine, glucagon, insulin, and norepinephrine); and assorted other molecules (acute phase proteins, IL-1Ra, leukotrienes, oxygen-free radicals, PAF, and prostaglandins). It is also recognized that TNF-α is not only involved in tissue inflammation and injury, but also appears to be a prominent ligand for the activation of programmed cell death through apoptosis (9). This latter function occurs not only during normal growth and development, as well as the re-establishment of homeostasis after an immune response, but may also result from pathologic conditions in which local and systemic production of TNF-α is increased. Exogenous administration of TNF-α to animals with experimentally implanted tumors produces anti-neoplastic activity secondary to its ability to induce apoptosis in selected tumor cell populations and through its inflammatory properties to disrupt neovascularization of solid cancers (52). Apoptosis of lymphoid cell populations associated with activation-induced cell death is also mediated in part by TNF-α (53).

TNF-α also plays an important role in the regulation of the TH1 immune response. This is particularly important in the pathogenesis of a number of chronic inflammatory diseases, including inflammatory bowel disease and rheumatoid arthritis, in which a positive feedback loop linking the autoimmune and the inflammatory or innate immune responses has been established (54). TNF-α induces the synthesis of IL-12 and IL-18, two cytokines that are potent inducers of IFN-γ. Therefore, TNF-α, by itself and through up-regulation of IL-12 and IL-18, amplifies the TH1 response, increasing CD4$^+$ T-cell activation and IFN-γ production. In turn, this leads to increased macrophage production of TNF-α and activation of the inflammatory response.

TNF-α SIGNALING THROUGH ITS TWO RECEPTORS

Biological responses to TNF-α are mediated by ligand binding via two structurally distinct receptors (Figs. 1 and 2): type I (TNF-RI; p60 or p55;CD120α) and type II (TNF-RII; p80 or p75; CD120β) (51). Both receptors are transmembrane glycoproteins that have multiple cysteine-rich domains (CRDs) in the extracellular N-terminal domain (16). TNF-RI and TNF-RII are present on all cell types except erythrocytes. Although the distribution of TNF-RI is more widespread, TNF-RII is present in greater amounts on endothelial and hematopoietically derived cells. TNF-RI expression is constitutive in most cell types, whereas expression of TNF-RII appears to be more inducible. Both TNF receptors are subject to proteolytic cleavage by members of the matrix metaloprotease family and are shed from the surface of cells in response to inflammatory signals such as TNF-α ligand-receptor binding (55). The shed extracellular domains of both receptors retain their ability to bind TNF-α and therefore may act as natural inhibitors of TNF-α bioactivity. During chronic and acute inflammatory conditions, the concentrations of both receptors increase dramatically, although the concentration of TNF-RII is generally more labile than is the concentration of TNF-RI. Both shed receptors are cleared by the kidney and excreted in the urine (56), usually immunologically intact (57). This shedding of the cellular receptors, their increased plasma concentrations, and their ability to bind TNF-α have led to the hypothesis that shed TNF receptors may serve either as natural antagonists or as delivery peptides (ligand passers) for circulating TNF-α, depending on their relative concentrations (58,59) (Fig. 3).

The two TNF receptors differ significantly in their binding affinities for TNF-α, as well as in their intracellular signaling pathways (51). These differences in ligand binding affinity and kinetics are presumed to reflect differences in the primary function for the two receptors. Early studies suggested that binding of TNF-α to both receptors appears to be of high affinity (60). However, more recent pulse-chase experiments demonstrate that the kinetics by which TNF-α binds to and is released from the two receptors differ significantly. TNF-α appears to bind both TNF-RI and TNF-RII with rapid association kinetics (1.1×10^9 and 1.5×10^9 M^{-1}min^{-1}, respectively) (61). However, these pulse-chase experiments suggest that binding of TNF-α to TNF-RI is nearly irreversible, due to very slow K_{off} kinetics (0.021 min^{-1}, $T_{1/2} = 33$ min) versus

TNF-RII, which had very rapid K_{off} kinetics (0.631 min^{-1}, $T_{1/2} = 1.1$ min).

The very different kinetics of binding of TNF-α to the two TNF receptors had originally raised speculation that, *in vivo*, the two receptors may have different functions (Fig. 4). TNF-RII may serve as a ligand passer, that is, a means to deliver or pass TNF-α to TNF-RI for signaling when concentrations of TNF-α are low (51). Supporting the hypothesis that TNF-RII functions primarily as a ligand passer is the observation that under *in vivo* conditions, the primary inflammatory responses to soluble 17-kDa TNF-α are mediated by TNF-RI, rather than by TNF-RII signaling (62–64).

TNF-α signaling through both the TNF-RI and TNF-RII is triggered by juxtaposition of the intracellular domains of receptor molecules following ligand binding (Fig. 5). Binding of a monomeric TNF-α to a single receptor is not sufficient to transduce a signal. Rather, homotrimeric TNF-α plays an essential role in this juxtaposition of the intracellular domains since oligomerization of the intracellular domains of the TNF receptors is required for signal transduction. It has been suggested that self-associations in the TNF-RI intracellular motifs contribute to the initiation and amplification of the signal. Interestingly, overexpression and oligomerization of the TNF-RI receptor can transduce a signal, even in the absence of ligand binding (65).

The intracellular signaling domains of TNF-RI actually share greater homology with the intracellular signaling domains of Fas (CD95) than they do with those of TNF-RII, particularly with regard to the highly conserved intracellular domain called the death domain (DD). This sequence of approximately 70 amino acids plays a pivotal role in the ability of TNF-α to trigger apoptosis in the cell (Fig. 5). Their intracellular death domains recruit other DD-containing and death effector domain (DED)–containing molecules, and initiate the intracellular signaling cascade. The recruitment of intracellular signaling molecules to the intracellular domain of the TNF-RI occurs via intermediate adaptor or docking proteins, most of which have no enzymatic (kinase) activity of their own. There are several of these docking proteins, including a protein called receptor interacting protein (RIP), which requires another DD-containing protein, TNF receptor I–associated death domain protein (TRADD) (66). TRADD can also interact with two other proteins, TRAF-1 and TRAF-2, from another family of signal-transducing proteins called TNF receptor–associated factors (TRAFs) (9). TRAF-2 is an intermediary in the activation of NFκB and JNK activation by TNF-α and its induction of pro-inflammation. TRADD lies at the bifurcation of the apoptotic and pro-inflammatory signaling pathways of TNF-α (Fig. 6).

The DD of TNF-RI is not the only region in the intracellular domain involved in signal transduction. Upstream of the DD in the membrane proximal region of TNF-RI, three proteins bind and are involved in signal transduction—FAN, TRAP2, and TRAP1. FAN appears to play a role in the activation of neutral sphongomyelinase responsible for the generation of ceramide (67,68). The functions of TRAP2 and TRAP1 are

26 kDa TNF-α Signaling

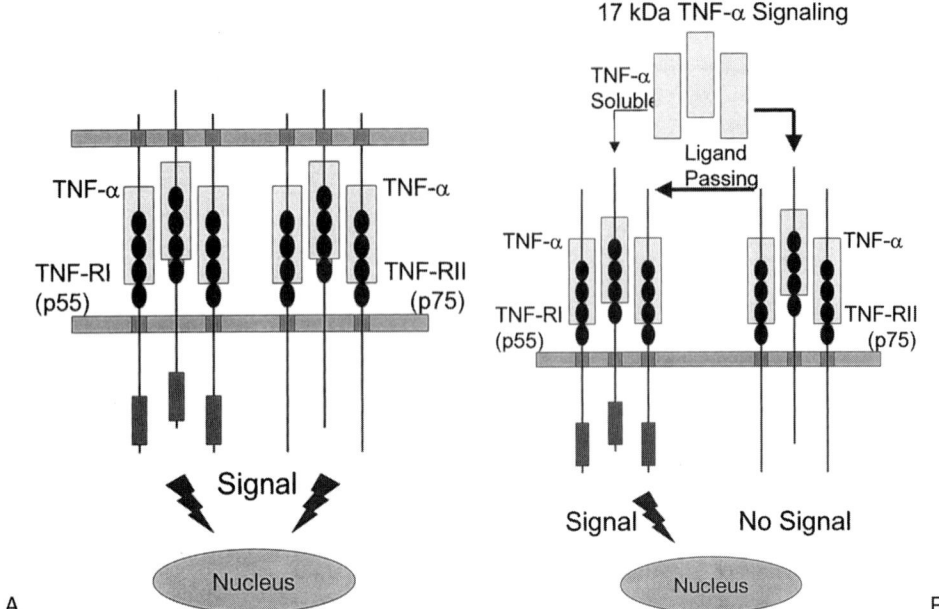

FIG. 4. Differences in TNF-α signaling between the two TNF-α receptors. Grell et al. (30) have speculated that due to the differences in the on-off kinetics for the two TNF receptors, the cell-associated and secreted forms of TNF-α may signal differently through the two receptors. Because of the rapid on–off kinetics of the TNF-RII, soluble TNF-α may be passed from the TNF-RII to the TNF-RI under conditions of low TNF-α conditions. In contrast, because of steric hindrance associated with the cell-associated forms, they may be preferential ligands for the TNF-RII receptor.

presently not known, although TRAP2 may be involved in the regulation of protease function (69).

TNF-RII may also participate in the pro-inflammatory signal of TNF-α via TRAF-2 (Fig. 6). Some investigators, however, have observed that TNF-RII agonists are able to induce apoptosis (70,71) despite the lack of a TRADD/FADD

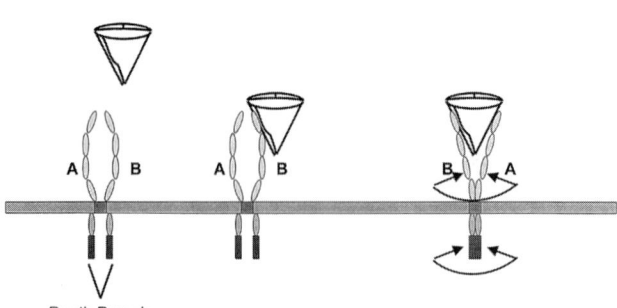

Death Domains

FIG. 5. One proposed model by which TNF receptor signaling occurs. Interactions between a trimeric form of TNF-α (as represented here by an inverted cone) with a dimeric TNF-RI complex (*A* and *B*) results in a conformational change in the intracellular domains bringing the "death domains" in proximity sufficient to interact with "death effector domains" on docking proteins such as TRADD. Adapted from Idriss and Naismith (13) with permission, based on Bazzoni and Beutler (32).

(Fas–associated death domain protein) binding region as found in TNF-RI. Induction of apoptosis by TNF-RII does not share the same pathways as TNF-RI, but seems to rely on the induction of TRAF-2. As with TNF-RI, TNF-RII has been found to associate with the C-terminus of TRAF-2, which mediates activation of NFκB. A protein kinase, NIK, which binds to TRAF-2 and stimulates NFκB activity, has been described (72,73).

The binding of TNF-α to its receptor can simultaneously initiate several signaling pathways, including those that promote and inhibit apoptosis. Intracellular mechanisms must exist, therefore, to define which pathway is activated and/or dominant. The apoptosis-inhibition pathway is NFκB dependent, as shown by studies demonstrating that TNF-α–induced apoptosis of malignant cells was inhibited by simultaneous activation of NFκB-dependent pathways and that inhibition of NFκB markedly increased the apoptotic response to TNF-α in several malignant tumor cell lines (74,75). The selection of the dominant pathway appears to rest with a "molecular switch" that acts in part through the intracellular concentration of cell-signaling intermediates. This has been best shown in T cells in which the intracellular concentration of RIP determines whether TNF-RII signaling occurs through apoptotic or NFκB-dependent pathways (76). Increases in the intracellular concentration of RIP, induced by IL-2, triggered cell death. Under the same conditions, depletion of RIP

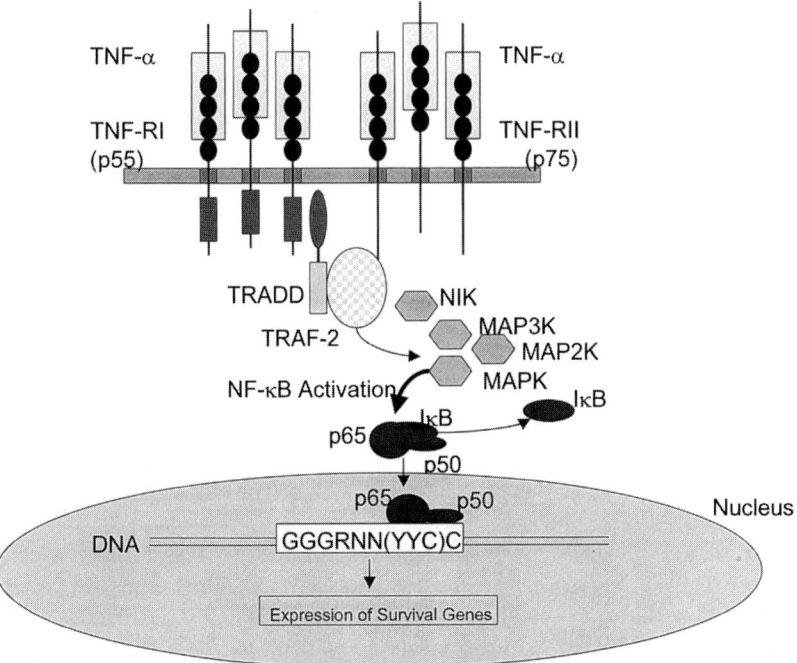

FIG. 6. Bifurcation of the TNF-RI signaling pathway that leads to apoptosis and through NFκB activation. TRADD can interact TRAF-2, which is an intermediary in the activation of NFκB and JNK activation by TNF-α and its induction of pro-inflammation. TRADD lies at the bifurcation of the apoptotic and pro-inflammatory signaling pathways of TNF-α. TRAF-2 activation is also involved in TNF-RII–mediated activation of NFκB.

reduced the susceptibility of the cell to TNF-α–dependent apoptosis. These findings suggest that the signaling outputs are regulated by intracellular factors. They may also help explain some of the conflicting data regarding the pro-apoptotic versus activating effects of TNF-α.

It should be noted, however, that much of the experimental data from *in vivo* and *in vitro* studies does not identify the quantitative importance of the individual receptor types in TNF-mediated signaling, particularly in response to secreted, homotrimeric 17-kDa TNF-α. For example, *in vitro* studies have revealed that upon binding of the ligand, both

TNF-RI and TNF-RII can transduce a signal for NFκB activation (73), whereas *in vivo* studies have suggested that TNF-RI is the receptor primarily responsible for the pro-inflammatory properties of TNF-α (Table 3). In fact, *in vivo* studies by Peschon et al. (77) and Nowak et al. (78) using TNF-RII knockout mice suggest that TNF-RII may function at times like a decoy receptor, since mice lacking a functional TNF-RII will often manifest an exaggerated inflammatory response. In addition, studies in baboons have shown that TNF-α muteins with specificity for TNF-RI are pro-inflammatory, whereas TNF-RII agonists are not (62–64). These primate

TABLE 3. *Inflammatory properties associated with TNF-RI and TNF-RII signaling*

TNF-RI	TNF-RII	Biological response
Yes	No (may actually be a decoy)	Induction of shock, hypotension, and tissue injury
Yes	No	Inflammation, proinflammatory cytokine expression, cell adhesion molecule expression
Yes	No	Tissue destruction associated with rheumatoid arthritis, signaling through both a secreted or cell associated TNF-α
Yes	No	Lymphocyte organogenesis, germinal center formation in secondary lymphatic organs
Yes	No	Hepatic acute-phase protein response, decrease in albumin synthesis
Yes	Yes	TNF-α–mediated hepatocyte injury, associated with concanavalin A
Yes	Unknown	Development of experimental EAE
No	Yes	T-cell proliferation, thymocyte proliferation, and T-cell apoptosis
Yes	No	Antimicrobial properties against intracellular bacterial and extracellular infections
Yes	Maybe	Antiviral properties, primarily TNF-R1
Yes	Yes	Antifungal properties

EAE, experimental autoimmune encephalomyelitis; TNF, tumor necrosis factor (R, receptor).

data are consistent with earlier studies performed using transgenic mice or receptor-specific antagonists. For example, antibodies that prevented TNF-α binding to TNF-RI, but not TNF-RII, protected mice from lethal endotoxic shock but blocked development of a protective response against *Listeria monocytogenes* infection (79). Similarly, transgenic mice lacking a functional TNF-RI are more resistant to TNF-α, but more susceptible to infection by *L. monocytogenes* (80,81). Although TNF-RII–deficient mice exhibit normal T-cell development and activity, these animals are also more resistant to TNF-α–induced death, suggesting that TNF-RII may have no intrinsic pro-inflammatory properties of its own, but can potentiate the actions of TNF-RI (82).

Based on observations that *in vivo* inflammatory responses to soluble 17-kDa TNF-α are mediated primarily by TNF-RI, and that TNF-α binding to TNF-RII is associated with very rapid on–off kinetics, it was postulated that TNF-α signaling was mediated primarily by binding of the 17-kDa ligand to TNF-RI. The proposal that *in vivo* TNF-α signaling of inflammation and apoptosis *in vivo* occurs principally through TNF-RI has been questioned (51). For example, Grell et al. (30) demonstrated that the secreted and cell-associated forms of TNF-α have markedly different affinities for the two TNF receptors. They propose that the principal ligand for TNF-RI is the 17-kDa secreted form of TNF-α, whereas cell-associated TNF-α is the primary signaling ligand for TNF-RII. The on–off kinetics of 17-kDa TNF-α with the type II receptor are very fast and thus, at low TNF-α concentrations, TNF-RII may serve only as a ligand passer for the type I receptor and increase TNF-α binding to TNF-RI. Conversely, because of the close juxtaposition of 26-kDa cell-associated TNF-α to TNF-RII that occurs during cell-to-cell contact, TNF-α/TNF-RII complexes may be generated with increased stability and signaling potential. Steric hindrance by cell-associated TNF-α would prevent ligand passing from TNF-RII and permit signal transduction to occur. These investigators propose that cell-associated TNF-α is the prime physiologic activator of TNF-RII, implying that TNF-RII contributes to the local TNF-α response in tissues, as occurs in experimental hepatitis and rheumatoid arthritis (83–85). Along these same lines, the investigators have demonstrated that overexpression of human TNF-RII can induce an exaggerated inflammatory response in several organs, suggesting that signaling through this receptor has the potential to directly induce tissue damage (86).

Data published to date suggest that the 17-kDa secreted TNF-α (and not the 26-kDa cell-associated form) is primarily responsible for mortality in endotoxin- or bacteremia-induced shock (87) (Table 3), and that this occurs primarily through TNF-RI signaling. Conversely, hepatocyte apoptosis, synovial inflammation, and joint erosion appear to be dependent, at least in part, on cell-associated TNF-α signaling, with involvement of TNF-RII. Using a novel transgenic mouse that expresses only a membrane-associated form of TNF-α, Alexopoulou et al. (84) have demonstrated that expression of the 26-kDa form of TNF-α was adequate by itself

to induce arthritis. These animals spontaneously developed a pattern of arthritic lesions similar to human rheumatoid arthritis at about 6 to 8 weeks of age. In addition, Williams et al. (88) noted that treatment of rheumatoid synovial explants with a matrix metaloprotease inhibitor blocked the processing of TNF-α and stabilized TNF receptors on cell membranes, but did not affect IL-1, IL-6, or chemokine release. In contrast, an antibody against TNF-α blocked the downstream induction of these other pro-inflammatory cytokines. The data suggest that cell-associated forms of TNF-α in synovial explants not inhibitable with matrix metaloprotease inhibitors may contribute to the local production of other pro-inflammatory cytokines.

These findings emphasize the complexity of the TNF-α signaling system and the multiple levels at which TNF-α signaling is regulated. Not only is the expression of TNF-α tightly controlled at the level of gene transcription and subsequent translation, but its processing from a cell-associated to a secreted form is regulated by protease activity. TNF-α signaling is also antagonized or aided by circulating extracellular domains of the TNF receptors, which, depending on their concentration, may serve as either inhibitors or ligand passers. Finally, the distribution of receptors on the target cells ultimately determines the responsiveness of a tissue to TNF-α.

LYMPHOTOXIN, NOT JUST ANOTHER TNF

TNF-α and lymphotoxin (LT) were first identified in the 1960s and 1970s based on their ability to kill various cell lines and tumor cells (2,4), with the primary difference being that lymphotoxin was the product of lymphocytes whereas TNF-α was the product of monocytes and macrophages. Like TNF-α, lymphotoxin-α is a structurally related homotrimeric protein of about 17 kDa. Both TNF-α and lymphotoxin-α3 can bind to both of the two TNF receptors, TNF-RI and TNF-RII. Because of the similar binding of these two ligands to the TNF receptors, the activities of these two proteins are assumed to be similar. The principal difference between the two species is that lymphotoxin-α3 is a predominantly secreted protein, whereas TNF-α is first synthesized as a cell-surface type II membrane protein that is only secreted as a result of TACE-mediated cleavage from the cell surface. Yet, it was quickly realized that lymphotoxin could also exist as a membrane-associated form, with a single lymphotoxin-α chain forming a heterotrimer with two copies of a structurally related type II transmembrane protein, designated lymphotoxin-β (89). The genes encoding TNF-α, lymphotoxin-α and lymphotoxin-β are genetically linked, adjacent to the major histocompatibility complex, probably resulting from tandem duplication of a common ancestral gene (32,90). Unlike TNF-α, the membrane-associated lymphotoxin heterotrimer (comprised of lymphotoxin-α1β2) does not undergo proteolytic cleavage and appears to exist only as a membrane-associated protein. Unlike lymphotoxin-α3, lymphotoxin-α1β2 does not bind to either the TNF-RI or TNF-RII receptor, but binds and signals through another receptor of the TNF receptor superfamily, designated the lymphotoxin-β receptor (91). The lymphotoxin-β receptor appears to be specific for lymphotoxin-$\alpha1\beta2$ and shows no measurable affinity for either homotrimeric TNF-α or lymphotoxin-$\alpha3$.

Thus, the TNF-α and the lymphotoxin families encode two sets of ligands: one membrane associated and one secreted (Fig. 2). The secreted forms of TNF-α and the lymphotoxin-$\alpha3$ both interact with the TNF-RI and TNF-RII receptors, whereas the membrane lymphotoxin-$\alpha1\beta2$ heterotrimer interacts with the lymphotoxin-β receptor. By signaling through the different intracellular domains of their receptors, these two sets of ligands and receptors would be expected to mediate independent sets of cellular and tissue responses.

There are also differences in the distribution of the two sets of receptors. As previously stated, the TNF-RI and TNF-RII receptors are expressed very broadly, whereas the lymphotoxin-β receptor is not expressed on lymphoid cells, but is expressed on stromal cells in various lymphoid tissues (92,93). Because the ligand for this receptor is membrane associated, it is likely that lymphotoxin-$\alpha1\beta2$–mediated responses require cell-to-cell contact between the lymphotoxin-expressing cell and its lymphotoxin-β receptor–bearing target.

Although many of the biological activities of lymphotoxin-$\alpha3$ overlap with TNF-α, lymphotoxin-$\alpha3$ and lymphotoxin-$\alpha1\beta2$ play unique roles in the genesis of secondary lymphoid organs, which is not seen with other members of the TNF superfamily, with perhaps the partial exception of LIGHT. Studies in mice with deletion of the lymphotoxin-α gene showed a profound defect in the formation of lymph nodes and the complete absence of Peyer's patches (94). Similar defects were not seen in either TNF-α–null mice or mice deficient in both TNF-RI and TNF-RII (95,96), suggesting that TNF-α signaling through the same receptors could not rescue lymphoid organ development. Furthermore, not all lymphotoxin-α–null mice failed to develop secondary lymph nodes; approximately 5% of the animals developed some modest mesenteric node.

It was immediately recognized that lymphotoxin-α was acting during some stage of ontogeny, but it was not originally clear whether the synthesis of homotrimeric lymphotoxin-$\alpha3$ or the heterotrimeric lymphotoxin-$\alpha1\beta2$ was required for lymph node development. It was actually some elegant studies by Rennert et al. (97) who blocked lymphotoxin-β receptor signaling with administration of a lymphotoxin-β receptor–immunoglobulin fusion protein. Treatment of mice in utero with these immunoadhesin ablated the appearance of Peyer's patches, and some lymph nodes, depending on when the immunoadhesin was administered. Surprisingly, there was a distinctly variable response by different lymph nodes to lymphotoxin-β receptor blockade. Later studies using lymphotoxin-β–null mice confirmed that genesis of Peyer's patches and peripheral lymph nodes required signaling through the lymphotoxin-β receptor, whereas mesenteric

and cervical lymph nodes were still present in these null mice (98,99). Rather, genesis of mesenteric and cervical lymph nodes appear to be dependent on signaling by lymphotoxin-α through the TNF receptors, since lymphotoxin-α–null mice lack mesenteric and cervical lymph nodes (94), and blocking TNF-RI signaling in lymphotoxin-β–null mice also eliminates cervical and mesenteric lymph nodes (98).

LIGHT OR HVEM LIGAND

LIGHT is homologous to lymphotoxins, exhibits inducible expression, and competes with HSV glycoprotein D for herpes virus entry mediator (HVEM), a receptor expressed by T-lymphocytes) or HVEM ligand. It is a newly described member of the TNF superfamily that shares homology with both Fas ligand and lymphotoxin-β (100). LIGHT is a 29-kDa type II transmembrane protein produced by activated T cells and other cells including dendritic cells, which also engages the lymphotoxin-β receptor, but does not form heteromeric complexes with either lymphotoxin-α or lymphotoxin-β. The herpes virus glycoprotein D inhibits the interaction of LIGHT with its second receptor, HVEM (100). Furthermore, the cytokine LIGHT and the herpes virus glycoprotein D interfere with HVEM-dependent cell entry by HSV1.

Since LIGHT binds to both the lymphotoxin-β receptor and HVEM, it would not be surprising that it shares some biological activities with lymphotoxin. By signaling through HVEM and the lymphotoxin-β receptor, LIGHT participates in multiple immunologic functions, similar to lymphotoxin and TNF-α. LIGHT mediates apoptosis in some tumor cell lines, leading to growth suppression in vitro and in vivo (101–103). LIGHT also serves as a co-stimulatory molecule for T-cell activation, leading to enhanced proliferation, as well as stimulating TH1-type cytokine production and NFκB translocation (104,105). Importantly, LIGHT plays a central role in fostering T-cell development as well as maintaining homeostasis of peripheral T cells. Signaling of LIGHT through the HVEM receptor also stimulates the maturation of dendritic cells in cooperation with CD40 signaling, resulting a mature phenotype consistent with increased expression of co-stimulatory molecules and cytokine production (106). Finally, LIGHT appears to play a complementary role with lymphotoxin in lymphoid organogenesis. Mice deficient in the lymphotoxin-β receptor (the receptor for both lymphotoxin-β and LIGHT) fail to develop any lymph nodes (LN) (98,107), whereas mice deficient in lymphotoxin-β, but have unaffected LIGHT expression still develop mesenteric and cervical lymph nodes (108). These differential responses suggest indirectly that LIGHT signaling through the lymphotoxin-β receptor may well play an important role in genesis of some lymph nodes.

FAS AND FAS LIGAND

Fas ligand (FasL), another member of the TNF cytokine superfamily, is both structurally and functionally related to

TNF-α and other members of its superfamily. Like TNF-α, FasL is synthesized and expressed first as a homotrimeric membrane-associated protein and is then processed further by matrix metaloproteases to a secreted form (109). Historically, FasL was presumed to have predominantly apoptosis-inducing properties that were associated primarily with its cell-associated form. Although it was noted that secreted FasL formed trimeric structures and retained its ability to engage the Fas receptor, it was unclear whether soluble FasL could induce apoptosis (110,111). These studies suggested that the soluble forms of FasL might actually be receptor antagonists of Fas and inhibit cell-associated FasL-mediated apoptosis.

The hypothesis that soluble FasL is strictly an inhibitor of Fas has recently been amended by several groups who have reported that soluble FasL is also chemotactic for neutrophils. Ottonello et al. (112) have demonstrated that human soluble FasL is also endowed with potent chemotactic properties for neutrophils at concentrations incapable of producing apoptosis. Furthermore, FasL did not appear to activate neutrophils, but only to recruit them, since neutrophil calcium flux, superoxide production, and degranulation were not affected. Other investigators have demonstrated that the chemotactic properties of FasL are separate and distinct from its apoptosis-inducing properties (113,114). The observation is significant in part because it suggests that FasL, like TNF-α and other members of the superfamily, may contribute to neutrophilic infiltration and recruitment as part of the host inflammatory response.

FasL was originally described for its ability to induce apoptosis in defined immune-privileged sites such as the eye, testis, and brain. It was recognized that immune cells entering these tissue compartments were rapidly killed, primarily through apoptotic processes mediated by FasL, and it was revealed that both inflammatory and noninflammatory cells expressing FasL were responsible, in part, for this elimination of immune cells. The concept of an immune-privileged site has been expanded by the recent observation that many tumors evade killing by tumor-infiltrating inflammatory or lymphoid cells through overexpression of FasL and are themselves resistant to Fas-mediated apoptosis (115).

Although FasL was originally thought to be expressed only by cells of the lymphoid or myeloid lineage, predominantly including T cells, B cells, phagocytes, and NK cells, it is now recognized that FasL can frequently be expressed by non-lymphoid cells (116,117). Fas, also called CD95 or Apo-1, is widely expressed on a variety of cell types. Fas shares structural homology with TNF-RI. The Fas apoptotic-signaling pathway, like that of TNF-RI, involves activation of caspase-8 via concatemerization of FADD and TRADD. However, there has been more recent evidence that Fas signaling can also lead to pro-inflammatory events through the activation of NFκB- and JNK-dependent pathways. NFκB-inducing kinase, which binds to TRAF-2 and induces the phosphorylation and activation of MAP kinases, is an intermediate in these

pathways (73). TRAF-2, a more proximal signal-transduction peptide, appears to be involved in both TNF-α– and FasL– induced pathways of NFκB activation and may be responsible for their chemotactic properties.

RANK LIGAND, RANK, AND OSTEOPROTEGERIN

The identification of the OPG/RANKL/RANK system as the predominant mediator of osteoclastogenesis represented a major advance in understanding the regulation of bone mass (51). It ended a long-standing search for the mediators produced by pre-osteoblastic stromal cells that were required for osteoclast development. It provided the common final mediators responsible for increased osteoclastic activity. The initial cloning and characterization of osteoprotegerin (OPG) as the soluble, decoy receptor belonging to the TNF receptor superfamily was the first step in this search that eventually led to more of a full understanding of this system (118). Soon thereafter, the protein blocked by OPG, initially called OPG-ligand/osteoclast differentiating factor (ODF) and subsequently termed RANK ligand, was identified as the key mediator of osteoclastogenesis. RANK ligand, in turn, was shown to bind its receptor, RANK, on osteoclast lineage cells (119).

The agonist in this pathway is a member of the TNF superfamily that has been named RANK ligand (120). It is also known as osteoprotegerin ligand (OPG ligand) (121) or osteoclast differentiation factor (ODF) (122,123). RANK ligand is expressed in at least two distinct forms, including the cell-associated peptide of 317 amino acids, as well as a truncated ectodomain created from the cell-bound form by cleavage of the extracellular domain by a TACE-like protease, and as a primary secreted form (121,124). While the cell-associated form is most common and is expressed by many cell types, activated T cells and some squamous cell carcinoma cell lines secrete the soluble form. Various cell types are capable of synthesizing RANK ligand, including stromal cells, osteoblasts, osteoclasts, mesenchymal periosteal cells, chondrocytes, and endothelial cells (120–122).

RANK ligand injected into mice induces mild hypercalcemia within 1 hour (125). Interestingly, RANK ligand may also have important immunomodulatory effects that indirectly affect bone mass, as well as other tissues, since transgenic mice deficient in RANK ligand have lymph node agenesis and thymic hypoplasia (126,127). In this latter regard, RANK ligand is also thought to play a role in T-cell and dendritic cell interactions, since RANK ligand was found to stimulate dendritic cell survival through up-regulation of Bcl-XL and to increase dendritic cell activation of T-cell proliferation (128–130).

Osteoprotegerin (OPG) is a specific antagonist of RANK ligand and is a secreted soluble member of the TNF receptor superfamily. *In vitro*, OPG has been shown to be a potent inhibitor of osteoclast differentiation, by blocking RANK ligand activity. Unlike other members of the TNF receptor superfamily, OPG exists only as a secreted, soluble decoy receptor, since the gene does not code for a membrane-bound form.

The importance of OPG and RANK ligand in normal physiology of bone has been revealed by targeted gene disruption. Mice lacking a functional OPG gene develop severe osteoporosis associated with skeletal deformities and fractures. Mice that are heterozygous for the defective OPG gene have a mild osteopenic phenotype (131). In contrast, mice that lack a functional gene for RANK ligand or its signaling receptor RANK have severe osteopetrosis with radiologically dense bones, failure of tooth eruption, and club-shaped long bones. These mice lack osteoclasts and suffer from a complete failure of bone resorption (132). Mice lacking the signaling receptor RANK have also been shown to be resistant to the hypercalcemic and osteoclastogenic effects of exogenous parathyroid hormone (PTH); parathyroid hormone-related protein (PTHrP); 1,25 dihydroxyvitamin D3 (1,25(OH)2D3); RANK ligand; IL-1β; and TNF-α. Only with TNF-α treatment was the formation of very occasional osteoclasts observed (132). These observations demonstrate an essential role for RANK ligand, RANK, and OPG in the regulation of osteoclast differentiation and in normal and pathologic bone resorption. Both OPG and RANK ligand are produced in the bone environment by stromal cells (fibroblast cells that support the hematopoietic cells of the marrow) and/or osteoblasts. Their expression is regulated by hormones, cytokines, and prostaglandins, as would be expected for mediators of the resorptive effects of these factors. For example, PGE2, which is known to increase bone resorption, increases RANK ligand expression and decreases OPG expression (132). On the other hand, cytokines such as TNF-α and IL-1 increase both OPG and RANK ligand expression (133). However, in this situation the expression of RANK ligand relative to OPG may be increased.

Since RANK ligand and its membrane-bound, signal-transducing receptor RANK are also expressed by activated T cells and dendritic cells, respectively, there may be a role for RANK ligand in both bone and non–bone-related immune responses, perhaps in modulating interactions between T cells and dendritic cells (123,134). The expression of RANK ligand by T cells raises the intriguing possibility that T cells in an inflammatory infiltrate could produce RANK ligand and directly enhance bone resorption. For example, OPG treatment of rats with adjuvant-induced arthritis resulted in almost complete protection of bone but had no effect on inflammation, as indicated by joint swelling and inflammatory cell infiltration of bone marrow (132).

TNF-RELATED APOPTOSIS-INDUCING LIGAND (TRAIL)

TRAIL, which has also been designated as Apo-2 ligand, represents another member of the TNF superfamily, with several unique twists (135–137). Like other members of the TNF superfamily, TRAIL is expressed primarily as a 33-kD type II membrane protein, and can also exist as a soluble form, although controversy exists regarding its biological activities. However, unlike other members of the TNF superfamily, the extracellular form of TRAIL contains a unique loop of 12 to 16 amino acids near its amino terminal end (138,139). In addition, TRAIL requires a zinc ion positioned at the interface of the trimer (at position Cys230), which is required for its structural integrity and function. Although many members of the TNF superfamily are involved in the regulation of cell proliferation and apoptosis, TRAIL is relatively unique in that it induces apoptosis specifically in transformed and cancer cells, whereas most normal cells appear to be resistant to TRAIL activation (137,140). Normal cells are believed to be resistant to TRAIL because they express higher levels of TRAIL decoy receptors TRID (DcR1) or TRUNDD (DcR2) on their cell surface (141–143), but this has been recently brought into question (144,145). Recent studies have investigated the potential role of TRAIL as an antineoplastic agent, and there is now accumulating evidence that systemic administration of TRAIL is relatively safe in mice (146), but perhaps not in humans (147). There is some concern that human hepatocytes, unlike those from rodents and primates (148), are sensitive to TRAIL mediated apoptotic cell death, which may limit its utility as anticancer therapeutic (149). TRAIL has been shown to be effective in killing some human breast and colon tumors when studied as xenografts, and prolongs the life of tumor-bearing mice (146,148) (Table 4).

Trail Receptors

TRAIL can interact with five distinct receptors, and all are members of the TNF receptor superfamily. Two of them contain cytoplasmic death domains and can be considered proapoptotic since ligation with TRAIL induces cell death in sensitive cell types. These two receptors, termed TRAIL-R1 or DR4 and TRAIL-R2 or DR5 (also called KILLER and TRICK2), interact through classical scaffolding proteins with death effector domains such as FADD, and signal in part through a prototypical caspase-8 extrinsic signaling pathway (135). In contrast, TRAIL can also bind to two other specific receptors, but these receptors lack traditional cytoplasmic death domains. TRAIL-R3 (also called decoy receptor-1 [DcR1], LIT, or TRID) is bound to the cell membrane through a GPI linker, and appears to function primarily to antagonize the activity of the death domain containing–receptors, DR4 and DR5 (137). Forced overexpression of TRAIL-R3 in sensitive cell lines protects them from the cytotoxic actions of TRAIL (141,150). The mechanism(s) of TRAIL-R3 protection is(are) still unresolved, since it is unclear whether the receptor acts simply by ligand depletion or whether TRAIL-R3 can act as a dominant negative repressor by forming inactive heterotrimeric complexes with DR4 and DR5 (for review, see Wajant et al. [136]). In contrast to TRAIL-R3, TRAIL-R4 (also called decoy receptor 2 [DcR2] or TRUNDD) contains

TABLE 4. *Tumor cell types that have been treated with tumor necrosis factor–related apoptosis-inducing ligand (TRAIL) in combination with chemotherapeutics*

Cell types	Chemotherapeutic
Colorectal cell lines	Sodium butyrate, nitroprusside, cyclohexamide, cisplatin, actinomycin D, doxorubicin, camptothecin, CPT-11
Multiple myeloma	Inhibitors of NFκB, doxorubicin
Glioma cells	Cyclohexyl, nitrosurea, diamino, dichloroplatinum
Breast and ovarian cancer	Herceptin, paclitaxel, cisplatin, doxorubicin, γ irradiation
Leukemia	Ultraviolet and γ irradiation
Neuroblastoma	5-aza-2′ deoxycytidine
Pancreatic cancer cell lines	Actinomycin D
Acute leukemia cells	STI-571
Chronic lymphocytic leukemia	Actinomycin D
Acute lymphocytic leukemia	Doxorubicin
Prostate cancer cell lines	Paclitaxel, doxorubicin
Renal cell carcinoma	Topotecan, 5-fluorouracil
Bladder cancer	Cisplatin
Hepatocellular carcinoma	Doxorubicin, camptothecin, actinomycin D
Ewing's sarcoma	MG-132

Modified from Wajant et al. (136).

a truncated cytoplasmic death domain that cannot transduce an apoptotic signal (142,143). Thus, it appears to act as a decoy receptor in a manner similar to TRAIL-R3, although there are controversial data in the literature that TRAIL-R4 signaling can inhibit TRAIL-mediated apoptosis by inducing NFκB pathways (145).

The final receptor that can bind to TRAIL is osteoprotegerin (OPG), the soluble member of the TNF receptor family that inhibits osteoclastogenesis by competitive binding to the RANK ligand (151). The importance of OPG as a decoy receptor for TRAIL and its ability to regulate TRAIL bioactivity remains unclear at the present time.

The potential use of TRAIL as an antineoplastic agent has generated some potentially interesting information about the relative specificity of soluble versus membrane-associated TRAIL for its pro-apoptotic receptors. At least for some of the recombinant forms of soluble TRAIL used in preclinical and clinical trials, there is growing evidence to suggest that soluble recombinant TRAIL has only limited activity on signaling through TRAIL-R2, whereas membrane-associated TRAIL is capable of stimulating both TRAIL receptors with similar effectiveness (136,152). Similar observations have been made for secreted and cell-associated TNF-α interactions with its two active receptors (30). Caution must be exercised, however, since little is known about whether the naturally occurring 20-kD soluble form of TRAIL has the same bioactivity of recombinant proteins.

Although TRAIL shares many similarities in its signaling pathways with other members of the TNF receptor superfamily, most notably FAS and TNF-R1, resolution of the signaling intermediates involved in TRAIL-mediated apoptosis has not been completed. Like other members of the TNF receptor superfamily, overexpression of TRAIL-R1 and TRAIL-R2 alone can induce signal transduction, suggesting that creation of the intracellular scaffolding and recruitment of adaptor proteins can be accomplished simply by recruit-

ment of the receptor proteins. There is also general agreement that TRAIL-induced cell death is mediated by apoptotic processes induced by proximal activation of caspase-8 and subsequent activation of the effector caspase, caspase-3 (153,154) (Fig. 7). What remains unclear, however, is the relative importance of the adaptor proteins FADD, DAP-3, and RIP in mediating this process.

Initially, it was presumed that TRAIL-induced apoptosis proceeded through a FADD-dependent process, analogous to TNF-R1 and FAS signaling. However, some investigators have shown that TRAIL-mediated apoptosis can proceed normally in some tissues from FADD-null mice (155), although more recent studies suggest that embryonic fibroblasts from FADD-null mice are resistant to TRAIL-mediated cell death (156). Similarly, Jurkat cells are sensitive to TRAIL-mediated death, but comparable FADD-deficient and caspase-8–deficient cells are resistant to the apoptotic effects of FADD (153,157).

However, other adaptor proteins also appear to be essential for TRAIL-induced apoptosis. For example, a mediator of interferon-α–induced cell death, DAP3 has been identified as an additional adaptor protein that binds to the death domains of TRAIL-R1 and TRAIL-R2, and to the death effector domain of FADD (158). It should be noted that in some cells, activation of caspase-8 is sufficient in itself to lead to a robust caspase-3 activation (type I cells) of cell death. However, in other cell types (most notably type II), TRAIL-mediated apoptosis can lead from a caspase-8 activation through a mitochondria-dependent amplification pathway; which promotes the release of cytochrome c (159,160). Cytoplasmic cytochrome c induces the formation of a complex, comprised of itself, Apaf-1, and caspase-9, which can activate caspase-3. In addition, Smac/Diablo released from the mitochondria, concomitant with cytochrome c antagonizes the actions of the caspase inhibitors cIAP1 and cIAP2 (161,162). This amplification pathway, as well as the direct

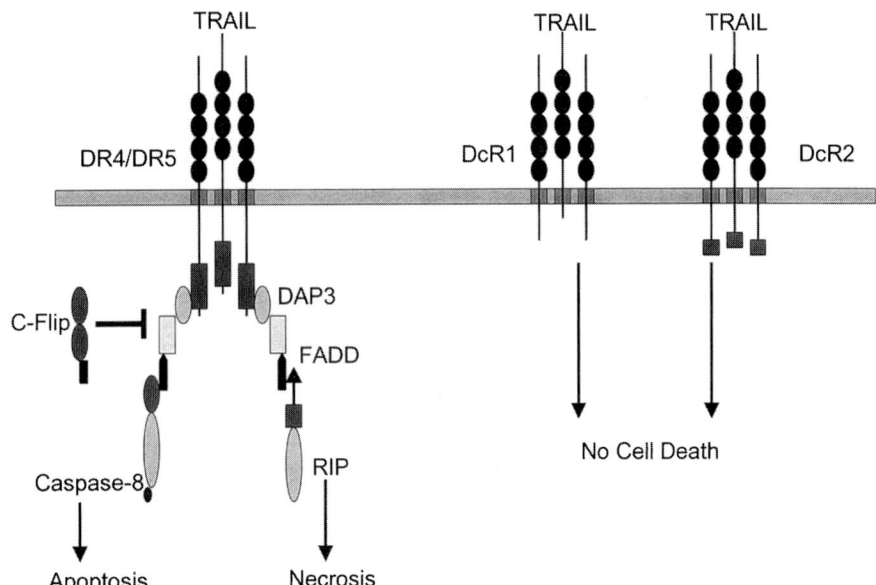

FIG. 7. Schematic representation of TRAIL signaling of cellular apoptosis or necrosis through caspase-8/caspase-3 or RIP-dependent pathways. In contrast to the DR4/DR5 (TRAIL-R1/TRAIL-R2) receptors, the decoy receptors DcR1 (TRAIL-R3) and DcR2 (TRAIL-R4) do not contain intracellular death domains, and therefore do not induce apoptosis. Adapted from from Srivastava (137), with permission.

signaling via caspase-8 induced by TRAIL is regulated by a large number of proteins including members of the Bcl-2 and cIAP families, as well as by the caspase-8 homologue (cFLIP or FLICE inhibitory protein).

TRAIL as a Cancer Chemotherapeutic

The overall goal of an effective cancer therapy is the ability to selectively kill neoplastic cells without interfering with the growth or viability of normal noncancer cells. It was originally proposed that the reduced TRAIL sensitivity by non-neoplastic cells was due to increased expression of decoy receptors in normal cells, with an absence or reduced expression of these receptors in transformed cells (140). However, as more and more cells and cell lines have been evaluated, the expression levels of both the pro-apoptotic and decoy receptors did not correlate with TRAIL sensitivity. Rather, there is growing consensus that resistance to TRAIL-mediated sensitivity is conferred intracellularly, and not at the level of cell receptors. More surprisingly, different forms of native and recombinant soluble and cell-associated TRAIL have been tested, and biological activity and cytotoxicity have varied considerably among the different preparations.

Development of TRAIL as a chemotherapeutic agent has been slowed by its apparent hepatotoxicity and the need to develop synthetic derivatives without systemic toxicity. The current limitation with this approach has been that with the advent of supposedly safe forms of TRAIL, antitumor activity has been dramatically reduced (for review, see Wajant et al. [136]). Further research has focused on increasing tumor sensitivity to TRAIL-mediated apoptosis through the use

of chemotherapy or radiation therapy induced increased expression of TRAIL receptors (TRAIL-R1 and TRAIL-R2) (Table 5). Another approach has been to modify the TRAIL ligand by fusing it with an antibody derivative, making it a better ligand for the TRAIL receptors that have restricted signaling capacity to soluble forms (163). Nevertheless, the potential role of TRAIL as an antineoplastic or antiviral agent has not been fully realized.

TWEAK

TWEAK is a recently identified member (1997) of the TNF superfamily that is expressed on interferon-γ, LPS, or cyclohexamide-stimulated monocytes and can induce apoptotic cell death in several tumor cell lines (164). However, more recent studies have demonstrated that TWEAK can have other biological activities, including the ability to stimulate proliferation of endothelial cells and angiogenesis (165), as well as induce the expression of other cytokines such as IL-8 (166,167). The putative TWEAK receptor (termed DR3, Apo-3, TRAMP, LARD, or WSLI) is a type I membrane protein (168–170). Like FAS and TNF-RI, DR3 contains a homologous death domain, and is thought to mediate apoptotic cell killing through traditional caspase-8 and caspase-3 extrinsic pathways (171). There remains a fair amount of controversy, however, about whether TWEAK-DR3 interactions are biologically significant for its apoptotic activities. Schneider et al. (172) reported that TWEAK-induced cell death in malignant Kym-1 cells was mediated not by DR3, but rather through the endogenous production of TNF-α and TNF-RI signaling. In a very recent report, Nakayama et al.

(173) noted that TWEAK induced multiple pathways of apoptosis and necrosis in several cancer cell lines, and in some cell lines, this appeared to be DR3 independent. Thus, at present, little is known regarding how TWEAK induces both its pro-apoptotic and pro-inflammatory responses.

T-LYMPHOCYTE CO-STIMULATORY MOLECULES: CD27, CD30, 4-1BB, AND OX40

Many of the members of the TNF ligand and TNF receptor superfamily are involved as co-stimulatory molecules for specific T-cell and B-cell populations. The diversity of these peptides and their relative specificity for individual T- and B-cell populations suggest that they have evolved for specific co-stimulatory functions independent of CD28 and B7. Many of these peptides are not constitutively expressed on either the effector or target cells, but their expression requires induction. Thus, it has been suggested that these molecules are not meant to replace the co-stimulatory properties of CD28 and the B7 family of peptides, but rather play complementary but independent functions (174). Most of these peptides share some structural homology to each other, as do their ligands. The receptors are most notable for the absence of any death domain in their cytoplasmic region and their lack of any pro-apoptotic activities. Rather, the primary signaling pathways of these members of the TNF receptor superfamily involve TRAF-2 and activation of NFκB and JNK signaling pathways.

CD27

CD27 is a lymphocyte-specific member of the TNF receptor superfamily that is expressed as a transmembrane homodimer with subunits of 55 kDa (175,176). In this regard, it differs from many other members of the TNF receptor superfamily that are predominantly trimers. Soluble forms of CD27 with an apparent mass of 32 kDa have also been detected, most likely via proteolytic cleavage of the surface molecule. The ligand for CD27 is a peptide identified as CD70 which is also cell associated (177). Although it is clear

that CD70 binding to CD27 enhances T-cell proliferation, the nature of this signal has not been well described (for review, see Lens et al. [178]). For example, CD27 ligation by CD70 does not induce IL-2 secretion, whereas surprisingly, it does augment TNF-α production by CD4$^+$ cells and enhances cytotoxicity by stimulated CD8$^+$ T cells (178). Part of the difficulty in describing the actions of CD27 ligation is because the co-stimulatory signal delivered by CD27 differs in varying T- and B-cell subsets. Whereas CD70–CD27 interactions are potent co-stimulatory signals for naive T cells (179), CD27–CD70 has only marginal effects on B-cell proliferation induced by *Staphylococcus aureus* and IL-2 (180). CD27's effects on B cells may be limited primarily to enhance immunoglobulin production and plasma cell differentiation into B cells (178).

Unlike most other members of the TNF receptor superfamily, CD27 exists primarily as a disulfide-linked homodimer. CD27 itself does not contain any death domains, but may associate with proteins that contain death domains similar to that seen in RIP and FADD. More importantly, the cytoplasmic domain of CD27 appears to associate with TRAF-2 and TRAF-5 (181,182). The coupling of TRAF-2 is significant, because this process is shared with other TNF receptor members that lack an intrinsic death domain (e.g., TNF-RII, CD30, CD40, OX40, and 4-1BB). The involvement of TRAF-2 in CD27-mediated NFκB and JNK activation, as well as the ability of TRAF-2 to bind cellular inhibitors of apoptosis (cIAP), is consistent with its capacity to enhance T-cell proliferation and B-cell differentiation (178,183).

CD30

CD30 was initially described as a surface antigen expressed on Reed–Sternberg cells in Hodgkin's disease (184). Later studies showed that CD30 was expressed on anaplastic large-cell lymphoma cells, but more importantly, was seen on activated lymphoid cells (185,186). Soluble CD30 was detected in patients with CD30-expressing neoplasms and during Th2-type immune responses (187,188) (Table 5). When CD30 was cloned and sequenced in 1992, it became clear

TABLE 5. *Expression of CD30, CD30 ligand, and soluble CD30*

Conditions associated with elevated sCD30	HIV, EBV, HTLV, and HBV infections; rheumatoid arthritis, systemic lupus erythematosus, Grave's disease, Hashimoto's thyroiditis, atopic dermatitis, systemic sclerosis, Wegener's granulomatosis, Omenn's syndrome, Hodgkin's disease, T-cell lymphoma, ALCL, ATL
Tissues/cells expressing CD30	*Resting:* CD8$^+$ T cells, lymph node cells, endometrial cells, and decidua *Activated:* T cells, B cells, virus-infected T cells, B cells *Malignant:* Reed-Sternberg cells, ALCL, ATL, NHL, embryonic carcinoma cells
Tissues/cells expressing CD30 ligand	*Resting:* neutrophils, eosinophils, B cells *Activated:* T cells, macrophages/monocytes *Malignant:* Burkitt lymphoma cells, AML, ALL cells

ALCL, anaplastic large cell lymphoma; ALL, acute lymphocytic leukemia; AML, acute myelogenous leukemia; ATL, adult T-cell leukemia; EBV, Epstein-Barr virus; HBV, hepatitis B virus; HIV, human immunodeficiency virus; HTLV, human T-cell leukemia/lymphoma virus; NHL, non-Hodgkins lymphoma.
Modified from Horie et al. (191).

that CD30 was a member of the TNF receptor superfamily (189). CD30 is a prototypical, type I glycosylated–membrane protein. Like other members of the TNF receptor superfamily that lack pro-apoptotic properties, CD30 lacks a cytoplasmic death domain, but contains sequences with binding to TRAF-2. Also, like other members of this superfamily, interactions with TRAF-2 appear to be responsible for the subsequent activation of NFκB and JNK signaling pathways that lead to proliferation, differentiation, and cytokine secretion. (For review, see Opat and Gaston [190] and Horie and Watanabe [191].)

CD30 is generally not expressed on resting lymphocytes, although expression has been detected on some resting peripheral blood CD8+ T cells (192). In lymph nodes, CD30 expression has been detected in cells around B-cell follicles and germinal centers (191). Under *in vitro* conditions, CD30 expression is inducible in T cells and B cells by stimulation with mitogens such as PHA, or by retroviruses such as HTLV and HIV (193–195). CD4+ T cells in particular will express CD30 when stimulated *in vitro*. It is now generally recognized that activation-induced expression of CD30 is dependent on either co-stimulation with CD28 or the addition of IL-4 (196,197). CD28 in particular induces CD30 expression through both IL-4–dependent and IL-4–independent mechanisms (Table 5).

Soluble forms of CD30 have been detected, and it appears to be a product of proteolytic cleavage of the cell membrane protein. Increased plasma concentrations of sCD30 have been detected in a number of pathologic conditions, including viral infections; autoimmune diseases such as rheumatoid arthritis, lupus, and systemic sclerosis; and hematolymphoid neoplasms (187,188,193,194,198,199). Unfortunately, the functions of sCD30 are unclear, although it may serve as a natural inhibitor of the membrane-associated CD30.

The CD30 ligand, or CD153, has been reported to be constitutively expressed by many hematologic cells, including neutrophils, eosinophils, B cells, monocytes, macrophages, dendritic cells, and megakaryocytes (200,201). CD30 ligand expression is also markedly up-regulated on CD4+ and CD8+ T cells after activation. CD30 ligand is a prototypical type II transmembrane protein, 40 kDa in mass, which forms a homotrimer when interacting with its receptor. In T cells, signaling through CD30 has been shown to induce NFκB, p42 MAP kinase/ERK2, and p38 MAP kinase activation. It has been recognized, however, that fine-tuning of the T-cell proliferative response involves a large number of different co-stimulatory molecules with differing specificity and functionality.

4-1BB

Many molecules have been identified as having co-stimulatory activity in T-cell activation. Of these, CD28 and its B7 ligands have been considered to be most critical for the T-cell proliferative response. However, it is clear that not all T-cell co-stimulatory signals are provided by CD28 and its ligands, and two additional members (besides CD27, CD30, and CD40) of the TNF superfamily and TNF receptor superfamily participate. These TNF superfamily members include 4-1BB and its ligand 4-1BB ligand and OX40 and its ligand OX40 ligand.

4-1BB was originally identified from activated mouse T-cell clones (202). The gene for 4-1BB resides on chromosome 1 in a cluster of other related TNF-receptor-family genes including CD30, OX40, TNFR II, HVEM, and DR3, suggesting that they all may have evolved through a localized gene duplication event (reviewed in Kwon et al. [203]). Like these other members of the TNF receptor superfamily, 4-1BB lacks a cytoplasmic death domain, and induces NFκB and JNK activation through TRAF2 signaling.

Expression of 4-1BB is inducible in T-lymphocytes by various stimuli for T-cell activation. 4-1BB is expressed primarily on activated CD4 and CD8 T cells, activated NK cells and activated NK T cells (204). In contrast, the ligand for 4-1BB is expressed primarily on antigen-presenting cells, such as mature dendritic cells, activated B cells, and activated macrophages (205,206). This expression pattern suggests that the relationship between 4-1BB and 4-1BB ligand is important for communication between antigen-presenting cells and T cells.

The co-stimulatory properties of 4-1BB are well demonstrated in T cells. 4-1BB is able to stimulate both T-cell proliferation and high production of IL-2 by resting T cells when the T cells are provided T-cell receptor signals. 4-1BB co-stimulation can be as effective as CD28 co-stimulation for the induction of IL-2 when the T-cell receptor signals are strong. 4-1BB is also able to replace CD28 in stimulating IL-2 production by resting T cells in the absence of CD28. The principal difference between the two is that CD28 is expressed constitutively, whereas 4-1BB expression must be induced, suggesting that 4-1BB and CD28 may play differential roles in the stages of the immune response. Whereas CD28 may play a greater role in the *induction* of the immune response, 4-1BB may be more important for *perpetuating* an established T-cell proliferative response. In fact, 4-1BB may play an important role in providing survival signals as well as co-stimulatory signals for activated T cells.

The 4-1BB ligand (CD137) is expectedly a member of the TNF ligand superfamily. Like the receptor, the gene for the 4-1BB ligand is clustered with those belonging to the TNF ligand superfamily such as CD27 ligand and CD40 ligand on chromosome 19 (207). Expression of 4-1BB has been detected on activated T cells, B cells, dendritic cells, and macrophages. 4-1BB is somewhat unique among members of the TNF ligand superfamily in that in addition to transmitting a signal through 4-1BB, it also receives a signal through ligation of 4-1BB. For example, cross-linking of 4-1BB ligand with a soluble 4-1BB immunoadhesin on activated T cells can inhibit their proliferation and promote cell death. Ligation of 4-1BB ligand also activates monocytes to produce TNF-α, IL-6, and IL-8, as well as induce apoptosis (206,208). These results suggest that in addition to providing a co-stimulatory

766 / CHAPTER 24

signal to 4-1BB, 4-1BB ligand may have broader functions on regulation of immune responses.

OX40 and OX40 Ligand

OX40, like many other cell-surface receptors discussed in this section was first identified on CD4$^+$ T cells activated with mitogens (for review, see Weinberg et al. [209]). Using initially an antibody to OX40 with antagonistic properties, it was readily shown that ligation of OX40 delivered a co-stimulatory signal to mature, differentiated CD4$^+$ T cells (210). Once the protein was cloned, it became evident that OX40 was a member of the TNF receptor superfamily and shared homology with CD40 (211,212). Expression of OX40 occurs on both human CD4$^+$ and CD8$^+$ T cells after stimulation with either PHA or Concanavalin A (213). The latter finding may be controversial since OX40 expression appears to be limited to CD4$^+$ T cells from lymph nodes of animals immunized with antigen and complete Freund's adjuvant (reviewed in Weinberg et al. [209]). Increased expression of OX40 can be induced in naïve or effector T cells solely by engagement of the T-cell receptor (214).

The ligand for OX40 was originally termed gp34 (215) and is also a type II membrane protein with some homology to other members of the TNF superfamily. Like other members of this family, OX40 ligand is found exclusively as a cell-associated protein, and its expression appears to be restricted to activated antigen-presenting cells. OX40 ligand appears to be involved in the amplification of co-stimulatory signals between antigen-presenting cells and T cells, since activation by CD40 of B cells and dendritic cells up-regulates OX40 ligand expression. However, cells expressing OX40 ligand may also receive a bi-directional signal from ligation with its receptor (216). This signal appears to promote differentiation of B cells and dendritic cells, and leads to increased production of IL-12, TNF-α, and IL-1β from dendritic cells (217). Thus, OX40/OX40 ligand may be involved in bi-directional communication between antigen-presenting cells and T cells.

Originally, OX40 ligation was shown to stimulate T-cell proliferation during the later stages of a mitogenic response (209,210). Importantly, there is evidence supporting the hypothesis that OX40 provides an alternate CD28-independent co-stimulatory pathway that drives antigen-specific T cells to proliferate. In combination with other co-stimulatory molecules, OX40 appears to play a role in sustaining a T-cell signal, which may promote more efficient T-cell memory (209).

BLyS AND APRIL: B-LYMPHOCYTE CO-STIMULATORS

The B-lymphocyte stimulator (also known as BAFF, THANK, TALL-1, and zTNF4) represents a newer recognized member of the TNF superfamily of ligands, and like APRIL, plays a critical role in B-cell immunity. APRIL and BlyS show considerable sequence homology between them-

selves, and lesser homology with other TNF ligand superfamily members including TNF-α, TRAIL, RANK ligand, and lymphotoxin-α (218,219). BLyS exists primarily as a type II membrane protein, but also exists as a soluble protein derived from the membrane-bound form by cleavage with a putative furin family protease. The soluble form consists of the extracellular domain, and BLyS circulates predominantly as a homotrimer, like many other members of this superfamily. Very recent data suggest that circulating BLyS may actually form very large "virus-like" particles comprised of multiple homodimers. This is mediated by a "flap" region that is not present in APRIL (220). These findings are controversial, however, since no proposed mechanism of how these large structures may interact with the receptor has been described. Furthermore, other investigators have not found soluble BLyS in any other form than a trimer (221,222). Interestingly, there is now some evidence that APRIL and BLyS can actually form heterotrimers when co-expressed in cell lines, and that biologically active heterotrimers may be present in serum samples from patients with systemic immune-based rheumatic diseases (223). If these recent data are substantiated, then BLyS/APRIL heterotrimers would represent only the second member of this superfamily (after lymphotoxin) not to form exclusively homotrimers.

BLyS expression is restricted to cells of the myeloid lineage, particularly macrophages and dendritic cells (Fig. 8) (218,221). Expression of BLyS is up-regulated by inflammatory mediators, most notably by interferon-γ and to a lesser extent IL-10 (224). In contrast, APRIL gene expression is seen in peripheral blood monocytes and macrophages as well as in peripheral blood lymphocytes. APRIL expression is also seen on a number of neoplastic cell lines, including malignant glioma cell lines, where it may be either a growth factor (225) or pro-apoptotic (226).

The search for the BLyS and APRIL receptors has yielded a number of candidates. TACI and BCMA were two receptors originally identified as members of the TNF receptor superfamily (227). It is now recognized that both BLyS and APRIL can signal through these two receptors. TACI was first described as a surface receptor on both B cells and T cells activated with ionomycin and phorbol esters. Collectively, this shared pattern of binding to the same receptors with the same affinity suggests that BLyS and APRIL may share a similar function, primarily affecting B cells and T cells to a lesser extent. This pattern, however, does not hold true for the BAFF receptor, which is expressed only on B cells and has BLyS as its only ligand (228). An analysis of the signaling events downstream of TACI and BCMA (and BAFF-R to a lesser extent) suggest that like other receptors of the TNF receptor superfamily, ligation of the receptor induces NFκB and JNK activation. In B-cell lines, the end product of this NFκB and JNK activation is the increased expression of a number of cell-survival genes, including Bcl-2 cFLIP and cIAP2. Not surprisingly, there is some indication that the TACI and BCMA receptors initiate NFκB activation through several members of the TRAF family, including TRAF-1,

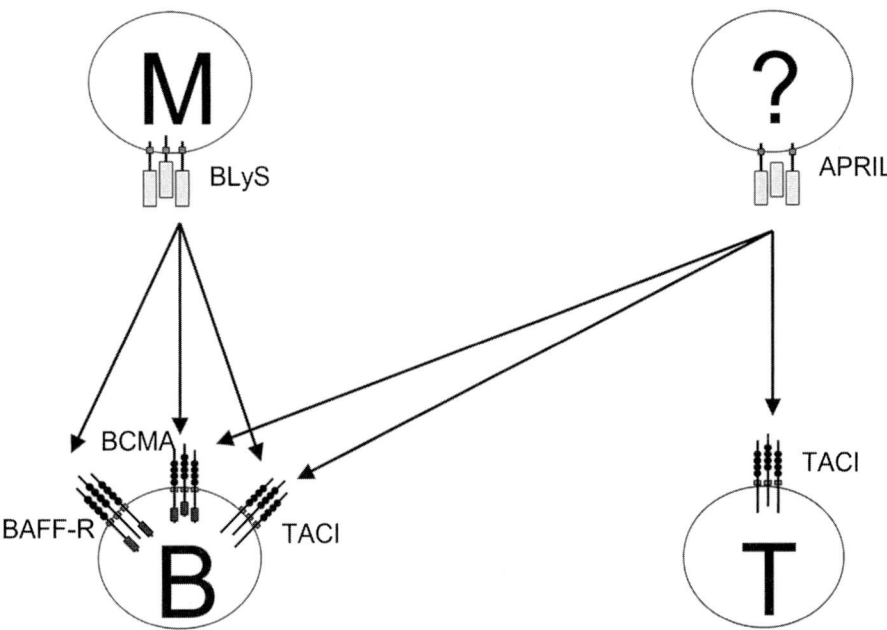

FIG. 8. Expression of BlyS/APRIL and their putative receptors. Although APRIL and BLyS can both signal through the BCMA and TACI receptors, only BLyS signals through the BAFF-R on B-cells (B). M, myeloid derived macrophages and dendritic cells; T, T cells. Adapted from Do and Chen-Kiang (231), with permission.

TRAF-2, TRAF-3, TRAF-5, and TRAF-6 (229,230). Some of the data remain unresolved over the relative contributions of these individual TRAF members, although there is little doubt that TRAFs play an important role in BLyS and APRIL signaling.

The actions of BLyS and APRIL are somewhat overlapping and serve to modulate B-cell responses. These cytokines appear to enhance the humoral immune response as a B-cell maturation agent, regulate antibody function, and inhibit B-cell apoptosis (231). BLyS signaling through the BAFF receptor appears to be critical to its role as a B-cell maturation agent.

ECTODYSPLASIN AND EDAR

One newly described member of the TNF superfamily was identified from studies cloning the genes responsible for ectodermal dysplasia syndrome (232), which is characterized by congenital defects in several organs including teeth, hair, and some exocrine glands. Positional cloning of the gene defective in the most common X-linked form of this ectodermal dysplasia led to the identification of a novel TNF family member, ectodysplasin or ED1. The autosomal form of this disease appears to result from mutations in the ED1 receptor, EDAR (233,234), or its downstream signaling mediators.

Interestingly, several splice variants have been observed for both the mouse and human forms of ED1. However, only one isoform actually encodes a TNF-like domain, suggesting that it is the only important isoform. It does share the characteristics of many TNF superfamily members; it is a glycosylated, homotrimeric membrane–associated type II protein. Where it differs from other family members, however, is that it contains two short collagen-like regions that are required for its biological activity.

EDAR (the ED1 receptor) is a protein containing 448 amino acids with one complete and two incomplete cysteine-rich repeats (233). EDAR shows the closest structural homology with TNFRSF19 members including TROY and TAJ. Like many other members of the family, the cytoplasmic domain of EDAR contains DD-like sequences, although EDAR signaling is not frequently associated with increased apoptosis. EDAR signaling leads to NFκB activation, possibly through TRAF-2 signaling (235,236).

ED1 and EDAR represent a ligand receptor pair in the TNF superfamily responsible for normal embryonic morphogenesis. These two proteins are expressed in partially overlapping or adjacent tissues in skin and are thus able to interact with each other.

CONCLUSIONS

There is remarkable diversity in the TNF superfamily of ligands and the TNF receptor superfamily. Although the ligands share some structural homology, they have evolved in diverse ways to fulfill specific niches in innate and acquired immunity and in organogenesis. However, when reviewing the family of ligands as a whole, there are some general commonalities that deserve mention. The ligands in general are membrane associated, although several can be processed from the cell membrane and are active in soluble form. The majority of these ligands form homotrimers that are required for their activity, although lymphotoxin and BLyS/APRIL can form heterotrimers. Nevertheless, it is this trimerization of the ligand that is required for their biological activities, since parallel oligomerization of the receptors is essential to construct the docking platforms required for signal transduction. As a group, there are two recurring themes in the actions of the receptors: the ability to interact with TRAF molecules to signal a pro-inflammatory response through NFκB, and to a lesser extent, JNK signaling, and the possession of death domains in the cytoplasmic region required for initiating apoptosis through extrinsic caspase-8–mediated pathways. Members of the receptor superfamily that contain death domains are primarily involved in apoptosis, while those containing regions that serve as platforms for the TRAF proteins are involved in inflammation, co-stimulatory activities, differentiation, and maturation. Many of these ligands serve both functions.

Members of the TNF superfamily contribute to the complexity of the innate and acquired immune responses. Each of the proteins has found an important niche where they serve to initiate, regulate, and terminate critical aspects of organogenesis and the immune response. In many cases, these functions are essential to appropriate developmental and immunologic response.

REFERENCES

1. Kwon B, Youn BS, Kwon BS. Functions of newly identified members of the tumor necrosis factor receptor/ligand superfamilies in lymphocytes. *Curr Opin Immunol* 1999;11:340–345.
2. Carswell EA, Old LJ, Kassel RL, et al. An endotoxin-induced serum factor that causes necrosis of tumors. *Proc Natl Acad SciU S A* 1975;72:3666–3670.
3. Green S, Dobrjansky A, Carswell EA, et al. Partial purification of a serum factor that causes necrosis of tumors. *Proc Natl Acad Sci U S A* 1976;73:381–385.
4. Kolb WP, Granger GA. Lymphocyte *in vitro* cytotoxicity: characterization of human lymphotoxin. *Proc Natl Acad Sci U S A* 1968;61:1250–1255.
5. Haranaka K, Carswell EA, Williamson BD, et al. Purification, characterization, antitumor activity of nonrecombinant mouse tumor necrosis factor. *Proc Natl Acad Sci U S A* 1986;83:3949–3953.
6. Aggarwal BB, Aiyer RA, Pennica D, et al. Human tumour necrosis factors: structure and receptor interactions. *Ciba Found Symp* 1987;131:39–51.
7. Pennica D, Hayflick JS, Bringman TS, et al. Cloning and expression in Escherichia coli of the cDNA for murine tumor necrosis factor. *Proc Natl Acad Sci U S A* 1985;82:6060–6064.
8. Beutler B, Cerami A. Cachectin and tumour necrosis factor as two sides of the same biological coin. *Nature* 1986;320:584–588.
9. Wallach D, Varfolomeev EE, Malinin NL, et al. Tumor necrosis factor receptor and Fas signaling mechanisms. *Annu Rev Immunol* 1999;17:331–67.:331–367.
10. Mackay F, Kalled SL. TNF ligands and receptors in autoimmunity: an update. *Curr Opin Immunol* 2002;14:783–790.
11. Zhou T, Mountz JD, Kimberly RP. Immunobiology of tumor necrosis factor receptor superfamily. *Immunol Res* 2002;26:323–336.
12. Griffith TS, Lynch DH. TRAIL: a molecule with multiple receptors and control mechanisms. *Curr Opin Immunol* 1998;10:559–563.
13. Idriss HT, Naismith JH. TNF alpha and the TNF receptor superfamily: structure–function relationship(s). *Microsc Res Tech* 2000;50:184–195.
14. Schluter D, Deckert M. The divergent role of tumor necrosis factor receptors in infectious diseases. *Microbes Infect* 2000;2:1285–1292.
15. Sedgwick JD, Riminton DS, Cyster JG, et al. Tumor necrosis factor: a master-regulator of leukocyte movement. *Immunol Today* 2000;21:110–113.
16. Locksley RM, Killeen N, Lenardo MJ, et al. The TNF and TNF receptor superfamilies: integrating mammalian biology. *Cell* 2001;104:487–501.
17. Fu YX, Chaplin DD. Development and maturation of secondary lymphoid tissues. *Annu Rev Immunol* 1999;17:399–433.
18. Hughes LB, Moreland LW. New therapeutic approaches to the management of rheumatoid arthritis. *BioDrugs* 2001;15:379–393.
19. Ksontini R, MacKay SL, Moldawer LL. Revisiting the role of tumor necrosis factor alpha and the response to surgical injury and inflammation. *Arch Surg* 1998;133:558–567.
20. Bodmer JL, Schneider P, Tschopp J. The molecular architecture of the TNF superfamily. *Trends Biochem Sci* 2002;27:19–26.
21. Cha SS, Sung BJ, Kim YA, et al. Crystal structure of TRAIL-DR5 complex identifies a critical role of the unique frame insertion in conferring recognition specificity. *J Biol Chem* 2000;275:31171–31177.
22. Hymowitz SG, O'Connell MP, Ultsch MH, et al. A unique zinc-binding site revealed by a high-resolution X-ray structure of homotrimeric Apo2L/TRAIL. *Biochemistry* 2000;39:633–640.
23. Shapiro L, Scherer PE. The crystal structure of a complement-1q family protein suggests an evolutionary link to tumor necrosis factor. *Curr Biol* 1988;8:335–338.
24. Kishore U, Reid KB. C1q: structure, function, receptors. *Immunopharmacology* 2000;49:159–170.
25. Naismith JH, Sprang SR. Tumor necrosis factor receptor superfamily. *J Inflamm* 1995;47:1–7.
26. Kriegler M, Perez C, DeFay K, et al. A novel form of TNF/cachectin is a cell surface cytotoxic transmembrane protein: ramifications for the complex physiology of TNF. *Cell* 1988;53:45–53.
27. Moss ML, Catherine-Jin SL, Milla ME, et al. Cloning of a disintegrin metalloproteinase that processes precursor tumor-necrosis factor-a. *Nature* 1997;385:733–736.
28. Peschon JJ, Slack JL, Reddy P, et al. An essential role for ectodomain shedding in mammalian development [see comments]. *Science* 1998;282:1281–1284.
29. Marino MW, Dunn A, Grail D, et al. Characterization of tumor necrosis factor–deficient mice. *Proc Natl Acad Sci U S A* 1997;94:8093–8098.
30. Grell M, Douni E, Wajant H, et al. The transmembrane form of tumor necrosis factor is the prime activating ligand of the 80 kDa tumor necrosis factor receptor. *Cell* 1995;83:793–802.
31. Eissner G, Kohlhuber F, Grell M, et al. Critical involvement of transmembrane tumor necrosis factor-alpha in endothelial programmed cell death mediated by ionizing radiation and bacterial endotoxin. *Blood* 1995;86:4184–4193.
32. Bazzoni F, Beutler B. The tumor necrosis factor ligand and receptor families. *N Engl J Med* 1996;334:1717–1723.
33. Beutler B, Krochin N, Milsark IW, et al. Control of cachectin (tumor necrosis factor) synthesis: mechanisms of endotoxin resistance. *Science* 1986;232:977–980.
34. Strieter RM, Remick DG, Lynch JP, et al. Differential regulation of tumor necrosis factor-alpha in human alveolar macrophages and peripheral blood monocytes: a cellular and molecular analysis. *Am. J. Respir. Cell Mol Biol* 1989;1:57–63.
35. Drouet C, Shakhov AN, Jongeneel CV. Enhancers and transcription factors controlling the inducibility of the tumor necrosis factor-alpha promoter in primary macrophages. *J Immunol* 1991;147:1694–1700.
36. Leitman DC, Mackow ER, Williams T, et al. The core promoter region of the tumor necrosis factor alpha gene confers phorbol ester responsiveness to upstream transcriptional activators. *Mol Cell Biol* 1992;12:1352–1356.
37. Leitman DC, Ribeiro RC, Mackow ER, et al. Identification of a tumor necrosis factor–responsive element in the tumor necrosis factor gene. *J Biol Chem* 1991;266:9343–9346.
38. Hensel G, Meichle A, Pfizenmaier K, et al. PMA-responsive 5′ flanking sequences of the human TNF gene. *Lymphokine Res* 1989;8:347–351.
39. Shakhov AN, Collart MA, Vassalli P, et al. Kappa B-type enhancers are involved in lipopolysaccharide-mediated transcriptional activation of the tumor necrosis factor alpha gene in primary macrophages. *J Exp Med* 1990;171:35–47.

40. Beutler B, Brown T. Polymorphism of the mouse TNF-alpha locus: sequence studies of the 3'-untranslated region and first intron. *Gene* 1993;129:279–283.

41. Han J, Brown T, Beutler B. Endotoxin-responsive sequences control cachectin/tumor necrosis factor biosynthesis at the translational level [published erratum appears in *J Exp Med* 1990;171:971–972]. *J Exp Med* 1990;171:465–475.

42. Dumitru CD, Ceci JD, Tsatsanis C, et al. TNF-alpha induction by LPS is regulated posttranscriptionally via a Tpl2/ERK-dependent pathway. *Cell* 2000;103:1071–1083.

43. Zhang T, Kruys V, Huez G, et al. AU-rich element-mediated translational control: complexity and multiple activities of trans-activating factors. *Biochem Soc Trans* 2001;30:952–958.

44. Baseggio L, Charlot C, Bienvenu J, et al. Tumor necrosis factor-alpha mRNA stability in human peripheral blood cells after lipopolysaccharide stimulation. *Eur Cytokine Netw* 2002;13:92–98.

45. Schindler R, Gelfand JA, Dinarello CA. Recombinant C5a stimulates transcription rather than translation of interleukin-1 (IL-1) and tumor necrosis factor: translational signal provided by lipopolysaccharide or IL-1 itself. *Blood* 1990;76:1631–1638.

46. Schindler R, Lonnemann G, Shaldon S, et al. Transcription, not synthesis, of interleukin-1 and tumor necrosis factor by complement. *Kidney Int* 1990;37:85–93.

47. Luedke CE, Cerami A. Interferon-gamma overcomes glucocorticoid suppression of cachectin/tumor necrosis factor biosynthesis by murine macrophages. *J Clin Invest* 1990;86:1234–1240.

48. Fiorentino DF, Zlotnik A, Mosmann TR, et al. IL-10 inhibits cytokine production by activated macrophages. *J Immunol* 1991;147:3815–3822.

49. Schumacher HRJ, Meng Z, Sieck M, et al. Effect of a nonsteroidal antiinflammatory drug on synovial fluid in osteoarthritis. *J Rheumatol* 1996;23:1774–1777.

50. Gonzalez E, de la Cruz C, de Nicolas R, et al. Long-term effect of nonsteroidal anti-inflammatory drugs on the production of cytokines and other inflammatory mediators by blood cells of patients with osteoarthritis. *Agents Actions* 1994;41:171–178.

51. Dinarello C, Moldawer LL. Proinflammatory and antinflammatory cytokines in rheumatoid arthritis. 3rd Edition, Amgen, Inc 2002.

52. Kido G, Wright JL, Merchant RE. Acute effects of human recombinant tumor necrosis factor-alpha on the cerebral vasculature of the rat in both normal brain and in an experimental glioma model. *J Neurooncol* 1991;10:95–109.

53. Wong B, Choi Y. Pathways leading to cell death in T cells. *Curr Opin Immunol* 1997;9:358–364.

54. Feldmann M, Brennan MF, Elliot MJ, et al. TNF alpha is a therapeutic target for rheumatoid arthritis. *Ann N Y Acad Sci* 1995;766:272.

55. Van Zee KJ, Kohno T, Fischer E, et al. Tumor necrosis factor soluble receptors circulate during experimental and clinical inflammation and can protect against excessive tumor necrosis factor alpha *in vitro* and *in vivo*. *Proc Natl Acad Sci U S A* 1992;89:4845–4849.

56. Seckinger P, Isaaz S, Dayer JM. A human inhibitor of tumor necrosis factor alpha. *J Exp Med* 1988;167:1511–1516.

57. Seckinger P, Vey E, Turcatti G, et al. Tumor necrosis factor inhibitor: purification, NH2-terminal amino acid sequence and evidence for anti-inflammatory and immunomodulatory activities. *Eur J Immunol* 1990;20:1167–1174.

58. Tartaglia LA, Pennica D, Goeddel DV. Ligand passing: the 75-kDa tumor necrosis factor (TNF) receptor recruits TNF for signaling by the 55-kDa TNF receptor. *J Biol Chem* 1993;268:18542–18548.

59. Aderka D, Engelmann H, Maor Y, et al. Stabilization of the bioactivity of tumor necrosis factor by its soluble receptors. *J Exp Med* 1992;175:323–329.

60. Higuchi M, Aggarwal BB. Differential roles of two types of the TNF receptor in TNF-induced cytotoxicity, DNA fragmentation, differentiation. *J Immunol* 1994;152:4017–4025.

61. Grell M, Wajant H, Zimmermann G, et al. The type 1 receptor (CD120a) is the high affinity receptor for soluble tumor necrosis factor. *Proc Natl Acad Sci U S A* 1998;95:570–575.

62. Welborn MB 3, Van Zee K, Edwards PD, et al. A human tumor necrosis factor p75 receptor agonist stimulates *in vitro* T cell proliferation but does not produce inflammation or shock in the baboon. *J Exp Med* 1996;184:165–171.

63. van der Poll T, Jansen PM, Van Zee KJ, et al. Tumor necrosis factor-alpha induces activation of coagulation and fibrinolysis in baboons

64. Van Zee KJ, Stackpole SA, Montegut MJ, et al. A human tumor necrosis factor (TNF) a mutant that binds exclusively to the p55 TNF receptor produces toxicity in the baboon. *J Exp Med* 1994;179:1185–1191.

65. Douni E, Kollias G. A critical role of the p75 tumor necrosis factor receptor (p75TNF-R) in organ inflammation independent of TNF, lymphotoxin alpha, or the p55TNF-R. *J Exp Med* 1998;188:1343–1352.

66. Tewari M, Dixit VM. Recent advances in tumor necrosis factor and CD40 signaling. *Curr Opin Genet Dev* 1996;6:39–44.

67. Segui B, Cuvillier O, Adam-Klages S, et al. Involvement of FAN in TNF-induced apoptosis. *J Clin Invest* 2001;108:143–151.

68. Adam-Klages S, Adam D, Wiegmann K, et al. FAN, a novel WD-repeat protein, couples the p55 TNF-receptor to neutral sphingomyelinase. *Cell* 1996;86:937–947.

69. Dunbar JD, Song HY, Guo D, et al. Two-hybrid cloning of a gene encoding TNF receptor-associated protein 2, a protein that interacts with the intracellular domain of the type 1 TNF receptor: identity with subunit 2 of the 26S protease. *J Immunol* 1997;158:4252–4259.

70. Grell M, Zimmermann G, Hülser D, et al. TNF receptors TR60 and TR80 can mediate apoptosis via induction of distinct signal pathways. *J Immunol* 1994;153:1963–1972.

71. Weiss T, Grell M, Hessabi B, et al. Enhancement of TNF receptor p60-mediated cytotoxicity by TNF receptor p80: requirement of the TNF receptor–associated factor-2 binding site. *J Immunol* 1997;158:2398–2404.

72. Natoli G, Costanzo A, Moretti F, et al. Tumor necrosis factor (TNF) receptor 1 signaling downstream of TNF receptor-associated factor 2. Nuclear factor kappaB (NFkappaB)-inducing kinase requirement for activation of activating protein 1 and NFkappaB but not of c-Jun N-terminal kinase/stress-activated protein kinase. *J Biol Chem* 1997;272:26079–26082.

73. Malinin NL, Boldin MP, Kovalenko AW, et al. MAP3K-related kinase involved in NF-kB induction by TNF, CD95 and IL-1. *Nature* 1997;385:540–544.

74. Baeuerle PA, Baltimore D. NF-KB: Ten years after. *Cell* 199;87:13–20.

75. Beg AA, Baltimore D. An essential role for NF-kappaB in preventing TNF-alpha-induced cell death [see comments]. *Science* 1996;274:782–784.

76. Pimentel-Muinos FX, Seed B. Regulated commitment of TNF receptor signaling: a molecular switch for death or activation. *Immunity* 1999;11:783–793.

77. Peschon JJ, Torrance DS, Stocking KL, et al. TNF receptor-deficient mice reveal divergent roles for p55 and p75 in several models of inflammation. *J Immunol* 1998;160:943–952.

78. Nowak M, Gaines GC, Rosenberg J, et al. LPS-induced liver injury in D-galactosamine-sensitized mice requires secreted TNF-alpha and the TNF-p55 receptor. *Am J Physiol Regul Integr Comp Physiol* 2000;278:R1202–R1209.

79. Sheehan KC, Pinckard JK, Arthur CD, et al. Monoclonal antibodies specific for murine p55 and p75 tumor necrosis factor receptors: identification of a novel *in vivo* role for p75. *J Exp Med* 1995;181:607–617.

80. Pfeffer K, Matsuyama T, Kundig TM, et al. Mice deficient for the 55 kd tumor necrosis factor receptor are resistant to endotoxic shock, yet succumb to *L. monocytogenes* infection. *Cell* 1993;73:457–467.

81. Rothe J, Lesslauer W, Lotscher H, et al. Mice lacking the tumour necrosis factor receptor 1 are resistant to TNF-mediated toxicity but highly susceptible to infection by Listeria monocytogenes. *Nature* 1993;364:798–802.

82. Erickson SL, de Sauvage FJ, Kikly K, et al. Decreased sensitivity to tumour-necrosis factor but normal T-cell development in TNF receptor-2–deficient mice. *Nature* 1994;372:560–563.

83. Kusters S, Tiegs G, Alexopoulou L, et al. *in vivo* evidence for a functional role of both tumor necrosis factor (TNF) receptors and transmembrane TNF in experimental hepatitis. *Eur J Immunol* 1997;27:2870–2875.

84. Alexopoulou L, Pasparakis M, Kollias G. A murine transmembrane tumor necrosis factor (TNF) transgene induces arthritis by cooperative p55/p75 TNF receptor signaling. *Eur J Immunol* 1997;27:2588–2592.

85. Probert L, Akassoglou K, Alexopoulou L, et al. Dissection of the pathologies induced by transmembrane and wild-type tumor necrosis factor in transgenic mice. *J Leukoc Biol* 1996;59:518–525.

through an exclusive effect on the p55 receptor. *Blood* 1996;88:922–927.

86. Douni E, Kollias G. A critical role of the p75 tumor necrosis factor receptor (p75TNF-R) in organ inflammation independent of TNF, lymphotoxin alpha, or the p55TNF-R. *J Exp Med* 1998;188:1343–1352.

87. Josephs MD, Bahjat FR, Fukuzuka K, et al. Lipopolysaccharide and D-galactosamine-induced hepatic injury is mediated by TNF-alpha and not by Fas ligand. *Am J Physiol Regul Integr Comp Physiol* 2000; 278:R1196–R1201.

88. Williams LM, Gibbons DL, Gearing A, et al. Paradoxical effects of a synthetic metalloproteinase inhibitor that blocks both p55 and p75 TNF receptor shedding and TNF alpha processing in RA synovial membrane cell cultures. *J Clin Invest* 1996;97:2833–2841.

89. Ruddle NH. Tumor necrosis factor (TNF-alpha) and lymphotoxin (TNF-beta). *Curr Opin Immunol* 1992;4:327–332.

90. Browning JL, Ngam-ek A, Lawton P, et al. Lymphotoxin beta, a novel member of the TNF family that forms a heteromeric complex with lymphotoxin on the cell surface. *Cell* 1993;72:847–856.

91. Gruss HJ. Molecular, structural, biological characteristics of the tumor necrosis factor ligand superfamily. *Int J Clin Lab Res* 1996;26:143–159.

92. Ngo VN, Korner H, Gunn MD, et al. Lymphotoxin alpha/beta and tumor necrosis factor are required for stromal cell expression of homing chemokines in B and T cell areas of the spleen. *J Exp Med* 1999; 189:403–412.

93. Endres R, Alimzhanov MB, Plitz T, et al. Mature follicular dendritic cell networks depend on expression of lymphotoxin beta receptor by radioresistant stromal cells and of lymphotoxin beta and tumor necrosis factor by B cells. *J Exp Med* 1999;189:159–168.

94. DeTogni P, Goellner J, Ruddle NH, et al. Abnormal development of peripheral lymphoid organs in mice deficient in lymphotoxin. *Science* 1994;264:703–707.

95. Matsumoto M, Mariathasan S, Nahm MH, et al. Role of lymphotoxin and the type I TNF receptor in the formation of germinal centers. *Science* 1996;271:1289–1291.

96. Pasparakis M, Alexopoulou L, Grell M, et al. Peyer's patch organogenesis is intact yet formation of B lymphocyte follicles is defective in peripheral lymphoid organs of mice deficient for tumor necrosis factor and its 55-kDa receptor. *Proc Natl Acad Sci U S A* 1997;94:6319–6323.

97. Rennert PD, Browning JL, Mebius R, et al. Surface lymphotoxin alpha/beta complex is required for the development of peripheral lymphoid organs. *J Exp Med* 1996;184:1999–2006.

98. Rennert PD, James D, Mackay F, et al. Lymph node genesis is induced by signaling through the lymphotoxin beta receptor. *Immunity* 1998;9:71–79.

99. Rennert PD, Browning JL, Hochman PS. Selective disruption of lymphotoxin ligands reveals a novel set of mucosal lymph nodes and unique effects on lymph node cellular organization. *Int Immunol* 1997;9:1627–1639.

100. Mauri DN, Ebner R, Montgomery RI, et al. LIGHT, a new member of the TNF superfamily, lymphotoxin alpha are ligands for herpesvirus entry mediator. *Immunity* 1998;8:21–30.

101. Harrop JA, McDonnell PC, Brigham-Burke M, et al. Herpesvirus entry mediator ligand (HVEM-L), a novel ligand for HVEM/TR2, stimulates proliferation of T cells and inhibits HT29 cell growth. *J Biol Chem* 1998;273:27548–27556.

102. Zhai Y, Guo R, Hsu TL, et al. LIGHT, a novel ligand for lymphotoxin beta receptor and TR2/HVEM induces apoptosis and suppresses *in vivo* tumor formation via gene transfer. *J Clin Invest* 1998;102:1142–1151.

103. Rooney IA, Butrovich KD, Glass AA, et al. The lymphotoxin-beta receptor is necessary and sufficient for LIGHT-mediated apoptosis of tumor cells. *J Biol Chem* 2000;275:14307–14315.

104. Tamada K, Ni J, Zhu G, et al. Cutting edge: selective impairment of CD8+ T cell function in mice lacking the TNF superfamily member LIGHT. *J Immunol* 2002;168:4832–4835.

105. Tamada K, Shimozaki K, Chapoval AI, et al. LIGHT, a TNF-like molecule, costimulates T cell proliferation and is required for dendritic cell-mediated allogeneic T cell response. *J Immunol* 2000;164:4105–4110.

106. Morel Y, Truneh A, Sweet RW, et al. The TNF superfamily members LIGHT and CD154 (CD40 ligand) costimulate induction of dendritic cell maturation and elicit specific CTL activity. *J Immunol* 2001;167:2479–2486.

107. Futterer A, Mink K, Luz A, et al. The lymphotoxin beta receptor controls organogenesis and affinity maturation in peripheral lymphoid tissues. *Immunity* 1998;9:59–70.

108. Alimzhanov MB, Kuprash DV, Kosco-Vilbois MH, et al. Abnormal development of secondary lymphoid tissues in lymphotoxin beta-deficient mice. *Proc Natl Acad Sci U S A* 1997;94:9302–9307.

109. Nagata S, Golstein P. The Fas death factor. *Science* 1995;267:1449–1455.

110. Schneider P, Holler N, Bodmer JL, et al. Conversion of membrane-bound Fas(CD95) ligand to its soluble form is associated with down-regulation of its proapoptotic activity and loss of liver toxicity. *J Exp Med* 1998;187:1205–1213.

111. Tanaka M, Suda T, Takahashi T, et al. Expression of the functional soluble form of human fas ligand in activated lymphocytes. *EMBO J* 1995;14:1129–1135.

112. Ottonello L, Tortolina G, Amelotti M, et al. Soluble Fas ligand is chemotactic for human neutrophilic polymorphonuclear leukocytes. *J Immunol* 1999;162:3601–3606.

113. Seino K, Iwabuchi K, Kayagaki N, et al. Chemotactic activity of soluble Fas ligand against phagocytes. *J Immunol* 1998;161:4484–4488.

114. Chen JJ, Sun Y, Nabel GJ. Regulation of the proinflammatory effects of Fas ligand (CD95L). *Science* 1998;282:1714–1717.

115. Walker PR, Saas P, Dietrich PY. Tumor expression of Fas ligand (CD95L) and the consequences. *Curr Opin Immunol* 1998;10:564–572.

116. Liles WC, Kiener PA, Ledbetter JA, et al. Differential expression of Fas (CD95) and Fas ligand on normal human phagocytes: implications for the regulation of apoptosis in neutrophils. *J Exp Med* 1996;184:429–440.

117. Kiener PA, Davis PM, Rankin BM, et al. Human monocytic cells contain high levels of intracellular Fas ligand: rapid release following cellular activation. *J Immunol* 1997;159:1594–1598.

118. Simonet WS, Lacey DL, Dunstan CR, et al. Osteoprotegerin: a novel secreted protein involved in the regulation of bone density [see comments]. *Cell* 1997;89:309–319.

119. Hsu H, Lacey DL, Dunstan CR, et al. Tumor necrosis factor receptor family member RANK mediates osteoclast differentiation and activation induced by osteoprotegerin ligand. *Proc Natl Acad Sci U S A* 1999;96:3540–3545.

120. Anderson DM, Maraskovsky E, Billingsley WL, et al. A homologue of the TNF receptor and its ligand enhance T-cell growth and dendritic-cell function. *Nature* 1997;390:175–179.

121. Lacey DL, Timms E, Tan HL, et al. Osteoprotegerin ligand is a cytokine that regulates osteoclast differentiation and activation. *Cell* 1998;93:165–176.

122. Yasuda H, Shima N, Nakagawa N, et al. Osteoclast differentiation factor is a ligand for osteoprotegerin/osteoclastogenesis-inhibitory factor and is identical to TRANCE/RANKL. *Proc Natl Acad Sci U S A* 1998;95:3597–3602.

123. Takahashi N, Udagawa N, Suda T. A new member of tumor necrosis factor ligand family, ODF/OPGL/TRANCE/RANKL, regulates osteoclast differentiation and function. *Biochem Biophys Res Commun* 1999;256:449–455.

124. Khosla S. Minireview: the OPG/RANKL/RANK system. *Endocrinology* 2001;142:5050–5055.

125. Burgess TL, Qian Y, Kaufman S, et al. The ligand for osteoprotegerin (OPGL) directly activates mature osteoclasts. *J Cell Biol* 1999; 145:527–538.

126. Dougall WC, Glaccum M, Charrier K, et al. RANK is essential for osteoclast and lymph node development. *Genes Dev* 1999;13:2412–2424.

127. Fata JE, Kong YY, J Li, et al. The osteoclast differentiation factor osteoprotegerin–ligand is essential for mammary gland development. *Cell* 2000;103:41–50.

128. Wong BR, Josien R, Lee SY, et al. TRANCE (tumor necrosis factor [TNF]–related activation-induced cytokine), a new TNF family member predominantly expressed in T cells, is a dendritic cell–specific survival factor. *J Exp Med* 1997;186:2075–2080.

129. Williamson E, Bilsborough JM, Viney JL. Regulation of mucosal dendritic cell function by receptor activator of NF-kappa B (RANK)/RANK ligand interactions: impact on tolerance induction. *J Immunol* 2002;169:3606–3612.

130. Green EA, Flavell RA. TRANCE-RANK, a new signal pathway involved in lymphocyte development and T cell activation. *J Exp Med* 1999;189:1017–1020.

131. Bucay N, Sarosi I, Dunstan CR, et al. Osteoprotegerin-deficient mice develop early onset osteoporosis and arterial calcification. *Genes Dev* 1998;12:1260–1268.

132. Kong YY, Yoshida H, Sarosi I, et al. OPGL is a key regulator of osteoclastogenesis, lymphocyte development and lymph-node organogenesis. *Nature* 1999;397:315–323.

133. Horwood NJ, Elliott J, Martin TJ, et al. Osteotropic agents regulate the expression of osteoclast differentiation factor and osteoprotegerin in osteoblastic stromal cells. *Endocrinology* 1998;139:4743–4746.

134. Suda T, Takahashi N, Udagawa N, et al. Modulation of osteoclast differentiation and function by the new members of the tumor necrosis factor receptor and ligand families. *Endocr Rev* 1999;20:345–357.

135. Abe K, Kurakin A, Mohseni-Maybodi M, et al. The complexity of TNF-related apoptosis-inducing ligand. *Ann N Y Acad Sci* 2000;926:52–63.

136. Wajant H, Pfizenmaier K, Scheurich P. TNF-related apoptosis inducing ligand (TRAIL) and its receptors in tumor surveillance and cancer therapy. *Apoptosis* 2002;7:449–459.

137. Srivastava RK. TRAIL/Apo-2L: mechanisms and clinical applications in cancer. *Neoplasia* 2001;3:535–546.

138. Cha SS, Sung BJ, Kim YA, et al. Crystal structure of TRAIL-DR5 complex identifies a critical role of the unique frame insertion in conferring recognition specificity. *J Biol Chem* 2000;275:31171–31177.

139. Cha SS, Kim MS, Choi YH, et al. 2.8 Angstrom resolution crystal structure of human TRAIL, a cytokine with selective antitumor activity. *Immunity* 1999;11:253–261.

140. Ashkenazi A, Dixit VM. Death receptors: signaling and modulation. *Science* 1998;281:1305–1308.

141. Pan G, Ni J, Wei YF, et al. An antagonist decoy receptor and a death domain–containing receptor for TRAIL [see comments]. *Science* 1997;277:815–818.

142. Pan G, J Ni, Yu G, et al. TRUNDD, a new member of the TRAIL receptor family that antagonizes TRAIL signalling. *FEBS Lett* 1998;424:41–45.

143. Marsters SA, Sheridan JP, Pitti RM, et al. A novel receptor for Apo2L/TRAIL contains a truncated death domain. *Curr Biol* 1997;7:1003–1006.

144. Griffith TS, Chin WA, Jackson GC, et al. Intracellular regulation of TRAIL-induced apoptosis in human melanoma cells. *J Immunol* 1998;161:2833–2840.

145. Degli-Esposti MA, Dougall WC, Smolak PJ, et al. The novel receptor TRAIL-R4 induces NF-kappaB and protects against TRAIL-mediated apoptosis, yet retains an incomplete death domain. *Immunity* 1997;7:813–820.

146. Walczak H, Miller RE, Ariail K, et al. Tumoricidal activity of tumor necrosis factor–related apoptosis-inducing ligand *in vivo*. *Nat Med* 1999;5:157–163.

147. Gores GJ, Kaufmann SH. Is TRAIL hepatotoxic? *Hepatology* 2001;34:3–6.

148. Ashkenazi A, Pai RC, Fong S, et al. Safety and antitumor activity of recombinant soluble Apo2 ligand. *J Clin Invest* 1999;104:155–162.

149. Jo M, Kim TH, Seol DW, et al. Apoptosis induced in normal human hepatocytes by tumor necrosis factor–related apoptosis-inducing ligand. *Nat Med* 2000;6:564–567.

150. Sheridan JP, Marsters SA, Pitti RM, et al. Control of TRAIL-induced apoptosis by a family of signaling and decoy receptors [see comments]. *Science* 1997;277:818–821.

151. Emery JG, McDonnell P, Burke MB, et al. Osteoprotegerin is a receptor for the cytotoxic ligand TRAIL. *J Biol Chem* 1998;273:14363–14367.

152. Wajant H, Moosmayer D, Wuest T, et al. Differential activation of TRAIL-R1 and -2 by soluble and membrane TRAIL allows selective surface antigen-directed activation of TRAIL-R2 by a soluble TRAIL derivative. *Oncogene* 2001;20:4101–4106.

153. Bodmer JL, Holler N, Reynard S, et al. TRAIL receptor-2 signals apoptosis through FADD and caspase-8. *Nat Cell Biol* 2000;2:241–243.

154. Sprick MR, Weigand MA, Rieser E, et al. FADD/MORT1 and caspase-8 are recruited to TRAIL receptors 1 and 2 and are essential for apoptosis mediated by TRAIL receptor 2. *Immunity* 2000;12:599–609.

155. Yeh WC, Pompa JL, McCurrach ME, et al. FADD: essential for embryo development and signaling from some, but not all, inducers of apoptosis. *Science* 1998;279:1954–1958.

156. Kuang AA, Diehl GE, Zhang J, et al. FADD is required for DR4- and DR5-mediated apoptosis: lack of trail-induced apoptosis in FADD deficient mouse embryonic fibroblasts. *J Biol Chem* 2000;275:25065–25068.

157. McAuliffe PF, Jarnagin WR, Johnson P, et al. Effective treatment of pancreatic tumors with two multimutated herpes simplex oncolytic viruses. *J Gastrointest Surg* 2000;4:580–588.

158. Miyazaki T, Reed JC. A GTP-binding adapter protein couples TRAIL receptors to apoptosis-inducing proteins. *Nat Immunol* 2001;2:493–500.

159. Li H, Zhu H, Xu CJ, et al. Cleavage of BID by caspase 8 mediates the mitochondrial damage in the Fas pathway of apoptosis. *Cell* 1998;94:491–501.

160. Luo X, Budihardjo I, Zou H, et al. Bid, a Bcl2 interacting protein, mediates cytochrome c release from mitochondria in response to activation of cell surface death receptors. *Cell* 1998;94:481–490.

161. Wu G, Chai J, Suber TL, et al. Structural basis of IAP recognition by Smac/DIABLO. *Nature* 2000;408:1008–1012.

162. Chai J, Du C, Wu JW, et al. Structural and biochemical basis of apoptotic activation by Smac/DIABLO. *Nature* 2000;406:855–862.

163. Muhlenbeck F, Schneider P, Bodmer JL, et al. The tumor necrosis factor–related apoptosis-inducing ligand receptors TRAIL-R1 and TRAIL-R2 have distinct cross-linking requirements for initiation of apoptosis and are non-redundant in JNK activation. *J Biol Chem* 2000;275:32208–32213.

164. Chicheportiche Y, Bourdon PR, Xu H, et al. TWEAK, a new secreted ligand in the tumor necrosis factor family that weakly induces apoptosis. *J Biol Chem* 1997;272:32401–32410.

165. Lynch CN, Wang YC, Lund JK, et al. TWEAK induces angiogenesis and proliferation of endothelial cells. *J Biol Chem* 1999;274:8455–8459.

166. Harada N, Nakayama M, Nakano H, et al. Pro-inflammatory effect of TWEAK/Fn14 interaction on human umbilical vein endothelial cells. *Biochem Biophys Res Commun* 2002;299:488–493.

167. Saas P, Boucraut J, Walker PR, et al. TWEAK stimulation of astrocytes and the proinflammatory consequences. *Glia* 2000;32:102–107.

168. Bodmer JL, Burns K, Schneider P, et al. TRAMP, a novel apoptosis-mediating receptor with sequence homology to tumor necrosis factor receptor 1 and Fas(Apo-1/CD95). *Immunity* 1997;6:79–88.

169. Kitson J, Raven T, Jiang YP, et al. A death-domain–containing receptor that mediates apoptosis. *Nature* 1996;384:372–375.

170. Chinnaiyan AM, O'Rourke K, Yu GL, et al. Signal transduction by DR3, a death domain–containing receptor related to TNFR-1 and CD95. *Science* 1996;274:990–992.

171. Marsters SA, Sheridan JP, Pitti RM, et al. Identification of a ligand for the death-domain–containing receptor Apo3. *Curr Biol* 1998;8:525–528.

172. Schneider P, Schwenzer R, Haas E, et al. TWEAK can induce cell death via endogenous TNF and TNF receptor 1. *Eur J Immunol* 1999;29:1785–1792.

173. Nakayama M, Ishidoh K, Kayagaki N, et al. Multiple pathways of TWEAK-induced cell death. *J Immunol* 2002;168:734–743.

174. Watts TH, DeBenedette MA. T cell co-stimulatory molecules other than CD28. *Curr Opin Immunol* 1999;11:286–293.

175. Borst J, Sluyser C, De VE, et al. Alternative molecular form of human T cell-specific antigen CD27 expressed upon T cell activation. *Eur J Immunol* 1989;19:357–364.

176. van Lier RA, Borst J, Vroom TM, et al. Tissue distribution and biochemical and functional properties of Tp55 (CD27), a novel T cell differentiation antigen. *J Immunol* 1987;139:1589–1596.

177. Goodwin RG, Alderson MR, Smith CA, et al. Molecular and biological characterization of a ligand for CD27 defines a new family of cytokines with homology to tumor necrosis factor. *Cell* 1993;73:447–456.

178. Lens SM, Tesselaar K, van Oers MH, et al. Control of lymphocyte function through CD27–CD70 interactions. *Semin Immunol* 1998;10:491–499.

179. Brown GR, Meek K, Nishioka Y, et al. CD27–CD27 ligand/CD70 interactions enhance alloantigen-induced proliferation and cytolytic activity in CD8+ T lymphocytes. *J Immunol* 1995;154:3686–3695.

180. Kobata T, Jacquot S, Kozlowski S, et al. CD27–CD70 interactions regulate B-cell activation by T cells. *Proc Natl Acad Sci U S A* 1995;92:11249–11253.

181. Akiba H, Nakano H, Nishinaka S, et al. CD27, a member of the tumor necrosis factor receptor superfamily, activates NF-kappaB and

stress-activated protein kinase/c-Jun N-terminal kinase via TRAF2, TRAF5, NF-kappaB–inducing kinase. *J Biol Chem* 1998;273:13353–13358.

182. Gravestein LA, Amsen D, Boes M, et al. The TNF receptor family member CD27 signals to Jun N-terminal kinase via Traf-2. *Eur J Immunol* 1998;28:2208–2216.

183. Rothe M, Pan MG, Henzel WJ, et al. The TNFR2–TRAF signaling complex contains two novel proteins related to baculoviral inhibitor of apoptosis proteins. *Cell* 1995;83:1243–1252.

184. Schwab U, Stein H, Gerdes J, et al. Production of a monoclonal antibody specific for Hodgkin and Sternberg–Reed cells of Hodgkin's disease and a subset of normal lymphoid cells. *Nature* 1982;299:65–67.

185. Ellis TM, Simms PE, Slivnick DJ, et al. CD30 is a signal-transducing molecule that defines a subset of human activated CD45RO+ T cells. *J Immunol* 1993;151:2380–2389.

186. Andreesen R, Osterholz J, Lohr GW, et al. A Hodgkin cell–specific antigen is expressed on a subset of auto- and alloactivated T (helper) lymphoblasts. *Blood* 1984;63:1299–1302.

187. Pizzolo G, Vinante F, Chilosi M, et al. Serum levels of soluble CD30 molecule (Ki-1 antigen) in Hodgkin's disease: relationship with disease activity and clinical stage. *Br J Haematol* 1990;75:282–284.

188. Caligaris-Cappio F, Bertero MT, Converso M, et al. Circulating levels of soluble CD30, a marker of cells producing Th2-type cytokines, are increased in patients with systemic lupus erythematosus and correlate with disease activity. *Clin Exp Rheumatol* 1995;13:339–343.

189. Durkop H, Latza U, Hummel M, et al. Molecular cloning and expression of a new member of the nerve growth factor receptor family that is characteristic for Hodgkin's disease. *Cell* 1992;68:421–427.

190. Opat S, Gaston JS. CD30:CD30 ligand interactions in the immune response. *Autoimmunity* 2000;33:45–60.

191. Horie R, Watanabe T. CD30: expression and function in health and disease. *Semin Immunol* 1998;10:457–470.

192. Agrawal B, Reddish M, Longenecker BM. CD30 expression on human CD8+ T cells isolated from peripheral blood lymphocytes of normal donors. *J Immunol* 1996;157:3229–3234.

193. Manetti R, Annunziato F, Biagiotti R, et al. CD30 expression by CD8+ T cells producing type 2 helper cytokines. Evidence for large numbers of CD8+CD30+ T cell clones in human immunodeficiency virus infection. *J Exp Med* 1994;180:2407–2411.

194. Pizzolo G, Vinante F, Morosato L, et al. High serum level of the soluble form of CD30 molecule in the early phase of HIV-1 infection as an independent predictor of progression to AIDS. *AIDS* 1994;8:741–745.

195. Chadburn A, Cesarman E, Jagirdar J, et al. CD30 (Ki-1) positive anaplastic large cell lymphomas in individuals infected with the human immunodeficiency virus. *Cancer* 1993;72:3078–3090.

196. Gilfillan MC, Noel PJ, Podack ER, et al. Expression of the costimulatory receptor CD30 is regulated by both CD28 and cytokines. *J Immunol* 1998;160:2180–2187.

197. Nakamura T, Lee RK, Nam SY, et al. Reciprocal regulation of CD30 expression on CD4+ T cells by IL-4 and IFN-gamma. *J Immunol* 1997;158:2090–2098.

198. Gerli R, Muscat C, Bistoni O, et al. High levels of the soluble form of CD30 molecule in rheumatoid arthritis (RA) are expression of CD30+ T cell involvement in the inflamed joints. *Clin Exp Immunol* 1995;102:547–550.

199. Giacomelli R, Cipriani P, Lattanzio R, et al. Circulating levels of soluble CD30 are increased in patients with systemic sclerosis (SSc) and correlate with serological and clinical features of the disease. *Clin Exp Immunol* 1997;108:42–46.

200. Pinto A, Aldinucci D, Gloghini A, et al. Human eosinophils express functional CD30 ligand and stimulate proliferation of a Hodgkin's disease cell line. *Blood* 1996;88:3299–3305.

201. Younes A, Consoli U, Zhao S, et al. CD30 ligand is expressed on resting normal and malignant human B lymphocytes. *Br J Haematol* 1996;93:569–571.

202. Kwon BS, Weissman SM. cDNA sequences of two inducible T-cell genes. *Proc Natl Acad Sci U S A* 1989;86:1963–1967.

203. Kwon BS, Moon CH, Kang S, et al. 4-1BB: still in the midst of darkness. *Mol Cells* 2000;10:119–126.

204. Vinay DS, Kwon BS. Role of 4-1BB in immune responses. *Semin Immunol* 1998;10:481–489.

205. Goodwin RG, Din WS, Davis-Smith T, et al. Molecular cloning of a ligand for the inducible T cell gene 4-1BB: a member of an emerging family of cytokines with homology to tumor necrosis factor. *Eur J Immunol* 1993;23:2631–2641.

206. DeBenedette MA, Shahinian A, Mak TW, et al. Costimulation of CD28⁻ T lymphocytes by 4-1BB ligand. *J Immunol* 1997;158:551–559.

207. Gruss HJ, Dower SK. Tumor necrosis factor ligand superfamily: involvement in the pathology of malignant lymphomas. *Blood* 1995;85:3378–3404.

208. Langstein J, Becke FM, Sollner L, et al. Comparative analysis of CD137 and LPS effects on monocyte activation, survival, proliferation. *Biochem Biophys Res Commun* 2000;273:117–122.

209. Weinberg AD, Vella AT, Croft M. OX-40: life beyond the effector T cell stage. *Semin Immunol* 1998;10:471–480.

210. Paterson DJ, Jefferies WA, Green JR, et al. Antigens of activated rat T lymphocytes including a molecule of 50,000 Mr detected only on CD4 positive T blasts. *Mol Immunol* 1987;24:1281–1290.

211. Mallett S, Fossum S, Barclay AN. Characterization of the MRC OX40 antigen of activated CD4 positive T lymphocytes—a molecule related to nerve growth factor receptor. *EMBO J* 1990;9:1063–1068.

212. Latza U, Durkop H, Schnittger S, et al. The human OX40 homolog: cDNA structure, expression and chromosomal assignment of the ACT35 antigen. *Eur J Immunol* 1994;24:677–683.

213. Baum PR, Gayle RB, Ramsdell F, et al. Molecular characterization of murine and human OX40/OX40 ligand systems: identification of a human OX40 ligand as the HTLV-1–regulated protein gp34. *EMBO J* 1994;13:3992–4001.

214. Gramaglia I, Weinberg AD, Lemon M, et al. Ox-40 ligand: a potent costimulatory molecule for sustaining primary CD4 T cell responses. *J Immunol* 1998;161:6510–6517.

215. Miura S, Ohtani K, Numata N, et al. Molecular cloning and characterization of a novel glycoprotein, gp34, that is specifically induced by the human T-cell leukemia virus type I transactivator p40tax. *Mol Cell Biol* 1991;11:1313–1325.

216. Stuber E, Neurath M, Calderhead D, et al. Cross-linking of OX40 ligand, a member of the TNF/NGF cytokine family, induces proliferation and differentiation in murine splenic B cells. *Immunity* 1995;2:507–521.

217. Ohshima Y, Tanaka Y, Tozawa H, et al. Expression and function of OX40 ligand on human dendritic cells. *J Immunol* 1997;159:3838–3848.

218. Moore PA, Belvedere O, Orr A, et al. BLyS: member of the tumor necrosis factor family and B lymphocyte stimulator. *Science* 1999;285:260–263.

219. Roth W, Wagenknecht B, Klumpp A, et al. APRIL, a new member of the tumor necrosis factor family, modulates death ligand–induced apoptosis. *Cell Death Differ* 2001;8:403–410.

220. Liu Y, Xu L, Opalka N, et al. Crystal structure of sTALL-1 reveals a virus-like assembly of TNF family ligands. *Cell* 2002;108:383–394.

221. Schneider P, Mackay F, Steiner V, et al. BAFF, a novel ligand of the tumor necrosis factor family, stimulates B cell growth. *J Exp Med* 1999;189:1747–1756.

222. Kanakaraj P, Migone TS, Nardelli B, et al. BLyS binds to B cells with high affinity and induces activation of the transcription factors NF-kappaB and ELF-1. *Cytokine* 2001;13:25–31.

223. Roschke V, Sosnovtseva S, Ward CD, et al. BLyS and APRIL form biologically active heterotrimers that are expressed in patients with systemic immune-based rheumatic diseases. *J Immunol* 2002;169:4314–4321.

224. Nardelli B, Belvedere O, Roschke V, et al. Synthesis and release of B-lymphocyte stimulator from myeloid cells. *Blood* 2001;97:198–204.

225. Hahne M, Kataoka T, Schroter M, et al. APRIL, a new ligand of the tumor necrosis factor family, stimulates tumor cell growth. *J Exp Med* 1998;188:1185–1190.

226. Kelly K, Manos E, Jensen G, et al. APRIL/TRDL-1, a tumor necrosis factor–like ligand, stimulates cell death. *Cancer Res* 2000;60:1021–1027.

227. Gross JA, Johnston J, Mudri S, et al. TACI and BCMA are receptors for a TNF homologue implicated in B-cell autoimmune disease. *Nature* 2000;404:995–999.

228. Thompson JS, Bixler SA, Qian F, et al. BAFF-R, a newly identified TNF receptor that specifically interacts with BAFF. *Science* 2001;293:2108–2111.

229. Hatzoglou A, Roussel J, Bourgeade MF, et al. TNF receptor family member BCMA (B cell maturation) associates with TNF receptor-associated factor (TRAF) 1, TRAF2, TRAF3 and activates NF-kappa B, elk-1, c-Jun N-terminal kinase, p38 mitogen-activated protein kinase. *J Immunol* 2000;165:1322–1330.

230. Shu HB, Johnson H. B cell maturation protein is a receptor for the tumor necrosis factor family member TALL-1. *Proc Natl Acad Sci U S A* 2000;97:9156–9161.

231. Do RK, Chen-Kiang S. Mechanism of BLyS action in B cell immunity. *Cytokine Growth Factor Rev* 2002;13:19–25.

232. Kere J, Srivastava AK, Montonen O, et al. X-linked anhidrotic (hypohidrotic) ectodermal dysplasia is caused by mutation in a novel transmembrane protein. *Nat Genet* 1996;13:409–416.

233. Headon DJ, Overbeek PA. Involvement of a novel TNF receptor homologue in hair follicle induction. *Nat Genet* 1999;22:370–374.

234. Monreal AW, Ferguson BW, Headon DJ, et al. Mutations in the human homologue of mouse dl cause autosomal recessive and dominant hypohidrotic ectodermal dysplasia. *Nat Genet* 1999;22:366–369.

235. Wisniewski SA, Kobielak A, Trzeciak WH, et al. Recent advances in understanding of the molecular basis of anhidrotic ectodermal dysplasia: discovery of a ligand, ectodysplasin A and its two receptors. *J Appl Genet* 2002;43:97–107.

236. Smahi A, Courtois G, Rabia SH, et al. The NF-kappaB signalling pathway in human diseases: from incontinentia pigmenti to ectodermal dysplasias and immune-deficiency syndromes. *Hum Mol Genet* 2002;11:2371–2375.

CHAPTER 25

Interleukin-1 Family of Ligands and Receptors

Charles A. Dinarello

Historical Background
The Interleukin-1 Ligand Superfamily
    Structures · Cells Producing Interleukin-1 Family Members · Transcriptional Regulation · Interleukin-1β Converting Enzyme · The P2X-7 Receptor and Secretion of Interleukin-1β and Interleukin-18 · Interleukin-1α as an Autocrine Growth Factor · Membrane Interleukin-1α · Autoantibodies to Interleukin-1α · Effects in Interleukin-1 Knockouts · Studies in Interleukin-1α–Deficient Mice · Differences between Interleukin-1α– and Interleukin-1β–Deficient Mice · Studies in Interleukin-1 Receptor Type I–Deficient Mice · Interleukin-1 Receptor Family · Interleukin-1 Receptor Type II · Gene and Surface Regulation of Interleukin-1 Receptor Type I · Interleukin-18 Binding Protein
Signal Transduction
    Associated or Intrinsic Kinases · Cytoplasmic Signaling Cascades · Characteristics of the Cytoplasmic Domain of the Interleukin-1 Receptor Type I · Recruitment of MyD88 and Interleukin-1 Receptor–Activating Kinases · Activation of Mitogen-Activated Protein Kinases after Interleukin-1 Receptor Binding · Human Abnormalities in Interleukin-1 Receptor Type I Expression
Blocking Interleukin-1 in Disease
    Blocking Interleukin-1 Receptor Type I in Disease · Effect of Interleukin-1 Soluble Receptor Type I in Humans
Interleukin-1 Receptor Antagonist
    Studies Using Interleukin-1 Receptor Antagonist in Animals and Humans · Interleukin-1 Receptor Antagonist (Anakinra) Treatment in Humans with Rheumatoid Arthritis
Conclusions
References

Unlike interleukin (IL)–2 and cytokines that affect primarily lymphocyte function and lymphocyte expansion, IL-1 and its related family members are primarily proinflammatory cytokines because of their ability to stimulate the expression of genes associated with inflammation and autoimmune diseases. The most salient and relevant properties of IL-1 in inflammation are the initiation of cyclooxygenase type 2 (COX-2), type 2 phospholipase A, and inducible nitric oxide synthase (iNOS). This accounts for the large amounts of prostaglandin E_2 (PGE_2), platelet-activating factor, and nitric oxide produced by cells exposed to IL-1 or in animals or humans injected with IL-1. Another important proinflammatory property of IL-1 is its ability to increase the expression of adhesion molecules such as intercellular adhesion molecule 1 on mesenchymal cells and vascular cell adhesion molecule 1 on endothelial cells. This latter property promotes the infiltration of inflammatory and *immunocompetent* cells into the extravascular space. IL-1 is also an angiogenic factor and plays a role in tumor metastasis and blood vessel supply. However, in addition to these and other proinflammatory properties, IL-1 is also an adjuvant during antibody production and acts on bone marrow stem cells for differentiation in the myeloid

series. Mice lacking IL-1 receptors fail to develop proliferative lesions of vascular smooth muscle cells in mechanically injured arteries. In humans with rheumatoid arthritis, the inflammatory and joint destructive nature of their disease is treated with systemic injections of the IL-1 receptor antagonist (IL-1Ra), a member of the IL-1 family that prevents IL-1 activity.

IL-1α, IL-1β, and IL-18 are unique in the cytokine families. Each is initially synthesized as precursor molecules without a signal peptide. After processing by the removal of N-terminal amino acids by specific proteases, the resulting peptides are called *mature* forms. The 31-kDa precursor form of IL-1β is biologically inactive and requires cleavage by specific intracellular cysteine protease called IL-1β converting enzyme (ICE). ICE is also termed caspase-1, the first member of a large family of intracellular cysteine proteases with important roles in programmed cell death. However, there is little evidence that ICE participates in programmed cell death (1). Rather, ICE seems to be used by the cell primarily to cleave the IL-1β and IL-18 precursors. As shown in Fig. 1, ICE cleaves both the IL-1β as well as the IL-18 precursors that immediately follow the aspartic acid in the P1

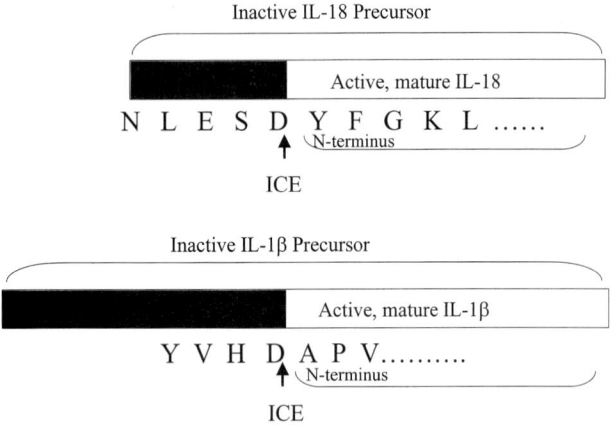

FIG. 1. Interleukin-1β converting enzyme (ICE, caspase-1) cleaves the IL-18 and IL-1β precursors at the aspartic acid in P1 position. (See text for discussion.)

position. As a result of cleavage, the mature form of IL-1β, a 17.5-kDa molecule, and that of IL-18, an 18-kDa peptide, are generated. Although ICE is responsible primarily for cleavage of the precursor intracellularly, other proteases such as proteinase-3 can process the IL-1β precursor extracellularly into an active cytokine (2).

In terms of the role of IL-1 in human disease, specific blockade of the IL-1 receptor type I (IL-1RI) (the ligand binding chain of the heterodimeric IL-1 receptor signaling complex) with the naturally occurring IL-1Ra in patients with rheumatoid arthritis has resulted in reduced disease activity and reduced joint destruction (3–5). To date, IL-1Ra has been approved for use in the United States, Canada, and Europe in the treatment of rheumatoid arthritis, and several thousand patients receive daily treatment; the results support the essential inflammatory and tissue remodeling functions of IL-1. However, IL-1 and IL-18 (a newly discovered member of the IL-1 family) are truly pleiotropic cytokines and affect the innate as well as the acquired immune systems.

Mice deficient in the IL-1RI, IL-1α, or IL-1β and those that are doubly deficient in IL-1α and IL-1β exhibit no phenotype different from the same-strain wild-type mice. A similar observation has been made with mice deficient in IL-18 or the IL-18 receptor. Thus, IL-1– and IL-18–deficient mice live in routine, microbially unprotected animal facilities. These observations show that these three agonist members of the IL-1 family, which play important roles in disease, are not essential for normal embryonic development, postnatal growth, homeostasis, reproduction, or resistance to routine microbial flora. These mice also do not exhibit evidence of spontaneous carcinogenesis, and their life span appears normal. Lymphoid organ architecture is also normal. Nevertheless, in the context of an inducible disease, a deficiency in any one of these three members of the IL-1 superfamily reveals a role in disease severity. In contrast, as described later, mice deficient in IL-1Ra do not exhibit normal reproduction, have stunted growth, and, in selected strains, develop spontaneous diseases

such as rheumatoid arthritis–like polyarthropathy and a fatal arteritis (6,7).

HISTORICAL BACKGROUND

The history of IL-1 begins with studies on the pathogenesis of fever. These were studies performed on the fever-producing properties of proteins released from rabbit peritoneal exudate cells by Menkin and Beeson in 1943 to 1948 and were followed by contributions of several investigators, who were interested primarily in the link between fever and infection/inflammation. In 1972, Waksman and Gery made an important contribution with the discovery that soluble factors augmented lymphocyte proliferation in response to antigenic or mitogenic stimuli. Kamschmidt also contributed to the "discovery phase" of IL-1 in describing macrophage products that induced the synthesis of acute phase proteins. The basis for the term *interleukin* was to streamline the growing number of biological properties attributed to soluble factors from macrophages and lymphocytes. IL-1 was the name given to the macrophage product, whereas IL-2 was used to define the lymphocyte product. At the time of the assignment of these names, there was no known amino acid sequence analysis, and the terms were used to define biological properties. In the field of rheumatoid arthritis, Krane and Dayer described IL-1 as an inducer of collagenases, and Saklatvala described IL-1 for its property to destroy cartilage. The large number of diverse multiple biological activities attributed to a single molecule engendered considerable skepticism in the scientific community, but with the cloning of IL-1 in 1984 (8,9), the use of recombinant IL-1 established that IL-1 was indeed a pleiotropic cytokine mediating inflammatory as well as immunological responses. With the use of targeted gene disruption, a more precise role for IL-1 in immune responses has been possible. For example, immunization with sheep red blood cells fails to elicit an antibody response in IL-1β–deficient mice, and hypersensitivity responses to antigens are suppressed in IL-1β–deficient mice.

THE INTERLEUKIN-1 LIGAND SUPERFAMILY

The intron–exon organization of the IL-1 genes suggests duplications of a common gene approximately 350 million years ago. Before this common IL-1 gene, there may have been another ancestral gene from which fibroblast growth factors (FGFs), such as acidic and basic FGF, also evolved, inasmuch as IL-1 and FGFs share significant amino acid homologies and, like IL-1, form an all–β-pleated sheet tertiary structure. To date, 10 individual members of the IL-1 gene *superfamily* have been described. Of these, four gene products have been thoroughly studied. The other six members have been shown to exist in various human tissues, but their role in health or disease is presently unknown. The four primary members of the IL-1 gene superfamily are IL-1α, IL-1β, IL-18, and IL-1Ra. IL-1α, IL-1β, and IL-18 are each agonists; IL-1Ra, on the other hand, is the specific receptor antagonist for

IL-1α and IL-1β but not for IL-18. When IL-1Ra occupies the IL-1 receptor, bona fide IL-1 cannot bind to the receptor, and there is no biological response to IL-1. The existence of a highly specific and naturally occurring receptor antagonist in cytokine biology appears to be unique to the IL-1 family. Recombinant IL-1Ra is approved in the United States and Europe for the treatment of patients with rheumatoid arthritis by reducing inflammation and joint destruction (3,4). As in the use of anti–tumor necrosis factor (TNF) α monoclonal antibodies or soluble TNF receptors, the beneficial effects of these anticytokine strategies is limited to amelioration of disease activity without affecting the dysfunctional autoimmune nature of rheumatoid arthritis.

Members of the IL-1 superfamily have been assigned a new nomenclature in which the expression IL-1F reflects their being part of a "family" of related ligands. Table 1 lists the current members of the IL-1 superfamily. In this chapter, the terms IL-1α, IL-1β, and IL-18, as well as IL-1Ra, are retained. Most members of the IL-1 superfamily are located on the long arm of chromosome 2. The intron–exon organization of the new members is also similar to that of the primary four members of the IL-1 superfamily. The six new members are closely related to IL-1β and IL-1Ra. From the intron–exon organization, some members represent gene duplications. In the case of IL-1F5, and possibly other newly described members, the duplication of the IL-1Ra gene has taken place (10). IL-1F7 and IL-1F9 are also closely related to IL-1Ra (11).

IL-1F5 shares 47% amino acid identity with IL-1Ra and is expressed in human monocytes activated by endotoxins. From the gene sequence, the predicted amino acid sequence of IL-1F5 does not have a leader peptide for secretion, which is in sharp contrast to the IL-1Ra (IL-1F3). IL-1F5 failed to exhibit agonist activity in studies of induction of IL-6 from fibroblasts, a well-described biological property of IL-1α and IL-1β (12). Furthermore, IL-1F5 did not block the IL-1α or IL-1β–induced IL-6 or IL-18–induced production of IFN-γ (12). Therefore, IL-1F5 possesses neither IL-1– or IL-18–like agonist activities nor the property to act as a receptor antagonist for IL-1, despite it close amino acid identity to IL-1Ra.

Although IL-1F7 (formerly IL-1ζ, IL-1H4, IL-1H, and IL-1RP1) is structurally related to IL-1Ra (36%), this IL-1 superfamily member binds to the IL-18 receptor α chain and therefore has attracted attention as being related to IL-18 (13). IL-1F7 has no leader peptide, and the recombinant form has been expressed with a N-terminal from a predicted ICE site (14). There are two forms of IL-1F7: a full-length peptide and a splice variant with an internal 40–amino acid deletion (13). The binding of IL-1F7 to the soluble IL-18R α chain has also been observed. However, in comparison with IL-18, recombinant IL-1F7 does not induce IFN-γ in whole human blood cultures, in peripheral blood mononuclear cells (PBMCs), or various cell lines. Therefore, it is unlikely that IL-1F7 is a true agonist for the IL-18 receptor. Whether IL-1F7 is a receptor antagonist for IL-18 remains to be determined.

IL-1F9 is constitutively expressed primarily in the placenta and the squamous epithelium of the esophagus. The three-dimensional folding of IL-1F9 is similar to that of IL-1Ra; therefore, IL-1F9 appears to be a possible IL-1Ra rather than an agonist. IL-1F10 shares 37% amino acid identity with the IL-1Ra and a similar three-dimensional structure (15). This cytokine is secreted from cells and is expressed in human skin, spleen, and tonsil cells. To date, recombinant IL-1F10 has been shown to bind to the isolated extracellular domains IL-1RI, but it is unclear whether IL-1F10 binds to complete cell surface–bound IL-1 receptors. Although these data suggest that IL-1F10 is likely to be a receptor antagonist, in comparison with IL-1Ra, its role in health and disease remains unclear.

In general, the functions of the newly described members of the IL-1 superfamily (IL-1F5-10) are currently unclear. It is unlikely that any possess proinflammatory properties, because recombinant forms have not revealed detectable effects in primary cells similar to those for IL-1α, IL-1β, or IL-18. Because most share significant amino acid identities with IL-1Ra, and because the intron–exon organization appears to reveal gene duplication of the IL-1Ra gene, these IL-1 superfamily members may be receptor antagonists. Whether these IL-1Ra–like homologs can block IL-18 is also currently unclear. Because deletion of only the IL-1Ra gene has resulted in a significant disease-producing phenotype in mice (see later discussion), the genes coding for the IL-1Ra homologs (IL-1F5-10) probably do not play a significant role in health. At present, the effect of deletion of IL-1F5 to Il-1F10 in mice is unknown.

Structures

The three-dimensional structure of the IL-1α is similar to those of IL-1β and IL-18 in that each cytokine forms an open-ended barrel composed of all β-pleated strands. Crystal structural analysis of the mature form of IL-1α is similar to that of IL-1β. IL-1α has two sites of binding to IL-1 receptor. There is a primary binding site located at the open top of its barrel, which is similar but not identical to that of IL-1β. IL-1Ra is structurally related to IL-1β rather than IL-1α. The unique structure of IL-1Ra that allows binding to the IL-1 receptor but without triggering signal transduction arises

TABLE 1. *Interleukin (IL)–1 superfamily members*

New name	Former name(s)	Property
IL-1F1	IL-1α	Agonist
IL-1F2	IL-1β	Agonist
IL-1F3	IL-1Ra	Antagonist
IL-1F4	IL-18; IFN-γ–inducing factor	Agonist
IL-1F5	IL-1Hy1, FIL1δ, IL-1H3, IL-1RP3, IL-1L1, IL-1δ	Unknown
IL-1F6	FIL-1ε, IL-1ε	Unknown
IL-1F7	FIL-1ζ, IL-1H4, IL-1RP1	Unknown
IL-1F8	FIL-1h, IL-1H2	Unknown
IL-1F9	IL-1H1, IL-1RP2	Unknown
IL-1F10	IL-1Hy2, FKSG75	Unknown

from the lack of a second binding site on the backside of the molecule (16). There are no data on the structure of IL-18 crystals. However, specific mutations in human IL-18 have revealed the importance of glutamic acid in position 35 and of lysine in position 89 for biological activity and binding to the IL-18 binding protein (17).

Cells Producing Interleukin-1 Family Members

The cells producing IL-1F5 to IL-1F10 were described previously. The primary sources of IL-1β are the blood monocyte, tissue macrophages, and dendritic cells. B-lymphocytes and natural killer cells are also sources. Keratinocytes produce IL-1β under inflammatory conditions, but there is no constitutive expression of IL-1β in these cells, in contrast to keratinocyte IL-1α. Fibroblasts and epithelial cells generally do not produce IL-1β. In health, the circulating human blood monocyte or bone marrow aspirate do not constitutively express IL-1β. However, there seems to be constitutive expression of IL-1β in the human hypothalamus (18). Nearly all microbial products induce IL-1β through the Toll-like receptor (TLR) family of receptors. TLR-4 is used by endotoxins to induce several cytokines, and the induction of IL-1β is particularly sensitive to low (1 to 10 pg/mL) concentrations of endotoxins. Depending on the stimulant, IL-1β messenger ribonucleic acid (mRNA) levels rise rapidly within 15 minutes but begin to decline after 4 hours. This decrease is likely caused by the synthesis of a transcriptional repressor or a decrease in mRNA half-life (19). However, using IL-1 itself as a stimulant of its own gene expression, IL-1β mRNA levels are sustained for more than 24 hours, in comparison with microbial stimulants. Raising intracellular cyclic adenosine monophosphate (cAMP) levels with histamine enhances IL-1α–induced IL-1β gene expression and protein synthesis (20). In human PBMCs, retinoic acid induces IL-1β gene expression, but the primary precursor transcripts fail to yield mature mRNA (21). Inhibition of translation by cycloheximide results in enhanced splicing of exons, excision of introns, and increased levels of mature mRNA (superinduction) by two orders of magnitude. Thus, synthesis of mature IL-1β mRNA requires an activation step to overcome an apparently intrinsic inhibition to process precursor mRNA.

Stimulants such as the complement component C5a, hypoxia, adherence to surfaces, or clotting of blood induce the synthesis of large amounts of IL-1β mRNA in monocytic cells without significant translation into the IL-1β protein (22). This dissociation between transcription and translation is characteristic of IL-1β but also of TNF-α. It appears that the aforementioned stimuli are not sufficient to provide a signal for translation despite a vigorous signal for transcription. Without translation, most of the IL-1β mRNA is degraded. Although the IL-1β mRNA assembles into large polyribosomes, there is little significant elongation of the peptide (23). However, adding bacterial endotoxin or IL-1 itself to cells with high levels of steady-state IL-1β mRNA results in augmented translation in somewhat the same manner as the removal of cycloheximide after superinduction. One explanation is that stabilization of the adenine/uracil-rich 3' untranslated region takes place in cells stimulated with lipopolysaccharide (LPS). These adenine/uracil-rich sequences are known to suppress normal hemoglobin synthesis. The stabilization of mRNA by microbial products may explain why low concentrations of LPS or a few bacteria or *Borrelia* organisms per cell induce the translation of large amounts of IL-1β (24).

Transcriptional Regulation

The promoter of IL-1α does not contain a clear TATA box, a typical motif of inducible genes. Inducible gene expression for IL-1α involves both a 4.2-kb upstream region and a proximal promoter region of 200 bp. A construct containing sequences −1,437 to +19 does not allow for stimulation of specific expression, but an additional 731 bp spanning exon I, intron I, and a segment of exon II controls a 20-fold increase in stimulation over background levels in murine macrophagic cells. Interestingly, with the same construct in human leukemic cells, only a twofold increase was observed. These additional 731 bp contain nuclear factor (NF) IL-6 and NFκB within intron I.

Unlike the promoter of IL-1α, the promoter region for IL-1β contains a clear TATA box. The half-life of IL-1β mRNA depends on the cell type and the conditions of stimulation. The most studied cells are freshly obtained human blood monocytes and macrophage cell lines derived from myelomonocytic leukemias. Endotoxin triggers transient transcription and steady-state levels of IL-1β mRNA, which accumulate for 4 hours, followed by a rapid fall caused by synthesis of a transcriptional repressor (25). Unlike most cytokine promoters, IL-1β regulatory regions can be found distributed over several thousand base pairs upstream and a few base pairs downstream from the transcriptional start site. The topic of IL-1β gene regulation has been reviewed in detail (26). The IL-1β promoter required for transcription has two independent enhancer regions (−2,782 to −2,729 and −2,896 to −2,846), which appear to act cooperatively. The latter contains a cAMP response element, whereas the former is a composite cAMP response element, NFIL-6, which is responsive to LPS. The 80-bp fragment (−2,782 to −2,729) is required for transcription and contains, in addition to a cAMP response element, an NFκB-like site. Activating protein 1 sites also participate in endotoxin-induced IL-1β gene expression.

Proximal promoter elements between −131 and +14 have also been identified, and sequences in this region contain the binding sites for the NFβA, which appears to be similar to NFβ1 and NFβ2. This proximal promoter is required for maximal IL-1β gene expression. Of importance is that the nucleotide binding sequences of NFβA were found to be identical to those of the transcription factor Spi-1/PU.1 (27), a well-established NF in cells that have myeloid and monocyte lineage. The requirement for Spi-1/PU.1 for IL-1β gene expression imparts tissue specificity, because not all cells constitutively express this NF. Human blood monocytes, which constitutively express Spi-1/PU.1, are exquisitely sensitive to gene expression of IL-1β by 1 to 10 pg/mL of LPS. Interestingly, the IL-1Ra promoter contains the proximal Spi-1/PU.1 site, which is also highly sensitive to LPS.

There is no constitutive gene expression for IL-1β in freshly obtained human PBMCs from healthy donors after more than 40 cycles of polymerase chain reaction (28); however, the same PBMCs express constitutive mRNA for IL-18. Constitutive expression was also observed in Western blot analysis for precursor IL-18 in lysates from the same PBMCs. However, there was no pro–IL-1β in the same cells. Constitutive IL-18 gene expression and the presence of precursor IL-18 protein were also observed in freshly obtained murine splenocytes (29). In these splenocytes, there was no constitutive expression of the IL-1β gene or protein. The promoter regions for IL-1β and IL-18 gene expression have been studied and may provide an insight into these observations. The promoter for IL-18 does not contain TATA, and IL-18 promoter activity upstream of exon 2 acts constitutively (30). The additional finding that the 3′ untranslated region of human IL-18 lacks the AUUUA destabilization sequence is also consistent with these observations. This would allow for more sustained levels of the polyadenylated species and translation into protein. Other than to distinguish differences between IL-1β and IL-18 in the same cells, the clinical significance of constitutive gene and protein expression for IL-18 in mononuclear cells remains unclear, but it certainly would focus on regulation's being at the level of processing the precursor and secretion of the mature form or forms. Osteoclasts also produce IL-18 (31), and regulation of bone density may be a property of IL-18, as it is for IL-1β.

IL-1α is also synthesized as a precursor molecule without a signal peptide; unlike IL-1β, the IL-1α precursor is biologically active. Processing of the IL-1α precursor yields a mature molecule of 17.5 kDa. Calpain, a calcium-activated cysteine protease associated with the plasma membrane, is responsible for cleavage of the IL-1α precursor into a mature molecule. It is unclear whether this process of calpain cleavage of the IL-1α is functional under physiological conditions, because IL-1α is rarely measured in the circulation. Even under conditions of cell stimulation, human blood monocytes do not process or readily secrete mature IL-1α. The 31-kDa IL-1α precursor is synthesized in association with cytoskeletal structures (microtubules), unlike most proteins, which are translated in the endoplasmic reticulum. It is unknown whether the IL-1α precursor is active intracellularly, and there is no appreciable accumulation of IL-1α in any specific organelle. Immunohistochemical studies of IL-1α in endotoxin-stimulated human blood monocytes revealed a diffuse staining pattern; in comparison, in the same cell, IL-1Ra, which has a signal peptide, is localized to the Golgi complex (32). In contrast to IL-1β, IL-1α is not commonly found in the circulation or in body fluids except during severe disease, in which case the cytokine may be released from dying cells.

IL-18 is also initially synthesized as an inactive precursor (24,000 kDa) and requires ICE cleavage for processing into a mature molecule of 18,000 kDa. ICE-deficient mice have been helpful in revealing non–ICE-mediated pathways of IL-18 processing. Following endotoxin, ICE-deficient mice do not exhibit circulating IFN-γ, because endotoxin-induced IFN-γ is IL-18 dependent (33). IL-12–induced IFN-γ is also ICE dependent (34), which again suggests that microbial toxins (through TLRs) require IL-18 for IFN-γ production. In general, processing of the IL-18 precursor is ICE dependent, but exceptions exist. Fas ligand stimulation results in release of biologically active IL-18 in ICE-deficient murine macrophages (35). As in IL-1β processing, proteinase-3 appears to activate processing to mature IL-18. In contrast to the agonists IL-1α, IL-1β, and IL-18, IL-1Ra has two prominent forms as a result of alternative mRNA splicing events. The IL-1Ra gene codes for a form with a strong signal peptide, but this signal peptide can be deleted, and the resulting ligand lacking a signal peptide remains intracellularly.

Although the blood monocyte and tissue macrophages are the primary sources of IL-1β, these cells in health do not constitutively express IL-1β. Expression of IL-1β mRNA in blood monocytes in health is caused by the activation of the IL-1β transcriptional process by surface contact (22). However, several malignant tumors express IL-1β as part of their neoplastic nature, particularly acute myelogenous leukemia, multiple myeloma, and juvenile myelogenous leukemia, each of which exhibits constitutive expression of IL-1β.

Interleukin-1β Converting Enzyme

ICE (caspase-1) is constitutively expressed in various cells as a primary transcript of 45 kDa (inactive precursor) requiring two internal cleavages before becoming the enzymatically active heterodimer composed of a 10-kDa chain and a 20-kDa chain. The active site cysteine is located on the 20-kDa chain. ICE itself contributes to autoprocessing of the ICE precursor by undergoing oligomerization with itself or homologs of ICE. In the presence of specific inhibitors of ICE, the generation and secretion of mature IL-1β is reduced and precursor IL-1β accumulates mostly inside the cell, but the precursor is also found outside the cell. This latter finding supports the concept that precursor IL-1β can be released from a cell independently of processing by ICE. Because of alternate RNA splicing, there are five isoforms of human ICE (ICE α, ICE β, ICE γ, ICE δ, and ICE ε); ICEα cleaves the ICE precursor and the IL-1β precursor. It is presumed that ICEβ and ICEγ also process precursor ICE. ICEε is a truncated form of ICE, which may inhibit ICE activity by binding to the p20 chain of ICE to form an inactive ICE complex.

In addition to ICE, the IL-1β precursor is cleaved by elastase, chymotrypsin, a mast cell chymase, proteinase-3, granzyme A, and a variety of proteases commonly found in inflammatory fluids. Some matrix metalloproteases (MMPs) commonly found in joint fluids from patients with rheumatoid arthritis also cleave the precursor of IL-1β into biologically active IL-1β. These MMPs include gelatinase-B, MMP-2, MMP-3 (stromelysin-1), and MMP-9. These alternative extracellular proteases may account for the observation that mice deficient in ICE can exhibit a full inflammatory response to subcutaneous turpentine, an IL-1β–dependent mode. As discussed later, the secretion of mature IL-1β is facilitated by a fall in the intracellular levels of potassium, which takes place when a cell is exposed to high levels of adenosine triphosphate (ATP) (36). The effect of ATP or nigericin, a potassium channel agonist, is caused by a net decrease in the intracellular levels of potassium. Increasing the extracellular level of potassium also results in the inhibition of caspases by preventing the formation of a large intracellular complex associated with activation of caspases (37).

The P2X-7 Receptor and Secretion of Interleukin-1β and Interleukin-18

The presence of millimolar concentrations of ATP results in the release of mature IL-1β from LPS-stimulated monocytes within minutes; a receptor-mediated event has been proposed as the reason. For ATP, this receptor is called a purinergic receptor (because adenosine is a purine). The purinergic receptor found on monocytes and macrophages is designated P2X-7. When triggered by millimolar concentrations of ATP, reversible pores form in the plasma membrane and, because of ion fluxes, the electrical potential of the membrane is transiently lost. In monocytes stimulated by LPS, this activation by ATP triggers the release of mature IL-1β (38). A monoclonal antibody to the P2X-7 receptor prevents the release of mature IL-1β from activated macrophages (39). Of importance is that the secretion of IL-1β through activation of the P2X-7 receptor by ATP is independent of ICE. For example, highly specific inhibitors of ICE prevent processing of the IL-1β precursor, and hence there is a build-up of the precursor intracellularly; however, the release of the IL-1β precursor or the release of lactic dehydrogenase takes place in cells stimulated with ATP (40). Triggering of the P2X-7 receptor is specific for the release of mature IL-1β and also IL-18 but does not result in the release of TNF-α. The effect of ATP or nigericin to stimulate the release of IL-1 and IL-18 is also observed in LPS-stimulated whole blood cultures (41). Convincing evidence for a role of the P2X-7 receptor in the secretion of IL-1β is found in mice deficient in this receptor. Like wild-type macrophages, P2X-7 receptor–deficient macrophages synthesize PGE$_2$ and the IL-1β precursor in response to LPS. However, when activated by ATP, P2X-7 receptor–deficient macrophages do not release IL-1β (42). *In vivo*, wild-type and P2X-7 receptor–deficient mice release the same amounts of IL-6 into the peritoneal cavity, but there is no release of mature IL-1β in P2X-7 receptor–deficient mice.

Interleukin-1α as an Autocrine Growth Factor

The concept that IL-1α acts as an autocrine growth factor takes into account three distinct observations: First, after synthesis, the IL-1α precursor remains inside the cell, where it has been shown to bind to the nucleus; second, the intracellular IL-1α precursor forms a complex with an intracellular pool of the IL-1RI; and third, either precursor IL-1α or mature IL-1α, when bound to surface IL-1RI, is internalized with subsequent translocation to the nucleus (similar to steroid receptors). Each mechanism has supporting experimental data. Some investigators have proposed that the intracellular IL-1α precursor regulates normal cellular differentiation, particularly in epithelial and ectodermal cells. This proposal is based on the finding that in keratinocytes, constitutive production of large amounts of precursor IL-1α is present in healthy human skin. The large amounts of precursor IL-1α in normal skin keratinocytes are thought to affect terminal differentiation. In support of the concept that precursor IL-1α functions as an intracellular messenger in certain cells, an antisense oligonucleotide to IL-1α reduces senescence in endothelial cells (43,44). In a murine T helper type 2 (Th2) cell line, IL-1α was proposed as an essential autocrine and paracrine growth factor through the use of an antisense IL-1α oligonucleotide or anti–IL-1α antibodies. Thymic epithelium also produces IL-1α constitutively, and a requirement for IL-1α has been demonstrated to regulate the expression of CD25 (IL-2 receptor α chain) and maturation of thymocytes. However, the concept that IL-1α acts as an autocrine growth factor for epithelial cells must be interpreted with the findings in mice deficient for IL-1α; in these mice, there are no demonstrable defects in growth and development, including processes involving the skin, fur, epithelium and gastrointestinal function (45). If there is a role for intracellular precursor IL-1α in normal cell function, this should be carefully regulated. One explanation for regulating the effect, if any, of IL-1α is the presence of large amounts of the intracellular form of the IL-1Ra (icIL-1Ra) (46). This form of the IL-1Ra also binds to the IL-1RI and prevents signal transduction. In fact, the icIL-1Ra is produced in the same cells expressing precursor IL-1α and is thought to compete with the intracellular pool of precursor IL-1α for nuclear binding sites. However, normal epithelial functions in the IL-1α–deficient mouse as well as in the IL-1Ra–deficient mouse do not support the concept that there is a natural role for IL-1α in epithelial growth and differentiation.

Membrane Interleukin-1α

Precursor IL-1α can be found on the surface of several cells, particularly on monocytes and B lymphocytes, where it is referred to as membrane IL-1α (47). Membrane IL-1α is biologically active; its biological activities are neutralized by anti–IL-1α but not by anti–IL-1β. Membrane IL-1α appears to be anchored to the cell membrane by a lectin interaction involving mannose residues. A mannose-like receptor appears to bind membrane IL-1α (48). The role of membrane IL-1α in disease remains unclear. *In vitro,* the amount of IL-1Ra needed to block membrane IL-1α was 10- to 50-fold greater than the amount required to block mature IL-1β (49).

Autoantibodies to Interleukin-1α

Neutralizing autoantibodies directed against IL-1α may function as natural buffers for IL-1α. Autoantibodies to IL-1α have been detected in healthy subjects as well as in patients with various autoimmune diseases. Autoantibodies to IL-1α are neutralizing immunoglobulin G (IgG) antibodies that bind natural precursor form of IL-1α as well as 17-kDa recombinant IL-1α (50). The incidence of these antibodies is increased in patients with autoimmune diseases. For example, in 318 patients with chronic arthritis, anti–IL-1α (but not anti–IL-1β or anti–TNF-α) IgG antibodies were detected in 18.9% of arthritis patients but in 9% of healthy subjects. Anti–IL-1α antibodies were present more commonly and at a higher level in patients with nondestructive arthritis. An inverse correlation has been observed between the levels of anti–IL-1α antibodies and the clinical disease activity.

Effects in Interleukin-1 Knockouts

The IL-1β–deficient mouse is without abnormal findings after 6 years of continuous breeding. However, upon challenge, IL-1β–deficient mice exhibit specific differences from their wild-type controls. The most dramatic is the response to local inflammation followed by a subcutaneous injection of turpentine (50 to 100 μL). Within the first 24 hours, IL-1β–deficient mice injected with turpentine do not manifest an acute-phase response, do not develop anorexia, and have no circulating IL-6 and no fever (51,52). These findings are consistent with those reported in the same model in which anti–IL-1RI antibodies were used in wild-type mice (51). IL-1β–deficient mice also have reduced inflammation after zymosan-induced peritonitis (53). Additional studies have also found that IL-1β–deficient mice have elevated febrile responses to IL-1β and IL-1α (54).

In contrast, IL-1β–deficient mice have nearly the same responses to LPS as do wild-type mice (55) with one notable exception: IL-1β–deficient mice injected with LPS have little or no expression of leptin mRNA or protein (56). In IL-1β pregnant mice, there is a normal response to LPS-induced premature delivery; however, in these mice, there are decreased numbers of uterine cytokines after LPS challenge (57). The reduction in LPS-induced cytokines is not found in nonpregnant IL-1β–deficient mice, which suggests that the combination of the hormonal changes in pregnancy and the state of IL-1β deficiency act together to reduce the responsiveness to LPS. The mechanism for the reduced cytokine production in pregnant IL-1β–deficient mice appears to be related to a reduction in the constitutive level of the p65 component of NFκB.

No differences were noted in plasma elevations of glucocorticoid steroids between IL-1β–deficient and wild-type mice after systemic injection of LPS, which indicates that IL-1β is not required for activation of the hypothalamic-pituitary-adrenal axis during endotoxemia. The overall data demonstrate that in the mouse, IL-1β is critical for the induction of fever and acute-phase changes caused by local inflammation induced by zymosan or turpentine. Another characterization of IL-1β deficiency is body temperature, activity, and feeding during live influenza virus infection. Body temperature and activity were lower in IL-1β–deficient mice (58). The anorexic effects of influenza infection were similar in both groups of mice. The mice deficient in IL-1β exhibited a higher rate of mortality from influenza infection than did the wild-type mice.

Studies in Interleukin-1α–Deficient Mice

Mice deficient in IL-1α are born healthy and develop normally. After subcutaneous injection of turpentine, which induces a local inflammatory response, wild-type and IL-1α–deficient mice develop fever and acute-phase proteins, whereas IL-1β–deficient mice do not (45). In addition, although the induction of glucocorticoids after turpentine injection was suppressed in IL-1β mice, this suppression was not observed in IL-1α–deficient mice. However, expression of IL-1β mRNA in the brain decreased 1.5-fold in IL-1α–deficient mice, whereas expression of IL-1α mRNA decreased more than 30-fold in IL-1β–deficient mice. These data suggest that IL-1β exerts greater control over production of IL-1α than does IL-1α over the production of IL-1β. In ICE-deficient mice, IL-1α production is also reduced (59), which suggests that production of IL-1α is under the control of IL-1β.

Differences between Interleukin-1α– and Interleukin-1β–Deficient Mice

Findings of studies on the effects of selective deficiency in IL-1β in mice are summarized in Table 2. Some of these findings are different from those of the same models in mice deficient in IL-1α. For example, mice deficient in IL-1α develop a normal immune response to immunization with sheep red blood cells, whereas mice deficient in IL-1β do not produce anti–sheep red blood cell antibodies, a T-dependent response (60). However, antibody production by T cell–independent antigens was normal in mice deficient in both IL-1α and IL-1, as was the proliferative response to anti-CD3. In mice deficient in IL-1Ra, there was an enhanced response (60). Also, mice deficient in IL-1α have a brisk inflammatory response to turpentine-induced inflammation, whereas IL-1β–deficient mice have nearly no response.

Studies in Interleukin-1 Receptor Type I–Deficient Mice

As stated previously, mice deficient in IL-1RI develop normally and exhibit no particular phenotype despite being housed in standard animal facilities (61). IL-1RI–deficient mice show no abnormal phenotype in health and exhibit normal homeostasis, similar to findings observed in IL-1β– or IL-1α–deficient mice (45,51) but distinctly different from mice deficient in IL-1Ra (62). They do, however,

TABLE 2. *Effects in interleukin (IL)–1β–deficient mice*

Disease model	Effect	Reference
Endotoxin fever	No effect	(55)
LPS-induced leptin	↓ Circulating leptin	(56)
Zymosan peritonitis	↓ Inflammation	
	↓ Mortality	
	↓ IL-6 and chemokines	(53)
Turpentine inflammation	↓ Inflammation	
	↓ Fever	
	↓ IL-6; ↓ SAA; ↓ cortisone	(51)
	↓ COX-2	(45)
IL-1α–induced fever	↑ Fever	
	↑ Cytokines	(54)
Hepatic melanoma	↓ Metastasis	(190)
Brain ischemia	↓ Neuronal death	(191)
Immune myasthenia gravis	Resistance to disease development	(192)
Fas-expressing tumors	↓ Neutrophil infiltration	(193)
LPS-induced shock lung	No effect on neutrophil infiltration	(194)
LPS-induced coagulopathy	Plasminogen activator inhibitor unchanged	(195)
Turpentine coagulopathy	↓ Plasminogen activator inhibitor	(195)
Contact hypersensitivity	↓ Delayed hypersensitivity	(69)
Contact hypersensitivity	↓ Langerhans cell activation	(196)
Steady-state p65 (NFκB)	↓ Levels and translocation	(57)

COX-2, cyclooxygenase-2; IL-6, interleukin-6; LPS, lipopolysaccharide; SAA, serum amyloid A.

exhibit reduced responses to challenge with inflammatory agents. When given a turpentine abscess, for example, IL-1RI–deficient mice exhibited an attenuated inflammatory response in comparison with wild-type mice (63). IL-1RI–deficient mice also had reduced delayed-type hypersensitivity responses. Like wild-type mice treated with anti–IL-1 antibodies or IL-1Ra, IL-1RI–deficient mice were susceptible to infection with *Listeria monocytogenes*. Lymphocytes from IL-1RI–deficient mice with major cutaneous leishmanial infection produced more IL-4 and IL-10, but less IFN-γ, than did those from wild-type mice.

Mice deficient in IL-1RI do not exhibit significant disruption of reproduction aside from a somewhat reduced litter size (64); in some laboratories, however, the body weights of the IL-1RI–deficient mice were 30% less than those of wild-type mice, whereas the TNF receptor p55–deficient mice weighed 30% more than wild-type mice of equivalent age (65). Although IL-1α is constitutively expressed in the skin, the barrier function of skin remains intact in mice deficient in IL-1RI (66). Similarly, mice deficient in IL-1 accessory protein receptor (IL-1R-AcP) appear normal but have no responses to IL-1 *in vivo* (67). However, cells deficient in IL-1R-AcP have normal binding of IL-1α and IL-1Ra (binding to the IL-1RI is intact in these mice) but a 70% reduction in binding of IL-1β (67). In these cells, there is no biological response to IL-1α despite binding of IL-1α to the type I receptor. The results suggest that IL-1R-AcP and not IL-1RI is required for IL-1β binding and biological response to IL-1.

Mice injected with LPS have been studied. IL-1RI–deficient mice exhibit the same decrease in hepatic lipase as do wild-type mice. However, injection of LPS directly into the eye of mice deficient in IL-1RI reveals a decrease in the number of infiltrating leukocytes, whereas there was no decrease in mice deficient in both TNF receptors (68). Not unexpectedly, IL-1RI–deficient mice failed to respond to IL-1 in a variety of assays, including IL-1–induced IL-6 and E-selectin expression and IL-1–induced fever. Like IL-1β–deficient mice, IL-1RI–deficient mice had a reduced acute-phase response to turpentine. Also like IL-1β–deficient mice (69), IL-1RI–deficient mice had a reduced delayed-type hypersensitivity response and were highly susceptible to infection by *Listeria monocytogenes*.

Mice deficient in IL-1RI did not develop trabecular bone loss after ovariectomy, in comparison with wild-type controls (70). Although mice deficient in both the TNF receptor types I and II develop experimental autoimmune encephalomyelitis (EAE) after immunization with central nervous system antigens, mice deficient in IL-1RI failed to develop inflammatory lesions in the central nervous system or evidence of clinical EAE. Although cells from IL-1R-AcP–deficient mice bound IL-1α, there was no activation of genes dependent on NFκB or activator protein-1 (67). In general, mice deficient in IL-1RI exhibit reduced disease severity, as do wild-type mice injected with pharmacological doses of IL-1Ra.

Interleukin-1 Receptor Family

The IL-1 receptor family now encodes nine distinct genes, of which some remain orphan receptors. As shown in Table 3, these receptors have been assigned a nomenclature in the order of their discovery. The IL-18 binding protein (IL-18BP) is not listed, because of its lack of being fixed to the cell through a transmembrane domain; however, the IL-18BP probably represents the former cell-bound decoy receptor for IL-18, similar to the decoy receptor for IL-1 [the IL-1 receptor type II (IL-1RII); see later discussion]. In fact, there is limited

TABLE 3. *Nomenclature of interleukin (IL)–1R family*

Name	New designation	Ligand
IL-1RI	IL-1R1	IL-1α, IL-1β, IL-1Ra
IL-1RII	IL-1R2	IL-1β, IL-1α, IL-1Ra
IL-1R Ac-P	IL-1R3	IL-1α, IL-1β
ST2/Fit-1	IL-1R4	Unknown
IL-18Rα/IL-1Rrp1	IL-1R5	IL-18
IL-1Rrp2	IL-1R6	IL-1ε, IL-1δ
IL-1R18β/IL-1RAcPL	IL-1R7	IL-18
IL-1RAPL	IL-1R8	Unknown
IL-R9	IL-1R9	Unknown

but significant amino acid homology between the IL-18BP and IL-1RII, particularly in the third domain (71). IL-1R1, IL-1R2, and IL-1R3 are the bona fide receptors for IL-1. IL-1R4 (also known as ST2 and Fit) remains an orphan receptor, although proteins that bind to this receptor have been reported (72). Despite a lack of a specific ligand for this receptor, a number of studies have examined the distribution and gene regulation of this receptor in mast cells (73). IL-1R5 was formerly an orphan receptor termed IL-1R related protein 1 (74) but was subsequently discovered to be the ligand-binding chain of the IL-18 receptor (75), now termed IL-18Rα chain. For the purposes of this chapter, the terms IL-1RI, IL-1RII, IL-1R-AcP, IL-18Rα, and IL-18Rβ are used, rather than the new nomenclature. However, the new nomenclature for the members of the family that remain orphan receptors is used.

The IL-1R–related protein 2 (IL-1R6) has been proposed to be the receptor for a novel member of the IL-1 family, IL-1F (76). The activity of this ligand for the IL-1R6 was demonstrated in a luciferase NFκB assay; another member of the IL-1 family, IL-1Fδ, appears to be its natural receptor antagonist for IL-1F binding to IL-1R6 (76). The IL-1R7, formerly the non–ligand-binding chain of the IL-18 receptor termed IL-1R AcPL (77), is now known as the IL-18Rβ chain. Like the IL-1R-AcP, the IL-18Rβ is essential for IL-18 signal transduction (77,78).

Two members of the IL-1 receptor family are particularly unique in that they are found on the X chromosome. These are IL-1R8 and IL-1R9, both of which are homologous to the IL-1 accessory protein receptor chains (IL-1R-AcP and IL-1R-AcPL). IL-1R9 (79) is highly homologous to IL-1R8 (80). Both forms have no known ligands and recerptor are found in the fetal brain. In fact, nonoverlapping deletions and a nonsense mutation in the IL-1R8 gene were found in patients with cognitive impairment (80), in which expression in the adult hippocampal area may play a role in memory or learning. The cytoplasmic domains of IL-1R8 and IL-1R9 are longer than the other accessory chains. The IL-1R9 may function as a negative receptor. This was shown in cells overexpressing this receptor as well as the IL-1RI and IL-1R-AcP in which IL-1β signaling was blocked with a specific antibody to the IL-1R-AcP. In the presence of the antibody,

IL-1β–induced luciferase was suppressed, which suggests that a possible complex of the type I receptor with IL-1β plus IL-1R9 results in a negative signal (79).

Interleukin-1 Receptor Type I

The first studies on the specific receptor for IL-1α and IL-1β were based on the identification of an 80-kDa glycoprotein on T cells and fibroblasts, which is now known as the IL-1RI (81–84). The molecular cloning of IL-1RI was first made in the mouse in 1988 (85) and then subsequently in the human (86). The extracellular segment of the IL-1RI and nearly all members of the IL-1 receptor family have three immunoglobulin-like domains. However, the cytoplasmic segment of the IL-1RI is unique in that it contains the Toll homology domain. This domain contains amino acids closely related to those of a gene found in *Drosophila* (87); the *Drosophila* gene is essential for the embryonic development of the fruit fly. The Toll homology domain is also found in the cytoplasmic domains of each member of the TLR, which transduce the signals of endotoxins, peptidoglycans, teichoic acids, and other microbial products in mammalian cells (88). In mammalian cells, the Toll homology domain of the IL-1R is necessary for signal transduction (89). For several years after the molecular cloning of the IL-1RI, IL-1 signal transduction was thought to occur when IL-1 bound to the single-chain IL-1RI. However, in 1995, Greenfeder et al. (90) discovered that IL-1 signal transduction was initiated by the formation of a heterodimer, in which a second receptor chain binds to the IL-1RI/IL-1 complex; this second chain is now known as IL-1R-AcP. There is considerable amino acid homology between the IL-1RI and IL-1R-AcP in the extracellular and cytoplasmic domains, including the Toll homology domain. Of importance is that IL-1R-AcP does not bind IL-1 itself but rather "wraps around" the complex of IL-1/IL-1RI (91). As shown by x-ray crystallization studies, IL-1RI exhibits a conformational change when binding IL-1β, and this shape change apparently allows the IL-1R-AcP to form the heterodimer.

The formation of the heterodimer of the IL-1RI with the IL-1R-AcP results in the physical approximation of the Toll homology domains of each chain in the cytoplasmic segments and initiates signal transduction (Fig. 2). A similar event of approximately Toll homology domains takes place when IL-18 binds to its receptor, the IL-18Rα chain (75), and recruits the IL-18Rβ chain (77) (see Fig. 3). The extracellular and cytoplasmic domains of the IL-1RI share homology with IL-18Rα chain (75), which was previously an orphan receptor in the IL-1R family (74). As with IL-1, IL-18 binding to the IL-18Rα chain recruits a second, non–ligand-binding chain (IL-18Rβ) (77). Thus, IL-1 and IL-18 signal transduction are initiated by similar if not identical physical approximation of the Toll homology domains, which initiates signal transduction for both cytokines. In both cases, the second chain, although not capable of binding the respective ligand, is essential for activity (77,78).

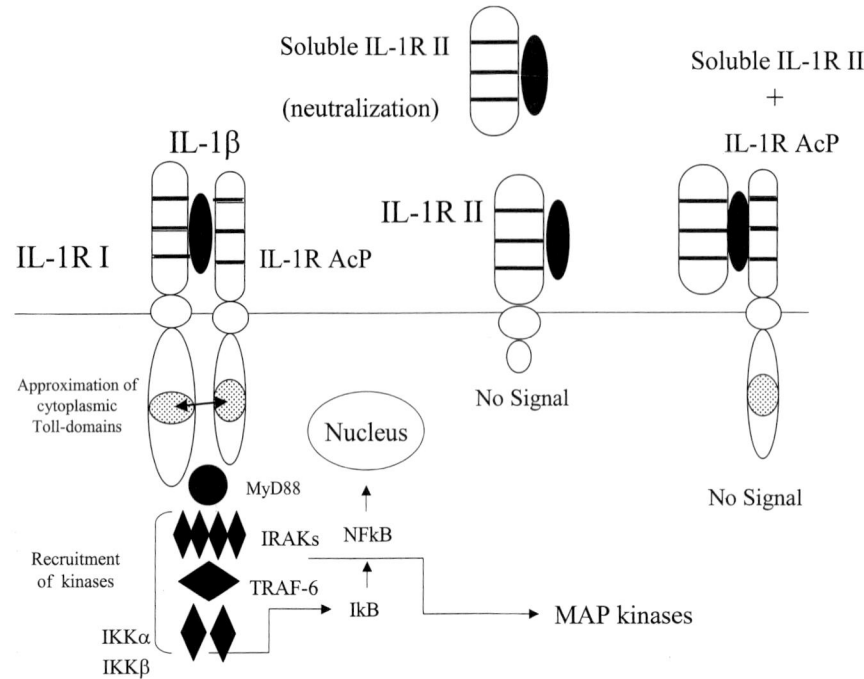

FIG. 2. Interleukin-1 signal transduction. (See text for discussion.)

Glycosylation of IL-1RI appears to be necessary for optimal activity. In fact, removing the glycosylation sites reduces the binding of IL-1. In general, IL-1 responsiveness is a more accurate assessment of receptor expression than is ligand binding (92). The failure to show specific and saturable IL-1 binding to cells is often a result of the low numbers of surface IL-1RI on primary cells. In cell lines, the number of IL-1RI can reach 5,000 per cell, but primary cells usually express fewer than 200 receptors per cell. In some primary cells, there are fewer than 50 per cell (93), and IL-1 signal transduction has been observed in cells expressing fewer than 10 type I receptors per cell (94).

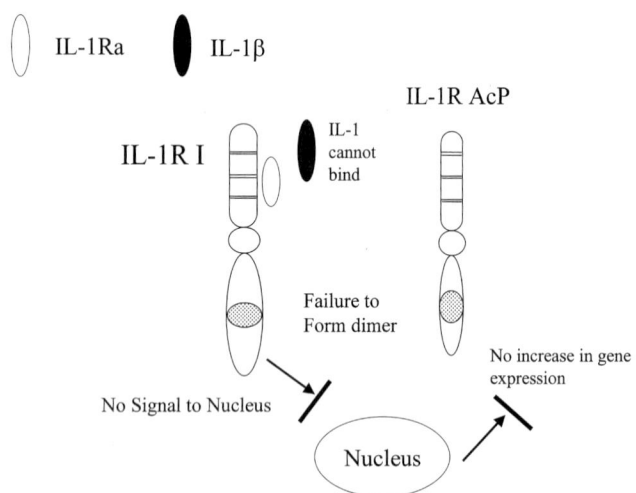

FIG. 3. Interleukin-18 signal transduction. (See text for discussion.)

Both chains of the IL-1 as well as IL-18 receptors are needed for signal transduction (see Fig. 3). For IL-1, this has been shown through the use of specific neutralizing antibodies to IL-1RI or IL-1R-AcP (95), and for IL-18, transfection of the IL-18Rβ chain provides responsiveness (77,78). The cytoplasmic segment of IL-1RI or IL-1R-AcP has no apparent intrinsic tyrosine kinase activity, but when IL-1 binds to only a few receptors, the remaining unoccupied receptors appear to undergo phosphorylation (96). However, the Toll homology domain is essential for biological activity of IL-1 (89,97). The TLRs have distinct extracellular domains that recognize microbial products such as endotoxins and peptidoglycans. In contrast, the intracellular domains of the TLR share significant sequences with the intracellular domains of IL-1RI and IL-1R-AcP. There are currently nine known TLRs. Therefore, it is not surprising that cellular responses to microbial products and to IL-1 are similar. For example, the portfolio of genes induced by endotoxins and that of genes induced by IL-1 are nearly the same.

Differences exist in the binding affinity, association and dissociation rates of the mature forms of each member of the IL-1 family and the cell-bound IL-1RI and soluble (extracellular domains) IL-1RI receptors (IL-1sRI). In some cells, there is a discrepancy between the dissociation constant of either form of IL-1 (usually 200 to 300 pM) and concentrations of IL-1 that elicit a biological response (10 to 100 fM) (98). In cells expressing large amounts of IL-1R-AcP, the high-affinity binding of the IL-1R/IL-1R-AcP complex may explain which two classes of binding have been observed. Human IL-1α binds to cell surface and IL-1sRI with approximately the same affinity (100 to 300 pM) as does IL-1Ra. If the binding of IL-1Ra is subjected to BIAcore analysis, the affinity is found to be even higher than that of IL-1α. IL-1Ra avidly binds to the surface type I receptor (50 to 100 pM). Although IL-1Ra binds to IL-1sRI, it is, nevertheless, a high-affinity binding.

Of the three members of the IL-1 family (IL-1α, IL-1β, and IL-1Ra), IL-1β has the lowest affinity for the cell-bound form of IL-1RI (500 pM to 1 nM). The greatest binding affinity of the three IL-1 ligands for the IL-1RI is that of the IL-1Ra. In fact, the "off" rate is slow, and binding of IL-1Ra to the cell-bound IL-1RI is nearly irreversible. In comparison with IL-1Ra, IL-1α binds to IL-1RI with affinities ranging from 100 to 300 pM, and IL-1β binds more avidly to the non–signal-transducing type II receptor (100 pM).

Interleukin-1 Receptor Type II

The IL-1RII was described by several investigators (99,100), and the ability of IL-1β to preferentially bind to B cells probably represents binding to the type II receptor (82,101). The amino acid sequence of the human IL-1RII was reported in 1991 (102). The concept that this receptor functioned as a negative or "decoy" receptor was demonstrated by Colotta et al. in 1993 (103,104). The extracellular segment of the IL-1RII has three typical immunoglobulin-like domains; there is a transmembrane segment and a short cytoplasmic domain (102). The short cytoplasmic domain is unable to initiate signal transduction because there is no Toll homology domain. Therefore, when IL-1 binds to the cell membrane, IL-1RII does not signal. Vaccinia and cowpox virus genes encode for a protein with a high amino acid homology to the type II receptor, and this protein binds IL-1β (105,106). These same viruses also code for IL-18–binding protein-like molecules (71). The viral form of the IL-1RII probably serves to reduce the inflammatory and immune response of the host to the virus. A soluble (extracellular) form of this receptor is released from the cell surface by the action of a protease, binds IL-1β, and neutralizes the biological effects of IL-1β (107). Although the short cytoplasmic domain in the rat is longer than in the human (108), this receptor does not signal. In the human and mouse, the cytoplasmic domain of IL-1RII consists of 29 amino acids; in the rat, there are an additional 6 charged amino acids (108).

As discussed previously, IL-1β binds with a greater affinity to the type II receptor than does IL-1α, and IL-1Ra binding to this receptor is with the lowest affinity of the three ligands (107,109,110). Although IL-1α binds to cell surface and IL-1sRI with approximately the same affinity (200-300 pM), IL-1α binding to surface and soluble type II receptors is with nearly 100-fold less (30 and 10 nM, respectively). In comparison, IL-1β binds avidly to the non–signal-transducing type II receptor (100 pM), and IL-1β binding to the soluble form of this receptor is also high, at 500 pM. Moreover, IL-1β binding to the soluble IL-1RII is nearly irreversible because of a long dissociation rate (2 hours) (107,109,111). The precursor form of IL-1β also preferentially binds to the soluble form of IL-1RII (99,100). The function of the type II receptor as a "decoy" receptor is based on the binding of IL-1β to the

cell surface form of this receptor, thus preventing the ability of the ligand to form a complex with the type I receptor and the accessory protein (103,104). Another and perhaps more efficient function of the decoy receptor is to form a trimeric complex made up of the IL-1β ligand with the type II soluble receptor and the IL-1R-AcP chain (112,113). This mechanism serves to deprive the functional receptor type I of the accessory chain.

Gene and Surface Regulation of Interleukin-1 Receptor Type I

The entire gene is distributed over 29 kb; the genomic organization of the human type I receptor reveals three distinct transcription initiation sites contained in three separate segments of the first exon. Each part of this first exon is thought to possess a separate promoter, which functions independently in different cells (114,115). Despite evidence that type I receptor gene expression can be up-regulated in vitro (116,117), the most proximal (5′) promoter region lacks a TATA or CAAT box (115). In fact, this promoter region for the human IL-1RI is strikingly similar to those of housekeeping genes rather than to highly regulated genes. The transcription initiation start site contains nearly the same motif as that for the terminal deoxynucleotide transferase gene (115). There is a guanosine-cytosine rich segment (75%) after the transcription initiation site of exon I that accounts for considerable secondary RNA structure. Low numbers of surface IL-1RI may, in fact, result from multiple secondary RNA structures, which reduce optimal translation of the mRNA (117).

Surface expression of IL-1RI clearly affects the biological response to IL-1. As with IL-1β, cells can express high steady-state levels of mRNA for IL-1RI but low levels of the protein. This may be because of the amount of secondary structure in each of the polyadenylated RNA species. Studies on IL-1R surface expression have used mostly binding of labeled ligands rather than assessment of surface receptor density with specific antibodies. Nevertheless, phorbol esters, PGE$_2$, dexamethasone, epidermal growth factor, IL-2, and IL-4 increase surface expression of IL-1RI. In cells that synthesize PGE$_2$, IL-1 up-regulates its own receptor through PGE$_2$; however, when PGE$_2$ synthesis is inhibited, IL-1 down-regulates IL-1RI in the same cells. Part of the immunosuppressive properties of TGF-β may result from down-regulation of the IL-1RI on T cells. In the case of Th2 lymphocytes, IL-1 down-regulates IL-1RI surface expression, and this is associated with a decrease in mRNA half-life. Therefore, despite the housekeeping nature of its promoters, IL-1RI is regulated in the context of inflammation and immune responses.

Interleukin-18 Binding Protein

There are limited amino acid homology between the IL-18BP (71) and the type II IL-1R, and both function as decoy receptors for their respective ligands. In many ways, the IL-18BP functions as a soluble receptor for IL-18 and, like the soluble form of the IL-1RII, neutralizes IL-18 (Fig. 3). It is possible that a putative transmembrane domain of the IL-18BP was deleted during evolution; however, the IL-18BP functions solely as a secreted protein. The IL-18BP has a single Ig-domain and limited homology to the IL-18Rα chain (118). Molecular modeling of IL-18 binding to IL-18BP has identified specific amino acids; when mutated, the ability of IL-18BP to bind and neutralize IL-18 is reduced (17). The affinity of IL-18 for IL-18BP is high (Kd of 400 pM), and plasma levels of 3 to 4 ng/mL are found in healthy subjects (119). It is likely that IL-18BP functions as a natural buffer against IL-18 and the T helper type 1 (Th1) response.

SIGNAL TRANSDUCTION

Associated or Intrinsic Kinases

Hopp (120) reported a detailed sequence and structural comparison of the cytosolic segment of IL-1RI with the Ras family of guanosine triphosphatases (GTPases). In this analysis, the known amino acid residues for GTP binding and hydrolysis by the GTPase family were found to align with residues in the cytoplasmic domain of the IL-1RI. These observations are consistent with the observations that GTP analogues undergo rapid hydrolysis when membrane preparations of IL-1RI are incubated with IL-1. Amino acid sequences in the cytosolic domain of the IL-1R-AcP also align with the same binding and hydrolytic regions of the GTPases. A protein similar to G protein–activating protein that associates with the cytosolic domain of the IL-1RI has been identified (121). This finding is consistent with the hypothesis that an early event in IL-1R signaling involves dimerization of the two cytosolic domains, activation of putative GTP binding sites on the cytosolic domains, binding of a G protein, hydrolysis of GTP, and activation of a phospholipase. It then follows that hydrolysis of phospholipids generates diacylglycerol or phosphatidic acids.

Cytoplasmic Signaling Cascades

Signal transduction of IL-1 depends on the formation of a heterodimer between IL-1RI and IL-1R-AcP (90). This interaction recruits MyD88, a cytoplasmic adapter molecule. This is followed by recruitment of the IL-1R activating kinase (IRAK) (122–125). Antibodies to IL-1RI block IL-1 activity. Although IL-1R-AcP does not bind IL-1, antibodies to IL-1R-AcP also prevent IL-1 activity (95). Both the extracellular domain of the IL-1R-AcP and its cytoplasmic segment share homology with the IL-1RI. There is a highly conserved protein kinase C acceptor site in both cytoplasmic domains, although agents activating protein kinase C do not mimic IL-1 signal transduction. Limited sequence homology of the glycoprotein 130 (gp130) cytoplasmic domain with those of IL-1RI and IL-1R-AcP suggest that complex formation of the IL-1R/IL-1/IL-1R-AcP transduces a signal similar to that observed with ligands, which cause the dimer-

ization of gp130. In fact, deletion of the gp130 shared sequences from the IL-1RI cytoplasmic domain results in a reduced response to IL-1. IL-1 shares some prominent biological properties with gp130 ligands; for example, fever, hematopoietic stem cell activation, and the stimulation of the hypothalamic-pituitary-adrenal axis are common to IL-1 and IL-6. Other biological activities of IL-1 and IL-6 are distinctly antagonistic.

High levels of IL-1R-AcP are expressed in murine and human brain tissue. The discovery and function of the IL-1R-AcP showed that IL-1 has receptor biology and signaling mechanisms into the same arena as other cytokines and growth factors. The IL-1R-AcP also explains previous studies' descriptions of low and high binding affinities of IL-1 to various cells. Although there is no direct evidence, a structural change may take place in IL-1, allowing for docking of IL-1R-AcP to the IL-1RI/IL-1 complex. However, the current view is that once IL-1β binds to the type I receptor, the membrane distal first domain folds over IL-1β and this exposes binding sites for the IL-1R-AcP. Once IL-1RI/IL-1β binds to IL-1R-AcP, high-affinity binding is observed. Antibodies to the type I receptor and to the IL-1R-AcP block IL-1 binding and activity. Therefore, IL-1 may bind to the type I receptor with low affinity, causing a structural change in the ligand, followed by recognition by the IL-1R-AcP.

Within a few minutes after binding to cells, IL-1 induces several biochemical events. It remains unclear which is the most "upstream" triggering event or whether several occur at the same time. No sequential order or cascade has been identified, but several signaling events appear to be taking place during the first 2 to 5 minutes. Some of the biochemical changes associated with signal transduction are probably cell specific. Within 2 minutes, hydrolysis GTP, phosphatidylcholine, phosphatidylserine, or phosphatidylethanolamine (126) and release of ceramide by neutral (127), not acidic, sphingomyelinase (128) have been reported. In general, multiple protein phosphorylations and activation of phosphatases can be observed with 5 minutes (129), and some are thought to be initiated by the release of lipid mediators. The release of ceramide has attracted attention as a possible early signaling event (130). Phosphorylation of phospholipase A₂ activating protein also occurs in the first few minutes (131), which would lead to a rapid release of arachidonic acid. Multiple and similar signaling events have also been reported for TNF.

Of special consideration to IL-1 signal transduction is the unusual discrepancy between the low number of receptors (fewer than 10 in some cells) and the low concentrations of IL-1, which can induce a biological response. This latter observation, however, may be clarified in studies on high-affinity binding with the IL-1R-AcP complex. A rather extensive "amplification" step takes place after the initial post–receptor-binding event. The most likely mechanism for signal amplification is multiple and sequential phosphorylations (or dephosphorylations) of kinases, which result in nuclear translocation of transcription factors and activation of proteins participating in translation of mRNA. IL-1RI is phosphorylated after IL-1 binding. It is unknown whether the IL-1R-AcP is phosphorylated during receptor complex formation. In primary cells, the number of IL-1 type I receptors is very low (fewer than 100 per cell), and a biological response occurs when only as few as 2% to 3% of IL-1 type I receptors are occupied (96,132). In IL-1–responsive cells, it is assumed that there is constitutive expression of the IL-1R-AcP.

With few exceptions, there is general agreement that IL-1 does not stimulate hydrolysis of phosphatidylinositol or an increase in intracellular calcium. Without a clear increase in intracellular calcium, early post-receptor binding events nevertheless include hydrolysis of a GTP (with no associated increase in adenyl cyclase), activation of adenyl cyclase (133,134), hydrolysis of phospholipids (92,135), release of ceramide (136), and release of arachidonic acid from phospholipids through cytosolic phospholipase A_2 after its activation by phospholipase A_2–activating protein (131). Some IL-1 signaling events are prominent in different cells. Post–receptor-signaling mechanisms may therefore provide cellular specificity. For example, in some cells, IL-1 is a growth factor, and signaling is associated with serine/threonine phosphorylation of the mitogen-activated protein (MAP) kinase p42/44 in mesangial cells (137). The MAP p38 kinase, another member of the MAP kinase family, is phosphorylated in fibroblasts (138), as is the p54α MAP kinase in hepatocytes (139).

Characteristics of the Cytoplasmic Domain of the Interleukin-1 Receptor Type I

The cytoplasmic domain of the IL-1RI does not contain a consensus sequence for intrinsic tyrosine phosphorylation, but deletion mutants of the receptor reveal specific functions of some domains. There are four nuclear localization sequences that share homology with the glucocorticoid receptor. Three amino acids (Arg-431, Lys-515, and Arg-518), also found in the Toll protein, are essential for IL-1–induced IL-2 production (89). However, deletion of a segment containing these amino acids did not affect IL-1–induced IL-8 (140). There are also two cytoplasmic domains in the IL-1RI that share homology with the IL-6–signaling gp130 receptor. When these regions are deleted, there is a loss of IL-1–induced IL-8 production (140).

The C-terminal 30 amino acids of the IL-1RI can be deleted without affecting biological activity (122). Two independent studies have focused on the area between amino acids 513 to 529. Amino acids 508 to 521 contain sites required for the activation of NFκB. In one study, deletion of this segment abolished IL-1–induced IL-8 expression, and in another study, specific mutations of amino acids 513 and 520 to alanine prevented IL-1–driven E-selectin promoter activity. This area is also present in the Toll protein domain associated with NFκB translocation and previously shown to be part of the IL-1 signaling mechanism. This area (513 to 520) is also responsible for activating a kinase, which associates with the receptor. This kinase, IL-1RI–associated kinase, phosphorylates a 100-

kDa substrate. Other authors have reported a serine/threonine kinase that coprecipitates with the IL-1RI (141). Amino acid sequence comparisons of the cytosolic domain of the IL-1RI have revealed similarities with a protein kinase C acceptor site. Because protein kinase C activators usually do not mimic IL-1–induced responses, the significance of this observation is unclear.

Recruitment of MyD88 and Interleukin-1 Receptor–Activating Kinases

An event that may be linked to the binding of G proteins to the IL-1 receptor complex is the recruitment of the cytosolic protein MyD88. This small protein has many of the characteristics of cytoplasmic domains of receptors, but MyD88 lacks any known extracellular or transmembrane structure. Mice deficient in MyD88 do not respond to IL-1 or IL-18. It is unclear exactly how this protein functions, because it does not have any known kinase activity. However, it may assist in the binding of the IRAKs to the complex and hence has been said to function as an adapter molecule. Currently, four IRAKs are known (142). In mice with a deletion in IRAK-4, there is reduced endotoxin as well as IL-1 signaling (142). The binding of IRAKs to the IL-1R complex appears to be a critical step in the activation of NFκB (122). The IL-1R-AcP is essential for the recruitment and activation of IRAK (124,143). In fact, deletion of specific amino acids in the IL-1R-AcP cytoplasmic domain results in loss of IRAK association (143). In addition, MyD88 appears to dock to the complex, allowing IRAK to become phosphorylated (122,125). IRAK then dissociates from the IL-1R complex and associates with TNF receptor–associated factor 6 (TRAF-6) (123). TRAF-6 then phosphorylates NFκB-inducing kinase (NIK) (144) and NIK phosphorylates the inhibitory κB kinases (IKK-1 and IKK-2) (145). Once phosphorylated, inhibitory κB is rapidly degraded by a ubiquitin pathway liberating NFκB, which translocates to the nucleus for gene transcription. Some studies suggest that NIK is not necessary for IL-1 signaling. However, in mice deficient in TRAF-6, there is no IL-1 signaling in thymocytes and the phenotype exhibits severe osteopetrosis and defective formation of osteoclasts (146).

IRAKs also associate with the IL-18R complex (147,148). This was demonstrated by using IL-12–stimulated T cells, followed by immunoprecipitation with anti–IL-18R or anti–IRAK (147). Furthermore, IL-18–triggered cells also recruited TRAF-6 (147). Like IL-1 signaling, MyD88 has a role in IL-18 signaling. MyD88-deficient mice do not produce acute-phase proteins and have diminished cytokine responses. Th1-developing cells from MyD88 deficient mice were shown to be unresponsive to IL-18–induced activation of NFκB and c-Jun N-terminal kinase (149). Thus, MyD88 is an essential component in the signaling cascade that follows IL-1 receptor as well as IL-18 receptor binding. It appears that the cascade of sequential recruitment of MyD88, IRAK, and TRAF-6, followed by the activation of NIK and degradation of IκBK and release of NFκB, is nearly identical for IL-1 and for IL-18. Indeed, in cells transfected with IL-18Rα and then stimulated with IL-18, translocation of NFκB takes is observed through electromobility shift assay (75). In IL-18–stimulated U1 macrophages, which already express the gene for IL-18Rα, there is translocation of NFκB and stimulation of the human immunodeficiency virus type 1 production (150).

Activation of Mitogen-Activating Protein Kinases after Interleukin-1 Receptor Binding

Multiple phosphorylations take place during the first 15 minutes after IL-1 receptor binding. Most consistently, IL-1 activates protein kinases that phosphorylate serine and threonine residues, targets of the MAP kinase family. An early study reported an IL-1–induced serine/threonine phosphorylation of a 65-kDa protein clearly unrelated to those phosphorylated through protein kinase C (151). As reviewed by O'Neill (152), before IL-1 activation of serine/threonine kinases, IL-1 receptor binding results in the phosphorylation of tyrosine residues (138,139). Tyrosine phosphorylation induced by IL-1 probably results from activation of MAP kinase kinase, which then phosphorylates tyrosine and threonine on MAP kinases.

After activation of MAP kinases, there are phosphorylations on serine and threonine residues of the epidermal growth factor receptor, heat-shock protein 27, myelin basic protein, and serine 56 and 156 of β-casein, each of which has been observed in IL-1–stimulated cells (153). TNF also activates these kinases. There are at least three families of MAP kinases. The p42/44 MAP kinase family is associated with signal transduction by growth factors, including Ras-Raf-1 signal pathways. In rat mesangial cells, IL-1 activates the p42/44 MAP kinase within 10 minutes and also increases *de novo* synthesis of p42 (137).

p38 Mitogen-Activating Protein Kinase Activation

The stress-activated protein kinase, which is molecularly identified as c-Jun N-terminal kinase, is phosphorylated in cells stimulated with IL-1 (154). In addition to p42/44, two members of the MAP kinase family (p38 and p54) have been identified as part of an IL-1 phosphorylation pathway and are responsible for phosphorylating heat-shock protein 27 (138,139). In rabbit primary liver cells, IL-1 selectively activates c-Jun N-terminal kinase without apparent activation of p38 or p42/p38 MAP kinases (155). These MAP kinases are highly conserved proteins homologous to the *HOG-1* stress gene in yeasts. In fact, when *HOG-1* is deleted, yeasts fail to grow in hyperosmotic conditions; however, the mammalian gene coding for the IL-1–inducible p38 MAP kinase (139) can reconstitute the ability of the yeast to grow in hyperosmotic conditions (156). In cells stimulated with hyperosmolar NaCl, LPS, IL-1, or TNF, indistinguishable phosphorylation of the p38 MAP kinase takes place (157). In human monocytes exposed to hyperosmolar NaCl (375 to

425 mOsm/liter), IL-8, IL-1β, IL-1α, and TNF-α gene expression and synthesis takes place and are indistinguishable from those induced by LPS or IL-1 (28,158). Thus, the MAP p38 kinase pathways involved in IL-1, TNF, and LPS signal transductions share certain elements that are related to the primitive stress-induced pathway. The dependency of Rho members of the GTPase family (see previous discussion) for IL-1–induced activation of p38 MAP kinases has been demonstrated (159). This latter observation links the intrinsic GTPase domains of IL-1RI and IL-1R-AcP with activation of the p38 MAP kinase.

Inhibition of p38 Mitogen-Activating Protein Kinase

The target for pyridinyl imidazole compounds has been identified as a homolog of the *HOG-1* family (160); its sequence is identical to that of the p38 MAP kinase–activating protein 2 (161). Inhibition of the p38 MAP kinase is highly specific for reducing LPS- and IL-1–induced cytokines (160). IL-1–induced expression of human immunodeficiency virus type 1 is suppressed by specific inhibition with pyridinyl imidazole compounds (162). As expected, this class of imidazoles also prevents the downstream phosphorylation of heat-shock protein 27 (163). Compounds of this class appear to be highly specific for inhibition of the p38 MAP kinase in that there was no inhibition of 12 other kinases. When one of these compounds was used, both hyperosmotic NaCl⁻- and IL-1α–induced IL-8 synthesis was inhibited (158). It has been proposed that MAP kinase–activating protein 2 is one of the substrates for the p38 MAP kinases and is the kinase that phosphorylates heat-shock protein 27 (163).

Human Abnormalities in Interleukin-1 Receptor Type I Expression

A case of a cortisol-secreting adrenal adenoma causing Cushing's syndrome in a 62-year-old woman has been described (164). The patient exhibited the classic clinical and laboratory findings of Cushing's syndrome, which abated once the tumor was removed. Examination of the tissue revealed high expression of IL-1RI. Moreover, unlike normal adrenal cells, the tumor did not respond to corticotropin-induced cortisol production but, rather, responded to IL-1β stimulation with cortisol production. In contrast to the patient's tumor, other adrenal tumors responded to corticotropin-induced cortisol production but not IL-1β. The abundant expression of the IL-1RI in the patient's tumor in comparison with other tumors was thought to account for these observations, and the induction of cortisol by IL-1β was thought to result in the pathological disease.

BLOCKING INTERLEUKIN-1 IN DISEASE

Blocking Interleukin-1 Receptor Type I in Disease

The administration of the extracellular domain of the type I receptor (IL-1sRI) has been used in several models of inflammatory and autoimmune disease. Administration of murine IL-1sRI to mice increased the survival of heterotopic heart allografts and reduced the hyperplastic lymph node response to allogeneic cells (165). In a rat model of antigen-induced arthritis, local instillation of the murine IL-1sRI reduced joint swelling and tissue destruction (107). When a dose of IL-sRI (1 μg) was instilled into the contralateral, unaffected joint, a reduction in the degree of tissue damage was observed in the affected joint. These data suggest that the amount of IL-1sRI given in the normal, contralateral joint was acting systemically. In a model of experimental autoimmune encephalitis, the IL-1sRI reduced the severity of this disease (166). Administration of IL-1sRI to animals has also been reported to reduce the physiological response to LPS, acute lung injury, and delayed-type hypersensitivity [reviewed by Dower et al. (107)].

However, there are also data suggesting that exogenous administration of IL-1sRI may act as carrier for IL-1α. In mice, an intravenous injection of IL-1sRI alone induced a rapid increase in circulating IL-1α but not of TNF-α or IL-1β (167). The soluble receptor did not interfere with the IL-1α assay. This observation is consistent with the view that IL-1sRI acts as a carrier for IL-1α. Treatment of mice with IL-1sRI improved length of survival during a lethal infection with *Candida albicans.*

In the accelerated model of autoimmune diabetes induced by cyclophosphamide in the nonobese diabetic mouse, repeated injections with IL-1sRI protected such mice from insulin-dependent diabetes mellitus in a dose-dependent manner; the incidence of diabetes was 53.3% among the mice treated with 0.2 mg/kg and only 6.7% in mice treated with 2 mg/kg. However, none of the doses of IL-1sRI reduced the extent of insulitis in nonobese diabetic mice. Splenic lymphoid cells from such mice treated with 2 mg/kg of IL-1sRI for 5 consecutive days showed a normal distribution of mononuclear cell subsets and maintained their capacity to secrete IFN-γ and IL-2 (168).

Effect of Interleukin-1 Soluble Receptor Type I in Humans

Recombinant human IL-1sRI has been administered intravenously to healthy humans in a phase I trial without side effects or changes in physiological, hematological, or endocrinological parameters. Thus, like infusions of IL-1Ra, infusions of IL-1sRI appear safe and reinforce the conclusion that IL-1 does not have a role in homeostasis in humans.

Human volunteers have also been injected with LPS after pretreatment with IL-1sRI. The basis for these studies is that in animal models, blocking IL-1 with IL-1Ra has reduced the severity of the response [reviewed by Dinarello (169)]. Pretreatment of subjects with 10 mg/kg of IL-1Ra before intravenous endotoxin resulted in a statistically significant but modest decrease (40%) in circulating neutrophils (170). Volunteers were also pretreated with IL-1sRI or placebo and then

challenged with endotoxin. No effects on fever or systemic symptoms were noted. Although there was a decrease in the level of circulating IL-1β in comparison to placebo-treated volunteers, there was also a decrease in the level of circulating IL-1Ra ($p < 0.001$) resulting from complexing of the soluble receptor to endogenous IL-1Ra (171). This decrease was dose-dependent and resulted in a 43-fold decrease in endotoxin-induced IL-1Ra. High doses of IL-1sRI were also associated with higher levels of circulating TNF-α and IL-8 as well as cell-associated IL-1β (171). These results support the concept that IL-1sRI binds endogenous IL-1Ra and reduces the biological effectiveness of this natural IL-1Ra in inhibiting IL-1. As discussed later, patients with rheumatoid arthritis treated with IL-1sRI do not exhibit improved clinical outcome, and the mechanism is likely to the to the binding of endogenous IL-1Ra with a reduction in its biological role.

IL-1sRI was administered subcutaneously to 23 patients with active rheumatoid arthritis in a randomized, double-blind, two-center study (172). Patients received subcutaneous doses of the receptor at 25, 250, 500, or 1,000 μg/m^2 per day or placebo for 28 consecutive days. Although four of eight patients receiving 1,000 μg/m^2 per day showed improvement in at least one measure of disease activity, only one of these four patients exhibited clinical improvement. As in the placebo-treated patients, lower doses of the receptor did not result in any improvement by acceptable criteria. Despite this lack of clinical or objective improvement in disease activity, cell surface monocyte IL-1α expression in all patients receiving IL-1sRI was significantly reduced. Other parameters of altered immune function in common in patients with rheumatoid arthritis were also reduced. One possible explanation for the lack of clinical response despite efficacy in suppressing immune responses could be the inhibition of endogenous IL-1Ra. This was observed in volunteers receiving IL-1sRI before challenge by endotoxin (171).

A phase I trial of IL-1sRI was conducted in patients with relapsed and refractory acute myeloid leukemia. IL-1sRI was well tolerated. Serum levels of IL-1β, IL-6, and TNF-α did not change. Circulating levels of IL-1sRI were elevated 360- and 25-fold after intravenous and subcutaneous administration, respectively. There were no complete, partial, or minor responses to treatment (173).

The goal of any anti–IL-1 strategy is to prevent IL-1 binding to surface receptors. Using IL-1sRI to block IL-1 activity in disease is similar to using neutralizing antibodies against IL-1 and distinct from using receptor blockade with IL-1Ra. Because the molar concentrations of circulating IL-1 in disease are relatively low, pharmacological administration of IL 1sRI to reach a 100-fold molar excess of the soluble receptor over that of IL-1 is feasible. The human trial of IL-1sRI in delayed hypersensitivity reactions supports the notion that low doses (100 μg per patient) can have anti-inflammatory effects. The fusion of two chains of extracellular domains of the type IL-1RI to the crystallized fragment portion of immunoglobulin enhances the binding

IL-1 over that of monomeric IL-1sRI (174) and may have a longer plasma half-life than the monomeric form. However, as shown in the study of IL-1sRI in rheumatoid arthritis, binding of the endogenous IL-1Ra worsened the disease. In contrast to neutralizing IL-1 itself, the goal of receptor blockade requires the condition of blocking all unoccupied IL-1 surface receptors, because triggering only a few evokes a response. Receptor blockade is a formidable task, partly because large amounts of IL-1Ra are necessary to reduce disease activity. The potential disadvantage of using IL-1sRI therapy is the possibility that these receptors will either prolong the clearance of IL-1 or bind the natural IL-1Ra.

The soluble form of IL-1RI and IL-1RII circulate in healthy humans at molar concentrations that are 10- to 50-fold greater than those of IL-1β measured in septic patients and 100-fold greater than the concentration of IL-1β after intravenous administration (175). Why do humans have a systemic response to an infusion of IL-1α (176) or IL-1β? One conclusion is that binding of IL-1 to the soluble forms of IL-1R types I and II exhibits a slow "on" rate in comparison with the cell-bound IL-1RI.

In addition, naturally occurring neutralizing antibodies to IL-1α are present in many persons and probably reduce the activity of IL-1α. Despite the portfolio of soluble receptors and naturally occurring antibodies, IL-1 produced during disease does, in fact, trigger the type I receptor, inasmuch as, in animals and humans, blocking receptors or neutralizing IL-1 ameliorates disease. These findings underscore the high functional level of only a few IL-1 type I receptors. They also imply that the post–receptor-triggering events are greatly amplified. It seems reasonable to conclude that treating disease on the basis of blocking IL-1R needs to take into account the efficiency of so few type I receptors in initiating a biological event.

INTERLEUKIN-1 RECEPTOR ANTAGONIST

Studies Using Interleukin-1 Receptor Antagonist in Animals and Humans

Because IL-1Ra exhibits no species specificity, much data have revealed a role for IL-1 in models of disease. As shown in Fig. 4, when IL-1Ra binds to the type I IL-1R, there is no formation of the heterodimer with the IL-1R-AcP chain. In the presence of IL-1β, there is no signal transduction, and hence there is classic competitive inhibition similar to other receptor antagonists. However, unlike small molecule receptor antagonists, IL-1Ra appears to be a pure receptor antagonist. Although not shown in the figure, IL-1Ra occupancy of the type I receptor also prevents the binding of IL-1α to the cell receptor. Because there is considerable evidence that the biological response of IL-1α is attributable to its membrane form, IL-1Ra nevertheless blocks the activities of membrane IL-1α.

IL-1Ra is used to treat patients with rheumatoid arthritis. The recombinant form of IL-1Ra produced in *Escherichia coli* is known by the generic name anakinra. Before IL-1Ra was approved for treating rheumatoid arthritis in humans, there were extensive preclinical trials in various animal models, particularly in models of autoimmune diseases and model of rheumatoid arthritis. Table 4 lists the effect of IL-1Ra in various animal models of disease.

The late Phillipe Seckinger, working in the laboratory of Jean-Michel Dayer, demonstrated that the urinary inhibitor of IL-1 prevented IL-1 binding to cells (177). A similar IL-1 inhibitor was induced by stimulating human blood monocytes with IgG (178). This IL-1 inhibitor was purified to homogeneity, and the amino acid sequence was used to clone the molecule from a monocyte cDNA library (179). The recombinant IL-1 inhibitor was renamed IL-1Ra and was shown

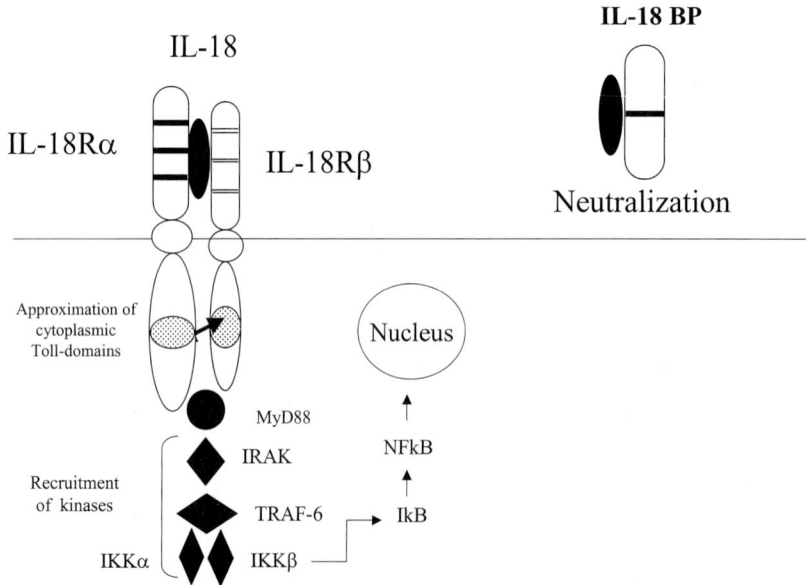

FIG. 4. Interleukin-1 receptor antagonist prevents interleukin-1 signaling. (See text for discussion.)

TABLE 4. *Effects of interleukin-1Ra*

Models of infection
Improved survival in LPS-induced shock in primates, mice, rats, and rabbits
Improved survival in *Klebsiella pneumoniae* infection in newborn rats
Reduction in shock and mortality in rabbits and baboons from *Escherichia coli* or *Staphylococcus epidermidis* bacteremia
Amelioration of shock and reduction in death after cecal ligation and puncture
Attenuation of LPS-induced lung nitric oxide activity
Decreased hypoglycemia, production of CSF, and early tolerance in mice after administration of endotoxin
Reduction in LPS-induced hyperalgesia
Protection against TNF-induced lethality in D-galactosamine–treated mice
Reduction in nematode-induced intestinal nerve dysfunction
Decreased circulating or cellular TNF production in models of sepsis
Decreased IL-6 production after LPS or enteric LPS administration
Protection from *Bacillus anthracis* toxin–induced lethality in mice
Decreased intestinal inflammation and bacterial invasion in shigellosis
Reversal of decreased survival by insulin-like growth factor–1 in sepsis
Decreased in live *E. coli*–induced thrombin, tissue plasminogen activator, plasminogen activator inhibitor, and elastase elevations
Models of local inflammation
Decreased neutrophil accumulation in inflammatory peritonitis in mice
Reduction in immune complex–induced neutrophil infiltration, eicosanoid production, and tissue necrosis in rabbit colitis
Reduction in acid-induced neutrophil infiltration and enterocolitis in rats
Decreased endotoxin-induced intestinal secretory diarrhea in mice
Inhibition of permanganate-induced granulomas in rats
Inhibition of LPS-induced intra-articular neutrophil infiltration
Decreased IL-1–induced synovitis and loss of cartilage proteoglycan
Reduced myocardial neutrophil accumulation after coronary occlusions in dogs
Reduced inflammation and mortality in acute pancreatitis
Decreased hepatic inflammation after hemorrhagic shock
Modest reduction in acetaminophen-induced liver damage
Decreased IL-8 and MCP-1 levels induced by intravitreal LPS
Reduction in hapten-induced intestestinal motor dysfunction and intestinal myeloperoxidase levels
Decreased cerulean-induced pancreatic inflammation
Models of acute or chronic lung injury
Decreased local LPS-induced neutrophil infiltration in rats
Inhibition of antigen-induced pulmonary eosinophil accumulation and airway hyperactivity in guinea pigs
Prevention of bleomycin- or silica-induced pulmonary fibrosis
Reduction in hypoxia-induced pulmonary hypertension
Reduction in carrageenan-induced pleurisy in rats
Decreased intratracheal IL-1–induced fluid leak (systemic administration)
Decreased albumin leak after systemic LPS
Inhibition of antigen-induced eosinophil accumulation in guinea pigs
Models of central nervous system functions
Decreased stress-induced hypothalamic-pituitary axis
Decreased immobilization-induced stress on hypothalamic-pituitary axis
Reduced astrocytosis after spinal cord transection
Increased survival after heat stroke in rats
Decreased cerebral ischemia–induced edema and infarct size
Reduced astrocytosis-mediated wound closure after brain damage
Decreased LPS-induced brain monoamine levels
Decreased in number of necrotic neurons in cerebral artery occlusion
Models of metabolic dysfunction
Reduction in hepatocellular damage after ischemia-reperfusion
Improved survival after hemorrhagic shock in mice
Inhibition of SAA gene expression and synthesis in high-dose IL-2 toxicity
Decreased muscle protein breakdown in rats with peritonitis due to cecal ligation
Reduced muscle protein breakdown in rats with chronic septic peritonitis
Inhibition of weight loss after muscle tissue injury
Decrease in bone loss in ovariectomized rats
Decreased multinucleated osteoclasts in ovariectomized rats
Reversal of LPS-induced CRF gene expression in the hypothalamus
Prevention of LPS-induced ACTH release
Decreased *E. coli*–induced chaperone protein–induced osteolytic activity in rat calvaria
Decreased LPS-induced bone resorption in mouse calvaria

(continued)

TABLE 4. *(Continued)*

Models of autoimmune disease
Diminution of *Streptococcus* cell wall-induced arthritis in rats
Reduction in collagen-induced arthritis in rats and mice
Suppression of anti–basement membrane glomerulonephritis
Delayed hyperglycemia in the diabetic BB rat
Decreased hyperglycemia in nonobese diabetic mice
Reduction in autoimmune myelin basic protein–induced encephalomyelitis
Reduction in elevated cortisone levels in allergic encephalomyelitis
Models of immune-mediated disease
Prevention of graft-versus-host disease in mice
Prolongation of islet allograft survival
Reduction in skin contact hypersensitivity to haptens
Decrease in coronary artery fibronectin deposition in heterotopic cardiac transplantation
Decreased adjuvant arthritis in rats
Reduction in streptozotocin-induced diabetes
Increased survival of corneal transplants
No effect on mitogen- or antigen-induced T-cell proliferation
Decreased IL-2–induced LAK cell generation
Decreased IL-2–induced LAK cell TNF production
Decreased phorbol ester–induced B-cell proliferation and IgG synthesis
Models of malignant disease
Reduction in the number and size of metastatic melanoma tumors
Reduction in growth of subcutaneous melanoma tumors
Reduced LPS-induced augmentation of metastatic melanoma
Reduction in tumor-mediated cachexia (intratumoral injection)
Reduced spontaneous proliferation, colony formation, and cytokine production of human AML and CML (adult and juvenile) leukemia cells
Reduced spontaneous IL-6 and PGE_2 production in multiple myeloma cells
Decreased spontaneous release of serotonin and histamine in rat basophilic leukemia cells
Decreased spontaneous blast proliferation and cytokine production
Effect of models of angiogenesis
Decreased new blood vessel growth after sciatic nerve injury in mice
Decreased vascularization of inflammatory polymers implanted subcutaneously in mice
Impairment of host responses
Increased mortality from *K. pneumoniae* in newborn rats (high dose)
Increased mortality from *Listeria* infection
Enhanced growth of *Mycobacterium avium* in organs
Worsening of infectious arthritis (late administration)
Increased vascular leakage in mice given high-dose IL-2
Effects on production of cytokines and other molecules
Reduced LPS-induced monocyte production of IL-1β, IL-1α, IL-6, IL-8
Decreased LPS-induced fibroblast production of IL-6
Decreased asbestos-stimulated IL-8 from mesothelial cells
Reduced spontaneous production of substance P by cultured neurons
Enhanced natural killer cell activity
Increased spontaneous PGE_2 production by cultured decidual cells
Increased smooth muscle cell proliferation
Other effects *in vitro*
Reduction in *Actinobacillus* LPS-induced bone resorption
Reduction in spleen cell colony-forming units after radiation
Decreased LPS-induced nitric oxide synthase in glial cells
Decreased *Clostridium difficile* toxin activity on hepatocytes
Reduced VCAM-1 and ICAM expresson induced by *Rickettsia* LPS on HUVEC
Decreased TSH-stimulated cAMP release in thyroid cells
Decreased *C. difficile* toxin A–induced intestinal secretory factor release
Decreased nitric oxide release and insulin production in rat islet cells after TNF stimulation
Decreased PDGF receptor expression in rat lung myofibroblasts after exposure to particulates

ACTH, adrenocorticotropic hormone; AML, acute myeloid leukemia; cAMP, cyclic adenosine monophosphate; CML, chronic myeloid leukemia; CRF, corticotropin-releasing factor; CSF, colony-stimulating factor; HUVEC, human umbilical vein endothelial cell; ICAM, intercellular adhesion molecule; IgG, immunoglobulin G; IL, interleukin; LAK, lymphokine-activated killer; LPS, lipopolysaccharide; MCP-1, monocyte chemoattractant protein–1; PDGF, platelet-derived growth factor; PGE_2, prostaglandin E_2; SAA, serum amyloid A; TNF, tumor necrosis factor; TSH, thyroid-stimulating hormone; VCAM-1, vascular cell adhesion molecule-1.

to block the binding of IL-1α as a receptor antagonist. The surprise for the entire IL-1 field was the discovery that the amino acid sequence of IL-1Ra was more homologous to the amino acid sequence of IL-1β than that of IL-1α was to that of IL-1β. There is only one IL-1Ra gene, but several isoforms exist. Unlike IL-1β, IL-1Ra has a classic leader peptide and is readily secreted. The other forms of IL-1Ra—namely, intracellular forms lacking a leader peptide but derived from the same gene—have been reported. When expressed as a mature recombinant molecule, intracellular IL-1Ra blocks IL-1 binding as well as does the secreted form.

The structural analysis of the IL-1RI/IL-1Ra complex with x-ray crystallography reveals that IL-1Ra contacts all three domains of IL-1RI. IL-1β has two sites of binding to IL-1RI. There is a primary binding site located at the open top of its barrel shape and a second site on the back side of the IL-1β molecule. IL-1Ra also has two binding sites, which are similar to those of IL-1β. However, the back side site of IL-1Ra is more homologous to that of IL-1β than is the primary binding site. Thus, the back side site of IL-1Ra binds to IL-1RI tightly and occupies the receptor. Because the second binding site is not available, IL-1Ra does not recruit the IL-1R-AcP to form the heterocomplex necessary to trigger a signal. After binding of IL-1Ra to IL-1RI–bearing cells, there was no phosphorylation of the epidermal growth factor receptor, a well-established and sensitive assessment of IL-1 signal transduction. Overwhelming evidence that IL-1Ra is a pure receptor antagonist comes from studies of intravenous injection of IL-1Ra into healthy humans. At doses 1,000,000-fold greater than that of IL-1α or IL-1β, IL-1Ra had no agonist activity in humans (180).

Mice deficient in IL-1Ra have low litter numbers and exhibit growth retardation in adult life (181). These animals also have elevated basal concentrations of plasma IL-6 and exhibit higher levels of hepatic acute-phase proteins in comparison with those of wild-type control mice. Injection of endotoxin or a turpentine abscess in IL-1Ra–deficient mice results in increased lethality. In a model of endotoxin-induced inflammation, IL-1Ra–deficient mice exhibit nearly twofold higher serum levels of sphingomyelinase than do wild-type mice. The most dramatic phenotype has been observed in IL-1Ra–deficient mice crossed from a C57BL/6 to a BALB/c genetic background (6). In these IL-1Ra–deficient mice, but not in IL-1Ra–deficient mice with the original C57BL/6 genetic makeup, a chronic inflammatory polyarthropathy developed spontaneously. The joints showed prominent synovial and periarticular infiltration of inflammatory cells, osteoclast activation, and structural erosion associated with the presence of granulation tissue. Overall, the histological pattern appeared similar to that of humans with rheumatoid arthritis. Elevated levels of anti-IgG1, but not anti–immunoglobulin M, were observed, as were elevated levels of rheumatoid factor and anti–double-strand DNA antibodies. Steady-state levels of COX-2, IL-1RI, IL-1β, IL-6, and TNF-α mRNA in the affected joints were also increased. Bone erosion with arthritis was present in the joints of IL-1Ra–deficient mice,

which was consistent with the observation that mice deficient in IL-1RI exhibited no significant trabecular bone loss after ovariectomy, in comparison with wild-type controls (70).

The finding that IL-1Ra–deficient mice spontaneously develop a destructive, inflammatory arthropathy strongly suggests that endogenous IL-1Ra functions to suppress inflammation in mice living in a normal environment. Furthermore, because IL-1Ra binds only IL-1 receptors, the results also implicate IL-1 as an essential cytokine in the pathological process. The onset of this autoimmune process requires a genetic background favoring the Th2 response, which produces antibodies rather than cytotoxic T cells in response to antigens. The immunological stimulus probably occurs when either an endogenous antigen or an antigen from the intestinal flora triggers a Th2 response, which, in the absence of IL-1 blockade, is uncontrolled.

IL-1Ra–deficient mice also develop a lethal arterial inflammation involving primary and secondary branch points of the aorta (7). These are stress points in the vessel wall as a result of blood flow and are also the same locations at which atherosclerotic plaques are commonly found. The lesions are characterized by transmural infiltration of neutrophils, macrophages, and CD4+ T cells. Death is caused by vessel wall collapse, stenosis, and organ infarction. Heterozygotes, which have reduced but detectable levels of endogenous IL-1Ra in comparison with wild-type controls, do not die from this severe arteritis but do develop small arterial lesions.

Numerous studies have implicated IL-1 in the pathogenesis of rheumatoid arthritis. Although the systemic administration of IL-1 or the instillation of IL-1 into a joint space provides supportive data, there are drawbacks to interpreting the effects of exogenously applied IL-1 as a preclinical model. The most convincing preclinical evidence for a pivotal role for IL-1 in rheumatoid arthritis is derived from experimental models in which specific blockade of IL-1 activity reduces one or more of the pathological processes that arise in the context of the naturally occurring disease. The administration of IL-1Ra reduces the inflammation as well as the loss of bone and cartilage in the rat adjuvant arthritis model and hence fulfills the criteria of reduction in disease severity in a complex model that mimics human rheumatoid arthritis. Rats with developing adjuvant arthritis were treated with IL-1Ra by continuous infusion. The results showed modest but significant reductions in swelling of the ankle joints and in paw weights and histological improvement of bone and cartilage lesions. However, marked inhibition (53%) of bone resorption was also observed, even at doses at which anti-inflammatory activity was not seen (182). A well-studied model for mimicking human rheumatoid arthritis is collagen-induced arthritis in which immunization with type II collagen is used. In this model, high levels of exogenous IL-1Ra completely suppress the disease (182). In the collagen-induced arthritis model in rats, methotrexate alone reduced bone erosions by 57%, but the combination of IL-1Ra with methotrexate reduced bone erosions by 97% (182). In addition, IL-1Ra treatment of rats with established collagen-induced arthritis resulted in nearly complete suppression of all parameters of the disease (182). Other methods of providing higher therapeutic levels of IL-1Ra have been investigated. For example, after transplantation of murine 3T3 fibroblasts transfected with the gene for human IL-1Ra, paws and knee joints were inspected to evaluate inflammation and cartilage destruction in a murine model of type II collagen-induced arthritis. The onset of collagen-induced arthritis was almost prevented in joints containing the transfected IL-1Ra–expressing cells, whereas joints containing cells transfected with the control (empty) vector showed severe inflammation and destruction of cartilage. In the paw ipsilateral to the IL-1Ra gene–expressing knees, reduced inflammation and joint destruction were observed (183). After instillation of endotoxin directly into the joints of rabbits, leukocyte infiltration and protein leak developed; however, administration of a neutralizing monoclonal antibody against rabbit IL-1Ra resulted in a 50% increase in the level of IL-1β and a 20% to 40% enhancement of leukocyte infiltration and protein leakage (184). It can be concluded that endogenous IL-1Ra functions as an anti-inflammatory cytokine in this model by limiting the production of IL-1β as well as the intensity of the inflammatory response.

Human chondrocytes can be cultured in the presence of a cartilaginous matrix and studied for the synthesis of proteoglycans. When synovial fibroblasts from patients with rheumatoid arthritis are added to this system, the cartilaginous matrix is destroyed in 10 to 18 days. The addition of IL-1Ra or anti–IL-1β monoclonal antibodies reduced the destruction of the matrix by 45% and 35%, respectively (185).

Interleukin-1 Receptor Antagonist (Anakinra) Treatment in Humans with Rheumatoid Arthritis

In a randomized, double-blind trial, anakinra was administered to 175 patients at 21 sites in the United States (186). During the first 3 weeks of the trial, patients received subcutaneous doses of 20, 70, or 200 mg of anakinra one, three, or seven times per week. To maintain the blindness of the study, patients received placebo injections on the days that anakinra was not administered. After 3 weeks, a statistically significant reduction in the swollen joint count was observed in patients receiving 70 or 200 mg per day ($p < 0.01$). Daily dosing was more effective than dosing three times per week, according to assessment by the number of swollen joints, the investigator and patient assessments of disease activity, pain score, and C-reactive protein (CRP) levels. CRP levels fell from a mean baseline of 4.7 μg/mL to 2.6 μg/mL after 3 weeks of daily therapy of 70 mg/day during the treatment phase. After this study, anakinra was evaluated in a double-blind, placebo-controlled European multicenter study in 472 patients (3). Patients had severe rheumatoid arthritis (disease duration, between 6 months and 8 years) and had discontinued use of disease-modifying drugs 6 weeks before entry into the study. Patients were randomly assigned to a 24-week course of therapy with placebo or one of three subcutaneous doses of anakinra: 30, 75, or 150 mg/day. After 24 weeks, 43% of the patients receiving 150 mg/day of anakinra exhibited a significant reduction in disease, in comparison with 27% of patients injected with placebo. In addition, there was a similar reduction in CRP levels and erythrocyte sedimentation levels at all doses, whereas CRP and erythrocyte sedimentation levels did not change in the placebo group.

The rate of radiologic progression of joint destruction in the patients receiving anakinra was significantly less than in the placebo group at 24 weeks (187). An additional evaluation of these patients revealed a decrease in the rate of progression in erosion and joint space narrowing in comparison with patients receiving placebo. These clinical findings are consistent with anakinra blocking the osteoclast activating factor property of IL-1 as has been reported using *in vitro* cultures (188). In fact, when purified to homogeneity, the amino terminal sequence of osteoclast activating factor revealed that osteoclast activating factor was, in fact, IL-1β (189). In patients who received anakinra, synovial biopsies before and after 24 weeks of daily treatment revealed evidence of decreased cellular infiltration and expression of E-selectin and vascular cell adhesion molecule 1, through immunohistochemical techniques (5). In addition, the numbers of macrophages and lymphocytes in the subintimal tissue were reduced in comparison with those found in biopsies from patients treated with injections of placebo. The study also found evidence of a reduction or arrest in cellular markers of progressive joint disease in the synovial membrane.

CONCLUSIONS

IL-1 and IL-2 were the first two cytokines cloned, and the availability of the recombinant molecules rapidly aided investigations. In the brief history of cytokines in relation to immune responses, IL-1 was originally thought to play a role as a nonspecific activator of lymphocyte responses to mitogens and antigens; IL-1 remains a nonspecific activator of lymphocytes during antigenic challenge. However, with the expanded studies of specifically blocking IL-1 and the use of IL-1 receptor–deficient mice, the role of IL-1 in disease appears more relevant to inflammation, and the cytokine exhibits a greater influence on tissue destruction rather than being required for a proper immune response. There is no question, however, that inflammation affects immune responses, but in the case of IL-1, the effect of the cytokine may be related to its ability to increase immune cell infiltration to an antigenic site. In addition, IL-1 may act as an immunosuppressive cytokine because of the ability of IL-1 to stimulate genes such as nitric oxide synthase and COX-2. On the other hand, IL-1β acts as an adjuvant and is required for the development of T-dependent antibodies to sheep red blood cells. Understanding the role of IL-1 in any immune response has been facilitated by blocking the IL-1 receptor with the IL-1Ra, which, because it exhibits no species specificity, has been used in various models of disease and immunological challenge. Thus, a better understanding of IL-1 has emerged for a role in affecting the pathogenesis of disease, particularly autoimmune diseases. Thousands of patients with rheumatoid arthritis are treated with IL-1Ra (the generic agent known as anakinra). The efficacy of IL-1Ra in reducing the severity of the disease and slowing the destructive processes of the joints is now well recognized and supports a broader role of this cytokine in immunobiology.

REFERENCES

1. Watanabe N, Kawaguchi M, Kobayashi Y. Activation of interleukin-1β converting enzyme by nigericin is independent of apoptosis. *Cytokine* 1998;10:645–653.
2. Coeshott C, Ohnemus C, Pilyavskaya A, et al. Converting enzyme-independent release of TNFα and IL-1β from a stimulated human monocytic cell line in the presence of activated neutrophils or purified proteinase-3. *Proc Natl Acad Sci U S A* 1999;96:6261–6266.
3. Bresnihan B, Alvaro-Gracia JM, Cobby M, et al. Treatment of rheumatoid arthritis with recombinant human interleukin-1 receptor antagonist. *Arthritis Rheum* 1998;41:2196–2204.
4. Jiang Y, Genant HK, Watt I, et al. A multicenter, double-blind, dose-ranging, randomized, placebo-controlled study of recombinant human interleukin-1 receptor antagonist in patients with rheumatoid arthritis: radiologic progression and correlation of Genant and Larsen scores. *Arthritis Rheum* 2000;43:1001–1009.
5. Cunnane G, Madigan A, Murphy E, et al. The effects of treatment with interleukin-1 receptor antagonist on the inflamed synovial membrane in rheumatoid arthritis. *Rheumatology (Oxford)* 2001;40:62–69.
6. Horai R, Saijo S, Tanioka H, et al. Development of chronic inflammatory arthropathy resembling rheumatoid arthritis in interleukin 1 receptor antagonist–deficient mice. *J Exp Med* 2000;191:313–320.
7. Nicklin MJ, Hughes DE, Barton JL, et al. Arterial inflammation in mice lacking the interleukin 1 receptor antagonist gene. *J Exp Med* 2000;191:303–312.
8. Auron PE, Webb AC, Rosenwasser LJ, et al. Nucleotide sequence of human monocyte interleukin 1 precursor cDNA. *Proc Natl Acad Sci U S A* 1984;81:7907–7911.
9. Lomedico PT, Gubler R, Hellmann CP, et al. Cloning and expression of murine interleukin-1 cDNA in *Escherichia coli*. *Nature* 1984;312:458–462.
10. Mulero JJ, Pace AM, Nelken ST, et al. IL1HY1: A novel interleukin-1 receptor antagonist gene. *Biochem Biophys Res Commun* 1999;263:702–706.
11. Busfield SJ, Comrack CA, Yu G, et al. Identification and gene organization of three novel members of the IL-1 family on human chromosome 2. *Genomics* 2000;66:213–216.
12. Barton JL, Herbst R, Bosisio D, et al. A tissue specific IL-1 receptor antagonist homolog from the IL-1 cluster lacks IL-1, IL-1ra, IL-18 and IL-18 antagonist activities. *Eur J Immunol* 2000;30:3299–3308.
13. Pan G, Risser P, Mao W, et al. IL-1H, an interleukin 1–related protein that binds IL-18 receptor/IL-1Rrp. *Cytokine* 2001;13:1–7.
14. Kumar S, McDonnell PC, Lehr R, et al. Identification and initial characterization of four novel members of the interleukin-1 family. *J Biol Chem* 2000;275:10308–10314.
15. Lin H, Ho AS, Haley-Vicente D, et al. Cloning and characterization of IL-1HY2, a novel interleukin-1 family member. *J Biol Chem* 2001;276:20597–20602.
16. Evans RJ, Bray J, Childs JD, et al. Mapping receptor binding sites in the IL-1 receptor antagonist and IL-1β by site-directed mutagenesis: identification of a single site in IL-1ra and two sites in IL-1β. *J Biol Chem* 1995;270:11477–11483.
17. Kim SH, Azam T, Yoon DY, et al. Site-specific mutations in the mature form of human IL-18 with enhanced biological activity and decreased neutralization by IL-18 binding protein. *Proc Natl Acad Sci U S A* 2001;98:3304–3309.
18. Breder CD, Dinarello CA, Saper CB. Interleukin-1 immunoreactive innervation of the human hypothalamus. *Science* 1988;240:321–324.
19. Fenton MJ, Clark BD, Collins KL, et al. Transcriptional regulation of the human prointerleukin 1 beta gene. *J Immunol* 1987;138:3972–3979.
20. Vannier E, Dinarello CA. Histamine enhances interleukin (IL)–1–induced IL-1 gene expression and protein synthesis via H2 receptors in peripheral blood mononuclear cells: comparison with IL-1 receptor antagonist. *J Clin Invest* 1993;92:281–287.
21. Jarrous N, Kaempfer R. Induction of human interleukin-1 gene expression by retinoic acid and its regulation at processing of precursor transcripts. *J Biol Chem* 1994;269:23141–23149.
22. Schindler R, Clark BD, Dinarello CA. Dissociation between interleukin-1β mRNA and protein synthesis in human peripheral blood mononuclear cells. *J Biol Chem* 1990;265:10232–10237.
23. Kaspar RL, Gehrke L. Peripheral blood mononuclear cells stimulated with C5a or lipopolysaccharide to synthesize equivalent levels of IL-1b mRNA show unequal IL-1b protein accumulation but similar polyribosome profiles. *J Immunol* 1994;153:277–286.
24. Miller LC, Isa S, Vannier E, et al. Live *Borrelia burgdorferi* preferentially activate IL-1b gene expression and protein synthesis over the interleukin-1 receptor antagonist. *J Clin Invest* 1992;90:906–912.
25. Fenton MJ, Vermeulen MW, Clark BD, et al. Human pro–IL-1 beta gene expression in monocytic cells is regulated by two distinct pathways. *J Immunol* 1988;140:2267–2273.
26. Auron PE, Webb AC. Interleukin-1: a gene expression system regulated at multiple levels. *Eur Cytokine Netw* 1994;5:573–592.
27. Fenton MJ, Lodie T, Buras J. NFbA is identical to the ETS family member PU.1 and is structurally altered following LPS activation. *Cytokine* 1994;6:558.
28. Shapiro L, Dinarello CA. Cytokine expression during osmotic stress. *Exp Cell Res* 1997;231:354–362.
29. Puren AJ, Fantuzzi G, Dinarello CA. Gene expression, synthesis and secretion of IL-1b and IL-18 are differentially regulated in human blood mononuclear cells and mouse spleen cells. *Proc Natl Acad Sci U S A* 1999;96:2256–2261.
30. Tone M, Thompson SAJ, Tone Y, et al. Regulation of IL-18 (IFN-γ–inducing factor) gene expression. *J Immunol* 1997;159:6156–6163.
31. Martin TJ, Romas E, Gillespie MT. Interleukins in the control of osteoclast differentiation. *Crit Rev Eukaryot Gene Expr* 1998;8:107–123.
32. Andersson J, Björk L, Dinarello CA, et al. Lipopolysaccharide induces human interleukin-1 receptor antagonist and interleukin-1 production in the same cell. *Eur J Immunol* 1992;22:2617–2623.
33. Gu Y, Wu J, Faucheu C, et al. Interleukin-1β converting enzyme requires oligomerization for activity of processed forms *in vivo*. *EMBO J* 1995;14:1923–1931.
34. Fantuzzi G, Reed DA, Dinarello CA. IL-12-induced IFNγ is dependent on caspase-1 processing of the IL-18 precursor. *J Clin Invest* 1999;104:761–767.
35. Tsutsui H, Kayagaki N, Kuida K, et al. Caspase-1–independent, Fas/Fas ligand–mediated IL-18 secretion from macrophages causes acute liver injury in mice. *Immunity* 1999;11:359–367.
36. Perregaux D, Barberia J, Lanzetti AJ, et al. IL-1b maturation: evidence that mature cytokine formation can be induced specifically by nigercin. *J Immunol* 1992;149:1294–1303.
37. Thompson GJ, Langlais C, Cain K, et al. Elevated extracellular K inhibits death-receptor and chemical-mediated apoptosis prior to caspase activation and cytochrome c release. *Biochem J* 2001;357:137–145.
38. Ferrari D, Chiozzi P, Falzoni S, et al. Extracellular ATP triggers IL-1 beta release by activating the purinergic P2Z receptor of human macrophages. *J Immunol* 1997;159:1451–1458.
39. Buell G, Chessell IP, Michel AD, et al. Blockade of human P2X7 receptor function with a monoclonal antibody. *Blood* 1998;92:3521–3528.
40. Perregaux DG, Gabel CA. Post-translational processing of murine IL-1: evidence that ATP-induced release of IL-1 alpha and IL-1 beta occurs via a similar mechanism. *J Immunol* 1998;160:2469–2477.
41. Perregaux DG, McNiff P, Laliberte R, et al. ATP acts as an agonist to promote stimulus-induced secretion of IL-1 beta and IL-18 in human blood. *J Immunol* 2000;165:4615–4623.
42. Solle M, Labasi J, Perregaux DG, et al. Altered cytokine production in mice lacking P2X(7) receptors. *J Biol Chem* 2001;276:125–132.
43. Maier JAM, Voulalas P, Roeder D, et al. Extension of the life span of human endothelial cells by an interleukin-1α antisense oligomer. *Science* 1990;249:1570–1574.

44. Maier JAM, Statuto M, Ragnotti G. Endogenous interleukin-1 alpha must be transported to the nucleus to exert its activity in human endothelial cells. *Mol Cell Biol* 1994;14:1845–1851.

45. Horai R, Asano M, Sudo K, et al. Production of mice deficient in genes for interleukin (IL)-1α, IL-1β, IL-1α/β, and IL-1 receptor antagonist shows that IL-1β is crucial in turpentine-induced fever development and glucocorticoid secretion. *J Exp Med* 1998;187:1463–1475.

46. Hammerberg C, Arend WP, Fisher GJ, et al. Interleukin-1 receptor antagonist in normal and psoriatic epidermis. *J Clin Invest* 1992;90:571–583.

47. Kurt-Jones EA, Beller DI, Mizel SB, et al. Identification of a membrane-associated interleukin-1 in macrophages. *Proc Natl Acad Sci U S A* 1985;82:1204–1208.

48. Brody DT, Durum SK. Membrane IL-1: IL-1α precursor binds to the plasma membrane via a lectin-like interaction. *J Immunol* 1989;143:1183.

49. Kaplanski G, Farnarier C, Kaplanski S, et al. Interleukin-1 induces interleukin-8 from endothelial cells by a juxtacrine mechanism. *Blood* 1994;84:4242–4248.

50. Bendtzen K, Svenson M, Jonsson V, et al. Autoantibodies to cytokines–friends or foes? *Immunol Today* 1990;11:167–169.

51. Zheng H, Fletcher D, Kozak W, et al. Resistance to fever induction and impaired acute-phase response in interleukin-1β deficient mice. *Immunity* 1995;3:9–19.

52. Fantuzzi G, Ku G, Harding MW, et al. Response to local inflammation of IL-1β converting enzyme–deficient mice. *J Immunol* 1997;158:1818–1824.

53. Fantuzzi G, Sacco S, Ghezzi P, et al. Physiological and cytokine responses in interleukin-1β–deficient mice after zymosan-induced inflammation. *Am J Physiol* 1997;273:R400–R406.

54. Alheim K, Chai Z, Fantuzzi G, et al. Hyperresponsive febrile reactions to interleukin (IL) 1alpha and IL-1beta, and altered brain cytokine mRNA and serum cytokine levels, in IL-1beta–deficient mice. *Proc Natl Acad Sci U S A* 1997;94:2681–2686.

55. Fantuzzi G, Zheng H, Faggioni R, et al. Effect of endotoxin in IL-1b–deficient mice. *J Immunol* 1996;157:291–296.

56. Faggioni R, Fantuzzi G, Fuller J, et al. IL-1b mediates leptin induction during inflammation. *Am J Physiol* 1998;274:R204–R208.

57. Reznikov LL, Shames BD, Barton HA, et al. Interleukin-1β–deficiency results in reduced NF-κB levels in pregnant mice. *Am J Physiol* 2000;278:R263–R270.

58. Kozak W, Kluger MJ, Soszynski D, et al. IL-6 and IL-1 beta in fever. Studies using cytokine-deficient (knockout) mice. *Ann N Y Acad Sci* 1998;856:33–47.

59. Kuida K, Lippke JA, Ku G, et al. Altered cytokine export and apoptosis in mice deficient in interleukin-1β converting enzyme. *Science* 1995;267:2000–2003.

60. Nakae S, Asano M, Horai R, et al. Interleukin-1 beta, but not interleukin-1 alpha, is required for T-cell–dependent antibody production. *Immunology* 2001;104:402–409.

61. Labow M, Shuster D, Zetterstrom M, et al. Absence of IL-1 signaling and reduced inflammatory response in IL-1 type I receptor–deficient mice. *J Immunol* 1997;159:2452–2461.

62. Hirsch E, Irikura VM, Paul SM, et al. Functions of interleukin-1 receptor antagonist in gene knockout and overproducing mice. *Proc Natl Acad Sci U S A* 1996;93:11008–11013.

63. Josephs MD, Solorzano CC, Taylor M, et al. Modulation of the acute phase response by altered expression of the IL-1 type 1 receptor or IL-1ra. *Am J Physiol Regul Integr Comp Physiol* 2000;278:R824–R830.

64. Abbondanzo SJ, Cullinan EB, McIntyre K, et al. Reproduction in mice lacking a functional type 1 IL-1 receptor. *Endocrinology* 1996;137:3598–3601.

65. Vargas SJ, Naprta A, Glaccum M, et al. Interleukin-6 expression and histomorphometry of bones from mice deficient in receptors for interleukin-1 or tumor necrosis factor. *J Bone Miner Res* 1996;11:1736–1744.

66. Man MQ, Wood L, Elias PM, et al. Cutaneous barrier repair and pathophysiology following barrier disruption in IL-1 and TNF type I receptor deficient mice. *Exp Dermatol* 1999;8:261–266.

67. Cullinan EB, Kwee L, Nunes P, et al. IL-1 receptor accessory protein is an essential component of the IL-1 receptor. *J Immunol* 1998;161:5614–5620.

68. Rosenbaum JT, Han YB, Park JM, et al. Tumor necrosis factor–alpha is not essential in endotoxin induced eye inflammation: studies in cytokine receptor deficient mice. *J Rheumatol* 1998;25:2408–2416.

69. Shornick LP, De Togni P, Mariathasan S, et al. Mice deficient in IL-1beta manifest impaired contact hypersensitivity to trinitrochlorobenzone. *J Exp Med* 1996;183:1427–1436.

70. Lorenzo JE, Naprta A, Rao Y, et al. Mice lacking the type I interleukin-1 receptor do not lose bone mass after ovariectomy. *Endocrinology* 1998;139:3022–3025.

71. Novick D, Kim S-H, Fantuzzi G, et al. Interleukin-18 binding protein: a novel modulator of the Th1 cytokine response. *Immunity* 1999;10:127–136.

72. Gayle MA, Slack JL, Bonnert TP, et al. Cloning of a putative ligand for the T1/ST2 receptor. *J Biol Chem* 1996;271:5784–5789.

73. Moritz D, Rodewald H-R, Gheysclinck J, et al. The IL-1 receptor–related T1 antigen is expressed on immature and mature mast cells an on fetal blood mast cell progenitors. *J Immunol* 1998;161:4866–4874.

74. Parnet P, Garka KE, Bonnert TP, et al. IL-1Rrp is a novel receptor-like molecule similar to the type I interleukin-1 receptor and its homologues T1/ST2 and IL-1R AcP. *J Biol Chem* 1996;271:3967–3970.

75. Torigoe K, Ushio S, Okura T, et al. Purification and characterization of the human interleukin-18 receptor. *J Biol Chem* 1997;272:25737–25742.

76. Debets R, Timans JC, Homey B, et al. Two novel IL-1 family members, IL-1 delta and IL-1 epsilon, function as an antagonist and agonist of NF-kappa B activation through the orphan IL-1 receptor–related protein 2. *J Immunol* 2001;167:1440–1446.

77. Born TL, Thomassen E, Bird TA, et al. Cloning of a novel receptor subunit, AcPL, required for interleukin-18 signaling. *J Biol Chem* 1998;273:29445–29450.

78. Kim SH, Reznikov LL, Stuyt RJ, et al. Functional reconstitution and regulation of IL-18 activity by the IL-18R beta chain. *J Immunol* 2001;166:148–154.

79. Sana TR, Debets R, Timans JC, et al. Computational identification, cloning, and characterization of IL-1R9, a novel interleukin-1 receptor–like gene encoded over an unusually large interval of human chromosome Xq22.2–q22.3. *Genomics* 2000;69:252–262.

80. Carrie A, Jun L, Bienvenu T, et al. A new member of the IL-1 receptor family highly expressed in hippocampus and involved in X-linked mental retardation. *Nat Genet* 1999;23:25–31.

81. Bird TA, Gearing AJ, Saklatvala J. Murine interleukin-1 receptor: differences in binding properties between fibroblastic and thymoma cells and evidence for a two-chain receptor model. *FEBS Lett* 1987;225:21–26.

82. Scapigliati G, Ghiara P, Bartalini A, et al. Differential binding of IL-1α and IL-1β to receptors on B and T cells. *FEBS Lett* 1989;243:394–398.

83. Savage N, Puren AJ, Orencole SF, et al. Studies on IL-1 receptors on D10S T-helper cells: demonstration of two molecularly and antigenically distinct IL-1 binding proteins. *Cytokine* 1989;1:23–25.

84. Qwarnstrom EE, Page RC, Gillis S, et al. Binding, internalization, and intracellular localization of interleukin-1 beta in human diploid fibroblasts. *J Biol Chem* 1988;263:8261–8269.

85. Sims JE, March CJ, Cosman D, et al. cDNA expression cloning of the IL-1 receptor, a member of the immunoglobulin superfamily. *Science* 1988;241:585–589.

86. Chizzonite R, Truitt T, Kilian PL, et al. Two high-affinity interleukin 1 receptors represent separate gene products. *Proc Natl Acad Sci U S A* 1989;86:8029–8033.

87. Gay NJ, Keith FJ. *Drosophila* Toll and IL-1 receptor. *Nature* 1991;351:355–356.

88. Beutler B. Autoimmunity and apoptosis. The Crohn's connection. *Immunity* 2001;15:5–14.

89. Heguy A, Baldari CT, Macchia G, et al. Amino acids conserved in interleukin-1 receptors and the *Drosophila* Toll protein are essential for IL-1R signal transduction. *J Biol Chem* 1992;267:2605–2609.

90. Greenfeder SA, Nunes P, Kwee L, et al. Molecular cloning and characterization of a second subunit of the interleukin-1 receptor complex. *J Biol Chem* 1995;270:13757–13765.

91. Casadio R, Frigimelica E, Bossu P, et al. Model of interaction of the IL-1 receptor accessory protein IL-1RAcP with the IL-1beta/IL-1R(I) complex. *FEBS Lett* 2001;499:65–68.

92. Rosoff PM, Savage N, Dinarello CA. Interleukin-1 stimulates

diacylglycerol production in T lymphocytes by a novel mechanism. *Cell* 1988;54:73–81.

93. Shirakawa F, Tanaka Y, Ota T, et al. Expression of interleukin-1 receptors on human peripheral T-cells. *J Immunol* 1987;138:4243–4248.

94. Stylianou E, O'Neill LAJ, Rawlinson L, et al. Interleukin-1 induces NFκB through its type I but not type II receptor in lymphocytes. *J Biol Chem* 1992;267:15836–15841.

95. Yoon DY, Dinarello CA. Antibodies to domains II and III of the IL-1 receptor accessory protein inhibit IL-1b activity but not binding: regulation of IL-1 responses is via type I receptor, not the accessory protein. *J Immunol* 1998;160:3170–3179.

96. Gallis B, Prickett KS, Jackson J, et al. IL-1 induces rapid phosphorylation of the IL-1 receptor. *J Immunol* 1989;143:3235–3240.

97. Guida S, Heguy A, Melli M. The chicken IL-1 receptor: differential evolution of the cytoplasmic and extracellular domains. *Gene* 1992;111:239–243.

98. Orencole SF, Dinarello CA. Characterization of a subclone (D10S) of the D10.G4.1 helper T-cell line which proliferates to attomolar concentrations of interleukin-1 in the absence of mitogens. *Cytokine* 1989;1:14–22.

99. Symons JA, Eastgate JA, Duff GW. Purification and characterization of a novel soluble receptor for interleukin-1. *J Exp Med* 1991;174:1251–1254.

100. Symons JA, Young PA, Duff GW. The soluble interleukin-1 receptor: ligand binding properties and mechanisms of release. *Lymphokine Cytokine Res* 1993;12:381.

101. Ghiara P, Armellini D, Scapigliati G, et al. Biological role of the IL-1 receptor type II as defined by a monoclonal antibody. *Cytokine* 1991;3:473(abst).

102. McMahon CJ, Slack JL, Mosley B, et al. A novel IL-1 receptor cloned form B cells by mammalian expression is expressed in many cell types. *EMBO J* 1991;10:2821–2832.

103. Colotta F, Dower SK, Sims JE, et al. The type II "decoy" receptor: a novel regulatory pathway for interleukin-1. *Immunol Today* 1994;15:562–566.

104. Colotta F, Re F, Muzio M, et al. Interleukin-1 type II receptor: a decoy target for IL-1 that is regulated by IL-4. *Science* 1993;261:472–475.

105. Alcami A, Smith GL. A soluble receptor for interleukin-1b encoded by vaccinia virus: a novel mechanism of virus modulation of the host response to infection. *Cell* 1992;71:153–167.

106. Spriggs MK, Hruby DE, Maliszewski CR, et al. Vaccinia and cowpox viruses encode a novel secreted interleukin-1 binding protein. *Cell* 1992;71:145–152.

107. Dower SK, Fanslow W, Jacobs C, et al. Interleukin-1 antagonists. *Therapeutic Immunol* 1994;1:113–122.

108. Bristulf J, Gatti S, Malinowsky D, et al. Interleukin-1 stimulates the expression of type I and type II interleukin-1 receptors in the rat insulinoma cell line Rinm5F; sequencing a rat type II interleukin-1 receptor cDNA. *Eur Cyokine Netw* 1994;5:319–330.

109. Arend WP, Malyak M, Smith MF, et al. Binding of IL-1α, IL-1β, and IL-1 receptor antagonist by soluble IL-1 receptors and levels of soluble IL-1 receptors in synovial fluids. *J Immunol* 1994;153:4766–4774.

110. Sims JE, Giri JG, Dower SK. The two interleukin-1 receptors play different roles in IL-1 activities. *Clin Immunol Immunopathol* 1994;72:9–14.

111. Symons JA, Young PA, Duff GW. Differential release and ligand binding of type II IL-1 receptors. *Cytokine* 1994;6:555(abst).

112. Lang D, Knop J, Wesche H, et al. The type II IL-1 receptor interacts with the IL-1 receptor accessory protein: a novel mechanism of regulation of IL-1 responsiveness. *J Immunol* 1998;161:6871–6877.

113. Neumann D, Kollewe C, Martin MU, et al. The membrane form of the type II IL-1 receptor accounts for inhibitory function. *J Immunol* 2000;165:3350–3357.

114. Sims JE, Painter SL, Gow IR. Genomic organization of the type I and type II IL-1 receptors. *Cytokine* 1995;7:483–490.

115. Ye K, Dinarello CA, Clark BD. Identification of the promoter region of the human interleukin 1 type I receptor gene: multiple initiation sites, high G+C content, and constitutive expression. *Proc Natl Acad Sci U S A* 1993;90:2295–2299.

116. Koch K-C, Ye K, Clark BD, et al. Interleukin 4 (IL) 4 up-regulates gene and surface IL-1 receptor type I in murine T helper type 2 cells. *Eur J Immunol* 1992;22:153–157.

117. Ye K, Vannier E, Clark BD, et al. Three distinct promoters direct transcription of different 5′ untranslated regions of the human interleukin 1 type I receptor: a possible mechanism for control of translation. *Cytokine* 1996;8:421–429.

118. Kim S-H, Eisenstein M, Reznikov L, et al. Structural requirements of six naturally occurring isoforms of the interleukin-18 binding protein to inhibit interleukin-18. *Proc Natl Acad Sci U S A* 2000;97:1190–1195.

119. Novick D, Schwartsburd B, Pinkus R, et al. A novel IL-18BP ELISA shows elevated serum IL-18BP in sepsis and extensive decrease of free IL-18. *Cytokine* 2001;14:334–342.

120. Hopp TP. Evidence from sequence information that the interleukin-1 receptor is a transmembrane GTPase. *Protein Sci* 1995;4:1851–1859.

121. Mitchum JL, Sims JE. IIP1: a novel human that interacts with the IL-1 receptor. *Cytokine* 1995;7:595(abst).

122. Croston GE, Cao Z, Goeddel DV. NFκB activation by interleukin-1 requires an IL-1 receptor–associated protein kinase activity. *J Biol Chem* 1995;270:16514–16517.

123. Cao Z, Xiong J, Takeuchi M, et al. Interleukin-1 receptor activating kinase. *Nature* 1996;383:443–446.

124. Huang J, Gao X, Li S, et al. Recruitment of IRAK to the interleukin 1 receptor complex requires interleukin 1 receptor accessory protein. *Proc Natl Acad Sci U S A* 1997;94:12829–12832.

125. Cao Z. Signal transduction of interleukin-1. *Eur Cytokine Netw* 1998;9:378(abst).

126. Rosoff PM. Characterization of the interleukin-1-stimulated phospholipase C activity in human T lymphocytes. *Lymphokine Res* 1989;8:407–413.

127. Schutze S, Machleidt T, Kronke M. The role of diacylglycerol and ceramide in tumor necrosis factor and interleukin-1 signal transduction. *J Leukoc Biol* 1994;56:533–541.

128. Andrieu N, Salvayre R, Levade T. Evidence against involvement of the acid lysosomal sphingomyelinase in the tumor necrosis factor and interleukin-1-induced sphingomyelin cycle and cell proliferation in human fibroblasts. *Biochem J* 1994;303:341–345.

129. Bomalaski JS, Steiner MR, Simon PL, et al. IL-1 increases phospholipase A2 activity, expression of phospholipase A2-activating protein, and release of linoleic acid from the murine T helper cell line EL-4. *J Immunol* 1992;148:155–160.

130. Kolesnick R, Golde DW. The sphingomyelin pathway in tumor necrosis factor and interleukin-1 signalling. *Cell* 1994;77:325–328.

131. Gronich J, Konieczkowski M, Gelb MH, et al. Interleukin-1α causes a rapid activation of cytosolic phospholipase A2 by phosphorylation in rat mesangial cells. *J Clin Invest* 1994;93:1224–1233.

132. Ye K, Koch K-C, Clark BD, et al. Interleukin-1 down regulates gene and surface expression of interleukin-1 receptor type I by destabilizing its mRNA whereas interleukin-2 increases its expression. *Immunol* 1992;75:427–434.

133. Mizel SB. Cyclic AMP and interleukin-1 signal transduction. *Immunol Today* 1990;11:390–391.

134. Munoz E, Beutner U, Zubiaga A, et al. IL-1 activates two separate signal transduction pathways in T helper type II cells. *J Immunol* 1990;144:964–969.

135. Kester M, Siomonson MS, Mene P, et al. Interleukin-1 generate transmembrane signals from phospholipids through novel pathways in cultured rat mesangial cells. *J Clin Invest* 1989;83:718–723.

136. Mathias S, Younes A, Kan C-C, et al. Activation of the sphingomyelin signaling pathway in intact EL4 cells and in a cell-free system by IL-1β. *Science* 1993;259:519–522.

137. Huwiler A, Pfeilschifter J. Interleukin-1 stimulates *de novo* synthesis of mitogen-activated protein kinase in glomerular mesangial cells. *FEBS Lett* 1994;350:135–138.

138. Freshney NW, Rawlinson L, Guesdon F, et al. Interleukin-1 activates a novel protein cascade that results in the phosphorylation of hsp27. *Cell* 1994;78:1039–1049.

139. Kracht M, Truong O, Totty NF, et al. Interleukin-1α activates two forms of p54a mitogen-activated protein kinase in rabbit liver. *J Exp Med* 1994;180:2017–2027.

140. Kuno K, Okamoto S, Hirose K, et al. Structure and function of the intracellular portion of the mouse interleukin-1 receptor (type I). *J Biol Chem* 1993;268:13510–13518.

141. Martin M, Bol GF, Eriksson A, et al. Interleukin-1–induced activation of a protein kinase co-precipitating with the type I interleukin-1 receptor in T-cells. *Eur J Immunol* 1994;24:1566–1571.

142. Suzuki N, Suzuki S, Duncan GS, et al. Severe impairment of interleukin-1 and Toll-like receptor signalling in mice lacking IRAK-4. *Nature* 2002;416:750–756.

143. Wesche H, Korherr C, Kracht M, et al. The interleukin-1 receptor accessory protein is essential for IL-1–induced activation of interleukin-1 receptor–associated kinase (IRAK) and stress-activated protein kinases (SAP kinases). *J Biol Chem* 1997;272:7727–7731.

144. Malinin NL, Boldin MP, Kovalenko AV, et al. MAP3K-related kinase involved in NF-kappaB induction by TNF, CD95 and IL-1. *Nature* 1997;385:540–544.

145. DiDonato JA, Hayakawa M, Rothwarf DM, et al. A cytokine-responsive I kappaB kinase that activates the transcription factor NF-kappaB. *Nature* 1997;388:548–554.

146. Lomaga MA, Yeh WC, Sarosi I, et al. TRAF6 deficiency results in osteopetrosis and defective interleukin-1, CD40, and LPS signaling. *Genes Dev* 1999;13:1015–1024.

147. Kojima H, Takeuchi M, Ohta T, et al. Interleukin-18 activates the IRAK-TRAF6 pathway in mouse EL-4 cells. *Biochem Biophys Res Commun* 1998;244:183–186.

148. Robinson D, Shibuya K, Mui A, et al. IGIF does not drive Th1 development but synergizes with IL-12 for interferon-γ production and activates IRAK and NFκB. *Immunity* 1997;7:571–581.

149. Adachi O, Kawai T, Takeda K, et al. Targeted disruption of the MyD88 gene results in loss of IL-1– and IL-18–mediated function. *Immunity* 1998;9:143–150.

150. Shapiro L, Puren AJ, Barton HA, et al. Interleukin-18 stimulates HIV type 1 in monocytic cells. *Proc Natl Acad Sci U S A* 1998;95:12550–12555.

151. Matsushima K, Kobayashi Y, Copeland TD, et al. Phosphorylation of a cytosolic 65-kDa protein induced by interleukin-1 in glucocorticoid pretreated normal human peripheral blood mononuclear leukocytes. *J Immunol* 1987;139:3367–3374.

152. O'Neill LAJ. Towards an understanding of the signal transduction pathways for interleukin-1. *Biochim Biophys Acta* 1995;1266:31–44.

153. Bird TA, Sleath PR, de Roos PC, et al. Interleukin-1 represents a new modality for the activation of extracellular signal-related kinases/microtubule-associated protein-2 kinases. *J Bio Chem* 1991;266:22661–22670.

154. Stylianou E, Saklatvala J. Interleukin-1. *Int J Biochem Cell Biol* 1998;30:1075–1079.

155. Finch A, Holland P, Cooper J, et al. Selective activation of JNK/SAPK by interleukin-1 in rabbit liver is mediated by MKK7. *FEBS Lett* 1997;418:144–148.

156. Galcheva-Gargova Z, Dérijard B, Wu I-H, et al. An osmosensing signal transduction pathway in mammalian cells. *Science* 1994;265:806–809.

157. Han J, Lee J-D, Bibbs L, et al. A MAP kinase targeted by endotoxin and hyperosmolarity in mammalian cells. *Science* 1994;265:808–811.

158. Shapiro L, Dinarello CA. Osmotic regulation of cytokine synthesis *in vitro*. *Proc Natl Acad Sci U S A* 1995;92:12230–12234.

159. Zhang S, Han J, Sells MA, et al. Rho family GTPases regulate p38 mitogen-activated protein kinase through the downstream mediator Pak1. *J Biol Chem* 1995;270:23934–23936.

160. Lee JC, Laydon JT, McDonnell PC, et al. A protein kinase involved in the regulation of inflammatory cytokine biosynthesis. *Nature* 1994;372:739–747.

161. Han J, Richter B, Li Z, et al. Molecular cloning of human p38 MAP kinase. *Biochim Biophys Acta* 1995;1265:224–227.

162. Shapiro L, Heidenreich KA, Meintzer MK, et al. Role of p38 mitogen-activated protein kinase in HIV type 1 production *in vitro*. *Proc Natl Acad Sci U S A* 1998;95:7422–7426.

163. Cuenda A, Rouse J, Doza YN, et al. SB 203580 is a specific inhibitor of a MAP kinase homologue which is stimulated by stresses and interleukin-1. *FEBS Letters* 1995;364:229–233.

164. Willenberg HS, Stratakis CA, Marx C, et al. Aberrant interleukin-1 receptors in a cortisol-secreting adrenal adenoma causing Cushing's syndrome. *N Engl J Med* 1998;339:27–31.

165. Fanslow WC, Sims JE, Sassenfeld H, et al. Regulation of alloreactivity *in vivo* by a soluble form of the interleukin-1 receptor. *Science* 1990;248:739–742.

166. Jacobs CA, Baker PE, Roux ER, et al. Experimental autoimmune encephalomyelitis is exacerbated by IL-1a and suppressed by soluble IL-1 receptor. *J Immunol* 1991;146:2983–2989.

167. Netea MG, Kullberg BJ, Boerman OC, et al. Soluble murine IL-1 receptor type I induces release of constitutive IL- 1 alpha. *J Immunol* 1999;162:4876–4881.

168. Nicoletti F, Di Marco R, Barcellini W, et al. Protection from experimental autoimmune diabetes in the non-obese diabetic mouse with soluble interleukin-1 receptor. *Eur J Immunol* 1994;24:1843–1847.

169. Dinarello CA. Biological basis for interleukin-1 in disease. *Blood* 1996;87:2095–2147.

170. Granowitz EV, Porat R, Mier JW, et al. Hematological and immunomodulatory effects of an interleukin-1 receptor antagonist coinfusion during low-dose endotoxemia in healthy humans. *Blood* 1993;82:2985–2990.

171. Preas HL 2nd, Reda D, Tropea M, et al. Effects of recombinant soluble type I interleukin-1 receptor on human inflammatory responses to endotoxin. *Blood* 1996;88:2465–2472.

172. Drevlow BE, Lovis R, Haag MA, et al. Recombinant human interleukin-1 receptor type I in the treatment of patients with active rheumatoid arthritis. *Arthritis Rheum* 1996;39:257–265.

173. Bernstein SH, Fay J, Frankel S, et al. A phase I study of recombinant human soluble interleukin-1 receptor (rhu IL-1R) in patients with relapsed and refractory acute myeloid leukemia. *Cancer Chemother Pharmacol* 1999;43:141–144.

174. Pitti RM, Marsters SA, Haak-Frendscho M, et al. Molecular and biological properties of an interleukin-1 receptor immunoadhesin. *Mol Immunol* 1994;31:1345–1351.

175. Crown J, Jakubowski A, Kemeny N, et al. A phase I trial of recombinant human interleukin-1β alone and in combination with myelosuppressive doses of 5-fluorouracil in patients with gastrointestinal cancer. *Blood* 1991;78:1420–1427.

176. Smith JW, Longo D, Alford WG, et al. The effects of treatment with interleukin-1α on platelet recovery after high-dose carboplatin. *N Engl J Med* 1993;328:756–761.

177. Seckinger P, Lowenthal JW, Williamson K, et al. A urine inhibitor of interleukin-1 activity that blocks ligand binding. *J Immunol* 1987;139:1546–1549.

178. Arend WP, Joslin FG, Massoni RJ. Effects of immune complexes on production by human monocytes of interleukin 1 or an interleukin 1 inhibitor. *J Immunol* 1985;134:3868–3875.

179. Eisenberg SP, Evans RJ, Arend WP, et al. Primary structure and functional expression from complementary DNA of a human interleukin-1 receptor antagonist. *Nature* 1990;343:341–346.

180. Granowitz EV, Porat R, Mier JW, et al. Pharmacokinetics, safety, and immunomodulatory effects of human recombinant interleukin-1 receptor antagonist in healthy humans. *Cytokine* 1992;4:353–360.

181. Hirsch E, Irikura VM, Paul SM, et al. Functions of interleukin 1 receptor antagonist in gene knockout and overproducing mice. *Proc Natl Acad Sci U S A* 1996;93:11008–11013.

182. Bendele A, McAbee T, Sennello G, et al. Efficacy of sustained blood levels of interleukin-1 receptor antagonist in animal models of arthritis: comparison of efficacy in animal models with human clinical data. *Arthritis Rheum* 1999;42:498–506.

183. Bakker AC, Joosten LA, Arntz OJ, et al. Prevention of murine collagen-induced arthritis in the knee and ipsilateral paw by local expression of human interleukin-1 receptor antagonist protein in the knee. *Arthritis Rheum* 1997;40:893–900.

184. Fukumoto T, Matsukawa A, Ohkawara S, et al. Administration of neutralizing antibody against rabbit IL-1 receptor antagonist exacerbates lipopolysaccharide-induced arthritis in rabbits. *Inflamm Res* 1996;45:479–485.

185. Neidhart M, Gay RE, Gay S. Anti–interleukin-1 and anti-CD44 interventions producing significant inhibition of cartilage destruction in an *in vitro* model of cartilage invasion by rheumatoid arthritis synovial fibroblasts. *Arthritis Rheum* 2000;43:1719–1728.

186. Campion GV, Lebsack ME, Lookabaugh J, et al. Dose-range and dose-frequency study of recombinant human interleukin-1 receptor antagonist in patients with rheumatoid arthritis. *Arthritis Rheum* 1996;39:1092–1101.

187. Genant HK, Bresnihan B, Ng E, et al. Treatment with anakinra reduces the rate of joint destruction and shows accelerated benefit in the second 6 months of treatment for patients with rheumatoid arthritis. *Ann Rheumat Dis* 2001;40(Suppl 1):169(abst).

188. Torcia M, Lucibello M, Vannier E, et al. Modulation of osteoclast-activating factor activity of multiple myeloma bone marrow cells by different interleukin-1 inhibitors. *Exp Hematol* 1996;24:868–874.

189. Dewhirst FE, Stashenko PP, Mole JE, et al. Purification and partial sequence of human osteoclast-activating factor: identity with interleukin 1 beta. *J Immunol* 1985;135:2562–2568.

190. Vidal-Vanaclocha F, Fantuzzi G, Mendoza L, et al. IL-18 regulates IL-1beta–dependent hepatic melanoma metastasis via vascular cell adhesion molecule–1. *Proc Natl Acad Sci U S A* 2000;97:734–739.

191. Boutin H, LeFeuvre RA, Horai R, et al. Role of IL-1alpha and IL-1beta in ischemic brain damage. *J Neurosci* 2001;21:5528–5534.

192. Huang D, Shi FD, Giscombe R, et al. Disruption of the IL-1beta gene diminishes acetylcholine receptor–induced immune responses in a murine model of myasthenia gravis. *Eur J Immunol* 2001;31:225–232.

193. Miwa K, Asano M, Horai R, et al. Caspase 1–independent IL-1beta release and inflammation induced by the apoptosis inducer Fas ligand. *Nat Med* 1998;4:1287–1292.

194. Parsey MV, Kaneko D, Shenkar R, et al. Neutrophil apoptosis in the lung after hemorrhage or endotoxemia: apoptosis and migration are independent of IL-1beta. *Clin Immunol* 1999;91:219–225.

195. Seki T, Healy AM, Fletcher DS, et al. IL-1beta mediates induction of hepatic type 1 plasminogen activator inhibitor in response to local tissue injury. *Am J Physiol* 1999;277:G801–G809.

196. Shornick LP, Bisarya AK, Chaplin DD. IL-1beta is essential for Langerhans cell activation and antigen delivery to the lymph nodes during contact sensitization: evidence for a dermal source of IL-1beta. *Cell Immunol* 2001;211:105–112.

CHAPTER 26

Chemokines

Philip M. Murphy

Introduction
A Brief History of Chemokines
Molecular Organization of the Chemokine System
  Structural Classification and Nomenclature · Immunologic Classification · Chemokine System Genes and Evolution · The Issue of Chemokine Redundancy
Chemokine Structural Biology
  The Chemokine Fold · Chemokine Receptor Structure · Chemokine Presentation Mechanisms
Leukocyte Responses to Chemokines
  Adhesion and Migration · Cytotoxicity · Proliferation and Apoptosis
Chemokine Signaling Pathways
  G Protein Signaling · Gi-Dependent Effectors · Gi-Independent Effectors · Mechanisms of Gradient Sensing · Cross Talk
Regulation of Chemokine Action
  Expression · Processing · Targeting · Receptor Deactivation
Chemokine Regulation of Hematopoiesis
  CXCL12 (SDF-1) in Myelopoiesis and B-Lymphopoiesis · Myelosuppressive Chemokines · T-Lymphopoiesis · Posting of Phagocytes in Peripheral Tissues
Chemokine Regulation of the Immune Response
  Innate Immunity · Adaptive Immunity
Chemokines and Disease
  Immunodeficiency/Infectious Disease · Acute Neutrophil-Mediated Inflammatory Disorders · Transplant Rejection · Autoimmunity · Atherosclerosis · Asthma · Cancer
Chemokine Mimicry in Infectious Disease
  Herpesvirus and Poxvirus Infection · HIV · Malaria
Therapeutic Applications
  Chemokines and Chemokine Receptors as Targets for Drug Development · Chemokines as Biological Response Modifiers
Conclusions
Acknowledgments
References
Appendices

INTRODUCTION

The immune system consists of diverse subpopulations of leukocytes, which unlike specialized cells in other physiologic systems must migrate through all tissues of the body for the whole system to work. At the molecular level, migration is coordinated in large part by the chemokines, a superfamily of specialized cytokines that directly and differentially chemoattract specific subsets of leukocytes. Some chemokines also regulate leukocyte development, differentiation, and effector functions, and some have functions unrelated to the immune system, such as organ development and regulation of angiogenesis. However, leukocytes are the most general target, migration the most general cellular response, and immunoregulation the most general biological function for these molecules. In addition to promoting normal host defense and repair, chemokines also have a dark side. They may act inappropriately and destructively as pathologic amplifiers of inflammation in the setting of immunologically mediated disease. They may also play a role in cancer through effects on tumor-cell proliferation, angiogenesis, and metastasis. In addition, many pathogens, including HIV, various herpesviruses and poxviruses, and the malaria-causing protozoan *Plasmodium vivax,* have evolved mechanisms to exploit or block the chemokine system to promote infection and disease. Together these pathologic roles have focused attention on chemokine receptors as potential drug targets. In addition, chemokines themselves have translational potential as biological response modifiers, for example as adjuvants in DNA vaccines. To date, over 100 chemokines, chemokine receptors, and viral chemokine mimics have been discovered, each having its own interesting place in immunology. This chapter will introduce the main principles of chemokine structure and function, and then focus on selected aspects of immunoregulation and disease in which individual chemokines have been found to play key roles *in vivo*. The figures and appendices provide core information about each chemokine and its receptor.

A BRIEF HISTORY OF CHEMOKINES

Chemokine research began quietly in 1977 with the discovery of CXCL4 (originally called platelet factor 4 [PF-4]), a protein stored in platelet α granules. From 1983 to 1987, several cDNAs encoding proteins related to CXCL4 were discovered by investigators searching for cell differentiation or activation genes, and were recognized as a structurally related molecular family before any functions were established (1–4). The discovery of CXCL8 (IL-8) in 1987 was the Big Bang in chemokine research and a landmark in immunology, because this molecule was the first leukocyte subtype–selective chemoattractant found, and the first chemokine shown to have chemotactic activity. This focused the search for chemokine function correctly on leukocyte chemotaxis and stimulated a search for new family members. Soon thereafter the first monocyte-, T cell-, and eosinophil-targeted chemokines were discovered in rapid succession. Database mining has been used as a powerful strategy to identify additional members of the family, which currently stands at 43 human members, the largest number of structurally related cytokines by far (5). Meanwhile, a conceptual model for how chemokines might work *in vivo* was formulated. Known as the multistep paradigm of leukocyte trafficking, this model postulates that chemoattractants and adhesion molecules coordinately regulate interactions between leukocytes and endothelial cells, thereby allowing both transendothelial migration and differential targeting to specific anatomic sites (6,7). The term "chemokine," a neologism derived from "chemotactic cytokine," was coined in 1993 to identify the superfamily and to distinguish its members from other types of leukocyte chemoattractants, such as the "classical chemoattractants" (complement protein C5a, N-formylpeptides such as fMet-Leu-Phe [fMLF], and the endogenous lipid mediators leukotriene B4 and platelet-activating factor) (8,9).

In the early 1990s, as the role of chemokines in regulating inflammation became more and more apparent, many investigators began to consider them as promising drug targets. This view was reinforced when chemokine receptors were found to be members of the 7-transmembrane domain (7TM) protein family of G protein–coupled receptors (GPCRs) (10), a class of receptors that unlike cytokine receptors is highly amenable to blockade with small organic molecules. In fact, GPCRs are disease targets for a high proportion of non-antibiotic prescription drugs (11).

By 1996 the early era of chemokine research, which was focused on phagocytes, inflammation and innate immunity, merged with the beginning of a second era focused on adaptive immunity (12–16). Also in 1996, interest in the field exploded in an unanticipated direction when chemokines were found to suppress HIV replication by blocking viral usage of chemokine receptors, particularly CXCR4 and CCR5, for cell entry (17,18). The idea that pathogens could exploit the chemokine system was reinforced by the discovery of viral chemokine and chemokine receptor mimics encoded by herpesviruses and poxviruses (19–21), and usage of the Duffy antigen receptor for chemokines (DARC) by *P. vivax* as a cell entry factor in malaria (22). More recently, knockout mice, neutralizing antibodies, and receptor antagonists have been developed to study the biological roles of individual chemokines and chemokine receptors in animal models of disease (23).

MOLECULAR ORGANIZATION OF THE CHEMOKINE SYSTEM

The chemokine system consists of chemokine ligands, chemokine receptors, nonsignaling chemokine binding proteins, and nonchemokine chemokine receptor ligands (Fig. 1). All four types of components are also encoded by microbes, mainly viruses, which are discussed in a later section.

Structural Classification and Nomenclature

Chemokines are defined by amino-acid–sequence relatedness, not by function. They are subclassified into two large (CC and CXC) and two small (C and CX3C) groups based on the number and positioning of the most highly conserved amino acids, which are cysteines (Fig. 2). All chemokines have at least two conserved cysteines, and all but two have at least four. In the four-cysteine group, the first two, which are located close to the N-terminus, are either adjacent (CC) or else separated by either one (CXC) or three (CX3C) nonconserved amino acids. The C chemokines are exceptional since they have only Cys-2 and Cys-4. In human, there are at the time of this writing 1, 2, 16, and 24 known members of the CX3C, C, CXC, and CC groups, respectively. Sequence similarity is low, at <30%, between members of different groups, but ranges from ~30% to 99% among CC and CXC chemokines considered separately. The cysteine motifs are used as roots followed by "L" for ligand and a number (e.g., CXCL1) in a systematic nomenclature that was established to deal with the problem of competing aliases (24). When older nonstandard names are used in scientific communication, the standard name is customarily indicated the first time the nonstandard name is mentioned.

The CC and CXC chemokine groups can be further divided by structural similarities into subgroups, some of which have clear-cut functional correlates (Figures 3 and 4). The

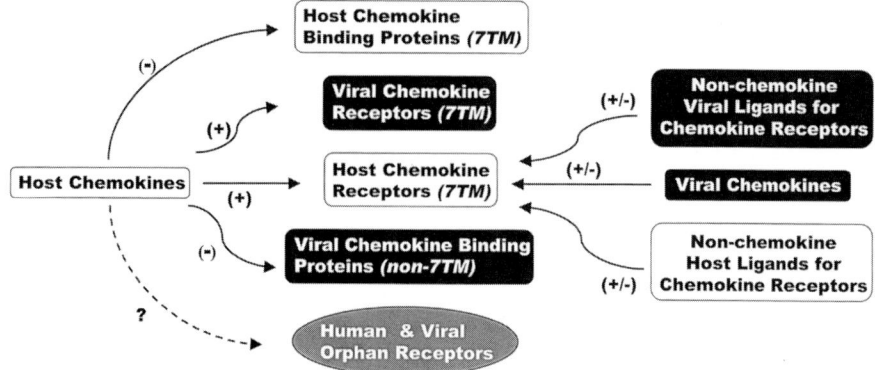

FIG. 1. Global organization of the chemokine network. Eight categories of molecules, four in vertebrates (*open boxes*) and four in viruses (*filled boxes*) have been identified. *Arrows* denote binding interactions; *(+)*, binding that leads to signal transduction and a cellular response; *(−)*, binding without cell signaling. Orphan receptors are theoretical proteins identified through genomics which have sequences that are most highly related to known chemokine receptors. (See text, tables, and appendices for properties of molecules in each category.)

strongest is the ELR subgroup of CXC chemokines (CXCL1, 2, 3, 5, 6, 7, and 8), which have >40% amino-acid identity, attract neutrophils, bind to the receptor CXCR2, and are angiogenic. ELR refers to a conserved Glu-Leu-Arg motif N-terminal to Cys-1, which is required for CXCR2 activation (25). Among the non–ELR-CXC chemokines, only CXCL12 (SDF-1 [stromal cell-derived factor-1]), which binds CXCR4, not CXCR2, attracts neutrophils; it is also angiogenic. CXCL9 (Mig [Monokine inducible by γ IFN]), CXCL10 (IP-10 [γ-IFN–inducible protein-10 kD]) and CXCL11 (I-TAC [interferon-inducible T cell α chemoattractant]) form a small subgroup with >40% amino acid identity that binds CXCR3 (26). They and CXCL4 (PF-4) are all strongly angiostatic (27).

The CC phylogenetic tree has two large subgroups, the MCPs (monocyte chemoattractant protein) and the MIPs (macrophage inflammatory protein), whose members typically chemoattract monocytes but not neutrophils, in addition to having differential cell targets (28). Two other subgroupings are not apparent from the phylogenetic tree. Members of the 6C subgroup (CCL7, 9, 15, 21, and 23) have two

additional cysteines, one in the C-terminal domain, the other either in the C-terminal domain or between conserved Cys-2 and Cys-3. CXCL16 and CX3CL1 (fractalkine) cross the cysteine motif boundary and form a unique multimodular subgroup. Each is comprised of an N-terminal chemokine domain, a mucin-like stalk, a transmembrane domain and a C-terminal cytoplasmic module (29). Shed forms exist for both. Tethered CX3CL1 functions as a direct adhesion molecule, and shed CX3CL1 is chemotactic.

Chemokine receptors are defined as molecules that modulate the activity of cellular signal transduction pathways upon binding chemokines. The 18 known human chemokine receptors and the classical chemoattractant receptors, but not receptors for other immunoregulatory cytokines, belong to the Type 1 rhodopsin family of 7TM GPCRs. (See *http://www.gpcr.org/7tm* for a website devoted to this superfamily.) Apart from odorant receptors, this is the largest known subfamily of GPCRs, itself the largest protein family from *C. elegans* to human.

In human, several chemokines and receptors pair monogamously, whereas the majority pair with varying degrees of

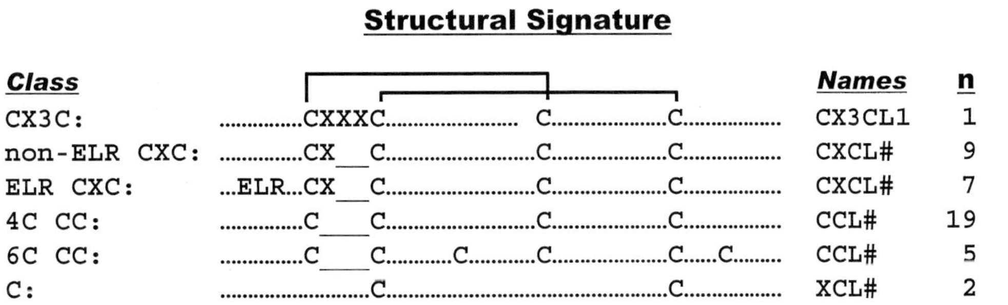

Structural Signature

Class		*Names*	n
CX3C:	...............CXXXC...................... C..................C................	CX3CL1	1
non-ELR CXC:	.............CX__C...................................C...................C................	CXCL#	9
ELR CXC:	...ELR...CX__C...............................C...................C................	CXCL#	7
4C CC:	.............C____C...............................C...................C................	CCL#	19
6C CC:	.............C____C.........C.........C...................C.....C........	CCL#	5
C:	..................................C.......................................C................	XCL#	2

FIG. 2. Chemokine classification and nomenclature. Chemokine classes are defined by the number and arrangement of conserved cysteines, as shown. *Brackets* link cysteines that form disulfide bonds. ELR, glu-leu-arg; X, an amino acid other than cysteine. The underscore is a spacer used to optimize the alignment. The N- and C-termini can vary considerably in length (not illustrated). For the molecules with four cysteines, there are approximately 24 amino acids between Cys-2 and Cys-3 and 15 amino acids between Cys-3 and Cys-4. At *right* are listed the nomenclature system and the number of human chemokines known in each class (n).

Classification		Nomenclature			Receptor	Main immunologic roles	Human chromosome
Family	Subgroup	Standard name	Common names				
			Human	Mouse			
CXC	ELR	CXCL1	GROα MGSA	KC and MIP-2	CXCR2	Innate immunity PMN-associated inflammation Angiogenic	4q21.1
		CXCL2	GROβ				
		CXCL3	GROγ				
	Non-ELR	CXCL4	PF-4	PF-4	ND	Angiostatic Procoagulant	
	ELR	CXCL5	ENA-78	LIX and ENA-78	CXCR2	Innate immunity PMN-associated Inflammation Angiogenic	
		CXCL6	GCP-2				
		CXCL7	NAP-2	Unknown			
		CXCL8	IL-8	Unknown	CXCR1 and CXCR2		
	Non-ELR	CXCL9	Mig	Mig	CXCR3	Th1 effector function Angiostatic	
		CXCL10	IP-10	CRG-2			
		CXCL11	I-TAC	I-TAC			
		CXCL12	SDF-1, PBSF	SDF-1, PBSF	CXCR4	Myelopoiesis B-lymphopoiesis Angiogenic	10q11.21
		CXCL13	BCA-1	BLC	CXCR5	B- and T-cell homing to follicles B1 cell homing to peritoneum, natural Ab production and body cavity immunity	4q21.1
		CXCL14	BRAK	BRAK	ND	MΦ migration	5q31.1
	ELR	CXCL15	Unknown	Lungkine	ND	Innate immunity PMN-associated inflammation	NA
		CXCL16	Sexckine	NA	CXCR6	T-cell and DC homing to spleen	17p13
CX3C	Non-ELR, multimodular	CX3CL1	Fractalkine	Neurotactin	CX3CR1	NK, MΦ and Th1 cell migration	16q13
C	NA	XCL1	Lymphotactin α	Lymphotactin	XCR1	CD62L^{lo} T effector cell migration	1q24.2
		XCL2	Lymphotactin β				

FIG. 3. The CXC, CX3C, and C chemokine families. Older and less commonly used synonyms can be found in Murphy et al. (31). NA, not applicable; ND, not determined. Acronyms are defined in text and in Appendix 1.

promiscuity (Appendix 1). The specificities of promiscuous ligand–receptor pairs may overlap considerably. However, each chemokine binds a unique set of receptors and each receptor binds a unique set of chemokines. Almost all chemokines are chemotactic agonists, but five have been reported that are agonists at one receptor and antagonists at another. CXCL9, 10, and 11 all activate CXCR3, which is associated with Th1 cells, but inhibit CCR3, which is associated with Th2 cells. The net result may be to favor a Th1 immune response. Conversely, CCL7 (MCP-3) and CCL11 (eotaxin) activate CCR3, but are antagonists at CCR5 and CCR2, respectively, which are associated with Th1 cells. The net result may be to favor a Th2 response.

The ligand binding, membrane anchoring, and signaling domains of chemokine receptors are all molded from a single polypeptide chain. Therefore, promiscuous ligands of a given receptor interact with the same receptor chain, which contrasts with other types of cytokines that share receptors,

such as IL-2, IL-13, and IL-15, where formation of multichain receptor complexes with shared signaling chains and unshared ligand binding chains is more typical (30). Receptor nomenclature, which is based on the fact that high-affinity ligands of promiscuous receptors are usually restricted to one chemokine subclass, is formulated as follows: ligand subclass root + R (for "receptor") + a number in order of discovery (31). An exception is the C chemokine receptor XCR1, where "X" distinguishes it from CR1, the previously assigned name for complement receptor 1. Accordingly, the XCR1 ligands are named XCL1 and XCL2 (lymphotactin α and β).

Three nonsignaling 7TM chemokine–binding proteins have been identified: Duffy, D6, and CCX CKR, the human homolog of the bovine gustatory receptor PPR1 (31,32). One theory is that these proteins function as anti-inflammatory chemokine buffers. Duffy is an extreme exception to the ligand rule since it binds with high affinity to many, but not all, CC and CXC chemokines.

Subgroup	Chemokine name			Receptors	Main immunologic roles	Human chromosome
	Standard name	Common names				
		Human	Mouse			
4 Cys	CCL1	I-309	TCA-3	CCR8	Th2 response	17q11-12
	CCL2	MCP-1	JE	CCR2	Innate immunity and Th2 effector response CD4$^+$ T cell differentiation	
	CCL3	MIP-1α LD78α MIP-1αS	MIP-1α	CCR1 CCR5	Innate immunity and Th1 effector response CD4 T cell differentiation	
	CCL3L1	LD78β MIP-1αP	Unknown	CCR1 CCR5	Probably similar to CCL3	
	CCL4	MIP-1β	MIP-1β	CCR5	Innate immunity and Th1 effector response	
	CCL5	RANTES	RANTES	CCR1, 3, 5	Innate immunity; Th1 and Th2 response	
	CCL6	Unknown	C10 MRP-1	CCR1	Th2 response	NA
6 Cys	CCL7	MCP-3	MARC	CCR1, 2, 3	Th2 response	17q11-12
4 Cys	CCL8	MCP-2	MCP-2	CCR1, 2, 3, 5	Th2 response	
6 Cys	CCL9/10	Unknown	MRP-2 CCF18	CCR1	ND	NA
4 Cys	CCL11	Eotaxin	Eotaxin	CCR3	Th2 response; eosinophil trafficking	17q11
	CCL12	NA	MCP-5	CCR2	Allergic inflammation	NA
	CCL13	MCP-4	Unknown	CCR1, 2, 3	Th2 response	17q11-12
	CCL14a	HCC-1	Unknown	CCR1, 5	ND	
	CCL14b	HCC-3	Unknown		ND	
6 Cys	CCL15	HCC-2, Lkn-1	Unknown	CCR1, 3	ND	
4 Cys	CCL16	HCC-4, LEC	Pseudogene	CCR1, 2, 5	ND	
	CCL17	TARC	TARC	CCR4	Th2 response	16q13
	CCL18	DC-CK1, PARC	Unknown	Unknown	DC attraction of naïve T cells	17q11.2
	CCL19	ELC, MIP-3β	ELC, MIP-3β	CCR7	T cell and DC homing to LN	9p13.3
	CCL20	LARC MIP-3α	LARC	CCR6	DC homing to Peyer's patch Humoral response	2q36.3
6 Cys	CCL21	SLC, 6Ckine	SLC	CCR7	T-cell and DC homing to lymph node	9p13.3
4 Cys	CCL22	MDC	ABCD-1	CCR4	Th2 response	16q13
6 Cys	CCL23	MPIF-1	Unknown	CCR1	ND	17q12
4 Cys	CCL24	Eotaxin-2, MPIF-2	Eotaxin-2	CCR3	Eosinophil migration	7q11.23
	CCL25	TECK	TECK	CCR9	Thymocyte migration Homing of T cells to gut	19p13.3
	CCL26	Eotaxin-3	Unknown	CCR3	Th2 response	7q11.23
	CCL27	CTACK, Eskine	CTACK, Eskine, ILC	CCR10	Homing of T cells to skin	9p13.3
	CCL28	MEC	MEC	CCR10	Homing of T cells to mucosal surfaces	5p12

FIG. 4. CC chemokine family. Older and less commonly used synonyms can be found in Murphy et al. (31). NA, not applicable; ND, not determined. Acronyms are defined in text and in Appendix 1.

Endogenous nonchemokine–chemokine receptor ligands have been identified. One example, tyrosyl tRNA synthetase, is normally involved in protein synthesis, but may also be involved in innate immunity since it has a cleavable subdomain containing an ELR motif that is able to specifically activate the CXCL8 receptor CXCR1 (33). A second, human β defensin 2 (HBD2), is an antimicrobial peptide released from activated neutrophils, but may also be involved in the transition from innate to adaptive immunity since it specifically chemoattracts immature dendritic cells via CCR6 (34). The immunoregulatory functions of these chemokine mimics have not been defined *in vivo*.

Immunologic Classification

With regard to leukocyte specificity, both broad- and narrow-spectrum chemokine–receptor pairs have been identified. Together they cover the full spectrum of leukocytes and can be divided into two main subsystems, *inflammatory* and *homeostatic,* according to whether they mainly control effector cell trafficking to inflamed sites or basal trafficking functions (Figures 3 and 4, Appendices 1 to 4).

In general, homeostatic chemokines, which are differentially and constitutively expressed in specific microenvironments of primary and secondary immune organs, differentially activate hematopoietic precursor cells, dendritic cells (DC) and lymphocytes via specific receptors (35–40). The inflammatory subsystem has separate components for innate and adaptive immunity. The innate components include ligands that are strongly induced by diverse tissue cells and leukocytes, and receptors that are constitutively expressed on myeloid cells and NK cells (41–43). In contrast, in the cellular arm of the adaptive immune system both the chemokine ligand and receptor tend to be strongly induced. Dynamic shifts in receptor expression occur during DC and NK-cell maturation and during B- and T-cell maturation, activation and differentiation. This is not an absolute classification, since constitutive chemokines may be further induced, and chemokines which are highly inducible in some cell types may be constitutively expressed in others. For example, CCL21 (SLC, secondary lymphoid tissue chemokine), which regulates T cell homing to lymph node via CCR7, can also be induced in damaged neurons and recruit microglial cells via CXCR3.

Chemokine System Genes and Evolution

Although the GPCR superfamily extends to yeast, chemokines have not been found earlier than lamprey (for updates and phylogenies see the Cytokine Family cDNA database at *http://cytokine.medic.kumamoto-u.ac.jp*). Both CC and CXC chemokines have been found in fish. Thus the chemokine system appears to have originated and rapidly diversified early in vertebrate evolution. Both ligand and receptor repertoires are large in the most thoroughly studied organisms, human and mouse, and their evolution is dynamic since there are numerous examples of lineage-specific genes (44). For example, mouse has only one copy of the genes

for CCL3 (MIP-1α) and CCL4 (MIP-1β), whereas multiple nonallelic human genes for CCL3 and CCL4 have been found that differ by as little as one amino acid in the open reading frame (ORF). Moreover, the number of these variants may differ among individuals.

Human chemokine genes are named using the formula SCY (for small cytokine) + a letter, "A," "B," "C," or "D," which corresponds to the CC, CXC, C, and CX3C chemokines, respectively, + a number, given in the order of discovery. Genes encoding inflammatory chemokines are found in two main clusters on human chromosomes 4q12-q21 (CXC) and 17q11-q21 (CC), whereas genes for homeostatic chemokines are scattered alone or in small clusters on chromosomes 1, 2, 5, 7, 9, 10 and 16 (44). The genes typically are ~4 kb long and usually have four exons in the case of CXC chemokines and three exons in the case of CC chemokines (45). The promoter is immediately upstream of exon 1, which encodes a leader sequence and a few amino acids of the mature peptide. Alternative splicing has been reported for several chemokines, but the significance is unknown. CCL14 (HCC-1, hemofiltrate CC chemokine-1) and CCL15 (HCC-2) are an exceptional example of tightly linked genes that give rise to a family of mono- and bicistronic transcripts.

The 18 chemokine receptor genes and 3 chemokine binding protein genes can be divided by chromosomal location into three groups: a large cluster on human chromosome 3p21-23 including multiple CCRs, CX3CR1, XCR1 and CXCR6, plus D6 and CCX CKR (n = 12); CXCR1, CXCR2 and one receptor pseudogene clustered on 2q34-q35; and CXCR3, 4 and 5, CCR6, 7 and 10 and Duffy, which are unclustered. With the exception of CCR9, genes in the two clustered groups lack introns in the ORF but have at least one and as many as 10 introns separating the promoter from the ORF. In contrast, an intron divides the N-terminus of the majority of unclustered receptor genes (CXCR3, 4 and 5; CCR6 and 10). Several of these undergo alternative splicing but the products appear to function similarly. CCR2 undergoes alternative splicing of a virtual intron in the C-terminal region of the ORF, but the two products have similar function and CCR2b appears to be the major expressed form.

The great majority of chemokine and chemokine receptor genes, like most other genes involved in immunity and inflammation, rank among the most rapidly evolving genes in phylogeny. The mechanism is unknown but positive selection due to pressures exerted by species-specific pathogens is a reasonable possibility (46). The concept of pathogen-shaped molecular evolution is not new, but it has been reinforced in the case of the chemokine system by the identification of the viral chemokine and chemokine receptor mimics (47).

With regard to horizontal evolution, variation in gene dosage among individuals has been observed for only a few chemokines (48). The *plt* locus (paucity of lymph node T cells) in mouse, which will be discussed in a later section, is an immunologically important example of this. In contrast, variation in gene sequence is common among individuals for most chemokine and chemokine receptors. However, the degree of polymorphism varies greatly among different genes. The most extreme and important example is the CCR2–CCR5 locus, in which combinations of common dimorphic single nucleotide polymorphisms (SNPs) in the CCR5 promoter with an SNP in the ORF of CCR2 named CCR2 V64I and a 32–base pair (bp) deletion in the ORF of CCR5 named CCR5Δ32 together form at least eight distinct haplotypes and in some cases affect HIV disease susceptibility (49,50).

The Issue of Chemokine Redundancy

Two chemokines that bind to the same receptor may still have highly specific biological roles. There are several potential explanations for this paradox. First, they may activate different signal transduction pathways through the same receptor, or, more likely, activate the same pathway with differential efficacy. Second, they may have additional differentially expressed receptors. Third, as the result of divergent regulatory elements in their promoters, they may each be expressed at different times and in different microenvironments (23,51–53). For example, CXCL7 (NAP-2, neutrophil-activating protein-2) and CXCL8 are both agonists for neutrophil CXCR2 but CXCL7 is stored in platelet α granules and released upon platelet activation, whereas CXCL8 is made by virtually all cell types upon gene induction by proinflammatory stimuli. There are few inflammatory processes in which only one chemokine is involved. They typically act cooperatively, on the same or separate cell types, but in a

hierarchical manner through promiscuous receptors. The net result is that there may be enough functional redundancy in the whole system such that loss of a single inflammatory chemokine or chemokine receptor, for example in a knock-out mouse, does not cause altered susceptibility to naturally acquired infections or other diseases, yet there may not be enough redundancy to handle a stronger stress when one particularly important component is missing. In contrast, homeostatic chemokines act much less redundantly and their loss has been associated with major defects in development and basal leukocyte homing.

CHEMOKINE STRUCTURAL BIOLOGY

The Chemokine Fold

Mature chemokine domains range from 66 to 111 amino acids in length. Variation is usually due to differences at the N- and C-termini, although some small insertions and deletions may also occur in more central parts of the sequence. Despite the wide range in primary structure, studies of representative C, CC, CXC, and CX3C chemokines, including one viral chemokine, have revealed a conserved compact globular tertiary structure composed of three antiparallel β sheets (β1, β2, and β3) folded into the shape of a Greek key, connected by short loops, and packed by hydrophobic interactions against an amphipathic C-terminal α helix (54) (Fig. 5). This helix is highly basic in most chemokines and may contain important

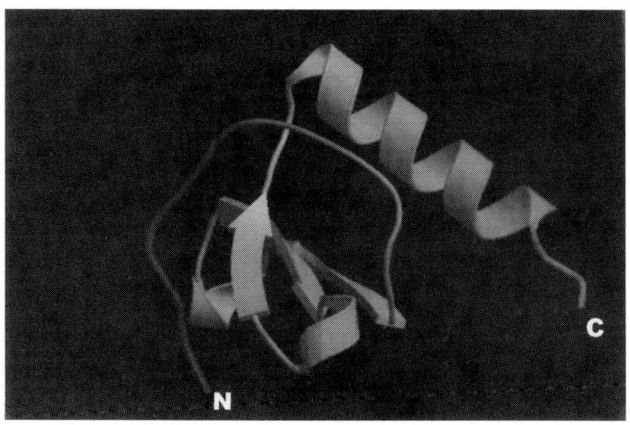
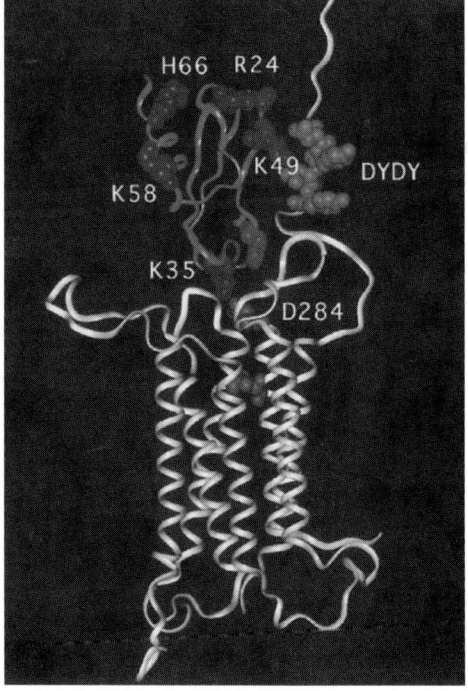

FIG. 5. Chemokine and chemokine receptor structure. **Left panel:** Ribbon structure of CXCL8 (from Protein Data Base [ID: 1IL8]). N, amino terminus; C, carboxy terminus. **Right panel:** Structure of CCL2 monomer (shaded structure at top) bound to a molecular model of CCR2 (white structure at bottom) (From ref 64, with permission). CCR2 amino acids important for ligand binding include DYDY in the N-terminus and D284 in TMD7. In the model, R24 and K49 of CCL2 bind to DYDY domain, K35 binds to D284 and H66 and K58 side chains point away from the structure for potential interaction with GAGs.

determinants of glycosaminoglycan (GAG) binding. The $\beta 1$-strand is preceded by 20 to 30 amino acids, which include Cys-1 and Cys-2. Preceding Cys-1 and Cys-2 is an unordered domain, designated the N-terminal domain, which is variable in length and critical for receptor activation. The ELR motif is located here. Between these cysteines and the $\beta 1$-sheet is the so-called N-loop region followed by a single turn of a 3_{10} helix, which are important for receptor binding. Cys-3 and Cys-4 are located in the $\beta 1$-$\beta 2$ loop and the $\beta 3$ strand, respectively.

Chemokines are very stable in biological fluids, in part because of disulfide bonds formed between Cys-1 and -3 and Cys-2 and -4 (55). Some members of the 6C subfamily of CC chemokines have a third disulfide bond tethering the C-terminal α helix to the β sheet, but this does not appear to be essential for folding or function (45). The single disulfide in XCL1 is sufficient to stabilize the fold (56).

Three major types of quaternary structure have been observed: monomers, dimers, and tetramers. Two distinct dimer types have been found: the compact CXCL8 type, common to many CXC chemokines, which consists of a six-strand antiparallel β sheet due to interaction between the $\beta 1$ strands of the monomers, and the extended CCL4 (MIP-1β) type, common to many CC chemokines, which consists of an antiparallel β sheet arrangement between the N-terminal domains and N-loops of the monomers. Although pure chemokines do not dimerize at concentrations close to the receptor binding constant, arguments in favor of the physiologic relevance of dimerization include evolutionary conservation of the dimerization interface, the ability of chemically forced dimers to function, and the ability of GAGs to promote dimerization at low chemokine concentrations (45,57). Recent evidence suggests that GAG induced dimerization of CCL2 may be critical for pro-inflammatory function *in vivo* (57a). Thus far, only one heteromultimer has been reported, a native heterodimer composed of CCL3 and CCL4 subunits purified from activated human monocytes and peripheral blood lymphocytes, but its structure is not defined (58).

Chemokine Receptor Structure

The protein sequences of chemokine receptors are colinear, and range between $\sim$340 to 370 amino acids in length and 25% to 80% in amino acid identity. Like other 7TM receptors, the N-terminus is extracellular, the C-terminus is intracellular, and there are seven predicted membrane spanning domains, three extracellular loops (ECL), and three intracellular loops (ICL). The least conserved amino acids segregate to the extracellular face of the receptor. Common features include an acidic and relatively short N-terminal segment; the sequence DRYLAIVHA (single letter code), or a variation of it, in ICL2; a short basic ICL3, and a cysteine in each of the four extracellular domains. None of these characteristics is unique to chemokine receptors, but the ensemble is uncommon in other types of GPCRs.

Four different post-translational modifications have been identified on chemokine receptors, some of which have been shown to affect function. Sulfation of a tyrosine in the N-terminal region of CCR5 is critical for ligand recognition (59). N-glycosylation motifs are commonly found in the N-terminus and ECL2. N-terminal N-glycosylation may be important for stable surface expression of CXCR2 (60), and for HIV strain specificity by CCR5 (61). On CCR5, the N-terminus is O-glycosylated. The C-terminal domain of CCR5 is palmitoylated, which tethers this domain to the plasma membrane forming a fourth ICL (62).

The tertiary structure of chemokine receptors is unknown, but a reasonable model can be constructed based on analogy with the crystal structure of rhodopsin (63). The TMDs are arranged like staves in a barrel in a counterclockwise orientation relative to the cell interior. Disulfide bonds, one linking ECL1 and ECL2, possibly another linking the N-terminus with ECL3, may stabilize the structure. The ICLs form a large docking surface for heterotrimeric G proteins and potentially other independent downstream effectors. The general model of the chemokine binding site features two functionally distinct subsites (Fig. 5). The first provides a docking site for the folded N-loop domain of the chemokine monomer, whereas the second, formed by the TMDs, accepts the chemokine's N-terminus when the first subsite is occupied, and is used for triggering. Subsite 1 accounts for high-affinity binding, which is the sum of multiple low-affinity interactions involving extracellular determinants on the receptor, which may vary in location for different ligands (64,65).

Chemokine Presentation Mechanisms

Most chemokines are produced locally and act locally, and are probably presented to receptors as tethered ligands bound to endothelial cells or extracellular matrix. A chemokine posted to an endothelial cell may have been directly produced by that cell or alternatively, as shown for CXCL8 and CCL19 (ELC [Epstein–Barr virus–induced receptor ligand chemokine]), it may have been produced by tissue cells and transcytosed through an endothelial cell (66,67). Thus, leukocytes are thought to crawl over tethered chemokines *in vivo*. Two main tethering mechanisms have been identified: GAGs and, in the case of the multimodular chemokines, intrinsic transmembrane domains. CCL3 and CCL5 (RANTES [regulated upon activation normal T cell expressed and secreted]), in particular, have been shown to be released from cytolytic granules of CD8$^+$ T cells precomplexed with GAGs, and GAGs modulate CXCL8 and CCL5 activity, but are not required for receptor binding (68,69). The chemokine-binding proteins could also conceivably present chemokines to receptors; however, this has not been demonstrated.

CELL RESPONSES TO CHEMOKINES

Adhesion and Migration

Adhesion and motility are both required for leukocyte migration out of the blood and lymphatics into and through tissue. These functions are mediated by combinations of selectins, $\beta 2$ integrins and chemokine receptors on the leukocyte, which together with their cognate ligands on endothelium have been proposed to form a molecular code directing leukocytes to specific microenvironments (6,7). Selectins and $\beta2$ integrins provide traction and the chemokine conveys direction as cells expressing only the appropriate set of receptors crawl between adjacent endothelial cells of high endothelial venules and through the tissue. First, the cell rolls across activated endothelium, a process mediated by weak, reversible binding of leukocyte selectins with their carbohydrate ligands on endothelial cells. Next, it encounters a chemokine posted on the surface of the endothelial cell, which induces activation and up-regulation of leukocyte $\beta2$ integrins. High-affinity binding of these molecules to ligands such as ICAM-1 on the endothelial cell causes the rolling cell to stop. The firmly adherent cell then becomes polarized as actin polymerizes at the leading edge (lamellipod), and motion is produced by coordinated cytoskeletal remodeling, myosin-based contraction at the trailing edge (uropod), release of the uropod from substrate, and membrane lipid movement. Transendothelial migration appears to be shear dependent and may require chemokine only on the luminal surface of the endothelial cell (70), whereas further navigation through tissue may require relays of chemokines. Chemotactic responses may be negative as well as positive, at least for CXCL12, which is a typical attractant at low concentrations, but may repel subpopulations of T cells at higher concentrations as a potential means of focusing the inflammatory response or for thymocyte emigration (71).

Cytotoxicity

Inflammatory chemokines may induce preformed mediator release and cytotoxic responses. In neutrophils, CXCL8 induces release of defensins and other antimicrobial proteins, as well as proteases such as elastase and collagenase that degrade extracellular matrix and amplify the inflammatory response. The non-ELR interferon (IFN)-γ–inducible CXC chemokines CXCL9, 10, and 11 have direct defensin-like antibacterial activity (72). Alone, CXCL8 is a weak activator of neutrophil oxidant production, but its potency can be increased by priming with cytokines and microbial products such as lipopolysaccharides (LPS). ELR-CXC chemokines as well as members of the MIP and MCP branches of the CC family are able to induce basophils to release histamine and eicosanoids (73), which are important vasoactive mediators in allergic responses. CCL2-5, CCL7 (MCP-3), CCL8 (MCP-2), CXCL10, and CX3CL1 (fractalkine) can promote NK-cell degranulation and a subset of these can promote tumor cell killing (43). Inflammatory chemokines injected at high concentrations directly into the bloodstream generally do not induce fever, changes in blood pressure, or other important systemic reactions.

Proliferation and Apoptosis

Chemokines have been reported to modulate both cell proliferation and death pathways. However, the importance of these effects *in vivo* is not known. One example is CXCL12, which stimulates pre–B cell and hematopoietic progenitor cell growth *in vitro* (74). The mechanism may involve autocrine/paracrine suppression of apoptosis and promotion of the G_0/G_1 transition in CD34$^+$ cells (75). Clonal deletion of T cells is critically dependent on apoptosis, which may be both positively and negatively regulated by chemokines *in vitro* (76–78). XCL1 has reciprocal effects on CD4$^+$ and CD8$^+$ T cells, directly promoting apoptosis of the former while stimulating proliferation of the latter. CXCL12 has also been reported to induce CD4$^+$ T-cell apoptosis *in vitro* by activating the Fas (CD95)/Fas ligand (CD95L) death pathway (76). Paradoxically, this pathway may induce an inflammatory response initiated by the release from pre-apoptotic resident tissue macrophages of proinflammatory mediators, including inflammatory chemokines, which have been reported to function as survival factors for neutrophils and monocytes (79). CX3CL1 promotes survival of rat microglial cells *in vitro* by up-regulating Bcl-2 (80). Several inflammatory chemokines (e.g., CCL2, CCL3) have also been reported to promote T-cell proliferation *in vitro* by acting as co-stimulatory factors during T-cell receptor activation (81,82), and CCL1 (I-309) has been reported to have anti-apoptotic effects.

CHEMOKINE SIGNALING PATHWAYS

Chemokines stimulate cellular responses by activating multiple intracellular signaling pathways regulated by diverse effectors, including phospholipases (PL) A2, C, and D, and phosphatidylinositol-3-kinaseγ (PI3Kγ). They may also activate effectors for classic growth-factor pathways, including protein tyrosine kinases (PTK) and phosphatases, low-molecular-weight GTPases (LMWG), and mitogen-activated protein (MAP) kinases, even in nondividing cells such as neutrophils (Fig. 6). The phospholipases and lipid kinases induce extensive remodeling of plasma membrane phospholipid and generate lipid second messengers.

The classic model of GPCR signaling, formation of a ternary complex composed of one molecule each of ligand, receptor, and G protein, has undergone extensive revision recently to include several novel concepts, including constitutive receptor signaling (83), receptor dimerization as a signaling intermediate (84), receptor-associated adaptors that assemble G-protein–independent signaling molecules (85), and formation of signaling assemblies in plasma membrane microdomains such as rafts (86). The available evidence suggests that these concepts may be relevant to at least some chemokine receptors. However, a consensus has not been reached (87).

G-Protein Signaling

G proteins form a family of evolutionarily conserved, plasma membrane-associated signal transducers composed of an α subunit, which binds the guanine nucleotides GDP or GTP, and a tightly associated $\beta\gamma$ heterodimer subunit. In mammals there are 20 α, 5 β, and 11 γ chains that combine to form

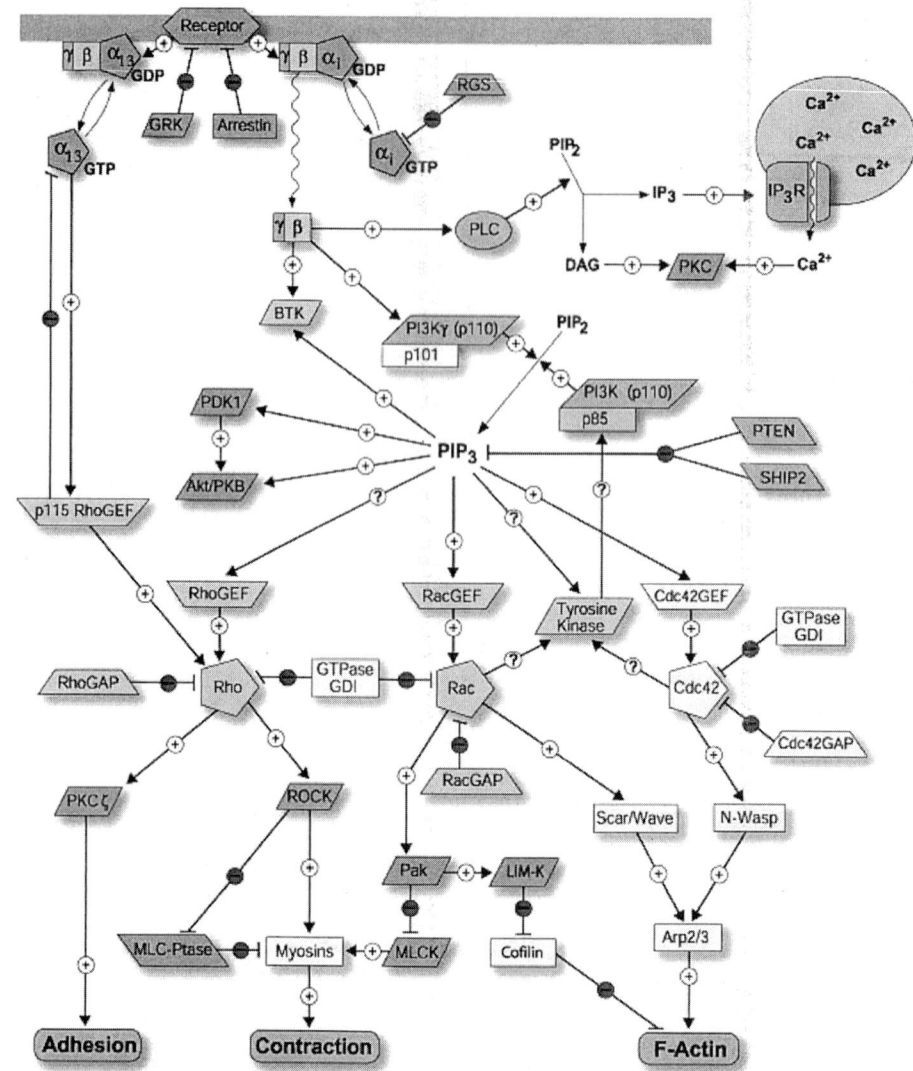

FIG. 6. Model of chemokine signal transduction pathway. This map is based primarily on studies of neutrophils and T cells. See text for details. From the Alliance for Cell Signaling (www.signaling-gateway.org), with permission. Contributors: H Bourne, O Weiner and F Wang.

many distinct G-protein subtypes. The α subunits, which are used to name the G protein, are divided by structure into four main subfamilies (αi, αq, αs, and α12/13). The classic test for Gi-dependent signaling is the ability of a pathway to be blocked by *Bordetella pertussis* toxin (PTX), which uncouples receptor from G protein by ADP ribosylating the αi subunit. This test, plus biochemical and genetic evidence in some cases, point to Gi as a key G protein coupled to almost all chemokine receptors in leukocytes. G16 and several other G proteins are able to couple to both CC and CXC chemokine receptors in model cotransfection systems and in leukocyte cell lines, and G16 is highly expressed in hematopoietic cells, but its exact role in chemokine signaling in primary cells is not fully defined.

In the classic G-protein activation cycle, agonist occupation converts the receptor into a GEF (guanine nucleotide exchange factor), which catalyzes the exchange of GDP for GTP on the α subunit. This causes the G protein to leave the receptor, to dissociate into α and $\beta\gamma$ subunits, which remain tethered to the plasma membrane by covalently attached lipid anchors on the α and γ chains, and to activate downstream intracellular effectors. The α subunit acts as a timer through its slow intrinsic GTPase activity, which can be accelerated by one or more RGS proteins (regulators of G-protein signaling), the GAPs (GTPase activating proteins) for heterotrimeric G proteins (88). The net result is restoration of the GDP-bound form of the α subunit, which then reassociates with $\beta\gamma$ subunits to return to fresh unoccupied receptors, thus completing the cycle. Studies in phagocytes suggest that the main signaling subunit for the chemotactic pathway is $\beta\gamma$ not α, and that $\beta\gamma$ must come specifically from Gi (89,90).

Gi-Dependent Effectors

Gi was originally named for its ability to inhibit adenylyl cyclase, but chemoattractants do not strongly inhibit this enzyme in leukocytes. The best-characterized immediate downstream effectors of $\beta\gamma$ in leukocytes are PLC subtypes $\beta2$ and $\beta3$, and PI3Kγ, all of which catalyze formation of distinct plasma-membrane–associated lipid second messengers from phosphorylated phosphatidylinositol (PI) substrates (91,92).

PLC hydrolyzes PI(4,5) bisphosphate (PIP$_2$) to form the second messengers 1,2-diacylglycerol (DAG) and inositol-1,4,5-trisphosphate (IP$_3$). IP$_3$ activates the IP$_3$ receptor on endoplasmic reticulum to induce Ca^{2+} release from intracellular stores. Ca^{2+} acts with DAG to activate protein kinase C (PKC) isoenzymes. Analysis of PLC $\beta2$ and $\beta3$ double knockout mice has established that these effectors are required for chemoattractant activation of neutrophil calcium flux and oxidant production, but not chemotaxis (93).

PI3Kγ phosphorylates PIP$_2$ at the three position to form PIP$_3$, which recruits proteins containing pleckstrin homology (PH) or Phox (PX) domains to the plasma membrane (94). Four PH domain-containing targets of PIP$_3$—Akt/PKB (protein kinase B), and the GEFs for the Rho family members Rac, Rho, and Cdc42—have been shown to modulate distinct phases of cell movement in various model systems (Fig. 6). Rho activates both PKCζ, which regulates cell adhesion and chemotaxis in leukocytes, and ROCK, which regulates contraction of myosin. Rho may also be required for activation of Akt/PKB in neutrophils. In fibroblasts, Rac and Cdc42 control lamellipod and filipod formation, respectively. In neutrophils, downstream targets of Rac include PAK1—which also regulates myosin contraction—and cytosolic components of the respiratory burst oxidase. ARF (ADP-ribosylation factor) GEF, another target of PIP$_3$, activates ARF, which together with PKC is involved in PLD activation. This effector, which catalyzes production of phosphatidic acid, has delayed and prolonged activation kinetics in neutrophils and has been implicated in degranulation and respiratory burst oxidase activation.

Analysis of PI3Kγ knockout mice has indicated that its importance in leukocyte migration depends on the specific subpopulation tested and the stimulus (93,95,96). *In vivo,* these mice exhibit neutrophilia whereas circulating lymphocyte levels are decreased. Neutrophil chemotactic responses are blunted *in vitro,* but the response to carrageenan installation in the peritoneal cavity is intact. In contrast, migration is severely reduced in macrophages. Chemoattractants fail to stimulate superoxide production in PI3K$\gamma^{-/-}$ neutrophils, whereas the response to particulate stimuli is unaffected. Rac2-deficient mice exhibit a similar phenotype (97). However, Rac2 activation appears to be intact in PI3K$\gamma^{-/-}$ neutrophils, raising questions about the pathway for activation of this mediator. In this regard, DOCK2, a CED family member expressed mainly in hematopoietic cells and an upstream activator of Rac, has been shown to be essential for chemokine-induced T-cell and B-cell migration, but not

for CCL2 (MCP-1) or CXCL12 recruitment of monocytes (98). Consistent with this, B cells from Rac2$^{-/-}$ mice are abnormally distributed *in vivo* and exhibit markedly depressed chemotactic responses to CXCL12 and CXCL13 *in vitro.*

Cytosolic and calcium-independent PLA2 are also Gi-dependent effectors and have been shown to be important for CCL2 activation of human monocyte chemotaxis (99). Both of these enzymes catalyze formation of arachidonic acid from membrane phospholipids.

Gi-Independent Effectors

Chemokines may activate effectors such as MAP kinases and nonreceptor protein tyrosine kinases (PTK) by Gi-independent mechanisms. Selective inhibitors of these pathways have been shown to block chemokine-induced chemotaxis, suggesting that nonoverlapping Gi-dependent and Gi-independent pathways must be activated in leukocytes in order to mediate chemokine-induced chemotaxis.

Several potential Gi-independent coupling mechanisms have been proposed. One involves direct coupling to a scaffold/adaptor protein, such as β arrestin or a PDZ domain protein, which brings sequentially acting PTKs and MAP kinases into proximity of each other and receptors (85). Consistent with this, CXCL8 activation of neutrophil degranulation may depend on β-arrestin activation of the PTK Hck (100). In addition, CCL3 stimulation of CCR5 has been reported to induce formation of a signaling complex consisting of focal adhesion–related PTK Pyk2, the Src-related PTK Syk, the phosphatase SHP1, and the adaptor protein Grb2 (101). A second mechanism involves receptor cross-activation by inducing ligands for growth factor receptors (102). A third mechanism proposed by Mellado et al. (103) involves a radical modification of the ternary complex model in which JAK2 acts upstream of Gi in the CCL2/CCR2 chemotactic pathway in T cells. Fourth, at high concentrations CCL5 forms fibrillar aggregates and acts as a T-cell mitogen through a PTK-dependent and PTX-insensitive mechanism (104).

Mechanisms of Gradient Sensing

In gradients of chemoattractants, leukocytes rapidly polarize and turn as the source of chemoattractant shifts position. Elegant imaging studies using fluorescently labeled molecules in living cells have shown that chemoattractant receptors from *Dictyostelium discoideum* amoebae and human phagocytes remain homogeneously distributed on the cell surface in gradients of chemoattractant (91). In contrast, there is dramatic but reversible recruitment of specific PH domain–containing proteins to areas of the plasma membrane adjacent to the point of highest concentration of chemoattractant. This suggests that lipid signaling is activated at the leading edge and that transformation of shallow chemoattractant gradients into steep PIP$_3$-dependent intracellular effector gradients may be a mechanism of polarization and directional sensing.

Other data disagree. For example, studies in T cells found that CCR2 clusters at the leading edge (105). Ultimately, any model must account for the fact that the cell can very rapidly reorient in response to changing the point of application of the chemoattractant, which implies that receptors cannot be completely redistributed to the leading edge. This implies that there may be global inhibitory factors that are opposed successfully by local stimulatory factors only at the point of maximal concentration (91).

Cross Talk

Chemoattractants are able to transmit signals which may reinforce or interfere with signals coming from other pathways. The classic example is the ability of chemoattractants to cross-desensitize each other's receptors (106). Others include the ability of hematopoietic growth factors such as GM-CSF to prime chemoattractant signaling by up-regulating receptors and Gi, and cross talk that occurs between CXCL8 and the EGF receptor (102). In addition, both B- and T-cell antigen receptors can down-regulate CXCR4 and inhibit CXCL12-dependent chemotaxis, which may represent a stop mechanism favoring formation of immunologic synapses (107,108). Conversely, CXCL12 has been reported to reduce tyrosine phosphorylation of the TCR effectors ZAP-70, SLP-76, and LAT, suggesting that it may reduce T-cell responsiveness to antigen (107). A particularly intriguing example of cross talk is the Eph receptor and its ligand ephrin-B, which signal bidirectionally in neurons and are involved in neuronal guidance during development. Reverse signaling by Eph activation of ephrin-B selectively inhibits CXCL12/CXCR4–induced chemotaxis of cerebellar granule cells. The mechanism involves a novel RGS protein that contains a PDZ domain that binds to ephrin B. Activation of ephrin B presumably activates RGS to accelerate inactivation of G protein and downstream chemotactic signaling induced by CXCL12 (109). The neuronal guidance factor Slit also inhibits chemokine signaling, by activation of its single transmembrane-domain receptor Robo on leukocytes (110).

REGULATION OF CHEMOKINE ACTION

Expression

Chemokine and chemokine-receptor gene expression is subject to complex positive and negative regulation by diverse factors, including pro-inflammatory cytokines, oxidant stress, viruses, bacterial products such as LPS and N-formylpeptides, cell adhesion, antigen uptake, T-cell costimulation, and diverse transcription factors. Pro-inflammatory cytokines such as IL-1, TNF, and IL-15 induce expression of many of the inflammatory chemokines involved in innate immunity such as CXCL8, whereas immunoregulatory cytokines such as IFN-γ and IL-4 are more tightly focused on Th1 (CXCL9, 10, and 11)- and Th2 (CCL11)-targeted chemokines, respectively. IFNs also suppress production of CXCL8 and related neutrophil-targeted chemokines. Glucocorticoids and anti-inflammatory cytokines (e.g., IL-10, TGF-β) also inhibit inflammatory chemokine gene expression.

Processing

Chemokines isolated from biological sources are polymorphic due mainly to differences in length of the N-termini (45,111). This can dramatically alter both potency and cell and receptor specificity, and in certain cases can convert agonists into antagonists, presumably as a mechanism for fine-tuning the nature and extent of the inflammatory response. Specific proteases have been identified that appear to account for this variability. Both broad-spectrum (e.g., CD26 [dipeptidyl peptidase IV] and matrix metalloproteinases [MMP]) and narrow-spectrum (e.g., TACE [the TNF α converting enzyme], plasmin, urokinase plasminogen activator and cathepsin G) chemokine proteases have been described (111–113). TACE is responsible for PMA-induced cleavage of the mucin-like stalk of CX3CL1, releasing its soluble, chemotactically active chemokine domain from the full-length, membrane-bound adhesive form of the molecule (113). CD26, which is expressed on T cells, cleaves N-terminal X-proline sites on CCL2, CCL5, CXCL11 and CXCL12 (111), which has differential effects on function. Several MMPs process the N-terminus of CCL7 and CXCL12.

Targeting

Leukocyte migration across mucosal surfaces may involve highly specialized mechanisms of chemokine gradient formation. For example, in the mouse neutrophil movement into the airway is dependent on epithelial cell release of a complex formed by syndecan-1 and the ELR+ CXC chemokine KC. The complex is released by cleavage of syndecan-1 by the matrix metalloproteinase matrilysin.

Chemokines may be diverted from active targets by chemokine-binding proteins (e.g., Duffy), endogenous receptor antagonists, receptor decoys, and autoantibodies. Specific cytokines have been identified that are able to convert a signaling receptor into a decoy (e.g., IL-10 inactivates CCR2 on monocytes) (114). Cell type–specific chemokine receptor cytoforms have also been described. In particular, CXCR4 cytoforms have been described on monocytes that may differ in HIV coreceptor activity (115). A given receptor may have different functions on different cell types. For example, CXCR2 is a classic chemotactic receptor on neutrophils but mediates only the adhesive part of this process for monocytes. In addition, chemokine receptor expression and/or function may change dramatically when leukocytes are harvested from the blood. For example, CCR1 appears to mediate human neutrophil migration in response to CCL3 in vivo, but it is poorly expressed and weakly coupled when purified neutrophils are studied in vitro.

Receptor Deactivation

Like other GPCRs, stimulation of chemokine receptors with agonists typically renders the receptor refractory to further stimulation, due to phosphorylation-dependent desensitization and internalization. Internalized receptors are dephosphorylated and a portion may be recycled to the cell surface, which is thought to be a mechanism for maintaining chemotactic responses in gradients of ligand. Receptor internalization is also a mechanism for suppression of HIV infection by chemokines.

Two major types of desensitization, homologous and heterologous, have been recognized depending on whether the stimuli given first and second activate the same or different receptors. Mechanisms have been worked out mainly for CXCR1, CXCR2, CXCR4, CCR2, and CCR5, and follow the general paradigm set for the $\beta 2$ adrenergic receptor (106). Homologous desensitization involves G-protein–independent recruitment of G-protein–coupled receptor kinases (GRKs) that phosphorylate serines and threonines located in the receptor C-terminal domain. This induces recruitment of β-arrestin, which prevents further coupling of receptor to G protein and serves with AP-2 and dynamin I as adaptors for binding to clathrin and initiation of endocytosis through clathrin-coated pits. A second, phosphorylation-independent internalization mechanism involving recruitment of Hsc-70 interacting protein (Hip) has also been described for CXCR2 and CXCR4, suggesting that chaperones may regulate internalization of these receptors (116). The mechanism of heterologous desensitization also involves receptor phosphorylation, but the relevant kinases appear to be PKC and PKA. Desensitization may also involve phosphorylation of downstream effectors such as PLC (106). Internalized receptors may be dephosphorylated—for example, by protein phosphatase 2A—and recycled, as shown for CXCR2 (117), or else ubiquitinated and sorted to lysosomes for degradation, as shown for CXCR4 (118).

CHEMOKINE REGULATION OF HEMATOPOIESIS

Cell counts are maintained at normal levels in the circulation in part by a balance between positive and negative factors acting on hematopoietic progenitor cells. The positive factors are well defined and can be divided into two major categories: late-acting factors such as G-CSF and M-CSF, which independently support proliferation of lineage-committed progenitor cells in colony-forming assays *ex vivo,* and early-acting factors, such as IL-3, GM-CSF, and SCF, which function in combination to support proliferation of stem cells and early myeloid progenitor cells (MPC). Most chemokines reported to modulate progenitor cell proliferation act early and are inhibitory. CXCL12 is an important exception.

CXCL12 (SDF-1) in Myelopoiesis and B-Lymphopoiesis

Originally identified as a pre–B-cell stimulatory factor made in bone marrow stromal cells, and later shown to stimu-late hematopoietic progenitor cell (HPC) colony formation *ex vivo,* CXCL12 is the most highly expressed chemokine in bone marrow. Consistent with this, mice lacking either CXCL12 or its receptor CXCR4 have the same severe defects in bone marrow myelopoiesis and B-cell lymphopoiesis (74). CXCL12 is the only chemokine able to chemoattract hematopoietic stem cells *in vitro.* Also, blocking CXCR4 on human hematopoietic stem cells prevents engraftment in severe combined immunodeficiency (SCID) mice (119). Together the data suggest that CXCL12 positively regulates hematopoiesis through multiple mechanisms, including stimulation of pre–B-cell growth, and generation, expansion, trafficking, positioning, and retention of $CD34^+$ early hematopoietic progenitor cells in marrow. In contrast, T-lymphopoiesis is normal in $CXCL12^{-/-}$ and $CXCR4^{-/-}$ mice, despite the fact that CXCR4 is expressed in functional form on developing thymocytes.

CXCR4 is also expressed in functional form on platelets, platelet precursors in the bone marrow, and most mature peripheral blood leukocytes (120). However, its precise importance in the actions of these cells has not been defined, in part because CXCL12 and CXCR4 knockout mice do not survive beyond the perinatal period. Although the exact cause of death has not been precisely delineated, the mice do have multiple developmental abnormalities that could contribute, including a ventricular septal defect, defective gastric vascularization, and defective cerebellar granule–cell positioning. This is consistent with CXCR4 expression on vascular endothelial cells and cerebellar granule cells, and the ability of CXCL12 to induce angiogenesis and chemotaxis of cerebellar granule cells *in vitro.* To date, all other chemokine and chemokine receptor knockout mice have been viable and fertile, and most appear normal under unstressed conditions. Thus, CXCL12 and CXCR4 comprise an essential chemokine–receptor pair with unusually pleotropic functions. Consistent with this, CXCL12 is the most structurally conserved chemokine and CXCR4 the most structurally conserved chemokine receptor.

Myelosuppressive Chemokines

When added to bone marrow culture systems *ex vivo,* many chemokines are able to suppress growth factor–dependent colony formation, apparently by acting directly on stem cells and early progenitors such as CFU-S, BFU-E, CFU-GM, and CFU-GEMM (35). In some cases, such as CCL3, colony formation *ex vivo* can also be reduced when the chemokine is injected *in vivo* into mice. While the physiologic importance of myelosuppressive chemokines is still not clear, they may have important clinical applications. For example, decreasing suppression by targeting a key chemokine or chemokine receptor with a blocking agent may be desirable in the setting of bone marrow transplantation to improve engraftment. Conversely, increasing suppression by administering a chemokine or a mimetic could theoretically spare stem cells by forcing them into the G_0 phase of the cell cycle in patients receiving cytoreductive therapy, thereby reducing the period of dangerous neutropenia. The latter application has been tested by British Biotech using a variant of CCL3 and by Human Genome Sciences using CCL23 (MPIF-1, myeloid progenitor inhibitory factor-1), both in phase 2 studies in cancer patients, but results were not considered sufficiently promising in either case to continue development. Myelosuppression may be counterbalanced to some extent by the ability of chemokines such as CCL3 to promote proliferation of more mature progenitor cells dependent on only a single growth factor and to promote mobilization of both mature and immature progenitor cell mobilization from bone marrow.

Studies with knockout mice have shown that suppression *ex vivo* by CXCL8 and its mouse homolog MIP-2 is mediated by CXCR2, and that CCR2 mediates CCL2 suppression, but that CCR1 does not mediate CCL3 suppression. CCR1, CCR2, and CCL3 knockout mice do not have major abnormalities in myelopoiesis *in vivo*. One explanation is that the suppressive factors may be differentially expressed, and each one may only be able to suppress a small subset of total progenitors *in vivo*. However, it is important to point out that unlike CXCL12, most other chemokines are not expressed constitutively in large amounts in bone marrow, the major source of progenitor cells. Moreover, while injection of CCL3 or other suppressive chemokines into mice may suppress both cycling and the absolute numbers of stem cells and progenitor cells that can be expanded from bone marrow and spleen, mature blood cell counts in the circulation are not significantly decreased.

One impressive result that is potentially explained by the myelosuppression hypothesis relates to the CXCR2$^{-/-}$ mouse, which when derived in a standard environment develops massive neutrophilia, splenomegaly, bone-marrow myeloid hyperplasia, and expansion of myeloid progenitor cells. Since this phenotype is not observed when the mice are derived under germ-free conditions, CXCR2-dependent suppression may be an important mechanism for opposing overstimulation of hematopoiesis induced by environmental flora. A competing or additional explanation is that CXCR2 might suppress production of enhancers by promoting immune surveillance, which is consistent with the severe defect in neutrophil migration found in CXCR2 knockout mice. These mice also develop lymph-node B-cell hyperplasia, which may occur by an indirect mechanism since CXCR2 has not been shown to be expressed on B cells or B-cell precursors.

Not all chemokine-induced suppression occurs via GPCRs: CXCL10 and CXCL4 in particular have been shown to displace hematopoietic growth factors from binding sites on GAGs. Moreover, suppressive chemokines, such as CXCL8 and CCL2, that do operate through their specific GPCRs, may use unusual PTX-resistant pathways. Another surprising finding is that other CXCR2 and CCR2 agonists such as CXCL1 (Groα [growth-related oncogene]), CXCL3 (Groγ), CXCL7, and CCL7 are not suppressive in colony assays (35). In summary, although myelosuppressive

chemokines clearly exist, much more work will be needed to understand their physiologic relevance, signaling mechanisms, and translational potential.

T-Lymphopoiesis

T-cell maturation requires sequential and orderly migration of T cells from the cortex to the medulla of the thymus, a process that is probably guided by specific chemokines. Exactly which chemokines are involved has been difficult to pinpoint since none of the 18 chemokine or chemokine-receptor knockout mice analyzed to date has had defects in thymic architecture or in T-cell development. However, since many chemokines are expressed in thymus, this is more likely to be due to functional redundancy than to lack of active chemokines in the thymus.

There is a suggestion that CCR9 and its ligand CCL25 (TECK [thymus-expressed chemokine]) may be important since competitive transplantation of CCR9$^{-/-}$ bone marrow is less efficient than normal marrow at repopulating the thymus of lethally irradiated Rag-1$^{-/-}$ mice (121). CCL25 is expressed by medullary dendritic cells and both cortical and medullary epithelial cells, and CCR9 is expressed on the majority of immature CD4$^+$CD8$^+$ thymocytes, but is downregulated during transition to the CD4$^+$ or CD8$^+$ single-positive stage (40,122). Thymocytes up-regulate the peripheral homing receptor L-selectin just before they are released to the periphery, by which time they no longer express CCR9 or respond chemotactically to CCL25. The transition from CD4$^+$CD8$^+$ thymocytes in the cortex to CD4 or CD8 single positive thymocytes in the medulla is also associated with up-regulation of CCR4 and CCR7, the receptors for CCL22 (MDC [macrophage-derived chemokine]) and CCL19 and CCL21 (ELC and SLC), respectively, which are expressed in the medullary stroma. Accordingly, *in vitro* these chemokines attract thymocytes between the late cortical and medullary stages of development. Neutralization studies suggest that egress of newly formed T cells from fetal thymus to the circulation is mediated by CCL19, which is selectively localized on endothelial cells of medullary venules and acts at CCR7 on mature thymocytes.

Phagocyte Positioning in Peripheral Tissue

The factors responsible for specific positioning of phagocytes in peripheral tissues after egress from bone marrow are not well defined. CXCL14 (BRAK [breast and kidney chemokine]) and CCR6 may be important in this regard. Like CXCL12, CXCL14 is a highly conserved (2-aa differences between human and mouse) CXC chemokine constitutively expressed in diverse human tissues and cell types (123). It is the only chemokine that exclusively chemoattracts monocytes, and since macrophages colocalize with CXCL14-producing fibroblasts *in vivo,* it may play a specialized role in homeostatic recruitment, retention, and development of resident tissue macrophages (124). Eosinophil distribution is controlled in part by the CCR3 ligand CCL11, since mice lacking CCL11 have increased eosinophils in spleen and markedly depleted levels in the gastrointestinal tract (125).

CCR6 had originally been thought to mediate positioning of immature DC, where it is selectively expressed, and in fact CCR6 knockout mice do have a selective deficiency in myeloid CD11c$^+$ CD11b$^+$ DC, in the subepithelial dome of Peyer's patches (126,127). This may explain in part why humoral immune responses within the gut mucosa of these animals are abnormal. However, CCR6 expression on B cells and subsets of T cells may also be responsible. The focal nature of the defect implies that other chemokines may control DC positioning in other organs.

CHEMOKINE REGULATION OF THE IMMUNE RESPONSE

The precise nature and magnitude of the immune response depends on the nature, dose, and entry site of the irritant, the type of antigen-presenting cell (APC), co-stimulatory factors and the genetic background of the host. Thus immunopathology is diverse, not monotonous. This diversity depends on graded action and interaction of the two major immune subsystems, innate and adaptive, deployed separately but brought together in part by specific sets of chemokines and dynamic changes in chemokine receptor expression on subsets of T cells and DC.

Innate Immunity

CXCL8 (IL-8) and Other Neutrophil-Targeted Chemokines

CXCL8 is a major mediator of neutrophil migration *in vivo*. Intradermal injection of CXCL8 in human causes rapid (<30 min) and selective accumulation of large numbers of neutrophils in perivascular regions of the skin without causing edema. Moreover, neutralizing CXCL8 in rabbits or its counterparts MIP-2 and KC in mice and CINC in rats, or genetically inactivating its receptor CXCR2 in rodents, is able to dramatically attenuate neutrophil-mediated inflammation and increase susceptibility to bacterial and fungal pathogens in disease models (128,129).

As was mentioned previously, the CXCL8 gene is normally silent in most cells, but can be rapidly induced in most if not all cell types. In a blister model of acute inflammation in human, endogenous CXCL8 peaks at nanomolar concentrations at ~24 hours, whereas C5a and leukotriene B4, which unlike CXCL8 do not require new gene expression but instead are formed enzymatically from precursor substrates, appear earlier (130). This suggests that orderly sequential expression of chemoattractants may control the evolution of the inflammatory response, and that the primary role of CXCL8 is not to initiate inflammation but amplify and direct it in the early stages. Moreover, tissue-specific transgenic overexpression of the mouse ELR-CXC chemokines KC and MIP-2, as well as other inflammatory chemokines such as CCL2, has sug-

gested that *in vivo* these factors may be responsible mainly for concentrating cells *in situ,* and may not be independently able to activate the cells and induce tissue damage.

In vitro CXCL8 appears to chemoattract human neutrophils by activating CXCR2 (131). It also binds with equal affinity to the closely related neutrophil receptor CXCR1, which in rat is expressed in macrophages but not neutrophils. In human, there is still disagreement about the relative functional importance of CXCR1. Six other ELR-CXC chemokines are also potent agonists at CXCR2 *in vitro,* but unlike CXCL8 have much lower potency and efficacy at CXCR1. *In vivo* this may provide a mechanism for graded navigation of neutrophils through tissue. CXCL1, 2, 3, 7, and 8 have also been reported to induce basophil chemotaxis and histamine release *in vitro* (73), which together with other factors such as complement-derived anaphylatoxins may promote vasodilatation during early stages of the innate immune response.

Apart from CXCL7, the ELR-CXC chemokines are all regulated at the level of transcription by the same factors previously mentioned to induce CXCL8; however, there are also differences. In mouse, blocking TNF-induced neutrophil extravasation requires neutralization of both MIP-2 and KC, the CXCL1-3 homologs of mice, indicating redundant function in this setting (132). In contrast, selective blockade of MIP-2 is sufficient to disrupt neutrophil migration into HSV-1–infected mouse cornea, even though both MIP-2 and KC are produced by corneal cells in this model (133). Thus, although these chemokines all act in innate immunity through a final common pathway, CXCR2, they may differ biologically due to temporal and spatial differences in expression.

CXCL15 (lungkine), a mouse chemokine that has no known human ortholog, is also a significant mediator of neutrophil migration (134). The selective and constitutive expression of CXCL15 mRNA in fetal and adult mouse lung, particularly in epithelial cells, is unique. The CXCL15 knockout mouse has normal lung development. Instead, it has increased susceptibility to *Klebsiella* pneumonia, indicating that CXCL15 functions in innate immunity. Consistent with this, CXCL15 is secreted into the air spaces, induces *in vitro* and *in vivo* migration of neutrophils, and is up-regulated in lung inflammation models. CC chemokines can also activate neutrophils in some cases. CCL3 is a potent neutrophil chemoattractant signaling through CCR1, and IFN-γ induces CCR2 expression in human neutrophils.

Made primarily during platelet development, stored in platelet α granules, and rapidly released during platelet degranulation, CXCL4 and CXCL7 may be among the first chemokines to appear at sites of tissue injury and infection, particularly when there is hemorrhage and vascular damage, and may reach extremely high concentrations (micromolar) (135). CXCL4 aggregates to form tetramers critical for binding to chondroitinsulfate proteoglycans, their major known binding sites. In contrast, CXCL7 is activated by sequential proteolysis of its N-terminus. The prepropeptide form, named platelet basic protein (92 aa), is trimmed during platelet maturation to produce the 85-aa major stored form, named connective tissue-activating peptide-III (CTAP-III), which is inactive on neutrophils. CTAP-III is further processed during degranulation to 81-aa β-thromboglobulin, also inactive. This is then cleaved by a cell-surface–bound, cathepsin G-like enzyme on neutrophils to form 70-aa CXCL7, which has high homology to CXCL4 (70% aa identity). Thus CXCL7 may function as an immediate, early mediator of neutrophil recruitment released from platelets at sites of inflammation. Although it is not a chemoattractant and does not induce degranulation of neutrophil lysosomal enzymes, CXCL4 is able to induce secondary granule exocytosis and release matrix-degrading enzymes that may facilitate neutrophil penetration of infected or injured tissues. Moreover, it mediates strong adhesion of neutrophils to endothelial cells by functional activation of LFA-1, unlike the ELR-CXC chemokines, which induce adhesion by up-regulating MAC-1.

NK Cells

Human NK-cell subsets express unique repertoires of chemokine receptors. The CD56^{dim}CD16^{+} subset, which is associated with high cytotoxic capacity and low cytokine production, expresses primarily CXCR1 and CX3CR1, whereas the minor subset of CD56^{bright}CD16^{dim} cells, which produce large amounts of cytokines but have low killing capacity, preferentially express CCR7 (42). The exact profile of chemokine receptor and chemokine expression can be modulated by adherence and stimulation *ex vivo* with IL-2 (LAK cells) (43). Chemokines for these receptors chemoattract appropriate subsets of NK cells, and promote NK-cell degranulation and killing. The importance of chemokines in NK-cell function *in vivo* is illustrated well by mouse cytomegalovirus (MCMV), a cause of hepatitis. MCMV induces CCL3 production in the liver, which is required for recruitment of NK cells. NK cells are the major source of IFN-γ in this model, and IFN-γ induces CXCL9, which is required for T cell recruitment and protection (136). Thus, a cytokine to chemokine to cytokine cascade is required for NK-cell–mediated host defense against this pathogen.

Mononuclear Phagocytes and Transition to the Adaptive Immune Response

Transition from the innate to the adaptive phase of the immune response involves entry of mononuclear phagocytes (resident tissue macrophages, blood-derived monocytes, and immature DC [iDC]) to inflamed sites in response to members of the inflammatory MCP or MIP subfamilies of CC chemokines, followed by contact with pathogens and other foreign matter via two major classes of receptors: the classic Fc and complement-dependent phagocytic receptors and the pattern recognition receptors (PRRs). The PRRs differentially bind a limited number of "pathogen-associated molecular patterns" (PAMPs), which provide a direct mechanism for differentiating pathogens from self (137).

Known PAMPs include LPS, flagellin, peptidoglycan, lipoproteins, and unmethylated CpG dinucleotides. PRRs include CD14, scavenger receptors and the family of Toll-like receptors (TLRs). Of these, the TLRs play a central role linking the innate to the adaptive immune response by converting phagocytes, particularly dendritic cells, from killers of pathogens into couriers of antigens, guided in part by specific chemokines. Each TLR has a specific PAMP preference— for example, TLR2 to peptidoglycan, TLR4 to LPS, TLR5 to flagellin, and TLR9 to CpGs. Although TLR–PAMP interaction appears to activate NFκB as a common signaling pathway, differential signaling is also evident since each TLR–PAMP pair activates specific sets of genes.

With regard to chemokines, both TLR2 and TLR4 induce expression of CCL3, CCL4, and CCL5, whereas TLR2 selectively induces CXCL8 and TLR4 selectively induces CXCL10 (138). CXCL8 may increase neutrophil migration to the site, whereas CXCL10 may enhance NK-cell or Th1-effector T-cell homing (Fig. 7). Thus, each pathogen through specific PAMPs may skew the nature and magnitude of the immune response in a specific direction. Resting peripheral blood neutrophils express mainly CXCR1, CXCR2, and CXCR4, whereas monocytes express most of the inflammatory chemokine receptors and CXCR4. Tissue macrophages may express differential subsets of these depending on the tissue source. Eosinophils express CCR3 and in some donors CCR1. The chemokine receptors expressed on DCs may vary depending on the nature of the inflammatory stimulus and type. For example, blood-derived plasmacytoid and myeloid DCs express a similar repertoire of inflammatory chemoattractant receptors, but they are functional only on myeloid DCs. CCL3, CCL4, and CCL5 may be particularly important for recruiting additional mononuclear phagocytes and DCs to sites of infection. This can amplify the late stage of the innate immune response, and in the extreme may devolve into endotoxic shock. Consistent with this idea, genetic disruption of the CCL3/CCL4/CCL5 receptor CCR5 renders mice relatively resistant to LPS-induced endotoxemia. CCR4$^{-/-}$ mice are also resistant to lethality induced by intraperitoneal administration of LPS, and this is associated with reduced macrophage extravasation to the peritoneum and production of the CCR4 ligand CCL17 (MDC, macrophage-derived chemokine), which can be produced by DCs (139). The innate immune response may also be amplified and connected to the adaptive response by neutrophil antimicrobial products such as defensins, which are able to chemoattract iDC by acting as a chemokine mimic at CCR6, and azurocidin and cathepsin G, which attract T cells (34).

ADAPTIVE IMMUNITY

Afferent Trafficking to Secondary Lymphoid Tissue

CXCR5 and CCR7 and their ligands have emerged as major regulators of the immune response, acting at the level

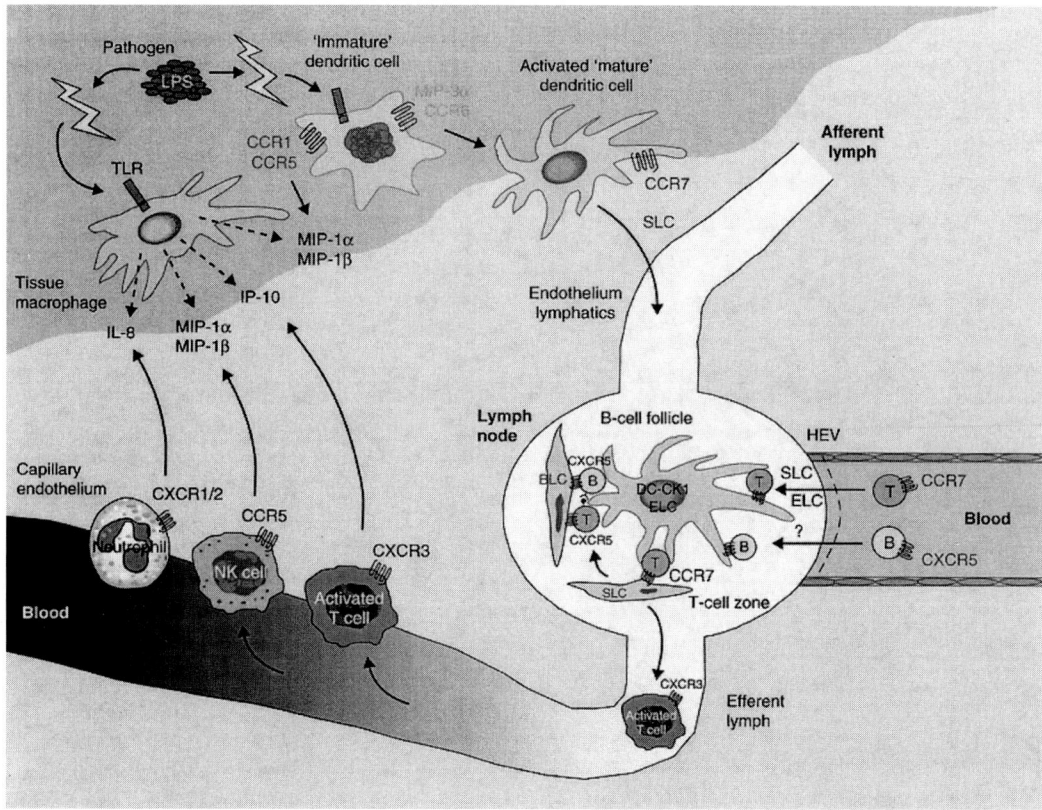

FIG. 7. Model of chemokine regulation of the immune response. From Luster (138), with permission. See text for description.

of B- and T-lymphocyte and DC trafficking to and within secondary lymphoid tissue (14,15,36). A model has been proposed in which DC maturation in peripheral tissues is associated with down-regulation of inflammatory receptors, which may be important for recruitment, migration, and retention in the periphery, associated with reciprocal up-regulation of CCR7, which is critical for migration of mature DCs through the afferent lymphatics to the draining lymph node. CCR7 is also expressed on naïve and activated T cells. Multiple lines of evidence have converged in support of this model. Other mechanisms may also be important. For example, expression of the inflammatory receptor CCR2 on Langerhans cells has been demonstrated to be critical for afferent trafficking in a mouse model of *Leishmania* infection (140).

The CCR7 ligand CCL21 is constitutively expressed on afferent lymphatic endothelium as well as on high endothelial venules (HEV), stromal cells, and interdigitating dendritic cells in T zones of lymph node, Peyer's patch, mucosa-associated lymphoid tissue, and spleen, but not in B zones or sinuses. Its expression is dependent on lymphotoxin $\alpha 1\beta 2$ (141). CCL19, another CCR7 ligand, is also restricted to the T zone and is expressed on interdigitating DCs.

Thus the CCR7 knockout mouse and the *plt* mouse, which is naturally deficient in CCL19 and a CCL21 isoform expressed in secondary lymphoid organs, have similar phenotypes: atrophic T zones populated by a paucity of naïve

T cells. This plus the failure of activated mDC to migrate to lymph node from the skin of these mice, explains why contact sensitivity, delayed type hypersensitivity and antibody production are severely impaired. Although they have not been reported to develop spontaneous infections, *plt* mice do have increased susceptibility to challenge with mouse hepatitis virus.

CXCR5 is expressed on all peripheral blood and tonsillar B cells, but only on a fraction of bone marrow B cells. Its ligand CXCL13 is expressed constitutively on follicular HEV and controls trafficking of CXCR5 positive B and T cells from the blood into follicles. Thus, CXCR5 knockout mice have a severe defect in normal B-cell migration and localization in lymph node, lack or have phenotypically abnormal Peyer's patches, and lack inguinal lymph nodes. CXCL13 is also required for B1 cell homing, natural antibody production, and body cavity immunity (142). CXCR5$^{-/-}$ mice are able to produce systemic antibody responses, perhaps in part because B cells and follicular DC, by an unknown mechanism, are able to form ectopic germinal centers within T zones of the periarteriolar lymphocyte sheath of spleen (143). Conversely, overexpression of CXCL13 in the pancreas of transgenic mice leads to B-cell accumulation and formation of ectopic lymphoid tissue (144).

CXCR5 and CCR7 are probably not the only chemokine receptors responsible for afferent trafficking of leukocytes to lymph node. CCL9 has been reported to mediate monocyte homing, suggesting a role for CXCR3 (145). CCR4 and CCR8 are expressed on a subset of human peripheral blood CD4$^+$CD25$^+$CTLA4$^+$ T cells, which are associated with suppression of T-cell responses and may be important in generation of tolerance (146). Mature DC are able to chemoattract these cells *in vitro* by secreting the CCR4 ligands CCL17 and CCL22 (TARC, thymus and activation related chemokine), suggesting a mechanism for trafficking to secondary lymphoid tissues and primary areas of antigen deposition. In addition, inflamed peripheral tissues may exert "remote control" over which leukocyte populations home to draining lymph nodes from the blood by "projecting" their local chemokine profile to HEVs of the draining lymph node (147). Migration of T cells to splenic red pulp may involve local production of CXCL16 (29). NK–T cells, and activated CD4$^+$ and CD8$^+$ T cells are found in this area and express the CXCL16 receptor CXCR6. CXCL16 is also made by DCs in the T zone, and CXCR6 is also found on intraepithelial lymphocytes. Thus, CXCL16 may function in T-cell–DC interactions and in regulating movements of activated T cells in the splenic red pulp and in peripheral tissues.

Positioning within Lymph Node

CXCR5 is also expressed on a subset of CD4$^+$ memory T cells, which account for the majority of CD4$^+$ memory cells in follicles of inflamed tonsils (15,148). These so-called follicular help T cells (T$_{FH}$) constitute the CD57$^+$ subset of CXCR5$^+$ T cells. These cells lack CCR7, which allows them to move from the T zone following activation to the follicles where they provide help for B-cell maturation and antibody production. They do not produce Th1 or Th2 cytokines upon activation. In a reciprocal manner, B cells activated by antigen in the follicles up-regulate CCR7 and move towards the T zone (149). Thus B–T interaction may be facilitated by reciprocal movement of these cells, which may be determined in part by the balance of chemokines made in adjacent lymphoid zones. CXCR4 signaling may also be important in naïve and memory B-cell trafficking to germinal centers.

Efferent Trafficking

A lymphocyte exiting from lymphoid tissue via efferent lymphatics has markedly different trafficking potential depending on whether or not it encountered antigen, which can be explained in part by the effects of antigen stimulation and the local lymphoid microenvironment on expression of specific adhesion molecules and chemokine receptors.

Naïve lymphocytes that do not encounter antigen continue to recirculate between the blood and secondary lymphoid tissue without acquiring any tissue-specific homing properties. Most antigen-stimulated T cells die by apoptosis. The survivors may be divided into functionally distinct subsets marked by characteristic patterns of chemokine receptor expression. In general, the trafficking properties of these cells

are not well-understood. Within the CD4$^+$ subpopulation, three memory subsets and two main effector subsets have been proposed. The memory subsets include T$_{FH}$ cells described in the previous section, and effector memory (T$_{EM}$) and central memory cells (T$_{CM}$) (14). T$_{EM}$ lack CCR7, and have been proposed to traffic through peripheral tissues as immune surveillance cells, rapidly releasing cytokines in response to activation by recall antigens. In contrast, T$_{CM}$ express CCR7 and lymph-node homing receptors, and traffic between the blood and secondary lymphoid organs, but are not polarized and lack immediate effector function. Instead, they may efficiently interact with DCs in lymph node and differentiate into T$_{EM}$ upon secondary stimulation. Both populations can be activated by APCs and antigen. CXCR5 is present on a subset of T$_{CM}$ cells in peripheral blood.

The two main effector subsets, Th1 and Th2, up-regulate inflammatory chemokine receptors. This switch renders the cells chemotactically responsive to cognate inflammatory chemokines, which are postulated to facilitate exit from lymph node via efferent lymphatics and homing to inflamed sites. The mechanisms that determine why different antigens and microenvironments may induce distinct effector responses, including differential chemokine receptor expression, have not been precisely delineated. *In vivo*, combinations of receptors rather than any single receptor appear to hold the strongest association with these functional subsets in the blood (39).

In vivo, Th1 cells, which by the simplest definition secrete IFN-γ but not IL-4 and control cellular and humoral immunity to intracellular pathogens, more frequently express CXCR3, CXCR6, CCR2, CCR5, and CX3CR1 than Th2 cells. In contrast, Th2 cells, which express IL-4 but not IFN-γ, and are associated with cellular and humoral immunity to extracellular pathogens and allergic inflammation, more frequently express CCR3, CCR4, and CCR8 than Th1 cells (39). CXCR3 expression has been most consistently associated with Th1 immune responses and Th1-associated disease. Consistent with this, its agonists CXCL9-11 are highly induced by IFN-γ but not by IL-4. Thus, in Th1 immunity there is the potential for a positive feedback loop in which IFN-γ induces production of CXCL9-11, which then recruit CXCR3$^+$ Th1 cells that produce IFN-γ. Strong evidence in favor of this model is that the CXCL10$^{-/-}$ mouse has impaired effector-Th1 immune responses and fails to mobilize effector T cells to brain when challenged with mouse hepatitis virus, resulting in increased viral replication and decreased demyelination. CXCL10 neutralization has a similar effect on susceptibility to this virus. The "Th1 chemokines" may also help maintain Th1 dominance, in part through their ability to block CCR3 (150). Specific cytokines, microenvironments, and inflammatory stresses may differentially regulate CXCL9, CXCL10, and CXCL11 expression, which may account for specialized biological roles. For example, detailed study of CXCL9 and CXCL10 during viral and protozoan infections of mice has revealed overlapping but distinct patterns of expression.

Conversely, research on chemokine expression and targets has led to a model of Th2 immunity in which IL-4 and IL-13 made at inflamed sites in the periphery may induce production of CCL7, CCL11, and other CCR3 ligands, the CCR4 ligands CCL17 and CCL22, and the CCR8 ligand CCL1. CCR3 is expressed on a small subset of Th2 T-lymphocytes as well as on eosinophils and basophils, the three major cell types associated with Th2-type allergic inflammation, and Th2 cells are associated with CCR4 and CCR8 expression. Arrival of Th2 cells amplifies a positive feedback loop through secretion of additional IL-4. Moreover, CCL7 and CCL11 may block Th1 responses by antagonizing CCR2, CXCR3, and CCR5 (151).

CD4$^+$ T-Cell Differentiation

Some chemokines appear to regulate not just trafficking but also differentiation of Th1 and Th2 cells (16). CCL2 and its receptor CCR2 have been most extensively studied in this regard, but the results are complex and appear at first glance contradictory since *in vivo* CCR2 is strongly associated with Th1 immune responses and CCL2 is associated with Th2 responses. For example, CCL2 transgenic mice and CCR2$^{-/-}$ mice, but not CCL2$^{-/-}$ mice, have increased susceptibility to lethal infection with *Mycobacterium tuberculosis*.

CCL2 appears to promote Th2 polarization directly, by inhibiting IL-12 production in monocytes, and by enhancing IL-4 but not IFN-γ production in memory and activated T cells. Thus, CCL2 influences both innate immunity through effects on monocyte trafficking, and adaptive immunity through control of T-helper cell polarization and trafficking. Why CCL2 and CCR2 have opposite effects on Th polarization is not yet resolved, but there are several possibilities. Most importantly, CCR2 can still be triggered by other CCR2 ligands in CCL2$^{-/-}$ mice, but none of these can activate CCR2 pathways in CCR2$^{-/-}$ mice. Also, CCR2 ligands that are normally depleted by CCR2 ligation may accumulate in CCR2$^{-/-}$ mice, thereby allowing triggering of alternative receptors such as CCR3 that, unlike CCR2, could be coupled to Th2 differentiation. Alternatively, CCL2 could act at a second receptor subtype. In the case of CCR2$^{-/-}$ mice, DC migration to draining lymph node after aerosol challenge with *M. tuberculosis* is markedly impaired, which preempts any direct effects of CCL2 on T cells.

The role of the inflammatory chemokine CCL3 and its receptors on T-cell polarization is also complex (16). CCL3 can directly enhance IFN-γ production in activated T cells, and CCL3 neutralization attenuates Th1-driven experimental autoimmune encephalomyelitis and Th1-dependent granuloma formation in mice. Nevertheless, mice lacking the CCL3 receptor CCR1 typically have reduced Th2 responses. This suggests a role for the CCL3 receptor CCR5 in mediating Th1-polarizing effects of CCL3, which is consistent with the role of this receptor in mediating CD8α^+ DC trafficking and IL-12 production in the spleen in mice injected with Stag, a soluble *Toxoplasma gondii* antigen preparation (152). Nevertheless,

CCR5$^{-/-}$ mice have also been reported to have enhanced delayed-type hypersensitivity reactions, and increased humoral responses to T-cell–dependent antigenic challenge, indicating a role for CCR5 in down-modulating certain T-cell–dependent immune responses (153).

Tissue-Specific Lymphocyte Homing

When lymphocytes encounter antigen in lymphoid tissue that drains mucosal surfaces or skin, they become programmed to home to the original tissue and to recirculate between it and its draining lymph nodes. This process probably evolved to help rapidly focus effector cells to inflamed and infected sites, as well as to optimize immune surveillance by confining memory cells to sites where repeat antigen encounter was most probable. In contrast, tissue-specific lymphocyte subsets for internal organs, which less frequently encounter foreign antigens, have not been found. The molecular determinants of homing and regional immunity, which were first shown to include tissue-specific adhesion molecules on lymphocytes, now appear to also include epithelial expression of homeostatic, tissue-specific chemokines and induction of their specific chemokine receptors on lymphocytes.

CLA$^+$ T-lymphocytes, which home to skin, preferentially express CCR4 and CCR10 (154). The CCR4 ligand CCL22 is made by resident dermal macrophages and DCs whereas the CCR10 ligand CCL27 (CTACK [cutaneous T-cell–associated chemokine]) is made by keratinocytes. Blocking both of these pathways, but not either one alone, has been reported to inhibit lymphocyte recruitment to the skin in a DTH (delayed-type hypersensitivity) model, implying that in this model these two molecules act redundantly and independently of inflammatory chemokines (155).

Homing to small intestine is determined in part by T-lymphocyte expression of the integrin $\alpha_4\beta_7$ and CCR9. The $\alpha_4\beta_7$ ligand MAdCAM-1 and the CCR9 ligand CCL25 colocalize on normal and inflamed small intestinal endothelium, and most T cells in the intraepithelial and lamina propria zones of the small intestine express CCR9. These cells, which are mainly $\gamma\delta$ TCR$^+$ or CD8$\alpha\beta^+$ $\alpha\beta$TCR$^+$, are reduced in small intestine from CCR9$^{-/-}$ mice (156).

CCL28 (MEC [mucosal epithelial cell chemokine]) may be important for homing to bronchus, colon, salivary gland, and mammary gland, where it is constitutively expressed at high levels. Although CCL28 also signals through the CCL27 receptor CCR10, CCR10$^+$ CLA$^+$ cells are not found in intestine because they lack $\alpha_4\beta_7$ integrin expression needed for gut homing.

As B cells differentiate into plasma cells, they also down-regulate CXCR5 and CCR7 and exit lymph node. B immunoblasts expressing IgG coordinately up-regulate CXCR4, which promotes homing to the bone marrow (37), whereas B immunoblasts expressing IgA specifically migrate to mucosal sites (157). Like gut-homing T cells, B immunoblasts that home to small intestine express $\alpha_4\beta_7$ integrin and CCR9 and respond to CCL25.

CHEMOKINES AND DISEASE

Although there is a vast literature correlating the presence of chemokines with human disease (2,158), direct proofs of important roles in pathogenesis exist for only four diseases: WHIM syndrome (warts, hypogammaglobulinemia, infection, and myelokathexis [neutropenia without maturation arrest]), heparin-induced thrombocytopenia, HIV/AIDS, and malaria (Table 1). The latter two examples fall into the category of microbial mimicry, which will be covered in the next section. The following discussion, which focuses on direct genetic tests of endogenous chemokine contributions to disease pathogenesis, is meant to be illustrative, not comprehensive, and is supplemented by Appendices 5 and 6 and by recent reviews (23,159–161).

Immunodeficiency/Infectious Diseases

Two naturally occurring mutations in the homeostatic chemokine system have been associated with increased susceptibility to pathogens. The first, a truncating mutation in the C-tail of CXCR4 that affects normal receptor desensitization processes, has been strongly linked by pedigree analysis to patients with WHIM syndrome, who are highly susceptible to papillomavirus infection (162). The exact pathogenetic mechanism has not yet been delineated. The second, which was discussed in the previous section, is the *plt* mutation in mouse, which is associated with increased susceptibility to mouse hepatitis virus (163).

Neutrophils from $CXCR2^{-/-}$ mice do not respond to any ELR-CXC chemokines and migrate mimimally in response to chemical irritants *in vivo*. Accordingly, the mice are more susceptible to infection when challenged with diverse bacterial, fungal, and helminth pathogens, summarized in Appendix 5, which all induce ELR-CXC chemokine production. Like CXCR2, CCR1 is important for resistance to lethal infection with *Aspergillus fumigatus*.

The situation is more complex for intracellular pathogens, where disease is driven by combined cytopathic effects from both the pathogen and the immune response. Influenza A, for example, induces the monocyte- and T-cell–targeted chemokines CCL2, CCL3, and CCL5, but not the neutrophil-targeted chemokines CXCL1 or CXCL8, and accordingly the cells present in the infected airway are macrophages and T cells, not neutrophils. As would be predicted, $CCL3^{-/-}$ and $CCR2^{-/-}$ mice have less pneumonitis, and higher viral titers (164). Yet, deficiency of CCR5, which is also present on macrophages and Th1 cells, is associated with worse pneumonitis and increased mortality rates in influenza infection. As with influenza, genetic disruption of CCL3 prevents the intense myocarditis that normally occurs in mice infected with Coxsackie B3 virus, but viral replication is unaffected. With regard to intracellular bacterial infection, mice lacking CCR2 are more susceptible to lethal infection with *Listeria monocytogenes* and *M. tuberculosis,* in both cases apparently due to defects in macrophage trafficking.

Acute Neutrophil-Mediated Inflammatory Disorders

Many neutrophil-mediated human diseases have been associated with the presence of CXCL8, including gout, acute glomerulonephritis, ARDS, rheumatoid arthritis, and ischemia-reperfusion injury. Systemic administration of neutralizing anti-CXCL8 antibodies is protective in diverse models of neutrophil-mediated acute inflammation in the rabbit (skin, airway, pleura, glomeruli), providing proof of concept that CXCL8 is a nonredundant mediator of innate immunity and acute pathologic inflammation in these settings (128,129). Moreover, CXCR2 knockout mice are less susceptible in a model of acute urate crystal-induced gouty synovitis (165), and SB-265610—a nonpeptide small molecule antagonist with exquisite selectivity for CXCR2—prevents neutrophil accumulation in the lungs of hyperoxia-exposed newborn rats (166). Together the results identify CXCL8 and its receptors as candidate drug targets for diseases mediated by acute neutrophilic inflammation.

Transplant Rejection

An advantage of transplant rejection over other animal models of human disease is that in both the human and animal

TABLE 1. *Members of chemokine system proven to be pathogenetic factors in human disease*

Molecule	Disease	Mechanism	Clinical manifestations
CXCL4	Autoimmune heparin-induced thrombocytopenia	AutoAb production to CXCL4-heparin complex, causing activation of platelets and microvascular endothelial cells	Thromboembolism in patients receiving heparin
CXCR4	HIV/AIDS	HIV coreceptor	HIV progression and AIDS
	WHIM syndrome	Loss of receptor desensitization due to mutation in CXCR4	Warts, hypogammaglobulinemia, infections, and myelokathexis (neutropenia without maturation arrest)
CCR5	HIV/AIDS	HIV coreceptor; CCR5Δ32 mutation is protective	HIV infection and AIDS
Duffy	*Plasmodium vivax* malaria	Cell entry; Duffy promoter mutation common in blacks abolishes RBC Duffy expression, thereby conferring resistance to disease	Anemia, fever

situation, the time of antigenic challenge is precisely known. The most extensive analysis of the role of chemokines in transplant rejection has been carried out in an MHC class I/II–mismatched cardiac allograft rejection model in the mouse, which is mediated by a Th1 immune response (159). Similar sets of inflammatory chemokines are found in the mouse model as in the human disease. ELR-CXC chemokines and CCL2 appear early, and are probably made by engrafted blood vessel endothelial cells. These are associated with neutrophil and mononuclear cell accumulation. On day 3 after engraftment, CCL2 is still present and the three CXCR3 ligands CXCL9 to CXCL11 and the CCR5 ligands CCL4 and CCL5 appear. Of the CXCR3 ligands, CXCL10 appears earliest and in largest amounts, probably in response to IFN-γ coming from NK cells. This phase is associated with transition to an adaptive immune response with accumulation of trafficking of recipient T cells, macrophages, and DCs to the graft followed by acute and chronic rejection. Graft arteriosclerosis, which is distinct from the lipid-driven disease, may be driven in part by CXCL10 and IFN-γ.

Analysis of knockout mice has demonstrated that multiple chemokine receptors contribute to rejection in this model by mediating leukocyte trafficking to and from the graft. There is a marked rank order: CXCR3>>CCR5>CCR1 = CX3CR1 = CCR2. Most impressively, rejection and graft arteriosclerosis do not occur if the recipient mouse, treated with a brief, subtherapeutic course of cyclosporin A, is CXCR3$^{-/-}$ or if the donor heart is CXCL10$^{-/-}$, identifying this axis as a potential drug target (167,168). Neutralization of CXCL9, a CXCR3 ligand that appears later than CXCL10, can also prolong cardiac allograft survival, and delay T-cell infiltration and acute rejection in class II MHC–disparate skin allografts (169). In rat, BX-471, a nonpeptide, small molecule antagonist of CCR1, was reported to be effective in heart transplant rejection (170).

In human, CCR5 may be important in chronic kidney allograft rejection, since individuals homozygous for the inactive CCR5Δ32 allele are underrepresented among patients with this outcome in a large German kidney transplantation cohort (171).

Autoimmunity

Two human diseases have been identified in which chemokines act as autoantigens for autoantibodies. The first, heparin-induced thrombocytopenia (HIT) is the only human autoimmune disease directly linked mechanistically to chemokines (172). An established risk factor for thromboembolic complications of heparin therapy, HIT occurs in 1% to 5% of patients treated with heparin and is the result of autoantibodies that bind specifically to CXCL4-heparin complexes in plasma. The second, autoimmune myositis, is associated with autoantibodies to histidyl tRNA synthetase, a protein synthesis factor that is also able to induce iDC chemotaxis, apparently by acting as an agonist at CCR5 (173). Its exact importance in promoting inflammation in myositis has not been established. As mentioned previously, tyrosyl tRNA

synthetase is also a nonchemokine chemokine receptor agonist, specific for CXCR1 (33).

In general, T-cell–dependent autoimmune diseases in human such as psoriasis, multiple sclerosis (MS), rheumatoid arthritis (RA), and type I diabetes mellitus are associated with inflammatory chemokines and tissue infiltration by T-lymphocytes and monocytes expressing inflammatory chemokine receptors (23,53,174,175). The relative importance of these is not yet known. Patients homozygous for the CCR5 null allele CCR5Δ32 have been reported who have MS, indicating that this receptor is not required for disease; however, heterozygotes have been reported to have delayed onset compared to patients lacking this allele. CCL2 and CCR2 and to a lesser extent CCL3 and CCR1 knockout mice have reduced disease in experimental allergic encephalomyelitis (EAE), a model of MS. Moreover, neutralization of CCL3 and CCL2 markedly reduced the early and relapsing phases of EAE, respectively. Interestingly, β-IFN, an approved treatment for MS, suppresses expression of these chemokines from T cells. MCP-1 (9-76), a dominant negative antagonist of CCL2, inhibits arthritis in the MRL-lpr mouse model of RA, suggesting a potential role for CCL2 and CCR2 (176). Met-RANTES, a chemically modified variant of CCL5 that blocks CCR1, CCR3, and CCR5, was beneficial in a collagen-induced arthritis model in DBA/I mice. In the NOD mouse model of diabetes, insulitis and hyperglycemia were reduced in CCL3 knockout mice (177).

Paradoxically, in some cases blocking chemokine receptors may lead to increased inflammation as shown for CCR1 and CCR2 in nephrotoxic nephritis and glomerulonephritis mouse models (178,179). This is associated with increased renal recruitment of CD4$^+$ and CD8$^+$ T cells and macrophages and enhanced Th1 immune responses; however, the exact mechanism is not defined.

Atherosclerosis

Atherosclerosis is a complex disease process with an inflammatory component that is probably regulated in part by inflammatory chemokines (23). Macrophages accumulate in atherosclerotic lesions and are associated with the presence of macrophage-targeted chemokines such as CCL2, CCL5, and CX3CL1. Both CCL2$^{-/-}$ and CCR2$^{-/-}$ mice have shown markedly reduced lesion size and delayed disease in diverse mouse models of atherosclerosis that appear to be due to reduced influx of macrophages into the vessel wall (180,181). CCL2 has also been shown to induce release of tissue factor from smooth muscle cells via an undefined but clearly CCR2-independent mechanism. Adoptive transfer studies with bone marrow from CXCR2$^{-/-}$ mice have also revealed a role for that receptor in promoting atherosclerosis in mouse models, apparently by promoting monocyte adhesion to early atherosclerotic endothelium through interaction with its mouse ligand KC and activation of the VLA-4/VCAM-1 adhesion system (182).

The CX3CR1 genetic variant CX3CR1-M280, which lacks normal CX3CL1-dependent adhesive function under conditions of physiologic flow (182a), has been associated with reduced risk of atherosclerotic vascular disease in man in three cohort studies, including a prospective study of the Framingham Heart Study Offspring Cohort (183,184). Consistent with this, CX3CR1 is expressed on monocytes, CX3CL1 is expressed in human atherosclerotic plaque, and CX3CR1$^{-/-}$ mice on an APOE$^{-/-}$ background have reduced susceptibility to atherosclerosis (184a,184b).

Asthma

Chemokine receptors associated with asthma include CXCR2 (185), CCR3 (186), CCR4, and CCR8 (187). CCR3 is present on eosinophils, basophils, mast cells, and some Th2 T cells, and CCR4 and CCR8 identify airway T cells of allergen-challenged atopic asthmatics. CCR8 knockout mice have reduced allergic airway inflammation in response to three different Th2-polarizing antigens: *Schistosoma mansoni* soluble egg antigen, ovalbumin, and cockroach antigen. The situation with the CCR4 axis is unsettled, since neutralization of the CCR4 ligand CCL22 was protective in a mouse model of airway hyperreactivity and eosinophilic inflammation, but CCR4 gene knockout was not. A role for the CCR3 axis in asthma has been supported by CCL11 neutralization in guinea pig, and CCR3 gene knockout in mouse. However, only one of three studies of CCL11 knockout mice found protection: ~40% reduction was found in airway eosinophils in ovalbumin sensitized/challenged mice, possibly due to compensation by other CCR3 ligands. The net effect of CCR3 knockout was expected to be more profound; however, the exact phenotype depends dramatically on the specific method of sensitization and challenge due to complex and opposite effects on eosinophil and mast cell trafficking. Thus, CCR3$^{-/-}$ mice sensitized ip have reduced eosinophil extravasation into the lung but an increase in mast cell homing to the trachea, with the net result being a paradoxical increase in airway responsiveness to cholinergic stimulation (188). Mast cell mobilization is not seen after epicutaneous sensitization, and these animals therefore have reduced airway eosinophilia on challenge and no increase in airway hyperresponsiveness (189). CCR6 also appears to play a role, since CCR6$^{-/-}$ mice have decreased allergic airway inflammation in response to sensitization and challenge with cockroach antigen, which is consistent with the induction of its ligand CCL20 in this model (190).

Cancer

Many chemokines have been detected *in situ* in tumors, and cancer cells have been shown to produce chemokines and express chemokine receptors. However, the exact role played by endogenous tumor-associated chemokines in recruiting tumor-infiltrating lymphocytes and tumor-associated macrophages and in promoting an antitumor immune response has not been delineated. On the contrary, there are data from mouse models suggesting that the overall

effect may be to promote tumorigenesis through additional effects on cell growth, angiogenesis, apoptosis, immune evasion, and metastasis. Controlling the balance of angiogenic and angiostatic chemokines may be particularly important (27). This has been shown in several instances, including human non–small-cell lung carcinoma (NSCLC), in which the ratio of ELR to non–ELR-CXC chemokine expression is high, and where in a SCID mouse model neutralization of endogenous tumor-derived CXCL8 (angiogenic) could inhibit tumor growth and metastasis by about 50% through a decrease in tumor-derived vessel density, without directly affecting tumor cell proliferation. Chemokine receptors on tumor cells have been shown to directly mediate chemokine-dependent proliferation, such as in the case of CXCL1 in melanoma (191,192), and metastasis, in the case of CXCR4 in a mouse model of breast cancer (193). It remains to be seen how general these effects are in other cancers.

Many chemokines, when delivered pharmacologically as recombinant proteins or by plasmid DNA or in transfected tumor cells, are able to induce immunologically mediated antitumor effects in mouse models and could be clinically useful. Mechanisms may differ depending on the model but may involve recruitment of monocytes, NK cells, and CD8$^+$ cytotoxic T cells to tumor. For example, induction of protective CD8$^+$ cellular immunity by IL-12 in a murine neuroblastoma model has been reported to depend entirely on endogenous CXCL10 (194). Also, CXCL10 transfection of a mouse B-cell–tumor cell line prevented establishment of tumor in a thymus-dependent manner. Synergistic effects of XCL1, CXCL9, and CXCL10 with cytokines such as IL-2 and IL-12 have been observed in various mouse models of cancer. Moreover, in SV40 large T-antigen transgenic mice, which develop spontaneous bilateral multifocal pulmonary adenocarcinomas, injection of recombinant CCL21 in the axillary lymph node region led to a marked reduction in tumor burden with extensive CD4$^+$ and CD8$^+$ lymphocytic and DC infiltration of the tumors, and enhanced survival (195). Chemokines may also function as adjuvants in tumor antigen vaccines. Chemokine tumor-antigen–fusion proteins represent a novel twist on this approach that facilitates uptake of tumor antigens by APCs via the normal process of ligand-receptor internalization (196). Non–ELR-CXC chemokines such as CXCL4 also exert antitumor effects through angiostatic mechanisms. Despite impressive antitumor effects in animal models, efforts to translate chemokines to patient therapy have been slow. In the only published study, a phase 1 trial of CXCL4 in colon cancer, the chemokine was well tolerated, but no efficacy was observed (197).

CHEMOKINE MIMICRY IN INFECTIOUS DISEASE

Herpesviruses, poxviruses, and retroviruses, have evolved diverse mechanisms to exploit and subvert the immune system through chemokine mimicry (19,47,198–200). These mimics represent a very high percentage of known viral homologs of host proteins in general, and immunoregulatory proteins in particular, and in some herpesviruses may occupy as much as 3% to 4% of the viral genome (Fig. 8). Three structural subclasses have been identified: proteins with unique structure of unknown ancestry, and chemokines and 7TM chemokine receptors that apparently were captured by the virus from the host. They can be divided into four major functional subclasses: chemoattractants, growth factors, cell entry factors, and antichemokines. The latter is a group of broad-spectrum chemokine scavengers and chemokine-receptor antagonists with diverse chemokine specificities that have been optimized during viral evolution to block chemokine action. Together these factors attest to the importance of the chemokine system in antiviral host defense.

Herpesvirus and Poxvirus Infection

The viral antichemokines are of particular interest because of their high potential for clinical application in immunologically mediated disease. Three unique secreted chemokine scavengers have been identified (198). vCKBP-I (viral chemokine binding protein-I) of myxoma virus, a rabbit poxvirus, is homologous to the mammalian IFNγ receptor. It binds and scavenges IFNγ, but also binds CXC, CC, and C chemokines. vCKBP-I has been shown to inhibit the early local inflammatory response in the skin of infected European rabbit hosts, and IV injection of recombinant vCKBP-I is safe and effective in blocking intimal hyperplasia after angioplasty injury in rats and rabbits. vCKBP-II is found in multiple poxviruses, including myxoma, vaccinia, variola, and cowpox. It is more specific for CC chemokines and is effective in attenuating airway inflammation in an allergen-induced asthma model (201). vCKBP-III of γ herpesvirus 68, a natural rodent pathogen, scavenges members of all chemokine classes (but not MIP-2 or KC) and is required for establishment of viral latency in B cells of mediastinal lymph node and spleen, acting in part by blocking CD8$^+$ T-cell suppression (202). It is also a virulence factor for neutrophilic meningitis, but not arteritis, in this model. The CC chemokine vMIP-II of HHV8 (human herpesvirus 8), a broad-spectrum chemokine-receptor antagonist that blocks members of all four receptor subfamilies, has been shown to block immune complex–induced glomerulonephritis in rats.

HHV8 encodes two other CC chemokines, vMIP-I and vMIP-III, as well as a constitutively active CC/CXC chemokine receptor named vGPCR, all of which are angiogenic and may contribute to the pathogenesis of Kaposi's sarcoma (KS), a highly vascular multicentric nonclonal tumor caused by HHV8, typically in the setting of immunosuppression such as in HIV/AIDS. Consistent with this, vGPCR induces KS-like tumors when expressed in transgenic mice (203). The mechanism may involve activation of NFκB and induction of angiogenic factors and proinflammatory cytokines (204). Thus, this virus appears to have converted a hijacked chemotactic receptor, probably CXCR2, into a regulator of gene expression.

Human cytomegalovirus (HCMV) encodes four GPCR homologs: UL33, UL78, US27, and US28, which are probably important virulence factors (21). UL33 and UL78 are conserved in all sequenced β herpesviruses. UL33 and UL78 are orphans, but probably are chemokine receptors since U12 and U51, their respective homologs in HHV6, are able to induce calcium flux in response to several CC chemokines. Both mouse and rat CMV UL33 homologs are critical for spread to salivary gland and are mortality factors. RCMV UL78 is also a mortality factor in vivo. HHV6 U51 expression in epithelial cells decreases transcription of CCL5, suggesting a novel mechanism of immune evasion. HCMV US28 is a multi-CC and CX3C receptor whose biological roles are not established. Its ability to sequester ligands in vitro suggests a role in immune evasion. Its ability to bind the adhesive chemokine CX3CL1 suggests that it may mediate cell–cell spread of the virus. US28 also mediates both ligand-dependent signaling, as well as constitutive activation of PLC and NFκB. It is also able to induce ligand-dependent chemokinesis and chemotaxis of smooth muscle cells, which points to a potential role in dissemination and in atherosclerosis, where HCMV has been implicated as an infectious cofactor. HCMV also encodes two CXC chemokines, named vCXC-1 and vCXC-2. vCXC-1, a potent neutrophil chemoattractant acting specifically at CXCR2, may facilitate immune evasion and/or viral dissemination. In this regard, m131/129, a CC chemokine encoded by mouse CMV, has been shown to promote both inflammation at the site of infection and viral dissemination to salivary gland, while delaying NK-cell and CD4$^+$ and CD8$^+$ T-cell–mediated viral clearance from spleen and liver.

The human poxvirus molluscum contagiosum virus (MCV) encodes a CC chemokine named MC148 that has been reported to block recruitment of neutrophils by CXCL8; monocytes by CCL2; and monocytes, T cells, and neutrophils by CXCL12. However, among the specific chemokine receptors tested, it selectively binds and blocks human CCR8 (199). The reason for this dichotomy is not known. Interestingly, vMIP-I and vMIP-III are agonists at CCR8, whereas this receptor may have only one high-affinity human ligand, CCL1. Of note, MCV infection characteristically is not associated with inflammation, perhaps in part due to antichemokine effects of MC148. Several other viral chemokines and chemokine receptors have been described but their properties in vivo have not been defined (Fig. 8).

HIV

The HIV envelope glycoprotein gp120 mediates fusion of viral envelope with the target-cell membrane by binding to CD4 and a chemokine receptor. This finding resulted from a remarkable convergence of three lines of investigation that were initially unrelated (17,205). The first addressed the question of why some HIV-infected individuals progress slowly to AIDS. One theory proposed that soluble suppressive factors made by CD8$^+$ T-lymphocytes were responsible, and in

Virus family	Virus	Molecule	Class	Ligands/receptors	Function
γ₂ Herpesviridae	H. saimiri	ECRF3 (ORF 74)	CXCR	Agonists: CXCL1, CXCL7, CXCL8	Calcium flux in frog oocytes
	HHV8 (KSHV)	vGPCR (ORF 74)	CCR and CXCR (constitutively active)	Agonists: CXCL1; Inverse agonists: vMIP-II, CXCL10, CXCL12	Transforms NIH 3T3 cells; Angiogenic; Induces Kaposi's Sarcoma-like tumors in transgenic mice; Activates NF-κB and pro-inflammatory cytokine and growth factor expression
		vMIP-I	CC chemokine	Agonist at CCR8	Angiogenic
		vMIP-II	CC chemokine	Agonist at CCR3 and CCR8; Antagonist at CCR1-5, 8, CXCR3, CXCR4, XCR1, CX3CR1 and US28; Inverse agonist at HHV8 vGPCR	Angiogenic; Suppresses X4 and R5 HIV; Th2 cell and eosinophil chemoattractant;
		vMIP-III	CC chemokine	Agonist at CCR4	Angiogenic; Th2 cell chemotaxis
	Mouse γHV68	vCKBP-III	C, CC, CXC, CX3C chemokine scavenger	Binds XCL1, CX3CL1, CXCL8, CCL5 and others	Anti-inflammatory; Latency factor; Virulence factor
	Equine HV2	E1	CCR	Agonists: Eotaxin	Chemotaxis
		E6	Putative CCR	ND	ND
		ORF 74	Putative CXCR	ND	ND
β Herpesviridae	Human CMV	US28	CCR and CX3CR	CCL2-5, CX3CL1	Chemokine sequestration; Smooth muscle cell motility; HIV coreceptor
		US27	Putative CCR	ND	ND
		UL33	Putative CCR	ND	ND
		UL78	Putative CCR	ND	ND
		vCXC-1 (ORF UL146)	CXC chemokine	CXCR2	Neutrophil chemotaxis and degranulation
		vCXC-2 (ORF UL147)	CXC chemokine	ND	ND
	Mouse CMV	MCK-2 (ORF m131/129)	CC chemokine	ND	Virulence factor; Anti-inflammatory
		M33	Putative CCR	ND	Virulence factor (targeting and replication in salivary gland)
		M78	Putative CCR	ND	ND
	Rat CMV	R33	Putative CCR	ND	Virulence factor (targeting and replication in salivary gland)
		R78	Putative CCR	ND	Virulence factor
	HHV6	U12	CCR	Agonists: CCL5	Calcium flux
		U51	CCR	ND	Downmodulation of CCL5 expression
		vCCL4(U83)	CC chemokine	CCR2 agonist	Chemotaxis
	HHV7	U12	Putative CCR	ND	ND
		U51	Putative CCR	ND	ND
α Herpesviridae	Marek's Disease Virus	v-IL-8	CXC chemokine	ND	ND
Poxviridae	Equine HV-1, Bovine HV-1, Bovine HV-5	vCKBP-4 (gG)	Chemokine binding protein	CC, C, CXC binding protein-different specificities for vCKBP-4 isoforms from different α herpesviruses	Membrane associated chemokine scavenger
	Molluscum Contagiosum Virus (MCV)	MC148R (MCC-1)	CC chemokine	Antagonist at CCR8	Blocks neutrophil, monocyte and T cell chemotaxis induced by multiple CC and CXC chemokines; Blocks human hematopoietic progenitor cell proliferation
	Ortho- and leporipoxviruses	vCKBP-II	CC chemokine binding protein	Binds multiple CC chemokines	Anti-inflammatory
	Myxoma	vCKBP-I	IFNγ and CC, C, and CXC chemokine–binding protein	Binds multiple CC and CXC chemokines and XCL1	Anti-inflammatory
Lentiviridae	HIV	Tat	CC and CXC chemokine mimic	Agonist at CCR2 and CCR3; Antagonist at CXCR4 and CCR8	Monocyte and neutrophil chemoattractant; HIV suppressive factor at CXCR4
		gp120	Chemokine mimic	CCR5, CXCR4	Chemotactic agonist at CCR5; Neuronal apoptosis via CXCR4; HIV-target cell fusion factor at CCR5, CXCR4, others

FIG. 8. Viral chemokines and chemokine receptors. Note that the following ORFs are syntenic: HHV6 U12, HHV7 U12; HCMV UL33, MCMV M33, and rat CMV R33; HCMV UL78, MCMV M78, rat CMV R78; HHV6 U51, and HHV7 U51. ND, not determined; vCKBP, viral chemokine binding protein; MCC, molluscum contagiosum virus CC chemokine; ORF, open reading frame.

1995, CCL3, CCL4, and CCL5 were reported to have this activity and to be selectively overproduced by PBMCs from individuals who were HIV-free despite repeated high-risk sexual activity.

The mechanism of suppression was identified through a second independent line of investigation aimed at the question of why many HIV strains, which can all infect PBMCs, are able to infect either primary macrophages (M-tropic HIV) or cultured T-cell lines (T-tropic HIV) *in vitro,* but not both. HIV cytotropism is important because, for reasons that are still not known, M-tropic strains but not T-tropic strains are transmitted in populations at risk, and persist, whereas T-tropic strains are found in a subset of patients, mainly during late stages of disease, and appear to be more virulent. The cytotropism problem was unequivocally solved in 1996 when Feng et al. (206) demonstrated that CXCR4 is used as a selective fusion cofactor with CD4 by T-tropic HIV. Later work proved that CCR5 plays an analogous role for M-tropic HIV, and the chemokine ligands for these receptors were shown to suppress HIV by blocking interaction of gp120 with chemokine receptor and promoting receptor down-regulation. Both CCR5 and CXCR4 physically associate with CD4 and gp120, and are therefore referred to as "HIV coreceptors." HIV strains are now functionally classified and named according to their specificity for CXCR4 (X4 strains), CCR5 (R5 strains), or both (R5X4 strains). Other chemokine receptors, several orphan receptors, the HCMV receptor US28, and the leukotriene B4 receptor are also HIV coreceptors; however, their activities are limited and at present there is little to no evidence that they are used by HIV to infect primary cells. The one clear exception is CXCR6, which in nonhuman primates replaces CXCR4 as the major HIV coreceptor for T-tropic SIV strains (17).

Proof of principle that CCR5 plays an important role in HIV disease was provided through discovery of the inactive CCR5Δ32 allele, which has a 32–base pair deletion in the ECL2 region of the ORF (50). This introduces a premature stop codon in TMD5 and causes massive truncation and intracellular retention of the protein. Consequently, PBMCs from CCR5Δ32 homozygotes are fully infectable by X4 HIV but cannot be infected by R5 strains, and CCR5Δ32 homozygotes are overrepresented in cohorts of exposed uninfected individuals but are almost never found among HIV+ individuals, regardless of the route of transmission. Together these *in vitro* and *in vivo* findings strongly support the conclusion that wild-type CCR5 is essential for efficient person-to-person transmission of HIV. Moreover, analysis of CCR5Δ32 heterozygotes has indicated that the level of CCR5 expression is a limiting factor for HIV replication and disease progression.

The evidence that CXCR4 regulates HIV pathogenesis is indirect. *In vitro,* all HIV-1 strains that cannot use CCR5 use CXCR4, and some strains use both. *In vivo,* X4 viruses are less common. They have been isolated from the few known HIV+ CCR5Δ32 homozygotes, suggesting that they are ca-

pable of transmitting disease, presumably by using CXCR4, and that ordinarily R5 strains in the transmitting inoculum generate factors that select against them. The appearance of X4 viruses in some patients late in disease is associated with an accelerated disease course, and, consistent with this, X4 strains are more cytopathic than R5 strains *in vitro.* The mechanism may simply involve target availability since CXCR4+ CD4+ T cells greatly exceed CCR5+ CD4+ T cells in both blood and lymph node (207). However, this only deepens the mystery of why X4 strains do not efficiently transmit infection. CXCR4+ CD4+ cells are found in rectal and vaginal mucosa, and in the blood, so that the major portals of HIV entry should support transmission by X4 strains.

Regulation of the precise level of coreceptor expression and function depends on the balance of both positive and negative factors, including cytokines, chemokines, viruses, bacterial products, and T-cell co-stimulation (208). CCR5 ligands can suppress R5 but enhance X4 HIV replication. Moreover, CCL5 can either suppress or enhance R5 HIV replication depending on the concentration used. Thus, the level of coreceptor ligands *in vivo* would also be predicted to modulate HIV replication. Numerous studies correlating chemokine levels with disease outcomes have been published; however, the results are not fully consistent. Additional HIV-suppressive chemokines include CCL22 and CCL2. CCL22 is the only one able to inhibit both R5 and X4 HIV, but the mechanism, which is unknown, does not involve direct binding to coreceptors. Additional CD8+ T-cell–derived HIV-suppressive activities have been identified that are independent of known chemokines.

Common genetic factors reported to be risk factors in HIV disease cohorts that may work by affecting the balance of coreceptor/chemokine expression and function include promoter variants for CCR5, CCL3, and CCL5; the structural variants CCR2 V64I and CX3CR1-M280; and the 3′-UTR variant SDF-1 3′A. However, additional cohorts will have to be studied and mechanisms rigorously defined to judge the significance (50). Combinations of "protective" alleles would be predicted to provide additive protection, and this was observed for CCR5Δ32 and CCR2 V64I in a large meta-analysis (209).

The mechanism of HIV fusion involves direct binding of CD4 to coreceptor, and gp120 to both CD4 and coreceptor (Fig. 9) (17). In the absence of CD4, gp120 binds with only low affinity to coreceptors. Coreceptor choice is determined by a small number of key residues in the V3 loop of gp120, and binding determinants have been mapped to multiple extracellular domains of coreceptors, including a sulfated tyrosine in the N-terminal domain of CCR5 (210). Efficiency is determined in part by the stoichiometry of CD4 and coreceptor and the cellular context (211). For example, monocytes and macrophages have been reported to have different molecular forms of CXCR4 and are differentially sensitive to X4 HIV infection. After gp120 binds, it undergoes a conformational change that releases a cryptic fusogenic peptide

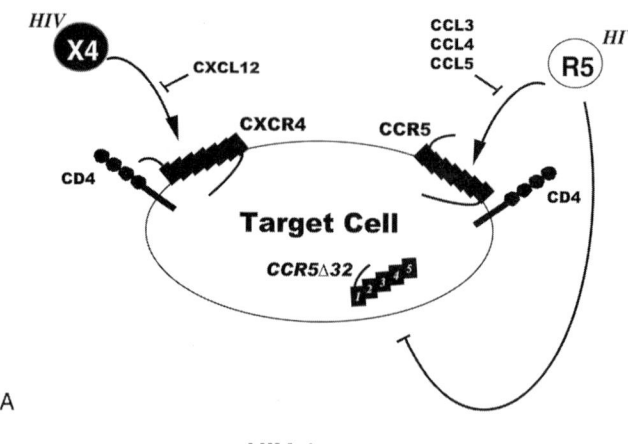

A

FIG. 9. Model of HIV coreceptor activity. **A:** HIV cytotropism is explained by differential usage of CXCR4 and CCR5 as coreceptors. The mutant receptor CCR5Δ32 is not expressed on the cell surface and cannot be used for cell entry by HIV. **B:** Model of HIV entry mechanism. See text for description.

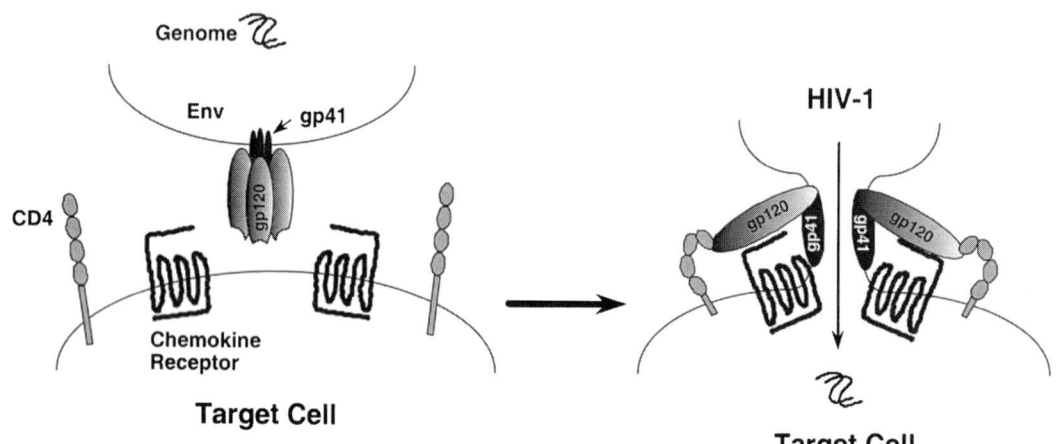

B

in gp41 that promotes fusion of the viral envelope and the target-cell membrane.

Coreceptor signaling is clearly not required for full fusion activity. Nevertheless, purified gp120 is able to act not just as a ligand but also as a potent agonist at CCR5 and CXCR4 and can induce calcium flux, chemotaxis, and activation of Pyk-2 and FAK. This could be a potential mechanism to attract additional target cells to the virus, or alternatively, just a method to facilitate fusion-pore penetration of the cytoskeleton. The effect of CCR5 signaling on X4 replication and concentration-dependent effects on R5 replication have been mentioned previously. In the case of CXCR4, signaling in response to purified X4 gp120 has been reported to induce apoptosis of human neurons, which may be important in the pathogenesis of HIV encephalitis and AIDS dementia. Finally, interaction of gp120 with CXCR4 on macrophages can induce apoptosis of $CD8^+$ T cells, which suggests that coreceptors may promote CTL suppression in trans, although the precise mechanism has not been delineated.

CCR5Δ32 is a common mutation: ~20% of North American Caucasians are heterozygous and 1% are homozygous. Since it is estimated to have originated in Caucasians recently, within the past ~3,000 years, it would take a narrow population bottleneck or a powerful positive selective pressure, such as another epidemic, to account for the high prevalence observed in populations today. Smallpox is a particularly attractive candidate since CCR5 (and several other chemokine receptors) have been reported to facilitate infection of target cells by myxoma, vaccinia, and several other related poxviruses (212).

The CCR5Δ32 genotype distribution is in Hardy–Weinberg equilibrium indicating that the allele has no intrinsic effect on fitness, which is consistent with the lack of any obvious health problems in the few homozygotes who have been examined and in unstressed CCR5 knockout mice. Thus, inactivating CCR5 with a drug should theoretically be safe and effective in preventing HIV infection. Two potent and selective small-molecule antagonists of CCR5 have been reported, SCH-C from Schering-Plough and TAK779 from Takeda Pharmaceuticals. SCH-C reduced HIV levels in infected SCID-hu mice and in a phase 1 study of patients (213). Escape mutants occurred when R5 tropic HIV strains were cultured in the presence of this compound *in vitro,* but the mechanism involved resistance to inhibition at CCR5, not expansion to usage of CXCR4. Potent CXCR4 small-molecule blocking agents include the polyarginine ALX40-4C, the bicyclam AMD3100, and the horseshoe-crab peptide T140. Targeting CXCR4 may be more hazardous than CCR5 since it is an essential gene, at least in mice, whereas CCR5 is dispensable in both human and mouse.

Malaria

Three years before the HIV coreceptors were discovered, Duffy, the 7TM promiscuous chemokine-binding protein of erythrocytes, had already been demonstrated to play a similar role in malaria (22). The key observation was that CXCL8 and several other chemokines could bind to erythrocytes from Caucasian but not African-American blood donors. This mimicked the racial distribution of the Duffy blood–group antigen, which is responsible for minor transfusion reactions and was already known to be the determinant of erythrocyte invasion by *P. vivax*. The chemokine and parasite determinants on erythrocytes both map to Duffy. The parasite ligand, which is named the *Plasmodium vivax* Duffy binding protein (PvDBP), is expressed in micronemes of merozoites and binds to the N-terminal domain of Duffy via a cysteine-rich domain. This interaction is required for junction formation during invasion, but not for initial binding or parasite orientation. Duffy deficiency, which is due mainly to an inherited single nucleotide substitution named −46C at an erythroid-specific GATA-1 site in the Duffy promoter (214), is fixed in sub-Saharan Africa but not in other malaria-endemic regions of the world. Accordingly, *P. vivax* malaria is rare in sub-Saharan Africa but common in Central and South America, India, and Southeast Asia. Fixation of the mutation in Africa presumably occurred because of positive selective pressure from malaria. Identification of the −46C mutation in the Melanesian Duffy allele among individuals living in a *P. vivax*–endemic region of Papua New Guinea provides an opportunity to test this hypothesis prospectively (215). Together with CCR5Δ32, Duffy −46C is the strongest genetic resistance factor known for any infectious disease in man.

The physiologic role of Duffy has not been clearly defined. In addition to erythrocytes, it is expressed on endothelial cells and Purkinje cells. Since it does not signal, it could either positively or negatively regulate inflammation, depending on whether it scavenges circulating chemokines or acts as a chemokine-tethering device on endothelial cells. Duffy deficiency in man and knockout mice is not associated with any known health problems. Study of Duffy knockout mice has not settled this question, since one group reported that these mice had reduced inflammation when challenged with LPS in the peritoneal cavity, whereas in a second line challenged with LPS systemically, inflammation was exaggerated in the lung and liver (216,217).

THERAPEUTIC APPLICATIONS

Chemokines and Chemokine Receptors as Targets for Drug Development

Although chemokine-targeted drug development is still in the early stages and there are no approved drugs, there are already two accomplishments that deserve special mention: First, chemokine receptors are the first cytokine receptors for which potent, selective, nonpeptide small-molecule antagonists have been identified that work *in vivo*; and second, targeting host determinants, as in the case of CCR5 and CXCR4 in HIV/AIDS, is a new approach in the development of antimicrobial agents. Other reasonable disease indications are Duffy in *P. vivax* malaria; CXCR2 in acute neutrophil-mediated inflammation; CXCR3 and CCR2 in Th1-driven disease; CCR2 and CX3CR1 in atherosclerosis; and CCR3 and possibly CCR4 and CCR8 in Th2 diseases such as asthma.

Potent and selective nonpeptide small-molecule antagonists of CCR5, CXCR4, CXCR2, CCR1, CCR2, and CCR3 have been reported. These molecules have in common a nitrogen-rich core and appear to block ligand binding by acting at a conserved allosteric site analogous to the retinal-binding site in the transmembrane region of rhodopsin. Although small molecules taken as pills are the main goal, other blocking strategies are also under consideration, such as ribozymes, modified chemokines (e.g., amino terminal–modified versions of CCL5) and intrakines, which are modified forms of chemokines delivered by gene therapy that remain in the endoplasmic reticulum and block surface expression of newly synthesized receptors.

The fact that viral antichemokines typically block multiple chemokines acting at multiple receptors may hint that the most clinically effective chemokine-targeted anti-inflammatory strategy will need to provide broad-spectrum coverage. In this regard, the viral antichemokines themselves may have a place therapeutically, although issues of antigenicity may be limiting. There is also proof of principle from work with a distamycin analog that broad-spectrum blockade is feasible with nonpeptide small molecules (11).

Chemokines as Biological Response Modifiers

Both inflammatory and homeostatic chemokines are being evaluated for therapeutic potential as biological response modifiers, acting mainly as immunomodulators or as regulators of angiogenesis. Studies to date have not revealed major problems with toxicity, and efficacy has been noted in models of cancer, inflammation, and infection. To date, clinical trials in cancer and stem cell protection have not produced an approved drug, as noted previously. Chemokines are also being developed as vaccine adjuvants, delivered either as pure protein, immunomodulatory plasmid (218), or as recombinant protein within antigen-pulsed DC. In this application, the chemokine may act at multiple different steps in the immune response—for example, to strengthen trafficking of specific classes of immune cells through the site of vaccination, or enhance uptake of antigen by APCs, or tilt the Th1/Th2 balance to a position that is optimal for a particular disease. Impressive efficacy in infectious disease, allergy, and tumor models has been observed in rodents (219). Chemokine gene administration has also been shown to induce neutralizing antibody against the encoded chemokine, to block immune responses and to ameliorate EAE and arthritis in rodent models.

CONCLUSIONS

Major progress has been made in our understanding of the chemokine system since it was discovered in the 1980s. The basic picture of chemokine structural biology, immunology, and biology is now in reasonably sharp focus. Recognition that chemokines play complex and prismatic roles in immune system development, differentiation, and activation has replaced an older, single-dimensional focus on cell migration. Major diseases of the hematopoietic system, HIV/AIDS and malaria, have been identified that are caused by microbial exploitation of chemokine receptors, and there is genetic proof of principle that blocking these receptors may safely and effectively prevent infection. Moreover, potent chemokine receptor antagonists have been developed and direct data indicate that some are safe and effective in diverse animal models of immunologically mediated disease.

Still, many chemokines have not yet been studied at the biological level (and were therefore not discussed in detail in this chapter). And our understanding of chemokine-signaling networks, *in vivo* gene-expression dynamics, and mechanisms of leukocyte migration, differentiation, and activation is still lacking in detail. With regard to clinical applications, it is still not clear whether chemokine blockade can effectively treat established immunologically-mediated disease, and most human disease indications for drug development now under consideration are still often based mainly on educated guesswork using inadequate small animal models. Finally, there are so far no chemokine-based therapeutics approved for use in the treatment or prevention of human disease. These are some of the major opportunities and challenges for future basic and applied research in this field.

ACKNOWLEDGMENTS

Thanks to Joshua Farber and Kevin Bacon for helpful comments on the manuscript. The author regrets that due to space limitations only a small fraction of relevant primary literature could be cited here.

REFERENCES

1. Baggiolini M, Walz A, Kunkel SL. Neutrophil-activating peptide-1/interleukin 8, a novel cytokine that activates neutrophils. *J Clin Invest* 1989;84:1045–1049.
2. Oppenheim JJ, Zachariae CO, Mukaida N, et al. Properties of the novel proinflammatory supergene "intercrine" cytokine family. *Annu Rev Immunol* 1991;9:617–648.
3. Schall TJ. Biology of the RANTES/SIS cytokine family. *Cytokine* 1991;3:165–183.
4. Wolpe SD, Cerami A. Macrophage inflammatory proteins 1 and 2: members of a novel superfamily of cytokines. *Faseb J* 1989;3:2565–2573.
5. Rossi D, Zlotnik A. The biology of chemokines and their receptors. *Annu Rev Immunol* 2000;18:217–242.
6. Springer TA. Traffic signals for lymphocyte recirculation and leukocyte emigration: the multistep paradigm. *Cell* 1994;76:301–314.
7. Butcher EC, Picker LJ. Lymphocyte homing and homeostasis. *Science* 1996;272:60–66.
8. Ye RD, Boulay F. Structure and function of leukocyte chemoattractant receptors. *Adv Pharmacol* 1997;39:221–289.
9. Le Y, Oppenheim JJ, Wang JM. Pleiotropic roles of formyl peptide receptors. *Cytokine Growth Factor Rev* 2001;12:91–105.
10. Murphy PM. The molecular biology of leukocyte chemoattractant receptors. *Annu Rev Immunol* 1994;12:593–633.
11. Cascieri MA, Springer MS. The chemokine/chemokine-receptor family:potential and progress for therapeutic intervention. *Curr Opin Chem Biol* 2000;4:420–427.
12. Sozzani S, Allavena P, Vecchi A, et al. The role of chemokines in the regulation of dendritic cell trafficking. *J Leukoc Biol* 1999;66:1–9.
13. Ansel KM, Cyster JG. Chemokines in lymphopoiesis and lymphoid organ development. *Curr Opin Immunol* 2001;13:172–179.
14. Sallusto F, Mackay CR, Lanzavecchia A. The role of chemokine receptors in primary, effector, and memory immune responses. *Annu Rev Immunol* 2000;18:593–620.
15. Moser B, Loetscher P. Lymphocyte traffic control by chemokines. *Nat Immunol* 2001;2:123–128.
16. Luther SA, Cyster JG. Chemokines as regulators of T cell differentiation. *Nat Immunol* 2001;2:102–107.
17. Berger EA, Murphy PM, Farber JM. Chemokine receptors as HIV-1 coreceptors:roles in viral entry, tropism, and disease. *Annu Rev Immunol* 1999;17:657–700.
18. Garzino-Demo A, DeVico AL, Conant KE, et al. The role of chemokines in human immunodeficiency virus infection. *Immunol Rev* 2000;177:79–87.
19. Rosenkilde MM, Waldhoer M, Luttichau HR, et al. Virally encoded 7TM receptors. *Oncogene* 2001;20:1582–1593.
20. Lalani AS, Barrett JW, McFadden G. Modulating chemokines: more lessons from viruses. *Immunol Today* 2000;21:100–106.
21. Vink C, Smit MJ, Leurs R, et al. The role of cytomegalovirus-encoded homologs of G protein-coupled receptors and chemokines in manipulation of and evasion from the immune system. *J Clin Virol* 2001;23:43–55.
22. Horuk R. The interleukin-8-receptor family: from chemokines to malaria. *Immunol Today* 1994;15:169–174.
23. Gerard C, Rollins BJ. Chemokines and disease. *Nat Immunol* 2001;2:108–115.
24. Zlotnik A, Yoshie O. Chemokines: a new classification system and their role in immunity. *Immunity* 2000;12:121–127.
25. Clark-Lewis I, Kim KS, Rajarathnam K, et al. Structure–activity relationships of chemokines. *J Leukoc Biol* 1995;57:703–711.
26. Farber JM. Mig and IP-10: CXC chemokines that target lymphocytes. *J Leukoc Biol* 1997;61:246–257.
27. Belperio JA, Keane MP, Arenberg DA, et al. CXC chemokines in angiogenesis. *J Leukoc Biol* 2000;68:1–8.
28. Van Coillie E, Van Damme J, Opdenakker G. The MCP/eotaxin subfamily of CC chemokines. *Cytokine Growth Factor Rev* 1999;10:61–86.
29. Matloubian M, David A, Engel S, et al. A transmembrane CXC chemokine is a ligand for HIV-coreceptor bonzo. *Nat Immunol* 2000;1:298–304.
30. Waldmann TA. T-cell receptors for cytokines: targets for immunotherapy of leukemia/lymphoma. *Ann Oncol* 2000;11:101–106.
31. Murphy PM, Baggiolini M, Charo IF, et al. International union of pharmacology. XXII. Nomenclature for chemokine receptors. *Pharmacol Rev* 2000;52:145–176.
32. Gosling J, Dairaghi DJ, Wang Y, et al. Cutting edge: identification of a novel chemokine receptor that binds dendritic cell– and T cell–active chemokines including ELC, SLC, and TECK. *J Immunol* 2000;164:2851–2856.
33. Wakasugi K, Schimmel P. Two distinct cytokines released from a human aminoacyl-tRNA synthetase. *Science* 1999;284:147–151.
34. Yang D, Chertov O, Oppenheim JJ. Participation of mammalian defensins and cathelicidins in anti- microbial immunity:receptors and activities of human defensins and cathelicidin (LL-37). *J Leukoc Biol* 2001;69:691–697.
35. Broxmeyer HE. Regulation of hematopoiesis by chemokine family members. *Int J Hematol* 2001;74:9–17.
36. Allavena P, Sica A, Vecchi A, Locati M, Sozzani S, Mantovani A. The chemokine receptor switch paradigm and dendritic cell migration:its significance in tumor tissues. *Immunol Rev* 2000;177:141–149.
37. Hargreaves DC, Hyman PL, Lu TT, et al. A coordinated change in chemokine responsiveness guides plasma cell movements. *J Exp Med* 2001;194:45–56.
38. Kunkel EJ, Boisvert J, Murphy K, et al. Expression of the chemokine

receptors CCR4, CCR5, and CXCR3 by human tissue-infiltrating lymphocytes. *Am J Pathol* 2002;160:347–355.

39. Kim CH, Rott L, Kunkel EJ, et al. Rules of chemokine receptor association with T cell polarization in vivo. *J Clin Invest* 2001;108:1331–1339.

40. Campbell JJ, Pan J, Butcher EC. Cutting edge: developmental switches in chemokine responses during T cell maturation. *J Immunol* 1999;163:2353–2357.

41. Youn BS, Mantel C, Broxmeyer HE. Chemokines, chemokine receptors and hematopoiesis. *Immunol Rev* 2000;177:150–174.

42. Campbell JJ, Qin S, Unutmaz D, et al. Unique subpopulations of CD56+ NK and NK-T peripheral blood lymphocytes identified by chemokine receptor expression repertoire. *J Immunol* 2001;166:6477–6482.

43. Robertson MJ. Role of chemokines in the biology of natural killer cells. *J Leukoc Biol* 2002;71:173–183.

44. Nomiyama H, Mera A, Ohneda O, et al. Organization of the chemokine genes in the human and mouse major clusters of CC and CXC chemokines:diversification between the two species. *Genes Immun* 2001;2:110–113.

45. Forssmann U, Magert HJ, Adermann K, et al. Hemofiltrate CC chemokines with unique biochemical properties: HCC-1/CCL14a and HCC-2/CCL15. *J Leukoc Biol* 2001;70:357–366.

46. Murphy PM. Molecular mimicry and the generation of host defense protein diversity. *Cell* 1993;72:823–826.

47. Murphy PM. Viral exploitation and subversion of the immune system through chemokine mimicry. *Nat Immunol* 2001;2:116–122.

48. Nakano H, Gunn MD. Gene duplications at the chemokine locus on mouse chromosome 4: multiple strain-specific haplotypes and the deletion of secondary lymphoid-organ chemokine and EBI-1 ligand chemokine genes in the plt mutation. *J Immunol* 2001;166:361–369.

49. Mummidi S, Bamshad M, Ahuja SS, et al. Evolution of human and non-human primate CC chemokine receptor 5 gene and mRNA. Potential roles for haplotype and mRNA diversity, differential haplotype-specific transcriptional activity, and altered transcription factor binding to polymorphic nucleotides in the pathogenesis of HIV-1 and simian immunodeficiency virus. *J Biol Chem* 2000;275:18946–18961.

50. O'Brien SJ, Moore JP. The effect of genetic variation in chemokines and their receptors on HIV transmission and progression to AIDS. *Immunol Rev* 2000;177:99–111.

51. Qiu B, Frait KA, Reich F, et al. Chemokine expression dynamics in mycobacterial (type-1) and schistosomal (type-2) antigen-elicited pulmonary granuloma formation. *Am J Pathol* 2001;158:1503–1515.

52. Gutierrez-Ramos JC, Lloyd C, Kapsenberg ML, et al. Non-redundant functional groups of chemokines operate in a coordinate manner during the inflammatory response in the lung. *Immunol Rev* 2000;177:31–42.

53. Karpus WJ, Ransohoff RM. Chemokine regulation of experimental autoimmune encephalomyelitis: temporal and spatial expression patterns govern disease pathogenesis. *J Immunol* 1998;161:2667–2671.

54. Stone MJ, Mayer KL. Three-dimensional structure of chemokines. In: Rothenberg ME, ed. *Chemokines in allergic disease* New York: Marcel Dekker, 2000:67–94.

55. Clore GM, Gronenborn AM. Three-dimensional structures of alpha and beta chemokines. *Faseb J* 1995;9:57–62.

56. Kuloglu ES, McCaslin DR, Kitabwalla M, et al. Monomeric solution structure of the prototypical 'C' chemokine lymphotactin. *Biochemistry* 2001;40:12486–12496.

57. Ali S, Palmer ACV, Fritchley SJ, et al. Multimerization of monocyte chemoattractant protein-1 is not required for glycosaminoglycan-dependent transendothelial chemotaxis. *Biochem J* 2001;358:737–745.

57a. Proudfoot AE, Handel TM, Johnson Z, et al. Glycosaminoglycan binding and oligomerization are essential for the in vivo activity of certain chemokines. *Proc Natl Acad Sci USA* 2003;100:1885–1890.

58. Guan E, Wang J, Norcross MA. Identification of human macrophage inflammatory proteins 1alpha and 1beta as a native secreted heterodimer. *J Biol Chem* 2001;276:12404–12409.

59. Bannert N, Craig S, Farzan M, et al. Sialylated O-glycans and sulfated tyrosines in the NH2-terminal domain of CC chemokine receptor 5 contribute to high affinity binding of chemokines. *J Exp Med* 2001;194:1661–1673.

60. Ludwig A, Ehlert JE, Flad HD, et al. Identification of distinct surface-expressed and intracellular CXC− chemokine receptor 2 glycoforms in neutrophils: N-glycosylation is essential for maintenance of receptor surface expression. *J Immunol* 2000;165:1044–1052.

61. Chabot DJ, Chen H, Dimitrov DS, et al. N-linked glycosylation of CXCR4 masks coreceptor function for CCR5-dependent human immunodeficiency virus type 1 isolates. *J Virol* 2000;74:4404–4413.

62. Blanpain C, Wittamer V, Vanderwinden JM, et al. Palmitoylation of CCR5 is critical for receptor trafficking and efficient activation of intracellular signaling pathways. *J Biol Chem* 2001;276:23795–23804.

63. Unger VM, Hargrave PA, Baldwin JM, et al. Arrangement of rhodopsin transmembrane alpha-helices. *Nature* 1997;389:203–206.

64. Hemmerich S, Paavola C, Bloom A, et al. Identification of residues in the monocyte chemotactic protein-1 that contact the MCP-1 receptor, CCR2. *Biochemistry* 1999;38:13013–13025.

65. Berson JF, Doms RW. Structure-function studies of the HIV-1 coreceptors. *Semin Immunol* 1998;10:237–248.

66. Middleton J, Neil S, Wintle J, et al. Transcytosis and surface presentation of IL-8 by venular endothelial cells. *Cell* 1997;91:385–395.

67. Baekkevold ES, Yamanaka T, Palframan RT, et al. The CCR7 ligand elc (CCL19) is transcytosed in high endothelial venules and mediates T cell recruitment. *J Exp Med* 2001;193:1105–1112.

68. Wagner L, Yang OO, Garcia-Zepeda EA, et al. Beta-chemokines are released from HIV-1-specific cytolytic T-cell granules complexed to proteoglycans. *Nature* 1998;391:908–911.

69. Burns JM, Lewis GK, DeVico AL. Soluble complexes of regulated upon activation, normal T cells expressed and secreted (RANTES) and glycosaminoglycans suppress HIV-1 infection but do not induce Ca(2+) signaling. *Proc Natl Acad Sci U S A* 1999;96:14499–14504.

70. Cinamon G, Grabovsky V, Winter E, et al. Novel chemokine functions in lymphocyte migration through vascular endothelium under shear flow. *J Leukoc Biol* 2001;69:860–866.

71. Poznansky MC, Olszak IT, Foxall R, et al. Active movement of T cells away from a chemokine. *Nat Med* 2000;6:543–548.

72. Cole AM, Ganz T, Liese AM, et al. Cutting edge: IFN-inducible ELR-CXC chemokines display defensin-like antimicrobial activity. *J Immunol* 2001;167:623–627.

73. Kaplan AP. Chemokines, chemokine receptors and allergy. *Int Arch Allergy Immunol* 2001;124:423–431.

74. Nagasawa T, Tachibana K, Kishimoto T. A novel CXC chemokine PBSF/SDF-1 and its receptor CXCR4: their functions in development, hematopoiesis and HIV infection. *Semin Immunol* 1998;10:179–185.

75. Lataillade JJ, Clay D, Bourin P, et al. Stromal cell-derived factor 1 regulates primitive hematopoiesis by suppressing apoptosis and by promoting G(0)/G(1) transition in CD34(+) cells:evidence for an autocrine/paracrine mechanism. *Blood* 2002;99:1117–1129.

76. Colamussi ML, Secchiero P, Gonelli A, et al. Stromal derived factor-1 alpha (SDF-1 alpha) induces CD4+ T cell apoptosis via the functional up-regulation of the Fas (CD95)/Fas ligand (CD95L) pathway. *J Leukoc Biol* 2001;69:263–270.

77. Cerdan C, Devilard E, Xerri L, et al. The C-class chemokine lymphotactin costimulates the apoptosis of human CD4(+) T cells. *Blood* 2001;97:2205–2212.

78. Youn BS, Kim YJ, Mantel C, et al. Blocking of c-FLIP(L)-independent cycloheximide-induced apoptosis or Fas-mediated apoptosis by the CC chemokine receptor 9/TECK interaction. *Blood* 2001;98:925–933.

79. Flad HD, Grage-Griebenow E, Petersen F, et al. The role of cytokines in monocyte apoptosis. *Pathobiology* 1999;67:291–293.

80. Boehme SA, Lio FM, Maciejewski-Lenoir D, et al. The chemokine fractalkine inhibits Fas-mediated cell death of brain microglia. *J Immunol* 2000;165:397–403.

81. Gu L, Tseng S, Horner RM, et al. Control of TH2 polarization by the chemokine monocyte chemoattractant protein-1. *Nature* 2000;404:407–411.

82. Nanki T, Lipsky PE. Cutting edge:stromal cell-derived factor-1 is a costimulator for CD4+ T cell activation. *J Immunol* 2000;164:5010–5014.

83. Lefkowitz RJ, Cotecchia S, Samama P, et al. Constitutive activity of receptors coupled to guanine nucleotide regulatory proteins. *Trends Pharmacol Sci* 1993;14:303–307.

84. Mellado M, Rodriguez-Frade JM, Manes S, et al. Chemokine signaling and functional responses: the role of receptor dimerization and TK pathway activation. *Annu Rev Immunol* 2001;19:397–421.

85. Miller WE, Lefkowitz RJ. Expanding roles for beta-arrestins as scaffolds and adapters in GPCR signaling and trafficking. *Curr Opin Cell Biol* 2001;13:139–145.

86. Manes S, Lacalle RA, Gomez-Mouton C, et al. Membrane raft microdomains in chemokine receptor function. *Semin Immunol* 2001; 13:147–157.

87. Thelen M, Baggiolini M. Is dimerization of chemokine receptors functionally relevant? *Sci STKE* 2001;E34.

88. Kehrl JH. Heterotrimeric G protein signaling: roles in immune function and fine-tuning by RGS proteins. *Immunity* 1998;8:1–10.

89. Neptune ER, Iiri T, Bourne HR. Galphai is not required for chemotaxis mediated by Gi-coupled receptors. *J Biol Chem* 1999;274:2824–2828.

90. Neptune ER, Bourne HR. Receptors induce chemotaxis by releasing the betagamma subunit of Gi, not by activating Gq or Gs. *Proc Natl Acad Sci U S A* 1997;94:14489–14494.

91. Rickert P, Weiner OD, Wang F, et al. Leukocytes navigate by compass: roles of PI3Kgamma and its lipid products. *Trends Cell Biol* 2000; 10:466–473.

92. Wu D, Huang CK, Jiang H. Roles of phospholipid signaling in chemoattractant-induced responses. *J Cell Sci* 2000;113:2935–2940.

93. Li Z, Jiang H, Xie W, et al. Roles of PLC-beta2 and -beta3 and PI3Kgamma in chemoattractant-mediated signal transduction. *Science* 2000;287:1046–1049.

94. Xu Y, Seet LF, Hanson B, et al. The Phox homology (PX) domain, a new player in phosphoinositide signalling. *Biochem J* 2001;360:513–530.

95. Hirsch E, Katanaev VL, Garlanda C, et al. Central role for G protein-coupled phosphoinositide 3-kinase gamma in inflammation. *Science* 2000;287:1049–1053.

96. Wymann MP, Sozzani S, Altruda F, et al. Lipids on the move: phosphoinositide 3-kinases in leukocyte function. *Immunol Today* 2000;21:260–264.

97. Roberts AW, Kim C, Zhen L, et al. Deficiency of the hematopoietic cell-specific Rho family GTPase Rac2 is characterized by abnormalities in neutrophil function and host defense. *Immunity* 1999;10:183–196.

98. Fukui Y, Hashimoto O, Sanui T, et al. Haematopoietic cell-specific CDM family protein DOCK2 is essential for lymphocyte migration. *Nature* 2001;412:826–831.

99. Carnevale KA, Cathcart MK. Calcium-independent phospholipase A(2) is required for human monocyte chemotaxis to monocyte chemoattractant protein 1. *J Immunol* 2001;167:3414–3421.

100. Barlic J, Andrews JD, Kelvin AA, et al. Regulation of tyrosine kinase activation and granule release through beta-arrestin by CXCRI. *Nat Immunol* 2000;1:227–233.

101. Ganju RK, Brubaker SA, Chernock RD, et al. Beta-chemokine receptor CCR5 signals through SHP1, SHP2, and Syk. *J Biol Chem* 2000; 275:17263–17268.

102. Venkatakrishnan G, Salgia R, Groopman JE. Chemokine receptors CXCR-1/2 activate mitogen-activated protein kinase via the epidermal growth factor receptor in ovarian cancer cells. *J Biol Chem* 2000;275:6868–6875.

103. Mellado M, Rodriguez-Frade JM, Aragay A, et al. The chemokine monocyte chemotactic protein 1 triggers Janus kinase 2 activation and tyrosine phosphorylation of the CCR2B receptor. *J Immunol* 1998; 161:805–813.

104. Appay V, Brown A, Cribbes S, et al. Aggregation of RANTES is responsible for its inflammatory properties. Characterization of nonaggregating, noninflammatory RANTES mutants. *J Biol Chem* 1999; 274:27505–27512.

105. Nieto M, Frade JM, Sancho D, et al. Polarization of chemokine receptors to the leading edge during lymphocyte chemotaxis. *J Exp Med* 1997;186:153–158.

106. Ali H, Richardson RM, Haribabu B, et al. Chemoattractant receptor cross-desensitization. *J Biol Chem* 1999;274:6027–6030.

107. Peacock JW, Jirik FR. TCR activation inhibits chemotaxis toward stromal cell-derived factor-1: evidence for reciprocal regulation between CXCR4 and the TCR. *J Immunol* 1999;162:215–223.

108. Guinamard R, Signoret N, Masamichi I, et al. B cell antigen receptor engagement inhibits stromal cell-derived factor (SDF)-1alpha chemotaxis and promotes protein kinase C (PKC)-induced internalization of CXCR4. *J Exp Med* 1999;189:1461–1466.

109. Lu Q, Sun EE, Klein RS, et al. Ephrin-B reverse signaling is mediated by a novel PDZ-RGS protein and selectively inhibits G protein-coupled chemoattraction. *Cell* 2001;105:69–79.

110. Wu JY, Feng L, Park HT, et al. The neuronal repellent Slit inhibits leukocyte chemotaxis induced by chemotactic factors. *Nature* 2001;410:948–952.

111. Van Damme J, Struyf S, Wuyts A, et al. The role of CD26/DPP IV in chemokine processing. *Chem Immunol* 1999;72:42–56.

112. McQuibban GA, Gong JH, Tam EM, et al. Inflammation dampened by gelatinase A cleavage of monocyte chemoattractant protein-3. *Science* 2000;289:1202–1206.

113. Tsou CL, Haskell CA, Charo IF. Tumor necrosis factor-alpha–converting enzyme mediates the inducible cleavage of fractalkine. *J Biol Chem* 2001;276:44622–44626.

114. Mantovani A, Locati M, Vecchi A, et al. Decoy receptors: a strategy to regulate inflammatory cytokines and chemokines. *Trends Immunol* 2001;22:328–336.

115. Baribaud F, Edwards TG, Sharron M, et al. Antigenically distinct conformations of CXCR4. *J Virol* 2001;75:8957–8967.

116. Fan GH, Yang W, Sai J, et al. Hsc/Hsp70 interacting protein (hip) associates with CXCR2 and regulates the receptor signaling and trafficking. *J Biol Chem* 2002;277:6590–6597.

117. Fan GH, Yang W, Sai J, et al. Phosphorylation-independent association of CXCR2 with the protein phosphatase 2A core enzyme. *J Biol Chem* 2001;276:16960–16968.

118. Marchese A, Benovic JL. Agonist-promoted ubiquitination of the G protein-coupled receptor CXCR4 mediates lysosomal sorting. *J Biol Chem* 2001;276:45509–45512.

119. Peled A, Petit I, Kollet O, et al. Dependence of human stem cell engraftment and repopulation of NOD/SCID mice on CXCR4. *Science* 1999;283:845–848.

120. Abi-Younes S, Sauty A, Mach F, et al. The stromal cell-derived factor-1 chemokine is a potent platelet agonist highly expressed in atherosclerotic plaques. *Circ Res* 2000;86:131–138.

121. Uehara S, Grinberg A, Farber JM, et al. A role for CCR9 in T lymphocyte development and migration. *J Immunol* 2002;168:2811–2819.

122. Zabel BA, Agace WW, Campbell JJ, et al. Human G protein-coupled receptor GPR-9-6/CC chemokine receptor 9 is selectively expressed on intestinal homing T lymphocytes, mucosal lymphocytes, and thymocytes and is required for thymus-expressed chemokine-mediated chemotaxis. *J Exp Med* 1999;190:1241–1256.

123. Hromas R, Broxmeyer HE, Kim C, et al. Cloning of BRAK, a novel divergent CXC chemokine preferentially expressed in normal versus malignant cells. *Biochem Biophys Res Commun* 1999;255:703–706.

124. Kurth I, Willimann K, Schaerli P, et al. Monocyte selectivity and tissue localization suggests a role for breast and kidney-expressed chemokine (BRAK) in macrophage development. *J Exp Med* 2001;194:855–861.

125. Rothenberg ME, Mishra A, Brandt EB, et al. Gastrointestinal eosinophils. *Immunol Rev* 2001;179:139–155.

126. Cook DN, Prosser DM, Forster R, et al. CCR6 mediates dendritic cell localization, lymphocyte homeostasis, and immune responses in mucosal tissue. *Immunity* 2000;12:495–503.

127. Varona R, Villares R, Carramolino L, et al. CCR6-deficient mice have impaired leukocyte homeostasis and altered contact hypersensitivity and delayed-type hypersensitivity responses. *J Clin Invest* 2001;107:37–45.

128. Harada A, Mukaida N, Matsushima K. Interleukin 8 as a novel target for intervention therapy in acute inflammatory diseases. *Mol Med Today* 1996;2:482–489.

129. Harada A, Sekido N, Akahoshi T, et al. Essential involvement of interleukin-8 (IL-8) in acute inflammation. *J Leukoc Biol* 1994;56:559–564.

130. Kuhns DB, DeCarlo E, Hawk DM, et al. Dynamics of the cellular and humoral components of the inflammatory response elicited in skin blisters in humans. *J Clin Invest* 1992;89:1734–1740.

131. White JR, Lee JM, Young PR, et al. Identification of a potent, selective non-peptide CXCR2 antagonist that inhibits interleukin-8-induced neutrophil migration. *J Biol Chem* 1998;273:10095–10098.

132. Tessier PA, Naccache PH, Clark-Lewis I, et al. Chemokine networks in vivo: involvement of C-X-C and C-C chemokines in neutrophil extravasation in vivo in response to TNF-alpha. *J Immunol* 1997;159:3595–3602.

133. Yan XT, Tumpey TM, Kunkel SL, et al. Role of MIP-2 in neutrophil migration and tissue injury in the herpes simplex virus-1-infected cornea. *Invest Ophthalmol Vis Sci* 1998;39:1854–1862.

134. Chen SC, Mehrad B, Deng JC, et al. Impaired pulmonary defense in mice lacking expression of the CXC chemokine lungkine. *J Immunol* 2001;166:3362–3368.

135. Brandt E, Petersen F, Ludwig A, et al. The beta-thromboglobulins and platelet factor 4:blood platelet-derived CXC chemokines with divergent roles in early neutrophil regulation. *J Leukoc Biol* 2000;67:471–478.

136. Salazar-Mather TP, Hamilton TA, Biron CA. A chemokine-to-cytokine-to-chemokine cascade critical in antiviral defense. *J Clin Invest* 2000;105:985–993.

137. Medzhitov R, Janeway C Jr. Innate immune recognition: mechanisms and pathways. *Immunol Rev* 2000;173:89–97.

138. Luster AD. The role of chemokines in linking innate and adaptive immunity. *Curr Opin Immunol* 2002;14:129–135.

139. Chvatchko Y, Hoogewerf AJ, Meyer A, et al. A key role for CC chemokine receptor 4 in lipopolysaccharide-induced endotoxic shock. *J Exp Med* 2000;191:1755–1764.

140. Sato N, Ahuja SK, Quinones M, et al. CC chemokine receptor (CCR)2 is required for langerhans cell migration and localization of T helper cell type 1 (Th1)-inducing dendritic cells. Absence of CCR2 shifts the Leishmania major-resistant phenotype to a susceptible state dominated by Th2 cytokines, b cell outgrowth, and sustained neutrophilic inflammation. *J Exp Med* 2000;192:205–218.

141. Ngo VN, Cornall RJ, Cyster JG. Splenic T zone development is B cell dependent. *J Exp Med* 2001;194:1649–1660.

142. Ansel KM, Harris RBS, Cyster JG. CXCL13 is required for B1 cell homing, natural antibody production, and body cavity immunity. *Immunity* 2002;16:67–76.

143. Voigt I, Camacho SA, de Boer BA, et al. CXCR5-deficient mice develop functional germinal centers in the splenic T cell zone. *Eur J Immunol* 2000;30:560–567.

144. Luther SA, Lopez T, Bai W, et al. BLC expression in pancreatic islets causes B cell recruitment and lymphotoxin-dependent lymphoid neogenesis. *Immunity* 2000;12:471–481.

145. Janatpour MJ, Hudak S, Sathe M, et al. Tumor necrosis factor-dependent segmental control of MIG expression by high endothelial venules in inflamed lymph nodes regulates monocyte recruitment. *J Exp Med* 2001;194:1375–1384.

146. Iellem A, Mariani M, Lang R, et al. Unique chemotactic response profile and specific expression of chemokine receptors CCR4 and CCR8 by CD4(+)CD25(+) regulatory T cells. *J Exp Med* 2001;194:847–853.

147. Palframan RT, Jung S, Cheng CY, et al. Inflammatory chemokine transport and presentation in HEV: a remote control mechanism for monocyte recruitment to lymph nodes in inflamed tissues. *J Exp Med* 2001;194:1361–1373.

148. Kim CH, Rott LS, Clark-Lewis I, et al. Subspecialization of CXCR5+ T cells: B helper activity is focused in a germinal center-localized subset of CXCR5+ T cells. *J Exp Med* 2001;193:1373–1381.

149. Reif K, Ekland EH, Ohl L, et al. Balanced responsiveness to chemoattractants from adjacent zones determines B-cell position. *Nature* 2002;416:94–99.

150. Loetscher P, Pellegrino A, Gong JH, et al. The ligands of CXC chemokine receptor 3, I-TAC, Mig, and IP10, are natural antagonists for CCR3. *J Biol Chem* 2001;276:2986–2991.

151. Ogilvie P, Bardi G, Clark-Lewis I, et al. Eotaxin is a natural antagonist for CCR2 and an agonist for CCR5. *Blood* 2001;97:1920–1924.

152. Aliberti J, Reis e Sousa C, Schito M, et al. CCR5 provides a signal for microbial induced production of IL-12 by CD8 alpha+ dendritic cells. *Nat Immunol* 2000;1:83–87.

153. Zhou Y, Kurihara T, Ryseck RP, et al. Impaired macrophage function and enhanced T cell-dependent immune response in mice lacking CCR5, the mouse homologue of the major HIV-1 coreceptor. *J Immunol* 1998;160:4018–4025.

154. Kunkel EJ, Butcher EC. Chemokines and the tissue-specific migration of lymphocytes. *Immunity* 2002;16:1–4.

155. Homey B, Alenius H, Muller A, et al. CCL27-CCR10 interactions regulate T cell–mediated skin inflammation. *Nat Med* 2002;8:157–165.

156. Uehara S, Song K, Farber JM, et al. Characterization of CCR9 expression and CCL25/thymus-expressed chemokine responsiveness during T cell development:CD3(high)CD69+ thymocytes and gammadeltaTCR+ thymocytes preferentially respond to CCL25. *J Immunol* 2002;168:134–142.

157. Bowman EP, Kuklin NA, Youngman KR, et al. The intestinal chemokine thymus-expressed chemokine (CCL25) attracts IgA antibody-secreting cells. *J Exp Med* 2002;195:269–275.

158. Baggiolini M, Dewald B, Moser B. Human chemokines: an update. *Annu Rev Immunol* 1997;15:675–705.

159. Hancock WW, Gao W, Faia KL, et al. Chemokines and their receptors in allograft rejection. *Curr Opin Immunol* 2000;12:511–516.

160. Strieter RM. Chemokines: not just leukocyte chemoattractants in the promotion of cancer. *Nat Immunol* 2001;2:285–286.

161. Strieter RM, Belperio JA, Keane MP. Cytokines in innate host defense in the lung. *J Clin Invest* 2002;109:699–705.

162. Hernandez PA, Gorlin RJ, Lukens JN, et al. Mutations in the chemokine receptor gene CXCR4 are associated with WHIM syndrome, a combined immunodeficiency disease. *Nat Genetics* 2003; epub.

163. Gunn MD, Kyuwa S, Tam C, et al. Mice lacking expression of secondary lymphoid organ chemokine have defects in lymphocyte homing and dendritic cell localization. *J Exp Med* 1999;189:451–460.

164. Dawson TC, Beck MA, Kuziel WA, et al. Contrasting effects of CCR5 and CCR2 deficiency in the pulmonary inflammatory response to influenza A virus. *Am J Pathol* 2000;156:1951–1959.

165. Terkeltaub R, Baird S, Sears P, et al. The murine homolog of the interleukin-8 receptor CXCR-2 is essential for the occurrence of neutrophilic inflammation in the air pouch model of acute urate crystal-induced gouty synovitis. *Arthritis Rheum* 1998;41:900–909.

166. Auten RL, Richardson RM, White JR, et al. Nonpeptide CXCR2 antagonist prevents neutrophil accumulation in hyperoxia-exposed newborn rats. *J Pharmacol Exp Ther* 2001;299:90–95.

167. Hancock WW, Lu B, Gao W, et al. Requirement of the chemokine receptor CXCR3 for acute allograft rejection. *J Exp Med* 2000;192: 1515–1520.

168. Hancock WW, Gao W, Csizmadia V, et al. Donor-derived IP-10 initiates development of acute allograft rejection. *J Exp Med* 2001; 193:975–980.

169. Miura M, Morita K, Kobayashi H, et al. Monokine induced by IFN-gamma is a dominant factor directing T cells into murine cardiac allografts during acute rejection. *J Immunol* 2001;167:3494–3504.

170. Horuk R, Clayberger C, Krensky AM, et al. A non-peptide functional antagonist of the CCR1 chemokine receptor is effective in rat heart transplant rejection. *J Biol Chem* 2001;276:4199–4204.

171. Fischereder M, Luckow B, Hocher B, et al. CC chemokine receptor 5 and renal-transplant survival. *Lancet* 2001;357:1758–1761.

172. Warkentin TE. Heparin-induced thrombocytopenia: a ten-year retrospective. *Annu Rev Med* 1999;50:129–147.

173. Howard OM, Dong HF, Yang D, et al. Histidyl-tRNA synthetase and asparaginyl-tRNA synthetase, autoantigens in myositis, activate chemokine receptors on T lymphocytes and immature dendritic cells. *J Exp Med* 2002;196:781–791.

174. Godessart N, Kunkel SL. Chemokines in autoimmune disease. *Curr Opin Immunol* 2001;13:670–675.

175. Huang D, Han Y, Rani MR, et al. Chemokines and chemokine receptors in inflammation of the nervous system: manifold roles and exquisite regulation. *Immunol Rev* 2000;177:52–67.

176. Gong JH, Ratkay LG, Waterfield JD, et al. An antagonist of monocyte chemoattractant protein 1 (MCP-1) inhibits arthritis in the MRL-lpr mouse model. *J Exp Med* 1997;186:131–137.

177. Cameron MJ, Arreaza GA, Grattan M, et al. Differential expression of CC chemokines and the CCR5 receptor in the pancreas is associated with progression to type I diabetes. *J Immunol* 2000;165:1102–1110.

178. Bird JE, Giancarli MR, Kurihara T, et al. Increased severity of glomerulonephritis in C-C chemokine receptor 2 knockout mice. *Kidney Int* 2000;57:129–136.

179. Topham PS, Csizmadia V, Soler D, et al. Lack of chemokine receptor CCR1 enhances Th1 responses and glomerular injury during nephrotoxic nephritis. *J Clin Invest* 1999;104:1549–1557.

180. Peters W, Charo IF. Involvement of chemokine receptor 2 and its ligand, monocyte chemoattractant protein-1, in the development of atherosclerosis:lessons from knockout mice. *Curr Opin Lipidol* 2001;12:175–180.

181. Aiello RJ, Bourassa PA, Lindsey S, et al. Monocyte chemoattractant protein-1 accelerates atherosclerosis in apolipoprotein E-deficient mice. *Arterioscler Thromb Vasc Biol* 1999;19:1518–1525.

182. Gerszten RE, Garcia-Zepeda EA, Lim YC, et al. MCP-1 and IL-8

trigger firm adhesion of monocytes to vascular endothelium under flow conditions. *Nature* 1999;398:718–723.

182a. McDermott DH, Fong AM, Yang Q, et al. Chemokine receptor mutant CX3CR1-M280 has impaired adhesive function and correlates with protection from cardiovascular disease in man. *J Clin Invest* 2003;111:1241–1250.

183. Moatti D, Faure S, Fumeron F, et al. Polymorphism in the fractalkine receptor CX3CR1 as a genetic risk factor for coronary artery disease. *Blood* 2001;97:1925–1928.

184. McDermott DH, Halcox JP, Schenke WH, et al. Association between polymorphism in the chemokine receptor CX3CR1 and coronary vascular endothelial dysfunction and atherosclerosis. *Circ Res* 2001;89:401–407.

184a. Lesnik P, Haskell CA and Charo IF. Decreased atherosclerosis in CX3CR1 −/− mice reveals a role for fractalkine in atherogenesis. *J Clin Invest* 2003;111:333–340.

184b. Combadiere C, Potteaux S, Gao JL, et al. Decreased atherosclerotic lesion formation in CX3CR1/Apo E double knockout mice. *Circulation* 2003;107:1009–1016.

185. Schuh JM, Blease K, Hogaboam CM. CXCR2 is necessary for the development and persistence of chronic fungal asthma in mice. *Journal of Immunology* 2002;168:1447–1456.

186. Fukunaga K, Asano K, Mao XQ, et al. Genetic polymorphisms of CC chemokine receptor 3 in Japanese and British asthmatics. *Eur Respir J* 2001;17:59–63.

187. Panina-Bordignon P, Papi A, Mariani M, et al. The C-C chemokine receptors CCR4 and CCR8 identify airway T cells of allergen-challenged atopic asthmatics. *J Clin Invest* 2001;107:1357–1364.

188. Humbles AA, Lu B, Friend DS, et al. The murine CCR3 receptor regulates both the role of eosinophils and mast cells in allergen-induced airway inflammation and hyperresponsiveness. *Proc Natl Acad Sci U S A* 2002;99:1479–1484.

189. Ma W, Bryce PJ, Humbles AA, et al. CCR3 is essential for skin eosinophilia and airway hyperresponsiveness in a murine model of allergic skin inflammation. *J Clin Invest* 2002;109:621–628.

190. Lukacs NW, Prosser DM, Wiekowski M, et al. Requirement for the chemokine receptor CCR6 in allergic pulmonary inflammation. *J Exp Med* 2001;194:551–555.

191. Richmond A. The pathogenic role of growth factors in melanoma. *Semin Dermatol* 1991;10:246–255.

192. Luan J, Shattuck-Brandt R, Haghnegahdar H, et al. Mechanism and biological significance of constitutive expression of MGSA/GRO chemokines in malignant melanoma tumor progression. *J Leukoc Biol* 1997;62:588–597.

193. Muller A, Homey B, Soto H, et al. Involvement of chemokine receptors in breast cancer metastasis. *Nature* 2001;410:50–56.

194. Pertl U, Luster AD, Varki NM, et al. IFN-gamma-inducible protein-10 is essential for the generation of a protective tumor-specific CD8 T cell response induced by single-chain IL-12 gene therapy. *J Immunol* 2001;166:6944–6951.

195. Sharma S, Stolina M, Luo J, et al. Secondary lymphoid tissue chemokine mediates T cell-dependent antitumor responses in vivo. *J Immunol* 2000;164:4558–4563.

196. Biragyn A, Surenhu M, Yang D, et al. Mediators of innate immunity that target immature, but not mature, dendritic cells induce antitumor immunity when genetically fused with nonimmunogenic tumor antigens. *J Immunol* 2001;167:6644–6653.

197. Belman N, Bonnem EM, Harvey HA, et al. Phase I trial of recombinant platelet factor 4 (rPF4) in patients with advanced colorectal carcinoma. *Invest New Drugs* 1996;14:387–389.

198. McFadden G, Murphy PM. Host-related immunomodulators encoded by poxviruses and herpesviruses. *Curr Opin Microbiol* 2000;3:371–378.

199. Moss B, Shisler JL, Xiang Y, et al. Immune-defense molecules of molluscum contagiosum virus, a human poxvirus. *Trends Microbiol* 2000;8:473–477.

200. Alcami A, Koszinowski UH. Viral mechanisms of immune evasion. *Immunol Today* 2000;21:447–455.

201. Dabbagh K, Xiao Y, Smith C, et al. Local blockade of allergic airway hyperreactivity and inflammation by the poxvirus-derived pan-CC-chemokine inhibitor vCCI. *J Immunol* 2000;165:3418–3422.

202. Bridgeman A, Stevenson PG, Simas JP, et al. A secreted chemokine binding protein encoded by murine gammaherpesvirus-68 is necessary for the establishment of a normal latent load. *J Exp Med* 2001;194:301–312.

203. Holst PJ, Rosenkilde MM, Manfra D, et al. Tumorigenesis induced by the HHV8-encoded chemokine receptor requires ligand modulation of high constitutive activity. *J Clin Invest* 2001;108:1789–1796.

204. Schwarz M, Murphy PM. Kaposi's sarcoma-associated herpesvirus G protein-coupled receptor constitutively activates NF-kappa B and induces proinflammatory cytokine and chemokine production via a C-terminal signaling determinant. *J Immunol* 2001;167:505–513.

205. Garzino-Demo A, DeVico AL, Cocchi F, et al. Beta-chemokines and protection from HIV type 1 disease. *AIDS Res Hum Retroviruses* 1998;14(suppl 2):177–184.

206. Feng Y, Broder CC, Kennedy PE, et al. HIV-1 entry cofactor: functional cDNA cloning of a seven-transmembrane, G protein-coupled receptor. *Science* 1996;272:872–877.

207. Grivel JC, Margolis LB. CCR5- and CXCR4-tropic HIV-1 are equally cytopathic for their T-cell targets in human lymphoid tissue. *Nat Med* 1999;5:344–346.

208. Kinter A, Arthos J, Cicala C, et al. Chemokines, cytokines and HIV: a complex network of interactions that influence HIV pathogenesis. *Immunol Rev* 2000;177:88–98.

209. Ioannidis JPA, Rosenberg PS, Goedert JJ, et al. Effects of CCR5-Delta 32, CCR2-641, and SDF-1 3′ A alleles on HIV-1 disease progression: an international meta-analysis of individual-patient data. *Ann Intern Med* 2001;135:782–795.

210. Farzan M, Mirzabekov T, Kolchinsky P, et al. Tyrosine sulfation of the amino terminus of CCR5 facilitates HIV-1 entry. *Cell* 1999;96:667–676.

211. Kuhmann SE, Platt EJ, Kozak SL, et al. Cooperation of multiple CCR5 coreceptors is required for infections by human immunodeficiency virus type 1. *J Virol* 2000;74:7005–7015.

212. Lalani AS, Masters J, Zeng W, et al. Use of chemokine receptors by poxviruses. *Science* 1999;286:1968–1971.

213. Strizki JM, Xu S, Wagner NE, et al. SCH-C (SCH 351125), an orally bioavailable, small molecule antagonist of the chemokine receptor CCR5, is a potent inhibitor of HIV-1 infection in vitro and in vivo. *Proc Natl Acad Sci U S A* 2001;98:12718–12723.

214. Tournamille C, Colin Y, Cartron JP, et al. Disruption of a GATA motif in the Duffy gene promoter abolishes erythroid gene expression in Duffy-negative individuals. *Nat Genet* 1995;10:224–228.

215. Zimmerman PA, Woolley I, Masinde GL, et al. Emergence of FY*A(null) in a Plasmodium vivax-endemic region of Papua New Guinea. *Proc Natl Acad Sci U S A* 1999;96:13973–13977.

216. Dawson TC, Lentsch AB, Wang Z, et al. Exaggerated response to endotoxin in mice lacking the Duffy antigen/receptor for chemokines (DARC). *Blood* 2000;96:1681–1684.

217. Luo H, Chaudhuri A, Zbrzezna V, et al. Deletion of the murine Duffy gene (Dfy) reveals that the Duffy receptor is functionally redundant. *Mol Cell Biol* 2000;20:3097–3101.

218. Scheerlinck JY. Genetic adjuvants for DNA vaccines. *Vaccine* 2001;19:2647–2656.

219. Murphy P. Chemokines: role as immunomodulators and potential as adjuvants for DNA vaccines. In: Ertl H. *DNA vaccines*. Georgetown, TX: Landes Bioscience, 2002:316–334.

APPENDIX 1. Chemokine specificities for human 7TM-chemokine receptors and chemokine-binding proteins

	CXCR1	CXCR2 (CD128)	CXCR3 (CD183)	CXCR4 (CD184)	CXCR5	CXCR6	CCR1	CCR2	CCR3	CCR4	CCR5 (CD195)	CCR6	CCR7 (CD197)	CCR8	CCR9	CCR10	XCR1	CX3CR1	CCX CKR	Duffy (CD234)	D6
CXCL1/Groα		+++																		+++	
CXCL2/Groβ		+++																			
CXCL3/Groγ		+++																			
CXCL4/PF-4																					
CXCL5/ENA-78	+	+++																			
CXCL6/GCP-2	++	+++																			
CXCL7/NAP-2		+++																		++	
CXCL8/IL-8	+++	+++																		++	
CXCL9/Mig			+++						Antag												
CXCL10/γ/IP-10			+++						Antag												
CXCL11/I-TAC			+++						Antag												
CXCL12/SDF-1				+++																	
CXCL13/BCA1			+		+++																
CXCL14/BRAK																					
*CXCL15/lungkine																					
CXCL16						+++															
CCL1/I-309														+++							
CCL2/MCP-1							+	+++												++	++
CCL3/MIP-1α							+++				+++										+++
CCL4/MIP-1β							Antag				+++			+							+++
CCL5/RANTES							+++		++		+++									++	+++
*CCL6/MRP-1																					
CCL7/MCP-3							+++	+++	++		Antag										+
CCL8/MCP-2							++	+++	++		+++										+++
*CCL9/10/MRP-2							++														
CCL11/eotaxin			Antag					Antag	+++		+										+
*CCL12/MCP-5								++													++
CCL13/MCP-4							+++	+++	+++		+++										+++
CCL14a/HCC-1							+++														+++
CCL14b/HCC-3																					
CCL15/HCC-2							+++		+++												
CCL16/HCC-4							+	+			+			+							
CCL17/TARC										+++				+							
CCL18/PARC																					
CCL19/ELC													+++						+		
CCL20/LARC												+++									
CCL21/SLC			+										+++						+		
CCL22/MDC										+++											
CCL23/MPIF-1							+++														
CCL24/eotaxin-2									+++												
CCL25/TECK															+++				+		
CCL26/eotaxin-3									++												
CCL27/CTACK																+++					
CCL28/MEC									+							+++					
XCL1/lymphotactin α																	+++				
XCL2/lymphotactin β																	+++				
CX3CL1/fractalkine																		+++			

Note: For each receptor, + indicates that the corresponding chemokine is an agonist, and "Antag" denotes an antagonist. For the 7TM chemokine-binding proteins CCX CKR, D6, and Duffy, the + signs indicate high-affinity binding without signaling. *Denotes mouse chemokines that may not have human counterparts. Commonly used nonstandard names are given with the standard name of each chemokine. Additional aliases can be found in Murphy et al. (31).

BCA, B-cell-activating chemokine; BRAK, B-cell- and kidney-associated chemokine; CTACK, cutaneous T-cell-associated chemokine; ELC, Epstein–Barr virus-induced receptor ligand chemokine; ENA-78, 78 amino–acid epithelial cell-derived neutrophil activator; GCP, granulocyte chemoattractant protein; GRO, growth-related oncogene; HCC, hemofiltrate CC chemokine; IL-8, interleukin-8; I-TAC, interferon-inducible T-cell-alpha chemoattractant; LARC, liver- and activation-related chemokine; MCP, monocyte chemoattractant protein; MDC, macrophage-derived chemokine; MEC, mucosal epithelium chemokine; Mig, monokine induced by IFNγ; MIP, macrophage inflammatory protein; MPIF, myeloid progenitor inhibitory factor; MRP, MIP-related protein; NAP, neutrophil-activating protein; PARC, pulmonary- and activation-related chemokine; PF-4, platelet factor-4; RANTES, regulated upon activation normal T-cell expressed and secreted; SDF, stromal cell-derived factor; SLC, secondary lymphoid tissue chemokine; TARC, thymus- and activation-related chemokine; TECK, thymus-expressed chemokine.

APPENDIX 2. *Specificities of functional human chemokine receptors for human leukocyte subsets*

	CXCR1	CXCR2	CXCR3	CXCR4	CXCR5	CXCR6	CCR1	CCR2	CCR3	CCR4	CCR5	CCR6	CCR7	CCR8	CCR9	CCR10	XCR1	CX3CR1
CD4−CD8− thymocytes				+														
CD4+CD8+ thymocytes				+														
CD4+CD8− thymocytes				+						+			+		+			
CD4−CD8+ thymocytes				+					+	+			+					
CD34+ HSC				+														
CD56dim CD16+ NK	+	+	+	+													+	+
CD56bright CD16− NK			+	+							+		+					
CD4 NK-T			+	+				+		+	+							
CD8 NK-T			+	+		+	+	+			+	+						
CD4−CD8− NK-T			+	+		+	+	+			+	+						
B cells			+	+	+		+	+				+	+					
Plasma cells				+		+			+							+		
IgA Ab-secreting cells				+											+	+		
Naïve T cells				+									+					
Follicular help T cells					+													
Central memory T cells			+							+		+	+					
Effector memory T cells						+	+		+		+							
Th1 Effector T cells			+			+		+			+	+	+					+
Th2 Effector T cells				+					+	+			+	+				
α4β7+ Gut-homing memory T cells			+								+	+			+			
CLA+ Skin-homing memory T cells				+						+		+	+			+		
CD4+CD25+ Regulatory T cells										+				+				
Immature DC	+			+			+	+			+	+						
Mature DC				+									+					
Monocytes		+		+			+	+			+			+				+
Basophils		+		+			+	+	+		+							
Eosinophils				+			+		+									
Neutrophils	+	+		+			+	+	+									
Platelets	+			+			+		+	+								

APPENDIX 3. *Immunoregulatory properties of CXC, CX3C, and C chemokines*

Chemokine	Cell sources	Regulators	Cell targets and responses
CXCL1/GROα CXCL2/GROβ CXCL3/GROγ	Constitutively made in many tumors, especially melanoma Inducible in most hematopoietic and tissue cells	*Pos:* IL-1, TNF, lps *Neg:* IL-10, IFNα and γ and glucocorticoids	PMN, Ba, Eo, Mo, L, and EC chemotaxis PMN degranulation and respiratory burst Melanoma cell, melanocyte, and EC growth MPC growth suppression
CXCL4/PF-4	Constitutively made in plt precursors and stored in mature plts	IL-6 Thrombin and other plt activators	PMN adhesion to EC via LFA-1 MPC growth suppression EC ctx and growth inhibition
CXCL5/ENA-78	Distinct from CXCL8: Inducible in epithelial cells, especially gut and lung, N, Mo, Plts, EC	*Pos:* IL-1, TNF, lps *Neg:* NO, IFNα and γ and glucocorticoids	PMN β2 integrin activation, ctx, and degranulation EC ctx and growth MPC growth suppression
CXCL6/GCP-2	Inducible in lung microvascular EC; Mo; alveolar epithelial cells, mesothelial cells, EC and MΦ; thymic and endometrial epithelial cells, and thymic fibroblasts	IL-1, lps, dsRNA	PMN ctx and release of gelatinase B EC ctx and growth MPC growth suppression
CXCL7/NAP-2	Inducible at low levels in Mo, PMN, T cells Constitutively made in large amounts in plt precursors and stored in mature plts	Thrombin and other plt activators	PMN ctx, degranulation, respiratory burst Mast cell and EC ctx Basophil histamine release MPC growth suppression Decreases tumor-specific CTL activity
CXCL8/IL-8	Inducible in most hematopoietic and tissue cells	*Pos:* IL-1, TNF, lps *Neg:* IL-4, IL-10, IFNα, and γ, TGFβ, vitamin D3 and glucocorticoids	PMN adhesion, ctx, transendothelial migration, degranulation, respiratory burst, and lipid mediator production Resting T cell, Ba and IL-5-stimulated Eo ctx Mo adhesion to EC EC ctx and growth MPC growth suppression
CXCL9/Mig	Inducible in PMN, MΦ, T cells, astrocytes, microglial cells, hepatocytes, EC, fibroblasts, keratinocytes, thymic stromal cells	IFNγ, TNF, lps	T-cell adhesion EC and MPC growth suppression CTX of TIL cells, activated CD4+ Th1 T cell, CD8+ T cell and NK cell
CXCL10/IP-10	Inducible in ECs, Mo, keratinocytes, respiratory and intestinal epithelial cells, astrocytes, microglia, mesangial cells, smooth muscle cells	IFNα/β, IFNγ, TNF, lps	Rapid adhesion of T cells EC and MPC growth suppression CTX of TIL cells, activated CD4+ Th1 T cell, CD8+ T cell and NK cell
CXCL11/I-TAC	Inducible in EC, Mo	IFNγ, TNF, lps	CTX of TIL cells, activated CD4+ Th1 T cell, CD8+ T cell and NK cell
CXCL12/SDF-1	Constitutively expressed in bone marrow stromal cells; most tissues also express CXCL12	Constitutively expressed	CTX of PMN, Mo, most T cells; CD34+ HPCs; cerebellar granule cells; and naïve and memory but not germinal center B cells; Pre–B-cell proliferation EC growth and ctx Plt degranulation MPC growth suppression HIV suppressive factor
CXCL13/BCA-1	Follicular HEV of secondary lymphoid tissue	Constitutively expressed	Mature B cell and CXCR5+ CD4 and CD8 T cell ctx
CXCL14/BRAK	Most tissues, breast and kidney tumors	Constitutively expressed	Mo ctx
CXCL15/Lungkine	Lung epithelial cells	Constitutively expressed	PMN ctx
CXCL16	Spleen; DCs of the T zone	Constitutively expressed	Splenic NK-T, CD4+ and CD8+ T cell ctx
CX3CL1/Fractalkine	Inducible on EC, neurons, Mo, DC	IL-1, TNF induce expression on EC	CX3CR1+ cell adhesion to EC and neurons NK, Mo, T cell ctx
XCL1/lymphotactin	γδ epidermal T cells, NK, NK-T, activated CD8+ and Th1 CD4+ T cells	MHC class I restricted T-cell activation	CD62lo CD4+ T cell ctx MPC growth suppression

Note: Information about cell sources and targets is restricted to primary cells and tissues. Detailed information about chemokine expression in cultured cell lines can be found at *www.RnDSystems.com.*

Ba, basophil; ctx, chemotaxis; DC, dendritic cell; EC, endothelial cell; Eo, eosinophil; HEV, high endothelial venule; MΦ, macrophage; Mo, monocyte; MPC, myeloid progenitor cell; plt, platelet; PMN, neutrophil.

APPENDIX 4. *Immunoregulatory properties of CC chemokines*

Chemokine	Cell sources	Regulators	Cell targets and responses
CCL1/I-309	Inducible in Mo and CD4$^+$ and CD8$^+$ $\alpha\beta$ and CD4$^-$ CD8$^-$ $\gamma\delta$ T cells	T-cell activation; Mo activation by lps, IL-1 and immobilized IgG	Th2>>Th1, Mo ctx Mouse thymoma cell line treated with dexamethasone: antiapoptotic MPC growth suppression
CCL2/MCP-1	Inducible in Mo, fibroblasts, keratinocytes, EC, PMN, synoviocytes, mesangial cells, astrocytes, lung epithelial cells and MΦ Constitutively made in splenic arteriolar lymphatic sheath and medullary region of lymph node, many tumors, and arterial plaque EC	*Pos:* IL-1, TNF, lps, PDGF, viruses, many others *Neg:* IL-4, IL-10, IL-13, TGFβ, glucocorticoids, estrogen, progesterone	Mo, CD45RO$^+$ T cell, Ba, DC, NK ctx Ba histamine release Mo, NK enzyme release Mo respiratory burst; $\beta2$ Integrin activation and VLA4-VCAM-1 adhesion; tumoricidal activity MPC growth suppression
CCL3/MIP-1αS	Inducible in Mo/MΦ, CD8$^+$ T cells, B cells, plts, PMN, Eo, Ba, DC, NK, mast cells, keratinocytes, fibroblasts, mesangial cells, astrocytes, microglial cells, epithelial cells	*Pos:* IL-1, TNF, lps, IL-15, IL-12, IFNγ, viruses including HIV, bacteria including TB, TCR crosslinking, CD40 activation *Neg:* IL-4, IL-10, IL-13, TGFβ, IFNγ, glucocorticoids	Mo, CD8$^+$ T cell, Th1 cell, TIL cell, Eo, B cell, Ba, DC, NK, mast cell, astrocyte, microglial cell, and osteoclast ctx and adhesion Mo, NK, Eo, and Ba degranulation Mo tumoricidal and microbicidal activity NK cell activation and cytolysis Promotes Th1 differentiation Costimulates activated T cells HPC, keratinocyte, and astrocyte growth suppression Suppresses R5 HIV infection
CCL3L1/MIP-1αP	Similar to CCL3	Similar to CCL3	Similar to CCL3
CCL4/MIP-1β	Similar to CCL3	Similar to CCL3	Similar to CCL3
CCL5/RANTES	Inducible in EC, T cells, epithelial cells, Mo, fibroblasts, mesangial cells, NK cells, DC Constitutively expressed and stored in plt and Eo granules	*Pos:* IL-1, TNF, IFNγ, thrombin *Neg:* IL-4	Mo, memory T cell, Eo, Ba, DC ctx Ag-independent T-cell activation at high concentrations Suppresses R5 HIV infection
CCL6/MRP-1	Inducible in bone marrow and peritoneal-derived MΦ	IL-3, IL-4, GM-CSF	Mo, B cell, NK, CD4$^+$ T-cell ctx MPC growth suppression
CCL7/MCP-3	Inducible in Mo, plts, fibroblasts, EC, skin, bronchial epithelial cells, astrocytes	IL-1, TNF, lps, PDGF, IFNγ	Mo, CD45RO$^+$ T cell, Eo, DC, NK ctx Ba histamine release Mo, NK enzyme release
CCL8/MCP-2	Inducible in fibroblasts, PMN, astrocytes Constitutively expressed in colon, small intestine, heart, lung, thymus, pancreas, spinal cord, ovary, placenta	IL-1, IFNγ	Mo, CD45RO$^+$ and RA$^+$ T cell, Ba, Eo, DC, NK ctx Ba histamine release Mo, NK enzyme release
CCL9/10/MRP-2	Constitutively expressed in all mouse organs except brain; highest in lung, liver, and thymus Induced in heart and lung	Lps	Mo, PMN, CD4$^+$ and CD8$^+$ T-cell ctx Pyrogenic when injected into rats
CCL11/eotaxin	Epithelial cells, EC, smooth muscle, cardiac muscle, Eo, dermal fibroblasts, mast cells, MΦ, Reed–Sternberg cells	*Pos:* IL-1, TNF, IL-4, IL-13 *Neg:* glucocorticoids, IFNγ	Th2 T cell, Eo, Ba, IFNγ-treated PMN ctx Eo respiratory burst and adhesion Ba degranulation and eukotriene generation
CCL12/MCP-5	Constitutive expression in lymph node and thymic stromal cells	Lps, IFNγ	Mo, T cell, B cell, Eo ctx
CCL13/MCP-4	Inducible in nasal and bronchial epithelial cells; dermal fibroblasts; PBMCs; atherosclerotic plaque EC and MΦ	IL-1, TNF, IFNγ	Mo, CD45RO$^+$ T cell, Ba, Eo, DC ctx Ba histamine release MPC growth suppression

(continued)

APPENDIX 4. *(Continued)*

Chemokine	Cell sources	Regulators	Cell targets and responses
CCL14a/HCC-1	Constitutively expressed in most organs; high plasma levels	Constitutively expressed in an inactive form in plasma. Activation requires proteolysis	Mo, Eo, T-lymphoblast ctx Enhances stem cell factor-treated CD34$^+$ bone-marrow cell proliferation HIV suppression
CCL14b/HCC-3	Same as CCL14b except absent from skeletal muscle and pancreas	Native protein not yet detected	ND
CCL15/HCC-2	Inducible in Mo and DC Constitutive RNA expression in liver, gut, heart, and skeletal muscle, adrenal gland, and lung leukocytes	TNF, lps, IFNγ, IL-4 induces mRNA in DC and Mo	Mo, T-cell, DC, Eo ctx MPC growth suppression
CCL16/HCC-4	Constitutively expressed in liver, possibly many other organs. Also, Mo, T cells and NK cells express mRNA	1.5 kb mRNA induced by IL-4	Mo, T-cell ctx MPC growth suppression
CCL17/TARC	Constitutive in normal DC and Reed–Sternberg cells of Hodgkin's disease	Constitutive	Th2-polarized CD4+CD45RO$^+$ memory T-cell ctx
CCL18/DC-CK-1 (PARC)	Constitutive in Mo/MΦ, germinal center DC	Constitutive	CD38^{neg} mantle zone B cell and CD45RA$^+$ T-cell ctx MPC growth suppression
CCL19/ELC	Constitutive on interdigitating DC in secondary lymphoid tissue	Constitutive	CCR7$^+$ naïve, memory, helper and cytotoxic T-cell, NK cell, B-cell and thymocyte ctx MPC growth suppression
CCL20/LARC	Constitutive in lymph nodes, peripheral blood leukocytes, thymus, and appendix Inducible in PBMC, HUVEC	TNF, lps	Immature DC ctx MPC growth suppression
CCL21/SLC	Constitutive in lymphatic EC, HEV, and interdigitating DC in T areas of secondary lymphoid tissue, thymic medullary epith cells and EC	Constitutive	Similar to CCL19 Angiostatic MPC growth suppression
CCL22/MDC	Constitutive in DC and MΦ Inducible in Mo, T and B cells	*Pos:* T cell activation B cells and DC: CD40L Mo: IL-4, IL-13 and GM-CSF *Neg:* IFNγ	HIV suppression
CCL23/MPIF-1	Constitutive in pancreas and skeletal muscle		PMN, Mo, T-cell ctx MPC growth suppression
CCL24/eotaxin-2	Inducible in Mo	Allergen challenge	Resting CD4$^+$ and CD8$^+$ T-cell, Eo, Ba, Mo ctx Ba histamine and leukotriene release MPC growth suppression
CCL25/TECK	Constitutive in thymic stromal cells and small intestine	Constitutive	Thymocyte, CCR9$^+$ T-cell and Mo ctx MPC growth suppression
CCL26/eotaxin-3	Constitutive in heart and ovary Inducible on dermal fibroblasts and EC	IL-4, IL-13 on EC	Eo and Ba ctx
CCL27/CTACK	Constitutive in placenta, keratinocytes, testis and brain	IL-1, TNF	CCR10$^+$ CLA$^+$ memory T-cell ctx
CCL28/MEC	Constitutive in epithelial cells of gut, airway	Constitutive	Resting CD4$^+$ and CD8$^+$ T-cell ctx

Note: Information about cell sources and targets is restricted to primary cells and tissues. Detailed information about chemokine expression in cultured cell lines can be found at *www.rndsystems.com*.

APPENDIX 5. *Immunologic phenotypes of chemokine receptor knockout mice*

Receptor	Phenotype		
	Infectious disease	Inflammation	Development

CXCR2	*Increased susceptibility to:*
	T. gondii
	Brain abscess
	Onchocerca volvulus
	E. coli pyelonephritis
		Reduced:
		  Wound healing
		  A. fumigatus AHR
		  Atherogenesis
		  Neutrophil extravasation
			Expansion of neutrophils and B cells in blood, marrow and lymphoid organs (not seen when derived in germ-free environment)

CXCR3	NR	Delayed cardiac allograft rejection	NR

CXCR4	NR	NR	Perinatal lethality
			Defective:
			  Ventricular septum
			  Bone marrow myelopoiesis
			  B-cell lymphopoiesis
			  Gastric vascularization
			  Cerebellar granule cell migration

CXCR5	NR	NR	Few Peyer's patches, no inguinal LN Defective germinal centers and B-cell homing to LN

CCR1	*Increased susceptibility to:*
	  T gondii
	  Pneumonia virus of mice
	  A. fumigatus
		Increased:
		  Th1 response and glomerular injury in nephrotoxic nephritis model
		  Th2 response to SEA
		Reduced:
		  Neutrophilic alveolitis in pancreatitis-ARDS model
		  Airway remodeling and Th2 response in *A. fumigatus* model
		  Th1 response and resistance to EAE
		  Th1 response to PPD
		  Delayed cardiac allograft rejection
			Reduced myeloid progenitor cells in spleen and blood

CCR2	*Increased susceptibility to:*
	  C. neoformans
	  Mouse hepatitis virus
	  L. monocytogenes
	  L. major
	  M. tuberculosis
	Resistance to:
	  L. donovani
	  Influenza A
		Decreased:
		  Th1 responses
		  EAE
		  Response to PPD
		  Atherosclerosis
		  Cardiac allograft rejection
		  AHR to CRA
		  Dextran sulfate-mediated colitis
		  Thioglycollate-induced peritonitis
		  FITC and bleomycin induced pulmonary fibrosis
		  MΦ recruited to injured nerve
		  DTH
		  Monocyte extravasation
		Increased:
		  AHR to OVA
		  AHR to *A. fumigatus*
		  Glomerulonephritis in antiglomerular basement membrane antibody model
			Enhanced myeloid progenitor–cell cycling and apoptosis

CCR3	NR	*ip OVA sensitization → OVA challenge:* Increased AHR and airway mast cells; decreased airway EOS trapped between elastic lamina and endothelial cells Epicutaneous OVA sensitization → OVA challenge: Protection from allergic skin inflammation and AHR. EOS and mast cells not recruited to skin or lung	NR

(continued)

APPENDIX 5. *(Continued)*

Receptor	Phenotype		
	Infectious disease	Inflammation	Development
CCR4	NR	Decreased susceptibility to lps	NR

CCR5	*Increased susceptibility to:*
	  L. monocytogenes
	  C. neoformans
	  T. gondii
	  Influenza A
	  L. major
	  LCMV
	Resistance to:
	  L. donovani
		Decreased:
		  Dextran sulfate-mediated colitis
		  Lps toxicity
		  Mouse hepatitis virus-induced demyelination due to decreased MΦ recruitment to CNS
		  Cardiac allograft rejection
		Increased:
		  DTH
		  Humoral response to T-dependent Ag
			NR

CCR6	NR	Defective CRA-induced allergic airway inflammation Increased contact hypersensitivity to 2,4-dinitrofluorobenzene Resistance to DTH to allogeneic splenocytes	Absent myeloid CD11b$^+$ CD11c$^+$ dendritic cells in subepithelial dome of Peyer's patches Increased T cells in intestinal mucosa Impaired humoral immune response to orally administered antigen and to rotavirus
CCR7	NR	Delayed humoral response Defective contact sensitivity Defective DTH	Defective lymphocyte and DC migration to LN Undeveloped T-cell zones Impaired trafficking of T cells and DC to LN
CCR8	NR	Defective SEA-induced granuloma formation Decreased OVA- and CRA-induced allergic airway inflammation	NR
CCR9	NR	NR	Decreased pre-pro–B cells, but normal T and B cells Decreased ratio of gut intraepithelial T-cell-to-epithelial cell ratio due to decreased $\gamma\delta$ T cells
CX3CR1	NR	Resistance to cardiac allograft rejection in cyclosporin A–treated animals Resistance to atherosclerosis	NR
Duffy	NR	Increased or decreased neutrophil mobilization, depending on the model	NR

AHR, airway hyperreactivity; CRA, cockroach antigen; DC, dendritic cell; DTH, delayed type hypersensitivity; LN, lymph node; NR, not reported; OVA, ovalbumin; SEA, Schistosoma mansoni soluble-egg antigen.

/ Chapter

APPENDIX 6. *Immunologic phenotypes of chemokine knockout mice*

Chemokine	Phenotype		
	Infectious disease	Inflammation	Development
CXCL10	NR	Delayed cardiac allograft rejection	NR
CXCL12	NR	NR	Identical to CXCR4$^{-/-}$ (see Appendix 5)
CXCL15	Increased susceptibility to *Klebsiella pneumoniae*	NR	NR
CCL2	Susceptible to *L. monocytogenes* Resistant to *M. tuberculosis* and *L. major*	*Decreased:* Atherosclerosis in LDL R deficient mice EAE NKT cells and Th1 response in lung after *C. neoformans* infection Tubular damage in nephrotoxic serum nephritis Monocyte extravasation Wound healing DTH Th2 response	Failure of Th2 Ig subclass switch
CCL3	*Increased susceptibility to:* Mouse CMV *Klebsiella pneumoniae* Respiratory syncytial virus *C. neoformans* in CNS *Resistance to:* Pneumonia virus of mice *L. donovani* Coxsacckie B3 virus myocarditis Influenza A pneumonia Herpes simplex keratitis	Resistance to diabetes in NOD mouse Decreased wound healing Decreased CD8$^+$ T cell recruitment in GVHD	NR
CCL11	NR	Resistance to Th2 oral Ag-induced eosinophil-associated gut disease Reduced early eosinophil recruitment after Ag challenge in models of asthma and stromal keratitis	Selective reduction of eos in blood, jejunum, thymus, and stroma of the pubertal and cycling uterus
CCL21 (=natural *plt* mutation)	Increased susceptibility to mouse hepatitis virus	NR	Undeveloped T-cell zones Impaired trafficking of T cells and DC to LN Impaired DTH and antibody production
CX3CL1	NR	NR	NR

AHR, airway hyperreactivity; CRA, cockroach antigen; DC, dendritic cell; DTH, delayed type hypersensitivity; LN, lymph node; NR, not reported; OVA, ovalbumin; SEA, Schistosoma mansoni soluble-egg antigen.

CHAPTER 27

Programmed Cell Death

Francis Ka-Ming Chan and Michael J. Lenardo

Introduction
Overview: Cellular Homeostasis and Programmed Cell Death in Multicellular Organisms
Programmed Cell Death and Immune Regulation
   Thymic Deletion: Positive and Negative Selection · PCD and the Homeostasis of Peripheral T Cells · Active or Antigen-Stimulated T-Lymphocyte Death · Passive or Lymphokine Withdrawal T-Cell Death · T-Cell Memory · B-Cell Homeostasis · Dendritic Cell Homeostasis · PCD as an Immune Effector Mechanism
Cellular and Molecular Mechanisms of PCD
   Apoptosis Initiation Mediated By Caspase Complexes: Two Principal Pathways · Special Role of the Mitochondrion · Programmed Necrosis
Families of Molecules Provide Precise Regulation of PCD
   Caspases · TNF-Receptor Superfamily Members · Bcl-2 Gene Family · Apaf Proteins
Structural Regulation of PCD
   TNF/TNFR Structure · Bcl-2 Homology Structures · The Hexahelical Bundle · Caspase Structure · PCD as Immune Therapy · PCD and Development of Lymphoid Malignancy
Conclusions
Acknowledgments
References

INTRODUCTION

Nontransformed cells have a finite life span. Most of our cells will die long before we do and evidence suggests that this is important for our health. However, in general, adult vertebrates, as well as their internal organs, stay a constant size, so a form of homeostasis is implied (1). In certain organs, this involves a constantly fluctuating dynamic equilibrium. A prime example is the immune system, which employs cell renewal, expansion, and elimination in carrying out its function (2–5). These changes can be systemic or localized to anatomic sites proximate to an antigen stimulus and may affect specific subsets of immune cells as dictated by the stimulus.

Programmed cell death (PCD) denotes a set of internal biochemical mechanisms that cause specific cells to die under defined conditions that are advantageous to the organism (6). Reasons for cell elimination include cell excess, improper cell differentiation, cell transformation, genetic damage to cells, and infection. Rather than using the title "Apoptosis" for this chapter, we chose "Programmed Cell Death" because increasing evidence suggests that nonapoptotic PCD could play an immunoregulatory role. The chapter has been organized so that we start with a broad overview of general immunoregulatory principles and then delve into the details of

molecules involved in apoptosis in specific sections at the end. Investigation into the molecular mechanism of PCD began in earnest about 1990. The development of an organized database of large sets of expressed sequence tags and bioinformatics tools by Boguski, Lipman, and colleagues at the U.S. National Center for Biotechnology Information in the mid-1990s, allowed extraordinary advances in identifying molecules involved in PCD (7). Although PCD is a large and contentious area of cell biology research, molecular advances have established a firm and tractable theoretical foundation. Remarkably, much of what we discuss in this chapter was completely unknown a mere decade ago. Yet these pathways are at work every day in our bodies to control responses to infectious agents, establish cellular homeostasis, prevent autoimmunity, and avert lymphoid malignancies.

OVERVIEW: CELLULAR HOMEOSTASIS AND PROGRAMMED CELL DEATH IN MULTICELLULAR ORGANISMS

Internal programs of death are likely to exist in all mammalian cells. Raff (8) has suggested that these internal programs must be constantly and actively suppressed. For

841

experimental investigation, it is thus important to discriminate between cellular demise caused by accident and that initiated or "programmed" by an internal biochemical mechanism. The term "apoptosis," a Greek word meaning "falling off" as in leaves from a tree, was introduced in 1972 by Kerr et al. (9) to describe the normal, presumably programmed, attrition of cells. It was defined as a microscopic appearance of cell death comprising cell shrinkage with nuclear and cytoplasmic condensation within an intact, but blebbed, cell membrane (10) (Fig. 1B and C). This cell phenotype has long been associated with cell death (11). Apoptosis is now mainly identified with the biochemical effects of the caspase family of proteases (12). Caspases are important in two respects. First, they are a feature of most if not all apoptosis pathways. Second, once activated, they usually represent a commitment to apoptosis that is not reversible, although there are suggestions that low-level caspase activation may occur during lymphocyte activation (13,14). For these reasons, caspases have been regarded as a final common pathway of apoptosis. In fact, the concept of PCD was significantly strengthened by the identification of caspases and other molecules that comprise dedicated internal biochemical death pathways. In general, the death machinery is preassembled and available without new gene transcription or protein synthesis (6). Caspases are constitutively expressed in the cytoplasm of the cell as zymogens. Once proteolytically activated, caspases

cause the morphologic changes of apoptosis culminating in cell death. The death program entrained to caspases includes cleavage of chromosomal DNA, nuclear chromatin condensation, exposure of phosphatidylserine on the exterior of the cell membrane, proteolysis of specific proteins including other caspases, and mitochondrial changes. These events are detectable by simple assays in tissue culture cells *in vitro* or, in some cases, *in vivo*. Protocols for these assays have been well described (15,16).

Cells that die without the characteristics of apoptosis undergo what is usually called "necrosis." While necrosis is often associated with accidental cell death, it may also result from programmed mechanisms. The appearance of a necrotic cell differs dramatically from apoptosis. Necrotic cells swell and lose the integrity of internal organelles and cell membrane, giving an enlarged "fractured" appearance under the microscope (Fig. 1D). Recently, various research groups have begun to define molecular programs resulting in necrotic death (17). Thus, we distinguish between "programmed" necrosis and necrosis due to accidental causes that are likely due to very different molecular events. It has been generally argued that apoptosis, which preserves membrane integrity, prevents inflammation from released cellular contents, whereas necrosis results in total cellular breakdown and content release, which causes an inflammatory response. There are contrasting views on whether remnants of apoptotic or necrotic cells are more immunogenic when engulfed by antigen-presenting cells, although exposure to necrotic cells can cause dendritic cell maturation (19–21). The distinct immunologic effects due to apoptosis and necrosis remain the subject of substantial experimental exploration.

As we argue below, the necessity of cellular homeostasis as well as the acute need to eliminate cells that are harmful or nonfunctional led to the early emergence of conserved cell-death mechanisms (11). Work by Metzstein and Horvitz (22) genetically identified several molecules essential for the death of specific cells during the development of the roundworm *C. elegans* that have subsequently been found to be homologs for mammalian PCD genes. It is clear from this simplified system that the molecular logic of one form of cell death was likely established early in evolution (23). PCD mechanisms are now evident in most contemporary multicellular organisms from plants to humans, although it is not clear whether convergent evolution or conservation of function is responsible. However, the molecular pathways in worms and other simple organisms are rudimentary compared with the complexity found in mammalian PCD systems. To understand how these mechanisms contribute to immunity, we focus on mice and humans, which are the subjects of most immunologic research.

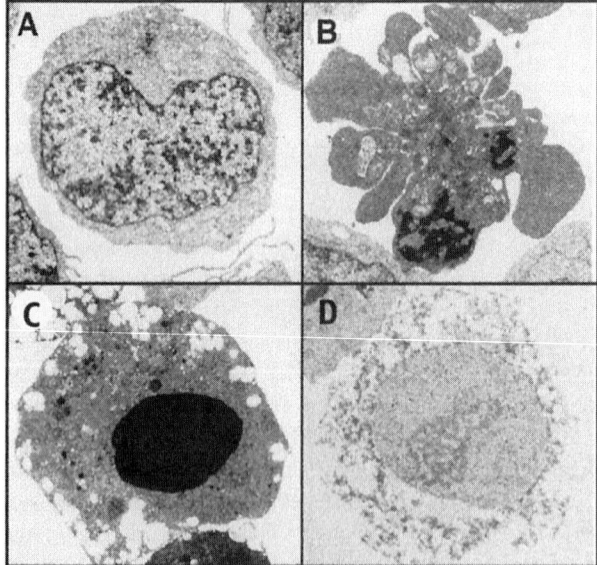

FIG. 1. Electron microscopy elucidates the morphology of different forms of PCD. **A:** A normal, unstimulated Jurkat leukemia cell. **B:** Jurkat cell undergoing apoptosis in response to Fas receptor stimulation. Note the condensed chromatin and the blebbing, but maintenance of plasma membrane integrity. **C:** Jurkat cell undergoing apoptosis in response to staurosporine treatment. Note the prominent nuclear condensation. **D:** Necrosis of human peripheral blood T-lymphocyte infected with HIV. Note the general loss of cellular integrity as well as the lack of chromatin condensation in the dying cell. Courtesy of D. Bolton and J. Orenstein.

PROGRAMMED CELL DEATH AND IMMUNE REGULATION

The fundamental unit of immune responsiveness is the cell. In considering the major immune cells, lymphocytes, each cell is distinguished by expressing a unique clonotypic antigen receptor. A large number of lymphocytes with different receptor specificities are generated during ontogeny—for example, the "immune repertoire"—and these cells can be programmed to expand or die throughout the life of the organism. Although the level of antigen presentation, the degree of lymphocyte responsiveness (vs. nonresponsiveness or anergy), and other factors also play important roles, the presence or absence of cells with specific recognition properties at any given time is a primary determinant of the quantitative response to any antigenic stimulus. The homeostasis of major lymphocyte populations is independently regulated such that deficits in B cells, T cells, or even major T-cell subpopulations ($\alpha\beta$ vs. $\gamma\delta$ or CD4 vs. CD8), do not prevent the normal homeostasis of the remaining populations. During development, lymphocytes respond to the antigenic environment with either survival or death (24). For the most part, developmental PCD eliminates lymphocytes that cannot recognize antigen appropriately or have dangerous self-reactivity (24,25). In the mature immune system, death is principally a negative feedback response that counterbalances proliferative responses to antigen (26). Although the clonal selection theory of F.M. Burnet encompassed clonal elimination during ontogeny, in the mature immune system, it allowed only selective expansion of antigen-stimulated lymphocytes. We have proposed that antigen-specific regulation of mature lymphocyte survival also powerfully controls immune responses and tolerance (5,26,53). Since the organism encounters an unpredictable universe of antigens in a lifetime, it is essential that there is feedback regulation of adaptive immune responses. Feedback is an essential element of any dynamic system in which final outcomes cannot be predicted from the starting conditions (27). In immunity, proliferation and death are coordinated by feedback regulation to provide measured responses by controlling the number of immunologic responsive cells.

Thymic Deletion: Positive and Negative Selection

Thymic selection represents one of the most intriguing examples of apoptosis induction in which the same receptor—the clonotypic T-cell receptor (TCR)—can lead to diametrically opposite outcomes depending on the level of stimulation (24,25). During development, at the stage when thymocytes express the TCR and both the CD4 and CD8 co-receptors (the "double-positive" stage), thymocytes will undergo apoptosis if they receive no TCR stimulation. This has been called "death by neglect" (28). This process will eliminate thymocytes that have not productively rearranged the TCR genes or have no capacity to recognize antigen in the context of self–major histocompatibility complex (MHC). "Low-level" stimulation of the TCR antagonizes death by neglect. This protective event ensures MHC-specific antigen recognition by T cells and is called "positive selection" (29). While weak TCR signals can deliver an anti-apoptotic stimulus, strong TCR engagement of double positive thymocytes delivers a

pro-apoptotic signal. This event, termed "negative selection" prevents the emergence of strongly autoreactive lymphocytes from the thymus (28). This deletion step is a major mechanism of central tolerance and the prevention of autoimmunity (30). These processes of selection employ caspase-dependent apoptosis and rapid phagocytosis of the dead thymocytes (31,32). Hence, thymocytes travel a narrow bridge of TCR avidity during development and will die if they deviate from it.

The differences among the neglect (or null), weak, and strong signals that result in life or death appear to be determined at early stages of TCR signaling (33,34). Death receptors (see below) appear not to be crucial; instead, there is a direct connection of the TCR-signaling apparatus to mitochondrial death pathways (35–38). Although there is not complete certainty about how the TCR dictates life or death at specific antigen levels, the answer to this puzzle will almost certainly reside in the complex signal pathways emanating from this receptor. TCR engagement that causes transient induction of the Erk kinase is associated with positive selection, whereas slow but constant Erk activity is associated with negative selection (39–41). Other distinctions in TCR signaling have been identified. Signaling through phosphotidylinositol-3 kinase, the anti-apoptotic Akt kinase, and the retinoid orphan receptor (ROR)-gamma may promote thymocyte survival. (For reviews, see Berg and Kang [33] and Kruisbeek and Amsen [42].) Gene knockouts in mice have revealed that several transcription factors, such as E2A, Id3, and IRF-1, can affect thymic cellularity, indicating that differential signaling may trigger transcriptional events that regulate cell survival (43–46). Finally, Huang and Strasser (47) and Bouillet et al. (48) have emphasized that various forms of physiologic cell death are likely to involve the subset of BH3-only proteins in the Bcl-2 family. The activation of proapoptotic BH3-only proteins such as Bak, Bid, and especially increased expression of the Bim gene, by TCR signals could initiate mitochondrial alterations leading to apoptosis during thymic selection processes. In sum, current evidence suggests a pathway wherein early TCR-induced signaling differences directly entrain distinct transcriptional events that modulate BH3-only regulators of the mitochondrial pathway of death. Hence, by intracellular communication with distinct apoptosis regulatory molecules, the TCR has a remarkable ability to signal life or death by the apparent strength of stimulus it receives.

PCD and the Homeostasis of Peripheral T Cells

Death of T cells in the periphery differs markedly from thymocyte selection in that PCD of mature lymphocytes occurs mainly in cells that have proven usefulness, that is, they have already been activated by antigen. This is because PCD of mature T cells is employed primarily to counter antigen-driven proliferation of activated T cells. In general, most naïve lymphocytes survive and circulate in the body in a resting state (G0 lymphocytes). The survival of such resting

T cells is constitutively maintained by the presence of contact with MHC, the lymphokine IL-7, and expression of the anti-apoptotic protein Bcl-2 (49–52). During an active immune response, T-lymphocyte proliferation can involve as much as a 1000-fold expansion within days. Such explosive proliferation is necessitated by the extraordinarily rapid propagation of microbial pathogens. However, these activated and cycling T cells are potentially damaging due to toxic effector functions and potential cross-reactivity with self-antigens. This expansion does not go unchecked and activated T cells are subjected to negative feedback in the form of death of the T cells involved in the immune response. However, because immune responses are directed at specific antigens, they must be independently regulated since some specific cell populations may be expanding while others are contracting. The immune system has developed propriocidal mechanisms to control independent populations of activated T cells. "Propriocidal regulation" refers to the various negative feedback death mechanisms that maintain homeostasis of mature peripheral T cells in an antigen-specific manner. These potently restrain the survival of antigen-activated T cells and tightly control lymphocyte numbers during and at the end of immune responses.

Propriocidal regulation of T cells is triggered by remarkably simple attributes of T-cell activation—the level of cell cycling and the level of antigen restimulation (26,53). These two features are ideally suited for triggering negative feedback death because they provide both a "sensing" mechanism for the level of active T-cell proliferation and a negative response mechanism to further antigen stimulation. There are essentially two different mechanisms: (a) active or antigen-stimulated PCD and (b) passive or lymphokine withdrawal PCD (Fig. 2) (5,54–56). These have different roles and occur at different times in immune responses as will be described in detail below. In some respects, it is paradoxical that lymphocytes that respond well to foreign antigen and presumably could have protective value are actively eliminated. However, it appears to be vital to constrain the number of activated T cells to prevent unhealthy effector or autoimmune reactions. It is possible that during a strong immune response, lymphocytes that cross-react with self-antigens will proliferate. The propriocidal mechanisms of programming these cells to die upon encountering self-antigens could be an important mechanism of preserving self-tolerance. By this formulation, tolerance is a quantitative effect that is due to the low number of significantly self-reactive lymphocytes in the naïve organism. Clonal expansion during immune responses can unleash dormant or infrequent self-reactive clones, called "forbidden clones" by Burnet, creating an autoimmune diathesis. Propriocidal death reduces these clones and thereby promotes tolerance. Active antigen-induced propriocidal death, which is induced by high or repeated doses of antigen, is especially well suited for the elimination of self-reactive clones since self-antigen is likely to be present in continuously high amounts (26,53).

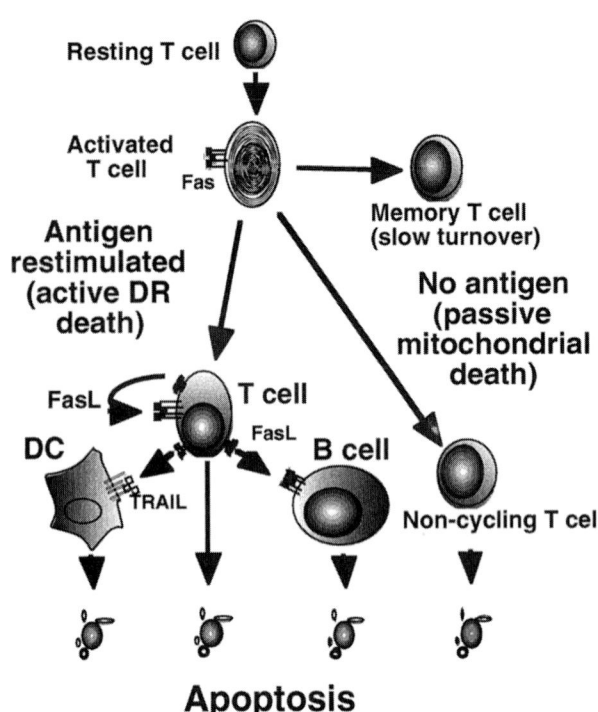

FIG. 2. Propriocidal regulation of immune cells. Shown are the apoptosis pathways that govern T-lymphocyte homeostasis by the antigen-restimulated (active DR death) and no-antigen (passive/lymphokine withdrawal [mitochondrial]) pathways of apoptosis. Also shown are the regulation of B cells by FasL expressed by T cells and DCs by TRAIL expressed by T cells.

Active or Antigen-Stimulated T-Lymphocyte Death

The active death mechanism involves apoptosis of mature T cells in response to antigen stimulation. This requires the T cells to be activated and cycling at the time that they undergo strong antigenic restimulation (26,53). The death is indirect in the sense that it requires the antigen-induced secretion of death ligands that engage specific apoptosis-inducing death receptors in the tumor necrosis factor–receptor (TNFR) superfamilies (Fig. 2) (57,58). Current evidence suggests that Fas ligand (FasL) as well as TNF are the key death ligands that mediate this process in mature CD4$^+$ and CD8$^+$ T cells (4,5,59). Watanabe-Fukunaga et al. (60,61) and Takahashi et al. (62) originally observed that the lymphoproliferative and autoimmune phenotype of lpr mice was due to genetic alterations of Fas and that a similar disease was due to a mutation in FasL. Defects in Fas (CD95) or FasL cause severe derangements of lymphocyte homeostasis and tolerance that will be detailed below in the section on Fas signaling. In humans, defects in Fas and FasL cause similar abnormalities in the autoimmune lymphoproliferative syndrome (ALPS), types Ia and Ib, respectively (63). An alternative mechanism of propriocidal regulation is via perforin, which is a chief mediator of cytolytic T-cell killing of target cells. Perforin defects in both mice and humans cause impaired clearance of activated CD8$^+$ T cells (64–67). Often these forms of death are called "activation-induced cell death" (AICD), but this is a misnomer whose use is not recommended (68). AICD has been used to describe any form of death of activated T cells, thus causing confusion among investigators working on molecularly distinct death pathways (5,69). Activation *per se* does not directly cause cell death; instead, death induction requires antigenic restimulation of activated T cells, that is, reengagement after the initial activation. For resting T cells, antigen encounter under co-stimulatory conditions leads to activation with very little cell death. Obviously, if the initial activation directly induced death, this would preclude immune responses. In fact, activated, cycling T cells do not spontaneously die by FasL or TNF unless they are strongly restimulated by antigen in the activated state, which causes up-regulation of the genes for these death cytokines and responsiveness to them (70).

Active death is a negative feedback mechanism, which explains why its primary triggers are lymphokine-induced cell cycling (usually caused by IL-2) and reengagement of the TCR. IL-2 induced cell cycling indicates that there has been a productive antigen response and the T cells are multiplying. Since T cells can expand rapidly to great numbers, a large fraction of cycling T cells dictates a need to down-regulate the response to any further antigen exposure. The presence of repeated or continuously high amounts of antigen would be a powerful stimulus to greater proliferation. Under these conditions, the system programs a fraction of the restimulated cells to undergo apoptosis by death ligand production or perforin. Unchecked, exponential T-cell expansion is thereby prevented by a simple and specific feedback loop. Like most negative feedback systems, the propriocidal response directly reverses the ongoing process of proliferation by programming activated T cells to die. Antigen-induced death provides an explanation for many historical observations in the literature that the reapplication or continuous presence of high concentrations of antigen can lead to suppression rather than augmentation of an immune response (reviewed in Critchfield et al. [53]).

Sensitivity to the active death mechanism is chiefly due to the effect of IL-2 in inducing cell-cycle progression into late G1 or S phase, which confers susceptibility to death (71–73). The requirement for cell-cycle progression has not been fully explained but appears to be necessary for apoptosis induced by TCR engagement or with direct Fas stimulation. Other cytokines that augment T-cell cycling, such as IL-4, IL-7, and IL-15, can also promote cell death to some degree but none with the potency of IL-2 (70). Hence, the theory of propriocidal regulation advanced the concept that IL-2 would have an important regulatory role in the elimination of activated T cells in addition to its previously known role in lymphocyte proliferation (53). This concept was later validated when genetic deficiencies of IL-2 and IL-2 receptor in mice were created and found to cause the accumulation of activated T cells and autoimmunity (74–76). This surprising property

of IL-2 is important to consider in the use of IL-2 as a therapeutic agent or vaccine adjuvant. It also underscores an important feature of feedback regulation: To achieve a maximal response for, say, a vaccine, more stimulation is not necessarily better. In a variety of test situations, active antigen-induced death decreases the number of T cells, but does not completely eliminate the T-cell immune response (26,77). In certain extraordinary conditions, such as high levels of a noncytopathic or chronic virus, essentially all responding T cells can be eliminated (78). FasL expressed on T cells also causes the death of B cells, which do not themselves express FasL (79). This causes a parallel regulation of the B-cell proliferative response by Fas-induced death that can be antagonized by B-cell receptor engagement (Fig. 2). Antigen-induced death therefore provides a mechanism to eliminate specific antigen-reactive lymphocytes under chronic stimulatory conditions when they might cause the host more harm than good.

Antigen-induced expression of death receptors and their ligands shunts a proportionate fraction of antigen-specific activated cells, but not bystander cells, into the death pathway. The activated T cells still carry out their effector function when re-stimulated by antigen, but their ultimate fate is death instead of proliferation (70,78). Since the agents of cell death, Fas and other TNFRs, have no inherent antigen specificity, it is important to consider how the clonal specificity of antigen-induced apoptosis is achieved (26). For the death of activated T cells, the simple engagement of Fas by its ligand is insufficient (80,81). Efficient death induction also requires a "competency" signal from the TCR delivered at the same time FasL binds Fas (81,82). However, these signals do not require new protein synthesis and are delivered rapidly in a few hours or less (80,81). The requirement for simultaneous engagement of Fas and TCR plays a critical role in establishing the antigen specificity of death. For example, it was shown that TCR stimulation of a specific subpopulation within a pool of Fas-expressing T-cell blasts, such as with agonistic anti-Vβ8 antibody, leads only to the death of that subpopulation despite the apparent exposure of other subtypes of T cells to the Vβ8-expressing cells that have been induced to express FasL (26,81). In addition, deletion *in vivo* is antigen specific (77). The molecular nature of the competency signal is presently unknown.

Passive or Lymphokine Withdrawal T-Cell Death

As much as it is important to avert overreaction during an immune response through active, TCR-induced death, it is equally important for the immune system to turn down the immune reaction after successful elimination of the pathogen. Lymphokine withdrawal death is a passive form of T-cell apoptosis that occurs naturally at the end of an immune response when the accumulation of effector cells becomes unnecessary and potentially damaging (83). When the trophic cytokine for activated T cells, typically IL-2, decreases because of reduced antigen stimulation, the excess T cells undergo apoptosis (84). This mechanism of cell death is readily modeled *in vitro* by simply removing IL-2 from T-cell cultures (85). This form of negative feedback death may affect specific classes of T cells, such as "effector" versus "memory" cells, although this distinction may be difficult to discern. Since most T cells in the expanded population are antigen specific, this represents clonotype-specific T-cell propriocidal regulation controlled by antigen and cell-cycle progression. The activated cells can "sense" decreased antigen drive and decreased trophic cytokine, which programs them for apoptosis. The elimination of the expanded pool of activated cells, except for a small number of memory cells, reestablishes homeostasis in T-cell numbers. It has been shown that if IL-2 is exogenously delivered at the end of a proliferative response to superantigen, the reactive T cells are not eliminated but persist as long as lymphokine is provided (86). Therefore, the lack of IL-2 is a key element in the feedback regulation of the cellular response. Antigen and IL-2 therefore carry out propriocidal regulation in the midst of an immune response and at its conclusion to down-regulate T-cell numbers.

Genetic studies reveal that the molecular mechanism of lymphokine withdrawal death is different than antigen-induced apoptosis (54,55). Although this event is often confused with active cell death mediated by Fas, death receptors are not involved. Rather, cytokine withdrawal for 2 to 4 hours commits the cell to a death pathway requiring new protein synthesis (85). Apoptosis is initiated through the mitochondrial pathway and can be effectively blocked by Bcl-2 and Bcl-X_L (see section below) (87). Also involved is the Bad protein, which is a death-inducing member of the Bcl-2 family. When the trophic cytokine is present, the Ser/Thr kinase Akt phophorylates Bad and it is then sequestered by the 14-3-3 scaffold protein (88,89). Death induction involves suppression of Akt, which causes the dephosphorylation of Bad and its insertion into the mitochondrial membrane, which initiates apoptosis (52). This likely involves complex formation between Bad and the anti-apoptotic members of the Bcl-2 family via the BH3 helices. How the molecular assembly with Bad can trigger apoptosis is unclear but appears to be due to a weakening or permeabilization of the outer mitochondrial membrane (OMM) (see below). It will be interesting to determine precisely how the withdrawal of trophic cytokines such as IL-2 and IL-3 regulate Akt and other molecules that participate in death induction. Such phenomena may be important in a variety of cell lineages since many cell types will die presumably from the lack of death-suppressing trophic influence when disaggregated from their parental organs (6).

T-Cell Memory

T cells, once activated, can persist as "memory" cells. One view is that the process involves an escape from apoptosis (50,90,91). Hence, such cells would have to avoid elimination by the propriocidal mechanisms. Increasing evidence supports the concept that memory is due to the long-term survival of antigen-specific T cells even without further antigen exposure. Several means to achieve such survival are possible. To escape killing by Fas and other death receptors, T cells could express c-FLIP (cellular FLICE inhibitory protein), which is a homolog of caspase-8 and caspase-10 that has no enzymatic function but can interpose itself into the death receptor complex and block caspase activation (174). This type of inhibition has been demonstrated in B cells by the ability of Ig stimulation, which up-regulates c-FLIP (92,93), to block Fas killing (94). Various inhibitors of apoptosis proteins (IAPs) might also interfere with death-receptor killing (95,96). Furthermore, the mitochondrial death pathway could be inhibited by up-regulation of Bcl-2 and Bcl-X_L, which have been shown to block lymphokine withdrawal apoptosis (87). The necessity of these inhibitory molecules for the persistence of a memory population of T cells is unknown. Another view is that long-term survival in a nonproliferative "resting" state characteristic of "virgin" T cells is never reestablished by memory cells. Recent work by Murali-Krishna et al. (97) and Ku et al. (98) suggests that there is continued low-level proliferation of memory CD8 T cells that is antigen dependent and probably maintained by IL-15. Also, the fraction of memory cells remains constant over time indicating that death is still taking place at some reduced rate. Hence, the balance of slow proliferation and slow death ensures memory cell maintenance. As the molecular mechanism of the memory state is further elucidated, the differing views of "memory" are likely to be reconciled.

B-Cell Homeostasis

We have focused most of our attention on T-lymphocyte apoptosis thus far because it has received the greatest experimental examination and more details are known. However, PCD also governs B-cell homeostasis and is regulated in ways that have both similarities and differences with T cells. Both death-receptor triggering and withdrawal of trophic stimuli contribute to B-cell elimination. Similar to T cells, developing B cells in the bone marrow undergo a series of proliferative expansion and apoptotic contraction events to shape the final B-cell repertoire (99). Immunoglobulin (Ig) gene rearrangement starting at the pro-B stage generates the B-cell receptor (BCR). The cytokine IL-7, which promotes the survival of developing thymocytes (100,101), is crucial in sustaining survival at the pro–B/pre–B juncture (102,103). Then a process of selection occurs for B cells that have undergone two developmental steps with successive gene rearrangements at the heavy- and light-chain Ig loci. B cells that fail to generate a productive BCR, due to abortive Ig gene rearrangements, are eliminated by PCD. At the other end of the spectrum, B cells that express BCRs directed against self-antigens are eliminated by apoptosis or undergo receptor editing to acquire new antigen specificity (104). The survival and antigen responsiveness of immature B cells can also be increased by LPS exposure, presumably to enhance B-cell production during infections (105). Fas, TNFR-1, or perforin are not involved in the death of developing B cells (reviewed in Hardy and Hayakawa [106]). Rather, death appears to be a consequence of a direct signaling event generated by the BCR (107).

In contrast to developing, immature B cells, mature B cells rely heavily on TNFR family receptors such as CD40 and Fas for regulating their survival and death. It is also clear that T cells control PCD of mature B cells. Rathmell et al. (108,109) have illustrated the importance of CD40 and Fas in the balance of life and death in B cells using the hen egg lysozyme (HEL)-transgenic and HEL-specific TCR-transgenic mice (108,109). Naïve, HEL-specific B cells undergo proliferation in the presence of HEL and HEL-specific CD4 T-cell help. Hence, proper B-cell activation requires triggering of the BCR as well as T-cell help in the form of CD40L expressed on activated T cells. The primary function of CD40L is to prevent death of the activated B cells and allow further differentiation and function (110). However, anergic HEL-specific B cells from HEL-transgenic animals undergo apoptosis in the presence of the same HEL-specific CD4 T-cell help. This antigen-specific B-cell death is absent in Fas-deficient B cells (108), thus establishing a role for Fas in causing the death of anergic antigen-specific B cells. Fas killing of mature B cells can also be abrogated by BCR engagement and IL-4, which promote antibody responses (111,112). An imbalance of CD40 and Fas signals might contribute to autoantibody production consequent to Fas and FasL mutations in both human and mouse.

The attenuation of B-cell responses at the end of an immune reaction is likely to involve cytokine withdrawal death similar to that of T cells, but is less well characterized. Cytokines such as IL-7 and IL-15, which enhance cellular survival through the up-regulation of Bcl-2 or Bcl-X$_L$, may be responsible (113). Lymphokine withdrawal death in B cells also requires de novo RNA/protein synthesis (114). Recently, a secreted lipocalin, identified through microarray analysis of an IL-3 dependent pro–B-cell line, was implicated as a potential mediator for IL-3 withdrawal death (115). Lipocalins are small extracellular peptide carriers of lipophilic ligands that have roles in cellular differentiation and proliferation (reviewed in Bratt [116]). However, it remains to be seen whether lipocalins or other similar molecules are involved in lymphokine withdrawal death in primary B or T cells. As we discuss later in this chapter, survival genes such as Bcl-2 can protect cells against lymphokine withdrawal death. Perhaps not too surprisingly, therefore, Bcl-2 assumes an important role in mature B-cell homeostasis. Moreover, Bcl-2 can also play a role in neoplastic B-lymphoid cell survival as revealed by the t(14:18) translocation of Bcl-2 to the Ig locus in follicular B-cell lymphomas (117).

Dendritic Cell Homeostasis

The regulation of dendritic cells (DCs) is still largely unexplored. However, emerging evidence suggests that these highly efficient antigen-presenting cells are also subject to homeostatic regulation by PCD. The natural turnover of DCs was demonstrated in the mouse by Ingulli et al. (118). Using elegant cell-labeling experiments, they showed that antigen-laden DCs stimulate the formation of a cluster of activated antigen-specific T cells and then disappear. This process was antigen- and T-cell–dependent. Later, it was shown that the TNF homolog TRAIL (TNF-related apoptosis inducing ligand), which is produced by activated T cells, could induce apoptosis in DCs (119), whereas FasL was incapable of killing DCs. This suggested the concept that there is homeostatic regulation of DCs involving recruitment and differentiation followed by their active elimination by stimulated T cells. Early removal of DCs has the benefit of allowing the activation of T cells but avoiding T-cell restimulation and propriocidal death too soon in the response to antigen. It is possible that additional regulation of DC elimination could be determined by different anatomical locations and exposure to other immune cells.

PCD as an Immune Effector Mechanism

Although this topic will be covered authoritatively elsewhere in the book, it is important to recognize that the same pathways that participate in homeostatic cell death also are used as immune effector mechanisms. The Fas pathway is now recognized as the principal Ca^{2+}-independent pathway of cytotoxic T-cell (CTL) killing (65). Fas ligand displayed by either CD4$^+$ or CD8$^+$ T cells can eliminate Fas-bearing cells that may be infected or malignant by inducing caspase-mediated apoptosis. Similarly, the Ca^{2+}-dependent CTL mechanism involving perforin and granzymes also can induce PCD in target cells. Granzyme B is the only serine protease capable of processing caspases (120–124). When perforin breaches the target-cell membrane, granzyme B gains access to the cytoplasm and proteolytically activates caspases leading to apoptosis. Although this cytoplasmic pathway of death does not emanate from the mitochondrion, the latter may amplify the death signal (125,126). Similarly, amplification of the death signal by Fas through the cleavage of Bid and activation of the mitochondrial pathway apparently also occur (127–129). These parallels may provide insight into why lymphocytes have evolved an indirect mechanism, involving the surface expression and/or secretion of FasL and subsequent interaction with cell surface Fas, or perforin/granzyme release to homeostatically control their numbers by apoptosis. This mechanism permits the T cell to regulate itself, other immune cells, and expunge nonlymphoid cells that require immune elimination such as those that are infected or malignant. Natural killer cells may also use PCD mechanisms for self-regulation and expunging infected or malignant cells (130,131). Hence, for mature T cells, the same molecules can subserve several death functions, perhaps even simultaneously. By contrast, a more direct connection of the TCR or BCR to death pathways is present in developing lymphocytes, which have no use for effector mechanisms or propriocidal regulation.

CELLULAR AND MOLECULAR MECHANISMS OF PCD

Apoptosis Initiation Mediated by Caspase Complexes: Two Principal Pathways

Caspases must be highly active within the cell cytoplasm to cause apoptosis. Like all proteases, these potentially destructive proteins are first produced as zymogens that are then proteolytically activated. In mammalian cells, the molecules and pathways regulating caspase activation are complex (Fig. 3). Elucidating these complex pathways provides a window into the myriad of molecular abnormalities of apoptosis that contribute to immunologic diseases and cancer. Fortunately, mammalian apoptosis can be described for didactic purposes by a few key concepts. Most importantly, the processing enzymes that activate caspases are caspases themselves. As explained below, autoprocessing occurs when caspase zymogens are brought into specific complexes. This is achieved by various types of adaptor molecules that specifically recruit and assemble caspases into complexes via death effector domains (DEDs) or caspase recruitment domains (CARD) (214,263). The DED and CARD are protein–protein interaction domains found in the caspase prodomains and other

adaptor molecules that mediate the specific intermolecular assemblies. The precise mechanism by which initiator caspases such caspase-8 or -10 become activated is unclear; however, it is likely to depend on a low level of proteolytic activity inherent in the caspase zymogen. When juxtaposed at the receptor complex, this proteolytic activity will cleave the zymogen, leading to the maturation of the enzyme through separation of the large and small enzymatic subunits. Autoprocessing also cleaves the enzymatic units from the prodomain, thereby liberating the highly active enzyme from the receptor complex. As discussed later in the chapter, structural studies reveal that active caspases are tetrameric species composed of two small and two large subunits. Hence, it is likely that autoprocessing and activation of caspases involves the cross-cleavage of at least two units of the unprocessed zymogen.

To initiate the caspase cascade, the enzyme must dock onto the appropriate adaptor molecules. The adaptor/caspase complex presumably provides a conformation that facilitates the initial autoprocessing step of the caspase zymogen. Adaptor/caspase complexes originate from two principal sites in the cell: the membrane (through death receptors) or the mitochondrion (Fig. 3). These are sometimes called the "outside-in" and the "inside-out" mechanisms, respectively (132).

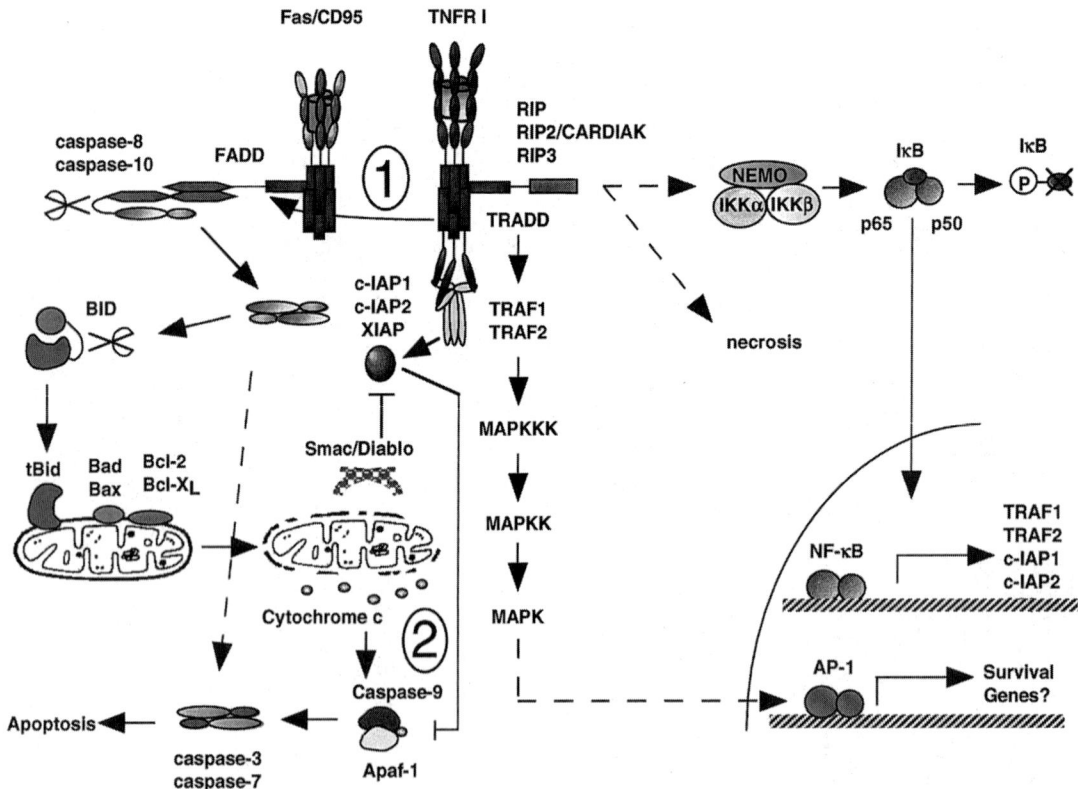

FIG. 3. Signal transduction pathways of death receptors. Shown are the two principal apoptosis pathways associated with death receptors (Fas and TNFR-1) shown by the *encircled number one* and that associated with the mitochondrial pathway of caspase-9 activation shown by the *encircled number two*. The *solid arrows* indicate direct association of the steps involved, whereas the *dashed arrows* indicate that multiple steps are involved. Inhibitory interactions are shown by a *barred line*.

However, this is misleading because many influences external to the cell, such as UV or ionizing irradiation, drugs such as glucocorticoids, etoposide, or staurosporine, DNA-damaging agents, and lymphokine withdrawal can trigger the mitochondrial pathway. Nevertheless, we will employ this primary dichotomy of receptor-induced and mitochondrial apoptosis since it recapitulates the two major forms of propriocidal regulation, antigen-induced and lymphokine withdrawal apoptosis, respectively.

Death-receptor engagement by cognate ligand causes the formation of the death-inducing signaling complex (DISC), which comprises the cytoplasmic tail of the receptor, the FADD adaptor protein, and caspase-8 or capase-10 (133,134). The recruitment of caspase-8 or -10 into the DISC triggers the processing of these proteases into their active form. An 80–amino-acid death domain (DD) present in the Fas cytoplasmic tail and FADD causes their interaction. The DD contains a "hexahelical bundle" that nucleates this complex, as described in greater detail below. There is likely to be 3:3 stoichiometry of the FADD adaptor protein and the Fas receptor. FADD recruits caspase-8 or -10 by homotypic interaction between DEDs present in each of these molecules. The DED has a hexahelical bundle structure homologous but not identical to DDs. Sensitive energy-transfer techniques showed that both caspases can enter the same receptor complex (135). The signal complex for TNFR-1 is not the same as for Fas since it includes the DD-containing adaptor TRADD in addition to FADD and caspase-8 and-10 (see below). Similar signaling complexes are likely formed with other DD-containing members of the TNFR superfamily including TNFR-1; death receptor (DR) 3; TRAIL receptors (TR)-1 and -2 (also called DR-4 and -5, respectively); and DR 6 (136–138). The physiologic significance of apoptosis mediated by any of these receptors besides Fas and TNFR-1 in immune regulation is unknown, although DR6 has been implicated in Th2 cell differentiation (139,140). It has been proposed that TR-1 and TR-2 may mediate the preferential killing of tumor cells (including lymphoid tumors) (141).

The mitochondrial death pathway mediates lymphokine withdrawal death. Activation of the mitochondrial pathway achieves the same end as DRs—caspase activation—by signal complex formation in a different way. The various inducers of death appear to converge on molecules within the OMM. Some molecules are well-defined members of the Bcl-2 protein family. Others are less well-defined regulators and/or are components of permeability complexes within the OMM. Alteration of these sentinel complexes by various apoptosis triggers leads to the release of the molecules between the mitochondrial membranes. The key factor released is cytochrome c. Once liberated into the cytosol, cytochrome c, Apaf-1, and caspase-9, together with ATP as a co-factor, associate into a signal complex termed the "apoptosome" (142, 143). This leads to caspase-9 autoactivation and apoptosis (reviewed in Shi [144] and Budihardjo [145]). There are specialized regulatory proteins for caspase-9 that provide additional levels of control: X-linked IAP (XIAP),

which inhibits caspase-9, and Smac/Diablo, which counteracts XIAP (146,147). The events at the OMM are tightly regulated and caspase-9 activation commits the cell to die.

Special Role of the Mitochondrion

A special role for the mitochondrion in apoptosis was first suggested by the finding that Bcl-2 and related molecules were anchored predominantly in the OMM. The inner membrane is devoted to energy conversion and ATP generation, but the OMM has emerged as a primary regulator of cell viability. A diversity of death inducers including trophic factor withdrawal, drugs such as staurosporine or steroids, or DNA damage, all generate signals that converge on the mitochondrion. Their principal effect is to cause the cytochrome c release which then coalesces with Apaf-1 and caspase-9 into a lethal proteolytic complex. How the OMM releases its mortal poison is not known, but the process may involve a selective increase in permeability or an actual bursting of the OMM. This process appears to be regulated and possibly coordinated by the large family of proteins related to Bcl-2.

A multiprotein complex at the junction between the inner and outer MM has been identified, called the permeability transition complex (PTC), which may play a key role in molecular release through the OMM and dissipation of the normal electrochemical gradient across the inner mitochondrial membrane. Kroemer (148) has argued that a variety of severe insults to the mitochondrion such as superoxides or inhibitors of the respiratory chain can cause a catastrophic event in which the mitochondrion releases apoptogenic proteins, but there is also a collapse in energy generation and disruption of the plasma membrane that can lead to necrosis of the cell (148). There may be a balance between these two series of events in response to mitochondrial insults that determines whether primary apoptotic and necrotic death occurs in any given cell. Of critical importance for determining cell fate is how the mitochondrion is affected by a death stimulus.

Studies of the mitochondrion have also focused on caspase-independent apoptosis mechanisms whose role in immune regulation is not fully understood. In general, this concept stemmed from examples of apoptosis that could not be blocked by small peptide caspase inhibitors such as zVAD (149,150). However, conclusions drawn from such experiments are limited by the short half-life of such inhibitors and the fact that they do not block all caspases. Recently, the cloning and genetic analysis of a protein called "apoptosis-inducing factor" (AIF) have given new impetus to mitochondria initiated death that is independent of Apaf-1 and caspase-9 (151,152). AIF is an oxidoreductase normally localized to the intermembrane space in the mitochondria. In response to apoptotic stimuli, AIF translocates from the mitochondria to the nucleus, causing DNA fragmentation and chromatin condensation (153). AIF is remarkably conserved across a broad spectrum of species, including plants, fungi, and bacteria (154). Genetic deficiency of this protein in mice inhibits the death of embryonic cells in response to serum starvation and appears to be responsible for embryonic morphogenesis and cavitation of the embryonic body. The observation that these processes did not depend on caspase-3, caspase-9, or Apaf-1 suggests that unlike *C. elegans,* not all programmed death in mammalian cells is dependent on caspases. Further work with conditional genetic deficiencies of AIF in immune cell lineages will be needed to determine if this mechanism has any role in immunity.

Another mitochondrial protein important in apoptosis is endonuclease G (EndoG). EndoG is a resident mitochondrial nuclease that is released and translocated to the nucleus upon apoptotic stimulation. Once situated in the nucleus, EndoG cleaves DNA into nucleosomal sizes independent of caspases, thus distinguishing itself from the caspase-dependent activation of another apoptotic nuclease CAD (155) (see below). Thus, the mitochondrion may participate in nuclear chromatin fragmentation, which is one of the chief effects of apoptosis.

Programmed Necrosis

While PCD has generally been equated with apoptosis, recent evidence suggests that necrotic or alternative forms of death may also result from internal death programs (149,150,156,157). This is different from secondary necrosis, which occurs in the late phase of apoptosis when membrane integrity is lost. Rather, PCD leading to a necrotic morphology without any intermediate stage of apoptosis or caspase activation, is now well documented (17,152). For example, it has been found that DRs can trigger necrotic death rather than apoptotic death under certain circumstances (149,150,157). Although TNF stimulation through TNFR-1 can trigger caspase-dependent classical apoptosis, necrosis may well be the dominant pathway for TNFR-1, at least in certain cell types (149,157). By contrast, Fas predominantly triggers apoptosis, but can also induce necrosis (17). A shift from apoptosis to necrosis can be induced by tetrapeptide-caspase inhibitors suggesting that a necrotic pathway may exist for cell elimination when apoptosis fails or is blocked (150). These observations have physiologic relevance since propriocidal death of mature T cells is partly refractory to inhibition by caspase blockers and can manifest features of necrosis (17). For these reasons, we have chosen to introduce the name "programmed necrosis" to describe the cases where cell death by necrosis (or at least a clearly nonapoptotic phenotype) is the result of activation of specific molecular pathways in a manner that appears to be advantageous to the host.

An interesting example of programmed necrosis has been investigated by Holler et al. (17), who have shown that necrosis can occur through strong Fas stimulation in a process that requires the receptor interacting protein (RIP). Originally identified by a yeast two–hybrid interaction screen using the DD of Fas as bait (158), RIP was later found to be an essential component of the TNFR-1 signaling complex that could induce the anti-apoptotic transcription factor NFκB (159–161). Besides a carboxy-terminal DD that is required for homophilic binding to the receptor-signaling complex, RIP also contains an amino-terminal serine/threonine kinase domain that is dispensable to its apoptosis-inducing activity, but is essential for its necrotic function. Both direct Fas engagement or TCR stimulation (which presumably indirectly triggers Fas by FasL induction) can stimulate necrosis *in vitro* (17). A similar form of RIP-dependent, caspase-independent necrosis has also been observed for TNFR-1 (F.K.M. Chan and M.J. Lenardo, *unpublished data,* 2002). Thus, RIP appears to be a bifunctional signaling molecule with stimulatory and necrosis-inducing effects. Paradoxically, RIP-deficient mice are severely runted and die shortly after birth, apparently due to increased TNF-induced death that correlates with a loss of NFκB induction (162). Since Fas-induced PCD has not been investigated extensively in RIP-deficient animals, it remains to be seen whether RIP-dependent programmed necrosis will have any role in normal physiology. Nevertheless, based on the available information, RIP appears to be the clearest talisman of a molecular pathway of programmed necrosis.

What is the potential role of DR-induced necrosis in immunity? Many viruses, particularly the poxviruses, encode inhibitors of caspases (163). Infection by poxviruses leads to blockade of caspase-dependent apoptosis. In fibroblasts, this results in the sensitization of the cells to TNF-induced necrosis (164). Therefore, programmed necrosis may serve to counteract the effects of viral anti-apoptotic mechanisms by eliminating virally infected cells. From an immunologic standpoint, necrotic cells may have a superior stimulatory activity than apoptotic cells for DC maturation (20,21). During viral infection, TNF-induced necrosis may indirectly enhance the CTL response to the virus by promoting the maturation of DCs. Programmed necrosis may therefore have an important immunostimulatory role in addition to any role in the direct elimination of virus-infected cells. Programmed necrosis may thereby serve as a "bridge" between the innate arm of immunity and the adaptive immune response.

Another important reason to further understand necrosis in the context of the immune system is that it may be responsible for the pathogenesis of viruses such as HIV. Although many claims have been made that HIV causes apoptosis—of either directly infected or bystander T cells—most infected cells that die during infection do not manifest hallmarks of apoptosis. Furthermore, these cells actually appear necrotic when examined by electron microscopy (Fig. 1) (164a). Hence, apoptosis does not appear to be the major mode of death. HIV-induced necrosis is not impaired by the absence of RIP, thus distinguishing it from DR-induced necrosis. Further studies on identifying the molecules involved in virally induced necrosis are needed to determine whether it involves a specific molecular program or simply lethal cell injury.

FAMILIES OF MOLECULES PROVIDE PRECISE REGULATION OF PCD

Caspases

A key concept in understanding PCD is that it was apparently so vital to the successful evolution of multicellular organisms that a specific set of genes was dedicated to the task. Chief among these genes were those encoding caspases. In 1993, Yuan et al. (165) first observed that a gene crucial for PCD in *C. elegans*, Ced-3, was related to a mammalian caspase, interleukin-1β–converting enzyme (ICE), thus implicating specific proteolytic events in the death program (165). The "caspase" moniker is a rubric indicating that these enzymes contain an active site cysteine, cleave substrates on the carboxyl side of aspartate residues, and are proteases. Caspases have been called the "executioners" of apoptosis because once activated, their cleavage of various cellular substrates, including other caspases, results in the morphologic features of apoptotic cell death. Earnshaw et al. (166) authoritatively discuss the detailed biochemical features of caspases and their substrates, which are beyond the scope of this chapter. There are 14 caspases in mammals. All appear to be involved in apoptosis except human caspase-1 (ICE) and caspase-4 (caspase-11 in the mouse), which serve to proteolytically process the precursors of cytokines such as interleukin-1β into their mature forms.

Because of the thermodynamic irreversibility of proteolysis, caspase activation is a commitment to death that cannot be undone. Hence, caspases are tightly regulated. This regulation is achieved by three principal means: (a) caspases are zymogens that require proteolytic processing; (b) certain caspases have a long "prodomains" that allow them to enter complexes with adaptor molecules that promote autoprocessing; and (c) specific inhibitors exist (6). How these mechanisms work is clear from the structures of caspases (Fig. 4). Caspases have an NH2-terminal "prodomain" that is removed in the active enzyme. The COOH-terminal protease domain comprises two catalytic subunits of the mature enzyme that are denoted by their processed molecular weights, such as p20 and p10. The processing sites between these parts occur at short specific tetrapeptide sequences ending in aspartate residues that dictate that the major processing enzymes are caspases themselves (166). For caspases with short prodomains, namely caspases 3, 6, and 7, this event is believed to be the primary mode of regulation. Those with long prodomains harbor protein-interaction domains that allow them to enter activating complexes for specific death pathways as described above. Caspase-8 and -10 have DEDs and caspases 1, 2, 4/11, 5, 9, 12 and 13 have CARD domains. How complex formation stimulates autoprocessing is not understood, but likely involves a stoichiometry in which multiple proenzymes come into close contact. Within such a complex, the proenzyme chains adopt a more active structure that may or may not resemble the final processed active structure. The liberated subunits form a heterotetramer of

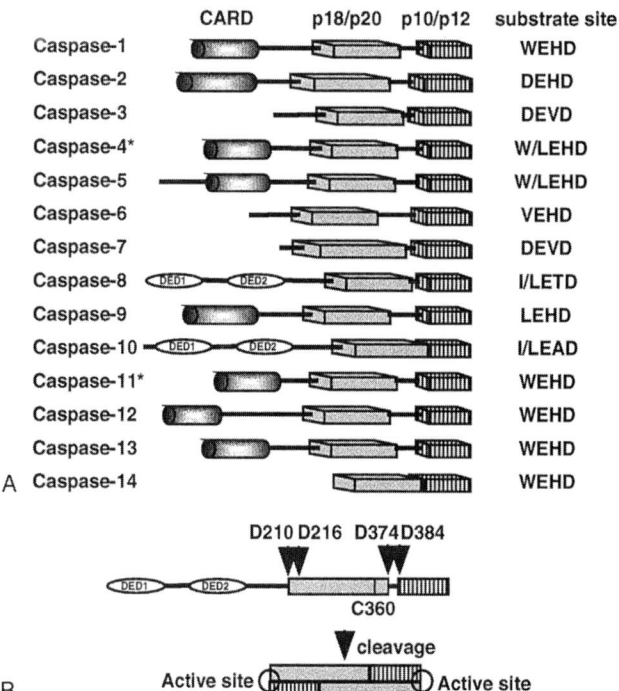

FIG. 4. Mammalian caspases. A: The structures of the 14 known mammalian caspases are shown. Many of the caspases contain at their NH2-terminal the CARD domain. Caspase-8 and caspase-10 contain a tandem copy of the DED at the NH2-terminal end of the pro-enzyme, which is essential for recruitment to the DISC. The large (p18/p20) and small (p10/p12) subunits near the COOH-terminals are also shown. The optimal tetrapeptide substrate specificity of each caspase is shown on the right hand column. Note that the caspase-4 and caspase-11 are human and mouse homologs, respectively (*asterisks*). B: Autoproteolytic cleavage of pro-caspases is crucial in activating the enzyme. Shown in the diagram by the *arrows* are the proteolytic cleavage sites of caspase-8 at aspartate residues 210, 216, 374, and 384, as well as the active site cysteine (C360) indicated by a *bar*. Two of each of the large and small subunits of the enzyme form the active enzyme in a head to tail conformation, resulting in a tetramer that contains two catalytic sites at the two ends of the molecule. The active sites of the enzyme, which are made up of residues from both the large and small subunits, are designated by the *circles* at the ends of the processed enzyme.

two large and two small enzyme subunits as reflected in the crystal structures of processed caspases (167–171). The consequences of subunit cleavage are dramatic—there is a 180° shift of the NH2 terminus of the small subunit to bring it into apposition with the catalytic cleft (172). To begin autoprocessing, an active intermediate pseudoconformation could be stabilized by internal hydrophobic interactions or by the action of chaperones. In the case of caspase zymogens recruited to a trimeric DR complex, an enzyme pseudostructure formed by two precursors could process a third proenzyme molecule. Subsequent subunit rearrangements could then lead to processing of additional unprocessed chains. Once a processed heterotetramer is formed, it will be thermodynamically stable and move out of the activating complex since it will be cleaved from the prodomain. If the stoichiometry of the activating complexes requires three proenzymes, this would match the symmetry of DRs (see below). Proteolytic activation is regulated by a variety of proteins. These inhibitors interact with the fully formed enzyme and remain bound as competitive inhibitors. Examples of such inhibitors are the CrmA protein, its homologs found in other viruses, and the IAP proteins (163,173). Other viral proteins that harbor DEDs can enter the DR-signaling complexes and inhibit cleavage of caspase-8 and -10 (174,175). Initially, it was thought that these inhibitors, termed v-FLIPs for viral FLICE (caspase-8) inhibitory proteins, inhibit apoptosis by competing with caspase-8 and -10 for entry into the DR complex. However, it is now clear that both proteins enter the complex together and the presence of v-FLIP in the complex prevents caspase autoactivation (T. Garvey and J. Cohen, *personal communication,* 2002). c-FLIP is structurally homologous to caspase-8 and -10 (indeed, it is encoded in the same locus on human chromosome 2 as these caspases), but has multiple mutations in the caspase domain that inactivate its protease function (92). It can also enter the Fas-signaling complexes and prevent caspase activation. However, this molecule can also induce apoptosis under certain conditions. The ability of antigen-receptor stimulation to block Fas-induced death is regulated in part by c-FLIP (94).

Another class of caspase regulators is the cellular IAPs (c-IAPs) that can directly inactivate mature caspases to avert the deleterious effects of inadvertent caspase activation (95,96). IAPs are characterized by the presence of up to three baculovirus IAP repeats (BIRs). Originally identified in baculoviruses, the BIR domains are characterized by the presence of cysteine and histidine residues in defined spacing arrangements ($Cx_2Cx_6Wx_3Dx_5Hx_6C$) (for review, see Deveraux and Reed [95]). The mechanisms of inhibition of IAPs on different caspases are quite distinct. For caspase-9, inhibition by XIAP depends on binding of the BIR3 domain with the tetrapeptide sequence ATPF at the NH_2-terminal of the p12 subunit that is exposed only in the mature enzyme. Hence, XIAP specifically inhibits active caspase-9, but not pro–caspase-9 (147). By contrast, XIAP inhibits caspase-7 and -3 by forming contacts in the catalytic groove with little involvement of the BIR domains (172). Interestingly, this mechanism of XIAP association is adopted by Smac/Diablo to inhibit the anti-apoptotic function of XIAP during the onset of mitochondrial PCD pathways (146). Smac/Diablo is a protein that resides in the intermembrane space of the mitochondria. It functions as an elongated dimer of α helices that adopts the shape of an arch. The NH_2-terminal sequences AVPI, generated from cleavage of the mitochondria-targeting sequence, are not well organized in the crystal structure. Nevertheless, they are critical for the inhibitory function of the protein as mutation of alanine to methionine abolished the inhibitory activity of Smac/Diablo on XIAP (146,147). The action of XIAP is flexible in order to carry out diverse functions.

Instead of the BIR3 domain, XIAP uses the linker region between BIR1 and BIR2 to interact with and inhibit the function of caspase-3 and caspase-7. In this case, the linker inserts into the catalytic groove of the caspase in reverse orientation to that of the tetrapeptide inhibitor DEVD-CHO. While BIR2 does not directly participate in the inhibitory activity, it may contribute to the stability of the association by making other contacts with caspase-3 (167,170,176).

The death-inducing effect of caspases is highly specific in that most proteins in the dying cell remain uncleaved. Lethality is therefore due to cleavage of a limited set of target substrates. Caspases have an absolute requirement for aspartate at the amino side of its cleavage sites (P1 site). Further specificity is dictated in part by the three amino acids preceding the obligatory aspartate in the substrate (P1–P4 positions) (166). Preferred tetrapeptides have been identified for each of the mammalian caspases so that, for example, caspase-3 is known to preferentially cleave at the sequence DEVD whereas caspase-8 prefers IETD (12,177,178). Nicholson and Thornberry (12) and Earnshaw et al. (166) have developed valuable tetrapeptide substrates and inhibitors based on these preferences, but they point out that in practice, these are not absolutely specific. In addition to primary amino-acid sequence, additional secondary structural features of target proteins may be recognized. For example, many proteins harboring a DVED sequence may not be cleaved at that sequence by caspase-3 (179). Thus, the tetrapeptide recognition sequences are required but not sufficient for apoptotic protein cleavage. Nevertheless, model caspase substrates and inhibitors based on short recognition peptides, such as zVAD- or DVED-fmk (fluoromethyl ketone), have been useful in assessing caspase function *in vitro* and *in vivo.*

Proteins known to be cleaved by caspases in the dying cells have been grouped according to apparent functional importance: (a) cytoskeletal proteins such as actin, gelsolin, α-fodrin, among others; (b) nuclear structure proteins, especially lamins A and B; (c) DNA metabolism and repair proteins such as PARP; (d) protein kinases such as various isoforms of PKC; and (e) signal transduction proteins such as STAT1, SREBP-1, and phospholipase C-γ1. More extensive discussions of identified caspase substrates have been published (166). A key point is that since PCD typically involves the elimination of somatic cells, there may be little evolutionary constraint on random cleavage sites. Hence, it has been difficult to distinguish functional versus adventitious sites. Key caspase substrates that have unequivocal roles in apoptosis include caspases themselves, Bcl-2 and Bcl-X_L, the ICAD inhibitor (inhibitor of caspase-activated deoxyribonuclease) of the DNase CAD, which is one enzyme causing apoptotic nuclear fragmentation, and the nuclear lamins (180,181). Cleavage of the nuclear lamins was shown by White (182) to be responsible for certain nuclear changes in apoptosis by experiments in which the aspartate cleavage sites were modified and the apoptotic changes were abrogated. This stringent test has been applied to very few proteins cleaved during apoptosis. In fact, evidence weighs against the role of many caspase substrates in apoptosis. The knockout of the PARP gene in mice revealed no abnormality of development, immunity, or apoptosis (183). Hence, further work is necessary to determine the importance of proteins cleaved during apoptosis.

Genetic analyses of human caspases have provided important information about their function. By contrast, homozygous deficiencies in mice have been associated with embryonic lethality or neurologic defects but have not yielded specific immunologic phenotypes (166). Inherited mutations of two caspases in humans cause prominent effects in the immune system. The first, an inherited mutation in caspase-10, was detected in the human disease ALPS, type II (119). Individuals with caspase-10 mutations exhibited defects in apoptosis triggered by multiple DRs affecting the homeostasis of T cells, B cells and DCs. The abnormal accumulation of immune cells leads to the formation of a variety of autoantibodies that cause autoimmune conditions including hemolytic anemia, thrombocytopenia, and others. Recently, individuals harboring mutations in caspase-8 have been identified (183a). These individuals also exhibit abnormal lymphocyte apoptosis and the accumulation of lymphocytes in secondary lymphoid tissues. However, unlike a caspase-10 mutant individual, the lack of caspase-8 does not lead to autoimmunity. Rather, the affected individuals exhibit immunodeficiency manifested as recurrent viral infections. This appears to be due to a deficiency in T- and B-lymphocyte activation as a consequence of the caspase-8 defect. The precise molecular mechanism by which caspase-8 plays a role of lymphocyte activation has not been determined. Nevertheless, these patients represent a novel clinical entity. Tentatively, the caspase-10 mutant individuals have been classified as ALPS, type IIa, and the caspase-8 mutant individuals as ALPS, type IIb.

TNF-Receptor Superfamily Members

The TNF-receptor superfamily constitutes a major class of cellular sensors to external physiologic cues that regulate PCD (184) (Fig. 5). The hallmark of these cell-surface receptors is the presence of the "cysteine-rich domains" (CRDs) in the extracellular region. Each receptor can contain between one (BCMA and TWEAK-R) (185,186) to six (CD30) CRDs. They can be further subdivided into two classes based on sequence homology within the cytoplasmic signaling domain. The DRs contain an 80-residue long DD that is essential for death signaling (134,187). The majority of the receptors, however, lack a DD but rather have a region that interacts with the TRAF (TNF-receptor–associated factors) proteins (188). Interestingly, some of the DRs, including TNFR-1, can indirectly recruit TRAF proteins and this may explain why there seems to be cross talk between certain DD-containing and DD-lacking receptors (189–191). In general, however, signals transduced by the non–DD-containing receptors are usually pro-survival, while that of the DRs are typically viewed as pro-apoptotic. In all, over 20 members of the TNF receptor

family in humans have been identified (57). With a few exceptions (EDAR and XEDAR), essentially all TNFRs play important regulatory roles in the immune system.

Signaling by the TNFRs is initiated when the trimeric ligand contacts the preformed receptor complex (reviewed in Chan et al. [192] and Siegel et al. [193]). Downstream signaling of DRs requires the recruitment of DD-containing and/or DED-containing proteins. For Fas, receptor engagement results in rapid recruitment of FADD and caspases-8 or -10 within the DISC as detailed above (133). Other DRs such as TNFR-1 may require recruitment of an additional adaptor molecule such as TRADD prior to the docking of FADD (194). These events eventually culminate in caspase activation. The non–DD-containing receptors mediate NFκB induction and the activation of c-Jun kinases through the recruitment of TRAF proteins, a property that is shared by some DRs such as TNFR-1. Recruitment of TRAF proteins by DRs may counter the pro-apoptotic response through their interactions with c-IAPs. "Knockout" analyses in mice reveal that many of these signaling intermediates, including TRAF2 (195), RIP (161), and components of the NFκB activation pathway (196–200), are essential for conferring protection against DR ligands. Deficiency of NFκB tends to sensitize cells to TNF-induced death (201–203). Both TRAF2 and NFκB induction through RIP may act in concert to promote survival in response to TNF (204). Interestingly, unlike the TNFR-1 and Fas-deficient mice, which are viable, knockout of the signaling components often results in embryonic lethality. The discordant results in knockout animals imply that TNFR signaling intermediates are involved in ontogenetic processes other than PCD. Alternatively, other TNFRs may mediate critical PCD events during development using the same set of signaling molecules. However, many other TNFRs-deficient animals, including Fas DR6 and multi-deficient animals (TNFR1$^{-/-}$, TNFR2$^{-/-}$, and Fas$^{lpr/lpr}$ together) are viable, thus arguing against the latter hypothesis (139,140,205).

Bcl-2 Gene Family

Bcl-2 and Bcl-X$_L$ are the prototypes of a diverse family of apoptosis-regulatory proteins whose filial relationships are conferred by four impressively short homology regions, termed BH-1 to BH-4 (Fig. 6) (52,206). Proteins in this family are classified as pro-apoptotic or anti-apoptotic by their effect principally on the mitochondrial death pathway. Bcl-2 was identified at the chromosomal breakpoint of t(14;18)-bearing, follicular B-cell lymphomas. Cleary et al. (117) and Raffeld et al. (207) demonstrated that the oncogenic effect of Bcl-2 could be attributed to enhanced cell survival rather than proliferation. Consequently, Bcl-2 represented a new class of death-preventing oncogenes that collaborates with growth-promoting oncogenes, such as Myc (208). It is not uncommon to find abnormal overexpression of Bcl-2 in lymphoid and nonlymphoid malignancies. Bcl-2 and Bcl-X$_L$ regulate various types of immune cell death caused by lymphokine

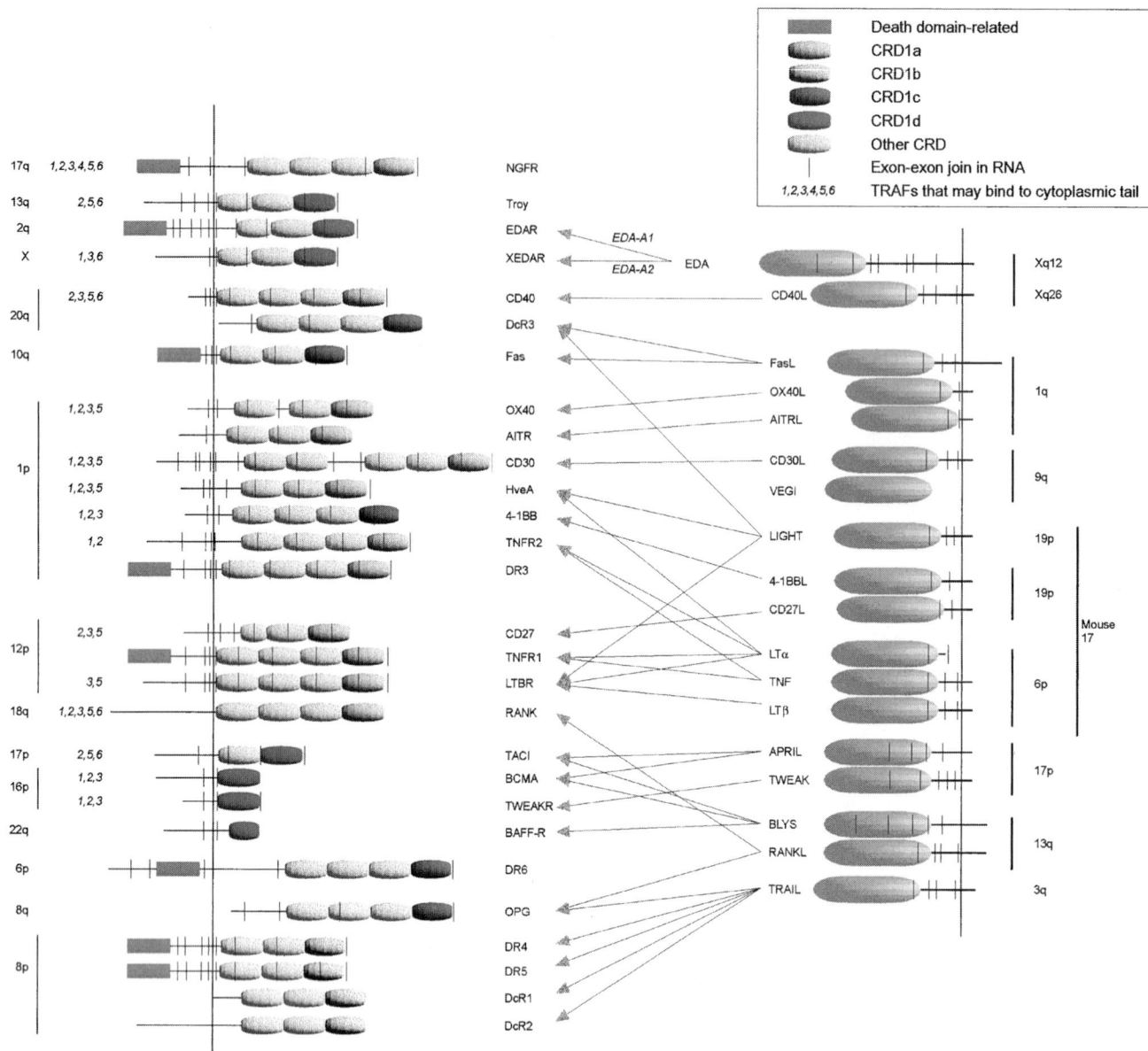

FIG. 5. Interacting proteins of the TNF/TNFR superfamily. TNFR- (**left**) and TNF-related (**right**) proteins, with *arrows* connecting ligand–receptor pairs. Cysteine-rich domains (CRDs) are shown as small ovals. The NH$_2$-terminal CRDs (CRD1a,1b,1c,1d) are grouped on the basis of sequence similarity as indicated by the use of different shades in the figure. Small vertical lines denote the locations of intron excision sites from the RNAs that encode the proteins (this information was not available for RANK, DcR1, and DcR2). *Red* boxes mark the locations of DD-related sequences in the cytoplasmic regions of the TNFR-related proteins. *Numbers* to the immediate left of the TNFR cytoplasmic regions denote known or inferred interactions with the indicated TRAFs. The locations of the human genes that encode the proteins are provided at the extreme left and right of the figure; the mouse cluster on chromosome 17 is also noted. Adapted from Locksley et al. (57), with permission.

withdrawal, γ-irradiation, and chemical death inducers such as glucocorticoids, phorbol esters, DNA-damaging agents, and ionomycin—all of which induce mitochondrial apoptosis (reviewed in Gross et al. [209]). Apoptosis induction is one means by which cancer chemotherapeutics exert an antitumor effect. Thus, since apoptosis antagonism may be as important in transformation as mitogenesis, new therapeutic

strategies aimed at antagonizing Bcl-2 may be effective in cancer therapy.

How Bcl-2 family proteins regulate cell death remains unsolved but several regulatory principles have been delineated (52). Key family members, including Bcl-2, Bcl-X$_L$, and Bax, associate with intracellular membranes, especially the OMM, via a COOH-terminal hydrophobic domain (210–213). Death

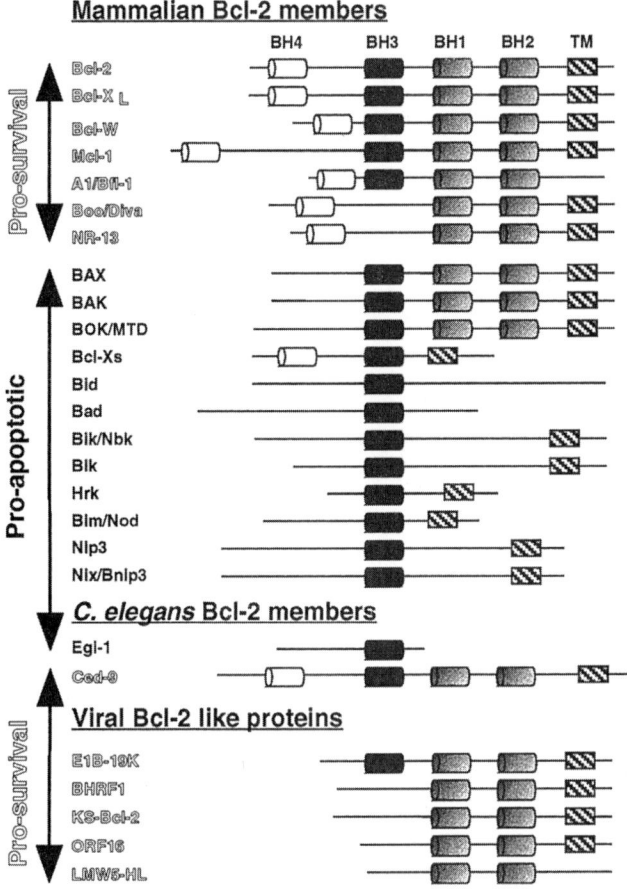

Mammalian Bcl-2 members

Pro-survival

Bcl-2
Bcl-X L
Bcl-W
Mcl-1
A1/Bfl-1
Boo/Diva
NR-13

Pro-apoptotic

BAX
BAK
BOK/MTD
Bcl-Xs
Bid
Bad
Blk/Nbk
Blk
Hrk
Bim/Nod
Nip3
Nix/Bnip3

C. elegans Bcl-2 members

Egl-1
Ced-9

Viral Bcl-2 like proteins

Pro-survival

E1B-19K
BHRF1
KS-Bcl-2
ORF16
LMW5-HL

FIG. 6. Schematic diagram of members of the Bcl-2 family. The cylinders represent the different Bcl-2 homology (BH) domains and the stippled boxes designate the hydrophobic transmembrane (TM) region that is required for insertion into the mitochondrial membrane.

regulation by the Bcl-2 family involves controlling the permeability and integrity of the OMM. Structural features suggest that Bcl-X$_L$ may form pores or channels in membranes, which could play a role in this process (214). Homotypic and heterotypic dimer complexes form between Bcl-2 family members and the balance between pro- and anti-apoptotic members determines cell fate probably through direct interactions with each other (215–219). The precise stoichiometry of these associations that lead to survival or death have not been defined. Regulation by these proteins appears to be "upstream" of caspase activation, but they may also govern a caspase-independent form of cell death (152). These proteins have their most important effects on mitochondrial death pathways and comparatively less effect on DR-initiated pathways. In particular, the pro-apoptotic family members such as Bax and Bak can cause mitochondrial release of cytochrome c and activation of cytosolic caspases (220). Diverse pathways, such as the transcriptional induction of Bcl-X$_L$ or phosphorylation of Bad, control the presence and biological activity of Bcl-2 family members (88,221).

Each of these principles has reported exceptions, but they constitute the current basis for our understanding of the Bcl-2 family of proteins.

The biological function of Bcl-2 family members has been examined in genetically engineered mice and tissue culture cells (for a review, see Chao and Korsmeyer [52]). Bcl-X$_L$-deficient mice die around embryonic day 13 due to massive neuronal apoptosis (222). By contrast, Bcl-2–deficient mice survive a few weeks postnatally but then develop polycystic kidney disease, hypopigmentation due to decreased melanocyte survival and, most importantly, massive apoptotic loss of all B- and T-lymphocytes (223). Thus, while Bcl-2 is not necessary for lymphocyte maturation, it is indispensable for the maintenance of mature lymphocytes. On the other hand, expression of Bcl-X$_L$ is required for the survival of DP (CD4$^+$CD8$^+$) thymocytes, B220$^+$ bone marrow cells, and mature B cells (52). Transgenic experiments in which Bcl-2 or Bcl-X$_L$ were overexpressed suggest, however, that the two proteins can functionally substitute for one another to some degree and may govern a final common death pathway (52). Selective transgenic overexpression of Bcl-2 in B or T cells leads to increased numbers of those cells and the late onset of lymphomas (224,225). Deficiency of the pro-apoptotic Bax protein has a surprisingly mild phenotype in mice, causing only abnormalities in testis development and sterility (226). Deficiency of the pro-apoptotic Bak protein also causes very little effect in mice; however, a combined deficiency of Bax and Bak causes multiple organ abnormalities due to failed apoptosis and perinatal death (227). This includes an accumulation of lymphocytes and other hematopoietic cells underscoring the importance of the Bax and Bak proteins for normal immune homeostasis.

Recent work has focused on the BH-3–only subset (Fig. 6). Structural analysis has revealed that a hydrophobic pocket is formed by the confluence of the BH-1, BH-2, and BH-3 helices through which Bcl-2 family members interact. The interactions among Bcl-2 family members have a characteristic selectivity and hierarchy that may depend principally on binding to the BH-3 helix (228). The BH-3–only proteins may access the other family members through interactions at the hydrophobic pocket. The BH-3–only subset includes Bid, Bad, Blk, Bim, and perhaps others since the BH-3 motif is only a 9- to 16–amino acid stretch of alpha helix. The activity of BH-3–only proteins is governed transcriptionally and post-transcriptionally in a highly regulated fashion according to their function. Bid is cleaved by caspase-8, myristoylated, and inserts itself into the mitochondrion, thereby connecting DR stimuli to the mitochondrial pathway of death (128,129,229,230). Following cleavage, a 15-kDa fragment inserts into mitochondrial membrane and triggers the oligomerization of Bax and Bak causing the release of cytochrome c and caspase activation (220,231). Phosphorylation of Bad and Bim can control their association with 14-3-3 proteins or the microtubule-associated dynein motor complex, respectively (88). When released,

Bad and Bim can induce apoptosis through the mitochondrial pathway. Genetic deficiency of Bim protects against a variety of death inducers, such as cytokine deprivation, gamma radiation, glucocorticoids, ionomycin, DNA, etoposide, and Taxol, but not FasL (48). Bim deficiency also significantly impairs TCR-induced thymocyte selection. These diverse forms of regulation allow a variety of different apoptosis inducers to converge on the mitochondrial pathway of death.

Apaf Proteins

Mammalian Apaf-1 constitutes another class of proteins that is critical for the mitochondrial pathway of apoptosis. Apaf-1 is structurally and functionally homologous to the *C. elegans* Ced-4 protein (232). Both Apaf-1 and Ced-4 contain an NH2-terminal CARD domain followed by a nucleotide-binding oligomerization domain (NOD). Ced-4 can complex with caspase-9 via the CARD domains present in both molecules. The NOD domain is essential for binding ATP and homo-oligomerization. In addition, Apaf-1 also contains WD-40 repeats at the COOH-terminal that bind cytochrome c released from damaged mitochondria. Interestingly, *C. elegans* Ced-4 contains no COOH-terminal WD-40 repeats and is not known for responding to mitochondrial insults (233). Apaf-1, cytochrome c and ATP are required to properly activate pro–caspase-9 (142,234). Genetic evidence from knockout animals revealed that Apaf-1 and caspase-9 are obligatory components of cellular response to DNA damage-induced apoptosis through p53 and other mitochondrial death events (235–237).

Other proteins with homology to Apaf-1/Ced-4 have been identified, most of which contain regions of homology to the NOD domain. One of these proteins, NOD2, has been mapped as a susceptibility gene for Crohn's disease (238,239). Human patients with NOD2 mutations have defects in NFκB induction in response to bacterial antigens. Since NOD2 also contains a CARD domain, this molecule may be involved in apoptosis as well as inflammatory responses. Many members of the TNFR superfamily such as TNFR-1 and Fas have divergent effects (such as cellular activation versus apoptosis) that are apparent at different times and depend on the context of the immune response. Hence, combinations of protein interaction motifs like the CARD, NOD, and other signaling domains in single adaptor proteins may allow bifurcation of biological responses from the same receptor.

STRUCTURAL REGULATION OF PCD

TNF/TNFR Structure

The recent determination of structures of components of the PCD pathways has led to a better physical sense of how these death programs work (Fig. 7). In almost all cases, the formation of specific stoichiometric protein complexes is crucial for apoptosis signaling. Receptor-mediated apoptosis involves

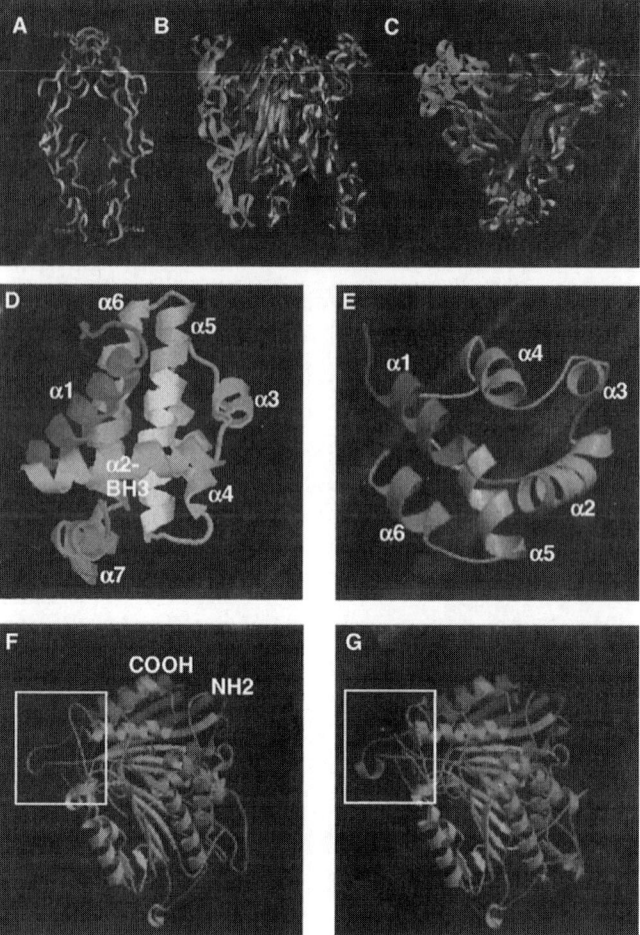

FIG. 7. Structural biology of apoptosis. A: Structure of the unliganded TNFR-1. B Side view of the TNFβ-bound TNFR-1 looking from plane of the membrane. Conserved disulfide bonds that are structurally essential are shown in *red*. C: Bird's eye view of the TNF/TNFR-1 structure looking down at the plane of the membrane. D: NMR structure of Bcl-XL. The BH3 (α2) domain runs perpendicularly across the molecule and the two central hydrophobic helices (α5 and α6) are buried in the middle portion of the molecule. E: Structure of the Fas DD, a prototypical hexahelical bundle. The bundle is composed of six helices, a structural scaffold that is conserved in also the DED and the CARD domain. The position of each of the helices is indicated. F: Structure of caspase-7 before proteolytic autoprocessing. G: Structure of caspase-7 after proteolytic autoprocessing. Note that the catalytic site (box) in the pro-enzyme is relatively "loose" (F). Processing of the pro-enzyme results in substantial "tightening" of the catalytic loops. The red-colored strand inside the boxed area in (G) denotes the position of the pseudosubstrate tetrapeptide DEVD.

DRs within the TNFR superfamily triggered by receptor-specific ligands within the TNF superfamily (57). The defining structural motif of the TNFR superfamily is the cysteine-rich pseudorepeat or the cysteine-rich domain (CRD). The CRD is a 40–amino-acid cluster of β strands folded back on themselves and pinned in place by three disulfide bonds formed by six cysteines in highly conserved positions

(Fig. 7A). Most of the TNFRs have multiple CRDs in the extracellular domain and these serve two primary functions. The membrane-proximal or central CRDs mediate ligand binding. For example, in TNFR-1, the two central CRDs, CRD2 and 3, provide the key ligand-binding contacts. The membrane distal CRD mediates receptor pre-assembly on the cell surface (240,241). This membrane distal CRD along with adjacent NH$_2$-terminal sequences is called the "pre-ligand assembly domain" or PLAD because it promotes the oligomerization of like receptor chains prior to ligand engagement. Pre-assembly of receptor chains into trimers or perhaps other oligomeric complexes is obligatory for both ligand binding and signal transduction. The PLAD has been identified in both TNFR superfamily members that mediate apoptosis such as Fas, TNFR-1, and TRAIL receptors as well as those that do not, such as TNFR-2 (240,241). The orientation of the receptor chains is likely to change drastically between the unliganded and liganded complexes as reflected in the extant crystal structures for unliganded and liganded TNFR-1 (see Fig. 7A and B). The receptor chains are initially attached at the membrane distal CRD and then these interactions fall apart as the receptor admits the ligand between three receptor chains to interact with the CRDs closer to the membrane. The discovery of the PLAD overturned the prevailing model that TNFR family members signal by the ligand "cross-linking" solitary receptor chains into a trimeric complex and replaced it with a model by which the ligand binds to and changes the configuration of pre-assembled receptor complexes. Hence, CRDs can regulate both intra- or inter-molecular associations critical to receptor function.

The ligands for TNFRs are typically obligate homotrimers that adopt a compact "jelly-roll" conformation with a hydrophobic face where the individual subunits stably interact with each other (57,242). Certain exceptions, such as Ltα and LTβ, can form heterotrimers. The ligand subunits are usually synthesized as type II transmembrane proteins and, following trimerization, may remain membrane bound or undergo metalloproteinase cleavage to a soluble form (243). Binding of the pre-assembled receptor complex with the trimeric ligand forms a symmetric 3:3 ligand-receptor complex that is evident in the crystal structures of the liganded TNFR1 and TRAIL receptors (244–248). Functionally, the ligand interaction appears to re-orient the receptor chains so that the intracellular domains adopt a specific juxtaposition that favors the binding of appropriate intracellular signaling proteins. The recently solved structure of the TRAIL trimer differs from the TNF structure in that it contains a loop insertion in the first β-strand that is critical for receptor association (245–248). In both the TNFR-1 and TRAIL-R2 crystals, ligand contacts appear to be restricted to the second and third CRDs. The extensive receptor–receptor interaction in the PLAD region found in the unliganded TNFR-1 receptor structure is absent in the ligand-bound receptor crystal structures (249–252). How the ligand initially contacts the preformed receptor complex and initiates chain rearrangement are important unresolved questions.

The fundamental three-fold symmetry of the ligands and receptors in the TNFR system is also conserved among the proximal signaling complexes. This includes the receptor–TRAF2 interaction (253,254), TRADD–TRAF2 interaction (255,256), and Fas–FADD interaction. The importance of the tri-fold symmetry in the receptor and signaling apparatus is highlighted by genetic mutations found in both human and mouse. For instance, heterozygous mutations in the cytoplasmic DD of Fas found in the lpr^{cg} (mouse) or Fas-defective form of ALPS resulted in a greater than 50% reduction in receptor signaling (257–259). This is likely due to the fact that inclusion of at least one bad subunit in the receptor trimer prevents the formation of a 3:3 Fas:FADD complex and thereby abrogates signaling (259).

The genetic effect by which a mutant allele encodes a protein that interferes with the protein encoded by the wild-type allele is called "dominant interference." Dominant interference is usually observed in proteins that carry out their function by forming oligomeric complexes, which is a common feature in PCD pathways. In the case of the trimeric Fas receptor, dominant interference was potent due to the fact that with equal expression of a wild-type and mutant allele, $(1/2)^3$ or 1/8 would be expected to have solely wild-type subunits and 7/8 of the complexes would have at least one bad subunit since the receptor chains randomly assort (257–259). To generalize, a dominant-interfering disease mechanism may be especially important in PCD disorders in outbred human populations, where most gene loci are heterozygous rather than homozygous. Thus, these studies of the Fas receptor have revealed that while higher-order symmetric signaling complexes may provide rapid and selective signaling in immune regulation, they also create a vulnerability to genetic disease.

Bcl-2 Homology Structures

Bcl-X$_L$ has the best-characterized structure and it has provided interesting hypotheses regarding the function of Bcl-2 family members (214). It contains a conserved nest of alpha helices including a backbone of two hydrophobic helices that are encircled by several amphipathic helices including the BH4 helix, which is a key interaction site for members of the Bcl-2 family (Fig. 7D). The structure has revealed a tantalizing similarity to pore-forming domains of bacterial toxins. This has stimulated a wealth of research into whether membrane pore formation is a key element of apoptosis modulation by Bcl-2 family proteins (260,261). It is interesting to consider that pore-forming toxins of bacteria have homology to regulatory proteins whose primary site of action is the mitochondria that is believed to have evolved as a bacteria-like organism subsumed into eukaryotic cells. The structure also reveals that the Bcl-2 homology regions—BH1, BH2, and BH3—that are widely spaced in the primary sequence are assembled closely together in a hydrophobic pocket. Through this pocket, the pro-apoptotic and anti-apoptotic members of the Bcl-2 family interact and cross-regulate one another.

Proteins with an amphipathic BH3 helix only can also interact with this pocket in the anti-apoptotic Bcl-2 family members and potentially nullify their protective function (214). The specific amino acids contained in this pocket confer a specific hierarchy of interactions between various members of the Bcl-2 family. Hence, the structure reveals a possible functional interaction with the mitochondrial membrane and functional associations between members of the Bcl-2 family that determine survival or death.

The Hexahelical Bundle

The DD, DED, and CARD domains are critical protein–protein interaction motifs in DR-mediated PCD. Interestingly, all three domains adopt a similar structural scaffold of a compact bundle of six antiparallel α-helices, which we will refer to as the "hexahelical bundle" (Fig. 7E). This structure is an ancient one that is related to the "ankyrin repeat," a protein interaction motif that is found in many proteins and conserved throughout phylogeny (57,214). Despite remarkable overall similarity, significant differences exist among the DD, DED, and CARD that likely account for their binding specificities. For example, while the surface of Fas DD is made up of mostly charged residues (262), that of FADD DED contains hydrophobic patches that are important for binding to caspase-8 (263). The six helices in the CARD domain of RAIDD form an acidic surface on one side of the molecule and a basic region on the other side of the molecule, which may be important for binding of the corresponding CARD domain in caspase-2 (264). Structural and mutagenesis data corroborate with the notion that helices 2 and 3 are critical contact regions for homophilic DD and DED interactions. In addition to the participation of $\alpha2$ and $\alpha3$, homophilic CARD–CARD interactions appears to involve electric dipole interactions between $\alpha2$, $\alpha3$, $\alpha5$ on one molecule and $\alpha1$, $\alpha4$ on the partner. Examination of the CARD domain from Apaf-1 yielded similar findings (265,266). Thus, specific molecular pathways are determined by defining residues in DD, DED, or CARDs that are presented by a common scaffold shared by all three. It is also important to recognize that DDs, DEDs, and CARDs are primarily protein–protein interaction domains, and that although they were initially discovered in apoptosis pathways, homologs of these motifs may be put to use by nature to associate proteins in pathways unrelated to apoptosis. In fact, a class of proteins containing the pyrin domain appears to adopt a similar structural scaffold to that found in the DDs, DEDs and CARDs (267–269). The pyrin domain was originally identified in a protein mutated in patients with familial Mediterranean fever, thus providing a tantalizing link between apoptosis and inflammatory diseases.

Caspase Structure

The recruitment of DD-, DED-, or CARD-containing proteins eventually leads to the recruitment and activation of caspases. The structures of caspase-1, -3, -7, -8, and -9 have been determined (146,167–172,176). The catalytic subunits of all caspases are similarly comprised of two p10/p20 heterodimers. Each p10/p20 heterodimer is folded into a compact cylindrical structure of six β strands and five α helices. The active site of the enzyme is formed by loops that come together at the top of the cylinder of β strands, which are contributed by both the p10 and p20 subunits. The two heterodimers are aligned in an antiparallel fashion where the β sheet forms the vertical axis of the tetrameric complex (Fig. 4 and Fig. 7F and G). Despite the overall structural similarity, distinct differences, especially in loops surrounding the catalytic active site, can be identified among the different caspases, which explain their respective substrate preferences.

Regulation of caspases by viral inhibitors has also been elucidated by structural studies. The baculovirus p35 is a potent inhibitor of many caspases that requires cleavage at its caspase recognition site D87 to manifest its inhibitory activity. Crystallographic studies reveal the formation of a thioester bond between the active site cysteine of caspase-8 (C360) and the aspartate of the amino-terminal cleavage product of p35 (D87). The thioester bond is shielded from hydrolysis through steric effects of the NH_2-terminal residues of p35 and is critical for the long-lasting inhibitory effect (270).

PCD as Immune Therapy

Because of its exquisite antigen specificity, the possibility of using antigen-induced death, particularly of T-lymphocytes, for the treatment of immunologic diseases has been suggested (271,272). In particular, the T-cell components of graft rejection, autoimmune diseases, and allergic reactions may be suppressed by antigen-induced cell elimination. This concept has been tested in both mice and monkeys with clearly beneficial effects on disease outcome. For example, it was found that the repetitive administration of a myelin basic-protein antigen could suppress experimental allergic encephalomyelitis by causing the elimination of disease-causing T cells in mice (77). This suggests that antigen-specific therapy is achievable if antigens relevant to the disease process are sufficiently well defined and that death of the culpable T cells can be triggered without exacerbation of symptoms (273). Studies are underway to evaluate the feasibility of this approach in human clinical trials.

PCD and Development of Lymphoid Malignancy

In this last section, we return to the question of why the mature immune system assiduously eliminates lymphocytes that have been activated by antigen and therefore have proven usefulness. Why can't the immune system adopt a laissez-faire economy of previously activated cells, which might have great value if the same pathogen is re-encountered? Several lines of evidence strongly suggest that in addition to potential loss of tolerance and autoimmunity, lymphoid malignancy is also promoted by defective apoptosis. Hence, the accumulation of excessive cells that have a propensity to proliferate and can undergo additional genetic changes may be deleterious to the organism. The association of translocations of the Bcl-2 gene with diffuse large-cell lymphoma suggested that somatic aberrations in apoptosis pathways might be important steps in the transformation process. Since then, somatic changes in a variety of apoptosis molecules including Fas, caspases, and Bcl-2 family members have been documented (274). By contrast, the well-known inheritable apoptosis defect in p53 in the Li-Fraumeni syndrome seems to cause predominantly solid tumors but not lymphomas. However, the study of large kindreds of patients with ALPS has revealed a 15-fold greater incidence of lymphomas. It is striking also that these families have several different classes of lymphoma, suggesting that Fas provides a protection against transformation not for a single cell type but generally for B- and T-lymphocytes (275). Thus, besides autoimmune manifestations, we can infer that protection against lymphoid malignancy dictates that strict control over the accumulation of activated lymphocytes is necessary.

CONCLUSIONS

The study of PCD has provided insights into many aspects of immune function, particularly in the establishment of central and peripheral tolerance and the numerical homeostasis of immune cells. Immune cells utilize conserved mechanisms of apoptosis and necrosis that are common to perhaps all mammalian cells and have been one of the most instructive model systems for understanding how these systems function. Finally, death is regulated by cues from the environment. For developing lymphocytes, the antigen environment determines cell survival and elimination. For mature cells, antigen and the growth cytokine IL-2 determine life or death. In this manner, the immune system can develop a wide repertoire of reactive cells, select the most useful members of the repertoire, and then expand and contract specific clonotypes as needed for specific immune responses. Such homeostatic control allows rapid cell proliferation in protective responses while preserving tolerance and avoiding autoimmunity and immune cell malignancies.

ACKNOWLEDGMENTS

We are grateful to Manzoor Ahmad, Wendy Davidson, Hao Wu, Sang-Mo Kang, Nigel Killeen, David Martin, Jan Paul Medema, John Monroe, Marcus Peter, David Scott, Gavin Screaton, Richard Siegel, and Lixin Zheng for thoughtful suggestions on the manuscript.

REFERENCES

1. Conlon I, Raff M. Size control in animal development. *Cell* 1999;96:235–244.
2. Green DR, Cotter TG. Introduction: apoptosis in the immune system. *Semin Immunol* 1992;4:355–362.
3. Cohen JJ. Apoptosis: mechanisms of life and death in the immune system. *J Allergy Clin Immunol* 1999;103:548–554.
4. Zheng L, et al. Mature T lymphocyte apoptosis in the healthy and diseased immune system. *Adv Exp Med Biol* 1996;406:229–239.
5. Lenardo M, et al. Mature T lymphocyte apoptosis—immune regulation in a dynamic and unpredictable antigenic environment. *Annu Rev Immunol* 1999;17:221–253.
6. Raff M. Cell suicide for beginners. *Nature* 1998;396:119–122.
7. Boguski MS, Tolstoshev CM, Bassett DE Jr. Gene discovery in dbEST. *Science* 1994;265:1993–1994.
8. Raff MC, et al. Programmed cell death and the control of cell survival. *Philos Trans R Soc Lond B Biol Sci* 1994;345:265–268.
9. Kerr JF, Wyllie AH, Currie AR. Apoptosis: a basic biological phenomenon with wide-ranging implications in tissue kinetics. *Br J Cancer* 1972;26:239–257.
10. Wyllie AH, Kerr JF, Currie AR. Cell death: the significance of apoptosis. *Int Rev Cytol* 1980;68:251–306.
11. Clarke PG, Clarke S. Nineteenth century research on naturally occurring cell death and related phenomena. *Anat Embryol (Berl)* 1996;193:81–99.
12. Nicholson D, Thornberry N. Caspases: killer proteases. *Trends Biochem Sci* 1997;22:299–306.
13. Kennedy NJ, et al. Caspase activation is required for T cell proliferation. *J Exp Med* 1999;190:1891–1896.
14. Alam A, et al. Early activation of caspases during T lymphocyte stimulation results in selective substrate cleavage in nonapoptotic cells. *J Exp Med* 1999;190:1879–1890.
15. Reed JC, ed. *Apoptosis*. Methods in enzymology, vol. 322. New York: Academic Press, 2000.
16. Coligan JE, ed. *Current protocols in immunology*. New York: Wiley, 1991 [loose-leaf].
17. Holler N, et al. Fas triggers an alternative, caspase-8–independent cell death pathway using the kinase RIP as effector molecule. *Nat Immunol* 2000;1:489–495.
18. Thompson CB. Apoptosis. In: Paul WE, ed. *Fundamental immunology*. 4th ed. Philadelphia: Lippincott-Raven, 1999:813–829.
19. Larsson M, Fonteneau JF, Bhardwaj N. Dendritic cells resurrect antigens from dead cells. *Trends Immunol* 2001;22:141–148.
20. Basu S, et al. Necrotic but not apoptotic cell death releases heat shock proteins, which deliver a partial maturation signal to dendritic cells and activate the NF-kappa B pathway. *Int Immunol* 2000;12:1539–1546.
21. Gallucci S, Lolkema M, Matzinger P. Natural adjuvants: endogenous activators of dendritic cells. *Nat Med* 1999;5:1249–1255.
22. Metzstein MM, Horvitz HR. The *C. elegans* cell death specification gene ces-1 encodes a snail family zinc finger protein. *Mol Cell* 1999;4:309–319.
23. Lodish H, Zipursky SL, Matsudaira P, et al. *Molecular cell biology*. 4th ed. New York: W. H. Freeman, 2000.
24. Ashton-Rickardt PG, Tonegawa S. A differential-avidity model for T-cell selection. *Immunol Today* 1994;15:362–366.
25. Ashton-Rickardt PG, et al. Evidence for a differential avidity model of T cell selection in the thymus [see comments]. *Cell* 1994;76:651–663.
26. Lenardo MJ. Interleukin-2 programs mouse alpha beta T lymphocytes for apoptosis. *Nature* 1991;353:858–861.
27. Weiner NL. Cybernetics, control and communication in the animal and machine. New York: MIT Press, 1961.
28. von Boehmer H, Teh HS, Kisielow P. The thymus selects the useful, neglects the useless and destroys the harmful. *Immunol Today* 1989;10:57–61.
29. Jameson SC, Hogquist KA, Bevan MJ. Positive selection of thymocytes. *Annu Rev Immunol* 1995;13:93–126.
30. Sprent J, Kishimoto H. The thymus and central tolerance. *Philos Trans R Soc Lond B Biol Sci* 2001;356:609–616.
31. Jiang D, Zheng L, Lenardo MJ. Caspases in T cell receptor-induced thymocyte apoptosis. *Cell Death Differ* 1999;6:402–411.
32. Sprent J, et al. The thymus and T cell death. *Adv Exp Med Biol* 1996;406:191–198.
33. Berg LJ, Kang J. Molecular determinants of TCR expression and selection. *Curr Opin Immunol* 2001;13:232–241.
34. Germain RN. The T cell receptor for antigen: signaling and ligand discrimination. *J Biol Chem* 2001;276:35223–35226.

35. Page DM, et al. TNF receptor-deficient mice reveal striking differences between several models of thymocyte negative selection. *J Immunol* 1998;160:120–133.

36. Sidman CL, Marshall JD, Von Boehmer H. Transgenic T cell receptor interactions in the lymphoproliferative and autoimmune syndromes of lpr and gld mutant mice. *Eur J Immunol* 1992;22:499–504.

37. DeYoung AL, Duramad O, Winoto A. The TNF receptor family member CD30 is not essential for negative selection. *J Immunol* 2000; 165:6170–6173.

38. Conte D, et al. Thymocyte-targeted overexpression of xiap transgene disrupts T lymphoid apoptosis and maturation. *Proc Natl Acad Sci U S A* 2001;98:5049–5054.

39. Alberola-Ila J, et al. Selective requirement for MAP kinase activation in thymocyte differentiation. *Nature* 1995;373:620–623.

40. Mariathasan S, Jones RG, Ohashi PS. Signals involved in thymocyte positive and negative selection. *Semin Immunol* 1999;11:263–272.

41. Werlen G, Hausmann B, Palmer E. A motif in the alphabeta T-cell receptor controls positive selection by modulating ERK activity. *Nature* 2000;406:422–426.

42. Kruisbeek AM, Amsen D. Mechanisms underlying T-cell tolerance. *Curr Opin Immunol* 1996;8:233–244.

43. Bain G, et al. E2A deficiency leads to abnormalities in alphabeta T-cell development and to rapid development of T-cell lymphomas. *Mol Cell Biol* 1997;17:4782–4791.

44. Rivera RR, et al. Thymocyte selection is regulated by the helix-loop-helix inhibitor protein, Id3. *Immunity* 2000;12:17–26.

45. Penninger JM, et al. The interferon regulatory transcription factor IRF-1 controls positive and negative selection of CD8+ thymocytes. *Immunity* 1997;7:243–254.

46. Williams O, Brady HJ. The role of molecules that mediate apoptosis in T-cell selection. *Trends Immunol* 2001;22:107–111.

47. Huang DC, Strasser A. BH3-only proteins—essential initiators of apoptotic cell death. *Cell* 2000;103:839–842.

48. Bouillet P, et al. Proapoptotic Bcl-2 relative Bim required for certain apoptotic responses, leukocyte homeostasis, to preclude autoimmunity. *Science* 1999;286:1735–1738.

49. Tanchot C, et al. Differential requirements for survival and proliferation of CD8 naive or memory T cells. *Science* 1997;276:2057–2062.

50. Sprent J, Tough DF. T cell death and memory. *Science* 2001;293:245–248.

51. Tan JT, et al. IL-7 is critical for homeostatic proliferation and survival of naive T cells. *Proc Natl Acad Sci U S A* 2001;98:8732–8737.

52. Chao DT, Korsmeyer SJ. BCL-2 family: regulators of cell death. *Annu Rev Immunol* 1998;16:395–419.

53. Critchfield JM, Boehme SA, Lenardo MJ. The regulation of antigen-induced apoptosis in mature T lymphocytes. In: Gregory CC, ed. *Apoptosis and the immune response.* New York: Wiley-Liss, 1995:55–114.

54. Reap EA, et al. bcl-2 transgenic Lpr mice show profound enhancement of lymphadenopathy. *J Immunol* 1995;155:5455–5462.

55. Strasser A, et al. Bcl-2 and Fas/APO-1 regulate distinct pathways to lymphocyte apoptosis. *EMBO J* 1995;14:6136–6147.

56. Van Parijs L, et al. Uncoupling IL-2 signals that regulate T cell proliferation, survival, Fas-mediated activation-induced cell death. *Immunity* 1999;11:281–288.

57. Locksley RM, Killeen N, Lenardo MJ. The TNF and TNF receptor superfamilies: integrating mammalian biology. *Cell* 2001;104:487–501.

58. Nagata S, Golstein P. The Fas death factor. *Science* 1995;267:1449–1456.

59. Zheng L, et al. Induction of apoptosis in mature T cells by tumour necrosis factor. *Nature* 1995;377:348–351.

60. Watanabe-Fukunaga R, et al. The cDNA structure, expression, chromosomal assignment of the mouse Fas antigen. *J Immunol* 1992;148:1274–1279.

61. Watanabe-Fukunaga R, et al. Lymphoproliferation disorder in mice explained by defects in Fas antigen that mediates apoptosis. *Nature* 1992;356:314–317.

62. Takahashi T, et al. Generalized lymphoproliferative disease in mice, caused by a point mutation in the Fas ligand. *Cell* 1994;76:969–976.

63. Straus SE, et al. An inherited disorder of lymphocyte apoptosis: the autoimmune lymphoproliferative syndrome. *Ann Intern Med* 1999; 130:591–601.

64. Kagi D, Odermatt B, Mak TW. Homeostatic regulation of CD8+ T cells by perforin. *Eur J Immunol* 1999;29:3262–3272.

65. Kagi D, et al. Fas and perforin pathways as major mechanisms of T cell-mediated cytotoxicity. *Science* 1994;265:528–530.

66. Stepp SE, et al. Perforin gene defects in familial hemophagocytic lymphohistiocytosis. *Science* 1999;286:1957–1959.

67. Spaner D, et al. A role for perforin in activation-induced T cell death *in vivo:* increased expansion of allogeneic perforin-deficient T cells in SCID mice. *J Immunol* 1999;162:1192–1199.

68. Budd RC. Activation-induced cell death. *Curr Opin Immunol* 2001; 13:356–362.

69. Lenardo MJ. The molecular regulation of lymphocyte apoptosis. *Semin Immunol* 1997;9:1–5.

70. Zheng L, et al. T cell growth cytokines cause the superinduction of molecules mediating antigen-induced T lymphocyte death. *J Immunol* 1998;160:763–769.

71. Boehme SA, Lenardo MJ. Propriocidal apoptosis of mature T lymphocytes occurs at S phase of the cell cycle. *Eur J Immunol* 1993;23:1552–1560.

72. Li QS, et al. Activation-induced T cell death occurs at G1A phase of the cell cycle. *Eur J Immunol* 2000;30:3329–3337.

73. Lissy NA, et al. A common E2F-1 and p73 pathway mediates cell death induced by TCR activation. *Nature* 2000;407:642–645.

74. Hunig T, Schimpl A. Systemic autoimmune disease as a consequence of defective lymphocyte death. *Curr Opin Immunol* 1997;9:826–830.

75. Willerford DM, et al. Interleukin-2 receptor alpha chain regulates the size and content of the peripheral lymphoid compartment. *Immunity* 1995;3:521–530.

76. Van Parijs L, et al. Functional responses and apoptosis of CD25 (IL-2R alpha)-deficient T cells expressing a transgenic antigen receptor. *J Immunol* 1997;158:3738–3745.

77. Critchfield JM, et al. T cell deletion in high antigen dose therapy of autoimmune encephalomyelitis. *Science* 1994;263:1139–1143.

78. Moskophidis D, et al. Virus persistence in acutely infected immunocompetent mice by exhaustion of antiviral cytotoxic effector T cells. *Nature* 1993;362:758–761.

79. Rothstein TL, et al. Protection against Fas-dependent Th1-mediated apoptosis by antigen receptor engagement in B cells. *Nature* 1995; 374:163–165.

80. Wong B, Arron J, Choi Y. T cell receptor signals enhance susceptibility to Fas-mediated apoptosis. *J Exp Med* 1997;186:1939–1944.

81. Hornung F, Zheng L, Lenardo MJ, Maintenance of clonotype specificity in CD95/Apo-1/Fas-mediated apoptosis of mature T lymphocytes. *J Immunol* 1997;159:3816–3822.

82. Combadiere B, et al. Differential TCR signaling regulates apoptosis and immunopathology during antigen responses *in vivo*. *Immunity* 1998;9:305–313.

83. Nahill SR, Welsh SM. High frequency of cross-reactive cytotoxic T lymphocytes elicited during the virus-induced polyclonal cytotoxic T lymphocyte response. *J Exp Med* 1993;177:317–327.

84. Razvi ES, et al. Lymphocyte apoptosis during the silencing of the immune response to acute viral infections in normal, lpr, Bcl-2-transgenic mice. *Am J Pathol* 1995;147:79–91.

85. Duke RC, Cohen JJ. IL-2 addiction: withdrawal of growth factor activates a suicide program in dependent T cells. *Lymphokine Res* 1986;5:289–299.

86. Kuroda K, et al. Implantation of IL-2-containing osmotic pump prolongs the survival of superantigen-reactive T cells expanded in mice injected with bacterial superantigen. *J Immunol* 1996;157:1422–1431.

87. Chao DT, et al. Bcl-XL and Bcl-2 repress a common pathway of cell death. *J Exp Med* 1995;182:821–828.

88. Zha J, et al. Serine phosphorylation of death agonist BAD in response to survival factor results in binding to 14-3-3 not BCL-X(L). *Cell* 1996;87:619–628.

89. Kelly E, et al. IL-2 and related cytokines can promote T cell survival by activating AKT. *J Immunol* 2002;168:597–603.

90. Callan MF, et al. CD8(+) T-cell selection, function, death in the primary immune response *in vivo*. *J Clin Invest* 2000;106:1251–1261.

91. Opferman JT, Ober BT, Ashton-Rickardt PG. Linear differentiation of cytotoxic effectors into memory T lymphocytes. *Science* 1999;283:1745–1748.

92. Irmler M, et al. Inhibition of death receptor signals by cellular FLIP. *Nature* 1997;388:190–195.

93. Hu S, et al. I-FLICE, a novel inhibitor of tumor necrosis factor receptor-1- and CD-95-induced apoptosis. *J Biol Chem* 1997;272:17255–17257.

94. Wang J, et al. Inhibition of Fas-mediated apoptosis by the B cell antigen receptor through c-FLIP. *Eur J Immunol* 2000;30:155–163.

95. Deveraux QL, Reed JC. IAP family proteins—suppressors of apoptosis. *Genes Dev* 1999;13:239–252.

96. Roy N, et al. The c-IAP-1 and c-IAP-2 proteins are direct inhibitors of specific caspases. *EMBO J* 1997;16:6914–6925.

97. Murali-Krishna K, et al. Persistence of memory CD8 T cells in MHC class I-deficient mice. *Science* 1999;286:1377–1381.

98. Ku CC, et al. Control of homeostasis of CD8+ memory T cells by opposing cytokines. *Science* 2000;288:675–678.

99. Norvell A, Mandik L, Monroe JG. Engagement of the antigen-receptor on immature murine B lymphocytes results in death by apoptosis. *J Immunol* 1995;154:4404–4413.

100. Akashi K, et al. Bcl-2 rescues T lymphopoiesis in interleukin-7 receptor-deficient mice. *Cell* 1997;89:1033–1041.

101. Maraskovsky E, et al. Bcl-2 can rescue T lymphocyte development in interleukin-7 receptor-deficient mice but not in mutant rag-1-/- mice. *Cell* 1997;89:1011–1019.

102. Grabstein KH, et al. Inhibition of murine B and T lymphopoiesis *in vivo* by an anti-interleukin 7 monoclonal antibody. *J Exp Med* 1993;178:257–264.

103. Namen AE, et al. Stimulation of B-cell progenitors by cloned murine interleukin-7. *Nature* 1988;333:571–573.

104. Sandel PC, Monroe JG. Negative selection of immature B cells by receptor editing or deletion is determined by site of antigen encounter. *Immunity* 1999;10:289–299.

105. Wechsler-Reya RJ, Monroe JG. Lipopolysaccharide prevents apoptosis and induces responsiveness to antigen receptor cross-linking in immature B cells. *Immunology* 1996;89:356–362.

106. Hardy RR, Hayakawa K. B cell development pathways. *Annu Rev Immunol* 2001;19:595–621.

107. King LB, Norvell A, Monroe JG. Antigen receptor-induced signal transduction imbalances associated with the negative selection of immature B cells. *J Immunol* 1999;162:2655–2662.

108. Rathmell JC, et al. CD95 (Fas)-dependent elimination of self-reactive B cells upon interaction with CD4+ T cells. *Nature* 1995;376:181–184.

109. Rathmell JC, et al. Expansion or elimination of B cells *in vivo*: dual roles for CD40- and Fas (CD95)-ligands modulated by the B cell antigen receptor. *Cell* 1996;87:319–329.

110. Choi MS, et al. The role of bcl-XL in CD40-mediated rescue from anti–mu-induced apoptosis in WEHI-231 B lymphoma cells. *Eur J Immunol* 1995;25:1352–1357.

111. Rothstein TL. Inducible resistance to Fas-mediated apoptosis in B cells. *Cell Res* 2000;10:245–266.

112. Foote LC, Marshak-Rothstein A, Rothstein TL. Tolerant B lymphocytes acquire resistance to Fas-mediated apoptosis after treatment with interleukin 4 but not after treatment with specific antigen unless a surface immunoglobulin threshold is exceeded. *J Exp Med* 1998;187:847–853.

113. Graninger WB, et al. Cytokine regulation of apoptosis and Bcl-2 expression in lymphocytes of patients with systemic lupus erythematosus. *Cell Death Differ* 2000;7:966–972.

114. Ishida Y, et al. Induced expression of PD-1, a novel member of the immunoglobulin gene superfamily, upon programmed cell death. *EMBO J* 1992;11:3887–3895.

115. Devireddy LR, et al. Induction of apoptosis by a secreted lipocalin that is transcriptionally regulated by IL-3 deprivation. *Science* 2001;293:829–834.

116. Bratt T. Lipocalins and cancer. *Biochim Biophys Acta* 2000;1482:318–326.

117. Cleary ML, Smith SD, Sklar J. Cloning and structural analysis of cDNAs for bcl-2 and a hybrid bcl-2/immunoglobulin transcript resulting from the t(14;18) translocation. *Cell* 1986;47:19–28.

118. Ingulli E, et al. In vivo detection of dendritic cell antigen presentation to CD4(+) T cells. *J Exp Med* 1997;185:2133–2141.

119. Wang J, et al. Inherited human Caspase 10 mutations underlie defective lymphocyte and dendritic cell apoptosis in autoimmune lymphoproliferative syndrome type II. *Cell* 1999;98:47–58.

120. Martin SJ, et al. The cytotoxic cell protease granzyme B initiates apoptosis in a cell-free system by proteolytic processing and activation of the ICE/CED-3 family protease, CPP32, via a novel two-step mechanism. *EMBO J* 1996;15:2407–2416.

121. Harvey NL, et al. Processing of the Nedd2 precursor by ICE-like proteases and granzyme B. *Genes Cells* 1996;1:673–685.

122. Zapata JM, et al. Granzyme release and caspase activation in activated human T-lymphocytes. *J Biol Chem* 1998;273:6916–6920.

123. Atkinson EA, et al. Cytotoxic T lymphocyte-assisted suicide. Caspase 3 activation is primarily the result of the direct action of granzyme B. *J Biol Chem* 1998;273:21261–21266.

124. Yang X, et al. Granzyme B mimics apical caspases. Description of a unified pathway for trans-activation of executioner caspase-3 and -7. *J Biol Chem* 1998;273:34278–34283.

125. Heibein JA, et al. Granzyme B-mediated cytochrome c release is regulated by the Bcl-2 family members bid and Bax. *J Exp Med* 2000;192:1391–1402.

126. Sutton VR, et al. Initiation of apoptosis by granzyme B requires direct cleavage of bid, but not direct granzyme B-mediated caspase activation. *J Exp Med* 2000;192:1403–1414.

127. Scaffidi C, et al. Two CD95 (APO-1/Fas) signaling pathways. *EMBO J* 1998;17:1675–1687.

128. Yin XM, et al. Bid-deficient mice are resistant to Fas-induced hepatocellular apoptosis. *Nature* 1999;400:886–891.

129. Gross A, et al. Caspase cleaved BID targets mitochondria and is required for cytochrome c release, while BCL-XL prevents this release but not tumor necrosis factor-R1/Fas death. *J Biol Chem* 1999;274:1156–1163.

130. Ortaldo JR, et al. Fas involvement in human NK cell apoptosis: lack of a requirement for CD16-mediated events. *J Leukoc Biol* 1997;61:209–215.

131. Ortaldo JR, Mason AT, O'Shea JJ. Receptor-induced death in human natural killer cells: involvement of CD16. *J Exp Med* 1995;181:339–344.

132. Strasser A, O'Connor L, Dixit VM. Apoptosis signaling. *Annu Rev Biochem* 2000;69:217–245.

133. Kischkel FC, et al. Cytotoxicity-dependent APO-1 (Fas/CD95)-associated proteins form a death-inducing signaling complex (DISC) with the receptor. *EMBO J* 1995;14:5579–5588.

134. Itoh N, Nagata S. A novel protein domain required for apoptosis. Mutational analysis of human Fas antigen. *J Biol Chem* 1993;268:10932–10937.

135. Wang J, et al. Caspase-10 is an initiator caspase in death receptor signaling. *Proc Natl Acad Sci U S A* 2001;98:13884–13888.

136. Kischkel FC, et al. Apo2L/TRAIL-dependent recruitment of endogenous FADD and caspase-8 to death receptors 4 and 5. *Immunity* 2000;12:611–620.

137. Sprick MR, et al. FADD/MORT1 and caspase-8 are recruited to TRAIL receptors 1 and 2 and are essential for apoptosis mediated by TRAIL receptor 2. *Immunity* 2000;12:599–609.

138. Kischkel FC, et al. Death receptor recruitment of endogenous caspase-10 and apoptosis initiation in the absence of caspase-8. *J Biol Chem* 2001;276:46639–46646.

139. Zhao H, et al. Impaired c-Jun amino terminal kinase activity and T cell differentiation in death receptor 6-deficient mice. *J Exp Med* 2001;194:1441–1448.

140. Liu J, et al. Enhanced CD4+ T cell proliferation and Th2 cytokine production in DR6-deficient mice. *Immunity* 2001;15:23–34.

141. Ashkenazi A, Dixit VM. Apoptosis control by death and decoy receptors. *Curr Opin Cell Biol* 1999;11:255–260.

142. Zou H, et al. An APAF-1. cytochrome c multimeric complex is a functional apoptosome that activates procaspase-9. *J Biol Chem* 1999;274:11549–11556.

143. Golstein P. Controlling cell death. *Science* 1997;275:1081–1082.

144. Shi Y. A structural view of mitochondria-mediated apoptosis. *Nat Struct Biol* 2001;8:394–401.

145. Budihardjo I, et al. Biochemical pathways of caspase activation during apoptosis. *Annu Rev Cell Dev Biol* 1999;15:269–290.

146. Wu G, et al. Structural basis of IAP recognition by Smac/DIABLO. *Nature* 2000;408:1008–1012.

147. Srinivasula SM, et al. A conserved XIAP-interaction motif in caspase-9 and Smac/DIABLO regulates caspase activity and apoptosis. *Nature* 2001;410:112–116.

148. Kroemer G. Mitochondrial control of apoptosis: an overview. *Biochem Soc Symp* 1999;66:1–15.
149. Vercammen D, et al. Inhibition of caspases increases the sensitivity of L929 cells to necrosis mediated by tumor necrosis factor. *J Exp Med* 1998;187:1477–1485.
150. Vercammen D, et al. Dual signaling of the Fas receptor: initiation of both apoptotic and necrotic cell death pathways. *J Exp Med* 1998; 188:919–930.
151. Susin SA, et al. Molecular characterization of mitochondrial apoptosis-inducing factor. *Nature* 1999;397:441–446.
152. Joza N, et al. Essential role of the mitochondrial apoptosis-inducing factor in programmed cell death. *Nature* 2001;410:549–554.
153. Daugas E, et al. Mitochondrio-nuclear translocation of AIF in apoptosis and necrosis. *Faseb J* 2000;14:729–739.
154. Lorenzo HK, et al. Apoptosis inducing factor (AIF): a phylogenetically old, caspase-independent effector of cell death. *Cell Death Differ* 1999;6:516–524.
155. Li LY, Luo X, Wang X. Endonuclease G is an apoptotic DNase when released from mitochondria. *Nature* 2001;412:95–99.
156. Wyllie AH, Golstein P. More than one way to go. *Proc Natl Acad Sci U S A* 2001;98:11–13.
157. Vercammen D, et al. Tumour necrosis factor-induced necrosis versus anti-Fas-induced apoptosis in L929 cells. *Cytokine* 1997;9:801–808.
158. Stanger BZ, et al. RIP: a novel protein containing a death domain that interacts with Fas/APO-1 (CD95) in yeast and causes cell death. *Cell* 1995;81:513–523.
159. Hsu H, et al. TNF-dependent recruitment of the protein kinase RIP to the TNF receptor-1 signaling complex. *Immunity* 1996;4:387–396.
160. Ting AT, Pimentel-Muinos FX, Seed B. RIP mediates tumor necrosis factor receptor 1 activation of NF-kappaB but not Fas/APO-1–initiated apoptosis. *EMBO J* 1996;15:6189–6196.
161. Kelliher MA, et al. The death domain kinase RIP mediates the TNF-induced NF-kappaB signal. *Immunity* 1998;8:297–303.
162. Lin Y, et al. The death domain kinase RIP is essential for TRAIL (Apo2L)-induced activation of IkappaB kinase and c-Jun N-terminal kinase. *Mol Cell Biol* 2000;20:6638–6645.
163. Shisler JL, Moss B. Immunology 102 at poxvirus U: avoiding apoptosis. *Semin Immunol* 2001;13:67–72.
164. Li M, Beg AA. Induction of necrotic-like cell death by tumor necrosis factor alpha and caspase inhibitors: novel mechanism for killing virus-infected cells. *J Virol* 2000;74:7470–7477.
164a. Lenardo MJ, Anleman SB, Bounkeua V, et al. Cytopathic killing of peripheral blood CD4+T lymphocytes by human immunodeficiency virus type I appears necrotic rather than apoptotic and does not require env. *J Virology* 2002;76:5082–5093.
165. Yuan J, et al. The C. elegans cell death gene ced-3 encodes a protein similar to mammalian interleukin-1 beta-converting enzyme. *Cell* 1993;75:641–652.
166. Earnshaw WC, Martins LM, Kaufmann SH. Mammalian caspases: structure, activation, substrates, functions during apoptosis. *Annu Rev Biochem* 1999;68:383–424.
167. Chai J, et al. Structural basis of caspase-7 inhibition by XIAP. *Cell* 2001;104:769–780.
168. Wei Y, et al. The structures of caspases-1, -3, -7 and -8 reveal the basis for substrate and inhibitor selectivity. *Chem Biol* 2000;7:423–432.
169. Watt W, et al. The atomic-resolution structure of human caspase-8, a key activator of apoptosis. *Structure (Camb)* 1999;7:1135–1143.
170. Riedl SJ, et al. Structural basis for the inhibition of caspase-3 by XIAP. *Cell* 2001;104:791–800.
171. Blanchard H, et al. The three-dimensional structure of caspase-8: an initiator enzyme in apoptosis. *Structure (Camb)* 1999;7:1125–1133.
172. Chai J, et al. Crystal structure of a procaspase-7 zymogen. *Mechanisms of activation and substrate binding. Cell* 2001;107:399–407.
173. Beidler DR, et al. The baculovirus p35 protein inhibits Fas- and tumor necrosis factor- induced apoptosis. *J Biol Chem* 1995;270:16526–16528.
174. Thome M, et al. Viral FLICE-inhibitory proteins (FLIPs) prevent apoptosis induced by death receptors. *Nature* 1997;386:517–521.
175. Bertin J, et al. Death effector domain-containing herpesvirus and poxvirus proteins inhibit both Fas- and TNFR1-induced apoptosis. *Proc Natl Acad Sci* 1997;94:1172–1176.
176. Huang Y, et al. Structural basis of caspase inhibition by XIAP: differential roles of the linker versus the BIR domain. *Cell* 2001;104:781–790.

177. Thornberry NA, et al. A combinatorial approach defines specificities of members of the caspase family and granzyme B. Functional relationships established for key mediators of apoptosis. *J Biol Chem* 1997;272:17907–17911.
178. Rano TA, et al. A combinatorial approach for determining protease specificities: application to interleukin-1beta converting enzyme (ICE). *Chem Biol* 1997;4:149–155.
179. Roy S, Nicholson DW. Criteria for identifying authentic caspase substrates during apoptosis. *Methods Enzymol* 2000;322:110–125.
180. Sakahira H, Enari M, Nagata S. Cleavage of CAD inhibitor in CAD activation and DNA degradation during apoptosis. *Nature* 1998;391:96–99.
181. Enari M, et al. A caspase-activated DNase that degrades DNA during apoptosis, its inhibitor ICAD. *Nature* 1998;391:43–50.
182. Rao L, Perez D, White E. Lamin proteolysis facilitates nuclear events during apoptosis. *J Cell Biol* 1996;135:1441–1455.
183. Wang ZQ, et al. PARP is important for genomic stability but dispensable in apoptosis. *Genes Dev* 1997;11:2347–2358.
183a. Chan HJ, Zheng L, Ahmad M, et al. Pleiotropic defects in lymphocyte activation caused by caspase-8 mutations lead to human immunodeficiency. *Nature* 2002;419:395–399.
184. Wallach D, et al. Tumor necrosis factor receptor and Fas signaling mechanisms. *Annu Rev Immunol* 1999;17:331–367.
185. Shu HB, Johnson H. B cell maturation protein is a receptor for the tumor necrosis factor family member TALL-1. *Proc Natl Acad Sci U S A* 2000;97:9156–9161.
186. Wiley SR, et al. A Novel TNF Receptor Family Member Binds TWEAK and Is Implicated in Angiogenesis. *Immunity* 2001;15:837–846.
187. Tartaglia LA, et al. A novel domain within the 55 kd TNF receptor signals cell death. *Cell* 1993;74:845–853.
188. Arch RH, Gedrich RW, Thompson CB. Tumor necrosis factor receptor-associated factors (TRAFs)—a family of adapter proteins that regulates life and death. *Genes Dev* 1998;12:2821–2830.
189. Rothe M, et al. A novel family of putative signal transducers associated with the cytoplasmic domain of the 75 kDa tumor necrosis factor receptor. *Cell* 1994;78:681–692.
190. Weiss T, et al. TNFR80-dependent enhancement of TNFR60-induced cell death is mediated by TNFR-associated factor 2 and is specific for TNFR60. *J Immunol* 1998;161:3136–3142.
191. Chan FK, Lenardo MJ. A crucial role for p80 TNF-R2 in amplifying p60 TNF-R1 apoptosis signals in T lymphocytes. *Eur J Immunol* 2000;30:652–660.
192. Chan KF, Siegel MR, Lenardo JM. Signaling by the TNF receptor superfamily and T cell homeostasis. *Immunity* 2000;13:419–422.
193. Siegel RM, et al. The multifaceted role of Fas signaling in immune cell homeostasis and autoimmunity. *Nat Immunol* 2000;1:469–474.
194. Hsu H, Xiong J, Goeddel DV. The TNF receptor 1-associated protein TRADD signals cell death and NF-kappa B activation. *Cell* 1995; 81:495–504.
195. Yeh WC, et al. Early lethality, functional NF-kappaB activation, increased sensitivity to TNF-induced cell death in TRAF2-deficient mice. *Immunity* 1997;7:715–725.
196. Li ZW, et al. The IKKbeta subunit of IkappaB kinase (IKK) is essential for nuclear factor kappaB activation and prevention of apoptosis. *J Exp Med* 1999;189:1839–1845.
197. Tanaka M, et al. Embryonic lethality, liver degeneration, impaired NF-kappa B activation in IKK-beta-deficient mice. *Immunity* 1999;10: 421–429.
198. Rudolph D, et al. Severe liver degeneration and lack of NF-kappaB activation in NEMO/IKKgamma-deficient mice. *Genes Dev* 2000;14:854–862.
199. Makris C, et al. Female mice heterozygous for IKK-gamma/NEMO deficiencies develope a dermatopathy similar to the human X-linked disorder incontinentia pigmenti. *Mol Cell* 2000;5:969–979.
200. Smahi A, et al. Genomic rearrangement in NEMO impairs NF-kappaB activation and is a cause of incontinentia pigmenti. The International Incontinentia Pigmenti (IP) Consortium. *Nature* 2000;405:466–472.
201. Beg AA, Baltimore D. An essential role for NF-kappaB in preventing TNF-alpha–induced cell death [see comments]. *Science* 1996; 274:782–784.
202. Van Antwerp DJ, et al. Suppression of TNF-alpha-induced apoptosis by NF-kappaB [see comments]. *Science* 1996;274:787–789.

203. Wang CY, Mayo MW, Baldwin AS Jr. TNF- and cancer therapy–induced apoptosis: potentiation by inhibition of NF-kappaB [see comments]. *Science* 1996;274:784–787.

204. Lee SY, et al. Stimulus-dependent synergism of the antiapoptotic tumor necrosis factor receptor-associated factor 2 (TRAF2) and nuclear factor kappaB pathways. *J Exp Med* 1998;188:1381–1384.

205. Adachi M, et al. Enhanced and accelerated lymphoproliferation in Fas-null mice. *Proc Natl Acad Sci U S A* 1996;93:2131–2136.

206. Hawkins CJ, Vaux DL. The role of the Bcl-2 family of apoptosis regulatory proteins in the immune system. *Semin Immunol* 1997;9:25–33.

207. Raffeld M, et al. Clonal evolution of t(14;18) follicular lymphomas demonstrated by immunoglobulin genes and the 18q21 major breakpoint region. *Cancer Res* 1987;47:2537–2542.

208. Vaux DL, Cory S, Adams JM. Bcl-2 gene promotes haemopoietic cell survival and cooperates with c-myc to immortalize pre-B cells. *Nature* 1988;335:440–442.

209. Gross A, McDonnell JM, Korsmeyer SJ. BCL-2 family members and the mitochondria in apoptosis. *Genes Dev* 1999;13:1899–1911.

210. Hockenbery D, et al. Bcl-2 is an inner mitochondrial membrane protein that blocks programmed cell death. *Nature* 1990;348:334–336.

211. de Jong D, et al. Subcellular localization of the bcl-2 protein in malignant and normal lymphoid cells. *Cancer Res* 1994;54:256–260.

212. Krajewski S, et al. Investigation of the subcellular distribution of the bcl-2 oncoprotein: residence in the nuclear envelope, endoplasmic reticulum, outer mitochondrial membranes. *Cancer Res* 1993;53:4701–4714.

213. Zamzami N, et al. Subcellular and submitochondrial mode of action of Bcl-2-like oncoproteins. *Oncogene* 1998;16:2265–2282.

214. Fesik SW. Insights into programmed cell death through structural biology. *Cell* 2000;103:273–282.

215. Oltvai ZN, Milliman CL, Korsmeyer SJ. Bcl-2 heterodimerizes *in vivo* with a conserved homolog, Bax, that accelerates programmed cell death. *Cell* 1993;74:609–619.

216. Korsmeyer SJ, et al. Bcl-2/Bax: a rheostat that regulates an antioxidant pathway and cell death. *Semin Cancer Biol* 1993;4:327–332.

217. Yin XM, Oltvai ZN, Korsmeyer SJ. Heterodimerization with Bax is required for Bcl-2 to repress cell death. *Curr Top Microbiol Immunol* 1995;194:331–338.

218. Yang E, et al. Bad, a heterodimeric partner for Bcl-XL and Bcl-2, displaces Bax and promotes cell death. *Cell* 1995;80:285–291.

219. Sedlak TW, et al. Multiple Bcl-2 family members demonstrate selective dimerizations with Bax. *Proc Natl Acad Sci U S A* 1995;92:7834–7838.

220. Wei MC, et al. Proapoptotic BAX and BAK: a requisite gateway to mitochondrial dysfunction and death. *Science* 2001;292:727–730.

221. Boise LH, et al. CD28 costimulation can promote T cell survival by enhancing the expression of Bcl-XL. *Immunity* 1995;3:87–98.

222. Motoyama N, et al. Massive cell death of immature hematopoietic cells and neurons in Bcl-x–deficient mice. *Science* 1995;267:1506–1510.

223. Veis DJ, et al. Bcl-2-deficient mice demonstrate fulminant lymphoid apoptosis, polycystic kidneys, hypopigmented hair. *Cell* 1993;75:229–240.

224. Strasser A, Harris AW, Cory S. E mu-bcl-2 transgene facilitates spontaneous transformation of early pre-B and immunoglobulin-secreting cells but not T cells. *Oncogene* 1993;8:1–9.

225. Linette GP, et al. Peripheral T-cell lymphoma in lckpr-bcl-2 transgenic mice. *Blood* 1995;86:1255–1260.

226. Knudson CM, et al. Bax-deficient mice with lymphoid hyperplasia and male germ cell death. *Science* 1995;270:96–99.

227. Lindsten T, et al. The combined functions of proapoptotic Bcl-2 family members bak and bax are essential for normal development of multiple tissues. *Mol Cell* 2000;6:1389–1399.

228. Sattler M, et al. Structure of Bcl-xL-Bak peptide complex: recognition between regulators of apoptosis. *Science* 1997;275:983–986.

229. Luo X, et al. Bid, a Bcl2 interacting protein, mediates cytochrome c release from mitochondria in response to activation of cell surface death receptors. *Cell* 1998;94:481–490.

230. Zha J, et al. Posttranslational N-myristoylation of BID as a molecular switch for targeting mitochondria and apoptosis. *Science* 2000;290:1761–1765.

231. Eskes R, et al. Bid induces the oligomerization and insertion of Bax into the outer mitochondrial membrane. *Mol Cell Biol* 2000;20:929–935.

232. Zou H, et al. Apaf-1, a human protein homologous to *C. elegans* CED-4, participates in cytochrome c-dependent activation of caspase-3. *Cell* 1997;90:405–413.

233. Inohara N, Nunez G. The NOD: a signaling module that regulates apoptosis and host defense against pathogens. *Oncogene* 2001;20:6473–6481.

234. Li P, et al. Cytochrome c and dATP-dependent formation of Apaf-1/caspase-9 complex initiates an apoptotic protease cascade. *Cell* 1997;91:479–489.

235. Fortin A, et al. APAF1 is a key transcriptional target for p53 in the regulation of neuronal cell death. *J Cell Biol* 2001;155:207–216.

236. Moroni MC, et al. Apaf-1 is a transcriptional target for E2F and p53. *Nat Cell Biol* 2001;3:552–558.

237. Soengas MS, et al. Apaf-1 and caspase-9 in p53-dependent apoptosis and tumor inhibition. *Science* 1999;284:156–159.

238. Hugot JP, et al. Association of NOD2 leucine-rich repeat variants with susceptibility to Crohn's disease. *Nature* 2001;411:599–603.

239. Ogura Y, et al. A frameshift mutation in NOD2 associated with susceptibility to Crohn's disease. *Nature* 2001;411:603–606.

240. Chan FK, et al. A domain in TNF receptors that mediates ligand-independent receptor assembly and signaling. *Science* 2000;288:2351–2354.

241. Siegel RM, et al. Fas preassociation required for apoptosis signaling and dominant inhibition by pathogenic mutations. *Science* 2000;288:2354–2357.

242. Jones EY, Stuart DI, Walker NP. Structure of tumour necrosis factor. *Nature* 1989;338:225–228.

243. McGeehan GM, et al. Regulation of tumour necrosis factor-alpha processing by a metalloproteinase inhibitor. *Nature* 1994;370:558–561.

244. Banner DW, et al. Crystal structure of the soluble human 55 kd TNF receptor-human TNF beta complex: implications for TNF receptor activation. *Cell* 1993;73:431–445.

245. Hymowitz SG, et al. Triggering cell death: the crystal structure of Apo2L/TRAIL in a complex with death receptor 5. *Mol Cell* 1999;4:563–571.

246. Cha SS, et al. Crystal structure of TRAIL-DR5 complex identifies a critical role of the unique frame insertion in conferring recognition specificity. *J Biol Chem* 2000;275:31171–31177.

247. Mongkolsapaya J, et al. Structure of the TRAIL-DR5 complex reveals mechanisms conferring specificity in apoptotic initiation. *Nat Struct Biol* 1999;6:1048–1053.

248. Cha SS, et al. 2.8 A resolution crystal structure of human TRAIL, a cytokine with selective antitumor activity. *Immunity* 1999;11:253–261.

249. Naismith JH, et al. Crystallographic evidence for dimerization of unliganded tumor necrosis factor receptor. *J Biol Chem* 1995;270:13303–13307.

250. Naismith JH, et al. Seeing double: crystal structures of the type I TNF receptor. *J Mol Recognit* 1996;9:113–117.

251. Naismith JH, et al. Structures of the extracellular domain of the type I tumor necrosis factor receptor. *Structure* 1996;4:1251–1262.

252. Naismith JH, Sprang SR. Modularity in the TNF-receptor family. *Trends Biochem Sci* 1998;23:74–79.

253. Park YC, et al. Structural basis for self-association and receptor recognition of human TRAF2. *Nature* 1999;398:533–538.

254. Ye H, et al. The structural basis for the recognition of diverse receptor sequences by TRAF2. *Mol Cell* 1999;4:321–330.

255. Park YC, et al. A novel mechanism of TRAF signaling revealed by structural and functional analyses of the TRADD-TRAF2 interaction. *Cell* 2000;101:777–787.

256. Tsao DH, et al. Solution structure of N-TRADD and characterization of the interaction of N-TRADD and C-TRAF2, a key step in the TNFR1 signaling pathway. *Mol Cell* 2000;5:1051–1057.

257. Kimura M, Matsuzawa A. Autoimmunity in mice bearing lprcg: a novel mutant gene. *Int Rev Immunol* 1994;11:193–210.

258. Fisher GH, et al. Dominant interfering Fas gene mutations impair apoptosis in a human autoimmune lymphoproliferative syndrome. *Cell* 1995;81:935–946.

259. Martin DA, et al. Defective CD95/APO-1/Fas signal complex formation in the human autoimmune lymphoproliferative syndrome, type Ia. *Proc Natl Acad Sci U S A* 1999;96:4552–4557.

260. Minn AJ, et al. Bcl-x(L) forms an ion channel in synthetic lipid membranes. *Nature* 1997;385:353–357.
261. Schendel SL, Montal M, Reed JC. Bcl-2 family proteins as ion-channels. *Cell Death Differ* 1998;5:372–380.
262. Huang B, et al. NMR structure and mutagenesis of the Fas (APO-1/CD95) death domain. *Nature* 1996;384:638–641.
263. Eberstadt M, et al. NMR structure and mutagenesis of the FADD (Mort1) death-effector domain. *Nature* 1998;392:941–945.
264. Chou JJ, et al. Solution structure of the RAIDD CARD and model for CARD/CARD interaction in caspase-2 and caspase-9 recruitment. *Cell* 1998;94:171–180.
265. Zhou P, et al. Solution structure of Apaf-1 CARD and its interaction with caspase-9 CARD: a structural basis for specific adaptor/caspase interaction. *Proc Natl Acad Sci U S A* 1999;96:11265–11270.
266. Qin H, et al. Structural basis of procaspase-9 recruitment by the apoptotic protease-activating factor 1. *Nature* 1999;399:549–557.
267. Fairbrother WJ, et al. The PYRIN domain: a member of the death domain-fold superfamily. *Protein Sci* 2001;10:1911–1918.
268. Bertin J, DiStefano PS. The PYRIN domain: a novel motif found in apoptosis and inflammation proteins. *Cell Death Differ* 2000;7:1273–1274.
269. Martinon F, Hofmann K, Tschopp J. The pyrin domain: a possible member of the death domain-fold family implicated in apoptosis and inflammation. *Curr Biol* 2001;11:118–120.
270. Xu G, et al. Covalent inhibition revealed by the crystal structure of the caspase-8/p35 complex. *Nature* 2001;410:494–497.
271. Harrison LC, Hafler DA. Antigen-specific therapy for autoimmune disease. *Curr Opin Immunol* 2000;12:704–711.
272. Waldmann TA, Dubois S, Tagaya Y. Contrasting roles of IL-2 and IL-15 in the life and death of lymphocytes: implications for immunotherapy. *Immunity* 2001;14:105–110.
273. Critchfield JM, Lenardo MJ. Antigen-induced programmed T cell death as a new approach to immune therapy. Clin *Immunol Immunopathol* 1995;75:13–19.
274. Evan G, Littlewood T. A matter of life and cell death. *Science* 1998;281:1317–1322.
275. Straus SE, et al. The development of lymphomas in families with autoimmune lymphoproliferative syndrome with germline Fas mutations and defective lymphocyte apoptosis. *Blood* 2001;98:194–200.

CHAPTER 28

Immunological Memory

David F. Tough and Jonathan Sprent

Longevity of Immunological Memory
Generation of Memory
  Generation of Memory T Cells · Generation of Memory B Cells
Identifying Memory Cells
  Identification of Memory T Cells · Identification of Memory B Cells
Factors Contributing to Memory
  Continued Expression of Effector Activity · Systemic Differences between the Memory and Naïve State · Altered Properties of Memory Cells on a Per-Cell Basis
Life Span and Turnover of Memory Cells
  Life Span of Memory T Cells · Life Span of Memory B Cells
Maintenance of Memory
  Maintenance of T-Cell Memory · Maintenance of B-Cell Memory
Concluding Remarks
References

The realization that surviving an infectious disease often leads to a state of specific immunity clearly pre-dates any knowledge of either the components of the immune system or the basis of infectious disease. Furthermore, procedures for inducing specific immune memory as a means of protection against infectious disease were practiced long before the basis of this protection was known. For example, for protection against smallpox, Edward Jenner's strategy of inducing immunity by vaccination with cowpox in 1796 was preceded for a long time by the practice of variolation (inoculation of virus taken from pustules of smallpox victims). Today, the term *immunity* remains synonymous with resistance to reinfection and hence with immunological memory.

Experimental observations on immunological memory, as evidenced by the altered characteristics of the secondary vs the primary response to immunization (once known as the "secondary stimulus phenomenon"), were also described before many of the fundamental components of the immune system became known. In this regard, a more rapid reaction to secondary immunization was reported first for antibody responses (1) and subsequently for "cellular" responses such as delayed type hypersensitivity reactions, graft rejection, and induction of cytotoxic T-lymphocytes (CTLs) (2–7). In addition to occurring faster, secondary responses were found to be more intense than primary responses and associated with production of higher affinity antibody.

Immunological memory can be considered broadly as any alteration in the response to an antigen induced by previous exposure to the same antigen. Strictly speaking, memory would include other phenomena such as partial or complete tolerance induction. However, this chapter focuses on the more classical view of memory as an enhanced (or primed) state of the immune system after exposure to antigen. By this definition, immune memory includes continued expression of effector activity, particularly antibody production, as well as the persistence of immune ("memory") T and B cells. To a large extent, immunological memory is a reflection of a greatly increased frequency of specifically reactive T and B cells in relation to unprimed animals. In addition, memory cells possess intrinsic functional differences from naïve cells that contribute to the enhanced nature of the secondary response. In this chapter, we discuss the current understanding of how immunological memory is generated and maintained as well as the cellular and molecular parameters contributing to memory.

LONGEVITY OF IMMUNOLOGICAL MEMORY

It is clear that immune-mediated protection against disease can be extremely long-lived after infection or vaccination. This is evident from the fact that lifelong resistance results from infections with childhood diseases such as chicken pox,

TABLE 1. *Longevity of immunological memory after virus infection*

Virus	Time since last exposure	Protection from disease	Antibodies present	T-cell memory present	Reference
Measles	65 years	Yes	NT, but protection is antibody mediated	NT	8
Yellow fever	75 years	Yes[a]	Yes	NT	9
Polio	40 years	NT	Yes	NT	10
Vaccinia	50 years	NT	NT	Yes	11

NT, not tested.
[a]Protection measured by injection of patients' serum into test animals followed by challenge infection of recipients.

mumps, and measles. However, because reexposure to the viruses that cause these diseases is a common occurrence, immunity might hinge on repeated boosting of memory cells through subsequent subclinical infection. Nevertheless, at least for certain viruses, a single exposure is sufficient to confer lifelong immunity (Table 1). This is apparent from studies of isolated human settlements, in which outbreaks of certain infectious diseases have occurred at infrequent and very defined intervals. One of the most informative studies of this type was conducted by the Danish physician Ludwig Panum (8), who recorded his observations on measles epidemics that occurred during the eighteenth and nineteenth centuries in the Faroe Islands. Of particular interest was the fate of people who survived two separate measles epidemics 65 years apart. Panum found that people who had been infected during the first epidemic did not suffer from disease during the second, whereas those who did not contract measles in the first outbreak did so in the second. Because the Faroe Islands had remained measles-free in the intervening years, it was clear that long-lasting immunity could result from a single infection.

Because protection from measles is largely antibody mediated, Panum's study implied that antibody production could continue for decades after recovery from infection and did not require reexposure to the pathogen. In support of this notion, protective antibodies against yellow fever virus were found in individuals who had suffered from yellow fever up to 75 years earlier but had had no further exposure to the disease (9). In another study, antibodies to poliovirus were examined in a group of Inuit people living in northern Alaska (10). According to clinical records of illness and death, this population had apparently been polio free for at least 20 years, a supposition that was supported by a failure to find polio-reactive antibodies in any people younger than 20 years. Of significance, however, was that high titers of anti-polio antibodies were observed in older individuals. Furthermore, antibodies specific for different strains of polio exhibited distinct age thresholds for their first appearance: Antibodies to one strain were found only in people older than 40.

Although T cell memory was not addressed in the studies just cited, there is evidence that this facet of memory is similarly long-lived. Perhaps the best example in which this was shown directly was the detection of vaccinia virus–specific CD4+ and CD8+ T cells in individuals vaccinated up

to 50 years before (11). Because there was virtually no chance that these people were subsequently exposed to vaccinia (or the cross-reacting smallpox virus, for which the vaccine was given), these observations implied that T-cell memory can persist for many decades after a single virus infection.

These data indicate that immunological memory in humans can be very long-lived at both the T-cell and B-cell level. These findings are supported by a large body of evidence derived from experimental animals (mainly mice) showing life-long antibody production and persistence of antigen-specific CD4+ and CD8+ T cells at high frequencies after infection (12). Although long-term memory is apparently not dependent on reinfection, it remains possible that intermittent contact between the immune system and antigen serves to boost the intensity of the secondary response. This issue is discussed in the following section.

GENERATION OF MEMORY

There are two main outcomes of a typical immune response: (a) generation of effector cells that act to clear the acute infection and (b) generation of immune memory, which provides long-term protection against reinfection. Although the distinction between these two phases of the immune response is not absolute (for example, long-term expression of effector activity probably contributes to immune memory, as outlined later), effector and memory responses typically exhibit considerable quantitative, qualitative, and temporal differences. Hence, the effector response is characterized by the generation of extremely high numbers of antigen-specific T and B cells that are in a highly activated state and have direct effector activity; the majority of these cells disappear once the infection is cleared (usually within 1 to 2 weeks of initiating the response) (12–15). Conversely, the frequency of antigen-specific lymphocytes among memory cells is much lower than that found during the acute response; moreover, most memory cells are in a less activated state than are effector cells. In addition, unlike the majority of effector lymphocytes, memory cells persist long after the infection is cleared (12,16).

Although the precise mechanisms involved in generating immune memory remain poorly understood, it is clear that both memory and effector cells are produced as a result of the activation of initially naïve lymphocytes in the specialized environment of secondary lymphoid tissues. In this section, we provide a brief description of the behavior of naïve lymphocytes, followed by a discussion of the cellular and molecular interactions occurring during the acute phase of the immune response, focusing on events that may play a role in determining whether antigen-activated lymphocytes become short-lived effectors or long-lived memory cells.

Generation of Memory T Cells

T cells are generated from immature precursors through a complex series of selection events in the thymus (see Chapter 9). During this process, immature thymocytes that lack T-cell receptor (TCR) specificity for self-peptides bound to major histocompatibility complex (MHC) molecules fail to receive a survival signal and die by apoptosis, whereas cells expressing a TCR with high affinity for self-MHC/self-peptide complexes are signaled to die. The outcome of these positive and negative selection events is the generation of a population of mature T cells expressing TCR with low but significant affinity for self-MHC/self-peptide complexes; cells with overt reactivity to these ligands are deleted (17).

Mature T cells are released from the thymus into the bloodstream in low numbers: approximately 1 to 2×10^6 cells per day (about 1% of total thymocytes) in young (<2-month-old) mice (18,19). Thymic output of T cells decreases considerably in older mice and humans, because of atrophy of the thymus at puberty in both species. Recent thymic emigrants are considered to be immunologically naïve, exposure to foreign antigens in the thymus being negligible.

Naïve T cells recirculate continuously between blood and lymph, entering into lymph nodes (LNs) via specialized high endothelial venules (HEV) before returning to the bloodstream through thoracic duct lymph (20–23). Naïve T cells maintain this pattern of recirculation through expression of a specific combination of adhesion molecules and chemokine receptors. In particular, naïve T cells express high levels of two LN homing receptors: (a) CD62L, which allows cells to adhere to specific ligands (vascular addressins) expressed in HEV, and (b) the CCR7 chemokine receptor, which controls responsiveness to chemokines (e.g., ELC) expressed in LN at sites of lymphocyte entry (24,25). Conversely, because of limited expression of other adhesion molecules and chemokine receptors, naïve T cells are unable to extravasate into peripheral, nonlymphoid tissues.

This pattern of recirculation through the lymphoid tissues is of key importance because it brings naïve T cells into continuous contact with specialized antigen-presenting cells (APCs), especially dendritic cells (DCs), which are present in the T-cell areas of lymph nodes and the spleen (26–28). DCs are positioned to capture antigen entering into secondary lymphoid organs via blood (i.e., in the spleen) or afferent lymph (in LNs). In addition, immature DCs present in peripheral tissues, such as Langerhans cells in skin, are induced to migrate to the T-cell areas of lymphoid organs after antigen capture. This homing property of antigen-bearing DCs allows naïve

T cells to scan the entire body for the presence of foreign antigens. The fact that DCs are the cell type scrutinized by naïve T cells in this surveillance operation is also highly significant, because DCs are the major, if not the only, APCs able to initiate the activation of naïve T cells (29).

T cells become activated in secondary lymphoid tissues upon recognition of MHC/peptide complexes to which their TCRs have high affinity. Optimal T-cell activation is dependent not only on triggering of the TCR but also on the delivery of a "second" signal, usually referred to as co-stimulation, by the APC (30–35). The best characterized co-stimulatory signal is that mediated by the binding of CD28 on the T cell to B7-1 (CD80) or B7-2 (CD86) molecules on APCs. This interaction has been shown to be crucially important in T-cell activation in vivo through a variety of studies of mice deficient in CD28 function [reviewed by Lenschow et al. (30)]. However, some T-cell responses can occur in the absence of CD28, which implies either that alternate co-stimulatory pathways are available for the activation of naïve T cells or that activation can occur in the absence of co-stimulation under certain circumstances (36–39). Other molecules on naïve T cells that are capable of delivering co-stimulatory signals include leukocyte function–associated antigen 1 (LFA-1) (CD11a/CD18), which binds to intercellular adhesion molecule (ICAM)–1, ICAM-2, or ICAM-3, and CD2, which binds to CD58 (humans) or CD48 (mouse) [reviewed by Watts and DeBenedette (40)]. The heat-stable antigen (HSA) (CD24), expressed on APCs, has also been shown to provide co-stimulation for T-cell activation, although its receptor on T cells has not been identified (41). In addition, a number of other co-stimulatory molecules are up-regulated after activation of T cells and APCs; as discussed later, these molecules may play an important role in amplifying or prolonging the response rather than in initiating T-cell activation (35,40).

It should be noted that overt T cell activation occurs only after recognition of antigen presented by activated APCs. DCs become activated after infection or exposure to a variety of infection-associated stimuli [e.g., lipopolysaccharide, bacterial deoxyribonucleic acid (DNA), double-stranded ribonucleic acid (RNA), type I interferon (IFN)] and also in response to "danger" signals [e.g., tumor necrosis factor α (TNF-α), heat-shock proteins expressed by necrotic cells] (27,42–52). Activated DCs possess a variety of properties that distinguish them from resting DCs, including increased expression of co-stimulatory molecules, cytokines, and chemokines involved in T-cell activation. Although T cells do respond to antigen presented by resting DCs, this response is abortive and is often followed by the induction of tolerance (53,54).

After activation, T cells enter cell cycle and undergo multiple rounds of cell division. From in vivo measurements, it has been estimated that CD8$^+$ T cells divide every 4.5 to 8 hours during the peak of the immune response (53,55). This rapid rate of division allows for massive clonal expansion of rare antigen-specific cells. During responses to certain viruses, such as lymphocytic choriomeningitis virus (LCMV) in mice and Epstein-Barr virus in humans, peak numbers of CD8$^+$ T cells can be extremely high; up to 50% of total CD8$^+$ T cells are specific for a single viral epitope. Because LCMV epitope–specific CD8$^+$ T cells are undetectable in naïve mice by current methods (i.e., less than 1 in 100,000 cells), reaching such numbers at the peak of the response would require at least a 50,000-fold expansion (or about 10 to 11 divisions) of the precursor cells. Although the frequencies of CD4$^+$ T cells, as well as that of CD8$^+$ T cells in more typical infections, may be 10- to 100-fold lower, it is clear that very large numbers of activated T cells are generated during this initial expansion phase. Most of these cells express direct effector activity (i.e., the ability to exert cytolytic activity or secrete cytokines upon TCR triggering).

The migratory behavior of T cells is markedly altered after contact with antigen. During the first 2 days of the response, antigen-specific T cells remain "trapped" in secondary lymphoid organs; thoracic duct lymph and peripheral blood are essentially devoid of antigen-responsive cells (56,57). Subsequently, activated T cells are released into the circulation. Many of these cells are able to enter into peripheral tissues at sites of inflammation by virtue of expressing a different set of adhesion and chemokine receptors from those expressed on naïve T cells. In addition, some activated CD4$^+$ T cells acquire the ability to migrate into B-cell areas of lymphoid tissues and provide help for antigen-specific B cells. Thus, the most prominent outcome of the acute immune response is the generation of tissue-homing effector T cells that either kill infected cells (for CD8$^+$ cells) or induce B cells to produce antibodies that bind to and facilitate the clearance of extracellular pathogens (for CD4$^+$ cells).

Once the pathogen has been cleared, it is no longer of benefit to the host to maintain the vast number of activated T cells generated in the immune response. Indeed, persistence of these cells en masse would probably have deleterious effects, because of both their capacity to secrete toxic cytokines and their occupation of available space; in addition, bulk persistence of effectors would deplete vital growth factors, thus compromising primary responses to new antigens. For these reasons, most activated T cells are removed at the end of the immune response. In secondary lymphoid organs, the disappearance of responding T cells is profound: The number of antigen-specific T cells is typically reduced by 95% or more in comparison to the peak of the response. The loss of cells is largely a reflection of cell death by apoptosis but is also caused in part by irreversible migration of cells into peripheral tissues (58). In this regard, studies have shown the disappearance of activated T cells to be much less extensive, or at least to occur much more slowly, in peripheral sites such as the intestine and the lung (59–62).

Of importance is that the disappearance of antigen-specific T cells at the end of immune responses is typically not complete, and the cells surviving this phase are generally considered to be memory T cells. These cells are maintained over a long term—for the lifetime of the host, in some animal models—at relatively constant frequencies. However,

the precise definition of memory T cells and a way to distinguish these cells from effector T cells are unclear. This is particularly relevant because some T cells with direct effector activity can be detected long after the primary infection has been cleared (as discussed later). With this in mind, it could be argued that the defining characteristic of a memory T-cell population is the ability to persist after the completion of the acute immune response. This definition incorporates the likelihood that memory T cells are heterogeneous with regard to activation and effector status.

In considering how T-cell memory is generated, the key question, therefore, is how a small proportion of cells is selected to withstand the dramatic purging of the activated T-cell population that occurs after clearance of antigen. In speculating how this is accomplished, it is worth noting that a correlation is often, although not always (see later discussion), observed between the number of activated T cells present at the peak of the response and the number of memory T cells generated (55,63–65). This implies that effector cell-promoting and memory T cell–promoting factors are often regulated in parallel. Three main mechanisms for the concomitant generation of effector and memory T cells during an immune response could be envisaged (Fig. 1). First, there could be distinct precursors present in the naïve T-cell pool that give rise to short-lived effectors versus long-lived memory cells. At present, there is no evidence that this is the case. Second, T cells destined to become long-lived memory cells might receive different initial activation signals from those delivered to short-lived effectors. Third, memory cells might selectively avoid death signals or receive survival signals late in the response. This third mechanism can be viewed as an extension of the second if the nature of initial T-cell activation is the factor that dictates the ability of the T cell to subsequently receive survival signals or avoid death signals. Conversely, delivery of survival/death signals could be completely random or at least be independent of initial T-cell activation. In this regard, the finding that the repertoires of memory and effector CD8$^+$ T cells are often very similar has been taken as evidence supporting a stochastic death process (65–69). However, these studies do not rule out the possibility that even members of the same T-cell clone could have received different early activation signals. Furthermore, other studies have shown that, in terms of fine specificity, the memory T-cell pool represents a restricted subset of the cells present at the peak of the acute response, which indicates that selection has occurred at some stage (70,71).

Compelling evidence that memory cells are selected from a unique subset of activated T cells comes from a novel transgenic mouse model (72). These mice were engineered to permanently express a reporter gene, placental alkaline phosphatase (PLAP), after activation of the granzyme B promoter. Because granzyme B is a key component of the lytic machinery of CTLs, PLAP was expected to serve as a marker for all activated and previously activated (i.e., memory) CD8$^+$ T cells. To test this idea, the mice were infected with LCMV, which induces a very strong CD8$^+$ cell response.

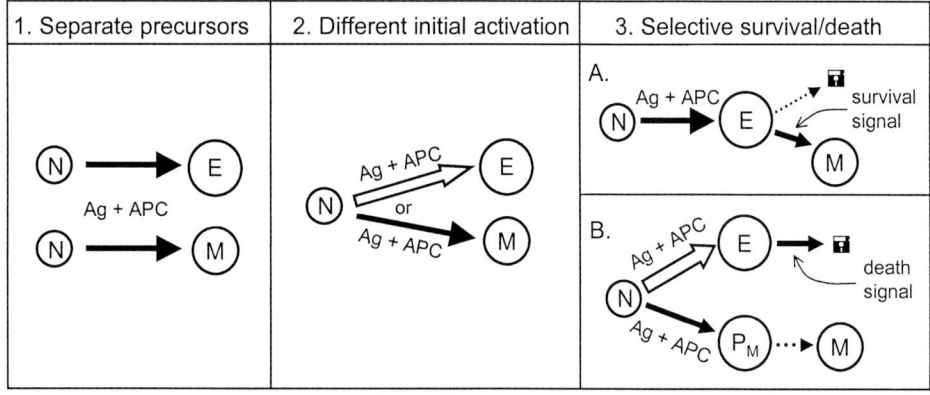

1. Separate precursors	2. Different initial activation	3. Selective survival/death

FIG. 1. Generation of effector and memory T cells during the immune response. Three possible mechanisms that could allow for production of short-lived effectors and long-lived memory cells are depicted: (a) Separate naïve precursors for effector and memory T cells could respond differently to the same initial activation stimulus. (b) Distinct conditions of initial activation could direct cells to become effector versus memory cells. (c) Memory cells are formed from a subset of activated T cells that either receives a survival signal or avoids being instructed to die. Survival of T cells into memory could be a stochastic process—that is, random survival from within a homogeneous population of activated cells—or could be selective on the basis of how the cells were initially activated. P_M, memory precursor; N, naïve T cell; E, effector T cell; M, memory T cell.

Surprisingly, only a small proportion of virus-specific CD8$^+$ T cells detected at the peak of the response expressed PLAP; CTLs were detected in both the PLAP$^+$ and PLAP$^-$ populations. A striking finding, however, was that when virus-specific CD8$^+$ T cells were examined 3 months after infection, the majority of cells were PLAP$^+$. Thus, memory cells appeared to have been selectively derived from the minority cell population that expressed PLAP early after activation. Although the reason for the heterogeneous and unexpected expression of the marker gene remains to be elucidated, it seems likely to be related to specific signals received during T-cell activation. This implies that the signals involved in generating short-lived effectors versus long-lived memory T cells may indeed be distinct.

Currently, the clearest evidence that the manner of T-cell activation influences the generation of T-cell memory has come from studies of a phenomenon known as *clonal exhaustion* (Fig. 2). The name refers to immune responses in which strong initial T-cell activation results not in memory but in deletion of essentially all responding T cells (73). This was shown to occur after immunization of mice with cells differing in expression of murine mammary tumor virus (Mtv) antigens (74). These molecules, which are encoded by endogenous retroviruses, are termed *superantigens* (SAgs) on the basis of their ability to activate all T cells bearing TCRs that include particular Vβ gene segments; SAgs activate T cells by binding simultaneously to class II MHC molecules (outside of the conventional peptide groove) and TCR Vβ regions (75). As shown by Webb et al. (74), injection of Mtv-7$^+$ cells into Mtv-7$^-$ recipients resulted in marked expansion of host Vβ6$^+$ CD4$^+$ T cells, followed by extensive deletion of these cells to levels below that seen in preimmune animals. Subsequent work has shown that similar deletion of

responding CD4$^+$ and CD8$^+$ T cells also occurs after injection of bacterial SAgs (76,77).

Although it could be argued that SAgs are atypical because of their manner of binding to the MHC, clonal exhaustion has also been shown to occur in response to conventional

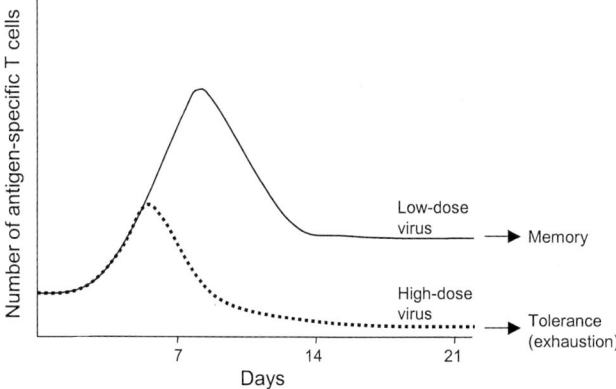

FIG. 2. Memory versus exhaustion as two opposite outcomes of the immune response. The disappearance of activated T cells at the end of typical immune responses is incomplete, leaving a higher frequency of antigen-specific cells in memory than existed in the naïve T cell pool. Under certain conditions, however, strong initial activation can lead to "exhaustion" of the responding T cells, in which essentially all responding cells are deleted. As a consequence of exhaustion, the host may be tolerant of subsequent challenge with antigen. T-cell exhaustion has been observed after injection of superantigens (39–42) or after high dose virus infection (43) (see text for details). In the latter situation, the T-cell expansion is of lower magnitude and peaks earlier than in a response to low-dose virus, indicating that excessive initial activation can result in an abortive T-cell response.

antigens. For these antigens, Moskophidis et al. (78) examined the response of a monoclonal population of CD8$^+$ T cells expressing a transgenic TCR specific for a peptide of LCMV. These cells were transferred in low numbers to syngeneic recipients with either a low or high dose of LCMV. When a low dose of virus was given, the transgenic cells expanded dramatically in number, cleared the virus, and then decreased in numbers to reach a memory level that was about 2% of that seen at the peak of the response. Conversely, when mice were infected with a high dose of LCMV, the transgenic CD8$^+$ T cells again underwent initial expansion in number (albeit to a lesser extent than in mice injected with a low dose of virus) but were unable to clear the infection. Of significance was that these cells declined to undetectable numbers after the initial response, which is consistent with clonal exhaustion and deletion. Whether the mechanisms involved in this process (see later discussion) are the same as those mediating deletion of SAg-reactive cells is unknown. The point to emphasize, however, is that the sparing of a small proportion of activated cells at the end of the immune response is not inevitable and can be limited or undetectable under certain conditions of T-cell activation.

During both SAg-induced exhaustion and high-dose virus–induced exhaustion, the amount of antigen presented, and hence the number of TCRs engaged per T cell, is probably very high. That a high dose of antigen is able to "exhaust" specific T cells is in keeping with a body of work showing that injection of large quantities of antigen or high doses of virus can lead to tolerance [reviewed by Moskophidis et al. (78)]. Therefore, one explanation for the clonal exhaustion phenomenon is that excessive or prolonged signaling through the TCR predisposes the responding T cells to die. If this idea can be extrapolated to memory cell generation in typical immune responses, it would follow that memory T cells represent cells that received less signaling through the TCR than the bulk of the responding population. However, it must be borne in mind that the strength of signal received by a T cell reflects a combination of the intrinsic TCR affinity for antigen, the number of peptide/MHC complexes engaged, and the duration of T-cell contact with antigen.

The available data do not support the idea that memory T cells are selected on the basis of low-affinity TCRs per se. Indeed, the converse may be true. Thus, it is generally accepted that memory T cells have a higher functional affinity for antigen than do naïve T cells. Evidence for such affinity maturation came originally from studies examining the ability of anti-CD8 antibodies to inhibit the cytolytic activity of alloreactive T cells isolated from either naïve or primed mice (79,80). Because CD8$^+$ cells from immunized mice were more resistant to anti-CD8 antibody, it was concluded that, on average, these cells had higher affinity TCRs than did naïve T cells. However, the heightened responsiveness of memory T cells may result from many factors other than TCR affinity (see later discussion). In particular, studies with TCR transgenic mice have shown that CD8$^+$ memory T cells are much more responsive to antigen than are naïve cells

expressing the same TCR (81–83). Nevertheless, more recent studies have provided direct evidence that, in normal mice, T cells (both CD4$^+$ and CD8$^+$) responding to secondary immunization express TCRs with higher affinity for antigen than do cells in the primary response (84,85). The caveat here is that selection for high affinity may have occurred not at the time of memory cell generation but during the secondary response. This could occur if antigen was cleared rapidly in the secondary response, which would thus lead to competition among memory T cells for a limited concentration of antigen.

Despite these findings, there is some evidence that high-affinity T cells can be selectively deleted during the primary immune response. In one study (86), the T-cell response against a specific peptide was assessed after immunization of mice with peptide analogues, bearing individual amino acid substitutions, which had a hierarchy of affinities for class II MHC. The interesting finding was that peptides with low affinity for class II MHC preferentially elicited T cells that had high affinity for the reference (nonsubstituted) peptide, whereas peptides that bound MHC with high affinity induced only low-affinity T cells. Furthermore, with the use of TCR transgenic CD4$^+$ T cells specific for the reference peptide, it was shown that injection of the high-affinity class II MHC–binding peptide actually led to deletion of high-affinity T cells. These results imply that, as for negative selection in the thymus, very strong signaling in mature T cells in certain situations can induce cell death.

As mentioned previously, the strength of signal delivered to the T cell through the TCR depends not only on its affinity for peptide/MHC complexes and the number of TCRs engaged but also on the duration of T-cell contact with antigen. It is likely that this third factor plays a role in some of the examples of exhaustion/deletion cited previously, particularly in the case of high-dose virus infections that are not cleared by the host and lead to persistent expression of antigen. Other evidence that prolonged TCR triggering has negative effects on responding T cells has come from the finding that, for TCR transgenic T cells, a single injection of peptide induces activation and expansion, whereas chronic administration induces marked deletion of the transgenic cells (87).

Further evidence that the initial conditions of T cell activation can influence the generation of memory T cells has come from *in vitro* studies. However, there are two obvious problems: (a) The conditions of T-cell activation *in vitro* are highly artificial and unlikely to correspond directly to how antigen is encountered *in vivo,* and (b) inferences about whether the T cells generated in response to antigen *in vitro* are "memory" cells or "effector" cells are imprecise and are based either on defining the surface markers on the cells or on examinations of the behavior of the cells after subsequent injection into mice. Nevertheless, as discussed later, there are several observations worth noting.

For human CD4$^+$ T cells, testing the functions and markers on these cells after antigen activation *in vitro* has led to the view that memory T cells come in two forms: "central" memory cells and "effector" memory cells (88). Central memory cells are regarded as primed cells that lack immediate effector activity and express the LN homing receptors CD62L and CCR7. In contrast, effector memory cells are highly polarized cells (i.e., expressing Th1 or Th2 cytokines), possess direct effector activity, and lack LN homing receptors. Effector memory cells are considered to be more differentiated than central memory cells, and these two subsets may play different roles in protecting the host against reinfection (see later discussion). With regard to how the two subsets of memory cells arise, strong TCR signaling (through prolonged contact with antigen) or the addition of certain cytokines to the culture or both are held to promote the generation of effector memory T cells, whereas activation with lower level TCR engagement or without added cytokines induces central memory cell generation (89–92). Differentiation may be partially linked to the number of cell divisions the activated T cell undergoes, inasmuch as CCR7 expression is markedly reduced in murine T cells after five divisions *in vitro* (93). Correlating with their CCR7 and CD62L phenotypes, CD4+ T cells activated with lower level stimuli migrated to LN after injection into mice, whereas cells activated for more prolonged periods were unable to do so (92).

These results led to the proposal by Lanzavecchia and Sallusto (94) that CD4+ T-cell differentiation follows a linear pathway, in which increasing levels of signaling induce a succession of memory T cells, effector T cells, and cell death (Fig. 3). This model takes into account previous observations that human T cells become increasingly susceptible to apoptosis with progressive differentiation after *in vitro* priming (95) and is consistent with the idea that memory T cells represent a population of T cells that were signaled less strongly than the bulk of the responding population on initial activation. However, the model leaves open the possibility that memory cells can be derived from fully differentiated effectors.

Direct evidence that effector cells can differentiate into memory cells has come from studies on the fate of *in vitro* activated CD8+ cells. In these studies, an apparently uniform population of effector CD8+ TCR transgenic T cells, in which all cells had undergone at least five cell divisions and expressed intracellular perforin, was generated by *in vitro* activation and then injected into antigen-free recipients (96). A significant finding was that CD8+ T cells with the characteristics of memory cells were present in these recipients 10 weeks after transfer, which indicates that memory CD8+ T cells could be derived from the progeny of cytolytic effectors.

Despite these findings, prior expression of overt effector activity does not seem to be an absolute requirement for the generation of memory CD8+ T cells. This is suggested by a study in which TCR transgenic CD8+ T cells were activated *in vitro* and then cultured in medium containing either interleukin (IL)–15 or IL-2 (97). Whereas the cells cultured in IL-2 differentiated into effector cells with potent cytolytic activity, IL-15–treated cells showed little if any effector activity. However, after transfer to syngeneic mice, a proportion of the IL-15–treated cells survived and mounted a rapid recall response 10 weeks later. The authors concluded that these cells had differentiated directly into memory cells, without an intervening effector cell stage. Interestingly, memory cells were also detected after transfer of cells from IL-2–containing cultures, although in lower numbers than were found after injection of IL-15–treated cells. The implication is therefore that, as for CD4+ cells (see previous discussion), CD8+ T-cell memory may be composed of two components: "central"

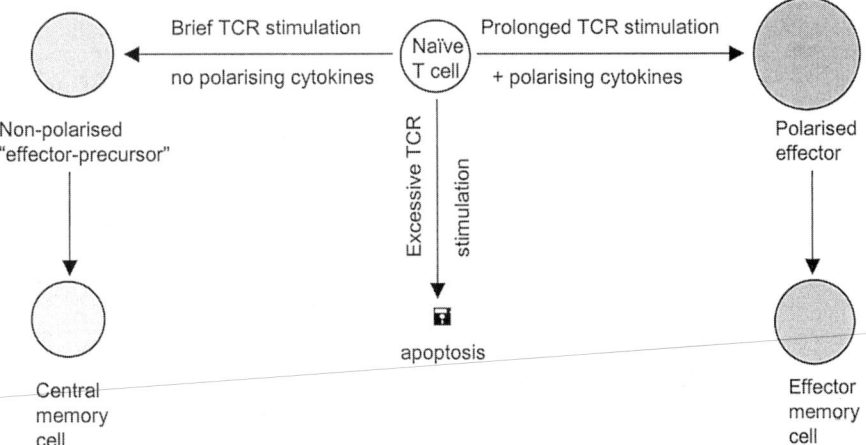

FIG. 3. Generation of central memory and effector memory T cells. Model proposed by Lanzavecchia and Sallusto (94), in which the fate of responding T cells is dictated by the duration of T-cell receptor (TCR) signaling and the presence or absence of polarizing cytokines. Relatively brief TCR signaling produces nonpolarized "effector-precursor" cells that may differentiate into central memory cells in the absence of further stimulation. More prolonged TCR stimulation in the presence of polarizing cytokines leads to the generation of polarized effector cells; these cells may give rise to effector memory cells. T cells receiving excessive stimulation die by apoptosis.

memory cells that are an early intermediate in the differentiation pathway and "effector" memory cells that arise from full-fledged effectors late in the response. Again, generation of these distinct types of memory cells may be affected by the extent of T-cell proliferation, because an increased number of cell divisions is associated with down-regulation of CD62L and acquisition of effector activity for mouse CD8$^+$ T cells *in vivo* (98). In this regard, it is worth noting that the cells generated in IL-15 but not IL-2 maintained expression of CD62L and CCR7 (97). Furthermore, IL-15– but not IL-2–treated cells localized in LN after injection into mice, whereas IL-2–treated cells were much more efficient at migrating to inflamed peritoneum (99). These findings are consistent with the differential migration patterns exhibited by central versus effector CD4$^+$ memory cells cited previously.

Further evidence that IL-15 can promote CD8$^+$ T cell memory has come from studies in mice expressing an IL-15 transgene under the class I MHC promoter (100). These mice have increased numbers of memory-phenotype CD8$^+$ T cells; in unimmunized mice, these cells are presumed to represent memory cells to environmental antigens (see later discussion). Higher numbers of memory-phenotype cells in IL-15 transgenic mice could reflect an enhancement in either the generation or the maintenance of memory cells. In this regard, experiments on antigen-specific T-cell responses in these mice are informative (101). IL-15 transgenic and control mice were infected with a bacterial pathogen, *Listeria monocytogenes,* and *Listeria* peptide–specific CD8$^+$ T cells were enumerated at different times after infection. Interestingly, similar numbers of *Listeria* peptide–specific cells were observed in control and IL-15 transgenic mice on day 7 after infection. However, the transgenic mice had considerably higher numbers of these cells 21 and 40 days after infection. These results have two main implications. First, the fact that similar numbers of specific cells were observed at the peak of the response (day 7) in control and transgenic mice indicates that IL-15 did not act by augmenting the initial expansion of the responding CD8$^+$ cells. Second, the finding that higher numbers of *Listeria*-specific cells were observed early in the "memory" phase of the response (day 21) suggests that IL-15 was in fact promoting the generation of memory cells. In this regard, the authors of this study proposed that IL-15 acted primarily by preventing the death of activated effectors, because expression of the antiapoptotic protein Bcl-2 in *Listeria*-specific cells on day 7 was considerably higher in the transgenic mice than in normal mice.

In addition to IL-15, other cytokines might also influence the generation of memory T cells. In this respect, data of Schluns et al. (102) suggested that IL-7 is important for the generation of memory CD8$^+$ T cells. In this study, IL-7R$^{+/+}$ or IL-7R$^{-/-}$ TCR transgenic T cells were adoptively transferred into congenic hosts, and the recipients were infected with a recombinant vaccinia virus expressing a specific antigen. The key finding was that, although both types of T cells exhibited similar initial proliferation, the IL-7R$^{-/-}$ CD8$^+$ cells were markedly underrepresented among memory cells.

Another cytokine that has been reported to have memory-promoting activity is IL-4 (103). In this study, TCR transgenic or polyclonal CD8$^+$ T cells were activated *in vitro* with or without the addition of various cytokines, and their ability to survive and persist as memory cells after injection into mice was examined. The striking finding was that addition of IL-4, but not IL-2 or IL-12, to the culture medium promoted the generation of long-lived memory cells. Although the mechanisms involved in this IL-4 effect remain to be determined, the authors reported the intriguing observation that CD8$^+$ T cells activated in IL-4–containing medium (but not IL-2–containing medium) expressed high levels of the IL-2 receptor β chain. Because IL-2Rβ (CD122) is a component of the receptor for IL-15 (as well as that for IL-2), the results support the view that IL-15 might play an important role in the generation of long-lived memory cells.

In considering the role of IL-4 in T-cell memory, it should be pointed out that CD8$^+$ memory responses are not impaired in IL-4–deficient mice (104). This finding indicates that IL-4 is not essential for the initiation of CD8$^+$ T-cell memory. A simple idea is that several different cytokines have overlapping roles in memory CD8$^+$ generation. This idea may not be applicable to CD4$^+$ cells, however, because generation of CD4$^+$ memory T cells is unimpaired in mice lacking the common γ chain, which forms a part of the receptor for a range of cytokines, including IL-4 and IL-15 (105). Whether CD8$^+$ memory is affected in these mice remains to be investigated.

In addition to TCR triggering and contact with cytokines, the strength of the signal received by the T cell during activation is affected by the extent of co-stimulation delivered by the APC. Hence, if the generation of memory T cells is favored by low-level signaling (see previous discussion), memory cells should be induced preferentially over effector T cells in conditions in which co-stimulation is limiting. In accordance with this idea, there is some evidence that the co-stimulatory requirements for the generation of memory CD8$^+$ T cells may be less stringent that those required to produce effector CTLs. Thus, infection of CD28-deficient mice with influenza virus was found to elicit memory CTL precursors but not effector CTL (39). Interestingly, memory CD8$^+$ cell generation in CD28-deficient mice was totally blocked after injection of an antibody against the co-stimulatory molecule, CD24. Likewise, injection of blocking antibodies against B7-1 and B7-2 blocked the development of CD8$^+$ memory in CD24-deficient mice. The implication is therefore that generation of effector cells in response to influenza virus is strictly dependent on CD28, whereas either B7-1– and B7-2–dependent or CD24-dependent co-stimulatory pathways can lead to memory cell development.

Even though memory CD8$^+$ cells can be generated under conditions of suboptimal co-stimulation, there is also evidence that strong co-stimulation can enhance production of memory cells. In this regard, the OX40 molecule appears to be important. OX40 is not expressed on resting T cells but is up-regulated 1 to 2 days after activation (106–109). Similarly, the ligand (OX40L) is expressed on APCs only after activation, the most potent signal for OX40L expression being ligation of CD40 on the APC (110–112). Hence, OX40–OX40L interaction is thought to provide co-stimulation late in the response, acting only after T cells have received initial activation signals through the TCR and CD28 and have up-regulated cell surface expression of CD40L and triggered CD40 expression on APCs. An important role for OX40 in CD4$^+$ T cell responses is suggested by the finding that OX40- or OX40L-deficient mice showed reductions in both the initial expansion of antigen-specific CD4$^+$ T cells and the generation of CD4$^+$ memory cells upon immunization (113–116). Conversely, injection of agonistic anti-OX40 antibodies during priming had the opposite effect: greater accumulation of antigen-specific CD4$^+$ T cells during the primary response and the generation of increased numbers of memory cells (116,117). Thus, OX40 signaling augments the generation of both short-lived effectors and memory cells. At face value, this observation appears to support the idea that memory cells are selected randomly from the activated population. However, it is also consistent with the possibility that OX40 is simply an amplifying signal that acts equally well on cells that were independently triggered toward effector or memory cell pathways.

Of note is that CD8$^+$ T-cell proliferative responses are relatively normal in OX40-deficient mice, which implies that OX40 may be a only requisite late co-stimulatory signal for CD4$^+$ cells (114). Another molecule that may play an analogous co-stimulatory role during CD8$^+$ T cell activation is 4-1BB (118). Like OX40, 4-1BB is expressed on T cells only after activation and binds to a ligand expressed on activated APCs. In vitro, ligation of 4-1BB augments responses of both CD4$^+$ and CD8$^+$ T cells (119). In vivo, however, targeted ablation of 4-1BBL expression appears to affect some CD8$^+$ responses but not others (120,121). Only a small reduction in antigen-specific CD8$^+$ T cells was observed after infection of 4-1BBL-deficient mice with influenza virus or LCMV. However, a much more prominent defect was observed after immunization with peptide, which implies that 4-1BB acts to augment suboptimal responses (122). With peptide immunization, 4-1BBL deficiency led to a reduction in both the number of antigen-specific CD8$^+$ T cells at the peak of the response (day 7) and in the number of memory cells present 2 months after vaccination. The implication is therefore that signals through 4-1BB do not specifically drive memory T-cell differentiation but, rather, act to amplify either committed or uncommitted precursors of both memory and effector cells.

Together, the data just described provide some indication that unique signals are involved in the generation of short-lived effectors versus long-lived memory T cells. In considering how this may be accomplished, it should be borne in mind that the defining property of memory cell–promoting stimuli is their ability to permit the survival of a small sub-population of activated cells in the context of massive cell death. In theory, this could result from either induction of prosurvival molecules or a failure to activate prodeath path-

ways (15). Therefore, understanding memory T-cell generation will depend on obtaining precise knowledge of the mechanisms mediating the death of effector cells at the end of an immune response and how these mechanisms are switched on and off.

Although it is currently unclear exactly why effector T cells die, there are considerable data regarding the termination of T-cell responses. In vitro, activated T cells are susceptible to a variety of death-inducing signals, involving molecules such as Fas, TNF-α, IL-2, and reactive oxygen species (123–127). In addition, accumulation of activated T cells is observed in mice deficient for many different molecules, including CTL-associated antigen 4 (CTLA-4) (128,129), IL-2 (130), CD25 (131,132), Fas (133,134), Fas ligand (133,134), CD122 (135), nuclear factor of activator T cells (136), transforming growth factor β receptor (137), and programmed cell death protein 1 (PD-1) (138). The implication is that several different, nonredundant mechanisms are involved in limiting the number of activated T cells, and loss of any one of these leads to T-cell hyperplasia. However, these mechanisms may operate at various stages of the immune response and might not contribute directly to the death of effectors at the end of an immune response. For example, CTLA-4 and PD-1, which are expressed by T cells and bind to B7 family members on APCs, probably inhibit the early activation and expansion of T cells (93). In fact, elimination of effector cells during immune responses appears to be normal in mice lacking CTLA-4, Fas, or TNF-α receptor (124,139–142). In contrast, deletion of effector T cells after clearance of antigen is reduced in IFN-$\gamma^{-/-}$ mice, which implicates this cytokine as a trigger for effector T-cell death (143–145).

As well as being actively signaled to undergo apoptosis, T cells may also die through a passive process initiated when they lose contact with life-sustaining cytokines or co-stimulatory molecules (146). In vitro, activated T cells can be rescued from passive cell death by IL-2 family cytokines that signal through the common γ chain (147). This prosurvival effect could be linked to the ability of these cytokines to induce up-regulation of Bcl-2, because enforced expression of Bcl-2 has been shown to reduce the death of activated CD4$^+$ T cells in vivo (139). Conversely, the same cytokines also cause T cells to up-regulate expression of Bcl-3, a member of the NFκB-IκB family that increases the survival of activated T cells in vitro and in vivo (148). Interestingly, Bcl-3 but not Bcl-2 is up-regulated by T cells in mice injected with adjuvants that reduce the death of activated T cells in vivo.

In summary, the mechanisms involved in the generation of memory T cells and the relationship between memory cells and effectors remain poorly understood. Part of the uncertainty may stem from the fact that memory T cells are heterogeneous, being broadly divisible into central memory and effector memory subpopulations. As discussed, these subtypes of memory cells might be produced via different pathways. Hence, central memory cells may arise under suboptimal stimulation conditions: namely, when antigen or polarizing cytokines, or both, are present only in low concentrations;

this setting may exist late in the immune response, when much of the antigen has been cleared and APCs are exhausted in terms of their ability to secrete cytokines (94,149). In contrast, the generation of effector memory cells may require a higher level of stimulation. Although this scenario is speculative, it implies that central and effector memory cells arise from different subpopulations of activated cells: central memory cells from effector precursors and effector memory cells from effector cells. Future studies in which phenotypic markers are used to distinguish between different types of memory T cells (e.g., CCR7, CD62L) should help elucidate the signals involved in memory generation and clarify the functional properties of memory T cells (see later discussion).

Generation of Memory B Cells

B cells can be divided broadly into a minority population of B-1 cells and a major population of conventional B-2 cells (see Chapter 6). The B-1 subset is located primarily in the pleural and peritoneal cavities (150), whereas B-2 cells are found mainly in defined B-cell zones in the spleen and LNs. This section focuses on the current understanding of memory generation among B-2 cells. Although there is some evidence that memory can be generated during B-cell responses to T cell–independent antigens (151,152), we review only the processes thought to occur during T cell–dependent B-cell responses.

B cells are produced throughout life in the bone marrow in an IL-7–dependent manner (153,154). It has been estimated that 10% to 20% of the immature B cells produced in the bone marrow enter the mature peripheral pool and that most of the loss occurs either in the bone marrow or during the migration of cells from the bone marrow to the spleen (155–157). Upon exiting the bone marrow, immature B cells enter the T-cell zones of secondary lymphoid organs before undergoing final maturation and entering B-cell follicles (158,159); newly produced B cells make up between 5% and 10% of splenic B cells (159).

Differences in the usage of immunoglobulin (Ig) variable region genes between peripheral B cells and pre–B cells in the bone marrow has been taken as evidence that, as in positive and negative selection of T cells in the thymus, the peripheral B cell repertoire is generated through ligand-mediated selection processes (160). In this regard, self-reactive B cells can either be deleted or undergo a change in their specificity through a process of receptor editing (161); whether the cells die or change their specificity seems to depend on when the cells first encounter antigen and whether the antigen is cell associated or soluble (162–166). Whether B cells undergo positive selection to self-ligands is unclear, although B-cell deficiencies in a variety of mutant mouse strains suggest that the transition of immature splenic B cells into follicular B cells is an active process (167–176). Of note is that relatively normal generation of immature B cells but poor production of mature B cells are evident in mice deficient for a number of molecules associated with signaling through the B-cell receptor (BCR), including the tyrosine kinase Syk (170), Bruton's tyrosine kinase (Btk) (169,171,173), Igα (168), CD45 (167), and CD22 (172). The implication is therefore that B cells must be triggered through the BCR before completing their maturation process, although it is possible that selection is not ligand driven but is simply dependent on proper assembly of all signaling components. If an external ligand is involved, it appears to be independent of foreign antigen, inasmuch as a stable pool of peripheral B cells is generated in germ-free mice (177). Furthermore, entry into the mature peripheral pool is not accompanied by somatic mutations of Ig variable region genes, which distinguishes this process from an overt B-cell response to foreign antigens (see later discussion) (178). Interestingly, immature B cells predominate in mice deficient for B-cell activation factor (BAFF), a member of the tumor necrosis family, or its receptor on B cells, which implies that BAFF may guide the final stages of B-cell maturation in the spleen (174,175).

As for T cells, naïve B cells recirculate continuously between blood and lymph, and B-cell responses are initiated in secondary lymphoid organs (179). In LNs and the spleen, naïve B cells are anatomically segregated from T cells and localize primarily in follicles. Although it is unclear where naïve B cells first encounter antigen, antigen-binding proliferating B cells can be detected in the outer T-cell zones of LNs and the spleen within 2 days of immunization (180–182). In these locations, B cells, which internalize antigen bound to their BCRs, present antigenic peptides in association with class II MHC to activated CD4$^+$ helper T (Th) cells. Cell membrane–associated and soluble signals delivered from Th cells promote further B cell activation. Subsequently, some of the B cells proliferate and differentiate to form foci of antibody-forming cells (AFCs) in the area adjacent to the T-cell zone (the red pulp in the spleen or the medullary cords in LNs) (181,183,184). These cells do not mutate their Ig variable region genes and are short-lived, dying by apoptosis within 2 weeks of immunization (185,186). At the same time, other B cells migrate to follicles and initiate the germinal center (GC) reaction. It is within the GC that both memory B cells and AFCs secreting high-affinity, isotype-switched antibodies are generated (Fig. 4) (181,187–193).

Each GC is founded by a small number (1 to 20) of activated B cells (182,194). These cells proliferate extensively, dividing every 6 to 7 hours to generate GCs containing about 10^4 cells within a few days (195,196). After the initial period of expansion, the GC polarizes, separating into "dark" and "light" zones. The dark zone is densely packed with rapidly proliferating, surface immunoglobulin (sIg)–negative B cells that are known as centroblasts. It is at this sIg$^-$ stage that somatic hypermutation of Ig variable region genes is thought to take place (188,191–193,197,198). Centroblasts give rise to sIg$^+$, nonproliferating centrocytes that migrate into the adjacent light zone. Here, the centrocytes are tested for their ability to bind antigen, which is retained on the surface of follicular dendritic cells (FDCs) in the form of antibody-antigen complexes. Centrocytes bearing sIg with high affinity for

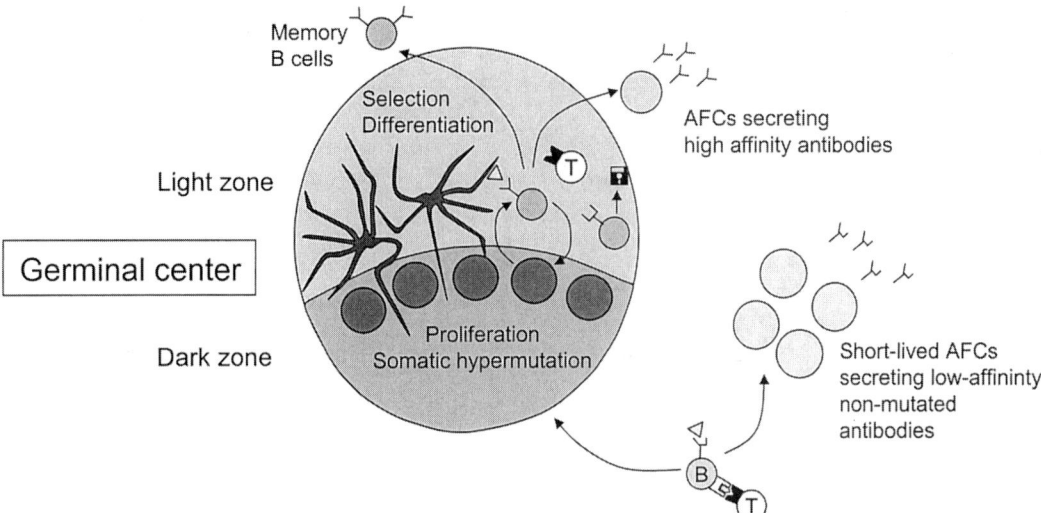

FIG. 4. Generation of memory B cells and antibody-forming cells (AFCs) during a T cell–dependent immune response. After internalization of antigen through the B-cell receptor and presentation of antigenic peptides to helper T cells, B cells either proliferate to form extrafollicular foci of AFCs or migrate to B-cell follicles and initiate the germinal center (GC) reaction. Within the dark zone of the GC, surface immunoglobulin–devoid (sIg⁻) centroblasts proliferate and introduce somatic mutations into their immunoglobulin variable region genes before giving rise to nonproliferating, sIg⁺ centrocytes in the light zone. Competition for antigen held on the surface of follicular dendritic cells (FDCs) leads to the selective survival of cells expressing sIg with high affinity for antigen; lower-affinity centrocytes die by apoptosis. On the basis of the signals derived from binding to antigen, and interactions with FDCs and helper T cells within the GC, high-affinity centrocytes differentiate into memory B cells or AFCs (see text for details).

antigen outcompete lower affinity cells and retrieve the FDC-bound antigen, which they subsequently internalize, process, and present in the form of class II MHC–associated peptides to Th cells within the GC (199). Survival signals are delivered to the B cell through sIg binding to antigen and from the Th cell (see later discussion). These cells may reenter the dark zone and undergo further rounds of mutation and selection or may differentiate into memory cells or AFCs and exit the GC, depending on other signals received (see later discussion). Centrocytes having insufficient affinity for antigen fail to receive survival signals and die by apoptosis (200), although some cells may reexpress the recombinase-activating genes in a final attempt to generate a useful immunoglobulin (201,202). B cells expressing sIg reactive with self-antigens are also deleted as a result of the absence of Th cells (203–205).

In contrast to the uncertainty surrounding the relationship between memory and effector T cells, it is clear that memory B cells and AFCs represent the products of distinct differentiation pathways. Thus, AFCs—which in their fully differentiated form exist as large sIg⁻ plasma cells—are nondividing cells specialized for secreting large quantities of antibody (206). These cells do not give rise to memory B cells, although memory B cells can further differentiate into AFCs upon secondary stimulation with antigen (207). The precise mechanisms governing the decision to form a memory B cell versus an AFC, however, are only poorly understood. Indeed, even the basic question of whether this decision is made before or after antigenic stimulation remains a matter of debate.

One theory for memory B cell generation holds that memory B cells and AFCs are derived from distinct precursors (208,209). Evidence supporting this idea has come largely from studies in which B cells from nonimmunized mice were fractionated on the basis of their cell surface expression of HSA and then challenged with antigen *in vitro* or *in vivo* (209–211). The key finding from this work was that the HSA^low population was enriched for progenitors of memory B cells and GC, whereas the HSA^int-high population contained mainly AFC precursors and was largely depleted of cells that could form GC. In addition, another study showed that HSA^low and HSA^high B cells differ in their use of Ig VH gene segments (212). In this study, investigation of the antiarsonate response in A/J mice, in which specific Ig idiotypes are associated with either the primary (CRI-C) or secondary (CRI-A) response, showed that transcripts for CRI-C and CRI-A were associated with HSA^high and HSA^low B cells, respectively, in unimmunized mice. Of importance is that the rearranged CRI-A genes were unmutated in naïve mice, which indicates that these cells represented memory cell precursors rather than preexisting memory B cells. Together, these findings imply that B cells may be committed toward a certain pathway of differentiation even before antigenic stimulation.

The more popular view is that memory B cells arise from the same precursor cells that produce AFCs (213). Support for this idea is provided by the demonstration of a common clonal origin of B cells proliferating in GC and extrafollicular foci (189). Nevertheless, this observation does not formally rule out the possibility that cell division yielding memory- versus AFC-committed precursors occurs before rather than after the response to antigen. If this were the case, however, there remains the question of what drives these cells to differentiate along these distinct developmental pathways.

More persuasive evidence that memory B cells and AFCs can arise from common precursors is derived from reports that different signals received by activated B cells can dictate cell fate. One signal that has been implicated in the generation of memory B cells is the ligation of CD40. Clear evidence of the importance of CD40–CD40 ligand (CD40L) interaction in T cell–dependent B-cell responses has come from studies showing that GC formation and memory B-cell generation fails to occur in CD40- or CD40L-deficient mice or in normal mice treated with reagents that block the CD40–CD40L interaction (214–220). At the same time, in vitro studies have suggested that at least one way in which CD40 ligation participates in memory B-cell generation is by acting at the level of GC B cells. Thus, it has been shown that treatment of GC B cells from human tonsils with anti-CD40 antibodies, trimeric CD40L, or CD40L-transfected cells promotes cell survival and the development of a memory B cell–like phenotype and simultaneously suppresses the differentiation of these cells into AFCs (221–225). Furthermore, it has been reported that CD4+ T cells present in GC light zones contain intracellular stores of preformed CD40L that can be rapidly expressed on the cell surface after T-cell activation (226). This is thought to occur when the T cells interact with centrocytes that have taken up antigen from the surface of FDC and presented the relevant peptide in association with class II MHC (199). Subsequent ligation of CD40 on the B cell may then lead to the delivery of a signal directing differentiation toward a memory B-cell fate. However, it is also possible that the memory-promoting CD40-mediated signal occurs before the GC reaction, inasmuch as T cells situated in the extrafollicular locations of initial T cell–B cell interaction also express CD40L (227). Consistent with this idea is the observation that treatment of mice with soluble CD40 immunoglobulin for the first 5 days after immunization blocked memory B-cell generation, whereas delaying the start of treatment until day 4 abrogated this effect (219).

Another B cell–signaling molecule that may participate in memory B-cell generation is CD19. CD19 associates with various other molecules on the B cell surface, including the type 2 complement receptor (CR2, CD21), CD81, Leu-13, and sIg (228–230). CD19 can function as a co-stimulatory molecule for B cells by lowering the threshold for B-cell activation through sIg (231). In addition, it is thought that CD19, which associates through its intracellular domain with the protein tyrosine kinases Lyn and Fyn, acts as a signal transducer for CR2, which has a very short cytoplasmic domain (232,233). Evidence that CD19 plays a key role in B-cell responses has come from studies in CD19-deficient mice, which exhibit impaired antibody responses and impaired GC formation in response to immunization with T cell–dependent protein antigens (234,235). Notably, these mice mount a strong primary antibody response and develop GC after infection with certain viruses (236). However, despite the presence of GC, memory B cells are greatly reduced in CD19-deficient mice, which implies that CD19 is essential for generation or maintenance of these cells, or both.

Differentiation of B cells into AFCs may involve signaling through OX40 ligand (OX40L), which is expressed on activated but not resting B cells (107). In support of this idea, initial studies showed that cross-linking OX40L on prestimulated murine B cells in vitro enhanced both proliferation and Ig secretion (111). Later, it was reported that injection of blocking antibodies against OX40 strongly inhibited the antihapten IgG response, although IgM production was not affected (237). Of note was that anti-OX40 treatment did not inhibit either GC formation or memory B-cell generation, which implies a specific role for OX40 in AFC differentiation rather than a more general role in B-cell activation. Furthermore, T cells expressing the highest levels of OX40 were detected 3 days after immunization and were situated close to antigen-specific B cells in the T-cell zones of the spleen.

However, subsequent work with gene-knockout mice has indicated that OX40 is in fact not required for generation of AFCs (113,114). Humoral immune responses, including generation of extrafollicular AFCs, were normal in both OX40- and OX40L-deficient mice. How can the differences between these results and the data derived from antibody injection experiments be reconciled? One possibility, suggested by Kopf et al. (114), is that anti-OX40 antibody does not simply block the OX40–OX40L interaction but rather may deliver a signal to Th cells. The authors proposed that such signaling may cause CD4+ T cells to migrate into B-cell follicles and thus inhibit the formation of extrafollicular foci of AFCs. In support of the idea that OX40 ligation induces T-cell migration to follicles, CD4+ T cells accumulate in B-cell areas after immunization of transgenic mice expressing OX40L on DCs (238).

In addition to cell-surface molecules, cytokines can have a marked influence on B-cell differentiation. In this respect, CD40-activated human B cells differentiate into AFCs after culture in the presence IL-3 and IL-10, whereas with IL-4, the cells proliferate extensively but do not form AFCs (223,239,240). In addition, IL-6 has been shown to stimulate terminal differentiation of B cells into AFCs, an activity that is associated with induction of cell cycle arrest (241).

Finally, differentiation of centrocytes into memory B cells versus AFCs may be dictated by interactions between B cells and particular APCs. Here, myeloid DCs are of interest because they promote the survival of splenic and LN plasmablasts and their differentiation into plasma cells (242). Likewise, FDCs could be important because, in addition to acting as a depot for antigen, FDCs are known to supply a variety of signals to GC B cells. Thus, GC B cell–FDC interaction promotes cross-linking of LFA-1 (CD11a/CD18), very late antigen 4 (CD49d), and CD21 on the B cell surface through contact with ICAM-1 (CD54), vascular cell adhesion molecule 1 (CD106), and CD23, respectively, expressed on the FDC (222,243–246). These interactions, as well as other undefined signals delivered by FDCs, have been shown to promote the survival or enhance the proliferation, or both, of GC B cells *in vitro* (247–249); the *in vitro* responses are thought to reflect the *in vivo* role of FDCs in maintaining the GC reaction. In addition, some FDC-associated signals have been shown to favor the production of AFCs from GC B cells *in vitro.* One of these is signaling through CD23, which was shown to promote AFC development when added in soluble form, together with IL-1α, to tonsillar GC B cells (222). More recently it was shown that an antibody raised against a novel FDC-expressed surface molecule (8D6) blocked the production of AFCs in cultures containing GC B cells and an FDC cell line, which implies a role for this molecule in directing the differentiation of B cells into AFCs (250).

In considering the *in vitro* data favoring a role for particular T cell or FDC molecules in dictating the fate of GC B cells, it should be borne in mind that these molecules could act largely by enhancing the survival of GC B cells that had previously received differentiation signals *in vivo* rather than by inducing differentiation per se. In this regard, it is notable that GC B cells are highly prone to apoptosis *in vitro.* This is associated with low-level expression of the antiapoptotic molecule Bcl-2 and high-level expression of proapoptotic proteins such as Fas, Bax, and p53 (251–253). The susceptibility of GC B cells to apoptosis *in vitro* is presumed to reflect a similar sensitivity *in vivo,* an idea that is supported by evidence of a high level of apoptosis within GC. It then follows that generation of memory B cells and AFCs is linked to a selection process that provides both survival and differentiation signals.

Although the precise pathways leading to death of GC cells *in vivo* are unknown, both Bcl-2 and Fas have been implicated in this process. A role for Bcl-2 in rescue of GC cells was originally suggested by the observation that there is an anatomical segregation of Bcl-2 expression in GC that is consistent with selective up-regulation of Bcl-2 in B cells that have received a survival signal (252). In this study, histochemical staining in tissue sections of human tonsils revealed that Bcl-2 expression in the GC was restricted to the apical light zone, a location in which selection of centrocytes expressing sIg with high affinity for antigen is thought to occur. Also in line with this idea are *in vitro* studies showing that expression of Bcl-2 is increased after treatment of GC B cells with various stimuli that support their survival *in vitro,* including antibodies to sIg, anti-CD40, and a combination of IL-1 and soluble CD23 (254). Furthermore, direct support for the participation of Bcl-2 in rescuing GC B cells from apoptosis *in vivo* has come from the analysis of mice expressing transgenic Bcl-2 in their B cells (255–258). In comparison with control mice, Bcl-2 transgenic mice have increased numbers of memory B cells and AFCs after immunization.

The fact that both memory B cells and AFCs are increased in Bcl-2 transgenic mice suggests that Bcl-2 can rescue cells of both lineages from apoptosis. This is consistent with either (a) action of Bcl-2 as an antiapoptotic factor for uncommitted centrocyte precursors or (b) Bcl-2 promotion of survival of centrocytes committed to both lineages. However, it is notable that an enrichment of low-affinity cells has been detected among memory B cells, but not among AFCs, in Bcl-2 transgenic mice (258). This observation has two important implications. First, it suggests that Bcl-2 can provide a survival signal for memory B cells that have failed to compete for access to antigen or Th cells. Second, the failure to generate low-affinity AFCs in these mice implies that either (a) differentiation into AFCs requires a strong signal through the BCR or (b) death of low-affinity cells of the plasma cell lineage may occur through a mechanism that cannot be rescued by Bcl-2. In this regard, it is interesting to note that there is an enrichment of AFCs that secrete low-affinity antibodies in mice with transgenic B-cell expression of another antiapoptotic Bcl-2 family member, Bcl-xL (259). Like Bcl-2, expression of Bcl-xL is increased after stimulation of B cells through cross-linking of sIg or CD40 (260,261). Furthermore, it has been shown that Bcl-xL is expressed in human GC centrocytes at the stage when clonal selection is thought to occur (262). Therefore, the available data imply that, both for memory B cells and AFC generation, expression of Bcl-2 or Bcl-xL can rescue GC B cells that would otherwise die through their inability to compete for antigen. Nevertheless, it should be emphasized that it remains unclear whether the results of artificially up-regulating Bcl-2 or Bcl-xL are applicable to B-cell selection in the normal GC reaction.

The participation of Fas in the death of GC B cells is suggested by the finding that human GC B cells appear to be poised for Fas-mediated death (263). Thus, Fas is associated intracellularly with a death-inducing signaling complex (DISC) in GC B cells. The preassembly of DISC components allows for the rapid delivery of an apoptotic signal upon triggering of Fas (264). Interestingly, however, DISC in freshly isolated GC B cells is in an inactive form, owing to its inclusion of the apoptosis-inhibiting molecule c-FLIP (265). Upon placement of the cells in culture, c-FLIP is rapidly lost from DISC, coincident with apoptosis of the cells. Of note is that dissociation of c-FLIP from DISC in GC B cells is prevented by ligation of CD40 or by coculture with FDCs (263,266); B cells can also acquire resistance to Fas-mediated death through engagement of the BCR (267). Furthermore, *in vivo* evidence that Fas-induced death may have a role in the selection of GC B cells has come from the finding that immunization of Fas-deficient lpr mice leads to higher numbers of memory B cells than in control mice (268). Of interest is that the memory B cells generated in lpr mice show an enrichment for heavily mutated Ig genes, which implies that clonal selection in the GC is altered in the absence of Fas.

Although the primary stimuli directing activated B cells toward a memory B cell or AFC fate remain to be elucidated, more is known about the downstream signaling events required for cellular differentiation. In particular, there is clear evidence for the involvement of specific transcription factors in this process. Two transcription factors that have been implicated in plasma cell differentiation are B-lymphocyte–induced maturation protein-1 and X-box–binding protein 1 (XBP-1) (269,270). Both of these factors are expressed in plasma cells and initiate plasma cell differentiation when introduced into B-lineage cells. Moreover, secretion of immunoglobulin and generation of plasma cells is largely absent after immunization of mice lacking functional expression of XBP-1 in lymphoid cells, even though B cells proliferate, secrete cytokines, and form GCs in normal numbers (270). This finding indicates that expression of XBP-1 may be mandatory for plasma cell differentiation. Conversely, another transcription factor, B cell–specific activator protein (BSAP), is expressed at all stages of B-cell differentiation except the plasma cell stage (271). BSAP has been shown to down-regulate expression of XBP-1, which suggests that BSAP actively blocks generation of plasma cells (272). In this regard, it is interesting to note that CD40L, which suppresses the development of AFCs, up-regulates expression of BSAP in B cells, whereas OX40L, which promotes the generation of AFCs, down-regulates BSAP expression (273).

In summary, it has been somewhat easier to study the mechanisms involved in the generation of B-cell memory than those in T-cell memory for two main reasons. First, B-cell memory is generated in a well-defined microenvironment within the secondary lymphoid tissues—namely, GC. This has allowed for direct examination of the memory B cell–generating response *in situ* as well as isolation of GC B cells and analysis of memory and AFC generation *in vitro*. Second, plasma cells and memory B cells exhibit clearly distinct phenotypes and represent separate outcomes of the immune response. For this reason, it has been possible to identify molecules expressed specifically by one lineage or the other and to investigate stimuli that influence this differentiation. Nevertheless, the key signals that determine whether a B cell will become a memory B cell or an AFC and the stage at which these signals are delivered remain poorly understood.

IDENTIFYING MEMORY CELLS

Identification of memory cells is clearly of crucial importance for understanding how these cells are generated and maintained and for examining their functional characteristics. The assumption that these cells can be identified as a discrete subset is based on the idea that memory cells carry a permanent imprint of having previously responded to antigen. For this reason, many of the cellular characteristics that have been employed as indicators for memory cells are surface marker changes that occur in response to lymphocyte activation. Although these markers have been useful for enriching memory cell populations, the discovery of definitive memory cell markers has so far been elusive. Five main facts have contributed to the difficulty in identifying memory cells: (a) Many of the markers that are expressed by previously activated lymphocytes do not distinguish between recently activated effectors and long-lived memory cells; (b) phenotypic changes that occur upon lymphocyte activation may be transient, with the result that memory cells revert to a naïve phenotype with time; (c) some cells may fail to acquire typical activation markers when stimulated with antigen; (d) naïve cells may express markers of activation without having responded to antigen; and (e) memory cells appear to be heterogeneous with regard to both phenotype and function.

These issues have particularly complicated the identification of memory T cells, but they also apply to B cells. Notwithstanding these difficulties, a brief description of the markers that have been associated with memory T and B cells is given as follows.

Identification of Memory T Cells

Attempts to discover markers for memory T cells have focussed on cell surface molecules that differ in expression between bona fide naïve T cells and previously activated T cells. By comparing the phenotypes of T cells that are presumed not to have encountered antigen (e.g., in umbilical cord blood or germ-free mice), T cells that have been acutely activated with antigen, and T cells that mediate a recall response in previously immunized individuals, a number of molecules have been identified as putative markers of memory cells. Extensive work over many years has shown that the utility of these markers varies with animal species, CD4+ versus CD8+ T cells, and even the specific immune response being studied.

Many of the molecules reported to be up-regulated on the surface of memory T cells are adhesion molecules. These include β1 (CD49d, CD49e, CD29) and β2 (CD11a, CD11b, CD18) integrins; CD2; CD44; CD54; and CD58 (79,274–283). To a degree, the detection of increased levels of adhesion molecules on "memory" T cells may reflect the presence of cells that have recently responded to antigen. In accordance with this idea, human memory-phenotype T cells express some markers of activation and are slightly larger than typical naïve T cells (280). However, at least one adhesion molecule, CD44, appears to be a long-term marker of memory T cells. Thus, murine memory CD8+ T cells retain a CD44hi phenotype indefinitely after adoptive transfer to recipient mice in the absence of antigen (284,285). For this reason, high surface expression of CD44 is commonly used as a marker of memory-phenotype CD8+ T cells in the mouse. CD44 is also used to distinguish between naïve and memory CD4+ T cells, although the stability of CD44 expression on memory CD4+ T cells is less certain; in at least one report, these cells reverted to a CD44lo phenotype (286).

Increased cell surface expression of adhesion molecules would be expected to influence the ability of memory T cells to interact with other cells and with the extracellular matrix. An increased ability to form such interactions may contribute to the migration pattern of memory T cells, which appears to differ substantially from that of naïve T cells (at least for a subset of memory cells, as discussed further later). Thus, rather than being restricted to entering LNs from the bloodstream through HEV, some memory-phenotype T cells are capable of extravasating into tissues before entering LNs through afferent lymph (278). This altered migration pattern is also influenced by other cell surface changes on memory T cells. In particular, both CD62L and CCR7 are down-regulated on some memory T cells (88,287–289). Loss of these molecules abrogates the ability of T cells to adhere to HEV and migrate into LNs in response to secondary lymphoid-tissue chemokine.

However, it should be pointed out that both CD62L and CCR7 are heterogeneously expressed among memory T cells (88,286–295). For CD62L, this heterogeneity appears to reflect reexpression of CD62L on cells that were negative or low for cell surface CD62L after their initial activation (286,293,296). In contrast, it is currently unclear whether the expression of CCR7 on a proportion of memory T cells is caused by phenotypic reversion of CCR7$^-$ cells or by variable retention of CCR7 on the surface of T cells after activation. Nevertheless, recent data provide strong support for the idea that reexpression of CCR7 can occur, at least on CD8$^+$ T cells (101). CCR7 was undetectable among antigen-specific CD8$^+$ T cells 7 days after infection of mice with *L. monocytogenes* but was expressed 21 days after infection. Because CCR7 expression was detected at the messenger RNA level in these experiments, the question of whether CCR7 was expressed by all or only a subset of memory CD8$^+$ cells was not addressed.

Whatever the mechanism, it is interesting to note that the CCR7$^-$ and CCR7$^+$ memory T cells detected in human peripheral blood express very different patterns of homing/adhesion molecules (88). In particular, CCR7$^-$ cells express high levels of β1 and β2 integrins and CLA, a molecule involved in lymphocyte homing to skin, as well as receptors for a number of inflammatory chemokines (CCR1, CCR3, CCR5). In contrast, CCR7$^+$ memory cells express lower levels of integrins, lack CLA, and express chemokine receptors involved in homing to lymphoid tissues (CCR4, CCR6, CXCR3). These findings have led to the proposal considered earlier that CCR7$^+$ central memory cells, like naïve T cells, recirculate through the lymphoid organs, whereas CCR7$^-$ effector memory cells migrate through inflamed tissues. In reality, the heterogeneity among memory T cells may be even more extensive, with cells specialized for particular effector functions or for homing to specific tissues exhibiting distinct phenotypes. This level of complexity is suggested by studies showing heterogeneous expression of different homing receptors and integrins on human T cells (297,298). In the future, characterizing unique combinations of chemokine receptors on memory cells may prove useful for defining the precise microenvironment in which these cells localize. In this regard, a subset of circulating CD4$^+$ memory T cells has been shown to express CXCR5 (299). Because a ligand for this receptor (B-lymphocyte chemoattractant) is expressed by stromal cells in B-cell follicles, CXCR5$^+$ memory cells may be specialized for homing to follicles and providing B-cell help (300–302).

Another cell surface molecule that has been commonly used to distinguish between naïve and memory T cells is CD45. The usefulness of CD45 as a memory marker stems from the fact that multiple isoforms of CD45 can be generated through differential splicing of three extracellular exons, A, B, and C (303), and that these isoforms are differentially expressed on naïve and memory T cells (276,278,287,304–310). Thus, in many species, naïve T cells express the highest molecular weight isoform of CD45, which contains all three variably spliced exons, whereas memory cells are enriched among cells expressing lower molecular weight forms (CD45RO in humans). Typically, the phenotype of T cells is described on the basis of reactivity with monoclonal antibodies specific for restricted (R) isoforms of CD45. For example, naïve and memory human T cells are considered to be CD45RA$^+$ and CD45RA$^-$ (CD45R0$^+$), respectively. Likewise, in mice, naïve T cells are CD45RB$^+$, whereas memory cells are typically CD45RB$^-$.

However, as for other putative memory markers, there is heterogeneity in the expression of low–molecular weight isoforms of CD45 on memory T cells (88,289,311–318). This appears to be largely a result of reexpression of high–molecular weight CD45 after its initial down-regulation, which occurs at different rates on CD4$^+$ versus CD8$^+$ cells and is species dependent (311,313,319–322). In the rat, in which loss of expression of CD45RC has been used as a memory marker, phenotypic reversion occurs very rapidly. Thus, CD45RC$^-$ CD4$^+$ T cells regain a CD45RC$^+$ phenotype within 1 week of injection into congenic rats in the absence of antigen (311,313). The implication here is that down-regulation of CD45RC is strictly dependent on recent contact with antigen. This is in contrast to the situation in mice, in which CD4$^+$ memory cells have been shown to maintain a CD45RB$^{lo/-}$ phenotype for at least 10 weeks in the absence of antigen (322).

For human memory T cells, reexpression of CD45RA may not be simply a reflection of loss of contact with antigen. Some CD45RA$^+$ CD8$^+$ T cells in peripheral blood exhibit the properties of activated effector cells (283). These cells, which express high levels of adhesion molecules but lack CD62L, CD28, and CD27, have high cytolytic activity without *in vitro* prestimulation. Their state of activation suggests that these cells have recently encountered antigen, although it remains unclear whether these cells have reexpressed CD45RA (despite continued antigenic stimulation) or simply retained expression from the time of activation. Interestingly, however, the number of CD28$^-$ CD45RA$^+$ CD8$^+$ T cells appears to increase with age, which suggests that cells with this phenotype may arise from chronic antigenic stimulation (323). In support of this idea, accumulation of CD28$^-$ CD45RA$^+$ CD8$^+$ T cells in the elderly is associated with seropositive responses to cytomegalovirus (324). Loss of CD27 expression has also been suggested to occur on chronically stimulated CD4$^+$ T cells, although these cells retain a CD45RA$^-$ phenotype (325). Nevertheless, equivalent responses to human rhinovirus among CD45RA$^+$ and CD45R0$^+$ CD4$^+$ T cells isolated from human tonsils suggest that CD45RA expression can be present on chronic or intermittently stimulated CD4$^+$ T cells (317).

In addition to the molecules just described, studies in mice have revealed a number of other cell surface markers that differ between naïve and memory T cells. The two phenotypic changes that appear to be most stable on memory cells are increased expression of Ly-6C and CD122; both of these serve as markers for CD8$^+$ but not CD4$^+$ T cells (326–329). Ly-6C is a low–molecular weight glycosylphosphatidylinositol-anchored cell surface protein that has been proposed to participate in intercellular adhesion, signaling, or both (330). At present, no ligand for this molecule has been identified, and its *in vivo* function remains unknown. As mentioned earlier, CD122 (IL-2Rβ) is a component of the receptors for both IL-2 and IL-15 (331). In view of the possible role of IL-15 in the generation (see previous discussion) or maintenance (see later discussion) of CD8$^+$ T cell memory, elevated expression of CD122 on memory cells may be of functional significance. Of note, however, is that a proportion (30%) of memory-phenotype CD8$^+$ T cells in normal mice are CD122^{lo}, and these cells predominate in IL-15–deficient mice (53).

Overall, the identification of memory T cells remains imprecise. This is in part because of the heterogeneity of memory cells, which is apparent at the level of cell surface phenotype. To what extent phenotypic heterogeneity reflects the existence of true subsets of differentiated memory T cells or, conversely, is an indicator of how recently cells have encountered antigen remains uncertain. In this regard, an inherent obstacle to the detection of memory T cells is an inability to distinguish these cells from effector cells (as discussed previously), because many of the cell surface markers for memory cells are expressed soon after T-cell activation. For CD8$^+$ cells, a change in surface glycosylation is proving useful for separating effector cells from resting memory cells. Thus, activation of CD8$^+$ cells is accompanied by desialylation of core 1 O-glycans and induction of core 2 O-glycan synthesis (332,333), whereas significant resialylation of core 1 O-glycans and a reduction in core 2 O-glycans occurs upon differentiation of activated CD8$^+$ cells into memory cells (334,335). On this basis, effector and memory CD8$^+$ cells can be distinguished by an antibody, 1B11, which binds to the CD43 molecule only when it has been modified by core 2 O-glycans (336). However, it is important to bear in mind that even in the absence of antigenic stimulation, memory T cells appear to be more metabolically active and less "resting" than typical naïve T cells, periodically entering cell cycle and undergoing activation in response to cytokines (see later discussion). Hence, even markers of recent activation may be insufficient to differentiate effector and memory T cells.

Another factor that complicates the identification of memory T cells is the fact that naïve T cells can, at least under experimental conditions, express a "memory phenotype" in the apparent absence of antigenic stimulation. This has been shown to occur after the adoptive transfer of small numbers of naïve T cells into lymphopenic recipients in several different mouse models (337–345). In this situation, naïve T cells exhibit a slow rate of proliferation that is dependent on their ability to interact with self-MHC/peptide complexes. This response, homeostatic proliferation, is distinct from that induced by antigenic stimulation in that the peptides being recognized represent low-affinity TCR ligands that may be related to the peptides involved in positive selection in the thymus (337,338,341). In addition to MHC and peptide, homeostatic proliferation is dependent on cytokines, particularly IL-7 and IL-4 (102,105,346). Notably, T cells proliferating in this way take on many of the characteristics of typical memory cells, including (for CD8$^+$ T cells) up-regulation of CD44, CD122, and Ly-6C and the ability to rapidly secrete IFN-γ and become cytotoxic effectors when stimulated with cognate antigen. Whether these changes are permanent or transient is an unresolved issue. In one study, the T cells stopped dividing and reacquired the characteristics of naïve T cells when the cellularity of the host lymphoid compartment was restored (342), whereas in another study, the transferred cells retained a memory phenotype indefinitely (344). More important, it is unclear whether homeostatic proliferation contributes to the formation of the pool of memory-phenotype T cells present in normal mice. However, very few memory-phenotype T cells are observed in germ-free mice (309) or in most TCR transgenic mice in the absence of challenge with specific antigen [for examples, see Rogers et al. (347), Saparov et al. (348), and Sepulveda et al. (349)], which would argue that most memory-phenotype T cells are generated through antigenic rather than homeostatic stimulation. Nevertheless, it remains possible that phenotypic conversion in the absence of antigen could make a substantial contribution to the memory pool during conditions of lymphopenia.

Identification of Memory B Cells

Identification of memory B cells is more straightforward than for memory T cells for two main reasons. First, memory B cells are clearly distinct from fully differentiated plasma cells. Thus, as described previously, these two cell types represent the products of separate differentiation pathways. Furthermore, memory B cells and plasma cells are phenotypically very different: Memory B cells are small and express surface immunoglobulin and class II MHC, whereas plasma cells are large and generally lack surface immunoglobulin and MHC class II (350,351).

Second, memory B cells are easily distinguished from naïve B cells by multiple parameters. For example, somatic hypermutation of Ig genes is prominent in memory B cells but largely undetectable in naïve B cells (193,352,353) [although in some species, such as sheep, hypermutation is involved in generating the primary Ig repertoire in an antigen-independent manner (354)]. Clearly, there are practical limitations to isolating memory B cells on the basis of sequencing rearranged Ig genes. Nevertheless, the fact that somatic mutation is a bona fide distinction between memory and naïve

B cells is useful for retrospective analysis of memory markers—that is, as evidence for the presence of memory B cells in cell populations separated on the basis of putative cell surface memory markers. One caveat to this approach, however, is that some cells exiting GC may bear unmutated Ig (BCR) genes (355), presumably because some germline-encoded BCR have sufficient affinity for antigen to compete successfully with mutated BCR.

Because most memory B cells undergo Ig class switching in response to antigen, typical memory B cells express Ig isotypes other than IgM or IgD (356–358). However, Ig class switching is not an inevitable consequence of B-cell activation. In this regard, work in mice (358–360), rats (361), and humans (362–366) has demonstrated the existence of sIgM+ memory B cells. In fact, in human peripheral blood, more than half of the B cells carrying mutated variable region genes are sIgM+ (366). Notably the majority of these cells also express sIgD.

In contrast, human B-cell expression of two other cell surface molecules, CD27 and CD148, correlates very closely with the presence of somatically mutated variable region genes, irrespective of sIg isotype; this was shown to be true for peripheral blood cells and splenic B cells (366,367). Of note is that there are very few CD27+ B cells in cord blood, which is consistent with the idea that expression of this molecule is dependent on prior exposure to antigen (368,369). Direct comparisons of CD27+ and CD27− B cells revealed that the former cells expressed lower levels of CD23 and higher levels of CD21, CD39, CD70, CD80, CD86, and sIgM or sIgA (366,367,369–371). In addition, CD27+ B cells are slightly larger than CD27− cells and have been shown to differentiate more rapidly into AFCs when stimulated *in vitro* (367,369,370); the latter property has been noted for memory B cells isolated from tonsils (372).

In mice, markers that have been used to identify memory B cells include CD44 (373) and HSA (374,375). As for T cells, CD44 is up-regulated upon B-cell activation and is expressed at high levels on short-term IgG-secreting cells as well as on long-term antigen-primed cells (373). Conversely, HSA expression increases after initial B-cell activation and

remains high on antibody-secreting cells, whereas memory B cells are HSA^{low} (374,375). In addition, changes in HSA expression appear to correlate with the history of antigen exposure: immature, recent bone marrow–emigrant B cells express very high levels of HSA (156,376), and overall HSA expression on B cells decreases as mice age (375). Of note is that HSA expression on B cells is maintained in germ-free and nude mice, which is consistent with the notion that HSA down-regulation is a result of T cell–dependent immune responses (375).

Although most memory B cells have an HSA^{low} phenotype, HSA expression may not be a definitive memory marker. As described earlier, some workers argue that precursors of memory B cells are HSA^{low} (208–211). Furthermore, studies have shown that some memory B cells express higher levels of HSA than naïve B cells (377). Clearly, other markers are needed to define memory B cells. On this point, it is notable that IgM−IgD−IgG+ memory B cells include both B-220^{hi}CD19+ and B-220−CD19− cells, whereas B-220− cells can be further divided into CD11b^{++}IgG+ and CD11b+IgE+ subsets (377,378). This finding implies that memory B cells show considerable phenotypic heterogeneity.

FACTORS CONTRIBUTING TO MEMORY

The factors contributing to the intensity of memory responses can be grouped into three categories: (a) continued expression of effector activity, (b) systemic differences between the memory and naïve state, and (c) altered properties of memory cells on a per-cell basis (Table 2). These factors are discussed in turn.

Continued Expression of Effector Activity

As discussed, antibody secretion can continue indefinitely after infection or vaccination. In addition, although most direct effector T-cell activity disappears after the resolution of the acute immune response, some T cells exhibiting the characteristics of effector T cells can be detected long after

TABLE 2. *Factors contributing to immunological memory*

Features	Naïve T and B cells	T memory Central	T memory Effector	Humoral immunity B memory	Humoral immunity Plasma cells
Distribution	Blood-to-lymph recirculation	Blood-to-lymph recirculation	Blood, spleen, mucosal tissues	Blood-to-lymph recirculation	Sessile (gut and marrow)
Frequency of cells specific for given antigen	Very low	High	High	High	High
Affinity for antigen	Low	High^a	High^a	High^b	High^b
Direct effector activity	−	−	+	−	+

^{a}Affinity maturation: selective expansion and survival of cells derived from high-affinity naïve precursors.
^{b}Somatic hypermutation: selective survival of high-affinity mutants.

the infection has been cleared (329,379–384). As discussed earlier, these cells are now commonly referred to as effector memory cells and are particularly prominent at mucosal sites (60,62,385). Whether such continued expression of effector activity should be classified as a "memory" function depends in part on the type of memory being considered. In terms of protection against reinfection, preexisting effector activity is of obvious importance for inducing an immediate response to the pathogen. Although not essential for the rapid generation of a secondary immune response, preexisting effectors may have important consequences for how the antigen is seen during the secondary response. For example, rapid clearance of the antigen/pathogen by effector T cells may dramatically reduce the amount of antigen seen by other immune cells, and binding of the antigen by high-affinity, isotype-switched antibodies influences its capture and presentation by APCs. Therefore, these factors need to be borne in mind in considering the contribution of continued effector activity to the secondary response.

Systemic Differences between the Memory and Naïve State

Two systemic features of memory cells cause secondary responses to pathogens to be more effective than primary responses. First, the frequency of antigen-specific T and B memory cells is much higher than that of naïve cells (12,14,15,34,386–392). This increase in frequency confers a strong kinetic advantage during the secondary response; thus, in contrast to the primary response, only a few cell divisions are needed to generate large numbers of effector cells in the secondary response. Second, unlike naïve T cells, effector memory T cells make rapid contact with pathogens, through their ability to migrate into inflamed tissues, and accumulate at mucosal sites (60,62,88,99,278,393,394). In this regard, it is well documented that subpopulations of memory T cells possess the capacity to migrate preferentially to different tissues: for example, the gut versus skin (297,298,393,395–398). This tissue-specific homing ability is linked to the expression of unique combinations of adhesion molecules and chemokine receptors and may be related to the initial conditions of activation (397–399).

Localization within peripheral tissues allows memory T cells to make immediate contact with pathogens at their site of entry. In view of the ability of effector memory cells to rapidly express effector activity (88,380) (see previous discussion), this type of local memory response presumably has a much shorter lag time between infection and T cell–mediated clearance of the pathogen than does a primary immune response, in which T cells must first respond and expand in secondary lymphoid organs before migrating to the periphery. In this respect, there is evidence that CD4+ memory T cells that persist in the lung after Sendai virus infection of mice mediate strong protection against secondary infection (394). Such protection is presumably a reflection of both

an increased frequency of antigen-specific cells and the less stringent activation requirements for T memory cells (see later discussion). Local responses by memory cells are likely to be restricted to the subset of effector memory cells. Like naïve T cells, central memory cells are relatively quiescent and need to be activated by antigens in the secondary lymphoid organs before contacting pathogens in mucosal sites.

Altered distribution of effector and memory cells in comparison with naïve cells is also a characteristic of B-cell memory. For AFCs, their localization is linked to their mode of effector activity, which differs from that of effector T cells in two key aspects. First, AFCs do not require contact with antigen in order to exert their effector activity; rather, they constitutively secrete antibodies. Second, because antibodies act systemically, AFCs do not require close contact with antigen. For these reasons, AFCs localize in highly vascularized regions that optimize systemic distribution of antibody, notably in the bone marrow, the red pulp of the spleen, the LN medulla, and the lamina propria of the gut (185,400–403).

Recall responses of memory B cells are dependent on T-cell help (404), thus restricting the generation of B-cell memory responses to secondary lymphoid organs. Nevertheless, the distribution of memory B cells within these organs is somewhat different than for naïve B cells. In particular, a population of somatically mutated memory B cells is found in the marginal zone of the spleen (which separates B-cell follicles from the red pulp) and also in extrafollicular areas of LN (361,367,405–408). The memory B cells in the splenic marginal zone apparently do not recirculate (409,410) but migrate rapidly to the T-cell zone after reexposure to antigen (182,361). Localization in the marginal zone may afford memory cells rapid access to blood-borne antigens, inasmuch as these areas of the spleen are perfused by blood sinusoids (411). Similarly, the marginal zone–like extrafollicular areas of LN enable rapid contact of memory B cells with antigen. In mucosal lymphoid organs, in which antigen influx occurs across a mucosal epithelium, memory B cells can be found in the intraepithelial areas (412,413).

Unlike the population of memory B cells resident in the marginal zone, other subsets of memory B cells recirculate between blood and lymph (414–420). As for memory T cells, there is heterogeneity in the expression of homing receptors among recirculating memory B cells, which suggests the existence of subpopulations of cells with preferential homing to different tissues (421–425). Thus, sIgA+ memory B cells express the $\alpha 4\beta 7$ integrin, a receptor for vascular mucosal addressin cell adhesion molecule 1, which is required for lymphocyte homing to Peyer's patches and intestinal lamina propria (426–428). Although homing to these sites is $\alpha 4\beta 7$ dependent, sIgA+ memory cells show heterogeneity in the expression of $\alpha 4\beta 7$ and other homing receptors, which suggests further subspecialization in their ability to home to different mucosal sites (425). Extensive recirculation through mucosal sites presumably allows memory B cells to make rapid contact with pathogens during secondary infection. In addition, memory B cells may be intrinsically more mobile than naïve B cells: In rats, memory B cells reenter the thoracic duct more rapidly than naïve B cells upon intravenous injection (415,417).

Altered Properties of Memory Cells on a Per-Cell Basis

In addition to the systemic differences in frequency and distribution just discussed, for T cells there is considerable evidence that memory cells respond to antigen in a qualitatively different way than do naïve cells. Much of the early work on this topic centered on comparing the responses of naïve- and memory-phenotype T cells to mitogens, mitogenic antibodies, or allogeneic stimuli; use of these surrogate antigens was necessary at the time because of the very low frequency of naïve T cells against any particular antigen. In general, these studies showed that memory-phenotype T cells were more easily activated, were less dependent on co-stimulation, and secreted a much broader range of cytokines than did naïve-phenotype cells (274,309,390,429–436). However, it was difficult to draw firm conclusions regarding the responsiveness of memory T cells from these experiments because of the relatively unphysiological stimuli employed and uncertainty surrounding the use of phenotypic markers to distinguish memory cells from effectors.

Subsequently, the availability of TCR transgenic mice has made it possible to isolate naïve T cells of known specificity in large numbers and to compare their response to antigen with that of memory T cells expressing the same TCR. Numerous studies utilizing this approach to characterize both CD4$^+$ and CD8$^+$ T cell responses (both *in vitro* and *in vivo*) have been reported. The most consistent observation, which applies to both CD4$^+$ and CD8$^+$ cells, is that memory T cells express effector functions (e.g., cytolytic activity or secretion of cytokines other than IL-2) much more rapidly than do naïve cells upon restimulation with antigen (329,383,437–441). Nevertheless, other proposed attributes of memory T cells, including a lower threshold for antigenic stimulation and an ability to enter cell cycle faster than naïve T cells after stimulation, are more questionable. For example, some studies reported that memory T cells can respond to lower concentrations of antigen than can naïve T cells (82,83,328,441,442), whereas others failed to detect any difference between these cells (437,438,440). Likewise, there are discrepancies on whether memory T cells proliferate faster (439,443) or with the same kinetics (440) as naïve T cells and whether the magnitude of the *in vivo* response of memory cells is greater than (81,443) or equivalent (440) to that of naïve cells.

Several factors may contribute to these discrepancies. First, because different TCR transgenics were utilized in these studies, the affinity of the TCRs for their respective peptide/MHC ligands may have varied considerably. This could contribute to the conflicting results if a lowered threshold of responsiveness is detected only when the TCR is of relatively low affinity. Second, the nature of the *in vivo* challenge may determine whether differences are observed in the response by naïve versus memory T cells. For example, a weak stimulus such as immunization with cells expressing a minor histocompatibility difference (e.g., H-Y) might be more likely to favor an enhanced response by memory cells than a would potent stimulus such as a virus infection. Finally, the properties of memory cells could be heavily influenced by how these cells were initially primed. As discussed previously, there appears to be considerable heterogeneity amongst memory T cells, which could be related to the particular conditions encountered during initial activation or the duration of contact with antigen. Hence, the response observed could depend crucially on the ratio of central and effector memory cells within the population being studied.

In this respect, it is of interest to determine whether the accelerated expression of effector activity that has been described for memory T cells applies to both central and effector memory cells or only to effector memory cells. Thus, the question of whether purified central memory cells can enter into cell cycle faster than naïve cells remains unresolved. In practice, however, the high precursor frequency of memory T cells is probably much more important than enhanced entry into cell cycle. For example, an increase in precursor frequency of 100-fold for T memory cells would reduce the number of cell divisions required to generate a given number of effector cells by sevenfold, in relation to naïve T cells. With a cell cycle time of 6 to 8 hours, this would shorten the response time by several days. In comparison, the difference noted between the times taken for naïve versus memory T cells to commence cell division is quite short (i.e., 27 vs. 12 hours). Nevertheless, in combination, both of these factors may ensure that the response of memory T cells is rapid and intense.

Notwithstanding the uncertainty surrounding the functional responsiveness of memory cells, some biochemical differences between naïve and memory T cells that could confer different biological properties on these cells have been described. For example, in relation to naïve cells, memory cells show differences in the phosphorylation and association of signaling components of the TCR/CD3 complex (444), expression of the linker/adapter molecule SLP-76 (445), the pattern of calcium influx in response to TCR stimulation (446), expression of the tyrosine kinase Lck and association of Lck with CD8 (83,447), and association of CD45 isoforms with the TCR and CD4 (448,449). In addition, memory T cells appear to be more metabolically active than naïve T cells, perhaps by remaining in the G1 rather than the G0 stage of the cell cycle (443,450), and may express messenger RNA for effector cytokines before secondary stimulation (439,443). Whether each of these attributes apply to all memory T cells or only to specific subpopulations remains to be investigated.

Another factor that may contribute to T-cell memory is affinity maturation. Thus, although TCRs apparently do not undergo somatic hypermutation, there is evidence that T cells expressing TCRs with higher affinity for antigen are recruited selectively during the immune response. This phenomenon is apparent during the primary response (66,451–454) but is most evident after repeated exposure of the host to the same antigen (65,84,85,451,455). Competition for limiting amounts of antigen favors the emergence of high-affinity cells (455–457). In this regard, it was reported that high-affinity T cells can actively down-modulate peptide/MHC complexes on APCs, thus reducing the amount of antigen available to lower affinity cells (458). At the structural level, TCR affinity maturation appears to result from the loss of cells expressing TCRs with the fastest dissociation rates for peptide/MHC binding (84,85). Therefore, the available data support the idea that memory T cells may represent a population of cells selected from the initial responding population on the basis of having a higher affinity for antigen. Any role for TCR affinity differences in the functional responsiveness of naïve versus memory cells would not have been apparent in the studies of TCR transgenic cells cited previously. Nevertheless, for polyclonal T cells, it should be noted that the increases in affinity observed for TCRs (twofold to fourfold) are relatively modest.

Like memory T cells, memory B cells exhibit functional differences from naïve B cells at the single-cell level. Of note is that memory B cells appear to be more easily stimulated *in vitro* than are naïve cells, responding to lower amounts of antigen and showing less dependence on T cells and cytokines such as IL-6 (208,459–461). It has also been reported that memory B cells differentiate into AFCs more rapidly than do naïve B cells (372). Thus, human tonsillar memory B cells give rise to many times more AFCs than do naïve B cells after stimulation with CD40L and cytokines, whereas naïve cells generate a larger number of nondifferentiated blast cells. The authors of this report proposed that this bias toward terminal differentiation might help prevent the accumulation of memory B cells with successive stimulations and could contribute to the enhanced production of antibodies during the secondary response.

As discussed earlier, the GC reaction during the primary response causes memory B cells to produce somatically mutated high-affinity antibodies (359,387-389,460,462–476). The capacity of memory B cells to synthesize high-affinity antibody, combined with the ability of these cells to rapidly differentiate into AFCs, causes secondary humoral responses to be much more effective than primary responses. Furthermore, the expression of high-affinity BCRs by memory B cells presumably enhances the sensitivity of these cells to antigen (477).

In addition to expressing sIg with high affinity for antigen, it was mentioned earlier that memory B cells frequently express Ig isotypes other than IgM or IgD (357,478,479). Hence, because of prior class switching, memory B cells lead to much earlier synthesis of IgG and IgA antibodies than do naïve B cells. Interestingly, one study indicated that cell surface expression of switched isotypes of immunoglobulin can enhance differentiation into antibody-secreting cells (480). In analysis of the *in vivo* response of B cells expressing trans-

genic immunoglobulin with identical high-affinity variable regions but differing in their cytoplasmic domains, it was shown that the cytoplasmic tail of IgG conferred a greatly increased production of AFCs. This appeared to be caused by a reduction in the loss of cells during clonal expansion rather than by increased proliferation.

LIFE SPAN AND TURNOVER OF MEMORY CELLS

Life Span of Memory T Cells

At a population level, mature T cells can survive for long periods of time in situations in which there is no possibility for the input of newly generated T cells: for example, in thymectomized animals or after adoptive transfer to T cell–deficient recipients (481–489). Under these conditions, memory T cells persist indefinitely. For naïve T cells, the life span of these cells in mice has been estimated to be approximately 6 months to a year, on the basis of the rate at which responsiveness to neoantigens is lost after thymectomy (481–483,485,490). However, in addition to death, the slow disappearance of naïve T cells may reflect conversion to memory cells as the result of exposure to environmental antigens. Furthermore, studies supporting a role for specific peptides in the maintenance of naïve T cells (see later discussion) suggest that naïve T cells of different specificities may be lost at different rates. Nevertheless, it is clear that both naïve and memory T cells are relatively long-lived at a population level.

In theory, T cells could be maintained through continuous cell proliferation and death (i.e., turnover) or by longevity at the single-cell level. However, it was evident from early experiments involving ^{3}H-thymidine infusion into rodents that the majority of T cells in peripheral lymphoid organs remain in interphase for weeks or months (491–495). From studies in mice, the life span (period of interphase) of T cells in thoracic duct lymph was calculated to be approximately 4 to 6 months (493), a period that is remarkably similar to the estimated half-lives of CD4$^+$ and CD8$^+$ T cells in human peripheral blood (87 and 77 days, respectively) obtained from studies of healthy subjects infused with ^{2}H-glucose (496).

The turnover of naïve- and memory-phenotype T cells has been examined in many different species by measuring the rate at which these cells incorporate DNA precursors. Through this approach, the common finding in mice (19), sheep (278), rhesus macaques (497) and humans (498) is that T cells with a memory phenotype are turning over much more rapidly than naïve-phenotype T cells. For example, the half-life of memory-phenotype (CD45R0$^+$) T cells in the peripheral blood of healthy humans was calculated to range from 22 to 79 days, whereas the half-life of naïve-phenotype (CD45RA$^+$) T cells is on the order of 116 to 365 days (498). These values are roughly similar to what has been obtained in other animals, which indicates that cell life span and turnover are intrinsic properties of T cells and not a function of the life span of the host.

These studies suggest that memory T cells are maintained through relatively frequent cell division, whereas naïve T cells are much more quiescent. However, a general classification of memory T cells as short-lived cells and naïve T cells as long-lived cells may be an oversimplification. In DNA labeling studies, there is considerable heterogeneity in the rate at which memory-phenotype T cells either incorporate label during the infusion period or lose label after the cessation of treatment (19,498). These data show that some memory-phenotype T cells can in fact remain in interphase for long periods of time, despite the rapid overall turnover of this population. The reason for this heterogeneity in kinetic behavior is currently unknown, but two non–mutually exclusive explanations are possible. First, heterogeneity in turnover among memory-phenotype T cells may reflect the diversity of cell types that can express "memory" markers. As discussed previously, these markers do not effectively discriminate between recently activated effectors and longer term memory cells. However, the possibility that memory-phenotype T cells exhibiting rapid turnover represent only recently activated cells has been excluded by studies in mice, in which "bona fide" memory T cells generated from TCR transgenic mice or detected by using MHC tetramers showed similar rates of cell division in vivo to memory-phenotype T cells in normal mice (285,379,499). Nevertheless, the possibility that central and effector memory cells exhibit different rates of turnover remains to be explored.

Second, different rates of cell division among memory T cells could reflect differences in the availability of proliferative stimuli for subpopulations of memory cells. Such a mechanism would be easiest to imagine if contact with antigen were the primary stimulus for memory T-cell turnover. Hence, memory T cells specific for antigens that persist would be periodically triggered through the TCR and divide, whereas memory cells against nonpersisting antigens would remain in a nondividing state. In this regard, studies in mice have yielded conflicting results regarding the possible role of antigen in promoting turnover of CD4+ versus CD8+ memory T cells. For CD8+ cells, TCR triggering does not appear to be necessary to drive cell division, inasmuch as CD8+ memory T cells continue to divide after adoptive transfer to MHC class I–deficient hosts (285,500). In contrast, it has been reported that CD4+ memory T cells (derived from Th2 effectors) exhibit only a very slow rate of proliferation after parking in class II MHC–deficient hosts (501). This observation suggests that contact with MHC may contribute to the rapid turnover of CD4+ memory T cells, although the question of whether recognition of specific antigen was required or whether contact with MHC plus self-peptide (see later discussion) was sufficient was not addressed. However, an alternative explanation for these data is that the particular memory cells examined in this study (i.e., Th2 effector memory cells) represent a slowly turning over subpopulation. Because turnover was not assessed after transfer of these cells to class II MHC–positive mice, this remains an open question.

Life Span of Memory B Cells

In vivo DNA labeling studies have shown that B cells in the periphery have an average life span of several weeks to months (155,156,179,493,502–506). These cells can be divided into a minor (10% to 15%) population of HSA^hi cells with a rapid turnover and a longer lived HSA^lo/int subset (156,376,504–506). The short-lived cells correspond to the transitional, immature B cells of the spleen; these cells either are selected into the peripheral recirculating pool or die within a few days of export from the bone marrow (see previous discussion). Their brief life span may be related to low expression of the antiapoptotic molecule A1, which is expressed at tenfold higher levels in the long-lived peripheral B cell pool (507).

Among mature B cells, there is only limited information available regarding the relative life spans of naïve versus memory B cells. In one study, it was reported that the cells expressing the lowest levels of HSA divide more slowly than HSA^int cells (508). Because low expression of HSA has been considered a marker of memory B cells, this result implies that memory B cells, unlike memory T cells, turn over more slowly than their naïve counterparts. However, because the HSA^lo phenotype has also been associated with memory B cell precursors (see previous discussion), this remains an open question. Nevertheless, direct analysis of antigen-binding, isotype-switched memory B cells in mice has provided evidence that memory B cells do in fact have a relatively slow rate of turnover (509). In this study, only 12% of memory B cells divided over a 5-week period when labeling was started 10 weeks after immunization with a protein antigen in adjuvant. Examination of memory B cell turnover in other systems, plus analysis of sIgM+ memory B cells, is necessary to confirm the generality of this finding.

There appears to be considerable heterogeneity in the life span of AFCs (185,510). Although plasma cells themselves are nondividing (206), a large proportion of AFCs is labeled rapidly upon infusion of DNA precursors, which indicates that these cells have been recently derived from dividing progenitors. A short life span (a few days) applies to most AFCs generated in the spleen and intestinal lamina propria during primary immune responses, although a small proportion of the cells in these locations may survive for several weeks (185,510). In contrast, there is strong evidence that a significant proportion of AFCs in the bone marrow can be very long-lived; some of these cells survive and secrete antibody for more than a year (511,512).

MAINTENANCE OF MEMORY

Maintenance of T-Cell Memory

Since 1990, considerable progress has been made toward understanding how T cell memory is maintained. During this time, much debate has centered on the issue of whether maintenance of memory requires periodic contact with antigen. Because many pathogens can persist at low levels in the host

(13), and because even nonreplicating antigens can remain trapped for substantial lengths of time on the surface of FDCs (513,514), it seems possible and perhaps even likely that persisting antigen could affect the behavior of memory cells. Thus, if memory T cells can gain access to antigen in recognizable form (i.e., as peptide/MHC complexes expressed on cells encountered during normal T-cell migration), intermittent contact with antigen may induce some degree of T-cell activation, possibly affecting cell life span, migration, and effector function. Furthermore, because memory T cells appear to be more easily triggered by cross-reactive antigens than are naïve T cells, this type of stimulation might not even require the original priming antigen (515,516).

However, despite the likelihood that reencounter with antigen affects the behavior of memory T cells, and despite evidence from a variety of studies that memory wanes more rapidly in the absence of antigen (517–520), it is now clear that memory T cells can survive long term in the complete absence of specific antigen. Both for CD4$^+$ and CD8$^+$ T cells, numerous studies in mice have shown that memory T cells of defined specificity survive indefinitely after transfer to antigen-free hosts (63,81,284,285, 439,443,501,521,522). Notably long-term survival also applies for CD4$^+$ and CD8$^+$ memory T cells transferred to recipients lacking expression of class II or class I MHC, respectively (285,501,523). These observations essentially rule out a fundamental requirement for cross-reactive antigens in maintaining T-cell memory and further indicate that memory T-cell survival is not dependent on signals derived from contact between the TCR and MHC plus self-peptides. On this point, memory T cells appear to differ from naïve T cells, which in many (285,500,524–526) but not all (527,528) studies have been shown to exhibit a greatly abbreviated life span in MHC-deficient hosts. Furthermore, memory T cells also proliferate after transfer to MHC-deficient mice (285,500,501). In fact, the rate of cell division among CD8$^+$ memory T cells was shown to be similar in MHC class I$^{+/+}$ and MHC class I$^{-/-}$ hosts, which implies that turnover, like survival, is regulated by signals independent of TCR triggering (285). In contrast, as mentioned previously, the turnover rate of CD4$^+$ memory T cells is considerably slower in class II MHC–deficient mice than in normal mice, although whether this finding is applicable to all CD4$^+$ memory cells or only to a subset of these cells is unclear (501).

Although the ability of memory T cells to survive in an antigen-independent manner is now widely accepted, it has been argued that maintaining a high frequency of memory cells may be insufficient to provide protective immunity against reinfection at peripheral sites (13,529–531). The proponents of this view argue that, at least for CD8$^+$ T cells, protective memory is dependent on periodic contact with persisting antigen, which confers on memory T cells the ability to migrate rapidly into peripheral tissues and generate effector activity. In this regard, it is currently unclear whether antigen-independent survival applies to both central and effector memory cells, although it was shown in one study that CD8$^+$ memory T cells parked in class I MHC–deficient hosts retained the ability to produce IFN-γ within 4 hours of restimulation (285). Further investigation is necessary to determine whether effector memory T cells persist, die, or return to a "resting" central memory phenotype and also whether the preferential accumulation of effector memory T cells in peripheral tissues is related to the presence of antigen or other factors at these sites.

Besides antigen, the other main factor that has been studied for its role in the maintenance of T cell memory is cytokine-mediated stimulation. Initial interest in the role of cytokines in regulating the life span of memory T cells stemmed from the finding that injection of either type I IFN or inducers of type I IFN into mice stimulated TCR-independent proliferation of memory-phenotype (CD44^{hi}) CD8$^+$ T cells (532,533). Subsequently, a number of other cytokines, including IL-12, IL-15, IL-18, and IFN-γ were found to have similar effects (327,534). Of the cytokines shown to promote T-cell proliferation *in vivo,* only IL-15 could induce CD44^{hi} CD8$^+$ T cells to divide when added to purified T cells *in vitro;* the selective responsiveness of CD44^{hi} CD8$^+$ cells among T cells was associated with high expression of the IL-2/IL-15 receptor β chain (CD122) by these cells. However, because type I IFN, IFN-γ, IL-12, and IL-18 were all capable of up-regulating IL-15 expression by APCs (the latter two through induction of IFN-γ), it was proposed that IL-15 acted as a common final effector in mediating this cytokine-driven "bystander" proliferation (327).

On the basis of the enhanced proliferation observed after systemic injection of cytokines or cytokine inducers, it was hypothesized that the high turnover rate of CD44^{hi} CD8$^+$ T cells in normal hosts might reflect intermittent contact of memory T cells with background levels of IL-15. In support of this idea, it was shown that injection of anti-CD122 antibodies into normal mice markedly reduced the proliferation of CD44^{hi} CD8$^+$ T cells (535). Although this antibody can block both IL-15– and IL-2–mediated signals, it is notable that injection of anti–IL-2 plus anti–IL-2Rα (which affects IL-2 but not IL-15 signaling) actually resulted in enhanced CD44^{hi} CD8$^+$ T cell proliferation. This finding implies that IL-15 and IL-2 have opposing effects on CD44^{hi} CD8$^+$ cell proliferation, IL-15 being stimulatory and IL-2 causing inhibition.

Further evidence that IL-15 contributes to T cell memory has come from the analysis of IL-15– and IL-15Rα–deficient mice (536,537). Both types of mice show a selective reduction in CD44^{hi} CD8$^+$ T cell numbers, which in IL-15$^{-/-}$ mice can be reversed by repeated treatment with IL-15. Conversely, transgenic mice overexpressing IL-15 have increased numbers of memory-phenotype CD8$^+$ T cells (100,538). Therefore, it appears that IL-15 is an important regulator of the population of CD44^{hi} CD8$^+$ T cells found in normal mice (Fig. 5), although definitive evidence of its importance for specific memory cells awaits the results of infection/immunization experiments in knockout mice.

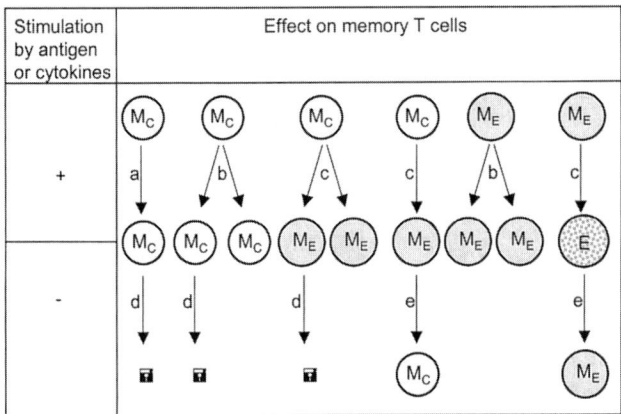

FIG. 5. Maintenance of T-cell memory. Persistence of memory T cells at relatively constant frequencies involves considerable cell turnover; periodic proliferation is balanced by cell death. Factors that may drive memory T-cell division include antigen, which could be either the original priming antigen or molecules possessing cross-reactive epitopes, and cytokines. Interleukin (IL)–15 appears to play an important role in maintaining CD8$^+$ memory T cells, but the participation of cytokines in regulating CD4$^+$ T cell memory is less certain. In addition to driving proliferation, antigen and cytokines may induce effector function in memory T cells, whereas cytokines such as IL-15 may also act as survival factors. As described in the text, the relationship between central memory (M$_C$), effector memory (M$_E$) and effector (E) T cells is unclear. In this figure, we speculate that interconversion between these functional states could occur depending on the cell's recent history of contact with antigen or cytokines. Possible outcomes of memory T-cell contact with cytokines or antigen or both include (a) cell survival without cell division or change in effector activity, (b) proliferation without change in effector activity, and (c) acquisition of effector activity, with or without cell division. When stimulation by cytokines/antigen is absent, memory T cells may die (d), or revert to a lower stage of activation (e).

It is currently unclear why lack of an IL-15 response leads to such a marked reduction in CD8$^+$ memory cells. If IL-15 is necessary simply to promote cell division, the assumption is that CD8$^+$ memory cells are intrinsically short-lived and therefore must be maintained through frequent division. However, as discussed previously, there is evidence that at least some memory T cells can persist for long periods of time in a nondividing state; this is particularly prominent among memory-phenotype CD8$^+$ T cells (19). Alternatively, IL-15 may also participate in the generation or survival of memory CD8 cells. In this regard, it is interesting to note that IL-15 up-regulates expression of the prosurvival factor Bcl-2 in CD8$^+$ T cells (539), and CD8$^+$ memory cells examined directly *ex vivo* express higher levels of Bcl-2 than do naïve T cells (539,540). If IL-15 promotes both proliferation and survival of memory-phenotype CD8$^+$ cells, this could account for the accumulation of these cells in IL-15 transgenic mice.

It should be pointed out that a small population of CD44^{hi} CD8$^+$ T cells is present in IL-15$^{-/-}$ mice (53). Interestingly,

these cells express low levels of CD122 and may correspond to a minor subset of CD44^{hi} CD8$^+$ T cells found in normal mice that fail to proliferate in response to IL-15 (327). In contrast to CD122^{hi} cells, the CD122^{lo} subset of CD44^{hi} CD8$^+$ cells may have an abbreviated life span. Thus, as discussed earlier, *in vitro* activated T cells expressing high levels of CD122 formed long-lived memory cells on adoptive transfer, whereas CD122^{lo} cells disappeared within a few weeks (103). Even though the stimulus used for CD122 up-regulation *in vitro*, IL-4, may have had other effects on the T cells, these results are consistent with the idea that activated CD122^{lo} CD8$^+$ T cells have only a short life span. Further support for this notion comes from the phenotype of the residual memory-phenotype cells present in IL-15R$\alpha^{-/-}$ mice (541): Unlike most CD44^{hi} CD8$^+$ T cells in normal mice, CD44^{hi} CD8$^+$ T cells in IL-15R$\alpha^{-/-}$ mice do not express higher levels of Bcl-2 than naïve CD8$^+$ T cells.

Another cytokine that has been reported to influence the kinetic behavior of memory-phenotype CD8$^+$ T cells is IL-2 (535,542). As mentioned previously, blocking the activity of IL-2 *in vivo* appears to enhance proliferation of CD44^{hi} CD8$^+$ T cells to IL-15. At face value, this finding appears paradoxical, because both IL-2 and IL-15 utilize common β and γ chains for signaling (331). However, it is possible that the inhibitory effects of IL-2 on T-cell proliferation *in vivo* are mediated indirectly, perhaps through the stimulation of another cell type, which then blocks CD8$^+$ T cell division. One possible mediator of the inhibitory effect of IL-2 is the so-called CD4$^+$ regulatory T cell, which is characterized by expression of the IL-2R α chain (CD25) (543,544). A prominent characteristic of these cells is their ability to inhibit T-cell proliferation, which may be mediated in part through production of transforming growth factor β (545,546). In this respect, it is notable that there is a massive expansion of CD44^{hi} CD8$^+$ T cells in mice expressing a dominant negative form of the type II transforming growth factor β receptor (137).

In addition to regulating their life span and turnover, cytokines may also have functional effects on memory T cells. For example, repeated injection of mice with IL-15 was shown to prolong protection against infection with *Toxoplasma gondii* (547). The increased resistance, which is mediated by CD8$^+$ T cells, was associated with an increased frequency of *Toxoplasma*-specific memory CD8$^+$ T cells. However, given that animals were challenged with a lethal dose of the pathogen, it is possible that IL-15 also promoted the survival or generation, or both, of effector memory cells, thus potentiating a rapid response to the infection. More support for this idea has come from an examination of the effects of cytokines on human CD4$^+$ T cells *in vitro* (548). In this study, it was shown that some central memory T cells acquired the characteristics of effector memory cells when cultured in the presence of a mixture of cytokines. This observation is corroborated by studies in mice, in which a combination of IL-12 and IL-18 was shown to induce expression of IFN-γ by CD44^{hi} CD8$^+$ T cells (549). These results raise the possibility that the preferential persistence of effector memory T cells in mucosal sites may be related to the cytokines expressed in these tissues.

Unlike the situation for CD8$^+$ T cells, there is currently little information regarding a possible role for cytokines in the maintenance of CD4$^+$ memory T cells. IL-15 induces only poor proliferation of memory-phenotype CD4$^+$ T cells *in vivo* and *in vitro,* and these cells are found in normal numbers in IL-15– and IL-15–deficient mice (327,536,537). Likewise, there is little effect on the turnover of CD44^{hi} CD4$^+$ T cells in mice after injection of a number of other cytokines and cytokine inducers that stimulate a marked response by CD44^{hi} CD8$^+$ T cells (532–534,550). Therefore, if CD4$^+$ memory T-cell life span is under the regulation of cytokines, the factors involved are clearly distinct from those affecting CD8$^+$ memory T cells. In addition, the generation of long-lived CD4$^+$ memory T cells from γ_c-deficient precursors implies that none of the cytokines using this receptor component (IL-2, IL-4, IL-7, IL-9, or IL-15) is essential for survival of CD4$^+$ memory cells (105). Currently, the best evidence for cytokine-driven bystander proliferation of CD4$^+$ memory cells comes from a study in which memory-phenotype CD4$^+$ T cells were shown to divide *in vivo* after activation of natural killer T cells, through a mechanism that is dependent on IL-12 or IFN-γ (551).

Maintenance of B-Cell Memory

There is less consensus concerning the possible role of persisting antigen in maintaining B-cell memory. As with T cells, it seems likely that intermittent contact with antigen by memory B cells modifies the behavior of these cells, but whether such contact is an absolute requirement for memory maintenance is a matter of debate. The ability of antigen to persist in an area that is accessible to B cells [i.e., on FDCs (513,514)], combined with the apparent short life span of many AFCs (185,510), contributed to the view that continued production of antibody is strictly dependent on persistence of antigen. Similarly, B cell memory appears to wane after adoptive transfer of cells from immune to naïve animals in the absence of antigen, which implicates a role for antigen in prolonging the survival of memory B cells (388,552). However, these long-held views have been challenged by two key findings. First, the discovery of a long-lived population of AFCs that can persist in the absence of antigen implies that at least a proportion of long-term antibody production is independent of persisting antigen (511,512,553). Second, an elegant *in vivo* system was used to show that memory B cells can survive for a long time in the absence of stimulation by the immunizing antigen (554). Here, the Cre recombinase system was used to switch the specificity of the sIg expressed on preexisting memory B cells so that these cells could no longer bind to the original priming antigen. In this model, the frequency of switching was less than 100%, so that memory B cells expressing the original specificity were also present in the same mice. The striking finding was that the life spans of the two

types of memory B cells were indistinguishable, and both antigen-binding and non–antigen-binding cells survived long-term. Although this experiment does not rule out the possibility that the switched memory B cells may have been stimulated by antigens that were cross-reactive with the new immunoglobulin, it clearly excludes an essential role for persistence of the priming antigen in the maintenance of memory B cells.

Little information is available concerning other factors that may control the survival of memory B cells, although it is clear that CD4$^+$ T cells are not required (555). The possible involvement of factors capable of inducing up-regulation of Bcl-2 is suggested by the greatly increased life span and accumulation of memory B cells expressing a Bcl-2 transgene (255). However, the nature of the stimuli involved and the relevance of these findings to normal memory B cell survival remain to be explored.

CONCLUDING REMARKS

Although the main features of immunological memory are now well understood, several fundamental questions remain, especially regarding the generation and maintenance of memory. Here, the chief problem is that immune memory is strictly an *in vivo* phenomenon and reflects the function of the immune system as a whole rather than of individual cells. Nevertheless, the application of molecular approaches to the study of *in vivo* immune responses is rapidly providing important insights into the elemental basis of immune memory; at the same time, these approaches are also revealing previously unrecognized levels of complexity in the immune system. Continuing these studies is clearly of great importance, both for the fundamental understanding of the immune system and for the rational design of vaccines.

REFERENCES

1. Glenny AT, Sudmersen HJ. Notes on the production of immunity to diphtheria toxin. *J Hygiene* 1921;20:176–220.
2. Perey DY, Cooper MD, Good RA. Normal second set wattle homograft rejection in agammaglobulinemic chickens. *Transplantation* 1967;5:615–623.
3. Pearson GR, Hodes RJ, Friberg S. Cytotoxic potential of different lymphoid cell populations against chromium-51 labelled tumor cells. *Clin Exp Immunol* 1969;5:273–284.
4. Ginzburg H. Graft versus host reaction in tissue culture. I. Lysis of monolayers of embryo mouse cells from strains differing in the H-2–histocompatibility locus by rat lymphocytes sensitized *in vitro*. *Immunol Lond* 1968;14:621–635.
5. Brunner KT, Nauel J, Cerottini J-C, et al. Quantitative assay of the lytic action of immune lymphoid cells on ^{51}CR-labelled allogeneic target cells *in vitro;* inhibition by isoantibody and by drugs. *Immunol Lond* 1968;14:181–196.
6. Benacerraf B. Cell associated immune reactions. *Cancer Res* 1968;28:1392–1398.
7. Canty TG, Wunderlich JR, Fletcher F. Qualitative and quantitative studies of cytotoxic immune cells. *J Immunol* 1971;106:200–208.
8. Panum PL. Beobachtungen uber das maserncontagium. *Virchows Arch* 1847;1:492–512.
9. Sawyer WA. The persistence of yellow fever immunity. *J Prev Med* 1931;5:413–428.

10. Paul JR, Riordan JT, Melnick JL. Antibodies to three different antigenic types of poliomyelitis virus in sera from north Alaskan Eskimos. *Am J Hygiene* 1951;54:275–285.

11. Demkowicz WEJ, Littaua RA, Wang J, et al. Human cytotoxic T-cell memory: long-lived responses to vaccinia virus. *J Virol* 1996;70:2627–2631.

12. Ahmed R, Gray D. Immunological memory and protective immunity: understanding their relation. *Science* 1996;272:54–60.

13. Zinkernagel RM, Bachmann MF, Kundig TM, et al. On immunological memory. *Annu Rev Immunol* 1996;14:333–367.

14. Dutton RW, Bradley LM, Swain SL. T cell memory. *Annu Rev Immunol* 1998;16:201–223.

15. Sprent J, Surh CD. Generation and maintenance of memory T cells. *Curr Opin Immunol* 2001;13:248–254.

16. Sprent J. T and B memory cells. *Cell* 1994;76:315–322.

17. Sebzda E, Mariathasan S, Ohteki T, et al. Selection of the T cell repertoire. *Annu Rev Immunol* 1999;17:829–874.

18. Scollay RG, Butcher EC, Weissman IL. Quantitative aspects of cellular traffic from the thymus to the periphery in mice. *Eur J Immunol* 1980;10:210–218.

19. Tough DF, Sprent J. Turnover of naïve- and memory-phenotype T cells. *J Exp Med* 1994;179:1127–1135.

20. Gowans JL, Knight EJ. The route of recirculation of lymphocytes in the rat. *Proc R Soc Lond (Biol)* 1964;159:257.

21. Sprent J. Recirculating lymphocytes. In: Marchalonis JJ, ed. *The lymphocytes: structure and function.* New York: Dekker, 1977:43–112.

22. Picker LJ, Butcher EC. Physiological and molecular mechanisms of lymphocyte homing. *Annu Rev Immunol* 1992;10:561–591.

23. Butcher EC, Picker LJ. Lymphocyte homing and homeostasis. *Science* 1996;272:60–66.

24. Berg EL, Robinson MK, Warnock RA, et al. The human peripheral lymph node vascular addressin is a ligand for LECAM-1, the peripheral lymph node homing receptor. *J Cell Biol* 1991;114:343–349.

25. Gunn MD, Tangemann K, Tam C, et al. A chemokine expressed in lymphoid high endothelial venules promotes the adhesion and chemotaxis of naïve T lymphocytes. *Proc Natl Acad Sci U S A* 1998;95:258–263.

26. Banchereau J, Steinman RM. Dendritic cells and the control of immunity. *Nature* 1998;392:245–252.

27. Banchereau J, Briere F, Caux C, et al. Immunobiology of dendritic cells. *Annu Rev Immunol* 2000;18:767–811.

28. Liu Y-J, Kanzler H, Soumelis V, et al. Dendritic cell lineage, plasticity and cross-regulation. *Nat Immunol* 2001;2:585–589.

29. Inaba K, Metlay JP, Crowley MT, et al. Dendritic cells as antigen presenting cells *in vivo*. *Int Rev Immunol* 1990;6:197–206.

30. Lenschow DJ, Walunas TL, Bluestone JA. CD28/B7 system of T cell costimulation. *Annu Rev Immunol* 1996;14:233–258.

31. Sperling AI, Bluestone JA. The complexities of T-cell co-stimulation: CD28 and beyond. *Immunol Rev* 1996;153:155–182.

32. Chambers CA, Allison JP. Co-stimulation in T cell responses. *Curr Opin Immunol* 1997;9:396–404.

33. McAdam AJ, Schweitzer AN, Sharpe AH. The role of B7 co-stimulation in activation and differentiation of CD4+ and CD8+ T cells. *Immunol Rev* 1998;165:231–247.

34. Whitmire JK, Ahmed R. Costimulation in antiviral immunity: differential requirements for CD4+ and CD8+ T cell responses. *Curr Opin Immunol* 2000;12:448–455.

35. Chambers CA. The expanding world of co-stimulation: the two-signal model revisited. *Trends Immunol* 2001;22:217–223.

36. Shahinian A, Pfeffer K, Lee KP, et al. Differential T cell costimulatory requirements in CD28-deficient mice. *Science* 1993;261:609–612.

37. Ronchese F, Hausmann B, Hubele S, et al. Mice transgenic for a soluble form of murine CTLA-4 show enhanced expansion of antigen-specific CD4+ T cells and defective antibody production *in vivo*. *J Exp Med* 1994;179:809–817.

38. Kundig TM, Shahinian A, Kawai K, et al. Duration of TCR stimulation determines costimulatory requirements of T cells. *Immunity* 1996;5:41–52.

39. Liu Y, Wenger RH, Zhao M, et al. Distinct costimulatory molecules are required for the induction of effector and memory cytotoxic T lymphocytes. *J Exp Med* 1997;185:251–262.

40. Watts TH, DeBenedette MA. T cell co-stimulatory molecules other than CD28. *Curr Opin Immunol* 1999;11:286–293.

41. Liu Y, Jones B, Sullivan K, et al. The heat-stable antigen is a co-stimulatory molecule for CD4 T cells. *J Exp Med* 1992;175:437–445.

42. Luft T, Pang KC, Thomas E, et al. Type I IFNs enhance the terminal differentiation of dendritic cells. *J Immunol* 1998;161:1947–1953.

43. Paquette RL, Hsu NC, Kiertscher SM, et al. Interferon-α and granulocyte-macrophage colony-stimulating factor differentiate peripheral blood monocytes into potent antigen presenting cells. *J Leuk Biol* 1998;64:358–367.

44. Sparwasser T, Koch ES, Vabulas RM, et al. Bacterial DNA and immunostimulatory CpG oligonucleotides trigger maturation and activation of murine dendritic cells. *Eur J Immunol* 1998;28:2045–2054.

45. Santini SM, Lapenta C, Logozzi M, et al. Type I interferon as a powerful adjuvant for monocyte-derived dendritic cell development and activity *in vitro* and in Hu-PBL-SCID mice. *J Exp Med* 2000;191:1777–1788.

46. Brightbill HD, Libraty DH, Krutzik SR, et al. Host defense mechanisms triggered by microbial lipoproteins through Toll-like receptors. *Science* 1999;285:732–736.

47. Gallucci S, Lolkema M, Matzinger P. Natural adjuvants: endogenous activators of dendritic cells. *Nat Med* 1999;5:1249–1255.

48. Rescigno M, Granucci F, Citterio S, et al. Coordinated events during bacteria-induced DC maturation. *Immunol Today* 1999;20:200–203.

49. Cella M, Salio M, Sakakibara Y, et al. Maturation, activation, and protection of dendritic cells induced by double-stranded RNA. *J Exp Med* 1999;189:821–829.

50. Klagge IM, Schneider-Schaulies S. Virus interactions with dendritic cells. *J Gen Virol* 1999;80:823–833.

51. Gagliardi MC, Sallusto F, Marinaro M, et al. Cholera toxin induces maturation of human dendritic cells and licences them for Th2 priming. *Eur J Immunol* 2000;30:2394–2403.

52. Le Bon A, Schiavoni G, D'Agostino G, et al. Type I interferons potently enhance humoral immunity and can promote isotype switching by stimulating dendritic cells *in vivo*. *Immunity* 2001;14:461–470.

53. Sprent J, Surh CD. T cell memory. *Annu Rev Immunol* 2002;20:551–579.

54. Kurts C, Kosaka H, Carbone FR, et al. Class I–restricted cross-presentation of exogenous self-antigens leads to deletion of autoreactive CD8+ T cells. *J Exp Med* 1997;186:239–245.

55. Murali-Krishna K, Altman JD, Suresh M, et al. Counting antigen-specific CD8 T cells: a reevaluation of bystander activation during viral infection. *Immunity* 1998;8:177–187.

56. Sprent J, Miller JF. Effect of recent antigen priming on adoptive immune responses. II. Specific unresponsiveness of circulating lymphocytes from mice primed with heterologous erythrocytes. *J Exp Med* 1974;139:1–12.

57. Sprent J. Role of H-2 gene products in the function of T helper cells from normal and chimeric mice *in vivo*. *Immunol Rev* 1978;42:108–137.

58. Sprent J. Fate of H-2–activated T lymphocytes in syngeneic hosts. I. Fate in lymphoid tissues and intestines traced with ^{3}H-thymidine, ^{125}I-deoxyuridine and ^{51}chromium. *Cell Immunol* 1976;21:278–302.

59. Reinhardt RL, Khoruts A, Merica R, et al. Visualizing the generation of memory CD4 T cells in the whole body. *Nature* 2001;410:101–105.

60. Masopust D, Vezys V, Marzo AL, et al. Preferential localization of effector memory cells in nonlymphoid tissue. *Science* 2001;291:2413–2416.

61. Marshall DR, Turner SJ, Belz GT, et al. Measuring the diaspora for virus-specific CD8+ T cells. *Proc Natl Acad Sci U S A* 2001;98:6313–6318.

62. Hogan RJ, Usherwood EJ, Zhong W, et al. Activated antigen-specific CD8+ T cells persist in the lungs following recovery from respiratory virus infections. *J Immunol* 2001;166:1813–1822.

63. Hou S, Hyland L, Ryan KW, et al. Virus-specific CD8+ T cell memory determined by clonal burst size. *Nature* 1994;369:652–654.

64. Vijh S, Pamer EG. Immunodominant and subdominant CTL responses to *Listeria monocytogenes* infection. *J Immunol* 1997;158:3366–3371.

65. Busch DH, Pilip I, Pamer EG. Evolution of a complex T cell receptor repertoire during primary and recall bacterial infection. *J Exp Med* 1998;188:61–70.

66. Maryanski JL, Jongeneel CV, Bucher P, et al. Single-cell PCR analysis of TCR repertoires selected by antigen *in vivo*: a high magnitude CD8 response is comprised of very few clones. *Immunity* 1996;4:47–55.

67. Callan MFC, Annels N, Steven N, et al. T cell selection during the evolution of CD8+ T cell memory *in vivo*. *Eur J Immunol* 1998;28:4382–4390.

68. Sourdive DJ, Murali-Krishna K, Altman JD, et al. Conserved T cell

receptor repertoire in primary and memory CD8 T cell responses to an acute viral infection. *J Exp Med* 1998;188:71–82.

69. Blattman JN, Sourdive DJ, Murali-Krishna K, et al. Evolution of the T cell repertoire during primary, memory, and recall responses to viral infection. *J Immunol* 2000;165:6081–6090.

70. Pantaleo G, Soudeyns H, Demarest JF, et al. Evidence for rapid disappearance of initially expanded HIV-specific CD8$^+$T cell clones during primary HIV infection. *Proc Natl Acad Sci U S A* 1997;94:9848–9853.

71. Callan MFC, Fazou C, Yang H, et al. CD8$^+$ T-cell selection, function, and death in the primary immune response *in vivo*. *J Clin Invest* 2000;106:1251–1261.

72. Jacob J, Baltimore D. Modelling T-cell memory by genetic marking of memory T cells *in vivo*. *Nature* 1999;399:593–597.

73. Simonsen M. Graft versus host reactions: their natural history and applicability as tools of research. *Prog Allergy* 1962;6:349–367.

74. Webb S, Morris C, Sprent J. Extrathymic tolerance of mature T cells: clonal elimination as a consequence of immunity. *Cell* 1990;63:1249–1256.

75. Li H, Llera A, Malchiodi EL, et al. The structural basis of T cell activation by superantigens. *Annu Rev Immunol* 1999;17:435–466.

76. Kawabe Y, Ochi A. Programmed cell death and extrathymic reduction of Vbeta8$^+$CD4$^+$T cells in mice tolerant to *Staphylococcus aureus* enterotoxin B. *Nature* 1991;349:245–248.

77. MacDonald HR, Baschieri S, Lees RK. Clonal expansion precedes anergy and death of V beta 8$^+$ peripheral T cells responding to staphylococcal enterotoxin B *in vivo*. *Eur J Immunol* 1991;21:1963–1966.

78. Moskophidis D, Laine E, Zinkernagel RM. Peripheral clonal deletion of antiviral memory CD8$^+$ T cells. *Eur J Immunol* 1993;23:3306–3311.

79. Budd RC, Cerottini J-C, MacDonald HR. Phenotypic identification of memory cytolytic T lymphocytes in a subset of Ly-2$^+$ cells. *J Immunol* 1987;138:1009–1013.

80. MacDonald HR, Glasebrook AL, Bron C, et al. Clonal heterogeneity in the functional requirement for Ly-2/3 molecules on cytolytic T lymphocytes (CTL): possible implications for the affinity of CTL antigen receptors. *Immunol Rev* 1982;68:89–115.

81. Bruno L, Kirberg J, Von Boehmer H. On the cellular basis of immunological T-cell memory. *Immunity* 1995;2:37–43.

82. Pihlgren M, Dubois PM, Tomkowiak M, et al. Resting memory CD8$^+$ T cells are hyperreactive to antigenic challenge *in vitro*. *J Exp Med* 1996;184:2141–2151.

83. Slifka MK, Whitton JL. Functional avidity maturation of CD8$^+$T cells without selection of higher affinity TCR. *Nat Immunol* 2001;2:711–717.

84. Busch DH, Pamer EG. T cell affinity maturation by selective expansion during infection. *J Exp Med* 1999;189:701–709.

85. Savage PA, Boniface JJ, Davis MM. A kinetic basis for T cell receptor repertoire selection during an immune response. *Immunity* 1999;10:485–492.

86. Anderton SM, Radu CG, Lowrey PA, et al. Negative selection during the peripheral immune response to antigen. *J Exp Med* 2001;193:1–11.

87. Mamalaki C, Tanaka Y, Corbella P, et al. T cell deletion follows chronic antigen specific T cell activation *in vivo*. *Int Immunol* 1993;5:1285–1292.

88. Sallusto F, Lenig D, Forster R, et al. Two subsets of memory T lymphocytes with distinct homing potentials and effector functions. *Nature* 1999;401:708–712.

89. Sad S, Mosmann TR. Single IL-2–secreting precursor CD4 T cell can develop into either Th1 or Th2 cytokine secretion phenotype. *J Immunol* 1994;153:3514–3522.

90. Iezzi G, Scotet E, Scheidegger D, et al. The interplay between the duration of TCR and cytokine signalling determines T cell polarization. *Eur J Immunol* 1999;29:4092–4101.

91. Langenkamp A, Messi M, Lanzavecchia A, et al. Kinetics of dendritic cell activation: impact on priming of TH1, TH2 and nonpolarized T cells. *Nat Immunol* 2000;1:311–316.

92. Iezzi G, Scheidegger D, Lanzavecchia A. Migration and function of antigen-primed nonpolarized T lymphocytes *in vivo*. *J Exp Med* 2001;193:987–993.

93. Doyle AM, Mullen AC, Villarino AV, et al. Induction of cytotoxic T lymphocyte antigen 4 (CTLA-4) restricts clonal expansion of helper T cells. *J Exp Med* 2001;194:893–902.

94. Lanzavecchia A, Sallusto F. Dynamics of T lymphocyte responses: intermediates, effectors and memory cells. *Science* 2000;290:92–97.

95. Salmon M, Pilling D, Borthwick NJ, et al. The progressive differentiation of primed T cells is associated with an increasing susceptibility to apoptosis. *Eur J Immunol* 1994;24:892–899.

96. Opferman JT, Ober BT, Ashton-Rickardt PG. Linear differentiation of cytotoxic effectors into memory T lymphocytes. *Science* 1999;283:1745–1748.

97. Manjunath N, Shankar P, Wan J, et al. Effector differentiation is not prerequisite for generation of memory cytotoxic T lymphocytes. *J Clin Invest* 2001;108:871–878.

98. Lauvau G, Vijh S, Kong P, et al. Priming of memory but not effector CD8 T cells by a killed bacterial vaccine. *Science* 2001;294:1735–1739.

99. Weninger W, Crowley MA, Manjunath N, et al. Migratory properties of naïve, effector, and memory CD8$^+$T cells. *J Exp Med* 2001;194:953–966.

100. Nishimura H, Yajima T, Naiki Y, et al. Differential roles of interleukin 15 mRNA isoforms generated by alternative splicing in immune responses *in vivo*. *J Exp Med* 2000;191:157–169.

101. Yajima T, Nishimura H, Ishimitsu R, et al. Overexpression of IL-15 *in vivo* increases antigen-driven memory CD8$^+$ T cells following a microbe exposure. *J Immunol* 2002;168:1198–1203.

102. Schluns KS, Kieper WC, Jameson SC, et al. Interleukin-7 mediates the homeostasis of naïve and memory CD8 T cells *in vivo*. *Nat Immunol* 2000;1:426–432.

103. Huang LR, Chen FL, Chen YT, et al. Potent induction of long-term CD8$^+$ T cell memory by short-term IL-4 exposure during T cell receptor stimulation. *Proc Natl Acad Sci U S A* 2000;97:3406–3411.

104. Villacres MC, Bergmann CC. Enhanced cytotoxic T cell activity in IL-4–deficient mice. *J Immunol* 1999;162:2663–2670.

105. Lantz O, Grandjean I, Matzinger P, et al. γ Chain required for naïve CD4$^+$T cell survival but not for antigen proliferation. *Nat Immunol* 2000;1:54–58.

106. Paterson DJ, Jefferies WA, Green JR, et al. Antigens of activated rat T lymphocytes including a molecule of 50,000 M detected only on CD4 positive T blasts. *Mol Immunol* 1987;24:1281–1290.

107. Calderhead DM, Buhlmann JE, van den Eerwegh AJ, et al. Cloning of mouse Ox40: a T cell activation marker that may mediate T–B cell interactions. *J Immunol* 1993;151:5261–5271.

108. Al-Shamkhani A, Birkeland ML, Puklavec M, et al. OX40 is differentially expressed on activated rat and mouse T cells and is the sole receptor for the OX40 ligand. *Eur J Immunol* 1996;26:1695–1699.

109. Gramaglia I, Weinberg AD, Lemon M, et al. Ox-40 ligand: a potent costimulatory molecule for sustaining primary CD4 T cell responses. *J Immunol* 1998;161:6510–6517.

110. Godfrey WR, Fagnoni FF, Harara MA, et al. Identification of a human OX-40 ligand, a costimulator of CD4$^+$T cells with homology to tumor necrosis factor. *J Exp Med* 1994;180:757–762.

111. Stuber E, Neurath M, Calderhead D, et al. Cross-linking of OX40 ligand, a member of the TNF/NGF cytokine family, induces proliferation and differentiation in murine splenic B cells. *Immunity* 1995;2:507–521.

112. Ohshima Y, Tanaka Y, Tozawa H, et al. Expression and function of OX40 ligand on human dendritic cells. *J Immunol* 1997;159:3838–3848.

113. Chen AI, McAdam AJ, Buhlmann JE, et al. Ox40-ligand has a critical costimulatory role in dendritic cell: T cell interactions. *Immunity* 1999;11:689–698.

114. Kopf M, Ruedl C, Schmitz N, et al. OX40-deficient mice are defective in Th cell proliferation but are competent in generating B cell and CTL responses after virus infection. *Immunity* 1999;11:699–708.

115. Murata K, Ishii N, Takano H, et al. Impairment of antigen-presenting cell function in mice lacking expression of OX40 ligand. *J Exp Med* 2000;191:365–374.

116. Gramaglia I, Jember A, Pippig SD, et al. The OX40 costimulatory receptor determines the development of CD4 memory by regulating primary clonal expansion. *J Immunol* 2000;165:3043–3050.

117. Maxwell JR, Weinberg A, Prell RA, et al. Danger and OX40 receptor signaling synergize to enhance memory T cell survival by inhibiting peripheral deletion. *J Immunol* 2000;164:107–112.

118. Vinay DS, Kwon BS. Role of 4-1BB in immune responses. *Semin Immunol* 1998;10:481–489.

119. Cannons JL, Lau P, Ghumman B, et al. 4-1BB ligand induces cell

division, sustains survival, and enhances effector function of CD4 and CD8 T cells with similar efficacy. *J Immunol* 2001;167:1313–1324.

120. DeBenedette MA, Wen T, Bachmann MF, et al. Analysis of 4-1BB ligand (4-1BBL)–deficient mice and of mice lacking both 4-1BBL and CD28 reveals a role for 4-1BBL in skin allograft rejection and in the cytotoxic T cell response to influenza virus. *J Immunol* 1999;163:4833–4841.

121. Tan JT, Whitmire JK, Ahmed R, et al. 4-1BB ligand, a member of the TNF family, is important for the generation of antiviral CD8 T cell responses. *J Immunol* 1999;163:4859–4868.

122. Tan JT, Whitmire JK, Murali-Krishna K, et al. 4-1BB costimulation is required for protective anti-viral immunity after peptide vaccination. *J Immunol* 2000;164:2320–2325.

123. Van Parijs L, Ibraghimov A, Abbas AK. The roles of costimulation and Fas in T cell apoptosis and peripheral tolerance. *Immunity* 1996;4:321–328.

124. Sytwu HK, Liblau RS, McDevitt HO. The roles of Fas/APO-1 (CD95) and TNF in antigen-induced programmed cell death in T cell receptor transgenic mice. *Immunity* 1996;5:17–30.

125. Hildeman DA, Mitchell T, Teague TK, et al. Reactive oxygen species regulate activation-induced T cell apoptosis. *Immunity* 1999;10:735–744.

126. Rathmell JC, Thompson CB. The central effectors of cell death in the immune system. *Annu Rev Immunol* 1999;17:781–828.

127. Leonardo M, Chan FKM, Hornung F, et al. Mature T lymphocyte apoptosis-immune regulation in a dynamic and unpredictable environment. *Annu Rev Immunol* 1999;17:221–253.

128. Tivol EA, Borriello F, Schweitzer AN, et al. Loss of CTLA-4 leads to massive lymphoproliferation and fatal multiorgan tissue destruction, revealing a critical negative regulatory role of CTLA-4. *Immunity* 1995;3:541–547.

129. Waterhouse P, Penninger JM, Timms E, et al. Lymphoproliferative disorders with early lethality in mice deficient in *Ctla-4*. *Science* 1995;270:985–988.

130. Kneitz B, Herrmann T, Yonehara S, et al. Normal clonal expansion but impaired Fas-mediated cell death and anergy induction in interleukin-2–deficient mice. *Eur J Immunol* 1995;25:2572–2577.

131. Van Parijs L, Biuckians A, Ibragimov A, et al. Functional responses and apoptosis of CD25 (IL-2R alpha)–deficient T cells expressing a transgenic antigen receptor. *J Immunol* 1997;158:3738–3745.

132. Tsunobuchi H, Nishimura H, Goshima F, et al. Memory-type CD8$^+$ T cells protect IL-2 receptor alpha–deficient mice from systemic infection with herpes simplex virus type 2. *J Immunol* 2000;165:4552–4560.

133. Cohen PL, Eisenberg RA. Lpr and gld: single gene models of systemic autoimmunity and lymphoproliferative disease. *Annu Rev Immunol* 1991;9:243–269.

134. Nagata S. Apoptosis by death factor. *Cell* 1997;88:355–365.

135. Suzuki H, Kundig TM, Furlonger C, et al. Deregulated T cell activation and autoimmunity in mice lacking interleukin-2 receptor beta. *Science* 1995;268:1472–1476.

136. Ranger AM, Oukka M, Rengarajan J, et al. Inhibitory function of two NFAT family members in lymphoid homeostasis and Th2 development. *Immunity* 1998;9:627–635.

137. Lucas PJ, Kim S-J, Melby SJ, et al. Disruption of T cell homeostasis in mice expressing a T cell-specific dominant negative transforming growth factor βII receptor. *J Exp Med* 2000;191:1187–1196.

138. Freeman GJ, Long AJ, Iwai Y, et al. Engagement of the PD-1 immunoinhibitory receptor by a novel B7 family member leads to negative regulation of lymphocyte activation. *J Exp Med* 2000;192:1027–1034.

139. Van Parijs L, Peterson DA, Abbas AK. The Fas/Fas ligand pathway and Bcl-2 regulate T cell response to model self and foreign antigens. *Immunity* 1998;8:265–274.

140. Bachmann MF, Waterhouse P, Speiser DE, et al. Normal responsiveness of CTLA-4–deficient anti-viral cytotoxic cells. *J Immunol* 1998;160:95–100

141. Reich A, Korner H, Sedgwick JD, et al. Immune down-regulation and peripheral deletion of CD8 T cells does not require TNF receptor–ligand interactions nor CD95 (Fas, Apo-1). *Eur J Immunol* 2000;30:678–682.

142. Nguyen LT, McKall-Faienza K, Zakarian A, et al. TNF receptor 1 (TNFR1) and CD95 are not required for T cell deletion after virus

143. Badovinac VP, Tvinnereim AR, Harty JT. Regulation of antigen-specific CD8$^+$ T cell homeostasis by perforin and interferon-γ. *Science* 2000;290:1354–1357.

144. Chu CQ, Wittmer S, Dalton DK. Failure to suppress the expansion of the activated CD4 T cell population in interferon gamma–deficient mice leads to exacerbation of experimental autoimmune encephalomyelitis. *J Exp Med* 2000;192:123–128.

145. Dalton DK, Haynes L, Chu CQ, et al. Interferon gamma eliminates responding CD4 T cells during mycobacterial infection by inducing apoptosis of activated CD4 T cells. *J Exp Med* 2000;192:117–122.

146. Van Parijs L, Abbas AK. Homeostasis and self-tolerance in the immune system: turning lymphocytes off. *Science* 1998;280:243–248.

147. Marrack P, Bender J, Hildeman D, et al. Homeostasis of alpha beta TCR$^+$ T cells. *Nat Immunol* 2000;1:107–111.

148. Mitchell TC, Hildeman D, Kedl RM, et al. Immunological adjuvants promote activated T cell survival *via* induction of Bcl-3. *Nat Immunol* 2001;2:397–402.

149. Sprent J. Immunological memory. *Curr Opin Immunol* 1997;9:371–379.

150. Stall AM, Wells SM, Lam K-P. B-1 cells: Unique origins and functions. *Semin Immunol* 1996;8:45–59.

151. Motta I, Portnoi D, Truffa-Bachi P. Induction and differentiation of B memory cells by a thymus-independent antigen, trinitrophenylated lipopolysaccharide. *Cell Immunol* 1981;57:327–338.

152. Colle JH, Motta I, Truffa-Bachi P. Generation of immune memory by haptenated derivatives of thymus-independent antigens in C57BL/6 mice. I. The differentiation of memory B lymphocytes into antibody-secreting cells depends on the nature of the thymus-independent carrier used for memory induction and/or revelation. *Cell Immunol* 1983;75:52–62.

153. Osmond DG, Nossal GJV. Differentiation of lymphocytes in mouse bone marrow. II. Kinetics of maturation and renewal of antiglobulin-binding cells studied by double labelling. *Cell Immunol* 1974;13:132–145.

154. Grabstein KH, Waldschmidt TJ, Finkelman FD, et al. Inhibition of murine B and T lymphopoiesis *in vivo* by an anti-interleukin 7 monoclonal antibody. *J Exp Med* 1993;178:257–264.

155. Gray D. Population kinetics of rat peripheral B cells. *J Exp Med* 1988;167:805–816.

156. Allman DM, Ferguson SE, Lentz VE, et al. Peripheral B cell maturation. II. Heat-stable antigen^{hi} splenic B cells are an immature developmental intermediate in the production of long lived marrow-derived B cells. *J Immunol* 1993;151:4431–4444.

157. Rolink AG, Melchers F, Andersson J. Characterization of immature B cells by a novel monoclonal antibody, by turnover and by mitogen reactivity. *Eur J Immunol* 1998;28:3738–3748.

158. Lortan JE, Roobottom CA, Oldfield S, et al. Newly-produced virgin B cells migrate to secondary lymphoid organs, but their capacity to enter follicles is restricted. *Eur J Immunol* 1987;17:1311–1316.

159. Chan EY-T, MacLennan ICM. Only a small proportion of splenic B cells in adults are short-lived virgin cells. *Eur J Immunol* 1993;23:357–363.

160. Gu H, Tarlinton D, Muller W, et al. Most peripheral B cells in mice are ligand selected. *J Exp Med* 1991;173:1357–1371.

161. Nemazee D. Receptor selection in B and T lymphocytes. *Annu Rev Immunol* 2000;18:19–51.

162. Nemazee DA, Burki K. Clonal deletion of auto-reactive B lymphocytes in a transgenic mouse bearing anti-MHC class I antibody genes. *Nature* 1989;337:562–566.

163. Hartley SB, Crosbie J, Brink RA, et al. Elimination from peripheral lymphoid tissues of self-reactive B lymphocytes recognising membrane-bound antigen. *Nature* 1991;353:765–769.

164. Cyster JG, Hartley SB, Goodnow CC. Competition for follicular niches excludes self-reactive cells from the recirculating B-cell repertoire. *Nature* 1994;371:389–395.

165. Cyster JG, Goodnow CC. Antigen-induced exclusion from follicles and anergy are separate and complementary processes that influence peripheral B cell fate. *Immunity* 1995;3:691–701.

166. Chen C, Nagy Z, Radic MZ, et al. The site and stage of anti-DNA B-cell deletion. *Nature* 1995;373:252–255.

167. Cyster JC, Healy JI, Kishihara K, et al. Regulation of B-lymphocyte

negative and positive selection by tyrosine phosphatase CD45. *Nature* 1996;381:325–328.

168. Torres RM, Flaswinkel H, Reth M, et al. Aberrant B cell development and immune response in mice with a compromised BCR complex. *Science* 1996;272:1804–1808.

169. Oka Y, Rolink AG, Andersson J, et al. Profound reduction of mature B cell numbers, reactivities and serum immunoglobulin levels in mice which simultaneously carry the XID and CD40-deficiency genes. *Int Immunol* 1996;8:1675–1685.

170. Turner M, Gulbranson-Judge A, Quinn ME, et al. Syk tyrosine kinase is required for the positive selection of immature B cells into the recirculating pool. *J Exp Med* 1997;186:2013–2021.

171. Klaus GG, Holman M, Johnson-Leger C, et al. A re-evaluation of the effects of X-linked immunodeficiency (xid) mutation on B cell differentiation and function in the mouse. *Eur J Immunol* 1997;27:2749–2756.

172. Otipoby KL, Andersson KB, Draves KE, et al. CD22 regulates thymus-independent responses and the lifespan of B cells. *Nature* 1996;384:634–637.

173. Rolink AG, Brocker T, Bluethmann H, et al. Mutations affecting either generation or survival of cells influence the pool size of mature B cells. *Immunity* 1999;10:619–628.

174. Gross JA, Dillon SR, Mudri S, et al. TACI-Ig neutralizes molecules critical for B cell development and autoimmune disease. Impaired B cell maturation in mice lacking BLyS. *Immunity* 2001;15:289–302.

175. Schiemann B, Gommerman JL, Vora K, et al. An essential role for BAFF in the normal development of B cells through a BCMA-independent pathway. *Science* 2001;293:2111–2114.

176. Thompson JS, Bixler SA, Qian F, et al. BAFF-R, a newly identified TNF receptor that specifically interacts with BAFF. *Science* 2001;293:2108–2111.

177. Forster I, Muller W, Schittek B, et al. Generation of long-lived B cells in germ-free mice. *Eur J Immunol* 1991;21:1779–1782.

178. Chies JAB, Lembezat MP, Freitas AA. Entry of B lymphocytes into the persistent cell pool in non-immunized mice is not accompanied by somatic mutation of VH genes. *Eur J Immunol* 1994;24:1657–1664.

179. Howard JC. The life-span and recirculation of marrow-derived small lymphocytes from the rat thoracic duct. *J Exp Med* 1972;135:185–199.

180. Claassen E, Kors N, Dijkstra CD, et al. Marginal zone of the spleen and the development and localization of specific antibody-forming cells against thymus-dependent and thymus-independent type-2 antigens. *Immunology* 1986;57:399–403.

181. Jacob J, Kassir R, Kelsoe G. In situ studies of the primary immune response to (4-hydroxy-3-nitrophenyl)acetyl. I. The architecture and dynamics of responding cell populations. *J Exp Med* 1991;173:1165–1175.

182. Liu Y-J, Zhang J, Lane PJL, et al. Sites of specific B cell activation in primary and secondary responses to T cell–dependent and T cell–independent antigens. *Eur J Immunol* 1991;21:2951–2962.

183. Kosco MH, Burton GF, Kapasi ZF, et al. Antibody forming cell induction during an early phase of germinal center development and its delay with aging. *Immunology* 1989;68:312–318.

184. Toellner K-M, Gulbranson-Judge A, Taylor DR, et al. Immunoglobulin switch transcript production *in vivo* related to the site and time of antigen-specific B cell activation. *J Exp Med* 1996;183:2303–2312.

185. Ho F, Lortan JE, MacLennan ICM, et al. Distinct short-lived and long-lived antibody-producing cell populations. *Eur J Immunol* 1986;16:1297–1301.

186. Smith KG, Hewitson TD, Nossal GJV, et al. The phenotype and fate of the antibody-forming cells of the splenic foci. *Eur J Immunol* 1996;26:444–448.

187. Coico RF, Bhogal BS, Thorbeck EJ. Relationship of germinal centres in lymphoid tissue to immunologic memory. VI. Transfer of B cell memory with lymph node cells fractionated according to their receptors for peanut agglutinin. *J Immunol* 1983;131:2254–2257.

188. Berek C, Berger A, Apel M. Maturation of the immune response in germinal centers. *Cell,* 1991;67:1121–1129.

189. Jacob J, Kelsoe G. *In situ* studies of the primary immune response to (4-hydroxy-3-nitrophenyl)acetyl. II. A common clonal origin for periarteriolar lymphoid sheath-associated foci and germinal centers. *J Exp Med* 1992;176:679–687.

190. Jacob J, Przylepa J, Miller C, et al. In situ studies of the primary immune response to (4-hydroxy-3-nitrophenyl)acetyl. III. The kinetics

191. Kuppers R, Zhao M, Hansmann M-L, et al. Tracing B cell development in human germinal centres by molecular analysis of single cells picked from histological sections. *EMBO J* 1993;12:4955–4967.

192. McHeyzer-Williams MG, McLean MJ, Lalor PA, et al. Antigen-driven B cell differentiation *in vivo*. *J Exp Med* 1993;178:295–307.

193. Pascual V, Liu Y-J, Magalski A, et al. Analysis of somatic mutation in five B cell subsets of human tonsil. *J Exp Med* 1994;180:329–339.

194. Kuppers R, Zhao M, Hansmann M-L, et al. Tracing B cell development in human germinal centres by molecular analysis of single cells picked from histological sections. *EMBO J* 1993;12:4955–4967.

195. MacLennan ICM. Germinal centers. *Annu Rev Immunol* 1994;12:117–139.

196. Kelsoe G. Life and death in germinal centers (redux). *Immunity* 1996;4:107–111.

197. Jacob J, Kelsoe G, Rajewsky K, et al. Intraclonal generation of antibody mutants in germinal centres. *Nature* 1991;354:389–391.

198. Leanderson T, Kallberg E, Gray D. Expansion, selection and mutation of antigen-specific B cells in germinal centers. *Immunol Rev* 1992;126:47–61.

199. Kosco MH, Szakal AK, Tew JG. *In vivo* obtained antigen presented by germinal center B cells to T cells *in vitro*. *J Immunol* 1988;140:354–360.

200. Liu Y-J, Joshua DE, Williams GT, et al. Mechanisms of antigen-driven selection in germinal centers. *Nature* 1989;342:929–931.

201. Papavasiliou F, Casellas R, Suh H, et al. V(D)J recombination in mature B cells: a mechanism for altering antibody responses. *Science* 1997;278:298–301.

202. Han S, Dillon SR, Zheng B, et al. V(D)J recombinase in a subset of germinal center B lymphocytes. *Science* 1997;278:301–305.

203. Pulendran B, Kannourakis G, Nouri S, et al. Soluble antigen can cause enhanced apoptosis of germinal-centre B cells. *Nature* 1995;375:331–334.

204. Shokat KM, Goodnow CC. Antigen-induced B-cell death and elimination during germinal centre immune responses. *Nature* 1995;375:334–338.

205. Han S, Zheng J, Porto D, et al. *In situ* studies of the primary immune response to (4-hydroxy-3-nitrophenyl)acetyl IV. Affinity-dependent, antigen-driven B cell apoptosis in germinal centers as a mechanism for maintaining self-tolerance. *J Exp Med* 1995;182:1635–1644.

206. Geldof AA, Rijnhart P, van de Ende M, et al. Morphology, kinetics and secretory activity of antibody-forming cells. *Immunobiology* 1984;166:296–307.

207. Decker DJ, Linton PJ, Zaharevitz S, et al. Defining subsets of naïve and memory B cells based on the ability of their progeny to somatically mutate *in vitro. Immunity,* 1995;2:195–203.

208. Klinman NR, Press JL, Pickard AR, et al. Biography of the B cell.In: Sercarz E, Williamson A, Fox CF, eds. *The immune system.* New York: Academic Press, 1974:357–365.

209. Linton PJ, Decker DJ, Klinman NR. Primary antibody-forming cells and secondary B cells are generated from separate precursor cell populations. *Cell* 1989;59:1049–1059.

210. Linton P-J, Lo D, Thorbecke GJ, et al. Among naïve precursor cell subpopulations only progenitors of memory B cells originate germinal centers. *Eur J Immunol* 1992;22:1293–1297.

211. Yin X-M, Vitetta ES. The lineage relationship between virgin and memory B cells. *Int Immunol* 1992;4:691–698.

212. Luko CM, Vansanten G, Ryelandt M, et al. Distinct VH repertoires in primary and secondary B cell lymphocyte subsets in the preimmune repertoire of A/J mice: the CRI-A idiotype is preferentially associated with the HSA^{low} B cell subset. *Eur J Immunol* 2000;30:2312–2322.

213. Byers VS, Sercarz EE. The X-Y-Z scheme of immunocyte maturation. IV. The exhaustion of memory cells. *J Exp Med* 1968;127:307–325.

214. Castigli E, Alt FW, Davidson L, et al. CD40-deficient mice generated by recombination-activating gene-2–deficient blastocyst complementation. *Proc Natl Acad Sci U S A* 1994;91:12135–12139.

215. Kawabe T, Naka T, Yoshida K, et al. The immune responses in CD40-deficient mice: impaired immunoglobulin class switching and germinal center formation. *Immunity* 1994;1:167–168.

216. Renshaw BR, Fanslow WC, Armitage RJ, et al. Humoral immune responses in CD40 ligand-deficient mice. *J Exp Med* 1994;180:1889–1900.

217. Xu J, Foy TM, Lamar JD, et al. Mice deficient for the CD40 ligand. *Immunity* 1994;1:423–431.

218. Foy TM, Lamar JD, Ledbetter JA, et al. gp39–CD40 interactions are essential for germinal center formation and the development of B cell memory. *J Exp Med* 1994;180:157–163.

219. Gray D, Dullforce P, Jainandunsing S. Memory B cell development but not germinal center formation is impaired by *in vivo* blockade of CD40–CD40 ligand interaction. *J Exp Med* 1994;180:141–155.

220. Han S, Hathcock K, Kheng B, et al. Cellular interaction in germinal centers. Roles of CD40 ligand and B7-2 in established germinal centers. *J Immunol* 1995;155:556–567.

221. Liu Y-J, Joshua JE, Williams GT, et al. Mechanism of antigen-driven selection in germinal centres. *Nature* 1989;342:929–931.

222. Liu Y-J, Cairns JA, Holder MJ, et al. Recombinant 25 kDa CD23 and interleukin 1α promote survival of germinal centre B cells: evidence for bifurcation in the development of centrocytes rescued from apoptosis. *Eur J Immunol* 1991;21:1107–1114.

223. Arpin C, Dechanet J, van Kooten C, et al. Generation of memory B cells and plasma cells *in vitro*. *Science* 1995;268:720–722.

224. Lane P, Burdet C, McConnell F, et al. CD40 ligand–independent B cell activation revealed by CD40 ligand–deficient T cell clones: evidence for distinct activation requirements for antibody formation and B cell proliferation. *Eur J Immunol* 1995;25:1788–1793.

225. Callard RE, Herbert J, Smith SH, et al. CD40 cross-linking inhibits specific antibody production by human B cells. *Int Immunol* 1995;7:1809–1815.

226. Casamayor-Palleja M, Khan M, MacLennan ICM. A subset of CD4+ memory T cells contains preformed CD40 ligand that is rapidly but transiently expressed on their surface after activation through the T cell receptor complex. *J Exp Med* 1995;181:1293–1301.

227. Van den Eertwegh AJM, Noelle RJ, Roy M, et al. *In vivo* CD40–gp39 interactions are essential for thymus dependent cytokines, and antibody production delineates sites of cognate T–B interactions. *J Exp Med* 1993;178:1555–1565.

228. Matsumoto AK, Kopicky-Burd J, Carter RH, et al. Intersection of the complement and immune systems: a signal transduction complex of the B lymphocyte–containing complement receptor type 2 and CD19. *J Exp Med* 1991;173:55–64.

229. Bradbury LE, Kansas GS, Levy S, et al. The CD19/CD21 signal transducing complex of human B lymphocytes includes the target of antiproliferative antibody-1 and Leu-13 molecules. *J Immunol* 1992;149:2841–2850.

230. Pesando JM, Bouchard LS, McMaster BE. CD19 is functionally and physically associated with surface immunoglobulin. *J Exp Med* 1989;170:2159–2164.

231. Carter RH, Fearon DT. CD19: lowering the threshold for antigen receptor stimulation of B lymphocytes. *Science* 1992;256:105–107.

232. Chalupny NJ, Aruffo A, Esselstyn JM, et al. Specific binding of Fyn and phosphatidylinositol 3-kinase to the B cell surface glycoprotein CD19 through their src homology 2 domains. *Eur J Immunol* 1995;25:2978–2984.

233. Myers DE, Jun X, Waddick KG, et al. Membrane-associated CD19-LYN complex is an endogenous p53-independent and Bcl-2–independent regulator of apoptosis in human B-lineage lymphoma cells. *Proc Natl Acad Sci U S A* 1995;92:9575–9579.

234. Engel P, Zhou LJ, Ord DC, et al. Abnormal B lymphocyte development, activation, and differentiation in mice that lack or overexpress the CD19 signal transduction molecule. *Immunity* 1995;3:39–50.

235. Rickert RC, Rajewsky K, Roes J. Impairment of T-cell–dependent B-cell responses and B-1 cell development in CD19-deficient mice. *Nature* 1995;376:352–355.

236. Fehr T, Rickert RC, Odermatt B, et al. Antiviral protection and germinal center formation, but impaired B cell memory in the absence of CD19. *J Exp Med* 1998;188:145–155.

237. Stuber E, Strober W. The T cell–B cell interaction via OX40–OX40L is necessary for the T cell–dependent humoral immune response. *J Exp Med* 1996;183:979–989.

238. Brocker T, Gulbranson-Judge A, Flynn S, et al. CD4 T cell traffic control: *in vivo* evidence that ligation of OX40 on CD4 T cells by OX40-ligand expressed on dendritic cells leads to the accumulation of CD4 T cells in B cell follicles. *Eur J Immunol* 1999;29:1610–1616.

239. Rousset F, Peyrol S, Garcia E, et al. Long-term cultured CD40-activated B lymphocytes differentiate into plasma cells in response to IL-10 but not IL-4. *Int Immunol* 1995;7:1243–1253.

240. Melville P, Dechanet J, Grouard G, et al. T-cell–induced B cell blasts differentiate into plasma cells in response to IL-10 but not IL-4. *Int Immunol* 1995;7:635–643.

241. Morse L, Chen D, Franklin D, et al. Induction of cell cycle arrest and B cell terminal differentiation by CDK inhibitor p18INK4c and IL-6. *Immunity* 1997;6:1–20.

242. Garcia De Vinuesa C, Gulbranson-Judge A, Khan M, et al. Dendritic cells associated with plasmablast survival. *Eur J Immunol* 1999;29:3712–3721.

243. Koopman G, Parmentier HK, Schuurman HJ, et al. Adhesion of human B cells to follicular dendritic cells involves both the lymphocyte function–associated antigen 1/intercellular adhesion molecule 1 and very late antigen 4/vascular cell adhesion molecule 1 pathways. *J Exp Med* 1991;173:1297–1304.

244. Kosco MH, Pflugfelder E, Gray D. Follicular dendritic cell–dependent adhesion and proliferation of B cells *in vitro*. *J Immunol* 1992;148:2331–2339.

245. Lindhout E, Mevissen ML, Kwekkeboom J, et al. Direct evidence that human follicular dendritic cells (FDC) rescue germinal centre B cells from death by apoptosis. *Clin Exp Immunol* 1993;91:330–336.

246. Koopman G, Keehnen RMJ, Lindhout E, et al. Adhesion through the LFA-1 (CD11a/CD18)–ICAM-1 (CD54) and the VKA-4 (CD49d)–VCAM-1 (CD106) pathways prevents apoptosis of germinal center B cells. *J Immunol* 1994;152:3760–3767.

247. Grouard G, de Bouteiller O, Banchereau J, et al. Human follicular dendritic cells enhance cytokine-dependent growth and differentiation of CD40-activated B cells. *J Immunol* 1995;155:3345–3352.

248. Wu J, Qin D, Burton GF, et al. Follicular dendritic cell–derived antigen and accessory activity in initiation of memory IgG responses *in vitro*. *J Immunol* 1996;157:3404–3411.

249. Tew JG, Wu J, Qin D, et al. Follicular dendritic cells and presentation of antigen and costimulatory signals to B cells. *Immunol Rev* 1997;156:39–52.

250. Zhang X, Li L, Jung J, et al. The distinct roles of T cell-derived cytokines and a novel follicular dendritic cell-signaling molecule 8D6 in germinal center–B cell differentiation. *J Immunol* 2001;167:49–56.

251. Pezzella F, Tse AG, Cordell JL, et al. Expression of the bcl-2 oncogene protein is not specific for the 14;18 chromosomal translocation. *Am J Pathol* 1990;137:225–232.

252. Hockenbery DM, Zutter M, Hickey W, et al. BCL2 protein is topographically restricted in tissues characterized by apoptotic cell death. *Proc Natl Acad Sci U S A* 1991;88:6961–6965.

253. Martinez-Valdez H, Guret C, de Bouteiller O, et al. Human germinal center B cells express the apoptosis-inducing genes Fas, c-myc, p53 and Bax but not the survival gene bcl-2. *J Exp Med* 1996;183:971–977.

254. Liu YJ, Mason DY, Johnson GD, et al. Germinal center cells express Bcl-2 protein after activation by signals which prevent their entry into apoptosis. *Eur J Immunol* 1991;21:1905–1910.

255. Nunez G, Hockenbery D, McDonnell TJ, et al. Bcl-2 maintains B cell memory. *Nature* 1991;353:71–73.

256. Strasser A, Whittingham S, Vaux DL, et al. Enforced BCL2 expression in B-lymphoid cells prolongs antibody responses and elicits autoimmune disease. *Proc Natl Acad Sci U S A* 1991;88:8661–8665.

257. Smith KGC, Weiss U, Rajewsky K, et al. Bcl-2 increases memory B cell recruitment but does not perturb selection in germinal centers. *Immunity* 1994;1:803–813.

258. Smith KGC, Light A, O'Reilly LA, et al. bcl-2 Transgene expression inhibits apoptosis in the germinal center and reveals differences in the selection of memory B cells and bone marrow antibody forming cells. *J Exp Med* 2000;191:475–484.

259. Takahashi Y, Cerasoli DM, Dal Porto JM, et al. Relaxed negative selection in germinal centers and impaired affinity maturation in bcl-xL transgenic mice. *J Exp Med* 1999;190:399–409.

260. Grillot DAM, Merino R, Pena JC, et al. bcl-x exhibits regulated expression during B cell development and activation and modulates lymphocyte survival in transgenic mice. *J Exp Med* 1996;183:381–391.

261. Choi MSK, Holman M, Atkins CJ, et al. Expression of bcl-x during mouse B cell differentiation and following activation by various stimuli. *Eur J Immunol* 1996;26:676–668.

262. Tuscano JM, Druey KM, Riva A, et al. Bcl-x rather than Bcl-2 mediates CD40-dependent centrocyte survival in the germinal center. *Blood* 1996;88:1359–1364.

263. Hennino A, Berard M, Krammer PH, et al. FLICE-inhibitory protein

is a key regulator of germinal center B cell apoptosis. *J Exp Med* 2001;193:447–458.

264. Kischkel FC, Hellbardt S, Behrmann I, et al. Cytotoxicity-dependent APO-1 (Fas/CD95)–associated proteins form a death-inducing signalling complex (DISC) with the receptor. *EMBO J* 1995;14:5579–5588.

265. Muzio M, Chinnaiyan AM, Kischkel FC, et al. FLICE, a novel FADD-homologous ICE/CED-3–like protease, is recruited to the CD95 (Fas/APO-1) death-inducing signaling complex. *Cell* 1996;85:817–827.

266. van Eijk M, Medema JP, de Groot C. Cutting edge: cellular Fas-associated death domain–like IL-1–converting enzyme–inhibitory protein protects germinal center B cells from apoptosis during germinal center reactions. *J Immunol* 2001;166:6473–6476.

267. Rothstein TL, Wang JKM, Panka DJ, et al. Protection against Fas-dependent Th1-mediated apoptosis by antigen receptor engagement in B cells. *Nature* 1995;374:163–165.

268. Takahashi Y, Ohta H, Takemori T. Fas is required for clonal selection in germinal centers and the subsequent establishment of the memory B cell repertoire. *Immunity* 2001;14:181–192.

269. Turner CA, Mack DH, Davis MM. Blimp-1, a novel zinc finger–containing protein that can drive the maturation of B lymphocytes into immunoglobulin-secreting cells. *Cell* 1994;77:297–306.

270. Reimold AM, Iwakoshi NN, Manis J, et al. Plasma cell differentiation requires the transcription factor XBP-1. *Nature* 2001;412:300–307.

271. Neurath MF, Stuber ER, Strober W. BSAP: a key regulator of B-cell development and differentiation. *Immunol Today* 1995;16:564–569.

272. Reimold AM, Ponath PD, Li YS, et al. Transcription factor B cell lineage–specific activator protein regulates the gene for human X-box binding protein 1. *J Exp Med* 1996;183:393–401.

273. Liu Y-J, Bancherau J. Regulation of B-cell commitment to plasma cells or to memory B cells. *Semin Immunol* 1997;9:235–240.

274. Budd RC, Cerottini JC, MacDonald HR. Selectively increased production of interferon-gamma by subsets of Lyt2+ and L3T4+ T cells identified by expression of Pgp-1. *J Immunol* 1987;138:3583–3586.

275. Tabi Z, Lynch F, Ceredig R, et al. Virus-specific memory T cells are Pgp-1+ and can be selectively activated with phorbol ester and calcium ionophore. *Cellular Immunology* 1988;113:268–277.

276. Sanders ME, Makgoba MW, Sharrow SO, et al. Human memory T lymphocytes express increased levels of three cell adhesion molecules (LFA-3, CD2, and LFA-1) and three other molecules (UCHL1, CDw29, and Pgp-1) and have enhanced IFN-γ production. *J Immunol* 1988;140:1401–1407.

277. Butterfield K, Fathman CG, Budd RC. A subset of memory CD4+ helper T lymphocytes identified by expression of Pgp-1. *J Exp Med* 1989;169:1461–1466.

278. Mackay CR, Marston WL, Dudler L. Naïve and memory T cells show distinct pathways of lymphocyte recirculation. *J Exp Med* 1990;171:801–817.

279. Buckle AM, Hogg N. Human memory T cells express intercellular adhesion molecule–1 which can be increased by interleukin 2 and interferon-γ. *Eur J Immunol* 1990;20:337–341.

280. Beverley PCL. Functional analysis of human T cell subsets defined by CD45 isoform expression. *Sem Immunol* 1992;4:35–41.

281. McFarland HI, Nahill SR, Maciaszek JW, et al. CD11b (Mac-1): a marker for CD8+ cytotoxic T cell activation and memory in virus infection. *J Immunol* 1992;149:1326–1333.

282. Okumura M, Fujii Y, Takeuchi Y, et al. Age-related accumulation of LFA-1high cells in a CD8+CD45RAhighT cell population. *Eur J Immunol* 1993;23:1057–1063.

283. Hamann D, Baars PA, Rep MHG, et al. Phenotypic and functional separation of memory and effector human CD8+T cells. *J Exp Med* 1997;186:1407–1418.

284. Lau LL, Jamieson BD, Somasundaram R, et al. Cytotoxic T cell memory without antigen. *Nature* 1994;369:648–652.

285. Murali-Krishna K, Lau LL, Sambhara S, et al. Persistence of memory CD8 T cells in MHC class I–deficient mice. *Science* 1999;286:1377–1381.

286. Andersen P, Smedegaard B. CD4+ T-cell subsets that mediate immunological memory to *Mycobacterium tuberculosis* infection in mice. *Infect Immun* 2000;68:621–629.

287. Swain SL, Bradley LM, Croft M, et al. Helper T-cell subsets: phenotype, function and the role of lymphokines in regulating their development. *Immunol Rev* 1991;123:115–144.

288. Bradley LM, Atkins GG, Swain SL. Long-term CD4+ memory T cells from the spleen lack MEL-14, the lymph node homing receptor. *J Immunol* 1992;148:324–331.

289. Hou S, Doherty PC. Partitioning of responder CD8+T cells in lymph node and lung of mice with Sendai virus pneumonia by LECAM-1 and CD45RB phenotype. *J Immunol* 1993;150:5494–5500.

290. Tedder TF, Matsuyama T, Rothstein D, et al. Human antigen-specific memory T cells express the homing receptor (LAM-1) necessary for lymphocyte recirculation. *Eur J Immunol* 1990;20:1351–1355.

291. Howard CJ, Sopp P, Parsons KR. L-selectin expression differentiates T cells isolated from different lymphoid tissues in cattle but does not correlate with memory. *Immunology* 1992;77:228–234.

292. Razvi ES, Welsh RM, McFarland HI. Characterization of a cycling cell population containing CTL precursors in immune mice. *J Immunol* 1995;154:620–632.

293. Tripp RA, Hou S, Doherty PC. Temporal loss of the activated L-selectin-low phenotype for virus-specific CD8+ memory T cells. *J Immunol* 1995;154:5870–5875.

294. Oehen S, Brduscha-Riem K. Differentiation of naïve CTL to effector and memory CTL: correlation of effector function with phenotype and cell division. *J Immunol* 1998;161:5338–5346.

295. Usherwood EJ, Hogan RJ, Crowther G, et al. Functionally heterogeneous CD8+T-cell memory is induced by Sendai virus infection of mice. *J Virol* 1999;73:7278–7286.

296. Jung TM, Gallatin WM, Weissman IL, et al. Downregulation of homing receptors after T cell activation. *J Immunol* 1988;141:4110–4117.

297. Picker LJ, Terstappen LW, Rott LS, et al. Differential expression of homing-associated adhesion molecules by T cell subsets in man. *J Immunol* 1990;145:3247–3255.

298. Horgan KJ, Luce GE, Tanaka Y, et al. Differential expression of VLA-alpha 4 and VLA-beta 1 discriminates multiple subsets of CD4+CD45RO+"memory" T cells. *J Immunol* 1992;149:4082–4087.

299. Forster R, Emrich T, Kremmer E, et al. Expression of the G-protein–coupled receptor BLR1 defines mature, recirculating B cells and a subset of T-helper memory cells. *Blood* 1994;84:830–840.

300. Breitfeld D, Ohl L, Kremmer E, et al. Follicular B helper T cells express CXC chemokine receptor 5, localize to B cell follicles, and support immunoglobulin production. *J Exp Med* 2000;192:1545–1552.

301. Mackay CR. Follicular homing T helper (Th) cells and the Th1/Th2 paradigm. *J Exp Med* 2000;192:F31–F34.

302. Schaerli P, Willimann K, Lang AB, et al. CXC chemokine receptor 5 expression defines follicular homing T cells with B cell helper function. *J Exp Med* 2000;192:1553–1562.

303. Thomas ML. The leukocyte common antigen family. *Annu Rev Immunol* 1989;7:339–369.

304. Merkenschlager M, Terry L, Edwards R, et al. Limiting dilution analysis of proliferative responses in human lymphocyte populations defined by the monoclonal antibody UCHL1: implications for differential CD45 expression in T cell memory formation. *Eur J Immunol* 1988;18:1653–1661.

305. Merkenschlager M, Beverley PCL. Evidence for differential expression of CD45 isoforms by precursors for memory-dependent and independent cytotoxic responses: human CD8 memory CTLp selectively express CD45RO (UCHL1). *Int Immunol* 1989;1:450–459.

306. Hayward AR, Lee J, Beverley PC. Ontogeny of expression of UCHL1 antigen on TcR+(CD4/8) and TCR d+T cells. *Eur J Immunol* 1989;189:19.

307. Birkeland ML, Johnson P, Trowbridge IS, et al. Changes in CD45 isoform expression accompany antigen-induced murine T-cell activation. *Proc Natl Acad Sci U S A* 1989;86:6734–6738.

308. Powrie F, Mason D. The MRC OX-22−CD4+T cells that help B cells in secondary immune responses derive from naïve precursors with the MRC OX-22+CD4+phenotype. *J Exp Med* 1989;169:653–662.

309. Lee WT, Yin XM, Vitetta ES. Functional and ontogenic analysis of murine CD45Rhi and CD45RloCD4+T-cells. *J Immunol* 1990;144:3288–3295.

310. Marvel J, Lightstone E, Samberg NL, et al. The CD45RA molecule is expressed in naïve murine CTL precursors but absent in memory and effector CTL. *Int Immunol* 1991;3:21–28.

311. Bell EB, Sparshott SM. Interconversion of CD45R subsets of CD4 T cells *in vivo*. *Nature* 1990;348:163–166.

312. Gahring LC, Ernst DN, Romball CG, et al. The expression of CD45RB on antigen-responsive CD4+lymphocytes: mouse strain

polymorphism and different responses to distinct antigens. *Cell Immunol* 1993;148:269–282.

313. Sparshott SM, Bell EB. Membrane CD45R isoform exchange on CD4 T cells is rapid, frequent and dynamic *in vivo*. *Eur J Immunol* 1994;24:2573–2578.

314. Pihlgren M, Lightstone L, Mamalaki C, et al. Expression *in vivo* of CD45RA, CD45RB and CD44 on T cell receptor–transgenic CD8+ T cells following immunization. *Eur J Immunol* 1995;25:1755–1759.

315. Pilling D, Akbar AN, Bacon PA, et al. CD4+CD45RA+ T cells from adults respond to recall antigens after CD28 ligation. *Int Immunol* 1996;8:1737–1742.

316. Richards D, Chapman MD, Sasama J, et al. Immune memory in CD4+ CD45RA+ T cells. *Immunology* 1997;91:331–339.

317. Wilamasundera S, Katz DR, Chain BM. Responses to human rhinovirus in CD45 T cell subsets isolated from tonsil. *Eur J Immunol* 1998;28:4374–4381.

318. Faint JM, Annels NE, Curnow SJ, et al. Memory T cells constitute a subset of the human CD8+CD45RA+ pool with distinct phenotypic and migratory characteristics. *J Immunol* 2001;167:212–220.

319. Rothstein DM, Yamada A, Schlossman SF, et al. Cyclic regulation of CD45 isoform expression in a long term human CD4+CD45RA+ T cell line. *J Immunol* 1991;146:1175–1183.

320. Warren HS, Skipsey LJ. Loss of activation-induced CD45RO with maintenance of CD45RA expression during prolonged culture of T cells and NK cells. *Immunology* 1991;74:78–85.

321. Fujii Y, Okumura M, Inada K, et al. Reversal of CD45R isoform switching in CD8+ T cells. *Cell Immunol* 1992;139:176–184.

322. Boursalian RE, Bottomly K. Stability of naïve and memory phenotypes on resting CD4 T cells *in vivo*. *J Immunol* 1999;162:9–16.

323. Nociari MM, Telford W, Russo C. Postthymic development of CD28−CD8+ T cell subset: age-associated expansion and shift from memory to naïve phenotype. *J Immunol* 1999;162:3327–3335.

324. Wikby A, Johansson B, Olsson J, et al. Expansions of peripheral blood CD8 T-lymphocyte subpopulations and an association with cytomegalovirus seropositivity in the elderly: the Swedish NONA immune study. *Exp Gerontol* 2002;37:445–453.

325. De Jon R, Brouer M, Hooibrink B, et al. The CD27− subset of peripheral blood memory CD4+ lymphocytes contains functionally differentiated T lymphocytes that develop by persistent antigenic stimulation *in vivo*. *Eur J Immunol* 1992;22:993–999.

326. Walunas TL, Bruce DS, Dustin L, et al. Ly-6C is a marker of memory CD8+ T cells. *J Immunol* 1995;155:1873–1883.

327. Zhang X, Sun S, Hwang I, et al. Potent and selective stimulation of memory-phenotype CD8+ T cells *in vivo* by IL-15. *Immunity* 1998;8:591–599.

328. Curtsinger JM, Lins DC, Mescher MF. CD8+ memory T cells (CD44high, Ly-6C+) are more sensitive than naïve cells (CD44low, Ly-6C−) to TCR/CD8 signaling in response to antigen. *J Immunol* 1998;160:3236–3243.

329. Cho BK, Wang C, Sugawa S, et al. Functional differences between memory and naïve CD8 T cells. *Proc Natl Acad Sci U S A* 1999;96:2976–2981.

330. Gumley TP, McKenzie IF, Sandrin MS. Tissue expression, structure and function of the murine Ly-6 family of molecules. *Immunol Cell Biol* 1995;73:277–296.

331. Waldmann TA, Tagaya Y. The multifaceted regulation of interleukin-15 expression and the role of this cytokine in NK cell differentiation and host response to intracellular pathogens. *Annu Rev Immunol* 1999;17:19–49.

332. Chervenak R, Cohen JJ. Peanut lectin binding as a marker for activated T-lineage lymphocytes. *Thymus* 1982;4:61–67.

333. Piller F, Piller V, Fox RI, et al. Human T-lymphocyte activation is associated with changes in O-glycan biosynthesis. *J Biol Chem* 1988;263:15146–15150.

334. Galvan M, Murali-Krishna K, Ming LL, et al. Alterations in cell surface carbohydrates on T cells from virally infected mice can distinguish effector/memory CD8+ T cells from naïve cells. *J Immunol* 1988;161:641–648.

335. Priatel JJ, Chui D, Hiraoka N, et al. The ST3Gal-I sialyltransferase controls CD8+ T lymphocyte homeostasis by modulating O-glycan biosynthesis. *Immunity* 2000;12:273–283.

336. Harrington LE, Galvan M, Baum LG, et al. Differentiating between memory and effector CD8 T cells by altered expression of cell surface O-glycans. *J Exp Med* 2000;191:1241–1246.

337. Goldrath AW, Bevan MJ. Low-affinity ligands for the TCR drive proliferation of mature CD8+ T cells in lymphopenic hosts. *Immunity* 1999;11:183–190.

338. Ernst B, Lee D-S, Chang JM, et al. The peptide ligands mediating positive selection in the thymus control T cell survival and homeostatic proliferation in the periphery. *Immunity* 1999;11:173–181.

339. Kieper WC, Jameson SC. Homeostatic expansion and phenotypic conversion of naïve T cells in response to self peptide/MHC ligands. *Proc Natl Acad Sci U S A* 1999;96:13306–13311.

340. Oehen S, Brduscha-Riem K. Naïve cytotoxic T lymphocytes spontaneously acquire effector function in lymphocytopenic recipients: a pitfall for T cell memory studies? *Eur J Immunol* 1999;29:608–614.

341. Viret C, Wong FS, Janeway CA Jr. Designing and maintaining the mature TCR repertoire: the continuum of self-peptide:self-MHC complex recognition. *Immunity* 1999;10:559–568.

342. Goldrath AW, Bogatzki LY, Bevan MJ. Naïve T cells transiently acquire a memory-like phenotype during homeostasis-driven proliferation. *J Exp Med* 2000;192:557–564.

343. Cho BK, Rao VP, Ge Q, et al. Homeostasis-stimulated proliferation drives naïve T cells to differentiate directly into memory T cells. *J Exp Med* 2000;192:549–556.

344. Murali-Krishna K, Ahmed R. Naïve T cells masquerading as memory cells. *J Immunol* 2000;165:1733–1737.

345. Muranski P, Chmielowski B, Ignatowicz L. Mature CD4+ T cells perceive a positively selecting class II MHC/peptide complex in the periphery. *J Immunol* 2000;164:3087–3094.

346. Boursalian TE, Bottomly K. Survival of naïve CD4 T cells: roles of restricting versus selecting MHC class II and cytokine milieu. *J Immunol* 1999;162:3795–3801.

347. Rogers PR, Huston G, Swain SL. High antigen density and IL-2 are required for generation of CD4 effectors secreting Th1 rather than Th0 cytokines. *J Immunol* 1998;161:3844–3852.

348. Saparov A, Kraus LA, Cong Y, et al. Memory/effector T cells in TCR transgenic mice develop via recognition of enteric antigens by a second, endogenous TCR. *Int Immunol* 1999;11:1253–1264.

349. Sepulveda H, Cerwenka A, Morgan T, et al. CD28, IL-2–independent costimulatory pathways for CD8 T lymphocyte activation. *J Immunol* 1999;163:1133–1142.

350. Abney ER, Cooper MD, Kearney JF, et al. Sequential expression of immunoglobulin on developing mouse B lymphocytes: a systematic survey that suggests a model for the generation of immunoglobulin isotype diversity. *J Immunol* 1978;120:2041–2049.

351. Halper J, Fu SM, Wang CY, et al. Patterns of expression of human Ia-like antigens during terminal stages of B cell development. *J Immunol* 1978;120:1480–1484.

352. MacLennan ICM, Gray D. Antigen-driven selection of virgin and memory B cells. *Immunol Rev* 1986;91:61–85.

353. Klein U, Kuppers R, Rajewsky K. Human IgM+IgD+ B cells, the major B cell subset in the peripheral blood, express V genes with no or little somatic mutation throughout life. *Eur J Immunol* 1993;23:3272–3277.

354. Reynaud CA, Garcia C, Hein WR, et al. Hypermutation generating the sheep immunoglobulin repertoire is an antigen-independent process. *Cell* 1995;80:115–125.

355. Smith KG, Light A, Nossal GJ, et al. The extent of affinity maturation differs between the memory and antibody-forming cell compartments in the primary immune response. *EMBO J* 1997;16:2996–3006.

356. Black SJ, Van der Loo W, Loken MR, et al. Expression of IgD by murine lymphocytes. Loss of surface IgD indicates maturation of memory B cells. *J Exp Med* 1977;147:984–996.

357. Coffman RL, Cohn M. The class of surface immunoglobulin on virgin and memory B lymphocytes. *J Immunol* 1977;118:1806–1815.

358. Teale JM, Lafrenz D, Klinman N, et al. Immunoglobulin class commitment exhibited by B lymphocytes separated according to surface isotype. *J Immunol* 1981;126:1952–1957.

359. Yefenof E, Sanders VM, Snow EC, et al. Preparation and analysis of antigen-specific memory B cells. *J Immunol* 1985;135:3777–3784.

360. White H, Gray D. Analysis of immunoglobulin (Ig) isotype diversity and IgM/D memory in the response to phenyl-oxazolone. *J Exp Med* 2000;191:2209–2220.

361. Liu Y-J, Oldfield S, MacLennan ICM. Memory B cells in T cell–dependent antibody responses colonize the splenic marginal zones. *Eur J Immunol* 1988;18:355–362.

362. Huang C, Stewart AK, Schwartz RS, et al. Immunoglobulin heavy

chain gene expression in peripheral blood lymphocytes. *J Clin Invest* 1992;89:1331–1343.

363. van Es JH, Meyling FH, Logtenberg T. High frequency of somatically mutated IgM molecules in the human adult blood B cell repertoire. *Eur J Immunol* 1992;22:2761–2764.

364. Klein U, Kuppers R, Rajewsky K. Evidence for a large compartment of IgM-expressing memory B cells in humans. *Blood* 1997;89:1288–1298.

365. Paramithiotis E, Cooper MD. Memory B lymphocytes migrate to the bone marrow in humans. *Proc Natl Acad Sci U S A* 1997;94:208–212.

366. Klein U, Rajewsky K, Kuppers R. Human immunoglobulin (Ig)M+IgD+ peripheral blood B cells expressing the CD27 cell surface antigen carry somatically mutated variable region genes: CD27 as a general marker for somatically mutated (memory) B cells. *J Exp Med* 1998;188:1679–1689.

367. Tangye SG, Liu Y-J, Aversa G, et al. Identification of functional human splenic memory B cells by expression of CD148 and CD27. *J Exp Med* 1998;188:1691–1703.

368. Maurer D, Holter W, Majdic O, et al. CD27 expression by a distinct subpopulation of human B lymphocytes. *Eur J Immunol* 1990;20:2679–2684.

369. Agematsu K, Nagumo H, Yang FC, et al. B cell subpopulations separated by CD27 and crucial collaboration of CD27+ B cells and helper T cells in immunoglobulin production. *Eur J Immunol* 1997;27:2073–2079.

370. Maurer D, Fischer GF, Fae I, et al. IgM and IgG but not cytokine secretion is restricted to the CD27+ B lymphocyte subset. *J Immunol* 1992;148:3700–3705.

371. Lens SMA, de Jong R, Hooibrink B, et al. Phenotype and function of human B cells expressing CD70 (CD27 ligand). *Eur J Immunol* 1996;26:2964–2971.

372. Arpin C, Banchereau J, Liu YJ. Memory B cells are biased towards terminal differentiation: a strategy that may prevent repertoire freezing. *J Exp Med* 1997;186:931–940.

373. Camp RL, Kraus TA, Birkeland ML, et al. High levels of CD44 expression distinguish virgin from antigen-primed B cells. *J Exp Med* 1991;173:763–766.

374. Bruce J, Symington FW, McKearn TJ, et al. A monoclonal antibody discriminating between subsets of T and B cells. *J Immunol* 1981;127:2496–2501.

375. Yin X-M, Lee WT, Vitetta ES. Changes in expression of J11d on murine B cells during activation and generation of memory. *Cell Immunol* 1991;137:448–460.

376. Allman DM, Ferguson SE, Cancro MP. Peripheral B cell maturation. I. Immature peripheral B cells in adults are heat-stable antigen^hi and exhibit unique signaling characteristics. *J Immunol* 1992;149:2533–2540.

377. McHeyzer-Williams LJ, Cool M, McHeyzer-Williams MG. Antigen-specific B cell memory: expression and replenishment of a novel B220– memory B cell compartment. *J Exp Med* 2000;191:1149–1166.

378. Driver DJ, McHeyzer-Williams LJ, Cool M, et al. Development and maintenance of a B220– memory B cell compartment. *J Immunol* 2001;167:1393–1405.

379. Zimmerman C, Brduscha-Riem K, Blaser C, et al. Visualization, characterization, and turnover of CD8+ memory T cells in virus-infected hosts. *J Exp Med* 1996;183:1367–1375.

380. Lalvani A, Brookes R, Hambleton S, et al. Rapid effector function in CD8+ memory T cells. *J Exp Med* 1997;186:859–865.

381. Selin LK, Welsh RM. Cytolytically active memory CTL present in lymphocytic choriomeningitis virus–immune mice after clearance of virus infection. *J Immunol* 1997;158:5366–5373.

382. Hawke S, Stevenson PG, Freeman S, et al. Long-term persistence of activated cytotoxic T lymphocytes after viral infection of the central nervous system. *J Exp Med* 1998;187:1575–1582.

383. Kedl RM, Mescher MF. Qualitative differences between naïve and memory T cells make a major contribution to the more rapid and efficient memory CD8+ T cell response. *J Immunol* 1998;161:674–683.

384. Ahmadzadeh M, Hussain SF, Farber DL. Effector CD4 T cells are biochemically distinct from the memory subset: evidence for long-term persistence of effectors *in vivo*. *J Immunol* 1999;163:3053–3063.

385. Masopust D, Jiang J, Shen H, et al. Direct analysis of the dynamics of the intestinal mucosa CD8 T cell response to systemic virus infection. *J Immunol* 2001;166:2348–2356.

386. Paul WE, Siskind GW, Benacerraf B, et al. Secondary antibody responses in hapten systems: cell population selection by antigen. *J Immunol* 1967;99:760–770.

387. Andersson B. Studies of the regulation of avidity at the level of the single antibody-forming cell. The effect of antigen dose and time after immunization. *J Exp Med* 1970;132:77–88.

388. Celada F. The cellular basis of immunologic memory. *Prog Allergy* 1971;15:223–267.

389. Davie JM, Paul WE. Receptors on immunocompetent cells. V. Cellular correlations of the "maturation" of the immune response. *J Exp Med* 1972;135:660–674.

390. Engers HD, MacDonald HR. Generation of cytolytic T lymphocytes *in vitro*. *Contemp Top Immunobiol* 1976;5:145–190.

391. MacDonald HR, Cerottini J-C, Ryser J-E, et al. Quantitation and cloning of cytolytic T lymphocytes and their precursors. *Immunol Rev* 1980;51:93–123.

392. Cerottini J-C, MacDonald HR. The cellular basis of T-cell memory. *Annu Rev Immunol* 1989;7:77–89.

393. Price PW, Cerny J. Characterization of CD4+ T cells in mouse bone marrow. I. Increased activated/memory phenotype and altered TCR Vβ repertoire. *Eur J Immunol* 1999;29:1051–1056.

394. Hogan RJ, Zhong W, Usherwood EJ, et al. Protection from respiratory virus infections can be mediated by antigen-specific CD4+ T cells that persist in the lungs. *J Exp Med* 2001;193:981–986.

395. Mackay CR, Marston WL, Dudler L, et al. Tissue-specific migration pathways by phenotypically distinct subpopulations of memory T cells. *Eur J Immunol* 1992;22:887–895.

396. Schweighoffer T, Tanaka Y, Tidswell M, et al. Selective expression of integrin α4β7 on a subset of human CD4+ memory T cells with hallmarks of gut-trophism. *J Immunol* 1993;151:717–729.

397. Austrup F, Vestweber D, Borges E, et al. P- and E-selectin mediate recruitment of T-helper-1 but not T-helper-2 cells into inflamed tissues. *Nature* 1997;385:81–83.

398. Campbell DJ, Butcher EC. Rapid acquisition of tissue-specific homing phenotypes by CD4(+) T cells activated in cutaneous or mucosal lymphoid tissues. *J Exp Med* 2002;195:135–141.

399. Gallichan WS, Rosenthal KL. Long-lived cytotoxic T lymphocyte memory in mucosal tissues after mucosal but not systemic immunisation. *J Exp Med* 1996;184:1879–1890.

400. Hall JG, Parry DM, Smith ME. The distribution and differentiation of lymph-borne immunoblasts after intravenous injection into syngeneic recipients. *Cell Tissue Kinet* 1972;5:269–281.

401. Parrott DM, Ferguson A. Selective migration of lymphocytes within the mouse small intestine. *Immunology* 1974;26:571–588.

402. Benner R, Hijmans W, Haaijman JJ. The bone marrow: the major source of serum immunoglobulins, but still a neglected site of antibody formation. *Clin Exp Med* 1981;46:1–8.

403. Slifka MK, Matloubian M, Ahmed R. Bone marrow is a major site of long-term antibody production after acute viral infection. *J Virol* 1995;69:1895–1902.

404. Mitchison NA. The carrier effect in the secondary response to hapten-protein conjugates. V. Use of antilymphocyte serum to deplete animals of helper cells. *Eur J Immunol* 1971;1:68–75.

405. Liu Y-J, Zhang J, Lane PJ, et al. Sites of specific B cell activation in primary and secondary responses to T cell–dependent and T cell–independent antigens. *Eur J Immunol* 1991;21:2951–2962.

406. Dunn-Walters DK, Isaacson PG, Spencer J. Analysis of mutations in immunoglobulin heavy chain variable region genes of microdissected marginal zone (MGZ) B cells suggests that the MGZ of human spleen is a reservoir of memory B cells. *J Exp Med* 1995;182:559–566.

407. Dunn-Walters DK, Isaacson PG, Spencer J. Sequence analysis of rearranged Ig V_H genes from microdissected human Peyer's patch marginal zone B cells. *Immunology* 1996;88:618–624.

408. Tierens A, Delabie J, Michiels L, et al. Marginal-zone B cells in the human lymph node and spleen show somatic hypermutations and display clonal expansion. *Blood* 1999;93:226–234.

409. Kumararatne DS, Bazin H, MacLennan ICM. Marginal zones: the major B cell compartment of rat spleens. *Eur J Immunol* 1981;11:858–864.

410. Gray D, MacLennan ICM, Bazin H, et al. Migrant μ+δ+ and static μ+δ– B lymphocyte subsets. *Eur J Immunol* 1982;12:564–569.

411. Herman P. Microcirculation of lymphoid tissues. *Monogr Allergy* 1980;16:126–142.

412. Spencer J, Finn T, Pulford KAF, et al. The human gut contains a novel

population of B lymphocytes which resemble marginal zone cells. *Clin Exp Immunol* 1985;62:607–612.

413. Liu YJ, Barthelemy C, de Bouteiller O, et al. Memory B cells from human tonsils colonize mucosal epithelium and directly present antigen to T cells by rapid upregulation of B7-1 and B7-2. *Immunity* 1995;2:239–248.

414. Gowans JL, Uhr JW. The carriage of immunological memory by small lymphocytes in the rat. *J Exp Med* 1966;124:1017–1030.

415. Strober S. Initiation of antibody responses by different classes of lymphocytes. V. Fundamental changes in the physiological characteristics of virgin thymus-independent ("B") lymphocytes and "B" memory cells. *J Exp Med* 1972;136:851–871.

416. Strober S, Dilley J. Biological characteristics of T and B memory lymphocytes in the rat. *J Exp Med* 1973;137:1275–1292.

417. Strober S, Dilley J. Maturation of B lymphocytes in the rat. I. Migration pattern, tissue distribution, and turnover rate of unprimed and primed B lymphocytes involved in the adoptive antidinitrophenyl response. *J Exp Med* 1973;138:1331–1344.

418. Strober S. Immune function, cell surface characteristics and maturation of B cell subpopulations. *Transplant Rev* 1975;24:84–112.

419. Tew JG, Mandel T. The maintenance and regulation of serum antibody levels: evidence indicating a role for antigen retained in lymphoid follicles. *J Immunol* 1978;120:1063–1069.

420. Bachmann MF, Kundig TM, Odermatt B, et al. Free recirculation of memory B cells versus antigen-dependent differentiation to antibody-forming cells. *J Immunol* 1994;153:3386–3397.

421. Kraal G, Weissman IL, Butcher EC. Memory B cells express a phenotype consistent with migratory competence after secondary but not short-term primary immunization. *Cell Immunol* 1988;115:78–87.

422. Farstad IN, Halstensen TS, Kvale D, et al. Topographic distribution of homing receptors on B and T cells in human gut-associated lymphoid tissue: relation of L-selectin and integrin alpha 4 beta 7 to naïve and memory phenotypes. *Am J Pathol* 1997;150:187–199.

423. Farstad IN, Norstein J, Brandtzaeg P. Phenotypes of B and T cells in human intestinal and mesenteric lymph. *Gastroenterology* 1997;112:163–173.

424. Williams MB, Rose JR, Rott LS, et al. The memory B cell subset responsible for the secretory IgA response and protective humoral immunity to rotavirus expresses the intestinal homing receptor, alpha4beta7. *J Immunol* 1998;161:4227–4235.

425. Rott LS, Briskin MJ, Butcher EC. Expression of alpha4beta7 and E-selectin ligand by circulating memory B cells: implications for targeted trafficking to mucosal and systemic sites. *J Leukoc Biol* 2000;68:807–814.

426. Berlin C, Berg EL, Briskin MJ, et al. $\alpha 4 \beta 7$ integrin mediates lymphocyte binding to the mucosal vascular addressin MAdCAM-1. *Cell* 1993;74:185–195.

427. Hamann A, Andrew DP, Jablonski-Westrich D, et al. Role of $\alpha 4$-integrins in lymphocyte homing to mucosal tissues *in vivo*. *J Immunol* 1994;152:3282–3293.

428. Bargatze RF, Jutila MA, Butcher EC. Distinct roles of L-selectin and integrins $\alpha 4 \beta 7$ and LFA-1 in lymphocyte homing to Peyer's patch-HEV *in situ*: the multistep model confirmed and refined. *Immunity* 1995;3:99–108.

429. Byrne JA, Butler JL, Cooper MD. Differential activation requirements for virgin and memory T cells. *J Immunol* 1988;141:3249–3257.

430. Byrne JA, Butler JL, Reinherz EL, et al. Virgin and memory T cells have different requirements for activation via the CD2 molecule. *Int Immunol* 1989;1:29–35.

431. Sanders ME, Makgoba MW, June CH, et al. Enhanced responsiveness of human memory T cells to CD2 and CD3 receptor-mediated activation. *Eur J Immunol* 1989;19:803–808.

432. Ehlers S, Smith KA. Differentiation of T cell lymphokine gene expression: the *in vitro* acquisition of T cell memory. *J Exp Med* 1991;173:25–36.

433. Akbar AN, Salmon M, Janossy G. The synergy between naïve and memory T cells during activation. *Immunol Today* 1991;12:184–188.

434. Luqman M, Bottomly K. Activation requirements for CD4+ T cells differing in CD45R expression. *J Immunol* 1992;149:2300–2306.

435. Fischer H, Gjorloff A, Hedlund G, et al. Stimulation of human naïve and memory T helper cells with bacterial superantigen. Naïve CD4+45RA+ T cells require a costimulatory signal mediated through the LFA-1/ICAM-1 pathway. *J Immunol* 1992;148:1993–1998.

436. Kuiper H, Brouwer M, de Boer M, et al. Differences in responsiveness

437. Constant S, Zain M, West J, et al. Are primed CD4+ T lymphocytes different from unprimed cells? *Eur J Immunol* 1994;24:1073–1079.

438. Bachmann MF, Barner M, Viola A, et al. Distinct kinetics of cytokine production and cytolysis in effector and memory T cells after viral infection. *Eur J Immunol* 1999;29:291–299.

439. Garcia S, DiSanto J, Stockinger B. Following the development of a CD4 T cell response *in vivo:* from activation to memory formation. *Immunity* 1999;11:163–171.

440. Zimmermann C, Prevost-Blondel A, Blaser C, et al. Kinetics of the response of naïve and memory CD8 T cells to antigen: similarities and differences. *Eur J Immunol* 1999;29:284–290.

441. Rogers PR, Dubey C, Swain SL. Qualitative changes accompany memory T cell generation: faster, more effective responses at lower doses of antigen. *J Immunol* 2000;164:2338–2346.

442. Kearney ER, Pape KA, Loh DY, et al. Visualization of peptide-specific T cell immunity and peripheral tolerance induction *in vivo*. *Immunity* 1994;1:327-339.

443. Veiga-Fernandes H, Walter U, Bourgeois C, et al. Response of naïve and memory CD8+ T cells to antigen stimulation *in vivo*. *Nat Immunol* 2000;1:47–53.

444. Farber DL, Acuto O, Bottomly K. Differential T cell receptor-mediated signalling in naïve and memory T cells. *Eur J Immunol* 1997;27:2094–2101.

445. Hussain SF, Anderson CF, Farber DL. Differential SLP-76 expression and TCR-mediated signaling in effector and memory CD4 T cells. *J Immunol* 2002;168:1557–1565.

446. Tanchot C, Guillaume S, Delon J, et al. Modifications of CD8+ T cell function during *in vivo* memory or tolerance induction. *Immunity* 1998;8:581–590.

447. Bachmann MF, Gallimore A, Linkert S, et al. Developmental regulation of Lck targeting to the CD8 coreceptor controls signaling in naïve and memory T cells. *J Exp Med* 1999;189:1521–1529.

448. Dianzani U, Luqman M, Rojo J, et al. Molecular associations on the T cell surface correlate with immunological memory. *Eur J Immunol* 1990;20:2249–2257.

449. Leitenberg D, Novak TJ, Farber D, et al. The extracellular domain of CD45 controls association with the CD4–T cell receptor complex and the response to antigen-specific stimulation. *J Exp Med* 1996;183:249–259.

450. Stout RD, Suttles J. T cells bearing the CD44hi "memory" phenotype display characteristics of activated cells in G1 stage of cell cycle. *Cell Immunol* 1992;141:433–443.

451. McHeyzer-Williams MG, Davis MM. Antigen-specific development of primary and memory T cells *in vivo*. *Science* 1995;268:106–111.

452. Zheng B, Han S, Zhu Q, et al. Alternative pathways for the selection of antigen-specific peripheral T cells. *Nature* 1996;384:263–266.

453. McHeyzer-Williams LJ, Panus JF, Mikszta JA, et al. Evolution of antigen-specific T cell receptors *in vivo:* preimmune and antigen-driven selection of preferred complementary-determining region 3 (CDR3) motifs. *J Exp Med* 1999;189:1823–1837.

454. Fasso M, Anandasabapathy N, Crawford F, et al. T cell receptor (TCR)–mediated repertoire selection and loss of TCR vβ diversity during the initiation of a CD4+ T cell response *in vivo*. *J Exp Med* 2000;192:1719–1730.

455. Rees W, Bender J, Teague TK, et al. An inverse relationship between T cell receptor affinity and antigen dose during CD4+ T cell responses *in vivo* and *in vitro*. *Proc Natl Acad Sci U S A* 1999;96:9781–9786.

456. Kedl RM, Rees WA, Hildeman DA, et al. T cells compete for access to antigen-bearing antigen-presenting cells. *J Exp Med* 2000;192:1105–1113.

457. van Bergen J, Kooy Y, Koning F. CD4-independent T cells impair TCR triggering of CD4-dependent T cells: a putative mechanism for T cell affinity maturation. *Eur J Immunol* 2001;31:646–652.

458. Kedl RM, Schaefer BC, Kappler JW, et al. T cells down-modulate peptide-MHC complexes on APCs *in vivo*. *Nat Immunol* 2002;3:27–32.

459. Klinman NR. The mechanism of antigenic stimulation of primary and secondary clonal precursor cells. *J Exp Med* 1972;136:241–260.

460. Yefenof E, Sanders VM, Uhr JW, et al. *In vitro* activation of murine antigen-specific memory B cells by a T-dependent antigen. *J Immunol* 1986;137:85–90.

461. Hilbert DM, Cancro MP, Scherle PA, et al. T cell derived IL-6 is differentially required for antigen-specific antibody secretion by primary and secondary B cells. *J Immunol* 1989;143:4019–4024.

462. Dixon FJ, Maurer PH, Deichmiller MP. Primary and specific anamnestic antibody responses of rabbits to heterologous serum protein antigens. *J Immunol* 1954;72:179–186.

463. Eisen HN, Siskind GW. Variations in affinities of antibodies during the immune response. *Biochemistry* 1964;3:996–1008.

464. Steiner L, Eisen HN. The relative affinity of antibodies synthesized in the secondary response. *J Exp Med* 1967;126:1185–1203.

465. Makela O, Karjalainen K. Inherited immunoglobulin idiotypes of the mouse. *Immunol Rev* 1977;34:119–138.

466. Reth M, Imanishi-Kari T, Rajewsky K. Analysis of the repertoire of anti-NP antibodies in C57BL/6 mice by cell fusion. II. Characterization of idiotopes by monoclonal anti-idiotope antibodies. *Eur J Immunol* 1979;9:1004–1013.

467. Berek C, Griffiths GM, Milstein C. Molecular events during maturation of the immune response to oxazolone. *Nature* 1985;316:412–418.

468. Clarke SH, Huppi K, Ruezinsky D, et al. Inter- and intraclonal diversity in the antibody response to influenza hemagglutinin. *J Exp Med* 1985;161:687–704.

469. Allen D, Cumano A, Dildrop R, et al. Genetic requirements and functional consequences of somatic hypermutation during B cell development. *Immunol Rev* 1987;96:5–22.

470. Blier PR, Bothwell A. A limited number of B cell lineages generates the heterogeneity of a secondary immune response. *J Immunol* 1987;139:3996–4006.

471. Duran LW, Metcalf ES. Clonal analysis of primary B cells responsive to the pathogenic bacterium *Salmonella typhimurium. J Exp Med* 1987;165:340–358.

472. Malipiero UV, Levy NS, Gearhart PJ. Somatic mutation in antiphosphorylcholine antibodies. *Immunol Rev* 1987;96:59–74.

473. Manser T, Wysocki LJ, Margolies MN, et al. Evolution of antibody variable region structure during the immune response. *Immunol Rev* 1987;96:141–162.

474. Berek C, Milstein C. The dynamic nature of the antibody repertoire. *Immunol Rev* 1988;105:5–26.

475. French DL, Laskov R, Scharff MD. The role of somatic hypermutation in the generation of antibody diversity. *Science* 1989;244:1152–1157.

476. McHeyzer-Williams MG, Nossal GJV, Lalor PA. Molecular characterization of single memory B cells. *Nature* 1991;350:502–505.

477. Batista FD, Neuberger MS. Affinity dependence of the B cell response to antigen: a threshold, a ceiling, and the importance of off-rate. *Immunity* 1998;8:751–759.

478. Okumura K, Julius MH, Tsu T, et al. Demonstration that IgG memory is carried by IgG-bearing cells. *Eur J Immunol* 1976;6:467–472.

479. Yuan D, Vitetta ES, Kettman JR. Cell surface immunoglobulin. XX. Antibody responsiveness of subpopulations of B lymphocytes bearing different isotypes. *J Exp Med* 1977;145:1421–1435.

480. Martin SW, Goodnow CC. Burst-enhancing role of the IgG membrane tail as a molecular determinant of memory. *Nat Immunol* 2002;3:182–188.

481. Taylor RB. Decay of immunological responsiveness after thymectomy in adult life. *Nature* 1965;208:1334–1335.

482. Metcalf D. Delayed effect of thymectomy in adult life on immunological competence. *Nature* 1965;208:1336.

483. Miller JFAP. Effect of thymectomy in adult mice on immunological responsiveness. *Nature* 1965;208:1337–1338.

484. Miller JFAP, Mitchell GF. Thymus and antigen-reactive cells. *Transplant Rev* 1969;1:3–42.

485. Kappler JW, Hunter PC, Jacobs D, et al. Functional heterogeneity among the T-derived lymphocytes of the mouse. I. Analysis by adult thymectomy. *J Immunol* 1974;113:27–38.

486. Jamieson BD, Ahmed R. T cell memory. Long-term persistence of virus-specific cytotoxic T cells. *J Exp Med* 1989;169:1993–2005.

487. Bell EB, Sparshott SM, Drayson MT, et al. The stable and permanent expansion of functional T lymphocytes in athymic nude rats after a single injection of mature T cells. *J Immunol* 1987;139:1379–1384.

488. Sprent J, Schaefer M, Hurd M, et al. Mature murine B and T cells transferred to SCID mice can survive indefinitely and many maintain a virgin phenotype. *J Exp Med* 1991;174:717–728.

489. Sprent J. Lifespans of naïve, memory and effector lymphocytes. *Curr Opin Immunol* 1993;5:433–438.

490. Di Rosa F, Ramaswamy S, Ridge JP, et al. On the lifespan of virgin T lymphocytes. *J Immunol* 1999;163:1253–1257.

491. Everett NB, Caffrey RW, Rieke WO. Recirculation of lymphocytes. *Ann N Y Acad Sci* 1964;113:887–897.

492. Everett NB, Tyler RW. Lymphopoiesis in the thymus and other tissues: functional implications. *Int Rev Cytol* 1967;22:205–237.

493. Sprent J, Basten A. Circulating T and B lymphocytes of the mouse II. Lifespan. *Cell Immunol* 1973;7:40–59.

494. Claesson MH, Ropke C, Hougen HP. Distribution of short-lived and long-lived small lymphocytes in the lymphomyeloid tissues of germfree NMRI mice. *Scand J Immunol* 1974;3:597–604.

495. Ropke C. Renewal rates of murine T-lymphocyte subsets. *Cell Immunol* 1990;128:185–197.

496. Hellerstein M, Hanley MB, Cesar D, et al. Directly measured kinetics of circulating T lymphocytes in normal and HIV-1 infected humans. *Nat Med* 1999;5:83–89.

497. Mohri H, Bonhoeffer S, Monard S, et al. Rapid turnover of T lymphocytes in SIV-infected rhesus macaques. *Science* 1998;279:1223–1227.

498. McCune JM, Hanley MB, Cesar D, et al. Factors influencing T-cell turnover in HIV-1–seropositive patients. *J Clin Invest* 2000;105:R1–R8.

499. Bruno L, von Boehmer H, Kirberg J. Cell division in the compartment of naïve and memory T lymphocytes. *Eur J Immunol* 1996;26:3179–3184.

500. Tanchot C, Lemonnier FA, Perarnau B, et al. Differential requirements for survival and proliferation of CD8 naïve or memory T cells. *Science* 1997;276:2057–2062.

501. Swain SL, Hu H, Huston G. Class II–independent generation of CD4 memory T cells from effectors. *Science* 1999;286:1381–1383.

502. Sprent J, Miller JFAP. Thoracic duct lymphocytes from nude mice: migratory properties and lifespan. *Eur J Immunol* 1972;2:384–387.

503. Forster I, Rjewsky K. The bulk of the peripheral B-cell pool in mice is stable and not rapidly renewed from the bone marrow. *Proc Natl Acad Sci U S A* 1990;87:4781–4784.

504. Fulcher DA, Basten A. Reduced life span of anergic self-reactive B cells in a double-transgenic model. *J Exp Med* 1994;179:125–134.

505. Fulcher DA, Basten A. Influences on the lifespan of B cell subpopulations defined by different phenotypes. *Eur J Immunol* 1997;27:1188–1199.

506. Kline GH, Hayden TA, Klinman NR. B cell maintenance in aged mice reflects both increased B cell longevity and decreased B cell generation. *J Immunol* 1999;162:3342–3349.

507. Tomayko MM, Cancro MP. Long-lived B cells are distinguished by elevated expression of A1. *J Immunol* 1998;160:107–111.

508. Morris SC, Moroldo M, Giannini EH, et al. *In vivo* survival of autoreactive B cells: characterisation of long-lived B cells. *J Immunol* 2000;164:3035–3046.

509. Schittek B, Rajewsky K. Maintenance of B-cell memory by long-lived cells generated from proliferating precursors. *Nature* 1990;346:749–751.

510. Mattioli CA, Tomasi TB. The life span of IgA plasma cells from the mouse intestine. *J Exp Med* 1973;138:452–460.

511. Manz RA, Thiel A, Radbruch A. Lifetime of plasma cells in the bone marrow. *Nature* 1997;388:133–134.

512. Slifka M, Antia R, Whitmire JK, et al. Humoral immunity due to long-lived plasma cells. *Immunity* 1998;8:363–372.

513. Mandel TE, Phipps RP, Abbot A, et al. The follicular dendritic cell: long-term antigen retention during immunity. *Immunol Rev* 1980; 53:29–59.

514. Tew JG, Kosco MH, Burton GF, et al. Follicular dendritic cells as accessory cells. *Immunol Rev* 1990;117:185–211.

515. Beverley PCL. Is T cell memory maintained by cross-reactive stimulation? *Immunol Today* 1990;11:203–205.

516. Amrani A, Serra P, Yamanouchi J, et al. Expansion of the antigenic repertoire of a single T cell receptor upon T cell activation. *J Immunol* 2001;167:655–666.

517. Feldbush TL. Antigen modulation of the immune response: the decline of immunological memory in the absence of continuing antigenic stimulation. *Cell Immunol* 1973;8:435–444.

518. Gray D, Matzinger P. T cell memory is short-lived in the absence of antigen. *J Exp Med* 1991;174:969–974.

519. Oehen S, Waldner H, Kundig TM, et al. Antivirally protective cytotoxic

T cell memory to lymphocytic choriomeningitis virus is governed by persisting antigen. *J Exp Med* 1992;176:1273–1281.

520. Gray D. Immunological memory. *Annu Rev Immunol* 1993;11:49–77.

521. Mullbacher A. The long-term maintenance of cytotoxic T cell memory does not require persistence of antigen. *J Exp Med* 1994;179:317–321.

522. Markiewicz MA, Girao C, Opferman JT, et al. Long-term T cell memory requires the surface expression of self-peptide/major histocompatibility complex molecules. *Proc Natl Acad Sci U S A* 1998;95:3065–3070.

523. Hu H, Huston G, Duso D, et al. CD4$^+$ T cell effectors can become memory cells with high efficiency and without further division. *Nat Immunol* 2001;2:705–710.

524. Takeda S, Rodewald H-R, Arakawa H, et al. MHC class II molecules are not required for survival of newly generated CD4$^+$ T cells, but affect their long-term life span. *Immunity* 1996;5:217–228.

525. Rooke R, Waltzinger C, Benoist C, et al. Targeted complementation of MHC class II deficiency by intrathymic delivery of recombinant adenoviruses. *Immunity* 1997;7:123–134.

526. Witherden D, van Oers N, Waltzinger C, et al. Tetracycline-controllable selection of CD4$^+$ T cells: half-life and survival signals in the absence of major histocompatibility complex class II molecules. *J Exp Med* 2000;191:355–364.

527. Clarke SRM, Rudensky AY. Survival and homeostatic proliferation of naïve peripheral CD4$^+$ T cells in the absence of self peptide:MHC complexes. *J Immunol* 2000;165:2458–2464.

528. Dorfman JR, Stefanova I, Yasutomo K, et al. CD4$^+$ T cell survival is not directly linked to self-MHC–induced TCR signalling. *Nat Immunol* 2000;1:329–335.

529. Kundig TM, Bachmann MF, Oehen S, et al. On the role of antigen in maintaining cytotoxic T-cell memory. *Proc Natl Acad Sci U S A* 1996;93:9716–9723.

530. Bachmann MF, Kundig TM, Hengartner H, et al. Protection against immunopathological consequences of a viral infection by activated but not resting cytotoxic T cells: T cell memory without "memory T cells"? *Proc Natl Acad Sci U S A* 1997;94:640–645.

531. Zinkernagel RM. What is missing in immunology to understand immunity? *Nat Immunol* 2000;1:181–185.

532. Tough DF, Borrow P, Sprent J. Induction of bystander T cell proliferation by viruses and type I interferon *in vivo*. *Science* 1996;272:1947–1950.

533. Tough DF, Sun S, Sprent J. T cell stimulation *in vivo* by lipopolysaccharide (LPS). *J Exp Med* 1997;185:2089–2094.

534. Tough DF, Zhang X, Sprent J. An IFN-γ–dependent pathway controls stimulation of memory phenotype CD8$^+$ T cell turnover *in vivo* by IL-12, IL-18, and IFN-γ. *J Immunol* 2001;166:6007–6011.

535. Ku CC, Murakami M, Sakamoto A, et al. Control of homeostasis of CD8$^+$ memory T cells by opposing cytokines. *Science* 2000;288:675–678.

536. Lodolce JP, Boone DL, Chai S, et al. IL-15 receptor maintains lymphoid homeostasis by supporting lymphocyte homing and proliferation. *Immunity* 1998;9:669–676.

537. Kennedy MK, Glaccum M, Brown SN, et al. Reversible defects in natural killer and memory CD8 T cell lineages in interleukin 15–deficient mice. *J Exp Med* 2000;191:771–780.

538. Marks-Konczalik J, Dubois S, Losi JM, et al. IL-2–induced activation–induced cell death is inhibited in IL-15 transgenic mice. *Proc Natl Acad Sci U S A* 2000;97:445–450.

539. Zhang X, Fujii H, Kishimoto H, et al. Aging leads to disturbed homeostasis of memory phenotype CD8$^+$ cells. *J Exp Med* 2002;195:283–293.

540. Grayson JM, Zajac AJ, Altman JD, et al. Cutting edge: increased expression of Bcl-2 in antigen-specific memory CD8$^+$ T cells. *J Immunol* 2000;164:3950–3954.

541. Wu T-S, Lee J-M, Lai Y-G, et al. Reduced expression of Bcl-2 in CD8$^+$ T cells deficient in the IL-15 receptor α-chain. *J Immunol* 2002;168:705–712.

542. Dai Z, Konieczny T, Lakkis FG. The dual role of IL-2 in the generation and maintenance of CD8$^+$ memory T cells. *J Immunol* 2000;165:3031–3036.

543. Suzuki H, Zhou TW, Kato M, et al. Normal regulatory alpha/beta T cells effectively eliminate abnormally activated T cells lacking the interleukin 2 receptor beta *in vivo*. *J Exp Med* 1999;190:1561–1572.

544. Annacker O, Burlen-Defranoux O, Pimenta-Araujo R, et al. Regulatory CD4 T cells control the size of the peripheral activated/memory CD4 T cell compartment. *J Immunol* 2000;164:3573–3580.

545. Neurath MF, Fuss I, Kelsall BL, et al. Experimental granulomatous colitis in mice is abrogated by induction of TGF-beta–mediated oral tolerance. *J Exp Med* 1996;183:2605–2616.

546. Powrie F, Carlino J, Leach MW, et al. A critical role for transforming growth factor–beta but not interleukin 4 in the suppression of T helper type 1–mediated colitis by CD45RB^{low}CD4$^+$ T cells. *J Exp Med* 1996;183:2669–2674.

547. Khan IA, Casciotti L. IL-15 prolongs the duration of CD8$^+$ T cell–mediated immunity in mice infected with a vaccine strain of *Toxoplasma gondii*. *J Immunol* 1999;163:4503–4509.

548. Geginat J, Sallusto F, Lanzavecchia A. Cytokine-driven proliferation and differentiation of human naïve, central memory, and effector memory CD4$^+$ T cells. *J Exp Med* 2001;194:1711–1719.

549. Lertmemongkolchai G, Cai G, Hunter CA, et al. Bystander activation of CD8$^+$ T cells contributes to the rapid production of IFN-gamma in response to bacterial pathogens. *J Immunol* 2001;166:1097–1105.

550. Tough DF, Sun S, Zhang X, et al. Stimulation of naïve and memory T cells by cytokines. *Immunol Rev* 1999;170:39–47.

551. Eberl G, Brawand P, MacDonald HR. Selective bystander proliferation of memory CD4$^+$ and CD8$^+$ T cells upon NK T or T cell activation. *J Immunol* 2000;165:4305–4311.

552. Gray D, Skarvall H. B-cell memory is short-lived in the absence of antigen. *Nature* 1988;336:70–73.

553. Manz RA, Lohning M, Cassese G, et al. Survival of long-lived plasma cells is independent of antigen. *Int Immunol* 1998;10:1703–1711.

554. Maruyama M, Lam KP, Rajewsky K. Memory B-cell persistence is independent of persisting immunizing antigen. *Nature* 2000;407:636–642.

555. Vieira P, Rajewsky K. Persistence of memory B cells in mice deprived of T cell help. *Int Immunol* 1990;2:487–494.

CHAPTER 29

Immunological Tolerance

Ronald H. Schwartz and Daniel L. Mueller

Introduction
Tolerance Is an Adaptive Process
Negative Selection during T-Cell Development
Stages of T-Cell Development at which Negative Selection Occurs · Antigen-Presenting Cells for Negative Selection · Biochemical Events in Thymocyte Clonal Deletion · Activation versus Tolerance Thresholds · T-Cell Tuning of Activation Thresholds
Negative Selection during B-Cell Development
Does Negative Selection Occur in the B-Cell Compartment? · Mechanisms of Negative Selection in the Bone Marrow · Antigen Characteristics Required for Negative Selection of B Cells · Immature B Cells Are Not Tolerizable Only
Tolerance to Peripheral Antigens
Tissue-Specific Peptide Antigens · Can Delivery to or Expression of Antigens in the Thymus Account for Tolerance to Peripheral Antigens? · Activation-Induced Cell Death and Homeostasis · T-Cell Anergy · CD4$^+$CD25$^+$ Suppressor T Cells · Pivotal Role of the Antigen-Presenting Cell in the Initiation of T-Cell Responses and Avoidance of Tolerance
Tolerance Induction in Mature B Cells
Receptor Blockade · B-Cell Anergy · Clonal Deletion · Thymic-Independent Antigens
Immunoregulation
Immune Deviation (Th1 versus Th2 CD4$^+$ Helpers) · CD4$^+$ T-Regulatory 1 Cells · Oral and Nasal Tolerance · CD8$^+$ Suppressor T Cells · CD8$^+$ Veto Cells · Antibody-Mediated Immunoregulation · Anti-Idiotypic B-Cell Regulation · Anti-Idiotypic T-Cell Regulation
Immune-Privileged Sites
Fetal–Maternal Relationship
Summary
References

INTRODUCTION

At the turn of the century, Ehrlich and Morgenroth (1) observed that goats they had injected with red blood cells from another goat always made hemolytic antibodies directed against the immunizing cells, but these antisera never reacted against the recipient's own red blood cells. Furthermore, they deliberately immunized a goat with its own red blood cells and also observed that no antibody response was elicited. They coined the Latin phrase "horror autotoxicus" to describe this situation. To them the term meant that the animals avoided self-destructive responses, although it has often been interpreted by others to mean a failure to make any immune responses against self-components. In this chapter, we retain Ehrlich's perspective. Hence, we define tolerance as a physiologic state in which the immune system does not react destructively against the components of an organism that harbors it or against antigens that are introduced to it. Destructive responses are prevented by a variety of mechanisms that operate during development of the immune system *and* during

the generation of each immune response. Pharmacologic manipulations are not included. This broad view allows one to consider immunoregulation as part of the tolerance process.

TOLERANCE IS AN ADAPTIVE PROCESS

Why didn't the goats make antibodies against their own red blood cells? The first observations that shed light on this issue were made by Owen (2) on dizygotic bovine twins and quintuplets. He analyzed the surface antigens of red blood cells from these cattle with alloantisera of the type raised by Ehrlich in goats and showed that each offspring possessed all antigens found in the parents, even though both parents did not express some of these determinants. In the quintuplets, this seemed highly unlikely to result from co-dominant heterozygosity, as the outbred parents would have had to be homozygous at multiple genetic loci. Instead, Owen was able to show in cytotoxicity assays that the offspring were chimeric, that is, their blood contained a mixture of cells with different

901

phenotypes. Based on the earlier work of Lillie, who had suggested that dizygotic cattle could exchange products through anastomoses of the blood vessels in their two placentas, Owen postulated that hemopoietic stem cells from each sibling migrated to the bone marrow of the others to create a stable chimeric state that persisted after the sibs were separated at birth. Because the chimerism of the antigenically disparate cells was not disturbed by an immune response, Owen described this state of peaceful coexistence as one of tolerance. These observations suggested that a foreign substance could be either reacted against or tolerated by an immune system depending on when the antigen was presented to it. These observations also suggested that there was no fundamental distinction between self-molecules (encoded by the host's genome) and foreign molecules in their ability to induce a tolerant state.

Burnet and Fenner (3) were strongly influenced by Owen's observations, as well as those of Traub, who demonstrated that a carrier state for the lymphocytic choriomeningitis virus (LCMV) could be induced in mice by natural exposure to this virus in utero or during the neonatal period. Their interpretation of both results was that the developing immune system was malleable and that if a foreign substance were introduced early enough, it would induce tolerance rather than immunity. The first experimental data to support this hypothesis were generated by Billingham et al. (4). The authors injected cell suspensions from mixed tissues of mouse strain A into neonatal or fetal mice of strain B and showed that as adults the strain B mice could accept skin grafts from a strain A mouse, although they would rapidly reject skin grafts from a third-party strain C mouse. The concept derived from this work, that tolerance was an acquired state, was confirmed by Hašek (5), who experimentally reproduced the observations of Owen by parabiosis of chick embryos. After separation at birth, the adult birds could not make an antibody response against each other's red blood cells (Ehrlich's experiment) and could not reject each other's skin grafts (Medawar's experiment). Burnet subsequently gave a theoretical framework to all of these results in his clonal selection theory, where he postulated that clones of lymphocytes with receptors on their surface specific for molecules present during the development of the immune system would be selectively eliminated by a deletion process (6).

Consistent with the idea that the immune system learns to be tolerant during its development was the subsequent experiment of Triplett (7). He removed the pituitary anlage from tree frog larvae and let them differentiate under the skin of other larvae. When the tadpoles went through metamorphosis, he gave back to the adult frogs their own pituitaries and found that the animals rejected the autografts. Partial hypophysectomized animals did not reject the grafts, arguing that the rejection was not caused by the acquisition of new antigens through either abnormal differentiation or carryover of the temporary host's tissues. Thus, even for self-antigens, tolerance appears to be an acquired state requiring the presence of the antigen to induce it.

The adaptive nature of tolerance is a fundamental property of the vertebrate immune system. Given the task of the system, which is to recognize and respond to unexpected molecules using the random structural diversity generated from rearranging T- and B-cell antigen-receptor genes, there is no way to genetically program it to know what molecules will lead to self-destructive responses. Instead, a series of steps must be undertaken somatically during which the environment is sampled and the system fine-tuned to avoid its own destruction. The nature of these steps in both the mature and developing immune system is the principal focus of this chapter.

NEGATIVE SELECTION DURING T-CELL DEVELOPMENT

The first demonstration of clonal deletion was published by Kappler and Marrack (8,9). They used a monoclonal antibody against the variable region of a T-cell receptor beta chain (anti-Vβ17a) to follow the fate of T cells expressing this chain. In mice expressing an E molecule encoded by MHC class II genes, Vβ17-bearing cells were eliminated. This process was later shown to be related to expression of an endogenous superantigen (the ORF gene product of mouse mammary tumor viruses 6, 8, or 9) (Mtv-6/8/9), which is capable of interacting with both Vβ17 and the E molecule. When E$^+$ and E$^-$ strains were crossed, the resulting F$_1$ animals also showed a deleted phenotype. This elimination process was shown to take place in the thymus. Cells expressing Vβ17 were found in only slightly reduced numbers in the immature CD4$^+$8$^+$ T-cell–receptor low population, but were greatly depleted among the more mature, single-positive (CD4$^+$8$^-$ and CD4$^-$8$^+$) thymocytes. The possibility that the cells had simply down-regulated their receptors was subsequently ruled out by showing that Vβ17 mRNA was also absent in mature T-cell populations. The actual deletion of the cells, however, was not observed until much later by other investigators. Similar observations were made by MacDonald and colleagues for Vβ6$^+$ T cells. Subsequent studies demonstrated that the deletion was occurring at the late double-positive stage when T-cell receptor expression is high and the CD4 and CD8 coreceptors have begun to down-modulate.

These observations were extended by Kisielow et al. (10) to a more conventional antigen system, the male-specific antigen H-Y. They took advantage of an α/β T-cell receptor (TCR$\alpha\beta^+$) transgenic mouse developed by Blüthmann and Steinmetz to follow the fate of a large cohort of T cells expressing the same anti–H-Y receptor, either in females, which do not express the antigen (controls), or in males that do. The male mice had a thymus of greatly reduced size (10% of normal) and a tremendous reduction in the percentage of double-positive thymocytes. Thus, the basic model postulated by Burnet appears to be correct for the standard TCR$\alpha\beta^+$ cell, that is, immature T cells encountering their antigen during development are clonally deleted. This process is referred to as "negative selection." More recent studies have shown that thymic negative selection also operates on other T-cell subsets including $TCR\gamma\delta^+$ cells, intraepithelial lymphocytes, and both the $CD4^-8^-$ and $CD4^+8^-$ $NK1.1^+$ $TCR\alpha\beta^+$ subpopulations.

Stages of T-Cell Development at which Negative Selection Occurs

The experiments involving tolerance to the H-Y antigen suggested that clonal deletion takes place at the early double-positive stage, whereas the experiments involving tolerance to superantigens suggested that clonal deletion takes place at the transition from the double-positive to the single-positive stage (11). It has been suggested by Singer that the early deletion seen in transgenic mice is a consequence of their premature expression of high levels of T-cell receptors and represents a different process akin to maturational arrest. However, a transgenic mouse developed by Pircher and colleagues, which carried a receptor specific for both a viral antigen and an Mtv-7 encoded superantigen deleted the double-positive cells when the mice carried the virus, but deleted only the single-positive cells when the mice were mated to animals expressing the Mtv-7 superantigen. Thus, it is likely that the nature of the antigen and where and how it is expressed for antigen presentation determine the stage at which the cells are deleted. Whether positive selection must take place as a necessary maturational step prior to negative selection is still not clear.

Evidence that clonal deletion can occur at the single-positive stage of T-cell development is also compelling. MacDonald and Lee observed that Mtv-7 superantigen-reactive $CD4^+8^-$ thymocytes disappear within the first few days of life. *In vitro* culture of these cells demonstrated that this was not just migration out of the thymus but an active death process that could be inhibited by low temperature, cycloheximide, or actinomycin D. *In vivo* experiments by Sprent and colleagues have suggested that it is the earliest HSA high $CD4^+8^-$ cells that are being deleted, by either a Fas-dependent mechanism for high doses of antigen or a Fas-independent mechanism for low doses of antigen. Thus, overall, it appears that thymocytes are susceptible to negative selection from the time that they first express their complete T-cell receptor up until the time that they are fully mature single-positive T cells.

Antigen-Presenting Cells for Negative Selection

Which cells are involved in presenting antigen for clonal deletion in the thymus has long been a point of contention (12). Consensus exists that bone marrow–derived cells play an important role, based initially on experiments with radiation-induced bone marrow chimeras. $(A \times B)F_1$ bone marrow transferred into a lethally irradiated strain-B recipient results in tolerance to both strain-A and strain-B peptide MHC complexes as measured in a mixed leukocyte culture. One bone marrow–derived cell involved in the deletion process is the dendritic cell. Donor-derived dendritic cells repopulate an irradiated thymus quickly, and Matzinger and Guerder showed that allogeneic dendritic cells from the spleen introduced into a thymic organ culture can induce tolerance to the alloantigens as measured in a CTL assay. Thus, a professional antigen-presenting cell (APC) capable of activating peripheral T cells, tolerizes thymocytes. Other experiments by Swat and colleagues with thymocyte suspensions from T-cell receptor transgenic mice showed directly that splenic antigen-presenting cells could induce deletion of $CD4^+8^+$ T cells. These observations suggest that it is the developmental stage of the T cell that determines the negative outcome of antigen presentation in the thymus, rather than a thymus-specific APC.

The role of thymic stromal (nonhematopoietic) cells in negative selection has been more controversial. Initial experiments with parental B bone marrow into $(A \times B)F_1$ irradiated hosts revealed alloreactivity against strain A APC. Similarly, deoxyguanosine-treated fetal thymuses (depleted of hematopoietic cells), when grafted into allogeneic nude mice, produced T cells that reacted in MLR and CML against the alloantigens of the thymus donor. The initial conclusion from these and other studies was that thymic stromal cells could not induce negative selection. A careful examination of the experiments, however, reveals that some negative effects did take place. For example, alloreactivity in the MLRs was often quantitatively diminished and the nude mice did not reject their thymus grafts. Subsequent experiments with T-cell receptor transgenic animals revealed strong evidence for thymic stromal cell-mediated deletion. Speiser and colleagues showed that transfer of TCR-transgenic bone marrow cells from a nondeleting strain into a virus-infected irradiated host, expressing on its stromal cells the MHC molecule required for virus-specific deletion, led to massive elimination of the cells in the thymus at the double-positive stage. Furthermore, Salaun and colleagues showed that grafts of allogeneic thymic anlagen (epitheliomesenchymal rudiment) induced tolerance to subsequent skin grafts, although not to allogeneic spleen cell stimulation *in vitro*. Thus, thymic stromal cells clearly can present antigens and induce tolerance although the mechanism is not always deletional (see below).

Subsequent studies using transgenic mice expressing MHC molecules under the control of tissue-specific promoters showed that both medullary and cortical epithelium can induce negative selection, but the latter cells appeared much less effective. How then does one account for the failure to completely induce tolerance by thymic (especially cortical) stromal-cell antigen presentation? One likely possibility is that the tolerance induced is tissue specific, that is, only for those peptides expressed by the stromal cells (13). Hence, MLR and CML assays in which splenic dendritic cells do the presenting will stimulate T cells, but only those specific for hematopoietic cell-derived peptides not expressed by the thymic stromal cells. When a second whole thymus graft is given, only the hematopoietic cells are rejected, not the stromal cells. The fate of other tissue grafts depends on how much peptide overlap there is between the thymus and those grafts. The second possibility is that only T cells with high-affinity receptors are deleted, leaving low-affinity clones to respond to strong dendritic cell presentation (14). Targeting of an MHC class I molecule to the thymic medullary epithelium with either a keratin IV promoter or an aberrantly expressed $E\mu$ promoter resulted in tolerance that was "spilt"; that is, the animals accepted skin grafts but manifested a CTL response *in vitro* in the presence of IL-2. Crossing the $E\mu$-K^b transgenic mouse to a $CD8^+$ TCR transgenic specific for this K^b MHC class I molecule deleted only T cells expressing high densities of the TCR, not those with lower densities as a consequence of endogenous $TCR\alpha$ chain expression.

Finally, a few reports suggest that even developing T cells can present antigen for tolerance induction. In the experiments by Shimonkevitz and Bevan, lethally irradiated syngeneic bone marrow-reconstituted mice were injected intrathymically with purified $Thy1^+$ $CD4^-8^-$ T cells that were haploidentical to the host [$(A \times B)F_1$ T cells into an A host]. Assay of host cells 50 days later showed specific tolerance to class I alloantigens of parent B as measured in a CTL response. This effect was not due to contaminating dendritic cells, because the host cells were not tolerant to MHC class II alloantigens in an MLR. Note that mouse T cells do not express class II molecules, whereas their dendritic cells do. Thus, the injected T cells appeared capable of inducing tolerance. A similar conclusion was reached by Pircher and colleagues from *in vitro* experiments using purified $CD4^+8^+$ thymocytes from a TCR transgenic mouse. These cells were killed when exposed to the peptide for which they were specific, presumably by recognizing peptide/MHC class I complexes on the surface of other T cells in the culture. This result suggests that T cells can directly induce clonal deletion of immature thymocytes.

Biochemical Events in Thymocyte Clonal Deletion

The fact that all types of antigen-presenting cells (APCs) induce tolerance in thymocytes indicates that the T cells at this stage of their development are tolerizable only (15). Burnet, as well as Lederberg, postulated that this occurs by signaling through the antigen-specific receptor followed by cell death. Histologic examination of the thymus does not reveal much evidence for ongoing cell death; yet kinetic labeling studies have demonstrated that over 95% of the cells generated in the thymus die there. More recent experiments, using a sensitive TUNEL assay to detect DNA strand breaks, showed that macrophages contain the debris of thymocytes that have died by apoptosis (16). In a TCR $V\beta5$ transgenic mouse expressing MHC class II E molecules and an endogenous $V\beta5$-reactive superantigen, the medulla of the thymus was found to contain aggregates of apoptotic cells that were engulfed by $MAC3^+$ macrophages.

While a consensus now exists that thymocytes can die by apoptosis during negative selection, the molecular mechanisms responsible for inducing apoptosis are not fully known

(11). Multiple experiments *in vitro* have shown that cross-linking the TCRs on isolated double-positive thymocytes is not sufficient to induce cell death. Instead, several studies have suggested that adding anti-CD28 to anti-TCR antibodies causes thymocyte death. The CD28 knockout mouse, however, has no problem with negative selection, suggesting that CD28 is not the only receptor capable of facilitating this process. *In vivo,* CD28 may only be involved in late-stage deletion, as its ligand, B7, is expressed in the medulla, but not in the cortex. Other T-cell surface molecules suggested to play a role are CD5 and CD43. All three of these molecules are known to be capable of affecting the strength of TCR signaling.

The molecular pathways that lead to apoptosis following TCR engagement are also not fully clear (15). Experiments with dominant negative and constitutively active transgenes, as well as pharmacologic inhibitors, have shown that activation of the mitogen-activated protein (MAP) kinase family of enzymes is necessary for negative selection to occur. Evidence supports a role for p38 and Jun N-terminal kinase (JNK) in the process, while data for the extracellular signal-regulated kinase (ERK) pathway is conflicting. The involvement of the calcium/calcineurin pathway is also controversial, but most of the evidence suggests that it plays no role in cases of strong deletion. Further downstream there is good evidence for the induction of the proapoptotic transcription factor Nur77; however, the Nur77 knockout mouse shows normal clonal deletion, again suggesting redundancy in the pathway that is possibly mediated by Nor-1, another member of the steroid nuclear receptor superfamily with homology to Nur77. Mutations in the Fas and Fas-ligand molecules have no effect on negative selection of double-positive thymocytes, although they do prevent deletion of HSA^{hi} $CD4^+$ thymocytes stimulated with high doses of antigen. Null mutations in the TNF and TNF-receptor molecules are also without effect. Only gene targeting by Mak and colleagues of the CD30 molecule, a member of the TNF/NGF cytokine receptor family, has been reported to influence negative selection. This mutation increased thymocyte numbers twofold and impaired anti–CD3-induced death of thymocytes *in vitro.* However, when crossed to either a $TCR\alpha\beta$ or a $TCR\gamma\delta$ transgenic mouse bearing a strong negative-selecting ligand, deletion was only partially reduced (mostly that seen at the early double-positive stage) and deletion by endogenous superantigens was unaffected. These results suggest that CD30 may be only one of several death receptors capable of mediating apoptosis in thymocytes. A more recent experiment by Schmitt-Verhulst and colleagues has found that double-positive thymocytes lack constitutive expression of protein kinase C epsilon, which may be required to induce or enhance $NF\kappa B$ activation during the negative selection process. This could be critical for shifting the molecular balance in these cells toward TNF family–member signaling for programmed cell death through the JNK pathway. On the other hand, Leiden and colleagues have shown that selective expression of a superinhibitory form of the $NF\kappa B$ inhibitory protein in the T-cell lineage using a CD2 promoter had no effect on the negative selection of two different CD8-restricted TCR transgenics. Finally, gene knockout experiments by Strasser and colleagues have shown that the BH3-only Bcl-2 family member Bim is required for complete negative selection. This protein is up-regulated in thymocytes following TCR ligation.

Activation versus Tolerance Thresholds

After T cells complete their maturation in the thymus, they are capable of responding to a foreign antigen when the concentration of peptide/MHC complexes derived from that antigen reach a certain critical threshold for activation (15,17). The relationship between this threshold and the concentration of intact antigen depends on processing and presentation requirements, in addition to the intrinsic affinity of the T-cell receptor for the peptide/MHC complex. An important question is the relationship between this threshold for activation and the one involved in negative selection. If a self-antigen presented in the thymus induces clonal deletion in only a subset of T cells, what happens if that antigen is subsequently expressed in peripheral tissues in increased amounts during tissue destruction in an inflammatory response? Will T-cell clones with low affinity for the self-peptide MHC complexes now become activated? This usually is not the case; that is, trauma rarely leads to autoimmunity. The question is, why? A similar problem should arise following T-cell priming when memory T cells become hyperresponsive to foreign antigens. Why don't they also become responsive to self-peptide MHC complexes?

Early observations by Palmer and colleagues on endogenous viral superantigens suggested that T cells bearing certain Vβs could be deleted in vivo if the mice carried the Mtv, but that cells developing in Mtv⁻ mice expressing these particular Vβ genes could not be stimulated in vitro to give a T-cell proliferative response by APCs expressing the Mtv. This suggested that tolerance induction in the thymus was achieved at a lower threshold than peripheral T-cell activation. The use of thymic organ cultures and TCR transgenic mice allowed a more quantitative analysis of this problem. Yagi and Janeway showed that deletion of TCR^hi Vβ8⁺ cells by staphylococcal enterotoxin B (SEB) in thymic organ culture occurred at concentrations that were 30- to 100-fold lower than those required to activate mature CD4⁺ cells to proliferate. For T-cell help, Mitchison and colleagues showed that exposure to the liver F protein during in vitro culture induced tolerance at a 10-fold lower concentration than that required for proliferation of mature T cells. Finally, for CTL responses, Pircher and colleagues compared variant LCMVs for their ability to elicit anti-viral responses in TCR transgenic mice and for their ability to induce neonatal tolerance in these mice. One viral variant could not activate a CTL response or be cleared by the animal over a 1,000-fold range of viral challenge doses; yet it was capable of inducing a partial deletion of transgenic TCR⁺ CD8⁺ T cells in the thymus after neonatal tolerization. Thus, all the experiments suggest that the concentration

threshold required for tolerance induction of immature T cells is lower than the threshold required by the mature T cell for activation.

In 1995, Ohashi and colleagues unexpectedly discovered a partial agonist peptide that was capable of mediating positive selection in thymic organ culture of thymocytes bearing a reactive transgenic TCR, but which at the same time eliminated the ability of the maturing T cells to respond to the selecting peptide, although not to a full agonist peptide. Lucas and Germain quantitated this effect using two analogs of a peptide from pigeon cytochrome c, one an agonist and the other a partial agonist, to stimulate the expression of CD69 in either DP thymocytes or peripheral CD4⁺ T cells. There was little or no difference in the response between cells from the two tissues using the high-affinity agonist; however, the lower-affinity partial agonist required a 10- to 30-fold higher antigen concentration to stimulate the peripheral CD4⁺ T cells to give CD69 expression comparable to that of the thymocytes. Biochemical experiments suggested that the observations could be accounted for by decreases in proximal TCR signaling of the mature cells affecting the level of tyrosine phosphorylation of ZAP 70 and the TCR zeta chain, possibly as a result of decreased mobilization of p56^lck to the receptor complex. Similar observations have been made by Jameson and colleagues for CD8⁺ T cells where the difference in activation thresholds between DP thymocytes and peripheral T cells has been attributed to differences in glycosylation of the CD8 molecule, which affect its ability to interact with the TCR during antigen recognition. The general conclusion is that T-cell maturation is accompanied by a large increase in the activation threshold of the cells, thus preventing reactivation of low-affinity clones in the periphery by small differences in concentration of self-peptide/MHC complexes.

T-Cell Tuning of Activation Thresholds

The male H-Y–specific TCR transgenic mouse deletes most of its CD8⁺ T cells in the thymus; yet some cells emerge unresponsive to H-Y with their level of expression of CD8 lower than normal (10). This phenomenon is enhanced if the H-Y antigen is only expressed on thymic epithelial cells. If, however, the H-Y transgenic mouse is crossed to a second transgenic mouse that constitutively expresses CD8, Robey and Fowlkes (12) showed that the T cells expressing low levels of endogenous CD8 disappear. Thus, either the increased CD8 levels during selection or an inability to down-regulate the CD8 transgene caused a complete deletion in the thymus. The low level of CD8 is a stable phenotype, because peripheral CD8 cells retain this level after polyclonal activation and proliferation. Also of interest is the observation by Schmitt-Verhulst and colleagues that T cells can exist with different levels of CD8, depending on the strength of the negative selection pressure. All these experiments suggest that individual T cells can sense when an antigenic signal in the thymus is too strong and to some extent adjust their threshold of activation to avoid deletion (15). This process has been referred to as "tuning of activation thresholds" by Grossman and Paul (18).

More recent experiments have suggested other tuning mechanisms that thymocytes may use to escape the process of negative selection. CD5 is a cell-surface molecule that negatively regulates TCR signaling via an ITIM motif in its cytoplasmic domain (19). Its expression increases during thymocyte development, and maximum levels, which are achieved at the double-positive stage, appear to roughly correlate with TCR avidity. Elimination of CD5 by gene targeting enhances the deletion of both CD4 and CD8 thymocytes from TCR transgenic mice, suggesting that CD5 might be involved in setting the threshold for clonal deletion. Another type of escape from negative selection results when the level of the T-cell receptor is lowered (14). This occurs in TCR transgenic mice through rearrangement and expression of endogenous α-chain genes, a process that is enhanced by presentation of high-affinity ligands on epithelial cells in the thymic cortex (17). In those cases in which the second expressed α-chain can pair with the transgenic β-chain, the T cell expresses to varying degrees two receptors on the cell surface. This lowers the surface density of the transgenic TCR, which can then allow the thymocyte to escape negative selection. Interestingly, Lanzavecchia's group found that many normal human T cells express two receptors, suggesting that they may have gone through such a tuning process. What variables control how the thymocyte chooses to adapt, via CD8, CD5, TCR, or some other form of adjustment, remains to be determined.

NEGATIVE SELECTION DURING B-CELL DEVELOPMENT

Does Negative Selection Occur in the B-Cell Compartment?

The introduction of fluorescein-tagged and radio-labeled antigens in the late 1960s allowed for the first time the quantitation of antigen-binding cells (8,20,21). Most of the cells detected were B cells as defined by the expression of surface immunoglobulin. When this technique was applied to tolerant animals, whether natural or acquired, the surprising observation was made that the animals had antigen-binding cells specific for the tolerogen. For example, cells binding thyroglobulin were observed repeatedly in human peripheral blood by Allison and colleagues, but cells specific for human serum albumin were not. This suggested that tolerance did not always involve deletion of clones as postulated by Burnet. Furthermore, when Möller and colleagues stimulated adult B cells with polyclonal activators such as the lipopolysaccharide (LPS) from *E. coli,* some of them differentiated into IgM-secreting plasma cells whose antibodies reacted against self-components. Such autoantibody-forming cells were then found without LPS stimulation in normal and germ-free mice as well as humans.

Evidence subsequently emerged which showed that negative selection for certain self-antigens existed only in the T-cell compartment and not in the B-cell compartment. The first example described by Iverson and Lindenmann was for the F protein from liver, which exists in two allelic forms (differing only by a single amino acid). Mouse strains expressing the right MHC haplotype (responders capable of binding the peptide to their class II molecules) could make an antibody response against the allelic product of F that they did not express. The antibodies elicited, however, reacted equally well with both forms of the F protein. These experiments were subsequently interpreted to mean three things: (a) the absence of T cells specific for the self-peptide derived from the variant region of the protein; (b) the presence of T cells with reactivity to the non–self-peptide encoded by the other allele; (c) and no negative selection at the B-cell level. A second example of no B-cell tolerance was observed by Haba and Nisonoff for IgE, which is nonimmunogenic on its own, but elicits a strong antibody response in syngeneic mice when coupled to a foreign carrier protein. Finally, Borel and colleagues reached the same conclusion with two congenic mouse strains expressing different amounts of the fifth component of complement (C5). In this case the B cells from the tolerant animal, with normal C5 levels, were capable of responding to a physiologic concentration of this self-antigen in the presence of T cells that had matured in the strain without C5 (and which therefore were not tolerant).

This series of experiments led many investigators to question whether negative selection existed at all in the B-cell compartment. Yet several lines of evidence clearly suggested that it must exist, at least to some degree. First, immunizations to produce xeno- and allo-antisera almost always yield antibodies that are specific for the foreign protein and that cross-react poorly if at all with the animal's own protein counterpart. This is true for cell-surface proteins such as MHC molecules as well as soluble protein antigens such as hemoglobin. The absence of antibodies against the self-proteins is not simply due to absorption by antigen in the animal, because hybridomas derived from these mice show the same preference for the foreign antigen. Second, the presence of antigen-binding cells and LPS-elicited IgM antibodies that react with self-proteins in *in vitro* assays could be explained by low-affinity interactions that might not be functionally relevant, that is, not adequate to lead to activation of the B cell in a physiologic situation. Thus, tolerance in the B-cell compartment might only affect high-affinity clones. Evidence in favor of this point of view came from the generation of a series of IgM-secreting hybridomas making anti–single-stranded DNA antibody (22). LPS-activated bone-marrow pre–B cells and mature splenic B cells yielded a similar percentage of these anti-DNA hybridomas; however, only 2% of the mature B-cell antibodies were of high affinity, while 17% of the pre–B-cell antibodies were of high affinity. These results suggest that some self-reactive cells are purged from the B-cell repertoire during the transition from the pre–B-cell to mature B-cell stage and that these B cells have on average a higher affinity for the antigen. The mechanism(s) of this purging was not clear from these experiments. Addressing this issue required the development of immunoglobulin receptor transgenic mice in order to provide an appropriate experimental tool to follow the fate of individual B cells during this transition.

Mechanisms of Negative Selection in the Bone Marrow

The first direct demonstration of negative selection at the B-cell level was made by Nemazee and Bürki (23–25). They constructed a transgenic mouse expressing an IgM B-cell receptor (BCR) reactive with the MHC class I molecules K^k and D^k. On the neutral MHC^d background, 25% to 50% of splenic B cells (B220$^+$, IgM$^+$) expressed this receptor and IgM antibody of this specificity was expressed in the serum. When crossed to an MHC^k mouse, however, both the peripheral B cells and the antibody disappeared. The site of negative selection appeared to be the bone marrow, as no transgenic receptor-bearing cells were detected in the spleen. In the bone marrow, IgM and receptor idiotype levels were low to undetectable, but B220 expression was normal. This suggested that the tolerance process might involve the down-modulation (patching, capping, and internalization) of the immunoglobulin receptor after antigen encounter. This is consistent with much earlier studies by Sidman and Unanue and Raff and colleagues, which showed that treatment of bone marrow or fetal liver B cells with high concentrations of anti-IgM antibody caused the permanent disappearance of Ig from the surface of the B cell.

There is now uniform agreement that sufficient engagement of the Ig receptor on immature B cells (B220$^+$, IgD$^-$, CD23$^-$) can lead to a state of maturational arrest. BCR transgenic bone marrow cells placed in culture with membrane-bound antigen or anti-κ antibody down-regulate their receptors and remain alive. If the cells come from double-transgenic animals expressing the BCR and the relevant antigen, then the *in vivo* arrested cells persist in culture in the presence of antigen. Interestingly, Goodnow's group showed that they come out of this state in the absence of antigen and differentiate into more mature B cells (B220^{hi}, IgD$^+$, CD23$^+$). Thus, the maturational arrest is reversible.

What is the function of this maturational arrest? Two groups, those of Weigert and Nemazee, have presented evidence suggesting that the B cells undergo a change in their Ig light chains, a process called "receptor editing." BCR transgenic bone-marrow cells arrested at the IgD$^-$, CD23$^-$ stage increase the level of their RAG enzymes and undergo endogenous light-chain gene rearrangements when stimulated with an anti-κ chain antibody. Similar results were observed *in vivo* when the BCR transgenic B cells encountered their antigen. Also, immature B cells from normal mice showed an increased percentage of λ-bearing cells (without undergoing cell division) following stimulation with an anti-κ antibody. The results suggest that feedback inhibition of light-chain gene rearrangements by a productively rearranged receptor

(allelic exclusion) does not take place, and that the immature B-cell can modify its receptor by light-chain exchange in order to escape silencing when it encounters self-antigens in the bone marrow.

What happens to the B cell if light-chain replacement fails to shift its specificity sufficiently away from autoreactivity? Weigert's group has some evidence for heavy chain editing as well. However, under inescapable conditions, such as stimulating immature B cells with anti-Ig *in vivo,* there is no reexpression of surface Ig, suggesting that the maturational arrest may eventually be followed by cell death. This was demonstrated directly by Monroe's laboratory (26), who showed that isolated immature B cells from the bone marrow undergo apoptosis when stimulated with high levels of anti-Ig. This observation is consistent with earlier *in vivo* experiments of Cooper and colleagues in which anti-μ antibodies, given to chickens or mice from birth, completely eliminated all B cells in the animal. In the BCR transgenic mice, exposure to the antigen during development also results in a depleted peripheral B-cell pool—at least in early adulthood before the receptor editing process has a chance to accumulate sufficient escapees to populate the periphery. All these results are consistent with Osmond's B-cell turnover studies, which showed that only 10% of the produced B cells ever leave the bone marrow. Thus, the bone marrow compartment has two mechanisms for dealing with autoreactive cells: One is a receptor selection process that allows cell survival following encounter with self antigens at an immature stage of development by exchange of light chains and some heavy chains; the other is a clonal deletion process by apoptosis, which ensues if the receptor is repeatedly occupied over a sufficient period of time without relief by receptor editing.

Antigen Characteristics Required for Negative Selection of B Cells

Insights into what characteristics of self-reactive B cells and of the autoantigen determine which B cells will be deleted can be inferred from early studies on B-cell tolerance induction to foreign antigens by Metcalf and Klinman (27–29). Using the *in vivo* limiting-dilution splenic-focus assay to study B-cell tolerance, they demonstrated that if immature hapten-specific B cells were exposed for 24 hours to the hapten in the absence of T-cell help, they become unresponsive to subsequent stimulation by the hapten in the presence of T-cell help. In order to induce tolerance in this system, the antigen had to be multivalent. DNP$_4$-ovalbumin was tolerogenic for DNP-specific B cells, but DNP$_1$-papain was not. This observation suggests that signaling through the immunoglobulin receptor requires cross-linking in order to induce tolerance. Thus, the MHC^k class I antigen in the BCR transgenic experiments described earlier, which is a transmembrane glycoprotein and therefore displayed on cell surfaces in a multimeric array, makes an excellent tolerogen. In contrast, when this BCR transgenic was crossed to a different transgenic mouse expressing a soluble form of the MHC K^k molecule, no deletion of the

B cells was observed. Although it is difficult to compare the levels of Ig receptor occupancy in these two models, the observations suggest that only self-antigens that can be presented to the B cell in a multivalent form will be tolerogenic. In a similar manner, Honjo's group showed that a transgenic mouse with an Ig receptor specific for a determinant on the surface of red blood cells negatively selects all of its conventional B-2 cells expressing this specificity (although the receptor was expressed in B-1 cells). Also consistent with the idea that surface-displayed antigens are good tolerogens is the general finding that many of the natural autoreactive antibodies are specific for intracellular molecules; only a few have been identified that react with cell-surface proteins, and these arise (as in the anti-RBC transgenic) from the B-1 subset of B cells, which may have different signaling properties.

Tolerance to secreted self-antigens is a more complex issue. From the in vitro experiments of Metcalf and Klinman, it is clear that in order to induce B-cell tolerance a molecule must not only be multivalent, but be present at a high enough concentration, and react with the Ig receptor with a high enough affinity. The importance of concentration has been confirmed in vivo in a series of transgenic mice that express hen egg-white lysozyme at different circulating levels (28). When the serum concentration was greater than 10^{-10} M, the animals were tolerant even if they were immunized in Freund's complete adjuvant with lysozyme coupled to a foreign carrier to provide T-cell help. The tolerance manifested itself as a markedly decreased plaque-forming cell response consisting only of B cells with low-affinity receptors. Below 10^{-10} M, the animals were still tolerant at the T-cell level but they could now make a normal high-affinity antibody response if given T-cell help. This model of natural tolerance is consistent with the original experiments of Chiller et al. (30) that were done with foreign antigens, and supports the notion that available antigen concentrations can produce situations in which only the T-cell compartment is unresponsive. Why the thresholds for B and T-cell negative selection should be different is not understood.

The absolute concentrations required to tolerize a particular set of B cells will obviously vary with the nature of the antigen. In the case of the C5 molecule discussed earlier, a circulating antigen concentration of 5×10^{-7} M was not adequate to induce tolerance, whereas in the case of lysozyme 10^{-10} M was. It should be noted, however, that the actual form of the antigen that induces the tolerance is not necessarily the free protein. For example, some evidence from Basten's group suggests that the tolerogenic form of lysozyme might be molecules bound to a high-molecular-weight serum protein, a modification that presumably gives lysozyme its tolerogenic efficacy by making it multivalent. When lysozyme was engineered to be expressed as a membrane-bound protein under the control of an MHC class I promoter, it led to negative selection of B cells in the bone marrow of a lysozyme-specific Ig-receptor transgenic mouse. Under these conditions lysozyme is a potent tolerogen because it is presented as a multimeric antigen at high local concentrations in the bone marrow.

Immature B Cells Are Not Tolerizable Only

T cells in the thymus presented with antigens on splenic dendritic cells are tolerized, consistent with the predictions of the clonal selection model. In contrast, when immature B cells are exposed to antigen in the presence of T-cell help, they make an antibody response (8,27,31,32). In these experiments, surface Ig⁻ bone marrow or neonatal spleen cells were transferred at limiting dilution to keyhole limpet hemocyanin (KLH) carrier-primed irradiated recipients. As the naïve B cells matured in splenic focus cultures in vitro, presentation of the DNP hapten coupled to KLH led to an IgM antibody response. In contrast, if the hapten was presented on another carrier (DNP-HGG) to which the T cells were not primed, then there was no antibody made to DNP. The antigen was recognized, however, because an initial 24-hour exposure to DNP-HGG prevented the antibody response to DNP-KLH. This showed that the developing immature B cells were tolerized to the hapten in the absence of T-cell help. Thus, the same B cells could be activated or tolerized depending on the presence of helper T cells.

Consistent with these early observations are more recent in vitro studies in which immature surface IgM⁺, IgD⁻ bone marrow–derived B cells were stimulated with anti-IgM antibodies (26). When the anti-μ was given alone, the B cells died by apoptosis, but if interleukin-4 (IL-4) was also added to the cultures, the apoptosis was prevented and the B cells proliferated. IL-4 is one of the known cytokines to participate in T-cell help. At a molecular level, the anti-IgM induced cyclin-dependent kinase (CDK)-4 and its regulatory subunit cyclin D2, which only allowed the cell to go from G0 to G1. With the addition of IL-4, however, the expression of cyclin E and CDK-2 was also induced, and this allowed the cell to transit into the S phase of the cell cycle. Thus, these experiments support the idea that tolerizable immature B cells can be rescued by T-cell help.

These observations are inconsistent with the clonal selection ideas proposed by Burnet, but fit nicely with the general model for B-cell activation originally proposed by Bretscher and Cohn (31,32). In an attempt to explain why immune responses require the recognition of two different determinants on the antigen and how the same antigen could both tolerize and immunize when given at different doses, they first suggested that antibody-forming cells must be tolerizable when stimulated through their antigen-specific receptor (this was referred to as signal one), but activated if they also received a second signal (referred to as signal two). This second signal was also postulated to be antigen specific, and both antigenic determinants were required to be linked together on the same molecule. In the original model, the second signal was delivered by antibody from another B-cell via an antigen bridge. With the subsequent discovery of T lymphocytes, the second signal became help from T cells specific for the same antigen. In today's way of thinking, the B-cell binds the antigen via its Ig receptor, which transduces the first signal into the cell via activation of tyrosine kinases, such as Syk and Lyn. The receptor-antigen complex is then internalized, the antigen processed, and peptide–MHC complexes displayed on the B-cell surface. If T cells exist with receptors that can recognize these peptide/MHC complexes, then the ensuing T-cell–B-cell interaction provides the second signals in the form of a CD40 ligand/CD40 interaction and the release of stimulatory cytokines such as IL-4 and IL-5 or IFN-γ. In this framework then, antigen stimulation of B cells in the absence of T-cell help leads to tolerance, while stimulation in the presence of antigen-specific T-cell help leads to proliferation and differentiation. Based on the experiments described above, it appears that these rules govern the response to antigens by immature B cells as well.

TOLERANCE TO PERIPHERAL ANTIGENS

At the completion of development, T and B cells emerge from the primary lymphoid organs and enter the recirculating pool of peripheral lymphocytes. One of the first things these naïve cells encounter in their fully mature state are antigens from various nonlymphoid organs that were thought to be restricted in their expression to a particular peripheral tissue. In this section we will discuss whether these tissue-restricted antigens are recognized by the immune system, whether the antigens are only expressed in the peripheral tissues, and whether the immune system is tolerant to them.

Tissue-Specific Peptide Antigens

When Medawar was asked if he could distinguish dizygotic from monozygotic bovine twins, he was certain this could be done by skin grafting; however, when his group attempted to test this, they found that most of the time (seven of eight) skin grafts exchanged between dizygotic twins were not rejected. This surprising result led to conclude that skin does not contain any unique transplantation antigens, that is, none other than those found on the hematopoietic cells for which the twins were chimeric. Thus, the concept emerged that blood cells tolerize for all tissues.

The first challenge to this intellectual framework came from the studies of Billingham and Brent (33) on neonatal tolerance in mice. They found that B6 newborn mice injected with inbred strain A spleen cells were not tolerant of strain A skin grafts. Boyse et al. (34) corroborated this finding in radiation-induced (A × B6)F$_1$ → B6 bone-marrow chimeras, where they were able to show that the recipient contained (A × B6)F$_1$ hematopoietic cells but still rejected A skin. Tolerance could be induced, however, if strain A epidermal cells were injected along with the F$_1$ bone marrow. They concluded that there must be a skin-specific transplantation antigen (Sk) expressed by A and not by B6 mice. Subsequent studies showed that two genes controlled the expression of this antigen(s) and that Sk antigens could be identified in other strain

combinations. These studies thus appeared at odds with the original Medawar results. A resolution of the contradiction was achieved by Emery and McCullagh. They repeated the early experiments of Medawar with a small technical modification. In the original study, skin grafts were prepared from the ears of the donor and placed on the back (whithers) of the recipient. Instead, Emery and McCullagh exchanged flank skin grafts. In this case, all dizygotic twins rejected their sib's graft. Repeating the technique of Medawar's group they confirmed that many animals did not reject under these conditions (50%). Thus, cattle also have skin-specific antigens.

The failure to elicit a rejection with ear skin grafts most likely relates to the "strength" of antigen presentation (e.g., the density of Langerhans cells), which has been shown by Chen and Silvers to vary in different areas of mouse skin. Although Medawar's group demonstrated that their ear skin grafts were antigenic across a complete MHC genetic disparity (i.e., outbred cattle), differences in skin-specific antigens between dizygotic twins is a situation in which the two immune systems are tolerant to all processed peptides derived from proteins of hematopoietic cells, but not to peptides derived from proteins unique to the skin. In the cases in which the gene encoding a skin protein exists in two allelic forms, the potential exists for peptides to be expressed by the graft tissue that are not present in the host's skin. To elicit an immune response such peptides have to be able to bind (one each) to the MHC class I and class II molecules, perhaps explaining why two genes "control" the expression of the Sk antigen. These three constraints—requirement for allelic polymorphism, requirement for peptide binding to MHC molecules (Ir gene control), and tolerance to minor histocompatibility antigens that are also expressed by hematopoietic cells—could explain why not all mouse strain combinations reveal an immune response to skin-specific antigens. Outbred animals such as cattle, however, should show this reactivity more frequently because of greater diversity in the genes encoding their skin-specific proteins.

The concept of tissue-specific antigens is not unique to skin. The experiment of Triplett (7) demonstrating that immunologic tolerance is an acquired state showed that frog pituitary also expresses tissue-specific antigens. Because an attempt to confirm that study for pituitary, thyroid, and eye in other species of frog failed, McCullagh (35) also readdressed this issue using the thyroid of fetal lambs. At 54 days of gestation, the lamb's immune system has not yet developed and the animal will accept allografts of adult skin. If the thyroid gland was removed at that time, implanted into a nude mouse for 5 to 9 weeks, and then reimplanted subcutaneously into the same lamb after birth, autoimmune thyroiditis developed. Partial thyroidectomized lambs did not get the disease, arguing that the immune response was specific for thyroid antigens and not any xenogeneic mouse tissue. These observations demonstrate that the immune system normally learns to become tolerant of other self-tissues and that it has mechanisms for dealing with the problem of tolerance to antigens that are predominantly synthesized in peripheral nonlymphoid tissues. These other mechanisms are the topics of the rest of this chapter.

Can Delivery to or Expression of Antigens in the Thymus Account for Tolerance to Peripheral Antigens?

The existence of tissue-specific antigens creates a problem for the immune system, because the primary mechanism for induction of tolerance in the T-cell compartment is by clonal deletion in the thymus. One possible solution to this problem is for these antigens to also be expressed in the thymus (36–38). The first hint that this might occur came from studies with transgenic mice expressing foreign antigens under the control of tissue-restricted promoters. In particular, the rat insulin promoter was found to sometimes express in the thymus in addition to the β cells of the pancreas. This expression was initially viewed as an artifact resulting from insertion of the transgene into regions of active chromatin; however, this expression was observed in the thymus by several groups, a similar phenomenon was also seen when using other promoters, and importantly was not observed very often in other nontarget tissues. In most cases, the expression levels in the thymus were very low (e.g., for the rat insulin promoter 10,000 times less than in the pancreas) and could only be detected at the message level by RT-PCR; yet this expression had clear immunologic effects. For example, von Herrath and Oldstone expressed the LCMV glycoprotein under the control of the rat insulin promoter and produced two types of transgenic founders, one with detectable expression in the thymus, the other not. The former showed only a slow onset of diabetes following LCMV infection, mediated by low-affinity CD8 T cells requiring CD4 help, while disease onset in the latter was rapid and independent of CD4 help. These observations suggested that the thymic expression had induced a partial state of tolerance. Convincing evidence that it is only the thymic expression that is responsible for the tolerance process was achieved in other models (lactalbumin, elastase, and C-reactive protein) in which the thymus from the transgenic mouse was transplanted to a normal recipient and found to induce the same tolerant state.

Subsequent studies using RT-PCR on human and normal murine thymuses revealed expression of many peripheral antigens, including somatostatin, insulin, myelin basic protein, glutamic acid decarboxylase (GAD) 67, glucagon, elastase, trypsin, astrocyte S100β, C-reactive protein, lactalbumin, and thyroglobulin, although a few proteins such as human GAD65 and mouse preproinsulin1 were not detected. Again, the expression was mostly confined to the thymus and the amounts expressed were small. In some cases, sensitive assays were used to detect protein expression. For insulin, Polychronakos and colleagues observed 100 to 1,000 fmol/g of wet weight in human thymus compared to 3×10^6 fmol/g in pancreas and <70 fmol/g in other tissues (skin, lung, kidney, heart). Which cell types in the thymus are expressing these proteins has been controversial. All investigators agree that they are rare cells mostly in the medulla. Some studies

from the labs of Hanahan and Pugliese suggest that they are MHC class II positive and express markers of the hemopoietic lineage. Both dendritic cells (N418[+]) and macrophages (F4/80[+]) have been implicated by Throsby et al. Studies from Kyewski's lab, however, have convincingly localized expression to medullary epithelial cells. Furthermore, bone marrow chimera experiments by Mellor et al. have shown that the cells expressing lactalbumin are radio-resistant. Experiments by Klein and Kyewski (38) using cell isolation and RT-PCR have found that almost all of the peripheral antigens are expressed in purified populations of medullary epithelial cells. A few antigens, such as elastase, trypsin, somatostatin, lens crystallin, and retinal S antigen, were also expressed in cortical epithelial cells.

No matter which thymus cells express these tissue-specific antigens, the important question that must be convincingly answered is whether the low levels of expression play a role in the tolerance process. Similar to the transgenes described above, detectable expression of the antigen in the thymus has been correlated with resistance to autoimmune disease induction among mouse and rat strains, such as for interphotoreceptor retinoid-binding protein in experimental autoimmune uveoretinits (EAU) by Gery and colleagues and for myelin basic protein in experimental autoimmune encephalomyelitis (EAE) by Voskuhl and colleagues. For EAE caused by immunization with proteolipid protein (PLP), Klein and Kyewski (38) found that the dominant immunogenic epitope is encoded by an exon that is not present in the mRNA splice variant expressed in the thymus, suggesting that the T cells responsive to all other potential epitopes have been tolerized by the thymic expression. Finally, an interesting correlation exists in the human population between a genetic susceptibility locus for diabetes (IDDM2) and proinsulin expression in the thymus. Both Pugliese and Polychronakos showed that variation in a minisatellite repeat element (VNTR) 0.5kb upstream of the human insulin gene gives the variation in proinsulin expression. The higher expressing alleles show a dominant form of protection with a three- to five-fold reduction in the risk of developing type 1 diabetes. This suggests an important biological effect for the thymic ectopic expression of this tissue-restricted antigen.

Another plausible mechanism for achieving central tolerance to molecules that are not normally expressed in the thymus is to bring them there. It has been speculated that dendritic cells can pick up peripheral antigens and take them to the thymus. However, veiled dendritic cells (activated Langerhans cells migrating from tissues to lymph nodes) have only been found in afferent and not efferent lymph and have never been demonstrated to migrate to the thymus following i.v. injection. To reach the thymus, however, APC migration would not be necessary for proteins and their fragments derived from peripheral tissues through secretion or cell necrosis. These molecules could easily enter the thymic medulla through its arterial circulation. Kyewski and Fathman showed that exogenous antigens injected intravenously can reach and be processed by thymic dendritic cells as well as presented on MHC class II molecules in a form that stimulates T-cell clones to proliferate. For peptides presented by MHC class I molecules, however, which largely derive from cytoplasmic proteins, this pathway would seem to be far less efficient at providing peripheral antigens for tolerance induction. Nonetheless, to test this idea, expression of allogeneic MHC class I and II molecules was carried out using tissue-restricted promoters. In contrast to soluble proteins, these MHC molecules must remain intact in order to present their tissue-specific peptides. In other words, if shed and processed by dendritic cells for presentation in the thymus, they would not tolerize T cells that are specific for the peptide/MHC complexes expressed in the peripheral tissue. The first transgenic model of this type from Lo and Flavell expressed the MHC class II E molecule either in β cells of the pancreas under the control of the rat insulin promoter or in acinar cells of the pancreas under the control of the elastase promoter. These animals were tolerant of the E molecule in a mixed leukocyte response, although they failed to delete certain Vβ-expressing T cells that are normally deleted when this E molecule is expressed in the thymus. Some of the cells expressing those Vβs were unresponsive when stimulated in culture with anti-Vβ antibodies immobilized on a plate. This tolerance process is referred to as anergy and is discussed further in a later section. The possibility that the tolerance was induced by low-level expression of the E molecule in the thymus was eliminated by introducing nontransgenic thymus grafts into adult thymectomized, lethally irradiated, and bone marrow–reconstituted (ATxBM) transgenic mice. Under these conditions the T cells mature in a thymic environment that does not endogenously express the transgene. These mice were also tolerant, arguing in favor of a peripheral mechanism for the tolerance induction. A similar series of experiments was done with MHC class I molecules expressed in a variety of peripheral tissues, as well as with different tissue-specific antigens, and the outcome was the same, although thymic transplant experiments were only performed in a few of these cases.

Overall, these experiments demonstrate that low-level expression of many tissue-restricted antigens occurs in the thymus and that this can diminish the immune response toward these antigens. Interestingly, the tolerance mechanism(s) involved in these situations are not always deletional. In the next sections of this chapter, we will examine the mechanisms of anergy and suppression in addition to activation-induced cell death (AICD) that are thought to be involved in this process.

Activation-Induced Cell Death and Homeostasis

The frequency of responding T cells in a mixed lymphocyte response (MLR) is quite high, ranging from 2% to 5% of the CD4$^+$ T-cell population. Proliferation following priming does not increase this frequency, suggesting that many of the dividing cells must die (39–44). Sprent and Miller followed the fate of the reactive cells in this assay by isolating 4-day blasts from the thoracic duct of F$_1$ mice injected with parental

cells, labeling the cells, and transferring them back to syngeneic parental hosts. These cells homed to the spleen and intestine and then most of them disappeared, appearing to die *in situ* and be degraded by macrophages or be excreted into the lumen of the gut over a 2-week period. Only a few survived to become memory cells that were capable of responding more rapidly.

Modern studies on the fate of T cells stimulated with superantigens have confirmed these early findings with alloreactive T cells. Injection of spleen cells expressing Mtv-7 into mice lacking Mtv-7 or injection of staphylococcal enterotoxin A or B into strains expressing Vβ8 and/or Vβ3 T cells, results in an initial expansion of the reactive T cells followed by extensive death via apoptosis. This is not simply a phenomenon observed with superantigens as transfer into male nude mice of spleen cells from a transgenic female mouse expressing the TCR$\alpha\beta$ anti–H-Y receptor resulted in a similar expansion and disappearance of CD8$^+$ T cells. The general pattern of response to all of these stimuli is shown in Fig. 1.

The biochemical pathway responsible for signaling the cell to die is initiated in some models by an Fas–Fas ligand interaction and in others by TNF and its receptor. Recent *in vivo* studies by Marrack and colleagues have suggested

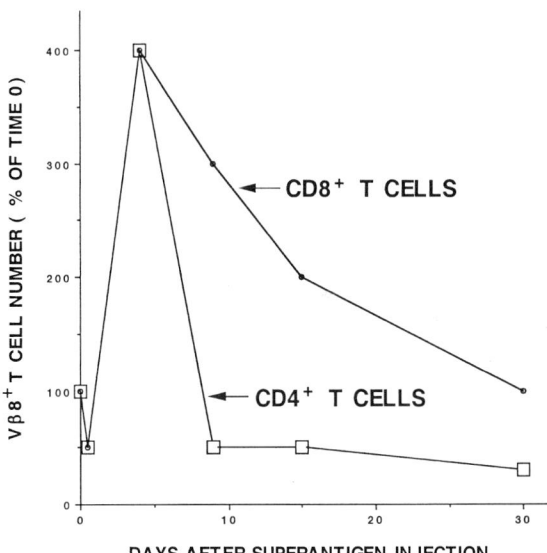

FIG. 1. The general pattern of *in vivo* responses of CD4$^+$ and CD8$^+$ T cells to superantigen and antigen stimulation. The response of Vβ8$^+$ T cells to staphylococcal enterotoxin B is shown as a model. The response occurs in four phases. During the first 12 hours, the massive release of cytokines from memory T cells can result in significant cell death in the stimulated cells. In the second phase, the remaining stimulated cells divide, increasing two- to eight-fold over a period of 4 days. In the third phase, CD4$^+$ T cells die off rapidly, but leave a residue of cells that appear to be anergized. In the fourth phase, the anergized cells slowly disappear. CD8$^+$ T cells, in contrast, slowly decrease in number from their peak expansion, returning to normal levels after 30 days. Whether these cells become anergic depends on the presence or absence of effective CD4$^+$ T-cell help.

that killing of CD4$^+$ T cells is instead mediated by reactive oxygen species via activation of bim. Also in an *in vitro* reactivation model, Cauley and Swain showed that IFNγ produced by activated CD4$^+$ cells could stimulate granulocytes to make nitrous oxides and reactive oxygen intermediates which in turn killed the activated CD4$^+$ cells. For Fas-mediated killing, the activated T cell is initially resistant to cell death, because the cells express a Fas-signaling antagonist called c-Flip and because the co-stimulation accompanying T-cell stimulation increases the synthesis of antiapoptotic Bcl-2 family members such as Bcl-X$_L$. When the latter decay and Flip is down-regulated following IL-2R signaling, the cell becomes vulnerable to Fas-mediated death. If restimulated through the antigen receptor, the surviving cells can also be killed by a rapid reexpression of the Fas ligand (the "propriocidal" effect of Lenardo). Other cells die simply when their growth factors are withdrawn. This last mechanism detailed by Thompson and colleagues involves down-regulation of the glucose transporter, atrophy of the cell, and mitochondrial changes leading to cytochrome C release and apoptosis.

Several recent experiments have demonstrated that the initial expansion phase of the T-cell response is started by the first encounter with antigen and that the cells are then programmed under optimum conditions to go through four to eight rounds of division without any restimulation. At the end of this period, they stop proliferating and then must receive further instructions to determine their fate. Death is only one possible outcome and all the quantitative parameters that influence the cell's fate at this point are not understood. CD28 signaling does not protect against the death induced by either the propriocidal effect or by superantigens. The experiments of Marrack and colleagues showed that only LPS or proinflammatory cytokines such as IL-1 and TNF-α prevent superantigen AICD. One way these molecules act is through up-regulation of the IκB family member Bcl-3, which in expression experiments was shown to have anti-apoptotic effects. Only the CD4$^+$ T cells die rapidly at day 4 following SEB injection; CD8$^+$ T cells do not. Thus, a completely different explanation for CD4$^+$ T-cell depletion has been proposed by Pernis and colleagues, who removed CD8$^+$ T cells from the mice prior to SEB injection, by treatment with anti-CD8 antibody, and prevented the rapid loss of CD4$^+$ T cells. They postulated that the activated CD8$^+$ T cells kill off the activated CD4$^+$ T cells by a perforin/granzyme-mediated cytotoxicity mechanism involving Qa-1.

One of the most interesting aspects of all these observations is that 90% of T cells responding to antigen or superantigen die. This is best understood in the context of homeostatic regulation of the immune system rather than antigen-specific tolerance *per se*. There is only so much space in the body for lymphocytes and room must be maintained for the influx of new naïve cells from the thymus as well as the preservation of memory T cells for an extended period of time. Transfer of splenic T cells into nude mice showed that the cells could expand only until a critical cell number is reached (approximately 2×10^8 cells per mouse). Surprisingly, memory T cells and naïve T cells were independently regulated; that is, each subpopulation did not influence the expansion of the other. Their half-lives were also controlled in different manners, as most naïve T cells were dependent on TCR recognition of self-MHC molecules for survival whereas memory T cells were not. In the immune response to a virus, Ahmed's group has shown that the frequency of the responding antigen-specific cells increases dramatically over an 8-day period, up to a frequency of 10% or more of the total CD8$^+$ T cells in the spleen. As these cells begin to effectively eliminate the virus, however, their frequency drops and in the memory phase of the response it becomes only 1/300 to 1/1000 of the total CD8$^+$ pool. Thus, homeostasis is maintained by allowing most of the generated new cells to die once the antigen is cleared.

Mature cells in the thymus can also undergo AICD via a Fas/Fas ligand (FasL)–mediated mechanism (11). Whether this mechanism is involved in cell loss seen during ectopic presentation of peripheral self-antigens in the thymus has not been clearly established. Transgenic mice made with human C-reactive protein (hCRP) express the molecule both in the liver and in medullary epithelial cells of the thymus. Crossing these mice to TCR transgenics specific for peptides from hCRP resulted in the absence of CD4$^+$ thymocytes (38). This was also seen in bone marrow chimeras in which the hCRP transgene was only expressed by radioresistant epithelial cells. Furthermore, it occurred even if the bone marrow was derived from MHC class II knockout mice so the donor-derived dendritic cells could not pick up and re-present the antigen. These results clearly demonstrate that a deletional mechanism can lead to tolerance in the thymus following antigen presentation by medullary epithelial cells.

T-Cell Anergy

The first experiments to explore the mechanism of tolerance induced by antigens expressed on thymic epithelial cells were done by Ramsdell and Fowlkes (42,45–49) using MHC class II E molecules and MMTV superantigens expressed by the irradiated host to tolerize reconstituting bone marrow–derived hemopoietic cells lacking the I-E molecules. Interestingly, the Vβ6$^+$, 17$^+$ CD4$^+$, and CD8$^+$ T cells interacting with the superantigens were not deleted, although these cells, either mature thymocytes or peripheral lymph node cells, appeared to be functionally unresponsive in a mixed leukocyte response *in vitro* as well as in a graft-versus-host response following adoptive transfer *in vivo*. Furthermore, attempts to directly stimulate the cells to proliferate using anti-Vβ antibodies on a plate were unsuccessful. Addition of exogenous IL-2 gave only a partial recovery of the proliferative response, suggesting that both IL-2 production and responsiveness to IL-2 were blocked. Subsequent experiments showed that the unresponsive state could be reversed if the T cells were cultured in the absence of antigen (either *in vitro* or *in vivo*), thus proving that the cells had not been deleted. This state of functional inactivation has been referred to as "anergy."

The first description of a CD4$^+$ T-cell anergic state was in clones and is now referred to as "T-cell clonal anergy." Activation of CD4$^+$ Th1 clones to proliferate requires live APCs. When the APCs were chemically treated with fixatives such as paraformaldehyde and used to present peptide antigens, the T cells did not proliferate. Instead, by 6 to 18 hours they had entered a new state in which they failed to make IL-2 or proliferate when restimulated with normal APC and antigen. The T cells were alive, as they could proliferate in response to added IL-2, and in fact this response brought them out of the state. Without IL-2, the unresponsiveness lasted for at least 2 weeks in the absence of any further antigen addition. Simultaneous studies using planar lipid membranes, composed of MHC class II molecules on a plastic surface and pulsed with peptide antigen, induced the same state. This suggested that TCR occupancy was all that was required to induce the state. Subsequent reconstitution experiments supported this idea. Addition of untreated, allogeneic APC (which could not present the peptide), along with chemically fixed syngeneic APC and peptide, prevented the induction of the unresponsive state. It also reconstituted the initial proliferative response. This suggested that the fixed cells were presenting antigen properly but that the fixation prevented other signals from being delivered by the APC. Addition of the allogeneic APCs allowed these second signals to be delivered in trans, although the process was relatively inefficient, requiring a 100-fold higher antigen concentration to achieve a comparable proliferative response. No soluble cytokines were ever effective in substituting for the allogeneic APC, and eventually the CD28 molecule was identified by Linsley and colleagues as a co-stimulatory receptor on the T-cell required for the IL-2 production. The ligand on the APC could be either B7-1 (CD80) or B7-2 (CD86). Subsequently other paired molecular interactions, such as LFA-1/ICAM-1, were also shown to provide co-stimulation for proliferation (see later discussion on co-stimulation).

In addition to induction by TCR occupancy in the absence of co-stimulation, clonal anergy was also achieved by stimulation with low-affinity peptide ligands (partial agonists) by Sloan-Lancaster and Allen or low doses of agonist peptides in the presence of co-stimulation by Sadegh-Nasseri and colleagues. Both these stimuli represent suboptimal activations that are inadequate to drive the cell into division, but adequate to induce a dominant biochemical feedback mechanism that blocks subsequent proliferative responses to normal activating stimuli. One biochemical block, described by the labs of Fitch and Mueller, is at the level of activation of the Ras/MAP kinase pathway by inhibiting the usual increase in GTP-p21^{Ras}. This prevents the induction and activation of certain transcription factors such as AP-1 that are required for transcription of the IL-2 gene. In the clonal anergy model described by Lamb and Feldmann, however, there is also a block in the calcium/calcineurin pathway. In this latter state all cytokine production is inhibited. In the former state only those responses involved in proliferation are blocked; for example, IL-4 production is unaffected in murine Th0 clones,

but the proliferative response to IL-4 is blocked. Chemokine production is unaffected and there is only a small effect on IFNγ production in Th1 clones. Finally, CD28 co-stimulation is not sufficient to prevent anergy induction. If the cells are stimulated with anti-TCR and anti-CD28 in the presence of rapamycin, a drug that blocks the cells from progressing from G1 into S phase of the cell cycle, the clones still become anergic. Thus, a major effect of co-stimulation is to produce enough T-cell growth factor(s) to drive the cells into cycle. This in turn counteracts the induction of anergy, possibly by degrading the newly synthesized proteins required to maintain the anergic state. Thus, clonal anergy in this case appears to be mainly a growth arrest state that maintains the cells in G1 even following full TCR stimulation.

Similar results have been obtained with primed or previously activated T cells from TCR transgenic mice; however, the extension of these findings to naïve T cells was harder to show. In many cases, naïve T cells could not be anergized by signal one alone. In those cases in which naïve cells were anergized, a strong TCR signal was required, such as several days of stimulation with anti-CD3 on a plate in the experiments of Lechler and colleagues, or addition of certain forms of co-stimulation by Webb and colleagues. The latter group showed that presentation of antigen to naïve CD4$^+$ T cells, using Drosophila cell lines transfected with murine MHC class II molecules, did not induce division or clonal anergy. If, however, the cell adhesion molecule ICAM-1 was also expressed as a form of co-stimulation, then the cells divided a few times and anergy was induced. If B7 molecules were expressed with or without ICAM-1 co-stimulation, then the T cells divided many times and ultimately ended up becoming primed. Division, however, is not a prerequisite for anergy induction. Using CFSE labeling to separate those cells that had not divided following stimulation with soluble anti-CD3 plus APC, in the presence of soluble CTLA-4Ig to block B7 co-stimulation, Wells and Turka showed that the recovered cells were still anergized. These results suggest that CD4$^+$ T cells need enough stimulation, either through a strong TCR signal or a weaker form of this signal plus a non–CD28-mediated form of co-stimulation, to induce a state of clonal anergy. Interestingly, if naïve CD4$^+$ T cells do not divide in the presence of B7 co-stimulation, they seem to go into an even deeper state of clonal anergy. Not only do these cells not make IL-2 or proliferate when restimulated, but they also do not proliferate when IL-2 is added. Induction of this "division arrest" form of anergy requires CTLA-4 signaling.

The first description of an anergic state *in vivo* was made in mice injected with superantigens by Rammensee and colleagues. In animals given SEB or Mtv7$^+$ spleen cells, there remains a population of Vβ8$^+$ CD4$^+$ T cells that fails to proliferate or produce IL-2 on restimulation with these antigens *in vitro* (Fig. 1). These cells stay in this functionally unresponsive state for weeks, especially if the animals have been thymectomized, but eventually the state reverses. These observations were extended to conventional antigens with

TCR transgenic mice either by crossing them to a mouse expressing the antigen they recognized or by transferring their mature T cells directly into this second mouse. In the H-Y transgenic model of Rocha and von Boehmer described earlier, the CD8$^+$ T cells become unresponsive when the cells are put into an environment in which the male antigen they recognize is highly expressed and cannot be eliminated, such as following transfer into a male nude mouse. If the CD8$^+$ T cells are removed from this environment and placed in a female nude mouse, they recover their function. Dependence of CD4$^+$ T-cell unresponsiveness on the persistence of antigen has also been reported by Tanchot and Schwartz. Also similar phenomena have been described by Jenkins and colleagues for CD4$^+$ transgenic T cells transferred to a syngeneic host and stimulated with a peptide ligand in the absence of a costimulatory signal such as LPS. Here a key role has been demonstrated for CTLA-4 signaling in the anergy induction process by Perez and Abbas, and the cells spontaneously come out of the anergic state several weeks after the antigen disappears. The unresponsive state for both CD4$^+$ and CD8$^+$ T cells involves a failure to produce IL-2 on restimulation with the antigen and APC; however, the production of other cytokines varies with the model. In some cases all cytokine production is inhibited, while in others the cells were found to make IL-10. Proliferation in most of these models is inhibited, and some also show a failure to respond to IL-2. It is not yet clear whether these differences relate to the depth of the anergic state induced, as discussed above for clonal anergy, or whether there are fundamental differences in the underlying biochemical mechanisms.

Only a few biochemical studies have been done with these *in vivo* models because of the difficulty of obtaining large numbers of cells for study. Nonetheless, if one pools all the data obtained so far in different systems, it appears as if *in vivo* anergy represents a block at the earliest steps of TCR-induced tyrosine phosphorylation (50). Activation-induced ZAP-70 phosphorylation is always reduced; also its downstream phosphorylation of the LAT adaptor molecule is inhibited. Interestingly, this results in a more profound inhibition of calcium mobilization than activation of the Ras/MAP kinase pathway, in contrast to some of the clonal anergy models. This may be explained by normal activation of the Slp-76 adaptor protein, which as shown by Madrenas can activate the Ras/MAP kinase pathway independent of LAT. The Src family kinases Lck and Fyn, which normally initiate Zap-70 activation by phosphorylating both the zeta chain of the TCR and ZAP-70, show definite changes in anergic cells. For example, there is often observed an increase in the levels of fyn and a decrease in the p23 isoform of phosphorylated TCR zeta. Gene targeting of Fyn partially restores the proliferative response of anergic cells by enhancing IL-2 receptor beta expression and cell survival, but it does not overcome the IL-2 production defect. Thus, overall it is still not clear how these changes cause the anergic phenotype. Finally, in those models where IL-2R signaling is also blocked, the CD25 α chain is usually normally up-regulated, but the mechanism of the downstream inhibition has not been identified.

The relationship between *in vivo* anergy models and *in vitro* T-cell clonal anergy is still not clear. There are some common threads. For example, all the states are antagonized by cell cycle progression, and inversely inhibition of progression from G1 to S phase by the drug rapamycin favors the development of anergy in both situations. Consistent with this notion is the demonstration that the major effect of anti-CTLA4 is to block cell cycle progression. Other parameters, however, suggest that the states are quite different. Clonal anergy is primarily a growth arrest state stemming from a block in the Ras/MAP kinase pathway, which can persist in the absence of antigen. CTLA4 plays no role in its induction or maintenance. By contrast, *in vivo* anergy is a desensitization state characterized by an early block in TCR signal transduction and a preferential block in the calcium pathway, which leads to inhibition of most cytokine production (with the notable exception of IL-10) in addition to blocking proliferation. *In vivo* anergy spontaneously reverses in the absence of the antigen. It generally arises following a proliferative expansion of the T cells and is maintained because the antigen signal persists. CTLA4 plays a critical role in determining the outcome (tolerance vs. priming) by influencing the amount of proliferation. These characteristics suggest that *in vivo* anergy is an adaptation of the cell to the persistence of antigen in its environment, consistent with the tunable activation threshold model of Grossman and Paul (18) discussed earlier for thymocyte development. The function of the anergic state in the periphery would be to retain a potentially useful cell in a harmless mode until a decision can be made as to whether it is autoreactive or critical for host defense. The half-life of these cells in the absence of other T cells is long; but in the presence of normal T cells the anergic cells more quickly disappear, possibly as suggested by Mostokides by a perforin and FasL-dependent mechanism. Premature entry into this state, however, can have deleterious effects such as impairment of an effective immune response to a viral infection as shown by Kundig and colleagues. However, if this state is induced in the thymus, it can serve as a mechanism for tolerance induction (45).

CD4$^+$CD25$^+$ Suppressor T cells

Nishizuka and Sakakura first showed that neonatal thymectomy of female mice at 3 days of age (but not at day 1 or 7) led to oophoritis and sterility (51–53). Subsequent studies showed that other organs could be affected such as the thyroid, stomach, prostate, and testis, and that the target tissue varied depending on the genetic background of the inbred mouse strain. Disease could be prevented either by thymus grafting or by injection of normal day 7 or adult spleen cells. A transfer model developed by Sakaguchi and Nishizuka eventually allowed the identification of the protecting cells as CD4$^+$ T cells and then much later as constitutively CD25$^+$ (the α chain of the IL-2 receptor).

The presence of CD4$^+$CD25$^+$ T cells in the thymus suggests that they develop there, although the possibility that the cells recirculate back from the periphery had to be considered.

The first convincing evidence that these regulatory cells arise in the thymus came from studies on embryonic epithelial grafts of thymic primordium by Le Douarin and Coutinho. These experiments were initially done in the chicken and then in the mouse. More recently, a mouse expressing MHC class II molecules only in the thymic cortex was shown by Laufer and colleagues to support the development of CD4+CD25+ immunoregulatory T cells, while mice deficient in all MHC class II molecules did not. Finally, a TCR transgenic mouse has been described by Caton and colleagues which gives rise to a high frequency of the CD4+CD25+ T cells at the transition from the double-positive to the single-positive thymocyte stage, but only when the animal also expresses the antigen for which the TCR is specific. Interestingly, another TCR transgenic with a lower-affinity receptor for the same antigen did not generate the regulatory T cells. These observations suggest that positive selection on cortical epithelial cells is all that is required for the development of the CD4+CD25+ T cells (i.e., dendritic cell interactions at the cortical/medullary junction are not necessary), and that a relatively high affinity for the selecting ligand is required to generate them.

The antigen recognition by CD4+CD25+ T cells appears to be organ specific, at least in the way the cells prevent autoimmune disease. For example, in the day-3 thymectomy models for orchitis and prostatitis, CD4+CD25+ suppressor T cells from the spleens of normal male mice are ten-fold more effective at preventing disease than spleen cells from either female mice or males that had been castrated at birth (and who therefore do not express antigens of the testes or the testes-dependent prostate). Tissue ablation experiments in adults by Seddon and Mason suggest that peripheral antigen expression is needed to sustain prolonged survival or expansion of the CD4+CD25+ T cells in the periphery. Whether the continued presence of these cells in the thymus requires ectopic antigen expression of peripheral antigens in epithelial cells of the thymic medulla remains to be investigated.

Peripheral and thymic CD4+CD25+ suppressor T cells have an activated phenotype. In addition to being CD25+, they express high levels of CD44, CD5, and CD54 and low levels of CD45RB. They also constitutively express CTLA4 (most of it intracellular) and much attention has been focused recently on whether this molecule plays any role in their function. The molecule is not essential, however, since CTLA4−/− gene-targeted mice show normal CD4+CD25+ T-cell development and function. Interestingly, the resting CD4+CD25+ T cells appear to be in a clonal anergic state. They do not make IL-2 or proliferate when stimulated through their TCR. The cells can proliferate if IL-2 is added to the cultures and this approach has been used to expand them in vitro. In vivo, their survival also seems to depend on IL-2 since as shown by Papiernik and others gene targeted mice deficient in either IL-2 or its co-signaling receptors, CD28 and CD40L, have fewer numbers of CD4+CD25+ cells.

In vitro studies by Shevach's group have shown that CD4+CD25+ cells function by suppressing the proliferative response of naïve CD4 and CD8 T cells through blocking of IL-2 production and arresting the cells in the G1 phase of the cell cycle. To do this, the regulatory cells must be activated through their TCRs and physically interact with the naïve T cells. Once activation is initiated by antigen or anti-TCR antibodies, the suppression becomes completely antigen independent. There is some controversy about whether an APC is also involved in the process and whether the mechanism of inhibition involves cytokines such as IL-10 and TGF-β. The suppressor cells clearly make these cytokines when they are stimulated, but again gene-targeted mice not expressing these cytokines or their receptors have normal numbers of functioning CD4+CD25+ T cells. In addition to preventing organ-specific autoimmune diseases, these cells have been found to play a significant role in preventing transplantation and tumor rejection.

Pivotal Role of the Antigen-Presenting Cell in Initiation of T-Cell Responses and Avoidance of Tolerance

It has generally been assumed that vertebrates evolved an adaptive immune system to respond to foreign antigens in order to identify and eliminate invading pathogens (54–56). For this reason, Dresser's (57) demonstration in the early 1960s that the infusion of a "deaggregated" form of a foreign protein into adult mice could lead to tolerance (an inability of the animal to make an antibody response to a subsequent rechallenge with the same antigen) was a surprising finding. He was also the first to show that deaggregated antigen could lead to the production of antibody when it is accompanied by substances like complete Freund's adjuvant. This experimental result suggested to him that antigen, in its simplest form, induces only a "paralysis" of the immune system rather than a productive immune response. Aware of Dresser's experimental work, as well as previous studies indicating the potency of bacterial endotoxins to act as adjuvants in vaccination studies, Claman (58) soon confirmed that a foreign protein antigen is immunogenic only when accompanied by a nonspecific stimulus such as endotoxin. Importantly, these findings led both investigators to propose the first (essentially similar) two-signal model of lymphocyte activation: specific antigen-receptor stimulation (signal one) of a naïve lymphocyte in the absence of a nonspecific immune stimulus (signal two, also called "adjuvanticity" by Dresser) fails to induce cell proliferation and instead leads to a durable tolerant state, whereas antigen stimulation in the presence of such a nonspecific proliferative stimulus is immunogenic and leads to both the clonal expansion and differentiation of the lymphocyte precursor.

A critical role for antigen uptake by macrophages in the initiation of an immune response was first considered by Thorbecke and colleagues who demonstrated that in vivo filtration of antigen in rabbits removed the aggregated material and converted an immunogen into a tolerogen. The antigen-presenting cell, however, did not achieve full-fledged importance until the discovery of T-cell MHC-restriction, and the accompanying acceptance of the notion that cell-cell interactions are required for antigen-presentation to T cells. Considering the problem of immune reactivity against allogeneic tissues, Lafferty and Woolnough suggested that a potent allogeneic reaction is initiated only in response to hematopoietic stimulatory cells carried within the allograft that possess both the specific alloantigen (signal one) as well as a nonspecific "inductive stimulus" (signal two) that they called "co-stimulation." They demonstrated that the metabolic inactivation of stimulatory leukocytes with ultraviolet irradiation eliminates only the nonspecific stimulus, without affecting the presentation of specific alloantigens to responder T cells. Using a similar approach of metabolic inactivation of antigen-presenting cells, Jenkins and Schwartz extended this work to the study of protein antigens, and demonstrated that cloned CD4$^+$T cells not only fail to produce growth factor and proliferate when confronted with chemically fixed antigen-bearing APC, but in fact develop a state of unresponsiveness to further antigen challenge. Consistent with Dresser's and Claman's original ideas, the loss of a nonspecific "co-stimulatory activity" following chemical treatment of the APCs accounted for the decrease in immunogenicity of the antigen and the induction of T-cell tolerance, since the addition of viable third-party activated B cells and macrophages (themselves incapable of presenting the peptide antigen) during the reaction promoted the proliferation of the T cells and prevented their development of unresponsiveness. Taken together, these *in vitro* studies provided the basis for our current thinking that APCs must provide both a stimulatory peptide/MHC complex as well as an antigen nonspecific co-stimulatory activity to promote T-cell clonal expansion and avoid the induction of tolerance in the antigen-specific responder population.

But how does this APC-derived co-stimulatory activity relate to the requirement for adjuvant or aggregation of protein antigen for productive engagement of the intact immune system? The solution to this problem was originally thought to be the existence of discrete populations of "professional" APCs. Matzinger coined this term to differentiate subpopulations of APCs capable of priming naïve T cells *in vivo* (e.g., dendritic cells) from those that could only stimulate previously activated T cells (e.g., B cells). *In vitro* experiments on spleen-derived interdigitating dendritic cells by Steinman and colleagues reinforced this premise, leading to the statement that dendritic cells were in fact "nature's adjuvant." This raised the question of how the administration of soluble foreign protein antigens *in vivo* could be naturally tolerogenic. Perhaps adjuvants or the presence of protein aggregates selectively promoted antigen presentation by stimulatory dendritic cells over other more tolerogenic cell types.

An alternative solution to the problem of tolerance induction in the absence of co-stimulatory signals was offered by Janeway. He suggested that the innate immune system evolved first to recognize and respond to certain characteristics or patterns common to infectious agents that were absent from the host. Only subsequently did the adaptive immune system evolve, with the recognition of foreign determinants

by antigen-specific receptors as a means to focus the immune response initiated by the recognition of pathogen-associated molecular patterns (PAMPs). In his model, the activation of pattern recognition receptors (PRRs) on innate immune cells leads to the up-regulation of co-stimulatory activities on APCs and the subsequent induction of second signals in T cells. Thus, the absence or presence of a PAMP becomes the critical determinant in peripheral self/non-self discrimination. The subsequent discovery by Janeway and others of multiple Toll-like receptors on innate immune cells capable of mediating this recognition of PAMPs (described below) now provides considerable support for this model.

One subsequent alteration in this theoretical framework was the concept that tissue injury and necrosis can also elicit an activation response in antigen-presenting cells that leads to an up-regulation of co-stimulatory signals and the avoidance of tolerance. In this "danger model" as proposed by Matzinger, tissue dendritic cells are activated by alarm signals generated by stressed or necrotic peripheral tissue cells. One could argue that such a response would have evolved because of the tight association that normally exists between tissue injury and infection. Once again, the effect of such recognition of dying or damaged cells by innate immune cells is the induction of co-stimulatory signals on APCs and the generation of second signals in the responding T-cell population, thus preventing the induction of tolerance. The unifying principal then is that resting dendritic cells present antigen in a tolerogenic mode, while activated dendritic cells initiate an immune response.

Toll-like Receptors, Nods, and Receptors for Heat-Shock Proteins Mediate Activation and Maturation of Dendritic Cells

Dendritic cells resident in peripheral nonlymphoid tissues sense the presence of pathogens by recognizing PAMPs such as microbial carbohydrates and lipids (e.g., peptidoglycan, lipoarabinomannan, lipopolysaccharides, lipoteichoic acid, lipoprotein) as well as nucleic acids (e.g., double-stranded RNA, unmethylated CpG DNA) through binding of PRRs such as the Toll-like receptor molecules and their associated adaptor protein MyD88 (59–61). Binding of PRRs on innate immune cells can lead to the activation of NFκB and secretion of proinflammatory cytokines such as IL-1, IL-6, IL-8, IL-12, and TNF-α, as well as the up-regulation of co-stimulatory ligands including CD80, CD86—all of which can contribute to the co-stimulatory activity of the antigen-presenting cell. There also exist a set of intracytoplasmic PRRs called Nods, which are members of the Apaf-1/Ced4 family of proteins. They can bind lipopolysaccharides and other PAMPs released into the cytoplasm by intracellular pathogens and activate the NFκB and JNK pathways by homodimerizing through their caspase recruitment domain (CARD) and then interacting with Rip2. The Nods have structural and sequence homology to the intracytoplasmic resistance (R) genes of plants. Their role in APC activation has yet to be studied.

There is also evidence to suggest that dendritic cells are highly sensitive to the presence of stressed or necrotic cells. Heat-shock proteins (HSPs) (e.g., gp96, hsp90, hsp70, calreticulin) normally are sequestered within tissue cells or synthesized only under stress. Consequently, cell necrosis is associated with the abnormal appearance of extracellular HSP. This is in contrast to apoptotic cell death, which does not lead to the release of HSP. Dendritic cells recognize and internalize protein complexes made up of HSP and antigens derived from the dying cell via the binding of CD91 molecules, allowing for the production of peptide/MHC complexes derived from these HSP-chaperoned antigens. In addition to transporting intracellular antigens from dying cells, extracellular HSPs induce the activation and maturation of dendritic cells, in part through their capacity to stimulate NFκB translocation to the nucleus. Thus, HSP binding and internalization by CD91 may be the molecular basis for the sensing of injury or "danger" by innate immune cells.

Recognition of microbial cell products also matures the dendritic cell in ways important to antigen presentation. Rapid uptake of antigens that normally occurs in immature dendritic cells by receptor- and clathrin-mediated endocytosis, macropinocytosis, and particulate phagocytosis, quickly ceases. Synthesis and transport of MHC class II molecules to the cell surface is transiently increased, and then shut off. As a consequence, newly formed peptide/MHC class II complexes are stabilized on the surface of the cells. MHC class I expression is also up-regulated, and "cross-presentation" of endocytic compartment antigens transported to the cytosol becomes efficient. Finally, expression of the CCR7 chemokine receptor is induced, leading to the trafficking of the maturing dendritic cell out of the infected tissue and through the afferent lymph to the T-cell–rich areas of the draining lymph node.

In Absence of Activation, Antigen-Presenting Cells Are Naturally Tolerogenic

Considered in the context of a dominant role for the innate immune system in the sensing of infection and injury, the capacity of adjuvants to promote the immunogenicity of a soluble protein antigen now appears to lie in their ability to provide or mimic PAMPs and extracellular HSPs and induce the expression of co-stimulatory molecules on APCs (63–66). Denatured protein aggregates also stimulate the production of the NFκB-dependent proinflammatory cytokines such as IL-1 by macrophages, suggesting a similar capacity to activate APCs and increase their co-stimulatory activity. In the absence of infection, injury, adjuvant, or protein aggregation, however, T-cell tolerance is elicited by exposure to foreign peptide/MHC complexes on APCs, because the resting APC is naturally tolerogenic for naïve T cells. Consistent with this, experiments designed by Finkleman and colleagues to target foreign protein antigens directly to IgD-bearing resting B cells using rabbit anti-mouse IgD antibody demonstrated that these B cells were competent to induce only tolerance in

responding naïve T cells. Similar results were obtained for foreign protein antigen targeted directly to splenic interdigitating dendritic cells using monoclonal antibodies against specific dendritic cell surface markers (33D1 or DEC-205). On the other hand, targeted dendritic cells became highly immunogenic when the antigen administration was accompanied by an agonistic CD40 mAb, a potent stimulator for NFκB activation. These results support the theory that the state of activation of the innate immune system plays a key role in determining the response to peptide/MHC complex recognition, rather than simply the identity or location of the APC controlling the outcome.

In fact, dendritic cells appear to be maintained in a "tolerogenic" state by the steady-state phagocytosis of apoptotic cell products. Unlike necrotic cells that promote the maturation of dendritic cells and increase their expression of co-stimulatory activities, apoptotic cell products phagocytosed by immature dendritic cells have been shown to inhibit the response of dendritic cells to proinflammatory stimuli and promote their production of anti-inflammatory substances such as IL-10, TGF-β1, and PGE2. The induction of this "anti-inflammatory" cell program occurs via the recognition and binding of apoptotic cell products by diverse surface-associated molecules such as phosphatidyl serine receptors, CD36, thrombospondin, the vβ3 and vβ5 integrins, pentraxins including serum amyloid P and C-reactive protein, collectins such as mannose-binding lectin, and the complement component C1q. Receptor tyrosine kinases of the Tyro3/Axl/Mer family have been shown by Lu and Lempke (67) to be necessary for the phagocytosis of these apoptotic cell products and they act as intermediates in the production of the immunosuppressive activities. Notably, mice that are genetically deficient for one or more of these kinases demonstrate evidence of spontaneous systemic autoimmunity.

"Two-Signal" Model of T-Cell Activation

Considerable data suggest that the APC regulates the induction of antigen-specific T-cell tolerance versus productive immunity through its expression of co-stimulatory activities (46,68–72). In the complete absence of co-stimulatory ligands, isolated TCR ligation by solid-phase high-affinity peptide Ag/MHC complexes (immobilized on plastic culture plates, latex beads, or gluteraldehyde-fixed mouse erythrocytes) has been shown to elicit a weak and transient proliferative response that is accompanied by suboptimal IL-2 secretion. Similarly, Frelinger and colleagues showed that high avidity peptide Ag/MHC class I tetramers can stimulate at least one round of cell division in single, isolated CD8+ T cells. Nevertheless, naïve T-cell growth factor production and proliferation induced by peptide Ag/MHC–bearing live APC generally requires the presence of co-stimulatory activity on the APC for a full immune response, with combinations of co-stimulatory ligands (e.g., ICAM-1 and B7) often demonstrating a synergistic enhancement. Furthermore, isolated peptide Ag/MHC complexes in planar lipid membranes can be a potent stimulus for the induction of clonal anergy (see above). These data have served as the basis for a general "two-signal" model of T-cell activation: namely, that TCR ligation alone (signal one) is insufficient for effective T-cell clonal expansion in response to antigen recognition, and that the recognition of additional co-stimulatory ligands on the APC (signal two) is required to elicit protective immunity and prevent the development of tolerance.

We have only just begun to understand the mechanisms by which co-stimulatory receptors regulate T-cell responsiveness to peptide Ag/MHC complexes. The binding of ICAM-1 to LFA-1 on the T cell leads to enhanced TCR serial engagements as measured by TCR down-modulation. However, LFA-1 co-stimulation is only a weak stimulus for cell cycle progression, in part because of its inability to efficiently promote the production of growth factors such as IL-2 and maintain survival. In fact, Webb and colleagues have shown the capacity of LFA-1 signaling to increase the likelihood of clonal anergy induction in the absence of CD28 signals. In contrast, CD28/B7 interactions promote naïve T-cell proliferation by lowering the threshold for cell activation in response to a given number of serial engagements by the TCR and its associated accessory molecules CD4 or CD8. CD28 co-stimulation induces the movement of lipid- and kinase-rich membrane raft microdomains to the interface between the T-cell and the APC (the "immunologic synapse"), leading to more effective and persistent tyrosine kinase activity, c-Jun N-terminal kinase activation, and NFκB translocation to the nucleus in response to continued TCR and CD28 engagement. As a consequence, CD28 co-stimulation has the capacity to enhance transcription of the IL-2 gene and increase the stability of resulting IL-2 transcripts, as well as induce Bcl-xL protein expression, leading to greater proliferation and improved T-cell survival. In addition, Allison and colleagues have shown that ligation of the CD28 molecule with a monoclonal antibody is sufficient to prevent the induction of clonal anergy in CD4+ T cells.

Thus, the two co-stimulatory pairs of molecules, LFA-1/ICAM-1 and CD28/B7, can act synergistically because they work through different mechanisms. As our understanding of the molecular aspects of co-stimulation becomes more refined, it seems clear that the time will come to abandon the simplified concept of a "two-signal" model for T-cell activation and instead to view the various types of co-stimulation as a series of additive amplifiers or modifiers of TCR signaling required to ensure a successful immune response. In a similar manner, negative signals through inhibitory receptors will also be integrated into the equation producing a net outcome of total stimulation that will determine the fate of the T-cell, on or off.

CD28/B7 and CD40/CD40L Co-stimulation Regulates Tolerance versus Productive Immunity

Despite our increased understanding of the biochemical nature of T-cell co-stimulatory signals, the establishment of any one or more of these molecules as crucial molecular reg-

ulators of tolerance versus immunity has been difficult (64, 73–77). TCR ligation is essential for the induction of tolerance as well as immunity; therefore, the capacity of a particular co-stimulatory receptor/ligand pair to influence TCR signaling does not in itself predict a role for these co-receptors in mediating the effects of PAMPs or "danger signals" on T cells. B7 molecules (CD80 and CD86) become more highly expressed on APC *in vivo* following exposure to bacterial adjuvants such as LPS. Taken together with the *in vitro* demonstrations of anergy avoidance in the presence of CD28 co-stimulation, these results have led to the paradigm that the induction of B7 molecules on professional APC during the course of an immune response against a pathogen provides a key co-stimulatory signal that promotes immunity and prevents the development of tolerance. Since CD28 co-stimulatory signals are a potent stimulus for T-cell proliferation, the result is consistent with the model that cell-cycle progression itself can antagonize the development of clonal anergy (see above). B7 molecules, however, can also interact with CTLA4, a receptor that inhibits proliferative expansion, and so the outcome of B7 presentation is not straightforward.

Extending the work of Dresser and Claman, Jenkins and colleagues observed that the i.v. administration of a chicken ovalbumin (OVA)-derived peptide Ag would induce only a transient clonal expansion of OVA-reactive TCR-transgenic CD4+ T cells that is soon followed by the contraction of the majority of the clone presumably as a consequence of programmed cell death, as well as the development of antigen-unresponsiveness in the survivors. Similar results were observed by Heath and colleagues for CD8+ T cells exposed to antigen in the draining lymph nodes of the kidney in mice expressing an OVA transgene, and by Mathis and Benoist for CD4+ T cells recognizing endogenous antigens from β islet cells in the draining pancreatic lymph nodes. In contrast, exposure to peptide Ag in the presence of bacterial LPS led to an enhanced and prolonged clonal expansion of the CD4+ T cells in the Jenkins model. Furthermore, as the Ag disappeared and the T-cell population underwent a significant contraction, the surviving T-cell numbers remained significantly higher and the Ag-responsiveness of the cells was preserved. In this model, studies using a CTLA-4/Fc fusion protein to antagonize the interaction of B7 molecules with their natural ligands *in vivo* suggested that the B7 co-stimulatory pathway was important for the clonal expansion of CD4+ T cells. Recently, Sharpe and Freeman (74) using gene-targeted mice lacking both B7-1 and B7-2 achieved more effective blockade. These mice fail to reject heart allografts, do not get experimental autoimmune encephalomyelitis following injection of myelin oligodendrocyte glycoprotein in CFA or allergic pulmonary inflammation following sensitization to OVA. When crossed onto the MRL/Mp-lpr/lpr background, the mice failed to develop autoimmunity. An analysis *in vitro* showed that B7-deficient APCs are impaired in stimulating IL-2 production and proliferation from both naïve and primed CD4+ T cells. In addition, the differentiation of naïve CD4+ T cells into IL-4 producers was impaired, although IFNγ production was not. CD8$^+$ T-cell–mediated contact sensitivity was also greatly impaired at low antigen doses. Finally, T cells residing in CD28-deficient mice were found to be resistant to the effects of LPS on clonal expansion, with defects observed in both growth factor production and proliferation. In addition, the T cells were more prone to tolerance induction following the recognition of antigen. Thus, CD28/B7 co-stimulation appears to be critical for the tolerance/immunity decision *in vivo*.

CD40L/CD40 interactions at the T-cell/APC interface during Ag priming can also act to amplify CD28 co-stimulatory signaling within CD4$^+$ T cells. TCR– and CD28– co-stimulated CD40L expression on T cells quickly occurs following Ag recognition, and subsequent binding of CD40 molecules on the APC then reinforces the priming of the T cells by promoting higher levels of expression of the B7 molecules. In the absence of CD40L, Ag-bearing APC remain only weak stimulators of CD4$^+$ T-cell growth and helper-cell differentiation. Consistent with this, mice treated with a neutralizing anti-CD40L mAb demonstrate only a suboptimal CD4$^+$ T-cell clonal expansion following immunization in the presence of Ag plus adjuvant. Furthermore, such T cells lose their responsiveness to recall Ag challenge. In addition, administration of anti-CD40L mAb prevents the induction of experimental arthritis in mice. T-cell tolerance induction in the presence of anti-CD40L mAb has also been used successfully to prevent the rejection of transplanted allogeneic skin, heart, kidney, and pancreatic islet-cell tissues in animals. Thus, the CD40L/CD40 amplification loop appears to be equally critical for effective co-stimulation.

OX40/OX40L and ICOS/ICOSL Co-stimulation as Secondary Amplification Signals

A large number of *in vivo* studies have now examined the role of OX40 (CD134)/OX40L co-stimulatory interactions in the regulation of T-cell activation (74,78–81). OX40 is expressed on activated T cells 1 to 3 days after stimulation with antigen and adjuvants such as LPS. This up-regulation is partially dependent on CD28 signaling and augmented by co-stimulation with cytokines such as IL-1. OX40L expression on dendritic cells also needs to be up-regulated during the cognate interaction with T cells. This comes about as a consequence of CD40 ligation by CD40L after it is induced on the T-cell. OX40L is also up-regulated on B cells following CD40 ligation in conjunction with BCR stimulation. Thus, the OX40/OX40L interaction represents a second wave of molecular co-stimulation following T-cell activation. During the response to antigen, Croft and colleagues showed that OX40 co-stimulation with an agonistic anti-OX40 mAb prolongs T-cell proliferation and reduces apoptosis by augmenting Bcl-xL and Bcl-2 expression and thus enhances the frequency of the resultant memory T-cell population. This anti-OX40 mAb also prevented the induction of T-cell anergy when co-administered with soluble peptide antigen *in vivo,* and restored the responsiveness of clonally anergic CD4$^+$ T cells *in vitro* when given at the time of antigen

rechallenge. As a consequence of this increased proliferation, survival, and avoidance of unresponsiveness, CD4$^+$ T cells primed in the presence of anti-OX40 mAb provide better help for antigen-specific IgG production. Genetic deficiency in OX40L expression leads to defective contact hypersensitivity as a consequence of poor naïve T-cell priming. Similarly, mice treated with a neutralizing anti-OX40L mAb show defective priming for T-cell proliferation and recall lymphokine production. Most remarkably, Powrie and colleagues showed that treatment of mice with ongoing inflammatory bowel disease using a blocking OX40/Fc fusion protein reduced both the number of T cells infiltrating the lamina propria as well as the amount of proinflammatory cytokine gene expression. The effect on migration is likely a consequence of OX40L expression on vascular endothelial cells where it facilitates adhesion and migration into tissues of activated T cells. Anti-OX40L Ab was also shown to ameliorate EAE by a similar mechanism. Perhaps surprisingly, OX40-deficient T cells demonstrate only modest impairment of T-cell clonal expansion in response to immunization with antigen in adjuvant. This suggests that there also may be an OX40 independent pathway by which OX40L expression on dendritic cells sustains the co-stimulation initiated by the original recognition of pathogens or necrotic cells.

A new CD28 homolog called ICOS was discovered by Hutloff et al. (82) and shown to be expressed on recently activated CD4$^+$ T cells. This receptor does not recognize B7; rather, it binds an ICOSL that is expressed by resting B cells and a number of nonlymphoid tissues following activation by TNF-α or bacterial LPS stimulation. Several studies of ICOS-deficient mice have suggested that it is a co-stimulatory receptor involved in Th2 cell differentiation. ICOS co-stimulation promotes the production of IL-4 and IL-10, although not IL-2 and IL-5. Accordingly, IL-4–dependent IgG1 and IgE isotype switching and secretion are reduced in ICOS$^{-/-}$ animals. However, Hancock and colleagues have shown that ICOS also plays a role in allograft and tumor rejection by enhancing secondary responses of CD8$^+$ T cells, including increasing IFNγ and TNF-α production. Interestingly, ICOS protein up-regulation appears to rely on CD28-mediated co-stimulatory signals, suggesting that like OX40 it is a second wave amplification system. Its impact, however, seems to be greatest on the T-cell's differentiation to effector functions.

CTLA-4 and PD-1 Coinhibition of T-Cell Activation

Several negative regulators of T-cell activation also appear to participate in the control of immune tolerance by antigen-bearing APC (42,43,49,68,74,83). Soon after activation, T cells express the CD28 homolog CTLA-4, and ligation of this receptor by B7 molecules on the APC promotes the activation of an associated SHP-2 tyrosine phosphatase, leading to reduced IL-2 production and inhibited progression through the cell-cycle. As shown by Abbas and colleagues this inhibition of cell-cycle progression is in part responsible for the anergy induction that occurs *in vivo* under conditions where B7 levels have not been sufficiently up-regulated by infection or injury. Similarly, as shown by Honjo and colleagues, the PD-1/PD-1L receptor/ligand pair inhibits T-cell activation by recruitment of the SHP-2 phosphatase to this receptor. The ligand is inducible on APCs with IFNγ but is constitutively expressed on many peripheral tissues, such as heart, lung, and kidney, and thus may be mostly involved in down-regulation of T cells during their effector phase. Interestingly, deficiency for either CTLA-4 or PD-1 leads to the development of a T-cell lymphoproliferative disorder that is associated with systemic autoimmunity in mice. Therefore, it is conceivable that in the absence of serious infection or injury, ligation of CTLA-4 and/or PD-1 by their respective ligands on APC limits T-cell cell-cycle progression and promotes the maintenance of tolerance.

Co-stimulation from T-Cell–T-Cell Interactions and Inflammatory Cytokines

Several of the co-stimulatory ligands, such as B7-1, are also expressed on activated T cells (84). Whether this up-regulation contributes to positive amplification loops in the immune response is still not clear. This does seem to be the case for the recently described TNF superfamily co-stimulatory pair, LIGHT and HVEM (84). The ligand LIGHT is only expressed on activated T cells and immature dendritic cells. It can interact with both the lymphotoxin beta receptor (LTβR) and the HVEM receptor. The latter is expressed on activated T cells, thus making a T-cell–T-cell interaction possible following activation. Blockade of LIGHT by Chen, Fu and colleagues with a soluble form of the LTβR inhibited anti-CD3 stimulated proliferation of purified T cells as well as a primary MLR. Inversely, an agonist LIGHT-Ig fusion protein enhanced the T-cell proliferative response to anti-CD3 by augmenting NFκB activation in a CD28-independent manner. IFNγ and GM-CSF production were also enhanced. Finally, blockade of LIGHT *in vivo* ameliorated graft-versus-host disease, while a transgenic mouse constitutively expressing LIGHT in the T-cell lineage developed T-cell hyperplasia and severe autoimmune disease. The LIGHT knockout mouse had defects in CD8+ T-cell expansion to superantigens, although surprisingly CD4+ T-cell expansion was normal. These results suggest that co-stimulatory molecules expressed by activated T cells can play an amplifying role in the immune response.

There is also strong evidence that proinflammatory cytokines secreted by APC or other nearby innate immune cells during the response to infection or injury can lead to a co-stimulatory effect in T cells (40,81,85). T cells demonstrate an enhanced life span *in vivo* if bacterial LPS is present during the antigen recognition event, most likely as a consequence of proinflammatory cytokine release by APCs, since as shown by Marrack and colleagues, the administration of TNF-α can substitute for LPS in this response. TNF-α has also been shown by Sha and colleagues to increase the expression of ICOSL on B cells and fibroblasts, similar to that observed with LPS treatment. As suggested earlier, IL-1 is secreted

by phagocytes in response to protein aggregates and PAMPs, and this cytokine can enhance CD4+ T-cell clonal expansion and protect against the development of tolerance. Interestingly, experiments carried out by Iwakura and colleagues with IL-1–deficient mice have indicated that IL-1 produced by activated APC induces CD4+ T cells (in concert with CD28 signaling) to express higher levels of CD40L and OX40 during the course of Ag-priming. Since T-cell–derived CD40L molecules stimulate APC to express the OX40L, IL-1 may be expected to have a profoundly enhancing effect on OX40 co-stimulation of T cells during antigen recognition. Taken together, the combination of OX40L and ICOSL ligation of their specific co-receptors on OX40+ICOS+CD4+ T cells that have recently been stimulated by B7-bearing APC in the presence of IL-1 may provide a potent co-stimulatory signal for the continued expansion and survival of the clone and the avoidance of tolerance. Finally, for CD8+ T cells, IL-12 production by APCs plays a pivotal role in the priming of naïve cells (see below).

Priming of CD8+ Cytotoxic T Cells Requires Three Signals

Naïve CD8+ T cells can be directly activated to proliferate by antigen and APC. Nevertheless, most cytotoxic responses depend on concomitant priming of CD4+ T cells in order to be sustained (86,87). Furthermore, in the Qa1 CTL model of Keene and Forman, both Matzinger and Singer showed that activation of the CD8+ cells in the absence of CD4+ T-cell help led to tolerance of the CD8+ cells (88,89). The nature of the help in this model was initially viewed as a three-cell interaction in which a single APC presented the antigen to activate both T cells in close proximity, and then the activated CD4+ T cell produced IL-2, which helped the CD8+ T cell to expand and differentiate. More recent studies have suggested that the information actually flows through two sequential two-cell interactions. Ridge et al. (89) showed that the need for CD4+ T-cell help could be bypassed by antibodies to CD40, which made the APC competent to present the antigen to naïve CD8+ T cells. B7 molecules were essential for effective stimulation, but they were not sufficient, suggesting the need for another form of co-stimulation. *In vitro* studies from Mescher's laboratory with a microbead presentation system have shown that IL-12 can synergize with antigen and either B7 or IL-2 to prime naïve CD8+ T cells for IFNγ production and CTL activity as well as stimulating proliferative expansion (90). Several labs have also shown *in vivo* that IL-12 can act as well as CFA as an adjuvant to prime naïve transgenic CD8+ T cells (90,91). Since, as Lanzavecchia and colleagues (62) showed, CD40L stimulation of APCs through CD40 greatly increases APC expression of IL-12, this molecule would seem to be a good candidate for the third required signal induced by CD4+ T-cell help. However, it is clearly not the only possible one since CD8+ T-cell priming can occur in IL-12 p40–deficient mice if they are stimulated with antigen in CFA. IL-1 is another possible candidate as it has some augmenting effect on human T cells, but in the mouse it only works on the CD4$^+$ T-cell subset. Another possible candidate is 4-1BB ligand on the APC, whose stimulation of the T cell through the inducible 4-1BB receptor (CD137) has been shown by Jone and colleagues to sustain CD8$^+$ T-cell proliferation and prevent apoptosis in long-term culture.

In the absence of a third signal, the naïve CD8$^+$ T cells are tolerized, even though the APCs express B7 (89). As shown by Albert et al. (91), the T cells undergo a weak expansion and then many of them die. The remaining cells appear to be anergic, that is, they fail to produce IL-2 on restimulation (90). Addition of IL-12, however, augments the amount of proliferation and thus helps prevent anergy induction. This model can also explain why CD8$^+$ T-cell priming occurs in certain viral infections in the absence of CD4$^+$ T-cell help (89). If the virus is capable of infecting the APC, the cell can turn on IL-12 production and B7 expression to provide the optimal co-stimulatory environment required for priming of CD8$^+$ T cells.

CD8$^+$ T cells are prone to one additional form of Ag-induced unresponsiveness. As shown by Mescher and colleagues (92), several days after optimal stimulation (in the presence of all three signals), CD8$^+$ T cells lose the capacity to proliferate in response to the continued presence of Ag. They also lose their ability to make IL-2, but retain effector functions such as IFNγ production and CTL activity. This activation-induced nonresponsiveness (AINR) biochemically resembles the clonal anergy of CD4$^+$ T cells in that activation of the MAP kinase pathways (ERK, JNK, and p38) is inhibited. Also similar is the fact that AINR can be overcome if large enough quantities of IL-2 are provided either by CD4$^+$ T-cell help or if IL-2 is added exogenously during the course of the immune response. The induction of AINR even in the presence of B7 co-stimulation and some division is presumably because the CD8$^+$ T cells cannot produce enough IL-2 (usually 1/10 of what a CD4$^+$ T-cell produces under optimal stimulation conditions) to drive sufficient rounds of cell cycle progression to reverse the unresponsive state (see earlier discussion for CD4$^+$ T cells). This phenomenon makes long-term CD8$^+$ T-cell expansion dependent on CD4$^+$ T-cell help.

TOLERANCE INDUCTION IN MATURE B CELLS

Receptor Blockade

The induction of tolerance to foreign antigens has a long experimental history, because of its importance for potentially treating autoimmune diseases and facilitating organ transplantation (93–97). One of the earliest bodies of work performed in this area was by Felton (93), who studied the immunogenicity of polysaccharides from *Pneumococcus pneumoniae* and found that doses of 0.5 mg paralyzed the immune system such that subsequent infection with the bacterium often led to death of the animal. The major immunologic effect

appeared to be an inhibition of the antibody response to an optimal dose (0.5 μg) of the polysaccharide. This paralysis was specific for the particular polysaccharide used, was induced in adult animals, and lasted for a long time, presumably because of the poor degradability of the molecules. Although Felton was sure that the effect was on antibody-forming cells, it was difficult at the time to rule out a masking of the antibody response by adsorption on the persisting antigen.

In the 1950s, a number of investigators extended these observations to protein antigens by showing that high doses of protein would paralyze the immune system and prevent it from making an antibody response to a subsequent immunogenic dose of the antigen. Subsequently, Katz and colleagues extended the polysaccharide experiments of Felton by examining haptens coupled to poorly degradable, synthetic D–amino acid copolymers. They showed that guinea pig B cells were directly affected by these antigens, even if the cells had been primed. Initially, it was thought that the B-cell unresponsiveness induced in these models might be due to receptor blockade by poorly degradable antigens stuck to the B-cell surface. Diener and Paetkau were the first to discover that antigen given to adult animals in tolerogenic doses could persist on the surface of lymphocytes. Such cells with bound antigen were also observed in the hapten IgG model of Aldo-Benson and Borel. Only tolerogenic conjugates such as DNP$_{12}$ IgG$_1$ produced these cells, not closely related nontolerogenic conjugates such as DNP$_{52}$ IgG$_3$. At high doses of tolerogen, the cells persisted for weeks, as did the tolerance, and when the tolerance waned, the cell-bound antigen was no longer detected. Culturing the cells *in vitro* allowed the antigen to be shed and the tolerance to disappear on adoptive transfer.

Physical properties of the antigen, such as size and hapten density were shown to be important variables in receptor blockade. In a rigorous series of experiments, Dintzis et al. (95) made linear polymers of acrylamide of various lengths, coupled with haptens at various densities, and found that large polymers with high hapten density were immunogenic, whereas small polymers with low hapten density were not. The latter, however, could block activation by the former. These results were interpreted as the need for B-cell receptors to be clustered into complexes of 10 to 15 receptors each in order to signal the cell. The small polymers with low hapten density could not achieve this configuration but they were able to tie up receptors in nonproductive complexes and therefore block activation by the larger polymers. This model provides one molecular mechanism for a receptor blockade.

Another mechanism emerged from the comparison of DNP$_{12}$ IgG$_1$ and DNP$_{52}$ IgG$_3$ by Waldschmidt et al. (96). The class of antibody turned out to be the critical variable in determining the outcome. TNP$_{11}$ IgG$_1$ induced tolerance, while TNP$_{11}$ IgG$_3$ was immunogenic. Furthermore, removal of the Fc portion of the antibody from human gamma globulin to make TNP$_{10}$F(ab')$_2$ created an immunogen out of a tolerogen. These results suggested that engagement of the Fc receptor on B cells might be responsible for the tolerance. More recent studies have shown that signaling through the BCR can be inhibited if Fc receptors are simultaneously engaged in the same complex, most typically brought about by the binding of antigen–antibody complexes (97).

B-Cell Anergy

The early studies of Katz and colleagues convincingly demonstrated that some forms of tolerance induction in adult B cells could be reversed by trypsination of the cells to remove bound antigen and the receptors, followed by receptor reexpression. Unresponsiveness in these cases was likely caused by receptor blockade without signaling. Tolerance induced by other antigens, however, could not be reversed by simply removing the surface molecules, indicating a requirement for active metabolic processes during induction. For example, the D co-polymers induced unresponsiveness at 37°C even if the B cells were subsequently trypsinized to clear the bound immunoglobulin receptors from the cell surface. In contrast, exposure of the cells to antigen at 4°C did not induce tolerance. The low temperature presumably prevented the necessary signaling to the cell required for the tolerance. In several other systems, stimulation with mitogens such as LPS was also required to reverse B-cell tolerance. These observations suggested that there might exist a stable but reversible unresponsive state for mature B cells in the short-term absence of antigen (98–104).

Because the total number of B cells capable of binding labeled antigen was not diminished in these models, the tolerant state was referred to by Nossal and Pike (98) as clonal anergy rather than clonal deletion or abortion. This was difficult to prove, however, because in a normal mouse only 1% to 3% of the antigen-binding cells (assayed at limiting dilution) were responsive to antigen or produced specific antibodies when stimulated with LPS. Thus, a small fraction of functionally important cells could have been deleted, but their absence may not have been detected amidst the mass of low-affinity antigen-binding cells. Subsequent limiting dilution experiments, with a more potent mitogenic mixture of dextran sulfate and LPS as a stimulant, revealed that some tolerized B cells could be stimulated to differentiate into antibody-forming cells when the BCR was bypassed. This reversal suggested that at least a portion of the cells had been rendered functionally unresponsive (anergized) rather than deleted.

A much clearer picture of the nature of B-cell anergy became possible with the introduction of BCR transgenic mice (99). A transgenic animal was created by Goodnow and colleagues that expressed on its B cells a high-affinity receptor (both IgM and IgD) specific for hen egg-white lysozyme. About 90% of the B cells in this mouse expressed the transgenic receptor. When this BCR transgenic was crossed with a second transgenic mouse constitutively expressing the lysozyme antigen, the double-transgenic offspring still expressed large numbers of transgenic, lysozyme-binding B cells in their spleens and lymph nodes. On immunization with lysozyme, these B cells failed to make an antibody or plaque-forming cell response. Because the failure to respond could have been caused by tolerance at the level of the T cells, spleen cells from these animals were transferred to irradiated nontransgenic recipients along with spleen cells from mice primed to horse or sheep red blood cells (RBC) as a source of T-cell help. The recipients were then boosted with lysozyme–RBC conjugates. Compared to control BCR transgenics, the B cells from double-transgenics made a 10- to 100-fold lower plaque-forming cell response. Thus, although the B cells had not been deleted, they appeared to be functionally hyporesponsive. Such an intrinsic, functionally unresponsive state has become the general definition for anergy.

The most striking characteristic of this anergic state was a 90% reduction of IgM on the surface of the B cells resulting from a block in IgM transport from the endoplasmic reticulum to the golgi (100). IgD levels were normal as were other surface markers such as B220 and J11d. The cells were also still capable of binding lysozyme and the antigen could be detected on the surface of B220$^+$ cells freshly isolated from both the bone marrow and the spleen, giving the appearance of receptor blockade. Interestingly, when the BCR transgenic was crossed to a different lysozyme transgenic, which expressed ten-fold lower levels of circulating antigen, the B cells were found not to be tolerant and no decrease in surface IgM was noted. If these animals were fed zinc in their drinking water, induction of the metalothionein promoter of the lysozyme transgene enhanced the circulating concentrations of lysozyme by 70-fold over a 4-day period. During this time, membrane IgM gradually decreased on the surface of all the transgenic BCR-bearing B cells, eventually reaching the low levels found in the initial double-transgenic mice described above. These mature cells appeared to have been tolerized as they failed to respond well to lysozyme–RBC conjugates when adoptively transferred into irradiated mice along with horse RBC-primed helper T cells. Similar results were observed when B cells from the Ig receptor transgenic mice were transferred into a lysozyme transgenic mouse expressing high levels of circulating antigen. Thus, the anergic state could be induced in mature adult B cells within 4 days.

The block in anergic B-cell activation appears to be entirely at the level of the Ig receptor, as activation for proliferation through CD40 or by LPS is unaffected in the absence of antigen (101). The Ig signaling block impairs the normal up-regulation of the B7 co-stimulatory molecules. In addition, it prevents uptake and antigen processing of new carrier determinants. Biochemically, the anergic block is at the earliest events in signal transduction, as tyrosine kinase activation is greatly reduced. This results in diminished calcium oscillations and a failure to activate the transcription factor NFκB as well as the Jun N-terminal kinase pathway. In contrast, activation of the NF-AT transcription factor and stimulation through the extracellular-signal regulated kinase pathway is normal. Finally, PKCδ has recently been shown by Tarakhovsky and colleagues to be required to achieve an anergic state as shown by the development of autoimmunity instead of anergy when a PKCδ-deficient mouse was crossed onto the HEL double-transgenic background.

The anergic state can be reversed in culture by stimulation with LPS (100). Although the initial proliferative response is somewhat less than for normal B cells, the anergic B cells fully reexpress surface IgM by 2 days, and after 3 days their antibody production increases. Interestingly, if antigen was included in the culture along with LPS, the B cells' ability to secrete antibody remained inhibited, even though they proliferated just as well during the treatment. This suggests that B-cell receptor occupancy by antigen is the critical signal for maintaining the state as well as inducing it.

The fate of anergic B cells in vivo was examined by bromodeoxyuridine labeling studies to determine the turnover of the cells (102). In contrast to normal mature B cells, which have a half-life of 4 to 5 weeks, anergic B cells were found to last for only 3 to 4 days and they tended not to enter into lymphoid follicles during their migration. The rate of emergence of B cells into the mature pool was similar for the two types of cells, suggesting that anergic B cells died more quickly. These events, however, occurred only in the presence of antigen. If the anergic B cells were adoptively transferred into irradiated, antigen-free recipients, the cells survived as long as normal B cells (100). Interestingly, their IgM levels returned to normal after 5 to 10 days, but when challenged with antigen, they still did not respond. Thus, decreased IgM serves as a marker for some anergic cells, but it is not an essential component of the unresponsiveness.

Surprisingly, the fate of the anergic cells in response to antigen and T-cell help turned out to be cell death (100). Nontolerant B cells from the BCR single transgenic mice proliferated and made antibodies against lysozyme when stimulated with antigen in the presence of CD4⁺ T cells from a lysozyme-specific TCR transgenic. In contrast, if the B cells came from a double-transgenic mouse where they had been exposed from early development to soluble circulating lysozyme, the anergic B cells underwent cell death by apoptosis in response to the same stimulus. Death was prevented on a CD95-deficient (lpr) background, suggesting that the Fas/FasL pathway was essential for the killing. Subsequent studies demonstrated that the CD40 receptor also had to be engaged in order to get B-cell death, because signaling through CD40 was required to up-regulate Fas expression on anergic B cells. Normal transgenic B cells did not die under the same circumstances and in fact required both CD40 ligation and FAS expression for optimal clonal expansion and antibody production as well as entry into the follicles (100,103). If, however, B-cell receptor occupancy by antigen was bypassed, by pulsing the B cells with the peptide recognized by T cells, then even nontolerant B cells were killed. These results suggest that for mature B cells signal 2 alone (as might occur in certain bystander

situations) can be tolerogenic. Thus, signaling through the BCR is critical for determining the outcome of helper T-cell/B-cell interactions, and, presumably, anergic B cells die because of their block in BCR signaling. Interestingly, two other research groups (101,103) were able to get the anergic B cells to make an antibody response in an in vivo adoptive transfer system by providing antigen-specific T-cell help. In the HEL system, they achieved this by immunizing with the antigen in complete Freund's adjuvant. One interpretation of this result is that the PAMPS and danger signals provided by the CFA were strong enough to induce the up-regulation of co-stimulatory molecules on the anergic B cells and that this led to enough enhancement of BCR signaling to shift the FAS signaling pathway away from the apoptosis.

Recently, a number of investigators have examined BCR transgenics specific for autoantigens involved in SLE pathogenesis such as single-stranded (ss) and double-stranded (ds) DNA and the ribonucleoprotein Smith antigen (Sm) (103,104). Several of these were placed on a Rag2⁻/⁻ or a Cκ⁻/⁻ background to eliminate complications in the phenotype stemming from receptor editing. These studies have revealed a spectrum of anergic states that the B-cell can adopt to suppress antibody production against self-antigens. At one extreme is a high-affinity BCR for ds-DNA studied by Erikson and colleagues in which many of the cells in the transgenic mouse are deleted in the bone marrow, but where a significant cohort of surviving cells make it to the spleen. The latter manifest an unusual surface phenotype which is immature for B-cell maturation markers—for example, HSAint—but show the presence of activation markers such as CD44hi. Their IgM levels are decreased ten-fold and the cells do not proliferate in vitro to either LPS or anti-IgM stimulation. They also do not differentiate into antibody-secreting cells. This anergic state can be partially overcome in vitro by stimulation with CD40 ligand and IL-4, which restores IgM expression, tyrosine phosphorylation of Syk, up-regulation of B7, and proliferation. However, the cells do not differentiate into antibody-forming cells even if IL-5 is added to the cultures. In vivo, the anergic cells are found only at the T–B interface of splenic follicles; they do not secrete antibodies, and they have a very fast turnover rate suggesting that they are dying quickly.

At the other end of the spectrum are transgenic mice from Erikson's lab with BCRs specific for ss-DNA and one from Borrero and Clarke's lab (104) with a low avidity BCR for Sm. In both cases, the B cells fully matured and had a normal follicular distribution and life span. IgM levels were normal or only slightly decreased and signaling for tyrosine phosphorylation of Syk and increases in intracellular calcium were intact. Nonetheless, the cells showed decreased antibody and proliferative responses to both LPS and anti-IgM stimulation in vitro and did not secret antibody in vivo. The proliferative block could be overcome by addition of CD40L and IL-4 to the anti-IgM, but antibody production was still impaired. This anergic state appears to be less profound than that observed for B cells in the HEL double-transgenic mice, while the HEL anergy is less repressive than the state for ds-DNA. Overall, these experiments suggest that B-cell anergy (like T-cell anergy) can exist at different levels, consistent with the tuning ideas of Grossman and Paul (18).

Clonal Deletion

The first experiments to show clonal deletion with BCR transgenic mice were done by Russell et al. (105) using a receptor specific for the K^b MHC class I molecule. This mouse was crossed to an MHC transgenic mouse expressing K^b in the liver, pancreas, and kidney, under the control of a metalothionein promoter. The double-transgenic offspring had only a few transgene-receptor positive B cells in the spleen and lymph node, although there were large numbers in the bone marrow. Because the number of $B220^+$ cells was also greatly reduced in the peripheral lymphoid tissues and because no mRNA encoding the transgenic receptor could be detected, it was concluded that the B cells had been deleted. Thus, B-cell recognition of K^b in certain peripheral tissues, even with very low affinity in this particular case, resulted in a tolerant state. The mechanism of this tolerance is likely to be clonal deletion, but cells undergoing apoptosis were not detected.

In general, once a B cell has been activated by a foreign antigen and divides, some of its progeny terminally differentiate into antibody-forming cells and die. This process is retarded in lpr and gld mice because of genetic defects in the Fas or Fas-ligand molecules required for cell death (106). These mice get an antibody-mediated autoimmune disease similar to Systemic Lupus Erythematosus in humans. B-cell death is also impaired in Bcl-2 transgenic mice that express the Bcl-2 protein at high levels in the B-cell lineage. These mice get B-cell lymphomas as well as autoimmunity. Based on these indirect experiments it is assumed that apoptotic cell death is a normal part of the B-cell response to foreign antigens and that this is at least in part Fas/FasL mediated. The observations also suggest that Fas-dependent death helps maintain self-tolerance by deleting peripheral B cells that have generated autoreactive receptors.

A fraction of the activated B cells also migrate to germinal centers where they undergo the process of somatic hypermutation. These B cells first remove the BCR from their surface, undergo several rounds of division, and then re-express mutated Ig receptors. The cells then undergo a selection process in which the antigen is provided to the BCR by antigen–antibody complexes from follicular dendritic cells. Survival requires the receptor to be of high enough affinity to outcompete the already circulating antibody and allow B-cell uptake and processing of antigen for display of peptides to primed helper T cells, which have also moved into the germinal centers. If the B cell receives T-cell help in addition to antigen stimulation through the BCR, it survives and is stimulated to undergo another round of expansion and differentiation. Alternatively, if T-cell help is not received the B cells can be-

come anergized or die by apoptosis. Apoptotic cell death was demonstrated by both Goodnow and colleagues and Nossal and colleagues (107) by giving large amounts of soluble antigen at the time of optimal germinal center formation. The antigen was selected to either lack the critical T-cell determinant required for help or deaggregated by ultracentrifugation (in the manner of Dresser) to reduce APC processing for T-cell activation. In each case, the high-affinity B cells, located in both the germinal centers and the nearby lymphoid zones rich in T cells, underwent apoptosis rather than the affinity maturation seen with T-cell help. Thus, as for immature and mature naïve B cells, signaling of memory B cells in the absence of T-cell help can result in deletional tolerance.

Thymic-Independent Antigens

There exists a class of antigens that elicit antibody responses in a T-cell independent (TI) manner (108). They are divided into two categories. TI-1 antigens represent haptens coupled to B-cell mitogens such as LPS. LPS bypasses the need for T-cell help and fully activates B cells through Toll receptors to proliferate and differentiate into antibody-forming cells, including Ig class switching. Under limiting conditions, TI-1 antigens can be targeted to specific B cells via high-affinity binding to Ig receptors that are specific for the hapten. Presumably, the response to TI-1 antigens represents a special adaptation to bypass the need for T-cell help in order to make a rapid response to certain infectious agents.

The TI-2 antigens represent a more puzzling class of molecules (109). These are not mitogenic for B cells and consist of large molecular-weight polymers such as polysaccharides composed of repeating antigenic determinants (95). They are usually poorly degradable and often capable of activating complement via the alternative pathway. They mostly stimulate mature B cells and often do not elicit responses in neonates or CBA/N mice (which have a genetic defect—Xid—in their Bruton's tyrosine kinase). Several models have been put forth to explain how these antigens work to activate without T-cell help. First, factors in addition to the TI-2 antigen are often required to get a response. For example, Scott and colleagues showed that cytokines from T cells, such as IL-2 and IL-5, can augment secretory responses to TI-2 antigens and prevent B-cell clonal deletion in certain model systems. Complement components such as C3d, which are activated by some TI-2 antigens, can bind to CR2 (CD21) receptors on B cells, and as shown by Fearon and colleagues, greatly enhance antibody responses by lowering the threshold for signaling through the Ig receptor. Even cytokines produced by the B cells themselves may play a role if the antigen stimulates their production. For example, TNF-α production by B cells has been shown by Boussiotis and colleagues to be involved in the B-cell proliferation stimulated by anti-Ig. B cells also have receptors (TACI, BCMA, and BAFF-R) for B-cell activating factor (BAFF) and a proliferation-inducing TNF family ligand expressed by APCs (APRIL), which facilitate B-cell expansion, maturation, and survival (110). Finally, IL-2 activated NK cells have been shown by Snapper and Mond (109) to augment Ig secretion induced by TI-2 antigens via an unknown mechanism.

A second possibility is that the repetitive array of antigenic determinants on TI-2 antigens engages the B-cell Ig receptor in a unique way which signals for activation instead of anergy or cell death (111). In the immune response to VSV, Bachmann and Zinkernagel showed that the early IgM neutralizing antibody to the glycoprotein (G) on the virus was elicited in a T-helper cell–independent manner. In contrast, immunization with VSV-G infected cells, which do not present an ordered lattice structure of the protein, led to an antibody response that was largely T-cell dependent. A search for cryptic second signals brought in by the viral particle failed to reveal any polyclonal B-cell stimulation, involvement of complement or TNF molecules, or activation of NK cells. Thus, it was concluded that the rigid paracrystalline structure of the virus particle with its determinant spacing of 5 to 10 nm, could activate rather than tolerize the B cell. Tolerance induction in this scenario is possibly mediated by the receptor blockade mechanisms mentioned earlier (95).

The third possibility (and the one most favored) is that the responding B cells represent a discrete subpopulation of cells (112). The response to some TI-2 antigens (e.g., Ficoll) has been localized by MacLennan and colleagues to the marginal zone (MZ) in the spleen, where the responding B cells are CD23$^-$, IgM^{bright}, IgD^{dull}, and express the complement receptors CD21/CD35 at high levels. A similar but separate subpopulation (B-1 cells) is located predominantly in the peritoneal cavity and often expresses CD5$^+$ in addition to the other markers (29). These cells are absent in the CBA/N mouse (the Btk mutant), which fails to respond to TI-2 antigens. Also, these cells are largely responsible for the low-affinity IgM autoreactive antibodies in normal mice and humans (discussed earlier). The B-1 cells are resistant to tolerization by anti-Ig *in vitro* (106) and can migrate from the peritoneal cavity to Peyer's patches in the mesenteric lymph nodes, where they undergo class switching to IgA and secrete into the lumen of the gut antibodies that react with cell walls of commensal bacteria (111).

The differentiation of B-1 cells in the bone marrow occurs only early in development (29) and seems to depend on the receipt of a strong signal through the BCR. In two of the Ig transgenic models described earlier (104,113), the presence of antigen in the developing environment prevented B-2 cell maturation, but allowed B-1 cell development and accumulation of the cells in the peritoneal cavity. In the anti-Sm transgenic model, transfer of a population of arrested transitional splenic B cells (CD23$^-$,CD43$^-$,CD5$^-$) to irradiated nontransgenic littermates showed that the cells could differentiate to B-1 cells (CD43$^+$,CD5$^+$) with little or no division. Furthermore, the B-1 cell differentiation could be augmented if the anti-Sm heavy-chain transgenic mouse was crossed onto a CD22$^{-/-}$ background, which generally augments

BCR signaling, and reduced if crossed onto a CD19$^{-/-}$ background, which generally impairs BCR signaling. The B-1 differentiation was also diminished when the transgenic heavy chain was paired with a transgenic V$_\kappa$8 light chain to produce a BCR of lower affinity. Finally, when the anti-Sm heavy-chain transgenic was transferred onto the autoimmune prone MRL/Mp-lpr/lpr background, the BCR no longer appeared in the peritoneal B-1 population and the animals were no longer tolerant to the Sm antigen. These results suggest that signaling of developing B cells whose receptor affinities are below that required for editing or deletion, but above that required for anergy induction, can sometimes preserve the BCR by allowing the cell to differentiate down the B-1 pathway. Why the MRL/Mp-lpr/lpr mouse cannot carry out this process is currently not understood.

Clear evidence that B-1 cells are positively selected and expanded by self-antigens *in vivo* was demonstrated by Hardy and Hayakawa (29) with a BCR heavy-chain transgenic capable of recognizing a carbohydrate determinant on the Thy-1 molecule. B-1 cells expressing this heavy chain paired with a unique light chain were expanded in mice expressing Thy-1, but they were not found in Thy-1–deficient mice. The knockout also lacked anti–Thy-1 antibodies in the serum, suggesting that stimulation of B-1 cells by self-antigens could also cause them to differentiate into antibody-secreting cells. How then does the immune system prevent autoimmunity? That this can be a problem was shown by the anti-RBC transgenic mouse of Honjo and colleagues (113) whose BCR ends up expressed in B-1 cells. These mice develop various degrees of hemolytic anemia depending on how strongly their B cells are stimulated. Interestingly, the B-1 cells can undergo an apoptotic cell death if large doses of RBC are injected into the peritoneal cavity. This B-1 tolerance mechanism is not universal, however, as thymocytes injected i.p. into the anti–Thy-1 transgenic did not induce apoptosis. The difference may relate to the nature of the BCR. The former was derived from a somatically mutated B-2 cell which following engineering ended up in the B-1 repertoire. In fact, only a few receptor-bearing cells escape the negative selection process that takes place in the bone marrow. The latter, by contrast, derived from a somatically unmutated B-1 BCR that naturally emerges. It is conceivable that the normal B-1 repertoire has been selected during evolution to release IgM antibodies following self-antigen stimulation, which cross react with polysaccharide coats on bacteria and fix complement to facilitate bacterial elimination. The self-cells would be protected by complement inhibitors such as decay accelerating factor (DAF) on their surface. Consistent with this idea is the observation that peritoneal B-1 cells do not undergo somatic hypermutation. In this scenario then, the population does not have to be tolerized. Instead, the major medical problem appears to be oncogenic transformation in old age (chronic lymphocytic leukemia) following persistent expansion and mutation from self-antigen stimulation. This is something that may not have been selected against during evolution.

IMMUNOREGULATION

Immune Deviation (Th1 versus Th2 CD4$^+$ Helpers)

The phenomenon of immune deviation was first described by Asherson and Stone (114). They injected guinea pigs with soluble or alum precipitated antigens two weeks prior to challenge with the same antigen in Freund's complete adjuvant. The pretreatment prevented the usual DTH response measured as 24-hour skin reactions on rechallenge. In contrast, antibody production was normal, although the class of antibody was deviated from IgG2 toward IgG1. Parish and Liew (115) subsequently discovered a general reciprocal relationship between antibody production and DTH reactions as a function of antigen dose. When small doses of antigen were administered, the immune response was predominantly DTH. As the antigen dose was increased, an antibody response was observed, while the DTH response diminished. At very high doses of antigen, the antibody response also declined and in some cases the DTH response reemerged. With the introduction of T-cell cloning technology, Mosmann and Coffman (116) discovered that fully differentiated mouse T-cell clones generally exhibit one of two discrete lymphokine production profiles. Th1 cells make IL-2, IFN-γ, and TNF-β, while Th2 cells make IL-4, IL-5, and IL-6. This cellular dichotomy provided a potential explanation for immune deviation because these two cell types can cross-regulate each other. Lymphokines produced by Th1 cells turned out to be primarily mediators for stimulating macrophage activation via induction of IFN-γ and complement fixing IgG$_{2a}$ antibodies, while those produced by Th2 cells were primarily mediators of helper T-cell function for B-cell IgG$_1$ and IgE antibody production. The cross-regulation is also mediated by these lymphokines. Thus, Gajewski and Fitch showed that IFN-γ produced by Th1 cells inhibits the proliferation of Th2 cells and Morel and colleagues showed that this was by blocking the co-stimulation of IL-1. In a reciprocal manner, Mosmann and colleagues showed that IL-10 produced by Th2 cells inhibits the stimulation of Th1 cells by blocking monocytic APC function and by preventing production of IL-2.

The forces that operate to determine the dominance of Th1 versus Th2 cells in any given immune response are not fully understood. The dose of antigen is critical and the genetic constitution of the responding individual determines which particular doses are perceived as high and low. In the *Leishmania major* parasite model, BALB/c mice make predominantly a nonprotective Th2 response, whereas C3H and C57BL/6 mice make predominantly a protective Th1 response (117). If, however, as shown by Bretscher, the BALB/c mice are inoculated with a minute number of parasites (<30), they become protected against a normal challenge dose due to deviation toward an IFN-γ response. The antigen specificity of the response is also a critical variable. A single immunodominant determinant of the Leishmania is recognized in the early response of the BALB/c mouse. Gleichenhaus and colleagues showed that if tolerance is induced to the protein containing this determinant, then the mouse mounts a protective Th1 immune response. Another critical parameter is the cytokine milieu. Seder and Paul showed that high concentrations of IL-4 deviate the response towards Th2, while Murphy and O'Garra showed that high concentrations of IL-12 deviate the response towards Th1. Furthermore, the molecular form of the antigen is also influential, with Hayglass and colleagues showing that particulate antigens favor macrophage uptake and IL-12 production, which skews the response towards a Th1 phenotype. Finally, even T-cell independent parameters have been shown to participate. Kamala and Matzinger found that the dissemination of the parasite from the local lesion to the major systemic organs such as the liver occurs more rapidly in BALB/c Rag$^{-/-}$ mice than it does in C57BL/6 Rag$^{-/-}$ mice.

CD4$^+$ T-Regulatory 1 Cells

T-regulatory 1 (Tr1) cells were first discovered by Roncarolo et al. (118) in SCID patients who had received HLA-mismatched hemopoietic stem cells and appeared to be tolerant. The cells were CD4$^+$ and produced IL-10 on stimulation with host APC. They also made TGF-β, IL-5, and IFN-γ, but not much IL-2 or IL-4. They did not proliferate well when stimulated through their TCR and were described as anergic. This clonal anergy also entailed a division arrest state as the cells failed to proliferate even in the presence of IL-2. Most interestingly, the cells were found to suppress the activation of other naïve and memory CD4$^+$ and CD8$^+$ T cells by indirectly inhibiting APC function, by down-regulating both MHC class II molecules and co-stimulatory molecules, as well as by directly inhibiting T-cell cytokine production (IL-2, TNF-α, and IL-5). Much of this suppression was of a bystander nature, mediated by the cytokines IL-10 and TGF-β released from the cells; however, in transwell experiments the suppression was only optimum if the two T cells were in contact, suggesting that there might also be cell-surface molecule(s) participating in the negative regulation. Thus, the cells have many properties in common with the CD4$^+$,CD25$^+$ regulatory T cells described earlier.

Stimulation of Tr1 clones with antigen leads to the rapid production of IL-10, peaking at 12 to 24 hours (118). Signaling through the calcium/calcineurin pathway seems to be intact and the cells up-regulate CD69 and CD40L normally. Surprisingly, signaling for phosphorylation of Erk and Raf-1 in the MAP kinase pathway was also reported to be normal leaving at this time no clear biochemical basis for the anergic phenotype. The cells express high levels of CTLA-4 that may contribute to the unresponsiveness, but the most prominent player is likely to be the IL-10, which is rapidly produced by the cell. In T-cell hybridomas, Becker and colleagues showed that IL-2 production inversely correlates with the level of IL-10 production, and Roncarolo et al. (118) showed that anti-IL-10 mAb will partially reverse the block in proliferation of stimulated Tr1 cells.

Tr1 cells negatively regulate many other cells in the immune system, including APCs, B cells, and T cells. In mouse models, they can suppress Th1-mediated colitis and EAE as well as Th2-mediated immediate hypersensitivity responses, the latter by blocking IgE production and Th2 cell priming. In humans, these cells have been observed in patients tolerant to kidney, liver, and bone marrow grafts, although a causal role in the tolerance process has not been established. In chronic infectious diseases caused by organisms such as the parasite *L. major,* the nematode *Onchocerca volvulus,* and the Lyme disease parasite *Borrelia burgdorferi,* the presence of Tr1 cells and their cytokine production (mostly IL-10) has been associated with persistence of the infection. Nonetheless, this can give rise to a state of concomitant immunity in which the host is resistant to rechallenge with the same parasite while still harboring the organism at a local site. This creates a state of equilibrium between host and parasite in which neither is completely destroyed by the other. In this regard, a number of pathogenic viruses (EBV, CMV, and pox) have also taken advantage of the negative regulation of Tr1 cytokines such as IL-10 by evolutionarily capturing and modifying these genes for their own use in down-regulating host immune responses.

Oral and Nasal Tolerance

The route of antigen introduction is a critical variable in determining the outcome of an immune response. Intravenous administration generally favors induction of tolerance, whereas subcutaneous administration favors immunity. Intravenous injection might allow antigen presentation by co-stimulatory molecule-deficient naïve B cells in the spleen, whereas subcutaneous injection would favor uptake and presentation by Langerhans cells, which following activation are very effective at initiating immune responses in the draining lymph nodes.

Oral and nasal administration of antigen has also been shown to favor tolerance induction (119,120). From the earliest studies of Wells in 1911 (121), it was clear that the oral route of administration induces some form of immunoregulation. Orally immunized animals usually make an initial systemic antibody response that subsequently diminishes. The tolerance state is often associated with large amounts of IgA production in the gut. In other cases (e.g., for myelin basic protein), where the antigen is administered in a form (peptides) preferentially recognized by T cells rather than B cells, the immunoregulation has been reported to be mediated either by T cells that secrete transforming growth factor β (TGF-β) on antigen stimulation or by induction of clonal anergy and deletion. The mechanism observed depends on the antigen dose, with high doses inducing direct inactivation of the antigen-specific T cells and low doses eliciting TGF-β–mediated immunoregulation. A role for γ/δ T cells secreting IL-10 has also been suggested by Hanninen and Harrison. Nasal administration of soluble proteins or peptides prevents and reduces ongoing Th1 IFN-γ responses by similar mechanisms.

The T cells in the gut, referred to as Th3 cells, are unusual in that they can make substantial amounts of TGF-β following antigen stimulation (119). This cytokine acts as a critical switch factor for B cells, favoring the production of IgA (122). TGF-β, however, is also an anti-inflammatory cytokine that blocks T-cell proliferation by inhibiting IL-2 production and cell cycle progression, although at the same time it also enhances T-cell survival. TGF-β–deficient mice, as well as mice harboring a dominant negative form of the receptor transgenically expressed in T cells, develop inflammatory bowel disease, suggesting that this cytokine, like IL-10, is critical for anti-inflammatory immune regulation. When activated Th3 cells leave the gut and migrate to other sites in the body—for example, the CNS in EAE—they can act as direct or indirect (bystander) suppressor cells if they recognize their peptide/MHC ligand at that site and release TGF-β. The relationship between Th3 cells and Tr1 cells has not been clearly established. Both these cell types, along with the CD4$^+$CD25$^+$ T cells, may represent a family of regulatory CD4$^+$ T cells whose members have differentiated in different places and times to produce (to varying degrees) the same set of inhibitory cytokines (IL-10 and TGF-β) and contact dependent T-cell interactions required to provide negative feedback regulation on T-cell immune responses.

CD8$^+$ Suppressor T Cells

Studies on CD8$^+$ suppressor T cells in immunoregulation and tolerance were a dominant theme in cellular immunology in the 1970s. Looking back at those systems now, it is possible to classify some of them as forms of immune deviation. For example, CD8$^+$ T cells are particularly good at making IFN-γ; thus they should be capable of functioning as potent suppressors of Th2 responses. Furthermore, recent experiments have demonstrated that Th2-like CD8$^+$ T cells (Tc2) can be generated and these could function as suppressors in CD4$^+$ Th1 DTH responses. Thus, regulatory cytokines could provide a sufficient explanation for many of the old experiments (123).

One exception to this idea is the human CD8$^+$ suppressor T cells first described in the early 1980s by several research groups (124). These cells inhibited either alloantigen or soluble-protein antigen-proliferative and antibody responses in an antigen-specific manner. The cells were subsequently shown to lack expression of the CD28 co-stimulatory molecule and to be separate from the cytotoxic subset of CD8$^+$ T cells. Recently their mechanism of action was shown by Chang et al. (125) to be through the APC. The CD8$^+$ T cell is first activated by recognizing peptide/MHC class I complexes on the APC. It then induces the expression of a pair of KIR-like inhibitory receptors, ILT3 and ILT4, on the APC surface, first described by Colonna et al. (126). Like inhibitory NK cell receptors, these monocyte and dendritic cell expressed molecules recognize HLA class I molecules on other cells, and when ligated and phosphorylated on the ITIM motif in their cytoplasmic tail, mobilize the SHP-1 tyrosine phosphatase to inhibit tyrosine phosphorylation and calcium mobilization in the APC. This prevents the activation of naïve CD4$^+$ T cells that recognize peptide/MHC class II molecules on this APC by preventing the up-regulation of B7 co-stimulatory molecules normally induced by CD40 signaling through the NFκB pathway. Instead, the CD4$^+$ T cells become anergic. This state appears to be clonal anergy as it could be overcome by the addition of IL-2. Finally, such CD8$^+$ CD28$^-$ suppressor T cells have been isolated from transplant patients who did not undergo acute rejection and these cells were shown *in vitro* to induce the up-regulation of ILT3/4 on MHC-matched APCs (125).

CD8$^+$ Veto Cells

A mechanism for tolerizing naïve CD8$^+$ precytotoxic T cells has been described by Miller (127), which involves negative immunoregulation by previously activated CD8$^+$ cells (T cells or NK cells). In this model system, a population of precultured MHC-incompatible CD8$^+$ T cells was recognized by unprimed allogeneic CD8$^+$ T cells and the former inactivated the latter; hence, the name "veto cells." These cells acted late in culture (after 20 hours), mediated their effects by cell–cell interaction (not secreted products), and did not compete for lysis of target cells in the CTL assay (as they could be eliminated prior to the assay with anti-MHC antibodies and complement without reversing the effect). The TCR specificity of the veto cell did not matter and engagement of its TCR was not required for its veto function. Instead, it was the recognition of cell-surface peptide/MHC class I antigens on the veto cell by the responding CD8$^+$ T-cell that led to the latter's inactivation. Evidence that the veto phenomenon can also operate *in vivo* has come largely from the experiments of Fink et al. (128). Injection of splenic CD8$^+$ T cells into mice differing at MHC class I loci resulted in inhibition of a subsequent *in vitro* CTL response by the recipient's T cells against donor class I molecules.

A molecular mechanism for vetoing has been described which involves signaling back through the MHC class I molecule following its interaction with CD8 on the veto cell (129). CD8 negative variants of clones otherwise capable of vetoing were found to lose their ability to veto. Furthermore, cell lines expressing the correct peptide/MHC complex, but which were not veto cells, became veto cells when transfected with a CD8 gene. Finally, a veto effect could be activated with peptide/MHC positive, CD8 negative cells by adding a monoclonal antibody against the α3 domain of the MHC class I molecule (the molecular region for CD8 binding). Conversely, a CD8$^+$ veto cell could be prevented from killing by a monoclonal antibody against CD8, which blocked its interaction with the MHC molecule. These results suggest that the veto signal is initiated by the interaction of CD8 on the veto cell with the α3 domain of an MHC class I molecule on the target cell, but only when the latter cell simultaneously becomes activated through its TCR via recognition of a peptide/MHC molecule on the veto cell. The effect of this dual

signaling by veto cells is to make the responding T cells susceptible to Fas/FasL-mediated apoptosis. The function of this mechanism in self-tolerance is not clear, but it may play a role in eliminating autoreactive CD8$^+$ T cells specific for blast antigens expressed on activated CTLs. In a clinical setting, CD8$^+$ veto cells raised against irrelevant third-party targets have been used by Reisner and colleagues to prevent graft rejection in allogeneic bone marrow transplantation using large doses of CD34$^+$ stem cells under minimal conditioning regimens.

Antibody-Mediated Immunoregulation

Passive transfer of antibodies into a naïve animal often prevents the priming of that animal with a subsequent injection of antigen (130). High-affinity antibodies are more effective than low-affinity ones. Some of this effect is due to formation and clearance of antigen–antibody complexes. The antibodies can also prevent the formation of particular peptides needed for T-cell recognition. The antigen–antibody complexes are also likely to be responsible for the phenomenon known as original antigenic sin, in which memory B cells, generated during a prior exposure to a cross-reacting antigen, prevent or down-regulate the response to the unique new determinants on the antigen. Memory B cells seem to have an advantage for rapid activation and this produces antibodies that feedback to inhibit the priming of naïve B cells possessing receptors that are specific for unique determinants of the second immunogen. This feedback mechanism is most likely mediated through antigen–antibody complexes that interact with the Fcγ RII B1 receptors on the naïve B cells and inhibit signal transduction through their IgM receptors by bringing phosphatases into the receptor complex (131).

Anti-Idiotypic B-Cell Regulation

In 1974, Jerne proposed that antibody production could be regulated by other antibodies that recognized unique idiotypic determinants in the V regions of the first antibody (132). He postulated that an increase in the production of the first antibody could negatively regulate the production of anti-idiotypic antibodies and vice versa. Because of the interconnected pathways in such a network, perturbation of one segment would be dampened by the presence of other segments and thus the original steady state would be buffered.

In recent years, studies have focused on the analysis of IgM hybridomas from nonimmunized neonatal mice or IgM antibodies derived from human-cord-blood EBV-transformed B cells. Interestingly, individual antibodies show the ability to react with several different self-ligands, many of which are intracellular proteins, such as cytoskeletal proteins. In both species their major source appears to be B1 and marginal zone B cells (133). The interesting aspect with regard to immunologic networks is that these antibodies also interact with other members of the set. Administration of such antibodies to neonatal mice perturbs the B-cell repertoire and affects the subsequent adult response to particular antigens (134). This effect is either positive or negative depending on the timing and the antibody. Whether the natural dominance of B cells expressing certain idiotypes is related to such network interactions, or is due to early exposure to commensural bacteria is still somewhat controversial. However, clonally dominant idiotypes emerge in germ-free animals and can be disrupted in their appearance by early antigen priming with heat-killed bacteria. Interestingly, these non–idiotype-positive antibodies elicited by the premature priming proved *not* to be protective for subsequent challenge with virulent bacteria, suggesting that the natural network derived antibodies could play a crucial role in host defense (134).

Anti-Idiotypic T-Cell Regulation

Standard T-cell activation involves recognition of antigenic peptides bound to MHC molecules. The generation of regulatory T cells that could suppress an immune response by recognizing the receptor on responding T cells requires the recognition of unique peptides derived from that TCR. Evidence that this might occur comes from studies of Vandenbark et al. (135) on experimental allergic encephalomyelitis. The CD4$^+$ T-cell response is dominated by cells expressing Vβ8 and Vα2 and 4. Animals immunized with a synthetic peptide corresponding to the CDR2 region of the TCR Vβ8 chain were protected against the demyelineating disease. Not all TCR peptides are effective, presumably because of the failure to bind to that animal's MHC molecules. The mechanism by which the regulatory process works is not totally clear, but CD4$^+$ regulatory T cells have been shown to secrete IL-10 on stimulation and effect bystander suppression. Another possible mechanism is that CD8$^+$ cytotoxic T cells are involved (136). Sun and Wekerle have produced lines of CD8$^+$ T cells from Lewis rats that can mediate resistance to disease induction *in vivo*. A comprehensive model integrating all these mechanisms has been proposed by Kumar and Sercarz (136). Clinical trials using this tolerance approach in multiple sclerosis patients have shown some ameliorating effects, but only in a subset of patients (135).

IMMUNE-PRIVILEGED SITES

Transplant surgeons have known for a long time that certain areas in the body are more favorable for grafting than others. In particular, the brain, the anterior chamber of the eye, and the testis seem to be privileged in their capacity to accept grafts readily (137). The idea thus emerged that antigens contained in these tissues could not be seen by the immune system because they were sequestered in some way, such as by the blood–brain barrier. Subsequent studies, however, showed that lymphocytes do migrate into these tissues. On the other hand, the nervous system does have a number of mechanisms for preventing the initiation of an immune response. The tissue has few if any dendritic cells. It also has no lymphatic drainage, which is normally required to bring antigen-bearing DCs to the lymph nodes for T-cell priming. Finally, neurons express few if any MHC molecules, and, even in the presence inflammatory cytokines, they only express low levels of MHC class I molecules.

Recent experiments have suggested an interesting mechanism by which a tissue may obtain privileged status even if exposed to activated T cells—namely, by expression of Fas ligand on its cells (138). The first nonlymphoid location where the presence of Fas Ligand was demonstrated by Belgrau and Duke was on the Sertoli cells of the testis. In a transplantation model, testis grafts from normal mice survived indefinitely under the kidney capsule of allogeneic recipients while similar grafts from mice carrying a mutation in the Fas ligand (gld) gene were rejected. In a tissue destruction model, Ferguson and colleagues showed that a viral infection of the anterior chamber of the eye of gld mice caused massive tissue damage, whereas the same infection in normal mice resulted in Fas/FasL–dependent killing of the inflammatory lymphoid cells. Fas ligand expression has been detected in corneal epithelial and endothelial cells.

Another mechanism that has been described to participate in the immune privilege of the eye is called anterior chamber-associated immune deviation (ACAID) (139). Injection of exogenous antigens into the anterior chamber results in a systemic impairment of the production of complement fixing antibodies and DTH to that antigen; that is, Th1 responses are blocked. The mechanism appears to be an effect of inhibitory cytokines such as TGF-β secreted from the iris and ciliary body cells in the eye as well as neuropeptides such as α MSH and VIP released by corneal nerves. These molecules alter the presentation properties of the APCs in the eye. The APCs then migrate to the thymus where they induce NK T cells to make IL-10. The NK T cells then migrate to the spleen where, along with $\gamma\delta$ T cells and B cells, they induce Qa-1 class Ib-restricted CD8$^+$ regulatory T cells. How these effector T cells suppress the CD4$^+$ DTH response in an antigen-specific manner has not yet been elucidated.

THE FETAL–MATERNAL RELATIONSHIP

A number of examples exist in the reproduction of vertebrates, in which one organism successfully grafts itself onto another as a parabiont, completely circumventing rejection by the host's immune system. Perhaps the most interesting example of this natural tolerance induction is in viviparous mammals, where the fetus successfully implants itself in the uterus (140–142). When any inbred mammalian strain A female is mated to a strain B male, the (A × B)F$_1$ fetus expresses histocompatibility antigens of the father to which the mother is not tolerant; yet the fetus is not rejected. This is also true for completely allogeneic fetuses that have been experimentally created by embryo transfer as shown by Heape and Mintz.

Witebski and Reich were the first to suggest that this protection from immune attack might exist because the placenta does not express histocompatibility antigens. Evidence to support this idea is very good in primates. Syncytiotrophoblasts of the human fetus do not express polymorphic MHC class I or class II molecules (with the exception of HLA-C). These cells are the closest in proximity to the maternal blood vessels in the villi of the placenta, and even when stimulated with IFN-γ, they do not express HLA-A and HLA-B class I molecules. The remaining cells, cytotrophoblasts, express only the relatively nonpolymorphic class Ib MHC molecule, HLA-G. Recent experiments by Strominger and colleagues have suggested that the major function of this molecule is to provide a ligand for the inhibitory receptor(s) on maternal NK cells and CD8$^+$ T cells, thus preventing them from killing the fetal cells. HLA-G is also expressed in thymic medullary epithelium, where it might ensure T-cell tolerance to this molecule. Finally, no cells expressing large amounts of class II molecules (dendritic cells) have been seen in the placenta. Possibly as a consequence of this limited MHC molecule expression, allogeneic fetuses do not prime for transplantation immunity as measured by subsequent skin grafting. One puzzling fact, however, is that rodent placental cells do express classical polymorphic MHC class I molecules, yet these animals routinely produce large litters. Hence other mechanisms must also play a role in fetal survival.

In the early experiments of Billingham and colleagues on multiparous rodents, allogeneic paternal skin grafts placed on mothers that had been mated several times to males of that allogeneic strain were rejected more slowly than the same grafts placed on mothers that had been mated to syngeneic males. More recently, an effect of the fetus on the mother's immune system was demonstrated clearly in TCR transgenic female mice whose CD8$^+$ T cells were specific for a paternal MHC class I molecule (K^b) (143). During pregnancy these cells were reduced in numbers and appeared to have down-regulated their receptor levels. They were also functionally impaired as the mother failed to reject K^b-bearing tumor grafts during this period. Following birth, the immune system returned to normal. Furthermore, these effects were antigen specific as they were not observed in syngeneic or non-K^b allogeneic pregnancies. In another study by Vecchio and colleagues, CD8$^+$ transgenic T cells specific for the male H-Y antigen were tolerized during pregnancy by mechanisms involving anergy and Fas-dependent deletion. In a similar manner, Langevin and colleagues showed that a B-cell receptor transgenic mouse specific for K^k deleted about 80% of its idiotype$^+$ B cells starting at midpregnancy and then reverting to normal levels at birth. Thus, pregnancy transiently results in a state of specific tolerance to paternal antigens.

Several mechanisms have been proposed for this transient tolerant state (141,142). One is expression of Fas ligand in the placenta, which, similar to its action in other privileged sites, would kill activated T cells entering the tissue. In the human placenta, Fas ligand is expressed early on cytotrophoblasts as well as at term in syncytiotrophoblasts. In the gld mouse, which lacks a functional Fas ligand, fetal resorption sites are common and litter sizes are small. A second mechanism is the production of cytokines and hormones by the placenta that would inactivate the T cells or deviate these cells away from a cell-mediated immune response. Progesterone, which is present in high concentrations in the placenta, has been shown by Stites and colleagues to prolong allogeneic skin graft survival and by Livi and colleagues to favor the development of Th2 responses from antigen-specific T-cell lines and clones. IL-4, IL-5, and IL-10 have been detected in the placenta as has an immunosuppressive cytokine related to TGF-β2. The latter is made by trophoblasts rather than immune cells, as is much of the IL-10 produced in the placenta. A study by Mosmann and colleagues of the effect of pregnancy on susceptibility to Leishmania infection in B6 mice, which normally resist the parasite with a vigorous Th1 response, showed an impaired clearance of the organism resulting from a general decrease in IFN-γ production. Reciprocally, infection with Leishmania enhanced both spontaneous abortion and failed implantation rates, as well as decreasing the production of IL-4 and IL-10 in the placenta. In humans, spontaneous abortions are also associated with an increased capability of producing IL-2 and IFN-γ and a decrease in IL-10 production. Finally, the excess fetal loss observed in the CBA and DBA/2 mouse-mating combination, which is mediated by activated NK cells and macrophages, is associated with decreased IL-4 and IL-10 production and can be reversed by administration of IL-10 or anti-IFN-γ antibody (144). Thus, the cytokine milieu of the placenta appears to play a critical role in the maternal acceptance of the fetus, and may provide another example of where immune deviation contributes to tolerance.

Often after multiple pregnancies the mother makes an antibody response to the father's histocompatibility antigens. Occasionally, the antibodies formed are harmful to the fetus, as in Rh incompatibility causing erythrocyte destruction, but for the most part the antibodies are not destructive. Several laboratories have demonstrated that many of these antibodies do not fix complement. When they do fix complement, cells in the placenta are equipped with molecules, such as DAF and membrane cofactor protein (MCP), which destroy or block the binding of complement. The importance of these protective mechanisms has been shown recently by Xu et al. (145) in a targeted mutation of a broadly distributed complement regulatory protein called Crry, a major complement inactivator in rodents. Homozygous knockout mice die in utero around embryonic day 10. The embryos at this time have C3 deposited in the placenta and the tissue is invaded with granulocytes. Crossing these mice to C3-deficient mice corrected the defect, demonstrating that the regulation of complement was an important variable in fetal survival.

Finally, the syncytiotrophoblasts synthesize the enzyme indoleamine 2,3-dioxygenase that breaks down the amino acid tryptophan. This enzyme has been shown to have negative effects on T-cell activation *in vitro* when produced by immunosuppressive human macrophages. Interestingly, a pharmacologic inhibitor of this enzyme administered by Mellor and colleagues (141) at the time of embryo implantation caused the loss of allogeneic fetuses in normal, but not Rag1-deficient mice. There was no effect on syngeneic litters.

TABLE 1. *Tolerance mechanisms*

Central lymphoid tissues	Peripheral lymphoid tissues
T cells in thymus Negative selection via clonal deletion by thymic dendritic cells expressing ubiquitous self-antigens Anergy or deletion resulting from self-peptide/MHC complex expression by thymic epithelial cells. This includes ectopically expressed tissue-specific antigens Generation of CD4$^+$ CD25$^+$ regulatory T cells that act in the periphery to inhibit self-antigen reactivity	**T cells in spleen and lymph nodes** Activation-induced cell death following persistent stimulation by antigen-bearing APCs Clonal anergy and *in vivo* anergy due to TCR occupancy that is unaccompanied by sufficient costimulation and/or cell-cycle progression to maintain Ag responsiveness Th1/Th2 immune deviation via cytokine regulatory effects Tr1/Th3 regulatory T cells acting via suppressive effects of IL-10 and TGF-β CD8$^+$ suppressor cells cause CD4 T-cell anergy by induction of inhibitory receptors on APC CD8$^+$ veto cells delete naïve CD8$^+$ T cells by engagement of its α3 domain of MHC class I molecules Anti-idiotypic CD8$^+$ T cells delete activated CD4$^+$ T cells by recognition of T-cell receptor peptides presented on Qa1 molecules
B cells in bone marrow Receptor editing as a consequence of growth arrest and immunoglobulin V-region substitution in response to polyvalent, high-concentration self-antigens Clonal deletion following persistent stimulation of high-affinity clones by polyvalent, high-concentration self-antigens leading to apoptosis Clonal anergy as a result of maturation arrest and subsequent loss of antigen responsiveness to soluble self-antigens Differentiation to B1 cells to allow survival of intermediate-affinity self-antigen reactive clones early in life	**B cells in spleen and lymph nodes** Clonal anergy due to a lack of T-cell help that leads to a maturation arrest, poor follicular entry, and functional unresponsiveness Clonal deletion by high-concentration, high-affinity, polyvalent antigens in the absence of T cell help Receptor blockade by smaller, soluble, low-valency antigens that tie up antigen receptors in nonfunctional clusters Antibody feedback inhibits naïve B-cell activation via Fc receptors Anti-idiotypic IgM antibody network regulates levels of natural antibodies

Conversely, feeding hamsters a high-tryptophan diet has been reported by Meier and Wilson to cause fetal loss. These observations suggest that tryptophan levels are important for regulating immunologic responses during pregnancy and show that in the absence of such placental regulatory mechanisms immune cells can respond to paternal antigens and reject the fetus.

SUMMARY

The immune system is often thought of as a protective device for responding to the dangers of pathogenic invaders and injury. However, one of the most serious threats to the organism is the immune system itself. Without the various phenomena referred to as tolerance, the system would surely self-destruct. Hence, the mechanisms required to guard against this possibility are numerous and not redundant (Table 1). First, in the primary lymphoid organs, cells reactive to available endogenous antigens are clonally deleted by an apoptotic process. In addition, editing allows B cells to replace their receptors in order to avoid autoreactivity. As the cells mature they next encounter peripheral antigens. Some of these are brought to the primary lymphoid organs by the bloodstream. Others are expressed ectopically in the medulla of the thymus. Here the cells are tolerized by a deletional or anergic process. In addition, CD4$^+$CD25$^+$ regulatory T cells are selected, which later can dampen immune

responses against tissue-specific antigens. Maturing transitional B cells can also be tolerized by an anergic process or they may be shunted into the B1 cell–differentiation pathway. Once the lymphoid cells have matured, their activation to antigen is still constrained by the requirement for two types of signaling, one antigen specific and the other co-stimulatory. APCs are normally in a quiescent state and thus only present antigens in a tolerogenic fashion (signal 1 alone). The cells may respond to this stimulation and even divide, but the process is ultimately abortive and the cells either die or become anergic. B cells require T-cell help as their form of co-stimulation, and antigen encounter without it leads to anergy or death. Finally, even following a strong immune response, the system can regulate itself by negative feedback mechanisms, which include various cells making IL-10 and TGF-β in response to antigen, cells killing effectors by recognizing idiotypic determinants or vetoing them, or by deviating the response towards a nonharmful state. B cells can be turned off by antibody signaling through Fc receptors. For B1 and marginal zone B cells, there exists regulation by an idiotypic network.

REFERENCES

1. Ehrlich P, Mogenroth J. On haemolysins: third and fifth communications. In: *The Collected Papers on Paul Ehrlich,* vol 2. London: Pergamon, 1957:205–212, 246–255.

2. Owen RD. Immunogenetic consequences of vascular ananstomoses between bovine twins. *Science* 1945;102:400–401.
3. Burnet FM, Fenner F. In: *The production of antibodies,* 2nd ed. London: Macmillan, 1949:102–105.
4. Billingham RE, Brent L, Medawar PB. Actively acquired tolerance of foreign cells. *Nature* 1953;172:603–606.
5. Hašek M. Parabiosis of birds during embryonic development. *Cesk Biol* 1953;2:265–270.
6. Burnet FM. A modification of Jerne's theory of antibody production using the concept of clonal selection. *Aust J Sci* 1957;20:67–69.
7. Triplett EL. On the mechanism of immunologic self recognition. *J Immunol* 1962;89:505–510.
8. Nossal GJ. Negative selection of lymphocytes. *Cell* 1994;76:229–239.
9. Kappler JW, Roehm N, Marrack P. T cell tolerance by clonal elimination in the thymus. *Cell* 1987;49:273–280.
10. Kisielow P, Blüthmann H, Staerz UD, et al. Tolerance in T-cell receptor transgenic mice involves deletion of nonmature CD4$^+$8$^+$ thymocytes. *Nature* 1988;333:742–746.
11. Kishimoto H, Sprent J. The thymus and negative selection. *Immunol Res* 2000;21:315–323.
12. Robey E, Fowlkes BJ. Selective events in T cell development. *Annu Rev Immunol* 1994;12:675–705.
13. Bonomo A, Matzinger P. Thymus epithelium induces tissue specific tolerance. *J Exp Med* 1993;177:1153–1164.
14. Hoffmann MW, Heath WR, Ruschmeyer D, et al. Deletion of high-avidity T cells by thymic epithelium. *Proc Natl Acad Sci U S A* 1995; 92:9851–9855.
15. Sebzda E, Mariathasan S, Ohteki T, et al. Selection of the T cell repertoire. *Annu Rev Immunol* 1999;17:829–874.
16. Surh CD, Sprent J. T-cell apoptosis detected in situ during positive and negative selection in the thymus. *Nature* 1994;372:100–103.
17. Hogquist KA. Signal strength in thymic selection and lineage commitment. *Curr Opin Immunol* 2001;13:225–231.
18. Grossman Z, Paul WE. Autoreactivity, dynamic tuning and selectivity. *Curr Opin Immunol* 2001;13:687–698.
19. Azzam HS, DeJarnette JB, Huang K, et al. Fine tuning of TCR signaling by CD5. *J Immunol.* 2001;166:5464–5472.
20. Rajewsky K. Clonal selection and learning in the antibody system. *Nature* 1996;381:751–758.
21. Rolink AG, Schaniel C, Andersson J, et al. Selection events operating at various stages in B cell development. *Curr Opin Immunol.* 2001;13:202–207.
22. Tsubata T, Nishikawa S, Katsura Y, et al. B cell repertoire for anti-DNA antibody in normal and lupus mice: differential expression of precursor cells for high and low affinity anti-DNA antibodies. *Clin Exp Immunol* 1988;71:50–55.
23. Radic MZ, Zouali M. Receptor editing, immune diversification, and self-tolerance. *Immunity* 1996;5:505–511.
24. Hertz M, Nemazee D. Receptor editing and commitment in B lymphocytes. *Curr Opin Immunol* 1998;10:208–213.
25. Nemazee DA, Bürki K. Clonal deletion of B lymphocytes in a transgenic mouse bearing anti-MHC class I antibody genes. *Nature* 1989;337:562–566.
26. Carman JA, Wechsler-Reya RJ, Monroe JG. Immature stage B cells enter but do not progress beyond the early G1 phase of the cell cycle in response to antigen receptor signaling. *J Immunol* 1996;156:4562–4569.
27. Metcalf ES, Schrater AF, Klinman NR. Murine models of tolerance induction in developing and mature B cells. *Immunol Rev* 1979;43:142–183.
28. Cornall RJ, Goodnow CC, Cyster JG. The regulation of self-reactive B cells. *Curr Opin Immunol* 1995;7:804–811.
29. Hardy RR, Hayakawa K. B cell development pathways. *Annu Rev Immunol* 2001;19:595–621.
30. Chiller JM, Habicht GS, Weigle WO. Kinetic differences in unresponsiveness of thymus and bone marrow cells. *Science* 1971;171:813–815.
31. Nossal GJ. Choices following antigen entry: antibody formation or immunologic tolerance? *Annu Rev Immunol* 1995;13:1–27.
32. Klinman NR. The "clonal selection hypothesis" and current concepts of B cell tolerance. *Immunity* 1996;5:189–195.
33. Billingham RE, Brent L. Quantitative studies on tissue transplantation immunity. IV. Induction of tolerance in newborn mice and studies on the phenomenon of runt disease. *Proc R Soc Lond B Biol Sci* 1959;242:439–477.
34. Boyse EA, Carswell EA, Scheid MP, et al. Tolerance of Sk-incompatible skin grafts. *Nature* 1973;244:441–442.
35. McCullagh P. Interception of the development of self tolerance in fetal lambs. *Eur J Immunol* 1989;19:1387–1392.
36. Miller JF, Flavell RA. T-cell tolerance and autoimmunity in transgenic models of central and peripheral tolerance. *Curr Opin Immunol* 1994;6:892–899.
37. Hanahan D. Peripheral-antigen-expressing cells in thymic medulla: factors in self-tolerance and autoimmunity. *Curr Opin Immunol* 1998; 10:656–662.
38. Klein L, Kyewski B. Self-antigen presentation by thymic stromal cells: a subtle division of labor. *Curr Opin Immunol* 2000;12:179–186.
39. Webb SR, Gascoigne NR. T-cell activation by superantigens. *Curr Opin Immunol* 1994;6:467–475.
40. Hildeman DA, Zhu Y, Mitchell TC, et al. Molecular mechanisms of activated T cell death in vivo. *Curr Opin Immunol* 2002;14:354–359.
41. Lenardo M, Chan KM, Hornung F, et al. Mature T lymphocyte apoptosis—immune regulation in a dynamic and unpredictable antigenic environment. *Annu Rev Immunol* 1999;17:221–253.
42. Walker LS, Abbas AK. The enemy within: keeping self-reactive T cells at bay in the periphery. *Nature Rev Immunol* 2002;2:11–19.
43. Alegre ML, Frauwirth KA, Thompson CB. T-cell regulation by CD28 and CTLA-4. *Nature Rev Immunol* 2001;1:220–228.
44. Tanchot C, Fernandes HV, Rocha B. The organization of mature T-cell pools. *Philos Trans R Soc Lond B Biol Sci* 2000;355:323–328.
45. Ramsdell F, Fowlkes BJ. Clonal deletion versus clonal anergy: the role of the thymus in inducing self tolerance. *Science* 1990;248:1342–1348.
46. Schwartz RH. T Cell Anergy. *Annu Rev Immunol* 2003;21:305–334.
47. Malvey EN, Telander DG, Vanasek TL, et al. The role of clonal anergy in the avoidance of autoimmunity: inactivation of autocrine growth without loss of effector function. *Immunol Rev* 1998;165:301–318.
48. Powell JD, Ragheb JA, Kitagawa-Sakakida S, et al. Molecular regulation of interleukin-2 expression by CD28 co-stimulation and anergy. *Immunol Rev* 1998;165:287–300.
49. Van Parijs L, Abbas AK. Homeostasis and self-tolerance in the immune system: turning lymphocytes off. *Science* 1998;280:243–248.
50. Utting O, Teh SJ, Teh HS. A population of in vivo anergized T cells with a lower activation threshold for the induction of CD25 exhibit differential requirements in mobilization of intracellular calcium and mitogen-activated protein kinase activation. *J Immunol* 2000;164: 2881–2889.
51. Coutinho A, Salaun J, Corbel C, et al. The role of thymic epithelium in the establishment of transplantation tolerance. *Immunol Rev* 1993;133:225–240.
52. Shevach EM. Regulatory T cells in autoimmmunity. *Annu Rev Immunol* 2000;18:423–449.
53. Sakaguchi S, Sakaguchi N, Shimizu J, et al. Immunologic tolerance maintained by CD25+ CD4+ regulatory T cells: their common role in controlling autoimmunity, tumor immunity, and transplantation tolerance. *Immunol Rev* 2001;182:18–32.
54. Lanzavecchia A, Sallusto F. The instructive role of dendritic cells on T cell responses: lineages, plasticity and kinetics. *Curr Opin Immunol* 2001;13:291–298.
55. Mellman I, Steinman RM. Dendritic cells: specialized and regulated antigen processing machines. *Cell* 2001;106:255–258.
56. Gallucci S, Matzinger P. Danger signals: SOS to the immune system. *Curr Opin Immunol* 2001;13:114–119.
57. Dresser DW. Specific inhibition of antibody production. II. Paralysis in adult mice by small quantities of protein antigen. *Immunology* 1962:5378–388.
58. Claman HN. Tolerance to a protein antigen in adult mice and the effect of nonspecific factors. *J Immunol* 1963;91:833–839.
59. Janeway CA Jr, Medzhitov R. Innate immune recognition. *Annu Rev Immunol* 2002;20:197–216.
60. Girardin SE, Sansonetti PJ, Philpott DJ. Intracellular vs extracellular recognition of pathogens—common concepts in mammals and flies. *Trends Microbiol* 2002;10:193–199.
61. Srivastava P. Roles of heat-shock proteins in innate and adaptive immunity. *Nature Rev Immunol* 2002;2:185–194.

62. Lanzavecchia A. Dendritic cell maturation and generation of immune responses. *Haematologica* 1999;84(suppl EHA-4):23–25.

63. Steinman RM, Nussenzweig MC. Avoiding horror autotoxicus: the importance of dendritic cells in peripheral T cell tolerance. *Proc Natl Acad Sci U S A* 2002;99:351–358.

64. Heath WR, Carbone FR. Cross-presentation, dendritic cells, tolerance and immunity. *Annu Rev Immunol* 2001;19:47–64.

65. Bellone M. Apoptosis, cross-presentation, and the fate of the antigen specific immune response. *Apoptosis* 2000;5:307–314.

66. Schwartzberg PL. Immunology. Tampering with the immune system. *Science* 2001;293:228–229.

67. Lu Q, Lemke G. Homeostatic regulation of the immune system by receptor tyrosine kinases of the Tyro 3 family. *Science* 2001;293:306–311.

68. Frauwirth KA, Thompson CB. Activation and inhibition of lymphocytes by costimulation. *J Clin Invest* 2002;109:295–299.

69. Bromley SK, Burack WR, Johnson KG, et al. The immunological synapse. *Annu Rev Immunol* 2001;19:375–396.

70. Krummel MF, Davis MM. Dynamics of the immunological synapse: finding, establishing and solidifying a connection. *Curr Opin Immunol* 2002;14:66–74.

71. Watts TH, DeBenedette MA. T cell co-stimulatory molecules other than CD28. *Curr Opin Immunol* 1999;11:286–293.

72. Gett AV, Hodgkin PD. A cellular calculus for signal integration by T cells. *Nat Immunol* 2000;1:239–244.

73. Jenkins MK, Khoruts A, Ingulli E, et al. In vivo activation of antigen-specific CD4 T cells. *Annu Rev Immunol* 2001;19:23–45.

74. Sharpe AH, Freeman GJ. The B7-CD28 superfamily. *Nature Rev Immunol* 2002;2:116–126.

75. Salomon B, Bluestone JA. Complexities of CD28/B7: CTLA-4 costimulatory pathways in autoimmunity and transplantation. *Annu Rev Immunol* 2001;19:225–252.

76. Foy TM, Aruffo A, Bajorath J, et al. Immune regulation by CD40 and its ligand GP39. *Annu Rev Immunol* 1996;14:591–617.

77. van Kooten C, Banchereau J. CD40-CD40 ligand. *J Leukoc Biol* 2000; 67:2–17.

78. Carreno BM, Collins M. The B7 Family of ligands and its receptors: new pathways for costimulation and inhibition of immune responses. *Annu Rev Immunol* 2002;20:29–53.

79. Weinberg AD, Vella AT, Croft M. OX-40: life beyond the effector T cell stage. *Semin Immunol* 1998;10:471–480.

80. Walker LS, Gulbranson-Judge A, Flynn S, et al. Co-stimulation and selection for T-cell help for germinal centres: the role of CD28 and OX40. *Immunol Today* 2000;21:333–337.

81. Liang L, Sha WC. The right place at the right time: novel B7 family members regulate effector T cell responses. *Curr Opin Immunol* 2002;14:384–390.

82. Hutloff A, Dittrich AM, Beier KC, et al. ICOS is an inducible T-cell co-stimulator structurally and functionally related to CD28. *Nature* 1999;397:263–266.

83. Nishimura H, Honjo T. PD-1: an inhibitory immunoreceptor involved in peripheral tolerance. *Trends Immunol* 2001;22:265–268.

84. Wang J, Lo JC, Foster A, et al. The regulation of T cell homeostasis and autoimmunity by T cell-derived LIGHT. *J Clin Invest* 2001;108:1771–1780.

85. Nakae S, Asano M, Horai R, et al. IL-1 enhances T cell-dependent antibody production through induction of CD40 ligand and OX40 on T cells. *J Immunol* 2001;167:90–97.

86. Mescher MF. Molecular interactions in the activation of effector and precursor cytotoxic T lymphocytes. *Immunol Rev* 1995;146:177–210.

87. Miller JF, Kurts C, Allison J, et al. Induction of peripheral CD8+ T-cell tolerance by cross-presentation of self antigens. *Immunol Rev* 1998;165:267–277.

88. Rees MA, Rosenberg AS, Munitz TI, et al. In vivo induction of antigen-specific transplantation tolerance to Qa1a by exposure to alloantigen in the absence of T-cell help. *Proc Natl Acad Sci U S A* 1990;87:2765–2769.

89. Ridge JP, Di Rosa F, Matzinger P. A conditioned dendritic cell can be a temporal bridge between a CD4+ T-helper and a T-killer cell. *Nature* 1998;393:474–478.

90. Schmidt CS, Mescher MF. Adjuvant effect of IL-12: conversion of peptide antigen administration from tolerizing to immunizing for CD8+ T cells in vivo. *J Immunol* 1999;163:2561–2567.

91. Albert ML, Jegathesan M, Darnell RB. Dendritic cell maturation is required for the cross-tolerization of CD8+ T cells. *Nat Immunol* 2001;2:1010–1017.

92. Tham EL, Mescher MF. Signaling alterations in activation-induced nonresponsive CD8 T cells. *J Immunol* 2001;167:2040–2048.

93. Felton LD. Significance of antigen in animal tissues. *J Immunol* 1949; 6:107–117.

94. Nossal GJV, Pike BL, Katz DH. Induction of B cell tolerance in vitro to 2,4-dinitrophenyl coupled to a copolymer of D-glutamic acid and D-lysine (DNP-D-GL). *J Exp Med* 1973;138:312–317.

95. Dintzis HM, Dintzis RZ, Vogelstein B. Molecular determinants of immunogenicity: the immunon model of immune response. *Proc Natl Acad Sci USA* 1976;73:3671–3675.

96. Waldschmidt TJ, Borel Y, Vitetta ES. The use of haptenated immunoglobulins to induce B cell tolerance in vitro. The roles of hapten density and the Fc portion of the immunoglobulin carrier. *J Immunol* 1983;131:2204–2209.

97. Daeron M. Fc receptor biology. *Annu Rev Immunol* 1997;15:203–234.

98. Nossal GJV, Pike BL. Clonal anergy: persistence in tolerant mice of antigen-binding B lymphocytes incapable of responding to antigen or mitogen. *Proc Natl Acad Sci USA* 1980;77:1602–1606.

99. Goodnow CC. Transgenic mice and analysis of B-cell tolerance. *Annu Rev Immunol* 1992;10:489–518.

100. Goodnow CC, Glynne R, Mack D, et al. Mechanisms of self-tolerance and autoimmunity: from whole-animal phenotypes to molecular pathways. *Cold Spring Harb Symp Quant Biol* 1999;64:313–322.

101. Eris JM, Basten A, Brink R, et al. Anergic self-reactive B cells present self antigen and respond normally to CD40-dependent T-cell signals but are defective in antigen-receptor-mediated functions. *Proc Natl Acad Sci U S A* 1994;91:4392–4396.

102. Fulcher DA, Basten A. B-cell activation versus tolerance—the central role of immunoglobulin receptor engagement and T-cell help. *Int Rev Immunol* 1997;15:33–52.

103. Seo SJ, Fields ML, Buckler JL, et al. The impact of T helper and T regulatory cells on the regulation of anti–double-stranded DNA B cells. *Immunity* 2002;16:535–546.

104. Borrero M, Clarke SH. Low-affinity anti-Smith antigen B cells are regulated by anergy as opposed to developmental arrest or differentiation to B-1. *J Immunol* 2002;168:13–21.

105. Russell DM, Dembic Z, Morahan G, et al. Peripheral deletion of self-reactive B cells. *Nature* 1991;354:308–311.

106. Donjerkovic D, Scott DW. Activation-induced cell death in B lymphocytes. *Cell Res* 2000;10:179–192.

107. Pulendran B, Kannourakis G, Nouri S, et al. Soluble antigen can cause enhanced apoptosis of germinal-centre B cells. *Nature* 1995;375:331–334.

108. Coutinho A, Moller G. Thymus-independent B-cell induction and paralysis. *Adv Immunol* 1975;21:113–236.

109. Vos Q, Lees A, Wu ZQ, et al. B-cell activation by T-cell-independent type 2 antigens as an integral part of the humoral immune response to pathogenic microorganisms. *Immunol Rev* 2000;176:154–170.

110. Laabi Y, Egle A, Strasser A. TNF cytokine family: more BAFF-ling complexities. *Curr Biol* 2001;11:1013–1016.

111. Zinkernagel RM, LaMarre A, Ciurea A, et al. Neutralizing antiviral antibody responses. *Adv Immunol* 2001;79:1–53.

112. Martin F, Kearney JF. B1 cells: similarities and differences with other B cell subsets. *Curr Opin Immunol* 2001;13:195–201.

113. Nisitani S, Honjo T. Breakage of B cell tolerance and autoantibody production in anti-erythrocyte transgenic mice. *Int Rev Immunol* 1999;18:259–270.

114. Asherson GL, Stone SH. Selective and specific inhibition of 24 hour skin reactions in the guinea-pig. I. Immune deviation: description of the phenomenon and the effect of splenectomy. *Immunology* 1965;9:205–217.

115. Parish CR, Liew FY. Immune response to chemically modified flagellin. 3. Enhanced cell-mediated immunity during high and low zone antibody tolerance to flagellin. *J Exp Med* 1972;135:298–311.

116. Mosmann TR, Coffman RL. Heterogeneity of cytokine secretion patterns and functions of helper T cells. *Adv Immunol* 1989;46:111–147.

117. Fowell DJ, Locksley RM. Leishmania major infection of inbred mice: unmasking determinants of infectious diseases. *Bioessays* 1999;21:510–518.

118. Roncarolo MG, Bacchetta R, Bordignon C, et al. Type 1 T regulatory cells. *Immunol Rev* 2001;182:68–79.

119. Faria AM, Weiner HL. Oral tolerance: mechanisms and therapeutic applications. *Adv Immunol* 1999;73:153–264.

120. Bai XF, Link H. Nasal tolerance induction as a potential means of immunotherapy for autoimmune diseases: implications for clinical medicine. *Clin Exp Allergy* 2000;30:1688–1696.

121. Wells HG. Studies on the chemistry of anaphylaxis (III). Experiments with isolated proteins, especially those of the hen's egg. *J Infect Dis* 1911;9:147–171.

122. Gorelik L, Flavell RA. Transforming growth factor-beta in T-cell biology. *Nature Rev Immunol* 2002;2:46–53.

123. Tada T, Inoue T, Asano Y. Suppression of immune responses by cloned T cells and their products. *Behring Inst Mitt* 1992;91:78–86.

124. Morimoto C, Distaso JA, Borel Y, et al. Communicative interactions between subpopulations of human T lymphocytes required for generation of suppressor effector function in a primary antibody response. *J Immunol* 1982;128:1645–1650.

125. Chang CC, Ciubotariu R, Manavalan JS, et al. Tolerization of dendritic cells by Ts cells: the crucial role of inhibitory receptors ILT3 and ILT4. *Nat Immunol* 2002;3:237–243.

126. Colonna M, Nakajima H, Cella M. A family of inhibitory and activating Ig-like receptors that modulate function of lymphoid and myeloid cells. *Semin Immunol* 2000;12:121–127.

127. Miller RG. The veto phenomenon and T cell regulation. *Immunol Today* 1986;7:112–114.

128. Fink PJ, Shimonkevitz RP, Bevan MJ. Veto cells. *Annu Rev Immunol* 1988;6:115–137.

129. Sambhara SR, Miller RG. Programmed cell death of T cells signaled by the T cell receptor and the alpha 3 domain of class I MHC. *Science* 1991;252:1424–1427.

130. Uhr JW, Moller G. Regulatory effect of antibody on the immune response. *Adv Immunol* 1968;8:81–127.

131. Amigorena S, Bonnerot C, Drake JR, et al. Cytoplasmic domain heterogeneity and functions of IgG Fc receptors in B lymphocytes. *Science, 131* 1992;256:1808–1812.

132. Coutinho A. The network theory: 21 years later. *Scand J Immunol* 1995; 42:3–8.

133. Pollok BA, Kearney JF. Identification and characterization of an apparent germline set of auto-anti-idiotypic regulatory B lymphocytes. *J Immunol* 1984;132:114–121.

134. Briles DE, Nahm M, Schroer K, et al. Antiphosphocholine antibodies found in normal mouse serum are protective against intravenous infection with type 3 streptococcus pneumoniae. *J Exp Med* 1981;153:694–705.

135. Vandenbark AA, Morgan E, Bartholomew R, et al. TCR peptide therapy in human autoimmune diseases. *Neurochem Res* 2001;26:713–730.

136. Kumar V, Sercarz E. An integrative model of regulation centered on recognition of TCR peptide/MHC complexes. *Immunol Rev* 2001; 182:113–121.

137. Barker CF, Billingham RE. Immunologically privileged sites. *Adv Immunol* 1977;25:1–54.

138. Green DR, Ferguson TA. The role of Fas ligand in immune privilege. *Nat Rev Mol Cell Biol* 2001;2:917–924.

139. Streilein JW, Takeuchi M, Taylor AW. Immune privilege, T-cell tolerance, and tissue-restricted autoimmunity. *Hum Immunol* 1997;52:138–143.

140. Medawar PB. Some immunological and endocrinological problems raised by the evolution of viviparity in vertebrates. *Symp Soc Exp Biol* 1953;7:320–338.

141. Mellor AL, Munn DH. Immunology at the maternal–fetal interface: lessons for T cell tolerance and suppression. *Annu Rev Immunol* 2000; 18:367–391.

142. Thellin O, Coumans B, Zorzi W, et al. Tolerance to the foeto-placental "graft": ten ways to support a child for nine months. *Curr Opin Immunol* 2000;12:731–737.

143. Tafuri A, Alferink J, Moller P, et al. T cell awareness of paternal alloantigens during pregnancy. *Science* 1995;270:630–633.

144. Chaouat G, Assal Meliani A, Martal J, et al. IL-10 prevents naturally occurring fetal loss in the CBA × DBA/2 mating combination, and local defect in IL-10 production in this abortion-prone combination is corrected by in vivo injection of IFN-tau. *J Immunol* 1995;154:4261–4268.

145. Xu C, Mao D, Holers VM, et al. A critical role for murine complement regulator crry in fetomaternal tolerance. *Science* 2000;287:498–501.

CHAPTER 30

Regulatory/Suppressor T Cells

Ethan M. Shevach

Historical Perspective
Identification of Regulatory/Suppressor T Cells
CD4⁺CD25⁺ Naturally Occurring Suppressor T Cells
 In Vitro Studies · Cellular Targets for Suppression · Role of Transforming Growth Factor β · Role of Cytotoxic T-Lymphocyte–Associated Antigen 4 · Regulating the Regulator · Thymic Origin of CD4⁺CD25⁺ T cells · Cytokine Requirements for the Generation and Maintenance of CD25⁺ T Cells · Molecular Analysis of Gene Expression by CD4⁺CD25⁺ T Cells
Induced Regulatory T Cells
 Oral Tolerance · T Regulatory 1 Cells · Pharmacological Induction of Regulatory T Cells · Regulatory Function of Anergic T-Cell Clones · Can CD4⁺CD25⁺–like T Cells Be Generated in the Periphery?
Control of Autoimmune Disease by Regulatory T Cells
 Autoimmune Gastritis · Inflammatory Bowel Disease · Autoimmune Thyroiditis · Insulin-Dependent Diabetes Mellitus · Antigenic Specificity of Regulatory T Cells in Autoimmunity · Lymphocyte Homeostasis and Autoimmunity
Control of Allograft Rejection and Graft-versus-Host Disease by Regulatory T Cells
Regulatory T Cells and Tumor Immunity
Regulatory T-Cell Control of Immunity to Infectious Agents
Other Types of Regulatory/Suppressor T Cells
 CD8⁺ Suppressor T Cells · Double Negative Suppressor T Cells · Natural Killer T Cells · CD4⁺CD25⁻ Immunoregulatory T Cells
Therapeutic Manipulation of Regulatory T-Cell Function
 Therapeutic Down-regulation of Suppressor T-Cell Function · Therapeutic Approaches to Enhancement of Regulatory T-Cell Function
References

T cells are crucial in the immune response because they can function as both effector cells in cell-mediated responses and as helper cells in both humoral and cell-mediated responses. Most biological systems are subject to complex regulatory controls, and the immune system is not an exception. In addition to T cells that up-regulate (help), other populations that down-regulate (suppress) the immune response must exist. Once a normal immune response is initiated by antigenic stimulation, mechanisms must be in place to control the magnitude of that response and to terminate it over time. Down-regulation should contribute to the homeostatic control of all immune responses serving to limit clonal expansion and effector cell activity in response to any antigenic stimulus. An active mechanism of T-cell suppression is also needed to control potentially pathogenic autoreactive T cells. The primary mechanism that leads to tolerance to self-antigens is thymic deletion of autoreactive T cells, but some autoreactive T cells may escape thymic deletion or recognize antigens that are expressed only extrathymically. T-cell anergy (1) and T-cell ignorance/indifference (2) have been proposed as the primary mechanisms used to control autoreactive T cells in the periphery, although these "passive" mechanisms for self-tolerance may not be sufficient to control potentially pathogenic T cells.

It was proposed in 1970 that a distinct subset of T cells is responsible for immune suppression (3). A suppressor T cell is functionally defined as a T cell that inhibits an immune response by influencing the activity of another cell type. Although a strong theoretical basis exists for T cell–mediated suppression, this area of immunological research has been plagued by controversy. Whereas the first two editions of this text extensively discussed T suppressor cells, they were only dealt with briefly in the third edition and barely mentioned in the fourth edition. Since publication of the fourth edition, there has been a resurgence of interest in the concept of T-cell suppression mediated by a distinct subset of T cells that are uniquely equipped to mediate suppressor activity.

HISTORICAL PERSPECTIVE

Suppressor T cells were first identified by Gershon and Kondo (3,4) during studies designed to understand the process of "high-zone" tolerance. Injection of supraoptimal doses of an antigen that included sheep red blood cells (SRBCs) resulted in specific tolerance or nonresponsiveness to subsequent challenge with that antigen. It was believed at that time that the antibody-producing B cell was rendered nonresponsive by exposure to the high concentration of antigen. To investigate whether B-cell tolerance was dependent on the presence of T cells, Gershon and Kondo injected high doses (2.5×10^{10}) of SRBCs into thymectomized, irradiated, bone marrow–reconstituted mice and then assayed the functional status of B cells from these mice by a secondary challenge with SRBCs in the presence of added thymocytes as a source of T-cell help. Surprisingly, nonresponsiveness as measured by deficient antibody production was induced in the B cells only of animals that had received thymocytes as well as bone marrow cells during the initial exposure to high dose antigen but not in mice that received bone marrow alone (Fig. 1). This result fulfilled Gershon and Kondo's prediction that, under certain conditions, antigen recognized by T cells can induce not only helper and effector cells but also cells that are able to suppress immune responses. Furthermore, when spleen cells from the tolerized animals were transferred into secondary recipients together with normal thymocytes and bone marrow cells, they were capable of suppressing the otherwise competent response of these animals to SRBCs. This suppression (or "infectious tolerance," as it was originally termed) was antigen specific, inasmuch as the immune response to an unrelated antigen, horse red blood cells, was not inhibited (4). T cells were necessary for the induction of B-cell tolerance, and these T suppressor cells were assumed to be a distinct

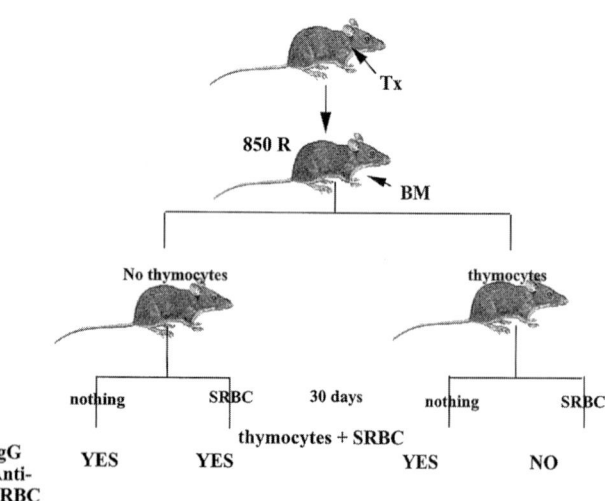

FIG. 1. First demonstration of suppressor T cells. BM, bone marrow reconstituted; IgG, immunoglobulin G; SRBC, sheep red blood cells; Tx, thymectomized. Adapted from Gershon and Kondo (3), with permission.

cell population with a fully differentiated gene program that allowed them to perform a very specialized function.

Other studies during the 1970s supported the existence of T cell–mediated suppression. Baker et al. (5) demonstrated that treatment of mice with antilymphocyte serum, which diminished immune responses to thymic-dependent antigens, paradoxically enhanced the immune response to thymic-independent antigens such as pneumococcal polysaccharide. A T suppressor cell was thought to be involved in this process. One potentially important function of T-cell suppression is the down-regulation of very vigorous or potentially harmful immune responses. Tada et al. (6) demonstrated that the immunoglobulin E (IgE) response of rats to immunization with dinitrophenylated (DNP)–*Ascaris* antigen peaked 1 week after antigen challenge. Thymectomy or sublethal irradiation resulted in a significantly enhanced peak IgE response, and high levels of IgE persisted for several weeks. These results suggested that a thymus-dependent mechanism might normally function to down-regulate the IgE response to DNP-*Ascaris* and to terminate that response over time. Suppression in this model was also transferable, because thymocytes from DNP-*Ascaris*–immunized rats suppressed the IgE responses of recipients that were irradiated at the time of their immunization with DNP-*Ascaris*. Again, the suppressor populations appeared to be antigen-specific, as only thymocytes from DNP-*Ascaris*–immunized rats inhibited the DNP-specific IgE responses after adoptive transfer (7).

Most of the early studies in these models demonstrated that the T cells mediating suppression were distinct from T cells mediating help because the former were CD8[+], whereas the latter were CD8[−]. The finding that T suppressor effector cells were CD8[+] distinguished them from helper cells but did not allow them to be distinguished from cytotoxic cells, which are also CD8[+]. It remained possible that suppressor T cells were actually cytotoxic cells that killed the helper or effector T cells. A cell surface marker that seemed to identify a suppressor cell–specific antigen was discovered in 1976. It was found that an antiserum raised by immunizing the congenic strains B10.A(3R) with cells from B10.A(5R) mice or vice versa gave rise to an antiserum that seemed to react exclusively with suppressor cells (8). CD8[+] suppressor cells were also shown to bind antigen in the absence of major histocompatibility complex (MHC) molecules. These experiments suggested that the suppressor effector cells differed from other T cells in that they were capable of binding antigen directly and did not recognize processed antigenic peptides in association with products of the MHC on the surface of antigen-presenting cells (APCs). Soon after the existence of T cell–mediated suppression was appreciated, some studies suggested that interactions among multiple distinct T-cell subpopulations might be involved. A CD4[+] cell that appeared to induce CD8[+] suppressor cells was described and was called the *suppressor-inducer cell*. Contrasuppressor T cells had no independent helper, suppressor, or cytotoxic activity on an immune response, but they enhanced immune responses by preventing the down-regulation mediated by suppressor cells.

Research in this area rapidly shifted from studies of the function of intact T cells to studies of their soluble products. One of the first demonstrations of such an antigen-specific suppressor factor was obtained by Tada and Okamura (9) in the model described previously in which sublethally irradiated rats immunized with DNP-*Ascaris* mounted an enhanced anti-DNP IgE response. When the thymus and spleen cells from these animals were sonicated, the lysate obtained was capable of suppressing an ongoing anti-DNP IgE response when injected into rats; the factor was antigen-specific. Tada and associates (9) later identified a keyhole limpet hemocyanin–specific suppressor factor in a mouse model. This second factor was not only antigen-specific but also MHC restricted. By the late 1970s, soluble factors from T suppressor cells had been described by several groups, and cloned T-cell hybridomas that produced such factors had been generated. T-cell suppression was regarded as being mediated by numerous soluble antigen-specific and -nonspecific factors that constituted a functionally unique network (10–12). The cascade involved antigen-specific, I-J–restricted $CD4^+$ suppressor inducer (Ts1) cells, $CD8^+$ anti–idiotype-specific (Ts2) cells, followed by $CD8^+$ antigen-specific effector (Ts3) cells, whose suppressor function was not restricted by the MHC. Some of these cells were capable of binding directly to immobilized antigen in the absence of MHC molecules. Connectivity in this cellular cascade was mediated by a series of soluble T-suppressor factors (TsF): TsF1 was idiotypic, antigen-specific, and restricted by the immunoglobulin heavy chain variable (VH) region. TsF2 was anti-idiotypic and required delivery by a macrophage. TsF3 acted totally nonspecifically. TsF1 and TsF2 required APCs, but TsF3 did not. Most of these factors were composed of two polypeptide chains, one of which was capable of binding native antigen and the other of which bore a determinant recognized by anti–I-J antibodies.

These elaborate, highly convoluted suppressor cell pathways and circuits fell out of favor in the mid-1980s for a number of important reasons. The existence of I-J was called into question by the finding that the region of the MHC complex to which I-J mapped did not contain a gene that could encode a unique I-J polypeptide (13). When the genes encoding the T cell receptor were isolated, they were completely unrelated to the genes encoding immunoglobulin heavy chains, thereby calling into question the existence of T-cell factors that expressed immunoglobulin VH region products. Many of the suppressor T-cell hybridomas that produced antigen-specific suppressor factors were found either to have unrearranged genes for the α or β chains of the T-cell receptor (TCR) or to have deleted genes for TCR β chain (14). No studies ever convincingly characterized at the molecular level any of suppressor T-cell factors. These studies, together with the inability to identify a marker specific for suppressor T cells and the inability to purify suppressor T cells, raised considerable

doubts about the existence of a distinct functional lineage of suppressor T cells.

In most of the studies in the 1970s that led to the discovery of soluble suppressor factors, investigators measured T suppressor activity by assaying delayed-type hypersensitivity responses *in vivo* or used plaque-forming cell assays for antibody production *in vitro*. Two completely different approaches to the demonstration of the importance of regulatory or suppressor T cells in the prevention of organ-specific autoimmunity were also developed in the 1970s. In one, mice that were thymectomized on the third day of life (d3Tx) were shown to develop organ-specific autoimmune diseases (Fig. 2). The specific disease that developed varied with the strain of mouse under study, and more than one organ could be involved in a given mouse. Most important, autoimmunity was not seen if the mouse was thymectomized on day 1 or day 7 of life, and disease could be completely prevented if the d3Tx mouse received a thymus transplant between days 10 and 15 of life (15). These observations led to the hypothesis that autoreactive T cells were exported from the thymus during the first 3 days of life and that, somewhat later in ontogeny, a population of suppressor cells that controlled the autoreactive T cells emigrated from the thymus. Removal of the thymus before the suppressor cells reached the periphery resulted in autoimmune disease. A number of other protocols (Table 1) that induced a lymphopenic state also resulted in the development of organ-specific autoimmunity. It was believed that these procedures resulted in a selective depletion of suppressor T cells but left the autoreactive effector populations intact. Subsequent studies demonstrated that the effector cells in this model were $CD4^+$ T cells. The suppressor T cells were also $CD4^+$ cells, and the development of autoimmune disease could be prevented by reconstitution of

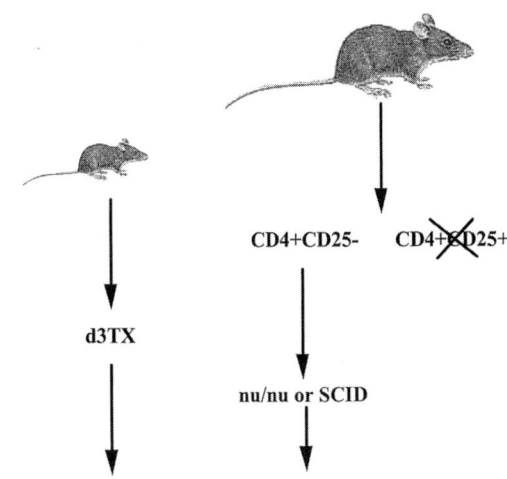

CD4+CD25-   CD4+CD25+

d3TX

nu/nu or SCID

ORGAN-SPECIFIC AUTOIMMUNITY

FIG. 2. Depletion of $CD4^+CD25^+$ T cells results in organ-specific autoimmunity. d3Tx, thymectomized on the third day of life; SCID, severe combined immunodeficient. Adapted from Nishizuka and Sakakura (15) and Sakaguchi et al. (21), with permission.

TABLE 1. *Lymphopenia results in organ-specific autoimmune disease*

d3Tx
Neonatal administration of cyclosporine
Thymectomy plus repeated low-dose irradiation
High-dose fractionated total lymphoid irradiation
Adult thymectomy plus cyclophosphamide
Single T-cell receptor α chain mice
Transfer of T cells to T-cell–deficient mice

Adapted from Sakaguchi and Sakaguchi (16), with permission.

the d3Tx animals with peripheral CD4$^+$ T cells from normal adult mice (16).

A second approach to define the role of regulatory T cells in the control of autoimmunity was described by Penhale et al. in the 1970s (17,18). They devised a procedure to deplete regulatory T cells from adult animals while leaving the helper population responsible for autoantibody production intact. The disease model was autoimmune thyroiditis because circulating antibody to thyroglobulin was believed to play an important pathogenic role. Spontaneous thyroiditis and circulating immunoglobulin G (IgG) autoantibodies developed in 60% of rats after the selective depletion of T cells by adult thymectomy followed by irradiation. Thymectomy was performed in rats between 3 and 5 weeks of age, and the rats were then given four to five repeated doses of 200 rad at 14-day intervals (Fig. 3). No evidence of thyroiditis was seen in rats that received only local irradiation to the thyroid region, which indicates that irradiation itself did not induce pathological changes. The conclusion drawn from these studies was that in the normal animal, B cells that recognized thyroid antigens were prevented from differentiating into autoantibody producing cells by an active controlling T-cell mechanism. It was assumed that the suppressor T-cell population was mediating its functions by acting directly on the B cell and not by regulating other T cells. The active role of T cells in preventing the development of autoimmunity in this model was confirmed by reconstituting, shortly after the final dose of irradiation, the Tx-irradiated mice with lymphoid cells from normal donors. Penhale et al. (19) also demonstrated that autoimmune diabetes would develop after the Tx-irradiation protocol in a strain of rats that was normally not susceptible to this disease. Together, the d3Tx model in the mouse and the Tx-irradiation model in the rat demonstrated that normally autoreactive helper and suppressor cells may coexist and that certain autoimmune responses are held in check by the equilibrium favoring suppressor activity.

IDENTIFICATION OF REGULATORY/ SUPPRESSOR T CELLS

An important extension of this hypothesis was that inhibition of autoreactive T cells by suppressor T cells was not a phenomenon unique to the neonate but that in the normal adult animal, autoreactive T cells are also under the constant control of the suppressor T cells. If the suppressor lineage was deleted, damaged, or compromised in the adult animal, autoimmune disease might develop. A number of studies suggested that the regulatory T cells in the normal adult animal might be identified by the expression of certain membrane antigens, such as high levels of CD5 (20); however, a major advance in the understanding of the role of regulatory T cells was the demonstration by Sakaguchi et al. (21,22) that a minor population of CD4$^+$ T cells (10%) that coexpressed the CD25 antigen [the interleukin (IL)–2 receptor α chain] appeared to function as regulatory T cells in the normal adult. When CD25$^+$ T cells were depleted from a population of normal adult CD4$^+$ T cells and the remaining CD4$^+$CD25$^-$ T cells transferred to an immunocompromised recipient such as a *nu/nu* mouse, the recipients developed a spectrum of autoimmune diseases that closely resembled those seen after d3Tx (Fig. 2). Cotransfer of the CD25$^+$ cells prevented the development of autoimmunity. Similarly, the induction of disease after d3Tx could also be prevented by reconstitution of the animals with CD4$^+$CD25$^+$, but not CD4$^+$CD25$^-$, normal adult T cells before day 14 of life (23). CD8$^+$CD25$^-$ T cells alone were not capable of inducing autoimmunity and enhanced the induction of disease by CD4$^+$CD25$^-$ T cells. These studies solidified the role of the CD4$^+$CD25$^+$ T cells as a major subset of cells that plays a unique role in the regulation of the immune response. The autoimmune diseases induced by depletion of CD4$^+$CD25$^+$ T cells are uniformly accompanied by the development of organ-specific autoantibodies, which suggests that this mode of loss of T-cell tolerance also results in the breakdown of B-cell tolerance as well. It is likely that the activated self-reactive T helper cells provide signals to self-reactive B cells, rescue them from apoptosis, and stimulate autoantibody production.

Powrie and Mason (24) were the first to identify cell surface markers that distinguished between regulatory and

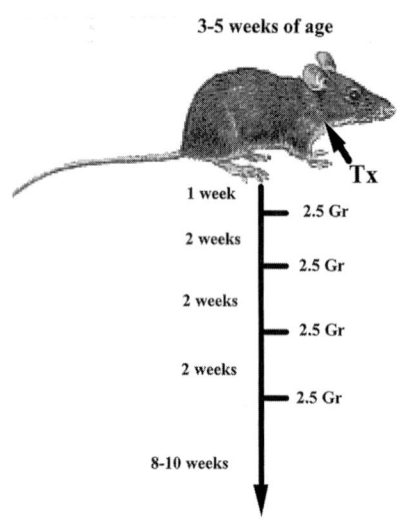

3-5 weeks of age

Tx

1 week — 2.5 Gr

2 weeks — 2.5 Gr

2 weeks — 2.5 Gr

2 weeks — 2.5 Gr

8-10 weeks

Organ-specific Autoimmunity

FIG. 3. Induction of organ-specific autoimmunity in rats by adult thymectomy (Tx) and irradiation. Adapted from Penhale et al. (17), with permission.

effector T cell populations in the rat. When athymic rats were reconstituted with small numbers of CD4$^+$CD45RC^{high} T cells, they developed a severe wasting disease characterized by extensive mononuclear cell infiltration in the lungs, liver, thyroid, stomach, and pancreas 6 to 10 weeks later. No disease developed in rats that received unseparated CD4$^+$ T cells or CD45RC^{low} cells. It seemed likely from these studies that the CD45RC^{low} subset controlled the capacity of the RC^{high} subset to mediate the wasting disease. The suppressive effect of the RC^{low} subset was directly demonstrated by Fowell and Mason (25) by using the thymectomy-irradiation model developed by Penhale. Transfer of RC^{low} CD4$^+$ T cells completely inhibited the development of diabetes and insulitis. RC^{low} T cells from long-term Tx donors could protect as efficiently as cells from normal donors, which demonstrated that the regulatory T cell is long-lived in the periphery. Subsequently, CD45RB^{low} subset in the mouse was shown to have regulatory properties similar to the CD4$^+$CD45RC^{low} subset of the rat (26). Taken together, these studies in mouse and rat model systems demonstrated for the first time that two-well characterized cell surface antigens (CD25 and CD45RC^{low}/CD4$^+$CD45RB^{low}) could be used to identify suppressor CD4$^+$ T-cell subpopulations present in normal animals. More recent studies have shown that the majority of the suppressor activity of the CD4$^+$CD45RB^{low} population is mediated by the CD25$^+$ T cells within that population (27).

CD4$^+$CD25$^+$ NATURALLY OCCURRING SUPPRESSOR T CELLS

CD4$^+$CD25$^+$ T cells typically represent 5% to 8% of the total population of T cells in the normal mouse lymph node, or 10% to 15% of mouse CD4$^+$ T cells (Fig. 4). CD4$^+$CD25$^+$ T cells can also be found in the thymus, where they repre-

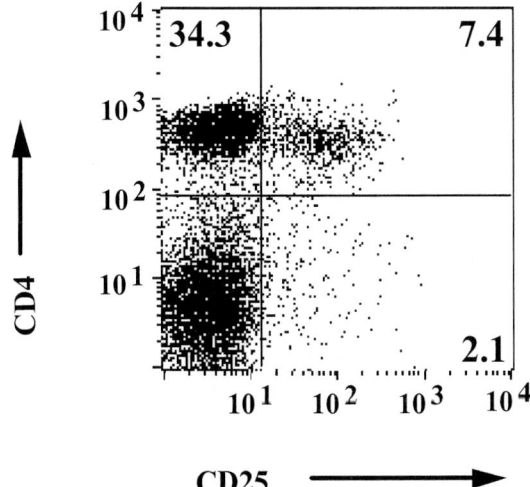

FIG. 4. Identification of CD4$^+$CD25$^+$ T cells in normal mouse lymph node. Adapted from Thornton and Shevach (37), with permission.

sent about 5% to 10% of the mature CD4$^+$CD8$^-$ population, or 0.5% of mouse thymocytes (21,28). A population with an identical phenotype has been identified in the rat, in human peripheral blood, and in the human thymus (29–36). In direct comparison with CD4$^+$CD25$^-$ T cells, CD4$^+$CD25$^+$ T cells express slightly higher levels of CD5, have a slightly higher proportion of CD62L^{low} cells, and have a higher proportion of CD69$^+$ cells. They express both intermediate and low levels of CD45RB and are completely absent from the CD45RB^{high} population (37). All of the CD4$^+$CD25$^+$ T cells express the TCR α/β receptor and are NK-1.1 negative. The distribution of expression of a given TCR Vα or Vβ specificity is similar on CD4$^+$CD25$^+$ and CD4$^+$CD25$^-$ T cells (28). One other unique property of CD25$^+$ T cells in both mouse and human is that they are the only nonactivated T-cell population that expresses high levels of the cytotoxic T-lymphocyte–associated antigen 4 (CTLA-4) intracellularly (27,38,39). The glucocorticoid-induced tumor necrosis factor (TNF)–like receptor (GITR) TNF receptor superfamily (TNFRSF) 18 has also been shown to be expressed on the majority of resting CD4$^+$CD25$^+$ T cells and to be expressed at very low levels on CD4$^+$CD25$^-$ T cells (40,41). The GITR is up-regulated on CD4$^+$CD25$^-$ T cells after TCR-mediated activation. Because the number of CD4$^+$CD25$^+$ T cells is remarkably constant in normal animals in the absence of perturbation of the immune system, they are referred to as "naturally occurring" or "endogenous" T suppressor cells (42).

In Vitro Studies

One of the major difficulties in the analysis of the mechanism of action of CD25$^+$ T cells is that the in vivo studies of autoimmune disease require weeks to months to perform. An in vitro model system has been established for the analysis of CD25$^+$ T cell function that allows rapid assays and offers some insights to the mechanism of action of CD25$^+$ T cell function in vivo (37,43–45). This approach also allows a comparison of the requirements for activation (co-stimulation, antigen concentration) of CD25$^+$ T cells in comparison with CD25$^-$ T cells. Purified CD25$^+$ T cells were completely unresponsive to high concentrations of IL-2 alone, to stimulation with plate-bound or soluble anti-CD3, or to the combination of anti-CD3 and anti-CD28. They could be induced to proliferate when stimulated with the combination of anti-CD3 and IL-2 but not when stimulated by endogenous IL-2 production with anti-CD28. The most striking property of the CD25$^+$ T cells is their ability to suppress proliferative responses of both CD4$^+$ and CD8$^+$ CD25$^-$ T cells (Fig. 5). The CD25$^+$ T cells must be activated through their TCR to suppress. No suppression was seen when CD25$^+$ T cells were separated by semipermeable membrane from the CD25$^-$ T cells. This finding demonstrates that cell contact between CD25$^+$ and CD25$^-$ T cells is required. Neutralization of the suppressor cytokines IL-4, IL-10, and transforming growth factor β (TGF-β) individually or in combination also had no effect on the CD25-mediated suppression. Similarly, CD25$^+$ T cells from mice deficient in IL-4, IL-10, or TGF-β

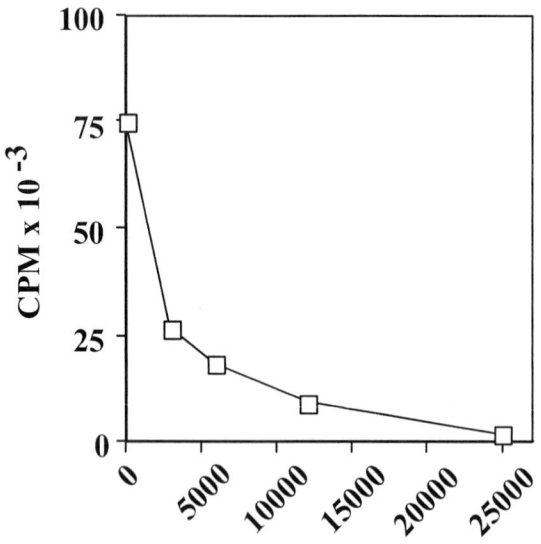

CPM x 10^{-3}

CD4+CD25+ CELLS

FIG. 5. CD4$^+$CD25$^+$ T cells suppress the proliferative response of CD4$^+$CD25$^-$ T cells. Graded numbers of CD4$^+$CD25$^+$ T cells were mixed with 5×10^4 CD4$^+$CD25$^-$ T cells, T-depleted spleen cells, and soluble anti-CD3. Proliferation was measured after 72 hours. CPM, counts per minute. Adapted from Thornton and Shevach (37), with permission.

were fully competent suppressors. Indo-1–loaded CD25$^+$ T cells did not flux calcium in response to TCR stimulation (46), which suggests that they have a block in proximal signaling similar to that seen in T cells rendered anergic *in vitro*.

CD25$^+$ T cells mediate suppression by inhibiting the induction of IL-2 messenger ribonucleic acid (mRNA) in the responder CD25$^-$ T cells. Thus, the trivial explanation for their suppressive properties, that they bind IL-2 and function as IL-2 "sinks" (47), is completely ruled out because no IL-2 is produced in the cocultures. Suppression can be abrogated by the addition of IL-2, thereby circumventing the block. The addition of anti-CD28 also overcomes suppression, presumably by potently stimulating the production of endogenous IL-2 and overriding the suppressive effects of the CD25$^+$ cells. CD25$^+$ T cells do not directly mediate the death of the responders but induce a cell-cycle arrest at the G1-S phase of the cell cycle. Such a cell-cycle arrest is often followed by cell death, and it is difficult to recover significant numbers of viable cells when the suppressors and responders are cocultured for periods longer than 48 hours. Suppression of T-cell proliferation is the exclusive property of CD25$^+$ T cells isolated from normal animals. The induction of CD25 expression by stimulating CD25$^-$ T cells through the TCRs does not render the stimulated cells suppressive. In this regard, it is important to emphasize that expression of CD25 does not indicate that a cell is likely to have suppressive properties. Indeed, the highest percentage of CD4$^+$ CD25$^+$ T cells (30% to 40%) is seen in mice that have un-

dergone d3Tx. When cells from these animals are tested *in vitro*, they fail to inhibit the proliferative responses of CD25$^-$ T cells (37). This population of CD4$^+$CD25$^+$ T cells probably represents autoreactive effector cells that express CD25 secondary to stimulation by autoantigens in the d3Tx host.

CD25$^+$ T cells can be easily propagated *in vitro* for 3 to 14 days by stimulation initially with anti-CD3 and IL-2 and then expansion in IL-2 alone (45). It has also been possible to clone murine CD25$^+$ T cells by repeated stimulation with anti-CD3 and IL-2 (41). After 7 to 14 days of activation and culture in IL-2, activated CD25$^+$ T cells remain nonresponsive and cannot be induced to proliferate when restimulated through their TCRs in the absence of IL-2. The activated CD25$^+$ T cells have more potent suppressor activity on a per-cell basis (threefold to fourfold) than freshly explanted CD25$^+$ T cells. CD25$^+$ T cells that appear to be antigen-specific can be identified in mice that express a transgenic TCR. In general, the percentage of CD25$^+$ cells is reduced in TCR transgenic mice (3% to 5%, in comparison with 10% in normal animals). More important, the population of CD25$^+$ T cells is barely detectable when the TCR transgenic mice are bred onto a recombination activation gene–deficient (RAG$^{-/-}$) background. This result suggests that expression of an endogenous TCR α chain is required for generation of the CD25$^+$ lineage (28). It is likely that antigen recognized by the endogenous α chain is the true physiological ligand of the CD25$^+$ T cell that is responsible for their differentiation in the thymus (see later discussion). The expression of the transgenic TCR α chain is a convenient tool that allows activation of the CD25$^+$ T cells with peptide/MHC ligand rather than with anti-CD3 (45). When T cells from TCR transgenic mice are activated with their peptide/MHC ligand and then expanded *in vitro* in IL-2, the activated suppressors are subsequently capable of suppressing the proliferative responses of fresh CD4$^+$CD25$^-$ T cells from mice that express a different transgenic TCR. There is no MHC restriction in the interaction of the activated suppressors and the CD25$^-$ responders. Therefore, the suppressor effector function of activated CD25$^-$ T cells is completely nonspecific (Table 2).

CD25-mediated suppression is highly sensitive to antigenic stimulation. For example, when CD25$^+$ and CD25$^-$ T cells are prepared from the same TCR transgenic mouse and stimulated with a specific peptide, the antigen concentration necessary to stimulate the CD25$^+$ T cells to suppress is 10- to 100-fold lower than that required for triggering the proliferation of the CD25$^-$ T-cell population (43). The partially activated phenotype of CD25$^+$ T-cell population, combined with their enhanced sensitivity to antigen stimulation, suggests that they are highly differentiated in their function and are ready to mediate their suppressive functions immediately upon encounter with their target antigens. Their capacity to rapidly suppress responses *in vitro* suggests that they have been continuously stimulated by self-antigens in the normal physiological state and continuously exert some degree of suppression *in vivo*.

TABLE 2. *The suppressor effector function of activated CD4$^+$CD25$^+$ T cells is completely nonspecific*

First culture		Second culture (TCR Tg CD4$^+$ CD25$^-$ T cells specific for)	Suppression
CD4$^+$CD25$^+$ from HA TCR Tg stimulated with HA$_{126-138}$ + IL-2 3–7 days	→	IA^d + HA$_{126-138}$	99%
		IE^d + HA$_{110-119}$	99%
		IE^k + PCC$_{88-104}$	95%
		IA^u + MBP$_{Ac1-11}$	91%

CD4$^+$CD25$^+$ T cells from mice expressing a TCR transgene specific for HA$_{126-138}$ were cultured with peptide, T cell–depleted spleen cells, and IL-2. They were then washed and mixed with CD4$^+$CD25$^-$ T cells from mice expressing the same or different TCR transgenes and then stimulated with the appropriate peptide.

HA, hemagglutinin; IL-2; interleukin-2; MBP, myelin basic protein; PCC, pigeon cytochrome C; TCR, T-cell receptor; Tg, transgenic.

Adapted From Thornton and Shevach (45), with permission.

CD25$^+$ T cells suppress the proliferative responses of CD8$^+$ T cells in a manner similar to that seen with CD4$^+$CD25$^-$ responders (48). Marked suppression of the effector cytokine, interferon (IFN)–γ, is also seen in the presence of CD25$^+$ T cells. Whereas suppression of the proliferation of CD4$^+$ responders by CD25$^+$ T cells can be completely reversed by the addition of IL-2 or anti-CD28, the suppression of CD8$^+$ T cell responses is not reversed by the addition of IL-2 or anti-CD28. The failure of IL-2 to abrogate suppression is secondary to a failure of full up-regulation of the expression of CD25 on the responder CD8$^+$ T cells. CD4$^+$CD25$^+$ T cells thereby prevent responses mediated by CD8$^+$ T cells both by inhibiting their ability to produce IL-2 and by inhibiting their ability to respond to IL-2, thus disrupting CD4$^+$ T cell help for CD8$^+$ T cells.

Cellular Targets for Suppression

In general, murine CD25$^+$ T cells failed to inhibit responses induced by plate-bound anti-CD3 but readily inhibited responses induced by soluble anti-CD3 (37). This finding raised the possibility that the cellular target of the CD25$^+$ T cell was the APC rather than the responder T cell, because responses to plate-bound anti-CD3 are relatively APC-independent. It was originally proposed that the CD25$^+$ T cells target APCs by inhibiting the induction of the expression of co-stimulatory molecules or perhaps by competition for co-stimulatory signals. In cocultures of CD4$^+$CD25$^+$ T cells, CD4$^+$CD25$^-$ T cells, and T-depleted spleen cells as APCs, the induction of expression of CD80, CD86, CD54, and CD40 on the APC (primarily B cells) appeared to be normal. CD25$^+$ T cells were also potent suppressors of T-cell proliferation when lipopolysaccharide (LPS)–activated APC were used, which suggests that they did not inhibit the expression of an unknown co-stimulatory molecule. Suppression was also observed when the LPS-activated APCs were fixed with paraformaldehyde. Last, suppression could not be overcome by adding an excess of LPS-activated APCs to the cocultures (45).

These studies strongly suggested that the APC was not the target of CD25-mediated suppression. To prove that the CD25$^+$ T cells were capable of acting directly on the responder T-cell population, the effects of the CD25$^+$ T cells on the responses of CD8$^+$ T cells to activation by soluble MHC tetramers in a completely APC-independent cell culture system were studied. Both T-cell proliferation and IFN-γ production were markedly inhibited by activated CD25$^+$ T cells in the complete absence of APCs. This result is most consistent with the view that CD25$^+$ T cells mediate suppression *in vitro* through a T-cell–T-cell interaction and that the APC is not directly required for delivery of the suppressive signal. Although similar conclusions were drawn in other studies in which CD25$^+$ T cells were shown to suppress responses of either mouse (49) or human (33) CD25$^-$ T cells induced by anti-CD3 coupled to beads in the absence of APCs, it is difficult to exclude the possibility that some of the suppressive effects of CD4$^+$CD25$^+$ T cells, particularly *in vivo*, might be mediated by the reduction of the stimulatory capacity of dendritic cells (DCs) or other types of APCs (50). CD25$^+$ T cells may turn off DCs presenting certain autoantigens, making them tolerogenic and thereby preventing the induction of naïve autoreactive T cells.

Role of Transforming Growth Factor β

Although the majority of studies with either human or murine CD25$^+$ T cells in which suppression of T cell activation *in vitro* has been examined have failed to identify a soluble suppressor cytokine, it is very difficult to rule out the involvement of a cytokine that acts over short distances or a cell-bound cytokine. Nakamura et al. (51) raised the possibility that TGF-β produced by CD25$^+$ T cells and then bound to their cell surface by an as yet uncharacterized receptor might mediate suppression in a cell contact-dependent manner. In their studies, TGF-β was detected on the surface of resting and activated CD25$^+$ T cells, and suppression could be reversed by high concentrations of anti–TGF-β monoclonal antibodies (mAbs). They postulated that latent (inactive) TGF-β, bound to the cell surface of activated CD25$^+$ T cells, is delivered directly to responder CD25$^-$ T cells and is then locally converted to its active form. High concentrations of neutralizing antibody would be required to reverse

TABLE 3. *CD4⁺CD25⁺ suppressor function occurs independently of TGF-β*

CD4⁺CD25⁺	CD4⁺CD25⁻	Suppression
Wild type	Wild type	Yes
Wild type	Wild type plus anti–TGF-β	Yes
TGF-β⁻/⁻	Wild type	Yes
Wild type	SMAD3⁻/⁻	Yes
SMAD3⁻/⁻	Wild type	Yes
Wild type	DNTGF βRII	Yes

CD4⁺CD25⁺ T cells were mixed with CD4⁺CD25⁻ T cells in the presence of T cell–depleted spleen cells and soluble anti-CD3 antibody.
Proliferation was measured at 72 hours.
TGF-β, transforming growth factor β.
Adapted from Piccirillo et al. (52), with permission.

suppression because of the need to penetrate the interface between the CD25⁺ and CD25⁻ T cells. In contrast to these studies, Piccirillo et al. (52) were unable to show a requirement for either the production of TGF-β or responsiveness to TGF-β in CD25-mediated suppression. CD25⁻ T cells from SMAD-3⁻/⁻ and from mice expressing a dominant negative form of the TGF-β receptor, which are completely resistant to the immunosuppressive effects of TGF-β, were readily suppressed by CD25⁺ T cells from wild-type mice (Table 3). CD25⁺ T cells from TGF-β⁻/⁻ mice were as efficient as CD25⁺ T cells from wild-type mice in mediating suppression of wild-type CD25⁻ T cells. High concentrations of anti–TGF-β did not reverse suppression, nor did anti–TGF-β or a soluble form of the TGF-β receptor inhibit suppression mediated by activated CD25⁺ T cells.

These studies strongly argue against a role for secreted or cell surface–associated TGF-β as a major mediator of the *in vitro* suppressive functions of CD25⁺ T cells. These results should be contrasted with the effects of anti–TGF-β in the reversal of CD25-mediated suppression in several *in vivo* models of organ-specific autoimmunity (see later discussion). An alternative possibility is that TGF-β plays a role in the induction or enhancement of CD25⁺ suppressor activity or in the development of suppressive functions in CD25⁻ T cells (53). Indeed, one of the most puzzling features of suppression mediated by CD25⁺ T cells is that only low numbers of suppressors are needed to profoundly produce 80% to 90% inhibition of T-cell proliferative responses. Suppression can be readily observed at ratios of 1 activated suppressor to 16 to 32 responders. One possibility is that the CD25⁺ T cells induce suppressor activity in the CD25⁻ responders as a form of infectious immunological tolerance. Indeed, it has been shown that human CD4⁺CD25⁺ T cells induce CD4⁺CD25⁻ T cells to become regulatory cells that are capable of suppressing by producing IL-10 (54) or TGF-β (55) and thereby mediating suppression of naïve CD4⁺ T cells. It is possible that the reversal of suppression produced by anti–TGF-β in some studies is mediated by neutralizing TGF-β produced by these recruited suppressor T cells.

Role of Cytotoxic T-Lymphocyte–Associated Antigen 4

Considerable controversy exists with regard to the significance of the expression of CTLA-4 on CD4⁺CD25⁺ T cells and its potential involvement in their suppressor function. Takahashi et al. (39) showed that the addition of the antigen-binding fragment (Fab) of anti-CTLA reverses suppression in cocultures of CD4⁺CD25⁺ and CD4⁺CD25⁻ T cells. This finding, together with the observation of Read et al. (27) that treatment of mice with anti–CTLA-4 abrogates suppression of inflammatory bowel disease (IBD) mediated by CD25⁺ T cells, has been interpreted as indicating that a co-stimulatory signal mediated by interaction of CTLA-4 with its ligands, CD80/CD86, is required for activation of CD25⁺ T cells to mediate their suppressive effects. Reversal of suppression by anti–CTLA-4 or its Fab *in vitro* has not been seen in all studies (31–37). In studies (49) in which CD25⁺ T cells suppress the activation of CD25⁻ T cells in the absence of APCs, the addition of anti–CTLA-4 or anti-CD80/CD86 did not reverse suppression, which suggests that engagement of CTLA-4 is not required for suppressor function. Furthermore, CD25⁺ T cells from CTLA-4⁻/⁻ mice are as efficient as CD25⁺ T cells in mediating suppressor function *in vitro*. Both the *in vitro* and *in vivo* actions of anti–CTLA-4 may be mediated, in part, on activated CD25⁻ effector T cells by raising their threshold for suppression. It remains possible that the interaction of CLTA-4 with antibody, or even Fab, may modulate the expression of CTLA-4 on the cell surface or inhibit its recycling and thereby block the TCR-mediated signals required for induction of suppressor activity. Further studies are needed to resolve these complex issues.

Regulating the Regulator

Although the mechanism by which CD4⁺CD25⁺ T cells mediate cell contact–dependent inhibition of T-cell activation remains unknown, one member of the TNFRSF, the GITR (TNFRSF18), has been shown to play an important role in regulation of T-cell suppressor activity. Deoxyribonucleic acid (DNA) microarray studies (see later discussion) revealed that the GITR was selectively expressed on resting CD4⁺CD25⁺ T cells. A polyclonal antiserum to the GITR was able to reverse suppression mediated by freshly isolated CD25⁺ T cells (40). Similarly, a mAb to the GITR was identified on the basis of its capacity to reverse suppression mediated by cloned CD4⁺CD25⁺ T cells (Fig. 6) (41). Anti-GITR was only minimally effective in neutralization of suppression mediated by preactivated CD4⁺CD25⁺ T cells. The GITR is expressed on two populations of cells (resting CD4⁺CD25⁺ cells and activated CD4⁺CD25⁻ cells) that do not manifest suppressor activity. It is therefore very unlikely that the GITR is the molecule responsible for mediating suppressor effector function. Surprisingly, culturing CD25⁺ T cells with the anti-GITR in the presence of IL-2, but in the absence of anti-CD3, resulted in a vigorous proliferative response. It appears

Anti-GITR Reverses CD+4+CD25+ Mediated Suppression

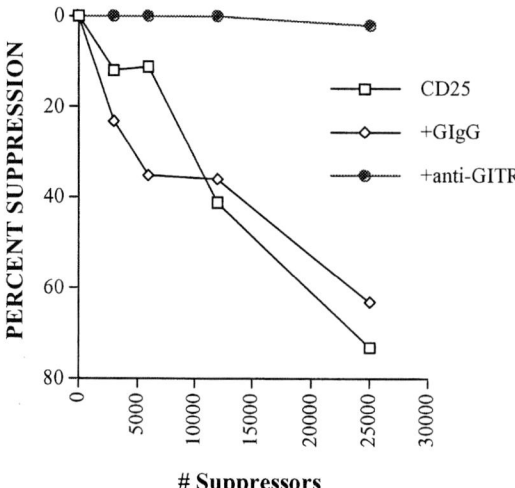

FIG. 6. CD4⁺CD25⁺ T cells were cultured with CD4⁺CD25⁻ T cells in the presence of T-depleted spleen cells and soluble anti-CD3. Normal goat immunoglobulin G (IgG) or polyclonal goat–anti-mouse glucocorticoid-induced tumor necrosis factor–like receptor (GITR) were added as indicated proliferation was measured at 72 hours. Adapted from McHugh et al. (40), with permission.

that the anti-GITR is capable of directly inducing a signal in the CD25⁺ T cells that reverses their inability of respond to IL-2. The anti-GITR is thereby functioning as an agonist for the GITR, resulting in a signal that instructs the CD4⁺CD25⁺ T cells not to mediate their suppressive functions. Very little is known about the GITR ligand (GITRL). One intriguing possibility is that engagement of the GITR by the GITRL during the course of a strong protective inflammatory response to an infectious agent may result in diminution of suppression.

Although the GITR/GITRL does not play the role of receptor/counterreceptor in CD25-mediated suppressor effector function, other known or unknown members of the TNFRSF/TNF family are logical candidates. It is also possible that an unknown ligand is induced on CD4⁺CD25⁺ T cells by TCR stimulation that then interacts with a cell surface molecule constitutively expressed or induced on the cell surface of CD4⁺CD25⁻ T cells. Such a receptor for the suppressive signal might contain an immunoreceptor tyrosine-based inhibitory motif with resultant activation of a phosphatase that mediates suppression. Other molecular pathways for cell contact–mediated inhibition are also possible.

Thymic Origin of CD4⁺CD25⁺ T Cells

The potential role of the thymus in the generation of regulatory T cells was first described in 1996 (56). In this study, *nu/nu* mice grafted with allogeneic fetal thymic epithelium devoid of hematopoietic precursors acquired donor-specific tolerance to heart and skin transplants but rejected third-

party grafts and donor-specific hematopoietic cells. CD4⁺ T cells from these mice could transfer tolerance to naïve *nu/nu* mice. The relationship of these suppressor T cells to CD4⁺CD25⁺ T cells is unknown. Most studies strongly support the view that the CD4⁺CD25⁺ T cell population is produced in the thymus as a functionally mature, distinct T-cell subpopulation. CD4⁺CD25⁺ T cells are not derived from peripheral CD4⁺CD25⁺ cells that have recirculated from the periphery to the thymus, because CD4⁺CD25⁺ T cells developed *in vitro* in organ cultures of the fetal thymus. CD4⁺CD25⁺ T cells are also detected in the newborn thymus, whereas they are not detected in the peripheral lymphoid tissues until three days of age. CD4⁺CD25⁺ thymocytes are nonresponsive and suppress T-cell activation *in vitro* in a manner similar to that of CD25⁺ T cells derived from the periphery (28). The capacity of CD25⁺ T cells to migrate from the thymus to the periphery was documented by injection of fluorescein isothiocyanate intrathymically. The percentages of CD4⁺CD25⁺ T cells within migrants and resident T cells were identical, which suggests that CD25⁺ T cells in the periphery can originate in the thymus (57). Thymectomy at 4 to 5 weeks of age did not modify the number of CD25⁺ T cells in the periphery even when the mice were tested 19 months later.

It is widely accepted that conventional CD4⁺ and CD8⁺ T cells develop in the thymus by a process of positive and negative selection. Positive selection is mediated by interaction of developing T cells with MHC antigens on thymic cortical epithelium. Negative selection is mediated both by DCs and by thymic medullary epithelium. It is not known whether CD4⁺CD25⁺ regulatory T cells are selected by a similar process. A number of studies have suggested that CD4⁺CD25⁺ T cells undergo a unique developmental process during their generation in the thymus. When TCR transgenic mice bearing a TCR specific for a determinant (S1) derived from influenza hemagglutinin (HA) in association with IEᵈ were crossed to mice expressing the HA transgene, the transgenic T cells were not deleted, and a large proportion of them expressed CD25 and functioned as regulatory T cells (58). Radioresistant elements of the thymus were shown to be both necessary and sufficient for the selection of CD25⁺ T cells in these doubly transgenic mice. Similar results were obtained when TCR transgenic mice bred on a RAG⁻/⁻ background were mated to the HA transgenic mice, which clearly indicates that thymocytes that can express only a single transgenic TCR can undergo selection to become regulatory cells.

A second group of TCR transgenic mice that recognized a variant determinant of HA but recognized the S1 determinant with 100-fold less affinity was generated. When these mice were bred to the HA transgenic mouse (S1), their offspring did not have an increased frequency of CD25⁺ T cells. Thus, thymocytes with a low intrinsic affinity for the S1 peptide did not develop into CD25⁺ thymocytes in response to HA. These data are consistent with a model in which selection of CD25⁺ T cells that express a transgenic TCR depends on a high-affinity interaction of the TCR with its ligand. It could not be determined from these studies whether this selection process occurs on cortical or medullary epithelial cells. It is also not clear why only 50% rather than 100% of the exported thymocytes express CD25. If selection of this one TCR by a high-affinity interaction with its selecting MHC/peptide is representative of all the TCRs expressed by CD25$^+$ T cells, all CD25$^+$ T cells in the periphery might have the potential to be highly reactive to, and specific for, self-peptides that might be encountered in the periphery.

To determine whether CD4$^+$CD25$^+$ T cells were generated on thymic cortical or medullary epithelial cells, Bensiger et al. (59) examined the selection of CD25$^+$ T cells in C57BL/6 mice in which class II MHC (IA^b) is expressed only on thymic cortical epithelium but not on medullary epithelium or bone marrow. Clonal deletion of CD4$^+$ T cells cannot be documented in these mice, and CD4$^+$ T cells respond to wild-type class II self-MHC (IA^b, C57BL/6) on bone marrow–derived APCs. In these mice, CD4$^+$ T cells in the thymus and the periphery expressed CD25. The CD25$^+$ T cells were both anergic and suppressive *in vitro* and *in vivo*. These data strongly demonstrate that selection on class II MHC positive cortical epithelium is sufficient for the complete development of CD25$^+$ T cells. Peripheral expression of class II MHC is not required for their maintenance in the periphery. CD25$^+$ T cells from the transgenic mice, but not normal C57BL/6 mice, could inhibit the mixed lymphocyte reactivity (MLR) of the transgenic T cells against C57BL/6. Thus, the repertoire of the CD25$^+$ cells from this strain of mice contains IA^b reactive cells, whereas the repertoire of C57BL/6 mice does not. These data indicate that a subset of CD25$^+$ T cells in wild-type C57BL/6 mice are negatively selected on hematopoietic APCs. Together, the results of these studies are most consistent with a model in which a high-affinity cognate interaction between developing T cells and self-peptides on thymic cortical epithelium leads to self-tolerance through the induction of CD4$^+$CD25$^+$ T cells.

Caution should be exercised in the interpretation of these studies because only a limited number of transgenic models have been studied, and it is also difficult to conclude that the differentiation of CD4$^+$CD25$^+$ T cells in normal mice strictly parallels what is seen in the TCR or nominal antigen transgenic mice. For example, Apostolou et al. (60) analyzed the process of regulatory T-cell differentiation in a model very similar to that used by others (58), except that the HA transgene was under the control of the Igκ promoter rather than the simian virus 40 promoter. In these mice, both TCR transgene–bearing CD25$^+$ and CD25$^-$ T cells exhibited regulatory T-cell function *in vitro* and *in vivo*. The relationship of the suppressor CD4$^+$CD25$^-$ T cells in this study to the CD4$^+$CD25$^+$ T cells found in normal mice remains to be determined. Studies in chimeric mice demonstrated that CD4$^+$CD25$^+$ regulatory T cells were generated primarily on thymic epithelium, whereas the generation of CD4$^+$CD25$^-$ regulatory T cells required that the HA be expressed on hematopoietic cells. It appears that multiple pathways

exist for the generation of regulatory cells. Important factors that influence this process include the affinity of the TCR for the selecting self-peptide, the cell type that expresses this peptide/MHC complex, and the level of expression of the complex on the selecting cell.

If the process of selection of CD4$^+$CD25$^+$ T cells is fundamentally different from that of CD4$^+$CD25$^-$ T cells, it might be predicted that their repertoire might be biased toward recognition of self-MHC. Romagnoli et al. (61) analyzed the frequency of CD25$^+$ T cells recognizing self- and non–self-MHC/peptide complexes expressed by professional APCs. The precursor frequency of CD4$^+$CD25$^-$ T cells that are specific for allogeneic MHC was higher than that for self-MHC, whereas the specificity of regulatory CD4$^+$CD25$^+$ T cells was strongly biased toward self-MHC. Although this result is consistent with the critical role of CD4$^+$CD25$^+$ T cells in the inhibition of autoimmunity, it is not consistent with results of more recent studies demonstrating the capacity of CD4$^+$CD25$^+$ T cells to potently suppress immune responses to foreign antigens such as complex infectious agents (see later discussion).

Other approaches (62) have suggested that the process of selection of CD4$^+$CD25$^+$ T cells is precisely the same as that involved in positive/negative selection of CD4$^+$CD25$^-$ T cells. Studies comparing the differentiation of CD4$^+$CD25$^+$ T cells in mice expressing a single or many different peptides coupled to class II MHC demonstrate that the proportion of CD25$^+$ T cells in the CD4$^+$CD8$^-$ T-cell pool remains constant and that their total number reflects the complexity of the class II MHC/peptide complexes. This result is not consistent with the hypothesis that the selection of CD4$^+$CD25$^+$ T cells requires a unique high-affinity interaction with MHC/peptide complexes but that CD4$^+$CD25$^+$ T cells are selected in a manner similar to selection of CD4$^+$CD25$^-$ T cells. Further studies on the pathways involved in the differentiation of CD4$^+$CD25$^+$ T cells in the thymus are needed to resolve the differences observed in these studies.

Cytokine Requirements for the Generation and Maintenance of CD25$^+$ T Cells

It was initially observed that CD4$^+$CD25$^+$ T cells were absent from the periphery and from the CD4$^+$CD8$^-$ thymocyte population of IL-2$^{-/-}$ mice (57). Partial or more profound defects both in the number and function of CD4$^+$CD25$^+$ T cells have been reported in mice deficient for CD28 (38), CD80/CD86, CD40 (63), CD40 ligand (64), CD122 (IL-2Rβ) (65), and STAT5a (66). The one common factor that characterizes these mice is that the products of all the deficient genes have important roles in the production or responsiveness to IL-2. Treatment of mice with anti–IL-2 or with CTLA-4 immunoglobulin to inhibit co-stimulatory signals also leads to a rapid decline in the number of CD4$^+$CD25$^+$ T cells (38). Because CD25$^+$ T cells do not produce IL-2, this deficiency may be secondary to the capacity of CD25$^-$

T cells to produce IL-2 or to some intrinsic defect in the CD25$^+$ T cells in their capacity to respond to IL-2. Many, but not all, of these strains develop an autoimmune syndrome associated with lymphoproliferation. Nonobese diabetic (NOD) mice have also been reported to have a defect in the numbers of CD25$^+$ T cells, but these cells appear to function normally (38). Blockade of the TNF-related activation-induced cytokine (TRANCE)–receptor-activator of NFκB (RANK) pathway also has been shown to inhibit the generation or function, or both, of CD4$^+$CD25$^+$ T cells in a model of autoimmune diabetes (67).

IL-2 could be required for the generation of CD4$^+$CD25$^+$ T cells in the thymus, for their maintenance and survival in the periphery, or for both. One study (67) that suggests that IL-2 plays a nonredundant role in the differentiation of CD4$^+$CD25$^+$ T cells in the thymus was performed in mice deficient for CD122. CD122$^{-/-}$ mice rapidly develop a lethal autoimmune syndrome. Transgenic expression of CD122 exclusively in the thymus prevents the development of autoimmunity and prolongs the life span of these mice from 8 to 12 weeks to 12 to 16 months. CD4$^+$CD25$^+$ T cells are barely detectable in the thymus and absent from the periphery of CD122$^{-/-}$ mice. In contrast, CD122$^{-/-}$ mice with thymic-only expression of CD122 had twofold higher numbers of CD4$^+$CD25$^+$ T cells in the thymus and lymph nodes than did wild-type mice. The CD4$^+$CD25$^+$ T cells from these mice were also fully capable of suppressing proliferative responses of T cells from wild-type mice. Because cells from the peripheral lymphoid tissues of these mice are completely unresponsive to IL-2, these results suggest that IL-2 may be required for the growth or survival of CD4$^+$CD25$^+$ T cells only in the thymus but not in the periphery. These results are also in conflict with those of other studies that suggest that IL-2 is also required in the periphery for survival of CD4$^+$CD25$^+$ T cells. It remains possible that other cytokines (e.g., IL-4) may in some circumstances be able to maintain CD4$^+$CD25$^+$ T cells in the periphery or that a higher output of CD4$^+$CD25$^+$ in the mice that express CD122 exclusively in the thymus may compensate for a lack of IL-2 in the periphery.

Molecular Analysis of Gene Expression by CD4$^+$CD25$^+$ T Cells

Both DNA microarray technology and serial analysis of gene expression (SAGE) technology have been used to compare patterns of gene expression between different cell types (40,46,68). These technologies have been applied to compare the patterns of gene expression in CD4$^+$CD25$^-$ T cells with CD4$^+$CD25$^+$ T cells and other cell types with regulatory functions. One major goal of this approach is to determine whether CD4$^+$CD25$^+$ cells simply represent a population of previously activated T cells or whether they display a unique pattern of gene expression that is correlated with their functional properties. Most of the results are consistent with the latter possibility. Only 29 genes are dif-

TABLE 4. *Genes selectively activated in CD4$^+$CD25$^+$ T cells*

Signaling: COS, SOCS-1, SOCS-2, SLAP-130
Secreted molecules: IL-10, IL-17, enkephalin, ETA-1, ECM-1, MIP-1α, MIP-1β
Cell surface molecules: CD2, OX40, CD25, CD122, GIR, GITR, Ly-6, Galectin-1, Thy-1

ECM, extracellular matrix protein-1; ETA-1, early T-cell activation antigen 1; GITR, glucocorticoid-induced tumor necrosis factor–like receptor; MIP, macrophage inflammatory protein; SLAP-130, Src-like adapter protein 130; SOCS, suppressor of cytokine signaling.
Adapted from McHugh et al. (40), with permission.

ferentially expressed between the resting CD25$^-$ and CD25$^+$ T cells, whereas 77 are differentially expressed after activation. Nine of these genes are shared between the resting and activated state, which makes the total number of genes differentially expressed 97 (Table 4). Four antigens—OX40, GITR, CD103, and CTLA-4—were readily detectable and exclusively expressed on the cell surface of resting CD4$^+$CD25$^+$ T cells but not CD4$^+$CD25$^-$ T cells. Several genes that encode cell surface antigens, including CTLA-4, Ly6, OX40, 4-1BB, CD103, and GITR, were differentially expressed in the CD25$^+$ subpopulation. Members of the TNF–nerve growth factor receptor (NGFR) superfamily (OX40, 4-1BB) may play a role in cell survival. As discussed previously, the GITR plays an important functional role in the regulation of suppressor cell activity. CD103 is expressed on only a minor (~30%) subpopulation of CD25$^+$ T cells, and the level of expression was not modulated by T-cell activation. Both CD25$^+$CD103$^+$ and CD25$^+$CD103$^-$ T cells were capable of inhibiting the activation of CD25$^-$ cells *in vitro,* but the CD103$^+$ cells displayed enhanced potency.

Several of the differentially expressed genes appear to be involved in maintenance of the anergic phenotype by the CD4$^+$CD25$^+$ population. Three members of the suppressors of cytokine signaling (SOCS) family—CIS, SOCS-1/JAB, and SOCS-2—appeared to be more highly induced after activation of the CD25$^+$ T cells. Because IL-2 is required for the survival/maintenance of the CD25$^+$ population, the SOCS proteins may be induced in response to this cytokine or other cytokines needed for the homeostatic control of these cells. CIS, like SOCS-1, is induced by IL-2, IL-3, and erythropoietin and inhibits STAT5 activation in response to these cytokines. IFN-γ is also a potent inducer of SOCS-1. Because large amounts of IFN-γ may be produced during an immune response to an infectious agent, the capacity of the CD25$^+$ T cells to preferentially up-regulate this inhibitor may diminish their suppressive function during protective immune responses and allow appropriate responses to foreign antigens. The increased levels of SOCS-2 suggest hyporesponsiveness to other factors, including insulin-like growth factor 1, growth hormone, IL-6, and leukemia inhibitory factor.

Because activated CD4$^+$CD25$^+$ T cells, but not CD4$^+$CD25$^-$ T cells, have suppressor effector function, approaches for the analysis of differential gene expression should also be useful for the identification of molecules (cell surface or secreted) that may be involved in the effector phase of suppression. Galectin-1 was highly expressed in the CD25+ subset, both in the resting state and after activation. This molecule has been shown to induce apoptosis and to inhibit TCR-induced IL-2 production and proliferation. T cells from mice deficient in N-acetylglucosaminyltransferase V (Mgat5), an enzyme involved in the N-glycosylation pathway that lack the glycans with affinity for galectin-1 binding, were as readily suppressed as wild-type CD4+CD25+ cells. This suggests that galectin-1 may not be critical for the suppressive function of the CD25+ population. Messenger RNA for the immunosuppressive cytokine IL-10, the inflammatory cytokine IL-17, enkephalin, and early T-cell activation antigen 1, a cytokine reported to regulate IL-12 and IL-10 expression in macrophages, were all elevated in activated CD4+CD25+ T cells. With the exception of IL-10, which plays an important role in immunosuppression by CD4+CD25+ T cells *in vivo,* the roles played by these secreted molecules in the function of CD25+ T cells remain to be defined. Although some of the data from the SAGE analysis (68) suggested that CD4+CD25+ T cells may be related to the subpopulation of T cells that secrete Th2 cytokines, on balance, the studies on global gene expression indicate that CD4+CD25+ T cells express a unique pattern of gene expression that contributes to their survival and anergic state. Continued studies of genes expressed by the CD25+ T cells will, it is hoped, yield more insights into the precise mechanism of their suppressor functions.

INDUCED REGULATORY T CELLS

Although CD4+CD25+ T cells represent a population of naturally occurring suppressor T cells, a number of different *in vivo* and *in vitro* protocols that result in populations of both CD4 and CD8 suppressor T cells that have certain properties in common with CD4+CD25+ T cells have been described. In some but not all studies, the possibility that these cells originate or are derived from the CD4+CD25+ T cells has been carefully ruled out by generating the suppressor population from highly purified CD4+CD25− T cells. It should be pointed out that CD25 cannot be used as a marker of these induced suppressor cells because many of the suppressor populations have been generated after exposure to antigen *in vivo* or after *in vitro* activation. This is a rapidly evolving area of investigation, and additional studies and specific cell surface markers are needed before the relationships between the various suppressor subpopulations can be clarified.

Oral Tolerance

One of the first approaches used for the induction of T regulatory cells was the administration of antigen via the oral route. Oral tolerance takes advantage of the normal physiological process that is needed to prevent systemic immune responses to ingested proteins. Oral administration of antigen at low doses induces populations of regulatory T cells that secrete suppressor cytokines, whereas higher antigen doses result in deletion or clonal anergy of autoreactive precursors. Pretreatment with orally administered antigen induced suppressor populations that suppressed disease in a number of different animal models of autoimmunity, including experimental allergic encephalomyelitis (EAE), collagen-induced arthritis, and uveitis (69). In the Lewis rat, the T cells induced by feeding myelin basic protein (MBP) were CD8+ and prevented disease by secreting TGF-β. Bulk T cells from orally tolerized animals can suppress active immune responses to other antigens in the microenvironment, a phenomenon called *antigen-driven bystander suppression.* Suppression is mediated primarily by TGF-β. A major advance in the understanding of the function of regulatory cells after oral tolerance was gained in the study by Chen et al. (70), who successfully isolated T-cell clones from the mesenteric lymph nodes of SJL mice that had been orally tolerized to MBP. These clones produced large amounts of TGF-β and varying amounts of IL-4 and IL-10. Most important, upon adoptive transfer to normal recipients, they suppressed EAE induced with either MBP or proteolipid protein. Their *in vivo* suppressive activity could be neutralized with anti–TGF-β.

The selective induction of regulatory T cells via the oral route is thought to be secondary to certain poorly characterized properties of the gut mucosal microenvironment, most likely the type of resident APCs (71). A well-developed mucosal immune system exists in both the gut and the respiratory tract, and certain immunological events occur when antigen contacts mucosal surfaces. T cells from the pulmonary compartment of mice administered antigen via the nasal route proliferated poorly when stimulated *in vitro* (72). Pulmonary DCs from treated animals had a decreased ability to activate CD4+ T cells *in vitro,* even though they appeared to express a mature phenotype. These pulmonary DCs could transfer tolerance to normal recipients in an IL-10–dependent manner. IL-10 producing DCs induced T cells that produced IL-10 and IL-4, but not IFN-γ. In contrast, DCs isolated from the mesenteric lymph nodes of animals that had been fed ovalbumin expressed increased amounts of TGF-β and induced TGF-β producing CD4+ T cells.

Although the oral administration of antigen represents a potentially easy way to induce regulatory T cells, progress in this area has been slow because it has been difficult to determine the concentration that is capable of inducing regulatory T cells but that does not induce deletion. It has also been very difficult to isolate the types of clones described previously in the EAE model in other systems. The therapeutic utility of orally administered antigens in autoimmunity has been demonstrated primarily in pretreatment protocols, and oral administration of antigen had been ineffective in treating animals once disease has been initiated. It is unlikely that oral tolerance will be a useful modality for the treatment of autoimmune disease in humans.

T Regulatory 1 Cells

One important lesson that can be derived from the experiments on oral tolerance is that the milieu in which T cells are primed is critically important in determining whether regulatory rather than effector T cells will be generated. Decreased expression of co-stimulatory molecules on APCs or the presence of suppressor cytokines such as IL-10 and TGF-β may generate suppressor T cells rather than effector T cells. The production of these suppressor cytokines by regulatory T cells may lead to the generation or expansion of additional regulatory cells through a positive feedback loop (Fig. 7).

One of the first studies demonstrating the potential importance of IL-10 in the generation of regulatory T cells was derived from an analysis (73) of patients with severe combined immunodeficiency (SCID) who received transplants of human leukocyte antigen (HLA)–mismatched hematopoietic stem cells. Complete immunological reconstitution was achieved in the absence of graft-versus-host disease (GVHD). CD4$^+$ T-cell clones reactive with host MHC antigens from these patients produced IL-10, but not IL-2, after antigen-specific stimulation *in vitro*. Proliferation was enhanced in the presence of neutralizing anti–IL-10, which suggests that high levels of endogenous IL-10 suppressed these cells. Levels of IL-10 mRNA were enhanced in the peripheral blood mononuclear cells of the patients, not only in T cells but also in the non–T cell fraction, which indicates that host cells also contributed to the high levels of IL-10 *in vivo*. T-cell clones derived from these patients produced IL-10 spontaneously, without TCR stimulation. It therefore seemed likely that endogenous IL-10 production in the transplant recipients was

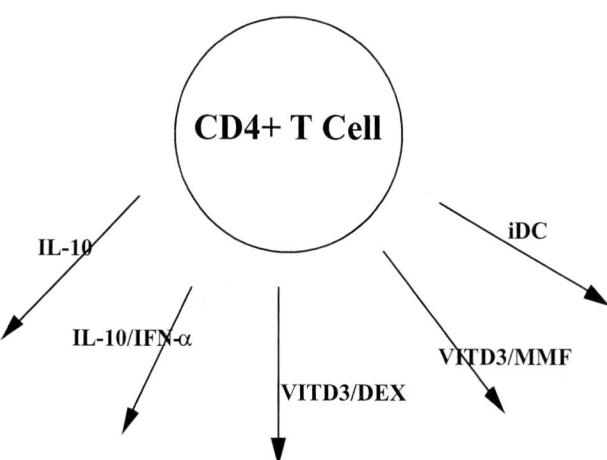

FIG. 7. Multiple factors can induce the differentiation of interleukin-10 (IL-10)–producing T cells. DEX, dexamethasone; iDC, immature dendritic cells; IFN-α, interferon α; MMF, mycophenolate mofetil; TR1, T regulatory 1; VITD3, 1,25(OH)$_2$D$_3$.

responsible for maintaining tolerance *in vivo*. The IL-10 may prevent the activation of host reactive T cells or suppress APC function and cytokine production by host APCs. The high IL-10 production *in vivo* may reflect a chronic activation of donor T cells and host monocytes.

IL-10 is a cytokine produced by numerous cell types, including activated T cells, mast cells, and macrophages, and acts primarily by inhibiting the maturation and function of APCs. The activation of CD4$^+$ human T cells in the presence of IL-10 renders them nonresponsive or anergic (74). Activation of human CD8$^+$ T cells with allogeneic APCs and IL-10 also results in reduced proliferation and cytotoxicity. T cells rendered anergic by the addition of exogenous IL-10 in an MLR become unable to respond to a repeat challenge with the same antigen. IL-10–induced anergy is strictly antigen specific because treated T cells retain normal proliferative and cytotoxic responses toward other protein antigens and third-party alloantigens. When murine T cells are stimulated in the presence of IL-10, T-cell proliferation is inhibited, but anergy is not induced. If TGF-β is added to the cultures in addition to the IL-10, the responder population is rendered anergic (75). Such T cells are markedly impaired in inducing GVHD in class II MHC–disparate recipients. With human T cells, endogenous TGF-β contributes to anergy induction by IL-10, and the addition of exogenous TGF-β is not required.

Collectively, these studies suggested that IL-10 itself is a major factor for the induction of suppressive IL-10–producing T cells. Culture of murine or human CD4$^+$ T cells with antigen or alloantigen in the presence of IL-10 results in the generation of IL-10–producing T-cell clones. Most of these T-cell clones produce high levels of IL-10 and TGF-β, moderate amounts of IFN-γ and IL-5, but no IL-2 or IL-4. CD4$^+$ T cells generated in this manner have been termed *T regulatory 1* (Tr1) cells (76). Tr1 cells proliferate poorly after polyclonal TCR-mediated or antigen-specific activation and do not expand significantly under standard T-cell culture conditions. This low proliferative capacity results in part from autocrine production of IL-10, inasmuch as anti–IL-10 mAbs partially restore proliferative responses. The intrinsic low proliferative capacity of Tr1 cells has been a major limitation and has hindered their detailed characterization. The ability to generate human Tr1 cells is enhanced by the addition of IFN-α (77). Tr1 cells can be generated from human cord blood with IFN-α alone, because cord blood T cells have the intrinsic ability to produce IL-10. IFN-α and IL-10 act not as general antiproliferative agents but rather as factors that induce the differentiation of Tr1 cells and inhibit the growth of non-Tr1 cells in the culture. TGF-β played no role in the induction of Tr1 cells in this model. A global suppression of all cytokine production was seen when TGF-β was added to the cultures.

Both human and mouse Tr1 clones suppress immune responses *in vitro*. Antigen-induced proliferation of naïve CD4$^+$ T cells was dramatically reduced after coculture with activated Tr1 clones that were separated from the responding cells by a trans-well insert. The capacity of either human or murine Tr1 clones to suppress CD4$^+$ T cells proliferation was reversed by the addition of anti–TGF-β and IL-10 mAbs (76). Human Tr1 cell clones also suppress the production of immunoglobulin by B cells, as well as the antigen-presenting capacity of monocytes and DCs. Most important, it was shown (76) that mouse Tr1 clones have regulatory effects *in vivo* and suppress Th1-mediated colitis induced by transfer of CD45RB^{hi} cells into SCID mice (see later discussion). Suppression was seen only if the Tr1 clones were activated by antigen-specific stimulation through their TCRs. Because the function of Tr1 cells is mediated by IL-10 and TGF-β, these studies imply that Tr1 clones can suppress active immune responses to unknown antigens in the microenvironment by an antigen-driven bystander suppression mechanism similar to the mechanism proposed for regulatory T cells in oral tolerance. Although IL-10 was originally described as a product of murine Th2 cells, Tr1 clones are also capable of regulating Th2 responses, including antigen-specific IgE production (78). Anti–IL-10 receptor antibodies reversed this inhibitory effect.

Pharmacological Induction of Regulatory T Cells

An alternative approach to the generation of T regulatory cells *in vitro* has involved pharmacological manipulation of the microenvironment during T-cell priming (79). The immunosuppressive drug 1,25(OH)$_2$D$_3$ (VitD$_3$) acts on APCs and activated T cells. VitD$_3$ inhibits antigen-induced T-cell proliferation, cytokine production, and the maturation of human DCs, leading to inhibition of the expression of CD40/CD80/CD86. It also appears to inhibit IL-12 production and prevents Th1 development but enhances IL-10 production by DCs. Similarly, the glucocorticoid, dexamethasone, inhibits key transcription factors involved in the regulation of a number of inflammatory cytokine genes. Glucocorticoids are among the most potent anti-inflammatory and immunosuppressive drugs available and are efficacious in the treatment of both Th1- and Th2-associated inflammatory diseases, including asthma and rheumatoid arthritis. VitD$_3$ and dexamethasone are known to inhibit transcription of nuclear factor of activated T cells (NF-AT), activator protein 1, and NFκB.

When naïve CD4$^+$ T cells were stimulated through their TCRs in the presence of the combination of VitD$_3$ and dexamethasone, the primed T cells produced IL-10 but not IFN-γ, IL-4, or IL-5 (79). The IL-10–producing cells developed independently of Th1 (IL-12, IFN-γ) and Th2 (IL-4) polarizing cytokines, and addition of these cytokines inhibited the development of the IL-10–producing cells. Although the induction of these regulatory cells could not be induced by IL-10, endogenous IL-10 production was required because addition of anti–IL-10 receptor antibodies substantially reduced the number of IL-10–producing T cells. One major difference between these regulatory T cells and those induced by culture in the presence of exogenous IL-10 is their lack of production

of the effector cytokines IFN-γ and IL-5. These cytokines have the potential to mediate inflammatory pathological processes. The development of the IL-10–producing T cells occurred under conditions in which the expression or activation, or both, of key transcription factors involved in Th1 (T-bet) and Th2 (GATA3) differentiation was minimal, which suggests that the IL-10 producers were completely unrelated to conventional Th1 or Th2 cells. Stimulation of CD4$^+$CD25$^-$ T cells with VitD$_3$ and dexamethasone also results in the generation IL-10–producing T cells, which indicates that these cells do not derive from CD25$^+$ T cells. VitD$_3$/dexamethasone-induced regulatory T cells are also capable of inhibiting the induction of Th1-mediated autoimmune disease *in vivo*. Marked suppression of the induction of EAE was seen when ovalbumin-specific regulatory T cells were transferred to normal recipients and then stimulated with ovalbumin intracranially but not intraperitoneally. Protection from EAE was dependent on recognition of the presence of the antigen by the regulatory cells and was abrogated if the mice were simultaneously treated with anti–IL-10 receptor mAbs.

Gregori et al. (80) combined the use of VitD$_3$ with a different immunosuppressive drug, mycophenolate mofetil (MMF), to induce transplantation tolerance. MMF inhibits T- and B-cell proliferation but also acts on DCs to inhibit IL-12 production and the expression of co-stimulatory molecules. VitD$_3$/MMF treatment of recipients induced donor-specific transplantation tolerance to transplantation of islet allografts. CD4$^+$ T cells from tolerant mice transferred into naïve syngeneic recipients prevented rejection of donor-type islet grafts. Graft acceptance was associated with impaired development of Th1 cells and an increased percentage of T cells expressing CD25$^+$ and CTLA-4 in the spleen and in the lymph nodes draining the transplantation. Transfer of these CD25$^+$ T cells from tolerant animals protected 100% of syngeneic recipients from islet allograft rejection. It is not clear, however, whether these CD25$^+$ T cells were derived from the naturally occurring population or from CD25$^-$ T cells. The role of suppressor cytokine production by the induced regulatory T cells was not investigated in this model.

One common theme to emerge from the studies on the *in vitro* induction of T regulatory cells, by the addition of either IL-10 or pharmacological agents, is that both of these modalities are likely to inhibit the maturation and activation of DCs and to generate what has been termed *tolerogenic DCs*. Potent regulatory T cells have also been generated by culturing human CD4$^+$ cord blood lymphocytes with allogeneic immature DCs (iDCs). Although stimulation with mature DCs resulted in expansion of alloreactive T cells of the Th1 phenotype, stimulation in the presence of iDCs resulted in the induction of poorly growing IL-10–producing T cells (81). These T cells suppressed the alloantigen-driven proliferation of syngeneic Th1 cells in cocultures in a cell contact–dependent manner. The suppressor effector function was nonspecific and was not mediated by IL-10 or TGF-β, but suppression could be partially be overcome by addition of IL-2. The suppressor population generated by stimulation with iDCs in many respects resembles the naturally occurring CD25$^+$ cells.

Regulatory Function of Anergic T-Cell Clones

One other mechanism that has been proposed for the induction of regulatory T cells during the course of a normal immune response is that antigen-specific effector T cells exposed to antigen in the absence of co-stimulation may be rendered anergic. Anergic T cells may be capable of mediating suppression by competing with responders for access to the cell surface of APCs, thereby depriving the effector cells of antigen, co-stimulatory signals, or paracrine stimulation by IL-2. Human T-cell clones rendered anergic by exposure to plate-bound anti-CD3 could suppress the proliferative responses of the same clone to antigen-bearing APCs (82). Suppression could be partially overcome by the addition of exogenous IL-2. Anergic T-cell clones could mediate "linked suppression" of the responses of T-cell clones specific for antigens unrelated to the one recognized by the anergic clone, if both antigens were displayed by the same APC. Similar results were seen by Chai et al. (83) with murine allospecific T-cell clones that were rendered unresponsive in vitro by stimulation with immobilized anti-CD3. These anergic clones manifested suppressor function in vivo, inasmuch as they were capable of delaying skin graft rejection upon adoptive transfer to naïve recipients.

Studies since 2000 have offered additional insight into the mechanisms by which anergic clones mediate their suppressive effects. When murine allospecific anergic T cells were cocultured with bone marrow–derived DCs, the capacity of these DCs to subsequently stimulate fresh responder T cells was markedly inhibited (84). After 48 hours of culture, expression of class I MHC and CD80/CD86 was reduced. Inhibition required cell contact, and antibodies to IL-4, IL-10, TGF-β, or Fas ligand had no effect on reversing the inhibition. Fully mature DCs were refractory to inhibition by the anergic clones. Similar studies with anergic human T-cell clones have shown that both immature and mature DCs were susceptible to suppressive signals (85). The suppressive effect on iDCs was mediated by down-regulation of their antigen-presenting capacity, whereas the effects on the mature DCs were mediated by apoptosis of the APCs, with subsequent deletion of the responder cells. The activation of the apoptotic pathway by anergic T cells is an antigen-specific phenomenon in which cognate recognition is required. Anergic T cells kill both APCs and responder T cells only when the three cell types come into contact. Apoptosis is mediated by Fas (CD95)/Fas ligand interactions. iDCs were resistant to apoptosis because they express high levels of Fas only at late stages of maturation. Similar results have been observed with anergic rat T-cell clones by Taams et al. (86). Exposure of APCs to anergic T-cell clones rendered them suppressive. The mechanism of inhibition of APC function was not determined in these studies, but down-regulation of MHC, co-stimulatory

molecules, or cytolysis was not observed. Suppression was not reversed by increasing the total number of peptide-pulsed APCs or by increasing the ligand density.

These studies suggest that anergic T-cell clones exert their suppressive effects by modulating the stimulatory capacity of APCs either by preventing their maturation or by cytolysis. The inhibition of the maturation of DCs by anergic T-cell clones may result in the generation of tolerogenic APCs, which may in turn mediate infectious tolerance by generating more suppressor cells (possibly suppressor cytokine–producing cells) from naïve precursors. In vivo, presentation of antigen to primed effector cells by nonprofessional APCs that lack co-stimulatory molecules may occur after inflammation has subsided and may result in the induction of a cohort of anergic T cells with the potential to inhibit the antigen-presenting capacity of newly recruited DCs. It has yet to be shown that anergic T cells capable of mediating this pathway of suppression are actually generated in vivo during the course of a normal or pathogenic immune response.

Can CD4$^+$CD25$^+$–like T Cells Be Generated in the Periphery?

Although suppressor populations that mediate their effects by producing suppressor cytokines can be generated in vitro, it remains unclear whether conventional CD4$^+$CD25$^-$ T cells can be converted to a cell population that resembles naturally occurring CD4$^+$CD25$^+$ T cells and that mediates suppression by the cell contact–dependent pathway (87,88). Thorstenson and Khoruts (87) administered either peptide antigen via the intravenous route or protein antigen via the oral route, two widely accepted methods for the induction of peripheral tolerance, to TCR transgenic mice bred onto the RAG background that lacked CD4$^+$CD25$^+$ T cells. CD25 was transiently expressed by antigen-specific T cells when antigen was administered in adjuvant. In contrast, late expression of CD25 was seen only if the antigen was administered under tolerogenic conditions. These cells resembled endogenous CD25$^+$ T cells in a number of ways. They were unable to produce IL-2, expressed high levels of CTLA-4, and suppressed IL-2 production and proliferation of responder cells of the same specificity. The capacity of these cells to produce suppressor cytokines was not analyzed. Mechanistic analysis of in vitro suppression was limited in this study, because very few cells expressed CD25 at the later time points, and recovery of CD25$^+$ T cells was low.

Apostolou et al. (60) transferred splenic CD4$^+$CD25$^-$ T cells specific for HA from RAG$^{-/-}$ mice to sublethally irradiated recipients that expressed HA under control of the immunoglobulin promoter. Two weeks later, 5% of the injected T cells were CD25$^+$, whereas the other 95% of the cells were CD25$^-$. Both populations were anergic and were able to suppress the response of naïve T cells expressing the transgenic TCRs. The mechanism by which these induced regulatory T cells suppressed was not explored. Together, these studies suggest that certain conditions of antigen exposure in the periphery may lead to both suppressor cytokine–producing regulatory cells and T cells resembling thymus-derived CD4⁺CD25⁺. There is one critical unanswered question: What percentage of the CD25⁺ pool in normal animals is thymus derived and what percentage may have been generated in the periphery (89)?

CONTROL OF AUTOIMMUNE DISEASE BY REGULATORY T CELLS

Autoimmune Gastritis

The role of regulatory T cells in the prevention of organ-specific autoimmune diseases has been studied in a number of different animals models. One of the best-studied models is autoimmune gastritis (AIG) that develops when BALB/c mice are subjected to d3Tx or when *nu/nu* mice bred on a BALB/c background are reconstituted with CD4⁺CD25⁻ T cells. A large body of evidence had implicated the major protein pump of the gastric parietal cell, the H,K-ATPase, as the target antigen for the CD4⁺ T cells that are responsible for inducing this disease (90). CD4⁺ T cells isolated from gastric lymph nodes demonstrated a vigorous proliferative response when stimulated in cultures with the purified ATPase (91). To evaluate whether CD25⁺ T cells could prevent disease induced by primed, fully differentiated effector cell populations, two H,K-ATPase–reactive T-cell lines were derived from d3Tx animals (23). Both of these lines were CD4⁺, IAᵈ restricted and recognized distinct peptides derived from the H,K-ATPase α-chain. One of the cell lines secreted Th1 cytokines and the other Th2, but both were equally pathogenic in inducing gastritis when transferred to immunocompromised recipients but not normal recipients. The gastric infiltrate seen after injection of Th2 cells was composed primarily of eosinophils and polymorphonuclear cells, whereas the infiltrate seen upon transfer of the Th1 clone was composed primarily of lymphocytes and monocytes. The capacity of both of these clones to transfer disease to *nu/nu* recipients could be inhibited by cotransfer of CD4⁺CD25⁺ T cells from normal BALB/c mice. Thus, CD4⁺CD25⁺ T cells are able to inhibit not only the initiation of disease after d3Tx, but also the function of fully activated effector cells. To address the possible involvement of cytokines in suppression of AIG, CD25⁺ T cells from a number of different cytokine deficient (−/−) mice were utilized to prevent induction of disease either after d3Tx or in *nu/nu* recipients of CD25⁻ T cells. CD4⁺CD25⁺ T cells from both IL-4 and IL-10⁻/⁻ mice were as efficient as CD4⁺CD25⁺ T cells in preventing the induction of disease (92,93). Furthermore, the protective capacity of CD25⁺ T cells from normal mice was not reduced when the reconstituted mice were treated with an antibody to TGF-β (52).

Inflammatory Bowel Disease

The differential expression of the CD45RB isoforms initially used to define effector and regulatory T cells in the rat was

extended to the mouse. Transfer of CD4⁺CD45RBʰⁱᵍʰ cells to SCID mouse recipients resulted in the development of a wasting disease and colitis 6 to 8 weeks after T-cell transfer. This disease was characterized pathologically by epithelial cell hyperplasia, goblet cell depletion, and transmural inflammation (94). There was a 20- to 30-fold accumulation of Th1 cells in the intestine in comparison to normal mice. Treatment of recipients with anti–IFN-γ, anti–TNF-α, or anti–IL-12 inhibited the induction of disease. Transfer of CD45RBˡᵒʷ cells did not induce colitis, and cotransfer of RBʰⁱᵍʰ and RBˡᵒʷ cells prevented the development of colitis. A ratio of 1:8 RBˡᵒʷ to RBʰⁱᵍʰ was able to prevent disease. When CD45RBˡᵒʷ cells were fractionated into CD25⁺ and CD25⁻ fractions, control of intestinal inflammation was mediated primarily by the CD25⁺ fraction (27). CD45RBˡᵒʷ CD25⁻ did exert some suppressive function when transferred at high cell concentrations.

Treatment of recipients of CD45RBʰⁱᵍʰ cells with IL-10 inhibited the development of colitis (Table 5). This treatment inhibited the accumulation of Th1 cells in the intestine but did not induce regulatory T cells, inasmuch as colitis developed when IL-10 administration ceased. RBʰⁱᵍʰ T cells from mice that expressed IL-10 under the control of the IL-2 promoter failed to induce colitis and were also able to prevent disease when cotransferred with RBˡᵒʷ cells. The administration of anti–IL-10R mAb abrogated the ability of regulatory T cells to inhibit colitis. Furthermore, CD45RBˡᵒʷ cells from IL-10⁻/⁻ mice were unable to protect recipients from colitis when cotransferred with CD45RBʰⁱᵍʰ cells and induced colitis when transferred alone (95). The ability of regulatory T cells to inhibit colitis did not involve IL-4 but was dependent on TGF-β, inasmuch as administration of anti–TGF-β abrogated the protective effect of these cells (96). The cellular source of the TGF-β is not yet known, although it has been assumed that it is produced by the CD4⁺CD25⁺ T cells. It should be emphasized that CD25-mediated suppression of AIG is mediated by a cell contact–dependent mechanism of

TABLE 5. *Role of cytokines in the pathogenesis and treatment of inflammatory bowel disease*

Treatment	Effect on disease
Anti–IFN-γ (days 1 and 4)	Substantial protection
Anti–TNF-α (days 1 and 4)	No protection
Anti-TNF (weekly)	Protection during treatment only
IL-10	Protection during treatment only
IL-4	No protection
CD4⁺CD25⁺ T Cells	Complete protection
CD4⁺CD25⁺ T Cells plus anti–IL-4	Complete protection
CD4⁺CD25⁺ T Cells plus anti–IL-10R	No protection
CD4⁺CD25⁺ T Cells plus anti–TGF-β	No protection

IFN, interferon; IL, interleukin; TGF, transforming growth factor; TNF, tumor necrosis factor.
Adapted from Powrie et al. (94,96) and Asseman et al. (95), with permission.

suppression, and IL-10 and TGF-β are not involved, whereas CD25-mediated suppression of IBD is abrogated by anti–IL-10 or anti–TGF-β or both. One reason for this difference is that the pathogeneses of AIG and IBD are quite distinct. Bacteria play a required role in IBD, whereas AIG can be induced by d3Tx in germ-free mice. It remains possible that suppression of IBD involves both the cell contact–dependent and the cytokine-mediated pathways of suppression. IL-10 and TGF-β are necessary to first dampen the inflammatory response induced by intestinal bacteria. Once this response is reduced, cell contact–mediated suppression can become operative.

Mice with colitis have an accumulation of activated CD4$^+$ T cells in the mesenteric lymph nodes and colon. This T-cell infiltrate is accompanied by an accumulation of DCs that, in the mesenteric lymph nodes but not the colon, express CD134 ligand (OX40 ligand). Binding of CD134 ligand to CD134 on T cells provides a co-stimulatory signal for T-cell activation. Administration of anti–CD134 ligand prevented the development of colitis (97). Blockade of CD134–CD134 ligand interactions does not inhibit signals involved in the early activation of pathogenic T cells, but it may inhibit amplification of the response. DCs may pick up intestinal antigens in the colon and transport them to the mesenteric lymph node, where they activate T effector cells. In the absence of regulatory T cells, CD134$^+$ DCs may magnify this response, leading to colitis. CD25$^+$ T cells may inhibit the migration of DCs to the lymph node or inhibit macrophage activation in the colon.

Autoimmune Thyroiditis

In more recent studies using the adult thymectomy-irradiation model for the induction of autoimmune thyroiditis, Seddon and Mason (98) demonstrated that disease could be prevented by the injection of CD4$^+$CD45RC^{low} peripheral T cells or by CD4$^+$CD8$^-$ thymocytes. In fact, the thymocytes were 10 times more potent that the regulatory T cells derived from the periphery. Similar results were observed in the autoimmune diabetes model that develops after use of this protocol. Suppression of thyroiditis mediated by both cell populations could be reversed by treatment of the recipients with either anti–IL-4 or anti–TGF-β. These studies strongly suggest that the mature CD4$^+$CD8$^-$ thymocyte population contains a high frequency of regulatory cells or regulatory cell precursors with the potential to differentiate in the periphery into regulatory cells that prevent organ-specific autoimmunity. One possibility is that IL-4 plays an important role in the growth or differentiation of regulatory T cells that produce TGF-β, which then functions as the major effector suppressor cytokine for thyroiditis in this rat model.

Further analysis of cell surface marker expression on rat CD45RC^{low} cells in the thymectomy-irradiation model for induction of diabetes demonstrated that depletion of CD25$^+$ T cells from the CD4$^+$CD45RC^{low} population resulted in loss of the ability of the remaining cells to protect thymectomized-irradiated recipients from diabetes

(36). CD4$^+$CD25$^+$ thymocytes were also shown to be protective. In addition, significant protective activity was present in the CD4$^+$CD45RC^{low}CD25$^-$ population of peripheral T cells. The presence of protective CD25$^-$ T cells could be seen only after removal of recent thymic emigrants. The origin of the CD25$^-$ regulatory T cells in this memory T cell pool is not clear. Because there are few data to suggest that the thymus exports CD4$^+$CD25$^-$ cells precommitted to a regulatory T-cell function, it is likely that the CD4$^+$CD25$^-$ T cells acquire their regulatory T-cell function in the periphery or are derived from CD25$^+$ T cells. These cells may also have been generated by recruitment or infectious tolerance.

Insulin-Dependent Diabetes Mellitus

The NOD mouse represents the best experimental model for autoimmune diabetes. It is widely accepted that CD4$^+$ regulatory T cells play a critical role in the regulation of disease in this animal model (99). The islets of Langerhans become rapidly infiltrated with immune cells several weeks before the onset of diabetes. Diabetes progression may relate to a subsequent failure in the maintenance of regulatory cell function. Because diabetes could be transferred from sick mice to normal syngeneic recipients only if the recipients were less than 5 weeks of age (female) or 3 weeks of age (male), it was assumed that regulatory T-cell function was deficient in young mice. Cyclophosphamide treatment, which may preferentially deplete regulatory T cells, accelerated the development of disease in young NOD mice. CD4$^+$ T cells from nondiabetic NOD mice could prevent the transfer of diabetes from overtly diabetic mice into sublethally irradiated NOD recipients. The protective cell population was not present in the spleen until mice were 3 weeks of age and reached its highest activity at 8 weeks of age; suppressor cells were present in the thymus of neonates, which may explain why thymectomy at weaning accelerated disease. Diabetes could also be efficiently transferred to nonirradiated adult NOD recipients, if they were Tx and depleted of CD4$^+$ T cells. Depletion of T cells alone was not sufficient for disease transfer, which suggests that thymectomy was needed to limit emergence of newly generated CD4$^+$ regulatory T cells from the thymus. Islet infiltrating T cells from young nondiabetic mice could transfer diabetes to NOD/SCID mice, but cotransfer of CD4$^+$CD45RB^{low} T cells from spleen from the same mice delayed the onset of disease. Some studies demonstrated that the regulatory T cells could also be separated from the effector T cells by differential expression of CD62 ligand.

Chatenoud et al. (100) examined whether CD4$^+$CD25$^+$ T cells play a protective role in the NOD mouse. Young NOD/SCID recipients were injected intravenously with mixtures of splenocytes from diabetic NOD mice and CD25$^+$ and CD25$^-$ T cells from the spleens of prediabetic NOD mice. CD25$^+$ T cells from young (6-week-old) prediabetic mice significantly protected against diabetes in this model. Protection could be reversed by treatment of the recipient mice with anti–TGF-β but not with anti–IL-4 or anti–IL-10.

Interestingly, anti–TGF-β did not reverse protection mediated by CD25$^+$ T cells derived from the thymus. CD4$^+$CD25$^-$ T cells from young NOD mice could also exert some degree of protection in adoptive transfer studies.

Analysis of regulatory T-cell function in the NOD mouse is difficult because not all animals develop disease and because it takes a long time for disease to develop. Green et al. (67) developed a model of insulin-dependent diabetes mellitus (IDDM) in which a regulatable TNF gene is expressed in the pancreatic islets. When these mice were crossed with mice expressing CD80 in their islets and TNF is expressed for 25 days from birth, diabetes is delayed. In contrast, if TNF expression is allowed to continue for 28 days, the regulatory mechanisms are overcome, and the animals rapidly develop diabetes. The autoreactive effector cells in this model are exclusively CD8$^+$ T cells. CD4$^+$CD25$^+$ T cells could be isolated from the islets and draining pancreatic node, but not from other nodes or the spleen, and they could suppress the development of disease in animals in which TNF was expressed for 28 days. These regulatory cells were extremely potent, and protection could be transferred with only 2×10^3 CD25$^+$ T cells. This site-specific accumulation of regulatory cells may be the result of localized production of chemokines that specifically recruit CD25$^+$ to the site of inflammation. Alternatively, the regulatory T cells in the draining node may be antigen-specific and generated *in situ* by stimulation by islet-derived antigens.

Antigenic Specificity of Regulatory T Cells in Autoimmunity

Very little progress has been made in the identification of the target antigen recognized by CD4$^+$CD25$^+$ regulatory T cells. Most of the current data have been derived from organ-specific autoimmunity models and suggest that suppressor T cells recognize a target antigen derived from the organ that is under autoimmune attack. Spleen cells from normal adult male mice were much more effective suppressors of autoimmune orchitis induced after d3Tx than were spleen cells from female mice or from male mice that had undergone a neonatal orchiectomy (101). In contrast, spleen cells from male and female mice exerted equivalent potency in protecting against gastritis. Taguchi et al. (102) showed that the suppressor cell population that was capable of inhibiting the induction of prostatitis was organ specific, because cells from male but not female mice or from male mice orchiectomized at birth inhibited disease after d3Tx. The d3Tx mice orchiectomized at birth also never develop prostatitis. Prostatitis did develop after treatment with testosterone, which indicates that expression of the prostate antigen responsible for evoking autoimmunity could be induced by hormonal stimulation. Spleen cells from these mice could prevent prostatitis when injected into d3Tx mice. Activation of these regulatory T cell takes place in the periphery because suppressor cells could be isolated from adult Tx hormone-treated mice. Other studies in autoimmune prostatitis suggested that

the differences were relative rather than absolute, inasmuch as protection could be achieved with 4×10^6 cells from normal male mice but only with 4×10^7 spleen cells from female mice. Moreover, normal male cells, normal female cells, and spleen cells from female mice that were oophorectomized at birth were found to suppress d3Tx-induced oophoritis with comparable efficiency (103).

A number of studies have shown that when the developing immune system is prevented from gaining access to a tissue-specific antigen, tissue-specific tolerance fails to develop. For example, when fetal rat thyroid glands were destroyed by exposure to radioactive iodine and syngeneic thyroid tissue was then implanted into the athyroid rats as adults, autoimmune thyroiditis developed in the grafted tissue (104). The development of thyroiditis in such rats could be prevented by parabiosis to normal syngeneic partners. Parabiosis was protective only if instituted at the time of thyroid grafting but not 1 to 2 weeks after graft implantation. This approach was extended by Seddon and Mason (105) to demonstrate that peripheral CD45RC^{low} T cells from rats rendered athyroid were unable to prevent thyroid-specific autoimmunity induced by the adult Tx-irradiation protocol. The loss of regulatory T cells was specific for the extirpated organ, inasmuch as T cells from the athyroid rats could prevent the development of diabetes. CD4$^+$CD8$^-$ thymocytes from the same athyroid donors were effective at preventing thyroiditis. It appears that regulatory T cells were normally generated in the thymus in the absence of the target organ but that the target organ was needed for their survival or expansion, or both, in the periphery.

Important insights into determining the antigenic specificity of regulatory T cells have also been derived from studies of the requirements for induction of organ-specific autoreactive effector cells (106). When susceptible strains of mice are immunized with the ovary-specific antigen, pZP3, 100-fold more pZP3 in completed Freund's adjuvant (CFA) was necessary to elicit the same pathogenic response in female mice as in male mice that had undergone grafting with an ovary. This differential responsiveness to stimulation by the autoantigen indicates that female mice have a certain level of tolerance to pZP3 that is dependent on the presence of physiologically expressed ZP3 antigen. Neonatal oophorectomy converts the female response to that of a male. Oophorectomy between the ages of 1 and 6 weeks also leads to conversion of the female to a male responsiveness profile when the ovaries are removed for more than 7 days, but not 3 days, before challenge with pZP3 in CFA. It remains to be determined whether tolerance in the female mice is mediated by suppressor T cells and whether continued expression of the endogenous antigen is required for the maintenance/survival of the suppressor T cells in the periphery.

Lymphocyte Homeostasis and Autoimmunity

Lymphocyte numbers in a normal adult animal remain stable throughout life. A homeostatic equilibrium exists between the numbers of newly produced cells, self-renewal of peripheral T cells, and the numbers of dying cells. The mechanism that controls the number of peripheral lymphocytes is unknown. The regulation of the numbers of naïve and memory CD4$^+$ and CD8$^+$ T cells is independently controlled. Most studies of the effects of regulatory T cells *in vivo* in the suppression of autoimmune disease involve the transfer of the effector populations to a T cell–deficient mouse (107). T-lymphocytes undergo a rapid, vigorous proliferative response when transferred to an immunodeficient recipient. The inhibitory effects of regulatory T cells in autoimmunity are presumably related to their ability to be specifically activated by autoantigens. An alternative possibility is that a major component of regulatory T-cell function is to nonspecifically inhibit lymphopenia-induced proliferation (108) and thereby prevent the development of autoimmune disease. CD4$^+$CD25$^+$ T cells might be potent inhibitors of lymphopenia-induced proliferation, but any T-cell population with an activated effector/memory phenotype might also be capable of mediating inhibition. Although activated CD4$^+$CD25$^+$, but not activated CD4$^+$CD25$^-$, T cells are suppressive *in vitro*, but *in vitro* assays do not mimic the migration of cells into different organs or the interaction of lymphocytes with other cell types.

Surprisingly, both CD4$^+$CD25$^-$ (including RB^{high} cells) T cells and CD25$^+$ T cells were capable of proliferating in a lymphopenic host, with proliferation beginning on days 3 to 4 after transfer and reaching as many as eight divisions by days 21 to 28 after transfer. CD4$^+$CD25$^+$ T cells did not inhibit this early phase of "homeostatic proliferation" of CD4$^+$CD25$^-$ T cells (109). Although CD4$^+$CD25$^+$ T cells have been shown to inhibit the accumulation of CD25$^-$ T cells 2 to 6 months after transfer to a RAG$^{-/-}$ recipient by an IL-10–dependent mechanism, this result must be interpreted with caution (110). The fact that CD25$^-$ T cells almost always induce some form of organ-specific autoimmune disease demonstrates that CD25$^-$ T cells have undergone some form of autoantigen-specific proliferation in addition to the lymphopenia-induced proliferation. As described previously, CD4$^+$CD25$^+$ T cells are highly efficient inhibitors of the induction of these autoimmune diseases. Transfer of CD25$^+$

T cells to immunodeficient mice results in loss of expression of CD25 by a majority of the transferred cells (46). The significance of this finding is unknown, inasmuch as the recovered CD25$^-$ T cells retain the ability to suppress T-cell activation *in vitro*.

CONTROL OF ALLOGRAFT REJECTION AND GRAFT-VERSUS-HOST DISEASE BY REGULATORY T CELLS

There is considerable evidence that regulatory/suppressor T cells exist in patients and animals with long-term surviving allografts (111). Analysis of the properties of these cells *in vitro* has been hampered because bulk populations of T cells from tolerant recipients proliferate normally when cultured *in vitro* with donor alloantigens and frequently secrete a proinflammatory Th1 pattern of cytokines. It appears that the regulatory T cells are masked by the presence of naïve T cells responding to alloantigens. In animal models, a number of protocols have been used to induce tolerance to allografts (Fig. 8). Tolerance of cardiac allografts in mice can be induced by pretreatment with a donor-specific blood transfusion combined with depleting or nondepleting anti-CD4 antibody. It is likely that the protective effects of this protocol were mediated by the induction of CD4$^+$ regulatory T cells, because complete depletion of CD4$^+$ T cells fails to induce tolerance. Pretreated mice accepted cardiac grafts, and cells from these mice could transfer tolerance to naïve recipients. CD4$^+$ T cells were responsible for both the induction and maintenance of tolerance.

In studies of allograft rejection across a full H-2 difference, the differential expression of CD45RB has facilitated separation of nontolerant naïve T cells from the induced regulatory T cells (112). RB^{high} cells from tolerant mice responded normally to challenge with alloantigen *in vitro* and were able to reject allogeneic skin grafts when transferred alone to T cell–deficient mice. In contrast, CD45RB^{low} cells failed to mount a proliferative response, to secrete cytokines in response to alloantigen *in vitro*, and to induce allograft rejection *in vivo*. The addition of CD45RB^{low} cells to an MLR with CD45RB^{high} cells as responders resulted in inhibition

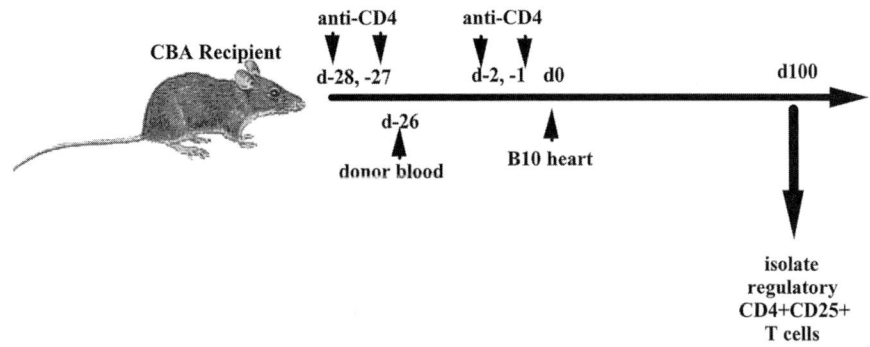

FIG. 8. Induction of regulatory T cells for tolerance to alloantigens. Adapted from Hara et al. (112), with permission.

of proliferation. CD45RB^{low} T cells from long-term tolerant mice were able to suppress responses to alloantigen *in vitro* only when the donor alloantigens were presented by the indirect pathway of allorecognition by the APCs present in the culture. One explanation for this result is that it is potentially advantageous for the regulatory T cells to respond to alloantigens via the indirect pathway because regulatory T cells may require constant stimulation to maintain their function. Passenger leukocytes rapidly migrate out of the graft, and the graft tissues lack co-stimulatory molecules. Donor-derived allopeptides must be presented by recipient APCs for stimulation of the regulatory T cells *in vivo* and for the detection of functional activity of these cells *in vitro*. All of the suppressive activity of the CD45RB^{low} cells was mediated by the CD4$^+$CD25$^+$ T-cell subset contained in that pool. The suppressive capacity of the regulatory T cells in this model *in vitro* and *in vivo* was reversed by anti–IL-10 receptor, but not by anti–IL-4.

Regulatory T cells can also be isolated from mice that were pretreated with donor alloantigen in combination with depleting anti-CD4 but did not receive an allograft transplant (113). These cells are fully competent in prolongation of cardiac graft survival when transferred to naïve recipients. Regulatory T cells can be isolated 28 days after pretreatment, and regulation is antigen-specific. Both treatments are required, and CD25$^+$ T cells from naïve donors do not prolong graft rejection. It is possible that the precursor frequency of alloantigen-specific regulatory CD25$^+$ T cells from naïve animals is too low for suppression to be observed at the cell doses used and that the pretreatment regimen serves to increase their frequency. No major increase in the percentage of CD25$^+$ cells is observed in the pretreated animals, and it remains to be proved that the CD25$^+$ T cells isolated from the pretreated animals are derived from the naturally occurring CD25$^+$ pool and not generated from CD25$^-$ T cells. In either case, it is likely that the pretreatment protocol maximizes the conditions for activation of regulatory T cells.

In studies examining induction of tolerance to minor histocompatibility antigens on allografts in accordance with protocols similar to those described previously, both CD4$^+$CD25$^+$ and CD4$^+$CD25$^-$ T cells from tolerant mice could mediate suppression, but suppression required 10 times more CD4$^+$CD25$^-$ T cells (114). Both populations may have a significant role in maintaining transplantation tolerance, inasmuch as the number of CD25$^-$ T cells is 10 times higher than CD25$^+$ T cells in the tolerant mouse. It is possible that some of the CD25$^+$ T cells have lost expression of CD25 during the tolerance induction protocol or that effector cell death in the CD25$^-$ T-cell pool unmasked the presence of regulatory T cells. In contrast to the results with a major MHC difference, CD4$^+$CD25$^+$ T cells from naïve mice could also prevent naïve T cells from rejecting skin grafts, although five times more cells were required than from tolerant donors. The enhanced potency of CD25$^+$ T cells from tolerant mice may be secondary to expansion of an alloantigen-specific population. The capacity of T cells from tolerant donors or CD25$^+$

T cells from normal mice to mediate their suppressive function could not be neutralized by anti–CTLA-4, by anti–IL-10, or by anti–IL-4.

When the generation of co-stimulatory signals are blocked in MLR cultures by the addition of anti–CD40 ligand or anti-CD80/CD86 (115), the surviving cells become specifically tolerant to class II MHC–bearing stimulator cells and have a greatly reduced capacity to induce GVHD *in vivo* (>30-fold). GVHD prevention was not mediated by skewing toward a Th2 phenotype. Both IL-4$^{-/-}$ and IL-10$^{-/-}$ T cells were susceptible to anergy induction. If CD4$^+$CD25$^+$ T cells were depleted from the responder population, tolerance was not induced, and all the recipients of CD4$^+$CD25$^-$ T cells died of GVHD 18 days after transfer (116). The most likely explanation for these results is related to the differential requirements for co-stimulation of the CD25$^+$ T cells in comparison with the CD25$^-$ T cells. CD25$^+$ T cells do not require co-stimulatory signals mediated by interactions of CD28/CLTA-4 with CD80/CD86 for induction of suppressor function, whereas activation of CD4$^+$CD25$^-$ T cell effectors is likely to be strongly dependent on co-stimulation. A major consequence of CD25-mediated suppression is the induction of cell cycle arrest in the CD25$^-$ responders. Because cell cycle arrest is normally followed by apoptotic cell death, it is highly likely that tolerance in this model is secondary to deletion of the CD4$^+$CD25$^-$ GVHD effectors. The only cells remaining in the cultures were the CD4$^+$CD25$^+$ suppressor cells.

The inability of T-cell populations containing large numbers of CD25$^+$ T cells to mediate GVHD raised the strong possibility that CD25$^+$ T cells might actually be capable of inhibiting CD25$^-$ effectors in cotransfer studies. Freshly isolated CD25$^+$ T cells only modestly inhibited GVHD when mixed with CD25$^-$ T cells in equal numbers, whereas alloantigen-stimulated, cultured CD25$^+$ T cells profoundly inhibited the capacity of CD25$^-$ T cells to inhibit rapidly lethal GVHD (117). Surprisingly, the best protection was observed with the culture method (allogeneic splenocytes, low-dose IL-2, and TGF-β) that resulted in the lowest rate of recovery. TGF-β may therefore function as a growth or differentiation factor for CD25$^+$ T cells, or it may render them more resistant to activation-induced cell death.

REGULATORY T CELLS AND TUMOR IMMUNITY

Studies by North and Bursuker (118) in the early 1980s demonstrated the role of suppressor T cells in the prevention of tumor immunity. In their studies, primed antitumor T cells were incapable of causing regression of a tumor when passively transferred into a normal host. If the tumor recipient was rendered T-cell deficient by thymectomy and lethal irradiation followed by bone marrow reconstitution combined with sublethal irradiation or treated with cyclophosphamide, the transferred cells could induce tumor regression. Cotransfer of T cells from tumor-bearing recipients prevented T cell–mediated tumor regression. T cells taken on day

6 after tumor implantation were capable of transferring protection to T cell–depleted recipients. By day 9 of tumor growth, the antitumor T cells were lost, and transfer of cells from the tumor-bearing animals suppressed antitumor immune effectors. Immediately after tumor implantation, mice developed concomitant immunity and would reject a challenge implant of cells of the same tumor given at another site; later in the course of tumor development, concomitant immunity decayed.

The suppressor T cells in the experiments of North and Bursuker were shown to be CD4+CD8− but were not characterized further (119). Their susceptibility to sublethal irradiation and cyclophosphamide is similar to that of CD4+CD25+ T cells. Because most tumor antigens are normal self-antigens, it is likely that the mechanisms maintaining immunological tolerance to self-antigens may impede the generation of effective tumor immunity against autologous tumor cells. In many cases, successful immunotherapy of cancer often leads to the appearance of autoimmunity because of cross-reactions between antigens expressed on tumors and normal tissue antigens. Onizuki et al. (120) were the first to suggest that naturally occurring CD4+CD25+ T cells played an important role in inhibiting tumor immunity. They first depleted CD4+CD25+ T cells by injecting a depleting anti-CD25 mAb and noted that this led to regression of a number of tumors that grew progressively in nondepleted mice. The depletion had to be performed no later than day 2 after injection of the tumor. Co-administration of anti-CD8 inhibited the tumor regression induced by anti-CD25 depletion, which suggests that CD8 T cells were responsible for tumor regression.

Similar conclusions were drawn by Shimizu et al. (121) who transferred CD25-depleted or CD25-containing spleen cells to *nu/nu* recipients and then challenged them with normally nonimmunogenic tumors. In the recipients of CD25-depleted cells, tumors grew but regressed; in contrast, all recipients of spleen cells containing CD25+ T cells died from rapidly growing tumors. Long-lasting tumor immunity to repeat challenge could also be demonstrated in the recipients of the CD25-depleted spleen cells. Conventional MHC-restricted CD8+ T cells mediated tumor rejection in this model. *In vitro* studies also indicated the presence of nonspecific killing mediated by CD4−CD8− natural killer (NK) cells. These investigators hypothesized that the large amounts of IL-2 produced by the CD25− T cells was responsible for the generation of the CD4−CD8− NK-like cells.

Together, the studies on depletion of CD4+CD25+ T cells and the transfer of CD4+CD25− T cells strongly suggest that the effectiveness of a tumor vaccine would be greatly enhanced by removal of CD4+CD25+ T-cell suppressor activity. Indeed, Sutmuller et al. (122) were able to demonstrate that antibody-mediated depletion of CD25+ T cells followed by vaccination with a granulocyte-macrophage colony-stimulating factor–transfected melanoma cell line resulted in enhanced tumor rejection. Tumor rejection was accompanied by skin depigmentation, which suggests

TABLE 6. *Depletion of CD4+CD25+ T cells augments the immune response to a tumor vaccine*

Treatment	% Surviving day 90
None	0
Anti-CD25 (day −4)	20
GM-CSF vaccine (days 0, 3, 6) plus anti-CD25 (day −4)	50
GM-CSF vaccine (days 0, 3, 6) plus anti–CTLA-4 (days 0, 3, 6)	50
GM-CSF vaccine (days 0, 3, 6) plus anti-CD25 (day −4) plus anti–CTLA-4 (days 0, 3, 6)	100

CTLA-4, cytotoxic T-lymphocyte–associated antigen 4; GM-CSF, granulocyte-macrophage colony-stimulating factor. Adapted from Sutmuller et al. (122), with permission.

that autoreactive immune responses are involved in this process. This group had previously shown that enhanced effectiveness of the tumor vaccine could also be induced by treatment of the mice with anti–CTLA-4. Because a number of studies have suggested that the anti–CTLA-4 targets CD4+CD25+ T cells, it was important to determine whether the enhancement of antitumor immunity by anti–CTLA-4 resulted from inhibition of CD25-mediated suppression. Depletion of CD25+ T cells followed by anti–CTLA-4 treatment and vaccination resulted in the most potent antitumor response (Table 6). Thus, CD25 depletion and anti–CTLA-4 treatment increase the immunogenicity of a tumor vaccine by distinct mechanisms involving nonredundant pathways. CTLA-4 blockade enhances the induction of antitumor effector cells by removing the normal inhibitory signals generated by CD80/CD86 interactions with CTLA-4.

Although these studies in well-characterized animals models demonstrate the role of CD4+CD25+ T cells in inhibiting tumor rejection, it is often difficult to extrapolate from tumor immunity studies in rodents to humans. Woo et al. (123) showed that CD4+CD25+ T cells exist in high proportions (~33%) in the tumor-infiltrating lymphocytes of patients with non–small cell lung cancer. These T cells were capable of suppressing the proliferative responses of autologous, but not allogeneic, T cells to suboptimal stimulation with anti-CD3. It is not known whether these tumor infiltrating CD4+CD25+ T cells arise from the naturally occurring CD4+CD25+ population or are generated from CD4+CD25− T cells. Nevertheless, these findings suggest that one component of the immune response to tumors in humans is the generation of tumor-specific suppressor T cells.

REGULATORY T-CELL CONTROL OF IMMUNITY TO INFECTIOUS AGENTS

Most of the studies of regulatory T cells have focused on their role in the suppression of the immune response to autoantigens, tumor antigens, or alloantigens. One of the most important roles of regulatory T cells may, in fact, involve modulation of the immune response to infectious agents to prevent the lethal consequences of an overwhelming inflammatory response during the course of a productive immune response to an invading microorganism (124). Regulatory and effector T cells must maintain equilibrium between no immunity at all and immunopathology. This critical role of regulatory T cells is well illustrated by the immune response of mice to infection with *Pneumocystis carinii*. When SCID mice chronically infected with *P. carinii* are reconstituted with CD4+CD25− T cells, they develop a severe inflammatory response in their lungs that is ultimately fatal. Animals injected with CD25+ T cells alone did not become moribund and manifested only transient weight loss. Cotransfer of CD25+ T cells prevented the development of the *P. carinii*–driven fatal pulmonary inflammation induced by CD25− T cells, but it also suppressed the elimination of *P. carinii* mediated by the CD25− T cells. Protective CD25+ T cells are needed to inhibit the lethal immunopathological response mediated by the *P. carinii*–specific CD4+CD25− T cells, but they also inhibited complete clearing of the organism (125). *P. carinii*–associated immunopathology is often seen in lymphopenic animals and humans, and this may reflect a relative deficiency in regulatory T cells.

The role of CD4+CD25+ T cells in the immune response to infection includes more than suppression of inflammation. CD4+CD25+ T cells also maintain persistence of infection and promote chronicity. The persistence of pathogens after clinical cure is a hallmark of certain viral, bacterial, and parasitic infections. In clinical and experimental forms of leishmaniasis, small numbers of viable organisms persist within lymphoid tissue and within the site of former skin lesions after self-cure or successful chemotherapy. Because low numbers of parasites persisting in the dermis can be efficiently transmitted back to their vector sandflies, the expansion or recruitment, or both, of regulatory T cells to the site of *Leishmania major* infection might reflect a parasite adaptive strategy to maintain its transmission cycle in nature. Despite the absence of sterilizing immunity, these individuals maintain strong lifelong immunity to reinfection, a status similar to the concomitant immunity described in tumor models (126).

In healed C57BL/6 mice, CD4+CD25+ regulatory T cells accumulate in sites of *L. major* infection in the skin (Fig. 9) (127). These cells are exclusively derived from naturally occurring CD25+ T cells and not from activated CD25− T cells. They suppress the expansion of and killing mediated by *L. major*–specific effector cells. Although IL-10 produced by CD25+ T cells is essential to the establishment of persistent infection, early in the infectious process CD25+ T cells can promote parasite survival and growth in an IL-10–independent manner. Later in the course of infection, IL-10 is absolutely required for development of the chronic lesion, inasmuch as recipients of CD25+ T cells from IL-10−/− mice ultimately healed and completely cleared the parasite from the site. IL-10 produced by regulatory T cells contributes directly to parasite persistence by modulating APC function, by inhibiting cytokine production by Th1 cells, or by rendering

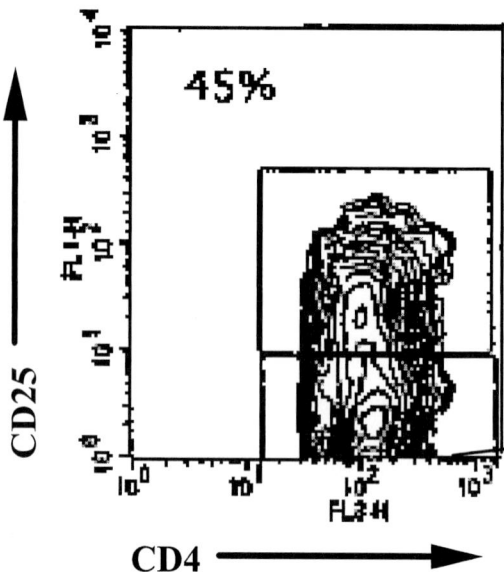

FIG. 9. CD4+CD25+ T cells constitute approximately 50% of the CD4+ T cells in chronic *Leishmania major* infection. Adapted from Belkaid et al. (127), with permission.

macrophages refractory to IFN-γ that is needed for intracellular killing.

Although one consequence of this regulation is parasite persistence and the potential for disease reactivation, parasite persistence itself is to the host a major benefit that is needed for lifelong immunity to reinfection. When repeat-challenge studies were performed in IL-10−/− mice or in wild-type mice that were treated during the chronic stage of their primary infection with anti–IL-10 receptor—conditions that result in complete clearance of parasites from the skin and draining lymph node—reinfection at a site distant from the initial infection resulted in parasite loads that were comparable with those after primary infection in naïve mice. Because healed mice treated with control antibody maintained strong immunity to reinfection, the maintenance of a residual source of infection, secondary to IL-10 production by CD25+ T cells at the lesion site, is required for preservation of acquired immunity to *L. major*.

Although certain pathogen-derived molecules such as bacterial DNA containing CpG motifs are powerful inducers of the differentiation of Th1 effector cells, other pathogen-derived components might induce the differentiation of regulatory T cells. Although Th1 effector cells are induced during the course of infection with *Bordetella pertussis* and ultimately play a critical role in the clearance of bacteria from the respiratory tract (128), antigen-specific Th1 responses in the lung and local lymph nodes are severely suppressed during the acute phase of infection. *B. pertussis* has evolved a number of strategies to circumvent protective immune responses. One bacterial component, filamentous hemagglutinin (FHA), is capable of inhibiting LPS-driven IL-12 production by macrophages and DCs and of stimulating IL-10 production. FHA may contribute to the suppressed Th1 responses during acute infection with *B. pertussis* by the induction of T cells with regulatory activity as a result of its interactions with cells of the innate immune system. Repeated stimulation of T cells from the lungs of mice acutely infected with *B. pertussis* resulted in the generation of Tr1 clones specific for FHA. Tr1 cells could be generated only from the lungs of infected animals and not from the spleen. These Tr1 cells secreted high levels of IL-10 and inhibited protective immune responses against *B. pertussis in vivo* and *in vitro*. Suppression was substantially reversed by anti–IL-10 *in vivo*. The capacity to induce Tr1 cells is thereby exploited by a respiratory pathogen to evade protective immunity and suppress protective Th1 responses at local sites of infection.

MacDonald et al. (129) took advantage of a unique accident in which a cohort of women were infected 20 years earlier with a single batch of immunoglobulin contaminated with a single genotype of hepatitis C virus (HCV). Analysis of cytokine production by T cells specific for the HCV core protein identified antigen-specific regulatory T cells that secreted IL-10 in addition to IFN-γ circulating Th1 cells; no IL-4–producing T cells were identified. IL-10 producing cells were detected in a higher proportion of patients with chronic infection than in those who had cleared the virus. One possibility for the selective induction of IL-10–producing regulatory T cells in HCV is that HCV infects the liver, and liver DCs secrete large amounts of IL-10, which in turn results in the generation of IL-10–producing regulatory T cells. Together with the studies on *L. major* and *B. pertussis,* these studies on HCV strongly support the general concept that many infectious agents have evolved mechanisms for selective activation of either naturally occurring CD25$^+$ T cells or the generation of IL-10–producing Tr1 cells from CD25$^-$ T cells. The ultimate result is perpetuation of the chronic infectious state with incomplete clearing of the infection. Depending on the extent of suppression of effector T cells in the host, the consequences of the chronic state may be protective immunity (*L. major*) or continued pathogen-mediated organ destruction (HCV).

Friend virus infection in mice has been used as an experimental model to study retrovirus-induced immunosuppression and may offer insights into our understanding of immunosuppression associated with human immunodeficiency virus. Mice chronically infected with Friend virus are unable to reject both Friend virus–induced and unrelated immunogenic tumors. CD4$^+$ but not CD8$^+$ T cells from infected mice can transfer suppression to normal mice and can inhibit the generation of cytotoxic T-lymphocytes in culture (130). The suppressive activity of the CD4$^+$ T cells was associated with a subpopulation that coexpressed the activation marker CD69. Suppression could be substantially reversed by the addition of anti–CTLA-4, but not anti–IL-10 receptor, to the cultures. The relationship of these virus-induced suppressor cells to either the naturally occurring CD4$^+$CD25$^+$ T cells or Tr1 cells is unclear at present. It also is unknown whether the regulatory T cells in chronically infected mice are specific for any viral proteins. Nevertheless, it appears that an important component of the generalized immunosuppression seen in retroviral infections involves the induction of suppressor T cells.

OTHER TYPES OF REGULATORY/ SUPPRESSOR T CELLS

CD8$^+$ Suppressor T Cells

Most of the early studies on T suppressor cells in the mouse demonstrated that they were confined to the CD8$^+$ subset. Although almost all of the more recent studies on suppressor/regulatory T cells in mouse or human have focused on CD4$^+$ T cells, a number of studies have suggested that potent CD8$^+$ suppressor cells may also exist. Repeated stimulation of human T cells in the MLR resulted in a progressive decrease of the capacity of CD4$^+$ T cells to proliferate when rechallenged with the APCs used for priming. The relative nonresponsiveness of the stimulated CD4$^+$ T cells could be restored by depletion of CD8$^+$CD28$^-$ but not CD8$^+$CD28$^+$ T cells from these cultures. The stimulated CD8$^+$CD28$^-$ T-cell population was devoid of cytotoxic activity for either CD4$^+$ T cells or the APCs used for priming. When the CD8$^+$CD28$^-$ T cells were added to mixtures of CD4 cells and APCs, they inhibited proliferation (131), but suppression was observed only when the stimulatory APCs shared at least one class I HLA allele with the original stimulator population. The regulatory effect of the CD8$^+$ suppressors was not restricted either by class I or class II MHC antigens expressed by the responder CD4$^+$ T cells. These CD8$^+$CD28$^-$ suppressor cells were clonally diverse, required IL-2 for proliferation, and proliferated in a manner similar to CD8$^+$CD28$^+$ T cells. CD8$^+$CD28$^-$ suppressors can also be generated *in vitro* by priming peripheral blood mononuclear cells with nominal antigens such as MHC antigens or with soluble protein antigens.

Suppression mediated by CD8$^+$CD28$^-$ T cells required cell–cell contact and was not reversed by antisuppressor cytokine antibodies. Co-incubation of the CD8 suppressors with CD4 responders had no effect, whereas co-incubation of the CD8 T cells with the APCs rendered the APCs unable to stimulate CD4 proliferation. Phenotypic analysis indicated that the CD8 suppressors blocked the up-regulation of co-stimulatory molecules such as CD80/CD86, CD54, and CD58 on the APCs (132). The mechanism by which the CD8 suppressors deactivate APC functions has been shown to involve up-regulation of the genes encoding immunoglobulin-like transcripts 3 and 4 (ILT3 and ILT4) (133). These inhibitory receptors are structurally and functionally related to killer cell inhibitory receptors (KIR). Both ILT3 and ILT4 have immunoreceptor tyrosine-based inhibitory motifs that mediate inhibition of cell activation by recruiting the tyrosine phosphatase SHP-1. The ligand for ILT3 is unknown, but ILT4 binds HLA-A, HLA-B, HLA-C, and HLA-G. A mAb to ILT3 or a combination of mAbs to ILT4 and class I HLA reversed suppression by 50%. In the presence of CD8$^+$CD28$^-$ suppressor cells, APCs have a reduced ability to signal through CD40 and to transcribe NFκB-dependent co-stimulatory molecules. Thus far, the biological activity of these CD8$^+$CD28$^-$ suppressor populations has been studied only *in vitro* in MLR cultures. Their potential roles in mediating immunosuppression *in vivo* and their relationship to CD4$^+$ suppressor cells remain to be explored.

Regulatory CD8$^+$ T cells have also been generated *in vitro* by stimulation with unique subpopulations of DCs (134). When naïve CD8$^+$ T cells were stimulated *in vitro* with CD40 ligand–activated monocyte-derived DCs (DC1), the primed CD8$^+$ T cells proliferated when restimulated with allogeneic targets, secreted large amounts of IFN-γ, and had potent cytotoxic activity. In contrast, when naïve CD8$^+$ T cells were stimulated with CD40 ligand–activated plasmacytoid DCs (DC2), the primed CD8$^+$ T cells proliferated poorly, displayed weak cytotoxic activity, and secreted primarily IL-10. DC2-primed CD8$^+$ T cells inhibited the ability of naïve CD8$^+$ T cells to proliferate to allogeneic monocytes, iDCs, or mature DCs. They could not inhibit the response of DC1-primed CD8$^+$ T cells. Both the generation of CD8$^+$ suppressor cells and their suppressor function could be markedly inhibited by anti–IL-10 but not by anti–TGF-β. DC2-induced CD8$^+$ suppressor cells inhibit bystander responses of naïve CD8$^+$ T cells if they are restimulated by their target alloantigen. The relationship of these CD8$^+$ suppressor cells to the CD8$^+$CD28$^-$ suppressor cells is not clear. The former can be isolated after only 6 days of culture, whereas the latter are seen only after multiple rounds of stimulation. CD8$^+$CD28$^-$ suppressor cells may represent an end stage of cytotoxic T-lymphocyte differentiation. DC2-induced CD8$^+$ suppressor cells have many similarities to CD4$^+$ Tr1 cells, including their poor responsiveness, their requirement for IL-10 for generation, and their use of IL-10 as the major mediator of their suppressive function.

Dhodapkar et al. (135) measured the ability of iDC to modulate the immune response *in vivo* in humans. Injection of iDCs pulsed with influenza matrix peptide resulted in an expansion of antigen-specific tetramer binding CD8$^+$ T cells. These CD8 cells were capable of proliferating when stimulated with antigen *in vitro* but were defective in IFN-γ secretion and lacked cytotoxic function. These findings indicate that iDCs can dampen preexisting antigen-specific effector function in humans. The potential suppressive function of the CD8$^+$ T cells that responded to the iDCs was not studied. The relationship of these CD8$^+$ T cells to those induced *in vitro* with DC2 is unknown. These studies raise the possibility that antigen-pulsed iDCs might be used to inhibit antigen-specific T cell function in autoimmunity and organ transplantation.

Double Negative Suppressor T Cells

CD4$^-$CD8$^-$ double negative (DN) T cells have also been shown to have immunoregulatory activity both *in vivo* and *in vitro*. These DN populations were derived after administration of donor antigens to induce tolerance of allografts

and are presumably derived from precursors present in normal peripheral lymphoid populations (136). DN suppressors generated in this way kill alloreactive CD4$^+$ and CD8$^+$ T responders that express functional Fas by a mechanism involving Fas–Fas ligand interactions. These activated DN cells were able to kill only syngeneic targets activated by the same alloantigenic stimulus. DN T cells also accumulate in lymphoproliferative (lpr) mice that develop autoimmune disease and have a mutation in the gene responsible for encoding Fas (137). DN T cells from B6/lpr mice can kill syngeneic CD8$^+$ and CD4$^+$ T cells from wild-type B6 mice through Fas–Fas ligand interactions both *in vivo* and *in vitro*. These DN T cells may accumulate in lpr mice because they are unable to undergo Fas-mediated apoptosis. In contrast to the DN suppressors generated *in vivo* by treatment with donor alloantigen, alloactivated DN suppressors from lpr mice were able to kill syngeneic T cells that were activated by either the same or a different alloantigen. They appear to display nonspecific suppressor effector function similar to that described for activated CD4$^+$CD25$^+$ T cells. The bystander killing may be secondary to their overexpression of Fas ligand. This discrepancy between *in vivo* activated and *in vitro* activated DN cells remains to be resolved.

Natural Killer T Cells

NK T cells are a unique subset of T cells that primarily express an invariant TCR (Vα14-Jα281 in the mouse and Vα24 in humans). NK T cells are deficient in NOD mice, and enhancement of their numbers by transgenic expression of Vα14-Jα281 can prevent IDDM in NOD mice (138). Deficiencies in the numbers of NK T cells have also been observed in humans with IDDM. Activation of NK T cells with their ligand, α-GalCer, results in inhibition of the development of IDDM (139). Prevention of disease correlated with the ability of α-GalCer to stimulate IL-4 production, elevate serum IgE, and promote the generation of islet antigen-specific Th2 cells. It has been proposed that the elevated production of IL-4, but not IFN-γ, after activation of NK T cells with α-GalCer facilitates the polarization of the anti–islet T cell responses to a protective Th2 type rather than a pathogenic Th1 type. Because α-GalCer has also been shown to inhibit the development of EAE by activation of NK T cells (140), it may prove to be useful as a therapeutic agent for treatment of multiple Th1-mediated autoimmune diseases.

CD4$^+$CD25$^-$ Immunoregulatory T Cells

The potential involvement of CD4$^+$CD25$^-$ T cells with suppressor activity in IBD, IDDM, allograft rejection, and thyroiditis has been discussed. The most convincing evidence for the existence of immunoregulatory T cells with this phenotype was seen in studies of the CD4$^+$ T cells that prevent spontaneous EAE. Mice expressing a transgenic TCR specific for MBP do not develop EAE spontaneously, whereas 100% of MBP-specific TCR transgenic mice bred on a RAG$^{-/-}$

TABLE 7. *Regulatory T cells expressing endogenous TCRs protect against EAE*

Anti-MBP TCR Tg RAG1$^{-/-}$ crossed to	EAE incidence (%)
TCR α^-/β^-	100
TCR α^-/β^+	95
TCR α^+/β^-	71
TCR α^+/β^+	0
TCR $\delta^{-/-}$	0
TCR β2m$^{-/-}$	0

EAE, experimental autoimmune encephalomyelitis; MBP, myelin basic protein; RAG-1, recombination activating gene 1; TCR, T-cell receptor; Tg, transgenic.
Adapted from Furtado et al. (142), with permission.

background develop EAE by the third month of life. Reconstitution of these TCR transgenic RAG$^{-/-}$ mice with a small number ($\sim$2 $\times$ 10^5) of splenic or thymic CD4$^+$ T cells from normal mice confers complete protection from EAE (141). Depletion of CD4$^+$CD25$^+$ T cells from the cell population used in these reconstitution studies did not diminish their protective capacity. The regulatory mechanisms that operate in these mice do not involve deletion of the MBP-specific effector cells, because severe EAE can be induced in the mice by immunization with MBP in adjuvant; MBP-specific T cells from these mice can also transfer disease to RAG$^{-/-}$ recipients. CD4$^+$ T cells expressing TCR $\alpha\beta$ chains were crucial for protection; CD8$^+$ T cells, NK T cells, and $\gamma\delta$ T cells played no role (Table 7). CD4$^+$ T cells from a mouse that expressed a TCR specific for ovalbumin on a RAG$^{-/-}$ background were unable to protect against EAE. Thus, the presence of a second TCR is not sufficient to generate regulatory T cells. CD4$^+$ T cells from mice deficient in terminal deoxynucleotide transferase, which express a fetal type repertoire lacking N nucleotides, effectively protected against EAE. T cells that expressed a single TCR α chain, obtained from MBP-specific TCR α chain–only mice, protected when crossed to the MBP-specific TCR transgenic mice on an α chain$^{-/-}$ background. Regulatory CD4$^+$CD25$^-$ T cells can be generated from a T-cell population expressing a single TCR α chain, if TCR β chain diversity is maintained (142). The mechanisms by which CD4$^+$CD25$^-$ T cells inhibit the development of spontaneous EAE in this TCR transgenic model have not yet been elucidated, although some evidence for a role for IL-10 has been obtained (142). As noted previously, the relationship of these CD4$^+$CD25$^-$ T cells to the CD4$^+$CD25$^+$ T-cell population is obscure, but it remains possible that CD4$^+$CD25$^-$ T cells are derived from CD4$^+$CD25$^+$ T cells. Some evidence for a protective role of CD4$^+$CD25$^+$ T cells in EAE has been obtained (143).

THERAPEUTIC MANIPULATION OF REGULATORY T-CELL FUNCTION

In this chapter, a number of distinct regulatory T-cell populations have been described, and their potential role in the regulation of the immune response in animal models of

disease has been reviewed. A large body of data supports the existence of CD4$^+$CD25$^+$ suppressor T cells in humans (29–36), and the *in vitro* characterization of human CD4$^+$CD25$^+$ T cells suggests that they are identical to their murine counterpart. Tr1 cells have been readily induced in cultures of human T cells, and a number of studies have supported the existence of cell populations with Tr1-like properties in humans (73,144,145). It is therefore appropriate to consider approaches to the modulation of regulatory T-cell function in humans as an adjunct to therapy of various diseases. The major question that must be addressed is whether more or less suppressor activity should be generated.

Therapeutic Down-regulation of Suppressor T-Cell Function

Because tumor antigens are most often autoantigens, the down-regulation of suppressor T cell function should result in enhanced immune responses to tumor cell vaccines. As previously stated, depletion of CD4$^+$CD25$^+$ T cells alone or combined with anti–CTLA-4 administration to enhance effector T cell function has resulted in potent antitumor immune responses in a mouse model. The only humanized anti-CD25 mAb approved for human use is nondepleting, and it blocks the binding of IL-2 to CD25 (146). It has proved efficacious in the treatment of autoimmune diseases such as uveitis and in preventing acute allograft rejection by blocking the utilization of IL-2 by effector T cells. The Fc fragment of this mAb could be modified so as to generate a depleting antibody. CD25 depletion could also be used in conjunction with poorly immunogenic vaccines as therapy for infectious agents such as human immunodeficiency virus, mycobacteria, or parasites. Although complete depletion of CD25$^+$ T cells may facilitate a vigorous immune response to an infectious agent that ultimately results in complete sterilization, the studies of the role of CD4$^+$CD25$^+$ T cells in infection by *L. major* also demonstrate a beneficial effect of regulatory T cells that is related to the persistence of a low level of chronic infection needed for long-lasting protective immunity. CD4$^+$CD25$^+$ T cells also play an important role in the modulation of the acute inflammatory response that is an integral part of the response to an infectious agent. In the absence of immunoregulatory T cells, the consequences of this exuberant response can be deleterious.

Studies in relatively young mice have indicated that depletion of CD4$^+$CD25$^+$ T cells is not permanent (109). Depending on the reagent, protocol, and age of the treated mouse, new CD4$^+$CD25$^+$ T cells begin to emigrate from the thymus and repopulate peripheral lymphoid tissues 2 to 4 weeks after cessation of therapy. No information is available on the output of CD4$^+$CD25$^+$ T cells from the thymus during adult life in mice or humans. Because the thymic output of the entire CD4$^+$ T-cell population decreases to low levels in humans older than 20, antibody-mediated depletion of CD25$^+$ T cells may be permanent in adult humans. It is possible only to speculate on negative effects of permanent depletion of CD25$^+$

T cells, but even in the mouse, depletion of CD4$^+$CD25$^+$ T cells does not usually result in the rapid development of autoimmune diseases. The autoreactive effector T cells need additional signals to become activated (109).

If future studies successfully define the cell surface molecules on CD4$^+$CD25$^+$ T cells that deliver the suppressive signal to the CD4$^+$CD25$^-$ responder cell, then an antibody to this molecule might be the ideal reagent for transiently inhibiting suppressor cell activity, facilitating immune responses to weak antigens. This interaction could also be targeted by small molecules. An alternative approach to the down-modulation of suppressor T cell function might be to target the GITR–GITR ligand interaction as means of inhibiting the function of CD4$^+$CD25$^+$ T cells. The simplest approach would be to inhibit suppressor function *in vivo* with an agonist anti-GITR antibody. Shimizu et al. (41) were able to induce AIG by repeated treatment of young BALB/c mice with a mAb to the GITR. A soluble GITR ligand–Fc fragment reagent might also have similar agonistic properties.

Therapeutic Approaches to Enhancement of Regulatory T-Cell Function

One common theme that has been discussed in this chapter is that the function or numbers of many types of regulatory T cells can be enhanced by antigenic stimulation under tolerogenic conditions: that is, with APCs that express low levels of co-stimulatory/adhesion molecules. Indeed, some of the therapeutic effects of blocking co-stimulation with anti-CD80/CD86 or CTLA-4 immunoglobulin may be secondary to the enhancement of regulatory T cell function. One of the roles of the suppressor cytokines IL-10 and TGF-β may be to down-regulate co-stimulation and thereby facilitate the activation of regulatory T cells. The production of these suppressor cytokines by regulatory T cells themselves may function in a positive feedback loop to generate more regulatory T cells.

Enhancement of either the numbers or the function of regulatory T cells represents a goal for the treatment of autoimmune and allergic diseases as well as for inhibition of allograft rejection. Either CD4$^+$CD25$^+$ T cells or Tr1 T cells might be expanded to generate sufficient numbers of cells for infusion back into patients. It has proved to be exceedingly difficult to grow either of these cells types in tissue culture. Although some modest growth is seen by stimulation with anti-CD3 in the presence of IL-2, other cytokines in combination with IL-2 might result in greater yields. IL-15 has been shown to enhance the growth of Tr1 cells (77). Ultimately, further studies of the molecular basis of their nonresponsiveness should yield important information that might facilitate their growth. For example, inhibition of the function of members of the SOCS family may be needed to achieve this goal. Because the GITR–GITR ligand interaction inhibits suppressor function, blocking this interaction with anti–GITR ligand might also enhance the activity of CD4$^+$CD25$^+$ T cells. If CD4$^+$CD25$^+$ T cells recognize organ-specific antigens, and

if these antigens can be identified, it may be possible to generate lines or clones of antigen-specific suppressor T cells *in vitro* that could be used therapeutically. These cells would home to the target organ and be activated by their target autoantigen but would mediate bystander suppression, because their effector function would be nonspecific.

REFERENCES

1. Schwartz RH. A cell culture model for T lymphocyte clonal anergy. *Science* 1990;248:1349–1356.
2. Miller JFAP, Heath WR. Self-ignorance in the peripheral T-cell pool. *Immunol Rev* 1993;133:131–150.
3. Gershon RK, Kondo K. Cell interactions in the induction of tolerance: the role of thymic lymphocytes. *Immunology* 1970;18:723–735.
4. Gershon RK, Kondo K. Infectious immunological tolerance. *Immunology* 1971;21:903–914.
5. Baker PJ, Barth RF, Stashak PW, et al. Enhancement of the antibody response to type III pneumococcal polysaccharide in mice treated with anti-lymphocyte serum. *J Immunol* 1970;104;1313–1315.
6. Tada T, Taniguchi M, Okumura K. Regulation of homocytotropic antibody response in the rat. II. Effect of x-irradiation. *J Immunol* 1971;106:1012–1018.
7. Okumura K, Tada T. Regulation of homocytotropic antibody in the rat. VI. Inhibitory effect of thymocytes on homocytotropic antibody response. *J Immunol* 1971;107:1682–1689.
8. Dorf ME, Benacerraf B. I-J as a restriction element in the suppressor cell system. *Immunol Rev* 1985;83:23–40.
9. Tada T, Okumura O. The role of antigen-specific T cell factors in the immune response. *Adv Immunol* 1979;28:1–87.
10. Germain RN, Benacerraf B. A single major pathway of T-lymphocyte interactions in antigen-specific immune suppression. *Scand J Immunol* 1981;13:1–10.
11. Green DR, Flood PM, Gershon RK. Immunoregulatory T-cell pathways. *Annu Rev Immunol* 1983;1:439–463.
12. Dorf ME, Benacerraf B. Suppressor cells and immunoregulation. *Annu Rev Immunol* 1984;2:127–158.
13. Murphy DB. The I-J puzzle. *Annu Rev Immunol* 1987;5:405–427.
14. Hedrick SM, Germain RN, Bevan MJ, et al. Rearrangement and transcription of a T-cell receptor β-chain gene in different T-cell subsets. *Proc Natl Acad Sci U S A* 1985;82:531–535.
15. Nishizuka Y, Sakakura T. Thymus and reproduction: sex-linked dysgenesia of the gonad after neonatal thymectomy in mice. *Science* 1969;166:753–755.
16. Sakaguchi S, Sakaguchi N. Thymus, T cells, and autoimmunity: various causes but a common mechanism of autoimmune disease. In: Coutinho A, Kazatchkine K, eds. *Autoimmunity: physiology and disease.* Wiley-Liss, 1994:203–227.
17. Penhale WJ, Farmer A, Irvine WJ. Thyroiditis in T cell-depleted rats: influence of strain, radiation dose, adjuvants and antilymphocyte serum. *Clin Exp Immunol* 1975;21:362–375.
18. Penhale WJ, Irvine WJ, Inglis JR, Farmer, A. Thyroiditis in T cell-depleted rats: suppression of the autoallergic response by reconstitution with normal lymphoid cells. *Clin Exp Immunol* 1976;25:6–16.
19. Penhale WJ, Stumbles PA, Huxtable CR, et al. Induction of diabetes in PVG/c strain rats by manipulation of the immune system. *Autoimmunity* 1990;7:169–179.
20. Sakaguchi S, Fukuma K, Kuribayashi K, et al. Organ-specific autoimmune diseases induced in mice by elimination of T cell subset. I. Evidence for the active participation of T cells in natural self-tolerance; deficit of a T cell subset as a possible cause of autoimmune disease. *J Exp Med* 1985;161:72–87.
21. Sakaguchi S, Sakaguchi N, Asano M, et al. Immunologic self-tolerance maintained by activated T cells expressing IL-2 receptor α-chains (CD25). *J Immunol* 1995;155:1151–1164.
22. Asano M, Toda M, Sakaguchi N, et al. Autoimmune disease as a consequence of developmental abnormality of a T cell subpopulation. *J Exp Med* 1996;184:387–396.
23. Suri-Payer E, Amar AZ, Thornton AM, et al. CD4$^+$CD25$^+$ T cells inhibit both the induction and effector function of autoreactive T cells

and represent a unique lineage of immunoregulatory cells. *J Immunol* 1998;160:1212–1218.

24. Powrie F, Mason D. OX-22^{high}CD4$^+$ T cells induce wasting disease with multiple organ pathology: prevention by the OX-22^{low} subset. *J Exp Med* 1990;172:1701–1708.

25. Fowell D, Mason D. Evidence that the T cell repertoire of normal rats contains cells with the potential to cause diabetes. Characterization of the CD4$^+$ T cell subset that inhibits this autoimmune potential. *J Exp Med* 1993;177:627–636.

26. Powrie F, Leach MW, Mauze S, et al. Phenotypically distinct subsets of CD4$^+$ T cells induce or protect from chronic intestinal inflammation in C.B-17 scid mice. *Int Immunol* 1993;5:1461–1471.

27. Read S, Malmstrom V, Powrie F. Cytotoxic T lymphocyte–associated antigen 4 plays an essential role in the function of CD25$^+$CD4$^+$ regulatory cells that control intestinal inflammation. *J Exp Med* 2000; 192:295–302.

28. Itoh M, Takahashi T, Sakaguchi N, et al. Thymus and autoimmunity: production of CD25$^+$CD4$^+$ naturally anergic and suppressive T cells as a key function of the thymus in maintaining immunologic self-tolerance. *J Immunol* 1999;162:5317–5326.

29. Baecher-Allan C, Brown JA, Freeman GJ, et al. CD4$^+$CD25^{high} regulatory cells in human peripheral blood. *J Immunol* 2001;167:1245–1253.

30. Stephens LA, Mottet C, Mason D, et al. Human CD4$^+$CD25$^+$ thymocytes and peripheral T cells have immune suppression activity. *Eur J Immunol* 2001;31:1247–1254.

31. Levings MK, Sangregorio R, Roncarolo MG. Human CD25$^+$CD4$^+$ T regulatory cells suppress naïve and memory T cell proliferation and can be expanded *in vitro* without loss of function. *J Exp Med* 2001; 193:1295–1301.

32. Jonuleit H, Schmitt E, Stassen M, et al. Identification and functional characterization of human CD4$^+$CD25$^+$ T cells with regulatory properties isolated from peripheral blood. *J Exp Med* 2001;193:1285–1294.

33. Dieckmann D, Plottner H, Berchtold S, et al. *Ex vivo* isolation and characterization of CD4$^+$CD25$^+$ T cells with regulatory properties from human blood. *J Exp Med* 2002;193:1303–1310.

34. Taams LA, Smith J, Rustin MH, et al. Human anergic/suppressive CD4$^+$CD25$^+$ T cells: a highly differentiated and apoptosis-prone population. *Eur J Immunol* 2001;31;1122–1131.

35. Ng WF, Duggan PJ, Ponchel F, et al. Human CD4$^+$CD25$^+$ cells: a naturally occurring population of regulatory T cells. *Blood* 2001;98:2736–2744.

36. Stephens LA, Mason D. CD25 is a marker for CD4$^+$ thymocytes that prevent autoimmune diabetes in rats, but peripheral T cells with this function are found in both CD25$^+$ and CD25$^-$ subpopulations. *J Immunol* 2001;165:3105–3110.

37. Thornton AM, Shevach EM. CD4$^+$CD25$^+$ immunoregulatory T cells suppress polyclonal T cell activation *in vitro* by inhibiting interleukin 2 production. *J Exp Med* 1998;188:287–296.

38. Salomon B, Lenschow DJ, Rhee L, et al. B7/CD28 costimulation is essential for the homeostasis of the CD4$^+$CD25$^+$ immunoregulatory T cells that control autoimmune diabetes. *Immunity* 12:431–440.

39. Takahashi T, Tagami T, Yamazaki S, et al. Immunologic self-tolerance maintained by CD25$^+$CD4$^+$ regulatory T cells constitutively expressing cytotoxic T lymphocyte–associated antigen 4. *J Exp Med* 2000; 192:303–309.

40. McHugh RS, Whitters MJ, Piccirillo CA, et al. CD4$^+$CD25$^+$ immunoregulatory T cells: gene expression analysis reveals a functional role for the glucocorticoid-induced TNF receptor. *Immunity* 2002; 16:311–323.

41. Shimizu J, Yamazaki S, Takahashi T, et al. Stimulation of CD25$^+$CD4$^+$ regulatory T cells through GITR breaks immunological self-tolerance. *Nat Immunol* 2002;3:135–142.

42. Shevach EM. Certified professionals: CD4$^+$CD25$^+$ suppressor T cells. *J Exp Med* 2001;193:F41–F45.

43. Takahashi T, Kuniyasu Y, Toda M, et al. Immunologic self-tolerance maintained by CD25$^+$CD4$^+$ naturally anergic and autoimmune disease by breaking their anergic/suppressive state. *Int Immunol* 1998; 10:1969–1980.

44. Read S, Mauze S, Asseman C, et al. CD38$^+$CD45RB^{low} T cells: a population of T cells with immune regulatory activities *in vitro*. *Eur J Immunol* 1998;28:3434–3447.

45. Thornton AM, Shevach EM. Suppressor effector function of CD4$^+$

46. Gavin MA, Clarke SR, Negrou E, et al. Homeostasis and anergy of CD4$^+$CD25$^+$ suppressor T cells *in vivo*. *Nat Immunol* 2002;3:33–41.

47. Palacios R, Moller G. T cell growth factor abrogates concanavalin A–induced suppressor cell function. *J Exp Med* 1981;153:1360–1365.

48. Piccirillo CA, Shevach EM. Cutting edge: control of CD8$^+$ T cell activation by CD4$^+$CD25$^+$ immunoregulatory cells. *J Immunol* 2000; 167:1137–1140.

49. Ermann J, Szanya V, Ford GS, et al. CD4$^+$CD25$^+$ T cells facilitate the induction of T cell anergy. *J Immunol* 2001;4271–4275.

50. Cederbom L, Hall H, Ivers F. CD4$^+$CD25$^+$ regulatory T cells down-regulate co-stimulatory molecules on antigen presenting cells. *Eur J Immunol* 2000;30:1538–1543.

51. Nakamura K, Kitani A, Strober W. Cell contact–dependent immunosuppression by CD4$^+$CD25$^+$ regulatory T cells is mediated by cell surface–bound transforming growth factor β. *J Exp Med* 2001; 194:629–644.

52. Piccirillo CA, Letterio JJ, Thornton AM, et al. CD4$^+$CD25$^+$ regulatory T cells can mediate suppressor function in the absence of transforming growth factor β1 production and responsiveness. *J Exp Med* 2002;196:1–10.

53. Yamagiwa S, Gray JD, Hashimoto S, et al. A role of TGF-β in the generation and expansion of CD4$^+$CD25$^+$-regulatory T cells from human peripheral blood. *J Immunol* 2001;166:7282–7289.

54. Dieckmann D, Bruett CH, Ploettner H, et al. Human CD4$^+$CD25$^+$ regulatory, contact-dependent T cells induce interleukin 10–producing, contact-independent type 1–like regulatory T cells. *J Exp Med* 2002: 196:247–253.

55. Jonuleit H, Schmitt E, Kakirman H, et al. Infectious tolerance: human CD25$^+$ regulatory T cells convey suppressor activity to conventional CD4$^+$ T helper cells. *J Exp Med* 2002;196:255–260.

56. Modigliani Y, Coutinho A, Pereira P, et al. Establishment of tissue-specific tolerance is driven by regulatory T cells selected by thymic epithelium. *Eur J Immunol* 1996;26:1807–1815.

57. Papiernik M, de Moraes ML, Pontoux C, et al. Regulatory CD4 T cells: expression of IL-2Rα chain, resistance to clonal deletion and IL-2 dependency. *Int Immunol* 1998;10:371–378.

58. Jordan MS, Boesteanu A, Reed AJ, et al. Thymic selection of CD4$^+$CD25$^+$ regulatory T cells induced by an agonist self-peptide. *Nat Immunol* 2001;2:301–306.

59. Bensinger SJ, Bandeira A, Jordan MS, et al. Major histocompatibility complex class II–positive cortical epithelium mediates the selection of CD4$^+$25$^+$ immunoregulatory T cells. *J Exp Med* 2001;194:427–438.

60. Apostolou I, Sarukhan A, Klein L, et al. Origin of regulatory T cells with known specificity for antigen. *Nat Immunol* 2002;3:756–763.

61. Romagnoli P, Hudrisier D, van Meerwijk JPM. Preferential recognition of self-antigens despite normal thymic deletion of CD4$^+$CD25$^+$ regulatory T cells. *J Immunol* 2002;168:1644–1648.

62. Pacholczyk P, Kraj P, Ignatowicz L. Peptide specificity of thymic selection of CD4$^+$CD25$^+$ T cells. *J Immunol* 2002:168:613–620.

63. Kumanogoh A, Wang X, Lee I, et al. Increased T cell autoreactivity in the absence of CD40–CD40 ligand interactions: a role of CD40 in regulatory T cell development. *J Immunol* 2001;166:353–360.

64. Singh B, Read S, Asseman C, et al. Control of inflammation by regulatory T cells. *Immunol Rev* 2001;182:190–200.

65. Malek TR, Yu A, Vincek V, et al. CD4 regulatory T cells prevent lethal autoimmunity in IL-2Rβ–deficient mice: implications for the nonredundant function of IL-2. *Immunity* 2002;17:167–178.

66. Kagami S-I, Nakajima H, Suto A, et al. Stat5a regulates T helper cell differentiation by several distinct mechanisms. *Blood* 2001;97:2358–2365.

67. Green EA, Choi Y, Flavell RA. Pancreatic lymph node–derived CD4$^+$CD25$^+$ Treg cells: highly potent regulators of diabetes that require TRANCE-RANK signals. *Immunity* 2002;16:183–191.

68. Zelenika D, Adams E, Humm S, et al. Regulatory T cells overexpress a subset of Th2 gene transcripts. *J Immunol* 2002;168:1069–1079.

69. Weiner HL, Friedman A, Miller A, et al. Oral tolerance: immunological mechanisms and treatment of animal and human organ-specific autoimmune diseases by oral administration of autoantigens. *Annu Rev Immunol* 1994;12:809–837.

70. Chen Y, Kuchroo VK, Inobe J-I, et al. Regulatory T cell clones induced by oral tolerance: suppression of autoimmune encephalomyelitis. *Science* 1994:265:1237–1240.

CD25$^+$ immunoregulatory T cells is antigen nonspecific. *J Immunol* 2000;164:183–190.

71. Weiner HL. The mucosal milieu creates tolerogenic dendritic cells and T_R1 and T_H3 regulatory cells. *Nat Immunol* 2001;2:671–672.

72. Akbari O, DeKruyff RH, Umetsu DT. Pulmonary dendritic cells producing IL-10 mediate tolerance induced by respiratory exposure to antigen. *Nat Immunol* 2001;2:725–731.

73. Bacchetta R, Bigler M, Touraine J-L, et al. High levels of interleukin 10 production *in vivo* are associated with tolerance in SCID patients transplanted with HLA mismatched hematopoietic stem cells. *J Exp Med* 1994;179:493–502.

74. Roncarolo MG, Bacchetta R, Bordignon C, et al. Type 1 regulatory cells. *Immunol Rev* 2001;182:68–79.

75. Zeller JC, Panoskaltsis-Mortari A, Murphy WJ, et al. Induction of CD4+ T cell alloantigen–specific hyporesponsiveness by IL-10 and TGF-β. *J Immunol* 1999;163:3684–3691.

76. Groux H, O'Garra A, Bigler M, et al. A CD4+ T-cell subset inhibits antigen-specific T-cell responses and prevents colitis. *Nature* 1997; 389:737–742.

77. Levings MK, Sangregorio R, Galbiati F, et al. INF-α and IL-10 induce the differentiation of human type 1 T regulatory cells. *J Immunol* 2001;166:5530–5539.

78. Cottrez F, Hurst SD, Coffman RL, et al. T regulatory cells 1 inhibit a TH2-specific response *in vivo*. *J Immunol* 2000;165:4848–4853.

79. Barrat FJ, Cua DJ, Boonstra A, et al. *In vitro* generation of interleukin 10–producing regulatory CD4+ T cells is induced by immunosuppressive drugs and inhibited by T helper type 1 (Th1)– and Th2-inducing cytokines. *J Exp Med* 2002;195:603–616.

80. Gregori S, Casorati M, Amuchastegui S, et al. Regulatory T cells induced by 1α,25-dihydroxyvitamin D_3 and mycophenolate mofetil treatment mediate transplantation tolerance. *J Immunol* 2001;167: 1945–1953.

81. Jonuleit H, Schmitt E, Schuler G, et al. Induction of interleukin 10–producing, nonproliferating CD4+ T cells with regulatory properties by repetitive stimulation with allogeneic immature human dendritic cells. *J Exp Med* 2000;192:1213–1222.

82. Lombardi G, Sidhu S, Batchelor R, et al. Anergic T cells as suppressor cells *in vitro*. *Science* 1994;264:1587–1589.

83. Chai J-G, Bartok I, Chandler P, et al. Anergic T cells act as suppressor cells *in vitro* and *in vivo*. *Eur J Immunol* 1999;29:686–692.

84. Vendetti S, Chai J-G, Dyson J, et al. Anergic T cells inhibit the antigen-presenting function of dendritic cells. *J Immunol* 2000;165:1175–1181.

85. Frasca L, Scotta C, Lombardi G, et al. Human anergic CD4+ T cells can act as suppressor cells by affecting autologous dendritic cell conditioning and survival. *J Immunol* 2002;168:1060–1068.

86. Taams LS, Boot EPJ, van Eden W, et al. Anergic T cells modulate the T-cell activating capacity of antigen-presenting cells. *J Autoimmun* 2000;14:335–341.

87. Thorstenson KM, Khoruts A. Generation of anergic and potentially immunoregulatory CD25+CD4+ T cells *in vivo* after induction of peripheral tolerance with intravenous or oral antigen. *J Immunol* 2001; 167:188–195.

88. Zhang X, Izikson L, Liu L, et al. Activation of CD25+CD4+ regulatory T cells by oral antigen administration. *J Immunol* 2001;167:4245–4253.

89. Taams LS, Vukmanovic-Stejic M, Smith J, et al. Antigen-specific T cell suppression by CD4+CD25+ regulatory T cells. *Eur J Immunol* 2002; 32:1621–1630.

90. Gleeson PA, Toh B-H, van Driel IR. Organ-specific autoimmunity induced by lymphopenia. *Immunol Rev* 1996;149:97–126.

91. Suri-Payer E, Amar AZ, McHugh R, et al. Post-thymectomy autoimmune gastritis: fine specificity and pathogenicity of anti-H/K ATPase–reactive T cells. *Eur J Immunol* 1999;29:669–677.

92. McHugh RS, Shevach EM, Thornton AM. Control of organ-specific autoimmunity by immunoregulatory CD4+CD25+ T cells. *Microbes Infect* 2001;3:919–927.

93. Suri-Payer E, Cantor H. Differential cytokine requirements for regulation of autoimmune gastritis and colitis by CD4+CD25+ T cells. *J Autoimmun* 2001;16:115–123.

94. Powrie F, Leach MW, Mauze S, et al. Inhibition of TH1 responses prevents inflammatory bowel disease in scid mice reconstituted with CD45RBhi T cells. *Immunity* 1994;1:553–562.

95. Asseman C, Mauze S, Leach MW, et al. An essential role for interleukin 10 in the function of regulatory T cells that inhibit intestinal inflammation. *J Exp Med* 1999;190:995–1003.

96. Powrie F, Carlino J, Leach MW, et al. A critical role for transforming factor-β but not interleukin 4 in the suppression of T helper 1–mediated colitis by CD45RBlowCD4+ T cells. *J Exp Med* 1996;183:2669–2674.

97. Malmstrom V, Shipton D, Singh B, et al. CD134L expression on dendritic cells in the mesenteric lymph nodes drives colitis in T cell restored SCID mice. *J Immunol* 2001;166:6972–6981.

98. Seddon B, Mason D. Regulatory T cells in the control of autoimmunity: the essential role of transforming growth factor β and interleukin 4 in the prevention of autoimmune thyroiditis in rats by peripheral CD4+CD45RC− cells and CD4+CD8− thymocytes. *J Exp Med* 1999;189:279–288.

99. Delovitch TL, Singh B. The non-obese diabetic mouse as a model of autoimmune diabetes: immune dysregulation gets the NOD. *Immunity* 1997;7:727–738.

100. Chatenoud L, Salomon B, Bluestone JA. Suppressor T cells—they're back and critical for regulation of autoimmunity! *Immunol Rev* 2001; 182:149–163.

101. Taguchi O, Nishizuka Y. Self-tolerance and localized autoimmunity. Mouse models of autoimmune disease that suggest tissue-specific suppressor T cells are involved in self-tolerance. *J Exp Med* 1987;165:146–156.

102. Taguchi O, Kontani K, Ikeda H, et al. Tissue-specific suppressor T cells involved in self-tolerance are activated extrathymically by self-antigens. *Immunology* 1994;82:365–369.

103. Smith H, Lou Y-H, Lacy P, et al. Tolerance mechanism in experimental ovarian and gastric autoimmune diseases. *J Immunol* 1992;149:2212–2218.

104. McCullagh P. The significance of immune suppression in normal self-tolerance. *Immunol Rev* 1996;149:127–153.

105. Seddon B, Mason D. Peripheral autoantigen induces regulatory T cells that prevent autoimmunity. *J Exp Med* 1999;189:877–881.

106. Tung KSK, Agersborg SS, Alard P, et al. Regulatory T cell, endogenous antigen and neonatal environment in the prevention and induction of autoimmune disease. *Immunol Rev* 2001;182:135–148.

107. Bonomo A, Kehn PJ, Shevach EM. Post-thymectomy autoimmunity: abnormal T-cell homeostasis. *Immunol Today* 1995;16:61–66.

108. Stockinger B, Barthlott T, Kassiotis G. T cell regulation: a special job or everyone's responsibility. *Nat Immunol* 2001;2:757–759.

109. McHugh RS, Shevach EM. Cutting edge: depletion of CD4+CD25+ regulatory T cells is necessary, but not sufficient, for induction of organ-specific autoimmune diseases. *J Immunol* 2002;168:5979–5983.

110. Annacker O, Pimenta-Araujo R, Burlen-Defranoux O, et al. CD25+ CD4+ T cells regulate the expansion of peripheral CD4 T cells through the production of IL-10. *J Immunol* 2001;166:3008–3018.

111. Waldmann H, Cobbold S. Regulating the immune response to transplants. A role for CD4+ regulatory cells? *Immunity* 2001;14:399–406.

112. Hara M, Kingsley CI, Niimi M, et al. IL-10 is required for regulatory T cells to mediate tolerance to alloantigens *in vivo*. *J Immunol* 2001; 166:3789–3796.

113. Kingsley CI, Karim M, Bushell AR, et al. CD25+CD4+ regulatory T cells prevent graft rejection: CTLA-4– and IL-10–dependent immunoregulation of alloresponses. *J Immunol* 2002;168:1080–1086.

114. Graca L, Thompson S, Lin C-Y, et al. Both CD4+CD25+ and CD4+CD25− regulatory cells mediate dominant transplantation tolerance. *J Immunol* 2002;168:5558–5567.

115. Taylor PA, Panoskaltsis-Mortari A, Noelle RJ, et al. Analysis of the requirements for the induction of CD4+ T cell alloantigen hyporesponsiveness by *ex vivo* anti-CD40 ligand antibody. *J Immunol* 2000; 164:612–622.

116. Taylor PA, Noelle PJ, Blazar BR. CD4+CD25+ immune regulatory cells are required for induction of tolerance to alloantigen via costimulatory blockade. *J Exp Med* 2001;193:1311–1317.

117. Taylor PA, Lees CJ, Blazer BR. The infection of *ex vivo* activated and expanded CD4+CD25+ immune regulatory cells inhibits graft-vs-host disease (GVHD) lethality. *Blood* 2002;99:4601–4609.

118. North RJ, Bursuker I. Generation and decay of the immune response to a progressive fibrosarcoma. I. Ly-1+2− suppressor T cells down-regulate the generation of Ly-1−2+ effector T cells. *J Exp Med* 1984; 159:1295–1311.

119. Awwad M, North RJ. Immunologically mediated regression of a murine lymphoma after treatment with anti-L3T4 antibody. A consequence of

removing L3T4+ suppressor T cells from a host generating predominantly Lyt-2+ T cell–mediated immunity. *J Exp Med* 1988;168:2193–2206.

120. Onizuka S, Tawara I, Shimizu J, et al. Tumor rejection by *in vivo* administration of anti-CD25 (interleukin-2 receptor α) monoclonal antibody. *Cancer Res* 1999;59:3128–3133.

121. Shimizu J, Yamazaki S, Sakaguchi S. Induction of tumor immunity by removing CD25+CD4+ T cells: a common basis between tumor immunity and autoimmunity. *J Immunol* 1999;163:5211–5218.

122. Sutmuller RPM, van Duivenvoorde LM, van Elsas A, et al. Synergism of cytotoxic T lymphocyte–associated antigen 4 blockade and depletion of CD25+ regulatory T cells in antitumor therapy reveals alternative pathways for suppression of autoreactive cytotoxic T lymphocyte responses. *J Exp Med* 2001;194:823–832.

123. Woo EY, Yeh H, Chu CS, et al. Cutting edge: regulatory T cells from lung cancer patients directly inhibit autologous T cell proliferation. *J Immunol* 2002;168:4272–4276.

124. Coutinho A, Hori S, Carvalho T, et al. Regulatory T cells: the physiology of autoreactivity in dominant tolerance and "quality control" of immune responses. *Immunol Rev* 2001;182:89–98.

125. Hori S, Carvalho TL, Demengeot J. CD25+CD4+ regulatory T cells suppress CD4+ T cell–mediated pulmonary hyperinflammation driven by *Pneumocystis carinii* in immunodeficient mice. *Eur J Immunol* 2002;32:1282–1291.

126. Belkaid Y, Hoffmann KF, Mendez S, et al. The role of interleukin (IL)–10 in the persistence of *Leishmania major* in the skin after healing and the therapeutic potential of anti–IL-10 receptor antibody for sterile cure. *J Exp Med* 2001;194:1497–1506.

127. Belkaid Y, Piccirillo CA, Mendez S, et al. CD4+CD25+ immunoregulatory T lymphocytes control *Leishmania major* persistence and immunity. *Nature* 2002;420:502–507.

128. McGuirk P, McCann C, Mills KHG. Pathogen-specific T regulatory 1 cells induced in the respiratory tract by a bacterial molecule that stimulates interleukin 10 production by dendritic cells: a novel strategy for evasion of protective T helper type 1 responses by *Bordetella pertussis*. *J Exp Med* 2002;195:221–231.

129. MacDonald AJ, Duffy M, Brady MT, et al. CD4 T helper type 1 and regulatory T cells induced against the same epitopes on the core protein in hepatitis C virus–infected persons. *J Infect Dis* 2002;185:720–727.

130. Iwashiro M, Messer RJ, Peterson KE, et al. Immunosuppression by CD4+ regulatory T cells induced by chronic retroviral infection. *Proc Natl Acad Sci U S A* 2001;98:9226–9230.

131. Liu Z, Tugulea S, Cortesini R, et al. Specific suppression of T helper alloreactivity by all–MHC class I–restricted CD8+CD28− T cells. *Int Immunol* 1998;10:775–783.

132. Li J, Liu Z, Jiang S, et al. T suppressor lymphocytes inhibit NF-κB-mediated transcription of CD86 gene in APC. *J Immunol* 1999;163:6386–6392.

133. Chang CC, Ciubotariu R, Manavalan JS, et al. Tolerization of dendritic cells by T(S) cells: the crucial role of inhibitory receptors ILT3 and ILT4. *Nat Immunol* 2002;3:237–243.

134. Gilliet M, Liu Y-J. Generation of human CD8 T regulatory cells by CD40 ligand–activated plasmacytoid dendritic cells. *J Exp Med* 2002;195:695–704.

135. Dhodapkar MV, Steinman RM, Krasovsky J, et al. Antigen-specific inhibition of effector T cell function in humans after injection of immature dendritic cells. *J Exp Med* 2001;193:233–238.

136. Zhang Z-X, Yang L, Young KJ, et al. Identification of a previously unknown antigen-specific regulatory T cells and its mechanism of suppression. *Nat Med* 2000;6:782–789.

137. Ford MS, Young KJ, Zhang Z, et al. The immune regulatory function of lymphoproliferative double negative T cells *in vitro* and *in vivo*. *J Exp Med* 2002;196:261–267.

138. Lehuen A, Lantz O, Beaudoin L, et al. Overexpression of natural killer T cells protects Vα14-Jα281 transgenic nonobese diabetic mice against diabetes. *J Exp Med* 1998;188:1831–1839.

139. Hong S, Wilson MT, Serizawa I, et al. The natural killer T-cell ligand α-galactosylceramide prevents autoimmune diabetes in non-obese diabetic mice. *Nat Med* 2001;7:1052–1056.

140. Jahng AW, Maricic I, Pederson B, et al. Activation of natural killer T cells potentiates or prevents experimental autoimmune encephalomyelitis. *J Exp Med* 2001;194:1789–1799.

141. Olivares-Villagomez D, Wensky AK, Wang Y, et al. Repertoire requirements of CD4+ T cells that prevent spontaneous autoimmune encephalomyelitis. *J Immunol* 2000;164:5499–5507.

142. Furtado GC, Olivares-Villagomez D, Curotto de Lafaille MA, et al. Regulatory T cells in spontaneous autoimmune encephalomyelitis. *Immunol Rev* 2001;182:122–134.

143. Hori S, Haury M, Coutinho A, et al. Specificity requirements for selection and effector functions of CD25+4+ regulatory T cells in anti–myelin basic protein T cell receptor transgenic mice. *Proc Natl Acad Sci U S A* 2002;99:8213–8218.

144. Khoo UY, Proctor IE, Macpherson AJS. CD4+ T cell down-regulation in human intestinal mucosa. *J Immunol* 1997;158:3626–3634.

145. VanBuskirk AM, Burlingham WJ, Jankowska-Gan E, et al. Human allograft acceptance is associates with immune regulation. *J Clin Invest* 2000:106:145–155.

146. Nussenblatt RB, Fortin E, Schiffman R, et al. Treatment of noninfectious intermediate and posterior uveitis with the humanized anti-Tac mAb: A phase I/II clinical trial. *Proc Natl Acad Sci U S A* 1999;96:7462–7466.

CHAPTER 31

The Mucosal Immune System

Jiri Mestecky, Richard S. Blumberg, Hiroshi Kiyono, and Jerry R. McGhee

---

Mucosal Barrier
  Epithelial Cells · Mucosal Microbiota
Mucosal Antibodies
  Distribution of Immunoglobulin Isotypes · Structure of Secretory Immunoglobulin A · Function · Origin and Transport of Mucosal Immunoglobulins
Inductive and Effector Sites of the Mucosal Immune System
  Organization of the Mucosal Immune System · Inductive Sites · Effector Sites · B-Cell Compartment · T-Cell Compartment and Regulation of Mucosal
  Immune System · Mucosal Cytotoxic T Cells · Intraepithelial Lymphocytes · Mucosal Cell Trafficking and Homing
Mucosal Immune Responses
  Intestinal Infections and Immunizations · Nasal and Upper Respiratory Tract Immunization · Immune Responses in the Genital Tract · Other Immunization
  Sites · Mucosal Adjuvants and Antigen-Delivery Systems
Mucosal Tolerance
  Basic Concepts · Mechanisms for Mucosal Tolerance
Mucosal Immunopathology
  Immunoglobulin A Deficiency · Human Immunodeficiency Virus Type 1 Infection and the Mucosal Immune System · Inflammatory Bowel
  Disease · Mucosal Allergies
Acknowledgments
References

The most important source of stimulation of the entire immune system is the external environment, which comprises indigenous mucosal microbiota, potential pathogenic microorganisms, abundant food antigens, and allergens, all of which are encountered mainly at the vast surface areas of mucosal membranes. This enormous and highly variable antigenic load has resulted in a strategic distribution of cells involved in the uptake, processing, and presentation of antigens; production of antibodies; and cell-mediated defenses at the front line of attack: Mucosal tissues and associated secretory glands. Quantitative data concerning the distribution of phagocytic cells, T and B lymphocytes, and antibody-producing cells illustrate the point: Mucosal tissues, particularly those of the intestinal tract, contain more macrophages, plasma cells, and T cells than any other lymphoid tissue of the entire immune system.

Notwithstanding the global importance of systemically acquired infections such as malaria and neonatal tetanus, the great majority of infectious diseases worldwide, including approximately 80% to 90% of human immunodeficiency virus (HIV) infections, either directly afflicts or is acquired through mucosal surfaces of the gastrointestinal (GI), respiratory, and genital tracts. Consequently, innate and adoptive immune mechanisms operational at mucosal surfaces are of considerable importance to the protection and survival of an animal in a hostile environment. The induction of preventive and protective immune responses to mucosal infectious agents and to inert food antigens and environmental allergens that would limit their absorption is usually the most emphasized functional aspect of the mucosal immune system. However, revived interest in the induction of systemic unresponsiveness to antigens applied first by the mucosal route, so-called oral or nasal (mucosal) tolerance, has directed the attention of immunologists working in the field of autoimmunity, transplantation, and hypersensitivity to the exploitation of this fundamental principle. Although limited in its clinical success, the phenomenon of mucosal tolerance is an essential feature and a critical functional component that efficiently prevents and suppresses otherwise unavoidable overstimulation of the entire immune system by the most common environmental antigens primarily of food and indigenous bacterial origins. The enhancement of protective mucosal responses to infectious agents that is sought by vaccinologists and the desired suppression of systemic immune responses to autoantigens and transplantation antigens may seem paradoxical. However, such outcomes are not mutually exclusive because of the hierarchy in the quality of immune responses induced by mucosal immunization: Mucosal immunity manifested by the appearance of secretory *antibodies* and systemic tolerance evaluated by diminished *cell-mediated* responses may be induced concomitantly. Therefore, the fundamental objectives of the mucosal immune system—(a) containment of the vast onslaught of environmental antigens without compromised integrity of mucosal barriers and (b) prevention of overstimulation of the systemic compartment—are achieved by concerted interactions of lymphoid and nonlymphoid cells, particularly epithelial cells, and their respective products as a mucosal internet of communication. Thus, an orchestrated mucosal immune system consisting of innate immunity, including an array of pattern recognition receptors and antimicrobial products as well as secretory immunoglobulin A (S-IgA) antibodies and mucosal cytotoxic T cells (CTLs), adds additional layers of host defense.

MUCOSAL BARRIER

Epithelial Cells

The epithelium of the mucosal-associated lymphoid tissues of the lung, gut, genitourinary tract, and probably other areas have been clearly shown to play an active role in both innate and adaptive types of mucosal immunity (1). Because of the physical proximity of the epithelial cell to the external milieu and, therefore, the primary site of initial antigen exposure, the epithelial cell may be a central cell type in both defining the antigens with which the mucosal immune system is confronted and regulating the ultimate responses to these antigenic exposures. These immunological functions of the epithelium can be considered partly in the context of epithelial

barrier function, which, in turn, captures the concept that the epithelial barrier is more than just a physical entity: It is a highly integrated immunological process that emanates from the epithelial cell per se and the epithelial cell in collaboration with subjacent cellular elements of the mucosal-associated lymphoid tissues and probably microbial components in the lumen. Together, these interactions between the commensal microbiota of the intestine, epithelium, and subjacent parenchymal cells (fibroblasts and mesenchymal cells and their connective tissue substances) and hematopoietic cells [macrophages, dendritic cells (DCs), polymorphonuclear leukocytes, and lymphocytes] function together to defend against invasion from pathogenic microorganisms.

Innate Functions of Epithelium

The innate immune functions of the epithelium include those that are intrinsic to the epithelial cell itself and those extrinsic factors that function outside but are derived from the epithelial cell to provide local barrier function (Fig. 1). The intrinsic factors associated with the epithelium involved in barrier functions are those that directly contribute to creating a barrier to reduce the promiscuous uptake of antigens from the lumen. Antigens can cross the epithelial barrier by three potential mechanisms: cellular (uptake, processing, presentation of luminal antigens), transcellular (transcytotic delivery of macromolecules), and paracellular (delivery of antigens from the lumen to the subjacent lamina propria between adjacent epithelial cells) (1). Prevention of paracellular transport is through cell–cell interactions at the juncture between adjacent epithelial cells that is mediated by physical structures associated with the epithelium, including the tight junctions and the subjacent desmosomes and adherence junctions (2). The

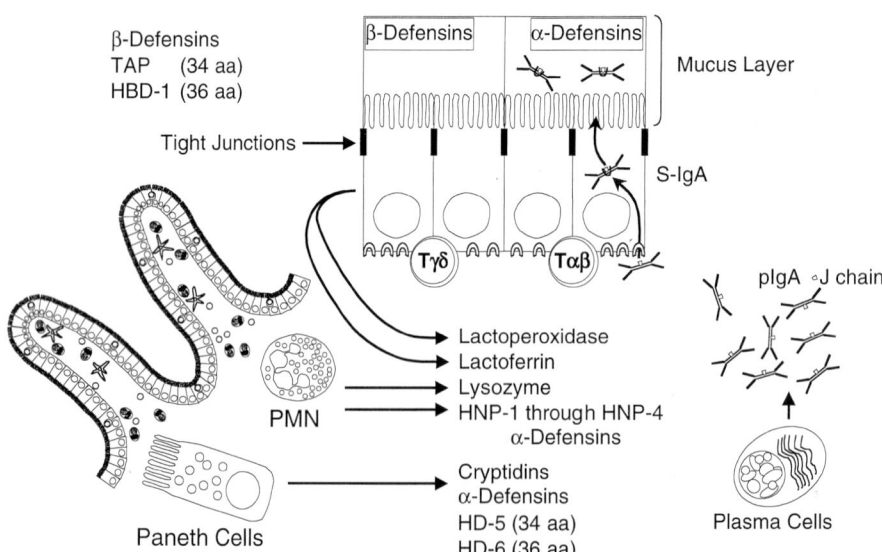

FIG. 1. Innate and antibody-mediated mucosal host defense mechanisms. Shown are soluble antimicrobial proteins lactoperoxidase, lactoferrin, and lysozyme, and the peptide defensins. Human neutrophil peptide (HNP) and Paneth cells in crypt regions produce α-defensins, whereas epithelial cells secrete β-defensins.

tight junctions are composed of a number of interacting cellular proteins, which include claudin, occludin, ZO-1, ZO-2, and cingulin, among others. Under normal circumstances, the tight junctions exclude antigens more than 6 to 12 Å($>$500 to 900 Da) in molecular diameter and are regulated by humoral factors associated with the immune system, growth factors, pharmacological agents, and bacterial toxins (3). As such, intrinsic barrier function as contributed by paracellular pathways, represents an immunologically regulated process. For example, cytokines such as transforming growth factor β (TGF-β), interleukin (IL)–10, and IL-15, increase paracellular resistance whereas proinflammatory cytokines such as interferon (IFN)–γ, IL-6, and tumor necrosis factor (TNF)–α diminish resistance. This has significant implications for understanding the pathogenesis of mucosal infection and inflammation, such as inflammatory bowel disease (IBD) and the possibility that the cytokine abnormalities defined in IBD model systems may have as their final common pathway effects on epithelial barrier function. Growth factors such as epidermal growth factor, fibroblast growth factor, hepatocyte growth factor, and intestinal trefoil factor peptides also regulate paracellular resistance through influencing the ability of epithelial cells to proliferate and repair physical defects in the barrier (4,5). In certain instances, these factors are derived from local immune cells and, in their absence, increase the susceptibility to infectious diseases and IBD (6).

The extrinsic barrier functions of the epithelium associated with innate immunity are those that arise from the ability of the epithelium to secrete a variety of factors into the lumen that are associated with resistance to invasion by pathogenic microorganisms. These secreted factors are either constitutively expressed or induced through the interaction of microbial factors with pattern recognition receptors, including the Toll-like receptor (TLR) family on the epithelium. However, because the epithelium exhibits immaturity in the absence of the normal commensal microbiota (7), it may be that all secreted factors from the epithelium associated with this type of innate immunity are induced through the interaction between components of the commensal microbiota and the epithelium. For example, lactobacilli species or activation of CD1d on epithelium is known to cause the secretion of IL-10 by epithelium, which is involved in paracrine regulation of barrier function (8,9). The epithelium also secretes the glycoproteins associated with the formation of intestinal mucus, complement components (including C3, C4, and factor B), a variety of antimicrobial peptides (including α-defensins and β-defensins), lysozyme, secretory phospholipase-A$_2$, lactoferrin, lactoperoxidase, and mucin, among others (10–14) (Fig. 1). The α-defensins secreted by intestinal epithelium are often called *cryptdins* to capture the fact that they are secreted primarily by a specialized type of epithelial cell, Paneth cells, within the intestinal crypt (15). The cryptdins, which exhibit significant homology to the defensins secreted by polymorphonuclear leukocytes, also exhibit potent and broad antimicrobicidal activity against a variety of pathogenic bacteria, including *Salmonella typhimurium* and *Listeria mono-*

cytogenes. Similarly, the human β-defensins 1 and 2, which also exhibit broad antimicrobial activity, are either constitutively expressed [human β-defensin 1 (hBD1)] or inducible by inflammatory cytokines such as IL-1 [human β-defensin 2 (hBD2)] (12). In addition, the epithelium is known to secrete peptide hormones with immunological function such as thyroid-stimulating hormone (TSH), which is important in regulation of conventional CD8$\alpha\beta^+$ T cells within the epithelium; nitrous oxide, through expression of constitutive and inducible nitric oxide synthetase; and a variety of prostaglandins, including prostaglandins E$_2$, D$_2$, F$_2\alpha$, and 6-keto-prostaglandin F$_1\alpha$ (1). Epithelial cells also directly contribute to barrier function through the secretion of a large number of chemokines and cytokines. Through the secretion of these soluble mediators, barrier function is enhanced by recruitment of other cell types: those that have potent antimicrobial activity (e.g., polymorphonuclear leukocytes) and those involved in adaptive immunity (e.g., macrophages, DCs, and T-lymphocytes) (16–18).

Thus, epithelial cells are considered a first line of defense, allowing for immediate responses and subsequent integration of downstream immunological events. The secretion of these factors is likely to be mediated initially in large part by interaction between components of microbes and pattern recognition receptors on the cell surface of the epithelium, which stimulate intracellular signals that initiate transcription of genes associated with the inflammatory cascade (19). Most prominent among these pattern recognition receptors that regulate innate immune responses of the epithelium is an array of TLRs. The TLRs have been appreciated to be expressed by epithelial cells and bind to microbial components such as bacterial lipopolysaccharide (LPS) of gram-negative bacteria (TLR-4), bacterial flagellin (TLR-5), microbial CpG motifs of deoxyribonucleic acid (DNA) (TLR-9), and lipoteichoic acids from gram-positive bacteria (TLR-3) (20). In the case of TLR-4, LPS recognition is coupled to CD14 binding of LPS, wherein LPS bound to CD14 interacts with a TL-4/MD-2 protein heterodimer. In the absence of CD14 expression by epithelial cells, CD14 might be provided by components within the lumen that contain, under certain circumstances (such as is the case in breast milk), soluble CD14 (21). The TLRs initiate intracellular signals that derive in a sequential manner from activation of myeloid differentiation marker 8 (MyD8), IL-1 receptor–associated kinase (IRAK), and TNF receptor–associated factor 6 (TRAF6), which culminate in nuclear translocation of activated NFκB. NFκB regulates both epithelial cell cycle and production of soluble mediators from the epithelium (22). As a result, epithelial cells are able to secrete a large number of chemokines in a temporally regulated manner, including IL-8, epithelial neutrophil activating peptide 78, growth-related oncogene α, macrophage inflammatory protein 1α, and monocyte chemoattractant protein, among others (16,17). Although, in general, it appears that production of these chemokines results largely from interactions between the epithelium and pathogenic microorganisms such as species of *Salmonella, Yersinia,* and *Shigella,* certain so-called commensal microbiota are probably able to do the same and, in addition, down-regulate the production of chemokines through regulation of NFκB pathways: for example, those induced by pathogenic microorganisms (23). In view of the enormous complexity of the microbial ecosystem, the final synthesis of these signals stimulated by ligation of pattern recognition receptors is likely to be complex but, presumably, ultimately integrated into providing a finely regulated first line of barrier function (7).

Cytokines and Cytokine Receptors

Epithelial cells are able to secrete a large number of inflammatory and regulatory cytokines both constitutively and inducibly. Through the use of epithelial cell lines, it has been shown that the epithelium can constitutively express proinflammatory cytokines such as IL-1α, IL-1β, IL-15, TNF-α, and IL-6 and anti-inflammatory and barrier-promoting cytokines such as TGF-β and IL-10, all of which may be further enhanced by interaction with pathogenic microorganisms and their toxic factors (24). The production of these cytokines by the epithelium probably plays an important role in promoting intestinal inflammation (e.g., IL-1 and TNF-α), regulating the activation and expansion of mucosal T cells within the epithelium (e.g., prostaglandin E, TSH, stem cell factor, IL-5, IL-7, and IL-15), regulating local B-cell production of immunoglobulins (e.g., TGF-β, IL-6, and IL-10), and, finally, regulating barrier function, per se (IL-10, IL-15, and TGF-β) (25,26). With regard to barrier function, epithelial cells also express a large number of cytokine receptors (27). Intestinal epithelial cell (IEC) lines and freshly isolated IECs express messenger ribonucleic acid (mRNA) for the common IL-2 receptor γ chain and specific α chains of the receptors for IL-2, IL-4, IL-7, IL-9, and IL-15. Epithelial cells also express receptors for TNF and IFN-γ, which not only regulate the expression of a wide variety of other immunologically important molecules, such as the polymeric immunoglobulin receptor (pIgR), but also tend to diminish epithelial barrier function. The expression of these cytokines and cytokine receptors thus further emphasizes the integration of the epithelium into the network of cellular interactions associated with the mucosa-associated lymphoid tissue. In this regard, bacterial infection can influence the interactions of IL-7/IL-7 receptor and IL-15/IL-15 receptor.

Transcellular Transport Functions of Epithelium

Another aspect of epithelial barrier function that represents a link between the epithelium and the adaptive components of the mucosa-associated lymphoid tissue is the ability of epithelium to transport macromolecules, especially immunoglobulins, transcellularly in a process termed *transcytosis,* which reflects the polarized nature of the epithelium. Two receptors for immunoglobulins have been shown to have such properties. The pIgR, whose itinerary is now well defined, transports polymeric immunoglobulins A and M (IgA and IgM) in a basal-to-apical direction with unloading of its cargo [S-IgA, polymeric IgA (pIgA), and IgM] in association with an extracellular proteolytic fragment of the pIgR receptor [secretory component (SC)] (28). This pathway not only is able to deliver large quantities of secretory immunoglobulins onto the mucosal surfaces but also is able to exclude antigens that have entered the secretory pathway either apically or basally (see later discussion). This type of defense, which takes advantage of a component of the adaptive immune response, is likely to be important in resistance against pathogenic viral infections. In a related but distinct manner, the epithelium also expresses the neonatal crystallized fragment (Fc) receptor for immunoglobulin G (FcRn). There is evidence that this molecule is expressed by adult human epithelium and macrophages of the intestine and, probably, other surfaces and is not strictly limited to neonatal life, as predicted by earlier studies in rodents wherein the FcRn was responsible for the passive acquisition of immunoglobulin G (IgG) neonatally (29,30). In the context of expression postnatally in adult humans, FcRn may therefore be in a position to provide luminal immunosurveillance against pathogenic exposure. FcRn binds IgG, its cargo, in a pH-dependent process (at a pH of 6, binding is on; at a pH of 7.4, binding is off) because of critical histine residues in the Fc-region of the IgG molecule. In contrast to the itinerary mediated by pIgR-associated transport, the transcytosis pathway associated with FcRn is bidirectional: both apical to basal and basal to apical (31). In addition, the FcRn does not require proteolytic cleavage, and this allows for reiterative rounds of transport. It is predicted, therefore, that the FcRn is at least in part responsible for the steady-state distribution of IgG on either side of an epithelial barrier, in view of the unlikely possibility that paracellular transport of this macromolecule results from the molecular exclusion of the tight junctions.

Adaptive Immune Functions of Epithelium

The epithelium is also likely to play an important role in adaptive immunity. The epithelium expresses a significant number of molecules in the cell surface that are associated with antigen presentation, leukocyte adhesion, and co-stimulation (Table 1) (32–43). Moreover, the intestinal epithelium and probably all epithelial cells associated with the mucosa-associated lymphoid tissue have residing at their basal surface distinct populations of intraepithelial lymphocytes (IELs), which are largely T cells, and of DCs (44,45). In view of the CD8$^+$ T-cell receptor (TCR) $\alpha\beta^+$ phenotype of most of these IELs, class I major histocompatibility complex (MHC)–related molecules are particularly likely to be especially important in these compartments, which raises a significant possibility that they have a major role in adaptive processes, in association with the epithelium, involving immunosurveillance of epithelial cell alterations and regulation of epithelial cell health. Under normal circumstances, the epithelium does not express classic co-stimulatory molecules such as CD80 and CD86, but it may do so, at least in the case of CD86,

TABLE 1. *Molecules associated with adaptive immunity on epithelium*

Molecules	Expression	References
Antigen-presenting molecules:		
HLA-class I/II	Basolateral > apical	35, 36
MICA/MICB	Apical > basolateral	37
CD1d	Apical > basolateral	38
HLA-E	ND	39
Co-stimulatory molecules:		
CD58	Basolateral	32
ICAM-1 (CD54)	Apical	40
CD40	ND	41
CEACAM1	Apical > basolateral	44
E-cadherin	Lateral	33
Receptors:		
FcRn	Apical > basolateral	30
pIgR	Basolateral > apical	27
DEC-205	ND	42
Ganglioside M1	Apical > basolateral	43

CEACAM1, carcinoembryonic antigen–related cell adhesion molecule 1; DEC- 205, dendritic cell receptor 205; FcRn, neonatal crystallized fragment receptor; HLA, human leukocyte antigen; ICAM, intracellular adhesion molecule; MICA, major histocompatibility complex (MHC) class IA; MICB, MHC class IB; ND, no data; pIgR, polymeric immunoglobulin receptor.

in the context of intestinal inflammation (46). On the other hand, the intestinal epithelium expresses a number of potential co-stimulatory molecules that, in certain circumstances, are functional. For example, lymphocyte function–associated antigen 3 (LFA-3), or CD58, is constitutively expressed on epithelial cells *in vivo* and *in vitro*, is up-regulated in response to inflammation, and may provide crucial co-stimulatory signals to mucosal T cells through its ligand, CD2, which is constitutively expressed on mucosal T cells (32,47). In general, mucosal T cells have down-regulated TCR/CD3 complex-mediated signaling but preserve signaling through CD58-CD2 pathways (33). The epithelial molecule E-cadherin, which is expressed in association with the tight junctions on the lateral surface of the epithelial cell, binds to the mucosal integrin, $\alpha^E\beta_7$, and provides important co-stimulatory signals to intestinal IEL, which are largely $\alpha^E\beta_7{}^+$ (34). Interestingly, mucosal T cells are also largely CD28⁻, especially the CD8⁺ cells within the epithelium (44). This raises the possibility that other molecules that are expressed on activated IELs, such as carcinoembryonic antigen–related cell adhesion molecule 1 (CEACAM1) (CD66a or biliary glycoprotein), may provide, through homophilic interactions with CEACAM1 on the epithelium, crucial positive and negative co-stimulatory signals (48).

Significant evidence also exists in support of a role for IECs in direct presentation of antigens, probably nonclassically in the absence of typical co-stimulatory molecules as described previously. Studies in *in vitro* model systems and in transgenic animal systems have provided evidence for class I, class II, and nonclassical class I MHC–restricted presentation to mucosal T cells. Expression of ovalbumin as a transgene under control of an IEC-specific promoter, for example, has allowed for the direct *in vivo* demonstration that IECs can present antigens to CD8⁺ transgenic T cells expressing TCRs

restricted to MHC class I (49). Similarly, direct evidence has been provided on both freshly isolated IECs from rodent intestine and transfected epithelial cell lines to present a soluble antigen in a class II MHC–restricted manner (35). Such presentation by class II MHC exhibits polarity with primarily apical uptake of antigen and basal presentation under normal noninflammatory conditions and with both basal uptake and basal presentation in inflammatory conditions, such as in the context of IFN-γ or up-regulation of the class II MHC machinery through expression of the class II MHC transactivator (CIITA) (36,50). This suggests that class II MHC–restricted presentation by epithelium may reveal novel epitopes during pathological conditions. Finally, nonclassical class I MHC–restricted presentation has been described in epithelium. IECs express CD1d constitutively, which is in turn regulated by IFN-γ, as are the classical class I and II MHC molecules (51). CD1d on intestinal epithelium can present model glycolipid antigens such as α-galactosylceramide to model natural killer (NK) T-cell clones; presentation is predominantly basal, which is consistent with the localization of CD1d-restricted T cells to this site (52). Low numbers of CD1d-restricted NK T cells have been defined in the epithelium with CD1d tetramers (52). Expression of other nonclassical class I MHC molecules on epithelium has, on the other hand, been directly linked to novel forms of co-stimulation. For example, expression of human leukocyte antigen (HLA)–E on the epithelium is associated with ligation of killer inhibitory-related receptors (CD94/NKG2) on activated mucosal T cells in human (53), and expression of the thymus leukemia antigen on rodent epithelium has been linked to ligation of CD8αα expressed on a subset of IELs that deliver a growth-promoting signal to these cells (54). In all cases in which antigen presentation has been described in the epithelium, it may be suggested that, in view of the predominant memory phenotype of mucosal T cells associated with the epithelium, the major role of these pathways is to either promote or regulate the activity of effector responses for the purposes of regional immunoregulation and surveillance for the benefit of both maintaining and repairing/restituting the barrier, including removal of epithelial cells altered as a consequence of infection, toxic exposures, or neoplastic transformation.

Mucosal Microbiota

Mucosal surfaces of the oral cavity, GI tract, genital tract, upper respiratory tract, and conjunctiva are populated by a large number of bacteria of more than 200 species with a characteristic distribution (55). The mucosal microbiota comprise approximately 10^{14} microorganisms, present mostly in the large intestine. In view of the relative numbers of host's eukaryotic cells and prokaryotic microorganisms, it is estimated that the mucosal microbiota outnumbers mammalian host cells by a factor of 10. Mutually beneficial coexistence of the mucosal microbiota with the effective mucosal immune system is one of the most interesting problems of mucosal immunology. Although the innate and specific immune factors present in mucosal secretions and tissues may limit the adherence of bacteria to mucosal epithelial cells and prevent penetration of such bacteria into the mucosal tissues with subsequent systemic dissemination, mucosal microbiota continue to survive with remarkable tenacity in the presence of an immune response manifested by corresponding antibodies (56). As a matter of fact, oral, intestinal, and probably other mucosal bacteria are coated *in vivo* with antibodies, particularly of the IgA isotype, that may prevent their adherence to the epithelial receptors but do not significantly interfere with their elimination and metabolism (57). Furthermore, it has been speculated that the long-lasting exposure of the mucosal immune system to such enormous numbers of bacteria may have resulted in diminished responsiveness to at least some microbial antigens (58).

The presence of mucosal microbiota has a profound influence on the evolution and functionality of the immune system. As evidenced by a large number of studies performed on gnotobiotic (germ-free) animals, the development of both mucosal and systemic lymphoid tissues and of the ensuing ability to respond to environmental antigens is, to a large extent, dependent on the previous exposure to mucosal microbiota (59). Specifically, in comparison to the lymphoid tissues of conventionally reared animals, those of germ-free animals are hypotrophic, lack well-developed germinal centers, display minute numbers of mucosal plasma cells, and respond poorly to mitogens and polyclonal stimulants. Upon colonization with even a few representative species of mucosal microbiota, a prompt development of lymphoid tissues and restoration of responsiveness to a plethora of antigens and other stimuli ensue. Of importance is that the development and responsiveness of both humoral and cell-mediated compartments of the immune system are profoundly affected by the mucosal microbiota, as documented by the presence

and numbers of B cells and ultimately antibody-forming cells in mucosal and nonmucosal tissues, the levels of mucosal and plasma antibodies, and T cells of various phenotypes in the IEL and lamina propria compartments of mucosal tissues and in the systemic secondary lymphoid tissues. In addition to immunologically effective microbial cell components (e.g., bacterial LPS), products generated as a result of fermentation by mucosal bacteria, such as butyric acid, are important sources of energy and carbon for IEC, which thus further stressing the immunological and physiological interdependence of the host on the mucosal microbiota (55).

Quantitative and Qualitative Aspects of Mucosal Microbiota

Quantitative data concerning the distribution of indigenous microbiota among mucosal surfaces of the oral cavity, conjunctiva, and upper respiratory, genital, and GI tracts indicate that of approximately 10^{14} bacteria, 99.9% are present in the large intestine (55). In this locale, bacteria are found free in the lumen and in feces, bound to the desquamated epithelial cells, entrapped in the mucus layer, and deep in intestinal crypts. Despite the inherent difficulties with representative sampling, culture conditions, identification of cultured bacteria, and obvious host variables (e.g., hormonal status, diet, use of antibiotics), hundreds of species in 40 to 50 bacterial genera have been described and identified. These studies revealed that gram-negative and gram-positive, spore- and non–spore-forming, and aerobic and strictly anaerobic bacteria are present and characteristically distributed in specific mucosal compartments. Although it is beyond the scope of this chapter to provide detailed information concerning specific species distribution of indigenous microbiota in individual mucosal compartments (55,59), a brief summary of colonic microbiota illustrates the most important points. Intestinal microbiota are acquired shortly after birth, and their composition is greatly influenced by the route of delivery (vaginal vs. cesarean section), by the environment, and, most profoundly, by the diet (breast-feeding vs. bottled formula and addition of solid food). Colonic microbiota changes from the dominant *Bifidobacterium* at the initial stage to other species, particularly *Bacteroides* and anaerobic cocci with a significant presence of coliforms, streptococci, and clostridia. Quantitative representation of bacteria in feces from adults indicates the dominance of bacteria of the genera *Bacteroides, Clostridium, Eubacterium, Lactobacillus, Streptococcus,* and *Bifidobacterium; Escherichia coli* constitutes only a minor contribution (∼1%) of the colonic microbiota.

Although humans have not been extensively studied, experiments performed in animals of various species (e.g., mice and pigs) colonized with well-defined microbiota indicate that the composition and succession of colonization with bacteria of various species have a profound influence on the maturation and responsiveness of the entire immune system to other mucosally or systemically administered antigens (59).

MUCOSAL ANTIBODIES

Distribution of Immunoglobulin Isotypes

Although immunoglobulin of all isotypes have been detected in human external secretions, their levels and relative proportions are markedly different from those measured in serum (Table 2). The dominance of antibodies of the IgA isotype is a characteristic feature of all secretions (except those from the female and male genital tracts and urine), including tears, saliva, colostrum, milk, and nasal and intestinal fluids. However, the levels of IgA and of immunoglobulins of other isotypes in individual secretions vary markedly (Table 2), partly as a reflection of the techniques used for their measurement, collection procedures, and humoral influences; this variation is especially pronounced in secretions of the female genital tract (60). Overall, the total immunoglobulin levels per milliliter of any external secretions are lower than those measured in serum. The dominance of IgA in secretions of normal individuals, that of IgM in secretions of some IgA-deficient patients, and that of IgG in the milk of several species (e.g., pigs, cows, horses) are the combined results of local tissues and glands, and selective, receptor-mediated transport (see later discussion).

Structure of Secretory Immunoglobulin A

In comparison with its serum counterpart, IgA in external secretions (S-IgA) displays unique structural features with regard to its molecular form, component chain composition, and IgA subclass distribution (61). In humans, almost all serum IgA is present in a monomeric (m) form (sedimentation constant 7S) and contains two heavy (α) and two light (κ and λ) chains; approximately 85% belongs to the IgA1 subclass, and approximately 15% to the IgA2 subclass. Only a small but variable fraction (1% to 10%) of serum IgA is found in a polymeric form and contains an additional polypeptide—the joining (J) chain. In contrast, approximately 90% of S-IgA occurs in a polymeric form (dimers and tetramers with sedimentation constants 11S and 15.5S, respectively), is associated with the J chain and SC acquired during the transepithelial transport (see later discussion), and, depending on individual secretions, contains an increased proportion of IgA2 subclass. The structure of a typical dimeric IgA molecule are shown in Fig. 2. Two mIgA molecules are mutually linked by disulfide bridges through their Fc regions; the J chain is bound to the penultimate Cys residues of α chains. Although SC interacts noncovalently with the Fc regions of both monomers, it is attached by disulfide bridges to only one of them, and there are no covalent bonds formed between the J chain and SC.

α Chains

Mammalian α chains with molecular mass of approximately 50 kDa contain one variable and three constant region domains. There are high numbers of Cys residues involved in the formation of intrachain and interchain disulfide bridges with another α chain, light and J chains, and SC. In addition, α chains can form complexes with a number of plasma and secretory proteins, including albumin, amylase, lactoferrin, glycosyltransferases, and proteolytic enzymes. An unusual hinge region is present in the middle of the α chain of IgA1, between Cα1 and Cα2 domains (61,62). This 13–amino acid–long region is reminiscent of mucin (high content

TABLE 2. *Levels of immunoglobulins in human external secretions (μg/ml)*

Secretion	IgA	IgG	IgM
Tears	80–400	Trace amounts–16	0–18
Nasal fluid	70–846	8–304	0
Parotid saliva[a]	15–319	0.4–5	0.4
Whole saliva	194–206	42	64
Bronchoalveolar fluid	3	13	0.1
Colostrum and breast milk	470–12,340	40–168	50–610
Hepatic bile	58–77	88–140	6–18
Gallbladder bile	92	12	46
Duodenal fluid	313	104	207
Jejunal fluid	32–276	4–340	2
Colonic fluid	240–827	1	Trace amounts–860
Intestinal fluid[b]	166	4	8
Urine	0.1–1.0	0.06–0.56	—
Semen	11–23	16–33	0–8
Cervical fluid	3–133	1–285	5–118
Vaginal fluid	35	52	—

High variability in immunoglobulin levels results from the method of collection; dilution of specimens by lavage fluids; methods of measurements, including the use of appropriate standards (secretory IgA vs. monomeric IgA), flow rates, and stimulation of secretions; hormonal status; and the health status of the individual.
[a]Unstimulated or stimulated.
[b]Whole gut lavage.
Data from Jackson et al. (60).

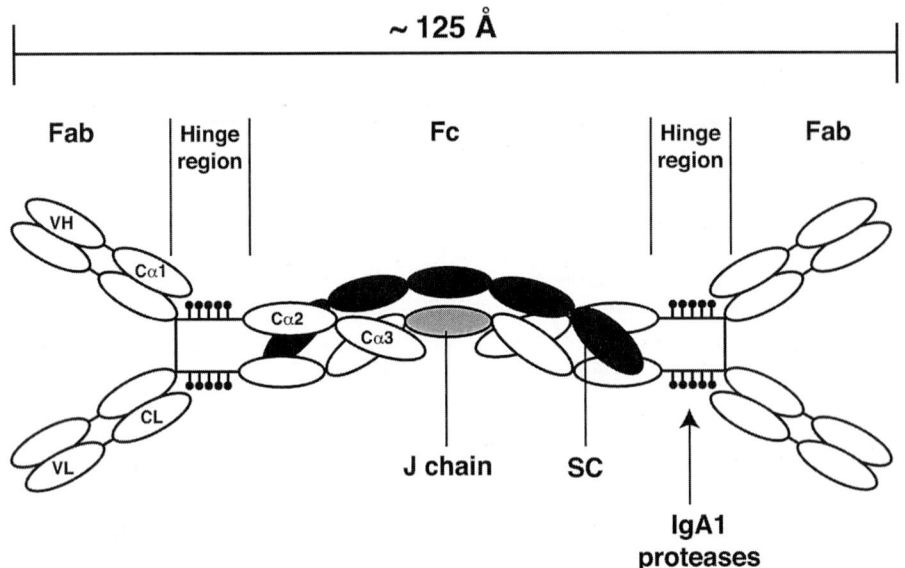

~ 125 Å

FIG. 2. Molecular dimensions, proteolytic fragments, and domain structure of the human dimeric secretory immunoglobulin A1 molecule.

of Pro, Ser, and Thr residues) and carries three to five *O*-linked oligosaccharide side chains (Fig. 2). Although IgA is quite resistant to common proteolytic enzymes, the hinge region contains peptide bonds susceptible to the cleavage by highly substrate-specific IgA1 proteases of bacterial origin (e.g., *Streptococcus pneumoniae, Neisseria meningitides, Neisseria gonorrhoeae, Haemophilus influenzae,*) (63). Comparative structural and genetic studies of IgA molecules from many species indicate that molecules of the IgA2 subclass represent phylogenetically older forms and that the IgA1 subclass arose in hominoid primates by insertion of a gene segment encoding the hinge region (64). The Fcα region and particularly its C terminal display a high degree of sequence homology to the μ chain of IgM, including the characteristic C terminal "tail" (an approximately 18–amino acid extension over the C terminals of γ, δ, and ε chains of corresponding immunoglobulin isotypes) involved in the polymerization and ability of α and μ chains to bind the J chain. Both IgA1 and IgA2 contain 6% to 8% of glycans associated in the form of approximately two to five *N*-linked side chains within the Fc region; the hinge region of IgA1 also contains *O*-linked glycans (61,64).

J Chain

The J chain is a characteristic polypeptide chain present in pIgA and IgM (61,65). It has a molecular mass of 15 kDa, has a single *N*-linked glycan chain, and displays an immunoglobulin domain folding pattern. Of eight Cys residues, six are involved in three intrachain disulfide bridges, and two participate in linkages to the penultimate Cys residues of α and μ chains. A very high degree of homology exists in the primary structures and antigenic cross-reactivities of mammalian and avian J chains, which indicates that the basic properties have

remained conserved through evolution (61). The incorporation of the J chain into pIgA and IgM is essential for the ability of these immunoglobulins to bind SC (66).

Secretory Component

The SC is the extracellular part of pIgR that remains associated with pIgA or IgM after epithelial transcytosis (see later discussion). It is a heavily glycosylated (~22%) polypeptide with a molecular mass of approximately 70 kDa that displays an immunoglobulin domain–like structure (67). Each of the five domains contain an intrachain disulfide bridge, and additional disulfides are present in domains 1 and 5; labile disulfide bonds in the latter domain participate in the covalent binding of SC to a single monomer of pIgA.

Assembly of Secretory Immunoglobulin A

Plasma cells in mucosal tissues and glands assemble pIgA intracellularly from monomeric IgA (mIgA) and the J chain as a last step before its externalization (61). Although the incorporation of the J chain is not absolutely required for polymerization (68), the ability of pIgA and IgM to interact with pIgR expressed on epithelial cells or SC depends on the presence of the J chain, as demonstrated *in vivo* in J chain knockout mice (69) and *in vitro* by binding experiments (65,70).

J chain–containing pIgA or IgM produced by plasma cells in mucosal tissues and glands is recognized by pIgR expressed on basolateral surfaces of adjacent epithelial cells, and the pIgA or IgM–pIgR complexes are transcytosed and released at the apical surface (see later discussion). Consequently, the resultant molecules of S-IgA or secretory IgM (S-IgM) are products of two cell types: plasma cells producing polymeric immunoglobulin with the J chain and epithelial cells that contribute SC to the assembled molecules.

Limited studies of IgG and immunoglobulins D and E (IgD, and IgE), which occur in small quantities in human external secretions, suggest that these immunoglobulins are structurally identical to their serum counterparts.

Function

Large amounts of immunoglobulin are delivered onto the mucosal surfaces as the result of receptor-mediated transepithelial transport and passive transudation of plasma-derived immunoglobulin. Depending on the species and type of secretions, IgA, IgM, and IgG are present in variable proportions (Table 3). Immunoglobulin of all of these isotypes provide, by different mechanisms, protection against pathogenic microorganisms, interact with commensal microbiota, and interfere with the absorption of undigested food antigens from the large surface area of the digestive tract (71).

The dominant S-IgA has several important functional advantages that render antibodies of this isotype and molecular form particularly suitable for functioning in the mucosal environment. Dimeric and tetrameric S-IgA and pentameric S-IgM display 4 to 10 antigen-binding sites. Although of lower affinity than for example IgG antibodies of the same specificity, this multi-valency of polymeric immunoglobulin enhances their effectiveness over monomeric immunoglobulins by at least one order of magnitude. The presence of such low-affinity IgA antibodies that are also "polyreactive" and

thus are capable of binding a variety of bacterial antigens and autoantigens has been demonstrated in human external secretions (72). Furthermore, the intrinsic resistance of IgA to proteolysis, enhanced by association with SC (73), is of functional advantage in secretions, particularly of the GI tract rich in proteolytic enzymes. Finally, because of the inability to activate complement and thus generate C3 and C5 fragments, IgA displays strong anti-inflammatory properties mediated by antibodies of other isotypes (74). This fact is of special importance in the GI tract, in which the external milieu rich in microbial and food antigens and the internal milieu are separated by only a single layer of epithelial cells.

As demonstrated in a number of studies, mucosal immunoglobulins inhibit the absorption of soluble and particulate antigens from mucosal surfaces by forming large immune complexes (71). Furthermore, endogenous commensal microorganisms are coated *in vivo* with corresponding antibodies that, in turn, prevent their adherence to epithelial receptors (56,57). The local protective effect of antibodies of IgA and IgG isotypes in the intestinal tract was most dramatically demonstrated in the newborn, colostrum-fed, and milk-deprived piglet model: animals given orally purified milk or serum immunoglobulins (after the closure of intestinal barrier so that these immunoglobulins are not absorbed) were fully protected against infection with *E. coli* that proved to be fatal in controls deprived of immunoglobulins (75). In addition, a direct protective effect of monoclonal IgA antibodies with specificity to relevant viral and bacterial antigens has been demonstrated in a murine model (71,76,77). Such antibodies have been applied directly onto a mucosal surface by instillation into the respiratory or GI tract before or together with an infectious inoculum. In another approach, preformed antigen-specific pIgA or hybridoma cells producing such antibodies were injected systemically into mice. In this species, circulating pIgA is effectively transported by the hepatobiliary route into the bile and ultimately into the gut lumen. Such animals were subsequently resistant to a challenge with corresponding pathogens, including Sendai virus, influenza, respiratory syncytial virus, rotavirus, reovirus, *S. pneumoniae, S. typhimurium,* or *Vibrio cholerae.* In this regard, mucosal antibodies and especially IgA may function by two independent mechanisms. Specific antibodies interact with corresponding antigens through the antigen-binding site. In addition, glycans that are abundant on S-IgA can aggregate bacteria on the basis of the interaction of bacterial glycan-binding lectins with glycan side chains present on IgA molecules (71,71a). Consequently, such IgA-coated bacteria are prevented from adhering to epithelial cells expressing analogous mannose-rich glycans on their luminal surfaces without the need for antigen-specific antibodies.

Biologically active antigens such as viruses, enzymes, and toxins can be effectively neutralized by mucosal antibodies. This neutralization activity that is operational in a fluid phase may also extend to the intracellular compartment. Using epithelial cell lines that on one hand express pIgR and thus internalize pIgA and on the other hand can be infected with

TABLE 3. *Functions/biological properties of IgA*

Protective functions in secretions
    Prevention of antigen absorption from mucosal surfaces as a result of the formation of Ag-IgA complexes
    Mucus trapping (IgA-mucin complexes entrap microorganisms)
    Virus neutralization (in some experiments, non-neutralizing antibodies may be also protective)
    Enzyme and toxin neutralization
    Enhancement of antimicrobial activities of innate factors (e.g., lysozyme, lactoperoxidase, and lactoferrin)
Biological activities in tissues
    Inhibition of complement activation in some experiments (polymeric IgA or glycan-altered IgA or both may activate complement by the alternative or lectin pathways)
    Enhancement (opsonization) or inhibition of phagocytosis
    Inhibition of type I and type II hypersensitivity reactions (e.g., anaphylaxis and Arthus reaction)
    Degranulation of eosinophils
    Intracellular virus neutralization
    Elimination of Ag-IgA immune complexes by epithelial cells and hepatocytes expressing IgA receptors
    Antibody-dependent cell-mediated cytotoxicity
    Inhibition of NK cell activity
    Inhibition of the release of inflammatory cytokines

Ag, antigen; IgA, immunoglobulin A; NK, natural killer.
Adapted from Russell et al. (71), with permission.

viruses, several investigators demonstrated that virus-specific pIgA also exhibit their *in vitro* neutralization activity intracellularly (71,78). Apparently, the transcytotic route of pIgA intercepts the pathways involved in virus assembly, which results in intracellular neutralization. Furthermore, elimination of immune complexes composed of noninfectious antigens, absorbed by epithelial cells and corresponding internalized pIgA antibodies, has been demonstrated *in vitro*. However, *in vivo* functionality and efficiency of this intracellular pathway of antigen disposal needs to be validated, as discussed elsewhere (71). Small circulating immune complexes containing soluble antigens and pIgA can be eliminated from the circulation into the bile by binding to hepatocytes that in some species (e.g., rats, mice, and rabbits) express pIgR (71). It appears that this mechanism of disposal of immune complexes is restricted primarily to species whose plasma IgA is dominated by pIgA, which in humans represents normally only a minor component (64). However, it is possible that immune complexes containing locally produced pIgA and absorbed antigens that may be formed within mucosal tissues are eliminated by this mechanism (Fig. 3).

The noninflammatory nature of IgA is probably of considerable importance for the maintenance of the structural and functional integrity of mucosal tissues (71,79). The concept that IgA antibodies are anti-inflammatory is exemplified by studies in which intact, native, and fully glycosylated human IgA antibodies failed to activate complement when complexed with antigens; actually in competition experiments, IgA effectively inhibited complement activation by IgM and IgG antibodies (71). Close examination of the frequently cited ability to activate complement reveals that this may result largely from artificial aggregation and conformational alterations caused by purification procedures and binding to hydrophobic surfaces in complement activation assays and aberrances in glycosylation frequently seen in IgA proteins (71). Indeed, specific IgA antibodies with modified

glycan moieties have been shown to activate the alternative and lectin pathways of complement activation (71,71b).

Although phagocytic cells, including monocytes/macrophages and polymorphonuclear neutrophils and eosinophils, express receptors for the Fc region of IgA (80), the ability of IgA alone to effectively promote phagocytosis of bacteria remains controversial and depends on the experimental system used in such studies (71). However, the binding of IgA and IgA-containing immune complexes to such receptors may provide transducing signals for cell activation and proliferation, oxidative metabolism, and prompt degranulation of eosinophils (81,82) with local inflammatory consequences and extensive tissue damage.

The function of mucosal S-IgA also depends on the subclass distribution of specific antibodies (61,71,83). Naturally occurring and immunization-induced antibodies to protein and glycoprotein antigens are present predominantly in the IgA1 subclass, whereas antibodies to polysaccharide antigens, LPS, and lipoteichoic acid are mainly of the IgA2 subclass. Because of its unique hinge region, IgA1 is susceptible to the cleavage by bacterial IgA1 proteases that are considered one of the virulence factors produced by *S. pneumoniae*, *H. influenzae*, *N. gonorrhoeae*, *N. meningitides*, and other microorganisms (63). *In vitro* studies indicate that bacteria coated with antigen-binding fragment α (Fabα) are refractory to IgM- and IgG-mediated and complement-dependent killing action caused by the blocking. The antibacterial activity of IgA may be further potentiated by cooperation with innate factors of immunity, including the peroxidase system, mucin, lactoferrin, and lysozyme (71).

Although S-IgA is the dominant isotype in most external secretion, the protective effects of antibodies of IgM and IgG isotypes are evident from many studies. In external secretions of some IgA-deficient individuals, S-IgM and IgG may functionally compensate for missing S-IgA (84). Furthermore, systemic immunization, particularly with conjugated polysaccharide-protein vaccines, induces vigorous and long-lasting IgG immune responses that protect children from infections with upper respiratory tract pathogens that cause otitis media and meningitis (*H. influenzae*, *N. meningitides*) (85). In animal species (e.g., horses, cows, pigs) in which prenatal transplacental active transport of IgG is not operational, consumption of milk rich in IgG is of lifesaving importance (86). Antibodies of this isotype are absorbed during the first 7 to 14 days of life from the gut into the circulation, presumably by the action of FcRn (see previous discussion). However, specific antibodies remaining in the gut are also protective, as convincingly demonstrated by passive immunization and bacterial challenge experiments.

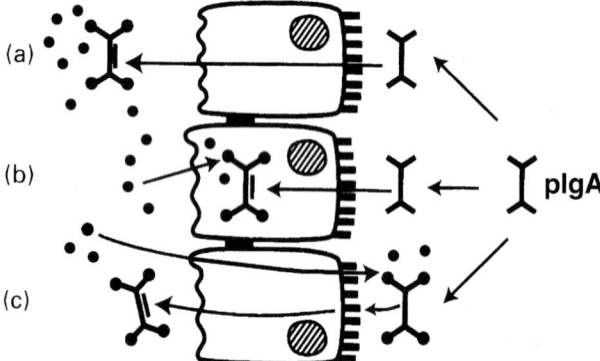

FIG. 3. Functions of immunoglobulin A (IgA) in external secretions and mucosal tissues. **A:** Secretory IgA can interact with luminal antigens and prevent their absorption or adherence to epithelial cells. **B:** Intracellular neutralization of biologically active antigens (e.g., viruses) that escape luminal exclusion or neutralization. **C:** Exclusion of antigen-IgA complexes formed within lamina propria by the polymeric immunoglobulin receptor–mediated mechanism.

Origin and Transport of Mucosal Immunoglobulins

Measurement of combined synthesis of immunoglobulin of all isotypes indicates that in a 70-kg individual, approximately 8 g are produced every day (61,87). With regard to individual isotypes, humans produce approximately 5 g of IgA, approximately 2.5 g of IgG, approximately 0.6 g of

IgM, and trace amounts of IgD and IgE per day. Approximately one half is internally catabolized mainly in the liver, and the second half is actively and passively transported into external secretions (61,87,88). It is estimated that approximately 50% to 70% of total IgA is selectively transported into external secretions (87); daily, more than 3 g of IgA is deposited on a large surface area of mucosal membranes. Studies that addressed the tissue origin of S-IgA convincingly demonstrated that approximately 99% is produced locally in mucosal tissues and glands (89–91). Intravenously injected pIgA appeared in minute quantities in saliva and intestinal fluid, and less than 1% of monoclonal IgA appeared in saliva of patients with multiple myeloma, whose plasma contained high levels of pIgA with the J chain. Parallel distribution of IgA1- and IgA2-producing cells in mucosal and nonmucosal tissues and of IgA1 and IgA2 in serum and various external secretions provided additional evidence for the local origin of S-IgA (88). These findings, combined with the marked differences in antigen specificities of serum and mucosal IgA antibodies induced by infection or mucosal and systemic immunizations, therefore provide strong evidence of a relative independence of the systemic and S-IgA compartments (61,87).

Structural and Cellular Interactions in an Effective Immunoglobulin A Transport

Detailed analyses of S-IgA structure and *in vitro* studies of molecular interactions have clearly indicated that a typical S-IgA molecule comprises two or four molecules of mIgA and one molecule each of the J chain and SC (61). As indicated previously, the incorporation of the J chain into intracellularly assembled pIgA is an essential requirement for its ability to interact with pIgR on epithelial cells and SC in a solution (66). In the absence of crystallographic data, the arrangement of component chains in the Fc region of S-IgA remains largely speculative. Nevertheless, it appears that the incorporation of the J chain in pIgA and IgM results in the generation of a pIgR- and SC-binding site on the α chain domains and perhaps also the J chain.

The receptor (pIgR) specific for the J chain–containing pIgA and IgM is expressed in humans on the basolateral surfaces of epithelial cells of the GI tract and endocervix and the acinar and ductal epithelia of the small and large secretory glands (e.g., lacrimal, mammary, and major and minor salivary glands) (66,67). In some species (rats, mice, and rabbits) pIgR is also expressed on hepatocytes (64,67). Structurally, pIgR comprises an extracellular region (called in its cleaved segment–SC) composed of five immunoglobulin domain–like structures with approximately 560 amino acids, a 23–amino acid membrane-spanning region, and a cytoplasmic region with approximately 103 amino acids; the molecular mass of pIgR with attached glycans is approximately 110 to 120 kDa. The similarity of the general structural features of pIgR from a number of mammalian species indicates that this receptor and its ability to interact with pIg are conserved in phylogeny (64,67).

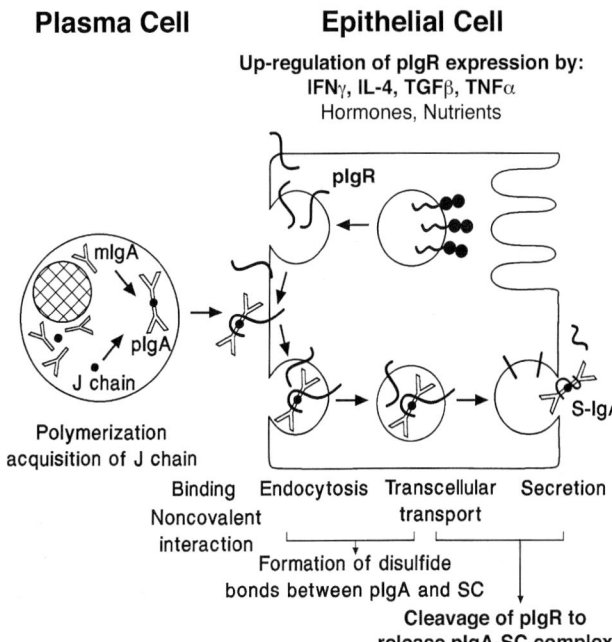

FIG. 4. Transcellular transport of polymeric immunoglobulin A (pIgA) by the polymeric immunoglobulin receptor (pIgR)–mediated mechanism and regulation of pIgR expression. Subepithelial plasma cells produce J chain–associated pIgA that interacts with the epithelial pIgR, and the pIgA-pIgR complex is transcytosed through the epithelial cells and released, after the proteolytic cleavage of pIgR, as secretory IgA (S-IgA).

The pIgA-binding site is present in the first, N-terminal domain of pIgR that interacts with Cα domains (67). The pIgA–pIgR complex is internalized, transcytosed, and finally released at the apical end of the epithelial cells; the entire process takes approximately 30 minutes (Fig. 4). Signals for basolateral targeting of pIgR, its endocytosis, and its transcytosis are encoded in the cytoplasmic region of pIgR, as revealed by deletion mutants. In the final steps, pIgR is proteolytically cleaved, thus releasing pIgA–SC complex; the intracellular and transmembrane regions are endocytosed and degraded or released from the apex. Of importance is that the intracellular sorting and trafficking of pIgR is not dependent on the presence of the ligand—pIgA or IgM: pIgR by itself is processed by the same pathway, and a proteolytically released extracellular region of pIgR appears in external secretions as free SC.

Regulation of Polymeric Immunoglobulin Receptor Expression

Unlike several other receptors, pIgR is not recycling; instead, it remains permanently associated with the ligand as bound SC (28,67). Therefore, the transport of pIgA and IgM is directly dependent on the availability of pIgR on epithelial cell (or hepatocyte) membrane. A number of substances of local and distant origin influence the pIgR expression (Fig. 4). Cytokines produced locally in mucosal tissues and glands upregulate, in an additive or synergistic pattern, the expression of pIgR on established epithelial cell lines, usually of intestinal or endometrial origin (28,67,88). The best-defined up-regulatory system involves the synergistic effect exhibited by IFN-γ and IL-4, two cytokines that in other effector systems usually display antagonistic actions (67). Other cytokines such as TNF-α, IL-1α, IL-1β, and TGF-β (in rat epithelia) also up-regulate pIgR expression (67).

Epithelial cells from the female genital tract and mammary gland express pIgR as a consequence of stimulation with hormones, particularly with estrogens, prolactin, and androgens (92,93). In addition, pIgR expression may be influenced by the incubation of epithelial cells with certain glycans (galactose), vitamin A, and microbial products (67).

Transepithelial and transhepatocytic transport of free pIgA is essential for the protection of enormous surface areas of mucosal membranes (see previous discussion). In addition, such transport is not restricted to free pIgA; low-molecular-weight immune complexes composed of protein, glycoprotein, and polysaccharide antigens and corresponding pIgA antibodies can be cleared from the circulation by pIgR expressed on hepatocytes of some species, and immune complexes found within mucosal tissues can probably be eliminated by an analogous mechanism (see previous discussion).

Other Immunoglobulin A Receptors

The Fc region of IgA can interact with other receptors expressed on structurally and functionally diverse cell populations, including monocytes, macrophages, mesangial cells, polymorphonuclear leukocytes, eosinophils, epithelial cells, hepatocytes, B- and T-lymphocytes, and plasma cells (67, 80,88,94). Some of these receptors have been structurally defined, and specific reagents are now available for their detection.

The best-characterized receptor expressed on monocytes, neutrophils, and eosinophils recognizes Fcα regions of both IgA1 and IgA2 with a certain degree of preference for pIgA, probably because of the presence of multiple binding site on pIgA. This Fcα receptor, designated FcαRI (CD89) and detectable by monoclonal antibodies, occurs in several isoforms and is heavily glycosylated (67,94–96). Most studies since 1990 (97) have indicated that CD89 is also present in minute quantities in the circulation in complexes with high-molecular-mass IgA. Detailed molecular properties of such complexes revealed that FcαRI and IgA are covalently linked, but the high-molecular-mass IgA complexes lack J chain; the authors speculated that the soluble FcαRI is linked to the binding site occupied in pIgA by J chain (97).

FcαRI isolated from cells display the molecular mass of 50 to 70 kDa. This variability results from the different degrees of glycosylation; removal of the six N-linked and O-linked glycans produces molecules with masses of 32 and 36 kDa. The protein core comprises two immunoglobulin-like domains, a 19–amino acid transmembrane segment, and 41–amino acid cytoplasmic tail.

Binding studies indicate that the site of interactions include the first extracellular domain of FcαRI and the boundary between Cα2 and Cα3 domains of IgA heavy chains (98). Cross-linking of FcαRI on cell surfaces triggers phagocytosis, generation of superoxide, and release of inflammatory mediators from neutrophils, eosinophils, monocytes, and macrophages. A novel receptor specific for the Fc regions of IgA and IgM has been described and designated as Fcα/μR (99). This receptor is expressed on murine cells of B-lymphocyte lineage and macrophages. A human homolog of this receptor has been identified on the basis of sequence homology, but its precise cell and tissue distribution remains to be determined. Structurally, Fcα/μR is a transmembrane glycoprotein composed of a single immunoglobulin-like domain. Although its function *in vivo* has not been determined, initial experiments indicate that Fcα/μR mediates endocytosis of IgM-coated microbes. Studies (100) have demonstrated that COS cells transfected with complementary DNA for Fcα/μR are capable of binding both human IgA and IgM but not IgG. Furthermore, the expression of Fcα/μR appears to be up-regulated by IL-1.

Previously reported transferrin receptor (CD71) is surprisingly effective in also binding IgA1 molecules, especially in their monomeric form (101). Because the binding of IgA1 is inhibitable by transferrin, it appears that this novel receptor binds two structurally highly dissimilar ligands: transferrin and IgA1. The receptor is expressed on human colonic carcinoma epithelial line HT-29, monomyelocytic cell line U937 cell, a B-lymphocyte cell line (DAUDI), and mesangial cells in kidneys of patients with IgA nephropathy. Structural studies indicate that under nonreducing conditions, CD71 displays a molecular mass of 180 kDa and is composed of two homologous 90-kDa chains. Although the function of this receptor remains to be determined, its expression on IECs may be involved in the appearance of mIgA in gut secretions.

The asialoglycoprotein receptor that is expressed abundantly on hepatocytes (102) is responsible for binding, internalization, and degradation of IgA and many other glycoproteins with terminal Gal and GalNAc residues that are recognized in the presence of Ca^{2+} (103,104). In addition to the free IgA1 and IgA2 molecules, the asialoglycoprotein receptor binds and internalizes immune complexes containing these two isotypes. Additional incompletely characterized receptors for IgA have been described on epithelial and mesangial cells (105,106).

INDUCTIVE AND EFFECTOR SITES OF THE MUCOSAL IMMUNE SYSTEM

Organization of the Mucosal Immune System

The mammalian host has evolved organized secondary lymphoid tissues in the upper respiratory and GI tract regions that facilitate antigen uptake, processing, and presentation for induction of mucosal immune responses. Collectively, these tissues are termed *inductive sites*. Although the gut-associated lymphoepithelial tissues (GALT), such as Peyer's patches (PP), the appendix, and smaller lymphoid aggregates called solitary lymph nodes appear to be major inductive sites in all of the most common experimental mammalian systems, the degree of bronchus-associated lymphoepithelial tissue (BALT) developed at airway branches for defense against intranasal/inhaled antigens differs considerably among species. In rabbits, rats, and guinea pigs, such BALT development is significant, whereas in humans and mice, it is negligible (107) unless chronic inflammation occurs (108). Instead, the major inductive tissues for intranasal/inhaled antigens in humans, primates, mice, and rats appear to be the palatine tonsils and adenoids (nasopharyngeal tonsils), which together form a physical barrier of lymphoid tissues termed the *Waldeyer's ring,* now more frequently referred to as a nasopharyngeal-associated lymphoepithelial tissue (NALT) (109). To summarize, then, NALT and GALT in humans and mice and possibly primates and NALT, BALT and GALT in other experimental mammalian systems comprise a mucosa-associated lymphoepithelial tissue (MALT) network (110,111) whose integration is only partly understood.

There are two major features that distinguish MALT from the other systemic lymphoid tissues. First, the epithelium that separates the tissue from the lumen contains a specialized cell type now called an M cell that is closely associated with lymphoid cells. This epithelial cell network is termed the *follicle-associated epithelial* (FAE) cell. Second, MALT contains organized regions that include a subepithelial area (dome), B-cell zones with germinal centers containing IgA-committed B cells [surface IgA$^+$ (sIgA$^+$) B cells], and adjacent T-cell regions with antigen-presenting cells (APCs)

and high endothelial venules (HEVs). Naïve, recirculating B- and T-lymphocytes enter MALT through HEVs. Antigen-activated and memory B- and T-cell populations then emigrate from the inductive environment via lymphatic drainage, circulate through the bloodstream, and home to mucosal *effector sites* (Fig. 5). These effector sites include more diffuse tissues in which antigen-specific T- and B-lymphocytes ultimately reside and perform their respective functions [i.e., cell-mediated immune (CMI), CTL, and regulatory functions or antibody synthesis, respectively] to protect mucosal surfaces.

Inductive Sites

Mucosal inductive sites of the GI tract include PP, the appendix, and solitary lymph nodules, which collectively constitute the GALT (110), whereas the tonsils and adenoids, or NALT, probably serve as the mucosal inductive sites for the upper respiratory tract, the nasal/oral cavity, and the genitourinary tract (109). The most extensively studied mucosal inductive tissues are the PP of the murine GI tract, although several groups have also characterized NALT, albeit to a lesser extent than GALT, and salient characteristics of both are presented.

Gut-Associated Lymphoepithelial Tissue

The initial steps involved in murine PP development have been studied in some detail in mice. A cluster of vascular cell adhesion molecule 1$^+$ (VCAM-1$^+$)/intracellular adhesion molecule 1$^+$ (ICAM-1$^+$) cells develops in the upper

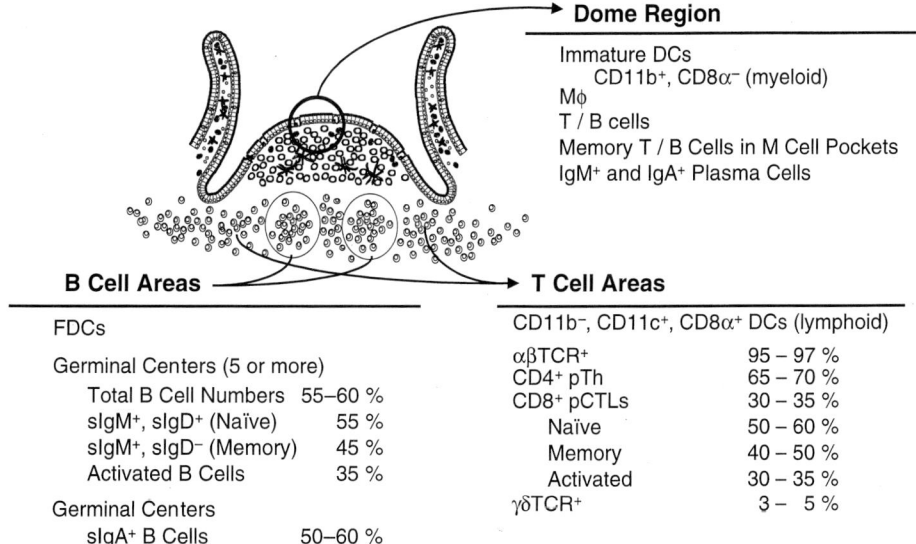

FIG. 5. The Peyer's patches or gut-associated lymphoepithelial tissues (GALT) consist of a follicle-associated epithelium with M cells and subepithelial dome (SED) region. Immature myeloid dendritic cells (DCs) are present in the SED, whereas mature lymphoid DCs characterize the T-cell areas. B cells in germinal centers are undergoing frequent switches to immunoglobulin A (IgA). Approximately two thirds of GALT T cells are CD4$^+$ precursors of T helper cells, whereas approximately one third are precursors of CD8$^+$ CTLs.

small intestine beginning at embryonic days 15 to 16, followed by the presence of cells expressing the IL-7 receptor (IL-7Rα⁺) at day 17.5 (112), which appear to be the anlage of the patch. Mice defective in IL-7Rα gene expression fail to form mature GALT (112). It now appears that IL-7–IL-7Rα triggering results in up-regulation of lymphotoxin (LT) α1β2 membrane expression by lymphoid cells, including those in developing PPs (113–116). Furthermore, mice that lack LTα or LTβ or that have been treated *in utero* with a fusion protein of LTβ receptor–immunoglobulin fail to develop PPs or systemic lymph nodes. In addition, lymphoplasia (*ala/ala*) mice, with a mutation in the NFκB-inducing kinase (117), which appears to act downstream of LTα1β2–LTβ receptor signaling, also fail to develop PPs (117). There is evidence that a lymphoid progenitor cell from the fetal liver expresses α4β7 and migrates to the PP anlage, where they ultimately develop into T, NK, dendritic, and LT-lineage cells (118). PPs develop during prenatal life in humans, as well as in sheep, pigs, dogs, and horses (119).

Murine PPs contain a dome, underlying follicles (B-cell zones with germinal centers), and parafollicular regions enriched with T cells (Fig. 5). Originally, the specialized epithelial cell covering MALT was called an FAE cell because it characterized the organized lymphoid tissues in the GI tract (120). However, the M cell was later named for its unique topical structure (microfold/membraneous) (121), and the entire epithelium covering MALT is now commonly described as an FAE type (122,123). The surface of the dome region is covered by the specialized FAE, 10% to 20% of which is composed of M cells that exhibit thin extensions around lymphoid cells (120–123). These extensions, which almost surround B- and T-lymphocytes and occasional macrophages (MØs), form an apparent pocket (122). The M cells, which have short microvilli, small cytoplasmic vesicles, and few lysosomes, are adept at uptake and transport of luminal antigens, including proteins and particulates such as viruses, bacteria, small parasites, and microspheres (123). Investigators in this field disagree on whether M cells are able to process and present antigen. Some believe that antigen uptake by M cells and transcellular passage results in delivery of intact antigen into the underlying lymphoid tissue (123). Others, however, contend that findings such as M-cell expression of class II MHC molecules and acidic endosomal-lysosomal compartments suggest that M cells may also be involved in antigen processing and presentation (124). It is possible that the nature of endocytosed antigen influences M-cell activation and their potential to express class II MHC molecules. In an important and elegant *in vitro* study, human Caco-2 cells, which are more immature enterocytes, differentiated into M-like cells when treated with mouse PP T and B cells or with a human B-cell line (Raji) (125). Mice that lack B cells (termed μMT) were also shown to exhibit fewer M cells and less well-developed FAE cells and PPs than did normal mice (126). These findings suggest that lymphocytes and especially B cells possess signaling molecules that induce M-cell differentiation.

In addition to serving as a means of transport for luminal antigens, the M cells also provide an entry way for pathogens. Invasive strains of *S. typhimurium* initiate murine infection by invading the M cells of the PPs (127). Although M cells are able to transport luminal antigen, noninvasive strains of *S. typhimurium* cannot penetrate M cells and thus are avirulent. Reoviruses also initiate infection of the mouse through the M cell (128), an ability that has been associated with the reovirus sigma protein (129). As discussed in more detail later, NALT also has a lymphoepithelium with M cells, and *Mycobacterium tuberculosis* uses this cell type for entry into the host, with subsequent uptake in draining lymph nodes (130). Identification of bacterial and viral virulence factors associated with invasion or infection of M cells may provide tools to construct more efficient attenuated bacterial or viral vectors (see later discussion) or to target mucosal vaccines to the inductive environment of MALT. Furthermore, it is possible that M cells are also involved in the induction of mucosally induced tolerance (e.g., oral tolerance).

The underlying dome region of the PP consists of sparse plasma cells, as well as B- and T-lymphocytes (111), and this suggests that immediate antigen presentation may occur in the dome area after antigen uptake. It is also possible that T- and B-cell interactions in the dome area provide necessary protection for the PP. The presence of MØs (131), including the tingible body type, suggests that significant apoptosis occurs, but this has not yet been proved. An immunohistological study has called into question whether dome MØs are indeed a major cell type (45,132). This important study has described a major APC population in the dome with characteristics of DCs (132). Interestingly, the dome DCs were N418⁺ (anti-CD11c) and could be differentiated from more classical DCs present in the interfollicular area (T cell zone), which demonstrates that two DC subsets occur in key antigen sampling areas of the PP (132). This study also suggested that fewer numbers of B220⁺ B cells occur in the dome area of mouse GALT. Studies of the lymphocyte populations associated with human M-cell pockets, the area where luminal antigen may first be recognized by T- and B-lymphocytes, have also provided evidence for a characteristic T-cell distribution. For example, M-cell pockets in human PPs contain approximately equal numbers of CD3⁺ T-lymphocytes and CD19⁺/CD20⁺ B-lymphocytes with fewer CD68⁺ MØs (122). Of the T cells in this location, approximately 75% exhibited a T helper (Th) cell phenotype.

Distinct follicles (B-cell zones) are located beneath the dome area of PPs and contain germinal centers in which significant B-cell division is seen. These germinal centers, which contain the majority of sIgA⁺ B cells (133–136), are considered to be sites at which frequent B-cell switches to IgA and affinity maturation occur. However, in contrast to immune lymph nodes and the spleen in the systemic compartment, plasma cell development does not occur at the germinal centers. All major T-cell subsets are found in the T cell–dependent areas adjacent to follicles (Table 4). The

TABLE 4. *Major mouse lymphocyte subpopulations associated with the mucosal immune system*

Mucosal sites	Example	Lymphocyte subsets	Distribution	Possible functions
Inductive tissues	Peyer's patches	CD3$^+$ T cells	35%–40%	
		CD4$^+$, CD8$^-$	65%	Major T helper cells for mucosal immunity
		CD4$^-$, CD8$^+$	30%	CTL precursors; regulatory/anergy
		CD4$^-$, CD8$^-$	2%–4%	Express $\gamma\delta$ TCRs
		Naïve	30%–40%	Circulate within the mucosal system
		Effector (activated)	30%–40%	Stimulated through M cell pathways
		Memory	30%–40%	Homing to effector sites
		B220$^+$ B cells	45%–47%	Include germinal center, where >60% are sIgA$^+$ B cells
		sIgA$^+$	~8%–10%	Committed to IgA
Effector tissues	Lamina propria lymphocytes	CD3$^+$ T cells	40%–50%	
		CD4$^+$, CD8$^-$	~60%–65%	Difficult to activate via TCR
		CD4$^-$, CD8$^+$	~30%–35%	Mature CTLs; other subset functions (?)
		CD4$^-$, CD8$^-$	~2%–5%	Express $\delta\gamma$ TCRs
		Memory	>90%	—
		sIgA$^+$ B cells	30%–50%	—
		IgA plasma cells	10%–15%	Highest numbers of plasma cells in the mammalian immune system
	Intraepithelial lymphocytes	CD3$^+$ T cells	85%–95%	
		CD4$^+$, CD8$^-$	~5%–8%	All express $\alpha\beta$ TCRs
		CD4$^-$, CD8$^+$	~75%–80%	Two thirds are CD8 $\alpha\alpha$; 50%, $\gamma\delta^+$; 50%, $\alpha\beta^+$
		CD4$^+$, CD8$^+$	~7%–10%	All express $\alpha\beta$ TCRs
		CD4$^-$, CD8$^-$	~5%–8%	All express $\gamma\delta$ TCRs
		No B cells/plasma cells	—	—

CTL, cytotoxic T-lymphocyte; IgA, immunoglobulin A; sIgA, secretory IgA; TCR, T-cell receptor.

parafollicular T cells are mature, and more than 97% of these T cells use the $\alpha\beta$ heterodimer form of the TCR. Approximately two thirds of PP $\alpha\beta$ TCR$^+$ T cells are CD4$^+$ and CD8$^-$ and exhibit properties of Th cells, including support for IgA responses (137). Approximately one third of the $\alpha\beta$ T cells in GALT are CD4$^-$ and CD8$^+$; this cell subset contains precursors of CTLs (138,139), whereas other CD8$^+$ T cell subsets appear to contribute to mucosally induced tolerance (see later discussion).

Nasal-Associated Lymphoepithelial Tissue

Although the mouse has been the major model used to study PPs, the human tonsils are the most accessible secondary lymphoid tissue for study of NALT, and a great deal is therefore known about the component cells (140). Although the palatine and nasopharyngeal tonsils (adenoids) are largely covered by a squamous epithelium and are often not appreciated as mucosal tissues, the palatine tonsils usually contain 10 to 20 crypts that increase their surface area. The deeper regions of these crypts contain M cells that may take up encountered antigens (140). The tonsils contain all major classes of APCs, including DCs and Langerhans cells, MØs, class II$^+$ B cells, and antigen-retaining follicular DCs in B-cell germinal centers. Tonsillar APCs are capable of inducing T-cell proliferative and cytokine responses after *in vitro* restimulation with appropriate vaccines such as tetanus and diphtheria toxoid and purified protein derivative (PPD) of *Mycobacterium*.

Approximately half of tonsillar cells are B-lymphocytes and are present mainly in follicles-containing germinal centers (140). Most human tonsillar B cells are actually surface IgG-positive (sIgG$^+$); however, significant numbers of surface IgM-positive (sIgM$^+$) and sIgA$^+$ B cells are also present. Furthermore, *in situ* staining of B-cell blasts/plasma cells indicate a predominance of IgG blasts in germinal centers and of plasma cells in the parafollicular area. The overall percentage of IgG$^+$ cells to IgA$^+$ cells was 65:30 (140). The human palatine tonsil also contains a distinct subepithelial B-cell population that differs from both germinal center and follicular mantle B cells (140). This subset may represent the homolog of the extrafollicular B cells of the splenic marginal zone (140). It is not accurate to suggest that the tonsils are only a mucosal IgA inductive site, because of the presence of B cells committed to other isotypes, especially for IgG subclasses. Approximately 40% of tonsillar cells are T cells, and more than 98% express the $\alpha\beta$ TCR. Furthermore, somewhat higher CD4-to-CD8 ratios are found in tonsils (3:1) in comparison with peripheral blood or murine GALT. In summary, the tonsils clearly exhibit not only features of mucosal inductive sites but also characteristics of effector sites with high numbers of plasma cells. The role of the tonsils in host mucosal immunity after intranasal immunization is not yet fully established.

In order to understand the precise contribution of NALT to the induction of IgA responses to inhaled antigens, studies in both mice and rats have established a NALT-like structure (109,141–143). The NALT consists of bilateral strips of nonencapsulated lymphoid tissue underlying the epithelium on the ventral aspect of the posterior nasal tract and exhibits a bell-like shape in cross sections (141–143). Although dense aggregates of lymphocytes have been observed in the NALT of normal mice, germinal centers are absent but could be induced by nasal application of antigen (136). Thus, uncommitted B cells (sIgM$^+$) have been found in high proportions (80% to 85%), whereas low numbers of sIgA$^+$ and sIgG$^+$ B cells (3% to 4% and 0% to 1%, respectively) have been noted in mononuclear cells isolated from NALT (142,143). In contrast to GALT, in which a high frequency (10% to 15%) of sIgA$^+$ B cells occur, NALT was found to contain fewer IgA$^+$ B cells. Despite this, nasal immunization induces much higher numbers of IgA$^+$ than IgG$^+$ NALT B cells in the memory compartment, which shows the propensity of NALT for mucosal S-IgA antibody responses (144). Characterization of isolated NALT mononuclear cells revealed that approximately 30% to 40% of these cells are CD3$^+$ T cells with a CD4/CD8 ratio of approximately 3.0 (143). The majority of NALT CD3$^+$ T cells coexpress CD45RB, which is suggestive of naïve, resting T cells. Because transcriptional single-cell analysis revealed the expression of mRNA for both Th1 and Th2 cytokines, the majority of CD4$^+$ T cells are considered Th0 types (143). Furthermore, stimulation through the TCR-CD3 complex resulted in differentiation of both Th1- and Th2-type cells. These results support the notion that NALT exhibits characteristics of mucosal inductive sites.

Other Potential Mucosal Inductive Sites in Humans

The follicular structures analogous to PPs found in the large intestine and especially in the rectum, known as rectal-associated lymphoepithelial tissue (RALT) (145,146), also show potential as an IgA-inductive site and as a source of IgA plasma cell precursors. As described in detail later in the section on mucosal immune responses, intrarectal immunization results in the induction of immune responses at both local and remote effector sites. Although local immune responses can be induced at mucosal sites devoid of organized lymphoepithelial tissues, analogous to PP, their magnitude is usually low. Thus, application or injection of antigens with or without appropriate adjuvants in the conjunctival sac, buccal mucosa, urinary bladder, vagina, lactating mammary gland, and salivary glands induces IgA and IgG immune responses at the site of immunization (147,148).

Effector Sites

After initial exposure to antigen in MALT, mucosal lymphocytes leave the inductive site and home to mucosal effector tissues (see later discussion). This pathway, which results in immunity at several mucous membrane sites, is referred to as the common mucosal immune system (Fig. 4). Effector sites for mucosal immune responses include the lymphoid cells in the lamina propria regions of the GI, upper respiratory, and reproductive tracts, as well as secretory glandular tissues such

as mammary, salivary, and lacrimal glands (110,111,147). In addition, most evidence suggests that the lymphocytes that reside in the epithelium (i.e., IELs) also serve as effector cells; however, it has been difficult to precisely define IEL functions (149) (see later discussion). Antigen-specific mucosal effector cells include IgA-producing plasma cells and B- and T-lymphocytes. IgA is the primary immunoglobulin involved in protecting mucosal surfaces and is locally produced in effector tissues (111). Again, the presence of antigen-specific S-IgA antibodies at mucosal surfaces other than the inductive site where antigen uptake initially occurred provides further evidence for the existence of the common mucosal immune system. Thus, it suggests that immunization of either NALT or GALT could induce mucosal immune responses in all mucosal effector tissues.

Effector mechanisms employed to protect mucosal surfaces include CTLs, as well as effector CD4$^+$ Th cells for CMI (Th1) and for humoral S-IgA antibody (Th2) responses (71,149,150). Indeed, both CTL and S-IgA responses have been associated with protection against infection at mucosal surfaces, and both may be important for resistance to or, more important, prevention of mucosal infection with viruses, including HIV (148). Although little information regarding protective CD4$^+$ Th1-CMI responses is available, mucosal CMI appears to be important in tolerance and in control of infections by intracellular pathogens.

However, effector sites, which must serve as a barrier against numerous environmental foreign antigens and mucosal pathogens with which the inductive sites need not contend, offer mechanisms of protection significantly different from those at the inductive sites. The high concentration of IgA plasma cells [estimated at more than 10^{10} IgA plasma cells per meter of human small intestine (151,152)] has traditionally been viewed as the most distinctive trait of the immunity offered at these effector sites. As discussed later, the murine GI lamina propria has an almost equal distribution of peritoneal B1 B cell–derived IgA plasma cells. Furthermore, the lamina propria of the gut also contains more than 50% IgA plasma cells that are B2 GALT B cell derived (see later discussion). However, as important, if not more so, are the large numbers of B- and T-lymphocytes (e.g., lamina propria lymphocytes), more than 60% of which are T cells (153,154).

When presented with an environmental antigen, epithelial cells endocytose it and, in some cases, themselves express class II MHC molecules, processing antigens with subsequent association of immunogenic peptides with class II MHC (155). It has also been shown that Langerhans-like cells occur on the luminal side of the intestine at epithelial junctions between epithelial cells that could also provide accessory functions (156). When confronted with microorganisms and even with soluble proteins that can transverse the tight junctions between epithelial cells, the APCs at the effector sites may process them and thereby induce B- and T-cell responses. Some investigators have suggested that MHC class II$^+$ sIgA$^+$ B cells may bind antigen through endocytic pathways and process and present peptides to CD4$^+$

Th cells. Macrophages in lamina propria regions could also function in this manner for more complex antigens. Freshly isolated mouse intestinal lamina propria CD4$^+$ T cells contain high numbers of IL-5–secreting Th2-type cells, in addition to IFN-γ–secreting Th1-type cells, which suggests that the effector regions of the mucosal immune system are somewhat biased toward a Th2 phenotype (157). Furthermore, findings obtained by a single-cell reverse-transcription polymerase chain reaction analysis of CD4$^+$ T cells from murine nasal passages revealed a high frequency of CD4$^+$ T cells expressing Th2 cytokine–specific mRNA (143). In summary, mucosal effector tissues contain all the necessary cellular components, including epithelial cells, Th1-/Th2-type CD4$^+$ T cells, CTLs, and IgA-producing cells, for a multilayer barrier against the numerous environmental foreign antigens and mucosal pathogens.

B-Cell Compartment

Quantitative studies of the distribution of T- and B-lymphocytes in the systemic pool versus mucosal tissues indicate that the majority of such cells is present in the latter compartment (151,152,158,159). This difference is particularly pronounced in the case of plasma cells: Mucosal tissues contain approximately two to three times more plasma cells than do the spleen, bone marrow, and lymph nodes (152). Furthermore, in this cell population, there are significant qualitative differences with regard to the distribution of immunoglobulin isotypes between systemic and mucosal tissues: There is a characteristic dominance of IgG-producing cells in the systemic compartment, and IgA-producing cells predominate in the mucosal compartment. In humans, immunoglobulins produced in the systemic pool remain mostly in the circulation and intestinal fluid and are catabolized in the liver (88); only relatively small quantities enter the external secretions (89–91). Immunoglobulins synthesized in mucosal tissues are selectively transported into external secretions, and only approximately 10% or less appears in the circulation. This typical distribution of particular IgA is less accentuated in other species such as mice, rats, and rabbits, in which IgA produced in mucosal tissues, especially in the gut, enters the circulation in large amounts and is selectively transported by a receptor-mediated mechanism through hepatocytes into the bile and then into the gut lumen (64). Thus, in this and other species, plasma IgA reinforces intestinal immunity.

Phenotypes of B-cell lineage are different in the inductive sites (i.e., PPs) and effector sites (i.e., intestinal lamina propria and secretory glands). Specifically, the former tissues contain large numbers of CD19$^+$ B cells but only a few differentiated CD38$^+$ cells. The CD19$^+$ cell population comprises surface IgD$^+$ (sIgD$^+$) (50%), sIgΛ^+ (30%), and sIgG$^+$ (14%) B-lymphocytes (152). In contrast, lamina propria B cells are represented mostly by large cells and express CD38 with the predominance of surface and cytoplasmic IgA (152). Although the precise determinations of lymphocytes of B- and T-cell lineages are technically difficult, mainly

because of the heterogeneity of B cells that are present at various differentiation stages, it appears that cells of both lineages are present in approximately equal proportions in the intestinal tissues.

Distribution of Immunoglobulin Isotypes in Effector Sites

Extensive studies of the distribution of immunoglobulin-producing cells in various mucosal tissues and glands by the immunofluorescence technique and enzyme-linked immunospot (ELISPOT) convincingly demonstrated a remarkable preponderance of IgA cells (151,152) in all such tissues. The only exception is the uterine cervix, in which the numbers of IgG-producing cells are equal or slightly exceed those of IgA-producing cells (160). However, there are tissue-specific differences in the proportions of IgA$^+$, IgG$^+$, IgM$^+$, and IgD$^+$ plasma cells (Fig. 6). For example, nasal mucosa contains, on average, 69% IgA$^+$ cells, 17% IgG$^+$ cells, 6% IgD$^+$ cells, and 6% IgM$^+$ cells, whereas in the large intestine, 90% of cells are positive for IgA, 6% for IgM, and 4% for IgG (151,152). Moreover, cells producing IgA1 or IgA2 also display a characteristic tissue distribution (83,151,152,161). Systemic lymphoid tissues (e.g., spleen, tonsils, lymph nodes, and bone marrow) and most of the mucosal tissues (nasal, gastric, and small intestinal mucosa and, to a lesser degree, glandular tissues) contain more IgA1- than IgA2-producing cells, whereas in the large intestine and the female genital tract tissues, IgA2-producing cells are more frequent than IgA1 cells. Although direct experimental evidence is not available, it has been speculated that this tissue-specific distribution of IgA1- or IgA2-producing cells is related to the differences in the origin of IgA1 and IgA2 precursors and perhaps to their distinct homing patterns (151,152). Alternatively, antigen-driven clonal expansion in various mucosal tissues may also be involved. For example, most of the naturally occurring S-IgA antibodies to bacterial endotoxin are associated with the IgA2 isotype (83). Thus, it is likely that endotoxin abundantly present in germ-negative bacteria in the large intestine induce clonal expansion of IgA2-producing cells in this locale.

Distribution of Polymeric or Monomeric Immunoglobulin A–Producing Cells

Analyses of molecular forms of IgA in supernatant of cells and tissue explants obtained from systemic and mucosal compartments, tissue perfusates, and immunohistochemical studies of such tissue demonstrated that separate populations of pIgA- and mIgA-secreting cells display a characteristic tissue distribution (61,151,152) (Fig. 6). Typically, almost all IgA-producing cells in the normal bone marrow produce mIgA (61). The admixture of peripheral blood in the bone marrow specimens grossly influences the results because peripheral blood lymphocytes secrete, especially after stimulation, predominantly pIgA and little mIgA (162). Supernatants collected from in vitro cultured human lymph nodes and spleen contained both forms, usually with the preponderance of

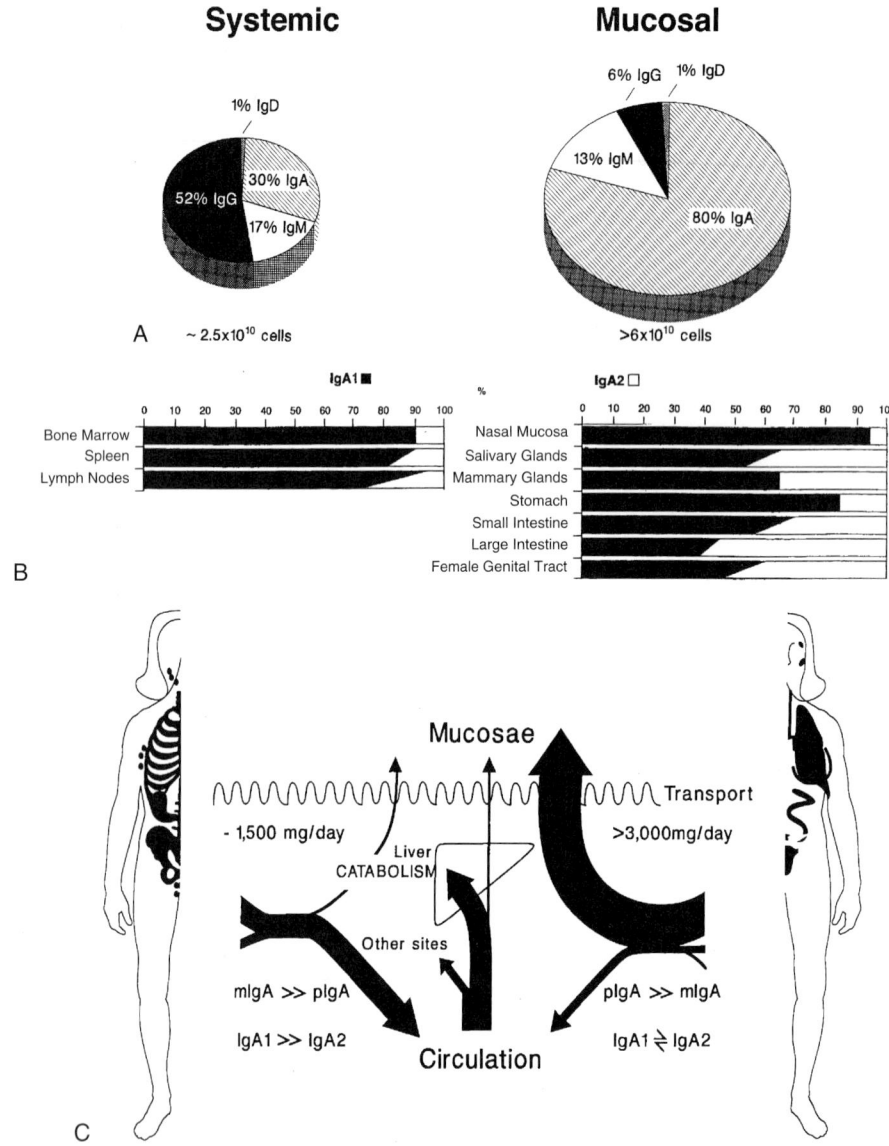

FIG. 6. Comparative distribution and B cells in systemic and mucosal compartments. **A:** Quantitative distribution and immunoglobulin isotypes. **B:** Distribution of immunoglobulin A (IgA) subclasses. **C:** Distribution and properties of IgA produced in the systemic and mucosal compartments.

mIgA (61). In contrast, such supernatants or perfusates of mucosal tissues, especially the gut, contained pIgA as the dominant form.

Examinations of sera and mucosal secretions, culture supernatants, and cell lysates and immunohistochemical studies of systemic and mucosal lymphoid tissues indicated that pIgA contains the J chain as a typical component and that J chain–containing pIgA is capable of binding to pIgR and its extracellular region, SC (61,151,152). Consequently, the presence of an intracellular J chain and the ability to bind SC have been taken as markers for pIgA- or IgM-producing cells (151). According to these criteria, almost all IgA plasma cells from mucosal tissues produced pIgA; in contrast, cells from the normal bone marrow produced mIgA (63). However, human

lymphoblastoid cell lines, *in vitro* mitogen-stimulated peripheral blood lymphocytes, bone marrow plasma cells from patients with multiple myeloma and B-cell leukemias, and cells from mucosal tissues produce the J chain irrespective of the immunoglobulin isotype (162–165). Thus, mucosal IgG- or IgD-producing cells are also J chain–positive (151,152). Furthermore, IgA and IgM may be produced in polymeric forms in the absence of the J chain (68,69). Obviously, the production of the J chain is regulated independently of the concomitant immunoglobulin production. Although the SC binding is indicative of the intracellular presence of J chain–containing pIgA or IgM, it does not necessarily prove that all intracellular IgA or IgM is polymeric. Comparative studies of culture supernatants and cell lysates of human lymphoblastoid cell lines, mitogen-stimulated peripheral blood cells, and cells from mucosal tissue and of murine cell lines clearly document that mIgA is the predominant *intracellular* form of IgA even in cells that secrete pIgA (163).

In summary, plasma cells in mucosal tissues differ from their systemic counterparts in a high level of expression of the J chain irrespective of the immunoglobulin isotype, dominant production of pIgA, and increased relative production of IgA2 in some tissues (large intestine and the uterine cervix). These structural differences in the properties of IgA may be related to the origin of cells (mucosal inductive sites as sources of IgA cells in effector sites), local regulatory mechanisms (e.g., arrays of cytokines produced by mucosal T cells and epithelial cells), expression of selective mucosal homing receptors on circulating B cells, and types of antigens present in the mucosal environment that may clonally expand specific antibody-secreting cells.

T-Cell Compartment and Regulation of Mucosal Immune System

The development of mucosal immunity, inflammation, or tolerance to protein-based vaccines, viral and bacterial pathogens, allergens, and autoantigens requires T cells, including CD4$^+$ Th1/Th2 cell subsets, CD8$^+$ CTLs, and T-cell subsets for induction of mucosal tolerance (158). Furthermore, these immune responses are also regulated by other cell subsets, termed T regulatory (Treg) cells. Of course, B-cell commitment ($\mu \rightarrow \alpha$ switching) and B–T interactions that result in the induction of plasma cells producing pIgA are of central importance to mucosal immunity. Cytokines produced by CD4$^+$ and CD8$^+$ T-cell subsets, by classical APCs (e.g., DCs, MØs, and B cells), and by nonclassical APCs (e.g., epithelial cells) contribute to all aspects of normal mucosal immunity, tolerance, and inflammation in the immune response.

Regulatory T Cells and Cytokines in the Mucosal Immune System

Treg cells that normally exhibit either a CD4$^+$ or CD8$^+$ phenotype, can be classified as (a) naïve, or those which have not yet encountered antigen; (b) activated (effector); and (c) memory, whereby both effector and memory T cells have engaged in the immune response (143,150,158). CD8$^+$ T cells are also classified in the same three subsets and are discussed later. The mucosal migration patterns of these three subsets, along with the homing of B-lymphocytes, form the cellular basis of the common mucosal immune system. Naïve CD4$^+$ precursors of Th cells (pTh) normally recognize foreign peptide in association with class II MHC on APCs and express an $\alpha\beta$ TCR$^+$, CD3$^+$CD4$^+$CD8$^-$ phenotype. On the other hand, precursor CTLs (pCTLs) express $\alpha\beta$ TCRs, which usually recognize foreign peptide in the context of class I MHC on target cells and normally exhibit a CD3$^+$CD4$^-$CD8$^+$ pheno-

type. Thus, encounter with foreign antigen (peptides) results in development of effector T cells that either are Th1 cells for cell-mediated responses and Th2 cells for antibody responses or lyse infected target cells (CTLs). Thus, the MALT can be considered as significant reservoirs of pTh cells and pCTLs so that encounter with bacterial or viral pathogens can result in the induction of effector CD4$^+$ Th cell responses and CD8$^+$ CTL responses.

Mucosal CD4$^+$ T Helper Cells

Th1 and Th2 Subsets

As CD4$^+$ Th cells mature in response to foreign antigens, they assume unique characteristics such as production of distinct cytokine arrays. The pTh cells first produce IL-2 in response to stimuli and develop into T cells that produce multiple cytokines (including both IFN-γ and IL-4), a stage often termed Th0 (166,167). The environment and cytokine milieu greatly influences the further differentiation of these Th0 cells (Fig. 7). For example, stimulation by certain pathogens such as intracellular bacteria leads to the differentiation of CD4$^+$ Th1 cells that produce IFN-γ, IL-2, and TNFs. These cells often develop after production of IL-12 by DCs or MØs (168,169) activated through the ingestion of intracellular pathogens (Fig. 7). There is compelling evidence that secreted IL-12 induces NK cells to produce IFN-γ (170), which, together with IL-12, up-regulates IL-12 receptor expression on differentiating Th1-type cells (Fig. 7). Furthermore, murine Th1-type responses are associated with development of CMI, as manifested by delayed-type hypersensitivity (DTH) and by B-cell antibody responses with characteristic patterns. For example, IFN-γ induces $\mu \rightarrow \gamma$2a switches (171) and production of complement-fixing IgG2a antibodies.

On the other hand, exogenous antigen in mucosal environments can trigger CD4$^+$ NK1.1$^+$ T cells (172) and other precursor cells that produce IL-4 for initiation of Th2-type responses. CD4$^+$ Th2-type cells also produce IL-4 for expansion of this subset, as well as IL-5, IL-6, IL-9, IL-10, and IL-13 (173,174) (Fig. 7). This Th2 cell array may include production of IL-4 with other Th2 cytokines; however, individual cytokines are regulated through different signal transduction pathways so that not all Th1 or Th2 cells produce the entire array of cytokines. The production of IL-4 by Th2 cells is supportive of B-cell switches from sIgM expression to IgG1 and to IgE (discussed later) (175–177). Furthermore, the Th2 cell subset is considered to be the major helper phenotype for supporting the IgA antibody isotype in addition to IgG1, IgG2b and IgE responses in the murine system (150).

Mucosal Helper T Cell Clones

Clones of antigen-specific PP Th cells were shown to support proliferation and differentiation of sIgA$^+$ B cells into IgA-producing plasma cells (178). These Th-cell clones were

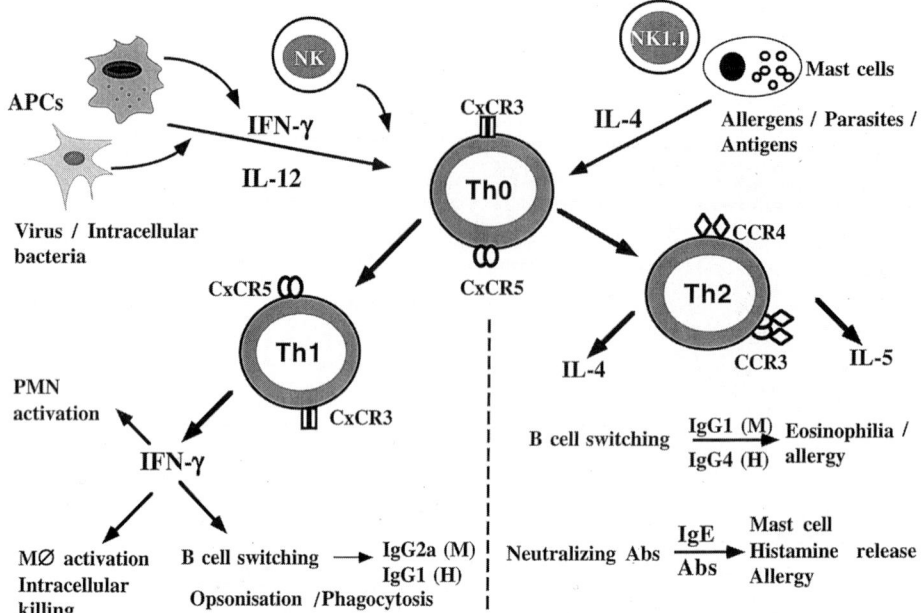

FIG. 7. T helper (Th) cell subset development. The cellular and cytokine environment induces Th0 cells to develop into either Th1 or Th2 cell subsets. Antigen-presenting cells (APCs) produce interleukin (IL)–12 in response to bacterial/viral infections and, together with interferon-γ (IFN-γ) produced by natural killer (NK) cells, induce mature Th1 cell formation. These Th1 cells express distinct chemokine receptors and, through IFN-γ synthesis, activate occasional macrophages (MØs) and induce opsonizing immunoglobulin-G2a (IgG2a) antibodies. Mast cells and NK1.1 cells respond to enterotoxins/allergens with IL-4 production, which induces Th0→Th2 switching with subsequent production of IL-4, IL-5, IL-6, IL-9, IL-10, and IL-13, which help regulate mucosal secretory IgA and serum antibody responses.

derived from PPs of mice fed sheep red blood cells (SRBCs), and SRBC-specific Th-cell clones were categorized on the basis of the antibody response induced. The first category supported IgM, IgG1, and high IgA anti-SRBC antibody responses, and although these studies preceded discovery of Th1 and Th2 subsets, these clones would, in retrospect, have properties of Th2-type cells. A second group of clones that supported only IgA anti-SRBC antibody responses (178) may be considered level 2 Th2-type cells. In this regard, it was suggested that CD4$^+$ Th cells preferentially producing IgA-enhancing cytokines (e.g., IL-6 and IL-10) were induced in a Th1-type dominant environment after oral immunization with recombinant *S. typhimurium* (179). This subset of Th2 cells was termed level 2 Th2-type cells, in contrast to level 1 CD4$^+$ T cells, which produced a full array of Th2 cytokines (IL-4, IL-5, IL-6, IL-10, and IL-13). Furthermore, several studies have shown that both PPs and effector site CD4$^+$ T cells produce IL-5, IL-6, and IFN-γ (157), and this cytokine array may also support induction of sIgA$^+$ B cells to differentiate into IgA-secreting plasma cells (see later discussion).

Mucosal Regulatory T Cells

It is now accepted that subpopulations of T cells that are CD3$^+$ $\alpha\beta$ TCR$^+$ and CD4$^+$ can regulate other T cell–mediated mucosal immune responses. All of the T cell subsets described as follows remain incompletely characterized in terms of antigen specificity, their pathway of development in the thymus, and their mode of regulation *in vivo*. The T regulatory (Tr) cells appear to control mucosal immunity, tolerance, and inflammation to a higher degree than comparable Tr cell types in peripheral lymphoid tissues. The areas in which their existence and function are best described are regulation of $\mu \rightarrow \alpha$ switching, oral tolerance induction, and normal control of intestinal homeostasis and prevention of IBD development. Unfortunately, the Tr cells that may mediate these functions have somewhat different regulatory characteristics and have been given separate designations [Th3 cells, and T regulatory 1 (Tr1) cells].

Helper Th3 Cells

As discussed later, cloned T "switch" (Tsw) cells induced sIgM$^+$ B cells to commit to sIgA expression (see later discussion). Since that early description, it has become clear that TGF-β1 is the major cytokine for $\mu \rightarrow \alpha$ switching (see later discussion). Interestingly, the finding of CD4$^+$ T-cell clones generated after induction of oral tolerance to myelin basic protein (MBP) clearly led to the description of a new phenotype of Tr cell. Clones of CD4$^+$ T cells were MBP specific, and of 48 clones assessed, 42 produced the active form of TGF-β1. Six clones produced high levels of TGF-β1 with essentially no IL-4 or IL-10 (180). On the other hand, five clones produced high IL-4 and IL-10, which, of course, is typical of Th2-type cells. The authors suggested the existence of a TGF-β1–producing Tr cell involved in control of mucosal immune responses and named it Th3 (180). This type of Tr cell is referred to in other sections of this chapter and book.

Tr1 Cells

In general, Tr cells do not proliferate well *in vitro;* this characteristic is reminiscent of anergic T cells. In fact, cloned anergic T cells can suppress immune responses *in vivo,* and this appears to be in part caused by effects on APCs (181,182). Thus, anergic T cells down-regulate DC expression of CD80 and CD86 in a contact-specific manner (181). Furthermore, anergic T cells have been shown to produce IL-10, which is a major characteristic of some CD4$^+$ CD25$^+$ Tr cells (183,184) (see later discussion). Thus, it appears that anergic T cells, through production of IL-10 (and perhaps through other mechanisms), become Treg cells that suppress immune responses to other antigens (184), a process sometimes termed *infectious tolerance* or *bystander suppression.* Despite their poor proliferative responses to antigen, it has been possible to induce populations of T-cell clones after incubation with IL-10 and alloantigen in humans (185) or to ovalbumin peptide in DO11.10 mice (186). The T-cell clones obtained had similar properties, including secretion of high levels of IL-10, some production TGF-β1, no IL-4 synthesis, and poor proliferative responses. Cells with these characteristics are now termed Tr1 cells (186,188). Thus far, Tr1 and Th3 cells have in common the production of TGF-β1 (Th3) or TGF-β1 plus IL-10 (Tr1) with suppressive-type properties.

CD4$^+$CD25$^+$ Tr Cells

Several groups have focused on naturally occurring "T suppressor" cells, using various models of organ-specific autoimmune or infectious diseases. In general, the suppressive activity is found in a rather large subset of CD3, αβTCR$^+$ CD4$^+$CD25$^+$ T cells (189). The study of this CD4$^+$CD25$^+$ Tr cell subset *in vivo* usually requires cell isolation and manipulation, followed by adoptive transfer into nude mice, mice with severe immunodeficiency disease (SCID), or mice with no recombination activating gene (RAG$^{-/-}$) (187). The CD4$^+$CD25$^+$ Tr cell subset can inhibit the development of experimental autoimmune encephalomyelitis (EAE) in MBP-transgenic mice (190,191) in a manner analogous to prevention of EAE by oral tolerance to MBP, and it is likely that Tr cells mediate some forms of oral tolerance (see later discussion). Likewise, CD4$^+$CD25$^+$ Tr cells, when cotransferred with pathogenic CD45RB^{hi} T cells that induce murine colitis (187,192), can prevent disease development (187). More details of mechanisms involved in Tr cell regulation of IBD are presented later. What is emerging from these studies is the finding that Th3, Tr1, and CD4$^+$CD25$^+$ Tr cells may

originate through a common lineage that includes anergy, TGF-β1 and IL-10 production, and prevention of autoimmune diseases.

T Cells and Cytokines for Immunoglobulin A Isotype Switching

B-cell isotype switching and gene rearrangements are discussed elsewhere in this book. In this section, we focused on the role of T cells and specific cytokines that are involved in switches to IgA. CD4$^+$ T cells and cytokines are essential for the generation of IgA-producing cells. For example, depletion of CD4$^+$ T cell subsets *in vivo* with monoclonal antibodies (mAbs) or by knockout of the CD4 co-receptor gene markedly affects mucosal immune responses (193,194). Loss of CD4$^+$ T cells is associated with diminished numbers of IgA plasma cells (193) and with deficient Th cell–regulated IgA responses (194). It is known that cytokines exert profound influences on B-cell switching from sIgM and sIgD expression to downstream isotypes, including IgG subclasses, IgE, and IgA. For B-cell terminal differentiation, IL-5 and especially IL-6, possibly in combination with other cytokines, appear essential for the continued presence of plasma cells undergoing high-rate secretion of IgA antibodies (195). Although many investigators presume that isotype switching to IgA (i.e., $\mu \rightarrow \alpha$) occurs in mucosal inductive sites such as GALT and that terminal differentiation into plasma cells producing IgA is a major event in effector sites, only indirect evidence is at hand to support these assumptions. In this regard, most studies of $\mu \rightarrow \alpha$ switching have been performed with nonmucosal lymphoid cells, such as splenic B cells, whereas *in vitro* studies of B-cell differentiation to IgA synthesis normally employ PP B cells (a mucosal inductive site) to support the idea that this also occurs in effector mucosal sites such as lamina propria and exocrine glands. Moreover, cytokine knockout mice have been studied to determine the relevance of particular cytokines for mucosal immunity, an approach discussed later. This dogma of $\mu \rightarrow \alpha$ switching occurring only in mucosal inductive sites is challenged by several findings. The activation-induced cytidine deaminase (AID) gene, initially discovered in germinal center B cells, has been cloned from B lymphoma cells stimulated with CD40 ligand, IL-4, and TGF-β that were undergoing $\mu \rightarrow \alpha$ switches (196). Overexpression of AID in μ^+ B lymphoma cells resulted in spontaneous class switching from IgM to IgA in the complete absence of TGF-β or other cytokines (197). Mice defective in the AID gene (AID$^{-/-}$) and humans with AID deficiency exhibit a hyper-IgM syndrome with no evidence of downstream switching (196,197). However, more recent studies revealed that AID$^{-/-}$ mice have a subset of B220$^+$ surface IgA$^+$ B cells in lamina propria (an effector site), and the presence of circles of "looped out" DNA suggests that $\mu \rightarrow \alpha$ switching had just occurred in this site (198). Along these lines, it was also revealed that B cell–deficient μMT mice also exhibit lamina propria IgA$^+$ plasma cells, which suggests that switches to IgA can occur even during pre–B cell development (199). These intriguing studies have used mouse models in which class switching in germinal centers is absent. Thus, $\mu \rightarrow \alpha$ B cell switches may occur throughout the mucosal immune system and in the complete absence of germinal centers.

T Cells for $\mu \rightarrow \alpha$ Switching

There is clear evidence that clones of T cells from murine GALT, when mixed with noncommitted sIgM$^+$ B cells, induce isotype switching to B cells expressing sIgA (200). The initial studies with murine Tsw cells used T-cell clones derived by mitogen stimulation and IL-2–supported outgrowth, and when Tsw cells were added to sIgM$^+$, sIgA$^-$ B-cell cultures resulted in marked increases in sIgA$^+$ cells (200). PP Tsw cells did not induce IgA synthesis, even when incubated with sIgA$^+$ B cell–enriched cultures; however, addition of B-cell growth and differentiation factors readily induced IgA secretion (200). Additional experiments showed that Tsw cells were autoreactive and suggested that continued uptake of gut luminal antigens in PPs resulted in a unique microenvironment for T–B cell interactions and subsequent IgA responses (200). This result suggests that cognate interactions between Tsw and B cells are required for induction of the IgA class switch. It is tempting to suggest that the Tsw cell is analogous to Th3 cells that produce high levels of TGF-β, perhaps in germinal centers of mucosal inductive sites.

Other studies have revealed that T–B cell interactions support B-cell switches and have postulated a major role for the CD40 receptor on germinal center B cells with CD40 ligand on activated T cells (201–203). In the presence of antigen, the B cells may alter the affinity and functions of the antibody receptor through somatic mutation of variable region genes, with cytokines such as IL-4 (for IgG1 and IgE) and TGF-β (for IgA) directing heavy chain (isotype) switching. Furthermore, the environment of the B cell may play a role in switching (136). Germane to this discussion are studies with an effective APC, the DC, which resides in the dome region and T-cell zones of PPs and influences switching to IgA. For example, coculture of activated T cells and DC from PPs with purified sIgM$^+$, sIgA$^-$ B cells resulted in the synthesis of large amounts of IgA, whereas DCs and T cells isolated from the spleen were less effective (204). Additional studies showed that the DC–T cell mixture from PPs also induced isotype switching to IgA in a pre–B cell line, whereas DC–T cell mixtures from the spleen had no effect. Although these studies purported to show that the DC was the major cell type promoting B-cell switches to IgA, it remains possible that the PP DC–T cell mixtures harbored contaminating B cells that produced IgA, and more definitive proof that the DC is directly involved in B-cell switches to IgA is thus required.

Evidence for Tsw cells in human IgA responses was presented in an earlier study with malignant T cells from a patient RAC (TRAC cells) who suffered from a mycosis fungoides/Sézary-like syndrome. The TRAC cells induced tonsillar sIgM$^+$ B cells to switch and secrete IgG and IgA

(205). Furthermore, TRAC cells, when added to B-cell cultures obtained from patients with hyper-IgM immunodeficiency, induced eight of nine cultures to secrete IgG and three of nine to produce IgA (205). T-cell clones have also been obtained from the human appendix, and these clones and their derived culture supernatants exhibited preferential help for IgA synthesis (206). There was also direct evidence that CD3$^+$CD4$^+$CD8$^-$ T cell clones induced $\mu \rightarrow \alpha$ B-cell switches and terminal differentiation of sIgA$^+$ B cells into IgA-producing plasma cells (150).

Cytokines that Induce Switches to Immunoglobulin A

Isotype switching involves the recombination between tandem repetitive DNA sequences [switch (S) regions] located 5′ of the respective heavy chain (CH) genes (see Chapter 5). Switching is an irreversible DNA deletional event in which recombination between upstream and downstream S regions forms a DNA circle containing the deleted intervening CH genes. Isotype switching can also be induced by cytokines in combination with activation signals provided by mitogens such as LPS or through the more physiological T-cell CD40 ligand and B-cell CD40 interactions discussed previously. The two best studied switch cytokines are IL-4, which induces switching to IgG1 and IgE in cultures of LPS-stimulated mouse splenic B cells (171,175), and TGF-β, which induces $\mu \rightarrow \alpha$ switches, discussed in detail later. Several tangible events, including demethylation of 5′ flanking region DNA, deoxyribonuclease hypersensitivity, and transcription of unrearranged CH genes, precede cytokine-induced switching. The germline transcripts correspond to the immunoglobulin isotype to which the B cell will switch, in which IL-4 will induce Cγ1 and Cϵ germline transcripts before the expression of either IgG1 or IgE in LPS-stimulated splenic B cells. IFN-γ has also been shown to induce germline Cγ2a transcription and isotype switching to IgG2a in murine splenic B-cell cultures (171). The germline transcription initiates 5′ of the targeted CH gene upstream of so-called I-region exons, which contain stop codons, in all translational reading frames; thus, the resulting transcripts are "sterile." I-region exons have been identified for all isotypes and subclasses; in general, their deletion—for example, in I-region exon–knockout mice—results in impaired switching to that isotype or subclass (207–209). An apparent exception has been observed for IgA switching, in which replacement of the Iα exon with an irrelevant human gene construct in the gene transcriptional orientation did not impair B-cell switching to IgA (210). These studies rule out a direct role for the I-region exon in controlling switch recombination. However, transcription of the Cα locus was found to be constitutive in the Iα-targeted mice, in contrast to other I-region knockout mice (207–209). It seems likely that cytokine-induced transcription of the germline transcripts themselves direct cytokine-regulated isotype switching.

The most definitive studies to date suggest that TGF-β is the major cytokine for B-cell switching to IgA (211–217).

The first studies showed that addition of TGF-β to LPS-triggered murine splenic B-cell cultures resulted in switching to IgA, and IgA synthesis was markedly enhanced by IL-2 (213) or IL-5 (217). The effect of TGF-β was on sIgM$^+$, sIgA$^-$ B cells and was not caused by selective induction of terminal B-cell differentiation. It was shown that TGF-β induced sterile Cα germline transcripts (211,213), an event that clearly precedes actual switching to IgA. Interestingly, Iα-deficient mice apparently lose their requirement for TGF-β-induced switching, presumably because the Cα locus is constitutively activated and LPS alone is sufficient for induction of $\mu \to \alpha$ B-cell switches (210). Subsequent studies showed that TGF-β induced human B cells to switch to either IgA1 or IgA2, an event clearly shown to be preceded by formation of Cα1 and Cα2 germline transcripts (214,215). It can be presumed that TGF-β induces $\mu \to \alpha$ switches in normal physiological circumstances, inasmuch as sIgM$^+$, sIgD$^+$ B cells triggered through CD40 were induced to switch to IgA by TGF-β and to secrete IgA in the presence of IL-10 (218,219).

It should be emphasized that almost all studies to date with TGF-β-induced switches have been done in B-cell cultures stimulated with mitogens or through co-receptor signaling (211–216,219). These studies reveal that only 2% to 5% of B cells actually switch to IgA, which makes it difficult to explain the high rate of switching that normally occurs in PP germinal centers (> 60%). This point was addressed in a system in which B cells were triggered with anti-CD40 and anti-dextran, both of which mimic T cell–dependent and T cell–independent stimuli, respectively. It was shown that TGF-β, together with IL-4 and IL-5, induced sIgA$^+$ B-cell populations of up to 15% to 20% (220). Although deletion of the TGF-β gene would be predicted to lead to a negative influence on the IgA immune system, the TGF-β gene knockout mice, unfortunately, die from a generalized lymphoproliferative disease 3 to 5 weeks after birth, which makes it difficult to use this model to investigate the role of TGF-β in IgA regulation *in vivo*. Nevertheless, TGF-$\beta^{-/-}$ mice exhibit low levels of IgA plasma cells in effector sites and low levels of S-IgA in external secretions (221), which provides evidence that TGF-β1 is also important for $\mu \to \alpha$ switching *in vivo*. In one study, conditional mutagenesis (Cre/loxP) was used to knock out the TGF-β receptor in B cells (222). Affected mice exhibited expanded peritoneal B-1 cells and B-cell hyperplasia in PPs and a complete absence of serum IgA (222).

Regulation of Mucosal Immunity by Helper T Cell Subsets

As discussed previously, there is clear evidence that CD4$^+$ Th cells and derived clones from mucosal inductive sites can support the IgA response (150,218). However, it still remains to be shown that immune responses to mucosally presented antigens belong to distinct classes of Th1- and Th2-type responses. Nevertheless, it is clear that Th1 and Th2 cells are sensitive to cross-regulation by the opposite cell type. For example, IFN-γ produced by Th1 cells inhibits proliferation of Th2 cells, is responsible for an isotype switch from IgM to IgG2a (171), and inhibits isotype switching induced by IL-4 (223). Th2 cells regulate the effects of Th1 cells by secreting IL-10, which inhibits cytokine secretion by Th1 cells (e.g., inhibition of IFN-γ secretion), in turn decreasing IFN-γ–mediated inhibition of Th2 cells. Therefore, it is important to determine the antigen-specific cytokine secretion profile, as well as the antigen-specific IgG subclasses and IgE and IgA responses, to fully characterize immune responses induced by mucosal antigens.

In addition to division of effector T cells into Th1- and Th2-types on the basis of cytokine expression profiles, it is also clear that both CD4$^+$ effector and memory T cells can be defined by their adhesion and chemokine receptor expression (224,225). These molecules direct T-cell subsets into their functional environments *in vivo*. This was illustrated by a study using the DO11.10 ovalbumin (OVA) transgenic mouse, in which OVA peptide–specific T cells are recognized by the mAb KJ1-26. An aliquot of KJ1-26$^+$ T cells was transferred to naïve BALB/c mice and then immunized with OVA and cholera toxin (CT) as adjuvant. Both B-cell help-type Th cells and those involved in inflammation were subsequently analyzed (226). As expected, CT induced anti-OVA antibodies of IgG1 subclass, which indicate Th2-type help. Of importance, the immune JK1-26 CD4$^+$ T cells were separable into distinct subsets on the basis of expression of adhesion molecules. Thus, one subset expressed an adhesion-chemokine receptor pattern consistent with inflammation, and a second subset a pattern associated with entry into B-cell follicles. The inflammatory T-cell phenotype exhibited poor B-cell help; however, these T cells produced higher levels of IFN-γ, which was consistent with their ability to mediate DTH responses in skin (226). Although this model has not yet been used for evaluation of mucosal DTH (CMI) or B-cell help-type responses, it is clear that nasal antigen plus CT induces CD4$^+$ T cells for high IFN-γ production and others providing help for IgE responses (227).

Earlier studies have shown that oral immunization with a combined vaccine containing protein antigens (e.g., tetanus toxoid) together with the mucosal adjuvant CT resulted in protein-specific CD4$^+$ T cells in GALT and the spleen that preferentially produce IL-4 and IL-5 but not IFN-γ or IL-2 (228). This immunization protocol also induces serum IgG responses characterized by high IgG1 titers with low or undetectable IgG2a antibodies and increased antigen-specific IgE responses (228). Co-administration of other antigens such as OVA or hen egg white lysozyme (HEL) with CT according to the same mucosal immunization schedule produced similar findings. It therefore appears that oral immunization with soluble proteins with CT as adjuvant results in the induction of Th2-type responses. Other investigators have also found that oral immunization of C3H/He, SWR/J, and DBA/1 mice with two doses of 200 to 1000 μg of the soluble protein HEL and 5 to 10 μg of CT separated by 3 weeks induces antigen-specific IgG (predominantly IgG1), IgA, and IgE responses (229). In addition, systemic challenge of orally immunized mice with HEL led to a fatal anaphylactic reaction caused by the high levels of antigen-specific IgE (229). Oral immunization of C57BL/6 mice with keyhole limpet hemocyanin (KLH), CT (0.5 μg), and B subunit of CT (CT-B) (10 μg) on three occasions at 10-day intervals resulted in both PP and lamina propria lymphocyte populations that produced low levels of IL-2 and IFN-γ and higher levels of IL-4 and IL-5. The results from this study support the conclusion that oral immunization with soluble protein antigen and CT as an adjuvant induces Th2-type immune responses.

In addition to CT, heat-labile toxin (LT) from enterotoxigenic *E. coli* is an effective immunogen and adjuvant for the induction and regulation of antigen-specific IgA responses (230,231). Oral immunization with LT resulted in the induction of antigen-specific serum IgG and mucosal IgA responses (232), and assessment of LT-specific IgG subclass responses revealed high levels of IgG1, IgG2a, and IgG2b, which contrasted with IgG subclass responses induced by CT (e.g., dominant IgG1 without IgG2a). Furthermore, lower IgE responses were observed after oral immunization with LT than with CT (232). With regard to the profile of isotype and subclass of antigen-specific responses induced by orally administered LT or CT, both bacterial enterotoxins supported mucosal IgA responses, although LT and CT behaved differently for the induction of serum IgG subclass and IgE responses. Large amounts of IFN-γ and IL-5 but little IL-4 were detected in LT-specific CD4$^+$ T cells from PPs and spleen cells of mucosally immunized mice. In marked contrast to CT, LT induced both Th1- and Th2-type responses. The production of IFN-γ by mucosally induced LT-specific Th1-type cells may lead to the induction of level 2 Th2-type cells, in which the IgA-enhancing cytokine IL-5 is produced without IL-4. In this regard, LT could be used as a mucosal adjuvant for induction of both Th1- and Th2-type responses after mucosal immunization, whereas CT could be considered as a selective Th2 inducer in the murine system. These findings suggest that the outcome of Th1- or Th2-type responses or both can be manipulated after mucosal immunization through the use of enterotoxins such as CT and LT.

Cytokine Regulation of Immunoglobulin A Production

Earlier studies revealed that addition of culture supernatants from DC–T cell clusters, T-cell clones, or T-cell hybridomas to cultures of PPs or splenic B cells resulted in enhanced secretion of IgA (233). One factor responsible for this activity was subsequently shown to be IL-5 (217,234–238). Removal of sIgA$^+$ B cells from PP B-cell cultures abrogated IgA synthesis, demonstrating that this cytokine affected postswitch IgA-committed B cells (237). No *in vitro* stimulus was required for PP B cells, and IL-4 did not further enhance the effect of IL-5 (233). If splenic B cells were used, these cells required stimulation with LPS before increased IgA secretion occurred. With LPS-stimulated splenic B cells, the IgA-enhancing effect of IL-5 could be further increased by addition of IL-2 or IL-4. Together, these results suggest that

IL-5 induces sIgA$^+$ B cells that are in cell cycle (blasts) to differentiate into IgA-producing cells. Interestingly, another B-cell population, the peritoneal cavity B-1 cells, has been shown to contain precursors of lamina propria IgA plasma cells (239). This population also contains cells that can be induced by IL-5 to secrete IgA (195). Human IL-5 is thought to act mainly as an eosinophil differentiation factor and thus may have little effect on B-cell isotype switching and differentiation. It has been reported, however, that human B cells, when stimulated with the bacterium *Moraxella (Branhamella) catarrhalis,* could be induced by IL-5 to secrete IgA and also to possibly undergo isotype switching to IgA (150,158,175–177). This effect could not be demonstrated with other more conventional B-cell mitogens; that finding demonstrates the importance of the primary *in vitro* activation signal for B-cell switching.

IL-6, when added to PP B cells in the absence of any *in vitro* stimulus, causes a marked increase in IgA secretion with little effect on either IgM or IgG synthesis (195). In these studies, IL-6 induced twofold to threefold more IgA secretion than did IL-5 (195). The removal of sIgA$^+$ B cells abolished the effect of IL-6, which demonstrates that, like IL-5, this cytokine also acted on postswitch B cells. In mice in which the IL-6 gene had been inactivated [IL-6 gene knockouts (IL-6$^{-/-}$)], the numbers of IgA$^+$ B cells in the lamina propria were markedly reduced, and antibody responses after mucosal challenge with OVA or vaccinia virus were greatly diminished. Although the findings from these studies demonstrate the *in vivo* importance of IL-6 for mucosal IgA responses (240), other studies have shown that IL-6$^{-/-}$ mice exhibit normal lamina propria distributions of IgA plasma cells and respond to oral protein when CT is used as mucosal adjuvant (241). The discrepancy in these results is difficult to explain; however, it is possible that compensatory pathways may become activated in IL-6$^{-/-}$ mice for support of IgA responses. Of relevance to this discussion was the finding that human appendix sIgA$^+$ B cells express IL-6 receptors, whereas other B cell subsets present do not. Furthermore, appendix B cells were induced by IL-6 to secrete both IgA1 and IgA2 in the absence of any *in vitro* activation (242). This effect was also shown in IgA-committed B cells, again demonstrating the importance of IL-6 for inducing the terminal differentiation of sIgA$^+$ B cells into IgA plasma cells.

An additional Th2 cytokine, IL-10, has also been shown to play an important role in the induction of IgA synthesis in humans (218,243,244). Stimulation of human B cells with anti-CD40 and *Staphylococcus aureus* Cowan (SAC) resulted in B-cell differentiation for IgM and IgG synthesis in patients with IgA deficiency. The addition of IL-10 to the anti-CD40$^-$ and SAC-stimulated B cell cultures induced IgA production (243). Cultured B cells from common variable immunodeficiency patients also produce IgA, in addition to IgM and IgG, in the presence of anti-CD40 and IL-10 (244). Furthermore, naïve sIgD$^+$ B cells could be induced to produce IgA after coculture with IL-10 in the presence of TGF-β and anti-CD40 (218). Together, these findings demonstrate that Th2 cytokines such as IL-5, IL-6, and IL-10 all play major roles in the induction of IgA responses.

Because IL-2 produced by pTh or Th1-type cells has been shown to enhance IgA synthesis in LPS-stimulated B-cell cultures, it would be too simplistic to conclude that Th2-type cells and their derived cytokines are the only cytokines important in the generation of IgA responses (218). IL-2 also synergistically augmented IgA synthesis in B-cell cultures in the presence of LPS and TGF-β (213). Although IFN-γ is not directly involved in the enhancement of IgA B-cell responses, this cytokine has been shown to enhance the expression of pIgR, an essential molecule for the transport of S-IgA (67). B cells activated through surface immunoglobulin in the presence of IFN-γ became potent APCs for T cells (245). In addition, IFN-γ enhances the expression of B7-2, which may be a key co-stimulatory molecule for the induction of Th2-type cells (246). In summary, an optimal relationship between Th1- and Th2-derived cytokines is essential for the induction, regulation, and maintenance of appropriate IgA responses in mucosa-associated tissues.

Mucosal Cytotoxic T Cells

In the mucosal setting, natural infection of the epithelium by enteric (e.g., rotavirus or reovirus) or respiratory [e.g., influenza, or respiratory syncytial virus (RSV)] viral pathogens leads to endogenous viral peptide processing that induces pCTLs to become effector (activated) and memory CTLs. Most virus-specific CTLs are CD8$^+$ $\alpha\beta$ TCR$^+$, and recognition of viral peptides is associated with class I MHC presentation by infected cells (139,247). In this regard, high numbers of CD8$^+$ T cells reside in the mucosal epithelium as a subpopulation of IELs (248,249). These CD8$^+$ IELs are thought to represent an important cytotoxic effector population that can eliminate virus-infected epithelial cells. When freshly isolated IELs were examined with a redirected cytotoxicity assay, these T-lymphocytes were found to constitutively possess lytic activity (250–252).

Significant progress is being made in areas related to the roles of APCs for induction of pCTLs and for mechanisms of perforin-mediated (252,253) or Fas–Fas ligand–associated killing of target cells (254). Remaining issues include the importance of class II MHC–restricted CD4$^+$ Th1-type (and Th2-type) cells for regulation of pCTL differentiation into effector and memory CTLs (247). This section briefly reviews the significant progress in the area of mucosal CTL induction and regulation as they pertain to viral infections. It should be noted that the same processes occur during host responses to intracellular bacteria and to tumor-associated antigens, and in certain mucosal parasite infestations. Although this focus is on CD8$^+$ CTLs, cell-mediated and antibody-mediated cytotoxicity and NK cell activity are major responses associated with IELs (139).

An obvious question is how a CTL immune response is initiated, because mucosal inductive sites, which harbor pCTLs, are separate from effector sites, such as infected epithelial cells in which activated CD8$^+$ CTLs function. A partial answer is that the M cell has specific receptors for mucosal viruses, best exemplified by reovirus. As described earlier, the reovirus sigma protein (123) enters the M cell in both NALT and GALT (128,255). It is likely, although less well documented, that other enteric viruses, such as rotavirus, and respiratory pathogens, such as influenza and RSV, also enter the mucosal inductive pathway through M cells (123,129). Furthermore, it is now established that administration of virus into the GI tract results in the induction of increased pCTL frequencies in PPs (138,256). For example, reoviruses localize to T-cell regions and are clearly associated both with increased CD8$^+$ pCTLs and with memory B-cell responses (139). Oral administration of vaccinia virus to rats results in the induction of virus-specific CTLs in PPs and mesenteric lymph nodes (257). These findings suggest that, after enteric infection or immunization, antigen-stimulated CTLs are disseminated from PPs into mesenteric lymph nodes via the lymphatic drainage (258). Furthermore, virus-specific CTLs are also generated in mucosa-associated tissues by oral immunization with reovirus and rotavirus (138,256). A high frequency of virus-specific CTLs was seen in PPs as early as 6 days after oral immunization. Moreover, virus-specific CTLs were also found among lamina propria lymphocytes, IELs, and spleen cells of mice mucosally immunized with reovirus or rotavirus (138,256,258). Although mucosal effector tissues such as intestinal epithelium contain high numbers of $\gamma\delta$ T cells in addition to $\alpha\beta$ T cells, virus-specific CTLs in IELs were associated with the latter T-cell subset (139). These studies suggest that oral immunization with live virus can induce antigen-specific CTLs in both mucosal inductive and effector tissues and in systemic lymphoid tissues.

The pCTLs induced by reovirus in GALT have been shown in kinetic studies to migrate to the systemic compartment (259,260). Such homing occurs to specialized effector compartments including the epithelium of the small intestine. Thus, reovirus-specific CD8$^+$ CTLs are present among IELs and are associated with the $\alpha\beta$ T-cell population (260). There also is clear that oral delivery of rotavirus induces increased pCTLs in GALT, which are then disseminated throughout the murine lymphoid system within 3 weeks (256). Furthermore, effector CTLs were shown to protect against gastritis in the suckling mouse model (261). In a series of elegant studies whose purpose was to define the host determinants of rotavirus immunity, it was shown that CD8$^+$ T cells mediated clearance of rotavirus infection of SCID mice (262). The murine system has been invaluable for discerning the pathways used by mucosal viruses and the importance of effector CTLs in immunity to infection. It should be kept in mind that CTLs do not function alone, and mucosal antibody responses are also of central importance in immunity. Indeed, both S-IgA antibodies and CD8$^+$ CTLs are of central importance in rotavirus immunity (263).

Detailed studies of immune responses after intranasal infection with influenza virus have also revealed that both humoral and cellular pathways are involved in virus clearance

(264–267). In this model, use of CD4–co-receptor knockouts or depletion of this subset did not affect induction of pCTLs or significantly alter the clearance of infection (264–267). It has been shown in mice that the lack of CD8$^+$ T cells (β_2-microglobulin knockout mice) or treatment with anti-CD8 mAbs did not alter clearance of influenza. These results support the presence of multiple pathways for immunity and suggest that CD4$^+$ Th-cell pathways are important for mucosal antibody responses and CD8$^+$ CTLs for respiratory tract immunity (265–267).

Several studies have also established that effector CTLs protect mice from RSV infection. In one, the RSV F determinant, a 22-kDa glycoprotein, was shown to induce protective CTLs (268,269). In a separate line of investigation, the murine RSV model was used to determine the relative importance of CD4$^+$ T cells, including Th1 and Th2 subsets, which resulted in inflammation versus immunity. These ongoing studies clearly suggest that CD4$^+$ IFN-γ–producing Th1 cells and CD8$^+$ T cells are associated with recovery, whereas CD4$^+$ Th2-type pathways are not (45,270). Interestingly, priming with inactivated RSV or F glycoprotein induced CD4$^+$ Th2 cells, whereas live RSV elicited the Th1-type pathway. In view of mucosal vaccine development for virus infections, these findings suggest that the outcome of Th1-type (including induction of CTLs) and Th2-type immune responses could be regulated by the nature and form of viral antigen used for immunization.

Intraepithelial Lymphocytes

The major interface between internal organs and outside environments is the columnar IEC layer in the GI tract. In addition to epithelial cells, the columnar epithelium includes a population of lymphocytes commonly termed *intraepithelial lymphocytes* (44,159,248,249). As their name implies, IELs reside between the basolateral surfaces of epithelial cells. It has been estimated that one IEL can be found for every six epithelial cells (149), which indicates that large numbers of lymphocytes are situated in the intestinal mucosal tissues. These lymphocytes are continuously exposed to antigens ingested via the epithelial layer. It is logical to assume that IELs are important lymphoid cells that participate in the induction and regulation of the mucosal immune response. Indeed, on the basis of new information, it is now well accepted that IELs play key roles in the induction and regulation of intestinal and mucosal immunity.

Origin and Development of Intraepithelial Lymphocytes

In general, the majority of human and murine IELs are classified as T cells because they express the CD3 molecule in association with two forms of TCRs: $\gamma\delta$ and $\alpha\beta$ (44,159,248). With regard to the expression of CD4 and CD8 by intraepithelial T cells, it has been shown that approximately 80% of these cells belong to the CD8 subset; however, a substantial number of IELs can be grouped as CD4-bearing cells, including CD4$^+$CD8$^-$ and CD4$^+$CD8$^+$ subsets (44,159,271–273). The

occurrence of large numbers of CD8$^+$ T cells among IELs is distinct from the case of T cells residing in other lymphoid tissues. In addition, it is now generally agreed that approximately equal numbers of TCR$\gamma\delta^+$ ($\gamma\delta$) and TCR$\alpha\beta^+$ ($\alpha\beta$) T cells develop in IELs of young adult mice (Fig. 8) (44,159,273–275).

The CD8 molecules expressed on IELs consist of either $\alpha\beta$ heterodimeric or $\alpha\alpha$ homodimeric chains. CD8$\alpha\beta^+$ IELs express Thy-1 and bear $\alpha\beta$ TCR. In contrast, CD8$\alpha\alpha^+$ IELs contain both TCR$\gamma\delta$ and TCR$\alpha\beta$ fractions, and the majority lack Thy-1 (276). Previous studies have shown that CD4$^-$CD8$\alpha\alpha^+$ IELs, but not CD4$^+$CD8$^-$ or CD4$^-$CD8$\alpha\beta^+$ IELs, also develop in nude mice (276). Furthermore, CD4$^-$CD8$\alpha\alpha^+$ can differentiate in thymectomized, lethally irradiated mice reconstituted with T cell–depleted bone marrow from normal mice. These findings indicate that CD4$^-$CD8$\alpha\alpha^+$ IELs develop via a thymus-independent pathway, whereas CD4$^+$CD8$^-$ and CD4$^-$CD8$\alpha\beta^+$ T-cell subsets develop in the thymus (Fig. 8).

In the case of $\gamma\delta$ IELs, a number of studies using athymic nude mouse bone marrow or fetal liver–reconstituted irradiation chimeras have demonstrated that significant numbers of intraepithelial $\gamma\delta$ T cells develop extrathymically (277–279). Furthermore, it has been shown that, before T-cell colonization of the mouse fetal thymus, rearrangements of the Vγ5 gene, the predominant Vγ region utilized by IELs, can be detected in the developing gut and liver (280). In addition, RAG1 is expressed by the subset of CD3$^-$ IELs (276, 281,282). Together, these results indicate that TCRγ-specific gene rearrangement can occur extrathymically (Fig. 8).

Studies have offered one explanation for the origin of extrathymic IELs. Clusters of lymphocytes that express c-kit, IL-7 receptor, Thy-1, and LFA-1 were found to be located in crypt lamina propria (cryptopatches) of the murine small

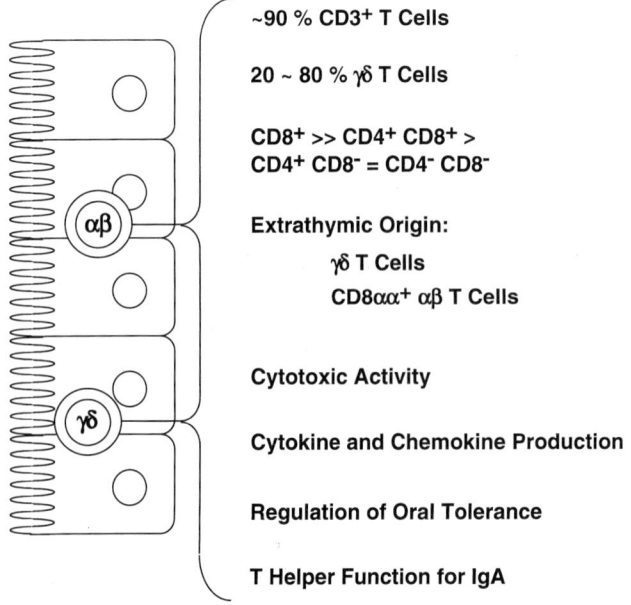

FIG. 8. Unique features of intraepithelial lymphocytes.

~90 % CD3$^+$ T Cells

20 ~ 80 % $\gamma\delta$ T Cells

CD8$^+$ >> CD4$^+$ CD8$^+$ > CD4$^+$ CD8$^-$ = CD4$^-$ CD8$^-$

Extrathymic Origin:
$\gamma\delta$ T Cells
CD8$\alpha\alpha^+$ $\alpha\beta$ T Cells

Cytotoxic Activity

Cytokine and Chemokine Production

Regulation of Oral Tolerance

T Helper Function for IgA

and large intestine, with a phenotype of CD3⁻, TCRαβ⁻, TCRγδ⁻, sIgM−, and B220⁻ (383). When c-kit⁺ but lineage marker–negative cells were isolated from these cryptopatches and adoptively transferred to SCID mice, they gave rise to intraepithelial γδ and αβ T cells in the intestinal epithelium (284), which indicates that the cryptopatch is a major source of mucosal IELs in the intestinal epithelium. In addition, this patch is an important nest for the development of extrathymic T cells associated with IELs.

Selection and Usage of T-Cell Receptors by Intraepithelial T-Lymphocytes

The influence of MHC antigens on TCRγδ usage in CD8⁺ IELs has been examined with the use of a panreactive and Vδ4 region–specific mAb, which showed that positive or negative selection of CD8⁺ γδ IELs can occur extrathymically (278). Interestingly, the selection of Vδ4⁺ intraepithelial T cells occurs in a class II MHC–dependent manner, although these cells express the CD8 molecule (278). In this regard, it has been shown that the selection of peripheral CD8⁺ αβ T cells by minor lymphocyte-stimulating (Mls) viral superantigens requires class II MHC expression (285). Interestingly, however, β₂-microglobulin–deficient mice possess a normal number of CD8⁺αα intraepithelial γδ T cells, whereas CD8⁺ αβ IELs are essentially absent (286), which suggests that class I MHC expression is not involved in the generation of γδ IELs. However, these findings do not preclude the possibility that this subset of IELs responds to antigens associated with class I MHC molecules.

As described, intraepithelial CD8αα⁺ αβ T cells are thought to develop extrathymically. Thus, certain Vβ regions (e.g., Vβ6, Vβ8.1, and Vβ11) that are not expressed in peripheral T cells of DBA/2 mice (Mlsᵃ, IE⁺) are expressed in their IELs (159). Furthermore, the forbidden V regions (e.g., Vβ3, Vβ6, and Vβ7) are expressed by CD8αα but not CD8αβ IELs (159), which suggests that CD8αα⁺ intraepithelial αβ T cells develop extrathymically. However, thymus grafting experiments on neonatally thymectomized mice with immature-phenotype αβ IELs have revealed that CD8αα⁺ αβ IELs can be thymus derived (159). It has also been shown that forbidden V-region expression is not strictly confined to the CD8αα⁺ subset. Comparison of TCRαβ V-region usage by CD4⁺CD8αα⁺ and CD4⁻CD8αα⁺ intraepithelial T-cell subsets in Mls-disparate, MHC-identical mouse strains revealed that in cases in which forbidden V regions are expressed by CD4⁻CD8αα⁺ IELs, the same TCRs are deleted from CD4⁺CD8αα⁺ IELs (159). These results suggest that lack of the β chain of the CD8 molecule is not solely responsible for forbidden V-region expression.

Mucosal Intranet Formed by Intestinal Epithelial Cells and Intraepithelial Lymphocytes

IECs are in constant contact with luminal flora and often become the target of microbial attachment and replication, leading to the establishment of infection. In view of the presence of immune and inflammatory cells within the epithelium and their obvious changes during infection or inflammation, it is worthwhile to consider the role of IECs in orchestrating these responses. Because IELs are adjacent to IECs, it is natural to assume that cell-to-cell communication, dynamically regulated by specific cytokines and corresponding receptor signaling, may occur between intraepithelial T cells and IECs during immunological reactions and changes at the epithelium.

Because certain IEL subsets (e.g., TCRγδ⁺ and TCRαβ⁺ CD8αα⁺) have been shown to develop extrathymically, several investigators have proposed the involvement of epithelial cells in the differentiation of IELs (159,287). For example, it is known that IECs constitutively express class II MHC molecules (44,159) and that IEC lines are capable of processing and presenting antigen to T cells (287). It has also been shown that class I MHC–like molecules such as CD1d and thymus leukemia antigen are predominantly expressed by IECs (288,289). Thymus leukemia antigen is also expressed on the cell surface of γδ and αβ IELs (289). These results suggest that these molecules may play important roles in the regulation of intestinal immune responses. In support of this hypothesis, an αβ IEL T-cell line established from human jejunum has been shown to exhibit CD1-specific cytotoxicity (290). However, a CD1-specific response of γδ IELs has not been reported.

IECs have been shown to produce a number of cytokines (see previous discussion). Although there are many potential cytokine–effector cell interactions, one of the best described responses that deserves some emphasis involves IELs and IL-7. To this end, it was shown that murine IECs express IL-7–specific mRNA (291), and human IECs are also capable of producing this cytokine (24). IL-7 supports the growth and development of intraepithelial γδ T cells, and a subset of γδ T cells isolated from murine epithelium expressed both IL-2– and IL-7–specific receptors (IL-2 and IL-7 receptors) (291). When the γδ T cells were incubated with an optimal concentration of IL-2 or IL-7, significant proliferative responses were noted (291). Other studies have also shown that mice that lack the common cytokine receptor γ chain (γ_c), a functional subunit of both IL-2 and IL-7 receptors (292), manifest complete loss of γδ T cells (293–295). These results indicate that IL-7 secreted by IEC is essential for the activation and growth of intraepithelial γδ T cells.

In addition to the IL-7 and corresponding receptor signaling cascade, stem cell factor and c-kit interactions have been shown to play important roles in the growth of intraepithelial T cells. Thus, although normal levels of IELs were detected in c-kit (W/Wv) or stem cell factor (SI/SId) mutant mice, the number of γδ IELs decreased beginning at 6 to 8 weeks of age (296), which indicates the importance of stem cell factor–c-kit interactions for IELs. Other studies have shown the effect of IL-15 on the proliferation and maintenance of intraepithelial γδ T cells. IECs and γδ IELs constitutively express high levels of IL-15 and IL-15 receptor α, respectively. Furthermore, γδ IELs proliferate in response to IL-15 more vigorously than do αβ IELs (297,298). Moreover, IL-15 receptor α gene–disrupted (IL-15R$\alpha^{-/-}$) mice are deficient in $\gamma\delta$ IELs (299). Together, these results indicate that the mucosal intrernet between epithelial cells and $\gamma\delta$ T cells via cytokine–cytokine receptor interactions could be an important communication link for the development of IELs.

With regard to the role of IELs in IEC development, it has been shown that $\gamma\delta$ but not $\alpha\beta$ T cells obtained from intestinal epithelium produce keratinocyte growth factor and promote the growth of epithelial cells (300). Furthermore, TCR$\gamma\delta^{-/-}$ mice have been shown to exhibit reduced epithelial cell turnover and down-regulated expression of class II MHC molecules (301). These studies provide evidence that intraepithelial $\gamma\delta$ T cells regulate the generation and differentiation of IECs.

Production of Helper T 1 and 2 Cells and Inflammatory Cytokines by Intraepithelial Lymphocytes

Analysis of cytokine expression by IELs has shown that both small and large intestinal IELs equally express mRNA for IL-1, IFN-γ, and TNF-α, whereas large intestinal IELs tend to produce higher levels of IL-2, IL-4, and IL-10 in comparison with small intestinal subsets (302). Both $\alpha\beta$ and $\gamma\delta$ IEL T cells synthesize an array of cytokines that includes IL-2, IL-3, IL-6, IFN-γ, TNF-α, and TGF-β (303). It has also been shown that freshly isolated CD4$^+$CD8$^-$ IEL T cells contain Th2-type cells, including high numbers of IL-5–secreting cells and cells secreting IL-4 and IL-6, whereas CD4$^+$CD8$^+$ T cells include IL-5– and IL-6–producing cells, which do not secrete IL-4 (304). In addition to Th2-type cytokine-producing T cells, both CD4$^+$ T-cell subsets contain IFN-γ–secreting Th1-type cells, but neither subset synthesizes IL-2. Stimulation of CD4$^+$CD8$^-$ and CD4$^+$CD8$^+$ IELs with anti-CD3 mAb resulted in production of IL-2 in addition to IFN-γ, IL-5, and IL-6, and this treatment stimulated CD4$^+$CD8$^+$ IELs to produce IL-4 (304). Other studies have shown that freshly isolated and activated TCR$\gamma\delta^+$ IEL T cells express high levels of mRNA specific for lymphotactin, a chemokine important for CD8$^+$ T-cell chemotaxis (305). Furthermore, human IELs have been shown to exhibit chemotactic activity in response to IL-8 and to chemokine regulated upon activation, normal T-cell expressed, presumably secreted (RANTES), whereas only a few lamina propria lymphocytes migrated toward IL-8, and none responded to RANTES (306). These results suggest that intraepithelial T cells actively produce cytokines and chemokines to provide specific immunological functions in the mucosal compartment (Fig. 8).

Role of Intraepithelial Lymphocytes in Mucosal Defense

Because mucosal surfaces are portals of entry of numerous pathogens, it is logical to consider that IELs represent an important first line of defense against external environmental challenge. Several studies have shown that freshly isolated murine and human CD8$^+$ IEL T cells are cytotoxic in the redirected lysis assay (159,306). In this assay, cells undergo reaction with an anti-TCR mAb and are then incubated with radiolabeled target cells, which allows polyclonally activated cells that exhibit cytotoxicity to be detected. Because splenic and lymph node CD8$^+$ T cells are not cytotoxic unless they have been previously activated (306), it is assumed that IELs are activated *in situ* as a result of the constant stimulation by environmental antigens. As discussed previously, freshly isolated IELs do spontaneously produce cytokines. Furthermore, cytotoxic activity is significantly reduced in IELs obtained from germ-free mice (306). These results support the notion that the presence of bacterial antigen is important for the induction of cytotoxic activity of IELs. However, other researchers have reported that this activity is also observable for IELs of germ-free mice (250). Therefore, it appears that cytotoxic activity of murine $\gamma\delta$ IELs was strain dependent and that the mucosal microbiota were not required to induce cytotoxic activity of $\gamma\delta$ (but not $\alpha\beta$) IELs (306). Thus, stimulation by bacterial antigens may not be required for cytolytic activity of $\gamma\delta$ IELs.

Another important aspect of the immune response at mucosal surfaces is the production of S-IgA antibodies. IELs produce a wide array of cytokines, including Th2-type cytokines such as IL-4, IL-5, and IL-6. Furthermore, a helper function of IELs has been proposed for support of IgA synthesis (271,304). Thus, IELs may be actively involved in the induction and regulation of S-IgA antibody responses at mucosal surfaces. It was shown that the number of IgA-producing cells in mucosa-associated tissues, such as the intestinal lamina propria of TCR$\gamma\delta^{-/-}$ mice, was significantly lower than that observed in control (TCR$\gamma\delta^{+/+}$) mice of the same genetic background (306). In contrast, identical numbers of IgM- and IgG-producing cells were found in systemic compartments of TCR$\gamma\delta^{-/-}$ and TCR$\gamma\delta^{+/+}$ mice. Furthermore, when TCR$\gamma\delta^{-/-}$ mice were orally immunized with tetanus toxoid (TT) plus CT as mucosal adjuvant, significantly lower IgA anti-TT antibody responses were induced in PPs and the lamina propria than in identically treated TCR$\gamma\delta^{+/+}$ mice (306). In addition, TT-specific serum IgA antibody titers were reduced in these TCR$\gamma\delta^{-/-}$ mice, which indicates that $\gamma\delta$ T cells are involved in the induction and regulation of antigen-specific IgA antibody responses in both mucosal and systemic compartments (306).

Mucosal Cell Trafficking and Homing

Several early studies demonstrated that lymphocytes circulated from blood to lymph nodes and that thoracic duct lymphocytes were retained primarily in the intestine. These findings have been reviewed (110,111,224,307–309).

A direct route for B-cell migration between PPs and the GI lamina propria was revealed by the finding that rabbit GALT B cells repopulated the gut with IgA plasma cells (307). Furthermore, the mesenteric lymph nodes of orally immunized animals were found to contain antigen-specific precursors of IgA plasma cells that repopulated the lamina propria of the gut and of mammary, lacrimal, and salivary glands (308). Studies of the origin, migration, and homing of lymphoid cells from mucosal inductive to effector sites were of basic importance for parallel attempts to induce specific immune responses. Consequently, specific antibodies in glandular secretions could be induced in human and animal experiments by oral or bronchial immunizations (309–311). These studies served as the basis for demonstrating the existence of a "common" mucosal immune system. This concept requires refinement because more recent studies have shown

that migration of cells into and from NALT adheres to different rules than does cell migration into and from GALT and the GI tract.

Lymphocyte Homing in the Gastrointestinal Tract

Lymphocytes enter mucosal or systemic lymphoid tissues from the blood through specialized HEVs, which consist of cuboidal endothelial cells (Fig. 9). In GALT, HEV are present

Lymphocyte Homing Into GALT

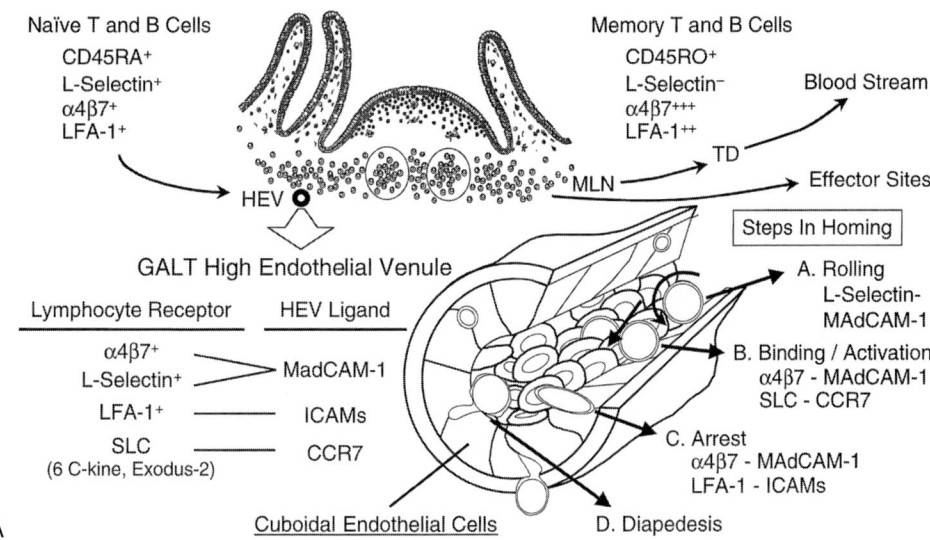

Lymphocyte Homing To Effector Sites Of The GI Tract

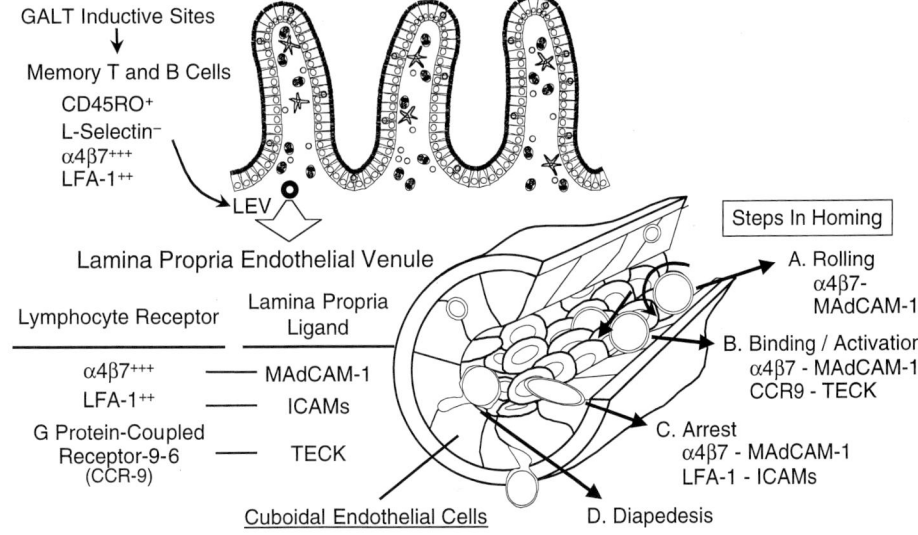

FIG. 9. Lymphocyte homing in the gastrointestinal tract. **A:** High endothelial venules (HEVs) in T-cell areas of gut-associated lymphoepithelial tissues (GALT) express ligands such as mucosal addressin cell adhesion molecule 1 (MAdCAM-1), intracellular adhesion molecule 1 (ICAM-1), and chemokine receptor 7 (CCR7). Naïve T- and B-lymphocytes express L-selectin and $\alpha 4\beta 7$, and lymphocyte function–associated antigen 1 (LFA-1) participate in rolling, binding-activation, arrest, and diapedesis into the HEV. Cells leaving GALT express $\alpha 4\beta 7^{+++}$ and LFA-1^{+++}. **B:** B- and T-lymphocyte receptors for ligands involved in homing into mucosal effector sites of the gastrointestinal tract. Essentially all T and B cells exhibit a memory phenotype with high expression of $\alpha 4\beta 7$ and LFA-1. The memory cells enter effector sites via the lamina propria endothelial venules (LPVs).

in the interfollicular zones rich in T cells (224,312). The endothelial venules in effector sites such as the lamina propria of the GI tract are less pronounced and tend to occur near villus crypt regions. Mucosal addressin cell adhesion molecule 1 (MAdCAM-1) is the most important addressin expressed by PP HEV or lamina propria endothelial venules (LPVs). Likewise, peripheral lymph node addressin (PNAd) and VCAM-1 are the principal addressins expressed by peripheral lymph node and skin HEVs, respectively.

The major homing receptors expressed by lymphocytes are the integrins, a large class of molecules characterized by a heterodimeric structure of α and β chains. In general, the type of homing receptor is determined by the integrin expressed with the $\alpha4$ chain; the $\beta1$ integrin characterizes the homing receptor for the skin, and the $\beta7$ integrin characterizes that for the gut. Thus, the pairing of $\alpha4$ with $\beta7$ represents the major integrin molecule responsible for lymphocyte binding to MAdCAM-1 expressed on HEVs in PP and GI tract LPVs (Fig. 9) (224,312).

In addition to $\alpha4\beta7$ integrin, the C-type lectin family of selectins that includes L-, E-, and P-selectins also serve as homing receptors. L-selectin has a high affinity for carbohydrate-containing PNAd, and this lectin-addressin is of central importance in peripheral lymph node homing of B and T cells. Despite this homing pair, L-selectin can also bind to carbohydrate-rich MAdCAM-1 and is an important initial receptor for homing into GALT HEVs. Interestingly, L-selectin is expressed on all naïve lymphocytes; however, memory T and B cells can be separated into $\alpha4\beta7^{hi}$, L-selectin$^+$, and L-selectin$^-$ subsets.

It is now clear that chemokines are directly involved in lymphocyte homing and that different chemokine-receptor pairs control migration into different lymphoid tissues. For example, loss of secondary lymphoid tissue chemokine results in lack of naïve T cell or DC migration into the spleen or PPs. Furthermore, the chemokine receptor CCR4, which responds to the thymus activation–regulated chemokine and macrophage-derived chemokine, mediates arrest of skin-homing T cells but does not affect $\alpha4\beta7^{hi}$ T-cell migration in the GI tract. On the other hand, human memory T-cell migration into the lamina propria of the GI tract is mediated by the thymus-expressed chemokine (TECK); more specifically, gut-homing $\alpha4\beta7^{hi}$ T cells express a TECK receptor, the CCR9 (313). Both human $\alpha E\beta7^+$ and $\alpha4\beta7^{hi}$ CD8 T cells express CCR9, which suggests that TECK-CCR9 is also involved in lymphocyte homing and arrest of IELs in the GI tract epithelium (Fig. 9).

PP and GALT contain both naïve and memory T- and B-cell subsets, whereas the lamina propria consists of memory T and B cells and terminally differentiated plasma cells (Table 4 and Fig. 9). Naïve B and T cells destined for GALT express L-selectin, moderate levels of $\alpha4\beta7$ ($\alpha4\beta7^+$), and LFA-1. Memory lymphocytes destined for the lamina propria express higher levels of $\alpha4\beta7$ ($\alpha4\beta7^{hi}$) and lack L-selectin. Initial rolling is dependent on $\alpha4\beta7$ interaction with MAdCAM-1 expressed on LPV. Activation-dependent binding and extravasation also require LFA-1–ICAM binding. Furthermore, it is clear that $\alpha E\beta7$ mediates binding to E-cadherin and that CCR9 expression may result in activation-dependent entry into the epithelial cell compartment (Fig. 9).

Cryosections of human tissues revealed naïve T and B cells in HEV that expressed both L-selectin and $\alpha4\beta7$, whereas memory T and B cells in efferent lymphatic vessels expressed $\alpha4\beta7$ but not L-selectin (314). The majority of cells in mesenteric lymph nodes, including B-cell blasts, was of memory phenotype, expressed $\alpha4\beta7$, and was L-selectin^{lo}. Of importance was that immunoglobulin-containing B-cell blasts expressed high levels of $\alpha4\beta7$.

The separation of naïve and memory T and B cells for entry into GALT HEVs or LPVs has important implications in vaccine development. There is strong evidence that peripheral blood mononuclear cells that are assumed to home to systemic lymphoid tissues are also destined for mucosal effector sites in the GI tract. For example, an oral cholera vaccine elicited transient IgA antibody-forming cells (AFCs) in blood and subsequent IgA anti-cholera toxin AFCs in duodenal tissues (315). In other studies, more than 80% of AFCs from parenterally immunized subjects but only 40% from subjects orally immunized with a live Ty21A vaccine were L-selectin$^+$ (316). In a separate study, most peripheral blood AFCs induced after parenteral immunization were L-selectin$^+$, whereas those induced after oral and rectal immunization were predominantly $\alpha4\beta7^+$ IgA AFCs but also included some IgG AFCs (317,318). It is now well established that epithelial cells in the GI tract produce TECK, and this molecule selectively chemoattracts committed IgA B cells to lamina propria regions (319,320). Interestingly, AFCs expressed both L-selectin and $\alpha4\beta7$ homing receptors after nasal immunization. These results indeed suggest that enteric immunization of GALT triggers $\alpha4\beta7^+$ memory B cells, which then migrate into the bloodstream. Antigen-specific $\alpha4\beta7^+$ human T cells also appear to be induced in GALT, inasmuch as oral immunization with KLH followed by systemic boosting yielded peripheral blood mononuclear cells with KLH-specific, $\alpha4\beta7^+$ T cells (321).

Lymphocyte Homing in Nasal-Associated Lymphoepithelial Tissue and Lung-Associated Tissues

Unlike PP HEVs, which are found in T-cell zones, murine NALT HEVs are found in B-cell zones and express PNAd either alone or associated with MAdCAM-1 (322). Furthermore, anti-L-selectin but not anti-MAdCAM-1 antibodies blocked the binding of naïve lymphocytes to NALT HEVs, which suggests predominant roles for L-selectin and PNAd in the binding of naïve lymphocytes to these HEVs.

Early induction of VCAM-1, E-selectin, and P-selectin in the pulmonary vasculature was reported during pulmonary immune responses with an initially increased expression of P-selectin ligand by peripheral blood CD4$^+$ and CD8$^+$ T cells (323). The number of cells expressing P-selectin ligand then declined in the blood as they accumulated in the bronchoalveolar lavage fluid. The very late antigen (VLA) 4 could be an important adhesion molecule involved in the migration of activated T cells into the lung, because migration of VLA-4$^+$ cells into bronchoalveolar fluid is impaired after treatment with anti-α4 antibodies. Other investigators have shown that antigen-specific L-selectin^{low} CTL effectors rapidly accumulate in the lung after adoptive transfer to naïve mice with reduced pulmonary viral titers early during infection.

An interesting approach used to address the homing of human cells in the NALT was the analysis of tissue-specific adhesion molecules after systemic, enteric, or nasal immunization (320). This study showed that, after systemic immunization, most effector B cells expressed L-selectin and only few cells expressed α4β7, whereas after enteric (oral or rectal) immunization, the opposite held true. Interestingly, effector B cells induced by nasal immunization displayed a more promiscuous pattern of adhesion molecules: A large majority of these cells expressed both L-selectin and α4β7 (322).

The existence of a common mucosal immune system has become almost a matter of dogma, and so the homing pattern that has been elucidated in the GI tract after immunization of GALT has been taken as a model for all mucosal immune sites. However, the more recent studies summarized previously suggest instead that the specific set of homing receptors and ligand addressins expressed in the GI tract are absent in NALT or associated lymph nodes. The failure of human tonsillar cells to demonstrate selective α4β7 expression and the lack of MAdCAM-1 expression on tonsil or adenoid HEVs make it likely that gut-homing does not extend to human NALT and associated lymph nodes. It is likely that memory T and B cells from the gut may enter NALT for additional priming and reprogramming of homing receptors. Likewise, memory T and B cells induced in NALT may traffic to lung and genitourinary tract tissues, as well as to the GI tract.

Thus, the rules for the homing of naïve T- and B-cell precursors into NALT as well as the homing program imprinted upon memory and effector lymphocytes, which supports their selective entry into the upper respiratory and genitourinary tracts, must be more clearly defined.

MUCOSAL IMMUNE RESPONSES

Mucosa-associated lymphoid tissues are the principal sites of continuous stimulation of the entire immune system with diverse environmental antigens of microbial and food origin. As a consequence of these constant exposures to environmental antigens, a broad spectrum of immune responses, including humoral and cellular immunity in both mucosal and systemic compartments, is induced (147,148). In addition to such responses mediated by mucosal and plasma antibodies and effector T cells, antigen ingestion profoundly influences systemic immunity. A state of systemic unresponsiveness called *mucosal tolerance* may also develop in parallel,

depending on the dose, frequency, type of antigen and delivery system, site of application, and species and age of the individual (324,325). As described later, mucosal tolerance is mediated by special subsets of Treg cells and their respective products. Mucosal surfaces are also the most frequent portals of entry of common viral, bacterial, fungal, and parasitic agents that cause both local and systemic infectious diseases. Therefore, numerous studies have been conducted to harness the enormous potential of the mucosal immune system to induce protective responses at the site of entry of infectious agents (147,148,326). However, because of the difficulties with dosing of relevant antigens, their limited absorption and proteolytic degradation, unique antigen delivery systems have been explored to avoid such problems (326). Although so far limited in their spectrum and frequency of use, mucosally administered vaccines are gaining in acceptance, particularly thanks to the remarkable advances in technologies applicable to the effective mucosal delivery of bacterial and viral proteins, glycoproteins, and DNA in combination with mucosal adjuvants. The route of infection or immunization, as well as the nature of antigen and the antigen-delivery system, greatly influences the magnitude and quality of the ensuing immune response. In general, the presence of mucosal inductive sites in a given locale, such as intestinal PPs, results in the stimulation of local and generalized mucosal immune responses, manifested by the parallel appearance of antibodies, predominantly of the IgA isotypes, at remote mucosal effector sites as a result of the dissemination of cells through the common mucosal immune system (147,148). In contrast, infection or immunization at sites devoid of the inductive lymphoepithelial structures (e.g., the conjunctiva and the female genital tract), the immune responses remain localized to the exposure site and are limited in their magnitude (147).

Intestinal Infections and Immunizations

The earlier appearance of specific antibodies in intestinal secretions rather than in plasma of individuals infected with intestinal pathogens (e.g., *Salmonella* or *Shigella* organisms) was noted in pioneering studies of Besredka (327). Stimulation of local and generalized mucosal immune responses can be achieved by ingestion of antigens or their introduction by the rectal route. The former route exploits the inductive potential of lymphoepithelial tissues distributed in the small intestine, whereas the latter route stimulates primarily cells accumulated in structures termed *rectal tonsils* (145,146). Interestingly, the rectal route appears to also be effective, at least in some experiments, in inducing humoral responses in the female genital tract secretions (328). A comparative study (318) of the immune responses to *S. typhi* Ty21a live attenuated vaccine given in the same dose orally or rectally demonstrated that administration via both routes resulted in the appearance of antibody-secreting cells in peripheral blood; the immune responses were similar with regard to the kinetics of appearance, the numbers of cells and their immunoglobulin isotypes, and the expression of the mucosal homing receptor α4β7.

Oral immunization elicited more pronounced responses in saliva and vaginal secretions, whereas rectal immunization was more effective in inducing specific antibodies in nasal and rectal secretions.

Extensive studies of oral immunization of humans and animals with killed bacteria and their products or with inactivated viruses clearly demonstrated that the antibody-secreting cells are easily detectable, for 1 week, in peripheral blood approximately 5 days after immunization, and specific antibodies become detectable 2 to 3 weeks later in parallel in tears, saliva, milk, and intestinal and genital tract secretions. However, the magnitude of responses in individual secretions may be substantially different; in some studies, serum antibodies were absent (147,148,324,325). Qualitatively and quantitatively different responses have been observed in studies using live viruses (e.g., polio virus) and bacteria or adjuvants that may accentuate both mucosal and systemic responses and alter the antibody isotypes (147,326). Because of the availability of not only various external secretions but also, most important, cells from all systemic and mucosal tissues that are furthermore amenable to detailed phenotypic and functional analyses, studies performed in animal models, particularly mice, have provided a much more comprehensive picture concerning the regulation of humoral and cellular immune responses (148,324).

The nature of the delivery system of antigen and the route of immunization influence the nature of Th cell subsets induced and markedly affect the outcome of systemic and mucosal immunity (325,326,329). For example, use of native CT or nontoxic mutants of CT with vaccines given orally or nasally tend to induce CD4$^+$ Th2-type cells with characteristic serum IgG1, IgG2b, IgE, and IgA and mucosal S-IgA responses (228). Both PPs and lamina propria lymphocytes, when restimulated with TT or KLH, produced significant quantities of IL-4 and IL-5, with minimal levels of IFN-γ and IL-2. Thus, several studies now support the notion that oral immunization with soluble proteins and CT as an adjuvant induce Th2-type responses that provide help for characteristic serum IgG1 and IgE and for mucosal S-IgA antibodies. On the other hand, oral immunization with recombinant bacteria (e.g., Salmonella)–expressing proteins tend to induce not only CD4$^+$ Th1-type cells and CMI but also characteristic CD4$^+$ Th2 cells. These CD4$^+$ Th2 cells produce cytokines such as IL-5, IL-6, and IL-10, which appear to support mucosal S-IgA responses (179).

Attenuated avirulent Salmonella strains have received considerable attention as mucosal vaccine delivery vectors for recombinant proteins associated with virulence (326,330,331). After oral administration, Salmonella organisms replicate directly in the mucosa-associated tissues (e.g., PPs) and thereafter disseminate via the GALT to systemic sites (e.g., spleen). This characteristic dissemination pattern of growth in both mucosal and systemic sites allows Salmonella organisms to induce broad-based immune responses, including cell-mediated and serum IgG and mucosal S-IgA anti-

body responses. Although a large number of genes from bacteria, viruses, parasites, and mammalian species have been expressed in attenuated Salmonella organisms, few studies have fully characterized both T- and B-cell responses to the expressed protein antigen. In particular, the balance between antigen-specific CD4$^+$, Th1, and Th2 cells and their subsequent influence on subclass-specific IgG and mucosal IgA responses has received little attention in these systems. Such clarity is paramount to the development of delivery protocols that will provide the appropriate immune response to a given pathogen.

Nasal and Upper Respiratory Tract Immunization

Immune responses induced by infections or immunization through the nasal mucosa and oropharyngeal lymphoid tissues (Waldeyer's ring) have been evaluated with particular emphasis on local respiratory tract pathogens such as influenza, parainfluenza, and RSV (332). Individuals naturally infected or locally immunized with attenuated viruses responded by formation of S-IgA and IgG antibodies in nasal secretions and also in saliva (332–335). In addition, virus-specific antibodies are also detectable in sera of infected and immunized individuals. In general, intranasal immunization, in contrast to intestinal administration, induces prominent systemic responses manifested by the presence of antibody-secreting cells in peripheral blood with mucosal and systemic homing receptors (320) and by serum antibody responses. Examination of other external secretions of nasally immunized humans and animals revealed another significant feature: the female genital tract secretions contained high levels of antimicrobial antibodies of IgA and IgG isotypes, which in some experiments were higher than those induced by local, oral, rectal, or systemic immunizations (328). Thus, it appears that the nasal exposure to antigens is the route of choice for the induction of female genital tract responses. Because levels of neither IgG nor IgA antibodies present in vaginal washes were correlated with serum antibody response, it is assumed that antibodies of both isotypes are produced locally by numerous IgG and IgA plasma cells dispersed mainly in the uterine cervix.

Several studies indicate that soluble vaccine components with mucosal adjuvants such as CT (as well as protein–CT-B conjugates) and use of attenuated vectors further enhance the magnitude of immune responses induced by nasal immunization. A series of extensive experiments using the influenza virus model demonstrated that nasal immunization with influenza virus vaccine provides more effective protective immunity than does oral immunization (326). Nasal immunization with trivalent vaccines in the presence of CT-B containing a trace amount of A subunit provided cross-protection against a broad range of viruses (326). It was also shown that nasal immunization with influenza virus vaccine with LT-B (containing a trace amount of LT) induces antigen-specific immune responses in humans (326).

These findings shown that an appropriate nasal vaccine with mucosal adjuvants can provide effective immunity against infection.

Several studies performed in animals can be used to illustrate principles associated with nasal immunization. In one study, nasal administration of inactivated RSV with CT resulted in nasal IgA and serum IgG anti-RSV responses (336). Analysis of IgG subclasses suggests that both IgG1 and IgG2a are induced. Interestingly, infection with RSV and subsequent Th1-type responses are characterized by a favorable outcome, whereas Th2-type responses are associated with significant disease (336). Nasal immunization with the C fragment of TT and with CT as adjuvant resulted in serum antibody responses characterized by comparable IgG1, IgG2a, and IgG2b anti-fragment C titers, which suggests that the use of CT as an adjuvant with fragment C induces a response characterized by both Th1- and Th2-type responses (337). However, when fragment C is administered nasally with pertussis toxin (PT) or a mutated form of PT known as PT-9K/129G as mucosal adjuvants, anti-fragment C IgG1 predominates, which suggests that an immune response biased toward the Th2 type has been induced. Direct comparisons between CT and PT or PT-9K/129 in this study are difficult because the use of CT is associated with much more potent anti–fragment C IgG responses.

Functional analogy between NALT and GALT is further manifested by the participation of both sites in the induction of mucosal tolerance. Soluble antigens administered nasally with or without suitable mucosal adjuvants result in systemic unresponsiveness (324,338). For example, in animal models of allergic encephalomyelitis, collagen-induced arthritis and diabetes, relevant antigens linked to CT-B and applied nasally before systemic immunization (which in the absence of mucosal immunization results in the development of respective autoimmune reaction) inhibited the development of disease (339). In comparison with antigen ingestion, nasal immunization has several important advantages. Because of the limited degradation by proteolytic enzymes abundant in the GI fluid, lower doses of antigens are required for nasal immunization to achieve the same results (induction of humoral responses or tolerance or both). Furthermore, because of the relative paucity of competing antigens in the nasal cavity in contrast to the plethora of food and microbial antigens in the gut, concomitantly used mucosal adjuvants enhance immunization with a much greater selectivity of responses to desired antigens without stimulating responses to bystander antigens.

It has been suggested that the tonsils may also serve as a source for precursors of IgA plasma cells found in the upper respiratory tract, the salivary glands, and perhaps the lactating mammary glands (140). Indeed, the immune response to the oral poliovirus vaccine in tonsillectomized children, whose secretions display reduced S-IgA levels, is inferior to that induced in children with intact tonsils (340). However, direct unilateral injection CT-B and TT into human tonsils resulted in the induction of dominantly local IgG response in the injected tonsil (341). Although anti–CT-B– and anti-TT–producing cells were detected in peripheral blood, the immune responses were not disseminated to remote mucosal effector sites.

Immune Responses in the Genital Tract

As described previously, the mucosal immune systems of the female and male genital tracts display several features distinct from other mucosal sites, such as the absence of lymphoepithelial structures analogous to intestinal PPs and dominance of IgG-producing cells in tissues and IgG in cervical mucus, vaginal washes, and semen (328). Furthermore, an inability or reduced ability to respond to allogeneic (in females) and autologous (in males) spermatozoa is of critical importance in the preservation of species.

Studies of immune responses to agents infecting the genital tract are hampered by problems associated with the acquisition of adequate samples, contamination with plasma, and technical difficulties with measurement of strictly mucosal antibodies. However, a common finding is beginning to emerge: Immune responses induced by genital tract infections and local immunization without adjuvants (e.g., CT or CT-B) are weak at best (328). For example, local infections with *N. gonorrhoeae, Chlamydia trachomatis,* human papilloma virus, and HIV-1 in genitally exposed but uninfected women are unimpressive or even absent, whether measured in terms of IgA and IgG antibodies in local secretions and serum, and cell-mediated responses (328,342–346). Obviously, repeated genital tract infections with *N. gonorrhoeae* do not confer desired immunity.

Numerous experiments concerning local induction of antibody responses in the female genital tract secretions of experimental animals yielded varying results, dependent on the species, type, site, frequency of antigen application, and use of adjuvants (328). Although repeated administration of antigens with adjuvants or infection with live viruses generated local immune responses (343,344,347–349), antibodies were absent or present in low levels in secretions of remote glands, probably because of the lack of organized inductive sites, equivalent to PPs, in the genital tract. However, systemic immunization followed by local mucosal booster or targeted immunization in the vicinity of local lymph nodes enhanced genital tract responses (348).

Remarkably, intranasal immunization performed in several animal species (mice, rats, rabbits, and rhesus macaques) and in humans, particularly with the use of adjuvants, proved to be effective in the induction of humoral responses in the female genital tract (328,343,350–353). Furthermore, sequential combination of several immunization routes (systemic, oral, rectal, vaginal, tracheal, or nasal) generated better results than repeated immunization at a single site (328). Oral or rectal immunizations of women without subsequent boosting by another mucosal route (including vaginal) or use of adjuvants has not been particularly effective in stimulating vigorous humoral responses (328,344).

Other Immunization Sites

Local application of antigens to the surface of the eye may induce antibody responses in all major isotypes, usually with dominance of IgA (147,354). However, the drainage of the conjunctival sac through the nasolacrimal duct may lead to the stimulation through NALT and perhaps GALT. Indeed nasal, oral, and even rectal immunizations may induce specific IgA and IgG antibodies in tears (318). Results of immunization studies to induce ocular immunity in humans and many animal species have been comprehensively reviewed (354).

Injection of antigens dispersed in various adjuvants into salivary and lactating mammary glands stimulates local humoral responses, often dominated by IgG rather than IgA, restricted to the immunized gland (147). Because of the commonly encountered local inflammatory response caused mostly by the adjuvants, the normal function of such a gland may be compromised. Retrograde immunization of mammary glands through teats of lactating cows with killed bacteria has been performed on experimental basis in veterinary medicine to prevent mastitis (147).

Mucosal Adjuvants and Antigen-Delivery Systems

Because of the proteolytic degradation of antigens and effective innate factors operational at mucosal surfaces, only minute quantities of antigens are taken up to generate immune responses. To circumvent these limitations, a number of strategies have been considered to enhance mucosal and systemic, humoral and cellular responses or to induce systemic unresponsiveness and mucosal tolerance (324–326). Some of the promising approaches are briefly described as follows.

Bacterial Enterotoxins and their Nontoxic Derivatives

Two bacterial enterotoxins (CT and LT) are now recognized as very effective mucosal adjuvants for the induction of both mucosal and systemic immunity to co-administered protein antigens. CT consists of two structurally and functionally separate A and B subunits (355). CT-B consists of five identical 11.6-kDa peptides that bind to GM1 gangliosides (Fig. 10). The binding of CT-B to GM1 gangliosides on epithelia allows the A subunit to reach the cytosol of target cells, where it binds to nicotinamide adenosyl dinucleotide phosphate and catalyzes the adenosine diphosphate (ADP) ribosylation of G protein sα. The latter guanosine triphosphate–binding protein activates adenyl cyclase with subsequent elevation of cyclic adenosine monophosphate in epithelial cells, followed by secretion of water and chloride ions into the intestinal lumen. LT from *E. coli* is closely related to CT, and the amino acid sequences of the two are 80% homologous (355). Although both CT and LT bind GM1 gangliosides, LT

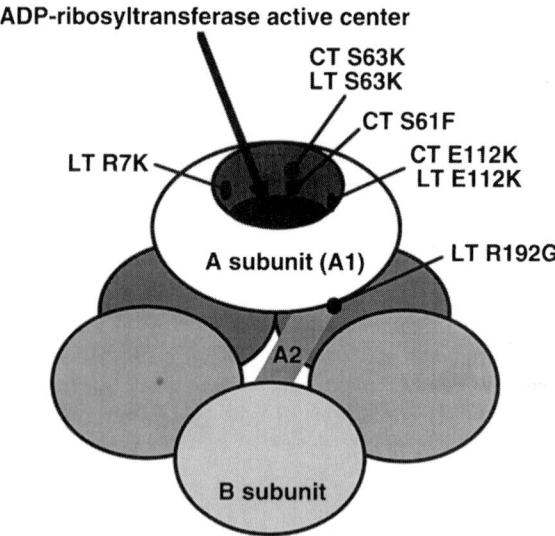

FIG. 10. Typical structure of cholera toxin (CT) of *Vibrio cholerae* or heat-labile toxin I (LT) of *Escherichia coli*. The positions indicate single amino acid substitutions of the mutants.

also exhibits an affinity for GM2 and asialo-GM1 (230,355). In order to circumvent toxicity linked to these enterotoxins, two strategies—(a) generation of mutant CT and mutant LT molecules devoid of their toxic activity (43,356–359), and (b) replacement of the toxic A subunit with an antigen (360)—have been developed. The first approach involves the introduction of single–amino acid substitutions in the active site (i.e., the site responsible for the ADP-ribosylation activity) of the A subunit of CT or LT or in the protease sensitive loop of LT.

Mutants of CT constructed by substitution of serine by phenylalanine at position 61 (CT-S61F) and glutamate by lysine at position 112 (CT-E112K) in the ADP-ribosyltransferase activity center of the CT gene from *V. cholerae* 01 strain GP14 display no ADP-ribosyltransferase activity or enterotoxicity (356) (Fig. 10). The levels of antigen-specific serum IgG and S-IgA antibodies induced by the mutants are comparable with levels of those induced by wild-type CT and significantly higher than levels of those induced by recombinant CT-B (356,357). Furthermore, the mutant CT-E112K, like mutant CT, induces Th2-type responses through a preferential inhibition of Th1-type CD4+ T cells. Mutations in other sites of the CT molecule were reported to induce nontoxic derivatives, but the adjuvant activity was also affected.

Mutant LT molecules, whether possessing a residual ADP-ribosyltransferase activity (e.g., LT-72R) or totally devoid of it (e.g., LT-7K and LT-6K3), can function as mucosal adjuvants when intranasally administered to mice together with unrelated antigens (358). However, discrepant results were reported when two nontoxic LT mutants were tested for their adjuvanticity after oral immunization of mice. Thus, although mutant LT-E112K (bearing a substitution in the active site of the A subunit) was unable to amplify the response to KLH when both were given orally to C57BL/6 mice, the mutant with a substitution in the protease-sensitive region, LT-R192G, retained the ability to act as a mucosal adjuvant (359). Whether the type of the substitution played a role in the reported discrepancies remains to be elucidated. Because LT induces a mixed $CD4^+$ Th1-type response (i.e., IFN-γ) and Th2-type response (i.e., IL-4, IL-5, IL-6 and IL-10) (232), the use of mutants of LT when both Th1- and Th2- type responses are desired might be envisioned.

Another novel strategy that exploits the binding potential of CT and CT-B to gangliosides on mucosal cells involves the genetic construction of recombinant chimeric proteins. Toxic subunit A of CT consists of two segments, A1 (carrier of toxicity) and A2, which interacts with B subunit. Genetic replacement of A1 segment with DNA encoding for desired antigen (e.g., antigen I/II of *Streptococcus mutans* results in the assembly of molecule composed of CTB/A2-antigen (360). When given intragastrically and especially intranasally, potent humoral immune responses were generated in mice.

Microbial Immunostimulatory DNA sequences

Plasmid DNA for gene vaccination can be functionally divided into two distinct units: a transcription unit and an adjuvant/mitogen unit [reviewed by Krieg (361)]. The latter unit contains immunostimulatory sequences consisting of short palindromic nucleotides around a CpG dinucleotide core, such as 5-purine-purine-CG-pyrimidine-pyrimidine-3'. The adjuvant effect of these sequences is mediated by bacterial (but not by eukaryotic) DNA because of its high frequency of CpG motifs and the absence of cytosine methylation. It is now clear that CpG motifs can induce B-cell proliferation and immunoglobulin synthesis, in addition to cytokine secretions (i.e., IL-6, IFN-α, IFN-β, IFN-γ, IL-12 and IL-18) by a variety of immune cells (361).

Because CpG motifs create a cytokine microenvironment favoring Th1-type responses, they can be used as adjuvants to stimulate antigen-specific Th1-type responses or to redirect harmful allergic or Th2-dominated autoimmune responses. Indeed, co-injection of bacterial DNA or CpG motifs with a DNA vaccine or with a protein antigen promotes Th1-type responses even in mice with a preexisting Th2-type of immunity (361). It has also been reported that CpG motifs can enhance systemic and mucosal immune responses when given nasally to mice (361).

Mucosal Cytokines, Chemokines, and Innate Factors as Adjuvants

Mucosal delivery of cytokine allowed the use of these molecules, which interact primarily with their corresponding receptors without the important adverse effects often asso-

ciated with the large and repeated parenteral cytokine doses generally required for the effective targeting of tissues and organs. After nasal delivery of IL-12, significant serum IL-12 levels, equivalent to approximately one tenth of those attained by parenteral injection, were achieved (362). Subsequent serum IFN-γ levels were tenfold lower in mice nasally treated with IL-12, which confirmed the biological activity of nasally administered IL-12. A nasal vaccine of TT given with either IL-6 or IL-12 induced serum TT–specific IgG antibody responses that protected mice against lethal challenge with TT, which suggests that both IL-6 and IL-12 can enhance protective systemic immunity to mucosal vaccines (362). Furthermore, nasal administration of TT with IL-12 as adjuvant induced high titers of S-IgA antibody responses in the GI tract, vaginal washes, and saliva.

A number of studies have addressed whether innate molecules secreted in the epithelium could provide signals to bridge the innate and adaptive mucosal immune systems. To prove this concept, protein antigens were given with IL-1 (363), α-defensins (i.e., human neutrophil peptides) (364), or lymphotactin (365). Nasal administration of protein antigens with these innate molecules enhanced systemic immune responses to co-administered antigens (363–365). However, although both IL-1 and lymphotactin enhanced mucosal S-IgA antibody responses, the α-defensins failed to do so (363–365). These studies show that inflammatory cytokines and molecules of the innate immune system can be effectively administered by mucosal routes to regulate both systemic and mucosal immune responses.

Antigen-Delivery Systems

Transgenic Plants

Novel molecular methods have allowed the production of subunit vaccines in transgenic plants (366). Plants can be engineered to synthesize and assemble one or more antigens that retain both T- and B-cell epitopes (366). Feeding of transgenic potato tubers was shown to induce systemic and mucosal immune responses in mice (366) and in humans (366). In order to circumvent potential denaturation of antigen during cooking, recombinant plants such as tomatoes, lettuce, and bananas have been developed.

Inert Microparticles

M cells present on the surfaces of mucosal inductive sites can take up soluble and, even more efficiently, particulate materials from mucosal surfaces (120,121,123,367). Consequently, strategies have been proposed and tested to exploit this potential in delivery of particles containing microbial antigens to stimulate mucosal and systemic immune responses (326,368). These particulate mucosal antigen-delivery systems include inert hydroxyapatite granules, biodegradable polymers of various compositions, cochleates, multiple emulsions, liposomes, and immunostimulating complexes.

Although detailed descriptions of individual approaches and technologies involved in the production and testing of immunogenicity with different vaccines in various species can be found elsewhere (326,368), a brief summary of advantages and disadvantages may be of relevance. Advantages are as follows: Antigens incorporated in some of these particles are usually well protected from proteolytic degradation by mucosal enzymes and acids; particles by themselves are nonimmunogenic; variation in their chemical compositions allow generation of particles with fast and slow degradation to stimulate long-lasting responses; several different antigens can be incorporated into a single preparation; other substances such as cytokines can be co-incorporated with antigens to show ensuing immune responses to a desired outcome; and some particulate vaccines can be stored at ambient temperatures and thus avoid refrigeration (326,368,369). These obviously attractive features are, however, counterbalanced by serious disadvantages. Specifically, the disappointingly low uptake from mucosal surfaces (<1%), the low rate of incorporation, the use of organic solvents that may denature antigens, and unexpectedly high species-dependent variabilities in immunogenicity represent serious problems. The last point is of particular concern. For example, biodegradable microspheres that generated promising results when used in mice were either poorly immunogenic or nonimmunogenic when tested in humans (326,368,370). Further technological improvements to enhance the uptake from mucosal surfaces are being pursued to exploit the potential of this attractive antigen-delivery system for human vaccinology.

Live Microbial Vectors

Recombinant bacterial and viral vectors containing genes from unrelated microbial species that encode important virulence factors and antigens have been explored in many experimental vaccines (330,371). The selection of a suitable vector usually involves consideration of its ability to selectively colonize specific mucosal locales to generate immune responses at desired sites. The generalization of the ensuing immune response through the common mucosal immune system and its specific compartments has been exploited in the context of the ability of individual vectors to colonize or infect specific inductive sites. Vectors that have been tested include (a) various species of attenuated bacteria, such as *Salmonella* and *Shigella* organisms, *E. coli, Lactobacillus* organisms, *Mycobacteria* organisms (bacille Calmette-Guérin), *Streptococcus* organisms, and *Vibrio* organisms, and (b) viruses, such as poliovirus, adenovirus, vesicular stomatitis, vaccinia virus and canarypox, Venezuelan equine encephalitis virus, rhinovirus, mengovirus, and influenza viruses (371–375). When expressed in viral vectors, relevant antigens are produced in host cells and therefore are likely to assume protein folding and glycosylation patterns analogous to the infection-induced antigens; this, however, may not be the case with antigens produced by bacteria. Unfortunately, live vectors themselves are antigenic, and the dominant immune response to the vec-

tor therefore diminishes the effectiveness of repeated immunization with the same vector. Promising results generated by mucosal immunization with recombinant vaccinia virus expressing other antigens (376,377) and performed in a murine model await evaluations in humans. Furthermore, the level of expression of the desired antigen in some vectors may be very low and nonetheless induce a substantial immune response. Because of a potential overattenuation of some vectors (e.g., salmonellae), their ability to colonize for an extended time is substantially limited because of the effective competition with endogenous microbiota. Thus, with most live microbial vectors, a critical balance among attenuation, ability to colonize, prevention of elimination by the immune response to the vector, and adequate expression and production of antigens with relevant properties (e.g., folding and glycosylation) and immunogenicity is often difficult to achieve.

MUCOSAL TOLERANCE

Basic Concepts

In addition to the beneficial induction of antigen-specific S-IgA and serum IgG antibody responses after mucosal vaccination, the mucosal route of antigen delivery can also induce systemic unresponsiveness, also called oral or mucosal tolerance (324,325,338,378). Thus, mucosal antigen delivery can either up-regulate or down-regulate systemic immune responses. As discussed previously, for the purpose of mucosal vaccine development against infectious diseases, the goal is induction of both mucosal and systemic immunity, in order to provide two layers of protection. In contrast, inhibition of antigen-specific immune responses in systemic compartments by mucosal antigen delivery is important for the prevention of overstimulation of responses and frequently encountered and hypersensitivity responses to food proteins and allergens (338). Furthermore, this system could potentially be applied to the prevention and treatment of autoimmune diseases by feeding relevant antigens (338).

Oral administration of a single high dose or repeated oral delivery of low doses of proteins have been shown to induce systemic unresponsiveness, presumably in the presence of mucosal IgA antibody responses (324,325,378). More recent studies have shown that the nasal administration of proteins also induces systemic unresponsiveness (379–384) and has led to the more general term *mucosal tolerance* to include nasal or oral antigen induction of unresponsiveness.

Mechanisms for Mucosal Tolerance

In the late 1970s and early 1980s, mucosal immunologists had already made attempts to investigate the possible mechanisms of oral tolerance at a time when the immune system was not characterized at the cellular and molecular levels. Although several possible mechanisms (e.g., B-cell tolerance, anti-idiotypic antibody, intestinal antigen-processing events for tolerogen and APCs) have been shown to be involved in the induction of oral tolerance (338), the most compelling evidence to date suggests that T cells are the major cell type involved in the induction of mucosally induced tolerance (Fig. 11). In earlier work, it was shown that systemic unresponsiveness was induced by adoptive transfer of T cells from rats orally fed bovine serum albumin. Subsequently, a large number of studies [reviewed by Mowat and Weiner (338)] demonstrated that oral immunization with protein antigen induces CD4[+] Th cells in mucosa-associated tissues that support IgA responses, whereas suppressor T cells were induced in systemic compartments such as splenic tissue that down-regulate antigen-specific IgM, IgG, and IgE responses (338). For example, oral feeding of OVA to mice led to the generation of Th cells supporting IgA responses and suppressor T cells for IgG and IgE responses in GALT (338). Furthermore, the former T cells for IgA responses remained in PPs, whereas the suppressor T cells migrated into the systemic compartment (e.g., the spleen). These observations were considered logical explanations for cellular mechanisms of oral tolerance whereby PP-derived CD4[+] Th cells supported IgA responses, whereas splenic T suppressor cells induced systemic unresponsiveness. These explanations must be reevaluated, because it has been shown that administration of a large dose of OVA to mice followed by attempts to orally immunize with OVA plus CT resulted in unresponsiveness in both mucosal and peripheral immune compartments (385).

Most investigators now agree that mucosal tolerance is mediated by T cells that are involved in the generation of active suppression or of clonal anergy or deletion or both (338). For example, high doses of antigen given via the oral route induced clonal deletion or anergy (386,387), charac-

terized by the absence of T-cell proliferation and diminished IL-2 production, and by IL-2 receptor expression. Frequently administered low doses of antigen, however, induced active suppression by CD4[+] or CD8[+] T cells that secreted cytokines such as TGF-β, IL-4, and IL-10 (338). It is interesting to note that the latter scenario involves cytokines that are also known to up-regulate IgA production (see previous discussion) and is thus compatible with the observation that mucosal immune responses and systemic tolerance may develop concomitantly (389,390). Because tolerance can be, in some experiments, transferred by serum from tolerized animals, it is possible that humoral antibodies (perhaps IgG and IgA, perhaps anti-idiotype antibody, perhaps immune complexes), circulating undegraded antigens, or tolerogenic antigen fragments and cytokines may act synergistically to confer T-cell unresponsiveness (338). Because oral tolerance is specific for the antigen initially ingested or inhaled and thus does not influence the development of systemic immune responses against other antigens, its manipulation has become an increasingly attractive strategy for preventing and possibly treating illnesses associated with or resulting from the development of untoward immunological reactions against specific antigens encountered or expressed (autoantigens) in nonmucosal tissues (324,338).

Role of Peyer's Patches in Oral Tolerance

The precise site of antigen uptake in the GI tract during oral tolerance induction has not been firmly established. At least three possibilities could be proposed, and no two are mutually exclusive (391). First, antigen may be pinocytosed into the epithelial cells themselves, and interactions with IELs may influence oral tolerance (see later discussion). Second,

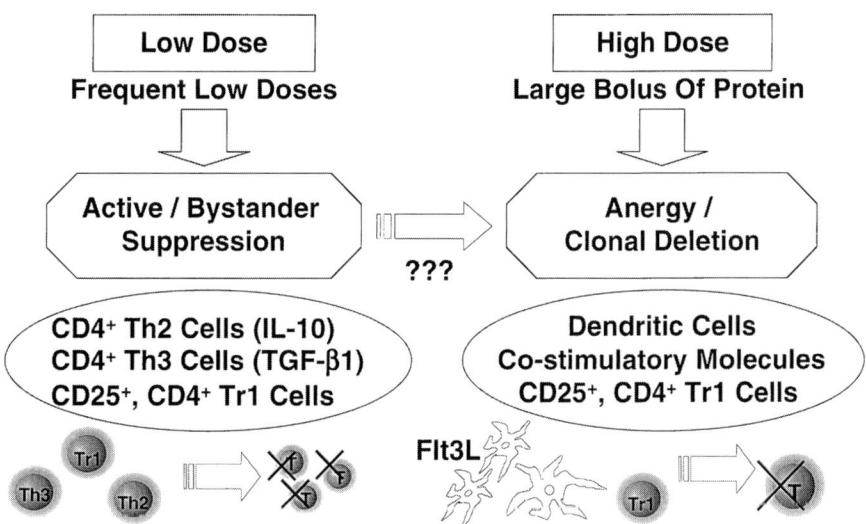

FIG. 11. Current concepts on the mechanisms regulating mucosal tolerance. Low, frequent doses of soluble proteins elicit active or bystander suppression that appears to be mediated by regulatory T cells. On the other hand, a large bolus of protein induces anergy, a process requiring dendritic cells and CD40–CD40 ligand interactions.

antigen may selectively enter the GALT via M cells (see previous discussion) and lead to APC–T cell interactions that down-regulate T- and B-cell responses. Finally, oral antigen may not perturb the GI tract immune system at all but simply enter and cross the epithelium in a paracellular manner and reach the bloodstream, in which tolerance would be induced. Some investigators have suggested that organized lymphoid tissue in the GI tract is not required for oral tolerance to OVA, inasmuch as B cell–defective mice, which contain poorly developed PPs, were fully tolerized at the level of T cells (392). Although those investigators claimed that GALT was absent, others have shown that some remnants of PPs are seen in μMT mice (126). Still others have shown that direct injection of antigen into PPs induced oral tolerance (393). The availability of mice without PPs has allowed reinvestigation of the notion that GALT may be involved in oral tolerance. In one study, it was shown that mice that lacked GALT but retained mesenteric lymph nodes could be orally tolerized to OVA (394). Other studies, however, showed that mice that lack PPs but retain mesenteric lymph nodes were resistant to oral tolerance to protein (395); however, these mice showed normal mucosal S-IgA antibody responses to oral protein given with CT as adjuvant (396). Although it cannot yet be concluded whether GALT is a strict requirement for oral tolerance to proteins, it is plausible to suggest that the nature of the antigen itself may influence the site of entry into the host.

CD4+ T Cells in Mucosal Tolerance

The $\alpha\beta$ T cells appear to be the major players in down-regulation of systemic immune responses to orally administered antigens (Fig. 11). It is generally agreed that the status of oral tolerance can be explained by (a) clonal anergy, (b) clonal deletion of T cells, or (c) active suppression by Treg cells through the secretion of inhibitory cytokines (338). Low doses of oral antigen tend to favor the third form of inhibition, whereas higher doses of feeding induce clonal anergy of immunocompetent T cells (338). These two forms of oral tolerance are not mutually exclusive and may occur simultaneously after oral administration of antigens.

T-Cell Anergy

Anergy is defined as a state of T-cell unresponsiveness characterized by the lack of both proliferation and IL-2 synthesis and by diminished IL-2 receptor expression (338), a condition reversed by preculturing T cells with IL-2 (338). Oral tolerance to a large dose of OVA induced anergy in OVA-specific T cells (386). Furthermore, oral MBP diminished IL-2 and IFN-γ synthesis (386). These findings suggest that Th1-type T cells may be susceptible to the induction of anergy after oral feeding. To support this, it has been shown that Th1-type cells appear to be more sensitive to the induction of tolerance *in vitro* than are Th2-type cells; *in vivo* evidence has demonstrated that Th1 cells are likely to be anergized in oral

tolerance (338). This may be an oversimplification, because it has been shown that oral tolerance can be induced in mice defective in Th1 cells (STAT4$^{-/-}$) or Th2 cells (STAT6$^{-/-}$) (338,397). Furthermore, in order to identify which lymphocyte compartment (e.g., CD4$^+$ vs. CD8$^+$ T cells) preferentially mediates the induction of oral tolerance, cell transfer experiments were performed with SCID and *nu/nu* mice (338). Adoptive transfer of splenic lymphocytes from mice orally tolerized to bovine α-casein resulted in the induction of tolerance in these immunocompromised mice. It was shown that oral tolerance was induced by anergized CD4$^+$ T cells but not CD8$^+$ T cells. Together, these findings show that a form of oral tolerance can be achieved by the induction of anergic CD4$^+$ T cells in the systemic compartment.

An Imbalanced Helper T 1/2 Cell–Cytokine Network

The induction of oral tolerance can also be explained by dysregulation of homeostasis between Th1- and Th2-type cells. For example, preferential activation of Th2 cells may lead to down-regulation of Th1-CMI responses by Th2 cytokines such as IL-4 and IL-10 (338). In addition, Th1 type cells are much more sensitive to anergy induction after oral administration of protein antigens. These findings suggest that oral tolerance is associated with selective down-regulation of Th1 cells by Th2 cells through their respective cytokines in the systemic immune compartment. This possibility is consistent with the fact that oral tolerance has more profound effects on Th1-regulated CMI responses than on Th2-mediated antibody responses. However, studies have shown that high doses of OVA inhibited production of both Th1 (IL-2 and IFN-γ) and Th2 (IL-4, IL-5, and IL-10) cytokines and resulted in the reduction of IFN-γ– and IL-4–dependent antigen-specific IgG2a and IgG1 antibody responses, respectively (338). These findings indicate that both subsets of Th cells are involved in the induction of oral tolerance and that both are down-regulated.

Oral OVA induced brisk IFN-γ production with inhibition of the IgG-enhancing cytokine IL-4 by Th2 cells, leading to reduced B-cell responses, whereas no oral tolerance was seen in IFN-γ knockout mice (338). Furthermore, repeated oral administration of high doses of OVA to OVA-specific TCR transgenic mice resulted in an IFN-γ–dominated immune responses in the PPs (338). Together, these findings indicate that the immunological consequences of systemic B-cell tolerance induced by a high dose of oral antigen could result from IFN-γ–mediated immune regulation, with significant suppression of Th2-type cells.

Regulatory T Cells in Oral Tolerance

In a hapten-induced model of colitis, it was shown that trinitrobenzene sulphonic acid (TNBS) coupled to mouse colonic (self-) proteins, when given orally, led to oral tolerance to hapten and a failure to induce TNBS-colitis (338). Interestingly, both PP and lamina propria CD4$^+$ T cells, when stimulated through the TCR, produced high levels of TGF-β, IL-4, and IL-10, which suggests that Th3 cells and possibly Tr1 cells regulate this type of tolerance. Direct evidence for intestinal tolerance to luminal bacteria in humans was provided by the finding that lamina propria CD4$^+$ T cells responded poorly to E. coli proteins, a condition reversed by anti–IL-10 or anti–TGF-β mAb treatment (398). The best direct evidence for induction of CD4$^+$CD25$^+$ Tr cells by oral antigen was provided by an adoptive transfer model of DO11.10 TCR OVA transgenic T cells. Transfer followed by either intravenous or oral OVA led to an increase in OVA-specific CD4$^+$CD25$^+$ T cells (399). It should be emphasized that this latter study used 25 mg of OVA in drinking water over an 18-hour period, which suggests a relatively high oral dose of antigen-induced Tr cells.

Role of Intraepithelial Lymphocytes in Mucosal Tolerance

Because mucosal $\gamma\delta$ T cells have been shown to be part of the network for the induction and regulation of IgA responses, it was important to examine whether these cells could also participate in mucosal tolerance. When intraepithelial $\gamma\delta$ T cells from mice orally tolerized with SRBCs were isolated and adoptively transferred to syngeneic mice with oral tolerance, the abrogation of antigen-specific systemic unresponsiveness was noted (271,338). Thus, these studies provided the first evidence that mucosal $\gamma\delta$ T cells are part of the essential Treg-cell network for the induction and maintenance of antigen-specific IgA immune response in the presence of systemic unresponsiveness induced by prolonged oral administration of protein antigens (271).

Interestingly, it has been shown that both anti-TCR$\gamma\delta$ mAb-treated wild-type and TCR$\gamma\delta^{-/-}$ mice fail to show systemic unresponsiveness after oral administration of antigens (400). Another study demonstrated that when either TCR$\delta^{-/-}$ or TCR$\delta^{+/+}$ mice were immunized orally with a high dose of OVA before parenteral challenge, systemic IgG and IgE antibody responses were markedly reduced in both types of mice (401). Reduced T-cell proliferative responses and DTH were seen in both TCR$\delta^{-/-}$ and TCR$\delta^{+/+}$ mice given high doses of OVA. In contrast, whereas oral tolerance associated with increased levels of IL-10 synthesis was induced by low-dose OVA in TCR$\delta^{+/+}$ mice, TCR$\delta^{-/-}$ mice were not tolerized and failed to produce IL-10 (401). These findings indicate that $\gamma\delta$ T cells play an important role in IL-10–mediated, low-dose oral tolerance induction but are not essential participants in the induction of systemic tolerance to orally introduced antigens given in large doses. It has been suggested that oral tolerance induced by repeated administration of small doses of antigens is mediated by T cells involved in the generation of active suppression, whereas systemic unresponsiveness induced by large doses of antigen is caused by clonal anergy or clonal deletion (338). Thus, it is likely that $\gamma\delta$ T cells play regulatory roles for the induction of active suppression, but they are not involved in the induction of clonal anergy or deletion. Nevertheless, additional

studies are required to establish whether $\gamma\delta$ T cells elicit active suppression in mucosally induced tolerance.

The $\gamma\delta$ T cells have also been shown to be involved in the regulation of IgE responses (338,402). For example, $\gamma\delta$ T cells from the spleens of nasally tolerized mice have been shown to suppress antigen-specific IgE responses. It has also been reported that IgE antibodies are significantly reduced in TCR$\delta^{-/-}$ mice exposed to aerosolized antigens after systemic challenge (402). Together, these findings suggest that mucosal $\gamma\delta$ T cells are involved in the regulation of IgA and IgE antibody responses and function as a part of the Treg-cell network in several different phases of mucosal tolerance.

Nasal Tolerance

The initial dogma that mucosal tolerance requires intestinal processing of the antigen was challenged by the observation that systemic unresponsiveness could be achieved by administration of the antigen via the nasal or aerosol routes (338). These routes were found to necessitate lower doses of antigens than did oral administration, a discrepancy that can be explained by the dilution effect and by the potential degradation of the antigen in the GI tract. The precise mechanism behind nasally induced tolerance is not yet known. It is possible that nasally administered antigens are processed in the mucosal inductive sites of the NALT, in which they generate regulatory Th2 and Th3 cells similar to those seen in PPs of the GI tract. In this regard, nasal passages were shown to be sites rich in Th2-type cells (403) and thus could favor the development of regulatory Th2 and Th3 cells for the induction of systemic unresponsiveness.

Oral Tolerance in Humans

Increasing attention is being paid to oral tolerance and the role it could play in the prevention or treatment of autoimmune diseases, including multiple sclerosis, rheumatoid arthritis, uveitis, type I diabetes, and contact hypersensitivity (338). Indeed, humans immunized with the neoantigen KLH by either the oral (404) or nasal (338,384) route developed systemic unresponsiveness, evaluated by DTH and T-cell proliferative responses. However, B-cell responses were primed in both systemic and mucosal sites. In more recent studies, humans naturally ingesting the dietary antigens bovine gamma globulin, OVA and soybean protein developed a T-cell tolerance characterized by anergy (405). Antigen-specific Th3 cells secreting TGF-β have been observed in the blood of patients with multiple sclerosis orally treated with a bovine myelin preparation (406), which demonstrates that oral administration of autoantigen can induce antigen-specific TGF-β–secreting cells in a human autoimmune disease.

Pilot clinical trials of oral tolerance have been conducted in patients with autoimmune diseases, and promising clinical benefits have been reported (338). Despite encouraging initial results regarding oral delivery of autoantigens for the treatment of human autoimmune diseases, a follow-up study did not demonstrate statistically significant beneficial effects. Furthermore, oral feeding of autoantigen in mice resulted in the generation of antigen-specific CD8$^+$ CTL responses that could lead to the aggravation of autoimmune disease (407). Thus, it must also be remembered that oral administration of autoantigen may induce undesirable CD8$^+$ CTLs that may worsen the disease instead of preventing the development of autoimmunity. However, one study provided new evidence that a temporary blockade of CD40 and CD40 ligand interactions can avoid the generation of unwanted CD8$^+$ CTLs during the induction of oral tolerance (408).

A description of extensive experiments and clinical studies based on the exploitation of principles of mucosal tolerance in the prevention and treatment of T and B cell–mediated hypersensitivity diseases (e.g., contact dermatitis and inhalation allergies), other autoimmune diseases (e.g., uveoretinitis, glomerulonephritis, and diabetes), and prolonged survival of allografts is beyond the scope of this review. However, these efforts have not yet reached fruition. Thus, the experience of most investigators is that once a systemic immune response has been induced, it is difficult to achieve a reversal through mucosal tolerance.

MUCOSAL IMMUNOPATHOLOGY

Immunoglobulin A Deficiency

Incidence and Immunological Features

Deficiency of IgA is the most common primary immunodeficiency disease in humans (84,409). Serological data indicate that in Western Europe and the United States, 1 in 400 to 700 individuals are affected; in Japan, the disease is far less frequent (1 in approximately 18,000). Deficiency of IgA frequently escapes detection, because a large percentage of afflicted individuals have no clinical symptoms. In an absolute majority of cases, both serum IgA1 and IgA2 are either deficient or present in low levels (<50 mg/100 mL). Although rare, selective deficiencies of IgA1 or IgA2 subclasses, caused by the deletion of Cα1 or Cα2 genes, have been described (84,410,411). A few cases of selective deficiencies of serum IgA with fairly intact S-IgA component have been observed (412). An important immunological finding concerns the presence of anti-IgA antibodies in sera of patients with total IgA deficiency (84). When these antibodies are present in the IgE and IgG isotypes, a transfusion of normal, IgA-containing blood or plasma to a patient with anti-IgA antibody may result in anaphylactic shock (84).

A relative absence of clinical symptoms in IgA-deficient individuals is usually explained by alternative compensatory mechanisms. In a large proportion of individuals, S-IgM is present in external secretions that functionally substitute for the deficient S-IgA (84,151,409,413). This is because J chain–containing pIgM is transported by the same pIgR-mediated pathway as pIgA and mucosal tissues, and secretory glands contain large numbers of IgM-producing plasma cells adjacent to pIgR-expressing epithelial cells (151,413).

Furthermore, IgA-deficient patients may have increased levels of IgG in sera and secretions and higher numbers of IgG-producing cells in mucosal tissues than do normal individuals (151,413). In IgA-deficient patients with clinical symptoms, additional immunological defects, such as concomitant deficiency of IgG subclasses, particularly IgG2 or IgG4, have been observed (409,411). Peripheral blood of IgA-deficient individuals contains a low number of sIgA$^+$ B cells and mucosal tissues, and glands display lower numbers of IgA-producing plasma cells (151,409). *In vitro* stimulation of peripheral blood lymphocytes with pokeweed mitogen reveals a defect in differentiation of cells toward IgA in some but not all patients (84). A defect in switching of B cells to IgA-producing cells is a common feature (84).

Molecular Basis

IgA deficiency is a heterogeneous disease with regard to the clinical symptoms and range of deficiency. Consequently, several mechanisms are likely to be involved in its development. A true deletion of genes encoding for the constant regions of α1 or α2 or both chains is extremely rare and accounts for selective IgA1 or IgA2 subclass deficiencies (84,410,411). Instead, it is obvious that regulatory defects in maturation of B-lymphocytes into IgA-secreting cells are main causes of this frequent disorder (84). Because the pokeweed mitogen–induced *in vitro* differentiation of peripheral blood lymphocytes into IgA-producing cells can be selectively suppressed by anti-IgA and by anti-IgA1 or anti-IgA2 reagents (414), it has been speculated that the development of IgA cells in the fetus can be suppressed before birth by transplacentally acquired IgG and anti-IgA antibodies present in plasma of IgA-deficient mothers (84,409). Reduced numbers of sIgA$^+$ cells present in peripheral blood of IgA-deficient patients suggests a defect in switching from sIgM$^+$ to sIgA$^+$ cells (84). Furthermore, an arrest in terminal differentiation into IgA-secreting plasma cells is an important feature of B cells from IgA-deficient patients. Many mechanisms may be involved in this defect, including the inability of T cells to produce cytokines required for differentiation of B cells, environmental factors, congenital viral infections, certain drugs, and genetic factors (84,409). Studies of families with members afflicted by IgA deficiency suggest the existence of a disease susceptibility candidate locus, designated *IGAD1,* which appears to be restricted to class II or, even more likely, class III MHC regions as its most probable location (415). A number of genes in these regions are implicated in lymphocyte activation.

Functional Abnormalities

It is well recognized that most IgA-deficient individuals are asymptomatic. However, it appears that, in comparison with normal individuals, patients with IgA deficiency have higher incidences of recurrent infections (particularly of the upper respiratory tract), allergic diseases, autoimmune disorders, and malignancies (particularly intestinal adenocarcinomas) (84,409). Absence or low levels of S-IgA antibodies to microbial and food antigens may result in higher rates of absorption of such antigens from mucosal surfaces (see previous discussion of the function of mucosal antibodies), induction of higher levels of corresponding antibodies in plasma, and formation of circulating immune complexes. Although S-IgM may replace S-IgA in IgA-deficient patients, it appears that S-IgM does not fully substitute for the IgA-associated functions (416). This situation may be ascribed partly to the anti-inflammatory nature of IgA, manifested by its inability to activate complement with potential inflammatory consequences (see previous discussion). In contrast, both IgM and IgG are potent complement activators, and it has been demonstrated that the formation of immune complexes composed of protein antigens and IgM or IgG within mucosal tissues leads to local damage and increased absorption of by-standard antigens (417). Diminished functional substitution of S-IgA with S-IgM is also apparent in frequency of viral and bacterial infections and in responses to vaccines (84,409).

Human Immunodeficiency Virus Type 1 Infection and the Mucosal Immune System

Mucosal tissues of the genital and intestinal tracts are the most important portals of entry of HIV (418). Epidemiological studies indicate that, worldwide, approximately 80% to 90% of HIV infections are acquired by mucosal routes through heterosexual and homosexual intercourse and by the vertical transmission route *in utero,* during the delivery, or by breast-feeding (418). Furthermore, application of simian immunodeficiency virus (SIV) on the surfaces of the vagina, penile urethra, or nasopharyngeal lymphoid tissues resulted in SIV infection in rhesus monkeys (419).

Several mucosal cell types may be involved in the initial uptake of HIV and SIV (418–420). In animal models, specialized epithelial M cells found in the intestinal PPs, in analogous lymphoepithelial structures of the rectum, and in tonsils are capable of internalization of HIV/SIV and presumably of passing the virus to adjacent infectible cells, including T cells, macrophages, and DCs (418–420). Human intestinal and oral epithelial cell lines and primary IECs internalize HIV and are infectible *in vitro* because of the expression of HIV receptors/co-receptors (CD4, galactosyl-ceramide, and the CC-chemokines, mainly CCR5 and perhaps CXCR4) on their surfaces (418–420). However, direct *in vivo* evidence for the presence of HIV in enterocytes is not available. In rhesus macaques intravaginally exposed to cell-free SIV, dendritic (Langerhans) cells dispersed in the stratified squamous vaginal epithelium were the first cells that were infected (419,421). Studies indicate that SIV and HIV primarily target and destroy mucosal CD4$^+$ cells, perhaps because of the selective expression of chemokine receptors (421). Isolated mucosal macrophages are less permissive of HIV infection than are phenotypically distinct blood monocytes, probably because of the reduced expression of HIV co-receptors (422).

Mucosal Immune Responses

HIV type 1 (HIV-1)–specific antibodies become detectable in sera shortly after the infection. In all seropositive individuals, these antibodies are of the IgG isotype; IgA antibodies are present less frequently and at much lower levels (423,424). Extensive studies of external secretions, including tears, saliva, nasal, intestinal and vaginal washes, semen, cervical mucus, milk, fecal extracts, and urine, yielded often controversial results with regard to the presence and isotypes of HIV-1–specific antibodies (345,346,424–426). Differences in the collection procedures, processing of samples, dilutions of some secretions by washing fluids (60), and methods used for antibody detection may account for some of these discrepancies. Surprisingly, HIV-1–specific antibodies of the IgG isotype are dominant in all secretions, despite the overwhelming levels of total IgA and the route of infection (systemic or mucosal) (423–428). For example, in human milk, intestinal fluid, and saliva, in which IgA represents approximately 98% to 99% and IgG only approximately 1% of total immunoglobulins, HIV-1–specific antibodies are present mainly in the IgG isotype. In external secretions of individuals with IgA HIV-1 antibodies, there is a pronounced restriction to the IgA1 subclass (429). Absence or presence of levels of HIV-1–specific IgA antibodies in external secretions does not result from the defect in the production of total IgA or unresponsiveness to viral antigens: IgA antibodies to, for example, influenza virus are readily detectable in secretions of HIV-1–infected individuals (424). Mechanisms involved in this diminished responsiveness to HIV-1 but not the influenza virus in the S-IgA isotype have not been clarified. The site of original infection and the presence of effective mucosal inductive sites in the upper respiratory tract (but not in the genital tract) may play a role. Initial reports (425,426) of the selective occurrence of HIV-1–specific antibodies in secretions of HIV-1–exposed but seronegative individuals have not been confirmed in other studies (345,346). Studies concerning the presence of cytotoxic lymphocytes in mucosal tissues of HIV-infected individuals are rather limited (418), mainly because of the unavailability of tissues to perform extensive analyses.

The progressive decline of immune functions in long-term HIV-1–infected and untreated individuals also compromises the mucosal immune system (418). An increased incidence of infections with mucosal opportunistic pathogens, including viruses, bacteria, fungi, and protozoa, and an increased incidence of mucosal neoplasms have been observed (418).

Inflammatory Bowel Disease

IBD represents a chronic, relapsing-and-remitting inflammatory condition of the GI tract that is manifested as one of two usually distinct but significantly overlapping clinical entities: ulcerative colitis and Crohn's disease, which predominantly affect the colon superficially or transmurally with the formation of granulomas, respectively. Increasing evidence suggests that IBD is a dysregulated mucosal immune response to components of the normal commensal luminal microbiota in a genetically susceptible host that is further modified by a variety of environmental factors (e.g., medication and tobacco use). As such, IBD represents a complex interaction among genetic susceptibility, environmental triggers, and mucosal immune dysregulation (430,431). The genetic basis for IBD in humans is supported by the facts that 10% to 30% percent of patients have a positive family history; there is an association between IBD and several genetic disorders (e.g., Turner's syndrome); the concordance rate for development of IBD among monozygotic twins is high, especially in Crohn's disease; and, finally, genome-wide searches for susceptibility genes utilizing microsatellite markers spanning the human genome have confirmed disease linkages on chromosomes 16 (IBD1), 12 (IBD2), 6 (IBD3), and 14 (IBD4) (432). The association with linkage on chromosome 16 (IBD1) has been defined as the NOD2 gene (433,434). NOD2 is related to the CED4/APAF1 superfamily of apoptosis regulators and to a class of plant resistance genes with expression restricted to monocytes. NOD2 contains caspase recruitment domains, a nucleotide-binding domain, and a leucine-rich region (LPS binding domain). The leucine-rich region of NOD2 regulates the NFκB-activating activity of NOD2 and, as a result, is considered an intracellular bacterial sensor. Mutations within the leucine-rich region of the NOD2 gene have been directly related to patients with Crohn's disease. Individuals who are homozygous for these particular substitutions, which create a truncated NOD2 gene product, exhibit a markedly increased risk for the development of Crohn's disease. This initial description of a genetic association between IBD and an intracellular bacterial sensor strongly emphasizes the importance of genetic regulation of mucosal immune responses to commensal organisms within the lumen and, moreover, the importance of innate immune responses in disease pathogenesis and mucosal immunoregulation.

Most of the understanding of IBD pathogenesis, however, is in clarification of the relationship between the mucosal immune system and its environmental triggers that initiate and drive the dysregulated response. The majority of these insights have come through a variety of animal models of IBD (430,431) (Table 5). The animal models of IBD include those that occur spontaneously and those that are induced by administration of exogenous agents, gene targeting through knockout or transgenic approaches, or transfer of cells into immunodeficient animals (432–451). These models have demonstrated that in IBD there appears to be a response to specific components of the commensal luminal microbiota that is distilled into a final common pathway of inflammation that is represented by an excess of either Th1 cytokines (e.g., CD45RB^{hi} transfer model, IL-10 deficiency) or Th2 cytokines (e.g., TCR-α deficiency, oxazolone hypersensitivity). This results in transmural (Th1 cytokine excess) and superficial (Th2 cytokine excess) inflammation which may mirror human Crohn's disease and ulcerative colitis, respectively. The data supporting this include the fact that the incidence of IBD in the animal models is reduced when bacterial colonization is eliminated through germ-free conditions or reduced, such as through antibiotic administration. However, not all bacteria are equal in this regard (452). For example, some groups of organisms are known to trigger colitis in genetically susceptible animal strains, such as the ability of *Bacteroides vulgatus* to stimulate colitis in HLA-B27 transgenic rats (453). On the other hand, some groups of organisms are able to prevent colitis, such as *Lactobacillus* species, which

TABLE 5. *Animal models of inflammatory bowel disease*

Induced			Spontaneous
Administration of exogenous agents	Gene targeting: knockout or transgenic	Transfer of cell populations into immunodeficient animals	
Enema	Cytokine/cytokine receptors and signaling pathways	CD4$^+$ CD45RBhi into *scid/scid* or RAG mice (447)	Cotton top tamarin (449)
Trinitrobenzene sulfonic acid (432)	IL-2$^{-/-}$ (440)	Bone marrow into Tgϵ26 mice (448)	C3H-HeJBir mouse (450)
Oxazalone (434)	IL-10$^{-/-}$ (441)		SAMP1/Yit mouse (451)
Acetic acid (435)	IL-7-Tg (442)		
Oral	T-cell function and development		
Carageenan (436)	Gαi2$^{-/-}$ (443)		
Dextran sodium sulfate (437)	TCR$\alpha^{-/-}$ (444)		
	N-WASP$^{-/-}$ (445)		
	HLA-B27 Tg rat (446)		
Other	IEC barrier function		
Cyclosporine (438)	Trefoil factor$^{-/-a}$(6)		
Peptidoglycan-polysaccharide (439)	N-cadherin dominant negative (433)		

HLA, human leukocyte antigen; IEC, intestinal epithelial cell; IL, interleukin; RAG, recombination activating gene; TCR, T-cell receptor; Tg, transgenic.

[a]Requires environmental stress, such as dextran sodium sulfate.

Adapted from Blumberg et al. (430), with permission.

are considered probiotics and are known to prevent colitis in genetically susceptible hosts such as IL-10 knockout mice (454). Moreover, in accordance with the polygenic nature of IBD as observed in humans, the responses to bacteria are genetically determined in such a way that even in a genetically susceptible mouse model, genetic strain differences are known to modify the final clinicopathological presentation of the disease (455). Not only do responses to specific organisms vary, but the bacterial constituents that appear to be responsible for initiating or driving the disease, or both, also appear to be restricted. Colitis in mouse models appears to be triggered by a subset of protein antigens that largely activate effector T cells, as manifested by the evidence of private and, to a lesser extent, public TCR motifs in bacterially driven disease models such as the CD45RB[hi] transfer model in SCID mice, which is consistent with observations in humans (456,457). Together, these findings indicate that, to the host that is genetically susceptible for the development of IBD, the normal commensal bacterial microbiota are inappropriately perceived by the mucosal immune system as if they were a pathogen (458). In other words, there appears to be a loss of immune tolerance to the autologous microbiota. In accordance with this, lamina propria mononuclear cells isolated from inflamed IBD intestine from both mouse and human exhibit responsiveness to autologous intestinal microbiota that is inhibited by blocking antigen presentation. Lamina propria mononuclear cells from noninflamed IBD intestine, IBD intestine in remission, and control intestine exhibit responsiveness only to heterologous intestinal microbiota (459). Interestingly, the response in the involved IBD intestine is associated with T-cell activation and production of Th1 (IFN-γ), Th2 (IL-4), and Treg cytokines (IL-10, TGF-β) (459). This is consistent with the concept that the final common pathway of excessive Th1 or Th2 cytokine production that underlies the pathogenesis of IBD is achieved either by excessive Th1 or Th2 effector T cells or by ineffective counterbalance of effector T cells by regulatory subsets of cells that secrete anti-inflammatory cytokines such as IL-10 and TGF-β (430,431). This has placed significant emphasis on defining the regulatory subsets of cells involved in blocking disease pathogenesis and has allowed for drawing significant similarities between and insights from mechanisms previously related to the study of oral tolerance. Indeed, oral tolerance has shown to be effective in the prevention of IBD through production of these regulatory cytokines in animal models (460,461). In this regard, cell types that can secrete these regulatory cytokines have been linked to ameliorating the pathogenesis of this disease. These include Th3 cells, which produce TGF-β; Tr1 cells, which produce IL-10; CD4$^+$ CD25$^+$ T cells, which secrete IL-10 and TGF-β; and regulatory B cells, which express CD1d and secrete IL-10 (189). It is thus the balance of T effector cells and regulatory cells—which are mostly T cells, within the GALT and probably originate in GALT (including PPs and cecal patches) through sampling of microbes and their components—that leads to the generation of a particular immunological

tone in a genetically susceptible host that is ultimately released into a pathogenic phenotype by a variety of potential triggers.

The animal models have also revealed that, in addition to perturbations of T-cell regulation and imbalanced cytokine production, mucosal barrier function and repair are important in the generation of IBD. Such an importance of barrier function in regulating antigen uptake in an appropriate manner had already been suggested by studies in humans before more definitive studies in mouse models. The mouse models have clearly shown that alterations of tight junction function through generation of a dominant negative N-cadherin transgenic animal model (462), alterations in the mucus and glycocalyx function through disruption of intestinal trefoil factor (6), or abrogation of enterocytes' ability to regulate the extrusion of luminal toxins through disruption of the *mdr1a* gene product (463) are all barrier dysfunctions that are channeled into a final pathological phenotype that is manifested as IBD. In addition, animals that lack $\gamma\delta$ T cells and thus are unable to generate keratinocyte growth factor exhibit increased susceptibility to the injury associated with TNBS administration (464). In the cases in which they have been examined, the enteric microbiota are important in driving or modifying the final disease process. These studies also suggest that a major initiating factor in the development of IBD may be leakiness of the mucosal barrier, which leads to a dysregulated immune response, resulting in up-regulation of inflammatory cytokines and membrane receptors, which, in turn, leads to endothelial activation, cellular recruitment and amplification, and, finally, the production of inflammatory mediators with reactive oxygen metabolites and metalloproteinases.

The central importance of luminal microbial-derived antigens as interpreted by the interactions between T cells and APCs has led to a dissection of the molecular events associated with promotion of Th1- and Th2-mediated inflammation. In addition to the important role played by cognate interactions, co-stimulatory events that up-regulate IL-12 and IL-18 production by macrophages are extremely important. Participants in these events include molecules such as CD40 (465), OX40 ligand (466), and CEACAM1 (467,468) and their counterligands on T cells. These interactions lead to the production of Th1-associated cytokines by CD4$^+$ T cells (TNF and IFN-γ) and inflammatory cytokines by the macrophage/DC through feedback regulation by T cell–derived IFN-γ, resulting in the production of TNF, IL-1-β, IL-8, and IL-6 by the macrophage/DC. TNF appears to be a particularly important proinflammatory cytokine in the Th1-associated colitis in animal models and in human IBD through its interactions with the TNF receptor that lead to activation of NFκB through phosphorylation of IκBα, an intracellular inhibitor of NFκB (469). NFκB elements are present on a wide variety of genes that are associated with promoting inflammation. Targeting TNF, IL-12, and their downstream events such as NFκB is therefore a major important avenue of anti-inflammation treatment in these diseases. Interestingly, IL-10 and standard therapies such as corticosteroids and

5-aminosalicylic acid block NFκB activation either through inducing the concentration of intracellular IκBα inhibitor or through diminishing its degradation, respectively (470). Less is known about the APC–T cell interactions involved in the development of Th2-mediated colitis. However, studies have suggested an important potential role for Epstein-Barr virus–induced gene 3, an IL-12 p40 homolog, that is known to be up-regulated in human ulcerative colitis and that, in its absence in animal models, may prevent the development of Th2-mediated colonic inflammation (471). Regulatory cytokines, on the other hand, function in the down-regulation of T-cell (TGF-β) activation (472) and macrophage (IL-10) activation (473).

Mucosal Allergies

The majority of allergic immunological diseases is of mucosal origin and in their clinical manifestations. The diseases tend to affect mainly the upper respiratory tract and lungs and the GI tract or to manifest as atopic dermatitis. Allergic diseases are now rampant in Western countries, and their incidence appears to be increasing. There is a general belief that this increase is due to "cleanliness" in the environment, so that exposure to allergens more often results in hypersensitivity and not classical immunity to infections such as tuberculosis, measles, or hepatitis A. The term *atopy* is used to describe a complex trait resulting in immune responses to "environmental" antigens in genetically susceptibility subjects (474,475). Asthma is the most common of the severe atopic diseases, which also include allergic rhinitis and atopic dermatitis. On the other hand, hypersensitivity in the GI tract emanates from ingestion of large amounts of food antigens, including cow's milk proteins (476,477). It occurs most frequently during the first year of life, and the syndrome that develops is termed *allergic gastroenteropathy* (AGE).

Asthma

The three hallmarks of asthma include (a) variable airflow obstruction, (b) airway hyperresponsiveness, and (c) airway inflammation. Airway inflammation includes a cell infiltrate into the airway wall of mast cells, eosinophils, and T and B cells (474). The sharp increase in asthma incidence since 1980 (more than 155 million cases in developed countries, 15 million in the United States alone) (478), with increased cost in treatment (more than $6 billion per year in the United States alone), has led to significant progress toward understanding the asthma syndrome (478). It is generally agreed that development of an IgE-mediated antibody response to common inhaled allergens is a major factor; however, genetic factors, discussed later, contribute to the atopy (474). In this scenario, termed *extrinsic asthma,* susceptible individuals (usually children) are repeatedly exposed to low antigen levels and develop specific IgE anti-allergen antibodies (474,479). Subsequent exposure to the allergen results in a two-tiered response. Within minutes, mucosal edema devel-

ops with airway narrowing and extensive mucosal mast cell degranulation (474). This early-phase response usually resolves within 1 hour. A late-phase response (beginning 3 to 6 hours later) may also develop. This latter response is characterized by infiltrations of neutrophils, eosinophils, and lymphocytes into the lung parenchyma and airway epithelium (474). Thus, mast cells may mediate the early-phase response to allergen, and eosinophils and mast cells may mediate the late-phase response. Eosinophils persist in the presence of IL-5 and granulocyte-macrophage colony-stimulating factor and in injury of airways and contribute to persistent airway inflammation. Not surprisingly, CD4+ T cells are of central importance in development of asthma. It is well established that higher CD4+ T-cell counts are seen in bronchoalveolar lavage, with decreases in blood CD4+ T-cell numbers (474). A general state of T-cell activation exists with expression of IL-2R (CD25), HLA-DR, and VLA-1 (474). In asthmatic patients, CD4+ T cells produce IL-4, IL-5, IL-13, and granulocyte-macrophage colony-stimulating factor (474,480,481), and the success of steroid treatment is correlated with increases in T cell-derived IFN-γ in bronchoalveolar lavage samples from patients (474,480,481). In addition, a direct correlation exists among activated CD4+ T cells, activated eosinophils, high exhalation, and more severe disease (474). As discussed in more detail later, there is evidence that CD4+ T cells producing Th1-type cytokines may set the stage for development of Th2-cell regulated IgE antibody responses.

Despite intensive investigation, the precise reason why asthmatic patients develop these CD4+ Th2-type profiles is not yet known. One possibility is that specific allergens may predispose them to the development of CD4+ Th cells through enzymatic reactions. One such allergen is a 25-kDa cysteine protease produced by the house dust mite *Dermatophagoides pteronyssinus,* termed Der p 1. Dust mites are common in Western culture, and Der p 1 is thought to penetrate into and through the respiratory epithelium. This cysteine protease cleaves CD25 expressed by activated T cells, resulting in decreased proliferation and IFN-γ synthesis (474). There is some evidence that Der p 1 cleaves CD23 (FcεRII) on B cells, a low-affinity IgE receptor ordinarily functioning to inhibit IgE response (474,482). Other potential polarizing elements may involve unique APC–T cell interactions for Th2-type responses. Asthmatic patients have increased numbers of DCs in bronchoalveolar lavage samples, and circulating monocytes are more potent accessory cells than are normal monocytes, which tend to be poor APCs (474). This fails to explain a disposition to Th2-type responses, however.

Perhaps a more plausible explanation is provided by genetic analysis. Asthma susceptibility is linked to multiple gene regions on chromosomes 5, 6 11, 14, and 12 (483–485). Chromosome 5 region q23–35 has the most candidate genes, including the IL-4 cytokine cluster, IL-9, and IL-12 p40 (483,484,486,487). The large size of the 5q region, which includes the genes for IL-4, IL-5, and IL-13, has made it difficult to study this coding region *in toto*. One study has provided a novel way to assess the asthmatic susceptibility genes by using BALB/c mice made congenic through backcrossing a small chromosomal region homologous to human chromosome 5q (488). This led to identification of a locus termed Tapr (T cell and airway phenotype regulator) that differed from the IL-4 gene cluster and from IL-12 p40. Through positional cloning, these investigators isolated a gene family encoding T-cell membrane proteins (TIMs), which co-segregated with Tapr (488). A human homolog of TIM-1 is the receptor for hepatitis A virus and could help explain the inverse relationship that exists between hepatitis A virus infection and failure to develop asthma. It should be emphasized that this highly significant finding still does not provide an explanation for the fact that lack of virus infection in genetically susceptible hosts leads to Th2-type allergic responses. However, genetic approaches like this one will clearly lead to identification, isolation, cloning, and diagnostic use of genes that regulate airway hyperresponsiveness in asthma. This picture of asthma may be too simplistic, inasmuch as murine models also support a CD4$^+$ Th1-type response in allergic inflammation. Use of adoptive transfer of OVA-specific, Th1- or Th2-polarized cells into an adoptive host challenged nasally with OVA leads to major accumulations of Th1-type cells early in airway responses (489,490). It appears that Th1-type cells actually potentiate the inflammatory response that later develops into a CD4$^+$ Th2 type, with IL-4–induced IgE and IL-5–elicited eosinophilia (491).

Gastrointestinal Allergy

During the first year of life, up to 6% to 8% of all infants can develop IgE antibody–mediated allergy to food (477), and 30% to 40% (or more) of these infants exhibit allergic responses to cow's milk (477). Affected infants most commonly show symptoms in both the GI and respiratory tracts, as well as rashes. Sensitization in 1- to 2-year-old children is traced to cow's milk- or soybean-based proteins used in their formula diet (477). Nevertheless, AGE is caused by maternal dietary proteins transferred to infants during breast-feeding (477,492). AGE from food proteins generally belongs to two categories: (a) disorders due to acute reactions [GI tract responses, urticaria, and asthma (see previous discussion)] or atopy associated with IgE antibodies and (b) disorders caused by T-cell responses, primarily in the GI tract, in the absence of IgE antibodies (493). These two forms can be further subdivided into enterocolitis syndrome, proctocolitis, enteropathy, and one form of allergic eosinophilic enteropathy (494).

The diagnosis of IgE-mediated AGE has improved, and one reason has been the use of a double-blind placebo–food ingestion test (495). In this test, infant histories are taken and used to tailor-design the food challenge. Skin testing is also commonly used. These methods have helped clarify the types of food most likely to induce AGE and the types of reactions to them that will occur. However, dietary alternatives for infants suffering from, for example, cow's milk AGE are somewhat limited. This has led to the development of pediatric amino acid–based formulas (494).

Progress in determining the pathogenesis of AGE has been made as a result of the development of several mouse models that mimic, at least in part, the symptoms of AGE. In one model, an OVA-specific, eosinophil-based allergy was induced in mice (496). Mice were given OVA with alum by the intraperitoneal route and then orally challenged with a large dose of OVA in enteric-coated beads (36). A CD4$^+$ Th2-type of response occurred with eosinophilia; however, this was ablated in the absence of the chemokine eotaxin. In another model (497), prior sensitization of C3H/HeJ mice with cow's milk allergen given orally with CT as adjuvant, which promotes Th2-type responses, induced a mast cell type of degranulation and anaphylaxis without marked eosinophil involvement. Finally, one of the authors' laboratories has developed a model in which BALB/c mice given OVA and complete Freund's adjuvant parenterally, followed by oral OVA, three times per week developed CD4$^+$ Th2-type cells in the colon with diarrhea. This eosinophil-based reaction was abrogated by anti–IL-4 mAb treatment, and disease failed to occur in STAT6-knockout mice (498). Despite these advances, there remain large gaps in the full understanding of AGE and therefore in effective treatment of this important mucosal disorder.

ACKNOWLEDGMENTS

We thank Mrs. Maria Crenshaw, Mrs. Janet Fox, and Ms. Sheila Turner for their assistance with the preparation of this chapter. Experimental work performed in authors' laboratories was supported by U.S. Public Health Service grants AI 28147, DK 44319, DK 51362, DK 53056, AI 18958, AI 43197, DK 44240, DC 04976, and DK 54781; by the Cancer Research Institute; and by the Harvard Digestive Disease Center.

REFERENCES

1. Christ AD, Blumberg RS. The intestinal epithelial cell: immunological aspects. *Springer Semin Immunopathol* 1997;18:449–461.
2. Anderson JM, Van Itallie CM. Tight junctions: closing in on the sea. *Curr Biol* 1999;9:R922–R924.
3. Madara JL. Epithelia: biologic principles of organization. In: Yamada T, ed. *Textbook of immunology*. Philadelphia: Lippincott-Raven, 1995:141–157.
4. Dignass AU, Podolsky DK. Cytokine modulation of intestinal epithelial cell restitution: central role of transforming growth factor beta. *Gastroenterology* 1994;376–383.
5. Nusrat A, Parkos CA, Bacarra AE, et al. Hepatocyte growth factor/scatter factor effects on epithelia. Regulation of intercellular junctions in transformed and nontransformed cell lines, basolateral polarization of c-met receptor in transformed and natural intestinal epithelia, and induction of rapid wound repair in a transformed model epithelium. *J Clin Invest* 1994;93:2056–2065.
6. Mashimo H, Wu DC, Podolsky DK, et al. Impaired defense of intestinal mucosa in mice lacking intestinal trefoil factor. *Science* 1996;274:262–265.
7. McCracken VJ, Lorenz RG. The gastrointestinal ecosystem: a precarious alliance among epithelium, immunity and microbiota. *Cell Microbiol* 2001;3:1–11.

8. Madsen K, Cornish A, Soper P, et al. Probiotic bacteria enhance murine and human intestinal barrier function. *Gastroenterology* 2001;121: 580–591.

9. Colgan SP, Hershberg RM, Furuta GT, Blumberg RS. Ligation of intestinal epithelial CD1d induces bioactive IL-10: critical role of the cytoplasmic tail in autocrine signaling. *Proc Natl Acad Sci U S A* 1999; 96:13938–13943.

10. Andoh A, Fujiyama Y, Bamba T, et al. Differential cytokine regulation of complement C3, C4, and factor B synthesis in human intestinal epithelial cell line, Caco-2. *J Immunol* 1993;151:4239–4247.

11. Eisenhauer PB, Harwig SS, Lehrer RI. Cryptdins: antimicrobial defensins of the murine small intestine. *Infect Immun* 1992;60:3556–3565.

12. O'Neil DA, Porter EM, Elewaut D, et al. Expression and regulation of the human β-defensins hBD-1 and hBD-2 in intestinal epithelium. *J Immunol* 1999;163:6718–6724.

13. Loomes KM, Senior HE, West PM, et al. Functional protective role for mucin glycosylated repetitive domains. *Eur J Biochem* 1999;266:105–111.

14. Kawasaki Y, Tazume S, Shimizu K, et al. Inhibitory effects of bovine lactoferrin on the adherence of enterotoxigenic *Escherichia coli* to host cells. *Biosci Biotechnol Biochem* 2000;64:348–354.

15. Ouellette AJ. Paneth cells and innate immunity in the crypt microenvironment. *Gastroenterology* 1997;113:1779–1784.

16. McCormick BA, Hofman PM, Kim J, et al. Surface attachment of *Salmonella typhimurium* to intestinal epithelia imprints the subepithelial matrix with gradients chemotactic for neutrophils. *J Cell Biol* 1995;11:599–608.

17. Jung HC, Eckman L, Yang SK, et al. A distinct array of proinflammatory cytokines is expressed in human colon epithelial cells in response to bacterial invasion. *J Clin Invest* 1995;95:56–65.

18. Reinecker HC, MacDermott RP, Mirau S, et al. Intestinal epithelial cells both express and respond to interleukin 15. *Gastroenterology* 1996;111:1706–1713.

19. Fearon DT, Locksley RM. The instructive role of innate immunity in the acquired immune response. *Science* 1996;272:50–53.

20. Akira S. Toll-like receptors and innate immunity. *Adv Immunol* 2001;78:1–56.

21. Labéta MO, Vidal K, Nores JER, et al. Innate recognition of bacteria in human milk is mediated by a milk-derived highly expressed pattern recognition receptor, soluble CD14. *J Exp Med* 2000;191:1807–1812.

22. Aradhya S, Nelson DL. NF-κB signaling and human disease. *Curr Opin Genet Dev* 2001;11:300–306.

23. Neish AS, Gewirtz AT, Zeng H, et al. Prokaryotic regulation of epithelial responses by inhibition of IκB-α ubiquitination. *Science* 2000;289:1483–1484.

24. Watanbabe M, Ueno Y, Yajima T, et al. Interleukin 7 is produced by human intestinal epithelial cells and regulates the proliferation of intestinal mucosal lymphocytes. *J Clin Invest* 1995;95:2945–2953.

25. Wang J, Whetsell M, Klein JR. Local hormone networks and intestinal T cell homeostasis. *Science* 1997;275:1937–1939.

26. Hata Y, Ota S, Nagata T, et al. Primary colonic epithelial cell culture of the rabbit producing prostaglandins. *Prostaglandins* 1993;45:129–141.

27. Reinecker HC, Podolsky DK. Human intestinal epithelial cells expression functional cytokine receptors sharing the common gamma c chain of the interleukin 2 receptor. *Proc Natl Acad Sci U S A* 1995;92:8353–8357.

28. Norderhaug IN, Johansen FE, Schjerven H, et al. Regulation of the formation and external transport of secretory immunoglobulins. *Crit Rev Immunol* 1999;19:481–508.

29. Israel EJ, Taylor S, Wu Z, et al. Expression of the neonatal Fc receptor, FcRn, on human intestinal epithelial cells. *Immunology* 1997;92:69–74.

30. Zhu X, Meng G, Dickinson BL, et al. MHC class I–related neonatal Fc receptor of IgG is functionally expressed in monocytes, intestinal macrophages, and dendritic cells. *J Immunol* 2001;166:3266–3277.

31. Dickinson BL, Badizadegan K, Wu Z, et al. Bidirectional FcRn-dependent IgG transport in a polarized human intestinal epithelial cell line. *J Clin Invest* 1999;104:903–911.

32. Kvale D, Krajci P, Brandtzaeg P. Expression and regulation of adhesion molecules ICAM-1 (CD54) and LFA-3 (CD58) in human intestinal epithelial cell lines. *Scand J Immunol* 1992;35:669–676.

33. Ebert EC. Proliferative responses of human intraepithelial lymphocytes to various T-cell stimuli. *Gastroenterology* 1989;97:1372–1381.

34. Cepek KL, Shaw SK, Parker CM, et al. Adhesion between epithelial cells and T lymphocytes mediated by E-cadherin and the $\alpha^E \beta_7$ integrin. *Nature* 1994;372:190–193.

35. Brandeis JM, Sayegh MH, Gallon L, et al. Rat intestinal epithelial cells present major histocompatibility complex allopeptides to primed T cells. *Gastroenterology* 1994;107:1537–1542.

36. Hershberg RM, Cho DH, Youakim A, et al. Highly polarized HLA class II antigen processing and presentation by human intestinal epithelial cells. *J Clin Invest* 1998;102:792–803.

37. Bauer S, Groh V, Wu J, et al. Activation of NK cells and T cells by NKG2D, a receptor for stress-inducible MICA. *Science* 1999;285:727–729.

38. Somnay-Wadgaonkar K, Nusrat A, Kim HS, et al. Immunolocalization of CD1d in human intestinal epithelial cells and identification of a β_2-microglobulin–associated form. *Int Immunol* 1999;11:383–392.

39. Jabri B, de Serre NP, Cellier C, et al. Selective expansion of intraepithelial lymphocytes expressing the HLA-E–specific natural killer receptor CD94 in celiac disease. *Gastroenterology* 2000;118:867–879.

40. Huang GT-J, Eckmann L, Savidge T, et al. Infection of human intestinal epithelial cells with invasive bacteria upregulates apical intercellular adhesion molecule–1 (ICAM-1) expression and neutrophil adhesion. *J Clin Invest* 1996;98:572–583.

41. Propst SM, Denson R, Rothstein E, et al. Proinflammatory and Th2-derived cytokines modulate CD40-mediated expression of inflammatory mediators in airway epithelia: implications for the role of epithelial CD40 in airway inflammation. *J Immunol* 2000;165:2214–2221.

42. Mahnke K, Guo M, Lee S, et al. The dendritic cell receptor for endocytosis, DEC-205, can recycle and enhance antigen presentation via major histocompatibility complex class II–positive lysosomal compartments. *J Cell Biol* 2000;151:675–684.

43. Arman AT, Fraser S, Merritt EA, et al. A mutant cholera toxin B subunit that binds GM1-ganglioside but lacks immunomodulatory or toxic activity. *Proc Natl Acad Sci U S A* 2001;98:8536–8541.

44. Lefrancois L, Fuller B, Huleatt JW, et al. On the front lines: intraepithelial lymphocytes as primary effectors of mucosal immunity. *Springer Semin Immunopathol* 1997;18:463–475.

45. Kelsall BL, Strober W. Dendritic cells of the gastrointestinal tract. *Springer Semin Immunopathol* 1997;18:409–420.

46. Blumberg RS, Hershberg, R. What's so (co)stimulating about the intestinal epithelium? *Gastroenterology* 1999;117:726–736.

47. Framson PE, Cho DH, Lee LY, et al. Polarized expression and function of the costimulatory molecule CD58 on human intestinal epithelial cells. *Gastroenterology* 1999;116:1054–1062.

48. Morales VM, Christ A, Watt SM, et al. Regulation of human intestinal intraepithelial lymphocyte cytolytic function by biliary glycoprotein (CD66a). *J Immunol* 1999;163:1363–1370.

49. Vezys V, Olson S, Lefrancois L. Expression of intestine-specific antigen reveals novel pathways of CD8 T cell tolerance induction. *Immunity* 2000;12:505–514.

50. Heshberg RM, Framson PE, Cho DH, et al. Intestinal epithelial cells use two distinct pathways for HLA class I antigen processing. *J Clin Invest* 1997;100:204–215.

51. Blumberg RS, Terhorst C, Bleicher P, et al. Expression of a nonpolymorphic MHC class I–like molecule, CD1d, by human intestinal epithelial cells. *J Immunol* 1991;147:2518–2524.

52. Matsuda JL, Naidenko OV, Gapin L, et al. Tracking the response of natural killer T cells to a glycolipid antigen using CD1d tetramers. *J Exp Med* 2000;192:741–754.

53. Roberts AI, Lee L, Schwarz E, et al. NKG2D receptors induced by IL-15 costimulate CD28-negative effector CTL in the tissue microenvironment. *J Immunol* 2001;167:5527–5530.

54. Leishman AJ, Naidenko OV, Attinger A, et al. T cell responses modulated through interaction between CD8 and the nonclassical MHC class I molecule, TL. *Science* 2001;294:1936–1939.

55. Savage DC. Mucosal microbiota. In: Ogra PL, Mestecky J, Lamm ME, et al., eds. *Mucosal immunology,* 2nd ed. San Diego, CA: Academic Press, 1999:19–30.

56. Shroff KE, Meslin K, Cebra JJ. Commensal enteric bacteria engender a self-limiting humoral mucosal immune response while permanently colonizing the gut. *Infect Immun* 1995;63:3904–3913.

57. Kroese FGM, deWaard R, Bos NA. B-1 cells and their reactivity with the murine intestinal microflora. *Semin Immunol* 1996;8:11–18.

58. Duchmann R, Kaiser I, Hermann E, et al. Tolerance exists towards resident intestinal flora but is broken in active inflammatory bowel disease (IBD). *Clin Exp Immunol* 1995;102:448–455.

59. Cebra JJ, Jiang H-Q, Sterzl J, et al. The role of mucosal microbiota in the development and maintenance of the mucosal immune system. In: Ogra PL, Mestecky J, Lamm ME, et al., eds. *Mucosal immunology,* 2nd ed. San Diego, CA: Academic Press, 1999:267–280.

60. Jackson S, Mestecky J, Moldoveanu Z, et al. Collection and processing of human mucosal secretions. In: Ogra PL, Mestecky J, Lamm ME, et al., eds. *Mucosal immunology,* 2nd ed. San Diego, CA: Academic Press, 1999:1567–1576.

61. Mestecky J, Moro I, Underdown BJ. Mucosal immunoglobulins. In: Ogra PL, Mestecky J, Lamm ME, et al., eds. *Mucosal Immunology,* 2nd ed. San Diego, CA: Academic Press, 1999:133–152.

62. Mattu TS, Pleass RJ, Willis AC, et al. The glycosylation pattern and structure of human serum IgA1, Fab and Fc regions and the role of *N*-glycosylation on Fc receptor interactions. *J Biol Chem* 1998;273:2260–2272.

63. Kilian M, Russell MW. Microbial evasion of IgA functions. In: Ogra PL, Mestecky J, Lamm ME, et al., eds. *Mucosal immunology,* 2nd ed. San Diego, CA: Academic Press, 1999:241–251.

64. Peppard JV, Russell MW. Phylogenetic development and comparative physiology of IgA. In: Ogra PL, Mestecky J, Lamm ME, et al., eds. *Mucosal immunology,* 2nd ed. San Diego, CA: Academic Press, 1999:163–179.

65. Mestecky J, Moro I. Joining (J) chain. In: Roitt IM, Delves PJ, eds. *Encyclopedia of immunology.* San Diego, CA: Academic Press, 1998; 1516–1518.

66. Brandtzaeg P. The role of J chain and secretory component in receptor-mediated glandular and hepatic transport of immunoglobulins in man. *Scand J Immunol* 1985;22:111–146.

67. Mostov K, Kaetzel C. Immunoglobulin transport and the polymeric immunoglobulin receptor. In: Ogra PL, Mestecky J, Lamm ME, et al., eds. *Mucosal immunology,* 2nd ed. San Diego, CA: Academic Press, 1999:181–211.

68. Sørensen V, Sundvold V, Michaelsen TE, et al. Polymerization of IgA and IgM: roles of Cys^{309}/Cys^{414} and the secretory tailpiece. *J Immunol* 1999;162:3448–3455.

69. Hendrickson BA, Rindisbacher L, Corthesy B, et al. Lack of association of secretory component with IgA in J chain–deficient mice. *J Immunol* 1996;157:750–754.

70. Vaerman JP, Langendries A, Giffroy D, et al. Lack of SC/pIgR-mediated epithelial transport of a human polymeric IgA devoid of J chain: *in vitro* and *in vivo* studies. *Immunology* 1998;95:90–96.

71. Russell MW, Kilian M, Lamm ME. Biological activities of IgA. In: Ogra PL, Mestecky J, Lamm ME, et al., eds. *Mucosal Immunology,* 2nd ed. San Diego, CA: Academic Press, 1999:225–240.

71a. Phalipon A, Corthesy B. Novel functions of the polymeric Ig receptor: well beyond transport of immunoglobulins. *Trends Immunol* 2003;24:55–58.

71b. Roos A, Bouwman LH, van Gijlswijk-Janssen DJ, et al. Human IgA activates the complement system via the mannan-binding lectin pathway. *J Immunol* 2001;167:2861–2868.

72. Quan CP, Berneman A, Pires R, et al. Natural polyreactive secretory immunoglobulin A autoantibodies as a possible barrier to infection in humans. *Infect Immun* 1997;65:3997–4004.

73. Crottet P, Corthesy B. Secretory component delays the conversion of secretory IgA into antigen-binding component F(ab')₂: a possible implication for mucosal defense. *J Immunol* 1998;161:5445–5453.

74. Russell MW, Sibley DA, Nikolova EB, et al. IgA antibody as a non-inflammatory regulator of immunity. *Biochem Soc Trans* 1997;25:466–470.

75. Rejnek JJ, Travnicek J, Kostka J, et al. Study of the effect of antibodies in the intestinal tract of germ-free baby pigs. *Folia Microbiol* 1968; 13:36–42.

76. Krachenbuhl J-P, Neutra MR. Monoclonal secretory IgA for protection of the intestinal mucosa against viral and bacterial pathogens. In: Ogra PL, Mestecky J, Lamm ME, et al., eds. *Handbook of mucosal immunology.* San Diego, CA: Academic Press, 1994:403–409.

77. Renegar KB, Small PA Jr. Passive immunization: systemic and mucosal. In: Ogra PL, Mestecky J, Lamm ME, et al., eds. *Mucosal immunology,* 2nd ed. San Diego, CA: Academic Press, 1999:729–738.

78. Mazanec M, Kaetzel CS, Lamm ME, et al. Intracellular neutralization of virus by immunoglobulin A antibodies. *Proc Natl Acad Sci U S A* 1992;89:6901–6905.

79. Russell MW, Sibley DA, Nikolova EB, et al. IgA antibody as a non-inflammatory regulator of immunity. *Biochem Soc Trans* 1997;25:466–470.

80. Kerr MA, Woof JM. Fcα receptors. In: Ogra PL, Mestecky J, Lamm ME, et al., eds. *Mucosal immunology,* 2nd ed. San Diego, CA: Academic Press, 1999:213–224.

81. Abu-Ghazaleh RI, Fujisawa T, Mestecky J, et al. IgA-induced eosinophil degranulation. *J Immunol* 1989;142:2393–2400.

82. Monteiro RC, Hostoffer RW, Cooper MD, et al. Definition of immunoglobulin A receptors on eosinophils and their enhanced expression in allergic individuals. *J Clin Invest* 1993;92:1681–1685.

83. Mestecky J, Russell MW. IgA subclasses. *Monogr Allergy* 1986;19: 277–301.

84. Burrows PD, Cooper MD. Ig A deficiency. *Adv Immunol* 1997;65:245–276.

85. Underdown BJ, Plotkin SA. The induction of mucosal protection by parenteral immunization. A challenge to the mucosal immunity paradigm. In: Ogra PL, Mestecky J, Lamm ME, et al., eds. *Mucosal immunology,* 2nd ed. San Diego, CA: Academic Press, 1999:729–738.

86. Mestecky J, Russell MW. Passive and active protection against disorders of the gut. *Vet Q* 1998;20:S83–S87.

87. Conley ME, Delacroix DL. Intravascular and mucosal immunoglobulin A: two separate but related systems of immune defense? *Ann Intern Med* 1987;106:892–899.

88. Mestecky J, Lue C, Russell MW. Selective transport of IgA: cellular and molecular aspects. *Gastroenterol Clin North Am* 1991;20:441–471.

89. Delacroix DL, Hodgson HJF, McPherson A, et al. Selective transport of polymeric immunoglobulin A in bile. Quantitative relationships of monomeric and polymeric immunoglobulin A, immunoglobulin M, and other proteins in serum, bile, and saliva. *J Clin Invest* 1982;70:230–241.

90. Jonard PP, Rambaud JC, Vaerman J-P, et al. Secretion of immunoglobulins and plasma proteins from the jejunal mucosa. Transport rate and origin of polymeric immunoglobulin A. *J Clin Invest* 1984;74:525–535.

91. Kubagawa H, Bertoli LF, Barton JC, et al. Analysis of paraprotein transport into the saliva by using anti-idiotype antibodies. *J Immunol* 1987;138:435–439.

92. Menge AC, Mestecky J. Surface expression of secretory component and HLA class II DR antigen on glandular epithelial cells from human endometrium and two endometrial adenocarcinoma cell lines. *J Clin Immunol* 1993;13:259–264.

93. Wira CR, Kaushic C, Richardson J. Role of sex hormones and cytokines in regulation of the mucosal immune system in the female reproductive tract. In: Ogra PL, Mestecky J, Lamm ME, et al., eds. *Mucosal immunology,* 2nd ed. San Diego, CA: Academic Press, 1999:1449–1461.

94. Morton HC, van Egmond M, van de Winkel JG. Structure and function of human IgA Fc receptors (FcαR). *Crit Rev Immunol* 1996;16:423–440.

95. Monteiro RC, Kubagawa H, Cooper MD. Cellular distribution, regulation, and biochemical nature of an Fcα receptor in humans. *J Exp Med* 1990;171:597–613.

96. Maliszewski CR, March CJ, Schoenborn MA, et al. Expression and cloning of a human Fc receptor for IgA. *J Exp Med* 1990;172:1665–1672.

97. van der Boog PJM, van Zandbergen G, deFijter JW, et al. FcαRI/CD89 circulates in human serum covalently linked to IgA in a polymeric state. *J Immunol* 2002;168:1252–1258.

98. Carayannopoulos L, Hexham JM, Capra JD. Localization of the binding site for the monocyte immunoglobulin (Ig) A-Fc receptor (CD89) to the domain boundary between Cα2 and Cα3 in human IgA1. *J Exp Med* 1996;183:1579–1586.

99. Shibuya A, Sakamoto N, Shimizu Y, et al. Fcα/μ receptor mediates endocytosis of IgM-coated microbes. *Nat Immunol* 2000;1:441–446.

100. McDonald KJ, Cameron AJM, Allen JM, et al. Expression of Fcα/μ receptor by human mesangial cells: a candidate receptor for immune complex deposition in IgA nephropathy. *Biochem Biophys Res Commun* 2002;290:438–442.

101. Moura IC, Centelles MN, Arcos-Fajardo M, et al. Identification of the transferrin receptor as a novel immunoglobulin (Ig) A1 receptor and its enhanced expression on mesangial cells in IgA nephropathy. *J Exp Med* 2001;194:417–425.

102. Stockert RJ. The asialoglycoprotein receptor: relationship between structure, function, and expression. *Physiol Rev* 1995;75:591–609.

103. Stockert RJ, Kressner MS, Collins JC, et al. IgA interaction with the asialoglycoprotein receptor. *Proc Natl Acad Sci U S A* 1982;79:6229–6231.

104. Tomana M, Kulhavy R, Mestecky J. Receptor-mediated binding and uptake of immunoglobulin A by human liver. *Gastroenterology* 1988;94:762–770.

105. Kitamura T, Garofalo RP, Kamijo A, et al. Human intestinal epithelial cells express a novel receptor for IgA. *J Immunol* 2000;164:5029–5034.

106. Novak J, Julian BA, Tomana M, et al. Progress in molecular and genetic studies of IgA nephropathy. *J Clin Immunol* 2001;21:310–327.

107. Pabst R. Is BALT a major component of the human lung immune system? *Immunol Today* 1992;13:119–122.

108. Sato A, Hayakawa H, Uchiyama H, et al. Cellular distribution of bronchus-associated lymphoid tissue in rheumatoid arthritis. *Am J Respir Crit Care Med* 1996;154:1903–1907.

109. Kuper CF, Koornstra PJ, Hameleers DM, et al. The role of nasopharyngeal lymphoid tissue. *Immunol Today* 1992;13:219–224.

110. Bienenstock J, McDermott M, Befus D, et al. A common mucosal immunologic system involving the bronchus, breast and bowel. *Adv Exp Med Biol* 1978;107:53–59.

111. Mestecky J, McGhee JR. Immunoglobulin A (IgA): Molecular and cellular interactions involved in IgA biosynthesis and immune response. *Adv Immunol* 1987;40:153–245.

112. Yoshida H, Honda K, Shinkura R, et al. IL-7 receptor α^+ CD3$^-$ cells in the embryonic intestine induces the organizing center of Peyer's patches. *Int Immunol* 1999;11:643–655.

113. DeTogni P, Goeilner J, Ruddle NH, et al. Abnormal development of peripheral lymphoid organs in mice deficient in lymphotoxin. *Science* 1994;264:703–707.

114. Alimzhanov MB, Kuprashi DV, Kosco-Vilbois MH, et al. Abnormal development of secondary lymphoid tissues in lymphotoxin β–deficient mice. *Proc Natl Acad Sci U S A* 1997;94:9302–9307.

115. Koni PA, Sacca R, Lawton P, et al. Distinct roles in lymphoid organogenesis for lymphotoxins α and β revealed in lymphotoxin β–deficient mice. *Immunity* 1997;6:491–500.

116. Futterer A, Mink K, Luz A, et al. The lymphotoxin β receptor controls organogenesis and affinity maturation in peripheral lymphoid tissues. *Immunity* 1998;9:59–70.

117. Shinkura R, Kitada K, Matsuda F, et al. Alymphoplasia is caused by a point mutation in the mouse gene encoding NF-κB–inducing kinase. *Nat Genet* 1999;22:74–77.

118. Yoshida H, Kawamoto H, Santee SM, et al. Expression of $\alpha4\beta7$ integrin defines a distinct pathway of lymphoid progenitors committed to T cells, fetal intestinal lymphotoxin producer, NK and dendritic cells. *J Immunol* 2001;167:2511–2521.

119. Griebel PJ, Hein WR. Expanding the role of Peyer's patches in B-cell ontogeny. *Immunol Today* 1996;17:30–39.

120. Bockman DE, Cooper MD. Pinocytosis by epithelium associated with lymphoid follicles in the bursa of Fabricius, appendix and Peyer's patches. An electron microscopic study. *Am J Anat* 1973;136:455–477.

121. Owen L, Jones AL. Epithelial cell specialization within human Peyer's patches: an ultrastructural study of intestinal lymphoid follicles. *Gastroenterology* 1974;66:189–203.

122. Farstad IN, Halstensen TS, Fausa O, et al. Heterogeneity of M-cell–associated B and T cells in human Peyer's patches. *Immunology* 1994;83:457–464.

123. Neutra MN, Kraehenbuhl J-P. Cellular and molecular basis for antigen transport across epithelial barriers. In: Ogra PL, Mestecky J, Lamm ME, et al., eds. *Mucosal immunology,* 2nd ed. San Diego, CA: Academic Press, 1999:101–114.

124. Allan C., Mendrick DL, Trier JS. Rat intestinal M cells contain acidic endosomal-lysosomal compartments and express class II major histocompatibility complex determinants. *Gastroenterology* 1993;104:698–708.

125. Kerneis S, Bogdanova A, Kraehenbuhl J-P, et al. Conversion by Peyer's patch lymphocytes of human enterocytes into M cells that transport bacteria. *Science* 1997;277:949–952.

126. Golovkina TV, Shlomchik M, Hannum L, et al. Organogenic role of B lymphocytes in mucosal immunity. *Science* 1999;286:1965–1968.

127. Jones BD, Ghori N, Falkow S. *Salmonella typhimurium* initiates murine infection by penetrating and destroying the specialized epithelial M cells of the Peyer's patches. *J Exp Med* 1994;180:15–23.

128. Wolf JL, Rubin DH, Finberg R, et al. Intestinal M cells: a pathway for entry of reovirus into the host. *Science* 1981;212:471–472.

129. Nibert ML, Furlong DB, Fields BN. Mechanisms of viral pathogenesis. Distinct forms of reoviruses and their roles during replication in cells and host. *J Clin Invest* 1991;88:727–734.

130. Teitelbaum R, Schubert W, Gunther L, et al. The M cell as a portal of entry to the lung for the bacterial pathogen *Mycobacterium tuberculosis*. *Immunity* 1999;10:641–650.

131. Sminia T, van der Ende MB. Macrophage subsets in the rat gut: an immunohistochemical and enzyme-histochemical study. *Acta Histochem* 1991;90:43–50.

132. Kelsall BL, Strober W. Distinct populations of dendritic cells are present in the subepithelial dome and T cell regions of the murine Peyer's patch. *J Exp Med* 1996;183:237–247.

133. Lebman DA, Griffin PM, Cebra JJ. Relationship between expression of IgA by Peyer's patch cells and functional IgA memory cells. *J Exp Med* 1987;166:1405–1418.

134. Butcher EC, Rouse RV, Coffman RL, et al. Surface phenotype of Peyer's patches germinal center cells: implications for the role of germinal centers in B-cell differentiation. *J Immunol* 1982;129:2698–2707.

135. George A, Cebra JJ. Responses of single germinal-center B cells in T-cell–dependent microculture. *Proc Natl Acad Sci U S A* 1991;88:11–15.

136. Weinstein PD, Cebra JJ. The preference for switching to IgA expression by Peyer's patch germinal center B cells is likely due to the intrinsic influence of their microenvironment. *J Immunol* 1991;147:4126–4135.

137. Kiyono H, McGhee JR, Wannemuehler MJ, et al. In vitro immune responses to a T cell–dependent antigen by cultures of disassociated murine Peyer's patch. *Proc Natl Acad Sci U S A* 1982;79:596–600.

138. London SD, Rubin DH, Cebra JJ. Gut mucosal immunization with reovirus serotype 1/L stimulates specific cytotoxic T-cell precursors as well as IgA memory cells in Peyer's patches. *J Exp Med* 1987;165:830–847.

139. London SD, Rubin DH. Functional role of mucosal cytotoxic lymphocytes. In: Ogra PL, Mestecky J, Lamm ME, et al., eds. *Mucosal immunology,* 2nd ed. San Diego, CA: Academic Press, 1999:643–653.

140. Bernstein JM, Gorfien J, Brandtzaeg P. The immunobiology of the tonsils and adenoids. In: Ogra PL, Mestecky J, Lamm ME, et al., eds. *Mucosal immunology,* 2nd ed. San Diego, CA: Academic Press, 1999:1339–1362.

141. Wu H-Y, Nikolova EB, Beagley KW, et al. Induction of antibody-secreting cells and T-helper and memory cells in murine nasal lymphoid tissue. *Immunology* 1996;88:493–500.

142. Wu H-Y, Nguyen HH, Russell MW. Nasal lymphoid tissue (NALT) as a mucosal immune inductive site. *Scand J Immunol* 1997;46:506–513.

143. Hiroi T, Iwatani K, Ijima H, et al. Nasal immune system: distinctive Th0 and Th1/Th2 type environments in murine nasal-associated lymphoid tissues and nasal passage, respectively. *Eur J Immunol* 1998;28:3346–3353.

144. Shimoda M, Nakamura T, Takahashi Y, et al. Isotype-specific selection of high affinity memory B cells in nasal-associated lymphoid tissue. *J Exp Med* 2001;194:1597–1607.

145. Langman JM, Rowland R. The number and distribution of lymphoid follicles in the human large intestine. *J Anat* 1986;194:189–194.

146. O'Leary AD, Swenney EC. Lympho-glandular complexes of the colon: structure and distribution. *Histology* 1986;10:267–283.

147. Mestecky J, Abram R, Ogra PL. Common mucosal immune system and strategies for the development of vaccines effective at the mucosal surfaces. In: Ogra PL, Mestecky J, Lamm M, et al., eds. *Handbook of mucosal immunology.* New York: Academic Press, 1994:357–372.

148. McGhee JR, Czerkinsky C, Mestecky J. Mucosal vaccines—an overview. In: Ogra PL, Mestecky J, Lamm ME, et al., eds. *Mucosal immunology,* 2nd ed. San Diego, CA: Academic Press, 1999:741–758.

149. Kiyono H, McGhee JR. Mucosal immunology: intraepithelial lymphocytes. *Advances in host defense mechanisms. Vol. 9: Mucosal immunology: intraepithelial lymphocytes.* New York: Raven Press, 1994.

150. McGhee JR, Mestecky J, Elson CO, et al. Regulation of IgA synthesis and immune response by T cells and interleukins. *J Clin Immunol* 1989;9:175–199.

151. Brandtzaeg P, Farstad IN. The human mucosal B-cell system. In: Ogra

PL, Mestecky J, Lamm ME, et al., eds. *Mucosal immunology,* 2nd ed. San Diego, Academic Press, CA: 1999:439–468.

152. Brandtzaeg P, Farstad IN, Johansen F-E, et al. The B-cell system of human mucosae and exocrine glands. *Immunol Rev* 1999;171:45–87.

153. James SP, Fiocchi C, Graeff AS, et al. Phenotypic analysis of lamina propria lymphocytes. Predominance of helper-inducer and cytolytic T-cell phenotypes and deficiency of suppressor-inducer phenotypes in Crohn's disease and control patients. *Gastroenterology* 1986;91:1483–1489.

154. Abreu-Martin, MT, Targan SR, Lamina propria lymphocytes: a unique population of mucosal lymphocytes. In: Kagnoff MF, Kiyono H, eds. *Essentials of mucosal immunology.* San Diego, CA: Academic Press, 1996:227–245.

155. Mayer L, Shlien R. Evidence for function of Ia molecules on gut epithelial cells in man. *J Exp Med* 1987;166:1471–1483.

156. Huang F-P, Platt N, Wykes M, et al. A discrete subpopulation of dendritic cells transports apoptotic intestinal epithelial cells to T cell areas of mesenteric lymph nodes. *J Exp Med* 2000;191:435–443.

157. Taguchi T, McGhee JR, Coffman RL, et al. Analysis of Th1 and Th2 cells in murine gut-associated tissues. Frequencies of CD4+ and CD8+ T cells that secrete IFN-γ and IL-5. *J Immunol* 1990;145:68–77.

158. James SP, Kiyono H. Gastrointestinal lamina propria T cells. In: Ogra PL, Mestecky J, Lamm ME, et al., eds. *Mucosal immunology,* 2nd ed. San Diego, CA: Academic Press, 1999:381–396.

159. Lefrancois L, Puddington L. Basic aspects of intraepithelial lymphocyte immunobiology. In: Ogra PL, Mestecky J, Lamm ME, et al., eds. *Mucosal immunology,* 2nd ed. San Diego, CA: Academic Press, 1999: 413–428.

160. Crowley-Nowick PA, Bell M, Edwards RP, et al. Normal uterine cervix: characterization of isolated lymphocyte phenotypes and immunoglobulin secretion. *Am J Reprod Immunol* 1995;34:241–247.

161. Crago SS, Kutteh WH, Moro I, et al. Distribution of IgA1-, IgA2-, and J chain–containing cells in human tissues. *J Immunol* 1984;132:16–18.

162. Kutteh WH, Koopman WJ, Conley ME, et al. Production of predominantly polymeric IgA by human peripheral blood lymphocytes stimulated *in vitro* with mitogens. *J Exp Med* 1980;152:1424–1429.

163. Moldoveanu Z, Egan ML, Mestecky J. Cellular origins of human polymeric and monomeric IgA: intracellular and secreted forms of IgA. *J Immunol* 1984;133:3156–3162.

164. Hajdu I, Moldoveanu Z, Cooper MD, et al. Ultrastructural studies of human lymphoid cells: μ and J chain expression as a function of B cell differentiation. *J Exp Med* 1983;158:1993–2006.

165. Kubagawa H, Burrows PD, Grossi CE, et al. Precursor B cells transformed by Epstein-Barr virus undergo sterile plasma-cell differentiation: J-chain expression without immunoglobulin. *Proc Natl Acad Sci U S A* 1988;85:875–879.

166. Weinberg AD, English M, Swain SL. Distinct regulation of lymphokine production is found in fresh versus *in vitro* primed murine helper T cells. *J Immunol* 1990;144:1800–1807.

167. Powers GD, Abbas AK, Miller RA. Frequencies of IL-2 and IL-4-secreting T cells in naïve and antigen-stimulated lymphocyte populations. *J Immunol* 1988;140:3352–3357.

168. Hsieh CS, Macatonia SE, Tripp CS, et al. Development of Th1 CD4+ T cells through IL-12 produced by *Listeria*-induced macrophages. *Science* 1993;260:547–549.

169. Trinchieri G. Interleukin-12: a proinflammatory cytokine with immunoregulatory functions that bridge innate resistance and antigen-specific adaptive immunity. *Annu Rev Immunol* 1995;13:251–276.

170. Chan SH, Perussia B, Gupta JW, et al. Induction of interferon gamma production by natural killer cell stimulatory factor: characterization of the responder cells and synergy with other inducers. *J Exp Med* 1991; 173:869–879.

171. Snapper CM, Paul WE. Interferon-gamma and B cell stimulatory factor–1 reciprocally regulate Ig isotype production. *Science* 1987; 236:944–947.

172. Yoshimoto T, Bendelac A, Watson C, et al. Role of NK1.1+ T cells in a Th2 response and in immunoglobulin E production. *Science* 1995;270:1845–1847.

173. Mosmann TR, Coffman RL. Th1 and Th2 cells: Different patterns of lymphokine secretion lead to different functional properties. *Annu Rev Immunol* 1989;7:145–173.

174. Coffman RL, Varkila K, Scott P, et al. Role of cytokines in the differentiation of CD4+ T-cell subsets *in vivo. Immunol Rev* 1991;123:189–207.

175. Coffman RL, Seymour BW, Lebman DA, et al. The role of helper T cell products in mouse B cell differentiation and isotype regulation. *Immunol Rev* 1988;102:5–28.

176. Esser C, Radbruch A. Immunoglobulin class switching: molecular and cellular analysis. *Annu Rev Immunol* 1990;8:717–735.

177. Finkelman FD, Holmes J, Katona IM, et al. Lymphokine control of *in vivo* immunoglobulin isotype selection. *Annu Rev Immunol* 1990;8: 303–333.

178. Kiyono H, Cooper MD, Kearney JF, et al. Isotype-specificity of helper T cell clones: Peyer's patch Th cells preferentially collaborate with mature IgA B cells for IgA responses. *J Exp Med* 1984;159:798–811.

179. VanCott JL, Staats HF, Pascual PW, et al. Regulation of mucosal and systemic antibody responses by T helper cell subsets, macrophages and derived cytokines following oral immunization with live recombinant *Salmonella. J Immunol* 1996;156:1504–1514.

180. Chen Y, Kuchroo VK, Inob J-I, et al. Regulatory T cell clones induced by oral tolerance: suppression of autoimmune encephalomyelitis. *Science* 1994;265:1237–1240.

181. Chai JG, Bartok I, Chandler P, et al. Anergic T cells act as suppressor cells *in vitro* and *in vivo. Eur J Immunol* 1999;29:686–692.

182. Vendetti S, Chai J-G, Dyson J, et al. Anergic T cells inhibit the antigen-presenting function of dendritic cells. *J Immunol* 2000;165:1175–1181.

183. Sundstedt A, Höidén I, Rosendahl A, et al. Immunoregulatory role of IL-10 during superantigen-induced hyporesponsiveness *in vivo. J Immunol* 1997;158:180–186.

184. Buer J, Lanoue A, Franzke A, et al. Interleukin 10 secretion and impaired effector function of major histocompatibility complex class II–restricted T cells anergized *in vivo. J Exp Med* 1998;187:177–183.

185. Groux H, Bigler M, de Vries JE, et al. Interleukin-10 induces a long-term antigen-specific anergic state in human CD4+ T cells. *J Exp Med* 1996;184:19–29.

186. Groux H, O'Garra A, Bigler M, et al. A CD4+ T-cell subset inhibits antigen-specific T-cell responses and prevents colitis. *Nature* 1997;389:737–742.

187. Maloy KJ, Powrie F. Regulatory T cells in the control of immune pathology. *Nat Immunol* 2001;2:816–822.

188. Shevach EM. Regulatory T cells in autoimmunity. *Annu Rev Immunol* 2000;18:423–449.

189. Roncarolo MG, Levings MK. The role of different subsets of T regulatory cells in controlling autoimmunity. *Curr Opin Immunol* 2000; 12:676–683.

190. Olivares-Villagomez D, Wang Y, Lafaille JJ. Regulatory CD4+ T cells expressing endogenous T cell receptor chains protect myelin basic protein–specific transgenic mice from spontaneous autoimmune encephalomyelitis. *J Exp Med* 1998;188:1883–1894.

191. Van de Keere F, Tonegawa S. CD4+ T cells prevent spontaneous experimental autoimmune encephalomyelitis in anti–myelin basic protein T cell receptor transgenic mice. *J Exp Med* 1998;188:1875–1882.

192. Read S, Malmstrom V, Powrie F. Cytotoxic T lymphocyte–associated antigen 4 plays an essential role in the function of CD25+ CD4+ regulatory cells that control intestinal inflammation. *J Exp Med* 2000;192: 295–302.

193. Mega J, Bruce MG, Beagley KW, et al. Regulation of mucosal responses by CD4+ T lymphocytes: effects of anti-L3T4 treatment on the gastrointestinal immune system. *Intern Immunol* 1991;3:793–805.

194. Hörnquist CE, Ekman L, Grdic KD, et al. Paradoxical IgA immunity in CD4-deficient mice. Lack of cholera toxin–specific protective immunity despite normal gut mucosal IgA differentiation. *J Immunol* 1995;155:2877–2887.

195. Beagley KW, Eldridge JH, Lee F, et al. Interleukins and IgA synthesis. Human and murine IL-6 induce high rate IgA secretion in IgA-committed B cells. *J Exp Med* 1989;169:2133–2148.

196. Muramatsu M, Kinoshita K, Fagarasan S, et al. Class switch recombination and hypermutation require activation-induced cytidine deaminase (AID), a potential RNA editing enzyme. *Cell* 2000;102:553–563.

197. Revy P, Muto T, Levy Y, et al. Activation induced cytidine deaminase (AID) deficiency causes the autosomal recessive form of the hyper-IgM syndrome (HIGM2). *Cell* 2000;102:565–575.

198. Fagarasan S, Dinoshita K, Muramatsu M, et al. *In situ* class switching and differentiation to IgA-producing cells in the gut lamina propria. *Nature* 2001;413:639–643.

199. Macpherson AJS, Lamarre A, McCoy K, et al. IgA production without

μ or δ chain expression in developing B cells. *Nat Immunol* 2001;
2:625–631.

200. Kawanishi H, Ozato K, Strober W. The proliferative response of cloned Peyer's patch switch T cells to syngeneic and allogenic stimuli. *J Immunol* 1985;134:3586–3591.
201. Fuleihan R, Ramesh N, Geha RS. Role of CD40–CD40-ligand interaction in Ig-isotype switching. *Curr Opin Immunol* 1993;5:963–967.
202. Banchereau J, Bazan F, Blanchard D, et al. The CD40 antigen and its ligand. *Annu Rev Immunol* 1994;12:881–922.
203. MacLennan IC. Germinal centers. *Annu Rev Immunol* 1994;12:117–139.
204. Spalding DM, Griffin JA. Different pathways of differentiation of pre–B cell lines are induced by dendritic cells and T cells from different lymphoid tissues. *Cell* 1986;44:507.
205. Mayer L, Kwan SP, Thompson C, et al. Evidence for a defect in "switch" T cell in patients with immunodeficiency and hyperimmunoglobulinemia M. *N Engl J Med* 1986;314:409–413.
206. Benson EB, Strober W. Regulation of IgA secretion by T cell clones derived from the human gastrointestinal tract. *J Immunol* 1988;140:1874–1882.
207. Jung S, Rajewsky K, Radbruch A. Shutdown of class switch recombinant by deletion of a switch region control element. *Science* 1993; 259:984–987.
208. Xu L, Groham B, Li SC, et al. Replacement of germ-line E promoter by gene targeting alters control of immunoglobulin heavy chain class switching. *Proc Natl Acad Sci U S A* 1993;90:3705–3709.
209. Bottaro A, Lansford R, Xu L, et al. S region transcription per se promotes basal IgE class switch recombination but additional factors regulate the efficiency of the process. *EMBO J* 1994;13:665–674.
210. Harriman GR, Bradley A, Das S, et al. IgA class switch in Iα exon–deficient mice. Role of germline transcription in class switch recombination. *J Clin Invest* 1996;97:477–485.
211. Coffman RL, Lebman DA, Schrader B. Transforming growth factor β specifically enhances IgA production by lipopolysaccharide-stimulated murine B lymphocytes. *J Exp Med* 1989;170:1039–1044.
212. Lebman DA, Nomura DY, Coffman RL, et al. Molecular characterization of germ-line immunoglobulin A transcripts produced during transforming growth factor type β–induced isotype switching. *Proc Natl Acad Sci U S A* 1990;87:3962–3966.
213. Lebman DA, Lee FD, Coffman RL. Mechanism for transforming growth factor β and IL-2 enhancement of IgA expression in lipopolysaccharide-stimulated B cell cultures. *J Immunol* 1990;144:952–959.
214. Islam KB, Nilsson L, Sideras P, et al. TGF-β1 induces germ-line transcripts of both IgA subclasses in human B lymphocytes. *Int Immunol* 1991;3:1099–1106.
215. Nilsson L, Islam KB, Olafsson O, et al. Structure of TGF-β1–induced human immunoglobulin Cα1 and Cα2 germ-line transcripts. *Int Immunol* 1991;3:1107–1115.
216. Stavnezer J. Regulation of antibody production and class switching by TGF-β. *J Immunol* 1995;155:1647–1651.
217. Sonoda E, Matsumoto R, Hitoshi Y, et al. Transforming growth factor β induces IgA production and acts additively with interleukin 5 for IgA production. *J Exp Med* 1989;170:1415–1420.
218. DeFrance T, Vanbervliet B, Briere F, et al. Interleukin 10 and transforming growth factor beta cooperate to induce anti-CD40–activated naïve human B cells to secrete immunoglobulin A. *J Exp Med* 1992;175:671–682.
219. Rousset F, Garcia E, Banchereau J. Cytokine-induced proliferation and immunoglobulin production of human B lymphocytes triggered through their CD40 antigen. *J Exp Med* 1991;173:705–710.
220. McIntyre TM, Kehry MR, Snapper CM. Novel *in vitro* model for high-rate IgA class switching. *J Immunol* 1995;154:3156–3161.
221. van Ginkel FW, Wahl SM, Kearney JF, et al. Partial IgA-deficiency with increased Th2-type cytokines in TGF-β1 knockout mice. *J Immunol* 1999;163:1951–1957.
222. Cazac BB, Roes J. TGF-β receptor controls B cell responsiveness and induction of IgA *in vivo*. *Immunity* 2000;13:443–451.
223. Gajewski TF, Fitch FW. Anti-proliferative effect of IFN-γ in immune regulation. I. IFN-γ inhibits the proliferation of Th2 but not Th1 murine helper T lymphocyte clones. *J Immunol* 1988;140:4245–4252.
224. Butcher E., Williams M, Youngman K, et al. Lymphocyte trafficking and regional immunity. *Adv Immunol* 1999;72:209–253.

225. Sallusto F, Lanzavecchia A. Understanding dendritic cell and T-lymphocyte traffic through the analysis of chemokine receptor expression. *Immunol Rev* 2000;177:134–140.
226. Campbell DJ, Kim CH, Butcher EC. Separable effector T cell populations specialized for B cell help or tissue inflammation. *Nat Immunol* 2001;2:8769–8781.
227. Jones HP, Hodge LM, Fujihashi K, et al. The pulmonary environment promotes Th2 cell responses after nasal-pulmonary immunization with antigen alone, but Th 1 responses are induced during instances of intense immune stimulation. *J Immunol* 2001;167:4518–4526.
228. Marinaro M, Staats HF, Hiroi T, et al. Mucosal adjuvant effect of cholera toxin in mice results from induction of T helper 2 (Th2) cells and IL-4. *J Immunol* 1995;155:4621–4629.
229. Snider DP, Marshall JS, Perdue MH, et al. Production of IgE antibody and allergic sensitization of intestinal and peripheral tissues after oral immunization with protein Ag and cholera toxin. *J Immunol* 1994;153:647–657.
230. Walker RI, Clements JD. Use of heat-labile toxin of enterotoxigenic *Escherichia coli* to facilitate mucosal immunization. *Vaccine Res* 1993; 2:1.
231. Spangler BD. Structure and function of cholera toxin and related *Escherichia coli* heat-labile enterotoxin. *Microbiol Rev* 1992;56:622–647.
232. Takahashi I, Marinaro M, Kiyono H, et al. Mechanisms for mucosal immunogenicity and adjuvant of *Escherichia coli* labile enterotoxin. *J Infect Dis* 1996;173:627–635.
233. Kiyono H, Mosteller-Barnum LM, Pitts AM, et al. Isotype-specific immunoregulation: IgA-binding factors produced by Fcα receptor+ T cell hybridomas regulate IgA responses. *J Exp Med* 1985;161:731–747.
234. Coffman RL, Shrader B, Carty J, et al. A mouse T cell product that preferentially enhances IgA production. I. Biologic characterization. *J Immunol* 1987;139:3685–3690.
235. Harriman GR, Kunimoto DY, Elliot JF, et al. The role of IL-5 in IgA B cell differentiation. *J Immunol* 1988;140:3033–3039.
236. Beagley KW, Eldridge JH, Kiyono H, et al. Recombinant murine IL-5 induces high rate IgA synthesis in cycling IgA-positive Peyer's patch B cells. *J Immunol* 1988;141:2035–2042.
237. Murray PD, McKenzie DT, Swain SL, et al. Interleukin 5 and interleukin 4 produced by Peyer's patch T cells selectively enhance immunoglobulin A expression. *J Immunol* 1987;139:2669–2674.
238. Lebman DA, Coffman RL. The effects of IL-4 and IL-5 on the IgA response by murine Peyer's patch B cell subpopulations. *J Immunol* 1988;141:2050–2056.
239. Kroese FG, Butcher EC, Stall AM, et al. Many of the IgA producing plasma cells in murine gut are derived from self-replenishing precursors in the peritoneal cavity. *Int Immunol* 1989;1:75–84.
240. Ramsay AJ, Husband AJ, Ramshaw IA, et al. The role of interleukin-6 in mucosal IgA antibody responses *in vivo*. *Science* 1994;264:561–563.
241. Bromander AK, Ekman L, Kopf M, et al. IL-6–deficient mice exhibit normal mucosal IgA responses to local immunizations and *Helicobacter felis* infection. *J Immunol* 1996;156:4290–4297.
242. Fujihashi K, McGhee JR, Lue C, et al. Human appendix B cells naturally express receptors for and respond to interleukin 6 with selective IgA1 and IgA2 synthesis. *J Clin Invest* 1991;88:248–252.
243. Briere F, Bridon JM, Chevet D, et al. Interleukin 10 induces B lymphocytes from IgA-deficient patients to secrete IgA. *J Clin Invest* 1994;94:97–104.
244. Nonoyama S, Farrington M, Ishida H, et al. Activated B cells from patients with common variable immunodeficiency proliferate and synthesize immunoglobulin. *J Clin Invest* 1993;92:1282–1287.
245. Morokata T, Kato T, Igarashi O, et al. Mechanism of enhanced antigen presentation by B cells activated with anti-μ plus interferon-γ: role of B7-2 in the activation of naïve and memory CD4$^+$ T cells. *Eur J Immunol* 1995;25:1992–1998.
246. Kuchroo VK, Das MP, Brown JA, et al. B7-1 and B7-2 costimulatory molecules activated differentially the Th1/Th2 developmental pathways: application to autoimmune disease therapy. *Cell* 1995;80:707–718.
247. Kägi D, Ledermann B, Bürki K, et al. Molecular mechanisms of lymphocyte-mediated cytotoxicity and their role in immunological protection and pathogenesis *in vivo*. *Annu Rev Immunol* 1996;14:207–232.

248. Ernst PB, Befus AD, Bienenstock J. Leukocytes in the intestinal epithelium: an unusual immunologic compartment. *Immunol Today* 1985;6:50–56.

249. Lefrancois L, Goodman T. *In vivo* modulation of cytolytic activity and Thy-1 expression in TCR-γδ+ intraepithelial lymphocytes. *Science* 1989;243:1716–1780.

250. Guy-Grand D, Malassis-Seris M, Briottet C, et al. Cytotoxic differentiation of mouse gut thymodependent and independent intraepithelial T lymphocytes is induced locally. Correlation between functional assays, presence of perforin and granzyme transcripts and cytoplasmic granules. *J Exp Med* 1991;173:1549–1552.

251. Viney JL, Kilshaw PL, MacDonald TT. Cytotoxic αβ+ and γδ+ T cells in murine intestinal epithelium. *Eur J Immunol* 1990;20:1623–1626.

252. Kägi D, Ledermann B, Bürki K, et al. Cytotoxicity mediated by T cells and natural killer cells is greatly impaired in perforin-deficient mice. *Nature* 1994;369:31–37.

253. Walsh CM, Matloubian M, Liu C-C, et al. Immune functions in mice lacking the perforin gene. *Proc Natl Acad Sci U S A* 1994;91:10854–10858.

254. Tartaglia LA, Ayres TM, Wong GH, et al. A novel domain within the 55 kd TNF receptor signals cell death. *Cell* 1993;74:845–853.

255. Morin MJ, Warner A, Fields BN. A pathway for entry of reoviruses into the host through M cells of the respiratory tract. *J Exp Med* 1994; 180:1523–1527.

256. Offit PA, Cunningham SL, Dudzik KI. Memory and distribution of virus-specific cytotoxic T lymphocytes (CTLs) and CTL precursors after rotavirus infection. *J Virol* 1991;65:1318–1324.

257. Issekutz TB. The response of gut-associated T lymphocytes to intestinal viral immunization. *J Immunol* 1984;133:2955–2960.

258. Offit PA, Dudzik KI. Rotavirus-specific cytotoxic T lymphocytes appear at the intestinal mucosal surface after rotavirus infection. *J Virol* 1989;63:3507–3512.

259. George A, Kost SI, Witzleben CL, et al. Reovirus-induced liver disease in severe combined immunodeficient (SCID) mice. A model for the study of viral infection, pathogenesis, and clearance. *J Exp Med* 1990; 171:929–934.

260. Cuff CF, Cebra CK, Rubin DH, et al. Developmental relationship between cytotoxic αβ T cell receptor–positive intraepithelial lymphocytes and Peyer's patch lymphocytes. *Eur J Immunol* 1993;23:1333–1339.

261. Offit PA, Dudzik KI. Rotavirus-specific cytotoxic T lymphocytes passively protect against gastroenteritis in suckling mice. *J Virol* 1990;64:6325–6328.

262. Franco MA, Tin C, Rott LS, et al. Evidence for CD8+ T cell immunity to murine rotavirus in the absence of perforin, fas, and gamma interferon. *J Virol* 1997;71:479–486.

263. Burns JW, Siadat-Pajouh M, Krishnaney AA, et al. Protective effect of rotavirus VP6–specific IgA monoclonal antibodies that lack neutralizing activity. *Science* 1996;272:104–107.

264. Allan W, Tabi Z, Cleary A, et al. Cellular events in the lymph node and lung of mice with influenza. Consequences of depleting CD4+ T cell. *J Immunol* 1990;144:3980–3986.

265. Eichelberger M, Allan W, Zijlstra M, et al. Clearance of influenza virus respiratory infection in mice lacking class I major histocompatibility complex–restricted CD8+ T cells. *J Exp Med* 1991;174:875–880.

266. Nguyen HH, van Ginkel FW, Vu HL, et al. Gamma interferon is not required for mucosal cytotoxic T-lymphocyte responses or heterosubtypic immunity to influenza A virus infection in mice. *J Virol* 2000;74:5495–5501.

267. Nguyen HH, van Ginkel FW, Vu HL, et al. Heterosubtypic immunity to influenza A virus infection requires B cells, but not CD8+ cytotoxic T lymphocytes. *J Infect Dis* 2001;183:368–376.

268. Muñoz JL, McCarthy CA, Clark ME, et al. Respiratory syncytial virus infection in C57BL/6 mice: clearance of virus from the lungs with virus-specific cytotoxic T cells. *J Virol* 1991;65:4494–4497.

269. Nicholas JA, Rubino KL, Levely ME, et al. Cytotoxic T cell activity against the 22-kDa protein of human respiratory syncytial virus (RSV) is associated with a significant reduction in pulmonary RSV replication. *Virology* 1991;182:664–672.

270. Graham BS, Bunton LA, Wright PF, et al. Role of T lymphocyte subsets in the pathogenesis of primary infection and rechallenge with respiratory syncytial virus in mice. *J Clin Invest* 1991;88:1026–1033.

271. Fujihashi K, Taguchi T, Aicher WK, et al. Immunoregulatory functions for murine intraepithelial lymphocytes: γ/δ T cell receptor-positive (TCR+) T cells abrogate oral tolerance, while α/β TCR+ T cells provide B cell help. *J Exp Med* 1992;175:695–707.

272. Mosley RL, Styre D, Klein JR. CD4+ CD8+ murine intestinal intraepithelial lymphocytes. *Int Immunol* 1990;2:361–365.

273. Taguchi T, Aicher WK, Fujihashi K, et al. Novel function for intestinal intraepithelial lymphocytes. Murine CD3+, γ/δ TCR+ T cells produce IFN-γ and IL-5. *J Immunol* 1991;147:3736–3744.

274. Bonneville M, Janeway CA, Ito K, et al. Intestinal intraepithelial lymphocytes are a distinct set of γδ T cells. *Nature* 1988;336:479–481.

275. Goodman T, Lefrancois L. Expression of the γ-δ T-cell receptor on intestinal CD8+ intraepithelial lymphocytes. *Nature* 1988;333:855–858.

276. Rocha B, Vassalli P, Guy-Grand D. The extrathymic T-cell development pathway. *Immunol Today* 1992;13:449–454.

277. Bandeira A, Itohara S, Bonneville M, et al. Extrathymic origin of intestinal intraepithelial lymphocytes bearing T-cell antigen receptor γδ. *Proc Natl Acad Sci U S A* 1991;88:43–47.

278. Lefrancois L, LeCorre R, Mayo J, et al. Extrathymic selection of TCR γδ+ T cells by class II major histocompatibility complex molecules. *Cell* 1990;63:333–340.

279. Mosley RL, Styre D, Klein JR. Differentiation and functional maturation of bone marrow–derived intestinal epithelial T cells expressing membrane T cell receptor in athymic radiation chimeras. *J Immunol* 1990;145:1369–1375.

280. Carding SR, Kyes S, Jenkinson EJ, et al. Developmentally regulated fetal thymic and extrathymic T-cell receptor γδ gene expression. *Genes Dev* 1990;4:1304–1315.

281. Lundqvist C, Baranov V, Hammarstrom S, et al. Intra-epithelial lymphocytes. Evidence for regional specialization and extrathymic T cell maturation in the human gut epithelium. *Int Immunol* 1995;7:1473–1487.

282. Lynch S, Kelleher D, McManus R, et al. RAG1 and RAG2 expression in human intestinal epithelium: evidence of extrathymic T cell differentiation. *Eur J Immunol* 1995;25:1143–1147.

283. Kanamori Y, Ishimaru K, Nanno M, et al. Identification of novel lymphoid tissues in murine intestinal mucosa where clusters of c-kit+ IL-7R+ Thy1+ lympho-hemopoietic progenitors develop. *J Exp Med* 1996;184:1449–1459.

284. Saito H, Kanamori Y, Takemori T, et al. Generation of intestinal T cells from progenitors residing in gut cryptopatches. *Science* 1998;280:275–278.

285. Chvatchko Y, MacDonald HR. CD8+ T cell response to Mls-1a determinants involves major histocompatibility complex class II molecules. *J Exp Med* 1991;173:779–782.

286. Correa I, Bix M, Liao NS, et al. Most γδ T cells develop normally in β2-microglobulin–deficient mice. *Proc Natl Acad Sci U S A* 1992;89:653–657.

287. Mayer L, Shlien R. Evidence for function of Ia molecules on gut epithelial cells in man. *J Exp Med* 1987;166:1471–1483.

288. Bleicher PA, Balk SP, Hagen SJ, et al. Expression of murine CD1 on gastrointestinal epithelium. *Science* 1990;250:679–682.

289. Hershberg R, Eghtesady P, Sydora B, et al. Expression of the thymus leukemia antigen in mouse intestinal epithelium. *Proc Natl Acad Sci U S A* 1990;87:9727–9731.

290. Balk SP, Ebert EC, Blumenthal RL, et al. Oligoclonal expansion and CD1 recognition by human intestinal intraepithelial lymphocytes. *Science* 1991;253:1411–1415.

291. Fujihashi K, Kawabata S, Hiroi T, et al. Interleukin 2 (IL-2) and interleukin 7 (IL-7) reciprocally induce IL-7 and IL-2 receptors on γδ T-cell receptor–positive intraepithelial lymphocytes. *Proc Natl Acad Sci U S A* 1996;93:3613–3618.

292. Noguchi M, Nakamura Y, Russell SM, et al. Interleukin-2 receptor γ chain: a functional component of the interleukin-7 receptor. *Science* 1993;262:1877–1880.

293. Cao X, Shores EW, Hu-Li J, et al. Defective lymphoid development in mice lacking expression of the common cytokine receptor γ chain. *Immunity* 1995;2:223–238.

294. He YW, Malek TR. Interleukin-7 receptor α is essential for the development of γδ+ T cells, but not natural killer cells. *J Exp Med* 1996; 184:289–293.

295. Maki K, Sunaga S, Komagata Y, et al. Interleukin 7 receptor–deficient mice lack γδ T cells. *Proc Natl Acad Sci U S A* 1996;93:7172–7177.

296. Puddington L, Olson S, Lefrancois L. Interactions between stem cell factor and c-Kit are required for intestinal immune system homeostasis. *Immunity* 1994;1:733–739.

297. Inagaki-Ohara K, Nishimura H, Mitani A, et al. Interleukin-15 preferentially promotes the growth of intestinal intraepithelial lymphocytes bearing $\gamma\delta$ T cell receptor in mice. *Eur J Immunol* 1997;27:2885–2891.

298. Kim JK, Takahashi I, Kai Y, et al. Influence of enterotoxin on mucosal intranet: selective inhibition of extrathymic T cell development in intestinal intraepithelial lymphocytes by oral exposure to heat-labile toxin. *Eur J Immunol* 2001;31:2960–2969.

299. Lodolce JP, Boone DL, Chai S, et al. IL-15 receptor maintains lymphoid homeostasis by supporting lymphocyte homing and proliferation. *Immunity* 1998;9:669–676.

300. Boismenu R, Havran WL. Modulation of epithelial cell growth by intraepithelial $\gamma\delta$ T cells. *Science* 1994;266:1253–1255.

301. Komano H, Fujiura Y, Kawaguchi M, et al. Homeostatic regulation of intestinal epithelia by intraepithelial $\gamma\delta$ T cells. *Proc Natl Acad Sci U S A* 1995;92:6147–6151.

302. Beagley KW, Fujihashi K, Lagoo AS, et al. Differences in intraepithelial lymphocyte T cell subsets isolated from murine small versus large intestine. *J Immunol* 1995;154:5611–5619.

303. Barrett TA, Gajewski TF, Danielpour D, et al. Differential function of intestinal intraepithelial lymphocyte subsets. *J Immunol* 1992;149:1124–1130.

304. Fujihashi K, Yamamoto M, McGhee JR, et al. Function of $\alpha\beta$ TCR$^+$ intestinal intraepithelial lymphocytes: Th1- and Th2-type cytokine production by CD4$^+$CD8$^-$ and CD4$^+$CD8$^+$ T cells for helper activity. *Int Immunol* 1993;5:1473–1481.

305. Boismenu R, Feng L, Xia YY, et al. Chemokine expression by intraepithelial $\gamma\delta$ T cells. Implications for the recruitment of inflammatory cells to damaged epithelia. *J Immunol* 1996;157:985–992.

306. Aranda R, Sydora BC, Kronenberg M. Intraepithelial lymphocytes: function. In: Ogra PL, Mestecky J, Lamm ME, et al., eds. *Mucosal immunology,* 2nd ed. San Diego, CA: Academic Press, 1999:429–437

307. Craig SW, Cebra JJ. Peyer's patches: an enriched source of precursors for IgA-producing immunocytes in the rabbit. *J Exp Med* 1971;134:188–200.

308. McDermott MR, Bienenstock J. Evidence for a common mucosal immunologic system. I. Migration of B immunoblasts into intestinal, respiratory, and genital tissues. *J Immunol* 1979;122:1892–1898.

309. Montgomery PC, Connelly KM, Cohn J, et al. Remote-site stimulation of secretory IgA antibodies following bronchial and gastric stimulation. *Adv Exp Med Biol* 1978;107:113–122.

310. Michalek SM, McGhee JR, Mestecky J, et al. Ingestion of *Streptococcus mutans* induces IgA and caries immunity. *Science* 1976;192:1238–1240.

311. Mestecky J, McGhee JR, Arnold RR, et al. Selective induction of an immune response in human external secretions by ingestion of bacterial antigens. *J Clin Invest* 1978;61:731–737.

312. Butcher EC. Lymphocyte homing and intestinal immunity. In: Ogra PL, Mestecky J, Lamm ME, et al., eds. *Mucosal immunology,* 2nd ed. San Diego, CA: Academic Press, 1999:507–522.

313. Zabel BA, Agace WW, Campbell JJ, et al. Human G protein–coupled receptor GPR-9-6/CC chemokine receptor 9 is selectively expressed on intestinal homing T lymphocytes, mucosal lymphocytes, and thymocytes and is required for thymus-expressed chemokine-mediated chemotaxis. *J Exp Med* 1999;190:1241–1255.

314. Farstad IN, Halstensen TS, Kvale D, et al. Topographic distribution of homing receptors on B and T cells in human gut-associated lymphoid tissue: relation of L-selectin and integrin alpha 4 beta 7 to naïve and memory phenotypes. *Am J Pathol* 1997;150:187–199.

315. Quiding M, Nordstrom I, Kilander A, et al. Intestinal immune responses in humans. Oral cholera vaccination induces strong intestinal antibody responses and interferon-gamma production and evokes local immunological memory. *J Clin Invest* 1991;88:143–148.

316. Kantele A, Kantele JM, Savilahti E, et al. Homing potentials of circulating lymphocytes in humans depend on the site of activation: oral, but not parenteral, typhoid vaccination induces circulating antibody-secreting cells that all bear homing receptors directing them to the gut. *J Immunol* 1997;158:574–579.

317. Quiding-Jarbrink M, Lakew M, Nordstrom I, et al. Human circulating specific antibody-forming cells after systemic and mucosal immuniza-

318. Kantele A, Hakkinen M, Moldoveanu Z, et al. Differences in immune responses induced by oral and rectal immunizations with *Salmonella typhi* Ty21a: evidence for compartmentalization within the common mucosal immune system in humans. *Infect Immun* 1998;66:5630–5635.

319. Bowman EP, Kukin NA, Youngman KR, et al. The intestinal chemokine thymus-expressed chemokine (CCL25) attracts IgA antibody-secreting cells. *J Exp Med* 2002;195:269–275.

320. Quiding-Jabrink M, Nordstrom I, Granstrom G, et al. Differential expression of tissue-specific adhesion molecules on human circulating antibody-forming cells after systemic, enteric, and nasal immunizations. A molecular basis for the compartmentalization of effector B cell responses. *J Clin Invest* 1997;99:1281–1286.

321. Kantele A, Zivny J, Häkkinen M, et al. Differential homing commitments of antigen-specific T cells after oral or parenteral immunization in humans. *J Immunol* 1999;162:5173–5177.

322. Csencsits KL, Jutila MA, Pascual DW. Nasal-associated lymphoid tissue: phenotypic and functional evidence for the primary role of peripheral node addressin in naïve lymphocyte adhesion to high endothelial venules in a mucosal site. *J Immunol* 1999;16:1382–1389.

323. Wolber FM, Curtis JL, Milik AM, et al. Lymphocyte recruitment and the kinetics of adhesion receptor expression during the pulmonary immune response to particulate antigen. *Am J Pathol* 1997;151:1715–1727.

324. Czerkinsky C, Anjuere F, McGhee JR, et al. Mucosal immunity and tolerance: relevance to vaccine development. *Immunol Rev* 1999;170:197–222.

325. McGhee JR, Lamm ME, Strober W. Mucosal immune responses. An overview. In: Ogra PL, Mestecky J, Lamm ME, et al., eds. *Mucosal immunology,* 2nd ed. San Diego, CA: Academic Press, 1999:485–506.

326. Kiyono H, Ogra PL, McGhee JR, eds. *Mucosal vaccines.* San Diego, CA: Academic Press, 1996.

327. Besredka A. *Local immunization.* Baltimore: Williams & Wilkins, 1927.

328. Russell MW, Mestecky J. Humoral immune responses to microbial infections in the genital tract. *Microbes Infect* 2002;4:667–677.

329. Holmgren J, Czerkinsky C, Lycke N, et al. Mucosal immunity: implications for vaccine development. *Immunobiology* 1992;184:157–179.

330. Curtiss R, III, Kelley SM, Hassan JO. Live oral avirulent *Salmonella* vaccines. *Vet Microbiol* 1993;37:397–405.

331. Chatfield S, Roberts M, Londono P, et al. The development of oral vaccines based on live attenuated *Salmonella* strains. *FEMS Immunol Med Microbiol* 1993;7:1–7.

332. Murphy BR. Mucosal immunity to viruses. In: Ogra PL, Mestecky J, Lamm ME, et al., eds. *Mucosal immunology,* 2nd ed. San Diego, CA: Academic Press, 1999:695–707.

333. Brown TA, Murphy BR, Radl J, et al. Subclass distribution and molecular form of immunoglobulin A hemagglutinin antibodies in sera and nasal secretions after experimental secondary infection with influenza A virus in humans. *J Clin Microbiol* 1985;22:259–264.

334. Moldoveanu Z, Clements ML, Prince SJ, et al. Human immune responses to influenza virus vaccine administered by systemic or mucosal routes. *Vaccine* 1995;13:1006–1012.

335. Sjölander S, Drane D, Davis R, et al. Intranasal immunization with influenza–ISCOM induces strong mucosal as well as systemic antibody and cytotoxic T-lymphocyte responses. *Vaccine* 2001;19:4072–4080.

336. Graham BS, Bunton LA, Wright PF, et al. Role of T lymphocyte subsets in the pathogenesis of primary infection and rechallenge with respiratory syncytial virus in mice. *J Clin Invest* 1991;88:1026–1033.

337. Roberts M, Bacon A, Rappuoli R, et al. A mutant pertussis toxin molecule that lacks ADP-ribosyltransferase activity, PT-9K/129G, is an effective mucosal adjuvant for intranasally delivered proteins. *Infect Immun* 1995;63:2100–2108.

338. Mowat AM, Weiner HL. Oral tolerance. In: Ogra PL, Mestecky J, Lamm ME, et al., eds. *Mucosal immunology,* 2nd ed. San Diego, CA: Academic Press, 1999:587–618.

339. Sun JB, Rask C, Olsson T, et al. Treatment of experimental autoimmune encephalomyelitis by feeding myelin basic protein conjugated to cholera toxin B subunit. *Proc Natl Acad Sci U S A* 1996;93:7196–7201.

340. Ogra PL. Effect of tonsillectomy and adenoidectomy on nasopharyngeal antibody response to polio virus. *N Engl J Med* 1971;284:59–64.

341. Quiding-Järbrink M, Granstrom G, Nordstrom I, et al. Induction of

compartmentalized B-cell responses in human tonsils. *Infect Immun* 1995;63:853–857.

342. Hedges SR, Mayo MS, Mestecky J, et al. Limited local and systemic antibody responses to *Neisseria gonorrhoeae* during uncomplicated genital infections. *Infect Immun* 1999;67:3937–3946.

343. Johansson E-L, Rask C, Fredriksson M, et al. Antibodies and antibody-secreting cells in the female genital tract after vaginal or intranasal immunization with cholera toxin B subunit or conjugates. *Infect Immun* 1998;66:514–520.

344. Kozlowski PA, Cu-Uvin S, Neutra MR, et al. Comparison of the oral, rectal, and vaginal immunization routes for induction of antibodies in rectal and genital tract secretions. *Infect Immun* 1997;65:1387–1394.

345. Dorrell L, Hessell AJ, Wang M, et al. Absence of specific mucosal antibody responses in HIV-exposed uninfected sex workers from the Gambia. *AIDS* 2000;14:1117–1122.

346. Skurnick JH, Palumbo P, DeVico A, et al. Correlates of non-transmission in US women at high risk of human immunodeficiency virus type 1 infection through sexual exposure. *J Infect Dis* 2002; 185:428–438.

347. Ashley RL, Corey L, Dalessio J, et al. Protein-specific cervical antibody responses to primary genital herpes simplex virus type 2 infections. *J Infect Dis* 1994;170:20–26.

348. Parr MB, Parr EL. Female genital tract immunity in animal models. In: Ogra PL, Mestecky J, Lamm ME, et al., eds. *Mucosal immunology,* 2nd ed. San Diego, CA: Academic Press, 1999:1395–1409.

349. Wassén L, Schön K, Holmgren J, et al. Local intravaginal vaccination of the female genital tract. *Scand J Immunol* 1996;44:408–414.

350. Wu H-Y, Russell MW. Induction of mucosal immunity by intranasal application of a streptococcal surface protein antigen with the cholera toxin B subunit. *Infect Immun* 1993;61:314–322.

351. Gallichan WS, Rosenthal KL. Specific secretory immune responses in the female genital tract following intranasal immunization with a recombinant adenovirus expressing glycoprotein B of herpes simplex virus. *Vaccine* 1995;13:1589–1595.

352. Russell MW, Moldoveanu Z, White PL, et al. Salivary, nasal, genital, and systemic antibody responses in monkeys immunized intranasally with a bacterial protein antigen and the cholera toxin B subunit. *Infect Immun* 1996;64:1272–1283.

353. Bergquist C, Johansson EL, Lagerfård T, et al. Intranasal vaccination of humans with recombinant cholera toxin B subunit induces systemic and local antibody responses in the upper respiratory tract and the vagina. *Infect Immun* 1997;65:2676–2684.

354. Sullivan DA. Ocular mucosal immunity. In: Ogra PL, Mestecky J, Lamm ME, et al., eds. *Mucosal immunology,* 2nd ed. San Diego, CA: Academic Press, 1999:1241–1281.

355. Spangler BD. Structure and function of cholera toxin and the related *Escherichia coli* heat-labile enterotoxin. *Microbiol Rev* 1992;56:622–647.

356. Yamamoto S, Takeda Y, Yamamoto M, et al. Mutants in the ADP-ribosyltransferase cleft of cholera toxin lack diarrheagenicity but retain adjuvanticity. *J Exp Med* 1997;185:1203–1210.

357. Yamamoto S, Kiyono H, Yamamoto M, et al. A nontoxic mutant of cholera toxin elicits Th2-type responses for enhanced mucosal immunity. *Proc Natl Acad Sci U S A* 1997;94:5267–5272.

358. Rappuoli R, Pizza M, Douce G, et al. Structure and mucosal adjuvanticity of cholera and *Escherichia coli* heat-labile enterotoxins. *Immunol Today* 1999;20:493–500.

359. Dickinson BL, Clements JD. Dissociation of *Escherichia coli* heat-labile enterotoxin adjuvanticity from ADP-ribosyltransferase activity. *Infect Immun* 1995;63:1617–1623.

360. Hajishengallis G, Hollingshead SK, Koga T, et al. Mucosal immunization with a bacterial protein antigen genetically coupled to cholera toxin A2/B subunits. *J Immunol* 1995;154:4322–4332.

361. Krieg AM. CpG motifs in bacterial DNA and their immune effects. *Annu Rev Immunol* 2002;20:709–760.

362. Boyaka PN, Marinaro M, Jackson RJ, et al. IL-12 is an effective adjuvant for induction of mucosal immunity. *J Immunol* 1999;162:122–128.

363. Staats HF, Ennis FA Jr. IL-1 is an effective adjuvant for mucosal and systemic immune responses when coadministered with protein immunogens. *J Immunol* 1999;162:6141–6147.

364. Lillard JW Jr, Boyaka PN, Chertov O, et al. Mechanisms for induction of acquired host immunity by neutrophil peptide defensins. *Proc Natl Acad Sci U S A* 1999;96:651–656.

365. Lillard JW Jr, Boyaka PN, Hedrick JA, et al. Lymphotactin acts as an innate mucosal adjuvant. *J Immunol* 1999;162:1959–1965.

366. Palmer KE, Arntzen CJ, Lomonossoff GP. Antigen delivery systems. Transgenic plants and recombinant plant viruses. In: Ogra PL, Mestecky J, Lamm ME, et al., eds. *Mucosal immunology,* 2nd ed. San Diego, CA: Academic Press, 1999:793–816.

367. Kato T, Owen RL. Structure and function of intestinal mucosal epithelium. In: Ogra PL, Mestecky J, Lamm ME, et al., eds. *Mucosal immunology,* 2nd ed. San Diego, CA: Academic Press, 1999:115–132.

368. Michalek SM, O'Hagan DT, Gould-Fogerite S, et al. Antigen delivery systems. Nonliving microparticles, liposomes, cochleates, and ISCOMS. In: Ogra PL, Mestecky J, Lamm ME, et al., eds. *Mucosal immunology,* 2nd ed. San Diego, CA: Academic Press, 1999:759–778.

369. Moureau C, Vidal P-L, Bennasser Y, et al. Characterization of humoral and cellular immune responses in mice induced by immunization with HIV-1 Nef regulatory protein encapsulated in poly (DL-lactide-co-glycolide) microparticles. *Mol Immunol* 2001;38:607–618.

370. Lambert JS, Keefer M, Mulligan M, et al. A phase I safety and immunogenicity trial of UBI microparticulate monovalent HIV-1 MN oral peptide immunogen with parenteral boost in HIV-1 seronegative human subjects. *Vaccine* 2001;19:3033–3042.

371. Nantman MJ, Hohmann EL, Murphy CG, et al. Antigen delivery systems. Development of recombinant live vaccines using viral or bacterial vectors. In: Ogra PL, Mestecky J, Lamm ME, et al., eds. *Mucosal immunology,* 2nd ed. San Diego, CA: Academic Press, 1999:779–791.

372. Fennelly GJ, Khan SA, Abad MA, et al. Mucosal DNA vaccine immunization against measles with a highly attenuated *Shigella flexneri* vector. *J Immunol* 1999;162:1603–1610.

373. Amara RR, Villinger F, Altman JD, et al. Control of a mucosal challenge and prevention of AIDS by a multi protein DNA/MVA vaccine. *Science* 2001;292:69–74.

374. Rose NF, Marx PA, Luckay A, et al. An effective AIDS vaccine based on live attenuated vesicular stomatitis virus recombinants. *Cell* 2001;106:539–549.

375. Crotty S, Miller CJ, Lohman BL, et al. Protection against simian immunodeficiency virus vaginal challenge by using Sabin poliovirus vector. *J Virol* 2001;75:7435–7452.

376. Meitin CA, Bender BS, Small PA Jr. Enteric immunization of mice against influenza with recombinant vaccinia. *Proc Natl Acad Sci U S A* 1994;91:11187–11191.

377. Belyakov IM, Moss B, Strober W, et al. Mucosal vaccination overcomes the barrier to recombinant vaccinia immunization caused by pre-existing poxvirus immunity. *Proc Natl Acad Sci U S A* 1999;96:4512–4517.

378. Strober W, Kelsall B, Marth T. Oral tolerance. *J Clin Immunol* 1998;18:1–30.

379. McMenamin C, Holt PG. The natural immune response to inhaled soluble protein antigens involves major histocompatibility complex (MHC) class I–restricted CD8+ T cell–mediated but MHC class II–restricted CD4+ T cell–dependent immune deviation resulting in selective suppression of immunoglobulin E production. *J Exp Med* 1993;178:889–899.

380. Hoyne GF, O'Hehir RE, Wraith DC, et al. Inhibition of T cell and antibody responses to house dust mite allergens by inhalation of the dominant T cell epitope in naïve and sensitized mice. *J Exp Med* 1993;178:1783–1788.

381. Metzler B, Wraith DC. Inhibition of experimental autoimmune encephalomyelitis by inhalation but not oral administration of the encephalitogenic peptide: influence of MHC binding affinity. *Int Immunol* 1993;5:1159–1165.

382. Ma CG, Zhang GX, Xiao BG, et al. Suppression of experimental autoimmune myasthenia gravis by nasal administration of acetylcholine receptor. *J Neuroimmunol* 1995;58:51–60.

383. Tian J, Atkinson MA, Clare-Salzler M, et al. Nasal administration of glutamate decarboxylase (GAD65) peptides induces Th2 responses and prevents murine insulin-dependent diabetes. *J Exp Med* 1996;183:1561–1567.

384. Waldo FB, van den Wall Bake AWL, Mestecky J, et al. Suppression of the immune response by nasal immunization. *Clin Immunol Immunopathol* 1994;72:30–34.

385. Kato H, Fujihashi K, Kato R, et al. Oral tolerance revisited: prior oral tolerization abrogates cholera toxin–induced mucosal IgA responses. *J Immunol* 2001;166:3114–3121.

386. Whitacre CC, Gienapp IE, Orosz CG, et al. Oral tolerance in experimental autoimmune encephalomyelitis III. Evidence for clonal anergy. *J Immunol* 1991;147:2155–2163.

387. Chen Y, Inobe J, Marks R, et al. Peripheral deletion of antigen-reactive T cells in oral tolerance. *Nature* 1995;376:177–180.

388. Melamed D, Friedman A. Direct evidence for anergy in T lymphocytes tolerized by oral administration of ovalbumin. *Eur J Immunol* 1993; 23:935–942.

389. Czerkinsky C, Holmgren J. The mucosal immune system and prospects for anti-infectious and anti-inflammatory vaccines. *Immunologist* 1995;3(3):97.

390. Challacombe SJ, Tomasi TB Jr. Systemic tolerance and secretory immunity after oral immunization. *J Exp Med* 1980;152:1459–1472.

391. Rubas W, Grass GM. Gastrointestinal lymphatic absorption of peptides and proteins. *Adv Drug Del Rev* 1991;7:15–69.

392. Alpan O, Rudomen G, Matzinger P. The role of dendritic cells, B cells, and M cells in gut-oriented immune responses. *J Immunol* 2001; 166:4843–4852.

393. Chen Y, Song K, Eck SL, et al. An intra-Peyer's patch gene transfer model for studying mucosal tolerance: distinct roles of B7 and IL-12 in mucosal T cell tolerance. *J Immunol* 2000;165:3145–3153.

394. Spahn TW, Fontana A, Faria AMC, et al. Induction of oral tolerance to cellular immune responses in the absence of Peyer's patches. *Eur J Immunol* 2001;31:1278–1287.

395. Fujihashi K, Dohi T, Rennert PD, et al. Peyer's patches are required for oral tolerance to proteins. *Proc Natl Acad Sci U S A* 2001;98:3310–3315.

396. Yamamoto M, Rennert P, McGhee JR, et al. Alternate mucosal immune system: organized Peyer's patches are not required for IgA responses in the gastrointestinal tract. *J Immunol* 2000;164:5184–5191.

397. Shi HN, Grusby MJ, Nagler-Anderson C. Orally induced peripheral nonresponsiveness is maintained in the absence of functional Th1 or Th2 cells. *J Immunol* 1999;162:5143–5148.

398. Khoo UY, Proctor IE, Macpherson JS. CD4$^+$ T cell down-regulation in human intestinal mucosa. Evidence for intestinal tolerance to luminal bacteria antigens. *J Immunol* 1997;158:3626–3634.

399. Thorstenson KM, Khoruts A. Generation of anergic and potentially immunoregulatory CD25$^+$ CD4 T cells *in vivo* after induction of peripheral tolerance with intravenous or oral antigen. *J Immunol* 2001; 167:188–195.

400. Ke Y, Pearce K, Lake JP, et al. $\gamma\delta$ T lymphocytes regulate the induction and maintenance of oral tolerance. *J Immunol* 1997;158:3610–3618.

401. Fujihashi K, Dohi T, Kweon MN, et al. $\gamma\delta$ T cells regulate mucosally induced tolerance in a dose-dependent fashion. *Int Immunol* 1999;11:1907–1916.

402. Seymour BW, Gershwin LJ, Coffman RL. Aerosol-induced immunoglobulin (Ig)–E unresponsiveness to ovalbumin does not require CD8$^+$ or T cell receptor (TCR)– γ/δ^+ T cells or interferon (IFN)–γ in a murine model of allergen sensitization. *J Exp Med* 1998;187:721–731.

403. Hiroi T, Iwatani K, Iijima H, et al. Nasal immune system: distinctive Th0 and Th1/Th2 type environments in murine nasal-associated lymphoid tissues and nasal passage, respectively. *Eur J Immunol* 1998; 28:3346–3353.

404. Husby S, Mestecky J, Moldoveanu Z, et al. Oral tolerance in humans. T cell but not B cell tolerance after antigen feeding. *J Immunol* 1994;152:4663–4670.

405. Zivny JH, Moldoveanu Z, Vu HL, et al. Mechanisms of immune tolerance to food antigens in humans. *Clin Immunol* 2001;101:158–168.

406. Fukaura H, Kent SC, Pietrusewicz MJ, et al. Induction of circulating myelin basic protein and proteolipid protein–specific transforming growth factor-beta1–secreting Th3 T cells by oral administration of myelin in multiple sclerosis patients. *J Clin Invest* 1996;98:70–77.

407. Blanas E, Carbone FR, Allison J, et al. Induction of autoimmune diabetes by oral administration of autoantigen. *Science* 1996;274:1707–1709.

408. Hänninen A, Martinez NR, Dewey GM, et al. Transient blockade of CD40 ligand dissociates pathogenic from protective mucosal immunity. *J Clin Invest* 2002;109:261–267.

409. Cunningham-Rundles C. Immunodeficiency and mucosal immunity. In: Ogra PL, Mestecky J, Lamm ME, et al., eds. *Mucosal immunology,* 2nd ed. San Diego, CA: Academic Press, 1999:939–948.

410. Lefranc MP, Hammarström L, Smith CIE, et al. Gene deletions in the human immunoglobulin heavy constant region locus: molecular and immunological analysis. *Immunodefic Rev* 1991;2:265–281.

411. Plebani A, Carbonara AO, Bottaro A, et al. Gene deletion as a cause of associated deficiency of IgA1, IgG2, IgG4, and IgE. *Immunodefic Rev* 1993;4:245–248.

412. Brandtzaeg P, Guy-Grand D, Griscelli C. Intestinal, salivary, and tonsillar IgA and J-chain production in a patient with severe deficiency of serum IgA. *Scand J Immunol* 1981;13:313–325.

413. Nilssen DE, Brandtzaeg P, Frøland SS, et al. Subclass composition and J-chain expression of the "compensatory" gastrointestinal IgG cell population in selective IgA deficiency. *Clin Exp Immunol* 1992;87:237–245.

414. Conley ME, Kearney JF, Lawton AR 3rd, et al. Differentiation of human B cells expressing the IgA subclasses as demonstrated by monoclonal hybridoma antibodies. *J Immunol* 1980;125:2311–2316.

415. Vorechovsky I, Cullen M, Carrington M, et al. Fine mapping of *IGAD1* in IgA deficiency and common variable immunodeficiency: identification and characterization of haplotypes shared by affected members of 101 multiple-case families. *J Immunol* 2001;164:4408–4416.

416. Savilahti E, Klemola T, Carlsson P, et al. Inadequacy of mucosal IgM antibodies in selective IgA deficiency: excretion of attenuated polio virus is prolonged. *J Clin Immunol* 1988;8:89–94.

417. Tolo K, Brandtzaeg P, Jonsen J. Mucosal penetration of antigen in the presence or absence of serum-derived antibody. An *in vitro* study of rabbit oral and intestinal mucosa. *Immunology* 1977;33:733–743.

418. Smith PD, Wahl SM. Immunobiology of mucosal HIV-1 infection. In: Ogra PL, Mestecky J, Lamm ME, et al., eds. *Mucosal immunology,* 2nd ed. San Diego, CA: Academic Press, 1999:977–989.

419. Lehner T. Mucosal infection and immune responses to simian immunodeficiency virus. In: Ogra PL, Mestecky J, Lamm ME, et al., eds. *Mucosal immunology,* 2nd ed. San Diego, CA: Academic Press, 1999: 963–976.

420. Meng G, Wei X, Wu X, et al. Primary intestinal epithelial cells selectively transfer R5 HIV-1 to CCR5$^+$ cells. *Nat Med* 2002;8:150–156.

421. Vaezey RS, Marx PA, Lackner AA. The mucosal immune system: primary target for HIV infection and AIDS. *Trends Immunol* 2001; 22:626–633.

422. Li L, Meng G, Graham MF, et al. Intestinal macrophages display reduced permissiveness to human immunodeficiency virus type 1 and decreased surface CCR5. *Gastroenterology* 1999;116:1043–1053.

423. Raux M, Finkielsztejn L, Salmon-Ceron D, et al. Comparison of the distribution of IgG and IgA antibodies in serum and various mucosal fluids of HIV type 1–infected subjects. *AIDS Res Hum Retroviruses* 1999;15:1365–1376.

424. Wright PF, Kozlowski PA, Rybczyk GK, et al. Detection of mucosal antibodies in HIV-infected individuals. *AIDS Res Hum Retroviruses* 2002;18:1291–1300.

425. Kaul R, Trabattoni D, Bwayo JJ, et al. HIV-1 specific mucosal IgA in a cohort of HIV-1–resistant Kenyan sex workers. *AIDS* 1999;13:23–29.

426. Mazzoli S, Lopalco L, Salvi A, et al. Human immunodeficiency virus (HIV)–specific IgA and HIV neutralizing activity in the serum of exposed seronegative partners of HIV-seropositive persons. *J Infect Dis* 1999;180:871–875.

427. Artenstein AW, VanCott TC, Sitz KV, et al. Mucosal immune response in four distinct compartments of women infected with human immunodeficiency virus type 1: a comparison by site and correlation with clinical information. *J Infect Dis* 1997;175:265–271.

428. Belec L, Dupre T, Prazuck T, et al. Cervicovaginal overproduction of specific IgG to human immunodeficiency virus (HIV) contrasts with normal or impaired IgA local response in HIV infection. *J Infect Dis* 1995;172:691–697.

429. Kozlowski P, Jackson S. Serum IgA subclasses and molecular forms in HIV infection: selective increases in monomer and apparent restriction of the antibody response to IgA1 antibodies mainly directed at Env glycoproteins. *AIDS Res Hum Retroviruses* 1992;8:1773–1780.

430. Blumberg RS, Saubermann LJ, Strober W. Animal models of mucosal inflammation and their relation to human inflammatory bowel disease. *Curr Opin Immunol* 1999;11:648–656.

431. Strober W, Fuss IJ, Blumberg RS. The immunology of mucosal models of inflammation. *Annu Rev Immunol* 2002;20:495–549.

432. Duerr RH. Genetics of IBD. In: Satsangi J, Sutherland LR, eds. *Inflammatory bowel disease,* 4th ed. Philadelphia: Elsevier, 2003; (in press).

433. Hugot J-P, Chamaillard M, Zouali H, et al. Association of NOD2 leucine-rich repeat variants with susceptibility to Crohn's disease. *Nature* 2001;411:599–603.

434. Boirivant M, Fuss IJ, Chu A, et al. Oxazalone colitis: A murine model of T helper cell type 2 colitis treatable with antibodies to interleukin 4. *J Exp Med* 1998;188:1929–1939.

435. Sharon P, Stenson WF. Metabolism of arachidonic acid in acetic acid colitis in rats: similarity to human inflammatory bowel disease. *Gastroenterology* 1985;88:55–63.

436. Abraham R, Fabian RJ, Goldberg L, et al. Role of lysosomes in carageenan-induced cecal ulceration. *Gastroenterology* 1974;1169–1181.

437. Ohkusa T. Production of experimental ulcerative colitis in hamsters by dextran sulfate sodium and change in intestinal microflora. *Jpn J Gastroenterol* 1985;82:1327–1336.

438. Glazier A, Tutschka PJ, Farmer ER, et al. Graft-versus host disease in cyclosporin A–treated rats after syngeneic and autologous bone marrow reconstitution. *J Exp Med* 1983:158:1–8.

439. Sartor RB, Cromartie WJ, Powell DW, et al. Granulomatous enterocolitis induced in rats by purified bacterial cell wall fragments. *Gastroenterology* 1985;89:587–595.

440. Sadlack B, Merz H, Schorle H, et al. Ulcerative colitis–like disease in mice with a disrupted interleukin-2 gene. *Cell* 1993;75:203–205.

441. Dieleman LA, Arends A, Tonkonogy SL, et al. *Helicobacter hepaticus* does not induce or potentiate colitis in interleukin-10–deficient mice. *Infect Immun* 2000:68:5107–5113.

442. Watanabe M, Ueno Y, Yamazaki M, et al. Mucosal IL-7–mediated immune responses in chronic colitis–IL-7 transgenic mouse model. *Immunol Res* 1999;20:251–259.

443. Rudolph U, Finegold MJ, Rich SS, et al. Gαi2 protein deficiency: a model of inflammatory bowel disease. *J Clin Immunol* 1995;15:1015–1055.

444. Mombaerts P, Mizoguchi E, Grusby MF, et al. Spontaneous development of inflammatory bowel disease in T cell receptor mutant mice. *Cell* 1993;75:275–282.

445. Hagemann TL, Kwan SP, Ferrini R, et al. Wiskott-Aldrich syndrome protein-deficient mice reveal a role for WASP in T but not B cell activation. *Immunity* 1998;9:81–91.

446. Hammer RE, Maika SD, Richardson JA, et al. Spontaneous inflammatory disease in transgenic rats expressing HLA-B27 and human β_2-m: an animal model of HLA-B27–associated human disorders. *Cell* 1990;63:1099–1112.

447. Powrie F, Correa-Oliveira R, Mauze S, et al. Regulatory interactions between CD45RB[high] and CD45RB[low] CD4[+] T cells are important for the balance between protective and pathogenic cell-mediated immunity. *J Exp Med* 1994;179:589–600.

448. Hollander GA, Simpson SJ, Mizoguchi E, et al. Severe colitis in mice with aberrant thymic selection. *Immunity* 1999;3:27–38.

449. Bertone ER, Giovannucci EL, King NW Jr, et al. Family history as a risk factor for ulcerative colitis–associated colon cancer in cotton-top tamarin. *Gastroenterology* 1998;114:669–674.

450. Sundberg JP, Elson CO, Bedigian H, et al. Spontaneous heritable colitis in a new substrain of C$_3$H/HeJ mice. *Gastroenterology* 1994;107;1726–1735.

451. Matsumoto S, Okabe Y, Setoyama H, et al. Inflammatory bowel disease–like enteritis and caecitis in a senescence accelerated mouse P1/Yit strain. *Gut* 1998;43:71–78.

452. Rath HC, Schultz M, Freitag R, et al. Different subsets of enteric bacteria induce and perpetuate experimental colitis in rats and mice. *Infect Immun* 2001;69:2277–2285.

453. Rath HC, Wilson KH, Sartor RB. Differential induction of colitis and gastritis in HLA-B27 transgenic rats selectively colonized with *Bacteroides vulgatus* or *Escherichia coli*. *Infect Immun* 1999;67:2969–2974.

454. Madsen KL, Doyle JS, Jewell LD, et al. *Lactobacillus* species prevents colitis in interleukin 10 gene–deficient mice. *Gastroenterology* 1999;116:1107–1114.

455. Mahler M, Bristol IJ, Sundberg JP, et al. Genetic analysis of susceptibility to dextran sulfate sodium–induced colitis in mice. *Genomics* 1999;55:147–156.

456. Aranda R, Sydora BC, McAllister PL, et al. Analysis of intestinal lymphocytes in mouse colitis mediated by transfer of CD4[+], CD45Rb[high] T cells to SCID recipients. *J Immunol* 1997;158:3464–3473.

457. Probert CS, Chott A, Turner JR, et al. Persistent clonal expansion of peripheral blood CD4[+] lymphocytes in chronic inflammatory bowel disease. *J Immunol* 1996;157:3183–3191.

458. Cong Y, Weaver CT, Lazenby A, et al. Colitis induced by enteric bacterial antigen-specific CD4[+] T cells requires CD40–CD40 ligand interactions for a sustained increase in mucosal IL-12. *J Immunol* 2000;165:2173–2182.

459. Duchmann R, May E, Heike M, et al. T cell specificity and cross reactivity towards enterobacteria, *Bacteroides*, *Bifidobacterium*, and antigens from resident intestinal flora in humans. *Gut* 1999;44:812–818.

460. Neurath MF, Fuss I, Kelsall BL, et al. Antibodies to interleukin 12 abrogate established experimental colitis in mice. *J Exp Med* 1995;182:1281–1290.

461. Neurath MF, Fuss IJ, Kelsall BL, et al. Experimental granulomatous colitis in mice is abrogated by induction of TGF-β–mediated oral tolerance. *J Exp Med* 1996;183:2605–2616.

462. Hermiston ML, Gordon JI. Inflammatory bowel disease and adenomas in mice expressing a dominant negative N-cadherin. *Science* 1995;270:1203–1207.

463. Panwala CM, Jones JC, Viney JL. A novel model of inflammatory bowel disease: mice deficient for the multiple drug resistance gene, mdr1a, spontaneously develop colitis. *J Immunol* 1998;161:5733–5744.

464. Hoffman JC, Peters K, Henschke S, et al. Role of T lymphocytes in rat 2,4,6-trinitrobenzene sulphonic acid induced colitis: increased mortality after $\gamma\delta$ T cell depletion and no effect of $\alpha\beta$ T cell depletion. *Gut* 2001;48:489–495.

465. Stüber E, Strober W, Neurath M. Blocking the CD40L–CD40 interaction *in vivo* specifically prevents the priming of T helper 1 cells through the inhibition of interleukin 12 secretion. *J Exp Med* 1996;183:693–698.

466. Higgins LM, McDonald SA, Whittle N, et al. Regulation of T cell activation *in vitro* and *in vivo* by targeting the OX40–OX40 ligand interaction: amelioration of ongoing inflammatory bowel disease with an OX40-IgG fusion protein, but not with an OX40 ligand–IgG fusion protein. *J Immunol* 1999;162:486–493.

467. Nakajima A, Iijima H, Neurath MF, et al. Activation-induced expression of carcinoembryonic antigen-cell adhesion molecule 1 regulates mouse T lymphocyte function. *J Immunol* 2002;168:1028–1035.

468. Kammerer R, Stober D, Singer BB, et al. Carcinoembryonic antigen-related cell adhesion molecule 1 on murine dendritic cells is a potent regulator of T cell stimulation. *J Immunol* 2001;166:6537–6544.

469. Kontoyiannis D, Pasparakis M, Pizarro T, et al. Impaired on/off regulation of TNF biosynthesis in mice lacking TNF AU-rich elements: implications for joint and gut-associated immunopathologies. *Immunity* 1999;10:387–398.

470. Kaiser GC, Yan F, Polk DB. Mesalamine blocks tumor necrosis factor growth inhibition and nuclear factor κB activation in mouse colonocytes. *Gastroenterology* 1999;116:602–609.

471. Christ AD, Stevens AC, Koeppen H, et al. An interleukin 12-related cytokine is upregulated in ulcerative colitis but not in Crohn's disease. *Gastroenterology* 1998;115:307–313.

472. Gorelik L, Flavell RA. Abrogation of TGFβ signaling in T cells leads to spontaneous T cell differentiation and autoimmune disease. *Immunity* 2000;12:171–181.

473. Florentino DF, Zlotnick A, Mosmann TR, et al. IL-10 inhibits cytokine production by activated macrophages. *J Immunol* 1991;147:3815–3822.

474. Wills-Karp M. Immunologic basis of antigen-induced airway hyperresponsiveness. *Annu Rev Immunol* 1999;17:255–281.

475. Hjern A, Haglund B, Hedlin G. Ethnicity, childhood environment and atopic disorder. *Clin Exp Allergy* 2000;30:521–528.

476. Ahmed T, Fuchs GJ. Gastrointestinal allergy to food: a review. *J Diarrhoeal Dis Res* 1997;15:211–223.

477. Mestecky J, Blair C, Ogra PL, eds. *Immunology of milk and the neonate*. New York: Plenum Press, 1991.

478. Smith DH, Malone DC, Lawson KA, et al. A national estimate of the economic costs of asthma. *Am J Respir Crit Care Med* 1997;156:787–793.

479. Sears MR, Burrows B, Flannery EM, et al. Relation between airway responsiveness and serum IgE in children with asthma and in apparently normal children. *N Engl J Med* 1991;325:1067–1071.

480. Del Prete GF, De Carli M, D'Elios MM, et al. Allergen exposure induces the activation of allergen-specific Th2 cells in the airway mucosa of patients with allergic respiratory disorders. *Eur J Immunol* 1993;23:1445–1449.

481. Robinson DS, Hamid Q, Ying S, et al. Predominant Th2-like bronchoalveolar T-lymphocyte population in atopic asthma. *N Engl J Med* 1992;326:298–304.

482. Shakib F, Schulz O, Sewell H. A mite subversive: cleavage of CD23 and CD25 by Der p 1 enhances allergenicity. *Immunol Today* 1998;19:313–316.

483. Marsh DG, Neely JD, Breazeale DR, et al. Linkage analysis of IL-4 and other chromosome 5q31.1 markers and total serum immunoglobulin E concentrations. *Science* 1994;264:1152–1156.

484. Postma DS, Bleecker ER, Amelung PJ, et al. Genetic susceptibility to asthma–bronchial hyperresponsiveness coinherited with a major gene for atopy. *N Engl J Med* 1995;333:894–900.

485. Hershey GK, Friedrich MF, Esswein LA, et al. The association of atopy with a gain of function mutation in the α subunit of the interleukin-4 receptor. *N Engl J Med* 1997;337:1710–1725.

486. Loots GG, Locksley RM, Blankespoor CM, et al. Identification of a coordinate regulator of interleukins 4, 13 and 5 by cross-species sequence comparisons. *Science* 2000;288:136–140.

487. Walley AJ, Wiltshire S, Ellis CM, et al. Linkage and allelic association of chromosome 5 cytokine cluster genetic markers with atopy and asthma associated tracts. *Genomics* 2001;72:15–20.

488. McIntire JJ, Umetsu SE, Akbari O, et al. Identification of *Tapr* (an airway hyperreactivity regulatory locus) and the linked *Tim* gene family. *Nat Immunol* 2001;2:1109–1116.

489. Byersdorfer CA, Chaplin DD. Visualization of early APC/T cell interactions in the mouse lung following intranasal challenge. *J Immunol* 2001;167:6756–6764.

490. Randolph DA, Carruthers CJL, Szabo SJ, et al. Modulation of airway inflammation by passive transfer of allergin-specific Th1 and Th2 cell in a mouse model of asthma. *J Immunol* 1999;162:2375–2383.

491. Hussain I, Randolph D, Brody SL, et al. Induction, distribution and modulation of upper airway allergic inflammation in mice. *Clin Exp Allergy* 2001;31:1048–1059.

492. Szepfalusi Z, Nentwich I, Gerstmayr M, et al. Prenatal allergen contact with milk proteins. *Clin Exp Allergy* 1997;27:28–35.

493. Sampson HA, Anderson JA. Summary and recommendations: classification of gastrointestinal manifestations due to immunologic reactions to foods in infants and young children. *J Pediatr Gastroenterol Nutr* 2000;30:S87–S94.

494. Sicherer SH, Noone SA, Koerner CB, et al. Hypoallergenicity and efficacy of an amino acid–based formula in children with cow's milk and multiple food hypersensitivities. *J Pediatr* 2001;138:688–693.

495. Bock SA. Evaluation of IgE-mediated food hypersensitivities. *J Pediatr Gastroenterol Nutr* 2000;30:S20–S27.

496. Hogan SP, Mishra A, Brandt EB, et al. A critical role for eotaxin in experimental oral antigen-induced eosinophilic gastrointestinal allergy. *Proc Natl Acad Sci U S A* 2000;97:6681–6686.

497. Li XM, Schofield BH, Huang CK, et al. A murine model of IgE-mediated cow's milk hypersensitivity. *J Allergy Clin Immunol* 1999;103:206–214.

498. Kweon M-N, Yamamoto M, Kajiki M, et al. Systemically derived large intestinal CD4$^+$ Th2 cells play a central role in STAT6-mediated allergic diarrhea. *J Clin Invest* 2000;106:199–206.

CHAPTER 32

Neural Immune Interactions in Health and Disease

Esther M. Sternberg and Jeanette I. Webster

Introduction
Effects of Immune Factors on CNS
    Effects of Immune Factors Expressed within CNS · Effects of Peripheral Immune Factors on CNS Function
CNS Regulation of Immune System
    Neuroendocrine Regulation of Immune System: Glucocorticoid Effects · Pathophysiologic Role of HPA Axis and GC Dysregulation in Pathogenesis of Immune-Mediated Diseases
Therapeutic Implications
Acknowledgments
References

INTRODUCTION

The traditional view of immune regulation has focused almost exclusively on molecular and cellular factors within the immune system as prime regulators of immune function and disease. However, a growing body of evidence indicates that many extraimmune factors including hormones, neuropeptides, and neurotransmitters derived from the nervous and endocrine systems, play an important physiologic role in modulating immune function at all levels. This extraimmune system modulation in turn plays a critical role in determining susceptibility and resistance to, as well as course, severity, and expression of a wide range of diseases mediated by the immune system, including inflammatory, autoimmune, allergic, and infectious diseases. Conversely, immune factors regulate the nervous system at molecular, cellular, organ, and system levels and thus play an important role in normal neuronal development, neuronal cell death and survival, and neuronal activity. Consequently, immune factors play an important role in the pathogenesis of neurodegenerative diseases, in neuroregeneration after trauma and in many brain functions, including mood, memory consolidation, and cognition. An in-depth understanding of the molecular, cellular, and system levels of these neural immune interactions therefore not only sheds light on normal physiologic responses and development, but also on pathogenesis of a wide variety of disease processes and provides new avenues for treatment of disease. This chapter will outline the many levels at which these two defense systems communicate, including molecular, cellular, organ, and system levels, the diseases that result when these regulatory connections are disrupted and potential new avenues for treatment derived from such understanding. Although the chapter will discuss both immune regulation of the nervous system and nervous system regulation of the immune system, it will focus in large part on the latter direction of this two-way regulatory communication (Fig. 1).

EFFECTS OF IMMUNE FACTORS ON CNS

The effects of immune factors on the central nervous system (CNS) can be considered in two compartments: (1) effects on nervous tissues of immune cells and molecules expressed within the nervous system; and (2) effects on CNS function of immune molecules produced outside the CNS. In the first case, immune factors act more like growth factors and affect neuronal cell death and survival. In the second case, immune factors act more like hormones, that is, molecules produced at a site distal to the organ whose function they affect. The next two sections outline these two very different effects of immune factors on the nervous system, the physiologic processes that they affect, and the diseases they impact, as well as new strategies for therapies that can be derived from understanding these modes of immune regulation of the nervous system.

Effects of Immune Factors Expressed within CNS

Cytokines are expressed during development and in resting physiologic conditions within the CNS in resident cells.

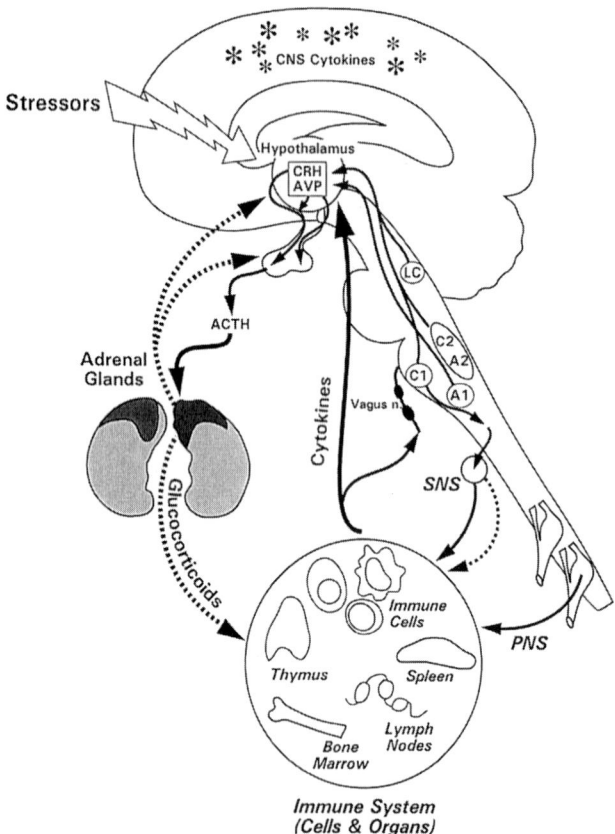

FIG. 1. Two-way communication between the immune and nervous systems. The immune system and the central nervous system (CNS) communicate with and regulate each other. Cytokines made in the periphery signal the CNS by several routes, including passage across the blood–brain barrier and via the vagus nerve. Peripheral cytokines affect many aspects of CNS function, including activation of the neuroendocrine stress response, or hypothalamic-pituitary-adrenal (HPA) axis. When activated, the hypothalamus releases corticotropin-releasing hormone (CRH) and arginine vasopressin (AVP) that together stimulate the pituitary gland to release adrenocorticotrophin (ACTH). This in turn stimulates the adrenal cortex to release glucocorticoids. These hormones suppress immunity at a molecular, cellular, and organ level. Other routes by which the CNS regulates immunity are through the sympathetic nervous system (SNS) and peripheral nervous system. Stress both activates the HPA axis to release these immunosuppressive hormones and also activates the SNS. The HPA axis and SNS communicate through brain stem routes that involve noradrenergic nuclei, including the locus ceruleus, C1, C2, A1, and A2. Cytokines are also expressed within the CNS and in this compartment play a role in neuronal cell death and survival.

Although mainly present in glia, astrocytes, and microglia, certain cytokines, including IL-6 (1) and IFN-γ (2), have been shown to be expressed in neurons, the latter under activated conditions. In pathologic conditions, increased quantities of cytokines are produced by resident glial cells or by invading cells of the peripheral immune system, including macrophages and lymphocytes (3–5) that traffic through the CNS. In addition to cytokine expression, CNS cells also express receptors for many cytokines (reviewed in Benveniste [5] and Sternberg [6]).

In general, cytokines expressed within the CNS play an important role in neuronal cell death and survival. Depending on the time of exposure to activated lymphocytes or macrophages in relation to nerve trauma, or the particular cytokine expressed, immune elements may either contribute to neuronal cell death or protect against it. Thus, a thorough understanding of the mechanisms and time course of cytokine and immune cell effects on neuronal cell death and survival are important for understanding the pathogenesis of diseases as disparate as neuroAIDS (7,8), toxoplasmosis, stroke (9), nerve trauma (10–12), and neurodegenerative diseases (13) in which cytokines mediate the final common pathway of neuronal death. In these conditions, immune manipulations, including the use of cytokine-receptor antagonists such as the endogenous interleukin-1 receptor antagonist (IL-1RA), nonsteroidal anti-inflammatory agents or carefully timed treatment with specific activated T cells, are being tested successfully in animal models and for potential treatment of human disease.

The pattern of cytokines produced in the CNS in pathologic conditions during infection or inflammation depends on the precise nature of the antigenic, proinflammatory, or infectious stimulus, as well as the cell source that is primarily activated. Cytokines produced by infiltrating lymphocytes or macrophages that traffic through the CNS from the periphery are a mechanism of exposure particularly relevant to infectious diseases of the brain, including neuroAIDS and toxoplasmosis (reviewed in Griffin [3], Persidsky et al. [4], and Kaul [7]). The resultant cytokine-induced neurodegeneration is responsible for the dementia seen in such conditions. Neuronal cell death after ischemic injury is also caused in part by the neurotoxic effects of IL-1. IL-1RA has thus been successfully used in animal models to reduce the area of ischemic injury by approximately 50%, suggesting potential novel therapeutic approaches for reduction of brain injury following stroke in humans (9). Cytokines and immune factors are not always neurotoxic, however. Specific activated T cells, at critical time periods after nerve trauma, promote neuroregeneration and prevent paralysis in rodents subjected to spinal cord crush injury (11).

Effects of Peripheral Immune Factors on CNS Function

In contrast to the growth factor–like effect of cytokines expressed within the CNS, peripheral cytokines—produced during immune activation in the course of infection or inflammation—act more like hormones to stimulate various brain functions. Cytokines produced within the CNS can also act like neuropeptides to affect certain neuronal cell functions. Thus, cytokines play a role in induction of fever, sleep, a characteristic set of behaviors seen in illness called "sickness behavior," alteration of mood, memory consolidation, cognition, and activation of the hormonal stress response. Interleukin-1 (IL-1), IL-6, tumor necrosis factor alpha

(TNF-α) and a variety of other cytokines have all been shown in animal models and in humans to activate some or all of these brain functions.

Routes of Access of Peripheral Immune Molecules to CNS

When these effects of peripheral cytokines were first described (14), even in relation to pure recombinant cytokines such as IL-1 (15), there was some resistance to the notion that peripheral immune molecules could directly affect brain function, in part because it was thought that such large molecules could not cross the blood–brain barrier (BBB). However, it is now known that there are many ways by which immune molecules in the periphery can either affect the CNS either directly, by crossing the BBB, or indirectly through second messenger signaling (16,17).

Thus, cytokines can cross the BBB passively at leaky areas such as the circumventricular organs, where the BBB is incomplete, or they may be actively transported in small amounts across portions of the BBB (18). Cytokines signal the brain through activation of endothelial-cell second messenger systems such as nitric oxide synthase (19) and cyclooxygenase (20,21), with resultant release of nitric oxide and prostaglandins. Such signaling may also induce secondary induction of expression of cytokines within the CNS (22). Finally, an important route by which peritoneally produced cytokines stimulate the brain is via the vagus nerve (23,24). It is likely that one or more of these mechanisms operate under different conditions, and the major or primary route by which cytokines activate the CNS in a given condition depends on the dose, route of administration (whether intravenous or intraperitoneal), or exposure, and the particular cytokine involved (25).

Blood–Brain Barrier

Most of the brain is protected from exposure to large peripheral blood molecules and cells by the BBB—an endothelial barrier composed of functionally and anatomically distinct brain capillary endothelial cells connected by tight junctions and with limited endocytotic vesicular activity resulting in limited paracellular flux (26,27) (Fig. 2). Under resting physiologic conditions, this structure excludes most molecules except small lipophilic ones. Hydrophilic molecules and essential nutrients are actively transported across the BBB.

Passive Transport across Circumventricular Organs

There are areas of the brain where the BBB is incomplete and therefore leaky even under normal physiologic conditions. These anatomical areas—the circumventricular organs—include the median eminence, the area postrema, the subfornical organ, the organum vasculosum of the lamina terminalis, and the choroid plexus. These areas tend to be rich in blood vessels that lack tight junctions and some, such as the median eminence located between the hypothalamus and pituitary glands, are areas into which many neurohormones are secreted. Thus, even large molecules in the range of 15 to 17 kD, such as interleukins, can cross from the blood to brain tissue in these areas.

Active Transport of Cytokines Across Blood–Brain Barrier

Although initially controversial, it has now been convincingly shown that small amounts of certain cytokines (IL-1 alpha, IL-1 beta, IL-1RA, GM-CSF, IL-6, TNF-α, and IFN-γ) are actively transported across the BBB, and that different

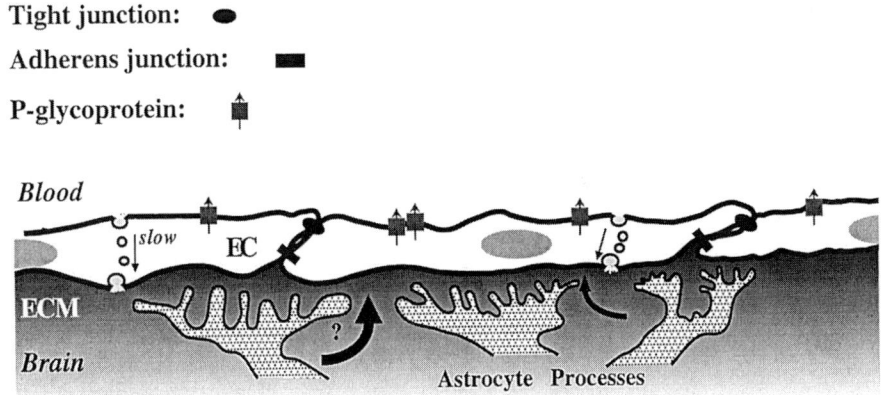

FIG. 2. Features of the blood–brain barrier. Adherens and tight junctions couple brain capillary endothelial cells (ECs). The multidrug transporter P-glycoprotein is expressed in the apical membranes of ECs and actively effluxes undesirable substances from the CNS. Transcytosis across the brain ECs is slow, minimizing transcellular movement into the CNS. Astrocyte processes ensheath the ECs. Their phenotype may be influenced by the extracellular matrix. The blood–brain barrier also contains transporters for essential nutrients, such as glucose and certain amino acids, and for macromolecules. From Rubin and Staddon (27), with permission.

cytokines may cross at different places (26,28,29). It is likely that both passive leaking across the BBB and active transport are routes that play an important role in CNS activation by intravascular cytokines.

Second Messenger Signaling

Probably the most common mechanism by which cytokines stimulate the CNS is through second messenger signaling. Thus, cytokines such as IL-1 bind to receptors in endothelial cells and activate second messenger systems including cyclooxygenase with production of prostaglandins (21), and nitric oxide synthase (NOS) (19,30) with production of nitric oxide. Such mechanisms play an important role in fever induction by peripherally produced cytokines. Treatment with nonsteroidal anti-inflammatory agents blocks these routes and thus prevents fever.

Vagus Nerve Stimulation

An important route by which cytokines produced in the peritoneum or liver may activate the brain is by stimulation of the vagus nerve (31,32). It has been proposed that a visceral chemosensory system exists in which cytokines, such as IL-1, bind to receptors expressed in paraganglia cells located in lymphoid tissue closely apposed to parasympathetic sensory ganglia (31). This, in turn, results in activation of the vagus nerve, and subsequent rapid activation through neural transmission of the nucleus of the tractus solitarius (NTS), the area in the brain stem that receives the vagus nerve's initial incoming signals. Thus, early gene activation of c-Fos has been shown in the NTS after intraperitoneal injection of IL-1, and cutting the vagus nerve prevents many of the functional effects of intraperitoneally IL-1 injected, including c-Fos expression (24). It is likely that this route is the principal one by which cytokines expressed in conditions of peritoneal inflammation activate the CNS.

Secondary Induction of Cytokine Production within CNS

It has recently been shown that peripheral cytokines can induce expression of cytokines centrally without crossing the BBB. Thus, peripheral injection of TNF-α is associated with production of IL-1 in certain brain regions (22). In this instance, the periphery and CNS use cytokines in a relay-like fashion to activate different functions in brain and immune system. The role that such CNS expression of interleukins plays in alterations of mood during illness and in non–illness-related mood disorders is currently being explored.

CNS Functions Induced by Peripherally Produced Cytokines

Just as hormones produced by glands affect a variety of functions of organs distal to their site of production, cytokines produced by peripheral immune cells at areas of inflamma-

tion or infection induce a variety of brain functions distal to their site of production. Included are induction of fever, sleep, and sickness behavior, and effects on mood, memory consolidation, and cognition, and activation of the neuroendocrine stress response. Early studies showing such CNS effects in animal models employed complex infectious or proinflammatory stimuli, including viruses (influenza, hepatitis) and bacteria as well as bacterial-wall lipopolysaccharide (LPS) (14). While such studies suggested that cytokines induced by infectious and inflammatory stimuli did affect brain function, it was not until pure recombinant cytokines became available in large enough quantities to test in animal models (15) that it could be proven that these were the direct biologic effects of cytokines rather than nonspecific effects of illness. With that evidence, subsequent research has focused on molecular mechanisms and neuroanatomical pathways by which cytokines induce these effects.

Fever

One of the most well-studied effects of peripheral cytokines on the brain is fever (33,34). Fever induction by bacterial cell wall products, such as LPS, occurs through monocyte activation and resultant release of pyrogenic cytokines IL-1, TNF-α, and IL-6. These cytokines then bind to endothelial cell receptors, in the case of IL-1 to the IL-1 receptor/Toll-like receptor (IL-1R/TLR Toll). While MyD88 is among the common signaling intermediates for IL-1R and TLR, it is not known whether this intermediate plays a role in fever. Signal transduction occurs through common pathways involving NFκB, p38 MAPK and Jun (33,35). LPS may also directly stimulate endothelial cells. Activation of endothelial cells results in induction of cyclooxygenase, with production of prostaglandins (PGs), and induction of nitric oxide synthase (NOS) with production of nitric oxide (NO). These second messengers diffuse into the brain parenchyma and induce fever through stimulation of temperature sensitive cells in the preoptic area of the hypothalamus. Neural pathways controlling physiologic responses important in heat conservation and generation are then activated, including vasoconstrictor and motor pathways governing shivering. This results in an increased body temperature set-point and thus increased body temperature, that is, fever.

Sleep

Normal sleep is characterized by cycles of phases defined by a combination of EEG and behavioral patterns. Sleep patterns are affected both by the cytokine stimulation arm and the neuroendocrine response arm of neural immune interactions. Thus, cytokines and infections disrupt sleep patterns; sleep deprivation alters neuroendocrine responses, which, in turn, alter sleep architecture; and disrupted sleep affects course and severity of infectious disease. The specific pattern of sleep that is induced in response to infection depends on a combination of factors related to the infectious agent (whether bacterial, viral, or parasitic) and the hosts' response patterns to the infection (36–38). This is in part related to the specific pattern of immune responses of the host, and the cell types involved in processing of the infectious agent, with resultant differential pattern of cytokines induced, as well as the presence of bacterial wall by-products, such as muramyl dipeptide, which in themselves alter sleep architecture. Several lines of evidence in animal models and humans indicate that many cytokines alter sleep architecture, and do so via specific cytokine receptors (39,40). Thus, cytokines such as IL-1, IL-2, IL-6, TNF-α, and IFN-α, IL-13, IL-15, IL-18, IFN-γ and TGF-β1 varyingly increase slow-wave sleep (SWS), reduce or increase rapid eye movement sleep (REMS), or produce fragmented sleep that reduces sleep efficiency and leads to daytime fatigue (39,41–43).

Furthermore, evidence from inbred strains of mice and rats, targeted mutant knockout mouse models and genetic linkage and segregation studies in mice, indicate that postinfectious and cytokine-induced sleep patterns depend upon not only the pattern and timing of cytokines produced in response to a given infectious agent, but also on other host genetic factors that include neuroendocrine stress and corticotrophin-releasing factor (CRH) responsiveness (39,44–46). Studies in inbred rat strains exhibiting differential CRH responsiveness indicate that hyper-CRH responders show less SWS and more REM sleep in response to IL-1 compared with hyporesponsive strains. Furthermore, intracerebroventricular administration of a CRH antagonist partially antagonizes this effect (46). Genetic linkage and segregation studies in mice have identified several linkage regions on mouse chromosomes 2, 5, 7, 17, and 19. The strength and presence of each specific linkage region is determined by the precise phenotype examined (whether circadian or infectious sleep patterns of SWS or REMS). One of these linkage regions contains several neuroendocrine related candidate genes that may potentially play a role in regulating sleep include the CRHR2 receptor and the growth hormone–releasing hormone receptor (GHRHR) (44). Furthermore, studies in GHRHR knockout mice show that the mutant mice sleep less at baseline, sleep less rather than more in response to influenza infection, and have a higher mortality to viral infection (47). While the association between sleep deprivation and greatly enhanced mortality from infection in animals has long been recognized, the mechanism of this effect is not known (48,49). The studies in GHRHR knockout mice suggest involvement of this receptor system in the phenomenon. All these lines of evidence indicate that genetic factors determining the set-point of the neuroendocrine stress response (see next section) interact with environmental exposures to pathogens, host responses in cytokine production to these pathogens to produce final overall outcome on sleep patterns and disease outcome.

Sickness Behavior

Intraperitoneally, intravenously, or intracerebroventricularly injected cytokines, including IL-1, IL-2, IL-6, and TNF-α, produce a set of behaviors that include decreased appetite (anorexia), decreased locomotion, loss of interest in sex, and depressed mood states. Together this pattern of behaviors, called sickness behavior, is thought to be protective from an evolutionary standpoint, as they allow the organism to conserve energy during infection. These behaviors can be blocked by cutting the vagus nerve, suggesting that activation of the vagus and vagally connected brainstem areas, including the NTS, may be a primary route by which peritoneal cytokines signal the brain. During illness rather than experimental conditions it is thought that cytokines produced by activated liver phagocytic cells such as macrophages or dendritic cells may stimulate the hepatic branches of the vagus nerve to induce sickness behaviors (31,32).

Mood

Peripheral cytokines also alter mood. Treatment of cancer or AIDS patients with IL-2 or IFN-α has been shown to profoundly affect mood, including serious depressive symptoms, as well as suicide (50–52). This side effect of treatment is the major limiting factor in the use of cytokines for treatment of immunosuppression in such patients. Patterns of symptomatology differ depending on the cytokine—in some cases (IL-2) suggesting BBB effects and some degree of organic brain syndrome, and in others (IFN-α) clinically resembling major depression. In the latter case, prophylactic treatment with antidepressants has been shown to be effective in melanoma patients treated with IFN-α (52). The effect of therapeutic doses of exogenous cytokines on mood has led some to hypothesize that endogenous CNS cytokine expression may play a pathophysiologic role in some cases of major depression.

Memory Consolidation

Cytokines such as IL-1 have been shown to play an important role in memory consolidation, particularly in forms of memory that involve the hippocampus. In such forms of memory, called context-conditioned fear learning, spatial cues provide the context for memory and for fearful events associated with place (53). Thus, IL-1 and agents that induce IL-1 impair hippocampal-dependent memory consolidation, and this impairment is prevented by treatment with IL-1 antagonists. At a cellular and electrophysiologic level, IL-1 has been shown to affect long-term potentiation, a critical component of neuronal function that occurs in the initial phases of learning and memory (54).

Activation of Neuroendocrine Stress Response

Early studies showed that the hypothalamic-pituitary-adrenal (HPA) axis was activated during viral infection or after intraperitoneal LPS injection in mice (14). Subsequent studies using recombinant IL-1 established that IL-1, injected intraperitoneally or intracerebroventricularly, induces hypothalamic production and secretion of the neuroendocrine stress hormone CRH into the hypothalamo-portal system of blood vessels (55–57). This in turn induces production and secretion from the pituitary gland of adrenocorticotropic hormone (ACTH), which in turn induces secretion of glucocorticoids (corticosterone in rodents and cortisol in humans) from the cortex of the adrenal glands (Fig. 1). Recognition that immune molecules activate specific brain regions to produce a cascade of neurohormones that ultimately suppress immune function permitted the recognition that such immune stimulation of the CNS might play an important role in physiologic regulation of the immune system. Identification of animal models in which dysregulations of this two-way communication are associated with enhanced or reduced susceptibility to autoimmune, inflammatory, allergic, or infectious disease further supported this concept. Finally, surgical or pharmacologic manipulations of neuroendocrine and neuronal response systems in animals resistant or susceptible to immune-mediated diseases confirmed the causal nature of this relationship.

CNS REGULATION OF IMMUNE SYSTEM

The nervous system regulates the immune system at multiple levels, through multiple anatomical routes and via many nervous system–derived molecules (6) (see Fig. 1). Together, the two arms of the neuroendocrine and neuronal stress, the HPA axis and the sympathetic nervous system (SNS) regulate the immune system through receptor-mediated effects of their effector molecules—neurohormones, neuropeptides, and neurotransmitters. Other components of the nervous system—including the parasympathetic nervous system and the peripheral nervous system—also provide a level of local and regional regulation of the immune system through similar receptor-mediated mechanisms.

Thus, glucocorticoid hormones (GC) secreted by the adrenal glands after HPA axis activation generally suppress immune function, providing a level of systemic negative feedback control to the immune system. At a regional level, GC are also synthesized in the thymus, and at this level play a role in lymphocyte selection during development. The autonomic nervous system regulates the immune system through sympathetic and parasympathetic nerve pathways, and innervation by these nerves of immune organs, including the spleen, lymph nodes, thymus, and bone marrow. At these sites, immune cells including lymphocytes, macrophages, dendritic cells, and mast cells may be found in close apposition to neurons that secrete neurotransmitters such as norepinephrine, acetylcholine, and serotonin. Such neurotransmitters affect immune cell function through receptor-mediated mechanisms, thus providing a regional level of regulation of immune responses. Finally, the peripheral nervous system regulates immune responses at a local level at sites of inflammation. Peripheral sensory nerves may be retrogradely activated to release neuropeptides into tissues, where these molecules also affect immune cell migration, activation, and mediator release.

Through this rich network of neuronal and hormonal connections in all tissues, the immune and nervous systems act in concert as a first-line defense against infectious, antigenic, or proinflammatory stimuli. Immune cells and neurons signal each other at all levels and with many molecules to provide a closely integrated and coordinated line of defense.

Neuroendocrine Regulation of Immune System: Glucocorticoid Effects

The final effector molecules released during activation of the HPA axis are the GC. While the anti-inflammatory effects of GC have been known since the Nobel Prize was awarded to Hench and Kendall for their discovery that GC suppress inflammation in rheumatoid arthritis, this effect was considered primarily a pharmacologic rather than physiologic one (58) until very recently. Several lines of evidence now indicate that GC play a physiologic role in immune regulation, including animal models in which GC feedback is disrupted, human studies showing an association between dysregulation of GC responses and altered immunity and *in vitro* studies examining the effects of physiologic concentrations of natural GC preparations on a variety of immune response end points. These are reviewed below and in Webster et al. (59).

Molecular Mechanisms of GC Action

The effects of GC on immunity occur through the glucocorticoid receptor (GR), an intracellular receptor that is part of the steroid hormone–receptor family of ligand-dependent transcription factors. These receptors are characterized by an N-terminal transactivation domain that includes the Tau1 domain, a DNA-binding domain, and a ligand-binding domain (Fig. 3). Once bound to ligand, the receptor dissociates from a heat-shock protein complex, translocates to the nucleus, dimerizes, binds to DNA, and activates transcription (Fig. 4). A detailed review of the effects of the molecular mechanisms and effects of GC on immunity is provided in Webster et al. (59).

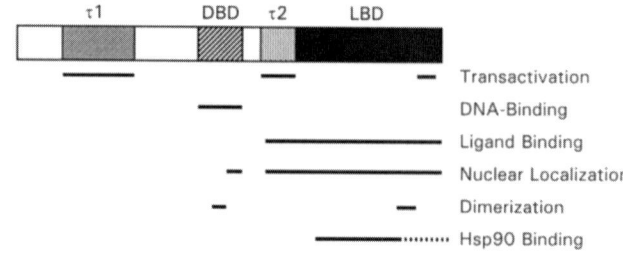

FIG. 3. Molecular structure of the glucocorticoid receptor. The areas associated with the functions of transactivation, DNA-binding, ligand binding, nuclear localization, dimerization, and Hsp90 binding are shown. From Webster et al. (59), with permission.

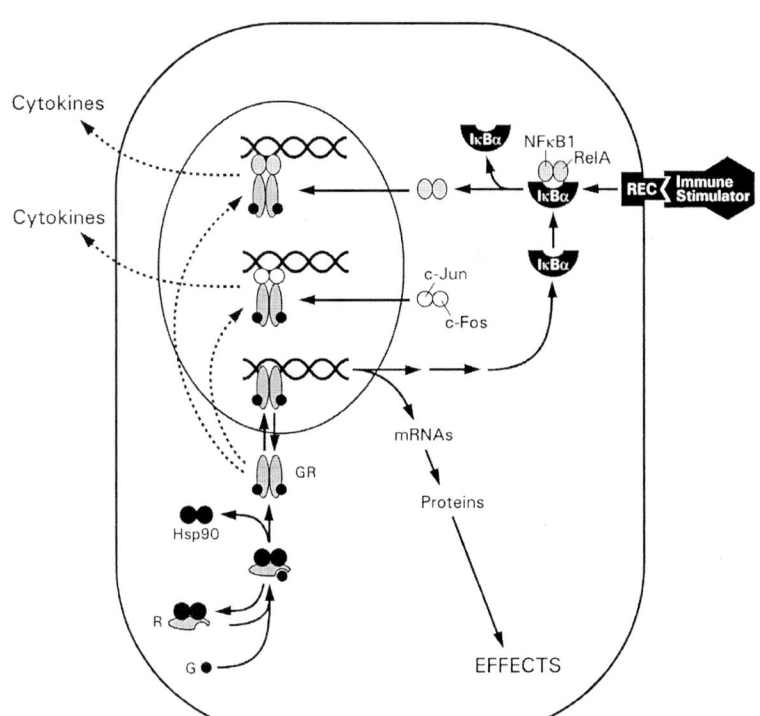

FIG. 4. Molecular mechanisms of glucocorticoid effects on immune cell function. Schematic diagram of the mechanism of action of the glucocorticoid receptor including interactions with the NFκB and AP-1 pathways. Dotted lines represent repressive pathways. From Webster et al. (59), with permission.

Effects of GC on Immune Cell Responses

In pharmacologic doses naturally occurring GC, such as corticosterone in rodents and cortisol in humans, and pharmacologic GC preparations such as dexamethasone suppress virtually every aspect of innate, as well as cellular and humoral acquired immunity (Figs. 5, 6, and 7). In physiologic concentrations, however, GC are not wholly immunosuppressive, but rather shift patterns of immune responses. The resultant effects on immunity include suppression of humoral and cellular immunity, with suppression of antibody production to immunization and delayed-type hypersensitivity. GC also alter immune cell trafficking through effects on vascular permeability, chemotaxis, and adhesion molecule expression. At a cellular level, GC alter immune cell activation, differentiation, and maturation, and play a role in apoptosis. Many of these effects are accomplished through GC effects on cytokine production.

Cytokines

GC affect the transcription of many cytokines, generally up-regulating anti-inflammatory cytokines and down-regulating proinflammatory cytokines. Thus, GC suppress the proinflammatory cytokines IL-1, IL-2, IL-6, IL-8, IL-11, IL-12, TNF-α, IFNγ, and GM-CSF and up-regulate the anti-inflammatory cytokines IL-4 and IL-10. These effects are largely mediated through repression of the transcription factor NFκB (60–62). The resultant shift from Th1 to Th2 immunity has been suggested to be due mainly to down-regulation of Th1 cytokines, allowing dominant expression of the Th2 cytokines.

Th1–Th2

Physiologic concentrations of GC shift the immune response from a Th1 to a Th2 pattern, with enhanced production of the anti-inflammatory cytokines IL-4 and IL-10 and decreased production of proinflammatory cytokines, including IFN-γ and IL-12 (63–66).

Th1 immunity or cellular immunity is characterized by expression of the proinflammatory cytokines IFN-γ, IL-2, and TNF-β. At a cellular level, a Th1 pattern is associated with differentiation of macrophages, natural killer (NK) cells and cytotoxic T cells that are involved in phagocytosis and destruction of bacteria. Th2 immunity or humoral immunity, characterized by production of the anti-inflammatory cytokines IL-4, IL-10, and IL-13, is associated with differentiation of eosinophils, mast cells, and B cells, and antibody-mediated defense against foreign antigens. IL-12, the main inducer of Th1 immunity, induces IFN-γ and inhibits IL-4. GC have also been shown to differentially affect the survival of Th1 and Th2 cells. Thus, Th2 NK1.1^{+} T cells that produce IL-4 are resistant to dexamethasone-induced apoptosis due to the expression of the proto-oncogene Bcl-2.

Cell Adhesion Molecules and Immune Cell Trafficking

GC reduce leucocyte trafficking to areas of inflammation via down-regulation of protein molecules involved in chemoattraction and adhesion. Thus, GC inhibit the expression of intracellular adhesion molecule 1 (ICAM-1), endothelial-leukocyte adhesion molecule 1 (ELAM-1) and vascular adhesion molecule 1 (VCAM-1), in part through GR-mediated repression of NFκB. GC also suppress expression of the

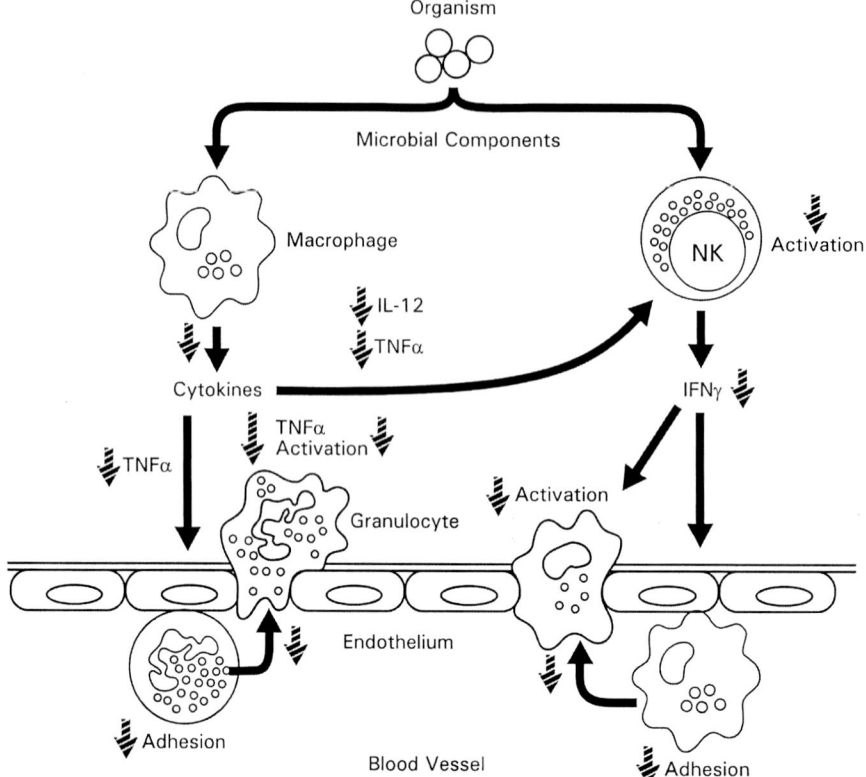

FIG. 5. Effects of glucocorticoids on innate immunity. Schematic diagram representing glucocorticoid effects on innate immunity. *Downward (hatched) arrows* show aspects of innate immunity that have been shown to be suppressed by glucocorticoids, including IL-12, IFNγ, and TNF-α production.

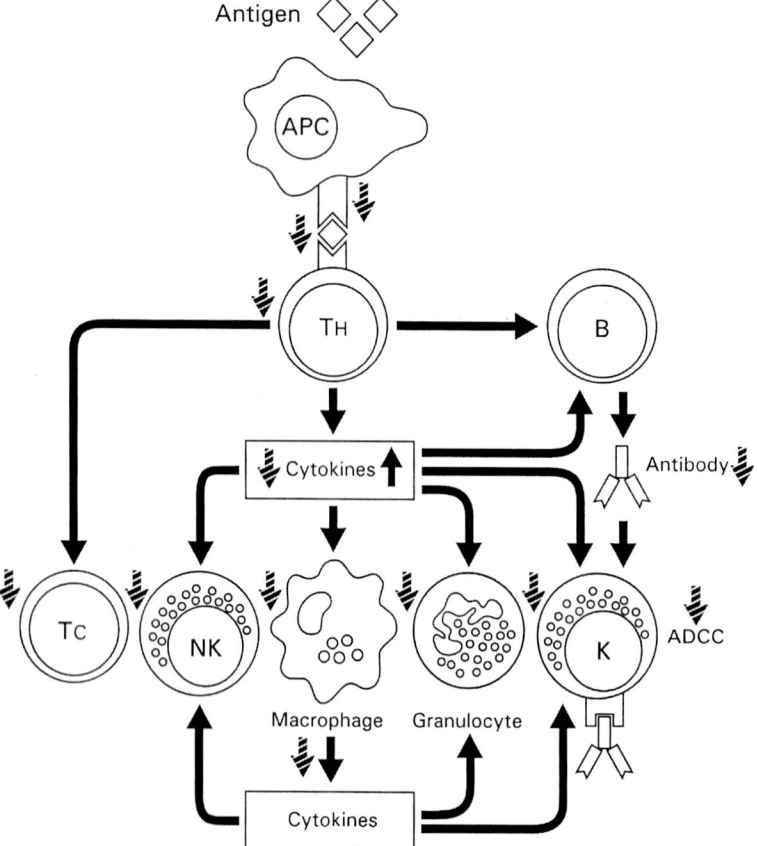

FIG. 6. Effects of glucocorticoids on cell-mediated immunity. Schematic diagram representing glucocorticoid effects on cell-mediated immunity. *Downward (hatched) arrows* show aspects of cell-mediated immunity that have been shown to be suppressed by glucocorticoids.

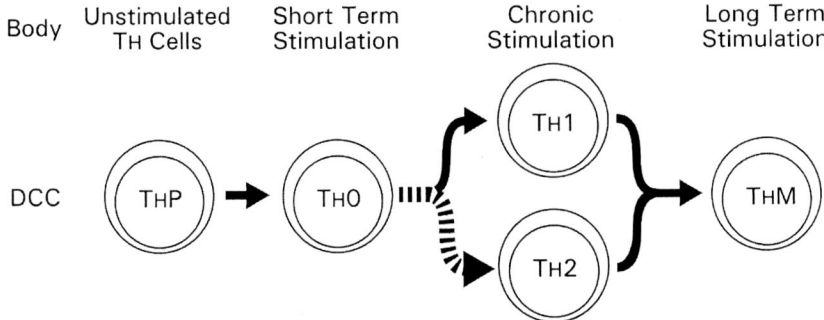

ThP	ThO	Th1	Th2	ThM
⇩IL-2	⇩INFγ ⇩IL-2 ⬆IL-4 ⬆IL-5 ⬆IL-10	⇩IFNγ ⇩IL-2	⬆IL-4 ⬆IL-5 ⇩IL-6 ⬆IL-10	⇩IL-2

Cytokines Released

FIG. 7. Effects of glucocorticoids on differentiation of T cells. Schematic diagram representing glucocorticoid (GC) effects on T-cell differentiation. *Downward (open) arrows* show cytokines that are suppressed by GC, including IL-2 and IL-6 and IFNγ. *Upward (closed) arrows* show cytokines that have been shown to be increased by GC, including IL-4, IL-5, and IL-10. This differential effect of GC causes a shift (*speckled arrow*) from a TH1 to a TH2 pattern of immunity.

endothelial cell-surface adhesion molecule E-selectin and bone-marrow and polymorphonuclear cell L-selectin (67–69).

Chemoattractants and Cell Migration

GC suppress a variety of molecules important in chemoattraction and cell migration. Thus, through suppression of IL-1β via NFκB, GC suppress cytokine-induced neutrophil chemoattractant (CINC)/growth-related oncogene (Gro), which is important for accumulating neutrophils at sites of inflammation (68). GC also suppress the eosinophil chemoattractants IL-5 in mast cells and T cells, RANTES in T cells, and Eotaxin in bronchial airways (70–72). The cytokines monocyte chemoattractant protein 1 (MCP-1), MCP-2, and MCP-3 have also been shown to be down-regulated by dexamethasone (73).

Production of Inflammatory Mediators

GC reduce production of inflammatory mediators including prostaglandins and nitric oxide by suppressing several enzymes involved in the synthesis of these molecules, including cytosolic PLA$_2$ and COX-2 mRNA (74), nitric oxide synthase II (NOS II), and inducible nitric oxide synthase (iNOS), the latter by the induction of IκB (75). In contrast to this suppressive effect of GC on proinflammatory mediators, GC increase externalization and synthesis of the anti-inflammatory molecule lipocortin 1 (or annexin 1). Lipocortin 1 is expressed in immune cells as well as in the neuroendocrine system, in the hypothalamus and pituitary, and exerts its anti-inflammatory action in the periphery by inhibition of arachadonic acid release and prostaglandin synthesis.

Neutrophils

GC affect neutrophil activation and function, including chemotaxis, adhesion, transmigration, apoptosis, and phagocytosis (76). Although these GC effects occur through regulation of many cytokines, lipocortin 1 plays a pivotal role in these effects on neutrophils. Pharmacologic doses suppress neutrophil activation and migration but increase circulating numbers of neutrophils through inhibition of apoptosis.

Monocytes

In contrast to their relative lack of effect on resting resident macrophages, GC suppress the protective and defense mechanisms of activated macrophages. Pharmacologic or stress levels of GC reduce circulating numbers of monocytes, inhibit secretion of IL-1, IL-6, TNF-α, and monocyte chemotractic-activating factors, and suppress components of macrophage activation, including collagenase, elastase, and tissue plasminogen–activator synthesis (77).

Eosinophils, Basophils, and Mast Cells

Pharmacologic doses of GC reduce circulating numbers of eosinophils through suppression of IL-5, IL-3, and GM-CSF, sequester eosinophils in primary and secondary lymphoid tissues, induce apoptosis, and inhibit eosinophil recruitment to areas of inflammation. GC reduce circulating numbers of basophils, inhibit basophil migration, reduce number of mast cells in airways, and impair basophil histamine and leukotriene release (78,79).

Resident Tissue Immune Cells

GC have been shown to affect resident tissue cells involved in antigen presentation and inflammation. Thus, GC reduce numbers of dendritic cells (80), inhibit the expression of cytokines, chemoattractants, and mediators of inflammation expressed in airway epithelial cells and inhibit the expression of MUC2 and MUC5AC in mucosal cells (81).

Effects of Glucocorticoids on Lymphocyte Selection at Cellular and Regional Immune Organ Level

In addition to these systemic effects of GC on most aspects of immune cell function in adults, GC also play an important regional role in regional lymphocyte selection in immune organs during development. This regional control occurs in part through local GC production within immune organs—for example, the thymus—and via several molecular and cellular mechanisms, including apoptosis and thymocyte differentiation. Fluctuations of systemic GC levels resulting from circadian physiologic variations and stress-induced increases in GC secretion are associated with shifts in patterns of immune response and effects on immune-mediated processes and diseases.

Apoptosis and Cell Cycle Arrest

GC induce G1 arrest and apoptosis (programmed cell death) in immune cells through several mechanisms, depending on the cell type. Cell cycle genes such as c-Myc, cyclin D3, and Cdk4, and the cyclin-dependent kinase inhibitor, p57^{Kip2}, mediate GC effects on cell cycle arrest (82–84). Glucocorticoid-induced apoptosis in proliferating and nonproliferating thymocytes is mediated via different mechanisms with some common features, including activation of caspases. Thus, GC-induced transcription of IκB or other similar inhibitory factors lead to apoptosis in T cells via repression of transcription of the c-Myc gene. In monocytes, increased expression of the death receptor, CD95, mediates GC-induced apoptosis through activation of a cascade involving caspase 8 and caspase 3 (85).

Thymic Regulation of T-Cell Selection

The thymus contains the entire enzymatic machinery for GC synthesis (86). Evidence from in vitro, knockout, and transgenic animal models indicate that this local GC production by thymic epithelial cells plays an important role in T-cell selection during development. It is not known whether intrathymic GC synthesis is under the same sort of regulatory control by the pituitary gland and hypothalamus as is adrenal GC synthesis. It has been suggested that GC regulate thymic

T-cell selection through a model of "mutual antagonism" in which GC up- or down-regulate the intensity of T-cell receptor (TCR) signaling (87). In this model, positive selection occurs when there is a balance between GC signaling and TCR avidity for self-antigen and MHC. The relative concentration of GC and antigen to which a T cell is exposed would then determine whether it dies by neglect or apoptosis. At higher concentrations of GC, a higher TCR avidity is needed for positive selection to occur. Negative selection occurs in the absence of such high TCR avidity and antigen. At lower levels of GC, cells that would otherwise have been positively selected die from apoptosis, as at these lower GC concentrations TCR signaling is enhanced.

Pathophysiologic Role of HPA Axis and GC Dysregulation in Pathogenesis of Immune-Mediated Diseases

Given the wide range of effects of GC on virtually all aspects of immunity, it is not surprising that these hormones play an important physiologic role in immune regulation, that when disrupted leads to disease. In physiologic situations GC effects on immune and inflammatory responses provide an extraimmune system level of control of immune responses, and a shut-off signal to prevent inflammation and immune activation from continuing once the initial stimulus has been cleared. Pathologic situations result when the GC response is insufficient or excessive. Thus, insufficient GC responses are associated with predisposition to inflammatory or autoimmune disease, and excess GC production, as occurs in chronic stress, predisposes to infectious diseases and other sequelae of immunosuppression (6,88).

Hypothalamic Pituitary Adrenal Axis

The physiologic level of GC is tightly controlled through secretion of a cascade of hormones initiated by secretion of corticotrophin-releasing hormone (CRH) from the paraventricular nucleus of the hypothalamus. CRH release into the pituitary portal–blood vessel system in turn results in secretion of ACTH from the anterior pituitary gland. This in turn stimulates secretion of cortisol (corticosterone in rodents) from the adrenal cortex. Hypothalamic CRH is the main CNS stress hormone, and the neurons of the paraventricular nucleus are closely connected to many other brain stress centers, including the brainstem noradrenergic system (89). These centers receive inputs from virtually all other parts of the brain, including sensory signals from the visual and auditory systems, signals from memory centers such as the hippocampus, and regions activated by peripheral cytokine signals (31,57). Through these pathways, plasma GC levels are continuously and exquisitely attuned to fluctuations in physical, psychological, and physiologic environmental stimuli. Such changes in the external environment to which the body must adapt are termed stressors, and can induce increases in plasma cortisol within 3 to 5 minutes. GC secretion also varies in a circadian fashion throughout the day, with its peak in the morning and nadir in the evening. This variation could contribute to daily fluctuations in immune responses seen in autoimmune/inflammatory illnesses such as rheumatoid arthritis, or changes in symptoms of such illnesses during stress.

Regulation of Immune Responses by HPA Axis under Physiologic Conditions

Animal and human studies have shown that various immune responses, including plasma cytokine levels, patterns of whole blood cytokine production, and T-cell subset and NK cell numbers and activity, vary in relation to both circadian and stress variations in plasma GC levels (90). Exercise is one physiologic condition that has been extensively used to study the effects on various aspects of immune function of controlled, graded, and quantitative HPA axis activation. In general, exercise is associated with shifts in numbers and ratios of CD4/CD8 lymphocytes in peripheral blood, shifts in patterns of cytokine production, and changes in NK cell activity (91,92). In addition to exercise, administration of physiologic preparations of GC, such as hydrocortisone, have also been shown to be associated in a dose-related manner with similar altered patterns of immune responses. In these conditions, it appears that some cytokines (IL-1 and TNF-α) are more sensitive than others to suppression by lower concentrations of GC (90). Circadian variations of GC levels, with high morning and low evening cortisol in humans are also associated with similar but less marked shifts in patterns of cytokine production, in concert with the smaller differences in GC levels that occur during circadian changes than during exercise.

It is difficult to evaluate the precise contribution of the HPA axis and GC alone to the mechanism of the effects of exercise on immune function, since exercise also activates many other stress response systems, including the adrenergic SNS, that are known to directly affect immune function. Furthermore, while studies of relationships between GC levels and patterns of immune responses are suggestive of the importance of these factors in regulating immune responses under normal physiologic conditions, they do not prove that GC fluctuations play a causal role in modulating immune responses under pathologic conditions.

Pathologic Conditions Associated with Dysregulation of HPA Axis: HPA Axis Hyporesponsiveness and Susceptibility to Autoimmune/Inflammatory Disease

The best evidence that HPA axis activation and resultant GC secretion plays a physiologic role in immune regulation is derived from animal models in which the HPA axis is disrupted on either a genetic basis or with pharmacologic or surgical interventions (93). The direct effects of such interventions on immune/inflammatory disease expression and susceptibility in these animal models suggests that the relationship between immune-mediated diseases and blunted or excessive GC secretion in humans is more likely causal than simply the result of coincidental association.

Insufficient activation of the HPA axis is associated with enhanced susceptibility to and severity of a variety of autoimmune/inflammatory diseases in both animal models and in humans. An association between blunted HPA axis responses and susceptibility to a wide range of autoimmune/inflammatory and allergic disease has been shown across species, in chickens, mice, rats, and humans. Thus, hypo-HPA axis responsiveness has been shown in chickens that develop spontaneous thyroiditis or a scleroderma-like illness (94), in certain strains of mice (MRL) that develop systemic lupus erythematosus (SLE) (95), and in rats that are susceptible to inflammatory arthritis, experimental allergic encephalomyelitis (EAE), thyroiditis, uveitis, adrenalitis, inflammatory bowel disease, and many other experimentally induced inflammatory diseases (96,97). Similarly blunted HPA axis responses have been shown in humans with SLE (98), rheumatoid arthritis (99–101), multiple sclerosis (102), Sjogren's syndrome (103), fibromyalgia, chronic fatigue syndrome (104,105), allergic dermatitis, and asthma (106) (Table 1).

In order to detect such differences in HPA axis responsiveness, it is necessary to stimulate the HPA axis and measure GC or ACTH responses over a full time period after stimulation. Single time–point measures and baseline unstimulated measures that do not activate the HPA axis or measure total hormone secretion over a given time period will not identify individual variations in responsiveness of the HPA axis. It is possibly for this reason that associations between a blunted HPA axis response and autoimmune/inflammatory disease went undetected for decades after the pharmacologic anti-inflammatory effects of GC were discovered.

In animals, immune/proinflammatory stimuli have been used to activate the HPA axis, including bacterial products such as LPS, streptococcal cell walls (SCW), and immune stimuli such as IL-1 (107). In addition, physiologic stimuli such as insulin hypoglycemia, and a variety of stressful stimuli including restraint, novel environments, swim stress, or startle have also been used. In humans, ovine CRH, insulin hypoglycemia, and psychologic stress of public speaking and mental arithmetic have all been used to activate the HPA axis response in subjects with autoimmune, allergic, or inflammatory disease.

TABLE 1. *Low hormonal stress response*

	Inflammatory/autoimmune disease
Chicken	Thyroiditis scleroderma
Mouse	SLE
Rat	Arthritis, EAE, septic shock, inflammation
Human	Rheumatoid arthritis, SLE, Sjogren's, dermatitis, asthma

EAE, experimental allergic encephalomyelitis; SLE, systemic lupus erthematosus.

Rat strains that have been shown to exhibit differential HPA-axis responsiveness include hyper-HPA axis-responsive Fischer (F344/N) and hypo-HPA axis-responsive Lewis (LEW/N) rats. Mouse strains that show such differential HPA axis responsiveness include hyper-HPA axis-responsive BALBc and relatively hypo-HPA axis-responsive C57BL/6J (108). It is important to note that in such studies the degree to which HPA axis responses vary between strains differs in relation to the precise nature and duration of the stressor. In studies in which HPA axis responsiveness has been compared to inflammatory disease susceptibility, animal strains susceptible to autoimmune/inflammatory disease or human subjects with a history of such illnesses, show a blunted HPA axis response compared to controls.

Genetic Animal Models of Blunted HPA Axis and Susceptibility to Autoimmune Inflammatory Disease

Genetic linkage and segregation studies have shown that susceptibility to autoimmune/inflammatory diseases such as inflammatory arthritis in rats, systemic lupus erythematosus in mice, and experimental allergic encephalomyelitis in rodents, is multigenic and polygenic. That is, many genes, each of which has small effect, contribute to susceptibility and resistance to such complex diseases. In the case of inflammatory arthritis, over 20 regions of 15 different chromosomes contribute to disease susceptibility (109). In murine models of SLE, four regions on four separate chromosomes contribute additively to the phenotype expression (110). That is, inheritance of such disease susceptibility–conferring regions contributes to disease expression in an almost dose-related manner, with inheritance of any combination of regions predisposing increasingly to disease expression as the number of regions inherited increases.

Genetic linkage and segregation studies in inflammatory-susceptible and -resistant inbred rat strains that also exhibit differential HPA axis responsiveness indicate an inflammatory resistance–linkage region on rat chromosome 10 (syntenic with human chromosome 17) that contains several interesting candidate genes involved in HPA axis regulation, including the CRH receptor type 1 and angiotensin-converting enzyme (ACE) (111,112). However, no mutation was identified in the coding region of the CRH receptor in these strains, and a mutation located near one active site of ACE did not functionally relate to the inflammatory resistance phenotype. Such findings indicate the complexity of relating disease-determining genetic factors in complex multigenic and polygenic illnesses such as inflammatory disease.

In such studies, in general approximately 35% of quantitative trait variance is related to genotypic factors, while approximately 65% of variance is related to environmental factors (111). Thus, the degree of susceptibility to autoimmune/inflammatory disease expression in any individual is determined by the load of disease predisposing and protective genes inherited, combined with the modifying effects of predisposing and protective environmental factors. Such factors may move an individual up or down a spectrum of disease expression toward or away from a threshold at which disease expression occurs (110).

In this context, neural and neuroendocrine factors are only a few of many genetic factors that determine susceptibility and resistance to autoimmune/inflammatory disease. However, since neural and neuroendocrine responses are so exquisitely responsive to environmental perturbations, they could play an important role in transducing many environmental variations to affect expression or susceptibility in such illness-prone individuals.

Surgical or Pharmacologic Interruption of Hypothalamic Pituitary Adrenal Axis: Effects on Autoimmune/Inflammatory Disease

Several animal models exist in which a blunted HPA axis response is associated with autoimmune/inflammatory disease. Obese chickens that develop spontaneous thyroiditis (94) and some strains of mice (MRL) that develop spontaneous SLE exhibit blunted HPA axis responses (95). It is, however, difficult to definitively prove the causal relationship between blunted HPA axis responses and disease expression in such models of spontaneous autoimmune/inflammatory disease, since inflammation itself can alter HPA axis responses. This confounding is avoided in animal models of experimentally induced autoimmune/inflammatory disease, in which healthy, noninflamed rats known to be susceptible to development of a range of proinflammatory or antigenically induced autoimmune/inflammatory diseases, also exhibit blunted HPA axis responses.

LEW/N rats are an inbred strain that is both highly susceptible to development of a range of autoimmune/inflammatory diseases and exhibits blunted HPA axis responses to a wide variety of proinflammatory and stress stimuli. In contrast, F344/N rats are largely histocompatible with LEW/N rats, exhibit hyper-HPA axis responses and are largely resistant to development of autoimmune inflammatory disease in response to the same antigenic or proinflammatory stimuli. The existence of such associations in inbred rodent strains allows genetic, pharmacologic, and surgical manipulations that can be used to precisely define and provide strong evidence for the causal relationship between interruptions of the HPA axis and susceptibility to autoimmune/inflammatory diseases.

Interruption of the HPA axis of the HPA hyperresponsive, inflammatory-resistant strains renders such animals highly susceptible to the proinflammatory effects of antigenic and proinflammatory stimuli, particularly to mortality from septic shock. Thus, hypophysectomy, adrenalectomy, or treatment with the GC receptor antagonist RU486 of resistant rats exposed to SCW, salmonella, or myelin basic protein results in greatly increased incidence of mortality from septic shock (up to 100%) (97,113,114). Surviving animals exhibit inflammatory disease. These effects of HPA axis blockade or disruption can be partially or wholly prevented in a dose-related manner by treatment with physiologic doses of GC. Similarly, the greatly increased mortality in GC-receptor antagonist-treated mice infected with MMCV virus is also reversed by treatment with GC (115). Finally, reconstitution of the HPA axis by intracerebroventricular transplantation of hypothalamic tissue from inflammatory-resistant F344/N rats into inflammatory-susceptible LEW/N rats results in more than 85% reduction in peripheral inflammation compared to controls in a carrageenan model of innate inflammation (116).

GC Resistance and Inflammatory/Autoimmune Disease

Another mechanism by which the immunosuppressive/anti-inflammatory effects of GC may be impaired is through GC resistance (117). This may result from inherited genetic mutations of GC-receptor or GR-associated factors and may also develop during chronic inflammation through increased expression of a nonfunctional soluble form of the GC receptor, GR-β. Thus, excess GR-β expression has been reported in chronic asthma in which GC resistance has developed (118,119). A mutation of the GR associated with increased stability of the GR-β is seen in rheumatoid arthritis and SLE patients in excess of controls and could potentially play a role in expression of these illnesses in some individuals (120).

Pathologic Conditions Associated with Dysregulation of HPA Axis: Excess HPA Axis Activity, Stress Effects on Immune-Mediated Diseases

While inadequate neuroendocrine stress responsiveness and subsequent lack of GC-negative feedback on immune responses predisposes to inflammation, excessive GC production—as occurs during stress—tends to suppress immune and inflammatory responses and predispose to infection. The effects of stress on immunity and immune-mediated diseases depend on several characteristics of the stressful stimulus dose (the intensity of the stressor), frequency, and duration. The total amount of stress sensed by an organism over a period of time has been termed "allostatic load" (121). The higher the intensity, the more frequent and the longer the duration of the stressful stimuli, the greater the allostatic load the individual will experience and the more likely it will be that the stressful situation will have an effect on health. Whether a given stressor will affect immune responses and health depends in part on duration of the stressful stimulus. Since the time course of activation of nervous system responses to external stimuli is on the order of milliseconds to seconds, while the time course of the effects of stress hormones on immune response systems occurs over minutes, hours, and days, it is more likely that a stressor of longer duration will have an effect on immunity and health.

In addition to these characteristics of the stressor, a number of characteristics of the host also play a role in determining the effects of stress on immune responses and disease. These include gender (122–124) and overall nutritional status. Initial studies on the effects of sex hormones and gender on both behavioral and physiologic aspects of stress responses indicate that these factors play an important role in overall stress response patterns and therefore will likely play an important role in the effects of stress on disease expression. Nutritional stress (loss of over 10% body weight in a period of weeks) compounds the deleterious effects of other stressors on suppression and infectious disease susceptibility (125).

In addition to these physiologic characteristics of stressors that determine their effects on immune responses and disease are the specific components of the stress response systems that become activated by different stressful stimuli. Thus, while when Hans Selye defined the term "stress" in the 1950s as a nonspecific response of the body to any demand, it is now clear that different kinds of stressful stimuli activate different neural pathways in a more specific manner than was previously thought (126,127). Thus, in rodent studies, physiologic stresses such as exercise and hemorrhage have been shown to activate different brain regions than psychogenic stress, such as pain. The degree to which the HPA axis and the other arm of the stress response, the SNS, are differentially activated by different sorts of stressors remains to be fully defined, especially in human studies (128,129).

Stress Effects on Viral or Bacterial Infection: Animal Models

Numerous animal studies have addressed the effects of stress on infection. The precise effect of activation of these stress response systems on the course of the viral infection is related to the mechanism by which the virus causes illness. If the illness is caused by the organism's inflammatory response to the viral infection, such as in influenza pneumonia, some degree of anti-inflammatory effects of GC may be beneficial, while excess immune suppression from excess GC will allow unrestrained viral replication and pathology related to increased viral load. Thus, adrenalectomized mice exposed to MMCV die from septic shock (115), and replacement of GC in physiologic doses prevents mortality and this excessive inflammatory response. Different kinds of stressful stimuli, such as physical (restraint) versus social stress, also exert differential effects on different kinds of viral infections, probably in relation to their differential activation of neuroendocrine, sympathetic, and other neural stress response systems (130,131). Thus, restraint stress in mice is associated with rapid death from influenza virus. In contrast, restraint stress has minimal effect on herpes viral infection in mice, while social stress is associated with exacerbation of herpes virus infection, in part through nerve growth factor–mediated mechanisms. Susceptibility and resistance to *Mycobacterium tuberculosis* is also affected by GC. In mycobacterial-resistant mice, GC accelerate mRNA decay of the mycobacterial-resistance gene Nramp1, thus leading to enhanced susceptibility to disease (132,133). These effects of GC and HPA axis activation on mycobacterial infection in animals are consistent with known effects of GC treatment in exacerbation and reactivation of tuberculosis in humans.

Stress Effects on Delayed Type Hypersensitivity: Animal Models

In contrast to the immunosuppressive effects of chronic stress or high-dose GC predisposing to infection, acute stress or low-dose GC enhance delayed-type hypersensitivity (DTH) (134,135). Thus, low-dose corticosterone treatment of adrenalectomized mice or acute stress enhanced the DTH skin reaction and increased numbers of sensitized T cells in draining lymph nodes, suggesting that acute stress may redirect lymphocyte trafficking to the skin. This effect may be in part mediated by IFN-γ (136).

Human Disease: Chronic Stress and Immune System–Mediated Disease

Animal and *in vitro* studies such as those outlined in the previous section provide mechanisms for and strengthen evidence that stress predisposes human subjects to greater susceptibility to and severity of infection. A number of interventional and survey studies indicate that chronic stress in humans is associated with increased susceptibility to and severity of viral infections (common cold, influenza), decreased antibody production to vaccine, and prolonged wound healing (137–141). In general, chronic or subacute stresses are more likely to be associated with such effects. Stressful situations that have been found to be associated with such effects include chronic caregivers of Alzheimer's patients, medical students undergoing exam stress, and army rangers undergoing extreme exercise training over a 3-week period (125,142). Acute studies of arguments between spouses show suppressive effects on immune cell function related to differences in duration of elevation of stress hormones. In this latter case, gender differences were observed in confrontation style, duration of hormone elevation and immune suppression, with females tending to show greater immune suppression associated with their more sustained hormone responses, which continued after the end of the argument (139).

Stress effects on allergic disease may be divided into acute and chronic effects. Chronic stress effects on asthma may include enhanced susceptibility to infection through mechanisms described above. In addition, during chronic inflammation in illnesses such as asthma, increased production of the GR-β is associated with development of some degree of GC resistance (119,143), and potentially less suppression of inflammation by either intrinsic or extrinsic GC. Hypersensitization of neuronal circuits exposed to allergens or inflammatory mediators (discussed in the next section) can lead to increased sensitivity to many stimuli and resulting increased bronchospasm in response to acute stress in asthma (144). Human studies provide evidence that such circuits do play a role in exacerbation of symptoms of asthma in children in relation to sad states, and improvement of symptoms during happy states induced by watching an emotionally uplifting movie (145) (see next section).

Autonomic Nervous System—Immune System Interactions

The CNS not only regulates the immune system through neuroendocrine routes but also via both sympathetic and parasympathetic nerves of the autonomic nervous system.

Sympathetic Nervous System

The SNS is composed of nerves that originate in the brain stem and synapse through ganglia located along the spinal cord. The main sympathetic neurotransmitter is norepinephrine, and the main sympathetic neuropeptide is neuropeptide Y (NPY). The adrenal medulla is a glandular component of the SNS that releases epinephrine (adrenalin) into the bloodstream during stress activation. Together, adrenalin released from the adrenal medulla, and norepinephrine and NPY released from nerve terminals, produce a variety of effects during stress. These include increased heart rate and peripheral vasoconstriction with resultant increased blood pressure and diversion of blood flow away from skin and to muscles—a pattern of cardiovascular response known as a "threat" pattern (146). The effects of activation of the SNS together with behavioral responses resulting from activation of the HPA axis produce the physiologic stress response commonly known as the "fight-or-flight" response.

Parasympathetic Nervous System

The system of nerves that make up the parasympathetic nervous system also originates in the brain stem, but synapse through ganglia located within or near organs they innervate. The major nerve of the parasympathetic nervous system is the vagus nerve and its main neurotransmitter is acetylcholine (ACh). The vagus nerve both sends signals to and receives signals from the CNS, and innervates the gut, liver, spleen, lungs, and heart. The parasympathetic nervous system also innervates the skin, sweat glands, and internal organs including the uterus and bladder. The vagus nerve is tonically active and provides a brake to the system, tending to slow heart rate and reduce blood pressure. Removal of the brake by inhibition of vagal tone, as occurs during a stress response, is the fastest way to increase heart rate and blood flow and activate the stress response (146). This occurs on the order of milliseconds, compared to sympathetic activation that occurs on the order of seconds, and HPA axis activation that occurs on the order of minutes. Frontal cortex brain regions projecting through descending pathways to brainstem vagal parasympathetic centers provide a route by which higher brain functions can alter cardiac performance and this component of the stress response (147). The pattern of enhanced cardiac performance and reduced peripheral resistance seen during vagal activation is known as a "challenge" response.

Autonomic Innervation of Immune Organs

Immune organs, including the spleen, thymus, lymph nodes, and bone marrow, are innervated by both the sympathetic and parasympathetic nervous system (148–151), although sympathetic noradrenergic and NPY innervation predominates in these lymphoid tissues. Within these organs immune cells are in close apposition to nerve endings. Evidence that neurotransmitters such as norepinephrine and ACh released from these nerves play an important role in regulating immune responses and disease expression is derived from both *in vitro* and *in vivo* pharmacologic studies, ablation studies, and studies in specific targeted mutant mice.

During stress, both circulating catecholamines (epinephrine) and norepinephrine and NPY released from nerve terminals within lymphoid organs, alter immune cell function through adrenergic receptors on the surface of these cells. This in turn affects the severity and course of diseases mediated by the immune system, including DTH and viral, mycobacterial, and bacterial infections (reviewed in Elenkov et al. [152]).

Autonomic Neurotransmitter Receptors on Immune Cells

Numerous studies show that virtually all immune cells, including macrophages and lymphocytes, express adrenergic receptors and cholinergic receptors. The effects of the adrenergic neurotransmitters norepinephrine and epinephrine are mediated through the various subtypes of alpha- and beta-adrenergic receptors (alpha-1 and -2 and beta-1, -2, and -3). These seven transmembrane protein receptors are G-protein subunit coupled receptors that activate protein kinase A and cAMP or PLC and inositol phospholipid metabolism.

In vivo and *in vitro* data indicate that the SNS and its neurotransmitters play a role in many aspects of immune cell development, activation, and function, including mitogen-induced T-lymphocyte proliferation; antigen-specific B-cell function; type 1–helper T-cell function; lymphocyte migration and trafficking; NK cell activity and macrophage phagocytosis; and chemotaxis, chemokine, cytokine, and nitric oxide production (153–155). Like GC, sympathetic neural factors, including norepinephrine, adrenalin, and the sympathetic neuropeptides, cause a shift of immune response pattern from a Th1- to a Th2-type response (152).

Sympathetic Nervous System Interruptions and Immune Disease

The role of regional immune organ–sympathetic innervation in immune-mediated disease is evidenced by studies in which the sympathetic innervation to such organs is disrupted by pharmacologic, chemical, or surgical ablation. In such cases, the effect depends on the location of the interruption (156–159)—systemic, regional, or local—as well as the method used to interrupt the SNS. Thus, systemic pharmacologic beta-adrenergic blockade is associated with decreased arthritis activity in adjuvant-treated rats (158). In contrast, regional interruption of sympathetic innervation to lymph nodes is associated with enhanced inflammation (160). Both experimental interruption of the sympathetic innervation of the spleen and the age-related dying back of splenic sympathetic nervous innervation are associated with blunted, splenic immune-cell responses (161). Conversely, reinnervation of splenic sympathetic nerves that occurs after treatment with tricyclic antidepressant deprenyl reconstitutes these impaired immune responses (162). The reasons for these discrepancies are not clear. In the case of chemical sympathectomy, the initial massive release of adrenergic neurotransmitters followed by depletion may alter subsequent immune cell sensitivity to adrenergic neurotransmitters. Dysregulation of beta-adrenergic responses have also been shown in human autoimmune/inflammatory illnesses and fatigue states, including juvenile rheumatoid arthritis (163,164) and chronic fatigue syndrome (165).

Relative Role of HPA Axis and Sympathetic Nervous System in Inflammation and Septic Shock

Activation of stress response systems also differentially affects the course of bacterial infections, depending on the organism's immune defense mechanisms that are recruited in response to the particular bacteria involved. Both GC responses and adrenergic responses appear to be involved in protection against inflammatory tissue damage and septic shock induced by a variety of gram-negative or gram-positive bacteria and other inflammatory agents. As described above, adrenalectomized or hypophysectomized rats or rats treated with GR antagonists, show greatly increased mortality rates in response to bacterial products such as salmonella, SCW, or bacterial LPS. Treatment with GC reverses this effect. Similarly, A2a-adenosine receptor–deficient knockout mice show greatly enhanced bacterial LPS-induced septic shock as well as greater hepatotoxicity when exposed to Con A or *Pseudomonas aeruginosa* exotoxin compared to wild-type controls. Pharmacologic agents that activate adenosine A2a receptors prevent both hepatic damage and increased macrophage TNF production in these knockout mice. Furthermore, adenosine A2a antagonists greatly enhance inflammatory tissue damage in wild-type mice (166). These data indicate that G-coupled adenosine receptors, including activation of beta-adrenergic receptors that stimulate cAMP accumulation, are an important natural termination signal for inflammation.

Pharmacologic studies in rodents using specific GC and adrenergic receptor antagonists indicate that both the HPA axis and SNS responses activated during stress alter the course, severity, and pattern of expression of viral infections, including influenza, hepatitis, and herpes virus (131,167,168). Thus, neither GR antagonists alone nor adrenergic antagonists alone completely block the effects of restraint stress on the course and severity of influenza infection in mice; however, together they prevent the increased mortality seen in mice subjected to restraint and simultaneously exposed to influenza virus.

Cholinergic Autonomic Nervous System Responses and Immune-Mediated Diseases

Cholinergic receptors are present on immune cells, and cholinergic agonists and antagonists alter immune cell function (169). The degree to which immune organs are innervated by cholinergic neurons and the role that such innervation may play in regulating immune function is not clear. However, recent studies suggest that parasympathetic autonomic neural circuits in both lung and gut may contribute to both enhanced sensitivity to inflammatory signals in these organs and enhanced responsiveness of these organs to autonomic stimulation (144) (Fig. 8).

In this paradigm, antigenic, allergic or proinflammatory stimuli in bronchial or gut lumen may retrogradely activate autonomic nerve endings resulting in release of autonomic neurotransmitters. Locally these neurotransmitters are generally proinflammatory. Simultaneously, action potentials are carried up to the CNS, activating a reflex loop through synapses in the brain stem. Action potentials then carried down the afferent arm of this loop activate not only neurons synapsing in autonomic ganglia, but also cause mast cell release of mediators within the ganglia. Mediators released,

such as histamine, further sensitize ganglionic neurons. Action potentials then propagated along autonomic nerves finally result in release of autonomic neurotransmitters into gut or bronchial smooth muscle, producing increased smooth muscle contractility of these organs. In this paradigm, hypersensitivity of both ascending and descending circuits due to excess release of these neurotransmitters contributes to and amplifies many of the motor symptoms of illnesses such as inflammatory and irritable bowel disease and bronchial asthma.

The contribution of brainstem centers such as Barrington's nucleus in these hyperirritable reflex loops has also been suggested (170). Barrington's nucleus lies close to the locus ceruleus, an important noradrenergic sympathetic center within the brain stem. The locus ceruleus becomes activated during stress and both receives signals from and sends signals to the hypothalamus through neuronal connections and CRH nerve pathways. Thus, these neural connections represent an area of convergence between the brain's neuroendocrine CRH-related stress centers and HPA axis and brainstem sympathetic nuclei, providing a neuroanatomical basis for coordination between these two major stress response systems. Barrington's nucleus also receives signals from and sends signals to the uterus, gut, and bladder, which suggests that it could be one of the brainstem areas that plays a role in coordination of pelvic viscera function. If hypersensitized reflex loops, such as those described above, develop in response to antigenic infectious agent or allergen exposure in these organs, such neural pathways could provide a neuroanatomical

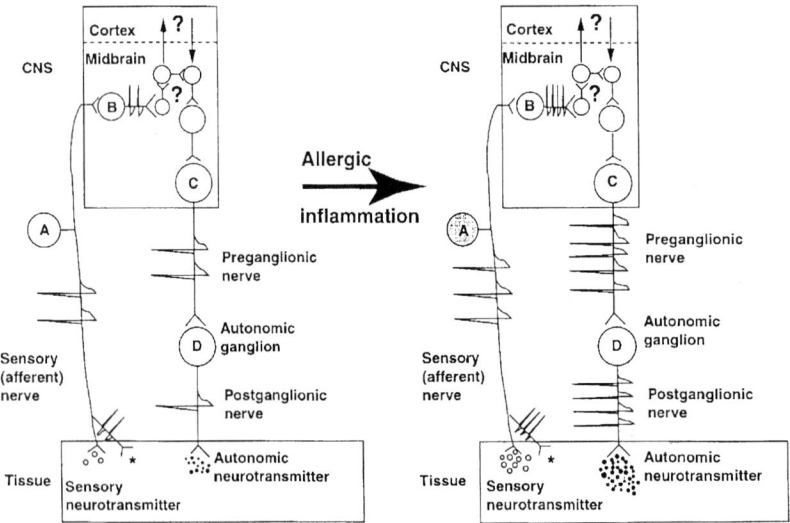

FIG. 8. Proposed pathways of immune factor activation of autonomic nervous system and autonomic nervous system effects on inflammation. A schematic diagram showing how an allergen challenge may affect and be affected by inflammation. A stimulatory input (indicated by the *asterisk [*]*) at a sensory nerve terminal results in a neuronal response and also in a "local reflex" release of a sensory neurotransmitter into the tissue (open circles). Action potentials carried along the sensory nerve *A* result in release of neurotransmitters in the CNS and stimulation of neuron *B* located in the midbrain with subsequent stimulation of the preganglionic nerve *C* and the postganglionic nerve *D* and release of autonomic neurotransmitters. During allergic inflammation (right hand side) the same stimulus may increase activity of neuron *A*, resulting in a greater stimulation of neuron *D* and an increased secretion of the neurotransmitter from the autonomic ganglion. From Undem et al. (144), with permission.

and neuropeptide basis for hypermotility symptoms in illnesses such as irritable bowel or irritable bladder syndrome (171–173).

Summary: Interruptions of HPA Axis and Sympathetic Nervous System and Immune-Mediated Diseases

Taken together these studies indicate that both the hormonal and neuronal stress response, that is, the HPA axis and autonomic nervous system, play an important role in mediating susceptibility to and course and severity of autoimmune, inflammatory, and allergic disease. In general, interruption of these neuronal and neuroendocrine responses predisposes to enhanced susceptibility to inflammation, and in extreme cases to septic shock in response to acute exposure to proinflammatory stimuli. Activation of autonomic circuits by inflammatory, antigenic, or allergenic stimuli may contribute to motor hypersensitivity in these illnesses. It is likely that in naturalistic genetic models and in humans highly predisposed to autoimmune inflammatory disease, multiple defects in these neural systems may occur simultaneously.

Peripheral Nervous System Regulation of Immunity

Neuropeptides and neurotransmitters released from peripheral nerves at sites of inflammation generally exert proinflammatory effects. Peripheral neuropeptides that have been extensively studied with regard to their effects on inflammation include substance P (SP) (174–176) and peripheral CRH and urocortin (177–181). Both the neuropeptides themselves and their receptors have been identified in immune tissues, including spleen, thymus, peripheral blood cells, lymphocytes, and lymphoma cell lines under basal- and inflammatory-stimulated conditions.

SP is a member of a family of tachykinins produced in both neural and non-neuronal cells that bind to a family of receptors called neurokinins (NK1, NK2). In the nervous system, SP is released from small, fast nerve fibers called C fibers that are the primary mode by which pain events in the periphery signal the CNS, and thus is one of the main neuropeptides involved in pain perception. When injected into tissues or released from peripheral nerve terminals at sites of inflammation, SP produces a wheal and flare and has been shown to induce mast cell release of histamine and induce mononuclear migration and neutrophil and eosinophil extravasation and accumulation in tissues. Lymphocytes also express NK receptors and generally show activation in response to tachykinins (182). Such effects are blocked by SP antagonists. Immune cells, including eosinophils and mononuclear cells, have also been shown to express SP, and this expression increases in response to infection and inflammation. SP neurons innervate immune organs including the thymus, spleen, and lymph nodes. SP is also expressed in Peyer's patches of the gut (183,184). Endothelial cells also produce SP and this expression also increases with inflammation. Thus, both the source and conditions of production of SP, its cellular receptor location, and cellular effects suggest that SP plays an important role in the coordinated sensory responses of pain and physiologic responses of hyperemia-mononuclear migration that occur at sites of inflammation.

When the neuropeptide CRH is produced centrally in a variety of brain regions, it initiates a set of behavioral responses to stress, and when released from the hypothalamus it acts as a neurohormone, initiating the HPA axis cascade, ultimately suppressing immune responses via the actions of the GC. However, when released at sites of inflammation from peripheral nerves (181) CRH has proinflammatory effects (185,186). CRH injected into tissues causes vascular leakiness and stimulates innate inflammatory responses, such as are seen in association with carrageenan injection. CRH acts through two receptors, CRH-R1 and CRH-R2, with different distributions. These are located in the pituitary gland (CRH-R1) (187), in blood vessels, heart and skeletal muscle (CRH-R2), and in the CNS (CRH-R1 and -R2) (188). In the immune system, CRH binding has been shown in monocytes, T-lymphocytes, endothelial cells, and resident splenic macrophages (189), and the CRH-R1 receptor has been shown in the spleen and during inflammation in both mature neutrophils and on granulocyte precursor cells. Both CRH-R1 and -R2 receptors have been shown in the thymus. The receptor specificity of the effects of these neuropeptides will be helpful in developing targeted therapeutic agents to modify their effects on CNS versus peripheral tissues.

THERAPEUTIC IMPLICATIONS

Many novel therapeutic applications can be derived from a detailed understanding of neural immune connections. Thus, recognition that interleukins and immune activation play a role in neurodegeneration has led to the application of immune agents for treatment of neurodegenerative diseases and nerve trauma. IL-1RA has been shown to be effective in animal models for reduction of brain damage in stroke (9), and nonsteroidal anti-inflammatory agents are being used in Alzheimer's dementia (5). The beneficial effect of specific activated T cells in neural repair suggests a novel approach to prevention of paralysis in spinal cord injury (11).

Conversely, the effects of neural factors on immune regulation suggest novel approaches to treatment of autoimmune and inflammatory diseases. The depressive effects of cytokines on mood in cytokine-treated patients can be prevented by the use of antidepressants (52). The tricyclic antidepressant deprenyl has been used to reverse the immunosuppression seen after splenic nerve ablation in rats (162,190–192), suggesting a novel treatment for immunosuppression of aging that is associated with dying back of splenic noradrenergic innervation. The anti-inflammatory effect of the phosphodiesterase-inhibitor antidepressant Rolipram has led to the use of this agent to inhibit plaque inflammatory activity in multiple sclerosis (193).

A nonpeptide CRH antagonist has been shown to effectively reduce inflammatory arthritis in rats by approximately

50% (194), suggesting that the target of action in this instance may be through inhibition of peripheral proinflammatory effects of CRH rather than the central anti-inflammatory effects derived from HPA axis activation. This latter example illustrates how the precise action of a novel therapeutic agent cannot be precisely predicted from *in vitro* data alone, and the overall effect in the whole animal will depend on the relative contribution of many systems to final disease expression.

At a broader level, elucidation of these interactions and their precise role in disease expression will identify conditions under which physical, physiologic, or psychological stressors can affect expression of different aspects of immune-mediated illness. Thus, elucidation of neural and neuroendocrine pathways activated differentially by physical, physiologic, psychological, or inflammatory/immune stimuli, will provide mechanisms by which such environmental perturbations, loosely defined as "stress," might affect disease outcome of inflammatory or infectious diseases. At a cellular and molecular level, understanding how neuroendocrine molecules released under such conditions affect different aspects of immune cell activation, trafficking, and function in response to immune or inflammatory stimuli will help to elucidate the role of such host factors in different stages of immune defense. In turn, this understanding will inform mechanisms by which popular alternative therapeutic approaches may affect disease. While research in this latter area is difficult to perform in humans, a thorough understanding of the neurobiology of stress and phenomena such as the placebo effect are essential for appreciating poorly understood phenomena, such as how writing about a stressful event in one's life can beneficially affect measures of disease activity in illnesses such as asthma and rheumatoid arthritis (195).

Thus, a thorough understanding of the molecular, cellular, and systemic mechanisms of communication between the immune and nervous systems will continue to shed light on these two systems' interdependent regulation and will suggest novel therapies for diseases in which these communications are disrupted.

ACKNOWLEDGMENTS

We are grateful to Socorro Vigil-Scott, Alexandra Knudson, and Kimberley Rapp for help in the preparation of this manuscript.

REFERENCES

1. Marz P, Cheng JG, Gadient RA, et al. Sympathetic neurons can produce and respond to interleukin 6. *Proc Natl Acad Sci U S A* 1998;95:3251–3256.
2. Neumann H, Schmidt H, Wilharm E, et al. Interferon gamma gene expression in sensory neurons: evidence for autocrine gene regulation. *J Exp Med* 1997;186:2023–2031.
3. Griffin DE. Cytokines in the brain during viral infection: clues to HIV-associated dementia. *J Clin Invest* 1997;100:2948–2951.
4. Persidsky Y, Zheng J, Miller D, et al. Mononuclear phagocytes mediate blood–brain barrier compromise and neuronal injury during HIV-1–associated dementia. *J Leukoc Biol* 2000;68:413–422.
5. Benveniste EN. Cytokine actions in the central nervous system. *Cytokine Growth Factor Rev* 1998;9:259–275.
6. Sternberg EM. Neural–immune interactions in health and disease. *J Clin Invest* 1997;100:2641–2647.
7. Kaul M, Garden GA, Lipton SA. Pathways to neuronal injury and apoptosis in HIV-associated dementia. *Nature* 2001;410:988–994.
8. Xiong H, Zeng YC, Lewis T, et al. HIV-1 infected mononuclear phagocyte secretory products affect neuronal physiology leading to cellular demise: relevance for HIV-1–associated dementia. *J Neurovirol* 2000;6(suppl 1):14–23.
9. Rothwell N, Allan S, Toulmond S. The role of interleukin 1 in acute neurodegeneration and stroke: pathophysiological and therapeutic implications. *J Clin Invest* 1997;100:2648–2652.
10. Eitan S, Solomon A, Lavie V, et al. Recovery of visual response of injured adult rat optic nerves treated with transglutaminase. *Science* 1994;264:1764–1768.
11. Moalem G, Leibowitz-Amit R, Yoles E, et al. Autoimmune T cells protect neurons from secondary degeneration after central nervous system axotomy. *Nat Med* 1999;5:49–55.
12. Schwartz M, Cohen IR. Autoimmunity can benefit self-maintenance. *Immunol Today* 2000;21:265–268.
13. McGeer PL, McGeer EG. Glial cell reactions in neurodegenerative diseases: pathophysiology and therapeutic interventions. *Alzheimer Dis Assoc Disord* 1998;12:1–6.
14. Fontana A, Weber E, Dayer JM. Synthesis of interleukin 1/endogenous pyrogen in the brain of endotoxin-treated mice: a step in fever induction. *J Immunol* 1984;133:1696–1698.
15. Besedovsky HO, Rey DA, Sorkin E, et al. Immunoregulatory feedback between interleukin-1 and glucocorticoid hormones. *Science* 1986;233:652–654.
16. Banks WA, Ortiz L, Plotkin SR, et al. Human interleukin (IL) 1a, murine IL-1a and murine IL-1b are transported from blood to brain in the mouse by a shared saturable mechanism. *J Pharmacol Exp Ther* 1991;259:988–1007.
17. Banks WA, Kastin AJ, Broadwell RD. Passage of cytokines across the blood–brain barrier. *Neuroimmunomodulation* 1995;2:241–248.
18. Banks WA. Anorectic effects of circulating cytokines: role of the vascular blood–brain barrier. *Nutrition* 2001;17:434–437.
19. Wong ML, Rettori V, al-Shekhlee A, et al. Inducible nitric oxide synthase gene expression in the brain during systemic inflammation. *Nat Med* 1996;2:581–584.
20. Breder CD, Saper CB. Expression of inducible cyclooxygenase mRNA in the mouse brain after systemic administration of bacterial lipopolysaccharide. *Brain Res* 1996;713:64–69.
21. Elmquist JK, Scammell TE, Saper CB. Mechanisms of CNS response to systemic immune challenge: the febrile response. *Trends Neurosci* 1997;20:565–570.
22. Bluthe RM, Pawlowski M, Suarez S, et al. Synergy between tumor necrosis factor alpha and interleukin-1 in the induction of sickness behavior in mice. *Psychoneuroendocrinology* 1994;19:197–207.
23. Bret DJ, Bluthe RM, Kent S, et al. Lipopolysaccharide and interleukin-1 depress food-motivated behavior in mice by a vagal-mediated mechanism. *Brain Behav Immun* 1995;9:242–246.
24. Goehler LE, Busch CR, Tartaglia N, et al. Blockade of cytokine induced conditioned taste aversion by subdiaphragmatic vagotomy: further evidence for vagal mediation of immune–brain communication. *Neurosci Lett* 1995;185:163–166.
25. Dantzer R, Konsman JP, Bluthe RM, et al. Neural and humoral pathways of communication from the immune system to the brain: parallel or convergent? *Auton Neurosci* 2000;85:60–65.
26. Banks WA. Cytokines, CVOs, and the blood–brain barrier. In: Ader R, Felten D, Cohen N, eds. *Psychoneuroimmunology*. San Diego: Academic Press, 2001:483–497.
27. Rubin LL, Staddon JM. The cell biology of the blood–brain barrier. *Annu Rev Neurosci* 1999;22:11–28.
28. Banks WA, Kastin AJ, Ehrensing CA. Blood-borne interleukin-1 alpha is transported across the endothelial blood-spinal cord barrier of mice. *J Physiol* 1994;479:257–264.
29. Maness LM, Kastin AJ, Banks WA. Relative contributions of a CVO and the microvascular bed to delivery of blood-borne IL-1 alpha to the brain. *Am J Physiol* 1998;275:207–212.
30. Scammell TE, Elmquist JK, Saper CB. Inhibition of nitric oxide

synthase produces hypothermia and depresses lipopolysaccharide fever. *Am J Physiol* 1996;271:333–338.

31. Goehler LE, Gaykema RP, Hansen MK, et al. Vagal immune-to-brain communication: a visceral chemosensory pathway. *Auton Neurosci* 2000;85:49–59.

32. Bluthe RM, Walter V, Parnet P, et al. Lipopolysaccharide induces sickness behaviour in rats by a vagal mediated mechanism. *Comptes Rendus Acad Sci III Sci Vie* 1994;317:499–503.

33. Dinarello CA, Gatti S, Bartfai T. Fever: links with an ancient receptor. *Curr Biol* 1999;9:147–150.

34. Saper CB, Breder CD. The neurologic basis of fever. *N Engl J Med* 1994;330:1880–1886.

35. O'Neill LA, Dinarello CA. The IL-1 receptor/toll-like receptor superfamily: crucial receptors for inflammation and host defense. *Immunol Today* 2000;21:206–209.

36. Moldofsky H, Dickstein JB. Sleep and cytokine-immune functions in medical, psychiatric and primary sleep disorders. *Sleep Med Rev* 1999;3:325–337.

37. Krueger JM, Majde JA. Cytokines and sleep. *Int Arch Allergy Immunol* 1995;106:97–100.

38. Dickstein JB, Moldofsky H. Sleep, cytokines and immune function. *Sleep Med Rev* 1999;3:219–228.

39. Fang J, Wang Y, Krueger JM. Effects of interleukin-1 beta on sleep are mediated by the type I receptor. *Am J Physiol* 1998;274:r655–660.

40. Rogers NL, Szuba MP, Staab JP, et al. Neuroimmunologic aspects of sleep and sleep loss. *Semin Clin Neuropsychiatry* 2001;6:295–307.

41. Kubota T, Brown RA, Fang J, et al. Interleukin-15 and interleukin-2 enhance non-REM sleep in rabbits. *Am J Physiol Regul Integr Comp Physiol* 2001;281:1004–1012.

42. Kubota T, Fang J, Brown RA, et al. Interleukin-18 promotes sleep in rabbits and rats. *Am J Physiol Regul Integr Comp Physiol* 2001; 281:828–838.

43. Kubota T, Fang J, Kushikata T, et al. Interleukin-13 and transforming growth factor-beta 1 inhibit spontaneous sleep in rabbits. *Am J Physiol Regul Integr Comp Physiol* 2000;279:r786–792.

44. Toth LA. Identifying genetic influences on sleep: an approach to discovering the mechanisms of sleep regulation. *Behav Genet* 2001;31: 39–46.

45. Chang F, Opp MR. Corticotropin-releasing hormone (CRH) as a regulator of waking. *Neurosci Biobehav Rev* 2001;25:445–453.

46. Opp MR, Imeri L. Rat strains that differ in corticotropin-releasing hormone production exhibit different sleep–wake responses to interleukin 1. *Neuroendocrinology* 2001;73:272–284.

47. Alt JA, Obal FJ, Trayor TR, et al. Alterations in EEG activity and sleep after influenza viral infection in GHRH receptor deficient mice. *J Appl Physics* (2003) in press.

48. Rechtschaffen A, Bergmann BM, Everson CA, et al. Sleep deprivation in the rat. X. Integration and discussion of the findings. *Sleep* 1989;12:68–87.

49. Benca RM, Kushida CA, Everson CA, et al. Sleep deprivation in the rat. VII. Immune function. *Sleep* 1989;12:47–52.

50. Valentine AD, Meyers CA, Kling MA, et al. Mood and cognitive side effects of interferon-alpha therapy. *Semin Oncol* 1998;25:39–47.

51. Janssen HL, Brouwer JT, van der Mast RC, et al. Suicide associated with alpha-interferon therapy for chronic viral hepatitis. *J Hepatol* 1994;21:241–243.

52. Musselman DL, Lawson DH, Gumnick JF, et al. Paroxetine for the prevention of depression induced by high-dose interferon alpha. *N Engl J Med* 2001;344:961–966.

53. Rachal Pugh C, Fleshner M, Watkins LR, et al. The immune system and memory consolidation: a role for the cytokine IL-1 beta. *Neurosci Biobehav Rev* 2001;25:29–41.

54. Schneider H, Pitossi F, Balschun D, et al. A neuromodulatory role of interleukin-1 beta in the hippocampus. *Proc Natl Acad Sci U S A* 1998;95:7778–7783.

55. Berkenbosch F, Oers VJ, Rey DA, et al. Corticotropin-releasing factor-producing neurons in the rat activated by interleukin-1. *Science* 1987;238:524–536.

56. Sapolsky R, Rivier C, Yamamoto G, et al. Interleukin-1 stimulates the secretion of hypothalamic corticotropin releasing factor. *Science* 1987;238:522–524.

57. Ericsson A, Kovacs KJ, Sawchenko PE. A functional anatomical analysis of central pathways subserving the effects of interleukin-1 on stress-related neuroendocrine neurons. *J Neurosci* 1994;14:897–913.

58. Cupps TR, Fauci AS. Corticosteroid-mediated immunoregulation in man. *Immunol Rev* 1982;65:133–155.

59. Webster JI, Tonelli L, Sternberg EM. Neuroendocrine regulation of immunity. *Annu Rev Immunol* 2002;20:125–163.

60. Baldwin AS Jr. The NF-kappa B and I kappa B proteins: new discoveries and insights. *Annu Rev Immunol* 1996;14:649–683.

61. Ghosh S, May MJ, Kopp EB. NF-kappa B and Rel proteins: evolutionarily conserved mediators of immune responses. *Annu Rev Immunol* 1998;16:225–260.

62. McKay LI, Cidlowski JA. CBP (CREB binding protein) integrates NF-kappa B (nuclear factor-kappa B) and glucocorticoid receptor physical interactions and antagonism. *Mol Endocrinol* 2000;14:1222–1234.

63. Franchimont D, Louis E, Dewe W, et al. Effects of dexamethasone on the profile of cytokine secretion in human whole blood cell cultures. *Regulat Peptides* 1998;73:59–65.

64. Elenkov IJ, Chrousos GP. Stress hormones, Th1/Th2 patterns, pro/anti-inflammatory cytokines and susceptibility to disease. *Trends Endocrinol Metab* 1999;10:359–368.

65. Nelms K, Keegan AD, Zamorano J, et al. The IL-4 receptor: signaling mechanisms and biologic functions. *Annu Rev Immunol* 1999;17:701–738.

66. Agarwal SK, Marshall GD Jr. Dexamethasone promotes type 2 cytokine production primarily through inhibition of type 1 cytokines. *J Interferon Cytokine Res* 2001;21:147–155.

67. Cronstein BN, Kimmel SC, Levin RI, et al. A mechanism for the antiinflammatory effects of corticosteroids: the glucocorticoid receptor regulates leukocyte adhesion to endothelial cells and expression of endothelial-leukocyte adhesion molecule 1 and intercellular adhesion molecule 1. *Proc Natl Acad Sci U S A* 1992;89:9991–9995.

68. Ohtsuka T, Kubota A, Hirano T, et al. Glucocorticoid-mediated gene suppression of rat cytokine-induced neutrophil chemoattractant CINC/gro, a member of the interleukin-8 family, through impairment of NF-kappa B activation. *J Biol Chem* 1996;271:1651–1659.

69. Nakagawa M, Bondy GP, Waisman D, et al. The effect of glucocorticoids on the expression of L-selectin on polymorphonuclear leukocyte. *Blood* 1999;93:2730–2737.

70. Sewell WA, Scurr LL, Orphanides H, et al. Induction of interleukin-4 and interleukin-5 expression in mast cells is inhibited by glucocorticoids. *Clin Diagn Lab Immunol* 1998;5:18–23.

71. Richards DF, Fernandez M, Caulfield J, et al. Glucocorticoids drive human CD8(+) T cell differentiation towards a phenotype with high IL-10 and reduced IL-4, IL-5 and IL-13 production. *Eur J Immunol* 2000;30:2344–2354.

72. Lilly CM, Nakamura H, Kesselman H, et al. Expression of eotaxin by human lung epithelial cells: induction by cytokines and inhibition by glucocorticoids. *J Clin Invest* 1997;99:1767–1773.

73. Pype JL, Dupont LJ, Menten P, et al. Expression of monocyte chemotactic protein (MCP)-1, MCP-2, and MCP-3 by human airway smooth-muscle cells. Modulation by corticosteroids and T-helper 2 cytokines. *Am J Respir Cell Mol Biol* 1999;21:528–536.

74. Perkins DJ, Kniss DA. Tumor necrosis factor-alpha promotes sustained cyclooxygenase-2 expression: attenuation by dexamethasone and NSAIDs. *Prostaglandins* 1997;54:727–743.

75. De Vera ME, Taylor BS, Wang Q, et al. Dexamethasone suppresses iNOS gene expression by upregulating I-kappa B alpha and inhibiting NF-kappa B. *Am J Physiol* 1997;273:1290–1296.

76. Goulding NJ, Euzger HS, Butt SK, et al. Novel pathways for glucocorticoid effects on neutrophils in chronic inflammation. *Inflamm Res* 1998;47(suppl 3):158–165.

77. Russo-Marie F. Macrophages and the glucocorticoids. *J Neuroimmunol* 1992;40:281–286.

78. Schleimer RP, Bochner BS. The effects of glucocorticoids on human eosinophils. *J Allergy Clin Immunol* 1994;94:1202–1213.

79. Hirai K, Miyamasu M, Takaishi T, et al. Regulation of the function of eosinophils and basophils. *Crit Rev Immunol* 1997;17:325–352.

80. Nelson DJ, McWilliam AS, Haining S, et al. Modulation of airway intraepithelial dendritic cells following exposure to steroids. *Am J Respir Crit Care Med* 1995;151:475–481.

81. Kai H, Yoshitake K, Hisatsune A, et al. Dexamethasone suppresses mucus production and MUC-2 and MUC-5AC gene expression by NCI-H292 cells. *Am J Physiol* 1996;271:484–488.

82. King KL, Cidlowski JA. Cell cycle regulation and apoptosis. *Annu Rev Med* 1998;60:601–617.

83. Planey SL, Litwack G. Glucocorticoid-induced apoptosis in lymphocytes. *Biochem Biophys Res Commun* 2000;279:307–312.

84. Samuelsson MK, Pazirandeh A, Davani B, et al. p57Kip2, a glucocorticoid-induced inhibitor of cell cycle progression in HeLa cells. *Mol Endocrinol* 1999;13:1811–1822.

85. Schmidt M, Lugering N, Lugering A, et al. Role of the CD95/CD95 ligand system in glucocorticoid-induced monocyte apoptosis. *J Immunol* 2001;166:1344–1351.

86. Ashwell JD, Lu FW, Vacchio MS. Glucocorticoids in T cell development and function*. *Annu Rev Immunol* 2000;18:309–345.

87. Vacchio MS, Lee JY, Ashwell JD. Thymus-derived glucocorticoids set the thresholds for thymocyte selection by inhibiting TCR-mediated thymocyte activation. *J Immunol* 1999;163:1327–1333.

88. Sternberg EM. Neuroendocrine regulation of autoimmune/inflammatory disease. *J Endocrinol* 2001;169:429–435.

89. Chrousos GP. The hypothalamic-pituitary-adrenal axis and immune-mediated inflammation. *N Engl J Med* 1995;332:1351–1362.

90. DeRijk R, Michelson D, Karp B, et al. Exercise and circadian rhythm-induced variations in plasma cortisol differentially regulate interleukin-1 beta (IL-1 beta), IL-6, and tumor necrosis factor-alpha (TNF alpha) production in humans: high sensitivity of TNF alpha and resistance of IL-6. *J Clin Endocrinol Metab* 1997;82:2182–2191.

91. DeRijk RH, Petrides J, Deuster P, et al. Changes in corticosteroid sensitivity of peripheral blood lymphocytes after strenuous exercise in humans. *J Clin Endocrinol Metab* 1996;81:228–235.

92. Deuster PA, Zelazowska EB, Singh A, et al. Expression of lymphocyte subsets after exercise and dexamethasone in high and low stress responders. *Med Sci Sports Exer* 1999;31:1799–1806.

93. Jafarian-Tehrani M, Sternberg EM. Animal models of neuroimmune interactions in inflammatory diseases. *J Neuroimmunol* 1999;100:13–20.

94. Wick G, Hu Y, Schwarz S, et al. Immunoendocrine communication via the hypothalamo-pituitary-adrenal axis in autoimmune diseases. *Endocrine Rev* 1993;14:539–563.

95. Shanks N, Moore PM, Perks P, et al. Alterations in hypothalamic-pituitary-adrenal function correlated with the onset of murine SLE in MRL +/+ and lpr/lpr mice. *Brain Behav Immun* 1999;13:348–360.

96. Sternberg EM, Young WS 3rd, Bernardini R, et al. A central nervous system defect in biosynthesis of corticotropin-releasing hormone is associated with susceptibility to streptococcal cell wall-induced arthritis in Lewis rats. *Proc Natl Acad Sci U S A* 1989;86:4771–4775.

97. Sternberg EM, Hill JM, Chrousos GP, et al. Inflammatory mediator-induced hypothalamic-pituitary-adrenal axis activation is defective in streptococcal cell wall arthritis-susceptible Lewis rats. *Proc Natl Acad Sci U S A* 1989;86:2374–2378.

98. Gutierrez MA, Garcia ME, Rodriguez JA, et al. Hypothalamic-pituitary-adrenal axis function and prolactin secretion in systemic lupus erythematosus. *Lupus* 1998;7:404–408.

99. Chikanza IC, Petrou P, Kingsley G, et al. Defective hypothalamic response to immune and inflammatory stimuli in patients with rheumatoid arthritis. *Arthritis Rheum* 1992;35:1281–1288.

100. Cash JM, Crofford LJ, Gallucci WT, et al. Pituitary-adrenal axis responsiveness to ovine corticotropin releasing hormone in patients with rheumatoid arthritis treated with low dose prednisone. *J Rheumatol* 1992;19:1692–1696.

101. Gutierrez MA, Garcia ME, Rodriguez JA, et al. Hypothalamic-pituitary-adrenal axis function in patients with active rheumatoid arthritis: a controlled study using insulin hypoglycemia stress test and prolactin stimulation. *J Rheumatol* 1999;26:277–281.

102. Michelson D, Stone L, Galliven E, et al. Multiple sclerosis is associated with alterations in hypothalamic-pituitary-adrenal axis function. *J Clin Endocrinol Metab* 1994;79:848–853.

103. Johnson EO, Vlachoyiannopoulos PG, Skopouli FN, et al. Hypofunction of the stress axis in Sjogren's syndrome. *J Rheumatol* 1998;25:1508–1514.

104. Crofford LJ. The hypothalamic-pituitary-adrenal stress axis in fibromyalgia and chronic fatigue syndrome. *Zeitschrift fur Rheumatologie* 1998;57:67–71.

105. Neeck G, Crofford LJ. Neuroendocrine perturbations in fibromyalgia and chronic fatigue syndrome. *Rheum Dis Clin North Am* 2000;26:989–1002.

106. Buske-Kirschbaum A, Jobst S, Psych D, et al. Attenuated free cortisol response to psychosocial stress in children with atopic dermatitis. *Psychosomal Med* 1997;59:419–426.

107. Turnbull AV, Rivier CL. Regulation of the hypothalamic-pituitary-adrenal axis by cytokines: actions and mechanisms of action. *Physiol Rev* 1999;79:1–71.

108. Shanks N, Griffiths J, Zalcman S, et al. Mouse strain differences in plasma corticosterone following uncontrollable footshock. *Pharmacol Biochem Behav* 1990;36:515–519.

109. Remmers EF, Longman RE, Du Y, et al. A genome scan localizes five non-MHC loci controlling collagen-induced arthritis in rats. *Nat Genet* 1996;14:82–85.

110. Wakeland EK, Wandstrat AE, Liu K, et al. Genetic dissection of systemic lupus erythematosus. *Curr Opin Immunol* 1999;11:701–707.

111. Listwak S, Barrientos RM, Koike G, et al. Identification of a novel inflammation-protective locus in the Fischer rat. *Mammalian Genome* 1999;10:362–365.

112. Jafarian-Tehrani M, Listwak S, Barrientos RM, et al. Exclusion of angiotensin I-converting enzyme as a candidate gene involved in exudative inflammatory resistance in F344/N rats. *Mol Med* 2000;6:319–331.

113. MacPhee IA, Antoni FA, Mason DW. Spontaneous recovery of rats from experimental allergic encephalomyelitis is dependent on regulation of the immune system by endogenous adrenal corticosteroids. *J Exp Med* 1989;169:431–445.

114. Edwards CK, Yunger LM, Lorence RM, et al. The pituitary gland is required for protection against lethal effects of *Salmonella typhimurium*. *Proc Natl Acad Sci U S A* 1991;88:2274–2277.

115. Ruzek MC, Pearce BD, Miller AH, et al. Endogenous glucocorticoids protect against cytokine-mediated lethality during viral infection. *J Immunol* 1999;162:3527–3533.

116. Misiewicz B, Poltorak M, Raybourne RB, et al. Intracerebroventricular transplantation of embryonic neuronal tissue from inflammatory resistant into inflammatory susceptible rats suppresses specific components of inflammation. *Exp Neurol* 1997;146:305–314.

117. DeRijk R, Sternberg EM. Corticosteroid resistance and disease. *Ann Med* 1997;29:79–82.

118. Bamberger CM, Bamberger AM, de Castro M, et al. Glucocorticoid receptor beta, a potential endogenous inhibitor of glucocorticoid action in humans. *J Clin Invest* 1995;95:2435–2441.

119. Leung DY, Hamid Q, Vottero A, et al. Association of glucocorticoid insensitivity with increased expression of glucocorticoid receptor beta. *J Exp Med* 1997;186:1567–1574.

120. Derijk RH, Schaaf MJ, Turner G, et al. A human glucocorticoid receptor gene variant that increases the stability of the glucocorticoid receptor beta-isoform mRNA is associated with rheumatoid arthritis. *J Rheumatol* 2001;28:2383–2388.

121. McEwen BS. Protective and damaging effects of stress mediators. *N Engl J Med* 1998;338:171–179.

122. Kirschbaum C, Kudielka BM, Gaab J, et al. Impact of gender, menstrual cycle phase, and oral contraceptives on the activity of the hypothalamus-pituitary-adrenal axis. *Psychosomal Med* 1999;61:154–162.

123. Harbuz MS, Rooney C, Jones M, et al. Hypothalamo-pituitary-adrenal axis responses to lipopolysaccharide in male and female rats with adjuvant-induced arthritis. *Brain Behav Immun* 1999;13:335–347.

124. Chrousos GP, Torpy DJ, Gold PW. Interactions between the hypothalamic-pituitary-adrenal axis and the female reproductive system: clinical implications. *Ann Intern Med* 1998;129:229–240.

125. Askew EW. Environmental and physical stress and nutrient requirements. *Am J Clin Nutr* 1995;61:631–637.

126. Imaki T, Nahan J, Rivier C, et al. Differential regulation of corticotropin-releasing factor mRNA in rat brain regions by glucocorticoids and stress. *J Neurosci* 1991;11:585–599.

127. Li HY, Ericsson A, Sawchenko PE. Distinct mechanisms underlie activation of hypothalamic neurosecretory neurons and their medullary catecholaminergic afferents in categorically different stress paradigms. *Proc Natl Acad Sci U S A* 1996;93:2359–2364.

128. Pacak K, Baffi JS, Kvetnansky R, et al. Stressor-specific activation of catecholaminergic systems: implications for stress-related hypothalamic-pituitary-adrenocortical responses. *Adv Pharmacol* 1998;42:561–564.

129. Pacak K, Palkovits M, Yadid G, et al. Heterogeneous neurochemical responses to different stressors: a test of Selye's doctrine of nonspecificity. *Am J Physiol* 1998;275:r1247–1255.

130. Sheridan JF, Feng NG, Bonneau RH, et al. Restraint stress differentially affects anti-viral cellular and humoral immune responses in mice. *J Neuroimmunol* 1991;31:245–255.

131. Padgett DA, Sheridan JF, Dorne J, et al. Social stress and the reactivation of latent herpes simplex virus type 1. *Proc Natl Acad Sci U S A* 1998;95:7231–7235.

132. Brown DH, Lafuse WP, Zwilling BS. Stabilized expression of mRNA is associated with mycobacterial resistance controlled by Nramp1. *Infect Immun* 1997;65:597–603.

133. Brown DH, Sheridan J, Pearl D, et al. Regulation of mycobacterial growth by the hypothalamus-pituitary-adrenal axis: differential responses of Mycobacterium bovis BCG-resistant and -susceptible mice. *Infect Immun* 1993;61:4793–4800.

134. Dhabhar FS, McEwen BS. Enhancing versus suppressive effects of stress hormones on skin immune function. *Proc Natl Acad Sci U S A* 1999;96:1059–1064.

135. Dhabhar FS, McEwen BS. Acute stress enhances while chronic stress suppresses cell-mediated immunity in vivo: a potential role for leukocyte trafficking. *Brain Behav Immun* 1997;11:286–306.

136. Dhabhar FS, Satoskar AR, Bluethmann H, et al. Stress-induced enhancement of skin immune function: a role for gamma interferon. *Proc Natl Acad Sci U S A* 2000;97:2846–2851.

137. Cohen S, Tyrrell DA, Smith AP. Psychological stress and susceptibility to the common cold. *N Engl J Med* 1991;325:606–612.

138. Kiecolt-Glaser JK, Glaser R, Shuttleworth EC, et al. Chronic stress and immunity in family caregivers of Alzheimer's disease victims. *Psychosomal Med* 1987;49:523–535.

139. Kiecolt-Glaser JK, Glaser R, Cacioppo JT, et al. Marital stress: immunologic, neuroendocrine, and autonomic correlates. *Ann N Y Acad Sci* 1998;840:656–663.

140. Marucha PT, Kiecolt-Glaser JK, Favagehi M. Mucosal wound healing is impaired by examination stress. *Psychosomal Med* 1998;60:362–365.

141. Glaser R, Kiecolt-Glaser JK, Bonneau RH, et al. Stress-induced modulation of the immune response to recombinant hepatitis B vaccine. *Psychosomal Med* 1992;54:22–29.

142. Kramer TR, Moore RJ, Shippee RL, et al. Effects of food restriction in military training on T-lymphocyte responses. *Int J Sports Med* 1997;18(suppl 1):84–90.

143. Hamid QA, Wenzel SE, Hauk PJ, et al. Increased glucocorticoid receptor beta in airway cells of glucocorticoid-insensitive asthma. *Am J Respir Crit Care Med* 1999;159:1600–1604.

144. Undem BJ, Kajekar R, Hunter DD, et al. Neural integration and allergic disease. *J Allergy Clin Immunol* 2000;106:213–220.

145. Miller BD, Wood BL. Influence of specific emotional states on autonomic reactivity and pulmonary function in asthmatic children. *J Am Acad Child Adolesc Psychiatry* 1997;36:669–677.

146. Thayer JF, Friedman BH, Borkovec TD, et al. Phasic heart period reactions to cued threat and nonthreat stimuli in generalized anxiety disorder. *Psychophysiology* 2000;37:361–368.

147. Jacob RG, Thayer JF, Manuck SB, et al. Ambulatory blood pressure responses and the circumplex model of mood: a 4-day study. *Psychosomal Med* 1999;61:319–333.

148. Felten DL, Felten SY. Sympathetic noradrenergic innervation of immune organs. *Brain Behav Immun* 1988;2:293–300.

149. Dahlstrom A, Zetterstrom BEM. Noradrenaline stores in nerve terminals of the spleen: changes during hemorrhagic shock. *Science* 1965;147:1583–1585.

150. Reilly FD, McCuskey RS, Meineke HA. Studies of the hemopoietic microenvironment. VIII. Andrenergic and cholinergic innervation of the murine spleen. *Anat Rec* 1976;185:109–117.

151. Tollefson L, Bulloch K. Dual-label retrograde transport: CNS innervation of the mouse thymus distinct from other mediastinum viscera. *J Neurosci Res* 1990;25:20–28.

152. Elenkov IJ, Wilder RL, Chrousos GP, et al. The sympathetic nerve—an integrative interface between two supersystems: the brain and the immune system. *Pharmacol Rev* 2000;52:595–638.

153. Stevens-Felten SY, Bellinger DL. Noradrenergic and peptidergic innervation of lymphoid organs. *Chem Immunol* 1997;69:99–131.

154. Ottaway CA, Husband AJ. The influence of neuroendocrine pathways on lymphocyte migration. *Immunol Today* 1994;15:511–517.

155. Benschop RJ, Rodriguez-Feuerhahn M, Schedlowski M. Catecholamine-induced leukocytosis: early observations, current research, and future directions. *Brain Behav Immun* 1996;10:77–91.

156. Felten SY, Madden KS, Bellinger DL, et al. The role of the sympathetic nervous system in the modulation of immune responses. *Adv Pharmacol* 1998;42:583–587.

157. Levine JD, Dardick SJ, Roizen MF, et al. Contribution of sensory afferents and sympathetic efferents to joint injury in experimental arthritis. *J Neurosci* 1986;6:3423–3429.

158. Levine JD, Coderre TJ, Helms C, et al. B2-adrenergic mechanisms in experimental arthritis. *Proc Nat Acad Sci U S A* 1988;85:4553–4556.

159. Green PG, Luo J, Heller PH, et al. Further substantiation of a significant role for the sympathetic nervous system in inflammation. *Neuroscience* 1993;55:1037–1043.

160. Felten DL, Felten SY, Bellinger DL, et al. Noradrenergic and peptidergic innervation of secondary lymphoid organs: role in experimental rheumatoid arthritis. *Eur J Clin Invest* 1992;22:37–41.

161. Madden KS, Stevens SY, Felten DL, et al. Alterations in T lymphocyte activity following chemical sympathectomy in young and old Fischer 344 rats. *J Neuroimmunol* 2000;103:131–145.

162. ThyagaRajan S, Madden KS, Stevens SY, et al. Restoration of splenic noradrenergic nerve fibers and immune reactivity in old F344 rats: a comparison between L-deprenyl and L-desmethyldeprenyl. *Int J Immunopharmacol* 2000;22:523–536.

163. Kuis W, de Jong-de Vos van Steenwijk C, Sinnema G, et al. The autonomic nervous system and the immune system in juvenile rheumatoid arthritis. *Brain Behav Immun* 1996;10:387–398.

164. Heijnen CJ, Rouppe van der Voort C, Wulffraat N, et al. Functional alpha 1-adrenergic receptors on leukocytes of patients with polyarticular juvenile rheumatoid arthritis. *J Neuroimmunol* 1996;71:223–226.

165. Kavelaars A, Kuis W, Knook L, et al. Disturbed neuroendocrine-immune interactions in chronic fatigue syndrome. *J Clin Endocrinol Metab* 2000;85:692–696.

166. Ohta A, Sitkovsky M. Role of G-protein–coupled adenosine receptors in downregulation of inflammation and protection from tissue damage. *Nature* 2001;414:916–920.

167. Hermann G, Tovar CA, Beck FM, et al. Restraint stress differentially affects the pathogenesis of an experimental influenza viral infection in three inbred strains of mice. *J Neuroimmunol* 1993;47:83–94.

168. Hermann G, Beck FM, Tovar CA, et al. Stress-induced changes attributable to the sympathetic nervous system during experimental influenza viral infection in DBA/2 inbred mouse strain. *J Neuroimmunol* 1994;53:173–180.

169. Rinner I, Schauenstein K. The parasympathetic nervous system takes part in the immuno-neuroendocrine dialogue. *J Neuroimmunol* 1991;34:165–172.

170. Valentino RJ, Kosboth M, Colflesh M, et al. Transneuronal labeling from the rat distal colon: anatomic evidence for regulation of distal colon function by a pontine corticotropin-releasing factor system. *J Comp Neurol* 2000;417:399–414.

171. Tache Y, Monnikes H, Bonaz B, et al. Role of CRF in stress-related alterations of gastric and colonic motor function. *Ann N Y Acad Sci* 1993;697:233–243.

172. Mayer EA, Naliboff B, Munakata J. The evolving neurobiology of gut feelings. *Prog Brain Res* 2000;122:195–206.

173. Tache Y, Martinez V, Million M, et al. Corticotropin-releasing factor and the brain–gut motor response to stress. *Can J Gastroenterol* 1999;13(suppl A):18–25.

174. Payan DG, Goetzl EJ. Substance P receptor–dependent responses of leukocytes in pulmonary inflammation. *Am Rev Respir Dis* 1987;136:39–43.

175. Stanisz AM, Scicchitano R, Payan DG, et al. In vitro studies of immunoregulation by substance P and somatostatin. *Ann N Y Acad Sci* 1987;496:217–225.

176. Maggi CA. The effects of tachykinins on inflammatory and immune cells. *Regulat Peptides* 1997;70:75–90.

177. Baigent SM. Peripheral corticotropin-releasing hormone and urocortin in the control of the immune response. *Peptides* 2001;22:809–820.

178. Radulovic M, Dautzenberg FM, Sydow S, et al. Corticotropin-releasing factor receptor 1 in mouse spleen: expression after immune stimulation and identification of receptor-bearing cells. *J Immunol* 1999;162:3013–3021.

179. Bamberger CM, Wald M, Bamberger AM, et al. Human lymphocytes produce urocortin, but not corticotropin-releasing hormone. *J Clin Endocrinol Metab* 1998;83:708–711.

180. Vaughan J, Donaldson C, Bittencourt J, et al. Urocortin, a mammalian neuropeptide related to fish urotensin I and to corticotropin-releasing factor. *Nature* 1995;378:287–292.

181. Crofford LJ, Sano H, Karalis K, et al. Local secretion of corticotropin-releasing hormone in the joints of Lewis rats with inflammatory arthritis. *J Clin Invest* 1992;90:2555–2564.

182. Kavelaars A, Jeurissen F, Heijnen CJ. Substance P receptors and signal transduction in leukocytes. *Immunomethods* 1994;5:41–48.

183. Weinstock JV. Neuropeptides and the regulation of granulomatous inflammation. *Clin Immunol Immunopathol* 1992;64:17–22.

184. Stanisz AM, Scicchitano R, Dazin P, et al. Distribution of substance P receptors on murine spleen and Peyer's patch T and B cells. *J Immunol* 1987;139:749–754.

185. Webster EL, Torpy DJ, Elenkov IJ, et al. Corticotropin-releasing hormone and inflammation. *Ann N Y Acad Sci* 1998;840:21–32.

186. Karalis K, Muglia LJ, Bae D, et al. CRH and the immune system. *J Neuroimmunol* 1997;72:131–136.

187. Turnbull AV, Smith GW, Lee S, et al. CRF type I receptor–deficient mice exhibit a pronounced pituitary–adrenal response to local inflammation. *Endocrinology* 1999;140:1013–1017.

188. Chalmers DT, Lovenberg TW, De Souza EB. Localization of novel corticotropin-releasing factor receptor (CRF2) mRNA expression to specific subcortical nuclei in rat brain: comparison with CRF1 receptor mRNA expression. *J Neurosci* 1995;15:6340–6350.

189. Webster EL, Tracey DE, Jutila MA, et al. Corticotropin-releasing factor receptors in mouse spleen: identification of receptor-bearing cells as resident macrophages. *Endocrinology* 1990;127:440–452.

190. Madden KS, Rajan S, Bellinger DL, et al. Age-associated alterations in sympathetic neural interactions with the immune system. *Dev Comp Immunol* 1997;21:479–486.

191. ThyagaRajan S, Felten SY, Felten DL. Restoration of sympathetic noradrenergic nerve fibers in the spleen by low doses of L-deprenyl treatment in young sympathectomized and old Fischer 344 rats. *J Neuroimmunol* 1998;81:144–157.

192. ThyagaRajan S, Madden KS, Kalvass JC, et al. L-deprenyl-induced increase in IL-2 and NK cell activity accompanies restoration of noradrenergic nerve fibers in the spleens of old F344 rats. *J Neuroimmunol* 1998;92:9–21.

193. Bielekova B, Lincoln A, McFarland H, et al. Therapeutic potential of phosphodiesterase-4 and -3 inhibitors in Th1-mediated autoimmune diseases. *J Immunol* 2000;164:1117–1124.

194. Webster EL, Barrientos RM, Contoreggi C, et al. Corticotropin-releasing hormone antagonist attenuates adjuvant-induced arthritis: evidence supporting major role for CRH in peripheral inflammation. *J Rheumatol* 2002;29:1252–1261.

195. Smyth JM, Stone AA, Hurewitz A, et al. Effects of writing about stressful experiences on symptom reduction in patients with asthma or rheumatoid arthritis: a randomized trial. *JAMA* 1999;281:1304–1309.

CHAPTER 33

Immunology of Aging

Dan L. Longo

Clinical Evidence of Immune Dysfunction in Aging Humans
Infectious Diseases Increase in Incidence and Severity in Aged · Cancer Increases in Incidence with Age · Autoimmune Disease Becomes More Prevalent in Aged · Decline in Response to Vaccination with Age · Increase in Graft-versus-Host Disease with Age · Implication of Immunity in Common Diseases of Aging and Longevity · Difficulty in Studying Immune Function
Age-Related Changes in Innate (or Natural) Immunity
Age-Related Changes in Barriers · Age-Related Changes in Complement · Age-Related Changes in Cells that Mediate Innate Immunity · Cytokines and Chemokines · What Does It All Mean?
Age-Related Changes in Adaptive Immunity
Age-Related Changes in T Cells · Age-Related Changes in Cell Biology of T Cells · Age-Related Changes in B-Cell Immunity · Age-Related Changes in Antigen Presentation
Age-Related Changes in Hematopoiesis
Interventions Aimed at Improving Immune Function in Aging
Vaccination · Exercise · Nutrition · Hormones · Immunotherapy
Summary
References

CLINICAL EVIDENCE OF IMMUNE DYSFUNCTION IN AGING HUMANS

Aging is a multifarious process that affects different individuals in different ways and affects discrete organ systems in distinct ways within an individual. Furthermore, within complex organ systems, different segments or portions of the system may be affected by the aging process at different rates and to different degrees. The heterogeneity of the aging process and its diverse manifestations generally invalidate nearly any categorical conclusion about the effects of aging on any system, the immune system in particular. A particular measure of a physiologic variable or organ system function plotted as function of age generally shows enormous scatter and wide individual differences within a particular age group with a statistical trend toward decline in function with age (see Fig. 1). Yet any particular value for the measured parameter is poor at discriminating young from old groups. However, the general consensus is that immune system function declines with age (reviewed in Miller [1], Ginaldi et al. [2], Franceschi et al. [3], Malaguarnera et al. [4] and Effros [5]).

The initial manifestations of the aging process usually involve a decline in physiologic reserve, the excess capacity of organ systems that is regulated by homeostatic mechanisms that permit the individual to adapt to environmental stress or change or danger. The loss of physiologic reserve is difficult

to differentiate from normal under usual circumstances. Such losses only appear under duress. The physiology of the organism involves interactions between the various organ systems such that the effects of aging on other systems, such as the endocrine system, and overt diseases involving other organ systems (e.g., renal failure) inevitably have an influence on immune function, and vice versa.

The main reasons for thinking that immune function declines with age are clinical observations (Table 1).

Infectious Diseases Increase in Incidence and Severity in Aged

Pneumonia and influenza are the fifth leading cause of death, but each of the entities ranked above them are chronic diseases in which infection often provides the coup de grace. Heart disease, the leading killer, includes infectious diseases such as endocarditis and rheumatic heart disease. About half of cancer deaths are complicated by infection. Chronic bronchitis and chronic obstructive pulmonary disease often become fatal as a consequence of infection. A 25% increase in deaths attributable to infectious organisms occurred between 1980 and 1992 for persons aged 65 years and older (6). Worldwide, infections cause at least one-third of deaths.

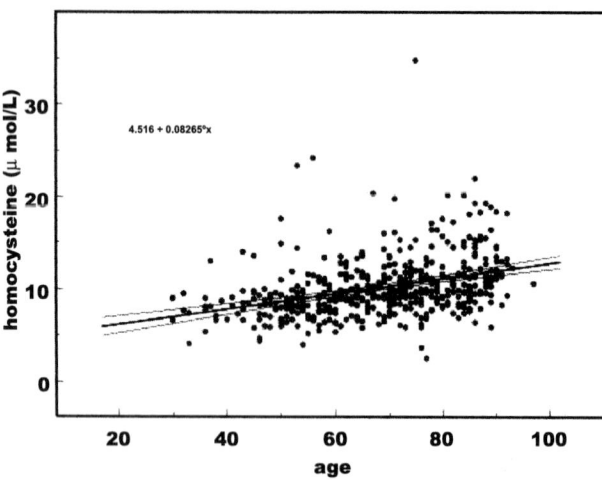

FIG. 1. Plot of serum level of homocysteine (μMol/L) versus age in years among healthy subjects in the National Institute on Aging's Baltimore Longitudinal Study of Aging. There is a significant increase in homocysteine levels with age; however, no particular value for the homocysteine level assists one in distinguishing old from young. This is a common feature of cross-sectional assessments of aging, probably due to the tight physiologic control over organ function in living humans. This observation makes it difficult to interpret the biologic significance of age-related changes in any organ system. With increasing age, the range of measured values is often expanded, suggesting less tight physiologic control with age. However, longitudinal data (generated by repeatedly measuring the same variable in a single person over time) are more informative but more difficult to obtain and are nearly absent from the literature on immune function. Data courtesy of Alan Zonderman, National Institute on Aging.

Aged humans usually do not become infected with opportunistic organisms such as those seen in patients with acquired immunodeficiency syndrome (AIDS). Older people become more susceptible to pathogenic organisms, rather than commensals. The most common sites of infection in the elderly are the lung, urinary tract, and skin. The seriousness of a particular type of infection can be heightened in the elderly

TABLE 1. *Clinical evidence for immunologic dysfunction in elderly*

Increased incidence of infections
  Bacterial infections (pneumonia, infections of urinary tract, skin, soft tissue, sepsis)
  Viral infections (reactivation of herpes zoster, increased morbidity and mortality from influenza, accelerated clinical course of HIV infection)
Increased incidence of cancer
Increased prevalence of autoimmune diseases
Diminished responses to vaccination and secondary vaccine challenges
Increased rate of graft-versus-host disease among older recipients of allogeneic T cells (contaminating T cells in stem-cell transplants, donor lymphocyte adoptive transfer)

because of an increased incidence, an increase in the fatality rate, or late recognition of the problem (7). Tuberculosis and pneumococcal pneumonia increase in incidence with age (8). Influenza and pneumococcal pneumonia are infections that have a higher fatality rate in older people than in younger people (9). Some infections, such as acute appendicitis or cholecystitis, are more serious in the elderly because they progress without detection for a longer period of time due to late recognition and delayed intervention. The difficulty of recognizing these serious infections can be related to a decline in the febrile response with age and the absence of localizing signs and symptoms in the elderly.

Tuberculosis and herpes zoster are infections that are increased in the elderly as a consequence of the reactivation of previously controlled infections. After age 60, probably under the influence of a decline in monocyte/macrophage production of tumor necrosis factor (10), tuberculosis infection can reactivate and the development of a cough could be a sign that the disease is once again transmissible. Persistent immunologic control of varicella virus leads to a chronic carrier state in which the virus resides in sensory nerve roots. Viral replication occurs periodically and is controlled by the immune memory cells. A decline in immunity with age can lead to spread of the virus and the development of herpes zoster (11). About 10% of individuals aged over 80 develop herpes zoster each year often accompanied by severe postherpetic neuralgia that may be debilitating (12).

HIV infection is said to run a more rapid course in older patients (13). However, older patients in this setting are defined as being over age 50 years and credible data on adequate numbers of older patients with AIDS are just emerging from ongoing studies. Human studies involving the deliberate infection of younger and older adults with respiratory syncytial virus have documented that older subjects produced significantly less interferon-γ on viral exposure than the younger subjects (14). Such information is in keeping with the impression that defects in immune function are associated with a greater frequency of infection and a more severe natural history as a consequence of the infection.

However, no specific defect has been identified in the immune response of older people that when corrected, alters the risk of infection. Furthermore, older people do not develop the clinical syndromes associated with congenital defects in one or another arm of the immune system. There is little evidence that the age-associated alterations of immune function measured *in vitro* play a causal role in clinical infections (15).

Cancer Increases in Incidence with Age

Cancer increases exponentially with age and is the second leading cause of death in the United States (16). People aged over 65 years account for over 60% of all cases of cancer and nearly 70% of cancer deaths (17). The decline in immune function with age has been posited to contribute to the increased incidence of cancer. However, there is little evidence of a direct causal link between immune senescence and most malignancies (18). Tumors are increased in patients with primary immunodeficiency diseases, but the spectrum of tumors is highly restricted to those with viral etiologies such as Epstein-Barr virus (EBV)–related lymphomas (49%), human herpesvirus-8–related Kaposi's sarcomas, and human papillomavirus–related vulvar and skin cancers (19). The common tumors of older adults (lung cancer, breast cancer, prostate cancer, colon cancer) do not appear to occur with increased frequency in severely immunodepressed people. The long-term iatrogenic immunosuppression associated with liver, kidney, or heart transplantation produces secondary cancers in 4% to 18% of cases (average 6%) but uncommon types of tumors such as lymphomas, Kaposi's sarcoma, and skin cancers predominate (20).

Yet a strong experimental link has been established between certain features of the immune system and resistance to cancer in animals. Even transplantable tumors are difficult to transplant into immunocompetent mice and the efficiency of tumor engraftment is greatly enhanced by using a strain of mouse defective in T-cell function or defective in both T-cell and B-cell function; tumor engraftment is further enhanced by depleting the host's NK cells (21,22). The immune system can mediate cancer prevention and regression in mice and people (e.g., Shankaran et al. [23], Karanikas et al. [24], and Bendandi et al. [25], and see Chapter 48 on tumor immunology), and cancers use diverse tactics to defeat the immune response, including down-regulating MHC molecules to prevent T-cell recognition (26); expressing Fas ligand to kill Fas-expressing T cells on contact (27); desensitizing chemokine receptors (28); and elaborating immunosuppressive factors that block immune activation (29); among others. Such evasive maneuvers are unlikely to develop without selective pressure.

However, the effects of the immune system on cancer are not entirely predictable. Chemokines can have both stimulatory and inhibitory effects on tumor regression (30) and immune stimulation of cancer growth has long been documented (31,32). Indeed, some have argued that the general tendency of cancers to grow more slowly in older people may be a direct consequence of the aged immune system producing fewer trophic factors and fewer vessels (33).

If the aging immune system is functionally compromised *in vivo*, as would be inferred from an enormous number of *in vitro* studies (see below), it retains sufficient function to resist the engraftment of allogeneic human tumors. In some studies of questionable ethical propriety from the 1950s, volunteers were injected subcutaneously with human tumor cells and those cells were universally rejected, even in older people with comorbid illnesses (34). These results imply that allogeneic recognition remains sufficiently strong in old people to reject a tumor graft.

Thus, the evidence is reasonably strong that the immune system may participate in the control of cancer in an individual. However, the increased risk of cancer in older people cannot be causally linked to a decline in immune function.

Autoimmune Disease Becomes More Prevalent in Aged

Autoimmune diseases can result when an immune attack damages normal tissues. Autoimmune disease may occur on an organ system level, as in endocrine (Hashimoto's thyroiditis, juvenile diabetes); hematopoietic (autoimmune hemolytic anemia, aplastic anemia, idiopathic thrombocytopenic purpura, pernicious anemia [which is actually due to gastric disease]); or neuromuscular (multiple sclerosis, myasthenia gravis) systems; or on a systemic level, as in rheumatoid arthritis, systemic lupus erythematosus, systemic sclerosis, Sjogren's syndrome, and dermatomyositis. The immune effectors most commonly involved in autoimmune disease are antibodies, antigen-antibody complexes, and T cells (see Chapters 44 and 45).

The process of generating normal T and B cells involves deleting cells expressing receptors with high affinity for self-antigens in the central lymphoid organs (thymus and bone marrow). However, T cells are positively selected on the basis of some (lower) affinity for self-MHC plus peptide and B cells with self-reactivity may be tolerized or may not see a sufficiently high level of antigen to crosslink the B-cell receptors that trigger deletion (see Chapters 6 and 9). T cells do not develop if they cannot recognize self-MHC. Thus, a large proportion of lymphocytes possess autoreactive potential and must be controlled. A substantial level of control over lymphoid cell activation is related to genetics (particularly the MHC genes) and to features of the peripheral environment. Antigens can be isolated from lymphocytes and antibodies anatomically through barriers of immune privilege (eye, brain, testis). Thresholds for activation can be regulated by other cell-surface molecules and cytokines. Lymphocyte populations can actively maintain control over autoreactive lymphocytes. Peripheral lymphocytes with autoreactivity may also be deleted or tolerized.

Not all autoimmune diseases increase in frequency with aging, but many do. Age and time may conspire to break down some of the systems that control autoreactive lymphocytes. Defective clearance mechanisms may result in an autoantigen lingering longer and at higher concentrations than normal and exceeding the threshold for lymphocyte activation. Anatomic barriers can break down or be altered by inflammation resulting in exposure to a sequestered autoantigen trigger. The aging process is associated with the accumulation of advanced glycation end (AGE) products that may trigger immune recognition (35). Other post-translational modifications of proteins that occur with age include isoaspartyl formation (36) and oxidation (37), both of which can trigger autoimmune responses to self-proteins with putative clinical ramifications (38). Infections can also be the trigger for autoimmune disease; *Klebsiella pneumoniae* is associated with ankylosing spondylitis, gastrointestinal infection with Yersinia, Salmonellae or Campylobacter species can be associated with reactive arthritis, and *Proteus mirabilis* infection can lead to rheumatoid arthritis (39). Other infectious triggers for autoimmune disease include group A streptococci (rheumatic fever), *Chlamydia trachomatis* (Reiter's syndrome), and *Borrelia burgdorferi* (Lyme disease). Furthermore, bacterial superantigens can trigger both T-cell (40) and B-cell (41) activation.

In addition to exposures that may alter the balance of control over self-reactive lymphocytes, it is also possible that the loss of regulatory T-cell function could result in the development of autoimmune disease. In a transgenic mouse model in which only T cells with specificity for myelin basic protein are produced, experimental autoimmune encephalomyelitis develops spontaneously unless normal splenic CD4$^+$ T cells are adoptively transferred into the host (42). These normal T cells can prevent autoimmune disease in a setting with abundant effectors exposed to self-antigen. It is possible that such regulatory cells decline in aging humans and permit autoreactive cells to be activated at a lower threshold.

However, it remains unclear what specific changes in the aging immune system, if any, predispose to autoimmune disease. The increased incidence could be entirely related to an accumulation of environmental exposures over time that select for an expansion of autoreactive cells on the appropriate predisposing genetic background. Additional study is necessary to tighten the link to the aging process.

Decline in Response to Vaccination with Age

A person who survives an episode of smallpox infection in childhood enjoys lifelong immunity from subsequent bouts of smallpox. This implies that memory cells generated from the initial infection must be capable of living many decades. How such cells survive through the life span and remain functional is unclear. Vaccines have been developed against a wide variety of bacterial and viral pathogens that elicit protective immunity, but surprisingly little is known about the duration of protection. In general, protection conveyed by vaccines is not lifelong. Data on persistence of vaccinia immunity are scarce and conflicting with one report suggesting anecdotal evidence of immunity lasting 50 years (43) and another finding no persistence beyond 15 years (44). The duration of immunity after vaccinia administration has become important in light of the threats of smallpox as an agent of bioterrorism. It is not known whether older people routinely vaccinated before 1970 remain protected. However, information on duration of protection is acutely needed to plan the best use of the available vaccine.

The main vaccines that older people should receive are influenza vaccine annually, pneumococcal vaccine periodically (current recommended periodicity is 5 years), and tetanus toxoid at least once every 10 years. In addition, those who deal with sick people or are exposed to blood products (e.g., those with chronic anemia on transfusion or with chronic

renal failure on hemodialysis) should receive hepatitis B vaccination. Travelers may have need for vaccination against other illnesses such as yellow fever, hepatitis A, Japanese encephalitis, and rabies, depending on the destination (45).

Older patients are said to respond less well to vaccinations. However, this is not a universal finding. Older people without chronic illness or malnutrition have been shown to respond similarly to younger people in some studies (46). Furthermore, increasing attention is now being paid to the nature of the immunization process and how it might need to be altered to afford protection to older people. For example, one group demonstrated that older patients required three doses of a tetanus vaccine to achieve antibody levels thought to be protective (47). Similarly, older people respond somewhat less well to three doses of hepatitis B vaccine than do younger people (48); 100% of young controls achieved protective levels of antibody compared to 42% of elderly. However, in another study, among hemodialysis patients who received a fourth dose, nearly 90% reached protective levels of antibody (49).

Similarly, older people respond less well than younger to the influenza vaccine (50). Efforts to understand the basis for the poor response have led to using the distribution of particular T-cell subsets as predictors of response; people with increased numbers of CD8$^+$CD28null cells were said to have little chance of responding (51). However, others have evaluated the effect of repeated vaccinations. Annual vaccination over 4 years increases the fraction of those vaccinated who achieve protective levels of antibody and develop cellular immunity to influenza virus (52). Furthermore, with improvements in vaccine formulation, both a combination of a trivalent inactivated egg-grown influenza vaccine (Wyeth) plus a live trivalent vaccine (53) and a trivalent inactivated vaccine grown in the Madin–Darby canine-kidney–derived cell line (54) produced protective antibody responses in 83% to 100% of those vaccinated regardless of age. Thus, the formulation of the vaccine can overcome what appear to be age-related defects in responsiveness. A population-based study of an immunogenic vaccine is now needed to prove efficacy in preventing influenza in the elderly.

The case of the pneumococcal vaccine is more complicated. The pneumococcal vaccine currently is a 23-valent polysaccharide vaccine that elicits a T-independent response mainly from the B-1 subset of B cells. No memory results from vaccination, and repeated exposure to the antigens does not produce a boost in antibody levels. The vaccine has been shown to be poor at stimulating antibody responses in older people (55). In murine models, the cellular basis of the poor response is related to a decline in antigen presentation in both splenectomized and old animals (56). The defect seems to be related to a quantitative decline in antigen-presenting macrophages; the response can be boosted in mice with IL-1, IL-4, or IL-5, but not IL-2 or IL-6. Despite this clear analysis and the failure of clinical studies to demonstrate efficacy of the pneumococcal vaccine in the elderly (57), and despite evidence that protective levels of antibody in responding patients decline within about 3 years (58), and despite the absence of any data supporting revaccination, the American College of Physicians–American Society of Internal Medicine recommends that pneumococcal vaccine be administered again and again every 5 years to adults, particularly those over age 65. Efforts are underway to evaluate the effects of revaccination. However, the major prospect for developing a protective vaccine in people is focused on eliciting a T-cell–dependent rather than a T-cell–independent response. Animal studies have shown protection of immunodeficient, splenectomized, and old mice with conjugate vaccines based on the antigen phosphorylcholine, a component of the cell wall of pneumococcus and a number of other bacteria (59). Conjugate T-dependent vaccines currently in clinical trial have shown some promising results, but at least one study involving elderly subjects found it to be no better than the polysaccharide vaccine (60). Additional improvements in pneumococcal vaccination are likely, however.

In conclusion, older people may not respond as briskly as younger people to a wide variety of vaccines. However, it appears that alterations in the number of inoculations or in the formulation of the vaccines are nonetheless likely to lead to protective immunity. Other strategies to improve vaccine efficacy are discussed later in this chapter.

Increase in Graft-versus-Host Disease with Age

It has long been established that older recipients of allogeneic bone marrow transplants experience greater morbidity and mortality from graft-versus-host disease (61). It is not clear whether this is related to the fact that the preparative regimens do more tissue damage to older patients and thus, elicit a greater response from transferred donor immunocompetent lymphocytes than the same level of treatment in younger patients. However, the seriousness of this complication limited the application of the procedure to patients aged less than 55 years until recently. In a murine model, heightened graft-versus-host disease was found to be related to enhanced stimulatory activity from the antigen-presenting cells of older hosts (61a).

Implication of Immunity in Common Diseases of Aging and Longevity

In recent years, common diseases of old age that have not routinely been considered to have an immune pathogenesis have been reconsidered in light of provocative experimental data suggesting a role for the immune response in disease progression. Atherosclerosis, the leading killer in the United States, has been thought to be an inflammatory disease exacerbated by infection with an intracellular pathogen, like chlamydia (62). Furthermore, immunization with oxidized low-density lipoproteins (LDLs) has been found to decrease the progression of atherosclerosis in several animal models, including

apolipoprotein-E knockout mice (63). Using malondialdehyde modified LDL as an immunogen, T-cell–dependent antibody responses were elicited that had a significant inhibitory effect on the development of plaques and also lowered serum cholesterol levels.

Similarly, Alzheimer's disease has been observed to have an inflammatory component. Indeed, cyclooxygenase-2 inhibitors are being tested for their effects on disease progression. However, in addition, using transgenic mice that mimic Alzheimer's disease in the development of cognitive defects and tissue pathology that resembles the human disease, another vaccine approach has been developed. Such mice vaccinated with amyloid-beta peptide showed dramatic decreases in the accumulation of amyloid in the brain and failed to develop the memory loss seen in unvaccinated controls (64). Human application of these results has been complicated by the development of brain inflammation in vaccine recipients. However, the development of a vaccine strategy to prevent or alter the progression of Alzheimer's disease remains an intense research focus.

Osteoporosis, a highly prevalent disease in older people, is responsible for significant morbidity that leads to mortality. The older person who breaks a hip, with that event leading to prolonged bed rest, further weakness, inanition, and fatal pneumonia or other complication is a common sequence of events at the end of life. The cytokine-regulated balance between osteoblastic and osteoclastic activity is increasingly recognized as a potential target for diminishing bone turnover in older people (65). Indeed, the phosphonates that are now widely used in the treatment of osteoporosis act in part by interfering with osteoclast activity. Additional manipulations of the cytokines involved in this regulation may further improve the control of osteoporosis.

Immune system function is also being linked to other significant problems of aging. Not all the connections between the immune system and other body systems have been elucidated. A growing body of evidence supports a connection with the central nervous system. Thymectomy has been reported to produce a decrease in learning and memory in mice (66). A few laboratories have worked diligently over the last 20+ years to demonstrate that immune stimulation and immune suppression can be regulated by operant conditioning for therapeutic effect (reviewed in Ader et al. [67]). The alteration of an immune response by exposure to a conditioned stimulus would be strong evidence for a central nervous system role in immune function. However, conditioning paradigms have not yet been defined that reproduce the animal findings convincingly in humans (68).

Much is written about the immunologic consequences of the hormonal changes that occur with aging, such as the alterations in sex hormone levels and the decline in growth hormone levels (69,70). Certainly dwarf mice that are defective in the production of anterior pituitary hormones have well-characterized immunologic defects that can be reversed largely by supplementation with the appropriate hormones

(71). However, the immunologic consequences of administering growth hormone to elderly normal people has not yet been fully assessed despite several clinical trials that assessed strength, body composition, and other endpoints. The use of hormones to promote immune function in the elderly will be more fully discussed below.

Confusing and mutually inconsistent hypotheses have been generated about the role of genetics in regulating the immune response, on one hand, and the relationship between excellent immune function and longevity, on the other hand. For example, a study of Biozzi mice that are bred to identify genes controlling high or low antibody responses has suggested that mouse strains that are high antibody producers have increased longevity and a lower incidence of spontaneous lymphomas than do low antibody producers (72). Similarly, the high producers appeared to maintain more successful DNA repair capacity than low producers, a finding that the authors link to the relationship between the helicase-containing Ku80 complex that functions both in DNA repair and in VDJ recombination. High levels of antibody production and longevity in these mice are both polygenic traits, but the number of genes involved is estimated to be small. Mice selected for low or high response to the T-cell mitogen, phytohemagglutinin, show differences in the incidence of tumors (lower incidence in high responders), but the high responders do not have increased life span (73).

By contrast, in humans, a variety of data suggest that individuals who maintain good in vitro T-cell proliferative responses may have improved longevity (see, for example, Murasko et al. [74], reviewed in Caruso et al. [75]). A longitudinal study of elderly Swedish people suggested that a poor T-cell proliferative response to mitogens, a high peripheral blood CD8+ T-cell count, and a low level of CD4+ T cells and CD19+ B cells were able to identify individuals significantly less likely to survive for 2 years (76). Efforts to identify genetic polymorphisms associated with better immune function and improved longevity in people have been plagued with methodologic problems, including small sample size, diverse methods of genotyping, different definitions of aged people, failure to correct for multiple comparisons, and several others. A number of HLA alleles have been implicated to influence longevity, but these have generally not been confirmed (75).

Important genetic studies are underway to assess genes that might account for age-related changes in immune function in mice (77) and genes that control longevity and rates of development of neoplastic and non-neoplastic diseases in mice (78). It remains unclear whether this work will elucidate important features of human immune function, aging and longevity in light of the very great differences in longevity and causes of death between mouse and human. Furthermore, the linkage between immune function and longevity is not completely clear. For example, the Snell–Bagg dwarf mouse that carries a mutation preventing production of anterior pituitary hormones has many defects in its immune function (79) but it lives 42% longer than normal mice with the same genetic

background (80). Longevity is a more complex trait than is implied by linking it to the function of a particular system.

Difficulty in Studying Immune Function

Defining the defects in the immune system that occur with aging is extremely difficult. Most other organ systems are assessable in straightforward, reliable, and reproducible ways. Renal function can be assessed by measuring glomerular filtration rate and studying the urine. Cardiac function can be assessed by physical examination, measuring blood pressure and heart rate; echocardiography can assess wall motion and stroke volume in situ. Reliable noninvasive or minimally invasive tests can assess function and physiologic reserve.

By contrast, we assess immune function very poorly. Most assaults on the body that elicit an immune response are regional and the system is developed to act locally. Those assaults that reach the bloodstream encounter additional protective systems in the blood, spleen, and reticuloendothelial systems. The immune system functions in tissues all over the body. There are no reliable methods of sampling the immune system or observing it in action in vivo. Measuring delayed-type hypersensitivity reactions to intradermal injection of antigen is as close as we come to in vivo assessment of immune function.

In vitro assessments distort physiologic interactions. No in vitro system can reproduce the ordered, sequential, and hierarchical features that contribute to the control of an infection in vivo. The tests we have developed tend to use cells obtained from the peripheral blood or some diseased lymphoid tissue that was removed because of chronic infections, such as the tonsils. However, the peripheral blood is not a lymphoid end organ. One can reliably assess the function of the hematopoietic system by quantitating red blood cells, white blood cells, and platelets circulating in the peripheral blood; however, lymphocytes in the peripheral blood do not reside there; they are on their way to somewhere else.

Add to this the great heterogeneity of immune function one encounters in a normal human population, the heterogeneity of the aging process and how it affects individuals, and the variability of measures of a particular test in an individual person based on daily (diurnal), seasonal, and hormonal variations, and nutritional influences. When one attempts to alter the immune system with therapeutic agents, it becomes a daunting task to demonstrate that a particular intervention had a particular biologic effect (81). Typically, a person needs to be compared to himself or herself rather than to other individuals thought to share characteristics. Baseline values need to be determined by performing at least three measurements clustered in time. Samples need to be taken from the same individual over time so that the impact of a single aberrant measurement can be assessed and overcome by drawing a time curve. Nearly none of the data discussed below were generated with such attention to detail.

The fundamental difficulty is that the work on age-related changes in the immune system is mainly descriptive. No one has yet identified an underlying pathophysiology or a correctable feature of immune dysfunction in aging that when corrected reverses the defect *in vivo* with the attendant decrease in infectious disease risk, cancer risk, and autoimmunity risk. None of the findings permit us to apply a diagnostic test to an asymptomatic person, detect a correctable defect, intervene on that basis, and alter disease risk. On the other hand, a number of available vaccines against a variety of pathogens appear to have at least some efficacy in older populations, but are underutilized. A variety of interventions aimed at promoting immune function will be discussed at the end of the chapter.

AGE-RELATED CHANGES IN INNATE (OR NATURAL) IMMUNITY

Innate immunity is that part of the host defense system that does not develop antigen-specific responses or adapt to the nature of the danger. The components of the innate system include local barriers, local secretions, cytokines and chemokines, complement, and cellular components that have no antigen specificity such as granulocytes, monocytes/macrophages, and natural killer (NK) cells. Today the dominant view is that the cellular components of innate immunity are largely conserved or at least less severely compromised in aging humans than is adaptive immunity (3,82,83). Nevertheless, important changes in local milieu contribute substantially to increased risk of pneumonia and skin infections, and alterations in mucosal immunity have been implicated in infectious diarrhea in the elderly.

Age-Related Changes in Barriers

At every interface between the individual and the environment, barriers exist to protect the individual. The skin is an important barrier against fluid loss, infection, and other dangers in the environment, but also has important roles to play in thermoregulation, absorption, pigment production, secretion, sensory perception, and the regulation of immune responses. Perhaps because of its accessibility, more information is available about its changing functions with age than other barrier sites such as the lung and gastrointestinal tract.

The skin loses Langerhans cells with age (84) more dramatically in sun-exposed than in sun-protected skin (85). Yet it is difficult to define a functional compromise in antigen presentation as a consequence of this loss (86). The skin becomes thinner with age, with loss of eccrine glands, slower growth of hair and nails, and reductions in the vascular network (reviewed in Ccrimele et al. [87]). The aging process is accelerated by sun exposure (particularly UVB radiation), neuropeptides released as a consequence of skin injury, and even psychological stress (reviewed in Giacomoni and Rein [88]). Wound healing is slower in older skin, a feature that correlates with slower kinetics of production of immune mediators such as monocyte chemoattractant protein 1 (MCP-1)

and a decrease in production of macrophage inhibitory proteins (MIP-1 α, MIP-1 β, MIP-2) that is associated with a reduction in phagocytic capacity (89). Dermal fibroblasts from aged human donors have increased synthesis of certain matrix metalloproteinases (particularly MMP1 and TIMP1, but not MMP2 or MMP9) and the aged fibroblasts migrate poorly *in vitro* at least in part due to decreased integrin expression and altered actin cytoskeleton organization (90). Altered production of or response to epidermal growth factor and keratinocyte growth factor may also influence the rate of wound healing (91).

The epidermal permeability barrier deteriorates with age as a consequence of a decrease in cholesterol synthesis that alters the optimal ratios of stratum corneum lipids (92), which leads to greater water loss and greater absorption of compounds in contact with the skin. The seasons further alter the barrier with an overall significant decrease in skin lipid synthesis in the winter (93). Topical mevalonic acid appears to reverse the age-related changes in barrier function in mice (94).

Innate immunity is also clinically relevant to the increased incidence of pneumonia in the elderly and possibly also to the increased incidence of asthma with age (reviewed in Meyer [95]). Defects in the swallowing mechanism and decreased gag reflex may lead to aspiration and introduction of bacteria into the tracheobronchial tree (96). Mucociliary clearance declines with age (97) and is further compromised by smoking (98). Respiratory mechanics are altered in the elderly with decreased cough strength, increased alveolar duct diameter, and smaller airway size (99). Respiratory secretions and bronchoalveolar lavage fluids have changes associated with age including increased numbers of CD4$^+$ memory T cells with increased expression of class II MHC molecules and increased concentrations of immunoglobulins, in keeping with the shift to a Th2-dominant pattern (more IL-4 and IL-10, less interferon-γ) of cytokine production in the elderly (see below) (95). Neutrophils are increased and levels of IL-6 and IL-8 are also elevated in bronchoalveolar lavage from clinically normal older individuals, in keeping with the low-grade inflammation seen systemically (100). In addition, animal studies have documented that alveolar macrophages are decreased in older rats, without compromise in their function (101). However, when challenged with bacteria, the alveolar macrophages from old rats produced significantly less nitric oxide (one of their strongest weapons) than did alveolar macrophages from young rats and this defect was associated with a higher mortality rate.

Oral and intestinal mucosal defenses are also altered with aging. Unlike the skin, Langerhans cell density is preserved in the oral mucosa (102). In patients with oral thrush, saliva may lose some its antibacterial and antifungal effects through decreased salivary flow rates and decreased content of IgA and lactoferrin (103). In addition, salivary neutrophils, like other neutrophils in aged subjects, produce less superoxide. It is unclear whether these changes are also present in older people without concomitant illness.

The activity of the gastrointestinal tract mucosal defense system has been assessed mainly in rats (reviewed in Schmucker [104]). The process can be broken down into four main steps:

1. Uptake of antigens by the specialized follicular epithelial M cells that distinguish dangerous bowel components from nondangerous ones and present antigens to dendritic cells for presentation to T cells.
2. Dendritic cells function to present antigen to T and B cells and promote isotype switching.
3. Homing and differentiation of IgA-secreting plasma cells from Peyer's patches to the lamina propria.
4. Local production of antibody in the intestinal wall.

There are no relevant studies of step 1; steps 2 and 4 appear normal in aged animals. However, homing of IgA immunoblasts appears to be compromised in old rats, even when young cells are adoptively transferred (105). Thus, the homing defects are related both to defects in migration of older cells and to the failure of old intestines to provide the proper chemoattractant signals. The putative changes in local defenses are listed in Table 2.

Additional studies are needed to understand local defense systems in the urinary tract (106), eyes (107), and other sites where older people are particularly susceptible to infection.

Age-Related Changes in Complement

Complement levels and activity have not been widely studied in aging humans; however, in general, no age-related complement defect has been noted (108). Genetic analysis of complement components has revealed that the null allele of factor B (so called C4B Q0) is reduced in frequency among

TABLE 2. *Changes in local and systemic innate immunity with aging*

Changes in integrity and structure of barriers, skin, and mucosa
Skin damage from sun (UV)
Decreased Langerhans cells in skin
Decreased gag reflex, abnormal swallowing, increased aspiration of infectious agents
Poor cough strength
Decreased mucociliary clearance (even worse in smokers)
Increased CD4$^+$ memory T cells, neutrophils, IL-6, IL-8, and immunoglobulins in BAL
Decreased number and nitric oxide production by alveolar macrophages
Decreased salivary flow rate and lower levels of salivary IgA and lactoferrin
Decreased migration of IgA immunoblasts to lamina propria
Increased sensitivity to LPS exposure manifested by increased production of IL-1, IL-6, IL-8
Altered macrophage function (see Table 3)
Altered PMN function (see Table 4)

BAL, bronchoalveolar lavage; PMN, polymorphonuclear neutrophil.

old people (109); however, this finding has not been reproduced or explained. Complement certainly plays a role in host defenses in older people, and abnormally high levels of complement components can be found in older people possibly related to systemic low-level inflammation (high C3a levels in the spinal fluid [110]) and as components of extracellular protein deposits in diseases such as macular degeneration and atherosclerosis (111). In aged mice, an age-related defect in the alternative complement pathway was found to result in defective phagocytosis of *Pseudomonas aeruginosa* (112) but no comparable studies have been done in humans.

Age-Related Changes in Cells that Mediate Innate Immunity

The diverse cell types that participate in innate immunity (monocytes/macrophages, polymorphonuclear leukocytes [PMNs], mast cells, NK cells, and hepatocytes) have a panoply of responses to encounters with pathogens that range from taking direct action to enlisting the aid of the adaptive immune system through antigen presentation to lymphoid cells. These cells express on their surface and secrete "pattern recognition" molecules (mannan-binding lectin, C-reactive protein, and serum amyloid protein) that recognize carbohydrate and lipid moieties on pathogens. The cell-surface receptors can then signal into the cell to activate particular effector pathways or their secreted products can facilitate opsonization, phagocytosis, complement and clotting cascade activation, or production of inflammatory cytokines that all act to control the pathogen in select circumstances (reviewed in Janeway et al. [113]). In particular, the growing Toll family of receptors (ten members so far) differ in ligand specificity, expression pattern, and target genes, and appear to be involved in recognition of pathogen-associated molecular patterns. Age-related changes in the function of these receptors likely would have consequences for the functional integrity of innate immunity; but the question has not yet been studied.

Macrophages/Monocytes

As noted in Chapter 16, macrophages play a key role in innate defenses mediating immediate responses to pathogens. Like other cell types involved in host defense, macrophages are difficult to study, as virtually anything one does to isolate them also activates them. A few studies have been done to assess their function in aging. Macrophages generated from bone marrow progenitors from old mice express less class II MHC protein (114), but it is not known whether they have altered capacity to present antigen to CD4+ T cells as a consequence. Studies of murine Kupffer cells suggest that in older mice the cells are less able to phagocytose colloidal carbon and phagocytosis elicits less oxygen consumption and reduced respiratory burst activity than in young mice (115). Peritoneal macrophages in young and old mice were studied for the influence of neuropeptide Y on adherence, chemotaxis, phagocytosis, superoxide anion production, and release of TNF and IL-1. De la Fuente et al. (116) argued that neuropeptide Y was capable of boosting peritoneal macrophage function, but a clear and biologically significant decline in function with age was not apparent.

In some animal models, macrophages from young and old animals function to a comparable degree, for example, in *Mycobacterium tuberculosis* infection (117). In contrast, an age-related decline in macrophage function appears to convey an increased susceptibility to parasitic infections, decreased wound-healing ability, and poorer capacity to kill tumor cells. Macrophages from old tumor-bearing mice appear to make less inducible nitric oxide synthase and oncostatin-M (118) and macrophages from old wounded mice produce smaller amounts of angiogenic cytokines like vascular endothelial growth factor and fibroblast growth factor-2 (119). Similarly, as noted above, rat alveolar macrophages from old mice make less nitric oxide than their younger counterparts (120). On the other hand, peritoneal macrophages from 18-month-old rats stimulated with lipopolysaccharide (LPS) make as much nitric oxide and produce more TNF and prostaglandin I than similar cells from young animals (121). One wonders whether the differences are related to technical issues rather than actual differences in how macrophages in different parts of the body work in old versus young animals.

A clear and reproducible age-related effect in human innate immunity is an increased sensitivity to exposure to LPS (122). Even the highly selected population of elderly patients fulfilling the rigid guidelines in the SENIEUR protocol (estimated to eliminate nearly 90% of the aged population at a given age because of comorbid illness and other confounding variables) (123) showed significantly greater production of monokines such as IL-1 beta, IL-6, and IL-8 after LPS stimulation compared to young donors. Differences between young and old in the production of cytokines is not a universal finding. Again, using rigid selection criteria (SENIEUR protocol), Ahluwalia et al. (124) found no differences between young and old healthy, well-nourished women in production of IL-2, IL-1, or IL-6 in whole blood cultures stimulated for 48 hours with phytohemagglutinin. Some researchers attribute a role to macrophages in atherosclerosis. Macrophages from aged persons have been shown to produce more prostaglandin E2 than those from younger persons; this is thought to be due to overexpression of COX-2 (125). Reduction of macrophage COX-2 activity is surmised to be a target for the therapeutic effects of vitamin E in some clinical settings; however, no data support that hypothesis.

The various defects that have been identified in macrophages from old animals or people are summarized in Table 3. However, it is unclear that any clinical manifestation of being old is attributable to a change in the function of monocytes/macrophages.

Neutrophils/PMNs

An early hint that polymorphonuclear neutrophils (PMNs) might be functionally compromised in older animals came

TABLE 3. *Age-related changes in macrophage function*

Increased susceptibility to parasitic infection in mice
Hyperresponsiveness to LPS
Decreased production of cytokines and growth factors (VEGF, FGF-2)
Increased production of TNF
Impaired tumor killing (decreased NO production, oncostatin-M)
Decreased respiratory burst
Increased PGE2 and arachidonic acid metabolites, increased COX-2
Defective presentation of polysaccharide antigens

from studies of *Staphylococcus aureus* infection in mice. PMNs are the cells that deal primarily with this organism and studies showed that staphylococcal infections were much more severe and more often fatal in older animals (126). Examination of bronchoalveolar lavage fluid from young and old people has demonstrated an increase in neutrophils (about 7,000/ml in 64- to 83-year-olds compared to 1,700/ml in 19- to 36-year-olds), and elevated levels of IL-8 and neutrophil elastase as well as elastase inhibitors (127). These results were interpreted as showing a low level of inflammation in older patients. By contrast, a study of experimental gingivitis in people demonstrated that gingival lesions in older people contained more B cells and fewer neutrophils compared to gingival infiltrates in younger people (128). This might suggest that neutrophils from older people are either decreased in number or have defects in migrating to sites of inflammation.

However, neutrophil numbers are normal in normal aging and increase normally in response to infection, but bone-marrow neutrophil precursors from older subjects have a somewhat lower proliferative response *in vitro* to G-CSF (129). Furthermore, migratory responses of neutrophils are normal in healthy aging (130,131) and the cells experience a normal delay in apoptosis and an extended half-life when they are recruited to the site of an infection (normal half-life of 6 to 10 hours is extended under the influence of bacterial components, complement, and proinflammatory cytokines). Thus, decreased appearance of neutrophils in a tissue site is mainly an indicator of defective production of chemotactic cytokines in the tissue.

In addition to migrating to sites of infection, neutrophils must phagocytose microorganisms and kill them (reviewed in Lord et al. [132]). Like macrophages, it is difficult to isolate neutrophils in their physiologic state in the circulation without activating them at least partially. However, in general, it appears that the capacity of neutrophils from older people to phagocytose microorganisms is reduced (133,134). Furthermore, neutrophils from older people express less CD16 on their surface (133) and generate lower levels of reactive oxygen species in response to stimulation with *Staphylococcus aureus* (134). Interestingly, the generation of reactive oxygen species was normal when the cells were stimulated with *Escherichia coli* exposure. The two major pathways for killing ingested organisms is the generation of reactive oxygen species and the release of cytotoxic proteases from their granules. Incomplete degranulation of neutrophils from elderly patients in response to f-metleuphe has been documented (135). However, most reports suggest that reactive oxygen species generation is unaffected or somewhat increased by aging.

The problem with phagocytosis is not due to a decrease in the number of cells capable of ingesting bacteria; however, each cell seems to ingest fewer organisms. The decline in CD16 levels could be a contributing factor to this phagocytosis defect. The reported decline in phagocytosis is not a universal finding. Miyaji et al. (136) noted that neutrophils from centenarians had increased phagocytic function and cytokine production and decreased generation of superoxide. Another unusual feature of these patients was that they had elevated serum levels of interferon-γ, a cytokine that most researchers report to be low in older people. Consistent with an interferon-γ effect, neutrophils in centenarians had increased CD64 in this series (136). However, it must be noted that survival to 100 years of age is not "normal," and to some extent, changes observed in the immune systems of centenarians are difficult to interpret. Are their immune systems affording the subjects better protection than that of a patient who died at age 90 from a car accident, or even from pneumonia? Or are these changes unrelated to the prolonged survival of the individual? Should we expect the immune function of centenarians to be similar to that of other older people, but shifted to the right on an age-versus-function curve? Are these individuals the elite group we need to emulate or do they define "abnormal aging"?

We speak of innate and adaptive immunity as if they are separate and distinct entities. However, it is clear that the systems interact intimately to regulate host defense. T-cell products are responsible for promoting neutrophil production, migration, activation, and survival. Changes in T-cell function with age (see below) thus can influence innate immunity in a direct way. With the shift to a Th2 pattern of cytokine production, interferon-γ levels (which augment Fc-receptor expression on neutrophils) and GM-CSF levels (which prevent apoptosis of neutrophils in tissues) decline, and TNF-α levels (which promote neutrophil apoptosis) increase (reviewed in Lord et al. [132]). Alterations reported in neutrophils from aged people are listed in Table 4.

TABLE 4. *Age-related changes in neutrophil function*

Normal endothelial adherence, chemotaxis, migration
Reduced entry into wounds
Possible decrease in survival in wounds related to
    decreased GM-CSF
Decreased bacterial phagocytosis
Decreased expression of CD16
Decreased ROS production to selected stimuli (e.g.,
    Staphylococcus aureus)
Defective bacterial killing perhaps related to impaired
    degranulation

NK Cells and NKT Cells

NK cells are much more heterogeneous than originally thought (see Chapter 12). Many insights have emerged in recent years regarding two new classes of regulatory receptors on NK cells that recognize class I MHC molecules (killer inhibitory receptors, Ly-49 family [137], and C-type lectin heterodimers of the immunoglobulin gene family [138]). These receptors are not clonally distributed and their expression defines subsets of cells. Unfortunately, no information has yet emerged on how these receptors are affected by the aging process. The alterations in NK number and function with age are shown in Table 5.

The percentage of peripheral blood lymphocytes expressing NK markers increases with age and the absolute numbers of NK cells increase (139,140). The percentage and absolute numbers of lymphocytes expressing CD3 decrease with aging roughly in proportion to the increase in NK cells such that total lymphocyte counts are the same or somewhat lower overall. In addition to an increase in CD56$^+$ cells, a new population of cells that coexpress CD3 and NK cell markers such as CD57 increases in older donors (141,142). Significant increases are seen with aging in cells coexpressing CD3, CD8, CD16, CD56, and CD57, with subsets within this group expressing more or less CD8 (143). Within the CD56$^+$ population of NK cells, some are CD56 bright and some are CD56 dim; it is said that the bright cells are proliferative, poorly cytotoxic, and less mature, while the dim cells do not proliferate, are cytotoxic, and are more mature (144). In the elderly, the main increase is in the mature CD56 dim cells and they express higher levels of HLA-DR and CD95 and lower levels of CD69 (which triggers cytotoxicity) (140).

Data regarding the cytotoxic activity of NK cells from elderly donors are conflicting; when health status is well controlled, cytotoxic capacity seems to be maintained (145,146), while less stringent selection of donors suggests that NK lytic capacity per cell declines with age (139,142). The basis of the decreased lytic activity per cell was not related to target binding or content or release of perforin or other lytic molecules. Instead, signal transduction within the NK cell after target binding was diminished. Specifically, the release

TABLE 5. *Age-related changes in NK cells*

Increased number in peripheral blood
Greater expression of HLA DR and CD95 (Fas), reduced
    CD69 on CD56dim subset
Increased number of cells expressing both CD3 and NK
    markers like CD57
Decreased killing per cell perhaps from defective signal
    transduction
Normal ADCC killing associated with normal signal
    transduction
Normal increase in NK killing in response to cytokines
Decreased induction of LAK activity by IL-2
Slower release of interferon-γ after IL-2 stimulation
Normal production of TNF and perforin in response to
    cytokines

of inositol triphosphate (IP3), a product of cleavage of phosphatidylinositol bisphosphate (PIP2) by phospholipase C-γ, is decreased (147). The basis of the defect is unknown, but it is restricted to spontaneous killing. Killing and signal transduction mediated by CD16 through antibody-dependent cellular cytotoxicity is normal in these same cells.

NK cells proliferate and augment their killing capacity in response to various cytokines. In general, NK-trophic cytokines (e.g., IL-2, IL-12, interferon-α and γ) continue to exert stimulatory effects on NK cell killing of NK-sensitive targets in cells from aged donors, but their capacity to develop lymphokine-activated killer (or LAK) activity directed against NK-resistant targets is compromised (146). Similarly, NK cells from older donors do not proliferate as much in response to IL-2 as do NK cells from younger donors (140). The kinetics of the production of cytokines in response to IL-2 are also altered in NK cells from older donors. Interferon-γ production within the first 18 hours of stimulation of older donor NK cells is decreased, but total amounts of the cytokine produced over 7 days of stimulation are normal (148). However, the production of TNF-α and perforin by NK cells are unaffected by aging. The basis for the defective response to IL-2 is unknown. No data have been generated regarding IL-15 responses in aged NK cells.

NK/T cells, the cells noted to express both T and NK cell markers, increase in the peripheral blood with age as noted above (141,142), but have not been well studied in either old mice or humans. It is not known whether they are increased in tissue sites, marrow, and lymph nodes. Fascinating work is being done on this cell type. The cells appear to be regulatory in function as they can express both Th1 and Th2 cytokine patterns. However, they influence CD4 T cells to become Th2-like in phenotype. It may be more than coincidence that the NK/T cells are increased in aging humans and these individuals also manifest a Th2-like cytokine pattern (see below). A subset of cells has an invariant Vα chain as part of the T-cell receptor (Vα14 in mice and Vα24 in humans) that recognizes a glycolipid, α-galactosylceramide, presented on CD1d molecules rather than class I MHC. The cells appear to be involved in regulating autoreactive T cells, mediating tumor regression, inducing rapid NK cell activation, and immunity to parasites. The role of NK/T cells in the aged immune system bears more thorough study.

Efforts have been made to relate NK cell number and activity to various other measures of well-being, to various disease states, and to life span. Natural killer activity is said to decrease in the face of low levels of triiodothyronine (149), to be positively correlated with serum concentrations of vitamin D (150), to decline in the setting of atherosclerosis (151), and to predict the risk of infection and death from infection in nursing home subjects (152). NK activity has also been promoted as a predictor of mortality (153). Increases in NK cell number are said to be compensatory for the decline in T-cell immunity seen with aging (see below) as a component of immune system "remodeling," a word with a perfectly clear definition in house decorating and bone turnover that is totally obscure when applied to the immune system. It remains a significant problem that the changes thought to be caused by aging cannot be reproduced in an experimental model with another stimulus under controlled conditions. Speculations about why decreased function is not really decreased function but a conscious effort on the part of the system to correct itself do not lead to testable hypotheses or to greater insights into altered immune function with age and how to improve it. Hypothesis-driven research has a chance to define whether the changes observed with aging are in response to something. Correctable problems can then be corrected first in animals and then in humans to see first if the system can be corrected and secondarily whether the correction influences the incidence or natural history of diseases. Descriptive research lacks this potential.

Cytokines and Chemokines

Immune cells and effector functions are largely regulated by soluble factors called cytokines and chemokines. These molecules act in groups on diverse cells and processes. Their biologic activity is directed in large part by the distribution of cellular receptors specific for them. Their action can vary with different target cells. Their production can be highly restricted to one or two cell types or they can be nearly universally produced. New cytokines and chemokines are being discovered at a rapid pace and their roles in normal homeostasis and disease are being defined (see Chapters 23 through 26). Descriptive studies of their changes in the course of aging are also burgeoning.

In general, the aging immune system is characterized by producing more Th2-type cytokines (IL-4, IL-10) than Th1-type cytokines (IL-2, interferon-γ), which is a reversal of the pattern seen earlier in adulthood, and by producing more proinflammatory cytokines such as IL-1, IL-6, IL-8, and TNF-α (154). These cytokines are noted in excess in a variety of tissues in the setting of diseases; in older people, they are also found to be increased in the blood and in places that are not obviously dysfunctional or manifesting pathology such as the lungs, skin, and joints. This has led to the notion that aging is associated with chronic low-grade inflammation manifested on a systemic level. Changes in cytokine and chemokine production in aging are listed in Table 6.

TABLE 6. *Changes in cytokine and chemokine production with age*

Increased serum levels of IL-6
Decreased production of IL-2 and interferon-γ from mitogen-stimulated mononuclear cells
Normal or increased production of IL-4, IL-6, tumor necrosis factor-α, IL-8, IL-10
Increased acute phase reactants (C-reactive protein, for example)
Serum elevations of monocyte chemoattractant protein-1 (MCP-1) and RANTES
More prolonged response to LPS

Under normal circumstances, circulating levels of cytokines are low. Tissue damage results in the production of TNF-α, IL-1, and IL-6, the prototypical proinflammatory cytokines, and these signals activate the acute phase response (proteins mainly produced in the liver), elicit fever, and stimulate granulocytosis, all of which are designed to isolate, wall off, and destroy pathogens and repair the damaged tissue. The proinflammatory cytokines also elicit counterbalancing anti-inflammatory cytokines like IL-10, soluble TNF receptor, and IL-1 receptor antagonist that limit the duration of TNF and IL-1 effects (reviewed in Bruunsgaard et al. [155]).

The main controversy in the field is whether this cascade is activated as a consequence of aging alone, or whether the detection of activation of the cascade is actually a manifestation of a subtle infection (e.g., *Helicobacter pylori,* chlamydia, periodontal inflammation), stress, smoking, obesity, or any of the myriad conditions that produce an increase in IL-6 levels. In a large study of 1,727 people over age 70 years, IL-6 levels increased with increasing age independent of disease states (156). Abundant data suggest that common age-related diseases such as Alzheimer's disease, Parkinson's disease, atherosclerosis, diabetes, and even sarcopenia are associated with increased levels of cytokines (reviewed in Bruunsgaard [155]). However, when the SENIEUR protocol is used to screen donors, IL-6 levels are not as obviously elevated (157). Furthermore, among a small number of randomly chosen old and young subjects, circulating IL-6 levels were low in the majority of both groups (158). Thus, the validity of the assertion that aging is associated with an increase in IL-6 levels is questioned.

However, IL-6 levels have been documented to increase with age in both mice and primates, and unstimulated human blood mononuclear cells have been shown to produce increased levels of IL-6 and IL-1 receptor antagonist (159). Some groups have not noted the production of IL-6 or other cytokines to be elevated in either unstimulated or stimulated peripheral blood mononuclear cells (158) and still others have found that TNF-α or IL-10 production increased but not other cytokines (160–162). Limited light can be shed on the controversy by studying peripheral blood cells given that these cytokines are produced by endothelial and other cell types in tissues all over the body. One study of IL-6 mRNA levels in tissues from young and old mice found that baseline levels of IL-6 mRNA expression were decreased in old mice but that old mice injected with LPS had greater induction of IL-6 mRNA expression in the tissues than did young mice (163).

Epidemiologic studies have intensified the relationship between high circulating inflammatory cytokines and morbidity and mortality. Among 675 healthy elderly subjects, those with the highest quartile of IL-6 levels in the serum had a twofold increased risk of death compared to the lowest quartile (164). People with three or four blood markers of ongoing inflammation (low albumin, low cholesterol, high IL-6 levels, high C-reactive protein levels) had a 6.6-fold increase in 3-year mortality than those without evidence of inflammation (164a). Another study of 880 high-functioning people aged

70 to 79 years found that IL-6 and C-reactive protein levels were lower in those with greater levels of moderate to strenuous exercise compared to less active individuals (165). Dividing the group in half on the basis of walking speed, those who walked faster had lower levels of IL-6 and C-reactive protein. When the strength and performance assessments were done on the same subjects 7 years later, the levels of IL-6 and C-reactive protein did not predict the level of decline in function over time, but those who died in the interim had significantly higher baseline IL-6 and C-reactive protein levels and slower walking speed.

What Does It All Mean?

Conclusions are difficult to reach from the published data and no consensus has been achieved. However, some *in vivo* studies in human subjects provide useful information that may help us to think of new experimental approaches to sort out the conundrum. Among 22 patients hospitalized with *Streptococcus pneumoniae* infection, TNF-α and soluble TNF receptor levels were higher in elderly than in young patients during the acute infection and IL-10 levels stayed elevated longer in elderly than in young patients (166). When nine healthy volunteers aged 61 to 69 years were given a human endotoxin challenge (intravenous LPS), plasma levels of TNF-α, IL-6, IL-10, IL-8, soluble TNF receptor, and IL-1 receptor antagonist increased markedly in both the healthy elderly and eight young controls and no significant difference was noted in the peak levels of these molecules between young and old groups (167). However, the elderly group showed larger initial increases in TNF-α and soluble TNF receptor, more prolonged increases in the levels of these molecules and C-reactive protein, and took longer to normalize their body temperature than the young subjects.

Thus, as is seen with aging in other organ systems, it appears that the immune system in the elderly has lost some homeostatic capacity. The system responds briskly to a perceived threat and takes longer to come back to normal after responding to the threat. At the moment, no compelling evidence exists to say that one cytokine or another is abnormally regulated in old people. That is, aging does not appear to be like a disease in which a particular cytokine or group of cytokines is autonomously overexpressed with health consequences. In the absence of such data, it is difficult to maintain the argument that such abnormal regulation is a primary event in aging. Instead, it appears that the innate immune system, which is responsible for the immediate response to pathogens and tissue damage, responds appropriately in the elderly (in the absence of chronic disease). However, because of possible defects in effector functions in the adaptive immune response (see below) resulting in less effective control of the threat (with attendant decreases in the anti-inflammatory or turn-off signals) or because of desensitization of the negative feedback system (or turn-off signals are sent but not received or the system may be reset to a different threshold for turn-off), inflammatory responses in the elderly are more prolonged. An imbalance between proinflammatory and anti-inflammatory cytokine levels has been suggested based on *in vitro* data on isolated blood cells that cannot be considered a reliable reflection of *in vivo* biology (160).

Data are beginning to emerge on changes in chemokine levels associated with aging. Numerous studies (see, for example, Clark and Peterson [168], Pulsatelli et al. [169], Mariani et al. [170,171]) report results on the production of chemokines *in vitro* after polyclonal stimulation of mixed cell populations, results that provide little insight into the aging immune system. Serum elevations in monocyte chemoattractant protein-1 (MCP-1) (172,173) and RANTES (173) have been noted in older subjects. The physiologic or pathophysiologic effects of circulating chemokines, which are generally released locally to act locally, are of some concern. CXC chemokines can increase brain inflammation and breakdown of the blood–brain barrier (174), possibly leading or predisposing to dementing illnesses like Alzheimer's disease (175–177).

Is aging caused or accelerated by chronic low-level systemic inflammation? Are the most significant diseases of aging mediated by uncontrolled inflammation? The widespread use of anti-inflammatory agents from aspirin to COX-2 inhibitors may be able to shed some light on these questions. However, a clinical trial addressing the hypothesis with specific disease and mortality endpoints seems impractical on a large scale. Perhaps animal models will provide a tool to address the question. Will animals fed an anti-inflammatory agent for a lifetime live longer? At the moment the only intervention that has reproducibly increased both mean and maximal lifespan in experimental animals is caloric restriction (see below). Yet the hypothesis that aging is worsened by chronic inflammation is testable and one or more rigorous tests seems preferable to what is currently being seen—a proliferation of papers hypothesizing on the issue as if it were a novel idea.

AGE-RELATED CHANGES IN ADAPTIVE IMMUNITY

Adaptive immunity involves the generation of antigen-specific responses to pathogens and immunogens. T cells and B cells are the effectors of adaptive immunity. These cells develop the capacity to generate specific antigen recognition receptors for the entire panoply of potential antigens and link recognition of antigen to the activation of a wide variety of protective functions. Adaptive immunity is the component of the immune system that is most affected by aging.

Age-Related Changes in T Cells

A variety of significant changes are noted in T-cell immunity with aging. Thymic involution, a shift to memory phenotype cells and away from naïve cells, an alteration in the antigen receptor repertoire, a shift from a Th1 to a Th2 pattern of cytokine production from CD4$^+$ T cells, altered

signal transduction within T cells, altered expression of costimulatory, adhesion, and growth factor receptors, and many other changes have been documented (reviewed in Linton and Thoman [178], Chakravarti and Abraham [179], Pawelec et al. [180], Globerson [181]). It is the development of defects in T-cell function that seems to be most clearly related to clinical events associated with aging such as shingles and reactivation of tuberculosis. Changes noted in T cells in aging are listed in Table 7.

Changes in T-Cell Development

Normal T-cell development is reviewed in Chapter 9. Here we shall focus on age-associated changes in T-cell development. The dominant maturation pathway for T cells is through the thymus, although a quantitatively smaller contribution to the peripheral T-cell pool can also be generated independent of the thymus through an extrathymic pathway (182). Thymic function has remained incompletely understood. Much has been inferred about thymic function from studies of manipulated animals. However, the capacity to identify and quantitate recent thymic emigrants has provided new insights into thymic function and how it changes with age (reviewed in Haynes et al. [183]).

Morphologists have clarified several long-standing misconceptions about the thymus (184,185). The thymus is comprised of two anatomic compartments: (a) the thymic epithelial space, in which thymopoiesis occurs, and (b) the perivascular space, the function of which is not known. The lymphoid component of the perivascular space increases in size from birth to age 20 to 25 years and then decreases; the lymphoid component of the thymic epithelial space begins to decrease shortly after birth, decreasing about 3% annually from age 35 through 45 and then decreasing about 1% annually through the rest of life. While the lymphoid component of the perivascular space decreases with age, the perivascular space itself increases, mainly as a consequence of fat accumulation (see Fig. 2).

TABLE 7. *Age-related changes in T cells*

Decreased thymopoiesis (thymic epithelial tissue declines in mass)
Decreased generation of naïve T cells
T-cell number maintained by antigen-driven expansion of post-thymic peripheral T cells
Decreased T-cell repertoire for foreign antigens
Altered peripheral blood T-cell subsets; decreased naïve CD4, increased memory CD4, decreased expression of CD28, increased coexpression of CD8 and CD56 and CD57
Distortion of repertoire; antigen-driven oligoclonal expansion, especially of CD8$^+$ T cells
Production of Th2 cytokines in preference to Th1 cytokines
Altered signal transduction; decreased calcium release; defective lipid raft formation; diminished downstream kinase activity and transcription factor (e.g., NFATc) activation

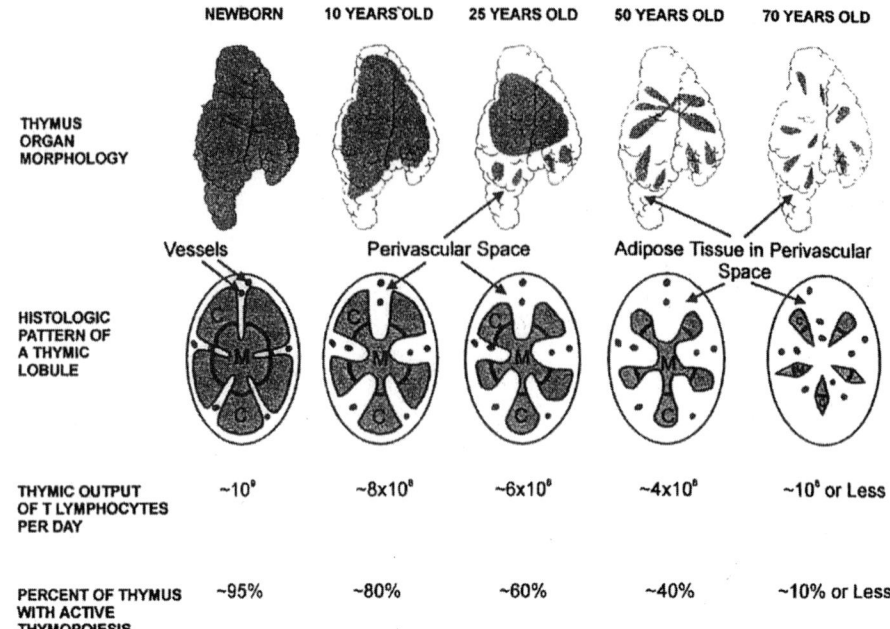

FIG. 2. The change in thymic epithelial cell mass with age is depicted. The thymus is comprised of thymic epithelial space, from which T cells are generated (shown in dark shade) and perivascular space (shown in light shade). With increasing age, thymic epithelial cell mass decreases to about 10% or less of the total thymic cell mass, the rate of T-lymphocyte production declines (but does not become zero) and the perivascular space is increasingly made up of fat. From Haynes et al. (183), with permission.

Recent thymic emigrants are thought to be identifiable by the presence of a fragment of DNA generated during the rearrangement of the antigen receptor genes. These fragments, called signal joint T-cell–receptor excision circles (sjTRECs or TRECs), are present in cells that have not yet encountered antigen and been required to divide (TRECs are lost on replication). Thus, TREC content is a reliable measure of the number of cell divisions that have occurred since the recombination event. To the extent that recent thymic emigrants have undergone relatively few cell divisions, TREC content can reflect thymus output. However, it must be noted that antigen-naïve T cells that have not yet been called upon to divide may also contain TRECs even if they emerged from the thymus a long time ago. Originally developed in the chicken (186), the technique has been adapted to humans (focusing on the α/δ gene locus) and used to demonstrate that TREC content in peripheral blood CD4 and CD8 T cells declines with age (187). However, generation of T cells containing TRECs continues into adulthood until at least the age of 50 years (188). More systematic study of older people is required but this finding alone alters the notion that thymopoietic activity paralleled thymic size and was essentially completed by age 30 years. The thymopoietic tissue does shrink with age; a 70-year-old has about 10% of the thymopoietic space of a child, yet thymic output of T cells continues, albeit at a reduced rate. The output declines as a function of thymopoietic tissue, but the production of new cells per gram of thymopoietic tissue remains relatively constant (183, 187–189).

If thymus function continues in adulthood and old age, the gland lacks the capacity to respond to a sudden decline in peripheral T cells with an increase in T-cell production. T-cell depletion is a common sequela of HIV infection, conventional dose chemotherapy for cancer, and high-dose (chemotherapy and radiation therapy) preparative regimens for allogeneic bone-marrow transplantation. HIV infection is associated with T-cell depletion and TRECs have been shown to increase with highly effective antiretroviral therapy (see Chapter 42) (187). The recovery of T-cell immunity, particularly the generation of naïve CD4$^+$ T cells, after high-dose preparative regimens and bone marrow transplantation is prolonged in older people and those without thymuses (190), even in recipients of autologous stem cells (191). However, in the setting of HIV infection and high-dose systemic therapy, interpretation of delayed T-cell recovery is complicated by the potential effects of the HIV and the preparative regimen on the thymus and its function. Is the lack of thymus recovery related to the aging process or a side effect of disease or its treatment?

The recovery of T cells after conventional dose chemotherapy is more likely to reflect the capacity of the thymus to respond to an increased demand because such therapy is less likely to do damage to the thymic epithelium itself, based on the resistance of other epithelial organs to chemotherapy effects. In 15 patients who underwent cancer chemotherapy, the CD4 T-cell count 6 months after the completion of therapy was inversely related to the age of the patient, and those patients who had some recovery of CD4 T-cell counts had evidence of thymic tissue on chest CT scans (192). Thymic hyperplasia has been identified in a number of children and young adults recovering from the effects of chemotherapy (193). Thus, the capacity of the thymus to augment its productivity physiologically in response to need appears to be greatly reduced after the age of 30 years. Indeed, little evidence exists to suggest that the thymus is sensitive to changes in the peripheral T-cell pool (194). Studies in animals have shown that the primary source of regenerated T cells in the absence of thymic function is the expansion of residual peripheral T cells, a process that is at least partially antigen driven and, as a consequence, results in an altered T-cell receptor repertoire (Mackall et al. [195], reviewed in Mackall and Gress [196]).

In contrast to situations producing profound peripheral T-cell depletion, the decline in thymic function with age is not associated with a dramatic decline in circulating T cells, although the subsets of T cells change (see below). The preservation of T-cell numbers with age appears to be largely related to the antigen-driven expansion of post-thymic mature T cells combined with less antigen-induced cell death (see below). What accounts for the decline in thymus function with age? Several hypotheses have been generated.

One idea is that the thymus involutes because of a decline in the supply of T-cell progenitors from the bone marrow. This notion was supported by early data using bone marrow from old donors to reconstitute young mice following lethal irradiation; such bone marrow was less efficient at repopulating the thymus than marrow from younger donors (197), a finding that has been reproduced (198). However, other groups found that the efficiency of old and young bone marrow at repopulating the thymus and spleen was comparable when given to mice of similar age (199). Furthermore, within the thymus of aged animals, the number of T-cell progenitors (200) and their function (201) appear to be normal, although others have found functional defects in the marrow progenitors (202). If there is a defect in the bone marrow progenitors of aged mice, it is not the controlling factor in the age-related decline in thymic function because even when older animals are provided with young bone-marrow stem cells, the thymi of the reconstituted old mice are small and generate significantly reduced numbers of splenic T cells compared to young recipients, although the subset distribution and capacity to mediate negative selection is intact in aged thymi (203). Furthermore, neonatal thymus grafts are as successful in old recipients as in young ones (196). Thus, it would appear that the thymus milieu rather than the extrathymic environment plays the greater role in thymic involution.

Another hypothesis is that the aged thymus acquires an altered environment that no longer supports T-cell development. Most of the specific ideas about the nature of the altered environment involve changes in cytokine expression. IL-7 was considered a prime candidate for a cytokine active in the thymus when it was shown to promote V(D)J rearrangement through induction of RAG-1 and RAG-2 genes in thymocytes from murine embryos (204). However,

investigation of changes in IL-7 expression in the aging thymus has produced inconsistent results. Aspinall and Andrew (201,205,206) claim that IL-7 production is decreased in the aging thymus, probably as a consequence of the loss of IL-7 expression in certain thymic epithelial cells, and suggest that administration of IL-7 to older mice augments thymic size and thymopoiesis. By contrast, Sempowski et al. (207) find that IL-7 is one of a group of cytokines (that includes IL-15 and GM-CSF) whose production is unaltered in the thymus with age (see Fig. 3). IL-2, IL-9, IL-10, IL-13, and IL-14 were cytokines whose expression declined with age and leukemia inhibitory factor (LIF), oncostatin M, IL-6, stem cell factor, and M-CSF were all expressed at increased levels with age in human thymi (207). All of the cytokines that increased with age except M-CSF (i.e., LIF, oncostatin M, IL-6, and stem cell factor) were shown to mediate thymic atrophy with loss of CD4$^+$CD8$^+$ (double-positive) cortical thymocytes when administered to mice intraperitoneally for 3 days (207). Furthermore, IL-7 administration was found to augment thymopoiesis (measured by an increased output of TREC-containing naïve T cells) in young mice but was ineffective in old mice (208). At the moment, the controversy is unresolved. However, given that IL-7 can restore immune responses in athymic hosts following peripheral T-cell depletion (209), it seems clear that IL-7 has pleiotropic effects including inhibiting apoptosis, improving co-stimulation, and improving efficiency of antigen presentation, all of which could look like an augmentation of thymus function. A plausible alternative to the simple view that thymic involution represents IL-7 deficiency is that an age-related increase in the expression of several cytokines that inhibit thymic function exert a dominant effect. It may be necessary to antagonize one or more of these cytokines in order to reap the full benefit of either endogenously produced or exogenous therapeutic IL-7. The role of chemokines in thymus function has not yet been studied.

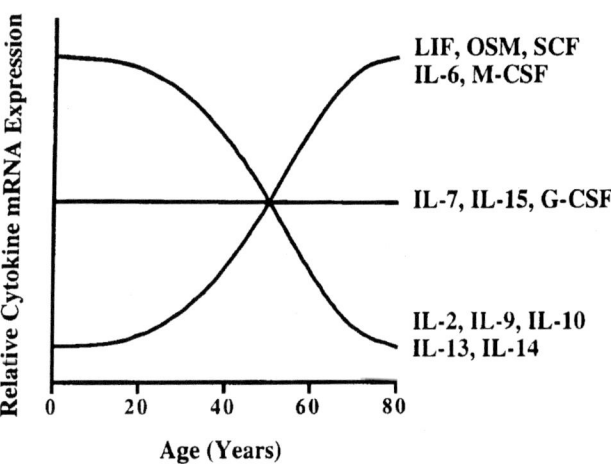

FIG. 3. The relative change in mRNA for various cytokines expressed in the thymus is illustrated as a function of age. From Haynes et al. (183), with permission.

It is somewhat surprising that the process of thymic involution has not been better studied with transgenic and knockout mice, given that the steps of T-cell development have been thoroughly elucidated by such studies. Many relevant animals have been generated, but usually not with thymus aging specifically in mind. Given the hypothesis that a key change in the aging thymus was the failure to rearrange the TCRβ chain genes (200), 12 month-old mice expressing a transgenic TCRβ chain were analyzed for their thymic function and found to undergo normal involution (210,211). Thus, supplying a rearranged TCRβ does not overcome the process of thymic atrophy, arguing that a defect in TCRβ rearrangement cannot be the signal for thymic involution.

Mice that do not express either MHC class I or MHC class II molecules do not undergo normal thymic involution (210). Their thymi stay the size of a normal young adult until at least 12 months of age. These organs cannot generate mature T cells and cannot mediate positive and negative selection. Thus, it is possible that something about the generation of mature T cells or some feature of positive or negative selection serves as a stimulus to thymus involution. Another crucial function of the thymus for the generation of CD4$^+$ T cells is the activity of cathepsin L; mice with cathepsin L knocked out (212) or with a natural mutation in the cathepsin L gene (Cts1) (213) fail to make CD4$^+$ T cells because cathepsin L is responsible for the degradation of the invariant chain (Ii), a chaperone for peptide-loaded class II MHC molecules. Mutations in cathepsin L result in failure of antigen presentation to and positive selection of CD4$^+$ cells by the thymic epithelium. Whether cathepsin L function in the thymus is affected by age is unknown.

A number of transgenic models have documented either premature thymic involution (human SOD-1 transgenic mice) (214) or delayed thymic involution (CD2-Fas transgenic mice [215]; human homeobox gene, HB24 transgenic mice [216]). However, these models have not led to insights about the physiologic changes that occur in the normal thymus with aging. Microarray analysis of changes in gene expression in the thymus with age is in progress and may lead to more revealing studies on the biology of thymic involution.

Endogenous thymic cytokine production is not the only control mechanism for thymic function. Hormones are well known to influence thymic function. Growth hormone declines with age, as does thymic function, and growth hormone has been shown to promote thymopoiesis in animals (71,217); human studies of growth hormone supplementation to older people have not been well designed to detect an immunologic effect (218). The thymic epithelium expresses androgen receptors (219). Castration of male rodents results in enlargement of the thymus, and androgen replacement reverses the effects (220). This may explain why peripheral blood from women contains significantly higher levels of TRECs per CD3 T cell than does blood from age-matched males (221). Although the CD3 levels are not different between men and women, women have considerably more recent thymic emigrants, a finding that has led to speculation about whether this

feature of preserved thymic function based on the absence of androgen effects on the thymus underlies the differences in life span between men and women. The T-cell and thymic function of men with prostate cancer treated with orchiectomy or medical castration (luteinizing hormone-releasing hormone) has not been well studied, but it is conceivable that antagonizing androgen action would prolong thymic function and have an immunostimulatory effect.

Glucocorticoids have a potent effect on the thymus. High blood levels such as those induced by stress, injury, or illness induce the death of cortical thymocytes (222). However, Vacchio and Ashwell (223) have suggested that the local endogenous production of a glucocorticoid signal is a key factor in mediating thymocyte survival; triggering a thymocyte through its antigen receptor can induce cell death, and exposure to glucocorticoids can induce cell death, but the two signals together result in cell survival. Whether a decline in the production of endogenous glucocorticoids could play a role in thymic involution has not been examined.

Neurotrophic hormones such as nerve growth factor (224), cholinergic (225), and adrenergic enervation (226), and a wide variety of "thymic hormones" have been proposed to regulate or "modulate" (the word we use when we do not see consistent changes) thymus function. Little work has been done on the neural regulation. However, an immense literature exists on various thymic hormones including thymosin, thymopoietin, thymulin, thymopentin, and other neuropeptides. I do not understand most of this work and cannot discern whether these factors play a role in thymic function in health, disease, or aging; however, I include a few references to assist the interested reader in gaining access to this literature (227–229).

Changes in T-Cell Subsets with Age

As noted above, total lymphocyte counts and total T-cell counts change little with age. However, conflicting reports claim a decline in lymphocyte and T-cell number. Most studies find that the number of CD4$^+$ T cells decreases with aging with naïve CD4$^+$ T cells (generally detected by coexpression of CD45RA) being more greatly reduced than memory CD4$^+$ T cells (detected by coexpression of CD45RO) and memory-type cells increasing over time; CD8$^+$ T-cell numbers are generally unchanged with aging; and cells coexpressing T-cell and NK cell markers (particularly CD56 and CD57) increase with aging in mice and in humans (230–236). γ/δ receptor-expressing T cells are also decreased in the elderly and express CD69, a marker of activation (237). Analysis of coexpression of other markers also shows age-related changes. For example, the CD4 T cells in older people are often CD7 negative (234,238) and the amount of CD4 expressed per cell is decreased on an expanding subset of CD4$^+$ T cells that also expresses a reduced level of CD3, CD95Fas, and CD28 (239). L-selectin expression (CD62L) declines with age (said to be a marker of naïve T cells) (240) and cells expressing the P-glycoprotein (241) and CD29 (242) increase with age. CD28, an important co-stimulatory molecule, is missing from an increasing fraction of T cells in older people (243,244), a change that has been correlated with signaling alterations (see below). Inconsistent with the theory that older people are under chronic immune stimulation, activation markers such as CD69, CD71, CD25, and HLA-DR are generally not expressed on peripheral blood T cells, although serum levels of cytokines and soluble CD25 may be elevated (see above).

CD31 has been shown to be expressed on a subset of naïve (CD45RA$^+$) T cells that are enriched for TRECs (245). When such cells are activated, CD31 disappears and the TREC levels decrease dramatically as a consequence of cell replication. Thus, in older people, the diminishing pool of naïve T cells has been found to have a larger subset that is CD31 negative and TREC depleted and a smaller subset that is CD31 positive and rich in TRECs. These data argue that expansion of the naïve cells has taken place by some mechanism, presumably by a stimulus that did not result in maturation to memory phenotype. This could reflect an effort to fill a CD4 niche by peripheral expansion in the face of decreasing thymic output.

It has been proposed that one can project the longevity of middle-aged mice by measuring peripheral blood levels of particular T-cell subsets; 8-month-old mice with lower levels of memory phenotype cells, higher levels of naïve CD4 T cells, and low levels of CD4 T cells expressing the p-glycoprotein lived about 6% longer than mice with higher levels of memory cells, lower levels of naïve CD4 T cells, and higher levels of CD4 T cells expressing p-glycoprotein (246). Such correlations are difficult to interpret. If one were able to alter the subsets experimentally in those with a shorter lifespan and find that survival had been prolonged, perhaps such results would have some meaning. The alleged correlation with survival cannot be interpreted as linking the variables (T-cell subsets and longevity) without additional data. Early data from the Swedish longitudinal study of octogenarians (OCTO) suggested a similar correlation in that 2-year survival was decreased in the group with low CD4:CD8 ratios, decreased CD4 cells, increased CD8 cells with NK cell markers, and decreased naïve cells; however, follow-up of the same cohort (236) and an additional cohort with median age of 90 years (NONA study) (247) found that the altered peripheral blood T-cell subsets were associated with CMV infections. Unknown environmental factors can influence the peripheral blood subsets and undermine the capacity to use such measures as a predictor of health status. Age-related reference intervals for lymphocyte subsets in the peripheral blood of healthy individuals have been described (248), but the quantitation of such subsets is of no established clinical value.

T-cell subset distribution has also been assessed in human tissues. In the bone marrow, overall cellularity decreases with age as the percentage of fat increases. There is some evidence of increased apoptosis in marrow cells from older people, but it is unclear whether this is restricted to lymphocytes (249).

In normal lungs, activated CD4$^+$ lymphocytes are increased with aging (250). CD4$^+$ T cells also increase in the tonsils with age as B-cell numbers and CD38$^+$ B cells (late-stage maturation) decline (251). CD8$^+$ T cells appear to decline in the spleen (252) but large numbers of CD4$^+$ CD8-$\alpha\alpha^+$ T cells—which are thought to be extrathymic in origin—accumulate in gut-associated lymphatic tissue (253). Studies in rats (254) and cynomolgus monkeys (255) have generally shown changes similar to those seen in humans.

Given the influence of adhesion molecules such as CD62L on lymphocyte migration (256) and the reported alterations of adhesion molecule expression on T cells from older patients (257,258) (memory T cells express less CD50 [ICAM-3] and naïve T cells express less CD62L), it is possible that T cells from old people do not migrate and recirculate normally. However, when trafficking of older lymphocytes was studied in vivo in mice, it was observed that they were equally capable of homing to young spleens and recirculating from that site elsewhere (259). By contrast, older spleens were less effective at taking up either young or old lymphocytes and once in the spleen, the cells tended to remain there. Thus, it would appear that, as noted in the aging thymus, any age-related problem in lymphocyte homing is a function of altered signals from the microenvironment rather than an intrinsic defect in old lymphocytes.

The decline in thymic function is most dramatically noted in the paucity of naïve phenotype CD4$^+$ T cells. The definition of naïve CD8$^+$ T cells is not as clearly demarcated by the expression of CD45RA as in CD4$^+$ T cells and thus, it is difficult to assess whether memory or naïve CD8$^+$ T cells are more affected by aging. In the absence of a functional thymus, the CD8$^+$ T cells recover more quickly than the CD4$^+$ T cells at least in part through the extrathymic generation of CD8$^+$ subsets that are CD8$^+$CD28$^-$ and CD8$^+$CD57$^+$. Both of these subsets of CD8$^+$ T cells also increase with age, suggesting that the preservation of CD8$^+$ T-cell number actually represents thymus-independent expansion of post-thymic cells.

Changes in T-Cell Antigen-Receptor Repertoire with Age

Studies of the expression of T-cell receptor gene families on the surface of lymphocytes using antibodies specific for particular receptor gene families, spectratyping, analysis of CDR3 length, and heteroduplex analysis have demonstrated that the distribution of receptor expression (typically a normal distribution of receptors from all gene families) is frequently altered in older mice (260–264) and human subjects (265–270). Both α/β- (260–269) and γ/δ-expressing (270) T cells can be affected. One or a few clones of cells expand to the point where a particular clone can represent one-third or more of all the T cells (269). CD8$^+$ T cells are usually affected; the involvement of CD4 T cells in oligoclonal expansion is debated, with some studies finding no alteration in the CD4 repertoire (260,265) and others finding similar expansions of certain CD4 clones (267,271), particularly in very old humans

(268). However, the CD8 subset is more often affected than the CD4. These expansions are not analogous to "monoclonal gammopathy of uncertain significance," that is, monoclonal expansions of a B-cell clone that occur in increased frequency with aging (see below). Unlike the B-cell disorder, which progresses to a frank B-cell malignancy at a rate of about 1% per year, oligoclonal T-cell expansions are not known to progress to malignancy. While particular clonal expansions of T cells have been shown to persist for up to 2 years in humans (267), they are more unstable in mice, disappearing after 2 to 4 months only to be replaced by another clone (268). However, the frequency of finding clonal expansions increases with age.

Most of the expansions were in the CD45RO (memory) subset, but some were seen in the CD45RA subset as well (268). The involvement of CD45RA-expressing cells in the CD8$^+$ CD28$^-$ subset may be a consequence of CD45RO memory cells reexpressing CD45RA rather than the involvement of authentic naïve cells (272). By what mechanism does a particular clone of cells expand? Similar alterations have been noted in people as a consequence of viral infection (273–275). In older people (and mice), the particular clone that is expanded is not the same in different individuals, and the same clone may not remain permanently expanded in the same individual, a finding that argues against the notion that a particular environmental antigen is the same trigger in all or most people.

In mice, the appearance of these clonal expansions can be hastened by thymectomy (263), arguing that they occur in the periphery (their development is not blocked by thymectomy) perhaps as a consequence of a decrease in thymic generation of naïve cells. Transfer of transgenic H-Y (male antigen)-specific autoreactive CD8$^+$ T cells from aged mice into male adoptive hosts demonstrates that older autoreactive T cells are less susceptible to peripheral tolerance induction than are younger autoreactive T cells (276). However, the clonal expansions in normal old people do not appear to be autoreactive or autoaggressive, making it difficult to relate the observation to defective self-tolerance. Clonal expansions can be identified in people with autoimmune disease (e.g., rheumatoid arthritis) (277); however, the prevalence of clonal expansions is much greater than the prevalence of autoimmune disease. The particular clone expanded can be affected by the presence of a chronic viral infection (278). For example, older C3H.HW (H-2b) mice from a mouse hepatitis virus–infected colony contained clonal expansion of Vβ7-expressing CD8 T cells; however, similarly exposed C57BL/10 mice did not show expansion of Vβ7-expressing cells (278). Thus, if the expansion is driven by a particular antigen/MHC–peptide presentation, it can be affected by undefined non–MHC-related genes. Clonal expansions are also less common in pathogen-free animals than in conventionally housed mice. These findings argue that clonal expansion is at least initiated as an antigen-driven event.

If clonal expansion is antigen driven, the response of the clone is unusual. The cells do not express activation markers.

On adoptive transfer to irradiated recipients, they are slow to emerge but they expand over time and measurement of *in vivo* turnover suggests that they are like normal T cells in their growth characteristics. Much of their expansion appears to be cytokine mediated (279). IL-2 seems to block expansion and IL-15 to promote expansion. Thus, the fate and size of the clones may be regulated by cytokine levels in the microenvironment rather than antigen exposure. It is tempting to speculate that the emergence of these clonal populations compromises the spectrum of antigen specificities recognized by the immune system. However, formal proof of that idea has not been generated by a comparison of receptor diversity in young and old animals or people. Whether clonal expansions underlie susceptibility to infection has not been proven.

CD4 T cells are generally less affected by clonal expansions during aging. In old mice whose T cells express the receptor specific for pigeon cytochrome c presented in the context of class II MHC (I-E), an antigen not encountered in the environment under normal circumstances, CD4 T cells maintain a naïve phenotype, although they have decreased antigen responsiveness (see below) (280). However, older mice generate more CD4 T cells that do not contain the transgenic receptor than do younger mice (i.e., generation of CD4 T cells is leaky), and these cells develop a memory phenotype and secrete IL-4 rather than IL-2 on antigen exposure. CD4 T cells that do not encounter antigen remain naïve in phenotype; those that encounter antigen develop age-associated defects in aged animals.

Based on these data and the experiments of Mackall et al. (281), who showed that skewed expansions of CD8$^+$ cells did not take place in mice deficient in expression of Class I MHC, it would appear that antigen presentation is at least involved in the initial selection of a clone for expansion. However, ongoing antigenic stimulation seems not to be necessary as long as appropriate cytokines (IL-15) are available to sustain the clone. The pattern of gene expression following IL-15 stimulation overlaps considerably with the pattern of gene expression following signal transduction through the antigen receptor in CD8$^+$-memory T cells (282).

Age-Related Changes in Cell Biology of T Cells

It has long and often been reported that polyclonal stimulation of peripheral blood T cells from old subjects results in less proliferation per cell than such cells from young subjects (see, for example, Nagel et al. [283]). The stimulated cells make less IL-2 than expected and express lower levels of IL-2 receptor in response to either lectins or antibodies that crosslink the antigen receptor and co-stimulatory receptors (anti-CD3, anti-CD28). The decreased proliferation appears to be associated with about half the cells progressing normally through the cell cycle and about half the cells arresting in mid-G1. The arrested cells do not down-regulate the cyclin-dependent kinase inhibitor p27Kip1 in the normal fashion, and unlike normal T cells, p27 expression is not down-regulated by IL-2

generations of lethally irradiated and marrow-reconstituted animals. The bone marrow cellularity changes with age in people; a larger percentage of the marrow cavity is occupied by fat (60% to 75%) and the number of lymphocytes, macrophages, and stromal cells declines somewhat (376). However, hemopoiesis is normal in healthy old people, and blood counts are normal in the absence of disease (377). Like lymphocytes, it appears that renewable hematopoietic stem cells are capable of regulating their telomere length in that the blood cell telomeres shorten a bit in the first year in transplant recipients compared to the donor but remain stable after that time (378). Older cancer patients may have somewhat greater sensitivity to the myelosuppressive effects of chemotherapy and radiation therapy and their recovery may be somewhat slower than the recovery in younger patients; however, full recovery is the rule in both age groups. Older people do not seem to run out of stem cell capacity even as a consequence of multiple cycles of myelotoxic therapy from which they must recover.

INTERVENTIONS AIMED AT IMPROVING IMMUNE FUNCTION IN AGING

Given that the defects that develop in the immune system with age do not seem to have a single reversible cause, a variety of interventions have been proposed to improve the function of the aging immune system (379). Vaccination has been demonstrated to induce protective immunity in certain settings in the elderly. However, no other interventions have been validated through prospective randomized clinical trials. Nevertheless, nutritional supplements, hormones, and cytokines are widely advocated in the absence of efficacy data.

Most of the therapeutic effort has been aimed at boosting T-cell immunity, the arm of the immune system most significantly and consistently compromised in aging. Appropriate assessment in future studies will need to include *in vivo* assessment of T-cell function, studies of signal transduction, and measurement of recent thymic emigrants.

Vaccination

Vaccination is discussed in detail in Chapter 43. In the elderly, repeated vaccination appears to be associated with greater efficacy for the influenza vaccine (380). Addition of adjuvants that improve antigen processing and presentation have been proposed and studied on a limited basis including GM-CSF, the hormone dehydroepiandrosterone (DHEA), novel oil-in-water emulsions, and lipid mixtures (380–382). More immunogenic formulations such as ISCOMs (immunostimulatory complexes formulated from antigen, cholesterol, phosphatidyl choline, and saponins) and DNA vaccines with adjuvant activity associated with the CpG content are also being tested, but have not yet become standard reagents (383,384). Variations in route of administration are also being explored; it is thought that mucosal (oral or nasal) administration may be more effective than subcutaneous administration

(385,386), although not all efforts at immunizing orally have been effective (387). Finally, new vaccines are being developed against other infectious agents (388) and cancer (389) in an effort to protect the elderly against common medical problems by boosting specific immunity.

Exercise

Moderate daily physical exercise has been shown to retard the development of age-associated defects in immune function in rats (390) and to enhance antigen-specific cytokine production in aged mice (391). However, human studies are less clear. Response depends on intensity, duration, and mode of exercise, hormone status, baseline levels of inflammatory cytokines, and many other factors (392). The most consistently observed change is an increase in NK cell number, activity, and responsiveness to interferon-α (393). It is not clear whether the beneficial effects of an ongoing exercise program are related to the exercise or the changes in body weight and fitness that accompany the exercise. Endurance training can produce elevations in inflammatory cytokines (TNF, IL-1, IL-6, IL-1RA, IL-10) that mimic sepsis (394), although actual increases in infection as a consequence of strenuous exercise–induced immune suppression have not been confirmed. Older subjects begin with baseline elevations in these cytokines and the levels and associated T-cell defects can be further increased by exercising to exhaustion (395). The benefits of moderate exercise on other organ systems outweigh any improvements seen in immune function (396).

Nutrition

The intervention that exerts the most powerful and consistent effects to increase both median and maximum life span in every species in which it has been tested is caloric restriction (reviewed in Pahlavani [397]). In addition to its effects on life span, caloric restriction has been shown to inhibit the age-related increase in TNF and IL-6 production (398), increase the expression of IL-2 and the activity of NFAT (399), and ameliorate the signaling defects in T cells in rats (400). Furthermore, caloric restriction enhanced the development of viral immunity to influenza in rats (401). However, calorie restriction in rhesus monkeys is associated with lymphopenia and reduced mitogen-induced proliferation (402). The mechanism of the effect of caloric restriction on longevity is not yet defined. The improvement in immune function in rodents may reflect a delay in the aging process. It remains unclear whether the effects on the immune system are related to the effects on longevity.

Older people are at risk for malnutrition, which can exert adverse effects on immune function (403). Meydani and colleagues have generated considerable data suggesting that vitamin E supplementation may be of benefit in modifying the defects in the aging immune system (404). Vitamin E deficiency may be noted in 5% to 15% of people in long-term care facilities. Vitamin E can augment Th1 cytokine responses in old mice infected with influenza (404) and increase IL-2 production from naïve T cells (405). The enhancing effects of Vitamin E on thymic activity have been hypothesized to be related to increased function of thymic epithelial cells mediated by up-regulation of ICAM-1 expression, which enhances binding to immature thymocytes (406). Administration of vitamin E (200 mg/d) improves DTH responses and primary responses to hepatitis B vaccine, but did not boost recall responses (407). No clinical studies have been powered to detect disease-related endpoints such as infection risk or days of illness.

Zinc and selenium supplements have also been suggested to be immune stimulants in aging (408,409), but clinical trials with immunologic endpoints are lacking. *In vitro* addition of antioxidant vitamins (particularly E and C) fail to correct the proliferative defects in T cells from aged people (410), and clinical studies of vitamin C supplementation do not confirm any immune stimulatory effect (403).

Japanese herbal medicine (kampo-hozai) (411) and a strain of *Lactobacillus casei* (412) have been found to stimulate immune function in aged rodents; the probiotic *Bifidobacterium lactis* HN019 was found to boost CD4$^+$ T-cell counts and cell-surface expression of IL-2 receptors in a small trial of healthy elderly people (413). However, alternative medicines are largely untested in this setting.

Hormones

Hormonal changes are among the most dramatic alterations that occur with aging. Growth hormone, sex steroids, melatonin, and a number of other hormones that decline with age have been implicated in the age-associated decline in immune function (414). Growth hormone has genuine stimulatory effect on murine thymus *in vivo* (71). However, human studies of growth hormone supplementation in aging have focused more on its effects on muscle strength and metabolism than on immune function. Growth hormone (415) and growth hormone–releasing hormone (416) need to be studied more carefully for their effects on immune function in humans. Dehydroepiandrosterone (DHEA), one of the principal adrenal steroids, decreases with age, and supplementation of people who have low levels of DHEA has been shown to increase the number of monocytes and B cells in the peripheral blood and augment B- and T-cell proliferative responses (417). Recent thymic emigrants and *in vivo* immunity have not been assessed in patients treated with DHEA.

Hormone replacement therapy appears to increase the number of peripheral blood B cells and produce higher levels of mitogen-induced T-cell proliferation in postmenopausal women compared to such women not taking hormone replacement (418). Decreased production of melatonin, a pineal hormone, has been implicated in the decline of immune function with aging; however, no clinical studies demonstrate significant immune stimulation as a consequence of melatonin ingestion in humans (419).

Immunotherapy

A number of recombinant cytokines merit clinical investigation for their influence on immune function in old people including IL-2, IL-7, IL-12, and IL-18. No relevant human studies have been conducted to date. Adoptive cellular therapy and thymus transplantation are also potential interventions. Little effort has been spent on developing immune interventions in the aged.

SUMMARY

Aging affects the immune system in diverse ways. The most consistent abnormalities are the presence of increased circulating levels of inflammatory cytokines, particularly IL-6, a decrease in the generation of CD4$^+$ T cells due to thymic involution, and an altered (mainly decreased) response of T cells to antigen. As with other organ systems, the immune system in aged individuals has less physiologic reserve and is slower at restoring homeostasis after encountering a stressor (for the immune system, this is most often an infectious agent) than the immune system in younger adults. However, it remains unclear how (or whether) the aging of the immune system contributes to the clinical illnesses that increase with age, including infections, cancer, atherosclerosis, Alzheimer's disease, and autoimmune disease. The immune system contains numerous functional redundancies that facilitate the preservation of host defenses but make interpretation of isolated abnormal findings, particularly *in vitro* abnormalities, extremely difficult. Thus, a high level of caution must be maintained in attempting to first describe and then understand the changes in the immune system with age, and finally to link those changes with susceptibilities to illness and ultimately to longevity. A better understanding of the pathogenesis of age-related immune defects may lead to hypothesis-driven interventions aimed at improving immune function and lowering the incidence and/or mortality of age-related diseases. Better tools to assess *in vivo* immune function would be of immense help in accomplishing this goal.

REFERENCES

1. Miller RA. The aging immune system: primer and prospectus. *Science* 1996;273:70–74.
2. Ginaldi L, DeMartinis M, D'Ostilio A, et al. Immunological changes in the elderly. *Aging* 1999;11:281–286.
3. Franceschi C, Bonafe M, Valensin S. Human immunosenescence: the prevailing of innate immunity, the failing of clonotypic immunity, and the filling of immunological space. *Vaccine* 2000;18:1717–1720.
4. Malaguarnera L, Ferlito L, Imbesi RM, et al. Immunosenescence: a review. *Arch Gerontol Geriatr* 2001;32:1–14.
5. Effros RB. Ageing and the immune system. *Novartis Found Symp* 2001;235:130–139.
6. Pinner RW, Teutsch SM, Simonsen L, et al. Trends in infectious diseases mortality in the United States. *JAMA* 1996;275:189–193.
7. Louria DB, Sen P, Sherer CV, et al. Infections in older patients: a systematic clinical approach. *Geriatrics* 1993;48:28–34.
8. Parsons HK, Dockrell DH. The burden of invasive pneumococcal disease and the potential for reduction by immunisation. *Int J Antimicrob Ag* 2002;19:85–93.

9. Neuzil KM. Influenza: new insights into an old disease. *Curr Infect Dis Rep* 2000;2:224–230.

10. Mohan VP, Scanga CA, Yu K, et al. Effects of tumor necrosis factor α on host immune response in chronic persistent tuberculosis: possible role for limiting pathology. *Infect Immun* 2001;69:1847–1855.

11. Schmader K. Herpes zoster in older adults. *Clin Infect Dis* 2001;32:1481–1486.

12. Schmader K. Postherpetic neuralgia in immunocompetent elderly people. *Vaccine* 1998;16:1768–1770.

13. Adler WH, Nagel JE. Acquired immunodeficiency syndrome in the elderly. *Drugs Aging* 1994;4:410–416.

14. Looney RJ, Falsey AR, Walsh E, et al. Effect of aging on cytokine production in response to respiratory syncytial virus infection. *J Infect Dis* 2002;185:682–685.

15. Castle SC. Clinical relevance of age-related immune dysfunction. *Clin Infect Dis* 2000;31:578–585.

16. Ershler WB, Longo DL. Aging and cancer: issues of basic and clinical science. *J Natl Cancer Inst* 1997;89:1489–1497.

17. Yancik R. Cancer burden in the aged: an epidemiological and demographic overview. *Cancer* 1997;80:1273–1283.

18. Burns EA, Leventhal EA. Aging, immunity and cancer. *Cancer Control* 2000;7:513–522.

19. Penn I. Depressed immunity and the development of cancer. *Cancer Detect Prev* 1994;18:241–252.

20. Penn I. Neoplastic complications of transplantation. *Semin Resp Dis* 1993;8:233–239.

21. Stutman O. Natural antitumor resistance in immune-deficient mice. *Exp Cell Biol* 1984;52:30–39.

22. Pawelec G. MHC unrestricted immune surveillance of leukemia. *Cancer Biother* 1994;9:265–288.

23. Shankaran V, Ikeda A, Bruce T, et al. Interferon-γ and lymphocytes prevent primary tumour development and shape tumor immunogenicity. *Nature* 2001;410:1107–1112.

24. Karanikas V, Colau D, Bairrain JF, et al. High frequency of cytolytic T lymphocytes directed against a tumor-specific mutated antigen detectable with HLA tetramers in the blood of a lung carcinoma patient with long survival. *Cancer Res* 2001;61:3718–3724.

25. Bendandi M, Gocke CD, Kobrin CB, et al. Complete molecular remissions induced by patient-specific vaccination plus granulocyte-monocyte colony-stimulating factor against lymphoma. *Nat Med* 1999;5:1171–1177.

26. Lassam N, Jay G. Suppression of MHC class I RNA in highly oncogenic cells occurs at the level of transcription. *J Immunol* 1989;143:3792–3797.

27. O'Connell J, O'Sullivan GC, Collins JK, et al. The Fas counterattack. Fas mediate T cell killing by colon cancer cells expressing Fas ligand. *J Exp Med* 1996;184:1075–1082.

28. Kurt RA, Baher A, Wisner KP, et al. Chemokine receptor desensitization in tumor-bearing mice. *Cell Immunol* 2001;207:81–88.

29. Ochoa AC, Longo DL. Alteration of signal transduction in T cells from cancer patients. *Important Adv Oncol* 1995;43–54.

30. Schneider GP, Salcedo R, Welniak LA, et al. The diverse role of chemokines in tumor progression: prospects for intervention. *Int J Mol Med* 2001;8:235–244.

31. Prehn RT. The immune reaction as a stimulator of tumor growth. *Science* 1972;176:170–171.

32. Schreiber H, Wu TH, Nachman J, et al. Immunologic enhancement of primary tumour development and its prevention. *Semin Cancer Biol* 2000;10:351–357.

33. Ershler WB. Explanations for reduced tumor proliferative capacity with age. *Exp Gerontol* 1992;27:551–558.

34. Southam CM, Moore AE. Induced immunity to cancer cell homografts in man. *Ann N Y Acad Sci* 1958;73:635–651.

35. Turk Z, Ljubic S, Turk N, et al. Detection of autoantibodies against advanced glycation end products and AGE-immune complexes in serum of patients with diabetes mellitus. *Clin Chem Acta* 2001;303:105–115.

36. Mamula MJ, Gee RJ, Elliott JI, et al. Isoaspartyl post-translation modification triggers autoimmune responses to self proteins. *J Biol Chem* 1999;274:22321–22327.

37. Allison ME, Fearon DT. Enhanced immunogenicity of aldehyde-bearing antigens: a possible link between innate and adaptive immunity. *Eur J Immunol* 2000;30:2881–2887.

38. Dotevall A, Hulthe J, Rosengren A, et al. Autoantibodies against oxidized low-density lipoprotein and C-reactive protein are associated with diabetes and myocardial infarction in women. *Clin Sci* 2001;101:523–531.

39. Ebringer A, Wilson C. HLA molecules, bacteria, and autoimmunity. *J Med Microbiol* 2000;49:305–311.

40. Macphail S. Superantigens: mechanism by which they may induce, exacerbate, and control autoimmune diseases. *Int Rev Immunol* 1999;18:141–180.

41. Zouali M. B-cell superantigens: implications for selection of the human antibody repertoire. *Immunol Today* 1995;16:399–405.

42. Furtado GC, Olivares-Villagomez D, Curotto De Lafaille MA, et al. Regulatory T cells in spontaneous autoimmune encephalomyelitis. *Immunol Rev* 2001;182:122–134.

43. Demkowicz WE Jr, Littaua RA, Wang J, et al. Human cytotoxic T-cell memory: long-lived responses to vaccinia virus. *J Virol* 1996;70:2627–2631.

44. Erickson AL, Walker CM. Class I major histocompatibility complex-restricted cytotoxic T-cell responses to vaccinia in humans. *J Gen Virol* 1993;74:751–754.

45. Leder K, Weller PF, Wilson ME. Travel vaccines and elderly persons: review of vaccines available in the United States. *Travel Med* 2001;33:1553–1566.

46. Carson PJ, Nichol KL, O'Brien J, et al. Immune function and vaccine responses in advanced elderly patients. *Arch Intern Med* 2000;160:2017–2024.

47. Mayas JM, Vilella A, Bertran MJ, et al. Immunogenicity and reactogenicity of the adult tetanus-diphtheria vaccine. How many doses are necessary? *Epidemiol Infect* 2001;127:451–460.

48. Looney RJ, Hasan MS, Coffin D, et al. Hepatitis B immunization of healthy elderly adults: relationship between naive CD4+ T cells and primary immune response and evaluation of GM-CSF as an adjuvant. *J Clin Immunol* 2001;21:30–36.

49. Tele SA, Martins RM, Lopes CL, et al. Immunogenicity of a recombinant hepatitis B vaccine (Euvax-B) in haemodialysis patients and staff. *Eur J Epidemiol* 2001;17:145–149.

50. Remarque EJ. Influenza vaccination in elderly people. *Exp Gerontol* 1999;34:445–452.

51. Goronzy JJ, Fulbright JW, Crowson CS, et al. Value of immunological markers in predicting responsiveness to influenza vaccination in the elderly. *J Virol* 2001;75:12182–12187.

52. Murasko DM, Bernstein ED, Gardner EM, et al. Role of humoral and cellular immunity in protection from influenza disease after immunization of healthy elderly. *Exp Gerontol* 2002;37:427–439.

53. Stepanova L, Naykhin A, Kolmskog C, et al. The humoral response to live and inactivated influenza vaccines administered alone and in combination to young adults and elderly. *J Clin Virol* 2002;24:193–201.

54. Halperin SA, Smith B, Mabrouk T, et al. Safety and immunogenicity of a trivalent, inactivated, mammalian cell culture–derived influenza vaccine in healthy adults, seniors, and children. *Vaccine* 2002;20:1240–1247.

55. Rubins JB, Puri AK, Loch J, et al. Magnitude, duration, quality, and function of pneumococcal vaccine responses in elderly adults. *J Infect Dis* 1998;178:431–440.

56. Garg M, Luo W, Kaplan AM, et al. Cellular basis of decreased immune responses to pneumococcal vaccines in aged mice. *Infect Immun* 1996;64:4456–4462.

57. Koivula I, Sten M, Leinonen M, et al. Clinical efficacy of pneumococcal vaccine in the elderly: a randomized single-blind population-based trial. *Am J Med* 1997;103:281–290.

58. Sankilampi U, Honkanen PO, Bloigu A, et al. Persistence of antibodies to pneumococcal capsular polysaccharide vaccine in the elderly. *J Infect Dis* 1997;176:1100–1104.

59. Fischer RT, Longo DL, Kenny JJ. A novel phosphocholine antigen protects both normal and X-linked immune deficient mice against Streptococcus pneumoniae. Comparison of the 6-O-phophocholine hydroxyhexanoate-conjugate with other phosphocholine-containing vaccines. *J Immunol* 1995;154:3373–3382.

60. Shelly MA, Jacoby H, Riley GJ, et al. Comparison of pneumococcal polysaccharide and CRM197-conjugated pneumococcal oligosaccharide vaccines in young and elderly adults. *Infect Immun* 1997;65:242–247.

61. Ringden O, Nilsson B. Death by graft-versus-host disease associated

with HLA mismatch, high recipient age, low marrow cell dose, and splenectomy. *Transplantation* 1985;40:39–44.

61a. Ordemann R, Hutchinson R, Friedman J, et al. Enhanced allostimulatory activity of host antigen-presenting cells in old mice intensifies acute graft-versus-host disease. *J Clin Invest* 2002;109:1249–1256.

62. Epstein SE, Zhu J, Burnett MS, et al. Infection and atherosclerosis: potential roles of pathogen burden and molecular mimicry. *Arterioscler Thromb Vasc Biol* 2000;20:1417–1420.

63. Zhou X, Caligiuri G, Hamsten A, et al. LDL immunization induces T-cell–dependent antibody formation and protection against atherosclerosis. *Arterioscler Thromb Vasc Biol* 2001;21:108–114.

64. Morgan D, Diamond DM, Gottschall PE, et al. A beta peptide vaccination prevents memory loss in an animal model of Alzheimer's disease. *Nature* 2000;408:982–985.

65. Ershler WB, Harman SM, Keller ET. Immunologic aspects of osteoporosis. *Dev Comp Immunol* 1997;21:487–499.

66. Nishiyama N. Thymectomy-induced deterioration of learning and memory. *Cell Molec Biol* 2001;47:161–165.

67. Ader R, Felton D, Cohen N. Interactions between the brain and the immune system. *Annu Rev Pharmacol Toxicol* 1990;30:561–602.

68. Longo DL, Duffey PL, Kopp WC, et al. Conditioned immune response to interferon-γ in humans. *Clin Immunol* 1999;90:173–181.

69. Burgess W, Liu Q, Zhou J, et al. The immune-endocrine loop during aging: role of growth hormone and insulin-like growth factor I. *Neuroimmunomodulation* 1999;6:56–68.

70. Mazzoccoli G, Correra M, Bianco G, et al. Age-related changes of neuro-endocrine-immune interactions in healthy humans. *J Biol Regul Homeost Agents* 1997;11:143–147.

71. Murphy WJ, Durum SK, Longo DL. Role of neuroendocrine hormones in murine T-cell development. Growth hormone exerts thymopoietic effects in vivo. *J Immunol* 1992;149:3851–3857.

72. Doria G, Frasca D. Genetic factors in immunity and aging. *Vaccine* 2000;18:1591–1595.

73. Doria G, Biozzi G, Mouton D, et al. Genetic control of immune responsiveness, aging, and tumor incidence. *Mech Ageing Dev* 1997;96:1–13.

74. Murasko DM, Weiner P, Kaye D. Association of lack of mitogen induced lymphocyte proliferation with increased mortality in the elderly. *Immunol Infect Dis* 1988;1:1–23.

75. Caruso C, Candore G, Colonna Romano G, et al. Immunogenetics of longevity. Is major histocompatibility complex polymorphism relevant to the control of human longevity? A review of literature data. *Mech Ageing Dev* 2001;122:445–462.

76. Ferguson G, Wikby A, Maxson P, et al. Immune parameters in a longitudinal study of a very old population of Swedish people: a comparison between survivors and nonsurvivors. *J Gerontol A Biol Sci Med Sci* 1995;50:B378–B382.

77. Mountz JD, Van Zant GE, Zhang H-G, et al. Genetic dissection of age-related changes of immune function in mice. *Scand J Immunol* 2001;54:10–20.

78. Miller RA, Chrisp C, Jackson AU, et al. Coordinated genetic control of neoplastic and nonneoplastic diseases in mice. *J Gerontol A Biol Sci Med Sci* 2002;57A:B3–B8.

79. Murphy WJ, Durum SK, Anver MR, et al. Immunologic and hematologic effects of neuroendocrine hormones. Studies on DW/J dwarf mice. *J Immunol* 1992;148:3799–3805.

80. Bartke A, Coschigano K, Kopchick J, et al. Genes that prolong life: relationships of growth hormone and growth to aging and life span. *J Gerontol A Biol Sci Med Sci* 2001;56A:B340–B349.

81. Urba WJ, Maluish AE, Longo DL. Strategies for immunologic monitoring. *Cancer Chemother Biol Resp Modif* 1987;9:484–501.

82. Ginaldi L, De Martinis M, D'Ostilio A, et al. The immune system in the elderly. III. Innate immunity. *Immunol Res* 1999;20:117–126.

83. Pawelec G, Solana R, Remarque E, et al. Impact of aging on innate immunity. *J Leukoc Biol* 1998;64:703–712.

84. Gilchrest BA, Murphy GF, Soter NA. Effect of chronologic aging an ultraviolet irradiation on Langerhans cells in human epidermis. *J Invest Dermatol* 1982;79:85–88.

85. Gilchrest BA, Szabo G, Flynn E, et al. Chronologic and actinically induced aging in human facial skin. *J Invest Dermatol* 1983;80(suppl):81s–85s.

86. Sprecher E, Becker Y, Kraal G, et al. Effect of aging on epidermal dendritic cell populations in C57BL/6J mice. *J Invest Dermatol* 1990;94:247–253.

87. Cerimele D, Celleno L, Serri F. Physiological changes in ageing skin. *Br J Dermatol* 1990;122(suppl 35):13–20.

88. Giacomoni PU, Rein G. Factors of skin ageing share common mechanisms. *Biogerontology* 2001;2:219–229.

89. Swift ME, Burns AL, Gray KL, et al. Age-related alterations in the inflammatory response to dermal injury. *J Invest Dermatol* 2001;117:1027–1035.

90. Reed MJ, Ferara NS, Vernon RB. Impaired migration, integrin function, and actin cytoskeletal organization in dermal fibroblasts from a subset of aged human donors. *Mech Ageing Dev* 2001;122:1203–1220.

91. Gibbs S, Silva Pinto AN, Murli S, et al. Epidermal growth factor and keratinocyte growth factor differentially regulate epidermal migration, growth, and differentiation. *Wound Repair Regen* 2000;8:192–203.

92. Ghadially R, Brown BE, Hanley K, et al. Decreased epidermal lipid synthesis accounts for altered barrier function in aged mice. *J Invest Dermatol* 1996;106:1064–1069.

93. Rogers J, Harding C, Mayo A, et al. Stratum corneum lipids: the effect of ageing and the seasons. *Arch Dermatol Res* 1996;288:765–770.

94. Haratake A, Ikenaga K, Katoh N, et al. Topical mevalonic acid stimulates de novo cholesterol synthesis and epidermal permeability barrier homeostasis in aged mice. *J Invest Dermatol* 2000;114:247–252.

95. Meyer KC. The role of immunity in susceptibility to respiratory infection in the aging lung. *Respir Physiol* 2001;128:23–31.

96. Aviv J. Effects of aging on sensitivity of the pharyngeal and supraglottic areas. *Am J Med* 1997;103(suppl 5A):74s–76s.

97. Puchelle E, Zahm JM, Bertrand A. Influence of age on bronchial mucociliary transport. *Scand J Respir Dis* 1979;60:307–313.

98. Thomson ML, Pavia D. Long-term tobacco smoking and mucociliary clearance from the human lung in health and respiratory impairment. *Arch Environ Health* 1973;26:86–89.

99. Gyetko MR, Toews GB. Immunology of the aging lung. *Clin Chest Med* 1993;14:379–391.

100. Meyer KC. Neutrophils and low-grade inflammation in the seemingly normal aging human lung. *Mech Ageing Dev* 1998;104:169–181.

101. Antonini JM, Roberts JR, Clarke RW, et al. Effect of age on respiratory defense mechanisms: pulmonary bacterial clearance in Fischer 344 rats after intratracheal instillation of Listeria monocytogenes. *Chest* 2001;120:240–249.

102. Cruchley AT, Williams DM, Farthing PM, et al. Langerhans cell density in normal human oral mucosa and skin: relationship to age, smoking and alcohol consumption. *J Oral Pathol Med* 1994;23:55–59.

103. Ueta E, Tanida T, Doi S, et al. Regulation of Candida albicans growth and adhesion by saliva. *J Lab Clin Med* 2000;136:66–73.

104. Schmucker DL. Intestinal mucosal immunosenescence in rats. *Exp Gerontol* 2002;37:197–203.

105. Thoreux K, Owen L, Schmucker DL. Intestinal lymphocyte number, migration, and antibody secretion in young and old rats. *Immunology* 2000;101:161–167.

106. Sobel JD. Pathogenesis of urinary tract infection. Role of host defenses. *Infect Dis Clin North Am* 1997;11:531–549.

107. Hazlett LD. Corneal and ocular surface histochemistry. *Prog Histochem Cytochem* 1993;25:1–60.

108. Bellavia D, Frada G, DiFranco P, et al. C4, BF, C3 allele distribution and complement activity in healthy aged people and centenarians. *J Gerontol A Biol Sci Med Sci* 1999;54:B150–B153.

109. Kramer J, Fulop T, Rajczy K, et al. A marked drop in the incidence of the null allele of the B gene of the fourth component of complement (C4B*Q0) in elderly subjects. C4B*Q0 as a probable negative selection factor for survival. *Hum Genet* 1991;86:595–598.

110. Loeffler DA, Brickman CM, Juneau PL, et al. Cerebrospinal fluid C3a increases with age, but does not increase further in Alzheimer's disease. *Neurobiol Aging* 1997;18:555–557.

111. Mullins RF, Russell SR, Anderson DH, et al. Drusen associated with aging and age-related macular degeneration contains proteins common to extracellular deposits associated with atherosclerosis, elastosis, amyloidosis, and dense deposit disease. *FASEB J* 2000;14:835–846.

112. Hazlett LD, Masinick-McClellan SA, Barrett RP. Complement defects in aged mice compromise phagocytosis of Pseudomonas aeruginosa. *Curr Eye Res* 1999;19:26–32.

113. Janeway C Jr, Medzhitov R. Innate immune recognition. *Annu Rev Immunol* 2002;20:197–216.

114. Herrero C, Sebastian C, Marques L, et al. Immunosenescence of macrophages: reduced MHC class II gene expression. *Exp Gerontol* 2002;37:389–394.

115. Videla LA, Tapia G, Fernandez V. Influence of aging on Kupffer cell respiratory activity in relation to particle phagocytosis and oxidative stress parameters in mouse liver. *Redox Rep* 2001;6:155–159.

116. De la Fuente M, Del Rio M, Medina S. Changes with aging in the modulation by neuropeptide Y of murine peritoneal macrophage functions. *J Neuroimmunol* 2001;116:156–167.

117. Rhoades ER, Orme IM. Similar responses by macrophages from young and old mice infected with Mycobacterium tuberculosis. *Mech Ageing Dev* 1998;106:145–153.

118. Khare V, Sodhi A, Singh SM. Age-dependent alterations in the tumoricidal functions of tumor-associated macrophages. *Tumour Biol* 1999;20:30–43.

119. Swift ME, Kleinman HK, DiPietro LA. Impaired wound repair and delayed angiogenesis in aged mice. *Lab Invest* 1999;79:1479–1487.

120. Koike E, Kobayashi T, Mochitate K, et al. Effect of aging on nitric oxide production by rat alveolar macrophages. *Exp Gerontol* 1999;34:889–894.

121. Yang Y, DiPietro L, Feng Y, et al. Increased TNF-α and PGI(2) but not NO release from macrophages in 18-month-old rats. *Mech Ageing Dev* 2000;114:79–88.

122. Gabriel P, Cakman I, Rink L. Overproduction of monokines by leukocytes after stimulation with lipopolysaccharide in the elderly. *Exp Gerontol* 2002;37:235–247.

123. Lightart GJ, Corberand JX, Geertzen HG, et al. Necessity of the assessment of health status in human immunogerontological studies: evaluation of the SENIEUR protocol. *Mech Ageing Dev* 1990;55:89–105.

124. Ahluwalia N, Mastro AM, Ball R, et al. Cytokine production by stimulated mononuclear cells did not change with aging in apparently healthy, well-nourished women. *Mech Ageing Dev* 2001;122:1269–1279.

125. Wu D, Hayek MG, Meydani SN. Vitamin E and macrophage cyclooxygenase regulation in the aged. *J Nutr* 2001;131:382–388.

126. Louria DB, Sen P, Buse M. Age-dependent differences in outcomes of infections, with special reference to experiments in mice. *J Am Geriatr Soc* 1982;30:769–773.

127. Meyer KC, Rosenthal NS, Soergel P, et al. Neutrophils and low-grade inflammation in the seemingly normal aging human lung. *Mech Ageing Dev* 1998;104:169–181.

128. Fransson C, Mooney J, Kinane DF, et al. Differences in the inflammatory response in young and old human subjects during the course of experimental gingivitis. *J Clin Periodontol* 1999;26:453–460.

129. Chatta GS, Andrews RG, Rodger E, et al. Hematopoietic progenitors and aging: alterations in granulocyte precursors and responsiveness to recombinant human G-CSF, GM-CSF and IL-3. *J Gerontol* 1993;48:207–213.

130. Phair JP, Kauffman CA, Bjornson A, et al. Host defense in the aged: evaluation of components of the inflammatory and immune responses. *J Infect Dis* 1978;138:67–76.

131. Esparza B, Sanchez M, Ruiz M, et al. Neutrophil function in elderly persons assessed by flow cytometry. *Immunol Invest* 1996;25:185–193.

132. Lord JM, Butcher S, Killampali V, et al. Neutrophil ageing and immunesenescence. *Mech Ageing Dev* 2001;122:1521–1535.

133. Butcher SK, Chahal H, Nayak L, et al. Senescence in innate immune responses: reduced neutrophil phagocytic capacity and CD16 expression in elderly humans. *J Leukoc Biol* 2001;70:881–886.

134. Wenisch C, Patruta S, Daxbock F, et al. Effect of age on human neutrophil function. *J Leukoc Biol* 2000;67:40–45.

135. Fulop T Jr, Komaromi I, Foris G, et al. Age-dependent variations of intra-lysosomal release from human PMN leukocytes under various stimuli. *Immunobiology* 1986;171:302–311.

136. Miyaji C, Watanabe H, Toma H, et al. Functional alteration of granulocytes, NK cells, and natural killer T cells in centenarians. *Hum Immunol* 2000;61:908–916.

137. Moretta A, Bissoni R, Bottino C, et al. Major histocompatibility complex class I-specific receptors on human natural killer and T lymphocytes. *Immunol Rev* 1997;155:105–117.

138. Colonna M, Navarro F, Bellon T, et al. A common inhibitory receptor for major histocompatibility complex class I molecules on human lymphoid and myelomonocytic cells. *J Exp Med* 1997;1809–1818.

139. Facchini A, Mariani E, Mariani AR, et al. Increased number of circulating Leu11+ (CD16) large granular lymphocytes and decreased NK activity during human ageing. *Clin Exp Immunol* 1987;68:340–347.

140. Borrego F, Alonso C, Galiani MC, et al. NK phenotypic markers and IL-2 response in NK cells from elderly people. *Exp Gerontol* 1999;34:253–265.

141. Solano R, Alonso MC, Pena J. Natural killer cells in healthy aging. *Exp Gerontol* 1999;34:435–443.

142. Solano R, Mariani E. NK and NK/T cells in human senescence. *Vaccine* 2000;18:1613–1620.

143. McNerlan SE, Rea IM, Alexander HD, et al. Changes in natural killer cells, the CD57CD8 subset, and related cytokines in healthy aging. *J Clin Immunol* 1998;18:31–38.

144. Baume DM, Robertson MJ, Levine H, et al. Differential responses to interleukin 2 define functionally distinct subsets of human natural killer cells. *Eur J Immunol* 1992;22:1–6.

145. Sansoni P, Cossarizza A, Brianti V, et al. Lymphocyte subsets and natural killer cell activity in healthy old people and centenarians. *Blood* 1993;82:2767–2773.

146. Kutza J, Murasko DM. Effects of aging on natural killer cell activity and activation by interleukin-2 and interferon-α. *Cell Immunol* 1994;155:195–204.

147. Mariani E, Mariani AR, Meneghetti A, et al. Age-dependent decreases of NK cell phosphoinositide turnover during spontaneous but not Fc mediated cytolytic activity. *Int Immunol* 1998;10:981–989.

148. Krishnaraj R, Bhooma T. Cytokine sensitivity of human NK cells during immunosenescence. 2. IL-2-induced interferon-γ secretion. *Immunol Lett* 1996;50:59–63.

149. Kmiec Z, Mysliwska J, Rachon D, et al. Natural killer activity and thyroid hormone levels in young and elderly persons. *Gerontology* 2001;47:282–288.

150. Mariani E, Ravaglia G, Meneghetti A, et al. Natural immunity and bone and muscle remodeling hormones in the elderly. *Mech Ageing Dev* 1998;102:279–292.

151. Bruunsgaard H, Pedersen AN, Schroll M, et al. Decreased natural killer cell activity is associated with atherosclerosis in elderly humans. *Exp Gerontol* 2001;37:127–136.

152. Ogata K, An E, Shioi Y, et al. Association between natural killer cell activity and infection in immunologically normal elderly people. *Clin Exp Immunol* 2001;124:392–397.

153. Ogata K, Yokose N, Tamura H, et al. Natural killer cells in the late decades of human life. *Clin Immunol Immunopathol* 1997;84:269–275.

154. Rink L, Cakman I, Kirchner H. Altered cytokine production in the elderly. *Mech Ageing Dev* 1998;102:199–210.

155. Bruunsgaard H, Pedersen M, Pedersen BK. Aging and proinflammatory cytokines. *Curr Opin Hematol* 2001;8:131–136.

156. Cohen HJ, Pieper CF, Harris T, et al. The association of plasma IL-6 levels with functional disability in community dwelling elderly. *J Gerontol A Biol Sci Med Sci* 1997;52:201–208.

157. Baggio G, Donazzan S, Monti D, et al. Lipoprotein(a) and lipoprotein profile in healthy centenarians: a reappraisal of vascular risk factors. *FASEB J* 1998;12:443–447.

158. Beharka AA, Meydani M, Wu D, et al. Interleukin-6 production does not increase with age. *J Gerontol A Biol Sci Med Sci* 2001;56:B81–B88.

159. Roubenoff R, Harris TB, Abad LW, et al. Monocyte cytokine production in an elderly population: effect of age and inflammation. *J Gerontol A Biol Sci Med Sci* 1998;53:M20–M26.

160. Saurwein-Teissl M, Blasko I, Zisterer K, et al. An imbalance between pro- and anti-inflammatory cytokines, a characteristic feature of old age. *Cytokine* 2000;12:1160–1161.

161. Spencer NFL, Norton SD, Harrison LL, et al. Dysregulation of IL-10 production with aging: possible linkage to the age-associated decline in DHEA and its sulfated derivative. *Exp Gerontol* 1996;31:393–408.

162. Mascaruccil P, Taub D, Saccani S, et al. Age-related changes in cytokine production by leukocytes in rhesus monkeys. *Aging* 2001;13:85–94.

163. Sharman K, Sharman E, Campbell A, et al. Reduced basal levels and enhanced LPS response of IL-6 mRNA in aged mice. *J Gerontol A Biol Sci Med Sci* 2001;56:B520–B523.

164. Harris TB, Ferrucci L, Tracy RP, et al. Associations of elevated

interleukin-6 and C-reactive protein levels with mortality in the elderly. *Am J Med* 1999;106:506–512.

164a. Reuben DB, Cheh AI, Harris TB, et al. Peripheral blood markers of inflammation predict mortality and functional decline in high-functioning community-dwelling older persons. *J Am Geriatr Soc* 2002;50:638–644.

165. Taafe DR, Harris TB, Ferrucci L, et al. Cross-sectional and prospective relationships of interleukin-6 and C-reactive protein with physical performance in elderly persons. MacArthur studies of successful aging. *J Gerontol A Biol Sci Med Sci* 2000;55:M706–M708.

166. Bruunsgaard H, Skinhoj P, Quist J, et al. Elderly humans show prolonged in vivo inflammatory activity during pneumococcal infections. *J Infect Dis* 1999;180:551–554.

167. Krabbe K, Bruunsgaard H, Hansen CM. Ageing is associated with a prolonged fever response in human endotoxemia. *Clin Diagn Lab Immunol* 2001;8:333–338.

168. Clark JA, Peterson TC. Cytokine production and aging: overproduction of IL-8 in elderly males in response to lipopolysaccharide. *Mech Ageing Dev* 1994;77:127–139.

169. Pulsatelli L, Meliconi R, Mazzetti I, et al. Chemokine production by peripheral blood mononuclear cells in elderly subjects. *Mech Ageing Dev* 2000;121:89–100.

170. Mariani E, Pulsatelli L, Meneghetti A, et al. Different IL-8 production by T and NK lymphocytes in elderly subjects. *Mech Ageing Dev* 2001;122:1383–1395.

171. Mariani E, Pulsatelli L, Neri S, et al. RANTES and MIP-1-α production by T lymphocytes, monocytes and NK cells from nonagenarian subjects. *Exp Gerontol* 2002;37:219–226.

172. Inadera H, Egashira K, Takemoto M, et al. Increase in circulating levels of monocyte chemoattractant protein-1 with aging. *J Interferon Cytokine Res* 1999;19:1179–1182.

173. Gerli R, Monti D, Bistoni O, et al. Chemokines, sTNF-Rs and sCD30 serum levels in healthy aged people and centenarians. *Mech Ageing Dev* 2000;121:37–46.

174. Anthony D, Dempster R, Fearn S, et al. CXC chemokines generate age-related increases in neutrophil-mediated brain inflammation and blood-brain barrier breakdown. *Curr Biol* 1998;8:923–926.

175. Paganelli R, Di Iorio A, Patricelli L, et al. Proinflammatory cytokines in sera of elderly patients with dementia: levels in vascular injury are higher than those of mild-moderate Alzheimer's disease patients. *Exp Gerontol* 2002;37:257–263.

176. Felzien LK, McDonald JT, Gleason SM, et al. Increased chemokine gene expression during aging in the murine brain. *Brain Res* 2001; 890:137–146.

177. Lue LF, Rydel R, Brigham EF, et al. Inflammatory repertoire of Alzheimer's disease and nondemented elderly microglia in vitro. *Glia* 2001;35:72–79.

178. Linton P-J, Thoman ML. T cell senescence. *Front Biosci* 2001;6: D248–D261.

179. Chakravarti B, Abraham GN. Aging and T-cell-mediated immunity. *Mech Ageing Dev* 1999;108:183–206.

180. Pawelec G, Remarque E, Barnett Y, et al. T cells and aging. *Front Biosci* 1998;3:D59–D99.

181. Globerson A. T lymphocytes and aging. *Int Arch Allergy Immunol* 1995;107:491–497.

182. Abo T, Watanabe H, et al. Extrathymic T cells stand at an intermediate phylogenetic position between natural killer cells and thymus-derived T cells. *Nature Immunol* 1995;14:173–187.

183. Haynes BF, Markert ML, Sempowski GD, et al. The role of the thymus in immune reconstitution in aging, bone marrow transplantation and HIV-1 infection. *Annu Rev Immunol* 2000;18:529–560.

184. Steinmann GG, Klaus B, Muller-Hermelink HK. The involution of the aging human thymic epithelium is independent of puberty. A morphometric study. *Scand J Immunol* 1985;22:563–575.

185. Steinmann GG. Changes in the human thymus during aging. *Curr Topics Pathol* 1986;75:43–88.

186. Kong F-K, Chen CH, Six A, et al. T cell receptor gene deletion circles identify recent thymic emigrants in the peripheral T cell pool. *Proc Natl Acad Sci USA* 1999;96:1536–1540.

187. Douek DC, McFarland RD, Keiser PH, et al. Changes in thymic function with age and during the treatment of HIV infection. *Nature* 1998;396:690–695.

188. Jamieson BD, Douek DC, Killian S, et al. Generation of functional thymocytes in the human adult. *Immunity* 1999;10:569–575.

189. Poulin J-F, Viswanathan MN, Komanduri KV, et al. Direct evidence for thymic function in adult humans. *J Exp Med* 1999;190:179–186.

190. Weinberg K, Annett G, Kashyap A, et al. The effect of thymic function on immunocompetence following bone marrow transplantation. *Biol Blood Marrow Transplant* 1995;1:18–23.

191. Mackall CL, Stein D, Fleisher TA, et al. Prolonged CD4 depletion after sequential autologous peripheral blood progenitor cell infusions in children and young adults. *Blood* 2000;96:754–762.

192. Mackall CL, Fleisher TA, Brown MR, et al. Age, thymopoiesis, and CD4+ T lymphocyte regeneration after intensive chemotherapy. *N Engl J Med* 1995;332:143–149.

193. Edington, H, Salwitz J, Longo DL, et al. Thymic hyperplasia masquerading as recurrent Hodgkin's disease: case report and review of the literature. *J Surg Oncol* 1986;33:120–123.

194. Gabor MJ, Scollay R, Godfrey DI. Thymic T cell export is not influenced by the peripheral T cell pool. *Eur J Immunol* 1997;27:1686–1693.

195. Mackall CL, Bare CV, Titus JA, et al. Thymic-independent T cell regeneration occurs via antigen driven expansion of peripheral T cells resulting in a repertoire that is limited in diversity and prone to skewing. *J Immunol* 1996;156:4609–4616.

196. Mackall CL, Gress RE. Thymic aging. *Immunol Rev* 1997;160:91–102.

197. Tyan ML. Impaired thymic regeneration in lethally irradiated mice given bone marrow from aged donors. *Proc Soc Exp Biol Med* 1976; 152:33–35.

198. Hirokawa K, Kubo S, Utsuyama M, et al. Age-related change in the potential of bone marrow cells to repopulate the thymus and splenic T cells in mice. *Cell Immunol* 1986;100:443–451.

199. Doria G, Mancini C, Utsuyama M, et al. Aging of the recipients but not of the bone marrow donors enhances autoimmunity in syngeneic radiation chimeras. *Mech Ageing Dev* 1997;95:131–142.

200. Aspinall R. Age-associated thymic atrophy in the mouse is due to a deficiency affecting rearrangement of the TCR during intrathymic T cell development. *J Immunol* 1997;158:3037–3045.

201. Aspinall R, Andrew D. Age-associated thymic atrophy is not associated with a deficiency in the CD44+CD25−CD3−CD4−CD8− thymocyte population. *Cell Immunol* 2001;212:150–157.

202. Globerson A. Thymocyte progenitors in ageing. *Immunol Lett* 1994; 40:219–224.

203. Mackall CL, Punt JA, Morgan P, et al. Thymic function in young/old chimeras: substantial thymic T cell regenerative capacity despite irreversible age-associated thymic involution. *Eur J Immunol* 1998;28:1886–1893.

204. Muegge K, Vila MP, Durum SK. Interleukin-7: a cofactor for V(D)J rearrangement of the T cell receptor beta gene. *Science* 1993;261:93–95.

205. Andrew D, Aspinall R. IL-7 and not stem cell factor reverses both the increase in apoptosis and the decline in thymopoiesis seen in aged mice. *J Immunol* 2001;166:1524–1530.

206. Andrew D, Aspinall R. Age-associated thymic atrophy is linked to a decline in IL-7 production. *Exp Gerontol* 2002:37:455–463.

207. Sempowski GD, Hale LP, Sundy JS, et al. Leukemia inhibitory factor, oncostatin M, IL-6, and stem cell factor mRNA expression in human thymus increases with age and is associated with thymic atrophy. *J Immunol* 2000;164:2180–2187.

208. Sempowski GD, Gooding ME, Liao HX, et al. T cell receptor excision circle assessment of thymopoiesis in aging mice. *Mol Immunol* 2002;38:841–848.

209. Fry TJ, Christensen BL, Komschlies KL, et al. Interleukin-7 restores immunity in athymic T-cell-depleted hosts. *Blood* 2001;97:1525–1533.

210. Lau LL, Spain LM. Altered aging-related thymic involution in T cell receptor transgenic, MHC-deficient, and CD4-deficient mice. *Mech Ageing Dev* 2000;114:101–121.

211. Lacorazza HD, Guevara Patino JA, Weksler ME, et al. Failure of rearranged TCR transgenes to prevent age-associated thymic involution. *J Immunol* 1999;163:4262–4268.

212. Nakagawa T, Roth W, Wong P, et al. Cathepsin L: critical role in Ii degradation and CD4 T cell selection in the thymus. *Science* 1998; 280:450–453.

213. Benavides F, Venables A, Poetschke Klug H, et al. The CD4 T cell-deficient mouse mutation nackt (nkt) involves a deletion in the cathepsin L (CtsI) gene. *Immunogenetics* 2001:53:233–242.

214. Nabarra B, Casanova M, Paris D, et al. Premature thymic involution, observed at the ultrastructural level, in two lineages of human-SOD-1 transgenic mice. *Mech Ageing Dev* 1997;96:59–73.

215. Zhou T, Edwards CK 3rd, Mountz JD. Prevention of age-related T cell apoptosis defect in CD2-fas-transgenic mice. *J Exp Med* 1995; 182:129–137.

216. Deguchi Y, Agus D, Kehrl JH. A human homeobox gene, HB24, inhibits development of CD4+ T cells and impairs thymic involution in transgenic mice. *J Biol Chem* 1993;268:3646–3653.

217. French RA, Broussard SR, Meier WA, et al. Age-associated loss of bone marrow hematopoietic cells is reversed by GH and accompanies thymic reconstitution. *Endocrinology* 2002;143:690–699.

218. Murphy WJ, Longo DL. Growth hormone as an immunomodulating therapeutic agent. *Immunol Today* 2000;21:211–213.

219. Olsen NJ, Olson G, Viselli SM, et al. Androgen receptors in thymic epithelium modulate thymus size and thymocyte development. *Endocrinology* 2001;142:1278–1283.

220. Greenstein BD, Fitzpatrick FT, Adcock IM, et al. Reappearance of the thymus in old rats after orchidectomy: inhibition of regeneration by testosterone. *J Endocrinol* 1986;110:417–422.

221. Pido-Lopez J, Imami N, Aspinall R. Both age and gender affect thymic output: more recent thymic migrants in females than males as they age. *Clin Exp Immunol* 2001;125:409–413.

222. Wylie AH. Glucocorticoid-induced thymocyte apoptosis is associated with endogenous endonuclease activation. *Nature* 1980;284:555–556.

223. Vacchio MS, Ashwell JD. Glucocorticoids and thymocyte development. *Semin Immunol* 2000;12:475–485.

224. Turrini P, Zaccaria ML, et al. Presence and possible functional role of nerve growth factor in the thymus. *Cell Mol Biol* 2001;47:55–64.

225. Bulloch K, Cullen MR, Schwartz RH, et al. Development of enervation within syngeneic thymus tissue transplanted under the kidney capsule of the nude mouse: a light and ultrastructural microscope study. *J Neurosci Res* 1987;18:16–27.

226. Madden KS, Felten DL. Beta-adrenoreceptor blockade alters thymocyte differentiation in aged mice. *Cell Mol Biol* 2001;47:189–196.

227. Kinoshita Y, Hato F. Cellular and molecular interactions of thymus with endocrine organs and nervous system. *Cell Mol Biol* 2001; 47:103–117.

228. Bodey B, Bodey B Jr, Siegel SE, et al. The role of the reticulo-epithelial (RE) cell network in the immuno-neuroendocrine regulation of intrathymic lymphopoiesis. *Anticancer Res* 2000;20:1871–1888.

229. Dardenne M. Role of thymic peptides as transmitters between the neuroendocrine and immune systems. *Ann Med* 1999;31(suppl 2):34–39.

230. Boersma WJA, Steinmeier FA, Haaijman JJ. Age-related changes in the relative numbers of Thy-1 and Lyt-2–bearing peripheral blood lymphocytes in mice: a longitudinal approach. *Cell Immunol* 1985;93:417–430.

231. Miller RA. Age-related changes in T-cell surface markers: a longitudinal analysis in genetically heterogeneous mice. *Mech Ageing Dev* 1997;96:181–196.

232. Rea IM, Stewart M, Campbell P, et al. Changes in lymphocyte subsets, interleukin 2, and soluble interleukin 2 receptor in old and very old age. *Gerontology* 1996;42:69–78.

233. Rink L, Seyfarth M. Characteristics of immunologic test values in the elderly. *Z Gerontol Geriatr* 1997;30:220–225.

234. Ginaldi L, De Martinis M, Modesti M, et al. Immunophenotypical changes of T lymphocytes in the elderly. *Gerontology* 2000;46:242–248.

235. Tarazona R, DelaRosa O, Alonso C, et al. Increased expression of NK cell markers on T lymphocytes in aging and chronic activation of the immune system reflects the accumulation of effector/senescent T cells. *Mech Ageing Dev* 2000;121:77–88.

236. Olsson J, Wikby A, Johansson B, et al. Age-related change in peripheral blood T-lymphocyte subpopulations and cytomegalovirus infection in the very old: the Swedish longitudinal OCTO immune study. *Mech Ageing Dev* 2000;121:187–201.

237. Colonna-Romano G, Potestio M, Aquino A, et al. Gamma/delta T lymphocytes are affected in the elderly. *Exp Gerontol* 2002;37:205–211.

238. Reinhold U, Abken H. CD4+ CD7– T cells: a separate subpopulation of memory T cells? *J Clin Immunol* 1997;17:265–271.

239. Bryl E, Gazda M, Foerster J, et al. Age-related increase of frequency of a new, phenotypically distinct subpopulation of human peripheral blood T cells expressing lowered levels of CD4. *Blood* 2001;98:1100–1107.

240. Ernst DN, Weigle WO, Noonan DJ, et al. The age-associated increase in IFN-γ synthesis by mouse CD8+ T cells correlates with shifts in the frequencies of cell subsets defined by membrane CD44, CD45RB, 3G11, and MEL-14 expression. *J Immunol* 1993;151:575–587.

241. Lerner A, Yamada T, Miller RA. PGP-1hi T lymphocytes accumulate with age in mice and respond poorly to concanavalin A. *Eur J Immunol* 1989;19:977–982.

242. Pilarski LM, Yacyshyn BR, Jensen GS, et al. Beta1 integrin (CD29) expression on human postnatal T cell subsets defined by selective CDE45 isoform expression. *J Immunol* 1991;147:830–837.

243. Effros RB, Boucher N, Porter V, et al. Decline in CD28+ T cells in centenarians and in long-term T cell cultures: a possible cause for both in vivo and in vitro immunosenescence. *Exp Gerontol* 1994;29:601–609.

244. Fagnoni FF, Vescovini R, Mazzola M, et al. Expansion of cytotoxic CD8+ CD28- T cells in healthy ageing people, including centenarians. *Immunology* 1996;88:501–507.

245. Kimmig S, Przybylski GK, Schmidt CA, et al. Two subsets of naive T helper cells with distinct T cell receptor excision circle content in human adult peripheral blood. *J Exp Med* 2002;195:789–794.

246. Miller RA. Biomarkers of aging: prediction of longevity by using age-sensitive T-cell subset determinations in a middle-aged, genetically heterogeneous mouse population. *J Gerontol A Biol Sci Med Sci* 2001;56A:B180–B186.

247. Wikby A, Johansson B, Olsson J, et al. Expansions of peripheral blood CD8 T-lymphocyte subpopulations and an association with cytomegalovirus seropositivity in the elderly: the Swedish NONA immune study. *Exp Gerontol* 2002;37:445–453.

248. McNerlan SE, Alexander HD, Rea IM. Age-related reference intervals for lymphocyte subsets in whole blood of healthy individuals. *Scand J Clin Lab Invest* 1999;59:89–92.

249. Ogawa T, Kitagawa M, Hirokawa K. Age-related changes of human bone marrow: as histometric estimation of proliferative cells, apoptotic cells, T cells, B cells and macrophages. *Mech Ageing Dev* 2000;117:57–68.

250. Meyer KC, Soergel P. Variation of bronchioalveolar lymphocyte phenotypes with age in the physiologically normal human lung. *Thorax* 1999;54:697–700.

251. Bergler W, Adam S, Gross HJ, et al. Age-dependent altered proportions in subpopulations of tonsillar lymphocytes. *Clin Exp Immunol* 1999;116:9–18.

252. Banerjee M, Sanderson JD, Spencer J, et al. Immunohistochemical analysis of ageing human B and T cell populations reveals an age-related decline of CD8 T cells in the spleen but not gut-associated lymphoid tissue (GALT). *Mech Ageing Dev* 2000;115:85–99.

253. Rozing J, de Geus B. Changes in the intestinal lymphoid compartment throughout life: implications for the local generation of intestinal T cells. *Int Rev Immunol* 1995;12:13–25.

254. Flo J, Massouh E. Age-related changes of naive and memory CD4 rat lymphocyte subsets in mucosal and systemic lymphoid organs. *Dev Compar Immunol* 1997;21:443–453.

255. Nam KH, Akari H, Terao K, et al. Age-related changes in major lymphocyte subsets in cynomolgus monkeys. *Exp Anim* 1998;47:159–166.

256. Steeber DA, Green NE, Sato S, et al. Lymphocyte migration in L-selectin–deficient mice. Altered subset migration and aging of the immune system. *J Immunol* 1996;57:1096–1106.

257. De Martinis M, Modesti M, Profeta VF, et al. CD50 and CD62L adhesion receptor expression on naive (CD45RA+) and memory (CD45RO+) T lymphocytes in the elderly. *Pathobiology* 2000;68:245–250.

258. De Martinis M, Modesti M, Loretor MF, et al. Adhesion molecules on peripheral blood lymphocyte subpopulations in the elderly. *Life Sci* 2000;68:139–151.

259. Albright JW, Mease RC, Lambert C, et al. Effects of aging on the dynamics of lymphocyte organ distribution in mice. Use of a radioiodinated cell membrane probe. *Mech Ageing Dev* 1998;101:197–211.

260. Callahan JE, Kappler JW, Marrack P. Unexpected expansions of CD8-bearing cells in old mice. *J Immunol* 1993;151:6657–6669.

261. Gonzalez-Quintial R, Baccala R, Balderas RS, et al. V beta gene

repertoire in the aging mouse: a developmental perspective. *Int Rev Immunol* 1995;12:27–40.

262. Hosono M, Toichi E, Hosokawa M, et al. Development of autoreactivity and changes of T cell repertoire in different strains of aging mice. *Mech Ageing Dev* 1995;78:197–214.

263. LeMaoult J, Messaoudi I, Manavalan JS, et al. Age-related dysregulation in CD8 T cell homeostasis. kinetics of a diversity loss. *J Immunol* 2000;165:2367–2373.

264. Blish CA, Gallay BJ, Turk GL, et al. Chronic modulation of the TCR repertoire in the lymphoid periphery. *J Immunol* 1999;162:3131–3140.

265. Posnett DN, Sinha R, Kabak S, et al. Clonal populations of T cells in normal elderly humans: the T cell equivalent to "benign monoclonal gammopathy." *J Exp Med* 1994;179:609–618.

266. Clarke GR, Humphrey CA, Lancaster FC, et al. The human T cell antigen receptor repertoire: skewed use of V beta gene families by CD8+ T cells. *Clin Exp Immunol* 1994;96:364–369.

267. Schwab R, Szabo P, Manavalan JS, et al. Expanded CD4+ and CD8+ T cell clones in elderly humans. *J Immunol* 1997;158:4493–4499.

268. Wack A, Cossarizza A, Heltai S, et al. Age-related modifications of the human αβ T cell repertoire due to different clonal expansions in the CD4+ and CD8+ subsets. *Int Immunol* 1998;10:1281–1288.

269. Van den Beemd R, Boor PP, van Lochem EG, et al. Flow cytometric analysis of the Vb repertoire in healthy controls. *Cytometry* 2000;40:336–345.

270. Giachino C, Granziero L, Modena V, et al. Clonal expansions of Vδ1+ and Vδ2+ cells increase with age and limit the repertoire of human γδ T cells. *Eur J Immunol* 1994;24:1914–1918.

271. Mosley RL, Koker MM, Miller RA. Idiosyncratic alterations of the TCR size distributions affecting both CD4 and CD8 T cell subsets in aging mice. *Cell Immunol* 1998;189:10–18.

272. Nociari MM, Telford W, Russo C. Postthymic development of CD28−CD8+ T cell subset: age-associated expansion and shift from memory to naive phenotype. *J Immunol* 1999;162:3327–3335.

273. Sourdive DJ, Murali-Krishna K, Altman JD, et al. Conserved T cell response repertoire in primary and memory CD8 T cell responses to an acute viral infection. *J Exp Med* 1998;188:71–82.

274. Weekes MP, Wills MR, Mynard K, et al. Large clonal expansions of human virus-specific memory cytotoxic T lymphocytes within the CD57+ CD28− CD8+ T cell population. *Immunology* 1999;98:443–449.

275. Maini MK, Gudgeon N, Wedderburn LR, et al. Clonal expansions in acute EBV infection are detectable in the CD8 and not the CD4 subset and persist with a variable CD45 phenotype. *J Immunol* 2000;165:5729–5737.

276. Hsu H-C, Zhou T, Shi J, et al. Aged mice exhibit in vivo defective peripheral clonal deletion of Db/H-Y reactive CD8+ T cells. *Mech Ageing Dev* 2001;122:305–326.

277. Hingorani R, Monteiro J, Furie R, et al. Oligoclonality of Vβ3 TCR chains in the CD8+ T cell population of rheumatoid arthritis patients. *J Immunol* 1996;156:852–858.

278. Ku CC, Kotzin B, Kappler J, et al. CD8+ T-cell clones in old mice. *Immunol Rev* 1997;160:139–144.

279. Ku CC, Kappler J, Marrack P. The growth of the very large CD8+ T cell clones in older mice is controlled by cytokines. *J Immunol* 2001;166:2186–2193.

280. Linton PJ, Haynes L, Klinman NR, et al. Antigen-independent changes in naive CD4 T cells with aging. *J Exp Med* 1996;184:1891–1900.

281. Mackall CL, Bare CV, Titus JA, et al. Thymic-independent T-cell regeneration occurs via antigen driven expansion of peripheral T cells resulting in a repertoire that is limited in diversity and prone to skewing. *J Immunol* 1996;156:4609–4616.

282. Liu K, Catalfamo M, Li Y, et al. IL-15 mimics T cell receptor cross linking in the induction of cellular proliferation, gene expression, and cytotoxicity in CD8+ memory T cells. *Proc Natl Acad Sci USA* 2002;99:6192–6197.

283. Nagel JE, Chopra RK, Chrest FJ, et al. Decreased proliferation, interleukin 2, synthesis, and interleukin 2 receptor expression are accompanied by decreased mRNA expression in phytohemagglutinin-stimulated cells from elderly donors. *J Clin Invest* 1988;81:1096–1102.

284. Kwon TK, Buchholz MA, Ponsalle P, et al. The regulation of p27Kip1

expression following the polyclonal activation of murine G0 T cells. *J Immunol* 1997;158:5642–5648.

285. O'Leary JJ, Fox R, Bergh N, et al. Expression of the human T cell antigen receptor complex in advanced age. *Mech Ageing Dev* 1988;45:239–252.

286. Fulop T, Gagne D, Goulet AC, et al. Age-related impairment of p56(lck) and ZAP-70 activities in human T lymphocytes activated through the TcR/CD3 complex. *Exp Gerontol* 1999;34:197–216.

287. Tamura T, Kunimatsu T, Yee ST, et al. Molecular mechanism of the impairment in activation signal transduction in CD4+ T cells from old mice. *Int Immunol* 2000;12:1205–1215.

288. Wakikawa A, Utsuyama M, Hirokawa K. Altered expression of various receptors on T cells in young and old mice after mitogenic stimulation: a flow cytometric analysis. *Mech Ageing Dev* 1997;94:113–122.

289. Miller RA, Jacobson B, Weil G, et al. Diminished calcium influx in lectin-stimulated T cells from old mice. *J Cell Physiol* 1988;132:337–342.

290. Whisler RL, Newhouse YG, Donnerberg RL, et al. Characterization of intracellular ionized calcium responsiveness and inositol phosphate production among resting and stimulated peripheral blood T cells from elderly humans. *Aging Immunol Infect Dis* 1991;3:27–36.

291. Philosophe B, Miller RA. Diminished calcium signal generation in subsets of T lymphocytes that predominate in old mice. *J Gerontol A Biol Sci Med Sci* 1990;45:B87–B93.

292. Philosophe B, Miller RA. T lymphocyte heterogeneity in old and young mice: functional defects in T cells selected for poor calcium signal generation. *Eur J Immunol* 1989;19:695–699.

293. Whisler RL, Beiqing L, Chen M. Age-related decreases in IL-2 production by human T cells are associated with impaired activation of nuclear transcriptional factors AP-1 and NF-AT. *Cell Immunol* 1996;152:96–109.

294. Garcia GG, Miller RA. Single-cell analyses reveal two defects in peptide-specific activation of naive T cells from aged mice. *J Immunol* 2001;166:3151–3157.

295. Pawelec G, Hirokawa K, Fulop T. Altered T cell signaling in ageing. *Mech Ageing Dev* 2001;122:1613–1637.

296. Haynes L, Linton PJ, Eaton SM, et al. Interleukin 2, but not other common γ chain-binding cytokines, can reverse the defect in generation of CD4 effector T cells from naive T cells of aged mice. *J Exp Med* 1999;190:1013–1024.

297. Pawelec G, Barnett Y, Mariani E, et al. Human CD4+ T cell clone longevity in tissue culture: lack of influence of donor age or cell origin. *Exp Gerontol* 2002;37:265–269.

298. Vallejo AN, Weyand CM, Goronzy JJ. Functional disruption of the CD28 gene transcriptional initiator in senescent T cells. *J Biol Chem* 2001;276:2565–2570.

299. Schrum AG, Wells AD, Turka LA. Enhanced surface TCR replenishment mediated by CD28 leads to greater TCR engagement during primary stimulation. *Int Immunol* 2000;12:833–842.

300. Ponnappan U. Ubiquitin-proteasome pathway is compromised in CD45RO+ and CD45RA− T lymphocyte subsets during aging. *Exp Gerontol* 2002;37:359–367.

301. Chrest FJ, Buchholz MA, Kim YH, et al. Anti-CD3-induced apoptosis in T cells from young and old mice. *Cytometry* 1995;20:33–42.

302. Pahlavani MA, Vargas DA. Aging but not dietary restriction alters the activation-induced apoptosis in rat T cells. *FEBS Lett* 2001;491:114–118.

303. Herndon FJ, Hsu H-C, Mountz JD. Increased apoptosis of CD45RO− T cells with aging. *Mech Ageing Dev* 1997;94:123–134.

304. Mountz JD, Wu J, Zhou T, et al. Cell death and longevity: implications of fas-mediated apoptosis in T-cell senescence. *Immunol Rev* 1997;160:19–30.

305. Monti D, Salvioli S, Capri M, et al. Decreased susceptibility to oxidative stress-induced apoptosis of peripheral blood mononuclear cells from healthy elderly centenarians. *Mech Ageing Dev* 2000;121:239–250.

306. Hsu H-C, Shi J, Yang P, et al. Activated CD8+ T cells from aged mice exhibit decreased activation-induced cell death. *Mech Ageing Dev* 2001;122:1663–1684.

307. Hathcock KS, Weng NP, Merica R, et al. Antigen-dependent regulation of telomerase activity in murine T cells. *J Immunol* 1998;190:5702–5708.

308. Son NH, Murray S, Yanovski J, et al. Lineage-specific telomere shortening and unaltered capacity for telomerase expression in human T and B lymphocytes with age. *J Immunol* 2000;165:1191–1196.

309. Batliwalla F, Monteiro J, Serrano D, et al. Oligoclonality of CD8+ T cells in health and disease: aging, infection, or immune regulation? *Hum Immunol* 1996;48:68–76.

310. Barnett YA, Barnett CR. DNA damage and mutation: contributors to the age-related alterations in T cell-mediated immune responses? *Mech Ageing Dev* 1998;102:165–175.

311. Doria G, Frasca D. Age-related changes of DNA damage recognition and repair capacity in cells of the immune system. *Mech Ageing Dev* 2001;122:985–998.

312. Bandres E, Merino J, Vazquez B, et al. The increase of IFN-γ production through aging correlates with the expanded CD8(+high) CD28(−)CD57(+) subpopulation. *Clin Immunol* 2000;96:230–235.

313. Yen CJ, Lin SL, Huang KT, et al. Age-associated changes in interferon-γ and interleukin-4 secretion by purified human CD4+ and CD8+ T cells. *J Biomed Sci* 2000;7:317–321.

314. Smith P, Dunne DW, Fallon PG. Defective in vivo induction of functional type 2 cytokine responses in aged mice. *Eur J Immunol* 2001;31:1495–1502.

315. Yamaguchi S, Kitagawa M, Inoue M, et al. Role of lymphoid cells in age-related change of susceptibility to Friend leukemia virus-induced leukemia. *Mech Ageing Dev* 2001;122:219–232.

316. Dong L, Mori I, Hossain MJ, et al. The senescence-accelerated mouse shows aging-related defects in cellular but not humoral immunity against influenza virus infection. *J Infect Dis* 2000;182:391–396.

317. Sambhara S, Kurich A, Miranda R, et al. Severe impairment of primary but not memory responses to influenza viral antigens in aged mice: costimulation in vivo partially reverses impaired primary immune responses. *Cell Immunol* 2001;210:1–4.

318. Koga T, McGhee JR, Kato H, et al. Evidence for early aging in the mucosal immune system. *J Immunol* 2000;165:5352–5359.

319. Ghia P, Melchers F, Rolink AG. Age-dependent changes in B lymphocyte development in man and mouse. *Exp Gerontol* 2000;35:159–165.

320. Nunez C, Nishimoto N, Gartland GL, et al. B cells are generated throughout life in humans. *J Immunol* 1996;156:866–872.

321. Huppert FA, Solomon W, O'Connor S, et al. Aging and lymphocyte subpopulations: whole-blood analysis of immune markers in a large population sample of healthy elderly individuals. *Exp Gerontol* 1998;33:593–600.

322. Klinman NR, Kline GH. The B-cell biology of aging. *Immunol Rev* 1997;160:103–114.

323. Kirman I, Zhao K, Wang Y, et al. Increased apoptosis of bone marrow pre–B cells in old mice associated with their low number. *Int Immunol* 1998;10:1385–1392.

324. Sherwood EM, Blomberg BB, Xu W, et al. Senescent BALB/c mice exhibit decreased expression of lambda5 surrogate light chains and reduced development within the pre–B cell compartment. *J Immunol* 1998;161:4472–4475.

325. Sherwood EM, Xu W, King AM, et al. The reduced expression of surrogate light chains in B cell precursors from senescent BALB/c mice is associated with decreased E2A proteins. *Mech Ageing Dev* 2000;118:45–59.

326. Szabo P, Shen S, Weksler ME. Age-associated defects in B lymphocyte development. *Exp Gerontol* 1999;34:431–434.

327. Stephan RP, Reilly CR, Witte PL. Impaired ability of bone marrow stromal cells to support B-lymphopoiesis with age. *Blood* 1998;91:75–88.

328. Stephan RP, Lill-Elghanian DA, Witte PL. Development of B cells in aged mice: decline in the ability of pro–B cells to respond to IL-7 but not to other growth factors. *J Immunol* 1997;158:1598–1609.

329. Yehuda AB, Wirtheim A, Abdulhai A, et al. Activation of the recombination activating gene-1 (RAG-1) transcript in bone marrow of senescent C57BL/6 mice by recombinant interleukin-7. *J Gerontol A Biol Sci Med Sci* 1999;54:B143–B148.

330. Szabo P, Zhao K, Kirman I, et al. Maturation of B cell precursors is impaired in thymic-deprived nude and old mice. *J Immunol* 1998;161:2248–2253.

331. Barrat FS, Lesourd BM, Louise AS, et al. Pregnancies modulate B lymphopoiesis and myelopoiesis during murine ageing. *Immunology* 1999;98:604–611.

332. Carvalho T, Mota-Santos T, Cumano A, et al. Arrested B lymphopoiesis and persistence of activated B cells in adult interleukin 7 (−/−) mice. *J Exp Med* 2001;194:1141–1150.

333. Okada S, Yoshida T, Hong Z, et al. Impairment of B lymphopoiesis in precocious aging (klotho) mice. *Int Immunol* 2000;12:861–871.

334. Fulcher DA, Basten A. B cell life span: a review. *Immunol Cell Biol* 1997;75:446–455.

335. Kline GH, Hayden TA, Klinman NR. B cell maintenance in aged mice reflects both increased B cell longevity and decreased B cell generation. *J Immunol* 1999;162:3342–3349.

336. Hayakawa K, Hardy RR. Development and function of B-1 cells. *Curr Opin Immunol* 2000;12:346–353.

337. Eaton-Bassiri AS, Mandik-Nayak L, Seo SJ, et al. Alterations in splenic architecture and the localization of anti-double-stranded DNA B cells in aged mice. *Int Immunol* 2000;12:915–926.

338. Hinkley KS, Chiasson RJ, Prior TK, et al. Age-dependent increase of peritoneal B-1b cells in SCID mice. *Immunology* 2002;105:196–203.

339. LeMaoult J, Delassus S, Dyall R, et al. Clonal expansions of B lymphocytes in old mice. *J Immunol* 1997;159:3866–3874.

340. Ben-Yehuda A, Szabo P, LeMaoult J, et al. Increased VH11 and VHQ52 gene use by splenic B cells in old mice associated with oligoclonal expansions of CD5+ B cells. *Mech Ageing Dev* 1998;103:111–121.

341. Li F, Jin F, Freitas A, et al. Impaired regeneration of the peripheral B cell repertoire from bone marrow following lymphopenia in old mice. *Eur J Immunol* 2001;31:500–505.

342. Van Arkel C, Hopstaken CM, Zurcher C, et al. Monoclonal gammopathies in aging mu, kappa-transgenic mice: involvement of the B-1 cell lineage. *Eur J Immunol* 1997;27:2436–2440.

343. Silverman GJ, Shaw PX, Luo L, et al. Neo-self antigens and the expansion of B-1 cells: lessons from atherosclerosis-prone mice. *Curr Top Microbiol Immunol* 2000;252:189–200.

344. Klonowski KD, Monestier M. Heavy chain revision in MRL mice: a potential mechanism for the development of autoreactive B cell precursors. *J Immunol* 2000;165:4487–4493.

345. Weksler ME. Changes in the B-cell repertoire with age. *Vaccine* 2000;18:1624–1628.

346. Nobrega A, Haury M, Gueret R, et al. The age-associated increase in autoreactive immunoglobulins reflects a quantitative increase in specificities detectable at lower concentrations in young mice. *Scand J Immunol* 1996;44:437–443.

347. Mattila PS, Tarkkanen J. Age-associated changes in the cellular composition of the human adenoid. *Scand J Immunol* 1997;45:423–427.

348. Lacroix-Desmazes S, Mouthon L, Kaveri SV, et al. Stability of natural self-reactive antibody repertoires during aging. *J Clin Immunol* 1999;19:26–34.

349. Geiger KD, Klein U, Brauninger A, et al. CD5-positive B cells in healthy elderly humans are a polyclonal B cell population. *Eur J Immunol* 2000;30:2918–2923.

350. Kyle RA, Therneau TM, Rajkumar SV, et al. A long-term study of prognosis in monoclonal gammopathy of undetermined significance. *N Engl J Med* 2002;346:564–569.

351. Cohen HJ, Crawford J, Rao MK, et al. Racial differences in the prevalence of monoclonal gammopathy in a community-based sample of the elderly. *Am J Med* 1998;104:439–444.

352. Stevenson FK, Sahota SS. B cell maturation in relation to multiple myeloma. *Pathol Biol* 1999;47:89–97.

353. Van Dijk-Hard I, Soderstrom I, Feld S, et al. Age-related impaired affinity maturation and differential D-JH gene usage in human VH6-expressing B lymphocytes from healthy individuals. *Eur J Immunol* 1997;27:1381–1386.

354. Rosner K, Winter DB, Kasmer C, et al. Impact of age on hypermutation of immunoglobulin variable genes in humans. *J Clin Immunol* 2001;21:102–115.

355. Rosner K, Winter DB, Tarone RE, et al. Third complementarity-determining region of mutated VH immunoglobulin genes contains shorter V, D, J, P, and N components than non-mutated genes. *Immunology* 2001;103:179–187.

356. Troutaud D, Drouet M, Decourt C, et al. Age-related alterations of somatic hypermutation and CDR3 lengths in human Vκ 4-expressing B lymphocytes. *Immunology* 1999;97:197–203.

357. Rosner K, Winter DB, Skovgaard GL, et al. Analysis of microsatellite instability and hypermutation of immunoglobulin variable genes in Werner syndrome. *Mech Ageing Dev* 2001;122:1121–1133.

358. Wang X, Stollar BD. Immunoglobulin VH gene expression in human aging. *Clin Immunol* 1999;93:132–142.

359. Borghesi C, Nicoletti C. In vivo and in vitro study of the primary and secondary antibody response to a bacterial antigen in aged mice. *Int J Exp Pathol* 1995;76:419–424.

360. Yang X, Stedra J, Cerny J. Relative contribution of T and B cells to hypermutation and selection of the antibody repertoire in germinal centers of aged mice. *J Exp Med* 1996;183:959–970.

361. Song H, Price PW, Cerny J. Age-related changes in antibody repertoire: contribution from T cells. *Immunol Rev* 1997;160:55–62.

362. Zheng B, Han S, Takahashi Y, et al. Immunosenescence and germinal center reaction. *Immunol Rev* 1997;160:63–77.

363. Szakal AK, Taylor JK, Smith JP, et al. Kinetics of germinal center development in lymph node of young and aging immune mice. *Anat Rec* 1990;227:475–485.

364. Buhl AM, Cambier JC. Co-receptor and accessory regulation of B-cell antigen receptor signal transduction. *Immunol Rev* 1997;160:127–138.

365. Souvannavong V, Lemaire C, Andreau K, et al. Age-associated modulation of apoptosis and activation in murine B lymphocytes. *Mech Ageing Dev* 1998;103:285–299.

366. Fernandez-Gutierrez B, Jover JA, De Miguel S, et al. Early lymphocyte activation in elderly humans: impaired T and T-dependent B cell responses. *Exp Gerontol* 1999;34:217–229.

367. Whisler RL, Newhouse YG, Grants IS, et al. Differential expression of the α and β isoforms of protein kinase C in peripheral blood T and B cells from young and elderly adults. *Mech Ageing Dev* 1995;77:197–211.

368. Whisler RL, Liu BQ, Newhouse YG, et al. Signal transduction in human B cells during aging: alterations in stimulus-induced phosphorylations of tyrosine and serine/threonine substrates and in cytosolic calcium responsiveness. *Lymphokine Cytokine Res* 1991;10:463–473.

369. Anspach J, Poulsen G, Kaattari I, et al. Reduction in DNA binding activity of the transcription factor Pax-5a in B lymphocytes of aged mice. *J Immunol* 2001;166:2617–2626.

370. O'Keefe TL, Williams GT, Batista FD, et al. Deficiency in CD22, a B-cell-specific inhibitory receptor, is sufficient to predispose to development of high affinity autoantibodies. *J Exp Med* 1999;189:1307–1313.

371. Hallgren HM, Buckley CE III, Gilbertsen VA, et al. Lymphocyte phytohemagglutinin responsiveness, immunoglobulins and autoantibodies in aging humans. *J Immunol* 1973;111:1101–1107.

372. Le Morvan C, Cogne M, Troutaud D, et al. Modification of HLA expression on peripheral lymphocytes and monocytes during ageing. *Mech Ageing Dev* 1998;105:209–220.

373. Saurwein-Teissl M, Romani N, Grubeck-Loebenstein B. Dendritic cells in old age: neglected by gerontology? *Mech Ageing Dev* 2000;121:123–130.

374. Szakal AK, Kapasi ZF, Masuda A, et al. Follicular dendritic cells in the alternative antigen transport pathway: microenvironment, cellular events, age and retrovirus related alterations. *Semin Immunol* 1992;4:257–265.

375. Globerson A. Hematopoietic stem cells and aging. *Exp Gerontol* 1999;34:137–146.

376. Ogawa T, Kitagawa M, Hirokawa K. Age-related changes of human bone marrow: a histometric estimation of proliferative cells, apoptotic cells, T cells, B cells, and macrophages. *Mech Ageing Dev* 2000;117:57–68.

377. Bagnara GP, Bonsi L, Strippoli P, et al. Hemopoiesis in healthy old people and centenarians: well-maintained responsiveness of CD34+ cells to hemopoietic growth factors and remodeling of cytokine network. *J Gerontol A Biol Sci Med Sci* 2000;55:B61–B66.

378. Brummendorf TH, Rufer N, Baerlocher GM, et al. Limited telomere shortening in hematopoietic stem cells after transplantation. *Ann N Y Acad Sci* 2001;938:1–7.

379. Hirokawa K Reversing and restoring immune functions. *Mech Ageing Dev* 1997;93:119–124.

380. Ben-Yehuda A, Danenberg HD, Zakay-Rones Z, et al. The influence of sequential annual vaccination and of DHEA administration on the efficacy of the immune response to influenza vaccine in the elderly. *Mech Ageing Dev* 1998;102:299–306.

381. Martin JT. Development of an adjuvant to enhance the immune response to influenza vaccine in the elderly. *Biologicals* 1997;25:209–213.

382. Swenson CD, Gottesman SR, Xue B, et al. The effect of aging on the immune response: influence of phosphatidylcholine-containing lipid on IgD-receptor expression and antibody formation. *Mech Ageing Dev* 1997;95:167–186.

383. Sambhara S, Kurichh A, Miranda R, et al. Enhanced immune responses and resistance against infection in aged mice conferred by Flu-ISCOMs vaccine correlate with up-regulation of costimulatory molecule CD86. *Vaccine* 1998;16:1698–1704.

384. Kovarich J, Bozzotti P, Tougne C, et al. Adjuvant effects of CpG oligodeoxynucleotides on responses against T-independent type 2 antigens. *Immunology* 2001;102:67–76.

385. Harrod T, Martin M, Russell MW. Long-term persistence and recall of immune responses in aged mice after mucosal immunization. *Oral Microbiol Immunol* 2001;16:170–177.

386. Wakabayashi A, Utsuyama M, Hosoda T, et al. Differential age effect of oral administration of an antigen on antibody response: an induction of tolerance in young mice but enhancement of immune response in old mice. *Mech Ageing Dev* 1999;109:191–201.

387. Fujihashi K, Koga T, McGhee JR. Mucosal vaccination and immune responses in the elderly. *Vaccine* 2000;18:1675–1680.

388. Trannoy E, Berger R, Hollander G, et al. Vaccination of immunocompetent elderly subjects with a live attenuated Oka strain of varicella zoster virus: a randomized controlled dose-response trial. *Vaccine* 2000;18:1700–1706.

389. Dranoff G. Cancer vaccines 2001. In: Chabner BA, Longo DL, eds. *Cancer chemotherapy and biotherapy: principles and practice.* 3rd ed. Philadelphia: Lippincott Williams & Wilkins, 2001:951–959.

390. Utsuyama M, Ichikawa M, Konno-Shirakawa A, et al. Retardation of the age-associated decline of immune function in aging rats under dietary restriction and daily physical exercise. *Mech Ageing Dev* 1996;91:219–228.

391. Kohut ML, Boehm GW, Moynihan JA. Moderate exercise is associated with enhanced antigenspecific cytokine, but not IgM antibody production in aged mice. *Mech Ageing Dev* 2001;122:1135–1150.

392. Nieman DC. Exercise immunology: practical applications. *Int J Sports Med* 1997;18(suppl 1):S91–S100.

393. Woods JA, Evans JK, Wolters BW, et al. Effects of maximal exercise on natural killer (NK) cell cytotoxicity and responsiveness to interferon-α in young and old. *J Gerontol A Biol Sci Med Sci* 1998;53:B430–B437.

394. Pedersen BK, Hoffman-Goetz L. Exercise and the immune system: regulation, integration, and adaptation. *Physiol Rev* 2000;80:1055–1081.

395. Shinkai S, Konishi M, Shephard RJ. Aging and immune response to exercise. *Can J Physiol Pharmacol* 1998;76:562–572.

396. Nieman DC. Exercise immunology: future directions for research related to athletes, nutrition, and the elderly. *Int J Sports Med* 2000;21(suppl 1):61–68.

397. Pahlavani MA. Caloric restriction and immunosenescence: a current perspective. *Front Biosci* 2000;5:D580–D587.

398. Spaulding CC, Walford RL, Effros RB. Calorie restriction inhibits the age-related dysregulation of the cytokines TNF-α and IL-6 in C3B10RF1 mice. *Mech Ageing Dev* 1997;93:87–94.

399. Pahlavani MA, Harris MD, Richardson A. The increase in the induction of IL-2 expression with caloric restriction is correlated to changes in the transcription factor NFAT. *Cell Immunol* 1997;180:10–19.

400. Pahlavani MA, Vargas DM. Influence of aging and caloric restriction on activation of Ras/MAPK, calcineurin, and CaMK-IV activities in rat T cells. *Proc Soc Exp Biol Med* 2000;223:163–169.

401. Webster RG. Immunity to influenza in the elderly. *Vaccine* 2000;18:1686–1689.

402. Weindruch R, Lane MA, Ingram DK, et al. Dietary restriction in rhesus monkeys: lymphopenia and reduced mitogen-induced proliferation in peripheral blood mononuclear cells. *Aging* 1997;9:304–308.

403. High KP. Nutritional strategies to boost immunity and prevent infection in elderly individuals. *Clin Infect Dis* 2001;33:1892–1900.

404. Han SN, Wu D, Ha WK, et al. Vitamin E supplementation increases T helper 1 cytokine production in old mice infected with influenza virus. *Immunology* 2000;100:487–493.

405. Adolfsson O, Huber BT, Meydani SN. Vitamin E-enhanced IL-2 production in old mice: naive but not memory T cells show increased cell division cycling and IL-2-producing capacity. *J Immunol* 2001;167:3809–3817.

406. Moriguchi S. The role of vitamin E in T-cell differentiation and the decrease of cellular immunity with aging. *Biofactors* 1998;7:77–86.

407. Meydani SN, Meydani M, Blumberg JB, et al. Vitamin E supplementation and in vivo immune response in healthy elderly subjects: a randomized controlled trail. *JAMA* 1997:277:1380–1386.

408. High KP. Micronutrient supplementation and immune function in the elderly. *Clin Infect Disease* 1999;28:717–722.

409. Mocchegiani E, Giacconi R, Muzzioli M, et al. Zinc, infections and immunosenescence. *Mech Ageing Dev* 2000;121:21–35.

410. Douziech N, Seres I, Larbi A, et al. Modulation of human lymphocyte proliferative response with aging. *Exp Gerontol* 2002;37:369–387.

411. Utsuyama M, Seidlar H, Kitagawa M, et al. Immunological restoration and anti-tumor effect by Japanese herbal medicine in aged mice. *Mech Ageing Dev* 2001:122:341–352.

412. Hori T, Kiyoshima J, Shida K, et al. Augmentation of cellular immunity and reduction of influenza virus titer in aged mice fed Lactobacillus casei strain Shirota. *Clin Diagn Lab Immunol* 2002;9:105–108.

413. Gill HS, Rutherford KJ, Cross ML, et al. Enhancement of immunity in the elderly by dietary supplemetation with the probiotic Bifidobacterium lactis HN019. *Am J Clin Nutr* 2001;74:833–839.

414. Straub RH, Cutolo M, Zietz B, et al. The process of aging changes the interplay of the immune, endocrine and nervous systems. *Mech Ageing Dev* 2001;122:1591–1611.

415. Gelato MC. Agina and immune function: a possible role for growth hormone. *Horm Res* 1996;45:46–49.

416. Khorram O, Yeung M, Vu L, et al. Effects of [norleucine27]growth hormone-releasing hormone (1-29)-NH2 administration in the immune system of aging men and women. *J Clin Endocrinol Metab* 1997;82:3590–3596.

417. Khorram O, Vu L, Yen SS. Activation of immune function by dehydroepiandrosterone (DHEA) in age-advanced men. *J Gerontol A Biol Sci Med Sci* 1997;52:M1–M7.

418. Porter VR, Greendale GA, Schocken M, et al. Immune effects of hormone replacement therapy in post-menopausal women. *Exp Gerontol* 2001;36:311–326.

419. Guardiola-Lemaitre B. Toxicology of melatonin. *J Biol Rhythms* 1997;12:697–706.

CHAPTER 34

Complement

Wolfgang M. Prodinger, Reinhard Würzner, Heribert Stoiber, and Manfred P. Dierich

Overview
Complement as a Functional System · Historical Roots · Phylogenetic Aspects · Nomenclature
Biosynthesis of Complement: Location and Regulation
Major Protein Families among Complement Components
Complement C3/α_2 Macroglobulin Superfamily · Proteins with Short Consensus Repeat Units · Proteins with a Serine Protease Module · Protein Motifs Found in Terminal Pathway Components
Complement Activation: Pivotal Role of C3
Activation via Classical Pathway
Activation of Classical Pathway · Regulation of Classical Pathway
Activation via Lectin Pathway
Activation of Lectin Pathway · Regulation of Lectin Pathway
Activation via Alternative Pathway
The C3b Amplification Loop · Initiation of Alternative Pathway via iC3 · Inactivation and Degradation of C3b and Control of Alternative Pathway
Terminal Pathway
Activation of C5 · Formation of Terminal Complement Complex · Control of Terminal Pathway · Biological Properties of Terminal Complement Complex
Complement Receptors
C3 Receptors · Anaphylatoxin Receptors C3aR and C5aR (CD88) · C1q Receptors
Complement as Pathogenic Factor in Disease
Complement in Renal Disease · Complement in Neurologic Disease
Complement in Defense against Infection
Evasion Strategies of Microorganisms · Mimicry of Complement Structures by Microorganisms
Complement Genetics
Complement Deficiencies
Complement as Target in Drug Therapy
Native or Modified Complement Regulators · Derivatives of Monoclonal Antibodies · Synthetic Molecules · Which Pathway to Block? · Exploitation of Complement Activation for Therapy or Prophylaxis
Summary and Conclusions
Acknowledgments
References

OVERVIEW

Complement as a Functional System

Complement, with its more than 35 plasma or membrane proteins (Table 1), serves as an auxiliary system in immunity and antimicrobial defense. Its activation as a whole is predominantly due to a cascade of proteolytic steps, performed by serine protease domains in some of the components. Three different pathways of activation are distinguished (Fig. 1), triggered by target-bound antibody (the classical pathway); microbial repetitive polysaccharide structures (the lectin pathway); or recognition of other "foreign"

surface structures (the alternative pathway). All three merge in the pivotal activation of C3 and, subsequently, of C5 by highly specific enzymatic complexes, the so-called convertases. The alternative pathway amplifies C3 activation triggered by the other pathways. In the common terminal pathway downstream of C5, additional complement components are activated in a nonproteolytic manner and assembled into the membrane attack complex (MAC). The entire powerful activation machinery is controlled redundantly by more than ten negative regulators.

In addition to direct killing of microbes through MAC formation, complement cooperates with other host defense

TABLE 1. *Complement components*

Component	Molecular weight in kD of intact protein (subunits)	Plasma concentration (μg/ml)	Chromosomal assignment
Alternative pathway			
C3	185 (α, 110; β, 75)	1200–1300	19p13
Factor B	93	200	6p21
Factor D	24	2	19
Properdin	Oligomers of 110, 165, 200 (monomer: 55)	25	Xp11
Classical pathway			
C1q	460 (6 subunits, each of 3 chains: A, 26; B, 26; C, 24)	150	3 genes at 1p34–1p36
C1r	85	50	2 genes at 12p13
C1s	85	50	
C4	205 (α, 97; β, 75; γ, 33)	300–600	6p21 (MHC-III region); two loci for C4: *C4A* and *C4B*
C2	102	20	
Lectin pathway			
MBL	200–600, i.e., 2–6 subunits (1 subunit = 3 chains, each 32 kD)	0.05–3	10q22
MASP-1	100	2–12	3q27–3q28 (splice variants of one gene)
MASP-3	42	n.d.	
MASP-2	76	n.d.	1p36 (splice variants of one gene)
sMAP/MAp19	19	n.d.	
Terminal pathway			
C5	190 (α, 115; β, 75)	80	9q33
C6	110	45	5p14–5p12 (MAC gene cluster)
C7	100	90	
C9	70	60	
C8	150 (α, 64; β, 64; γ, 22)	55	α, β: 1p22 γ: 9q22–9q32
Control proteins (in plasma)			
Factor I	88	35	4q25
C1-INH	105	240	11q12–11q13
Factor H	150	300–450 ⎤	
FHL-1	42	5–20 ⎟	*RCA* gene cluster at 1q32.
C4bp	550 (7 α chains, each 70; 1 β-chain, 45)	250 ⎦	
S protein (vitronectin)	84	500	17q11
Clusterin (SP-40,40)	70 (2 × 35)	50	8p21–8p12
Carboxy-peptidase N	280 (2 × 83 and 2 × 50)	35	83-kD subunit: 8p23–8p22; 50-kD subunit: chromosome 10
Membrane-bound complement control proteins			
CR1 (CD35)	190–280 (due to isoforms)	— ⎤	
DAF (CD55)	70	— ⎟	*RCA* gene cluster at 1q32
MCP (CD46)	45–70 (due to glycosylation)	— ⎦	
CD59	18–20	—	11p13
Complement proteins with unclear function			
FHR-1	39 and 42 (due to glycosylation)	60 ⎤	
FHR-2	24 and 29 (due to glycosylation)	40 ⎟	*RCA* gene cluster at 1q32
FHR-3	55	n.d. ⎟	
FHR-4	86	n.d. ⎦	
FHR-5	80	5	1q22–1q23

C1-INH, C1 inhibitor; C4bp, C4-binding protein; CR, complement receptor; DAF, decay-accelerating factor; FHL, factor H–like protein; FHR, factor H-related protein; MAC, membrane attack complex; MASP, MBL-associated serine protease; MBL, mannan-binding lectin; MCP, membrane cofactor protein; MHC, major histocompatability complex; n.d., not determined; sMAP/MAp19, small MBL-associated protein or MBL-associated protein of 19 kD.

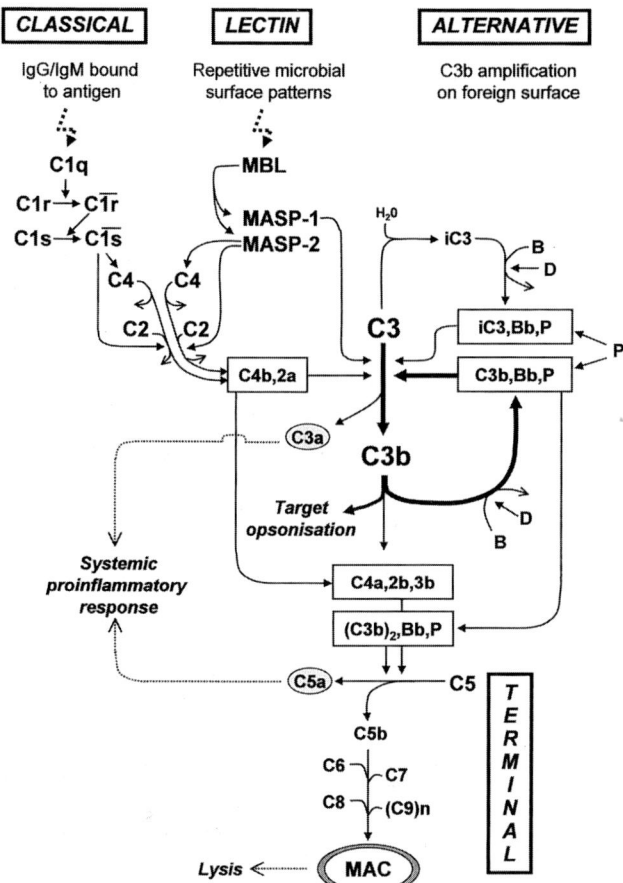

FIG. 1. Overview of complement activation pathways. The C3 or C5 convertases of the pathways are boxed. The alternative pathway amplification loop of C3b generation is indicated by *thick arrows*. Note the systemic action of the anaphylatoxins in contrast to the effect of opsonisation or lysis via membrane attack complex that occurs on the target surface.

mechanisms (Fig. 2). Opsonisation with complement, in particular with C3-fragments, enhances uptake of microbes into phagocytic cells via complement receptors. The solubility of immune complexes and the immunogenicity of antigens are also enhanced by C3-fragment deposition. At the C3 and C5 activation steps, powerful cleavage products (the anaphylatoxins C3a and C5a) are generated, which set the stage for inflammation systemically.

Historical Roots

In the second half of the 19th century, a first concept of complement emerged with the distinction of "alexin," a heat-labile fraction in normal serum necessary for killing of bacteria in addition to antibody. The term "complement" was introduced by Paul Ehrlich in 1899. In the 1950s, Louis Pillemer advanced the concept of complement, which at that time comprised primarily the classical pathway, by postulating an antibody-independent mechanism of activation (1), which is now referred to as the alternative pathway. Like in archaeological excavations, however, the oldest layer is discovered last: the third and phylogenetically old lectin pathway was discovered a little more than 10 years ago and, despite recent cloning of several new components, remains incompletely understood.

Phylogenetic Aspects

A complement system with three C3 activation pathways and a common lytic pathway is found only in jawed vertebrates. These are capable of an adaptive immune response, and that new trigger became purposefully connected to older defense mechanisms (see Chapter 18). Thus, the lectin and alternative pathways can be seen as descendants of a primordial surveillance system for microbes that has existed long before adapted immunity evolved. In the higher vertebrates, this system has developed into a major effector mechanism for the

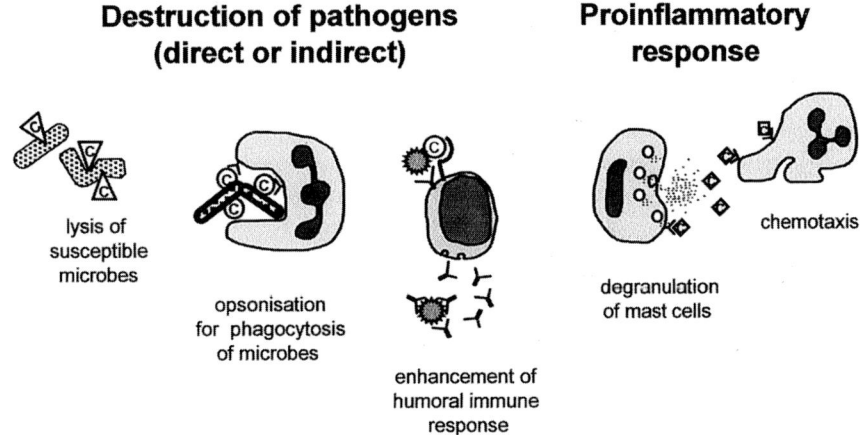

Destruction of pathogens (direct or indirect)

lysis of susceptible microbes

opsonisation for phagocytosis of microbes

enhancement of humoral immune response

Proinflammatory response

degranulation of mast cells

chemotaxis

FIG. 2. Overview of contribution of complement activation to antimicrobial defense.

powerful humoral immune system, when the classical pathway was "added." This extension involved gene duplication events and subsequent functional divergence leading to pairs of related genes in the old (lectin or alternative) and new (classical) pathways (e.g., factor B and C2) (2).

The presence of single genes characterizes the primitive complement systems of jawless vertebrates (cyclostomes or invertebrate deuterostomes). A central C3-like opsonin interacts with primordial C3-receptors on phagocytes and with molecules that resemble mannan-binding lectin (MBL), MASP-1 (mannose-binding protein–associated serine protease 1), or factor B, suggesting that a C3 activation mechanism that combines lectin and alternative pathway functions (3). However, even protostomes such as Limulus or the dipterans Drosophila and Anopheles possess proteins of the C3/α_2-macroglobulin superfamily of thioester proteins, which are either homologs of α_2-macroglobulin (and thus unspecific protease inhibitors) or opsonins (and as such up-regulated during infectious challenges). One of the latter, the *Anopheles gambiae* protein aTEP-1 already shows more similarity to C3 than to α_2-macroglobulin in the thioester part, although it cannot bind covalently to substrates (4).

Nomenclature

Classical and terminal pathway components were early designated C1 through C9. Notably, the activation sequence of the cascade (determined later on) is C1-C4-C2-C3-C5-C6-C7-C8-C9. Alternative pathway components are called "factors" and distinguished by letters (factors B, D, H, I, P). Proteolytic activation of C2 through C5 produces smaller fragments and larger ones remaining in a complex required for the next activation step. The small, liberated fragments are denoted by the letter "a" (e.g., for C4, C4a), and the larger ones by "b" (e.g., C4b), the notable exception being C2 (i.e., C2a is the large active fragment). Inactivation of C3b or C4b yields even smaller fragments (C4c, C4d, etc.). These must not be confused with the subunits of C3 and C4 (e.g., C4α, C4β, C4γ) or isotypic proteins (e.g., C4A and C4B derived from two genetic C4 loci).

BIOSYNTHESIS OF COMPLEMENT: LOCATION AND REGULATION

The liver is the major site of production for complement proteins. About 90% of the plasma complement components are synthesized in the liver (5), exceptions being C1 (produced in the intestinal epithelium, monocytes, and macrophages) and factor D (produced in adipose tissue). C7 of hepatic origin was found to contribute less than 60% to plasma C7 with bone marrow–derived cells, in particular granulocytes, representing an alternative major source (6,7). The main source for plasma properdin has not yet been identified.

In addition to the liver, complement components are synthesized in many cell types, such as endothelial cells, lymphocytes, renal epithelium, reproductive organs, and others.

Notably, production of virtually all components has been observed in monocytes/macrophages and in astrocytes (8). Extrahepatic complement production appears to be important—as for astrocytes or other glial cells, it is the only source for complement behind an intact blood–brain barrier. Hence, the role of complement in the brain is an emerging field of interest in several, primarily noninfectious, diseases. Second, activated macrophages at sites of infection or in lymphatic tissue produce effective levels of complement locally. C3-deficient mice reconstituted with wild-type bone marrow show local synthesis of C3 by macrophages in the spleen. Macrophage C3 production started on antigenic challenge and proved sufficient for the enhancement of the humoral immune response otherwise observed at normal C3 plasma levels (9).

The production of plasma complement components is augmented in the acute-phase response. This pertains to most components, although the extent of induction varies substantially (from about 3- to 50-fold). The main common transcriptional inducer of complement genes is IFN-γ, others being IL-1- and IL-6-type cytokines (i.e., IL-1α, IL-1β, IL-6, IL-11, and others) (10). Cell-surface–bound complement regulators are expressed on a variety of tissues (5). The observation that DAF or MCP expression is down-regulated after ischemic injury of endothelial cells may explain the importance of complement for the extent of ischemic tissue damage (11).

MAJOR PROTEIN FAMILIES AMONG COMPLEMENT COMPONENTS

Complement C3/α_2 Macroglobulin Superfamily

C3, C4, and C5, are central components in the complement system (Figs. 1 and 3). They are derived from one ancestral protein that may have served as a multispecific protease inhibitor. The central feature of these proteins is an internal thioester formed during biosynthesis in C3, C4, and the structurally related α_2-macroglobulin between a cysteine and a glutamine residue three positions apart (see Fig. 4) (12). C5 has lost this function during evolution. C3, C4, and C5, are activated by proteolytic cleavage at a conserved peptide bond and undergo a gross conformational change associated with the exposition of new epitopes. The protected thioester of C3 or C4 becomes exposed, leading to the formation of a reactive intermediate that enables the glutamyl residue to form a covalent ester or amide bond with water or with NH_2- or OH-residues of surrounding molecules. C3 and the C4B isotype of C4 possess a histidine positioned in close proximity to the thioester (13), which acts as the catalyst for the formation of ester bonds. In contrast, the C4A isotype lacks this histidine and preferentially forms amide bonds (14).

Proteins with Short Consensus Repeat Units

Short consensus repeats (SCRs) or, according to another preferred designation, complement control protein (CCP)

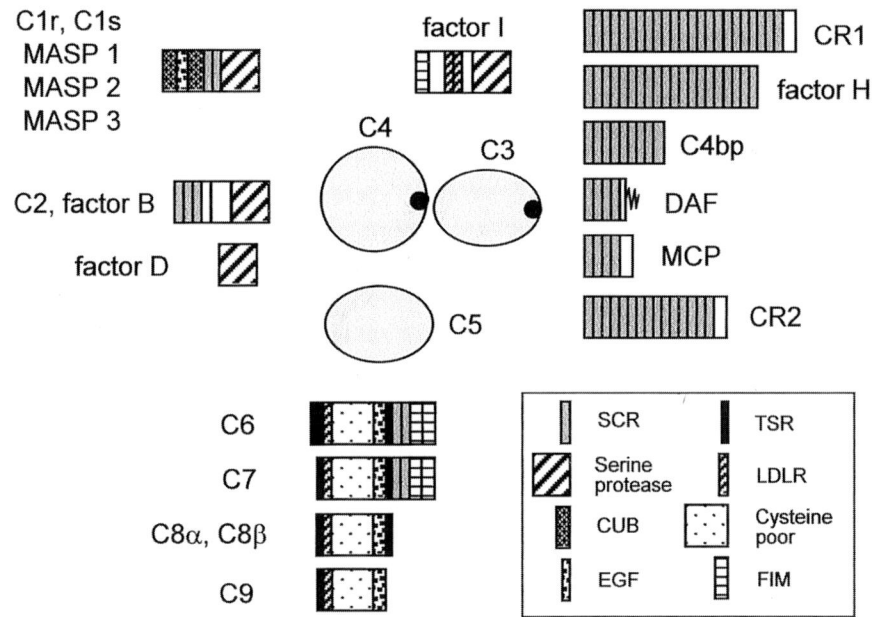

FIG. 3. Motifs and molecular families common among complement proteins. Components with serine protease domains important in proteolytic activation steps (**left**), regulatory proteins of the RCA gene cluster based on SCRs (**right**), and terminal pathway mosaic proteins (**below**), are grouped around the homologous proteins with a thioester region (*black dot* representing formed thioester). GPI anchors are symbolized by *zigzag line*. Domains not mentioned in the text or unspecified protein parts are left *white*. (For domain abbreviations, see text.)

modules, are individually folding domains of about 60 amino acids displaying a β barrel structure (15,16) and distinct conserved residues (e.g., tryptophane, prolines) and, most importantly, four cysteines that form two disulfide bonds (Cys_1 to Cys_3 and Cys_2 to Cys_4) (17). Although SCRs can be found in various noncomplement proteins (e.g., in the selectins), proteins that consist predominantly of SCRs are encoded by genes in the "regulator of complement activation" (RCA) gene cluster. The *RCA* comprises the genes for factor H and the factor–H family proteins, for C4bp, DAF, CR2, CR1, and MCP (18). The number of SCRs in the proteins ranges from 4 to 34, and some proteins possess transmembrane and short intracytoplasmic parts (CR1, CR2, MCP) or glycosylphosphatidylinositol (GPI) anchors. RCA proteins are elongated in shape; for instance, CR1 extends 90 nm from the cell membrane.

The RCA is thought to have evolved from one ancestral prototypic SCR by duplication and gene conversion events as a family of genes for proteins controlling C3 and C4 activation. Nevertheless, the binding of activated C3 or C4 can be attributed to distinct, often adjacent, SCRs in each member. Few SCRs are present in mosaic proteins such as factor B, C2, C1r, C1s, MASP-1, MASP-2, MASP-3, C6, and C7, all of which interact with thioester proteins.

Proteins with a Serine Protease Module

Proteins with serine protease activity are crucially involved in the early, amplifying steps of complement activation. Serine

protease domains are present in the two homologous proteins C2 and factor B, as well as in factor I, factor D, and in the members of the MASP-like family (i.e., C1r, C1s, MASP-1, MASP-2, MASP-3). The latter proteins contain a serine protease domain together with two CUB domains, an EGF-like domain, and two SCRs. (CUB domains are widespread protein modules and found, among others, in complement C1r/C1s, sea urchin EGF [uEGF], and bone morphogenetic protein-1.)

Protein Motifs Found in Terminal Pathway Components

C6 through C9 have an amphiphilic character that allows them to act in plasma and on lipid membranes, an important feature for MAC formation. As true mosaic proteins they assemble a variety of modules in a characteristic sequence (Fig. 3): thrombospondin type 1 repeats (TSRs) also found in the extracellular matrix protein thrombospondin and in properdin, a low-density lipoprotein receptor (LDLR) domain, a conserved cysteine-poor region (19) also found in perforin, an epidermal growth factor (EGF) module, SCRs, and factor I modules (FIMs). Functional activity is preserved even in absence of the latter (20).

COMPLEMENT ACTIVATION: PIVOTAL ROLE OF C3

All three activation pathways merge into activation of C3 (Fig. 1). The physiologically relevant activators of C3 are

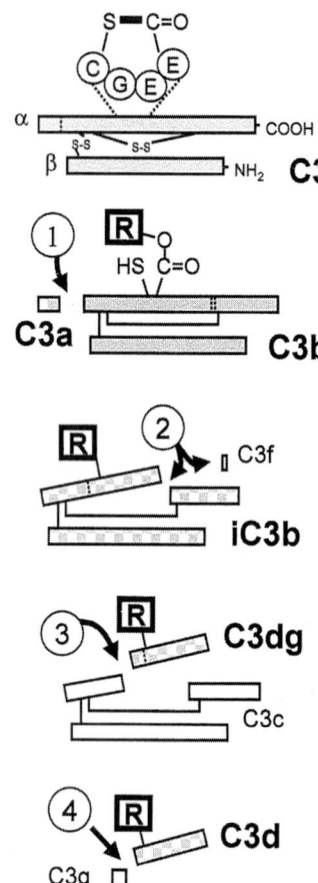

FIG. 4. Activation and inactivation of C3. The thioester bond (*thick line*) formed between Cys and Glu is shown for native C3 (amino acids of the thioester region are in *circles*). **(1)** Activation of native C3 by C3 convertases yields C3a and C3b bound to an acceptor R (here via ester linkage). **(2)** C3b inactivation by factor I and a cofactor. **(3)** iC3b is further degraded by factor I and CR1. **(4)** Acceptor-bound C3dg is trimmed by unspecific plasma proteases to C3d. C3 fragments that are biologically active, but do not participate in complement activation are *hatched*.

the C3 convertases, although proteases like plasmin can activate C3 *in vitro*. The following four distinct protein entities act on C3 or its fragments.

- Homologous C3 convertases C3b,Bb and C4b,2a, consisting of proteins with an activated serine protease domain in complex with C3b or C4b. They cleave C3 into C3a and C3b.
- Factor I, a constitutively active plasma serine protease specific for C3b and C4b. It inactivates C3b and C4b by cleaving it into iC3b (and iC4b). Factor I requires one out of several potential cofactors.
- RCA family proteins composed of SCRs. They negatively regulate C3 and C4 activation by disintegrating the C3 convertases and serving as cofactors for factor I.
- Receptors for fragments of C3, a heterogeneous group comprising integrins, seven-transmembrane receptors, and

RCA family members. They use C3 activation products to mediate induction of phagocytosis or chemotaxis.

The native C3 molecule becomes cleaved at a conserved arginine residue in the α chain into C3a and C3b. The peptide C3a (77 amino acids) is a potent anaphylatoxin and exerts its effects distant from the site of C3 activation in circulation. The large "nascent" C3b has a half-life of 60 μs during which it changes its conformation, exposes the internal thioester bond and binds through the now highly reactive thioester to nearby nucleophils (e.g., OH groups of any surrounding molecule, including H_2O).

ACTIVATION VIA CLASSICAL PATHWAY

The proteins forming the activation cascade of the classical pathway comprise C1, C4, C2, and C3 (in this order). C1-INH, C4bp, CR1, factor I, DAF, and MCP function as control proteins. C1 consists of one C1q molecule noncovalently bound to two C1r and two C1s molecules (Fig. 5). Calcium ions are required for formation of the stable C1 complex. About 70% of the C1 components in plasma are present in C1 complexes at a given time. The C1q protein is assembled from six identical subunits each of which consists of three homologous chains (A, B, and C). These chains form a globular domain at the C-terminus, followed by the "neck" and a coil in the "stalk." The six subunits are held together by the collagenous stalk parts (giving rise to the comparison of C1q with a "bunch of six tulips"). The stalks also interact with the $C1r_2C1s_2$ tetramer assembled in a linear chain (21). Each C1s and C1r possesses a serine protease domain (catalytic domain) and a contact domain, and before activation, all four catalytic domains are placed inside the cone-shaped stalk of C1q (22) (Fig. 5).

Activation of Classical Pathway

The physiologically most important activation of C1 is initiated by binding of the globular domains of C1q to

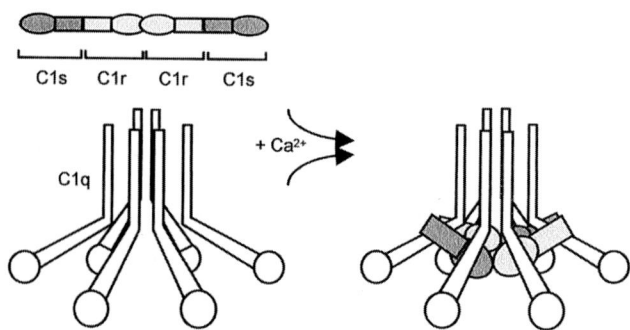

FIG. 5. The C1 complex. The model for the C1 complex proposes that the folding of the rod-like $C1r_2$-$C1s_2$ around the arms of C1q causes the catalytic domains of C1s to contact the catalytic domains of C1r. Inactivation of C1 occurs by covalent binding of C1r and C1s to C1-inhibitor (C1-INH).

antigen-bound IgG or IgM. C1q must bind to at least two of the conformationally altered Fc portions, implying that only one IgM, but at least two IgG molecules in sufficient proximity (i.e., <40 nm apart) are required. This restricts C1 activation by IgG to substrates with a critical density of bound antibody. The C1q binding potential of human IgG subclasses increases in the order IgG4<IgG2<IgG1<IgG3 which is important with regard to the humanization of murine monoclonal antibodies. (Some mouse IgG subclasses—for example, IgG2a, but not IgG1—can also activate human complement which is exploited for selective *in vitro* killing of human cells by monoclonal antibodies.)

Other triggers of C1 activation include bacterial lipopolysaccharide, polyanionic compounds, myelin, the acute-phase reactant C-reactive protein (CRP), and viral envelopes (e.g., of HIV-1). Recent data suggest a new role of C1q binding followed by classical pathway activation for the clearance of apoptotic cells through phagocytosis by macrophages (23,24). This mechanism may explain the strong association of systemic lupus erythematodes with complete deficiencies of classical pathway components, especially C1q (25,26).

Binding of C1q to its substrates induces a conformational change in C1q and subsequently a change in position of the two C1r serine esterase domains relative to each other. This allows for reciprocal cleavage of the C1r molecules. Such activated C1r in turn cleaves and activates C1s, which is the enzyme to activate C4 and C2. Cleavage of C1r and C1s does not liberate proteolytic fragments. Altogether, one active C1 molecule can produce about thirty-five C4b molecules due to its low K_m value and the high plasma concentration of C4 (27).

C4 is cleaved into the small C4a and the large C4b fragment (termed nascent C4b), which undergoes a gross conformational change. The internal thioester in C4b becomes exposed and able to form covalent bonds with surrounding molecules. These reactions take place within microseconds (12), and most nascent C4b is lost by reacting with water.

About 5% of the C4b become covalently attached to the surface, clustered around the activating Ig–C1 complex.

Due to the lower plasma concentration of C2, C2 activation proceeds slower than C4 activation (about four C2 are cleaved per active C1) (28). As free C2 is infrequently cleaved by C1s, it forms a complex with C4b in a Mg^{2+}-dependent manner and becomes easily accessible for cleavage by C1s into C2a (larger fragment) and C2b (released smaller fragment). C2b exhibits kinin activity and is thus responsible for the generation of the pathogenic peptide in hereditary angioedema (see below). C2a is the enzymatically active fragment in the C4b,2a complex, termed the classical pathway C3 convertase. C2a is active only as long as associated with C4b and, once dissociated, cannot bind to C4b again. With the C3 convertase formation, the classical pathway leads into the common step of C3 activation (see below).

Regulation of Classical Pathway

C1s and C1r are tightly controlled by C1-INH, a member of the serpine family (serine protease inhibitors) that inactivates serine proteases by a suicide substrate mechanism: their active site forms a covalent bond with the active serine of the substrate protease domain. C1-INH is already associated with the native C1 molecule that tends towards autoactivation. Activated C1r and C1s are rapidly bound by C1-INH in a stoichiometric relation, yielding two C1rC1s(C1-INH)$_2$ molecules per C1. Notably, C1-INH, unlike other complement inhibitors, is not redundant and may become a limiting factor in situations like septic shock that require extensive complement activation control. Inhibitors farther downstream are C4bp, DAF, and CR1 (see Table 2). Interestingly, because C4bp can bind seven C4b, it has been used for multimerization of recombinant proteins (29). C4b,2a disassembles spontaneously, but its decay is accelerated by CR1 or DAF, and C4b is inactivated through factor I (Table 2).

TABLE 2. *Mode of action of complement control proteins*

Regulator	Site of action	Mode of action			
		Binds covalently to active C1s, C1r, MASPs			
		Decay acceleration		Cofactor activity	
		C3b,Bb	C4b,2a	C3b	C4b
C1-INH	Plasma				
Factor H	Plasma, nonactivators	+	−/+[a]	+	−
C4bp	Plasma	−	+	−	+
CR1	(Homologous) cell membrane[b]	+	+	+	+
MCP	(Homologous) cell membrane[b]	−	−	+	+
DAF	(Homologous) cell membrane[b]	+	+	−	−
S protein; clusterin	Plasma	Bind to soluble C5b-7 and block its integration into membranes			
CD59	(Homologous) cell membrane	Inhibits binding of C9 and its polymerization			

[a]Decay acceleration of classical pathway C5 convertase, but not of classical pathway C3 convertase.
[b]CR1 has a narrow tissue distribution, in contrast to DAF, MCP, and CD59.
C1-INH, C1 inhibitor; C4bp, C4-binding protein; CR, complement receptor; DAF, decay-accelerating factor; MCP, membrane cofactor protein.

ACTIVATION VIA LECTIN PATHWAY

The concept of the lectin pathway of complement activation has emerged relatively recently and therefore not all details are already fully understood. Its main constituent is the plasma protein mannan-binding lectin or mannose-binding lectin, MBL (reviewed in Petersen et al. [30]). (The terms "mannan-binding protein" or "mannose-binding protein," which abbreviate to MBP, should not be used for MBL to avoid confusion with myelic basic protein.) MBL is a member of the collectins, proteins with collagen-like stalk parts and lectin domains (reviewed in Holmskov [31]). Other non-complement collectins are lung-surfactant proteins SP-D and SP-A. Human MBL is expressed from a single gene, in contrast to MBL in other species. It is made up of subunits that consist of three polypeptide chains, each with an N-terminal cross-linking region followed by a collagen-like region, a neck part and a globular carbohydrate recognition domain (CRD). The three collagenous parts form a coil structure and this subunit structure is stabilized by interchain disulfide bonds and hydrophobic interactions. Two to six subunits (i.e., 6 to 18 CRDs), held together by disulfide bonds in the cross-linking region, form an MBL oligomer with multipronged appearance. Plasma MBL is a mixture of these oligomers, but the complement-activating potential is associated only with the higher oligomeric forms.

MBL plasma levels among presumably normal individuals differ substantially (up to 1,000-fold) and are largely dependent on the allelic form of the *MBL* gene. Different point mutations in exon 1 lead to disruption of the coil in the subunit or in the oligomerization of subunits, resulting in three *MBL* variant alleles (B, C, D variants) associated with low MBL plasma levels as compared to the wild-type *MBL* allele (A variant) (32). Additionally, promoter polymorphisms such as the H/L and Y/X variants influence MBL plasma levels, the haplotypes HY and LX being associated with high and low MBL levels, respectively. Nevertheless, there is still considerable variation in MBL plasma levels even among individuals with the same genotype. MBL levels increase relatively weakly during an acute-phase response.

The complement-activating properties of MBL became clear when MBL deficiency was found to be associated with "defective yeast opsonisation," a functional defect of some patients' sera (33). Currently, many studies underline that MBL plasma levels and allotypes influence the predisposition to infections (34). Although isolated MBL deficiency is not considered a major risk factor, it may coexist with other common deficiencies in the immune system (e.g., partial C4-deficiency or IgG subclass deficiencies). A population-based prospective study showed twice as many acute respiratory infections in infants with MBL deficiency, although that risk is largely confined to a "window of vulnerability" at the age of 6 to 18 months, when maternal antibody disappears (35). Administration of MBL to deficient patients, either prophylactically or during infection episodes, may be a new therapeutic approach, and has been successfully undertaken in isolated cases. Controlled clinical trials have not yet been performed.

MBL in plasma is found in complexes with the proenzymes MBL-associated serine proteases, MASP-1, MASP-2, and MASP-3. A large proportion of the MASPs in circulation, however, is not complexed with MBL. The nature and sequence of MASP activation and the functional relevance of the individual MASPs are not fully understood to date. MBL–MASP complexes in plasma can be separated by density gradient centrifugation (36): MASP-2 and MASP-3 are associated with a larger form of MBL (MBL-II), whereas a smaller MBL (MBL-I) is in complex with MASP-1 and the proteolytically inactive protein MAp19/sMAP (Table 1).

Activation of Lectin Pathway

The CRDs of MBL function as C-type lectins as they recognize carbohydrates like N-acetylglucosamine or mannose, but not galactose or sialic acid, in a Ca^{2+}-dependent manner. The affinity of a single CRD to these ligands is low ($K_d = 10^{-3}M$); therefore, multiple CRDs have to interact for avid binding, which is best achieved with repetitive carbohydrate structures found as common constituents of bacterial, viral, fungal, and parasitic surfaces (37). MBL is thus a prototypic pattern recognition molecule of the innate immune system. Upon CRD ligand binding, MASPs are activated in an unknown manner. The MBL-II/MASP-2/MASP-3 complex appears to be the main activator of C4 and C2, leading to C1-independent formation of the C3 convertase C4b,2a (36). Active MASP-2 is the major C4- and C2-cleaving enzyme (38), and its activity is competitively inhibited by MASP-3 (36). MBL-I complexes (via active MASP-1) were found to directly cleave C3. Although much less efficient than C3 cleavage through the convertases, this mechanism has been hypothesized to provide an initial source for amplification of surface-deposited C3b by alternative pathway activation (30).

In addition to MBL, two serum ficolins (ficolin/p35 and Hakata antigen) can activate the lectin pathway. Ficolins are lectins with a fibrinogen-like and a collagen-like domain. MASP proteins as well as MAp19 were co-purified with ficolin/p35 from plasma (39). The role of ficolins in complement activation remains to be determined.

Regulation of Lectin Pathway

Control of the lectin pathway seems to be exerted mainly through covalent binding of C1-INH to active MASPs and to be very similar to control of the classical pathway in general, although the effects of synthetic inhibitors suggest that differences do exist (40). Furthermore, altered mammalian cell membranes can trigger lectin pathway activation via MBL in situations like ischemia followed by reoxygenation (41). Complement activation does not appear to be the only contribution of MBL to host defense. An MBL receptor or collectin receptor has long been postulated (42), but not identified unequivocally (see below). An MBL receptor is thought to mediate a C3b-independent opsonic effect on phagocytes that may also attribute a new role to the noncomplement-activating forms of MBL.

ACTIVATION VIA ALTERNATIVE PATHWAY

The proteins participating in alternative pathway activation are C3 (and C3b), the factors B, D, and properdin. In the first place, alternative pathway activation is a positive feedback mechanism to increase C3b ("C3b-amplification loop"). The starting C3b is generated through either of the other two pathways. Besides, the alternative pathway may also be triggered directly via iC3.

The C3b Amplification Loop

Surface structures that allow alternative pathway activation are called activator surfaces, whereas those effectively limiting activation are termed nonactivators. Whether a given structure (e.g., a cell membrane, viral envelope, bacterial polymer) is an activator or nonactivator, depends on the relative affinity of factor H for C3b deposited on that structure (Figs. 6,7) and whether other regulators are present. When a first C3b becomes covalently attached to an activator surface, factor B subsequently associates with this C3b in the presence of Mg^{2+}. In this complex, the zymogen factor B is accessible to cleavage by factor D, a serine protease present in plasma in minute amounts. Factor D is brought into its active conforma-

tion through recognition of its substrates, C3b,B or iC3,B, and returns to its "inactive" state after the cleaved Ba fragment is released from B (43). The enzymatically active Bb fragment remains attached to C3b and forms the C3 convertase of the alternative pathway, C3b,Bb (Fig. 6). Surface-attached C3b,Bb activates additional C3 molecules and more nascent C3b will attach to the same surface. C3b,Bb remains active as long as Bb remains bound to C3b (half-life 90 seconds), and properdin stabilizes the convertase against decay by binding to both Bb and C3b. A microbe may thus become covered within minutes with a coat of C3b, which is slowly (i.e., relatively inefficient as compared to C3b on nonactivators) turned into iC3b.

Initiation of Alternative Pathway via iC3

A longstanding conceptual problem was to explain the generation of the first C3b and thus whether the alternative pathway can be triggered on its own. The concept of "C3 tickover" provided such an explanation (28). Plasma C3 constantly reacts at a low rate into inactive C3 (iC3 or "C3b-like" C3) through spontaneous reaction of the C3 internal thioester bond with H_2O. iC3 can be described as uncleaved C3 in a C3b-like conformation that accounts for 0.5% of total plasma C3. Like C3b, iC3 can associate with factor B in an Mg^{2+}-dependent reaction, thus forming iC3,B. It is thought that this initial C3 convertase of the alternative pathway is constantly formed, but rapidly inactivated in plasma. Nevertheless, by this mechanism nascent C3b molecules randomly attach onto nearby microbes and trigger the amplification loop. Whether this mechanism or the low-rate, but targeted, generation of

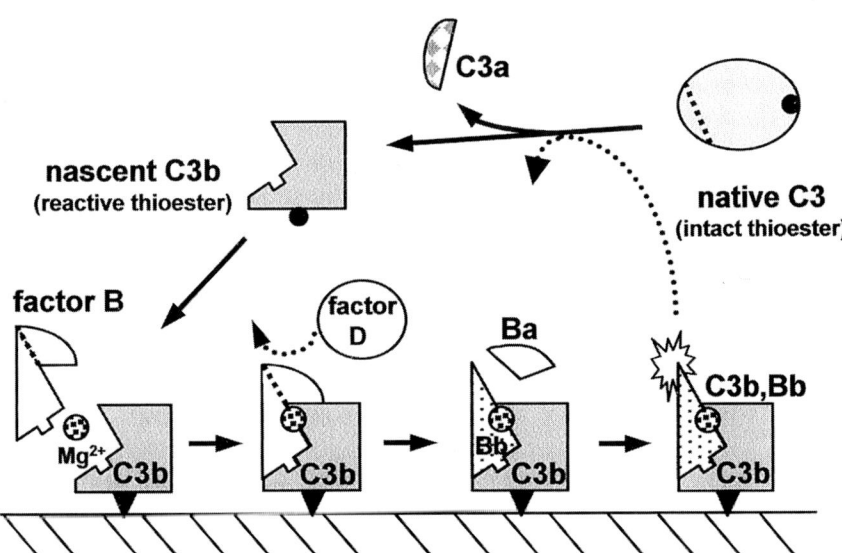

FIG. 6. Generation of the alternative pathway C3 convertase. Upon cleavage of C3 to C3b, the reactive thioester (*full black circle*) is exposed and forms covalent bonds to activator surface molecules (*black arrowheads*). C3b associates with B in the presence of Mg^{2+}, which is then cleaved by factor D. Bb bound to C3b is the proteolytically active part of the convertase C3b,Bb. *Dotted-line arrows* represent enzymatic action; *dotted lines within molecules* indicate cleavage sites for enzymes.

FLUID PHASE:

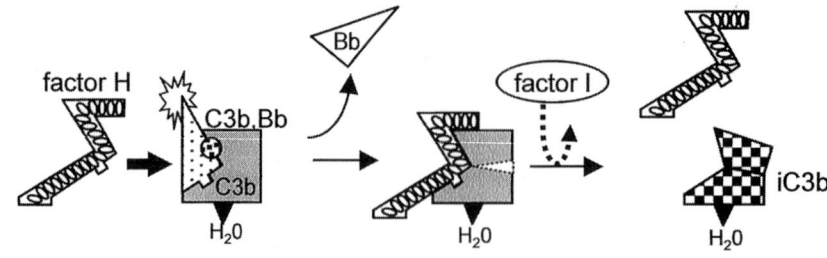

ACTIVATOR SURFACE: NONACTIVATOR SURFACE:

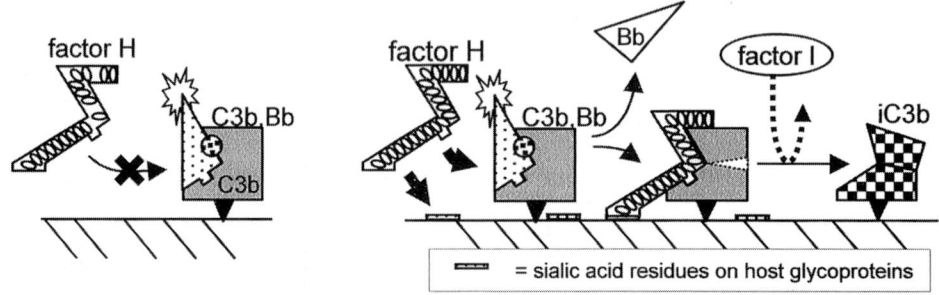

FIG. 7. Control of C3b amplification by factor H depends on its binding affinity to the respective C3b target. **Upper part:** In the fluid phase, C3b,Bb is rapidly disassembled through high-affinity factor H binding. C3b cleavage through factor I (and factor H as cofactor) generates iC3b, which has no complement-activating potential. **Lower part:** Factor H binding to C3b is low on activator surfaces such as microbial cell walls, and C3b,Bb remains active. On nonactivator surfaces, such as host cells with sialic acid residues, factor H has a high affinity to C3b, and binding is followed by convertase dissociation and C3b inactivation.

the first C3b via MBL/MASP-1 complexes is more relevant *in vivo* is not fully understood at present.

Inactivation and Degradation of C3b and Control of Alternative Pathway

Through its self-amplifying capacity, C3b circulating in plasma is subject to tight control (Table 2). The spontaneous decay of C3 convertases (approximate half-life, 2 minutes) is accelerated by CR1, factor H, or DAF, an activity termed decay acceleration. Cleavage of C3b prevents formation of a new convertase. Considerable redundancy in control proteins exists for these steps, although CR1 can actually substitute for all other regulatory RCA proteins in this respect. The inactivation of C3b relies on factor I and its cofactors. Due to the high plasma concentration of factor H, virtually all C3b or iC3 present in plasma quickly binds to H and the low K_m of factor I for C3b,H permits an efficient cleavage of C3b (and iC3). Factor I inactivates C3b into iC3b, which is split into the biologically inert C3c and the smaller C3dg fragment remaining bound to the target (see Fig. 4). Thus, C3b degradation eliminates the complement-activating C3b, but produces new biologically active fragments. Notably, control proteins of other species normally have no effect on human complement components.

In this respect, the physiologic role of the increasing family of factor H-like– or factor H–related proteins (FHRs) (Table 1) is incompletely understood (44). FHL-1 (reconectin) represents the N-terminal seven SCRs of factor H and has cofactor and decay-accelerating activity. It may play a role in cell–extracellular matrix interaction. All FHR share homology with the factor H C-terminus that binds C3b. FHR-1, FHR-2, and FHR-4 are constituents of lipoproteins, and FHR-3 binds to heparin. For FHR-3 and FHR-4, interaction with C3b and thus a potential role in C3b regulation was proposed (44).

TERMINAL PATHWAY

Activation of C5

The same complexes as for C3 activation are employed for the cleavage of C5. C3 convertases with an additional C3b molecule covalently deposited in the immediate vicinity form the C5 convertases C3b,Bb,C3b and C4b,2a,3b, respectively. The (second) C3b acts like an anvil for C5: it interacts with C5 and presents C5 in the correct conformation for cleavage by the C2a or Bb enzyme. Cleavage of C5 in the α chain generates the 11-kD C5a peptide, whereas C5b starts the membrane-attack complex formation. It has to be noted that the classical C3 convertase together with another C4b was shown to cleave C5 directly to some extent (45).

Formation of Terminal Complement Complex

After cleavage of C5 the terminal complement components C6, C7, C8, and C9 are sequentially, but nonenzymatically, activated, resulting in the formation of the terminal complement complex (TCC) (46). On a cellular target membrane, TCC can be generated as potentially membranolytic membrane attack complex (MAC), or in extracellular fluids as nonlytic SC5b-9 in the presence of S protein (vitronectin). Both forms consist of C5b and the complement proteins C6, C7, C8, and C9. After cleavage of C5, C5b undergoes conformational changes and exposes a binding site for C6. The ability of C5b—staying near the C5 convertase on the target surface—to bind C6 decays rapidly, but once bound, C5b6 forms a stable bimolecular complex. C5b6 binds C7 resulting in the exposure of membrane binding sites and incorporation into target membranes. If C7 concentrations near the site of complement activation are limiting, the stable bimolecular C5b6 complex dissociates from the C5-activating complex and accumulates in solution. In the presence of C7, fluid phase C5b-7 is formed, which will not necessarily stay soluble as it has a transient ability to attach to membranes, bind C8 and C9, and initiate lysis, a process called "reactive lysis" (47). Both the membrane-bound C5b-7 complex as well as the fluid-phase C5b-7 complex can bind C8. C8 consists of three nonidentical polypeptide chains: the α- and γ chain are covalently linked by a disulfide bond and the β chain is attached by noncovalent forces. Nascent C5b-7 binds to C8β via C5b. The C8 γ chain has no apparent function in complement lysis, probably because it does not lie adjacent to the membrane but faces the extracellular plasma (Fig. 8).

Efficient lysis is dependent on an interaction of the C8 α moiety with C9, although some lytic activity is expressed already by the C5b-8 complex alone. C5b-8 acts as a polymerizing agent for C9. The first C9 bound to C5b-8 undergoes major structural changes enabling formation of an elongated molecule and allows binding of additional C9 molecules and insertion of C9 cylinders into the target membrane (Fig. 8). Whereas only one molecule of each C5b, C6, C7, and C8, is involved in TCC formation, the number of C9 molecules varies from 1-3 in the fluid phase and from 1-12 in the membrane-bound form, although polymers containing up to fifteen C9 molecules are also possible, if sufficient amounts of C9 are provided. Due to the different number of C9 molecules involved, the tubular structure is not homogeneous. In solution, C9 is also capable of polymerizing with itself without binding to C5b-8 and this tendency toward polymerization can be increased by the presence of metal ions.

Two mutually nonexclusive hypotheses have been proposed to explain the precise mechanism of terminal complement–mediated cytotoxicity after insertion of C9.

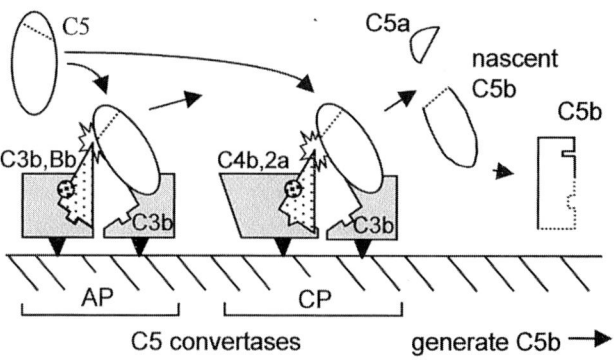

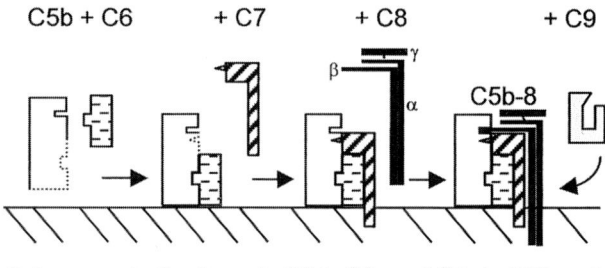

Subsequent attachment of C6, C7, and C8, to C5b →

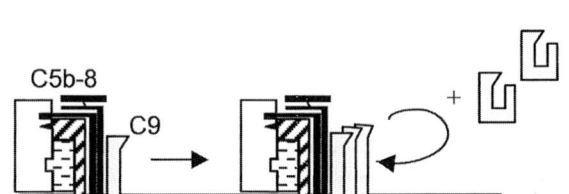

C9 unfolds   Formation of poly-C9 on C5b-8

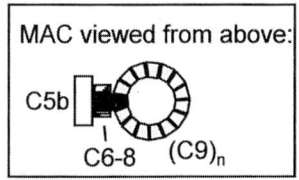

FIG. 8. Activation of C5 and terminal complement pathway. C5 is activated by C5 convertases of the classical (CP) or alternative (AP) pathway. Nascent C5b interacts sequentially with C6, C7, and C8, and attaches to lipid membranes. C9 polymerization on C5b-8 completes the membrane attack complex (MAC).

According to one model, the polar domains of inserted complement proteins, particularly C9, cause local distortion of the phospholipid bilayer resulting in "leaky patches" (48). The other theory postulates that the terminal complement proteins form a hydrophilic channel ("pore") through the membrane with consequent disruption of the cell (49).

Control of Terminal Pathway

Control is executed before the integration of the assembling MAC into the membrane and at the stage of pore formation, that is, association of C8 and polymerization of C9 (Table 2). A number of different membrane and plasma molecules are involved in modulating TCC assembly, of which C8 is probably the most important. It represents not only an essential component of the lytic complex but, paradoxically, also prevents membrane damage by binding to the nascent C5b-7 complex in the fluid phase, thereby precluding its firm insertion into the membrane.

Not only C8 but also the abundant S protein, clusterin, lipoproteins, antithrombin III, and proteoglycans such as heparin and protamine are able to bind to nascent C5b-7 and to prevent its membrane insertion. The final step of MAC assembly, subsequent to C5b-7 insertion, when the MAC becomes more firmly inserted into the lipid bilayer, is safeguarded by cell membrane proteins, termed "homologous restriction factors" showing some degree of species restriction of preventing lysis by autologous complement (50): (a) a well-characterized 18- to 20-kD glycolipid-anchored membrane molecule (CD59) that protects against complement-mediated lysis by interfering with the particular C9 interaction site on the C8 α chain that is needed for membrane insertion and subsequent polymerization of C9; and (b) a 65- to 68-kD molecule (C8bp, HRF, MIP), which remains less well characterized and which is supposed to predominantly bind to C8.

Membrane perforation by complement is not a unique feature. Damage to mammalian cells by proteins that destroy target membranes can be also caused by perforin, which is contained in the cytoplasmic granules of cytotoxic T-lymphocytes and natural killer cells (see Chapters 36 and 12) and actually shows a strong homology with C9 (51). Bacterial proteins also destroy cellular membranes by a similar action (see "Evasion strategies by microorganisms").

Biological Properties of Terminal Complement Complex

The MAC deposited on cells may either exert lytic properties that are important in host defense (Fig. 8) (see below) or may induce so called sublytic effects on nucleated cells that are not unequivocally identified as "non-self" (52). The term "sublytic" refers to the fact that nucleated cells can withstand single (and erroneous) attacks, unlike erythrocytes. Furthermore, previous sublytic effects even protect these cells from additional, otherwise lytic doses, favoring the host cells that are constantly in contact with complement (53). Sublytic attack also stimulates protein synthesis and arachidonic acid metabolism and activates attacked polymorphonuclear leukocytes. In particular, sublytic TCC on nucleated cells transiently increases intracellular Ca^{2+}, activates protein kinase C and G-proteins (54) and induces procoagulant and proinflammatory activities. Likewise, the presence of TCC on the surface of viable immune cells suggests a modulating role in the physiology of cells to which it attaches (55). Thus, the main biological functions of the terminal complement cascade as an important humoral effector arm of host defense thus extend far beyond those originally described. Whether SC5b-9 represents simply the inactivated form of the TCC or whether it plays a role in immune defense remains controversial. It has been recently shown that cytolytically inactive TCC activates endothelial cells to express adhesion molecules and tissue factor procoagulant activity (56).

COMPLEMENT RECEPTORS

The consequences of complement activation as described above encompass changes in cellular functions. Central activated complement proteins or their fragments are recognized by specific receptors found on a variety of different cell types (Table 3). A primary function of the interaction of complement fragments with their receptors is the enhancement of innate immune responses to increase removal of foreign material by phagocytosis of pathogens or modulation of cellular responses. The best-studied complement receptors (CR) so far are CR1 to CR4. A common feature of these C3 receptors is the recognition of the C3 fragments covalently bound to surfaces upon complement activation (Fig. 9).

The anaphylatoxin receptors C3aR and C5aR (ligands are C3a, C5a, and $C5a_{desArg}$), in contrast, belong to the rhodopsin family of G-coupled proteins with seven transmembrane domains. Most recently, a growing number of intracellular and cellular surface receptors for C1q were identified, which are discussed as modulators of cell responses after ligand binding. This group of receptors includes cloned proteins such as $C1qR_p$, $gC1qbp$, $cC1qR$, also termed calreticulin or collectin receptor, or a putative $C1qR_{O2}^-$. Another less well-characterized cell-surface protein is the factor H receptor supposed to be expressed on B cells, neutrophils, and monocytes.

C3 Receptors

Antigen–antibody complexes or pathogens that have C3 fragments covalently linked to their surface are immunologic tags for phagocytes and other immunocompetent cells. Uptake of such opsonized particles and subsequent activation of intracellular pathways is the main function of C3 receptors (i.e., CR1 through CR4).

Complement Receptor Type 1 (CR1, C3b/C4b Receptor, CD35)

Human CR1 is a large and multifunctional glycoprotein belonging to the family of complement regulator proteins (57). A common feature of these proteins are repeats of tandemly arranged modules of about 60 amino acids, referred to as short consensus repeats (SCRs). Within the CR1, larger structural elements are formed, called long homologous repeats (LHRs), each consisting of seven SCRs. The four known

TABLE 3. *Complement receptors*

Type	Ligand	Structure, MW	Distribution	Function
CR1 (CD35)	C3b>C4b>iC3b	Single-chain glycoprotein, 160–250 kD; allotypes A through D with 30, 37, 23, or 44 SCRs	Monocytes, macrophages, neutrophils, eosinophils, erythrocytes, B and T cells, FDC, mesangium cells in glomeruli	Immune complex clearance, immune complex localization to germinal centers, regulator of C3 and C5 activation
CR2 (CD21)	C3dg/C3d, iC3b, EBV, human CD23, IFNα	Single-chain glycoprotein, 140–145 kD; two isoforms: CD21S or CD21L (15 or 16 SCRs)	B cells, activated T cells, epithelial cells, FDC (CD21L)	B-cell activation, immune complex localization to germinal centers, rescue of germinal center cells from apoptosis
CR3 (CD11b/CD18)	iC3b, ICAM-1, LPS, fibrinogen, clotting factor X; carbohydrates	Heterodimeric glycoprotein $\alpha + \beta$ chain: 165 + 95 kD	Monocytes, macrophages, neutrophils, NK cells, FDC, T cells, mast cells	Phagocytosis, cell adhesion, signal transduction, oxidative burst
CR4 (CD11c/CD18)	iC3b, fibrinogen	Heterodimeric glycoprotein $\alpha + \beta$ chain: 165 + 95 kD	Monocytes, macrophages, neutrophils, NK cells, T cells, mast cells	Phagocytosis, cell adhesion
C3aR	C3a	Single chain of 48 kD, G-protein–linked receptor	Mast cells, basophils, smooth muscle cells, lymphocytes	Increases vascular permeability, triggers serosal-type mast cells
C5aR (CD88)	C5a, C5a$_{\text{desArg}}$	Single chain of 48 kD, G-protein–linked receptor	Mast cells, basophils, neutrophils, monocytes, macrophages, endothelial cells, smooth muscle cells, lymphocytes	Increases vascular permeability, triggers serosal-type mast cells, promotes chemotaxis
C1qR$_{\text{p}}$	C1q (collagenous part), MBL, SP-A	Single chain of 126 kD, highly glycosylated	Monocytes, macrophages, neutrophils, endothelial cells, microglia	Phagocytosis
cC1qR, "collectin-receptor"	C1q (collagenous part), MBL, SP-A, CL-43	Single chain of 60 kD, acidic glycoprotein	B cells, monocytes, macrophages, platelets, endothelial cells, fibroblasts	Phagocytosis, localization of immune complexes; enhances ADCC, oxidative metabolism
gC1qR	C1q (globular heads)	Tetramer of 33-kD subunits, acidic protein	B cells, monocytes, macrophages platelets, endothelial cells, neutrophils	Inhibition of complement activation, phagocytosis

ADCC, antibody-dependent cellular cytotoxicity; EBV, Epstein–Barr virus; FDC, follicular dendritic cells; MBL, mannan-binding lectin; NK, natural killer; SCR, short consensus repeat.

polymorphic forms of human CR1 differ not only in the number of SCRs (up to 34) or LHRs and therefore in their molecular size, but also in their respective allele frequencies (e.g., 0.83 for *CR1*1* and less than 0.01 for *CR1*4*). The ligand-binding sites for C3b and C4b are localized in LHR B (SCR 8–10) and LHR C (SCR 15–17). LHR A harbors an additional C4b-binding region and decay-accelerating activity for both C3 convertases (57). This modular arrangement provides the basis for multivalent CR1–C3b/C4b interactions. In addition to C3b and C4b, CR1 also binds iC3b, although with low affinity. The tissue distribution of CR1 covers a broad spectrum of peripheral blood cells, except platelets, NK cells, and

some T cells. CR1 is also found on follicular dendritic cells (FDC). Due to the numerical predominance of erythrocytes, about 90% of CR1 is found on this cell type.

A main function of CR1 on erythrocytes is its ability to serve as an immune adherence receptor for transport of C3b/C4b opsonized immune complexes (IC), which, after binding, are transported to the liver and spleen. In these organs, IC are transferred to phagocytic cells for removal. On cytokine- or C5a-activated phagocytes, such as neutrophils or macrophages, CR1 mediates phagocytosis of opsonized pathogens. On nonactivated cells, CR1 cooperates with FcR or CR3 to bind and ingest foreign material. Interaction with

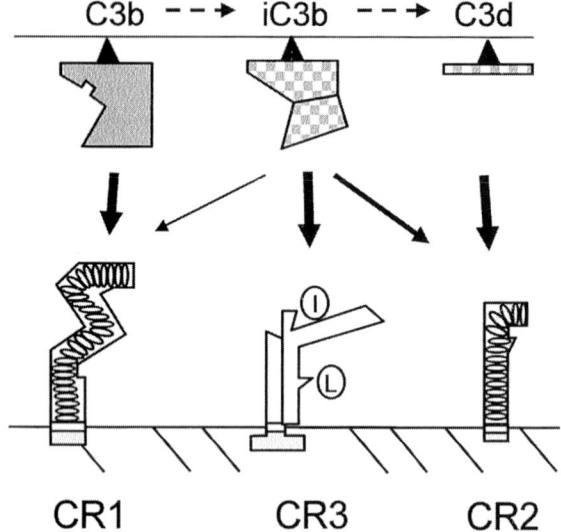

FIG. 9. Binding of the main C3 fragments C3b, iC3b, and C3d to complement receptors CR1, CR2, and CR3, respectively. CR1 and CR2 are single, membrane-spanning, proteins consisting of SCRs (drawn as *ovals*), whereas CR3 is a heterodimeric protein of the integrin superfamily. A relatively higher affinity of a C3-fragment to a given CR is indicated by a *thicker arrow*.

CR1 results in activation of phospholipase D, which mediates phosphorylation of the receptor, followed by Ca^{2+} mobilization and further downstream the signaling cascade by NFκB translocation. The possible C1q-mediated binding of IC to CR1 for clearing of IC seems to be of minor physiologic importance, since patients lacking single complement components downstream of C1q are unable to clear IC via CR1–C1q interactions (58). On B cells, CR1 is suggested to participate in B-cell proliferation and differentiation. In germinal centers of the lymphoid follicles, FDC express CR1, which may be of importance in the induction of immunologic memory. CR1 has decay-accelerating activity for the C3 and C5 convertases and cofactor activity for factor I–mediated cleavage of C3b and iC3b. This broad regulatory activity is the basis for the anticomplement therapeutic strategies that use recombinant CR1 (see below).

Complement Receptor Type 2 (CR2, C3d Receptor, CD21)

Similar to CR1, CR2 is assembled from tandem repeat motifs and consists of 15 or 16 SCRs (59), termed CD21S and CD21L, respectively. CD21L comprises an additional exon, which encodes for an additional SCR 10a (60). CD21L seems to be selectively expressed on FDC, while CD21S is mainly found on B cells, but is also expressed to a small extent on activated T cells and epithelial cells. CR2 interacts with C3d, C3dg, and iC3b, and is the receptor for the Epstein–Barr virus (EBV), facilitating virus entry into B cells and epithelial cells. The EBV envelope protein gp350/220 interacts with the first two SCRs of CR2. The EBV–binding site overlaps with, but is not identical to, the C3d site, and both can be effectively blocked (61). The latter has been assigned to SCR

2 by solution of the crystal structure for the CR2–C3d complex (62). Unlike human CR1 and CR2, the mouse homologs result from alternative splicing of one common gene, *Cr2* (63). As in the mouse, human CR1 and CR2 colocalize on B cells. Only human CR2 has been reported to interact with CD23, the low-affinity receptor for IgE, which is thought to be involved in regulation of IgE production (64).

The most important role of CR2 is bridging parts of innate and adaptive immunity (65), since it is involved in antibody maturation and induction of B-cell memory. On the surface of human B cells, CD21 is associated with CD19 and CD81, forming a trimolecular co-receptor complex (66). Through C3d-opsonized antigens, the CR2/CD19/CD81 complex is cross-linked with the B-cell receptor complex (BCR), a process, which is stabilized in lipid rafts (67). As shown in detail in Chapter 7, BCR-associated kinases can phosphorylate cytoplasmic tyrosines of CD19. This generates binding sites for Vav and PI3' kinase and allows activation of downstream kinases, such as Erk2, Jnk, or Btk (68). Altogether, cross-linking of the CD19/CR2/CD81 and the BCR complexes lowers the threshold for B-cell activation by the specific antigen by two orders of magnitude, as compared to antigen alone (66). The amount of antigen-bound C3d molecules determines the increase in specific Ig (69), a basis for development of new adjuvants (see below). CR2 on FDC in germinal centers is important for development of an antibody response and for B-cell memory as it helps to retain opsonized Ag–Ab complexes (Notably, this CR2 trap on FDC also works with whole infectious agents like HIV [70].) Whereas centroblasts undergo apoptosis in the absence of FDC contact and T-cell help, CR2-positive cells gain easier access to (C3d-coated) antigen, even if their antibody is of lower affinity (71). CR2 may also be involved in maintenance of B-cell tolerance (72). Normally, self-reactive B cells are either deleted or become anergic. In mice deficient in C4 or CD21/CD35, self-antigens are not efficiently localized in the bone marrow or in germinal centers, which contributes to keeping B cells reactive against soluble self-antigens.

Complement Receptor Type 3 (CR3, Mac-1, Mo-1, $\alpha_M\beta_2$, CD11b/CD18)

Together with LFA-1 (CD11a/CD18) and CR 4 (CD11c/CD18), CR3 belongs to the family of β_2 integrins (73). The heterodimeric CR3 consists of a 165 kD α chain (CD11b) and a 95 kD β chain (CD18). A remarkable feature of CR3 is its promiscuous interaction with numerous ligands, including the C3 fragment iC3b, ICAM-1 and -2, proteins of the clotting system, or molecules of microbial origin, such as from Leishmania, *Klebsiella pneumoniae, Mycobacterium tuberculosis, Candida albicans* or *Saccharomyces cerevisiae* (73).

Most ligands investigated so far bind to a specialized region in the α chain, referred to as I (for "inserted") domain in a Ca^{2+}-dependent manner (74). In addition, a C-terminal extracellular domain of CD11b has been identified as a high-affinity interaction site for β glucans that may interact with carbohydrate structures of different pathogens (75). CR3 is found on mononuclear phagocytes, neutrophils, mast and NK-cells, FDC, and T-cell subsets. The crucial role of CD11b/CD18 as complement receptor in phagocytosis has been recognized in patients with reduced or absent expression of β_2 integrins, known as leukocyte adhesion deficiency (76), and in CR3 knockout mice (77). Evidence exists that interaction of iC3b-coated particles with CR3 is not sufficient to induce phagocytosis, and that in addition, coligation of the CR3 lectin site by microbial surface polysaccharides is required (75). Instead of engaging the lectin site, CR3 can cooperate with other phagocytic receptors such as FcγRIII, FcαRI, or the LPS receptor CD14. CR3 has been shown to be associated on the cell surface with these GPI-anchored surface proteins and may be used as adaptor for intracellular signaling (78).

Phagocytosis induces activation of small GTPases of the Rho family (Rho, Rac, Cdc42) that regulate integrin-mediated cytoskeletal rearrangements. FcR-mediated phagocytosis depends on Rac and Cdc42, while CR3-mediated uptake of microbes activates Rho. This divergence may account for different cellular responses, such as absent respiratory burst in case of CR3-dependent phagocytosis, since Rac, but not Rho, is involved in NADPH oxidase activation.

Complement Receptor Type 4 (CR4, p150/95, $\alpha_X\beta_2$, CD11c/CD18)

CR4 belongs to the same β_2 integrin subfamily as CR3 (Table 3). Ligand specificities of CR4 tested so far seem to be similar to CR3. Also, tissue distribution of CD11c is comparable to CR3, even if CR4 seems to be more prominent on distinct dendritic cell subsets.

Anaphylatoxin Receptors C3aR and C5aR (CD88)

As discussed above, cleavage of C3, C4, and C5 results in generation of the small fragments C3a, C4a, and C5a with a C-terminal arginine residue, which are termed anaphylatoxins (AT). While C4a is thought to be inactive, C3a and C5a are powerful mediators of inflammation when bound to their specific receptors C3aR and C5aR (CD88), respectively (79). Both are seven-transmembrane receptors of the rhodopsin superfamily of G-coupled receptors (80). C3aR is slightly larger than C5aR, due to a longer second extracellular loop. Expression of C3Ra and C5aR was thought to be restricted to cells of myeloid origin, until recent studies demonstrated the presence of C5aR on epithelial, endothelial, and parenchymal cells. Most recently, evidence for the expression of C5a on B- and T-lymphocytes was provided.

C5a is the best-characterized AT. It is a potent proinflammatory mediator that induces chemotactic migration, enhances cell adhesion, stimulates the oxidative burst, and induces the release of various inflammatory mediators such as histamine or cytokines (79). C3a is spasmogenic, stimulates the release of PGE$_2$ from macrophages, induces degranula-

tion and chemotaxis of eosinophils, attracts mast cells, and exhibits proinflammatory characteristics which overlap with C5a-induced responses (81). The binding of AT mainly activates the G$_{i2}$ protein-inducing PIP$_2$ hydrolysis and activation of the MAP kinase pathway (82). Recent studies suggest that the phosphorylation of AT receptors is a key event that regulates their biological function (83). Since excessive inflammation may result in tissue damage, the biological activities of C3a and C5a are tightly controlled. Carboxypeptidase N, a plasma enzyme, rapidly removes the C-terminal arginine residue from C3a and C5a, thereby converting the AT into the desArg form. C5a$_{desArg}$ exerts still some proinflammatory effects, although in smaller extent as compared to C5a. In contrast, C3a$_{desArg}$ is generally regarded to be biologically inactive, since it does not bind to C3aR.

C1q Receptors

The best-characterized immunologic function of C1q is its role in the classical pathway. However, several reports indicate that C1q binds to a variety of different cell types, presumably via distinct receptors, and mediates enhanced phagocytosis or oxidative burst metabolism (84). However, the definition and function of these C1q receptors or C1q-binding proteins are still confusing. The best-characterized C1q receptor is C1qR$_p$, whereas the existence of a C1q receptor triggering superoxidative burst (C1qR$_{O2}{}^-$) is controversial (58). The collagen-like tail of C1q is thought to interact with C1qR$_p$, a putative C1qR$_{O2}{}^-$, cC1qR, or CR1 (73), while the globular region of C1q is interacting with gC1qR (85) (Table 3).

C1q Receptor Triggering Phagocytosis (C1qR$_p$)

The N-terminal domain is similar to C-type lectins and harbors a carbohydrate recognition motif. This region is followed by five epidermal growth factor motifs that represent a putative Ca^{2+} binding region. Juxtaposed, a serine–threonine-rich mucin-like domain was identified, which is followed by a transmembrane stretch 25 amino acids long. The C-terminus harbors a tyrosine kinase–binding motif. Monoclonal antibodies against C1qR$_p$ are capable to block C1q-mediated enhancement of phagocytosis in human monocytes and macrophages. The receptor was also localized on human endothelial cells. The mouse homolog was recognized as a stem-cell marker; however, its role in this context is presently unclear.

Collagen C1q Receptor (cC1qR, Calreticulin, Collectin Receptor)

Ligands of cC1qR besides C1q appear to be the collectins MBL and the surfactant protein SpA. Therefore, cC1qR is also referred to as collectin receptor. cC1qR is identical with calreticulin (CRT), a chaperone and Ca^{2+}-dependent signaling molecule most abundant in the endoplasmic reticulum. Additionally, CRT is found on the membrane of other cellular organelles, on the cell surface and released as soluble protein. It is unclear how CRT may become associated with the cell surface, but together with CD91, surface CRT is involved in uptake and removal of cell remnants (86) when opsonized with C1q.

Globular Head C1q Receptor (gC1qR, Identical to Tat-Associated Protein)

Immunoprecipitation experiments provided evidence that gC1qR is associated with cC1qR on the cell surface (86). gC1qR has no transmembrane domain or a known binding site for cellular anchor molecules, but it seems to be located on the surface of fibroblasts, neutrophils, endothelial cells, and platelets. However, the majority of gC1qR is found in intracellular vesicles and on mitochondria. Besides C1q, gC1qR interacts with the plasma proteins thrombin, S protein, factor XII, and high-molecular-weight kininogen, and with bacterial and viral proteins, such as HIV Tat.

COMPLEMENT AS PATHOGENIC FACTOR IN DISEASE

Complement may become a pathogenic factor in disease by "complementing" the destructive action of antibodies via an activation of the whole cascade system, but it is often only one of several factors involved in pathogenesis. In addition, complement may contribute to diseases if its physiologic actions are not performed well: one of the most important tasks of the complement system is a proper immune complex processing and disposal, namely the clearance of complement-coated immune complexes from the circulation. There are probably two ways in which complement fixation influences the fate of immune complexes (87). First, the fixation of C4 and C3 fragments into the antigen–antibody lattice significantly reduces the size of the single immune complex (step 1), giving rise to a larger number of small complexes ("detergent-like" effect of complement). Second, and probably more important, the presence of C4b and C3b on the immune complexes facilitates efficient fixation of these smaller immune complexes to complement receptors, predominantly erythrocyte CR1, and ensures transportation and sequestration into the liver and spleen (step 2), where antigenic material can be removed by reticulohistiocytic cells, followed by degradation of the antigen (step 3).

Consequently, pathophysiologically detrimental effects of complement become apparent when a failure in this clearance system occurs. A defect interfering with this mechanism at any stage will lead to an uptake of these immune complexes by endothelial cells and their sequestration into various organs or tissues ("trapping"), giving rise to more inflammation and immune complex formation with concomitant destruction of surrounding tissue. These pathological conditions are listed below.

- Inherited, often complete, classical pathway complement deficiency (C1q or C4 deficiency)
- Acquired complement consumption due to constant activation on continuously generated immune complexes as in autoimmune diseases (membranoproliferative glomerulonephritis [MPGN] type I, systemic lupus erythematosus with or without associated lupus nephritis) or chronic bacteremia (step 1 compromised: complement fixation failure)
- Inherited or acquired low CR1 per erythrocyte ratio as in active lupus, or low red-cell count (step 2 compromised: transportation failure)
- Extensive liver or spleen disease, impairing the removal of the antigen (step 3 compromised: stripping failure)

Clinically, the step 1 failures are the most relevant and common ones. As immune complexes are in particular trapped in small capillaries of the skin or the renal glomeruli, clearance disorders predominantly manifest in the skin and the kidney. Complement also contributes to inflammation and tissue damage in neurodegenerative and autoimmune diseases and also in ischemia and reperfusion injury or in shock (Table 4).

The application of activation-specific monoclonal antibodies (preferably in EIA) helps to monitor complement activation in biological fluids during the course of these diseases to reveal exacerbations or to evaluate the success of a treatment (88).

Complement in Renal Disease

Preformed immune complexes are often trapped in the kidneys in case of a clearance disorder. The hypocomplementemia, which characterizes these diseases, is usually due

TABLE 4. *Human diseases with a contribution of complement to pathogenesis and/or perpetuation*

Biocompatibility/shock	Neurological	Rheumatological
Postbypass syndrome	Myasthenia gravis	Rheumatoid arthritis
Acute respiratory distress syndrome	Multiple sclerosis	Systemic lupus erythematosus
Anaphylaxis	Cerebral lupus erythematosus	Behcet's syndrome
Tissue incompatibility/transplantation	Guillain–Barré syndrome	Juvenile rheumatoid
Pre-eclampsia	Alzheimer's disease	Sjogren's syndrome
Dermatological	**Renal**	**Other diseases**
Pemphigus vulgaris/Pemphigoid	Lupus nephritis	Atheroma
Phototoxic reactions	Membranproliferative glomerulonephritis	Thyreoiditis
Vasculitis	Membranous nephritis	Infertility

Adapted from Morgan (150), with permission.

to systemic complement activation in the circulation, whereas the intraglomerular complement activation has only a minimal, if any, effect on serum complement levels. C3 and TCC, however, are frequently found in glomerular deposits. These are usually accompanied by local production of cytokines, prostaglandins, proteolytic enzymes, and reactive oxygen metabolites that create, together with leukocytes, an extended area of inflammation. The crucial role of complement for this inflammation is long known from animal studies showing that complement-deficient or -depleted animals do not develop nephritis deliberately produced by an antiglomerular basement-membrane antibody (89).

A second important role of complement in renal disease with increased complement-related inflammation, such as in membranoproliferative glomerulonephritis (MPGN), is due to so-called nephritic factors, which are circulating IgG autoantibodies of which the most prominent member (NFa) is directed against the alternative pathway C3 convertase (89). By binding to the convertase, NFa stabilizes it in the fluid phase as well as after binding to mesangium cells, slowing down its physiologic decay by more than ten-fold. Interestingly, NFa increases the turnover (cleavage) of C3 directly without activating the classical or terminal complement cascade. The respective clinical conditions are MPGN type II and partial lipodystrophy, an acute condition characterized by loss of fat from the face and upper body often triggered by a viral infection. It has been shown that, pathophysiologically, the dysregulated complement activation by NFa sera directly leads to adipocyte lysis via the alternative pathway (90).

Stabilizing autoantibodies directed against the alternative pathway C5 convertase or the classical pathway C3 convertase are also known. The spontaneous formation of the former may be less frequent *in vivo,* accounting for slow conversion *in vitro* ("slow nephritic factor"). The latter is probably not spontaneously formed and augments C3 conversion only in cases of classical pathway activation (89). It is not clear whether the nephritic factors themselves are nephritogenic, and thus involved in pathogenesis, or whether they represent epiphenomena. An important argument for the former is that the stabilizing effect of nephritic factors is, at least in part, due to a prevention of the physiologic dissociation of the convertase by factor H. In this respect NeFs have the same consequence as a dysfunctional or missing factor H.

Complement in Neurologic Disease

The human brain is immunologically an isolated tissue and sheltered by the tight and selective blood–brain barrier from cells and proteins of the immune system. Nevertheless, all major cell types in the brain including astrocytes, microglia, neurons, and oligodendrocytes were shown to produce at least some complement proteins, including regulators and receptors for the complement protein fragments (91). Of these cell types, astrocytes, the most abundant glial cells, are the major source of complement in the brain, thereby providing immune defense against invading pathogens but also contributing to brain cell damage in some diseases. Activation of complement was found in brain-associated pathologic conditions such as multiple sclerosis and Alzheimer's disease. For these situations, a harmful role for complement in tissue destruction was implicated.

Alzheimer's disease is characterized by neuronal loss, neuritic dystrophy, and the accumulation of senile plaque in the brain. Activation of the complement system has been widely investigated as a potential mechanism for these processes. The main protein component of senile plaque is the β-amyloid peptide that has been demonstrated to exert very heterogeneous functions such as support of neuronal survival and growth and the induction of neurotoxicity. The function correlates with the assembly state of the peptide: whereas solubilized amyloid peptide induces neurite outgrowth, aggregated peptide results in neuron cytotoxicity. This fibrillar amyloid-β protein has been found to be involved in the pathogenesis of the disease because of its ability to activate complement via the classical pathway by binding specifically to the collagen-like domain of C1q (92). Thus, activation products of the classical pathway complement components C1q, C3, and C4 can be found in the fibrillar β-amyloid plaque in cerebral cortex and hippocampus of Alzheimer patients (93). Consecutive complement-dependent processes will likely contribute to neuronal injury in the proximity of these fibrillar β-amyloid plaque.

Multiple sclerosis is an inflammatory autoimmune disease characterized by demyelination of axons. In addition, failure in remyelination and loss of oligodendrocytes, the main myelinating cells of the central nervous system, are observed. The demyelination process not only results from an autoimmune response against myelin components and subsequent activation of the classical pathway, but also from direct binding of complement factors to myelin. The myelin moiety directly interacting with C1q has been identified as myelin oligodendrocyte glycoprotein (MOG), located at the most external layer of the myelin sheath (94). MOG harbors a (protein) domain similar to the C1q-binding sequence previously identified in IgG antibodies. Complement activation results in lysis of oligodendrocytes and chemo attraction of phagocytes that accumulate at the site of inflammation and degrade the myelin sheath. This recruitment of macrophages and the phagocytosis of myelin are mediated by complement receptor CR3 present on the phagocyte surface and induce production of local inflammatory substances like TNF-α and nitric oxide (95).

COMPLEMENT IN DEFENSE AGAINST INFECTION

Complement plays a major role in the innate immune system as important first-line defense of higher vertebrates against invading microorganisms. First, it recognizes foreign material immediately after infection as a primitive surveillance system independent from antibodies or immune cells, and second, it serves as an executor of antibody-mediated immunity.

Microorganisms invading the human body are usually classified by the immune system as "non-self." Non-self structures activate the alternative and lectin pathways (triggered by the surface composition of the invader, such as lipopolysaccharides, sialic acids, glycoproteins, and peptidoglycans). Microorganisms, however, may also directly activate the classical pathway, mainly via C1q-binding moieties. Stimulation of phagocytic cells by generated anaphylatoxins, attracts them to the site of infection (chemotaxis). Generation of C3 fragments, mainly C3b and iC3b (opsonization), on the microbial surface and their recognition via complement receptors on phagocytic cells, mainly CR1 and CR3 (see below), followed by phagocytosis or lysis of the microbe, mostly lead to a control of the infection. Meanwhile, intracellular processing in phagolysosomes and presentation of phagocytosed material on the cell surface by professional antigen-presenting cells (see Chapter 20) will initiate adaptive immune responses and trigger production of specific antibodies targeted toward the intruder, thereby linking innate immunity to adaptive response (see Chapters 38–41).

Whereas lysis is effective against some viruses and gram-negative bacteria, chemotaxis followed by opsonophagocytosis represents probably the main mechanism for destruction of most viruses, bacteria, and fungi that cannot be lysed by complement (96,97).

Not only the number of C3-fragment molecules deposited on the invader, but also the amount of C5b-9 inserted into the target membrane is decisive for host defense. The latter strongly correlates with bactericidal activity and inversely with complement resistance. The debate on how lysis is brought about—that is, by producing a physical hole or by generating membrane perturbations (see above)—is in particular interesting in the light of immune defense against *Neisseria meningitidis*. The particularly frequent occurrence of terminal complement deficiencies in patients with meningococcal infections suggests that the cytolytic activity of complement is important in resistance to gram-negative bacteria (98). It is established that the terminal pathway damages the LPS-containing cell wall. However, it is still unclear how the "inner" cell membrane is destroyed. Two possibilities are via induction of injurious processes or directly by bacteria-derived lysozyme or bacterially generated ATP. Alternatively, additional terminal components, entering the periplasmic space via the outer membrane attack leaks, may insert into the inner membrane as MACs (99) or even as polymerized or single C9 alone (100).

Evasion Strategies of Microorganisms

Evolution of both host and microorganisms has created a commensal relationship between humans and microbes, so that in many cases potentially infectious microorganisms are not attacked and live in symbiosis with the host. Most of them only cause disease when the host defense is considerably weakened.

A different type of relationship is medically very important and scientifically the most interesting: microorganisms that are highly pathogenic but nevertheless either evade appropriate recognition or constrain suitable attack and destruction (101). To achieve these goals, a range of strategies has been developed by microorganisms during evolution including both biochemical or biophysical measures to (a) avoid complement activation; (b) resist C3-dependent opsonophagocytosis; or (c) prevent complement-mediated cytolytic damage or the remarkable mimicking of complement-like structures or functions (101). Microorganisms may initiate infection in two ways: (a) commonly, they have refined complement-activating properties that lead to a mere attachment of C3 fragments on their surface in a way that does not allow an appropriate recognition by polymorphonuclear phagocytes (disguise); and (b) even more sophisticated, some microorganisms display proteins antigenically and/or functionally mimicking C3 that can bind to complement receptors mediating uptake in a complement-independent manner, that is, the uptake does not rely on prior opsonisation of the invader (mimicry). By both means, disguise and mimicry, the pathogen avoids destruction by complement and antibody and can harness the cellular machinery for its own reproduction. However, it should be stressed that complement resistance may depend on molecules other than proteins.

An interesting additional feature is the proteolytic degradation of complement proteins by microorganisms protecting them from opsonisation and/or lysis (101). Cleavage of C1-INH by proteases, for example, leads to constant activation (and also consumption) of C1. Microorganisms evading complement by consuming it at a secure distance from their cellular membranes must ensure that enough (for sufficient consumption) but not too much detrimental complement activation occurs that could lead to a bystander attack on themselves. This is also true for pathogens using a particular receptor for their entry into the host cells. Cleavage of complement proteins has to be very accurate so that most of the surface-deposited C3 is present in the optimum form (C3b or iC3b) for receptor binding.

Another mechanism is the use of complement proteins provided by the host. When HIV-1 buds from an infected cell, it is encoated by a lipid bilayer obtained from the host cell membrane, and as a consequence carries, in addition to viral, also host cell membrane proteins. Of the latter, especially DAF and CD59 are of particular importance as they protect HIV-1 from complement lysis (102). Attachment of factor H to C3b on the virus and to several sites on the external portion of gp41 and to one site on gp120 (103) confers an additional protective effect against efficient destruction (104). Similarly, binding of factor H to streptococcal M protein was shown to protect these pathogens from complement-mediated lysis.

Mimicry of Complement Structures by Microorganisms

During evolution alongside their obligate hosts, several pathogenic microorganisms have evolved functional properties identical to those used by normal mammalian cells preventing destruction by complement. In particular, a number of distinct microbial proteins have been identified which share structural or genetic similarities (antigenic cross-reactivity, sequence homology) with complement proteins or receptors. Such "molecular mimicry" not only enables the pathogens to avoid destruction by complement but also facilitates complement-mediated infection via complement receptors (105). Under certain circumstances mimicry can even lead to development of autoimmunity.

Furthermore, in some instances only a certain principle is adopted. Several microorganisms attack human cells by drilling holes into their lipid bilayer using polymerization and cylinder formation of specific cytolysins: streptococcal streptolysin-O, *Escherichia coli* hemolysin, or staphylococcal α-toxin (106). The presence of these pore-forming proteins is strongly associated with the virulence of their carriers. However, although using a similar biological principle as C9, these microbial toxins do not exhibit structural homology on the amino acid sequence level to each other or to C9. A number of lysis-inducing molecules have been identified (107).

The question is how these molecules have evolved. Teleologically, some of the complement-like molecules facilitating attachment, penetrating into host cells or escaping from lysis became the basis for selection (107). Others, such as the vaccinia-virus complement-control protein (VCP), a functionally CR1-like and structurally C4bp-like protein, were presumably originally acquired from the host and have evolved to retain only the most essential domains, as any additional manipulation of the small viral protein results in loss of function, indicating that the gene has achieved maximum efficiency to encode a protein with the minimum number of amino acids (108). In other pathogens, molecular mimicry may represent the conservation of ancestral molecular recognition motifs. Many are related to mammalian CR1, DAF, MCP, or C4bp, confirming the importance of C3- and C4-fragment–binding molecules.

The overall homology of HIV envelope proteins gp41 and gp120 with complement proteins is very low; however, in certain short stretches remarkable similarities were discovered. These sites appear to be involved in complement binding and may facilitate virus uptake via complement receptors or play a role in the noncovalent association between gp41 and gp120 (103).

The trematode *Schistosoma mansoni* has a highly elaborated anticomplement arsenal: first, it can modify its surface sialic acids, thus modulating activation; second, it can acquire DAF to accelerate decay of surface-bound C3; third, it can bind and cleave C4 and C3 mimicking in part CR1; fourth, it can cleave C9, preventing MAC assembly; and fifth, but probably not last, it encodes a protein mimicking CD59 that inhibits membrane attack (109).

The yeast *C. albicans* possesses an integrin/CR3-like molecule on its surface (110) that is involved in inducing morphology changes. Furthermore, it appears to facilitate cellular adherence like all members of the human integrin gene family. Interestingly, this molecule is not only functionally (110) but also antigenically and structurally related to human CR3. There is strong evidence that HIV-1 is able to bind to candida directly, possibly via C3-like regions on gp41 and the CR3-like molecule on candida (111). This interaction enhances fungal proteinase release and suppresses phagocytosis by PMNs (112). Thus, the concerted mimicry of both pathogens may contribute to the virulence of both candida and HIV (111).

It has been proposed that sites of molecular mimicry may represent useful sites for vaccine development (109). However, considering the multiple as yet unrevealed interactions, a detrimental effect of such a vaccine cannot be excluded.

COMPLEMENT GENETICS

The study on genetics of complement proteins was initiated by the discovery of complement deficiencies in animals and humans. It has been used to detect both homozygous-deficient individuals and heterozygous carriers in family studies and to compile additional evidence for disease associations with certain complement alleles. However, complement genetics has also been a valuable tool to investigate plasma protein genetics in general and their evolution. The chromosomal locations of the genes coding for complement proteins are given in Table 1. These genes are not scattered around the chromosomes but form linkage groups of structurally homologous components, confirming previous assumptions based on homology studies at the protein level that the majority of complement proteins has evolved by duplication and diversion events from only a small number of precursor genes (113).

Because complement receptors and certain regulatory proteins are expressed on erythrocytes, they also represent blood group antigens: for example, the Knops, McCoy, Swain-Langley, and York antigens are on CR1. Variations in the DAF antigen are responsible for the Cromer blood group system with the rare Inab phenotype lacking DAF altogether. Chido and Rogers blood-group antigens are associated with C4 (113). In this respect, complement genetics has been widely applied to anthropological investigations and forensic medicine.

Progress in DNA work has facilitated the characterization of complement allotypes on the molecular level. Both phenotypical assessments of protein variants (phenotyping) and characterizations of genomic DNA (genotyping) are currently used (114). Phenotyping is performed by analysis of electrophoretic mobility or the isoelectric point of proteins in agarose or polyacrylamide gels. In addition, monoclonal antibodies have been described that distinguish among certain complement allotypes (114). Phenotyping has the advantage that the presence and, depending on the method applied, even the functional activity of a protein can be ascertained. Genotyping by the RFLP or PCR methods followed by enzymatic digestion or sequencing does not allow identification of silent or null alleles as such; however, once a mutation is known, a defective gene may be traced in family studies, providing a basis for genetic counseling for the afflicted family.

COMPLEMENT DEFICIENCIES

Complete or subtotal inherited deficiencies have been described for most complement components and regulatory proteins. These abnormalities are relatively rare and usually inherited in an autosomal recessive manner, which means that only homozygous subjects are readily detected and susceptible to disease. The important exception is hereditary angioedema (see below), which is inherited as an autosomal dominant trait. Complement deficiencies may be considered as important *in vivo* "experiments" of nature, defining the role of the particular components in the immune system that give insights into their normal function. Two mutated alleles of a particular gene are usually responsible for deficiencies that, however, are not necessarily identical—that is, several compound deficiencies for C6 or C7 have been described that have two different mutations each.

Complement defects can be ascertained by the traditional total hemolytic complement assays (CH_{50}, $APCH_{50}$) followed by radial immunodiffusion (Mancini), electroimmunodiffusion (rocket electrophoresis, Laurell) or enzyme immunoassays (EIAs) (115). The latter are of particular importance as so-called subtotal deficiencies, where residual functionally active amounts can only be detected by sensitive EIAs, may have a different clinical picture and prognosis (116). For example, low concentrations of terminal components can be tested for their ability to incorporate into the TCC by EIAs based on neoepitope-specific anti-C9 monoclonal antibodies (88). None of these quantitative assays allow, although widely practiced, the assumption that approximately half-normal concentrations indicate heterozygous deficiency: heterozygous subjects may present with almost normal concentrations of the component in question.

The incidence of complement deficiency states has been difficult to ascertain. Large numbers of individuals need to be screened, and data available now suggest that the incidence varies considerably depending on the ethnic and geographical background for each component. Genealogical studies and population screening have also led to the identification of a relatively large number (up to 10% to 20%, depending on the component) of (still?) healthy deficient individuals.

However, complement-deficient subjects are usually detected because of their increased propensity to infection or, especially for deficiencies of the early classical pathway components, in association with systemic lupus erythematosus (SLE) (Table 5). As only *C4* and *C2* are located on the same chromosome (within the MHC-III region; Table 1), the possibility that these deficiencies are all linked to a disease-susceptibility gene has to be excluded. In contrast, it is the absent "detergent-like" effect of complement (see below) that leads to an impaired clearance of immune complexes and to their sequestration at peripheral sites, giving rise to more inflammation and immune complex formation. Thus, early classical pathway deficiency can be regarded as one of the very few examples where a single defect is sufficient (however, not necessary) for the development of an autoimmune disease (87).

In individuals with homozygous C3 deficiency, pyogenic infections with encapsulated bacteria are severe, recurrent, and life threatening, usually starting in early childhood. Deficiencies of either factor I or factor H are associated with the inability to degrade C3b, leading to uncontrolled amplification of cleavage of C3 by C3b,Bb and resulting in a state of acquired, severe C3 deficiency (117). Interestingly, the disease associations are not uniform, as factor H deficiency, in contrast to C3 or factor I deficiency, predisposes also to glomerulonephritis, which is supported by studies on pig factor H deficiency. Deficiency in the factor H–related protein FHR-1 is commonly encountered, but has not been linked to any disease (118).

TABLE 5. *Complement deficiency states*

Component	No. of reported patients	Functional defect	Disease associations[a]
C1	50–100	Impaired immune complex handling	SLE, bacterial infections
C4	20–50	Impaired immune complex handling	SLE, bacterial infections
C2	>100	Impaired immune complex handling	SLE, bacterial infections
C3	20–50	Impaired opsonisation	Bacterial infections
C1-INH	>>100	Excessive C2 and kininogen activation	HAE
B	None	—	Incompatible with life?
D	3	Impaired alternative pathway activation	Bacterial infections?
P	50–100	Impaired alternative pathway activation	Meningococcal infections
H	<20	Excessive alternative pathway activation	Meningococcal infections, glomerulonephritis
I	20–50	Excessive alternative pathway activation	Bacterial infections
C5	20–50	Impaired chemotaxis, absent lytic activity	Meningococcal infections
C6, C7, C8	>100 each (independent)	Absent lytic activity	Meningococcal infections
C9	>100	Impaired lytic activity	Meningococcal infections

[a]Only established disease associations are listed (i.e., >50% of deficient subjects suffering from disease).
C1-INH, C1 inhibitor; HAE, hereditary angioedema; SLE, systemic lupus erythematosus.

While deficiencies of properdin predispose to (usually singular) meningococcal infections, deficiencies of a terminal complement component lead to recurrent infections by gram-negative bacteria due to an inability to generate a bactericidal membrane attack complex. Recurrent infection or infection with uncommon serogroups should alert the clinician in nonendemic regions, whereas recurrent disease is the important indicator in endemic areas (116). The incidence of gonococcal infections is not increased in deficient subjects, possibly because infections by gonococci usually remain restricted to the local mucous membrane. Associations of terminal complement deficiencies with susceptibility to autoimmune diseases or non-neisserial infections are likely the result of ascertainment artifacts (116). SLE, for example, is found among homozygous terminal complement–deficient subjects, but the frequency is very low and not significantly higher than that found for complement-competent patients.

Several features of terminal complement deficiency have been accumulated in recent years.

1. Low amounts of functionally active terminal complement proteins (i.e., subtotal deficiency) may be sufficient for preventing meningococcal disease, suggesting that there is a wide safety margin.
2. Although the incidence of meningococcal infection is much higher, the case fatality rate and the percentage of fulminant cases appears to be lower in terminal complement–deficient subjects, when compared to normal subjects. A failure to generate the membrane attack complex with the consequent inability to lyse bacteria may lead to a milder form of disease because of lower endotoxin concentrations. In addition, fewer organisms are required for systemic infection. However, in many families of patients investigated, there are often unaccounted deaths of siblings in early childhood, and the possibility of ascertainment artifacts cannot be excluded.
3. The mean age of the first meningococcal attack in complement-deficient individuals tends to be higher than in complement-sufficient patients and the percentage of deficient subjects among meningococcal patients is highest in areas where *N. meningitidis* infections are rare. This reveals that terminal complement deficiency is less likely to be detected in situations where meningococcal infection is common (e.g., in early childhood, and in "meningitis belt countries" like the Sahel zone) and shows that TCC is only one of the means to successfully tackle meningococci.

Hereditary angioedema (HAE), the clinically most relevant, by far most acute and, if untreated, potentially lethal complement deficiency, is the clinical manifestation of an inherited or acquired C1-inhibitor deficiency (119). Control of C1 activation consumes C1 inhibitor, and if there is no sufficient back-up of C1 inhibitor, this leads to consumption of complement proteins (especially C4 and C2) by unimpeded C1s activity. The C2b fragment (or split products thereof) and/or bradykinin generated by concomitant contact system activation are held primarily responsible for the classical symptoms of HAE: the affected patients intermittently suffer from multiple edemas, predominantly in the skin, gastrointestinal tract, or oropharynx, usually when the patient experiences minor traumas or infections that trigger unrestricted complement activation. Especially in the larynx, these oedemas cause life-threatening situations (i.e., danger of suffocation). Despite its relatively slow development—in contrast to an allergic larynx oedema—HAE is even today associated with a high mortality rate. The frequent association with abdominal colics may also delay the correct diagnosis. The acute treatment of HAE consists of replacement of C1 inhibitor in purified form or, if unavailable, as fresh frozen plasma. Testosterone derivatives (e.g., danazol) have been successfully used for the long-term prevention of attacks.

A particular deficiency, which is primarily not a complement deficiency, is paroxysmal nocturnal hemoglobinuria (PNH). Mutations in the *PIG-A* gene affect the synthesis of a competent glycosylphosphatidylinositol (GPI) anchor, which leads to failure of expression of all molecules attached to the membrane via this anchor, including CD55 and CD59. The lack of these two complement control proteins is responsible for the extreme susceptibility of PNH erythrocytes to lysis by complement that is either activated by the alternative pathway or via acidic generation of C56, that is, the activation of C6 without cleavage of C5, especially at the physiologically lower blood pH at nighttime (120).

COMPLEMENT AS TARGET IN DRUG THERAPY

The cloning of the complement components and the determination of their functional domains have made it feasible to generate substances that interfere with complement in pathophysiologic settings. Other than organic molecules occurring in nature, or relatively unspecific, synthetic complement inhibitors (reviewed in Makrides [121]) described earlier, the substances currently undergoing clinical testing are (a) native or modified complement regulators such as C1-INH, CR1, DAF, or CD59; (b) derivates of monoclonal antibodies; or (c) synthetic small molecules, all of which can specifically inhibit key activation steps. Several such substances that have been studied in clinical settings or animal models of disease and are currently being developed are listed in Table 6.

Native or Modified Complement Regulators

Native regulatory proteins generally have the advantages of perfect specificity and low antigenicity. Recombinant soluble CR1 (sCR1) is particularly interesting as it exerts the inhibitory potential of the natural regulators C4bp and factor H, respectively, but at a much lower concentration (122,123). However, such proteins are expensive to produce, need parenteral application, and are rapidly cleared from the circulation. New inhibitors therefore have different approaches to target the compound to the site of action, that is, the vascular tissue of a transplanted or inflamed organ. Chemical

TABLE 6. *Inhibitors of complement activation*

Target	Inhibitor substance	(Presumed) indication	Type of studies	Reference
C1-INH effect on active C1r/C1s and active MASPs	C1-INH (from human plasma)	Substitution in acute crises of HAE or AAE	(Current standard therapy)	(119)
		Capillary leak syndrome, septic shock	Open uncontrolled studies	(125)
		Myocardial infarction with reperfusion therapy	Preclinical (animal models)	(125)
	C1-INH (rec., soluble)	As above; increased stability of C1-INH	Preclinical	(138)
	C1-INH (rec., GPI-anchored)	Perfusion of donor organs	Preclinical	(139)
Active C1s	C1s-INH 248	Myocardial IRI	Preclinical (animal models)	(126)
Factor D	TNX-224 (antifactor D mAb)	Myocardial IRI during surgery (CABG)	Preclinical (animal models)	(133)
CR1 effect on the C3/C5 convertases, C3b, and C4b	TP10 (full-length sCR1)[a]	IRI, transplant rejection, ARDS	Stopped after phase II trial	(122,140)
	TP20 (full-length sCR1 with sialyl Lewis^x glycosylation)[a]	IRI (neuronal, myocardial, lung tissue)	Preclinical (animal models)	(141,142)
	APT070 (SCRs 1–3 of CR1 fused to a membrane insertion peptide)[a]	Rheumatoid arthritis (application: intraarticular); renal transplant IRI (application: perfusion of donor organ)	Phase II clinical trial; Phase IIa clinical trial	(124)
C3 activation	Compstatin (synthetic tridecapeptide)	Transplantation: organ preservation *ex vivo*, hyperacute rejection (xenotransplantation)	Preclinical (animal models)	(132)
C3 convertase	DAF expressed on viral envelope	Protection of viral vectors in gene therapy	Preclinical	(143)
	Soluble, membrane-targeted DAF	Xenotransplantation	Animal model	(144)
C5 activation	Pexelizumab (humanized anti-C5 scFv)[a]	Myocardial IRI during surgery (CBP, CABG), myocardial infarction	Phase I, II, IIb, III clinical trials	(145,146)
	Eculizumab[a]	Membraneous nephritis, rheumatoid arthritis	Phase I, II, IIb clinical trials	(147)
	Anti-C5 RNA-aptamer	As above	Preclinical	(148)
C3a receptor	SB 290157 (C3a antagonist)	Allergic asthma	Preclinical	(129)
C5a receptor	AcF-(OPdChaWR) and MeF-(OPdChaWR)	Anti-inflammation (e.g., in septic shock or immune complex disease)	Preclinical (animal models)	(130)
	CGS 32359 (rec. C5a antagonist)	IRI	Preclinical (animal models)	(131)
	ΔpIII-A8 (rec. C5a antagonist)	IRI, immune complex disease	Preclinical (animal models)	(149)

[a]For current status of development, see *http://www.avantimmune.com* (on TP10, TP20); *http://www.adprotech.co.uk* (on APT070); and *http://www.alexionpharmaceuticals.com* (on Pexelizumab).

AAE, acquired angioedema; ARDS, acute respiratory distress syndrome; CABG, coronary artery bypass graft; CPB, cardiopulmonary bypass; CR, complement receptor; DAF, decay-accelerating factor; HAE, hereditary angioedema; IRI, ischemia/reperfusion injury; mAb, monoclonal antibody; MASP-1, mannose-binding lectin–associated serine protease 1; rec., recombinant; sCR1, soluble CR1; scFv, single-chain fragment variable antibody; SCR, short consensus report.

coupling of (parts of) recombinant CR1, DAF, or CD59 to a membrane-targeting substance consisting of a positively charged peptide and a fatty acid moiety resulted in soluble proteins integrating effectively, although indiscriminately, into endothelial cell surfaces (124). Another elegant approach was undertaken by expressing sCR1 in cells adding high amounts of the sialyl Lewis^x (sLex) carbohydrate, the ligand for E-selectin (CD62E). The resulting sCR1sLex compound

(TP20) becomes targeted to E-selectin, which is up-regulated on inflamed endothelium, and in this manner blocks the L-selectin–mediated attachment of neutrophils to that site. TP20 showed additional benefits over the unmodified sCR1 (TP10) in a murine model of stroke and in a rat-lung transplantation model.

Plasma-derived C1-INH has been used for standard substitution therapy in hereditary or acquired angioedema, but also favorably influences the outcome in life-threatening conditions associated with a relative deficiency of functional C1-INH (reviewed in Caliezi et al. [125]). The inhibition of other serpins in addition to C1r/C1s and the MASPs may contribute to the observed C1-INH effects. Although C1-INH substitution has been used with success in several animal models or open uncontrolled clinical trials in septic shock, capillary leak syndrome, or ischemia/reperfusion injury larger randomized, controlled clinical trials are still awaited. A recombinant, more stable C1-INH protein and C1s-INH 248, a recently published small molecule inhibitor of C1s acting faster than administered C1-INH (126), are newly developed promising inhibitors of the classical and lectin pathways.

Derivatives of Monoclonal Antibodies

Anti-C5 monoclonal antibodies are the best-studied inhibitors of that class of anticomplement drugs. Following an initial observation that an anti-C5 monoclonal can efficiently block both TCC assembly and C5a release (127), humanized scFv have been generated, and among them pexelizumab is the most advanced candidate. They bind to C5 with high affinity and prevent C5 cleavage and thus MAC formation and C5a generation, but notably allow C3 activation and deposition. These drugs are being developed against tissue damage accompanying surgical interventions requiring cardiopulmonary bypass and thus contact of blood with artificial surfaces. Anti-C5 had a dose-dependent beneficial effect on the myocardial tissue damage in patients receiving coronary artery bypass grafts and/or valve replacements as measured by CK-MB release and death rate after 30 days in these patients. The effect of anti-C5 in other clinical settings such as rheumatoid arthritis is also being investigated. Surprisingly, data presented with the anti–factor D antibody TNX-224 showed quite effective suppression of complement activation, neutrophil activation, and IL-8 production in rats, obviously due to the inactivation of the alternative pathway alone.

Synthetic Molecules

The number of small synthetic molecules that have been designed to inhibit complement activation is still comparably low. Compstatin, a synthetic 13-residue cyclic peptide (128) that binds to native C3 of primates and inhibits its cleavage by C3 convertases, can inhibit the activation of C3 and downstream pathways in animal models for extracorporeal circulation or xenotransplantation, respectively. Compstatin may serve as a starting point for the design of an orally applied drug.

The role of the complement-split products C3a and C5a in anaphylaxis, sepsis, and adverse reactions in extracorporeal circulation or dialysis, has led to the generation of selective inhibitors for the interaction of the peptides with their respective G-protein coupled receptors.

In vitro, SB 290157, a small C3aR antagonist, inhibited C3a-triggered and Ca^{2+}-mediated effects of the C3aR at IC_{50}

of 2×10^{-8} M and showed C3a-dependent anti-inflammatory activity in animal models (129). The compound will not only be valuable to define the physiologic roles of C3a and its receptor, but is a first candidate to interfere with complement-dependent mechanisms in the pathogenesis of asthma. The cyclic hexapeptide F-(OPdChaWR), acetylated or methylated on the N-terminus, was designed to competitively inhibit the C5a/C5aR interaction. Its solution structure was determined by NMR spectroscopy and it was found to inhibit hallmarks of inflammation like neutrophil emigration or vascular leakage in the reverse-passive Arthus reaction (130). Another C5a antagonist, the dimeric recombinant mutant C5a protein CGS 32359, showed an attenuation of neutrophil activation and a reduction of infarct size in a porcine model of cardiac ischemia/reperfusion (131).

Which Pathway to Block?

In principle, two "schools of thought" (132) may be distinguished regarding the targeted steps: those acting early on the activation of C3 (and all downstream effects including C3b opsonization) and those acting later on activation of C5 (i.e., C5a generation and MAC formation only). Deposition of C3b is considered to contribute substantially to surveillance of gram-negative bacteria, and patients with C3 deficiency suffer from repeated pyogenic infections. The question of which of the three pathways to block has not been finally resolved, and indeed amazingly similar results have been obtained in animal studies by the selective blocking of the alternative pathway (133) or the classical pathway (126). The fact that each of the three pathways can lead to activation of others (132), especially the alternative pathway serving as the subsequent amplification loop, may explain this observation.

Exploitation of Complement Activation for Therapy or Prophylaxis:

A gene therapy strategy has proposed delivery of a Gal(α-1,3)galactosyl transferase gene into cancer cells (134). Cell membranes with the unusual Gal(α-1,3) galactose residues would activate complement through natural IgM and be destroyed, just as it occurs with endothelial cells in xenografts. Another strategy to exploit complement activation makes use of C3 deposition. The C3d fragment, via binding to the CR2/CD19/CD81 B-cell co-receptor complex, can serve as an adjuvant in immunization (69). Recombinantly or chemically attached C3d has been shown to enhance the immune response against prominent pathogens such as measles virus, influenza virus, or pneumococci (135–137). Various vaccine formulations including C3d—for example, against the *Plasmodium falciparum* merozoite antigen MSP-1.19—are under development. C3d attachment may not only lead to higher antibody titers, but may help to raise an effective immune response against such poorly immunogenic but protective antigens.

SUMMARY AND CONCLUSIONS

Complement comprises plasma proteins (i.e., substrates and regulators of the activation cascades) and cell-membrane proteins (i.e., receptors and cell-protecting regulators). Complement activation, triggered by bound antibody or microbial patterns directly, proceeds in three intertwined pathways (classical, lectin, and alternative) and either directly leads to destruction of foreign structures through insertion of a lytic pore, or contributes to their elimination, such as through promotion of phagocytosis and antibody formation.

Recent findings have advanced our understanding of complement, especially of the ways that it can be dealt with in clinical therapy. The MBL genotype, standing for the activity of the lectin pathway, was shown to correlate widely with disposition to infection. The three-dimensional structures of core components (e.g., the thioester region in C3) have been solved. Finally, several specific complement inhibitors (chimeric constructs derived from natural regulators, monoclonal antibodies, or small molecules found by combinatorial approaches) are in advanced stages of clinical trials. Ischemic and inflammatory diseases, including ischemia/reperfusion injury in surgery and transplantation, are particularly interesting for therapeutic complement inhibition.

ACKNOWLEDGMENTS

We would like to acknowledge the Austrian Science Fund and the Ludwig Boltzmann Society for support of our research.

REFERENCES

1. Pillemer L, Blum L, Lepow IH. The properdin system and immunity. I. Demonstration and isolation of a new serum protein, properdin, its role in immune phenomena. *Science* 1954;120:279–285.
2. Nonaka M. Evolution of the complement system. *Curr Opin Immunol* 2001;13:69–73.
3. Smith LC, Azumi K, Nonaka M. Complement systems in invertebrates. The ancient alternative and lectin pathways. *Immunopharmacology* 1999;42:107–120.
4. Levashina EA, Moita LF, Blandin S, et al. Conserved role of a complement-like protein in phagocytosis revealed by dsRNA knockout in cultured cells of the mosquito, Anopheles gambiae. *Cell* 2001;104:709–718.
5. Morgan BP, Gasque P. Extrahepatic complement biosynthesis: where, when and why? *Clin Exp Immunol* 1997;107:1–7.
6. Würzner R, Joysey VC, Lachmann PJ. Complement component C7. Assessment of in vitro synthesis after liver transplantation reveals that hepatocytes do not synthesize the majority of the C7. *J Immunol* 1994;152:4624–4629.
7. Naughton MA, Walport MJ, Würzner R, et al. Organ-specific contribution to circulating C7 levels by the bone. *Eur J Immunol* 1996;26:2108–2112.
8. Morgan BP, Gasque P. Expression of complement in the brain: role in health and disease. *Immunol Today* 1996;17:461–466.
9. Fischer MB, Ma M, Hsu NC, et al. Local synthesis of C3 within the splenic lymphoid compartment can reconstitute the impaired immune response in C3-deficient mice. *J Immunol* 1998;160:2619–2625.
10. Volanakis JE. Transcriptional regulation of complement genes. *Annu Rev Immunol* 1995;13:277–305.
11. Kilgore KS, Friedrichs GS, Homeister JW, et al. The complement system in myocardial ischaemia/reperfusion injury. *Cardiovasc Res* 1994;28:437–444.
12. Law SKA, Dodds AW. The internal thioester and the covalent binding properties of the complement proteins C3 and C4. *Protein Sci* 1997;6:263–274.
13. Nagar B, Jones RG, Diefenbach RJ, et al. X-ray crystal structure of C3d: a C3 fragment and ligand for complement receptor 2. *Science* 1998;280:1277–1281.
14. Carroll MC, Fathallah DM, Bergamaschini L, et al. Substitution of a single amino acid (aspartic acid for histidine) converts the functional activity of human complement C4B to C4A. *Proc Natl Acad Sci U S A* 1990;87:6868–6872.
15. Barlow PN, Steinkasserer A, Norman DG, et al. Solution structure of a pair of complement modules by nuclear magnetic resonance. *J Mol Biol* 1993;232:268–284.
16. Casasnovas JM, Larvie M, Stehle T. Crystal structure of two CD46 domains reveals an extended measles virus-binding surface. *EMBO J* 1999;18:2911–2922.
17. Janatova J, Reid KB, Willis AC. Disulfide bonds are localized within the short consensus repeat units of complement regulator proteins: C4b-binding protein. *Biochemistry* 1989;28:4754–4761.
18. Heine-Suner D, Diaz-Guillen MA, Pardo F, et al. A high resolution map of the regulator of the complement activation gene cluster on 1q32 that integrates new genes and markers. *Immunogenetics* 1997;45:422–427.
19. Hobart MJ, Fernie BA, DiScipio RG. Structure of the human C7 gene and comparison with the C6, C8A, C8B, C9 genes. *J Immunol* 1995;154:5188–5194.
20. Würzner R, Hobart MJ, Fernie BA, et al. Molecular basis of subtotal complement C6 deficiency. A carboxy-terminally truncated but functionally active C6. *J Clin Invest* 1995;95:1877–1883.
21. Tschopp J, Villiger W, Fuchs H, et al. Assembly of subcomponents C1r and C1s of the first component of complement: electron microscopic and ultracentrifugal studies. *Proc Natl Acad Sci U S A* 1980;77:7014–7018.
22. Arlaud GJ, Rossi V, Thielens NM, et al. Structural and functional studies on C1r and C1s: new insights into the mechanisms involved in C1 activity and assembly. *Immunobiology* 1998;199:303–316.
23. Taylor PR, Carugati A, Fadok VA, et al. A hierarchical role for classical pathway complement proteins in the clearance of apoptotic cells in vivo. *J Exp Med* 2000;192:359–366.
24. Navratil JS, Watkins SC, Wisnieski JJ, et al. The globular heads of C1q specifically recognize surface blebs of apoptotic vascular endothelial cells. *J Immunol* 2001;166:3231–3239.
25. Navratil JS, Korb LC, Ahearn JM. Systemic lupus erythematosus and complement deficiency: clues to a novel role for the classical complement pathway in the maintenance of immune tolerance. *Immunopharmacology* 1999;42:47–52.
26. Botto M. Links between complement deficiency and apoptosis. *Arthritis Res* 2001;3:207–210.
27. Ziccardi R. Activation of the early components of the classical complement pathway under physiologic conditions. *J Immunol* 1981;126:1769–1773.
28. Müller-Eberhard HJ. Molecular organization and function of the complement system. *Annu Rev Biochem* 1988;57:321–347.
29. Libyh MT, Goossens D, Oudin S, et al. A recombinant human scFv anti-Rh(D) antibody with multiple valences using a C-terminal fragment of C4-binding protein. *Blood* 1997;90:3978–3983.
30. Petersen SV, Thiel S, Jensenius JC. The mannan-binding lectin pathway of complement activation: biology and disease association. *Mol Immunol* 2001;38:133–149.
31. Holmskov UL. Collectins and collectin receptors in innate immunity. *Acta Pathol Microbiol Immunol Scand* 2000;100(suppl):1–59.
32. Madsen HO, Garred P, Kurtzhals JA, et al. A new frequent allele is the missing link in the structural polymorphism of the human mannan-binding protein. *Immunogenetics* 1994;40:37–44.
33. Super M, Thiel S, Lu J, et al. Association of low levels of mannan-binding protein with a common defect of opsonisation. *Lancet* 1989;2(8674):1236–1239.
34. Turner MW and Hamvas RM. Mannose-binding lectin: structure, function, genetics and disease associations. *Rev Immunogenet* 2001;2:305–322.
35. Koch A, Melbye M, Sorensen P, et al. Acute respiratory tract infections and mannose-binding lectin insufficiency during early childhood. *JAMA* 2001;285:1316–1321.

36. Dahl MR, Thiel S, Matsushita M, et al. MASP-3 and its association with distinct complexes of the mannan-binding lectin complement activation pathway. *Immunity* 2001;15:127–135.

37. Iobst ST, Wormald MR, Weis WI, et al. Binding of sugar ligands to Ca(2+)-dependent animal lectins. I. Analysis of mannose binding by site-directed mutagenesis and NMR. *J Biol Chem* 1994;269:15505–15511.

38. Thiel S, Vorup-Jensen T, Stover CM, et al. A second serine protease associated with mannan-binding lectin that activates complement. *Nature* 1997;386:506–510.

39. Matsushita M and Fujita T. Ficolins and the lectin complement pathway. *Immunol Rev* 2001;180:78–85.

40. Petersen SV, Thiel S, Jensen L, et al. Control of the classical and the MBL pathway of complement activation. *Mol Immunol* 2000;37:803–811.

41. Collard CD, Vakeva A, Morrissey MA, et al. Complement activation after oxidative stress: role of the lectin complement pathway. *Am J Pathol* 2000;156:1549–1556.

42. Malhotra R, Willis AC, Jensenius JC, et al. Structure and homology of human C1q receptor (collectin receptor). *Immunology* 1993;78:341–348.

43. Volanakis JE and Narayana SVL. Complement factor D, a novel serine protease. *Protein Sci* 1996;5:553–564.

44. Zipfel PF, Jokiranta TS, Hellwage J, et al. The factor H protein family. *Immunopharmacology* 1999;42:53–60.

45. Masaki T, Matsumoto M, Yasuda R, et al. A covalent dimer of complement C4b serves as a subunit of a novel C5 convertase that involves no C3 derivatives. *J Immunol* 1991;147:927–932.

46. Müller-Eberhard HJ. The membrane attack complex of complement. *Annu Rev Immunol* 1986;4:503–528.

47. Thompson RA, Lachmann PJ. Reactive lysis: the complement-mediated lysis of unsensitized cells. I. The characterization of the indicator factor and its identification as C7. *J Exp Med* 1970;131:629–641.

48. Esser AF. Big MAC attack: complement proteins cause leaky patches. *Immunol Today* 1991;12:316–318.

49. Bhakdi S, Tranum Jensen J. Complement lysis: a hole is a hole. *Immunol Today* 1991;12:318–320.

50. Lachmann PJ. The control of homologous lysis. *Immunol Today* 1991;12/9:312–315.

51. Peitsch MC, Amiguet P, Guy R, et al. Localization and molecular modelling of the membrane-inserted domain of the ninth component of human complement and perforin. *Mol Immunol* 1990;27:589–602.

52. Morgan BP. Complement membrane attack on nucleated cells: resistance, recovery and non-lethal effects. *Biochem J* 1989;264:1–14.

53. Reiter Y, Ciobotariu A, Fishelson Z. Sublytic complement attack protects tumor cells from lytic doses of antibody and complement. *Eur J Immunol* 1992;22:1207–1213.

54. Niculescu F, Rus H, Shin ML. Receptor-independent activation of guanine nucleotide-binding regulatory proteins by terminal complement complexes. *J Biol Chem* 1994;269:4417–4423.

55. Würzner R, Xu H, Franzke A, et al. Blood dendritic cells carry terminal complement complexes on their cell surface as detected by newly developed neoepitope-specific monoclonal antibodies. *Immunology* 1991;74:132–138.

56. Tedesco F, Pausa M, Nardon E, et al. The cytolytically inactive terminal complement complex activates endothelial cells to express adhesion molecules and tissue factor procoagulant activity. *J Exp Med* 1997;185:1619–1627.

57. Krych-Goldberg M, Atkinson JP. Structure-function relationships of complement receptor type 1. *Immunol Rev* 2001;180:112–122.

58. Eggleton P, Tenner AJ, Reid KB. C1q receptors. *Clin Exp Immunol* 2000;120:406–412.

59. Moore MD, Cooper NR, Tack BF, et al. Molecular cloning of the cDNA encoding the Epstein-Barr virus/C3d receptor (complement receptor type 2) of human B lymphocytes. *Proc Natl Acad Sci U S A* 1987;84:9194–9198.

60. Liu YJ, Xu JC, Debouteiller O, et al. Follicular dendritic cells specifically express the long CR2/CD21 isoform. *J Exp Med* 1997;185:165–170.

61. Prodinger WM, Schwendinger MG, Schoch J, et al. Characterization of C3dg binding to a recess formed between short consensus repeats 1 and 2 of complement receptor type 2 (CR2; CD21). *J Immunol* 1998;161:4604–4610.

62. Szakonyi G, Guthridge JM, Li D, et al. Structure of complement receptor 2 in complex with its C3d ligand. *Science* 2001;292:1725–1728.

63. Carroll MC. The role of complement and complement receptors in induction and regulation of immunity. *Annu Rev Immunol* 1998;16:545–568.

64. Aubry JP, Pochon S, Graber P, et al. CD21 is a ligand for CD23 and regulates IgE production. *Nature* 1992;358:505–507.

65. Chen Z, Koralov SB, Kelsoe G. Regulation of the humoral immune responses by CD21/CD35. *Immunol Rev* 2000;176:194–204.

66. Fearon DT, Carroll MC. Regulation of B lymphocyte responses to foreign and self-antigens by the CD19/CD21 complex. *Annu Rev Immunol* 2000;18:393–422.

67. Cherukuri A, Cheng PC, Sohn HW, et al. The CD19/CD21 complex functions to prolong B cell antigen receptor signaling from lipid rafts. *Immunity* 2001;14:169–179.

68. Tedder TF, Inaoki M, Sato S. The CD19-CD21 complex regulates signal transduction thresholds governing humoral immunity and autoimmunity. *Immunity* 1997;6:107–118.

69. Dempsey PW, Allison MED, Akkaraju S, et al. C3d of complement as a molecular adjuvant: bridging innate and acquired immunity. *Science* 1996;271:348–350.

70. Chen Z, Koralov SB, Gendelman M, et al. Humoral immune responses in Cr2−/− mice: enhanced affinity maturation but impaired antibody persistence. *J Immunol* 2001;164:4522–4532.

71. Kacani L, Prodinger WM, Sprinzl GM, et al. Detachment of human immunodeficiency virus type 1 from germinal centers by blocking complement receptor type 2. *The Journal of Virology,* 2000;74:7997–8002.

72. Carroll MC. The lupus paradox. *Nat Genet* 1998;19:3–4.

73. Ehlers MR. CR3: a general purpose adhesion-recognition receptor essential for innate immunity. *Microbes Infect* 2000;2:289–294.

74. Diamond MS, Garcia-Aguilar J, Bickford JK, et al. The I domain is a major recognition site on the leukocyte integrin Mac-1 (CD11b/CD18) for four distinct adhesion ligands. *J Cell Biol* 1993;120:1031–1043.

75. Thornton BP, Vetvicka V, Pitman M, et al. Analysis of the sugar specificity and molecular location of the beta-glucan–binding lectin site of complement receptor type 3 (CD11b/CD18). *J Immunol* 1996;156:1235–1246.

76. Hogg N, Stewart MP, Scarth SL, et al. A novel leukocyte adhesion deficiency caused by expressed but nonfunctional beta2 integrins Mac-1 and LFA-1. *J Clin Invest* 1999;103:97–106.

77. Coxon A, Rieu P, Barkalow FJ, et al. A novel role for the beta 2 integrin CD11b/CD18 in neutrophil apoptosis: a homeostatic mechanism in inflammation. *Immunity* 1996;5:653–666.

78. Stockinger H. Interaction of GPI-anchored cell surface proteins and complement receptor type 3. *Exp Clin Immunogenet* 1997;14:5–10.

79. Gerard NP, Gerard C. The chemotactic receptor for human C5a anaphylatoxin. *Nature* 1991;349:614–617.

80. Ames RS, Li Y, Sarau HM, et al. Molecular cloning and characterization of the human anaphylatoxin C3a receptor. *J Biol Chem* 1996;271:20231–20234.

81. Hugli TE. Structure and function of C3a anaphylatoxin. *Curr Top Microbiol Immunol* 1990;153:181–208.

82. Boulay F, Naik N, Giannini E, et al. Phagocyte chemoattractant receptors. *Ann N Y Acad Sci* 1997;832:69–84.

83. Ahamed J, Haribabu B, Ali H. Cutting edge: differential regulation of chemoattractant receptor-induced degranulation and chemokine production by receptor phosphorylation. *J Immunol* 2001;167:3559–3563.

84. Eggleton P, Reid KB, Tenner AJ. C1q—How many functions? How many receptors? *Trends Cell Biol* 1998;8:428–431.

85. Ghebrehiwet B, Lim BL, Kumar R, et al. gC1q-R/p33, a member of a new class of multifunctional and multicompartment cellular proteins, is involved in inflammation and infection. *Immunol Rev* 2001;180:65–77.

86. Henson PM, Bratton DL, Fadok VA. The phosphatidylserine receptor: a crucial molecular switch? *Nat Rev Mol Cell Biol* 2001;2:627–633.

87. Lachmann PJ. Complement. In: McGee JOD, Isaacson PG, Wright NA, eds. *Oxford textbook of pathology.* Oxford: Oxford University Press, 1992:259–266.

88. Würzner R, Mollnes TE, Morgan BP. Immunochemical assays for complement components. In: Johnstone AP, Turner MW, eds. *Immunochemistry 2: a practical approach.* Oxford: Oxford University Press, 1997:197–223.

89. West C. Complement and glomerular disease. In: Volanakis JE, Frank MM, eds. *The human complement system in health and disease.* New York: Marcel Dekker, 1998:571–596.

90. Mathieson PW, Würzner R, Oliveria DB, et al. Complement-mediated adipocyte lysis by nephritic factor sera. *J Exp Med* 1993;177:1827–1831.

91. Gasque P, Dean YD, McGreal EP, et al. Complement components of the innate immune system in health and disease in the CNS. *Immunopharmacology* 2000;49:171–186.

92. Jiang H, Burdick D, Glabe CG, et al. Beta-amyloid activates complement by binding to a specific region of the collagen-like domain of the C1q A chain. *J Immunol* 1994;152:5050–5059.

93. Veerhuis R, Janssen I, Hack CE, et al. Early complement components in Alzheimer's disease brains. *Acta Neuropathol (Berl)* 1996;91:53–60.

94. Johns TG, Bernard CC. Binding of complement component C1q to myelin oligodendrocyte glycoprotein: a novel mechanism for regulating CNS inflammation. *Mol Immunol* 1997;34:33–38.

95. van der Laan LJ, Ruuls SR, Weber KS, et al. Macrophage phagocytosis of myelin in vitro determined by flow cytometry: phagocytosis is mediated by CR3 and induces production of tumor necrosis factor-alpha and nitric oxide. *J Neuroimmunol* 1996;70:145–152.

96. Petry F, Loos M. Bacteria and complement. In: Volanakis JE, Frank MM, eds. *The human complement system in health and disease.* New York: Marcel Dekker, 1998:375–391.

97. Cooper NR. Complement and viruses. In: Volanakis JE, Frank MM, eds. *The human complement system in health and disease.* New York: Marcel Dekker, 1998:393–407.

98. Figueroa JE, Densen P. Infectious diseases associated with complement deficiencies. *J Clin Microbiol Rev* 1991;4:359–395.

99. Hänsch GM. Defense against bacteria. In: Rother K, Till GO, Hänsch GM, eds. *The complement system.* 2nd rev. ed. Berlin, New York: Springer, 1998:285–301.

100. Taylor PW. Complement-mediated killing of susceptible gram-negative bacteria: an elusive mechanism. *Exp Clin Immunogenet* 1992;9:48–56.

101. Würzner R. Evasion of pathogens by avoiding recognition or eradication by complement, in part via molecular mimicry. *Mol Immunol* 1999;36:249–260.

102. Marschang P, Sodroski J, Würzner R, et al. Decay-accelerating factor (CD55) protects human immunodeficiency virus type I from inactivation by human complement. *Eur J Immunol* 1995;25:285–290.

103. Stoiber H, Schneider R, Janatova J, et al. Human complement proteins C3b, C4b, factor H and properdin react with specific sites in gp120 and gp41, the envelope protein of HIV-1. *Immunobiology* 1995;193:98–113.

104. Stoiber H, Pinter C, Siccardi AG, et al. Efficient destruction of human immunodeficiency virus in human serum by inhibiting the protective action of complement factor H. *J Exp Med* 1996;183:307–310.

105. Cooper NR. Complement evasion strategies of microorganisms. *Immunol Today* 1991;12:327–331.

106. Bhakdi S, Tranum Jensen J. Damage to cell membranes by pore-forming bacterial cytolysins. *Prog Allergy* 1988;40:1–43.

107. Fishelson Z. Complement-related proteins in pathogenic organisms. *Springer Semin Immunopathol* 1994;15:345–368.

108. Kotwal GJ. The great escape: immune evasion by pathogens. *Immunologist* 1997;4:157–164.

109. Fishelson Z. Complement evasion by parasites: search for "Achilles' heel." *Clin Exp Immunol* 1991;86(suppl 1):47–52.

110. Heidenreich F, Dierich MP. Candida albicans and Candida stellatoidea, in contrast to other Candida species, bind iC3b and C3d but not C3b. *Infect Immun* 1985;50:598–600.

111. Würzner R, Gruber A, Stoiber H, et al. Human immunodeficiency virus type I gp41 binds to Candida albicans via complement C3-like regions. *J Infect Dis* 1997;176:492–498.

112. Gruber A, Lukasser-Vogl E, Borg-von Zepelin M, et al. Human immunodeficiency virus type 1 gp160/gp41 binding to Candida albicans enhances candidal virulence in vitro. *J Infect Dis* 1998;177:1057–1063.

113. Schneider PM, Rittner C. Complement genetics. In: Dodds A, Sim RB, eds. *Complement—a practical approach.* Oxford: Oxford University Press, 1997:165–198.

114. Mauff G, Würzner R. Complement genetics. In: Herzenberg LA, Weir DM, Blackwell C, eds. *Weir's handbook of experimental immunology.* Malden, MA: Blackwell Science, 1997:77.1–77.11.

115. Kirschfink M. The clinical laboratory: testing the complement system. In: Rother K, Till GO, Hänsch GM, eds. *The complement system.* Berlin, New York: Springer, 1998:522–547.

116. Würzner R, Orren A, Lachmann PJ. Inherited deficiencies of the terminal components of human complement. *Immunodeficiency Rev* 1992;3:123–147.

117. Morgan BP, Walport MJ. Complement deficiency and disease. *Immunol Today* 1991;12:301–306.

118. Feifel E, Prodinger WM, Molgg M, et al. Polymorphism and deficiency of human factor H-related proteins p39 and p37. *Immunogenetics* 1992;36:104–109.

119. Carugati A, Pappalardo E, Zingale LC, et al. C1-inhibitor deficiency and angioedema. *Mol Immunol* 2001;38:161–173.

120. Bessler M, Schaefer A, Keller P. Paroxysmal nocturnal hemoglobinuria: insights from recent advacnes in molecular biology. *Transfus Med Rev* 2001;15:255–267.

121. Makrides SC. Therapeutic inhibition of the complement system. *Pharmacol Rev* 1998;50:59–87.

122. Weisman HF, Bartow T, Leppo MK, et al. Soluble human complement receptor type 1: in vivo inhibitor of complement suppressing post-ischemic myocardial inflammation and necrosis. *Science* 1990;249:146–151.

123. Kalli KR, Hsu P, Fearon DT. Therapeutic uses of recombinant complement protein inhibitors. *Springer Semin Immunopathol* 1994;15:417–431.

124. Smith GP, Smith RAG. Membrane-targeted complement inhibitors. *Mol Immunol* 2001;38:249–255.

125. Caliezi C, Wuillemin WA, Zeerleder S, et al. C1-Esterase inhibitor: an anti-inflammatory agent and its potential use in the treatment of diseases other than hereditary angioedema. *Pharmacol Rev* 2000;52:91–112.

126. Buerke M, Schwertz H, Seitz W, et al. Novel small molecule inhibitor of C1s exhibits cardioprotective effects in ischemia-reperfusion injury in rabbits. *J Immunol* 2001;167:5375–5380.

127. Würzner R, Schulze M, Happe L, et al. Inhibition of terminal complement complex formation and cell lysis by monoclonal antibodies. *Complement Inflamm* 1991;8:328–340.

128. Morikis D, Assa Munt N, Sahu A, et al. Solution structure of Compstatin, a potent complement inhibitor. *Protein Sci* 1998;7:619–627.

129. Ames RS, Lee D, Foley JJ, et al. Identification of a selective nonpeptide antagonist of the anaphylatoxin C3a receptor that demonstrates anti-inflammatory activity in animal models. *J Immunol* 2001;166:6341–6348.

130. Strachan AJ, Woodruff TM, Haaima G, et al. A new small molecule C5a receptor antagonist inhibits the reverse-passive Arthus reaction and endotoxic shock in rats. *J Immunol* 2000;164:6560–6565.

131. Riley RD, Sato H, Zhao ZQ, et al. Recombinant human complement C5a receptor antagonist reduces infarct size after surgical revascularization. *J Thorac Cardiovasc Surg* 2000;120:350–358.

132. Sahu A, Lambris JD. Complement inhibitors: a resurgent concept in anti-inflammatory therapeutics. *Mol Immunol* 2000;49:133–148.

133. Fung M, Loubser PG, Undar A, et al. Inhibition of complement, neutrophil, platelet activation by an anti-factor D monoclonal antibody in simulated cardiopulmonary bypass circuits. *J Thorac Cardiovasc Surg* 2001;122:113–122.

134. Jager U, Takeuchi Y, Porter C. Induction of complement attack on human cells by Gal(alpha1, 3)Gal xenoantigen expression as a gene therapy approach to cancer. *Gene Ther* 1999;6:1073–1083.

135. Green TD, Newton BR, Rota PA, et al. C3d enhancement of neutralizing antibodies to measles hemagglutinin. *Vaccine* 2001;20:242–248.

136. Ross TM, Xu Y, Bright RA, et al. C3d enhancement of antibodies to hemagglutinin accelerates protection against influenza virus challenge. *Nat Immunol* 2000;1:127–131.

137. Test ST, Mitsuyoshi J, Connoly CC, et al. Increased immunogenicity and induction of class switching by conjugation of complement C3d to pneumococcal serotype 14 capsular polysaccharide. *Infect Immun* 2001;69:3031–3040.

138. Eldering E, Huijbregts CC, Nuijens JH, et al. Recombinant C1 inhibitor P5/P3 variants display resistance to catalytic inactivation by stimulated neutrophils. *J Clin Invest* 1993;91:1035–1043.

139. Matsunami K, Miyagawa S, Yamada M, et al. A surface-bound form

of human C1 esterase inhibitor improves xenograft rejection. *Transplantation* 2000;69:749–755.

140. Zimmerman JL, Dellinger RP, Straube RC, et al. Phase I trial of the recombinant soluble complement receptor 1 in acute lung injury and acute respiratory distress syndrome. *Crit Care Med* 2000;28:3149–3154.

141. Huang J, Kim LJ, Mealey R, et al. Neuronal protection in stroke by an sLex-glycosylated complement inhibitory protein. *Science* 1999;285:595–599.

142. Mulligan MS, Warner RL, Rittershaus CW, et al. Endothelial targeting and enhanced antiinflammatory effects of complement inhibitors possessing sialyl Lewis^x moieties. *J Immunol* 1999;162:4952–4959.

143. Huser A, Rudolph M, Hofmann C. Incorporation of decay-accelerating factor into the baculovirus envelope generates complement-resistant gene transfer vectors. *Nat Biotechnol* 2001;19:451–455.

144. Kroshus TJ, Salerno CT, Yeh CG, et al. A recombinant soluble chimeric complement inhibitor composed of human CD46 and CD55 reduces acute cardiac tissue injury in models of pig-to-human heart transplantation. *Transplantation* 2000;69:2282–2289.

145. Thomas TC, Rollins SA, Rother RP, et al. Inhibition of complement activity by humanized anti-C5 antibody and single-chain Fv. *Mol Immunol* 1996;33:1389–1401.

146. Fitch JC, Rollins SA, Matis LA, et al. Pharmacology and biological efficacy of a recombinant, humanized, single-chain antibody C5 complement inhibitor in patients undergoing coronary artery bypass graft surgery with cardiopulmonary bypass. *Circulation* 1999;100:2499–2506.

147. Wang Y, Hu Q, Madri JA, et al. Amelioration of lupus-like autoimmune disease in NZB/WF1 mice after treatment with a blocking monoclonal antibody specific for complement component C5. *Proc Natl Acad Sci U S A* 1996;93:8563–8568.

148. Biesecker G, Dihel L, Enney K, et al. Derivation of RNA aptamer inhibitors of human complement C5. *Immunopharmacology* 1999;42:219–230.

149. Heller T, Hennecke M, Baumann U, et al. Selection of a C5a receptor antagonist from phage libraries attenuating the inflammatory response in immune complex disease and ischemia/reperfusion injury. *J Immunol* 1999;163:985–994.

150. Morgan BP. Clinical complementology: recent progress and future trends. *Eur J Clin Invest* 1994;24:219–228.

CHAPTER 35

Phagocytosis

Eric J. Brown and Hattie D. Gresham

Genetic Approaches to Understanding Phagocytosis
Types and Derivations of Phagocytes
Cell Biology of Phagocytosis
　　Recognition of the Phagocytic Target · Mechanisms of Phagocytosis · Signaling Events in Fcγ Receptor–Mediated Phagocytosis · Signaling Events in Complement Receptor Phagocytosis · Macropinocytosis and Phagocytosis · Cytoskeleton in Phagocytosis · Phagosome and Phagolysosome Formation · Consequences of Phagocytosis · Regulation of Phagocytosis
Microbes and Phagocytosis
　　Phagocytosis by "Nonprofessionals" · Microbial Subversion of Professional Phagocytes
Conclusions
References

Phagocytosis is the process by which a single cell can internalize and digest particulate material. In amebae and other free-living unicellular eukaryotes, this is primarily a feeding mechanism. This process of bulk uptake of particulates (primarily bacteria) for nutrition has been co-opted by Metazoa to provide a mechanism for uptake, destruction, and removal of unwanted or dangerous particulates, and its role in providing nutrition to the organism has decreased. In mammals, phagocytosis is the primary mechanism for removing invading microorganisms, dead and dying cells, tissue debris, protein aggregates, and foreign bodies. Phagocytosis is essential for host defense against infectious diseases, for organ remodeling in embryonic development, for tissue repair after injury, and for removal of aging and senescent cells. Because these functions are essential for survival and homeostasis, complex signaling pathways have evolved both to regulate the engulfment process and to link uptake of particulate material with appropriate cellular responses. For example, the engulfment of an invading bacterial pathogen is linked to the development and delivery of host-derived bactericidal molecules into the digestive vacuole. This link of engulfment to response is dictated by plasma membrane receptors that sense either specific molecular structures on the surface of the target or host components that have coated the particle. Because in many cases the cellular response can result in the production of potentially host-damaging products, ingestion and its consequences must be closely regulated. Both positive and negative regulatory mechanisms exist to ensure that the rate and extent of engulfment and the downstream cellular responses occur at

an appropriate level. It is the goal of this chapter to explain the molecular mechanisms involved in receptor function during phagocytosis, in the process of ingestion, and in the linkage of ingestion to specific cellular responses.

The term *phagocytosis* is generally reserved for ingestion of targets that are more than 1 μm in diameter, because at this size the mechanisms for internalization clearly differ from those used for endocytosis of soluble material. Phagocytosis was first described by Elie Metchnikoff, who in the 1880s first observed cells in starfish larvae capable of ingesting a deliberately introduced foreign substance. Metchnikoff extended these studies to higher organisms and was the first to describe the ability of the white blood cells in vertebrate animals and humans to migrate to sites of infection and to ingest and destroy live bacteria. This led him to propose the hypothesis that phagocytosis by these cells was an essential aspect of host defense (1). In 1922, Ludwig Aschoff recognized that there was a network of highly phagocytic cells throughout the organs of the body that was extremely important in host defense and immunity, which he called the reticuloendothelial system and later was renamed the mononuclear phagocyte system (2,3). The identical origins of Aschoff's fixed phagocytic cells and Metchnikoff's wandering phagocytes were elucidated over the next decade, as was the realization that both were necessary for appropriate defense against infection. By the 1960s, the ability of antibody and complement to contribute to pathogen uptake by phagocytes had been recognized, and the concept of opsonization by serum components was promulgated (4). However, no detailed investigations of the process of phagocytosis were made until the 1970s, when Silverstein's laboratory began a systematic study of immunoglobulin G (IgG)–mediated ingestion. On the basis of these experiments, Silverstein et al. (5) proposed the "zipper hypothesis," according to which phagocytosis requires repeated interactions between ligands on the target particle and receptors on the phagocytic cell. In this model, membrane protrusions of the phagocytic cell move over the target like a zipper, with a requirement for repeated interactions between ligands on the phagocytic target and receptors on the host cell. Interactions between the phagocytic cell and target were postulated to be close at the leading edge (front) of the zipper and more distant at the base of the phagocytic cup. An important feature of this model was that the membrane events that lead to engulfment must be very localized. A variety of experimental evidence in favor of the model was generated in the ensuing decade, but the molecular basis for the localized changes was not elucidated. Moreover, it became clear that zippering could not be the only mechanism for phagocytosis: As early as 1976, a morphologically distinct mechanism of phagocytosis in which membrane zippering did not play an obvious role (6) was described. Finally, studies of the phenomenon of macropinocytosis, in which macrophages internalize ("drink") large amounts of their surrounding medium, revealed that it had many biochemical similarities to phagocytosis, but because there was no phagocytic target, there was no possibility of repeated target-phagocyte interaction as envisioned by the zipper hypothesis. These data have forced a reexamination of the process of phagocytosis since 1990 that has led to the elucidation of important molecular mechanisms underlying this essential cellular function and its control. It is very clear that phagocytosis is an extremely complex process that requires cellular integration of dynamic changes in plasma membrane, cytoskeleton, vesicular traffic, signaling cascades, and effector molecules. In addition, it has become clear since 1990 that a variety of microorganisms can exploit this process to establish infection in hosts, leading to intracellular infections that present special challenges for host defense and immunity. In this chapter, we review current understanding of the various molecular and cell biological processes that result in internalization of particulate material.

GENETIC APPROACHES TO UNDERSTANDING PHAGOCYTOSIS

Phagocytosis as a cell biological process is conserved from amebae to the wandering and fixed phagocytes of mammals. Elucidation of the common mechanisms underlying this complex but evolutionarily conserved process by which diverse cell types and organisms carry out ingestion thus represent a problem of fundamental importance in cell biology and immunology. Because of the complexity of the process and its required coordination with other effector mechanisms in the ingesting cells, a nonbiased approach to understanding the molecular mechanisms of the process is extremely important for identifying the proteins and other cellular components involved. The advent of available elegant genetic screens in simple eukaryotes has made a genetic approach to this problem possible. Random mutagenesis has been used in Dictyostelium species, in Caenorhabditis elegans, and, to a more limited extent, in Drosophila species to investigate phagocytic mechanisms. In many ways, Dictyostelium discoideum is the ideal model organism for studying phagocytosis by ameboid cells (which include polymorphonuclear leukocytes and macrophages of vertebrates), because it is actively phagocytic and genetically manipulatable. For this reason, Dictyostelium has been used increasingly to understand the genes involved in the process of ingestion; at least 25 gene mutations that affect phagocytosis have been identified (7). These genes can be classified generally as cytoskeletal proteins; signaling proteins regulating cytoskeletal rearrangements; and proteins involved in or regulating membrane fusion. In addition, calreticulin and calnexin, both calcium-binding proteins of the endoplasmic reticulum, are essential for efficient phagocytosis in Dictyostelium (8). These proteins may provide calcium for optimal actin polymerization around the phagocytic cup and, in addition, may indicate that the endoplasmic reticulum is an important source of membrane for the forming phagosome. Calreticulin and calnexin, as well as other endoplasmic reticulum proteins, have been detected on phagosomes purified from mammalian phagocytes (9). A current model for phagocytosis based on these studies in Dictyostelium is shown in Fig. 1.

Genetic investigations of phagocytosis in C. elegans have the longest history, on the basis of the requirement for phagocytosis of apoptotic cells during normal development. Seven mutant C. elegans genes that lead to failure to phagocytose apoptotic cells have been identified (10). Six of these have homologs that also function in phagocytosis of apoptotic cells in mammals. Although some of these genes, such as the apparent receptor for apoptotic cells and an adenosine triphosphate (ATP) binding cassette (ABC)–type transporter, may function specifically in recognition and uptake of apoptotic cells, several of the gene products probably have a wider role in phagocytosis because they are involved in regulation of the cytoskeleton. These include adapter proteins CrkII, DOCK180, and Elmo and the low-molecular-weight guanosine triphosphatase (GTPase) Rac (11,12).

Drosophila species have been increasingly used as a genetically tractable model for studying both removal of apoptotic cells and phagocytosis in the context of infection (13,14). The importance of Drosophila species as a model for innate immunity in general was established by the initial identification of the central role of Toll and Toll-like receptors in host defense against infection in the fruit fly (15). Although studies in this organism have not yet led to a comprehensive model for the genes involved in phagocytosis, it is likely that Drosophila species will be increasingly used to study the genetics of host defense.

The basic molecular mechanisms of ingestion are probably quite similar through evolution, but there are many specializations that have occurred as the process has changed from

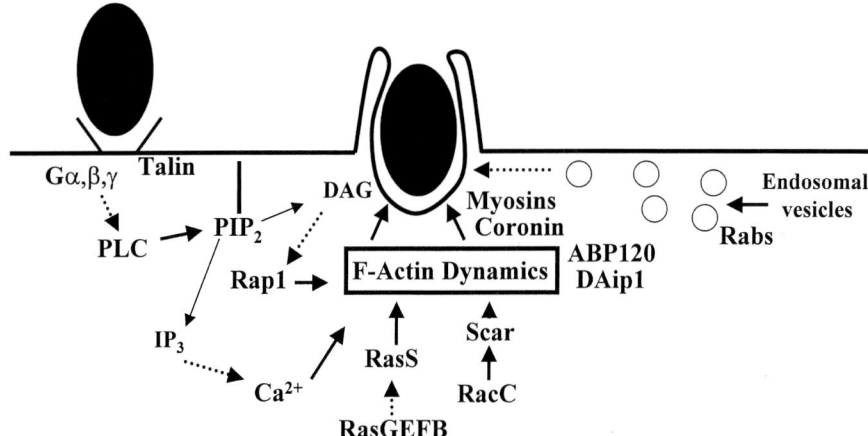

FIG. 1. The genetics of phagocytosis in *Dictyostelium*. *Dictyostelium discoideum* has been used as a genetically tractable model organism to understand the molecular basis of phagocytosis. The genes shown to be involved in phagocytosis by this approach include those for proteins involved in signal transduction, cytoskeletal rearrangements, and delivery of membranes to the forming phagosome. From Cardelli (7), with permission.

one involved primarily in nutrient uptake to one involved in host defense and as the mechanisms for the function of innate and adaptive immunity have grown more complex. For this reason, a focus on the role of phagocytosis in the context of the immune system necessitates a detailed consideration of the cells of higher vertebrates; the remainder of the chapter focuses on phagocytosis in mammalian cells.

TYPES AND DERIVATIONS OF PHAGOCYTES

As an essential element of host defense, phagocytosis is a part of the mechanism by which most potential pathogens are ultimately destroyed. The host defense aspects of phagocytosis require recognition of potential pathogens and are a function primarily of specialized leukocytes, the myeloid cells known as polymorphonuclear neutrophils (PMNs); mast cells; and monocytes, macrophages, and their differentiated derivatives specialized for interaction with lymphocytes, known as dendritic cells. All phagocytes are bone marrow-derived. PMNs and monocytes migrate through blood and tissues, surveying for disruptions of homeostasis that necessitate repair. Macrophages and mast cells are resident in all tissues of the body, in which they are involved in normal tissue turnover and wound repair as well as in host defense against infection. Dendritic cells are resident in tissues as well as in lymph nodes and spleen; an important part of their function is to bring antigens derived from tissue infections to local lymph nodes, where lymphocytes can be recruited to initiate specific immunity.

Myeloid granulocytes are divided on the basis of staining properties of their granules into neutrophils, eosinophils, and basophils. PMNs are the most abundant, constituting about 95% of the total granulocytes. PMNs mature from committed precursors for 6 days in the bone marrow and then are released into the vasculature to circulate for only a few hours, after

which they enter various tissues, where they ultimately undergo programmed cell death and are efficiently removed by resident macrophages. During infection, PMNs are released from the bone marrow in greater numbers and sometimes before full maturation. The existence of increased numbers of PMNs or immature PMNs, or both, in the blood has been used clinically for many years as a sign of infection. Mature PMNs contain at least three classes of granules, termed primary, secondary, and tertiary, which differ in their contents. In general, the granules contain lysosomal enzymes and other bacteriostatic or bacteriocidal molecules and act as a repository for membrane molecules that can be rapidly mobilized to the cell surface for use in host defense. The regulated secretion of granule contents is a critical component of host defense, as demonstrated by the marked increase in susceptibility to infection in patients lacking one or more classes of neutrophil granules.

Mononuclear phagocytes are released from the bone marrow as monocytes, which migrate into different tissues, in which they further differentiate into mature macrophages. The phenotype of these macrophages is highly dependent on their environment in tissue. In the absence of inflammation, a major role for tissue macrophages is to remove dead and damaged cells and particulate matter from tissues. As Kupffer cells in the liver, they remove senescent erythrocytes, fibrin degradation products, immune complexes, and bacteria from the portal circulation, which perfuses the intestine. As alveolar macrophages, they ingest and remove inhaled particles small enough to reach the terminal air ways. When inflammation is present, the rate of migration of monocytes into the site of inflammation is increased, and the numbers of macrophages present begins to increase within a few hours and can remain elevated until inflammation is resolved. Inflammatory macrophages differ from resident tissue macrophages by expression of myeloperoxidase, increased phagocytic capacity, and enhanced ability to generate toxic oxygen and nitrogen metabolites.

Also resident in tissues are immature dendritic cells, which are highly phagocytic and extremely important in the response to infection. Indeed, dendritic cells may be more capable of destruction of certain invading pathogens than are tissue macrophages. Phagocytosis by dendritic cells provides a major route for interaction between innate and acquired immunity, because dendritic cells are specialized for presentation of ingested antigens to T and B cells. After phagocytosis of pathogens in peripheral tissues, dendritic cells migrate to lymph nodes, where they become much less phagocytic but are particularly efficient at activating T cells for initiation of specific immunity.

A specialized phagocytic cell related to the macrophage, the microglial cell, exists in the brain. Microglia are derived from bone marrow derived, express many of the phagocytic receptors of macrophages, and have been implicated in the removal of apoptotic cells and cell debris in a variety of pathological conditions in the brain. Like macrophages and dendritic cells, microglia can present antigens to lymphocytes; this property may be important in the pathogenesis of various brain inflammatory diseases, including multiple sclerosis and experimental allergic encephalomyelopathy. Phagocytosis of pathological material by microglia and the subsequent induction of inflammation have been implicated in the pathophysiology of a variety of neurodegenerative diseases, including Alzheimer's disease.

CELL BIOLOGY OF PHAGOCYTOSIS

Phagocytosis can be modeled as occurring in four basic steps (Fig. 2). The initial event is recognition of the target by the phagocytic cell. Recognition of a phagocytic target can be either direct, through interaction with molecular motifs expressed by the target that the phagocyte recognizes as "foreign," or through the process of opsonization. Opsonization occurs when soluble host proteins, present in plasma and extracellular fluids, interact with invading pathogens, apoptotic cells, or cellular debris. In the second step of phagocytosis, receptor–ligand interactions cause specific cellular responses through signal transduction pathways. These responses are required for membrane and cytoskeletal changes that lead to engulfment and can also be accompanied by other aspects of inflammation, such as enzyme secretion, adhesion, degranulation, and activation of the respiratory burst. The third step is the actual process of internalization, which requires one or more membrane fusion events in the phagocytic cell to bring the target from the extracellular milieu to the intracellular vesicular network. As discussed later, there are several distinct mechanisms for engulfment. Finally, the ingested particle enters the lysosomal system in the phagocyte, where it is degraded. The study of the response to both model particles and to infectious organisms, and the mechanisms by which virulent organisms evade ingestion and killing, have helped elucidate these steps of phagocytosis.

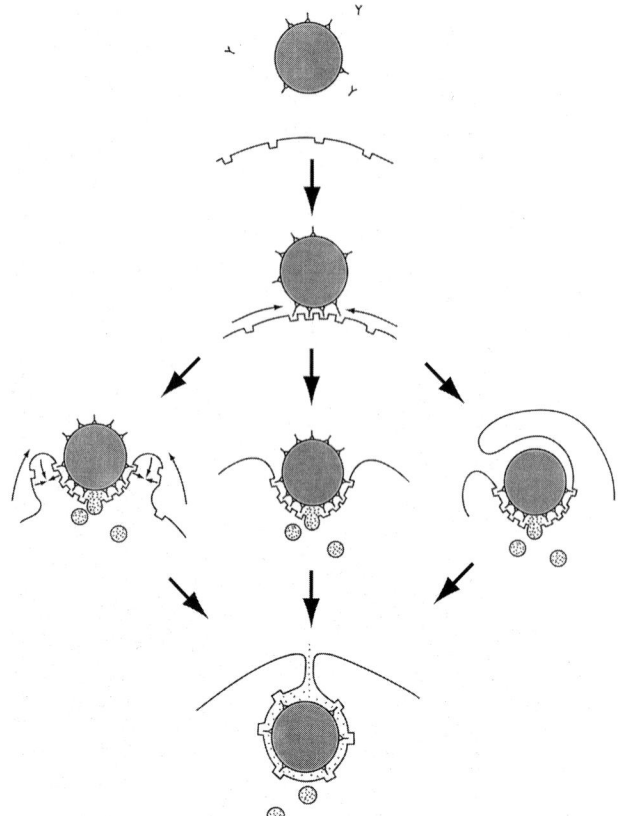

FIG. 2. The four steps of phagocytosis. Phagocytosis can be modeled as occurring in four steps. Initially, the phagocyte interacts with the target of ingestion either through specific receptors for opsonin (as depicted) or through receptors that directly recognize biochemical attributes of the surface of the target. Attachment of the target initiates signal transduction in the phagocyte, often through ligation and clustering of the recognition receptors, which begins the process of ingestion. Ingestion can occur through three morphologically distinct processes: "zippering," in which the membrane of the phagocyte extends around the target through protrusion of pseudopods in close apposition to the target of ingestion; "sinking," in which the plasma membrane of the phagocyte remains in close apposition to the target but pseudopods are not extended and the target appears to sink into the phagocytic cell; and "induced uptake," in which the target causes an increase in membrane ruffling in the phagocyte, leading to its uptake by a mechanism resembling macropinocytosis. Induced uptake often occurs because the target injects specific effectors into the cytoplasm of the phagocyte, rather than because of signaling from the recognition receptors. Finally, all three morphologically distinct mechanisms of ingestion lead to fusion of the phagosome with intracellular vesicular compartments, including endosomes and lysosomes, which can deliver antimicrobial effectors to the intracellular compartment containing a potential pathogen.

Recognition of the Phagocytic Target

Nonopsonic Recognition

The initial event of phagocytosis is recognition of the particle to be ingested by the phagocytic cell. In "professional phagocytes," this occurs because of expression on the phagocytic cell of a set of receptors that have evolved to recognize invading organisms and devitalized cells or tissues. The target motifs are called pathogen-associated molecular patterns (PAMPs); conversely, the phagocytic receptors that recognize these PAMPs are called pattern recognition receptors (PRRs). A number of these receptors recognize specific features that differentiate the target from normal cells or tissue. For example, there are phagocyte receptors for bacterial lipopolysaccharide, for peptidoglycan, for certain carbohydrates, for denatured proteins, and for phosphatidylserine (a surface-exposed component of apoptotic cells). The Toll-like receptors (TLRs) have been described as extremely important PRRs in innate immunity (16). TLRs are a family of receptors that recognizes a variety of molecules specific to pathogens, including surface components such as lipopolysaccharide, peptidoglycan, lipoarabinomannan, lipoteichoic acid, and bacterial deoxyribonucleic acid. Toll, the original family member, is a *Drosophila* membrane receptor essential in host defense against fungi and in embryonic dorsal-ventral patterning. Toll and the mammalian TLRs all are able to activate the NFκB pathway of gene transcription that regulates synthesis of numerous molecules involved in the inflammatory response. TLRs are recruited to phagosomes containing ingested targets (17). However, there is no evidence that the TLRs can themselves initiate phagocytosis. There is no homology between the intracytoplasmic domains of TLRs and receptors known to initiate phagocytosis. In addition, TLRs are widely expressed on cell types such as epithelia and endothelia that are not professional phagocytes. Thus, it is likely that TLRs localized to phagosomes act primarily to signal NFκB activation from PAMPs generated by degradation of an already internalized pathogen in a phagolysosome. In this way, the TLRs are essential for linking phagocytosis to other effector functions of innate immunity.

Other receptors that can interact directly with bacteria and fungi can initiate phagocytosis. For example, CR3, an integrin receptor expressed on phagocytic cells, can bind directly to lipopolysaccharide, *Histoplasma capsulatum, Neisseria gonorrhoeae,* and other pathogens. Cell surface proteins in the scavenger receptor family recognize a wide variety of ligands, including modified proteins; polyanions, including nucleic acids; and acidic phospholipids, including lipopolysaccharides of gram-negative bacteria and lipoteichoic acids of gram-positive bacteria. Other receptors that can mediate nonopsonic recognition of pathogens include CD66 (for Opa-52 on *N. gonorrhoeae*); the integrins $\alpha v\beta 3$ (for *Bordetella pertussis* and *Coxiella burnetii*) and $\alpha 5\beta 1$ (for *H. capsulatum*); and mannose receptor (for multiple organisms, including various *Mycobacteria* species, *Pneumocystic carinii,* and *Borrelia burgdorferi*). Ingestion of apoptotic cells also may involve direct recognition, especially of phosphatidylserine, a lipid not present in the outer leaflet of the plasma membrane unless cell death has occurred. Scavenger receptors can recognize phosphatidylserine. There is evidence that CD36, a class B scavenger receptor, is involved in phagocytosis of apoptotic cells (18), and receptors for apoptotic cells in

C. elegans and *Drosophila* species have homology to scavenger receptors. A mammalian receptor for phosphatidylserine with homology to *C. elegans* and *Drosophila melanogaster* receptors has been identified and demonstrated to participate in phagocytosis of apoptotic cells (19). In general, efficient initiation of phagocytosis by direct recognition of either pathogen or apoptotic targets may require simultaneous engagement of more than one type of receptor. This could provide a level of control in this process of ingestion that might both inhibit undesirable ingestion of host cells and provide a better regulation of the coupling of ingestion to the inflammatory response than could occur if only a single receptor type mediated the entire process of ingestion and initiation of inflammation.

Opsonin Receptors

Successful homeostasis has required the evolution of other mechanisms for recognition and destruction of invaders or damaged tissue. The host response to this challenge has been to evolve a series of soluble proteins that recognize invaders and in turn are recognized by specific receptors on phagocytic cells. These plasma proteins increase the range of microbes recognized as potential pathogens, or extracellular debris recognized as damaged or defective, and they engage potentially more efficient mechanisms for signaling the removal and destruction of the targets to which they attach than do receptors involved in direct recognition of pathogens. The plasma proteins are called *opsonins,* from the Greek *opson,* meaning "to prepare to eat." The classic opsonins of plasma are immunoglobulin and complement, for which there are various receptors on phagocytic cells. It has become clear that there are other opsonins in plasma or other body fluids, including collectins and pentraxins, which may be very important for triggering or regulating phagocytosis.

Immunoglobulin (Ig) Fc Receptors

Fc receptors bind to the Fc portion (immunoglobulin domains C2 to C3 of the heavy chain) of IgG and immunoglobulins A and E (IgA and IgE) molecules. IgG receptors (FcγR) and IgA receptors (FcαR) are widely expressed on professional phagocytes, whereas the high-affinity IgE receptor is expressed exclusively on mast cells and basophils. The phagocytic function of the FcγR has been the most extensively studied. These receptors are immunoglobulin family members with three (FcγRIA) or two (other FcR) extracellular immunoglobulin domains, a single transmembrane segment, and a relatively short cytoplasmic tail, except for human FcγRIIIB, which is anchored to the membrane through a glycosyl-phosphoinositol (GPI) linkage and thus lacks transmembrane and intracellular domains. All phagocyte Fcγ receptors are located within a small region of chromosome 1 in both humans and mice. Most likely is that the different genes evolved from a single ancestral FcγR by a series of duplications. Whereas FcγRI can bind monomeric IgG with nanomolar affinity, FcγRII and FcγRIII are mainly receptors for polyvalent IgG, such as occurs in immune complexes or on antibody-coated bacteria, viruses, or cellular debris. The affinity of different Fcγ receptors differs considerably for immune complexes made with different IgG subclasses. The major histocompatibility complex–related placental Fcγ receptor, which mediates transfer of maternal IgG to the fetus and, because of expression on endothelial cells, regulates IgG lifetime in blood, is not expressed on phagocytes.

FcγRI. FcγRI, with its three immunoglobulin domains, is a high-affinity (1- to 10-nmol) receptor for IgG. There are three FcγRI genes: FcγRIA, FcγRIB, and FcγRIC. FcγRIA is normally expressed on macrophages and monocytes; expression of the protein products of the other two genes is not certain. FcγRI is not normally expressed on PMNs but can be induced by interferon-γ or granulocyte colony-stimulating factor (G-CSF). Like the high-affinity IgE receptor FcεRI FcγRIA is associated with an additional membrane molecule, the γ chain dimer. The γ chain, named because of its association with the α and β chains of FcεRI, is a relative of the ζ chain of the T-cell antigen receptor and of the death-associated protein (DAP)–12 chain of myeloid and natural killer cells. Like ζ and DAP-12, γ mediates receptor signaling via immune-tyrosine activation motifs [ITAMs (20)] and binding of Syk family tyrosine kinases. In contrast to FcεRI, T-cell antigen receptor, and FcγRIIIA (see later discussion), FcγRIA surface expression is not dependent on expression of the signaling γ chain. However, association with γ chain does increase affinity for monomeric IgG about threefold, perhaps by increasing receptor dimerization (21). FcγRI is the only FcγR that has sufficient affinity for ligand to bind monomeric IgG well. Although it can initiate phagocytosis of IgG-coated targets, FcγRI is saturated with monomeric IgG on circulating monocytes. Thus, it may additionally function as a cytophilic antibody similar to FcεRI on basophils and mast cells, requiring only dimeric antigen to induce cell activation.

FcγRII. FcγRII is a medium-affinity Fcγ receptor. As with FcγRI, there are three gene loci that end-code FcγRII proteins: FcγRIIA, FcγRIIB, and FcγRIIC. In human phagocytes, PMNs express only FcγRIIA. Monocytes and macrophages express some FcγRIIB, but FcγRIIA predominates. FcγRIIC has not been detected at the protein level. A polymorphism in the membrane proximal immunoglobulin domain (H131R) of human FcγRIIA leads to an isoform with substantially reduced affinity for IgG2. This may affect host defense, inasmuch as homozygosity for the high-affinity 131H allele is associated with a lower incidence of infections with encapsulated bacteria, for which IgG2 is required for optimal host defense (22).

There are significant differences in function between FcγRIIA and FcγRIIB because of differences in sequence in the cytoplasmic tails of the two receptors. Whereas particle attachment via FcγRIIA leads to phagocytosis, attachment via FcγRIIB does not. Ligation of FcγRIIA with an IgG-opsonized target activates the tyrosine kinase Syk and subsequent signaling events, including the initiation of actin polymerization (23). Although FcγRIIA may, like other phagocyte Fcγ receptors, associate with the ITAM-containing γ chain dimer, its signaling activity critically depends on two of the three tyrosines in its own cytoplasmic tail. These two tyrosines are in ITAM-like motifs, although the spacing between the two critical tyrosines is greater than in a typical ITAM. Nonetheless, Syk appears to bind directly to FcγRIIA and to be activated when these tyrosines are phosphorylated, which suggests that FcγRIIA does have a functional ITAM (24). Also, FcγRIIA functions normally when expressed on macrophages that lack γ chain because of a genetic deletion (25). In contrast, FcγRIIB fails to activate the tyrosine kinase Syk, which is essential for phagocytosis. FcγRIIB does not have an ITAM sequence; instead, its phosphorylated tyrosine is within a sequence that binds the inhibitory Src homology 2 domain–containing inositol 5′-phosphatase (SHIP) (26). SHIP diminishes phagocytosis by counteracting the signaling of phosphatidylinositol 3-kinase (PI3K), and so coligation of FcγRIIB with other Fcγ receptors actually decreases ingestion. In addition, FcγRIIB is constitutively associated with actin microfilaments, which may exclude it from membrane domains active in phagocytosis or may inhibit the actin rearrangements required for ingestion. Thus, ligation of FcγRIIA and ligation of FcγRIIB have opposite effects, inasmuch as the former activates phagocytes and the latter diminishes cell activation.

There is a distinction between murine and human physiology in the function of FcγRII, inasmuch as mouse phagocytes express only the inhibitory FcγRIIB. Thus, the only activating receptors in murine cells are FcγRI and FcγRIII. There is no obvious difference in phagocytosis or other Fcγ receptor functions between murine and human cells, despite this difference in Fcγ receptor representation.

FcγRIII. FcγRIII is encoded by two nearly identical genes: FcγRIIIA and FcγRIIIB. FcγRIIIA is a transmembrane protein with two immunoglobulin domains. There are nine nucleotide differences between the genes encoding FcγRIIIA and FcγRIIIB. A single nucleotide change leads to substitution of Phe at amino acid 185 in FcγRIIIA with Ser in FcγRIIIB, a difference that creates a signal for addition of a GPI anchor rather than a transmembrane domain in FcγRIIIB. FcγRIIIA has intermediate affinity for IgG (30 nmol), whereas FcγRIIIB binds monomeric IgG very poorly, which suggests that the γ chain association of FcγRIIIA may affect ligand affinity, as it does for FcγRI. Macrophages, some monocytes, natural killer cells, and some T-lymphocytes express FcγRIIIA. Only neutrophils constitutively express FcγRIIIB, which is also expressed on eosinophils after exposure to interferon-γ. FcγRIIIA has a sequence in its transmembrane segment that leads to retention in the endoplasmic reticulum unless it is associated with the γ chain. Thus both its signaling and its surface expression are dependent on association with γ chain. In this way, it differs from FcγRI and FcγRII. The

GPI-linked FcγRIIIB is not present in the mouse genome, and so murine leukocytes express only FcγRIIIA. In humans, loss of FcγRIIIB through chromosomal deletion does not cause an obvious increase in susceptibility to bacterial infections (27).

Soluble Fc Receptors. Several Fcγ receptors can be secreted after synthesis from alternatively spliced messenger ribonucleic acids or released from the cell surface by proteolytic cleavage (28). These soluble products are increased in inflammatory diseases and in situations in which phagocyte numbers or turnover is increased. Although these proteins *in vitro* can inhibit immune complex–mediated phagocyte activation by blocking immune complex interaction with cellular Fcγ receptors, the *in vivo* significance of these receptor fragments is unclear.

FcαR. FcαR is expressed on monocytes and PMNs. This receptor has nanomolar affinity for IgA and associates with the γ chain homodimer, like Fcγ receptors. Like FcγRI and FcγRIIA, FcαR expression is not dependent on γ chain association. Because of its relatively high affinity for IgA and its γ chain association, FcαR may have functions similar to those of FcγRI. Although FcαR-mediated phagocytosis has been reported, its phagocytic capacity has not been studied extensively. IgA antibody to some bacteria and viruses actually increases susceptibility to systemic infection and blocks opsonization and phagocytosis *in vitro*, which suggests that IgA does not have a potent opsonic effect. A possible resolution of this dilemma is the discovery that inflammatory mediators can induce FcαR expression on Kupffer cells, the macrophages of the liver that are important for removal of gastrointestinal bacteria that have penetrated intestinal barriers (29). When induced on Kupffer cells, FcαR can mediate the removal of bacteria opsonized with serum (but not secretory) IgA. Expression of FcαR also differs between mouse and human, inasmuch as mice apparently lack this gene (30). The polymeric immunoglobulin receptor, which transports IgA across mucosal barriers, is essential for normal host defense but is not expressed on phagocytes.

Complement Receptors

The complement component C3 is the second major opsonin of serum. During complement activation, C3 is cleaved to C3b and then further to inactivated C3B (iC3b), both of which are covalently attached to the complement-activating surface. Phagocytes express receptors for both of these C3 fragments, and these complement receptors may initiate phagocytosis. Unlike Fc receptors, however, complement receptors are not competent for ingestion in unactivated cells. Instead, phagocytes ingest C3-opsonized targets efficiently only after cell activation, both *in vivo* and *in vitro*. Thus, the capacity of these receptors for ingestion is not constitutive but depends on many other cellular events. Because the primary role of phagocytosis in host defense is at sites of infection and inflammation, where activating stimuli abound, it is likely that at these sites, complement receptors make an important contribution to the phagocytic potential of the responding cells.

Complement Receptor Type 1

Complement receptor type 1 (CR1) is a single-chain type 1 transmembrane protein that is expressed on erythrocytes and glomerular podocytes, as well as on phagocytes and some lymphocytes. CR1 recognizes C3b. The CR1 molecule consists of multiple loose repeats of an approximately 60–amino acid disulfide-bonded domain, known as the short consensus repeat. There are allelic polymorphisms in the number of short consensus repeats expressed by CR1, which have been associated with differences in immune complex clearance and with autoimmunity, but these do not affect the phagocytic function of CR1. Phagocytosis of many complement-opsonized bacteria and other targets is partly inhibited by antibody to CR1, because the complement opsonins on the bacterial surface are a mixture of C3b and iC3b. It is likely that CR1 functions primarily as a receptor that mediates adhesion of the opsonized target to the phagocytic cell, whereas the integrin complement receptors (see below) are responsible primarily for the ingestion signals.

Integrin Complement Receptors

Two phagocyte-specific integrins of the β2 (CD18) family act as receptors for the iC3b fragment of C3. These two are αMβ2 [also known as complement receptor 3 (CR3), Mac1, and CD11b/CD18] and αXβ2 [also known as complement receptor 4 (CR4), p150,95 or CD11c/CD18]. αMβ2 has a special and central role in many PMN adhesion–dependent functions, such as phagocytosis, because its expression is required for multiple other receptors to interact appropriately with the phagocyte cytoskeleton for adhesion and ingestion (31). The central role of this integrin on PMNs is best appreciated by the phenotype of humans, cows, dogs, or transgenic mice with leukocyte adhesion deficiency type I, a complete or almost complete absence of expression of the β2 integrin chain. These patients and animals have severe recurrent infections because of both the failure of PMNs to migrate to sites of infection and the failure of the few cells that do migrate to activate and phagocytose efficiently (32). Migration appears to depend more on the related integrin αLβ2, which is also absent in leukocyte adhesion deficiency; activation and phagocytosis at the site of activation is a property of αMβ2 (33). In the absence of αMβ2, PMNs fail to phagocytose IgG or complement-opsonized targets appropriately; to secrete leukotriene B4 normally after immune complex binding; to generate a normal increase in intracytoplasmic Ca^{2+} in response to FcγR ligation; to make a respiratory burst in response to many inflammatory stimuli; or to phosphorylate the cytoskeleton and adapter protein paxillin (34,35). The ability of integrins to link to cytoskeleton through their cytoplasmic tails suggests that these various effects of αMβ2 on PMN activation may be intimately linked to its effects on cytoskeleton organization in these cells. An additional function of $\alpha M\beta 2$ may be to mediate lateral interactions with other receptors in the phagocyte plasma membrane (36). These lateral interactions have been studied most intensively for Fcγ receptors and the urokinase-plasminogen activator receptor (uPAR), which, like FcγRIIIB, is anchored to the membrane by a GPI link. $\alpha M\beta 2$ cocaps with FcγRIIIB and uPAR in PMNs. When FcγRIIIB is transfected into fibroblasts, cotransfection of $\alpha M\beta 2$ is necessary to make it competent for IgG-mediated phagocytosis (37). Both fluorescence resonance energy transfer and diffusion experiments suggest an intimate association of FcγRIIIB and uPAR with $\alpha M\beta 2$. The link of $\alpha M\beta 2$ with other membrane receptors is not limited to GPI-linked receptors, inasmuch as a variety of evidence demonstrates an association with FcγRIIA and FcαR as well. Together, these data support a model in which the role of $\alpha M\beta 2$ in phagocyte effector mechanisms extends beyond its function as a complement receptor to a general role as an essential component of the adhesive and phagocytic functions of diverse phagocyte plasma membrane receptors.

This more general role in adhesive and phagocytic function may explain another remarkable feature of $\alpha M\beta 2$: the large number of ligands thought to bind to it. These include ICAM-1; fibrinogen; factor X; various bacterial components, including lipopolysaccharide and lipopeptides; denatured proteins; heparan sulfates; and yeast glucans, in addition to iC3b. Because many of these potential ligands have been defined by antibody inhibition of adhesion to ligand-coated particles and surfaces, the more fundamental role for $\alpha M\beta 2$ in PMN adhesion and cytoskeleton-dependent activation may require that these results be interpreted with caution.

$\alpha X\beta 2$ is less abundant than $\alpha M\beta 2$ on PMNs and monocytes but increases in expression as monocytes differentiate into macrophages *in vitro* and in tissues. Like $\alpha M\beta 2$, $\alpha X\beta 2$ binds iC3b and fibrinogen, although there is no evidence that it interacts with any other of the wide spectrum of potential CR3 ligands. Like $\alpha M\beta 2$, $\alpha X\beta 2$ can mediate phagocytosis, but its other physiological functions may differ. For example, ligation of $\alpha X\beta 2$, but not $\alpha M\beta 2$, induces a respiratory burst in human PMNs (38). In mice, $\alpha X\beta 2$ is present on many dendritic cells and some tissue T cells but not on most tissue macrophages. To date, a detailed comparison of the roles of $\alpha X\beta 2$ and $\alpha M\beta 2$ in phagocytosis has not been undertaken.

Activation of Complement Receptors for Phagocytosis

As discussed previously, complement receptors on unactivated cells bind opsonized targets but do not initiate phagocytosis. A fundamental question about their function is how they gain the ability to ingest when phagocytes are activated by cytokines, chemoattractants, lipid messengers, extracellular matrix proteins, or other signals present at sites of inflammation. How the integrin complement receptors activate has been much better studied than CR1. There are two distinct properties of the integrins that are altered by cell activation. First, affinity for ligand increases; second, there is increased

clustering of these receptors within the plasma membrane. It is very likely that both these changes contribute to activation of phagocytosis. A general property of leukocyte integrins is the requirement for cell activation to induce high affinity for their ligands, a phenomenon called *inside-out activation.* The conformational change in the integrin induced by inside-out activation that leads to increased affinity is now determined at the atomic level for integrins, such as CR3 and CR4, which contain an inserted ligand-binding domain known as an I domain. An α helix in the integrin I domain moves away from the ligand binding site, making it more accessible to ligand. This conformational change has been estimated to increase affinity of $\alpha L\beta 2$, an integrin closely related to $\alpha M\beta 2$ and $\alpha X\beta 2$, for its ligand ICAM-1 by 10,000-fold (39). Similar affinity measurements have not yet been made for the phagocyte integrin complement receptors. How the conformational change in the I domain, distant from the plasma membrane, is induced by intracellular signaling is not yet known.

Second, integrin clustering occurs on cell activation. The initiation of clustering involves release of unclustered integrins from cytoskeletal constraint to diffusion, perhaps through regulation of microtubule function by activation of the GTPase Rho (40,41). These integrins are now free to diffuse and can become clustered, perhaps through the interaction of ligated integrins with cytoskeletal and adapter proteins [e.g., Fyb/SLAP130 (42,43)]. Integrin clustering may result from a conformational change in the extracellular domain, inasmuch as $\alpha L\beta 2$ missing its I domain spontaneously clusters (44). Integrin clustering can induce adhesion to ligand-coated substrates and targets. Integrin diffusion and clustering as a result of inside-out signaling is likely to be very important in activation of complement-mediated phagocytosis. Enhanced receptor diffusion was shown to be necessary for complement-mediated phagocytosis in experiments in the 1970s (45), but the role of receptor clustering was not tested in those early experiments because the molecular identity of the complement receptor was not yet known. How the potentially independent processes of affinity modulation and clustering each contribute to induction of phagocytic competence of C3 receptors is not yet determined. This is clearly an area in which thorough study would lead to improved understanding of cellular regulation of phagocytosis.

Collectins and Their Receptors

Collectins (named for for *col*lagenous *lectins*) are oligomeric C-type lectins covalently associated with collagen-like domains that initiate their multimerization by forming triple helices. Collectins can bind to a variety of bacterial carbohydrates to initiate host defense. Two collectins, surfactant proteins A and D, are found only on mucosal surfaces in the lung and the gastrointestinal tract; three others—mannose-binding lectin (MBL), conglutinin, and collectin-43—are serum proteins synthesized in the liver (46). To date, conglutinin and collectin-43 have been found only in cattle; thus, most studies on the role of collectins in host defense have focused on MBL and the surfactant proteins. The surfactant proteins can act as opsonins to enhance phagocytosis by alveolar macrophages and can also act as macrophage chemoattractants. This is thought to be a major mechanism of innate host defense at mucosae, especially in the lung. MBL apparently can initiate phagocytosis by two distinct mechanisms (47). First, it can opsonize bacteria for direct recognition and ingestion. The molecular nature of the receptor or receptors that recognize MBL is controversial; both CR1 (the C3b receptor) and a heavily glycosylated type I membrane protein termed C1qRP have been shown to have this property. Second, MBL bound to bacteria can initiate the classical pathway of complement activation through a serine protease, MBL-associated serine protease (MASP)–2, related to the proteolytic (C1r and C1s) subunits of the first component of complement. From this perspective, it is not surprising that C1q, the third subunit of C1 is closely related structurally to collectins. Like MBL, C1q binds to both CR1 and C1qRP (48). Thus, from the point of view of a phagocytic cell, both C1q and MBL can directly opsonize bacteria and can amplify bacteria-phagocyte interaction by initiating the deposition of C3b and iC3b.

Pentraxins and Their Receptors

Pentraxins are so named because they consist of a radially symmetric arrangement of five identical, noncovalently linked chains in a pentagonal array. Two pentraxins, serum amyloid P component (SAP) and C-reactive protein (CRP), are rapidly produced in the liver in response to inflammation through activation of their transcription by a variety of cytokines. In humans, CRP levels in particular respond to inflammation, increasing as much as 1,000-fold within hours of acute infection. In the mouse, SAP appears to be more responsive than CRP to inflammatory signals. The pentraxin bind their ligand—which includes a diverse array of substances such as phosphocholine, fibronectin, chromatin, histones, and ribonucleoprotein—in a calcium-dependent manner (49). Like collectins, CRP can activate complement through the classical pathway and also has a cell surface receptor. Evidence has been presented that both CRP and SAP can bind to Fcγ receptors, especially FcγRI and FcγRIII, although there are differences between human and murine receptors (50). In addition, CRP may bind to human FcγRIIA on neutrophils; however, this view has been challenged (51). Thus, pentraxins, like both collectins and immunoglobulin, can induce recognition of pathogenic organisms by two mechanisms, direct interaction with a phagocyte cell surface receptor and activation of complement, which result in deposition of C3-derived opsonins on the surface of the invader.

Mechanisms of Phagocytosis

The Zipper Hypothesis

In 1977, Silverstein et al. (5) proposed a model for phagocytosis that has guided much of the research in the field.

According to their zipper hypothesis, phagocytosis requires repeated interactions between ligands on the target particle and receptors on the phagocytic cell, and interruption of the formation of new interactions at any point prevents ingestion of the particle. In this model, the phagocytic cell moves over the target like a zipper. Most of the data in favor of the model have been obtained from studies of Fc receptor–mediated phagocytosis. During phagocytosis of IgG-coated particles, the phagocyte plasma membrane protrudes around the target. Interaction between the plasma membrane of the phagocytic cell and the ingestion target is close at the leading edge of these protrusions but more distant at the base of the phagocytic cup. Actin microfilaments polymerize and organize at the leading edge of the zipper as well, whereas the actin at the base of the phagocytic cup is less organized. This depolymerization may be necessary to allow fusion of the forming phagosome with intracellular vesicles, both as a source of membrane for completion of the phagocytic event and as a source of enzymes involved in killing and destruction of invading pathogens. An implication of the zipper hypothesis is that the signal transduction involved in phagocytosis is very localized, because the processes that occur at the leading edge of the membrane protrusion and those at the base of the phagocytic cup are quite different. The localized nature of the membrane events was demonstrated elegantly in an experiment in which Griffin and Silverstein (52) showed that unactivated macrophages (which have nonphagocytic complement receptors) that had both complement-coated pneumococci and IgG-coated erythrocytes bound to their surfaces ingested only the IgG-coated particles, even though the pneumococci and erythrocytes were contiguous on the macrophage plasma membrane. There is some evidence that phagocytosis is localized to membrane rafts, specialized regions of the plasma membrane enriched in glycosphingolipids, cholesterol, GPI-anchored proteins, and certain signaling molecules (53). This requirement for raft association could explain the confinement of phagocytic signals to small regions of the plasma membrane. However, this hypothesis remains controversial, in part because the nature and functions of the raft domains in cells remain difficult to manipulate experimentally.

Morphological Differences between Crystallized Fragment and Complement Receptor Phagocytosis

Since the 1970s, it has been clear that ingestion of complement-coated particles (by activated macrophages) and IgG-coated targets are morphologically distinguishable (6,54,55). As mentioned, in Fcγ receptor–mediated phagocytosis, membrane protrusion around the target is a prominent feature; in complement-mediated ingestion, in contrast, the target appears to sink into the macrophage. This morphological difference suggests there may be a difference in mechanism of ingestion and has led to questions about whether the zipper hypothesis and its implication of localized signaling are true for all phagocytosis or just for Fc receptor–mediated ingestion. In fact, basic questions about the mechanism of complement receptor–mediated ingestion remain unanswered. No study of whether repeated interactions between target cell ligands and complement receptors are required for ingestion, the *sine qua non* of the zipper hypothesis, has been reported. As discussed later, certain biochemical differences between complement receptor phagocytosis and Fcγ receptor phagocytosis have been described, but whether these result in fundamental changes in mechanism is not known.

Signaling Events in Fcγ Receptor–Mediated Phagocytosis

The Tyrosine Kinase Syk Is Critical for Initiation of Phagocytosis

The evolution of phagocytosis through receptor engagement and clustering, actin polymerization, membrane addition and extension, and, finally, membrane fusion suggests that there must be an evolution of signaling events that accompany these processes. This possibility has been studied in some detail for Fc receptor–mediated ingestion. When Fc receptors are ligated and clustered, tyrosine kinases are activated. The cytoplasmic domains of the phagocytic Fc receptors contain tyrosines within ITAMs. As shown by mutagenesis studies, these tyrosines are required for phagocytosis. ITAM-mediated activation requires the tyrosine kinase Syk; in accordance with this model, Syk is required for Fc receptor–mediated ingestion, as shown by pharmacological inhibition, antisense, and gene-disruption experiments (56,57). Whether Syk activation is the earliest signaling event in Fc receptor phagocytosis is debated. Syk activation apparently requires phosphorylation of the tyrosines within the ITAM, and, in many circumstances, ITAM tyrosines are phosphorylated by members of the Src family of kinases. However, genetic deletion of Hck, Fgr, and Lyn, the three major Src family kinases of macrophages, delays but does not inhibit Fc receptor–mediated ingestion (58). Thus, it is possible that Syk itself, which can associate with Fc receptors in the absence of ITAM phosphorylation, can phosphorylate the Fc receptor ITAM when the receptors are sufficiently clustered by ligand. In this model, Src family kinases can accelerate, but are not required for, the process.

A number of signaling events relevant to phagocytosis occur as a result of Syk activation. Syk can act not only as a kinase but also as a docking molecule for other signaling effectors. Syk activation leads to actin polymerization, apparently through activation of PI3K, the Rho family GTPases, and p21-activated kinase (PAK), which in turn can activate the Wiskott-Aldrich syndrome protein (WASP) and the Arp2/3 complex, which together increase the number of nucleation sites for actin polymerization (59). Syk activation also leads to activation of phospholipase C, which in turn generates the mediators diacylglycerol and IP3. Although the increase in cytoplasmic Ca^{2+} that results from IP3 generation apparently is not absolutely required for phagocytosis, the diacylglycerol is. Diacylglycerol released by Fc receptor ligation activates both classical and novel protein kinase C (PKC) isoforms (60), and the novel isoforms δ and ε are required for phagocytosis. Protein kinase Cα, on the other hand, apparently links Fc receptor ligation to effector mechanisms of inflammation, such as activation of the respiratory burst and generation of lipid mediators of inflammation. Exactly why protein kinase C is required for phagocytosis is not known; it may influence both actin polymerization and delivery of membrane to the nascent phagosome.

Phosphatidylinositols in Crystallized Fragment Receptor–Mediated Phagocytosis

The phosphatidylinositol lipids phosphatidylinositol 4,5-bisphosphate (PIP2) and phosphatidylinositol 3,4,5-trisphosphate (PIP3) play critical roles in phagocytosis. PIP3 is generated from PIP2 by PI3K. There is probably more than one role for PI3K in phagocytosis. As mentioned previously, PIP3 is required for the activation of actin polymerization, and studies with pharmacological inhibitors of the enzyme demonstrate that pseudopod extension, which depends on actin polymerization, is inefficient in cells with inhibited PI3K (61). PI3K inhibitors also block membrane closure and retraction events required for phagocytosis (62), which suggests the potential involvement of the enzyme both in recruitment of myosin and in the final fusion events of phagosome formation. Furthermore, PI3K is present on some intracellular membrane vesicular compartments and may be required for vesicle fusion with plasma membrane-derived phagosomes (63), which suggests that it may have a role in delivery of membrane to nascent phagosomes as well. In the absence of membrane delivery from intracellular vesicles, phagocytosis is blocked (64).

The central role for PI3K in so many steps of ingestion represents an apparent challenge to the central tenet of the zipper hypothesis: that signaling is localized in space. Because the product of PI3K is a lipid, it appears to be able to diffuse rapidly from its site of synthesis. Plextrin homology domain–containing proteins that interact with PIP3 would not obviously be confined to the membrane at the site of ingestion. However, PIP3 appears not to diffuse away from its site of formation, apparently because of a marked restriction of diffusion at the site of Fc receptor ligation (65). This mechanism for this very important aspect of Fc receptor signaling, central to the validity of the zipper hypothesis, is unknown. It is possible that plextrin homology domain–containing cytoskeletal proteins that simultaneously bind PIP3 and microfilaments can restrict diffusion of the lipid.

The plasma membrane lipid PIP2 has been recognized as important in phagocytosis as well (66). The PIP2 concentration increases rapidly at sites of Fc receptor ligation, where it is presumably restricted by mechanisms similar to those that restrict PIP3. The increase in PIP2 is thought to be dependent on local recruitment of phosphatidylinositol 4-phosphate 5-kinase and can be temporally correlated with the increase in F-actin at the nascent phagocytic cup. PIP2

phagocytosis and focal contact formation may represent specializations of a general adhesion apparatus common to both functions. However, differences between the two events may be equally relevant, because there is no evidence for receptor alignment or actin stress fibers (prominent features of focal adhesions) in phagocytosis and no evidence for delivery of intracellular membranes and membrane fusion (necessary features of phagocytosis) in focal contact formation.

Regulation of F-Actin Organization

The dynamic regulation of the three-dimensional structure of the cytoskeletal complexes that associate with phagosomes is complex. Actin filaments within the extending pseudopods that arise during FcγR phagocytosis are arranged in parallel arrays, cross-linked by several actin-bundling proteins such as ABP-120, L-plastin, and α-actinin. At the base of the phagocytic cup, the actin filaments are less ordered. Actin polymerization occurs primarily at the extending tips of the pseudopod, and there is net depolymerization at the base of the forming phagosome. Presumably, depolymerization aids fusion with intracellular vesicles and may be required for further steps in phagosome maturation. Despite its importance, little is understood about this aspect of phagosome-cytoskeleton interaction.

Localization of Signaling Proteins to the Phagosome

The analogy between phagosomes and focal adhesions extends to interactions between signaling molecules and the cytoskeleton. In focal adhesions, the cytoskeleton can form a scaffold for recruitment of signaling molecules such as kinases and phosphatases, lipid-modifying enzymes, and many adapter and regulatory proteins that are important for coordination of the events of phagocytosis. This provides a mechanism to bring phagocytic receptors, "activatable" enzymes, and their substrates into close proximity at the forming phagosome. Because multiple, sequential interactions are required for some kinds of phagocytosis, the relevant molecular events that arise from receptor–ligand interaction must be regulated very locally, so that the signals are confined to the immediate vicinity of the receptor. Both the cytoskeleton and the membrane environment of the phagosome may contribute to containment of these signals. It is intriguing that, although the events that pertain to ingestion remain quite local, phagocytosis can give rise to signals that affect gene expression in the nucleus; thus there must be exquisite control over which signals are "contained" and which "escape" the local environment of the phagocytic receptor.

Generation of the Forces Necessary for Engulfment

There exist three models that may explain the generation of forces required to extend pseudopodia and engulf particles during phagocytosis. The first model predicts that the forces generated by actin polymerization are sufficient to cause membrane extension. This is quite analogous to current models for generation of the force of locomotion (95). However, this model cannot account for the contractile force necessary for internalization of the phagosome. The second model adds actin cross-linking and gel-osmotic forces to actin polymerization in linking actin polymerization to the membrane protrusions. There is evidence for NHE1 activation during phagocytosis, occurring both with FcγR ligation and with CR3 ligation (96); this could lead to localized osmotic changes necessary for the cytoplasmic gel to cause membrane protrusion (97). However, there has been no direct test of whether NHE1 activation is required for phagocytosis. The third model predicts that actin-myosin complexes generate a motor force that drives phagocytosis. In accordance with this hypothesis, inhibitors of both the myosin ATPase and myosin light-chain kinase block FcγR-mediated phagocytosis (98). The nature of the myosin required for phagocytosis is uncertain. Involvement of myosin light chain suggests that "conventional" nonmuscle myosin (myosin II) is involved in the process, whereas genetic evidence from *Dictyostelium* organisms demonstrates important roles for myosin I and myosin VII rather than myosin II in phagocytosis. Myosin I appears to regulate actin polymerization during phagocytosis, whereas myosin VII regulates attachment of ingestion targets (99). Myosin I isoforms also have been implicated in *Entamoeba histolytica* phagocytosis by erythrocytes and in macrophage FcγR-mediated ingestion.

Phagosome and Phagolysosome Formation

The efficient engulfment of a phagocytic target requires delivery of intracellular membranes to the site of ingestion. If this did not occur, the surface area of a phagocyte would decrease during phagocytosis. However, careful measurements have demonstrated that the surface area of macrophages actually increases during the phagocytic process. The processes of exocytosis and membrane recycling are required for the addition of intracellular membranes to the cell surface during phagocytosis and depend on similar cell machinery [e.g., N-ethylmaleimide-sensitive fusion protein (NSF) and vesicle-associated soluble NSF attachment protein receptors (v-SNAREs)] as other exocytic processes. Blockade of rapid recycling of intracellular vesicles back to the plasma membrane inhibits phagocytosis. In macrophages, the GTPase Rab11 participates in the recruitment of a rapid recycling endocytic compartment to the plasma membrane during phagocytosis, and this recruitment is essential for optimal ingestion (100). In addition, the GTPase dynamin 2 recruits additional membrane to the nascent phagosome (101). In neutrophils, it is clear that regulated exocytosis leads to fusion of primary and secondary granules with the nascent phagosome that has not yet budded off the plasma membrane. This leads to leakage of contents of these granules into the extracellular space during robust ingestion. Thus, the initial phagosome is formed from plasma membrane and membranes of exocytic vesicles.

When fluid phase endocytosis occurs, there is an ordered fusion of the endocytic vesicle with a variety of intracellular vesicles, with sorting of intravesicle contents into different pathways, leading to recycling of some components of the endosome to the plasma membrane and eventual delivery of other endocytosed components to the lysosomal compartment for degradation. In macrophages, phagosomes appear to follow a similar pathway to fusion with lysosomes as the endocytic vesicles destined for lysosomal degradation. In endosome maturation, the Rab small GTPases are important in the fusion of endosomes with specific intracellular vesicles so that orderly maturation is maintained. This appears to be true for phagosomes as well, because Rab5 mediates fusion of early endosomes with phagosomes and Rab7 mediates fusion with late endosomes (102). Some intracellular pathogens specifically block phagosome-endosome fusion at discrete steps along this cascade, presumably to create a more amenable environment for survival (see later discussion). Fusion of late phagosomes (i.e., after interaction with the endosome pathway) with lysosomes appears to be calcium dependent, unlike the earlier fusion events. In neutrophils, phagosome maturation may occur through different mechanisms, because they have a small endocytic compartment and no true lysosomes. Instead, the primary (azurophil) granule substitutes for a lysosome and fuses directly with the base of the phagosome as it develops. Whether Rabs regulate this fusion event is unknown.

The identification of approximately 140 proteins associated with phagosomes in macrophages by a proteomic two-dimensional gel analysis has provided a glimpse into the complexity of phagolysosome biogenesis and intriguing possibilities for linking phagocytosis to subsequent cellular responses (9) (Fig. 3). Many proteins expected to be present were identified, including hydrolases, proteins involved in membrane fusion, actin-binding proteins, and proton pump subunits. Other, unexpected proteins were also detected. These included proteins involved in signaling apoptosis, the lipid-raft associated protein flotillin, and a complex of proteins from the endoplasmic reticulum, including calnexin and calreticulin. The presence of these proteins suggests that the phagosome may function as a platform for the recruitment of signaling pathways linking ingestion to downstream effectors.

Consequences of Phagocytosis

When phagocytic receptors are engaged, intracellular signals are generated not only to initiate ingestion but also to activate effector functions appropriate to the physiological circumstances. During infection and inflammation, engagement of phagocytic receptors may activate degranulation, respiratory burst, and metabolic pathways, leading to generation of inflammatory mediators such as leukotrienes, cytokines, and chemokines and of molecules involved in cross-talk between the innate immune system and effectors of specific immunity, such as B cells and T cells. Phagocytosis of apoptotic cells, in contrast, occurs during resolution of inflammation or

development, situations in which activation of inflammatory cascades could be harmful. Thus, it might be expected that the consequences of ingestion of apoptotic cells are quite distinct from those of phagocytosis of bacteria, necrotic cells, foreign bodies, or tissue debris. Very often, the signaling cascades that activate these effector mechanisms during phagocytosis are distinct from those involved in the ingestion process itself. For example, extracellular signal–regulated protein kinase (ERK) activation is a prominent consequence of $Fc\gamma R$-mediated phagocytosis and is important for both degranulation and activation of transcription of proinflammatory genes; however, ERK inhibition does not affect the ingestion process itself.

Phagocytosis of IgG-opsonized targets is the prototype of a proinflammatory signal. In general, the signaling cascades activated to induce these proinflammatory functions are distinct from those involved in phagocytosis itself, although, like phagocytosis itself, all are initiated by Syk. $Fc\gamma R$-mediated phagocytosis is associated with activation of the reduced nicotinamide adenine dinucleotide phosphate (NADPH) oxidase, through a pathway requiring activation of the α isoform of protein kinase C. This may represent a distinct signaling pathway from the involvement of protein kinase C in the ingestion process, which apparently involves the atypical isoforms of protein kinase C, δ and ϵ. Ligation of $Fc\gamma$ receptors also is associated with activation of phospholipase A_2, with consequent release and metabolism of arachidonic acid to leukotriene B_4 and generation of platelet-activating factor from lysophosphatidic acid. All these products are proinflammatory. $Fc\gamma R$ ligation also activates tumor necrosis factor α (TNF-α) production, apparently through activation of an ERK (103). The combined effects of TNF-α and $Fc\gamma R$ ligation also can activate the NFκB pathway for expression of inflammatory gene products (104). NFκB activation during IgG-mediated phagocytosis may require activation of the NADPH oxidase as an intermediate step. Another potential pathway to NFκB activation during phagocytosis is through TLRs, which can activate NFκB through a pathway similar to that of IL-1. Whether this pathway is activated during phagocytosis of intact bacteria, fungi, or other pathogens is not yet known.

Phagocytosis of apoptotic cells is the opposite extreme from $Fc\gamma R$-mediated ingestion, because it not only does not elicit proinflammatory effectors but also actively suppresses these events, which is concordant with its role in the resolution of inflammation. Phagocytosis of apoptotic cells induces secretion of transforming growth factor β (TGF-β), which appears to be the mechanism for suppression of inflammation (11). A number of macrophage receptors have been implicated in recognition and phagocytosis of apoptotic cells, including scavenger receptors, the integrin $\alpha v\beta 3$, CD14, and a cloned receptor for phosphatidylserine. Which of these is important for signaling TGF-β synthesis is not certain. Ligation of αv integrins or the phosphatidylserine receptor on macrophages can induce TGF-β secretion, and so these are leading candidates for involvement in this mechanism of

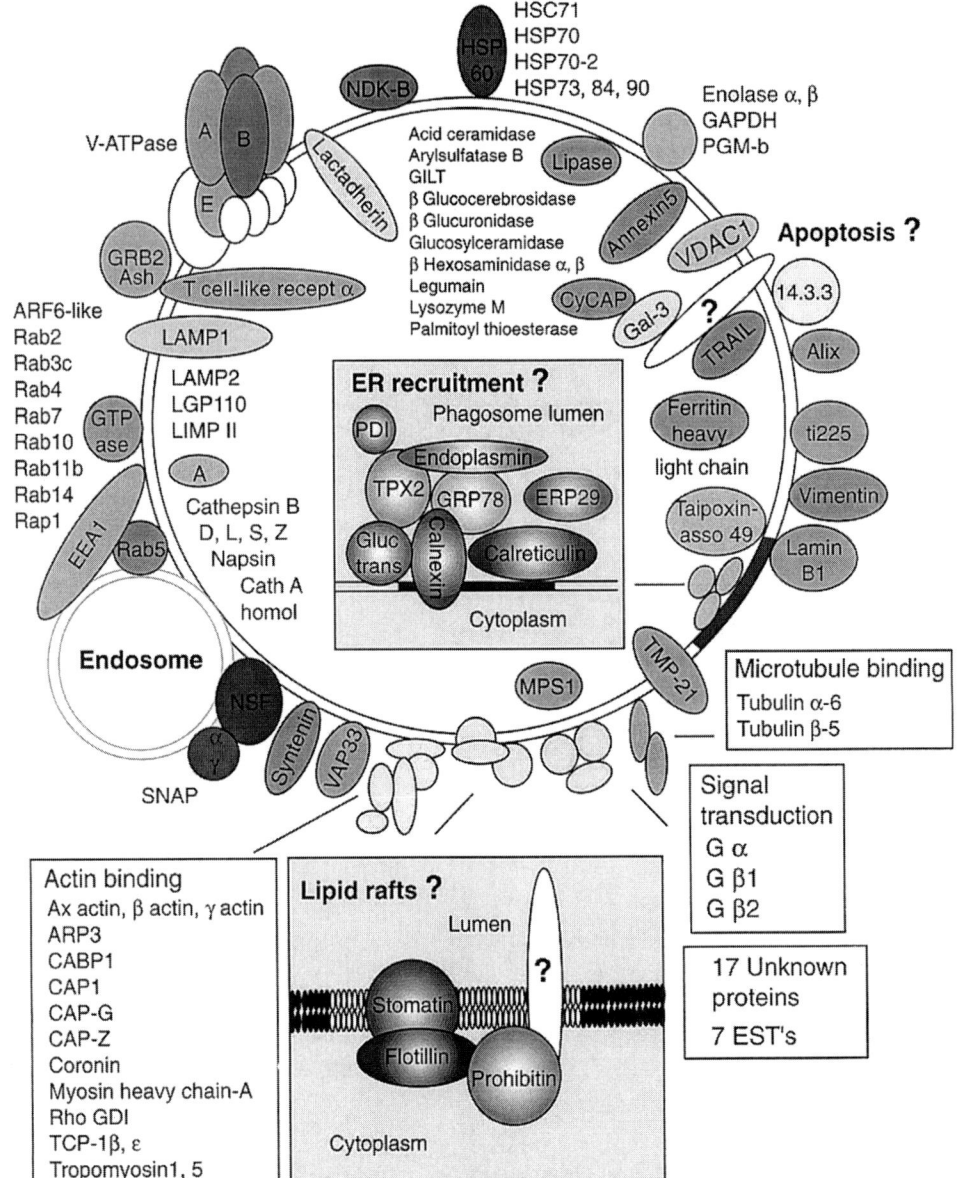

FIG. 3. The virtual phagosome. Proteomic approaches have led to the identification of numerous phagosome-associated molecules, which provides new insights into the function, formation, and dynamic changes of the phagolysosome. From Garin et al. (9), with permission.

suppression of inflammation (19,105). However, nothing is known of the signaling pathways that might lead from these receptors to induction of TGF-β.

Phagocytosis through CR3 lies between the extremes of IgG-mediated ingestion and phagocytosis of apoptotic cells. Unlike phagocytosis of apoptotic cells, it clearly does not suppress inflammation. On the other hand, its connection to proinflammatory effector mechanisms is less absolute than for FcγR. In some instances, CR3-mediated ingestion does not lead to activation of the respiratory burst or generation of arachidonate metabolites, whereas in other cases, it does. The reason for this difference in effect of engagement of the same receptor may depend on the site on the receptor engaged, the

extent of cross-linking of the receptor, engagement of additional cell surface receptors, or the state of activation of the cell. TNF-α pretreatment of neutrophils enhances CR3-mediated activation of the respiratory burst through recruitment of Syk, which is otherwise not engaged during CR3 phagocytosis (106).

Another consequence of phagocytosis in mammalian phagocytes involves nutrient uptake that is necessary for lipid-mediated signaling. Like CR3-mediated ingestion, the mechanisms for nutrient uptake may activate both non-inflammatory and proinflammatory signaling pathways. CD14, a GPI-anchored protein expressed by phagocytes that mediates recognition and ingestion of apoptotic cells (noninflammatory) (107) and delivery of lipopolysaccharide from gram-negative bacteria to TLR4 (proinflammatory), also internalizes phosphatidylinositol, which monocytes and macrophages use as a major source of arachidonate for leukotriene synthesis (108). CD14-mediated uptake of phosphatidylinositol does not lead to activation of the cells. In contrast, macrophage uptake of lipoproteins associated with extracellular matrix is a key step in the proinflammatory events leading to atherogenesis (109). Although the receptors involved in uptake of matrix-bound lipoprotein have not been characterized, the mechanism is known to involve cytoskeleton and Rho family GTPases, which thus demonstrates similarity to more conventional phagocytic processes. It is intriguing to speculate that the lipid-recognition receptors involved in bacterial lipoprotein and lipopolysaccharide activation of phagocytes are also involved in this process, linking phagocytosis to atherogenesis.

Regulation of Phagocytosis

Because uptake of nutrients into a digestive vacuole is at the core of the phagocytic process, phagocytosing cells logically express receptors that sense the environment and inform the cell of the presence of appropriate particulate nutrients. This is exemplified by the promotion of feeding behavior in *Dictyostelium* organisms by environmental folic acid signaling through a specific G protein–coupled receptor that stimulates uptake of nutrient bacteria (110). In response to this signal, the ameba moves efficiently toward the nutrient source and maximally activates the cell machinery necessary for optimal uptake. Similarly, bacterial formylated peptides stimulate both the migration toward bacteria and the phagocytic activity of mammalian neutrophils through G protein–coupled receptors (111). These and other environmental cues regulate phagocytic responses (a) through effects on efficiency and extent of ingestion by phagocytic cells and (b) by modulation of the signaling pathways engaged by phagocytic receptors. Whereas the marking of phagocytic targets by opsonins has long been recognized to engage specific receptor-mediated signaling pathways, the contribution of environmental signals to the alteration of these pathways is less well understood. Environmental regulation is composed of both positive and negative signals that act to tune the phagocytic response to an appropriate threshold. This homeostatic control limits the release of self-damaging products generated by the phagocytic process to the site of infection or inflammation. Thus, unactivated circulating phagocytes are capable of only minimal ingestion, and they develop their full phagocytic potential after exposure to additional signals, such as bacterial peptides, fragments of complement, clotting proteins, arachidonate metabolites, and cytokines that predominate at sites of infection and inflammation. One important function of these positive signals is to overcome negative signals that act as constitutive brakes on ingestion. Negative signals are important for raising the threshold of phagocyte activation, terminating overwhelming inflammatory responses, and dis-

criminating between an appropriate target and a host cell that are marked for uptake. Host cells express molecules that send a "don't eat me" signal through these negative regulatory mechanisms. Both positive and negative signals must be coordinated with the signals provided by the primary opsonin receptor ("eat me") to provide fine control of the phagocytic response. Thus, the overall milieu in which a phagocyte exists directly affects its phagocytic potential.

Positive Regulation

A major mechanism to enhance the rate and extent of phagocytosis by neutrophils and monocytes is adhesion to extracellular matrix proteins. Teleologically, phagocytes contact extracellular matrix in tissues only after exodus from the blood, and this acts to inform these cells that they have migrated out of the vasculature and are present at a site of infection or tissue injury in which their full phagocytic potential is required. Demonstrated initially for fibronectin-induced enhancement of both FcγR- and complement-mediated ingestion by monocytes (112), this mechanism been extended to include neutrophils, multiple opsonins, and additional adhesive proteins, including entactin, laminin, collagen, fibrinogen, and vitronectin. The signal for enhanced phagocytosis by many of these adhesive proteins is mediated by a short peptide sequence, Arg-Gly-Asp, contained within these molecules. Although this peptide is a recognition motif for multiple members of the integrin receptor family, αvβ3 integrin expressed by both monocytes and neutrophils plays an essential role in adhesive protein-amplified phagocytic responses (113,114). Phagocyte activation by this receptor has been studied in depth; it involves the physical association of αvβ3 with an immunoglobulin superfamily member, CD47 (integrin-associated protein) (115). That these two proteins function as a signal transduction unit for enhancement of phagocytosis was confirmed by the failure of neutrophils from CD47-deficient mice to enhance IgG-dependent ingestion when stimulated with an Arg-Gly-Asp peptide mimic (116). In addition to αvβ3, some β1 integrins expressed by monocytes and neutrophils can also send a signal that stimulates phagocytosis through IgG and complement receptors.

Chemotactic peptides and certain cytokines, including G-CSF, granulocyte-macrophage colony-stimulating factor, and TNF-α, also stimulate phagocytosis. The first description of a cytokine-stimulating phagocytic potential was the demonstration that CR3 on macrophages could be converted from a primarily attachment-promoting receptor to a fully phagocytic receptor after exposure of the cells to an as yet uncharacterized T-lymphocyte–derived cytokine (117). Subsequent work in neutrophils revealed that exposure to cytokines and chemotactic peptides could enhance FcγR-mediated ingestion as well. These studies gave rise to the concept that neutrophils express two distinct molecular mechanisms for FcγR-mediated phagocytosis that use distinct signal transduction pathways (111) and distinct effector mechanisms, distinguished by their dependence or independence of β2 integrin function (73). These studies and others assessing the role of the αvβ3/CD47 complex in the activation of αMβ2 (118,119) clearly implicate αMβ2 function in the ability of matrix proteins, chemotactic peptides, and cytokines to positively regulate phagocytosis independently of the primary opsonin receptor. Involvement of αMβ2 involves its activation by the cytokines and chemokines, through affinity modulation and clustering, as described previously. Although the precise intracellular signals that lead to αMβ2 activation are poorly understood, seem to be at least two distinct pathways (120). Whatever the molecular mechanism involved, it is intriguing to speculate that cooperative signaling from multiple receptors may recruit additional signals for remodeling of the cytoskeleton. Because distinct Rho family GTPases have been implicated in FcγR- and αMβ2-mediated ingestion (see previous discussion), it is possible that cytokine or matrix protein activation of αMβ2 could enhance FcγR-mediated phagocytosis by recruiting additional GTPase function for maximal actin remodeling.

Negative Regulation

There has emerged a paradigm that negative regulation of leukocyte activation is essential for homeostasis and therefore is necessary for normal initiation, amplification, and termination of immune and inflammatory responses (121). Although negative signals, and the pathological sequelae of their absence, have been best studied in B-lymphocytes, natural killer cells, and mast cells, it is clear that they also play an important role in regulating phagocytosis. Phagocytic signals can be limited or attenuated by either of two inhibitory signaling receptors, FcγRIIb (122,123) and signal regulatory protein α (SIRPα) (also known as SHPS-1, BIT, or P84) (124,125) expressed by the phagocyte. These plasma membrane receptors are two members of an expanding family of immune inhibitory receptors that contains more than 20 members and can be identified by a consensus amino acid sequence, the immunoreceptor tyrosine-based inhibitory motif (ITIM), in the cytoplasmic domain. This motif contains a tyrosine surrounded by five amino acids (the prototype being Ile/Val/Leu/Ser-X-Tyr-X-X-Leu/Val); most immune inhibitory receptors contain between one and four ITIMS. Receptor clustering results in tyrosine phosphorylation within the ITIM, most probably by an Src kinase family member, providing a docking site for the recruitment of cytoplasmic phosphatases that have an Src homology 2 domain. One tyrosine phosphatase, SHP-1, and a lipid phosphatase, SHIP, have been demonstrated to negatively regulate both FcγR- and αMβ2-mediated phagocytosis (124,126).

Inhibition of phagocytosis by FcγRIIb derives from its ability to bind the same IgG-opsonized target recognized by an activating FcγR. Thus, both positive and negative signals are generated anytime a phagocyte encounters an IgG-opsonized target, and all FcγR-mediated signals in addition to phagocytosis are attenuated. This pairing of an activating

and an inhibiting receptor by ligand cross-linking raises the threshold necessary to observe a phagocytic response and thereby limits tissue injury caused by FcγR activation. For example, mice that lack FcγRIIb are more susceptible to immune complex–induced injury than are normal mice (122). In contrast to its role in inhibiting immune complex disease, FcγRIIb has no effect on FcγR-mediated uptake of IgG1-opsonized autologous red blood cells by splenic macrophages in a murine model of autoimmune hemolytic anemia (127). This suggests that additional regulatory mechanisms must exist on splenic macrophages to prevent uptake of autologous red blood cells. In this regard, SIRPα inhibits uptake of either unopsonized or opsonized autologous red blood cells by the spleen (125,128). Unlike FcγRIIb, SIRPα recognizes not an activating ligand but rather a cell adhesion molecule, CD47, expressed on the surface of the red blood cell (129). In this manner, CD47 expression by the target cell delivers a "don't eat me" signal to the macrophage through ligation of SIRPα. Thus, CD47 and SIRPα function as two components of a cell recognition system whose interaction negatively regulates destruction of autologous cells by activated phagocytes. SIRPα and FcγRIIb differ not only in their ligand recognition and their mechanism of action but also in which phosphatases they recruit; SIRPα recruits SHP-1, which acts to decrease tyrosine phosphorylation stimulated by the activating receptor (124), and FcγRIIb recruits SHIP, which limits phagocytosis by suppressing PI3K-dependent pathways (126). In macrophages, the Src family kinase Fgr potentiates SHP-1 recruitment to SIRPα in a kinase-independent manner but has no effect on FcγRIIB-mediated inhibition of phagocytosis (130). Presumably, this difference in phosphatase recruitment underlies the different pathological mechanisms regulated by these two receptors.

Phagocytes express many additional members of the inhibitory receptor family, and it is not known whether these molecules also negatively regulate phagocytic responses or other functions of phagocytes such as migration, adhesion, and cytokine production. Because some activating receptor family members are almost exclusively expressed on phagocytes present at sites of infection and inflammation (e.g., TREM-1) (131), there may well be inhibitory receptor family members whose expression and function are limited to phagocytes at sites of tissue injury. This possibility reinforces the concept that the milieu surrounding the phagocyte directly affects its phagocytic potential.

MICROBES AND PHAGOCYTOSIS

Phagocytosis by "Nonprofessionals"

The "professional phagocytes"—neutrophils, macrophages, dendritic cells, and the bone marrow-derived organ-specific macrophage-like cells in the skin, liver, brain, and so forth—are the cells most important for phagocytosis in host defense and immunity. However, fibroblasts and epithelial cells also are capable of ingestion, albeit less efficiently than the professionals. In general, those cells lack the specialized mechanisms for pathogen destruction that characterize professional phagocytes. As a result, several bacteria have exploited the phagocytic ability of those cells as a way to evade normal host barriers to infection or other mechanisms of host defense. Because epithelial cells are devoid of receptors for IgG or complement opsonins, the standard recognition mechanisms of professional phagocytes are unavailable to initiate uptake. Instead, the bacteria interact with other cell-surface molecules to initiate uptake. For example, *Listeria monocytogenes* binds to E-cadherin to initiate its uptake by epithelial cells (132), and *S. pneumoniae* can interact with the polymeric IgA receptor on the apical surface of polarized epithelia (133). Other organisms, such as *Yersinia* and *Shigella* species, can bind to epithelial integrins to initiate uptake (134). For some infecting organisms, the recognition mechanism involves receptors specifically expressed on M cells, specialized cells of the epithelial monolayer overlying Peyer's patches. Because they are very endocytic and a very efficient transcytosis pathway, M cells increase the efficiency with which antigens on the epithelial surface are presented to the immune system. Bacteria that can bind to M cells can exploit this property to evade the epithelial barrier to infection.

The mechanisms of uptake induced by pathogens fall into two general categories: zippering, which resembles conventional IgG-mediated phagocytosis, and triggering, which resembles macropinocytosis. Uptake by zippering characterizes invasion by *Yersinia* pseudotuberculosis, which expresses a virulence gene, invasin, that binds to $\beta1$ integrins, which are present on the apical membranes of M cells and the basolateral membranes of other epithelial cells. On binding to the integrin, phagocytosis is induced, in association with the accumulation of actin and actin-binding proteins. Once through the epithelial barrier, *Yersinia* organisms live within lymph nodes as extracellular bacteria. To do this, they produce and secrete into host cells specific proteins that inhibit phagocytosis by blocking required signaling events. Thus, to successfully invade a mammalian host, *Yersinia* organisms induce phagocytosis by nonprofessional phagocytes to initiate invasion but then avoid phagocytosis by professional phagocytes in order to survive extracellularly within the host.

The classic example of microbial invasion by a triggering mechanism rather than zippering phagocytosis is that of *Salmonella typhimurium* (135). *S. typhimurium* binds to an unknown receptor present on many cells and then injects specific proteins into the epithelial cell cytoplasm to initiate a wave of actin polymerization that leads to markedly enhanced macropinocytosis, facilitating uptake of the organism. This wave of actin polymerization resembles that which occurs after growth factor signaling. In fact, uptake of nonpathogenic *Salmonella* organisms can be induced by simultaneous incubation with epidermal growth factor. Thus, both zippering and triggering mechanisms of bacterial invasion exploit normal host cellular mechanisms to the benefit of the invading bacteria.

Microbial Subversion of Professional Phagocytes

The examples just discussed represent microbes that have exploited phagocytosis as a mechanism for crossing the epithelial mechanical barrier to infection. A group of microbes, known as intracellular pathogens, have subverted phagocytosis to enhance their ability to survive within a host (Fig. 4). These organisms generally reside within host cells, especially macrophages, to evade recognition and destruction by other elements of innate or acquired immunity. Often, because of the difficulty in eliminating these organisms, chronic infection occurs. The ability to survive within the seemingly hostile macrophage is a common feature of such pathogens, but the strategies used to subvert the microbicidal activities of the phagocyte are quite diverse. Some, such as *Listeria, Shigella,* and *Rickettsia* organisms, express hemolysins, which dissolve the phagosome, allowing the bacteria to escape into the cytosol, where they can grow effectively and are free of the potentially damaging acidic and proteolytic environment of the phagolysosome. In contrast, some organisms (e.g., *Coxiella, Histoplasma,* and *Leishmania*) can withstand the intravacuolar environment of the phagolysosome. Still others (e.g., *Mycobacterium tuberculosis, Legionella* species, *Toxoplasma* species, and *Legionella* species) remain within the phagosome but prevent its maturation within the endosomal network and fusion with lysosomes. This has been well studied for *M. tuberculosis.* The organism is able to prevent the docking of the GTPase Rab7 and the PI3K hVPS34 on the maturing phagosome, ultimately blocking the ability of lysosomes to fuse with the *Mycobacteria*-containing phagosome

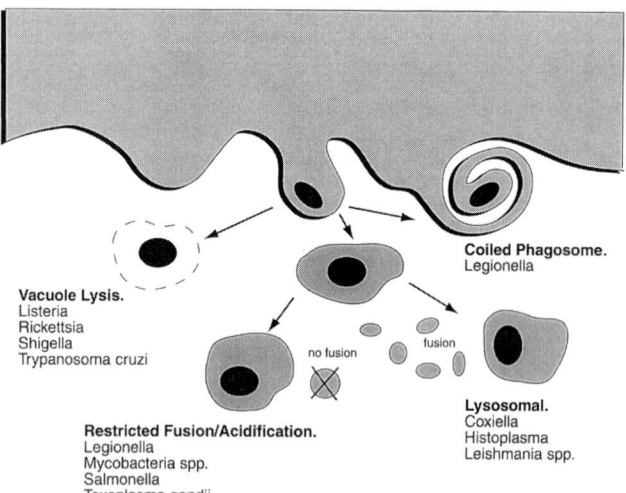

FIG. 4. Macrophage invasion and survival strategies of intracellular pathogens. Intracellular pathogens in macrophages can protect themselves from normal host defense in several ways, including altering the mode of phagocytosis (coiling phagocytosis), escape from the phagosome, and inhibition of phagolysosome maturation, leading to defective acidification and delivery of microbicidal effectors to the phagosome. Other organisms can survive within phagolysosomes.

(63,136). Although this clearly depends on specific and unique components of the mycobacterial cell wall, a detailed understanding of the molecular mechanisms by which *Mycobacteria* or other intraphagosomal pathogens interrupt the normal cell biology of the phagosome awaits further investigation.

CONCLUSIONS

The targets of phagocytosis, their recognition motifs, the receptors essential for their uptake, and the intracellular signals necessary for their entry into phagosomes are as diverse as the biological processes that depend on the function of professional phagocytes for homeostasis, such as nutritional uptake, tissue remodeling during development, removal of apoptotic cells, wound repair, and innate and adaptive immunity. Central to all this diversity is the formation of the phagosome, which is proving to be a key, dynamic organelle in all of these processes. The source of membrane necessary for its formation, how it acquires the effectors necessary to perform its function, how it communicates information to the nucleus and other downstream pathways, how its maturation differs among professional phagocytes, and how pathogens subvert this process are all subjects of intense investigation. *In vitro* application of proteomic and genomic analyses to these areas will significantly increase the depth of understanding about this important organelle. However, *in vivo*, professional phagocytes exist in a complex milieu in which they continually receive signals from contact with other cells, matrix components, hormones, growth factors, and various cytokines. Because these external signals can both positively and negatively regulate phagocytic mechanisms, elucidation of these regulatory cascades is essential in order to exploit phagocytosis as a target for amelioration of disease. The future holds the hope that further understanding of the molecular mechanisms underlying both primary phagosome biogenesis and secondary regulatory signals will allow clinically relevant pharmacological regulation of diseases as diverse as autoimmunity, atherosclerosis, and chronic infection.

REFERENCES

1. Weissmann G. Inflammation: historical perspective. In: Gallin JI, Goldstein IM, Snyderman R, eds. *Inflammation.* New York: Raven Press, 1988:5–8.
2. Burnet M. The role of macrophages, eosinophils and other auxiliary agents in relation to adaptive immunity. In: *Cellular immunology.* Carlton, Victoria, Australia: Melbourne University Press, 1969:147–162.
3. Van Furth R, Cohn ZA, Hirsch JG, et al. The mononuclear phagocyte system: a new classification of macrophages, monocytes, and their precursor cells. *Bull WHO* 1972;46:845–852.
4. Ruddy S, Gigli I, Austen KF. The complement system of man. I. *N Engl J Med* 1972;287:489–495.
5. Silverstein SC, Steinman RM, Cohn ZA. Endocytosis. *Annu Rev Biochem* 1977;46:669–722.
6. Munthe-Kaas AC, Kaplan G, Seljelid R. On the mechanism of inter-nalization of opsonized particles by rat Kupffer cells *in vitro. Exp Cell Res* 1976;103:201–212.
7. Cardelli J. Phagocytosis and macropinocytosis in *Dictyostelium*: phosphoinositide-based processes, biochemically distinct. *Traffic* 2001;2:311–320.
8. Muller-Taubenberger A, Lupas AN, Li H, et al. Calreticulin and calnexin in the endoplasmic reticulum are important for phagocytosis. *EMBO J* 2001;20:6772–6782.
9. Garin J, Diez R, Kieffer S, et al. The phagosome proteome: insight into phagosome functions. *J Cell Biol* 2001;152:165–180.
10. Gumienny TL, Hengartner MO. How the worm removes corpses: the nematode *C. elegans* as a model system to study engulfment. *Cell Death Differ* 2001;8:564–568.
11. Fadok VA, Henson PM. Apoptosis: getting rid of the bodies. *Curr Biol* 1998;8:R693–R695.
12. Gumienny TL, Brugnera E, Tosello-Trampont AC, et al. Ced-12/Elmo, a novel member of the Crkii/Dock180/Rac pathway, is required for phagocytosis and cell migration. *Cell* 2001;107:27–41.
13. Elrod-Erickson M, Mishra S, Schneider D. Interactions between the cellular and humoral immune responses in *Drosophila. Curr Biol* 2000; 10:781–784.
14. Bangs P, Franc N, White K. Molecular mechanisms of cell death and phagocytosis in *Drosophila. Cell Death Differ* 2000;7:1027–1034.
15. Imler JL, Hoffmann JA. Toll receptors in innate immunity. *Trends Cell Biol* 2001;11:304–311.
16. Akira S, Takeda K, Kaisho T. Toll-like receptors: critical proteins linking innate and acquired immunity. *Nat Immunol* 2001;2:675–680.
17. Ozinsky A, Underhill DM, Fontenot JD, et al. The repertoire for pattern recognition of pathogens by the innate immune system is defined by cooperation between Toll-like receptors. *Proc Natl Acad Sci U S A* 2000; 97:13766–13771.
18. Platt N, Da Silva RP, Gordon S. Recognizing death: the phagocytosis of apoptotic cells. *Trends Cell Biol* 1998;8:365–372.
19. Fadok VA, Bratton DL, Rose DM, et al. A receptor for phosphatidyl-serine-specific clearance of apoptotic cells. *Nature* 2000;405:85–90.
20. Weiss A, Littman DR. Signal transduction by lymphocyte antigen receptors. *Cell* 1994;76:263–274.
21. Harrison PT, Allen JM. High affinity IgG binding by FcgammaRI (CD64) is modulated by two distinct IgSF domains and the transmembrane domain of the receptor. *Protein Eng* 1998;11:225–232.
22. van der Pol W, van de Winkel JG. IgG receptor polymorphisms: risk factors for disease. *Immunogenetics* 1998;48:222–232.
23. Indik ZK, Park JG, Hunter S, et al. The molecular dissection of Fcgamma receptor mediated phagocytosis. *Blood* 1995;86:4389–4399.
24. Mitchell MA, Huang M-M, Chien P, et al. Substitutions and deletions in the cytoplasmic domain of the phagocytic receptor FcgammaRIIA: effect on receptor tyrosine phosphorylation and phagocytosis. *Blood* 1994;84:1753–1759.
25. McKenzie SE, Taylor SM, Malladi P, et al. The role of the human Fc receptor Fc gamma RIIA in the immune clearance of platelets: a transgenic mouse model. *J Immunol* 1999;162:4311–4318.
26. Ono M, Bolland S, Tempst P, et al. Role of the inositol phosphatase SHIP in negative regulation of the immune system by the receptor Fc(gamma)RIIB. *Nature* 1996;383:263–266.
27. De Haas M, Kleijer M, Van Zwieten R, et al. Neutrophil FcgammaRIIIb deficiency, nature, and clinical consequences: a study of 21 individuals from 14 families. *Blood* 1995;86:2403–2413.
28. Koene HR, De Haas M, Roos D, et al. Soluble FcgRIII: biology and clinical implications. In: Van de Winkel JGJ, Capel PJA, eds. *Human IgG Fc receptors.* Austin, TX: RG Landes, 1996:181–194.
29. van Egmond M, van Garderen E, van Spriel AB, et al. FcalphaRI-positive liver Kupffer cells: reappraisal of the function of immunoglobulin A in immunity. *Nat Med* 2000;6:680–685.
30. van Egmond M, Damen CA, van Spriel AB, et al. IgA and the IgA Fc receptor. *Trends Immunol* 2001;22:205–211.
31. Brown EJ. Complement receptors and phagocytosis. *Curr Opin Immunol* 1991;3:76–82.
32. Anderson DC, Schmalstieg FC, Arnaout MA, et al. Abnormalities of polymorphonuclear leukocyte function associated with a heritable deficiency of high molecular weight surface glycoproteins (GP138): common relationship to diminished cell adherence. *J Clin Invest* 1984; 74:536–551.

33. Prince JE, Brayton CF, Fossett MC, et al. The differential roles of LFA-1 and Mac-1 in host defense against systemic infection with *Streptococcus pneumoniae*. *J Immunol* 2001;166:7362–7369.

34. Graham IL, Lefkowith JB, Anderson DC, et al. Immune complex–stimulated neutrophil LTB$_4$ production is dependent on beta2 integrins. *J Cell Biol* 1993;120:1509–1517.

35. Graham IL, Anderson DC, Holers VM, et al. Complement receptor 3 (CR3, Mac-1, integrin alpha-M beta-2, CD11b/CD18) is required for tyrosine phosphorylation of paxillin in adherent and nonadherent neutrophils. *J Cell Biol* 1994;127:1139–1147.

36. Petty HR, Todd RF 3rd. Integrins as promiscuous signal transduction devices. *Immunol Today* 1996;17:209–212.

37. Krauss JC, Poo H, Xue W, et al. Reconstitution of antibody-dependent phagocytosis in fibroblasts expressing Fc gamma receptor IIIB and the complement receptor type 3. *J Immunol* 1994;153:1769–1777.

38. Berton G, Laudanna C, Sorio C, et al. Generation of signals activating neutrophil functions by leukocyte integrins: LFA-1 and gp150/95, but not CR3, are able to stimulate the respiratory burst of human neutrophils. *J Cell Biol* 1992;116:1007–1017.

39. Shimaoka M, Lu C, Palframan RT, et al. Reversibly locking a protein fold in an active conformation with a disulfide bond: integrin alphaL I domains with high affinity and antagonist activity *in vivo*. *Proc Natl Acad Sci U S A* 2001;98:6009–6014.

40. Rodriguez-Fernandez JL, Sanchez-Martin L, Rey M, et al. Rho and Rho-associated kinase modulate the tyrosine kinase PYK2 in T-cells through regulation of the activity of the integrin LFA-1. *J Biol Chem* 2001;276:40518–40527.

41. Zhou X, Li J, Kucik DF. The microtubule cytoskeleton participates in control of beta 2 integrin avidity. *J Biol Chem* 2001;276:44762–44769.

42. Peterson EJ, Woods ML, Dmowski SA, et al. Coupling of the TCR to integrin activation by Slap-130/Fyb. *Science* 2001;293:2263–2265.

43. Griffiths EK, Krawczyk C, Kong YY, et al. Positive regulation of T cell activation and integrin adhesion by the adapter Fyb/Slap. *Science* 2001;293:2260–2263.

44. Leitinger B, Hogg N. Effects of I domain deletion on the function of the beta2 integrin lymphocyte function–associated antigen–1. *Mol Biol Cell* 2000;11:677–690.

45. Griffin FM Jr, Mullinax PJ. Augmentation of macrophage complement receptor function *in vitro*. III. C3b receptors that promote phagocytosis migrate within the plane of the macrophage plasma membrane. *J Exp Med* 1981;154:291–305.

46. Kishore U, Reid KB. Structures and functions of mammalian collectins. *Results Probl Cell Differ* 2001;33:225–248.

47. Gadjeva M, Thiel S, Jensenius JC. The mannan-binding–lectin pathway of the innate immune response. *Curr Opin Immunol* 2001;13:74–78.

48. Eggleton P, Tenner AJ, Reid KB. C1q receptors. *Clin Exp Immunol* 2000;120:406–412.

49. Westhuyzen J, Healy H. Review: biology and relevance of C-reactive protein in cardiovascular and renal disease. *Ann Clin Lab Sci* 2000;30:133–143.

50. Mold C, Gresham HD, Du Clos TW. Serum amyloid P component and C-reactive protein mediate phagocytosis through murine Fc gamma Rs. *J Immunol* 2001;166:1200–1205.

51. Saeland E, van Royen A, Hendriksen K, et al. Human C-reactive protein does not bind to FcgammaRIIa on phagocytic cells. *J Clin Invest* 2001;107:641–643.

52. Griffin FM Jr, Silverstein SC. Segmental response of the macrophage plasma membrane to a phagocytic stimulus. *J Exp Med* 1974;139:323–336.

53. Gatfield J, Pieters J. Essential role for cholesterol in entry of mycobacteria into macrophages. *Science* 2000;288:1647–1650.

54. Kaplan G. Differences in the mode of phagocytosis with Fc and C3 receptors in macrophages. *Scand J Immunol* 1977;6:797–807.

55. Allen LAH, Aderem A. Molecular definition of distinct cytoskeletal structures involved in complement- and Fc receptor–mediated phagocytosis in macrophages. *J Exp Med* 1996;184:627–637.

56. Matsuda M, Park JG, Wang DC, et al. Abrogation of the Fc gamma receptor IIA–mediated phagocytic signal by stem-loop Syk antisense oligonucleotides. *Mol Biol Cell* 1996;7:1095–1106.

57. Kiefer F, Brumell J, Al Alawi N, et al. The Syk protein tyrosine kinase is essential for Fcgamma receptor signaling in macrophages and neutrophils. *Mol Cell Biol* 1998;18:4209–4220.

58. Fitzer-Attas CJ, Lowry M, Crowley MT, et al. Fcgamma receptor–mediated phagocytosis in macrophages lacking the Src family tyrosine kinases Hck, Fgr, and Lyn. *J Exp Med* 2000;191:669–682.

59. Takenawa T, Miki H. WASP and WAVE family proteins: key molecules for rapid rearrangement of cortical actin filaments and cell movement. *J Cell Sci* 2001;114:1801–1809.

60. Larsen EC, DiGennaro JA, Saito N, et al. Differential requirement for classic and novel PKC isoforms in respiratory burst and phagocytosis in RAW 264.7 cells. *J Immunol* 2000;165:2809–2817.

61. Cox D, Tseng CC, Bjekic G, et al. A requirement for phosphatidylinositol 3-kinase in pseudopod extension. *J Biol Chem* 1999;274:1240–1247.

62. Araki N, Johnson MT, Swanson JA. A role for phosphoinositide 3-kinase in the completion of macropinocytosis and phagocytosis by macrophages. *J Cell Biol* 1996;135:1249–1260.

63. Fratti RA, Backer JM, Gruenberg J, et al. Role of phosphatidylinositol 3-kinase and Rab5 effectors in phagosomal biogenesis and mycobacterial phagosome maturation arrest. *J Cell Biol* 2001;154:631–644.

64. Hackam DJ, Rotstein OD, Sjolin C, et al. v-SNARE–dependent secretion is required for phagocytosis. *Proc Natl Acad Sci U S A* 1998;95:11691–11696.

65. Marshall JG, Booth JW, Stambolic V, et al. Restricted accumulation of phosphatidylinositol 3-kinase products in a plasmalemmal subdomain during Fc gamma receptor–mediated phagocytosis. *J Cell Biol* 2001;153:1369–1380.

66. Botelho RJ, Teruel M, Dierckman R, et al. Localized biphasic changes in phosphatidylinositol-4,5-bisphosphate at sites of phagocytosis. *J Cell Biol* 2000;151:1353–1368.

67. Woodside DG, Obergfell A, Leng L, et al. Activation of Syk protein tyrosine kinase through interaction with integrin beta cytoplasmic domains. *Curr Biol* 2001;11:1799–1804.

68. Miranti CK, Leng L, Maschberger P, et al. Identification of a novel integrin signaling pathway involving the kinase Syk and the guanine nucleotide exchange factor Vav1. *Curr Biol* 1998;8:1289–1299.

69. Greenberg S. Diversity in phagocytic signalling. *J Cell Sci* 2001;114:1039–1040.

70. Serrander L, Fallman M, Stendahl O. Activation of phospholipase D is an early event in integrin-mediated signalling leading to phagocytosis in human neutrophils. *Inflammation* 1996;20:439–450.

71. Caron E, Hall A. Identification of two distinct mechanisms of phagocytosis controlled by different Rho GTPases. *Science* 1998;282:1717–1721.

72. May RC, Machesky LM. Phagocytosis and the actin cytoskeleton. *J Cell Sci* 2001;114:1061–1077.

73. Gresham HD, Graham IL, Anderson DC, et al. Leukocyte adhesion deficient (LAD) neutrophils fail to amplify phagocytic function in response to stimulation: evidence for CD11b/CD18-dependent and -independent mechanisms of phagocytosis. *J Clin Invest* 1991;88:588–597.

74. Graham IL, Gresham HD, Brown EJ. An immobile subset of plasma membrane CD11b/CD18 (Mac-1) is involved in phagocytosis of targets recognized by multiple receptors. *J Immunol* 1989;142:2352–2358.

75. Swanson JA. Phorbol esters stimulate macropinocytosis and solute flow through macrophages. *J Cell Sci* 1989;94:135–142.

76. Nobes C, Marsh M. Dendritic cells: new roles for Cdc42 and Rac in antigen uptake? *Curr Biol* 2000;10:R739–R741.

77. Francis CL, Ryan TA, Jones BD, et al. Ruffles induced by *Salmonella* and other stimuli direct macropinocytosis of bacteria. *Nature* 1993;364:639–642.

78. Galan JE, Bliska JB. Cross-talk between bacterial pathogens and their host cells. *Annu Rev Cell Dev Biol* 1996;12:221–255.

79. Simonsen A, Wurmser AE, Emr SD, et al. The role of phosphoinositides in membrane transport. *Curr Opin Cell Biol* 2001;13:485–492.

80. May RC, Caron E, Hall A, et al. Involvement of the Arp2/3 complex in phagocytosis mediated by FcgammaR or CR3. *Nat Cell Biol* 2000;2:246–248.

81. Evangelista M, Klebl BM, Tong AH, et al. A role for myosin-I in actin assembly through interactions with Vrp1p, Bee1p, and the Arp2/3 complex. *J Cell Biol* 2000;148:353–362.

82. Lechler T, Jonsdottir GA, Klee SK, et al. A two-tiered mechanism by which Cdc42 controls the localization and activation of an Arp2/3-activating motor complex in yeast. *J Cell Biol* 2001;155:261–270.

83. Lee WL, Bezanilla M, Pollard TD. Fission yeast myosin-I, Myo1p, stimulates actin assembly by Arp2/3 complex and shares functions with WASp. *J Cell Biol* 2000;151:789–800.

84. Maniak M, Rauchenberger R, Albrecht R, et al. Coronin involved in phagocytosis: dynamics of particle-induced relocalization visualized by a green fluorescent protein Tag. *Cell* 1995;83:915–924.

85. Serrander L, Skarman P, Rasmussen B, et al. Selective inhibition of IgG-mediated phagocytosis in gelsolin-deficient murine neutrophils. *J Immunol* 2000;165:2451–2457.

86. Witke W, Li W, Kwiatkowski DJ, et al. Comparisons of CapG and gelsolin-null macrophages: demonstration of a unique role for CapG in receptor-mediated ruffling, phagocytosis, and vesicle rocketing. *J Cell Biol* 2001;154:775–784.

87. Aizawa H, Fukui Y, Yahara I. Live dynamics of *Dictyostelium* cofilin suggests a role in remodeling actin latticework into bundles. *J Cell Sci* 1997;110:2333–2344.

88. Nagaishi K, Adachi R, Matsui S, et al. Herbimycin A inhibits both dephosphorylation and translocation of cofilin induced by opsonized zymosan in macrophagelike U937 cells. *J Cell Physiol* 1999;180:345–354.

89. Matsui S, Adachi R, Kusui K, et al. U73122 inhibits the dephosphorylation and translocation of cofilin in activated macrophage-like U937 cells. *Cell Signal* 2001;13:17–22.

90. Defacque H, Egeberg M, Habermann A, et al. Involvement of ezrin/moesin in *do novo* actin assembly on phagosomal membranes. *EMBO J* 2000;19:199–212.

91. Denker SP, Huang DC, Orlowski J, et al. Direct binding of the Na—H exchanger NHE1 to ERM proteins regulates the cortical cytoskeleton and cell shape independently of H(+) translocation. *Mol Cell* 2000;6:1425–1436.

92. Aderem A. The MARCKS brothers: a family of protein kinase C substrates. *Cell* 1992;71:713–716.

93. Zhu Z, Bao Z, Li J. MacMARCKS mutation blocks macrophage phagocytosis of zymosan. *J Biol Chem* 1995;270:17652–17655.

94. Underhill DM, Chen J, Allen LA, et al. MacMARCKS is not essential for phagocytosis in macrophages. *J Biol Chem* 1998;273:33619–33623.

95. Condeelis J. How is actin polymerization nucleated *in vivo? Trends Cell Biol* 2001;11:288–293.

96. Fukushima T, Waddell TK, Grinstein S, et al. Na$^+$/H$^+$ exchange activity during phagocytosis in human neutrophils: role of Fcgamma receptors and tyrosine kinases. *J Cell Biol* 1996;132:1037–1052.

97. Condeelis J. Life at the leading edge: the formation of cell protrusions. *Annu Rev Cell Biol* 1993;9:411–444.

98. Mansfield PJ, Shayman JA, Boxer LA. Regulation of polymorphonuclear leukocyte phagocytosis by myosin light chain kinase after activation of mitogen-activated protein kinase. *Blood* 2000;95:2407–2412.

99. Titus MA. A class VII unconventional myosin is required for phagocytosis. *Curr Biol* 1999;9:1297–1303.

100. Cox D, Lee DJ, Dale BM, et al. A Rab11-containing rapidly recycling compartment in macrophages that promotes phagocytosis. *Proc Natl Acad Sci U S A* 2000;97:680–685.

101. Gold ES, Underhill DM, Morrissette NS, et al. Dynamin 2 is required for phagocytosis in macrophages. *J Exp Med* 1999;190:1849–1856.

102. Jahraus A, Tjelle TE, Berg T, et al. *In vitro* fusion of phagosomes with different endocytic organelles from J774 macrophages. *J Biol Chem* 1998;273:30379–30390.

103. Rose DM, Winston BW, Chan ED, et al. Fc gamma receptor crosslinking activates p42, p38, and JNK/SAPK mitogen-activated protein kinases in murine macrophages: role for p42MAPK in Fc gamma receptor–stimulated TNF-alpha synthesis. *J Immunol* 1997;158:3433–3438.

104. Muroi M, Muroi Y, Suzuki T. The binding of immobilized IgG2a to Fc gamma 2a receptor activates NF-kappa B via reactive oxygen intermediates and tumor necrosis factor–alpha 1. *J Biol Chem* 1994;269:30561–30568.

105. Freire-de-Lima CG, Nascimento DO, Soares MB, et al. Uptake of apoptotic cells drives the growth of a pathogenic trypanosome in macrophages [published erratum appears in *Nature* 2000;404:904]. *Nature* 2000;403:199–203.

106. Forsberg M, Lofgren R, Zheng L, et al. Tumour necrosis factor–alpha potentiates CR3-induced respiratory burst by activating p38 MAP kinase in human neutrophils. *Immunology* 2001;103:465–472.

107. Devitt A, Moffatt OD, Raykundalia C, et al. Human CD14 mediates recognition and phagocytosis of apoptotic cells. *Nature* 1998;392:505–509.

108. Wang PY, Munford RS. CD14-dependent internalization and metabolism of extracellular phosphatidylinositol by monocytes. *J Biol Chem* 1999;274:23235–23241.

109. Sakr SW, Eddy RJ, Barth H, et al. The uptake and degradation of matrix-bound lipoproteins by macrophages require an intact actin cytoskeleton, Rho family GTPases, and myosin ATPase activity. *J Biol Chem* 2001;276:37649–37658.

110. Maeda M, Firtel RA. Activation of the mitogen-activated protein kinase ERK2 by the chemoattractant folic acid in *Dictyostelium. J Biol Chem* 1997;272:23690–23695.

111. Rosales C, Brown EJ. Neutrophil receptors and modulation of the immune response. In: Abramson JS, Wheeler JG, eds. *The neutrophil.* Oxford, UK: IRL Press, 1993:23–62.

112. Pommier CG, Inada S, Fries LF, et al. Plasma fibronectin enhances phagocytosis of opsonized particles by human peripheral blood monocytes. *J Exp Med* 1983;157:1844–1854.

113. Brown EJ. Signal transduction from leukocyte integrins. In: Hemler ME, Mihich E, eds. *Cell adhesion molecules.* New York: Plenum Press, 1993:105–126.

114. Gresham HD, Goodwin JL, Anderson DC, et al. A novel member of the integrin receptor family mediates Arg-Gly-Asp–stimulated neutrophil phagocytosis. *J Cell Biol* 1989;108:1935–1943.

115. Brown EJ, Lindberg FP. Leucocyte adhesion molecules in host defence against infection. *Ann Med* 1996;28:201–208.

116. Lindberg FP, Bullard DC, Caver TE, et al. Decreased resistance to bacterial infection and granulocyte defects in IAP-deficient mice. *Science* 1996;274:795–798.

117. Griffin JA, Griffin FM Jr. Augmentation of macrophage complement receptor function *in vitro.* I. Characterization of the cellular interactions required for the generation of a T-lymphocyte product that enhances macrophage complement receptor function. *J Exp Med* 1979;150:653–675.

118. Zhou M-J, Brown EJ. Leukocyte response integrin and integrin associated protein act as a signal transduction unit in generation of a phagocyte respiratory burst. *J Exp Med* 1993;178:1165–1174.

119. Van Strijp JAG, Russell DG, Tuomanen E, et al. Ligand specificity of purified complement receptor type 3 (CD11b/CD18, Mac-1, alphaM beta2): indirect effects of an Arg-Gly-Asp sequence. *J Immunol* 1993;151:3324–3336.

120. Jones SL, Knaus UG, Bokoch GM, et al. Two signaling mechanisms for activation of $\alpha M\beta 2$ avidity in polymorphonuclear neutrophils. *J Biol Chem* 1998;273:10556–10566.

121. Hoek RM, Ruuls SR, Murphy CA, et al. Down-regulation of the macrophage lineage through interaction with OX2 (CD200). *Science* 2000;290:1768–1771.

122. Clynes R, Maizes JS, Guinamard R, et al. Modulation of immune complex-induced inflammation *in vivo* by the coordinate expression of activation and inhibitory Fc receptors. *J Exp Med* 1999;189:179–185.

123. Hunter S, Indik ZK, Kim MK, et al. Inhibition of Fcgamma receptor–mediated phagocytosis by a nonphagocytic Fcgamma receptor. *Blood* 1998;91:1762–1768.

124. Gresham HD, Dale BM, Potter JW, et al. Negative regulation of phagocytosis in murine macrophages by the Src kinase family member, Fgr. *J Exp Med* 2000;191:515–528.

125. Oldenborg PA, Gresham HD, Lindberg FP. CD47-signal regulatory protein alpha (SIRPalpha) regulates Fcgamma and complement receptor-mediated phagocytosis. *J Exp Med* 2001;193:855–862.

126. Cox D, Dale BM, Kashiwada M, et al. A regulatory role for Src homology 2 domain–containing inositol 5′-phosphatase (SHIP) in phagocytosis mediated by Fc gamma receptors and complement receptor 3 (alpha(M)beta(2); CD11b/CD18). *J Exp Med* 2001;193:61–71.

127. Schiller C, Janssen-Graalfs I, Baumann U, et al. Mouse FcgammaRII is a negative regulator of FcgammaRIII in IgG immune complex–triggered inflammation but not in autoantibody-induced hemolysis. *Eur J Immunol* 2000;30:481–490.

128. Oldenborg PA, Zhelezynak A, Fang YF, et al. Role of CD47 as a marker of self on red blood cells. *Science* 2000;288:2051–2054.

129. Jiang P, Lagenaur CF, Narayanan V. Integrin-associated protein is a ligand for the P84 neural adhesion molecule. *J Biol Chem* 1999;274:559–562.

130. Vines CM, Potter JW, Xu Y, et al. Inhibition of beta2 integrin receptor and Syk kinase signaling in monocytes by the Src family kinase Fgr. *Immunity* 2001;15:507–519.

131. Bouchon A, Facchetti F, Weigand MA, et al. TREM-1 amplifies inflammation and is a crucial mediator of septic shock. *Nature* 2001; 410:1103–1107.

132. Mengaud J, Ohayon H, Gounon P, et al. E-cadherin is the receptor for internalin, a surface protein required for entry of *L. monocytogenes* into epithelial cells. *Cell* 1996;84:923–932.

133. Zhang JR, Mostov KE, Lamm ME, et al. The polymeric immunoglobulin receptor translocates pneumococci across human nasopharyngeal epithelial cells. *Cell* 2000;102:827–837.

134. Kerr JR. Cell adhesion molecules in the pathogenesis of and host defence against microbial infection. *Mol Pathol* 1999;52:220–230.

135. Raupach B, Mecsas J, Heczko U, et al. Bacterial epithelial cell cross talk. *Curr Top Microbiol Immunol* 1999;236:137–161.

136. Via LE, Deretic D, Ulmer RJ, et al. Arrest of mycobacterial phagosome maturation is caused by a block in vesicle fusion between stages controlled by rab5 and rab7. *J Biol Chem* 1997;272:13326–13331.

CHAPTER 36

Cytotoxic T-Lymphocytes

Pierre A. Henkart and Michail V. Sitkovsky

Cytotoxic Lymphocytes Are Defined by Their *In Vitro* Functional Activity
Basic Properties of Lymphocyte-Mediated Cytotoxicity
Distinguishing the Two Major Mechanisms of Lymphocyte-Mediated Cytotoxicity
Cytotoxic Lymphocyte Secretory Granules
  Cytotoxic T-Lymphocyte Secretory Pathways: Cytotoxicity and Cytokines · Properties of Cytotoxic T-Lymphocyte Granules · Components of Cytotoxic Lymphocyte Granules · Other Lysosomal Enzymes · Other Granule Membrane Proteins
Functional Steps in the Granule Exocytosis Cytotoxic Mechanism
  Adhesion · Effector Polarization · Signaling Exocytosis · Exocytosis · The Role of Granzymes in Target Death through Granule Exocytosis · Perforin-Mediated Granzyme Entry into Target Cells · Caspase-Dependent and -Independent Pathways of Cytotoxic T-Lymphocyte–Induced Target Death · Cytotoxic T-Lymphocyte Detachment · Self-Protection of Cytotoxic Lymphocytes
Differentiation-Dependent Expression of Cytotoxic Mediators
  In Vivo versus *In Vitro* Studies of Cytotoxic T-Lymphocyte–Mediated Cytotoxicity: The Role of Oxygen · Extracellular Adenosine as a Physiological Signal to Trigger the Down-regulation of Immune Response
***In Vivo* Role of Perforin- and Fas-Mediated Cytotoxicity**
  Homeostasis of the Immune System · Cytotoxic T-Lymphocytes in Host Defense against Infection · Cellular Cytotoxicity Pathways in Antitumor Cytotoxic T-Lymphocyte Activity · Cytotoxic Lymphocytes in Control of Viral Infections · Cytotoxic T-Lymphocytes in Disease Pathogenesis · Cytotoxic T-Lymphocytes and Autoimmunity · Cytotoxic Lymphocytes and Graft-versus-Host Disease · Cytotoxic Mediators in Contact Hypersensitivity · Role of Different Cytotoxic T-Lymphocyte Subsets in Delayed-Type Hypersensitivity · Cytotoxic Lymphocyte-Induced Inflammation in Liver Carcinogenesis · Therapeutic Modulation of Cytotoxic T-Lymphocyte Effector Functions · Localization of Cytotoxic T-Lymphocytes *In Vivo*
Conclusions
References

Lymphocytes share with macrophages the unusual cellular property of being able to rapidly destroy other cells *in vitro*. Not surprisingly, this activity must be tightly controlled in order to prevent harm to the host, and this chapter summarizes the current understanding of the cytotoxic mechanisms used by lymphocytes, emphasizing cytotoxic T-lymphocytes. Natural killer (NK) cells use similar mechanisms but a largely different set of receptors to trigger cytotoxicity, as described in Chapter 12.

Cytotoxic lymphocytes are also important producers of cytokines such as interferon (IFN)–γ, and, *in vivo,* such inflammatory cytokines can activate macrophages to become cytotoxic. However, cytokine secretion by cytotoxic lymphocytes appears to be basically similar to that by other lymphocytes and is not emphasized in this chapter. The question of whether the readily observable lymphocyte *in vitro* cytotoxic activities are important *in vivo* has been traditionally difficult to address, but the development of mice deficient in cytotoxic mediators has allowed direct testing of this issue.

These studies have confirmed that the cytotoxic mediators defined for their functional importance *in vitro* are indeed vital to *in vivo* immune responses, not only in the destruction of pathogens but also in the maintenance of immune homeostasis *in vivo*.

CYTOTOXIC LYMPHOCYTES ARE DEFINED BY THEIR *IN VITRO* FUNCTIONAL ACTIVITY

Cytotoxicity assays are conveniently carried out by short-term (4- to 18-hour) microcultures in which cytotoxic effector cells are mixed with target cells at varying ratios, followed by assessment of target cell death. The most common death assessment is based on target cell lysis, as measured by the chromium release assay. Target cells are loaded with the isotope chromium 51 (^{51}Cr) by preincubation with tracer levels of the oxidant $^{51}Cr_2O_7^{-2}$, which becomes reduced to $^{51}Cr^{+3}$ intracellularly and is stably complexed with intracellular polyanions (1,2). Upon lysis, released $^{51}Cr^{+3}$ complexes are not taken up by living cells and can therefore be readily quantitated by sampling the supernatant for radioactivity. Comparably sensitive nonradioactive techniques for quantitating target lysis have been developed, including some that measure release of preloaded, impermeant, soluble fluorescent dyes (3) or that measure release of chelators detectable by time-resolved fluorescence of rare earth complexes (4).

Alternative target cell death measurements are based on apoptotic properties, particularly deoxyribonucleic acid (DNA) fragmentation. Fragmented DNA is released from nuclei, which allows its release into detergent lysates (5) or through automated cell harvesters (6). Lysis and DNA fragmentation readouts typically correlate well (7), although DNA fragmentation represents a commitment to target cell death that can sometimes be measured earlier than lysis (8).

Measurements of target cell death by these approaches do not allow for direct comparisons of the cytotoxic potency of different effector cell populations because target cell death is not linearly related to the input of cytotoxic cells. A practical means of comparing the cytotoxic capacity of different populations is to compare the number of effector cells necessary to achieve a given level of target lysis in a given assay system. The results are expressed in "lytic units," which are inversely related to the effector cell number required (9).

BASIC PROPERTIES OF LYMPHOCYTE-MEDIATED CYTOTOXICITY

Many elegant studies of cytotoxic lymphocyte mechanisms were carried out before the recognition of several different molecular pathways of target cell damage, but these older studies must be interpreted cautiously. Nevertheless, such studies clearly established that cytotoxic lymphocytes have the ability to kill target cells quickly, sequentially, and selectively. Bystander cells lacking antigen intimately mixed with lysed target cells are generally spared destruction (10), although low levels of cytotoxic T-lymphocyte (CTL) bystander lysis can be detected in some systems (11,12). In time-lapse cinematography studies of the cytotoxic process, CTLs have been observed to bind target cells and inflict visible injury within a few minutes, with target death in some cases following within another few minutes (13). Such studies show that single CTLs can kill multiple target cells within a few hours, as also seen by examination of CTL-target clusters (14). The rapid CTL-induced death process was not blocked by inhibitors of protein synthesis (15), which suggests the existence of preformed lytic mediators. One of the most striking aspects of CTL-induced cytotoxicity has been its generally strict T-cell receptor (TCR)–defined specificity, and the phenomenon of major histocompatibility complex (MHC) restriction can be clearly demonstrated by using cytotoxicity as a rapid and convenient readout of TCR recognition (16). Use of interleukin (IL)–2 and other cytokines has allowed the culture of cloned CTL lines that exhibit a potent cytotoxicity capable of completely destroying target cells within a few hours when mixed at less than a 1:1 ratio (17).

During the 1970s, studies of CTL-mediated target lysis defined three distinct phases of the process (18,19). The first is CTL-target adhesion, defined as formation of a firm attachment that cannot be disrupted by mild shearing forces. This adhesion step requires several minutes at 37°, occurs in the absence of calcium if magnesium is provided, and is blocked by cold temperatures and a range of drugs. This is followed by a second step, "lethal hit" or "programming for lysis," which also requires several minutes. Its hallmark property is a requirement for calcium in the medium, and, like adhesion, it is blocked by cold temperatures and a range of drugs. The final stage of CTL cytotoxicity, "target cell disintegration," ends with lysis and is the most prolonged, with a mean half-life of 1.7 hours. This stage involves only the target cell, inasmuch as it is unaffected if CTLs are eliminated (e.g. by complement treatment). It is characterized by its independence of divalent cations, and no drugs that effectively block lysis of the lethally injured target cell have been found.

DISTINGUISHING THE TWO MAJOR MECHANISMS OF LYMPHOCYTE-MEDIATED CYTOTOXICITY

As schematically shown in Fig. 1 and described in detail later, CTLs use two distinct cytolytic pathways in 4- to 6-hour assays *in vitro*: the perforin-dependent granule exocytosis pathway and the Fas ligand/Fas pathway. Because distinct effector molecules are required for the function of each pathway, it is possible to block each pathway selectively and thus assess their relative importance to particular CTL-target combinations. The Fas ligand/Fas pathway can be selectively blocked by several approaches: (a) use of CTL effectors from *gld* mutant mice lacking functional Fas ligand; (b) use of Fas-negative targets, particularly those derived from *lpr* mutant mice; and (c) use of non–cross-linking anti-Fas antibody or soluble Fas constructs to block Fas ligand–Fas binding. Inhibitors of transcription and translation provide another possible approach (20), but, in addition to problems with side effects of such drugs, CTLs express preexisting Fas ligand in granules (21). The perforin-dependent granule exocytosis pathway can be blocked most cleanly by using effector cells from perforin-knockout mice (22,23). A useful pharmacological approach to blocking the granule exocytosis pathway is treatment of effector cells with concanamycin A (24) (see below).

With target cells bearing fully functional Fas, the Fas ligand/Fas pathway can contribute as much as half the cytotoxicity in a 4- to 6-hour assay. However, for most CTL-target combinations, target death in short-term assays is dominated by the granule exocytosis pathway (22,23). When both pathways are blocked, CTLs lose all detectable cytotoxicity in short-term assays. For assays of 12 to 20 hours' duration, the Fas ligand/Fas mechanism can be more prominent in the death of Fas-bearing target cells. For such longer term assays, a third mechanism utilizing tumor necrosis factor (TNF) produced

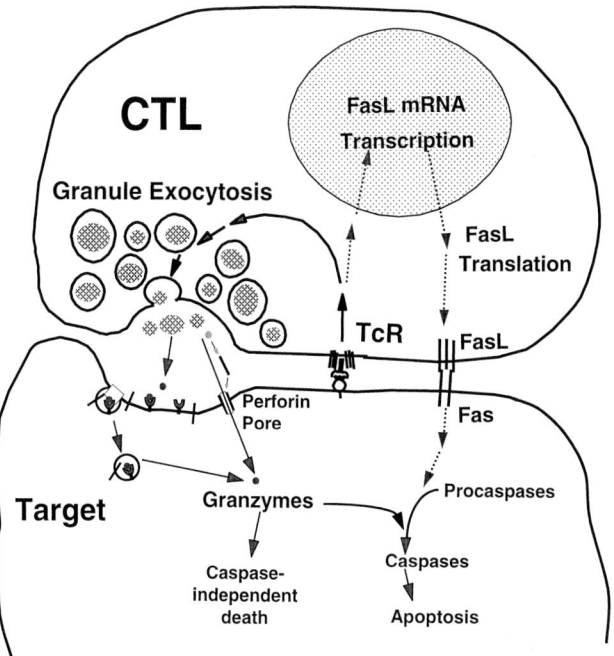

CTL

FasL mRNA Transcription

Granule Exocytosis

FasL Translation

TcR

FasL

Perforin Pore

Fas

Target

Granzymes — Procaspases

Caspase-independent death

Caspases

Apoptosis

FIG. 1. The two cytotoxicity pathways used by cytotoxic T-lymphocytes (CTLs) *in vitro.* Both pathways are initiated via T-cell receptor cross-linking by target cell antigen, which is made possible by adhesive interactions between the cells. Within the CTL, common initial signaling steps are shared by both pathways, which then diverge. The granule exocytosis pathway on the left side is a typical receptor-controlled secretion process resulting in the release of perforin and granzymes from the granule cores into the synapse-like junctional region between the CTL and its target. Granzyme entry into target cells may occur through receptor-mediated endocytosis (left), in which case perforin serves to "permeabilize" the endosome, allowing granzymes to enter the cytoplasm. Alternatively, granzymes might enter the target cells via perforin pores. Granzymes cause caspase activation and apoptosis either directly or through mitochondrial damage. However, granzymes can also mediate target death through a caspase-independent pathway. The Fas ligand/Fas pathway on the right requires *de novo* transcription of Fas ligand messenger ribonucleic acid and its subsequent surface expression on the CTL, where it cross-links target cell Fas. (Fas ligand has also been shown to be expressed in granules, so that this effector molecule can also utilize the granule exocytosis pathway). Fas cross-linking on target cells leads to caspase activation and apoptosis.

by CTLs can also contribute to cytotoxicity of TNF-sensitive target cells (25).

CYTOTOXIC LYMPHOCYTE SECRETORY GRANULES

Cytotoxic T-Lymphocyte Secretory Pathways: Cytotoxicity and Cytokines

Cellular secretion occurs through a membrane fusion process, termed *exocytosis,* in which an intracellular vesicle or granule membrane fuses with the plasma membrane, thus releasing material enclosed within the granule to the extra-

cellular space. Such secretion has been categorized as either regulated, if the exocytosis occurs with preformed granules in response to a membrane signal, or constitutive, if vesicles containing newly synthesized proteins undergo exocytosis without delay (26). Most lymphocyte protein secretion (antibodies, cytokines) is constitutive, inasmuch as it occurs without detectable intracellular storage of newly secreted proteins. This secretion is greatly stimulated in response to lymphocyte activation and differentiation, especially as B-lymphocytes mature into plasma cells, and in this sense, the "constitutive" secretory pathway is highly regulated in lymphocytes. The "regulated" secretory pathway is prominent in many nonlymphoid cell types and is characterized by an initial vesicular transport of newly synthesized proteins to larger secretory granules, where they are stored for indefinite periods. Degranulation is typically triggered by a plasma membrane receptor.

CTLs use both regulated and constitutive secretory pathways. Cytokines such as IFN-γ are secreted by CTL via the constitutive pathway (27). Even cytotoxic mediators principally secreted by the regulated pathway are secreted by the constitutive pathway immediately after antigen triggering of cloned CTL (28), and such constitutive secretion may mediate some bystander killing.

The presence of secretory granules in lymphocytes is not always obvious because they are few in number in comparison with granulocytes or mast cells. Sensitive immunostaining for the major granule component perforin shows that resting naïve $\alpha\beta$ TCRs have few if any granules, whereas most resting $\gamma\delta$ TCRs, NK T cells, and NK cells have detectable granules (29,30). Antigen-triggered activation results in granule formation in CD8$^+$ and, to some extent, CD4$^+$ T cells, and granules are detectable in most blood CCR7$^-$ memory CD8$^+$ T cells (31).

Cytokine secretion by CTLs is similar to that of T helper (Th) cells, and after activation of naïve CD8$^+$ T cells, they can differentiate into at least two subsets of CTLs with different cytokine-secreting patterns: CTLs that are similar to Th1 cells in that they secrete IL-2 and IFN-γ are designated T cytotoxic–1 (Tc1) cells; CTLs secreting IL-4, IL-5, and IL-10 are designated Tc2 cells. Both Tc1 and Tc2 cells are cytotoxic *in vitro* (32).

Properties of Cytotoxic T-Lymphocyte Granules

Electron microscopy of CTL granules shows they are typically 0.5 to 1 μm in diameter and have a heterogeneous structure consisting of two components. The first component, the core, is a densely staining homogeneous region that shows some similarity to cores of granules of mast cells. In some granules, the cores are surrounded by a double membrane, whereas in other cases, the cores are not bound by membranes (33). The second granule component is multivesicular, composed of numerous membrane vesicles ranging from 30 to 150 nm in diameter. Granules have been classified on the basis of the dominance of these components: Type I granules are defined as those dominated by cores, with only a small cortical rim of the multivesicular component; in contrast, type II granules contain only the multivesicular component with no cores. These appear similar to late endosomes or prelysosomes in other cells. Intermediate granules contain both components, with smaller cores than those in type I granules.

Electron micrograph studies with immunogold staining have revealed that the granule cores contain perforin, granzymes, and proteoglycan, whereas the multivesicular regions contain lysosomal enzymes and lysosomal membrane markers. Evidence that the vesicles are derived from the plasma membrane by endocytosis comes from electron micrograph studies in which immunogold staining showed the presence of TCR, CD8, and class I MHC molecules (33). These proteins are oriented with the normally extracellular domains facing the lumen of the granules, as expected from an endocytic origin. In conjunction with microscopy, weak base pH probes show that CTL granules have an acidic interior, with an estimated internal pH of 5.4 (34). Similar estimates have been obtained for secretory granules in other cell types.

Components of Cytotoxic Lymphocyte Granules

Cytotoxic lymphocyte granules have been purified from homogenates of cloned lymphocytes grown *in vitro*. When analyzed biochemically, such granules show a limited number of prominent protein bands. The most abundant proteins are perforin and the granzymes, components that have been studied for their functional role in target cell death. The biochemical properties of these components are discussed in this section, and their functional roles in cytotoxicity are described as follows.

Perforin (Cytolysin, PFP)

Perforin appears to be uniquely expressed in cytotoxic lymphocyte granules and is required for the function of the granule exocytosis pathway of cytotoxicity. It is a 555–amino acid glycoprotein of 65 to 75 kDa that, in the presence of calcium, has the ability to insert into lipid bilayer membranes, polymerize, and form structural and functional pores, which can lead to cell lysis (35). Although perforin is a water-soluble protein after careful isolation from granules, exposure to calcium concentrations normally found extracellularly appears to trigger a conformational change that exposes hydrophobic groups and renders it amphipathic. In the presence of calcium, perforin inserts into pure lipid membranes and self-associates into stable polymeric forms that appear by electron microscopy to be pore-like structures with striking homology to those formed by complement (Fig. 2). The internal diameter of these structures is larger for perforin than for complement, but the overall shapes are similar. Such pore-like structures can be detected on the surface of target cells killed by large granular lymphocytes or CTL (36–38), which provides evidence that effector cell degranulation accompanies target cell death.

As shown in Fig. 2, cloning and sequence analysis of perforin from three mammalian species has revealed two regions of sequence homology of probable functional importance: (a) a complement homology domain related to proteins of the complement "membrane attack" complex (C6, C7, C8a, C8b, and C9), which associate to form lytic pores (39,40), and (b) a C2 domain related to those in other calcium-binding lipid-interacting proteins (41). These domains are connected by a short cysteine-rich region. The amino terminal third of the molecule does not show significant homology to database proteins. The COOH terminal peptide is removed by proteolytic processing of the newly synthesized perforin molecule between the Golgi apparatus and granules, activating the C2 domain for phospholipid binding (42). C2 domains are found in other proteins that show a calcium-dependent interaction with lipids, including phospholipase C, protein kinase C, and vesicle-associated soluble N-ethylmaleimide–sensitive fusion protein attachment protein receptors (v-SNAREs). However, how lipid binding by perforin leads to pore formation remains unclear. Typical membrane-spanning motifs of about 20 hydrophobic amino acids characteristic of α helical transmembrane domains are absent. The functional implications of the complement homology remain open to question, and it is tempting to speculate that polymerization of monomers leads to assembly of a β barrel, as described for staphylococcal α toxin (43).

The pore-like structure of aggregated perforin on membranes immediately suggests a central hydrophilic core surrounded by protein molecules lining the membrane (Fig. 2). However, such fully aggregated pore-like structures may not be necessary to form smaller pores capable of allowing passage of ions and small molecules. Electrical studies of planar lipid bilayers show that perforin pores induce large ion-permeable channels that are heterogeneous in size (44). Studies examining the ability of labeled macromolecules to cross perforin-treated cell membranes show that it forms functional pores capable of allowing passage of proteins and dextrans with diameters of up to 10 to 14 nm—that is, globular proteins of more than 100 kDa (45,46). These estimates are thus in reasonable agreement with the 14-nm inner diameter of the pore structure seen in the electron micrograph.

In the presence of calcium, perforin is extremely potent when assayed for red blood cell lysis or for its ability to render liposomes permeable. Studies of perforin's lytic activity on nucleated cells show that approximately 10 to 100 times more perforin is required to achieve lysis in comparison with red blood cells (47). This has been found for other pore-forming agents and presumably results from membrane repair mechanisms present in nucleated cells. As discussed later, CTL-delivered perforin pores appear not to lyse nucleated target cells directly but rather to function by rendering target cells permeable to granzymes. Although complement and perforin lyse red cell targets by a colloid osmotic mechanism, this does not explain their action on nucleated target cells (48).

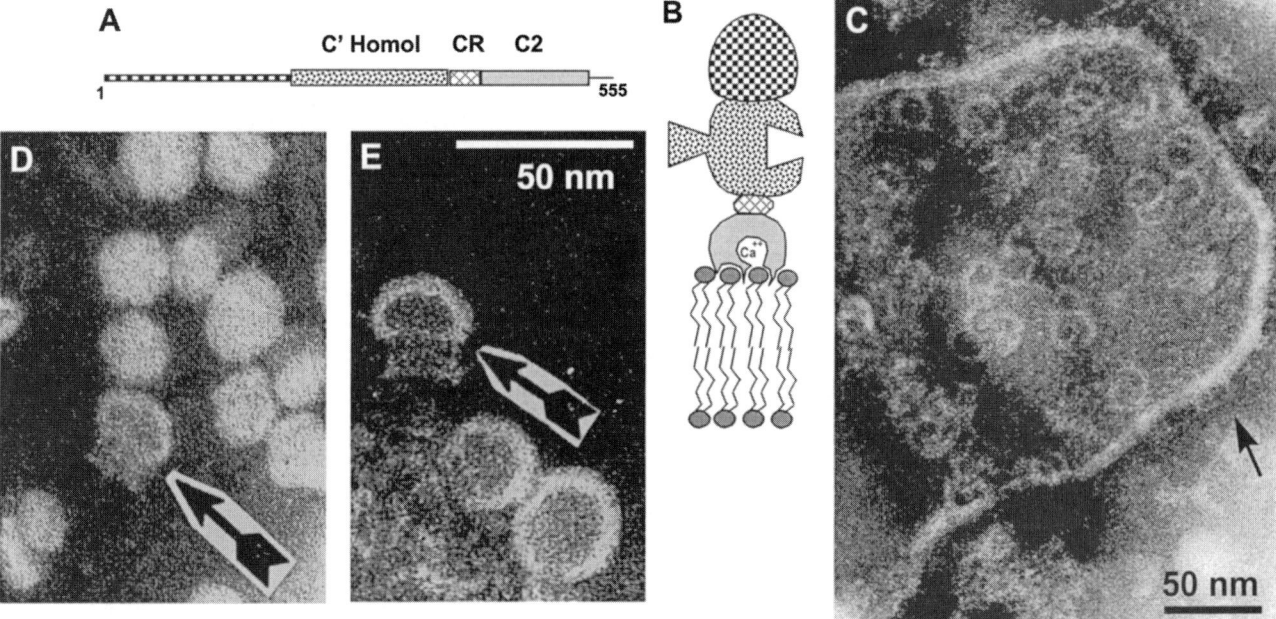

FIG. 2. Perforin sequence and pore-like structures. **A:** Schematic view of perforin protein sequence. The amino terminal portion of the molecule shows no homology to database proteins. The stippled central region (C′ Homol) shows significant but distant homology to complement components C6, C7, C8a, and C9 and contains a putative amphipathic helix at its left end. This is followed by a short, cysteine-rich (CR) region of unknown significance, then by the C2 homology domain implicated in calcium-dependent phospholipid interactions, and finally by the COOH peptide, which is removed by processing before granule storage. **B:** A speculative schematic depiction of the perforin domains in the monomer bound to membrane before its polymerization and membrane insertion. The C2 domain is shown binding calcium and phospholipid head groups. The C′ homology domain is shown with motifs that allow self-aggregation, inasmuch as C9 forms polymers and the other complement proteins bind other homologous proteins in forming the membrane attack complex. The regions of membrane interaction after aggregation and insertion remain unknown. **C:** Electron micrographic images of negative stained perforin pore-like structures on the surface of resealed red blood cell ghosts attacked by human large granular lymphocytes in antibody-dependent cell-mediated cytotoxicity (ADCC) (36). Similar but slightly smaller structures had been previously described from red blood cells lysed by complement. *Arrow* points to edge view of the pore-like structure, which suggests that they are short cylinders embedded in the membrane. In this ADCC system, previous functional experiments with this system had indicated a pore-like sieving behavior of released marker proteins (45). Micrograph courtesy of Robert Dourmashkin. **D:** Small unilamellar liposomes treated with low concentration of purified perforin in the presence of calcium. Under these conditions, soluble markers were released from these liposomes. *Arrow* shows one liposome with the perforin pore-like structure inserted in its membrane. This liposome has become permeable to the dark negative stain. From Blumenthal et al. (234), with permission. **E:** Liposomes treated with a higher concentration of purified perforin releasing a high percentage of trapped marker. *Arrow* shows pore-like structure inserted into lipid bilayer. From Blumenthal et al. (234), with permission.

Several properties of perforin help explain its function in cytotoxic lymphocytes. Its lytic activity drops off rapidly as the pH diminishes below 7 (47), so that it would not be expected to make pores in the acidic granule membranes. Its functional activity is efficiently inhibited by hydrophobic substances, including lipoproteins and membranes. Thus, the postsecretion amphipathic form arising after exposure to calcium and neutral pH rapidly inserts into any hydrophobic surface nearby, which raises the issue of CTL self protection, discussed later.

The mechanism by which newly synthesized perforin is sorted to granules after passage through the Golgi apparatus is unknown. This protein does not have covalently attached mannose-6-phosphate groups, as is the case with granzymes and lysosomal proteins. However, lysosomal proteins appear to also utilize an uncharacterized second system for sorting, and it is likely that perforin shares this feature. It is also not clear which perforin properties are important to its ability to form the granule core complexes with proteoglycan and granzymes, although cationic regions of the sequence can be identified.

Granzymes

Granzymes are serine proteases present in the granules of cytotoxic lymphocytes and show minimal expression in other sites or in the granules of other tissues (49). Their protein sequence shows clear homology to serine proteases, including conservation of the amino acids of the classical serine protease catalytic triad. On the basis of sequence homology, granzymes form a monophyletic subfamily of serine proteases along with granule proteases of mast cells, macrophages, and neutrophils (50). This subfamily is characterized by a conserved PHRPSYM motif near the amino terminal of the mature enzyme. The term *granzyme* has been used for the members of this subfamily expressed in lymphocytes. Granzymes are highly positively charged proteins, forming electrostatic complexes with granule proteoglycans. Biochemical properties of granzymes are described in this section; their contributions to target death are described in the following section.

Although the physiological substrates of granzymes remain a matter of speculation, synthetic peptide substrates have been found for some of these proteases, allowing biochemical studies (51). Table 1 summarizes properties of the known granzymes. Murine granzymes A and B are the only ones detectable in the highly cytolytic CTLs found in the peritoneal cavity after alloimmunization, and these two proteases are expressed within a few days of activation of CD8$^+$ CTLs *in vitro* (52). It is interesting that these two proteases have enzymatic specificities that are distinctly different from each other and from most of the remaining granzymes.

Granzyme B has a substrate specificity unique among mammalian serine proteases in that it requires aspartic acid as the P1 amino acid (i.e., cleavage leaves a carboxyl-terminal aspartic acid). The peptide cleavage preferences of granzyme B beyond the P1 position have been defined by a combinational approach (53), and the three-dimensional structure of the protein has been determined (54,55). Granzyme B is a potent activator of caspases-3, -7, -8, -9, and -10 (but not of caspases-1 or -2), thus inducing target cell apoptosis. However, granzyme B can also trigger caspase-dependent or caspase-independent target death by inducing mitochondrial damage through cleavage of Bid (56–59), in conjunction with Bak (60). Granzyme B also can induce DNA fragmentation through its ability to cleave a cytoplasmic nuclease inhibitor (61). Because a number of clinically important autoantigens

are cleaved by granzyme B, it has been suggested that such cleavage is important in the induction of autoimmunity (62).

In contrast to granzyme B, granzyme A cleaves substrates with arginine or lysine at the P1 amino acid, a "tryptase" activity, which is conveniently monitored by following the cleavage of BLT (benzoyl lysine thioester). Several protein substrates for granzyme A have been described (63,64), including nuclear proteins (64–67). Although it has generally been assumed that protease activity is important to the functional role of granzymes, enzymatically inactive granzyme A can induce cytolysis when loaded into tumor cells with sublytic perforin (68).

Upon culture *in vitro*, CD8$^+$ CTLs express other granzymes. For all granzymes studied, enzymatic activity is maximal at neutral pHs rather than at the acidic pH of the granules. It is thus unlikely that the granzyme functional substrates are intragranular, inasmuch as they appear designed to operate in the neutral pH environment after exocytosis.

Like many other proteases, granzymes are synthesized as inactive proenzymes and must be proteolytically processed in order to become enzymatically active. All known granzymes contain an "activation dipeptide" after the signal sequence before the consensus amino terminal sequence IIGG of the mature enzyme. The activation dipeptide is removed within the granule.

Dipeptidyl Peptidase I (Cathepsin C)

The lysosomal cysteine protease dipeptidyl peptidase I (DPPI) cleaves an amino terminal dipeptide from progranzymes to produce the mature and enzymatically active proteases. Coexpression of both DPPI and granzymes in nonhematopoietic cells allows expression of enzymatically active granzymes (69). Chemical inhibition of DPPI impairs lymphocyte cytotoxicity (70), as confirmed by genetic deletion of this enzyme (71).

Proteoglycan

Proteoglycans are found in secretory granules of many hematopoietic cells (72) and are known to play an important role in binding other granule components to form an insoluble

TABLE 1. *Lymphocyte granzymes*

Granzyme	P1 amino acid at cleavage	Expressed in	Species	Other features
A	Lys/Arg	CD8$^+$ CTL, NK, $\gamma\delta$	M, H, R	SS dimer
B	Asp	CD8$^+$ CTL, NK, $\gamma\delta$	M, H, R	Glycosylation variable
C	Unknown	CD8$^+$ CTL clones	M, R	Not glycosylated
D	Lys/Arg	CD8$^+$ CTL clones	M	Highly glycosylated
E	Unknown	CD8$^+$ CTL clones	M	Highly glycosylated
F	Unknown	CD8$^+$ CTL clones	M	Highly glycosylated
G	Unknown	CD8$^+$ CTL clones	M	—
H	Hydrophobic	CD8$^+$ CTL clones	H	—
K	Lys/Arg	CD8$^+$ CTL clones	R, H	—
Met-1	Met/Leu	NK	M, H, R	—

CTL, cytotoxic T lymphocyte; NK, natural killer (cells).

complex visualized as the granule core. CTL and NK granule proteoglycans are heterogeneous molecules composed of a serglycin protein backbone with a variable number of covalently attached glycosaminoglycan chains. The serglycin protein backbone is a 17- to 20-kDa protein containing an unusual interior domain with the repeat sequence (ser-gly)$_n$, where $n = 9$ to 24, depending on the species. These serines are substituted with 50- to 85-kDa chondroitin sulfate chains to form high-molecular-weight proteoglycans. The sulfate groups of chondroitin sulfate maintain their negative charge even at the low intragranular pH, thus allowing the formation of an ionic complex with the cationic granzymes, as well as binding perforin by less defined forces (73). Evidence for such an ionic complex among proteoglycans, granzymes, and perforin comes from the isolation of an insoluble complex from granules in low salt and its dissociation at physiological pH and salt. After exocytosis, perforin and granzymes are released as a large electrostatic complex that may be involved in cytotoxic effects (74,75).

Other Lysosomal Enzymes

A variety of normal lysosomal enzymes are detectable in granules of cytotoxic lymphocytes by histochemical and biochemical techniques. This has led to their characterization as "secretory lysosomes," which also describes mast cell granules, azurophilic granules of neutrophils, and platelet granules, as well as a subpopulation of lysosomes in fibroblasts and endothelial cells (76). Lysosomes with a classical appearance are rare in CTLs, and it appears that their normal internal digestive functions take place largely in the secretory granules. Because lysosomal enzymes have a low optimal pH or are unstable at neutral pH, or both, they are generally considered unlikely to participate in target cell damage after exocytosis. The protease cathepsin D has been localized to the cortical region of CTL granules between the membrane vesicles, where it is found with endocytosed bovine serum albumin (77).

Fas Ligand

Although TCR-induced Fas ligand expression on the plasma membrane often requires *de novo* transcription and was generally assumed to occur via the constitutive pathway, experiments have shown that Fas ligand is localized in CTL granules (21). Transfection of rat basophilic leukemia (RBL) mast cell tumor cells with Fas ligand–green fluorescent protein (GFP) constructs resulted in a granule localization, which domain-swapping experiments showed was attributable to its cytoplasmic tail. Subsequent studies have defined an unusual proline-rich domain within this tail as responsible for granule localization and provided evidence that Fas ligand does not arrive in granules through endocytosis (78). However, because CTLs from degranulation-deficient *ashen* mice appear to have normal Fas-mediated cytotoxicity (79), it remains unclear whether all CTL effector Fas ligand is granule derived.

Other Granule Membrane Proteins

Granule membrane proteins can be divided into several categories. The lysosomal membrane proteins LAMP1, LAMP2 (CD107a and b), CD63 (granulophysin), and the cation-independent mannose-6-phosphate receptor are found on both the vesicles and the internal surface of the outer granule membrane. LAMP1 and LAMP2 become exposed on the cell surface after exocytosis but are rapidly removed by endocytosis (80). The second category of membrane proteins in granules comprises normal surface proteins that are present on the cortical vesicles of CTL granules. They include the TCR, CD8, and class I MHC (77). These appear to arise as a result of the budding processes of compound endocytosis that may be part of the lysosomal functions of these granules.

The low intragranular pH is maintained by a membrane proton pump termed the *vacuolar-type adenosine triphosphatase* (V-ATPase) (81). This pump is selectively inhibited by the macrolide antibiotic concanamycin A, which neutralizes CTL granules and triggers a degradation of intragranular perforin but not of granzymes, with concomitant loss of cytotoxic activity (82).

TIA-1 is a protein component unique to CTL granules that is localized in the outer granule membranes with the protein domain exposed to the cytoplasm (83). TIA-1 can also be localized to the interior of some of the intragranular vesicles derived from these membranes by budding. The protein is expressed as two isoforms. The 15-kDa form is the dominant isoform in CTL granules and is composed of the carboxyl-terminal third of the other form, the 40-kDa protein.

Granulysin (NK-Lysin/519)

Granulysin is a small protein present in CTL granules (84) and is homologous to NK-lysin in porcine T and NK cell granules (85). Granulysin occurs in two forms: a 15-kDa form, present only in immature granules, and a further processed 9-kDa form, which is secreted in response to TCR cross-linking and is present in both mature and immature granules. The 9-kDa protein sequence shows homology to the amoebapore family of membranolytic proteins, and purified granulysin can disrupt model membranes. Accordingly, granulysin has *in vitro* lytic activity against tumor targets and bacteria (86,87), although granulysin's contribution to target cell injury by cytotoxic lymphocytes is still unclear.

Because granulysin is bactericidal, it has attracted attention as a potential effector molecule in the T cell–mediated killing of intracellular bacteria, particularly mycobacteria (88). In the case of intracellular *Mycobacterium tuberculosis*, T cells required granule exocytosis for their *in vitro* bactericidal activity, and a combination of perforin and granulysin was shown to be effective (89). However, other studies have questioned the role of perforin in the *in vitro* T cell–mediated killing of intracellular *M. tuberculosis* (90).

Calreticulin

Calreticulin is an acidic 46-kDa protein known as a calcium-binding protein and a molecular chaperone expressed in the endoplasmic reticulum of most cells. It was identified as a CTL granule component on the basis of its copurification with perforin in granule extracts (91). It appears likely that calreticulin binds to perforin at least in part because of its lectin-like function in binding carbohydrates that have not been terminally processed by endoplasmic reticulum glycosidases (92). Immunolocalization studies show that calreticulin resides in CTL granules as well as in the endoplasmic reticulum, and it is secreted in response to TCR stimulation, but its functional role remains unclear.

Chemokines

Cloned human CTL specific for human immunodeficiency virus (HIV) have been shown to rapidly secrete the chemokines MIP-1α, MIP-1β, and regulated upon activation, normal T-cell expressed, presumably secreted (RANTES) chemokine through the granule exocytosis pathway after TCR ligation (74). Secreted chemokines were present in the medium as complexes with proteoglycan, which were capable of inhibiting HIV replication in monocytes in vitro. Immunolocalization of chemokines in CTLs showed them to be in granules that partially colocalized with granzyme A and underwent polarization in response to TCR ligation.

FUNCTIONAL STEPS IN THE GRANULE EXOCYTOSIS CYTOTOXIC MECHANISM

Figure 1 illustrates the basic properties of the granule exocytosis pathway for lymphocyte cytotoxicity, showing discrete steps that have been defined in varying levels of detail, as discussed later. The essential feature of this mechanism is the exocytosis step, in which preformed mediators in secretory granules are released locally from the polarized CTLs into a synapse-like region formed between the CTL and its bound target cell. A number of important molecular details of this cytotoxic pathway remain to be elucidated, including the terminal steps leading to target lysis. Although all short-term in vitro target cell cytotoxicity via this pathway is perforin dependent, other noncytotoxic physiological mediators such as chemokines may be rapidly secreted by the granule exocytosis pathway.

Adhesion

Time-lapse cinematography observations of CTLs interacting with target cells show CTLs moving on the substrate in apparently random motion before encountering other cells (13,93–95). When contact is made through fine membrane processes, a firmer adhesion involving membrane-membrane contact appears to follow rapidly; the CTLs sometimes move along the surface of the typically larger cells (Fig. 3). In some cases, the CTLs soon detach and resume their random motion, even with target cells of appropriate specificity. In other cases, the adhesion is maintained for minutes to hours until signs of target cell damage can be observed. Electron micrographs of CTLs bound to target cells show considerable areas of close membrane–membrane contact with some gaps in the center of this contact area (Fig. 4).

CTL-target adhesion has been studied by isolation of "conjugates," which are CTL-target clusters observed after CTLs have been centrifuged into contact with nonadherent tumor target cells and gently resuspended (96). By varying the ratio of CTLs and targets, clusters containing more than one target or CTL can be observed. Study of isolated 1:1 conjugates between allogeneic tumor target cells and potent in vivo CTLs showed that target cells were killed within 2 hours of further incubation (14). Classically, conjugates have been enumerated by microscopic counting, with target cells identified by use of a prelabeled fluorescent marker, but two-color flow cytometry has more recently been used for such studies (97). When potent in vivo–derived CTLs from the peritoneal exudate after rejection of allogeneic tumors are used, the specificity of conjugate formation generally reflects TCR recognition, with a variable background of nonspecific conjugates that are not lysed. However, when cloned CTLs grown in long-term in vitro cultures are used, this nonspecific conjugate formation may dominate (98), apparently because of the stronger expression of adhesion molecules such as leukocyte function–associated antigen (LFA) 1 and CD2 on such CTLs.

Specific CTL-target conjugate formation requires a few minutes of incubation at 37° after CTL-target contact to achieve the stability necessary to survive the isolation-induced shear forces. This adhesion does not take place in the cold, can be blocked by inhibitors of intracellular energy generation, and requires magnesium in the medium (99). The requirement for magnesium appears to result from the interaction of the CTL adhesion molecule CD11a (LFA-1) with its target cell ligands intracellular adhesion molecule (ICAM)–1 or ICAM-2, which also requires magnesium. A temperature-sensitive strengthening of the adhesion of specific CTL-target pairs can be measured by varying the shear forces necessary to disrupt binding (100).

Specific CTL-target conjugate formation (as well as cytotoxicity) can be blocked by antibodies against adhesion molecules, and this approach led to the identification of the two pairs of "nonspecific" adhesion molecules: CD11a on the CTL surface, which interacts with ICAM molecules on target cells, and CD2 on the CTL surface, which interacts with LFA-3 on target cells (101). The dependence of such "nonspecific" adhesive interactions for successful CTL-target interactions appears to vary with the CTL (102).

Adhesion Strengthening and Membrane Mixing

The simplest view of adhesion molecules is that they provide additional adhesive forces between interacting cell

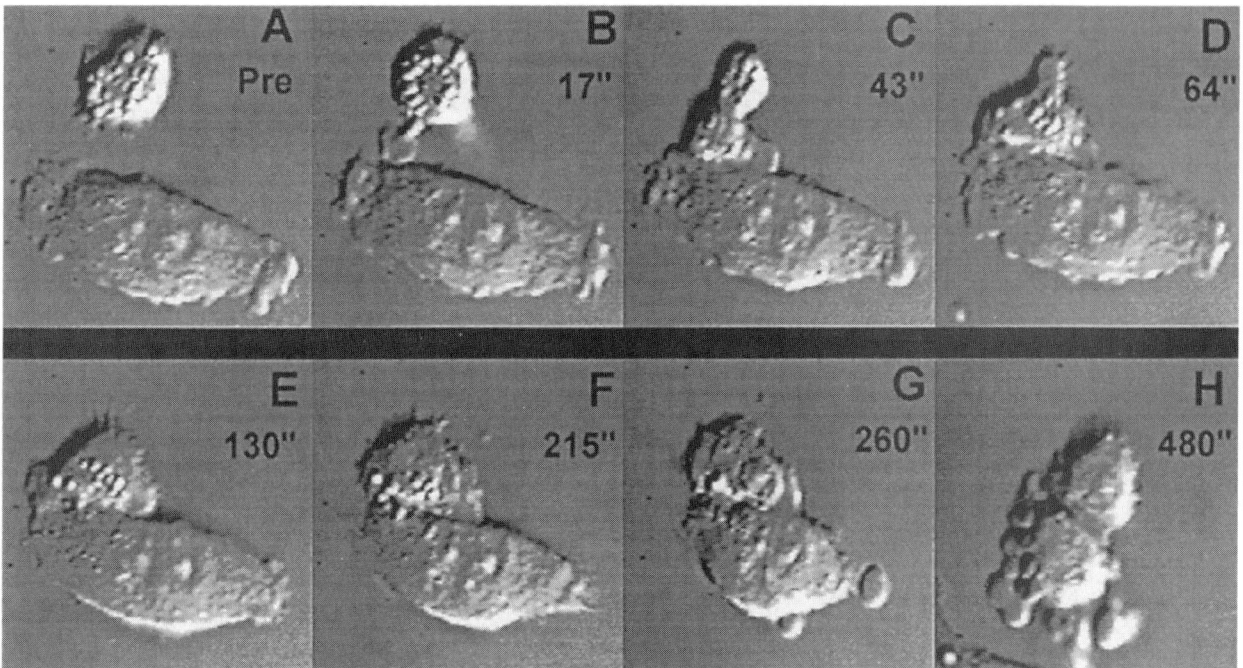

FIG. 3. Time-lapse frames of cytotoxicity by a cloned class I major histocompatibility complex (MHC)–allospecific CD8+ cytotoxic T-lymphocyte (CTL) on a fibroblast target cell as seen with differential interference contrast microscopy. **A:** The CTL approaching the target cell before contact, with random ruffling and extension of small lamellae. **B** to **H:** Sequential images after contact, with the time in seconds after contact indicated. A single large lamella connects the CTL and target (**B**), followed by the extension of membrane-membrane contact along the target surface (**C** to **D**). Granule movement from the initially dispersed array toward the bound target cell is seen in **D** to **G**, followed by granule disappearance in **F** to **H**. Membrane blebbing, a sign of target injury, is first seen in **G** and becomes more dramatic in **H**. Images provided by Dr. Klaus Hahn, Scripps Clinic and Research Foundation, from Hahn et al. (110), with permission.

membranes and hence allow a more efficient interaction of the specific receptor–ligand interactions. However, there is considerable evidence for a more complex set of interactions among the TCR–MHC/peptide interaction, CD8/MHC interaction, and the engagement of CTL adhesion molecules with their target ligands. It has become clear that the adhesion molecules and CD8 are capable of generating signals within the CTL and that TCR engagement leads to a strengthening of the avidity of the CD11a–ICAM interaction as well as the CD8–MHC interaction (103,104). Thus, the initial weak interactions between CTL adhesion molecules and target ligands promote interaction between TCR and target MHC/peptide. This in turn induces a further strengthening of CD11a–ICAM and CD8–MHC interaction that provides strong adhesion. The cytoskeleton may play a role in these interactions because cytochalasins block conjugate formation. Because CTL-target conjugates form stable adhesion in the absence of extracellular calcium, a functionally useful definition of the adhesion and adhesion-strengthening phase of the CTL lytic process is that this is the calcium-independent, magnesium-dependent step.

During CTL-target interaction, membrane proteins, including class I MHC/peptide complexes and lipid probes

are rapidly acquired by the CTL from the target (105–107). Although the molecular mechanism of this transfer remains unclear, electron micrograph observations show regions of membrane fusion between the two cells, which appears independent of target cytotoxicity (108). The membrane molecules acquired by the CTL can subsequently be endocytosed, but enough remain on the surface to allow fratricidal recognition by other CTLs. Such fratricide may contribute to the *in vivo* perforin-dependent downregulation of T-cell numbers after antigen challenge (see later discussion).

Effector Polarization

Microscopic studies of CTL-target conjugates reveal that a pronounced polarization exists within CTLs that are bound to specific target cells, as can be seen in Fig. 3 (109). Under favorable circumstances, polarization can be observed within 1 minute after CTL-target contact (110). The microtubule organizing center is the first CTL component seen to be polarized, followed by recruitment of talin, Lck, and protein kinase C-θ to the submembranous cytoplasm opposite the target cell, followed in turn by the granules (108). It appears that,

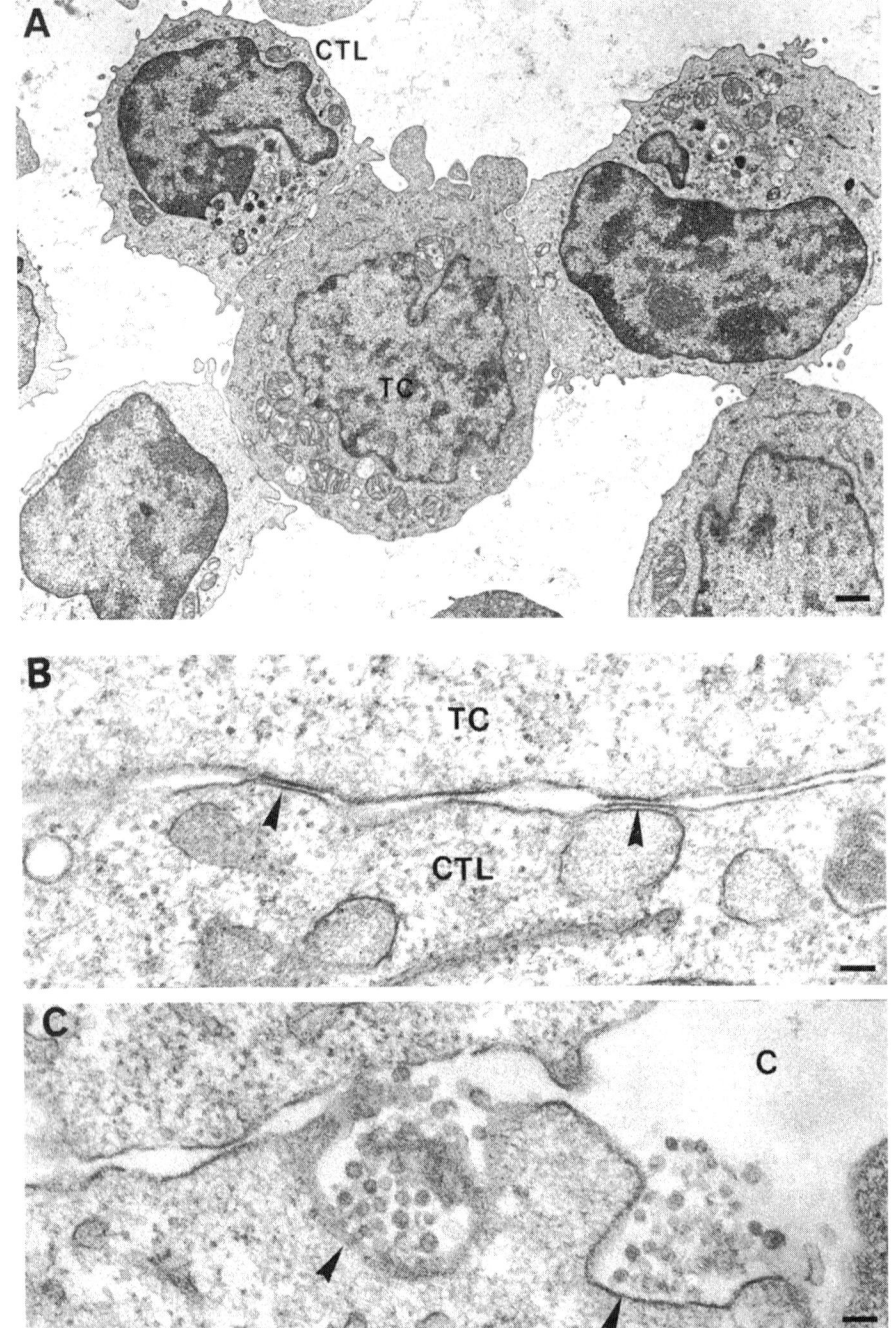

FIG. 4. Rapid polarization and exocytosis induced by target cells in a human cytotoxic T-lymphocyte (CTL) clone. **A:** Three CTLs adherent to one target cell (TC) fixed 1 minute after the two cell types were mixed. Polarization is seen only in the CTL in the upper left (labeled *CTL*). Size bar, 1 μm. **B:** CTL-target interface fixed at 1 minute after mixing at higher power, showing two sites of close apposition of CTL and target cell plasma membranes (*arrowheads*). Size bar, 0.1μm. **C:** CTL-target interface fixed 10 minutes after mixing, showing exocytosis of granules containing membrane vesicles. Granule cores are not seen in this section. Size bar, 0.1μm. From Peters et al. (77), with permission, courtesy of Dr. Peter Peters, Dutch Cancer Institute.

ultimately, most of the cytoplasmic organelles are coordinately moved in response to target recognition.

CTL polarization by target cells requires calcium in the medium, and nonpolarized conjugates formed in the absence of calcium subsequently polarize when calcium is added (111). Effector polarization is also blocked by microtubule-disrupting drugs (112). The demonstration of kinesin-dependent movement of isolated CTL granules along microtubules provides insights into the mechanism of CTL polarization (113).

Signaling Exocytosis

A rearrangement of interacting membrane proteins at the CTL-target interface to form the "immunological synapse" appears generally similar to that described between CD4+ T cells and antigen-presenting cells (108). Within the contact plane, CD11a forms an outer ring in parallel with the CTL cytoplasmic protein talin. Central to this ring is a highly concentrated domain containing the signaling kinases Lck and protein kinase C-θ. It is hard to determine precisely which aspects of synapse formation are critical to signaling exocytosis. Protein kinases have been implicated in CTL signaling, such as from the strong stimulatory effect of the protein kinase C activator PMA on CTL degranulation in the presence of calcium ionophores (27). Anti-TCR antibody stimulation of CTL induces tyrosine phosphorylation of a discrete set of substrates, including p56[Lck], with additional substrates phosphorylated upon CD8 binding to class I (114). These results show that CD8 engagement provides co-stimulation signals via protein kinases. However, TCR-induced protein kinase activation was found to be stronger in CD8-dependent CTLs than in CD8-independent CTLs (115). In this system, TCR engagement increased the association of p56[Lck] with CD8 and recruited ZAP70 to the TCR complex. These studies of protein kinases in CTL activated by target recognition suggest TCR signaling pathways similar to those found in other T cells, covered elsewhere (Chapter 11). However, it is not yet clear at what point signaling for cytoplasmic polarization and degranulation diverges from signaling for gene expression (e.g., Fas ligand and IFN-γ).

CTL signaling also involves an increase in intracellular calcium, which accompanies many examples of T-cell activation (116). Through the use of single-cell imaging with intracellular calcium-sensitive fluorescent dyes, CTLs were shown to undergo a rapid cytoplasmic calcium increase after engagement of specific target cells (117,118). Resting CTL calcium levels of approximately 100 nM rose to a mean of approximately 500 nM within a few minutes before declining to baseline over the course of about 20 minutes. Multiple cycles of intracellular calcium increase were sometimes seen (119). The antigen-induced intracellular calcium increase was blunted and transient if extracellular calcium was removed, which suggests an influx of external calcium through the plasma membrane as the major source. However, the calcium channel blocker verapamil does not inhibit this increase, which occurs via a potential-sensitive calcium channel activated in response to depletion of intracellular calcium stores (120,121). The target cell–induced calcium increase in CTLs is correlated with the calcium-requiring lethal hit phase of the CTL mechanism, described from functional measurements earlier.

Exocytosis

Secretion is the result of a membrane fusion event between the granule membrane and plasma membrane, termed *exocytosis,* resulting in a continuity between the granule interior and the extracellular space. Many examples of polarized secretion can be found in cell biology, but few if any follow a rapid induced polarization such as that which occurs after target binding by cytotoxic lymphocytes. Basic molecular aspects of the final critical exocytosis process are still poorly understood. Images from high-resolution time-lapse cinematographic studies of CTL-induced cytotoxicity show what appears to be granule exocytosis after CTL-target contact (94,95). In these images, visible granules close to the CTL membrane disappear shortly after reorientation but before visible target injury. Electron microscopic images such as those of Fig. 4 strongly suggest granule exocytosis into a restricted volume between the CTL and the bound target cell and transfer of the CTL granule contents into this space (108,122). Confocal microscopy shows the granules apparently inserting within the outer ring of CD11a molecules, adjacent to the protein kinases in the plane of interaction between CTL and target (108).

CTL exocytosis can be measured by assessing the release of granule components into the medium. By this approach, degranulation of CTL is observed within a few hours of culture in the presence of target cells, on immobilized antibodies against the TCR complex, or in response to stimulatory lectins such as concanavalin A. In common with most other forms of secretion via the regulated secretory pathway, CTL degranulation triggered by anti-TCR antibodies and antigen is blocked by removal of extracellular calcium (123). Granzyme A secretion is not blocked by inhibitors of ribonucleic acid (RNA) and protein synthesis (in striking contrast to that of IFN-γ in the same CTL), but TCR cross-linking can be replaced by a combination of the calcium ionophore and the protein kinase C activator phorbol myristyl acetate (27).

According to work in both human and mouse genetic defects, CTL and NK cell granule exocytosis requires the Rab family small guanosine triphosphatase protein Rab-27a (79,124,125). Defects in Rab-27a lead to a failure of the granule exocytosis cytotoxicity pathway but not the Fas pathway. After TCR ligation, CTLs with defective Rab-27a fail to degranulate, although they secrete IFN-γ normally. Unlike the case of melanosomes in melanocytes, Rab-27a does not appear to play a role granule movement, inasmuch as CTL cytoplasmic polarization in response to antigen is normal. Thus, Rab-27a is required for a late step in the granule exocytosis pathway. This is compatible with one of the major described functions of Rab proteins: promoting tethering of the granule membrane to the plasma membrane at the terminal exocytosis step (126).

The Role of Granzymes in Target Death through Granule Exocytosis

Evidence implicating particular molecules as cytotoxic mediators comes from several approaches. The requirement for perforin in target death *in vitro* was made clear from studies of cytotoxic lymphocytes in perforin-knockout mice, which are completely lacking the granule exocytosis cytotoxicity pathway *in vitro* (22,23,127). However, several lines of evidence argue convincingly that, in addition to perforin, granzymes are also required to induce death in nucleated target cells (128).

Cytotoxic lymphocytes from granzyme B–deficient mice show slightly deficient target lysis and a more profound deficiency in target DNA fragmentation (129,130). Cytotoxic lymphocytes from granzyme A knockout mice displayed no detectable defects in either target lysis or DNA fragmentation (131), although it seems possible that granzymes A and K have redundant function (132). Cytotoxic lymphocytes from granzyme A/B double-knockout mice give markedly reduced target DNA damage (133,134), but their ability to cause target lysis is reduced only marginally. Loss of the granzyme-processing enzyme DPPI gave rise to lymphocytes with inactive granzymes (71), which also showed markedly reduced ability to induce target DNA damage. Thus, the granzyme knockout results show that granzyme B contributes significantly to target cell nuclear damage, whereas considerable target lysis occurs in the absence of both granzymes A and B.

A complementary approach to knocking out mediator expression was taken in experiments in which lymphocyte granule mediators were expressed in the RBL mast cell tumor line. These cells have an intact granule exocytosis pathway triggered by the immunoglobulin E receptor. Although RBL cells transfected with perforin alone acquired a potent hemolytic activity, their ability to kill nucleated targets was negligible. For cytolytic activity comparable with that of CTLs, including DNA fragmentation, expression of both granzymes A and B was required, along with perforin (135,136). Analysis of transfectant clones showed their cytolytic activity on tumor targets was quantitatively correlated with granzyme but not perforin expression levels (although perforin expression was required for activity).

Another approach has been to analyze the effects of purified mediator proteins on target cells. Perforin's lytic activity is not accompanied by apoptotic DNA fragmentation (137). When added to the medium, granzymes are not toxic to cells, although granzyme B is internalized by receptor-mediated endocytosis (138). Granzyme A causes DNA fragmentation in cells rendered permeable by detergent (139), and granzymes A, B, and K show this activity in cells treated with sublytic doses of perforin (140), with a synergistic effect between perforin and granzymes in promoting target nuclear damage and lysis. A noninfectious adenovirus, bacterial toxins, or direct microinjection can also be used to allow granzymes to access target cytoplasm with accompanying apoptotic DNA fragmentation (138,141,142).

If granzymes are cytotoxic mediators that work after introduction into target cytoplasm, expression of cytoplasmic granzyme inhibitors should block target death. The general serine protease inhibitor aprotinin was found to block target lysis when loaded into the target cell cytoplasm (143) or coupled to the target membrane (144) but not in the medium,

and blocking was not seen with effectors expressing perforin only. The granzyme B inhibitor PI-9 is an intracellular member of the serpin family present in cytotoxic lymphocytes and other cells that can protect tumor cells against CTL-induced death *in vitro* and *in vivo* (145–148).

Perforin-Mediated Granzyme Entry into Target Cells

Electron micrograph observations of complement-like, pore-like structures on target cells attacked by cytotoxic large granular lymphocytes and CTLs strongly suggested that analogous membrane damage was responsible for target cell killing by both complement and cytotoxic lymphocytes (36–38). Subsequent studies have raised a number of issues that have forced a significant revision of this paradigm. Both complement and isolated perforin at high concentrations can cause the death of nucleated target cells within a few minutes at 37° (149,150), but target cells lethally injured by CTL require an average of 1.7 hours between infliction of the lethal damage and target lysis (18). It has become recognized that nucleated cells have a cytoplasmic system of repair of membrane injury. This has been characterized in studies with complement as resulting from a calcium-dependent shedding of vesicles containing pore-like structures into the medium (48) and in studies with physical wounding of cell membranes as resulting from a calcium-dependent exocytosis of internal membranes (151). Such repair mechanisms can explain the ability of cells to recover within minutes from the permeability increases induced by sublytic perforin concentrations (152) and the cross-protection from lysis observed among different channel forming agents (153).

Because pore-forming agents, including purified perforin, induce a nonapoptotic death (137), perforin "permeabilization" cannot explain the apoptotic phenotype seen in most target cells killed by CTLs or NK cells (154). Studies with noncytolytic RBL mast cell tumors show that perforin expression confers a very potent cytolytic activity against red blood cell targets but only a very modest lytic activity against tumor targets, which was not accompanied by DNA fragmentation (155). These results argue that nucleated cells, unlike mammalian erythrocytes, have defensive systems that can normally repair the membrane damage from pore formation induced by high local concentrations of perforin after degranulation. However, because perforin is absolutely required for rapid lethal damage of Fas-negative cells induced by CTLs and NK cells, it appears that the primary role for perforin is to allow granzymes access to the target cytoplasm.

There are two general mechanisms by which perforin could allow granzymes access to the cytoplasm. The simplest case would be that granzymes transit through perforin's large membrane pores, as suggested by results with resealed red blood cell ghost targets and the electron micrographic images of large aqueous pores (36,45). However, direct experimental evidence for this entry route is lacking. An alternative proposal is that granzymes are taken up with perforin into endosomes and that perforin subsequently causes a breakdown in the endosomal membrane, releasing granzymes into the cytoplasm, where apoptosis is triggered. This model was suggested by experiments in which cells were first exposed to granzyme B and then washed. When this was followed by addition of perforin or other "permeabilizing" agents, apoptosis was induced (138,141), which clearly suggests that perforin renders endosomes permeable to release granzyme B into the cytoplasm. Further evidence for this model comes from studies supporting a role for the mannose-6-phosphate receptor in apoptosis induced by addition of noninfectious adenovirus and granzyme B (156). These studies showed that a cell line lacking the cation-independent mannose-6-phosphate receptor was resistant to apoptosis by granzyme B and adenovirus, to CTL-mediated DNA damage (although not lysis), and to CTL-mediated allograft rejection *in vivo*. These studies suggest that granzyme B enters the target cells through receptor-mediated endocytosis, although the mechanism by which perforin "permeabilizes" endosomes remains unclear.

Caspase-Dependent and -Independent Pathways of Cytotoxic T-Lymphocyte–Induced Target Death

Observations of apoptotic structure (157) and DNA fragmentation (154) in CTL targets suggested that CTLs trigger target cell apoptosis, although double-strand DNA cleavage is not invariably found (158). The role of nuclear damage in CTL-induced target cell death was addressed in experiments using enucleated cytoplasts. Such targets could be fully lysed by CTLs through both the granule exocytosis and Fas death pathways, and the tenfold increase in effector potency resulting from granzyme expression in RBL effector cells was seen in such targets (159). These results are parallel to some other apoptotic death inducers that also do not require target nuclei (160), and they show that apoptotic nuclear damage is not required for CTL-induced target cell lysis.

The ability of granzyme B to proteolytically process and hence activate caspases is well documented. Purified granzyme B can process and activate caspases-3, -7, -8, -9, and -10 but not caspases-1 or -2. Furthermore, CTLs have been shown to specifically induce the processing of caspase-3 in target cells (161), which does not occur with CTL lacking granzyme B (162). The mechanisms by which granzymes trigger death has been pursued with the use of purified granzyme B in cells that have been rendered permeable. Labeled granzyme B localizes in the nucleus of "permeabilized" target cells, which correlates with induction of apoptosis (163,164), but inhibition of caspases blocks this nuclear localization without blocking killing (165).

The role of caspases in CTL-induced cytotoxicity has been tested with caspase inhibitors, which block most apoptotic death in a variety of *in vitro* and *in vivo* systems (166). Both cell-permeant peptide-based caspase inhibitors and the protein inhibitor baculovirus p35 effectively block the lysis and apoptotic nuclear damage induced by the CTL Fas ligand/Fas pathway in several different target cell types. Through the

granule exocytosis pathway, CTL-induced lysis of these targets was unaffected by either of these types of caspase inhibitors, which is compatible with the idea that granzyme B activates caspases that trigger nuclear damage but not lysis. Caspase inhibitors also fail to block CTL-induced blebbing, mitochondrial depolarization, or phosphatidyl serine flipping by the granule exocytosis pathway, although they did block the increased target endocytosis induced by CTL degranulation (167). Thus, it is clear that, although CTLs do trigger target caspase activation, death can also occur by caspase-independent pathways. Whether the known extranuclear substrates of granzymes (56) account for this death remains unclear.

The Bcl-2 family of intracellular proteins contains members that oligomerize with each other and interact with mitochondrial membranes to give both proapoptotic and antiapoptotic functional effects (168). Antiapoptotic members of the Bcl-2 family, such as Bcl-2 and Bcl-x, protect against many different death inducers, but for CTL-induced death, these antiapoptotic proteins have a variable effect, protecting in some cases but not others. Bcl-2 has been reported by different laboratories to inhibit or have no effect on the CTL Fas ligand/Fas and granule exocytosis death pathways (59,169–171), and it blocks the nuclear accumulation of granzymes (172). Proapoptotic members of this family have been implicated in granzyme B–mediated apoptosis. Bid can be cleaved directly by granzyme B to a truncated form with potent proapoptotic activity through mitochondrial damage (57,173), and this appears to be the major granzyme B–induced death pathway, in at least some cells (as opposed to direct procaspase processing). Granzyme B–induced mitochondrial damage by Bid requires another proapoptotic member of this family, Bak (60), which is compatible with the known tendency of these family members to associate with each other. It is still unclear whether such mitochondrial damage can also explain caspase-independent death induced by CTLs.

Cytotoxic T-Lymphocyte Detachment

Time-lapse cinematography of CTL-induced cytotoxicity shows that CTLs detach from target cells, move away, and subsequently kill more neighboring target cells. The mechanism of this detachment is unclear, and it is also unclear whether the CTLs remain attached until target lysis or if an active decision is made before lysis but after the lethal injury has been delivered (174).

Self-Protection of Cytotoxic Lymphocytes

A major question facing the granule exocytosis model has always been why the effector cells are not themselves lysed after degranulation releases lethal mediators at high local concentrations. Microscopic studies established that CTLs can kill multiple target cells without suffering detectable damage themselves. Numerous subsequent investigations addressed the question of whether CTLs are themselves susceptible targets to attack by other CTLs. Early studies found that uncloned CTLs were inactivated by other CTLs, and it was assumed that they were killed. However, more recent studies indicate that such "target" CTLs are not necessarily killed when other CTLs inactivate them (175). Cloned CTLs have frequently been found to be highly resistant to lysis after recognition by other CTLs (176–178). Thus, CTLs appear to express a permanent global resistance to their own lethal mediators. CTLs are resistant to perforin-induced lysis, in relation to other lymphoid cells (179,180). Such resistance is not absolute, and it is not clear that CTLs are uniquely resistant to perforin lysis, because there is a wide range of resistance among non-CTL targets. Protective membrane proteins have been proposed to be responsible for this resistance—for example, by binding perforin molecules before membrane insertion or before inserted molecules aggregate and form functional pores (181)—but satisfactory molecular identification and functional experiments establishing their role in CTL self-protection have not been carried out. Another explanation for CTL perforin resistance is that they have a particularly active system of removing inserted perforin from their membranes, as discussed previously.

In spite of this evidence in favor of a global system of CTL self-protection, a variety of studies show that CTLs can kill other CTLs, which implies that the resistance just described can be overcome. Thus, enriched populations of *in vivo*–derived CTLs are lysed by other CTLs, hapten-specific cloned CTLs kill other hapten-specific cloned CTLs, and peptide-specific cloned CTLs kill each other in the presence of peptide (182,183). These findings continue to pose a challenge for the granule exocytosis model and suggest that other local or temporary protective systems exist in CTLs to prevent self-destruction after degranulation. Because granule membrane components become locally incorporated into the plasma membrane after exocytosis, they are one class of candidates. Another possibility is a transient global protection triggered by target recognition. These speculative possibilities have been difficult to test experimentally.

Cytotoxic T-Lymphocyte–Mediated Induction of Target Fas

Perforin-deficient CTLs have been found to lyse Fas-negative target cells slowly *in vitro*. The mechanism for this cytotoxicity was revealed to be a CTL-mediated induction of Fas expression in the target (184). CTL degranulation was not required for this inductive effect, but the nature of the inductive signal generated in the target cell remains unknown.

DIFFERENTIATION-DEPENDENT EXPRESSION OF CYTOTOXIC MEDIATORS

A general survey of normal tissues for expression of perforin messenger RNA or protein shows that it is expressed exclusively in lymphoid tissue, and closer examination reveals that its expression is highly correlated with lymphocyte cytotoxic activity. For example, in normal human peripheral blood, perforin protein was detected in more than 95% of the $CD56^+$ NK cells and in more than 97% of the $\gamma\delta$ T cells (29). Both of these populations show cytolytic activity with redirected lysis. Although blood $CD4^+$ T cells were negative for perforin expression and cytotoxicity, $CD8^+$ cells with memory phenotype showed substantial cytotoxic activity and perforin expression. Naïve and cord blood $CD8^+$ T cells were shown to lack detectable perforin expression (185). After *in vitro* activation, $CD4^+$ T cells remained negative for perforin expression and cytotoxicity, whereas $CD8^+$ T cells increased their perforin expression and cytotoxicity (29).

Granzyme messenger RNA and protein expression are not detectable in resting peripheral T-lymphocytes (in contrast to resting NK cells) (52,186). *In vitro* activation increases expression of all granzymes in both $CD4^+$ and $CD8^+$ T cells, as well as in NK cells. Granzyme A and B messenger RNA expression is detectable in immature thymocytes but declines at the $CD4^+CD8^+$ stage (187). In $CD4^-CD8^+$ thymocytes, granzyme A messenger RNA and enzymatic activity is detectable.

Murine peritoneal exudate lymphocytes induced by allostimulation have been a classical source of highly potent CTLs (96). These cells express perforin and granzymes but at lower levels than do CTLs grown *in vitro* (188). After *in vitro* culture in IL-2, such CTLs acquire higher levels of these granule mediators, but there is no evidence that this enhances cytotoxic function.

There remain many questions regarding differences in expression of lytic mediators among naïve, effector, and different subtypes of memory $CD8^+$ T cells. Indeed, surprisingly little is known about molecules that control expression of cytolytic machinery in CTLs. It was proposed (189) that CD30 may represent one such molecule by virtue of inhibiting effector cell cytotoxicity. It was shown in studies of the granular lymphoma line YT that CD30-mediated signaling caused strong inhibition of cytotoxicity by blocking the expression of such crucial cytotoxic molecules as perforin, Fas ligand, and granzyme B. Additional *in vivo* studies demonstrated CD30-mediated suppression, which suggests that CD30-mediated signaling may function *in vivo* by down-regulating CTL effector functions and proliferation while enabling CTLs to home to lymph nodes.

In Vivo versus In Vitro Studies of Cytotoxic T-Lymphocyte–Mediated Cytotoxicity: The Role of Oxygen

CTLs are exposed to different extracellular signaling molecules in normal and inflamed local tissue as they differentiate and function in primary, secondary, and tertiary lymphoid organs with different infrastructure, vasculature, and cell metabolism. In addition to encountering immunologically relevant signaling molecules (e.g., TCRs, lymphokines), CTLs experience diverse biochemical and biophysical local environments, in which they are exposed to different repertoires of physiologically abundant "non-immune" molecules, capable of affecting lymphocyte and antigen-presenting cell physiology.

One example of such a molecule is molecular oxygen. Immune cells and their progenitors could be exposed to both relatively high (normoxia) and low oxygen tensions [hypoxia, as low as 4 to 34 mm Hg, which is 0.5% to 4.5% O_2 (percent volume of solute)] as they travel between blood and different tissues in lymphoid organs (190). To test whether lymphocyte adaptation to changes in oxygen tension may have an effect on their functions, CTL differentiation and functions were compared at very low (1% O_2) and low (2.5% O_2) oxygen tensions versus routinely used (20% O_2) oxygen tensions. It was found that physiologically relevant hypoxic conditions have different effects on CTL lethal hit delivery and secretion of cytokines. The differentiated CTLs deliver Fas ligand and perforin-dependent lethal hits equally well under both hypoxic and normoxic conditions, thereby extending the reach of CTL-mediated lethal hits to all local tissue environments and preventing escape of infected cells to hypoxic "niches."

However, naïve $\alpha\beta$ T cells differentiate poorly into CTLs at 1% O_2, and CTL development is delayed at 2.5% oxygen in comparison with 20% O_2. Interestingly, the CTLs that developed at hypoxic conditions were much more lytic, whereas their accumulation was accelerated at 20% oxygen. These experiments show that the routinely used conditions of in vitro CTL incubation with ambient 20% O_2 tension in the presence of reducing agent is well suited for immunological specificity and cytotoxicity studies, but oxygen dependence should be taken into account in immunophysiological studies of CTL activation, expansion, and cytokine production.

Extracellular Adenosine as a Physiological Signal to Trigger the Down-regulation of Immune Response

Inflamed local tissue environments are associated with accumulation of extracellular adenosine, and this fact led to studies of the possible role of adenosine receptors in regulation of CTLs. It was shown that extracellular adenosine is an interesting candidate for being endogenous regulator of CTL functions, because CTLs express A2a adenosine receptors and are inhibitable by extracellular adenosine (191). Adenosine suppressed all tested TCR-triggered effector functions, including cytotoxicity, via both granule exocytosis/perforin- and Fas ligand–mediated pathways and by cytokine secretion. Even brief exposure to adenosine was sufficient to observe inhibition of TCR-triggered effector functions. Such "memory" of T cells to adenosine exposure is explained by the long-lasting increased levels of intracellular cyclic adenosine monophosphate even after the extracellular adenosine has been degraded.

Further studies are necessary to understand the functioning of adenosine receptor–mediated CTL down-regulation in different models of immune response in vivo, including anti-tumor CTL activity. Studies using adenosine receptor gene–deficient mice provided in vivo evidence for the nonredundant role of extracellular adenosine and adenosine receptors as negative regulators of NK T cell–, T cell–, and macrophage-mediated immune response in vivo: Extensive tissue damage and higher and longer lasting levels of proinflammatory cytokines were observed in A2a adenosine receptor–deficient animals in comparison with wild-type animals (192). Thus, it appears that extracellular concentrations of adenosine in inflamed areas are sufficiently high to activate A2a receptors on CTLs and that adenosine receptors may contribute to the negative feedback mechanism of down-regulation of CTLs in vivo.

IN VIVO ROLE OF PERFORIN- AND FAS-MEDIATED CYTOTOXICITY

The description of perforin as a cytolytic molecule and cloning of the perforin gene not only facilitated studies and led to better understanding of cytotoxic cells functions but has also provided tools for identifying the genetic basis of some human immunological disorders. In vivo, CTL-mediated cytotoxicity can be mediated not only by the rapid mechanisms of lethal hit delivery involving perforin or Fas ligand but also by slower processes resulting from activities of soluble mediators such as TNF-α. The development of knockout mice lacking individual effector molecules allows assessment of their importance to various in vivo processes. A series of studies have compared wild-type mice with Fas- and Fas ligand–deficient and perforin-deficient mice and mice with combinations of these deficiencies in order to evaluate the role of these cytotoxic mechanisms in vivo. These studies revealed defects ranging from impaired immune surveillance and defense against pathogens to autoimmunity.

Homeostasis of the Immune System

Several studies using different approaches have concluded that perforin plays a significant role in the homeostasis of the immune system, requiring elimination of expanded numbers of antigen-specific T cells after the peak of the immune response (193). Previous studies had shown that deficiency of Fas and Fas ligand is associated with lymphoproliferative autoimmune diseases (194), and it is generally accepted that the Fas-mediated destruction of antigen-presenting cells by T helper cells plays an important role in a negative feedback regulation of generation and expansion of both CD4+ and CD8+ T cells to protect from excessive tissue destruction by immune cells (195). The role of perforin has been suggested by studies showing the early death and infiltration of liver and kidney by CD8+ T cells in perforin-deficient mice (196).

Another example showing perforin involvement in down-regulation of CD8+ cells was provided by the demonstration that antigen-exposed perforin-deficient mice are defective in down-regulation of peripheral CD8 T cells but not of CD4+ cells. The important role of perforin in homeostasis of CD8+ T cells was subsequently confirmed in studies of Listeria *monocytogenes*–infected mice lacking perforin and IFN-γ (197). This suggests that perforin plays a critical role in limiting the life span of $CD8^+$ CTLs *in vivo*. Thus, there is an emerging consensus about the dual role of CTLs and antimicrobial cytokines that function as both pathogen-destroying effectors and down-regulators of expanded immune T cells.

The unexpected finding that the fatal human disease familial hemophagocytic lymphohistiocytosis (FHL) is caused by defective perforin expression (198) has confirmed animal studies showing perforin's role in homeostatic regulation of the immune system. FHL is characterized by uncontrolled activation of T cells and macrophages and high levels of proinflammatory cytokines, which were convincingly shown to be caused by missense and homozygous nonsense mutations in the perforin gene in unrelated patients with FHL (198). Lymphocytes of these patients had no cytolytic activity, and no perforin protein was detected in granules.

Observations of immune abnormalities in double–cytotoxic mechanism–deficient mice (Fas ligand$^{-/-}$, perforin$^{-/-}$), which are more severe than in single Fas ligand– or perforin-knockout mice, support the view that perforin and death-signal transducing receptors function as both redundant and complementary mechanisms of homeostatic control (199).

CTL-mediated cytotoxicity against CTLs (fratricide) is also implicated in control of numbers of CTLs *in vivo*. For example, virus-induced liver injury attributable to CTL damage declined as the number of virus-specific CTLs diminished. In this system, the death of $CD8^+$ T cells accounting for complete elimination of virus-specific CTL requires Fas but not the perforin or TNF-α pathways (200).

The importance of perforin/Fas ligand pathways in maintenance of homeostasis is illustrated by pathological processes in perforin/Fas ligand double-deficient mice, which die early of severe pancreatitis. Such female mice are infertile and have hysterosalpingitis (199). The tissue destruction probably results from infiltration with monocytes/macrophages, which is accompanied by the expansion of $CD8^+$ T cells. The role of macrophages is consistent with observations of healing effects of monocyte/macrophage inactivation by carrageenan *in vivo*. The accumulation of disease-causing macrophages is explained by the inability of perforin/Fas ligand–deficient $CD8^+$ or $CD4^+$ T cells to destroy cognate antigen-presenting cells and thereby provide negative feedback homeostatic regulation of the immune processes.

Cytotoxic T-Lymphocytes in Host Defense against Infection

Antigen-specific CTLs have been shown to be involved in the immunity against intracellular pathogens such as *L. monocytogenes* and *Trypanosoma cruzi,* which are able to escape from phagocytic vacuoles into the cytoplasm of infected cells, as well as in the immunity against microorganisms which stay within the vacuoles (e.g., *Salmonella typhimurium, Escherichia coli,* and *M. tuberculosis*) (201).

Study findings have provided a potential explanation of the mechanism by which CTLs directly destroy microbial pathogens residing in intracellular compartments (89,202). The bactericidal granule protein granulysin has been proposed to be critically responsible for the death of intracellular mycobacteria. This protein is expressed in skin lesions from leprosy patients. The authors hypothesized that perforin ensures the delivery of granule-located proteins, thereby enabling granulysin's access to intracellular compartments in order to kill a pathogen. A role for granulysin in immunity to leprosy was suggested by experiments showing that $CD4^+$ T cells localized in skin lesions in leprosy patients express granulysin, and T-cell lines derived from such lesions used granule exocytosis to suppress intracellular *M. leprae in vitro* (203). However, the critical role of these mediators in immune protection against mycobacteria *in vivo* remains unclear, inasmuch as immune protection appears normal in perforin-knockout mice (204,205).

Cellular Cytotoxicity Pathways in Antitumor Cytotoxic T-Lymphocyte Activity

Studies of perforin gene–deficient mice after injection with different tumors, chemical carcinogens, and oncogenic viruses strongly suggest that perforin-dependent cytotoxicity is functional in antitumor CTL and NK surveillance during both viral and chemical carcinogenesis. The lack of perforin was associated with decreased tumor surveillance (127,206). Striking evidence for the role of cytotoxic lymphocytes in control of tumor growth was provided by testing the prediction that the incidence of tumors in tumor-prone p53-deficient mice would be increased or accelerated if these mice were also deficient in perforin expression (207). It was shown that disseminated lymphoma is likely to be controlled by perforin in CTLs, because increased lymphomagenesis was observed in perforin-deficient mice. Together with other indirect evidence, studies of perforin-deficient mice suggest that CTLs may indeed participate in the mechanisms of host resistance to spontaneous tumors.

The role of granzymes in antitumor immunity remains unclear, because mice lacking granzymes A and B were as efficient as wild-type mice in their abilities to reject tumors *in vivo* (208).

Cytotoxic Lymphocytes in Control of Viral Infections

Studies of the role of individual components of cytotoxic machinery in immune response to different viral infections suggest that control of viral replication requires granule exocytosis/perforin-mediated cytotoxicity (127). Different combinations of molecules in cytotoxic granules may be necessary to control replication of different viruses. It was demonstrated in studies of mouse cytomegalovirus (MCMV) infection of wild-type C57BL/6 (B6) mice and of mice lacking recombination activating gene 2 (RAG2), perforin, granzyme A, or granzyme B in different combinations, that both perforin- and granzyme-mediated pathways are involved in control of viral replication (209). The authors concluded that CD8$^+$ T cells and NK cells are absolutely necessary and that perforin and granzymes A and B do contribute in the control of MCMV infection of salivary gland. However, experiments with gene-deficient mice revealed that viral elimination proceeds even in the absence of one of each of these effector molecules, which thereby suggests their redundant roles in an antiviral response.

In contrast to these observations of salivary gland infection by MCMV, studies of the natural mouse pathogen ectromelia established that mice deficient in granzymes A and B fail to control primary infections by this virus, in spite of normal perforin expression and CTL activity *in vitro* (210). Thus, in some viral infections granzymes are absolutely indispensable and are required together with perforin for protection of the host animal. These findings are in contrast with earlier observations showing normal protection against *L. monocytogenes* and lymphocytic choriomeningitis virus (LCMV) infections in granzyme A–deficient mice (131).

Cytotoxic T-Lymphocytes in Disease Pathogenesis

The well-established concept of CTLs as a double-edged sword capable of both killing infected cells and inflicting collateral tissue damage (211) is further supported by studies of the role of cytotoxic mechanisms in LCMV clearance and tissue damage (212). To address the question as to which cytotoxicity mechanism is involved in the viral clearance versus tissue damage during viral hepatitis pathogenesis, mice deficient in either individual Fas ligand or perforin pathways of cytotoxicity were used. It was found that perforin-mediated granule exocytosis pathway is required for viral clearance but that both Fas ligand and perforin/granule exocytosis pathways must be activated in order to observe liver damage. These observations may suggest the therapeutic strategies for avoiding liver damage while maintaining efficient antiviral CTL response.

Interesting insights into mechanisms of antiviral effector functions of CTLs were gained in studies of hepatitis B virus (HBV) antigen–specific CTLs in HBV-transgenic mice (213). It is believed that antigen-activated CTLs secrete proinflammatory cytokines (including IFN-γ) and that this, in turn, results in noncytopathic inhibition of HBV replication in most infected hepatocytes. In contrast, perforin- and Fas ligand–triggered apoptosis affects only a very small proportion of infected hepatocytes. It has been assumed that CTL-induced apoptosis of virus-infected cells also destroys replicating viral nucleic acids through the activation of proteases and endonucleases in apoptotic cells. It was discovered in studies of HBV-transgenic mice that, at least in the case of HBV infection, the virus-specific CTLs do trigger apoptosis in a small proportion of HBV-infected hepatocytes, but this is not accompanied by the destruction of replicative DNA containing cytoplasmic HBV nucleocapsids.

These studies provided an example of pathological CTL-mediated inflammatory tissue damage and destruction of infected cells that is not accompanied by complete destruction of the pathogen and is not sufficient on its own to accomplish viral clearance. The authors concluded that HBV nucleocapsids are very resistant to proteases and endonucleases and that the proapoptotic effector functions of HBV-specific CTLs are not sufficient on their own for clearance of this viral infection. Accordingly, the explanation of efficient control of HBV infection *in vivo* must involve not only CTLs but also cytokines and cells of the innate immune system.

Cytotoxic T-Lymphocytes and Autoimmunity

CTLs have been implicated in destruction of pancreatic β cells during the course of autoimmune type 1 diabetes, and studies were conducted to evaluate the contribution of CTL-mediated cytotoxic mechanisms in pathogenesis of this disease. Experiments were performed with transgenic mice expressing LCMV antigen in β cells. These mice rapidly became diabetic after an LCMV injection induced a CTL response against the antigen.

The critical role of perforin in these processes is shown by the absence of diabetes after LCMV infection in perforin-deficient mice with the LCMV transgene. Thus, perforin-mediated cytotoxicity is crucial for β-cell destruction, exceeding the importance of other potential inflammatory cytotoxic molecules (214). These conclusions were reinforced in subsequent studies in which CTL-mediated, perforin-dependent cytotoxicity is strongly implicated in autoimmune diabetes by observations of the delay in the onset of the disease and of decreased incidence of spontaneous and cyclophosphamide-induced diabetes in perforin-deficient mice that were backcrossed with the nonobese diabetes mouse strain (215).

In experimental autoimmune encephalomyelitis, studies with mice defective in both perforin- and Fas-mediated cytotoxicity have shown that the latter defect is required for the major pathological effects in this disease model (216).

Cytotoxic Lymphocytes and Graft-Versus-Host Disease

Perforin- and Fas ligand–deficient mice also allowed experiments addressing the long-standing question as to the mechanism of complex tissues damage processes. It was shown that transplantation of Fas ligand–deficient T cells into lethally irradiated recipient mice resulted in cachexia but not in significant levels of cutaneous or liver graft-versus-host disease (GVHD) (217). In contrast, an acute, although delayed, GVHD was observed in mice that received perforin-deficient T cells. The authors concluded that perforin-mediated cytotoxicity may influence the time course of GVHD development but is not required for tissue damage. Thus, different tissue damage is inflicted by Fas ligand– and perforin-dependent mechanisms during the course of GVHD, and Fas ligand–mediated cytotoxicity is responsible for hepatotoxicity and cutaneous GVHD. This model may provide a convenient assay for future studies of regulation of CTLs in pathogenesis of GVHD *in vivo*.

These observations are in agreement with an independent study (218) in which a similar question was addressed; Fas ligand, but not perforin, was found to have the major role in pathogenesis of class II MHC–restricted acute GVHD. In contrast, the perforin-mediated pathway, but not Fas ligand–mediated cytotoxicity, is required for class I-restricted acute murine GVHD. The authors suggested selectively inhibiting the granule exocytosis/perforin pathway as a novel anti-GVHD therapeutic strategy and showed that inhibitors of this pathway do not interfere with posttransplantation hematopoietic reconstitution. However, more recent studies of mice doubly deficient in Fas ligand- and perforin have demonstrated that both effector pathways play a role in GVHD (219). The double cytotoxic deficiency resulted in a decrease in numbers of donor CD4 T cells and a delay in GVHD-associated death and weight loss, which suggests that GVHD-induced tissue injury is mediated by cytotoxic effects of donor CD4 T cells.

Cytotoxic Mediators in Contact Hypersensitivity

Although cytotoxic CD8$^+$ T cells were long considered to be involved largely in antitumor and antiviral activities, CTL have also been shown to mediate other pathological processes, such as delayed-type hypersensitivity (DTH) reactions. The availability of Fas- and perforin-deficient mice allowed a test of whether these molecules are involved in the CD8$^+$ T cell-mediated cutaneous hypersensitivity, whereby a skin inflammation is induced by cutaneously applied haptens (220). It was found that mice doubly deficient in Fas and perforin developed hapten-specific CD8$^+$ T cells lacking cytotoxic activity, but the same mice did not develop contact hypersensitivity (CHS). This strongly suggests that both Fas-mediated and perforin-mediated CD8$^+$ CTL-dependent cytotoxicities are required for CHS. Because CHS has been observed in mice deficient in only Fas or perforin, it was concluded that CHS-mediating CTLs could utilize either Fas or perforin interchangeably. An additional lesson of these studies is that mice with deficiencies in individual lytic molecules are not sufficient to clarify the role of these molecules in an *in vivo* pathogenic processes.

Role of Different Cytotoxic T-Lymphocyte Subsets in Delayed-Type Hypersensitivity

The description of Tc1 and Tc2 subsets of CTLs (221) led to the evaluation of their role in DTH (222). It was shown that when injected into animals, CD4 Th1 cells induce DTH more effectively than do Th2 cells. However, both Tc1 and Tc2 cells induced similar antigen-specific footpad swelling, as well as similar accumulation of macrophages and neutrophils.

Because the perforin-deficient Tc1 or Tc2 cells were also effective in induction of DTH, it was concluded that perforin-mediated cytotoxicity of CD8 T cells is not essential and that both Tc1- and Tc2-derived cytokines produce similar levels of DTH (222).

CTL persistence and effector functions are regulated by cytokines, which suggests the possibility of autocrine regulation of CTLs. It was shown, for example, that IL-4 inhibits the production of IL-2, IFN-γ, TNF-α, and IL-10 by differentiated Tc1 cells in response to antigenic stimulation, without changing their cytotoxic potential (223). These studies provide yet another example of dissociation of cytokine-secreting and cytotoxic functions, inasmuch as normal short-term lytic effects *in vitro* and adoptively transferred DTH in recipient mice *in vivo* were observed in assays of Tc1 cells with impaired cytokine synthesis. However, the inability to produce IL-2 and, therefore, defective proliferation/expansion of IL-4–treated CTLs was invoked to explain the decrease of their long-term antitumor capacities.

Cytotoxic Lymphocyte–Induced Inflammation in Liver Carcinogenesis

One example of pathogenic CTL effector functions is provided by the processes leading to the development of hepatocellular carcinoma, which often represents a complication of chronic HBV infection. Antiviral T cells are believed to be crucial in the control of HBV infection, but the inefficient T-cell response to HBV in persistently infected patients is proposed to contribute to the pathogenesis of chronic hepatitis. According to current views, the cytotoxic T cell–induced death of infected liver cells is accompanied by hepatocyte regeneration in an inflamed hepatic environment, thereby increasing probabilities of neoplastic transformation and hepatocellular carcinoma in patients with chronic hepatitis (224).

Therapeutic Modulation of Cytotoxic T-Lymphocyte Effector Functions

The potential use of CTLs for tumor therapy has long been recognized, but many problems remain before this approach can become a practical reality. Studies of T-cell activation and of negative regulators of CTL-mediated cytotoxicity coupled with identification of tumor antigens that can be recognized by CTLs have improved chances for successful manipulation of antitumor CTLs (225). As described previously, CTLs were shown to participate in antitumor immune response through the perforin-dependent mechanism of cytotoxicity. Promising approaches to enhancing CTL antitumor activity without deleterious autoimmune effects include inhibition of immunoinhibitory CTL-association antigen 4 (CTLA-4)–CD28 interactions (226) and inhibition of CD25$^+$ regulatory T cells (227). Depletion of either one of these two natural immunoregulatory mechanisms improves antitumor CTL activity, but the best result was observed when these treatments and strategies were combined.

It was shown in studies of experimental B16 melanoma that the optimal CD8⁺ CTL-mediated tumor rejection is accomplished by depletion of CD25⁺ regulatory T cells when accompanied by blockade of CTLA-4. In addition, the ability of T cells to penetrate and destroy solid tumors was exploited in the development of the "T-body" approach, which involves CTLs that express chimeric receptors, enabling the recognition and killing of cancer cells (228,229).

Localization of Cytotoxic T-Lymphocytes *In Vivo*

CTLs migrate between the lymphoid compartment and tissues in the course of immunological surveillance, and they exert their cytotoxic function after recognition and triggering by antigen; for example, memory CTL migrate through different tissues and reside in secondary lymphoid organs (230,231). The efficiency of the CTL-mediated response also results from the dramatic increases in numbers of antigen-specific CTLs after the antigen/TCR-driven proliferation and expansion. After elimination of the pathogen, the number of CTLs decreases, and only memory CTLs remain. An interesting exception to observations of CTL cytotoxicity development was provided in studies of intestinal intraepithelial lymphocytes (IELs). IELs represent an unusual subset of CTLs because they possess strong constitutive cytotoxic activity. In studies of mechanisms of cytotoxicity of naïve versus primed IEL CTLs, it was shown that they switch from Fas ligand–mediated to perforin-mediated cytotoxicity mechanisms as they mature (232). It was shown in assays of naïve CD8αβ IELs that antigen activation triggers Fas ligand–mediated, constitutive cytotoxic activity that can be detected in long-term assays. In contrast, it was the perforin-dependent exocytosis that mediated strong cytotoxicity of primed CD8αβ IELs. These observations demonstrate that priming of CTLs may trigger a switch from a pathway that depends on target Fas expression and function to the more generally applicable perforin pathway, against which resistance may be more difficult.

An important question about the localization and functions of CTLs during and after antimicrobial response *in vivo* was clarified in studies of CD8⁺ T-cell distribution. It had been assumed that CTLs localize mostly in lymphoid tissues, but the direct enumeration of CD8⁺ CTLs in different organs during and after infections within total tissue lymphocyte population, through the use of class I MHC tetramers coupled to antigenic peptide, revealed a significant proportion of long-lived memory CTLs not only in lymphoid tissues but also in nonlymphoid tissues such as those of the lung, fat pad, liver, kidney, bone marrow, and peritoneal cavity (233). In contrast to splenic CTLs, these non–lymphoid tissue–located CTLs were able to deliver a lethal hit immediately *ex vivo*. The presence of such an "immediate early response" CTL population is likely to provide the most efficient mechanism of counteracting the pathogens *in vivo*.

CONCLUSIONS

This chapter summarizes studies of molecular mechanisms of target cell death induced by cytotoxic T cells *in vitro* and related studies of the *in vivo* implications of these mechanisms for immune surveillance and disease pathogenesis. Currently, there is considerable detailed knowledge of two different death pathways induced by CTLs: the granule exocytosis pathway and the Fas/Fas ligand pathway. Although some steps in these death pathways are still not well understood, they account for virtually all cytotoxicity demonstrable by lymphocytes *in vitro*. The identification of unique molecules that function critically in these pathways has led to the creation of knockout mice specifically lacking them and to subsequent studies of their *in vivo* role in various immune phenomena. Such studies clearly implicate both *in vitro*–defined death pathways as important for *in vivo* immune function, in which cell death is difficult to measure directly. In some cases, such as graft rejection, it appears that the two *in vitro*–defined death pathways cannot explain all the phenomena, and other, as yet undefined pathways may contribute. These results point out that *in vitro* systems cannot faithfully recreate the complex and long-term *in vivo* conditions, and it is therefore likely that some important immunological mediators of cytotoxicity *in vivo* are still to be discovered. The identification of human genetic diseases manifested by defects in the two cytotoxicity pathways adds another level of understanding. It was particularly instructive that perforin-defective humans suffer from pathological processes not fully expected from studies of laboratory-reared mice with similar molecular defects. Nevertheless, it is clear that the current understanding of cytotoxicity is sufficiently advanced to allow for the beginning of attempts to exploit it for therapeutic benefit.

REFERENCES

1. Martz E. The ⁵¹Cr release assay for CTL-mediated target cell lysis. In: Sitkovsky MV, Henkart PA, eds. *Cytotoxic cells: recognition, effector function, generation, and methods.* Boston: Birkhauser, 1993:457–467.
2. Sanderson CJ. The uptake and retention of chromium by cells. *Transplantation* 1976;21:526–529.
3. Lichtenfels R, Biddison WE, Schulz H, et al. CARE-LASS (calcein-release assay), an improved fluorescence-based test system to measure cytotoxic T lymphocyte cytotoxicity. *J Immunol Methods* 1994;172:227–239.
4. Blomberg K, Hautala R, Lovgren J, et al. Time-resolved fluorometric assay for natural killer activity using target cells labelled with a fluorescence enhancing ligand. *J Immunol Methods* 1996;193:199–206.
5. Russell JH, Masakowski V, Rucinsky T, et al. Mechanisms of immune lysis. III. Characterization of the nature and kinetics of the cytotoxic T lymphocyte–induced nuclear lesion in the target. *J Immunol* 1982;128:2087–2094.
6. Matzinger P. The JAM test. A simple assay for DNA fragmentation and cell death. *J Immunol Methods* 1991;145:185–192.
7. Russell JH, Masakowski VR, Dobos CR. Mechanisms of immune lysis. I. Physiological distinction between target cell death mediated by cytotoxic T lymphocytes and antibody plus complement. *J Immunol* 1980;124:1100–1105.
8. Duke RC, Chervenak R, Cohen JJ. Endogenous endonuclease-induced

DNA fragmentation: an early event in cell-mediated cytolysis. *Proc Natl Acad Sci U S A* 1983;80:6361–6365.

9. Bryant J, Day R, Whiteside TL, et al. Calculation of lytic units for the expression of cell-mediated cytotoxicity. *J Immunol Methods* 1992;146:91–103.

10. Cerottini JC, Nordin AA, Brunner KT. Specific *in vitro* cytotoxicity of thymus-derived lymphocytes sensitized to alloantigens. *Nature* 1970; 228:1308–1309.

11. Fleischer B. Lysis of bystander target cells after triggering of human cytotoxic T lymphocytes. *Eur J Immunol* 1986;16:1021–1024.

12. Kojima H, Eshima K, Takayama H, et al. Leukocyte function–associated antigen–1–dependent lysis of Fas$^+$ (CD95$^+$/Apo-1$^+$) innocent bystanders by antigen-specific CD8$^+$ CTL. *J Immunol* 1997;159: 2728–2734.

13. Rothstein TL, Mage M, Jones G, et al. Cytotoxic T lymphocyte sequential killing of immobilized allogeneic tumor target cells measured by time-lapse microcinematography. *J Immunol* 1978;121:1652–1656.

14. Zagury D, Bernard J, Thiernesse N, et al. Isolation and characterization of individual functionally reactive cytotoxic T lymphocytes: conjugation, killing and recycling at the single cell level. *Eur J Immunol* 1975;5:818–822.

15. Thorn RM, Henney CS. Studies on the mechanism of lymphocyte-mediated cytolysis. VI. A reappraisal of the requirement for protein synthesis during T cell–mediated lysis. *J Immunol* 1976;116:146–149.

16. Zinkernagel RM, Doherty PC. The discovery of MHC restriction. *Immunol Today* 1997;18:14–17.

17. Gillis S, Smith KA. Long term culture of tumor specific cytotoxic T cells. *Nature* 1977;268:154–156.

18. Martz E. Mechanism of specific tumor cell lysis by alloimmune T lymphocytes: resolution and characterization of discrete steps in the cellular interaction. *Contemp Top Immunobiol* 1977;7:301–361.

19. Golstein P, Smith ET. Mechanism of T-cell–mediated cytolysis: the lethal hit stage. *Contemp Top Immunobiol* 1977;7:273–300.

20. Lowin B, Mattman C, Hahne M, et al. Comparison of Fas(Apo-1/CD95)– and perforin-mediated cytotoxicity in primary T lymphocytes. *Int Immunol* 1996;8:57–63.

21. Bossi G, Griffiths GM. Degranulation plays an essential part in regulating cell surface expression of Fas ligand in T cells and natural killer cells. *Nat Med* 1999;5:90–96.

22. Kagi D, Vignaux F, Ledermann B, et al. Fas and perforin pathways as major mechanisms of T cell–mediated cytotoxicity. *Science* 1994; 265:528–530.

23. Lowin B, Hahne M, Mattmann C, et al. Cytolytic T-cell cytotoxicity is mediated through perforin and Fas lytic pathways. *Nature* 1994; 370:650–652.

24. Kataoka T, Shinohara N, Takayama H, et al. Concanamycin A, a powerful tool for characterization and estimation of contributed of perforin- and Fas-based lytic pathways in cell-mediated cytotoxicity. *J Immunol* 1996;156:3678–3686.

25. Ratner A, Clark WR. Role of TNF-α in CD8$^+$ cytotoxic T lymphocyte–mediated lysis. *J Immunol* 1993;150:4303–4314.

26. Burgess TL, Kelly RB. Constitutive and regulated secretion of proteins. *Annu Rev Cell Biol* 1987;3:243–293.

27. Fortier AH, Nacy CA, Sitkovsky MV. Similar molecular requirements for antigen receptor-triggered secretion of interferon and granule enzymes by cytolytic T lymphocytes. *Cell Immunol* 1989;124:64–76.

28. Isaaz S, Baetz K, Olsen K, et al. Serial killing by cytotoxic T lymphocytes: T cell receptor triggers degranulation, re-filling of the lytic granules and secretion of lytic proteins via a non-granule pathway. *Eur J Immunol* 1995;25:1071–1079.

29. Nakata M, Kawasaki A, Azuma M, et al. Expression of perforin and cytolytic potential of human peripheral blood lymphocyte subpopulations. *Int Immunol* 1992;4:1049–1054.

30. Ohkawa T, Seki S, Dobashi H, et al. Systematic characterization of human CD8$^+$ T cells with natural killer cell markers in comparison with natural killer cells and normal CD8$^+$ T cells. *Immunology* 2001;103:281–290.

31. Sallusto F, Lenig D, Forster R, et al. Two subsets of memory T lymphocytes with distinct homing potentials and effector functions. *Nature* 1999;401:708–712.

32. Mosmann TR, Li L, Sad S. Functions of CD8 T-cell subsets secreting different cytokine patterns. *Semin Immunol* 1997;9:87–92.

33. Peters PJ, Borst J, Oorschot V, et al. Cytotoxic T lymphocyte granules are secretory lysosomes, containing both perforin and granzymes. *J Exp Med* 1991;173:1099–1109.

34. Burkhardt JK, Hester S, Lapham CK, et al. The lytic granules of natural killer cells are dual-function organelles combining secretory and prelysosomal compartments. *J Cell Biol* 1990;111:2327–2340.

35. Young JD, Cohn ZA, Podack ER. The ninth component of complement and the pore-forming protein (perforin 1) from cytotoxic T cells: structural, immunological, and functional similarities. *Science* 1986;233(4760):184–190.

36. Dourmashkin RR, Deteix P, Simone CB, et al. Electron microscopic demonstration of lesions on target cell membranes associated with antibody-dependent cytotoxicity. *Clin Exp Immunol* 1980;43:554–560.

37. Podack ER, Dennert G. Assembly of two types of tubules with putative cytolytic function by cloned natural killer cells. *Nature* 1983;302:442–445.

38. Dennert G, Podack ER. Cytolysis by H-2 specific T killer cells. Assembly of tubular complexes on target membranes. *J Exp Med* 1983; 157:1483–1495.

39. Shinkai Y, Takio K, Okumura K. Homology of perforin to the ninth component of complement (C9). *Nature* 1988;334:525–527.

40. Lowrey DM, Aebischer T, Olsen K, et al. Cloning, analysis, and expression of murine perforin 1 cDNA, a component of cytolytic T-cell granules with homology to complement component C9. *Proc Natl Acad Sci U S A* 1989;86:247–251.

41. Nalefski EA, Falke JJ. The C2 domain calcium-binding motif: structural and functional diversity. *Protein Sci* 1996;5:2375–2390.

42. Uellner R, Zvelebil MJ, Hopkins J, et al. Perforin is activated by proteolytic cleavage during biosynthesis which reveals a phospholipid binding domain. *EMBO J* 1997;16:7287–7296.

43. Valeva A, Weisser A, Walker B, et al. Molecular architecture of a toxin pore: a 15-residue sequence lines the transmembrane channel of staphylococcal alpha-toxin. *EMBO J* 1996;15:1857–1864.

44. Young JD, Nathan CF, Podack ER, et al. Functional channel formation associated with cytotoxic T-cell granules. *Proc Natl Acad Sci U S A* 1986;83:150–154.

45. Simone CB, Henkart P. Permeability changes induced in erythrocyte ghost targets by antibody-dependent cytotoxic effector cells: evidence for membrane pores. *J Immunol* 1980;124:954–963.

46. Sauer H, Pratsch L, Tschopp J, et al. Functional size of complement and perforin pores compared by confocal laser scanning microscopy and fluorescence microphotolysis. *Biochim Biophys Acta* 1991;1063:137–146.

47. Henkart PA, Millard PJ, Reynolds CW, et al. Cytolytic activity of purified cytoplasmic granules from cytotoxic rat LGL tumors. *J Exp Med* 1984;160:75–93.

48. Kim SH, Carney DF, Papadimitriou JC, et al. Effect of osmotic protection on nucleated cell killing by C5b-9: Cell death is not affected by the prevention of cell swelling. *Mol Immunol* 1989;26:323–331.

49. Smyth MJ, O'Connor MD, Trapani JA. Granzymes: a variety of serine protease specificities encoded by genetically distinct subfamilies. *J Leukoc Biol* 1996;60:555–562.

50. Lutzelschwab C, Pejler G, Aveskogh M, et al. Secretory granule proteases is rat mast cells. Cloning of 10 different serine proteases and a carboxypeptidase A from various rat mast cell populations. *J Exp Med* 1997;185:13–29.

51. Kam CM, Hudig D, Powers JC. Granzymes (lymphocyte serine proteases): characterization with natural and synthetic substrates and inhibitors. *Biochim Biophys Acta* 2000;1477:307–323.

52. Garcia-Sanz JA, MacDonald HR, Jenne DE, et al. Cell specificity of granzyme gene expression. *J Immunol* 1990;145:3111–3118.

53. Thornberry NA, Rano TA, Peterson EP, et al. A combinatorial approach defines specificities of members of the caspase family and granzyme B. Functional relationships established for key mediators of apoptosis. *J Biol Chem* 1997;272:17907–17911.

54. Estebanez-Perpina E, Fuentes-Prior P, Belorgey D, et al. Crystal structure of the caspase activator human granzyme B, a proteinase highly specific for an Asp-P1 residue. *Biol Chem* 2000;381:1203–1214.

55. Rotonda J, Garcia-Calvo M, Bull HG, et al. The three-dimensional structure of human granzyme B compared to caspase-3, key mediators of cell death with cleavage specificity for aspartic acid in P1. *Chem Biol* 2001;8:357–368.

56. Andrade F, Roy S, Nicholson D, et al. Granzyme B directly and efficiently cleaves several downstream caspase substrates: implications for CTL-induced apoptosis. *Immunity* 1998;8:451–460.

57. Sutton VR, Davis JE, Cancilla M, et al. Initiation of apoptosis by granzyme B requires direct cleavage of bid, but not direct granzyme B–mediated caspase activation. *J Exp Med* 2000;192:1403–1414.

58. Alimonti JB, Shi L, Baijal PK, et al. Granzyme B induces BID-mediated cytochrome c release and mitochondrial permeability transition. *J Biol Chem* 2001;276:6974–6982.

59. Pinkoski MJ, Waterhouse NJ, Heibein JA, et al. Granzyme B–mediated apoptosis proceeds predominantly through a Bcl-2–inhibitable mitochondrial pathway. *J Biol Chem* 2001;276:12060–12067.

60. Wang GQ, Wieckowski E, Goldstein LA, et al. Resistance to granzyme B–mediated cytochrome c release in Bak-deficient cells. *J Exp Med* 2001;194:1325–1337.

61. Sharif-Askari E, Alam A, Rheaume E, et al. Direct cleavage of the human DNA fragmentation factor-45 by granzyme B induces caspase-activated DNase release and DNA fragmentation. *EMBO J* 2001;20:3101–3113.

62. Casciola-Rosen L, Andrade F, Ulanet D, et al. Cleavage by granzyme B is strongly predictive of autoantigen status: implications for initiation of autoimmunity. *J Exp Med* 1999;190:815–826.

63. Beresford PJ, Kam CM, Powers JC, et al. Recombinant human granzyme A binds to two putative HLA-associated proteins and cleaves one of them. *Proc Natl Acad Sci U S A* 1997;94:9285–9290.

64. Beresford PJ, Zhang D, Oh DY, et al. Granzyme A activates an endoplasmic reticulum-associated caspase-independent nuclease to induce single-stranded DNA nicks. *J Biol Chem* 2001;276:43285–43293.

65. Pasternack MS, Blier KJ, McInerney TN. Granzyme A binding to target cell proteins. Granzyme A binds to and cleaves nucleolin *in vitro*. *J Biol Chem* 1991;266:14703–14708.

66. Zhang D, Beresford PJ, Greenberg AH, et al. Granzymes A and B directly cleave lamins and disrupt the nuclear lamina during granule-mediated cytolysis. *Proc Natl Acad Sci U S A* 2001;98:5746–5751.

67. Zhang D, Pasternack MS, Beresford PJ, et al. Induction of rapid histone degradation by the cytotoxic T lymphocyte protease granzyme A. *J Biol Chem* 2001;276:3683–3690.

68. Beresford PJ, Xia Z, Greenberg AH, et al. Granzyme A loading induces rapid cytolysis and a novel form of DNA damage independently of caspase activation. *Immunity* 1999;10:585–594.

69. Smyth MJ, McGuire MJ, Thia KY. Expression of recombinant human granzyme B. A processing and activation role for dipeptidyl peptidase I. *J Immunol* 1995;154:6299–6305.

70. Thiele DL, McGuire MJ, Lipsky PE. A selective inhibitor of dipeptidyl peptidase I impairs generation of CD8+ T cell cytotoxic effector function. *J Immunol* 1997;158:5200–5210.

71. Pham CT, Ley TJ. Dipeptidyl peptidase I is required for the processing and activation of granzymes A and B *in vivo*. *Proc Natl Acad Sci U S A* 1999;96:8627–8632.

72. Kolset SO, Gallagher JT. Proteoglycans in haemopoietic cells. *Biochim Biophys Acta* 1990;1032:191–211.

73. Masson D, Peters PJ, Geuze HJ, et al. Interaction of chondroitin sulfate with perforin and granzymes of cytolytic T cells is dependent on pH. *Biochemistry* 1990;29:11229–11235.

74. Wagner L, Yang OO, Garcia-Zepeda EA, et al. Beta-chemokines are released from HIV-1 specific cytolytic T cell granules complexed to proteoglycans. *Nature* 1998;391:908–911.

75. Galvin JP, Spaeny-Dekking LH, Wang B, et al. Apoptosis induced by granzyme B–glycosaminoglycan complexes: implications for granule-mediated apoptosis *in vivo*. *J Immunol* 1999;162:5345–5350.

76. Rodriguez A, Webster P, Ortego J, et al. Lysosomes behave as Ca+2-regulated exocytic vesicles in fibroblasts and epithelial cells. *J Cell Biol* 1997;137:93–104.

77. Peters PJ, Geuze HJ, van der Donk HA, et al. Molecules relevant for T cell–target cell interaction are present in cytolytic granules of human T lymphocytes. *Eur J Immunol* 1989;19:1469–1475.

78. Blott EJ, Bossi G, Clark R, et al. Fas ligand is targeted to secretory lysosomes via a proline-rich domain in its cytoplasmic tail. *J Cell Sci* 2001;114:2405–2416.

79. Haddad EK, Wu X, Hammer JA, et al. Defective granule exocytosis in Rab27a-deficient lymphocytes from *ashen* mice. *J Cell Biol* 2001;152:835–841.

80. Kannan K, Stewart RM, Bounds W, et al. Lysosome-associated membrane proteins h-LAMP1 (CD107a) and h-LAMP2 (CD107b) are activation-dependent cell surface glycoproteins in human peripheral blood mononuclear cells which mediate cell adhesion to vascular endothelium. *Cell Immunol* 1996;171:10–19.

81. Mellman I, Fuchs R, Helenius A. Acidification of the endocytic and exocytic pathways. *Annu Rev Biochem* 1986;55:663–700.

82. Kataoka T, Takaku K, Magae J, et al. Acidification is essential for maintaining the structure and function of lytic granules of CTL: Effect of concanamycin A, an inhibitor of vacuolar type H+-ATPase, on CTL-mediated cytotoxicity. *J Immunol* 1994;153:3938–3947.

83. Anderson P. TIA-1: structural and functional studies on a new class of cytolytic effector molecule. *Curr Top Microbiol Immunol* 1995;198:131–143.

84. Krensky AM. Granulysin: a novel antimicrobial peptide of cytolytic T lymphocytes and natural killer cells. *Biochem Pharmacol* 2000;59:317–320.

85. Andersson M, Gunne H, Agerberth B, et al. NK-lysin, a novel effector peptide of cytotoxic T and NK cells. Structure and cDNA cloning of the porcine form, induction by interleukin 2, antibacterial and antitumour activity. *EMBO J* 1995;14:1615–1625.

86. Kaspar AA, Okada S, Kumar J, et al. A distinct pathway of cell-mediated apoptosis initiated by granulysin. *J Immunol* 2001;167:350–356.

87. Pardo J, Perez-Galan P, Gamen S, et al. A role of the mitochondrial apoptosis-inducing factor in granulysin-induced apoptosis. *J Immunol* 2001;167:1222–1229.

88. Stenger S, Rosat JP, Bloom BR, et al. Granulysin: a lethal weapon of cytolytic T cells. *Immunol Today* 1999;20:390–394.

89. Stenger S, Hanson DA, Teitelbaum R, et al. An antimicrobial activity of cytolytic T cells mediated by granulysin. *Science* 1998;282:121–125.

90. Canaday DH, Wilkinson RJ, Li Q, et al. CD4(+) and CD8(+) T cells kill intracellular *Mycobacterium tuberculosis* by a perforin and Fas/Fas ligand–independent mechanism. *J Immunol* 2001;167:2734–2742.

91. Dupuis M, Schaerer E, Krause KH, et al. The calcium-binding protein calreticulin is a major constituent of lytic granules of cytolytic T lymphocytes. *J Exp Med* 1993;177:1–7.

92. Helenius A, Trombetta ES, Hebert DN, et al. Calnexin, calreticulin and the folding of glycoproteins. *Trends Cell Biol* 1997;7:193–200.

93. Sanderson CJ. The mechanism of T cell mediated cytotoxicity. II. Morphological studies of cell death by time-lapse microcinematography. *Proc R Soc Lond* 1976;192:241–255.

94. Yannelli JR, Sullivan JA, Mandell GL, et al. Reorientation and fusion of cytotoxic T lymphocyte granules after interaction with target cells as determined by high resolution cinemicrography. *J Immunol* 1986;136:377–382.

95. Waters JB, Oldstone MBA, Hahn KM. Changes in the cytoplasmic structure of CTLs during target cell recognition and killing. *J Immunol* 1996;157:3396–3403.

96. Berke G. Interaction of cytotoxic T lymphocytes and target cells. *Prog Allergy* 1980;27:69–133.

97. Perez C, Albert I, DeFay K, et al. A nonsecretable cell surface mutant of tumor necrosis factor (TNF) kills by cell-to-cell contact. *Cell* 1990;63:251–258.

98. Martz E. LFA-1 and other accessory molecules functioning in adhesions of T and B lymphocytes. *Human Immunology* 1987;18:3–37.

99. Martz E. Immune T lymphocyte to tumor cell adhesion. Magnesium sufficient, calcium insufficient. *J Cell Biol* 1980;84:584–598.

100. Hubbard BB, Glacken MW, Rodgers JR, et al. The role of physical forces on cytotoxic T cell–target cell conjugate stability. *J Immunol* 1990;144:4129–4138.

101. Martz E, Davignon D, Kurzinger K, et al. The molecular basis of cytolytic T lymphocyte function: analysis with blocking monoclonal antibodies. *Adv Exp Med Biol* 1982;146:447–468.

102. Springer TA, Davignon D, Ho M-K, et al. LFA-1 and Lyt-2,3, molecules associated with T lymphocyte–mediated killing; and Mac-1, an LFA-1 homologue associated with complement receptor function. *Immunol Rev* 1982;68:171–195.

103. Berg NN, Ostergaard HL. Characterization of intercellular adhesion molecule–1 (ICAM-1)–augmented degranulation by cytotoxic T cells. ICAM-1 and anti-CD3 must be co-localized for optimal adhesion and stimulation. *J Immunol* 1995;155:1694–1702.

104. Mescher MF. Molecular interactions in the activation of effector and precursor cytotoxic T lymphocytes. *Immunol Rev* 1995;146:177–210.

105. Huang JF, Yang Y, Sepulveda H, et al. TCR-mediated internalization of peptide–MHC complexes acquired by T cells. *Science* 1999;286:952–954.

106. Hwang I, Huang JF, Kishimoto H, et al. T cells can use either T cell receptor or CD28 receptors to absorb and internalize cell surface molecules derived from antigen-presenting cells. *J Exp Med* 2000; 191:1137–1148.

107. Hudrisier D, Riond J, Mazarguil H, et al. Cutting edge: CTLs rapidly capture membrane fragments from target cells in a TCR signaling-dependent manner. *J Immunol* 2001;166:3645–3649.

108. Stinchcombe JC, Bossi G, Booth S, et al. The immunological synapse of CTL contains a secretory domain and membrane bridges. *Immunity* 2001;15:751–761.

109. Kupfer A, Singer SJ. Cell biology of cytotoxic and helper T cell functions: immunofluorescence microscopic studies of single cells and cell couples. *Annu Rev Immunol* 1989;7:309–337.

110. Hahn K, DeBiasio R, Tishon A, et al. Antigen presentation and cytotoxic T lymphocyte killing studied in individual, living cells. *Virology* 1994;201:330–340.

111. Kupfer A, Dennert G, Singer SJ. The reorientation of the Golgi apparatus and the microtubule-organizing center in the cytotoxic effector cell is a prerequisite in the lysis of bound target cells. *J Mol Cell Immunol* 1985;2:37–49.

112. Kupfer A, Dennert G, Singer SJ. Polarization of the Golgi apparatus and the microtubule-organizing center within cloned natural killer cells bound to their targets. *Proc Natl Acad Sci U S A* 1983;80:7224–7228.

113. Burkhardt JK, McIlvain JM, Sheetz MP, et al. Lytic granules from cytotoxic T cells exhibit kinesin-dependent motility on microtubules *in vitro*. *J Cell Sci* 1993;104:151–162.

114. Anel A, O'Rourke AM, Kleinfeld AM, et al. T cell receptor and CD8-dependent tyrosine phosphorylation events in cytotoxic T lymphocytes: activation of p56lck by CD8 binding to class I protein. *Eur J Immunol* 1996;26:2310–2319.

115. Anel A, Martinez-Lorenzo MJ, Schmitt-Verhulst AM, et al. Influence on CD8 of TCR/CD3-generated signals in CTL clones and CTL precursor cells. *J Immunol* 1997;158:19–28.

116. Lewis RS. Calcium signaling mechanisms in T lymphocytes. *Annu Rev Immunol* 2001;19:497–521.

117. Poenie M, Tsien RY, Schmitt-Verhulst AM. Sequential activation and lethal hit measured by [Ca^{2+}] in individual cytolytic T cells and targets. *EMBO J* 1987;6:2223–2232.

118. Gray LS, Gnarra JR, Engelhard VH. Demonstration of a calcium influx in cytolytic T lymphocytes in response to target cell binding. *J Immunol* 1987;138:63–69.

119. Gray LS, Gnarra JR, Sullivan JA, et al. Spatial and temporal characteristics of the increase in intracellular Ca^{2+} induced in cytotoxic T lymphocytes by cellular antigen. *J Immunol* 1988;141:2424–2430.

120. Gray LS, Gnarra JR, Russell JH, et al. The role of K$^+$ in the regulation of the increase in intracellular Ca^{2+} mediated by the T lymphocyte antigen receptor. *Cell* 1987;50:119–127.

121. Densmore JJ, Haverstick DM, Szabo G, et al. A voltage-operable current is involved in Ca^{2+} entry in human lymphocytes whereas ICRAC has no apparent role. *Am J Physiol* 1996;271:C1494–C1503.

122. David A, Bernard J, Thiernesse N, et al. Le processus d'exocytose lysosomale localisee: est il responsable de l'action cytolytique des lymphocytes T tuers? *C R Seances Acad Sci D* 1979;288:441–444.

123. Takayama H, Trenn G, Sitkovsky MV. A novel cytotoxic T lymphocyte activation assay. Optimized conditions for antigen receptor triggered granule enzyme secretion. *J Immunol Methods* 1987;104:183–190.

124. Menasche G, Pastural E, Feldmann J, et al. Mutations in RAB27A cause Griscelli syndrome associated with haemophagocytic syndrome. *Nat Genet* 2000;25:173–176.

125. Stinchcombe JC, Barral DC, Mules EH, et al. Rab27a is required for regulated secretion in cytotoxic T lymphocytes. *J Cell Biol* 2001;152:825–834.

126. Zerial M, McBride H. Rab proteins as membrane organizers. *Nat Rev Mol Cell Biol* 2001;2:107–117.

127. Kagi D, Ledermann B, Burki K, et al. Cytotoxicity mediated by T cells and natural killer cells is greatly impaired in perforin-deficient mice. *Nature* 1994;369:31–37.

128. Trapani JA, Davis J, Sutton VR, et al. Proapoptotic functions of cytotoxic lymphocyte granule constituents *in vitro* and *in vivo*. *Curr Opin Immunol* 2000;12:323–329.

129. Heusel JW, Wesselschmidt RL, Shresta S, et al. Cytotoxic lymphocytes require granzyme B for the rapid induction of DNA fragmentation and apoptosis in allogeneic target cells. *Cell* 1994;76:977–987.

130. Shresta S, MacIvor DM, Heusel JW, et al. Natural killer and lymphokine-activated killer cells require granzyme B for the rapid induction of apoptosis in susceptible target cells. *Proc Natl Acad Sci U S A* 1995;92:5679–5683.

131. Ebnet K, Hausmann M, Lehmann-Grube F, et al. Granzyme A–deficient mice retain potent cell-mediated cytotoxicity. *EMBO J* 1995; 14:4230–4239.

132. Shresta S, Goda P, Wesselschmidt R, et al. Residual cytotoxicity and granzyme K expression in granzyme A–deficient cytotoxic lymphocytes. *J Biol Chem* 1997;272:20236–20244.

133. Simon MM, Hausmann M, Tran T, et al. *In vitro*– and *ex vivo*–derived cytolytic leukocytes from granzyme A × B double knockout mice are defective in granule-mediated apoptosis but not lysis of target cells. *J Exp Med* 1997;186:1781–1786.

134. Shresta S, Graubert TA, Thomas DA, et al. Granzyme A initiates an alternative pathway for granule-mediated apoptosis. *Immunity* 1999;10: 595–605.

135. Shiver JW, Su L, Henkart PA. Cytotoxicity with target DNA breakdown by rat basophilic leukemia cells expressing both cytolysin and granzyme A. *Cell* 1992;71:315–322.

136. Nakajima H, Park HL, Henkart PA. Synergistic roles of granzymes A and B in mediating target cell death by RBL mast cell tumors also expressing cytolysin/perforin. *J Exp Med* 1995;181:1037–1046.

137. Duke RC, Persechini PM, Chang S, et al. Purified perforin induces target cell lysis but not DNA fragmentation. *J Exp Med* 1989;170:1451–1456.

138. Froelich CJ, Orth K, Turbov J, et al. New Paradigm for lymphocyte granule-mediated cytotoxicity. Target cells bind and internalize granzyme B, but an endosomolytic agent is necessary for cytosolic delivery and subsequent apoptosis. *J Biol Chem* 1996;271:29073–29079.

139. Hayes MP, Berrebi GA, Henkart PA. Induction of target cell DNA release by the cytotoxic T lymphocyte granule protease granzyme A. *J Exp Med* 1989;170:933–946.

140. Shi L, Kam CM, Powers JC, et al. Purification of three cytotoxic lymphocyte granule serine proteases that induce apoptosis through distinct substrate and target cell interactions. *J Exp Med* 1992;176:1521–1529.

141. Pinkoski MJ, Hobman M, Heibein JA, et al. Entry and trafficking of granzyme B in target cells during granzyme B- perforin-mediated apoptosis. *Blood* 1998;92:1044–1054.

142. Browne KA, Blink E, Sutton VR, et al. Cytosolic delivery of granzyme B by bacterial toxins: evidence that endosomal disruption, in addition to transmembrane pore formation, is an important function of perforin. *Mol Cell Biol* 1999;19:8604–8615.

143. Nakajima H, Henkart PA. Cytotoxic lymphocyte granzymes trigger a target cell internal disintegration pathway leading to cytolysis and DNA breakdown. *J Immunol* 1994;152:1057–1063.

144. Wagner L, Avery RK, Bensinger L, et al. Inhibition of cytotoxic T-lymphocyte–triggered apoptosis by target cell surface–coupled aprotinin. *Mol Immunol* 1995;32:853–864.

145. Sun J, Bird CH, Sutton V, et al. A cytosolic granzyme B inhibitor related to the viral apoptotic regulator cytokine response modifier A is present in cytotoxic lymphocytes. *J Biol Chem* 1996;271:27802–27809.

146. Bladergroen BA, Strik MC, Bovenschen N, et al. The granzyme B inhibitor, protease inhibitor 9, is mainly expressed by dendritic cells and at immune-privileged sites. *J Immunol* 2001;166:3218–3225.

147. Buzza MS, Hirst CE, Bird CH, et al. The granzyme B inhibitor, PI-9, is present in endothelial and mesothelial cells, suggesting that it protects bystander cells during immune responses. *Cell Immunol* 2001;210:21–29.

148. Medema JP, de Jong J, Peltenburg LT, et al. Blockade of the granzyme B/perforin pathway through overexpression of the serine protease inhibitor PI-9/SPI-6 constitutes a mechanism for immune escape by tumors. *Proc Natl Acad Sci U S A* 2001;98:11515–11520.

149. Morgan BP. Complement membrane attack on nucleated cells: resistance, recovery, and non-lethal effects. *Biochem J* 1989;264:1–14.

150. Henkart PA, Henkart M, Millard P, et al. Isolation and cytolytic activity of granule from naturally occurring LGL tumors. In: Hondo H, ed. *Proceedings of the International Symposium on Natural Killer Activity and Its Regulation.* Tokyo: Excerpta Medica, 1983:150–155.

151. Miyake K, McNeil PL. Vesicle accumulation and exocytosis at sites of plasma membrane disruption. *J Cell Biol* 1995;131:1737–1745.

152. Bashford CL, Menestrina G, Henkart PA, et al. Cell damage by cytolysin: spontaneous recovery and reversible inhibition by divalent cations. *J Immunol* 1988;141:3965–3974.

153. Reiter Y, Ciobotariu A, Jones J, et al. Complement membrane attack complex, perforin, and bacterial exotoxins induce in K562 cells calcium-dependent cross-protection from lysis. *J Immunol* 1995;155:2203–2210.

154. Russell JH. Internal disintegration model of cytotoxic lymphocyte-induced target damage. *Immunol Rev* 1983;72:97–118.

155. Shiver JW, Henkart PA. A noncytotoxic mast cell tumor line exhibits potent IgE-dependent cytotoxicity after transfection with the cytolysin/perforin gene. *Cell* 1991;62:1174–1181.

156. Motyka B, Korbutt G, Pinkoski MJ, et al. Mannose 6-phosphate/insulin-like growth factor II receptor is a death receptor for granzyme B during cytotoxic T cell–induced apoptosis. *Cell* 2000;103:491–500.

157. Sanderson CJ, Glaueret AM. The mechanism of T cell mediated cytotoxicity. V. Morphological studies by electron microscopy. *Proc R Soc Lond* 1977;198:315–323.

158. Sellins KS, Cohen JJ. Cytotoxic T lymphocytes induce different types of DNA damage in target cells of different origins. *J Immunol* 1991;147:795–803.

159. Nakajima H, Golstein P, Henkart PA. The target cell nucleus is not required for cell-mediated granzyme- or Fas-based cytotoxicity. *J Exp Med* 1995;181:1905–1909.

160. Jacobson MD, Burne JF, Raff MC. Programmed cell death and Bcl-2 protection in the absence of a nucleus. *EMBO J* 1994;13:1899–1910.

161. Darmon AJ, Nicholson DW, Bleackley RC. Activation of the apoptotic protease CPP32 by cytotoxic T cell–derived granzyme B. *Nature* 1995;377:446–448.

162. Darmon AJ, Ley TJ, Nicholson DW, et al. Cleavage of CPP-32 by granzyme B represents a critical role for granzyme B in the induction of target cell DNA fragmentation. *J Biol Chem* 1996;271:21709–21712.

163. Pinkoski MJ, Winkler U, Hudig D, et al. Binding of granzyme B in the nucleus of target cells—recognition of an 80-kilodalton protein. *J Biol Chem* 1996;271:10225–10229.

164. Shi L, Mai S, Israels S, et al. Granzyme B (GraB) autonomously crosses the cell membrane and perforin initiates apoptosis and GraB nuclear localization. *J Exp Med* 1997;185:855–866.

165. Trapani JA, Jans DA, Jans PJ, et al. Efficient nuclear targeting of granzyme B and the nuclear consequences of apoptosis induced by granzyme B and perforin are caspase-dependent, but cell death is caspase-independent. *J Biol Chem* 1998;273:27934–27938.

166. Sarin A, Williams MS, Alexander-Miller MA, et al. Target cell lysis by CTL granule exocytosis is independent of ICE/Ced-3 family proteases. *Immunity* 1997;6:209–215.

167. Sarin A, Haddad EK, Henkart PA. Caspase dependence of target cell damage induced by cytotoxic lymphocytes. *J Immunol* 1998;161:2810–2816.

168. Martinou JC, Green DR. Breaking the mitochondrial barrier. *Nat Rev Mol Cell Biol* 2001;2:63–67.

169. Chiu VK, Walsh CM, Liu C-C, et al. *Bcl*-2 blocks degranulation but not *fas*-based cell-mediated cytotoxicity. *J Immunol* 1995;154:2023–2032.

170. Lee RK, Spielman J, Podack ER. bcl-2 Protects against fas-based but not perforin-based T cell–mediated cytolysis. *Int Immunol* 1996;8:991–1000.

171. Schroter M, Lowin B, Borner C, et al. Regulation of Fas(Apo-1/CD95)– and perforin-mediated lytic pathways of primary cytotoxic T lymphocytes by the protooncogene bcl-2. *Eur J Immunol* 1995;25:3509–3513.

172. Jans DA, Sutton VR, Jans P, et al. BCL-2 blocks perforin-induced nuclear translocation of granzymes concomitant with protection against the nuclear events of apoptosis. *J Biol Chem* 1999;274:3953–3961.

173. Heibein JA, Goping IS, Barry M, et al. Granzyme B–mediated cytochrome c release is regulated by the bcl-2 family members bid and Bax. *J Exp Med* 2000;192:1391–1402.

174. Martz E. Overview of CTL-target adhesion and other critical events in the cytotoxic mechanism. In: Sitkovsky MV, Henkart PA, eds. *Cytotoxic cells: recognition, effector function, generation, and methods.* Boston: Birkhauser, 1993:9–45.

175. Gorman K, Liu CC, Blakely A, et al. Cloned cytotoxic T lymphocytes as target cells. II. Polarity of lysis revisited. *J Immunol* 1988;141:2211–2215.

176. Luciani MF, Brunet JF, Suzan M, et al. Self-sparing of long-term *in vitro*–cloned or uncloned cytotoxic T lymphocytes. *J Exp Med* 1986;164:962–967.

177. Bensussan A, Leca G, Corvaïa N, et al. Selective induction of autocytotoxic activity through the CD3 molecule. *Eur J Immunol* 1990;20:2615–2619.

178. Kranz DM, Eisen HN. Resistance of cytotoxic T lymphocytes to lysis by a clone of cytotoxic T lymphocytes. *Proc Natl Acad Sci U S A* 1987;84:3375–3379.

179. Verret CR, Firmenich AA, Kranz DM, et al. Resistance of cytotoxic T lymphocytes to the lytic effects of their toxic granules. *J Exp Med* 1987;166:1536–1547.

180. Shinkai Y, Ishikawa H, Hattori M, et al. Resistance of mouse cytolytic cells to pore-forming protein–mediated cytolysis. *Eur J Immunol* 1988;18:29–33.

181. Persechini PM, Young JD, Almers W. Membrane channel formation by the lymphocyte pore-forming protein: comparison between susceptible and resistant target cells. *J Cell Biol* 1990;110:2109–2116.

182. Su MW-C, Walden PR, Eisen HN, et al. Cognate peptide–induced destruction of CD8+ cytotoxic T lymphocytes is due to fratricide. *J Immunol* 1993;151:658–667.

183. Suhrbier A, Burrows SR, Fernan A, et al. Peptide epitope induced apoptosis of human cytotoxic T lymphocytes. Implications for peripheral T cell deletion and peptide vaccination. *J Immunol* 1993;150:2169–2178.

184. Simon MM, Waring P, Lobigs M, et al. Cytotoxic T cells specifically induce Fas on target cells, thereby facilitating exocytosis-independent induction of apoptosis. *J Immunol* 2000;165:3663–3672.

185. Berthou C, Legros-Maida S, Soulie A, et al. Cord blood T lymphocytes lack constitutive perforin expression in contrast to adult peripheral blood T lymphocytes. *Blood* 1995;85:1540–1546.

186. Smyth MJ, Browne KA, Kinnear BF, et al. Distinct granzyme expression in human CD3− CD56+ large granular- and CD3− CD56+ small high density-lymphocytes displaying non–MHC-restricted cytolytic activity. *J Leukoc Biol* 1995;57:88–93.

187. Ebnet K, Levelt CN, Tran TT, et al. Transcription of granzyme A and B genes is differentially regulated during lymphoid ontogeny. *J Exp Med* 1995;181:755–763.

188. Berke G, Rosen D. Highly lytic *in vivo* primed cytolytic T lymphocytes devoid of lytic granules and BLT-esterase activity acquire these constituents in the presence of T cell growth factors upon blast transformation *in vitro*. *J Immunol* 1988;141:1429–1436.

189. Muta H, Boise LH, Fang L, et al. CD30 signals integrate expression of cytotoxic effector molecules, lymphocyte trafficking signals, and signals for proliferation and apoptosis. *J Immunol* 2000;165:5105–5111.

190. Caldwell CC, Kojima H, Lukashev D, et al. Differential effects of physiologically relevant hypoxic conditions on T lymphocyte development and effector functions. *J Immunol* 2001;167:6140–6149.

191. Koshiba M, Kojima H, Huang S, et al. Memory of extracellular adenosine A2A purinergic receptor–mediated signaling in murine T cells. *J Biol Chem* 1997;272:25881–25889.

192. Ohta A, Sitkovsky M. Role of G-protein–coupled adenosine receptors in downregulation of inflammation and protection from tissue damage. *Nature* 2001;414:916–920.

193. de Saint Basile G, Fischer A. The role of cytotoxicity in lymphocyte homeostasis. *Curr Opin Immunol* 2001;13:549–554.

194. Takahashi T, Tanaka M, Brannan CI, et al. Generalized lymphoproliferative disease in mice, caused by a point mutation in the Fas ligand. *Cell* 1994;76:969–976.

195. Ashany D, Song X, Lacy E, et al. Th1 CD4+ lymphocytes delete activated macrophages through the Fas/APO-1 antigen pathway. *Proc Natl Acad Sci U S A* 1995;92:11225–11229.

196. Kagi D, Odermatt B, Mak TW. Homeostatic regulation of CD8+ T cells by perforin. *Eur J Immunol* 1999;29:3262–3272.

197. Badovinac VP, Tvinnereim AR, Harty JT. Regulation of antigen-specific CD8+ T cell homeostasis by perforin and interferon-gamma. *Science* 2000;290:1354–1358.

198. Stepp SE, Dufourcq-Lagelouse R, Le Deist F, et al. Perforin gene defects in familial hemophagocytic lymphohistiocytosis. *Science* 1999;286:1957–1959.

199. Spielman J, Lee RK, Podack ER. Perforin/Fas-ligand double deficiency is associated with macrophage expansion and severe pancreatitis. *J Immunol* 1998;161:7063–7070.

200. Liu ZX, Govindarajan S, Okamoto S, et al. Fas-mediated apoptosis causes elimination of virus-specific cytotoxic T cells in the virus-infected liver. *J Immunol* 2001;166:3035–3041.

201. Kaufmann SH, Hug E, De Libero G. *Listeria monocytogenes*–reactive T lymphocyte clones with cytolytic activity against infected target cells. *J Exp Med* 1986;164:363–368.

202. Stenger S, Modlin RL. Cytotoxic T cell responses to intracellular pathogens. *Curr Opin Immunol* 1998;10:471–477.

203. Ochoa MT, Stenger S, Sieling PA, et al. T-cell release of granulysin contributes to host defense in leprosy. *Nat Med* 2001;7:174–179.

204. Cooper AM, D'Souza C, Frank AA, et al. The course of *Mycobacterium tuberculosis* infection in the lungs of mice lacking expression of either perforin- or granzyme-mediated cytolytic mechanisms. *Infect Immun* 1997;65:1317–1320.

205. Laochumroonvorapong P, Wang J, Liu CC, et al. Perforin, a cytotoxic molecule which mediates cell necrosis, is not required for the early control of mycobacterial infection in mice. *Infect Immun* 1997;65:127–132.

206. van den Broek M, Kagi D, Ossendorp F, et al. Decreased tumor surveillance in perforin-deficient mice. *J Exp Med* 1996;184:1781–1790.

207. Smyth MJ, Thia KY, Street SE, et al. Perforin-mediated cytotoxicity is critical for surveillance of spontaneous lymphoma. *J Exp Med* 2000;192:755–760.

208. Davis JE, Smyth MJ, Trapani JA. Granzyme A and B–deficient killer lymphocytes are defective in eliciting DNA fragmentation but retain potent *in vivo* anti-tumor capacity. *Eur J Immunol* 2001;31:39–47.

209. Riera L, Gariglio M, Valente G, et al. Murine cytomegalovirus replication in salivary glands is controlled by both perforin and granzymes during acute infection. *Eur J Immunol* 2000;30:1350–1355.

210. Mullbacher A, Waring P, Tha Hla R, et al. Granzymes are the essential downstream effector molecules for the control of primary virus infections by cytolytic leukocytes. *Proc Natl Acad Sci U S A* 1999;96:13950–13955.

211. Doherty PC, Zinkernagel RM. T-cell–mediated immunopathology in viral infections. *Transplant Rev* 1974;19:89–120.

212. Balkow S, Kersten A, Tran TT, et al. Concerted action of the FasL/Fas and perforin/granzyme A and B pathways is mandatory for the development of early viral hepatitis but not for recovery from viral infection. *J Virol* 2001;75:8781–8791.

213. Pasquetto V, Wieland S, Chisari FV. Intracellular hepatitis B virus nucleocapsids survive cytotoxic T-lymphocyte–induced apoptosis. *J Virol* 2000;74:9792–9796.

214. Kagi D, Odermatt B, Ohashi PS, et al. Development of insulitis without diabetes in transgenic mice lacking perforin-dependent cytotoxicity. *J Exp Med* 1996;183:2143–2152.

215. Kagi D, Odermatt B, Seiler P, et al. Reduced incidence and delayed onset of diabetes in perforin-deficient nonobese diabetic mice. *J Exp Med* 1997;186:989–997.

216. Malipiero U, Frei K, Spanaus KS, et al. Myelin oligodendrocyte glycoprotein-induced autoimmune encephalomyelitis is chronic/relapsing in perforin knockout mice, but monophasic in Fas- and Fas ligand–deficient lpr and gld mice. *Eur J Immunol* 1997;27:3151–3160.

217. Baker MB, Altman NH, Podack ER, et al. The role of cell-mediated cytotoxicity in acute GVHD after MHC-matched allogeneic bone marrow transplantation in mice. *J Exp Med* 1996;183:2645–2656.

218. Graubert TA, DiPersio JF, Russell JH, et al. Perforin/granzyme-dependent and independent mechanisms are both important for the development of graft-versus-host disease after murine bone marrow transplantation. *J Clin Invest* 1997;100:904–911.

219. Jiang Z, Podack E, Levy RB. Major histocompatibility complex–mismatched allogeneic bone marrow transplantation using perforin and/or Fas ligand double-defective CD4(+) donor T cells: involvement of cytotoxic function by donor lymphocytes prior to graft-versus-host disease pathogenesis. *Blood* 2001;98:390–397.

220. Kehren J, Desvignes C, Krasteva M, et al. Cytotoxicity is mandatory for CD8(+) T cell-mediated contact hypersensitivity. *J Exp Med* 1999;189:779–786.

221. Mosmann TR, Sad S. The expanding universe of T-cell subsets: Th1, Th2 and more. *Immunol Today* 1996;17:138–146.

222. Li L, Sad S, Kagi D, et al. CD8Tc1 and Tc2 cells secrete distinct cytokine patterns *in vitro* and *in vivo* but induce similar inflammatory reactions. *J Immunol* 1997;158:4152–4161.

223. Sad S, Li L, Mosmann TR. Cytokine-deficient CD8+ Tc1 cells induced by IL-4: retained inflammation and perforin and Fas cytotoxicity but compromised long term killing of tumor cells. *J Immunol* 1997;159:606–613.

224. Nakamoto Y, Guidotti LG, Kuhlen CV, et al. Immune pathogenesis of hepatocellular carcinoma. *J Exp Med* 1998;188:341–350.

225. Chambers CA, Kuhns MS, Egen JG, et al. CTLA-4–mediated inhibition in regulation of T cell responses: mechanisms and manipulation in tumor immunotherapy. *Annu Rev Immunol* 2001;19:565–594.

226. Kuhns MS, Epshteyn V, Sobel RA, et al. Cytotoxic T lymphocyte antigen-4 (CTLA-4) regulates the size, reactivity, and function of a primed pool of CD4+ T cells. *Proc Natl Acad Sci U S A* 2000;97:12711–12716.

227. Sutmuller RP, van Duivenvoorde LM, van Elsas A, et al. Synergism of cytotoxic T lymphocyte–associated antigen 4 blockade and depletion of CD25(+) regulatory T cells in antitumor therapy reveals alternative pathways for suppression of autoreactive cytotoxic T lymphocyte responses. *J Exp Med* 2001;194:823–832.

228. Eshhar Z. Tumor-specific T-bodies: towards clinical application. *Cancer Immunol Immunother* 1997;45:131–136.

229. Bolhuis RI, Willemsen R, Gratama J. Clinical applications of redirected cytotoxicity. In: Sitkovsky M, Henkart PA, eds. *Cytotoxic cells: mechanisms and medical applications*. Philadelphia: Lippincott Williams & Wilkins, 2000:423–441.

230. Murali-Krishna K, Altman JD, Suresh M, et al. Counting antigen-specific CD8 T cells: A reevaluation of bystander activation during viral infection. *Immunity* 1998;6:177–187.

231. Harty JT, Tvinnereim AR, White DW. CD8+ T cell effector mechanisms in resistance to infection. *Annu Rev Immunol* 2000;18:275–308.

232. Corazza N, Muller S, Brunner T, et al. Differential contribution of Fas- and perforin-mediated mechanisms to the cell-mediated cytotoxic activity of naïve and *in vivo*–primed intestinal intraepithelial lymphocytes. *J Immunol* 2000;164:398–403.

233. Masopust D, Vezys V, Marzo AL, et al. Preferential localization of effector memory cells in nonlymphoid tissue. *Science* 2001;291:2413–2417.

234. Blumenthal R, Millard PJ, Henkart MP, et al. Liposomes as targets for granule cytolysin from cytotoxic LGL tumors. *Proc Natl Acad Sci U S A* 1984;81:5551–5555.

CHAPTER 37

Inflammation

Helene F. Rosenberg and John I. Gallin

Historical Perspective and Overview
The "Double-Edged Sword" of Inflammation
Initiation of the Acute Inflammatory Response
  Vasodilation · Increased Vascular Permeability · Neutrophil Recruitment and Activation · Fever
Molecular Mediators of the Acute Inflammatory Response
  The Plasma Proteases · Lipid Mediators · Peptides and Amines · Nitric Oxide · Acute-Phase Reactants · Proinflammatory Cytokines · Novel Mediators: Leptin and Lipocalins
Cellular Mediators of the Acute Inflammatory Response
  Neutrophils · Monocytes and Macrophages · Eosinophils · Platelets and Lymphocytes · Endothelial and Epithelial Cells
Allergy and Inflammation
Human Model Systems of Inflammation
  Response to Intravenous Endotoxin · Temporal Analysis of Soluble Mediators in Blister Fluid
Mouse Models of Inflammation
Resolution of the Acute Inflammatory Response
  Cell Senescence or Apoptosis · Anti-inflammatory Mediators · Hypothalamic-Pituitary-Adrenocortical Axis · Wound Repair and Angiogenesis
Chronic Inflammation
Future Directions: Novel Anti-inflammatory Therapies
References

HISTORICAL PERSPECTIVE AND OVERVIEW

Inflammation is the physiological process by which vascularized tissue responds to injury. During the inflammatory process, soluble mediators and cellular components work together in a systematic manner in the attempt to contain and to eliminate the agents causing physical distress. Although inflammation is crucial to maintaining the health and integrity of an organism, the inflammatory process, when poorly controlled, can result in massive tissue destruction. This chapter presents a limited overview of the cellular and molecular events related to the inflammatory response; a more thorough discussion of these topics can be found in the textbook *Inflammation: Basic Principles and Clinical Correlates* (1).

The first observations on the inflammatory response are credited to Cornelius Celsus, who described the cardinal clinical signs of inflammation during the first century of the Common Era. His signs—rubor (redness), dolor (pain), calor (heat), and tumor (swelling)—remain focal points for study today. Another early contributor to this field was John Hunter (2), who in 1793 was the first to appreciate inflammation as a host defense, as opposed to a disease process.

In the 1800s, Julius Cohnheim (3) provided the first microscopic descriptions of the inflammatory process. Paul Ehrlich contributed to the overall understanding of the inflammatory process with his observations on the role of antibodies, as did Elie Metchnikoff, with his observations on phagocytosis; both were awarded the 1908 Nobel Prize for their work. Other crucial discoveries included those of Wright, who described the plasma proteins (opsonins) that coat and tag foreign substances for phagocytic destruction, and Dale and Laidlaw (4), who demonstrated the vasoactive role of histamine. In more recent history, many investigators have contributed observations on roles of soluble proinflammatory mediators, including chemokines, interleukins, interferons, and their specific receptors in modulating nearly every event characteristic of the inflammatory response.

Inflammation has traditionally been categorized into acute and chronic responses. Acute inflammation is the rapid, short-lived (minutes to days), relatively uniform response to acute injury and is characterized by accumulations of fluid, plasma proteins, and granulocytic leukocytes. In contrast, chronic inflammation is of longer duration and includes influx of lymphocytes and macrophages and fibroblast growth.

The highlights of the events characteristic of acute and chronic inflammation are depicted in Fig. 1 and described as follows:

1. An injuring agent evades or destroys primary barriers—specifically, epithelial or endothelial cells and their specialized structures—and thereby initiates the acute inflammatory response. Examples of injurious agents include pathogens (bacteria, viruses, parasites), foreign bodies from exogenous (asbestos) or endogenous (urate crystals, immune complexes) sources, and physical (fire) and chemical agents.

2. Tissue damage initiates a series of molecular events that result in the production of proinflammatory mediators. Working together, these mediators promote the hallmark physical signs of inflammation, which include increased blood flow and vascular permeability, migration of leukocytes from the peripheral blood into the tissues, accumulation of these leukocytes at the inflammatory focus, and activation the leukocytes to destroy and (if possible) to eliminate the foreign substance. These soluble mediators include the plasma protease systems, lipid mediators, and proinflammatory peptides and cytokines, all

discussed in detail later. Additional mediators secreted by activated leukocytes can serve to prolong the inflammatory response.

3. If the initiating agent is eliminated, anti-inflammatory agents then take over and act to limit damage to the tissues surrounding the inflammatory focus. If there is only incomplete destruction or incomplete elimination of the foreign substance, the inflammatory process persists and expands its repertoire of soluble mediators and cellular components; this process is referred to as *chronic inflammation.*

This chapter describes the physical, cellular, and molecular events underlying acute and chronic inflammation in some detail. Included are descriptions of several of clinical disorders in which deficient or deranged inflammatory responses play a crucial role in disease pathogenesis. References have been selected to include up-to-date reviews and textbook chapters that cover the individual topics in greater depth.

THE "DOUBLE-EDGED SWORD" OF INFLAMMATION

The "double-edged sword" is an important and useful metaphor for understanding the role of inflammation in higher organisms, because inherent in it is the recognition that the inflammatory response can mediate both beneficial and detrimental contributions to the health and welfare of the host. There are no unique and separable "beneficial" and "detrimental" inflammatory responses; inflammatory cells participating in innate host defense and the signals to which they respond are, simply, somewhat primitive in terms of specificity, and together they are not as skilled at definitive pathogen targeting as the cells and signals participating in the acquired immune response. The responses that were designed to provide host defense can, under certain circumstances, also result in significant tissue damage and functional pathological processes. For example, although neutrophilic leukocytes are clearly effective at mediating host defense against bacterial and fungal pathogens through degranulation, phagocytosis, and production of reactive oxygen species, the dysregulation of these essential, beneficial responses can lead to reperfusion injury and adult respiratory distress syndrome (5,6). The same is likely to be true for the beneficial and detrimental responses of eosinophils (7).

INITIATION OF THE ACUTE INFLAMMATORY RESPONSE

The way in which the inflammatory process is initiated depends in part on the nature and portal of entry of the foreign substance and, to some degree, the nature and circumstances of a particular individual. Pathogens can initiate inflammation by a number of distinct and idiosyncratic mechanisms, including activation of the plasma protease systems by interaction with degradation products of the bacterial cell walls

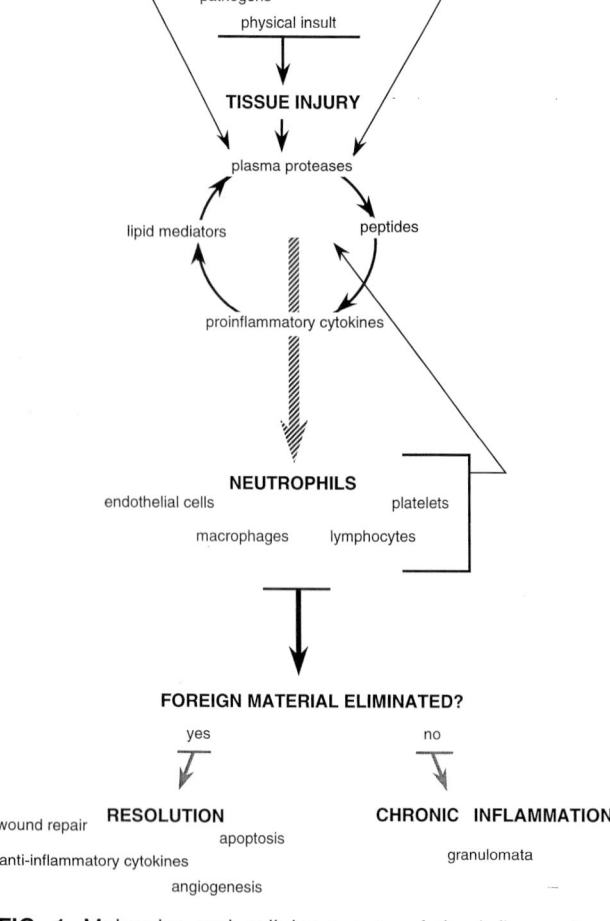

FIG. 1. Molecular and cellular events of the inflammatory response.

and by secretion of toxins that can activate the inflammatory response directly (8). Injured cells themselves can release degradation products that initiate one or more of the plasma protease cascades and can augment expression of proinflammatory cytokines that promote the inflammatory process.

Regardless of the initiating agent, the physiological changes accompanying acute inflammation encompass four main features: vasodilation, increased vascular permeability, neutrophil recruitment and activation, and fever.

Vasodilation

Vasodilation, often preceded by a brief period of vasoconstriction, is among the earliest physical responses to acute tissue injury. The arterioles are the first to be involved, followed by the capillary beds, and this results in a net increase in blood flow. The increased blood flow results in the characteristic heat and redness (calor and rubor) associated with foci of acute inflammation.

Increased Vascular Permeability

Under normal conditions, the vascular endothelial cells function as a semipermeable membrane, restricting the plasma proteins to the intravascular space. In response to inflammatory stimuli, endothelial cells lining the venules contract, widening the intercellular junctions to produce gaps that permit passage of plasma proteins. This results in characteristic pain (dolor) and swelling (tumor) in the affected region (9). More severe injury is associated with endothelial cell necrosis and increased leakage of plasma proteins and blood cells.

Neutrophil Recruitment and Activation

One of the initial and most crucial responses to acute inflammation is the recruitment of leukocytes (primarily neutrophils) from the blood stream and ultimately from the bone marrow to the focus of inflammatory activity. The first step observed in this process is margination, as the neutrophils appear to "roll" slowly along the periphery of the blood vessel. This is followed by a more definitive adherence stage. Neutrophils then migrate into the tissue. Under the influence of multiple soluble chemotactic agents, neutrophils are targeted to the site of inflammation. At this site, the neutrophils ingest pathogenic material by a process known as phagocytosis and detoxify and digest these substances by the actions of endogenous oxidants and proteolytic enzymes.

Fever

Fever remains the most poorly understood of the acute inflammatory responses. Agents producing fever, or pyrogens, are released from leukocytes in response to specific stimuli, including bacterial endotoxin. Pyrogens exert their actions through the temperature-regulating mechanism of the hypothalamus. A number of soluble proinflammatory mediators (discussed later and in Chapters 23 to 25) have been implicated in this process, including interleukin (IL)–1, tumor necrosis factor α (TNF-α), and prostaglandins. The beneficial role of fever with regard to the acute inflammatory response remains a mystery.

MOLECULAR MEDIATORS OF THE ACUTE INFLAMMATORY RESPONSE

The physiological features of the inflammatory process just described are initiated, regulated, and ultimately eliminated by the actions of numerous proinflammatory mediators. Some of these mediators are stored within cells in inactive form and are activated by products of acute inflammation; others are synthesized or released from cellular sources, or both, also in response to the products of acute inflammation, or by other soluble inflammatory mediators. Although these mediators are discussed as separate components, it is important to appreciate that they perform their functions through an interplay of coordinately regulated and mutually augmenting pathways.

The Plasma Proteases

Among the central components of the inflammatory response are the three interacting groups of plasma proteases. Through the actions of plasma proteins as they convert one another from inactive to active forms, many of the major soluble mediators of inflammation are generated.

Complement

This group of plasma proteins was initially identified on the basis of their ability to "complement" the bactericidal activities of antibodies. At current count, 30 to 40 proteins are recognized as participants in the complement cascade. By serial and sequential proteolytic cleavage, the complement proteins become activated, bind to foreign organisms, and thereby enhance their recognition by phagocytic cells. Several components also function by increasing vascular permeability, by serving as chemoattractants for inflammatory cells, and by creating lytic multiprotein complexes (10–14). Host cells in turn protect themselves through expression of complement-inhibitory cell-surface receptors, including CD46, decay-activating factor (CD55), Crry, and CD59 (15). The classical pathway of complement was the first to be described; this cascade is activated by antigen-bound antibodies of the immunoglobulin M or G class, now recognized as a significant bridge between innate, inflammatory pathways and the systems promoting acquired immunity. The first complement component, C1, undergoes autocatalytic cleavage to produce C1s, which in turn catalyzes a specific cleavage of C4 to C4b and C4a; C4b then binds to the target antigen, and C4a combines with C2a (product of the proteolytic cleavage of C2 by C1s) to create a protease specific for the component C3, and so on. The alternative pathway is used by other initiating agents (e.g., bacterial endotoxin) and converges with the classical pathway at the cleavage of C3; in addition, proteases from bacteria and damaged tissue, as well as plasmin generated by the fibrinolytic system (see later discussion), can catalyze the cleavage of C3. From this point, the cleavage product C3b goes on to create proteolytic products of C5, and serial proteolysis leads to activation of proteins C6 through C9, which are recognized as the membrane attack complex. In addition to their role in host defense, complement components have been recognized for promoting rapid clearance of apoptotic host cells (16). Inherited deficiencies in individual components of the complement system can result in increased susceptibility to infection, rheumatic disorders, or angioedema (17,18), and several strains of complement transgenic and gene-deleted mice have been described (19,20). A more complete discussion of complement deficiencies, and the disorders to which they relate, can be found in Chapter 34.

Kinins

Among the ultimate products of the kinin cascade is bradykinin, an agent known to induce smooth muscle contraction, vasoconstriction, and increased permeability of smaller blood vessels (21). The kinin cascade is initiated by a number of by-products of tissue damage, including collagen, cartilage, and basement membranes, as well as by endotoxin and inorganic materials, which serve to activate factor XII (or Hageman factor, better known as a participant in the clotting cascade, as described later). Factor XII mediates the cleavage of prekallikrein to kallikrein, which not only serves to activate more factor XII but also cleaves the proenzyme kininogen to produce bradykinin. Factor XII represents a crucial intersection between these pathways, inasmuch as it can also be activated by plasmin, a product of proteolytic cleavage among the fibrinolytic proteins, and by kallikrein, another protein of the kinin group. The proinflammatory effects of neurokinins (substance P, neurokinins A and B) provide a link to the peripheral nervous system (22,23). Research has focused on specific kinin receptors (24–27), particularly those expressed by neutrophils (28), and on the role of receptor antagonists (29) in modulating the inflammatory response.

Clotting/Fibrinolytic Proteins

In addition to the roles played by these proteins in hemostasis, they contribute significantly to the amplification of the inflammatory response through the direct activation of factor XII, as just described. Proteolytic cleavages initiated by activated factor XII ultimately result in the cleavage of fibrinogen to fibrin and to smaller fibrinopeptides that serve as inflammatory modulators. Activated factor XII similarly activates the fibrinolytic system by generating the protease plasmin. Similar to factor XII, plasmin represents an important intersecting locus for all three protease systems, because its activity proceeds in a number of directions. Plasmin activity can generate

fibrin split products, which are also inflammatory mediators, but, of more importance, plasmin activity augments the production of activated factor XII and results in direct activation of the complement pathway through proteolytic cleavage of factor C3 (30–35).

Lipid Mediators

Lipid mediators are a complex group of chemicals that also participate in augmenting the inflammatory response. This group includes the prostaglandins, leukotrienes, and platelet-activating factor. A fourth group of lipid mediators, including lipoxin and 15-epi-lipoxin, promote inflammatory resolution (36,37).

Prostaglandins

Prostaglandins are oxidized derivatives of the fatty acid arachidonate that mediate a number of the cardinal signs of inflammation, including fever, pain, and vascular permeability (38). The major sources of prostaglandin in acute inflammation include mononuclear phagocytes, endothelial cells, and platelets. Prostaglandin synthesis is augmented during inflammation by a number of stimuli, including bacterial endotoxin, immune complexes, complement component C3a, bradykinin, and IL-1, and they mediate their proinflammatory effects through specific receptors (39–42). Research in this field has focused on the prostaglandin synthetic enzymes cyclooxygenases 1 and 2 (COX-1 and COX-2) and on the findings relating to the COX-2 isoform as the major producer of proinflammatory prostaglandins (43–45). Although specific COX-2–selective inhibitors have been introduced as gastrointestinal-sparing anti-inflammatory agents (46), there is evidence that administration of these agents may result in delayed resolution of detrimental inflammatory sequelae (47,48).

Leukotrienes

Leukotrienes are also oxidation products of arachidonate that are synthesized in and released from neutrophilic and, to a lesser extent, eosinophilic leukocytes (49). Leukotriene A_4 (LTA$_4$) and its synthetic products leukotrienes B$_4$ and C$_4$ (LTB$_4$ and LTC$_4$) are synthesized and exported from these cells; LTA$_4$ can then be taken up by erythrocytes, platelets, and endothelial cells, in which conversion to LTB$_4$ and LTC$_4$ can also take place. Leukotrienes D$_4$ and E$_4$ are additional metabolic conversion products of LTC$_4$. Although evidence for the existence of specific receptors for individual leukotrienes exists, these receptors remain as yet undefined. Together, leukotrienes mediate a large array of proinflammatory activities, including vasoconstriction, increased vascular permeability, and increased endothelial adhesiveness, as well as neutrophil chemotaxis and activation (50–52). Most recently, leukotrienes have received attention as contributors to the pathophysiology of asthma (53–58).

Platelet-Activating Factor

Platelet-activating factor (59–63) is a substituted derivative of glycerol phosphate that exists in both circulating and cellular forms. In its cellular form in endothelial cells, platelet-activating factor has been shown to enhance neutrophil–endothelial cell adhesion. Specific receptors for platelet-activating factor have been identified on neutrophils (64), and numerous antagonists that may have potential for clinical use have been identified (65–69).

Peptides and Amines

Histamine and Serotonin

Histamine, a decarboxylated derivative of histidine, was among the earliest of the soluble inflammatory mediators to be discovered (70–82). Tissue mast cells and basophils synthesize and store histamine, which is released in response to variety of physical and chemical stimuli. Histamine diffuses rapidly through tissues and into the blood stream and promotes many of the sequelae of acute inflammation, including vasodilation, increased vascular permeability, and interactions with the peripheral nervous system. Histamine binds to three distinct G protein–coupled receptors: H1, H2 and H3. Serotonin, a derivative of tryptophan, is stored in platelets, mast cells, and enterochromaffin cells of the gastrointestinal tract and is released through degranulation. Like histamine, serotonin has receptor-mediated vasoactive properties, although its role in acute inflammation is not well defined (83).

Neuropeptides

Neuropeptides are among the many aspects of the connection between the nervous system and the inflammatory response. As a group, neuropeptides are inflammatory mediators released from neurons in response to local tissue damage. This group of mediators includes substance P, vasoactive intestinal peptide, somatostatin, and calcitonin gene–related peptide (84–88). Although numerous immunomodulatory activities have attributed to these mediators, the determination of their true physiological roles and their overall effects is currently under study. Neutral endopeptidase, a member of the nephrolysin family of proteolytic enzymes, limits inflammation by specific degradation of neuropeptides. Its activity is reduced in the presence of respiratory irritants (89–91).

Nitric Oxide

Although its role as an inflammatory mediator has been clearly established in mouse model systems, the role of nitric oxide in human host defense remains controversial. The best-characterized responses are the production of nitric oxide in murine macrophages, mediating host defense against bacterial, fungal, parasitic, and viral pathogens and mediating vascular tone (92–101). Unlike most other mediators, nitric oxide does not mediate its effects through specific membrane receptors; it is a small molecule that diffuses readily across cell membranes and activates a variety of enzymes and enzyme systems intracellularly, in addition to functioning as a free radical both directly or through its interactions with superoxide anions.

Acute-Phase Reactants

C-reactive protein, serum amyloid A, and fibrinogen are among the best characterized of the group of serum proteins known as acute-phase reactants, plasma proteins produced in the liver in increased quantities in response to inflammatory stimuli (102–104). Numerous proinflammatory activities have been attributed to C-reactive protein, including the induction of cytokine synthesis, and C-reactive protein has received significant attention as a marker for the inflammation associated with advanced coronary artery disease. Similarly, serum amyloid A has been shown to induce cellular chemotaxis and adhesion. In addition to its role in hemostasis, fibrinogen has been shown to activate stimulated human neutrophils to produce the proinflammatory chemokine IL-8 (105) and to stimulate chemokine secretion from macrophages through the Toll-like receptor (TLR) 4 (106). The kinetics of the production of these proteins *in vivo* are depicted in Fig. 2 (107).

Proinflammatory Cytokines

The identification and characterization of these soluble mediators constitute one of the most active fields in current

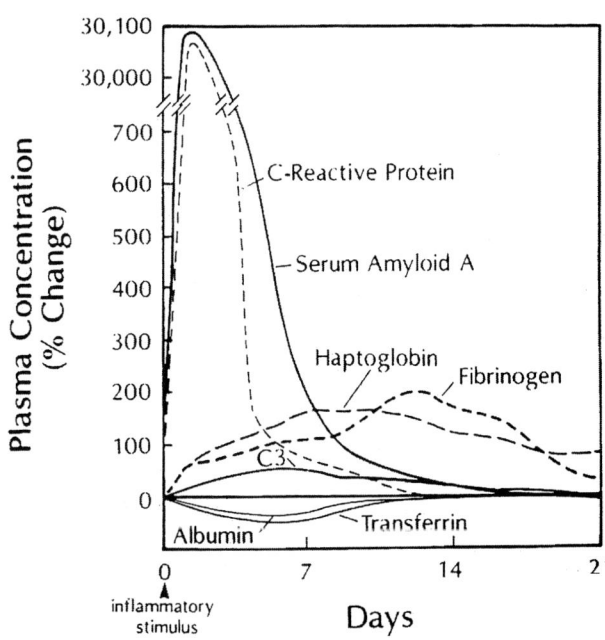

FIG. 2. Plasma concentrations of acute-phase reactant proteins *in vivo* in response to an inflammatory stimulus. From Kushner (107), with permission.

inflammation research. A comprehensive discussion of individual proinflammatory cytokines and their interactions can be found in Chapters 23 to 25.

Novel Mediators: Leptin and Lipocalins

Leptin, a protein derived from adipocytes that was initially recognized for its role in regulating food intake, has been shown to regulate several features characteristic of the inflammatory response, including macrophage activation and cytokine production as well as wound healing and angiogenesis. Increased production of leptin has been reported as a component of the acute-phase response to inflammatory stimuli; its secretion is regulated by the proinflammatory mediator TNF-α (108,109).

Lipocalins are a diverse group of small, primarily secreted proteins that form complexes with hydrophobic ligands. They share significant sequence homology with one another and are found in virtually all major kingdoms of life. In mammals, many of the best-characterized animal dander allergens are among the lipocalins, as well as the "immunocalins" α_1-acid glycoprotein, α_1-microglobulin, the γ chain of complement factor 8, and neutrophil gelatinase–associated lipocalin (110,111).

CELLULAR MEDIATORS OF THE ACUTE INFLAMMATORY RESPONSE

In one sense, the entire interconnecting network of proinflammatory responses can be viewed as a means of facilitating the recruitment of neutrophils to the site of tissue injury. Neutrophils respond to soluble inflammatory mediators by migrating to sites of tissue injury and by ingesting and destroying invading pathogens and damaged tissue, leading the way to resolution and ultimately, tissue repair. Other participants in the acute response include platelets, lymphocytes, and endothelial cells, as discussed later.

Neutrophils

Neutrophilic leukocytes are crucial to both immunity and inflammation, and prolonged neutropenia leads inevitably to an organism's demise as a result of overwhelming infection (112–114). Neutrophils normally represent between 40% and 50% of the circulating leukocyte population and are easily recognized on Wright's stained blood smear by their size, their characteristic multilobed nuclei, and the presence of fine stippling representing granules throughout the cytoplasmic compartment (Fig. 3). Primary and secondary granules contain their own distinct sets of proinflammatory mediators. There are several well-characterized neutrophil dysfunctional states and diseases that serve as "experiments of nature," elucidating the roles played by these leukocytes and their individual components in inflammation and host defense against infection (115,116).

Development in the Bone Marrow

Neutrophils develop from undifferentiated precursors present in the bone marrow (117). The myeloblast is the first

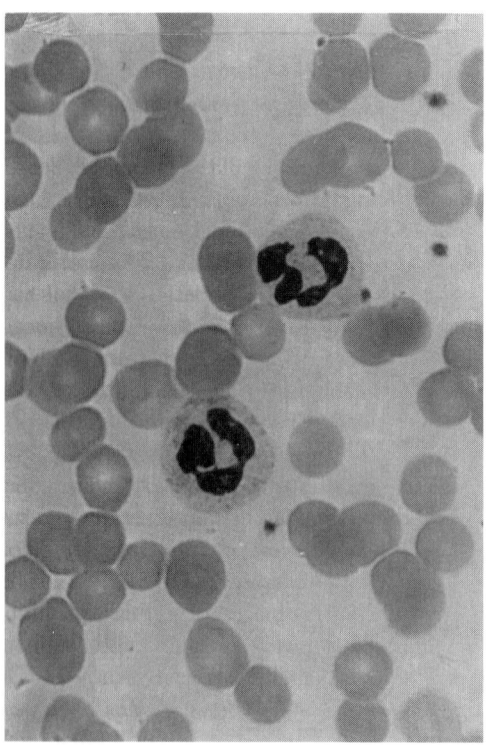
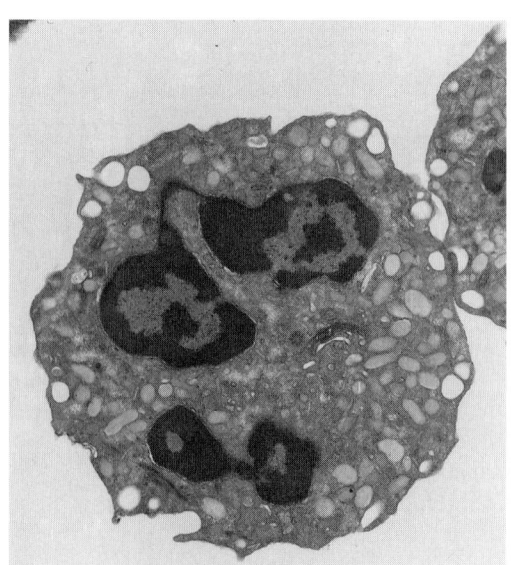

FIG. 3. Light (**A**) and electron (**B**) microscopic views of a mature human peripheral blood neutrophil. Photographs courtesy of Dr. Douglas Kuhns.

morphologically identifiable precursor of the neutrophil lineage, followed by the promyelocyte, myelocyte, metamyelocyte, and band form, which directly precedes the mature neutrophil (Fig. 4). Several products of activated T-lymphocytes, including granulocyte-macrophage colony-stimulating factor (GM-CSF), IL-3, and granulocyte colony-stimulating factor (G-CSF), participate in the process of neutrophil maturation by direct interactions with their respective receptors, which have been identified on neutrophil precursor cells. When mature, neutrophils are released into the circulation, from which they are recruited to sites of inflammation by the actions of soluble mediators, most notably IL-8. Neutropenia may be related to chemotherapeutic agents, autoantibodies, or infections that are often reversible; in contrast, familial neutropenias are chronic, inherited disorders of neutrophil metabolism (118–122). Similarly, there is evidence that familial Mediterranean fever and related disorders are primarily disorders of neutrophil homeostasis (123,124).

Activation/Priming

Neutrophils in the circulation are quiescent cells with the potential to mediate a wide range of inflammatory activities. This potential is realized when neutrophils are activated (125,126). Neutrophils can be activated by a large (and increasing) number of specific agents (Table 1). As a group, these activating agents transmit signals to the neutrophils through interaction with specific cell-surface receptors (112,127–130), many of which interact with intracellular G proteins. G proteins catalyze the hydrolysis of guanosine triphosphate to guanosine diphosphate and inorganic phosphate and thereby initiate activation of phospholipase C, calcium fluxes, and membrane depolarization. Once activated, neutrophils are able to adhere to endothelial cells, migrate through the endothelial barrier, and ingest and at least attempt to destroy pathogens, foreign bodies, and remnants of tissue damage. An intriguing aspect of neutrophil activation is the phenomenon of priming. Neutrophils primed by brief exposure to activating agents (endotoxin, IL-1, f-Met-Leu-Phe, GM-CSF) exhibit an enhanced response to subsequent stimuli. Both short-term responses (including changes in cell shape and in oxidative and phagocytic capacity) and long-

TABLE 1. *Agents promoting neutrophil activation*

Agent	Function stimulated
Leukotriene B$_4$	Chemoattractant, enhances adherence to endothelial cells, activates degranulation and NADPH oxidase activity
Complement fragment C5a	Chemoattractant, induces degranulation and adherence
Platelet activating factor	Induces aggregation and adherence, chemoattractant degranulation
Histamine	Concentration-dependent changes in chemotaxis priming, degranulation
Interferon γ	Increases antibody-dependent cytotoxicity, priming
Granulocyte-CSF	Increases antibody-dependent cytotoxicity, priming; enhances phagocytosis; stimulates maturation within bone marrow
Granulocyte-macrophage CSF	Priming, stimulates maturation within bone marrow
Tumor necrosis factor-α	Chemoattractant, priming, enhances phagocytosis and antibody-dependent cytotoxicity
Interleukin-8 (IL-8)	Chemoattractant, induces degranulation and NADPH oxidase activity
f-Met-Leu-Phe	Chemoattractant, induces aggregation, degranulation, and NADPH oxidase activity
Fibrinogen	Primes neutrophil IL-8 synthesis in response to f-Met-Leu-Phe and LTB4

CSF, colony-stimulating factor; NADPH, nicotinamide adenine dinucleotide phosphate, reduced form.

term responses (prolonged cell viability) to priming agents have been observed. Overall, the phenomenon of priming suggests that neutrophil activation is a two-step process, requiring an initial switch from a nonreceptive to a receptive state. The molecular basis for this switch is currently under investigation. Among the most intriguing investigations are those pursuing the role of TLRs, which mediate phagocyte

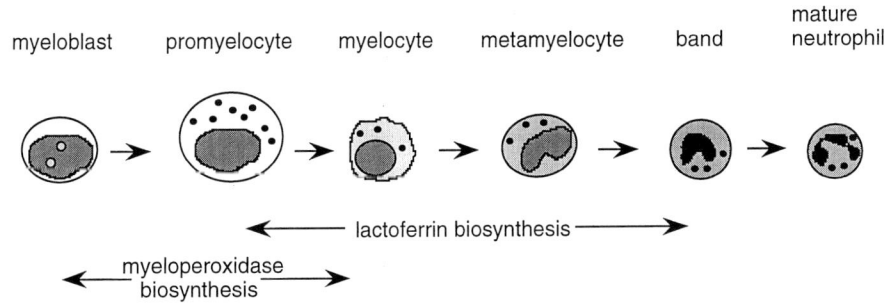

FIG. 4. Stages of neutrophil maturation in the bone marrow, from myeloblast to mature neutrophil. The *large black circles* represent the primary granules, and the *dark shading* represents the secondary granules. The stages at which the proinflammatory mediators myeloperoxidase and lactoferrin are synthesized are as indicated by the *arrows*. Adapted from Rosenberg and Gallin (113), with permission.

responses to bacterial lipopolysaccharide (131–133). The TLR family is ancient and highly conserved, and its members function in host defense through specific recognition of motifs and patterns conserved among pathogens.

Adherence

In order to participate effectively in the inflammatory process, neutrophils must ultimately leave the blood stream and migrate into the tissues. The initial step in this process is adherence to the vascular endothelium. Neutrophil adherence is a two-step process, the first involving a class of cell-surface molecules known as selectins (134–143). Selectins mediate the process in which neutrophils "roll" or "slow down" before their actual activation-dependent adherence to the endothelial cells. Three classes of selectins have been identified: L-selectins, which have been identified on all leukocytes; E-selectin, on the surface of activated endothelial cells; and P-selectin, found on endothelial cells and platelets. Selectins function by binding to carbohydrate ligands present on the adhering cell. The ligand for the endothelial E-selectin is sialylated Lewis X antigen, found on the neutrophil, which, when absent, results in a marked immunodeficiency state.

The second part of the adherence process is the tight binding mediated by integrins (144–151). The leukocyte integrins are a subgroup of an extensive family of proteins that mediate a wide range of interactions between cells and between cells and the extracellular environment. The leukocyte integrins—leukocyte function–associated antigen 1 (LFA-1) (CD11a/CD18), Mac-1 (CD11b/CD18), and p150,95 (CD11c/CD18)—are heterodimeric proteins with distinct α and shared β polypeptide chains. Mac-1 in particular has several well-characterized roles in the inflammatory process. Mac-1 is stored in the secondary granule compartment and brought to the cell surface in conjunction with neutrophil activation. In addition to mediating specific adherence, Mac-1 participates in signal transduction, phagocytosis, and chemotaxis and in production of reactive oxygen species. Intercellular cell adhesion molecule (ICAM)–1, a cell-surface protein found on endothelial cells, has been identified as a ligand for Mac-1.

Two forms of inherited defects of neutrophil adhesion have been identified: Leukocyte adhesion deficiency I (LAD I) involves a genetic defect in the biosynthesis of CD18, the shared β chain for all three leukocyte adhesion molecules (152–157). The defect is autosomal recessive, and has been mapped to human chromosome 22q22.3. Individuals with this disorder have frequent and recurrent skin and soft tissue infections, poor wound healing, and severe periodontal disease. In contrast, leukocyte adhesion deficiency II (LAD II) is a glycosylation defect that results in the inability to synthesize the sialyl-Lewis X carbohydrate ligand for E- and P-selectins (158–160). This condition results in a defect in neutrophil "rolling" that occurs before and facilitates neutrophil adherence to endothelial cells, and affected individuals likewise suffer from frequent severe bacterial infections.

Chemotaxis

As part of the activation process, neutrophils are capable of sensing and responding to concentration gradients of the activating agents that are highlighted in Table 1. By "crawling" across a surface, neutrophils can be seen to migrate toward a higher concentration of attractant. At the subcellular level, cell motility requires alterations in the neutrophil cytoskeleton, which is composed primarily of actin filaments. Although the precise mechanism by which signals are transmitted directly to the cytoskeleton is unclear, there is evidence that several actin-binding proteins (including profilin, cofilin, and gelsolin) participate in altering the actin filament structure, permitting net movement of the cell in response to a chemoattractant gradient (161–164).

Phagocytosis

Phagocytosis, or engulfment of foreign or damaged material, is central to the inflammatory process and discussed in detail in Chapter 35 (165,166). In order to engulf a particle, neutrophils extend pseudopodia that encircle the offending material; the pseudopodia then fuse, trapping the material inside the cell in a compartment known as a phagosome. Particles coated with immunoglobulins (or opsonized) are phagocytosed in a highly efficient manner, inasmuch as they are recognized by and bind directly to the crystallized fragment receptors present on the neutrophil cell surface. Particles opsonized by proteolytic products of complement are similarly phagocytosed in a specific, receptor-mediated manner, involving complement receptors 1 and 3 (CR1 and CR3). Studies have focused on the involvement of Rho proteins in this process (167).

Degranulation

The primary and secondary granules of neutrophils contain a number of distinct effector proteins, listed in Table 2. As part

TABLE 2. *Major components of neutrophil primary and secondary granules*

Primary granules	Secondary granules
Myeloperoxidase	Lactoferrin
Defensins	Gelatinase
BPI	Collagenase
Cathepsin G	Vitamin B_{12} binding protein
Lysozyme	Lysozyme
Elastase	Cytochrome b558
Alkaline phosphatase	f-MLP receptor
Proteinase 3	CD11b/CD18, CD11c/CD18 (integrins)
β-glucuronidase	Complement receptor 3 (CR3)
α-fucosidase	Histaminase
Phospholipases A2, C, D	Plasminogen activator
α-mannosidase	

BPI, bacterial permeability–increasing protein; f-MLP, f-Met-Leu-Phe.

of the activation process, the cytoplasmic membrane-bound granules fuse with the phagosome, placing the effector proteins in direct contact with the ingested material. Among the highlights of the components of the primary (also known as azurophil) granules are lysozyme, which can digest the peptidoglycan component of most bacterial cell walls, and cathepsin G, defensins, and bacterial permeability-increasing protein, all with inherent antibacterial activity. Goldman et al. (168) showed that human β-defensin-1 is inactivated in patients with cystic fibrosis and thus may be related to the pathogenesis of bacterial infections in such patients. Also among the more prominent components is myeloperoxidase, which converts hydrogen peroxide generated by the reduced nicotinamide adenine dinucleotide phosphate (NADPH) oxidase and hydrochloric acid to hypochlorous acid, another antimicrobial agent.

The secondary (or specific) granules contain several proteins whose role in the inflammatory response remains a bit mysterious. Among these proteins is lactoferrin, an iron-binding protein with some antibacterial activity (169). The secondary granules also contain stored sources of CR3 and other receptors for neutrophil activation agents, as well as stored membrane components of the NADPH oxidase.

Chédiak-Higashi syndrome is a disorder in which neutrophils demonstrate abnormal structure, abnormal chemotaxis, and failure to degranulate, and affected patients are subject to recurrent severe bacterial and fungal infections. Three independent groups have reported the identification of the genetic defect in Chédiak-Higashi syndrome, residing on human chromosome 1q42–43 (170,171). Another rare disorder of neutrophils is specific granule deficiency, in which the secondary, or specific, granules are absent or, alternatively are present but without the granule protein components (172–175). Myeloperoxidase deficiency is a fairly common disorder resulting from a variety of missense mutations in the coding sequence of the gene encoding this granule protein (176–180). The resulting defect in microbicidal activity is present but is not as clinically severe as that observed in chronic granulomatous disease (discussed later).

NADPH Oxidase

A crucial component of the neutrophil host-defense mechanism is the NADPH oxidase enzyme complex (Fig. 5) (181–187). This enzyme assembles on the phagosomal membrane from two integral membrane components (gp91-phox and p22-phox, for *p*hagocyte *ox*idase) and three cytosolic components (p47-phox, p67-phox, and Rac) to catalyze the production of superoxide anion from molecular oxygen and free electrons. Superoxide is then converted to the toxic metabolite hydrogen peroxide by the actions of superoxide dismutase or to hypochlorous acid, by the primary granule protein myeloperoxidase, as described previously.

Although the ability to generate toxic oxygen metabolites is crucial to host defense, these agents represent the sharpest part of the "double-edged sword" of inflammation. Superoxide anion is readily diffusible through membranes and can be converted to toxic metabolites outside the restricted locale of the phagosome. Products of oxygen radicals can create enlarged foci of tissue damage, thereby enhancing and

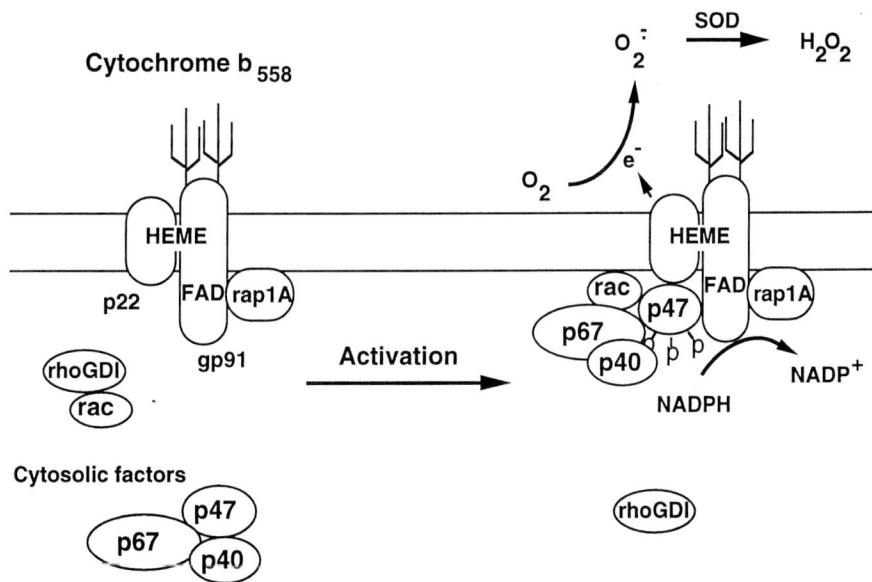

FIG. 5. Schematic of the protein components of the phagocyte reduced nicotinamide adenine dinucleotide phosphate (NADPH) oxidase. Upon activation, the cytoplasmic components Rac, p67-phox, p47-phox, and p40-phox are translocated to the cell membrane to form the catalytic complex. Once formed, the complex can catalyze the conversion of molecular oxygen (O_2) to superoxide (O_2^-) that is then converted to the toxic oxygen metabolite hydrogen peroxide (H_2O_2) by the actions of superoxide dismutase (SOD). The proteins associate through specific SH3 domain recognition sites (183). Drawing courtesy of Dr. Thomas Leto.

augmenting the inflammatory process far beyond what was necessary to contain the initial insult. Similarly, oxidative injury has been implicated in the pathogenesis of cardiovascular, neoplastic, arthritic, and neurodegenerative disease.

Chronic granulomatous disease is an inherited disorder in which neutrophils are rendered incapable of generating toxic oxygen metabolites (188–191). This results in an inability to mount an effective defense against bacteria (particularly catalase-positive strains) and fungi, and many affected patients have recurrent, life-threatening infections. Inherited defects in any one of the four oxidase proteins can disable the enzyme complex and result in disease. Standard therapies for this disorder include prophylactic antibiotics and injections of the inflammatory modulating agent interferon (IFN)–γ. In rare patients, the disease has been corrected with bone marrow transplantation (191), and gene therapy is under investigation (192).

Protein Biosynthesis

Although neutrophils are generally perceived as "end-stage" cells, they have been shown to be capable of significant biosynthetic activity. The proteins expressed *de novo* in neutrophils include components of the NADPH oxidase and specific membrane receptors and antigens. Several proinflammatory mediators are released by activated neutrophils, including IL-1, TNF-α, IL-6, IL-8, GM-CSF, G-CSF, and plasminogen activator (112,193–197). Kuhns and Gallin (198) showed that IL-8 is actively synthesized by exudate neutrophils. These mediators can "feed back" on the system and augment the overall inflammatory response.

Monocytes and Macrophages

Monocytes are also phagocytic cells, and they migrate into the tissues in response to local stimuli, like the neutrophils (199,200). Activated macrophages, like neutrophils, are capable of phagocytosis and release antibacterial proteins and proinflammatory mediators. Macrophage functions complement those of neutrophils during the acute response and take on a more central role during chronic inflammation. The biology and physiology of macrophages are covered in detail in Chapter 16.

Eosinophils

Eosinophils are primarily tissue-dwelling granulocytes that are also recruited to sites of acute inflammation, seen most prominently in response to respiratory, gastrointestinal, and dermatological allergens and in response to generalized infection with helminthic parasites (201–205). Like neutrophils, eosinophils develop in the bone marrow, have receptor-mediated responses to specific activating agents [including the chemokine regulated upon activation, normal T-cell expressed presumably secreted (RANTES), macrophage inflammatory protein (MIP)–1α, eotaxin, and

IL-5], and contain cytoplasmic granules with oxidative and cationic proteins. In contrast to neutrophils, eosinophils are ineffective phagocytes and release the contents of their granules to the extracellular milieu. Interestingly, the detrimental features of eosinophils, particularly their contributions to the pathogenesis of reactive airway disease (206–208), are among the best characterized, whereas the beneficial aspects of eosinophils in the inflammatory response remain poorly understood. Studies have suggested a role for eosinophils in host defense against respiratory virus pathogens, which in turn suggests the possibility that asthma and respiratory allergy represent the detrimental side of what has been designed as innate, eosinophil-mediated antiviral host defense (7,209).

Platelets and Lymphocytes

Platelets contribute to the inflammatory response by several mechanisms (210). Platelets contain and can release numerous inflammatory mediators, including fibrinogen, plasminogen, and other components, including lipids and serotonin, that participate in the plasma protease systems. Several of these mediators released from platelets are direct activating agents for neutrophils, and, conversely, mediators released by activated neutrophils (oxygen metabolites, granule proteins, lipids) serve to alter platelet function. Platelets interact with lymphocytes, providing the cell contact and reagents for prostaglandin synthesis. Platelets also interact with fibroblasts, stimulating collagen and fibronectin synthesis during resolution.

The complex biology of T- and B-lymphocytes and their role in specific immunity are discussed in detail in Chapters 3 to 13; the role of immunoglobulins in augmenting the inflammatory response and enhancing neutrophil phagocytosis has been discussed previously. It is also important to emphasize that many of the soluble mediators (interleukins, IFN-γ) are produced by activated T-lymphocytes, as are a number of the anti-inflammatory mediators to be discussed.

Endothelial and Epithelial Cells

The role of endothelial cells in providing a base for neutrophil adherence has already been discussed. More recently appreciated is the fact that endothelial and epithelial cells synthesize and release numerous proinflammatory mediators (211–217).

ALLERGY AND INFLAMMATION

Allergy is also a form of inflammation. The central components of this type of the allergic response are immunoglobulin E (IgE), IgE receptors on basophils and mast cells, and histamine released from these cells upon IgE receptor–mediated interaction. The role of allergy in host defense remains controversial, and research is focused on the role of IgE and mucosal mast cells in the defense against gastrointestinal parasites (218–220); understandably, most of the literature on allergy focuses on its more clear-cut detrimental features.

HUMAN MODEL SYSTEMS OF INFLAMMATION

Two model systems have provided insight into the temporal appearance and importance of mediators in the various processes of inflammation in humans. In one model, small amounts of the lipid-A derivative of endotoxin are administered intravenously to normal human subjects, and mediator accumulation in peripheral blood is monitored (221). In the other model, mediator accumulation is monitored locally in the skin after creation of skin blisters by suction (222,223).

Response to Intravenous Endotoxin

After intravenous endotoxin, a characteristic change in body temperature and white blood cell count is observed. Body temperature begins to increase after about 1 hour and reaches a maximum after about 4 hours. The leukocyte count shows a characteristic decrease after about 30 minutes, as a result of neutrophil and monocyte adherence to endothelial cells in the lungs and spleen. This is followed by a leukocytosis, characterized by the presence of immature neutrophils at about 4 hours, which can persist throughout 24 hours with a gradual return to baseline by 48 hours. The leukocytosis is predominantly caused by mobilization of immature neutrophils from the bone marrow. The critical components of the inflammatory response—fever, neutrophil margination in the circulatory vessels, and then mobilization from the bone marrow—are associated with readily detected changes in circulating levels of certain mediators of inflammation. For example, TNF-α peaks within 2 hours (224) and is probably the predominant pyrogen associated with the febrile response. Plasma levels of the chemoattractant IL-8 increase early and peak by 4 hours. Early increases in IL-8 may relate to the transient decrease in the neutrophil count at 30 minutes (margination), because administration of intravenous chemoattractants in experimental animals is associated with a rapid neutropenia, probably a result of increased neutrophil expression of adhesion receptors (CR3) (225). In this regard, it is of interest that significant increases in plasma C5a and LTB$_4$ were not detected after administration of intravenous endotoxin to humans, which reinforces the notion of the crucial role of IL-8 in the process of neutrophil margination. Plasma concentrations of IL-6 also increased 2 to 4 hours after intravenous administration of endotoxin. In addition to not detecting increases in plasma C5a, LTB$_4$, or IL-1, no increases in circulating IL-2, IL-3, IL-4, IFN-γ, transforming growth factor (TGF-) β, or nitrate/nitrite were detected after intravenous administration of endotoxin; this emphasizes the specificity of the responses observed. Kuhns et al. (226) described a patient with recurrent bacterial infections who displayed hyporesponsiveness to both endotoxin and IL-1, which was attributable to a defect in signal transduction. Although the precise molecular basis of endotoxin activity has not yet been determined, there is evidence that endotoxin interacts with the cell surface antigen CD14 on the surface of phagocytes (227,228) and modulates the expression of nuclear factor κB (NFκB), a factor that promotes the transcription of numerous proinflammatory mediators, through TLR4. Similarly, there are several reports describing a novel X-linked immunodeficiency disorder related to mutations in IKK-γ (NEMO) that result in impaired NFκB signaling (229–231).

Temporal Analysis of Soluble Mediators in Blister Fluid

Soluble mediator accumulation at local inflammatory processes can be detected in raised skin blisters induced in normal volunteers (222). Mediators detected in blister fluid within 3 to 5 hours of the inflammatory response included LTB$_4$, C5a, IL-8, and IL-6. In contrast, IL-1β, GM-CSF and TNF-α were not detected until after 8 hours in the blister. Although IFN-γ was reported by Zimmerli and Gallin (222) to be an early mediator in skin blister fluid, these results have not been repeated in subsequent studies (D. B. Kuhns and J. I. Gallin, unpublished results 2002).

Small amounts of IL-4 accumulated in the skin blisters, but IL-2 and IL-1α were not detected. Thus, the endotoxin and skin blister models of inflammation demonstrate that there are clear differences in the mediators that can be detected systemically and locally.

MURINE MODELS OF INFLAMMATION

Mouse models of human disease are powerful tools for the study of specific inflammatory responses. Because of the power and widespread availability of gene-deletion technology, there now exist many strains of mice in which genes encoding one or more proinflammatory mediators have been eliminated. Although these strains of mice have added substantially to the understanding of the role of various proinflammatory mediators *in vivo*, it is important to keep in mind that no one rodent model is absolutely perfect at all times and for all questions (232–241). Whereas inflammatory responses to chemical and physical trauma may be somewhat stereotyped, the selection of agents for studies of responses to pathogen infection require significant consideration. This is of particular importance in attempts to draw conclusions from the work on human pathogens studied in mice, because the evolutionary divergence of mammalian host defense proteins is quite extensive (242,243) and relatively large, nonphysiological inocula are often necessary to initiate cross-species infections. This can lead to remarkable difficulties in attempts to determine which responses are to infection and which responses are to acute presentation of what is essentially an antigen bolus. A carefully selected natural rodent pathogen studied in a rodent host can provide a model of innate and acute inflammatory responses that is superior to the model for a related human pathogen (244,245).

RESOLUTION OF THE ACUTE INFLAMMATORY RESPONSE

Resolution, or the way in which the acute inflammatory response is gradually diminished, is currently an area of active research. The mediators promoting inflammatory resolution may ultimately be used as therapeutic agents in limiting the injurious aspects of acute inflammation.

Cell Senescence or Apoptosis

A concept that has been appreciated only since the 1990s, apoptosis, or programmed cell death, is an active process in which cells, responding to specific stimuli, undergo a stereotypical pattern of morphological changes (nuclear condensation, deoxyribonucleic acid "laddering") before their eventual demise. Granulocyte apoptosis as a means of inflammatory resolution is an intriguing avenue of current research (246–252). Several cytokines have been reported to modulate neutrophil apoptosis *in vitro,* including TNF-α, eicosanoids, IL-10, and antioxidants (253–257); the role of these mediators in the resolution of acute inflammation awaits future study (see also Chapter 27).

Anti-inflammatory Mediators

In addition to the proinflammatory effects described previously, IL-4 down-regulates IL-6 production and is involved in the down-regulation of neutrophil superoxide production (258) (see also Chapters 23 to 25). TGF-β promotes several anti-inflammatory effects, including suppression of hematopoiesis, reduction in production of proinflammatory cytokines, and inhibition of leukocyte adhesion (259–261). Perhaps most dramatic is the finding that TGF-β1 knockout mice develop severe inflammation in multiple tissues, which suggests TFG-β's primary role as an anti-inflammatory mediator (262,263). TGF-β is produced in many cell types, including platelets, macrophages, and T- and B-lymphocytes. IL-10 is produced by macrophages and CD8+ T lymphocytes and has been shown to inhibit the activation of specific macrophage subsets, including inhibiting the production of proinflammatory cytokines and interfering with the macrophage-mediated antigen presentation. IL-10 is also implicated in host response to both Epstein-Barr virus and human immunodeficiency virus infections (264–267). IL-13 has been observed to induce IL-4–independent IgE synthesis and to induce proliferation and differentiation of human B cells activated by the CD40 ligand (268). Ohta and Sitkovsky (269) demonstrated an important role for G protein–coupled adenosine receptors in the down-regulation of the inflammatory response.

Hypothalamic-Pituitary-Adrenocortical Axis

One of the more intriguing avenues of investigation is the connection among the central nervous system, the adrenal cortex, and the resolution of inflammation (270–276). An appreciation of this phenomenon relates to the observation that glucocorticoids, produced by the adrenal cortex, mediate immunosuppression and thus may down-regulate the acute inflammatory response. Numerous studies have suggested that IL-1, IL-6, and TNF-α promote marked increases in hypothalamic stimulation, leading to increases in serum adrenocorticotropic hormone and corticosterone in experimental animal systems; prostaglandins have also been implicated in this process.

Wound Repair and Angiogenesis

Several morphological stages of wound repair have been described (277–282). Neutrophils and macrophages carry out the initial débridement, including removal of foreign material and cellular debris. Fibroblasts, epithelial cells, and endothelial cells, responding to multiple inflammatory mediators, grow and divide to create new tissue and restore function. Angiogenesis is the process by which new tissue is revascularized. The formation of capillaries has been shown to proceed through several well-defined morphological events, including vasodilation of the parent venule or capillary, removal of the preexisting basement membrane, migration and proliferation of endothelial cells, and formation of a new lumen. These events are promoted by numerous soluble mediators, including epidermal growth factor, keratinocyte growth factor, platelet-derived growth factor, fibroblast growth factors, TGF-α and TGF-β, and cellular mediators (macrophages, platelets, keratinocytes, endothelial cells, and mast cells).

CHRONIC INFLAMMATION

When acute inflammation persists, either through incomplete clearance of the initial inflammatory focus or as a result of multiple acute events occurring in the same location, it becomes chronic inflammation. In contrast to acute inflammation, which is characterized by a primarily neutrophil influx, the histological findings in chronic inflammation include accumulation of macrophages and lymphocytes and the growth of fibroblasts and vascular tissue. These latter two features result in the tissue scarring that is typically seen at sites of prolonged or repeated inflammatory activity.

Among the most interesting sequelae of chronic inflammation is the formation of tissue granulomas (283–290). A granuloma is a collection of inflammatory cells—principally macrophages and lymphocytes, which are eventually surrounded by a fibrotic wall—that forms in tissues as part of the inflammatory response to a persistent irritant. Several unusual cell types are characteristic of granulomas, including epithelioid cells, which are macrophage derivatives, and multinuclear giant cells, which are fusions of epithelioid cells and macrophages (Fig. 6). Although the precise mechanism of granuloma formation and resolution is not yet clear, the actions of specifically sensitized T cells and their soluble mediators (including TNF-α and IFN-γ) participate in the formation and maintenance of granulomas in their active

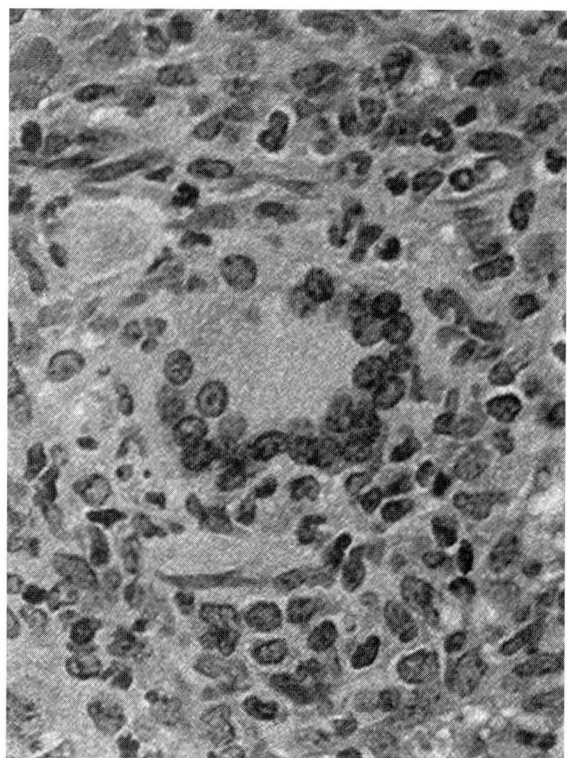

FIG. 6. Light microscopic image of a tissue granuloma from the murine chronic granulomatous disease (p47-phox knockout) model (186). Lymphocytes constitute the central core, which is surrounded by macrophages and fibroblasts.

state. Several conditions predispose to an individual to granuloma formation, most notably the presence of intracellular bacteria (e.g., tuberculosis; see Chapter 40), inorganic antigens (e.g., berylliosis), and abnormal regulation of granulomatous formation (as in chronic granulomatous disease of childhood and Wegener's granulomatosis).

Work on the molecular mechanisms underlying chronic inflammation has focused on the role of NFκB, a transcription factor originally identified as a central regulator of the expression of the murine κ light chains. NFκB activation has been associated with endotoxin, cytokines, viruses, and oxidants, and NFκB has been shown to regulate expression of adhesion molecules, E-selectin, and numerous chemotactic cytokines (291–293).

FUTURE DIRECTIONS: NOVEL ANTI-INFLAMMATORY THERAPIES

The goal of anti-inflammatory therapy is to eliminate the undesirable aspects of the "double-edged sword": tissue destruction beyond what is absolutely necessary for containing and eliminating the injuring agent. At the same time, anti-inflammatory therapy must be sufficiently short-lived or selective, or both, so as to avoid rendering the host immunocompromised. To this end, several generalized anti-inflammatory agents (e.g., glucocorticoids, nonsteroidal anti-inflammatory

agents) have been recognized for their broad scope of effectiveness. Specific agents on the horizon may be more effective at pinpointing specific aspects of the inflammatory response that might be more carefully controlled. Specific agents in use or under study include inhibitors of complement component C1, IL-1 and leukotriene receptors, TNF-α, NFκB activation, and the prostaglandin-synthetic enzyme cyclooxygenase 2; these are described in greater detail in other references (294–310). In the not-too-distant future, gene replacement therapy may emerge as an option, once the genetic bases of the complex inflammatory disorders have been identified and elucidated.

REFERENCES

1. Gallin JI, Snyderman R, eds. *Inflammation: basic principles and clinical correlates,* 3rd ed. Philadelphia: Lippincott Williams & Wilkins, 1999.
2. Hunter J. *A treatise of the blood inflammation, and gunshot wounds,* vol 1. London: J. Nicoll, 1794.
3. Cohnheim J. *Lectures in general pathology* (McKee AD, Trans.), vol. 1. London: New Sydenham Society, 1889.
4. Dale HH, Laidlaw PP. The physiologic action of beta-imidazolylethylamine. *J Physiol* 1911;41:318–344.
5. Babior BM. Phagocytes and oxidative stress. *Am J Med* 2000;109:33–44.
6. Svanborg C, Godaly G, Hedlund M. Cytokine responses during mucosal infections: role in disease pathogenesis and host defence. *Curr Opin Microbiol* 1999;2:99–105.
7. Rosenberg HF, Domachowske JB. Eosinophils, eosinophil ribonucleases and their role in host defense against respiratory virus pathogens. *J Leukoc Biol* 2001;70:691–698.
8. Musher D, Cohen M, Baker C. Immune responses to extracellular bacteria. In: Rich RR, Fleisher TA, Schwartz, BD, et al., eds. *Clinical immunology: principles and practice,* vol. 1. St. Louis: Mosby–Year Book, 1996:479–502.
9. Robbins SL, Cotran RS. Inflammation and repair. In: *Pathologic basis of disease,* 2nd ed. Philadelphia: WB Saunders, 1979:59–63.
10. Barrington R, Zhang M, Fischer M, et al. The role of complement in inflammation and adaptive immunity. *Immunol Rev* 2001;180:5–15.
11. Cooper NR. Biology of the complement system. In: Gallin JI, Snyderman R, eds. *Inflammation: basic principles and clinical correlates,* 3rd ed. Philadelphia: Lippincott Williams & Wilkins, 1999:267–280.
12. Sim RB, Laich A. Serine proteases and the complement system. *Biochem Soc Trans* 2000;28:545–550.
13. Walport MJ. Complement. First of two parts. *N Engl J Med* 2001;344:1058–1071.
14. Walport MJ. Complement. Second of two parts. *N Engl J Med* 2001;344:1140–1144.
15. Hourcade D, Holers VM, Atkinson JP. The regulators of complement activation (RCA) gene cluster. *Adv Immunol* 1989;45:381–416.
16. Fishelson Z, Attali G, Mevorach D. Complement and apoptosis. *Mol Immunol* 2001;38:207–219.
17. Frank MM. Complement deficiencies. *Pediatr Clin North Am* 2000;47:1339–1354.
18. Ratnoff WD. Inherited deficiencies of complement in rheumatic diseases. *Rheum Dis Clin North Am* 1996;22:75–94.
19. Mold C. Role of complement in host defense against bacterial infection. *Microbes Infect* 1999;1:633–638.
20. Sahul A, Lambris JD. Complement inhibitors: a resurgent concept in anti-inflammatory therapeutics. *Immunopharmacology* 2000;48:133–148.
21. Kaplan AP, Joseph K, Shibayama Y, et al. Bradykinin formation: plasma and tissue pathways and cellular interactions. In: Gallin JI, Snyderman R, eds. *Inflammation: basic principles and clinical correlates,* 3rd ed. Philadelphia: Lippincott Williams & Wilkins, 1999:331–348.
22. Granstein RD. Neuropeptides in inflammation and immunity. In: Gallin JI, Snyderman R, eds. *Inflammation: basic principles and clinical*

correlates, 3rd ed. Philadelphia: Lippincott Williams & Wilkins, 1999: 397–404.

23. Campos MM, Calixto JB. Neurokinin mediation of edema and inflammation. *Neuropeptides* 2000;34:314–322.

24. Couture R, Harrisson M, Vianna RM, et al. Kinin receptors in pain and inflammation. *Eur J Pharmacol* 2001;429:161–176.

25. Mahabeer R, Bhoola KD. Kallikrein and kinin receptor genes. *Pharmacol Ther* 2000;88:77–89.

26. Bock MG, Longmore J. Bradykinin antagonists: new opportunities. *Curr Opin Chem Biol* 2000;4:401–406.

27. Marceau F, Bachvarov DR. Kinin receptors. *Clin Rev Allergy Immunol* 1998;16:385–401.

28. Bockmann S, Paegelow I. Kinins and kinin receptors: importance for the activation of leukocytes. *J Leukoc Biol* 2000;68:587–592.

29. Ozturk Y. Kinin receptors and their antagonists as novel therapeutic agents. *Curr Pharm Des* 2001;7:135–161.

30. Carmeliet P, Collen D. Gene targeting and gene transfer studies of the biological role of the plasminogen/plasmin system. *Thromb Haemost* 1995;74:429–436.

31. Altieri DC. Inflammatory cell participation in coagulation. *Semin Cell Biol* 1995;6:269–274.

32. Mosesson MW, Siebenlist KR, Meh DA. The structure and biological features of fibrinogen and fibrin. *Ann N Y Acad Sci* 2001;936:11–30.

33. Esmon CT. Does inflammation contribute to thrombotic events? *Haemostasis* 2000;30:(Suppl 2):34–40.

34. Salgado A, Boveda JL, Monasterio J, et al. Inflammatory mediators and their influence on haemostasis. *Haemostasis* 1994;24:132–138.

35. Vaday GG, Lider O. Extracellular matrix moieties, cytokines and enzymes: dynamic effects on immune cell behavior and inflammation. *J Leukoc Biol* 2000;67:149–159.

36. Serhan CN. Lipoxins and aspirin-triggered 15-epi-lipoxins. In: Gallin JI, Snyderman R, eds. *Inflammation: basic principles and clinical correlates,* 3rd ed. Philadelphia: Lippincott Williams & Wilkins, 1999: 373–385.

37. McMahon B, Mitchell S, Brady HR, et al. Lipoxins: revelations on resolution. *Trends Pharmacol Sci* 2001;22:391–395.

38. Griffiths RJ. Prostaglandins and inflammation. In: Gallin JI, Snyderman R, eds. *Inflammation: basic principles and clinical correlates,* 3rd ed. Philadelphia: Lippincott Williams & Wilkins, 1999:349–360.

39. Serhan CN, Oliw E. Unorthodox routes to prostanoid formation: new twists in cyclooxygenase-initiated pathways. *J Clin Invest* 2001;107: 1481–1489.

40. Tilley SL, Coffman TM, Koller BH. Mixed messages: modulation of inflammation and immune responses by prostaglandins and thromboxanes. *J Clin Invest* 2001;108:15–23.

41. Ushikubi F, Sugimoto Y, Ichikawa A, et al. Roles of prostanoids revealed from studies using mice lacking specific prostanoid receptors. *Jpn J Pharmacol* 2000;83:279–285.

42. Breyer RM, Kennedy CR, Zhang Y, et al. Structure-function analyses of eicosanoid receptors. Physiologic and therapeutic implications. *Ann N Y Acad Sci* 2000;905:221–231.

43. Morteau O. Prostaglandins and inflammation: the cyclooxygenase controversy. *Arch Immunol Ther Exp* 2000;48:473–480.

44. van Ryn J, Trummlitz G, Pairet M. COX-2 selectivity and inflammatory processes. *Curr Med Chem* 2000;7:1145–1161.

45. Everts B, Wahrborg P, Hedner T. COX-2–specific inhibitors—the emergence of a new class of analgesic and anti-inflammatory drugs. *Clin Rheum* 2000;19:331–343.

46. Buttar NS, Wang KK. The "aspirin" of the new millennium: cyclooxygenase-2 inhibitors. *Mayo Clin Proc* 2000;75:1027–1038.

47. Colville-Nash PR, Gilroy DW. Potential adverse effects of cyclooxygenase-2 inhibition: evidence from animal models of inflammation. *BioDrugs* 2001;15:1–9.

48. Willoughby DA, Moore AR, Colville-Nash PR, et al. Resolution of inflammation. *Int J Immunopharmacol* 2000;22:1131–1135.

49. Penrose JF, Austen KF, Lam BK. Leukotrienes: biosynthetic pathways, release, and receptor-mediated actions with relevance to disease states. In: Gallin JI, Snyderman R, eds. *Inflammation: basic principles and clinical correlates,* 3rd ed. Philadelphia: Lippincott Williams & Wilkins, 1999:361–372.

50. Serhan CN, Prescott SM. The scent of a phagocyte: advances on leukotriene B$_4$ receptors. *J Exp Med* 2000;192:F5–F8.

51. Bulger EM, Maier RV. Lipid mediators in the pathophysiology of critical illness. *Crit Care Med* 2000;28:N27–N36.

52. Dahlen SE. Pharmacological characterization of leukotriene receptors. *Am J Respir Crit Care Med* 2000;161:S41–S45.

53. O'Byrne PM. Why does airway inflammation persist? Is it leukotrienes? *Am J Respir Crit Care Med* 2000;161:S186–S187.

54. Bisgaard H. Pathophysiology of the cysteinyl leukotrienes and effects of leukotriene receptor antagonists in asthma. *Allergy* 2001; 56(Suppl 66):7–11.

55. Crowther SD, Rees PJ. Current treatment of asthma—focus on leukotrienes. *Expert Opin Pharmacopther* 2000;1:1021–1040.

56. Leff AR. Regulation of leukotrienes in the management of asthma: biology and clinical therapy. *Annu Rev Med* 2001;52:1–14.

57. Nicosia S, Capra V, Rovati GE. Leukotrienes as mediators of asthma. *Pulm Pharmacol Ther* 2001;14:3–19.

58. Calabrese C, Triggiani M, Marone G, et al. Arachidonic acid metabolism in inflammatory cells of patients with bronchial asthma. *Allergy* 2000;55(Suppl 61):27–30.

59. Prescott SM, Zimmerman GA, Stafforini DM, et al. Platelet-activating factor and related lipid mediators. *Annu Rev Biochem* 2000;69:419–445.

60. Marathe GK, Harrison KA, Murphy RC, et al. Bioactive phospholipid oxidation products. *Free Radic Biol Med* 2000;28:1762–1770.

61. Baker RR. Lipid acetylation reactions and the metabolism of platelet-activating factor. *Neurochem Res* 2000;25:677–683.

62. Ishii S, Shimizu T. Platelet-activating factor (PAF) receptor and genetically engineered PAF receptor mutant mice. *Prog Lipid Res* 2000; 39:41–82.

63. Zimmerman, GA, Prescott SM, McIntyre TM. Platelet-activating factor: a phospholipid mediator of inflammation. In: Gallin JI, Snyderman R, eds. *Inflammation: basic principles and clinical correlates,* 3rd ed. Philadelphia: Lippincott Williams & Wilkins, 1999:387–396.

64. Dent G, Ukena D, Chanez P, et al. Characterization of PAF receptors on human neutrophils using the specific antagonist, WEB 2086. *FEBS Lett* 1989;244:365–368.

65. Hilger RA, Koller M, Konig W. Inhibition of leukotriene formation and IL-8 release by the PAF-receptor antagonist SM-12502. *Inflammation* 1996;20:57–70.

66. Catalan RE, Martinez AM, Aragones MD, et al. PCA-4248, a PAF receptor antagonist, inhibits PAF-induced phosphoinositide turnover. *Eur J Pharmacol* 1995;290:183–188.

67. Canz MJ, Weg VG, Walsh DT, et al. Differential effects of the PAF receptor antagonist UK-74, 505 on neutrophil and eosinophil accumulation in guinea-pig skin. *Br J Pharmacol* 1994;113:513–521.

68. Yokota Y, Inamura N, Asano M, et al. Effect of FR128998, a novel PAF receptor antagonist on endotoxin-induced disseminated intravascular coagulation. *Eur J Pharmacol* 1994;258:239–246.

69. Underwood SL, Lewis SA, Raeburn D. RP 59227, a novel PAF receptor antagonist: effects in guinea pig models of airway hyperreactivity. *Eur J Pharmacol* 1992;210:97–102.

70. Nilsson G, Costa JJ, Metcalfe DD. Mast cells and basophils. In: Gallin JI, Snyderman R, eds. *Inflammation: basic principles and clinical correlates,* 3rd ed. Philadelphia: Lippincott Williams & Wilkins, 1999:97–117.

71. MacDonald SM. Histamine-releasing factors. *Curr Opin Immunol* 1996;8:778–783.

72. Gurish MF, Austen KF. The diverse role of mast cells. *J Exp Med* 2001; 194:F1–F5.

73. Greaves MW, Sabroe RA. Histamine: the quintessential mediator. *J Dermatol* 1996;23:735–740.

74. Gothert M, Garbarg M, Hey JA, et al. New aspects of the role of histamine in cardiovascular function: identification, characterization and potential pathophysiological importance of H3 receptors. *Can J Physiol Pharmacol* 1995;73:558–564.

75. Hart PH. Regulation of the inflammatory response in asthma by mast cell products. *Immunol Cell Biol* 2001;79:149–153.

76. Falcone FH, Haas H, Gibbs BF. The human basophil: a new appreciation of its role in immune responses. *Blood* 2000;96:4028–4038.

77. Nielsen HJ. Histamine-2 receptor antagonists as immunomodulators: new therapeutic views? *Ann Med* 1996;28:107–113.

78. Bochner BS. Systemic activation of basophils and eosinophils: markers and consequences. *J Allergy Clin Immunol* 2000;106:S292–S302.

79. Leurs R, Smit MJ, Timmerman H. Molecular pharmacological aspects of histamine receptors. *Pharmacol Ther* 1995;66:413–463.

80. Weltman JK. Update on histamine as a mediator of inflammation. *Allergy Asthma Proc* 2000;21:334.

81. Arrang JM, Drutel G, Garbarh M, et al. Molecular and functional diversity of histamine receptor subtypes. *Ann N Y Acad Sci* 1995;757:314–323.

82. Holgate ST. The role of mast cells and basophils in inflammation. *Clin Exp Allergy* 2000;30(Suppl 1):28–32.

83. Mossner R, Lesch KP. Role of serotonin in the immune system and neuroimmune interactions. *Brain Behav Immun* 1998;12:249–271.

84. Chancellor-Freeland C, Zhu GF, Kage R, et al. Substance P and stress-induced changes in macrophages. *Ann N Y Acad Sci* 1995;771:472–484.

85. Hanesch U. Neuropeptides in dural fine sensory nerve endings—involvement in neurogenic inflammation? *Prog Brain Res* 1996;113:299–317.

86. Said SI. Vasoactive intestinal peptide and nitric oxide: divergent roles in relation to tissue injury. *Ann N Y Acad* 1996;805:379–387.

87. Weinstock JV. Vasoactive intestinal peptide regulation of granulomatous inflammation in murine schistosomiasis *mansoni. Adv Neuroimmunol* 1996;6:95–105.

88. Reichlin S. Neuroendocrine-immune interactions. *N Engl J Med* 1993;329:1246–1253.

89. Turner AJ, Brown CD, Carson JA, et al. The neprilysin family in health and disease. *Adv Exp Med Biol* 2000;477:229–240.

90. Di Maria GU, Belloriore S, Geppetti P. Regulation of airway neurogenic inflammation by neutral endopeptidase. *Eur Respir J* 1998;12:1454–1462.

91. van der Velden VH, Naber BA, van Hal PT, et al. Peptidases in the asthmatic airways. *Adv Exp Med Biol* 2000;477:413–430.

92. Brunet LR. Nitric oxide in parasitic infections. *Int Immunopharmacol* 2001;1:1457–1467.

93. Bogdan C. Nitric oxide and the immune response. *Nat Immunol* 2001;2:907–916.

94. Laroux FS, Lefer DJ, Kawachi S, et al. Role of nitric oxide in the regulation of acute and chronic inflammation. *Antioxid Redox Signal* 2000;2:391–396.

95. Forsythe P, Gilchrist M, Kulka M, et al. Mast cells and nitric oxide: control of production, mechanisms of response. *Int Immunopharmacol* 2001;1:1525–1541.

96. Hickey MJ. Role of inducible nitric oxide synthase in the regulation of leucocyte recruitment. *Clin Sci* 2001;100:1–12.

97. Weinberg JB. Nitric oxide synthase 2 and cyclooxygenase 2 interactions in inflammation. *Immunol Res* 2001;22:319–341.

98. Granger DL, Hibbs JB Jr. High-output nitric oxide: weapon against infection? *Trends Microbiol* 1996;4:46–47.

99. Gentiloni Silveri N, Mazzone M, Portale G, et al. Nitric oxide. A general review about the different roles of this innocent radical. *Minerva Med* 2001;92:167–171.

100. Schneemann M, Schoedon G, Hofer S, et al. Nitric oxide synthase is not a constituent of the antimicrobial armature of human mononuclear phagocytes. *J Infect Dis* 1993;167:1358–1363.

101. van der Vliet A, Eiserich JP, Cross CE. Nitric oxide: a pro-inflammatory mediator in lung disease? *Respir Res* 2000;1:67–72.

102. Kushner I, Rzewnicki D. Acute phase response. In: Gallin JI, Snyderman R, eds. *Inflammation: basic principles and clinical correlates,* 3rd ed. Philadelphia: Lippincott Williams & Wilkins, 1999:317–330.

103. Ebersole JL, Cappelli D. Acute-phase reactants in infections and inflammatory diseases. *Periodontol* 2000;23:19–49.

104. Koenig W. Inflammation and coronary heart disease: an overview. *Cardiol Rev* 2001;9:31–35.

105. Kuhns DB, Nelson EL, Alvord WG, et al. Fibrinogen induces IL-8 synthesis in human neutrophils stimulated with formyl-methionyl-leucyl phenylalanine or leukotriene B$_4$. *J Immunol* 2001;167:2869–2878.

106. Smiley ST, King JA, Hancock WW. Fibrinogen stimulated macrophage chemokine secretion through Toll-like receptor 4. *J Immunol* 2001;167:2887–2894.

107. Kushner I. Regulation of the acute phase response by cytokines. In: Oppenheim J, Rossio J, Gearing A, eds. *Clinical applications of cytokines: role in pathogenesis, diagnosis and therapy.* New York: Oxford University Press, 1993:27–34.

108. Fantuzzi G, Faggioni R. Leptin in the regulation of immunity, inflammation, and hematopoiesis. *J Leukoc Biol* 2000;68:437–446.

109. Finck BN, Johnson RW. Tumor necrosis factor-alpha regulates secretion of the adipocyte-derived cytokine, leptin. *Microsc Res Tech* 2000;50:209–215.

110. Akerstrom B, Flower DR, Salier J-P. Lipocalins: unity in diversity. *Biochim Biophys Acta* 2000;1482:1–8.

111. Logdberg, L, Wester L. Immunocalins: a lipocalin subfamily that modulates immune inflammatory responses. *Biochim Biophys Acta* 2000;1482:284–297.

112. Smith JA. Neutrophils, host defense, and inflammation: a double-edged sword. *J Leukoc Biol* 1994;56:672–686.

113. Rosenberg HF, Gallin JI. Neutrophils. In: Frank MM, Austen KF, Claman HN, et al., eds. *Samter's immunologic diseases,* 6th ed. Boston: Little, Brown and Company, 2001:216–220.

114. Domachowske JB, Malech HL. Phagocytes. In: Rich, RR, Fleisher TA, Schwartz BD, et al., eds. *Clinical Immunology: principles and practice.* St. Louis: Mosby–Year Book, 1996:392–407.

115. Lekstrom-Himes JA, Gallin JI. Immunodeficiency diseases caused by defects in phagocytes. *N Engl J Med* 2000;343:1703–1714.

116. Malech HL, Nauseef WM. Primary inherited defects in neutrophil function: etiology and treatment. *Semin Hematol* 1997;34:279–290.

117. Bainton DF. Developmental biology of neutrophils and eosinophils. In: Gallin JI, Snyderman R, eds. *Inflammation: basic principles and clinical correlates,* 3rd ed. Philadelphia: Lippincott Williams & Wilkins, 1999:13–34.

118. Sievers EL, Dale DC. Non-malignant neutropenia. *Blood Rev* 1996;10:95–100.

119. Kim SK, Demetri GD. Chemotherapy and neutropenia. *Hematol Oncol Clin North Am* 1996;10:377–395.

120. Bernini JC. Diagnosis and management of chronic neutropenia during childhood. *Pediatr Clin North Am* 1996;43:773–792.

121. Welte K, Dale D. Pathophysiology and treatment of severe chronic neutropenia. *Ann Hematol* 1996;72:158–165.

122. Souid AK. Congenital cyclic neutropenia. *Clin Pediatr* 1995;34:151–155.

123. Scholl PR. Periodic fever syndromes. *Curr Opin Pediatr* 2000;12:563–566.

124. Centola M, Aksentijevich I, Kastner DL. The hereditary periodic fever syndromes: molecular analysis of a new family of inflammatory diseases. *Hum Mol Genet* 1998;7:1581–1588.

125. Cohen MS. Molecular events in the activation of human neutrophils for microbial killing. *Clin Infect Dis* 1994;18(Suppl 2):S170–S179.

126. Yoshie O, Imai T, Nomiyama H. Chemokines in immunity. *Adv Immunol* 2001;78:57–110.

127. Sengelov H. Complement receptors in neutrophils. *Crit Rev Immunol* 1995;15:107–131.

128. McDermott DH, Murphy PM. Chemokines and their receptors in infectious disease. *Springer Semin Immunopathol* 2000;22:393–415.

129. Wells TN, Lusti-Narasimhan M, Chung CW, et al. The molecular basis of selectivity between CC and CXC chemokines: the possibility of chemokine antagonists as anti-inflammatory agents. *Ann N Y Acad Sci* 1996;796:245–256.

130. Baggiolini M. Chemokines in pathology and medicine. *J Intern Med* 2001;250:91–104.

131. Akira S. Toll-like receptors: lessons from knockout mice. *Biochem Soc Trans* 2000;28:551–556.

132. O'Neill L. The Toll–interleukin-1 receptor domain: a molecular switch for inflammation and host defence. *Biochem Soc Trans* 2000;28:557–563.

133. Muzio M, Polentarutti N, Bosisio D, et al. Toll-like receptor family and signaling pathway. *Biochem Soc Trans* 2000;28:563–566.

134. Symon FA, Wardlaw AJ. Selectins and their counter receptors: a bitter sweet attraction. *Thorax* 1996;51:1155–1157.

135. Crockett-Torabi E, Fantone JC. The selectins: insights into selectin-induced intracellular signalling in leukocytes. *Immunol Res* 1995;14:237–251.

136. Kansas GS. Selectins and their ligands: current concepts and controversies. *Blood* 1996;88:3259–3287.

137. Vestweber D. Ligand-specificity of the selectins. *J Cell Biochem* 1996;61:585–591.

138. Tedder TF, Steeber DA, Chen A, et al. The selectins: vascular adhesion molecules. *FASEB J* 1995;9:866–873.

139. Kubes P, Ward PA. Leukocyte recruitment and the acute inflammatory response. *Brain Pathol* 2000;10:127–135.

140. Meager A. Cytokine regulation of cellular adhesion molecule expression in inflammation. *Cytokine Growth Factor Rev* 1999;10:27–39.

141. Gonzalez-Amaro R, Sanchez-Madrid F. Cell adhesion molecules: selectins and integrins. *Crit Rev Immunol* 1999;19:389–429.

142. Pober JS. Immunobiology of human vascular endothelium. *Immunol Res* 1999;19:225–232.

143. Hartwell DW, Wagner DD. New discoveries with mice mutant in endothelial and platelet selectins. *Thromb Haemost* 1999;82:850–857.

144. Madri JA, Graesser D. Cell migration in the immune system: the evolving inter-related roles of adhesion molecules and proteinases. *Dev Immunol* 2000;7:103–116.

145. Edwards SW. Cell signalling by integrins and immunoglobulin receptors in primed neutrophils. *Trends Biochem Sci.* 1995;20:362–367.

146. Kerr JR. Cell adhesion molecules in the pathogenesis of and host defense against microbial infection. *Mol Pathol* 1999;52:220–230.

147. Kishimoto TK, Rothlein R. Integrins, ICAMs and selectins: role and regulation of adhesion molecules in neutrophil recruitment to inflammatory sites. *Adv Pharmacol* 1994;25:117–169.

148. Roebuck KA, Finnegan A. Regulation of intercellular adhesion molecule-1 (CD54) gene expression. *J Leukoc Biol* 1999;66:876–888.

149. Harris ES, McIntyre TM, Prescott SM, et al. The leukocyte integrins. *J Biol Chem* 2000;275:23409–23412.

150. Chapman HA, Wei Y, Simon DI, et al. Role of urokinase receptor and caveolin in regulation of integrin signaling. *Thromb Haemost* 1999;82:291–297.

151. Sendo F, Araki Y. Regulation of leukocyte adherence and migration by glycosylphosphatidyl-inositol–anchored proteins. *J Leukoc Biol* 1999;66:369–374.

152. Bauer TR Jr, Hickstein DD. Gene therapy for leukocyte adhesion deficiency. *Curr Opin Mol Ther* 2000;2:383–388.

153. Lakshman R, Finn A. Neutrophil disorders and their management. *J Clin Pathol* 2001;54:7–19.

154. Papadaki HA, Palmblad J, Eliopoulos GD. Non-immune chronic idiopathic neutropenia of adult: an overview. *Eur J Haematol* 2001;67:35–44.

155. Anderson DC, Springer TA. Leukocyte adhesion deficiency and inherited defect in the Mac-1, LFA-1, and p150,95 glycoproteins. *Annu Rev Med* 1987;38:175–194.

156. Etzioni A, Doerschuk CM, Harlan JM. Similarities and dissimilarities between humans and mice looking at adhesion molecule defects. *Adv Exp Med Biol* 2000;479:147–161.

157. Kishimoto TK, Hollander N, Roberts TM, et al. Heterogeneous mutations in the beta subunit common to the LFA-1, Mac-1 and p150,95 glycoproteins cause leukocyte adhesion deficiency. *Cell* 1987;50:193–202.

158. Etzioni A, Frydman M, Pollack S, et al. Brief report: recurrent severe infections caused by a novel leukocyte adhesion deficiency. *N Engl J Med* 1992;327:1789–1792.

159. Becker DJ, Lowe JB. Leukocyte adhesion deficiency type II. *Biochim Biophys Acta* 1999;1455:193–204.

160. Etzioni A, Tonetti M. Leukocyte adhesion deficiency II—from A to almost Z. *Immunol Rev* 2000;178:138–147.

161. Stossel TP, Condeelis J, Cooley L, et al. Filamins as integrators of cell mechanics and signaling. *Nat Rev Mol Cell Biol* 2001;2:138–145.

162. Southwick FS, Stossel TP. Contractile proteins in leukocyte function. *Semin Hematol* 1984;30:305–310.

163. Jones GE. Cellular signaling in macrophage migration and chemotaxis. *J Leukoc Biol* 2000;68:593–602.

164. Stossel TP. Mechanical responses of white blood cells. In: Gallin JI, Snyderman R, eds. *Inflammation: basic principles and clinical correlates*, 3rd ed. Philadelphia: Lippincott Williams & Wilkins, 1999:661–680.

165. Greenberg S. Biology of phagocytosis. In: Gallin JI, Snyderman R, eds. *Inflammation: basic principles and clinical correlates*, 3rd ed. Philadelphia: Lippincott Williams & Wilkins, 1999:681–702.

166. Allen LA, Aderem A. Mechanisms of phagocytosis. *Curr Opin Immunol* 1996;8:36–40.

167. Chimini G, Chavrier P. Function of the Rho family proteins in actin dynamics during phagocytosis and engulfment. *Nat Cell Biol* 2000;2:E191–E196.

168. Goldman MJ, Anderson GM, Stolzenberg ED, et al. Human beta-defensin-1 is a salt-sensitive antibiotic in lung that is inactivated in cystic fibrosis. *Cell* 1997;88:553–560.

169. Lonnerdal B, Iyer S. Lactoferrin: molecular structure and biological function. *Annu Rev Nutr* 1995;15:93–110.

170. Nagle DL, Karim MA, Woolf EA, et al. Identification and mutation analysis of the complete gene for Chédiak-Higashi syndrome. *Nat Genet* 1996;14:307–311.

171. Barbosa MD, Nguyen QA, Tchernev VT, et al. Identification of the homologous beige and Chédiak-Higashi syndrome genes. *Nature* 1996;382:262–265.

172. Barrat FJ, Auloge L, Pastural E, et al. Genetic and physical mapping of the Chédiak-Higashi syndrome on chromosome 1q42–43. *Am J Hum Genet* 1996;59:625–632.

173. Gallin JI. Neutrophil specific granule deficiency. *Annu Rev Med* 1985;36:263–274.

174. Lomax KJ, Gallin JI, Rotrosen D, et al. Selective defect in myeloid cell lactoferrin gene expression in neutrophil specific granule deficiency. *J Clin Invest* 1989;83:514–519.

175. Lekstrom-Himes JA, Dorman SE, Kopar P, et al. Neutrophil-specific granule deficiency results from a novel mutation with loss of function of the transcription factor CCAAT/enhancer binding protein epsilon. *J Exp Med* 1999;189:1847–1852.

176. Parry MF, Root RK, Metcalf JA, et al. Myeloperoxidase deficiency: prevalence and clinical significance. *Ann Intern Med* 1981;95:293–301.

177. Nauseef WM, Brigham S, Cogley M. Hereditary myeloperoxidase deficiency due to a missense mutation of arginine 569 to tryptophan. *J Biol Chem* 1994;269:1212–1216.

178. Nauseef WM, Cogley M, McCormack S. Effect of R569W missense mutation on the biosynthesis of myeloperoxidase. *J Biol Chem* 1996;271:9546–9549.

179. Petrides PE. Molecular genetics of peroxidase deficiency. *J Mol Med* 1998;76:688–698.

180. Lanza F. Clinical manifestation of myeloperoxidase deficiency. *J Mol Med* 1998;76:676–681.

181. DeLeo FR, Quinn MT. Assembly of the phagocyte NADPH oxidase: molecular interaction of the oxidase proteins. *J Leukoc Biol* 1996;60:677–691.

182. Leusen JH, Verhoeven AJ, Roos D. Interactions between the components of the human NADPH oxidase: intrigues in the Phox family. *J Lab Clin Med* 1996;128:461–476.

183. Leto TL, Adams AG, de Mendez I. Assembly of the phagocyte NADPH oxidase: binding of Src homology 3 domains to proline-rich targets. *Proc Natl Acad Sci U S A* 1994;91:10650–10654.

184. Henderson LM, Chappel JB. NADPH oxidase of neutrophils. *Biochim Biophys Acta* 1996;1273:87–107.

185. Segal AW. The NADPH oxidase and chronic granulomatous disease. *Mol Med Today* 1996;2:129–135.

186. Jackson SH, Gallin JI, Holland SM. The p47 phox mouse knockout model of chronic granulomatous disease. *J Exp Med* 1995;182:751–758.

187. Bokoch GM. Regulation of the human neutrophil NADPH oxidase by the Rac GTP-binding proteins. *Curr Opin Cell Biol* 1994;6:212–218.

188. Mardiney MM, Jackson SH, Spratt SK, et al. Enhanced host defense after gene transfer in the murine p47-phox–deficient model of chronic granulomatous disease. *Blood* 1997;89:2268–2275.

189. Segal BH, Leto TL, Gallin JI, et al. Genetic, biochemical, and clinical features of chronic granulomatous disease. *Medicine* 2000;79:170–200.

190. Winkelstein JA, Marino MC, Johnston RB Jr, et al. Chronic granulomatous disease. Report on a national registry of 368 patients. *Medicine* 2000;79:155–169.

191. Horwitz ME, Barrett AJ, Brown MR, et al. Treatment of chronic granulomatous disease with nonmyeloablative conditioning and a T-cell–depleted hematopoietic allograft. *N Engl J Med* 2001;344:881–888.

192. Malech HL. Progress in gene therapy for chronic granulomatous disease. *J Infect Dis* 1999;179(Suppl 2):S318–S325.

193. Lloyd AR, Oppenheim JJ. Poly's lament: the neglected role of the polymorphonuclear neutrophil in the afferent limb of the immune response. *Immunol Today* 1992;13:169–172.

194. Granelli-Piperno A, Vassalli JD, Reich E. Secretion of plasminogen activator by human polymorphonuclear leukocytes. *J Exp Med* 1977;149:284–289.

195. Shirafuji N, Matsuda S, Ogura H, et al. Granulocyte colony-stimulating factor stimulates human mature neutrophilic granulocytes to produce interferon-alpha. *Blood* 1990;75:17–19.

196. Tiku K, Tiku ML, Skosey JL. Interleukin 1 production by human polymorphonuclear neutrophils. *J Immunol* 1986;136:3677–3685.

197. Hughes V, Humphreys JM, Edwards SW. Protein synthesis is activated in primed neutrophils: a possible role in inflammation. *Biosci Rep* 1987;7:881–889.

198. Kuhns DB, Gallin JI. Increased cell-associated IL-8 in human exudative and A23187-treated peripheral blood neutrophils. *J Immunol* 1995;154:6556–6662.

199. Gordon S. Development and distribution of mononuclear phagocytes: relevance to inflammation. In: Gallin JI, Snyderman R, eds. *Inflammation: basic principles and clinical correlates*, 3rd ed. Philadelphia: Lippincott Williams & Wilkins, 1999:35–48.

200. Laskin DL, Pendino KJ. Macrophages and inflammatory mediators in tissue injury. *Annu Rev Pharmacol Toxicol* 1995;35:655–677.

201. Rosenberg HF. Eosinophils. In: Gallin JI, Snyderman R, eds. *Inflammation: basic principles and clinical correlates*, 3rd ed. Philadelphia: Lippincott Williams & Wilkins, 1999:61–76.

202. Gleich GJ. Mechanisms of eosinophil-associated inflammation. *J Allergy Clin Immunol* 2000;105:651–663.

203. Rothenberg ME, Mishra A, Brandt EB, et al. Gastrointestinal eosinophils in health and disease. *Adv Immunol* 2001;78:291–328.

204. Makino S, Fukuda T. *Eosinophils: biological and clinical aspects.* Boca Raton, FL: CRC Press, 1993.

205. Wardlaw AJ. Eosinophils in the 1990s: new perspectives on their role in health and disease. *Postgrad Med J* 1994;70:536–552.

206. Wardlaw AJ. Molecular basis for selective eosinophil trafficking in asthma: a multistep paradigm. *J Allergy Clin Immunol* 1999;104:917–926.

207. Foster PS, Mould AW, Yang M, et al. Elemental signals regulating eosinophil accumulation in the lung. *Immunol Rev* 2001;179:173–181.

208. Lee NA, Gelfand EW, Lee JJ. Pulmonary T cells and eosinophils: co-conspirators of independent triggers of allergic respiratory pathology? *J Allergy Clin Immunol* 2001;107:945–957.

209. Rosenberg HF, Domachowske JB. Eosinophils, ribonucleases and host defense: solving the puzzle. *Immunol Res* 1999;20:261–274.

210. Marcus AJ. Platelets: their role in hemostasis, thrombosis and inflammation. In: Gallin JI, Snyderman R, eds. *Inflammation: basic principles and clinical correlates*, 3rd ed. Philadelphia: Lippincott Williams & Wilkins, 1999:77–96.

211. Tonnel AB, Gosset P, Molet S, et al. Interactions between endothelial cells and effector cells in allergic inflammation. *Ann N Y Acad Sci* 1996;796:9–20.

212. Kubes P, Granger DN. Leukocyte-endothelial cell interactions evoked by mast cells. *Cardiovasc Res* 1996;32:699–708.

213. Malik AB, Lo SK. Vascular endothelial adhesion molecules and tissue inflammation. *Pharmacol Rev* 1996;48:213–229.

214. Luscinskas FW, Gimbrone MA Jr. Endothelial-dependent mechanisms in chronic inflammatory leukocyte recruitment. *Annu Rev Med* 1996;47:413–421.

215. Garcia JG, Pavalko FM, Patterson CE. Vascular endothelial cell activation and permeability responses to thrombin. *Blood Coagul Fibrinolysis* 1995;6:609–626.

216. Bevilacqua MP, Nelson RM, Mannori G, et al. Endothelial-leukocyte adhesion molecules in human disease. *Annu Rev Med* 1994;45:361–378.

217. Granger DN, Kubes P. The microcirculation and inflammation. Modulation of leukocyte-endothelial cell adhesion. *J Leukoc Biol* 1994;55:662–675.

218. Jarrett E, Bazin H. Elevation of total serum IgE in rats following helminth parasite infection. *Nature* 1974;251:541–543.

219. Jarrett E. Stimuli for the production and control of IgE in rats. *Immunol Rev* 1978;41:52–76.

220. Hussain R, Ottesen EA. IgE responses in human filariasis. 3. Specificities of IgE and IgG antibodies compared by immunoblot analysis. *J Immunol* 1985;135:1415–1420.

221. Brown CC, Malech HL, Gallin JI. Intravenous endotoxin recruits distinct subset of human neutrophils, defined by monoclonal antibody 31D8, from bone marrow to the peripheral circulation. *Cell Immunol* 1989;123:294–306.

222. Zimmerli W, Gallin JI. Monocytes accumulate on Rebuck skin window coverslips but not in skin chamber fluid. *J Immunol Methods* 1987;96:11–17.

223. Kuhns DB, DeCarlo E, Hawk DM, et al. Dynamics of the cellular and humoral components of the inflammatory response elicited in skin blisters in human. *J Clin Invest* 1992;89:1734–1740.

224. Martich GD, Danner RL, Ceska M, et al. Detection of interleukin-8 and tumor necrosis factor in normal humans after intravenous endotoxin: the effects of anti-inflammatory agents. *J Exp Med* 1991;173:1021–1024.

225. Kishimoto TK, Anderson DC. The role of integrins in inflammation. In: Gallin JI, Goldstein IM, Snyderman R, eds. *Inflammation*, 2nd ed. New York: Raven Press, 1992:353–406.

226. Kuhns DB, Long Priel DA, Gallin JI. Endotoxin and IL-1 hyporesponsiveness in a patient with recurrent bacterial infections. *J Immunol* 1997;158:3959–3964.

227. Haziot A, Tsuberi BZ, Goyert SM. Neutrophil CD14: biochemical properties and role in the secretion of tumor necrosis factor alpha in response to lipopolysaccharide. *J Immunol* 1993;150:5556–5565.

228. Frey EA, Miller DS, Jahr TG, et al. Soluble CD14 participates in the response of cells to lipopolysaccharide. *J Exp Med* 1992;176;1665–1671.

229. Doffinger R, Smahi A, Bessia C, et al. X-linked anhidrotic ectodermal dysplasia with immunodeficiency is caused by impaired NF-kappaB signaling. *Nat Genet* 2001;27:277–285.

230. Zonana J, Elder ME, Schneider LC, et al. A novel X-linked disorder of immune deficiency and hypohidrotic ectodermal dysplasia is allelic to incontinentia pigmenti and due to mutations in IKK-gamma (NEMO). *Am J Hum Genet* 2000;67:1555–1562.

231. Schmidt-Supprian M, Block W, Courtois D, et al. NEMO/IKK gamma–deficient mice model incontinentia pigmenti. *Mol Cell* 2000;5:981–992.

232. Behm CA, Ovington KS. The role of eosinophils in parasitic helminth infections: insights from genetically modified mice. *Parasitol Today* 2000;16:202–209.

233. Pastor CM, Frossard JL. Are genetically modified mice useful for the understanding of acute pancreatitis? *FASEB J* 2001;15:893–897.

234. Patterson JB, Manchester M, Oldstone MB. Disease model: dissecting the pathogenesis of the measles virus. *Trends Mol Med* 2001;7:85–88.

235. Reardon CA, Getz GS. Mouse models of atherosclerosis. *Curr Opin Lipidol* 2001;12:167–173.

236. Joe B, Griffiths MM, Remmers EF, et al. Animal models of rheumatoid arthritis and related inflammation. *Curr Rheumatol Rep* 1999;1:139–148.

237. Stotland PK, Radzioch D, Stevenson MM. Mouse models of chronic lung infection with *Pseudomonas aeruginosa*: models for the study of cystic fibrosis. *Pediatr Pulmonol* 2000;30:413–424.

238. Holland CV, Cox DM. *Toxocara* in the mouse: a model for parasite-altered host behaviour? *J Helminthol* 2001;75:125–135.

239. Barry CE. *Mycobacterium smegmatis*: an absurd model for tuberculosis? *Trends Microbiol* 2001;9:473–474.

240. Clark S, Duggan J, Chakraborty J. Ts1 and LP-BM5: a comparison of two murine retrovirus models for HIV. *Viral Immunol* 2001;14:95–109.

241. Denzler KL, Borchers MT, Crosby JR, et al. Extensive eosinophil degranulation and peroxidase-mediated oxidation of airway proteins do not occur in a mouse ovalbumin-challenge model of pulmonary inflammation. *J Immunol* 2001;167:1672–1682.

242. Murphy PM. Molecular mimicry and the generation of host defense protein diversity. *Cell* 1993;72:823–826.

243. Rosenberg HF, Dyer KD, Tiffany HL, et al. Rapid evolution of a unique family of primate ribonuclease genes. *Nat Genet* 1995;10:219–223.

244. Domachowske JB, Bonville CA, Gao JL, et al. The chemokine MIP-1α and its receptor CCR1 control pulmonary inflammation and anti-viral host defense in paramyxovirus infection. *J Immunol* 2000;165:2677–2682.

245. Mahalingam S, Karupiah G, Takeda K, et al. Enhanced resistance in STAT6-deficient mice to infection with ectromelia virus. *Proc Natl Acad Sci U S A* 2001;98:6812–6817.

246. Anderson GP. Resolution of chronic inflammation by therapeutic induction of apoptosis. *Trends Pharmacol Sci* 1996;17:438–442.

247. Savill J, Haslett C. Granulocyte clearance by apoptosis in the resolution of inflammation. *Semin Cell Biol* 1995;6:385–393.

248. Bellamy CO, Malcomson RD, Harrison DJ, et al. Cell death in health and disease: the biology and regulation of apoptosis. *Semin Cancer Biol* 1995;6:3–16.

249. Savill J. Apoptosis in disease. *Eur J Clin Invest* 1994;24:715–723.

250. Haslett C, Savill JS, Whyte MK, et al. Granulocyte apoptosis and the control of inflammation. *Philos Trans R Soc Lond B Biol Sci* 1994; 345:327–333.

251. Simon HU, Yousefi S, Blaser K. Tyrosine phosphorylation regulated activation and inhibition of apoptosis in human eosinophils and neutrophils. *Int Arch Allergy Immunol* 1995;107:338–339.

252. Liles WC, Klebanoff SJ. Regulation of apoptosis in neutrophils—Fas track to death? *J Immunol* 1995;155:3289–3291.

253. Cox G. IL-10 enhances resolution of pulmonary inflammation *in vivo* by promoting apoptosis of neutrophils. *Am J Physiol* 1996;27:L566–L571.

254. Gelrud AK, Carper HT, Mandell GL. Interaction of tumor necrosis factor-alpha and granulocyte colony-stimulating factor on neutrophil apoptosis, receptor expression, and bactericidal function. *Proc Assoc Am Physicians* 1996;108:455–456.

255. Gon S, Gataga T, Sendo F. Involvement of two types of TNF receptor in TNF-alpha induced neutrophil apoptosis. *Microbiol Immunol* 1996;40:463–465.

256. Hebert MJ, Takano T, Holthofer H, et al. Sequential morphologic events during apoptosis of human neutrophils. Modulation by lipoxygenase-derived eicosanoids. *J Immunol* 1996;157:3105–3115.

257. Oishi K, Machida K. Inhibition of neutrophil apoptosis by antioxidants in culture medium. *Scand J Immunol* 1997;45:21–27.

258. Abramson SL, Gallin JI. Interleukin-4 inhibits superoxide production by human mononuclear phagocytes. *J Immunol* 1990;144:625–630.

259. Lawrence DA. Transforming growth factor-beta: a general review. *Eur Cytokine Netw* 1996;7:363–374.

260. Kolodziejczyk SM, Hall BK. Signal transduction and TGF-beta superfamily receptors. *Biochem Cell Biol* 1996;74:299–314.

261. Kingsley DM. The TGF-beta superfamily: new members, new receptors, and new genetic tests of function in different organisms. *Genes Dev* 1994;8:133–146.

262. Letterio JJ, Geiser AG, Kulkarni AB, et al. Autoimmunity associated with TGF-beta1–deficiency in mice is dependent on MHC class II antigen expression. *J Clin Invest* 1996;98:2109–2119.

263. Dang H, Geiser AG, Letterio JJ, et al. SLE-like autoantibodies and Sjögren's syndrome-like lymphoproliferation in TGF-beta knockout mice. *J Immunol* 1995;155:3205–3212.

264. Moore KW, O'Garra A, deWaal Malefyt R, et al. Interleukin-10. *Annu Rev Immunol* 1993;11:165–190.

265. Klein SC, Kube D, Abts H, et al. Promotion of IL-8, IL-10, TNF-alpha and TNF-beta production by EBV infection. *Leuk Res* 1996;20:633–636.

266. Schuitemaker H. IL-4 and IL-10 as potent inhibitors of HIV-1 replication in macrophages *in vitro*. A role for cytokines in the *in vivo* virus host range? *Res Immunol* 1994;145:588–592.

267. Mosmann TR. Properties and functions of interleukin 10. *Adv Immunol* 1994;56:1–26.

268. Mossman T. Cytokines and immune regulation. In: Rich RR, Fleisher TA, Schwartz BD, et al., eds. *Clinical Immunology: principles and practice.* St. Louis: Mosby–Year Book, 1996:217–230.

269. Ohta A, Sitkovsky M. Role of G-protein–coupled adenosine receptors in downregulation of inflammation and protection from tissue damage. *Nature* 2001;414:916–920.

270. Sternberg EM. Neuroendocrine factors in susceptibility to inflammatory disease: focus on the hypothalamic-pituitary-adrenal axis. *Horm Res* 1995;43:159–161.

271. Buckingham JC, Loxley HD, Christian HC, et al. Activation of the HPA axis by immune insults: roles and interactions of cytokines, eicosanoids and glucocorticoids. *Pharmacol Biochem Behav* 1996;54:285–298.

272. Derjik R, Sternberg EM. Corticosteroid action and neuroendocrine-immune interactions. *Ann N Y Acad Sci* 1994;746:33–41.

273. Gaillard RC. Interaction between the hypothalamo-pituitary-adrenal axis and the immunological system. *Ann Endocrinol* 2001;62:155–163.

274. Jessop DS, Harbuz MS, Lightman SL. CRH in chronic inflammatory stress. *Peptides* 2001;22:803–807.

275. Chikanza IC, Petrous P, Chrousos G. Perturbations of arginine vasopressin secretion during inflammatory stress. Pathophysiologic implications. *Ann N Y Acad Sci* 2000;917:825–834.

276. Jafarian-Tehrani M, Sternberg EM. Neuroendocrine and other factors in the regulation of inflammation. Animal models. *Ann N Y Acad Sci* 2000;917:819–824.

277. Martin P. Wound healing—aiming for perfect skin regeneration. *Science* 1997;276:75–81.

278. Chettibi S, Ferguson MWJ. Wound repair: an overview. In: Gallin JI, Snyderman R, eds. *Inflammation: basic principles and clinical correlates,* 3rd ed. Philadelphia: Lippincott Williams & Wilkins, 1999:865–882.

279. Arenberg DA, Streiter RM. Angiogenesis. In: Gallin JI, Snyderman R, eds. *Inflammation: basic principles and clinical correlates,* 3rd ed. Philadelphia: Lippincott Williams & Wilkins, 1999:851–864.

280. Crowther M, Brown NJ, Bishop ET, et al. Microenvironmental influence on macrophage regulation of angiogenesis in wounds and malignant tumors. *J Leukoc Biol* 2001;70:478–490.

281. Gillitzer R, Goebeler M. Chemokines in cutaneous wound healing. *J Leukoc Biol* 2001;69:513–521.

282. Lingen MW. Role of leukocytes and endothelial cells in the development of angiogenesis in inflammation and wound healing. *Arch Pathol Lab Med* 2001;125:67–71.

283. Wynn TA, Cheever AW. Cytokine regulation of granuloma formation in schistosomiasis. *Curr Opin Immunol* 1995;7:505–511.

284. Kaye P. Granulomatous diseases. *Int J Exp Pathol* 2000;81:289–290.

285. Mornex JF, Leroux C, Greenland T, et al. From granuloma to fibrosis in interstitial lung diseases: molecular and cellular interactions. *Eur Respir J* 1994;7:779–785.

286. Kunkel SL, Lukacs NW, Strieter RM, et al. Th1 and Th2 responses regulate experimental lung granuloma development. *Sarcoidosis Vasc Diffuse Lung Dis* 1996;13:120–128.

287. Hansch HC, Smith DA, Mielke ME, et al. Mechanisms of granuloma formation in murine *Mycobacterium avium* infection: the contribution of CD4$^+$ T cells. *Int Immunol* 1996;8:1299–1310.

288. Chensue SW, Warmington KS, Ruth JH, et al. Cytokine function during mycobacterial and schistosomal antigen–induced pulmonary granuloma formation. Local and regional participation of IFN-gamma, IL-10, and TNF. *J Immunol* 1995;154:5969–5976.

289. Di Perri G, Bonora S, Allegranzi B, et al. Granulomatous inflammation and transmission of infectious disease. *Immunol Today* 1999;20:337–338.

290. Saunders BM, Cooper AM. Restraining mycobacteria: role of granulomas in mycobacterial infections. *Immunol Cell Biol* 2000;78:334–341.

291. Barnes PJ, Karin M. Nuclear factor kappa-B—a pivotal transcription factor in chronic inflammatory diseases. *N Engl J Med* 1997;336:1066–1071.

292. Magnani M, Crinelli R, Bianchi M, et al. The ubiquitin-dependent proteolytic system and other potential targets for the modulation of nuclear factor κB (NF-κB). *Curr Drug Targets* 2000;1:387–399.

293. Silverman N, Maniatis T. NF-kappaB signaling pathways in mammalian and insect innate immunity. *Genes Dev* 2001;15:2321–2342.

294. Aradhya S, Nelson DL. NF-kappaB signaling and human disease. *Curr Opin Genet Dev* 2001;11:300–306.

295. Gelfand EW. Antibody-directed therapy: past, present, and future. *J Allergy Clin Immunol* 2001;108:111S–116S.

296. Kirschfink M, Mollnes TE. C1-inhibitor: an anti-inflammatory reagent with therapeutic potential. *Expert Opin Pharmacother* 2001;2:1073–1083.

297. Bjermer L. History and future perspectives of treating asthma as a systemic and small airways disease. *Respir Med* 2001;95:703–719.

298. Grover JK, Vats V, Gopalakrishna R, et al. Thalidomide: a re-look. *Natl Med J India* 2000;13:132–141.

299. Dinarello CA. The role of interleukin-1–receptor antagonist in blocking inflammation mediated by interleukin-1. *N Engl J Med* 2000;343:732–734.

300. Ulevitch RJ. New therapeutic targets revealed through investigations of innate immunity. *Crit Care Med* 2001;29:S8–S12.

301. Fassbender K, Masters C, Beyreuther K. Alzheimer's disease: molecular concepts and therapeutic targets. *Naturwissenschaften* 2001;88:261–267.

302. Surh YJ, Chun KS, Cha HH, et al. Molecular mechanisms underlying chemopreventive activities of anti-inflammatory phytochemicals: down-regulation of COX-2 and iNOS through suppression of NF-kappa B activation. *Mutat Res* 2001;480–481:243–268.

303. Barnes PJ. Cytokine-directed therapies for asthma. *J Allergy Clin Immunol* 2001;108:S72–S76.
304. FitzGerald GA, Patrono C. The coxibs, selective inhibitors of cyclo-oxygenase-2. *N Engl J Med* 2001;345:433–442.
305. Wardle N. New vistas in anti-inflammatory therapy. *Nephron* 2001; 88:289–295.
306. Haraoui B, Strand V, Keystone E. Biologic agents in the treatment of rheumatoid arthritis. *Curr Pharm Biotechnol* 2000;1:217–233.
307. Gardenerova M, Banque R, Gardner CR. The use of TNF family ligands and receptors and agents which modify their interaction as therapeutic agents. *Curr Drug Targets* 2000;1:327–364.
308. Aldred A. Etanercept in rheumatoid arthritis. *Expert Opin Pharmacother* 2001;2:1137–1148.
309. Panaccione R. Infliximab for the treatment of Crohn's disease: review and indications for clinical use in Canada. *Can J Gastroenterol* 2001: 15:371–375.
310. Sandborn WJ. Transcending conventional therapies: the role of biologic and other novel therapies. *Inflamm Bowel Dis* 2001;7(Suppl 1): S9–S16.

CHAPTER 38

The Immune Response to Parasites

Alan Sher, Thomas A. Wynn, and David L. Sacks

Parasites and the Immune System
    The Nature and Global Health Importance of Parasitic Pathogens · Some Hallmarks of the Immune Response to Parasites
Innate Recognition and Host Defense
    Innate Barriers to Infection · Role of Antigen-Presenting Cells in Innate Recognition and Initiation of Adaptive Immunity · Mechanisms Underlying Th1/Th2 Response Selection
Effector Mechanisms of Host Resistance
    Intracellular Parasites · Extracellular Parasites
Mechanisms of Immune Evasion and Latency
    Evasion of Immune Recognition · Evasion by Immune Suppression · Immune Suppression and Latency
Immunopathologic Mechanisms and Their Regulation
    The Quest for Homeostasis in the Anti-Infective Immune Response · Pathogenesis of Chronic Th1 Responses · Pathogenesis of Chronic Th2 Responses
Parasite Vaccine Strategies
    B-Cell Vaccines · T-Cell Vaccines
Conclusions
Acknowledgments
References

PARASITES AND THE IMMUNE SYSTEM

The Nature and Global Health Importance of Parasitic Pathogens

Although used loosely to describe all infectious agents, for historical reasons the term "parasite" has been formally reserved as a designation for eukaryotic single-cell and metazoan pathogens, the most highly evolved and biologically sophisticated invaders encountered by the vertebrate immune system. Despite their phylogenetic diversity, parasites share certain biologic characteristics. They frequently (although not always) display complex life cycles consisting of morphologically and antigenically distinct stages and produce long-lived chronic infections to ensure transmission among their hosts. The induction of morbidity and mortality is rarely part of their design. However, in the tropics where transmission persists, the low frequency of disease translates into a major global health and economic problem because of the sheer numbers exposed as well as the confounding issues of malnutrition, overpopulation, and co-infection. As illustrated by the recent outbreaks in North America of disease caused by protozoa, the *Giardia, Cryptosporidia, Cyclospora,* and *Toxoplasma* parasites also represent a continuing threat to populations in wealthier countries. The current AIDS epidemic has also increased the impact of parasitic disease in developed regions since immunocompromised hosts become highly susceptible to some normally tolerated parasites such as *Cryptosporidia, Toxoplasma gondii,* and *Leishmania.* Finally, parasitic disease remains an important problem in livestock, causing annual economic losses in the billions and, in the case of trypanosomiasis, limiting the agricultural development of huge areas of potential grazing lands on the African continent.

The immune system plays a central role in determining the outcome of parasitic infection by establishing a critical balance meant to ensure both host and pathogen survival. As with other infectious agents, disease emerges when the scales tip toward either a deficient or excessive immune response. Manipulation of that response by means of vaccination or immunotherapy remains a key approach for global intervention in parasitic disease. A list of the most important parasitic infections of humans, along with estimates of their prevalence, annual mortality, health impact (measured in disability-adjusted life years) and current control methods, is presented in Table 1. The data testify to the continued enormity of the problem reflected in the numbers of people annually infected and dying of diseases such as malaria and trypanosomiasis, as well as the high level of morbidity in

TABLE 1. *Global impact of parasitic disease and current control measures[a]*

	Estimated prevalence (millions)	Disease burden DALYs (thousands)[b]	Annual deaths (thousands)	Control methods currently utilized
Malaria	300–500	44,998	1086	Vector control, chemotherapy
Lymphatic filariasis	120	4918	0	Vector control, chemotherapy
African trypanosomiasis	0.5	2048	66	Vector control
Leishmaniasis	12	1983	57	Vector control, chemotherapy
Schistosomiasis	200	1932	280[c]	Chemotherapy, hygiene
Onchocerciasis	18	1085	0	Vector control, chemotherapy
Chagas' disease	18	676	21	Vector control

[a]Data compiled from World Health Organization Tropical Disease Burden Data Sources *(http://www.who.int/tdr/kh/res_link.html#diseases)* and Morel (238). [b]Disability-adjusted life years, a parameter that measures the difference between a population's health and a normative goal of living in full health (239). [c]Schistosomiasis mortality figures are based on recent estimates (240).

those surviving. A striking situation reflected in the data is the complete absence of effective vaccines for protecting human populations. In the case of malaria, the need for a global immunization strategy has become particularly acute as drug resistance spreads worldwide. Clearly, the development of vaccines to prevent parasitic diseases remains one of the major unachieved goals of modern immunology and one of its greatest and most difficult challenges.

Although the study of the immune response to parasites was once considered a backwater, this is no longer the case. Years of concerted effort employing modern immunologic and molecular techniques have now been devoted to the quest for parasite vaccines. Of particular note are the recently initiated government- and private foundation–sponsored programs for malaria vaccine development. The difficulties appear to lie then not with the lack of workers and tools needed to tackle this problem but with the extraordinary complexity of parasites as immunologic targets and their remarkable adaptability to immunologic pressure. The field of immunoparasitology is focused on developing a basic understanding of this important host–pathogen interface for the ultimate purpose of intervention. At the same time, the work in this area—particularly in recent years—has provided immunology with a series of major insights concerning effector and regulatory responses as they occur *in vivo*. Indeed, because of their years of close encounter with and adaptation to the vertebrate immune system, parasites can be thought of as the "ultimate immunologists" and there is much to be learned from them about the fundamental nature of immune responses.

Some Hallmarks of the Immune Response to Parasites

The interaction of parasites with the immune system has several distinguishing features that are of special interest to fundamental immunologists. Most parasitic pathogens are able to survive the initial host response and produce long-lasting chronic infections designed to promote transmission. In the case of many protozoa (e.g., *Toxoplasma, Leishmania*),

chronicity is characterized by a state of *latency* in which replication of the parasite is minimal and infection cryptic. The development of chronicity depends not only on the ability of the parasite to escape protective immune responses (immune evasion) but on the generation of finely tuned mechanisms of immunoregulation that serve both to prevent parasite elimination and suppress host immunopathology. As discussed in detail later in this chapter, the study of these immunomodulatory pathways in both human and experimental parasitic infections has yielded important insights concerning the mechanisms by which regulatory T cells and cytokines control immune effector functions *in vivo*.

An additional prominent feature of the immune response to parasites is Th1/Th2 polarization. For reasons that are not entirely clear, parasitic infections often induce CD4+ T-cell responses that are highly polarized in terms of their Th1/Th2 lymphokine profiles. This phenomenon is particularly striking in the case of helminths, which in contrast to nearly all other pathogens, routinely trigger strong Th2 responses leading to high IgE levels, eosinophilia, and mastocytosis. At the opposite pole, many intracellular protozoa (in common with their bacterial counterparts) induce CD4+ T-cell responses with Th1-dominated lymphokine secretion patterns. This striking difference presents a beautiful example of immunologic class selection. Interestingly, in murine *Leishmania major* infection, CD4+ cells polarize to either Th1 or Th2 depending on the strain of mouse infected, and the association of these responses with healing or exacerbation (1,2) provided the first demonstration of a functional role for this dichotomy. The *L. major*–infected mouse has subsequently become the most widely utilized experimental model for studying Th1/Th2 differentiation *in vivo*, although the originally observed genetic-based dichotomy is now known to be restricted to only certain laboratory strains of this *Leishmania* species (3).

Parasite models have also been used to reveal new effector functions such as the ability of eosinophils to kill pathogens and, as discussed below, are now being used extensively to study microbial innate recognition and immune response initiation. This ability to uncover and investigate basic immune mechanisms while studying the host response to a group of phylogenetically unique pathogens of global importance is perhaps the most engaging and rewarding aspect of research in immunoparasitology.

INNATE RECOGNITION AND HOST DEFENSE

It is becoming increasingly clear that events occurring during the early contact of parasites with the immune system can play a critical role in determining the character of the ensuing host–parasite relationship. Thus, innate immune defenses must be overcome for infections to establish, while the nature of the initial contact of parasites with antigen-presenting cells (APC) can dictate both the magnitude and class of adaptive immune responses that emerge.

Innate Barriers to Infection

Humoral Mechanisms

Innate resistance against parasitic infection is mediated in part by preexisting, soluble factors that recognize and destroy invading developmental stages or target them for killing by effector cells. The alternative pathway of complement activation provides a first line of defense against extracellular parasites. Invading forms of many of these pathogens lack the complement regulatory factors that normally promote the degradation of C3b on the surface of host cells. The resulting activation of the complement cascade leads to formation of the potentially lytic membrane attack complex (MAC) as well as opsonic recognition by C3 receptors on phagocytes. In addition, other products of complement activation are chemotactic and attract immune cells to the site of infection. There is also a lectin-mediated pathway in which recognition of mannose residues on parasite surfaces by a mannan-binding protein triggers the complement cascade.

Because the complement system represents such an important first line of defense in resistance to pathogens, successful parasites have developed a variety of developmentally regulated strategies to subvert complement-mediated attack (4). For example, while the epimastigote stage of *Trypanosoma cruzi,* found in the insect vector, is susceptible to the alternative pathway of complement, infective metacyclic and bloodstream trypomastigotes are resistant. In this case, evasion of complement appears to be due to expression by the trypomastigote of a 160-kDa glycoprotein (gp160), which is a homolog of the host complement regulatory protein, decay-accelerating factor (DAF) (5). Like DAF, gp160 can bind to C3b and C4b and inhibit the uptake of subsequent members of the complement cascade, thus preventing convertase formation and lysis of the parasite. Importantly, whereas complement-sensitive epimastigotes fail to express gp160, epimastigotes transfected with gp160 are resistant to complement-mediated lysis (6). *Schistosoma*

mansoni also appears to utilize DAF-mediated regulation to avoid complement-mediated attack. In the case of this helminth, however, the DAF molecules are not synthesized by the parasite but instead are acquired from the host and incorporated into the worm tegument (7).

Another interesting strategy is deployed by *Leishmania* sp, which evade complement-mediated lysis while using complement activation as a mechanism for targeting host cells. As insect-stage procyclic promastigotes develop into infective metacyclic forms, their membrane is altered to prevent the insertion of the lytic C5b-C9 complex (8). This correlates with their expression of a modified surface lipophosphoglycan (LPG) approximately twice as long as the form on procyclic promastigotes, and which may act as a barrier for the insertion of the MAC into the surface membrane of the parasite (9). Another developmental change that occurs during generation of metacyclics is the increased expression of the surface proteinase gp63 (10), which can cleave C3b to the inactive iC3b form, thus preventing deposition of the lytic C5b-C9 complex (11). However, iC3b will opsonize the parasites for phagocytosis through the complement receptors Mac-1 and CR1, thereby targeting the parasite to the macrophage, its host cell of choice (12). Tissue-invasive strains of *Entamoeba histolytica* also activate complement but are resistant to MAC deposited on the membrane surface. The *E. histolytica* Gal/GalNAc lectin, which mediates adherence of trophozoites to host cells, is involved in avoidance of lysis by MAC via its ability to bind to C8 and C9 terminal components (13). Interestingly, the lectin shares sequence similarities with CD59, a membrane inhibitor of MAC in human blood cells.

In addition to complement, other soluble mediators are being uncovered that provide a barrier to parasitic infection. Best studied are the primate-specific Trypanosome lysis factors (TLF) that contribute to the innate resistance of humans to *Trypanosome brucei* infection. Biochemical analysis of the activity present in human serum revealed that high-density lipoproteins are part of the substance that mediates cytolysis of the parasite and initial studies demonstrated that this complex, Trypanosome lysis factor 1 (TLF1), is composed of several common apoplipoproteins, as well as a haptoglobin-related protein (Hpr) (14,15). A second cytolytic complex, TLF2, has also been identified that shares many of the components of TLF1 but contains a unique IgM component, and a lower lipid content (14). To mediate cytotoxicity, TLF has to undergo receptor-mediated uptake and enter an intracellular acidic compartment; the peroxidase activity associated with TLF suggests that lysis of trypanosomes may be due to oxidative damage (15). Whereas TLF is capable of killing *T. brucei*, the species that infect humans, *T. b. gambiense* and *T. b. rhodesiense* are both refractory to TLF-mediated cytolysis. This resistance has been correlated with the expression of a serum resistance associated (SRA) gene that is homologous to the variant surface glycoprotein (16). Importantly, transfection of SRA from *T. b. rhodesiense* into *T. brucei* confers resistance to lysis by human serum, arguing that its expression may have been a critical step in the adaptation of the former parasite for infection of primates (17).

Cellular Mechanisms

Phagocytosis by macrophages represents an innate first line of defense against protozoan pathogens. Once taken up by these cells, frequently as a consequence of complement-mediated opsonization, parasites must confront a potential respiratory burst as well as a hostile lysosomal environment. Therefore, evasion of phagocytic defenses is a critical adaptation to the mammalian host. The ability of *Leishmania* sp to gain access to the macrophage via CR1 and CR3, which fail to trigger the respiratory burst, is likely an important step allowing them to successfully invade and persist within these cells. Similarly, the intracellular survival of *T. cruzi* is dependent on the ability of the parasite to escape from the phagolysosome, a process facilitated by this protozoan's expression of a homolog of C9 that can disrupt the phagosome membrane allowing egress of the parasite into the cytoplasm (18). The capacity of *T. gondii* to actively invade cells enables it to form a parasitophorous vacuole that fails to undergo acidification. If instead the parasite is forced to enter the cell by a phagocytic pathway, it is exposed to the normal phagolysosomal system and is killed (19).

Unlike protozoa, helminths are too big to be engulfed by phagocytes and can only be killed by these cells when the latter have been activated by products of the adaptive immune response (20). Recent studies suggest instead that eosinophils, which frequently accumulate in tissues soon after worm invasion, may play a role in innate defense against this type of parasitic pathogen. Thus, L3 larvae of *Strongyloides stercoralis* are killed within 72 hours when implanted in millipore chambers into wild-type (WT) mice. Eosinophils are prominent amongst the cells infiltrating the chambers. Larval attrition is greatly reduced when worms are transferred instead into IL-5–deficient mice, which lack mature eosinophils (21). Discharge of the eosinophil granule's major basic protein and eosinophil cationic protein is the likely explanation of the larvacidal activity observed. This nonspecific eosinophilic response may represent a barrier that limits invasion of tissue-dwelling helminths.

In contrast to intracellular killing by phagocytes and extracellular killing by eosinophils, most innate cellular defenses do not eliminate parasites directly but instead trigger other effector cells to do so. Perhaps the best-studied example of this form of innate immunity is the NK cell pathway of IFN-γ production. Although NK cells appear unable to directly recognize and kill parasites, their numbers and nonspecific lytic activity are clearly increased as a consequence of a variety of parasitic infections. The discovery that these cells can be triggered to produce high levels of IFN-γ and TNF-α suggested that they could provide a T-lymphocyte independent pathway for cytokine-mediated defense, and as such, serve to prevent parasites from overwhelming the host prior to the development of adaptive responses. In support of this concept, *Leishmania* promastigotes as well as subcellular components of *T. gondii* were shown to activate human peripheral blood NK cells to produce IFN-γ. Later studies in both bacterial and protozoan systems established that NK cell IFN-γ is triggered by monokines produced by adherent cells in response to microbial products. The critical monokine that stimulates this NK cell function was shown to be IL-12 (22,23), although optimal IFN-γ production also depends on TNF and IL-1 (24). The response is also positively regulated by co-stimulatory interaction of parasite-induced B7 on APC with CD28 on NK cells (25). Both IL-10 and TGF-β have been shown to serve as negative regulators of NK cell IFN-γ production by means of their suppression of monokine and B7 expression by APC or, in the case of TGF-β by directly affecting NK cell function (26,27). Such suppression may be important in protecting the host against the tissue damaging defects of excessive NK-derived IFN-γ and TNF.

Parasite-driven NK-cell IFN-γ production has been described in a variety of different protozoan infections, including *Leishmania*, *Toxoplasma*, *T. cruzi*, *E. histolytica*, *Cryptosporidium parvum* and *Plasmodium chabaudi* (28). Although its protective function is assumed, it is equally clear that in many situations adaptive T-cell immunity is sufficient to control infection even in the absence of this early NK response (e.g., Bregenholt et al. [29]).

Two other cell populations that may function to provide a rapid cytokine response to invading parasites are $\gamma\delta$ lymphocytes and NK T cells. These "unconventional T-lymphocytes" express T-cell receptor chains of limited diversity, which may be designed for innate recognition of microbial structures or self-components revealed by infection of host cells. While the function of NK T cells in innate resistance to parasites is currently under debate (see below), there is considerable evidence supporting a protective role for $\gamma\delta$ T cells. Although the latter cells represent a small percentage of lymphocytes in the periphery, they are abundant in epithelial and mucosal tissues, the sites of initial host invasion by many parasites. Moreover, their numbers increase in peripheral blood in response to a number of different protozoan and helminth infections (e.g., Kasper et al. [30] and Scalise et al. [31]). $\gamma\delta$ T cells can respond to heat-shock proteins (HSP) and since invasion and intracellular replication by different parasites results in increased expression of HSP, this may provide a mechanism that allows $\gamma\delta$ T cells to nonspecifically restrict infection either by direct host cell lysis or more likely by the production of IFN-γ and other effector lymphokines. Studies in murine models of *Toxoplasma* and malaria infection, several of which involve direct analysis of host resistance in $\alpha\beta$ and $\gamma\delta$ T-cell–deficient mice, have provided experimental support for the above concept (e.g., Hisaeda et al. [32] and Tsuji et al. [33]). Nevertheless, rather than being essential for host resistance, it is likely that $\gamma\delta$ T-lymphocytes (in common with NK cells) provide an adjunct to conventional $\alpha\beta$ CD4 and CD8 cells, restricting parasite growth during the vulnerable period when the adaptive responses mediated by these effectors are emerging.

Role of Antigen-Presenting Cells in Innate Recognition and Initiation of Adaptive Immunity

In addition to providing a natural barrier that limits infection, there is growing evidence that the innate immune system plays a critical role in the initial recognition of parasites and the triggering of adaptive immunity. Antigen-presenting cells are the major sentinels in this process and their ability to recognize and discriminate among pathogens is thought to be determined by pattern recognition receptors (PRR) that recognize pathogen-associated molecular patterns (PAMPS) shared by different groups of microbes (34). An exciting new research area is the delineation of these PRR/PAMP receptor–ligand interactions in the parasite–host interaction.

In the case of protozoa, an important set of PAMPS are the glycosylphosphatidylinositols (GPI) lipid anchors present on many parasite surface proteins (Fig. 1). Thus, GPIs from *T. brucei, Leishmania mexicana,* and *Plasmodium falciparum* can stimulate macrophages to up-regulate iNOS and produce TNF and IL-1. Similarly, the GPI anchor fraction of mucin-like molecules from *T. cruzi* trypomastigotes stimulates macrophage production of IL-12 and TNF (35,36). Interestingly, the GPI from insect-stage epimastigotes are unable to stimulate cytokine production. This inactivity appears to correlate with the absence of additional galactose residues and unsaturated fatty acids present in the GPI anchors isolated from trypomastigotes (36) (Fig. 1). Recent data suggest that Toll-like receptor-2 (TLR-2) is the PPR that recognizes these GPI structures on *T. cruzi* glycoconjugates. Thus, macrophages from TLR-2–deficient mice failed to produce IL-12, TNF-α, and nitric oxide (NO) in response to GPI stimulation (36). A further role for protozoan GPI in the stimulation of innate immunity is suggested by the evidence that these structures, when presented by CD1d molecules, may be recognized by NK 1.1$^+$ CD4$^+$ T cells and that this pathway results in MHC-independent stimulation of anti-GPI IgG antibodies (37). This hypothesis, however, was challenged in a later study in which CD1d-deficient mice were found to mount normal IgG antibody titers to the GPI-linked circumsporozoite (CS) Ag, while MHC class II knockout (KO) mice were nonresponsive (38).

At present, it is not clear to what extent TLR serve as PRR for parasites and whether other as yet unidentified receptors exist that are specialized for recognition of eukaryotic pathogens. Such a unique pattern recognition system is most likely to be directed at helminths because these parasites trigger Th2 responses that are not normally associated with TLR signaling (39). Many worm proteins are heavily glycosylated and these carbohydrate side chains could provide unique molecular patterns for initiation of the innate response. For example, schistosome egg antigens are potent Th2 response inducers and this property has been associated with the presence of the oligosaccharides, lacto-N-fucopentaose III

(LNFPIII) and lacto-N-neotetraose (LNnT). These structures were shown to induce IL-10 production by both B1-lymphocytes and macrophages, and to bias *in vitro* lymphocyte responses in a Th2 direction (40). Nevertheless, it is not known whether the receptors that recognize such helminth moieties are representative of a PRR family analogous to TLR, or whether they play a similar sentinel function in the induction of host responses to these extracellular pathogens.

Parasite-derived molecules, in addition to triggering APC function, also play a major role in its positive and negative regulation. *T. gondii* induces a potent IL-12 response leading to IFN-γ production by NK cells and T-lymphocytes, and control of infection. Studies in a model system involving injected tachyzoite extract (STAg) indicated that CD8α^+ DC can serve as a major initial source of this cytokine in spleen and that these cells undergo a dramatic redistribution into T-cell areas following such stimulation (41). Further investigation revealed that the CC chemokine receptor CCR5 plays an important role not only in DC migration but also in the regulation of IL-12 triggering. Thus, DC purified from spleens of CCR5-deficient mice produced only a small fraction of the IL-12 stimulated by STAg in DC from control animals (42). Recent studies indicate that this CCR5-dependent up-regulation of IL-12 synthesis is stimulated by a parasite-derived protein that functions as a CCR5 ligand mimic (42a).

In addition to up-regulating APC function, parasite products can also dampen their activity either as a mechanism of immune evasion or for the purpose of protecting the host against an uncontrolled immune response. Although IL-12 is essential for the development of protective immunity to leishmaniasis, early studies indicated that promastigotes of *L. major* do not activate macrophages to produce IL-12 (43), and that infected macrophages have an impaired ability to produce this cytokine in response to even strong stimuli such as IFN-γ and LPS (44). Instead, it is now recognized that in contrast to macrophages, dendritic cells have the capacity to make IL-12 following uptake of *Leishmania* amastigotes and promastigotes (45–47), and thus may provide the initial source of IL-12 during *Leishmania* infection. In contrast to the activating effects of many parasite GPI, the LPG and GIPLS of *Leishmania* have been shown to inhibit signaling pathways in macrophages, resulting in impaired production of proinflammatory cytokines, including IL-12 (e.g., Piedrafita et al. [48]). A related structure expressed by *E. histolytica,* termed lipophosphopeptidoglycan, was also found to be anti-inflammatory and, in fact, down-regulated TLR-2 gene expression in human monocytes (49). Thus, it appears that variation in structure of parasite GPI imparts different properties of signal transduction upon this class of glycolipid (Fig. 1).

In addition to their suppressive effects on macrophages, parasite products can also negatively regulate dendritic cell function. For example, CCR5-dependent IL-12 production by splenic DC is rapidly suppressed following initial *in vivo* stimulation with *T. gondii* (STAg) and cannot be restimulated

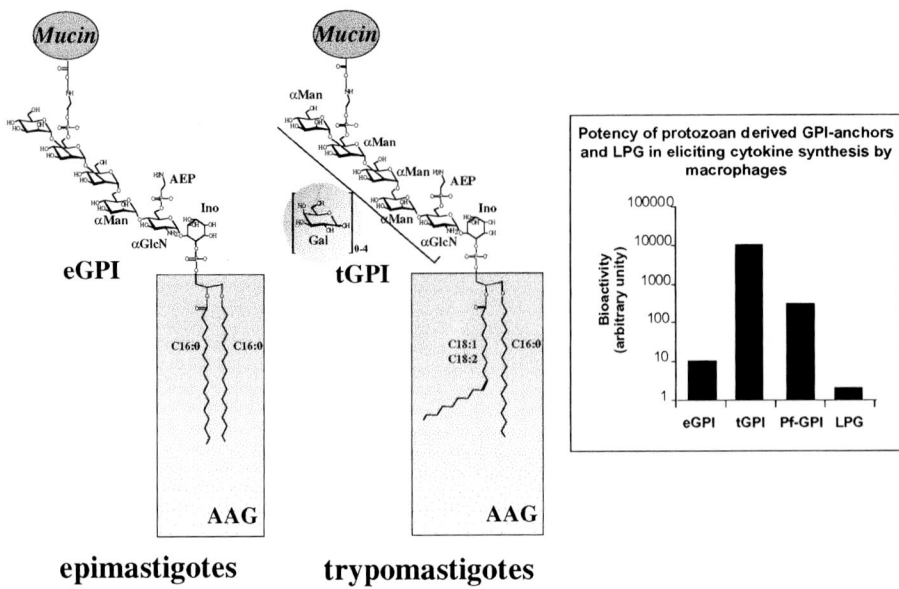

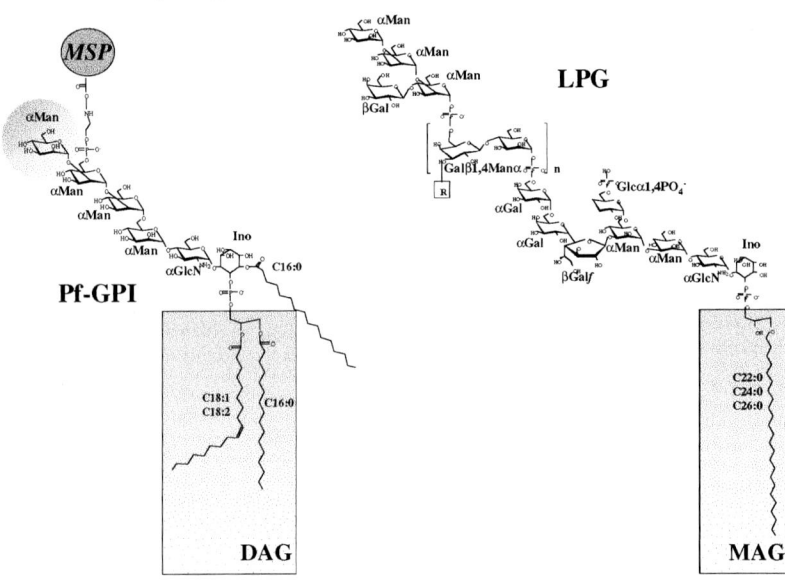

FIG. 1. Primary structures of protozoan-derived glycosylphosphatidylinositol (GPI) anchors and their cytokine-inducing activity in murine macrophages. GPI anchors from *T. cruzi* mammalian cell-derived trypomastigote mucin (tGPI) and invertebrate vector-derived epimastigote mucins (eGPI), *Plasmodium falciparum* merozoite surface protein (MSP) (Pf-GPI), and *Leishmania major*–derived lipophosphoglycan (LPG) are shown. The hydrophobic moiety of each GPI is depicted inside a *shaded rectangle*. The *insert* depicts potency of the different protozoan-derived GPI anchors in activating macrophages. The bioactivity is indicated by arbitrary units based on studies published by various groups. In the case of tGPI, eGPI, and Pf-GPI, the macrophage stimulatory activity is attributed to the GPI anchor and dependent on the phospho-inositol glycerolipid (*shaded box*) as well as extra carbohydrates (*shaded circle*) linked to the main glycan core from GPI anchor. In contrast, the repeating disaccharide-phosphate unit (within *brackets*) in the LPG is thought to be responsible for macrophage deactivation exhibited by some Leishmania species. Note the developmental change in the *T. cruzi* mucin as the parasite develops from the insect epimastigote to the vertebrate trypomastigote stage along with the accompanying acquisition of cytokine-inducing function. Key: *m*-Ins, myo-inositol; GlcN, glucosamine; 0Man, mannose; Gal*f* galacto-furanose; AEP, aminoethylphosphonate; EtNP, ethanolaminephosphate; AAG, alkylacylglycerol; MAG, mono- or *lyso*-alkylglycerol. Courtesy of R.T. Gazzinelli and colleagues (Federal University of Minas Gerais, Belo Horizonte, Brazil).

for approximately 1 week thereafter. Recent studies (e.g., Aliberti et al. [50]) indicate that this inhibition is due the induction by parasite products of lipoxin A4, an arachadonic acid metabolite that down-regulates both CCR5 expression on DC as well as IL-12 production by the same cells.

Mechanisms Underlying Th1/Th2 Response Selection

In addition to initiating the adaptive immune response, the interaction of invading pathogens with the innate immune system strongly influences the class of adaptive response induced. Because parasites often stimulate CD4$^+$ T-cell responses that are highly polarized in either the Th1 or Th2 direction, parasitic infection models have become important tools for studying the cellular basis of Th1/Th2 subset selection. Indeed, as noted above, the first direct demonstrations of the relevance of the Th1/Th2 paradigm to the regulation of disease outcome *in vivo* were made in studies on the *L. major*/ mouse model (1,2). Infection with *L. major* causes resolving cutaneous leishmaniasis in humans and in the majority of WT mouse strains. In BALB/c mice, however, the infection does not resolve and disseminates to visceral sites.

Landmark experiments performed during the late 1980s showed that resistance to *L. major* is associated with the development of a marked Th1-like response, with IFN-γ playing the role of the major effector cytokine owing to its ability to activate macrophages to kill the intracellular *Leishmania* parasites. The ability of resistant mouse strains to generate this protective IFN-γ response was in turn shown to require IL-12. In direct contrast, BALB/c mice develop a strong Th2 response following infection due in large part to the absence of a macrophage-activating type 1 cytokine (IFN-γ) in combination with the production of the macrophage-deactivating type 2 cytokines (e.g., IL-4) (51). In BALB/c mice, *L. major* is able to stimulate a burst of IL-4 production in the draining LN as early as 16 hours following subcutaneous infection (52). The critical role played by early IL-4 production in determining exacerbation of infection is supported by the observation that anti-IL-4–treated BALB/c mice exhibit a healing phenotype (51). There is evidence that other Th2 cytokines— for example, IL-13 and IL-10—contribute to the polarized response and that, depending on the parasite substrain, inhibition of IL-4 alone is not a sufficient condition to reverse susceptibility (3).

The mechanisms controlling the polarized Th2 response in BALB/c mice have been of enormous interest. A key finding was that much of the early IL-4 derives from an oligoclonal population of CD4 cells with the Vβ4 Vα8 TCR that recognize the *Leishmania* antigen LACK (52). The critical importance of this population of cells is supported by the observation that infected Vβ4-deficient BALB/c mice mount stronger Th1 responses and control their lesions. Moreover, BALB/c mice tolerant to LACK as a result of the transgenic expression of the protein were also found to control *L. major* infections and to mount diminished Th2 responses (53). Nonetheless, because LACK-reactive cells are present at

similar frequencies in resistant and susceptible mouse strains, the underlying mechanism that controls CD4$^+$ subset selection in this model remains unresolved. It has been suggested that LACK-specific Vβ4 Vα8 CD4$^+$ T cells may represent a unique lineage in BALB/c mice that are precommitted to releasing large amounts of IL-4 (54). There is also evidence, however, that the function of these cells is plastic with respect to IL-4 or IFN-γ (55) and that the aberrant Th2 response in BALB/c mice reflects a default pathway, secondary to an intrinsic defect in their ability to mount or sustain an effective Th1 response.

BALB/c mice do not appear to have a generalized defect in the capacity of their DC to prime Th1 cells in response to *L. major*, because *L. major*–infected fetal skin-derived DC from BALB/c mice produced IL-12 *in vitro* and primed for a protective Th1 response following syngeneic transfer to naïve mice (56). Of more likely relevance is the observation that under conditions of neutral priming, IL-12Rβ2 expression is not maintained during Th development in BALB/c mice (57). It has also been reported that in contrast to resistant B10.D2 mice, BALB/c mice select for low-affinity as opposed to high-affinity LACK-reactive cells (58), with the latter having a greater tendency to develop a Th1 phenotype. This might provide an explanation for the observation that BALB/c mice develop stable resistance to small parasite inocula (59), if one assumes that low parasite numbers and thus low determinant densities selectively activate cells that bear high-affinity clonotypic receptors. Why the inoculation of identical numbers of parasites in resistant versus susceptible mice should activate low- versus high-affinity T cells is not known, but may be related to the finding that the dissemination of parasite antigens from the site of inoculation to the draining lymph nodes and spleen occurs early in BALB/c mice, whereas early parasite containment is observed in resistant mice (60). These differences in parasite dissemination also raise the possibility that distinct populations of DC, with the capacity to induce preferential priming for either Th1 or Th2 cells, become activated in resistant versus susceptible mice. Such populations might not represent distinct APC lineages, but may instead reflect modulation of APC function by specific tissue environments. That the site of antigen delivery can influence T-cell priming has been clearly demonstrated in the *L. major* model; parasites delivered intravenously, intranasally, or even to different skin environments, can elicit Th2 responses and nonhealing infections in normally resistant mice (61,62).

The concept that the early production of the CD4 T-cell– polarizing cytokines IL-12 and IL-4 is only one of several factors influencing Th1/Th2 subset selection, is also supported by observations in other host–parasite models. Mice deficient in IL-4, IL-4R or the Th2 promoting transcription factor STAT-6, when infected with the helminth parasites *Nippostrongylus brasiliensis* or *S. mansoni*, develop diminished but still physiologically significant Th2 responses. In the case of the IL-4 deficient mice, such residual Th2 cytokine secretion was shown to mediate, through the action of IL-13, protective or immunopathologic effects against *N. brasiliensis* or *S. mansoni,* respectively (63–65). Although these findings argue that IL-4R/STAT-6 signaling is not essential for priming of IL-4+CD4$^+$ T-lymphocytes, it is clear that IL-4 plays a critical role in the maturation and stabilization of Th2 cells once their phenotype has been decided. For example, STAT-6–deficient animals exposed to a helminth stimulus display not only diminished numbers of Th2 cells but also an expanded population of Th1 cells (66) that appears to be IL-12 independent. This observation supports data from other studies arguing that an important function of the IL-4R/STAT-6 pathway may be to silence IFN-γ gene expression, a mechanism that would indirectly lead to elevated Th2 frequencies (63).

Because autocrine IL-4 produced by CD4 T-lymphocytes has been shown to be sufficient to drive Th2 differentiation (67), it is perhaps not surprising that the presence of this cytokine during initial T-cell priming is not essential for subset polarization. In contrast, IL-12 is produced mainly by antigen-presenting cells and not T-lymphocytes and thus would be predicted to play a primarily initiative function in Th1 differentiation. Recent findings in protozoan infection models indicate that this concept is oversimplified. In both *T. gondii* and *Leishmania* infections continuous IL-12 signaling has now been shown to be required for the maintenance of host resistance even in the chronic state (e.g., Park et al. [68] and Yap et al. [69]). Also contrary to accepted dogma is the evidence that IL-12 signaling is not obligatory for initial Th1 subset selection. Thus, in studies in which parasite-induced CD4$^+$ T-lymphocyte responses were analyzed at a single cell level, WT and IL-12–KO mice exposed to *T. gondii* developed comparable frequencies of splenic IFN-γ^+CD4$^+$ T cells, despite different levels of IFN-γ detected in the culture supernatants, suggesting that IL-12 may be more important for Th1 effector competence rather than for Th1 cell priming per se (63,70). Together, the above findings argue that IL-12 and IL-4, while strongly influencing Th polarization and stabilizing Th1 and Th2 effector populations, are not the sole determinants of Th subset selection.

Because of their critical role in T-cell priming, DC are thought to be an important source of the signals that determine CD4 T-cell effector choice. The role of DC in Th polarization is best understood for Th1 responses. Both *T. gondii* and *Leishmania* have been shown to activate DC resulting in upregulated expression of IL-12 and co-stimulatory molecules. In the case of *T. gondii,* these parasite-conditioned DC have been shown to promote Th1 differentiation *in vitro*. One of the co-stimulatory molecules induced on such DC is CD40. Interestingly, when this up-regulated CD40 on DC interacts with CD40L on T cells, both IL-12 p40 and, more dramatically, p35 synthesis, are enhanced providing a positive feedback loop for Th1 induction (71). As discussed above, however, it is clear that in addition to IL-12 there are other signals provided by protozoan-conditioned DC that influence Th1 effector choice. These yet to be defined factors may be other co-stimulatory molecules or cytokines (e.g., IL-18).

In the opposing direction, DC conditioned by exposure to helminth products (*Brugia* or *Schistosoma*) have been shown to polarize naïve T cells toward a Th2 phenotype (72,73). In this case, however, activation of DC as judged by the upregulation of prototypic MHC and co-stimulatory markers appears to be minimal—nor is enhanced IL-12 or IL-4 production detected. The latter observations are consistent with a model of Th effector choice in which Th2 differentiation represents the default pathway, followed by CD4$^+$ T cells primed by DC in the absence of IL-12 stimulation. However, such defaulting to Th2 is not observed when IL-12–deficient mice are infected with either *T. gondii* or *Leishmania* (see above). Therefore, it is more likely that helminth-conditioned DC provide a set of positive signals that result in Th2 priming. The elucidation of these Th2 promoting signals induced by helminths in DC is an exciting area for future research that should have broad implications for the fields of both T-cell immunobiology and allergy.

EFFECTOR MECHANISMS OF HOST RESISTANCE

Once parasites have successfully evaded innate host defenses and had their antigens processed by APC, adaptive cellular and humoral immune responses are invariably induced, usually against a wide array of antigenic constituents of each pathogen. The problem is that because of the nature of the host–parasite adaptation, few and sometimes none of these responses are capable of killing parasites or restricting their growth. The design of successful immune intervention strategies depends on the identification of relevant target antigens but even more importantly on an understanding of the type of immune response and protective mechanism that must be induced. These effector mechanisms can be broadly classified based on the type of parasite (intracellular or extracellular) against which they are directed.

Intracellular Parasites

Because of their primary habitat within host cells, intracellular parasites are thought to be susceptible mainly to cell-mediated immune effector mechanisms. Nevertheless, during their initial host invasion as well as their transit to new cells they are potential targets for antibody-mediated attack. Similarly, while immunity to intracellular parasites (nearly all protozoa) has been traditionally thought to involve Th1 (or Tc1) effector function, this distinction is not absolute and there is also evidence for the participation of Th2- (or Tc2-) directed protective mechanisms.

Cell-mediated immunity against intracellular protozoa often involves a mixture or succession of CD4$^+$ and CD8$^+$ T-cell responses. The extent of CD8 involvement appears to be partially related to the degree of class II versus class I MHC expression on the host cells infected. CD8$^+$ T cells are especially critical effector cells for the control of *T. cruzi* or *T. gondii* infections, since these parasites can infect many nucleated cell types that express only MHC class I molecules.

Nevertheless, even in *Leishmania* infection where parasites reside almost exclusively in macrophages, CD8$^+$ T cells can be highly protective, particularly in acquired resistance to challenge exposure (74). One mechanism by which CD8$^+$ T cells could control intracellular parasitic infection is through the lysis of host cells. This might be of particular benefit to the host if the target cells from which viable parasites are released are themselves defective in intracellular killing (e.g., fibroblasts, DC), and if the parasites are subsequently made available for uptake by cells that are more responsive to activation signals (e.g., macrophages). In every protozoan infection analyzed, however, including *T. gondii* (75), malaria (76), and *T. cruzi* (77), mice deficient in the lytic molecules perforin or granzyme B show no or minimal loss of host resistance. The above observations suggest that as already noted for NK cells (see above), the protective functions of CD4 and CD8 T cells against intracellular parasites are mediated primarily through lymphokine production rather than target-cell lysis.

IFN-γ is the key lymphokine involved in control of intracellular protozoan parasites, as demonstrated by the extreme susceptibility of IFN-γ–deficient mouse strains to infections involving *Leishmania* (78), *T. cruzi* (79), *T. gondii* (80), and even *C. parvum* (81), which dwells in epithelial cells inside the gut. Its mechanism of action is perhaps clearest in the case of *Leishmania,* which replicate primarily, if not exclusively, in macrophages—a cell type readily activated by this cytokine. The major function of IFN-γ in restricting parasite growth appears to be the induction of inducible nitrogen oxide synthase (NOS2) and the subsequent generation of toxic reactive nitrogen intermediates (RNI) within infected macrophages. Thus, disruption of the NOS2 gene in a normally resistant strain leads to a susceptible phenotype, and macrophages from the same KO strain show defective IFN-γ-induced control of parasite growth (82).

The up-regulation of iNOS and subsequent production of RNI by activated macrophages has in many systems been considered to be TNF dependent. However, it is now clear that in *L. major*–infected macrophages, RNI can be produced in a TNF-independent manner, since IFNγ- and/or LPS-activated macrophages taken from mice lacking TNF receptors (83) can make NO and kill *Leishmania* parasites *in vitro*. Recent studies suggest that in this situation, RNI is triggered by alternative signals such as IFN-α/β or by CD40 L and LFA-1 produced by parasite-induced CD4$^+$ T cells (83). Interestingly, whereas TNFR 1– and 2–deficient mice are able to control *L. major* infection, TNF KO mice on the same genetic background develop rapidly fatal disease (84), suggesting that TNF can signal through a third receptor and that this signaling is needed to confer protection. The production of RNI by IFN-γ–activated macrophages is inhibited by IL-4, IL-10, IL-13, and TGF-β (85), and this is likely to be a major but not sole mechanism by which the Th2 response prevents healing of *Leishmania*.

In contrast to *Leishmania*, most intracellular protozoa, including *T. cruzi, T. gondii, Cryptosporidium, Eimeria,* and *Plasmodium* sp, primarily invade nonprofessional phagocytes not traditionally thought to possess microbicidal mechanisms that can be activated by IFN-γ. In the case of these pathogens, the role of RNI or respiratory oxygen intermediates (ROI) in IFN-γ–mediated control of parasite growth is more tissue restricted. A good example is the role of IFN-γ in immunity against the exoerythrocytic stages of malaria. IFN-γ produced primarily by CD8 T cells in response to vaccination induces RNI within hepatocytes invaded early after sporozoite challenge and restricts further pathogen development (86). However, when malaria parasites escape the liver they take up residence in erythrocytes, which in contrast to hepatocytes are unable to produce RNI.

A more complicated scenario occurs in IFN-γ–mediated control of *T. gondii* infection. IFN-γ plays a critical role in restricting the growth of this pathogen in the acute tachyzoite stage, as well as later in preventing reactivation of infection from dormant cysts. This immunity cannot be attributed solely to activated macrophages as originally thought, because reciprocal bone marrow chimera experiments performed with IFN-γ receptor–deficient and WT mice indicate that IFN-γ signaling is required in cells of both hemapoietic and nonhemapoietic origin (87). Accordingly, the role of RNI in resistance has been shown to be limited, functioning in the effector mechanism of resistance against chronic but not acute infection (88). An important clue concerning the mechanism controlling acute infection comes from recent studies in mice deficient for members of the IGTP family of GTP-binding proteins. These molecules, many of which possess known GTPase activity, are induced by IFN-γ in a variety of hemapoietic as well as nonhemapoietic cell types. Mice deficient in either IGTP or a second family member, LRG-47, were found to be highly susceptible to infection with *T. gondii,* while developing a normal IFN-γ response (89). Although the role played by these molecules in host resistance is unclear, their membrane association suggests a possible role in parasitophorous vacuole trafficking or function. Another candidate IFN-γ–dependent mechanism, which can limit *T. gondii* replication in human but not mouse nonhemapoietic cells, is the induction of indolamine 2,3 dioxygenase, an enzyme that catabolizes tryptophan, an essential amino acid for growth of this protozoan (90). The above examples underscore the concept that the induction of RNI is only one of a number of IFN-γ–dependent effector mechanisms that act against parasites in different host cells.

Although resistance to the erythrocytic stages of malaria is thought to be mediated primarily by humoral mechanisms, the observation of naturally acquired blood-stage immunity in B-cell–deficient mice and its transfer with defined CD4$^+$ T-cell lines and clones suggests that cell-mediated effector mechanisms must also exist (91). Even when the role of antibody is clear, as with the passive transfer of immunity, the extent of protection is reduced by prior splenectomy or T-cell depletion. There is growing evidence that the relevant pathways function through cytokine (e.g., IFN-γ, TNF) activation of macrophages that phagocytose and destroy infected RBC in spleen. In support of this concept, resistance to human malaria has been correlated with T-cell production of IFN-γ and generation of NO (92) *in vitro*. The identification of the effector mechanism involved is important as it could lead to new and potentially more effective strategies for malaria vaccination (see below).

Intracellular protozoa live briefly in the extracellular milieu during initial host infection and when they invade new cells during their *in vivo* multiplication. During this period they are vulnerable to attack by antibody. In addition, while not directly killing free parasites, antibodies can block their invasion of new cells thereby suppressing infection. These forms of humoral immunity appear to develop gradually in hosts naturally exposed to protozoa and are of special interest in vaccine development.

In humans living in areas endemic for *P. falciparum*, there is evidence for the slow development of immunity. The Ab-based nature of this resistance was demonstrated in experiments in which sera from adults were transferred to children, resulting in a temporary but highly significant reduction in parasitemia (93). This form of immunity is directed against asexual blood stages and probably develops gradually because of the need to recognize multiple-variant antigens expressed by the parasite. The mechanism of action of the protective antibodies is not entirely clear but probably involves agglutination of parasitized RBC, inhibition of cytoadherence to small blood vessels and/or blocking of red cell invasion by free merozoites (91). Additionally, an *in vitro* mechanism has been described called Ab-dependent cellular inhibition (ADCI), in which IFN-γ–dependent cytophilic IgG1 and IgG3 in donor sera interact with monocytes or granulocytes via FcR, thereby triggering them to produce TNF, which is proposed to be inhibitory for parasite development (94). Arguing against the latter mechanism, however, are the observations in mouse malaria models that protective monoclonal antibodies can transfer resistance in Fc receptor–deficient mice and that Fab fragments of such mAbs are also fully active *in vivo*. Moreover, it is clear that both Th1 and Th2 Ab isotypes can confer protection against blood stages (86,91). These observations argue that multiple mechanisms of Ab-mediated blood-stage immunity must exist, and/or that the critical determinant of protection is the antigenic fine specificity of the Ab induced together with the range of parasite variants recognized.

Naturally acquired humoral immunity against parasite invasive stages is generally inefficient and in most circumstances must work together with cell-mediated immunity to confer complete protection. A well-studied example is the antibody response against the circumsporozoite (CS) protein present on preerythrocytic stages of malaria (95). Monoclonal Abs directed against CS prevent the invasion and development of *P. falciparum* in cultured human hepatocytes or, as in the case of *Plasmodium yoelii*, directly neutralize sporozoites resulting ultimately in the disappearance of infected hepatocytes from culture. *In vivo*, antibody-mediated protective immunity against *Plasmodium berghei, P. yoelii, Plasmodium vivax* or *Plasmodium knowlesi* sporozoite challenge has been demonstrated in passive transfer studies in mice and monkeys (86,96). However, since the extracellular sporozoites invade the hepatocyte within 2 to 30 minutes of inoculation, antisporozoite antibodies must be present in circulation at high titers and exert their activity within minutes of infection. Incomplete sporozoite neutralization or inhibition of hepatocyte invasion allows the development of forms that can infect red cells and result in disease. Thus, the induction of antibodies against CS and other sporozite surface Ag is unlikely by itself to result in effective vaccination against malaria (97).

While the role of Abs in resistance to most intracellular protozoa is limited, there is a growing awareness that immune effector mechanism previously thought to be purely cell mediated in nature can have a humoral component. For example, although resistance to *T. gondii* is highly dependent on IFN-γ–mediated effector mechanisms, B-cell–deficient mice succumb at 3 to 4 weeks of infection despite the normal induction of IFN-γ and other Th1-associated cytokines. Passive transfer of anti–*T. gondii* Ab protects these animals from mortality (98). Such observations along with recent findings in helminth models (see below) testify to the complexity of antiparasitic effector mechanisms and the shortsightedness of many of the established paradigms that categorize them.

Extracellular Parasites

Extracellular parasites comprise a large group of diverse organisms. Because they exhibit variability in size, tissue tropism, and mechanisms of immune evasion, it is probably not surprising that resistance against many of these pathogens often requires both cellular and humoral mechanisms. Unique antiparasite effector strategies are employed in most cases involving a variety of host cells and immune mediators that include, but are not limited to, T cells, eosinophils, mast cells, basophils, macrophages, and antibodies. Resistance is mediated by an armament that includes ADCC, killing by activated macrophages, activation of mast cells, changes in mucus production, and alterations in gut physiology. Immunity is manifested by a variety of strategies that include direct killing by toxic mediators, alterations in parasite migration, expulsion from host tissues, and the inhibition of egg production, among others. Such complex mechanisms are needed against helminth parasites because they live in the gut, blood, lymphatics, and a variety of other host tissues. As with the intracellular parasites, the preferential activation of a type 1 versus type 2 immune response appears to play a central role in the regulation of immunity.

Helminth parasites induce strong Th2 responses that contribute to the mast cell, eosinophil, giant cell, IgE/IgA, and mucosal responses that are typically associated with these infections. For the intestinal helminths in particular, it is clear that elements of the type 2 response are crucial for resistance to infection. Several worms have been studied in detail in this regard: *Trichuris muris,* a natural parasite of the mouse and closely related to human whipworm; *Heligomosoides polygyrus; Trichinella spiralis; N. brasiliensis,* the rat hookworm; and *Strongyloides stercoralis.* However, while Th2 cytokines are clearly involved in resistance to intestinal nematodes, the roll of Th2 immunity is much less obvious with many of the filarial (*Brugia malayi* and *Wuchereria bancrofti*) (99–102) and schistosome species (103).

Both *T. muris* and *H. polygyrus* are transmitted by the oral-fecal route independently of an intermediate host and, in some strains of mice, they cause chronic infections. In the case of the *T. muris,* susceptibility depends on the mouse strain, with some animals rejecting the parasite shortly after exposure and others developing long-lived infections (102). In this system, resistant mice express type 2 responses, susceptible mice mount type 1 responses, and IL-12 (104) causes a switch from a protective type 2 to an infection-permissive type 1 response. Similarly, in normally susceptible strains, *in vivo* depletion of IFN-γ or IL-12 (102) allows the expansion of type 2 responses and effective clearance of infection. Most mouse strains are susceptible to a primary *H. polygyrus* infection, but following drug clearance the animals exhibit a strong type 2 response and are highly resistant to a secondary infection. For both *H. polygyrus* and *T. muris,* CD4 cells are required for the induction and/or expression of immunity (104). IL-4 can cure primary infections with both *T. muris* and *H. polygyrus,* anti-IL-4R blocks resistance to both, and IL-4$^{-/-}$ mice are unable to resist a challenge infection with *H. polygyrus* or a primary infection with *T. muris* (100, 102). The role of IL-4, however, appears to depend on the background of the mouse because C57BL/6 IL-4 KO mice develop chronic *T. muris* infections, while some BALB/c IL-4 KO mice clear their infections (105–107). This suggests an IL-4–independent role for IL-13 in resistance, which was confirmed by treating BALB/c IL-4–deficient mice with a soluble IL-13 receptor protein (106) that blocks IL-13 function. Chronic infections are also established in IL-13–deficient mice, despite the fact that they develop relatively normal type 2 responses (105). Similarly, anti-TNF treated mice also develop normal type 2 responses, yet are unable to expel the parasite, which suggests an important role for TNF in the regulation of IL-13–mediated immunity (107). In contrast, IL-18–deficient mice develop stronger IL-13 responses and are much more resistant to *T. muris* infection. In support of this conclusion, rIL-18 was found to down-regulate IL-13 and promote chronic infection in normally resistant mice (108). Chronic *T. muris* infections are also established in IL-10 and IL-10/IL-4 double-deficient mice; however, in contrast to the inhibitory effects of IL-18, which are clearly IFN-γ independent (108), IL-10 promotes immunity by down-regulating IFN-γ and IL-12 levels (109). IL-10–deficient mice also display marked morbidity and mortality following infection, suggesting a critical role for IL-10 in immunity to *T. muris* infection. Mortality correlates with increased inflammation, loss of Paneth cells, and absence of

mucus in the cecum. Survival is enhanced, however, if IL-10 and IL-10/4–deficient mice are treated with a broad-spectrum antibiotic, suggesting that an outgrowth of opportunistic bacteria contributes to the high degree of morbidity and mortality of infected IL-10–deficient animals (109).

Although IL-4 can lead to the expulsion of *N. brasiliensis* from infected severe combined immunodeficient (SCID) or CD4 cell–depleted mice (which normally are unable to expel the usually short-lived adult *N. brasiliensis* parasites), it clearly controls a redundant protective mechanism as anti–IL-4 mAb-treated and IL-4$^{-/-}$ mice are as resistant to infection as WT animals (110). The redundant mechanism is dependent upon the IL-4 receptor alpha chain and Stat6-dependent signaling, strongly suggesting a role for IL-13, which was again proven with a soluble antagonist of IL-13 (110). IL-4/IL-13–deficient mice are also severely impaired in their ability to expel the parasite, further emphasizing the redundant roles played by IL-4 and IL-13. Exogenous IL-4 and IL-13 can expel *N. brasiliensis* in immunodeficient mice, demonstrating that type 2 cytokines must stimulate nonlymphoid cells and, as recent evidence suggests, IL-4 receptor expression by non–bone marrow-derived gut cells is required to expel the parasites (111). With *T. spiralis,* worm expulsion is almost normal in IL-4–deficient mice but substantially delayed in STAT6-deficient (112, 113) and anti-IL-4R–treated mice (100), again strongly suggesting that IL-13 plays a protective role.

While it is now tempting to extrapolate the findings from these various experimental systems and state that resistance to intestinal nematodes requires Th2-mediated responses, it remains unclear how type 2 responses actually function to mediate protection. The most simple explanation, and one predicted over many years, that IgE is protective against intestinal helminths, has either been refuted following intensive investigation using mouse models, or at least received little direct confirmation (114). The possibility exists, however, that there are host species differences in this regard because in rats the "rapid expulsion" (speedy rejection of a secondary *T. spiralis* infection) can be transferred to naïve animals with IgE (115). How IL-4 and IL-13 mediate protection against gastrointestinal nematodes is unclear at present. In uninfected mice IL-4 has dramatic effects on intestinal physiology causing decreased peristalsis, increased mucosal permeability, and reduced sodium-linked glucose absorption (114,116). Muscle hypercontractility and goblet-cell hyperplasia are also regulated in the gut by type 2 cytokines and attenuated by IL-12 treatment, possibly implicating them in the resistance mechanism (109,113,117). For the most part, these responses appear to be T-cell and mast cell dependent (114). Their net effect is to trap parasites in mucus within the gut lumen, increase intestinal fluid content, and accelerate peristalsis, phenomena whose contribution to parasite rejection remains to be fully elucidated.

Eosinophils, elevated numbers of which are usually associated with helminth infections—the production and activation of which are stimulated by the type 2 cytokine IL-5 and inhibited by anti–IL-5 mAb—do not appear to play any role in protective responses to *T. muris, H. polygyrus,* or *N. brasiliensis* (114). However, there is evidence from the use of anti–IL-5, IL-5 transgenic mice and/or IL-5R α-chain KO mice, that eosinophils can be important in protective immune responses directed against tissue-invasive larval forms of *Strongyloides* sp (118,119) and *Angiostrongylus cantonensis* (119,120). IL-5–deficient mice have also been shown to exhibit impaired muscle hypercontractility and host defense against primary *T. spiralis* infection (121). Moreover, there is a body of literature primarily from studies in rats and humans that suggests that eosinophils play a role in protection against (non-gut dwelling) schistosomes (122)—although anti–IL-5 treated mice can develop immunity to this parasite, again suggesting host species differences. Overall, despite the prevailing dogma, the record does not strongly support an indispensable role for eosinophils in immunity to most helminth parasites.

Additional prominent components of the type 2 response induced by intestinal helminths are increased IgG1 production and intestinal mastocytosis (114). While IgG1 may play a role in immunity to *T. spiralis* and *H. polygyrus* (114), it plays no obvious protective role in the other intestinal helminthiases. Mast cells, which are implicated in the effects of IL-4 on intestinal physiology, appear to play an important role in immunity to *T. spiralis,* as mice treated with mAbs against stem cell factor (SCF, a non–T-cell derived cytokine) or c-kit, its receptor (both of which play a central role in mast cell development) are unable to expel worms (123). In the latter experiments, there was no effect from the treatment on the CD4 response and once the mAb treatment was stopped, the parasites were expelled. These data, together with other findings in this system, suggest that a CD4 cell–dependent response cooperates with SCF to promote a mast cell response that mediates parasite expulsion. Several cytokines made by CD4 cells, including IL-3, IL-4, and IL-9 (64), have been implicated in mastocytosis. Consistent with this, IL-9, when expressed at high levels from a transgene, allows mice to expel *T. spiralis* (124) and *T. muris* (125) even more rapidly than is usual, and anti–IL-9 antibodies prevent expulsion of *T. muris* (126). Moreover, the IL-9 transgenic mice exhibit an enhanced Th2 response raising the possibility that IL-4 from mast cells is feeding back to enhance Th2 differentiation (125) (as has been proposed for IL-4 from basophils in schistosome infected mice [127]).

In addition to playing a role in immunity to gastrointestinal helminths, there is growing epidemiologic evidence that type 2 responses, particularly in the form of Ag-specific IgE, mediate the resistance to infection with schistosomes that develops with age in endemic areas (122). While the exact mechanism by which IgE Ab would mediate protection is unclear, it is possible that they cooperate with eosinophils or macrophages in an ADCC mechanism (122). Consistent with this general hypothesis, data from field studies in Brazil indicate that the ability to resist infection is influenced by a major

gene that localizes to a region of chromosome 5 that encodes type 2 cytokines (128). In addition, studies from rodent models suggest that vaccine-induced antischistosome immunity is controlled by both cell-mediated (20) and humoral mechanisms (129,130). However, the requirement for a polarized, type 2 cytokine response (and thus, IgE and eosinophils) appears to be less important in these vaccine models (131). The latter conclusion may also extend to lymphatic filariasis, where both type 1 and type 2 responses may be needed to clear infection (132).

Resistance to protozoan trypanosomes also appears to require elements of both cell-mediated and humoral immunity. The African trypanosomes are tsetse-transmitted parasites that inhabit the extracellular compartment of their host's blood and avoid detection by the humoral immune system by switching among antigenically distinct variant surface glycoproteins (VSGs) (see below). Trypanosome-infected hosts typically do not produce antibodies that destroy the parasite, other than those that are VSG specific. Parasitemias manifest as recurring waves and are cleared following development of VSG-specific Ab. The primary component of the antibody response to VSG is a T-cell–independent IgM response. However, T-cell–dependent B-cell responses are also involved in eliciting VSG-specific IgG. Nevertheless, because the VSG-specific antibody response takes several days to develop and because the doubling time of the parasite is approximately 7 hours, the host can develop quite high parasitemias, severe trypanosomiasis-associated pathology, generalized immunodepression, and, in some circumstances, debilitating secondary infections (133). Interestingly, overproduction of IFN-γ and NO appears to be the root cause of these deleterious side effects (134). It is clear, however, that both innate and acquired responses contribute to trypanosome control (133), and experimental models suggest that IFN-γ, but not IL-4, is linked to host resistance (135).

Another important extracellular protozoan, *Giardia,* is a flagellated intestinal parasite, which causes both acute and chronic diarrheal disease in many parts of the world. Despite its intestinal habitat, *Giardia* appears to be controlled by mechanisms distinct from those mediating resistance to most gastrointestinal nematodes. Several lines of evidence, including results from murine models and studies of natural resistance in humans, suggest that both antibodies and T cells are required for control of *Giardia* infections. Nevertheless, in contrast to the situation with gut nematodes, neither a Th2- or Th1-dominated CD4 T-cell response appears necessary for restriction of parasite growth (136). While a T-cell–dependent mechanism is clearly essential for resistance to acute infections (136), numerous studies have suggested that antibodies, particularly of the IgA isotype, are required to control chronic *Giardia lamblia* infections (reviewed in Faubert [137]).

The above examples stress that while intracellular and extracellular parasites often stimulate distinct immune response profiles, their immune control may involve overlapping immunologic effector arms.

MECHANISMS OF IMMUNE EVASION
AND LATENCY

Pathogens that rely on an insect vector to complete their life-cycle, or are only sporadically transmitted from one host to another, are under strong evolutionary pressure to prolong their survival within the mammalian host. As the adaptive immune response is the principal barrier to the persistence of pathogens in the mammalian host, parasites have evolved diverse strategies to evade immune control mechanisms, either by evading immune recognition or by suppressing the immune response. The former strategy refers to the ability of some parasites to sequester within sites that are inaccessible to immune attack, to mask themselves with host antigens, to shed their own target antigens, or most notably, to undergo antigenic variation.

Evasion of Immune Recognition

The asexual blood stage of malaria would seem the most obvious example of a well-hidden parasite. Its ability to invade mature erythrocytes, which lack either class I or class II histocompatibility molecules, protects it from recognition by antibodies or effector T cells. Thus, while some parasitized erythrocytes might be cleared from the circulation, taken up by DC, and elicit a malaria-specific T-cell response, this response will do little to limit the enormous expansion of asexual-stage merozoites remaining within blood cells that have escaped clearance. Other intracellular protozoa appear to hide within immunologically privileged sites. The persistence of T. cruzi within heart or skeletal muscle, which is believed to underlie the pathogenesis of Chagas disease, occurs despite the fact that parasites are cleared from most other tissue (138). Infected muscle cells may be only poorly recognized as targets for CTL, poorly accessible to their homing, or they may have intrinsic defects in immune-mediated killing mechanisms. A similar form of sequestration has been proposed to explain the long-term persistence of Leishmania within fibroblasts and dendritic cells following their efficient killing by activated macrophages during the acute stage of infection (139). While persistent low-level infection of host cells has been proposed as an explanation for latency in T. gondii infection, the major parasite reservoir during chronic infection is undoubtedly provided by the tissue cyst, essentially a modified host cell carrying a specialized dormant parasite stage, the bradyzoite. Helminths (with the exception of Trichinella) do not invade host cells and therefore cannot use this strategy for evading immune recognition. Furthermore, because most multicellular helminth parasites do not replicate themselves within their mammalian hosts, they are not equipped to evade immune recognition by undergoing antigenic variation. Instead, they employ alternative mechanisms such as disguising their surfaces with host molecules and rapidly shedding membrane (tegument)-bound immune complexes (140). In addition, helminths have evolved a series of elaborate processes for inactivating antibody, complement,

and cellular effector elements that threaten the parasite surface (141). Interestingly, recent data suggest that helminths may exploit host T-lymphocyte and cytokine signals as developmental triggers and if these signals are in low abundance or lacking in vivo, parasite growth may be aborted or severely attenuated (142,143).

Antigenic variation is an important mechanism of immune evasion shared by diverse classes of pathogenic protozoa, including African trypanosomes, Giardia, and malaria (reviewed in Deitsch et al. [144]). In each case, the antigens involved are highly immunogenic but poorly cross-reactive, and are encoded by large families of nonallelic genes. The best-studied example of antigenic variation in parasites is that of African trypanosomes, the etiologic agents of sleeping sickness. These organisms, such as T. brucei, produce waves of parasitemia by generating subpopulations that express antigenically different forms of the major surface variant-specific glycoprotein (VSG). These molecules are so densely packed together that they prevent antibody from binding to subsurface epitopes of the VSG coat or to any other components of the plasma membrane. The growth of trypanosomes in the bloodstream results in a strong B-cell response to exposed VSG epitopes, leading to the elimination of organisms expressing the relevant VSG and the selection of organisms that have switched expression to another VSG. This switching occurs independent of antibody and at relatively high frequency. In addition to antibody-dependent variant-specific clearance of trypanosomes in the vascular compartment, parasite control within the extravascular tissue compartment has been shown to involve a parasite antigen-specific Th1 response, associated with IFN-γ-dependent activation of macrophages (135). An internal subregion of the VSG appears to be the major epitope driving the Th1 response, and this region is also highly variable.

G. lamblia also undergoes surface antigenic variation. In this case, the antigens belong to a family of variant-specific cysteine-rich zinc finger proteins (VSPs). After inoculation into mice of a single G. lamblia clone, the original VSP is expressed for approximately 2 weeks and then is gradually replaced by other VSP, coincident with the appearance of variant-specific antibodies (reviewed in Nash [145]). Mice that are unable to make antibodies, however, are still able to control acute G. lamblia infection and, even in immunodeficient mice or gerbils, certain clones of G. lamblia are selected for or against, depending on the parasite clone and the host species (146). Thus, in addition to immune evasion, antigenic variation may be involved in other aspects of biologic selection, such as diversifying the host range of the parasite.

The generally accepted explanation for the slow acquisition of naturally acquired immunity to malaria is the fact that resistance is strain specific, and that an individual becomes immune only after being exposed to a large number of strains circulating in an endemic community. While allelic polymorphisms were originally thought to account for strain-specific immunity, it is now recognized that clonal antigenic variation is largely responsible for immune escape by blood-stage malaria parasites (147,148). Variable forms of parasite-derived protein at the surface of infected erythrocytes elicit antibodies that mediate a significant component of the strain-specific, host-protective response in both animal models and in human infection. For *P. falciparum*, these molecules are termed *P. falciparum* erythrocyte membrane protein-1 (PfEMP-1), and are encoded by members of the *var* family of genes (reviewed in Newbold [149]). The products of *P. falciparum var* genes are transported to the surface of infected erythrocytes and localized in electron-dense structures termed "knobs." These structures confer on the infected red cell the ability to adhere to vascular endothelium via a variety of host receptors. When the brain or the placenta are the preferred targets of vascular adhesion, then the severe clinical forms of cerebral and pregnancy malaria may result. Cytoadherence is thought to have evolved in *P. falciparum* to prevent the passage of infected erythrocytes through the spleen, where they would be recognized as damaged or as foreign and removed from the circulation. Since antibodies against PfEMP-1 will prevent cytoadherence, then the purpose of antigenic variation is to ensure that parasites expressing new *var* gene products will continue to sequester and to avoid splenic clearance.

Evasion by Immune Suppression

Generalized immunodepression, which is a feature of many chronic parasitic infections, including malaria, African trypanosomiasis, and visceral leishmaniasis, appears in most instances to be secondary to other immune evasion strategies, and results from a variety of immune dysfunctions that high systemic parasite burdens can produce. These include disruption of normal lymphoid architecture, or the accumulation of parasite-derived metabolic products that are directly inhibitory to lymphocyte function, or that induce suppressor cell activities such as prostaglandin production by macrophages. The examples of immune suppression referred to below are thought to operate as more primary escape mechanisms that help parasites become well established within their mammalian hosts.

Because most helminths do not replicate themselves within their mammalian hosts, parasite loads usually increase only as a result of prolonged survival and accumulated exposure. In addition to masking or shedding their target antigens, a consistent picture of immune suppression has been established in human helminth infections. Peripheral blood T cells from patients with filariasis show impaired antigen-specific proliferative responses that do not necessarily reflect immune deviation toward a Th2 bias, since Th2 proliferation can also be inhibited by filarial antigens (150). Metabolic products of *S. mansoni* adult worms have also been shown to strongly inhibit lymphocyte proliferation, including primary and secondary Th2 responses (151). More recent findings indicate that alteration of antigen-presenting cell function may be a

major mechanism of helminth-induced immunosuppression (152). Further intriguing data suggest that helminths may manipulate immune responses by mimicking host cytokine and cytokine receptors (150).

With regard to immunosuppressive antigens derived from parasitic protozoa, there are a surprising number of examples of variant antigens that may promote parasite survival, not by avoiding immune recognition but by modulating the immune response. The simultaneous presence of variant CSP T-cell epitopes (also referred to as altered peptide ligands), as might occur in African children infected with multiple allelic variants of malaria, was found to deliver an altered signal to the responding T cells that induced nonresponsiveness to its target agonist epitope (153). In the case of *T. cruzi*, which can express and secrete multiple members of the highly polymorphic surface sialidase superfamily at one time, epitope-specific T-cell responses are suppressed either by altered peptide ligand inhibition or because immune recognition is flooded with competing targets (154). An alternative role for variant PfEMP-1 and its equivalent in other malaria species that do not cytoadhere to endothelial cells has been proposed, based on the observation that infected erythrocytes adhere to dendritic cells and inhibit their maturation (155). In these studies, erythrocytes infected with parasite lines that do not express PfEMP-1 failed to adhere to dendritic cells or to affect their function. Thus, expression of variant parasite antigens at the surface of infected red cells may have evolved to suppress the development of protective immunity.

Lymphocyte polyclonal activation is a generalized mechanism of immune evasion among parasitic protozoa, including blood and tissue trypanosomes, *Leishmania donovani*, *Toxoplasma gondii*, and rodent malarias. These organisms possess mitogenic or superantigenic moieties that trigger polyclonal lymphocyte responses, resulting in a generalized depression of antigen-specific responses (156). The mechanism by which this occurs is not well defined; hyperstimulation may result in a state of clonal exhaustion, although it is also commonly associated with the presence of cells and cytokines with suppressive activities. Most pathogenic trypanosomes possess powerful B-cell mitogens, resulting in hypergammaglobulinemia, lymphocyte proliferation, and induction of nonspecific and autoreactive antibodies. The *T. cruzi* B-cell mitogen has been cloned and characterized as a eukaryotic proline racemase (157). Both T-cell–dependent and –independent forms of polyclonal B-cell activation have been described. In the case of rodent malarias, mitogenic activation of T cells appears necessary for the amplification of B cells.

Immune Suppression and Latency

Immune suppressive mechanisms have also been shown to account for the persistence of parasites in their hosts following clinical cure of the disease. These are individuals that have therefore developed effective immunity to primary infection and that in many cases maintain strong immunity to reinfection despite the fact that they harbor persistent parasites. The ability to establish latency is a hallmark of many parasites and can have severe consequences in terms of reactivation disease, such as can occur under conditions of immunocompromise, as in HIV co-infection. In clinical and experimental forms of leishmaniasis, small numbers of viable organisms persist within lymphoid tissue and within the site of the former skin lesion following self-cure. IL-10 was revealed to play an essential role in chronicity because the parasite was unable to establish latency in IL-10 KO mice (158). In addition, sterile immunity was achieved in WT mice treated during the chronic phase with anti–IL-10 receptor antibody (Fig. 2). A high frequency of the CD4$^+$ T cells found in sites of chronic infection released IL-10 and were CD25/CTLA-4 positive (159), a phenotype that is consistent with the recently described T regulatory or "suppressor" subset (159a). The activation of these regulatory cells, while undoubtedly exploited by the parasite to prolong its survival within the immune host, is also host beneficial because they modulate the

immunopathology that in many cases is the defining character of the disease.

IMMUNOPATHOLOGIC MECHANISMS AND THEIR REGULATION

Immune pathology is generally viewed as the result of an inappropriate or excessive host response, but with many parasites it may be an inevitable outcome of persistent infection, which is often the case for many of the parasitic diseases. In terms of naturally stimulated host resistance, the most obvious type of protective immune response is that which allows an infected animal to clear its parasites. In reality, as discussed above, most parasites through their elaborate evasion strategies produce infections that are chronic or persistent in nature and are seldom completely eliminated by host immunity. The more usual situation is that the immune response is able to partially protect the host, thereby preventing lethal infection; however, in the process it may stimulate various types of immune-mediated pathology. Nonspecific immune responses such as fever and inflammation provide an essential first line of host defense against a variety of infectious pathogens. In ideal circumstances, this is a transient phase that terminates as soon as the host has acquired specific effector mechanisms such as antibodies or lymphokine-producing T-lymphocytes. If such protective mechanisms do not develop, or if they are not effective in eradicating the infection, then persistent inflammation and other nonspecific responses may be the only way of limiting the infection. This is the case for many parasitic diseases and it carries an inevitable risk of pathologic side effects.

This does not mean that all infections with the same parasite species lead to the same immune pathology. One of the most striking features of human parasitic disease is the great variability in clinical outcome, ranging from asymptomatic infection to fatal disease. Esophageal disease due to *T. cruzi*, portal hypertension due to *S. mansoni*, and nephrotic syndrome due to *Plasmodium malariae* are a few examples of the many immunopathologic complications that may occur in some infected individuals but not others. Part of this variability is determined by host genetics, while other potential determinants include parasite virulence factors, infectious dose, and the prior level of immunity. The picture may be complicated by coinfection with other infectious agents: for example, the severity of *P. falciparum* malaria appears to be increased by concomitant bacteremia but reduced by concomitant *P. vivax* infection, although the underlying mechanisms remain poorly understood (160). Similarly, coinfections of *T. gondii* and *S. mansoni* have also proven highly lethal in rodents, with liver damage being the primary cause of the enhanced morbidity (161). Even more striking is the recent data demonstrating that LPS derived from an endosymbiotic *Wolbachia* bacteria appears to be almost entirely responsible for the chronic inflammation and river blindness induced by filarial infection (162,163).

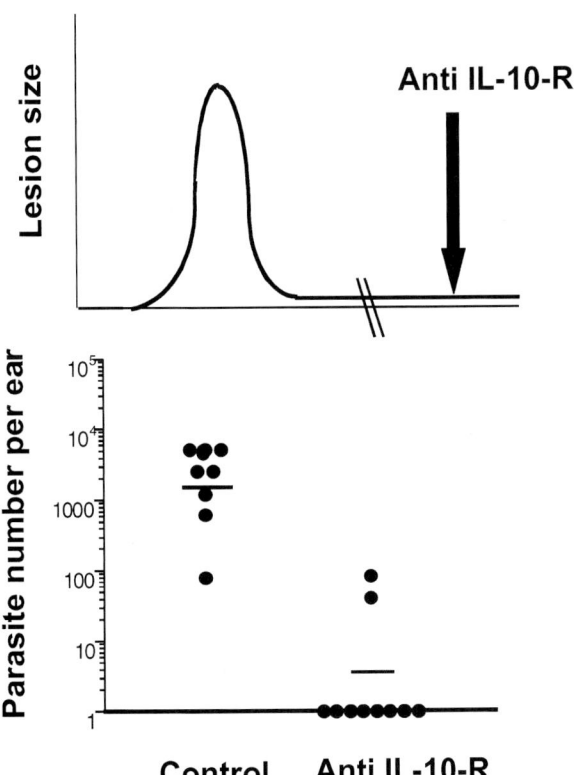

FIG. 2. IL-10 receptor blockade as immunotherapy for latent infection. Following healing of their cutaneous lesions, *L. major*–resistant C57Bl/6 mice were treated with anti–IL-10 receptor or control antibody (*top*). Two weeks later, the number of parasites in the dermis was quantitated (*bottom*). Parasite numbers per individual ear are shown, indicating that IL-10 receptor blockade results in rapid clearance of persistent parasites from the skin and sterile cure.

It is impossible to do justice to the remarkably broad range of immunologic mechanisms that contribute to the pathology of parasitic disease. Twenty years ago, much of the research in this field concerned the role of immune complexes, complement, and anaphylaxis. These areas remain important but the focus has shifted to the molecular basis of cellular processes such as inflammation, granuloma formation, and fibrosis. An important issue is how the host maintains the fine balance between a protective immune response and one that is liable to cause pathologic complications. It is becoming increasingly clear that this is one of the most critical determinants of a successful host–parasite relationship and, as such, it is of considerable importance for vaccinologists. Interestingly, in many parasitic infections this balance appears to be regulated by the coordinated actions of a few essential immunoregulatory cytokines.

This section focuses primarily on the question of how the balance between immune protection and immune pathology is regulated. The issue is both quantitative (e.g., the optimal amount of proinflammatory cytokines required when a parasite is first encountered by the immune system) and qualitative (e.g., the optimal balance between the Th1 response that promotes cell-mediated immunity and the Th2 response that promotes antibody generation and tissue remodeling). A fundamental biological dilemma is that the host has to deal with many different infectious pathogens and, even for a single species of parasite, with different strains. For example, a strain of *P. falciparum* or *T. gondii* that replicates slowly, releasing highly proinflammatory factors, may require a different regulatory response to a fast-replicating strain with little proinflammatory activity (160). In such circumstances, there may be no single optimal response and, however well the system is regulated, a certain proportion of natural infections will have a pathologic outcome.

The Quest for Homeostasis in the Anti-Infective Immune Response

Whereas a proinflammatory Th1 response is usually required to control intracellular infections, there is also a need to balance the response. The various effector molecules, particularly those associated with the Th1 pathway, are nonspecific in their action and can be detrimental if produced for too long, in excess, or in the wrong place. The potentially harmful molecules include NO, ROI, IL-1, IFNγ, and TNF, which often operate in a synergistic fashion. Therefore, it is important to produce a sufficiently potent type 1 response to control the infection, while producing at the same time just enough of a type 2 or immunosuppressive response to prevent the protective response from causing pathology. IL-10, TGF-β, and to a lesser extent IL-4, appear to be important in preventing the Th1 response from overshooting during infection.

There are also several examples wherein Th2 responses appear to be detrimental. Strong antibody responses may lead to the formation of antigen–antibody complexes or complement activation resulting in bystander lysis (164). Eosinophils, typically associated with the Th2 response, are involved in hypersensitivity reactions to the filarial worm *Onchocerca volvulus* (165). Th2 responses appear to be the primary cause of hepatic fibrosis, portal hypertension, and chronic morbidity in *S. mansoni*–infected mice (166). The available data suggest that IFN-γ, IL-12, and IL-10 cooperate to keep Th2 responses in check. Thus, it is now clear that both type 1 and type 2 responses, under inappropriate conditions, can initiate tissue damage during infection. In summary, a successful resolution to infection requires precise titration of Th1 and Th2 responses, appropriate to the type of pathogen. This is not just in terms of amount but also where, when, and for how long these responses occur.

Pathogenesis of Chronic Th1 Responses

Control of intracellular pathogens such as *Leishmania* sp, *T. gondii,* and *T. cruzi* requires the coordinated activation of both antigen-specific cells (T-lymphocytes) and less specific responses (NK cells, neutrophils, and macrophages) with IFN-γ and TNF playing critical roles by up-regulating macrophage activation and NO production (167). In *L. monocytogenes*–infected mice, IL-10 is induced simultaneously with IFN-γ and TNF and promotes bacterial growth by down-regulating the host protective cell-mediated immune response. IL-10–deficient mice are highly resistant to *L. monocytogenes,* while mice treated with exogenous IL-10 succumbed to infection (168). Proinflammatory cytokine expression is increased and the rapid elimination of the organism in mice deficient in IL-10 decreases the number and size of granulomatous lesions in the liver and spleen, thus reducing the marked tissue destruction that is typically seen late in infection. Thus, in this intracellular infection, IL-10 potently inhibits both innate and acquired immunity and promotes development of tissue pathology. In contrast, IL-10–deficient mice inoculated with a normally virulent *T. gondii* strain or with a virulent strain of *T. cruzi,* succumb to infection within the first 2 weeks of infection (169,170). In both of these infections, animals lacking IL-10 show increased suppression of parasite growth and, in the case of *T. cruzi,* inflammation and necrosis within the endocardium and interstitium of the myocardium is reduced. The increase in mortality appears to be caused by high systemic levels of IFN-γ, TNF, and IL-12, produced in large part by activated CD4$^+$ lymphocytes and macrophages. The livers of both *T. gondii* and *T. cruzi*–infected mice show numerous prominent foci of necrosis and increased cellular infiltration, composed of lymphocytes, macrophages, and necrotic cellular debris. Levels of IL-12 and IFN-γ in sera of infected IL-10–deficient animals are four- to six-fold higher than in sera from control mice, as are mRNA levels of several proinflammatory cytokines (169). Similarly, macrophages from the mutant mice activated *in vitro* or *in vivo* with *T. gondii* secrete higher levels of TNF, IL-12, and inducible NO than macrophages from control animals. The clinical manifestations of weight loss, hypothermia, hypoglycemia, and increased liver-derived enzymes in the blood, together with hepatic necrosis, suggest that the IL-10 KO mice die in response to an overwhelming systemic immune response, resembling that observed during septic shock. In support of this conclusion, administration of anti-CD4, anti–IL-12, or anti–TNF Abs reduces mortality in IL-10 KO mice (169,170). Thus, in these models, IL-10 plays a major role in protecting the host against an excessive and lethal type 1–cytokine response.

The above findings indicate that IL-10 can be either protective or detrimental. A possible explanation for the somewhat unexpected lethal outcome observed with *T. gondii* or *T. cruzi*–infected IL-10–deficient mice, is that both pathogens infect virtually all nucleated cells and are characterized by an acute phase in which the parasite disseminates throughout the body. This induces an overwhelming systemic immune response in the absence of the immunoregulatory cytokine IL-10. In contrast, when WT or IL-10–deficient mice are infected with *L. monocytogenes* or *L. major,* macrophages serve as the primary host cells and the infection is localized within granulomatous foci. In these circumstances, systemic cytokine levels remain relatively low (170), and the absence of IL-10 boosts the protective type 1 cytokine response, but not to the extent that it induces damage to host tissues (158). Thus, depending on timing, dose, and strain of parasite, the production of a particular set of cytokines can be either protective or detrimental, and this may be largely dictated by the nature of the host–parasite interaction.

Interestingly, mortality of *T. gondii*–infected IL-10–deficient mice is prevented by either systemically priming mice with soluble *T. gondii* antigens prior to infection (171) or by simultaneously blocking the CD28-B7 and CD40-CD40L co-stimulatory pathways (172). In both situations, the mutant mice mount impaired type 1 cytokine responses and are protected from infection-induced immunopathology. The production of IL-12 is markedly decreased in the antigen-sensitized IL-10–deficient mice. These findings suggest that the immunoprotective effect of IL-10 in this model is mediated through its ability to regulate the functional activity of dendritic cells or other antigen-presenting cells.

In studies where infection is initiated with peroral administration of *T. gondii* cysts, the natural route of infection, it has become apparent that there is great potential for an unregulated type 1 response to cause fatal inflammatory disease in the intestine. This was particularly well demonstrated in a comparison of the outcome of infection with the ME49 strain of *T. gondii* in C57BL/6 and BALB/c mice (173). When challenged perorally with a high dose of cysts, C57BL/6 mice develop a potent type 1 response and severe ileal inflammation that can be averted by a mAb that neutralizes IFN-γ. In contrast, the type 1 response in BALB/c mice was more subdued and the animals avoided intestinal damage. IL-4 and/or other anti-inflammatory cytokines such as IL-10 play a role in controlling the magnitude of the type 1 response because in a mouse strain that is resistant to peroral infection, the absence of a functional IL-4 gene leads to increased mortality. Interestingly, in the latter situation, IL-4$^{-/-}$ mice that survive the acute intestinal disease, subsequently exhibit reduced brain pathology and parasite burdens. Similarly, IL-10–deficient mice perorally infected with *T. gondii* also succumb rapidly to infection, but in contrast to intraperitoneal infections, mortality is attributed to type 1–mediated intestinal rather than hepatic pathology (174).

Much has been written about the pathologic consequences of excessive proinflammatory cytokine production in malaria (175). In experimental murine models of malaria, the proinflammatory response may be either protective or pathologic in various circumstances. During the preerythrocytic stage in the liver, when parasite burden is relatively low and the infection is clinically asymptomatic, there is evidence that IL-12, IFN-γ, and NO each play an important role in preventing the infection from progressing further (176). Once the parasites invade erythrocytes and grow to large numbers, the risk–benefit equation is less clear. Although TNF, IL-12, and IFN-γ have been shown to inhibit blood-stage parasites and thereby exert a protective function (176), at this stage the cytokine response is systemic and some pathologic side effects are inevitable. The most common clinical consequence in humans is fever, while life-threatening complications, such as profound anemia and cerebral malaria occur in a proportion of infections due to *P. falciparum,* but not other species. Mice with malaria do not develop fever but, depending on the specific host–parasite combination, they may develop profound anemia, fatal neurologic symptoms, or multiorgan failure; TNF has been the cytokine most consistently associated with severe pathology in most of these models (175). Moreover, polymorphisms of the promoter regions of TNF (177) have been associated with susceptibility to severe complications of *P. falciparum* malaria in African children. One interpretation of these findings is that a strong early proinflammatory cytokine response is protective while a strong late response is pathologic (178).

Recent experimental studies suggest that IL-10 and TGF-β cooperate to down-regulate potentially pathogenic proinflammatory cytokine responses in malaria (179). IL-10–deficient mice infected with *P. chabaudi chabaudi* showed increased mortality compared with normal WT litter mates, although peak parasitemias did not differ markedly. Instead, acute infection was characterized by an enhanced type 1 cytokine response (180). The IFN-γ response was retained in the chronic phase of infection, whereas control mice ultimately developed a dominant type 2 cytokine response. Thus, susceptibility of IL-10–deficient mice to an otherwise nonlethal infection results not from fulminant parasitemia but from a sustained and enhanced proinflammatory cytokine response.

Evidence for a protective role for TGF-β in blood-stage infection comes from a murine model of *P. berghei* infection, where susceptible strains of mice show increased IFN-γ and reduced TGF-β mRNA expression compared with resistant strains (179). Treatment of infected mice with a neutralizing antibody to TGF-β exacerbated the virulence of *P. berghei* and caused *P. c. chabaudi* infection, which normally resolves spontaneously, to become lethal. Although administration of rTGF-β to *P. berghei*–infected mice slowed the rate of parasite proliferation, this was accompanied by a marked decrease in serum TNF-β levels, and it was concluded that the protective effects of this cytokine are less due to its effects on parasite growth than to its down-regulation of inflammatory responses (178). These observations are consistent with the role of TGF-β as an immunosuppressive cytokine. TGF-β was shown to directly induce IL-10 expression in macrophages and it has been proposed that this may explain its protective effects, down-regulating potentially pathogenic type 1 responses and TNF production in favor of a Th2-type profile.

Pathogenesis of Chronic Th2 Responses

Schistosomiasis is caused by three major species of helminth parasites, *S. mansoni*, *Schistosoma haematobium*, and *Schistosoma japonicum*. Upon infection, adult parasites of *S. mansoni* migrate to the mesenteric veins where they live up to 10 years or more, laying hundreds of eggs per day. Some of the eggs become entrapped in the microvasculature of the liver and once there, induce a granulomatous response (181). Subsequently, fibrosis and portal hypertension may develop, which is the primary cause of morbidity in infected individuals and in some cases may be lethal. Consequently, much of the symptomatology of schistosomiasis is attributed to the egg-induced granulomatous inflammatory response and associated pathology.

Granulomas are pathogenic, primarily not because they cause hepatic failure in the short term, but rather because they precipitate fibrosis, increased portal blood pressure, and the development of portal systemic shunts (181). Th cells are essential for granuloma formation, while all other lymphocyte types examined so far (including B cells, CD8 cells, NK T cells, and $\gamma\delta$ T cells) are not (181). It is interesting to note, however, that B-cell–deficient (μMT) mice mount an exacerbated granulomatous response and, unlike WT animals, fail to down-modulate pathology late in infection (182). Moreover, perinatal exposure to specific anti-SEA idiotypes has been shown to induce long-term effects on survival, pathology, and immune response patterns in mice subsequently infected with *S. mansoni* (183), further suggesting that Ab-mediated signaling events strongly influence the magnitude of the granulomatous response. The importance of Th2 cells in these pathologic processes was shown by experiments in which mice vaccinated with egg Ag plus IL-12 to induce an egg-specific Th1 response upon subsequent infection, developed smaller granulomas and less severe fibrosis than did nonvaccinated infected controls (184). Decreased fibrosis was associated with a diminished Th2 response and accentuated type 1 cytokine production. Additionally, mAb anti–IL-4 treatment of infected mice tends to reduce granuloma size and fibrosis (181), although the same outcome is not always observed when different strains of IL-4$^{-/-}$ mice are studied (185). It is important to note, however, that Th1 cytokines (IL-2, IFN-γ)

also contribute to granuloma formation but their role is more prominent in the early stages of the response where they affect peak granuloma size but not the formation of fibrotic pathology (184,186).

While granulomas are widely thought to be detrimental to the infected host, it is clear that the egg-induced lesions also serve a requisite host-protective function during infection, particularly in *S. mansoni* infections. In chronically infected hosts, schistosome eggs provide a continuous antigenic stimulus for the immune response. If these antigens are not sequestered or neutralized effectively, they may damage host tissues, with the liver being particularly sensitive. In support of this conclusion, T-cell–deprived, nude, SCID, and egg-tolerized mice infected with *S. mansoni* die earlier than comparably infected, immunologically intact control mice because they are unable to satisfactorily mount a granulomatous response (187,188). Widespread microvesicular hepatic damage induced by toxic egg products contributes to the poorer survival of infected immunosuppressed mice. Presumably, the chronic detrimental effects associated with granulomas represent a better alternative (for host and parasite) than that of the host dying soon after parasite egg production begins. Granuloma formation therefore seems to be a compromise solution to allow the host to live with the infection.

During granuloma development, the dominant CD4$^+$ T-cell response changes from a Th1 response of short duration to a sustained Th2 response that is most prominent at the height of granulomatous activity. The development of the Th2 response is highly dependent on IL-4; therefore, it was expected that IL-4–deficient mice might develop less severe disease. Nevertheless, consistent with the requirement to form granulomas, studies with IL-4–deficient mice indicate that Th2 responses play an essential host protective role during infection with *S. mansoni* (185,189). Unlike WT mice that develop chronic disease when infection intensities are moderate, infected Th2-response–defective, C57BL/6 IL-4–deficient mice suffer from an acute disease, which is characterized by cachexia and significant mortality. The primary cause of morbidity in the infected IL-4$^{-/-}$ animals appears to be due to the formation of numerous nonhemorrhagic lesions on the mucosal surface of the small intestine (185). Little change in hepatic pathology was detected in these mice. Evidence suggests that IL-4 is required for the efficient passage of eggs through the intestinal wall (188). Consequently, eggs are trapped in the intestine, causing significant intestinal inflammation and ultimately increased systemic exposure to bacterial toxins. This combined with the decreased Th2- and enhanced Th1-type response results in an increase in proinflammatory cytokine expression that contributes to the significant weight loss and death of the IL-4–deficient mice (185,188).

These observations suggest that development of the egg-specific Th2 response is required to prevent the deleterious effects of sustained proinflammatory cytokine expression. Indeed, morbidity can be partially ameliorated in IL-4–deficient animals with a neutralizing antibody against TNF, and disease severity can be correlated with the level of NO made *in vitro* by their LPS-activated spleen cells (189). Interestingly, IL-10 plays a role similar to IL-4 during infection with *S. mansoni* (166) and has been postulated to be a central regulator of both IFN-γ and proinflammatory cytokine production in human schistosomiasis (190). In mouse studies, marked increases in IFN-γ, TNF, and iNOS expression are detected in infected IL-10–deficient animals, and this correlates with the development of significant morbidity and mortality. Even greater mortality is observed in mice exhibiting deficiencies in both IL-4 and IL-10 (166). These double cytokine–deficient animals uniformly die between week 7 and 9 postinfection and at a rate that far exceeds the mortality observed in their single cytokine–deficient counterparts. The double cytokine–deficient animals also develop the strongest and most highly polarized Th1-type response, and elevated serum aspartate transaminase levels suggest that mortality is attributable in part to acute hepatotoxicity. cDNA microarray experiments conducted on granulomatous tissues suggest that neutrophils and an altered pattern of apoptosis in the liver may also contribute to the severe pathology of the infected type 1 polarized mice (191). Still other studies suggest that IL-4, and perhaps IL-10, protect the host by down-regulating the generation of reactive oxygen and nitrogen intermediates that damage the liver (192). Regardless of the exact mechanisms involved, these observations clearly demonstrate that IL-4 and IL-10 are both required to prevent Th1 responses from overshooting and becoming pathologic during infection with *S. mansoni*.

While the studies described above confirm a protective role for type 2–associated cytokines, other studies indicate that these mediators also contribute to the development of hepatic fibrosis, the primary cause of chronic morbidity in schistosomiasis. Specifically, the Th2-associated cytokine IL-13 was shown to act as the dominant fibrogenic mediator in this disease (193) (Fig. 3). Perhaps even more striking is the

recent observation that infected IL-13–deficient mice survive longer than WT control animals. These findings confirm that IL-13 contributes to the morbidity of the infected host. Recombinant IL-13 stimulates collagen synthesis in fibroblasts; therefore, the detrimental effects of IL-13 may be mediated directly through its profibrogenic activity (193). Type-2 cytokines were also recently shown to induce the arginase-dependent production of proline in macrophages, an essential amino acid involved in collagen production; thus, providing additional mechanistic explanation for the pathogenic potential of persistent type 2 cytokine responses (194). These results, when combined with the findings from IL-4–deficient mice, suggest that IL-4 is host-protective while IL-13 is host-damaging during chronic murine schistosome infection. This conclusion is supported by recent studies conducted in IL-10/IL-12 and IL-10/IFN-γ–deficient mice that develop exacerbated type 2 cytokine responses (166,195). These double cytokine–deficient animals develop ten times as many egg-specific IL-13–producing cells than do similarly infected WT controls and, consequently, hepatic fibrosis is increased significantly. The double cytokine–deficient mice also show significant morbidity and mortality at the chronic stage of infection. Interestingly, however, their pathologic reaction is distinct from the acute hepatotoxic tissue response observed in the type 1–polarized, IL-10/IL-4–deficient mice (166). Indeed, blood is frequently found in their intestines, which suggests these type 2–exaggerated animals develop portal hypertension and collateral blood circulation that ultimately contributes to their death. Together, these observations demonstrate that IL-10, IL-12, and IFN-γ are all required to prevent the overshooting of Th2 responses during infection with *S. mansoni*. Thus, in schistosomiasis, distinct but equally detrimental forms of lethal tissue pathology develop when the immune response is biased toward an extreme Th1- or Th2-type phenotype. Therefore, co-dominant but controlled

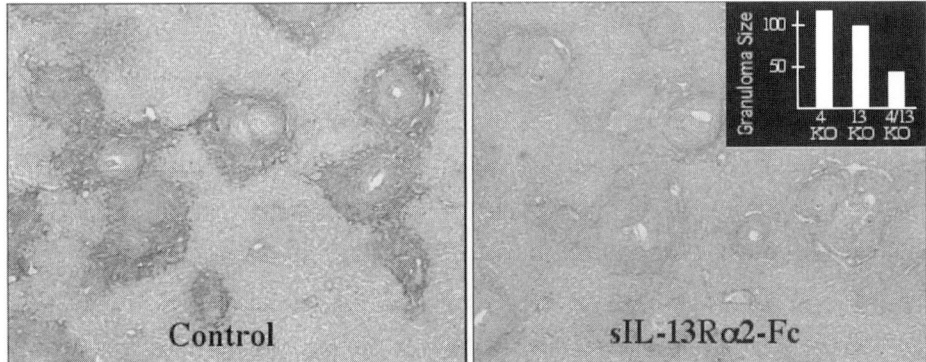

FIG. 3. Pivotal role of IL-13 in schistosome egg–induced hepatic fibrosis. C57BL/6 mice were infected with *S. mansoni* cercariae and treated with sIL-13Rα2-Fc or control Ig on week 6 through week 12 postinfection. Mice were sacrificed and liver sections stained with picrosirius red (dark-staining areas around granulomas) to identify collagen and examined at 25-X magnification. Note the presence of granulomas in the liver of sIL-13Rα2–treated mice, yet absence of significant collagen staining. The *insert* in the second panel shows the relative change in granuloma size in animals deficient in IL-4, IL-13, or simultaneously deficient in IL-4 and IL-13, relative to wild-type mice. Note that granuloma size decreases only in mice deficient in both cytokines.

Th1/Th2 responses may provide the best protection from severe egg-induced immunopathology.

PARASITE VACCINE STRATEGIES

There is as yet no safe, uniformly effective vaccine against any human parasitic infection. The lack of progress in this field is due to many factors, including the low priority that has historically been given to development of vaccines against diseases confined mainly to the developing world. The greater impediments, however, may be related to the nature of parasitic infections themselves. In contrast to those bacterial and viral infections for which highly effective vaccines exist, and for which there is complete immunity induced by primary infection, most antiparasite vaccines will need to outperform the immune response to natural infection. Further, virtually all bacterial or viral vaccines that are currently in use mediate their protection by inducing a strong, long-lived humoral response that inhibits attachment or invasion, promotes clearance, or neutralizes released toxins. By contrast, there are no vaccines that are uniformly effective against diseases caused by intracellular pathogens that require cellular immunity to mediate protection. Thus, the manner in which potentially protective antigens can be administered to generate and maintain appropriate T-cell responses has yet to be proven in a clinical setting; there are no empiric models for these sorts of vaccines. Consequently, for the development of vaccines against intracellular protozoa—for example, malaria, *Leishmania, T. cruzi,* and toxoplasma—simply identifying target antigens will not be sufficient; novel and rational approaches to vaccine design and delivery will need to be explored. The vaccination strategies that are currently being explored to meet these challenges are considered in the general context of B- and T-cell antiparasite vaccines. Note that the examples provided are by no means exhaustive, but reflect general principles of vaccination against extracellular and intracellular targets.

B-Cell Vaccines

Vaccination against Intestinal Protozoa

Parasitic protozoa that have an exclusive extracellular lifestyle in their mammalian hosts and are sensitive to antibody mediated control include the intestinal pathogens *E. histolytica* and *G. lamblia.* Most deaths from *E. histolytica* arise from amebic liver abscess, the major extraintestinal manifestation of disease. An amebic serine–rich protein (SREHP) is a highly immunogenic surface antigen of *E. histolytica,* containing multiple tandem octapeptide and dodecapeptide repeats. Passive immunization with antibodies to SREHP protects SCID mice from amebic liver abscess. Parenteral immunization with recombinant SREHP, or with a SREHP-based DNA vaccine, was highly effective in protecting gerbils against amebic liver abscess (196). Specific serum and mucosal antibodies targeting surface antigens are also known to

be important in elimination of *Giardia* from the host intestine. *Giardia* vaccines containing whole trophozoite preparations protected animals even when challenged with heterologous strains (197). Thus, an immune response to variant surface antigens, which are known to be targets of cytotoxic antibodies, appears not to be essential for control of acute infection, and supports an alternative role for antigenic variation in, for example, diversifying the host range of the parasite (146).

Vaccines Targeting Extracellular Stages of Malaria

Because both preerythrocytic- and erythrocytic-stage malaria parasites are at least transiently exposed to humoral antibody, vaccine strategies based on eliciting high-titered antibodies that can inhibit their invasion of red blood cells or hepatocytes have long been favored vaccine candidates. Antibodies that inhibit the invasion of erythrocytes by the extracellular merozoite stage of malaria *in vitro* are found in some, but not all, individuals living in malaria endemic regions. Although the significance of these inhibitory antibodies to naturally acquired resistance remains unclear, their target antigens nonetheless remain the prime candidates for asexual malaria vaccines (reviewed in Miller et al. [198] and Richie and Saul [199]) (Fig. 4). One of the main targets of invasion-inhibitory antibodies is merozoite surface protein (MSP1), which was the first purified malaria protein to be used as a vaccine (200). The 19-kDa C-terminal fragment of MSP1 is the only part of the larger molecule to be taken into the red cell during invasion. Native and recombinant forms of *P. falciparum* $MSP1_{19}$ and a longer fragment $MSP1_{42}$ have been demonstrated to protect *Aotus* monkeys (201). $MSP1_{42}$ is currently in clinical trials. A recombinant protein 190LCS.T3 from the N-terminal half of MSP1 has also protected *Aotus* monkeys against challenge (202). While MSP1 proteins from different isolates of *P. falciparum* show considerable allelic polymorphism, the regions corresponding to the 19-kDa fragment and to 190LCS.T3 are relatively conserved. Other antigen targets of antibodies that inhibit *P. falciparum* growth *in vitro* include MSP2 and RESA, also known as Pf155, that is discharged from dense granules in the merozoite apical region during invasion. A vaccine formulated from recombinant fragments of each of the molecules significantly decreased parasite density in children from an endemic area of Papua New Guinea (203). It is important to note that the efficacy of vaccines targeting conserved epitopes expressed by extracellular asexual-stage malaria parasites is dependent on the induction of high antibody titers that may not be maintained by natural exposure.

By contrast, blood-stage antigens that appear to be under strong selection pressure in the field are the variant antigens present on infected erythrocytes that mediate adhesion to endothelial cells. Clinical data are consistent with the idea that the accumulation of a large repertoire of PfMEP1 variant-specific antibody responses, as is found in immune adults, is necessary for clinical immunity to malaria. Thus, a vaccine that will confer solid blood-stage immunity in children will be extremely difficult to develop because it would need to

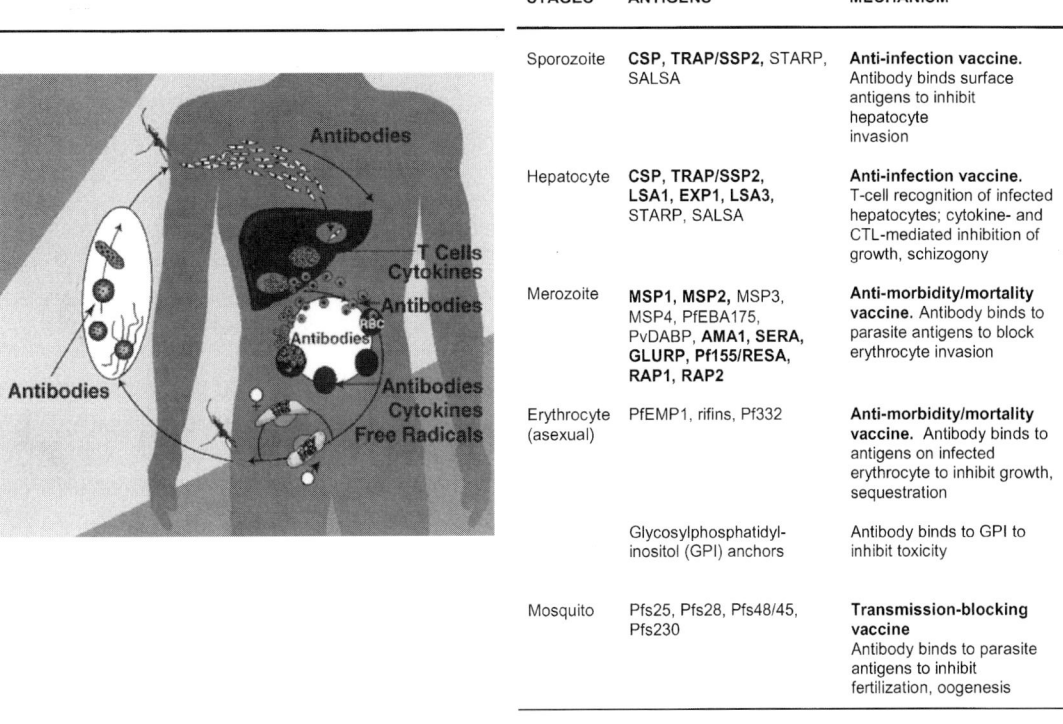

STAGES	ANTIGENS [a]	MECHANISM
Sporozoite	**CSP, TRAP/SSP2,** STARP, SALSA	**Anti-infection vaccine.** Antibody binds surface antigens to inhibit hepatocyte invasion
Hepatocyte	**CSP, TRAP/SSP2, LSA1,** EXP1, **LSA3,** STARP, SALSA	**Anti-infection vaccine.** T-cell recognition of infected hepatocytes; cytokine- and CTL-mediated inhibition of growth, schizogony
Merozoite	**MSP1, MSP2,** MSP3, MSP4, PfEBA175, PvDABP, **AMA1, SERA, GLURP, Pf155/RESA, RAP1, RAP2**	**Anti-morbidity/mortality vaccine.** Antibody binds to parasite antigens to block erythrocyte invasion
Erythrocyte (asexual)	PfEMP1, rifins, Pf332	**Anti-morbidity/mortality vaccine.** Antibody binds to antigens on infected erythrocyte to inhibit growth, sequestration
	Glycosylphosphatidyl-inositol (GPI) anchors	Antibody binds to GPI to inhibit toxicity
Mosquito	Pfs25, Pfs28, Pfs48/45, Pfs230	**Transmission-blocking vaccine** Antibody binds to parasite antigens to inhibit fertilization, oogenesis

[a] Antigens in **bold type** represent those currently in clinical trial

FIG. 4. Stage-specific vaccine targets in malaria parasites. **Left:** Figure depicts the life cycle of malaria and the immune effector mechanisms that target the various developmental forms of the parasite. From Malaria Vaccine Initiative website, *www.malariavaccine.org/mal-what_is_malaria.htm,* with permission. **Right:** The table lists the major candidate vaccine antigens identified at these stages and the proposed mechanism by which immunization would act against each target. Adapted from Richie and Saul (199), with permission.

contain an enormous number of as yet undefined variant antigens. However, recent epidemiologic data also suggest that the risk of severe manifestations of the disease are reduced after only a very few clinical episodes (204) and that parasites causing severe disease tend to express a subset of variant surface antigens (205). Thus, a finite number of variant antigens might be sufficient to elicit broad immunity against severe disease. The general malaria vaccine candidates that are currently being investigated contain two structural domains, termed DBLα CIDR1α, chosen because they appear in the semiconserved head structure of all PfEMP1 molecules sequenced to date (206). A similar approach is being used to develop a vaccine against pregnancy-associated malaria. The variant antigens of parasites sequestered in the placenta during pregnancy have been shown to be distinctive in both their adhesive and antigenic properties (207). The pregnancy malaria vaccine would theoretically work by targeting the DBLγ domain that mediates binding of infected erythrocytes to the placenta.

Studies in the 1980s demonstrated that the sporozoite coat protein, the circumsporozoite protein (CSP), was the target of protective antibodies (reviewed in Nussenzweig and Nussenzweig [95] and Nussenzweig and Zavala [208]). The dominant antibody epitope was represented by the CSP central repeat sequences (NANPn in *P. falciparum*). Vaccines targeting the immunodominant CS protein B-cell epitope have been extensively tested to induce preerythrocytic immunity in malaria (Fig. 4). The induction of anti-CS antibodies alone, however, is not adequate to confer sterilizing immunity against malaria liver stages, and vaccines targeting the CD4 and CD8 epitopes contained within the CS protein are currently being developed (see below).

Effective transmission-blocking immunity works primarily by an antibody-mediated mechanism that acts against the extracellular sexual stages of the parasite within the midgut of a blood-feeding mosquito (reviewed in Carter et al. [209]) (Fig. 4). Transmission-blocking immunity has been induced *in vivo* by immunization with gametes of avian, rodent, and monkey malarias. A series of potential transmission-blocking vaccine candidates have been identified and the genes encoding these surface proteins have now been isolated and sequenced. Although *in vitro* data suggest that antibodies against such antigens may block transmission (210), the high levels of antibodies required will not be maintained by natural boosting since their target antigens are confined to invertebrate stages of the parasite.

Clearly, an optimal vaccine against malaria would need to target multiple antigens and induce immunity against all stages. However, by targeting certain antigens confined to asexual blood stages, the induction of an adult-like immune status among high-risk infants in Sub-Saharan Africa could greatly diminish severe disease and death caused by *P. falciparum*.

T-Cell Vaccines

Vaccination against Leishmaniasis

Vaccines against intracellular parasites will need to induce long-lived cellular immune responses. As already discussed, for diseases such as malaria, leishmaniasis, Chagas disease, and toxoplasmosis, Th1 and/or CD8$^+$ T-cell responses are the effector mechanisms required for protective immunity. An inherent problem with most nonliving vaccines is their relative inefficiency in generating these sorts of cellular responses. A major advance in T-cell vaccine development was the demonstration that proteins derived from *L. major* could elicit a powerful Th1 response and protective immunity if given with recombinant IL-12 as adjuvant (211). IL-12– or IL-12–inducing adjuvants such as BCG, CpG-oligodinucleotides (CpG-ODN), or CD40L, have since been used repeatedly in Leishmania models to potentiate the efficacy of whole-cell killed or recombinant protein vaccines (212). More recently, however, a serious shortcoming of this approach has been appreciated. When mice were challenged with *L. major* 3 months as opposed to 2 weeks after immunization, the protein plus rIL-12 vaccine was no longer effective (213). In contrast, a DNA vaccine encoding the same antigen remained effective, as did the protein given with IL-12 DNA as adjuvant. These results suggest that for the cellular immunity induced by T-cell vaccines to be durable, then persistence of antigen and/or regulatory cytokines may be crucial. Similar findings have recently been reported (214) in which transfer of immune cells from subclinical mice could protect naïve BALB/c mice against a pathogenic challenge and could completely clear the parasite, leaving the mice susceptible to a rechallenge infection. This susceptibility was associated with the disappearance of both parasite-specific effector and memory T cells from secondary lymphoid organs. Such loss of memory T cells following antigen clearance might well explain the repeated failures of a whole-cell killed *L. major* vaccine plus BCG to reduce the incidence of cutaneous leishmaniasis in individuals living in areas of relatively low transmission, where natural boosting is unlikely to have occurred.

These results are somewhat surprising in light of a number of adoptive transfer studies that have clearly demonstrated that both CD4$^+$ and CD8$^+$ memory T cells can be sustained in the absence of antigen. The data might be reconciled, however, in the context of more refined notions about memory T cells as representing heterogeneous populations of central as distinct from effector/memory cells (215). Whereas the former are small, resting, recirculating cells that need to be restimulated with antigen and reeducated with IL-12 to differentiate into IFNγ–producing or cytolytic effectors, the latter

are larger, tissue-seeking cells that readily secrete cytokine or have direct cytolytic activity *ex vivo*. Most importantly, it is effector/memory cells that are likely to be required for protection, and persistent antigen appears necessary to maintain a population of these cells.

The requirement for persistent antigens places major constraints on the development of T-cell vaccines using killed cells or recombinant proteins, and reinforces the rationale for live vaccines. The only vaccination strategy against leishmaniasis that has worked in humans is leishmanization, which is based on the life-long convalescent immunity that is acquired following induction of a lesion at a selected site with small doses of a cutaneous strain. Unfortunately, leishmanization using virulent strains can be associated with severe pathology, and the practice has been discontinued. The generation of safe, live attenuated vaccines using molecular genetic approaches has been accomplished by targeted deletion of genes involved in parasite survival or virulence. Promastigotes lacking the DHFR gene were able to persist in macrophages for several days and provided partial protection against cutaneous leishmaniasis (216). Promastigotes deleted of genes encoding a family of cysteine proteinases were completely attenuated and also produced partial protection against cutaneous disease (217). However, as live parasite vaccines will be extremely difficult to standardize and to deliver in field settings, there has been considerable interest in developing DNA vaccination strategies because, as already indicated, they are capable of eliciting long-lived humoral and cellular immune responses *in vivo*. Protective immunity against cutaneous or visceral leishmaniasis has been demonstrated in mice using single or multivalent DNA vaccines encoding a diversity of leishmania antigens, including gp63, LACK, PSA-2, cysteine proteinase, TSA, LmST11, and histones (reviewed in Handman [212]). Importantly, the DNA vaccines could be administered subcutaneously or intramuscularly and they did not require adjuvants.

Another advantage of DNA vaccines is their ability to elicit specific CD8$^+$ T cells. While CD8$^+$ T cells contribute to leishmania resistance, they are especially important to the control of infections involving *T. cruzi* and *T. gondii*, which require effector CD8$^+$ T cells to kill parasites within cells lacking MHC class II molecules. Furthermore, because *T. cruzi* escapes from the parasitophorous vacuole and becomes cytoplasmic, many of its released antigens have access to the class I processing pathway. Immunization using plasmid DNA encoding the trypomastigote surface antigen (TSA-1) elicited long-lasting class I–restricted CTL and protected mice against lethal *T. cruzi* infection (218). Similarly, immunization with plasmid DNA encoding the *T. gondii* dense granule protein GRA4 induced high levels of specific antibodies and cellular responses and protected mice against a lethal oral challenge with *T. gondii* cysts (219).

Vaccination against Malaria Liver Stages

Because certain stages of malaria parasites infect and replicate in hepatocytes, which express MHC class I, infected hepatocytes are targets of CD8$^+$ T-cell responses, and both CTL and IFN-γ producing CD8$^+$ cells have been implicated in preerythrocytic liver stage immunity (Fig. 4). Irradiated *Plasmodium* sporozoites, which can infect hepatocytes but do not progress to a blood-stage infection, have been shown to protect rodents, monkeys, and humans against malaria by inducing CD8$^+$ T-cell responses against preerythrocytic antigen (reviewed in Hoffman and Doolan [220]). Similar to that described following sterile cure in leishmaniasis, immunity using irradiated sporozoites was lost in rats that were treated with a drug that eliminated parasites in the liver prior to rechallenge (221). Efforts to mimic the protection generated by irradiated sporozoites using nonliving protein- and DNA-based vaccines have yielded encouraging results. A synthetic peptide representing the 102-amino acid–long C-terminal region of the *P. falciparum* CS protein elicited strong CD8$^+$ and CD4$^+$ T cells responses as well as antisporozoite antibodies, in human volunteers, particularly when given with the water-in-oil adjuvant Montanide ISA-720 (222). A construct consisting of a recombinant hybrid particle that includes 19 NANP repeats and the C-terminus of CS fused to the hepatitis-B surface antigen coexpressed in yeast with unfused HbsAg (RTS,S) and incorporating a new oil in water adjuvant (ASO2) induced strong antibody and T-cell responses in adults already primed to CS by preexposure to malaria. Most significantly, vaccine efficacy during the first 9 weeks of follow-up was 71%, but decreased to 0% over the next 6 weeks (223). DNA vaccination strategies are being pursued with a view toward improving the durability and potency of the cellular response. Intramuscular injection of mice with plasmid DNA encoding the *P. yoelii* CSP induced high levels of antibodies and cytotoxic T-lymphocytes against the *P. yoelii* CSP, and the mice had significant reduction in liver-stage parasite burden after challenge (224). In a seminal study, immunization of malaria-naïve volunteers with a *P. falciparum* homolog of this DNA vaccine elicited antigen-specific CD8$^+$ T cells with CTL activity (225). A mixture of five plasmids encoding distinct *P. falciparum* antigens expressed by irradiated sporozoites in hepatocytes, including CS, TRAP, exported protein 2, and liver-stage antigen 1, is being tested in clinical trials (220). However, as the responses to plasmid alone has been relatively weak even after repeated immunizations, the use of sequential immunizations using various heterologous prime/boost protocols are being tested to enhance the effectiveness of preerythrocytic vaccines (reviewed in Schneider et al. [226]). Priming with plasmid DNA encoding CSP and boosting with recombinant adenovirus or pox virus, such as modified vaccinia virus Ankara (MVA), has induced complete protection and very high levels of IFN-γ–secreting CD8$^+$ T cells. Clinical trials of the vaccinia vector used alone and in the prime/boost combination have been initiated.

Vaccination to Prevent Pathology

In many parasitic infections, disease is not directly induced by the parasite but instead is a consequence of the host immune response. Because these pathogens are so well adapted to their hosts, it may therefore be easier and more efficient to design immune interventions that prevent parasite-induced immunopathology rather than the infection itself. While this approach will not lead to eradication of the parasite, it would likely reduce or alleviate the health consequences of infection. The feasibility of an antipathology vaccine was demonstrated in a murine model of schistosomiasis (184). Because disease in schistosomiasis is largely due to the granulomatous pathology that develops around parasite eggs trapped in target host tissues, a valid approach toward immunoprophylaxis for schistosomiasis is to vaccinate to minimize granulomatous pathology. In WT mice, granuloma size and collagen deposition are correlated with the intensity of the type 2 response, and immunologic interventions, such as the administration of IL-4 and IL-13 antagonists, reduces both the size of granulomas and magnitude of fibrosis (discussed above) (181,193). In extensions of these studies, mice immunized with parasite egg antigens plus IL-12 (227) or CpG oligonucleotides (228) to induce an egg-antigen–specific type 1 response, upon subsequent infection, exhibited far less severe egg-associated liver disease than did infected nonimmunized controls. Importantly, several immunodominant egg antigens have been described in recent studies (229,230), thus it may be possible to design recombinant antipathology vaccines that duplicate the promising results produced with these crude parasite extracts.

Vaccines against Helminths

Infection with helminthic parasites remains a significant health problem in many tropical countries. While control measures are available in some areas, in most cases, patients living in endemic regions are quickly reinfected. Therefore, vaccines that reduce parasite and/or egg burdens would be a valuable tool to complement existing disease prevention programs and could represent a less costly and more practical approach than repeated chemotherapy. Nevertheless, while many subunit vaccines have been described and tested in various animal models, suboptimal levels of protection have hindered the development of all but a few of these candidate vaccines (231). Significant advances in vaccination technology over the past decade have made it possible to engineer vaccines that elicit strong cellular and humoral immunity. Novel DNA vectors, improved delivery systems, new adjuvants, and immunomodulatory cytokines allow significant augmentation of the immune response to vaccines and preferential induction of specific effector mechanisms, including antibody isotypes, T helper (Th)–cell subsets and cytotoxic T cells. However, in order to effectively harness and implement these advances, it will be necessary to first better elucidate the immune mechanisms responsible for killing helminth parasites.

The best examples of successful immunization against helminths are provided by vaccine models utilizing radiation-attenuated larval parasites. With the irradiated schistosome vaccine, while complete sterilizing immunity appears to be an unachievable goal, immunity approaching 60% to 80% is clearly possible, and has served as the "gold standard" for schistosome vaccine development (232). The cumulative evidence from vaccine studies conducted in numerous gene KO mice suggest that irradiated parasites can induce protection via both Th1- and Th2-dependent pathways (103). Of interest, however, the protective mechanisms evoked may depend on the time and number of immunizations. Thus, a single vaccination with attenuated parasites induces protection that is highly dependent on IFN-γ and IL-12 (129,232), while mice immunized multiple times develop immunity that operates through Th1- and Th2-dependent pathways (103,233). In each case, however, studies conducted in IFN-γ–deficient and B-cell–deficient mice clearly demonstrate that humoral and cellular mechanisms are both required for the generation of optimal immunity (130,234). Interestingly, while high IgE and IgA isotype levels often correlate with immunity in humans, vaccine studies conducted in IgE-deficient mice have revealed no specific requirement for an IgE Ab response (235).

While there has been extensive research on defined vaccines against helminth infection (reviewed recently by Maizels et al. [236]), none of the candidate antigens have yet to be shown to be protective in humans. Based on antibody responses in schistosome-vaccinated mice, a set of six vaccine candidate antigens has been put forward for phase I trials and at least one of the antigens (GST) has completed phase I and is entering phase II trial. These antigens include glutathione-S-transferase (P28/GST), paramyosin (Sm97); IrV5 (myosin-like 62-kDa protein); triose phosphate isomerase (TPI); Sm23, integrated membrane protein; and Sm14, fatty acid–binding protein (237). A number of filarial vaccine candidates have also been described and are being tested, which include chitinase, tropomyosin, paramyosin, and several larval antigens called the "abundant larval transcript family" (ALT) (236). While these accomplishments represent a significant advance for the field of helminthology, it is important to note that all of the candidate antischistosome vaccine antigens have, at best, provided only partial immunity, with none consistently reaching a required threshold of 40% protection. It is hoped, however, that ongoing improvements in vaccination technology, combined with greater knowledge of the mechanisms controlling resistance, will allow development of more efficacious and better-defined vaccines for these complex organisms.

CONCLUSIONS

The period since the publication of the last version of this chapter in *Fundamental Immunology* has been a time of both intense activity and reflection for the field of immunoparasitology. During this period, public recognition of the importance of malaria as one of three major global infectious diseases (along with AIDS and tuberculosis) has resulted in the launching of major government and private foundation supported vaccine programs aimed primarily at moving candidate immunogens into clinical trials. In addition to its

urgent public health importance, this research should deepen our understanding of protective immune responses against parasites in humans and hopefully stimulate the creation of similar vaccine programs directed against other parasitic diseases.

The last 4 years have also seen a rapid expansion in research dealing with innate determinants of the immune response to parasites and in innate effector functions. This work has important implications not only for understanding the basis of Th subset selection by parasites but also for providing insights useful in the design of new adjuvants and immunomodulators. While the latter is a potential benefit of studies on the innate immune response to all microbial agents, the extreme immune response polarization induced by parasites offers some special advantages. In particular, studies on helminth infections provide a unique opportunity to decipher the innate determinants of the Th2 response and should represent an exciting research area in coming years. At the core of these, as well as investigations on the initiation of immunity to protozoa, will be studies on the nature of DC parasite interactions, a field that has already provided a series of intriguing observations on the functional regulation of this important APC population.

The study of immunoregulatory mechanisms in parasitic infection has also seen important progress in recent years with much of this work testifying to the multilayered complexity and tightly balanced interaction of antiparasitic immune responses. This work has forced us to rethink many of the paradigms concerning polarized effector functions and their regulation in parasitic infection. Thus, it is becoming increasingly evident that rather than being the product of a single arm of the immune response, effective immune control of parasites involves the coordination of both humoral and cellular elements dependent on both Th1 and Th2 cytokines. Moreover, the recent demonstration (159) that T$_{reg}$ cells can markedly inhibit protozoan-induced Th1 function has established that such suppression need not depend on cross-regulation by Th2 cells. While by no means negating the Th1/Th2 paradigm, such observations suggest that its scope in explaining immunoregulatory mechanisms in parasitic infection may be more limited than envisioned in the past.

Although the field still lacks many of the important tools (e.g., transgenesis for helminths) available to those studying less complex prokaryotic pathogens, the enormous advances and sophisticated insights of past decades have placed immunoparasitology back into the mainstream of infectious disease immunology. Although in one sense an extremely positive development, this trend is forcing the field to redefine its own identity and uniqueness. We have sought to emphasize what we believe are the key elements. Of these, the most important are the intricate evolution-based co-adaptation of parasites and the immune system, and the exciting challenge of designing interventions that disrupt this balance in the favor of the host. Clearly, immunologists have many more lessons to learn from studying the host–parasite relationship and it is perhaps only with these lessons that we will achieve the long sought after goal of effective vaccines for preventing parasitic disease.

ACKNOWLEDGMENTS

We are grateful to Allan Saul, Ricardo Gazzinelli, Denise Doolan, Ed Pearce, Chris Hunter, Tom Nutman, Rick Tarleton, Carole Long, and Stephanie James for their invaluable advice in the preparation of this chapter.

REFERENCES

1. Scott P, Natovitz P, Coffman RL, et al. Immunoregulation of cutaneous leishmaniasis. T cell lines that transfer protective immunity or exacerbation belong to different T helper subsets and respond to distinct parasite antigens. *J Exp Med* 1988;168:1675–1684.
2. Heinzel FP, Sadick MD, Holaday BJ, et al. Reciprocal expression of interferon gamma or IL4 during the resolution or progression of murine leishmaniasis. Evidence for expansion of distinct helper T cell subsets. *J Exp Med* 1989;169:59–72.
3. Noben-Trauth N, Paul WE, Sacks DL. IL-4- and IL-4 receptor–deficient BALB/c mice reveal differences in susceptibility to *Leishmania major* parasite substrains. *J Immunol* 1999;162:6132–6140.
4. Joiner KA. Complement evasion by bacteria and parasites. *Annu Rev Microbiol* 1988;42:201–230.
5. Norris KA, Bradt B, Cooper NR, et al. Characterization of a *Trypanosoma cruzi* C3 binding protein with functional and genetic similarities to the human complement regulatory protein, decay-accelerating factor. *J Immunol* 1991;147:2240–2247.
6. Norris KA. Stable transfection of *Trypanosoma cruzi* epimastigotes with the trypomastigote-specific complement regulatory protein cDNA confers complement resistance. *Infect Immun* 1998;66:2460–2465.
7. Pearce EJ, Hall BF, Sher A. Host-specific evasion of the alternative complement pathway by schistosomes correlates with the presence of a phospholipase C–sensitive surface molecule resembling human decay accelerating factor. *J Immunol* 1990;144:2751–2756.
8. Puentes SM, Da Silva RP, Sacks DL, et al. Serum resistance of metacyclic stage *Leishmania major* promastigotes is due to release of C5b-9. *J Immunol* 1990;145:4311–4316.
9. Saraiva EM, Pimenta PF, Brodin TN, et al. Changes in lipophosphoglycan and gene expression associated with the development of *Leishmania major* in *Phlebotomus papatasi*. *Parasitology* 1995;111:275–287.
10. Kweider M, Lemesre JL, Santoro F, et al. Development of metacyclic *Leishmania* promastigotes is associated with the increasing expression of GP65, the major surface antigen. *Parasite Immunol* 1989;11:197–209.
11. Brittingham A, Morrison CJ, McMaster WR, et al. Role of the Leishmania surface protease gp63 in complement fixation, cell adhesion, and resistance to complement-mediated lysis. *J Immunol* 1995;155:3102–3111.
12. Mosser DM, Edelson PJ. The mouse macrophage receptor for C3bi (CR3) is a major mechanism in the phagocytosis of *Leishmania* promastigotes. *J Immunol* 1985;135:2785–2789.
13. Braga LL, Ninomiya H, McCoy JJ, et al. Inhibition of the complement membrane attack complex by the galactose-specific adhesion of *Entamoeba histolytica*. *J Clin Invest* 1992;90:1131–1137.
14. Raper J, Fung R, Ghiso J, et al. Characterization of a novel trypanosome lytic factor from human serum. *Infect Immun* 1999;67:1910–1916.
15. Smith AB, Esko JD, Hajduk SL. Killing of trypanosomes by the human haptoglobin-related protein. *Science* 1995;268:284–286.
16. De Greef C, Hamers R. The serum resistance-associated (SRA) gene of *Trypanosoma brucei rhodesiense* encodes a variant surface glycoprotein-like protein. *Mol Biochem Parasitol* 1994;68:277–284.
17. Xong HV, Vanhamme L, Chamekh M, et al. A VSG expression site–associated gene confers resistance to human serum in *Trypanosoma rhodesiense*. *Cell* 1998;95:839–846.
18. Andrews NW. The acid-active hemolysin of *Trypanosoma cruzi*. *Exp Parasitol* 1990;71:241–244.
19. Joiner KA, Fuhrman SA, Miettinen HM, et al. *Toxoplasma gondii:* fusion competence of parasitophorous vacuoles in Fc receptor-transfected fibroblasts. *Science* 1990;249:641–646.
20. James SL, Sher A, Lazdins JK, et al. Macrophages as effector cells of protective immunity in murine schistosomiasis. II. Killing of newly transformed schistosomula in vitro by macrophages activated as a consequence of *Schistosoma mansoni* infection. *J Immunol* 1982;128:1535–1540.
21. Herbert DR, Lee JJ, Lee NA, et al. Role of IL-5 in innate and adaptive immunity to larval *Strongyloides stercoralis* in mice. *J Immunol* 2000;165:4544–4551.
22. Gazzinelli RT, Hieny S, Wynn TA, et al. Interleukin 12 is required for the T-lymphocyte–independent induction of interferon gamma by an intracellular parasite and induces resistance in T-cell–deficient hosts. *Proc Natl Acad Sci U S A* 1993;90:6115–6119.
23. Tripp CS, Wolf SF, Unanue ER. Interleukin 12 and tumor necrosis factor alpha are co-stimulators of interferon gamma production by natural killer cells in severe combined immunodeficiency mice with listeriosis, and interleukin 10 is a physiologic antagonist. *Proc Natl Acad Sci U S A* 1993;90:3725–3729.
24. Hunter CA, Chizzonite R, Remington JS. IL-1 beta is required for IL-12 to induce production of IFN-gamma by NK cells. A role for IL-1 beta in the T cell-independent mechanism of resistance against intracellular pathogens. *J Immunol* 1995;155:4347–4354.
25. Hunter CA, Ellis-Neyer L, Gabriel KE, et al. The role of the CD28/B7 interaction in the regulation of NK cell responses during infection with *Toxoplasma gondii*. *J Immunol* 1997;158:2285–2293.
26. Scharton-Kersten TM, Sher A. Role of natural killer cells in innate resistance to protozoan infections. *Curr Opin Immunol* 1997;9:44–51.
27. Hunter CA, Bermudez L, Beernink H, et al. Transforming growth factor-beta inhibits interleukin-12–induced production of interferon-gamma by natural killer cells: a role for transforming growth factor-beta in the regulation of T cell-independent resistance to Toxoplasma gondii. *Eur J Immunol* 1995;25:994–1000.
28. Hunter CA, Sher A. Innate immunity to parasitic infections. In: Kaufman S, Sher A, Ahmed R, eds. *The immunology of infectious disease.* Washington, DC: ASM Press, 2001:111–125.
29. Bregenholt S, Berche P, Brombacher F, et al. Conventional alpha beta T cells are sufficient for innate and adaptive immunity against enteric *Listeria monocytogenes*. *J Immunol* 2001;166:1871–1876.
30. Kasper LH, Matsuura T, Fonseka S, et al. Induction of gammadelta T cells during acute murine infection with *Toxoplasma gondii*. *J Immunol* 1996;157:5521–5527.
31. Scalise F, Gerli R, Castellucci G, et al. Lymphocytes bearing the gamma delta T-cell receptor in acute toxoplasmosis. *Immunology* 1992;76:668–670.
32. Hisaeda H, Nagasawa H, Maeda K, et al. Gamma delta T cells play an important role in hsp65 expression and in acquiring protective immune responses against infection with *Toxoplasma gondii*. *J Immunol* 1995;155:244–251.
33. Tsuji M, Mombaerts P, Lefrancois L, et al. Gamma delta T cells contribute to immunity against the liver stages of malaria in alpha beta T-cell–deficient mice. *Proc Natl Acad Sci U S A* 1994;91:345–349.
34. Janeway CA Jr. Approaching the asymptote? Evolution and revolution in immunology. *Cold Spring Harb Symp Quant Biol* 1989;54:1–13.
35. Ropert C, Gazzinelli RT. Signaling of immune system cells by glycosylphosphatidylinositol (GPI) anchor and related structures derived from parasitic protozoa. *Curr Opin Microbiol* 2000;3:395–403.
36. Almeida IC, Gazzinelli RT. Proinflammatory activity of glycosylphosphatidylinositol anchors derived from *Trypanosoma cruzi:* structural and functional analyses. *J Leukoc Biol* 2001;70:467–477.
37. Schofield L, McConville MJ, Hansen D, et al. CD1d-restricted immunoglobulin G formation to GPI-anchored antigens mediated by NKT cells. *Science* 1999;283:225–229.
38. Molano A, Park SH, Chiu YH, et al. Cutting edge: the IgG response to the circumsporozoite protein is MHC class II–dependent and CD1d-independent: exploring the role of GPIs in NK T cell activation and antimalarial responses. *J Immunol* 2000;164:5005–5009.
39. Schnare M, Barton GM, Holt AC, et al. Toll-like receptors control

activation of adaptive immune responses. *Nat Immunol* 2001;2:947–950.

40. Velupillai P, Harn DA. Oligosaccharide-specific induction of interleukin 10 production by B220+ cells from schistosome-infected mice: a mechanism for regulation of CD4+ T-cell subsets. *Proc Natl Acad Sci U S A* 1994;91:18–22.

41. Sousa CR, Hieny S, Scharton-Kersten T, et al. In vivo microbial stimulation induces rapid CD40 ligand-independent production of interleukin 12 by dendritic cells and their redistribution to T cell areas. *J Exp Med* 1997;186:1819–1829.

42. Aliberti J, Reis e Sousa C, Schito M, et al. CCR5 provides a signal for microbial induced production of IL-12 by CD8 alpha+ dendritic cells. *Nat Immunol* 2000;1:83–87.

42a. Aliberti J, Valenzuela JG, Carruthers VB, et al. Molecular mimicry of a CCR5 binding-domain in the microbial activation of dendritic cells. *Nature Immunology* 2003 in press (May).

43. Reiner SL, Zheng S, Wang ZE, et al. Leishmania promastigotes evade interleukin 12 (IL-12) induction by macrophages and stimulate a broad range of cytokines from CD4+ T cells during initiation of infection. *J Exp Med* 1994;179:447–456.

44. Belkaid Y, Butcher B, Sacks DL. Analysis of cytokine production by inflammatory mouse macrophages at the single-cell level: selective impairment of IL-12 induction in Leishmania-infected cells. *Eur J Immunol* 1998;28:1389–1400.

45. Gorak PM, Engwerda CR, Kaye PM. Dendritic cells, but not macrophages, produce IL-12 immediately following *Leishmania donovani* infection. *Eur J Immunol* 1998;28:687–695.

46. Konecny P, Stagg AJ, Jebbari H, et al. Murine dendritic cells internalize *Leishmania major* promastigotes, produce IL-12 p40 and stimulate primary T cell proliferation in vitro. *Eur J Immunol* 1999;29:1803–1811.

47. von Stebut E, Belkaid Y, Jakob T, et al. Uptake of *Leishmania major* amastigotes results in activation and interleukin 12 release from murine skin-derived dendritic cells: implications for the initiation of anti-Leishmania immunity. *J Exp Med* 1998;188:1547–1552.

48. Piedrafita D, Proudfoot L, Nikolaev AV, et al. Regulation of macrophage IL-12 synthesis by Leishmania phosphoglycans. *Eur J Immunol* 1999;29:235–244.

49. Maldonado C, Trejo W, Ramirez A, et al. Lipophosphopeptidoglycan of *Entamoeba histolytica* induces an antiinflammatory innate immune response and downregulation of toll-like receptor 2 (TLR-2) gene expression in human monocytes. *Arch Med Res* 2000;31:S71–S73.

50. Aliberti J, Hieny S, Sousa CR, et al. Lipoxin-medited inhibition of IL-12 production by DCs: a mechanism for the regulation of microbial immunity. *Nat Immunol* 2002;3:76–82.

51. Reiner SL, Locksley RM. The regulation of immunity to *Leishmania major*. *Annu Rev Immunol* 1995;13:151–177.

52. Launois P, Maillard I, Pingel S, et al. IL-4 rapidly produced by V beta 4 V alpha 8 CD4+ T cells instructs Th2 development and susceptibility to *Leishmania major* in BALB/c mice. *Immunity* 1997;6:541–549.

53. Julia V, Rassoulzadegan M, Glaichenhaus N. Resistance to *Leishmania major* induced by tolerance to a single antigen. *Science* 1996;274:421–423.

54. Bix M, Wang ZE, Thiel B, et al. Genetic regulation of commitment to interleukin 4 production by a CD4(+) T cell–intrinsic mechanism. *J Exp Med* 1998;188:2289–2299.

55. Maillard I, Launois P, Himmelrich H, et al. Functional plasticity of the LACK-reactive Vbeta4-Valpha8 CD4(+) T cells normally producing the early IL-4 instructing Th2 cell development and susceptibility to *Leishmania major* in BALB / c mice. *Eur J Immunol* 2001;31:1288–1296.

56. von Stebut E, Belkaid Y, Nguyen BV, et al. *Leishmania major*-infected murine langerhans cell-like dendritic cells from susceptible mice release IL-12 after infection and vaccinate against experimental cutaneous leishmaniasis. *Eur J Immunol* 2000;30:3498–3506.

57. Guler ML, Gorham JD, Hsieh CS, et al. Genetic susceptibility to Leishmania: IL-12 responsiveness in TH1 cell development. *Science* 1996;271:984–987.

58. Malherbe L, Filippi C, Julia V, et al. Selective activation and expansion of high-affinity CD4+ T cells in resistant mice upon infection with *Leishmania major*. *Immunity* 2000;13:771–782.

59. Bretscher PA, Wei G, Menon JN, et al. Establishment of stable, cell-mediated immunity that makes "susceptible" mice resistant to *Leishmania major*. *Science* 1992;257:539–542.

60. Laskay T, Diefenbach A, Rollinghoff M, et al. Early parasite containment is decisive for resistance to *Leishmania major* infection. *Eur J Immunol* 1995;25:2220–2227.

61. Constant SL, Lee KS, Bottomly K. Site of antigen delivery can influence T cell priming: pulmonary environment promotes preferential Th2-type differentiation. *Eur J Immunol* 2000;30:840–847.

62. Nabors GS, Nolan T, Croop W, et al. The influence of the site of parasite inoculation on the development of Th1 and Th2 type immune responses in (BALB/c × C57BL/6) F1 mice infected with *Leishmania major*. *Parasite Immunol* 1995;17:569–579.

63. Jankovic D, Sher A, Yap G. Th1/Th2 effector choice in parasitic infection: decision making by committee. *Curr Opin Immunol* 2001; 13:403–409.

64. Finkelman FD, Urban JF Jr. The other side of the coin: the protective role of the TH2 cytokines. *J Allergy Clin Immunol* 2001;107:772–780.

65. Chiaramonte MG, Schopf LR, Neben TY, et al. IL-13 is a key regulatory cytokine for Th2 cell–mediated pulmonary granuloma formation and IgE responses induced by *Schistosoma mansoni* eggs. *J Immunol* 1999;162:920–930.

66. Jankovic D, Kullberg MC, Noben-Trauth N, et al. Single cell analysis reveals that IL-4 receptor/Stat6 signaling is not required for the in vivo or in vitro development of CD4+ lymphocytes with a Th2 cytokine profile. *J Immunol* 2000;164:3047–3055.

67. Schmitz J, Thiel A, Kuhn R, et al. Induction of interleukin 4 (IL-4) expression in T helper (Th) cells is not dependent on IL-4 from non-Th cells. *J Exp Med* 1994;179:1349–1353.

68. Park AY, Hondowicz BD, Scott P. IL-12 is required to maintain a Th1 response during *Leishmania major* infection. *J Immunol* 2000; 165:896–902.

69. Yap G, Pesin M, Sher A. Cutting edge: IL-12 is required for the maintenance of IFN-gamma production in T cells mediating chronic resistance to the intracellular pathogen, *Toxoplasma gondii*. *J Immunol* 2000;165:628-631.

70. Jankovic D, Kullberg MC, Hieny S, et al. In the absence of IL-12 CD4+ T cell responses to intracellular pathogens fail to default to a Th2 pattern and are host protective in an IL-10−/− setting. *Immunity* 2002;16:429–439.

71. Schulz O, Edwards DA, Schito M, et al. CD40 triggering of heterodimeric IL-12 p70 production by dendritic cells in vivo requires a microbial priming signal. *Immunity* 2000;13:453–462.

72. MacDonald AS, Straw AD, Bauman B, et al. CD8(−) Dendritic cell activation status plays an integral role in influencing Th2 response development. *J Immunol* 2001;167:1982–1988.

73. Whelan M, Harnett MM, Houston KM, et al. A filarial nematode-secreted product signals dendritic cells to acquire a phenotype that drives development of Th2 cells. *J Immunol* 2000;164:6453–6460.

74. Muller I, Pedrazzini T, Farrell JP, et al. T-cell responses and immunity to experimental infection with *Leishmania major*. *Annu Rev Immunol* 1989;7:561–578.

75. Denkers EY, Yap G, Scharton-Kersten T, et al. Perforin-mediated cytolysis plays a limited role in host resistance to *Toxoplasma gondii*. *J Immunol* 1997;159:1903–1908.

76. Doolan DL, Hoffman SL. The complexity of protective immunity against liver-stage malaria. *J Immunol* 2000;165:1453–1462.

77. Kumar S, Tarleton RL. The relative contribution of antibody production and CD8+ T cell function to immune control of *Trypanosoma cruzi*. *Parasite Immunol* 1998;20:207–216.

78. Belosevic M, Finbloom DS, Van Der Meide PH, et al. Administration of monoclonal anti–IFN-gamma antibodies in vivo abrogates natural resistance of C3H/HeN mice to infection with *Leishmania major*. *J Immunol* 1989;143:266–274.

79. Torrico F, Heremans H, Rivera MT, et al. Endogenous IFN-gamma is required for resistance to acute *Trypanosoma cruzi* infection in mice. *J Immunol* 1991;146:3626–3632.

80. Scharton-Kersten TM, Wynn TA, Denkers EY, et al. In the absence of endogenous IFN-gamma, mice develop unimpaired IL-12 responses to *Toxoplasma gondii* while failing to control acute infection. *J Immunol* 1996;157:4045–4054.

81. McDonald V. Host cell-mediated responses to infection with Cryptosporidium. *Parasite Immunol* 2000;22:597–604.

82. Wei XQ, Charles IG, Smith A, et al. Altered immune responses in mice lacking inducible nitric oxide synthase. *Nature* 1995;375:408–411.

83. Nashleanas M, Scott P. Activated T cells induce macrophages to produce NO and control *Leishmania major* in the absence of tumor necrosis factor receptor p55. *Infect Immun* 2000;68:1428–1434.

84. Wilhelm P, Ritter U, Labbow S, et al. Rapidly fatal leishmaniasis in resistant C57BL/6 mice lacking TNF. *J Immunol* 2001;166:4012–4019.

85. Bogdan C, Rollinghoff M, Diefenbach A. Reactive oxygen and reactive nitrogen intermediates in innate and specific immunity. *Curr Opin Immunol* 2000;12:64–76.

86. Good MF, Doolan DL. Immune effector mechanisms in malaria. *Curr Opin Immunol* 1999;11:412–419.

87. Yap GS, Sher A. Effector cells of both nonhemopoietic and hemopoietic origin are required for interferon (IFN)-gamma- and tumor necrosis factor (TNF)-alpha–dependent host resistance to the intracellular pathogen, *Toxoplasma gondii*. *J Exp Med* 1999;189:1083–1092.

88. Scharton-Kersten TM, Yap G, Magram J, et al. Inducible nitric oxide is essential for host control of persistent but not acute infection with the intracellular pathogen *Toxoplasma gondii*. *J Exp Med* 1997;185:1261–1273.

89. Collazo CM, Yap GS, Sempowski GD, et al. Inactivation of LRG-47 and IRG-47 reveals a family of interferon gamma–inducible genes with essential, pathogen-specific roles in resistance to infection. *J Exp Med* 2001;194:181–188.

90. Pfefferkorn ER, Eckel M, Rebhun S. Interferon-gamma suppresses the growth of *Toxoplasma gondii* in human fibroblasts through starvation for tryptophan. *Mol Biochem Parasitol* 1986;20:215–224.

91. Good MF. Towards a blood-stage vaccine for malaria: are we following all the leads? *Nat Rev Immunol* 2001;1:117–125.

92. Anstey NM, Weinberg JB, Hassanali MY, et al. Nitric oxide in Tanzanian children with malaria: inverse relationship between malaria severity and nitric oxide production/nitric oxide synthase type 2 expression. *J Exp Med* 1996;184:557–567.

93. Cohen S, McGregor IA, Carrington S. Gamma globulin and acquired immunity to malaria. *Nature* 1961;192:733–737.

94. Druihle P, Perignon JL. Mechanisms of defence against P. falciparum asexual blood stages in humans. *Immunol Lett* 1994;41:115–120.

95. Nussenzweig V, Nussenzweig RS. Circumsporozoite proteins of malaria parasites. *Cell* 1985;42:401–403.

96. Hoffman SL, Franke ED. Inducing protective immune responses against the sporozoite and liver stages of Plasmodium. *Immunol Lett* 1994;41:89–94.

97. Good MF, Kaslow DC, Miller LH. Pathways and strategies for developing a malaria blood-stage vaccine. *Annu Rev Immunol* 1998;16:57–87.

98. Kang H, Remington JS, Suzuki Y. Decreased resistance of B cell–deficient mice to infection with *Toxoplasma gondii* despite unimpaired expression of IFN-gamma, TNF-alpha, and inducible nitric oxide synthase. *J Immunol* 2000;164:2629–2634.

99. Nutman TB, Kumaraswami V. Regulation of the immune response in lymphatic filariasis: perspectives on acute and chronic infection with *Wuchereria bancrofti* in South India. *Parasite Immunol* 2001;23:389–399.

100. Finkelman FD, Wynn TA, Donaldson DD, et al. The role of IL-13 in helminth-induced inflammation and protective immunity against nematode infections. *Curr Opin Immunol* 1999;11:420–426.

101. King CL. Transmission intensity and human immune responses to lymphatic filariasis. *Parasite Immunol* 2001;23:363–371.

102. Grencis RK. Cytokine regulation of resistance and susceptibility to intestinal nematode infection - from host to parasite. *Vet Parasitol* 2001;100:45–50.

103. Wynn TA, Hoffmann KF. Defining a schistosomiasis vaccination strategy—is it really Th1 versus Th2? *Parasitol Today* 2000;16:497–501.

104. Bancroft AJ, Else KJ, Sypek JP, et al. Interleukin-12 promotes a chronic intestinal nematode infection. *Eur J Immunol* 1997;27:866–870.

105. Bancroft AJ, McKenzie AN, Grencis RK. A critical role for IL-13 in resistance to intestinal nematode infection. *J Immunol* 1998;160:3453–3461.

106. Bancroft AJ, Artis D, Donaldson DD, et al. Gastrointestinal nematode expulsion in IL-4 knockout mice is IL-13 dependent. *Eur J Immunol* 2000;30:2083–2091.

107. Artis D, Humphreys NE, Bancroft AJ, et al. Tumor necrosis factor alpha is a critical component of interleukin 13–mediated protective T helper cell type 2 responses during helminth infection. *J Exp Med* 1999;190:953–962.

108. Helmby H, Takeda K, Akira S, et al. Interleukin (IL)-18 promotes the development of chronic gastrointestinal helminth infection by downregulating IL-13. *J Exp Med* 2001;194:355–364.

109. Schopf LR, Hoffmann KF, Cheever AW, et al. IL-10 is critical for host resistance and survival during gastrointestinal helminth infection. *J. Immunol* 2002; In press.

110. Urban JF Jr, Noben-Trauth N, Donaldson DD, et al. IL-13, IL-4Ralpha, and Stat6 are required for the expulsion of the gastrointestinal nematode parasite *Nippostrongylus brasiliensis*. *Immunity* 1998;8:255–264.

111. Urban JF Jr, Noben-Trauth N, Schopf L, et al. Cutting edge: IL-4 receptor expression by non-bone marrow–derived cells is required to expel gastrointestinal nematode parasites. *J Immunol* 2001;167:6078–6081.

112. Urban JF Jr, Schopf L, Morris SC, et al. Stat6 signaling promotes protective immunity against *Trichinella spiralis* through a mast cell– and T cell–dependent mechanism. *J Immunol* 2000;164:2046–2052.

113. Khan WI, Vallance BA, Blennerhassett PA, et al. Critical role for signal transducer and activator of transcription factor 6 in mediating intestinal muscle hypercontractility and worm expulsion in *Trichinella spiralis*–infected mice. *Infect Immun* 2001;69:838–844.

114. Finkelman FD, Shea-Donohue T, Goldhill J, et al. Cytokine regulation of host defense against parasitic gastrointestinal nematodes: lessons from studies with rodent models. *Annu Rev Immunol* 1997;15:505–533.

115. Bell RG. The generation and expression of immunity to Trichinella spiralis in laboratory rodents. *Adv Parasitol* 1998;41:149–217.

116. Shea-Donohue T, Sullivan C, Finkelman FD, et al. The role of IL-4 in *Heligmosomoides polygyrus*-induced alterations in murine intestinal epithelial cell function. *J Immunol* 2001;167:2234–2239.

117. Khan WI, Blennerhassett PA, Deng Y, et al. IL-12 gene transfer alters gut physiology and host immunity in nematode-infected mice. *Am J Physiol Gastrointest Liver Physiol* 2001;281:G102–110.

118. Rotman HL, Yutanawiboonchai W, Brigandi RA, et al. *Strongyloides stercoralis*: eosinophil-dependent immune-mediated killing of third stage larvae in BALB/cByJ mice. *Exp Parasitol* 1996;82:267–278.

119. Korenaga M, Hitoshi Y, Takatsu K, et al. Regulatory effect of anti-interleukin-5 monoclonal antibody on intestinal worm burden in a primary infection with *Strongyloides venezuelensis* in mice. *Int J Parasitol* 1994;24:951–957.

120. Yoshida T, Ikuta K, Sugaya H, et al. Defective B-1 cell development and impaired immunity against *Angiostrongylus cantonensis* in IL-5R alpha-deficient mice. *Immunity* 1996;4:483–494.

121. Vallance BA, Blennerhassett PA, Deng Y, et al. IL-5 contributes to worm expulsion and muscle hypercontractility in a primary T. spiralis infection. *Am J Physiol* 1999;277:G400–408.

122. Dombrowicz D, Capron M. Eosinophils, allergy and parasites. *Curr Opin Immunol* 2001;13:716–720.

123. Donaldson LE, Schmitt E, Huntley JF, et al. A critical role for stem cell factor and c-kit in host protective immunity to an intestinal helminth. *Int Immunol* 1996;8:559–567.

124. Faulkner H, Humphreys N, Renauld JC, et al. Interleukin-9 is involved in host protective immunity to intestinal nematode infection. *Eur J Immunol* 1997;27:2536–2540.

125. Faulkner H, Renauld JC, Van Snick J, et al. Interleukin-9 enhances resistance to the intestinal nematode *Trichuris muris*. *Infect Immun* 1998;66:3832–3840.

126. Richard M, Grencis RK, Humphreys NE, et al. Anti–IL-9 vaccination prevents worm expulsion and blood eosinophilia in *Trichuris muris*–infected mice. *Proc Natl Acad Sci U S A* 2000;97:767–772.

127. Kullberg MC, Berzofsky JA, Jankovic DL, et al. T cell-derived IL-3 induces the production of IL-4 by non-B, non-T cells to amplify the Th2-cytokine response to a non-parasite antigen in *Schistosoma mansoni*-infected mice. *J Immunol* 1996;156:1482–1489.

128. Marquet S, Abel L, Hillaire D, et al. Genetic localization of a locus controlling the intensity of infection by *Schistosoma mansoni* on chromosome 5q31-q33. *Nat Genet* 1996;14:181–184.

129. Wynn TA, Reynolds A, James S, et al. IL-12 enhances vaccine-induced immunity to schistosomes by augmenting both humoral and cell-mediated immune responses against the parasite. *J Immunol* 1996;157:4068–4078.

130. Jankovic D, Wynn TA, Kullberg MC, et al. Optimal vaccination

against *Schistosoma mansoni* requires the induction of both B cell–and IFN-gamma–dependent effector mechanisms. *J Immunol* 1999; 162:345–351.

131. Hoffmann KF, James SL, Cheever AW, et al. Studies with double cytokine-deficient mice reveal that highly polarized Th1- and Th2-type cytokine and antibody responses contribute equally to vaccine-induced immunity to *Schistosoma mansoni. J Immunol* 1999; 163:927–938.

132. Babu S, Ganley LM, Klei TR, et al. Role of gamma interferon and interleukin-4 in host defense against the human filarial parasite Brugia malayi. *Infect Immun* 2000;68:3034–3035.

133. Black SJ, Seed JR, Murphy NB. Innate and acquired resistance to African trypanosomiasis. *J Parasitol* 2001;87:1–9.

134. Sternberg JM. Immunobiology of African trypanosomiasis. *Chem Immunol* 1998;70:186–199.

135. Hertz CJ, Filutowicz H, Mansfield JM. Resistance to the African trypanosomes is IFN-gamma dependent. *J Immunol* 1998;161:6775–6783.

136. Singer SM, Nash TE. T-cell–dependent control of acute *Giardia lamblia* infections in mice. *Infect Immun* 2000;68:170–175.

137. Faubert G. Immune response to *Giardia duodenalis. Clin Microbiol Rev* 2000;13:35-54,

138. Tarleton RL, Zhang L. Chagas disease etiology: autoimmunity or parasite persistence? *Parasitol Today* 1999;15:94–99.

139. Bogdan C, Gessner A, Solbach W, et al. Invasion, control and persistence of Leishmania parasites. *Curr Opin Immunol* 1996;8:517–525.

140. Pearce EJ, Sher A. Mechanisms of immune evasion in schistosomiasis. *Contrib Microbiol Immunol* 1987;8:219–232.

141. Maizels RM, Bundy DA, Selkirk ME, et al. Immunological modulation and evasion by helminth parasites in human populations. *Nature* 1993;365:797–805.

142. Davies SJ, Grogan JL, Blank RB, et al. Modulation of blood fluke development in the liver by hepatic CD4$^+$ lymphocytes. *Science* 2001;294:1358–1361.

143. Wolowczuk I, Nutten S, Roye O, et al. Infection of mice lacking interleukin-7 (IL-7) reveals an unexpected role for IL-7 in the development of the parasite *Schistosoma mansoni. Infect Immun* 1999;67: 4183–4190.

144. Deitsch KW, Moxon ER, Wellems TE. Shared themes of antigenic variation and virulence in bacterial, protozoal, and fungal infections. *Microbiol Mol Biol Rev* 1997;61:281–293.

145. Nash TE. Antigenic variation in *Giardia lamblia* and the host's immune response. *Philos Trans R Soc London B Biol Sci* 1997;352:1369–1375.

146. Singer SM, Elmendorf HG, Conrad JT, et al. Biological selection of variant-specific surface proteins in *Giardia lamblia. J Infect Dis* 2001;183:119–124.

147. Brown KN, Brown IN. Immunity to malaria: antigenic variation in chronic infections of *Plasmodium knowlesi. Nature* 1965;208:1286–1288.

148. Howard RJ, Barnwell JW, Kao V. Antigenic variation of *Plasmodium knowlesi* malaria: identification of the variant antigen on infected erythrocytes. *Proc Natl Acad Sci U S A* 1983;80:4129–4133.

149. Newbold CI. Antigenic variation in *Plasmodium falciparum:* mechanisms and consequences. *Curr Opin Microbiol* 1999;2:420–425.

150. Maizels RM, Gomez-Escobar N, Gregory WF, et al. Immune evasion genes from filarial nematodes. *Int J Parasitol* 2001;31:889–898.

151. Langlet C, Mazingue C, Dessaint JP, et al. Inhibition of primary and secondary IgE-response by a schistosome-derived inhibitory factor. *Int Arch Allergy Appl Immunol* 1984;73:225–230.

152. MacDonald AS, Loke P, Allen JE. Suppressive antigen-presenting cells in helminth infection. *Pathobiology* 1999;67:265–268.

153. Gilbert SC, Plebanski M, Gupta S, et al. Association of malaria parasite population structure, HLA, and immunological antagonism. *Science* 1998;279:1173–1177.

154. Millar AE, Wleklinski-Lee M, Kahn SJ. The surface protein superfamily of *Trypanosoma cruzi* stimulates a polarized Th1 response that becomes anergic. *J Immunol* 1999;162:6092–6099.

155. Urban BC, Ferguson DJ, Pain A, et al. *Plasmodium falciparum*–infected erythrocytes modulate the maturation of dendritic cells. *Nature* 1999;400:73–77.

156. Greenwood BM. Possible role of a B-cell mitogen in hypergammaglobulinaemia in malaria and trypanosomiasis. *Lancet* 1974;1:435–436.

157. Reina-San-Martin B, Degrave W, Rougeot C, et al. A B-cell mitogen from a pathogenic trypanosome is a eukaryotic proline racemase. *Nat Med* 2000;6:890–897.

158. Belkaid Y, Hoffmann KF, Mendez S, et al. The role of interleukin (IL)-10 in the persistence of *Leishmania major* in the skin after healing and the therapeutic potential of anti-IL-10 receptor antibody for sterile cure. *J Exp Med* 2001;194:1497–1506.

159. Belkaid Y, Piccirillo CA, Mendez S, et al. CD4+ CD25+ regulatory T cells control *Leishmania major* persistence and immunity. *Nature* 2002;420:502–7.

159a. Shevach EM. Certified professionals: CD4(+)CD25(+) suppressor T cells. *J Exp Med* 2001;193:41–46.

160. Wynn TA, Kwiatkowski D. Pathology and Pathogenesis of Parasitic Disease. In: Kaufmann S, Sher, A. and Ahmed, ed. *Immunology of infectious diseases.* Washington DC: ASM Press, 2001;293–306.

161. Marshall AJ, Brunet LR, van Gessel Y, et al. Toxoplasma gondii and *Schistosoma mansoni* synergize to promote hepatocyte dysfunction associated with high levels of plasma TNF-alpha and early death in C57BL/6 mice. *J Immunol* 1999;163:2089–2097.

162. Taylor MJ, Cross HF, Bilo K. Inflammatory responses induced by the filarial nematode *Brugia malayi* are mediated by lipopolysaccharide-like activity from endosymbiotic Wolbachia bacteria. *J Exp Med* 2000;191:1429–1436.

163. Saint Andre A, Blackwell NM, Hall LR, et al. The role of endosymbiotic *Wolbachia bacteria* in the pathogenesis of river blindness. *Science* 2002;295:1892–1895.

164. Infante-Duarte C, Kamradt T. Th1/Th2 balance in infection. *Springer Semin Immunopathol* 1999;21:317–338.

165. Kaifi JT, Diaconu E, Pearlman E. Distinct roles for PECAM-1, ICAM-1, and VCAM-1 in recruitment of neutrophils and eosinophils to the cornea in ocular onchocerciasis (river blindness). *J Immunol* 2001; 166:6795–6801.

166. Hoffmann KF, Cheever AW, Wynn TA. IL-10 and the dangers of immune polarization: excessive type 1 and type 2 cytokine responses induce distinct forms of lethal immunopathology in murine schistosomiasis. *J Immunol* 2000;164:6406–6416.

167. Yap GS, Sher A. Cell-mediated immunity to *Toxoplasma gondii:* initiation, regulation and effector function. *Immunobiology* 1999; 201:240–247.

168. Dai WJ, Kohler G, Brombacher F. Both innate and acquired immunity to *Listeria monocytogenes* infection are increased in IL-10-deficient mice. *J Immunol* 1997;158:2259–2267.

169. Gazzinelli RT, Wysocka M, Hieny S, et al. In the absence of endogenous IL-10, mice acutely infected with *Toxoplasma gondii* succumb to a lethal immune response dependent on CD4$^+$ T cells and accompanied by overproduction of IL-12, IFN-gamma and TNF-alpha. *J Immunol* 1996;157:798–805.

170. Holscher C, Mohrs M, Dai WJ, et al. Tumor necrosis factor alpha-mediated toxic shock in *Trypanosoma cruzi*-infected interleukin 10-deficient mice. *Infect Immun* 2000;68:4075–4083.

171. Reis e Sousa C, Yap G, Schulz O, et al. Paralysis of dendritic cell IL-12 production by microbial products prevents infection-induced immunopathology. *Immunity* 1999;11:637–647.

172. Villegas EN, Wille U, Craig L, et al. Blockade of costimulation prevents infection-induced immunopathology in interleukin-10–deficient mice. *Infect Immun* 2000;68:2837–2844.

173. Liesenfeld O, Kosek J, Remington JS, et al. Association of CD4$^+$ T cell-dependent, interferon-gamma-mediated necrosis of the small intestine with genetic susceptibility of mice to peroral infection with *Toxoplasma gondii. J Exp Med* 1996;184:597–607.

174. Suzuki Y, Sher A, Yap G, et al. IL-10 is required for prevention of necrosis in the small intestine and mortality in both genetically resistant BALB/c and susceptible C57BL/6 mice following peroral infection with *Toxoplasma gondii. J Immunol* 2000;164:5375–5382.

175. Kwiatkowski D, Perlmann P. *Inflammatory processes in the pathogenesis of malaria.* Harwood Academic Publishers; 1999.

176. Li C, Seixas E, Langhorne J. Rodent malarias: the mouse as a model for understanding immune responses and pathology induced by the erythrocytic stages of the parasite. *Med Microbiol Immunol (Berl)* 2001;189:115–126.

177. Knight JC, Udalova I, Hill AV, et al. A polymorphism that affects OCT-1 binding to the TNF promoter region is associated with severe malaria. *Nat Genet* 1999;22:145–150.

178. Omer FM, Kurtzhals JA, Riley EM. Maintaining the immunological

balance in parasitic infections: a role for TGF-beta? *Parasitol Today* 2000;16:18–23.

179. Omer FM, Riley EM. Transforming growth factor beta production is inversely correlated with severity of murine malaria infection. *J Exp Med* 1998;188:39–48.

180. Li C, Corraliza I, Langhorne J. A defect in interleukin-10 leads to enhanced malarial disease in *Plasmodium chabaudi chabaudi* infection in mice. *Infect Immun* 1999;67:4435–4442.

181. Cheever AW, Yap GS. Immunologic basis of disease and disease regulation in schistosomiasis. *Chem Immunol* 1997;66:159–176.

182. Jankovic D, Cheever AW, Kullberg MC, et al. CD4$^+$ T cell-mediated granulomatous pathology in schistosomiasis is downregulated by a B cell-dependent mechanism requiring Fc receptor signaling. *J Exp Med* 1998;187:619–629.

183. Montesano MA, Colley DG, Eloi-Santos S, et al. Neonatal idiotypic exposure alters subsequent cytokine, pathology, and survival patterns in experimental *Schistosoma mansoni* infections. *J Exp Med* 1999;189:637–645.

184. Wynn TA, Cheever AW, Jankovic D, et al. An IL-12-based vaccination method for preventing fibrosis induced by schistosome infection. *Nature* 1995;376:594–596.

185. Brunet LR, Finkelman FD, Cheever AW, et al. IL-4 protects against TNF-alpha-mediated cachexia and death during acute schistosomiasis. *J Immunol* 1997;159:777–785.

186. Rutitzky LI, Hernandez HJ, Stadecker MJ. Th1-polarizing immunization with egg antigens correlates with severe exacerbation of immunopathology and death in schistosome infection. *Proc Natl Acad Sci U S A* 2001;98:13243–13248.

187. Fallon PG, Dunne DW. Tolerization of mice to *Schistosoma mansoni* egg antigens causes elevated type 1 and diminished type 2 cytokine responses and increased mortality in acute infection. *J Immunol* 1999;162:4122–4132.

188. Fallon PG, Richardson EJ, Smith P, et al. Elevated type 1, diminished type 2 cytokines and impaired antibody response are associated with hepatotoxicity and mortalities during *Schistosoma mansoni* infection of CD4-depleted mice. *Eur J Immunol* 2000;30:470–480.

189. Pearce EJ, La Flamme A, Sabin E, et al. The initiation and function of Th2 responses during infection with *Schistosoma mansoni*. *Adv Exp Med Biol* 1998;452:67–73.

190. King CL, Medhat A, Malhotra I, et al. Cytokine control of parasite-specific anergy in human urinary schistosomiasis. IL-10 modulates lymphocyte reactivity. *J Immunol* 1996;156:4715–4721.

191. Hoffmann KF, McCarty TC, Segal DH, et al. Disease fingerprinting with cDNA microarrays reveals distinct gene expression profiles in lethal type 1 and type 2 cytokine-mediated inflammatory reactions. *FASEB J* 2001;15:2545–2547.

192. La Flamme AC, Patton EA, Bauman B, et al. IL-4 plays a crucial role in regulating oxidative damage in the liver during schistosomiasis. *J Immunol* 2001;166:1903–1911.

193. Chiaramonte MG, Donaldson DD, Cheever AW, et al. An IL-13 inhibitor blocks the development of hepatic fibrosis during a T-helper type 2–dominated inflammatory response. *J Clin Invest* 1999; 104:777–785.

194. Hesse M, Modolell M, La Flamme AC, et al. differential regulation of nitric oxide synthase-2 and arginase-1 by type 1/type 2 cytokines in vivo: granulomatous pathology is shaped by the pattern of l-arginine metabolism. *J Immunol* 2001;167:6533–6544.

195. Vaillant B, Chiaramonte MG, Cheever AW, et al. Regulation of hepatic fibrosis and extracellular matrix genes by the Th response: New insight into the role of tissue inhibitors of matrix metalloproteinases. *J Immunol* 2001;167:7017-7026.

196. Zhang T, Stanley SL Jr. DNA vaccination with the serine rich Entamoeba histolytica protein (SREHP) prevents amebic liver abcess in rodent models of disease. *Vaccine* 1999;18:868–874.

197. Olson ME, Ceri H, Morck DW. Giardia vaccination. *Parasitol Today* 2000,16:213–217.

198. Miller LH, Good MF, Kaslow DC. Vaccines against the blood stages of falciparum malaria. *Adv Exp Med Biol* 1998;452:193–205.

199. Richie TL, Saul A. Progress and challenges for malaria vaccines. *Nature* 2002;415:694–701.

200. Holder AA, Freeman RR. Immunization against blood-stage rodent malaria using purified parasite antigens. *Nature* 1981;294:361–364.

201. Stowers AW, Chen L-H, Zhang Y, et al. A recombinant vaccine expressed in the milk of transgenic mice protects Aotus monkeys from a lethal challenge with *Plasmodium falciparum*. *Proc Natl Acad Sci U S A* 2002;99:339–344.

202. Herrera MA, Rosero F, Herrera S, et al. Protection against malaria in Aotus monkeys immunized with a recombinant blood-stage antigen fused to a universal T-cell epitope: correlation of serum gamma interferon levels with protection. *Infect Immun* 1992;60:154–158.

203. Genton B, Betuela I, Felger I, et al. A recombination blood-stage malaria vaccine reduces *Plasmodium falciparum* density and exerts selective pressure on parasite populations in a Phase I/IIb trial in Papua New Guinea. *J Infect Dis* 2002;185:820–827.

204. Gupta S, Snow RW, Donnelly CA, et al. Immunity to non-cerebral severe malaria is acquired after one or two infections. *Nat Med* 1999; 5:340–343.

205. Bull PC, Kortok M, Kai O, et al. Plasmodium falciparum–infected erythrocytes: agglutination by diverse Kenyan plasma is associated with severe disease and young host age. *J Infect Dis* 2000;182:252–259.

206. Duffy PE, Craig AG, Baruch DI. Variant proteins on the surface of malaria-infected erythrocytes—developing vaccines. *Trends Parasitol* 2001;17:354–356.

207. Duffy PE, Fried M. Malaria during pregnancy: parasites, antibodies and chondroitin sulphate A. *Biochem Soc Trans* 1999;27:478–482.

208. Nussenzweig RS, Zavala F. A malaria vaccine based on a sporozoite antigen. *N Engl J Med* 1997;336:128–130.

209. Carter R, Mendis KN, Miller LH, et al. Malaria transmission-blocking vaccines—how can their development be supported? *Nat Med* 2000;6:241–244.

210. Stowers AW, Keister DB, Muratova O, et al. A region of *Plasmodium falciparum* antigen Pfs25 that is the target of highly potent transmission-blocking antibodies. *Infect Immun* 2000;68:5530–5538.

211. Afonso LC, Scharton TM, Vieira LQ, et al. The adjuvant effect of interleukin-12 in a vaccine against Leishmania major. *Science* 1994;263:235–237.

212. Handman E. Leishmaniasis: current status of vaccine development. *Clin Microbiol Rev* 2001;14:229–243.

213. Gurunathan S, Prussin C, Sacks DL, et al. Vaccine requirements for sustained cellular immunity to an intracellular parasitic infection. *Nat Med* 1998;4:1409–1415.

214. Uzonna JE, Wei G, Yurkowski D, et al. Immune elimination of Leishmania major in mice: implications for immune memory, vaccination, and reactivation disease. *J Immunol* 2001;167:6967–6974.

215. Seder RA, Hill AV. Vaccines against intracellular infections requiring cellular immunity. *Nature* 2000;406:793–798.

216. Titus RG, Gueiros-Filho FJ, de Freitas LA, et al. Development of a safe live Leishmania vaccine line by gene replacement. *Proc Natl Acad Sci U S A* 1995;92:10267–10271.

217. Alexander J, Coombs GH, Mottram JC. Leishmania mexicana cysteine proteinase-deficient mutants have attenuated virulence for mice and potentiate a Th1 response. *J Immunol* 1998;161:6794–6801.

218. Wizel B, Garg N, Tarleton RL. Vaccination with trypomastigote surface antigen 1-encoding plasmid DNA confers protection against lethal *Trypanosoma cruzi* infection. *Infect Immun* 1998;66:5073–5081.

219. Desolme B, Mevelec MN, Buzoni-Gatel D, et al. Induction of protective immunity against toxoplasmosis in mice by DNA immunization with a plasmid encoding *Toxoplasma gondii* GRA4 gene. *Vaccine* 2000;18:2512–2521.

220. Hoffman SL, Doolan DL. Malaria vaccines-targeting infected hepatocytes. *Nat Med* 2000;6:1218–1219.

221. Scheller LF, Azad AF. Maintenance of protective immunity against malaria by persistent hepatic parasites derived from irradiated sporozoites. *Proc Natl Acad Sci U S A* 1995;92:4066–4068.

222. Lopez JA, Weilenman C, Audran R, et al. A synthetic malaria vaccine elicits a potent CD8(+) and CD4(+) T lymphocyte immune response in humans. Implications for vaccination strategies. *Eur J Immunol* 2001;31:1989–1998.

223. Bojang KA, Milligan PJ, Pinder M, et al. Efficacy of RTS,S/AS02 malaria vaccine against *Plasmodium falciparum* infection in semi-immune adult men in The Gambia: a randomised trial. *Lancet* 2001; 358:1927–1934.

224. Hoffman SL, Sedegah M, Hedstrom RC. Protection against malaria

by immunization with a *Plasmodium yoelii* circumsporozoite protein nucleic acid vaccine. *Vaccine* 1994;12:1529–1533.

225. Wang R, Doolan DL, Le TP, et al. Induction of antigen-specific cytotoxic T lymphocytes in humans by a malaria DNA vaccine. *Science* 1998;282:476–480.

226. Schneider J, Gilbert SC, Hannan CM, et al. Induction of CD8$^+$ T cells using heterologous prime-boost immunisation strategies. *Immunol Rev* 1999;170:29–38.

227. Wynn TA, Eltoum I, Oswald IP, et al. Endogenous interleukin 12 (IL-12) regulates granuloma formation induced by eggs of *Schistosoma mansoni* and exogenous IL-12 both inhibits and prophylactically immunizes against egg pathology. *J Exp Med* 1994;179:1551–1561.

228. Chiaramonte MG, Hesse M, Cheever AW, et al. CpG oligonucleotides can prophylactically immunize against Th2-mediated schistosome egg-induced pathology by an IL-12-independent mechanism. *J Immunol* 2000;164:973–985.

229. Chen Y, Boros DL. Polarization of the immune response to the single immunodominant epitope of p38, a major *Schistosoma mansoni* egg antigen, generates Th1- or Th2-type cytokines and granulomas. *Infect Immun* 1999;67:4570–4577.

230. Asahi H, Osman A, Cook RM, et al. Schistosoma mansoni phosphoenolpyruvate carboxykinase, a novel egg antigen: immunological properties of the recombinant protein and identification of a T-cell epitope. *Infect Immun* 2000;68:3385–3393.

231. Hagan P, Doenhoff MJ, Wilson RA, et al. Schistosomiasis vaccines: a response to a devils' advocate's view. *Parasitol Today* 2000;16:322–323.

232. Wilson RA, Coulson PS. Strategies for a schistosome vaccine: can we manipulate the immune response effectively? *Microbes Infect* 1999;1:535–543.

233. Anderson S, Shires VL, Wilson RA, et al. In the absence of IL-12, the induction of Th1-mediated protective immunity by the attenuated schistosome vaccine is impaired, revealing an alternative pathway with Th2-type characteristics. *Eur J Immunol* 1998;28:2827–2838.

234. Anderson S, Coulson PS, Ljubojevic S, et al. The radiation-attenuated schistosome vaccine induces high levels of protective immunity in the absence of B cells. *Immunology* 1999;96:22–28.

235. El Ridi R, Ozaki T, Kamiya H. *Schistosoma mansoni* infection in IgE-producing and IgE-deficient mice. *J Parasitol* 1998;84:171–174.

236. Maizels RM, Holland MJ, Falcone FH, et al. Vaccination against helminth parasites—the ultimate challenge for vaccinologists? *Immunol Rev* 1999;171:125–147.

237. Bergquist NR, Colley DG. Schistosomiasis Vaccines: Research to Development. *Parasitol Today* 1998;14:99–104.

238. Morel CM. Reaching maturity–25 years of the TDR. *Parasitol Today* 2000;16:522–528.

239. Murray CJ, Lopez AD. Progress and directions in refining the global burden of disease approach: a response to Williams. *Health Econ* 2000;9:69–82.

240. van der Werf MJ, de Vlas SJ, Looman CW, Nagelkerke NJ, Habbema JD, Engels D. Associating community prevalence of *Schistosoma mansoni* infection with prevalence of signs and symptoms. *Acta Tropica* 2002;82:127–137.

CHAPTER 39

Viral Immunology

Hildegund C. J. Ertl

Obstacles to Viral Entry and Early Replication
Recognition of Viruses by the Innate Immune System
Non–Antigen-Specific Antiviral Defense Mechanisms
Induction of Antigen-Specific Immune Responses
  Presentation of Viral Antigens to the Immune System · Antigen Processing for Activation of CD4$^+$ T Cells · Antigen Processing for Activation of CD8$^+$ T Cells · Activation of B Cells
The Effector Functions of Antigen-Specific Immune Mechanisms
Immunological Memory
The Mucosal Immune System
Persistent Virus Infections
Autoimmunity after Virus Infections
Viral Superantigens
Viral Subversion of Immune Responses
  Escape by Mutations · Escape by Hiding · Escape by Latency · Escape by Destruction of Immune Cells · Escape by Subverting Antigen Processing and Antigen Presentation · Inhibition of T Cell–Mediated Target Cell Lysis · Inhibition of Natural Killer Cell Activity · Inhibition of Complement Activation · Interference of Cytokine Functions · Crystallized Fragment (Fc) Receptor Mimetics
Summary
References

The essence of all viruses, a heterogenous group of small genetic entities surrounded by proteinous structures that facilitate transfer of the genome across cell membranes, is their uncompromising parasitism. Unlike other pathogens their propagation, the ultimate driving force in nature, is absolutely dependent on cells of animals, plants, or bacteria. Viruses can be subdivided, depending on their genome, into ribonucleic acid (RNA) and deoxyribonucleic acid (DNA) viruses. RNA viruses are divided into single-strand (negative or positive) or double-strand RNA viruses. DNA viruses are either single- or double-strand. RNA viruses are further classified into segmented and nonsegmented viruses, and both RNA and DNA viruses are, moreover, distinguished into those that are enveloped and those that are not. The taxonomy of viruses includes orders, families and subfamilies, and genera and species. For example, the order Mononegavirales includes the family Rhabdoviridae, the genus *Lyssavirus,* and the species of rabies virus (Table 1). Of the more than 70 viral families identified to date, 24 contain viruses that infect humans. Altogether, more than 400 viruses cause disease in their human hosts, and more than 100 of those belong to the *Rhinovirus* genus (Table 2). Considering the multitude of viruses that are

pathogenic in humans, it is not surprising that, in spite of advances in modern medicine, viral infections are still among the leading causes of human morbidity and mortality worldwide.

By the 1970s, infectious diseases in developing countries had markedly declined and were no longer considered a major threat. Vaccines to many of the common childhood infectious diseases were available, and improved hygiene and antibiotics had diminished the impact of bacterial infections. At the same time, a number of new viruses made their appearance. In 1967, factory workers at a German pharmaceutical company and a veterinarian and his wife in Belgrade in the former Yugoslavia died of a hemorrhagic disease caused by a new virus, the Marburg virus (1). In 1976, an epidemic with a related virus, the Ebola virus, occurred in Yandongi in Zaire with a mortality rate exceeding 90% of those infected (2). In 1993, a new strain of *Hantavirus* called Muerto Canyon caused an outbreak in the Four Corners region in the United States with a mortality rate of over 70%; young and otherwise healthy adults were commonly afflicted (3).

In 1999, West Nile virus appeared in New York City (4). The following year, the virus spread into New Jersey and

TABLE 1. *Taxonomy of viruses: examples*

Family	Genus	Species	Genome	Envelope structure
Picornaviridae	Enterovirus	Poliovirus (serotypes 1–3)	ss RNA (+), 7–8 kb	Spherical, non-enveloped
	Hepatovirus	Hepatitis A virus		
	Rhinovirus	Rhinovirus (serotypes 1–100)		
Togaviridae	Rubivirus	Rubella virus	ss RNA (+), 10 kb	Icosahedral, enveloped
Flaviviridae	Hepaciviruses	Hepatitis C virus	ss RNA (+), 11 kb	Spherical, enveloped
	Flaviviruses	Dengue virus (serotypes 1–4)		
		West Nile encephalitis virus		
		Yellow fever virus		
Rhabdoviridae	Lyssaviruses	Rabies virus	ss RNA (−), 11 kb	Bullet-shaped, enveloped
Filoviridae	Ebola-like viruses	Ebola virus Zaire	ss RNA (−), 19 kb	Pleomorphic, enveloped
		Ebola virus Reston		
	Marburg-like viruses	Marburg virus		
Paramyxoviridae	Subfamily Paramyxovirinae		ss RNA (−), 15–19 kb	Spherical or pleiomorphic, enveloped
	Respirovirus	Human parainfluenza virus (serotypes 1–3)		
	Morbillivirus	Measles virus		
	Rubulavirus	Mumps virus		
		Human parainfluenza virus (serotypes 2, 4)		
	Subfamily Pneumovirinae			
	Pneumovirus	Human respiratory syncytial virus		
Orthomyxoviridae	Orthomyxovirinae	Influenza virus (serotypes A–C)	Segmented ss RNA (−), ~14 kb	Spherical, enveloped
Bunyaviridae	Hantavirus	Hantaan virus	Segmented ss RNA (−), 10–20 kb	Spherical, enveloped
Arenaviridae	Arenavirus	Lymphocytic choriomeningitis virus	Segmented ss RNA (−), ~3.5 kb	Pleomorphic, enveloped
		Lassa fever virus		
Reoviridae	Rotavirus	Human Rotavirus (serotypes A–C)	Segmented ds RNA, ~24 kb	Icosahedral, enveloped
Retroviridae	Deltaretroviruses	Human T lymphotropic viruses	ds RNA, 7–13 kb	Spherical, enveloped
	Lentivirus	Human immunodeficiency virus 1		
		Simian immunodeficiency virus		
	Spumavirus	Human foamy virus		
Polyomaviridae	Papillomaviruses	Human papilloma virus (serotypes 1–80)	Circular ds DNA, ~8 kb	Icosahedral, non-enveloped
Adenoviridae	Mastadenovirus	Human adenovirus (serotypes 1–49)	ds DNA, 40–160 bp	Icosahedral, non-enveloped
Herpesviridae	Subfamily Alphaherpesvirinae		ds DNA, 145–170 kb	Icosahedrical, enveloped
	Simplexvirus	Herpes simplex virus (HHV1)		
	Varicellovirus	Varicella zoster virus (HHV3)		
	Subfamily Gammavirinae			
	Cytomegalovirus	Human cytomegalovirus (HHV4)		
	Lymphocryptovirus	Epstein Barr virus (HHV8)		
Poxviridae	Orthopoxvirus	Vaccinia virus	ds DNA, ~150–200 kb	Rectangular, enveloped
		Ectromelia virus		
		Cowpoxvirus		
	Leporipoxvirus	Myxoma virus		
	Molluscipoxvirus	Molluscum contagiosum		
Hepadnaviridae	Hepadnavirus	Human hepatitis B virus	ds DNA, 3.2 kb	Spherical and filamentous, enveloped

ds, double-strand; DNA, deoxyribonucleic acid; HHV, human herpesvirus; RNA, ribonucleic acid; ss, single-strand.

TABLE 2. *Viruses pathogenic in humans*

Virus	Transmission	Site of entry	Disease	Fatality rate
Hepatitis A virus	Fecal–oral from human to human	Intestinal tract	Acute hepatitis	2%–3%
Poliomyelitis virus	Fecal–oral from human to human	Intestinal tract	None (90%), mild febrile symptoms (4%), aseptic meningitis (1%), paralysis (0.5%)	
Rubella virus	Aerosols from human to human Maternal—fetal	Respiratory tract Transplacental	Rash, low-grade fever, arthralgia, hearing loss, congenital heart disease	<0.1%
West Nile fever virus	Bite by an infected mosquito	Skin	Headache, fever, encephalitis in elderly patients	<1%
Rabies virus	Bite by a rabid mammal	Muscle, skin, mucosa	Encephalitis, paralysis, coma	>99%
Ebola virus Zaire	Unknown, human to human	Parenteral, aerosols (?)	Fever, hemorrhagic shock	~80%
Mumps virus	Close human-to-human contact	Respiratory tract	Parotitis, meningoencephalitis, orchitis	0.02%
Measles virus	Casual human-to-human contact	Respiratory tract	Fever, rash, pneumonitis, lymphopenia	Up to 6%
Influenza A virus	Casual human-to-human contact	Respiratory tract	Fever, pneumonia	0.05%–0.3%
Hantavirus	Mouse urine or feces to human	Respiratory tract	Fever, capillary leakage, pulmonary edema	<1%–70%
Lassa fever virus	Rodents to human	Respiratory tract	Fever, sore throat, capillary leakage	15%–20%
Rotavirus	Fecal–oral from human to human	Intestinal tract	Diarrhea	<0.1%
Cytomegalovirus	Human to human Maternal–fetal	Mucosal surfaces	Mononucleosis; in infant, microcephaly, hearing loss, optic atrophy	
Hepatitis B virus	Human to human Mother to newborn	Parenteral, mucosa	Acute and chronic hepatitis, hepatocarcinoma	0.2%–0.5%

Pennsylvania, and by 2001, the virus had gained a foothold along the East Coast of North America.

Vaccines are available thus far for only a fraction of the identified human viral pathogens. They provide the most efficacious medical intervention to reduce the incidence of virus-associated morbidity and mortality. Smallpox virus, which had decimated populations in Asia and Europe for centuries, was eradicated in the 1970s through a global vaccination campaign started in 1967 under the guidance of the World Health Organization (5). Complete elimination of this virus was feasible because an efficacious inexpensive vaccine that provided protective immunity after a single noninvasive application was available against this strictly human pathogen, which was not sheltered by an animal reservoir. Poliovirus, which also infects only humans and for which an inexpensive, efficacious vaccine is at hand, is expected to become extinct soon.

Infections with some viruses can be treated with antiviral drugs, which suppress viral replication. Such drug treatment successfully decreases the viral burden in patients infected with the human immunodeficiency virus type 1 (HIV-1) and prolongs or even prevents progression to the acquired immunodeficiency syndrome (AIDS).

Although modern medicine with its vaccines and drugs has dramatically reduced the impact of viral infections on human health, new viruses emerge constantly and, with increased global travel, spread far too rapidly for medicinal interventions to keep ahead. The immune system thus remains the body's prime source of defense against viruses. Viruses, which mutate more speedily than mammalian genomes, are constantly adapting to the defense mechanisms of their unwilling hosts to ensure their own survival. Some viruses induce acute disease, which ends with the elimination of all infected cells. Other viruses establish persistent infections by dodging the hosts' immune system. Some of those, such as papillomaviruses, adenoviruses, retroviruses, and some hepadnaviruses, integrate into the genome of the host cells. This can lead to the transformation of cells either through viral oncoproteins, such as the E6 and E7 of oncogenic types of human papillomaviruses that inactivate p53 and retinoblastoma gene product, respectively, or through activation of cellular oncoproteins. Herpesviruses can persist within the host indefinitely by establishing a stage of latency in permissive cells when viral protein synthesis is virtually shut off, thus allowing the virus to escape immune surveillance. Details on pathways that permit viruses to dodge elimination by the immune system are described in more detail in the section on viral subversion of immune responses in this chapter.

OBSTACLES TO VIRAL ENTRY AND EARLY REPLICATION

Most viruses infect their hosts through the mucosal surfaces of the airways, the conjunctivae, the gastrointestinal tract, or the urogenital tract. Others invade through the skin or through direct inoculation into a tissue. The first layer of defense against an invading pathogen is provided not by the immune system but rather by nonspecific barriers, such as the nearly impenetrable keratinous outer layer of the skin or the acidic environment of the upper intestinal and the female genital tracts. Once viruses overcome these obstacles, they enter cells upon binding to specific receptors, either by fusion or by endocytosis. The CD4 molecule on T-lymphocytes serves as a receptor for HIV, which further uses CCR5 and CXCR4 chemokine receptors as co-receptors (6). Humans who lack the CCR5 chemokine receptor have increased resistance to progression of HIV-1 infections (7). Sialic acids permit entry of influenza viruses (8), and herpesviruses utilize heparan sulfate (9). Some receptors are expressed only on specialized cells such as CD21 and C3d on B cells, utilized by Epstein-Barr virus (10,11) or the Coxsackie adenovirus receptor (CAR) that is put to use by adenoviruses and Coxsackie viruses (12). Sendai virus, a paramyxovirus, can penetrate the host cell wall by fusion. Many viruses can infect cells through multiple pathways. For example, adenoviruses infect CAR-positive cells very efficiently through binding of the viral fiber to CAR. The virus can also infect CAR-negative cells, albeit less efficiently, through interactions between the viral penton with cell surface integrins (13). The use of specific receptors commonly determines the tropism of the virus. It can also form the basis for the species specificity of some viruses. For example, polioviruses infect only human cells but can be propagated in transgenic mice genetically engineered to carry the human poliovirus receptor (14,15).

Another nonspecific defense mechanism employed by some cells such as epithelial cells and neutrophils are so-called defensins, which are a family of antimicrobial peptides 29 to 47 amino acids in length (16,17). Cationic defensins form pores in membranes rich in anionic phospholipids and have demonstrated antimicrobial activity against enveloped viruses, as well as against bacteria and fungi.

Upon entering the cells, the virus particles disassemble, releasing the viral genome, which is then transcribed either in the cytoplasm or, more commonly, in the nucleus. Most viruses rely strictly on the host cell machinery for production of new progeny. Some of the larger DNA viruses, such as poxviruses, which replicate in the cytoplasm, provide their own polymerases to facilitate early host cell-independent transcription. DNA viruses that reach the cytoplasm and, upon uncoating, release their genome into the nucleus encounter another cellular defense mechanism called nuclear domain 10 (ND10) (18). ND10 is a complex of nuclear proteins, including the nuclear autoantigen Sp100 and the promyelocytic leukemia gene product. They form distinct dotlike structures in which DNA viruses such as herpes simplex virus type I, simian virus 40, and human adenovirus of the serotype 5 start their transcription and replication (19). The amount of ND10 per nucleus is up-regulated by interferon. An increase of ND10 results in reduced viral replica-

tion through pathways not yet defined. Some viruses, such as those of the Alphaherpesvirinae and Betaherpesvirinae subfamilies, trigger dispersions of the proteins of the ND10 complex, which, again, indicates that these structures are part of a cellular defense system against foreign genetic material and that evasion thereof provides a survival advantage to viral pathogens (20).

RECOGNITION OF VIRUSES BY THE INNATE IMMUNE SYSTEM

Viruses that enter an organism are recognized as foreign and thus potentially dangerous because of their expression of pathogen-associated molecular patterns (PAMPs). PAMPs are recognized by an array of different receptors, called pattern recognition receptors, expressed on cells of the innate immune system and on epithelial cells that form the host's boundary to the environment (21). Such receptors, studied mainly within the context of bacterial and protozoan infections, include the evolutionary highly conserved Toll-like receptors (TLRs) (22). TLRs are expressed on the cell surface and in the phagosomes of cells, which suggests that they serve to sample the content of phagocytosed material, which includes debris of dead cells. Ten types of TLRs have been identified to date that function as homodimers, heterodimers, or upon binding with co-receptors such as CD14 and MD-2a small protein that associates with TLR-4 (23). Ligand binding to different TLRs activates the same signal transduction pathways, which results through a cascade of events in phosphorylation and degradation of IκB, leading to release of NFκB, which, upon translocation into the nucleus, induces transcription of its target genes such as those encoding proinflammatory cytokines (Fig. 1). This in turn promotes activation of type 1 immune responses, which promote the induction of CD8$^+$ T-lymphocytes. Pattern recognition receptors that led to the induction of type 2 immune responses, best suited to combat infections with parasites such as helminthic infections, remain to be identified. Triggering of TLRs such as TLR-4 also causes up-regulation of co-stimulatory molecules on dendritic cells, as does ligand binding to TLR-2 by bacterial lipopeptides. Endogenous proteins such as heat-shock protein 60 may bind to the TLR-4, inducing a T helper type 1 (Th1)–type inflammatory reaction, including secretion of tumor necrosis factor α (TNF-α), interleukin (IL)–6, IL-12, and IL-15 (24). The fusion protein of respiratory syncytial virus has been suggested to bind to TRL-4 and CD14, a previously described receptor for bacterial lipopolysaccharides (25). Other viral proteins that carry PAMPs and interact with TLRs remain to be identified. Infectious viruses can also trigger a type 1 immune response by double-strand RNA, a common intermediate product of viral replication, which signals through TLR-3. One of the open reading frame products of vaccinia virus A52R, was shown to antagonize TLR-4 signaling (26). This strongly suggests that the TLR-4 pathway serves the hosts' defense against this viral pathogen. In

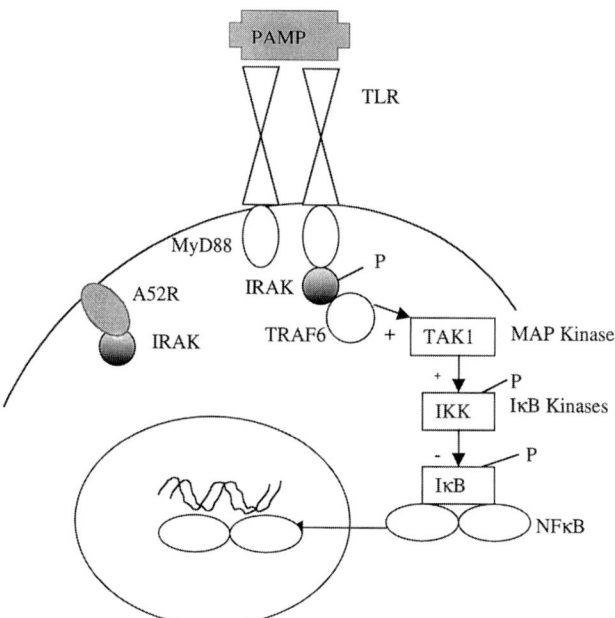

FIG. 1. Signaling through Toll-like receptors (TLRs). Viral products [pathogen-associated molecular patterns (PAMPs)], upon binding to TLRs, initiate signal transduction that leads to activation of NFκB and transcription of NFκB-controlled genes. The A52R protein of poxvirus interferes with this signaling pathway by inactivation of interleukin-1 receptor activating kinase.

turn, vaccinia virus may have evolved to counteract TLR-4 signaling, thus increases its chance of survival. Unmethylated CpG sequences, uncommon in mammalian genomes but present in the genomes of bacteria (27), and some viruses such as Ebola virus bind to the TLR-9 receptor. This, within minutes, causes an increase in reactive oxygen species and inducible nitric oxygen synthetase and in induction of mitogen-activated protein kinases and NFκB. In B cells, macrophages, and dendritic cells, this leads to expeditious production of Th1-linked cytokines such as IL-12 and IL-18, which in turn induce production of interferon (IFN)–γ (28), one of the most potent antiviral cytokines. Most viruses have suppressed contents of immunostimulatory CpG sequences, which reflects frequencies of CpG motifs below that expected from random codon usage. Other viruses contain immunoinhibitory CpG motifs, which counterbalance immunostimulatory motifs (29). It is possible that strong evolutionary forces favored viruses that avoid this pathway of immune activation. Ebola virus, a rather recent addition to the potpourri of human viral pathogens first identified in the mid-1970s, has a high content of immunostimulatory CpG sequences. This fledging virus, despite its zest to rapidly kill most of its hosts, has not yet succeeded in causing more than a few self-limited outbreaks in Central Africa. It thus still has to master the art of becoming a successful pathogen by causing more sustained infections while at the same time avoiding destruction by the immune system. Ebola viruses, like other viruses, will undoubtedly adapt to its new human host by rapid mutations and selections.

NON–ANTIGEN-SPECIFIC ANTIVIRAL DEFENSE MECHANISMS

One of the best known antiviral mediators is interferon. Interferon is subdivided into type I interferons, which include IFN-α, IFN-β, IFN-σ, and IFN-τ, and type II interferon, also called immune interferon or IFN-γ. Monocytes/macrophages, lymphoblastoid cells, fibroblasts, and a number of additional cell types produce IFN-α, which consists of at least 23 variants. IFN-σ shows sequence homology and functional similarity to IFN-α (30) IFN-τ has been identified only in cattle and sheep (31). Mainly fibroblasts and epithelial cells produce IFN-β, which is encoded by a single gene. Both IFN-α and IFN-β use the same receptor and have thus interchangeable functions. Double-strand RNA present in the viral genome or generated as an intermediate product of viral synthesis seems to be the main inducer of type I interferons (32). Viral glycoproteins can also induce production of interferons (33). Binding of a type I interferon to its receptor leads to phosphorylation of the tyrosine kinase 2 (TYK2) and Janus kinase 1 (Jak1). This in turn causes tyrosine phosphorylation of signal transducer and activator of transcription (STAT)–1 and STAT2 proteins, which, upon translocation into the nucleus, form a complex with other proteins, leading to activation of interferon-inducible genes (34). IFN-γ is produced mainly by natural killer cells and subpopulations of activated T-lymphocytes in response to exogenous stimuli, such as components of viruses or bacteria, or endogenous inducers, such as IL-12 or IL-18. IFN-γ, which binds to a receptor different from that for type I interferons, also leads via Janus kinases to the phosphorylation of STAT1 (35). Type I interferons are generally 10 to 100 times more potent as antiviral agents than is IFN-γ. Both types of interferons affect viral multiplication at several levels. They can inhibit entry of the viruses into host cells by reducing expression of the viral receptors. Type I interferons induce production of the Mx protein that, through an as-yet ill-defined pathway, inhibits transcription of influenza viruses (36). Both types of interferon down-regulate viral regulatory elements such as the early promoter of cytomegalovirus (37). Both trigger expression of 2'5'-oligoadenylsynthase and double-strand RNA kinase, which inhibit production of viral progeny. For some viruses, IFN-γ can promote transcription. For example, the long terminal repeat of HIV-1 is activated by IFN-γ (38). IFN-γ induces nitric oxide synthases, which converts L-arginine to L-citrulline and nitric oxide. The latter has direct effects on poxviruses and herpesviruses by inhibiting DNA replication, synthesis of late viral proteins, and viral assembly. Production of early viral proteins is not affected by nitric oxide (39). In addition to their antiviral activity, interferons play a dominant role in other host defense mechanisms. They activate macrophages and natural killer cells.

They promote Th1-type immune responses. They drive maturation of dendritic cells, induce or augment expression of class I and II major histocompatibility complex (MHC) determinants, co-stimulatory molecules of the B7 family, and proteins involved in antigen processing. Interferon-knockout mice show increased susceptibility to some viral infections. IFN-α has been licensed for treatment of chronic infections with hepatitis B (40) and C viruses (41) and for treatment of human papillomavirus–associated genital warts (condyloma acuminatum) (42).

In addition to inducing synthesis of interferons, many viruses stimulate production of other cytokines and chemokines, which elicit an inflammatory reaction at the site of infection. These cytokines include TNF-α, IL-1, IL-6, IL-12, IL-15, IL-18, colony-stimulating factors, and a myriad of chemokines, including IL-8, macrophage inflammatory protein (MIP)–1α, MIP-1β, and monocyte chemotactic protein–1, a subset of cytokines that control lymphocyte trafficking. Other chemokines such as monokine induced by IFN-γ (MIG) and interferon-inducible protein (IP)–10 are induced by IFN-γ.

Through the induction of IL-12 and type I interferons, viruses activate natural killer (NK) cells. Type I interferons induce NK cells primarily with lytic activity, whereas IL-12 triggers production of IFN-γ by NK cells. NK cells have a number of activating receptors. These receptors, unlike those on α/β receptor–positive T cells, lack antigen specificity, thus increasing the chance for inadvertent killing of normal cells. Therefore, as a safeguard, NK cells carry inhibitory receptors that bind partly to MHC determinants, which are expressed on most normal cells (43). Down-regulation of MHC determinants upon infection with some viruses such as adenoviruses both decreases their resistance to killing by CD8+ T cells and augments their susceptibility to NK cell–mediated killing. NK cells express a number of different invariant receptors that, upon their interaction with their ligands, cause release of perforin and lysis of the ligand-expressing cells (Fig. 2). The ligands have not yet been characterized, but it is tempting to speculate that they recognize PAMPs.

INDUCTION OF ANTIGEN-SPECIFIC IMMUNE RESPONSES

Stimulation of cells of the adaptive immune system—that is, CD4+ and CD8+ T cells and B cells—takes at least 4 to 5 days. Viruses can replicate in a 12- to 24-hour cycle, and each individual virus particle can produce more than 100 progeny. A single virus growing without any hindrance could thus, within a 4-day period, produce 10^{16} or more new virus particles, which is well in excess of the number of cells present in a human body, let alone of what the immune system could possibly contain. The innate immune system, together with other nonimmunological defense mechanisms, restrains viral propagation without affecting its complete elimination, thus providing sufficient time for activation of T and B cells.

Presentation of Viral Antigens to the Immune System

Induction of antigen-specific immune responses of the adaptive immune system requires presentation of viral antigens by professional antigen-presenting cells, which are, in general, dendritic cells (44). Dendritic cells, which are derived from bone marrow progenitors, are dispersed throughout an organism. They are exceptionally common in tissues that form the boundary to the outside world, such as the skin and mucosal surfaces. Dendritic cells within these tissues are immature. They constantly take up antigen, but they are ill suited to present the antigen to naïve T cells. Their class II MHC molecules, which must be expressed at the cell surface for presentation of antigenic peptides to CD4+ T helper cells, are localized mainly within intracellular compartments. They carry only low levels of co-stimulatory signals, and they lack CCR7 receptor expression, which promotes homing to lymphoid tissues, in which activation of T cells takes pace. They express other chemokine receptors, such as CCR1, CCR2, CCR5, and CXCR1, which leads to their recruitment to inflammatory sites, where MIP-1α, MIP-1β, and the "chemokine regulated upon activation, normal T-cell expressed, presumably secreted" (RANTES) are produced. Invasion of pathogens triggers maturation of dendritic cells. Maturation after an infection can be mediated by direct binding of substances derived from the pathogen to the dendritic cells' pattern recognition receptors (45). Alternatively, maturation of dendritic cells can be a consequence of the induction of proinflammatory cytokines or of cell damage or cell death after viral infection. Cell damage or death causes the

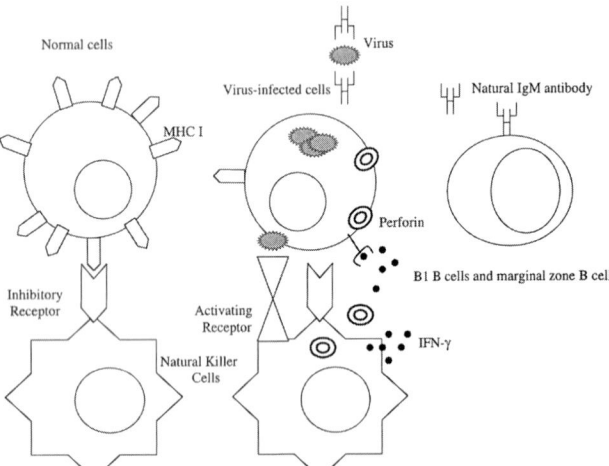

FIG. 2. Early immune defense mechanisms. Infections of cells with some viruses causes reduced expression of class I major histocompatibility complex (MHC) determinants. Natural killer (NK) cells become activated in absence of class I MHC molecules that on normal cells bind to inhibitory receptors. Once activated, NK cells secrete interferon (IFN)–γ or perforin. Marginal zone B cells and B1 cells secrete immunoglobulin M (IgM) antibodies with low affinity to an array of pathogens. Such antibodies can bind and neutralize circulating virus.

release of heat-shock proteins, shown to bind to TLR-4 (46). During maturation, dendritic cells initially increase and then gradually decrease antigen uptake. Dendritic cells internalize antigen through phagocytosis, receptor-mediated endocytosis, or pinocytosis. Some viruses, such as adenoviruses, can directly infect dendritic cells, partly through receptor-facilitated uptake. Other viruses such as paramyxoviruses enter dendritic cells through fusion of the viral envelope with the cell membranes. Some viruses such as *Lyssavirus* species cannot infect dendritic cells directly. Their presentation relies either on phagocytosis of viral particles or on pinocytosis of antigen released from infected cells. Once dendritic cells receive a maturation signal, they initially up-regulate and then down-regulate expression of CCR1, CCR5, and CXCR1 and thus at first become more sensitive and then resistant to recruitment by proinflammatory chemokines. While down-regulating CCR1, CCR5, and CXCR1, they increase expression of CCR7. CCR7 renders cells responsive to secondary lymphoid tissue chemokine and EB11-ligand chemokine, two CCR7-binding ligands that are produced in T cell–rich areas of lymphoid tissues, to which mature dendritic cells migrate (47). Early after activation, dendritic cells transiently secrete increased levels of chemokines, such as MIP-1α and MIP-2, that are chemoattractants for immature dendritic cells (48). Upon maturation, dendritic cells up-regulate expression of cell surface–expressed class II MHC and co-stimulatory molecules. At a later time after maturation, dendritic cells produce macrophage-derived chemoattractant, which attracts already activated T cells (49).

These delicately orchestrated changes after a maturation signal optimize the dendritic cells' ability to detect an incoming invasion of a pathogenic entity and to inform the adaptive immune system of the nature of such pathogens (50) (Fig. 3). Dendritic cells are localized at the boundaries that are the most common ports of entry for a viral invasion. They carry an array of receptors that can recognize a pathogen or a stress signal from an insulted cell. Once these receptors encounter their ligands, dendritic cells start to mature. They first increase their uptake of antigens to improve their ability to inform lymphocytes with the appropriate specificity of the nature of the invader. They recruit additional immature dendritic cells to further optimize communication with the adaptive immune system. Once this is achieved, they retreat from the site of invasion to lymph nodes to activate the adaptive immune system.

Dendritic cells determine the type of the induced T-cell response (Fig. 4). In humans, dendritic cells are divided into myeloid, or type 1, dendritic cells and plasmacytoid, or type 2, dendritic cells [reviewed by Liu et al. (51)]. Human type 1 dendritic cells, upon activation, secrete IL-12, thus sponsoring activation of Th1 responses. Type 2 dendritic cells produce markedly lower amounts of IL-12 and favor activation of T helper type 2 (Th2) cells. In mice, the situation is reversed: Lymphoid dendritic cells secrete large amounts of IL-12, whereas myeloid dendritic cells produce more modest amounts of IL-12. Depending on the stimulus and the surrounding cytokine milieu, human type 1 dendritic cells can induce Th2 responses. The density of dendritic cells affects the outcome of the induced type of the immune response: High concentration favors activation of Th1 responses. The duration of activation of the dendritic cells plays a role; shortly after activation, dendritic cells produce IL-12. After prolonged activation, dendritic cells cease to synthesize IL-12 and then favor induction of Th2 responses, commonly observed during chronic viral infections. Dendritic cells isolated from different tissues act differently: Those from the spleen favor activation of Th1 responses, whereas those from the liver or intestinal tract sponsor Th2 responses. Upon virus infection,

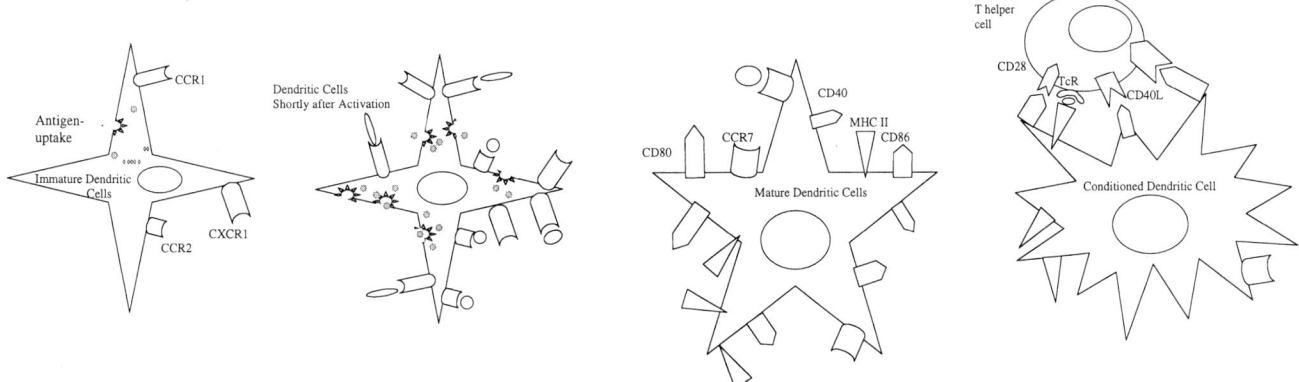

FIG. 3. Maturation of dendritic cells. **A:** Immature dendritic cells sample antigen and express CCR1, CXCR1, and CCR2. **B:** Shortly after activation, dendritic cells show increased uptake of antigen and expression of CCR1, CXCR1, and CCR2. **C:** Mature dendritic cells down-regulate expression of CCR1, CCR2, and CXCR and are no longer recruited to sites of inflammation. They up-regulate CCR7 and are recruited to lymph nodes. They up-regulate expression of class II major histocompatibility complex (MHC), CD40, and co-stimulatory molecules such as CD80 and CD86. **D.** Within lymph nodes, mature dendritic cells interact with T helper cells. Interaction of CD40 on dendritic cells and CD40 ligand on T helper cells causes further changes of dendritic cells, which are now able to activate naïve CD8+ T cells.

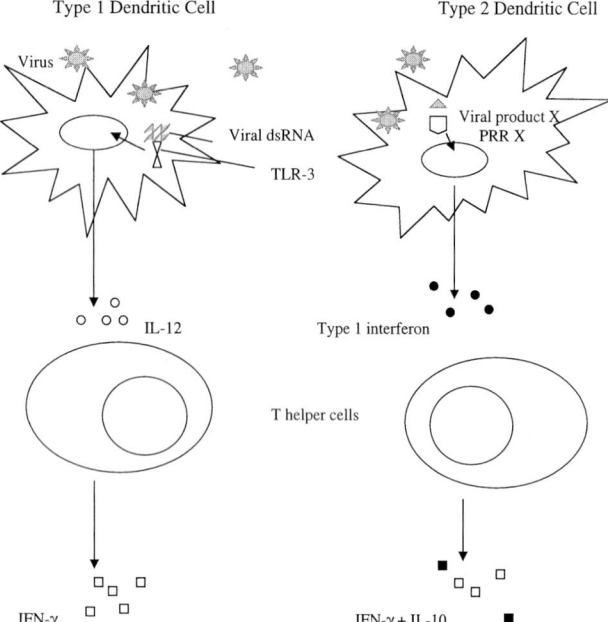

FIG. 4. Interactions between viruses and dendritic cells. Type 1 dendritic cells carry Toll-like receptor 3 (TLR-3), which binds to double-strand viral ribonucleic acid (RNA). This in turn causes release of interleukin-12 (IL-12), which promotes activation of a T helper type 1 (Th1)–type immune response. Type 2 dendritic cells do not carry TLR-3 receptors. Yet-to-be-identified viral products bind to thus far uncharacterized pattern recognition receptors, initiating release of type I interferon.

murine type 2 dendritic cells produce large amounts of type I interferon, which facilitates maturation of dendritic cells and induces T helper cells independently of IL-12 to produce IFN-γ and IL-10. Virus infection of type 1 dendritic cells causes release of IL-12, which also induces T helper cells to produce IFN-γ but not IL-10. Most virus infections induce mixed responses that are predominantly but not exclusively of the Th1 type, which suggests that both type 1 and type 2 dendritic cells may be activated upon viral infections. Immature human type 1 dendritic cells express high levels of TLR-1, TLR-2, and TLR-3; low levels of TLR-5, TLR-6, TLR-8, and TLR-10; and no TLR-4, TLR-7, or TLR-9. Immature type 2 dendritic cells, in contrast, express high levels of transcript for TLR-7 and TLR-9; low levels of TLR-1, TLR-6 and TLR-10; but no TLR-2, TLR-3, TLR-4, TLR-5, or TLR-8 (52). TLR-3, which binds to double-strand viral RNA, is expressed in type 1 and not type 2 dendritic cells, which suggests that viral infections activate mainly human myeloid dendritic cells, which in general favor activation of Th1 responses. Additional viral PAMPs remain to be identified to elucidate a role for type 2 dendritic cells in the activation of antiviral immune responses.

Antigen Processing for Activation of CD4+ T Cells

Upon maturation, antigen-expressing dendritic cells migrate to the T cell–rich areas of lymph nodes, where they initially activate CD4+ T cells, which are pivotal to provide help for stimulation of B cells and CD8+ T cells. CD4+ T cells are stimulated by peptides presented by class II MHC molecules (53). Class II MHC molecules, upon synthesis of α and β subunits, assemble in the endoplasmic reticulum with invariant chain. This polypeptide stabilizes the overall structure of the complexes. The invariant chain contains a peptide sequence, class II–associated invariant peptide, that promiscuously binds to the groove of class II MHC dimers, thus preventing binding of other peptides within the endoplasmic reticulum. The class II MHC/invariant chain complexes are translocated to an endosomal/lysosomal storage area called class II MHC–enriched compartments, which are abundant in immature dendritic cells. During maturation of dendritic cells, the invariant chain is degraded by cathepsin S, which in immature dendritic cells is inhibited by cystatin C and whose synthesis is induced by proinflammatory cytokines. Antigen taken up by dendritic cells progresses from early to late endosomes and then to lysosomes, in which they are broken down by disulfide reduction and enzymatic proteolysis. Class II MHC dimers released from the invariant chains enter a later compartment, the so-called class II MHC vesicles. Loading of peptides derived from exogenous proteins can take place in this compartment, which then fuses with the cell membrane displaying the class II MHC/peptide complexes on the cell surface. Immature dendritic cells constantly synthesize class II MHC molecules to replace those that are degraded in the class II MHC–enriched compartments. Mature dendritic cells shut off synthesis of class II MHC molecules and rely on the long-half life of cell surface expressed (more than 10 hours) and recycled class II MHC molecules to present antigen to CD4+ T cells.

Naïve CD4+ T cells, whose T-cell receptors (TCRs) are complementary to the class II MHC/peptide complex displayed by the dendritic cells in the context of co-stimulatory signals, become activated, proliferate, and differentiate into effector cells (54). CD4+ T cells mature either into Th1- or Th2-type cells (55). The choice of pathway may be influenced partly by the nature of the antigen-presenting dendritic cells (56). Th1 cells release IFN-γ and lymphotoxin, aid activation of CD8+ T cells, and, in mice, promote generation of antibodies of the immunoglobulin (Ig) G2a isotype. Th2 cells secrete IL-4, IL-5, and IL-10; promote B cells that secrete IgG1, IgE, or IgA; and activate mast cells and eosinophils. The cytokine milieu during CD4+ T cell activation determines whether they develop into Th1 or Th2 cells. IL-12 promotes activation of Th1 cells (57), whereas IL-4 sponsors differentiation into Th2 cells. If both are present concomitantly, IL-4 overrides the functions of IL-12. IL-10 inhibits the activity of IL-12 and thus favors generation of Th2 cells (58). Upon recognition of pathogens, the innate immune system presumably determines the type of the T helper cells best suited to protect an organism. Most viruses trigger release of interferons from NK and dendritic cells and thus generate a Th1 response. Most immune responses are not exclusively of one type or the other but, rather, reflect mixed responses in which one type of T helper cell predominates. Measles virus in humans, for example, induces an early Th1 response that, during the late course of the infection, switches to a Th2 response, which persists for several weeks. The apparent immunosuppression after a measles virus infection affects mainly Th1-linked immune responses and may result from the prolonged Th2 response and its dampening effect on activation of Th1 cells (59).

Antigen Processing for Activation of CD8$^+$ T Cells

CD8$^+$ T cells recognize antigenic peptides associated with class I MHC determinants that, unlike class II MHC molecules, are expressed on the majority of cells. Viruses have evolved a number of mechanisms to interfere with the class I MHC antigen-presentation pathway, which stresses the importance of this T-cell subset in the organism's defense against viral infections. Class I MHC molecules, unlike class II MHC molecules, associate mainly with peptides derived from de novo synthesized proteins, constantly reporting intracellular events to the outside. Newly synthesized class I MHC heavy chains associate in the endoplasmic reticulum with calnexin, which promotes appropriate folding of the protein. The folded heavy chain then binds β_2-microglobulin. The correct folding of the class I MHC heavy chain is facilitated by calreticulin. The resulting complex binds to tapasin, providing a link to the transporter associated with antigen presentation (TAP), which connects the endoplasmic reticulum with the cytoplasm, in which viral proteins are being synthesized (60). Newly produced proteins that are faulty or incorrectly folded are degraded in the cytoplasm by a complex of proteolytic enzymes that assemble into a proteasome complex (61). Synthesis and posttranslational modifications of this complex are affected by IFN-γ (62). Peptides that are derived upon enzymatic cleavage of proteins are transported into the endoplasmic reticulum though TAP (63). TAP shows preference for peptides of 8 to 13 amino acids in length and, depending on the species of the host cell, for peptides with certain motifs such as hydrophobic carboxyl terminals (64). Once peptides reach the endoplasmic reticulum, they bind to the groove of class I MHC determinants (65), provided they carry the appropriate anchor residues (66). It has been estimated that each class I MHC molecule has the potential to bind any of 10,000 peptides. Nevertheless, upon virus infection, a CD8$^+$ T-cell population that recognizes one or two epitopes commonly dominates the response (67).

Upon binding of peptides, the class I MHC heavy chain/β_2-microglobulin complex releases calreticulin and tapasin and is transported through the Golgi apparatus to the cell surface. Dendritic cells can also present exogenous antigen in the context of class I MHC determinants, which is crucial for the activation of CD8$^+$ T cells against viruses that fail to directly infect dendritic cells (68). Presentation of exogenous antigen is dependent on proteasome and TAP and takes place in the endoplasmic reticulum. Peptides that contain a signal sequence can cross from the cytoplasm into the endo-

plasmic reticulum independently of TAP. Upon reaching the endoplasmic reticulum, these peptides are degraded further by peptidases until they reach a size that is compatible with binding to the cleft of class I MHC molecules. Nonclassical class I MHC molecules such as CD1 (69) or H-2M3 (70) can also present antigen—in part, nonpeptide antigen such as lipids—to the immune system. The role of these alternative pathways for antiviral defense is not yet understood.

Dendritic cells that display antigenic peptides in association with class I MHC molecules can activate CD8$^+$ T cells with the corresponding receptors. Induction of CD8$^+$ T cells to most viruses depends on CD4$^+$ T helper cells. T-cell help does not require concomitant binding of activated CD4$^+$ T cells and naïve CD8$^+$ T cells to dendritic cells displaying the CD4$^+$ T cells' antigen in the context of class II MHC molecule and the CD8$^+$ T cells' epitopes associated with class I MHC molecules. Such a simultaneous meeting among three rare cells (i.e., an antigen expressing dendritic cell, a specific CD4$^+$ T cell, and a CD8$^+$ T cell with the appropriate TCR) would be infrequent and thus not guarantee efficient activation of CD8$^+$ T cells. It is more likely that such interaction occurs sequentially (71). Dendritic cells, upon binding of T helper cells, receive an additional activation signal through CD40 expressed on the surface of T cells binding to the dendritic cells' CD40 ligand (72). Dendritic cells thus conditioned can now stimulate naïve CD8$^+$ T cells directly without further cognate interactions with CD4$^+$ T cells. Some viruses such as influenza virus, Sendai virus, or adenovirus induce CD8$^+$ T-cell responses in CD4- or class II MHC–deficient mice. Upon infection of dendritic cells, these viruses presumably furnish the same activation signals that are otherwise provided by CD40–CD40 ligand interactions. Induction of a cytolytic T-cell response in absence of T-cell help indicates that CD4$^+$ T cell–derived growth factors are not absolutely required for activation of CD8$^+$ T cells. Nevertheless, T helper cells commonly augment the CD8$^+$ T-cell response even to viruses that can induce CD8$^+$ T cells independently of CD4$^+$ T cells. CD8$^+$ T cells proliferate far more vigorously than CD4$^+$ T cells upon encountering their antigen. At the height of the immune response, depending on the antigen, up to 20% to 40% of all central CD8$^+$ T cells are those with specificity to a single epitope of the pathogen (73). Upon activation, CD8$^+$ T cells proliferate, partly in response to growth factors provided by T helper cells. IL-2 sponsors mainly proliferation of T cells (74), and IL-1 indirectly increases proliferation of T cells by up-regulating expression of the IL-2 receptor (75). IL-15 and IL-21 serve as growth factors for activated T cells (76,77).

Activation of B Cells

B cells are induced by soluble antigen. Activation of B cells is achieved most effectively by antigen complexed by natural antibodies to the crystallized fragment (Fc) γ receptor on follicular dendritic cells. Activation of B cells is facilitated by co-stimulatory signals from T helper cells. Once B cells encounter their antigen, they proliferate. The immunoglobulin hypervariable region mutates, and B cells, which secrete high-affinity antibodies proliferate. B cells with immunoglobulin mutations that result in loss of affinity undergo programmed cell death (78). Isotype switching is controlled by T helper cells. B cells proliferate in response to a number of cytokines such as IL-1, IL-2, IL-4, IL-6, IL-10, IL-13, IL-15, and IL-21 (79). IL-4 promotes B-cell maturation, which is enhanced by ligation of CD40 (80). IL-5 acts synergistically with IL-4 by enhancing CD40 expression. IL-13 has an effect similar to that of IL-4; together, these two cytokines also block programmed cell death of B cells. Proliferation of B cells is inhibited by transforming growth factor β. In mice, isotype switching of B cells toward IgE and IgG1 is mediated by IL-4 and IL-13, switching toward the IgG2a isotype is favored by IFN-γ, and switching toward IgA is facilitated by transforming growth factor β (81).

B cells can be separated according to their anatomical location into B1 cells, which are found in the peritoneal cavity, and conventional B2 cells, found in lymphoid tissues (82). B cells in the spleen can be subdivided into marginal zone B cells and follicular B cells (83). B1 cells are the source of natural antibodies that facilitate activation of antigen-specific B cells in lymphoid tissues. Natural antibodies may play a crucial role in impairing early viral dissemination (84). They are able to form complexes with a wide variety of viral pathogens. Such complexes are selectively retained in lymphoid tissues, thus reducing the spread of the pathogen to other vital organs.

Marginal zone B1 cells have a preactivated phenotype and, like B2 cells, respond very rapidly to viral pathogens by secretion of IgM antibodies, which in general have low affinity to the antigen. This response, which is independent of T helper cells, peaks after 3 to 4 days and is then followed by antibodies originating from follicular B cells in lymph nodes and spleens. Once B1 cells or marginal zone B cells become activated, they terminally differentiate into plasma cells. They do not contribute to the memory response but undergo programmed cell death. B cells have thus evolved to respond very rapidly with "unedited" antibodies of low affinity to an incoming pathogen (Fig. 2). These antibodies are secreted without further input from T helper cells that are not yet fully activated at this early stage after an infection. A T helper cell–independent B-cell response has an increased risk for cross-reactivity with self-antigen. To lessen the threat of permanent damage from autoantibodies, the B cells that provide early antibodies are not destined to become part of the memory B-cell pool. Follicular B cells respond later, and their activation is controlled by T helper cells. Some viruses induce potent IgG responses independently of T helper cells (85). Several avenues that cause T helper cell–independent activation of B cells can be envisioned. Viruses with complex structures that carry repetitions of a pattern may activate B cells directly by cross-linking of the immunoglobulin receptors (86). A subset of NK cells that expresses T-cell markers, termed NK1.1 cells, responds to viral infection with release of copious amounts of cytokines (87), which may facilitate

differentiation and proliferation of B cells. Other viruses may express epitopes that have sequence similarity to common environmental antigens that trigger a memory rather than a primary B-cell response.

THE EFFECTOR FUNCTIONS OF ANTIGEN-SPECIFIC IMMUNE MECHANISMS

Upon activation, antibody-secreting B cells home to the bone marrow and, to a lesser extent, to the spleen. T cells are recruited to the sites of inflammation, where the virus replicates. Activated T cells express different chemokine receptors and have a higher density of certain types of adhesion molecules (leukocyte function–associated antigen 1 or integrin $\alpha4$) than do naïve T cells; these features allow them to leave blood vessels and to enter inflamed tissues (88). Once activated, T cells that reach an area of inflammation interact through their adhesion molecules with P- and E-selectins, intracellular and vascular cell adhesion molecules, and CD34 that are expressed at increased levels on vascular endothelial cells in presence of cytokines such as IL-1 or TNF-α. These interactions initially cause a loose attachment of the lymphocytes, followed by their rolling along the vessel walls (89). Chemokines secreted at the site of inflammation carry heparin-binding sites that cause them to be retained in the extracellular matrix close to their site of origin. Once the lymphocytes reach an area rich in chemokines corresponding to their receptors, they bind firmly to the vascular endothelial cells and eventually emigrate out of the vessels into the tissue. Recruitment of activated T cells is driven by chemokines and not by the antigen specificity of the TCRs (90). Thus, all activated T cells are recruited to an inflammatory site. T cells that at these sites encounter their specific antigen commence effector functions, whereas T cells recruited serendipitously either down-regulate expression of their chemokine receptors and depart from the tissue or undergo activation-induced cell death (91). Unlike naïve T cells, T cells at the effector cell stage respond to antigen presented by MHC determinants without further need for co-stimulatory signals. Otherwise, recognition of antigen follows the same rules seen during the induction phase. Antibodies secreted by activated B cells bind to extracellular intact antigen or to proteins expressed on the cell surface. CD8$^+$ T cells react to peptides from *de novo* synthesized proteins displayed by class I MHC molecules. CD4$^+$ T cells recognize peptides from processed exogenous antigen displayed by class II MHC molecules that are expressed only on specialized cells such as dendritic cells, macrophages, and B cells. This recognition pattern determines the role of the different antigen-specific immune effector mechanisms in clearing a virus infection. Antibodies act best against soluble antigen, such as viruses released from dying cells. Antibodies to certain viral surface proteins can neutralize the virus by impairing its ability to infect other cells. Nonneutralizing antibodies to structural viral proteins can facilitate phagocytosis of the virus particles. Antibodies of the IgG1 isotype in humans or the IgG2a isotype in mice that bind viral proteins expressed on the surface of infected cells can recruit complement and thus affect the demise of the infected cells. Because such proteins are commonly expressed only late in infection, which is when virus replication is partly completed, this can actually facilitate rather than inhibit the spread of the virus. Although antibodies, especially those that are neutralizing, are undeniably the most effective immune mechanisms for preventing or lessening a viral invasion, they are less suited to completely clear an already established infection. Viruses, being obligatory intracellular pathogens, are best combated by CD8$^+$ T cells, which evolved to recognize antigen synthesized within a cell displayed by class I MHC molecules. All nucleated cells, with the exception of neurons, express such class I MHC molecules. Although neurons, at least *in vitro*, can be induced to express class I MHC determinant upon treatment with IFN-γ, production of IFN-γ by T cells *in vivo* requires their initial receptor engagement with peptide-class I MHC determinants. Strictly neurotropic viruses such as rabies virus thus successfully evade recognition by CD8$^+$ T cells. The central nervous system is otherwise shielded from the immune system by the blood–brain barrier, which is impermeable to resting lymphocytes or larger molecules such as antibodies, and by the lack of a lymphatic draining system. This state of immune privilege presumably provides an advantage to the host. Neurons are irreplaceable, and their destruction by a potent CD8$^+$ T cell response may be more troublesome for the well-being of the afflicted individual than is a neuronal infection with a noncytopathic virus. The disadvantage of such an immunologically privileged status is a lack of defense against highly virulent neurotropic viruses such as rabies virus, which can readily overwhelm an organism once it successfully establishes an intracerebral infection.

CD8$^+$ T cells can eliminate virus-infected cells through a number of mechanisms. They can kill them by the release of perforin (92), a membrane pore-forming protein similar to complement. Perforin-knockout mice show an increased susceptibility to certain virus infections (93). Activated CD8$^+$ T cells express Fas ligand (CD95L) on their surface. Interactions of CD95L with Fas (CD95) expressed on virus-infected cells induce the infected cells' death by apoptosis (94,95). Activated T cells also express TNF-related apoptosis-inducing ligand (TRAIL), which, upon binding to the corresponding receptor such as the apoptosis-inducing proteins DR4 or DR5, instigates programmed cell death. CD4$^+$ T cell–mediated lysis through TRAIL has been demonstrated for tumor cells and antigen-presenting cells (96). The role of this death pathway in antiviral immunity remains to be elucidated.

Upon engagement of their receptors, most CD8$^+$ T cells release IFN-γ, which not only reduces viral replication but also clears persistent infection with certain viruses such as lymphocytic choriomeningitis virus (LCMV) (97) or hepatitis B virus (HBV) (98). CD8$^+$ T cells, unlike CD4$^+$ T cells and antibodies, recognize predominantly viral antigens that are produced early during viral propagation (99). This may relate to the inhibition of cellular protein synthesis upon viral infection, which may interfere with the class I MHC antigen–

processing pathways and in turn favor presentation of early viral proteins that are produced before the cellular machinery is taken over by the virus. Recognition of early viral antigens by CD8$^+$ T cells is advantageous for the host because it allows lysis of infected cells before new viral progeny have been assembled, thus very efficiently preventing further spread of the virus. Upon infections with certain viruses, especially those inclined to establish persistent infections, CD4$^+$ T cells, in addition to CD8$^+$ T cells, are necessary to control the spread of the virus (100). This may in part relate to the ability of CD4$^+$ T cells to secrete IFN-γ and TNF-α to activate macrophages and to promote activation of CD8$^+$ T cells.

Once the effector phase has been terminated upon removal of the infectious agent, most of the virus-specific CD8$^+$ T cells undergo activation-induced cell death (101,102). Frequencies of antigen-specific CD8$^+$ T cells decline sharply until they reach the steady-state level during the immunological memory phase (103). Frequencies of virus-specific CD4$^+$ T cells also decline. Because this population does not expand upon activation as dramatically as CD8$^+$ T cells do, their decline is equally less pronounced (104). The absolute frequencies of the virus-specific T cells at the height of the effector phase depend on a number of parameters, such as the antigenic load, interactions between the virus and the antigen-presenting cells, the type of the ensuing immune response (Th1/Th2), and the duration of antigen presentation (Fig. 5). This has been studied in part with recombinant viral vaccines that encode the same transgene product but differ in characteristics of the carrier. For example, E1-deleted adenoviral recombinants that are noncytopathic and thus persist in transduced cells until they are eliminated by CD8$^+$ T effector cells induce markedly higher frequencies of CD8$^+$ T cells to the transgene product than do vaccinia virus recombinants, which rapidly kill the infected cells (105).

IMMUNOLOGICAL MEMORY

The adaptive immune system, unlike the innate immune system, establishes memory, which, upon reencounter of the same pathogen, mounts an accelerated and enhanced response of B and T cells that generally eliminate the virus before the infection becomes clinically apparent. The existence of immunological memory was already appreciated in ancient Greece. In 631 B.C., a plague struck Athens, and the year-long epidemic left Athenians so demoralized that they ended up defeated by the far less advanced Spartans. Thucydides, a wealthy young philosopher, chronicled that year, observing that survivors of the plague were rendered resistant for life against this bacterial disease, whose etiology at that time was obscure (106). In 1781, a measles epidemic struck the isolated Faroe Islands (107). Once the epidemic ran its natural course, the Faroe Islanders did not reencounter this pathogen until 65 years later, when a new epidemic infected nearly all its inhabitants except for the elderly population, which had been infected more than six decades earlier. Immunological

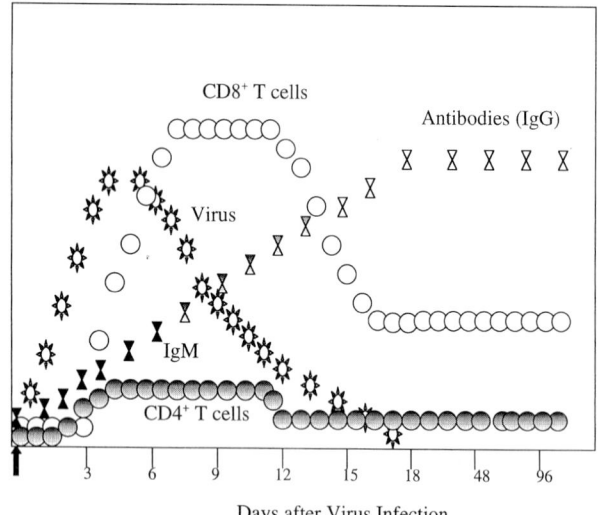

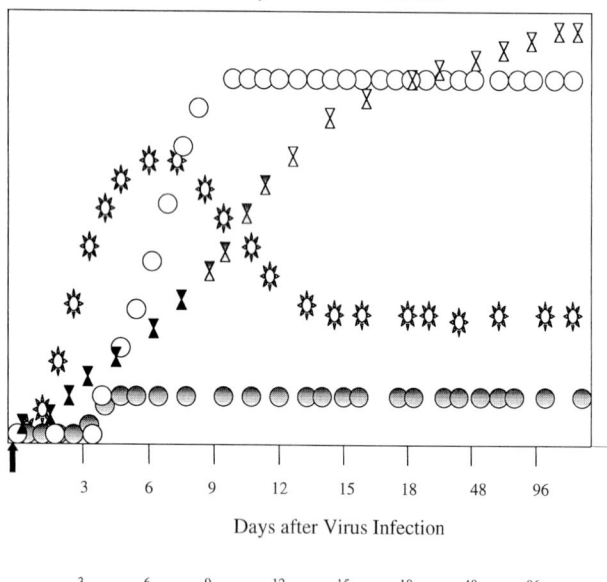

FIG. 5. Kinetics of immune response during acute viral infection. This is a virtual kinetic of an acute immune response after an infection. Kinetics of T- and B-cell responses differ, depending on the virus.

memory is thus long-lived and provides protection against some pathogens for life. In addition, this natural experiment on a remote island demonstrates that protective memory is maintained without periodic encounter of the antigen.

Memory T cells carry phenotypic markers that distinguish them from naïve T cells. Naïve T cells are CD44^{low}, whereas memory T cells are CD44^{high}. Memory T cells are distinct from effector T cells in that the former are low in CD25 and CD69, which are expressed highly on activated effector T cells (108,109). Memory T cells of a given specificity are present at higher frequencies than naïve T cells to an individual epitope. The memory T-cell population is maintained at remarkably stable levels; dying cells are replaced by cell divisions, which for CD8^{+} T cells are driven by IL-15 (110). Persistence of memory T cells is independent of anti-

gen (111); a maintenance of CD8^{+} T cell memory appears to depend on CD4^{+} T cells. Memory T helper cells are committed to become either Th1 or Th2 cells upon reactivation (112). Although the threshold for reactivation of memory T cells is lower than that for initiation of naïve T cells, memory T cells still must reencounter the antigen expressed in the context of MHC-restricting elements and co-stimulatory signals. Proliferation of memory T cells upon antigenic challenge takes place within lymphatic tissues. Memory T cells differentiate into effector cells more rapidly than do naïve T cells (113); however, this process nevertheless takes 3 to 4 days. Because viruses can overwhelm an organism during this time span, the role of memory T cells in providing protection to a reinfection with a pathogen has been considered as being marginal. Studies (114) have shown that memory CD8^{+} T cells can be subdivided into two anatomically separated populations. The first, central memory CD8^{+} T cells, are found in lymph nodes, in the spleen, and in peripheral blood. They are CCR7^{+}, which forms the basis for their preferential homing to lymphatic tissues. The second subset of CD8^{+} memory T cells, which is CCR7^{-}, homes to nonlymphoid tissues and to the spleen (115). These T cells, which can be found in the liver, fatty tissue, the peritoneal cavity, the kidneys, and other organs and tissues, are maintained at surprisingly high frequencies. Unlike the central CCR7^{+} memory CD8^{+} T cells, the CCR7^{-} subset retains effector function. CCR7^{-} memory CD8^{+} T cells lyse target cells and release cytokines without further activation or expansion. This subset of memory CD8^{+} T cells, effector-memory cells, may thus represent a crucial first line of defense against an invasion with a familiar pathogen.

Antibodies, which persist for a lengthy time after a primary infection, provide a crucial barrier to reinfection. Antibody titers are maintained by periodic reactivation of B cells through antigen released from antigen-antibody complexes on follicular dendritic cells (116). Systemic antibody titers can persist for decades. Antibodies secreted at mucosal surfaces are relatively short-lived (117). This may reflect a difference in life span between bone marrow plasma cells, which produce the antibodies found in serum, and plasma cells, which secrete mucosal antibodies. Once antigen-antibody depots are depleted from lymphoid tissues, the antibody response declines. Maintenance of memory B cells at a quiescent stage is apparently independent of antigen (118). Upon reencounter of the antigen, memory B cells proliferate rapidly and produce antibodies with already mature affinity as a result of hypermutation and selection during the primary response, thereby providing a qualitatively improved defense against the invading pathogen (119).

THE MUCOSAL IMMUNE SYSTEM

The immune system can be subdivided roughly into two separate, albeit interactive, entities: a central immune system localized in the spleen and lymph nodes, which patrols the inner tissues and organs, and a mucosal immune system, which covers in humans a total surface area of approximately 400 m² of mucosa of the airways, the intestines, and the urogenital tract, which are the most common ports of entry for pathogens. Mucosal surfaces, such as those of the intestinal tract or the airways, are constantly bombarded with "harmless" antigens, including those present in food, that are best tolerated. The inner tissues and organs, however, are in a sterile environment, which warrants more stringent control against foreign antigens. The two immune systems that control the central organism and the mucosal surfaces are thus faced by different challenges and have, as a result, distinct characteristics. The central immune system has been extremely well characterized since the early 1970s. Less is known about the mucosal immune system.

The mucosal immune system consists anatomically of (a) local inductive sites, called organized mucosa-associated lymphoid tissue (O-MALT), such as tonsils, Peyer's patches, and the appendix, and (b) effector sites present directly in the mucosal epithelium, called diffuse mucosa-associated lymphoid tissue (D-MALT) [reviewed by Neutra et al. (120)]. Some mucosal surfaces, such as those of the vagina, lack an O-MALT system. Therefore, lymphocyte stimulation upon vaginal infection relies on antigen transport to local lymph nodes. The epithelium that covers the mucosal surfaces differs, depending on the anatomical location: For example, the intestine is covered by a single epithelial layer, whereas the vagina is covered by a multilayered squamous epithelium that varies in thickness with the menstrual cycle. Transport of antigen from the mucosal surface to the O-MALT system or the local lymph nodes occurs in the intestine and the airways by M cells, whereas mucosal surfaces covered by a squamous epithelium rely on local dendritic cells for transport of antigen to the inductive sites (120). Mucosal dendritic cells may differ functionally from those in the central immune system (121). A potential role of M cells in antigen presentation also remains to be resolved (122).

Not only is the anatomy of the mucosal immune system different from that of the systemic immune system, but also the individual immune cells show distinct characteristics (123). The best studied population is that of the intraepithelial lymphocytes (IELs) of the intestine. They appear relatively late in development [approximately 2 to 4 weeks after birth in mice (124)] and initially are composed mainly of T cells expressing the γ/δ receptor (125). These γ/δ T cells are eventually joined by T cells carrying the α/β receptor. The number of IELs increases substantially between 6 and 20 weeks; by 20 weeks, most of the intraepithelial T cells express α/β receptors (125). Some of the α/β T cells are double positive for CD4 and CD8; such T cells are not found in the spleen or lymph nodes. Most of the double-positive mucosal T cells carry homodimers of the CD8 α chain, rather than heterodimers of α and β, which are found on CD8⁺ T cells of the central immune system. T cells that carry the γ/δ TCR and are single positive for CD8 also lack CD8 β chain expression (123). Some of the intraepithelial T cells (both α/β and γ/δ TCR⁺) develop within the mucosal immune

system independently of the thymus (126). Antigen recognition by double-positive CD8 α/α and TCR γ/δ T cells is different from that by single-positive and α/β TCR-expressing T cells; double-positive CD8 γ/δ T cells of the mucosal immune system fail to respond to activation with anti-TCR antibodies and, furthermore, express potentially autoreactive antigen receptors (127). This has led to the conclusion that this T-cell subset might be immature and functionally inactive. T cells that express the γ/δ receptor have been shown to have effector functions; for example, they have antimicrobial activity (128), secrete cytokines (129), and promote the development of IgA-secreting B cells (130). Mice that lack γ/δ T cells fail to develop IgA-secreting B cells in Peyer's patches and the intestinal lamina (130). Many of the γ/δ T cells seem to recognize antigen, including nonprotein structures, directly without the need for presentation by classical MHC determinants (131). T cells expressing either the γ/δ or the α/β receptor are present in vaginal epithelium. The γ/δ T cells have a distinctive phenotype that in some aspects resembles that of those cells in the skin: they are CD4⁻CD8⁻ and CD45⁺ and express an invariant TCR (Vγ4 and Vδ1) (132). Not only is a portion of the T cells of the mucosal immune system of primordial origin, predating "modern" single-positive α/β-expressing T cells by approximately 200 million years, but also some of the B cells (so-called B1 cells) belong to a more primitive system. A portion of gut B cells (which can also be found in the pleural and peritoneal cavity) are phenotypically IgM^high, B220^low, CD23⁻, Mac-1⁺, and Ly-1⁺, as opposed to "modern" B cells, which are Ly-1⁻ and B220^high. Although "modern" B cells secrete high-affinity antibodies with exquisite specificity, the B1 cells secrete mainly IgM and IgA with low affinity and broad cross-reactivity. B cells derive from the bone marrow, whereas B1 cells are capable of self-renewal.

Oral immunization causes activation of Th2-type cells at mucosal surfaces, which secrete IL-4 and IL-5 but not IL-2 or IFN-γ in response to antigen (129,133). Cytokines are released by both double-positive and CD4⁺CD8⁻ TCR α/β^+ IELs. Although targeting of antigen to mucosal surfaces generally favors stimulation of Th2 cells, some antigens, such as those presented by a recombinant *Salmonella* species, give rise to Th1-type responses (134), which suggests that the nature of the antigen and its carrier affects the type of the response. The mucosal immune response can also be shifted toward a Th1-type pathway by concomitant oral application of IL-12, which was shown to redirect the T-cell response both in the spleen and in Peyer's patches without affecting IgA secretion at mucosal surfaces (135). Some studies addressed activation of cytolytic T cells by using redirected lysis. These studies showed that both γ/δ and α/β intraepithelial T cells have lytic capabilities (136).

PERSISTENT VIRUS INFECTIONS

Many viruses cause an acute disease during their replication, resulting in activation of adaptive immune responses that successfully eliminate all virus-infected cells. Examples of such acute infections include those with orthomyxoviruses (influenza virus), paramyxoviruses (mumps virus, measles virus, respiratory syncytial virus), reoviruses (rotavirus), and picornaviruses (poliovirus, hepatitis A virus, rhinoviruses). Some of these viruses, such as poxviruses or adenoviruses, are cytopathic. Cytopathic viruses cause the death of the infected cells, whereas noncytopathic viruses, such as LCMV, propagate without killing their host cells. Cytopathic viruses either are completely eliminated by the immune system or kill the infected organism. Noncytopathic viruses, on the other hand, can establish very long-lasting infections and successfully evade complete destruction by immune effector mechanisms. Different viruses establish different types of chronic infections, and each provides a unique challenge to the immune system.

Treatment of persistent viral infections predates modern medicine, as shown by the following citation from Mark Twain's *Tom Sawyer* about warts that are caused by infections with some types of human papillomaviruses (HPV). Huckleberry Finn's remedies were unorthodox and imaginative but probably nevertheless effective:

> "You take and split the bean, and cut the wart as to get some blood, and then you put the blood on one piece of the bean and take and dig a hole and bury it 'bout midnight at the crossroads in the dark of the moon..." or "You take your cat and go and get in the graveyard 'long about midnight when somebody that was wicked has been buried; and when it's midnight a devil will come, or maybe two or three, but you can't see 'em, you can only hear something like the wind, or maybe hear 'em talk; and when they are taking the feller away you heave your cat after 'em and say 'Devil follow corpse, cat follow devil, wart follow cat, I'm done with you!' That'll fetch any wart."

Huckleberry Finn's proposed cure for HPV-infected skin lesions by cutting the wart until blood is drawn may actually have an immunological basis. The injury of the wart initiates an inflammatory reaction, especially if it is done with a dirty pocketknife at some crossroad in the middle of the night by a child. This in turn causes maturation of resident dendritic cells, which, upon processing some of the viral proteins released from the infected cells, induce activation of a T-cell response to HPV, which could clear the infected cells and thus induce regression of the warts. The efficacy of Huck's alternative therapy may just be another example of the effect of the conscious/subconscious mind on the immune system.

A typical example of a viral family that establishes persistent infections is that of retroviruses such as the HIV, described in detail in Chapter 42. Other human retroviruses include human T-cell leukemia viruses (HTLV) types 1 and 2, which cause adult T-cell leukemia. HTLV-1 infections are most commonly found in Japan, the Caribbean, and parts of Africa and South America. HTLV-2–associated adult T-cell leukemia is restricted to certain ethnic groups in the Americas and in Africa. Patients develop both B- and T-cell responses to the antigens of HTLV, which control disease progression but are incapable of completely eradicating the virally transformed cells (137).

Rabies virus, a cytopathic virus can cause symptoms in humans within 10–14 days, which inevitably progress to eventually fatal encephalitis. In other patients, rabies virus that is generally transmitted through the bite of an infected mammal such as a dog, fox, raccoon, or bat leads to encephalitis 20 to 30 years after exposure. The time of exposure to rabies virus can be tracked quite accurately. Rabies virus strains prevailing in different countries and in different mammalian species show sufficient sequence variability to pinpoint the geographic origin of the infection. Patients residing in the United States have been reported to develop a rabies virus infection caused by a virus prevalent in dogs of Asia but not North America. The patients' histories revealed that they visited or emigrated from Asia more than 20 years earlier, where they contracted an infection with rabies virus that remained clinically asymptomatic for decades. During the incubation time, such patients fail to develop immunity to rabies virus. It is currently unknown where the virus remains dormant and what ultimately causes its reactivation. The long latency between infection and disease does not reflect a typical persistent infection, inasmuch as rabies virus most probably fails to replicate during these long incubation periods.

Adenoviruses, which produce generally mild infections of the respiratory or intestinal tract, can persist in lymphoid tissues for several years (138). Although adenoviruses, like many of the complex DNA viruses, have developed a number of pathways to evade the immune system, the underlying basis for their persistence is currently not understood.

Certain Arenaviridae entities such as LCMV establish lifelong infections upon inoculation into neonatal rodents or upon maternal–fetal transmissions (139). LCMV antigens are expressed within the thymus, causing T-cell tolerance in immunologically immature animals. Infected animals develop vigorous antibody responses, which fail to clear the virus but rather lead to immunocomplex disease such as glomerulonephritis and eventual kidney failure (140). Adoptive transfer of CD8$^+$ T cells to LCMV clears the infection in carrier mice, which implies that the unresponsiveness of this T-cell subset is the reason for the viral persistence (141). Inoculation of adult mice with high doses of some strains of LCMV can establish persistent infections by leading to exhaustion of peripheral CD8$^+$ T LCMV antigen-specific T cells (142). Apparently, the overwhelming number of virus-infected cells causes activation of all available CD8$^+$ T cells to LCMV-associated antigens, including those destined for the memory T-cell pool. Upon activation to effector cells, the CD8$^+$ T cell eventually undergo programmed cell death, causing complete elimination of CD8$^+$ LCMV antigen-specific T cells. Infection of thymic epithelial cells with LCMV induces tolerance of new T cells derived from bone marrow progenitors. This form of immunological exhaustion has not been observed with other persistent viral infections that perpetually provide potent stimulation to CD8$^+$ T cells, such as HIV-1.

Herpesviruses establish persistent infections that follow a lytic/latent life cycle. Viral latency is characterized by decreased viral gene expression and is another mechanism by which viruses avoid immune surveillance and establish persistent infections. Upon the initial infection of host cells, they commence production of new viral progeny, which results in the death of the infected cells. This is referred to as the lytic cycle of the virus. Viruses derived from the primary site of infection either can produce more viral progeny upon infection of additional cells or can establish a latent infection during which viral protein production is virtually shut off (143). T cells can recognize herpesvirus antigens during the lytic cycle of the virus but fail to detect a target during latency. Upon reactivation of herpesviruses as a result of stress such as ultraviolet light exposure or hormonal imbalance, the virus reenters a lytic cycle, during which newly synthesized viral proteins reactivate antigen-specific CD8$^+$ and CD4$^+$ T cells, which eventually control the recurrent infection (144). Different types of herpesvirus differ in their tropism and hence in their pathogenicity. Herpes simplex viruses initially infect epithelial cells and then, upon retrograde axonal transport, establish latent infections in neurons. Upon reactivation, the virus is transported back to the skin or mucosa, where it replicates (145). Epstein-Barr virus (EBV), a potentially oncogenic herpesvirus, infects B cells. It can cause lymphoproliferative disease and lymphomas in immunosuppressed individuals (146). This can be treated in transplant recipients by lowering of the immunosuppressive regimen, which allows resurgence of T cells that eliminate the EBV-infected B cells. Patients with X-linked hyperproliferative disease are prone to develop fulminant infections with EBV (147). These patients have a mutation of the signaling lymphocyte-activation molecule (SLAM)–associated protein (SAP). SAP-knockout mice are impaired in their ability to develop Th2 responses and generate enhanced CD8$^+$ T cell responses to viral challenge, which indicates that the SAP signal transduction pathway is an inhibitor for CD8$^+$ T-cell proliferation (148). EBV can cause Burkitt's lymphoma, which is prevalent in North Africa and South America. The EBV remains immunologically silent in Burkitt's lymphoma by means of evasive actions of the virus. Nevertheless, the slight increase of the incidence of Burkitt's lymphomas in patients with AIDS suggests that a competent immune system can at least partly control the development of the EBV-associated malignancies (149).

Cytomegalovirus persists in cells of the bone marrow, and, again, immunosuppressed individuals are at increased risk for fatal infections after viral reactivation (150). Other herpesviruses such as varicella-zoster virus or human herpesviruses 6, 7, or 8 (the last being associated with Kaposi's sarcoma) also cause severe disease primarily in immunocompromised individuals (151), which indicates that, in general, a competent immune system successfully controls herpesvirus reactivation.

HPVs can establish persistent infections upon integration into the host cells' genome. Most HPVs cause harmless, albeit unattractive, proliferation of keratinocytes in the skin or the genital mucosa. Skin warts, which are common in children, often regress spontaneously, presumably upon activation of an immune response. Genital warts are highly infectious but can be treated either surgically or by topical application of interferon (152). Most patients rapidly clear genital infections with oncogenic types of HPV through cellular immune responses to the early viral proteins. Some patients develop persistent infections, which after years of latency can lead to cervical cancer (153). HPV-associated genital malignancies remain the second most common type of cancer in women worldwide. Immunosuppressed women have a significantly higher incidence of cervical cancer (154). This indicates that adaptive immune responses either clear virus-infected cells early before they transform or alternatively eliminate the transformed cells, which express the viral E6 and E7 oncoproteins, before the malignancy reaches a size that is diagnosed.

Hepatitis C virus, a flavivirus, and HBV, a hepadnavirus, can establish persistent hepatic infections that cause chronic inflammatory liver disease and liver failure or hepatocellular carcinoma (155). It is currently not clear why a fraction of patients develop persistent infections but others clear the virus completely during the acute infection. Patients chronically infected with HBV have relatively weak CD8$^+$ T-cell responses to this virus (156), which may contribute to the inability to eradicate it completely. In contrasts, carriers of hepatitis C virus have vigorous CD8$^+$ T-cell responses to multiple viral antigens (157). Hepatitis C virus mutates more rapidly than HBV, and the resulting viral variants may continuously escape immune-mediated destruction (158). During chronic infections, CD8$^+$ T cells control the viral load while at the same time contributing to liver injury (159). Patients with chronic hepatitis virus infections are currently treated with type I interferon, which in some but not all patients results in clearance of the virus-infected cells.

In rare cases, measles virus can cause subacute sclerosing panencephalitis after a 7- to 10-year delay after the primary infection (160). In this disease, a small amount of virus particles enters neurons and slowly spreads throughout the central nervous system. Because the central nervous system and especially class I MHC–negative neurons provide a safe haven for viruses, the immune system remains ignorant of the simmering infection.

During chronic infections, viruses may escape the immune system by mutation of T-cell epitopes. Although the T-cell repertoire may contain cells with receptors that optimally fit these mutants' epitopes, the immune system may fail to take advantage of such cells. This phenomenon, called "original antigenic sin," was initially described for B-cell responses to influenza virus (161). Individuals infected with an influenza virus of a given serotype generate high-affinity antibodies to this virus. Upon reencounter with a variant of the original virus, the individual's immune system mounts a secondary B-cell response. The B cells secrete antibodies that have a perfect fit for the initial virus but markedly lower affinity for the virus causing the ongoing infection. The immune system thus remembers but is unable to adjust to the changed needs of the infected individual. Cytolytic T cells can fall into the same trap, which can lead to impaired clearance of viral mutants that arise during the course of a chronic infection (162).

AUTOIMMUNITY AFTER VIRUS INFECTIONS

Virus infections can lead to the development of autoimmune diseases (163). This can be attributed to molecular mimicry, in which a viral antigen shows sequence homology with a self-protein (164); to epitope spreading (165); or to abnormal regulation of T-cell responses (166).

Many proteins derived from pathogens show sequence homology with proteins of the hosts. The immune system is tolerant of the hosts' proteins. Tolerance against self-proteins is maintained through clonal deletion of autoreactive lymphocytes, anergy, ignorance, or an active form of suppression. Ignorant or anergic T cells can become autoreactive if stimulated within the context of an infection with a virus expressing cross-reactive epitopes that are produced at higher concentrations, at an unusual location, or within the context of a cytokine-rich environment. For example, a monoclonal antibody to Coxsackie B4 virus was found to cross-react with a protein present in heart muscle, which implicates autoimmunity as an underlying reason for cases of idiopathic myocarditis after Coxsackie virus infections (167).

Epitope spreading is implicated in causing acute disseminated encephalomyelitis after measles infection. This rare complication is associated with an immune response to myelin basic protein similar to that seen in experimental allergic encephalitis or multiple sclerosis. Theiler's murine encephalitis virus induces a $CD4^+$ T cell–mediated demyelinating disease that also resembles experimental allergic encephalitis or multiple sclerosis. The virus initially damages the central nervous system, which causes the release of sequestered antigens such as myelin basic protein. Within an inflammatory environment, epitopes of myelin basic protein became processed by antigen-presenting cells, which leads to the induction of autoreactive $CD4^+$ T cells, which in turn perpetuates the disease. This form of virus-induced autoimmune reaction is called *epitope spreading;* this term reflects the fact that the damage caused by the virus infections allows the induction of immune responses to self-proteins that are otherwise ignored by the immune system.

VIRAL SUPERANTIGENS

Superantigens are proteins or polypeptides that cause massive activation of $CD4^+$ T cells expressing a given TCR $V\beta$ chain. This activation, which can be fatal for the host as a result of the toxicity of the resulting, often overwhelming, cytokine production, eventually leads to elimination of the induced $CD4^+$ T-cell population. Superantigens best characterized for bacterial products bind to the lateral face of class II MHC molecules distant from the peptide-binding groove. The superantigen then interacts with the $V\beta$ chain of the TCRs, causing activation of all T cells expressing the corre-

sponding TCR chain. This initially leads to vigorous proliferation of the T cells, followed by their activation-induced cell death. At the end, the organism is virtually depleted of T cells expressing this $V\beta$ chain. Superantigens are expressed by murine type B retroviruses such as mouse mammary tumor viruses, which induce massive negative selection of T cells in the thymus and in the periphery (168). A number of human viral pathogens have been postulated to carry superantigens, but this has been demonstrated with some certainty only for rabies virus. The rabies virus nucleoprotein, which is the most abundant protein of the viral capsid, binds to the MHC determinants of different murine or human haplotypes. In susceptible humans, the rabies virus nucleoprotein causes proliferation and then deletion of T cells expressing $V\beta8$ TCR (169); in mice, T cells expressing $V\beta7$ or $V\beta6$ receptor are affected (170). Depletion of these T-cell subsets apparently provides a survival advantage to the host. Mice depleted of T cells expressing the $V\beta6$ and $V\beta7$ TCR show increased resistance to an infection with rabies virus. They also fail to develop the pronounced paralysis observed in mice that carry these T cells. In humans, an infection with rabies virus can lead either to a paralytic form, indicative of spinal cord and peripheral nervous system damage, or to an encephalitic form, also called furious rabies, reflecting damage of the central nervous system (171). The paralytic form of rabies may be linked to an autoimmune reaction after hyperactivation of the immune system by the superantigen activity of the nucleoprotein.

VIRAL SUBVERSION OF IMMUNE RESPONSES

Viruses, especially the large, more complex DNA viruses have a number of strategies for evading the hosts' immune system. One strategy is to obscure their identity by mutations. Viruses can also hide in cells inaccessible to the immune system, or they can assume a state of latency in which they cannot be recognized. Some viruses infect and kill immune cells, they can down-regulate immune responses by altering the cells' antigen processing pathway, or they can interfere with the activity of cytokines. Poxviruses, herpesviruses, and adenoviruses encode a large number of proteins that interfere with activation of innate and adaptive immune responses. Many of these proteins show homology with cellular proteins of their hosts. In view of the size limitations of viral genomes, the multitude of genes that serve to subvert immune responses must clearly provide an evolutionary advantage to the virus. For immunologists, these proteins and their mode of action reveal the soft spots of viruses that are most suited for a successful attack by the immune system.

Escape by Mutations

Viruses mutate far more rapidly than mammalian cells. In the presence of a neutralizing antibody response, viral variants that have lost or modified the antibody's targets are selected. Such mutations most commonly affect viral surface proteins that provide epitopes for neutralizing antibodies, but they can also be seen on internal viral proteins in which selection is prompted by the activity of T cells (172).

Escape by Hiding

As mentioned earlier, the central nervous system is an immunologically privileged site in which viruses are relatively sheltered from the immune system. A number of viruses take advantage of this and establish neuronal infections. A typical example is rabies virus, which multiplies in neurons. Once the virus is ready to be transmitted to the next host, it spreads via axonal flow to the periphery to infect cells of the salivary gland. The neuronal damage changes the behavior of the infected animal so that it becomes aggressive and inclined to attack others, thus further facilitating the spread of the virus. Although effector or memory T-lymphocytes can cross the blood–brain barrier, the immune system lacks the needed signals in the periphery to activate rabies virus–specific T cells and is thus incapable of controlling the infection.

Escape by Latency

As discussed previously, upon infection of cells, herpesviruses can shut off viral protein synthesis and enter a state of latency. The immune system remains ignorant of latently infected cells that do not express viral antigens. This allows the virus to evade complete destruction during the height of an acute immune response. Once the immune system assumes a more relaxed stage of memory, the virus can reactivate and replicate unhindered for a few days until T cells convert from memory cells back to effector cells. These short bursts of viral replication suffice to produce ample amounts of virus to allow its spread to other organisms.

Escape by Destruction of Immune Cells

A number of viruses infect cells of the adaptive immune system, leading to the demise of those cells. The best example is HIV-1 virus, which infects and destroys CD4$^+$ T cells, as described in more detail in another chapter.

Rather than directly infecting immune cells, viruses can kill such cells indirectly and focus more specifically on those that are directed against their antigens. For example, HBV can establish persistent infections. Although this is more common in maternal–fetal transmission, in which the immature immune system becomes tolerant of the viral antigens, some adults are also incapable of completely clearing an HBV infection. It is speculated that HBV-infected cells actively kill HBV-specific CD8$^+$ T cells. Inflammatory cytokines can induce Fas expression on hepatocytes, the main target of HBV (173). T effector cells not only express Fas in order to induce programmed cell death of infected Fas ligand–positive cells, but they themselves also carry Fas ligand, which eventually triggers their own apoptosis. Although expression of Fas ligand on effector T cells is vital to negatively regulate

an immune response, it also renders T cells susceptible to a premature death by cells that express Fas. Some type of tumor cells express Fas and thus successfully evade destruction of cytolytic T cells. HBV-infected Fas-positive hepatocytes may have the same effect on CD8$^+$ T cells that, upon recognition of their target antigen, are killed before they can deliver a lethal hit against the virus-producing cells. This would also explain the discrepancy of the CD8$^+$ T-cell responses during acute, as opposed to chronic, HBV infections. During the acute phase of the infection, patients have a vigorous CD8$^+$ T-cell response against HBV-infected cells; this response is markedly lower in viral carriers. Other mechanisms such as immunological exhaustion or induction of tolerance may contribute to this lowered T-cell response (174).

Escape by Subverting Antigen Processing and Antigen Presentation

A number of viruses have devised strategies to impair presentation of their antigens by the class I MHC pathway, thus reducing activation of antigen-specific CD8$^+$ T cells. This again stresses the importance of this cell subset for antiviral defense. Nearly every step of the class I MHC presentation pathway can be interfered with, and some viruses encode multiple proteins that act at different levels of the class I MHC processing pathway (Fig. 6, Table 3) (175). Interference of class II MHC processing is less common but has also been described (176).

Inhibition of Class I or II Major Histocompatibility Complex Synthesis

The Vpu and Tat proteins of lentiviruses can interfere with synthesis of class I MHC molecules (177,178). Human cytomegalovirus (HCMV) can impair class II MHC expression through two distinct pathways (Fig. 7). Class II MHC molecules are expressed only on a subset of cells, and its expression is regulated at the transcriptional level through control elements that include those that allow both constitutive and cytokine-induced transcription of the class II MHC genes. The class II MHC transactivator (CIITA) is essential for constitutive and induced transcription and is the rate-limiting factor of class II MHC production (179). One of the four promoters controlling CIITA production is activated by IFN-γ, which, upon binding to its receptors, triggers through Janus kinases a signal transduction cascade that eventually results in transcription of interferon-inducible genes. HCMV inhibits the up-regulation of class II MHC expression by IFN-γ by decreasing the amount of Janus kinases (180). In addition, HCMV can interfere further downstream with the CIITA promoter (181).

Inhibition of Peptidases

The metalloproteases CD10 and CD13 serve as amino peptidases that trim peptides to a size that allows their binding to

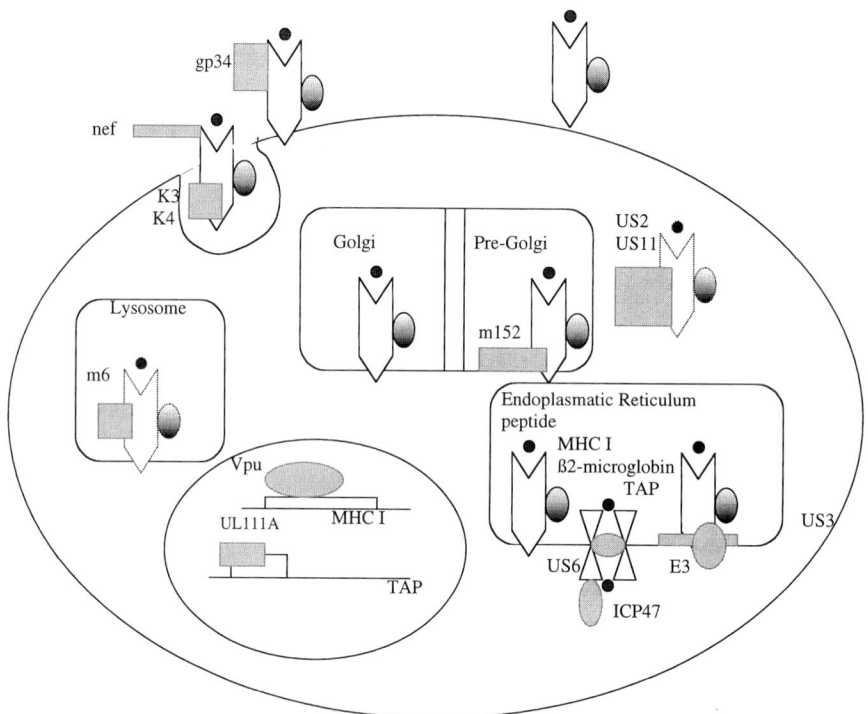

FIG. 6. Inhibition of antigen presentation by class I major histocompatibility complex (MHC) molecules. A number of viral proteins (*gray outline*) interfere with the class I MHC presentation pathway.

TABLE 3. *Inhibition of antigen presentation through the class I MHC pathway*

Virus	Viral product(s)	Function
Lentivirus	Vpu	Inhibits class I MHC synthesis
HCMV	US6	Inhibits TAP
HSV	ICP47	Inhibits TAP
EBV	IL-10 homolog	Inhibits expression of TAP
HCMV	UL111A	IL-10 homolog, inhibits expression of TAP
HCMV	US3	Retains class I MHC in the ER
Adenovirus	E3-19K	Retains class I MHC in the ER
MCMV	m152	Retains class I MHC in the pre-Golgi compartment
HCMV	US11, US2	Dislocates class I MHC to the cytoplasma
MCMV	m6/gp48	Dislocates class I MHC to lysosomes
MCMV	gp34	Binds to cell surface expressed class I MHC molecules
HIV-1	nef	Augments endocytosis of class I MHC molecules
HHV-8	K3, K4	Enhance endocytosis of class I MHC molecules

EBV, Epstein Barr virus; ER, endoplasmic reticulum; HCMV, human cytomegalovirus; HHV-8, human herpesvirus 8; HIV-1, human immunodeficiency virus 1; HSV, herpes simplex virus; ICP47, infected cell protein 47; IL-10, interleukin-10; MCMV, murine cytomegalovirus; MHC, major histocompatibility complex; TAP, transporter associated with antigen processing.

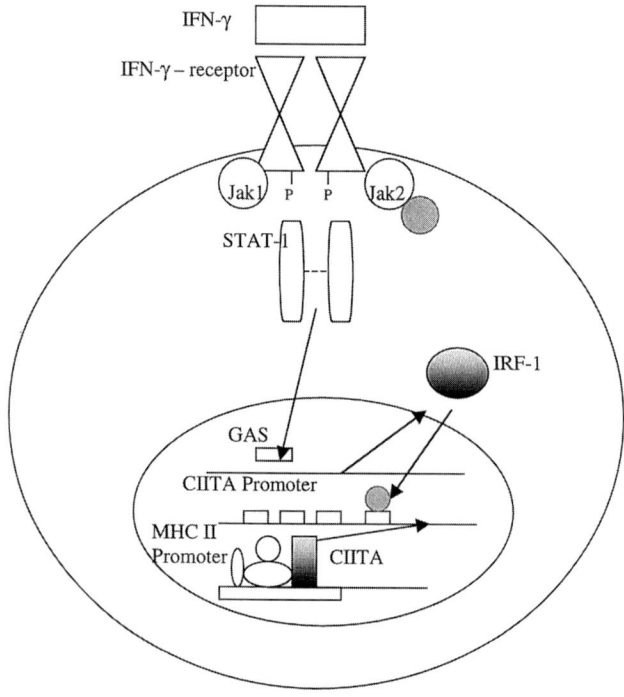

FIG. 7. Inhibition of class II major histocompatibility complex (MHC) synthesis. Cytomegalovirus proteins (*gray outline*) inhibit synthesis of class II MHC determinants.

the groove of class I or II MHC molecules. Proteins of HCMV block the activity of CD10 and CD13 (182). Whereas CD10 expression is apparently blocked at the transcriptional or translational level, CD13 seems to be retained within the endoplasmic reticulum.

Inhibition of Transporter Associated with Antigen Processing

The peptide transporter TAP is needed to shuttle peptides from the cytoplasm to the endoplasmic reticulum, in which they associate with class I MHC determinants. TAP peptide transport is inhibited by a protein of HCMV, US6, which acts from the luminal site of the endoplasmic reticulum. This protein binds to TAP and prevents binding of adenosine triphosphate, which is needed for peptide transport (183). ICP47 polypeptide from herpes simplex virus inhibits TAP by binding to TAP's peptide binding site, thus preventing its association with other peptides. This results in an insufficient number of peptides in the endoplasmic reticulum for binding to class I MHC molecules (184). TAP-independent peptide loading of class I MHC molecules is not affected by US6 or ICP47. EBV encodes a protein that weakly binds the IL-10 receptor. Like cellular IL-10, the EBV protein reduces expression of TAP and of class II MHC (185). Another IL-10 homolog, UL111A, is encoded by HCMV (186).

Retention of Class I Major Histocompatibility Complex Molecules in the Endoplasmic Reticulum

Once class I MHC molecules have bound peptide, they must be transported to the cell surface to present the peptides to CD8$^+$ T cells. A number of viral products interfere with this transport by either retaining or destroying class I MHC molecules within the endoplasmic reticulum. The US3 protein of HCMV (187) and the E3-19K protein of adenovirus (188,189) bind to polymorphic parts of class I MHC within the endoplasmic reticulum. Upon binding of these viral proteins the class I MHC molecules are unable to leave the endoplasmic reticulum. Neither of these proteins interferes with peptide loading.

Retention of Class I Major Histocompatibility Complex in a Pre-Golgi/Golgi Compartment

The m152 gene of murine cytomegalovirus (MCMV), which encodes a 40-kDa glycoprotein (gp), affects retention of peptide-loaded class I MHC molecules in a pre-Golgi compartment (190). Direct binding of m152/gp40 to class I MHC molecules has not been demonstrated thus far.

Dislocation of Class I Major Histocompatibility Complex into the Cytoplasm

US11 and US2 proteins of HCMV dislocate the class I MHC molecules from the endoplasmic reticulum to the cytoplasm,

in which they are rapidly degraded (191). In the presence of US2 protein, the intracellular half-life of class I MHC is reduced from approximately 6 hours to less than 2 minutes; this demonstrates that this pathway of class I MHC destruction is highly efficient. US2 protein in the endoplasmic reticulum binds to class I MHC molecules while they are being glycosylated, causing them to fold incorrectly. The complex is then transported through Sec61 pores back into the cytoplasm, in which, upon deglycosylation, both proteins—the class I MHC molecule and the viral protein—are degraded. The US11 protein has a similar mode of action but, unlike US2, does not become demolished upon translocation into the cytoplasm.

Dislocation of Class I Major Histocompatibility Complex Molecules into Lysosomes

The m6/gp48 protein of MCMV binds to class I MHC β_2-microglobulin complexes in the endoplasmic reticulum. During transport of the complex to the cell surface, the m6/gp48 protein, whose cytoplasmic tail has a two-leucin motif, targets the complex to lysosomes, in which they are proteolytically digested (192).

Interference with Surface-Expressed Class I Major Histocompatibility Complex/Peptide Complexes

The MCMV-encoded gp34 is transported to the cell surface upon forming a complex with class I MHC molecules (193). It is not yet known whether binding of gp34 interferes with binding of TCRs to the class I MHC peptide complexes. The Nef protein of HIV-1 binds to the AP-2 adaptor protein and augments endocytosis of class I MHC molecules, thus reducing their overall numbers on the cell surface (194). The K3 and K4 proteins of the herpesvirus HHV8 also lower expression of cell surface class I MHC molecules by enhancing their endocytosis (195). Both proteins show specificity for certain human leukocyte antigen (HLA) types; K3 reduces expression of HLA-A, HLA-B, HLA-C, and HLA-E, whereas K5 affects mainly HLA-A and HLA-B. K3 shows sequence homology with IE1 of bovine herpesvirus 4, and K5 resembles the open reading frame 12 of herpes simplex virus. All these proteins carry a zinc finger motif with an internal hydrophobic domain. These proteins translocate to membranes and may sponsor ubiquination of cell membrane–associated proteins, which leads to their proteolytic degradation (196).

Inhibition of T Cell–Mediated Target Cell Lysis

T cells kill virus-infected target cells through induction of programmed cell death. A number of viral proteins prevent apoptosis (Fig. 8) and thus preserve the cells that support their replication. Apoptosis can be triggered by Fas–Fas ligand (CD95) interactions. The intracellular domain of CD95 contains a death effector domain. These domains bind to corresponding death effector domains on adaptor proteins such

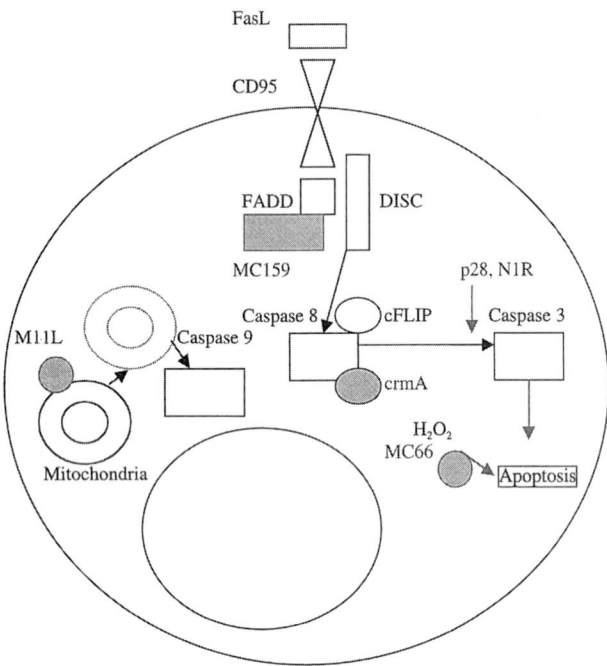

FIG. 8. Inhibition of apoptosis by viral antigens. A number of viral proteins (*gray outline*) inhibit apoptosis, thus preventing T cell–mediated lysis of infected cells before new viral progeny has been assembled.

as Fas-associated death domain. Upon binding of the extracellular part of the receptor, the cytoplasmic tail binds to death-inducing signal complex, which contains caspase-8 (FLICE). This results in activation of FLICE, which in turn activates caspase-3, which, through cleavage of cellular proteins, induces cell apoptosis. Activation of FLICE is inhibited by cellular FLICE-like inhibitor proteins (197). Another apoptotic pathway involves mitochondrial damage, which, upon "permeabilization" of the mitochondrial membrane, causes activation of caspase-9.

Poxviruses inhibit apoptosis of infected cells through a number of pathways. They produce either a serine protease inhibitor–like molecule, cytokine response modifier A (CrmA) (cowpox), or SPI-2 (vaccinia virus). CrmA inhibits the activity of caspases such as IL-1β–converting enzyme and caspase-8, which are part of the death pathway (198). In addition, both proteins bind to granzyme B, a serine protease that is part of the lytic granules that are secreted by cytolytic T cells upon recognition of their target (199). SPI-1 is another serine protease produced by orthopoxviruses. This protein does not inhibit Fas-mediated cell death. It binds to cathepsin G, a cellular serine protease of the chymotrypsin family (200).

The MC159 protein of molluscum contagiosum virus is a c-FLIP homolog that binds to Fas-associated death domain and the precursor form of caspase-8, thus inhibiting its activation (201). Some herpesviruses such as HHV8 encode a FLICE inhibitory protein, termed v-FLIP, that prevents recruitment and activation of FLICE (202). Intracellular reactive oxygen

intermediates, which trigger apoptotic cell death, can be reduced by cellular enzymes such as glutathione peroxidase, a selenocysteine-containing protein. The MC66 of molluscum contagiosum virus shows 74% sequence homology to this enzyme (203) and was shown to protect cells from death caused by reactive oxygen intermediates (204). MC66 does not interfere with apoptosis induced through Fas.

The p28 protein of ectromelia virus (mousepox) (205) and the N1R protein of Shope fibroma virus have a RING zinc finger motif that inhibits apoptosis induced by ultraviolet light. The M11L protein of myxomavirus localizes to mitochondrial membranes and prevents their "permeabilization" upon cell damage, thus inhibiting activation of caspase-9 (206). The MT4 of myxomavirus localizes to the endoplasmic reticulum and was shown to inhibit apoptosis through an as yet undefined pathway (207).

Inhibition of Natural Killer Cell Activity

NK cells, unlike T cells, can commence effector function without prior editing through negative selection. To prevent uncontrolled killing of vital cells, NK lymphocytes carry receptors that, upon recognition of class I MHC molecules, inhibit cytokine synthesis or release of toxic substances. Cells infected with viruses that down-regulate class I MHC surface expression thus become susceptible to lysis by NK cells. In order to avoid this destruction by NK cells, cytomegalovirus encodes two proteins, m144 and UL18, which serve as class I MHC decoys (208,209) (Fig. 9). HCMV down-regulates the expression of most type of HLA molecules without strongly impairing HLA-E expression. Cell-surface expression of

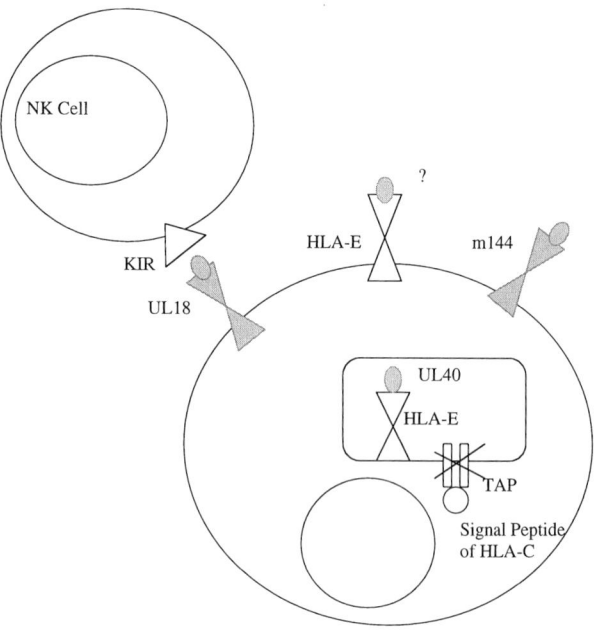

FIG. 9. Inhibition of natural killer (NK) cell functions. Viral products (*gray outline*) inhibit NK cell activity by providing class I major histocompatibility complex (MHC) decoys.

HLA-E is generally TAP dependent. In uninfected cells, HLA-E presents a peptide present in the signal sequence of HLA-C. Processing of this peptide, needed for its transport into the endoplasmic reticulum for binding to HLA-E, requires TAP, which is inhibited in HCMV-infected cells. The signal sequence of UL40, another HCMV-encoded protein, carries a sequence with a potential binding motif to HLA-E (210). It is feasible, albeit not yet proved, that this peptide associates with HLA-E independently of TAP, thus allowing its translocation to the cell surface. Expression of HLA-E in turn inhibits NK cell–mediated lysis.

Inhibition of Complement Activation

Complement can directly inactivate some viruses or affect lysis of virus-infected cells upon binding of antibodies to cell surface–expressed viral antigens. Complement is activated through the alternative pathway as a direct consequence of viral infection or later on through the traditional pathway upon formation of antigen-antibody complexes. Both pathways converge after formation of the C3 complex. A family of proteins, which carry a consensus motif, negatively regulates the activation of complement. The VCP protein of vaccinia virus contains four copies of this motif and can inhibit both pathways of complement activation at several levels. VCP binds C3b and C4b, thus inhibiting their function and causing their accelerated degradation (211).

Interference of Cytokine Functions

Viruses have developed three mechanisms that affect the activity of cytokines (Table 4). They can produce proteins that mimic cytokines and bind to the same receptors. They can produce antigens that mimic cytokine receptors and thus neutralize the corresponding factors. Finally, they can directly interfere with the synthesis of cytokines.

Cytokine Mimetics

EBV produces an IL-10–like molecule (212) that inhibits synthesis of IL-12 and thus the generation of Th1 immune responses. Similarly, the UL111A open reading frame of HCMV has sequence homology with IL-10 (213). UL146 and 147 of HCMV encode an IL-8–like molecule that may affect lymphocyte trafficking (214).

Receptor Mimetics

Herpesviruses and poxviruses encode a number of secreted proteins that bind chemokines or cytokines, thus preventing their binding to the corresponding cellular receptors. Four proteins of HCMV (UL33, UL78, US27, and US28) show homology with the CCR1 receptor (215). MC148 protein of *Molluscipox* virus shows similarity to the CCR8 chemokine receptor (216). The protein lacks the signaling domain and thus functions as an antagonist. Both *Leporipoxvirus* and

TABLE 4. *Interference of Cytokine Functions*

Virus	Viral product	Function
EBV	BCRF1	IL-10 homolog
HCMV	UL111A	IL-10 homolog
HCMV	UL146, 147	IL-8 homolog
HCMV	UL33, 78, 27, 28	CCR1 receptor homolog
Molluscipox	MC148	CCR8 homolog (antagonist)
Leporipoxvirus	M-T1	CC-1 chemokine inhibitor
Orthopoxvirus	p35	CC-1 chemokine inhibitor
Poxvirus	M104L	MIG homolog
Vaccinia virus	B8R	IFN-γ homolog
Vaccinia virus	B18R	Type 1 IFN homolog, inhibits IL-1β
Myxoma virus	M135R	Inhibits IL-1β
Myxoma virus	MT-7	IFN-γ receptor homolog
Poxvirus	GIF	Binds GM-CSF and IL-2
HCMV	UL144	TNFR homolog
Shope fibroma virus	T2	TNFR homolog
Orthopoxviruses	CrmB, CrmC, CrmD	TNFR homolog

CCR, chemokine receptor; EBV, Epstein Barr virus; GM-CSF, granulocyte-macrophage colony-stimulating factor; HCMV, human cytomegalovirus; IFN, interferon; IL, interleukin; MIG, monokine induced by γ interferon; TNFR, tumor necrosis factor receptor.

Orthopoxvirus species encode secreted proteins (M-T1 and p35, respectively) that have functional homology to chemokine receptors and thus interfere with lymphocyte trafficking (217). The M104L protein of poxvirus shows some similarity to MIG (218), an interferon induced monokine of the CXC chemokine family. The B8R protein of vaccinia virus binds to IFN-γ (219), whereas B18R binds to type I interferons (220). The poxvirus-encoded GIF binds to both GM-CSF and IL-2 (221). HCMV encodes UL144, which is a homolog of the TNF receptor supergene family (222). Its functions are currently unknown. Shope fibroma virus and myxomavirus encode a single TNF receptor homolog called T2 (223), whereas *Orthopoxvirus* species encode one to three different TNF receptor homologs, called CrmB, CrmC, and CrmD (224). T2, CrmB, and CrmD bind TNF-α and lymphotoxin A, whereas CrmC associates only with TNF-α. T2, CrmC, and CrmD block TNF-α–mediated cell lysis. The T2 protein in addition prevents apoptosis of CD4$^+$ T cells. This activity is independent of TNF-α. Poxviruses encode M135R (myxomavirus) and B18R (vaccinia virus), two proteins that bind and consequently inhibit IL-1β (225).

Inhibition of Interleukin-1 Cleavage

IL-1β is synthesized as a precursor that requires cleavage by caspase-1 to gain functional activity. The same caspase also cleaves the precursor molecule of IL-18. Cowpoxvirus encodes a serine protease inhibitor, CrmA, that inhibits the function of caspase-1 (226). The activity of CrmA is not restricted to caspase-1 but also affects additional caspases involved in apoptosis (227).

Inhibition of Interferons

Viruses of two distinct families, the paramyxoviruses and human papillomaviruses, inhibit transcriptional activation by interferons (Fig. 10). Type I interferons are produced early after infection, whereas immune interferon is synthesized later by activated T cells. Both have potent antiviral activities, which are mediated partly through downstream pathways upon induction of synthesis of other proteins. Type I interferons and immune interferon bind to different receptors. Binding of type I interferons leads to phosphorylation of Jak1/TYK2 kinases, whereas binding of the immune interferon receptor causes phosphorylation of Jak1 and Jak2. Jak1/TYK2, once activated, phosphorylate STAT1 and STAT2, which form a heterodimer, whereas Jak1/Jak2 phosphorylate only STAT1, causing its homodimerization. The STAT dimers translocate to the nucleus, where they assemble with other proteins into a transcriptional activating complex. This complex contains interferon responsive factors (IRFs), which bind to motifs present on interferon-inducible promoters.

Viruses of the paramyxovirus family, which is composed of a number of different viruses, including Sendai virus, human parainfluenza virus types 2 and 3, simian virus 5, and

mumps virus have several strategies to abrogate interferon signaling. The simian virus 5 V protein causes proteolytic degradation of STAT1, thus inhibiting both signaling through type I and immune interferons (228). Human parainfluenza virus type 2 interferes only with STAT2, thus inhibiting the activity of type I interferon without affecting that of IFN-γ (229). Normal levels of both STAT1 and STAT2 are detectable in Sendai virus or human parainfluenza virus type 3–infected cells. Nevertheless, in infected cells, both STAT proteins show lack of serine 727 phosphorylation, which is needed for their optimal transcriptional activity.

HPVs inhibit the activity of interferon through the early proteins E6 and E7 that, in oncogenic types of papillomavirus, interfere with cell cycle regulation. The E6 protein binds and inactivates IRF-3 (230). The E7 protein binds to IRF-1 and histone deacetylase, thus silencing the activity of the transactivator on IFN-inducible promoters.

Other viral proteins act downstream on the activity of interferon-induced proteins (231). The M-T7 protein of myxoma virus and the B8R protein of vaccinia virus (both of which belong to the poxvirus family) show sequence homology with the IFN-γ receptor. Both proteins bind to IFN-γ, inhibiting its ligation to its receptor. Vaccinia virus also encodes a type I interferon inhibitor that shows sequence homology with the type I interferon receptor.

The protein kinase R is induced by interferons. It negatively regulates protein synthesis through phosphorylation of the translation initiation factor eIF-2. The E3L protein of vaccinia virus inhibits activation of protein kinase R. The K3L protein of vaccinia virus is a homolog of eIF-2, which serves as a decoy for activated protein kinase R.

Inhibition of Interleukin-18

IL-18 is a cytokine that, like IL-12, induces IFN-γ production and thus sponsors NK and Th1 cell activation. Molluscum contagiosum virus, as well as *Orthopoxvirus* species, secrete IL-18–binding proteins, which prevent the interaction of the cytokine with its natural receptor. IL-18 is produced as a precursor molecule that is cleaved by caspase-1 into its active form. The CrmA protein of vaccinia virus inhibits the activity of this caspase (232).

Crystallized Fragment (Fc) Receptor Mimetics

MCMV encodes a crystallized fragment (Fc) γ receptor–like molecule that subverts antibody-mediated lysis of infected cells (233).

SUMMARY

Understanding how the immune system copes with viruses, the smallest of all genetic entities that cause transmittable diseases in humans, is crucial to eventually lessening their toll on human well-being. Viruses come in many forms. They

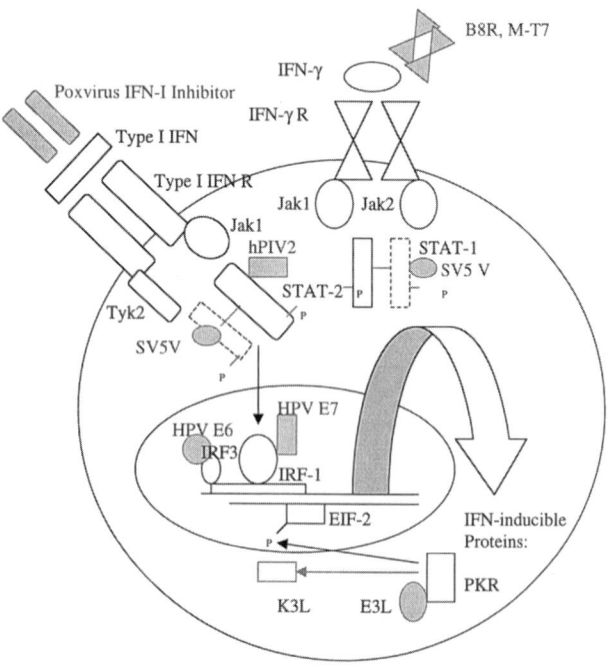

FIG. 10. Inhibition of interferons by viral proteins. Viral proteins (*gray outline*) inhibit the functions of interferons (IFNs).

change rapidly, and new types of viruses are constantly arising or crossing species barriers. The immune system remains the best defense against viral infections. Understanding the complex interactions between the immune system of the host and the invading viral pathogen will eventually enable researchers to devise better strategies for annihilating viral diseases. In the meantime, it is sobering to realize that these small genetic entities seem to understand and dodge the immune system far better than the people who have devoted their time to studying it.

REFERENCES

1. Martini GA, Siegert R. *Marburg virus disease.* Berlin: Springer-Verlag, 1971.
2. Ebola haemorrhagic fever in Zaire, 1976. *Bull World Health Organ* 1978;56:271–293.
3. Nichol ST, Spiropoulou CF, Morzunov S, et al. Genetic identification of a hantavirus associated with an outbreak of acute respiratory illness. *Science* 1993;262:914–917.
4. Garmendia AE, Van Kruiningen HJ, French RA. The West Nile virus: its recent emergence in North America. *Microbes Infect* 2001;3:223–229.
5. Fenner F. The eradication of smallpox. *Prog Med Virol* 1977;23:1–21.
6. Pleskoff O, Treboute C, Brelot A, et al. Identification of a chemokine receptor encoded by human cytomegalovirus as a cofactor for HIV-1 entry. *Science* 1997;276:1874–1878.
7. Winkler C, Modi W, Smith MW, et al. Genetic restriction of AIDS pathogenesis by an SDF-1 chemokine gene variant. ALIVE Study, Hemophilia Growth and Development Study (HGDS), Multicenter AIDS Cohort Study (MACS), Multicenter Hemophilia Cohort Study (MHCS), San Francisco City Cohort (SFCC). *Science* 1998;279:389–393.
8. Weis W, Brown JH, Cusack S, et al. Structure of the influenza virus haemagglutinin complexed with its receptor, sialic acid. *Nature* 1988;333:426–4231.
9. Shieh MT, WuDunn D, Montgomery RI, et al. Cell surface receptors for herpes simplex virus are heparan sulfate proteoglycans. *J Cell Biol* 1992;116:1273–1281.
10. Nemerow GR, Siaw MF, Cooper NR. Purification of the Epstein-Barr virus/C3d complement receptor of human B lymphocytes: antigenic and functional properties of the purified protein. *J Virol* 1986;58:709–712.
11. Nemerow GR, Mullen JJ 3rd, Dickson PW, et al. Soluble recombinant CR2 (CD21) inhibits Epstein-Barr virus infection. *J Virol* 1990;64:1348–1352.
12. Bergelson JM, Cunningham JA, Droguett G, et al. Isolation of a common receptor for Coxsackie B viruses and adenoviruses 2 and 5. *Science* 1997;275:1320–1323.
13. Wickham TJ, Mathias P, Cheresh DA, et al. Integrins alpha v beta 3 and alpha v beta 5 promote adenovirus internalization but not virus attachment. *Cell,* 1993;73:309–319.
14. Mendelsohn C, Johnson B, Lionetti KA, et al. Transformation of a human poliovirus receptor gene into mouse cells. *Proc Natl Acad Sci U S A* 1986;83:7845–7849.
15. Mendelsohn CL, Wimmer E, Racaniello VR. Cellular receptor for poliovirus: molecular cloning, nucleotide sequence, and expression of a new member of the immunoglobulin superfamily. *Cell* 1989;56:855–865.
16. Tang YQ, Yuan J, Osapay G, et al. A cyclic antimicrobial peptide produced in primate leukocytes by the ligation of two truncated alpha-defensins. *Science* 1999;286:498–502.
17. Yang D, Chertov O, Bykovskaia SN, et al. Beta-defensins: linking innate and adaptive immunity through dendritic and T cell CCR6. *Science* 1999;286:525–528.
18. Maul GG. Nuclear domain 10, the site of DNA virus transcription and replication. *Bioessays* 1998;20:660–667.
19. Tang Q, Bell P, Tegtmeyer P, et al. Replication but not transcription of simian virus 40 DNA is dependent on nuclear domain 10. *J Virol* 2000;74:9694–9700.
20. Bell P, Lieberman PM, Maul GG. Lytic but not latent replication of Epstein-Barr virus is associated with PML and induces sequential release of nuclear domain 10 proteins. *J Virol* 2000;74:11800–11810.
21. Ozinsky A, Underhill DM, Fontenot JD, et al. The repertoire for pattern recognition of pathogens by the innate immune system is defined by cooperation between Toll-like receptors. *Proc Natl Acad Sci U S A* 2000;97:13766–13771.
22. Medzhitov R, Janeway C Jr. The Toll receptor family and microbial recognition. *Trends Microbiol* 2000;8:452–456.
23. Shimazu R, Akashi S, Ogata H, et al. MD-2, a molecule that confers lipopolysaccharide responsiveness on Toll-like receptor 4. *J Exp Med* 1999;189:1777–1782.
24. Ohashi K, Burkart V, Flohe S, et al. Cutting edge: heat shock protein 60 is a putative endogenous ligand of the Toll-like receptor–4 complex. *J Immunol* 2000;164:558–561.
25. Kurt-Jones EA, Popova L, Kwinn L, et al. Pattern recognition receptors TLR4 and CD14 mediate response to respiratory syncytial virus. *Nat Immunol* 2000;1:398–401.
26. Bowie A, Kiss-Toth E, Symons JA, et al. A46R and A52R from vaccinia virus are antagonists of host IL-1 and Toll-like receptor signaling. *Proc Natl Acad Sci U S A* 2000;97:10162–10167.
27. Bauer S, Kirschning CJ, Hacker H, et al. Human TLR9 confers responsiveness to bacterial DNA via species-specific CpG motif recognition. *Proc Natl Acad Sci U S Am* 2001;98:9237–9242.
28. Krieg AM. The role of CpG motifs in innate immunity. *Curr Opin Immunol* 2000;12:35–43.
29. Krieg AM, Wu T, Weeratna R, et al. Sequence motifs in adenoviral DNA block immune activation by stimulatory CpG motifs. *Proc Natl Acad Sci U S A* 1998;95:12631–12636.
30. Adolf GR. Human interferon omega—a review. *Mult Scler* 1995;1(Suppl 1):S44–S47.
31. Martal JL, Chene NM, Huynh LP, et al. IFN-tau: a novel subtype I IFN1. Structural characteristics, non-ubiquitous expression, structure-function relationships, a pregnancy hormonal embryonic signal and cross-species therapeutic potentialities. *Biochimie* 1998;80:755–777.
32. Tiwari RK, Kusari J, Sen GC. Functional equivalents of interferon-mediated signals needed for induction of an mRNA can be generated by double-stranded RNA and growth factors. *EMBO J* 1987;6:3373–3378.
33. Taira H, Kanda T, Omata T, et al. Interferon induction by transfection of Sendai virus C gene cDNA. *J Virol* 1987;61:625–628.
34. Taniguchi T, Takaoka A. A weak signal for strong responses: interferon-alpha/beta revisited. *Nat Rev Mol Cell Biol* 2001;2:378–386.
35. Darnell JE Jr. Studies of IFN-induced transcriptional activation uncover the Jak-Stat pathway. *J Interferon Cytokine Res* 1998;18:549–554.
36. Zurcher T, Pavlovic J, Staeheli P. Nuclear localization of mouse Mx1 protein is necessary for inhibition of influenza virus. *J Virol* 1992;66:5059–5066.
37. Harms JS, Splitter GA. Interferon-gamma inhibits transgene expression driven by SV40 or CMV promoters but augments expression driven by the mammalian MHC I promoter. *Hum Gene Ther* 1995;6:1291–1297.
38. Warfel AH, Belsito DV, Thorbecke GJ. Activation of an HIV-LTR-CAT transgene in murine macrophages by interferon-gamma in synergism with other cytokines or endotoxin. *Adv Exp Med Biol* 1995;378:489–492.
39. Karupiah G, Xie QW, Buller RM, et al. Inhibition of viral replication by interferon-gamma–induced nitric oxide synthase. *Science* 1993;261:1445–1448.
40. Malik AH, Lee WM. Chronic hepatitis B virus infection: treatment strategies for the next millennium. *Ann Intern Med* 2000;132:723–731.
41. Lauer GM, Walker BD. Hepatitis C virus infection. *N Engl J Med* 2001;345:41–52.
42. Gross G. Therapy of human papillomavirus infection and associated epithelial tumors. *Intervirology* 1997;40:368–377.
43. Long EO, Burshtyn DN, Clark WP, et al. Killer cell inhibitory receptors: diversity, specificity, and function. *Immunol Rev* 1997;155:135–144.
44. Mellman I, Steinman RM. Dendritic cells: specialized and regulated antigen processing machines. *Cell* 2001;106:255–258.

45. Hertz C, Kiertscher S, Godowski P, et al. Microbial lipopeptides stimulate dendritic cell maturation via Toll-like receptor 2. *J Immunol* 2001; 166:2444–2450.

46. Kuppner MC, Gastpar R, Gelwer S, et al. The role of heat shock protein (hsp70) in dendritic cell maturation: hsp70 induces the maturation of immature dendritic cells but reduces DC differentiation from monocyte precursors. *Eur J Immunol* 2001;31:1602–1609.

47. Sallusto F, Lanzavecchia A. Understanding dendritic cell and T-lymphocyte traffic through the analysis of chemokine receptor expression. *Immunol Rev* 2000;177:134–140.

48. Vissers JL, Hartgers FC, Lindhout E, et al. Quantitative analysis of chemokine expression by dendritic cell subsets *in vitro* and *in vivo*. *J Leukoc Biol* 2001;69:785–793.

49. Vulcano M, Albanesi C, Stoppacciaro A, et al. Dendritic cells as a major source of macrophage-derived chemokine/CCL22 *in vitro* and *in vivo*. *Eur J Immunol* 2001;31:812–822.

50. Dieu MC, Vanbervliet B, Vicari A, et al. Selective recruitment of immature and mature dendritic cells by distinct chemokines expressed in different anatomic sites. *J Exp Med* 1998;188:373–386.

51. Liu YJ, Kanzler H, Soumelis V, et al. Dendritic cell lineage, plasticity and cross-regulation. *Nat Immunol* 2001;2:585–589.

52. Kadowaki N, Ho S, Antonenko S, et al. Subsets of human dendritic cell precursors express different Toll-like receptors and respond to different microbial antigens. *J Exp Med* 2001;194:863–869.

53. Pieters J. MHC class II–restricted antigen processing and presentation. *Adv Immunol* 2000;75:159–208.

54. Jenkins MK, Khoruts A, Ingulli E, et al. *In vivo* activation of antigen-specific CD4 T cells. *Annu Rev Immunol* 2001;19:23–45.

55. Dong C, Flavell RA. Th1 and Th2 cells. *Curr Opin Hematol* 2001;8:47–51.

56. Jankovic D, Liu Z, Gause WC. Th1- and Th2-cell commitment during infectious disease: asymmetry in divergent pathways. *Trends Immunol* 2001;22:450–457.

57. Trinchieri G. Immunobiology of interleukin-12. *Immunol Res* 1998;17:269–278.

58. O'Garra A. Cytokines induce the development of functionally heterogeneous T helper cell subsets. *Immunity* 1998;8:275–283.

59. Karp CL, Wysocka M, Wahl LM, et al. Mechanism of suppression of cell-mediated immunity by measles virus. *Science* 1996;273:228–231.

60. Cresswell P, Bangia N, Dick T, et al. The nature of the MHC class I peptide loading complex. *Immunol Rev* 1999;172:21–28.

61. York IA, Goldberg AL, Mo XY, et al. Proteolysis and class I major histocompatibility complex antigen presentation. *Immunol Rev* 1999; 172:49–66.

62. Pamer E, Cresswell P. Mechanisms of MHC class I–restricted antigen processing. *Annu Rev Immunol* 1998;16:323–358.

63. Abele R, Tampe R. Function of the transport complex TAP in cellular immune recognition. *Biochim Biophys Acta* 1999;1461:405–419.

64. Cresswell P, Androlewicz MJ, Ortmann B. Assembly and transport of class I MHC–peptide complexes. *Ciba Found Symp* 1994;187:150–162; discussion, 162–169.

65. Murray N, McMichael A. Antigen presentation in virus infection. *Curr Opin Immunol* 1992;4:401–407.

66. Falk K, Rotzschke O, Stevanovic S, et al. Allele-specific motifs revealed by sequencing of self-peptides eluted from MHC molecules. *Nature* 1991;351:290–296.

67. Fairchild PJ, Wraith DC. Lowering the tone: mechanisms of immunodominance among epitopes with low affinity for MHC. *Immunol Today* 1996;17:80–85.

68. Heath WR, Carbone FR. Cytotoxic T lymphocyte activation by cross-priming. *Curr Opin Immunol* 1999;11:314–318.

69. Benlagha K, Bendelac A. CD1d-restricted mouse V alpha 14 and human V alpha 24 T cells: lymphocytes of innate immunity. *Semin Immunol* 2000;12:537–542.

70. Chiu NM, Chun T, Fay M, et al. The majority of H2-M3 is retained intracellularly in a peptide-receptive state and traffics to the cell surface in the presence of *N*-formylated peptides. *J Exp Med* 1999;190:423–434.

71. Ridge JP, Di Rosa F, Matzinger P. A conditioned dendritic cell can be a temporal bridge between a CD4+ T-helper and a T-killer cell. *Nature* 1998;393:474–478.

72. Bennett SR, Carbone FR, Karamalis F, et al. Help for cytotoxic-T-cell responses is mediated by CD40 signalling. *Nature* 1998;393:478–480.

73. Gallimore A, Glithero A, Godkin A, et al. Induction and exhaustion of lymphocytic choriomeningitis virus-specific cytotoxic T lymphocytes visualized using soluble tetrameric major histocompatibility complex class I–peptide complexes. *J Exp Med* 1998;187:1383–1393.

74. Smith KA. T-cell growth factor. *Immunol Rev* 1980;51:337–357.

75. O'Garra A. Interleukins and the immune system 1. *Lancet* 1989;1:943–947.

76. Sprent J, Zhang X, Sun S, et al. T-cell proliferation *in vivo* and the role of cytokines. *Philos Trans R Soc Lond Ser B Biol Sci* 2000;355:317–322.

77. Vosshenrich CA, Di Santo JP. Cytokines: IL-21 joins the gamma(c)-dependent network? *Curr Biol* 2001;11:R175–R177.

78. Brack C, Hirama M, Lenhard-Schuller R, et al. A complete immunoglobulin gene is created by somatic recombination. *Cell* 1978;15:1–14.

79. Kehry MR, Yamashita LC, Hodgkin PD. B-cell proliferation and differentiation mediated by Th-cell membranes and lymphokines. *Res Immunol* 1990;141:421–423.

80. Grandien A, Bras A, Martinez C. Acquisition of CD40 expression during murine B-cell differentiation. *Scand J Immunol* 1996;43:47–55.

81. Aversa G, Cocks BG, Punnonen J, et al. Contact-mediated signals and cytokines involved in B-cell activation and isotype switching in pre-B and mature B cells. *Res Immunol* 1994;145:222–226; discussion, 244–249.

82. Stall AM, Wells SM, Lam KP. B-1 cells: unique origins and functions. *Semin Immunol* 1996;8:45–59.

83. Martin F, Oliver AM, Kearney JF. Marginal zone and B1 B cells unite in the early response against T-independent blood-borne particulate antigens. *Immunity* 2001;14:617–629.

84. Ochsenbein AF, Fehr T, Lutz C, et al. Control of early viral and bacterial distribution and disease by natural antibodies. *Science* 1999;286:2156–2159.

85. Burns W, Billups LC, Notkins AL. Thymus dependence of viral antigens. *Nature* 1975;256:654–656.

86. Bachmann MF, Hengartner H, Zinkernagel RM. T helper cell-independent neutralizing B cell response against vesicular stomatitis virus: role of antigen patterns in B cell induction? *Eur J Immunol* 1995; 25:3445–3451.

87. Brinkmann V, Kristofic C. Massive production of Th2 cytokines by human CD4+ effector T cells transiently expressing the natural killer cell marker CD57/HNK1. *Immunology* 1997;91:541–547.

88. Faveeuw C, Di Mauro ME, Price AA, et al. Roles of alpha(4) integrins/VCAM-1 and LFA-1/ICAM-1 in the binding and transendothelial migration of T lymphocytes and T lymphoblasts across high endothelial venules. *Int Immunol* 2000;12:241–251.

89. Li X, Abdi K, Rawn J, et al. LFA-1 and L-selectin regulation of recirculating lymphocyte tethering and rolling on lung microvascular endothelium. *Am J Respir Cell Mol Biol* 1996;14:398–406.

90. Kowalczyk DW, Wlazlo AP, Blaszczyk-Thurin M, et al. A method that allows easy characterization of tumor-infiltrating lymphocytes. *J Immunol Methods* 2001;253:163–175.

91. Janssen O, Sanzenbacher R, Kabelitz D. Regulation of activation-induced cell death of mature T-lymphocyte populations. *Cell Tissue Res* 2000;301:85–99.

92. Jenne DE, Tschopp J. Granzymes, a family of serine proteases released from granules of cytolytic T lymphocytes upon T cell receptor stimulation. *Immunol Rev* 1988;103:53–71.

93. Kagi D, Seiler P, Pavlovic J, et al. The roles of perforin- and Fas-dependent cytotoxicity in protection against cytopathic and noncytopathic viruses. *Eur J Immunol* 1995;25:3256–3262.

94. Topham DJ, Cardin RC, Christensen JP, et al. Perforin and Fas in murine gammaherpesvirus-specific CD8(+) T cell control and morbidity. *J Gen Virol* 2001;82:1971–1981.

95. Topham DJ, Tripp RA, Doherty PC. CD8+ T cells clear influenza virus by perforin or Fas-dependent processes. *J Immunol* 1997;159:5197–5200.

96. Kaplan MJ, Ray D, Mo RR, et al. TRAIL (Apo2 ligand) and TWEAK (Apo3 ligand) mediate CD4+ T cell killing of antigen-presenting macrophages. *J Immunol* 2000;164:2897–2904.

97. Planz O, Ehl S, Furrer E, et al. A critical role for neutralizing-antibody-producing B cells, CD4(+) T cells, and interferons in persistent and acute infections of mice with lymphocytic choriomeningitis virus:

implications for adoptive immunotherapy of virus carriers. *Proc Natl Acad Sci U S A* 1997;94:6874–6879.

98. Guidotti LG, McClary H, Loudis JM, et al. Nitric oxide inhibits hepatitis B virus replication in the livers of transgenic mice. *J Exp Med* 2000;191:1247–1252.

99. Koszinowski U, Ertl H. Role of early viral surface antigens in cellular immune response to vaccinia virus. *Eur J Immunol* 1976;6:679–683.

100. Ghiasi H, Wechsler SL, Cai S, et al. The role of neutralizing antibody and T-helper subtypes in protection and pathogenesis of vaccinated mice following ocular HSV-1 challenge. *Immunology* 1998;95:352–359.

101. Ju ST, Matsui K, Ozdemirli M. Molecular and cellular mechanisms regulating T and B cell apoptosis through Fas/FasL interaction. *Int Rev Immunol* 1999;18:485–513.

102. Budd RC. Activation-induced cell death. *Curr Opin Immunol* 2001;13:356–362.

103. Blattman JN, Sourdive DJ, Murali-Krishna K, et al. Evolution of the T cell repertoire during primary, memory, and recall responses to viral infection. *J Immunol* 2000;165:6081–6090.

104. Whitmire JK, Murali-Krishna K, Altman J, et al. Antiviral CD4 and CD8 T-cell memory: differences in the size of the response and activation requirements. *Philos Trans R Soc Lond Ser B Biol Sci* 2000;355:373–379.

105. He Z, Wlazlo AP, Kowalczyk DW, et al. Viral recombinant vaccines to the E6 and E7 antigens of HPV-16. *Virology* 2000;270:146–161.

106. Thucydides. The plague in Athens. Thucydides. The history of the Peloponnesian War. Translated by Thomas Hobbes. *N C Med J* 1980;41:230–232.

107. Rhodes CJ, Anderson RM. A scaling analysis of measles epidemics in a small population. *Philos Trans R Soc Lond Ser B Biol Sci* 1996;351:1679–1688.

108. Beverley P. Immunological memory in T cells. *Curr Opin Immunol* 1991;3:355–360.

109. Galvan M, Murali-Krishna K, Ming LL, et al. Alterations in cell surface carbohydrates on T cells from virally infected mice can distinguish effector/memory CD8+ T cells from naïve cells. *J Immunol* 1998;161:641–648.

110. Bruno L, von Boehmer H, Kirberg J. Cell division in the compartment of naïve and memory T lymphocytes. *Eur J Immunol* 1996;26:3179–3184.

111. Lau LL, Jamieson BD, Somasundaram T, et al. Cytotoxic T-cell memory without antigen. *Nature* 1994;369:648–652.

112. Asnagli H, Murphy KM. Stability and commitment in T helper cell development. *Curr Opin Immunol* 2001;13:242–247.

113. Swain SL, Bradley LM, Croft M, et al. Helper T-cell subsets: phenotype, function and the role of lymphokines in regulating their development. *Immunol Rev* 1991;123:115–144.

114. Masopust D, Vezys V, Marzo AL, et al. Preferential localization of effector memory cells in nonlymphoid tissue. *Science* 2001;291:2413–2417.

115. Sallusto F, Langenkamp A, Geginat J, et al. Functional subsets of memory T cells identified by CCR7 expression. *Curr Top Microbiol Immunol* 2000;251:167–171.

116. Szakal AK, Tew JG. Follicular dendritic cells: B-cell proliferation and maturation. *Cancer Res* 1992;52:5554s–5556s.

117. Ahmed R, Gray D. Immunological memory and protective immunity: understanding their relation. *Science* 1996;272:54–60.

118. Maruyama M, Lam KP, Rajewsky K. Memory B-cell persistence is independent of persisting immunizing antigen. *Nature* 2000;407:636–642.

119. MacLennan IC. Germinal centers. *Annu Rev Immunol* 1994;12:117–139.

120. Neutra MR, Pringault E, Kraehenbuhl JP. Antigen sampling across epithelial barriers and induction of mucosal immune responses. *Annu Rev Immunol* 1996;14:275–300.

121. Holt PG, Stumbles PA, McWilliam AS. Functional studies on dendritic cells in the respiratory tract and related mucosal tissues. *J Leukoc Biol* 1999;66:272–275.

122. Hathaway LJ, Kraehenbuhl JP. The role of M cells in mucosal immunity. *Cell Mol Life Sci* 2000;57:323–332.

123. Poussier P, Julius M. Thymus independent T cell development and selection in the intestinal epithelium. *Annu Rev Immunol* 1994;12:521–553.

124. Ferguson A, Parrott DM. The effect of antigen deprivation on thymus-dependent and thymus-independent lymphocytes in the small intestine of the mouse. *Clin Exp Immunol* 1972;12:477–488.

125. Yoshikai Y, Ishida A, Murosaki S, et al. Sequential appearance of T-cell receptor gamma delta– and alpha beta–bearing intestinal intraepithelial lymphocytes in mice after irradiation. *Immunology* 1991;74:583–588.

126. Bandeira A, Itohara S, Bonneville M, et al. Extrathymic origin of intestinal intraepithelial lymphocytes bearing T-cell antigen receptor gamma delta. *Proc Natl Acad Sci U S A* 1991;88:43–47.

127. Poussier P, Edouard P, Lee C, et al. Thymus-independent development and negative selection of T cells expressing T cell receptor alpha/beta in the intestinal epithelium: evidence for distinct circulation patterns of gut- and thymus-derived T lymphocytes. *J Exp Med* 1992;176:187–199.

128. Rosat JP, MacDonald HR, Louis JA. A role for gamma delta+ T cells during experimental infection of mice with *Leishmania major.* *J Immunol* 1993;150:550–555.

129. Beagley KW, Fujihashi K, Black CA, et al. The *Mycobacterium tuberculosis* 71-kDa heat-shock protein induces proliferation and cytokine secretion by murine gut intraepithelial lymphocytes. *Eur J Immunol* 1993;23:2049–2052.

130. Fujihashi K, McGhee JR, Kweon MN, et al. gamma/delta T cell–deficient mice have impaired mucosal immunoglobulin A responses. *J Exp Med* 1996;183:1929–1935.

131. Chien YH, Jores R, Crowley MP. Recognition by gamma/delta T cells. *Annu Rev Immunol* 1996;14:511–532.

132. Nandi D, Allison JP. Phenotypic analysis and gamma delta–T cell receptor repertoire of murine T cells associated with the vaginal epithelium. *J Immunol* 1991;147:1773–1778.

133. Hiroi T, Fujihashi K, McGhee JR, et al. Polarized Th2 cytokine expression by both mucosal gamma delta and alpha beta T cells. *Eur J Immunol* 1995;25:2743–2751.

134. Wu S, Pascual DW, Lewis GK, et al. Induction of mucosal and systemic responses against human immunodeficiency virus type 1 glycoprotein 120 in mice after oral immunization with a single dose of a *Salmonella*-HIV vector. *AIDS Res Hum Retroviruses* 1997;13:1187–1194.

135. Boyaka PN, Marinaro M, Jackson RJ, et al. IL-12 is an effective adjuvant for induction of mucosal immunity. *J Immunol* 1999;162:122–128.

136. Cuff CF, Cebra CK, Rubin DH, et al. Developmental relationship between cytotoxic alpha/beta T cell receptor–positive intraepithelial lymphocytes and Peyer's patch lymphocytes. *Eur J Immunol* 1993;23:1333–1339.

137. Bangham CR, Hall SE, Jeffery KJ, et al. Genetic control and dynamics of the cellular immune response to the human T-cell leukaemia virus, HTLV-I. *Philos Trans R Soc Lond Ser B Biol Sci* 1999;354:691–700.

138. Israel MS. The viral flora of enlarged tonsils and adenoids. *J Pathol Bacteriol* 1962;84:169–172.

139. Buchmeier MJ, Welsh RM, Dutko FJ, et al. The virology and immunobiology of lymphocytic choriomeningitis virus infection. *Adv Immunol* 1980;30:275–331.

140. Buchmeier MJ, Oldstone MB. Virus-induced immune complex disease: identification of specific viral antigens and antibodies deposited in complexes during chronic lymphocytic choriomeningitis virus infection. *J Immunol* 1978;120:1297–1304.

141. Hoffsten PE, Oldstone MB, Dixon FJ. Immunopathology of adoptive immunization in mice chronically infected with lymphocytic choriomeningitis virus. *Clin Immunol Immunopathol* 1977;7:44–52.

142. Moskophidis D, Lechner F, Hengartner H, et al. MHC class I and non–MHC-linked capacity for generating an anti-viral CTL response determines susceptibility to CTL exhaustion and establishment of virus persistence in mice. *J Immunol* 1994;152:4976–4983.

143. Fraser NW, Spivack JG, Wroblewska Z, et al. A review of the molecular mechanism of HSV-1 latency. *Curr Eye Res* 1991;10(Suppl):1–13.

144. Liu T, Khanna KM, Chen X, et al. CD8(+) T cells can block herpes simplex virus type 1 (HSV-1) reactivation from latency in sensory neurons. *J Exp Med* 2000;191:1459–1466.

145. Halford WP, Gebhardt BM, Carr DJ. Mechanisms of herpes simplex virus type 1 reactivation. *J Virol* 1996;70:5051–5060.

146. Hsieh WS, Lemas MV, Ambinder RF. The biology of Epstein-Barr virus in post-transplant lymphoproliferative disease. *Transpl Infect Dis* 1999;1:204–212.

147. Yasuda N, Lai PK, Rogers J, et al. Defective control of Epstein-Barr

virus–infected B cell growth in patients with X-linked lymphoproliferative disease. *Clin Exp Immunol* 1991;83:10–16.

148. Schuster V, Kreth HW. X-linked lymphoproliferative disease is caused by deficiency of a novel SH2 domain–containing signal transduction adaptor protein. *Immunol Rev* 2000;178:21–28.

149. Okano M, Gross TG. A review of Epstein-Barr virus infection in patients with immunodeficiency disorders. *Am J Med Sci* 2000;319:392–396.

150. Guiloff RJ, Tan SV. Central nervous system opportunistic infections in HIV disease: clinical aspects. *Baillieres Clin Neurol* 1992;1:103–154.

151. Huang LM, Chao MF, Chen MY, et al. Reciprocal regulatory interaction between human herpesvirus 8 and human immunodeficiency virus type 1. *J Biol Chem* 2001;276:13427–13432.

152. Jablonska S. Traditional therapies for the treatment of condylomata acuminata (genital warts). *Australas J Dermatol* 1998;39(Suppl 1):S2–S4.

153. Durst M, Gissmann L, Ikenberg H, et al. A papillomavirus DNA from a cervical carcinoma and its prevalence in cancer biopsy samples from different geographic regions. *Proc Natl Acad Sci U S A* 1983;80:3812–3815.

154. Marais DJ, Vardas E, Ramjee G, et al. The impact of human immunodeficiency virus type 1 status on human papillomavirus (HPV) prevalence and HPV antibodies in serum and cervical secretions. *J Infect Dis* 2000;182:1239–1242.

155. Koike K. Role of hepatitis viruses in multistep hepatocarcinogenesis. *Dig Liver Dis* 2001;33:2–6.

156. Chisari FV, Ferrari C. Hepatitis B virus immunopathogenesis. *Annu Rev Immunol* 1995;13:29–60.

157. Koziel MJ, Dudley D, Wong JT, et al. Intrahepatic cytotoxic T lymphocytes specific for hepatitis C virus in persons with chronic hepatitis. *J Immunol* 1992;149:3339–3344.

158. Weiner A, Erickson AL, Kansopon J, et al. Persistent hepatitis C virus infection in a chimpanzee is associated with emergence of a cytotoxic T lymphocyte escape variant. *Proc Natl Acad Sci U S A* 1995;92:2755–2759.

159. Moriyama T, Guilhot S, Klopchin K, et al. Immunobiology and pathogenesis of hepatocellular injury in hepatitis B virus transgenic mice. *Science* 1990;248:361–364.

160. Billeter MA, Cattaneo R, Spielhofer P, et al. Generation and properties of measles virus mutations typically associated with subacute sclerosing panencephalitis. *Ann N Y Acad Sci* 1994;724:367–377.

161. De St Groth F, Webster R. Disquisitions on original antigenic sin. I. Evidence in man. *J Exp Med* 1966;124:331–345.

162. Klenerman P, Zinkernagel RM. Original antigenic sin impairs cytotoxic T lymphocyte responses to viruses bearing variant epitopes. *Nature* 1998;394:482–485.

163. Whitton JL, Fujinami RS. Viruses as triggers of autoimmunity: facts and fantasies. *Curr Opin Microbiol* 1999;2:392–397.

164. Oldstone MB. Molecular mimicry and autoimmune disease. *Cell* 1987;50:819–820.

165. Miller SD, Vanderlugt CL, Begolka WS, et al. Persistent infection with Theiler's virus leads to CNS autoimmunity via epitope spreading. *Nat Med* 1997;3:1133–1136.

166. Horwitz MS, Sarvetnick N. Viruses, host responses, and autoimmunity. *Immunol Rev* 1999;169:241–253.

167. Srinivasappa J, Saegusa J, Prabhakar BS, et al. Molecular mimicry: frequency of reactivity of monoclonal antiviral antibodies with normal tissues. *J Virol* 1986;57:397–401.

168. Huber BT. Mls superantigens: how retroviruses influence the expressed T cell receptor repertoire. *Semin Immunol* 1992;4:313–318.

169. Lafon M, Lafage M, Martinez-Arends A, et al. Evidence for a viral superantigen in humans. *Nature* 1992;358:507–510.

170. Lafon M, Scott-Algara D, Marche PN, et al. Neonatal deletion and selective expansion of mouse T cells by exposure to rabies virus nucleocapsid superantigen. *J Exp Med* 1994;180:1207–1215.

171. Lafon M, Galelli A. Superantigen related to rabies. *Springer Semin Immunopathol* 1996;17:307–318.

172. Ertl HC, Dietzschold B, Gore M, et al. Induction of rabies virus–specific T-helper cells by synthetic peptides that carry dominant T-helper cell epitopes of the viral ribonucleoprotein. *J Virol* 1989;63:2885–2892.

173. Galle PR, Hofmann WJ, Walczak H, et al. Involvement of the CD95 (APO-1/Fas) receptor and ligand in liver damage. *J Exp Med* 1995;182:1223–1230.

174. Chisari FV. Cytotoxic T cells and viral hepatitis. *J Clin Invest* 1997;99:1472–1477.

175. Lorenzo ME, Ploegh HL, Tirabassi RS. Viral immune evasion strategies and the underlying cell biology. *Semin Immunol* 2001;13:1–9.

176. Abendroth A, Arvin AM. Immune evasion as a pathogenic mechanism of varicella zoster virus. *Semin Immunol* 2001;13:27–39.

177. Howcroft TK, Strebel K, Martin MA, et al. Repression of MHC class I gene promoter activity by two-exon Tat of HIV. *Science* 1993;260:1320–1322.

178. Kerkau T, Bacik I, Bennink JR, et al. The human immunodeficiency virus type 1 (HIV-1) Vpu protein interferes with an early step in the biosynthesis of major histocompatibility complex (MHC) class I molecules. *J Exp Med* 1997;185:1295–1305.

179. Chang CH, Roys S, Gourley T. Class II transactivator: is it a master switch for MHC class II gene expression? *Microbes Infect* 1999;1:879–885.

180. Miller DM, Rahill BM, Boss JM, et al. Human cytomegalovirus inhibits major histocompatibility complex class II expression by disruption of the Jak/Stat pathway. *J Exp Med* 1998;187:675–683.

181. Le Roy E, Muhlethaler-Mottet A, Davrinche C, et al. Escape of human cytomegalovirus from HLA-DR–restricted CD4(+) T-cell response is mediated by repression of gamma interferon–induced class II transactivator expression. *J Virol* 1999;73:6582–6589.

182. Phillips AJ, Tomasec P, Wang EC, et al. Human cytomegalovirus infection downregulates expression of the cellular aminopeptidases CD10 and CD13. *Virology* 1998;250:350–358.

183. Hewitt EW, Gupta SS, Lehner PJ. The human cytomegalovirus gene product US6 inhibits ATP binding by TAP. *EMBO J* 2001;20:387–396.

184. Galocha B, Hill A, Barnett BC, et al. The active site of ICP47, a herpes simplex virus–encoded inhibitor of the major histocompatibility complex (MHC)–encoded peptide transporter associated with antigen processing (TAP), maps to the NH2-terminal 35 residues. *J Exp Med* 1997;185:1565–1572.

185. Qin L, Ding Y, Tahara H, et al. Viral IL-10–induced immunosuppression requires Th2 cytokines and impairs APC function within the allograft. *J Immunol* 2001;166:2385–2393.

186. Lockridge KM, Zhou SS, Kravitz RH, et al. Primate cytomegaloviruses encode and express an IL-10–like protein. *Virology* 2000;268:272–280.

187. Tortorella D, Gewurz BE, Furman MH, et al. Viral subversion of the immune system. *Annu Rev Immunol* 2000;18:861–926.

188. Beier DC, Cox JH, Vining DR, et al. Association of human class I MHC alleles with the adenovirus E3/19K protein. *J Immunol* 1994;152:3862–3872.

189. Feuerbach D, Etteldorf S, Ebenau-Jehle C, et al. Identification of amino acids within the MHC molecule important for the interaction with the adenovirus protein E3/19K. *J Immunol* 1994;153:1626–1636.

190. Ziegler H, Muranyi W, Burgert HG, et al. The luminal part of the murine cytomegalovirus glycoprotein gp40 catalyzes the retention of MHC class I molecules. *EMBO J* 2000;19:870–881.

191. Jones TR, Sun L. Human cytomegalovirus US2 destabilizes major histocompatibility complex class I heavy chains. *J Virol* 1997;71:2970–2979.

192. Reusch U, Muranyi W, Lucin P, et al. A cytomegalovirus glycoprotein re-routes MHC class I complexes to lysosomes for degradation. *EMBO J* 1999;18:1081–1091.

193. Kleijnen MF, Huppa JB, Lucin P, et al. A mouse cytomegalovirus glycoprotein, gp34, forms a complex with folded class I MHC molecules in the ER which is not retained but is transported to the cell surface. *EMBO J* 1997;16:685–694.

194. Riggs NL, Craig HM, Pandori MW, et al. The dileucine-based sorting motif in HIV-1 Nef is not required for down-regulation of class I MHC. *Virology* 1999;258:203–207.

195. Ishido S, Wang C, Lee BS, et al. Downregulation of major histocompatibility complex class I molecules by Kaposi's sarcoma–associated herpesvirus K3 and K5 proteins. *J Virol* 2000;74:5300–5309.

196. Gewurz BE, Gaudet R, Tortorella D, et al. Virus subversion of immunity: a structural perspective. *Curr Opin Immunol* 2001;13:442–450.

197. Cohen GM. Caspases: the executioners of apoptosis. *Biochem J* 1997;326:1–16.

198. Komiyama T, Ray CA, Pickup DJ, et al. Inhibition of interleukin-1 beta converting enzyme by the cowpox virus serpin CrmA. An example of cross-class inhibition. *J Biol Chem* 1994;269:19331–19337.

199. Quan LT, Caputo A, Bleackley RC, et al. Granzyme B is inhibited by the cowpox virus serpin cytokine response modifier A. *J Biol Chem* 1995;270:10377–10379.

200. Moon KB, Turner PC, Moyer RW. SPI-1–dependent host range of rabbitpox virus and complex formation with cathepsin G is associated with serpin motifs. *J Virol* 1999;73:8999–9010.

201. Shisler JL, Moss B. Molluscum contagiosum virus inhibitors of apoptosis: the MC159 v-FLIP protein blocks Fas-induced activation of procaspases and degradation of the related MC160 protein. *Virology* 2001;282:14–25.

202. Grundhoff A, Ganem D. Mechanisms governing expression of the v-FLIP gene of Kaposi's sarcoma–associated herpesvirus. *J Virol* 2001;75:1857–1863.

203. Senkevich TG, Bugert JJ, Sisler JR, et al. Genome sequence of a human tumorigenic poxvirus: prediction of specific host response-evasion genes. *Science* 1996;273:813–816.

204. Shisler JL, Senkevich TG, Berry MJ, et al. Ultraviolet-induced cell death blocked by a selenoprotein from a human dermatotropic poxvirus. *Science* 1998;279:102–105.

205. Brick DJ, Burke RD, Minkley AA, et al. Ectromelia virus virulence factor p28 acts upstream of caspase-3 in response to UV light-induced apoptosis. *J Gen Virol* 2000;81(Pt 4):1087–1097.

206. Everett H, Barry M, Lee SF, et al. M11L: a novel mitochondria-localized protein of myxoma virus that blocks apoptosis of infected leukocytes. *J Exp Med* 2000;191:1487–1498.

207. Hnatiuk S, Barry M, Zeng W, et al. Role of the C-terminal RDEL motif of the myxoma virus M-T4 protein in terms of apoptosis regulation and viral pathogenesis. *Virology* 1999;263:290–306.

208. Cretney E, Degli-Esposti MA, Densley EH, et al. m144, a murine cytomegalovirus (MCMV)–encoded major histocompatibility complex class I homologue, confers tumor resistance to natural killer cell–mediated rejection. *J Exp Med* 1999;190:435–444.

209. Chapman TL, Heikeman AP, Bjorkman PJ. The inhibitory receptor LIR-1 uses a common binding interaction to recognize class I MHC molecules and the viral homolog UL18. *Immunity* 1999;11:603–613.

210. Ulbrecht M, Martinozzi S, Grzeschik M, et al. Cutting edge: the human cytomegalovirus UL40 gene product contains a ligand for HLA-E and prevents NK cell–mediated lysis. *J Immunol* 2000;164:5019–5022.

211. Sahu A, Isaacs SN, Soulika AM, et al. Interaction of vaccinia virus complement control protein with human complement proteins: factor I–mediated degradation of C3b to iC3b1 inactivates the alternative complement pathway. *J Immunol* 1998;160:5596–5604.

212. Hsu DH, de Waal Malefyt R, Fiorentino DF, et al. Expression of interleukin-10 activity by Epstein-Barr virus protein BCRF1. *Science* 1990;250:830–832.

213. Kotenko SV, Saccani S, Izotova LS, et al. Human cytomegalovirus harbors its own unique IL-10 homolog (cmvIL-10). *Proc Natl Acad Sci U S A* 2000;97:1695–1700.

214. Penfold ME, Dairaghi DJ, Duke GM, et al. Cytomegalovirus encodes a potent alpha chemokine. *Proc Natl Acad Sci U S A* 1999;96:9839–9844.

215. Bodaghi B, Jones TR, Zipeto D, et al. Chemokine sequestration by viral chemoreceptors as a novel viral escape strategy: withdrawal of chemokines from the environment of cytomegalovirus-infected cells. *J Exp Med* 1998;188:855–866.

216. Luttichau HR, Stine J, Boesen TP, et al. A highly selective CC chemokine receptor (CCR)8 antagonist encoded by the poxvirus molluscum contagiosum. *J Exp Med* 2000;191:171–180.

217. Graham KA, Lalani AS, Macen JL, et al. The T1/35kDa family of poxvirus-secreted proteins bind chemokines and modulate leukocyte influx into virus-infected tissues. *Virology* 1997;229:12–24.

218. Barrett JW, Cao JX, Hota-Mitchell S, et al. Immunomodulatory proteins of myxoma virus. *Semin Immunol* 2001;13:73–84.

219. Verardi PH, Jones LA, Aziz FH, et al. Vaccinia virus vectors with an inactivated gamma interferon receptor homolog gene (B8R) are attenuated *in vivo* without a concomitant reduction in immunogenicity. *J Virol* 2001;75:11–18.

220. Liptakova H, Kontsekova E, Alcami A, et al. Analysis of an interaction between the soluble vaccinia virus–coded type I interferon (IFN)–receptor and human IFN-alpha1 and IFN-alpha2. *Virology* 1997;232:86–90.

221. Deane D, McInnes CJ, Percival A, et al. Orf virus encodes a novel secreted protein inhibitor of granulocyte-macrophage colony-stimulating factor and interleukin-2. *J Virol* 2000;74:1313–1320.

222. Benedict CA, Butrovich KD, Lurain NS, et al. Cutting edge: a novel viral TNF receptor superfamily member in virulent strains of human cytomegalovirus. *J Immunol* 1999;162:6967–6970.

223. Schreiber M, Sedger L, McFadden G. Distinct domains of M-T2, the myxoma virus tumor necrosis factor (TNF) receptor homolog, mediate extracellular TNF binding and intracellular apoptosis inhibition. *J Virol* 1997;71:2171–2181.

224. Loparev VN, Parsons JM, Knight JC, et al. A third distinct tumor necrosis factor receptor of orthopoxviruses. *Proc Natl Acad Sci U S A* 1998;95:3786–3791.

225. Smith GL, Symons JA, Khanna A, et al. Vaccinia virus immune evasion. *Immunol Rev* 1997;159:137–154.

226. Ray CA, Black RA, Kronheim SR, et al. Viral inhibition of inflammation: cowpox virus encodes an inhibitor of the interleukin-1 beta converting enzyme. *Cell* 1992;69:597–604.

227. Komiyama T, Quan LT, Salvesen GS. Inhibition of cysteine and serine proteinases by the cowpox virus serpin CRMA. *Adv Exp Med Biol* 1996;389:173–176.

228. Young DF, Chatziandreou N, He B, et al. Single amino acid substitution in the V protein of simian virus 5 differentiates its ability to block interferon signaling in human and murine cells. *J Virol* 2001;75:3363–3370.

229. Parisien JP, Lau JF, Rodriguez JJ, et al. The V protein of human parainfluenza virus 2 antagonizes type I interferon responses by destabilizing signal transducer and activator of transcription 2. *Virology* 2001;283:230–239.

230. Ronco LV, Karpova AY, Vidal M, et al. Human papillomavirus 16 E6 oncoprotein binds to interferon regulatory factor–3 and inhibits its transcriptional activity. *Genes Dev* 1998;12:2061–2072.

231. Mossman K, Upton C, McFadden G. The myxoma virus–soluble interferon-gamma receptor homolog, M-T7, inhibits interferon-gamma in a species-specific manner. *J Biol Chem* 1995;270:3031–3038.

232. Xiang Y, Moss B. IL-18 binding and inhibition of interferon gamma induction by human poxvirus-encoded proteins. *Proc Natl Acad Sci U S A* 1999;96:11537–11542.

233. Thale R, Lucin P, Schneider K, et al. Identification and expression of a murine cytomegalovirus early gene coding for an Fc receptor. *J Virol* 1994;68:7757–7765.

CHAPTER 40

Immunity to Intracellular Bacteria

Stefan H. E. Kaufmann

Introduction
General Principles of Pathogenicity and Virulence of Intracellular Bacteria
  Characteristic Features of Intracellular Bacteria · Hallmarks of an "Idealized" Intracellular Bacterium · Two Types of Intracellular Bacteria: Facultative and Obligate Intracellular
Specific Features and Examples
  M. tuberculosis and Tuberculosis · *L. monocytogenes* and Listeriosis · *S. enterica* and Salmonellosis
Entry into, Killing by, and Survival within Host Cells
  Adhesion and Invasion · Recognition Receptors for Microbes · Invasion of Nonprofessional Phagocytes · Phagosome Maturation, Acidification, and Phagosome–Lysosome Fusion · Intracellular Iron · Tryptophan Degradation · Toxic Effector Molecules · Evasion of Killing by ROI and RNI · Evasion into Cytoplasm · Cell-to-Cell Spreading · Apoptosis
Professional Phagocytes
  Mononuclear Phagocytes · Polymorphonuclear Granulocytes
Central Role of Acquired Immune Response
  Dendritic Cells · T-Cell Subpopulations · CD1 Molecules and Antigen Presentation · Multiple Roles of β2 Microglobulin
T-Cell Functions during Course of Infection
  T-Cell Functions · Contribution of Conventional and Unconventional T Cells to Protection: Implications for Vaccine Design · Kinetics of Infection
Cytokines in Antibacterial Defense
  Leukocyte Recruitment · Granuloma Formation · Macrophage Activation · Induction of Protective T-Cell Response · Down-Regulation of Antibacterial Host Response to Avoid its Harmful Sequelae
Predominance of Th1 over Th2 Cell Activities in Intracellular Bacterial Infections: Influence of Innate Immune System
Death of Infected Cells
Granulomatous Lesion
  "Idealized Granuloma" · Leukocyte Extravasation · Granuloma formation · Tuberculosis · Experimental Listeriosis · Leprosy
Delayed-Type Hypersensitivity
Genetic Control of Resistance against Intracellular Bacteria
  Control of Innate Antibacterial Resistance by the Nramp1 Gene · Vitamin D Receptor · MHC Control of Severity and Form of Disease
Conclusions and Outlook
Acknowledgments
References

INTRODUCTION

This chapter focuses on infections with intracellular bacteria, emphasizing in particular the general immune mechanisms underlying protection and pathogenicity. Intracellular bacteria comprise numerous pathogens, some of which are of utmost medical importance whereas others play only an inferior role. Ancient (but still existent) as well as newly emerging diseases are caused by intracellular bacteria. Of paramount significance for humans are *Mycobacterium tuberculosis, Mycobacterium leprae, Salmonella enterica* serovar Typhi, and *Chlamydia trachomatis,* the etiologic agents of tuberculosis,

leprosy, typhoid, and trachoma, respectively, which, together, afflict more than 600 million people. An association of *Chlamydia pneumoniae* with cardiovascular diseases has been claimed. Some opportunistic pathogens such as *Mycobacterium avium/Mycobacterium intracellulare* are gaining increasing significance with the growing number of immunodeficient patients, such as acquired immune deficiency syndrome (AIDS) sufferers.

As can be deduced from their name, intracellular bacteria live inside host cells for most of their lives. Intracellular living implies coexistence with the abused host cells; accordingly, many intracellular bacteria are of low toxicity by themselves.

These characteristic features have direct consequences for the immune response evoked. Because of their intracellular location, these pathogens are relatively well shielded from humoral immunity. However, during intracellular living, microbial proteins are processed and peptides presented in the context of major histocompatibility complex (MHC) molecules, thus promoting activation of T-lymphocytes. Accordingly, acquired resistance against and pathogenesis of intracellular bacterial infections crucially depend on T-lymphocytes. Although CD4 T-lymphocytes are central to acquired resistance, recent evidence suggests contribution by CD8 T cells as well as additional unconventional T cells. Moreover, while macrophage activation by interferon γ (IFN-γ) is crucial for antibacterial protection, additional functions are often required for clearance of infection.

GENERAL PRINCIPLES OF PATHOGENICITY AND VIRULENCE OF INTRACELLULAR BACTERIA

Characteristic Features of Intracellular Bacteria

Bacterial pathogens are microorganisms that cause disease in a given host species. The term pathogenicity embodies the quality of a whole microbial species comprising several strains of varying virulence—that is, of varying disease-causing strength. Only rarely is infectious disease the direct and invariable consequence of an encounter between host and pathogen. Rather, it is the eventual outcome of complex interactions between them. Because this is particularly relevant to our understanding of infections with intracellular bacteria, the principal steps are discussed briefly.

Some intracellular bacteria, in particular *Rickettsia* sp, are introduced directly into the bloodstream by insect bites from where they have ready access to internal tissues. Most intracellular bacteria, however, enter the host through the mucosa, and bacterial entry is frequently initiated by adhesion to cells of the epithelial mucosa (1). Major ports of entry are the lung for airborne pathogens such as *M. tuberculosis* and *Legionella pneumophila,* and the intestine for food-borne pathogens such as *S. enterica* and *Listeria monocytogenes.* Subsequently, intracellular bacteria pass through the epithelial layers. Either they actively induce transcytosis (i.e., endo- and exo-cytosis) through the epithelial cells or they are passively translocated within macrophages. Bacteria may be removed by nonspecific defense mechanisms such as mucociliary movements and gut peristalsis, or they may be destroyed by professional phagocytes without necessitating the specific attention of the immune system. Cells that survive these nonspecific defense reactions colonize deeper tissue sites and stably infect a suitable niche. At this stage, the host generally pays sufficient attention to the infectious agent as indicated by the development of a specific acquired immune response.

Infection is abortive when the immune system succeeds in eliminating the pathogen before overt clinical disease develops. Alternatively, tissue damage increases to a significant level before the immune system succeeds in controlling the pathogen effectively and clinical disease develops. This is the case with many extracellular bacteria that cause diseases of acute type, but less common in the case of intracellular bacteria. Finally, it is possible that the immune response restrains the infectious agent but fails to completely eradicate it. Under these conditions, a long-lasting equilibrium between microbial persistence and the immune response unfolds. This balance, however, remains labile and can be tipped in favor of the pathogen at a later time, converting infection into disease.

The time lapse between host entry and expression of clinical disease is often termed incubation time and from what has been said above, it follows that in many intracellular bacterial infections the incubation times are long-lasting to lifelong. By improving the immune response or by impairing bacterial growth (typically accomplished by chemotherapy), or both, disease can be overcome. Ideally, bacterial eradication is achieved; alternatively, some dormant bacteria continue to persist in niches poorly accessible to the immune response.

To reemphasize the relevant steps leading to diseases caused by intracellular bacteria:

- Commonly, infection is clearly separated from disease, and the immune response is already induced at the stage of infection.
- Infection persists in face of dynamic interactions between pathogen and immune mechanisms.
- The host–pathogen relationship represents a highly sophisticated form of parasitism that does not necessarily lead to disease but rather allows for long-lasting coexistence.
- Infection includes the potential to harm the host severely at a later stage, and pathogenesis is strongly influenced by the immune response.

Hallmarks of an "Idealized" Intracellular Bacterium

Although this chapter focuses on general mechanisms underlying immunity to intracellular bacteria, it is important to emphasize that this group is extremely heterogeneous despite several commonalities. Therefore, the major hallmarks of intracellular bacterial infections will first be described for a nonexistent "idealized" intracellular bacterium and compared with an "idealized" extracellular bacterium (Table 1).

TABLE 1. *Hallmarks of intracellular bacterial infections*

Essential
Intracellular habitat
T-cell–mediated protection
Delayed-type hypersensitivity
Granulomatous tissue reaction
Conditional
Low intrinsic toxicity/immune pathology
Labile balance between infection and protective immunity
Protracted incubation time/chronic disease
Dissociation of infection from disease

Subsequently, characteristics of selected intracellular bacteria will be specified.

Hallmark 1. As implied by the name, the intracellular lifestyle represents the distinguishing feature of intracellular bacteria. Yet, invasion of host cells is not restricted to these pathogens, and transient trespassing through epithelial cells is a common invasion mechanism of both intracellular and extracellular pathogens.

Hallmark 2. T cells are the central mediators of protection against intracellular bacterial infections. These T cells do not interact with microbes directly, but instead interact with the infected host cell. In contrast, antibodies that recognize microbial antigens directly are of exquisite importance for defense against extracellular bacteria.

Hallmark 3. Infections with intracellular bacteria are accompanied by delayed-type hypersensitivity (DTH), which expresses itself after local administration of soluble antigens as a delayed-tissue reaction mediated by T cells and effected by macrophages.

Hallmark 4. Tissue reactions against intracellular bacteria are granulomatous; and protection against, as well as pathology caused by, intracellular bacteria are centered on these lesions. Rupture of a granuloma promotes bacterial dissemination and formation of additional lesions at distinct tissue sites. In contrast, tissue reactions against extracellular bacteria are purulent and lead to abscess formation or systemic reactions.

Hallmark 5. Intracellular bacteria express little or no toxicity for host cells by themselves, and the pathology is primarily a result of immune reactions, particularly those mediated by T-lymphocytes. In contrast, extracellular bacteria produce various toxins that are directly responsible for tissue damage.

Hallmark 6. Intracellular bacteria coexist with their cellular habitat for long periods of time. A labile balance develops between persistent infection and protective immunity, resulting in long incubation time and in chronic disease. Accordingly, infection is clearly dissociated from disease. In contrast, extracellular bacteria typically cause acute diseases that develop soon after their entry into the host and are terminated once the immune response has developed. Thus, the transition of infection into clinical disease occurs rapidly.

Hallmarks 1 to 4 should be considered essential, and hallmarks 5 and 6 conditional, criteria for defining intracellular bacteria.

Of course, the ideal intracellular bacterium as characterized above does not exist. *M. tuberculosis* probably resembles it most. Yet, at the height of active tuberculosis, tubercle bacilli replicate extracellularly in the detritus of dissolved host cells in an unrestricted way (2). Experimental listeriosis of mice fulfills many criteria (though not all) but takes an acute course of disease (3). In typhoid, antibodies participate in the protective immune response, and in leprosy they contribute to pathogenesis (4).

Two Types of Intracellular Bacteria: Facultative and Obligate Intracellular

With respect to their preferred habitat, intracellular bacteria can be divided into two groups: Those pathogens which do not essentially depend on the intracellular habitat include *M. tuberculosis, M. bovis, M. leprae, S. enterica, Brucella* sp, *L. pneumophila, L. monocytogenes,* and *Francisella tularensis* (Table 2) (2,3,5–10). Although these pathogens favor mononuclear phagocytes (MP) as their biotope, other types of host cells are infected as well. *M. leprae,* for example, lives in numerous host cell types, notably in Schwann cells and hepatocytes serve as an important reservoir for *L. monocytogenes.* Although *M. tuberculosis* can infect a variety of mammalian cells *in vitro, in vivo* it seems to restrict itself to macrophages.

So-called obligate intracellular bacteria fail to survive outside host cells. These bacteria prefer nonprofessional phagocytes as their habitat—for example, endothelial and epithelial cells. Nevertheless, they are sometimes found in MP as well. Rickettsiae and chlamydiae are representatives of this group. They include *Rickettsia prowazekii, Rickettsia*

TABLE 2. *Major infections of humans caused by facultative intracellular bacteria*

Pathogen	Disease	Preferred target cell	Preferred location in host cell	Preferred port of entry
Mycobacterium tuberculosis	Tuberculosis	Macrophages	Early phagosome	Lung
Mycobacterium leprae	Leprosy	Macrophages, Schwann cells, other cells	Phagolysosome (?)	Nasopharyngeal mucosa
Salmonella enterica serovar *Typhi*	Typhoid fever	Macrophages	Spacious phagosome	Gut
Brucella sp	Brucellosis	Macrophages	Phagolysosome	Mucosa
Legionella sp	Legionnaire's disease	Macrophages	Autophagosome	Lung
Listeria monocytogenes	Listeriosis	Macrophages, hepatocytes	Cytosol	Gut
Francisella tularensis	Tularemia	Macrophages	Phagosome	Skin, lung, mucosa

TABLE 3. *Major infections of humans caused by obligate intracellular bacteria*

Pathogen	Disease	Preferred target cell	Preferred location in host cell	Preferred port of entry
Rickettsia rickettsii	Rocky Mountain spotted fever	Endothelial cells, smooth muscle cells	Cytosol	Blood vessel (tick bite)
Rickettsia prowazekii	Endemic typhus	Endothelial cells	Cytosol	Broken skin, mucosa
Rickettsia typhi	Typhus	Endothelial cells	Cytosol	Blood vessel (flea bite)
Rickettsia tsutsugamushi	Scrub typhus	Endothelial cells	Cytosol	Blood vessel (mite bite)
Coxiella burnetii	Q-fever	Macrophages, lung parenchyma cells	Late phagosome	Lung
Chlamydia trachomatis	Urogenital infection, conjunctivitis, trachoma, lymphogranuloma, venerum (different serovars)	Epithelial cells	Phagosome	Eye, urogenital mucosa
Chlamydia psittaci	Psittacosis	Macrophages, lung parenchyma cells	Phagosome	Lung
Chlamydia pneumoniae	Pneumonia, coronary heart disease	Lung parenchyma cells	Phagosome	Lung

rickettsii, Rickettsia typhi, Rickettsia tsutsugamushi, and *Coxiella burnetii,* the etiologic agents of louse-borne typhus, Rocky Mountain spotted fever, typhus, scrub typhus, and Q-fever, respectively (11). Various biovars of *Chlamydia trachomatis,* which are responsible for trachoma, conjunctivitis, urogenital infections, and lymphogranuloma venerum, as well as *C. psittaci* and *C. pneumoniae,* causative agents of psittacosis or rare types of pneumonia, respectively, also belong to this group (Table 3) (12). *C. pneumoniae* infection is considered a cofactor in the development of atherosclerotic cardiovascular disease (13).

Preferential living in macrophages does not depend on specific invasion mechanisms but rather on highly sophisticated intracellular survival strategies. Yet, most facultative intracellular bacteria express specific invasion factors if only to cross epithelial layers. In contrast, selection of nonprofessional phagocytes as habitat essentially depends on invasion molecules whereas survival inside these cells is generally less hazardous.

Because this chapter focuses on general mechanisms underlying the immune response to intracellular bacteria, some selectivity is required and major emphasis is given to (a) experimental listeriosis of mice because this model has proven most productive in the exploration of the immune mechanisms responsible for acquired resistance against intracellular bacteria; (b) tuberculosis, which not only represents the paradigm of intracellular bacterial infections but also is of paramount medical importance; and (c) *S. enterica* infection, which is increasingly used for elucidating the intracellular lifestyle of bacteria. Where appropriate, other infections will be included in the discussion. The genomes of *L. monocytogenes, M. tuberculosis, S. enterica* (serovars Typhi and Typhimurium) have been sequenced, providing new insights into the molecular strategies that these pathogens use for infection (14–17).

SPECIFIC FEATURES AND EXAMPLES

M. tuberculosis and Tuberculosis

This paradigmatic intracellular bacterium is an acid-fast bacillus with a replication time of more than 20 hours. Tubercle bacilli are obligate aerobes and hence prefer tissue sites with high oxygen pressure such as the lung. *M. tuberculosis* as well as other mycobacteria contain abundant lipids, glycolipids, and waxes that are responsible not only for the hydrophobic character of the mycobacteria, but also for their acid fastness, strong adjuvanticity (mycobacteria are the crucial components of Freund's complete adjuvant), resistance against complement lysis, and resistance against acids, alkalines, and simple disinfectants. Most importantly, these glycolipids are central to intracellular survival inside activated MP. More recent findings have revealed that certain mycobacterial glycolipids serve as antigenic targets for a small population of unconventional T cells in humans. The importance of glycolipids is reflected by the large number of *M. tuberculosis* genes encoding enzymes involved in fatty acid metabolism and catabolism. *M. tuberculosis* and, to a lesser extent, *M. bovis* cause tuberculosis, which is of paramount medical importance globally (18,19). The disease is characterized by long incubation time, dormant infection, and protracted course. Consistent with this, the genome of *M. tuberculosis* comprises several genes that enable survival under nutrient deprivation and low oxygen pressure, which may play a role during mycobacterial persistence.

It is estimated that every year 8 million new cases arise and 2 million people die of this disease, making *M. tuberculosis* one of the major killers. On the other hand, it has been estimated that one-third of the entire world population (2 billion people) are infected with *M. tuberculosis*. Infected individuals harbor *M. tuberculosis* inside small granulomas at sequestered tissue sites. Persistence of *M. tuberculosis* in these seclusions does not remain unrecognized by the immune system; rather, it is controlled by T cells (20). Hence, the vast majority (>90%) of infected people remain healthy, and only a minority develop disease following weakening of the immune response. Primary infection generally proceeds via the aerosol route, and the lung remains the principal site of infection as well as disease. Nevertheless, any other tissue site can be infected following reactivation of dormant foci and hematogenic/lymphogenic dissemination. Tuberculosis of adults primarily develops through reactivation of dormant foci; only rarely does reinfection of individuals already harboring dormant *M. tuberculosis* cause disease. In 1927, Calmette and Guérin developed an attenuated strain of *M. bovis,* termed Bacille Calmette Guérin (BCG). At present, this strain is the most widely used viable vaccine globally. Although BCG is efficacious in preventing miliary tuberculosis in young children, its protective efficacy against pulmonary tuberculosis in adults is insufficient. Whole genome DNA microarray analyses have led to the identification of 129 genes present in *M. tuberculosis* but absent from BCG (21). These genes are considered central to the virulence of *M. tuberculosis,* and may also comprise important antigens.

L. monocytogenes and Listeriosis

This bacterium is a gram-positive, non–spore-forming, facultatively anaerobic rod. Recent molecular biology analyses have revealed several virulence factors of *L. monocytogenes* that are instrumental for cell invasion, intracellular replication, and cell-to-cell spread (5,14). Listeriolysin is a sulfhydril-activated, pore-forming cytolysin that is active at the low pH existing in the phagosome and promotes escape from the phagosomal into the cytoplasmic compartment. Two different phospholipase C molecules and a lecithinase contribute to the escape of *L. monocytogenes* into the cytoplasm and to cell-to-cell spread. Transition from the phagosome into the cytosol not only is essential for virulence, but also markedly influences the type of T-cell response evoked, because it promotes loading of MHC class I molecules with antigenic peptides. The ActA gene product is involved in intracellular movements and promotes cell-to-cell spreading, while intracellular survival may be further facilitated by a metalloprotease. Several internalins and p60-like proteins encoded by the Iap gene are involved in invasion of nonphagocytic host cells and crossing of the intestinal barrier. The PrfA gene positively regulates expression of several virulence factors such as listeriolysin, lecithinase, and phospholipase C. Listeriosis is primarily a disease of sheep and cattle and only rarely occurs in humans. *L. monocytogenes* infection of experimental mice has provided an extremely helpful tool for elucidating the mechanisms central to our understanding of immunity to intracellular bacteria (3). Despite the capacity of *L. monocytogenes* organisms to survive in resting macrophages, they are readily killed once macrophages are activated. Therefore, murine listeriosis is an acute infection that is easily terminated following T-cell activation. Even in the absence of

T cells, listeriosis is quite efficiently if incompletely controlled. These features must be kept in mind in interpreting data from murine listeriosis experiments.

S. enterica and Salmonellosis

According to the latest nomenclature, all salmonellae belong to a single species termed *S. enterica* (4,22). This species encompasses more than 2,000 serovars including *S. enterica* serovar Typhi, the causative agent of human typhoid, and *S. enterica* Typhimurium, which is responsible for a similar disease in mice. The salmonellae are widespread in nature and infect a vast variety of animals, including mammals, reptiles, and birds. Some salmonellae, such as *S. enterica* Typhimurium have a broad host range; others are highly restricted, such as *S. enterica* Typhi, which is almost exclusively restricted to humans. Comparison of the genomes of *S. enterica* Typhimurium and Typhi revealed that approximately 10% of the genes of Typhimurium are missing in Typhi, suggesting that they are important for the broader host spectrum of the former (15,16). The genome of *S. enterica* comprises several insertions termed the Salmonella pathogenicity islands (SPI), which, as the name suggests, encode genes central to pathogenicity. This includes secretion systems, virulence factors, and ion transporters. Typically, salmonellosis is food-borne, and in the susceptible host the pathogens cause diseases ranging from mild enterocolitis to severe diarrhea. Some salmonellae, having passed through the gut epithelium, can cause bacteremia, which sometimes results in enteric fever or typhoid. Although human typhoid is now much better controlled than it was in the past, it still causes severe health problems globally, with approximately 16 million new cases every year, resulting in 600,000 deaths. The diarrheal diseases caused by various *S. enterica* serovars are a major threat to humankind as well. Findings, described in the remaining part of this chapter, are almost exclusively derived from experiments in mice with *S. enterica* Typhimurium. Although this model reflects numerous aspects of human typhoid, it must be kept in mind that some of these findings cannot be extrapolated to other serovars of *S. enterica,* including Typhi.

ENTRY INTO, KILLING BY, AND SURVIVAL WITHIN HOST CELLS

For intracellular bacteria, entry into host cells represents the central requirement for survival in, as well as elimination by, the host. Host-cell–directed uptake, called "phagocytosis," is a feature of the so-called professional phagocytes that comprise polymorphonuclear granulocytes (PNG) and MP. Entry induced by the pathogen is termed invasion: It allows entry into nonphagocytic cells (nonprofessional phagocytes). Contact between host cells and pathogens proceeds either directly via receptor–ligand interactions or indirectly via deposition on the surface of the pathogen of host molecules for which physiologic receptors exist on the target cell.

Depending on the cellular target, the final outcome of host cell entry varies markedly.

1. Nonprofessional phagocytes are nonphagocytic, and hence entry depends on expression of surface receptors that can be misused for invasion. Because of their low antibacterial activities, they primarily serve as a habitat.
2. PNG are short-lived. Because they are highly phagocytic and express potent antibacterial activities constitutively, uptake by PNG is generally fatal for the pathogen.
3. MP are phagocytic and express medium to high antibacterial activities depending on their activation status. Accordingly, they serve both as habitat and as effector cell.

In the following, the major steps from uptake to bacterial elimination by, or survival in, host cells will be described with emphasis on the major target of intracellular bacteria, the MP (Fig. 1).

Adhesion and Invasion

Adhesion to mammalian cells is a common feature of bacterial pathogens. It is a prerequisite for extracellular colonization and for host cell invasion. Bacterial adhesins that solely expedite adhesion to host cells are expressed by numerous extracellular bacteria. In contrast, invasion-inducing molecules are a feature of bacteria that permanently or transiently enter host cells. The intracellular bacteria covered here live in host cells permanently, whereas other pathogens, such as *Shigella* sp and *Yersinia* sp intrude host cells transiently (23).

Although induced by the bacterium, invasion is ultimately a function of the host cell. Following adhesion, invasion can be induced in either of the following two ways: First, cell signaling by host cell receptors that were the target of

adhesion induces uptake; second, uptake is induced independently from the molecules that mediate adhesion (23). The term "zipper mechanism" has been suggested for the highly selective receptor-mediated bacterial entry, whereas the term "trigger mechanism" has been proposed for indiscriminate, apparently adhesion-independent, uptake (24).

Entry by Zipper Mechanisms

Host cell invasion by *Yersinia* sp and *L. monocytogenes* are examples of invasion via the "zipper mechanism" (23). Invasion of *Yersinia* sp is specific for an integrin receptor. Its binding induces phagocytic mechanisms in nonprofessional phagocytes similar to those that are constitutively operative in MP. Host entry of *L. monocytogenes* through the intestinal epithelia is mediated by internalin on the surface of this pathogen and E cadherin on human epithelial cells (23,25). Murine E cadherin does not serve as a receptor for internalin due to an amino acid substitution in position 16 (26). Schwann cells, a major target of *M. leprae,* are shielded by a basal lamina composed of laminin, collagen, and proteoglycans. The unique tropism of *M. leprae* for peripheral nerves appears to be due to bacterial binding to laminin. This molecule, which serves as natural ligand for integrins, thus provides a link between pathogen and Schwann cell (27).

Entry by Trigger Mechanisms

Different molecules and mechanisms participate in host cell entry by *S. enterica*. Interactions between *S. enterica* with host cells causes "membrane ruffling" at the site of attachment followed by bacterial entry (23). Ruffling induces indiscriminate uptake even of other particles in the vicinity of *S. enterica*. This process has been termed macropinocytosis. *S. enterica* triggers its uptake by exploiting the signaling machinery of the host cell, thus inducing cytoskeletal rearrangements. In certain mouse cells, *S. enterica* induces phosphorylation of the receptor for the epidermal growth factor (EGF) (28). Yet, *S. enterica* can also enter cells that do not express the EGF receptor. This pathogen possesses two type III secretion systems that allow it to directly manipulate intracellular molecules within host cells (29,30). SopE (Salmonella outer proteins) are secreted into the host cells rapidly after contact. SopE activate the small GTP binding protein CDC42 of the Ras superfamily, which, in turn, induces the reorganization of the actin cytoskeleton, promoting bacterial invasion through membrane ruffling. A homolog of SopE (termed SopE2) performs similar functions, and hence the two molecules may partly compensate each other's functions. The transiently intracellular pathogen *Shigella* sp utilizes similar mechanisms for uptake via membrane ruffling (31).

Recognition Receptors for Microbes

Professional phagocytes express receptors for conserved molecular structures on microbial pathogens that are normally absent from the mammalian host. These structures are

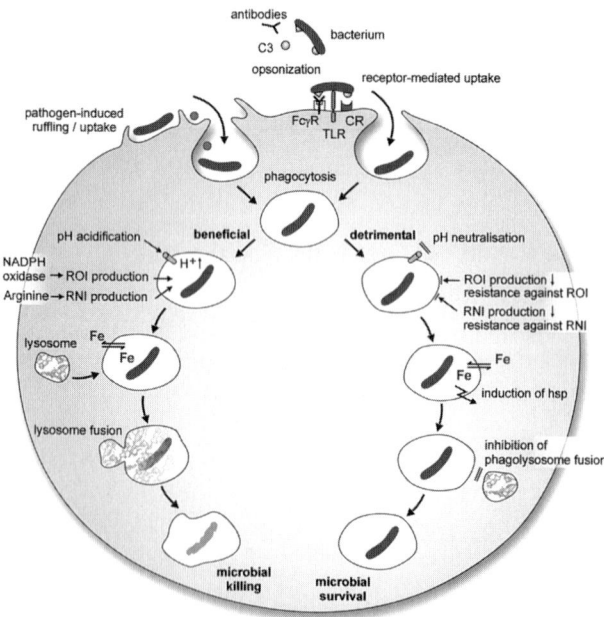

FIG. 1. The multiple encounters between mononuclear phagocytes and intracellular bacteria.

termed "pathogen-associated microbial patterns" (PAMP). The broad spectrum of microbes is recognized in this manner by a limited number of host receptor molecules (32). Binding to these receptors induces a variety of biological responses in host cells. By means of these so-called "pattern recognition receptors" (PRR), host cells expressing these receptors, such as professional phagocytes, promptly identify and respond to bacterial invaders (33). The type of microbial phagocytosis, the type of immediate effector response of professional phagocytes and the type of inflammation are determined in this manner. Moreover, the early inflammatory milieu markedly influences the type of the ensuing acquired immune response. These PRR are described below.

- The Toll-like receptor (TLR) family, which senses distinct structures unique for microbes encompassing glycolipds, lipoproteins, heat-shock proteins, flagella, and oligodeoxynucleotides that induce intracellular signaling and host cell activation (Fig. 2) (34–36)
- Lectin-like glycoproteins with specificity for sugars commonly expressed on the bacterial cell surface that induce microbial uptake (37)
- Surface molecules, notably CD14, with specificity for glycolipids, such as lipopolysaccharide (LPS) of gram-negative bacteria and certain lipoarabinomannans (LAM) of mycobacteria (38,39)

In addition, the following receptors for host-derived molecules promote microbial recognition either directly through cross reactivity, or indirectly: scavenger receptors, Fc receptors (FcR), complement receptors (CR), and fibronectin receptors (FnR). Some of these receptors promote binding and endocytosis only whereas others also activate host cells and hence are central for the immediate activation of the immune system following pathogen escape. The former group comprises CD14, mannose receptors, and scavenger receptors, while the latter comprises FcR and, most notably, TLR.

Pattern Recognition Receptors that Mediate Signaling

Recent interest in the signals that rapidly trigger the immune system to respond to infection has focused on TLR. The mammalian TLR family comprises at least 10 members named TLR-1 to TLR-10 (Fig. 2). These TLR not only interact with PAMP, but are also capable of transducing signals into the cell causing rapid activation. Signal transduction pathways utilized by TLR follow a common sequence shared with the IL-1 receptor signaling pathway, which ultimately leads to the phosphorylation of NFκB. Stimulation via TLR results in rapid activation of innate host defense mechanisms such as secretion of proinflammatory cytokines and production of reactive nitrogen intermediates (RNI). Moreover, TLR-mediated activation causes release of IL-12, promoting the induction of protective T-cell responses (34–36,40). TLR are particularly abundant on professional phagocytes and professional antigen-presenting cells (primarily MP and dendritic cells [DC]), and hence are well suited to both activating the immune system and determining the type of the ensuing immune response. In addition, TLR are found on various other host cells, such as endothelial cells and intestinal epithelial cells. Ligands for several TLR have been defined recently. TLR-2 respond to LAM and lipoproteins, for example, from *M. tuberculosis*. TLR-3 responds to double-stranded RNA as a molecular pattern of numerous viruses. TLR-4 is specific for LPS from many gram-negative bacteria. TLR-5 interacts with bacterial flagellin from both gram-positive (e.g., *L. monocytogenes*) and gram-negative bacteria (e.g., *S. enterica*). TLR-9 recognizes oligonucleotides comprising unmethylated CpG nucleotides characteristic for bacterial DNA. TLR are not restricted to microbial PAMP, and can also respond to some host components indicative of inflammation, such as the heat-shock proteins (Hsp), which interact with TLR-4. Some TLR form heterodimers, further broadening the spectrum of recognized ligands. Thus, TLR-2 and TLR-6 heterodimers react with peptidoglycan from gram-positive bacteria and zymosan from yeast. Generally, TLR interact with their ligands in the phagosome, therefore depending on prior recognition of the respective ligand and induction of microbial engulfment by

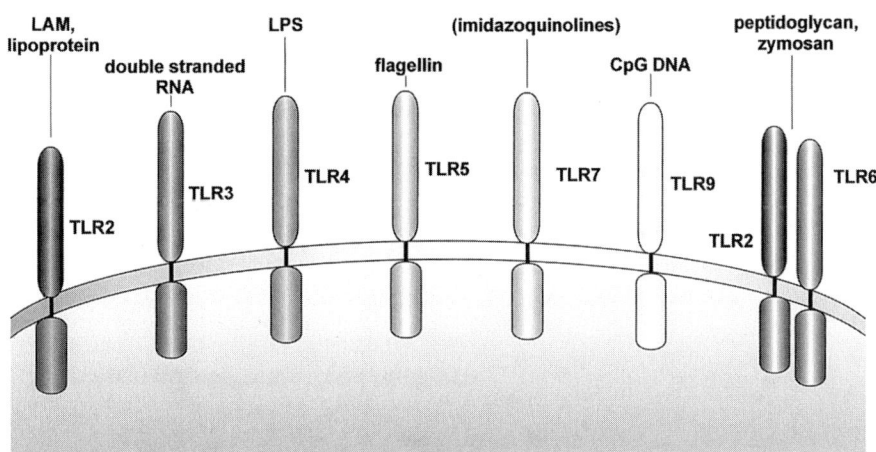

FIG. 2. The Toll-like receptor family.

additional receptors. This, for example, explains cooperation between CD14 and TLR-4 in LPS stimulation.

Pattern Recognition Receptors that Mediate Microbial Binding and Uptake

Three types of lectin-like receptors can be distinguished (32,37,41): the mannose-type receptor recognizes N-acetylglucosamine, mannose, glucose, and L-fucose; the galactose-type receptor is specific for N-acetylgalactosamine and galactose; and the fucose-type receptor is specific for L-fucose. Broad distribution of these sugars on various microbes guarantees the broad target spectrum of professional phagocytes. LAM with terminal mannan (ManLAM) is primarily recognized by the mannose type receptor. In contrast, LAM lacking these mannose caps and having terminal arabinose cannot be recognized through these receptors. Evidence has been presented that CD14 is involved in recognition of these AraLAM moieties (42).

Pattern Recognition Receptors that Recognize Host Molecules

A group of receptors, which are collectively termed scavenger receptors, react with host serum lipoproteins (43,44). Some of these receptors also bind microbial surface molecules and circumstantial evidence suggests that they may participate in host defense against bacterial infection.

Indirect recognition of bacteria by professional phagocytes involves immunoglobulin G (IgG), breakdown products of the complement component C3, or fibronectin as ligands; and the FcR and the complement receptors, CR1, CR3, and CR4 or the FnR, respectively, on the part of the host cell (45–47). Binding of specific IgG antibodies to bacteria promotes phagocytosis via FcR and—after complement activation—by CR1, CR3, or CR4, in addition. FcR binding generally activates the respiratory burst, resulting in the activation of reactive oxygen intermediates (ROI) (48). Many intracellular bacteria such as *M. tuberculosis, M. leprae,* and *L. pneumophila* induce breakdown of C3 and, as a corollary, their own uptake. The phenolic glycolipid of *M. leprae* and the major outer-membrane protein of *L. pneumophila,* for example, promote uptake via CR through C3 fixation. C3 fixation and activation by *M. leprae* surface glycolipid either proceed through the antibody-independent alternative pathway or are promoted by low concentrations of cross-reactive serum antibodies through the classical pathway of complement activation. C3b deposition on the cell wall of the pathogenic mycobacteria *M. tuberculosis, M. leprae,* and *M. avium* is promoted by the natural complement component C2a. Apparently, these microbes first cleave serum C2 to become the C3 convertase, C2a, which then causes formation from C3 of C3b and its fixation (49). Some intracellular bacteria directly bind to CR3 independent of C3 activation. Direct binding to CR3 involves either the RGD sequence or a lectin-like binding site for β-glucan. Thus, CR3 serves as both PRR and

as a receptor for host molecules. CR-promoted uptake may interfere with the generation of ROI in MP and hence may represent a bacterial evasion mechanism. CR3-deficient mice and wild-type animals, however, control tuberculosis equally well (50). Some intracellular bacteria, such as *L. pneumophila* and *C. psittaci,* enter MP by an unusual engulfment process called "coiling phagocytosis" (51). Coiling is promoted by C3 breakdown products and does not stimulate ROI secretion. In contrast, FcR-facilitated uptake of *L. pneumophila* is normal and induces neither coiling nor interference with the ROI burst. CR-mediated uptake of particles does not trigger the oxidative burst, suggesting that it represents a general evasion mechanism that facilitates intracellular survival.

Fibronectin binds to FnR through an RGD sequence, so that intracellular bacteria expressing fibronectin-binding molecules may be taken up via this pathway. For example, *M. tuberculosis* secretes a family of 32-kD molecules with fibronectin-binding activity. Fibronectin, however, appears to be a weak and inefficient inducer of phagocytosis that requires additional internalization mechanisms (45,52). In fact, members of the 32-kD molecular complex act primarily as mycolyl transferases and thus are involved in cell wall biosynthesis rather than in host cell adhesion of mycobacteria (53). Probably, intracellular bacteria misuse a variety of other proteins present in serum or secretion. Thus, *M. tuberculosis* was found to bind to heparin or to surfactant protein, which may promote adhesion and perhaps uptake by epithelial cells in the lung (54–56).

Invasion of Nonprofessional Phagocytes

Intracellular bacteria generally do not attempt to avoid phagocytosis; rather, they often promote their own engulfment. Microbe-directed uptake allows entry into nonphagocytic cells and hence can be seen as an evasion mechanism from phagocytosis by professional phagocytes. The target spectrum of intracellular bacteria ranges from very broad to highly specific. *M. leprae* is found in a large variety of host cells and hence shows a broad target cell spectrum. *L. monocytogenes* enters the host through the gut epithelium and its major target besides MP is the hepatocyte; *M. tuberculosis* is almost, if not exclusively, restricted to MP, although pneumocytes have been proposed as a safe "first niche" in the lung. Note that intracellular bacteria are often capable of entering a variety of the *in vitro* cell lines. These *in vitro* experiments do not necessarily reflect the *in vivo* situation, and care should be taken in extrapolating from them. For the obligate intracellular bacteria, nonprofessional phagocytes rather than MP represent the preferred habitat. These bacteria are primarily found in endothelial and epithelial cells (12).

Phagosome Maturation, Acidification, and Phagosome–Lysosome Fusion

Phagocytosis of inert particles initiates a series of events that ultimately lead to the formation of a phagolysosome

(Fig. 1) (46,57). The following three major stages can be distinguished.

- Early phagosome characterized by a slightly acidic to neutral pH and membrane markers, such as mannose receptor, the tryptophane aspartate-containing coat protein (TACO), and the transferrin receptor with its ligand transferrin
- Late phagosome characterized by pH <5.5 and the acquisition of the vacuolar ATPase proton pump
- Phagolysosome as the result of fusion between phagosomes and lysosomes characterized by pH <5.5, high density of lysosome-associated membrane proteins (LAMP) and typical lysosomal enzymes

It should be kept in mind that the three stages are not distinctly separated, but rather form a continuum involving the sorting of membrane proteins, as well as budding of and fusion with other vesicles. During this dynamic process, the phagosomes successively interact with the corresponding endosomes and subsequently with lysosomes (58).

Acquisition of a vacuolar ATPase proton pump plays a central role in acidification (59). Immediately after phagocytosis, the phagosome becomes alkaline for a short time before acidification is initiated. The basic milieu is optimal for the activity of defensins and basic proteins, whereas the acidic pH is optimal for lysosomal enzymes. Defensins are small (3.5–4.0 kD) peptides rich in arginine and cysteine (60,61). They are abundant in PNG and present in some, though not all, MP (depending on species and tissue location). Purified defensins are microbicidal for certain intracellular bacteria such as *S. enterica* and *L. monocytogenes*. A virulence factor of *S. enterica* for mice, phoP, has been implicated in resistance against defensins (4). Contribution of lysosomal enzymes to bacterial killing is small. Their major task is the degradation of already killed bacteria. These enzymes reside in the lysosome and are delivered into the phagosome during maturation through several independent waves and they reach their optimum activity during later stages, that is, in the phagolysosome.

Most intracellular bacteria interfere with phagosome maturation and alter the phagosome in order to facilitate and support their own survival (46,57,62). These include *L. pneumophila*, *M. tuberculosis*, *S. enterica*, and *C. psittaci*. Although mechanistically incompletely understood, mycobacterial sulfatides and some mycobacterial glycolipids impede phagolysosome fusion. Antibody-coated *M. tuberculosis* organisms lose their capacity to block discharge of lysosomal enzymes, suggesting an auxiliary function of antibodies in cell-mediated protection against tuberculosis (63). Finally, the robust, lipid-rich cell wall of mycobacteria renders them highly resistant against enzymatic attack. *M. tuberculosis* as well as *M. avium* arrest phagosome maturation at an early stage. They restrict phagosome acidification via the exclusion of the proton pump from the phagosome. Additional mechanisms may contribute to this event, such as NH_4^+ production by *M. tuberculosis*. Consistent with intraphagosomal NH_4^+ production, the urease of *M. tuberculosis* is active at low pH. It has been known for long that NH_4^+ also interferes with phagosome lysosome fusion. Recently, exogenous ATP has been shown to promote phagolysosome fusion resulting in concomitant death of macrophages and killing of *M. bovis* BCG (64,65).

Phagosome maturation is somewhere arrested between the early and the late stage by *M. tuberculosis*, *M. bovis* BCG, *L. pneumophila*, *S. enterica*, and *C. trachomatis*, all of which replicate in nonacidified vacuoles. Phagosomes containing *S. enterica*, *M. bovis* BCG, or *C. trachomatis* appear uncoupled from the maturation process through which phagosomes containing inert particles proceed (46). *S. enterica* remains in the spacious membrane-bound phagosome that is formed after uptake by the trigger mechanism. The vacuole containing *C. trachomatis*, which lacks any specific phagosome markers, is loaded with ATP by an unknown mechanism that is required by *C. trachomatis*. The *L. pneumophila*–containing phagosome is surrounded by mitochondria, and later by ribosomes connected with the endoplasmic reticulum. Evidence has been presented that *L. pneumophila* exploits an intracellular compartment with some features of autophagosomes.

Intracellular Iron

Intracellular bacteria require iron, and production of ROI and RNI also depends on iron. Thus, competition for the intracellular iron pool between the intracellular pathogen and the host cell markedly influences the outcome of their relationship (66–68). To improve their iron supply, mammalian cells utilize specific molecules. In the extracellular host milieu, iron is tightly bound to transferrin and lactoferrin, and the transferrin–iron complex is taken up by host cells via transferrin receptors. The lactoferrin–iron complex is not taken up into the cell. Iron is released from the transferrin–transferrin receptor complex under the reducing conditions of the early phagosome. This event is controlled by Hfe (the product of the hereditary hemachromatosis gene). Hfe reduces iron uptake either by inhibiting transferrin receptor internalization or by blocking iron release from transferrin in the early phagosome. The Nramp system is involved in iron transport from the phagosome to the cytosol, where iron is bound to ferritin. Accordingly, iron availability is controlled in multiple ways, including transferrin receptor expression on the cell surface, lactoferrin concentration in the extracellular space, and intracytosolic ferritin concentrations. Many intracellular bacteria, including *M. tuberculosis* and *S. enterica*, accommodate themselves in the early phagosomes, where the abundance of iron-loaded transferrin guarantees a high availability of iron. In order to successfully compete for iron, these bacteria possess a variety of iron-binding proteins. These include iron chelators (siderophores), transferrin-binding proteins, heme-like proteins, and ABC transporters. Expression of genes involved in iron uptake is controlled by a conserved mechanism involving the Fur protein. IFN-γ–activated MP down-modulate transferrin receptor expression and intracellular ferritin, resulting in reduced iron availability within the phagosome. The iron content of the phagosome in the resting MP seems to be sufficient for *L. pneumophila*. However, the available iron is markedly reduced in IFN-γ–activated MP and, as a consequence, *L. pneumophila*, which lacks efficient iron uptake mechanisms, starves from iron deprivation in activated macrophages. In contrast, *M. tuberculosis* possesses a potent iron acquisition system comprising exochelins and mycobactins. The exochelins successfully compete for iron under limiting conditions and transfer it to mycobactins in the cell wall (69,70).

Tryptophan Degradation

Increased degradation of the amino acid tryptophan has been associated with killing of *C. psittaci* and the intracellular protozoan pathogen, *Toxoplasma gondii* (71,72). Although it is possible that limiting the intracellular availability of essential amino acids provides a potent antimicrobial mechanism, little is known about its general role in resistance against intracellular bacteria.

Toxic Effector Molecules

Killing of intracellular bacteria by MP and/or PNG is primarily accomplished by highly reactive toxic molecules, particularly ROI and RNI (48,73–75).

Many bacteria are susceptible to ROI *in vitro*. Yet, the contribution of ROI to killing of intracellular bacteria by MP remains unclear; in murine macrophages, RNI appear more important. Consistent with a central role of RNI in antibacterial defense, gene knockout (KO) mice with a deficient inducible NO synthase (iNOS) (which is responsible for RNI production, as discussed below) suffer from slightly worsened listeriosis and markedly exacerbated tuberculosis (76,77). In the mouse, ROI and RNI act consecutively to defend against *S. enterica* infection (78,79). On the other hand, production of RNI by human MP at levels sufficiently high for bacterial killing remains controversial (80). However, evidence is accumulating to the effect that human MP from the site of intracellular bacterial infection possess the potential to produce RNI. Using antibodies with exquisite specificity for human iNOS, for example, this enzyme could be detected in a large proportion of alveolar macrophages from tuberculosis patients (81). ROI production is initiated by a membrane-bound NADPH oxidase, which is activated by IFN-γ and by IgG–FcR binding:

$$O_2 + NADPH \xrightarrow{\text{NADPH oxidase}} NADP + O_2^- + H^+$$

O_2^- is further metabolized by superoxide dismutase (SOD):

$$O_2^- + H^+ \xrightarrow{\text{SOD}} O_2 + H_2O_2$$

In the presence of appropriate iron catalysts, the Haber–Weiss reaction takes place:

$$O_2^- + Fe^{3+} \longrightarrow O_2 + Fe^{2+}$$

$$H_2O_2 + Fe^{2+} \longrightarrow {}^\bullet OH + OH^- + Fe^{3+}$$

$$O_2^- + H_2O_2 \longrightarrow {}^\bullet OH + OH^- + O_2$$

In addition, O_2^- is transformed into ${}^1O_2$. The ${}^1O_2$ and ${}^\bullet OH$ radicals are short-lived powerful oxidants with high antibactericidal activity causing damage to DNA, membrane lipids, and proteins. (Note: O_2^-, hyperoxide anion; ${}^\bullet OH$, hydroxyl radical containing a free electron; ${}^1O_2$, singlet oxygen, a highly reactive form of O_2.)

Granulocytes and blood monocytes, but not tissue macrophages, possess myeloperoxidase (MPO), thus allowing halogenation of microbial proteins (48):

$$H_2O_2 + Cl^- \xrightarrow{\text{MPO}} OCl^- + H_2O$$

In addition to hypochlorous acid, chloramines are formed and both agents further increase the bactericidal power of the ROI system by destroying biologically important proteins through chlorination.

Nitric oxide is exclusively derived from the terminal guanidino-nitrogen atom of L-arginine (Fig. 3). This reaction is catalyzed by iNOS, which leads to the formation of L-citrulline and NO${}^\bullet$.

NO${}^\bullet$ can act as oxidizing agent alone or it interacts with O_2^- to form the unstable peroxynitrite (ONOO$^-$). This then may be transformed to the more stable anions, NO_2^- and NO_3^-, or decomposed to NO${}^\bullet$:

$$O_2^- + NO^\bullet \longrightarrow ONOO^-$$

$$ONOO^- + H^+ \longrightarrow NO_2^- + {}^\bullet OH$$

$$NO_2^- + {}^\bullet OH \longrightarrow NO_3^- + H^+$$

$$ONOO^- + H^+ \longrightarrow {}^\bullet OH + NO^\bullet$$

NO${}^\bullet$ and ONOO$^-$ are highly reactive antimicrobial agents. NO${}^\bullet$ may be transformed to nitrosothiols expressing the most potent antimicrobial activity. In contrast, NO_2^- and NO_3^- are without notable effects on microorganisms.

Production of NO${}^\bullet$ is NADPH dependent and requires tetrahydrobiopterin as co-factor. Three distinct NOS isoenzymes are known. The two constitutive NOS (cNOS) exist in various host cells and account for basal NO synthesis, whereas iNOS is primarily found in professional phagocytes and is responsible for microbial killing. Its induction is

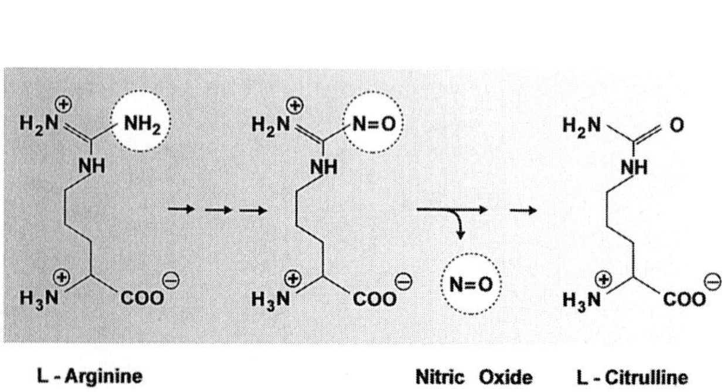

FIG. 3. Generation of nitric oxide from L-arginine.

controlled by exogenous stimuli such as IFN-γ. This iNOS stimulation results in a burst of high RNI concentrations required for microbial killing, whereas the low NO levels produced by cNOS perform physiologic functions. The RNI exert their bactericidal activities by directly inactivating iron-sulfur containing enzymes, by S-nitrosylating proteins, by damaging DNA, or by synergizing with ROI.

Evasion of Killing by ROI and RNI

Binding to CR1/CR3 does not induce the respiratory burst and ROI production (47). The CR therefore provide a less dangerous way of entry for intracellular bacteria. Low-molecular-weight fractions, particularly of mycobacteria, such as phenolic glycolipid 1 of *M. leprae,* scavenge ROI. Some intracellular bacteria may block the respiratory burst by interfering with protein kinase C activity. *S. enterica* mutants deficient in SPI2 (Salmonella pathogenicity island 2) are susceptible to ROI (82). SPI2 enables *S. enterica* to exclude NADPH oxidase from the phagosomal membrane, thus interfering with ROI release into the Salmonella phagosome. Such a mechanism also affects iNOS activity. Finally, many intracellular bacteria produce superoxide dismutase and catalase that detoxify O_2 and H_2O_2, respectively. Production of ROI-detoxifying molecules by intracellular bacteria is not constitutive; rather, expression of these enzymes is controlled by regulators such as soxR or oxyR that sense for concentrations of O_2 or H_2O_2, respectively. Accordingly, several transposon mutants of *S. enterica* that fail to survive inside murine MP are highly sensitive to ROI *in vitro*. Although less is known about specific mechanisms by which intracellular bacteria may interfere with killing by RNI, catalase and other antioxidative enzymes may indirectly inhibit RNI functions. ROI- and RNI-detoxifying gene products have been identified in *M. tuberculosis* (83). Because both ROI and RNI also affect host molecules, excess generation of these effector molecules is dangerous for the host as well.

Evasion into Cytoplasm

Evasion from the phagosomal into the cytoplasmic compartment represents a highly successful microbial survival strategy because bacterial killing is focused on the phagolysosome in order to limit self-damage of MP. This egression has been extensively studied in *L. monocytogenes,* but may also be utilized by other intracellular pathogens (5). Such experiments, however, need to be interpreted with care, and current evidence argues against perforation of the phagolysosome membrane by *M. tuberculosis* (18).

Cytoplasmic invasion by *L. monocytogenes* depends on listeriolysin, an SH-activated cytolysin. Deletion of the responsible gene renders *L. monocytogenes* avirulent. Other cytolysins such as phospholipases and lecithinase are likely involved in membrane transition but are insufficient on their own. Evasion of *L. monocytogenes* into the cytoplasmic compartment is, however, markedly reduced in IFN-γ–

activated macrophages in which the microbe entrapped in the phagosome rapidly succumbs to attack by ROI, RNI, and/or defensins.

Cell-to-Cell Spreading

L. monocytogenes is cleared from the blood by Kupffer cells, and from here it spreads to adjacent hepatocytes without reentering the extracellular milieu. This mechanism of cell-to-cell spreading has been carefully studied *in vitro* (84). Having entered the cytoplasm, *L. monocytogenes* is surrounded by fibrillar material that subsequently forms a tail composed of actin filaments. In this way, *L. monocytogenes* is pushed forward to the outer regions of the cell, where it induces pseudopod formation. Intracellular movement is achieved by coordinated actin polymerization at, and polarized release from, the bacterial surface (85). The ActA gene encodes a 90-kD protein located on the bacterial surface, which is responsible for these actin-based movements (5). A host cytosolic complex composed of eight polypeptides has been identified which, on binding ActA, induces actin polymerization (86). The pseudopod-containing *L. monocytogenes* is engulfed by the adjacent cell, and the microbe reaches the phagosome of the recipient cell still enclosed by the cytoskeletal material from the donor cell. The two plasma membranes of the host and recipient cell apparently fuse, thereby allowing the introduction of *L. monocytogenes* into the cytoplasm of the recipient cell. Thus, *L. monocytogenes* can infect numerous cells without contacting extracellular defense mechanisms. *Shigella* sp use similar mechanisms for evasion and intracellular movement, and a similar spreading mechanism seems to be employed by *S. enterica* and by *R. rickettsii,* but not by *R. prowazekii* and *R. typhi.*

Apoptosis

Death of mammalian cells occurs by two different forms: accidental and programmed cell death, resulting in necrosis or apoptosis, respectively (87–89). Necrosis is the result of cell destruction caused by various exogenous effector mechanisms, including those mediated by complement and cytolytic T-lymphocytes (CTL). Apoptosis, in contrast, is initiated by intrinsic mechanisms within the dying cell itself. This programmed cell death involves a series of tightly controlled enzymatic events, notably intracellular caspases. Several bacterial pathogens, including *M. tuberculosis, S. enterica* and *L. monocytogenes,* can activate the apoptotic machinery in cells after their uptake. The responsible molecules and mechanisms are incompletely understood in these cases. Perhaps the formation of small pores by listeriolysin from *L. monocytogenes* and by SipB of *S. enterica* initiate apoptosis. Apoptosis induced by *Shigella flexneri* has been studied in more detail, and it was found that its virulence factor, IpaB, not only participates in pore formation, but also interacts with the apoptotic machinery by binding to and activating caspases. Depending on the situation, either the host or the pathogen can primarily benefit from apoptosis. Exogenous ATP causes death of host cells harboring *M. bovis* BCG which, in turn, results in mycobacterial killing (64,65). Although this macrophage death has some resemblance to apoptosis, it is also distinct from conventional apoptosis induced through CD95 and mediated by caspases.

PROFESSIONAL PHAGOCYTES

Mononuclear Phagocytes

Metchnikoff (90) was the first to realize the importance of professional phagocytes in resistance against bacterial infections. He observed that leukocytes accumulated at the site of inflammation and bacterial growth, where they were heavily engaged in microbial engulfment and destruction. Metchnikoff distinguished two types of phagocytes: (a) the early-appearing and short-lived microphages that are now called PNG, and (b) the later-appearing long-lived macrophages still known under this name. The preferential localization of tubercle bacilli inside macrophages as already discovered by Koch (91) and Metchnikoff (90) pointed to the central role of these phagocytes in defense against intracellular bacteria. Metchnikoff also observed that during infection, macrophages are nonspecifically activated. Macrophage activation as an important factor of acquired resistance against bacterial infections was further substantiated by Lurie (92) and shown to be under the control of lymphocytes by Mackaness (3). Later, cytokines were identified as the mediator of macrophage activation (93,94).

It is now clear that many of the antibacterial activities described above are not constitutively expressed in MP. Rather, expression of full antibacterial activities by MP depends on appropriate stimulation by cytokines, with IFN-γ being of paramount importance (95,96). Furthermore, significant differences exist among MP of different maturation status or from different species. For example, human blood monocytes, but not tissue macrophages, possess myeloperoxidase activity. High RNI levels are produced by murine MP and probably by human MP under certain conditions. Activation of MP coincides with increased phagocytosis, elevated CR, and reduced FcR expression, and a higher overall metabolic rate, to name but a few inducible activities. Most importantly, during macrophage activation, iNOS and NADPH oxidase, which initiate RNI or ROI production, respectively, are stimulated. In other words, activation by cytokines results in transition of MP from habitat supporting microbial replication into an effector cell capable of terminating, or at least restricting, microbial survival (97).

Polymorphonuclear Granulocytes

Although the role of PNG in intracellular bacterial infections has often been neglected, their high antibacterial potential allows them to kill many intracellular bacteria (98). However, PNG are short-lived and intracellular bacteria are sequestered in intracellular niches; hence, the overall contribution of PNG to defense against chronic infections remains small. Yet, during the early acute inflammatory response they help to reduce the initial bacterial load. This is particularly evident in experimental listeriosis, which is an acute disease: The first day of infection is characterized by extensive PNG infiltration at sites of listerial growth (99) and elimination of PNG by mAb treatment remarkably exacerbates listeriosis (100,101). While the listerial burden in the liver of mAb-treated mice was dramatically increased, the burden in the spleen remained virtually unchanged. This finding shows an organ-specific role of PNG in early antilisterial resistance. The central role of PNG in defense against *S. enterica* has been established in a similar experimental setting. In contrast, depletion of PNG apparently does not affect experimental tuberculosis in mice (102). PNG are also potent secretors of ROI and hypochlorous acid as well as of proteolytic enzymes such as elastase (a serine proteinase), collagenase, and gelatinase (48,102a,102b). Such proteases express potent microbicidal activity. In particular, elastase has been shown to specifically destroy the virulence proteins of Shigella, Salmonella, and Yersinia organisms (102a,102b). These secretion products also act as mediators of tissue destruction. In the extracellular milieu, protease inhibitors are normally present, preventing tissue damage by these proteases. However, the concomitant secretion of hypochlorous acid inactivates these proteinase inhibitors, thus promoting cell lysis. Accordingly, PNG have been shown to cause inflammatory liver damage by destroying infected hepatocytes during early listeriosis (99). MP are less potent secretors of proteinases and fail to produce the major inactivator of proteinase inhibitors, hypochlorous acid. Thus, established granulomas, such as productive granulomas in chronic tuberculosis, are dominated by MP and are characterized by necrosis and fibrosis and lack signs of tissue liquefaction. During reactivation, however, PNG may eventually be recruited to tuberculous granulomas and then contribute to granuloma caseation and liquefaction.

CENTRAL ROLE OF ACQUIRED IMMUNE RESPONSE

Acquisition of resistance against intracellular bacteria crucially depends on T-lymphocytes that, ideally, accomplish sterile bacterial eradication. When a "normal" immune status is provided, bacterial clearance is rapidly achieved in the case of susceptible bacteria such as *L. monocytogenes*. In the case of resistant pathogens such as *M. tuberculosis,* clearance frequently remains incomplete and is arrested at the stage of bacterial containment to, and growth control at, distinct foci. Bacterial containment and eradication occur in granulomatous lesions. The longer the struggle between host and microbial pathogen continues, the more essential the granuloma becomes. Granuloma formation and perpetuation are orchestrated by T-lymphocytes. The cross talk in the granuloma between T-lymphocytes, MP, and the other cells is promoted by cytokines.

The T-cell requisite is probably best exemplified by the high incidence of tuberculosis and other intracellular bacterial infections in patients suffering from T-cell deficiencies, particularly AIDS. It is not contradicted by experiments showing transient resistance of nu/nu and severe combined immunodeficient (SCID) mice against experimental listeriosis. Although these T-cell–deficient mice are capable of controlling experimental listeriosis for relatively long periods of time, primarily by means of highly activated natural killer (NK) cells that produce IFN-γ, they ultimately fail to eradicate their pathogens (103). In the long run, therefore, these animals succumb to disseminated listeriosis.

At the same time, T-lymphocytes are an unavoidable element of the pathogenesis of intracellular bacterial infections. First, expanding granulomas impair tissue functions by occupying space and affecting surrounding cells. Second, the physiologic functioning of infected host cells may be affected by specific T-lymphocytes.

Dendritic Cells

MP not only serve as major habitat for intracellular bacteria, they are also potent antigen-presenting cells. However, MP are not the most efficacious antigen-presenting cells, and their capacity may even be reduced during infection. DC comprise a heterogeneous leukocyte population that share the common feature of being the most efficacious antigen-presenting cells (104–108). DC endocytose-soluble proteins efficiently, but have a poor phagocytic capacity. Nevertheless, recent evidence points to a critical role of DC in infections with intracellular bacteria. First, DC themselves can be infected by intracellular bacteria, and can thus readily present accessible

antigens from their resident microbes. Second, the transport of microbial antigens from infected MP to bystander DC can combine the high phagocytic and degradative capacity of MP with the high antigen-presenting capacity of DC.

The superior antigen-presenting capacity of DC can be deduced to three major features: abundant MHC and CD1 molecules to present antigens to T cells, abundant TLR to rapidly sense infection, and co-stimulatory molecules and cytokines that influence T-cell activation and differentiation. DC comprise different populations of both myeloid and lymphoid origin, and express high plasticity. During their development they express different functional capacities. In response to infection and inflammation, monocyte-derived DC migrate into draining lymph nodes where they differentiate into CD11$^+$ cells that stimulate various T-cell populations that participate in the immune response against intracellular bacteria. The role of the CD11$^-$ lymphoid DC cells in immunity to intracellular bacteria remains to be established. In sum, despite their relatively poor phagocytic and degradative activity, DC are central regulators of the acquired immune response to intracellular bacteria.

T-Cell Subpopulations

The peripheral T-cell system comprises several phenotypically distinct and stable populations (Table 4). T-lymphocytes expressing the $\alpha\beta$ T-cell receptor (TCR) make up >90% of all T cells in secondary lymphoid organs and peripheral blood of humans and experimental mice. They are further subdivided into (a) CD4 $\alpha\beta$ T cells that recognize antigenic peptides

TABLE 4. *Conventional and unconventional T cells in antibacterial immunity*

| Group | T-cell population | Antigen-presenting molecule | | | Ligand | Site of ligand loading |
		Type	Tissue distribution	Polymorphism		
1	CD4 $\alpha\beta$ T cell	MHC class II	Restricted (APC)	High	12–20mer peptide	Phagosome
2	CD8 $\alpha\beta$ T cell	MHC class I (+ β2m)	Broad	High	Nonapeptide	Phagosome
3	CD8 $\alpha\beta$ T cell	MHC class Ib (+ β2m)	Broad	Low	N-f-met-pentapeptide	Cytosol, phagosome
4	DN (CD8) $\alpha\beta$ T cell	Group 1 CD1 (+ β2m)	Restricted (APC)	Low	Glycolipid	Phagosome
5	CD4 (DN) $\alpha\beta$ T cell	Group 2 CD1 (+ β2m)	Intermediate	Low	Glycolipid	Phagosome
6	DN $\gamma\delta$ T cell	No presentation molecule known	Not applicable	Not applicable	Phospholigand and others	?

Group	Species	Major *in vitro* function	Role in antibacterial protection	Comment
1	Human, murine	IFN-γ, CTL	Proven	Control of "endosomal pathogens"
2	Human, murine	CTL, IFN-γ	Proven	Control of "cytosolic pathogens"
3	Murine	CTL, IFN-γ	Proven	Well characterized in murine listeriosis
4	Human	CTL, IFN-γ	Likely	Specificity for mycobacteria (and related species); known ligands: mycolic acid, LAM
5	Human, murine	IL-4, IFN-γ	Unknown (regulatory ?)	N-galactosyl-ceramide (sponge), phosphatidyl-inositol tetramannoside (mycobacteria)
6	Human	IFN-γ, CTL	Proven (compensatory, regulatory)	Human system: isopentenyl-pyrophosphate and alkyl derivatives (present in prokaryotes and eukaryotes); murine $\gamma\delta$ T cells with reactivity for phospholigands unknown

presented by gene products of the MHC class II, and (b) CD8 $\alpha\beta$ T cells that interact with antigenic peptides in the context of MHC class I molecules.

Undoubtedly, these conventional $\alpha\beta$ T cells are of primary importance for antibacterial resistance, although good evidence exists that unconventional T cells also participate in control of intracellular bacteria (97). These unconventional T-cell populations are listed below.

• CD8 $\alpha\beta$ T cells that recognize bacterial peptides presented by nonclassical MHC class Ib molecules
• Double-negative (DN), CD4, or CD8 $\alpha\beta$ T cells that recognize bacterial glycolipids presented by group 1 CD1 molecules
• CD4 or DN $\alpha\beta$ T cells that generally coexpress the NK cell marker and are specific for group 2 CD1 molecules
• $\gamma\delta$ T-lymphocytes with specificity for antigenic ligands presented in different manners

Conventional CD4 and CD8 $\alpha\beta$ T Cells

Both MHC class II–restricted CD4 $\alpha\beta$ T cells and MHC class I–restricted CD8 $\alpha\beta$ T cells participate in acquired resistance against intracellular bacteria. Most intracellular bacteria reside in the phagosomal compartment of MP and hence pathogen-derived peptides have ready access to the MHC class II presentation pathway (Fig. 4). However, some microbes are capable of egressing into the cytosol. Accordingly, intracellular bacteria can be grouped as "phagosomal pathogens" or "cytosolic pathogens" (109). The phagosomal pathogens encompass most intracellular bacteria with the exception of *Rickettsia* sp and *L. monocytogenes,* which are clearly cytosolic pathogens. Obviously, antigens from

cytosolic pathogens can be readily introduced into the MHC class I processing pathway, thus promoting activation of CD8 T cells (110,111). Yet, CD8 T cells have also been isolated from mice infected with phagosomal pathogens, such as *M. tuberculosis* and *S. enterica.* The following, speculative and not mutually exclusive, pathways for the introduction of antigen to MHC class I, independent from bacterial egression into the cytosol, are conceivable.

1. Some intracellular bacteria possess cytolysins that would permit translocation into the cytosol of secreted proteins or peptides without requiring bacterial egression from the phagosome.
2. The early phagosome retains MHC class I molecules, which may allow direct loading of peptides from bacteria such as *M. tuberculosis* and *S. enterica* that reside in this compartment.
3. Some phagosomal bacteria, such as *S. enterica,* possess a specific secretion apparatus that translocates proteins into the cytosol of host cells (112).
4. Bacteria containing phagosomes have thorough exchange with corresponding endosomes, which may allow peptide loading of vacuolar MHC class I molecules (113).
5. Antigens from bacteria that persist in the phagosome may leak into the cytosolic compartment (114).
6. Antigenic peptides from phagosomal bacteria are loaded to surface-expressed MHC class I molecules by regurgitation (113). This pathway may involve sensitization of bystander cells.
7. Numerous intracellular bacteria induce apoptosis in their host cells. Apoptosis results in the formation of vesicles containing antigenic cargo that can be shuttled to bystander cells. Engulfment of these antigen-loaded vesicles

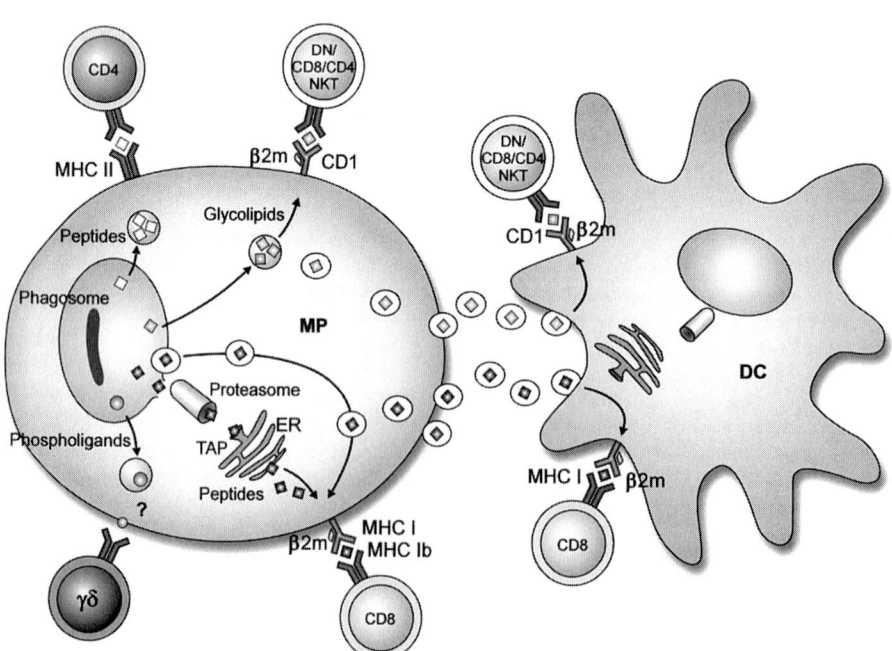

FIG. 4. Multiple antigen processing pathways for stimulation of T cells during bacterial infections.

results in stimulation of MHC class I–restricted CD8 T cells (18,115).

Alternatives 6 and 7 could also explain the efficient antigenic presentation by DC via cross-priming (116). While macrophages are the preferred habitat of intracellular bacteria, their antigen-presenting capacity is weaker than that of DC. Hence, the transport of antigens from infected macrophages to bystander DC would improve antigen presentation during infection (Fig. 4).

It is now beyond doubt that various pathways of MHC class I antigen presentation exist. Yet, the antigen-processing pathways for MHC class I remarkably differ in their efficacy. The most efficacious means for antigen introduction into the MHC class I processing machinery are bacterial egression into the cytosol. Accordingly, cytosolic pathogens are the most potent stimulators of CD8 T cells, whereas CD4 T-lymphocytes are primarily stimulated by phagosomal pathogens. Reciprocally, phagosomal or cytosolic pathogens are primarily controlled by CD4 or CD8 T cells, respectively.

Intracellular bacteria also invade nonprofessional phagocytes, some of which do not express MHC class II molecules constitutively. Consequently, such cells remain unrecognized by CD4 T-lymphocytes and provide a hiding place for intracellular bacteria—a situation that has consequences for the course of disease. Because MHC class I molecules are expressed by almost every cell, CD8 T-lymphocytes have the potential of surveying the whole body. This is particularly important for those intracellular bacteria that hide in MHC class II⁻ host cells. Obviously, recognition of these cells depends on CD8 T-lymphocytes (and perhaps unconventional T cells, as discussed below). *L. monocytogenes,* on the one hand, resides in nonprofessional phagocytes with low antibacterial potential and, on the other hand, promotes MHC class I presentation of its antigens. This may explain the predominance of MHC class I–restricted CD8 T-lymphocytes in defense against experimental listeriosis both by number and by biological relevance. In contrast, *M. bovis* BCG is primarily restricted to MP and remains in the phagosome. This is compatible with its preferential control by MHC class II–restricted CD4 T-lymphocytes. Although *M. tuberculosis* primarily resides in MP, its high resistance to antibacterial effector mechanisms may require the concerted action of both CD4 and CD8 T cells (20). In this situation, a discrepancy may arise between strong dependence on CD8 T cells and insufficient activation of these cells.

Unconventional T Cells

During recent years, several populations of unconventional T-lymphocytes have been identified, some of them showing unique specificity for bacterial ligands. Some of these T cells do not follow the rule of MHC/peptide recognition by the TCR and recognize unusual ligands either directly or in the context of nonclassical MHC class Ib or CD1 molecules. In some cases, unconventional T cells recognize ligands unique

to bacteria suggesting an important role for these T cells in antibacterial resistance. This also provides strong evidence that these unconventional T cells are the end result of a long-lasting coevolution between bacterial pathogens and their mammalian host. It is conceivable that specificity for ligands that are unique to bacteria provides a powerful means for distinguishing foreign invaders from self-antigens.

MHC Class Ib–Restricted CD8 T Cells

In the mouse, CD8 T cells with protective activity have been identified that are restricted by nonclassical MHC class Ib molecules (110,111). In murine salmonellosis, these CD8 T cells are restricted by Qa-1 (117). In murine listeriosis, these T cells recognize N-formyl-methionine (N-f-met)–containing peptides presented by H-2M3 (118). In mammalian cells, only a few N-formylated proteins exist, these being of mitochondrial origin. In contrast, many bacterial proteins contain the N-f-met sequence (Table 4). (Furthermore, N-f-met–containing peptides have proinflammatory activity for MP and PNG, as discussed below.) Thus, it appears that MHC class Ib gene products are specialized for presentation of these bacterial antigens (119). The peptide-binding groove of H2-M3 has room for small peptides only. Consistent with this, the recently identified N-f-met peptides from *L. monocytogenes* are penta- or hexa-peptides, as compared to the nonapeptides typically presented by classical MHC class I molecules. While the nonclassical MHC class Ib molecules are noncovalently bound to β2m on the cell surface as are classical MHC class I molecules, N-f-met peptide presentation seems to originate in the phagosome (Fig. 4) (120). Consistent with this notion, killed listeriae are a source of N-f-met peptides for H2-M3 presentation. Yet, it seems likely that N-f-met peptides can also be loaded to H2-M3 from listeriae residing in the cytosol. Nonclassical MHC class Ib–restricted CD8 T cells specific for N-f-met peptides have also been isolated from mice infected with *M. bovis* or *M. tuberculosis* and their role in protection has been revealed recently (121,122). Thus, activation of MHC class Ib–restricted, N-f-met peptide–specific CD8 T cells may be a general phenomenon of intracellular bacterial infections in mice. It remains to be established, however, whether a similar type of unconventional CD8 T cells also exists in humans.

CD1 Molecules and Antigen Presentation

Although the CD1 polypeptides share several features with MHC class I or Ib molecules, they are encoded outside of the MHC (123). On the one hand, CD1 and MHC class I or Ib heavy chains have some homologies, and both CD1 and MHC class I molecules are generally surface expressed in association with β2m. On the other hand, their unique functional features and their genomic location outside the MHC define CD1 polypeptides as a distinct family of nonpolymorphic antigen-presenting molecules. In humans, four major types of CD1 molecules can be distinguished (CD1a to CD1d), which in turn fall into two groups: group1 encompasses CD1a/b/c, and group 2 comprises CD1d. The group 1 CD1 molecules, which are primarily expressed on conventional antigen-presenting cells, are capable of presenting mycobacterial glycolipids to T cells (Fig. 4). The distribution and functional role of group 2 CD1 molecules is less well understood. However, group 2 CD1 molecules have been identified on numerous host cells. Only group 2 CD1 molecules exist in the mouse. These CD1d molecules are recognized by murine NK T cells described below (124). CD1 molecules form a bifurcated hydrophobic cleft in which two hydrophobic lipid tails can be accommodated (125).

Group 1 CD1–Restricted DN, CD4, or CD8 T Cells

In humans, unconventional $\alpha\beta$ T cells of DN, CD4, or CD8 phenotype have been described with the unique capacity to recognize mycobacterial glycolipids presented by group 1CD1 molecules (126). Several mycobacterial ligands have been identified so far, including mycolic acids and LAM, both of which are abundant components of the mycobacterial cell wall (Table 4). The lipid tails of these antigens are anchored in the hydrophobic cleft of the CD1 molecule, whereas the carbohydrate part is recognized by the TCR. Variations in the carbohydrate structure therefore account for different T-cell specificities. The group 1 CD1 molecules CD1 a, b, and c meet their antigenic ligands in different intracellular compartments (127). Glycoplipids are introduced to CD1b in the late phagosome and phagolysosome, whereas CD1a is found mainly at the cell surface and probably also in the early phagosome. CD1c is localized both on the cell surface and in phagosomes at different stages of maturation. *M. tuberculosis* arrests phagosome maturation at an early stage. However, cell wall glycolipids are shed from mycobacteria and transported to lysosomal vesicles where they can interact with CD1b molecules. Moreover, mycobacterial glycolipids have been identified in apoptotic vesicles, where they could be transferred from infected macrophages to bystander DC. In contrast to DC, macrophages are virtually devoid of surface-expressed group 1 CD1 molecules (127). Hence, the transfer of mycobacterial glycolipids from infected macrophages to bystander DC appears to be an essential prerequisite for glycolipid presentation to T cells (Fig. 4).

The unconventional glycolipid specific $\alpha\beta$ T cells produce IFN-γ and lyse target cells, strongly suggesting that they participate in anti-infective immunity. Similar T-lymphocytes have been identified in guinea pigs but not in mice, due to the lack of group 1 CD1 molecules in the latter. In the absence of an appropriate mouse model, a clear role for group 1 CD1–restricted T cells in antibacterial immunity has not yet been shown. Nevertheless, the data obtained with the human T cells demonstrate the impact of bacterial pathogens on the evolution of the T-lymphocyte system that apparently resulted in a highly specialized T-cell population with specificity for components highly abundant in the mycobacterial cell wall.

NK T Cells with Specificity for Group 2 CD1 Molecules

In mice, lymphocytes have been identified which coexpress the $\alpha\beta$ TCR and the NK cell marker, NK1 (124). The NK T cells are specific for group 2 CD1d (the only CD1 molecules that exist in mice). Binding of highly hydrophobic peptides, α-galactosyl ceramide from a sponge or N-glycosylceramides from malaria plasmodia to CD1d and T-cell recognition of this complex has been described. The recent identification of phosphatidylinositol tetramannoside as a CD1d-presented antigen of mycobacterial origin provides further evidence for the role of these T cells in the immune response to tuberculosis (Table 4). Use of a restricted repertoire and of an invariant Vα14-Jα281 chain would be consistent with recognition of highly conserved antigenic ligands. CD1d-deficient KO mice do not suffer from exacerbated tuberculosis, but treatment of mice with anti-CD1d monoclonal antibodies has been found to transiently ameliorate listeriosis and exacerbate tuberculosis (128–130). Moreover, NK T cells have been shown to be involved in granuloma formation induced by mycobacterial glycolipids (131). Hence, the role of these T cells in antibacterial immunity remains elusive. Although characterization of NK T cells was mostly done in the mouse system, CD1d-restricted T-lymphocytes expressing a homologous invariant Vα chain have been described in humans. Thus, similar cells exist in humans.

Multiple Roles of β2 Microglobulin

Experiments with β2m KO mice have been widely used to analyze the role of CD8 T-lymphocytes in protection against intracellular bacteria. This strategy is based on the notion that the development of conventional CD8 T cells requires antigen presentation by MHC class I molecules, the surface expression of which depends, in turn, on β2m. The β2m KO mice therefore lack functional CD8 T cells. However, β2m also controls the surface expression of various other molecules, including nonclassical MHC class Ib and CD1 molecules (Fig. 4 and Table 4). As described above, unconventional T cells controlled by these presentation molecules contribute to the antibacterial immune response. Moreover, β2m is involved in the surface expression of Hfe (hereditary hemachromatosis gene product), which regulates iron uptake, and of FcRn, which regulates Ig transport through intestinal epithelial cells. While the role of FcRn in antibacterial immunity is unknown, iron levels in the early phagosome are critical for bacteria residing in this cellular compartment. Hence, β2m controls a variety of mechanisms central to protection against intracellular bacteria. Consistent with this notion, β2m KO mice are far more susceptible to infection with the intracellular bacteria *M. tuberculosis*, *L. monocytogenes*, and *S. enterica* than KO mice deficient in MHC class I heavy chain (20,110,132). In light of these recent findings, experiments extrapolating β2m deficiency to CD8 T-cell deficiency must be interpreted with care.

$\gamma\delta$ T Cells

A minor T-cell population in the peripheral blood and lymphoid organs of humans expresses an alternative TCR made up of a γ and a δ chain. Although the role of these $\gamma\delta$ T cells in antibacterial immunity has not been fully revealed, recent years have witnessed compelling evidence that $\gamma\delta$ T cells play a prominent role in antibacterial immunity (133, 134).

$\gamma\delta$ T cells from the peripheral blood of healthy individuals are strongly reactive to mycobacterial components *in vitro*. The responsible entities have been identified as small-molecular-weight nonproteinaceous molecules, of which phosphate is an essential component (135,136). Isopentenyl pyrophosphate and alkyl derivatives thereof have been defined as natural ligands, but other components, including phosphosugars, phospho-esters, and nucleotides, serve as antigenic ligands as well (Table 4). These phospholigands stimulate the major subset of $\gamma\delta$ T cells in humans expressing the Vγ2Vδ2 TCR combination with high junctional diversity. Despite this oligoclonal activation, a conserved TCR binding site is required for stimulation. The isopentenyl pyrophosphate represents a ubiquitous precursor of various metabolites, both in prokaryotes and eukaryotes. Apparently, the most active phospholigands are intermediates of isoprenoid biosynthesis from nonmevalonate precursors, which occurs in certain microorganisms such as *M. tuberculosis* and is absent in eukaryotes (137,138). In addition, these phospholigands are apparently presented to $\gamma\delta$ T cells on the host cell membrane independently from known antigen-presenting molecules encoded by MHC or CD1 genes (Fig. 4). The most likely explanation for these findings is direct recognition of phospholigands by the TCR$\gamma\delta$. In contrast to the human system, murine $\gamma\delta$ T cells are not stimulated by these phospholigands.

Studies with $\gamma\delta$ T-cell–deficient gene-deletion mutant mice or with mice treated with anti-$\gamma\delta$ TCR mAb suggest an auxiliary role of $\gamma\delta$ T cells in antilisterial protection. The $\gamma\delta$ T-cell–deficient KO mice die from a high inoculum of *M. tuberculosis,* but are not affected when confronted with a low inoculum of this pathogen (139,140). At present, it is safe to state that $\gamma\delta$ T cells participate in antibacterial immunity, and that they do so by controlling inflammation. In most cases, this appears to be an auxiliary rather than an essential function. Increased numbers of $\gamma\delta$ T cells have been frequently identified at sites of inflammation. In particular, an increased proportion of $\gamma\delta$ T cells has been noted in lesions of leprosy patients during reactional stages and at the sites of DTH reaction to lepromin. In TCRδ KO mice infected with the intracellular bacteria *L. monocytogenes* or *M. tuberculosis,* the characteristic granulomas do not develop. Instead, inflammatory abscess-like lesions emerge, reminiscent of the characteristic tissue response to purulent extracellular pathogens. Taken together, these findings indicate a role for $\gamma\delta$ T cells in inflammation, and particularly in the formation of lesions at the site of bacterial infection.

Because $\gamma\delta$ T cells are activated prior to $\alpha\beta$ T cells, they could fill a gap between early, nonspecific resistance mediated by the innate immune system and the later highly specific acquired immune responses mediated by $\alpha\beta$ T cells.

Although $\gamma\delta$ T cells represent a minor population of all T cells in peripheral blood and lymphoid organs, bacterial pathogens can stimulate high numbers of $\gamma\delta$ T cells. Oligoclonal stimulation of approximately 80% of all $\gamma\delta$ T cells by phospholigands as compared to clonal stimulation of antigen-specific $\alpha\beta$ T cells accounts for this phenomenon. Finally, in the complete absence of $\alpha\beta$ T cells, $\gamma\delta$ T cells can assume biological effector functions that are performed by $\alpha\beta$ T cells under normal conditions. Thus, $\gamma\delta$ T cells possess a high compensatory plasticity.

The $\gamma\delta$ T cells make up a large proportion of all T cells in mucosal epithelia, both in human and mouse (134,141). Because mucosal epithelia represents the major port of entry for many intracellular bacteria, a role in first-line defense of intraepithelial $\gamma\delta$ T cells in gut and lung can be assumed. Although this is an intriguing assumption, convincing evidence to support this hypothesis is still missing.

T-CELL FUNCTIONS DURING COURSE OF INFECTION

T-Cell Functions

Generally speaking, T-lymphocytes perform three major functions: cytolytic functions and helper functions of Th1 and Th2 cells. Th cells produce various cytokines with Th1 cells being characterized by potent IL-2 and IFN-γ secretion and Th2 cells by potent IL-4 and IL-5 production (142,143). The cytolytic T-lymphocytes (CTL) lyse infected target cells by direct cell contact (110,144). Although each of the T-cell populations, as described above, can in principle perform numerous biological functions, some preference can be observed. CD8 T cells (either MHC class I– or MHC class Ib–restricted) are preferentially cytolytic. A role for CTL in immunity against *L. monocytogenes* has been demonstrated by the use of KO mice with deficient CTL functions (110). CD4 T cells as well as $\gamma\delta$ T cells are typically cytokine-producing Th cells. Similarly, the CD1-restricted $\alpha\beta$ T cells are potent cytokine producers. IFN-γ–producing Th1 cells are of paramount importance for acquired immunity against intracellular bacteria. In contrast to Th1 cells, Th2 cells do not contribute to acquired resistance against intracellular bacteria measurably and if default Th2 cell activation occurs, disease is exacerbated.

Contribution of Conventional and Unconventional T Cells to Protection: Implications for Vaccine Design

The findings described above emphasize that a number of distinct T-lymphocyte populations participate in the antibacterial host response. Without doubt, a hierarchy exists regarding the contribution of T-cell sets, with the conventional CD4 and CD8 $\alpha\beta$ T cells being of highest importance. Yet, unconventional T cells that make up only a minor population are probably required for efficient control to occur. This may be particularly important for combat of highly resistant bacteria such as *M. tuberculosis*. In principle, each of the different T-cell populations is capable of expressing various biological functions relevant to antibacterial immunity. Thus, other differences must exist if one considers high functional redundancy an insufficient explanation. These differences are summarized below.

- Differential tissue expression of the restricting elements (MHC class I being broadly distributed, MHC class II and group 1 CD1 having a restricted tissue expression with preference for antigen-presenting cells)
- Differential origin of the antigen-processing pathway (MHC class I starting in the cytosol; MHC class II, MHC class Ib, and CD1 originating in the endosome)
- Differential physicochemical nature of the ligands (peptides being presented by MHC class I and MHC class II, glycolipids being presented by CD1, phospholigands being recognized by $\gamma\delta$ T cells directly)
- Differential kinetics of activation ($\gamma\delta$ T cells, NK T cells, and N-f-met–specific T cells frequently preceding conventional $\alpha\beta$ T cells)
- Differential expression of nonclonal co-stimulatory receptors that control TCR-independent activation or inhibition by microbial pathogens. Examples of activating or inhibiting receptors are CD28 or CTLA-4, respectively

Identification of the spectrum of T-cell sets involved in antibacterial immunity as well as characterization of the stimulatory antigenic ligands form the basis for rational design of effective vaccines directed against intracellular bacteria. With regard to activation of conventional CD4 and CD8 T cells, two major issues deserve particular consideration (Fig. 5). First, localization of the bacterial pathogen within the host cell influences the relative contribution of CD4 or CD8 T cells

to antibacterial protection. Consequently, the use of vaccines, which are preferentially localized in the endosome and, thus, predominantly activate CD4 T cells, may be insufficient for control of microbial pathogens that are primarily defeated by CD8 T cells. Such discrepancy may explain the low efficacy of BCG against tuberculosis. Yet, as discussed above, alternative pathways exist that allow introduction of antigens from endosomal vaccines into the MHC class I processing machinery. Second, a profound impact of antigen display in secreted or somatic form on vaccine efficacy has been described (145,146). *S. enterica* or BCG vaccine carriers expressing the same listerial antigens confer protection against *L. monocytogenes* infection only when the vaccine displays the antigens in secreted form or on the surface. Because intracellular bacteria only survive within resting macrophages, secreted or surface-expressed proteins are already available for antigen processing in the initial phase of infection. Accordingly, only T cells directed against such antigens can be activated. Once MP have been activated by T cells, they can kill and degrade the intracellular pathogens and, thus, somatic proteins become available for antigen processing. Accordingly, at later times of infection, T-cell responses against somatic antigens arise. Because efficacious vaccines must activate the T-cell response promptly after infection, secreted proteins are superior vaccine antigen candidates over somatic ones.

The nonpolymorphic nature of MHC class Ib and CD1 gene products circumvents problems associated with genetic variations among vaccines, as is the case for peptides presented by the highly polymorphic classical MHC molecules. On the other hand, experiments in the mouse suggest that MHC Ib (H2-M3)– and CD1 (CD1d)–restricted T cells do not develop memory responses (147). Obviously, uncovering the rules underlying antigen processing and activation of distinct T-cell subsets will promote rational design of vaccines against intracellular bacteria (18).

Kinetics of Infection

The course of infection with intracellular bacteria can be conveniently separated into three stages (Fig. 6). At each stage, cytokines are produced that perform two functions: First, they execute effector functions directed at reducing the microbial burden, and second, they express regulatory functions that influence the subsequent course of infection. The *early stage* is initiated within minutes after microbial entry and dominated by cells of the innate immune system, in particular PNG and MP, which are attracted to the site of bacterial replication by chemokines and proinflammatory cytokines. Phagocytosis and intracellular killing of bacterial pathogens by PNG and MP probably represents the predominant effector function at this early stage. At the same time, monocytes immigrating to the site of microbial deposition differentiate to DC, mature and migrate to draining lymph nodes. These DC as well as resident DC produce proinflammatory and immunoregulatory cytokines, notably IL-12, and thus influence the subsequent stages by promoting induction

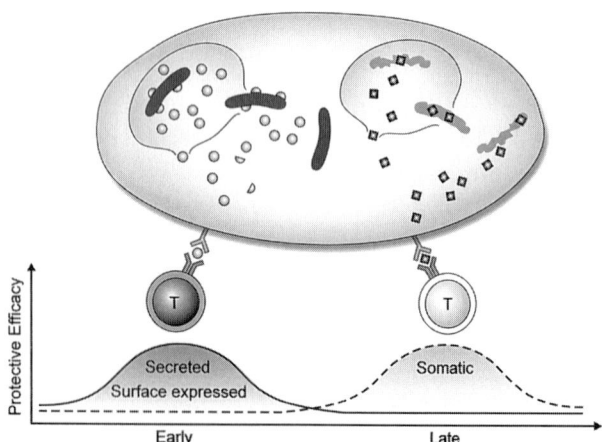

FIG. 5. Influence of intracellular localization and antigen display on the protective T-cell response.

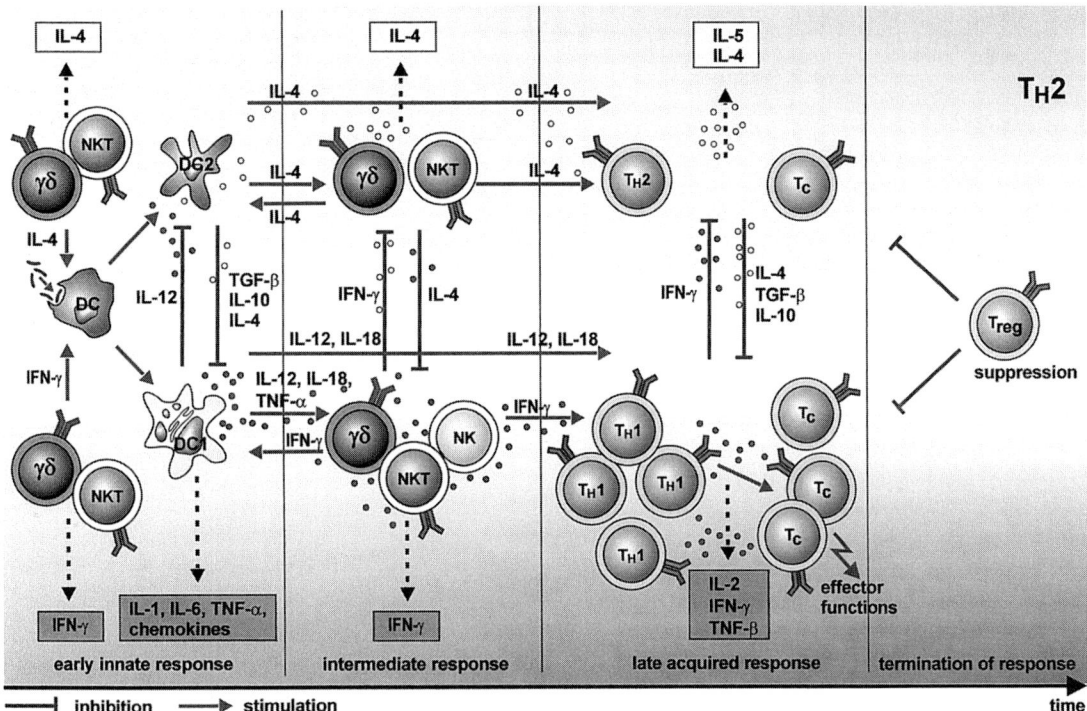

FIG. 6. Predominance of Th1 over Th2 cell activities at the three stages of the immune response against intracellular bacteria. The role of regulatory T cells (T reg) in the down-regulation of agents of the immune response remains to be established.

of the protective acquired immune response. The *intermediate stage* is characterized by NK cells, NK T cells, and $\gamma\delta$ T cells, all of which produce IFN-γ. Although NK T cells express a clonally distributed TCR, they recognize a limited set of antigens and hence lack the diversity of conventional T cells governing the late stage. Moreover, the cells operative at the intermediate stage can be activated via non-clonally distributed receptors such as TLR. The intermediate stage links the early (innate) with the late (acquired) immune response. At the *late stage,* conventional $\alpha\beta$ T cells with unique specificity are operative, which mobilize and sustain host defense mechanisms primarily in granulomatous lesions that result in effective control and ideally sterile eradication of the pathogen. Recent technical achievements have allowed a quantitative assessment of antigen-specific CD4 and CD8 T-cell populations that predominate in the late stage of infection (148,149). In the *L. monocytogenes* model, construction of tetrameric complexes comprising MHC class I molecules with an antigenic peptide revealed that during primary responses, 1% of all CD8$^+$ T cells respond to single listerial epitopes.

During secondary responses, these populations expand to up to 10% of the CD8$^+$ T-cell population. Hence, the proportion of antigen-specific T-lymphocytes activated during infection is far greater than previously assumed (147).

The length and importance of each stage are markedly influenced by the type of intracellular pathogen. In experimental listeriosis of mice, the complete sequence of host response lasts for less than 10 days, whereas in tuberculosis of humans

it may endure for several years. The early stage is particularly important for control of *L. monocytogenes* organisms that divide rapidly and, at the same time, are highly susceptible to intracellular killing. The more robust and slowly dividing *M. tuberculosis* organisms are less vulnerable to this early stage of response. The relevance of the intermediate stage to microbial control is significantly influenced by the strength of the innate and the acquired immune response. The broader the window between these two stages is, the more important the intermediate stage becomes. In T-cell–deficient mice (e.g., nu/nu mice, SCID mice, or RAG-1 KO mice), the late stage fails to develop and, accordingly, the intermediate stage has to compensate for this lack (103). Such mice, therefore, provide a useful model for analyzing the role of NK cells in antibacterial immunity. Upon secondary infection, the conventional T cells are activated more rapidly from the pool of memory T cells. The early and intermediate stages become largely dispensable because invading pathogens are rapidly confronted with the late-stage immune response. Suffice it to say that this is the major principle of vaccination.

CYTOKINES IN ANTIBACTERIAL DEFENSE

Cytokines are central to resistance against intracellular bacteria (Table 5). At all stages, cytokines are produced that perform regulator and/or effector functions. Although cytokines are essential for control of infection, they can also cause harm to the host. To avoid such harmful consequences, down-regulation of the immune response is required at later

TABLE 5. *Cytokines in antibacterial immunity*

Cytokine	Contribution to antibacterial protection
Chemokines	The important role of some members proven
IL-1	Important role proven
IL-6	Essential role proven
TNF-α	Essential role proven
LT-α3	Important role proven
IFN-γ	Essential role proven
IL-12	Important role proven
IL-18	Likely
IL-4	Exacerbation
IL-10	Exacerbation
TGF-β	Exacerbation

stages of infection. Neutralization of cytokines with specific antibodies and application of KO mice lacking defined cytokine or cytokine receptor genes have provided deep insights into the role of single cytokines. Identification of cytokines in lesions, in particular those from leprosy patients, has provided further information about the role of cytokines in antibacterial immunity. The highly intertwined steps of the anti-infectious host response controlled by cytokines are listed below.

- Leukocyte recruitment to the site of bacterial deposition
- Formation of granulomatous lesions
- Activation of antibacterial functions in MP
- Induction of a protective T-cell response
- Down-regulation of the antibacterial host response to avoid harmful sequelae of an exaggerated immune response

Leukocyte Recruitment

Influx of inflammatory phagocytes occurs prior to the appearance of specific T-lymphocytes, and accordingly the relevant cytokines are primarily produced by MP, as well as by epithelial and endothelial cells in response to microbial invasion. Early produced cytokines with effector functions include the proinflammatory cytokines, TNF, IL-1, IL-6, and macrophage migration inhibitory factor (MIF), as well as chemokines (150–154). The chemokine superfamily encompasses more than 50 related small-molecular-weight polypeptides (155). Four subgroups can be distinguished on the basis of a conserved cysteine motif: the CC chemokines with two unseparated terminal cysteine residues; the CXC chemokines with nonconserved amino acids separating the two terminal cysteine residues; the CX$_3$C chemokines with several amino acids separating the cysteine residues; and the C chemokine with only one terminal cysteine (C chemokine). Grouping of the large chemokine family can be further extended on the basis of different chemokine receptors (154,155). The CC chemokines preferentially act on MP, whereas PNG are primarily activated by CXC chemokines. Other leukocytes, including lymphocytes, eosinophils, and basophils may also be stimulated by these chemokines. The C and CX$_3$C chemokines primarily recruit NK cells and lymphocytes.

Chemokines as a group play an important role in early mobilization of host defense. KO mice lacking the receptor for the CC chemokine MCP-1 are more susceptible to listeriosis than controls (156). KO mice deficient in CC chemokine receptor 2 (CCR2) succumb to tuberculosis infection. In these mutants, the recruitment of macrophages, DC, and T cells to the lung is impaired (157). On the other hand, MCP-1–deficient KO mice control *M. tuberculosis* infection similarly to wild-type animals. MCP-1 acts through the CCR2 receptor like MCP-3 and MCP-5. It therefore appears that these chemokines are essential for antibacterial protection but compensate for each other (158). Experiments in other systems have revealed a central role of chemokines in early inflammation, in particular PNG and monocyte extravasation (Fig. 7). In addition, some chemokines activate professional phagocytes and in this way probably promote early reduction of the bacterial load. The proinflammatory cytokines, IL-1, IL-6, TNF, and MIF are also involved in the early accumulation of inflammatory phagocytes at the site of bacterial growth. The essential role of IL-6 and TNF in antibacterial immunity is demonstrated by the exacerbated susceptibility to listeriosis and tuberculosis of KO mice with a deficient IL-6 or TNF type 1 receptor (TNF-R1) gene. Similarly, KO mice deficient in MIF suffer from exacerbated *S. enterica* infection (159). The proinflammatory cytokines, when produced in high amounts, cause acute-phase responses by inducing release of various plasma proteins from hepatocytes. However, they serve as endogenous pyrogens that stimulate fever, and TNF is also responsible for cachexia, the characteristic feature of wasting in infections with many intracellular bacteria, notably tuberculosis. Clinical trials showing that detrimental effects of excessive TNF production in tuberculosis and leprosy patients can be ameliorated by treatment with thalidomide emphasize the double-sided role of TNF in chronic infections (159a,160).

Granuloma Formation

Experiments utilizing the respective KO mice emphasize a role of IFN-γ, TNF-α, and lymphotoxin (LT)-α3 in granuloma formation and maintenance during tuberculosis (161–164). Hereditary IFN-γR deficiency has been described in humans and these immunodeficient patients severely suffer and ultimately die of infections with intracellular bacteria (165–167). This high susceptibility was accompanied by impaired granuloma formation. The critical role of TNF-α in the containment of *M. tuberculosis* in humans was impressively demonstrated by the increased risk of the reactivation of tuberculosis in rheumatoid arthritis patients undergoing treatment with anti–TNF-α mAb (168,169).

Conversely, evidence has been presented that transforming growth factor beta (TGF-β) and IL-10 counteract granuloma development (170,171). These cytokines probably minimize immunopathology by preventing formation of extensive lesions. Premature inhibition of granuloma formation, however, may interfere with optimum protection. The relatively

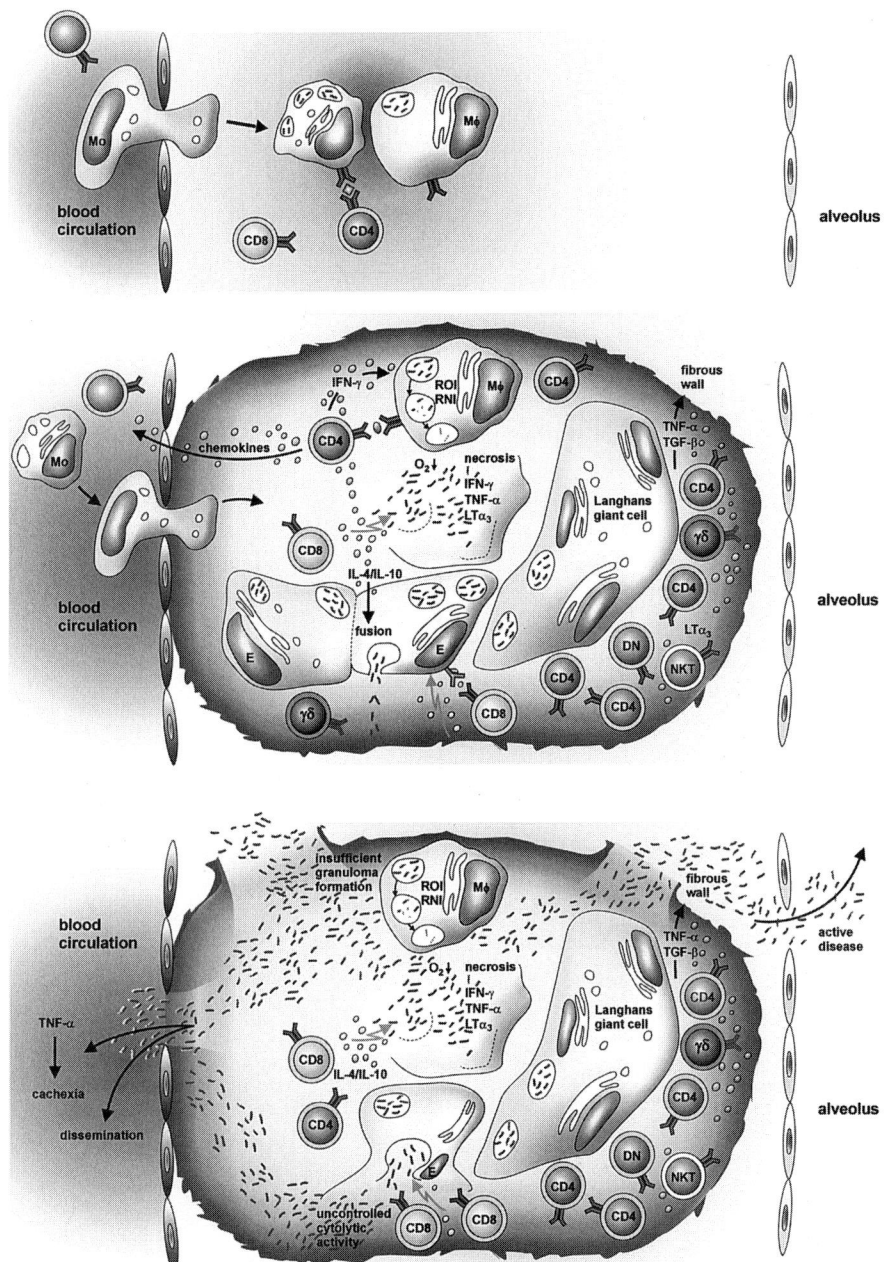

FIG. 7. Cellular interactions in an "idealized" granuloma. Mo, monocyte; Mø, macrophage.

easy access to clinical leprosy lesions has provided complementary insights into the function of cytokines in granulomatous lesions (172). Analysis of cytokine mRNA patterns in tuberculoid leprosy lesions has revealed abundant IL-1, TNF, granulocyte–macrophage colony-stimulating factor (GM-CSF), TGF-β, IL-6, IL-2, IL-12, and IFN-γ mRNA, indicating an involvement of these cytokines in the control of granuloma perpetuation (173). In contrast, IL-4, IL-5, and IL-10 mRNA levels are low to undetectable in these granulomas but relatively high in lepromatous lesions, suggesting a role of these cytokines in granuloma down-regulation. The recent development of DNA chip technology has facilitated the global analysis of host immune response at the level of the

transcriptome. Although these experiments have been thus far restricted to *in vitro* analysis (174), in the near future valuable information about the signature response in granulomatous lesions can be expected.

Macrophage Activation

The activation of antibacterial macrophage properties by cytokines represents a central step in acquired resistance against intracellular bacteria. This step has been extensively studied *in vitro* using murine macrophages, and IFN-γ has been identified as the major cytokine of MP activation. IFN-γ–activated macrophages rapidly kill susceptible intracellular bacteria, such as *L. monocytogenes*. Although the question as to whether IFN-γ–stimulated MP actually kill *M. tuberculosis* remains a matter of controversy, they markedly inhibit growth of these pathogens. RNI and ROI are the major effectors of bacteriostatic/bactericidal MP activities against most intracellular bacteria (46,175). IFN-γ–stimulated MP often produce TNF, which synergizes with IFN-γ in the activation of antibacterial macrophage functions. Consistent with such a central role of IFN-γ in antibacterial immunity, IFN-γ– or IFN-γR–deficient KO mice rapidly succumb to infections with *L. monocytogenes, M. tuberculosis, S. enterica,* and other intracellular pathogens (20,162,163). The activation by cytokines of antibacterial functions in human MP is less well understood. First, the production of high levels of RNI by human MP remains a matter of debate, although more recent data consolidate profound RNI synthesis by MP from patients with infectious disease (73). Second, IFN-γ fails to consistently induce tuberculostasis in human macrophages. Some tuberculostasis has been achieved in human MP by co-stimulation with IFN-γ and TNF and maximum tuberculostasis can apparently be achieved by addition of 1,25-dihydroxyvitamin D3, the biologically active metabolite of vitamin D3 (176,177). This latter steroid is either taken up in the diet or produced in the skin after exposure to ultraviolet (UV) light (178). By 1α-hydroxylation, vitamin D3 is converted to its circulating metabolite, 1α-hydroxyvitamin D3. Further hydroxylation at C25 yields 1,25-dihydroxyvitamin D3, the biologically active component. Macrophages possess 1α-hydroxylase activity, which is controlled by IFN-γ. It is therefore likely that *in situ* IFN-γ can induce the autocrine 1,25-dihydroxyvitamin D3 production that may be missing in certain *in vitro* systems. Further support for the central role of IFN-γ in control of intracellular bacterial infections in humans stems from the identification of hereditary IFN-γR deficiency in young children who succumbed to infections with various intracellular bacteria or even to *M. bovis* BCG vaccination (165–167). Conversely, IFN-γ treatment in adjunct to chemotherapy has been used successfully in the treatment of leprosy, tuberculosis, and atypical mycobacteriosis (179). Hence, IFN-γ also plays a central role in host defense against intracellular bacteria in humans. This cytokine is produced by various cells that infiltrate the lesion in a sequential order. These are NK cells, γδ T cells, αβ T cells of CD4, CD8 or DN phenotype, and even MP (180). In experimental listeriosis of mice, NK cells produce IFN-γ 1 day after infection, IFN-γ–producing γδ T cells appear by day 2, and IFN-γ–secreting CD4 and CD8 αβ T cells are demonstrable by day 5 (Fig. 6).

Induction of a Protective T-Cell Response

The type of immune response and hence the course and ultimate fate of infection are determined soon after bacterial entry into the host (143,181). IL-12 is the crucial promoter of the protective immune response (182,183). It is rapidly produced by DC and MP in response to infection, activates NK cells,

and stimulates maturation of Th1 cells. In either case, IFN-γ production is the end result. TNF-α produced by infected macrophages synergizes with IL-12 for NK cell activation and IFN-γ from activated NK cells further promotes IL-12 secretion via a positive feedback mechanism (103). In infections with microbes of weak stimulatory potential, IFN-γ may be required for appreciable IL-12 secretion (184,185). In murine listeriosis, IL-12 is apparently essential for the generation of a protective primary immune response, whereas secondary challenge with *L. monocytogenes* of previously vaccinated mice shows partial IL-12 independence (186). Similarly, IL-12 seems to be an important, but not absolute, requirement for immunity against tuberculosis (187). These findings argue against exclusive IL-12 dependency of IFN-γ induction. Probably the more recently identified cytokine IL-18 is responsible for this partial IL-12 independence (188). Consistent with studies in the mouse system, patients with an intrinsic IL-12 defect suffer from lowered IFN-γ titers accompanied by disseminated BCG and *M. avium* complex infections (167,189–191).

Down-Regulation of Antibacterial Host Response to Avoid its Harmful Sequelae

Generally, IL-4–producing Th2 cells are not significantly activated in intracellular bacterial infections. Nevertheless, counterregulatory cytokines are produced during infection. IL-10 is secreted rapidly after infection and probably serves to control Th1 cell development (192–195). Both murine and human macrophages produce IL-10 concomitantly with IL-12 in response to bacterial infections, and in both systems IL-10 was found to decrease IL-12 secretion and, as a corollary, IFN-γ production (196). Consistent with a down-regulatory role of IL-10 in antibacterial immunity, IL-10–deficient KO mice control listeriosis more efficiently, this being correlated with elevated production of numerous cytokines of relevance to protection, including IL-12 and IFN-γ (192). Precedent exists in murine toxoplasmosis for the importance of IL-10 in the control of antimicrobial immunity by preventing immunopathology caused by exaggerated IL-12 and IFN-γ responses. Once the bacterial pathogen is successfully defeated, the ongoing immune response must be confined to avoid severe harm to the host. In certain systems, IL-4–producing Th2 cells have been detected at later stages of chronic infections with bacterial pathogens, probably to counteract IFN-γ–producing Th1 cells (Fig. 6) (197,198). Macrophage deactivation and Th1 cell inhibition by TGF-β and IL-10 may further contribute to this event (170,171,199). Evidence from other experimental models suggests that a discrete regulatory T-cell population of CD4+25+ phenotype is critical for the down-regulation of immune responses (Fig.6). Research of the impact of these cells on the termination of immunity to infectious agents is a challenging task for the future (199a). Although down-regulation of the anti-infective immune response has been largely ignored, it is probably essential for bringing back the activated immune response to normal levels. On the other hand, premature mobilization of down-regulatory immune mechanisms prior to successful pathogen defeat may cause disease exacerbation. Such an aberrant situation may lead to the lepromatous form of leprosy.

PREDOMINANCE OF TH1 OVER TH2 CELL ACTIVITIES IN INTRACELLULAR BACTERIAL INFECTIONS: INFLUENCE OF INNATE IMMUNE SYSTEM

The kind of infectious agent has a decisive influence on the type of cytokine-producing Th cells that develop as most appropriate defense mechanisms (Fig. 6) (142,181,200). The two Th populations that arise, Th1 cells characterized by IFN-γ and IL-2 secretion and Th2 cells typically producing IL-4 and IL-5, are derived from a common precursor cell, designated Th0 cell (143). Th1 cells combat intracellular pathogens, including bacteria, protozoa, and fungi, while Th2 cells are responsible for control of helminths (142,181,200). Microbes and virions present in the extracellular milieu are also controlled by antibodies and hence Th2 cells. Conversely, uncontrolled Th1 or Th2 responses have been made responsible for autoimmune or allergic diseases, respectively. The distinction between Th1 and Th2 cells is made operationally on the basis of the type of cytokines produced and is, by no means, absolute. Stable surface markers that distinguish Th1 and Th2 cells have not been identified unequivocally. The $\beta2$ chain of the IL-12 receptor (IL-12Rβ2) is distinctive for Th1 cells in the human and murine systems (201,202). Reciprocally, the IL-1 receptor family member T1/ST2 is considered indicative of murine Th2 cells (203). Finally, Th1 and Th2 cells can be distinguished on the basis of their chemokine receptors (204).

As was said above, in infections with the vast majority of intracellular bacteria, potent Th1 responses develop and Th2 responses are virtually absent. The prominent Th1 response caused by these infections has even been claimed to antagonize development of allergic diseases (205). Only in the case of leprosy, profound polarization towards a resistant tuberculoid or susceptible lepromatous pole occurs and some evidence suggests that a Th1/Th2 dichotomy underlies this polarization—at least in part.

How is the predominant Th1 response achieved at the different stages of anti-infective immunity? At the early stage of infection, IL-12 and IL-18 are produced rapidly after microbial entry into the host, which serve as the central signal for Th1 cell development. In contrast, prompt IL-4 and IL-10 secretion is low and short-lived. Evidence has been presented suggesting that Th1/Th2 cell polarization is directed by DC, which rapidly differentiate into DC1 and DC2 cells upon encounter with invading pathogens. Stimulation of DC precursors by bacterial components (PAMP) via TLR results in the development of DC1 cells that produce IL-12 and IL-18, thus promoting Th1 cell polarization. Components from helminths that are still not well defined stimulate the develop-

ment of IL-4–producing DC2 cells, and hence promote Th2 cell polarization (104). NK T cells and $\gamma\delta$ T cells that rapidly produce the Th1- or Th2-cell–promoting cytokines IFN-γ or IL-4 following TCR stimulation by conserved microbial ligands could support DC polarization at this early stage (Fig. 6).

Th1 and Th2 cell differentiation progresses through several stages that are initiated promptly after microbial entry into the host (Fig. 6). Under the counterregulatory influence of Th1 and Th2 cytokines, gradually polarization becomes more stable. By promptly reacting to microbial components, the innate immune system determines the generation of the appropriate immune response. Default recognition of the infectious agent by the innate immune system, therefore, results in development of an inappropriate immune response, thus causing exacerbation of, rather than protection from, pathology. This has been best studied in the model of experimental infection of mice with the intracellular protozoal pathogen, *Leishmania major* (206). When challenged with *L. major*, C57BL/6 mice build up a potent Th1 response and are protected. In contrast, BALB/c mice develop a Th2 response accompanied by increased susceptibility to leishmaniasis.

IL-12 does not only act on Th1 cells, but also on NK cells and $\gamma\delta$ T cells, the central players at the intermediate stage of infection. Activation of both cell types profits from co-stimulation with TNF-α that is secreted by activated macrophages concomitantly with IL-12. The IFN-γ from NK cells further increases IL-12 production by macrophages via a positive feedback loop, thus greatly enhancing IL-12 production. Under the concerted action of IFN-γ and IL-12, stable Th1 cell development is achieved. Conventional CD4 and CD8 T cells as well as MHC class Ib–restricted CD8 T cells, CD1 controlled T cells, and $\gamma\delta$ T cells acquire a Th1 phenotype during intracellular bacterial infections.

Although cytokines are the prime signal transmitters in Th-cell activation and polarization, cognate receptor interactions participate in this process. The most important ones are the CD40–CD154 system and the B7–CD28–CTLA-4 system (207,208). The CD40–CD154 system was originally identified as an important regulator of B-cell activation and Ig class switching. Later it was found that interactions between CD40 on MP and DC with its ligand CD154 on T cells provides a bi-directional cross talk that participates in activation of either partner cell. The major function of CD40–CD154 interactions is to support IL-12 production induced by PAMP and by Th1 cytokines, notably IFN-γ. Thus, during the whole course of the anti-infective Th1 response—from its initiation to the execution of effector functions—CD40–CD154 interactions may participate. In KO mice with deficient CD40 or CD154 genes, IL-12 and IFN-γ secretion are impaired resulting in increased susceptibility to the intracellular protozoan parasite, *L. major* (209). Such disease exacerbation has not been observed in experimental listeriosis of CD154-deficient mutant mice (210). However, CD40 signaling has been found to improve vaccine-induced immunity against *L. monocytogenes* (211). In these experiments, vaccination with killed organisms together with an agonistic anti-CD40 monoclonal antibody stimulated potent protection mediated by both CD4 and CD8 T cells. The B7 system comprises the B7-1 (CD80) and the B7-2 (CD86) molecules on macrophages and DCs and the CD28 and CTLA-4 (CD152) receptors on T cells (208). The cross talk between B7 and CD28 supports the induction of primary T-cell responses. CTLA-4 interacts with B7 as well, but it inhibits T-cell activation. Consistent with a co-stimulatory role of CD28 in antibacterial protection, KO mice deficient in CD28 are highly susceptible to *S. enterica* infection and even fail to control infection with auxotrophic *S. enterica* vaccine strain (212). *L. monocytogenes* infection is also less well controlled in these mice (213). Microbial PAMP regulate surface expression of B7 molecules via TLR signaling, and the relative densities of B7-1 and B7-2 molecules on the surface of antigen-presenting cells appear to influence the maturation of Th0 cells toward either the Th1 or the Th2 pole (208). The B7-1 and B7-2 molecules are expressed in the vicinity of MHC molecules, and hence promote antigen-specific T-cell stimulation (107).

Employing both cytokines and cognate interactions provides the means for balanced amplification and tight control of the anti-infective immune response. Cytokines promote the broad-spectrum signaling that is required for accumulation and activation of leukocytes at the site of microbial replication. Cognate interactions between cell-surface receptors are more restricted and hence avoid activation of bystander cells that may cause undesirable tissue reactions or even activation of autoimmune responses. The coexistence of activating (e.g., CD28) and inhibitory (e.g., CTLA-4) molecules that compete for the same ligands (B7) allows further fine-tuning of the system. Finally, human polarized Th1 and Th2 cells express differential patterns of chemokine receptors that facilitate preferential attraction of Th1 cells to sites of bacterial growth, providing an additional control mechanism during infection (204).

DEATH OF INFECTED CELLS

Several lines of evidence suggest that the death of infected cells plays an important role in protection against and pathogenesis caused by intracellular bacteria. First, several intracellular bacteria, including *S. enterica, Mycobacterium* sp, and *L. monocytogenes,* have exploited ways to induce apoptosis in infected host cells. Apoptosis of infected macrophages as an important means of antigen presentation by bystander DC deserves further investigation. Subsequently, different host cells with killer potential enter the stage in succession. These are, in order of appearance, PNG, NK cells, $\gamma\delta$ T cells, and $\alpha\beta$ T cells. PNG rapidly infiltrate the *L. monocytogenes*–infected liver where they not only contribute to listerial killing but also to hepatocyte damage (100). Elimination of these PNG markedly exacerbates listeriosis (101). Hepatocytes are highly permissive to listerial growth and both *L. monocytogenes*–induced apoptosis and PNG-mediated lysis of these host cells appears to play an important role in

early antilisterial defense. NK cells are activated during intracellular bacterial infections (103). *In vitro,* activated NK cells lyse MP infected with a variety of intracellular bacteria, leaving uninfected target cells unaffected. Activated $\gamma\delta$ T cells and CD1-restricted $\alpha\beta$ T cells are also capable of lysing bacteria-infected target cells. MHC I– and MHC Ib–restricted CD8 T cells as well as MHC class II–restricted CD4 T cells from mice infected with intracellular bacteria rapidly express cytolytic activities after restimulation *in vitro.* Similarly, CD8 and CD4 T cells expressing specific cytolytic activity have been isolated from patients suffering from bacterial infections. A role of CTL in antilisterial resistance has been corroborated by the finding that perforin-deficient KO mice with impaired CTL activity suffer from exacerbated listeriosis (110). At the same time, evidence has been presented that CD8 T cells cause liver damage in experimental listeriosis. CD4 and CD8 T cells in lesions of tuberculoid leprosy patients express phenotypic markers indicative for cytolytic activities (214). CTL generally employ two forms of killer mechanism: apoptosis through Fas/FasL interactions and lysis via perforin-dependent mechanisms (144). Using human CTL clones expressing either form of cytolytic mechanism, evidence was presented that perforin-dependent, but not apoptotic, macrophage death participates in bacterial growth inhibition (215). This antibacterial activity is probably caused by granulysin. Purified granulysin has potent bacteriocidal activity *in vitro* (216). Moreover, granulysin is expressed in granulomatous lesions of leprosy patients (214). It is most likely that an attack of MP by CTL coexpressing perforin and granulysin results in the killing of intracellular bacteria (172,217). Perforin creates pores in the membranes of infected host cells, thus facilitating the translocation of granulysin to the intracellular microbes that are subsequently killed by the latter. Using mouse mutants, no major role for conventional CTL activity mediated by perforin or Fas/FasL interactions in the control of tuberculosis has been found thus far (218,219). However, macrophage death caused by ATP has been shown to result in mycobacteriostasis (64,65). CTL can induce cell death via secretion of ATP, and in this way they may participate in mycobacteriostasis (220). Binding of exogenous ATP to the P2Z receptor apparently causes fusion of phagosomes harboring mycobacteria within lysosomes and this fusion results in both cell death and mycobacteriostasis, independent from RNI and ROI.

Altogether, these findings suggest the participation of cell-destructive mechanisms in intracellular bacterial infections. The concerted action of perforin and granulysin can cause direct killing of intracellular bacteria, and by facilitating release from uncapacitated host cells (be they nonprofessional phagocytes or deactivated MP), lysis promotes bacterial killing by more potent effector mechanisms. Thus, bacteria taken up by blood monocytes immediately after their release from incapacitated cells could be killed more efficiently (221). On the other hand, death of nonprofessional phagocytes may contribute to pathogenesis by affecting physiologic organ functions. In addition, lysis of MP in the absence of bacterial killing is potentially harmful because it can facilitate microbial dissemination.

GRANULOMATOUS LESION

"Idealized Granuloma"

The encounter between intracellular bacteria and host defense is a local event centered on the granulomatous lesion that forms the focus of antibacterial protection (172,222). Failure to develop a granuloma or breakdown of an organized granuloma generally leads to disease exacerbation, often with fatal consequences. At the same time, expanding granulomas impair physiologic tissue function and, therefore, are central to pathogenesis. The "idealized" granuloma is a well-structured and organized lesion composed of T-lymphocytes of diverse phenotype and MP at differing maturation and differentiation stages (Fig. 7). These include multinucleated giant cells, epithelioid cells, freshly immigrant monocytes, and mature MP, among which numerous CD4 T cells are interspersed. The whole is surrounded by an outer mantle primarily composed of CD8 T-lymphocytes. Microorganisms are located inside the granuloma MP. As a result of necrotic death of the inner cells, a caseous, but still solid, center develops. Eventually the lesion is encapsulated by fibrosis and calcification. In the following, the development of an "idealized" granuloma is first described; subsequently, various forms of granulomatous lesions are discussed.

Leukocyte Extravasation

In the early phase of granuloma formation, extravasation of (and invasion by) PNG and, subsequently, blood monocytes is induced by proinflammatory signals mediated by bacterial components (N-f-met–containing peptides, such as f-Met-Leu-Phe or ligands for TLR), complement components (C5a), and cytokines (Fig. 8). Infected MP produce numerous proinflammatory cytokines, such as IL-1, IL-6, and TNF-α, as well as various chemokines that stimulate local endothelial cells and blood phagocytes. In the lung, substance P, a neuropeptide produced by sensory neuronal cells, and MIF may further promote the inflammatory process (223). The inflamed endothelium around the primary lesion expresses elevated levels of adhesion molecules, thus promoting extravasation of inflammatory phagocytes (Fig. 8) (224). Extravasation is mediated by interactions between leukocytes and endothelial cells by means of adhesion molecules (223,224). These include selectins, integrins, and members of the immunoglobulin (Ig) superfamily (Fig. 8).

The L-selectins are found on leukocytes, whereas the P- and E-selectins are expressed by endothelial cells. Selectins are lectins that bind to carbohydrate ligands on the corresponding cell type. The integrins are heterodimers expressed on many cell types, including leukocytes and endothelial cells. At least six different integrins on leukocytes mediate binding to endothelial cells, notably LFA-1, Mac-1,

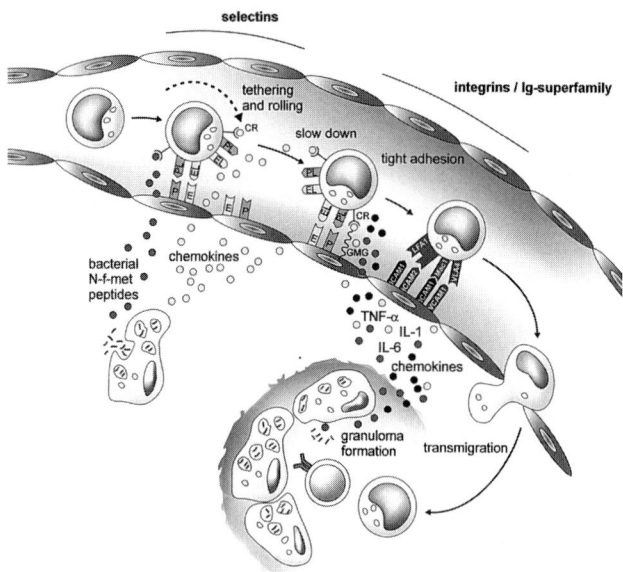

FIG. 8. Influx of phagocytes and T-lymphocytes from the blood to the site of bacterial growth. Selectins and their receptors: E, E-selectin; P, P-selection; EL, E-selectin ligand; PL, P-selectin ligand; integrins: LFA-1, Mac-1, VLA-4; Ig superfamily molecules: ICAM-1, ICAM-2, VCAM-1; CR, chemokine receptor; CMG, glycosaminoglycan.

and VLA-4. The ICAMs are members of the Ig superfamily that include ICAM-1, ICAM-2, ICAM-3, VCAM-1, and PECAM-1. ICAM-1 is strongly induced on leukocytes and endothelial cells. Endothelial cells constitutively express ICAM-2, VCAM-1, and PECAM-1, whereas resting leukocytes bear ICAM-3 and PECAM-1 on their surface. ICAM-1 interacts with the integrins LFA-1 and Mac-1, ICAM-2 and ICAM-3 with LFA-1, VCAM-1 with VLA-4, and PECAM-1 is engaged in homophilic interactions.

Contact between leukocytes and endothelial cells is initiated when the blood vessel is suddenly broadened in diameter at inflammation sites (224). Activated endothelial cells and leukocytes up-regulate surface expression of adhesion molecules and thus promote leukocyte binding to the endothelium. This sets into motion the cascade of adhesion events. Selectin-mediated interactions result in leukocyte tethering and rolling. Subsequently, integrin interactions with Ig superfamily molecules cause tight leukocyte adhesion to endothelial cells. Once leukocytes firmly adhere to the endothelium, transmigration to the inflammatory focus occurs. Up-regulation of P- and E-selectin expression primarily promotes PNG extravasation. In contrast, the L-selectins are constitutively expressed on virtually all leukocytes. Activated and memory T cells as well as inflammatory phagocytes, however, express higher levels of integrins such as LFA-1 and VLA-4 and activated endothelial cells show elevated expression of Ig superfamily molecules. ICAM-1 and VCAM-1 up-regulation is primarily important for monocyte and T-cell transmigration to inflammatory foci. Recent findings have pointed to chemokine receptors as decisive factors for selective T-cell migration (154,204). Differential expression of chemokine receptors on human Th1 and Th2 cells, as well as naïve versus memory T cells, direct preferential migration of Th1 cells to the site of inflammation (204,225). Chemokines can bind to glycosaminoglycans bound to the endothelial surface without loss of biological activity. Interactions between chemokine receptors on lymphocytes and chemokines bound to endothelial cells further promote selective T-cell migration (226). The lack of CCR7 (receptor type 7 for CC chemokines) combined with the low expression of CD62L and the high expression of LFA and of $\alpha4\beta1$ integrin seems characteristic for effector memory Th1 cells that migrate to sites of inflammation. In summary, tethering and rolling, which is then succeeded by tight adhesion and subsequent extravasation of leukocytes, results in leukocyte accumulation at the site of microbial colonization, which forms the basis for granuloma formation.

Granuloma Formation

Although inflammatory PNG and MP restrict bacterial replication, they frequently fail to eradicate their pathogens. At the same time, these phagocytes release proteolytic enzymes that cause tissue damage. The early lesion, therefore, is often exudative. Eventually specific T-lymphocytes are activated in the draining lymph nodes. Recirculating T-lymphocytes passing by the inflammatory lesion are recruited by proinflammatory cytokines and chemokines through mechanisms described above.

Gradually, infiltrating cells become organized and form a granuloma predominantly consisting of MP. Although TNF and IFN-γ participate in this event, LTα3 appears to be of particular importance. Although $\alpha\beta$ T cells are the dominant T-lymphocyte population throughout all stages of granuloma formation, a significant proportion of $\gamma\delta$ T cells has been observed in the initial phase (134). These $\gamma\delta$ T cells apparently play a role in the organization of a tight and well-structured granulomatous lesion because in their absence more loosely structured or even abscess-like lesions develop that represent the characteristic tissue reactions against purulent bacteria. Moreover, evidence has been presented for the participation of group 2 CD1–restricted NK T cells with reactivity for microbial glycolipids in the formation of granulomatous lesions. Finally, group 1 CD1–restricted $\alpha\beta$ T cells have been isolated from skin lesions of leprosy patients indicating their participation in this tissue reaction. Upon antigen-specific interactions with infected MP and DC, T-lymphocytes produce IFN-γ, thus activating antimicrobial macrophage functions.

Granulomas are at the forefront of protection by restricting bacterial replication at, as well as confining pathogens to, discrete foci (Fig. 7). This is achieved by the following: activated MP capable of inhibiting bacterial growth, encapsulation promoted by fibrosis and calcification, and necrosis leading to reduced nutrient and oxygen supply. However, frequently microbial pathogens are not fully eradicated, and

some microorganisms survive in a dormant form. A labile balance between microbial persistence and antibacterial defense develops, which lasts for long periods of time.

Macrophage activation strongly relies on IFN-γ, which is sufficient in the mouse but requires support by TNF and 1,25-dihydroxyvitamin D3 in the human system. Fibrosis and necrosis are primarily promoted by TNF (151). MP are deactivated by various microbial components. Under the influence of these factors, immigrant blood monocytes mature into epithelioid cells and multinucleated giant cells. Sequestering of bacteria in these granuloma MP protects them from host cell attack. Release of these bacteria from lysed MP may facilitate their eradication by more proficient immigrant monocytes. Furthermore, release into the nutrient- and oxygen-deficient necrotic center may restrict bacterial survival. Although the granulomatous lesion may impair tissue functions, detriment to the host usually remains limited and infection does not necessarily cause clinical disease.

Tuberculosis

The productive and proliferative granuloma that effectively controls *M. tuberculosis* best resembles the "idealized" granuloma described above. This lesion can then progress in five directions as described below.

1. The labile balance between microbial persistence and local protection remains equilibrated and succeeds in perpetuating stable immunity in the absence of disease. In more than 90% of *M. tuberculosis*–infected individuals, the microorganism becomes dormant and infection enters into a latent stage (227,228). Recent studies in the mouse point to TNF-α, IFN-γ, and RNI in the maintenance of latent infection. Both CD4 and CD8 T cells contribute to latency, and evidence has been presented that CD4 T cells perform critical functions in addition to IFN-γ secretion resulting in RNI production (229).
2. In very rare cases, the proliferative granuloma succeeds in fully eradicating the microbial pathogens and disappears; an abortive infection has occurred.
3. In the face of a strong immune response, necrotic reactions prevail, thereby extending tissue injury. Extensive secretion of fibrogenic cytokines, including TNF and TGF-β, may then lead to lung fibrosis. Yet, bacteria frequently remain restricted within the necrotic lesion. The clinical disease is thus confined to the affected organ (typically the lung), takes a more benign form, and is usually noncontagious.
4. Provided that cell destructive mechanisms endure, the granuloma becomes exudative and subsequently liquefies. Although mostly attributed to necrotic mechanisms, apoptosis also occurs in granulomatous lesions. In the liquefied cellular detritus, *M. tuberculosis* grows in an uncontrolled manner and extensive tissue damage markedly impairs the affected organ. It is in this cell detritus in which huge numbers (up to 10^9) of *M. tuberculosis* organisms emerge

from which multidrug-resistant tubercle bacilli develop under incomplete chemotherapy. Microbial dissemination through blood circulation promotes infection of secondary organs, and rupture into the bronchoalveolar system facilitates spreading into the environment. Excessive TNF may be released into the circulation and cause cachexia (230). The disease takes a malignant form and is highly contagious.

5. In cases of insufficient or deficient T-cell immunity, the granuloma remains incomplete or breaks down and bacteria are disseminated. In cases of severe immunodeficiency as seen in AIDS patients or in newborn, productive granulomas do not develop at all and infection directly progresses to disseminated, generally fatal, miliary tuberculosis.

Experimental Listeriosis

In experimental listeriosis, development of lesions is arrested at the stage of infiltration by inflammatory phagocytes and specific T-lymphocytes. Because *L. monocytogenes* is rapidly eradicated, a highly structured granuloma does not develop. In fact, formation of lesions is not essentially required for elimination of *L. monocytogenes*. On the other hand, infiltration of PNG, MP, and T cells causes hepatocyte damage, which impairs liver function. Hence, in experimental listeriosis, lesions have a strong pathologic component.

Leprosy

The lesions in tuberculoid leprosy have much resemblance to those in tuberculosis. Toward the lepromatous pole, suppressive mechanisms dictate the fate of the granuloma. Lepromatous leprosy lesions are characterized by the presence of abundant *M. leprae* organisms and deactivated MP, such as foamy macrophages, as well as few T-lymphocytes expressing phenotypic markers characteristic for regulatory T cells with suppressive functions. Evidence for involvement of Th2-like activities in lepromatous leprosy lesions has been presented.

DELAYED-TYPE HYPERSENSITIVITY

An individual immune to an intracellular bacterium will develop a skin reaction at the site of local administration of soluble antigens from this agent. The reaction is characterized by monocyte infiltration and develops after 24 to 72 hours; that is, it is delayed. The first description of a DTH reaction against bacterial antigens was given in 1890 by Koch (91), who showed that guinea pigs infected with *M. tuberculosis* develop a specific inflammatory response against locally applied soluble culture filtrate, which he called tuberculin. In the 1930s, F. Seibert (cited in Kaufmann and Young [231]) produced a purified protein derivative (PPD) by removing the bulk of carbohydrates and enriching for proteins and peptides; PPD is still widely used.

It is now clear that DTH to antigens of intracellular bacteria is mediated by T cells primarily of the CD4 phenotype. Because soluble protein antigens generally fail to enter the MHC class Ia pathway, contribution of conventional CD8 T cells to the DTH reaction must be considered low to absent. An auxiliary role of $\gamma\delta$ T cells, however, appears likely (134). It is not yet clear whether these $\gamma\delta$ T cells respond to specific antigens or whether they are nonspecifically activated by inflammatory stimuli. Although the DTH reaction, like the granulomatous lesion, primarily consists of MP and is dependent on T-lymphocytes, it is a short-lived response lasting for the few days it takes for the proteins to have been degraded. Accordingly, pathology of a DTH reaction is generally minimal. Application of high antigen doses into the skin of individuals with active tuberculosis, however, can cause marked necrotic reactions leading to significant tissue damage.

GENETIC CONTROL OF RESISTANCE AGAINST INTRACELLULAR BACTERIA

Resistance against intracellular bacteria is genetically controlled, and inherited factors are of particular importance in chronic infections with broad clinical spectrum, such as tuberculosis and leprosy. Although the impact of host genetic mechanisms on the outcome of infectious disease has been recognized for a long time, our understanding of the underlying factors remains fragmented. First, resistance to infections is highly polygenic. Second, a marked heterogeneity exists within populations. Third, variability in the genome of the pathogen, as well as environmental factors such as the availability of nutrients, further affect the outcome of the host–pathogen relationship.

The significance of genetic factors was perhaps most dramatically illustrated by the Luebeck disaster, which occurred in 1927 when 251 babies had been vaccinated accidentally with viable *M. tuberculosis* instead of BCG. At the end of the 6-year observation period, six children (2%) still suffered from tuberculosis, 129 (51%) had become ill but recovered, 77 (31%) had died, and in 39 children (16%) clinical signs of tuberculosis had never developed (232). The marked influence of ethnic differences on the prevalence of tuberculosis further supports the role of genetic factors (233).

In the 1940s, Lurie studied native resistance to tuberculosis in rabbits, and by selective inbreeding he succeeded in establishing strains of rabbits that differed remarkably in their susceptibility to infection with *M. tuberculosis* (92). Similarly, congenic mouse strains that differ in their susceptibility to experimental infection with several intracellular bacteria have been developed (234).

At least three levels of the host–pathogen relationship serve as potential targets for genetic control. These three are briefly described below.

1. Genetic factors decide whether infection becomes abortive or establishes itself in a stable form. Convincing evidence for genetic control mechanisms at this level does not exist.

2. Genetic factors control transition from infection to disease. This control step segregates "susceptible" from "resistant" individuals. Such inherited influences are well proven in mice and are most likely in the human population.
3. Severity and/or form of disease are controlled by genetic factors. It is generally accepted that MHC class II–encoded factors influence the development of leprosy towards the tuberculoid or the lepromatous pole.

Control of Innate Antibacterial Resistance by the Nramp1 Gene

Studies in the mouse system have revealed a single dominant autosomal gene on chromosome 1, which is responsible for resistance against *M. bovis* BCG, *M. lepraemurium*, *M. avium/M. intracellulare*, *S. enterica*, and the protozoan pathogen *Listeria donovani*. In contrast, murine resistance against other intracellular bacteria, most remarkably *M. tuberculosis*, is apparently not controlled by this gene (234). Positional cloning led to the identification of a full-length cDNA sequence. The responsible gene has been named Nramp1 for natural-resistance–associated macrophage protein (235,236). The gene belongs to a family of genes that also encompasses Nramp2 on mouse chromosome 15. The human syntenic genes Nramp1 and Nramp2 have been identified on chromosomes 2q and 12q, respectively (237). The Nramp1 gene product shows 85% identity/92% similarity with its murine cognate.

The functional importance of Nramp1 could be proven using transfected macrophage cell lines and by the generation of gene-disruption mutant mice (238,239). Differential susceptibility of Nramp1^s and Nramp1^r mouse strains can be traced to a single, nonconservative glycine to aspartic acid substitution at position 169 of the Nramp1 gene product. Importantly, transfer of the glycine 169 allele of Nramp1 into animals of susceptible background reestablishes resistance to *M. bovis* BCG infection.

Expression of the Nramp1 gene product is restricted to professional phagocytes, whereas the Nramp2 product is found in various cell types (240). The Nramp1 polypeptide is an integral membrane protein that contains several phosphorylation sites. It is found in the late endosome rather than on the outer surface of macrophages (241). Because it has characteristic features of transporter molecules, it is likely that Nramp1 participates in ion transport in and out of the phagosome. The role of Nramp1 in controlling infectious diseases in humans remains controversial (167,242,243). Linkage of Nramp1 and leprosy has been reported for the Vietnamese population but not for populations in India and Africa. However, an association of Nramp1 with increased susceptibility to tuberculosis has been described recently in patients from African populations (244). These highly divergent results underline the highly polygenic nature of resistance to tuberculosis, comprising both host and exogenous factors.

Vitamin D Receptor

As discussed previously, 1,25-dihydroxyvitamin D3 participates in the activation of antibacterial capacities in human macrophages. Evidence for a role of the vitamin D–receptor polymorphism in resistance to pulmonary tuberculosis has been described in certain populations (242,245,246). The availability of 1,25-dihydroxyvitamin D3 depends on uptake of the precursor and its conversion under the influence of UV light. Hence, susceptibility is influenced by both genetic and environmental factors, further complicating comparisons of different populations.

MHC Control of Severity and Form of Disease

Human malaria caused by the protozoan parasite *Plasmodium* sp represents the best example of the impact of MHC molecules on the severity of disease. Moreover, these studies emphasize the profound influence of natural selection against infection on MHC polymorphism (167,242). Segregation analyses in various human populations also indicate linkage of human leukocyte antigen (HLA) types with severity of tuberculosis and leprosy. Strong evidence exists to suggest an influence of the HLA on the development towards the tuberculoid or the lepromatous pole of leprosy. Although some linkage with MHC class I molecules has been observed in certain populations, MHC class II control appears to be more important (242). Originally, it was found that HLA-DR2 subtypes are linked with increased incidences of lepromatous leprosy, and that HLA-DR3 represents a linkage marker for tuberculoid leprosy. Recent population-based association studies, however, have provided evidence for an association between distinct HLA-DR2 alleles and susceptibility to tuberculoid leprosy. In tuberculosis, evidence for association of HLA-DR2 subtypes with pulmonary tuberculosis has been found. With more data from various population groups being available, it is becoming increasingly clear that HLA-DR associations with distinct disease forms differ among population groups, thus making it often impossible to extrapolate from one population to another. Again, these discrepancies underline the polygenic nature of resistance to infectious diseases.

CONCLUSIONS AND OUTLOOK

It is hoped that the reader of this chapter not only has become familiar with the principal mechanisms underlying immunity against intracellular bacteria but also realizes the great complexity of this system. Understanding intracellular bacterial infections requires knowledge not only of immunology, but also of molecular biology of the infectious agent and biology of the target cell. *In vitro* analyses can only provide incomplete answers to the questions relevant to antibacterial immunity and must be complemented by *in vivo* experiments.

Despite the high degree of complexity, such interdisciplinary research efforts almost certainly will provide rewards.

First, understanding the performance of the immune system in bacterial infections can provide clues to questions pertinent to basic immunology. Knowledge of the rules underlying the extraordinary plasticity and adaptability of the immune system required for coping with transmutable "viable antigens" that developed during millennia of coexistence will provide deeper insights into the immunoregulation and evolution of the immune system. Second, applied questions will benefit equally well from these approaches. With the increasing inadequacy of chemotherapy in the control of bacterial infections, the need for adjunctive immune measures is gaining further importance. Rational strategies toward vaccination and immunotherapy will benefit from the deeper understanding of the immune mechanisms operative in intracellular bacterial infections. With the elucidation of the genomes of all major intracellular pathogens, and the elucidation of the human and murine genomes nearing completion, this type of interdisciplinary research has, in fact, entered a new phase. Global analyses at the transcriptome and proteome levels will undoubtedly provide a comprehensive view of this dynamic interplay in the near future. The reader may find it ironic that the spirit of these investigations remains the same as it was at the early beginnings of immunology, which started as an approach to the intervention of bacterial infections.

ACKNOWLEDGMENTS

I would like to acknowledge financial support from the German Science Foundation, the Bundesministerium für Bildung und Forschung, the World Health Organization, the European Community, and Fonds Chemie. I am grateful to T. Ulrichs for drawing some of the figures, L. Lom-Terborg for her excellent assistance with the manuscript, and D. Schad for graphics work.

REFERENCES

1. Neutra MR, Kraehenbuhl JP. Regional immune response to microbial pathogens. In: Kaufmann SHE, Sher A, Ahmed R, eds. *Immunology of infectious diseases.* Washington, DC: ASM Press, 2002:191–206.
2. Schlossberg D. *Tuberculosis.* 3rd ed. New York: Springer, 1988.
3. Mackaness GB. Cellular resistance to infection. *J Exp Med* 1962; 116:381–406.
4. Kaufmann SHE, Raupach B, Finlay BB, eds. Microbiology and immunology: lessons learned from Salmonella. *Microbes Infect* 2001;3: 1177–1375.
5. Vazquez-Boland JA, Kuhn M, Berche P, et al. Listeria pathogenesis and molecular virulence determinants. *Clin Microbiol Rev* 2001;14:584–640.
6. Cianciotto N, Eisenstein BI, Engleberg NC, et al. Genetics and molecular pathogenesis of Legionella pneumophila, an intracellular parasite of macrophages. *Mol Biol Med* 1989;6:409–424.
7. Hastings RC. *Leprosy.* 2nd ed. Edinburgh: Churchill Livingstone, 1994.
8. Sandstrom G. The tularaemia vaccine. *J Chem Technol Biotechnol* 1994;59:315–320.
9. Smith LD, Ficht TA. Pathogenesis of Brucella. *Crit Rev Microbiol* 1990;17:209–230.
10. Marre R, Abu Kwaik Y, Bartelt C, et al., eds. *Legionella.* Washington: ASM Press, 2001.
11. Hackstadt T. The biology of rickettsiae. *Infect Agents Dis* 1996;5:127–143.
12. Moulder JW. Interaction of chlamydiae and host cells in vitro. *Microbiol Rev* 1991;55:143–190.
13. Dunne M. The evolving relationship between Chlamydia pneumoniae and atherosclerosis. *Curr Opin Infect Dis* 2000;13:583–591.
14. Glaser P, Frangeul L, Buchrieser C, et al. Comparative genomics of Listeria species. *Science* 2001;294:849–852.
15. McClelland M, Sanderson KE, Spieth J, et al. Complete genome sequence of Salmonella enterica serovar Typhimurium LT2. *Nature* 2001;413:852–856.
16. Parkhill J, Dougan G, James KD, et al. Complete genome sequence of a multiple drug resistant Salmonella enterica serovar Typhi CT18. *Nature* 2001;413:848–852.
17. Cole ST, Brosch R, Parkhill J, et al. Deciphering the biology of Mycobacterium tuberculosis from the complete genome sequence. *Nature* 1998;393:537–544.
18. Kaufmann SHE. How can immunology contribute to the control of tuberculosis? *Nat Rev Immunol* 2001;1:20–30.
19. Kaufmann SH. Is the development of a new tuberculosis vaccine possible? *Nat Med* 2000;6:955–960.
20. Flynn JL, Chan J. Immunology of tuberculosis. *Annu Rev Immunol* 2001;19:93–129.
21. Behr MA, Wilson MA, Gill WP, et al. Comparative genomics of BCG vaccines by whole-genome DNA microarray. *Science* 1999;284: 1520–1523.
22. Le Minor L. Typing of Salmonella species. *Eur J Clin Microbiol Infect Dis* 1988;7:214–218.
23. Finlay BB, Cossart P. Exploitation of mammalian host cell functions by bacterial pathogens. *Science* 1997;276:718–725.
24. Swanson JA, Baer SC. Phagocytosis by zippers and triggers. *Trends Cell Biol* 1995;5:89–92.
25. Mengaud J, Ohayon H, Gounon P, et al. E-cadherin is the receptor for internalin, a surface protein required for entry of L. monocytogenes into epithelial cells. *Cell* 1996;84:923–932.
26. Lecuit M, Vandormael-Pournin S, Lefort J, et al. A transgenic model for listeriosis: role of internalin in crossing the intestinal barrier. *Science* 2001;292:1722–1725.
27. Rambukkana A, Salzer JL, Yurchenco PD, et al. Neural targeting of Mycobacterium leprae mediated by the G domain of the laminin-alpha2 chain. *Cell* 1997;88:811–821.
28. Galan JE, Pace J, Hayman MJ. Involvement of the epidermal growth factor receptor in the invasion of cultured mammalian cells by Salmonella typhimurium. *Nature* 1992;357:588–589.
29. Jones BD, Falkow S. Salmonellosis: host immune responses and bacterial virulence determinants. *Annu Rev Immunol* 1996;14:533–561.
30. Hansen-Wester I, Hensel M. Salmonella pathogenicity islands encoding type III secretion systems. *Microbes Infect* 2001;3:549–559.
31. Parsot C, Sansonetti PJ. Invasion and the pathogenesis of Shigella infections. *Curr Top Microbiol Immunol* 1996;209:25–42.
32. Brown DG, Gordon S. Phagocytosis and anti-infective immunity. In: Kaufmann SHE, Sher A, Ahmed R, eds. *Immunology of infectious diseases.* Washington, DC: ASM Press, 2002:79–92.
33. Janeway CA Jr. The immune system evolved to discriminate infectious nonself from noninfectious self. *Immunol Today* 1992;13:11–16.
34. Akira S, Takeda K, Kaisho T. Toll-like receptors: critical proteins linking innate and acquired immunity. *Nat Immunol* 2001;2:675–680.
35. Krutzik SR, Sieling PA, Modlin RL. The role of Toll-like receptors in host defense against microbial infection. *Curr Opin Immunol* 2001;13:104–108.
36. Medzhitov R. Toll-like receptors and innate immunity. *Nat Rev Immunol* 2001;1:135–145.
37. Stahl PD. The mannose receptor and other macrophage lectins. *Curr Opin Immunol* 1992;4:49–52.
38. Ulevitch RJ, Tobias PS. Receptor-dependent mechanisms of cell stimulation by bacterial endotoxin. *Annu Rev Immunol* 1995;13:437–457.
39. Fenton MJ, Golenbock DT. LPS-binding proteins and receptors. *J.Leukoc.Biol* 1998;64:25–32.
40. Aderem A, Ulevitch RJ. Toll-like receptors in the induction of the innate immune response. *Nature* 2000;406:782–787.
41. Ofek I, Sharon N. Lectinophagocytosis: a molecular mechanism of recognition between cell surface sugars and lectins in the phagocytosis of bacteria. *Infect Immun* 1988;56:539–547.
42. Schlesinger LS. Role of mononuclear phagocytes in M. tuberculosis pathogenesis. *J Investig Med* 1996;44:312–323.

43. Pearson AM. Scavenger receptors in innate immunity. *Curr Opin Immunol* 1996;8:20–28.

44. Krieger M, Herz J. Structures and functions of multiligand lipoprotein receptors: macrophage scavenger receptors and LDL receptor-related protein (LRP). *Annu Rev Biochem* 1994;63:601–637.

45. Ruoslahti E. Fibronectin and its receptors. *Annu Rev Biochem* 1988;57:375–413.

46. Schaible UE, Collins HL, Kaufmann SH. Confrontation between intracellular bacteria and the immune system. *Adv Immunol* 1999; 71:267–377.

47. Carroll MC. The role of complement and complement receptors in induction and regulation of immunity. *Annu Rev Immunol* 1998;16:545–568.

48. Elsbach P, Weiss J. A reevaluation of the roles of the O2-dependent and O2-independent microbicidal systems of phagocytes. *Rev Infect Dis* 1983;5:843–853.

49. Schorey JS, Carroll MC, Brown EJ. A macrophage invasion mechanism of pathogenic mycobacteria. *Science* 1997;277:1091–1093.

50. Hu C, Mayadas-Norton T, Tanaka K, et al. Mycobacterium tuberculosis infection in complement receptor 3-deficient mice. *J Immunol* 2000;165:2596–2602.

51. Horwitz MA. Phagocytosis of the Legionnaires' disease bacterium (Legionella pneumophila) occurs by a novel mechanism: engulfment within a pseudopod coil. *Cell* 1984;36:27–33.

52. Hynes RO. *Fibronectins*. New York: Springer Verlag, 1990.

53. Belisle JT, Vissa VD, Sievert T, et al. Role of the major antigen of Mycobacterium tuberculosis in cell wall biogenesis. *Science* 1997;276:1420–1422.

54. Menozzi FD, Rouse JH, Alavi M, et al. Identification of a heparin-binding hemagglutinin present in mycobacteria. *J Exp Med* 1996;184: 993–1001.

55. Downing JF, Pasula R, Wright JR, et al. Surfactant protein a promotes attachment of Mycobacterium tuberculosis to alveolar macrophages during infection with human immunodeficiency virus. *Proc Natl Acad Sci U S A* 1995;92:4848–4852.

56. Pethe K, Alonso S, Biet F, et al. The heparin-binding haemagglutinin of M. tuberculosis is required for extrapulmonary dissemination. *Nature* 2001;412:190–194.

57. Pieters J. Evasion of host cell defense mechanisms by pathogenic bacteria. *Curr Opin Immunol* 2001;13:37–44.

58. Mellman I. Endocytosis and molecular sorting. *Annu Rev Cell Dev Biol* 1996;12:575–625.

59. Sturgill-Koszycki S, Schlesinger PH, Chakraborty P, et al. Lack of acidification in Mycobacterium phagosomes produced by exclusion of the vesicular proton-ATPase. *Science* 1994;263:678–681.

60. Selsted ME, Quellette AJ. Defensins in granules of phagocytic and non-phagocytic cells. *Trends Cell Biol* 2001;5:114–119.

61. Ganz T, Lehrer RI. Defensins and cathelicidins: antimicrobial peptide effectors of mammalian innate immunity. In: Kaufmann SHE, Sher A, Ahmed R, eds. *Immunology of infectious diseases*. Washington, DC: ASM Press, 2002:105–110.

62. Galan JE. Alternative strategies for becoming an insider: lessons from the bacterial world. *Cell* 2000;103:363–366.

63. Armstrong JA, Hart PD. Response of cultured macrophages to Mycobacterium tuberculosis, with obervation on fusion lysosomes with phagosomes. *J Exp Med* 1971;134:713–740.

64. Lammas DA, Stober C, Harvey CJ, et al. ATP-induced killing of mycobacteria by human macrophages is mediated by purinergic P2Z (P2X7) receptors. *Immunity* 1997;7:433–444.

65. Molloy A, Laochumroonvorapong P, Kaplan G. Apoptosis, but not necrosis, of infected monocytes is coupled with killing of intracellular bacillus Calmette–Guerin. *J Exp Med* 1994;180:1499–1509.

66. Lieu PT, Heiskala M, Peterson PA, et al. The roles of iron in health and disease. *Mol Aspects Med* 2001;22:1–87.

67. Andrews NC. Iron metabolism: iron deficiency and iron overload. *Annu Rev Genomics Hum Genet* 2000;1:75–98.

68. Ehrlich R, Lemonnier FA. HFE—a novel nonclassical class I molecule that is involved in iron metabolism. *Immunity* 2000;13:585–588.

69. Gobin J, Moore CH, Reeve JR Jr, et al. Iron acquisition by Mycobacterium tuberculosis: isolation and characterization of a family of iron-binding exochelins. *Proc Natl Acad Sci U S A* 1995;92:5189–5193.

70. Gobin J, Horwitz MA. Exochelins of Mycobacterium tuberculosis remove iron from human iron–binding proteins and donate iron to mycobactins in the M. tuberculosis cell wall. *J Exp Med* 1996; 183:1527–1532.

71. Byrne GI, Lehmann LK, Landry GJ. Induction of tryptophan catabolism is the mechanism for gamma-interferon–mediated inhibition of intracellular Chlamydia psittaci replication in T24 cells. *Infect Immun* 1986;53:347–351.

72. Pfefferkorn ER. Interferon gamma blocks the growth of Toxoplasma gondii in human fibroblasts by inducing the host cells to degrade tryptophan. *Proc Natl Acad Sci U S A* 1984;81:908–912.

73. MacMicking J, Xie QW, Nathan C. Nitric oxide and macrophage function. *Annu Rev Immunol* 1997;15:323–350.

74. Raupach B, Kaufmann SH. Immune responses to intracellular bacteria. *Curr Opin Immunol* 2001;13:417–428.

75. Bogdan C. Nitric oxide and the immune response. *Nat Immunol* 2001; 2:907–916.

76. MacMicking JD, Nathan C, Hom G, et al. Altered responses to bacterial infection and endotoxic shock in mice lacking inducible nitric oxide synthase. *Cell* 1995;81:641–650.

77. MacMicking JD, North RJ, LaCourse R, et al. Identification of nitric oxide synthase as a protective locus against tuberculosis. *Proc Natl Acad Sci U S A* 1997;94:5243–5248.

78. Mastroeni P, Vazquez-Torres A, Fang FC, et al. Antimicrobial actions of the NADPH phagocyte oxidase and inducible nitric oxide synthase in experimental salmonellosis. II. Effects on microbial proliferation and host survival in vivo. *J Exp Med* 2000;192:237–248.

79. Vazquez-Torres A, Jones-Carson J, Mastroeni P, et al. Antimicrobial actions of the NADPH phagocyte oxidase and inducible nitric oxide synthase in experimental salmonellosis. I. Effects on microbial killing by activated peritoneal macrophages in vitro. *J Exp Med* 2000;192:227–236.

80. Chan ED, Chan J, Schluger NW. What is the role of nitric oxide in murine and human host defense against tuberculosis? Current knowledge. *Am J Respir Cell Mol Biol* 2001;25:606–612.

81. Nicholson S, Bonecini-Almeida M, Lapa e Silva JR, et al. Inducible nitric oxide synthase in pulmonary alveolar macrophages from patients with tuberculosis. *J Exp Med* 1996;183:2293–2302.

82. Vazquez-Torres A, Xu Y, Jones-Carson J, et al. Salmonella pathogenicity island 2-dependent evasion of the phagocyte NADPH oxidase. *Science* 2000;287:1655–1658.

83. Ehrt S, Shiloh MU, Ruan J, et al. A novel antioxidant gene from Mycobacterium tuberculosis. *J Exp Med* 1997;186:1885–1896.

84. Lasa I, Cossart P. Actin-based bacterial motility: towards a definition of the minimal requirements. *Trends Cell Biol* 1996;6:109–114.

85. Sanders MC, Theriot JA. Tails from the hall of infection: actin-based motility of pathogens. *Trends Microbiol* 1996;4:211–213.

86. Welch MD, Iwamatsu A, Mitchison TJ. Actin polymerization is induced by Arp2/3 protein complex at the surface of Listeria monocytogenes. *Nature* 1997;385:265–269.

87. Majno G, Joris I. Apoptosis, oncosis, and necrosis. An overview of cell death. *Am J Pathol* 1995;146:3–15.

88. Navarre WW, Zychlinsky A. Pathogen-induced apoptosis of macrophages: a common end for different pathogenic strategies. *Cell Microbiol* 2000;2:265–273.

89. Weinrauch Y, Zychlinsky A. The induction of apoptosis by bacterial pathogens. *Annu Rev Microbiol* 1999;53:155–187.

90. Metchnikoff M. *Immunity to infectious diseases*. London: Cambridge University Press, 1905.

91. Koch R. Weitere Mitteilungen über ein Heilmittel gegen Tuberkulose. *Dtsch Med Wochenschr* 1890;16:1029–1032.

92. Lurie MB. *Resistance to tuberculosis*. Cambridge, MA: Harvard University Press, 1964.

93. Bloom BR, Bennett B. Mechanism of a reaction in vitro associated with delayed-type hypersensitivity. *Science* 1966;153:80–82.

94. David JR. Delayed hypersensitivity in vitro: its mediation by cell-free substances formed by lymphoid cell-antigen interaction. *Proc Natl Acad Sci U S A* 1966;56:72–77.

95. Bach EA, Aguet M, Schreiber RD. The IFN gamma receptor: a paradigm for cytokine receptor signaling. *Annu Rev Immunol* 1997;15:563–591.

96. Boehm U, Klamp T, Groot M, et al. Cellular responses to interferon-gamma. *Annu Rev Immunol* 1997;15:749–795.

97. Kaufmann SH. Immunity to intracellular bacteria. *Annu Rev Immunol* 1993;11:129–163.

98. Haslett C, Savill JS, Meagher L. The neutrophil. *Curr Opin Immunol* 1989;2:10–18.

99. Conlan JW, North RJ. Neutrophil-mediated dissolution of infected host cells as a defense strategy against a facultative intracellular bacterium. *J Exp Med* 1991;174:741–744.

100. Rogers HW, Unanue ER. Neutrophils are involved in acute, non-specific resistance to Listeria monocytogenes in mice. *Infect Immun* 1993;61:5090–5096.

101. Conlan JW, North RJ. Neutrophils are essential for early anti-Listeria defense in the liver, but not in the spleen or peritoneal cavity, as revealed by a granulocyte-depleting monoclonal antibody. *J Exp Med* 1994;179:259–268.

102. Seiler P, Aichele P, Raupach B, et al. Rapid neutrophil response controls fast replicating intracellular bacteria, but not slow replicating Mycobacterium tuberculosis. *J Infect Dis* 2000;181:671–688.

102a. Reeves EP, Lu H, Jacobs HL, et al. Killing activity of neutrophils is mediated through activation of proteases by K+ flux. *Nature* 2002; 416:291–297.

102b. Weinrauch Y, Drugan D, Shapiro SD, et al. Neutrophil elastase targets virulence factors of enterobacteria. *Nature* 2002;417:91–94.

103. Unanue E. Innate immunity in bacterial infections. In: Kaufmann SHE, Sher A, Ahmed R, eds. *Immunology of infectious diseases.* Washington, DC: ASM Press, 2002:93–104.

104. Reis e Sousa C. Dendritic cells as sensors of infection. *Immunity* 2001;14:495–498.

105. Banchereau J, Steinman RM. Dendritic cells and the control of immunity. *Nature* 1998;392:245–252.

106. Lanzavecchia A, Sallusto F. The instructive role of dendritic cells on T cell responses: lineages, plasticity and kinetics. *Curr Opin Immunol* 2001;13:291–298.

107. Lanzavecchia A, Sallusto F. Regulation of T cell immunity by dendritic cells. *Cell* 2001;106:263–266.

108. Banchereau J, Briere F, Caux C, et al. Immunobiology of dendritic cells. *Annu Rev Immunol* 2000;18:767–811.

109. Reimann J, Kaufmann SH. Alternative antigen processing pathways in anti-infective immunity. *Curr Opin Immunol* 1997;9:462–469.

110. Harty JT, Tvinnereim AR, White DW. CD8+ T cell effector mechanisms in resistance to infection. *Annu Rev Immunol* 2000;18:275–308.

111. Pamer E, Cresswell P. Mechanisms of MHC class I–restricted antigen processing. *Annu Rev Immunol* 1998;16:323–358.

112. Russmann H, Shams H, Poblete F, et al. Delivery of epitopes by the Salmonella type III secretion system for vaccine development. *Science* 1998;281:565–568.

113. Pfeifer JD, Wick MJ, Roberts RL, et al. Phagocytic processing of bacterial antigens for class I MHC presentation to T cells. *Nature* 1993; 361:359–362.

114. Kovacsovics-Bankowski M, Rock KL. A phagosome-to-cytosol pathway for exogenous antigens presented on MHC class I molecules. *Science* 1995;267:243–246.

115. Yrlid U, Wick MJ. Salmonella-induced apoptosis of infected macrophages results in presentation of a bacteria-encoded antigen after uptake by bystander dendritic cells. *J Exp Med* 2000;191:613–624.

116. den Haan JM, Bevan MJ. Antigen presentation to CD8+ T cells: cross-priming in infectious diseases. *Curr Opin Immunol* 2001;13:437–441.

117. Lo WF, Woods AS, DeCloux A, et al. Molecular mimicry mediated by MHC class Ib molecules after infection with gram-negative pathogens. *Nat Med* 2000;6:215–218.

118. Lenz LL, Bevan MJ. H2-M3 restricted presentation of Listeria monocytogenes antigens. *Immunol Rev* 1996;151:107–121.

119. Lindahl KF, Byers DE, Dabhi VM, et al. H2-M3, a full-service class Ib histocompatibility antigen. *Annu Rev Immunol* 1997;15:851–879.

120. Lenz LL, Dere B, Bevan MJ. Identification of an H2-M3-restricted Listeria epitope: implications for antigen presentation by M3. *Immunity* 1996;5:63–72.

121. Chun T, Serbina NV, Nolt D, et al. Induction of M3-restricted cytotoxic T lymphocyte responses by N-formylated peptides derived from Mycobacterium tuberculosis. *J Exp Med* 2001;193:1213–1220.

122. Rolph MS, Kaufmann SH. Partially TAP-independent protection against Listeria monocytogenes by H2-M3–restricted CD8+ T cells. *J Immunol* 2000;165:4575–4580.

123. Porcelli SA, Modlin RL. The CD1 system: antigen-presenting molecules for T cell recognition of lipids and glycolipids. *Annu Rev Immunol* 1999;17:297–329.

124. Park SH, Bendelac A. CD1-restricted T-cell responses and microbial infection. *Nature* 2000;406:788–792.

125. Moody DB, Besra GS. Glycolipid targets of CD1-mediated T-cell responses. *Immunology* 2001;104:243–251.

126. Beckman EM, Porcelli SA, Morita CT, et al. Recognition of a lipid antigen by CD1-restricted alpha beta+ T cells. *Nature* 1994;372:691–694.

127. Schaible UE, Kaufmann SH. CD1 and CD1-restricted T cells in infections with intracellular bacteria. *Trends Microbiol* 2000;8:419–425.

128. Behar SM, Dascher CC, Grusby MJ, et al. Susceptibility of mice deficient in CD1D or TAP1 to infection with Mycobacterium tuberculosis. *J Exp Med* 1999;189:1973–1980.

129. Szalay G, Ladel CH, Blum C, et al. Cutting edge: anti-CD1 monoclonal antibody treatment reverses the production patterns of TGF-beta 2 and Th1 cytokines and ameliorates listeriosis in mice. *J Immunol* 1999;162:6955–6958.

130. Szalay G, Zugel U, Ladel CH, et al. Participation of group 2 CD1 molecules in the control of murine tuberculosis. *Microbes Infect* 1999;1:1153–1157.

131. Apostolou I, Takahama Y, Belmant C, et al. Murine natural killer T (NKT) cells contribute to the granulomatous reaction caused by mycobacterial cell walls. *Proc Natl Acad Sci U S A* 1999;96:5141–5146.

132. Rolph MS, Raupach B, Kobernick HH, et al. MHC class Ia-restricted T cells partially account for beta2-microglobulin–dependent resistance to Mycobacterium tuberculosis. *Eur J Immunol* 2001;31:1944–1949.

133. Kaufmann SH. gamma/delta and other unconventional T lymphocytes: what do they see and what do they do? *Proc Natl Acad Sci U S A* 1996;93:2272–2279.

134. Hayday AC. γδ cells: a right time and a right place for a conserved third way of protection. *Annu Rev Immunol* 2000;18:975–1026.

135. Constant P, Davodeau F, Peyrat MA, et al. Stimulation of human gamma delta T cells by nonpeptidic mycobacterial ligands. *Science* 1994;264:267–270.

136. Tanaka Y, Morita CT, Tanaka Y, et al. Natural and synthetic nonpeptide antigens recognized by human gamma delta T cells. *Nature* 1995;375:155–158.

137. Altincicek B, Moll J, Campos N, et al. Cutting edge: human gamma delta T cells are activated by intermediates of the 2-C-methyl-D-erythritol 4-phosphate pathway of isoprenoid biosynthesis. *J Immunol* 2001;166:3655–3658.

138. Belmant C, Espinosa E, Poupot R, et al. 3-Formyl-1-butyl pyrophosphate: a novel mycobacterial metabolite-activating human gammadelta T cells. *J Biol Chem* 1999;274:32079–32084.

139. Ladel CH, Blum C, Dreher A, et al. Protective role of gamma/delta T cells and alpha/beta T cells in tuberculosis. *Eur J Immunol* 1995; 25:2877–2881.

140. D'Souza CD, Cooper AM, Frank AA, et al. An anti-inflammatory role for gamma delta T lymphocytes in acquired immunity to Mycobacterium tuberculosis. *J Immunol* 1997;158:1217–1221.

141. Sim GK. Intraepithelial lymphocytes and the immune system. *Adv Immunol* 1995;58:297–343.

142. Abbas AK, Murphy KM, Sher A. Functional diversity of helper T lymphocytes. *Nature* 1996;383:787–793.

143. Mosmann TR, Fowell DJ. The Th1/Th2 paradigm in infections. In: Kaufmann SHE, Sher A, Ahmed R, eds. *Immunology of infectious diseases.* Washington, DC: ASM Press, 2002:163–174.

144. Liu CC, Young LH, Young JD. Lymphocyte-mediated cytolysis and disease. *N Engl J Med* 1996;335:1651–1659.

145. Hess J, Gentschev I, Miko D, et al. Superior efficacy of secreted over somatic antigen display in recombinant Salmonella vaccine induced protection against listeriosis. *Proc Natl Acad Sci U S A* 1996;93:1458–1463.

146. Grode L, Kursar M, Fensterle J, et al. Cell-mediated immunity induced by recombinant Mycobacterium bovis Bacille-Calmette–Guérin strains against an intracellular bacterial pathogen: importance of antigen secretion or membrane-targeted antigen display as lipoprotein for vaccine efficacy. *J Immunol* 2002;168:1869–1876.

147. Busch DH, Kerksiek K, Pamer EG. Processing of Listeria monocytogenes antigens and the in vivo T-cell response to bacterial infection. *Immunol Rev* 1999;172:163–169.

148. Kerksiek KM, Pamer EG. T cell responses to bacterial infection. *Curr Opin Immunol* 1999;11:400–405.

149. Bousso P. Generation of MHC-peptide tetramers: a new opportunity for dissecting T-cell immune responses. *Microbes Infect* 2000;2:425–429.

150. Dinarello CA. Role of interleukin-1 in infectious diseases. *Immunol Rev* 1992;127:119–146.

151. Vassalli P. The pathophysiology of tumor necrosis factors. *Annu Rev Immunol* 1992;10:411–452.

152. Taga T, Kishimoto T. Gp130 and the interleukin-6 family of cytokines. *Annu Rev Immunol* 1997;15:797–819.

153. Metz CN, Bucala R. Role of macrophage migration inhibitory factor in the regulation of the immune response. *Adv Immunol* 1997;66:197–223.

154. Yoshie O, Imai T, Nomiyama H. Chemokines in immunity. *Adv Immunol* 2001;78:57–110.

155. Zlotnik A, Yoshie O. Chemokines: a new classification system and their role in immunity. *Immunity* 2000;12:121–127.

156. Kurihara T, Warr G, Loy J, et al. Defects in macrophage recruitment and host defense in mice lacking the CCR2 chemokine receptor. *J Exp Med* 1997;186:1757–1762.

157. Peters W, Scott HM, Chambers HF, et al. Chemokine receptor 2 serves an early and essential role in resistance to Mycobacterium tuberculosis. *Proc Natl Acad Sci U S A* 2001;98:7958–7963.

158. Lu B, Rutledge BJ, Gu L, et al. Abnormalities in monocyte recruitment and cytokine expression in monocyte chemoattractant protein 1-deficient mice. *J Exp Med* 1998;187:601–608.

159. Koebernick H, Grode L, David JR, et al. Macrophage migration inhibitory factor (MIF) plays a pivotal role in immunity against Salmonella typhimurium. *Proc Natl Acad Sci USA* 2002;99:3681–3686.

159a. Tramontana JM, Utaipat U, Molloy A, et al. Thalidomide treatment reduces tumor necrosis factor alpha production and enhances weight gain in patients with pulmonary tuberculosis. *Mol Med* 1995;1:384–397.

160. Sampaio EP, Kaplan G, Miranda A, et al. The influence of thalidomide on the clinical and immunologic manifestation of erythema nodosum leprosum. *J Infect Dis* 1993;168:408–414.

161. Flynn JL, Goldstein MM, Chan J, et al. Tumor necrosis factor-alpha is required In the protective immune response against Mycobacterium tuberculosis in mice. *Immunity* 1995;2:561–572.

162. Cooper AM, Dalton DK, Stewart TA, et al. Disseminated tuberculosis in interferon gamma gene–disrupted mice. *J Exp Med* 1993;178:2243–2247.

163. Flynn JL, Chan J, Triebold KJ, et al. An essential role for interferon gamma in resistance to Mycobacterium tuberculosis infection. *J Exp Med* 1993;178:2249–2254.

164. Roach DR, Briscoe H, Saunders B, et al. Lymphotoxin, Tnf, tuberculosis, granuloma, lung. Secreted lymphotoxin-alpha is essential for the control of an intracellular bacterial infection. *J Exp Med* 2001;193:239–246.

165. Jouanguy E, Altare F, Lamhamedi S, et al. Interferon-gamma–receptor deficiency in an infant with fatal bacille Calmette–Guerin infection. *N Engl J Med* 1996;335:1956–1961.

166. Newport MJ, Huxley CM, Huston S, et al. A mutation in the interferon-gamma–receptor gene and susceptibility to mycobacterial infection. *N Engl J Med* 1996;335:1941–1949.

167. Abel L, Casanova J-L. Immunogenetics of the host response to bacteria and parasites in humans. In: Kaufmann SHE, Sher A, Ahmed R, eds. *Immunology of infectious diseases*. Washington, DC: ASM Press, 2002:395–406.

168. Keane J, Gershon S, Wise RP, et al. Tuberculosis associated with infliximab, a tumor necrosis factor alpha–neutralizing agent. *N Engl J Med* 2001;345:1098–1104.

169. Maini R, St Clair EW, Breedveld F, et al. Infliximab (chimeric anti-tumour necrosis factor alpha monoclonal antibody) versus placebo in rheumatoid arthritis patients receiving concomitant methotrexate: a randomised phase III trial. *Lancet* 1999;354:1932–1939.

170. Hirsch CS, Hussain R, Toossi Z, et al. Cross-modulation by transforming growth factor beta in human tuberculosis: suppression of antigen-driven blastogenesis and interferon gamma production. *Proc Natl Acad Sci U S A* 1996;93:3193–3198.

171. Lin YG, Zhang M, Hofman FM, et al. Absence of a prominent Th2 cytokine response in human tuberculosis. *Infect Immun* 1996;64:1351–1356.

172. Stenger S, Modlin RL. Pathology and pathogenesis of bacterial infections. In: Kaufmann SHE, Sher A, Ahmed R, eds. *Immunology of infectious diseases*. Washington, DC: ASM Press, 2002:281–292.

173. Yamamura M, Uyemura K, Deans RJ, et al. Defining protective responses to pathogens: cytokine profiles in leprosy lesions. *Science* 1991;254:277–279.

174. Ehrt S, Schnappinger D, Bekiranov S, et al. Reprogramming of the macrophage transcriptome in response to interferon-gamma and Mycobacterium tuberculosis. Signaling roles of nitric oxide synthase-2 and phagocyte oxidase. *J Exp Med* 2001;194:1123–1140.

175. Collins HL, Kaufmann SHE. Acquired immunity against bacteria. In: Kaufmann SHE, Sher A, Ahmed R, eds. *Immunology of infectious diseases*. Washington, DC: ASM Press, 2002:207–222.

176. Crowle AJ. Immunization against tuberculosis: what kind of vaccine? *Infect Immun* 1988;56:2769–2773.

177. Rook GA, Taverne J, Leveton C, et al. The role of gamma-interferon, vitamin D3 metabolites and tumour necrosis factor in the pathogenesis of tuberculosis. *Immunology* 1987;62:229–234.

178. Rigby WF. The immunobiology of vitamin D. *Immunol Today* 1988;9:54–58.

179. Holland SM. Therapy of mycobacterial infections. *Res Immunol* 1996;147:572–581.

180. Wang J, Wakeham J, Harkness R, et al. Macrophages are a significant source of type 1 cytokines during mycobacterial infection. *J Clin Invest* 1999;103:1023–1029.

181. Fearon DT, Locksley RM. The instructive role of innate immunity in the acquired immune response. *Science* 1996;272:50–53.

182. Trinchieri G, Gerosa F. Immunoregulation by interleukin-12. *J Leukoc Biol* 1996;59:505–511.

183. Gately MK, Renzetti LM, Magram J, et al. The interleukin-12/interleukin-12–receptor system: role in normal and pathologic immune responses. *Annu Rev Immunol* 1998;16:495–521.

184. Flesch IE, Hess JH, Huang S, et al. Early interleukin 12 production by macrophages in response to mycobacterial infection depends on interferon gamma and tumor necrosis factor alpha. *J Exp Med* 1995;181:1615–1621.

185. Hayes MP, Wang J, Norcross MA. Regulation of interleukin-12 expression in human monocytes: selective priming by interferon-gamma of lipopolysaccharide-inducible p35 and p40 genes. *Blood* 1995;86:646–650.

186. Tripp CS, Gately MK, Hakimi J, et al. Neutralization of IL-12 decreases resistance to listeria in SCID and C.B–17 mice. Reversal by IFN-gamma. *J Immunol* 1994;152:1883–1887.

187. Cooper AM, Magram J, Ferrante J, et al. Interleukin 12 (IL-12) is crucial to the development of protective immunity in mice intravenously infected with Mycobacterium tuberculosis. *J Exp Med* 1997;186:39–45.

188. Nakanishi K, Yoshimoto T, Tsutsui H, et al. Interleukin-18 regulates both Th1 and Th2 responses. *Annu Rev Immunol* 2001;19:423–474.

189. Ottenhoff TH, Kumararatne D, Casanova JL. Novel human immunodeficiencies reveal the essential role of type-I cytokines in immunity to intracellular bacteria. *Immunol Today* 1998;19:491–494.

190. de Jong R, Altare F, Haagen IA, et al. Severe mycobacterial and Salmonella infections in interleukin-12 receptor–deficient patients. *Science* 1998;280:1435–1438.

191. Altare F, Durandy A, Lammas D, et al. Impairment of mycobacterial immunity in human interleukin-12 receptor deficiency. *Science* 1998;280:1432–1435.

192. Tripp CS, Wolf SF, Unanue ER. Interleukin 12 and tumor necrosis factor alpha are costimulators of interferon gamma production by natural killer cells in severe combined immunodeficiency mice with listeriosis, and interleukin 10 is a physiologic antagonist. *Proc Natl Acad Sci U S A* 1993;90:3725–3729.

193. Flesch IE, Kaufmann SH. Role of macrophages and alpha beta T lymphocytes in early interleukin 10 production during Listeria monocytogenes infection. *Int.Immunol* 1994;6:463–468.

194. Gong JH, Zhang M, Modlin RL, et al. Interleukin-10 downregulates Mycobacterium tuberculosis-induced Th1 responses and CTLA-4 expression. *Infect Immun* 1996;64:913–918.

195. Moore KW, de Waal MR, Coffman RL, et al. Interleukin-10 and the interleukin-10 receptor. *Annu Rev Immunol* 2001;19:683–765.

196. Trinchieri G. Interleukin-12: a proinflammatory cytokine with immunoregulatory functions that bridge innate resistance and antigen-specific adaptive immunity. *Annu Rev Immunol* 1995;13:251–276.

197. Orme IM, Roberts AD, Griffin JP, et al. Cytokine secretion by CD4 T lymphocytes acquired in response to Mycobacterium tuberculosis infection. *J. Immunol* 1993;151:518–525.

198. Surcel HM, Troye-Blomberg M, Paulie S, et al. Th1/Th2 profiles in tuberculosis, based on the proliferation and cytokine response of blood lymphocytes to mycobacterial antigens. *Immunology* 1994;81:171–176.

199. Toossi Z, Ellner JJ. Mechanisms of anergy in tuberculosis. *Curr Top Microbiol Immunol* 1996;215:221–238.

199a. Shevach EM. Regulatory T cells in autoimmunity. *Annu Rev Immunol* 2000;18:423–449.

200. Kaufmann SH. Immunity to intracellular microbial pathogens. *Immunol Today* 1995;16:338–342.

201. Rogge L, Barberis-Maino L, Biffi M, et al. Selective expression of an interleukin-12 receptor component by human T helper 1 cells. *J Exp Med* 1997;185:825–831.

202. Szabo SJ, Dighe AS, Gubler U, et al. Regulation of the interleukin (IL)–12R beta 2 subunit expression in developing T helper 1 (Th1) and Th2 cells. *J Exp Med* 1997;185:817–824.

203. Lohning M, Stroehmann A, Coyle AJ, et al. T1/ST2 is preferentially expressed on murine Th2 cells, independent of interleukin 4, interleukin 5, and interleukin 10, and important for Th2 effector function. *Proc Natl Acad Sci U S A* 1998;95:6930–6935.

204. Sallusto F, Mackay CR, Lanzavecchia A. The role of chemokine receptors in primary, effector, and memory immune responses. *Annu Rev Immunol* 2000;18:593–620.

205. Shirakawa T, Enomoto T, Shimazu S, et al. The inverse association between tuberculin responses and atopic disorder. *Science* 1997;275:77–79.

206. Reiner SL, Locksley RM. The regulation of immunity to Leishmania major. *Annu Rev Immunol* 1995;13:151–177.

207. Noelle RJ. CD40 and its ligand in host defense. *Immunity* 1996;4:415–419.

208. Salomon B, Bluestone JA. Complexities of CD28/B7: CTLA-4 costimulatory pathways in autoimmunity and transplantation. *Annu Rev Immunol* 2001;19:225–252.

209. Campbell KA, Ovendale PJ, Kennedy MK, et al. CD40 ligand is required for protective cell-mediated immunity to Leishmania major. *Immunity* 1996;4:283–289.

210. Grewal IS, Borrow P, Pamer EG, et al. The CD40–CD154 system in anti-infective host defense. *Curr Opin Immunol* 1997;9:491–497.

211. Rolph MS, Kaufmann SH. CD40 signaling converts a minimally immunogenic antigen into a potent vaccine against the intracellular pathogen Listeria monocytogenes. *J Immunol* 2001;166:5115–5121.

212. Mittrucker HW, Kohler A, Mak TW, et al. Critical role of CD28 in protective immunity against Salmonella typhimurium. *J Immunol* 1999;163:6769–6776.

213. Mittrucker HW, Kursar M, Kohler A, et al. Role of CD28 for the generation and expansion of antigen-specific CD8(+) T lymphocytes during infection with Listeria monocytogenes. *J Immunol* 2001;167:5620–5627.

214. Ochoa MT, Stenger S, Sieling PA, et al. T-cell release of granulysin contributes to host defense in leprosy. *Nat Med* 2001;7:174–179.

215. Stenger S, Mazzaccaro RJ, Uyemura K, et al. Differential effects of cytolytic T cell subsets on intracellular infection. *Science* 1997;276:1684–1687.

216. Stenger S, Hanson DA, Teitelbaum R, et al. An antimicrobial activity of cytolytic T cells mediated by granulysin. *Science* 1998;282:121–125.

217. Kaufmann SHE. Killing vs suicide in antibacterial defence. *Trends Microbiol* 1999;7:59–61.

218. Laochumroonvorapong P, Wang J, Liu CC, et al. Perforin, a cytotoxic molecule which mediates cell necrosis, is not required for the early control of mycobacterial infection in mice. *Infect Immun* 1997;65:127–132.

219. Cooper AM, D'Souza C, Frank AA, et al. The course of Mycobacterium tuberculosis infection in the lungs of mice lacking expression of either perforin- or granzyme-mediated cytolytic mechanisms. *Infect Immun* 1997;65:1317–1320.

220. Blanchard DK, Wei S, Duan C, et al. Role of extracellular adenosine triphosphate in the cytotoxic T-lymphocyte–mediated lysis of antigen presenting cells. *Blood* 1995;85:3173–3182.

221. Kaufmann SH. CD8+ T lymphocytes in intracellular microbial infections. *Immunol Today* 1988;9:168–174.

222. Dannenberg AM Jr. Delayed-type hypersensitivity and cell-mediated immunity in the pathogenesis of tuberculosis . *Immunol Today* 1991; 12:228–233.

223. Colten HR, Krause JE. Pulmonary inflammation—a balancing act. *N Engl J Med* 1997;336:1094–1096.

224. Salmi M, Jalkanen S. How do lymphocytes know where to go: current concepts and enigmas of lymphocyte homing. *Adv Immunol* 1997;64:139–218.

225. Ahmed R, Lanier JG, Pamer E. Immunological memory and infection. In: Kaufmann SHE, Sher A, Ahmed R, eds. *Immunology of infectious diseases.* Washington, DC: ASM Press, 2002:175–190.

226. Loetscher P, Moser B, Baggiolini M. Chemokines and their receptors in lymphocyte traffic and HIV infection. *Adv Immunol* 2000;74:127–180.

227. Munoz-Elias EJ, McKinney JD. Bacterial persistence: strategies for survival. In: Kaufmann SHE, Sher A, Ahmed R, eds. *Immunology of infectious diseases.* Washington, DC: ASM Press, 2002:331–356.

228. Wayne LG, Sohaskey CD. Nonreplicating persistence of mycobacterium tuberculosis. *Annu Rev Microbiol* 2001;55:139–163.

229. Mohan VP, Scanga CA, Yu K, et al. Effects of tumor necrosis factor alpha on host immune response in chronic persistent tuberculosis: possible role for limiting pathology. *Infect Immun* 2001;69:1847–1855.

230. Tracey KJ, Cerami A. Cachectin/tumor necrosis factor and other cytokines in infectious disease. *Curr Opin Immunol* 1989;1:454–461.

231. Kaufmann SH, Young DB. Vaccination against tuberculosis and leprosy. *Immunobiology* 1992;184:208–229.

232. Reiter H, ed. *Die Säuglingstuberkulose in Lübeck.* Berlin: Julius Springer, 1935.

233. Stead WW. Racial differences in suceptibility to infection by Mycobacterium tuberculosis. *N Engl J Med* 1990;322:422–427.

234. Gros P, Schurr E. Immunogenetics of the host immune response to bacteria in mice. In: Kaufmann SHE, Sher A, Ahmed R, eds. *Immunology of infectious diseases.* Washington, DC: ASM Press, 2002:407–420.

235. Cellier M, Govoni G, Vidal S, et al. Human natural resistance–associated macrophage protein: cDNA cloning, chromosomal mapping, genomic organization, and tissue-specific expression. *J Exp Med* 1994;180:1741–1752.

236. Vidal SM, Malo D, Vogan K, et al. Natural resistance to infection with intracellular parasites: isolation of a candidate for Bcg. *Cell* 1993;73:469–485.

237. Blackwell JM, Barton CH, White JK, et al. Genomic organization and sequence of the human NRAMP gene: identification and mapping of a promoter region polymorphism. *Mol Med* 1995;1:194–205.

238. Govoni G, Vidal S, Gauthier S, et al. The Bcg/Ity/Lsh locus: genetic transfer of resistance to infections in C57BL/6J mice transgenic for the Nramp1 Gly169 allele. *Infect Immun* 1996;64:2923–2929.

239. Vidal S, Tremblay ML, Govoni G, et al. The Ity/Lsh/Bcg locus: natural resistance to infection with intracellular parasites is abrogated by disruption of the Nramp1 gene. *J Exp Med* 1995;182:655–666.

240. Blackwell JM, Searle S, Goswami T, et al. Understanding the multiple functions of Nramp1. *Microbes Infect* 2000;2:317–321.

241. Gruenheid S, Pinner E, Desjardins M, et al. Natural resistance to infection with intracellular pathogens: the Nramp1 protein is recruited to the membrane of the phagosome. *J Exp Med* 1997;185:717–730.

242. Hill AV. The genomics and genetics of human infectious disease susceptibility. *Annu Rev Genomics Hum Genet* 2001;2:373–400.

243. Abel L, Sanchez FO, Oberti J, et al. Susceptibility to leprosy is linked to the human NRAMP1 gene. *J Infect Dis* 1998;177:133–145.

244. Bellamy R. Variations in the Nramp1 gene and susceptibility to tuberculosis in West Africans. *N Engl J Med* 1998;338:640–644.

245. Bellamy R. Tuberculosis and chronic hepatitis B virus infection in Africans and variation in the vitamin D receptor gene. *J Infect Dis* 1999;179:721–724.

246. Wilkinson RJ. Influence of vitamin D deficiency and vitamin D receptor polymorphisms on tuberculosis among Gujarati Asians in west London: a case-control study. *Lancet* 2000;355:618–621.

CHAPTER 41

Immunity to Extracellular Bacteria

Moon H. Nahm, Michael A. Apicella, and David E. Briles

Bacterial Surface Structure of Gram-Positive and Gram-Negative Bacteria
Bacterial Virulence Factors
Bacterial Invasion of the Host
Antigen-Nonspecific Host Defense Response
   Mucosal Defense · Local Response to Bacterial Invasion (Acute Inflammation) · Systemic Response to Bacterial Invasion
Antigen-Specific Host Defense Response
   Responses of the Host (B-Cell) Immune System to Bacteria · Protective Mechanisms of Antibodies · Responses by T-Cell Immune System to the Extracellular Bacteria
Deleterious Host Response
   Antigen-Nonspecific Deleterious Response · Antigen-Specific Deleterious Response
Summary
References

Human interactions with bacteria are complex. A consortial relationship has developed between humans and microbes. Humans are composed of 10^{12} human cells and are inhabited by 10^{14} bacteria representing innumerable species. Relatively few of these bacteria are harmful in any way to humans. Little is known about the innate or acquired immune mechanisms that maintain this equilibrium. In large part, many diseases caused by bacteria are mistakes in which this consortial relationship breaks down and lines are crossed. The innate and adaptive responses to these transgressions can lead to dire consequences. In *Lives of the Cell: Notes of a Biology Watcher*, Lewis Thomas (1) pointed out that

> "The microorganisms that seem to have it in for us in the worst way—the ones that really appear to wish us ill—turn out on close examination to be rather more like bystanders, strays, strangers in from the cold. They will invade and replicate if they get the chance, and some of them will get into our deepest tissues and set forth in the blood, but it is our response to their presence that makes the disease. Our arsenals for fighting off bacteria are so powerful, and involve so many different defense mechanisms, that we are in more danger from them than from the invaders. We live in the midst of explosive devices; we are mined."

Although certain bacterial species are classified as pathogens, they can live in harmony on mucosal surfaces for long periods and never cause disease. The bacteria that can cause human disease are quite diverse. On the basis of

the pathogenesis of infection and the resulting immune response, these bacteria can be categorized into two general types: those causing intracellular infections and those causing extracellular infections. Most bacteria causing intracellular infections avoid being killed after phagocytosis by either interfering with phagosome-lysosome fusion or by escaping from the phagosome and into the cytoplasm. Cellular immunity is critical against intracellular bacteria, as is described in Chapter 40. In contrast, the bacteria causing extracellular infections survive in the host by avoiding phagocytosis. They do this by presenting a surface that minimizes the opsonic and lytic effects of antibody and complement. Although extracellular bacteria do have the ability to enter and pass through cells as a means of moving from one *in vivo* environment to another, they are readily killed once captured by phagocytes. Accordingly, the host-defense against extracellular bacteria is critically dependent on humoral immunity complement and the production of specific antibody. Table 1 lists many of the important bacteria that can cause extracellular infections in humans, together with the diseases they cause and some of their major virulence factors. In this chapter, we describe the surface structures of many of these bacteria and provide examples of how they are able to infect their hosts and cause disease. We also describe the salient aspects of the innate immunity and antigen-induced immunity important in the host's defense against these bacteria.

TABLE 1. *Extracellular bacteria commonly associated with diseases*

Species	Disease	Important virulence structures/molecules	Special adaptations critical to host infection
Neisseria gonorrhoeae	Urethritis, cervicitis, salpingitis, endometritis, prostatitis, arthritis, proctitis, pharyngitis	Lipopolysaccharide, fimbria, peptidoglycan, Opa protein, unidentified adhesins and invasins	Phase and antigenic variation, molecular mimicry of human antigens
Neisseria meningitidis	Meningitis, meningococcemia, arthritis, pneumonia, asymptomatic carriage	Capsular polysaccharide, lipopolysaccharide, fimbria, membrane proteins, unidentified adhesins and invasins	Phase and antigenic variation, molecular mimicry of human antigens
Haemophilus influenzae type b	Meningitis, sepsis, arthritis, epiglottitis, asymptomatic carriage	Capsular polysaccharide, lipopolysaccharide, fimbria, peptidoglycan	Asymptomatic colonization, phase and antigenic variation, molecular mimicry of human antigens
Nontypeable *Haemophilus influenzae*	Otitis media, bronchitis, pneumonia, neonatal sepsis, endometritis, asymptomatic carriage	Lipopolysaccharide, fimbria, adhesive fibrils, peptidoglycan	Phase and antigenic variation, molecular mimicry of human antigens
Haemophilus ducreyi	Genital ulcer disease	Lipopolysaccharide (?), adhesive fibrils, hemolysin	Molecular mimicry of human antigens
Bordetella pertussis	Whooping cough in children, chronic cough syndrome in adults	Pertussis toxin, pertactin, filamentous hemagglutinin, fimbria, ciliary toxin	Coordinate regulation of toxin expression
Pseudomonas aeruginosa	Infections in compromised hosts, pneumonia, sepsis	Lipopolysaccharide, proteases, lipases, lecithinases, exotoxin A, elastase	Relatively large genomic size (~6 Mb) allows considerable adaptability to changes in environmental conditions
Escherichia coli	Urinary tract infection, sepsis, traveler's diarrhea, dysentery, meningitis, hemolytic-uremic syndrome	Capsular polysaccharide, lipopolysaccharide, fimbria, toxins	Antigenic heterogeneity of capsule and lipopolysaccharide
Vibrio cholera	Diarrhea	Cholera toxin, fimbria	Bacterial dispersal through cholera toxin, which induces copious watery diarrhea
Helicobacter pylori	Peptic ulcer disease	Urease, flagella, CagA	Ability to survive at low pH provides a niche lacking bacterial competition or efficient immune surveillance
Treponema pallidum	Local genital ulcer disease, disseminated infection, tertiary disease	Endoflagella, rare outer membrane proteins	Limited exposed antigenic sites
Streptococcus pneumoniae	Pneumonia, otitis media, meningitis, sinusitis	Capsule, PspA, pneumolysin, neuraminidase, PsaA, hyaluronidase, teichoic acids	Asymptomatic colonization, genetic transformation permitting continual generation of new genotypes
Staphylococcus aureus	Impetigo, folliculitis, boils, cellulitis, wound infections, toxic shock, osteomyelitis, endocarditis, bacteremia, pneumonia, food poisoning	Tissue-degrading enzymes, alpha toxin and other membrane-damaging toxins, epidermolytic toxins, enterotoxins, capsule	Resistant to dehydration, asymptomatic colonization, regulation of virulence factor expression
Streptococcus pyogenes	Acute pharyngitis, scarlet fever, necrotizing fasciitis, streptococcal toxic shock syndrome, rheumatic fever, and glomerulonephritis	Hyaluronic acid capsule, M protein, streptococcal pyogenic exotoxins, streptolysin O, streptolysin S	Molecular mimicry of human antigens, high diversity of M proteins, phage-associated virulence properties
Streptococcus agalactiae	Bacteremia, pneumonia, otitis media, and other focal infections	Capsule, beta hemolysin, hyaluronidase	Asymptomatic colonization, acquisition by infants during parturition
Corynebacterium diphtheria	Diphtheria (pharyngitis/tonsillitis)	Diphtheria toxin	Toxin gene contained in temperate phage and expression regulated by iron concentration
Clostridium tetani	Tetanus (lockjaw)	Tetanus toxin (affects central nervous system)	Opportunistic infection by a spore-forming soil anaerobe
Clostridium perfringens	Gas gangrene, anaerobic cellulitis, endometritis, food poisoning	More than 10 exotoxins	Opportunistic infection of wounds

CagA, cytotoxin-associated gene A; Opa, outer membrane opacity; PsaA, pneumococcal surface adhesin A; PspA, pneumoccal surface protein A.

BACTERIAL SURFACE STRUCTURE OF GRAM-POSITIVE AND GRAM-NEGATIVE BACTERIA

Extracellular, as well as intracellular, pathogenic bacteria can be divided into two major tribes (gram-negative and gram-positive) on the basis of their staining characteristics with Gram's stain. To illustrate the surface of bacteria in the two tribes, the surface structures of *Streptococcus pneumoniae* and *Neisseria meningitidis* are shown in Fig. 1. Three layers are commonly recognized: cytoplasmic membrane, cell wall, and outer layer. Although these layers are described later in detail, it is important to note that these definitions are operational and that, in reality, the layers are not entirely distinct. Molecules anchored in the cytoplasmic membrane or cell wall may extend into or through other layers. Thus, there are molecules other than peptidoglycan and capsular polysaccharide (PS) in the cell wall and the outer layer, respectively. It is also important to note that the capsule, O-antigens, and cell wall are not contiguous shields but are open enough to be permeable to secreted products and nutrients, as well as some immunological factors (e.g., antibodies and complement) (Fig. 1).

All bacteria have a cytoplasmic membrane, which is a phospholipid bilayer containing various proteins. This membrane is an osmotic barrier and forms a barrier for most molecules. The lipid bilayer is composed mainly of phospholipid and does not contain sterols. Many membrane

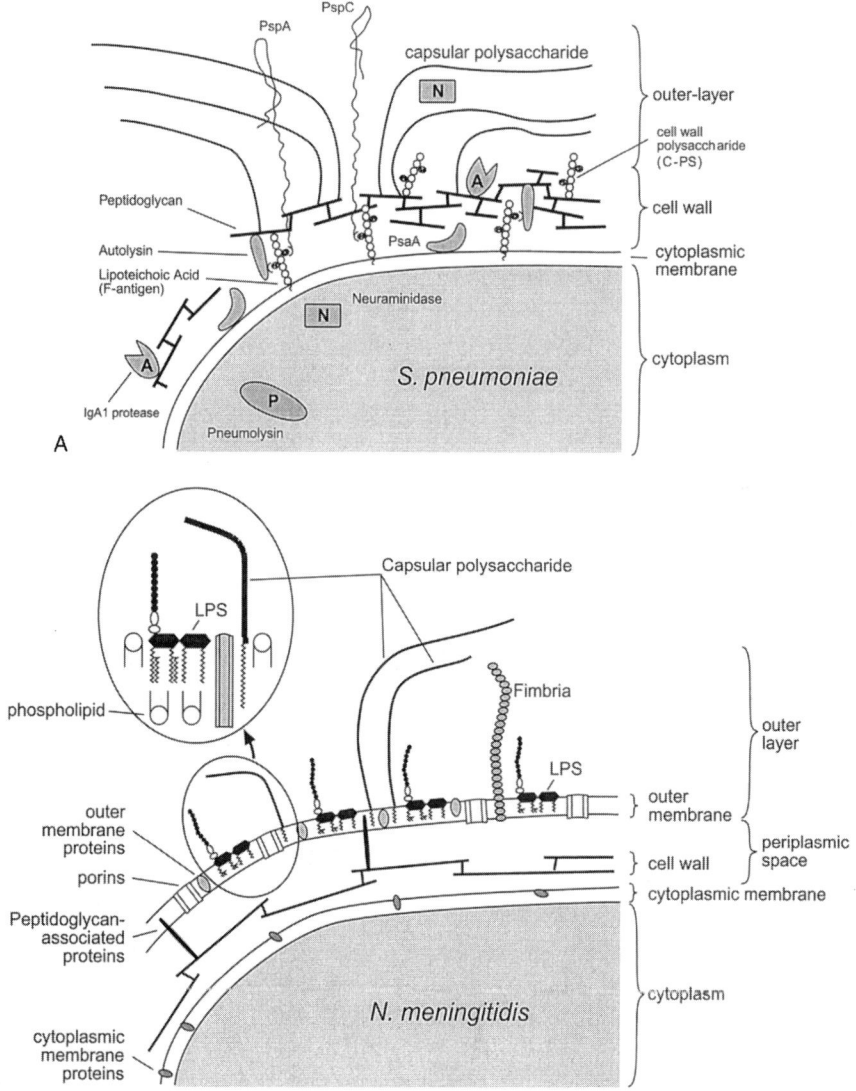

FIG. 1. Schematic representation of the surfaces of *Streptococcus pneumoniae* (**A**) and *Neisseria meningitidis* (**B**) as examples of gram-positive and gram-negative bacteria, respectively. The cell wall polysaccharide of *S. pneumoniae* is often called C-polysaccharide. The inset in B shows lipopolysaccharide anchored to the outer leaflet of the outer membrane.

proteins are transport proteins, and many physical connections between the cell wall and the membrane can be visualized by electron microscopy.

A cell wall is found in all of the pathogenic bacteria of both tribes, with the exception of Mollicute organisms (which include mycoplasmas). The cell wall surrounds the cytoplasmic membrane and is made of peptidoglycan, which is a highly cross-linked polymer of amino sugars (N-acetyl glucosamine and muramic acid) and amino acids. The peptidoglycan polymerization is performed by enzymes, many of which are also referred to as penicillin-binding proteins. In comparison with gram-negative bacteria, gram-positive organisms have a thicker (20- to 30-nm vs. 2- to 4-nm) cell wall layer and can thus retain the Gram's stain better. The cell walls help protect the bacteria from the extremes of the environment (especially differences in osmolarity). The thick cell wall of the gram-positive bacteria may be responsible for their resistance to complement-mediated lysis.

In addition to peptidoglycan, many gram-positive bacteria have PS associated with their cell walls, and this cell wall PS often extends into the capsular area. The cell wall PS of gram-positive bacteria varies among different bacteria, and the structure of the cell wall PS has been used to distinguish many different species of streptococci (i.e., groups A, B, C, and so forth) (2,3). Cell wall PS often has a phosphate group in the repeating unit, and it is then called a teichoic acid. In the pneumococcus, the teichoic acid is C-polysaccharide (C-PS), which is relatively invariant among pneumococcal strains (4,5). In gram-positive bacteria, teichoic acid is often linked to lipid molecules, and this is then called lipoteichoic acids, which is attached to the cytoplasmic membrane and extends out through the cell wall (6). In pneumococci, the overall PS structures of lipoteichoic acid (also called F-antigen) and cell wall teichoic acid are very similar. They are thought to differ only in their mode of attachment to the bacterial surface (7).

The cell wall and outer layer of gram-positive bacteria are the locations of a number of cell-surface proteins involved in a variety of functions, including, but not limited to, adherence, enzyme activity against host substrates, nutrient transport, and interference with complement deposition. For instance, S. pneumoniae has pneumococcal surface protein A (PspA) (8,9), pneumococcal surface protein C (PspC) (10,11), pneumococcal surface adhesin A (PsaA) (12), autolysin (13), immunoglobulin A1 (IgA1) protease (14,15), C3 protease (16), and other less well-characterized proteins (17,18). C3 protease is able to inactivate native C3 in serum. PspA may also interfere with complement fixation (19,20) and may play a role in colonization (21). PspA, autolysin, and PsaA have all been shown to elicit protective immune responses in mice (12,22,23). PspC, which is also known as CbpA, SpsA, or C3-binding protein (24,25), plays an important role in bacterial adhesion to host cells because it binds to the secretory component of immunoglobulin A (IgA) or to the receptor for the platelet-activation factor (PAFR) (26). In addition to pneumococci, many other extracellular bacteria,

including Neisseria and Haemophilus organisms, produce an IgA1 protease (IgA1 is the most common form of human secretory IgA) (14,15). Streptococcus pyogenes has highly variable and strain-specific M proteins, which can interfere with complement activation (27).

In the pneumococcus, many of the proteins presently identified in the cell wall and outer layer have choline binding sites through which they attach to phosphocholine residues in the teichoic and lipoteichoic acids (19,28). In other gram-positive bacteria, such as group A streptococci and staphylococci, most surface proteins have a peptide motif of LPXTGX, which precedes a hydrophobic stretch referred to as a stop-transfer sequence. In staphylococci, the LPXTGX sequence is cleaved in the carboxyl direction to the threonine and covalently linked to the free amino group of a pentaglycine crossbridge in the bacterial cell wall (29,30), thus covalently attaching the protein to the cell wall. Some of these surface proteins have become candidates for the development of new protein-based vaccines (31). In contrast, few proteins are bound to the surface through this mechanism in pneumococci (32).

Gram-negative bacteria typically have thinner cell walls than do gram-positive bacteria. Another major difference in surface structure between gram-negative and gram-positive bacteria is the presence of an outer membrane on gram-negative bacteria. The outer membrane is an asymmetrical bilayer. The inner leaflet is primarily phospholipid. The outer, but not the inner, leaflet contains the lipid A component of lipopolysaccharide (LPS). In addition to enclosing the cell, the outer membrane contains proteins, enzymes, invasins, adhesins, and toxins, which are important in pathogenesis. These molecules are also recognition targets for the host cells, antibodies, bacteriophages, and bacterial conjugation. Although the outer membrane is a selective barrier, it is more permeable to ions than the cytoplasmic membrane and is relatively resistant to osmotic rupture. The space between the cell wall and the outer membrane is called periplasmic space and contains a variety of enzymes and proteins that act to bind and transport substrates against a gradient and form disulfide bonds. These proteins are generally hydrophobic and insert into the periplasmic membrane through hydrophobic–hydrophobic interactions. This space also contains cytoplasmic membrane–derived oligosaccharides, which help regulate cellular osmolarity.

The outer membrane of gram-negative bacteria contains LPS. LPS, also called endotoxin, is an amphipathic molecule with four distinct regions: lipid A, the inner core, the outer core and, in some species, the O-antigen. Lipid A is composed of a dihexosamine backbone to which between five and seven saturated (12- to 16-carbon) fatty acids are attached through amide and ester linkages. Lipid A is the principal toxin associated with most gram-negative bacteria. Lipid A is the major lipid component of the outer leaflet, and the acyl portion of lipid A is embedded in the phospholipid inner leaflet. The carbohydrate portion of the LPS is attached to the lipid A through a molecule unique to gram-negative bacteria called keto-deoxyoctanoate. This molecule, with its heptose moieties, forms the inner core of the LPS. The outer core is composed of 7 to 10 monosaccharide units whose arrangement is relatively conserved among gram-negative species (33).

In most gram-negative bacteria, the outer core of LPS is connected to a polysaccharide, called the O-antigen. It has repeating units containing 4–6 monosaccharides. The O-antigen forms a hydrophilic shield around the bacterium and forms a barrier to complement deposition on the bacterial cell surface. The O-antigen is variable in length, antigenically diverse, and confers serotypic specificity. The O-antigens of *Escherichia coli*, *Klebsiella* species, and *Salmonella* species have as many as 30 repeating units composed of four to six sugars each (33). In the case of the pathogenic *Neisseria* organisms, *Haemophilus influenzae*, and *Haemophilus ducreyi*, the LPS lacks O-antigens and the size of the carbohydrate region does not exceed 7,000 Da. The LPSs of these organisms have been called lipo-oligosaccharides to distinguish them from their longer relatives (34).

In addition to LPS, a number of proteins are found in the outer membrane. *E. coli* and *Neisseria* organisms have 20 to 30 distinct proteins in the outer membrane, whereas the *Treponema pallidum* outer membrane has very few. A major group of outer membrane proteins are porins, which facilitate the diffusion of small hydrophilic molecules through the outer membrane. The basic porin structure is a homotrimer arranged to form a channel with a discrete pore size through the outer leaflet. Although most porins are nonselective, some porins are components in transport systems for specific metabolites [e.g., the LamB porin of *E. coli* which mediates maltose transport (33)]. The expression of selective porins is generally regulated by the presence or absence of substrate in the environment. Some proteins in the outer leaflet form components of the pumping systems for removal of hydrophobic compounds (e.g., tetracycline) or form a specialized pore through which pili exit the membrane (33,35).

For most gram-positive and gram-negative bacteria, PS dominates the outer layer. *S. pneumoniae* has capsular PS that is covalently attached to the cell wall. In gram-negative bacteria, the outer layer is composed mainly of LPS and capsular PS. An exception to this general rule is *Bacillus anthracis*, whose capsule is poly-D-glutamic acid rather than a PS (36). The capsule PS is anchored to the outer membrane by acyl chains in *N. meningitidis* (37) or *H. influenzae* type b (Hib) (38).

The outer layer is well developed in bacteria that cause extracellular infections and has many features that help the bacteria circumvent the host immune system. First, the outer layer has properties that reduce the attachment of extracellular bacteria to eukaryotic surfaces, including those of phagocytes. In general, the PS capsules render the bacteria hydrophilic and negatively charged, like eukaryote cell surfaces, which are rich in sialic acid. The negatively charged surface makes the bacteria partly resistant to the alternative pathway of complement fixation by enhancing the degradation of C3b (39) (Chapter 34). Second, in some cases, elicitation of anti-

body is minimized because the capsular PS or LPS mimics host antigens, as is more fully described later in the section on antigen-specific host defense response. This mimicry may also reduce interactions between the bacteria and host surfaces. Third, the outer layer can physically mask most of the other bacterial surface components and thus minimize the number of exposed epitopes that can be recognized by the antibody and complement. Although the capsule is porous to antibodies and complement, the binding of antibodies and fixation of complement beneath the capsule surface are relatively ineffective at promoting opsonophagocytosis and blood clearance (40).

Finally, the shielding function of the outer layer is further augmented by the presence of proteins that can interfere with complement deposition. Examples of these proteins are PspA and the C3-binding protein in *S. pneumoniae* (20,41) or M protein of *S. pyogenes* (27). Extracellular bacteria (including *Neisseria* organisms, *H. influenzae*, group B streptococci, and *S. pneumoniae*) can modify their cell surfaces in order to adapt to different host environments, such as the natural environment independent of a host, the mucosa of a host, or more invasive host environments (42–46). For instance, bacteria may shut down the synthesis of capsular PS upon contact with the epithelial surface (47). This change facilitates the bacterial adhesion to the epithelial cells, perhaps by exposing the bacterial adhesion proteins. By decreasing capsule production, the bacteria become less hydrophilic and less negatively charged. This change facilitates their entry to the epithelial cells and their subsequent invasion into deeper tissues. Upon the emergence of the bacteria from the epithelial cells in the submucosa, capsule synthesis is resumed. The principal genetic mechanism for the reversible phenotype changes appears to be "phase variation," caused by either slip-strand mispairing or recombinational events within the bacterial genome. The flexibility to express different surface properties helps bacteria successfully evade the host immune system and survive in many niches inside the host.

BACTERIAL VIRULENCE FACTORS

Extracellular bacteria often elaborate many molecules useful to their survival and proliferation in the host. These molecules are called virulence factors. Sequencing of the entire genomes of bacteria has shown that the genes for the virulence factors have generally originated from other organisms and exist as a part of large blocks of deoxyribonucleic acid (DNA)–containing multiple genes. These DNA blocks are called pathogenicity islands (PAIs). For instance, *Helicobacter pylori* has a PAI that is 41-kb long, contains 31 genes, and codes for type IV secretory pathway (48). Pathogenic bacteria usually contain one or two PAIs, but some (e.g., *Salmonella* organisms) contain up to five PAIs (49).

The best-known virulence factors are toxins, which are highly toxic to the host and can be responsible for the symptoms caused by the bacterial infection. The toxins can be grouped on the basis of their molecular structure and their mechanism of action (49). The largest group is called A-B toxins, which have two subunits. The A subunit has enzymatic activity, and the B subunit targets the A subunit to the host cells. This group includes diphtheria toxin, cholera toxin, pertussis toxin, and two anthrax toxins (lethal factor and edema factor). For instance, lethal factor of *B. anthracis* behaves as the A subunit and requires a B subunit protein, "protective antigen," to enter into target cells. In some cases, the toxic effect of toxins can almost completely account for the detrimental symptoms of their respective infections. For example, cholera toxin blocks the uptake of sodium in the intestine and is responsible for severe diarrhea, causing dehydration that, if not treated, can kill people. Tetanus toxin causes central nervous system paralysis (50). Staphylococcal enterotoxin A, which is one of five membrane-damaging toxins produced by staphylococci, is the primary cause of staphylococcal food poisoning and plays a major role in invasive infections (51). Some strains of *E. coli* produce verotoxin, which may damage the microvasculature of the kidney and cause hemolytic uremic syndrome (52,53).

One group of virulence factors helps bacteria to acquire essential nutrients. Mucosal fluid and blood are low in free iron because of the presence of iron-binding proteins such as lactoferrin and transferrin. To successfully compete with the host for this vital metabolite, *N. meningitidis, Neisseria gonorrhoeae,* and *H. influenzae* have complex surface transport systems that can obtain iron from human transferrin, lactoferrin, and hemoglobin (54–57). Pneumococci, which can also survive in blood and other body fluids, do not get iron from transferrin or lactoferrin but acquire iron from heme and hemoglobin released from lysed cells (58). *E. coli* and *Salmonella* organisms use a different mechanism to acquire iron. They secrete a low-molecular-weight iron chelator, called a siderophore, which removes iron from human proteins in the environment surrounding the bacteria. The iron–siderophore complex is then taken up by the bacterium, and the siderophore is degraded so that the iron can be freed for utilization (59,60).

Another important class of virulence factor is involved in the adherence of bacteria to the host cells. Nasopharyngeal carriage of pneumococci is mediated largely by adherence to the host molecules *N*-acetyl-D-glucosamine β1-3 galactose or *N*-acetyl-D-glucosamine β1-4 galactose (26,61). In the lower respiratory tract, pneumococci can use phosphocholine to bind to PAFR without triggering the cell-signaling pathway (62). In contrast, nontypeable *H. influenzae* binds to and signals through PAFR. This occurs by the interaction of a nontypeable *H. influenzae* lipo-oligosaccharide glycoform-containing phosphocholine with the receptor (63,64). Many bacteria use a pilus for adhesion. The Pap pilus of *E. coli* binds the Galα1-4 Gal unit of cell-surface globoside in urethral epithelial cells (65). The *Vibrio cholerae* pilus allows attachment of the bacterium to the enterocyte for efficient toxin delivery (66,67). *Bordetella pertussis* has three adherence factors—a filamentous hemagglutinin, pertactin, and a pilus (fimbriae)—that allow it to attach to ciliated respiratory epithelial cells in the trachea and bronchi and thus enable it to resist the cleansing action of mucus flow (68,69).

Another class of virulence factor neutralizes host defenses. Pneumolysin from *S. pneumoniae* is a cytoplasmic protein, which is released during pneumococcal growth, and possibly also by autolysis of some of the bacteria (70). It can consume complement at a distance from the pneumococci and can interfere with the function of phagocytes (9,71). Its presence also appears to impair the development of protective host responses against pneumococci (72). *S. pyogenes* and group B streptococci produce C5 peptidases that inhibit chemotaxis of host phagocytes to the sites of infections (73,74). Some bacteria also produce C3 protease (75) or IgA1 protease (14,15,76). *H. pylori* produces urease, which can generate ammonia that can neutralize acid in the stomach and thereby promotes the survival of *H. pylori*.

Production of virulence factors is often closely regulated by bacteria in order to accommodate the changes in the environmental stimuli. In staphylococci, it has been shown that the amount of capsule is regulated in response to environmental stimuli (77,78). One of the best studied of such regulatory systems is the BvgAS, a two-component regulatory system in *B. pertussis* (79). This system regulates the expression of adhesins, toxins, and other virulence factors. The system is controlled by external signals, including Mg^{2+}, temperature, and nicotinic acid. Two proteins, BvgS and BvgA, are involved in this regulatory system. BvgS, the sensor, is a kinase and is able to phosphorylate itself in response to the environmental signal. BvgA is in turn phosphorylated by BvgS. Phosphorylated BvgA is able to activate transcription of virulence genes through a change in its interaction with a 70-bp consensus sequence repeated in Bvg-regulated promoters (79). Two-component regulatory systems are frequently used to regulate the expression of genes associated with virulence (80).

Bacteria-to-bacteria signaling is another important mechanism for the control of virulence factors. This phenomenon, "quorum sensing" (81), has been shown to be operative in a large number of gram-negative and gram-positive species. The signal transmitted between the bacteria can be an acylated molecules (e.g., homoserine lactone) in gram-negative bacteria or a peptide in gram-positive bacteria. Quorum sensing has been shown to be important in biofilm formation in a number of bacterial species and for the expression of a number of virulence factors (81,82). Biofilms are communities of one or multiple bacterial species, adherent to each other and to a target surface.

In gram-positive bacteria, virulence factor genes generally encode for a signal sequence that permits the export of their product from the bacteria. Gram-negative bacteria have four specialized pathways for secreting virulence factors (49,83). Each pathway requires multiple molecules encoded by linked genes and shares similarity among different bacterial species. Although they are used for secreting virulence factors, these pathways were derived from the apparatuses used to perform their physiological functions. For instance, pathways III and IV are derived from pathways used for the export of flagella and conjugative pilus components, respectively. In some cases, bacteria use the pathway to inject virulence factors directly into the host cells. For instance, *H. pylori* injects cytotoxin-associated gene A (CagA) molecules directly into the host cells with a type IV secretory pathway. CagA is then phosphorylated by the host cells, and the phosphorylated CagA alters host cell structure (83,84).

An important characteristic of the virulence factors is their structural polymorphism. For instance, there are at least 100 different serological types of M proteins of *S. pyogenes* (85). Similarly, pneumococci have 90 serologically distinct capsular PSs (86), and more than 20 non–cross-reactive groups of pneumococci are common in human disease (87). Other serologically variable proteins include IgA1 protease and PspA of pneumococci. Lipo-oligosaccharides of *N. gonorrhoeae* are unusual in that they can be modified by the host enzymes and host substances (88).

The polymorphism in the structure of many virulence factors allows the bacteria making them to avoid the antigen-specific host immunity. For instance, antibodies to one serotype of M protein do not cross-react with M proteins of other serotypes and do not provide protection against strains expressing other serotypes (89). Similarly, newly invading pneumococci can escape recognition by anticapsular antibodies produced in response to previous pneumococcal infections with other serotypes.

The polymorphism in virulence factors is achieved by various genetic mechanisms. Variation in M proteins is the result of sequence differences in the N-terminal (but not C-terminal) half of M proteins (90). *S. pneumoniae* has the genes for synthesizing capsular PS as a "genetic cassette" that can be exchanged among different strains (91) and may result in the shift in the serotype distribution after the use of vaccines, eliciting serotype-specific protection (92–94). *Neisseria* organisms have genetic machinery for rapid gene rearrangement (95), and this enables an individual bacterium to produce progeny expressing pili with different antigenic characteristics very quickly. The number of potential pilus-antigen variants within the progeny of a single organism is estimated to be more than 100,000 (96). In addition, *N. gonorrhoeae* expresses outer membrane surface proteins, designated Opa proteins, which can facilitate the internalization of the bacterium into an epithelial cell (46). The gene for each Opa protein has a series of CTCTT within the opa open reading frame. Recombination between CTCTT sequences varies the number of repeats (97); the number of repeats determines the translational frame of the gene and the ultimate expression of the complete protein. This slip-strand mispairing enables rapid variation in the Opa proteins, and the progeny of a single bacterium can express many variant Opa proteins on the surface.

BACTERIAL INVASION OF THE HOST

Both the keratinized skin and mucosal surfaces have inherent nonimmune defense mechanisms that modulate bacterial

growth and minimize the risk of invasion. Healthy human skin is an effective physical barrier to infection by most human extracellular and intracellular pathogens. The keratinization of fully differentiated skin epithelium results in a relatively impermeable surface. In addition, lysozymes, toxic lipids and hydrogen ions secreted by cutaneous glands offer bacteriostatic protection for cutaneous pores and hair follicles (98). Occasionally, this defense can be breached by extracellular bacteria such as *S. pyogenes* or *Staphylococcus aureus,* causing cellulitis and abscess. More commonly, bacterial invasion through intact skin requires physical damage, such as abrasions, burns, or other trauma. For instance, cutaneous anthrax develops when *B. anthracis* enters the body through a break in the skin. *Staphylococcus epidermidis,* a member of the commensal skin flora, can infect indwelling catheters by spreading through the puncture site in the skin and may lead to bacteremia or colonization of prosthetic devices, including artificial heart valves and shunts. A major factor that enables these bacteria to cause disease is their ability to elaborate within the bacterial population a biofilm induced by quorum sensing (described previously), which facilitates its adhesion, is antiphagocytic, and acts as a barrier to antibiotic penetration (99).

Unlike the skin, the mucosal epithelium is not keratinized. Instead, mucosal areas, such as the gastrointestinal tract, nasopharynx, upper airway, and vagina, are moist and nutritionally rich. Thus, it is not surprising that mucosal areas contain a large number of bacteria. In oral secretions and gastrointestinal products, 10^8 and 10^{11} bacteria per milliliter, respectively, may be found. To ensure their survival in the mucosal environment, extracellular bacteria elaborate many virulence factors required for acquisition of essential nutrients or for adherence to the host cells. In some cases, bacteria may subvert the host inflammatory response. *Salmonella* species can block the activation of NFκB and subsequent activation of the inflammatory response. They achieve this by preventing the degradation of IκB, which is essential for the translocation of NFκB from the cytoplasm to the nucleus (100,101). In some cases, pathogens locate in a less protected microenvironment within the mucosal areas. *H. pylori* survives in the very acidic stomach by burying itself in the mucus, which protects it from direct exposure to the acid and from the phagocytes. In other cases, collaboration among bacteria is essential for their successful colonization. For instance, bacterial collaboration can lead to the formation of biofilm that is critical for their survival (102).

Mucosal sites have diverse species of bacteria. Most of the bacteria species found at the mucosal sites are harmless. In addition, reverse-transcription polymerase chain reaction studies of 16S ribosomal ribonucleic acid (RNA) suggest the presence of many additional unidentified (and, so far, unculturable) bacterial species on the mucosal surface (103). Many potentially pathogenic bacterial strains are also often found in the mucosal areas of healthy individuals without causing symptoms. *S. pneumoniae, N. meningitidis, H. influenzae,* and *S. aureus* are examples of pathogenic extracellular bacteria that are frequently carried in the nasopharynx of a healthy individual. The carriage rate of the pathogenic bacteria can be relatively high, as shown by the fact that 50% to 60% of healthy young children may carry *S. pneumoniae* in their throats (92). Maintenance of the diverse species is dynamic. Bacterial species compete and regulate diversity among themselves. Many bacterial species produce molecules that suppress the growth of other bacterial species (104). The host may also control the diversity of colonizing bacteria by controlling the pH or other environmental conditions in the mucosal area. The presence of the host control is suggested by a striking example found among invertebrates in which the light organ of the bobtail squid is colonized by a single bacterial species, *Vibrio fischeri* (105). At present, little is known about how the host may regulate bacterial populations.

Because pathogenic bacteria are readily found in the mucosal area, several explanations have been advanced to explain the absence of the diseases they normally cause. One explanation is that the maintenance of diverse bacterial population is responsible for the prevention of the disease. For instance, the destruction of the normal gastrointestinal bacterial flora with a number of antibiotics can be associated with a selective expansion of *Clostridium difficile* and development of pseudomembranous colitis (106). Another explanation may be that the pathogenic bacteria carried in healthy persons are different from those isolated from patients. For instance, during nonepidemic periods, approximately 5% to 10% of the population are carriers of *N. meningitidis*, which is mostly nonencapsulated (107). During epidemics, 30% to 60% of the population may carry meningococci, which are mostly encapsulated and the majority of which are of the same capsular type as the case strain causing the epidemic (108). A third explanation is that the pathogenic bacteria are frequently confined to mucosal area. Group B streptococci are carried asymptomatically in the lower intestine and the female genital tract but can be acquired by infants during parturition and cause life-threatening bacteremia and sepsis (109).

Another explanation centers on the differences among hosts. It has long been known that the presence of *N. gonorrhoeae* in the female genital tract is frequently asymptomatic, whereas its presence in boys and men is generally symptomatic and often associated with a deleterious disease (110,111). Investigations have shown that the mechanisms of pathogenesis of infection used by *N. gonorrhoeae* are different in men than in women (112–114). In women, initial attachment of *N. gonorrhoeae* to urethral and cervical epithelial cells is accomplished through pili (115). Infection of cervical cells is facilitated when their cell surface becomes ruffled in response to the interaction between gonococci and the complement receptor type 3 (CR3) on the surface of the cervical cells (113,114). The CR3 interaction may serve to downregulate the inflammatory response during cervical gonorrhea. In men, clathrin-dependent, receptor-mediated endocytosis occurs by the interaction of a terminal galactose on gonococcal lipo-oligosaccharide with the human asialoglycoprotein receptor on the urethral epithelial cell. The epithelial cells are capable of evoking an inflammatory cytokine response that results in the recruitment of neutrophils (116). In addition, gonococci have been shown to bind to human sperm through the same receptor present on sperm.

Although the pathogenic extracellular bacteria can exist asymptomatically in the mucosa, they can more or less passively enter into less defended sites and cause focal infections. For instance, *E. coli*, normally present in the gut, may enter the urogenital tract and cause urinary tract infections. *S. pneumoniae* and Hib are often carried in the nasopharyngeal space, but they can invade nearby normally sterile cavities (e.g., the lungs and middle ear) and cause focal infections. Aspiration of bacteria from the nasopharynx into the lung undoubtedly occurs frequently with no ill effects; however, aspiration may lead to an infection when there is a pulmonary blockage (such as aspirated food), damage to the epithelial surface (such as that caused by smoking), or viral infection (respiratory syncytial virus or influenza) (3,117). Viral infections are important because they can lead to host expression of molecules, which are adhesive to pneumococci, in addition to the loss of host ciliary action (3,118). Some bacteria produce molecules that modify the host cell surfaces and reduce bacterial clearance from the upper airways. Some gram-positive bacteria produce hyaluronidase, neuraminidase, or both (119–121), which modify the host cell surfaces, release host sugars to the bacteria, and destroy host tissues important for drainage. Staphylococci and *S. pyogenes* are effectively cleared from the blood but can cause transient bacteremia as a result of breaks in the mucosal surface or in the skin. These circulating bacteria can, under rare conditions, cause focal infections, including cellulitis, in damaged (or bruised) tissue when the blood flow is interrupted (122).

Bacteria can actively invade deeper tissues by multiple pathways. They can enter through specialized cells (M cells) in the gut. Alternatively, they can breach a cellular barrier (epithelium or endothelium) by going through (transcytosis) or between (paracellular pathway) the cells (123). *Porphyromonas gingivalis*, an organism associated with adult periodontitis, may breach the epithelial layer by the paracellular pathway and produces enzymes useful in digesting the tight junction (124). *Shigella* organisms may breach the gut mucosa primarily by transcytosing through the M cells (123). Two mechanisms of transcytosis have been described for pneumococci. In one, pneumococci may cross the bronchial epithelial cells by binding polymeric immunoglobulin receptor of the epithelial cells with CbpA (PspC) and traveling through the IgA secretory pathway in reverse (125). In the other, pneumococci may use phosphocholine to bind to PAFR, which is abundant on activated endothelial cells, epithelial cells, or pneumocytes (26,126). Nonencapsulated pneumococci appear to be more efficient in these processes than are encapsulated pneumococci, and the physiological significance of these mechanisms is still unclear. In many cases, the bacterial adhesion triggers changes in the host cell function, and this change can assist transcytosis. For instance, nontypeable *H. influenzae* can bind to PAFR on endothelial cells with lipo-oligosaccharide glycoform–containing phosphocholine and signal through the receptor (63,64). The bacteria enter vacuoles, but little is known about their trafficking within the epithelial cell.

ANTIGEN-NONSPECIFIC HOST DEFENSE RESPONSE

To protect itself from infections caused by highly adaptable bacteria, the host employs a multilayered defense. This includes the mechanical barriers and iron sequestration described previously, as well as phagocytes, complement fixation, lysozyme, and cytokine-mediated local inflammation. In addition, the host is protected with antigen-specific antibody (see the section on antigen-specific host defense response) and T cell–mediated cellular immunity. Antigen-specific immunity, although powerfully protective, takes from several days to weeks to develop after exposure to a pathogen. Consequently, the primary defense against bacteria during the early phase of infection remains the antigen-nonspecific host immunity. The importance and significance of nonspecific immunity is readily demonstrated by the relative ease with which colonies of mice with severe combined immunodeficiency, which lack antigen-specific immunity, can be maintained (127). This section describes several antigennonspecific host defense mechanisms, but for additional information, see Chapter 17.

Mucosal Defense

Although mucosal areas are rich in nutrients for bacteria, the proliferation of bacteria in the mucosal areas is largely held in check by mechanical cleansing actions and the lack of available iron. In the gastrointestinal tract, normal peristaltic motility, the secretion of mucus, and the detergent action of bile limit the number of bacteria. The movements of cilia along the bronchial tree continually remove aspirated bacteria, along with the mucus from the lower respiratory tract. Normal epithelial and tissue architecture are essential for the draining and expulsion of bacteria, and disruption of this mechanism by smoking, viral infections (e.g., influenza), or bacterial infection (e.g., pertussis) makes the host markedly susceptible to infection by bacteria that normally colonize just the upper airway. The increased frequency of lower respiratory tract infections in the elderly population results, in large part, from loss of function of the mucociliary elevator and increased aspiration of secretions containing bacteria from the upper respiratory tract (128,129).

In addition to the removal of bacteria by mucus flow, mucosal fluid contains many antibacterial products such as lactoferrin, lactoperoxidase, mucin, lysozyme, and defensins (130). Lactoferrin, found in various body fluids, such as milk, saliva, and tears, binds iron and lowers the level of available iron (especially in areas with low pH) (131,132). Mucin traps the microbes and facilitates their removal. IgA antibodies in mucosal fluid may inhibit colonization by blocking microbial adherence sites and by inactivating toxins. Lysozyme reduces bacterial load by cleaving 1-4 linkage of *N*-acetyl muramic acid in the bacterial peptidoglycan. Many bactericidal peptides, including defensins, disrupt the bacterial membrane and kill the bacteria (133). In the lung, surfactants such as SP-A and SP-D may be important in host defense by opsonizing bacteria for alveolar macrophages (134). SP-A–deficient mice were shown to be more susceptible than normal mice to group B streptococci infection in the lung (135).

Local Response to Bacterial Invasion (Acute Inflammation)

Upon entry into the host, many bacterial products initiate local inflammatory processes. The list of the bacterial products initiating these processes includes peptidoglycan, LPS, formyl-methionyl peptides (e.g., f-Met-Leu-Phe), lipoteichoic acid, exotoxins, lipoproteins, and glycolipids (136). Most of these molecules appear to bind a new class of pathogen pattern-recognition molecules, called Toll-like receptors (TLRs) (see Chapter 17). Lipoproteins or peptidoglycans stimulate the host cells by binding to TLR-2. Although LPS binds to CD14 and lipid binding proteins, it requires binding to TLR-4 for cell signaling, because mice with a mutated TLR-4 gene are unresponsive to LPS. Bacterial DNA, rich in unmethylated CpG motif, was shown to bind TLR-9. Double-strand RNA can bind TLR-3 and activate NFκB in the target cells (137). Bacterial flagellin can bind TLR-5 (138). In addition to the TLR molecules, many components of bacteria (e.g., peptidoglycan) can enhance the inflammatory process by activating complement through the alternative pathway (139) and generating inflammatory fragments.

During the initial phase of inflammation after a bacterial invasion, many cell types residing in the mucosa or skin (e.g., keratinocytes) may produce molecules important in controlling infections. Several studies revealed that mast cells are among the important resident host cells. Mast cells are abundant along the bronchial tree and epidermis of the skin and are classically known for their stores of histamine and serotonin (140). They are now known to contain preformed tumor necrosis factor α (TNF-α), as well as to be a major source of various cytokines. Mast cells account for 90% of interleukin (IL)–4– and IL-6–producing cells in the nasal cavity (141). Upon exposure to various bacterial products (e.g., LPS), mast cells release these cytokines, which are essential for the recruitment of neutrophils to the site of inflammation. The absence of mast cells can increase the susceptibility of animals to bacterial infections in the peritoneum or the lung, and their absence can be partially compensated for by administration of TNF-α (142,143).

As the inflammatory process persists, additional cell types come to the site of inflammation. In the case of experimental pneumococcal pneumonia, neutrophils come to the lung in 12 to 24 hours, followed by the appearance of monocytes and macrophages in 48 hours (144). Few lymphocytes are observed in the lung during this time. Neutrophils and macrophages become activated by the bacterial products (e.g., LPS) and cytokines upon their arrival at the site of infection. Neutrophils and macrophages can rapidly phagocytize and kill the bacteria (see Chapter 35 for a detailed description of phagocytosis). Phagocytosis can occur by recognizing certain native molecular structures of the bacteria such as lectins, PS, and peptides (RGD sequence) (145), or by recognizing the host opsonins on the bacterial surface with CR3 and crystallized fragment (Fc) receptors.

Inflammatory processes trigger the cascade of chemokine and cytokine release at the site of inflammation. Sequential appearance of chemokines has been noted in the pneumonia model (144). The peak levels of chemokines MIP-2 and KC are achieved in the lung less than 6 hours after infection. The peak levels of MIP-1a and MCP-1 are observed in 12 to 24 hours. Neutralizing MIP-1a and MCP-1 along with RANTES reduces macrophage recruitment. f-Met-Leu-Phe from bacteria may be also important in recruiting monocytes and neutrophils, because its antagonist can reduce the entry of these cells to the lung. The cytokines produced during acute inflammation can be divided into two groups: proinflammatory cytokines (e.g., IL-1 and TNF-α) and anti-inflammatory cytokines (e.g., IL-4). The molecules produced during inflammation can induce the expression of endothelial cell, intracellular, and vascular cell adhesion molecules on endothelial cells and selectins and integrins in leukocytes (see Chapter 37), thereby modifying the properties of the cells at the site of inflammation (e.g., cell adhesion, vascular permeability).

Systemic Response to Bacterial Invasion

Once bacteria enter the systemic circulation, they are largely removed by the spleen or the liver (40,146). Persons lacking splenic function (because of sickle cell disease or splenectomy) are at increased risk of pneumococcal sepsis (147,148). Clearance of bacteria from the blood by these organs is facilitated because phagocytes are abundant and blood circulates slowly in these organs, because preexisting cross-reactive antibodies can fix complement (149), and because the alternative pathway or mannose-binding lectin can fix complement nonspecifically. The bacteria release many inflammatory bacterial products into the systemic circulation and trigger many systemic changes, such as fever and accumulation of leukocytes at the sites of infection.

Cytokines (e.g., IL-6, IL-1) and glucocorticoids trigger the acute-phase response by stimulating hepatocytes to produce and secrete a variety of molecules termed acute-phase reactants, such as coagulation factors, serum amyloid A protein, C-reactive protein (CRP), and collectins (150). Collectin molecules have a C-type lectin motif and a collagen-like motif, and they can bind to the surface of bacteria, activate complement along the classical pathway, and opsonize bacteria. For instance, mannose-binding lectin, a collectin, binds bacterial surface glycoproteins that contain mannose and N-acetyl glucosamine. Increased incidence of infection has been associated with low serum levels of mannose-binding lectin (151,152).

Because CRP was shown to protect animals from pneumococcal infections (153,154), explanations for the observations were sought. CRP can bind to phosphocholine, which is expressed on many pathogens. Because many pathogens appear to use phosphocholine to bind to the host cells (26,64), CRP may inhibit bacterial adhesion. Also, CRP can bind Fc receptor (FcR) expressed on the cell (155,156) and fix complement (157) and therefore may function like anti-phosphocholine antibodies. Indeed, CRP can kill H. influenzae in vitro in the presence of complement. Studies in transgenic mice confirmed that CRP is protective against microbial pathogens (158). This is consistent with its ability in vitro to bind microbes, activate the complement classical pathway, and engage FcγRI and FcγRII (159). In transgenic mice, however, protection also requires the alternative pathway of complement, and FcγRI is dispensable.

One systemic response to infection is to lower the serum concentration of iron (131). This is achieved by an increase in the transferrin concentration in serum and by an increase in iron storage of tissues. Iron at the site of inflammation may be reduced by neutrophil-secreted lactoferrin. The reduction in the amount of iron available to bacteria can be a significant defensive measure (160). Moreover, even moderate reduction of iron intake (161) or use of an iron chelator (162) has been shown to be beneficial against infections by extracellular bacteria. In contrast, iron excess may predispose a person to infections (163).

In the past, study of molecules for their role in host defense in vivo was limited by the availability of a few natural mutations (or alleles). With the widespread use of targeted gene deletion and transgenic technology, many new molecules have been investigated for their in vivo role. Some of these studies relevant to extracellular bacterial infections are listed in Table 2. Although the story is still evolving, these studies have begun to show the complexity of host defense in molecular detail. For instance, studies have revealed unexpected relevance of some molecules to protection against bacterial infections. Lipoproteins are shown to be relevant to bacterial infections because lipoproteins can bind and neutralize LPS. Surfactant molecules are also important, and their mechanisms are under investigation. These studies further illustrate the differences in the protective mechanisms used against different groups of bacteria. C9 deficiency predisposes a person to infection by gram-negative organisms such as N. meningitidis but not to infection by gram-positive bacteria. This information has supported the understanding that bactericidal killing is not the major protective mechanism against gram-positive bacteria.

Several additional mutations are found to predominantly affect the defense against gram-negative organisms (164).

TABLE 2. *Genes associated with the changes in the susceptibility to extracellular bacterial infections*

Genes involved	Susceptible	Reference
LDL Receptor	Gram-negative bacteria (LPS)	(288)
C3	Group B streptococcus	(289)
C4	Group B streptococcus	(289)
C9	*Neisseria meningitidis*	(290)
SP-A	Group B streptococcus	(135)
TNFRI	*Streptococcus pneumoniae*	(291)
IL-6	*Escherichia coli*	(292)
IFN-g	*Brucella abortus*	(293)
IL-10	*E. coli* (fewer bacteria but more damage)	(169)
TNFRI and type 1 IL-1R	*E. coli*	(294)
bcl-3	*S. pneumoniae*	(164)
P50 unit of NFκB	*S. pneumoniae Listeria monocytogenes*	(295)
Nude mice	*Helicobacter pylori*	(296)
Btk	*S. pneumoniae*	(209)
TLR-4	*E. coli*	(267)
CXCL15	*Klebsiella pneumoniae*	(297)
CXCR2	*Pseudomonas aeruginosa*	(298)
IL-8R murine homolog	*E. coli*	(299)
LFA-1 (CD11a/CD18)	*S. pneumoniae*	(300)
Mac-1 (CD11b/CD18)	*S. pneumoniae*	(300)
Mrp-1	More resistant to *S. pneumoniae*	(170)

Btk, Bruton's tyrosine kinase; CXCL15, chemokine ligand 15; CXCR2, chemokine receptor 2; IFN, interferon; IL, interleukin; LDL, low-density lipoprotein; LFA-1, leukocyte function–associated antigen 1; LPS, lipopolysaccharide; Mrp-1, macrophage inflammatory protein–related protein 1; SP-A, surfactant protein A; TLR, Toll-like receptor; TNFRI, tumor necrosis factor receptor type I.

The IL-1β gene is allelic at various locations, but only the allelic homozygosity at position −511 of IL-1β gene is associated with increased fatal outcome to *N. meningitidis* infections in humans, in comparison with heterozygosity at that position (165). The fact that heterozygous individuals are more protected than homozygotes also complicates the potential explanations. In addition, *in vivo* manifestations of the same genetic defect can be different in different genetic backgrounds. The effect of the btk mutation is largely limited to production of antibodies to PS antigens in mice (166), but the same mutation produces agammaglobulinemia in humans (167). Interestingly, an immunodeficient human patient with the inability to produce antibodies to PS (but not protein) antigens was found to have a mutation at btk (168), which further emphasizes that background genes can have a profound effect on the *in vivo* role of one mutation. Last, phenotypic changes are complex. IL-10 gene deletion results in fewer bacteria but more tissue damage after an infection (169). Mrp-1 deletion results in an increased resistance to pneumococcal infections (170). As additional information becomes available, a more comprehensive picture will emerge. This should help expand the use of immunoregulators (e.g., TNF-α antagonist) for treating autoimmune diseases (171) without compromising the patient's ability to combat infections.

ANTIGEN-SPECIFIC HOST DEFENSE RESPONSE

In addition to antigen-nonspecific responses, the host mounts an adaptive, antigen-specific immune response. For protective responses to extracellular bacteria, B cell (not T cell)–mediated immune responses are critical, as shown by the clinical observations of patients with Bruton's agammaglobulinemia. These patients, who have relatively normal T-cell function but lack B cells, suffer mostly from infections by extracellular bacteria and can be treated very successfully with passive administration of pooled gamma globulin (172). Protective B-cell responses are described in detail as follows.

Responses of the Host (B-Cell) Immune System to Bacteria

After an asymptomatic exposure or an infection, the host develops antibodies to many different bacterial antigens. For instance, the level of antibodies to various pneumococcal antigens increases in young children as they age, even without clinical infections (173). An infection, when it occurs, presents the host with a large load of antigens, especially free PS antigen. In fact, PS is readily detectable in the urine of many patients (174,175) and may be sufficient to neutralize the anti-PS antibodies in the host. Bacterial toxins are generally proteins and induce strong immune responses in a conventional T cell–dependent manner. In contrast, PS capsules are often elusive targets for the host immune system. PS antigens generally stimulate a subset of B cells (176) with minimal help from T cells (177). PS does not bind MHC class II molecules as protein antigens do (178) and may actually interfere with the presentation of protein antigens (179). PS antigens do not usually induce the formation of germinal centers (180,181), they elicit poor immune memory (182), and they easily tolerize B cells (182,183).

PS antigens commonly elicit oligoclonal antibodies, which utilize a restricted number of V-region genes (184–187) even among genetically unrelated humans (188,189). In addition, the antibodies to PS exhibit few somatic mutations (189,190) and generally have low affinity (191,192). However, because the capsular PS and LPS O-antigens present repeating epitopes, even low-affinity antibody can bind with enough avidity to fix complement and cause opsonization and bacteriolysis.

The poor immunogenicity of PS antigens in comparison with protein antigens (193) contributes to the ability of surface PS to shield bacteria from the host immune system. Children do not produce antibodies to most PS antigens until they are several years old (87), and they are particularly susceptible during the first few years of life to infections by encapsulated bacteria (194).

Although young children respond poorly to pure PS antigens, they readily produce antibodies to PS conjugated to a protein carrier. The clinical use of the "conjugate" vaccines inducing antibodies to Hib PS in young children has virtually eliminated Hib meningitis (195), as well as oropharyngeal colonization by Hib (196). Similar "conjugate" vaccine approaches have been used to produce a seven-valent pneumococcal vaccine and a meningococcal conjugate vaccine. Both vaccines were shown to be effective in clinical trials (197,198); however, the new pneumococcal conjugate vaccine is complex and relatively expensive.

Not all PS antigens are presented to the host as free PS molecules, and some PS antigens remain associated with the bacteria. When the bacteria enter the blood circulation, they localize at the marginal zone of the spleen (199). Bacterial PS antigens then stimulate the marginal zone B cells, which rapidly (within 2 to 3 days) become antibody-producing plasma cells. Marginal zone B cells have several unique characteristics. They have distinct phenotypes (CD21^{hi}, CD23$^-$), have unique response characteristics to polyclonal activators (200), and uniquely require a proline-rich tyrosine kinase (Pyk-2) for their development (201). In accordance with these findings, immune responses to the PS attached to bacteria have additional distinct features that indicate an involvement of T cells (202). Unlike free PS, the response to the PS attached to bacteria appears to require cofactors such as B7-2 (203) and CD40 (203,204). Also, the immune response to bacterial PS could be reduced with simultaneous injection of anti-CD4 and anti-CD8 antibodies, although the immune response was intact in mice lacking the T-cell receptor genes (205,206). In addition, other bacterial molecules would participate in this antibody response as adjuvant.

Preimmune animals have antibodies that cross-react with many structurally unrelated antigens. These antibodies are often labeled "natural antibodies." The majority of these antibodies are of the immunoglobulin M (IgM) isotype and frequently bind autologous antigens. Various studies have suggested that natural antibodies are from B1 cells, which are found primarily in the peritoneum. Studies also suggest that these natural antibodies are important in the early phase of infections by bacteria or viruses (207). Anti-phosphocholine antibodies may be an example of natural antibodies. Anti-phosphocholine antibodies react with a phosphocholine epitope found on *S. pneumoniae, H. influenzae,* and *Wuchereria bancrofti* (a tissue nematode) (208–210). Anti-phosphocholine antibodies may reduce the susceptibility of mice to pneumococcal infections (209). Deletion of the V-region gene, used to produce anti-phosphocholine antibodies, renders a mouse susceptible to pneumococcal infections (211).

In addition to natural antibodies, animals often have preexisting antibodies to a PS that often cross-react with structurally similar PS (212–214). This often occurs because many PS molecules have very similar structures. Sometimes it is difficult to distinguish the usual "anti-PS antibody" from the "natural antibodies." Cross-reactions may play an important role in protecting the host against their first exposure to a bacterial species. For instance, human adults carry detectable amounts of antibodies to the Hib PS, even in the absence of vaccination, and are relatively resistant to *H. influenzae* infections (194). Although some of the antibodies may be the result of immunization by subclinical infections, the majority of human preimmune (but not postimmune) anti–Hib PS antibody cross-reacts with *E. coli* K100, whose PS capsule is an isopolymer of Hib PS (215). Experimental colonization of rats with *E. coli* K100 can protect them against Hib (216). About 1% of human immunoglobulin G (IgG) binds a carbohydrate epitope (Galα1→3Gal) (217), and this antibody can kill *Trypanosoma* and *Leishmania in vitro* (218). Cross-reactive antibodies binding the LPS core components are thought to be responsible for the protection from bacteremic dissemination of gonococci in nonimmune patients (149), although they cannot prevent infection of the genital tract (149).

Normal gut flora may be the antigenic stimulus for many of the cross-reactive anti-PS antibodies. About 1% of the population carries *E. coli* K100 in the gut at any time (219). Antibodies to (Galα1→3Gal) are found to bind many species of bacteria isolated from normal stool specimens (217). The gut flora may have additional interesting effects on the immune system. In some transgenic mice, inflammatory bowel diseases develop in the presence of normal intestinal flora but not in the absence of gut flora. In some animals, such as chickens and rabbits, microbial colonization of the gut appears to be necessary for the normal development of antibody V-region repertoires (220). Bacteria should therefore be considered as active participants in shaping the host immune system.

Protective Mechanisms of Antibodies

Antibodies to virulence factors may act by neutralizing their function. Antitoxin antibodies can protect a host by blocking their action or by increasing the removal rate of the toxins (e.g., blocking the binding to the host cell receptors). Antibodies to an *E. coli* adhesin can prevent experimental infections of *E. coli* (221), and antibodies to PsaA may inhibit its adhesion function. Antibody to M protein neutralizes its ability to interfere with complement and provides protection against infections by *S. pyogenes*. Antibodies to PspA, pneumolysin, autolysin, or PspC (CbpA) can protect animals from fatal pneumococcal sepsis. Although these antigens are being investigated as potential replacements for the expensive pneumococcal conjugate vaccines, the protective mechanisms are still unclear. The most recent hypothesis suggests that antibodies to PspA may alter the complement fixation on pneumococci (19,20). Antibodies to IgA1 protease or iron-transport systems (55–57) can also protect against bacterial infections, most probably by neutralizing their normal functions.

Another mechanism of protection by antibodies may be the facilitation of *in vivo* removal of bacteria from circulation by enhancing the clearance of bacteria by the reticuloendothelial system. In the presence of the antibody, bacterial removal by the liver increases significantly (40). This enhancement is not observed in C3-deficient animals, which demonstrates the need for C3.

Antibodies to the capsule PS can provide protection by fixing complement on the surface of bacteria and by inducing bacteriolysis or opsonization. The bacteriolysis pathway can be significant *in vivo* in protection against gram-negative bacteria, as illustrated by the fact that persons with deficiencies of C5 to C9 components are susceptible to the infections by *N. meningitidis* (222). In contrast, antibodies and complement do not lyse gram-positive bacteria but opsonize them for phagocytic killing, as explained later (139). Host phagocytes cannot readily recognize and kill the intact encapsulated gram-positive bacteria. However, once they are coated with antibodies and complement fragments, the host phagocytes can readily recognize the bacteria with various recognition receptors and engulf the bacteria for intracellular killing. An FcR (CD16b) and a complement receptor (CR3) are some of the important recognition receptors. CR3, an integrin molecule, is a heterodimer of CD11b and CD18. Protection mediated by this antibody/complement-mediated opsonization is probably very important *in vivo*, because both complement deficiency and agammaglobulinemia predispose individuals to infections by many different extracellular bacteria (172,222). To be effective for opsonization, the epitope of the surface antigens must be exposed on the surface of the bacteria. Effective antibodies to the porins of *N. meningitidis* recognize the surface loop of the molecule (223). In most pneumococci, C-PS is mostly buried underneath the PS capsule. Although antibodies to the C-PS can fix complement (40), anti–C-PS are not as effective against most *S. pneumoniae* as antibodies to capsular PS (224). Antibodies to C-PS are much more protective, however, against capsular type 27 pneumococci, in which the capsule itself contains C-PS epitopes (225).

Because antibody-mediated opsonization and bacteriolysis are dependent on the complement-fixing properties of the Fc region, the relative efficacies of antibodies of different immunoglobulin isotypes have been compared. IgM antibodies are produced early in the course of infections and should be important in the early phase of infections, because they fix complement very efficiently and can opsonize the bacteria. Selective deficiency of IgM antibodies was found to increase susceptibility to bacterial infections (226). Studies revealed that specific IgM antibodies agglutinate erythrocytes, fix complement, and lyse erythrocytes more readily than do IgG antibodies (227), and IgM antibodies are more effective in complement-mediated bacteriolysis (228,229); however, IgG antibodies are more effective than IgM antibodies at preventing infection of mice with pneumococci (230,231) or in opsonizing Hib *in vitro* (232). Moreover, some IgG subclasses have been reported to be more protective against specific viral (233) and fungal (234) infections than are antibodies to other subclasses. These results suggest that optimal opsonization requires not only complement receptors but also FcRs for IgG. In the absence of inflammation, IgM antibodies are confined to the intravascular space, whereas IgG antibodies can enter the extracellular space. Inflammation can make the vessels at the infection site permeable, however, and antibodies of all isotypes may enter the site of infection. In comparison with IgM antibodies, IgG antibodies may be especially efficient at neutralizing toxins, inasmuch as they have a longer half-life, generally have a higher affinity, and are already present in extravascular spaces before infection (235).

IgG subclasses differ in their ability to fix complement and to bind FcRs (236,237). It was also reported that IgG1 mouse monoclonal antibody is protective against *Cryptococcus neoformans*, but IgG3 mouse antibody is not (234). Consequently, the fact that antibodies to bacterial PS are found to be largely restricted to a single IgG subclass (IgG2 in humans and IgG3 in mice) has led to many studies of differences in the protective properties of anti-PS antibodies of different isotypes. Mouse IgG3 (but not other IgG subclasses) antibodies can associate with each other through their Fc regions (238), and this feature may make the IgG3 antibodies to PS with low affinity more effective in binding the antigen than are antibodies of other isotypes of the same affinity. Although these observations provide a theoretical advantage for mouse IgG3, the same aggregation phenomenon has not been observed for human IgG2 antibodies. The full significance of IgG3 aggregation is not clear, however, inasmuch as anti-PS antibodies of the IgG3 isotype have not been observed to be any more efficacious against pneumococcal infections than antibodies of other isotypes (239).

Moreover, in contrast to expectations, many studies found that human IgG1 antibodies are slightly more effective than human IgG2 antibodies for opsonization and bacteriolysis (237,240–242). Neither of these isotypes appears to be essential, however, inasmuch as individuals lacking IgG1 and IgG2 subclass genes are healthy (243). Furthermore, human IgG2 antibodies bind less strongly to CD16, CD32, and CD64 than do IgG1 or IgG3 (244) and may not be effective for opsonization by neutrophils from the individuals homozygous for a specific CD32 allele (242). Together, these observations strongly suggest that human IgG2 (or mouse IgG3) subclass may not provide any unique advantage in defense against bacteria.

IgG (but not IgM and IgA) antibodies are transported across the placenta to the fetus during the late phase of gestation. The maternal antibodies provide significant amounts of protection to the neonates from many extracellular bacterial infections. Neonates with Bruton's agammaglobulinemia are generally healthy for about 6 to 9 months, until their maternal antibodies are catabolized. Among IgG subclasses, IgG1 concentration in the cord blood is higher (1.8-fold) than that in mother's blood, whereas IgG2 concentrations in both sites are comparable (245). Studies have suggested that IgG antibodies are actively transported across the placenta by neonatal FcR, which is structurally similar to the MHC class I molecules (246). This molecule may also be responsible for the rescue of the antibody molecules from intracellular catabolism (247).

IgA is highly heterogeneous in structure (it can exist as a monomer, as a polymer, or in secretory forms), and its function is still unclear. Although it has been reported that IgA can opsonize (248), fix complement (249), and facilitate the lysis of *N. meningitidis* (250), other studies have found that IgA does not fix complement *in vitro* (251) and may even inhibit the IgG-mediated complement-dependent killing (252,253). The ability of IgA to fix complement may also depend on its denaturation or its glycosylation status (229,254). Nevertheless, studies have indicated that IgA antibodies may fix complement by the mannose-binding lectin pathway (255), and human IgA antibodies against pneumococcal capsular PS can opsonize pneumococci for killing by polymorphonuclear neutrophils (256).

Bacteria that commonly colonize or infect mucosal areas often produce IgA1 protease, and IgA antibody has been found to provide protection in at least some cases (257). These findings suggest that IgA may play an important role as a part of the complex mucosal immune defense. It may function by aggregating the bacteria and facilitating their expulsion from mucosal areas. IgA may also block the invasion of bacteria through the mucosal epithelial cells, inasmuch as endocytosed IgA was found to block the transport of virus through the epithelial cells (258). IgA-deficient persons and mice are relatively healthy, however, and IgA-deficient mice could elicit normal protective immunity to experimental infections with influenza virus. IgM antibodies may function as secretory antibodies in IgA-deficient individuals (259).

Responses by T-Cell Immune System to the Extracellular Bacteria

Although the response to toxins from extracellular bacteria is T cell–dependent, antibodies to the toxins mediate protection and therefore the protective immunity against extracellular bacteria is clearly centered on the B-cell responses. Studies have, however, suggested additional roles for T cells in responses to extracellular bacteria and their products.

Zwitterionic capsular PS of *Bacteroides fragilis* and *S. pneumoniae* serotype 1 can stimulate CD4$^+$ T cells in the presence of antigen-presenting cells (260). It is also well established that PS associated with lipid can stimulate T cells in association with CD1 molecule (261). This may be relevant because capsular PS of gram-negative bacteria (38) and lipoteichoic acid of gram-positive bacteria are associated with lipid. Last, studies of vaccines against *H. pylori* in experimental animals suggested that the protection is associated with CD4$^+$ T cells and not with the level of antibodies (262). Future studies will undoubtedly reveal additional roles for T cells in responses to extracellular bacteria.

The following experience showed that bactericidal anticapsular antibodies are the key factor in protection from systemic infections with Neisseria organisms (285–287). In the past, meningococcal epidemics were common among the military recruits. Gotschlich et al. were studying the military trainees at the U.S. Army basic training center at Fort Dix, New Jersey. As a part of their study, these investigators obtained blood samples from all of the recruits (more than 15,000 men) at the time of their arrival at the camp and obtained nasopharyngeal cultures from them at regular intervals during their training. During the study, an epidemic of meningococcal disease occurred, and eventually five cases of *N. meningitidis* serogroup C infection were identified among members of the same training battalion. Nasopharyngeal cultures obtained before the outbreak indicated that 53 recruits were colonized with *N. meningitidis* serogroup C, considered to be the case strain. Of these colonized recruits, 13 lacked bactericidal antibody to the case strain. The five cases of systemic meningococcal infection occurred among the 13 recruits who lacked this bactericidal antibody and had nasopharyngeal colonization with the case strain. Thus, in a meningococcal epidemic situation, if a person acquires the case strain in the nasopharynx and lacks bactericidal antibody, the risk of serious infection is approximately 30% to 40%. These findings led to the development and use of a tetravalent meningococcal capsular vaccine in military recruits, which has prevented epidemics in basic training centers since 1973.

DELETERIOUS HOST RESPONSE

Inflammatory response by the host inevitably causes some tissue damage, and in some bacterial infections, such as pneumonia and meningitis, this damage plays a significant role in disease pathological processes and symptoms. For instance, it has been shown with animal models of meningitis that inflammation associated with bacterial products (primarily cell walls) is the primary cause of neurological damage. Treatment of animals with antibiotics alone can eradicate the bacteria but does not prevent neurological damage. In contrast, it was shown that when inflammation was controlled by steroids administered along with the antibiotic, the amount of neurological damage was considerably reduced (263).

Antigen-Nonspecific Deleterious Response

Uncontrolled inflammation at the systemic level can produce septic shock, which can be triggered by several factors, including exotoxins (e.g., staphylococcal enterotoxin B) of gram-positive bacteria or LPS of gram-negative bacteria. Staphylococcal enterotoxin B binds the host's class II molecules of the MHC region and can stimulate large numbers of helper T cells to release cytokines. Such toxins are termed *superantigens,* because they are often able to stimulate all T cells expressing one particular $V\beta$ TCR family. Septic shock can also be initiated when LPS from gram-negative bacteria binds CD14 and a TLR and stimulates macrophages or monocytes to secrete inflammatory cytokines (see Chapter 17). In addition to cytokines, the stimulation of host cells by bacterial products leads to the release of other mediators of inflammation, such as arachidonic acid metabolites, activation of complement cascade, and activation of coagulation cascade. Excess release of the mediators leads to the failure of the vascular system and, finally, the failure of multiple organ systems. Studies using transgenic mice with defective genes have identified several molecules critical in developing the septic shock, such as TNF-α, one of its receptors (TNFRI), IL-1-converting enzyme, and intracellular adhesion molecule–1 (264). This approach also showed that CD14 and TLR-4 are critical for LPS-induced septic shock and CD28, a T-cell co-stimulation molecule, is necessary for superantigen-induced septic shock (264).

Another example of uncontrolled host response is found with anthrax infections. Lethal factor binds the protective antigen immobilized on the macrophages and then stimulates the cells to secrete cytokines and reactive oxygen intermediates. These macrophage products are thought to kill the host, because the host dies even when the proliferation of the bacteria is controlled. When macrophage cells are removed from animals, the animals are resistant to anthrax toxins (265). This suggests that the macrophage response to the toxins is actually responsible for the death of the host.

Although inflammation is a significant cause of morbidity and mortality, it must also be regarded as the host's primary protection from bacterial infections. Evidence for this hypothesis comes from studies with TLR-4–deficient mice, which, although nonreactive to LPS and completely resistant to LPS shock, are more susceptible to infection with gram-negative bacteria than are normal mice (266,267). Perhaps LPS is "toxic" because the host has evolved to use this common bacterial component as a trigger for host responses.

Antigen-Specific Deleterious Response

Many bacterial antigens express the epitopes cross-reactive with host antigens and thus have the potential to elicit antibodies during infections that cross-react with host tissue. For instance, the PS capsule of *N. meningitidis* group B mimics epitopes expressed in the central nervous system (268), such as *N*-acetylneuraminic acid epitope in the embryonic neural cell adhesion molecule (269). The LPS of many strains of *N. meningitidis, N. gonorrhoeae, H. influenzae,* and *H. ducreyi* express the epitope of a blood group antigen, p^K (270). The LPS of *Campylobacter jejuni* and *H. pylori* express epitopes mimicking other host antigens, such as ganglioside and Lewis X, respectively (270). Epidemiological studies associated *C. jejuni* infections with the development of an autoimmune disease, Guillain-Barré syndrome (271). Studies with experimental animals found that immunization with *S. pneumoniae* can elicit antibodies to C-PS that can react with mouse kidney glomerulus and cause proteinuria (272). Further studies of this observation suggest that the B cells producing antibodies that cross-react with autoantigens may normally be eliminated by apoptosis (273).

Although the association between the previously noted examples of cross-reacting bacterial antigens and autoimmunity is unclear, *S. pyogenes* infection is associated with rheumatic fever and acute glomerulonephritis. Studies revealed that *S. pyogenes* can be divided into two classes with a monoclonal antibody to M protein (274) and that rheumatic fever develops only after an infection of *S. pyogenes* with class I strains (274). Class I and class II strains of *S. pyogenes* can also be readily distinguished by the linkage relationship of the M protein genes with the genes encoding related surface proteins (274,275). M proteins from some class I *S. pyogenes* express epitopes highly cross-reactive with epitopes of cardiac myosin, tropomyosin, vimentin, laminin, and keratin (276–278). An antibody molecule may bind to all of these protein molecules, because a major portion of these proteins is coiled-coil α helix (278). The polyreactive antibodies to M protein may directly damage myocardial and endothelial cells (279). In addition to antibodies, CD4$^+$ and CD8$^+$ T cells are found at the rheumatic heart valves (280), and the T cells proliferate in response to M protein peptides and heart proteins (281). These observations suggest that the T cells with cross-reactivity between M protein and myosin may be involved in the pathogenesis of rheumatic fever as well.

In addition to M protein, group A PS of *S. pyogenes* has been shown to express epitopes that are cross-reactive with myosin. This antibody to group A PS also binds M protein and other α helical molecules (278,282,283) and may be cytotoxic to cardiac myocardium and endothelium. Interestingly, the V region of antibodies to group A PS with myosin cross-reactivity is encoded by the same germline V-region genes used for antibodies binding only group A PS (284).

SUMMARY

Because extracellular bacteria can grow rapidly and produce toxins, some are potent pathogens. To combat these bacteria, higher organisms have developed a facet of the immune system centered on antibody molecules, complement, and phagocytes. This facet of the immune system is composed of multiple layers of protection. In the early stage of an infection, complement, phagocytes, and natural antibodies cross-reacting with many antigens are important in host defense. During the late stage of an infection, pathogen-specific antibodies appear. These antibodies generally mediate the ultimate protection against extracellular bacteria by triggering the protective effects of complement and phagocytes. Although antibody molecules are central to the process, host defense requires a broad diversity of molecules (including CRP, TLRs, and transferrin), and antibody molecules may cause damage instead of protection. A better understanding of how this facet of the immune system protects against each pathogen will aid in the development of more effective preventive and therapeutic measures against these pathogens.

REFERENCES

1. Thomas L. *The lives of a cell: notes of a biology watcher.* New York: Bantam Books, 1974.
2. McCarty M. The streptococcal cell wall. *Harvey Lect* 1971;65:73.
3. Gray BM. Streptococcal infection. In: Brachman PE, ed. *Bacterial infection.* New York: Plenum Publishing, 1997.
4. Tomasz A. Choline in the cell wall of a bacterium: novel type of polymer-linked choline in pneumococcus. *Science* 1967;157:694.
5. Brundish DE, Baddiley J. Pneumococcal C-substance, a ribitol teichoic acid containing choline phosphate. *Biochem J* 1968;110:573.
6. Fischer W. Teichoic acid and lipoglycans. *New Compr Biochem* 1994; 27:199.
7. Fischer W, Behr T, Hartmann R, et al. Teichoic acid and lipoteichoic acid of *Streptococcus pneumoniae* possess identical chain structures. A reinvestigation of teichoic acid (C-polysaccharide). *Eur J Biochem* 1993;215:851.
8. Briles DE, Hollingshead SK, King J, et al. Immunization of humans with recombinant pneumococcal surface protein A (rPspA) elicits antibodies that passively protect mice from fatal infection with *Streptococcus pneumoniae* bearing heterologous PspA. *J Infect Dis* 2000;182:1694.
9. Briles DE, Paton JC, Nahm MH, et al. Immunity to *Streptococcus pneumoniae.* In: Cunningham MW, Fujinami RS, eds. *Effects of microbes on the immune system.* Philadelphia: Lippincott-Raven, 1999:263.
10. Brooks-Walter A, Briles DE, Hollingshead SK. The pspC gene of *Streptococcus pneumoniae* encodes a polymorphic protein, PspC, which elicits cross-reactive antibodies to PspA and provides immunity to pneumococcal bacteremia. *Infect Immun* 1999;67:6533.
11. Rosenow C, Ryan P, Weiser JN, et al. Contribution of novel choline-binding proteins to adherence, colonization and immunogenicity of *Streptococcus pneumoniae. Mol Microbiol* 1997;25:819.
12. Briles DE, Ades E, Paton JC, et al. Intranasal immunization of mice with a mixture of the pneumococcal proteins PsaA and PspA is highly protective against nasopharyngeal carriage of *Streptococcus pneumonia. Infect Immun* 2000;68:796.
13. Canvin JR, Marvin AP, Sivakumaran M, et al. The role of pneumolysin and autolysin in the pathology of pneumonia and septicemia in mice infected with a type 2 pneumococcus. *J Infect Dis* 1995;172: 119.
14. Wani JH, Gilbert JV, Plaut AG, et al. Identification, cloning, and sequencing of the immunoglobulin A1 protease gene of *Streptococcus pneumoniae. Infect Immun* 1996;64:3967.
15. Poulsen K, Reinholdt J, Kilian M. Characterization of the *Streptococcus pneumoniae* immunoglobulin A1 protease gene and its translation product. *Infect Immun* 1996;64:3957.
16. Nandiwada LS, Hostetter MK, Dunny GM. Genetic analysis of a C3 degrading proteinase in *Streptococcus pneumoniae.* Presented at the 96th General Meeting of the American Society of Microbiology, New Orleans 1996;177(abst B).
17. Adamou JE, Heinrichs JH, Erwin AL, et al. Identification and characterization of a novel family of pneumococcal proteins that are protective against sepsis. *Infect Immun* 2001;69:949.
18. Wizemann TM, Heinrichs JH, Adamou JE, et al. Use of a whole genome approach to identify vaccine molecules affording protection against *Streptococcus pneumoniae* infection. *Infect Immun* 2001;69:1593.
19. Briles DE, Hollingshead SK, Swiatlo E, et al. PspA and PspC: their potential for use as pneumococcal vaccines. *Microb Drug Resist* 1997; 3:401.
20. Tu AH, Fulgham RL, McCrory MA, et al. Pneumococcal surface protein A inhibits complement activation by *Streptococcus pneumoniae. Infect Immun* 1999;67:4720.
21. Wu H-Y, Nahm MH, Guo Y, et al. Intranasal immunization of mice with PspA (pneumococcal surface protein A) can prevent intranasal carriage, pulmonary infection, and sepsis with *Streptococcus pneumoniae. J Infect Dis* 1997;175:839.
22. Lock RA, Hansman D, Paton JC. Comparative efficacy of autolysin and pneumolysin as immunogens protecting mice against infection by *Streptococcus pneumoniae. Microb Pathog* 1992;12:137.
23. Tart RC, McDaniel LS, Ralph BA, et al. Truncated *Streptococcus pneumoniae* PspA molecules elicit cross-protective immunity against pneumococcal challenge in mice. *J Infect Dis* 1996;173:380.
24. Briles DE, Paton JC, Swiatlo E, et al. Pneumococcal vaccines. In: Fischetti VA, Novick RP, Ferretti JJ, et al., eds. *Gram-positive pathogens.,* Washington, DC: ASM Press, 2000:244.
25. Madsen M, Lebenthal Y, Cheng Q, et al. A pneumococcal protein that elicits interleukin-8 from pulmonary epithelial cells. *J Infect Dis* 2000;181:1330.
26. McCullers JA, Tuomanen EI. Molecular pathogenesis of pneumococcal pneumonia. *Front Biosci* 2001;6:D877.
27. Horstmann RD, Sievertsen HJ, Knobloch J, et al. Antiphagocytic activity of streptococcal M protein: selective binding of complement control protein factor H. *Proc Natl Acad Sci U S A* 1988;85:1657.
28. Briese T, Hakenbeck R.. Interaction of the pneumococcal amidase with lipoteichoic acid and choline. *Eur J Biochem* 1985;146:417.
29. Schneewind O, Fowler A, Faull KF. Structure of cell wall anchor of cell surface proteins in *Staphylococcus aureus. Science* 1995;268:103.
30. Fischetti VA, Pancholi V, Schneewind O. Conservation of a hexapeptide sequence in the anchor region of surface proteins from gram-positive cocci. *Mol Microbiol* 1990;4:1603.
31. Dale JB, Chiang EY, Lederer JW. Recombinant tetravalent group A streptococcal M protein vaccine. *J Immunol* 1993;151:2188.
32. Janulczyk R, Iannelli F, Sjoholm AG, et al. Hic, a novel surface protein of *Streptococcus pneumoniae* that interferes with complement function. *J Biol Chem* 2000;275:37257.
33. Nikaido H. Outer membrane. In: Neidhardt FC, ed. *Escherichia coli and Salmonella: cellular and molecular biology.* Washington, DC: ASM Press, 1996:29.
34. Preston A, Mandrell RE, Gibson BW, et al. The lipooligosaccharides of pathogenic gram-negative bacteria. *Crit Rev Microbiol* 1996;22:139.
35. Jap BK, Walian PJ. Structure and function of porins. *Physiol Rev* 1996;76:1073.
36. Ezzell JW, Welkos SL. The capsule of *Bacillus anthracis,* a review. *J Appl Microbiol* 1999;87:250.
37. Gotschlich EC, Fraser BA, Nishimura O, et al. Lipid on capsular polysaccharides of gram-negative bacteria. *J Biol Chem* 1981;256: 8915.
38. Kuo JS-C, Doelling VW, Graveline JF, et al. Evidence for covalent attachment of phospholipid to the capsular polysaccharide of *Haemophilus influenzae* type b. *J Bacteriol* 1985;163:769.
39. Kazatchkine MD, Fearon DT, Austen KF. Human alternative complement pathway: membrane-associated sialic acid regulates the competition between B and beta 1H for cell-bound C3b. *J Immunol* 1979; 122:75.
40. Brown EJ, Hosea SW, Hammer CH, et al. A quantitative analysis of the interactions of antipneumococcal antibody and complement in experimental pneumococcal bacteremia. *J Clin Invest* 1982;69:85.
41. Cheng Q, Finkel D, Hostetter MK. Novel purification scheme and functions for a C3-binding protein from *Streptococcus pneumoniae. Biochemistry* 2000;39:5450.
42. Gray BM, Pritchard DG. Phase variation in the pathogenesis of group B streptococcal infections. *Zbl Bakt Suppl* 1992;22:452.
43. Jonsson AB, Nyberg G, Normark S. Phase variation of gonococcal pili by frameshift mutation in pili C, a novel gene for pilus assembly. *EMBO J* 1991;10:477.
44. Weiser JN, Markiewicz A, Tuomanen EI, et al. Relationship between phase variation in colony morphology, intrastrain variation in cell wall

physiology, and nasopharyngeal colonization by *Streptococcus pneumoniae*. *Infect Immun* 1996;64:2240.

45. Weiser JN. Relationship between colony morphology and the life cycle of *Haemophilus influenzae:* the contribution of lipopolysaccharide phase variation to pathogenesis. *J Infect Dis* 1993;168:672.

46. Bos MP, Grunert F, Belland RJ. Differential recognition of members of the carcinoembryonic antigen family by Opa variants of *Neisseria gonorrhoeae*. *Infect Immun* 1997;65:2353.

47. Hammerschmidt S, Muller A, Sillmann H, et al. Capsule phase variation in *Neisseria meningitidis* serogroup B by slipped-strand mispairing in the polysialyltransferase gene (siaD): correlation with bacterial invasion and the outbreak of meningococcal disease. *Mol Microbiol* 1996;20:1211.

48. Covacci A, Telford JL, Del Giudice G, et al. *Helicobacter pylori* virulence and genetic geography. *Science* 1999;284:1328.

49. Finlay BB, Falkow S. Common themes in microbial pathogenicity revisited. *Microbiol Mol Biol Rev* 1997;61:136.

50. Salyers AA, Whitt DD. *Bacterial pathogenesis.* Washington, DC: ASM Press, 1994:47.

51. Barg NL, Harris T. Toxin-mediated syndromes. In: Crossely KB, ed. *The staphylococci.* New York: Churchill Livingston, 1997:527.

52. Noel JM, Boedeker EC. Enterohemorrhagic *Escherichia coli:* a family of emerging pathogens. *Dig Dis* 1997;15:67.

53. Lingwood CA. Verotoxin-binding in human renal sections. *Nephron* 1994;66:21.

54. Stojiljkovic I, Srinivasan N. *Neisseria meningitidis* tonB, exbB and exbD genes: Ton-dependent utilization of protein-bound iron in *Neisseriae*. *J Bacteriol* 1997;179:805.

55. Lewis LA, Gray E, Wang YP, et al. Molecular characterization of hpuAB, the haemoglobin-haptoglobin–utilization operon of *Neisseria meningitidis*. *Mol Microbiol* 1997;23:737.

56. Pettersson A, Poolman JT, van der Ley P, et al. Response of *Neisseria meningitidis* to iron limitation. *Antonie Van Leeuwenhoek* 1997; 71:129.

57. Thomas CE, Sparling PF. Isolation and analysis of a fur mutant of *Neisseria gonorrhoeae*. *J Bacteriol* 1996;178:4224.

58. Tai SS, Lee CJ, Winter RE. Hemin utilization is related to virulence of *Streptococcus pneumoniae*. *Infect Immun* 1993;61:5401.

59. Earhart CF. Uptake and metabolism of iron and molybdenum. In: Neidhardt FC, ed. Escherichia coli *and* Salmonella: *cellular and molecular biology.* Washington DC: ASM Press, 1996:1075.

60. Neilands JB. Siderophores: structure and function of microbial iron transport compounds. *J Biol Chem* 1995;270:26723.

61. Andersson B, Dahmen J, Frejd T, et al. Identification of an active disaccharide unit of a glycoconjugate receptor for pneumococci attaching to human pharyngeal epithelial cells. *J Exp Med* 1983;158:559.

62. Cundell DR, Gerard NP, Gerard C, et al. *Streptococcus pneumoniae* anchor to activated human cells by the receptor for platelet-activating factor. *Nature* 1995;377:435.

63. Swords WE, Ketterer MR, Shao J, et al. Binding of the non-typeable *Haemophilus influenzae* lipooligosaccharide to the PAF receptor initiates host cell signalling. *Cell Microbiol* 2001;3:525.

64. Swords WE, Buscher BA, Ver Steeg K II, et al. Non-typeable *Haemophilus influenzae* adhere to and invade human bronchial epithelial cells via an interaction of lipooligosaccharide with the PAF receptor. *Mol Microbiol* 2000;37:13.

65. Striker R, Nilsson U, Stonecipher A, et al. Structural requirements for the glycolipid receptor of human uropathogenic *Escherichia coli*. *Mol Microbiol* 1995;16:1021.

66. Sengupta TK, Sengupta DK, Ghose AC. A 20-kDa pilus protein with haemagglutination and intestinal adherence properties expressed by a clinical isolate of a non-01 *Vibrio cholerae*. *FEMS Microbiol Lett* 1993;112:237.

67. Chiang SL, Taylor RK, Koomey M, et al. Single amino acid substitutions in the N-terminus of *Vibrio cholerae* TcpA affect colonization, autoaggregation, and serum resistance. *Mol Microbiol* 1995;17: 1133.

68. Brennan MJ, Shahin RD. Pertussis antigens that abrogate bacterial adherence and elicit immunity. *Am J Respir Crit Care Med* 1996;154:S145.

69. Geuijen CA, Willems RJ, Bongaerts M, et al. Role of the *Bordetella pertussis;* minor fimbrial subunit, FimD, in colonization of the mouse respiratory tract. *Infect Immun* 1997;65:4222.

70. Balachandran P, Hollingshead SK, Paton JC, et al. The autolytic enzyme LytA of *Streptococcus pneumoniae* is not responsible for releasing pneumolysin. *J Bacteriol* 2001;183:3108.

71. Paton JS. The contribution of pneumolysin to the pathogenicity of *Streptococcus pneumoniae*. *Trends Microbiol* 1996;4:103.

72. Benton KA, Everson MP, Briles DE. A pneumolysin-negative mutant of *Streptococcus pneumoniae* causes chronic bacteremia rather than acute sepsis in mice. *Infect Immun* 1995;63:448.

73. Ji Y, Carlson B, Kondugunta A, et al. Intranasal immunization with C5a peptidase prevents nasopharyngeal colonization of mice by the group A streptococcus. *Infect Immun* 1997;65:2080.

74. Bohnsack JF, Widjaja K, Ghazizadeh S, et al. A role for C5 and C5a-ase in the acute neutrophile response to group B streptococcal infections. *J Infect Dis* 1997;175:847.

75. Angel CS, Ruzek M, Hostetter MK. Degradation of C3 by *Streptococcus pneumoniae*. *J Infect Dis* 1994;170:600.

76. Kilian M, Mestecky J, Kulhavy R, et al. IgA1 proteases from *Haemophilus influenzae, Streptococcus pneumoniae, Neisseria meningitidis,* and *Streptococcus sanguis:* comparative immunochemical studies. *J Immunol* 1980;124:2596.

77. Dassy B, Hogan T, Foster TJ, et al. Involvement of the accessory gene regulator (agr) in expression of type-5 capsular polysaccharide by *Staphylococcus aureus*. *J Gen Microbiol* 1993;139:1301.

78. Lee JC, Takeda S, Livolsi PJ, et al. Effects of *in vitro* and *in vivo* growth conditions on expression of type-8 capsular polysaccharide by *Staphylococcus aureus*. *Infect Immun* 1993;61:1853.

79. Uhl MA, Miller JF. Autophosphorylation and phosphotransfer in the *Bordetella pertussis* BvgAS siganl transduction cascade. *Proc Natl Acad Sci U S A* 1994;91:1163.

80. Hoch JA, Silhavy TJ. *Two-component signal transduction.* Washington DC: ASM Press, 1995:488.

81. de Kievit TR, Iglewski BH. Bacterial quorum sensing in pathogenic relationships. *Infect Immun* 2000;68:4839.

82. Withers H, Swift S, Williams P. Quorum sensing as an integral component of gene regulatory networks in gram-negative bacteria. *Curr Opin Microbiol* 2001;4:186.

83. Covacci A, Rappuoli R. Tyrosine-phosphorylated bacterial proteins: Trojan horses for the host cell. *J Exp Med* 2000;191:587.

84. Asahi M, Azuma T, Ito S, et al. *Helicobacter pylori* CagA protein can be tyrosine phosphorylated in gastric epithelial cells. *J Exp Med* 2000;191:593.

85. Fischetti VA. Streptococcal M protein: molecular design and biological behavior. *Clin Microbiol Rev* 1989;2:286.

86. Henrichsen J. Six newly recognized types of *Streptococcus pneumoniae*. *J Clin Microbiol* 1995;33:2759.

87. Robbins JB, Austrian R, Lee CJ, et al. Considerations for formulating the second-generation pneumococcal capsular polysaccharide vaccine with emphasis on the cross-reactive types within groups. *J Infect Dis* 1983;148:1136.

88. Mandrell RE, Apicella MA. Lipo-oligosaccharides (LOS) of mucosal pathogens: molecular mimicry and host-modifications of LOS. *Immunobiology* 1993;187:382.

89. Lancefield RC. Current knowledge of the type specific M antigens of group A streptococci. *J Immunol* 1962;89:307.

90. Fischetti VA, Bessen DE, Schneewind O, et al. Protection against streptococcal pharyngeal colonization with vaccines composed of M protein conserved regions. *Adv Exp Med Biol* 1991;303:159.

91. Dillard JP, Vandersea MW, Yother J. Characterization of the cassette containing genes for type 3 capsular polysaccharide biosynthesis in *Streptococcus pneumoniae*. *J Exp Med* 1995;181:973.

92. Mbelle N, Huebner RE, Wasas AD, et al. Immunogenicity and impact on nasopharyngeal carriage of a nonavalent pneumococcal conjugate vaccine. *J Infect Dis* 1999;180:1171.

93. Dagan R. Treatment of acute otitis media—challenges in the era of antibiotic resistance. *Vaccine* 2000;19(Suppl 1):S9.

94. Dagan R, Melamed R, Muallem M, et al. Reduction of nasopharyngeal carriage of pneumococci during the second year of life by a heptavalent conjugate pneumococcal vaccine. *J Infect Dis* 1996;174:1271.

95. Zhang QY, DeRyckere D, Lauer P, et al. Gene conversion in *Neisseria gonorrhoeae:* evidence for its role in pilus antigenic variation. *Proc Natl Acad Sci U S A* 1992;89:5366.

96. Seifert HS. Questions about gonococcal pilus phase and antigenic variation. *Mol Microbiol* 1997;21:433.

97. Stern A, Meyer TF. Common mechanisms controlling phase and antigenic variation in pathogenic *Neisseria*. *Mol Microbiol* 1987;1:5.

98. Salyers AA, Whitt DD. *Bacterial pathogenesis, a molecular approach.* Washington, DC: ASM Press, 1994:3.

99. Rupp ME, Archer GL. Coagulase-negative staphylococci: pathogens associated with medical progress. *Clin Infect Dis* 1994;19:231.

100. Neish AS, Gewirtz AT, Zeng H, et al. Prokaryotic regulation of epithelial responses by inhibition of IkappaB-alpha ubiquitination. *Science* 2000;289:1560.

101. Xavier RJ, Podolsky DK. Microbiology. How to get along—friendly microbes in a hostile world. *Science* 2000;289:1483.

102. Davey ME, O'Toole GA. Microbial biofilms: from ecology to molecular genetics. *Microbiol Mol Biol Rev* 2000;64:847.

103. Edwards C. Problems posed by natural environments for monitoring microorganisms. *Mol Biotechnol* 2000;15:211.

104. Pericone CD, Overweg K, Hermans PW, et al. Inhibitory and bactericidal effects of hydrogen peroxide production by *Streptococcus pneumoniae* on other inhabitants of the upper respiratory tract. *Infect Immun* 2000;68:3990.

105. McFall-Ngai MJ. Negotiations between animals and bacteria: the "diplomacy" of the squid—*Vibrio* symbiosis. *Comp Biochem Physiol A Mol Integr Physiol* 2000;126:471.

106. Bartlett JG, Chang TW, Taylor NS, et al. Colitis induced by *Clostridium difficile*. *Rev Infect Dis* 1979;1:370.

107. Caugant DA, Hoiby EA, Magnus P, et al. Asymptomatic carriage of *Neisseria meningitidis* in a randomly sampled population. *J Clin Microbiol* 1994;32:323.

108. Kuhns DM, Nelson CT, Feldman HA, et al. The prophylactic value of sulfadiazine in the control of meningococcic meningitis. *JAMA* 1943;123:335.

109. Zangwill KM, Schuchat A, Wenger JD. Group B streptococcal disease in the United States, 1990: report from a multistate active surveillance system. *MMWR CDC Surveill Summ* 1992;41:25.

110. Rein MF. Epidemiology of gonococcal infections. In: Roberts RB, ed. *The gonococcus*. New York: John Wiley and Sons, 1977:1.

111. Handsfield HH, Lipman TO, Harnisch JP, et al. Asymptomatic gonorrhea in men: diagnosis, natural course, prevalence, and significance. *N Engl J Med* 1974;290:117.

112. Apicella MA, Ketterer M, Lee FKN, et al. The pathogenesis of gonococcal urethritis in men: confocal and immunoelectron microscopic analysis of urethral exudates from men infected with *Neisseria gonorrhoeae*. *J Infect Dis* 1996;173:636.

113. Edwards JL, Shao JQ, Ault KA, et al. *Neisseria gonorrhoeae* elicits membrane ruffling and cytoskeletal rearrangements upon infection of primary human endocervical and ectocervical cells. *Infect Immun* 2000;68:5354.

114. Edwards JL, Brown EJ, Ault KA, et al. The role of complement receptor 3 (CR3) in *Neisseria gonorrhoeae* infection of human cervical epithelia. *Cell Microbiol* 2001;3:611.

115. Swanson J, Kraus SJ, Gotschlich EC. Studies on gonococcus infection. I. Pili and zone of adhesion: their relation to gonococcal growth patterns. *J Exp Med* 1971;134:886.

116. Ramsey KH, Schneider H, Cross AS, et al. Inflammatory cytokines produced in response to experimental human gonorrhea. *J Infect Dis* 1995;172:186.

117. Musher DM. Infections caused by *Streptococcus pneumoniae*: clinical spectrum, pathogenesis, immunity, and treatment. *Clin Infect Dis* 1992;14:801.

118. Tuomanen EI. The biology of pneumococcal infection. *Pediatr Res* 1997;42:253.

119. Berry AM, Lock RA, Paton JC. Cloning and characterization of nanB, a second *Streptococcus pneumoniae* neuraminidase gene, and purification of the NanB enzyme from recombinant *Escherichia coli*. *J Bacteriol* 1996;178:4854.

120. Berry AM, Lock RA, Thomas SM, et al. Cloning and nucleotide sequence of the *Streptococcus pneumoniae* hyaluronidase gene and purification of the enzyme from recombinant *Escherichia coli*. *Infect Immun* 1994;62:1101.

121. Lin B, Hollingshead SK, Coligan JE, et al. Cloning and expression of the gene for group B streptococcal hyaluronate lyase. *J Biol Chem* 1994;269:30113.

122. Swartz MN. Skin and soft tissue infections. In: Mandell GL, Bennett JE, Dolin R, eds. *Principles and practice of infectious diseases*. New York: Churchill Livingstone, 1995:909.

123. Kazmierczak BI, Mostov K, Engel JN. Interaction of bacterial pathogens with polarized epithelium. *Annu Rev Microbiol* 2001;55:407.

124. Katz J, Sambandam V, Wu JH, et al. Characterization of *Porphyromonas gingivalis*–induced degradation of epithelial cell junctional complexes. *Infect Immun* 2000;68:1441.

125. Zhang JR, Mostov KE, Lamm ME, et al. The polymeric immunoglobulin receptor translocates pneumococci across human nasopharyngeal epithelial cells. *Cell* 2000;102:827.

126. Cundell DR, Weiser JN, Shen J, et al. Relationship between colonial morphology and adherence of *Streptococcus pneumoniae*. *Infect Immun* 1995;63:757.

127. Bancroft GJ, Kelly JP. Macrophage activation and innate resistance to infection in SCID mice. *Immunobiology* 1994;191:424.

128. Musher DM. *Streptococcus pneumoniae*. In: Mandell GL, Bennett JE, Dolin R, eds. *Principles and practice of infectious diseases*. New York: Churchill Livingstone, 1995:1811.

129. Donowitz GR, Mandell GL. Acute pneumonia. In: Mandell GL, Bennett JE, Dolin R, eds. *Principles and practice of infectious diseases*. New York: Churchill Livingstone, 1995:619.

130. Pruitt KM, Rahemtulla F, Mansson-Rahemtulla B. Innate humoral factors. In: Ogra PL, ed. *Handbook of mucosal immunology*. New York: Academic Press, 1994:53.

131. Weinberg ED. Iron withholding: a defense against infection and neoplasia. *Physiol Rev* 1984;64:65.

132. Vorland LH. Lactoferrin: a multifunctional glycoprotein. *APMIS* 1999;107:971.

133. Fellermann K, Stange EF. Defensins—innate immunity at the epithelial frontier. *Eur J Gastroenterol Hepatol* 2001;13:771.

134. Crouch E, Wright JR. Surfactant proteins a and d and pulmonary host defense. *Annu Rev Physiol* 2001;63:521.

135. LeVine AM, Bruno MD, Huelsman KM, et al. Surfactant protein A–deficient mice are susceptible to group B streptococcal infection. *J Immunol* 1997;158:4336.

136. Henderson B, Poole S, Wilson M. Bacterial modulins: a novel class of virulence factors which cause host tissue pathology by inducing cytokine synthesis. *Microbiol Rev* 1996;60:316.

137. Alexopoulou L, Holt AC, Medzhitov R, et al. Recognition of double-stranded RNA and activation of NF-kappaB by Toll-like receptor 3. *Nature* 2001;413:732.

138. Hayashi F, Smith KD, Ozinsky A, et al. The innate immune response to bacterial flagellin is mediated by Toll-like receptor 5. *Nature* 2001;410:1099.

139. Frank MM, Fries LF. The role of complement in defense against bacterial disease. *Baillieres Clin Immunol Allergy* 1988;2:335.

140. Galli SJ. New concepts about the mast cell. *N Engl J Med* 1993;328:257.

141. Bradding P, Feather IH, Wilson S, et al. Immunolocalization of cytokines in the nasal mucosa of normal and perennial rhinitic subjects. The mast cell as a source of IL-4, IL-5, and IL-6 in human allergic mucosal inflammation. *J Immunol* 1993;151:3853.

142. Malaviya R, Ross EA, MacGregor JI, et al. Mast cell phagocytosis of fimH-expressing enterobacteria. *J Immunol* 1994;152:1907.

143. Malaviya R, Ikeda T, Ross E, et al. Mast cell modulation of neutrophil influx and bacterial clearance at sites of infection through TNFα. *Nature* 1996;381:77.

144. Fillion I, Ouellet N, Simard M, et al. Role of chemokines and formyl peptides in pneumococcal pneumonia–induced monocyte/macrophage recruitment. *J Immunol* 2001;166:7353.

145. Ofek I, Goldhar J, Keisari Y, et al. Nonopsonic phagocytosis of microorganisms. *Annu Rev Microbiol* 1995;49:239.

146. Brown EJ, Hosea SW, Frank MM. The role of complement in the localization of pneumococci in the splanchnic reticuloendothelial system during experimental bacteremia. *J Immunol* 1981;126:2230.

147. Styrt B. Infection associated with asplenia: risks, mechanisms, and prevention. *Am J Med* 1990;88:33N.

148. Van Wyck DB, Witte MH, Witte CL. Synergism between the spleen and serum complement in experimental pneumococcemia. *J Infect Dis* 1982;145:514.

149. Apicella MA, Westerink MAJ, Morse SA, et al. Bactericidal antibody response of normal human serum to the lipooligosaccharide of *Neisseria gonorrhoeae*. *J Infect Dis* 1986;153:520.

150. Steel DM, Whitehead AS. The major acute phase reactants: C-reactive protein, serum amyloid P component and serum amyloid A protein. *Immunol Today* 1994;15:81.

151. Turner MW. Mannose-binding lectin: the pluripotent molecule of the innate immune system. *Immunol Today* 1996;17:532.

152. Lau YL, Chan SY, Turner MW, et al. Mannose-binding protein in

preterm infants: developmental profile and clinical significance. *Clin Exp Immunol* 1995;102:649.

153. Mold C, Nakayama S, Holzer TJ, et al. C-reactive protein is protective against *Streptococcus pneumoniae* infection in mice. *J Exp Med* 1981;154:1703.

154. Yother J, Volanakis JE, Briles DE. Human C-reactive protein is protective against fatal *Streptococcus pneumoniae* infection in mice. *J Immunol* 1982;128:2374.

155. Marnell LL, Mold C, Volzer MA, et al. C-reactive protein binds to Fc gamma RI in transfected COS cells. *J Immunol* 1995;155:2185.

156. Bharadwaj D, Stein MP, Volzer M, et al. The major receptor for C-reactive protein on leukocytes is fcgamma receptor II. *J Exp Med* 1999; 190:585.

157. Agrawal A, Shrive AK, Greenhough TJ, et al. Topology and structure of the C1q-binding site on C-reactive protein. *J Immunol* 2001;166: 3998.

158. Szalai AJ. The antimicrobial activity of C-reactive protein. *Microbes Infect* 2002;4:201.

159. Szalai AJ, Agrawal A, Greenhough TJ, et al. C-reactive protein: structural biology and host defense function. *Clin Chem Lab Med* 1999; 37:265.

160. Bullen JJ. *Iron and infection.* New York: John Wiley and Sons, 1999.

161. Weinberg ED, Weinberg GA. The role of iron in infection. *Curr Opin Infect Dis* 1997;8:164.

162. Jones RL, Peterson CM, Grady RW, et al. Effects of iron chelators and iron overload on *Salmonella* infection. *Nature* 1977;267:63.

163. Patruta SI, Horl WH. Iron and infection. *Kidney Int Suppl* 1999;69: S125.

164. Schwarz EM, Krimpenfort P, Verma IM. Immunological defects in mice with a targeted disruption in Bcl-3. *Genes Dev* 1997;11:187.

165. Read RC, Camp NJ, di Giovine FS, et al. An interleukin-1 genotype is associated with fatal outcome of meningococcal disease. *J Infect Dis* 2000;182:1557.

166. Perlmutter RM, Nahm M, Stein KE, et al. Immunoglobulin subclass-specific immunodeficiency in mice with an X-linked B-lymphocyte defect. *J Exp Med* 1979;149:993.

167. Kinnon C, Hinshelwood S, Levinsky RJ, et al. X-linked agammaglobulinemia—gene cloning and future prospects. *Immunol Today* 1993; 14:554.

168. Wood PM, Mayne A, Joyce H, et al. A mutation in Bruton's tyrosine kinase as a cause of selective anti-polysaccharide antibody deficiency. *J Pediatr* 2001;139:148.

169. Sewnath ME, Olszyna DP, Birjmohun R, et al. IL-10–deficient mice demonstrate multiple organ failure and increased mortality during *Escherichia coli* peritonitis despite an accelerated bacterial clearance. *J Immunol* 2001;166:6323.

170. Schultz MJ, Wijnholds J, Peppelenbosch MP, et al. Mice lacking the multidrug resistance protein 1 are resistant to *Streptococcus pneumoniae*–induced pneumonia. *J Immunol* 2001;166:4059.

171. Firestein GS, Zvaifler NJ. Anticytokine therapy in rheumatoid arthritis. *N Engl J Med* 1997;337:195.

172. Lederman HM, Winkelstein JA. X-linked agammaglobulinemia: an analysis of 96 patients. *Medicine* 1985;64:145.

173. Rapola S, Jäntti V, Haikala R, et al. Natural development of antibodies to pneumococcal surface protein A, pneumococcal surface adhesion A, and pneumolysin in relation to pneumococcal carriage and acute otitis media. *J Infect Dis* 2000;182:1146.

174. Mayer ME, Geiseler PJ, Harris B. Coagglutination for detection and serotyping of bacterial antigens: usefulness in acute pneumonias. *Diagn Microbiol Infect Dis* 1983;1:277.

175. Scott JA, Hannington A, Marsh K, et al. Diagnosis of pneumococcal pneumonia in epidemiological studies: evaluation in Kenyan adults of a serotype-specific urine latex agglutination assay. *Clin Infect Dis* 1999;28:764.

176. Herzenberg LA, Stall AM, Lalor PA, et al. The LY-1 B cell lineage. *Immunol Rev* 1986;93:81.

177. Humphrey JH, Parrott DMV, East J. Studies of globulin and antibody production in mice thymectomized at birth. *Immunology* 1964;7: 419.

178. Harding CV, Roof RW, Allen PM, et al. Effects of pH and polysaccharides on peptide binding to class II major histocompatibility complex molecules. *Proc Natl Acad Sci U S A* 1991;88:2740.

179. Leyva-Cobian F, Unanue ER. Intracellular interference with antigen presentation. *J Immunol* 1988;141:1445.

180. Weissman IL, Gutman GA, Friedberg SH, et al. Lymphoid tissue ar-

chitecture. III. Germinal centers, T cells, and thymus-dependent vs thymus-independent antigens. *Adv Exp Med Biol* 1976;66:229.

181. Davies AJS, Carter RL, Leuchars E, et al. The morphology of immune reactions in normal, thymectomized and reconstituted mice III. Response to bacterial antigens: salmonellar flagellar antigen and pneumococcal polysaccharide. *Immunology* 1970;19:945.

182. Baker PJ, Stashak PW, Amsbaugh DF, et al. Characterization of the antibody response to type III pneumococcal polysaccharide at the cellular level. I. Dose-response studies and the effect of prior immunization on the magnitude of the antibody response. *Immunology* 1971;20:469.

183. Klaus GGB, Humphrey JH. The immunological properties of haptens coupled to thymus-independent carrier molecules. I. The characteristics of the immune response to dinitrophenol-lysine–substituted pneumococcal polysaccharide (SIII) and levan. *Eur J Immunol* 1974; 4:370.

184. Crews S, Griffin J, Huang H, et al. A single V_H gene segment encodes the immune response to phosphorylcholine: somatic mutation is correlated with the class of the antibody. *Cell* 1981;25:59.

185. Carroll WL, Adderson EE, Lucas AH, et al. Molecular basis of antibody diversity. In: Ellis RW, Granoff DM, eds. *Development and clinical uses of Haemophilus b conjugate vaccines.* New York: Marcel Dekker, 1994:207.

186. Claflin JL, Hudak S, Maddalena A. Anti-phosphocholine hybridoma antibodies. I. Direct evidence for three distinct families of antibodies in the murine response. *J Exp Med* 1981;153:352.

187. Briles DE, Davie JM. Clonal dominance. I. Restricted nature of the IgM antibody response to group A streptococcal carbohydrate in mice. *J Exp Med* 1975;141:1291.

188. Insel RA, Kittelberger A, Anderson P. Isoelectric focusing of human antibody to the *Haemophilus influenzae* b capsular polysaccharide: restricted and identical spectrotypes in adults. *J Immunol* 1985; 135:2810.

189. Scott MG, Crimmins DL, McCourt DW, et al. Clonal characterization of the human IgG antibody repertoire to *Haemophilus influenzae* type b polysaccharide. III. A single VKII gene and one of several JK genes are joined by an invariant arginine to form the most common L chain V region. *J Immunol* 1989;143:4110.

190. Gearhart PJ, Johnson ND, Douglas R, et al. IgG antibodies to phosphorylcholine exhibit more diversity than their IgM counterparts. *Nature* 1981;291:29.

191. Sharon J, Kabat EA, Morrison S. Association constants of hybridoma antibodies specific for alpha (1-6) linked dextran determined by affinity electrophoresis. *Mol Immunol* 1982;19:389.

192. Hetherington SV. The intrinsic affinity constant (K) of anticapsular antibody to oligosaccharides of *Haemophilus influenzae* type b. *J Immunol* 1988;140:3966.

193. Mond JJ, Lees A, Snapper CM. T cell–independent antigens type 2. *Annu Rev Immunol* 1995;13:655.

194. Fothergill LD, Wright J. Influenzal meningitis: the regulation of age incidence to the bactericidal power of blood against the causal organism. *J Immunol* 1933;24:273.

195. Adams WG, Deaver KA, Cochi SL, et al. Decline of childhood *Haemophilus influenzae* type b (Hib) disease in the Hib vaccine era. *JAMA* 1993;269:221.

196. Takala AK, Eskola J, Leinonen M, et al. Reduction of oropharyngeal carriage of *Haemophilus influenzae* type b (Hib) in children immunized with an Hib conjugate vaccine. *J Infect Dis* 1991;164:982.

197. Shinefield HR, Black S. Efficacy of pneumococcal conjugate vaccines in large scale field trials. *Pediatr Infect Dis J* 2000;19:394.

198. Miller E, Salisbury D, Ramsay M. Planning, registration, and implementation of an immunisation campaign against meningococcal serogroup C disease in the UK: a success story. *Vaccine* 2001; 20(Suppl 1):S58.

199. Martin F, Oliver AM, Kearney JF. Marginal zone and B1 B cells unite in the early response against T-independent blood-borne particulate antigens. *Immunity* 2001;14:617.

200. Oliver AM, Martin F, Gartland GL, et al. Marginal zone B cells exhibit unique activation, proliferative and immunoglobulin secretory responses. *Eur J Immunol* 1997;27:2366.

201. Guinamard R, Okigaki M, Schlessinger J, et al. Absence of marginal zone B cells in Pyk-2–deficient mice defines their role in the humoral response. *Nat Immunol* 2000;1:31.

202. Briles DE, Nahm M, Marion TN, et al. Streptococcal group A carbohydrate has properties of both a thymus-independent (TI-2) and a thymus-dependent antigen. *J Immunol* 1982;128:2032.

203. Wu ZQ, Vos Q, Shen Y, et al. *In vivo* polysaccharide-specific IgG isotype responses to intact *Streptococcus pneumoniae* are T cell dependent and require CD40– and B7–ligand interactions. *J Immunol* 1999;163:659.

204. Hwang Y, Nahm M, Briles D, et al. Acquired, but not innate, immune responses to *Streptococcus pneumoniae* are compromised by neutralization of CD40L. *Infect Immun* 2000;68:511.

205. Wu ZQ, Khan AQ, Shen Y, et al. B7 requirements for primary and secondary protein- and polysaccharide-specific Ig isotype responses to *Streptococcus pneumoniae*. *J Immunol* 2001;165:6840.

206. Snapper CM, Shen Y, Khan AQ, et al. Distinct types of T-cell help for the induction of a humoral immune response to *Streptococcus pneumoniae*. *Trends Immunol* 2001;22:308.

207. Bouvet J, Dighiero G. From natural polyreactive autoantibodies to à la carte monoreactive antibodies to infectious agents: is it a small world after all? *Infect Immun* 1998;66:1.

208. Lal RB, Paranjape RS, Briles DE, et al. Circulating parasite antigen(s) in lymphatic filariasis: use of monoclonal antibodies to phosphocholine for immunodiagnosis. *J Immunol* 1987;138:3454.

209. Briles DE, Nahm M, Schroer K, et al. Antiphosphocholine antibodies found in normal mouse serum are protective against intravenous infection with type 3 *Streptococcus pneumoniae. J Exp Med* 1981;153:694.

210. Weiser JN, Shchepetov M, Chong ST. Decoration of lipopolysaccharide with phosphorylcholine: a phase-variable characteristic of *Haemophilus influenzae. Infect Immun* 1997;65:943.

211. Mi QS, Zhou L, Schulze DH, et al. Highly reduced protection against *Streptococcus pneumoniae* after deletion of a single heavy chain gene in mouse. *Proc Natl Acad Sci U S A* 2000;11:6031.

212. Heidelberger M, Rebers PA. Immunochemistry of the pneumococcal types II, V, and VI. The relation of type VI to type II and other correlations between chemical constitution and precipitation in antisera to type VI. *J Bacteriol* 1960;80:145.

213. MacPherson CFC, Heidelberger M, Alexander HE, et al. The specific polysaccharides of types A, B, C, D, and F *Haemophilus influenzae. J Immunol* 1946;52:207.

214. Heidelberger M, Bernheimer AW. Cross-reactions of polysaccharides of fungi, molds, and yeasts in anti-pneumococcal and other antisera. *Proc Natl Acad Sci U S A* 1984;81:5247.

215. Lucas AH, Langley RJ, Granoff DM, et al. An idiotypic marker associated with a germ-line encoded kappa light chain variable region that predominates the vaccine-induced human antibody response to the *Haemophilus influenzae* b polysaccharide. *J Clin Invest* 1991;88:1811.

216. Moxon ER, Anderson P. Meningitis caused by *Haemophilus influenzae* in infant rats: protective immunity and antibody priming by gastrointestinal colonization with *Escherichia coli. J Infect Dis* 1979;140:471.

217. Galili U, Mandrell RE, Hamadeh RM, et al. Interaction between human natural anti–alpha-galactosyl immunoglobulin G and bacteria of the human flora. *Infect Immun* 1988;56:1730.

218. Avila JL, Rojas M, Galili U. Immunogenic Gal-alpha-1—3Gal carbohydrate epitopes are present on pathogenic American *Trypanosoma* and *Leishmania. J Immunol* 1989;142:2828.

219. Ginsburg CM, McCracken GH Jr, Schneerson R, et al. Association between cross-reacting *Escherichia coli* K100 and disease caused by *Haemophilus influenzae* type b. *Infect Immun* 1978;22:339.

220. Knight KL, Crane MA. Generating the antibody repertoire in rabbit. *Adv Immunol* 1994;56:179.

221. Langermann S, Palaszynski S, Barnhart M, et al. Prevention of mucosal *Escherichia coli* infection by FimH-adhesin–based systemic vaccination. *Science* 1997;276:607.

222. Winkelstein JA. The complement system. In: Gorbach SL, Bartlett JG, Blacklow NR, eds. *Infectious diseases.* Philadelphia: WB Saunders, 1992:37.

223. Van der Lay P, Heckels JE, Virji M, et al. Topology of outer membrane porins in pathogenic *Neisseria* spp. *Infect Immun* 1991;59:2963.

224. Nielsen SV, Sorensen UBS, Henrichsen J. Antibodies against pneumococcal C-polysaccharide are not protective. *Microb Pathog* 1993;14:299.

225. Briles DE, Forman C, Horowitz JC, et al. Antipneumococcal effects of C-reactive protein and monoclonal antibodies to pneumococcal cell wall and capsular antigens. *Infect Immun* 1989;57:1457.

226. Boes M, Prodeus AP, Schmidt T, et al. A critical role of natural immunoglobulin M in immediate defense against systemic bacterial infection. *J Exp Med* 1998;188:2381.

227. Cooper NR. The classical complement pathway: activation and regulation of the first complement component. *Adv Immunol* 1985;37:151.

228. Mostov KE. Transepithelial transport of immunoglobulins. *Annu Rev Immunol* 1994;12:63.

229. Nikolova EB, Tomana M, Russell MW. All forms of human IgA antibodies bound to antigen interfere with complement (C3) fixation induced by IgG or by antigen alone. *Scand J Immunol* 1994;39:275.

230. McDaniel LS, Benjamin WH, Forman C, et al. Blood clearance by anti-phosphocholine antibodies as a mechanism of protection in experimental pneumococcal bacteremia. *J Immunol* 1984;133:3308.

231. Briles DE, Claflin JL, Schroer K, et al. Mouse IgG3 antibodies are highly protective against infection with *Streptococcus pneumoniae. Nature* 1981;294:88.

232. Schreiber JR, Barrus V, Cates KL, et al. Functional characterization of human IgG, IgM, and IgA antibody directed to the capsule of *Haemophilus influenzae* type b. *J Infect Dis* 1986;153:8.

233. Schlesinger JJ, Foltzer M, Chapman S. The Fc portion of antibody to yellow fever virus NS1 is a determinant of protection against YF encephalitis in mice. *Virology* 1993;192:132.

234. Yuan R, Casadevall A, Spira G, et al. Isotype switching from IgG3 to IgG1 converts a nonprotective murine antibody to *Cryptococcus neoformans* into a protective antibody. *J Immunol* 1995;154:1810.

235. Possee RD, Schild GC, Dimmock NJ. Studies on the mechanism of neutralization of influenza virus by antibody: evidence that neutralizing antibody inactivates influenza virus by inhibiting virion transcriptase activity. *J Gen Virol* 1997;58:373.

236. Jefferis R, Pound J, Lund J, et al. Effector mechanisms activated by human IgG subclass antibodies: clinical and molecular aspects. *Ann Biol Clin (Paris)* 1994;52:57.

237. Burton DR, Woof JM. Human antibody effector function. *Adv Immunol* 1992;51:1.

238. Cooper LJ, Shikhman AR, Glass DD, et al. Role of heavy chain constant domains in antibody–antigen interaction. Apparent specificity differences among streptococcal IgG antibodies expressing identical variable domains. *J Immunol* 1993;150:2231.

239. Briles DE, Forman C, Hudak S, et al. The effects of subclass on the ability of anti-phosphocholine antibodies to protect mice from fatal infection with *Streptococcus pneumoniae. J Mol Cell Immunol* 1984;1:305.

240. Amir J, Scott MG, Nahm MH, et al. Bactericidal and opsonic activity of IgG1 and IgG2 anticapsular antibodies to *Haemophilus influenzae* type b. *J Infect Dis* 1990;162:163.

241. Weinberg GA, Granoff DM, Nahm MH, et al. Functional activity of different IgG subclass antibodies against type b capsular polysaccharide of *Haemophilus influenzae. J Immunol* 1986;136:4232.

242. Bredius RGM, de Vries CEE, Troelstra A, et al. Phagocytosis of *Staphylococcus aureus* and *Haemophilus influenzae* type b opsonized with polyclonal human IgG1 and IgG2 antibodies. *J Immunol* 1993;151:1463.

243. Lefranc M, Lefranc G, Rabbitts TH. Inherited deletion of immunoglobulin heavy chain constant region genes in normal human individuals. *Nature* 1982;300:760.

244. Ravetch JV, Kinet J. Fc Receptors. *Annu Rev Immunol* 1991;9:457.

245. Einhorn MS, Granoff DM, Nahm MH, et al. Concentrations of antibodies in paired maternal and infant sera: relationship to IgG subclass. *J Pediatr* 1987;111:783.

246. Leach JL, Sedmak DD, Osborne JM, et al. Isolation from human placenta of the IgG transporter, FcRn, and localization to the syncytiotrophoblast: Implications for maternal-fetal antibody transport. *J Immunol* 1996;157:3317.

247. Ravetch JV, Margulies DH. New tricks for old molecules. *Nature* 1994;372:323.

248. Gorter A, Hiemstra PS, Leijh PCJ, et al. IgA- and secretory IgA-opsonized *S. aureus* induce a respiratory burst and phagocytosis by polymorphonuclear leucocytes. *Immunology* 1987;61:303.

249. Hiemstra PS, Gorter A, Stuurman ME, et al. Activation of alternative pathway of complement by human serum IgA. *Eur J Immunol* 1987;17:321.

250. Jarvis GA, Griffiss JM. Human IgA1 initiates complement-mediated killing of *Neisseria meningitidis. J Immunol* 1989;143:1703.

251. Imai H, Chen RJ, Wyatt RJ, et al. Lack of complement activation by human IgA immune complexes. *Clin Exp Immunol* 1988;73:479.

252. Jarvis GA, Griffiss JM. Human IgA1 blockade of IgG-initiated lysis of *Neisseria meningitidis* is a function of antigen-binding fragment binding to the polysaccharide capsule. *J Immunol* 1991;147:1962.

253. Griffiss JM, Bertram MA. Immunoepidemiology of meningococcal disease in military recruits. II. Blocking of serum bactericidal activity by circulating IgA early in the course of invasive disease. *J Infect Dis* 1977;136:733.

254. Russell MW, Mansa B. Complement-fixing properties of human IgA antibodies. Alternative pathway complement activation by plastic-bound, but not specific antigen-bound, IgA. *Scand J Immunol* 1989; 30:175.

255. Roos A, Bouwman LH, van Gijlswijk-Janssen DJ, et al. Human IgA activates the complement system via the mannan-binding lectin pathway. *J Immunol* 2001;167:2861.

256. Janoff EN, Fasching C, Orenstein JM, et al. Killing of *Streptococcus pneumoniae* by capsular polysaccharide-specific polymeric IgA, complement, and phagocytes. *J Clin Invest* 1999;104:1139.

257. Michetti P, Mahan MJ, Slauch JM, et al. Monoclonal secretory immunoglobulin A protects mice against oral challenge with the invasive pathogen *Salmonella typhimurium. Infect Immun* 1992;60:1786.

258. Lamm ME. Interaction of antigens and antibodies at mucosal surfaces. *Annu Rev Microbiol* 1997;51:311.

259. Brandtzaeg P, Fjellanger I, Gjeruldsen ST. Immunoglobulin M: local synthesis and selective secretion in patients with immunoglobulin A deficiency. *Science* 1968;160:789.

260. Tzianabos AO, Finberg RW, Wang Y, et al. T cells activated by zwitterionic molecules prevent abscesses induced by pathogenic bacteria. *J Biol Chem* 2000;275:6733.

261. Sieling PA, Chatterjee D, Porcelli SA, et al. CD1-restricted T cell recognition of microbial lipoglycan antigens. *Science* 1995;269:227.

262. Sutton P. Progress in vaccination against *Helicobacter pylori. Vaccine* 2001;19:2286.

263. Bhatt SM, Cabellos C, Nadol JB, et al. The impact of dexamethasone on hearing loss in experimental pneumococcal meningitis. *Pediatr Infect Dis J* 1995;14:93.

264. Gutierrez-Ramos JC, Bluethmann H. Molecules and mechanisms operating in septic shock: lessons from knockout mice. *Immunol Today* 1997;18:329.

265. Hanna PC, Acosta D, Collier RJ. On the role of macrophages in anthrax. *Proc Natl Acad Sci U S A* 1993;90:10198.

266. O'Brien AD, Rosenstreich DL, Scher I, et al. Genetic control of susceptibility to *Salmonella typhimurium* in mice: role of the Lps gene. *J Immunol* 1980;124:20.

267. Hagberg L, Briles DE, Eden CS. Evidence for separate genetic defects in C3H/HeJ and C3HeB/FeJ mice that affect susceptibility to gram-negative infections. *J Immunol* 1985;134:4118.

268. Finne J, Leinonen M, Makela PH. Antigenic similarities between brain components and bacteria causing meningitis. Implications for vaccine development and pathogenesis. *Lancet* 1983;2:355.

269. Rougon G, Dubois C, Buckley N, et al. A monoclonal antibody against meningococcus group B polysaccharides distinguishes embryonic from adult N-CAM. *J Cell Biol* 1986;103:2429.

270. Moran AP, Prendergast MM, Appelmelk BJ. Molecular mimicry of host structures by bacterial lipopolysaccharides and its contribution to disease. *FEMS Immunol Med Microbiol* 1996;16:105.

271. Rees JH, Soudain SE, Gregson NA, et al. *Campylobacter jejuni* infection and Guillain-Barré syndrome. *N Engl J Med* 1995;333:1374.

272. Limpanasithikul W, Ray S, Diamond B. Cross-reactive antibodies have both protective and pathogenic potential. *J Immunol* 1995;155:967.

273. Ray SK, Putterman C, Diamond B. Pathogenic autoantibodies are routinely generated during the response to foreign antigen: a paradigm for autoimmune disease. *Proc Natl Acad Sci U S A* 1996;93:2019.

274. Bessen D, Jones KF, Fischetti VA. Evidence for two distinct classes of streptococcal M protein and their relationship to rheumatic fever. *J Exp Med* 1989;169:269.

275. Hollingshead SK, Bessen DE. Evolution of the emm gene family: virulence gene clusters in group A streptococci. *Dev Biol Stand* 1995;85:163.

276. Cunningham MW, McCormack JM, Fenderson PG, et al. Human and murine antibodies cross-reactive with streptococcal M protein and myosin recognize the sequence gln-lys-ser-lys-gln in M protein. *J Immunol* 1989;143:2677.

277. Cunningham MW, Antone SM, Gulizia JM, et al. Alpha-helical coiled-coil molecules: a role in autoimmunity against the heart. *Clin Immunol Immunopathol* 1993;68:118.

278. Cunningham MW. Streptococci and rheumatic fever. In: Friedman H, Rose NR, Bendinelli M, eds. *Microorganisms and autoimmune disease.* New York: Plenum Publishing, 1996:13.

279. Cunningham MW, Antone SM, Gulizia JM, et al. Cytotoxic and viral neutralizing antibodies crossreact with streptococcal M protein, enteroviruses and human cardiac myosin. *Proc Natl Acad Sci U S A* 1992;89:1320.

280. Chow LH, Yuling Y, Linder J, et al. Phenotypic analysis of infiltrating cells in human myocarditis. An immunohistochemical study in paraffin-embedded tissue. *Arch Pathol Lab Med* 1989;113:1357.

281. Guilherme L, Chuna-Neto E, Coelho V, et al. Human heart-infiltrating T cell clones from rheumatic heart disease patients recognize both streptococcal and cardiac proteins. *Circulation* 1995;92:415.

282. Shikhman AR, Greenspan NS, Cunningham MW. A subset of mouse monoclonal antibodies cross-reactive with cytoskeletal proteins and group A streptococcal M proteins recognizes *N*-acetyl-β-D-glucosamine. *J Immunol* 1993;151:3902.

283. Shikhman AR, Cunningham MW. Immunological mimicry between *N*-acetyl-β-D-glucosamine and cytokeratin peptides. *J Immunol* 1994;152:4375.

284. Quinn A, Adderson EE, Shackelford PG, et al. Autoantibody germline gene segment encodes VH and VL regions of a human anti-streptococcal Mab recognizing streptococcal M protein and human cardiac myosin epitopes. *J Immunol* 1994;154:4203.

285. Gotschlich EC, Goldschneider I, Artenstein MS. Human immunity to the meningococcus. V. The effect of immunization with meningococcal group C polysaccharide on the carrier state. *J Exp Med* 1969; 129:1385.

286. Gotschlich EC, Goldschneider I, Artenstein MS. Human immunity to the meningococcus. IV. Immunogenicity of group A and group C meningococcal polysaccharides in human volunteers. *J Exp Med* 1969;129:1367.

287. Gotschlich EC, Liu TY, Artenstein MS. Human immunity to the meningococcus. III. Preparation and immunochemical properties of the group A, group B, and group C meningococcal polysaccharides. *J Exp Med* 1969;129:1349.

288. Netea MG, Demacker PN, Kullberg BJ, et al. Low-density lipoprotein receptor–deficient mice are protected against lethal endotoxemia and severe gram-negative infections. *J Clin Invest* 1996;97:1366.

289. Wessels MR, Butko P, Ma M, et al. Studies of group B streptococcal infection in mice deficient in complement component C3 or C4 demonstrate an essential role for complement in both innate and acquired immunity. *Proc Natl Acad Sci U S A* 1995;92:11490.

290. Ross SC, Densen P. Complement deficiency states and infection: epidemiology, pathogenesis and consequences of neisserial and other infections in an immune deficiency. *Medicine (Baltimore)* 1984;63: 243.

291. OBrien DP, Briles DE, Szalai A, et al. Tumor necrosis factor alpha receptor I is important for survival from *Streptococcus pneumoniae* infections. *Infect Immun* 1999;67:595.

292. Khalil A, Tullus K, Bartfai T, et al. Renal cytokine responses in acute *Escherichia coli* pyelonephritis in IL-6–deficient mice. *Clin Exp Immunol* 2000;122:200.

293. Murphy EA, Sathiyaseelan J, Parent MA, et al. Interferon-gamma is crucial for surviving a *Brucella abortus* infection in both resistant C57BL/6 and susceptible BALB/c mice. *Immunology* 2001;103:511.

294. Mizgerd JP, Spieker MR, Doerschuk CM. Early response cytokines and innate immunity: essential roles for TNF receptor 1 and type I IL-1 receptor during *Escherichia coli* pneumonia in mice. *J Immunol* 2001;166:4042.

295. Sha WC, Liou HC, Tuomanen EI, et al. Targeted disruption of the p50 subunit of NF-kappa B leads to multifocal defects in immune responses. *Cell* 1995;80:321.

296. Engstrand L. Potential animal models of *Helicobacter pylori* infection in immunological and vaccine research. *FEMS Immunol Med Microbiol* 1995;10:265.

297. Chen SC, Mehrad B, Deng JC, et al. Impaired pulmonary host defense in mice lacking expression of the CXC chemokine lungkine. *J Immunol* 2001;166:3362.

298. Tsai WC, Strieter RM, Mehrad B, et al. CXC chemokine receptor CXCR2 is essential for protective innate host response in murine *Pseudomonas aeruginosa* pneumonia. *Infect Immun* 2000;68:4289.

299. Frendeus B, Godaly G, Hang L, et al. Interleukin 8 receptor deficiency confers susceptibility to acute experimental pyelonephritis and may have a human counterpart. *J Exp Med* 2000;192:881.

300. Prince JE, Brayton CF, Fossett MC, et al. The differential roles of LFA-1 and Mac-1 in host defense against systemic infection with *Streptococcus pneumonia. J Immunol* 2001;166:7362.

CHAPTER 42

Immunology of HIV Infection

Mark Dybul, Mark Connors, and Anthony S. Fauci

Introduction
Clinical Aspects of HIV Infection
  Epidemiology · Spectrum of HIV Infection and Development of Disease · Antiretroviral Therapy
Reservoirs of HIV Infection
  Lymphoid Tissue · Resting CD4$^+$ T Cells · Peripheral Blood Dendritic Cells · Monocytes/Macrophages · Central Nervous System · Reproductive Tract
Immune Dysfunction Caused by HIV Infection
  CD4$^+$ T Cells · CD8$^+$ T Cells · Dendritic Cells · B-Lymphocytes · Polymorphonuclear Leukocytes · Monocytes/Macrophages · Natural Killer Cells
HIV-Specific Immune Responses
  Humoral Immune Responses · Cellular Immune Responses
Genetic Factors in HIV Pathogenesis
Long-Term Nonprogressors
  Host Genetic Factors · Host Immune-Response Factors · Virologic Factors
Vaccines
Role of Cellular Activation in HIV Pathogenesis
Cytokines, Chemokines, and HIV
  Effect of Cytokines on HIV Replication · Effect of HIV on Cytokine Production and Networks · HIV Infection and Cytokine Network in Central Nervous System
Conclusions
Acknowledgments
References

INTRODUCTION

The human immunodeficiency virus (HIV) was first identified in 1983 and was shown to be the cause of acquired immunodeficiency syndrome (AIDS) in 1984 (1–3). HIV infection is characterized by the depletion of the CD4$^+$ helper/inducer subset of T-lymphocytes, leading to severe immune deficiency, constitutional symptoms, neurologic disease, and opportunistic infections and neoplasms (reviewed in Fauci and Lane [4]). As of December 2002, 42 million people are living with HIV throughout the world; more than 20 million have died. Between 1981, when the first AIDS patients were described, and 2000, approximately 1.4 million cases of HIV infection have been diagnosed in the United States. HIV is transmitted by sexual contact, parenteral (and rarely mucosal) exposure to blood or blood products during pregnancy or the perinatal period, and by breast-feeding. Rectal or vaginal trauma and the presence of ulcerative genital lesions increase the risk of HIV transmission during sexual contact.

HIV infection is predominantly an infection of the human immune system; its mechanisms of pathogenesis are intricately intertwined with normal immune processes. The introduction of effective antiretroviral therapy has resulted in extraordinary clinical benefits while contributing greatly to the understanding of important virologic and immunologic aspects of HIV infection. Although a wide array of immune system defects are associated with the advanced stages of HIV infection, including abnormalities in the function of all limbs of the immune system, including T- and B-lymphocytes, antigen-presenting cells, natural killer cells, and neutrophils, the loss of immune competence during the course of HIV disease progression can be gauged by the sequential loss of *in vitro* proliferative responses of peripheral blood lymphocytes to recall antigens, alloantigens, and finally, to mitogens (5). In addition to the progressive loss of immune function in general, recent investigations have advanced significantly our understanding of the evolution of HIV-specific immune responses during the course of infection. Insights into aspects of HIV-specific immune responses that may contribute to the *in vivo* control of HIV replication and dissemination are critical to the efforts to develop effective vaccines and, potentially, to therapeutically enhance HIV-specific immunity in HIV-infected individuals. In addition, advances in knowledge regarding the role of cellular activation and the expression and secretion of cytokines in HIV replication and disease progression may provide insights into novel immunomodulatory therapies for the treatment of HIV infection.

CLINICAL ASPECTS OF HIV INFECTION

Epidemiology

The HIV epidemic has occurred in multiple waves, depending on the timing of introduction of the virus into a population and the demographics of the population in question. In certain regions of the world the incidence of infection has recently plateaued, while in other regions incidence rates continue to rise. In 16 African countries, the prevalence of HIV infection among adults aged 15 to 49 exceeds 10% (6); similar rates may be seen in the near future in regions of Asia where the epidemic is accelerating. In the Unites States, male-to-male sexual contact remains the most common mechanism of HIV transmission over the entire course of the epidemic; however, heterosexual transmission and injection drug use account for an increasing proportion of cases of HIV over the past few years.

Globally, different subtypes of HIV, commonly referred to as clades, have been identified. Phylogenetic analysis of HIV proviral sequences reveals two major genetic groups of HIV, the M (major) and O (outlier) groups. The relatively rare O group viruses are concentrated in West Africa, and may elude detection by standard antibody tests for HIV-1. Within the M group, related HIV variants are classified as subtypes (currently designated A to J) according to their degree of genetic similarity. The biochemical basis for the generation of viral diversity is the relative infidelity of the viral reverse transcriptase (RT) enzyme. At the nucleotide level, there is a range of viral diversity among the subtypes; for example, subtypes may diverge up to 14% in their *Gag* (viral core) coding sequences, and by about 30% in their envelope coding sequences. Subtype A viruses are prevalent in central Africa and are also found in East Asia, Europe, Russia, and South America. Subtype B viruses comprise the overwhelming majority of viruses isolated in the United States. Subtype B viruses also are prevalent in Europe, Australia, and South America; variant subtype B viruses have been isolated in Thailand, China, Malaysia, Brazil, and Japan. Subtype C viruses are the most common worldwide; they are prevalent in Southern Africa, Ethiopia, Malawi, Botswana, India, and southern provinces of China, and are also found in Europe, East Asia, and areas of Brazil. Subtype D viruses circulate primarily in Central Africa, while subtype E viruses are isolated predominantly in the rapidly expanding epidemic in Southeast Asia. HIV viral subtypes G, H, and J have been isolated in Africa; however, all three of these subtypes are un-

common. Finally, subtype I viruses have been isolated from patients in Cyprus, although these viruses may actually be recombinants of other viral subtypes. In this regard, recombinant strains of HIV are increasingly recognized throughout the world.

Spectrum of HIV Infection and Development of Disease

Primary Infection

Approximately 3 to 6 weeks following exposure and primary infection with HIV, at least 50% of individuals experience an acute, self-limited syndrome of variable severity that typically persists from one to several weeks and usually resolves spontaneously (reviewed in Tindall and Cooper [7]). This acute HIV syndrome is associated with a burst of viremia; concomitantly, the level of CD4$^+$ T cells in peripheral blood declines, sometimes precipitously. CD4$^+$ T-cell levels frequently rebound to near normal or moderately decreased levels following resolution of the acute syndrome; however, markedly decreased levels may persist and worsen subsequent to the immediate period of primary infection (Fig. 1). In some cases the initial transient decline in CD4$^+$ T-cell levels is so profound, and the levels of plasma viremia so high, that opportunistic infections have occurred during the period of primary infection. The levels of CD8$^+$ T cells and B cells also decline during primary infection; however, the levels of CD8$^+$ T cells usually rise to normal or higher-than-normal levels within 3 to 4 weeks following the onset of illness. Because the CD8$^+$ T-cell count rebounds faster than the CD4$^+$ T-cell level, an inversion of the normal CD4:CD8 ratio occurs during the later phases of primary infection and is maintained following resolution of the acute phase of infection even in the unusual setting of a normal CD4$^+$ T-cell count (4). Despite the fact that much of the data concerning immunologic changes during primary HIV infection have been collected on patients who were brought to the attention of their physicians because of symptoms associated with the acute retroviral syndrome, it is likely that these changes occur to a greater or lesser degree in most patients following primary HIV infection, even in the absence of clinical symptoms.

Primary infection with HIV is followed by a series of events including rapid dissemination of virus throughout the body and the subsequent induction of immune responses that partially control viral replication (reviewed in Pantaleo et al. [8]) (see discussion of HIV-specific immune responses below). The events that occur during primary HIV infection involve both viral and host factors, and are important in determining the course of HIV disease. Depending on the route of exposure, the mechanisms of initial infection may vary, although there are no obvious differences in manifestations of disease in individuals infected by blood-borne versus mucosal routes, suggesting that even if the initial target cells of HIV infection are different, the subsequent rounds of viral spread occur ultimately in similar cells with a similar outcome.

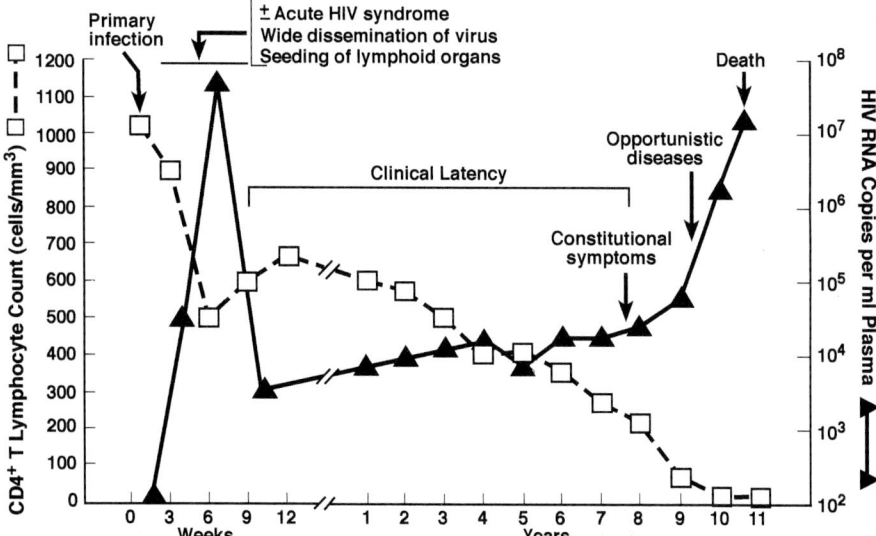

FIG. 1. The typical clinical course of an HIV-infected individual. After primary infection, a burst of plasma viremia occurs in concert with a transient decline in the CD4+ T-cell count. Partial immune control over virus replication ensues, resulting in a variable period of clinical latency. As the CD4+ T-cell count declines, the risk of developing constitutional symptoms and opportunistic diseases increases. Adapted from Fauci et al. (234), with permission.

Chronic/Persistent Infection

HIV is a lentivirus, a family of viruses characterized by chronic persistent infection with development of pathologic consequences in the later stages of disease. Similar to other lentiviruses, and despite potent cellular and humoral immune responses that develop following primary infection, HIV is not completely cleared from the body. Ongoing virus replication can be detected consistently in the blood and in lymphoid tissue during the course of chronic infection. This situation differs from certain other viral infections (e.g., herpesvirus infections) that have a microbiologically latent phase wherein the viral genome is present but significant amounts of viral RNA, DNA, and proteins are not made. In HIV disease, chronic infection is the norm and a completely protective immune response has not been identified. Important factors in the ability of the virus to avoid immune clearance are the extraordinary replication kinetics of HIV (9), and the high error rate of reverse transcriptase (RT) (10), which allow for the constant generation and accumulation of genomic mutations.

Chronic HIV disease comprises a spectrum from the asymptomatic state to advanced immunodeficiency and clinical disease. The median time between primary HIV infection and the development of AIDS is approximately 10 years (11). During this period, CD4+ T-cell counts usually decrease gradually until they reach a level at which the risk of opportunistic diseases is high (12) (Fig. 1). Prior to the onset of opportunistic diseases, HIV-infected individuals may experience various constitutional signs and symptoms (4). Neurologic disease in the form of AIDS encephalopathy may occur in HIV-infected individuals in the absence of opportunistic diseases.

Advanced HIV Disease (AIDS)

Progression of HIV disease is associated with depletion of CD4+ T cells and consequent increased risk for the development of opportunistic AIDS-defining diseases (12). The loss of integrity of immune function, particularly cell-mediated immune responses, allows ubiquitous environmental organisms with limited virulence (e.g., *Pneumocystis carinii* and *Mycobacterium avium*) to become life-threatening pathogens. A number of severe conditions indicative predominantly of depressed cell-mediated immunity due to HIV infection constitute the Centers for Disease Control and Prevention (CDC) surveillance case definition of AIDS (13). These conditions include fungal infections (e.g., esophageal or pulmonary candidiasis; extrapulmonary Cryptococcosis, Histoplasmosis, or Coccidioidomycosis; and pulmonary or extrapulmonary *P. carinii* infection); viral infections (e.g., cytomegalovirus retinitis, esophagitis, pneumonia, myelitis, pancreatitis, or adrenalitis; and herpes simplex virus bronchitis, pneumonia, esophagitis, or chronic skin ulcers); bacterial and mycobacterial infections (e.g., pulmonary tuberculosis, extrapulmonary infection due to any mycobacterium, recurrent bacterial pneumonia, and recurrent *Salmonella* septicemia); protozoal infections (e.g., gastrointestinal syndromes due to infection with *Cryptosporidium* or *Isospora,* and toxoplasmic encephalitis); neoplasia (e.g., invasive cervical cancer; Burkitt's, immunoblastic, or primary central-nervous-system [CNS] lymphoma; and Kaposi's sarcoma); HIV-related encephalopathy, progressive multifocal leukoencephalopathy (due to reactivation of JC virus); and wasting syndrome. Nearly all of these HIV-associated illnesses, including the malignancies, are now known to be caused by infection with or reactivation of opportunistic organisms. In this regard, human papillomaviruses, Epstein–Barr virus, and human herpesvirus-8 appear to play causative roles in the AIDS-defining malignancies, cervical cancer, lymphomas, and Kaposi's sarcoma, respectively (14,15).

The degree to which an infection can be considered opportunistic can be inferred by the CD4$^+$ T-cell counts at which it occurs (12,16). These observations have provided an extraordinary "experiment of nature" whereby the relationship between a measurable degree of immune dysfunction (i.e., the level of CD4$^+$ T-cell count) and the probability of contracting a particular opportunistic infection has become apparent. For example, oral candidiasis and tuberculosis tend to occur as the CD4$^+$ T-cell count falls into the 250 to 500 cells/μL range. Cryptosporidiosis generally does not occur until the CD4$^+$ T-cell count is less than 200 cells/μL. *P. carinii* pneumonia, disseminated *M. avium* complex infection, cryptococcosis, and toxoplasmosis are indicative of more severe immunodeficiency. At the more extreme end of the opportunistic disease spectrum, cytomegalovirus (CMV) retinitis is usually diagnosed after the CD4$^+$ T-cell count has fallen below 50 cells/μL. The steep increase in the risk of developing AIDS-defining illnesses associated with a CD4$^+$ T-cell count of less than 200 cells/μL led to the 1993 revision of the CDC definition of AIDS, which now includes a low CD4$^+$ T-cell count (less than 200 cells/μL) as an AIDS-defining criterion (13).

The clinical management of HIV-infected patients with advanced-stage disease requires intense vigilance since complications directly related to HIV or opportunistic diseases may affect virtually any organ system. The combination of multidrug antiretroviral therapy, prophylaxis against opportunistic infections, and aggressive treatment of opportunistic diseases as they occur has led to a significant increase in survival and quality of life after diagnosis of AIDS (17).

Long-term Nonprogression

In a small percentage of HIV-infected individuals, no evidence of disease progression can be detected over an extended period of time (18,19). Studies of such "long-term nonprogressors" have contributed to our understanding of the pathogenesis of disease progression and have increased optimism that some forms of protective immunity may indeed exist in HIV infection. For a complete discussion, see discussion of long-term nonprogressors below.

Antiretroviral Therapy

Recent progress in understanding the pathogenesis of HIV disease combined with the development of potent antiretroviral agents have resulted in an abundance of treatment options for HIV-infected individuals. Combination therapy with at least three different agents, known as highly active antiretroviral therapy (HAART), has resulted in suppression of plasma HIV RNA and a significant increase in CD4$^+$ T-cell counts

in a majority of patients (20). This salutary effect on laboratory parameters has a direct clinical correlate; there has been a significant decrease in morbidity and a 60% reduction in mortality in the United States since the introduction of HAART. However, due to toxicities of the drugs and difficulty adhering to complex regimens, in studies in community clinics, success rates in terms of maintaining suppression of plasma HIV RNA at 52 weeks approximate 50% (21). There appears to be a degree of immune restoration with effective antiretroviral therapy. It is now clear that patients who experience an increase in CD4$^+$ T cells to a certain level while receiving HAART may safely discontinue secondary and/or primary prophylactic medications against certain opportunistic pathogens, such as *P. carinii* and cytomegalovirus (22). In addition, HAART can prevent the appearance of Kaposi's sarcoma as well as lead to a regression of existing lesions in certain individuals. Unfortunately, the immune restoration observed with HAART does not seem to extend to HIV-specific immune responses, at least not in the short term (see discussion of HIV-specific immune responses below).

RESERVOIRS OF HIV INFECTION

It has been clearly demonstrated that in the vast majority of HIV-infected individuals there is persistent HIV replication despite highly effective therapy. HIV proviral DNA and mRNA can be detected in CD4$^+$ T cells in individuals who have maintained "undetectable" plasma viremia (<50 copies of HIV RNA/ml) for prolonged periods of time while receiving HAART (23). In addition, continual evolution in HIV envelope and protease genes occurs in individuals who have been effectively treated indicating persistent HIV replication (24). Finally, it has been demonstrated using ultrasensitive assays with a limit of detection of <3 copies/ml that many individuals with "undetectable" (<50 copies/ml) plasma HIV by standard assays have persistent low-level plasma viremia (25). However, the most dramatic evidence for the inability of HAART to eradicate HIV infection comes from *in vivo* studies of individuals who began antiretroviral therapy during the chronic stage of HIV infection, achieved and maintained suppression of plasma HIV RNA for up to 2 years, and subsequently interrupted therapy. Interruption of antiretroviral therapy resulted in a rapid rebound of plasma viremia in 95% of individuals (26). Furthermore, individuals whose HAART was interrupted and who remained off therapy for 4 to 6 weeks experienced increases in the plasma HIV RNA to the same level that was reached prior to the initiation of HAART. These data suggest that HAART neither eradicates HIV infection nor does it substantially alter the post-therapy replication kinetics of the virus. Thus, there are reservoirs of ongoing HIV replication that persist in the presence of effective antiretroviral therapy. Important HIV reservoirs sites include lymphoid tissue and resting CD4$^+$ T cells that circulate in the blood. Putative reservoir sites include the reproductive and gastrointestinal tract, the reticuloendothelial system, bone marrow, peripheral blood dendritic cells and monocytes,

TABLE 1. *Potential reservoirs of HIV infection*

Lymphoid tissue, including lymph nodes, gastrointestinal
  tissue, retriculoendothelial system
Resting CD4+ T cells in peripheral blood
Dendritic cells
Monocytes/macrophages
Central nervous system
Reproductive tract

and microglial cells of the CNS (Table 1). Genetic variability has been demonstrated in HIV isolated simultaneously from the plasma and several reservoir sites, indicating that there may be compartmentalization of HIV in different sites. Such compartmentalization may provide a sanctuary for HIV that may be relatively impenetrable by antiretroviral drugs; however, it is unclear if these sanctuary sites contribute significantly to ongoing HIV replication in the presence of HAART.

It remains unclear which cell type in the blood, lymphoid tissue, spleen, or mucosa is the first to actually become infected with HIV. However, in studies of macaques exposed to SIV intravaginally, bone marrow–derived DCs in the vaginal mucosa are the first cells to contain SIV DNA, which is detectable 2 days after exposure. In subsequent examinations of lymphoid organs, the pattern of appearance and spread of SIV mirrored the course that DCs take upon migrating from peripheral tissues to lymphoid organs (27). DCs function by binding antigens in the peripheral tissues, processing them into peptides that are associated with MHC antigens, migrating to lymphoid organs via afferent lymphatics into the paracortical regions, and activating T cells (see Chapter 15). DCs are capable of retaining infectious virus on their

surface for extended periods of time. Thus, their role in the initiation of HIV infection likely includes capturing virions at sites of entry, carrying them to the paracortical regions of lymphoid organs, and delivering virus to CD4+ T cells that become activated through their interaction with DCs (Fig. 2).

The precise nature of the early events during primary HIV and SIV infection that lead to viral replication in lymphoid tissue have not been elucidated. DCs express low levels of CD4, and it is generally agreed that these cells can be infected by HIV only at a low level. Although study of DC infection in lymphoid organs has been more limited, in one investigation the frequency of HIV-infected splenic DCs was approximately 2 logs less than that observed in CD4+ T cells from the same individuals (28). In an analysis of lymph node biopsies, tissue sections from HIV-infected individuals at various stages of disease were stained for DC markers by immunohistochemistry and for HIV RNA by *in situ* hybridization. No cells that stained for both DC markers and HIV were observed, suggesting that DCs in these organs were rarely, if ever, infected with HIV at any stage of disease. *In vitro* studies have demonstrated that DCs and CD4+ T cells form conjugates and active viral replication takes place within these conjugates (29). Similar conjugates of DCs and CD4+ T cells containing HIV antigen have been identified *in vivo* in tonsillar biopsy specimens obtained from individuals infected with HIV (30), in the peripheral blood at low quantities (31), and in the submucosal tissue after vaginal exposure to SIV (27). Recently, it has been shown that dendritic cell–specific ICAM-3 grabbing nonintegrin (DC-SIGN), a protein expressed on DCs in the T-cell area of tonsils, lymph nodes, and spleen, and in the lamina propria of mucosal tissues, may

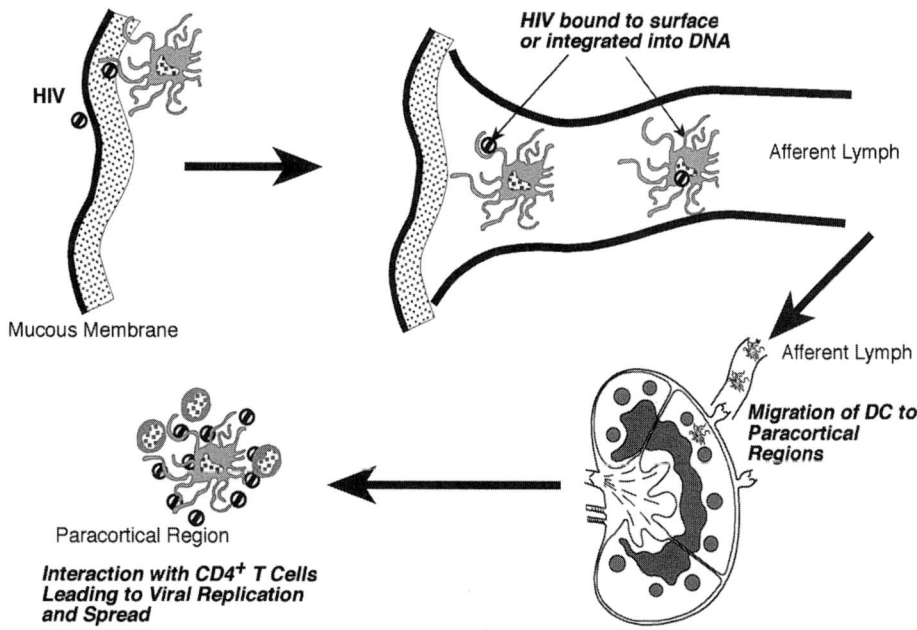

FIG. 2. The role of DCs in the initiation of HIV replication. DCs at the site of exposure transport HIV to the paracortical regions of draining lymphoid tissues, leading to infection of CD4+ T cells. From Weissman and Fauci (127), with permission.

be important in the attachment of HIV to DCs and may be an important factor in the transmission of HIV from DCs to T cells (32). It is likely that DCs carry HIV from tissues in which the initial rounds of viral replication occur to the regional lymph nodes, where $CD4^+$ T cells become infected after contact with DCs. This leads to subsequent rounds of virus replication and spread in the absence of HIV-specific immune responses. Thus, lymphoid tissue plays a key role in the initiation and dissemination of HIV infection.

Lymphoid Tissue

In addition to its central role during primary infection, lymphoid tissue is a major site of HIV replication and plays a role in the progression of disease throughout all stages of infection. In the absence of antiretroviral therapy, the early chronic stage of HIV disease is characterized by a dichotomy in viral load between peripheral blood and lymphoid tissue. In this regard, the frequency of infected cells in lymphoid tissue exceeds that in peripheral blood by five- to ten-fold; differences in levels of viral replication are generally 10- to 100-fold (33). Embretson et al. (34) utilized *in situ* PCR to demonstrate that up to 25% of $CD4^+$ T-lymphocytes present in lymph node germinal centers harbor HIV DNA, further emphasizing the role of lymphoid tissue as a critical reservoir for HIV *in vivo*. The continuous state of rapid high-level turnover of plasma viremia discussed previously derives in large measure from viral replication in lymphoid tissue (35).

The dichotomy in viral burden and replication between lymphoid tissue and peripheral blood is created in part by the normal process of follicular hyperplasia within lymphoid germinal centers following antigenic challenge (35). The expansion of the follicular dendritic cell (FDC) network within hyperplastic lymphoid follicles is an efficient mechanism for viral trapping via interactions between antibody and complement-coated virions with the complement receptor molecules C3b and C3d on the surface of FDCs. In addition to this mechanical phenomenon, immunologic mechanisms may play a major role in maintaining the dichotomy between lymphoid tissue and peripheral blood. The microenvironment of lymphoid tissue is ideally suited to maintain a high degree of immune activation. Cell-to-cell contact among immune effector cells and the resultant high levels of proinflammatory cytokines produced in lymphoid tissues that harbor trapped virions favors viral replication in several ways. Activated $CD4^+$ T-lymphocytes migrating through lymphoid tissue in response to antigens serve as ideal targets for *de novo* infection with HIV. Activation signals such as those delivered by proinflammatory cytokines, found in abundance within activated lymphoid tissue, are potent inducers of HIV replication in $CD4^+$ T cells harboring HIV DNA and also are able to increase the pool of activated HIV-susceptible cells (see discussion below of resting $CD4^+$ T cells) (reviewed in Fauci [36]). Another example of the ability of HIV to subvert the immune system for its own replicative advantage is the aberrant hyperactivation of immune competent cells induced

by the virus itself (37). Sequestration of HIV-infected cells within lymphoid tissue may also contribute to the dichotomy between lymph node and peripheral blood. This sequestration may result from defective egress of cells due to histopathologic abnormalities and/or cytokine imbalances.

During the stage of dichotomy in viral burden between lymphoid tissue and peripheral blood, there is a progressive shift in the lymphoid histopathologic pattern from follicular hyperplasia to follicular involution. This shift in histopathology is associated with important changes in distribution of virus within tissue and in peripheral blood. Disruption of the FDC network is characteristic during the transition from follicular hyperplasia to involution, leading to a decrease in the efficiency of viral trapping in germinal centers and a resultant increase in plasma viremia (38). Sequestration of infected cells within lymphoid tissue also becomes less efficient during follicular involution. Thus, changes in the levels of viral burden between lymphoid tissue and peripheral blood may be dependent, at least in part, on the physical redistribution of viral load between these two compartments.

As the $CD4^+$ T-lymphocyte count falls below 200 cells/μL, there is a tendency for viral load to increase more rapidly in the peripheral blood compartment leading to equilibration between lymphoid tissue and peripheral blood. As noted above, disruption of the FDC network and the consequent loss of the ability to trap virions may contribute significantly to the process of equilibration of viral load between these compartments. Destruction of lymphoid tissue certainly is a major mechanism responsible for the severe immune dysfunction and the observed loss of ability to inhibit viral replication in advanced-stage HIV disease. The ability to maintain an effective immune response to HIV is severely impaired in the absence of intact lymphoid tissue architecture. In this regard, increased cell-associated viral RNA is evident in the paracortical regions of lymph nodes, reflecting increased viral replication. Thus, during progression of HIV disease there is a reversal in the predominant forms of virus in lymphoid tissue, with progressive diminution of the extracellular form (i.e., trapped virus) and an increase in cell-associated virus (i.e., cells expressing HIV) (reviewed in Pantaleo et al. [38]).

The significant role of lymphoid tissue in ongoing HIV replication during all stages of disease in the absence of antiretroviral therapy suggest that it may play a significant role in ongoing HIV replication in the presence of HAART. There is a rapid decrease in lymph node viral burden following the initiation of HAART; within 24 weeks, the majority of HIV RNA is detected by *in situ* hybridization is eliminated and it is uncommon to detect HIV RNA in the germinal centers (39). There is a commensurate decrease in HIV RNA as quantified by RT-PCR per gram of tissue or in isolated lymph node mononuclear cells. However, it is almost universally possible to detect "burst" cells producing HIV RNA in the subcortical regions of lymph nodes despite prolonged antiretroviral therapy; the precise identity of these cells remains unknown (39). In addition, low-level HIV RNA is detected by a variety of quantification techniques despite prolonged periods of plasma HIV RNA levels less than 50 copies/ml (39). Lymphoid tissue other than lymph nodes may serve as important reservoirs of HIV infection. Gastrointestinal lymphoid tissue harbors HIV that is not completely cleared with antiretroviral therapy. In addition, the variability in the genetic composition of HIV isolated from plasma and gut-associated lymphoid tissue in certain individuals suggests that the latter may serve as a sanctuary site for HIV (40). However, the contribution of non–lymph node lymphoid tissue to persistent HIV replication in the presence of HAART remains unknown.

Resting CD4+ T cells

The presence of replication-competent HIV in resting CD4+ T cells was initially demonstrated in HIV-infected individuals who were not receiving HAART (41). At that time, the understanding of viral latency was largely limited to the concept of preintegration latency. HIV may enter resting CD4+ T cells, at which point a limited degree of reverse transcription of the HIV genome may occur in these cells (42,43). This period of preintegration latency may last hours to days; in the absence of an activation signal, unintegrated proviral DNA loses its capacity to initiate a productive infection. If these cells become activated, however, reverse transcription proceeds to completion, followed by nuclear translocation and integration of proviral DNA into cellular DNA (42,43). Using rigorous cell purification methods and a selective PCR technique that detects only integrated forms of HIV DNA, it has been shown that less than 0.1% of resting CD4+ T cells carry integrated provirus (postintegration latency). In this form, the DNA that has been reverse transcribed from the genomic RNA of the virus is integrated into the cellular DNA and can remain transcriptionally silent. Among the total pool of resting CD4+ T cells that harbor viral DNA in infected individuals who are untreated or treated with a less than optimal regimen of one or two antiretroviral drugs, only a fraction carry replication-competent HIV (44). Upon activation in vitro, these cells can produce high levels of infectious HIV. Shortly after it was established that such a population of latently infected cells exists and may serve as a long-term viral reservoir in infected individuals, this initial observation was extended to patients who were receiving HAART. In this regard, it has been clearly demonstrated that the pool of resting CD4+ T cells that carry replication-competent HIV persists in essentially all infected individuals who were receiving HAART and in whom plasma viremia was suppressed below levels of detectability (23,45,46). In addition, this HIV reservoir is established during the earliest stages of HIV infection. The initiation of HAART as early as 10 days following infection with HIV does not prevent the establishment of the resting CD4+ T-cell reservoir of HIV.

It has been demonstrated that cytokines that are naturally produced in the lymphoid tissue microenvironment, particularly IL-2, IL-6, and tumor necrosis factor (TNF)-α, are potent inducers of viral replication in HIV-infected resting CD4+ T cells (47). Recently, it has been suggested that the lymphoid tissue microenvironment may also provide subtle activation signals that promote HIV replication in resting CD4+ T cells in the absence of inducing the cells to express classical markers of activation (A. Kinter, personal communication). These data suggest that resting CD4+ T cells that carry replication-competent HIV may contribute in a significant way to ongoing HIV replication in the presence of HAART in vivo. In this regard, several investigators have reported that in a proportion of HIV-infected individuals who have maintained plasma viremia below the limits of detection (<50 copies/ml) while receiving HAART and who subsequently interrupt therapy, the rebound plasma HIV RNA is genetically similar to the HIV that was isolated from the resting CD4+ T-cell reservoir prior to treatment interruption (48). Thus, the pool of HIV-infected resting CD4+ T cells is a clinically relevant reservoir of HIV.

Peripheral Blood Dendritic Cells

DCs derived from the peripheral blood of normal volunteers were initially found to be highly infectable with HIV in vitro, and DCs from HIV-infected individuals were found to be HIV-infected in vivo; however, these early studies used relatively impure populations of cells (reviewed in Knight and Macatonia [49]). Follow-up studies of DCs from uninfected normal volunteers were discordant in their results: some groups found that DCs obtained by negative selection from peripheral blood were easily and productively infected in vitro with multiple strains of HIV, whereas other groups found that peripheral blood DCs isolated by similar methods were not infectable. Identification of multiple populations of cells with dendritic morphology in peripheral blood is a likely reason for these differing results (31,50,51). When three different populations of peripheral blood DCs were analyzed for infectability with HIV, only one was easily and productively infected in vitro with HIV (31). Studies of DCs from HIV-infected individuals have yielded similarly conflicting results: some authors found high levels of infection in DCs isolated ex vivo from peripheral blood, while others did not.

A number of studies have demonstrated that productive infection of tissue DCs with HIV is rare. There is general agreement that Langerhans cells (LC, dendritic cells resident in the epidermis) from the skin of HIV-infected individuals are occasionally infected; however, such infection occurs at a very low frequency, rarely approaching the level of infection found in peripheral blood CD4+ T cells and often 10 to 100 times less (28). LCs from normal skin appear to be infectable with HIV, although viral production is very low (52).

Monocytes/Macrophages

Monocytes/macrophages may be important in HIV infection as reservoirs of infection. Peripheral blood monocytes are generally normal in number in HIV-infected individuals. Since monocytes express CD4 and numerous HIV co-receptors including CCR5, CXCR4, and CCR3 on their surface (53), they are potential targets of HIV infection. Unlike infection of CD4$^+$ T cells, which generally results in cell lysis, HIV cytopathicity for cells of the monocyte lineage is low and HIV can replicate extensively in these cells (54). Circulating monocytes are rarely found to be infected *in vivo* and are difficult to infect *in vitro* in the undifferentiated state (55). However, there is persistent infection of peripheral blood monocytes following effective antiretroviral therapy (56). Unlike the situation with monocytes, HIV infection can readily be demonstrated in tissue macrophages, including resident microglial cells in the brain, pulmonary alveolar macrophages, and mature macrophages derived from blood monocytes *in vitro* (57).

Central Nervous System

In advanced HIV disease, high numbers of HIV-infected CNS microglial cells can be detected in brain tissue (57). These cells are not killed by acute HIV infection and may become viral reservoirs. However, recent data in the SIV model in macaques suggest that infection of parenchymal microglial cells occurs relatively late in the course of infection. In the early stages of disease, the SIV-infected macrophage cells were confined to the perivascular areas of the brain. HIV detected in the cerebral spinal fluid of individuals is rapidly decreased following the initiation of HAART (59). However, in certain individuals, there is genetic variability in HIV isolated from the plasma and the CNS (59); this suggests that there may be compartmentalization of HIV in the CNS and thus this site may serve as a sanctuary for HIV. However, the contribution of the CNS to ongoing HIV replication in the presence of HAART remains unknown.

Reproductive Tract

Since the major mode of HIV transmission is through sexual contact, it is not surprising that HIV can be isolated from the fluids as well as the cells of the reproductive tract. However, in certain individuals there is discordance in the response to effective antiretroviral therapy in genital secretions and plasma (60). In addition, there can be genetic variability in the HIV isolated from genital secretions and plasma (61). These data suggest that there may be compartmentalization of HIV in the reproductive tract and that the reproductive tract may serve as a sanctuary site of HIV. However, the contribution of the reproductive tract to ongoing HIV replication in the presence of HAART remains unknown.

IMMUNE DYSFUNCTION CAUSED BY HIV INFECTION

Dysfunction of virtually every component of the immune system can be demonstrated during the course of HIV infection. Ultimately, the immunodeficiency induced by HIV must be considered in the context of the microenvironment in which immune responses are generated. The advanced stages of HIV infection are marked by striking disruption of lymphoid tissue architecture (62). Follicular involution, hypervascularity, and fibrosis are some of the pathologic changes evident in lymph nodes from patients with advanced HIV disease. The loss of FDCs, resulting in follicular involution, has important implications with regard to the pathogenesis of HIV-related immunodeficiency. The ability to mount immune responses against new antigens and the ability to maintain memory responses are severely impaired in the absence of an intact FDC network (63). This loss of functional substrate for the generation and maintenance of immune responses results in loss of containment of HIV replication and enhanced susceptibility to opportunistic infections.

In the advanced stage of disease there is almost total dissolution of lymphoid tissue architecture. Follicular involution, fibrosis, frank lymphocyte depletion, and fatty infiltration herald complete loss of functional lymphoid tissue, contributing to the state of immunodeficiency and the dramatically enhanced susceptibility to opportunistic infections.

Disruption of the lymphoid microenvironment during the course of HIV infection remains an enigmatic process with considerable implications for future therapeutic interventions. Productive infection of FDCs by HIV may occur, particularly in the late stages of HIV infection; however, most data suggest that productive infection of FDCs is rare during the period of intermediate stage disease when dissolution of the FDC network begins (64). Direct toxicity to cells by viral gene products may contribute to loss of FDC network integrity. Tat and/or gp120 have been shown to be capable of disrupting normal intracellular signaling (65) as well as inducing apoptosis (66,67), although these effects have been studied largely in CD4$^+$ T cells and little is known regarding the normal physiology of FDCs and their interactions with HIV proteins. Tat, Nef, and Vpu have been found to downregulate MHC class I expression (64,68), which may interfere with normal cell–cell interactions in the lymphoid microenvironment. Depletion of CD4$^+$ T cells during the course of HIV disease could also lead to withdrawal of a trophic factor necessary for FDC survival. Induction of tissue-damaging gene products by HIV may contribute to disruption of the FDC network over time; candidate mediators include nitric oxide (69) and matrix metalloproteinases (MMP) such as MMP-9 (70). An "innocent bystander" phenomenon is also a possibility, wherein cells such as CD8$^+$ T cells or macrophages infiltrating into hyperplastic lymph nodes elaborate substances such as TNF-α that may be toxic at high, sustained concentrations.

Because CD4$^+$ T cells play a critical role in the orchestration of normal immune responses, it is not surprising that many of the immune defects observed during HIV disease are secondary to the progressive decline in the number and function of CD4$^+$ T cells. CD4$^+$ T-lymphocytes and cells of the monocyte lineage are the principal targets of HIV infection. However, virtually any cell that expresses the CD4 molecule together with an appropriate co-receptor molecule can potentially be infected with HIV. In addition, HIV has been reported to infect *in vitro* a wide range of primary cells and cell lines that may or may not express CD4 or HIV co-receptors. These include follicular dendritic cells (FDCs), microglial cells, megakaryocytes, eosinophils, CD8$^+$ T cells, B cells, natural killer cells, thymus and bone marrow stromal cells, astrocytes, oligodendrocytes, renal epithelial cells, cervical cells, trophoblastic cells, rectal and bowel mucosal cells, and parenchymal cells from a variety of organs such as heart, muscle, liver, lung, salivary gland, eye, testis, prostate, and adrenal gland. However, *in vivo* the only cells unequivocally shown to be infected with HIV are CD4$^+$ T-lymphocytes and cells of the monocyte/macrophage lineage, suggesting that the clinical relevance of *in vitro* infection of other cell types may be marginal.

CD4$^+$ T cells

CD4$^+$ T-cell dysfunction and depletion are the hallmark of HIV disease. The opportunistic infections observed with advancing disease are primarily due to defects in CD4$^+$ T-cell number and function that result directly or indirectly from HIV infection. Direct effects of HIV on CD4$^+$ T cells include infection and loss of absolute cell numbers. Indirect effects of HIV infection result in decreased CD4$^+$ T-cell proliferation and differentiation, dysregulation, and decreased production of IL-2 and other cytokines, decreased IL-2 receptor expression, and defective colony formation and other precursor defects.

A relentless loss of CD4$^+$ T-cell function is observed with progression of HIV disease. Among the first abnormalities noted are a loss of response to common recall antigens such as tetanus toxoid, and decreased IL-2 production, followed by defects in T-cell proliferative responses to alloantigens. Subsequently, with the continued decline in CD4$^+$ T cells, defects in response to mitogenic stimulation occur (5). A more incisive view of the qualitative nature of the immunodeficiency that occurs in the late stages of HIV infection is provided by study of the CD4$^+$ T-cell receptor Vβ repertoire. Polymerase chain reaction (PCR) amplification across the CDR3 region of the T-cell receptor with primers specific for the T-cell receptor Vβ families yields products of different lengths depending upon the recombination of variable, diversity, and junctional gene segments. An abnormal distribution of these products within a Vβ family indicates disruption or skewing of the Vβ repertoire. Such disruptions are seen with increased frequency in CD4$^+$ T cells from patients in advanced stage HIV disease, particularly with CD4$^+$ T-cell counts of less than 200 cells/μL (72). Interestingly, increases in CD4$^+$ T-cell counts associated with antiretroviral or IL-2 therapy do not result in restoration of the normal pattern of the disrupted Vβ repertoire (72).

The mechanisms responsible for the CD4$^+$ T-cell defects are only partially understood. Viral proteins have been demonstrated to directly alter T-cell function. gp41 has been observed to inhibit antigen- and mitogen-induced proliferation of peripheral blood mononuclear cells (PBMC) (73). Circulating gp120 molecules may deliver aberrant immuno-

logic signals and dysregulate expression of co-stimulatory molecules in uninfected CD4$^+$ cells, rendering these cells anergic and/or variably dysfunctional (65,74,75).

T cells from HIV-infected individuals manifest a variety of phenotypic abnormalities. The percentage of CD4$^+$ T cells expressing CD28, the ligand for B-7 and a major coactivation signal necessary for activation of T cells, is reduced compared to uninfected individuals (68% in cells from AIDS patients versus 96% in cells from healthy, uninfected subjects) (76). CD28$^-$ cells do not respond to activation signals, including anti-CD3 monoclonal antibodies or mitogens, and express markers of terminal activation, including human leukocyte antigen (HLA)-DR, CD38, and CD45RO (77). HIV-infected individuals develop an increase in CD45RO expressing memory cells and a loss of naïve, CD45RA expressing cells. Of note, the CD45RO cells appear to be the main source of HIV replication *in vivo* and produce much more HIV *in vitro* compared to CD45RA cells (78).

Mechanisms of CD4$^+$ T-Cell Depletion

It has been clearly demonstrated that HIV infection results in a significant loss of total body CD4$^+$ T cells. In this regard, it is estimated that HIV-infected individuals with <200 CD4$^+$ T cells/μL have a total body count of approximately 1×10^{11} mature CD4$^+$ T cells; this is half the expected count for an uninfected male under age 30 years (reviewed in McCune [79]). However, there is considerable controversy regarding the relative contribution of various mechanisms for the depletion of CD4$^+$ T cells during the course of HIV infection. As with many other areas of HIV immunopathogenesis, evaluations of patients who initiate, and subsequently withdraw, effective antiretroviral therapy have provided fundamental insights into the understanding of the potential contributions of increased destruction, decreased production, and redistribution as mechanisms for CD4$^+$ T-cell depletion in HIV-infected individuals (Table 2).

Increased Destruction

Virus-Mediated Killing. The observations that CD4$^+$ T cells are the principal targets of HIV infection *in vivo* (80) and that HIV infection of CD4$^+$ T cells *in vitro* causes cytopathicity (81–83) led to a reasonable assumption that

TABLE 2. *Potential mechanisms of CD4$^+$ T-cell depletion*

Increased destruction
  Cytolysis; direct HIV effect or immune mediated
  Apoptosis
  Autoimmune mediated
Decreased production
  Dysregulation or destruction of CD34$^+$ progenitor cells
  Thymic dysregulation and destruction
Redistribution
  Homing of CD4$^+$ T cells from peripheral blood to lymphoid tissue

direct infection of CD4⁺ T cells *in vivo* results in their depletion. However, quantitative studies of the frequency of HIV-infected cells *in vivo* suggest that single-cell killing by direct infection with HIV may not be the predominant mechanism of CD4⁺ T-cell depletion. In this regard, the proportion of HIV-infected, peripheral-blood CD4⁺ T cells in individuals in the early asymptomatic stage of HIV infection is typically in the range of 1 in 1,000 to 1 in 10,000 (reviewed in Pantaleo et al. [84]). Although this frequency increases with disease progression, the proportion of HIV-infected peripheral blood CD4⁺ T cells rarely exceeds 1 in 100 even in patients with advanced HIV disease (85). In the early stages of disease, the frequency of HIV-infected cells in lymphoid tissue exceeds that in peripheral blood by 0.5 to 1 log. In the advanced stage of disease, equilibration in viral burden between these compartments is seen (33). In lymphoid tissue, the percentage of cells harboring HIV DNA and actively expressing viral mRNA is generally less than 1%. Although viral burden and expression are clearly far greater than earlier estimates based on standard *in situ* hybridization methods, the data illustrate the difficulty in accounting for CD4⁺ T-cell depletion solely by direct mechanisms.

Multiple mechanisms of cell death appear to be operative after infection of a CD4⁺ T-cell with HIV. Early events in the viral life cycle, such as accumulation of reverse-transcribed viral DNA in the cytoplasm, have been associated with cell death in other retroviral systems (86) and may also contribute to cell killing in HIV infection (81); however, accumulation of unintegrated DNA is clearly not the sole mechanism responsible for single-cell killing by HIV. High levels of viral RNA and aberrant RNA molecules also are present in the cytoplasm of infected cells, and possibly interfere with normal cellular RNA processing (87).

The intracellular concentration of envelope gp120 molecules is high during the process of virion assembly in an HIV-infected cell. Several studies have suggested that intracellular gp120 may interact with intracellular CD4 molecules, and that this interaction may induce cell death (88). The mechanism of cell death as a consequence of this intracellular gp120–CD4 interaction may be autofusion events that disrupt the integrity of the cell membrane. Cell membrane integrity also may be compromised by the budding of virions from an infected cell (89) and by HIV-induced increases in the concentration of intracellular monovalent cations (90).

Immune-Mediated Killing. HIV-infected cells also may die as a consequence of viral-specific immune responses that occur before the cell succumbs directly to viral infection. Multiple effector mechanisms may be involved in the killing of HIV-infected cells, including cytotoxic T-lymphocyte responses, antibody-dependent cellular cytotoxicity (ADCC), and NK cell responses (see discussion of HIV-specific immune responses below).

Since the frequency of HIV-infected CD4⁺ T cells is relatively low, investigators have evaluated the destruction of HIV-uninfected cells as a contributory mechanism to the loss of CD4⁺ T cells during the course of infection. Immune

responses that target HIV determinants on infected cells may also contribute to elimination of uninfected cells bearing HIV proteins (e.g., gp120) on their surface. Targeting of such "innocent bystander" cells by antibody and cellular immune responses has been described (91). In addition, fusion between infected and uninfected cells, resulting in multinucleated giant cells, or syncytia has long been observed *in vitro* (92). Other molecules implicated in syncytium formation include LFA-1 (93), CD7 (94), and HLA class I molecules (95). Syncytia have been observed only rarely in tissues obtained from HIV-infected individuals (96); thus, it is unlikely that syncytium formation is a major pathogenic mechanism of CD4⁺ T-cell depletion *in vivo*.

Apoptosis. Ascher and Sheppard (97) suggested in 1990 that HIV pathogenesis was largely caused by the inappropriate signals delivered to T cells by HIV envelope molecules. Subsequently, Ameisen and Capron (98) proposed in 1991 that apoptosis may be a pathogenic mechanism of CD4⁺ T-cell depletion during HIV infection. Apoptosis is the morphologic description of a form of programmed cell death critical to physiologic homeostasis in virtually every organ system (reviewed in Thompson [99]). Apoptotic cell death is characterized by plasma membrane blebbing, nuclear condensation, DNA fragmentation, and release of cellular contents in the form of small, dense apoptotic bodies. Ingestion of apoptotic bodies by phagocytes completes the apoptotic death process without the inflammation associated with spillage of cellular contents that occurs in nonphysiologic necrotic cell death. A wide array of physiologic stimuli serves as positive and negative regulators of apoptosis. Important inhibitors of apoptosis include growth factors, extracellular matrix, and CD40 ligand, while important activators of apoptosis include CD95 (Fas) ligand, TNF, transforming growth factor (TGF)-β, neurotransmitters, and withdrawal of growth factor. The discoveries that the *Bcl-2* gene plays an important pathogenic role in lymphomagenesis through its ability to prevent cells from undergoing apoptosis, and that the p53 gene is necessary for initiation of apoptosis, established the paradigm that diseases associated with increased cell survival or increased cell death may result from dysregulation in normal pathways of apoptosis (reviewed in Thompson [99].

Acute infection of T cells with HIV *in vitro* was shown to induce apoptosis, and T cells from HIV-infected patients were demonstrated to undergo enhanced rates of apoptosis *in vitro* compared with normal T cells, particularly following activation (100). Cross-linking of CD4 followed by ligation of the T-cell receptor is sufficient to induce apoptosis, suggesting that uninfected CD4⁺ T cells could be depleted inappropriately upon encountering antigen if CD4 had been cross-linked by gp120 (101). HIV envelope-mediated apoptosis may be enhanced through activation of caspase-3 and caspase-6 (102). In addition, cells from HIV-infected individuals may be anergic and undergo apoptosis in response to CD4 cross-linking more readily than do cells from normal individuals (66). The viral Tat protein can also lead to apoptotic cell death, possibly by up-regulation of CD95 ligand

and/or by enhancing activation of cyclin-dependent kinases (66). HIV viral protein R (Vpr) may induce apoptosis through G2/M cycle arrest (103).

It remains uncertain whether HIV-induced apoptosis plays an important role *in vivo* in CD4$^+$ T-cell depletion. The frequency of apoptotic CD4$^+$ and CD8$^+$ T cells as well as B cells is significantly higher in lymphoid tissue from HIV-infected individuals compared with uninfected controls (104). The intensity of apoptosis is related to the degree of immune activation and is observed predominantly in uninfected "bystander" cells (104). Although some data support a positive correlation between the stage of HIV disease and susceptibility of peripheral blood T cells to apoptosis, another study found no such correlation; Muro-Cacho et al. (105) found that the intensity of apoptosis in lymphoid tissue was independent of the peripheral CD4$^+$ T-cell count and level of plasma viremia. Perhaps the most compelling evidence that apoptosis may play a role in HIV pathogenesis is that an increased frequency of apoptosis in CD4$^+$ T cells is seen in HIV-infected humans and in primates infected with pathogenic strains of SIV, but not in primates infected with nonpathogenic strains of SIV (106).

Autoimmune Phenomena. Autoimmune phenomena occur in HIV-infected individuals and may contribute to CD4$^+$ T-cell depletion. Autoimmunity may occur as a result of molecular mimicry by viral components, and by abnormal release of nuclear antigens from cells dying by apoptosis. Highly homologous regions exist in the carboxy terminus of the HIV-1 envelope glycoprotein and the amino terminal domains of different HLA-DR and DQ alleles. Monoclonal antibodies generated using the HIV envelope peptide as immunogen can recognize native gp160 and MHC class II molecules (107). Sera from one-third of HIV-infected individuals were found to react with the gp41 and MHC class II determinants: these sera were capable of inhibiting normal antigen-specific proliferative responses and also eliminated class II-bearing cells by ADCC (107). Similar instances of molecular mimicry between HIV-1 envelope constituents and host proteins that may result in pathogenic autoimmune responses include the collagen-like region of complement component C1q-A (282); MHC class I heavy chains; HLA-DR4 and DR2 alleles; variable regions of the T-cell receptor alpha, beta, and gamma chains; Fas; functional domains of IgG and IgA; denatured collagen; and a number of nuclear antigens (108).

Lymphocyte Turnover. Mathematical models of lymphocyte turnover derived through analysis of immediate changes in circulating CD4$^+$ T-cell counts in individuals following the initiation of HAART led to estimates that approximately 2×10^9 CD4$^+$ T cells are destroyed, and replenished, each day (9). However, studies utilizing a variety of techniques to measure lymphocyte proliferation—including Ki-67, BrdUrd, and 2H-glucose—to evaluate the effects of HIV on T-cell turnover have yielded mixed results. Several investigators have demonstrated that there is an increase in CD4$^+$ T-cell proliferation in both HIV and SIV infections (reviewed

in Lempicki et al. [109]). In certain studies, the enhanced T-cell proliferation that was observed during active disease was significantly decreased following the initiation of antiretroviral therapy, and proliferation increased again in parallel with plasma viremia following the cessation of treatment in these individuals (109). These data suggest that HIV infection results in a high turnover of CD4$^+$ T cells, perhaps as a consequence of destruction of CD4$^+$ T cells through certain of the mechanisms reviewed above. However, several investigators have had contrary results and have suggested that HIV replication blocks the ability of new CD4$^+$ T cells to regenerate (reviewed in McCune [79]).

Decreased Production

Failure of normal hematopoiesis is an obvious candidate mechanism to account for depletion of CD4$^+$ T cells during HIV infection. A subset of CD34$^+$ progenitor cells express CD4 and are infectable *in vitro* with HIV-1 (110). It is controversial whether CD34$^+$ progenitor cells represent a substantial *in vivo* reservoir for HIV. A number of studies have failed to detect HIV-infected CD34$^+$ progenitor cells in most HIV-infected individuals (111). However, a large study showed that a substantial minority of HIV-infected patients with severe CD4$^+$ T-cell depletion have a reservoir of HIV-infected CD34$^+$ progenitor cells. Recent reports demonstrating expression of CXCR4 on CD34$^+$ progenitor cells (112) suggest that the CD4$^+$ subset of CD34$^+$ cells may be infectable with CXCR4-utilizing strains of HIV (i.e., strains that predominate in the later stages of HIV disease), further substantiating the earlier findings.

Although the role of direct infection of CD34$^+$ progenitor cells in HIV pathogenesis remains controversial, a large body of evidence suggests that viral proteins and HIV-induced cytokines can impair the survival and clonogenic potential of these cells. CD34$^+$ cells cultured in the presence of HIV exhibit defective clonogenic potential; uninfected CD34$^+$ cells purified from bone marrow of HIV-infected patients also manifest defective clonogenic potential, and are committed to apoptotic death in culture (113). The HIV envelope gp120 and Tat proteins have been implicated in these effects on CD34$^+$ progenitor cells, possibly due to gp120 and Tat-mediated up-regulation of TGF-β, or gp120-mediated up-regulation of TNF-α.

Disruption of the thymic microenvironment (114) and HIV-induced thymocyte depletion may also contribute to the failure of CD4$^+$ T-cell replenishment. Thymic epithelial cells normally secrete IL 6, which can in turn increase HIV replication in infected cells. Subpopulations of thymic CD3$-$CD4$-$CD8$^-$ cells are susceptible to infection with HIV *in vitro* (315), and thymic CD3$-$CD4$+$CD8$^-$ progenitor cells from HIV-infected patients are infected *in vivo*. Finally, uninfected thymocytes from HIV-infected individuals are primed for apoptotic death, suggesting that indirect mechanisms of defective thymopoiesis are operative as well. There are *in vivo* correlates of these deleterious effects of HIV on the thymus. Circulating CD4$^+$ and CD8$^+$ naïve (CD45RA$^+$CD62L$^+$) T cells decrease as a result of HIV infection. In addition, Douek et al. (116) have demonstrated that recent thymic emigrants in HIV-infected individuals are significantly decreased as a consequence of HIV infection. The percent of circulating and lymph node naïve CD4$^+$ T cells carrying signal-joint TCR excision circle (TREC) gene products, a marker of recent thymic emigration was significantly reduced in HIV infection compared to age-matched controls. In addition, initiation of effective antiretroviral therapy resulted in a significant increase in signal-joint TRECs in CD4$^+$CD45RO-CD27$^+$ naïve T cells in the periphery; the latter finding suggested that the thymus remained functional in these individuals who were past adolescence and may contribute to immune reconstitution. Subsequently, several investigators have demonstrated that, contrary to previously held beliefs, the thymus remains capable of producing substantial quantities of immune-competent cells for decades in many individuals (117). Zhang et al. (118) found similar decreases in TRECs in certain HIV-infected individuals. However, although there was an increase in TRECs in these individuals following the initiation of HAART, the numerical increase was not sufficient to account for the rise in levels of naïve CD4$^+$ T cells.

Redistribution

Data from both HIV and SIV infections indicate that there is significant trafficking of CD4$^+$ T cells from the peripheral blood to lymphoid tissue in acute and chronic infection (reviewed in McCune [79]). The trafficking of lymphocytes is mediated, in part, through the expression of homing receptors, such as CD62L on CD4$^+$ T cells. As circulating T cells expressing homing markers cross-link their ligands on endothelial venule cells, the T cells extravasate from the peripheral blood to the lymph nodes. Since CD62L expression on CD4$^+$ T cells is up-regulated following HIV infection, it is possible that redistribution contributes to the depletion of circulating CD4$^+$ T cells observed during the course of disease. In support of this view, several investigators have suggested that redistribution of CD4$^+$ T cells from lymphoid tissue to the peripheral blood contributes significantly to the increase in CD4$^+$ T cells following the initiation of HAART (reviewed in McCune [79]). However, other investigators have developed models in which redistribution is not an important component of the increase in CD4$^+$ T cells observed in these patients (119). In these latter scenarios, CD4$^+$ T cells that have trafficked to lymphoid tissues are destroyed by apoptosis or other mechanisms and, therefore, they are not available for redistribution following the initiation of HAART.

CD8$^+$ T Cells

Levels of circulating CD8$^+$ T cells vary throughout the course of HIV disease. Following acute primary infection, CD8$^+$ T-cell counts usually rebound in the peripheral blood to supernormal levels and may remain elevated for prolonged periods. Increases in CD8$^+$ T cells during all but the late stages of disease may, in part, reflect the expansion of HIV-specific CD8$^+$ CTLs. As with CD4$^+$ T cells, as a result of HIV infection there is a significant decrease in naïve CD8$^+$ T cells (CD45RA$^+$CD62L$^+$) carrying signal TRECs compared to age-matched controls (116).

HIV-specific CD8$^+$ CTLs have been identified in HIV-infected individuals early in the course of disease and their activity can be measured in peripheral blood lymphocytes without prior *in vitro* stimulation (120). During HIV disease progression, CD8$^+$ T cells assume an abnormal phenotype characterized by the expression of certain activation markers and the absence of expression of the CD25 molecule (IL-2 receptor alpha chain). Alterations in the phenotype of CD8$^+$ T cells in HIV-infected individuals may have prognostic significance. In particular, individuals whose CD8$^+$ T cells express HLA-DR but not CD38 after seroconversion experience a stabilization of their CD4$^+$ T-cell counts and a less fulminant disease course, while individuals whose CD8$^+$ T cells express both HLA-DR and CD38 experience a more aggressive course with rapid CD4$^+$ T-cell depletion and a poorer prognosis (121). CD8$^+$ T cells lacking CD28 expression are also increased in HIV disease, possibly reflecting expansion of the CD8$^+$CD28$^-$CD57$^+$ T-cell subset containing *in vivo* activated CTLs (122). The loss of CTL activity with disease progression is not restricted to HIV-specific CTLs: a loss of cytotoxic activity to other common antigens including EBV and *Mycobacterium tuberculosis* has also been observed (123).

In addition to CTL activity, other CD8$^+$ T-cell functions are impaired during HIV disease progression, including loss of noncytolytic non–MHC-restricted CD8$^+$ T-cell–derived HIV suppression. Analyses of factors released by CD8$^+$ T cells demonstrate that in certain *in vitro* systems the CD8$^+$ T-cell–associated suppressor activity termed CD8 antiviral factor (CAF) decreases with disease progression (124). In contrast, levels of macrophage inflammatory protein (MIP)-1α, MIP-1β, and RANTES, factors produced by CD8$^+$ T cells that also suppress HIV replication, are not reduced with progression of HIV disease (125).

For a complete discussion of HIV-specific CD8$^+$ T-cell responses, see discussion of HIV-specific immune responses below.

Dendritic Cells

The question of depletion and dysfunction of DCs in HIV disease follows the same controversy as discussed above for infectability. Studies of the number of DCs present in peripheral blood of HIV-infected individuals compared to uninfected individuals have demonstrated a decrease, increase, or no change. Most studies have found no decrease in the percentage of LC in skin cell preparations when comparing infected with uninfected individuals or when comparing HIV-infected individuals at various stages of disease (reviewed in Blauvelt and Katz [126]). In a study of lymphoid organs, sections of lymph node tissue from HIV-infected individuals at various stages of disease were stained for DC markers and examined by light microscopy. Visual analysis did not suggest a selective loss in the number of DCs populating the paracortical regions of the lymph node; rather, loss of DCs from the lymph node occurred in parallel with the loss of lymphoid architecture and the development of fibrosis (127).

With regard to DC function, studies of the effect of HIV infection on the ability of DCs to activate T cells have also yielded conflicting results. Several studies found that peripheral blood DCs from HIV-infected individuals were much less efficient in activating T cells than DCs from uninfected individuals (128), while another report (129) found no difference in the ability of peripheral blood DCs from HIV-infected versus uninfected individuals to activate allogeneic CD4$^+$ T cells. All of these studies used peripheral blood DCs that have the confounding variables of a requirement for *in vitro* maturation, long purification processes, and the existence of multiple subpopulations. In a study using identical twins discordant for HIV infection, DCs were obtained from each sibling and co-cultured with their own CD4$^+$ T cells, the CD4$^+$ T cells of their sibling, or allogeneic CD4$^+$ T cells. No defects were found in the ability of the DCs from the HIV-infected sibling to present antigen to the uninfected T cells as compared to the DCs from the uninfected sibling. The only defect observed in DCs from the HIV-infected sibling was a decreased ability to activate allogeneic T cells (126). Further studies will be required to clarify the possible role of DC depletion and dysfunction in the pathogenesis of HIV disease.

B-Lymphocytes

Dysregulation of B-cell activation and the decreased ability of these cells to respond to antigen are likely responsible in part for the increase in certain bacterial infections seen in advanced HIV disease in adults, as well as for the morbidity and mortality associated with bacterial infections in HIV-infected children who cannot mount an adequate humoral response to common bacterial pathogens. The number of circulating B cells may be decreased in primary HIV infection; however, this is usually a transient phenomenon and likely reflects, at least in part, a redistribution of cells into lymphoid tissues. Soon after the resolution of acute HIV infection, hypergammaglobulinemia and B-lymphocyte hyperactivation are noted. The increase in immunoglobulins occurs for all classes of antibody. A large component of the immunoglobulin specificity, at least in early-stage disease, is directed against HIV antigens. It has been suggested that a majority of activated B cells produce antibodies directed against HIV during this stage of infection (reviewed in Amadori and

Chieco-Bianchi [130]). B cells isolated from patients with high levels of HIV plasma viremia have been shown to be defective in their proliferative responses to various stimuli (131). Substantial plasma viremia was also associated with the appearance of a subpopulation of B cells that expressed reduced levels of CD21. Upon fractionation into CD21 high- and low-expressing B cells, the CD21-low fraction showed dramatically reduced proliferation in response to B-cell stimuli and enhanced secretion of immunoglobulins when compared to the CD21-high fraction. Electron microscopic analysis of each fraction revealed cells with plasmacytoid features in the CD21-low B-cell population but not in the CD21-high population. These results indicate that HIV viremia induces the appearance of a subset of B cells whose function is impaired and which may be responsible for the hypergammaglobulinemia associated with HIV disease. The phenotypic and functional aberrations were reversed upon reduction of HIV plasma viremia by antiretroviral therapy, suggesting that control of viremia may contribute to the restoration of the humoral arm of the immune system (131).

B cells from HIV-infected individuals secrete increased amounts of TNF-α and IL-6, cytokines known to enhance HIV replication (132), and express surface-bound TNF-α that can induce the production of HIV from infected CD4$^+$ T cells (133). The secretion of proinflammatory cytokines and the expression of surface-bound TNF-α by B cells in the lymphoid microenvironment may contribute to T-cell activation and HIV replication in these tissues. HIV gp120 has been observed to directly bind to an immunoglobulin variable chain (VH3) and activate these B cells in much the same manner as a superantigen (134). This antigen-independent polyclonal activation leads in part to the hypergammaglobulinemia and B-lymphocyte hyperactivation of HIV infection. Other portions of HIV, including gp41, directly activate B cells in a nonsuperantigen-mediated manner. Correlates of B-cell dysfunction observed in HIV-infected individuals include an increase in spontaneous EBV transformation *in vitro* and may contribute to the observed increased frequency of EBV-induced lymphomas (135).

Several studies have found an overall increase in IgE levels among HIV-infected individuals, likely reflecting a spectrum of IgE regulatory dysfunction. The mechanisms of this increase are unclear but may include B-cell hyperactivation and cytokine dysregulation. Levels of IgE continue to increase with disease progression. An increase in aeroallergen-specific IgE has not been associated with the increase in total IgE; in one study, allergen-specific IgE decreased with HIV disease progression in all but the subgroup with the highest total IgE level (136). An overall increase in IgE levels was noted in pediatric HIV infection without an increase in allergen-specific IgE, suggesting polyclonal activation. An association between elevated levels of IgE and emergence of syncytium-inducing viruses was also noted. In HIV-infected children, an expanded minor population of B-lymphocytes has been identified that does not express CD23 (IgE receptor) and CD62L (L-selectin), and may be involved in the pathogenesis of IgE dysregulation (137).

Polymorphonuclear Leukocytes

Defects in neutrophil function have been observed at all stages of HIV disease. Neutrophils isolated from asymptomatic HIV-infected individuals have an increase in nitroblue tetrazolium reduction suggesting a state of increased cellular activation (138). Plasma from these individuals activates neutrophils from healthy, uninfected individuals, suggesting the presence of a soluble neutrophil activating factor. In addition, plasma from the same individuals was found to be low in N-acetyl cysteine, indicating that depletion of antioxidants may occur due to increased oxygen radical production (139). The oxidative capacity of neutrophils after priming with granulocyte/macrophage (GM)-colony–stimulating factor (CSF) also was increased in HIV-infected individuals with CD4$^+$ T-cell counts >200/μL. There is some controversy regarding neutrophil defects in HIV infection; this may be due to differences in in vitro preparation and analysis of cells. In a flow cytometric analysis of neutrophils in whole blood, which obviates the need for purification, neutrophils from HIV-infected subjects demonstrated increased expression of adhesion molecules, decreased expression of CD62L, and increased actin polymerization and H$_2$O$_2$ production (138), indicating activation of neutrophils. Opsonizing activity of neutrophils was significantly impaired and this correlated with disease progression. Neutrophils from AIDS patients also undergo apoptosis at an increased rate compared to those from normal controls. Unlike the neutrophil activating factor described above, serum from HIV-infected individuals could not transfer the increased apoptosis activity to neutrophils from healthy, uninfected individuals. The addition of GM-CSF to the assay system significantly decreased apoptosis in neutrophils from AIDS patients (140). Neutrophils from HIV-infected individuals also produce more TNF-α and IL-6 in response to lipopolysaccharide (LPS) or Candida antigen compared to neutrophils from normal donors.

Dysfunction of neutrophils in HIV-infected individuals has several clinical implications. HIV infection, especially in women, is characterized by an increase in the incidence and severity of Candida infections. In a study comparing the ability of neutrophils from HIV-infected patients and normal controls to phagocytize and kill Candida albicans, neutrophils from AIDS patients showed an increased ability to phagocytize the organism, a similar ability to generate reactive oxygen, but a decreased ability to kill Candida, suggesting a defect in nonoxidative killing. A potential mechanism for the decreased ability of neutrophils to kill Candida organisms has been suggested by the finding that IL-10, shown in some studies to be increased in HIV disease, inhibits neutrophil killing of Candida (141).

Abnormalities in eosinophils also have been observed in HIV infection. Eosinophil counts in HIV-infected individuals are preserved in the setting of decreases in other blood cells;

however, they may be increased in a subgroup of patients. Eosinophils express low levels of CD4 and are infectable with HIV in vitro, leading to productive infection and apoptosis (142). The significance of eosinophil infection in vivo, if it in fact occurs, is unclear at present.

Monocytes/Macrophages

Treatment of normal monocytes in vitro with HIV gp120 or Tat leads to abnormal activation of these cells. In vitro infection of monocytes from healthy individuals leads to a decrease in ADCC and killing of intracellular Candida pseudotropicalis as well as to a decrease in Fc- and C3-mediated phagocytosis. Monocytes isolated from HIV-infected subjects exhibit a number of functional abnormalities as well. A decrease in the oxidative burst has been observed in individuals with both early- and advanced-stage disease (143). In addition, impairment of chemotaxis and migration has been observed in monocytes from patients with AIDS (144). Finally, infection of monocytic precursors in bone marrow may be directly or indirectly responsible for certain of the hematologic abnormalities observed in HIV-infected individuals.

Natural Killer Cells

The presumed role of NK cells is to provide immunosurveillance against virus-infected cells, certain tumor cells, and allogeneic cells (see Chapter 12). Abnormalities of NK cells are observed throughout the course of HIV disease and these abnormalities increase with disease progression. Most studies report that NK cells are normal in numbers and phenotype in HIV-infected individuals; however, decreases in numbers of the CD16$^+$/CD56$^+$ subpopulation of NK cells with an associated increase in activation markers has been reported. NK cells from HIV-infected individuals are defective in their ability to kill typical NK target cells as well as gp160-expressing cells. The abnormality in NK cell lysis is thought to occur after binding of the NK cell to its target. Nonetheless, the NK lytic machinery appears to be capable of functioning normally since NK cells from HIV-infected individuals are able to mediate ADCC (145). A possible mechanism for defective NK activity includes a lack of cytokines necessary for optimal function. Addition of IL-2, IL-12, or IFN-α to cultures enhances the defective in vitro NK cell function of HIV-infected individuals (146).

HIV-SPECIFIC IMMUNE RESPONSES

Although the immune response to HIV has been extensively studied, many fundamental issues remain unclear. In this regard, the mechanisms by which HIV evades control by the human immune system require further elucidation. New technologies for inducing or measuring cellular and humoral immune responses and new models of immune system–mediated protection or control of virus replication are permitting the dissection of what constitutes an effective immune response against HIV in greater detail than was previously possible. One animal model that has been particularly useful for the study of lentivirus-specific immunity and vaccine development is SIV infection of macaques. SIV is closely related to HIV-2 and causes an acute infection that leads to CD4$^+$ T-cell depletion, immunodeficiency, opportunistic infections, and death in susceptible animals. In addition, humoral immunity to HIV can be evaluated by the study of macaques infected with SIV-HIV chimeras (SHIV) that encode the HIV envelope surface glycoprotein. Through passive transfer or depletion studies in experimental animals, and correlative studies in humans, it is now known that humoral immune responses can protect against lentiviral infection and cellular immune responses can control viral replication. Elucidation of the breadth and magnitude of HIV-specific immune responses, the HIV protein targets of these responses and the precise mechanisms by which protection or control occur may provide insights for the development of novel prophylactic or therapeutic vaccines.

Humoral Immune Responses

Antibodies that bind the viral core protein p24 or the viral surface envelope glycoprotein can be detected in the plasma within weeks of HIV infection coincident with the decline of plasma viremia. Although antibodies that bind several HIV proteins are detected by ELISA early in HIV infection, most individuals do not develop antibodies capable of neutralizing the autologous viral isolate until well after plasma viremia has declined (147). Sera of chronically infected patients commonly contain some neutralizing activity against viruses that have undergone laboratory passage. However, high levels of antibodies that are capable of neutralizing viruses that have not undergone laboratory passage (primary isolates) are only rarely detected, typically in long-term nonprogressors (19). In addition, the breadth of the neutralizing antibody response is greater in some patients with nonprogressive disease. The structure, diversity, and immunogenicity of the envelope protein likely contribute to the lack of antibodies that neutralize broad classes of viral isolates in most chronically infected individuals.

Of the spectrum of antibodies directed against HIV-1 encoded proteins, only antibodies directed against surface envelope glycoprotein are thought to be important in protective immunity. Epitope mapping using monoclonal antibodies and study of x-ray crystallographic structures have permitted some estimation of the structural constraints of the envelope glycoprotein in its dissociated and oligomeric conformations (148,149). The envelope protein (gp160) exists in a trimeric structure with six subunits (three gp120s and three gp41s) and it is heavily glycosylated with N- and O-linked sugars. The CD4 binding site on gp120 is located within a depression of this oligomeric structure. In addition to CD4, HIV also binds CC or CXC chemokine receptors as co-receptors to mediate viral entry. The co-receptor binding surface on

gp120 is located within another depression separate from the CD4 binding site (150). Both the CD4 and co-receptor binding sites are well conserved among known viral isolates. They are also not glycosylated and for these reasons are thought to be targets of neutralizing antibodies. The description of monoclonal antibodies derived from a single patient with broadly cross-neutralizing antibodies that bind to the CD4 binding site has led to the hypothesis that generation of antibodies specific to these sites may be a prerequisite for neutralization (151). It is thought that these sites remain masked in the native conformation and that access of antibody to these sites may require the conformational changes induced by CD4 binding. However, there is not general agreement regarding the necessity to target these sites for effective neutralization (reviewed in Parren and Burton [152]). In this regard, antibodies capable of protecting rhesus macaques against SIV challenge were specific for HLA-DR that is included in the virus envelope upon budding from the host cell. In addition, the amount of antibody bound to virus particles has been correlated with neutralization regardless of the epitope specificity. Thus, antibodies that bind the virus particle but do not bind the CD4 or co-receptor binding site may be capable of interfering with the virus-cell interaction and mediating neutralization of HIV.

The genetic diversity between HIV isolates is also thought to contribute to the difficulty in neutralizing the virus. The level of genetic variation of HIV is high within geographically defined populations and even within a single infected patient (see discussion of epidemiology above). Mutations that occur during the reverse transcription process generate highly diverse viral sequences that coexist in the plasma. Although more recent estimates place the error rate of HIV reverse transcriptase close to the error rates of RNA polymerases of other RNA viruses, high levels of replication and prolonged duration of infection with HIV are major contributors to viral diversity (153). The level of diversity of HIV is much higher than most human RNA viruses and is likely a major contributor to the lack of cross-neutralizing antibodies. It is known for some respiratory viruses, for example, that changes in only a few amino acids within the surface glycoproteins can result in loss of cross-neutralization between virus isolates. By comparison, HIV viral sequences may vary between 10% and 16% in the plasma of an individual. It is thought that these diverse circulating envelope sequences may represent a constantly evolving target that contributes to the ability of HIV to evade the humoral immune response.

Cellular Immune Responses

Cytotoxic T-Lymphocytes

Immune Control

Classical MHC class I–restricted, HIV-specific, CD8$^+$ cytotoxic (CTL) responses have been demonstrated in the peripheral blood within the first few months of HIV infection and are detected during the chronic phases of infection in most

HIV-infected individuals (120,154). HIV-specific CD8$^+$ T cells specific for each of the known HIV-1 gene products have been detected in the peripheral blood by bulk CTL assays, limiting dilution assays for cytolysis, interferon-γ secretion, or tetramer staining. Several lines of evidence suggest that HIV-specific CD8$^+$ T cells play a critical role in restriction of virus replication. The peak of the HIV-specific CTL response occurs shortly after the peak of viremia (Fig. 1). This temporal association between the emergence of an HIV-specific CTL response and decrease of viremia following acute infection is thought to represent the effect of virus-specific CTL in restricting HIV replication in humans. Further indirect evidence of an important role of CD8$^+$ T cells in restriction of HIV replication in humans comes from strong associations between restriction of virus replication and certain MHC class I alleles and functional links with epitopes presented by these alleles (see discussion of genetic factors below). More direct evidence for the role of CD8$^+$ T cells in restriction of lentiviral replication *in vivo* is provided by several recent studies in experimental animals. CD8$^+$ T-cell depletion by exogenous monoclonal antibodies has been shown to abrogate restriction of virus replication in both SHIV-infected and SIV-infected monkeys (155,156). In addition, it has been shown that animals infected with live attenuated SIV vaccines are able to resist SIV challenge through antibody and chemokine independent mechanisms (157). It now appears clear that CD8$^+$ T cells are an important component in the restriction of virus replication that is induced by chronic virus infections in each of these model systems. It is likely that CD8$^+$ T cells play a similar role in the restriction of HIV replication in humans. However, although HIV-specific CTL likely exert some control over HIV replication, this restriction is generally poor with viral RNA levels reaching 10^3 to 10^6 copies/ml plasma in the vast majority of HIV-infected individuals during the chronic phase of infection in the absence of antiretroviral therapy. Many different mechanisms have been proposed to explain the inability of cell-mediated immunity to control HIV replication. These include viral factors and quantitative and qualitative factors within the HIV-specific CD8$^+$ T-cell pool (Table 3).

Immune Escape

Several viral factors distinguish HIV from other animal viruses; these factors likely contribute to the ability of HIV to evade the cellular immune response. Mutations produced during the reverse transcription process combined with high levels of replication over a prolonged period result in a highly diverse population of viruses that circulate in a given patient (see discussion of humoral immune responses above). It is thought that this extraordinary level of viral diversity may permit development of mutant viruses that escape immune recognition. Selection of "escape" mutations has been documented in HIV-infected humans and SIV-infected macaques. Longitudinal studies of viral sequences and CTL responses to known motifs have shown the appearance of single or

TABLE 3. *Proposed mechanisms by which HIV evades immune system–mediated restriction of virus replication*

Virus mediated
Broad genetic diversity resulting in CTL "escape" mutations
MHC down-regulation causing diminished recognition of HIV-infected cells
Quantitative defects in CD8$^+$ T cell responses
Insufficient numbers of HIV-specific CTL
Diminished numbers of HIV-specific CTL secondary to loss of "CD4$^+$ T-cell help"
Qualitative defects in CD8$^+$ T-cell responses
Loss of "CD4$^+$ T cell help" resulting in CD8$^+$ T-cell dysfunction
Insufficient maturation of HIV-specific T cells
Diminished avidity
Perforin defect

CTL, cytotoxic T-lymphocytes.

clustered mutations that no longer bind to the MHC class I molecule and are associated with dominance of these sequences in the quasispecies in the peripheral blood (158). Certain well-characterized mutations have been shown to occur with epitopes presented by HLA-B27 (159). Single or clustered mutations cause *Gag* peptides to no longer be presented by the B-27 molecule. These mutants accumulate in the peripheral blood and are associated with diminished responses to the nonmutated sequence. In addition, evidence for the selection of escape mutants was found in a single patient that was treated with high numbers of an autologous *Nef*-specific CTL clone (160). This treatment resulted in the selection of variant viruses in which the targeted region of *Nef* was deleted. Examples of escape mutations that alter HLA-binding and -dominant viral sequences have also been observed for HLA B8, A3, and B4. However, it should be noted that these host–virus dynamics are extraordinarily complex given the large number of permutations of viral epitopes, timing of gene expression during the viral replication cycle, and complement of MHC class I alleles. The host CTL response is constrained by the ability of the MHC class I alleles to bind to various viral epitopes, while the virus is constrained by the degree to which an escape mutation impairs viral replicative capacity or "fitness." In addition, the CD8$^+$ T-cell response to each of the viral proteins in the context of each of a single patient's MHC alleles is very broad. Although escape mutations may be found within a single epitope, it is likely that other conserved epitopes within the same gene remain as targets. Thus, it remains uncertain whether these mutations cause true escape from immune system surveillance or escape mutations at single epitopes occur in the context of high levels of virus replication. Although escape mutations clearly occur, the relative importance of these mutations in the pathogenesis of HIV infection remains incompletely understood.

In addition to the high levels of diversity generated during HIV infection, there are other viral factors that that may contribute to the poor ability of the immune system to control HIV replication. HIV *Nef, Tat* and *Vpu* are each capable of down-regulating surface expression of MHC class I molecules necessary for recognition of infected cells). This occurs by either removal or rerouting for endosomal degradation in clatherin-coated pits (161). The effect of *Nef* is mediated by the sequence motif in the cytoplasmic tail of HLA A and B molecules. HLA C and E lack this motif and are not down-regulated. It has been proposed that these effects may permit infected cells to escape lysis by HLA-A– or HLA-B–restricted T cells which dominate the cellular immune response, yet avoid lysis by NK cells expressing inhibitory receptors that recognize HLA C or E (162). However, there is not uniform agreement that this is a predominant mechanism by which HIV avoids the cellular immune response. Demonstrations of HIV-specific CD8$^+$ T cells that are unable to lyse infected cells that express *Nef* yet lyse cells infected with *Nef* deleted viruses were performed using CD8$^+$ T-cell clones. Certain clones maintained the ability to lyse cells infected with *Nef*-expressing or *Nef*-deleted viruses. Several investigators have demonstrated the ability of autologous HIV-infected cells to stimulate cytokine secretion or perforin-mediated lysis by class I–restricted HIV-specific CD8$^+$ T cells (163). However, HLA-A and -B down-regulation may play a role in avoiding recognition by low-avidity HIV-specific CD8$^+$ T cells.

It has been proposed that the low numbers of HIV-specific CD8$^+$ T cells may be the reason that HIV escapes immune control. Inverse correlations were found between the frequency of CD8$^+$ T cells specific for two putative immunodominant A*0201-restricted HIV epitopes and plasma viral RNA (164). Others have found associations between higher numbers of HIV-specific CD8$^+$ T cells and the presence of a CD4$^+$ T-cell proliferative response to HIV antigens, suggesting that the frequency of HIV-specific CD8$^+$ T cells falls due to a lack of CD4$^+$ T-cell help. However, several studies that examined a broad range of HIV epitopes in the context of multiple HLA alleles have not found an inverse correlation between plasma viral RNA and the frequency of HIV-specific CD8$^+$ T cells. In this regard, HIV-specific CD8$^+$ T cells that respond to a broad array of HIV peptides persist in the range of 1% to 22% in most untreated patients with relatively high-level plasma viremia (165,166).

One parameter of the HIV-specific CD8$^+$ T-cell response that might confer significant restriction of virus replication is the preferential targeting of genes that are expressed early in the virus replication cycle prior to budding of mature virions. Several publications have described responses to *Tat* or *Rev* gene products in infected humans or their SIV homologs in macaques, and certain reports have associated these responses with better outcomes. It has been shown previously that several patients with nonprogressive HIV infection have HLA B 57–restricted responses specific for *Tat* or *Rev* (167). However, in other studies responses of *Tat*- or *Rev*-specific CD8$^+$ T cells did constitute a large portion of the overall response in patients with progressive or nonprogressive disease (163,166). Although responses to these early genes is

of theoretical importance, at present their role in restricting viral replication in infected individuals remains unclear.

Another parameter of the CD8$^+$ T-cell response that may confer enhanced restriction of virus replication is the breadth or number of HIV peptides to which a patient may respond. During acute infection, expansion of HIV-specific CD8$^+$ T cells is restricted to a relatively small number of clones. In certain cases these expansions are monoclonal, and this monoclonality carries a poor prognosis (168). However, several reports describe a narrowly focused CD8$^+$ T-cell response in nonprogressors or in individuals treated with HAART during acute infection and who have restricted virus replication (163,169). A highly focused response in nonprogressors may appear somewhat unexpected given previous descriptions of greater breadth of CD8$^+$ T-cell expansions during acute infection in patients that go on to nonprogressive disease, the protective effect of heterozygosity at MHC loci, or associations of broader HIV-specific CD8$^+$ T-cell responses with lower viral loads. However, it is possible that a highly focused response is the result, not the cause, of effective restriction of virus replication in nonprogressors or patients treated during acute infection. In this view, restriction of virus replication would not allow the expansion of subdominant clones with specificities for other peptides restricted by other MHC alleles. In addition, since, as noted above, HIV-specific CD8$^+$ T cells of chronically HIV-infected patients with relatively high-level plasma viremia persist at high levels and respond to a broad array of HIV peptides, it remains unclear whether inadequate breadth of the response alone is a major contributor to poor restriction of virus replication during chronic infection.

Several lines of evidence have suggested that the inability of CD8$^+$ T cells to control HIV may lie not in the quantity of these cells but rather in qualitative properties. CD3 molecules have been shown to be down-regulated in the HIV-specific CD8$^+$ T cells of infected individuals and to have a diminished capacity to lyse autologous infected cells. It has also been shown that HIV-specific CD8$^+$ T cells may contain less perforin compared to CMV-specific cells. Progressively diminished secretion of interferon-gamma by HIV-specific CD8$^+$ T cells during late-stage disease also has been observed. More recently, it was found that HIV-specific CD8$^+$ T cells may have a phenotype that is skewed such that they do not develop a fully mature effector phenotype (170) compared to CMV-specific cells. Although each of these observations must be confirmed, as noted above, the persistence of high frequencies of HIV-specific CD8$^+$ T cells in both nonprogressors and patients with progressive disease strongly suggests that some qualitative parameters likely underlie the vast differences in the abilities of their CD8$^+$ T cells to restrict viral replication.

Soluble CD8$^+$ T-Cell Secreted Factors

In addition to classical MHC-restricted cytolysis, other mechanisms of CD8$^+$ T-cell–mediated antiviral activities have been described in HIV infection. CD8$^+$ T cells of HIV-infected patients are able to inhibit viral replication via soluble factors in the absence of cell killing. Noncytolytic antiviral activity was initially described *in vitro* using CD8$^+$ T cells from HIV-infected patients (171). Although these cells show characteristics of activated CD8$^+$ CTL, this antiviral activity can be observed in the absence of HLA match or cell contact. This suppressive activity was shown to be mediated in part by the CC chemokines, MIP-1α, MIP-1β, and RANTES (172). These chemokines are natural ligands for *CCR5,* a co-receptor for certain strains of HIV-1, and inhibit viral replication primarily at the level of cell entry. Although the CC chemokines exert their effect at HIV entry into CD4$^+$ T cells and macrophages, additional factor(s) act after viral entry to suppress HIV transcription in infected cells. These additional factor(s), which remain poorly characterized, have been termed CD8$^+$ T-cell antiviral factors (CAF). HLA compatibility between CD8$^+$ T cells and target CD4$^+$ T cells is not required for this suppressive activity but maximal suppression is observed under conditions when cell contact is maintained and cells are HLA matched (173). Although this suppressive activity has been shown to be greater in PBMC of HIV-infected patients than uninfected controls, it remains unclear whether they are secreted in an antigen-specific manner.

CD4$^+$ T-Cell Responses

Several animal models of viral pathogenesis have demonstrated that virus-specific CD4$^+$ T cells are critical in induction or maintenance of an effective CD8$^+$ CTL response that mediates restriction of virus replication. Acute or chronic virus infections in humans or experimental animals typically result in induction of CD4$^+$ T-cell responses that can be demonstrated by proliferation to virus antigens *in vitro* long after elimination or control of infection due to the persistence of memory CD4$^+$ T cells. In most individuals, untreated HIV infection is characterized by poorly restricted virus replication, the loss of CD4$^+$ T cells, and progressive immunologic dysfunction (see discussion above of immune dysfunction caused by HIV infection). In addition, HIV infection is characterized by the early disappearance of CD4$^+$ T-cell–mediated proliferative responses to HIV antigens; this response typically remains absent in the untreated individual.

However, loss of HIV-specific CD4$^+$ T-cell responses during infection is not universal (165). In certain long-term nonprogressors who restrict HIV replication in the absence of antiretroviral therapy, HIV-specific proliferative responses are maintained. Recently, proliferative responses to the *Gag* p24 antigen were also shown in patients who initiated effective antiretroviral therapy during acute HIV infection (174,175). Because HIV infects CD4$^+$ T cells, it is believed that the early loss of these proliferative responses may be the result of deletion of HIV-specific cells early in infection when they encounter the virus. However, there is not uniform agreement that all HIV-specific CD4$^+$ T cells are deleted in patients with

progressive disease. Although proliferative responses are almost universally lost, in several studies using a 6-hour assay for intracellular IFN-γ, HIV antigen-specific CD4$^+$ T cells were found to remain present in some patients with progressive disease, albeit at lower levels than long-term nonprogressors (166,176,177). In addition, proliferation of HIV-specific CD4$^+$ T cells was abrogated during an interruption of antiviral therapy, suggesting that diminished proliferation of these cells may be, in part, a result of high levels of HIV antigen; this event would be similar to that observed during viremia with other human viruses. Furthermore, HIV antigen-specific proliferative responses have been demonstrated *in vitro* after addition of CD40 ligand and IL-12 or anti–CD28 antibody, indicating that HIV-specific cells with proliferative capacity remain in patients with progressive disease. Although HIV-specific CD4$^+$ T cells may be present, it has been suggested that they are present in numbers too low to be detected by certain assays such as lymphocyte proliferation. In four separate studies, 0.1% to 2.0% of CD4$^+$ T cells in the peripheral blood of patients with progressive disease were HIV specific. This number is approximately ten-fold lower than the frequency of CMV-specific cells, yet it is similar to those specific for VZV or EBV.

GENETIC FACTORS IN HIV PATHOGENESIS

A number of host genetic factors influence the rate of disease progression in HIV infection (reviewed in Paxton et al. [178]). *CCR5* is a major co-receptor for strains of HIV-1. A mutant allele of the *CCR5* gene, which contains an internal 32–base-pair deletion resulting in a truncated nonfunctional co-receptor for HIV fusion, is associated with slower rates of HIV disease progression. Since *CCR5*-utilizing HIV is almost universally responsible for primary infection, homozygosity for the *CCR5* mutation results in near-total protection from HIV-1 infection. Heterozygosity for the *CCR5* mutation results in decreased expression of *CCR5* on the cell surface and reduced infectability of T cells of these patients compared with cells from *CCR5* wild-type individuals. Although heterozygosity for *CCR5* does not appear to afford protection against HIV-1 infection, it may result in partial protection against disease progression in HIV-infected individuals. Protection against disease progression in *CCR5* heterozygotes is due in part to the lower levels of HIV replication after seroconversion, and a slower rate of CD4$^+$ T-cell depletion compared with *CCR5* wild-type individuals. In addition, heterozygosity for the *CCR5* mutation is significantly more common in cohorts of HIV-infected long-term nonprogressors compared with HIV-infected control populations (see discussion of long-term nonprogressors below).

The most extensively studied of genetic factors that might affect disease progression are associations between HLA alleles and disease progression. A large number of conflicting or unconfirmed reports have described MHC alleles, including classes I, II, and III, that may influence the pathogenesis and course of HIV disease. The MHC alleles that are most consistently associated with nonprogression are HLA B27 and B57 (reviewed in Carrington et al. [179]). In one large population study, these two alleles were those most associated with slower disease progression. Several alleles have also been associated with a more severe disease course. In this regard, the A1-B8-DRB3 haplotype has been associated with more rapid progression of disease. The allele that has been most consistently associated with rapid disease progression is HLA B35. A subsequent study has shown that almost all of the increased risk of disease progression is attributable to a subset of HLA B35 molecules that segregate from other alleles based on binding motifs that may affect presentation of HIV peptides. More rapid progression was also observed in individuals who are homozygous in class I alleles. This observation is thought to suggest that the diminished breadth of the $CD8^+$ T-cell response afforded by homozygosity may favor diminished control of virus replication. Of class II alleles the DRB1*-DQB1*06 haplotype has been associated with improved outcome. Transporter-associated with antigen-presenting (TAP) genes, which are members of the MHC class III family of alleles, also have been observed to play a role in determining the rate of disease progression in HIV infection or have been found to be significantly increased in individuals who have been exposed to HIV-1 but who do not become infected.

LONG-TERM NONPROGRESSORS

The mean time between infection with HIV and development of AIDS is approximately 10 years; however, rates of disease progression vary widely among individuals. In recent years, it has become clear that in a small percentage of untreated HIV-infected individuals, no evidence of disease progression can be detected over a long period of time (18,19). In addition to nonprogressors, other individuals who remain uninfected and seronegative despite multiple exposures to HIV have been identified, suggesting that immunologic elements of protection exist but may not be readily detectable by standard measures of immune response. This group is likely heterogeneous with regard to the mechanisms of resistance to HIV infection (reviewed in Shearer et al. [180]). Studies of both "long-term nonprogressors" and "exposed uninfected patients" have contributed to our understanding of the pathogenesis of disease and have increased optimism that some forms of protective immunity may indeed exist in HIV infection.

Definitions of long-term nonprogressors have varied. One early definition that was widely used included documented HIV infection for more than 7 years; $CD4^+$ T-cell count greater than 600 cells/μL without significant decline over time; no symptoms of HIV disease; and no history of antiretroviral therapy. Because definitions of long-term nonprogressors were created empirically, it is not surprising that such individuals constitute a heterogeneous group. Many individuals who were defined by these clinical criteria have now gone on to progressive disease. However, there remains a small subgroup of untreated long-term nonprogressors who

have now been infected for 20 years and maintain normal $CD4^+$ T-cell counts and plasma viral RNA at <50 copies/ml of plasma (163). Long-term nonprogressors have been identified in all HIV risk groups and no demographic features reliably distinguish them from typical progressors. Mechanisms that may determine a nonprogressive course during HIV infection include host genetic factors, effective immunologic control of virus replication, and/or infection with an attenuated strain of HIV (Table 4). Compared with individuals with progressive HIV disease, nonprogressors tend to have lower viral loads, and more vigorous antiviral humoral and cell-mediated immune responses. However, measurement of any of these parameters in nonprogressors reveals a great deal of heterogeneity as well as some degree of overlap with measurements in progressors. Although patients with normal $CD4^+$ T-cell counts and low levels of plasma virus are a heterogeneous group, a small subset of patients with truly nonprogressive HIV infection and control of virus replication in the absence of antiretroviral therapy are likely to hold important clues to the basis of an effective immune response to HIV.

Host Genetic Factors

As mentioned above, an HIV-infected individual's MHC alleles play an important role in determining the rate of disease progression (see discussion above of genetic factors in HIV pathogenesis). Because definitions of nonprogressors and frequency of these patients has varied between studies, several large population studies have not consistently found associations between HLA alleles and nonprogression. In one study, B57 was second to B27 as the allele most commonly associated with nonprogression. In two other large studies, only B14 and C8 were significantly associated with nonprogression, or only weak protective effects of individual class I alleles were found. However, recent reports, heavily enriched for patients

TABLE 4. *Possible mechanisms of long-term nonprogression with HIV infection*

Host genetic factors
  Slow progressor HLA profile
  Heterozygosity for 32-bp deletion in chemokine receptor CCR5
  Mannose binding lectin alleles
  Tumor necrosis factor c2 microsatellite alleles
  Gc vitamin D–binding factor alleles
Host immune response factors
  Effective CTL responses
  Secretion of CD8 antiviral factor
  Secretion of chemokines that block HIV entry co-receptors CCR5 (e.g., MIP-1α, MIP-1β, and RANTES) and CXCR4 (e.g., SDF-1)
  Secretion of IL-16
  Effective humoral immune response
  Maintenance of functional lymphoid tissue architecture
Virologic factors
  Infection with attenuated strains of HIV

that meet more stringent definitions of nonprogression based upon plasma viral RNA (<50 copies/ml), have found much stronger associations with HLA B 5701 or HLAB27 alleles (163). In addition, the HIV-specific CD8$^+$ T-cell response in these B 5701$^+$ patients is highly focused on B57-restricted peptides, which suggests that although the precise mechanisms of this effect remain unclear, the B57 molecule plays a direct role in restriction of virus replication in these individuals.

In addition, the chemokine receptor genotype has an impact on rates of progression of HIV-induced disease. For example, individuals who harbor one copy of the mutant *CCR5-Δ 32* allele have an increased chance of experiencing a slow rate of disease progression compared with individuals who inherit only the wild-type alleles (see discussion above of genetic factors in HIV pathogenesis). In addition, some *CCR2* alleles have been associated with slower rates of disease progression, although this association is not as strong as that of *CCR5*. Despite the association between *CCR5* genotype and nonprogressive HIV infection, this factor does not appear to be a dominant influence in determining the state of long-term nonprogression. In this regard, although the frequency of *CCR5* heterozygotes is increased twofold among non-progressors compared with HIV-infected controls, less than 50% of nonprogressors are *CCR5* heterozygotes (Carrington et al. [179]). The possibility that *CCR5* heterozygotes might constitute a subgroup among nonprogressors with the lowest viral loads and most preserved CD4$^+$ T-cell counts was investigated; however, the immunologic and virologic profile of *CCR5* wild-type and *CCR5* heterozygous nonprogressors was indistinguishable (181). These data indicate that although *CCR5* heterozygotes have an increased chance of becoming nonprogressors, HIV-infected *CCR5* wild-type individuals may arrive at the same phenotype by other means.

Host Immune-Response Factors

It is likely that HIV-specific CTLs play a major role in the maintenance of low viral load and the state of nonprogression. In the vast majority of long-term nonprogressors, *CCR5* mutations and attenuated viruses have not been found. In addition, strong MHC class I associations and the likely role of CTLs in reducing levels of plasma viremia during primary HIV infection and the association of progression to AIDS with late viral escape from long-lived (9 to 12 years) immunodominant CTL responses (158) suggest the importance of HIV-specific CTL in nonprogression (see discussion above of HIV-specific immune responses). Further support for the salutary role of CTLs comes from a longitudinal study in which maintenance of HIV *Gag*-specific CTL precursors was associated with nonprogression, whereas loss of these CTLs was associated with rising viral load and CD4$^+$ T-cell depletion. Although data from experimental animals and humans strongly suggest that HIV-specific CD8$^+$ T cells play an important role in restricting virus replication in long-term nonprogressors, clear and consistent *in vitro* correlates or mecha-

nisms of such an effect have not been demonstrated. Precursor frequencies of HIV-specific CTLs have intermittently been detected at higher levels in long-term nonprogressors compared with progressors. However, a number of recent studies using more quantitative techniques that examine the response to a broad array of HIV gene products have not found higher frequencies of HIV-specific CD8$^+$ T cells in nonprogressors. In many cases, the frequencies of HIV-specific CTLs were lower in nonprogressors than in progressors, likely reflecting lower levels of viral antigen in nonprogressors. Because antiretroviral therapy lowers the frequency of HIV-specific CD8$^+$ T cells to levels at or below detection, the maintenance of modest frequencies of HIV-specific CTLs in the face of low or undetectable levels of plasma viremia indicates that HIV replication is occurring in HIV reservoirs in long-term nonprogressors, but at a level that is not sufficient to result in substantial levels of plasma viremia (see discussion above of HIV reservoirs). Whether the apparent ability of CD8$^+$ T-cell responses of some long-term nonprogressors to restrict viral replication is due to viral factors (e.g., a lack of escape mutations) or other qualitative aspects of the host response (see CD8$^+$ T-cell responses above) remains unclear.

The relationship between humoral immune responses to HIV and disease progression remains uncertain. Nonprogressive HIV infection has been associated with lack of an antibody response to an epitope (residues 503 to 528) within the carboxy terminus of gp120, with maintenance of high levels of p24-specific antibodies, and with maintenance of neutralizing antibodies. Sei et al. (182) showed that the presence of HIV IIIB–neutralizing antibodies correlated with a more favorable prognosis. Subsequent studies demonstrated that the presence of neutralizing antibodies to primary HIV isolates and to autologous virus was associated with nonprogression. Furthermore, viral escape from neutralizing antibody responses is associated with the emergence of highly pathogenic HIV and with disease progression. Although HIV-infected long-term nonprogressors tend to maintain antibody responses that can neutralize a broad panel of primary isolates and autologous virus isolates, they are a heterogeneous group with regard to these neutralizing antibody responses. Whether the maintenance of neutralizing antibodies in nonprogressors is simply a marker for a relatively intact immune system, or whether these antibodies actually play an active role in determining the state of nonprogression remains unclear.

The morphologic abnormalities of lymphoid tissue associated with HIV disease progression are important determinants of immunodeficiency (see discussion above of immune dysfunction caused by HIV infection). Despite the long period of HIV infection in long-term nonprogressors, histopathologic examination of lymph node biopsies from these individuals reveals only mild HIV-related abnormalities such as follicular hyperplasia (18). The degree of follicular hyperplasia seen in nonprogressors is significantly less than that seen in progressors and is qualitatively distinct as well, without evidence of large geographic germinal centers extending into the nodal medulla. It is likely that preservation of lymphoid architecture in nonprogressors is a reflection of the lower levels of viral replication over time. Regardless of the mechanisms responsible for lower levels of viral replication in nonprogressors, preservation of lymphoid tissue architecture is a critical component of their immunocompetence. This further highlights the need to understand the mechanisms responsible for the destruction of lymphoid tissue architecture during progression of HIV disease.

Virologic Factors

Infection with attenuated strains of HIV may result in nonprogression in a small subset of individuals. The strongest evidence for an association of attenuated viral strains and nonprogression comes from an Australian cohort of nonprogressors who were infected by transfusion from a common donor, himself a nonprogressor (183). Viruses from these individuals frequently contained deletions in the *Nef* gene and in the *Nef*/U3 LTR overlap region, as well as duplications and rearrangements of NFκB/SP-1 sites in the viral LTR. Another isolated nonprogressor with viruses containing deletions within the *Nef* gene was reported by Kirchhoff et al. (184). Although these cases argue strongly that nonprogression may be due to infection with viral strains containing attenuated *Nef* genes, this scenario appears to be quite uncommon even among long-term nonprogressors. Other anecdotes implicate defective *Env, Gag, Rev, Vif, Vpr, Vpu,* and *Tat* genes in the pathogenesis of nonprogression; however, such instances appear to be the exception rather than the rule.

VACCINES

There is an urgent need to develop a safe and effective prophylactic vaccine for HIV infection. However, there are significant logistic and scientific obstacles to achieving that goal. Several aspects of HIV infection itself contribute to the difficulties in designing an effective vaccine. First, although the precise infectious dose in humans is not known, data from animal models indicates that it is likely to be quite low. Doses in the range of 100 TCID$_{50}$ of SHIV administered intravaginally (185) or doses as low as 200 TCID$_{50}$ of SIV atraumatically placed on the tonsil of naïve macaques (186) result in viremia and rapid progression of disease. In addition, latency is rapidly established during SIV infection of macaques, and likely during HIV infection of humans, within only a few rounds of replication. Thus, an effective vaccine must be capable of inducing potent immune responses to a relatively small inoculum and it must do so rapidly before latency is established. In addition, there are aspects of HIV itself that contribute to the challenges facing the development of a vaccine. The diversity of HIV envelope requires an effective global vaccine to span a wide range of HIV strains. Finally, the mechanisms of protective immunity to HIV are unknown. There are only rare examples of natural immunity that might clearly indicate the parameters to be measured or

mechanisms to be exploited in a prophylactic or therapeutic vaccine and there are no known examples of eradication of infection once it has been established in humans or experimental animals. These factors, in addition to the difficulties in generating and maintaining effective immune responses, have posed extraordinary obstacles to development of safe, effective immunogens.

Given the obstacles to developing a preventive vaccine, and the general failure of available vaccines to prevent infection, there may be more modest goals with significant clinical relevance. These include prevention or slowing of disease progression following infection, prevention of person-to-person spread by lowering levels of viral replication after natural infection, and therapeutic immunization of chronically infected patients. Whether attenuation of disease alone rather than complete protection from infection is a more realistic goal of immunization is a matter of considerable discussion. Nonetheless, our current understanding of the immune response in infected humans and data from recent animal model studies indicate that some form of vaccine-induced immunity in humans may be feasible (reviewed in Moore et al. [187] and Nabel [188]). It is likely that maximal protection will be provided through combined induction of primed cellular and humoral immune responses. However, a number of formidable challenges to induction and maintenance of such responses remain.

A wide variety of vaccine candidates are in clinical or preclinical development. There is now a large experience with several purified proteins, whole killed virus, live recombinant viruses, and live attenuated viruses in experimental animals or humans. In addition, several recent advances in primate models, and the ability to measure cellular immune responses in these models and to correlate these responses with protection from infection or restriction of challenge virus replication, have provided important insights into factors that may contribute to the development of effective immunogens. Although progress is incremental, a number of vaccine approaches in macaque models have provided results that are encouraging for induction of an immune response that appears to be capable of restricting HIV replication and disease progression.

Vaccines using viral proteins alone or in various delivery vectors have now been extensively tested in experimental animals and in phase I/II clinical trials. Two phase III clinical trials of a gp120 monomer are currently being conducted. The first generation of candidate HIV vaccines was composed of recombinant envelope proteins derived from HIV-LAV, the prototypic T-cell–line-tropic strain of HIV. The predominant immune response to these immunizations in uninfected individuals was humoral (reviewed in Moore et al. [187]), and antibodies induced by these immunogens varied in the level of their neutralizing activity. A major drawback of these initial vaccine candidates was that the antibodies induced could only neutralize CXCR4-utilizing viruses and were typically ineffective against primary HIV-1 strains. A number of studies of envelope structure either in its native trimeric virion-associated state or during the interaction with target cell receptors have led to the development of new immunogens intended to generate antibodies capable of neutralizing primary HIV isolates. Some of these vaccine candidates are designed to more closely mimic native trimeric gp160; alternatively, other vaccine candidates expose epitopes not accessible on virion-associated gp160 prior to the conformational changes induced by the interaction with target cell receptors.

The most encouraging results have been observed in studies of candidate vaccines that are live recombinant-vector viruses. A large number of these vaccine approaches are being evaluated in primate models, such as poxviruses; adenovirus; poliovirus (189,190); the herpesvirus family; Venezuelan equine encephalitis virus; and vesicular stomatitis virus (reviewed in Nabel et al. [188]). One candidate canarypox vector that encodes multiple HIV proteins is currently in phase II clinical trials. The poxvirus-based vaccines appear to be safe and have induced modest cellular immune responses in primates and humans. A number of live recombinant vaccines are being tested in combination with purified protein- or DNA-based vaccines in "prime-boost" strategies, and have proven to be much more immunogenic than most earlier vaccine approaches. Intramuscularly or intradermally injected, plasmid DNA-encoding viral antigens are transcribed, and the expressed proteins are processed and presented in the secondary lymphoid tissue, resulting in the induction of cellular and humoral responses. In one recent study (191), macaques immunized with a recombinant DNA plasmid vaccine and boosted with recombinant MVA (modified vaccinia Ankara) encoding SIV *Gag, Pol,* and 89.6 *Env,* restricted replication of a intrarectal challenge with a pathogenic SHIV. This effect was observed even though the challenge was administered 7 months after the final booster immunization. Similar levels of restriction of pathogenic SHIV challenge have recently been observed in the absence of live recombinant vectors, using DNA that encode an IL-2 immunoglobulin fusion protein or in combination with the fusion protein itself (192).

Vaccines that induce antibody responses also may play a role in strategies to attenuate HIV replication following initial infection. However, a number of obstacles persist in the development of vaccines that may mediate their effect through neutralizing antibodies. Several studies have suggested that extraordinarily high levels of neutralizing antibodies would be required to prevent infection. A neutralizing antibody b12 was shown to protect hu-PBL-SCID mice against challenge with primary isolate viruses only when extremely high levels of this neutralizing antibody were present at the time of challenge (188). The potential for neutralizing antibodies to provide protection from infection has been demonstrated by several passive transfer studies using SIV-HIV chimeras that express HIV envelopes (SHIV) (193). In these studies, neutralizing polyclonal chimpanzee-derived antibodies or cocktails of monoclonal antibodies with polyclonal human anti-HIV preparations (HIVIG) were passively transferred. In each case, extremely high levels of neutralizing antibodies sufficient to neutralize essentially all of the challenge virus

were required to protect macaques from intravenous SHIV challenge. These levels of neutralizing antibodies are thought to be unattainable by any current vaccine candidates. However, a number of other recent studies have suggested that protection from oral or vaginal challenge is easier to achieve and levels of neutralizing antibodies required for this protection may be closer to that required for protection from other viruses (185). Serum neutralizing antibody titers on the order of 1:400 achieved by passive transfer have provided complete protection from vaginal challenge with SHIV. This level is similar to levels known to protect in other virus systems. In addition, there is some suggestion that titers in the range of 1:100, although not providing complete protection, may attenuate peak viremia and provide significant benefit. However, the relatively poor immunogenicity of HIV-envelope glycoprotein makes even these lowered goals of neutralizing antibody levels difficult to achieve with current immunogens. In addition, because only low levels of neutralizing antibodies are induced by natural infection or current vaccines, division of highly diverse clades of virus into serotypes has not been achieved. Neutralization appears to be highly strain-specific and examples of broadly cross-neutralizing antibodies have only infrequently been demonstrated. If neutralizing antibodies to prevent infection cannot be generated, it may be possible to generate sterilizing immunity to control infection. Utilizing a novel technique of screening random peptide libraries with sera from HIV-infected individuals, Chen and colleagues identified antigenic and immunogenic mimics of HIV epitopes (194). Upon immunization with the mimotopes together with QS21 adjuvant, rhesus macaques generated antibody responses that cross-reacted with HIV envelope proteins. The mimotope-immunized animals, a control group of monkeys immunized with wild-type phages or vaccine-naïve animals were challenged with intravenous SHIV-89.6PD, a virus commonly used in vaccine research in macaques. During 10 months of observation, monkeys in the control groups experienced high peaks of viremia, an irreversible decline of CD4$^+$ T cells and AIDS-like syndromes. The mimotope-immunized monkeys were not protected against infection; however, four out of five animals showed significantly reduced levels of peak viremia compared to control animals with a subsequent spontaneous decrease in viremia to low or undetectable levels. In addition, the CD4$^+$ T-cell count in the mimotope-immunized macaques remained relatively stable and there was no evidence of AIDS-like syndromes.

One of the earliest demonstrations of the ability to protect against a pathogenic challenge virus was provided by the use of live attenuated viruses. Macaques infected with an SIV lacking the *Nef* gene developed a nonpathogenic infection and were protected against a subsequent challenge with a pathogenic SIV containing an active *Nef* gene (195). The mechanism of protection of the attenuated *Nef*-deleted SIV is unknown but it is believed to be mediated in large part by a cellular immune response. Use of a live attenuated virus may have an advantage over other approaches in that it may intermittently or continuously restimulate a cellular immune response. However, enthusiasm for development of live attenuated approaches has diminished. Of note, when the attenuated *Nef*-deleted virus was given to neonatal macaques, a pathogenic infection ensued (196), suggesting that under certain circumstances the attenuated virus is pathogenic. In addition, members of a cohort infected by blood transfusion from a single donor that carried a *Nef*-deleted virus have ultimately developed progressive disease, although direct comparisons with an engineered live attenuated virus cannot be drawn. Nonetheless, the potent restriction of challenge virus that is induced by a chronically expressed vaccine antigen has led to a continued interest in other viral vectors that persist in the host but that lack the safety concerns of live attenuated HIV. HIV genes inserted into vectors that chronically or intermittently express antigens of interest, such as members of the herpesvirus family, are currently being tested in experimental primates.

ROLE OF CELLULAR ACTIVATION IN HIV PATHOGENESIS

The primary function of the immune system is to recognize foreign antigens, mobilize a response to pathogenic substances, clear them, and then return to a resting state in order to respond efficiently to other antigens or to a second challenge of the same antigen with increased efficiency (anamnestic response). In HIV infection, the immune system is chronically activated in response to persistent HIV replication. HIV subverts the immune system by inducing immune activation and utilizing this milieu toward its own replicative advantage (reviewed in Fauci [197]). Manifestations of an activated immune system include hyperactivation of B cells leading to hypergammaglobulinemia; spontaneous lymphocyte proliferation; activation of monocytes; an increase in the expression of activation markers on CD4$^+$ and CD8$^+$ T cells; lymphoid hyperplasia, particularly early in the course of disease; increased secretion of proinflammatory cytokines; elevated levels of neopterin, β2-microglobulin, acid-labile interferon, and soluble IL-2 receptors; and autoimmune phenomena (see above discussion of immune dysfunction caused by HIV infection).

A number of experiments suggest that HIV replication *in vivo* is dependent on antigen-driven activation of CD4$^+$ T cells. HIV-infected individuals who had intercurrent infections, or who were immunized with various vaccines, experienced transient increases in plasma viremia that correlated with the degree of immune activation that was induced; similar observations have been made in SIV-infected macaques (reviewed in Goletti et al. [198] and Stanley et al. [199]). The amount of viral replication observed after vaccination with influenza vaccine or tetanus toxoid, or during active infection with *M. tuberculosis,* correlated inversely with the stage of HIV disease. Individuals with late-stage HIV disease had a moderate increase in viral replication, while individuals with early-stage disease had a much greater increase in plasma viremia over baseline, suggesting a correlation

between the ability of the immune system to respond to antigen and the magnitude of viral induction. Furthermore, when PBMC from tetanus toxoid–immunized, HIV-infected individuals were stimulated *in vitro* with tetanus antigen, or when PBMC from purified protein derivative (PPD)–positive, HIV-infected individuals were stimulated *in vitro* with PPD or live *M. tuberculosis,* subjects with early-stage disease manifested a much stronger proliferative response to the respective antigens with a larger increase in viral replication *in vitro* than did individuals with advanced-stage disease. These studies suggest that the level of viral replication correlates with the level of immune system activation in response to an antigen. Other experiments have analyzed lymphoid tissue from HIV-infected individuals. Within individual splenic white pulps, a restricted number of individual antigen-specific immune responses occurred (defined by the analysis of T-cell receptor Vβ gene usage), and each of the immune responses contained a single or limited number of HIV quasispecies (see HIV reservoirs above). These data support the theory that within the context of individual antigen-specific immune responses, a single quasispecies of HIV, which was present at the initiation of the reaction, spread among the newly activated T cells. Thus, it is likely that the continuous daily production of HIV occurs in newly activated CD4$^+$ T cells that are being driven by antigen-specific activation.

The potential deleterious consequences of chronic immune activation are numerous. From an immunologic standpoint, activation of the immune system in response to antigenic stimuli is critical for normal immune function. However, chronic, persistent exposure of the immune system to a particular antigen over an extended period of time may lead to a decreased ability to maintain an adequate immune response to the antigen in question. Additionally, the functional capability of the aberrantly activated immune system to respond to a broad spectrum of antigens may be compromised. From a virologic standpoint, although quiescent CD4$^+$ T cells can be infected with HIV, reverse transcription, integration, and virus spread are much more efficient in activated cells. In addition, it has been demonstrated that cellular activation induces expression of virus in latently infected CD4$^+$ T cells. These observations highlight the extraordinary capacity of HIV to exploit immune activation for its own replicative advantage.

CYTOKINES, CHEMOKINES, AND HIV

Cytokines (see Chapters 23, 24, and 25) are the soluble mediators of inflammation, activation, differentiation, and chemotaxis. They have complex effects on the replication of HIV (reviewed in Fauci [200], Poli and Fauci [201], and Cohen et al. [202]) (Fig. 3); certain cytokines (e.g., TNF-α) can directly induce HIV expression through the activation of NFκB while others act by altering the state of activation or differentiation of target cells. HIV infection induces the production of TNF-α and IL-6, as well as other cytokines, which act in an autocrine and paracrine manner to up-regulate HIV

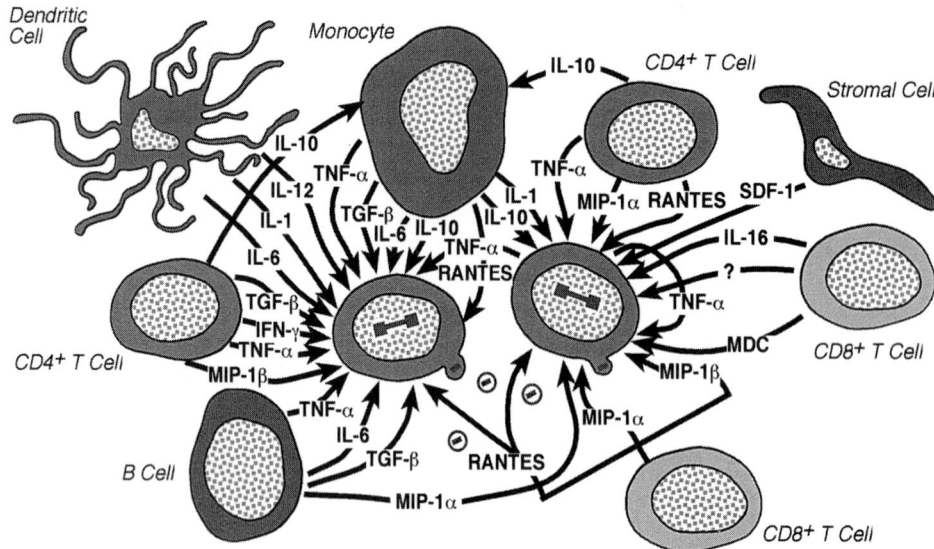

FIG. 3. Cytokine and chemokine regulatory networks that affect HIV. Endogenous cytokines regulate viral replication in CD4+ T cells. Numerous cytokines, particularly the proinflammatory cytokines TNF-α, IL-1β, and IL-6, strongly up-regulate viral replication. TGF-β and IL-10 down-regulate viral replication; in the case of IL-10, this effect is at least in part due to the down-regulation of proinflammatory cytokines. The β-chemokines, which are secreted by a variety of cell types, including CD8+ and CD8− mononuclear cells, strongly inhibit infection by CCR5-utilizing strains of HIV, whereas SDF-1 inhibits infection with CXCR4-utilizing strains. Adapted from Fauci (200), with permission.

replication. HIV envelope proteins also can directly induce the release of many cytokines, suggesting that HIV infection of a cell is not required to induce the release of certain cytokines. *In vitro* studies in a variety of model systems have assigned general HIV regulatory activities to individual cytokines; certain of these cytokines can either induce or suppress HIV, depending on the *in vitro* system used. The *in vivo* effects of a cytokine on HIV replication are difficult to predict because most *in vitro* systems reflect a small fraction of the possible interactions in an entire immune system. However, it is likely that cytokines are important modulators of HIV replication *in vivo* and that the balance between HIV-inductive and HIV-suppressive cytokines is important

in determining the steady-state level of viral replication that occurs in an HIV-infected individual (Fig. 4). Alterations in cellular activation and the resultant change in the cytokine milieu, as well as the administration of anti-inflammatory cytokines, have been shown to have substantial effects on HIV replication.

Effect of Cytokines on HIV Replication

Multiple cytokines—including IL-1β, IL-2, IL-3, IL-6, IL-8, IL-12, IL-15, TNF-α and β, macrophage (M)-CSF, and GM-CSF—induce HIV replication in *in vitro* systems. Other cytokines including IL-4, TGF-β, IL-10, and IFN-γ, have dual

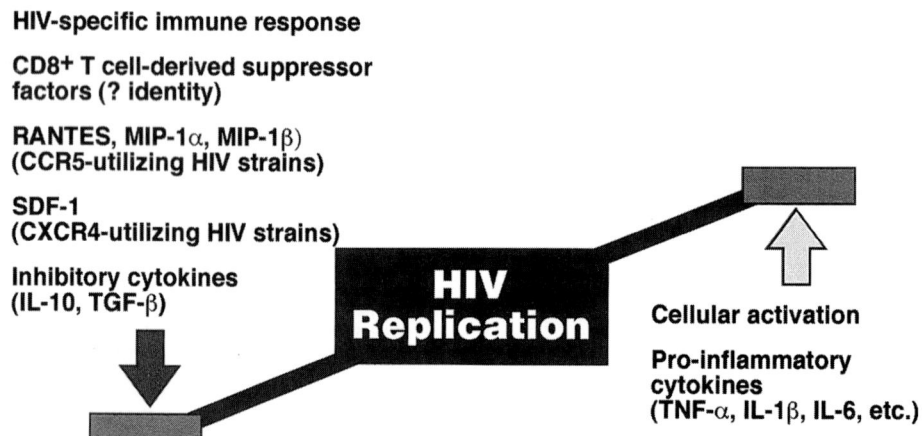

FIG. 4. A delicate balance of host factors determines the net rate of HIV replication. Several of the HIV-inductive and HIV-suppressive factors are depicted. Adapted from Fauci (200), with permission.

TABLE 5. Cytokine, chemokine and cytokine-related molecules with regulatory effects on HIV replication

Cytokine/chemokine	Effects on	
	T cells	Macrophages
IL-1β	↑	↑
IL-2	↑	nd
IL-3	nd	↑
IL-4	↑	↑↓
IL-6	↑	↑
IL-8	↑	↑
IL-10	↓	↑↓
IL-12	↑	nd
IL-13	nd	↓
IL-15	↑	nd
IL-18	↓	nd
IFN-α	↓	↓
IFN-γ	↑↓	↑↓
TGF-β	↑↓	↑↓
GM-CSF	nd	↑
M-CSF	nd	↑
TNF-α/β	↑	↑
CD30 (ligand)	↑	↑
MIP1α	↑↓	↑↓
MIP1β	↑↓	↑↓
RANTES	↑↓	↑↓
GRO-α	↑	↑

↑, enhancement of HIV replication; ↓, suppression of HIV replication; nd, not tested or no substantial effects have been reported.

effects depending on the system employed in their study, and some cytokines, including IFN-α and IFN-β, IL-13 and IL-18, have only been observed to suppress HIV replication (reviewed in Poli et al. [203]) (Table 5). The α and β chemokines also have profound effects on virus replication. Most of these effects are suppressive; however, under certain circumstances these cytokines can up-regulate virus replication (reviewed in Fauci [619]). Cell culture systems employed to study cytokine regulation can be broadly divided into transformed cell lines and primary cells. These can be further divided into acute infection systems, where HIV is added to uninfected cell lines or to cells from healthy, uninfected individuals, and endogenous infection systems, where chronically infected cell lines or cells from HIV-infected subjects are used and the virus that replicates is produced by the infected cells. A number of *in vitro* model systems of chronically infected monocytic or T-cell lines, primary cultures of peripheral-blood or lymph-node mononuclear cells from HIV-infected individuals, and acutely infected primary cell cultures have been utilized to demonstrate the role of cytokines in the regulation of HIV expression. In addition, modulation of HIV expression has been demonstrated either by manipulating endogenous cytokines or by adding exogenous cytokines to culture.

Proinflammatory Cytokines

The best-studied activators of HIV replication are the proinflammatory cytokines, TNF-α, IL-1β, and IL-6. HIV infection directly up-regulates TNF-α production *in vitro* and TNF-α increases HIV replication in multiple *in vitro* systems

(reviewed in Poli et al. [203]). Initial studies of the effect of TNF-α on HIV were conducted in cell lines chronically infected with HIV with low levels or no baseline level of virus production. The addition of TNF-α to these cell lines resulted in an increase in viral RNA, protein, and virion production. This enhancement of HIV replication was found to be due to TNF activation of NFκB proteins, which bind to tandem NFκB sites on the viral LTR and increase transcription. Addition of exogenous TNF-α to monocyte-derived macrophages (MDM) or activated PBMC also resulted in enhancement of HIV replication; inhibition of the endogenously produced TNF-α by the addition of neutralizing antibodies or soluble receptors resulted in inhibition of HIV replication. Another member of the TNF receptor family, CD30, can stimulate HIV replication in a chronically infected T-cell line in an NFκB-dependent, TNF-independent manner.

IL-1β directly activates HIV replication in monocytic cell lines by transcriptional and post-transcriptional mechanisms independent of NFκB. It synergizes with multiple cytokines, including IL-4 and IL-6, to induce HIV expression in the chronically HIV-infected promonocytic U1 cell line; this effect can be inhibited with IL-1 receptor antagonist (ra) (reviewed in Poli et al. [203]). Inhibition of endogenously produced IL-1β in activated PBMC by the addition of neutralizing antibodies or IL-1ra to the culture leads to inhibition of viral replication. IL-6 induces HIV replication in chronically infected monocytic cell lines and synergizes with other cytokines including TNF-α. In the U1 promonocytic cell line, the mechanism of IL-6 action on HIV appears to be mainly post-transcriptional; however, when IL-6 was added to TNF-α–stimulated cells, enhancement of transcription was also observed. Inhibition of endogenously produced IL-6 in cultures of stimulated PBMC results in a decrease in viral replication.

IL-2 is the most potent stimulator of HIV replication in activated CD4$^+$ T cells, due to the dependence of HIV replication on T-cell proliferation (1,3). IL-2 does not appear to have an enhancing effect on HIV in the absence of T-cell proliferation. The addition of IL-2 to acutely infected PBMC or CD8$^+$ T-cell–depleted PBMC from HIV-infected individuals results in the production of multiple cytokines, including IL-1β, IL-6, TNF-α, and IFN-γ. Neutralization of these endogenous cytokines blocks viral replication, suggesting that IL-2 can induce an autocrine and paracrine loop of HIV-inductive cytokines. However, IL-2 also can increase HIV replication in systems that are relatively independent of proinflammatory cytokines, suggesting multiple mechanisms of IL-2–induced HIV replication. Although IL-2 can increase the expression of the HIV co-receptor *CCR5* on CD4$^+$ T cells (204), it does not result in a net increase in plasma viremia when administered to HIV-infected subjects, as discussed below.

IL-15 is produced by antigen-presenting cells including monocyte/macrophages and DCs, and uses portions of the IL-2 receptor (the β and γ chains) for signaling. In both HIV$^+$ and HIV-negative individuals, IL-15 induces many of the same LAK-activating and IFN-γ enhancing activities as does IL-2. Similarly, both cytokines induce HIV replication in PBMC, although some reports suggest that IL-15 induces less p24 production compared to that induced by IL-2 (205). It has also been suggested that IL-15 plays a role in the hypergammaglobulinemia observed in HIV-infected subjects (206).

Anti-Inflammatory Cytokines

IL-4, IL-10, IL-13, TGF-β, and IL-1ra all have anti-inflammatory activities, in that they inhibit the production and/or action of the inflammatory mediators IL-1β, IL-6, and TNF-α. In addition to their anti-inflammatory effect, each has different and partially overlapping immune activities and each can modulate expression of HIV. IL-4 has both enhancing and suppressing activities on HIV infection of MDM depending on the culture conditions. IL-4, either alone or in combination with IL-2, is a very potent stimulator of HIV replication in CD4$^+$ T cells, likely by increasing the growth rate of these cells through its T-cell growth factor activities. IL-10 potently inhibits HIV replication in acute and endogenous infection systems of CD4$^+$ T cells. One of its mechanisms of action is an inhibition of activation and proliferation of T cells (207). IL-10 also inhibits HIV replication in MDM (208). At high concentrations, IL-10 inhibits the release of HIV-induced TNF-α and IL-6; exogenous supplementation of these cytokines restores viral replication. At lower concentrations of IL-10, inhibition of TNF-α and IL-6 is incomplete, no inhibition of HIV replication is observed, and modest enhancement may be seen (209). In the chronically HIV-infected U1 cell line, IL-10 alone has no effect on HIV replication; however, it can synergize with multiple cytokines, including IL-1β, IL-4, IL-6, TNF-α, and GM-CSF to increase viral production (210). IL-13 has been found to inhibit HIV infection of MDM by unknown mechanisms; this effect may be dependent on the stage of maturation of the infected cells (211). TGF-β has dichotomous effects on HIV replication in acutely infected MDM, depending on when the cytokine is added to the culture relative to infection (212). In chronically infected monocytic cell lines, TGF-β blocks phorbol 12-myristate, 13-acetate (PMA)– or IL-6–induced production of HIV. IL-1ra inhibits HIV replication in IL-2-stimulated PBMC through its blockade of IL-1β. In addition, IL-4, IL-13, and TGF-β inhibit HIV expression in LPS- and GM-CSF-stimulated, chronically infected monocytic cell lines by increasing the ratio of expression of endogenous IL-1ra to IL-1β (213). Thus, although each of these anti-inflammatory cytokines has multiple effects on HIV replication in different systems, they share the ability to inhibit at least a portion of the proinflammatory cytokine response, thereby inhibiting HIV production.

Colony-Stimulating Factors

GM-CSF and M-CSF are both potent stimulators of HIV replication in MDM. Initial studies of MDM infection with HIV used M-CSF and GM-CSF to promote the *in vitro* mat-

uration of the macrophages and allow for efficient infection (214). GM-CSF has been used in clinical trials for leukopenia in advanced HIV disease; it resulted in a greater than twofold increase in total leukocytes, monocytes, and neutrophils that was maintained throughout therapy, and no adverse events or significant increases in plasma viremia were detected. Likewise, a study of GM-CSF therapy in HIV-infected children found similar increases in leukocyte and neutrophil counts (215). Thus, although GM-CSF has been demonstrated to be a potent inducer of HIV replication in MDM *in vitro*, no increases in viral replication were noted in adults or children receiving this cytokine. This observation may be due to the fact that most patients were concomitantly receiving antiretroviral therapy.

Interferons

Interferons have potent effects on HIV replication in various *in vitro* systems. IFN-α and IFN-β suppress HIV replication at multiple steps in the viral life cycle in both activated CD4$^+$ T cells and MDM. In acute infection systems of activated T cells and monocytes, the major level of blockade occurs prior to formation and integration of the provirus. In chronically infected cell lines, at least two mechanisms of inhibition have been identified. One is a block in viral assembly and release, and the second is the inhibition of viral transcription. IFN-γ enhances HIV replication in CD4$^+$ T cells in an autocrine manner. In MDM and chronically infected monocytic cell lines, it enhances viral replication when added prior to infection and inhibits replication when added following infection (216). Inhibition of viral replication occurs by a mechanism similar to that observed for the alpha interferons (217). IL-18 suppresses HIV replication in T cells *in vitro* by enhancing the antiviral effects of IFN-γ (218). Clinical trials with IFN-α, generally used to treat Kaposi's sarcoma, have not generally shown a favorable impact on progression of HIV disease (219).

Chemokines

MIP-1α, MIP-1β, and RANTES inhibit *CCR5*-utilizing HIV infection of CD4$^+$ T cells by blocking the interaction of gp160 with *CCR5* and subsequent fusion of the virus with the cell membrane. However, these chemokines also can enhance viral replication of viruses that use CXCR4 for entry into cells (220). They also enhance the replication of *CCR5*-utilizing virus in MDM (221). Levels of MIP-1α, MIP-1β, and RANTES have varied from individual to individual in most studies; however, no significant differences in plasma levels or in levels from mitogen-stimulated PBMCs were noted among HIV-infected individuals at various stages of disease (see above discussion on HIV-specific immune responses). SDF-1, a ligand for CXCR4 (a co-receptor for certain strains of HIV), has been shown to block infection of CXCR4-utilizing viruses by blocking fusion and entry of the virus. There are numerous effects in terms of both up-regulation and down-regulation of cytokines on the expression of *CCR5* and CXCR4 that may contribute to enhancement or suppression of HIV replication (reviewed in Kinter et al. [222]). The CXC chemokines IL-8 and growth-regulated oncogene alpha (GRO-α) stimulate replication in MDM and T-lymphocytes in a paracrine/autocrine fashion (223). Exposure of MDM to HIV results in increased production of both IL-8 and GRO-α that then act to enhance HIV replication in both MDM and T cells. In addition, compounds that inhibit the interaction of these chemokines with their receptors, CXCR1 and CXCR2, prevent the enhanced replication that is induced by IL-8 and GRO-α.

Effect of HIV on Cytokine Production and Networks

HIV has multiple effects on cytokine production *in vivo* and *in vitro*. These include direct effects due to infection of cells or binding of the virus to the cell surface, and indirect effects mediated by responses to the viral infection. Soluble viral proteins can also directly induce certain cytokines. The role of HIV-induced dysregulation of cytokine networks in disease pathogenesis is likely multifactorial; many of the alterations in cytokine production, such as the increases in proinflammatory cytokines, favor HIV replication while others, such as the decrease in IL-2 production, have effects that are less clear (reviewed in Cohen et al. [202]).

As noted above, HIV infection of cells *in vitro* induces the secretion of TNF-α, IL-1β, and IL-6. These proinflammatory cytokines then act on the cell to increase HIV replication, forming an autocrine/paracrine loop. Production of these cytokines is not dependent on infection, as the addition of HIV envelope protein alone induces these cytokines through ligation of cell surface CD4 on monocytes and MDM (209). During acute infection with HIV in humans and SIV in macaques, elevated levels of both TNF-α and IL-6 have been observed. During the clinically latent stages of disease, levels of TNF-α, IL-1β, IFN-γ, and IL-6 have been observed to be elevated in some but not all studies. PBMC, CD4$^+$ T cells, monocyte/macrophages, and alveolar macrophages from HIV-infected subjects produce more TNF-α *in vitro* compared to cells from healthy, uninfected control subjects (224). Certain studies have demonstrated that, with disease progression, levels of TNF-α increase suggesting a pathogenic role for this cytokine.

Dysregulation of IL-2 production has long been recognized as a characteristic of HIV infection (reviewed in Poli and Fauci [201]). HIV infection of CD4$^+$ T cells *in vitro* results in a decreased ability to produce IL-2; indeed, CD4$^+$ T cells isolated from HIV-infected individuals produce abnormally low levels of IL-2 in response to mitogenic or antigenic stimulation. A decrease in IL-2 production and loss of antigen-specific T cells are hallmarks of the immune deficiency of HIV infection. IL-2 protein and mRNA levels are reduced in both PBMC and lymph node cells from HIV-infected individuals compared to levels found in healthy, uninfected control subjects. Loss of IL-2 secretion in response to mitogens,

alloantigens, and recall antigens correlates with the loss of CD4$^+$ T cells and disease progression.

T helper (Th)-1 cells are characterized by the secretion of IL-2 and IFN-γ and favor cell-mediated immune responses, while Th2 cells secrete IL-4, IL-5, and IL-6, and preferentially support humoral immune responses, although clones of each type can support either activity. While it is clear that the Th1 limb of cellular immune responses is impaired during the course of HIV infection, controversy surrounds the proposed dominance of Th2-like responses (i.e., secretion of IL-4, IL-5, and IL-10) during progression of HIV disease. Clerici et al. (reviewed in Clerici and Shearer [225]) showed that stimulated PBMC from HIV-infected patients exhibit a preferential Th2 pattern of cytokine secretion with disease progression; however, other investigators have found a skewing of the cytokine secretion pattern of T cells from HIV-infected patients toward a Th0 state (i.e., secretion of cytokines characteristic of both Th1 and Th2 patterns) rather than toward a Th2 state. In either case, the finding that HIV replication is more efficient in Th0 compared to Th1 clones highlights the potential importance of impaired Th1 responses in the pathogenesis of HIV disease. In this regard, IL-12 plays an important role in Th1 immune responses by enhancing production of IFN-γ. Several intracellular pathogens, including HIV, subvert the development of cell-mediated immunity to themselves by inhibiting the production of IL-12 (226). The mechanisms for this dysregulation of Th1 responses remain unknown.

In vitro studies of the effect of various cytokines on HIV replication provide models to understand possible pathogenic mechanisms; however, the complexity of the *in vivo* cytokine network renders the interpretation of the role of individual cytokines in HIV pathogenesis quite difficult. In this regard, a number of cytokines have been used therapeutically in HIV-infected individuals, including IL-2, IL-4, IL-10, IFN-α, and GM-CSF.

IL-2 is currently being studied in clinical trials using a regimen of continuous intravenous or daily subcutaneous dosing for 3 to 5 days followed by a rest period of approximately 8 weeks. In phase I/II studies, many subjects had a significant increase in their CD4$^+$ T-cell counts, often to ranges of 800 to 1,000/μl (227) (Fig. 5). Administration of IL-2 was associated with multiple, transient adverse effects that correlated in part with IL-2–induced secretion of TNF-α. A transient increase in plasma viremia that returned to baseline was also noted in the acute setting of IL-2 administration. All patients who received IL-2 were also receiving some form of antiretroviral therapy, and levels of baseline viremia were no different from those in comparable patients who were receiving antiretroviral therapy without IL-2. In subjects with low CD4$^+$ T-cell counts (i.e., <200 cells/μL) who received IL-2, CD4$^+$ T-cell counts failed to increase and levels of plasma viremia increased. This latter finding likely relates to the fact that patients with lower CD4$^+$ T-cell counts were more likely to harbor a virus that was resistant to the antiretroviral drugs that they were receiving. In addition, patients with advanced-stage HIV disease have

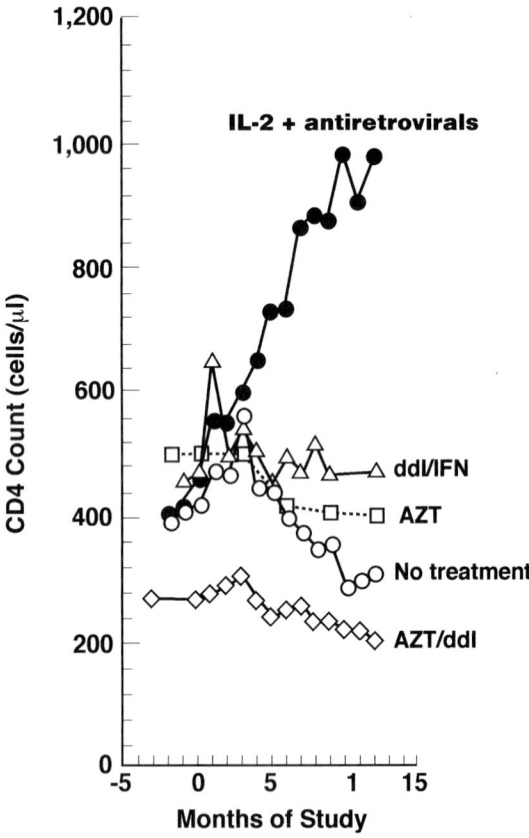

FIG. 5. IL-2 administration in combination with antiretroviral agents induces sustained increases in CD4+ T-cell counts compared with antiretroviral therapy alone or no treatment.

substantial depletion of multiple CD4+ T-cell clones, a situation apparently not reversed by IL-2 therapy. In cells isolated from patients with moderate immunodeficiency, IL-2 *in vitro* selectively and preferentially induces the noncytolytic CD8 suppressor effect, rather than increasing virus replication (202). The addition of combination antiviral therapy to IL-2 therapy resulted in a more sustained increase in CD4+ T-cell counts, a blunted transient burst in plasma viremia, and increases in CD4+ T-cell counts in patients with initial counts below 200 cells/μL. Increases in CD4+ T cells during IL-2 therapy appear to result from extrathymic expansion of the existing CD4+ T-cell repertoire, since PCR analysis of the T-cell receptor repertoire indicate that deleted clones are not regenerated and that the repertoire remains skewed as it expands. In addition, the increase in CD4+ T cells is a result of a balance between destruction induced by IL-2–mediated apoptosis and an increase in CD4+ T cells from peripheral expansion through enhanced proliferation (228).

IL-10 has been used in phase I clinical trials in HIV-infected subjects. Despite the strong effect on HIV replication *in vitro,* there has been no significant decrease in plasma viremia in HIV-infected patients *in vivo* (229). IL-4 has been used in the treatment of Kaposi's sarcoma. No in-

creases in plasma viral load were observed during treatment, again demonstrating the differences between *in vitro* systems and *in vivo* activity.

Cytokines may play an important role as adjuvant therapy in the development of effective vaccines against HIV. In a study utilizing DNA vaccines expressing SIVmac239 Gag and HIV-1 89.6P Env, macaques receiving the DNA vaccines augmented by the administration of purified fusion protein consisting of IL-2 and the Fc portion of IgG demonstrated potent secondary CTL responses, stable CD4+ T-cell counts, and persistent suppression of plasma viremia following challenge with SHIV 89.6P (192). In contrast, animals that were not vaccinated, or that were vaccinated in the absence of adjuvant therapy, had a significantly less pronounced response to vaccination and a worse clinical course following challenge. In addition, IL-12 and GM-CSF have been observed to synergistically induce CTL and protect against mucosal viral transmission when administered with HIV peptide and cholera toxin (230).

HIV Infection and Cytokine Network in Central Nervous System

HIV-induced CNS disease likely is a result of the complex interaction of cytokine networks and activation of the targets of HIV infection, including microglial cells. HIV infection of brain microglial cells, derived from the monocytic lineage, may lead to certain of the manifestations of HIV nervous system disease. HIV infection of microglial cells, like that of CD4+ T cells, results in a higher level of cytopathicity than that seen in macrophages (231). The manifestations of HIV infection of microglial cells include encephalopathy and neuropathy, astrocytosis, and cerebral vasculitis. IL-1β and TNF-α, both induced by HIV, have neurotoxic activities (232). TGF-β, an anti-inflammatory cytokine, has been demonstrated to have both a neuroprotective and a neurotoxic effect. IL-10 has a macrophage-deactivating and antiproinflammatory effect on CNS microglia, resulting in a decrease in neurotoxin release.

New insights into the pathogenesis of AIDS-associated CMV encephalitis highlight the complex interactions among cytokines, HIV co-receptors, and HIV. Bernasconi et al. (233) reported that levels of the chemokine monocyte chemotactic protein (MCP)-1, were markedly elevated in the cerebrospinal fluid of AIDS patients with CMV encephalitis. Subsequently, it was shown that CMV encodes a chemokine receptor, US28, that is homologous to CCR2. This receptor is triggered by MCP-1 and can also be used by HIV as a co-receptor for cell entry. Thus, the high levels of MCP-1 that are found in cerebrospinal fluid during CMV encephalitis may be responsible for recruitment and activation of monocytes; these cells can elaborate proinflammatory cytokines and thereby enhance HIV replication and induce neuropathologic disease. Furthermore, expression of US28 on CMV-infected cells may provide HIV with an expanded range of target cells for infection.

CONCLUSIONS

Great strides have been made in the clinical management of HIV disease. Although these advances have greatly improved the quality of life for many HIV-infected individuals, it is likely that further advances will be dependent on a fuller understanding of the immunopathogenesis of HIV infection. In this regard, the discovery that certain chemokine receptors function as co-receptors for cellular entry by HIV has greatly expanded the range of host factors that can be targeted for therapeutic intervention. As more is learned about the expression and regulation of these chemokine receptors in tissues, and about the complex effects that these receptors and their ligands have on the trafficking of cells that may play central roles in the pathogenesis of HIV disease, no doubt more opportunities for therapeutic intervention will arise. Many other questions linger regarding the pathogenesis of HIV disease. The dynamics of CD4$^+$ T-cell production, trafficking, and death during the course of HIV infection and following initiation of antiretroviral therapy remain enigmatic. Many mechanisms of HIV-induced CD4$^+$ T-cell death appear to be operative *in vitro;* however, debate continues regarding the precise mechanisms of CD4$^+$ T-cell depletion *in vivo.* Studies of individuals who are frequently exposed to HIV infection yet remain uninfected, and HIV-infected long-term nonprogressors should yield important insights into the nature of protective immunity in HIV infection. Answers to these central questions in HIV pathogenesis will facilitate the rational development of vaccines, antiretroviral agents, and immunorestorative strategies.

ACKNOWLEDGMENTS

The authors gratefully acknowledge helpful discussions with Greg Folkers, and the expert editorial assistance of Mary Rust.

REFERENCES

1. Gallo R, Salahuddin S, Popovic M, et al. Frequent detection and isolation of cytopathic retroviruses (HTLV-III) from patients with AIDS and at risk for AIDS. *Science* 1984;224:500–503.
2. Levy JA, Hoffman AD, Kramer SM, et al. Isolation of lymphocytopathic retroviruses from San Francisco patients with AIDS. *Science* 1984;225:840–842.
3. Barre-Sinoussi F, Chermann JC, Rey F, et al. Isolation of a T-lymphotropic retrovirus from a patient at risk for acquired immune deficiency syndrome (AIDS). *Science* 1983;220:868–871.
4. Fauci AS, Lane HC. Human immunodeficiency virus (HIV) disease: AIDS and related disorders. In: Fauci AS, Braunwald BE, Isselbacher KJ, eds. *Harrison's principles of internal medicine,* 14th ed., New York: McGraw-Hill, 1998:1791–1856.
5. Clerici M, Stocks NI, Zajac RA, et al. Detection of three distinct patterns of T helper cell dysfunction in asymptomatic, human immunodeficiency virus-seropositive patients independent of CD4+ cell numbers and clinical settings. *J Clin Invest* 1989;84:1892–1899.
6. Joint United Nations Programme on HIV/AIDS. *Report on the global HIV/AIDS epidemic: December 2000.* Geneva: UNAIDS, 2000.
7. Tindall B, Cooper DA. Primary HIV infection: host responses and intervention strategies. *AIDS* 1991;5:1–14.
8. Pantaleo G, Graziosi C, Fauci AS. Virologic and immunologic events in primary HIV infection. *Springer Semin Immunopathol* 1997;18:257–266.
9. Ho DD, Neumann AU, Perelson AS, et al. Rapid turnover of plasma virions and CD4 lymphocytes in HIV-1 infection. *Nature* 1995;373:123–126.
10. Roberts JD, Benbenek K, Kunkel TA. The accuracy of reverse transcriptase from HIV-1. *Science* 1988;242:1171–1173.
11. Lemp GF, Payne SF, Rutherford GW, et al. Projections of AIDS morbidity and mortality in San Francisco. *JAMA* 1990;263:1497–1501.
12. Masur H, Ognibene F, Yarchoan R, et al. CD4 counts as predictors of opportunistic pneumonias in human immunodeficiency virus (HIV) infection. *Ann Intern Med* 1989;111:223–231.
13. Centers for Disease Control and Prevention. 1993 revised classification system for HIV infection and expanded surveillance case definition for AIDS among adolescents and adults. *MMWR Morb Mortal Wkly Rep* 1992;41:1–19.
14. Moore PS, Chang Y. Detection of herpesvirus-like DNA sequences in Kaposi's sarcoma in patients with and without HIV infection. *N Engl J Med* 1995;332:1181–1185.
15. Schalling M, Ekman M, Kaaya EE, et al. A role for a new herpes virus (KSHV) in diffeent forms of Kaposi's sarcoma. *Nat Med* 1995;1:707–708.
16. Crowe S, Carlin J, Stewart K, et al. Predictive value of CD4 lymphocyte numbers for the development of opportunistic infections and malignancies in HIV-infected persons. *J Acquir Immune Defic Syndr* 1991;4:770–776.
17. Graham N, Zeger S, Park L, et al. The effects on survival of early treatment of human immunodeficiency virus infection. *N Engl J Med* 1992;326:1037–1042.
18. Pantaleo G, Menzo S, Vaccarezza M, et al. Studies in subjects with long-term nonprogressive human immunodeficiency virus infection. *N Engl J Med* 1995;332:209–216.
19. Cao Y, Qin L, Zhang L, et al. Virologic and immunologic characterization of long-term survivors of human immunodeficiency virus type 1 infection [see comments]. *N Engl J Med* 1995;332:201–208.
20. Hammer S, Squires K, Hughes M, et al. A controlled trial of two nucleoside analogues plus indinavir in persons with human immunodeficiency virus infection and CD4 cell counts of 200 per cubic millimeter or less. *N Engl J Med* 1997;337:725–733.
21. Lucas GM, Chaisson RE, Moore RD. Highly active antiretroviral therapy in a large urban clinic: risk factors for virologic failure and adverse drug reactions. *Ann Intern Med* 1999;131:81–87.
22. Whitcup SM, Fortin E, Lindblad AS, et al. Discontinuation of anticytomegalovirus therapy in patients with HIV infection and cytomegalovirus retinitis. *JAMA* 1999;282:1633–1637.
23. Chun TW, Stuyver L, Mizell SB, et al. Presence of an inducible HIV-1 latent reservoir during highly active antiretroviral therapy. *Proc Natl Acad Sci U S A* 1997;94:13193–13197.
24. Furtado MR, Callaway DS, Phair JP, et al. Persistence of HIV-1 transcription in peripheral-blood mononuclear cells in patients receiving potent antiretroviral therapy. *N Engl J Med* 1999;340:1614–1622.
25. Dornadula G, Zhang H, VanUitert B, et al. Residual HIV-1 RNA in blood plasma of patients taking suppressive highly active antiretroviral therapy. *JAMA* 1999;282:1627–1632.
26. Davey RT Jr, Bhat N, Yoder C, et al. HIV-1 and T cell dynamics after interruption of highly active antiretroviral therapy (HAART) in patients with a history of sustained viral suppression. *Proc Natl Acad Sci U S A* 1999;96:15109–15114.
27. Spira AI, Marx PA, Patterson BK, et al. Cellular targets of infection and route of viral dissemination after an intravaginal inoculation of simian immunodeficiency virus into rhesus macaques. *J Exp Med* 1996;183:215–225.
28. McIlroy D, Autran B, Cheynier R, et al. Infection frequency of dendritic cells and CD4(+) T lymphocytes in spleens of human immunodeficiency virus-positive patients. *J Virol* 1995;69:4737–4745.
29. Pope M, Betjes MG, Romani N, et al. Conjugates of dendritic cells and memory T lymphocytes from skin facilitate productive infection with HIV-1. *Cell* 1994;78:389–398.
30. Frankel SS, Wenig BM, Burke AP, et al. Replication of HIV-1 in dendritic cell-derived syncytia at the mucosal surface of the adenoid. *Science* 1996;272:115–117.
31. Weissman D, Li Y, Ananworanich J, et al. Three populations of cells with dendritic morphology exist in peripheral blood, only one of which

is infectable with human immunodeficiency virus type 1. *Proc Natl Acad Sci U S A* 1995;92:826–830.

32. Geijtenbeek TBH, Kwon DS, Torensma R, et al. DC-SIGN, a dendritic cell-specific HIV-1–binding protein that enhances trans-infection of T cells. *Cell* 2000;100:587–597.

33. Pantaleo G, Graziosi C, Demarest JF, et al. HIV infection is active and progressive in lymphoid tissue during the clinically latent stage of disease. *Nature* 1993;362:355–358.

34. Embretson J, Zupancic M, Ribas JL, et al. Massive covert infection of helper T lymphocytes and macrophages by HIV during the incubation period of AIDS. *Nature* 1993;362:359–362.

35. Haase AT, Henry K, Zupancic M, et al. Quantitative image analysis of HIV-1 infection in lymphoid tissue. *Science* 1996;274:985–989.

36. Fauci AS. The human immunodeficiency virus: infectivity and mechanisms of pathogenesis. *Science* 1988;239:617–622.

37. Ott M, Emiliani S, VanLint C, et al. Immune hyperactivation of HIV-1–infected T cells mediated by tat and the CD28 pathway. *Science* 1997;275:1481–1485.

38. Pantaleo G, Graziosi C, Demarest J, et al. Role of lymphoid organs in the pathogenesis of human immunodeficiency virus (HIV) infection. *Immunol Rev* 1994;140:105–130.

39. Cavert W, Notermans DW, Staskus K, et al. Kinetics of response in lymphoid tissues to antiretroviral therapy of HIV-1 infection. *Science* 1997;276:960–963.

40. Poles MA, Elliott J, Vingerhoets J, et al. Despite high concordance, distinct mutational and phenotypic drug resistance profiles in human immunodeficiency virus type 1 RNA are observed in gastrointestinal mucosal biopsy specimens and peripheral blood mononuclear cells compared with plasma. *J Infect Dis* 2001;183:143–148.

41. Chun TW, Finzi D, Margolick J, et al. In vivo fate of HIV-1–infected T cells: quantitative analysis of the transition to stable latency. *Nat Med* 1995;1:1284–1290.

42. Zack JA, Arrigo SJ, Weitsman SR, et al. HIV-1 entry into quiescent primary lymphocytes: molecular analysis reveals a labile, latent viral structure. *Cell* 1990;61:213–222.

43. Bukrinsky MI, Stanwick TL, Dempsey MP, et al. Quiescent T lymphocytes as an inducible virus reservoir in HIV-1 infection. *Science* 1991;18:423–427.

44. Chun TW, Carruth L, Finzi D, et al. Quantification of latent tissue reservoirs and total body viral load in HIV-1 infection [see comments]. *Nature* 1997;387:183–188.

45. Finzi D, Hermankova M, Pierson T, et al. Identification of a reservoir for HIV-1 in patients on highly active antiretroviral therapy [see comments]. *Science* 1997;278:1295–1300.

46. Wong JK, Hezareh M, Gunthard HF, et al. Recovery of replication-competent HIV despite prolonged suppression of plasma viremia. *Science* 1997;278:1291–1295.

47. Chun TW, Engel D, Mizell SB, et al. Induction of HIV-1 replication in latently infected CD4(+) T cells using a combination of cytokines. *J Exp Med* 1998;188:83–91.

48. Chun T-W, Davey RTJ, Engel D, et al. Re-emergence of HIV after stopping therapy. *Nature* 1999;401:874–875.

49. Knight SC, Macatonia SE. Dendritic cells and viruses. *Immunol Lett* 1988;19:177–181.

50. O'Doherty U, Steinman RM, Peng M, et al. Dendritic cells freshly isolated from human blood express CD4 and mature into typical immunostimulatory dendritic cells after culture in monocyte-conditioned medium. *J Exp Med* 1993;178:1067–1076.

51. Thomas R, Lipsky PE. Human peripheral blood dendritic cell subsets—isolation and characterization of precursor and mature antigen-presenting cells. *J Immunol* 1994;153:4016–4028.

52. Ramazzotti E, Marconi A, Re MC, et al. In vitro infection of human epidermal Langerhans' cells with HIV-1. *Immunology* 1995;85:94–98.

53. He J, Chen Y, Farzan M, et al. CCR3 and CCR5 are co-receptors for HIV-1 infection of microglia. *Nature* 1997;385:645–649.

54. Weinberg JB, Mathews TJ, Cullen BR, et al. Productive human immunodeficiency virus type1 (HIV-1) infection of nonproliferating human monocytes. *J Exp Med* 1991;174:1477–1482.

55. Schnittman SM, Psallidopoulos MC, Lane HC, et al. The reservoir for HIV-1 in human peripheral blood is a T cell that maintains expression of CD4. *Science* 1989;245:305–308.

56. Lambotte O, Taoufik Y, de Goer MG, et al. Detection of infectious HIV in circulating monocytes from patients on prolonged highly active antiretroviral therapy. *J Acquir Immune Defic Syndr* 2000;23:114–119.

57. Koenig S, Gendelman HE, Orenstein JM, et al. Detection of AIDS virus in macrophages in brain tissue from AIDS patients with encephalopathy. *Science* 1986;233:1089–1093.

58. Williams KC, Corey S, Westmoreland SV, et al. Perivascular macrophages are the primary cell type productively infected by simian immunodeficiency virus in the brains of macaques: implications for the neuropathogenesis of AIDS. *J Exp Med* 2001;193:905–915.

59. Stingele K, Haas J, Zimmermann T, et al. Independent HIV replication in paired CSF and blood viral isolates during antiretroviral therapy. *Neurology* 2001;56:355–361.

60. Barroso PF, Schechter M, Gupta P, et al. Effect of antiretroviral therapy on HIV shedding in semen. *Ann Intern Med* 2000;133:280–284.

61. Gupta P, Leroux C, Patterson BK, et al. Human immunodeficiency virus type 1 shedding pattern in semen correlates with the compartmentalization of viral Quasi species between blood and semen. *J Infect Dis* 2000;182:79–87.

62. Pantaleo G, Graziosi C, Demarest JF, et al. HIV infection is active and progressive in lymphoid tissue during the clinically latent stage of disease [see comments]. *Nature* 1993;362:355–358.

63. Tew JG, Burton GF, Kupp LI, et al. Follicular dendritic cells in germinal center reactions. *Adv Exp Med Biol* 1993;329:461–465.

64. Schmitz J, van Lunzen J, Tenner-Racz K, et al. Follicular dendritic cells retain HIV-1 particles on their plasma membrane, but are not productively infected in asymptomatic patients with follicular hyperplasia. *J Immunol* 1994;153:1352–1359.

65. Hivroz C, Mazerolles F, Soula M, et al. Human immunodeficiency virus gp120 and derived peptides activate protein tyrosine kinase p56lck in human CD4 T lymphocytes. *Eur J Immunol* 1993;23:600–607.

66. Li CJ, Friedman DJ, Wang C, et al. Induction of apoptosis in uninfected lymphocytes by HIV-1 Tat protein. *Science* 1995;268:429–431.

67. Westendorp MO, Frank R, Ochsenbauer C, et al. Sensitization of T cells to CD95-mediated apoptosis by HIV-1 Tat and gp120. *Nature* 1995;375:497–500.

68. Howcroft TK, Strebel K, Martin MA, et al. Repression of MHC class I gene promoter activity by two-exon Tat of HIV. *Science* 1993;260:1320–1322.

69. Bukrinsky M, Nottet H, Schmidtmayerova H, et al. Regulation of nitric oxide synthase activity in human immunodeficiency virus type 1 (HIV-1)–infected monocytes: Implications for HIV-associated neurological disease. *J Exp Med* 1995;181:735–745.

70. Lafrenie RM, Wahl LM, Epstein JS, et al. HIV-1-Tat modulates the function of monocytes and alters their interactions with microvessel endothelial cells. A mechanism of HIV pathogenesis. *J Immunol* 1996;156:1638–1645.

71. Levy J, Shimabukuro J, McHugh T, et al. AIDS-associated retroviruses (ARV) can productively infect other cells besides human T helper cells. *Virology* 1985;147:441–448.

72. Connors M, Kovacs JA, Krevat S, et al. HIV infection induces changes in CD4+ T-cell phenotype and depletions within the CD4+ T-cell repertoire that are not immediately restored by antiviral or immune-based therapies. *Nat Med* 1997;3:533–540.

73. Chen YH, Christiansen A, Dierich MP. HIV-1 gp41 selectively inhibits spontaneous cell proliferation of human cell lines and mitogen- and recall antigen-induced lymphocyte proliferation. *Immunol Lett* 1995;48:39–44.

74. Linette GP, Hartzman RJ, Ledbetter JA, et al. HIV-I–infected T cells show a selective signaling defect after perturbation of CD3/antigen receptor. *Science* 1988;241:573–576.

75. Chirmule N, McCloskey TW, Hu R, et al. HIV gp120 inhibits T cell activation by interfering with expression of costimulatory molecules CD40 ligand and CD80 (B7-1). *J Immunol* 1995;155:917–924.

76. Choremi-Papadopoulou H, Viglis V, Gargalianos P, et al. Downregulation of CD28 surface antigen on CD4+ and CD8+ T lymphocytes during HIV-1 infection. *J Acquir Immune Defic Syndr* 1994;7:245–253.

77. Borthwick NJ, Bofill M, Gombert WM, et al. Lymphocyte activation in HIV-1 infection. II. Functional defects of CD28− T cells. *AIDS* 1994;8:431–441.

78. Schnittman SM, Lane HC, Greenhouse J, et al. Preferential infection of CD4+ memory T cells by human immunodeficiency virus type 1: evidence for a role in the selective T-cell functional defects observed in infected individuals. *Proc Natl Acad Sci U S A* 1990;87:6058–6062.

79. McCune JM. The dynamics of CD4+ T-cell depletion in HIV disease. *Nature* 2001;410:974–979.

80. Schnittman SM, Psallidopoulos MC, Lane HC, et al. The reservoir for HIV-1 in human peripheral blood is a T cell that maintains expression of CD4. *Science* 1989;245:305–308.

81. Shaw GM, Hahn BH, Arya SK, et al. Molecular characterization of human T-cell leukemia (lymphotropic) virus type III in the acquired immune deficiency syndrome. *Science* 1984;226:1165–1171.

82. Lifson JD, Reyes GR, McGrath MS, et al. AIDS retrovirus induced cytopathology: giant cell formation and involvement of CD4 antigen. *Science* 1986;232:1123–1127.

83. Lifson JD, Feinberg MB, Reyes GR, et al. Induction of CD4-dependent cell fusion by the HTLV-III/LAV envelope glycoprotein. *Nature* 1986;323:725–728.

84. Pantaleo G, Graziosi C, Butini L, et al. Lymphoid organs function as major reservoirs for human immunodeficiency virus. *Proc Natl Acad Sci U S A* 1991;88:9838–9842.

85. Schnittman SM, Greenhouse JJ, Psallidopoulos MC, et al. Increasing viral burden in CD4+ T cells in pateitns with human immunodeficiency virus (HIV) infection reflects rapidly progressive immunosuppression and clinical disease. *Ann Intern Med* 1990;113:438–443.

86. Weller SK, Joy AE, Temin HM. Correlation between cell killing and massive second round superinfecton by members of some subgroups of avian leukosis virus. *J Virol* 1980;33:494–506.

87. Somasundaran M, Robinson HL. Unexpectedly high levels of HIV-1 RNA and protein synthesis in a cytocidal infection. *Science* 1988; 242:1554–1557.

88. Koga Y, Lindstrom E, Fenyo EM, et al. High levels of heterodisperse RNAs accumulate in T cells infected with human immunodeficiency virus and in normal thymocytes. *Proc Natl Acad Sci U S A* 1988;85:4521–4525.

89. Leonard R, Zagury D, Desportes I, et al. Cytopathic effect of human immunodeficiency virus in T4 cells is linked to the last stage of virus infection. *Proc Natl Acad Sci U S A* 1988;85:3570–3574.

90. Voss TG, Fermin CD, Levy JA, et al. Alteration of intracellular potassium and sodium concentrations correlates with induction of cytopathic effects by human immunodeficiency virus. *J Virol* 1996;70:5447–5454.

91. Weinhold KJ, Lyerly HK, Stanley SD, et al. HIV-1 GP120-mediated immune suppression and lymphocyte destruction in the absence of viral infection. *J Immunol* 1989;142:3091–3097.

92. Lifson JD, Feinberg MB, Reyes GR, et al. Induction of CD4-dependent cell fusion by the HTLV-III/LAV envelop glycoprotein. *Nature* 1986;323:725.

93. Pantaleo G, Butini L, Graziosi C, et al. Human immunodeficiency virus (HIV) infection in CD4+ T lymphocytes genetically deficient in LFA-1: LFA-1 is required for HIV-mediated cell fusion but not for viral transmission. *J Exp Med* 1991;173:511–514.

94. Sato AI, Balamuth FB, Ugen KE, et al. Identification of CD7 glycoprotein as an accessory molecule in HIV-1–mediated syncytium formation and cell free infection. *J Immunol* 1994;152:5142–5152.

95. deSantis C, Robbioni P, Longhi R, et al. Role of HLA class I in HIV type 1–induced syncytium formation. *AIDS Res Hum Retroviruses* 1996; 12:1031–1040.

96. Sharer LR, Cho ES, Epstein LG. Multinucleated giant cells and HTLV-III in AIDS encephalopathy. *Hum Pathol* 1985;16:760.

97. Ascher MS, Sheppard HW. AIDS as immune system activation, a model for pathogenesis. *Clin Exp Immunol* 1988;73:165–167.

98. Ameisen JC, Capron A. Cell dysfunction and depletion in AIDS: the programmed cell death hypothesis. *Immunol Today* 1991;12:102–105.

99. Thompson CB. Apoptosis in the pathogenesis and treatment of disease. *Science* 1995;267:1456–1462.

100. Meyaard L, Otto SA, Jonker RR, et al. Programmed death of T cells in HIV-1 infection. *Science* 1992;257:217–219.

101. Oyaizu N, McCloskey TW, Coronesi M, et al. Accelerated apoptosis in peripheral blood mononuclear cells (PBMCs) from human immunodeficiency virus type-1 infected patients and in CD4 cross-linked PBMCs from normal individuals. *Blood* 1993;82:3392–3400.

102. Cicala C, Arthos J, Rubbert A, et al. HIV-1 envelope induces activation of caspase-3 and cleavage of focal adhesion kinase in primary human CD4(+) T cells. *Proc Natl Acad Sci U S A* 2000;97:1178–1183.

103. Gozlan J, Lathey JL, Spector SA. Human immunodeficiency virus type 1 induction mediated by genistein is linked to cell cycle arrest in G2. *J Virol* 1998;72:8174–8180.

104. Finkel TH, Tudor-Williams G, Barda NK, et al. Apoptosis occurs predominantly in bystander cells and not in productively infected cells of HIV- and SIV-infected lymph nodes. *Nat Med* 1995;1:129–134.

105. Muro-Cacho C, Pantaleo G, Fauci AS. Analysis of apoptosis in lymph nodes of HIV-infected persons. Intensity of apoptosis correlates with the general state of activation of the lymphoid tissue and not with stage of disease or viral burden. *J Immunol* 1995;154:5555–5566.

106. Estaquier J, Idziorek T, DeBels F, et al. Programmed cell death and AIDS: signficance of T-cell apoptosis in pathogenic and nonpathogenic primate lentiviral infections. *Proc Natl Acad Sci U S A* 1994;91:9431–9435.

107. Golding H, Shearer G, Hillman K, et al. Common epitope in human immunodeficiency virus (HIV)1 gp41 and HLA class II elicits immunosuppressive autoantibodies capable of contributing to immune dysfunction in HIV 1–infected individuals. *J Clin Invest* 1989;83:1430–1435.

108. Silvestris F, Williams RC, Dammacco F. Autoreactivity in HIV-1 infections: the role of molecular mimicry. *Clin Immunol Immunopathol* 1995;75:197–205.

109. Lempicki RA, Kovacs JA, Baseler MW, et al. Impact of HIV-1 infection and highly active antiretroviral therapy on the kinetics of CD4+ and CD8+ T cell turnover in HIV-infected patients. *Proc Natl Acad Sci U S A* 2000;97:13778–13783.

110. Folks TM, Kessler SW, Orenstein JM, et al. Infection and replication of HIV-1 in purified progenitor cells of normal human bone marrow. *Science* 1988;242:919–922.

111. Neal TF, Holland HK, Baum CM, et al. CD34+ progenitor cells from asymptomatic patients are not a major reservoir for human immunodeficiency virus-1. *Blood* 1995;86:1749–1756.

112. Deichmann M, Kronenwett R, Haas R. Expression of the human immunodeficiency virus type-1 coreceptors CXCR-4 (fusin, LESTR) and CKR-5 in CD34+ hematopoietic progenitor cells. *Blood* 1997;89: 3522–3528.

113. Re MC, Zauli G, Gibellini D, et al. Uninfected haematopoietic progenitor (CD34+) cells purified from the bone marrow of AIDS patients are committed to apoptotic cell death in culture. *AIDS* 1993;7:1049–1055.

114. Stanley S, McCune J, Kaneshima H, et al. Human immunodeficiency virus infection of the human thymus and disruption of the thymic microenvironment in the SCID-hu mouse. *J Exp Med* 1993;178:1151–1163.

115. Valentin H, Nugeyre MT, Vuillier F, et al. Two subpopulations of human triple-negative thymic cells are susceptible to infection by human immunodeficiency virus type 1 in vitro. *J Virol* 1994;68:3041–3050.

116. Douek DC, McFarland RD, Keiser PH, et al. Changes in thymic function with age and during the treatment of HIV infection. *Nature* 1998;396:690–695.

117. Jamieson BD, Douek DC, Killian S, et al. Generation of functional thymocytes in the human adult. *Immunity* 1999;10:569–575.

118. Zhang L, Lewin SR, Markowitz M, et al. Measuring recent thymic emigrants in blood of normal and HIV-1–infected individuals before and after effective therapy. *J Exp Med* 1999;190:725–732.

119. Hengel RL, Jones BM, Kennedy MS, et al. Lymphocyte kinetics and precursor frequency-dependent recovery of CD4(+)CD45RA(+) CD62L(+) naïve T cells following triple-drug therapy for HIV type 1 infection. *AIDS Res Hum Retroviruses* 1999;15:435–443.

120. Walker BD, Chakrabarti S, Moss B, et al. HIV specific cytotoxic T lymphocytes in seropositive individuals. *Nature* 1987;328:345.

121. Giorgi JV, Ho H-N, Hirji K, et al. CD8+ Lymphocyte activation at human immunodeficiency virus type 1 seroconversion: development of HLA-DR+ CD38− CD8+ cells is associated with subsequent stable CD4+ cell levels. *J Infect Dis* 1994;170:775–781.

122. Vingerhoets JH, Vanham GL, Kestens LL, et al. Increased cytolytic T lymphocyte activity and decreased B7 responsiveness are associated with CD28 down-regulation on CD8+ T cells from HIV-infected subjects. *Clin Exp Immunol* 1995;100:425–433.

123. Carmichael A, Jin X, Sissons P, et al. Quantitative analysis of the human immunodeficiency virus type 1 (HIV-1)-specific cytotoxic T lymphocyte (CTL) response at different stages of HIV-1 infection: differential CTL responses to HIV-1 and Epstein–Barr virus in late disease. *J Exp Med* 1993;177:249–256.

124. Mackewicz CE, Yang LC, Lifson JD, et al. Non-cytolytic CD8 T-cell anti-HIV responses in primary HIV-1 infection. *Lancet* 1994; 344:1671–1673.

125. Zanussi S, D'Andrea M, Simonelli C, et al. Serum levels of RANTES and MIP-1a in HIV-positive long-term survivors and progressor patients. *AIDS* 1996;10:1431–1432.

126. Blauvelt A, Katz SI. The skin as target, vector, and effector organ in human immunodeficiency virus disease. *J Invest Dermatol* 1995; 105:122S–126S.

127. Weissman D, Fauci AS. Role of dendritic cells in immunopathogenesis of human immunodeficiency virus infection. *Clin Microbiol Rev* 1997;10:358–367.

128. Macatonia SE, Gompels M, Pinching AJ, et al. Antigen-presentation by macrophages but not by dendritic cells in human immunodeficiency virus (HIV) infection. *Immunology* 1992;75:576–581.

129. Cameron PU, Forsum U, Teppler H, et al. During HIV-1 infection most blood dendritic cells are not productively infected and can induce allogeneic CD4+ T cells clonal expansion. *Clin Exp Immunol* 1992;88:226–236.

130. Amadori A, Chieco-Bianchi L. B-cell activation and HIV-1 infection: deeds and misdeeds. *Immunol Today* 1990;11:374–379.

131. Moir S, Malaspina A, Ogwaro KM, et al. HIV-1 induces phenotypic and functional perturbations of B cells in chronically infected individuals. *Proc Natl Acad Sci U S A* 2001;98:10362–10367.

132. Kehrl JH, Rieckmann P, Kozlow E, et al. Lymphokine production by B cells from normal and HIV-infected individuals. *Ann N Y Acad Sci* 1992;651:220–227.

133. Macchia D, Almerigogna F, Parronchi P, et al. Membrane tumour necrosis factor-alpha is involved in the polyclonal B-cell activation induced by HIV-infected human T cells. *Nature* 1993;363:464–466.

134. Berberian L, Goodglick L, Kipps TJ, et al. Immunoglobulin VH3 gene products: natural ligands for HIV gp120. *Science* 1993;261:1588–1591.

135. Monroe JG, Silberstein LE. HIV-mediated B-lymphocyte activation and lymphomagenesis. *J Clin Immunol* 1995;15:61–68.

136. Goetz DW, Webb EL Jr, Whisman BA, et al. Aeroallergen-specific IgE changes in individuals with rapid human immunodeficiency virus disease progression. *Ann Allergy Asthma Immunol* 1997;78:301–306.

137. Rodriguez C, Thomas JK, O'Rourke S, et al. HIV disease in children is associated with a selective decrease in CD23+ and CD62L+ B cells. *Clin Immunol Immunopathol* 1996;81:191–199.

138. Elbim C, Prevot MH, Bouscarat F, et al. Impairment of polymorphonuclear neutrophil function in HIV-infected patients. *J Cardiovasc Pharmacol* 1995;25(suppl 2):S66–S70.

139. Jarstrand C, Akerlund B. Oxygen radical release by neutrophils of HIV-infected patients. *Chem Biol Interact* 1994;91:141–146.

140. Pitrak DL, Tsai HC, Mullane KM, et al. Accelerated neutrophil apoptosis in the acquired immunodeficiency syndrome. *J Clin Invest* 1996; 98:2714–2719.

141. Tascini C, Baldelli F, Monari C, et al. Inhibition of fungicidal activity of polymorphonuclear leukocytes from HIV-infected patients by interleukin (IL)-4 and IL-10. *AIDS* 1996;10:477–483.

142. Weller PF, Marshall WL, Lucey DR, et al. Infection, apoptosis, and killing of mature human eosinophils by human immunodeficiency virus-1. *Am J Respir Cell Mol Biol* 1995;13:610–620.

143. Muller F, Rollag H, Froland SS. Reduced oxidative burst responses in monocytes and monocyte-derived macrophages from HIV-infected subjects. *Clin Exp Immunol* 1990;82:10–15.

144. Poli G, Botazzi B, Acero R, et al. Monocyte function in intravenous drug abusers with lymphadenopathy syndrome and in patients with acquired immunodeficiency syndrome: selective impairment of chemotaxis. *Clin Exp Immunol* 1985;62:136–142.

145. Ahmad A, Menezes J. Antibody-dependent cellular cytotoxicity in HIV infections. *FASEB J* 1996;10:258–266.

146. Ullum H, Gotzsche PC, Victor J, et al. Defective natural immunity: an early manifestation of human immunodeficiency virus infection. *J Exp Med* 1995;182:789–799.

147. Pilgrim AK, Pantaleo G, Cohen OJ, et al. Neutralizing antibody responses to human immunodeficiency virus type 1 in primary infection and long-term nonprogressive infection. *J Infect Dis* 1997;176:924–932.

148. Kwong PD, Wyatt R, Robinson J, et al. Structure of an HIV gp120 envelope glycoprotein in complex with the CD4 receptor and a neutralizing human antibody. *Nature* 1998;393:648–659.

149. Saphire EO, Parren PW, Pantophlet R, et al. Crystal structure of a neutralizing human IGG against HIV-1: a template for vaccine design. *Science* 2001;293:1155–1159.

150. Rizzuto CD, Wyatt R, Hernandez-Ramos N, et al. A conserved HIV gp120 glycoprotein structure involved in chemokine receptor binding. *Science* 1998;280:1949–1953.

151. Burton DR, Pyati J, Koduri R, et al. Efficient neutralization of primary isolates of HIV-1 by a recombinant human monoclonal antibody. *Science* 1994;266:1024–1027.

152. Parren PW, Burton DR. The antiviral activity of antibodies in vitro and in vivo. *Adv Immunol* 2001;77:195–262.

153. Coffin JM. HIV population dynamics in vivo: implications for genetic variation, pathogenesis, and therapy [see comments]. *Science* 1995;267:483–489.

154. Koup RA, Safrit JT, Cao Y, et al. Temporal association of cellular immune responses with the initial control of viremia in primary human immunodeficiency virus type 1 syndrome. *J Virol* 1994;68:4650–4655.

155. Schmitz JE, Kuroda MJ, Santra S, et al. Control of viremia in simian immunodeficiency virus infection by CD8+ lymphocytes. *Science* 1999;283:857–860.

156. Matano T, Shibata R, Siemon C, et al. Administration of an anti-CD8 monoclonal antibody interferes with the clearance of chimeric simian/human immunodeficiency virus during primary infections of rhesus macaques. *J Virol* 1998;72:164–169.

157. Gundlach BR, Reiprich S, Sopper S, et al. Env-independent protection induced by live, attenuated simian immunodeficiency virus vaccines. *J Virol* 1998;72:7846–7851.

158. Goulder PJ, Phillips RE, Colbert RA, et al. Late escape from an immunodominant cytotoxic T-lymphocyte response associated with progression to AIDS. *Nat Med* 1997;3:212–217.

159. Nowak MA, May RM, Phillips RE, et al. Antigenic oscillations and shifting immunodominance in HIV-1 infections [see comments]. *Nature* 1995;375:606–611.

160. Koenig S, Conley AJ, Brewah YA, et al. Transfer of HIV-1-specific cytotoxic T lymphocytes to an AIDS patient leads to selection for mutant HIV variants and subsequent disease progression. *Nat Med* 1995; 1:330–336.

161. Le Gall S, Erdtmann L, Benichou S, et al. Nef interacts with the mu subunit of clathrin adaptor complexes and reveals a cryptic sorting signal in MHC I molecules. *Immunity* 1998;8:483–495.

162. Cohen GB, Gandhi RT, Davis DM, et al. The selective downregulation of class I major histocompatibility complex proteins by HIV-1 protects HIV-infected cells from NK cells. *Immunity* 1999;10:661–671.

163. Migueles SA, Sabbaghian MS, Shupert WL, et al. HLA B*5701 is highly associated with restriction of virus replication in a subgroup of HIV-infected long term nonprogressors. *Proc Natl Acad Sci U S A* 2000;97:2709–2714.

164. Ogg GS, Jin X, Bonhoeffer S, et al. Quantitation of HIV-1–specific cytotoxic T lymphocytes and plasma load of viral RNA. *Science* 1998;279:2103–2106.

165. Gea-Banacloche JC, Migueles SA, Martino L, et al. Maintenance of large numbers of virus specific CD8+ T cells in HIV infected progressors and long term nonprogressors. *J Immunol* 2000;165:1082–1092.

166. Betts MR, Ambrozak DR, Douek DC, et al. Analysis of total HIV-specific CD4+ and CD8+ T cell responses: relationship to viral load in untreated HIV infection. *J Virol* 2001;75:11983–11991.

167. van Baalen CA, Pontesilli O, Huisman RC, et al. Human immunodeficiency virus type 1 Rev– and Tat–specific cytotoxic T lymphocyte frequencies inversely correlate with rapid progression to AIDS. *J Gen Virol* 1997;78:1913–1918.

168. Pantaleo G, Demarest JF, Soudeyns H, et al. Major expansion of CD8+ T cells with a predominant V beta usage during the primary immune response to HIV [see comments]. *Nature* 1994;370:463–467.

169. Altfeld M, Rosenberg ES, Shankarappa R, et al. Cellular immune responses and viral diversity in individuals treated during acute and early HIV-1 infection. *J Exp Med* 2001;193:169–180.

170. Champagne P, Ogg GS, King AS, et al. Skewed maturation of memory HIV-specific CD8 T lymphocytes. *Nature* 2001;410:106–111.

171. Walker CM, Moody DJ, Stites DP, et al. CD8+ Lymphocytes can control HIV infection in vitro by suppressing virus replication. *Science* 1986;234:1563–1566.

172. Cocchi F, DeVico A, Garzino-Demo A, et al. Identification of RANTES, MIP-1a, and MIP-1b as the major HIV suppressive factors produced by CD8+ T cells. *Science* 1995;270:1811–1815.

173. Chun TW, Justement JS, Moir S, et al. Suppression of HIV replication in the resting CD4+ T cell reservoir by autologous CD8+ T cells:

Implications for the development of therapeutic strategies. *Proc Natl Acad Sci U S A* 2001;98:253–258.

174. Rosenberg ES, Billingsley JM, Caliendo AM, et al. Vigorous HIV-1-specific CD4+ T cell responses associated with control of viremia. *Science* 1997;278:1447–1450.

175. Rosenberg ES, Altfeld M, Poon SH, et al. Immune control of HIV-1 after early treatment of acute infection. *Nature* 2000;407:523–526.

176. Pitcher CJ, Quittner C, Peterson DM, et al. HIV-1–specific CD4+ T cells are detectable in most individuals with active HIV-1 infection, but decline with prolonged viral suppression [see comments]. *Nat Med* 1999;5:518–525.

177. McNeil AC, Shupert WL, Iyasere CA, et al. High level HIV-1 viremia suppresses viral antigen-specific CD4+ T cell proliferation. *Proc Natl Acad Sci U S A* 2001;98:13878–13883.

178. Paxton WA, Kang S, Koup RA. The HIV type 1 coreceptor CCR5 and its role in viral transmission and disease progression. *AIDS Res Hum Retroviruses* 1998;14(suppl 1):S89–S92.

179. Carrington M, Nelson G, O'Brien SJ. Considering genetic profiles in functional studies of immune responsiveness to HIV-1. *Immunol Lett* 2001;79:131–140.

180. Shearer GM, Clerici M, Clerici M, et al. Protective immunity against HIV infection: has nature done the experiment for us? HIV-specific T-helper activity in seronegative health care workers exposed to contaminated blood. *Immunol Today* 1996;17:21–24.

181. Cohen O, Vaccarezza M, Lam G, et al. Heterozygosity for a defective gene for CC chemokine receptor 5 is not the sole determinant for the immunologic and virologic phenotype of HIV-infected long term nonprogressors. *J Clin Invest* 1997;100:1581–1589.

182. Sei Y, Tsang PH, Roboz JP, et al. Neutralizing antibodies as a prognostic indicator in the progression of acquired immune deficiency syndrome (AIDS)–related disorders: a double-blind study. *J Clin Immunol* 1988;8:464–472.

183. Deacon NJ, Tsykin A, Solomon A, et al. Genomic structure of an attenuated quasi species of HIV-1 from a blood transfusion donor and recipients. *Science* 1995;270:988–991.

184. Kirchhoff F, Greenough TC, Brettler DB, et al. Brief report: absence of intact nef sequences in a long-term survivor with nonprogressive HIV-1 infection [see comments]. *N Engl J Med* 1995;332:228–232.

185. Parren PW, Marx PA, Hessell AJ, et al. Antibody protects macaques against vaginal challenge with a pathogenic R5 simian/human immunodeficiency virus at serum levels giving complete neutralization in vitro. *J Virol* 2001;75:8340–8347.

186. Stahl-Hennig C, Steinman RM, Tenner-Racz K, et al. Rapid infection of oral mucosal-associated lymphoid tissue with simian immunodeficiency virus. *Science* 1999;285:1261–1265.

187. Moore JP, Parren PW, Burton DR. Genetic subtypes, humoral immunity, and human immunodeficiency virus type 1 vaccine development. *J Virol* 2001;75:5721–5729.

188. Nabel GJ. Challenges and opportunities for development of an AIDS vaccine. *Nature* 2001;410:1002–1007.

189. Crotty S, Miller CJ, Lohman BL, et al. Protection against simian immunodeficiency virus vaginal challenge by using Sabin poliovirus vectors. *J Virol* 2001;75:7435–7452.

190. Crotty S, Lohman BL, Lu FX, et al. Mucosal immunization of cynomolgus macaques with two serotypes of live poliovirus vectors expressing simian immunodeficiency virus antigens: stimulation of humoral, mucosal, and cellular immunity. *J Virol* 1999;73:9485–9495.

191. Amara RR, Villinger F, Altman JD, et al. Control of a mucosal challenge and prevention of AIDS by a multiprotein DNA/MVA vaccine. *Science* 2001;292:69–74.

192. Barouch DH, Santra S, Schmitz JE, et al. Control of viremia and prevention of clinical AIDS in rhesus monkeys by cytokine-augmented DNA vaccination. *Science* 2000;290:486–492.

193. Shibata R, Igarashi T, Haigwood N, et al. Neutralizing antibody directed against the HIV-1 envelope glycoprotein can completely block HIV-1/SIV chimeric virus infections of macaque monkeys [see comments]. *Nat Med* 1999;5:204–210.

194. Chen X, Scala G, Quinto I, et al. Protection of rhesus macaques against disease progression from pathogenic SHIV-89.6 PD by vaccination with phage-displayed HIV-1 epitopes. *Nat Med* 2001;7:1225–1231.

195. Daniel MD, Kirchhoff F, Czajak SC, et al. Protective effects of a live attenuated SIV vaccine with a deletion in the nef gene [see comments]. *Science* 1992;258:1938–1941.

196. Ruprecht RM, Baba TW, Liska V. Attenuated HIV vaccine: caveats. *Science* 1996;271:1790–1792.

197. Cohen OJ, Kinter A, Fauci AS. Host factors in the pathogenesis of HIV disease. *Immunol Rev* 1997;159:31–45.

198. Goletti D, Weissman D, Jackson RW, et al. Effect of Mycobacterium tuberculosis on HIV replication. Role of immune activation. *J Immunol* 1996;157:1271–1278.

199. Stanley S, Ostrowski MA, Justement JS, et al. Effect of immunization with a common recall antigen on viral expression in patients infected with human immunodeficiency virus type 1 [see comments]. *N Engl J Med* 1996;334:1222–1230.

200. Fauci A. Host factors and the pathogenesis of HIV-induced disease. *Nature* 1996;384:529–534.

201. Poli G, Fauci A. Role of cytokines in the pathogenesis of human immunodeficiency virus infection. In: Aggarwal B, Puri R, eds. *Human cytokines: their role in disease and therapy.* Cambridge, MA: Blackwell Science, 1995:421–449.

202. Cohen OJ, Kinter A, Fauci AS. Host factors in the pathogenesis of HIV disease. *Immunol Rev* 1997;159:31–48.

203. Poli G, Kinter AL, Vicenzi E, et al. Cytokine regulation of acute and chronic HIV infection in vitro: from cell lines to primary mononuclear cells. *Res Immunol* 1994;145:578–582.

204. Bleul C, Wu L, Hoxie J, et al. The HIV coreceptors CXCR4 and CCR5 are differentially expressed and regulated on human T lymphocytes. *Proc Natl Acad Sci U S A* 1997;94:1925–1930.

205. Lucey DR, Pinto LA, Bethke FR, et al. In vitro immunologic and virologic effects of interleukin 15 on peripheral blood mononuclear cells from normal donors and human immunodeficiency virus type 1–infected patients. *Clin Diagn Lab Immunol* 1997;4:43–48.

206. Kacani L, Stoiber H, Dierich MP. Role of IL-15 in HIV-1–associated hypergammaglobulinaemia. *Clin Exp Immunol* 1997;108:14–18.

207. Weissman D, Daucher J, Barker T, et al. Cytokine regulation of HIV replication induced by dendritic cell-CD4-positive T cell interactions. *AIDS Res Hum Retroviruses* 1996;12:759–767.

208. Kollmann TR, Pettoello-Mantovani M, Katopodis NF, et al. Inhibition of acute in vivo human immunodeficiency virus infection by human interleukin 10 treatment of SCID mice implanted with human fetal thymus and liver. *Proc Natl Acad Sci U S A* 1996;93:3126–3131.

209. Weissman D, Poli G, Fauci AS. Interleukin 10 blocks HIV replication in macrophages by inhibiting the autocrine loop of tumor necrosis factor alpha and interleukin 6 induction of virus. *AIDS Res Hum Retroviruses* 1994;10:1199–1206.

210. Weissman D, Poli G, Fauci AS. IL-10 synergizes with multiple cytokines in enhancing HIV production in cells of monocytic lineage. *J Acquir Immune Defic Syndr Hum Retrovirol* 1995;9:442–449.

211. Naif HM, Li S, Ho-Shon M, et al. The state of maturation of monocytes into macrophages determines the effects of IL-4 and IL-13 on HIV replication. *J Immunol* 1997;158:501–511.

212. Poli G, Kinter AL, Justement JS, et al. Transforming growth factor beta suppresses human immunodeficiency virus expression and replication in infected cells of the monocyte/macrophage lineage. *J Exp Med* 1991;173:589–597.

213. Goletti D, Kinter AL, Hardy EC, et al. Modulation of endogenous IL-1 beta and IL-1 receptor antagonist results in opposing effects on HIV expression in chronically infected monocytic cells. *J Immunol* 1996;156:3501–3508.

214. Koyanagi Y, O'Brien WA, Zhao JQ, et al. Cytokines alter production of HIV-1 from primary mononuclear phagocytes. *Science* 1988;241:1673–1675.

215. Zuccotti GV, Plebani A, Biasucci G, et al. Granulocyte-colony stimulating factor and erythropoietin therapy in children with human immunodeficiency virus infection. *J Int Med Res* 1996;24:115–121.

216. Poli G, Biswas P, Fauci AS. Interferons in the pathogenesis and treatment of human immunodeficiency virus infection. *Antiviral Res* 1994;24:221–233.

217. Poli G, Orenstein JM, Kinter A, et al. Interferon-alpha but not AZT suppresses HIV expression in chronically infected cell lines. *Science* 1989;244:575–577.

218. Choi HJ, Dinarello CA, Shapiro L. Interleukin-18 inhibits human immunodeficiency virus type 1 production in peripheral blood mononuclear cells. *J Infect Dis* 2001;184:560–568.

219. Kovacs J, Bechtel C, Davey RJ, et al. Combination therapy with didanosine and interferon-alpha in human immunodeficiency virus–infected patients: results of a phase I/II trial. *J Infect Dis* 1996;173:840–848.

220. Kinter A, Catanzaro A, Monaco J, et al. CC-chemokines enhance the replication of T-tropic strains of HIV-1 in CD4(+) T cells: role of signal transduction. *Proc Natl Acad Sci U S A* 1998;95:11880–11885.

221. Schmidtmayerova H, Sherry B, Bukrinsky M. Chemokines and HIV replication. *Nature* 1996;382:767.

222. Kinter A, Arthos J, Cicala C, et al. Chemokines, cytokines and HIV: a complex network of interactions that influence HIV pathogenesis. *Immunol Rev* 2000;177:88–98.

223. Lane BR, Lore K, Bock PJ, et al. Interleukin-8 stimulates human immunodeficiency virus type 1 replication and is a potential new target for antiretroviral therapy. *J Virol* 2001;75:8195–8202.

224. Israel-Biet D, Cadranel J, Beldjord K, et al. Tumor necrosis factor production in HIV-seropositive subjects. Relationship with lung opportunistic infections and HIV expression in alveolar macrophages. *J Immunol* 1991;147:490–494.

225. Clerici M, Shearer GM. The Th1-Th2 hypothesis of HIV infection: new insights. *Immunol Today* 1994;15:575–581.

226. Sutterwala FS, Mosser DM. The taming of IL-12: suppressing the production of proinflammatory cytokines. *J Leukoc Biol* 1999;65: 543–551.

227. Kovacs JA, Vogel S, Albert JM, et al. Controlled trial of interleukin-2 infusions in patients infected with the human immunodeficiency virus. *N Engl J Med* 1996;335:1350–1356.

228. Sereti I, Herpin B, Metcalf JA, et al. CD4 T cell expansions are associated with increased apoptosis rates of T lymphocytes during IL-2 cycles in HIV infected patients. *AIDS* 2001;15:1765–1775.

229. Angel JB, Jacobson MA, Skolnik PR, et al. A multicenter, randomized, double-blind, placebo-controlled trial of recombinant human interleukin-10 in HIV-infected subjects. *AIDS* 2000;14:2503–2508.

230. Belyakov IM, Ahlers JD, Clements JD, et al. Interplay of cytokines and adjuvants in the regulation of mucosal and systemic HIV-specific CTL. *J Immunol* 2000;165:6454–6462.

231. Watkins BA, Dorn HH, Kelly W, et al. Specific tropism of HIV-1 for microglial cells in primary human brain cultures. *Science* 1990;249:549–553.

232. Giulian D, Vaca K, Noonan CA. Secretion of neurotoxins by mononuclear phagocytes infected with HIV-1. *Science* 1990;250:1593–1596.

233. Bernasconi S, Cinque P, Peri G, et al. Selective elevation of monocyte chemotactic protein-1 in the cerebrospinal fluid of AIDS patients with cytomegalovirus encephalitis. *J Infect Dis* 1996;174:1098–1101.

234. Fauci AS. Immunopathogenic mechanisms of HIV infection. *Ann Intern Med* 1996;124:654–663.

CHAPTER 43

Vaccines

G. J. V. Nossal

Historical Perspectives
The Jennerian Era · Dawn of Immunological Science (1875–1910): Pasteur, Koch, von Behring, and Ehrlich · Early Bacterial Vaccines, Toxins, and Toxoids (1910–1930) · Early Viral Vaccines: Yellow Fever and Influenza (1930–1950) · The Tissue Culture Revolution: Poliomyelitis, Measles, Mumps, and Rubella (1950–1970) · Dawn of the Molecular Era: Hepatitis B, *Pneumococcus,* and *Haemophilus influenzae* B (1970–1990)
Public Health Triumphs, Past and Present
Smallpox Eradication · Expanded Program on Immunization · Poliomyelitis Eradication · Global Eradication of Measles? · The Global Alliance for Vaccines and Immunization
Classification of Vaccines
Live Attenuated Vaccines · Vaccines Consisting of Killed Microorganisms · Toxoids · Molecular Vaccines: Protein · Molecular Vaccines: Carbohydrate and Conjugate · Combination Vaccines
New Approaches to Vaccine Design
Vectored Vaccines · Nucleic Acid Vaccines · Peptide Vaccines · Mucosal Vaccines · Transdermal Vaccines · Edible Vaccines · Prime-Boost Strategies
Adjuvants
New Insights into Antigen-Presenting Cell Activation · Empirical Approaches to Design of Adjuvants · Aluminum Compounds as Adjuvants · Emulsions as Adjuvants · Microparticles, Including Immunostimulatory Complexes, Liposomes, Virosomes, and Viruslike Particles · Other Methods of Rendering Antigens Particulate · Oligonucleotides, Especially CpG Motifs · Other Chemical Adjuvants · Microencapsulation of Antigens · Cytokines as Adjuvants · Molecular Targeting of Antigens · Mucosal Adjuvants
Standard Immunization Schedules
Bacterial Vaccines
Diphtheria, Acellular Pertussis, and Tetanus · Diarrheal Disease Vaccines: Typhoid, Cholera, and Shigellosis · *Helicobacter pylori* Vaccines · Vaccines against Encapsulated Organisms · Intracellular Pathogens, Especially Tuberculosis and Leprosy · Vaccines against Group A Streptococci
Viral Vaccines
Hepatitis A, B, and C · Rotavirus Vaccines · Respiratory Syncytial Virus Vaccine · Influenza Vaccines · Prophylactic Vaccines against Human Immunodeficiency Virus · Therapeutic Human Immunodeficiency Virus Vaccines
Vaccines against Parasitic Disease
Malaria Vaccines · Leishmaniasis Vaccines · Schistosomiasis Vaccines · Vaccines against Other Parasitic Diseases
Vaccines and Bioterrorism
Vaccines in Fields Other Than Communicable Diseases
Adverse Effects of Vaccines
Vaccination of the Very Young and the Old
Conclusions
Acknowledgments
References

Vaccines are history's most cost-effective public health tools and have so reduced the prevalence of many infectious diseases as to engender a dangerous complacency in many communities. Furthermore, in our rapidly changing society, there is a tendency for yesterday's miracle to become today's commonplace. The triumph of polio immunization is taken for granted, but the medical community's incapacity yet to immunize against the human immunodeficiency virus (HIV) and acquired immunodeficiency syndrome (AIDS) is

criticized. The devastating impact of the AIDS pandemic has certainly increased interest in vaccine research and has led to improved funding for the whole area from both public and private sources, and so an overview of the vaccine field is timely. However, vaccinology, positioned as it is at the interface of medical microbiology, public health, and immunology, is not an area that fundamental immunologists traditionally warm to. This chapter attempts to point out how much our new knowledge of the molecular and cellular regulation of immune responses can contribute to rational design of vaccines and adjuvant formulations. However, this technical material is interwoven with practical questions such as how to avoid a plethora of injections for infants, how to cope with vaccine-related adverse events, and how to ensure that the benefits of vaccines reach the citizens of the poorer countries without delay.

The chief focus, of course, is on vaccines to prevent infections, but other possible uses need to be explored. Can a vaccine approach treat an established infection, providing immunotherapy rather than immunoprophylaxis? Can there be "negative" vaccines such as in autoimmunity, allergy, or transplantation? What about vaccines in cancer and birth control vaccines? These concepts are briefly explored.

This chapter is not meant as a compendium of current or probable future vaccines. There are excellent recent works that fulfill this purpose (1,2). Rather, the examples of vaccines described are meant to be illustrative both of the diverse processes capable of leading to protection and of the immense public benefits obtainable. The fact that it has been necessary to cite quite a few diseases reflects the protean nature and rich promise of the field.

HISTORICAL PERSPECTIVES

Early civilizations that left written records, such as those of Egypt, India, Greece, and China, made references to infectious diseases, but the accuracy of diagnosis is frequently questionable. For example, it is now believed that the "leprosy" referred to in the Bible may well have represented a dermatological condition such as psoriasis. In their monumental work on smallpox and its eradication, Fenner et al. (3) concluded that "unmistakable descriptions of smallpox did not appear until the fourth century A.D. in China." Nevertheless, the specificity of immunity and its frequent lifelong duration were known, for example, to the ancient Greeks. The word *immunity* was first used in the fourteenth century with reference to plague. In the absence of knowledge of the microbial origin of infections, including epidemics, little could be done to make use of the concept.

One exception was the practice of variolation as a procedure to prevent smallpox. This most feared of diseases caused a case-fatality rate of 20% to 30% and left its other victims scarred for life. As early as the tenth century A.D., the pustular fluids from smallpox lesions, or the dried scabs from healing sores, were given to susceptible individuals to make them immune. In India, inoculation was into the skin, but in China, it was into the nose. For reasons that are not entirely clear, variolation resulted in less severe disease than natural infection. There was usually a nasty lesion at the inoculation site, some satellite blisters, frequently a mild rash, and constitutional symptoms. However, the mortality rate, at 1% to 2%, was relatively low, and there was much less scarring than after a regular attack. There were other serious constraints. For example, persons in contact with variolated people frequently developed the full, natural infection. Despite this, no

less august a body than the Royal Society of London debated the subject in the early eighteenth century. There is no doubt that variolation worked, in the sense of conferring immunity. Nevertheless, the medical profession as a whole remained skeptical.

Lady Mary Montagu is usually credited for introducing variolation into Great Britain, although the importance of her promotional work has been called into question. As the wife of the British Ambassador in Constantinople, she had been sufficiently impressed with the common local practice to have her own 6-year-old son variolated in 1718. Returning to London, she interested several prominent members of the Royal College of Physicians in the practice as they struggled with the terrible smallpox epidemic of 1721. The President of the College, Sir Hans Sloane, became a convert after some experiments on convicted felons and arranged the variolation of two royal princesses. Despite several successes, variolation never became a truly widespread practice in Britain or Europe. However, certain failures of variolation to take effect ushered in the vaccine era.

The Jennerian Era

In the 1760s and 1770s, several physicians drew attention to the fact that milkmaids were rarely pockmarked. Frequently, they developed sores on their hands because they had caught an infection from the teat of a cow. The relevant cow disease bore some similarity to human smallpox. It was found that these milkmaids could not be successfully variolated. Several people—for example, farmer Benjamin Justy—claimed to have inoculated cowpox material into their children because of this series of observations. Be that as it may, it was Edward Jenner (4) who not only published first but also actually tested immunity by challenge with smallpox. Sarah Nelmes donated a little fluid from her cowpox-infected hands, and on 14 May 1796, Jenner inoculated James Phipps with this material, which "took" at the inoculation site. As Jenner noted, "Notwithstanding the resemblance which the pustule, thus excited on the boy's arm, bore to variolous inoculation, yet as the indisposition attending it was barely perceptible, I could scarcely persuade myself the patient was secure from the smallpox. However, on his being inoculated some months afterwards, it proved that he was secure" (5). A further challenge with smallpox material 5 years later confirmed maintenance of immunity. Jenner failed to get his work into the *Transactions of the Royal Society* and published his "Inquiry" privately. Soon after, vaccination, as the practice came to be called, became popular. It spread to Europe, to the United States, and thence throughout the world. Vaccination became compulsory in several European countries in the early years of the nineteenth century, and, as a result, the number of smallpox deaths fell dramatically. For example, in Sweden, there were 5,126 deaths per million population in 1800 but 100-fold fewer by 1821. In Britain, vaccination became compulsory in 1853. The source of vaccine material changed from human to calf-derived in the second half of the nineteenth century, and revaccination also became popular. In 1896, Britain extensively celebrated the centenary of the James Phipps experiment, secure in the knowledge that vaccination had proven brilliantly successful. The final chapter in the smallpox drama is so compelling that it requires a section of its own. At this point, it is simply recorded that the Gloucestershire general practitioner has been recognized by statues and memorials in many parts of the world. He sits in state in Kensington Gardens, London, the statue there representing a focal point for the extensive 1996 bicentenary celebrations. The plaque under the statue refers to "the country doctor who benefited mankind." Who could have guessed that more than 80 years had to elapse before the next big advance in immunization?

Dawn of Immunological Science (1875–1910): Pasteur, Koch, von Behring, and Ehrlich

Jenner had no overarching theory for how vaccination provided immunity to smallpox. Two great giants of the medical profession, Louis Pasteur (1822–1895) and Robert Koch (1843–1910), established the true etiological cause of infectious diseases and thus set the scene for a better understanding of the specificity of immunity. Pasteur (6) destroyed the spontaneous generation theory of bacteria, and Koch, his archrival and debating opponent, enunciated his famous postulates that, if fulfilled, established an agent as the cause of a disease. Pasteur made the critically important observation that bacteria grown for substantial periods in artificial media lost their virulence. For example, *Pasteurella septica,* the cause of fowl cholera, when attenuated *in vitro,* no longer caused disease. Rather, injection of such attenuated bacteria protected chickens from the effects of fresh, virulent cultures (7). With surprising speed, the idea was tested in a real-life setting. In 1881, the first tests of an attenuated anthrax vaccine were run and in 1882, 85,000 sheep were immunized. Pasteur coined the word *vaccine* as a general one for immunizing preparations in homage to Edward Jenner and his use of vaccinia virus. Even though Pasteur did not know that rabies was caused by a virus rather than a bacterium and had to attenuate it in rabbit spinal cord rather than through culture, his introduction of rabies immunization on little Jacob Meister had a galvanic effect and was soon widely practiced. Monarchs from all over the world came to pay honor to Pasteur, and he was able to build the Pasteur Institute in Paris entirely from benefactions. Founded in 1888, this institute is of huge historic significance because it was the first human institution entirely devoted to biomedical research.

Pasteur originally believed that microbes had to be alive to engender immunity, but after Koch's discovery of *Vibrio cholerae,* killed whole-cell bacterial vaccines were introduced as early as 1896. Essentially similar, very reactogenic vaccines against typhoid fever and plague were shown to be at least partially effective. It is amazing that it took another 60 years for controlled trials to show that this type of vaccine

could confer significant short-term protection. However, immunity research soon took quite a different direction. Émile Roux and Alexandre Yersin discovered that certain bacteria, notably diphtheria and tetanus bacilli, produced powerful soluble exotoxins, and Emil von Behring and Shibasaburo Kitasato discovered antibodies in 1890 and had some success in the passive immunotherapy of diphtheria, with antidiphtheria toxin antibodies from horses. This resulted in the awarding of the first ever Nobel Prize in Medicine. Antitoxin could be mixed with the relatively crude toxin preparations available from culture supernatants, and the first active immunization against diphtheria or tetanus involved toxin–antitoxin mixtures. However, quantitation was poor, and the results were variable. It took the genius and tenacity of Paul Ehrlich to bring rigor to the field. His development of quantitative methods for the measurement of antibody levels made von Behring's passive immunotherapy workable, and his theories on the cellular and molecular basis of immune phenomena gave the field tremendous intellectual thrust.

It could be argued that the first golden age of immunology (approximately 1880–1910) was accompanied by a certain degree of hubris. There was a time when it appeared that almost all that was needed to conquer communicable diseases was to isolate the causative agent, establish Koch's postulates, attenuate or kill the agent, and immunize. However, from the earliest trials, such as those of Pasteur on rabies, there was controversy. Levine et al. (1) noted a number of historic disasters arising from vaccines, and it is clear that several of the early preparations were neither as safe nor as protective as their proponents claimed. It must be remembered that neither production facilities nor regulatory agencies were well developed at that time, and the design of many of the clinical trials left much to be desired. In the main, particular triumphs notwithstanding, the early promise of vaccines was not fully realized in the first golden age. There were significant professional reservations about vaccines and, in certain quarters, a distinctly antagonistic community reaction. The author was born in 1931, and it is quite clear that at that time, educated parents were by no means convinced about the advantages of immunization as a whole.

Early Bacterial Vaccines, Toxins, and Toxoids (1910–1930)

The flame of the live attenuated vaccine never died in the Pasteur Institute, and after Koch's isolation of the tubercle bacillus, the search for a tuberculosis vaccine began. Calmette and Guérin (8) started with an isolate of tuberculosis from a cow. After an amazing series of 213 subcultures over a period of 13 years, they intrepidly tried the culture orally in a newborn infant. Thus, the bacille Calmette-Guérin (BCG) was born. It was soon given intradermally rather than orally and was clearly effective in infants for the prevention of miliary tuberculosis and tuberculous meningitis, although its capacity to prevent adult pulmonary tuberculosis, the real killer in tuberculosis infection, is much more controversial.

World War I gave increased opportunity for the killed whole-cell bacterial vaccines to make their mark, especially in the case of typhoid, for which systematic use did seem to control the disease despite the absence of a formal clinical trial. Another killed bacterial vaccine used fairly widely in the 1920s was that against *Bordetella pertussis.*

In 1923, Glenny and Hopkins (9) discovered that formalin treatment of diphtheria toxin could render it harmless while preserving its immunogenic potential. At the Pasteur Institute, Gaston Ramon conducted similar studies. It was soon realized that these so-called toxoids were much more satisfactory as vaccines than were the chancy toxin–antitoxin mixture, and their progressive introduction into the industrialized countries from about 1930 markedly lowered the impact of both diphtheria and tetanus. The decrease in the United States is over 99%.

Early Viral Vaccines: Yellow Fever and Influenza (1930–1950)

In the 1920s, the differences between viruses and bacteria became clear, and the 1930s was a heady period for isolation of disease-causing viruses, but tissue culture was still the realm of very few practitioners. An important development was Ernest Goodpasture's discovery of and Macfarlane Burnet's improvement of techniques for growing viruses and *Rickettsiae* in embryonated hen's eggs. Max Theiler's safe and effective live attenuated yellow fever vaccine, 17D, hails from this period, as do first-generation killed whole-virus influenza vaccines and vaccines against typhus that were important for troops in World War II. Formalin-killed mouse brain–derived Japanese B encephalitis vaccine was also effective.

The Tissue Culture Revolution: Poliomyelitis, Measles, Mumps, and Rubella (1950–1970)

The revolution in antiviral vaccines really began with the development of tissue culture as a way of growing viruses. The paper by Enders et al. (10) on the cultivation of the Lansing strain of the poliomyelitis virus in 1949 was a watershed. It is difficult now to reconstruct the fear that surrounded poliomyelitis before 1955. Although the disease was epidemic in nature, waxing and waning with the summer seasons of maximum spread, it never disappeared. During a high-incidence year, parents feared sending their children to the cinema or the swimming pool. Polio was a dreaded enemy. In the United States, for example, there were typically 20,000 or more cases of paralytic poliomyelitis per year. On April 12, 1955, the tenth anniversary of the death of Franklin D. Roosevelt, perhaps the most famous polio victim, a press conference at the University of Michigan revealed to the world that Jonas Salk's formalin-treated whole virus vaccine provided protection. Between 1955 and 1961, 300 million doses of the vaccine were administered, and the incidence of polio declined dramatically. A major setback was the infamous

Cutter Incident, in which faulty production techniques allowed two lots of vaccine to slip through with inadequate formalin inactivation, resulting in 149 cases of polio, a disaster that lent impetus to the development of the live attenuated oral poliomyelitis vaccine of Albert Sabin, first introduced in 1961. By 1965, this latter vaccine had essentially replaced the Salk vaccine in the United States and, soon after, in most countries, although not in The Netherlands, Iceland, or Sweden. Being orally active, it was more convenient to use, and because it contained far fewer virions, it was also much cheaper. It is somewhat ironic that the very rare reversions to neurovirulence, particularly in poliomyelitis virus type 3 (estimated at one case of acute flaccid paralysis per 2.7 million doses of oral poliomyelitis vaccine administered) have now prompted U.S. health authorities to recommend injectable poliomyelitis vaccine again to obviate this very rare but extremely serious problem. The late Jonas Salk campaigned tirelessly for this reversion, the rivalry between him and Albert Sabin being legendary.

The great adventure of polio eradication is discussed in a later section, but there is no doubt that the dramatic success of polio immunization paved the way for a number of other live attenuated virus vaccines, which were dependent on the principle of attenuation in tissue culture. Enders' original Edmondston strain of measles vaccine first introduced in 1963, was a little bit risky. When the author's younger son was born in 1964, the recommendation was to use this vaccine but to co-administer gamma globulin containing antimeasles antibodies! The problem was solved through the introduction of the more attenuated Moraten and Schwartz derivatives of the original Enders strain. This excellent measles vaccine was followed by a mumps vaccine, first introduced in 1967, and a live attenuated rubella vaccine, introduced in 1968. Hilleman (11) recorded that a combined measles-mumps-rubella vaccine was the realization of a long-term dream, achieved in 1969 and licensed in 1971. Development of a measles-mumps-rubella-varicella quadrivalent vaccine is currently expected. The potential to eliminate all four diseases from the industrialized countries is real. In several European countries, measles, mumps, and rubella transmission appears to have ceased, apart from imported cases.

Dawn of the Molecular Era: Hepatitis B, *Pneumococcus,* and *Haemophilus influenzae* B (1970–1990)

Hepatitis B vaccine represented a watershed from several points of view. Although the toxoids and polysaccharide meningococcal vaccines are molecular or subunit vaccines from one point of view, use of the surface antigen of the hepatitis B virus (HBsAg) represented a new degree of purity of a single protein as a vaccine. It was also the first vaccine manufactured through recombinant deoxyribonucleic acid (DNA) technology. This protein had the tendency for self-assembly into 22-nM virion-like particles, which greatly aided immunogenicity. Less obvious was that it was the first time that a vaccine was introduced to the market as an expensive "boutique" vaccine for special risk groups such as doctors, nurses, and blood bank workers, later to become a much cheaper public health tool of immense significance for developing countries. Because there are 250 million carriers of hepatitis B worldwide, and because 20% to 25% of carriers develop chronic liver disease and, in a substantial proportion of these, the disease progresses to primary hepatocellular carcinoma, the hepatitis B vaccine is considered the first anticancer vaccine in history. It is also unique in that the relevant antigen was originally thought to represent a protein polymorphism (Australia antigen) (12) and only later was recognized as a viral component (13).

The great success of the hepatitis B vaccine has stilled many of society's fears about the use of recombinant DNA products and has certainly helped usher in the new era in which genetic engineering approaches have become the norm in vaccine research and development. It is hoped that the 18-year gap between Blumberg's (13) discovery of Australia antigen and the development of the first-generation blood-derived vaccine will not be repeated. Indeed, the time gap between cloning HBsAg and the yeast-derived vaccine was much shorter (14), and expression systems have improved enormously since that time.

Molecular vaccines of a different character were the subunit capsular polysaccharide vaccines against *Streptococcus pneumoniae, Neisseria meningitidis,* and *Haemophilus influenzae* type B (Hib). These were licensed in the 1970s and early 1980s. Unfortunately, these vaccines do not work well in young infants, and so another major molecular breakthrough was the conjugation of the carbohydrate antigens to a protein carrier, usually diphtheria or tetanus toxoid. This allowed effective T-cell help and immunological memory to develop. Various Hib conjugates were licensed in the late 1980s, effectively bringing us to the modern era.

PUBLIC HEALTH TRIUMPHS, PAST AND PRESENT

No discussion of the history of vaccines would be complete without reference to the very real efforts that the world has made to bring the benefits of vaccines to the developing countries. Because some of these are very recent, both past triumphs and ongoing struggles are considered.

Smallpox Eradication

By the mid-1960s, the societal skepticism about vaccines had largely evaporated; the polio success was in the vanguard in reshaping public opinion. However, no matter how successful any vaccine had been, there was no example of a disease having actually been eradicated from the globe. Interestingly, Edward Jenner had speculated about this with regard to smallpox. However, despite the good efforts of many countries, global eradication was not a subject of much discussion before the formation of the World Health Organization (WHO). Because Europe had essentially beaten this scourge by 1953 and, similarly, North and Central America had beaten it by

1951, global eradication seemed feasible. Progress in many of the countries of Asia was also good, but by 1960 smallpox was still a serious matter in Africa and most of the Indian subcontinent.

A heady decision was taken by the Twelfth World Health Assembly in May 1959. Global eradication of smallpox was set as a new goal for the WHO. At that time, 977 million people lived in smallpox endemic areas. The preamble to the 1959 resolution mentioned a wildly optimistic timetable of 4 to 5 years. In any event, little happened between 1959 and 1966, but at last a significant budgetary allocation was made for a major WHO effort to begin on January 1, 1967. The plan of that time called for 220 million people to be vaccinated in 1967 at a total cost of some U.S. $180 million (including indigenous country costs). Dr. D. A. Henderson was appointed Head of the Smallpox Eradication Unit at the WHO in 1966, with Dr. Isao Arita as his Medical Officer. Setting themselves a target of a decade for eradication, and with an external budget averaging U.S. $7 million per year (in addition to the countries' own efforts), the team attacked their ambitious goal, realizing the vital challenges in vaccine requirements and quality control, disease surveillance, data collection, training programs needed for mass vaccination campaigns, the requirements for WHO's own reference laboratories, and a host of similar practical problems. Sufficient progress toward global eradication had been made by 1971 for both the United States and the United Kingdom to cease their routine vaccination programs. Africa and the Indian subcontinent still remained problematic. This led to a greatly intensified effort in these regions in 1973, and by 1975, the virus was eliminated from Asia; Ethiopia remained the only real problem area. War broke out between Ethiopia and Somalia, and smallpox reestablished itself in the latter. A large-scale emergency effort was made to resolve the problem, and the last case of naturally occurring smallpox was recorded in Merca, Somalia, on October 26, 1977.

The certification of smallpox eradication was no easy task. A Global Commission had to tread warily amid the sensitivities of several countries. On December 9, 1979, the Global Commission certified that eradication had been achieved (Fig. 1). Unfortunately, in the Birmingham, United Kingdom, outbreak of 1978, a medical photographer died from the disease; she had apparently caught it somehow from the smallpox laboratory one floor below her in the medical school. This highlighted the danger of variola virus stocks in laboratories. The 49-year-old head of the smallpox laboratory, Prof. H. S. Bedson, died soon after, apparently of suicide. At the time of writing, the last stocks of smallpox virus remaining in the United States and Russia have still not been destroyed. Furthermore, there is good evidence of stocks being held for bioterrorism. Nevertheless, the eradication of the natural disease, many centuries after its first appearance, and 181 years after the first use of an effective vaccine, counts as one of humanity's noblest achievements. The total costs of smallpox eradication to industrialized and developing countries together have been estimated as U.S. $300 million over an

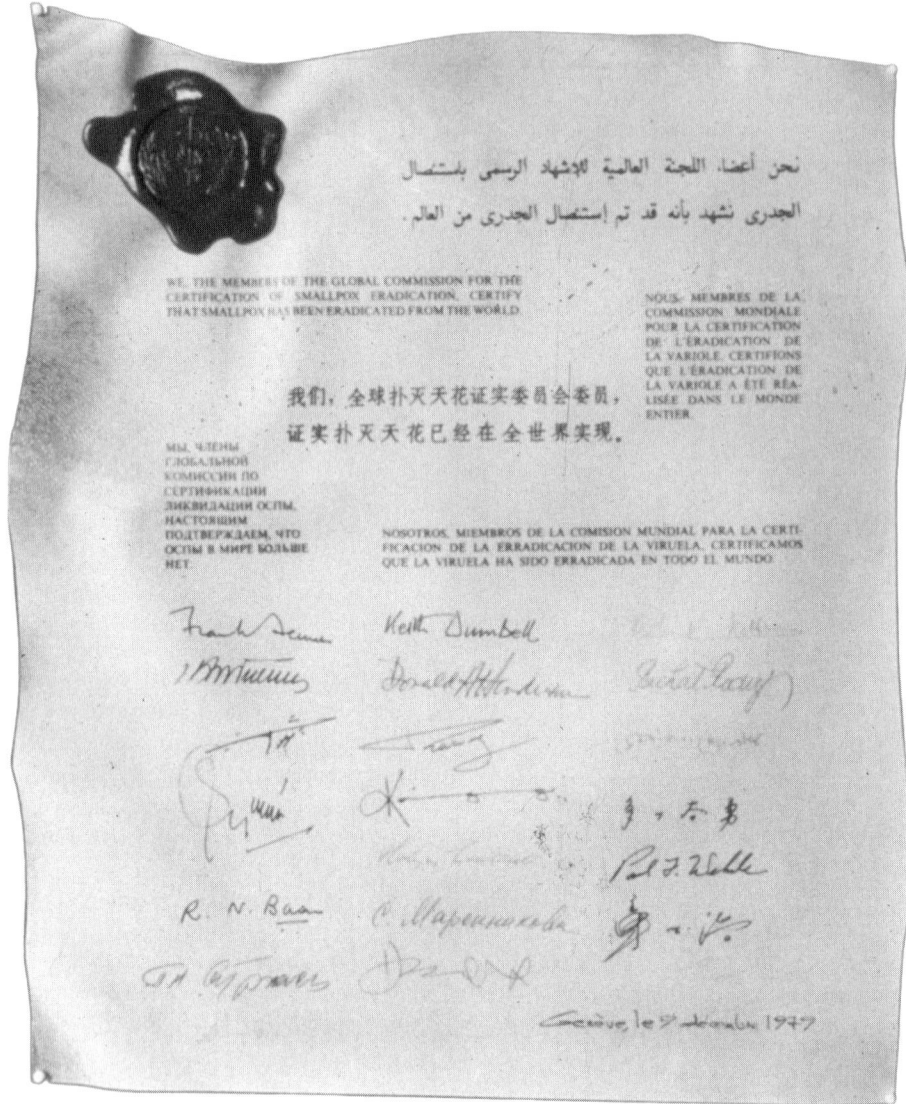

FIG. 1. Frontispiece picture of the official parchment certifying the global eradication of smallpox. From the World Health Organization, with permission.

11-year period. This compares with an annual cost of smallpox to the world of U.S. $1,350 million per annum in 1967 dollars (Fig. 2)

Expanded Program on Immunization

The planned and coordinated determined action of the smallpox eradication campaign required a logical successor, and so the WHO and its partner organizations launched the Expanded Program on Immunization (EPI) with Dr. Ralph H. Henderson (no relation to D. A. Henderson of smallpox fame) as its head. The object was to provide the six commonest infant vaccines (diphtheria, pertussis, tetanus, poliomyelitis, measles, and BCG for tuberculosis) for the total global birth cohort of over 130 million children. Before the launching of the EPI, only 5% of children in developing countries were reached. It took some time for the EPI to swing into full gear,

but in 1984 a historic meting was held in Bellagio, Italy, where key organizations, including the WHO, the United Nations Children's Fund (UNICEF), the World Bank, the United Nations Development Programme (UNDP), major foundations, government development agencies, and prominent nongovernmental organizations embraced the concept of universal childhood immunization. Dr. James Grant, the Executive Director of UNICEF, is generally given most of the credit for raising the $100 million per annum for vaccine purchase, although Rotary International, with its special emphasis on polio, has made a major contribution. By 1990, almost 80% of infants were being immunized, although not necessarily with the full schedule. (Fig. 3) This was an undoubted triumph, saving some 3 million lives per year. By 1990, however, some problems arose with the global immunization effort. It appeared that the 80% figure represented some kind of a plateau; despite much effort, the global figure

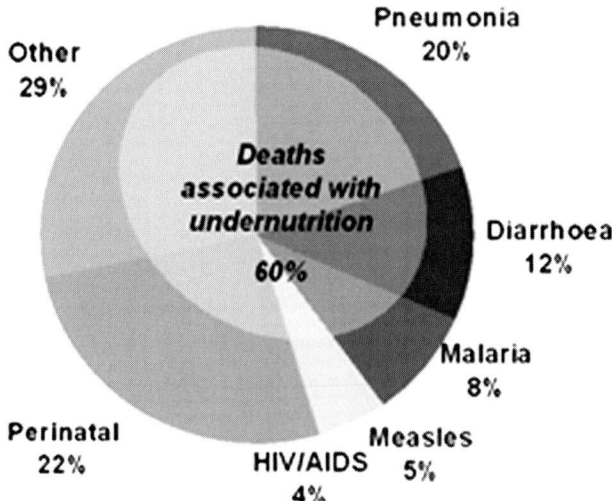

FIG. 2. Communicable diseases are still the main cause of deaths in children younger than 5 years. Frequently, malnutrition is a co-factor. World Health Organization estimates with year 2000 data. From the World Health Organization, with permission.

did not rise, and in sub-Saharan Africa, the coverage remained below 50%. Questions about the accuracy of the coverage reporting were raised. Pleas by the World Health Assembly that hepatitis B and yellow fever vaccines be added in appropriate countries went largely unheeded because of lack of funding. Brilliant new vaccines such as Hib could not even be considered. Donor fatigue was certainly evident. Before the world's current response is described, however, a further major triumph should be discussed.

Poliomyelitis Eradication

The smallpox triumph showed that the total eradication of a disease from the globe was possible. If there are an effective vaccine, no infected animal or other reservoir in the biosphere, and a genuine worldwide commitment, eradication

of quite a number of diseases should prove possible. Perhaps the first century of the third millennium will be the time when humanity takes this issue seriously.

In 1985, 11 years after the EPI was launched, the Pan-American Health Organization adopted the goal of polio eradication. There were three overarching elements to the strategy (15): first, achieving and maintaining high oral polio vaccine immunization levels; second, effective surveillance and accurate diagnosis; and, third, area-wide vaccination around all new cases. Cuba was the first country to mount a major national campaign. By 1989, an 86% decline had been achieved in all the Americas from the 1986 incidence, and by 1990, only 18 cases were reported. "Operation Mop-up" started in 1989, involving special house-to-house campaigns in areas deemed still at risk. In any event, the last case of polio occurred in Peru in August 1991, and in 1994, an International Commission certified that polio had been eradicated from the Western Hemisphere.

The WHO has set its cap at the global eradication of poliomyelitis by the year 2005. Immunization of about 80% of infants in their first 6 months of life is being achieved, but this alone will not do the job. An extremely valuable tool has been the establishment of National Immunization Days (NIDs). These are particular days—usually in winter, when natural transmission of polio is at its seasonal low—when a whole country mobilizes a massive effort to immunize all children younger than 5 years, regardless of previous immunization history; the aim is to catch those normally hard to reach and thus not yet immunized. These NIDs have been spectacularly successful and are a great credit to the health officials and political leaders in the relevant countries; to Rotary International, which, through its Polio Plus campaign, has privately raised hundreds of millions of dollars and has played a big role in mobilizing local voluntary support; and to the literally millions of volunteers involved in the effort.

One aspect of great importance in achieving eradication is disease surveillance. This involves a reporting system for all cases of acute flaccid paralysis as well as a network

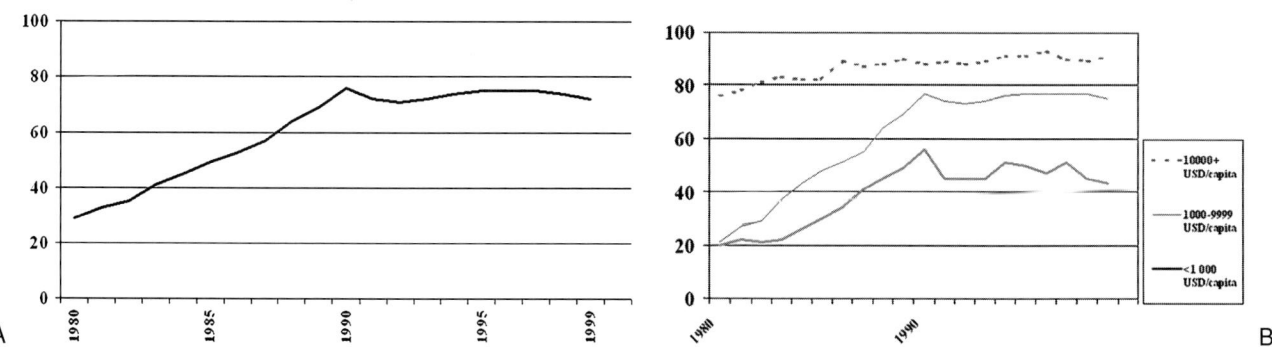

FIG. 3. The Expanded Program on Immunization (EPI) had a major effect on immunization coverage rates, as measured by the third dose of DTP (**A**) but coverage varied greatly between countries and remains <50% in countries with gross domestic product (GDP) per head less than U.S. $1,000. From the World Health Organization, with permission.

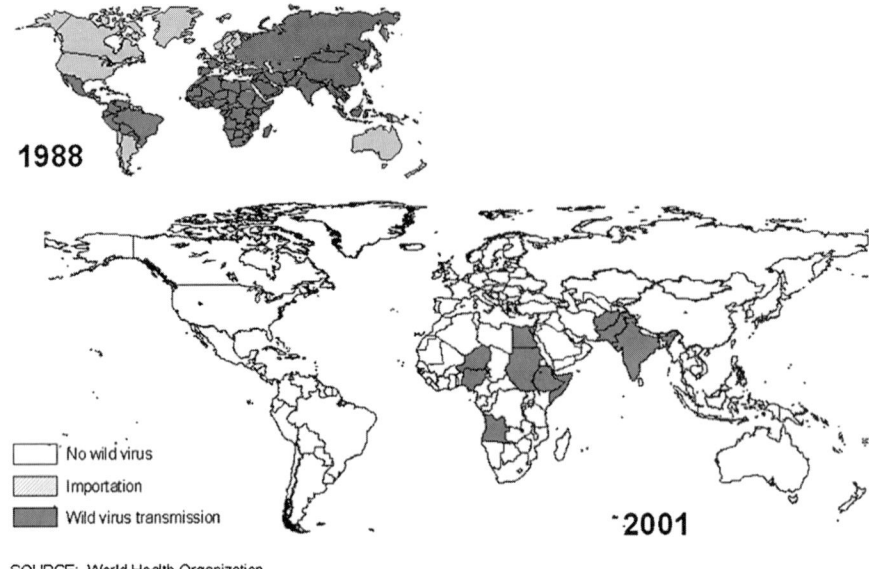

FIG. 4. Wild polio virus in 2001 (10 endemic countries, as of January 15, 2002). The polio eradication campaign has been extremely effective; only 10 countries reported wild polio virus transmission as of January 2002. From the World Health Organization, with permission.

of laboratories to provide confirmation of the diagnosis by examination of stool samples. Good surveillance is necessary for the intensive "mopping up" immunizations necessary when chains of transmission are confined to a few geographic pockets. Follow-up surveillance for several years is required when transmission has ceased, in order to be sure that the disease is really no longer occurring, before eradication can be certified.

With the quadruple strategy (high infant immunization coverage, NIDs, good acute flaccid paralysis surveillance, and "mop-up" campaigns surrounding the last few index cases), polio has also been eradicated in the Western Pacific region, the European region, and in many countries of the other regions (Eastern Mediterranean, South-East Asian and African). Even in India, with its 1.1 billion people and NIDs involving an unbelievable 100 million children, progress has been spectacular, with very few cases except in two northern states. Figure 4 shows the progress that has been made.

An 18-nation grouping from the Middle East, the Caucasus, and the Central Asian Republics (MECACAR) also achieved a success rate of over 95% in most of the countries in their NIDs. In Africa, during the 1996–1997 winter, Nelson Mandela assumed the presidency of the "Kick Polio Out of Africa" campaign, with 42 countries running NIDs under the auspices of the Organization for African Unity and the strong backing of the African Regional Office of the WHO.

The chief emphasis in 2002 was on 10 countries with residual considerable polio transmission. Some, such as Angola, the Democratic Republic of Congo, Afghanistan, the Sudan, and Somalia, are affected by war or civil strife. Others, such as Nigeria or Pakistan, have high population density and extensive poverty. For the countries in conflict, "Days of Tran-

quility" have been organized in which the guns are put down while a NID proceeds! With adequate resources, it should be possible to meet the 2005 goal (Fig. 5).

Eventually, it is hoped that immunization can cease, and there has been much discussion of a "polio dividend," the

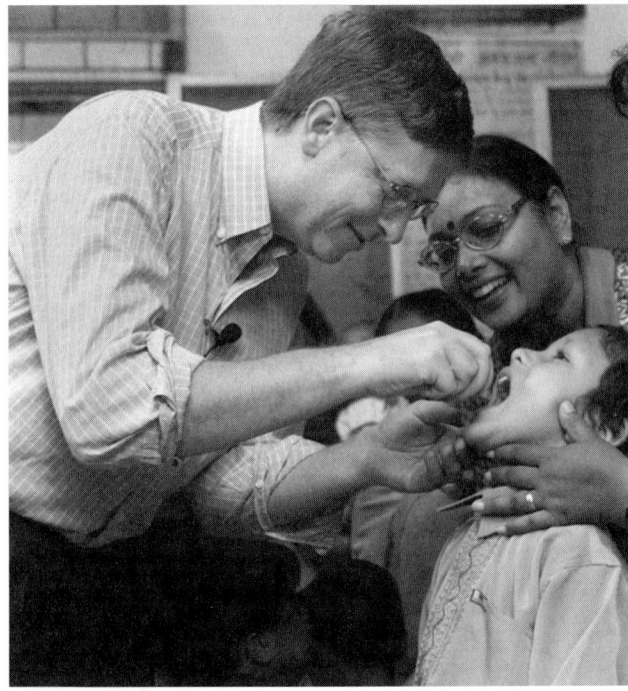

FIG. 5. Mr. William H. Gates III, aided by Ms. Mahdu Krishna, giving live attenuated oral poliomyelitis vaccine to a child in India. From the Bill and Melinda Gates Foundation, with permission.

estimated global savings being $1.5 billion annually. However, despite the extreme rarity of reversion to virulence, sustained circulation of vaccine-derived polioviruses can occur and cause outbreaks. The last case of polio caused by the wild-type virus in the Americas occurred in 1991, but between July 2000 and January 2001, a polio outbreak occurred on the island of Hispaniola, with 14 cases in the Dominican Republic and 3 in Haiti. The vaccine-derived virus spread because of low routine immunization coverage. This is the second such outbreak documented, the first being in Egypt in the 1980s. At the time of writing, a third possible outbreak in the Philippines is under investigation. These examples complicate the polio "end-game" and reaffirm the need to maintain high population immunity even when the virus has been eliminated from a country. There is as yet no consensus as to the best end-game strategy; the principal options are coordinated global pulse immunization with the Sabin vaccine before cessation and a transition to routine immunization with the Salk vaccine for some time. It now looks as though the oral vaccine will be needed at least until 2010.

Global Eradication of Measles?

Despite the great infectiousness of measles, many of the lessons learned from polio eradication can be applied to this disease. The WHO Regional Office for the Americas has made measles eradication a goal, and in many countries, a 95% coverage rate has been achieved in infants. Already transmission has ceased in Cuba, the English-speaking Caribbean countries, and Chile. Measles, mumps, and rubella transmission has ceased in some of the Scandinavian countries. One experience in the United Kingdom is worth recording. In 1993, small outbreaks of measles among children in secondary school, and epidemiological study of the probable pool of susceptible subjects with reasonable assumptions about vaccine efficacy rates, suggested the possibility of a brisk epidemic among schoolchildren. Accordingly, in November 1994, a national immunization campaign was mounted, targeted at children aged 5 to 16 years, who received a measles/rubella vaccine. This achieved more than 90% coverage; 8 million children were immunized by a mobilized workforce of nurses. Reports of serious adverse reactions were very rare, at 7 per 100,000. As a result, measles has very nearly disappeared from the United Kingdom; the very rare cases that have been confirmed since have arisen in persons from overseas.

An Australian experience is also of interest (16). The realization that an 83% coverage rate left a large cohort of susceptible persons led to a multipronged campaign starting in 1998. The first stage was aimed at mass school-based immunization [with measles-mumps-rubella (MMR) vaccine, to be discussed] of 5- to 12-year-old children, plus some supplementary methods to ensure that as many people younger than 18 as possible had received two doses of MMR. In all, 1.7 million doses of vaccine were used, and 8,783 schools were covered. As a result, seropositivity rose from a previous

84% to 94%, and the number of measles cases in the 5- to 12-year age group fell markedly. The next stage of the campaign is targeting older age groups. Of special interest was the low incidence of adverse events, and this is described fully in a later section. The success of this campaign and certain financial incentives put in place by the Australian government has had a remarkable effect on citizens. In October 2001, it was reported that 95.5% of infants had been correctly immunized by 1 year of age. Of the 4.5% not immunized, it appears that about half had parents with some concerns about immunization, which suggests that the "hard core" of immunization dissenters is only about 2% of the population.

Despite some of these encouraging statistics, it is by no means certain that the WHO will embark on global measles eradication when the polio job is complete. Resources would represent a great problem, and mass campaigns are much more difficult with an injectable rather than an oral preparation. Because the current vaccine is not effective in children younger than 9 months of age, some experts feel that a population of susceptible persons aged between 4 to 6 months (when maternally derived passive immunity wanes) and 9 months may frustrate eradication efforts. For this reason, research is being directed at vaccine formulations that are effective even in the presence of maternal antibodies.

Eradication efforts and NIDs have been criticized as representing vertical programs with the possibility of drawing resources away from more broadly based health initiatives. In many instances, however, NIDs have also given opportunities for extended activities, such as provision of vitamin A supplements or administration of vaccines other than the target one. Moreover, the social mobilization required for NIDs tends to raise a community's health consciousness, which is of benefit to regular health programs. The author's preference would be to support Dr. Ciro de Quadro's hope of measles eradication by 2015.

The Global Alliance for Vaccines and Immunization

An influential World Bank report concluded in 1993 that vaccines represented one of the most cost-effective of all medical interventions in terms of disability-adjusted life-years saved per dollar spent. However, rhetoric and advocacy alone did not unlock the extra funding that was needed to put routine global immunization back on track, let alone to make newer vaccines available. Three events in 1998 heralded the beginnings of a new approach. First, the WHO appointed a dynamic new Director-General, Dr. Gro Harlem Brundtland. Second, the President of the World Bank convened a Vaccine Summit meeting in Washington, D.C., embracing leaders of United Nations organizations as well as key industry leaders, senior academics, health bureaucrats, and prominent philanthropists. Third, William H. Gates III and his wife, Melinda French Gates, made the first of a series of extraordinary donations which, at the time of writing, total U.S. $1.4 billion for research on vaccines for diseases in developing nations, improvement of immunization infrastructure in the poorest countries, and purchase of newer vaccines such as hepatitis B and Hib. There followed a period of nearly 2 years of intensive consultations, and in January 2000, the Global Alliance for Vaccines and Immunization (GAVI) was launched (17). At its center is the Global Children's Vaccine Fund with $750 million from the Bill and Melinda Gates Foundation and substantial donations from a number of other nations. This fund addresses the needs of all countries with a gross domestic product less than U.S. $1,000 per head of population, with a clearly articulated policy for infrastructure development and vaccine purchase, rewarding the countries that increase their immunization coverage year by year. GAVI is also active in advocacy, in within-country coordination, in raising public sector and private sector funds, and in the delineation of research and development priorities. Although formally separate from GAVI, a series of research grants by the Bill and Melinda Gates Foundation dealing with vaccines for malaria, HIV/AIDS, tuberculosis, various diarrheal diseases, meningitis, pneumococcal disease, and Japanese B encephalitis, among others, form part of the new overall global thrust. The nongovernmental organization PATH plays an important coordinating role in much of this work.

The vaccine industry is fully supportive of GAVI, although many issues regarding pricing of vaccines and intellectual property rights require constant attention. The debate about cost-effective technology transfer to developing country manufacturers is also a lively one.

The most vexing of all the issues facing GAVI is sustainability. It would be most unwise to assume that philanthropic donations will go on forever. In the long run, the cost burden must eventually fall on the developing countries' own health budgets. It is hoped that the substantial childhood health gains achieved over the next decade will persuade the governments concerned.

CLASSIFICATION OF VACCINES

The purpose of a vaccine is to stimulate the immune response without subjecting an individual to the risk of actual infection. An ideal vaccine would confer the same degree of immunity as natural infection for diseases against which immunity is solid, or it would do better than nature for diseases in which immunity is not solid. Because most vaccines fall short of this ideal, it is frequently necessary to give vaccines more than once, making use of the phenomenon of immunological memory: namely, the capacity to respond more strongly to an antigen on reexposure to it. Vaccines can elicit every kind of immune response, including antibody formation, T helper 1 and 2 (Th1 and Th2)–type $CD4^+$ T-cell responses and $CD8^+$ T-cell responses, but most vaccine development programs for currently licensed vaccines have relied on the vaccine's capacity to evoke antibody formation. This will change as more ambitious targets are set and as capacity to guide immune responses down particular pathways improves. In particular, much more interest is being taken in whether a vaccine can led to Th1-type and cytotoxic $CD8^+$ T-cell responses.

Vaccines are designed primarily to prevent infection, although one of the first vaccines, that against rabies, was given after infection had been initiated. There is now increasing research on therapeutic vaccines—that is, vaccines administered after infection has been established. Such vaccines are designed to strengthen an immune response that is inadequate, particularly in cases of chronic or recurrent disease.

Obviously, microorganisms possess thousands of molecules that are foreign to a host animal or person and that are thus antigenic. Immune responses against the majority of these are entirely irrelevant to the prevention of infection. Therefore, increasing attention is being given to the identification, purification, and, frequently, molecular cloning of the antigens that evoke host-protective responses. With more complex pathogens such as parasites, it is not immediately apparent which antigens these are, and detective work needs to be done to establish correlates of immunity. The full genome sequence of many pathogens has been determined, and a new strategy is to search for likely transmembrane proteins and then to conduct trials of these in mice for possible vaccine efficacy. Identification of the correct antigens is not the end of the story, however, because many pure, soluble proteins are poorly immunogenic. In fact, there is the need to balance the greater immunogenicity of whole microorganisms against the lower reactogenicity and greater conceptual elegance of molecular vaccines. This situation needs to be dissected on a case-by-case basis, although with more recent vaccines, such as Hib and acellular pertussis, the balance appears to be swinging in the latter direction.

Vaccines have potential usefulness beyond communicable diseases, such as anticancer vaccines, birth control vaccines, and vaccines aimed at lowering immune responses, such as in autoimmunity or allergy. These uses fall outside the scope of this chapter.

Classifications of vaccines are presented in Table 1 for licensed vaccines and in Table 2 for experimental vaccines.

Live Attenuated Vaccines

Ever since Jenner's smallpox vaccine, live attenuated vaccines have occupied a special place in the pantheon of vaccinology. Many viral vaccines of this type have an efficacy of more than 90%, and protection frequently lasts for many years. This is perhaps not surprising, because the multiplication of the pathogen in the host creates an antigenic stimulus not unlike that of a natural infection in terms of antigen amount, character, and location. This key advantage is also the source of potential disadvantage, as the "mini-version" of the relevant disease can assume dangerous proportions: for example, generalized vaccinia or BCG spread in immunodeficient or immunosuppressed children. In some vaccines, the mutations causing loss of virulence are not known. Furthermore, mutations can restore virulence, as noted in the case of poliomyelitis. Much research has centered on more rationally planned attenuation based on an understanding of the molecular determinants of virulence. Relevant genetic engineering

TABLE 1. *Classification of licensed vaccines*

Types of vaccine	Examples
Live attenuated virus	Poliomyelitis (Sabin), measles, mumps, rubella, rabies, varicella, vaccinia, yellow fever
Live attenuated bacterium	Bacille Calmette-Guérin for tuberculosis or leprosy, Ty21a for typhoid fever
Killed whole virus	Poliomyelitis (Salk), influenza, hepatitis A, rabies
Killed whole cell bacterium	Pertussis, cholera, anthrax
Toxoids	Diphtheria, tetanus
Molecular vaccines: protein	Acellular pertussis, subunit influenza, hepatitis B
Molecular vaccines: carbohydrate	*Haemophilus influenzae* type B (Hib), Vi typhoid, meningococci, pneumococci
Molecular vaccines: carbohydrate-protein conjugate	Hib, meningococci, pneumococci
Combination vaccines	Diphtheria, pertussis, tetanus (DPT); measles, mumps, rubella (MMR); DPT-Hib

TABLE 2. *Newer approaches to vaccine design*

Approach	Purpose
Vectored vaccines	To employ an attenuated virus or bacterium with limited replication potential to carry a gene or genes for antigens from a pathogen into the body
Nucleic acid vaccines	To use a plasmid containing genes coding for one or more antigens from a pathogen so that the body itself becomes a factory for the antigen(s) in question; there are variations on this theme
Peptide vaccines	To construct a polymer out of a number of peptides, frequently T cell epitopes, thereby creating an immunogen
Mucosal vaccines	To administer an antigen not by injection but through a mucosal surface (e.g., orally or intranasally), so as to engage the mucosal immune system in protection
Transdermal vaccines	To administer the antigen through the skin
Edible vaccines	To genetically engineer a plant so that it comes to contain antigen(s) in a form that is immunogenic when eaten
Prime-boost strategies	To administer two separate versions of a vaccine sequentially, typically a DNA vaccine followed by a vectored vaccine, or either of these followed by a protein vaccine

can result in improved vaccines in which reversion to virulence is impossible.

It must be recognized that the success of live attenuated vaccines poses some problems as to correct maintenance of immune status. For example, in many countries, measles vaccine is given only once, and nowhere is it mandated more than twice. Will this confer the same life-long immunity as an attack of measles? We cannot be sure, and until disease eradication is achieved, we must maintain a level of alertness about booster doses in adult life. This has not been a priority area for live attenuated or any other kind of vaccine but is currently the subject of much debate. There are instances in which public health regulations mandate regular boosters: for example, the yellow fever vaccine for travelers to affected countries. Another vexing question is whether repeated environmental exposure to a common microbe provides a kind of natural booster. If so, problems may arise as a disease becomes uncommon in a community.

Vaccines Consisting of Killed Microorganisms

Because these are nonreplicating antigens, booster doses are essential. Some are excellent vaccines with high efficacy and safety, such as the Salk injectable poliomyelitis vaccine or the hepatitis A vaccine. Others are of poor efficacy and short duration, such as the whole-cell killed injectable cholera vaccine, which has been all but abandoned. Others are partially effective but require improvement in terms of percentage of protection or duration of immunity or both. These include the older killed influenza and typhoid vaccines. Many of these vaccines have already been overtaken by new and improved versions, including subunit vaccines and orally active preparations.

Toxoids

When disease pathological processes are caused predominantly by a powerful exotoxin or enterotoxin, vaccines provoking antitoxin antibodies make good sense. In some cases, an exotoxin is a bacterium's device for creating sufficient tissue destruction to permit a rich growth medium to develop. That is the case in tetanus, diphtheria, and gas gangrene. For these cases, the relevant toxoids make good vaccines. Toxoids from enterotoxins have, in general, been less successful. However, a genetically detoxified derivative of the heat-labile enterotoxin (LT) of enterotoxigenic *Escherichia coli* is showing promise as a possible vaccine against traveler's diarrhea (18). This has been achieved through site-directed mutagenesis to inactivate the adenosine diphosphate–ribosyltransferase activity of the A subunit of LT. Equivalent mutants of cholera toxin (CT) may eventually prove important.

As Rappuoli (19) pointed out, the current conventional diphtheria and tetanus vaccines contain many impurities; furthermore, the formaldehyde treatment needed to turn the toxins into toxoids also causes cross-linkage of beef peptides present in the culture medium, resulting in the presence of unnecessary antigens in the final preparation. Scientifically, one could mount an argument for a mutant, nontoxic pure molecule, such as CRM197, as a new vaccine. CRM197 is a material cross-reacting to diphtheria toxin and containing a single glycine to glutamic acid substitution at position 52 and rendering the toxin inactive. Despite scientific attractiveness, there is not much commercial pressure for changing vaccines that are working well. Doubtless, if the acellular pertussis component of diphtheria toxoid, whole-cell pertussis, and tetanus toxoid (DPT) vaccine continues to impress with its lack of reactogenicity, more pressure may build up for the diphtheria and tetanus components to be free of side effects, and so ongoing research should be encouraged.

Molecular Vaccines: Protein

The recombinant DNA era has yielded a plethora of antigenic molecules that are pure and that have been chosen in animal models through their capacity to provoke an immune response that is host protective. Some subunit vaccines, such as Hib and acellular pertussis, result from extremely elegant research that warrants description in its own right. Whereas some subunit vaccines, such as HBsAg, are highly immunogenic at low doses, others have been of disappointing strength and require adjuvants more powerful than the aluminum salts currently used to adsorb pure proteins onto small particles. As a group, subunit vaccines have been more expensive than older vaccines. This major barrier to developing country use can be partially countered by programs such as GAVI that create a very large demand, whereby high volumes drive down costs of production.

Molecular Vaccines: Carbohydrate and Conjugate

The capsular polysaccharides of encapsulated bacteria are powerfully immunogenic and can make good vaccines. However, they suffer from three drawbacks. Usually, the carbohydrates are serotype specific, and an effective vaccine may have to be a "cocktail" of many different carbohydrate molecules. Thus, the Merck pneumococcal vaccine has 23 separate components. Second, these vaccines work poorly or not at all in very young infants. For a disease such as meningitis, in which the greatest rate of mortality is among children younger than 1 year, this represents a serious limitation. Third, being T-independent antigens, the vaccines engender suboptimal immunological memory. Therefore, the conjugation of these carbohydrates to protein carriers that engender T-cell help represented a major step forward, which is described in detail in a later section.

Combination Vaccines

As more effective vaccines are developed, the question of the number of needle pricks to which young infants are subjected becomes an urgent one. Among the traditional vaccines, the DPT combination was standard for a long time; whole-cell pertussis has been replaced by the subunit acellular pertussis in many countries. As already mentioned, MMR is an extremely successful combination, and it is very likely that varicella will be successfully added to this (MMR-V), but at the time of writing, this combination has not yet been licensed. Considering DPT as a "platform," one can see logical additions to this, such as the addition of one or more of Hib, injectable killed polio (Salk) vaccine, and hepatitis B. Doubtless, formulation issue will have to be faced and, sooner or later, antigenic competition may become manifest. Already the addition of Hib to DPT has caused problems for some manufacturers in the levels of antibodies reached. As successful vaccines for other types of meningitis become more popular (e.g., against *N. meningitidis* type C), the question of whether to add these or whether to create a second "meningitis/pneumonia" package will have to be faced. At least two companies are considering the possibility of heptavalent combinations, such as DPT–HiB–hepatitis B–meningitis A/C.

NEW APPROACHES TO VACCINE DESIGN

Table 2 outlines the main new approaches to vaccine design. In thinking about these, it is important to remember that established public health practice is not easy to change, and it appears likely that the newer approaches will find more favor with regard to diseases for which no vaccine currently exists, such as HIV/AIDS or malaria, than in situations in which current vaccines are reasonably satisfactory.

Vectored Vaccines

Bernard Moss and Enzo Paoletti independently opened up a major chapter in vaccinology when they demonstrated that genes for important antigens could be introduced into the vaccinia virus without perturbing its replication and could be expressed in host cells in which the virus was dividing (20,21). This "Trojan Horse" concept, whereby harmless microorganisms act as vectors for antigen genes, has been extended in innumerable directions. Among other important vectors in use experimentally are vaccinia variants; avipoxviruses; adenoviruses; polioviruses; herpesviruses; *Salmonella, Shigella,* and BCG bacterial species; and doubtless many more. The power of the concept is that it combines the best of two worlds: the force of a live attenuated vaccine and the scientific precision of the rational subunit vaccine approach. Furthermore, in view of the large size of the vaccinia genome or, for that matter, the genomes of some of the other vectors, it is feasible to consider the insertion of quite a few antigen genes, thus covering several diseases at once. It is also straightforward to incorporate one or more cytokine genes in the construct, should this be desirable for either the strength of the immune response or the direction it should take.

Although the concept was first introduced in the early 1980s, no relevant vaccine has yet come on the market.

Clinical investigation has been somewhat limited so far, but, as discussed later, has accelerated in the context of the so-called "prime-boost" strategy. There are understandable reservations about the use of unmodified vaccinia, particularly at a time when HIV is rife, because it can be dangerous in people with an ineffective T-cell system, a reservation that could be partially countered by the inclusion of the interleukin (IL)–2 gene in the construct, which prevents athymic nude mice from succumbing to vaccinia (22). A number of vaccinia strains lacking genes that contribute to virulence have been prepared and are in clinical trial: for example, modified vaccinia Ankara (MVA). Also, nonreplicating viral vectors, such as canarypox or fowlpox in humans, can be considered. The field has doubtless been slowed up somewhat by poor responses in early clinical trials of experimental HIV and malaria vaccines. Nevertheless, the overwhelming weight of preclinical data, with disease protection against at least 20 pathogens in at least 15 species, suggests that further research must eventually be crowned with success. It should be noted that the approach is designed to induce excellent T-cell, including cytotoxic T-cell, immunity.

Experimentation with bacterial vectors is not yet as far advanced, but examples are taken up when enteric and intracellular pathogens are discussed.

Nucleic Acid Vaccines

Few areas of experimental vaccinology have emerged as surprisingly and developed as explosively as that of nucleic acid vaccines. Two preludes to the actual discovery warrant mention. Wolff et al. (23), using plasmid DNA coding for a reporter gene, found that DNA injected as a saline solution and without the adjunct agents normally used for transfection could cause synthesis of the reporter protein in the recipient animal. This surprising finding came from a control group in which the real hope for the experimental group was uptake of liposomes containing DNA. Of various injection sites tested, intramuscular injection worked best. The total number of myotubes transfected within the injection region is 1% to 5%. The second prelude relates to a DNA delivery system, originally developed by an agricultural firm, Agrecetus, first used as a means of transfecting plant cells. This Accell gene delivery system, also termed the "gene gun," consists of a helium gas pressure–driven device capable of delivering into very superficial layers of tissue tiny gold particles coated with plasmid DNA. These DNA-coated microprojectiles could, for example, be delivered to the skin of mice, resulting in the synthesis of the relevant protein (24). It was not long before each of these two approaches was used to elicit immune responses in the mouse. The gene gun approach induced antibody formation against human growth hormone and human α_1-antitrypsin in the first demonstration that DNA immunization could work (25). Furthermore, the prolonged persistence of encoded protein in the serum signaled the probability of continued antigenic stimulation. The first demonstration of a host-protective immune response came from the intramus-

cular injection approach (26). Mice were injected with plasmids encoding the nucleoprotein of influenza A virus. They developed both antibodies and class I major histocompatibility complex (MHC)–restricted cytotoxic T-lymphocytes (CTLs). Upon challenge with a virulent influenza A strain, PR/8, 100% of treated mice survived, whereas 100% of controls were dead by day 9. Almost simultaneously, Fynan et al. (27) also protected mice against PR/8 by using the gene gun and DNA encoding the relevant hemagglutinin as the antigen. After these two striking results, the field really took off. A scant 4 years later, Donnelly et al. (28) were able to review an extraordinary range of preclinical studies showing humoral and T-cell responses protective against a wide range of viruses, bacteria, and parasites, as well as various tumor models.

What are the essential features of nucleic acid vaccines? The key difference from the live vector approach is that the DNA encoding the antigen of interest cannot replicate in the human or animal body. The plasmids concerned are usually grown in *E. coli*. Their origin of replication is not suitable for mammalian cells. It is important to include a strong promoter element suitable for high-level gene expression in mammalian cells; for example, the immediate/early promoter of the human cytomegalovirus works well. The construct should also have an appropriate messenger ribonucleic acid (RNA) transcript termination/polyadenylation sequence. After intramuscular injection, the DNA enters the cytoplasm and then the nucleus of the myocyte, but it is not integrated into the genome. Neither muscle cells nor the dendritic cells, which are the targets of the gene gun approach, have a high rate of division, nor do they show extensive homology with the plasmid, and so homologous recombination is highly unlikely. Random integration remains a formal possibility, but, so far, no adverse effects have been noted. Gene expression is not at a high level. Antigen leaks out of myocytes for a considerable period and, in the case of the gene gun, the gold particles deposited in the epidermis soon find their way into Langerhans cells, which then make their way to local lymph nodes. In the case of intramuscular injection, it is clear that the myocyte itself is not the inducer of immune responses. This was approached by Fu et al. (29) in an ingenious experiment. Parental into F1 bone marrow chimeric mice were prepared in such a way that the myocytes carried both parental MHC haplocytes but the professional antigen-presenting cells (APCs) such as dendritic cells, being (after an appropriate period) bone marrow derived, carried only the bone marrow donor parental haplotype. After reconstitution, the chimeric mice were given plasmid DNA coding for influenza virus nucleoprotein to generate CTLs. According to the rules of MHC restriction, because the mice possessed the thymic epithelial framework of the F1, their peripheral T cells, although of parental genotype, should be capable of recognizing antigen in the context of *both* parental haplotypes. However, when the CTLs were tested *in vitro*, they were clearly restricted only by the MHC alleles of the bone marrow donor. Had myocytes been the APCs creating the CTLs *in vivo*, this would not have been the case. Furthermore, in further chimeras, transplantation studies were done with an NP gene–transfected myoblast cell line. With appropriate choice of strains, it could be shown that H2-incompatible myoblasts could induce CTL responses, but these, when analyzed, were restricted to the MHC haplocyte not of the myoblast donor but of the bone marrow donor. This clearly showed that the myoblasts acted as a source of antigen that was somehow transferred to APCs in a way that allowed processing for the class I MHC pathway. This apparent exception to the dual pathway rules is an example of "cross-priming," which has also been noted in other systems. The efficacy of DNA vaccines in generating CTLs has been a common feature of most examples so far studied in mice.

The potential advantages of nucleic acid vaccines are numerous. The subunit approach to pure molecular vaccines can be seriously hampered by incorrect folding or glycosylation of antigens, which can present formidable problems and add to the cost of such vaccines. This should be largely obviated in DNA vaccines. Once an appropriate DNA vaccine has been engineered, it should be stable, and batch variation should be minimal, facilitating quality control procedures. In terms of actual manufacturing procedure, nucleic acid vaccines should be relatively cheap. Multivalency could be achieved either by co-injection of a mixture of plasmids or by constructing complex plasmids.

A variation on the theme is the use of positive-strand RNA viruses such as alphaviruses, which self-replicate within non-dividing host cells and can be engineered to deliver inserted RNA coding for the antigen in question. It is also possible to engineer replicons in which the antigen-encoding RNA is substituted for viral structural genes and replicons can be packaged into infectious particles with helper viruses or split-genome packaging cell lines. DNA/RNA replicons can also be engineered and in some circumstances are more immunogenic than plasmid-based DNA vaccines.

Despite the justifiable excitement about nucleic acid vaccines, it has become clear that the responses achieved in subhuman primates and in humans are much lower than those in mice. In part, this may be a dosage question, because a human weighs 3,000 times more than a mouse, and it has not been practical to increase dosage commensurately. Considerable effort has therefore gone into enhancing the efficacy of DNA vaccines. Uptake of DNA has been enhanced by in vivo electroporation. DNA has been incorporated into microparticles or liposomes or has been given with an oil-in-water emulsion. Co-injection of cytokines or engineering the DNA to encode for a cytokine represents another approach. Of particular interest is the concept of encoding together with the DNA for the antigen DNA for a ligand that can target the fusion protein to an appropriate site. Boyle et al. (30) used L-selectin to target the antigen to high endothelial venule receptors, thus enhancing the amount going to lymphoid tissue, or CTL-associated antigen 4 to target the antigen to the counterstructures CD80 and CD86 on the surface of APCs. This strategy greatly increased antibody responses and improved

protective efficacy in an influenza virus model. Moreover, the approach worked in a large animal, the sheep. Pig skin is believed to be a reasonable model for human skin, and when CTL-associated antigen 4–antigen fusion constructs were delivered into pig skin by the gene gun, the targeting strategy markedly enhanced the speed and magnitude of the antibody response.

Further aspects of nucleic acid vaccines are discussed later in the section on prime-boost strategies and in the specific context of HIV/AIDS and malaria vaccines.

It is clear that something as novel as nucleic vaccines will present substantial problems for the regulatory agencies. In addition to the carcinogenicity/insertional mutagenesis possibility, the conjectural hazards include autoimmunity to DNA or as a result of immune-mediated destruction of antigen-expressing cells. The latter could lead to damage directly or could occasion the release of intracellular antigens that would then provoke autoimmunity. In practice, however, induction of autoimmunity to autologous constituents is quite difficult and proceeds only with the use of strong adjuvants such as Freund's complete adjuvant. Another objection that has been raised is the possibility that a constant leak of small quantities of antigen over a prolonged period of time could lead to immunological tolerance, thus making the recipient incapable of responding to the antigen in question. This has not been encountered in any situation so far.

Peptide Vaccines

Peptide vaccines can be either synthetically prepared or encoded by DNA. Frequently, the plan is to include a multiplicity of epitopes, particularly T-cell epitopes: for example, from several different antigens of a pathogen. The approach can also deal with serotype variation of antigens, epitopes being chosen from multiple strains. Peptide vaccines suffer from the constraint that many antibodies are directed to conformational determinants. The most interesting peptide vaccine research is in HIV, malaria, and tumor immunology.

An interesting variant involving highly polymerized peptides is considered in the section on adjuvants in the discussion of rendering antigens particulate.

Mucosal Vaccines

It has been estimated that the combined surface area of the mucosae of the gastrointestinal, respiratory, and urogenital tracts is 400 m^2. The total lymphocyte complement of the mucosal immune system is greater than that of the lymph nodes and spleen. The mucosal immune system includes organized collections of lymphoid tissue such as the tonsils, adenoids, Peyer's patches, and appendix and also single lymphoid follicles. These collections contain macrophages and dendritic cells, sample antigens, and generate both T- and B-cell responses, including germinal center formation. There is a high proportion of immunoglobulin A (IgA) in the antibody formed. There is also extensive infiltration of epithelia and the lamina propria with lymphocytes and plasma cells. It is believed that these represent effector cells and that there is no immune induction within these latter sites.

Two types of antigen-capturing cells are of importance in mucosal immunity: the intraepithelial dendritic cells and M cells. In stratified or pseudostratified epithelia, the dendritic cells serve much the same function as skin Langerhans cells and extend right to the surface. In tracheal epithelium, for example, there are up to 700 such cells per mm^2, forming an almost contiguous network (31). As in the case of Langerhans cells, these dendritic cells take antigens to draining lymph nodes for immune induction. The M cells are unique features of the mucosal immune system. They exist in the epithelium overlying organized collections such as Peyer's patches. Their job is to take up antigens from the mucosa and to deliver them to the mucosal lymphoid tissue via a specialized pocket in the epithelium. M cells are active in taking up both macromolecular antigens and particulate antigens such as bacteria and essentially serve to channel them to professional APCs in the lymphoid collections beneath. M-cell membranes contain the glycolipid GM1, to which CT can bind, and a variety of other carbohydrate structures with selective binding activity. Bacteria and viruses can also exploit this capacity of M cells to take them up efficiently to infect mucosae. This exploitation probably includes sexual transmission of HIV.

The lymphocyte traffic pattern differs for the mucosal immune system and the conventional immune system (32). There is a distinct tendency for mucosa-associated cells to home back to mucosal tissue but not necessarily to the same mucosa. The possibility therefore exists that immunization could occur via one mucosal surface but an unrelated one could be protected. Nevertheless, there is some compartmentalization within the system. It is of interest, for example, that nasal immunization induces IgA production in a wider range of mucosal tissues, including the genital tract, than does oral immunization. In contrast, vaginal immunization of monkeys yields good antibody formation in cervical and vaginal mucosa but not in other mucosal compartments.

Stimulation of immune responses via mucosal surfaces, leading to local IgA production and a variety of systemic B- and T-cell effects, suffers from two difficulties: Most nonreplicating antigens lead to immune responses only after large and multiple antigen doses, and these responses are of short duration. Even natural infection may lead to shorter lived immunity than in the case of a systemic infection. This is why the field of mucosal adjuvants is particularly important.

Mucosal adjuvants, which are considered later, include any substance or process that enhances uptake of antigen by mucosal lymphoid tissue. For example, bacteria are capable of recruiting large numbers of dendritic cells into tracheal epithelium, and these dendritic cells are critical to the induction of an immune response (33). Similarly, viruses can bring dendritic cells into epithelia and can stimulate subsequent migration to draining lymph nodes. It has been argued that the increased susceptibility of neonates to respiratory infections results from the hyporesponsiveness of their immature dendritic cells to such signals. In more mature individuals, the inherent immunogenicity of microorganisms suggests that the use of live vectors, be they bacterial or viral, engineered to express the antigen of interest, may in itself provide sufficient adjuvanticity, albeit perhaps with a limited duration of immunity.

Enteric and acute respiratory infections represent major public health problems, and HIV infection is frequently acquired through mucosal routes; therefore, vaccines protecting mucosal surfaces are highly desirable. With regard to their construction, it must be noted that mucosal surfaces are normally colonized by a rich flora of commensal bacteria. Remarkably little is known about what permits these commensals to remain but not to overgrow. To the extent that they are tolerated, there may well be some degree of immunological tolerance at work. Also, oral tolerance is a well-established phenomenon. At the same time, overgrowth and invasion would appear likely were there not some level of immune response. For the intelligent design of mucosal vaccines, better understanding of this balanced situation is required. Tolerance-including strategies may be valuable as well: for example, in autoimmune situations.

Cell-mediated immune responses within mucosal tissue must also be considered. These doubtless contribute to clearance of both bacteria and viruses from mucosal areas after infection: Holmgren and Rudin (34) made the point that with some infections, such as *V. cholerae* or enterotoxigenic *E. coli*, the infection is so superficial that neither the bacteria nor their toxins penetrate into the epithelial cells, and in that case, antibodies alone (ideally mucosal IgA) are required for protection, whereas other pathogens, such as *Salmonella* and *Shigella* infections, penetrate deeper, where IgA but also systemic immunoglobulins M and G (IgM and IgG) antibodies may be important, as may the T-cell component (34). Ideally, a mucosal vaccine should protect both against toxins produced by pathogens and against antigens involved in adhesion to epithelial cells (e.g., fimbriae) or invasion of tissue. In the case of viruses, $CD8^+$ $\alpha\beta$ TCR^+ cytotoxic T cells that are present intraepithelially clearly contribute to protection.

At the time of writing, only five vaccines that can be considered mucosal vaccines have been licensed (although not in all countries). These are the oral Sabin-type polio vaccine; the oral killed cholera vaccine, given with cholera toxin B subunit (CT-B); the oral live attenuated typhoid vaccine; an oral tetravalent live attenuated rotavirus vaccine (which was subsequently withdrawn); and an intranasal influenza vaccine. In view of the power of the approach, it is hoped that more mucosal vaccines will follow. Much effort is going into the use of live recombinant microorganisms as mucosal delivery systems, such as live attenuated *Salmonella* bacteria given orally or adenoviruses given intranasally, but none of these have progressed very far.

Further aspects of the mucosal approach is discussed in the section on HIV/AIDS vaccines.

Transdermal Vaccines

It has been known for decades that antigens applied directly to the skin can cause an immune response, for that is exactly what contact sensitization represents. On the other hand, the realization that direct topical application of vaccines to the skin can cause systemic T- and B-cell responses is relatively novel (35). It is noteworthy that the Langerhans type of dendritic cell is really quite superficial in the epidermis, and once antigen has reached them, the question of their activation and consequent migration to the draining lymph node depends very much on the type of stimulus. For example, if the vaccine in question is administered together with an adjuvant such as CT, the immune cascade is initiated. Simple admixture with, for example, influenza virus hemagglutinin, suffices to initiate a boostable immune response involving both the systemic and mucosal compartments. Other exotoxins, including detoxified mutants, also work well. Simple skin manipulation, such as cleansing with alcohol or hydration of the skin, may enhance responses, and patches, gels, creams, and ointments are also under investigation.

Edible Vaccines

Mason et al. (36) were stimulated by the call at the 1990 World Summit for Children for a radical new approach to vaccines for developing nations, so they set about creating transgenic plants that expressed putative vaccine antigens. The long-range idea was the possibility that a readily available food, such as bananas, might come to constitute a cheap source of edible vaccines. Apart from the considerable technical hurdles involved in expression of genes for antigens in edible portions of plants, a series of immunological questions needed to be addressed. These included the avoidance of oral tolerance, ensuring sufficient oral immunogenicity, ensuring some degree of protection against enzymatic degradation of vaccines, and determining adequate dosage. Despite these constraints, progress has actually been remarkably rapid. A start was made with HBsAg in tobacco plants. Successful engineering resulted in the accumulation of viruslike particles in the tobacco leaf. Similar success was achieved with viruslike particles of Norwalk virus capsid protein. Next, potato plants were engineered to express the B subunit of heat-labile *E. coli* enterotoxin (LT-B), in the hope that a cheap source of a mucosal adjuvant would eventually result. Mice fed 5-g samples of raw potatoes on four occasions developed serum IgG and mucosal IgA specific for LT-B. The author had the pleasure of being a visiting professor in Dr Myron Levine's laboratory in the University of Maryland on the very day that the first clinical trial of feeding raw, engineered potatoes to human volunteers was initiated. Both mucosal and systemic antitoxin immune responses were induced. Of course, it is not anticipated that potatoes will be used in the long run, because they need to be cooked. Rather, the aim is to engineer fruit that can be fed raw to infants and small children. To that end, a transformation system for bananas has been developed.

Active research is being pursued on edible vaccines against hepatitis B, cholera, measles, and human papilloma virus.

It is envisaged that edible vaccines either will contain a mucosal adjuvant or will consist of viruslike particles. Either of these strategies should militate against oral tolerance. Co-expression of cytokine genes could also be envisaged. It is hoped that the plant cell wall, consisting of cellulose, pectins, and proteins, will be a partial barrier to enzymatic degradation of the enclosed antigen, allowing some to reach the small intestine, a major inductive site of mucosal immunity. Clearly, dosage in infants of various ages will have to be the subject of extensive research. The long-term hope of a multisubunit edible vaccine, cheap and acceptable in a developing country setting, now seems much less fanciful since even the previous edition of this book.

Prime-Boost Strategies

Most vaccines have to be administered on more than one occasion to achieve a satisfactory level of disease prophylaxis. Normally, booster vaccines are identical to the priming vaccines except that one or more components of a combination may be dropped. The initial impetus for a different approach came because of early disappointments with HIV envelope protein–based vaccines, which failed to produce antibodies capable of neutralizing primary isolates of HIV and failed to induce significant levels of HIV-specific CD8[+] CTLs. This prompted a search for alternative approaches. First, recombinant vaccinia virus engineered to express *env* was given as a primary dose to mice, followed by a booster dose of recombinant glycoprotein (gp) 160 (37). This endeavor was soon broadened to include priming with other vectored vaccines and boosting with either pure protein or viruslike particles. It gradually evolved into a variety of mixed-modality approaches, some of which are summarized in Table 3. The favorite viral vectors have been various modified vaccinia variants of diminished virulence and poxviruses of birds such as canarypox and fowlpox, which do not complete their replication cycle in mammalian hosts and yet express inserted genes. Less commonly, alphaviruses, adenoviruses, and polioviruses have been used.

Prime-boost strategies can markedly enhance antibody formation but, more important, can engender strong CD8[+] and CD4[+] T-lymphocyte responses. Just why the mixed-modality approach works so well is not entirely clear. "Focused

TABLE 3. *Some examples of "prime-boost" strategies of immunization*

Priming entity	Boosting entity
Viral vector	Recombinant protein
Naked DNA	Recombinant protein
Naked DNA	Viral vector
Viral vector	Naked DNA[a]
Viral vector	Different viral vector

[a]In general, not very effective.

priming" of T cells by naked DNA has been invoked, a CD8$^+$ T-cell response to one or a few immunodominant epitopes then being strongly amplified by, for example, a poxvirus boost. Certainly if the only antigen shared between the priming entity and the boosting entity is the antigen of interest, it seems logical that the immune system would react in a secondary manner to only that antigen. With DNA priming and protein boosting, it has been postulated that the low doses of protein associated with priming engender a high-affinity antibody response. Different mechanisms probably underlie the different regimens. There is, however, no doubt that the prime-boost approach has conferred excellent protection in animal models of various diseases and in some early clinical trials in the malaria field. The matter is examined in more detail in the sections dealing with HIV/AIDS and malaria. A useful review of prime-boost strategies was published by Ramshaw and Ramsay (38).

ADJUVANTS

Many foreign proteins are poorly or not at all immunogenic when injected in soluble, monomeric form but, when administered together with an immune-stimulating entity (i.e., an adjuvant), cause a satisfactory immune response. Furthermore, the nature of the adjuvant controls the type of immune response, which may be biased toward antibody formation or cell-mediated immunity and toward particular antibody isotypes or T-cell subsets. Now that pathogen genomics as well as conventional vaccine research have yielded such a plethora of candidate antigens, it could be argued that the right adjuvant has become the "Holy Grail" of vaccinology.

New Insights into Antigen-Presenting Cell Activation

To understand the complex field of adjuvants, it is necessary to examine the intimate relationships between the innate and the adaptive immune systems. The innate immune system is evolutionarily as old as multicellular life itself, around 2 billion years, but its central molecular basis has been elucidated only as recently as 2000 (39). From the viewpoint of the current discussion, its most important elements are the scavenger cells, especially macrophages and dendritic cells, which in higher species are referred to as APCs. The adaptive immune system, arising first in the cartilaginous fishes about 300 million years ago, is composed essentially of three types of cells—APCs, T-lymphocytes, and B-lymphocytes—and their diverse molecular products. Thus, APCs constitute an important link between the systems. It has long been known that T cells and B cells must be activated to exert their defensive functions. An important insight was the suggestion (reviewed in Janeway, ref. 39a) that APCs were not constitutively in an active state but needed special stimuli to do their job, be this phagocytosis, cytokine or chemokine secretion, up-regulation of lymphocyte co-stimulator molecules, or movement toward secondary lymphoid organs. Because APCs normally initiate the adaptive immunoproliferative

cascade, what is it that actually activates the APCs? Janeway postulated receptors on APCs capable of recognizing patterns found only on evolutionarily distant organisms such as bacteria, ligation of which would activate the APCs.

The strange saga of the Toll-like receptors (TLRs) began when it was found that the cytoplasmic domain of the IL-1 receptor was homologous to a gene known as Toll, which was involved in dorsal-ventral polarization of the *Drosophila* embryo (40). The IL-1 receptor can initiate a cascade of cellular signals that leads to activation of the NFκB transcription factor pathway and of mitogen-activated protein kinases. This in turn regulates the expression of genes involved in inflammation, immunity, and tissue repair. Not surprisingly, therefore, the insect scientists began to look for possible defense functions of the Toll gene. It was soon found that Toll was essential for protecting adult *Drosophila* from fungal infection (41). A search for further mammalian homologs of Toll has, so far, identified 10 genes that have come to be known as TLRs. These can indeed recognize a variety of important pathogen-derived materials.

TLR-4, the first of the family for which the ligand was found, is highly specific for the lipopolysaccharide (LPS) of gram-negative bacteria; claims that TLR-4 also recognizes heat-shock protein 60 and respiratory syncytial virus proteins are regarded as controversial (39). TLR-4 appears to function as a homodimer, and signaling is dependent on the coexpression of the glycophosphatidylinositol (GPI)–linked protein CD14, the two molecules acting as co-receptors. In contrast, TLR-2 agonists are more varied (42). They include mycobacterial glycolipids AraLAM and PIM, peptidoglycans, LPS from gram-positive bacteria, and a variety of lipoproteins. This promiscuity may result from the fact that TLR-2 can form heteromers with TLR-1 or TLR-6, associations that impart differing ligand specificities. It is not yet clear how general heteromer formation is among the 10 or more TLRs. If it is, quite a large repertoire of unique specificities can be imagined.

Another interesting specificity is that of TLR-9, which senses bacterial DNA, especially nonmethylated CG-rich DNA (43). As discussed later, this has implications for the design of a new generation of adjuvants. The author was particularly fascinated by the discovery of the ligand for TLR-5, bacterial flagellin (44). Forty-five years earlier, the author's group had used *Salmonella* flagellin as a model antigen, marveling at the fact that picogram amounts could be immunogenic without use of any adjuvant. Association with TLR-5 and subsequent APC activation may well be the reasons. At the moment, the six other known mammalian TLRs are "orphans," but the field is moving so quickly that their ligand specificities may soon be identified.

If the TLRs are indeed innate immune sensors, they are the oldest transducers of microbial systems in nature. In the mouse, the effects of TLR ligation on APCs include upregulation of class II MHC and of CD80, CD86, and CD83, as well as NFκB activation and cytokine production. The TLRs thus appear to be a hard-wired strategy for detecting pathogen-associated molecular patterns. The associations are not of high affinity, hence perhaps the need for co-receptors such as CD14 and CD11b/CD18 to assist in activation (42). It is tempting to think that TLR ligation–induced APC activation is the first step signaling to the mammalian immune system that the body is in danger. However, this view was challenged by Matzinger (45), who believed that the ultimate controlling "danger" signal may be endogenous and may emanate from stressed or damaged tissues. She saw products of injured cells as activating the APC. From that viewpoint, work by Li et al. (46) is of interest. They showed that necrotic cells, but not apoptotic cells, release materials that can stimulate APCs via TLR-2, leading to NFκB activation. Both mitochondrial and nuclear fractions work. Moreover, when apoptotic cells are artificially lysed, they too can activate NFκB in a TLR-2–dependent manner, showing that it is the maintenance of cell membrane integrity that prevents physiologically dying cells from alerting the immune system. Whether the "danger" hypothesis is ultimately vindicated or not, the proinflammatory action of necrotic cells could certainly augment the immune cascade in many "real-life" situations.

Finally, TLR-mediated signals do not necessarily all lead to the same end result. For example, whereas TLR-4 signaling by E. coli LPS induces considerable production of IL-6, IL-12, and interferon (IFN)–γ in macrophages, Porphyromonas gingivalis activation via the TLR-2 receptor does not. Moreover, a given agonist can have differing effects on different types of APCs. This leads to the hope that when we understand the TLRs sufficiently well, we may be able to use that knowledge to devise adjuvants capable of guiding immune responses down different paths. There certainly exists the possibility that different TLRs transmit different signals.

Empirical Approaches to Design of Adjuvants

Long before the TLRs were recognized, a great deal of empirical research had resulted in a variety of adjuvants that are now understood a little better. For example, it was realized that particulate antigens, readily scavenged by APCs, were much more immunogenic than soluble antigens. As early as 1926, Glenny et al. (47) noted that alum precipitation of diphtheria toxoid, creating a microparticulate antigen, increased immunogenicity considerably. It was found that killed bacteria could nonspecifically raise immune responsiveness, and Mycobacterium tuberculosis was very effective. Freund and McDermott (48) combined killed tubercle bacteria with the absorption-delaying effects of mineral oil, creating the strong and widely used Freund's adjuvant. This caused local and systemic reactions far too serious for human use, and in many countries, it is no longer deemed appropriate for experimental animals either; this has prompted a search for less toxic bacteria-derived products retaining adjuvant properties. It was realized even in Freund's day that the adjuvant could guide the direction of the immune response. Freund's adjuvant promotes both antibody formation and delayed-type hypersensitivity reactions, but when the mycobacteria are

omitted, as in Freund's incomplete adjuvant, only antibody formation results.

The empirical tradition has produced a large number of adjuvant formulations, but only aluminum phosphate and aluminum hydroxide to which protein antigens are adsorbed have enjoyed widespread human use in all countries. Two reasons underlie this somewhat disappointing situation. First, it has proved very difficult to dissociate the immunogenic from the toxic properties of bacterial products or other chemical adjuvants. This may change as knowledge of the TLRs increases. Second, commercial interests have dictated that the major firms involved in vaccine manufacture have gone with their own particular experimental adjuvants, with little collaboration between groups and few head-to-head comparisons, a circumstance that is unlikely to change soon.

In experimental immunology, various bacteria other than killed M. tuberculosis are used as adjuvants. It appears that if a killed bacterial preparation is itself highly antigenic, the adjuvant power spills over to the response to an antigen co-administered with it. Some guidance may also be given to the response. Killed B. pertussis organisms are a strong Th2/antibody formation adjuvant for pure protein antigens. Corynebacterium parvum is more of a Th1 adjuvant. A parasite, Nippostrongylus brasiliensis, has long been used to elicit powerful immunoglobulin E (IgE) responses.

A rational classification of adjuvants is difficult because, in practice, most adjuvants make use of several different principles. These include rendering antigens particulate or polymeric or both; creating water-in-oil or oil-in-water emulsions; encapsulating antigens in biodegradable microcapsules; including bacteria, bacterial products, or other immunostimulatory chemicals; adding immunostimulatory cytokines; or chemically coupling the antigen in question to an agent that targets it to APCs. Table 4 illustrates some of the relevant principles.

This section focuses on the most promising approaches and those closest to human application. For a fuller analysis of all the variables, the reader is referred to an excellent book (49).

TABLE 4. *Some principles underlying the design of adjuvants*

Uptake of antigens by APCs is vital; hence, rendering antigens polymeric or particulate helps
Activation of APCs is essential; hence, agents that engage TLR work well
Depot effects and delayed absorption can enhance immunity; hence, emulsions and biodegradable microparticles underlie many adjuvant approaches
Bacteria and bacterial products were found early to stimulate immunity; many pure derivatives have resulted
A heterogeneous collection of natural or synthetic chemicals has been found empirically to enhance immunity
Many cytokines increase immune responses
Molecular targeting of antigens to APCs through conjugation of ligands can enhance immune responses

APC, antigen-presenting cell; TLR, Toll-like receptor.

Aluminum Compounds as Adjuvants

Aluminum hydroxide and aluminum phosphate are the two most commonly used adjuvants. Two chief methods underlie alum adjuvants: either *in situ* precipitation of aluminum compounds in the presence of antigen or adsorption of antigen onto preformed aluminum gel. The latter is now more commonly used because alum precipitation is quite demanding and batch-to-batch variation is a significant problem. The insoluble particles that result are less than 10 μm in diameter and may be as small as 0.1 μm. Alum adjuvants promote good antibody formation but little or no delayed-type hypersensitivity or CD8$^+$ T cell–mediated cytotoxicity. They can lead to significant IgE responses, which on the one hand may be advantageous for antiparasite vaccines but, on the other hand, can lead to hypersensitivity to the antigen in question. Overall, the safety record is good, but local reactions are occasionally troublesome. Properly formulated alum adjuvants are thus very satisfactory for diseases that can be prevented by serum IgG antibodies.

Emulsions as Adjuvants

Emulsions and emulsifying reagents have been central to adjuvant research. Incomplete Freund's adjuvant was used in the 1950s for the human influenza vaccine but never passed the regulatory hurdles. Companies have continued to improve their formulations, which may also contain one or more chemical promoters of immunogenicity. Both water-in-oil and oil-in-water emulsions can be used, and the oil can be of mineral, vegetable, animal, or synthetic origin. Stabilization by a surfactant is important, as is the nature of the emulsifying agent.

The firm SEPPIC has been promoting water-in-oil emulsions for human use: namely, Montanide ISA51 and Montanide ISA720, which have been used in numerous phase I and II trials. Montanide ISA720 is of special interest because it has been used in HIV, malaria, and cytomegalovirus vaccine trials. The adjuvant contains a natural, metabolizable oil and a highly refined mannide oleate emulsifier. Seventy parts of adjuvant are mixed with 30 parts of the aqueous, antigen-containing medium and homogenized, yielding watery droplets 0.3 to 3 μm in diameter, the emulsion being stable at 4°C for at least 2 years. The adjuvant promotes antibody formation and significant cytotoxic T-cell activity.

The firm Chiron has clinical experience since the early 1990s with an oil-in-water emulsion known as MF59. This is now registered in Italy for use with an influenza vaccine (Fluad) and has been used in about 1 million doses. It has been found to be very safe and effective. The droplets of the metabolizable oil squalene are about 0.15 μm in diameter, and the other components are polysorbate 80, sorbitan trioleate, trisodium citrate dihydrate, and citric acid monohydrate. The preparation is surprisingly nonviscous, and thus easy to use, and minimally reactogenic. The emulsion is stable at 2°C to 8°C for at least 3 years. MF59 is a good promoter of antibody formation and of Th2 type CD4$^+$ T-cell responses but not of cytotoxic T cells in subhuman primates or human subjects.

The Syntex adjuvant formulation (SAF) is another oil-in-water emulsion but is noteworthy for also containing the immunostimulatory compound threonyl-muramyl dipeptide (threonyl-MDP) (50). This agent has an interesting history, going back to the early days of the search for the immunopotentiating chemicals in bacteria. Ellouz et al. (51), searching for the minimal structural requirements needed for the adjuvant properties of bacterial peptidoglycans, found that *N*-acetyl-muramyl-*L*-analyl-*D*-isoglutamine, or MDP, powerfully promoted both antibody formation and cell-mediated immunity. There have been variations on the theme; Allison and Byars (50) claimed that the threonyl derivative is less toxic and more powerful. The SAF emulsion vehicle also contains the non-ionic block polymer surfactant poloxamer 401, which has adjuvant properties in its own right. The metabolizable oil is squalene, and the emulsifier is polysorbate 80. The adjuvant has elicited both cell-mediated and humoral immune responses with a variety of antigens. However, it does not appear to be progressing rapidly to clinical use, perhaps because the MDP component is, after all, too reactogenic.

One of the most interesting oil-in-water emulsions is the adjuvant AS02A, being promoted by the company GlaxoSmithKline. It is hoped that this preparation will be useful for vaccines against the three most dreaded diseases of developing countries: HIV/AIDS, malaria, and tuberculosis. This adjuvant has been administered to more than 1,300 volunteers and has raised no serious safety concerns. The special feature of AS02A is that it contains two separate chemical immunostimulants, known as 3D–monophosphoryl lipid A (MPL) and QS21. MPL is the best product remaining from an important line of work. This sought to take the LPS endotoxins of gram-negative bacteria such as *Escherichia, Pseudomonas,* or *Salmonella* and to extract from them less toxic adjuvants. MPL is modified from lipid A and is much less toxic (52) but powerfully immunostimulatory; 3D-MPL is a further derivative. QS21 is an adjuvant derived from the bark of the South American tree *Quillaja saponaria.* Crude extracts consisting of a mixture of tannins, polyphenolics, and triterpene glycoside saponins were found to be immunostimulatory. A saponin mixture known as Quill A was a somewhat purer preparation, and when it was fractionated by high-performance liquid chromatography into at least 23 components, QS21 emerged as the saponin with the most power and least toxicity (53). QS21 strongly stimulates both T cell–dependent and T cell–independent antibody formation and also cell-mediated immunity, including CD8$^+$ T-cell cytotoxicity.

Not surprisingly, therefore, AS02A proved to be a powerful adjuvant in rodents, subhuman primates, and humans. In human malaria vaccine trials (see also later discussion), it caused rapid and strong antibody formation, Th1 T-cell proliferation with IFN-γ production, and CD8$^+$ CTL responses (54). In HIV vaccine studies in Rhesus monkeys, the same results were obtained, and T-cell immunity was impressive with two *M. tuberculosis* antigens in the same species.

Microparticles, Including Immunostimulatory Complexes, Liposomes, Virosomes, and Viruslike Particles

Again, early immunologists were quick to realize that poorly immunogenic proteins could cause antibody formation as microparticles or microaggregates, such as through mild heat aggregation of serum proteins. Similarly, the property of physiological self-asssembly was found useful. Soluble flagellin self-assembles into flagella-like strands of polymerized flagellin and HBsAg into virus-like particles. In each case, the particulate preparation is more immunogenic than the soluble monomeric protein.

Immunostimulating complexes (ISCOMs) are a variation on this theme. These are microparticles consisting of lipids, saponins, and antigens that form spontaneously under the correct conditions (55). They are cagelike structures—that is, hollow, spherical particles of approximately 40 nm diameter. Typically, the saponin would consist of Quill A, the lipids would be a mixture of cholesterol and either phosphatidyl choline or phosphatidylethanolamine, and the antigen would be a protein possessing a transmembrane domain. These amphipathic molecules are incorporated into the lipid-saponin structure when the detergent is removed. Incorporation of hydrophilic proteins can be achieved with acid treatment, although this represents an association rather than true insertion. ISCOMS promote antibody formation, delayed-type hypersensitivity, and CTLs. Like liposomes, some ISCOMS appear to enter the APCs without going through the endocytic pathway. Thus, they achieve the necessary class I MHC–restricted antigen presentation. Because of this efficacy in multiple limbs of immunity, ISCOMS have proved valuable in many experimental animal models, including vaccines against viruses, bacteria, and parasites. There is a registered veterinary ISCOM-based vaccine for equine influenza, and CSL, Ltd., in Australia has commenced phase I clinical trial work in humans with an ISCOM-influenza vaccine.

Liposomes have some but not all of the features of ISCOMS. Alving et al. (56), using liposomes with cholera and malaria antigens, obtained a good adjuvant effect. They have also obtained quite promising results by using envelope protein peptides in a simian immunodeficiency virus (SIV) trial with macaque monkeys. The liposomes contain dimyristoyl phosphatidyl choline, dimyristoyl phosphatidyl glycerol, cholesterol, and monophosphoryl lipid A. In some experiments, liposomes were alum-adsorbed. Liposomes have also acted as adjuvants for diphtheria toxoid, tetanus toxoid, and a variety of hepatitis antigens. There is a great capacity to vary the particle size of liposomes, from approximately 20 nm up to more than 10 μm in diameter. In general, liposomes are best used together with some other adjuvant.

Virosomes are multimeric aggregates of virus-derived transmembrane proteins (e.g., influenza hemagglutinin) and proteosomes are similar multimers of bacterial transmembrane proteins. They consist of 60- to 100-nm vesicles or membrane vesicle fragments. Amphipathic immunogens can be incorporated into these structures. These agents do not induce cell-mediated immunity unless an appropriate further adjuvant is added. Glück et al. (58), of the Swiss Serum and Vaccine Institute, are a strong proponents of the virosome approach. They used influenza virus virosomes as a delivery system for, for example, hepatitis A and B or diphtheria and tetanus antigens (57) or as a mucosal vaccination strategy against influenza itself. In the latter case, hemagglutinin and neuraminidase were extracted from influenza virus, and phosphatidylcholine liposomes also containing the mucosal adjuvant *E. coli* heat-labile toxin at 1 μg per dose were prepared. Two nasal spray immunizations induced good humoral responses in adult human volunteers, with significant salivary IgA. Elderly subjects also tolerated the vaccine well.

Viruslike particles (VLPs) are the results of self-assembly of virus capsid proteins. The considerable success of the hepatitis B vaccine owes much to the strong immunogenicity of the HBsAg particles. Similarly, the major capsid protein of the human papilloma virus is strongly immunogenic as a VLP. It has also been possible to incorporate other proteins into HBsAg VLPs and thus to enhance their immunogenicity.

Other Methods of Rendering Antigens Particulate

There are other ways of effecting a polymerization of antigens such as association with polymers. Non-ionic block copolymers, usually used as additives to adjuvants employing an emulsion, are polymers of polyoxypropylene and polyoxyethylene with which antigen can be associated. They have been used as components of complex adjuvant formulations by both Syntex and Ribi Chemical Co. These formulations induce a good Th1 response.

Carbohydrate polymers of mannose (e.g., mannan) or of β1-3 glucose (e.g., glucan) have been used in a similar manner. It is possible to conjugate peptides to mannan by means of an aminocaproic spacer and thereby produce a good antibody response. Mannan can also enhance the adjuvant properties of LPS. Part of the action may result from the stimulation of macrophages, which have a mannan-binding receptor.

O'Brien-Simpson et al. (59) reported a generic method for the assembly of multipeptide polymers that results in highly antigenic preparations. The basic principle is that peptides are synthesized in the solid phase, the N-terminal residue is acryloyated, and, after cleavage, the derivatized peptides are polymerized by free radical–induced polymerization. The peptides used can be the same or different. Multiple B- and T-cell epitopes can be incorporated into the final construct. The approach has been validated with peptides from influenza virus, malaria and other parasites, tetanus toxin, protein hormones, and various model proteins. Furthermore, the geometry of the synthetic peptide-based immunogen is important because branched configurations are more efficient at stimulating T-cell clones (through dendritic cells) and at eliciting antibody formation (60). They are also more stable in serum. Although many peptide dendrimers are good immunogens, when polymerizing separate, defined epitopes, chemoligation through thioether bond formation was preferable to oxime bond formation or disulfide bond formation (61).

Oligonucleotides, Especially CpG Motifs

There is a long history of attempting to use nucleic acids as adjuvants. In the 1960s, there was quite a vogue for using the polynucleotides polyinosine:polycytidylic acid (polyI:C) and polyadenylate:polyuridylate (polyA:U), known stimulators of interferon production, as experimental immunostimulators. The field took on an altogether different and more promising dynamic as a result of the work of Tokunaga et al. (62). These investigators were interested in the antitumor potential of BCG, noted that much of it was in the DNA fraction, and drew attention to particular sequences of oligodeoxyribonucleotides. Subsequently, using shorter oligodeoxyribonucleotides, they discovered that palindromic hexamers, each of which contains nonmethylated CpG dinucleotides, are responsible for immune activation, measured in their case by induction of interferon production by natural killer cells (63). Krieg et al. (64) established that the minimal immunostimulatory sequence was unmethylated 5'-Pur-Pur-CpG Pyr-Pyr-3'. Methylation of the cytosine was found to reduce activity. Because mammalian DNA contains fourfold fewer CpG dinucleotides than would be anticipated in mammalian genomic DNA on the basis of the frequency of the bases, and because 70% of these are methylated, whereas bacterial cytosines rarely are, there arose the speculation that the mammalian innate immune system evolved to recognize the bacteria-specific pattern (65). This was well before the recognition of the TLR-9 receptor as the relevant counterstructure for CpG motifs, as already discussed.

Two commercial firms have performed extensive research on CpG oligonucleotides as immune stimulants. Coley Pharmaceuticals has experimented with quite a number of sequences, chiefly in the context of conventional adjuvants for vaccines. For example, the compound 1826, consisting of 5'-TCCATGACGTTCCTGACGTT-3', strongly enhanced antibody formation to recombinant HBsAg (66) and acted as a powerful mucosal adjuvant when given intranasally with recombinant glycoprotein B of herpes simplex type 1 in a mouse model (67). The 24-mer compound 2006 (5'-TCGTCGTTTTGTCGTTTTGTCGTT-3') was a strong Th1-type adjuvant in orangutans (67).

This firm considers that a CpG motif is $X_1X_2CGY_1Y_2$, in which X_1 is a purine, X_2 is not C, Y_1 is preferably T and not G, and Y_2 is T. Furthermore, there is some degree of species specificity, GACGTT being optimal for mice and GTCGTT for humans. The oligonucleotides act on natural killer cells, dendritic cells, monocytes, and macrophages, but also directly on B cells. Apart from IFN-γ, other cytokines and chemokines are induced, and markers such as class II MHC, CD80, and CD86 are up-regulated. Thus, CpG

oligonucleotides used alone can stimulate innate immunity and protect against pathogens for short periods. Used as an adjuvant, the compound 7909 raises the anti-HBsAg titer 10- to 35-fold in human volunteers, in comparison with antigen alone, and is well tolerated.

The company Dynavax Technologies tends to term its products *immunostimulatory sequences* (ISS). Apart from infectious diseases, in which targets include hepatitis B, hepatitis C, and HIV, Dynavax is especially interested in allergy; ISS covalently linked to allergens are seen as a possible treatment. The motif AACGTTCG is considered superior to the hexamer AACGTT, and Dynavax has published extensively on the compound 1018, which is 5'-TGACTGTGAACGTTCGAGATGA-3', but has also used other oligonucleotides. When 1018 was covalently coupled to the ragweed pollen antigen Amb a 1, the conjugate included a strong Th1-type response in mice, in contrast to Amb a 1, alone which led to a Th2 response (68). Moreover, when peripheral blood mononuclear cell cultures from ragweed-allergic subjects were stimulated *in vitro* with the conjugate, the resulting cytokine profile was IFN-γ dominated, and even when the cells had been prestimulated with Amb a 1 (leading to a Th2 response), the conjugate induced IFN-γ production and partially inhibited IL-4 and IL-5 production (69).

Because of these promising results, Dynavax went on to a phase II clinical trial in 27 hay fever sufferers, achieving good allergen-specific IgG levels. Randomized, placebo-controlled phase III trials have started. A phase I/II clinical trial of HBsAg linked to the ISS molecule has also begun.

It therefore appears that the CpG oligonucleotides have a promising future in both immunoprophylaxis and immunotherapy of various kinds.

Other Chemical Adjuvants

A wide variety of other chemicals, both natural and synthetic, have been found to stimulate immune responses. Cytokines are discussed further later. Bacterial products not yet mentioned include *Klebsiella pneumoniae* glycoprotein, heat-labile enterotoxins, trehalose dimycolate, tripalmitoyl-S-glycerine cysteine, and Detox, prepared from mycobacterial cell walls. Other surface active agents include dimethyl dioctadecyl ammonium bromide, avridine, and polyphosphazenes. Carbohydrate polymers with adjuvant properties include mannans, as mentioned previously; glucans; and dextrans. An interesting parasite-derived adjuvant is the *Leishmania* protein LeIF. This list is by no means exhaustive.

Microencapsulation of Antigens

This idea combines several desirable principles for adjuvants. Biodegradable microcapsules are particulate. They can enclose immunostimulatory molecules as well as antigen. They delay absorption of antigen and act as long-term depots. Best of all, they offer the hope that different chemical compositions will create particles that release their antigen as a pulse at various defined times after injection. Variables that affect the timing of release include particle size and the composition of the polymer. An ideal preparation would be a mixture of particles dissolving at intervals to mimic a primary dose and two booster doses.

Several laboratories share the credit for the development of controlled-release vaccine through encapsulation. The idea of biodegradable microcapsules containing antigens was promoted by Chang (70) and put into practice by Langer (71). The currently most popular material, the polymer poly(lactide-co-glycolide) (PLG), was first used by O'Hagan et al. (72) and by Eldridge et al. (73). This material was a happy choice because PLG has been used for many years as a biodegradable suture material. In that context, it has shown itself to be safe and nonreactogenic. PLG degrades by hydrolysis. How long this takes is determined both by chain length and by the ratio of lactide to glycolide in the polymer. The WHO has sponsored a considerable amount of work on PLG, in the hope of coming up with a "one shot" formulation, which in the first instance could be applied to the problem of neonatal tetanus in developing countries. Because infant immunization rates were low for women now of childbearing age, the WHO programs aim to immunize pregnant women with tetanus toxoid so that the newborn infants would be protected by antibodies crossing the placenta. However, it is difficult to persuade these women to make three trips to their local health center, which may require hours of walking. Once the controlled-release strategy has been perfected for this purpose, it could be adapted to other vaccines, such as hepatitis B or Hib.

Many frustrating problems were encountered in this endeavor, but they are gradually being overcome one by one. The most important one relates to stability of antigens in microparticles, both during the manufacturing process and *in vivo*. Furthermore, although the lactide-to-glycolide ratio in PLG affects degradation rate, it was found in practice that a mixture of two different sets of microcapsules resulted not in sharp peaks of antigen release but rather in continuous release over a period. This seems to produce satisfactory antibody responses (74). It is now clear that, in preclinical studies, one injection of antigen in microcapsules can lead to higher and more sustained antibody formation than can two injections of antigen adsorbed onto alum.

Macdonald et al. (75) at CSL, Ltd., in Australia have come up with an experimental "one-shot" method in their formulation of a single-dose but two-component experimental influenza vaccine. There is an immediate-release component that is produced by spray-drying the antigen, with or without adjuvant, in the presence of a stabilizer, such as trehalose. The delayed-release component consists of antigen that is encapsulated in a PLG matrix. An aqueous solution of influenza A/PR8 virus, ISCOMS, and trehalose is emulsified into a solution of PLG in methylene chloride. The resultant water-in-oil emulsion is also spray-dried. Shortly before use, the two components are mixed and suspended in buffer with 0.1% Tween 80. Such a formulation significantly outperformed a single injection of a liquid preparation and in fact resembled two spaced doses in efficacy.

Cyanoacrylates are another form of biodegradable polymer. For example, poly(butyl-2-cyanoacrylate) has been used as an adjuvant for oral immunization. Poly(methylmethacrylate) nanoparticles constitute another biodegradable adjuvant. The antigen can be either incorporated into the nanoparticles or adsorbed onto previously formed particles.

The use of PLG and other microparticles is under extensive investigation for the mucosal administration of vaccines. Particles of very small size (nanoparticles) may be even more suitable. Digestion in the stomach needs to be combated, perhaps by enteric-coated polymers, and coating with substances that increase intestinal absorption may be necessary. Delivery via the respiratory tract—for example, via intranasal immunization or aerosol administration—is a good possibility for respiratory pathogens. Rectal and vaginal delivery is also possible. Because there is a great deal of "cross-talk" between the various components of the mucosal immune system, and because oral delivery is by far the most practical, this deserves full experimental exploration in the first instance.

Biodegradable microparticles can induce T-cell immunity, including $CD8^+$ CTLs, as well as just antibody formation. For example, HIV envelope proteins contained in PLG particles induced HIV-specific $CD4^+$ and $CD8^+$ T-cell responses in mice. Similarly, microparticles outperformed incomplete Freund's adjuvant in promoting Th1 $CD4^+$ T-cell responses with a subunit antigen from *M. tuberculosis* (76). The addition of cytokines or chemical adjuvants to further enhance these T-cell effects remains to be explored.

Cytokines as Adjuvants

Cytokines have profound regulatory effects on all three cell types (APCs, T cells, and B cells) involved in immune responses, and so it is natural to ask whether they might find a use in adjuvant preparations, particularly inasmuch as some cytokines are noteworthy for guiding the immune response down particular pathways. This being so, it is interesting to note that the field of cytokines as adjuvants has not yet made much progress. Of course, cytokines are quite expensive and also can exhibit marked, although dose-dependent, toxic effects. A variation on the theme explored in a later discussion is cytokine gene constructs as components of vectored or DNA vaccines, an approach that would have the advantage that the cytokine is delivered to the same milieu as the antigen, as opposed to systemically administered cytokines.

Several cytokines act on APCs. IFN-γ and tumor necrosis factor α recruit and activate macrophages and help T cells develop antiviral effector functions, and IL-1α and IL-1β are also strongly proinflammatory. These cytokines have been assessed for their capacity to improve the response of mice to an inactivated rabies vaccine (77). All of them increased virus-specific IgG responses, IFN-γ raised resistance to challenge infection, and IFN-γ and IL-2 acted synergistically. Limited clinical trials have shown IFN-γ to accelerate the response of humans to hepatitis B vaccines. Granulocyte-macrophage colony-stimulating factor (GM-CSF) and FLT-3 ligand are strong stimulators of dendritic cells; each has been claimed to have adjuvant properties in soluble form, and each has been used to stimulate dendritic cells in various approaches to cell-based anticancer vaccines (78). The FLT-3 ligand stimulates both CD8α^+ (lymphoid type) and CD8α^- (myeloid type) dendritic cells in the mouse and both CD11c$^+$ (monocytoid) and CD11c$^-$ (plasmacytoid) dendritic cells in the human, whereas GM-CSF stimulates only the latter in each case. The former dendritic cell type tends to produce Th1 stimulating cytokines and the latter a Th2 bias. The differential mobilization of distinct dendritic cell subsets may have some potential in guiding immune responses. An early trial of FLT-3 ligand as an adjuvant in combination with alum failed to show an increase in the already strong immune response.

IL-2 has been explored most extensively (79). It can be highly effective in restoring immune responsiveness in mice with a deficient T-cell system or in overcoming immune response gene-mediated low titers. Its effects in healthy animals are less impressive, although some enhanced protection in a variety of infectious disease models has been noted. IL-2 can improve survival in a variety of cancer immunotherapeutic models. One noteworthy clinical effect is its capacity to convert lepromatous leprosy into tuberculoid leprosy when injected directly into the lesions of patients. IL-4 and IL-10 have received some attention through their capacity to send the immune response veering into a Th2 direction, but currently the focus is on Il-10 as a possible therapy in autoimmunity rather than as an adjuvant. IL-12 can promote Th1 development, an effect that has been beneficial in a trial *Leishmania* vaccine. One does not detect a great thirst within pharmaceutical industry to use soluble cytokines as adjuvants. In the longer term, it is conceivable that one or more could find a place in either vectored or DNA vaccines, as a gene construct rather than a finished product.

Molecular Targeting of Antigens

Antigens have to be brought to APCs, which in turn have to be activated to begin the adaptive immune response. Getting antigens to APCs by linking them to ligands for which the APCs have a counterstructure is a good first step. For example, fusing a protein antigen with C3d can increase murine anti–hen egg lysozyme responses by up to 10,000-fold (80), yielding responses much higher than with Freund's complete adjuvant. In mucosal immunity, coupling antigens covalently to a mucosal adjuvant can have profound effects as discussed previously. Now that the TLRs are being rapidly unraveled, one can anticipate more experimentation on antigens coupled to their various ligands, and certainly new knowledge on dendritic cells will be of equal relevance (81).

The reader by now has gathered that the field of adjuvants is not too rich in simplifying or overarching paradigms. It seems likely that empirical research will continue to dominate for some time. It may be well to end on a positive note. Com-

binations of the principles discussed seems the way of the future. There have been any number of disappointing clinical trials of a malaria vaccine based on the *Plasmodium falciparum* circumsporozoite protein (CS). When and only when three separate principles of adjuvanticity were combined did a vaccine capable of protecting six of seven volunteers against mosquito-bite challenge result (54).

That is not to extol AS02A ahead of its competitors but to make the point that the production of a virus-like particle, incorporation in an oil-in-water emulsion, and the use of two strong immune stimulants, MPL and QS21, conspired together to achieve the desired result. Perhaps malaria or HIV will represent the challenge to get the best out of the many competitive approaches and to arrive at a satisfactory end result.

Mucosal Adjuvants

While conventional adjuvants can be considered for mucosally delivered vaccine preparations, there is a special class of lectin-like molecules endowed with immunostimulatory properties that are uniquely involved in enhancing mucosal responses. CT is the most powerful mucosal adjuvant yet developed. The CT-B retains much of the adjuvant property but not the toxicity. *E. coli* LT is active and Fragment C of tetanus toxin has similar effects.

Obviously, the toxicity of CT and LT limits their usefulness as adjuvants. A clever strategy was developed by Pizza et al. (18), involving genetic modification of CT and LT, which resulted in derivatives that are still able to assemble into a holotoxin but have greatly diminished toxicity. These mutants act not only as mucosal immunogens but also as adjuvants for co-administered bystander antigens. Two equivalent derivatives of CT and LT, known as CTK63 and LTK63, have been prepared by substitution of a single, identical amino acid. The substitution is near the nicotinamide adenine dinucleotide (NAD) binding cleft. Interestingly, LTK63 worked much better than CTK63 both for the facilitation of serum antibody and as a co-inducer of IgA in nasal or lung lavages of mice, being only slightly inferior to CT itself (82). The reasons for this difference are currently entirely obscure. Indeed, the mechanisms whereby the toxins mediate immunity are poorly understood. The nature of the co-administered antigen is clearly important; there is a hierarchy of immunogenicity as for injected antigens. Capacity of the adjuvant to bind to M cells is obviously essential.

Interestingly, when CT-B is covalently coupled to an antigen and is then given by a mucosal route, CT-B induces a strong mucosal IgA response to itself and, frequently, the conjugated antigen, but it actually causes systemic or peripheral immunological tolerance (83,84). Moreover, far less antigen is required than for normal mucosal immunity or tolerance induction. Furthermore, the strategy works even in the presence of an already established state of systemic immunity. Impressive results have been obtained in animal models of autoimmune disease, including autoimmune encephalomyelitis, collagen-induced arthritis, and nonobese diabetes–insulin-dependent diabetes mellitus. One possible mechanism may be the induction of T cells producing immunosuppressive cytokines such as transforming growth factor β and IL-10. Interestingly, even trace amounts of co-administered CT prevent tolerance induction.

STANDARD IMMUNIZATION SCHEDULES

A prominent role of health departments in various countries is to establish and promulgate a schedule of immunizations considered optimal for that country. This schedule varies, depending on burden of disease, local experience, particular preferences of in-country experts, and (unfortunately) ability to pay. Furthermore, the way that vaccines are combined is constantly changing. Table 5 shows the schedule of a typical industrialized country.

BACTERIAL VACCINES

The particular vaccines discussed in this section are not a comprehensive list of important vaccines. Rather, they are chosen to reveal major research achievements and to highlight future challenges.

Diphtheria, Acellular Pertussis, and Tetanus

Historically, the DPT combination has come to be well accepted; only about 2% of the population harbor serious reservations. In view of its importance in a developing nation and the fact that health systems are geared to it, DPT has been regarded as a "platform" on which further vaccines, such as hepatitis B, Hib, and injectable poliomyelitis vaccines, and

TABLE 5. *A typical standard immunization schedule*[a]

Age	Vaccines
Birth	Hepatitis B
2 months	Diphtheria, tetanus, acellular pertussis, *Haemophilus influenzae* type B, hepatitis B, poliomyelitis[b]
4 months	Same as at 2 months
6 months	Same as at 2 months
12 months	Measles, mumps, rubella, varicella,[c] *Haemophilus influenzae* type B, hepatitis B
18 months	Diphtheria, tetanus, acellular pertussis
4 years	Diphtheria, tetanus, acellular pertussis, measles, mumps, rubella, polio
15–19 years[d]	Tetanus, adult diphtheria, polio
50 years	Tetanus, adult diphtheria
65 years	Pneumococcal vaccine, then every 5 years; influenza vaccine, then yearly

[a]Some vaccines given in combination.
[b]Injectable polio vaccine now preferred in the United States; Sabin-type oral polio vaccine still used in most other countries.
[c]Boosters in later life depend on current research aiming to determine whether these can prevent herpes zoster.
[d]Tetanus boosters are recommended with penetrating injuries. Ten-yearly booster would be a good idea.

perhaps others, could be placed. Different countries follow different schedules for a primary course of DPT, such as at 2, 3, or 4 months of age; 2, 4, and 6 months of age; or, in the setting of a developing country, 6, 10, and 14 weeks. It is generally agreed that three doses should be administered by 6 months of age. There is also variability between countries on the timing of a booster dose, such as at 18 month or diphtheria toxoid only at 3 to 5 years. Tetanus toxoid plus a low dose of diphtheria toxoid is advised again at school leaving age, and, ideally, a further booster should be given if a person suffers a penetrating wound (for tetanus) or travels to an epidemic or endemic area (for diphtheria). With regard to tetanus, five doses are regarded as conferring life-long immunity but this may not be correct. For diphtheria, a major epidemic in the countries of the former United Soviet Socialist Republic, including many cases among adults, has shown that initial immunization had been inadequate, that immunity does wane with time, or both. In the United Kingdom, 25% of blood donors aged 20 to 29 but 53% of those aged 50 to 59 were found to have inadequate antibodies to diphtheria toxin. Relatively little attention has been given to adult reimmunization, but a movement for more aggressive immunization of older persons has begun. Boosters of diphtheria and tetanus every 10 years would be a very good idea.

It has already been mentioned that genetic detoxification of diphtheria and tetanus toxins is possible but that there has been little pressure to modify the traditional toxoid vaccines. Nevertheless, the mutant diphtheria protein CRM197 has been popular as the protein component of conjugate vaccines. Pertussis, however, has a reputation for being reactogenic and perhaps for causing rare more serious side effects. Whole killed *B. pertussis* organisms are irritating and do cause local reactions and pyrexia in a significant proportion of infants.

For these reasons, there has been pressure for a subunit vaccine containing not killed bacteria but pure antigens derived from the bacteria. In fact, acellular pertussis vaccines have been in routine use in Japan since 1981. Renewed interest in the United States and in Europe has resulted in the testing of no fewer than 13 acellular pertussis vaccines. The key antigen is pertussis toxoid (PT), and other important antigens for protection are filamentous hemagglutinin and pertactin. Typical of the extensive clinical research that has been done on acellular pertussis vaccines is a trial in Italy, where immunization rates are low (around 40%); two acellular vaccines from SmithKlineBeecham and Chiron Biocine (renamed Chiron Vaccines in 1996) were compared with a whole-cell vaccine from Connaught Laboratories. The double-blind, randomized controlled trial involved 14,751 infants enrolled over a 1-year period in 1992–1993 (85). It involved 62 public health clinics and follow-up for an average of 17 months. Pertussis infection was confirmed by culture and quantitative serological tests. Unfortunately, the Connaught vaccine behaved quite atypically, giving only 36% protection. The two acellular vaccines behaved equivalently, giving 84% protection. Local and systemic adverse events were significantly less frequent with the two acellular vaccines, and their incidences were similar to those of a diphtheria toxoid vaccine without the pertussis component.

The chief difference between these two vaccines was that in the SmithKlineBeecham vaccine, the PT was detoxified by chemical treatment, whereas the Chiron Biocine vaccine contained a mutated, nontoxic form of PT that had been genetically detoxified. Site-directed mutagenesis introduced two point mutations (Arg 9→Lys and Glu 129→Gly) in the enzymic site of the PT. This vaccine caused a higher anti-PT response than that containing chemically inactivated PT, and continued blinded observation for a further year revealed significantly fewer pertussis cases in the Chiron Biocine group. A brief review by Rappuoli (86) gives a sobering insight into what is involved in bringing a new vaccine to the market. The project started in 1984. The cloning and sequencing of the PT gene was achieved in 1985; the amino acids that needed to be changed to remove toxicity were identified in 1987; the filamentous hemagglutinin was cloned in 1988; and the *B. pertussis* strain producing the nontoxic PT was constructed in 1989. Phased clinical trials were started as follows: phase I, in 1989; phase II, in 1990; phase III, in 1992; end of phase III, in 1995; filing of worldwide product license application world-wide, in 1996. Introduction of new and improved vaccines is not for the faint-hearted!

An analysis of six acellular pertussis vaccines from nine trials was presented by Klein (87). In all of these, the acellular vaccine was either statistically no different from or more protective than the whole cell vaccine. In three of the trials, the acellular vaccine was about 10% less protective (84% vs. 93%, 89% vs. 98%, 85% vs. 96%), but the differences did not reach statistical significance. The author is not aware of any meta-analysis of these data. However, an interesting review of all available clinical trial data was presented by Hewlett and Cherry (88). They reached the tentative conclusion that a five-component vaccine—including not only pertussis toxin, filamentous hemagglutinin, and pertactin but also fimbrial antigens 2 and 3—gave the greatest protection. These last two proteins are not the primary adhesins for the target cell surface but, rather, may serve to sustain attachment. Among other questions, it remains to be determined how long protection lasts with these newer vaccines. At the moment, there is no major push to switch over to these more expensive vaccines in developing countries, but the trend to the less reactogenic preparations is marked in the industrialized world and probably will prove irresistible globally.

Pertussis affects persons of all ages, although morbidity and mortality rates are highest among children younger than 1 year. Because antibiotics appear to be of little use when symptoms are fully established, the intravenous administration of high-titered pertussis immune globulin in hospitalized children is currently the subject of a phase III controlled trial that is fully enrolled.

There are some doubts about the duration of immunity to pertussis, even with regard to the natural disease itself, and there is increasing evidence of this organism as a cause of prolonged cough illnesses in adolescents and adults. This raises the issues of regular booster immunization, not currently practiced, and of the highest possible infant coverage to achieve eventual herd immunity.

Diarrheal Disease Vaccines: Typhoid, Cholera, and Shigellosis

Vaccines consisting of killed whole typhoid or cholera bacilli were among the earliest developed. However, efficacy was distinctly suboptimal, and local reactions at the injection site and within draining lymph nodes were marked. This approach has been all but abandoned, and much progress has been made toward orally active vaccines, although much more is needed.

Typhoid Vaccines

Typhoid fever, which is far more than a diarrheal disease because *Salmonella typhi* is an invasive organism that causes severe parenteral toxicity, remains a serious public health problem. There are an estimated 33 million cases annually, with more than 500,000 deaths. In endemic countries, the majority of patients are aged between 5 and 19, which makes school-based immunization an attractive possibility. Unfortunately, routine immunization is not yet occurring, and the reasonably effective present-day vaccines are almost entirely confined to use by travelers and armed services personnel.

The live attenuated orally administered *S. typhi* strain Ty21a has been licensed in the United States since 1991. This was derived from the wild-type strain Ty2, which has been maintained in the laboratory since 1918 and doubtless contains many mutations. Ty21a has been extensively tested in Egypt and Chile. Three to five spaced oral doses are required, it has been found to be very safe, and efficacy varies from fair to good in different trials. The current alternative is a single dose by injection of the Vi antigen. This is a linear homopolymer of galacturonic acid and forms a part of the capsular polysaccharide of the organism. Clinical trials in South Africa and Nepal have shown efficacy varying from 55% to 80%. The WHO would like to see a head-to-head comparison of these two vaccines.

Because these two vaccines are fairly but not overwhelmingly good, the search is on for more immunogenic but still well-tolerated vaccines. This involves further manipulation of living typhoid bacteria or conjugate versions of the Vi vaccine. As early as 1981, Hoiseth and Stocker (89) demonstrated that aromatic-dependent *Salmonella* bacteria such as *Salmonella typhimurium* are nonvirulent but nevertheless efficient immunogens. Precise deletion mutations can be engineered: for example, in the genes *aro* C and *aro* D, which render the bacteria nutritionally dependent on substrates para-aminobenzoic acid and 2,3-dihydroxy-benzoate, which are not present in high concentrations in human tissues. Such mutants and others like them have been the subject of extensive research, not only for the creation of vaccines against the organism but also as potential vectors for other antigen genes.

One attenuated *S. typhi* strain of this type is CVD908, which has been the subject of early clinical trials (90). A dose of 5×10^7 bacteria gives impressive rises in anti–O antibody titers in serum as well as inducing intestinal IgA formation. However, it also induce silent, asymptomatic, and time-limited vaccinemias, a characteristic shared by the early strains of Stocker. A modified strain, CVD 908-*htr* A, a deletion mutant lacking a particular serine protease, was developed by Chatfield et al. (91) on the basis of experimentation in an *S. typhimurium* mouse model. This attenuated variant does not cause vaccinemia but is equally immunogenic and thus appears particularly promising as a typhoid vaccine candidate.

Both CVD908 and CVD908 *htr*A can be used as live vectors for other antigens. For example, important antigens of enterotoxigenic *E. coli* have been successfully inserted (92), and other successes have involved the carriage of tetanus, diphtheria, *Schistosoma,* and malaria antigens. Furthermore, oral feeding of CVD908 can induce cellular immunity, including CD8+ CTLs. It seems that this strain could prove to be a highly versatile vector with oral activity.

Further vaccines of the same general type include the triple deletion of the genes *cya, crp,* and *cdt* or a double deletion of *phoP* and *phoQ*. These are in early stage clinical trial.

As far as Vi is concerned, it has been shown that immunogenicity can be increased by conjugating the Vi polysaccharide to a protein carrier. Good early results have been obtained when the protein is mutant heat-labile toxin of *E. coli,* and this strategy is being pursued with the hope that antitoxin immunity may also provide some protection against enterotoxigenic *E. coli.*

Cholera Vaccines

Cholera is a much-feared disease caused by the waterborne and highly infectious bacterium *V. cholerae,* which has caused devastating epidemics in many parts of the world. Although oral rehydration represented a real breakthrough, case-fatality rates can still reach 20%; the very young and the very old are most susceptible. Through the decades, there has been much strain variation. Since 1961, the biotype El Tor of serogroup 01 has been dominant, and since 1992, the new and more virulent variant 0139 has been a threat (see later discussion). Cholera accounts for an estimated 120,000 deaths each year.

Humans are the only known natural host for *V. cholerae,* although it is also known to be able to survive in water for very long periods. Transmission results from fecal contamination of water or food, and direct transmission from person to person is thought to be rare. Invasion does not occur, and pathological processes are caused by the toxin and the profuse watery diarrhea that it induces. Protection is through mucosal antibodies.

In a troubled world, a cholera vaccine would take on new significance. Refugee camps represent populations at special risk. In this situation, vaccination should be undertaken preemptively. Once an epidemic is under way, it is probably too late.

More than 100 years after Koch's discovery of the cholera bacterium, there is still no cholera vaccine that has gained wide acceptability. This is a pity, as a natural infection can produce fairly solid immunity of substantial duration. However, progress has been heartening, and the competition appears to be between two orally active types of preparation, featuring either live or attenuated *Vibrio* organisms.

Extensive work has been done on a Swedish vaccine consisting of a mixture of the CT-B and killed whole bacteria. In a large clinical trial in Bangladesh conducted among 62,285 children and women, involving three doses, a 5-year follow-up showed 49% efficacy of the vaccine, but, interestingly, the whole-cell vaccine without CT-B performed just as well (93). This result was different from what was noted in the first 6 months, when the combined vaccine worked much better. Protection was evident only during the first 3 of the 5 years, with protection better in the first 2 years than in the third. In fact, protection against *V. cholerae* 01 was 85% for 6 months and 60% for 3 years with the combined vaccine. Since this trial was initiated, a further variant of cholera has emerged in Madras, India. This variant, *V. cholerae* serogroup 0139, has spread rapidly in India, Bangladesh, and adjacent countries and has reached as far as Malaysia, Thailand, and China. Accordingly, formalin-killed 0139 *Vibrio* organisms were added to the existing 01 vaccine, and intestinal and systemic immune responses against both strains were elicited in a majority of human volunteers. This suggests that the development of a bivalent vaccine will be relatively straightforward.

Beautiful work has been done under difficult circumstances in Vietnam. Trach et al. (94) reported on an oral killed whole-cell *V. cholerae* vaccine, consisting of two doses of a mixture of Inaba and Ogawa strains, that was subjected to trials in 134,453 people in Vietnam. This vaccine was locally produced in Hanoi and was quite inexpensive, at about U.S. 10 cents per dose. During an epidemic about 8 months after immunization, it proved 66% protective. Despite some admitted limitations in the trial protocol, the results are promising.

Several live attenuated strains of *V. cholerae* have reached clinical trial. All these have been constructed to possess known genetic deletions to reduce virulence. The most advanced strain is CVD103-HgR, a live oral cholera vaccine strain constructed by recombinant DNA methods from a classical Inaba strain in which the A subunit of CT has been deleted. This was safe and immunogenic in North American volunteers and provides significant protection against experimental challenge (95), and in 1993 a large-scale, randomized, placebo-controlled field trial was initiated in North Jakarta involving a single oral dose of vaccine. About 67,000 subjects aged 2 to 42 were involved. Unfortunately, in a 4-year follow-up, the vaccine could not be shown to be efficacious. The results were somewhat confounded by an unexpectedly low incidence of cholera during the first year of the trial. Although the results showed 60% protection over the first 6 months and 24% protection during the first year, the low numbers make these results uncertain. Some good results did come out of this trial, however. The vaccine was well tolerated, even in infants as young as 3 months, and it did not interfere with the oral typhoid vaccine Ty21a. Further work on CVD103-HgR is in progress. It is reasonable to conclude that it is a good vaccine for travelers, because protection is evident already 7 days after a single dose. Convincing protection in field situations remains to be demonstrated. An attenuated 0139 live oral vaccine, known as CD112, has also been prepared and confers good protection against challenge with wild-type 0139.

Pearson et al. (96) constructed a new series of live attenuated oral cholera vaccines that are based on the deletion of a whole "virulence cassette." Instead of deleting just the CT gene, additional associated virulence factors are deleted. These include the genes for zona occludens toxin, auxiliary cholera enterotoxin, and core-encoded pilus. Certain sequences encouraging recombination were also deleted to prevent the strain from regaining CT genes. Furthermore, mobility-deficient variants were found to be less reactogenic. Volunteer studies with two of these, Peru-15 for *V. cholerae* 01 and Bengal-15 for *V. cholerae* 0139, look promising for a one-dose oral vaccine.

Shigellosis Vaccines

The author was probably among the majority of medical graduates when he was surprised to learn that shigellosis or bacillary dysentery was a bigger public health problem than either typhoid or cholera. It is one of the most serious diarrheal diseases in the world. Kotloff et al. (97) estimated that there are 175 million episodes per annum throughout the world and 1.1 million deaths. The WHO's more cautious estimate is 800,000 deaths. The most important organisms are *Shigella flexneri, Shigella sonnei, Shigella boydii,* and *Shigella dysenteriae. S. flexneri* predominates in developing countries, and *S. sonnei* in industrialized countries, the latter type of country accounting for fewer than 1% of episodes. Each species has multiple serotypes; there are about 30 serotypes altogether. Usually, a given serotype predominates in a given area at a given time.

Clinical findings of shigellosis include diarrhea, which can vary from mild to extremely severe with ulcerative lesions of the colon and significant blood in the motions. Fever, dehydration, and metabolic disturbances are common, and hemolytic uremic syndrome is a serious complication.

Shigella is, in fact, a facultative intracellular parasite that invades the colonic and rectal mucosa. Invasion of M cells and other APCs occurs, and lymphoid collections can be rapidly destroyed. Systemic and mucosal humoral immune responses are elicited by an infection, and the LPS of the organism is of great importance, because antibodies to it can protect against bacterial challenge. Thus, much of the search for an effective vaccine has centered on the LPS O antigen and on the development of orally administered live attenuated vaccines. However, parenteral vaccines are also under consideration, as in an intranasal proteosome population.

Among the live attenuated orally active vaccines, much work has been done by Sansonetti and Phalipon (98) on a deletion mutant of *S. flexneri* serotype 2a strain SC602. This carries both an auxotrophic mutation (deletion of *ivcA*) and one diminishing virulence (deletion of *icsA,* also known as *virG*). An attractive feature of this vaccine is that oral administration of as few as 10^3 to 10^4 live organisms elicits a good local response to L73S. After a single dose of 10^4 colony-forming units, it provided 100% protection against severe diarrhea in seven North American volunteers homologously challenged. This group has also developed a candidate vaccine for *S. dysenteriae* type 1, again with a *virG* deletion as well as two auxotrophic mutations.

Kotloff et al. (99) promoted the live attenuated strains CVD 1203 and CVD 1207. Both are deletion mutants, the second being less reactogenic because of deletions that prevent the bacterium from synthesizing enterotoxin. In a phase I clinical trial in 35 healthy adult volunteers, it was found that CVD 1207 was remarkably well tolerated at doses up to 10^8 colony-forming units. The vaccine engendered a dose-dependent mucosal IgA response specific for *S. flexneri* 2a LPS. This vaccine invades gut epithelial cells, although to a much lesser degree than wild-type bacteria, but undergoes only very limited intracellular proliferation and spread. Backup candidates from this group include CVD 1204, CVD 1208 and CVD 1211. A major challenge is to gain sufficiently broad protection among species and serotypes. There is some cross-protection among *S. flexneri* serotypes, but a final multivalent *Shigella* vaccine will probably have to have about three *S. flexneri* serotypes as well as *S. sonnei* and *S. dysenteriae* components.

Parenteral vaccination represents a different alternative. The laboratory of Dr. John Robbins at the U.S. National Institutes of Health, which was so prominent in Hib conjugate vaccines, is pioneering efforts to link detoxified *Shigella* LPS covalently to proteins, and encouraging results have been obtained both in Israeli army volunteers and in young children. After a single intramuscular injection, significant antibody to both *S. sonnei* and *S. flexneri* 2a was generated in over 90% of cases. In the adults, challenge with virulent organisms showed good protection.

The final approach involves *S. flexneri* LPS noncovalently coupled to purified meningococcal outer membrane proteins. Hydrophobic interactions result in a multimolecular vesicular structure, which can be given intranasally. This is reasonably protective against severe diarrhea after challenge with 500 colony-forming units of virulent bacteria.

Helicobacter pylori Vaccines

In 1983, one of those rare true breakthroughs in medicine occurred. Peptic ulcer, a classical and common disease, had been thought to be caused by stress and hyperacidity. Instead, Marshall and Warren (100) attributed it to a spiral bacterium, soon identified as *Helicobacter pylori.* This discovery from Australia was greeted with great skepticism but was supported by Marshall's brave attempt to fulfill Koch's postulates through infecting himself, which resulted in gastritis and re-isolation of the organism, after which he cured himself with antibiotics. It is now generally accepted that *H. pylori* accounts not only for the majority of gastric and duodenal ulcers but also for acute gastritis, chronic active gastritis, a significant proportion of gastric adenocarcinomas, and essentially 100% of B-cell lymphomas of gastric mucosa–associated lymphoid tissue (MALT). Although the WHO had classified *H. pylori* as a class I carcinogen in 1994, it was only in 2001 that Uemura et al. (101) put the issue beyond doubt with a long-term, prospective study of 1,526 Japanese patients with dyspepsia who were monitored for a mean period of 7.8 years. Of these, 1,246 had *H. pylori* infection and 280 did not. Within the study period, 36 gastric cancers developed, of which 23 were intestinal-type cancers and 13 were diffuse-type cancers. Every single cancer occurred among the infected patients ($p < 0.001$). Kaplan-Meier analysis showed the gastric cancer risk to be 5% in the infected group at 10 years.

Infection is acquired mostly during childhood and persists chronically if not treated, but it is reasonably easily cured by so-called "triple therapy" consisting of a proton-pump inhibitor and two antibiotics (e.g. metronidazole and ampicillin).

Many aspects of the epidemiology of *H. pylori* remain mysterious. Transmission is believed to be oral, through vomitus or diarrheal feces. Infection may result in a brief period of acute gastritis, after which the carrier has few or no symptoms for years or even decades. Infection is incredibly common, typically 40% in industrialized countries and up to 90% in developing countries. However, of these infected people, only 15% to 20% eventually develop severe gastric or duodenal disease. The degree to which these bacteria represent a public health problem is still not generally appreciated. In the United States, it has been estimated that up to 25 million persons are ill with this infection at some stage of their lives. In these cases, reinfection after cure is rare, perhaps 1% per year, but in developing countries, it could be expected to be much higher. In such settings, a prophylactic vaccine would be especially desirable.

H. pylori is a gram-negative spiral, microaerophilic, flagellated bacterium that produces an amazing amount of the enzyme urease, which can make up 5% to 10% of the bacterium's protein. This converts gastric fluid urea to ammonia and carbon dioxide, a very efficient buffering system against stomach acid. Urease-negative *H. pylori* strains appear unable to colonize the stomach. We know much too little about why only some infected people develop chronic gastric disease. The best hint (102) comes from strain variation in the bacteria. Specifically, strains of type I possess a 40-kb fragment of

DNA that comprises 31 genes and constitutes a pathogenicity island. Important within this area are the antigen CagA and genes that encode a secretion machinery that allows the active transfer of molecules from the bacterium to the gastric epithelial cell on which the bacteria reside. So-called type I strains express CagA (and appear to be more virulent), whereas type II strains do not. Furthermore, type II strains are sometimes low expressers of another gene, that for the vacuolating cytotoxin VacA, which is thought to be important in pathogenesis. More work needs to be done on strain subtyping.

Neutrophil infiltration is a prominent feature in biopsy specimens from *H. pylori*–infected stomachs. An *H. pylori* 15-kDa protein that is chemotactic for neutrophils and monocytes and is a strong inducer of the production of reactive oxygen intermediates in neutrophils has been identified. This has been termed *neutrophil-activating protein* (NAP). Other possible candidate antigens of *H. pylori* include flagellin, various adhesins, heat-shock proteins, and LPS.

Animal models have provided proof of principle that both prophylactic and therapeutic *H. pylori* vaccines are feasible. Lee et al. (103) isolated a gastric spiral bacterium from cats, and this organism, *Helicobacter felis,* can colonize the mouse stomach and cause gastritis and even lymphoma. With this model in place, it was soon shown that a sonicate of *H. felis* was a protective vaccine in mice, providing 96% protection against oral challenge (104). A further important development was that of adapting fresh clinical isolates of *H. pylori* to grow in the mouse stomach by biweekly serial passage through specific pathogen-free mice. This resulted in the development of (a) one strain, derived from a type I clinical isolate, that caused gastric pathological processes mimicking those in the human and (b) of another strain, derived from a type II clinical isolate, that caused only a mild inflammatory infiltrate without erosive lesions.

These considerations naturally led to the possibility of subunit vaccines. *H. pylori* urease was the first antigen in clinical trial, because it confers protection in animal models. The results of the first studies were not too impressive, although there was some reduction in the bacterial load. Both CagA and VacA are being assessed as possible oral immunogens in the *H. pylori* mouse model, with the addition of the genetically detoxified *E. coli* heat-labile enterotoxin, LTK63, as a mucosal adjuvant. Early results appear encouraging, as do those with CagA, VacA, and NAP in combination.

What about therapeutic intervention? Doidge et al. (105) achieved eradication of *H. felis* in infected mice with an oral administration of *H. felis* sonicate and CT as a mucosal adjuvant. Similarly, Corthesy-Theulaz et al. (106) successfully used the *H. pylori* urease B subunit as an oral treatment in mice. These results give encouragement for the early commencement of clinical therapeutic vaccine trials. It is probable that Th1 T cells are responsible for much of the inflammatory damage in the stomach, and a change in the balance towards a greater proportion of Th2 cells may be helpful. This accentuates the importance of a safe and effective adjuvant suitable for human use.

A beagle model of *H. pylori* infection has been developed, enabling serial gastric biopsies and thus dynamic evaluation of progressive pathological processes (107). In this model, encouraging results have been obtained with systemic immunization with a variety of recombinant proteins, including VacA, CagA, and NAP, simply adsorbed onto alum. In view of the relatively low rate of acquisition of infection in industrialized countries, it is likely that any subunit combination vaccine arising from this research will have to be tested in areas with high transmission rates, such as in less developed countries or high-susceptibility ethnic minorities.

If a safe, effective vaccine conferring a substantial period of protection can be developed, the approximately 1% lifetime risk of gastric cancer would, by itself, justify universal use; in view of the additional severe morbidity arising from chronic gastritis, gastric dysplasia, and peptic ulcer disease, the case becomes very strong indeed.

Vaccines against Encapsulated Organisms

Haemophilus influenzae *Type B, Meningococci, and Pneumococci*

Vaccines traditionally available for encapsulated organisms such as those just described have been prepared from purified capsular polysaccharide antigen. These vaccines suffer from two major disadvantages. First, being polysaccharide in nature, they do not engage the T-cell limb of the immune response. This means that the antibodies are chiefly IgM, affinity maturation does not occur, and, most important, young infants do not respond well. Because the incidence of Hib meningitis peaks at around 10 to 11 months of age, a vaccine that is not really effective before the ages of 18 to 24 months is far from ideal.

The first-generation Hib vaccine, based on the polyribosylribitol phosphate (PRP) capsule, was developed almost simultaneously by Anderson et al. (108) and Rodrigues et al. (109). An extensive clinical trial involving 130,178 Finnish children was performed by Peltala et al. (110). No protection was noted in children younger than 18 months, even in those given a booster dose, but just a single dose in children aged 18 months to 5 years of age gave good protection against invasive Hib disease.

The second problem for these vaccines is that, in each case, there are multiple serotypes. With Hib, six capsular serotypes, a to f, are capable of causing disease in humans; fortunately, 99% of typeable strains causing invasive disease are type b. With pneumococci, on the other hand, there are 84 capsular types. Although 8 to 10 cause 70% of the serious infections, the present carbohydrate vaccine is a cocktail of no fewer than 23 serotypes! This covers more than 90% of serious infections. With *N. meningitidis,* there are five main antigenically distinct groups, of which groups A, B, and C

are the most important. Group B strains account for about two thirds of cases of meningococcal meningitis in industrialized countries. Group A strains cause epidemic disease, particular in the "meningitis belt" of sub-Saharan Africa. For example, the 1996 epidemic caused more than 200,000 cases, with 20,000 deaths, and this is probably a vast underestimate. Polysaccharide outer capsule vaccines are available for group A and C organisms and have been used in outbreak control.

The same groups that pioneered the carbohydrate vaccine were involved in the breakthrough that yielded the extremely effective Hib conjugate vaccine (111,112). These researchers made use of the principle of conjugating antigenic Hib PRP saccharides to protein carriers in order to induce a T cell–dependent response, which matures much earlier in the human than does the T cell–independent response to saccharides alone. Different-length saccharides and different carriers were used by different companies; small, medium, and large polysaccharides were attached, with or without linkers, to diphtheria toxoid, the diphtheria toxin variant CRM197, tetanus toxoid, or the group B meningococcal outer membrane complex. Eskola et al. (113) led the way with a clinical trial in Finland in 1986–1987 in which the vaccine was 83% effective and also eliminated oropharyngeal carriage. A further trial with an improved vaccine in 1988–1990 showed higher, more persistent antibody levels and better efficacy. From about 1990 on, there has been an increasing number of countries with national vaccination programs, and the result has been a dramatic decline in invasive Hib disease because of immunity, herd immunity, and lowered pathogen carriage rates. Already by 1991, meningitis incidence had decreased by 82% in the United States. In many countries, Hib meningitis is simply not seen any more. It may not be too early to hope for the eventual control and near-eradication of this pathogen. Particularly encouraging is the fact that the conjugate vaccine works well in the setting of a developing country. Mullholland et al. (114) performed a double-blind randomized trial in The Gambia involving 42,848 infants who were given either DPT alone at 2, 3, and 4 months or DPT mixed with Hib polysaccharide-tetanus protein (PRP-T). Hib meningitis, Hib pneumonia, and five other forms of invasive Hib disease were evaluated over a 3-year period. Among the children (83%) who received all three doses, the efficacy of the vaccine for the prevention of all invasive Hib disease was 95%; for the prevention of Hib pneumonia, 100%; and of meningitis, 92%. Furthermore, there was a 21.1% reduction of *all* cases of radiologically defined pneumonia. In view of the importance of acute respiratory disease as a killer of infants in developing countries, this is an important finding. It is probable that the conjugate Hib vaccine will become the ninth vaccine recommended for all children in most parts of the world, although perhaps not Asia. Some developing Latin American countries have already begun to deploy it.

Through the GAVI program, Hib vaccine is now being made available to many poor countries that request it, chiefly in Africa. It has long been suspected that Hib is less of a problem in Asia than in Africa, and a series of studies is under way to examine this matter in detail. Early unpublished results are hinting that the anecdotal evidence may be correct, in which case universal deployment of Hib vaccine may not be cost effective in these countries.

Through a major grant from the Bill and Melinda Gates Foundation, a large program has been mounted to counter epidemic meningitis in Africa. This involves the development and deployment of a conjugate *Meningococcus* A vaccine, the current plan calling for mass immunization of 1- to 29-year-olds with a single dose, followed by repeated mass immunization of 1- to 5-year-olds every 4 to 5 years until a sufficiently satisfactory routine infant program comprising two or three doses can be established. At a later stage, it is hoped that a heptavalent vaccine that includes *Meningococcus* A and C will be used to immunize infants. The distinguished physician Dr. Mark la Force has recently assumed directorship of this Meningitis Vaccine Project Partnership.

After the outstanding success of the introduction of Hib immunization, the United Kingdom decided in 1999 to commence mass immunization against *N. meningitidis* serogroup C (115). This was in the presence of great public anxiety and intense press interest, with 40% of bacterial meningitis cases being caused by this organism. It was estimated that if nothing were done, there would have been 1,530 cases annually with 150 deaths. The experience with Hib suggested that a conjugate *Meningococcus* C vaccine would work well. The involvement of manufacturers was critical, and three went on to develop products; the licensing authorities were persuaded to expedite the regulatory process. In any event, in the first year, 87% of infants received the vaccine at 2, 3, and 4 months of age, and a catch-up campaign targeted at 1- to 18-year-olds reached 85% of the population. As a result, there were more than an 80% reduction in confirmed cases and a 90% reduction in deaths within 18 months of the start of the program. Interestingly, in nonimmunized groups, the attack rate has fallen by two thirds, which hints at the possibility of herd immunity. Surveillance studies have shown no evidence of any capsular switching to serogroup B during the first 18 months of the program. The cost of the program has been estimated at U.K. £4,000 per life-year saved, which is less cost effective than many other vaccines but well within what is acceptable in an industrialized country.

There is currently no *N. meningitidis* serogroup B vaccine licensed in the United States. Unlike the other meningococcal polysaccharides, that of group B is poorly immunogenic in adults, possibly because of immunological tolerance occasioned by cross-reaction with mammalian oligosaccharides; effective immunization might raise fears of autoimmune phenomena. This suggests the need for other approaches, such as protein-based vaccines: for example, porins from the outer membrane of the bacteria. A Cuban vaccine based on outer membrane proteins was 74% effective in individuals aged 4 and older but less effective in infants.

There still remains the problem of untypeable and non–type B serotypes of *H. influenzae*. A promising vaccine candidate outer membrane protein known as D15 has been cloned by Thomas et al. (116). It is present in sarcosyl-insoluble outer membrane protein preparations in every one of 36 *H. influenzae* isolates tested. Affinity-purified antibodies against cloned D15 were protective in a rat pup model. There is 98% conservation among all serotypes in this 778–amino acid, 85-kDa molecule (W. R. Thomas, personal communication 1992). No homologous protein has been found in data banks. This protein could represent a "universal" candidate vaccine against recurrent otitis media.

Obviously, the same issues that have been raised for Hib and meningococci come up with the enormously important pathogen *S. pneumoniae* and with *Pneumococcus*. At least four companies are involved in the development of pneumococcal conjugate vaccines, and, furthermore, several promising initial attempts have been made to develop broadly reactive protein-based vaccines. A large-scale phase III clinical trial involving 37,000 Californian infants, with a seven-valent conjugate, resulted in 22 cases of invasive disease with pneumococci of serotypes included in the vaccine in the control group but 0 cases in the immunized group ($p < 0.0001$). This 100% efficacy raised ethical concerns with regard to further trials. There is also evidence in both industrialized and developing countries for a lowering of nasopharyngeal carriage rates after immunization, which raises hopes of herd immunity in the longer term. At least four efficacy trials of conjugate vaccines are ongoing in developing countries. At the same time, it must be recognized that conjugate vaccines comprising so many valencies (probably at least 9 to 11) will be quite expensive. Therefore, research on protein vaccines should be strongly encouraged. There is broad agreement that a pneumococcal vaccine is of very high priority for developing countries.

Intracellular Pathogens, Especially Tuberculosis and Leprosy

Bacteria that exploit the scavenger cell system and successfully learn to live inside cells present special challenges to the vaccine developer. Organisms of this sort include *M. tuberculosis*, *Mycobacterium leprae*, and *Listeria monocytogenes*. Robust T-cell responses are the key to immune protection in these cases, involving Th1-type CD4$^+$ cells and CD8$^+$ CTLs, as well as γ/δ T cells and natural killer cells, each of which has been shown to be of importance in animal models. Because of its great public health importance, we shall consider mainly tuberculosis.

Tuberculosis is one of the greatest communicable disease killers in the world. An astonishing 2 billion people harbor the bacterium in latent form; of these people, fewer than 10% develop active disease. However, there are about 8 million new active cases each year and about 2 to 3 million annual deaths. Two huge threats are (a) combined infection with HIV and tuberculosis, in which death can occur within weeks of infection, and (b) the increased prevalence of strains of *M. tuberculosis* that are resistant to one or more antimicrobial agents. For example, in the United States, 13% of new cases of tuberculosis are resistant to at least one first-line drug, and 3% are resistant to both isoniazid and rifampicin, the two most important drugs.

BCG was introduced in 1921 and reaches nearly 90% of the world's children, being the most widely used EPI vaccine. Its protective efficacy in childhood tuberculosis, such as tuberculosis meningitis and miliary tuberculosis, ranges from 50% to 80% in various trials. Its capacity to prevent adult pulmonary tuberculosis is more controversial; reasonably good early European results contrast with poor results in developing countries, including an entirely negative large trial in India. One possible reason relates to the presence of cross-reacting *Mycobacteria* species in the setting of a developing country, which may already have caused some immunity without BCG.

There is no shortage of good ideas in this field. Three broad areas of research are commanding most attention: DNA vaccines, subunit vaccines, and genetically engineered *Mycobacteria* species, including BCG and *M. tuberculosis*. In 1998, the whole of the *M. tuberculosis* genome was sequenced, providing (in principle at least) a vast number of potential candidate molecules for a subunit vaccine. Even without this new information, there are several strong candidates. Among them are a secreted molecule, ESAT6, expressed only in virulent mycobacterial strains and absent in BCG, which is an effective vaccine in mice and guinea pigs. A combination of BCG priming and boosting with MVA engineered to express Ag85 is slated to enter clinical trials, the guinea pig model again showing good vaccine efficacy. Another candidate is HSP60 from *M. leprae,* a DNA vaccine that appears to give good protection. Other interesting antigens include the 36-kDa proline-rich mycobacterial antigen, mycobacterial cell wall mycolic acids, and HSP65, which, as a DNA vaccine, shows promise in a therapeutic vaccine model.

Genetic engineering of mycobacterial species continues apace. BCG has been modified to express cytokines or to overexpress Ag85 or other protective antigens. Auxotrophic mutants of BCG or of *M. tuberculosis* have been developed in the hope of finding a vaccine suitable for immunocompromised people. As genomics further defines virulence determinants in *M. tuberculosis,* rational attenuation should become feasible.

As with malaria vaccines, the big problem will be clinical trials. The Sequella Global Tuberculosis Foundation was created in 1997 to help to fill this gap and has been helped by a U.S. $25 million grant from the Bill and Melinda Gates Foundation. Its hope is to get three candidate vaccines to phase I trials by early 2003. Even so, phase III trials will be vastly expensive.

M. leprae has many similarities to *M. tuberculosis.* Some of the urgency has gone out of the search for a leprosy vaccine because of the remarkable success of multidrug therapy. There is good evidence that BCG itself is a moderately protective vaccine against leprosy, and Convit's vaccine, consisting of killed, armadillo-derived *M. leprae* plus live BCG, appears

to be better. Other mycobacteria vaccines such as killed *Mycobacterium w* appear to be modestly effective. The subunit vaccine approach is not being actively pursued. One candidate is a 35-kDa protein that is a major target of the human T-cell response to *M. leprae*. Sequencing of the *M. leprae* genome is now complete and may in time provide further candidate molecules.

Vaccines against Group A Streptococci

Somewhat amazingly, since the development of penicillin during World War II, rheumatic fever and rheumatic heart disease nevertheless remain common in many developing countries, the prevalence being up to 20 per 1000. *Streptococcus pyogenes* infections can also be followed by acute and chronic glomerulonephritis and otitis media. A good vaccine candidate would be the M protein, a coiled-coil α helical surface protein of the bacterium. However, the vaccine developer faces two major hurdles. First, there are more than 100 serotypes of group A streptococci, and much of the variation is in the immunity-inducing but highly variable N-terminal portion of the M protein. Second, the major complications are almost certainly autoimmune in nature, and it would be a disaster if immunization triggered the very events that the vaccine is supposed to prevent. Brandt et al. (117) first identified a conserved, non–host cross-reactive peptide from the C-terminal half of the M protein and then linked this (in a manner that maintained the peptide's helical conformation) with a multiepitopic peptide consisting of seven N-terminal portions from seven different, relatively common serotypes, targeting northern Australian aboriginal isolates. The polymer technology, already described in the section on adjuvants, ensured full immunogenicity of all components. The vaccine was strongly immunogenic and protective in mice against a wide variety of strains and was not cross-reactive with any of many host self-proteins. The nature of the polymer backbone would allow peptides from other, non–M protein–derived vaccine candidates to be added as well. Such candidates include C5a peptidase, cysteine protease, and other streptococcal pyrogenic exotoxins. Some of these toxins can be rendered harmless through mutagenesis of the relevant genes. Another candidate is the major streptococcal adhesin, a protein known as sfbI.

Various formulations of these candidates, including parenteral injection, intranasal inoculation, and expression on the surface of *Streptococcus gordonii,* a commensal organism of the oral cavity, are in preclinical research. As antibiotic resistance becomes more of a problem, the pressure will build to take some of these candidates to the clinic.

VIRAL VACCINES

Viral vaccine research has produced both triumphs and tribulations. The triumphs include success against poliomyelitis, measles, mumps, rubella, varicella, hepatitis B, and, to a lesser extent, hepatitis A. The tribulations include struggles with HIV/AIDS and hepatitis C. Influenza and rotavirus are poised in between. It is not possible to run through the whole gamut of viral vaccines. Rather, the author wishes to highlight some of the complexities and remaining challenges and draw some lessons from them.

Hepatitis A, B, and C

These three viruses show an interesting spectrum of solved and unsolved problems that confront the vaccinologist. Hilleman (118) cited literature suggesting that contagious jaundice has been known to occur since the fifth century B.C. It became clear in the 1950s that "infectious hepatitis" and "homologous serum jaundice" had differing features, and this difference was cemented in the 1960s. Since the isolation of hepatitis A and B viruses and good serological tests for their recent presence, other forms of fecal-oral and of blood transmission of hepatitis have been discovered, of which the most important enterically transmitted agent is hepatitis E, and the most important parenterally transmitted is hepatitis C.

Hepatitis A is one of a group of diseases that also includes infectious mononucleosis, which is mild or entirely asymptomatic in young children but more severe in adolescents and adults. In rare cases, it causes fulminant hepatitis but is usually less severe, although it causes illness for up to several months. It is now only moderately common in industrialized countries but very common in many developing countries. Immunization is a good idea for travelers, and both active immunization, giving long protection, and passive immunization with immune serum globulin, giving 3 months' protection, work well.

The virus initially proved very difficult to grow, and early studies depended on its identification in fecal extracts by electron microscopy. It was eventually grown in marmoset liver cells and a human hepatoma cell line, after which many types of cells were successfully infected. Growth of the virus in LLC-MK2 cells and availability of a marmoset model for vaccine testing led to a formalin-inactivated killed whole-virus vaccine, which, however, was not acceptable at that time because malignant cells were involved in growing the virus. Two groups eventually succeeded in obtaining growth in human diploid lung fibroblasts, and the resultant vaccines from SmithKlineBeecham and Merck Sharp & Dohme work well. However, because virus yields are not enormous, hepatitis A is an expensive vaccine, and a live attenuated vaccine would be most beneficial in a developing nation. Several candidate vaccines exist; one has been extensively tested in China and found to be highly effective, but none has yet made it through to full registration.

Hepatitis B carrier rates vary from less than 0.1% to 15% of the population in different countries. Altogether, 2 billion people have serological evidence of past infection, and 350 million people are chronically infected. One million people die each year of cirrhosis or hepatocellular carcinoma. The acute attack is mild or insignificant. Hepatitis B virus does not grow in tissue culture, and there are two sources of

vaccine: HBsAg isolated from chronic carriers of the virus and the same material molecularly cloned in yeast or Chinese hamster ovary cells. The carrier-derived vaccine was, for a long time, far cheaper and has been widely used in developing countries. Now the recombinant vaccine is becoming much cheaper. Some recent tenders for the public sector in developing countries have come in at around U.S. 30 cents per dose. Recombinant vaccine may eventually replace the human-derived material. Both vaccines are about equally effective; response rates to protective levels of antibody vary from 85% to 95% in different studies. Protection may be achieved with lower levels of antibody than those generally believed to be protective, perhaps because of CD8$^+$ T-cell effects. One worry is that some vaccinated people become carriers of what have been called "escape mutants," which persist despite the presence of good antibody levels to the native virus. The most common change is an arginine-for-glycine substitution in the *a* loop, against which antibodies are usually directed. Although it is not yet certain that the mutation changes the virus to one of lower infectivity, M. H. Kane (personal communication 1996) pointed out that there is no evidence yet of escape mutants having spread from one person to another. There is therefore no need yet to worry about the univalency of the current vaccine. Presumably, if escape mutants become a problem, but if the number of different serotypes is limited, the variants could be included in a recombinant vaccine. It is encouraging to note that universal infant immunization is now being adopted very widely.

The hepatitis C virus was the first of the non-A, non-B viruses identified, but it has not been grown in tissue culture or visualized in the electron microscope. Hepatitis C is transmitted in the same way as hepatitis B but is an even nastier disease, inasmuch as about 80% of people who contract the infection become chronic carriers and the majority of these go on to develop chronic liver disease. Furthermore, a significant proportion develop hepatocellular carcinoma; in Japan, where about 2% of people are carriers, hepatitis C is a more common cause of liver cancer than is hepatitis B.

Because of the frustrations surrounding the difficulty of isolating this virus, the cloning of the virus by Choo et al. (119) was considered a major triumph, particularly because it soon led to the development of an assay for antibodies useful in screening blood donations. However, development of a vaccine against hepatitis C faces difficulties. The virus is a rapidly mutating RNA virus with a single open reading frame encoding a polyprotein of about 3,000 amino acids. There are two putative envelope proteins, E1 and E2, identified by analogy with other flaviviruses, which presumably are produced by proteolytic cleavage. Study of these by genomic analysis of hepatitis C cloned from patients in different parts of the world shows a great degree of structural (and therefore presumably antigenic) diversity. Furthermore, experimentation on vaccine candidates is rendered difficult by the fact that the only animal model is the chimpanzee. This makes it hard to characterize and quantitate neutralizing antibodies, although it is known that plasma from a chronic carrier can protect chimpanzees from infection. An assay that shows great promise as a surrogate neutralization assay has been developed (120): the neutralization of binding (NOB) assay. Hepatitis C virus (HCV) recombinant envelope antigen E2 was expressed in HeLa or CHO cells, and it bound with high affinity to MOLT-4 cells, a human cell line that may allow low-level replication of HCV. The degree of binding can be readily assessed through the use of a sandwich fluorescent antibody technique to detect E2 antigen. Unknown serum can then be assayed for its ability to neutralize this binding. Chimpanzees immunized with E1 and E2 show varying degrees of protection to challenge. It was found that the degree of protection correlated with the NOB titer. Also, the assay showed cross-neutralization of binding between greatly disparate isolates, leading to the hope that binding (and hence presumably neutralization) is at least partly independent of E2 antigenic variation. It has further been found that high titers of NOB antibodies correlate with resolution of HCV infection in patients. Of 34 patients with acute hepatitis C, 29 developed chronic hepatitis, but in 7 of these, the disease gradually resolved. In 6 of these 7, the emergence and persistence of high serum titers of NOB antibodies coincided with virus clearance and clinical resolution, whereas patients with continuing chronic disease not showing resolution had low or undetectable NOB antibody levels. This was quite different from enzyme-linked immunosorbent assays against HCV structural proteins, which showed no such correlation. T-lymphocyte responses, particularly to the core antigen, may also be critical for a benign course of an HCV infection. These correlations should be helpful to the design of further experiments seeking a vaccine against this important pathogen. Clinical trials of an E1/E2 vaccine are in progress. DNA vaccines using envelopes as well as core protein constructs are being tested in chimpanzees.

Progress has been made in the therapy of HCV, through both a combination of interferon-α and ribavirin and, perhaps, the use of polyclonal immune globulin. Nevertheless, there is much interest in a possible therapeutic vaccine. A tissue culture model replicating nonintegrated nonstructural viral proteins should prove helpful for the screening of new drugs, such as the protease or the helicase.

Rotavirus Vaccines

In 1973, Bishop et al. (121) in Australia discovered 70-nm virus particles possessing a distinctive double-shelled outer capsid in duodenal epithelium and stool filtrates from children with acute gastroenteritis. These so-called rotaviruses turned out to be an extremely important cause of diarrheal illness. In industrialized countries, rotavirus accounts for about a third of the hospitalizations of infants and young children for diarrhea. Although the mortality rate is quite low because of intravenous rehydration, both the cost and distress are high. It has been estimated that 2 to 7 million children in the United States suffer rotavirus diarrhea each year, which results in 500,000 physician visits, 50,000 hospitalizations, and

$274 million in direct medical costs. In developing countries, rotavirus is devastating, causing over 800,000 deaths per year. In a developing country like Bangladesh, it has been estimated that up to 1% of all children die of rotavirus diarrhea. The disease is widespread around the world, infection being via the fecal-oral route. By the age of 5 years, 95% of children have encountered the virus. Natural immunity develops. Severe diarrhea is rare on second infection. This is interesting, because there are four commonly encountered strains, and so some degree of cross-protection is likely (121). The virus has 11 segments of double-strand RNA, each of which encodes a protein. The outer capsid (against which protection is required) consists of G and P proteins, both of which induce neutralizing antibodies. The 10 known G proteins and the 8 known P proteins of the human virus could theoretically reassort into 80 different serotypes, but only four strains—P8G1, P8G3, P8G4, and P4G2—are globally important. For the future, two nonstructural proteins could emerge as vaccine candidates: a putative enterotoxin NSP4 and the inner capsid protein VP6. Rarer serotypes are not to be entirely neglected and crop up in some surveys.

Early vaccine trials were with a live attenuated bovine rotavirus and were predicated on the view that animal and human rotaviruses shared a common group antigen. Next, a Rhesus rotavirus was tested. These early vaccines gave variable results. Then a Rhesus–human reassortant vaccine was generated by co-infecting cell cultures with a Rhesus rotavirus possessing G serotype 3 and three different human rotaviruses of G serotypes 1, 2, and 4. The three reassortants possessing a Rhesus genetic background but the human capsid protein 1, 2, or 4 were combined with the G3 Rhesus strain to create a tetravalent vaccine. Each of the four viruses was tested at 10^4 and later 10^5 plaque forming units (PFU), vaccine being administered in three oral doses, and the final vaccine submitted for licensure contained 10^5 PFU of each virus, thus 4×10^5 PFU per dose, all told. In clinical trials involving about 10,000 infants, no major adverse events were noted, except one to be discussed. Vaccine efficacy was 48% to 60% in terms of all disease but 61% to 100% against severe disease. In the United States, 80% of very severe episodes and 100% of dehydrating rotavirus illnesses were prevented. The vaccine, produced by Wyeth-Lederle, was duly licensed in August 1998. It was recommended for all children in the United States, to be given orally at 2, 4, and 6 months. By July 1999, 1.5 million doses had been given to 800,000 children.

In the 27 prelicensing trials of candidate rotavirus vaccines, five cases of a rare form of bowel obstruction were noted. In this syndrome, known as intussusception, a portion of bowel prolapses into a more distal portion, and peristalsis propels it further, causing a painful and potentially fatal blockage. The incidence was 0.05%, in comparison with a 0.02% incidence in the placebo control group; this difference did not reach statistical significance but was sufficient to warrant listing in the manufacturer's product insert. In any event, 15 cases of intussusception were reported between September 1998 and July 1999, which led to a suspension of the use of the vaccine. The Centers for Disease Control performed a case–control analysis of 429 infants with intussusception (122) and reached the view that there was an increased risk 3 to 14 days after immunization, particularly after the first dose, and the probability of a causal relationship. They estimated one extra case of intussusception for every 4,670 to 9,474 infants vaccinated. A larger study on 1,450 cases of intussusception in New York State found that the overall incidence of the disease fell from 6.1 cases per 10,000 in 1989 to 3.9 per 10,000 in 1998 (123). Over the 9-month period of rotavirus vaccination, there were 81 cases, in comparison with 78 during the same period in the prevaccination year, which cast doubt on the causal relationship. The most recent figure from the National Immunization Program is 1 in 12,000 "caused" intussusceptions. This is not a huge burden, inasmuch as intussusception is readily treated medically (with an air enema) or surgically, with a case-fatality rate of only 2.1 per 1,000. At the moment, it is not clear whether the risk observed is truly an excess or whether the vaccine was simply triggering intussusception in children who might have had a predisposition for it and in whom it thus might have developed later. It is possible that enlargement of Peyer's patches in the terminal ileum, frequently a leading edge for intussusception, constituted a trigger. In any case, the Wyeth-Lederle vaccine has been withdrawn, and the search for an alternative vaccine is in progress.

Because rotavirus is so much more serious a problem in developing countries, one might well ask whether the vaccine should have been deployed there despite the possible rare complication. Apart from cost, there is a political question here. It would simply not be possible for a Prime Minister of such a country to explain to his or her people that a vaccine deemed to be too dangerous for American children was nevertheless fine for his or her country's children, whatever the logic may be. A fine way out could be a new vaccine actually developed in a developing nation, say in India, China, or Indonesia. Significant effort is currently going into this. Obviously any trial would have to be very large, and thus expensive, to pin the intussusception risk down.

Merck, Inc., together with National Institutes of Health scientists, is developing a tetravalent bovine–human reassortant vaccine with genes coding for G1, G2, G3, and P8. Phase II studies show it to be similar in efficacy to the Wyeth-Lederle vaccine, although it may cause a little less fever. This vaccine has not yet been submitted for licensing.

Several investigators, including Dr. Ruth Bishop, the codiscoverer of the virus, are evaluating so-called nursery strains, isolates from naturally infected, asymptomatic infants in a nursery, that have been further attenuated by growth in tissue culture. Two viruses from India are of special interest. Both strains are safe and immunogenic, but neither causes any vaccine-induced fever. This might indicate less inflammation of Peyer's patches and, therefore, conceivably no intussusception.

Further ideas being explored are parenteral injection of baculovirus-expressed viruslike particles containing structural rotavirus proteins from multiple serotypes; DNA vaccines; or incorporating rotavirus into microspheres for use as an oral mucosal vaccine. Rotavirus genes have also been inserted into Sabin poliovirus and into vaccinia viruses.

The intussusception saga illustrates some of the very real problems in vaccine development. Rare complications can be quite significant when a whole population is the object of study. The more clinical prelicensure work needs to be done, the greater the research and development costs for the manufacturer and the more the pressure to charge a high price. The higher the price, the lower is the likelihood of extensive use in developing nations. Clearly, risk–benefit and cost–benefit analyses will need to form a prominent part of the landscape for the vaccines of the future.

Respiratory Syncytial Virus Vaccine

Respiratory syncytial virus (RSV) is a widespread, highly contagious virus that infects the respiratory tract of infants and young children. In the upper respiratory tract, it causes symptoms of coryza, but danger emerges when it reaches the lower respiratory tract, in which it represents the single most important viral cause of acute infections. Worldwide, it ranks as a major killer; especially in developing countries, it is commonly complicated by bacterial infection, such as with Hib or pneumococci. Children with bronchopulmonary diseases (such as cystic fibrosis), HIV/AIDS, iatrogenic or congenital immunodeficiency, or congenital heart disease and premature infants are at special risk. By 2 years of age, 90% of children have been infected with this virus, and most disease occurs among children between 6 weeks and 6 months of age. Primary infection does not give lifelong immunity, although subsequent infections tend to be less severe. Frail elderly persons constitute another high-risk group. The virus is a frequent cause of the distressing form of wheezing known as croup.

RSV is an enveloped RNA virus of the family Paramyxoviridae; the genome consists of a single, nonsegmented strand of RNA encoding 11 major proteins. Of these, the envelope glycoproteins G (attachment) and F (fusion) are the most important from a vaccine viewpoint because they induce neutralizing antibody. Two strain subgroups, A and B, have been identified, and although subgroup A usually causes more severe disease, a successful vaccine would have to encompass both. The search for a vaccine was substantially set back when a formalin-inactivated whole-virus RSV vaccine investigated in the 1960s actually caused an increased number and increased severity of lower respiratory tract infections on subsequent natural exposure to the virus. One theory holds that this resulted from the vaccine priming for a Th2-type response after exposure to RSV, whereas a Th1 response and CD8$^+$ cytotoxic T cells may be necessary to protect the lower respiratory tract. More recently, efforts to produce a vaccine have been renewed.

One line of work involves a live attenuated vaccine designed to be given intranasally (124). A candidate strain was derived by passaging in heterologous hosts, extensive cold passage in tissue culture followed by chemical mutagenesis and selection of temperature-sensitive mutants. This was found to be greatly attenuated, infectious, immunogenic, and well tolerated, but it caused nasal congestion in 1- to 2-month-old infants. Current efforts involve reverse genetics to introduce further attenuating mutations and deletion of certain genes. Furthermore, F and G envelope genes of subgroup B can be substituted into the attenuated A prototype, creating a second strain with identical attenuation characteristics but the required second subgroup specificity. Early clinical trials have shown that these novel strains are safe and well tolerated.

A second approach involves a subunit vaccine consisting of purified F protein or chimeric FG protein [reviewed by Patel and Simoes (125)]. There have been a number of small clinical trials, including one in children with cystic fibrosis, and the vaccines appear to be safe and immunogenic and do not cause enhanced disease; however, they do not appear to be enormously effective in preventing lower respiratory tract infection. Further clinical trials with QS21 adjuvant are under way, as are preclinical studies of recombinant IL-12. One interesting possibility involves use of the subunit vaccine in women in the third trimester of pregnancy to protect newborn infants. DNA vaccines coding for RSV F or G or both proteins provide good neutralizing antibodies in mice. Vectored vaccines incorporating F or G proteins re also in preclinical research.

One challenge is to find a vaccine that would work in very young infants. Therefore, the work of Siegrist et al. (126) is of special interest. This work involves the recombinant vaccine candidate BBG2Na. The conserved central domain of the G protein of RSV (G2Na) is fused to the albumin-binding region of streptococcal protein G (BB), enhancing *in vivo* exposure time. This is immunogenic in neonatal mice and is currently in phase I clinical trial with the long-range goal of assessing protection of RSV when given to very young infants.

High-risk infants and children can now be helped in another way. The firm MedImmune developed a humanized anti-RSV monoclonal IgG1 antibody, palivizumab (Synagis), that binds to an epitope on the F protein. Given once a month, it has a significant protective effect, lowering hospitalization rates in United States by a factor of about 5. This success of passive immunization is an encouraging sign for the eventual development of a successful vaccine.

Influenza Vaccines

It is easy to underestimate influenza, inasmuch as most attacks in the industrialized countries are self-limited. However, it can be the prelude to fatal pneumonia in elderly patients, and we should never forget the devastation caused by the so-called "swine" flu pandemic in 1918–1919, with between 20 and 40 million deaths. Currently, approximately 200 million doses of influenza vaccine are used annually, and so it is an important vaccine.

The influenza virus is an RNA virus; the genome consists of eight segments of single-strand RNA. The most important antigen for neutralization is the hemagglutinin (HA), one of two dominant surface proteins; antibodies to the other, the neuraminidase, can also be neutralizing. The big problem in influenza immunization is the virus's capacity to change its antigenic type. This happens in two ways. Point mutations in the HA occur with a frequency of $10^{-5.5}$ per generation. These lead to subtle but important changes in HA epitopes. This tendency to mutate away from antibody attack is referred to as *drift*. It means that the antibodies made one winter may not be as effective against the next winter's flu. Accordingly, an elaborate system of monitoring and nomenclature has arisen around the world; several WHO Collaborating Centers are responsible for providing seed lots of vaccine twice a year that reflect the most recent and dominant antigenic types. Influenza viruses also infect animals, such as pigs and horses; birds, such as geese, ducks, and chickens; and marine mammals. There are 15 distinct HA types in influenza A, and only some are infectious for humans. There are nine distinct neuraminidase types, only some of which occur in humans. Thus, influenza A viruses are frequently referred to by their serotype (e.g., H3N1). Influenza B virus is also highly adapted to humans. This virus has no subtypes, and the infections on the whole tend to be less severe.

The segmented nature of the viral genome and the existence of a variety of animal hosts makes for the possibility of co-infection of cells with human-adapted and animal-adapted strains, in turn leading to the emergence of novel strains with the sudden appearance of a new antigenic subtype. Such a major change is referred to as antigenic *shift*. There may be little or no cross-reactivity with antibody provoked by previously circulating strains. The stage is then set for a major pandemic. In the twentieth century, there were three such pandemics: the so-called swine flu of 1918–1919, the "Asian" flu of 1957, and the "Hong Kong" flu of 1969. The latter two pandemics killed an estimated 1 million people each, older adults accounting for the great majority of deaths. It would appear that the risk for such reassortants is greatest in areas where humans and animals such as pigs (or birds such as chickens) live in close contact. History suggests about three pandemics per century.

Just to illustrate how real and present the danger for a shift variant is, consider the 1997 outbreak of H5N1 influenza in Hong Kong. This chicken influenza killed thousands of birds and also infected a total of 18 people, all closely involved in chicken husbandry. Six of these people died in spite of modern medical care. Imagine if a virus with this 33% case-fatality rate had acquired the capacity to spread from human to human, easily possible with further reassortments. The authorities promptly killed more than 1 million chickens, at great economic cost, and thus averted further disaster. The probable sequence here was goose to duck to chicken to human. Ducks certainly represent a serious reservoir. Hong Kong is closely monitoring flu viruses in wild birds and commercial poultry.

The standard influenza vaccine consists of formalin-inactivated whole virus, still grown in fertile hen's eggs and frequently rendered less reactogenic by "splitting" through ether or detergent treatment. The adjuvant used is alum; in Italy, a vaccine incorporating MF59 adjuvant is registered. The standard vaccine is reasonably effective, but protection is of short duration. A typical study resulted in 53% prevention of infection and 68% prevention of deaths in a population of persons older than 65 years. Helpful though such a vaccine is, the search for better vaccines is lively.

Obvious areas to explore are live attenuated vaccines and mucosal administration. These are combined in the efforts of Aviron with their preparation FluMist. Cold-adapted viruses, initially developed in the University of Michigan, are produced in specific pathogen-free eggs, and a trivalent preparation consisting of 2A and 1B strains has been delivered to volunteers via a nasal spray–syringe delivery system. When given once, it has been proved safe and effective in a number of clinical studies. The largest trial achieved 93% efficacy in the first year and 100% efficacy against strains included in the vaccine and 86% against the emergent mismatched strain A/Sydney/05/97 (H3N2) in the second year. If the vaccine passes certain U.S. Food and Drug Administration–mandated safety tests, which are just about completed at the time of writing, it should be licensed, possibly by the time this volume appears.

The intranasal virosomal influenza vaccine of Glück has already been mentioned in the section on adjuvants. This is a subunit vaccine prepared by extracting HA and neuraminidase from influenza virus and incorporating it into the membranes of liposomes composed of phosphatidylcholine, with *E. coli* heat-labile toxin as a mucosal adjuvant. Administered intranasally, it produces protective anti-HA antibody titers. This vaccine has been used fairly widely in Switzerland. Another interesting approach, promoted by CSL, Ltd. (127), involves intranasal administration of influenza vaccines in ISCOMS. This has proved protective in preclinical studies, and early clinical trials have shown faster antibody production, good CD8$^+$ T-cell responses, and excellent T helper responses. There seems little doubt that one or more of these newer approaches will provide a better vaccine than the current one, in which case one could foresee flu vaccines being much more widely used.

Prophylactic Vaccines against Human Immunodeficiency Virus

The HIV-1 has developed some devilishly clever strategies to foil the human immune response. It exhibits an astonishing rate of mutation, particularly in the portion of its envelope protein that is involved in infectivity, allowing the virus to escape the antibody response. It finds several levels of "safe haven" refuges unreachable by antibodies: for example, persistence within macrophages and dendritic cells or penetration into the brain. Furthermore, integration of provirus DNA into the host cell genome, with no external evidence of the

virus's presence, represents an escape resistant to CTL attack. It targets the first lymphocyte in the immune cascade, the CD4$^+$ T cell, which may delay an effective immune response and will certainly facilitate the disastrous upsurge in viral load late in the disease, because T-cell levels fall so low that resistance essentially disappears. It has an extraordinarily high rate of replication. We now know that the immune system is a pitched battleground from the first entry of the virus. Large numbers of CD4$^+$ lymphocytes are infected, die, and are replaced. CD8$^+$ CTLs help to control the early infection and bring the virus load down to one thousandth of the peak level, but the repeated cycle of infection and death of CD4$^+$ cells and CD8$^+$ cell activation to control infected cell numbers continues (128). In fact, the degree to which the virus load can be driven down is an important prognostic factor. At the same time, high rates of HIV replication continue in lymphatic tissues.

The global research community can hardly be accused of indolence with regard to HIV/AIDS vaccines. Serious preclinical work has been done on about 100 candidate vaccines, and, in the United States alone, 27 of these progressed to early clinical trials between 1987 and 1999 in 52 preventive vaccine studies involving 3,000 people. Since then, the number has expanded still further. All in all, collaboration among the academic community, governmental funding agencies, the philanthropic sector, and industry has been good, although one could argue that the industry input could have been more intense and focused.

Early attempts to develop an AIDS vaccine followed the classical path of seeking to induce antibodies to the most prominent antigens on the viral surface: namely, the envelope (*env*) glycoproteins gp160 or the products it yields, the exterior viral protein gp120, and the transmembrane glycoprotein gp41. The first part of this review goes into some detail about *env* interactions with the target cell surface and makes the point that "all is not lost" with regard to antibody as a possible component of anti-HIV defense. The second part, however, reveals that many investigators believe that a robust T-cell response, particularly of HIV-specific CD8$^+$ CTLs, is a more critical component of the host response, particularly after a decision taken in 1994 not to go ahead with a large phase III trial of gp160 or gp120. This decision was made because of two unfortunate findings from phase II trials of recombinant *env* antigens. First, the data showed a small number of "breakthrough" infections despite immunization; second, antibodies engendered by immunization, although capable of neutralizing HIV grown in transformed T-cell lines, were much less effective against freshly isolated virus grown in peripheral blood mononuclear cells. This led to a period of pessimism about envelope-based vaccines and serum antibodies, which might turn out to be somewhat premature. Nevertheless, most investigators now believe that an ideal vaccine should engender effective defense by both T and B cells.

Since those early days, we have learned a great deal about the details of how HIV infects its target cells. After cleavage of gp160, gp120 and gp41 are assembled into oligomeric spikes and remain noncovalently associated on the viral surface. These heteromeric spikes facilitate viral entry by the sequential binding of gp120 to the primary viral receptor, CD4, and subsequently to one of two co-receptors, CCR5 and CXCR-4. These co-receptors are members of the chemokine receptor family. They are seven-transmembrane G protein–coupled receptors. A small subset of viruses can use other seven-transmembrane domain receptors as well.

It is believed that gp120 undergoes an allosteric conformational change involving displacement of the V1/V2 loop after binding to CD4. This permits high-affinity binding of gp120 to the chemokine co-receptors through amino acids in the V3 loop and the C4 region. Then a further conformational change leads to insertion of a hydrophobic amino-terminal fusion peptide of gp41 into the target cell membrane. Cross-linking through gp41 finally results in membrane fusion and viral entry.

Crystal structure studies have shown that the CD4-binding domain of gp120 is somewhat recessed and, moreover, that heavy glycosylation may further help create a barrier to the entry of antibodies to the actual binding site. This has led to attempts to create a more effective recombinant immunogen through deletions of amino acids in the V1 and V2 loops. Furthermore, selective removal of carbohydrate groups is a helpful stratagem in an SIV model. Both the actual CD4-binding area of gp120 and the fusion-inducing area of gp41 are more conserved between viral subtypes than are the more immunodominant V loops. Indeed, if highly conserved, functionally important portions of envelope proteins were used as immunogens, HIV sequence diversity might not represent an absolute obstacle to the eventual development of broadly protective HIV vaccines.

HIV-1 virus tropism depends, *inter alia,* on co-receptor utilization (129). Strains that can infect primary T cells and macrophages, known as R5 or M-tropic viruses, use CCR5, whereas strains that can infect primary cells and transformed T-cell lines, known as T-tropic or X4 viruses, use CXCR4. In addition, many virus strains are dual-tropic (i.e., R5X4). R5 viruses tend to be mainly involved in transmission and the early phases of infection, whereas R5X4 viruses are found mainly in the later stages of the disease. To emphasize the importance of CCR5, the 1% of white persons who are homozygous for a polymorphism resulting in failure to transport CCR5 to the cell surface are highly resistant to HIV-1 infection.

In view of the extremely high mutation rates of RNA viruses in general and HIV-1 in particular, the classification and nomenclature of HIV isolates is somewhat of a nightmare. More than 170 HIV strains have been subjected to full-length genome sequencing, and at least 200 times more than that have been subjected to sequencing of the C2V3 segment of gp120. HIV-1 is divided into groups M, N, and O, and group M is further divided into subtypes or classes. Some newer data have allowed the recognition that subtypes B and D of group M should have been classified as a single subtype

and that a new subtype, found most commonly in Senegal, should be added as subtype L. Moreover, intersubtype recombination is frequent, and circulating recombinant forms can be very prevalent in some countries. Currently, the subtypes A, B+D, C, E, F, G, H, J, K, and L and the circulating recombinant forms AB, AE, AG, and BC are widely recognized, although this nomenclature is sure to change again.

Correlation between these HIV genotypes and immunotypes remains controversial. Clearly, we face a complex matrix of partial cross-reactivities in both humoral and cellular responses, and at present some authors prefer the idea of diffuse immunotypes with the highest cross-reactivity to different isolates from the same subtype and weaker cross-reactivity as genetic distance increases, whereas others favor the progressive identification of discrete immunotypes, each of which might contain several genotypes. The argument depends very much on which antigen or portion of an antigen is the focus of interest. There is certainly no straightforward correlation between genetic subtypes of HIV and *in vitro* virus neutralization pattern.

A great deal of work has been done on the antibodies of HIV-infected individuals to see whether and when antibodies capable of neutralizing primary isolates appear. The suggestion has come forward that the presence of neutralizing antibodies of sufficiently broad specificity may indicate a more favorable prognosis. Neutralizing antibodies tend not to appear before 6 to 8 months after infection, and the response subsequently broadens. Not surprisingly, the breadth of neutralizing activity induced by a subtype-specific immunization is less than that of antibodies from individuals. Nevertheless, some vaccines display significant cross-reactivities, leaving open the possibility that a defined mixture of immunogens might lead to a broadly protective vaccine.

The firm VaxGen is preparing a recombinant gp120 vaccine, AIDSVAX, for a phase III clinical trial. This is in accordance with studies suggesting that bivalent, dual-specificity *env* vaccines presented as oligomeric preparations could induce antibodies capable of neutralizing both R5 and X4 viruses. Two large, randomized, double-blind, placebo-controlled trials are under way. The first involves two largely non–cross-reactive B subtype *env* proteins. It is being conducted in 5,400 men who have sex with men or female professional sex workers at 61 clinical sites in North America. This trial was fully enrolled in October 1999. With an annual infection rate of about 1.5% in this population, the results should be available in early 2003. The second involves a bivalent subtype B/subtype E formulation and is being tested in Thailand in 17 clinical trial sites, the subjects being intravenous drug users. Because the annual infection rate is about 6% in such a population, 2,500 was deemed an adequate enrollment, and this was completed in August 2000. Results should be available in late 2003.

A lively discussion at the time of writing concerns the question of two further trials involving VaxGen's gp120 as a boost after Aventis Pasteur's canarypox-based priming regimen involving gene constructs for *gag, env,* and protease together with, in one case, *pol* and *nef* (130). The problem is that these two trials together would involve 27,000 subjects and cost at least U.S. $95 million, some of this necessarily being taxpayers' money. Final decisions are expected early in 2002.

There are good reasons to believe that CD8$^+$ T cells play a critical role in the control of HIV. Relevant findings include a close correlation between CTL appearance and a fall in virus levels in HIV-1–infected Rhesus macaque monkeys and the detection of significant numbers of HIV-specific CTLs in a variety of seronegative individuals at high risk, such as babies born to HIV-positive mothers, a small proportion of female African professional sex workers, and a proportion of subjects with needlestick injuries. Among seropositive individuals, those who do not progress or progress slowly to AIDS have robust CTL responses. In view of this evidence, it is important to include in a vaccine virally encoded proteins produced in the cytosol of the infected cell, so that peptide fragments of such proteins could be presented at the surface of the infected cell in association with class I MHC molecules. Furthermore, it would be advantageous to use adjuvants or other techniques known to favor CD8$^+$ T-cell production. Use of a multiplicity of antigens might counteract mutations occurring in any single component within the virus-infected cells that should be eliminated. Finally, a procedure evoking mucosal as well as lymph node and splenic CTLs would be ideal.

In a resurgent and now well-financed AIDS vaccine effort, a large number of antigens or genes for antigens have been the subject of intensive research. These include *env, gag, pol, nef, rev, tat,* and HIV protease. Furthermore, an incredible variety of vector systems has been included in preclinical research. Among these are vaccinia; vaccinia modified to be less aggressive (e.g., MVA); avipox viruses, including canarypox and fowlpox; and (although less frequently) other viruses, including recombinant avirulent poliovirus, mengovirus, herpesvirus, Venezuelan equine encephalitis virus, Semliki Forest virus, adenovirus, and influenza virus. Possible bacterial vectors include *Salmonella*, BCG, *Shigella, Listeria,* and *Lactobacillus.* Many of these have been through a variety of animal models of protection with a measure of success.

Among the 100 or so vaccine candidates, there is no doubt that the prime-boost strategies described earlier hold pride of place (131–133). Increasing use is being made of a sophisticated macaque monkey model of AIDS with viral constructs known as SHIV. This is a genetically engineered hybrid between HIV and SIV, which causes a disease similar in many ways to HIV/AIDS in humans. The SHIV virus possesses an HIV envelope and an SIV core.

There is by now substantial literature on virtually every conceivable variation on this prime-boost scheme, with many preclinical successes. A constant undercurrent in the literature is strong CD8$^+$ CTLs as a signpost of promise. Among the many additions to prime-boost strategies, a recurring theme is either strong adjuvants accompanying particularly a

protein boost or co-administration of cytokine gene expression cassettes with DNA immunogens.

Some other quite novel approaches are also being developed. For example, it has been possible to "freeze" the fusion conjugate of HIV *env* with its receptor and co-receptor, and this mixture induces antibodies capable of neutralizing a wide diversity of HIV strains, presumably because the newly exposed antigenic determinants of *env* are relatively conserved.

It has been hypothesized that the configuration of antigenic determinants that is displayed by HIV at the moment of fusion of HIV *env* with both the receptor and the co-receptor must be relatively well conserved between clades. Attempts to capture this configuration—for example, by fixing the fusion conjugate—are under way.

A mucosal approach is also being pursued in a variety of ways. Mucosal surfaces are a major natural route of HIV entry, and protection through the mucosal immune system would therefore be valuable. Berzofsky et al. (134) have long been championing the idea of a multideterminant peptide vaccine comprising epitopes for both T helper cells and CTLs. The mucosal study (135) focused on the antigens *env, pol,* and *gag,* using *env* from HIV and *pol* and *gag* from SIV. The study design involved macaque monkeys and a challenge with virulent SHIV intrarectally. The investigators compared two vaccine approaches: a subcutaneous injection with Montanide ISA51 as an adjuvant versus intrarectal inoculation of the vaccine with a mutant heat-labile *E. coli* toxin as a mucosal adjuvant. The latter provided significantly better protection, because (at least in part) of a strong intestinal mucosal CTL response. This group is also exploring the concept of epitope enhancement: that is, slightly modifying T helper cell epitope sequences in order to increase epitope affinity for class II MHC. This results in more effective helper T cells and also more CTLs (136). It must be remembered, however, that appropriate systemic immunization can also raise enough CTLs to protect against rectal challenge. For example, a prime-boost regimen consisting of priming with a cytokine-augmented DNA vaccine and boosting with a recombinant MVA construct, each vaccine containing multiple viral antigens, completely protected against intrarectal SHIV challenge in the same macaque model.

Although many preclinical studies have been encouraging, the picture for human studies is not quite so rosy. Of course, in the absence of clear-cut correlates of protection, no definitive verdict can be given, but it is widely assumed that a potent CTL response is important. So far, most virus vector priming–protein-boosting regimens have given HIV-specific CTL responses in only one third to one half of volunteer subjects. It is urgent to get more vaccine candidates into clinical trial; in that regard, two generously funded United States–based initiatives are to be commended: the AIDS Vaccine Evaluation Group of the National Institute for Allergy and Infectious Diseases, and the nongovernmental International Aids Vaccine Initiative, initially spun out of the Rockefeller Foundation. Both bodies are seeking to accelerate the pathway of the most promising basic research into sponsored clinical trials.

The author has been tempted into a largely optimistic overview of the landscape, but the formidable problems remaining before a prophylactic vaccine emerges should not be underestimated. Perhaps the greatest practical problem in HIV vaccine research is where to go after encouraging phase 1 and 2 studies. Large prophylactic studies are horrendously expensive. Results would be most rapidly obtained in developing countries because of the high rate of carriage, but such trials are beset with practical and ethical problems. Practically, will it be possible to conduct trials the results of which meet U.S. Food and Drug Administration standards? Ethically, will it be possible to give trial participants sufficient safe sex education? Will it be possible to guarantee to developing country governments that, if the trial in which their citizens have taken part is successful, the relevant vaccine will be made available to the population at an affordable price? Clearly, the eventual development of a successful vaccine remains an immense scientific and humanitarian challenge.

Therapeutic Human Immunodeficiency Virus Vaccines

Because AIDS is the end result of a lengthy pitched battle between HIV and the human host's immune defenses, it is legitimate to ask whether an HIV vaccine has a role to play not in prophylaxis but in therapy, particularly during the long latent period during which the subject is seropositive but clinically well. This question becomes more urgent in a sense now that the prognosis for seropositive individuals is so much better because of highly active antiretroviral therapy (HAART). There is a beguiling logic to the idea that drug therapy should knock the virus load down to a very low level, after which immunotherapy finishes the job. Conceptually, the issues are somewhat similar to those in cancer immunotherapy. That said, the amount of clinical work that has been done on therapeutic vaccines is very small. Phase I and phase II trials have shown augmented T helper and CTL responses but not yet clear-cut evidence of clinical benefit. In animal models, there are some promising data demonstrating synergy between chemotherapy and therapeutic vaccination. The one sizable clinical study is with the candidate therapeutic vaccine Remune, which is based on inactivated, gp120-depleted, whole HIV virions. Postinfection immunization induced T helper cell responses that cross-reacted to several subtypes of HIV-1. There was also some stimulation of β-chemokines and a down-regulation of CCR-5 receptors on T cells. Clinical efficacy of this candidate is under investigation. A small prime-boost clinical trial with canarypox vector priming and gp160 boosting involving a substantial cocktail of antigens showed promising results in terms of viral load reduction in 10 patients identified early after acute infection.

An ancillary role of therapeutic vaccination might be to strengthen HIV-specific immunity in patients in whom the antigenic load has fallen so far because of HAART that the risk of rebound resurgence of viral multiplication upon cessation or interruption of therapy is major. Indeed, there have been some protagonists of the idea that there should be structured treatment interruptions, which would result in a viral rebound, which in turn would provide a kind of autoimmunization with boosting of flagging anti-HIV responses. To the degree that this idea has validity, it should be possible to design less dangerous antigenic boosters not involving actual living and virulent virus.

In broad terms, the candidates that have come forward as possible therapeutic vaccines do not, on the whole, differ from those aiming at primary prophylaxis. If there is a difference, it is an even increased emphasis on the importance of CTL stimulation.

It is impossible to conclude an analysis of HIV vaccines without stressing the need to make a successful candidate available to the developing countries with a minimum of delay. There are more than 35 million people living with HIV/AIDS, 95% of them in developing countries, with 6 million new infections each year and nearly 3 million deaths annually (2.3 million in 1998). Students of this volume should keep a good watch on a new program that has the personal backing of the Secretary-General of the United Nations, Nobel Laureate Kofi Annan. It is the Global Fund for AIDS, Malaria and Tuberculosis, targeted primarily at control within African and other poor developing countries. Although drugs will undoubtedly be important, vaccines will be essential for true global control.

VACCINES AGAINST PARASITIC DISEASES

If viruses and bacteria have evolved elaborate strategies to defeat the vertebrate immune system, parasites, with their much larger complement of DNA, possess an even wider and more diverse range. Although no vaccine against any human parasitic disease has been licensed, the feasibility of such vaccines has been demonstrated in the veterinary field, in which a range of successful vaccines is in use to deal with both protozoan and metazoan infestations. The difficulty of overcoming all the necessary hurdles for human vaccines is evidenced by the fact that since the mid-1970s, some of the best minds in vaccinology have applied themselves to the problem, but only in malaria has one vaccine moved to the stage of phase III trials, and that with dubious success. Nevertheless, parasitism is so important from a public health viewpoint, and the progress in understanding of parasite molecular biology and genetics so significant, that the research effort must continue. Moreover, the progressive resistance of some parasites to chemotherapy and of vectors to insecticides highlights the importance of vaccines for disease control.

Malaria Vaccines

Malaria is the most prevalent vector-borne disease in the world. It is caused by protozoa of four species of *Plasmodium*.

It threatens 2 billion people in 90 countries and causes approximately 500 million clinical cases and 2 million deaths per year. Overwhelmingly, the worst continent for malaria is Africa, where 90% of the deaths occur, chiefly in children younger than 5 years. *P. falciparum* is by far the most dangerous of the four species that affect humans, and cerebral malaria, in which parasitized erythrocytes develop cytoadherence antigens and block up cerebral arterioles, is the most prominent cause of death. It is known that antibodies can be therapeutic, and the hope that a vaccine will eventually be developed is sustained by the observation that inhabitants of endemic areas eventually become relatively immune to attacks, although this immunity is not sterilizing, small quantities of parasites being left in the host.

The next most important species is *Plasmodium vivax,* famous for attacks that can recur long after exposure. From a practical point of view, a vaccine that could protect against both *P. falciparum* and *P. vivax* would have much to commend it. Industry could then charge highly for a traveler's vaccine in industrialized countries. However, the preclinical research is being pursued separately for the two species with a heavy concentration on the bigger killer.

In view of the considerable amount of research that has been done, it is legitimate to ask why no effective malaria vaccine yet exists. This involves both theoretical and practical considerations. The best vaccines are for diseases in which nature provides solid immunity if an individual survives a first attack. This is not the case in malaria, in which immunity in endemic areas is tenuous at best and easily lost if the individual leaves to live in a malaria-free country. Clearly, the parasite has evolved powerful strategies to evade the host immune response. From a practical viewpoint, the parasite is difficult to grow; *P. falciparum* requires human blood, and *P. vivax* does not even replicate *in vitro* in red blood cells. Investigators are thus driven to recombinant DNA technology with all of the difficulties of choice of antigen among hundreds of candidates and correct refolding of every candidate. Add to this the fact that no animal model is a really good imitation of the human disease, and the difficulties for the investigator mount.

Among the evolutionary strategies of the parasite, two stand out. The first is high mutability in most of the antigens that have been studied, resulting in extensive allelic polymorphism, so that multiple forms of the antigen exist in the parasite population as a whole, which presumably reflects selection of mutants because parental forms are eliminated by antibody. Second, a very key antigen of *P. falciparum,* the so-called *P. falciparum* erythrocyte membrane protein 1 (PfEMP1), which is prominent on the surface of infected red blood cells, is represented in the genome by approximately 50 variant copies (137). As a clone of parasites emerges and reaches a sufficient size to strongly signal the immune system, eliminating most parasites, a variant expressing a different PfEMP1 arises, grows, reaches a critical size, and in turn is eliminated by antibody, and so the cycle repeats itself until, eventually, immunity to all the forms of PfEMP1 is achieved.

Life Cycle of **Plasmodium falciparum**

With these preliminary considerations out of the way, we should now look at the parasite's life cycle (with *P. falciparum* as the model) in order to determine where the different points of attack might be. Figure 6 shows this schematically. Invasion of the human is initiated when the female anopheline mosquito bites the human subject, thereby injecting a mobile form known as a sporozoite into the skin. The dominant surface antigen of the sporozoite is the CS, first identified by the Nussenzweigs (138) in the early 1980s and cloned soon thereafter. This candidate vaccine antigen has been the subject of intensive research. The sporozoite rapidly and efficiently invades hepatocytes. Two to ten sporozoites can initiate infection within 5 to 30 minutes, probably involving an interaction between CS and the glycosaminoglycan chains of heparin sulfate proteoglycans (139). A second sporozoite surface protein, the thrombospondin-related adhesion protein (TRAP), has a region highly homologous to a part of CS and is probably also involved in binding to hepatocyte heparin sulfate proteoglycans. TRAP is required for sporozoite mobility and infectivity.

Within the hepatocyte, each sporozoite develops into a schizont containing 10,000 to 30,000 merozoites. Over this period, the hepatocyte presents on its surface peptides from

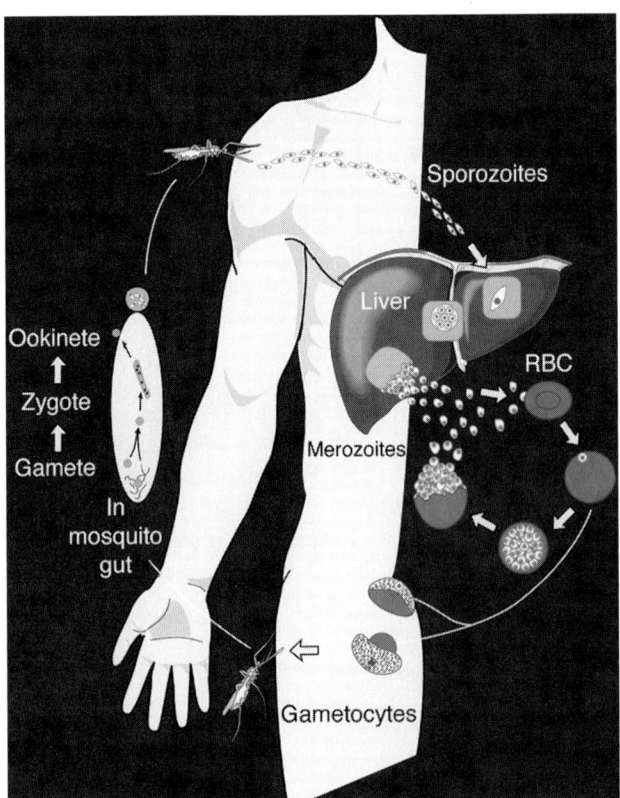

FIG. 6. The life cycle of *Plasmodium falciparum.* A vaccine might eventually include antigens/epitopes from all four stages: sporozoites, liver cell surface T-cell epitopes, merozoites, and gametocytes.

a number of pre-erythrocytic stage proteins. A CD8$^+$ cytotoxic T-cell attack on infected liver cells could materially lower the number of merozoites formed and thus lessen the attack on erythrocytes. As long as the parasite is confined to the liver, there are no clinical symptoms of malaria. Within 10 days or less, the liver schizont ruptures, and the merozoites are released and begin to invade erythrocytes, there to undergo another asexual amplification. The erythrocytic cycle is responsible for disease manifestation, inasmuch as development, rupture, and re-invasion initiate a vicious cycle (Fig. 7).

Merozoite invasion of erythrocytes is a complex process involving multiple steps. The merozoite attaches to the erythrocyte, reorients itself so that its apical end faces the red blood cell, after which a tight junction develops, and parasite organelles known as rhoptries discharge their contents onto the red blood cell membrane. A progressively deeper vacuole forms and eventually closes to surround the engulfed parasite. The best studied erythrocyte surface receptor for a parasite ligand is the Duffy blood group antigen for *P. vivax*. In contrast, *P. falciparum* seems capable of using multiple pathways for invasion, including sialic acids on glycophorins A, B, and C, as well as peptide sequences on glycophorins. As for the parasite ligands, a Duffy binding-like (DBL) superfamily has been defined. For *P. vivax*, the most important member is a 140-kDa Duffy-binding protein (PvDBP) (140) and for *P. falciparum*, EBA-175 appears to be the prototype. But additional merozoite proteins play a role in invasion, inasmuch as quite a number of monoclonal antibodies against them can block invasion *in vitro*. These include various merozoite surface proteins (MSPs) and proteins translocated from the apical organelles, the rhoptries and the micronemes, to the surface before invasion.

An important event in clinical malaria is the adherence of infected erythrocytes to vascular endothelium. When this occurs in small vessels in the brain, blockage can follow, resulting in cerebral malaria and death. The chief molecular mediator of cytoadherence is the variant surface antigen

PfEMP1, as already mentioned (137). The receptors for adherence are various and include CD36, intracellular adhesion molecule 1, vascular cell adhesion molecule 1, E-selectin, and chondroitin sulfate A.

In addition to producing merozoites, the erythrocytic cycle is also responsible for the production of the sexual forms known as gametocytes. These are taken up by the mosquito and mature into gametes. A vaccine capable of producing antigametocyte antibodies could destroy them in the blood of the vaccinee or could interfere with their maturation in the mosquito, or both. The life cycle of the parasite is, of course, completed in the mosquito, in which sexual union occurs, sporozoites emerge from mature oocysts 10 to 14 days after an infective blood meal, and invasion of salivary glands occurs soon thereafter.

Possible Vaccine Approaches

Because of the complexity of this life cycle, many observers believe that a final malaria vaccine will contain key molecules from various and perhaps all stages. However, it is necessary to consider the best candidates from each stage in turn. Much knowledge has accumulated since the early 1980s [reviewed by Doolan and Hoffman (141) and Good et al. (142)].

The sporozoite stage is an attractive target, inasmuch as a 100% effective vaccine would prevent infection completely and a partially effective one would lower the eventual invasive merozoite burden. Like most malarial antigens, the CS presents as dominant-antigen multiple tandem repeats, in this case of the sequence NANP, which can absorb a large proportion of the anti-CS antibodies both of the serum of patients and of CS (or irradiated sporozoite) immunized persons. However, early attempts to gain protection by using this epitope proved disappointing. Although there was at first great excitement about a vaccine developed by Patarroyo et al. (143) known as SPf66, which was a multipeptide vaccine that included epitopes from both CS and blood-stage antigens, this failed to protect in hyperendemic areas and is not proceeding further. A more promising area is the vaccine known as RTS,S, given with the adjuvant AS02 (144). RTS,S is a fusion protein of the carboxy-terminal half of CS (which includes both part of the tandem repeat, thus R, and also important T-cell epitopes, thus T) fused to the HBsAg. This is coexpressed in yeast with (nonfused) HBsAg (thus, S), which self-assembles into virionlike structures, aiding immunogenicity. The adjuvant AS02, already described, has strong T and B cell–stimulatory properties. In a human challenge model, this significantly protected malaria-naïve volunteers, although immunity was of short duration. In a field study in a rural area of The Gambia involving 306 men aged 18 to 45 years, the vaccine was safe and well-tolerated although fairly reactogenic, evoked strong anti-CS antibody and T-cell responses, and clearly gave partial protection in that it significantly delayed *P. falciparum* infection and reduced symptomatic malaria. Again, immunity waned rather quickly, but some immunological memory resulted,

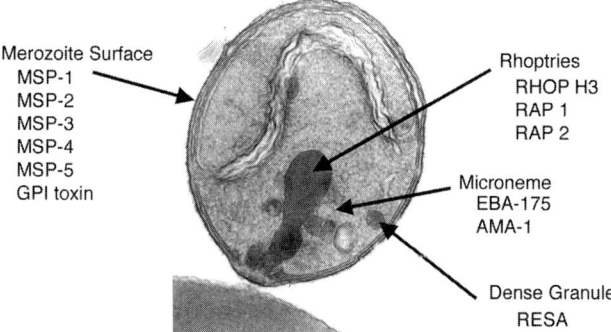

FIG. 7. Transmission electron micrograph of a merozoite invading an erythrocyte. Note electron-dense material at the attachment site, possibly representing proteins secreted by the rhoptries or the micronemes. Merozoite surface antigens are further obvious candidate vaccine antigens.

inasmuch as a booster dose given the following year reduced the incidences of infection and of symptomatic malaria. It is now planned to assess this vaccine in children.

There is a plethora of blood stage antigens at various stages of testing. The subject of the largest amount of work has been the protein MSP-1, a 195-kDa major merozoite protein, and various fragments of it. Considerable protective efficacy has been shown in murine and simian vaccine trials, although in the human the highly polymorphic nature of this antigen may prove problematic. Efforts are being directed toward defining conserved protective epitopes of MSP-1. Other significant merozoite surface candidates are MSP-2, MSP-3, MSP-4, and MSP-5. The combination 4/5 looks attractive because it is relatively less polymorphic (145).

As noted, rhoptry-associated proteins (RAPs) perform as yet ill-defined tasks in merozoite invasion of erythrocytes. The antigens RAP-1 and RAP-2 show less polymorphism and have been partially successful in a Saimiri monkey model. The apical merozoite antigen 1 (AMA-1) is strongly protective in murine and simian trials, has been in phase I human trials, and is in continuing clinical development (146). Because this antigen has 16 conserved cysteine residues and exhibits a three-domain structure, correct refolding after expression is essential and presents a challenge.

In view of the importance of the initial docking events involving PvDBP for *P. vivax* and EBA-175 for *P. falciparum,* these represent further interesting candidates. For PvDBP, the cysteine-rich amino-terminal region II is conserved and constitutes the receptor-binding domain. This fragment, PvRII, when correctly refolded, represents an interesting *P. vivax* candidate. The same may be true for a homologous region of EBA-175.

Although the highly variant surface antigen family PfEMP1, which mediates cytoadherence, also exhibits Duffy binding-like domains, it remains to be determined whether there is enough conservation in the RII domain for a polypeptide vaccine to hold promise.

Sexual Stage Vaccines

Sexual stage vaccines would not protect the individual vaccinee but could have profound effects at the community level if widely deployed. Antibodies to gametocytes, gametes, or ookinetes could prevent development of sporozoites within the mosquito. Such transmission-blocking vaccines would have to be combined with other pre-erythrocytic or erythrocytic stage vaccines. One gametocyte-derived protein, Pfs25, looks promising in preclinical models, and other antigens are under development.

Deoxyribonucleic Acid Vaccines, Prime-Boost Strategies, and Combination Approaches

There is considerable evidence that T cells are importantly involved in immunity to malaria, and this has led to efforts for a DNA vaccine and prime-boost strategies. A group at Oxford University led by A. V. S. Hill has systematically exam-

ined various immunization regimens against a CS-derived, liver stage–expressed CD8[+] T-cell epitope in a *Plasmodium berghei* murine model (147). Best results for protection against sporozoite challenge were obtained with DNA priming followed by boosting with MVA in which both the naked plasmid and the MVA contained inserted sequences coding for a string of CD8[+] T-cell epitopes or the full CS. Priming with yeast-derived Ty virus–like particles (Ty VLPs) carrying the inserted sequence and boosting with recombinant MVA also worked well, but the reverse-sequence MVA followed by Ty VLPs was totally ineffective. Repeated immunization with Ty VLPs alone, naked plasmid DNA alone, or recombinant MVA alone was also of little effect, showing the power of the prime-boost approach. Now the group is exploring the polyepitope string fused to the TRAP gene, or CS-TRAP combination.

A group formerly headed by S. L. Hoffman has explored DNA immunization against 15 well-characterized *P. falciparum* antigens, five pre-erythrocytic stage proteins expressed in infected hepatocytes, and 10 blood stage antigens. The project has been entitled MuStDO, for *Multi*stage *Malaria DNA-based Vaccine Operation* (141). Phase I clinical trials of DNA vaccines containing some of these genes proved to be safe and well tolerated, and some T-cell responses were obtained, but the results were suboptimal. Accordingly, several stratagems to enhance the immune response are under way. These include prime-boost, using priming with DNA, and boosting with either recombinant poxvirus or with purified recombinant proteins in various adjuvants. Furthermore, codon-optimized versions of DNA more closely resembling human genes are being prepared, and the addition of plasmids expressing cytokines such as GM-CSF, co-stimulatory molecules, or chemokines is being studied.

The Australian group is exploring various combinations of blood stage antigens in subjects in Papua New Guinea. The combination MSP-1/MSP-2/RESA looked promising in phase II studies, and further trials involving AMA-1 and RAP-2 are planned for 2002.

Antidisease Vaccines: Glycophosphatidylinositol Toxin of Malaria as a New Candidate Vaccine Molecule

An imaginative new approach to malaria immunization is being investigated by Schofield (148). This is predicated on the idea that much of the pathological processes in malaria result from an inflammatory cascade initiated by a malarial toxin. GPI of parasite origin is the candidate and an oligosaccharide of the *P. falciparum* GPI glycan was synthesized, conjugated to a protein carrier, and injected into mice, together with Freund's adjuvant. This protocol substantially reduced severe pathological processes, cerebral malaria, and mortality in a *P. berghei* challenge model. There is also evidence that GPIs are the dominant proinflammatory molecules of *Trypanosoma cruzi* and *Trypanosoma brucei.* They constitute tumor necrosis factor, IL-1, and nitric oxide–inducing molecules in diverse parasite systems.

The Gates Malaria Vaccine Initiative

The analysis just described, which is by no means exhaustive, shows that the malaria vaccine field fairly bristles with promise. A critical block has been the capacity to take candidate molecules that look interesting on the basis of preclinical research to phase I and phase II clinical trials. Therefore, a new Malaria Vaccine Initiative funded by the Bill and Melinda Gates Foundation and directed by Dr. Regina Rabinovich is highly welcome. It will fund the preparation of vaccine pilot lots in accordance with Good Manufacturing Practice criteria, improve facilities for clinical and field trials, and provide coordination and cooperation between various major groups, thus optimizing their potential. This is not to deny the many hurdles that must still be overcome before this badly needed vaccine emerges.

Leishmaniasis Vaccines

Leishmania parasites are vector-borne protozoa that cause a variety of serious diseases that, together, represent a formidable global public health problem, affecting about 12 million people. Six *Leishmania* species are pathogenic for humans: *L. donovani, L. major, L. tropica, L. aethiopica, L. braziliensis,* and *L. mexicana.* In general, some species (e.g., *L. major*) are chiefly involved with skin lesions, whereas others (e.g. *L. donovani,* which invades the liver, spleen, and bone marrow, causing the serious disease kala azar) migrate chiefly to visceral organs. However, the distinction is by no means absolute. Strains normally confined to the skin occasionally invade the viscera, and in some patients with kala azar, the skin can become a target. Mucocutaneous leishmaniasis is well recognized and can cause extensive disfigurement. Moreover, subclinical infection is frequent: The individual has no symptoms, but disease flares up when T cells fail, as in AIDS. As with HIV and tuberculosis, a combination of leishmaniasis and HIV is truly disastrous.

Immunological interest in leishmaniasis was first aroused by the realization that cutaneous leishmaniasis (tropical sore) caused solid immunity to reinfection when it eventually healed. On the other hand, visceral leishmaniasis causing kala azar is frequently progressive and fatal. A second fascinating observation in leishmaniasis arises from the murine model, which yielded some of the first evidence that Th1-type immunity helps cure but Th2-type immunity leads to increasing lesions and death (149).

In a procedure reminiscent of variolation, an ancient practice known as leishmanization, material from an active lesion was used to produce a self-limited sore on normal people. Prophylactic immunization with killed *Leishmania* was used in the 1940s. Animal experimentation showed the feasibility of live attenuated vaccines, and work is continuing on an attenuated *L. major* lacking the dihydrofolate reductase/thymidylate synthetase gene. However, subunit vaccines are receiving the most attention, not only in a variety of adjuvants but also in the vectored and DNA delivery approaches.

It must be admitted that none of the approaches has progressed very far, in part because of a lack of commercial interest. To analyze the various molecular vaccine candidates, it is important to consider the parasite's life cycle. A sandfly bite introduces 100 to 1,000 mobile promastigotes into the skin that attach to macrophages and are taken up into a phagolysosome, in which intracellular multiplication takes place, yielding nonmotile amastigotes. When an infected macrophage eventually ruptures, the amastigotes reinfect other mononuclear cells. The life cycle is completed when the fly takes a blood meal containing monocytes and amastigotes. A poorly understood maturation process leads to the appearance and maturation of promastigotes. Unlike malaria, leishmaniasis is a zoonosis, and various mammalian animal hosts constitute a reservoir of infection. In most cases, humans are accidental hosts.

Two antigens on the surface of *Leishmania* promastigotes are parasite ligands for macrophage receptors (150). One is a 65-kDa membrane glycoprotein with protease activity, present in promastigotes of all species, known as gp63. Parasite mutants lacking gp63 are avirulent. The second is a glycoconjugate, the *Leishmania* lipophosphoglycan (LPG). Both can induce good protection in a mouse model. It is known that fragments of LPG can be presented to T cells by a specialized subset of class I MHC proteins, CD1. Both gp63 and LPG remain viable vaccine candidates.

A further interesting antigen is a membrane protein of unknown function known as gp46 or parasite antigen 2 (PSA-2). This is present in promastigotes of all species but in amastigotes of only some. Yeast-derived recombinant PSA-2 is an effective vaccine in the murine model and confers partial cross-species protection. A leishmanial ribosomal protein known as LeIF is of both theoretical and practical interest. This molecule has particular adjuvant properties in that it powerfully promotes IL-12 production in mice and humans and thus steers the immune response in a Th1 direction, just the type of response required for immunity to leishmaniasis. It therefore represents a vaccine candidate with built-in adjuvanticity.

Amastigote antigens can be thought of as being like merozoite antigens in malaria, and a variety have proved efficacious in the murine model. Among them are antigens known as A2, P4, P8 and Lcr1. A further approach to the identification of potential amastigote candidates has been the elution of peptides from APCs and using their sequence to identify and clone the relevant parasite genes (151).

In summary, the potential is considerable, the complexities are major, and the prospects for a licensable vaccine in the medium term are not especially good.

Schistosomiasis Vaccines

Schistosomiasis or bilharziasis, also known as snail fever, is the second most important human parasitic disease and the most prevalent caused by a metazoan parasite. Six to eight hundred million people in 74 countries are exposed to the risk of infection, and 200 million are actually infected, of whom 20 million exhibit serious morbidity and 200,000 die each year from the disease. Schistosomiasis is caused by five species of *Schistosoma,* of which the three most important are *S. mansoni, S. hematobium,* and *S. japonicum.* Freshwater snails are the intermediate host for the parasite, and they release free-swimming cercariae, which penetrate human skin. There are also plentiful animal hosts; schistosomiasis is a zoonosis, which makes control of transmission much harder. In quite a complex migratory process, adult worms eventually develop and lodge in the veins, the predominant organs depending on the species. The male and female conjugate, and the female lays up to thousands of eggs per day. These ova are the real inducers of immunopathological processes. They penetrate the tissues and reach the gastrointestinal tract or the urinary tract, thus being excreted in feces or urine. The life cycle is completed if water sources are contaminated and snails become infested. At the same time, ova lodge in organs such as the liver or the bladder and cause granuloma formation and fibrosis. Induction of cirrhosis of the liver caused by *S. japonicum* is the most fatal manifestation of *schistosomiasis.* Because the adult worms consume blood, anemia is a complication. Bladder cancer associated with schistosomiasis is common in young men in Egypt.

Control of the snail intermediate host and greater care with feces and urine represent important intervention strategies. Beyond that, the community-wide introduction and use of the safe and effective drug praziquantel (152) offer the hope of control. However, rapid reinfection after drug treatment and the ever-present risk of drug resistance make the development of a vaccine most desirable. Combined with the other measures just mentioned, it could reduce reinfection rates and lower disease burden.

By far the most advanced vaccine candidate is the molecule Sm28GST, being promoted by the group of Capron (153). This is a 28-kDa recombinant protein initially cloned from a complementary DNA library of *S. mansoni,* which is the enzyme glutathione S-transferase (GST). Yeast-derived recombinant GST has been extensively tested as a vaccine candidate in various experimental models, including extensive trials in rodents, cattle, and subhuman primates with *S. mansoni, S. haematobium, S. japonicum,* and *S. bovis.* Consistently, it is only partially effective in preventing infection, typically reducing the worm burden by 40% to 60%. However, there is a more profound effect on female worm fecundity and egg viability, in which reductions varying from 75% to 94% in various models have been achieved. Moreover, whereas there is no cross-protection as far as the anti-infective immunity is concerned, the reduction in egg production and viability crosses species barriers, offering the hope that Sm28GST might be broadly effective. How protection is achieved is far from clear; one possibility is that GST is involved in prostaglandin biosynthesis and female worm reproductive physiology.

After more than a decade's preclinical work, Capron's group decided to embark on clinical trials using *S. haematobium* GST (Sh28GST) (154). The chief reasons were the capacity to study egg burden easily by means of urine

filtration and the opportunity to monitor bladder lesion development by noninvasive ultrasonography. Sh28GST has been produced under Good Manufacturing Practice conditions and named Bilhvax. Phase I trials involving 24 white adults and 24 noninfected Senegalese children, injecting three doses of 100 μg of Bilhvax in alum hydroxide, showed no adverse reactions and strong anti-GST responses with no cross-reactivity to human GST. Further studies have been completed in which infected adults have been given Bilhvax in association with chemotherapy, and no adverse effects have been noted. Phase III efficacy studies began in 2001.

Other vaccine candidates are not as far advanced. They include the enzyme triose phosphate isomerase; two parasite muscle proteins (paramyosin and a myosin-like protein); a 23-kDa protein and a 38-kDa protein, both of unknown function; and a molecule called calpain. Each has been effective in one animal model or another.

As in other fields, experimentation is under way to investigate GST and other antigens with a variety of adjuvants, as vectored and DNA vaccines, and as mucosal vaccines. Preliminary results have been encouraging.

Vaccines against Other Parasitic Diseases

Toxoplasmosis is a disease, predominantly of the central nervous system, that affects the developing fetus or premature babies and also represents a major opportunistic infection in patients with AIDS. A major surface antigen of *Toxoplasma gondii* called p30 has been cloned and is protective in a murine model.

Amebiasis, caused by the invasion of the intestinal wall by the protozoan parasite *Entamoeba histolytica,* kills 100,000 people per year. A lectin on the parasite surface helps in the adherence of the parasite to the colonic mucosa. The active sites or domains of this lectin could have potential as a recombinant vaccine.

Hydatid disease caused by the metazoan parasite *Echinococcus granulosus* is still a threat in parts of the world where there is close contact between humans and infected dogs, which release eggs in their feces. An antigen known as EG95, derived from the egg or oncosphere, has been the subject of several years of intensive research by Lightowlers (155). It has proved remarkably effective in sheep: Two injections of recombinant protein give 96% to 98% protection in sheep, an intermediate host, as is (less commonly) the human. This could lead to a sheep vaccine and, conceivably, one useful for humans at special risk. An oncosphere antigen with distinct amino acid homology has been identified in various *Taenia* species and could constitute a vaccine against cysticercosis.

In conclusion, parasitism is so grave a problem that it must be tackled on many fronts simultaneously. Protection from vectors is obviously important, as is chemical and biological control of vectors. Drug therapy is highly effective in many cases but always fraught with the danger of development of resistance. Vaccines are still in many ways a distant dream but one that must be sustained.

VACCINES AND BIOTERRORISM

The terrorist attacks of September 11, 2001, and the mysterious mailings of powder containing anthrax spores that followed soon after have put a new spotlight on bioterrorism, biological warfare, and defense against them. Clearly, vaccines have a role to play. Even before September 11, the United States had made a decision to stockpile 40 million doses of smallpox vaccine for control of any outbreaks that might occur after an attack, and it has been decided that this stockpile will be made much larger, to 300 million doses. It appears likely that about 10 countries have active offensive biological warfare programs, and some terrorist organizations have certainly shown an interest in the field as well. The range of microorganisms and toxins on which research has been done is extensive. Anthrax, smallpox, and botulinum toxin appear on most lists, but plague, tularemia, Venezuelan equine encephalitis, influenza, Marburg virus, Ebola virus, Lassa fever, cholera, typhoid, brucellosis, Q fever, and aflatoxins all appear to have been the subject of research in various countries at various times.

Vaccines against many of these agents have been licensed. However, some are clearly not satisfactory. The licensed anthrax vaccine, consisting of a crude mixture of toxins, is safe but fairly reactogenic, and at present, six doses are recommended because it is not very immunogenic. Smallpox vaccine was previously derived from calf lymph, but this is clearly not satisfactory in the modern era, and tissue culture–derived material, now being used, is more expensive, at about U.S. $1.00 per dose. The standard vaccinia strains are rather reactogenic; it is by no means clear that the modified strains, such as are being used as vectors for other antigens, would be as protective. The formalin-killed whole plague bacillus vaccine is effective against the bubonic but not the pneumonic form of the disease. There exist a formalin-inactivated whole-cell vaccine against Q fever and a live attenuated tularemia vaccine. Inactivated vaccines exist against some of the encephalitogenic α viruses. Who will pay the research costs required to improve and validate such vaccines? Which, if any, should be stockpiled? What plans can be forged to increase production capacity rapidly after at attack? These difficult issues must be faced in the broad context of the present war against terrorism. As this book goes to press, the U.S. government is making major resources available to tackle the subject, including significant new money for vaccine research. In the meantime, there is a pressing need for more broad-scale education of physicians and emergency services on outbreak control, for stockpiling of antibiotics and perhaps antiviral drugs, and for research on every aspect of the problem.

VACCINES IN FIELDS OTHER THAN COMMUNICABLE DISEASES

Manipulation of the immune system offers opportunities beyond the field of communicable diseases. The vital field of vaccines against cancer is covered elsewhere in this volume. "Negative" vaccines—that is, antigens delivered for the purpose of preventing, inhibiting, or modulating an immune response—offer rich promise in both autoimmune and allergic diseases, and readers are referred to the relevant chapters. Birth control vaccines offer potential for a new approach to contraception. Some of these, such as those used to block the activity of human chorionic gonadotrophin, are long-acting but reversible and thus potentially very valuable in the setting of a developing country. Others offer the possibility of targeting men rather than women. Immunological approaches to inhibit the deposition of amyloid β peptide deposits in the brain by immunizing with amyloid β is one of the most exciting new developments in the murine model of Alzheimer's disease. Although these are beyond the scope of this chapter, they surely will gain prominence in future editions of this volume.

ADVERSE EFFECTS OF VACCINES

Three considerations dictate that adverse effects of vaccines must be taken very seriously. First, vaccines are normally given to healthy individuals, as opposed to most other biopharmaceuticals, which are given to the sick. Second, most vaccines are given to infants and young children, deemed to be both very precious and very vulnerable. Third, in the industrialized countries, the very success of immunization programs, combined with good personal hygiene, environmental sanitation, and improved living conditions, has made epidemic disease seem like something unfamiliar and perhaps something with which antibiotics and other medical treatments can cope. In other words, opponents of immunization can be excused for not understanding the risk-benefit equation of vaccines because of a lack of personal experience. This has to be countered by good education.

Fortunately, serious adverse events are very rare with currently used vaccines. This creates what at first seems a curious problem. Because nearly all children get quite a few vaccine injections in the first year of life, a reasonable proportion of all infants coming down with some rare complaint, such as encephalitis, will have had an immunization within, for example, a week of that illness. The assumption of a causative rather than coincidental relationship is quite human and can be contested only by statistical arguments, which are unfamiliar to most people. The more serious claimed side effects are considered first.

The most controversial vaccine from the viewpoint of side effects has been DPT, containing whole killed pertussis bacteria. Reactions such as fever, irritability, local redness, swelling and pain, anorexia, and drowsiness are quite common, although of short duration and easily ameliorated by a drug such as paracetamol. Febrile convulsions occur in about 1 case in 2,000 to 3,000 and cause no long-term harm. Follow-up study has shown no evidence of neurological damage or intellectual impairment. The question of serious acute neurological illness, such as encephalopathy, has caused the most concern. The incidence was put at 1 case per 330,000 vaccine doses in the United Kingdom in 1981, but reanalysis of the data, coupled with a large study in the United States by the Institute of Medicine, challenged this conclusion. The American Academy of Pediatrics found that, although "the data accumulated to date may not prove that pertussis vaccine can never cause brain damage, they indicate that if it does so, such occurrences must be exceedingly rare" (156). The Institute of Medicine concluded that the risk of serious neurological complications was somewhere between 0 and 1 per 200,000. Because the number of cases of whooping cough has fallen by a factor of 50 in the United States since the introduction of the vaccine, and because the disease is accompanied by permanent brain damage in about 1% of cases and by death in 0.1% to 4% of cases, depending on the study, the risk-benefit equation is still enormously on the side of vaccination, even with the worst assumptions about brain damage from vaccination.

The acellular pertussis vaccine has certainly caused less acute reactogenicity, as measured by the superficial parameters of local pain, swelling, redness, and so forth. It will, however, take a great deal of experience in the actual deployment phase of this vaccine to determine whether the alleged serious side reactions are less frequent with this purer vaccine.

The Institute of Medicine study determined that the following alleged adverse events of the DTP (whole-cell pertussis) were *not* supported by the evidence: infantile spasms, hypsarrhythmia, Reye's syndrome, and sudden infant death syndrome. However, an association with "protracted, inconsolable crying" as a rare complication seems established.

The next important area of concern is poliomyelitis. Adverse reactions to this vaccine are of particular importance because there have been no cases of wild poliomyelitis in the industrialized countries for many years. In fact, poliomyelitis transmission ceased in the Western Hemisphere in 1991. Thus, even a single case of vaccine-associated poliomyelitis is a real tragedy. Unfortunately, a reversion to neurovirulence of the Sabin poliovirus, although excessively rare, is not absolutely unknown. It appears that for approximately 2.7 million doses of the oral poliovirus vaccine, there is one case of paralytic polio, most commonly of Sabin type 3. On average, there have been about five such cases in the United States per year. Some have been in vaccinees and some in their contacts.

A major survey of paralytic poliomyelitis in England and Wales between 1985 and 1991 was reported by Joce et al. (157). In total, 21 confirmed cases were found. Thirteen were vaccine-associated, nine being in vaccinees and four in contacts. Five were imported cases, and three were cases whose source of infection was unknown. The estimated risk of vaccine-associated paralysis was 1.46 per million for the first dose but 0.49 per 106 for the second and 0 for the third and fourth. In all, nine cases of paralysis arose from 18.4 million doses of vaccine administered over 7 years, with a risk of paralysis of 0.49% per 10^6 immunizations, which is remarkably similar to the U.S. figure of 1 per 2.7 million. Two vaccine-associated cases occurred in immunodeficient

children, for whom inactivated poliomyelitis vaccine should have been offered.

Whereas the risks of oral polio vaccine are truly minuscule, the United States suggested that, beginning in the year 2000, there should be a complete switch to injectable, Salk-type vaccine. We have already discussed the special problem of mini-epidemics caused by circulation of vaccine-associated strains, some of which have recombined with other enteroviruses, in communities with low vaccination coverage. Expert opinion has, as yet, not reached a consensus as to how these strains will affect the polio "end game" and the hoped-for capacity to cease immunization.

One can draw up a panoply of other "accusations" against vaccines. Live attenuated virus vaccines can certainly cause damage in immunodeficient or immunosuppressed children; generalized vaccinia was probably the worst example. Now that smallpox has been eradicated, this risk has disappeared. If a vaccinia variant is rescued as a vaccine vector, it will be one of lessened virulence.

One can examine the existing vaccines one by one and identify claims for side reactions. Mild measles rash can follow the measles vaccine. Certainly, measles is a nasty disease for the unimmunized, with a case-fatality rate in developing nations of about 2% to 3% in unimmunized infants. In the industrialized world, the measles case-fatality rate is vastly lower, at 0.01% to 0.02%. However, nonfatal complications are common, including otitis media, pneumonia, and subacute sclerosing pan-encephalitis. As far as the live attenuated vaccine is concerned, encephalitis and similar problems are very occasionally reported, but their origins have been hard to pin down, and the feasibility of reducing these rare, conjectural complications, as well as the acknowledged commoner ones (e.g., febrile convulsions), remains problematic at this stage.

Both the measles vaccine and its companions (mumps, rubella, and soon, perhaps, varicella) have good track records in *not* causing serious complications. Suffice it to say that these are live attenuated vaccines, which can cause problems in particular patients. Reactions are mild and include malaise, fever, mild rash, and (rarely) febrile convulsions. One report (158) surveyed the incidence of thrombocytopenic purpura after MMR vaccination. The incidence was 1 per 500,000 for measles or rubella alone, 1 per 120,000 for measles and rubella, and 1 per 105,000 for the combined MMR vaccine. The syndrome resembled the purpura that can occur after natural measles or rubella infections. Complete recovery occurred in 89.5% of cases; normalization followed by relapse was noted in 7%. No deaths have been reported. This French study accords with conclusions reached in several other countries. Although a plausible causal relationship can be argued, the usually favorable outcome ensures that this rare complication does not modify the risk-benefit equation significantly. The mumps vaccine occasionally causes aseptic meningitis.

A good opportunity to examine adverse reactions to MMR immunization came up in Australia (16). The Australian measles control campaign targeted primary school children, and 1.7 million doses of MMR were given, chiefly at school, over a brief period in 1998. A major effort was made to document all adverse events after immunization, and all commencing within 30 days of vaccination were closely analyzed. There were 89 adverse events (5 per 100,000), no sequelae, and no deaths. The commonest reactions were syncopal episodes (24%), allergic reactions that did not include anaphylaxis (12%), and illnesses resembling mumps or measles (11%). There were six reports of neurological reactions, including one case of encephalopathy and three cases of arthritis or arthralgia. These low rates constitute a truly remarkable safety record.

From time to time, somewhat exotic claims of adverse events are made. For example, measles vaccination was claimed to cause autism and Crohn's disease. Nine studies have now refuted this. The hepatitis B vaccine was supposed to cause multiple sclerosis; exhaustive analysis has failed to support the association. No matter how bizarre, each claim must be examined carefully.

Vaccinia, although used, was a reasonably reactogenic vaccine and quite dangerous in immunodeficient/immunosuppressed children. Fortunately, this has no longer been a problem since smallpox eradication. In general, severe reactions against BCG, varicella, measles, or other live vaccines can occur in such individuals.

Excipients in the vaccine or adjuvant substances can occasion side reactions varying from inflammation to abscess formation. More seriously, vaccines can occasionally cause anaphylaxis, thrombocytopenia, or acute arthritis. These serious complications occur in fewer than 1 case in 100,000.

In summary, vaccines that have been through the current stringent regulatory process are incredibly safe. This fact deserves to be widely promulgated, and the media in particular need to be educated through a consistent and nonconfrontational effort.

VACCINATION OF THE VERY YOUNG AND THE OLD

Both extremes of age offer special challenges for the designer of new and improved vaccines. Some vaccines should be delivered very early in life, such as at birth, to be maximally useful. These include vaccines for diseases carried by the mother, such as hepatitis B, hepatitis C, HIV, or cytomegalovirus. Traditionally, BCG has also been given within a few days of birth in developing countries. Other vaccines are recommended for the elderly, including (in many countries) influenza and pneumococcal vaccines. There has been an upsurge of interest in protecting the elderly.

Although much more mature than that of the newborn mouse, the newborn infant's immune system is not yet hugely responsive, and neonatal immunization does not generally lead to extensive antibody formation. This is particularly the case for bacterial capsular polysaccharide antigens. However, neonatal immunization can lead to useful priming of both B- and T-cell memory responses and thus serve a useful purpose (159). There appears to be somewhat of a Th2 bias in the neonate: Work on mice and on infant subhuman primates suggests that if first immunization is with a DNA vaccine or with a Th1-promoting adjuvant such as CpG-containing oligonucleotides, this bias can be overcome (160). This suggests that a prime-boost strategy might work very well in neonates. Of course, the introduction of any new adjuvant for immunization of human newborns would face considerable regulatory hurdles.

Preclinical studies suggest that the immaturity is not so much in $CD4^+$ or $CD8^+$ T cells themselves but rather in APCs and the APC–T cell interaction. This again suggests that suitable adjuvant formulations could overcome the problem. Another feature of neonates is that they appear deficient in the capacity to form long-lived, bone marrow–seeking, antibody-forming plasma cells.

Maternally acquired antibodies can interfere with primary active immune responses. This is a serious point for many infant vaccines, including live and nonlive preparations, although it appears not to be an issue for hepatitis B. Inhibition is highly epitope specific and is much more important for B-cell than for T-cell responses. From a practical viewpoint, each case must be investigated specifically. For the most important vaccines of the future, maternal antibodies should not be a problem for HIV or tuberculosis, but for malaria, in which antibodies are of at least equal importance to T cells, the matter may be more germane.

At the other end of life, several factors militate against robust immune responses. The thymic cortex is largely replaced by fat, and few or no new T cells are exported from there. Thus, T cell immunity to new antigens must depend on cross-reactions with previously encountered ones. Similarly, the number of progenitors of B cells in the bone marrow is also reduced, although not as markedly. Interestingly, dendritic cells from the peripheral blood of individuals older than 65 years are present in somewhat *increased* numbers, are normal in appearance and surface markers, and are unimpaired in antigen-presenting function. This may partly militate against the reduced proliferative capacity of aged T cells. Overall, the capacity to mount a serum antibody response may be reduced by up to tenfold in old age.

It is well known that the elderly are relatively more susceptible to infections such as tuberculosis, influenza, and pneumonia. An interesting although infrequent problem relates to tetanus. It has been estimated that only 25% to 40% of the healthy elderly have protective levels of antitetanus antibodies in their serum, as opposed to 92% in subjects younger than 30 years. This is mainly the result of a failure to receive the recommended booster injections every 10 years. It is possible, however, that the frequency of boosters may have to be greater after 70 years of age. The fact that immunization against influenza and pneumococci significantly reduces the burden of these infections in the elderly should prompt an examination of other vaccines that might be useful in this age group, in view of the emergence of many antibiotic-resistant strains of bacteria and the ever-present threat of many viruses. For example, the effects of boosting with the varicella vaccine on the later incidence of herpes zoster is the subject of a large phase III trial, the results of which are eagerly awaited.

As more vaccines become available, and as the lowered impact of epidemic diseases prompts complacency in the minds of many, health authorities will have to give much more thought to the whole question of booster immunizations in adult life. In terms of policy, this area is currently a bit of a mess. It should not be left to the vagaries of choices by travelers.

CONCLUSIONS

There is no doubting the current renaissance in vaccinology. The field veritably bristles with new and exciting possibilities, and although the commercial potential is not as great as for prescription drugs, the healthy percentage sales growth of the sector has not gone unnoticed in the board rooms of the big pharmaceutical companies. Of the new vaccination approaches discussed, DNA vaccines, superior adjuvant formulations, microencapsulation, and mucosal immunity are among the more promising. Despite his great enthusiasm for them, the author is also aware of the fact that changes to national immunization programs can be made only after very extensive clinical research, particularly in cases in which an effective vaccine already exists. The future therefore represents a judicious balance between conservatism in a measure already regarded skeptically by a minority and cautious activism as thorough research documents the value of each new and improved vaccine. Nor should a healthy pluralism be opposed. Some countries will move faster on some vaccines because of their particular perspectives and problems. All of this means that the widespread introduction of the rich panoply of vaccines coming from the research sector will probably be slower than the scientific community would like. In the long run, however, the approach to many communicable diseases will be revolutionized by the new vaccinology. The legacy of Jenner and Pasteur is in good hands.

ACKNOWLEDGMENTS

The author thanks Ms. Jill Van Es and Ms. Pamela Dewhurst for their careful typing of the manuscript; Ms. Josephine Marshall and Ms. Wendy Hertan for help with references; and both the WHO and the Bill and Melinda Gates Foundation for permission to reproduce the figures.

REFERENCES

1. Levine MM, Woodrow GC, Kaper JB, et al. *New generation vaccines,* 2nd ed. New York: Marcel Dekker, 1997.
2. Gerber MA, ed. *The Jordan report 2000. Accelerated development of vaccines.* Rockville, MD: Division of Microbiology & Infectious Diseases, National Institute of Allergy and Infectious Diseases, National Institutes of Health, 2000.
3. Fenner F, Henderson DA, Arita I, et al. *Smallpox and its eradication.* Geneva: World Health Organization, 1988.
4. Jenner E. *An inquiry into the causes and effects of the variolae vaccinae, a disease discovered in some of the western counties of England, particularly Gloucestershire, and known by the name of cow pox.* London: Edward Jenner, 1778.
5. Jenner E. *The origin of the vaccine inoculation.* London: DN Shury, 1801.
6. Pasteur L, Joubert J, Chamberland C. The germ theory of disease. *C R Hebd Seances Acad Sci* 1878;86:1037–1052.
7. Pasteur L. De l'attenuation du virus du cholera des poules. *C R Acad Schi Paris* 1880;91:673–680.
8. Calmette LCA, Guérin C, Weill-Hallé B. Essai d'immunisation contre l'infection tuberculeuse. *Bull Acad Med (Paris)* 1924;91:787–796.
9. Glenny AT, Hopkins BE. Diptheria toxoid as an immunising agent. *Br J Exp Pathol* 1923;4:283–288.
10. Enders JF, Weller TH, Robbins RC. Cultivation of the Lansing strain of poliomyelitis virus in cultures of various human embryonic tissues. *Science* 1949;109:85–87.
11. Hilleman MR. The development of live attenuated mumps virus vaccine in historic perspective and its role in the evolution of combined measles-mumps-rubella. In: Fantini B, Plotkin S, eds. *Vaccinia, vaccination and vaccinology: Jenner, Pasteur and their successors.* Paris: Elsevier, 1996:283–292.
12. Blumberg BS, Alter HJ, Visnich S. A "new" antigen in leukemia sera. *JAMA* 1965;191:541–546.
13. Blumberg BS. Australia antigen, hepatitis, and leukemia. *Tokyo J Med Sci* 1968;76:1.
14. Valenzuela P, Medina A, Rutter WJ, et al. Synthesis and assembly of hepatitis B virus surface antigen particles in yeast. *Nature* 1982;298:347–350.
15. de Quadros CA, Andrus JK, Olivé J-M, et al. Polio eradication from the Western Hemisphere. *Annu Rev Public Health* 1992;13:239–252.
16. Turnbull FM, Burgess MA, McIntyre PB, et al. The Australian Measles Control Campaign 1998. *Bull World Health Organ* 2001;79:882–888.
17. Nossal GJV. The Global Alliance for Vaccines and Immunization—a millennial challenge. *Nat Immunol* 2000;1:5–8.
18. Pizza M, Fontana MR, Giuliani MM, et al. A genetically detoxified derivative of heat-labile *Escherichia coli* enterotoxin induces neutralizing antibodies against a subunit. *J Exp Med* 1994;180:2147–2153.
19. Rappuoli R. New and improved vaccines against diphtheria and tetanus. In: Levine MM, Woodrow GC, eds. *New generation vaccines.* New York: Marcel Dekker, 1990:251–68.
20. Mackett M, Smith GL, Moss B. Vaccinia virus: a selectable eukaryotic cloning and expression vector. *Proc Natl Acad Sci U S A* 1982;79:7415–7419.
21. Panicali D, Paoletti E. Construction of pox viruses as cloning vectors: insertion of the thymidine kinase gene from herpes simplex virus into the DNA of infectious vaccinia virus. *Proc Natl Acad Sci U S A* 1982;79:4927–4931.
22. Ramshaw IA, Andrew ME, Phillips SM, et al. Recovery of immunodeficient mice from a vaccinia/Il-2 recombinant infection. *Nature* 1987;329:545–546.
23. Wolff JA, Malone RW, Williams P, et al. Direct gene transfer into mouse muscle *in vivo*. *Science* 1990;247:1465–1468.
24. Williams RS, Johnstone SA, Reidy M, et al. Introduction of foreign genes into tissues of living mice by DNA-coated microprojectiles. *Proc Natl Acad Sci U S A* 1991;88:2726–2730.
25. Tang DC, Devit M, Johnston SA. Genetic immunization is a simple method for eliciting an immune response. *Nature* 1992;356:152–154.
26. Ulmer JB, Donnelly JJ, Parker SE, et al. Heterologous protection against influenza by injection of DNA encoding a viral protein. *Science* 1993;259:1745–1749.
27. Fynan EF, Webster RG, Fuller DH, et al. DNA vaccines—protective immunizations by parenteral, mucosal and gene-gun innoculations. *Proc Natl Acad Sci U S A* 1993;90:11478–11482.
28. Donnelly JJ, Ulmer JB, Shiver JW, et al. DNA vaccines. *Annu Rev Immunol* 1997;15:617–648.
29. Fu TM, Ulmer JB, Caufield MJ, et al. Priming of cytotoxic T lymphocytes by DNA vaccines: requirement for professional antigen presenting cells and evidence for antigen transfer from myocytes. *Mol Med* 1997;3:362–371.

30. Boyle JS, Brady JL, Lew AM. Enhanced responses to a DNA vaccine encoding a fusion antigen that is directed to sites of immune induction. *Nature* 1998;392:408–411.

31. Holt PG, Schon-Hegrad MA, McMenamin PG. Dendritic cells in the respiratory tract. *Int Rev Immunol* 1990;6:139–149.

32. Picker LJ, Butcher EC. Physiological and molecular mechanisms of lymphocyte homing. *Annu Rev Immunol* 1994;62:561–569.

33. McWilliam AS, Nelson D, Thomas JA, et al. Rapid dendritic cell recruitment is a hallmark of the acute inflammatory response at mucosal surfaces. *J Exp Med* 1994;179:1331–1336.

34. Holmgren J, Rudin A. Mucosal immunity and bacteria. In: Ogra P, Mestecky J, Lamm M, et al., eds. *Mucosal immunology*. San Diego: Academic Press, 1999:685–693.

35. Glenn GM, Scharton-Kersten T, Vassell R, et al. Transcutaneous immunization with bacterial ADP-ribosylating exotoxins as antigens and adjuvants. *Infect Immun* 1999;67:1100–1106.

36. Mason HS, Lam DM, Arntzen CJ. Expression of hepatitis B surface antigen in transgenic plants. *Proc Natl Acad Sci U S A* 1992;89:11745–11749.

37. Hu SL, Klaniecki J, Dykers T, et al. Neutralizing antibodies against HIV-1 Bru and Sf2 isolates generated in mice immunized with recombinant vaccinia virus expressing HIV-1 (Bru) envelope glycoproteins and boosted with homologous gp160. *AIDS Res Hum Retroviruses* 1991;7:615–620.

38. Ramshaw IA, Ramsay AJ. The prime-boost strategy: exciting prospects for improved vaccination. *Immunol Today* 2000;21:163–165.

39. Beutler B. The Toll-like receptors as the primary sensors of the innate immune system. *The Immunologist* 2000;8:123–130.

39a. Janeway CR. A trip through my life with an immunological theme. *Annu Rev Immunol* 2002;20:1–28.

40. Gay NJ, Keith FJ. Drosophila Toll and Il-1 receptor. *Nature* 1991;351:355–356.

41. Lemaitre B, Nicholas E, Michaut L, et al. The dorsoventral regulatory gene cassette Spatzle/Toll/Cactus controls the potent antifungal response in *Drosophila* adults. *Cell* 1996;86:973–983.

42. Heldwein KA, Golenbock DT, Fenton MJ. Recent advances in the biology of the Toll-like receptors. *Mod Aspects Immunobiol* 2001;1:249–252.

43. Hemmi H, Takeuchi O, Kawai T, et al. A Toll-like receptor recognizes bacterial DNA. *Nature* 2000;408:740–745.

44. Hayashi F, Smith KD, Ozinsky A, et al. The innate immune response to bacterial flagellin is mediated by Toll-like receptor 5. *Nature* 2001;410:1099–1103.

45. Matzinger P. Essay 1: the danger model in its historical context. *Scand J Immunol* 2001;54:4–9.

46. Li M, Carpio DF, Zheng Y, et al. An essential role of the Nf-Kappa β/Toll-like receptor pathway in induction of inflammatory and tissue-repair gene expression by necrotic cells. *J Immunol* 2001;166:7128–7135.

47. Glenny AT, Pope CG, Waddington H, et al. The antigenic value of toxoid precipitated by potassium alum. *J Pathol Bacteriol* 1926;29:38–45.

48. Freund J, McDermott K. Sensitization to horse serum by means of adjuvants. *Proc Soc Exp Biol Med* 1942;49:548–553.

49. O'Hagan DT, ed. *Vaccine adjuvants*. Totowa, NJ: Humana Press, 2000.

50. Allison AC, Byars NE. An adjuvant formulation that selectively elicits the formation of antibodies of protective isotypes and of cell-mediated immunity. *J Immunol Methods* 1986;95:157–168.

51. Ellouz F, Adam A, Ciorbaru R, et al. Minimal structural requirements for adjuvant activity of bacterial peptigoglycans. *Biochem Biophys Res Commun* 1974;59:1317–1325.

52. Johnson AG, Tomai M, Solem L, et al. Characterization of a nontoxic monophosphoryl lipid A. *Rev Infect Dis* 1987;9(Suppl 5):S512–S516.

53. Kensil CR, Patel U. Lennick M, et al. Separation and characterization of saponins with adjuvant activity from *Quillaja saponaria* Molina cortex. *J Immunol* 1991;146:431–437.

54. Stoute JA, Slaoui M, Heppner DG, et al. A preliminary evaluation of a recombinant circumsporozoite protein vaccine against *Plasmodium falciparum* malaria. RTS,S Malaria Vaccine Evaluation Group. *N Engl J Med* 1997;336:86–91.

55. Morein B, Sundquist B, Höglund S, et al. ISCOM, a novel structure for antigenic presentation of membrane proteins from enveloped viruses. *Nature* 1984;308:457–460.

56. Alving CR, Detrick B, Richards RL, et al. Novel adjuvant strategies for experimental malaria and AIDS vaccines. *Ann N Y Acad Sci* 1993;690:265–275.

57. Mengiardi B, Berger R, Just M, et al. Virosomes as carriers for combined vaccines. *Vaccine* 1995;13:1306–1315.

58. Glück U, Gebbers JO, Glück R. Phase 1 evaluation of intranasal virosomal influenza vaccine with and without *Escherichia coli* heat-labile toxin in adult volunteers. *J Virol* 1999;73:7780–7786.

59. O'Brien-Simpson NM, Ede NJ, Brown LE, et al. Polymerization of unprotected synthetic peptides: a view towards synthetic peptide vaccines. *J Am Chem Soc* 1997;119:1183–1188.

60. Fitzmaurice CJ, Brown LE, Kronin V, et al. The geometry of synthetic peptide–based immunogens affects the efficiency of T cell stimulation by professional antigen-presenting cells. *Int Immunol* 2000;12:527–535.

61. Zeng WS, Ghosh S, Macris M, et al. Assembly of synthetic peptide vaccines by chemoselective ligation of epitopes: influence of different chemical linkages and epitope orientations on biological activity. *Vaccine* 2001;19:3843–3852.

62. Tokunaga T, Yamamoto H, Shimada S, et al. Antitumor activity of deoxyribonucleic acid fraction from *Mycobacterium bovis* BCG. I. Isolation, physicochemical characterization, and antitumor activity. *J Natl Cancer Inst* 1984;72:955–962.

63. Yamamoto S, Yamamoto T, Kataoka T, et al. Unique palindromic sequences in synthetic oligonucleotides are required to induce IFN and augment IFN-mediated natural killer activity. *J Immunol* 1992;148:4072–4076.

64. Krieg AM, Yi AK, Matson S, et al. CpG motifs in bacterial DNA trigger direct B-cell activation. *Nature* 1995;374:546–549.

65. Medzhitov R, Janeway CA Jr. Innate immunity: the virtues of a nonclonal system of recognition. *Cell* 1997;91:295–298.

66. Malanchère-Brès E, Payette PJ, Mancini M, et al. CpG oligodeoxynucleotides with hepatitis B surface antigen (HBsAg) for vaccination in HBsAg-transgenic mice. *J Virol* 2001;75:6482–6491.

67. Gallichan, WS, Woolstencroft RN, Guarasci T, et al. Intranasal immunization with CpG oligodeoxynucleotides as an adjuvant dramatically increases IgA and protection against herpes simplex virus–2 in the genital tract. *J Immunol* 2001;166:3451–3457.

68. Tighe H, Takabayashi K, Schwartz D, et al. Conjugation of immunostimulatory DNA to the short ragweed allergen Amb a 1 enhances its immunogenicity and reduces its allergenicity. *J Allergy Clin Immunol* 2000;106:124–134.

69. Marshall JD, Abtahi S, Eiden JJ, et al. Immunostimulatory sequence DNA linked to the Amb a 1 allergen promotes T(H)1 cytokine expression while downregulating T(H)2 cytokine expression in PBMCs from human patients with ragweed allergy. *J Allergy Clin Immunol* 2001;108:191–197.

70. Chang TMS. Biodegradable, semi-permeable microcapsules containing enzymes, hormones, vaccines, and other biologicals. *J Bioeng* 1976;1:25–32.

71. Langer R. Polymers for the sustained release of macromolecules: their use in a single-step method of immunization. *Methods Enzymol* 1981;73:57–75.

72. O'Hagen DT, Rahman D, McGee JP, et al. Biodegradable microparticles as controlled release antigen delivery systems. *Immunology* 1991;73:239–242.

73. Eldridge JH, Staas JK, Meulbroek JA, et al. Biodegradable and biocompatible poly(Dl-lactide-co-glycolide) microspheres as an adjuvant for staphylococcal enterotoxin B toxoid which enhances the level of toxin-neutralizing antibodies. *Infect Immun* 1991;59:2978–2986.

74. McGee JP, Davis SS, O'Hagan DT. The immunogenicity of a model protein entrapped in poly(lactide-co-glycolide) microparticles prepared by a novel phase-separation technique. *J Cont Rel* 1994;31:55–60.

75. Macdonald L, Kleinig M, Cox J. A single dose (two component) experimental influenza vaccine. *Proc Intern Symp Control Rel Bioact Mater* 1997;24:1–2.

76. Vordermeier HJ, Coombes AG, Jenksins P, et al. Synthetic delivery system for tuberculosis vaccines: immunological evaluation of the *M. tuberculosis* 38 kDa protein entrapped in biodegradable PLG microparticles. *Vaccine* 1995;13:1576–1582.

77. Schijns VE, Claasen IJ, Vermeulen AA, et al. Modulation of antiviral immune responses by exogenous cytokines: effects of tumour necrosis factor–alpha, interleukin-1 alpha, interleukin-2 and interferon-gamma

on the immunogenicity of an inactivated rabies vaccine. *J Gen Virol* 1994;75:55–63.

78. Pulendran B, Palucka K, Banchereua J. Sensing pathogens and tuning immune responses. *Science* 2001;293:253–256.

79. Giedlin MA. Cytokines as vaccine adjuvants: the use of interleukin-2. In: O'Hagan DT, ed. *Vaccine adjuvants. Preparation methods and research protocols.* Totowa, NJ: Humana Press, 2000:283–297.

80. Dempsey PW, Allison ME, Akkaraju S, et al. C3d of complement as a molecular adjuvant: bridging innate and acquired immunity. *Science* 1996;271:348–350.

81. Pulendran B, Palucka K, Banchereau J. Dendritic cells in the spleen and lymph nodes. In: Lotze MT, Thomson AW, eds. *Dendritic cells: biology and clinical applications.* San Diego: Academic Press, 2001:357–370.

82. Douce G, Fontana M, Pizza M, et al. Intranasal immunogenicity and adjuvanticity of site-directed mutant derivatives of cholera toxin. *Infect Immun* 1997;65:2821–2828.

83. Sun J-B, Holmgren J, Czerkinsky C. Cholera toxin B subunit: an efficient transmucosal carrier-delivery system for induction of peripheral immunological tolerance. *Proc Natl Acad Sci U S A* 1994;91:10795–10799.

84. Rask C, Fredriksson M, Lindblad M, et al. Mucosal and systemic antibody responses after peroral or intranasal immunization: effects of conjugation to enterotoxin B subunits and/or of co-administration with free toxin as adjuvant. *APMIS* 2000;108:178–186.

85. Greco D, Salmaso S, Mastrantonio P, et al. A controlled trial of two acellular vaccines and one whole-cell vaccine against pertussis. Progetto Petrosse Working Group. *N Engl J Med* 1996;334:341–348.

86. Rappuoli R. Rational design of vaccines. *Nat Med* 1997;3:374–376.

87. Klein D. Pertussis vaccines: a continuing saga. In: PJ Baker, ed. *The Jordan report. Accelerated development of vaccines.* Bethesda, MD: Division of Microbiology and Infectious Diseases, National Institute of Allergy and Infectious Diseases, National Institutes of Health, 1996;29–32.

88. Hewlett EL, Cherry D. New and improved vaccines against pertussis. In: Levine MM, Woodrow GC, Kaper JB, et al., eds. *New generation vaccines,* 2nd ed. New York: Marcel Dekker, 1997:387–416.

89. Hoiseth SK, Stocker BA. Aromatic-dependent *Salmonella typhimurium* are non-virulent and effective as live vaccines. *Nature* 1981;291:238–239.

90. Tacket CO, Hone DM, Losonsky GA, et al. Clinical acceptability and immunogenicity of CVD 908 *Salmonella typhi* vaccine strain. *Vaccine* 1992;10:443–446.

91. Chatfield SN, Strahan K, Pickard D, et al. Evaluation of *Salmonella typhimurium* strains harbouring defined mutations in *htrA* and *aroA* in the murine salmonellosis model. *Microb Pathog* 1992;12:145–151.

92. Gomez-Duarte OG, Galen J, Chatfield SN, et al. Expression of fragment C of tetanus toxin fused to a carboxyl-terminal fragment of *Diphtheria* toxin in *Salmonella typhi* CVD 908 vaccine strain. *Vaccine* 1994;13:1596–1602.

93. van Loon FPL, Clemens JD, Chakraborty J, et al. Field trial of inactivated oral cholera vaccines in Bangladesh: results from 5 years of follow-up. *Vaccine* 1996;14:162–166.

94. Trach DD, Clemens JD, Ke NT, et al. Field trial of a locally produced, killed, oral cholera vaccine in Vietnam. *Lancet* 1997;349:231–235.

95. Tacket CO, Losonsky G, Nataro JP, et al. Onset and duration of protective immunity in challenged volunteers after vaccination with live oral cholera vaccine CVD 103-HgR. *J Infect Dis* 1992;166:837–841.

96. Pearson GD, Woods A, Chiang SL, et al. CTX genetic element encodes a site-specific recombination system and an intestinal colonization factor. *Proc Natl Acad Sci U S A* 1993;90:3750–3754.

97. Kotloff KL, Winickoff JP, Ivanoff B, et al. Global burden of *Shigella* infections: implications for vaccine development and implementation of control strategies. *Bull World Health Organ* 1999;77:651–666.

98. Sansonetti P, Phalipon A. Shigellosis: from molecular pathogenesis of infection to protective immunity and vaccine development. *Res Immunol* 1996;147:595–602.

99. Kotloff KL, Noriega FR, Samandari T, et al. *Shigella flexneri* 2a strain CVD 1207, with specific deletions in *virG, sen, set,* and *guaBA,* is highly attenuated in humans. *Infect Immun* 2000;68:1034–1039.

100. Marshall BJ, Warren JR. Unidentified curved bacilli in the stomach of patients with gastritis and peptic ulceration. *Lancet* 1983;1:1311–1315.

101. Uemura N, Okamoto S, Yamamoto S, et al. *Helicobacter pylori* infection and the development of gastric cancer. *N Engl J Med* 2001;345:784–789.

102. Del Giudice G, Covacci A, Telford JL, et al. The design of vaccines against *Helicobacter pylori* and their development. *Annu Rev Immunol* 2001;19:523–563.

103. Lee A, Hazell SL, O'Rourke J, et al. Isolation of a spiral-shaped bacterium from the cat stomach. *Infect Immun* 1988;56:2843–2850.

104. Chen M, Lee A, Hazell S. Immunization against gastric *Helicobacter* infection in a mouse/*Helicobacter felis* model. *Lancet* 1992;339:1120–1121.

105. Doidge C, Crust I, Lee A, et al. Therapeutic immunization against *Helicobacter* infection. *Lancet* 1994;343:914–915.

106. Corthesy-Theulaz I, Porta N, Glauser M, et al. Oral immunization with *Helicobacter pylori* urease B subunit as a treatment against *Helicobacter* infection in mice. *Gastroenterology* 1995;109:115–121.

107. Rossi G, Fortuna D, Pancotto L, et al. Immunohistochemical study of lymphocyte populations infiltrating the gastric mucosa of beagle dogs experimentally infected with *Helicobacter pylori*. *Infect Immun* 2000;68:4769–4772.

108. Anderson P, Peter G, Johnston RB Jr, et al. Immunization of humans with polyribophosphate, the capsular antigen of *Haemophilus influenzae,* type B. *J Clin Invest* 1972;51:39–44.

109. Rodrigues LP, Schneerson R, Robbins JB. Immunity to *Haemophilus influenzae* type B. I. The isolation, and some physicochemical, serologic and biologic properties of the capsular polysaccharide of *Haemophilus influenzae* type B. *J Immunol* 1971;107:1071–1080.

110. Peltala H, Käyhty H, Sivonen A, et al. *Haemophilus influenzae* type B capsular polysaccharide vaccine in children: a double-blind field study of 100,000 vaccines 3 months to 5 years of age in Finland. *Pediatrics* 1977;60:730–737.

111. Anderson P. Antibody responses to *Haemophilus influenzae* type B and diphtheria toxin induced by conjugates of oligosaccharides of the type B capsule with the non-toxic protein Crm197. *Infect Immun* 1983;39:233–238.

112. Schneerson R, Robbins JB, Chu C, et al. Semi-synthetic vaccines composed of capsular polysaccharides of pathogenic bacteria covalently bound to proteins for the prevention of invasive diseases. *Prog Allergy* 1983;33:144–158.

113. Eskola J, Kayhty H, Takala AK, et al. A randomized, prospective field trial of a conjugate vaccine in the protection of infants and young children against invasive *Haemophilus influenzae* type B disease. *N Engl J Med* 1990;323:1381–1387.

114. Mullholland K, Hilton S, Adegbola R, et al. Randomised trial of *Haemophilus influenzae* type-B tetanus protein conjugate vaccine for prevention of pneumonia and meningitis in Gambian infants. *Lancet* 1997;349:1191–1197.

115. Miller E, Salisbury D, Ramsay M. Planning, registration and implementation of an immunisation campaign against meningococcal serogroup C disease in the UK: a success story. *Vaccine* 2002;20:S58–S67.

116. Thomas WR, Callow MG, Dilworth RJ, et al. Expression in *Escherichia coli* of a high-molecular-weight protective surface antigen found in nontypeable and type B *Haemophilus influenzae*. *Infect Immun* 1990;58:1909–1913.

117. Brandt ER, Sriprakash KS, Hobb RI, et al. New multi-determinant strategy for a group A streptococcal vaccine designed for the Australian aboriginal population. *Nat Med* 2000;6:455–459.

118. Hilleman MR. Hepatitis and hepatitis a vaccine: a glimpse of history. *J Hepatol* 1993;18:S5–S10.

119. Choo QL, Richman KH, Han JH, et al. Genetic organization and diversity of the hepatitis C virus. *Proc Natl Acad Sci U S A* 1991;88:2451–2455.

120. Rosa D, Campagnoli S, Moretto C, et al. A quantitative test to estimate neutralizing antibodies to the hepatitis C virus: cytofluorometric assessment of envelope glycoprotein 2 binding to target cells. *Proc Natl Acad Sci U S A* 1996;93:1759–1763.

121. Bishop RF, Barnes GL, Cipriani E, et al. Clinical immunity after neonatal rotavirus infection. A prospective longitudinal study in young children. *N Engl J Med* 1983;309:72–76.

122. Murphy TV, Gargiullo PM, Massoudi MS, et al. Intussusception among infants given an oral rotavirus vaccine. *N Engl J Med* 2001;344:564–572.

123. Chang H-G. Smith PF, Ackelsberg J, et al Intussusception, rotavirus

diarrhea, and rotavirus vaccine use among children in New York State. *Pediatrics* 2001;108:54–60.

124. Wright PF, Karron RA, Bleshe RB, et al. Evaluation of a live, cold-passaged, temperature-sensitive, respiratory syncytial virus vaccine candidate in infancy. *J Infect Dis* 2000;182:1331–1342.

125. Patel RM, Simoes EAF. Respiratory syncytial virus infection: pathogenesis and its implications for prevention. In: David TJ, ed. *Recent advances in paediatrics.* Edinburgh: Churchill Livingstone, 2001:197–210.

126. Siegrist CA, Plotnicky-Gilquin H, Cordova M, et al. Protective efficacy against respiratory syncytial virus following murine neonatal immunization with BBG2Na vaccine: influence of adjuvants and maternal antibodies. *J Infect Dis* 1999;179:1326–1333.

127. Rimmelzwaan GF, Nieuwkoop N, Brandenburg A, et al. A randomized, double blind study in young healthy adults comparing cell mediated and humoral immune responses induced by influenza ISCOM vaccines and conventional vaccines. *Vaccine* 2000;19:1180–1187.

128. Ho DD, Neumann AU, Perelson AS, et al. Rapid turnover of plasma virions and CD4 lymphocytes in HIV-1 infection. *Nature* 1995;373:123–126.

129. Rucker J, Doms RW. Chemokine receptors as HIV coreceptors: implications and interactions. *AIDS Res Hum Retroviruses* 1998;14(Suppl 3):S241–S246.

130. Francis DP, Gregory T, McElrath MJ, et al. Advancing AIDSVAX[TM] to phase 3. Safety, immunogenicity, and plans for phase 3. *AIDS Res Hum Retroviruses* 1998;14(Suppl 3):S325–S331.

131. Letvin NL, Montefiori DC, Yasutomi Y, et al. Potent, protective anti-HIV immune responses generated by bimodal HIV envelope DNA plus protein vaccination. *Proc Natl Acad Sci U S A* 1997;94:9378–9383.

132. Amara RR, Villinger F, Altman JD, et al. Control of a mucosal challenge and prevention of AIDS by a multiprotein DNA/MVA vaccine. *Science* 2001;292:69–74.

133. Barouch DH, Santra S, Schmitz JE, et al. Control of viremia and prevention of clinical aids in Rhesus monkeys by cytokine-augmented DNA vaccination. *Science* 2000;290:486–492.

134. Berzofsky JA, Ahlers JD, Derby MA, et al. Approaches to improve engineered vaccines for human immunodeficiency virus and other viruses that cause chronic infections. *Immunol Rev* 1999;170:151–172.

135. Belyakov IM, Hel Z, Kelsall B, et al. Mucosal AIDS vaccine reduces disease and viral load in gut reservoir and blood after mucosal infection of macaques. *Nat Med* 2001;7:1320–1326.

136. Ahlers JD, Belyakov IM, Thomas EK, et al. High-affinity T helper epitope induces complementary helper and APC polarization, increased CTL, and protection against viral infection. *J Clin Invest* 2001;108:1677–1685.

137. Biggs BA, Anders RF, Dillon HE, et al. Adherence of infected erythrocytes to venular endothelium selects for antigenic variants of *Plasmodium falciparum. J Immunol* 1992;149:2047–2054.

138. Nussenzweig V, Nussenzweig RS. Circumsporozoite proteins of malaria parasites. *Cell* 1985;42:401–403.

139. Frevert U, Sinnis P, Cerami C, et al. Malaria circumsporozoite protein binds to heparan sulfate proteoglycans associated with the surface membrane of hepatocytes. *J Exp Med* 1993;177:1287–1298.

140. Singh S, Pandey K, Chattopadhayay R, et al. Biochemical, biophysical and functional characterization of bacterially expressed and refolded receptor binding domain of *Plasmodium vivax* Duffy-binding protein. *J Biol Chem* 2001;276:17111–17116.

141. Doolan DL, Hoffman SL. DNA-based vaccines against malaria: status and promise of the multi-stage malaria DNA vaccine operation. *Int J Parasitol* 2001;31:753–762.

142. Good MF, Kaslow DC, Miller LH. Pathways and strategies for developing a malaria blood-stage vaccine. *Annu Rev Immunol* 1998;16:57–87.

143. Patarroyo ME, Amador R, Clavijo P, et al. A synthetic vaccine protects humans against challenge with asexual blood stages of *Plasmodium falciparum* malaria. *Nature* 1988;332:158–161.

144. Bojang KA, Milligan PJM, Pinder M, et al. Efficacy of RTS,S/AS02 malaria vaccine against *Plasmodium falciparum* infection in semi-immune adult men in The Gambia: a randomised trial. *Lancet* 2001;358:1927–1934.

145. Kedzierski L, Black CG, Coppel RL. Immunization with recombinant *Plasmodium yoelii* merozoite surface protein 4/5 protects mice against lethal challenge. *Infect Immun* 2000;68:6034–6037.

146. Anders RF, Saul A. Malaria vaccines. *Parasitol Today* 2000;16:444–447.

147. Schneider J, Gilbert SC, Blanchard TJ, et al. Enhanced immunogenicity for CD8+ T cell induction and complete protective efficacy of malaria DNA vaccination by boosting with modified vaccinia virus Ankara. *Nat Med* 1998;4:397–402.

148. Schofield L. Antidisease vaccines. In: Perlmann P, Troye-Blomberg M, eds. *Malaria immunology.* Basel: Karger, 2002:322–342.

149. Locksley RM, Louis JA. Immunology of leishmaniasis. *Curr Opin Immunol* 1992;4:4213–4218.

150. Handman E. Leishmaniasis: current status of vaccine development. *Clin Microbiol Rev* 2001;14:229–243.

151. Campos-Neto A, Soong L, Cordova JL, et al. Cloning and expression of a *Leishmania donovani* gene instructed by a peptide isolated from major histocompatibility complex class II molecules of infected macrophages. *J Exp Med* 1995;182:1423–1433.

152. Stelma FF, Talla I, Sow S, et al. Efficacy and side effects of praziquantel in an epidemic focus of *Schistosoma mansoni. Am J Trop Med Hyg* 1995;53:167–170.

153. Capron A. Schistosomiasis: forty years' war on the worm. *Parasitol Today* 1998;14:379–384.

154. Capron A, Capron M, Dombrowicz, et al. Vaccine strategies against schistosomiasis: from concepts to clinical trials. *Int Arch Allergy Immunol* 2001;124:9–15.

155. Lightowlers MW, Flisser A, Gauci CG, et al. Vaccination against cysticercosis and hydatid disease. *Parasitol Today* 2000;16:191–196.

156. American Academy of Pediatrics Committee on Infectious Diseases. The relationship between pertussis vaccine and brain damage: reassessment. *Pediatrics* 1991;88:397–400.

157. Joce R, Wood D, Brown D, et al. Paralytic poliomyelitis in England and Wales 1985–1991. *BMJ* 1992;305:79–82.

158. Jonville-Béra AP, Autret E, Galy-Eyraud C, et al. Thrombocytopenic purpura after measles, mumps and rubella vaccination: a retrospective survey by the French Regional Pharmacovigilance Centres and Pasteur-Mérieux Sérums et Vaccins. *Pediatr Infect Dis J* 1996;15:44–48.

159. Siegrist CA. Neonatal and early life vaccinology. *Vaccine* 2001;19:3331–3346.

160. Kovarik JP, Bozzetti L, Love-Homan L, et al. CpG oligodeoxynucleotides can circumvent the Th2 polarization of neonatal responses to vaccines but may fail to fully redirect Th2 responses established by neonatal priming. *J Immunol* 1999;162:1611–1617.

CHAPTER 44

Systemic Autoimmunity

Philip L. Cohen

Introduction
Historical
Nonpathologic Systemic Autoimmunity
Autoimmunity and Tolerance
   T-Cell Tolerance in Systemic Autoimmunity · B-Cell Tolerance in Systemic Autoimmunity
Nature of Autoantigens
General Characteristics of Autoantibodies
Genetics of Systemic Autoimmune Disease
Role of T Cells in Systemic Autoimmune Disease
   Nature of T-Cell Help for Autoantibody Formation · Regulatory T-Cell Abnormalities
Cytokines in Systemic Autoimmune Disease
Environmental Influences on Systemic Autoimmunity
Apoptosis Abnormalities in Systemic Autoimmune Disease
Autoimmunity and Malignancy
Features of Human Systemic Autoimmune Disorders
   Systemic Lupus Erythematosus · Rheumatoid Arthritis · Reactive Arthritis and Spondyarthritides · Systemic Vasculitis · Sjögren's Syndrome · Chronic Graft versus Host Disease · Scleroderma (Systemic Sclerosis)
Commonly Used Animal Models of Systemic Autoimmune Disease
   lpr and gld Mice · NZB and NZB/NZW F1 Mice · BXSB Mice · Induction of Systemic Lupus-like Syndrome in Mice through Injection of Pristane · Systemic Autoimmunity Induced by Idiotype Infusion · Viable Moth-eaten Mouse
Severe Autoimmune Disease in Knockout and Transgenic Strains
Tight-skin Mouse
Models of Rheumatoid Arthritis
Immune Injury in Systemic Autoimmune Disease
Approaches to Treatment of Systemic Autoimmune Disease
Conclusions
References

INTRODUCTION

The study of systemic autoimmune disease has held the interest of many immunologists for two important reasons. First, human systemic autoimmune diseases are an important cause of suffering and shortening of life. Second, the aberrations that lead to autoreactivity against multiple self-antigens must hold the keys to understanding important aspects of the fundamental basis of self–non-self discrimination.

Some of the mystery surrounding the genesis of systemic autoimmune disease has been dispelled by careful analysis of autoantigens and self-reactive T cells and B cells. Little about the structure of autoantigens sets them apart from conventional proteins or nucleic acids. Autoantibody responses use immunoglobulin and T-cell receptor genes in a fashion similar to that used in ordinary responses, and the latter display a degree of somatic mutation expected for chronic, antigen-selected secondary responses. T–B collaboration is required for autoantibody responses, and the accessory molecules involved in this process appear similar to those used in responses to exogenous antigen.

Many potential etiologies have been put forth to explain systemic autoimmune disease. It seems unlikely that a single explanation is adequate to account for the diverse phenomena described in this chapter, yet there are common issues regarding self-reactive immune responses, regardless of the inciting causes. The comments regarding overall mechanisms of autoimmune disease may not apply to all diseases or models, but are intended to place systemic autoreactivity into the context of basic immunology and to focus future thought about mechanisms.

Systemic autoimmunity encompasses autoimmune conditions in which autoreactivity is not limited to a single organ or organ system. Included under this definition are systemic lupus erythematosus (SLE), systemic sclerosis (scleroderma), rheumatoid arthritis (RA), chronic graft-versus-host (GVH) disease, and the various forms of vasculitis. While autoimmune phenomena are prominent in these conditions, the formal demonstration that autoimmunity is a cause of a disease or one of its features is especially difficult for systemic disease, as it requires the replication of disease manifestations by transfer of antibody or T-lymphocytes. The inference that a systemic disease is autoimmune is usually based on the presence of autoantibodies and the localization in diseased tissue of antibody, complement, and T-lymphocytes. Many animal models have been helpful in testing hypotheses about human systemic autoimmune disease, and in gaining insights into fundamental mechanisms; yet some models may not be representative of human diseases. The growing number of mouse strains whose autoimmunity occurs following deletion of immune system genes has at once generated many important basic insights yet at the same time raised questions about whether lesions in the targeted pathways are responsible for spontaneous autoimmune diseases.

Certain general features of systemic autoimmune diseases stand out as clues to their etiologies. The first is their variable course from person to person (or even from inbred mouse to inbred mouse) and their tendency to wax and wane in severity over time. In a single individual, disease activity can vary from life threatening to asymptomatic, even without medical intervention. This suggests the operation of potent forces that can down-regulate the autoimmune process.

A second characteristic of most systemic autoimmune conditions is the increased susceptibility of the female sex (1). Women are at least ten-fold more likely to develop SLE, for instance (2). Increased female disease incidence and severity is seen in many animal models as well. Efforts to understand the female tendency to develop autoimmune disease have not been entirely successful, but hormonal influences play a major role and endocrinologic abnormalities have been described (3,4).

A third feature of autoimmune disease is usually referred to as "overlap," the finding in certain individual patients of features of multiple systemic autoimmune diseases (5), and even of coexisting organ-specific autoimmune disease. This leads to taxonomic confusion; for example, some patients have an autoimmune disease sometimes termed "mixed connective tissue disease," which has features of SLE, scleroderma, and polymyositis (6).

It seems paradoxical that humans and animals with systemic autoimmune disease, despite their high immunoglobulin and autoantibody levels, respond poorly when immunized with exogenous antigens, as if their immune systems were preoccupied with responses to self-antigens (7). Cell-mediated immunity is particularly impaired (8), in part reflecting the lymphocytopenia characteristic of SLE (9). This immunosuppression may be further exacerbated by medical efforts to suppress autoantibody formation; infection due to immunosuppression is a regrettably common feature in patients suffering from systemic autoimmune disease (10).

HISTORICAL

The notion that autoantibodies or self-reactive cellular immunity could ever occur met with considerable resistance throughout the development of immunology as a discipline. Ehrlich and Morgenroth (11) and others proposed that the consequences of the formation of self-antibodies were so severe ("horror autotoxicus") that the immune system stringently prohibited its occurrence. Although investigators as early as Donath observed clear evidence of anti–self-agglutinins, it was not until the 1950s that the general acceptance of the concept that autoantibodies could cause immune injury came from the experiments of Harrington in human idiopathic thrombocytopenic purpura (ITP), where the profoundly low platelet counts of the ITP patients were reproduced in the investigator and his colleagues by transfer of patient serum (12); and from the pioneering work of Rose and Witebsky (13) in rabbit experimental thyroiditis. An important intellectual figure of the era was Burnet (14), whose the clonal selection theory postulated the elimination of self-reactive antibody producing cells.

NONPATHOLOGIC SYSTEMIC AUTOIMMUNITY

Autoimmune disease must be distinguished from the many instances of nonpathologic self-recognition by the immune system. These include the ready isolation of self–class II reactive T-lymphocytes (15) and the existence in normal individuals of low levels of autoantibodies to certain self-proteins (16). The use of binding assays like ELISA further complicates the definition of autoantibodies, as low-titer, low-affinity autoantibodies can be readily detected in the sera of normal individuals using almost any assay system of sufficient sensitivity. Even when threshold values are set to exclude low-titer positives, antinuclear antibodies and rheumatoid factor are seen in small but significant numbers of normal humans (17) and become more prevalent among the aged and among hospitalized patients (18).

Autoantibodies to some self-proteins may serve important physiologic functions. This has been best shown for rheumatoid factor (RF), which is autoantibody against IgG. RF is mainly of the IgM isotype, and a substantial fraction of IgM-bearing lymphocytes express this specificity (19,20). RF levels rise promptly after immunization with foreign antigens (21,22), and the antibody is commonly observed in the sera of patients with chronic infections (23), especially hepatitis C (24). RF probably serves to eliminate immune complexes; its affinity for monomeric IgG is low, yet is much higher for the multimeric IgG that exists in complexes. The binding of

RF to complexes very likely expedites their removal from the circulation via the mononuclear phagocyte system.

RF-bearing B cells may also serve an important function in presenting foreign antigens by virtue of their binding of antigen–antibody complexes (25). Mice expressing a human RF transgene produce little circulating RF; their RF-producing B cells are found in primary B-cell follicles and in the mantle zone of secondary splenic follicles (26). Spleen cells from these RF transgenic mice present human IgG antitetanus toxoid immune complexes with high efficiency. The resulting wave of T-cell help may serve to amplify the immune response, and its subsequent down-regulation may be related to deletion of many of the RF-bearing cells (26).

As depicted in Fig. 1, low-affinity IgM antibodies against other self-antigens have been observed in unimmunized animals (27,28). These antibodies may help shape the repertoire reactive against exogenous antigens. The fetal repertoire is rich in such antibodies, which are derived from a small set of VH and VL genes with limited somatic mutation (29). In mice expressing transgenic natural autoantibodies, neither deletion nor anergy of self-reactive B cells occurs, although these cells are functionally capable of deletion (30).

The B1 subset of B-lymphocytes, which in rodents is concentrated in the peritoneal cavity, may have as its primary function the production of IgM autoantibodies such as RF (31). In mice, B1 cells are responsible for production of certain antierythrocyte autoantibodies (32), but they are not the source of antichromatin antibodies or RF in the lpr model (33), nor do they produce such antibodies in GVH

disease (34). In SLE, both B1 and B2 cells secrete anti-DNA, but high-affinity autoantibody is derived from the B2 cells (35–37).

Autoantibodies to idiotypes are another form of nonpathogenic humoral autoimmunity. Anti-idiotypes arise after immunization and have been shown to mediate both negative and positive feedback of humoral responses, in some systems via regulatory T cells (38–40).

AUTOIMMUNITY AND TOLERANCE

The establishment and maintenance of immunologic tolerance is a key feature of the immune system, and is discussed in depth in Chapter 29. The occurrence of autoimmunity may reflect the imperfect nature of the tolerance generated in the developing T- and B-cell repertoires. Very likely, peripheral tolerance mechanisms prevent the emergence of systemic autoimmunity in adult life. In this regard, stra-13, a recently identified member of the basic helix-loop-helix family of transcription factors, may be critical for ongoing negative selection of both T and B cells, as its absence leads to an SLE-like disorder (41).

T-Cell Tolerance in Systemic Autoimmunity

No spontaneous systemic autoimmune disorders have thus far been shown to involve deficits in thymic negative selection and autoimmune diseases typically do not occur in the neonatal period, when one would anticipate the most intense

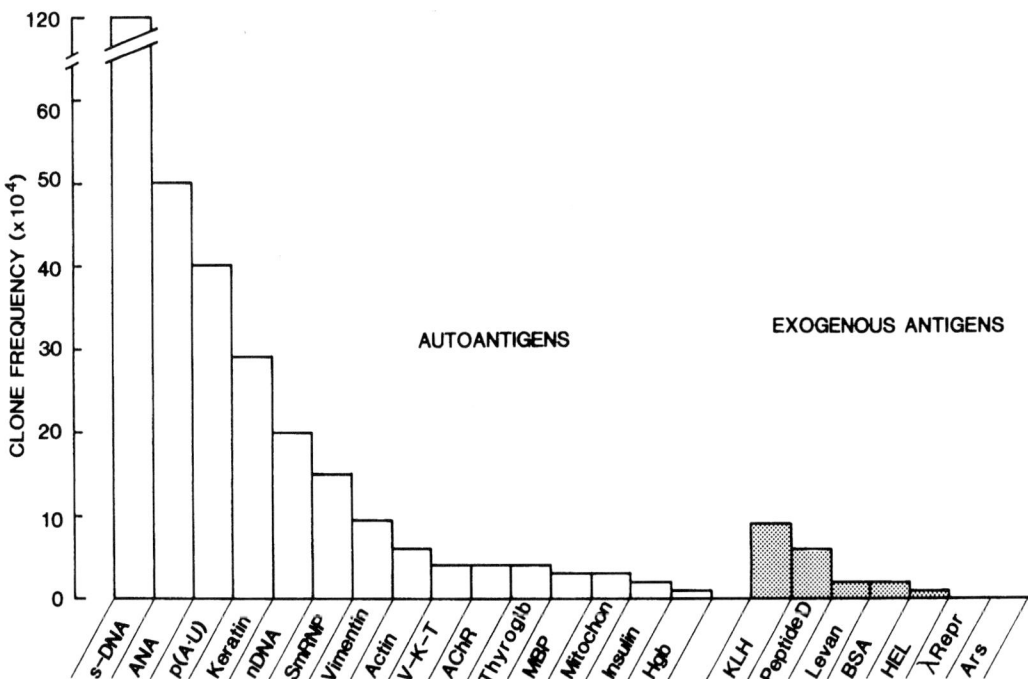

FIG. 1. The natural autoantibody repertoire in normal mice. Antibodies produced by 11,800 hybridomas prepared from splenic B cells of unimmunized 6-week-old A/J mice were screened for reactivity against a panel of autoantigens and foreign antigens. Note the high frequency of antibodies against nuclear and cytoskeletal antigens. (From Souroujon et al. (357), with permission.)

shaping of the T-cell repertoire. Lupus-like autoimmune disease provoked by the cardiac antiarrhythmic drug procainamide, however, has been shown to involve a lowered threshold for intrathymic positive selection, leading to export of chromatin-reactive T-lymphocytes (42). Such a mechanism might account for autoimmunity associated with other drugs or environmental agents.

Additional data show that intrathymic tolerance is of potential importance in establishing tolerance to nuclear antigens (43). Further, mice engineered to express class II MHC antigens only on epithelial cells fail to tolerize intrathymic CD4$^+$ T cells normally. T cells transferred from these animals into hosts with normal class II expression develop systemic autoimmunity, demonstrating that establishment of intrathymic tolerance as a necessary process to prevent autoimmunity (44).

B-Cell Tolerance in Systemic Autoimmunity

B-cell tolerance to protein antigens is abnormal in certain autoimmune disease models (45,46). Impaired B-cell tolerance may be more important than T-cell autoreactivity in the pathogenesis of NZB autoimmunity (47). The critical role of maintenance of B-cell tolerance in preventing systemic autoimmunity is further illustrated by a number of murine models in which deletion or addition of genes resulting in heightened B-cell activation leads not only to diffuse B-cell activation but also to autoantibodies and systemic autoimmunity. Overexpression of CD19, for example, leads to hyperglobulinemia, autoantibodies, and autoimmune disease, apparently due to a lower threshold of B-cell activation (48). Mice with targeted deletion of Lyn, which plays a key role in regulation of B-cell signaling, also develop systemic autoimmune disease, though the mechanism may be more complex (49). Animals rendered deficient in PD-1, which normally down-regulates B-cell function through immunoreceptor tyrosine-based inhibitory motifs, suffer a progressive systemic autoimmune syndrome (50), as do animals lacking CD22 (51), TGF β (52), the inhibitory wedge of CD45 (53), the B-cell inhibitory Fc γ RIIb (54), and SHP-1 (55). All of these genes appear to act constitutively to down-regulate B cells and thereby prevent systemic autoimmunity. The role of aberrations in these genes in spontaneous autoimmune diseases remains to be established, but there is evidence in humans correlating expression of genes leading to heightened B-cell activation with autoimmune disease (56).

While disordered tolerance is key to the pathogenesis of autoimmunity, the self-reactivity observed in most of these disorders argues for more than a global loss of tolerance. Instead, there is a selective autoimmune response directed primarily against intracellular autoantigens, and especially against components of the nucleus (57). A persistent question has been why these sequestered antigens become apparently immunogenic in individuals with SLE and other systemic autoimmune diseases. Exposure during apoptosis,

post-translational modification, and other mechanisms have been proposed to explain this bias toward nuclear antigens (58).

NATURE OF AUTOANTIGENS

Unlike immune responses arising from deliberate immunization, it is not obvious that autoimmunity is initiated or perpetuated by self-antigen. Other mechanisms can be conceived, and some have been seriously put forth. For instance, the diffuse activation of B cells by LPS leads to limited systemic autoimmunity (chiefly IgM antibodies to DNA and RF) and may be a good model for the autoimmunity that accompanies certain infections (e.g., Epstein–Barr virus [EBV] and mycoplasma [59]). It is also possible that aberrations in the web of idiotypes and anti-idiotypes could result in autoimmunity without the need for autoantigen as immunogen. Yet considerable evidence supports the view that self-antigens themselves act as immunogens for autoantibody responses.

Autoimmunity against nuclear protein complexes such as the snRNP spliceosome is directed against multiple components of the autoantigen, as might be expected from an immune response to the intact particle (60). Analysis of the fine specificity of these responses has revealed a further complexity consistent with what might be expected from a high-affinity, antigen-driven response (61,62). Administration to autoimmune-prone mice of a dominant peptide derived from the Sm autoantigen accelerates autoantibody production and disease, suggesting dependence of autoimmune responses on a supply of antigen (63).

A number of protein autoantigens have been shown to have undergone post-translational modification (64). For example, patients with rheumatoid arthritis frequently have antibodies to citrullinated proteins, which can be demonstrated in inflamed synovium (65). Many SLE-associated autoantigens undergo cleavage during apoptosis, and it has been argued that this process and also phosphorylation (66) render these proteins immunogenic (67).

Antigens seem to be necessary but not sufficient for significant autoantibody production: immunization of normal individuals with purified nuclear antigens in general yields weak responses and requires adjuvant, such as in the case of Ro antigen (68); and administration to mice of apoptotic cells results in only transient and low-level antinuclear antibody production (69). In contrast, immunization of rabbits and mice with small peptide fragments of certain autoantigens has been reported to result in antigen not only to the immunogenic epitope, but also to other epitopes on the same antigen and even to autoantibodies to other nuclear antigens and clinical evidence of SLE (70), although this finding may be difficult to reproduce (71,72). The peptide most intensively studied is found in EBV, suggesting a possible provocative agent (73). Autoimmunity may reflect epitope spreading, that is, the recruitment of T cells reactive to additional epitopes on the autoantigen. As tolerance usually does not extend to all such "cryptic" epitopes, a mechanism that might be capable of enlisting progressively more autoreactive T cells might amplify any initial breakage of tolerance. The impetus for such responses might come from immunization with autoantigens from another species, which could elicit T-cell help against bona fide foreign determinants, along with the generation of antibody against the foreign antigen (74). B cells expressing antibody cross-reactive with self-determinants could then selectively take up autoantigens, process them, and express autoantigenic peptides, including cryptic epitopes. The physical association of many autoantigens, such as Ro and La (75) or the many components of the snRNP complex, could lead to further diversification of an autoimmune response initiated by the breaking of tolerance to only a single autoantigen (76). For the La nuclear antigens, a hierarchy of immunogenic cryptic epitopes with differing potential for driving a full autoimmune response has been identified using peptide fragments of the intact antigen (77).

Immunization of animals with mammalian DNA generally does not lead to autoantibody production unless the DNA is complexed to a cationic protein such as methylated bovine serum albumin (78). DNA that has been damaged by UV irradiation or by reactive oxygen species is much more immunogenic than unaltered DNA, which may be relevant to UV-induced SLE exacerbations (79). Recently, much interest has focused on the potential of bacterial DNA to activate B cells and provoke autoimmune responses, through CpG motifs not found in mammalian DNA (80). Exposure to bacterial DNA also accelerates genetically predetermined autoimmune disease in NZB/NZW mice (81). Although it is possible that microbial DNA is an immunogen in SLE, the bulk of the small amount of circulating DNA in SLE has been shown to be of human origin and mostly in the form of small complexes bound to histone (82,83).

If nuclear antigens, normally sequestered behind two membranes, serve as immunogens, how do they become available for recognition by the immune system? Events related to cell death seem related to the release of self-antigens, although this area has been controversial. Autoantigens are released from senescent cells; they can be demonstrated in blebs on the surface of cells undergoing programmed cell death (84). It has been proposed that nuclear antigens in this form may serve autoimmunogens. As discussed above, proteolytic cleavage during apoptosis may render nuclear antigens particularly immunogenic, although not all SLE-related nuclear antigens behave in this manner (67).

It seems doubtful that the apoptotic cell itself can serve as a competent antigen-presenting cell for nuclear autoantigens; rather, it seems more likely that specialized APC present these molecules, perhaps the same cells which so avidly phagocytose apoptotic cells. Evidence for such cross-presentation by dendritic cells of antigens has been reported for the class I pathway (85). Macrophages bear the major burden of ingestion of apoptotic cells, a process facilitated by an array of receptors, and generally leading to the release of nonin-

flammatory cytokines such as TGF-β and IL-10, in contrast to TNF-α and other "inflammatory" cytokines stimulated by phagocytosis of yeast or particulate antigens (86). As a consequence, apoptotic debris generally does not provoke immune responses. When apoptotic cells are administered with LPS or other adjuvant, the altered macrophage cytokine profile leads to induction of co-stimulatory molecules and the generation of T-cell responses (87,88). Thus, apoptotic debris may be necessary but not sufficient to trigger autoreactivity. Adjuvant-like effects might come from infections or noxious environmental stimuli.

The elution of peptides from both class I and class II MHC molecules provides further reason to believe that nuclear autoantigens are presented to the immune system. Both in rodents and in humans, MHC molecules have been found to have peptides derived from such nuclear antigens as histone on their cell surfaces, presumably through the processing of nuclear debris (89). It is also possible that these peptides are derived from autoantigens are processed from within normal antigen processing cells using a class II pathway, although examples of such "inside-out" class II processing are uncommon (90). MHC class II molecules from autoimmune MRL/lpr mice appear to bind a more complex array of self-peptides than nonautoimmune controls, suggesting some selectivity among class II antigen-presenting cells in processing self-antigens (91).

GENERAL CHARACTERISTICS OF AUTOANTIBODIES

With some notable exceptions, the autoantibodies characteristic of systemic autoimmune disease are high-titer IgG antibodies (92). The genetic basis of autoantibodies has been best studied in mice, where hybridomas have been useful for sequence analysis (93). For individual autoimmune mice, anti-DNA and other autoantibodies recovered from hybridomas are usually clonally related, with extensive somatic mutation (94). Many clones show dual reactivity for DNA and other nuclear antigens, implying a common ancestry for some of these specificities (95). The binding site of antinuclear autoantibodies is dictated neither by the VH nor the VL hypervariable regions, but usually by a combination of both (96). In mice, there appears to be little bias in the use of heavy chains for antinuclear antibodies (97), while in humans certain VH genes may be predisposed to generate autoantibodies (98,99). Anti-DNA antibodies may arise from point mutations in the hypervariable regions of antibodies to exogenous antigens (100).

Extensive epitope mapping studies have been undertaken for many antinuclear antibodies. In most cases, it appears that the antibodies recognize multiple conformationally dependent, often discontinuous, epitopes of nuclear proteins (101,102). There is a predilection for binding to the active site of nuclear proteins. Thus the function of certain enzymes and other autoantigens may be inhibited by autoantibody containing sera. Antibodies to RNA are often found together with antibodies to the protein components of the snRNP particle, as well in sera containing antibody to other RNA-binding proteins (103). Autoantibodies in systemic autoimmune disease usually bind with greater avidity to antigen derived from the same species, emphasizing their derivation through affinity maturation, and their probable origin from immunization with self-proteins (104).

Isotype switching from IgM to IgG has been observed for some but not all autoantibodies. Anti-DNA antibodies in NZB/NZW mice undergo this process (105), as do certain serial samples of human sera. Autoantibodies in human and murine SLE are mostly of the highly T-dependent IgG (human IgG1, and mouse IgG2a and IgG2b) subclasses, probably reflecting their T-cell dependence (106,107).

Individuals with autoimmune diseases frequently have autoantibodies to multiple components of subcellular particles, such as ribosomal proteins, nucleoli, or snRNPs (108,109). This is suggestive of immunization by the particle itself. Autoantibodies also tend to be directed against nuclear antigens that are present in greater amounts in cells undergoing proliferation. For instance, proliferating cell nuclear antigen (PCNA), the centromeric proteins, and the nuclear mitotic apparatus protein NuMa are present in greatly increased concentrations during S and G2 phases of the cell cycle (110). Perhaps nuclear antigens are more available as immunogens at such times.

Antinuclear antibody levels can be quite high. In exceptional patients, 30% or more of the total antibody repertoire can be directed against a single specificity (111). Certain autoantibody levels fluctuate with disease activity (antinative DNA is the best-known example), but in the more usual case, antibody levels are fairly constant over time. Autoantibodies in SLE and SLE models occur in the midst of diffuse polyclonal B-cell activation. Antibodies to haptens, such as DNP, and to viral antigens are increased on the order of five- to ten-fold (112,113). In contrast, the levels of specific autoantibodies, such as antibodies to snRNP, or to Ro and La, are elevated far out of proportion to the polyclonal B-cell activation, and are not uncommonly thousands or millions of times greater than the weak binding that might be found in normal control serum (Fig. 2)

Certain SLE serologic specificities are seen in a variety of autoimmune and inflammatory diseases, and do not connote diagnostic specificity. Examples include antihistone and anti-DNA antibodies. Other autoantibodies, such as anti–double-stranded DNA, anti-Sm, and anti-Ro, are highly specific for the diagnosis of SLE and must in some way be linked to its

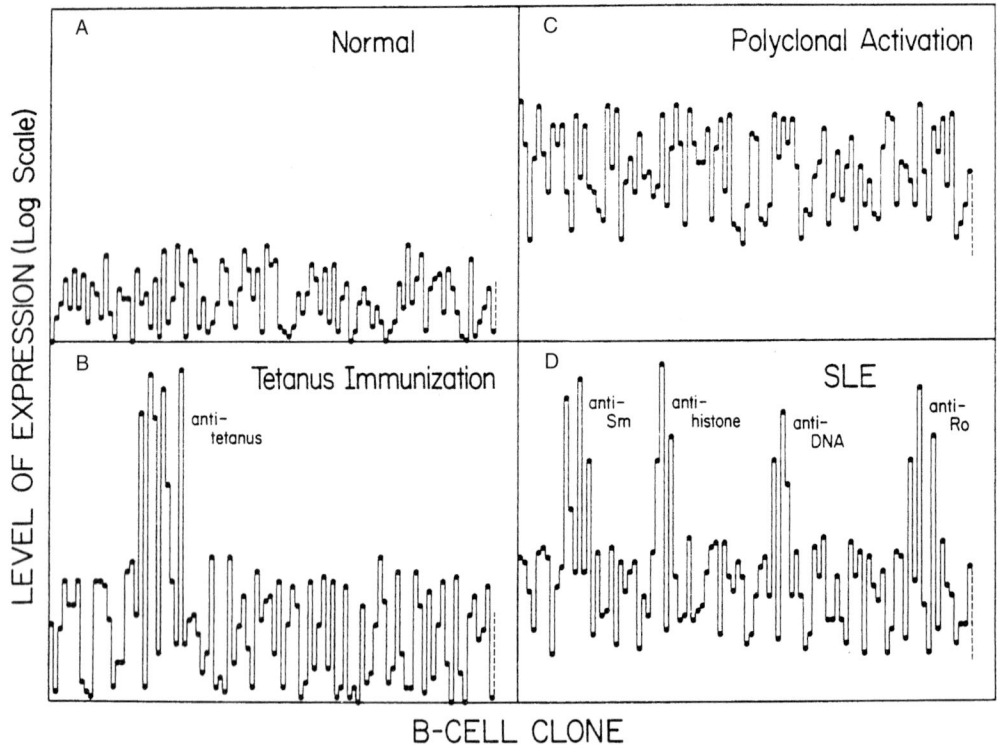

FIG. 2. Nature of autoantibody production in SLE. **A:** This panel depicts antibody arising from multiple B-cell clones in a normal individual. **B:** Tetanus toxoid immunization is shown to provoke a group of tetanus-specific B-cell clones, along with a modest degree of polyclonal activation. **C:** Effect of diffuse polyclonal activation resulting from exposure to bacterial lipopolysaccharide or other polyclonal B-cell activator. **D:** In contrast to *C,* illustrates the usual situation in SLE and other systemic autoimmune diseases, namely, a background of polyclonal B-cell activation together with large amounts of autoantibody arising from a discrete number of clones of defined specificity. From Eisenberg and Cohen (358), with permission.

TABLE 1. *Autoantibodies to nuclear proteins in systemic autoimmune disease*

Specificity	Antigen recognized	Disease association
Sm	U1, U2, U4-6 snRNPs	SLE
RNP	U1 snRNP	SLE, MCTD
Ro (SS-A)	60-kD RNA-binding protein	SLE, Sjögren's syndrome
La (SS-B)	50-kD RNA-binding protein	SLE, Sjögren's syndrome
Histone	H1, H2a, H2b, H3 (native)	SLE
Jo-1	Histidyl tRNA synthetase	Myositis
Scl-70	DNA topoisomerase I	Scleroderma
PCNA (cyclin)	DNA polymerase delta	SLE
Alu	Signal recognition particle	SLE, myositis
PL-7	Threonyl tRNA synthetase	Myositis
tRNA-1	Alanyl tRNA synthetase	Myositis, SLE, JRA
RNA polymerase I		Scleroderma
DNA (native)	Double-stranded DNA	SLE
DNA (denatured)	Single-stranded DNA	SLE, RA, inflammation
Centromere	CENP A, B, C	Raynaud's syndrome, CREST

RA, rheumatoid arthritis; SLE, systemic lupus erythematosus.

pathogenesis (Table 1). Some marker autoantibodies serve as excellent diagnostic correlates of scleroderma (antitopoisomerase I, or Scl-70) (114), of myositis (antihistidyl tRNA synthetase (115), or of Sjögren's syndrome (anti-Ro and anti-La) (116). Some of these autoantibodies are exquisitely specific for their autoantigens, and are hard if not impossible to generate by deliberate immunization of rabbits or other experimental animals (117).

Individual patients with SLE tend to have distinctive profiles of autoantibodies that usually remain stable throughout the course of the illness. While the patient-to-patient variability in antibody spectrum is undoubtedly due in part to genetic diversity, it is surprising that even genetically homogeneous inbred mice show considerable differences in their autoantibody levels. Inbred mice maintained in the same colony under the same conditions have sharp differences in their autoantibody specificities. The anti-Sm response of MRL/lpr may give insight into the genesis of SLE autospecificities. Only about 25% of these mice develop anti-Sm, regardless of the colony from which they are derived. Antibody levels show a true bimodal distribution, that is, anti-Sm negative MRL/lpr mice have negligible amounts of anti-Sm, comparable to normal mice. When the lineage and microenvironment of anti-Sm positive mice were traced, no genetic or environmental clustering could explain the appearance of autoantibody in certain mice but not others. The occurrence of the anti-Sm specificity in only a minority of mice was not due to the use of an uncommon V gene, nor to unusual gene rearrangements. The individual variability in the laboratory and perhaps the clinical manifestations of SLE and other autoimmune diseases may arise from poorly understood stochastic influences (118).

GENETICS OF SYSTEMIC AUTOIMMUNE DISEASE

Susceptibility to SLE is strongly influenced by genetics. In studies of identical twins with SLE, the concordance rate has been reported to be between 28% and 57% (119,120). Multiple genes are involved in determining SLE susceptibility; even in inbred mouse models, the genetics are complex, contributions from multiple genes. Genes that alone do not cause disease may interact with other genes to result in disease, and inhibitory genes further complicate the picture (121). Neither the NZB nor the NZW parent strains develop renal disease or antinative DNA antibodies, yet the F1 hybrid resulting from their crossing develops severe SLE-like renal disease and antinative DNA. The most important NZW genetic contribution to murine SLE is linked to the MHC, probably MHC class II genes. Much progress has been made in characterizing the three most important non-MHC linked genes derived from this strain, termed *Sle-1*, *Sle-2*, and *Sle-3*. *Sle-1* results in impaired tolerance to nuclear antigens, while *Sle-2* renders B cells mores susceptible to activation (122). *Sle-3* controls CD4 T-cell regulation. These genes interact to produce an SLE phenotype. The *Sle-1* locus itself is subdivided into three loci. One of these appears to encode a defective form of CR1 that results in reduced C3d binding and signaling (123).

NZB contributes a chromosome 4–linked gene that is most important for nephritis, but at least seven other genes have been reported to contribute. Surprisingly, the chromosome 4 gene determining nephritis susceptibility does not affect the levels of anti-DNA, antihistone, and antichromatin (124). Microarray analysis of B cells from congenic mouse strains has produced strong evidence that the interferon-inducible gene Ifi-202 is involved (125), possibly through the action of variant forms on apoptosis and cell proliferation.

Microsatellite markers analysis of sib pairs with SLE has defined a region of human chromosome 1 linked to disease susceptibility (126). This region may be syntenic to the region of mouse chromosome 1 previously shown to determine renal disease and mortality in NZB mice. While the region encompassed by these studies is large and remains to be defined further, candidate genes include those for Fc receptor γ II and III (127).

Genetic deficiencies of complement result in increased risk of SLE (128). C2-deficient individuals are at greatly increased risk of developing SLE, as are those with absent C1q. Several possibilities could explain the link between C deficiency and lupus. First, as discussed elsewhere, C assists the removal of apoptotic cells and its absence might lead to an increased amount of apoptotic debris. Next, C deficiency might predispose to certain infections which might trigger lupus. Finally, especially because several C genes are located within the major histocompatibility complex, the SLE association might reflect linkage to other genes.

Other disorders of the innate immune system may also represent risk factors for SLE. Mutations in the mannose-binding lectin have been reported to be increased in SLE and other autoimmune disorders (129).

ROLE OF T CELLS IN SYSTEMIC AUTOIMMUNE DISEASE

Nature of T-Cell Help for Autoantibody Formation

A diverse body of evidence supports the notion that T-lymphocytes are required for the generation of systemic autoimmune disease. In spontaneous SLE animal models, administration of anti–T-cell antibody ameliorates disease and reduces autoantibody levels, as does blocking of T-cell costimulatory molecules (130–132). Mice lacking T cells as a result of thymic extirpation, via genetic restriction of the T-cell repertoire by receptor gene deletion, or by imposition of transgenes have much reduced autoimmunity (133). In humans, therapy directed against T cells, such as cyclosporine A, mycophenolate mofetil, and cyclophosphamide, leads to improvement of SLE and other systemic autoimmune conditions. Although thymectomy in SLE may lead to exacerbation or remission of disease (134), HIV infection of SLE patients, with its depletion of CD4-bearing T cells, has been reported to induce remissions in SLE activity (135,136), further supporting a role for a continuing source of T-cell help for SLE autoantibodies.

Indirect evidence for T-cell participation in SLE comes from analysis of the isotype and extent of somatic mutation of autoantibodies. In general, autoantibody responses are high-affinity IgG responses (137), which appear to have undergone affinity maturation, a process that requires T cells. Their pattern of extensive replacement mutations in hypervariable regions underlies this increase in antibody affinity.

Defining the specificity of autoreactive T cells required for spontaneous autoimmunity in humans and in animal models has been a challenging problem. It is not difficult to find evidence of T-cell autoreactivity to class II MHC antigens (138), even in normal individuals. The degree to which this represents autoreactivity to self-peptides compared to reactivity to the class II MHC molecule itself is uncertain. Self–Ia-reactive T cells are less abundant in human and murine systemic autoimmunity (139), and this defect may vary with disease activity. Such autoreactive T cells cloned from diseased individuals, on the other hand, have been shown to induce pathology under some circumstances. They elicit lesions typical of the inflammatory skin disease lichen planus (140) and are present among the hyperproliferative T cells found in mice expressing the lpr Fas mutant gene (141). Whether cells capable of provoking an autologous mixed lymphocyte reaction are involved in providing help for autoantibody production is unknown.

Beside any role as helpers, T cells may provoke direct cellular injury in systemic autoimmunity. In chronic GVH disease, CD4- and CD8-bearing T cells cause inflammatory infiltrates in skin, intestine, and elsewhere (142). There is evidence that T cells in systemic lupus are spontaneously activated, as judged by increased expression of activation antigens (143,144). T-lymphocytes are found in inflammatory skin lesions (145) and may be responsible for some of the other nonrenal manifestations of the illness (146,147). For the most part, however, autoimmunity mediated directly by T cells seems to be more characteristic of organ-specific autoimmune disease, such as experimental allergic encephalomyelitis (EAE), than it is of systemic autoimmune disease.

Even in patients with high titer autoantibodies, T-cell proliferation to most nuclear autoantigens has been difficult to demonstrate, though reactivity against several *bona fide* SLE autoantigens has been documented (148,149). Weak T-cell responses, despite high levels of autoantibodies to SLE autoantigens, may reflect recognition of proteins (some perhaps not yet recognized) that may be linked to those autoantigens recognized by B cells, as has been suggested to explain the low magnitude of patient T-cell responses to nested peptides from the entire La molecule (150).

Some of the most extensive work on specificity of T-helper cells in systemic autoimmunity comes from analysis of clones of SLE T cells that provide help for anti-DNA autoantibody production. These cells have charged motifs in their T-cell receptor CDR3s, presumably promoting binding to peptides derived from charged DNA-binding nucleosomal proteins (high-mobility group and histones). Anti–DNA-specific B cells probably bind to the DNA, complexed with associated proteins, thus leading to the internalization and to the processing of these proteins for presentation to CD4$^+$ T cells (151). SLE mouse models have allowed *in vivo* experiments to define the role of T cells. Treatment of NZB/NZW mice with anti–Thy 1 or anti-CD4 prevents autoantibody production and renal disease (131,152). Thymectomy of these mice, on the other hand, exacerbates autoimmunity in males but ameliorates disease in females, reflecting complex T-cell interactions early in life (153). In the lpr model, thymectomy prevents disease if done within 72 hours of birth (154,155), and antibody depletion of T cells prevents both autoantibody formation and lymphoid hyperplasia.

Even in these defined genetic models, the precise role of T cells and the amount of nonspecific versus specific help for autoantibody production has been elusive. The T-cell repertoire of NZB/NZW mice, despite its content of autoantigen specific T cells, shows polyclonal and not oligoclonal T-cell activation (156). In MRL/lpr mice, disease fails to develop in animals in which a source of normal T cells is provided and in which lpr T cells have been depleted, indicating that the T cells provide more than just a passive source of cytokines or nonspecific help and that they participate actively as helpers for autoantibody-producing B cells (157). The extreme restriction of the TCR repertoire imposed by expression of a TCR Vβ transgene has been reported to result in lower autoantibody levels and increased survival in MRL/lpr mice (158), suggesting again that autoantigen-specific T-cell help is required for autoantibody production.

The transgenic studies could be confounded by the ability of such mice to express endogenous α or β chains. MRL/lpr mice transgenic for both the α and β chains of a pigeon cytochrome C hybridoma and lacking endogenous α and β chains, have been constructed (159). Hypergammaglobulinemia and autoantibodies to IgG, DNA, and snRNPs developed despite the lack of autoantigen-specific T-cell help in these mice. Lymphadenopathy, renal, salivary, and cutaneous disease were absent, suggesting that more specific T-cell help was required for these manifestations. These studies indicate that both antigen-specific and antigen-nonspecific T-cell help are required for full development of the MRL/lpr SLE syndrome. In this regard, chimera studies in which lpr mice have been constructed using congenic donors in which T–B interactions could be analyzed have shown that the T help required for autoantibody production is MHC restricted: in other words, autoreactive T cells must share class II MHC determinants with autoreactive B cells in order for autoantibody production to occur (160).

The role of $\gamma\delta$ T cells has also been evaluated in MRL/lpr mice by comparing disease manifestations and autoimmunity in mice lacking $\gamma\delta$ T cells (161). In the absence of the latter, mice developed a more severe autoimmune syndrome, suggesting a regulatory role for $\gamma\delta$ T cells. In the converse situation, mice lacking $\alpha\beta$ T cells had only an attenuated SLE syndrome, implying that $\gamma\delta$ T cells were capable of providing significantly less help for autoantibody production than $\alpha\beta$ T cells.

T cells reactive to nuclear proteins have been further studied in murine models. For MRL mice, which are prone to develop antibodies to the snRNP complex, snRNP-reactive T cells can be demonstrated in draining lymph nodes after immunization with purified snRNPs (162). While normal mice can generate T cells reactive to foreign snRNP, only MRL mice and mice expressing certain MHC alleles can recognize snRNP of murine origin (163). The ability of normal mice to generate T cells reactive to self-antigens after immunization with foreign nuclear antigen may reflect "epitope spreading." This process entails the recruitment of T cells reactive to self-peptides as a result of the presentation of self-antigen by B cells cross-reactive with self-proteins.

T cells reactive to overlapping core histone peptides have been described in SLE-prone SWR X NZB F1 mice (164). These antigenic determinants are apparently protected in intact chromatin, as responses to whole histone are usually not measurable. Interestingly, these T-cell antigenic regions of histones overlap with determinants recognized by antihistone autoantibodies. Chromatin-reactive T cells have been reported in procainamide-induced SLE, and are able to transfer disease (165).

T-cell help for autoantibody production may also be mediated through T cells specific for variable regions of autoantibody molecules. NZB/NZW mice develop T cells that recognize peptides corresponding to the variable regions of anti-DNA antibodies (166). Presumably there is presentation to T cells of peptides derived from the processing of self-immunoglobulin by B cells. The resulting helper T cells can provide autoantibody-specific help, and interference with their action has been reported to ameliorate autoimmune disease.

CD40 ligand (CD40L) may play a critical role in regulating autoantibody production in SLE. Expression of this T-cell activation-related molecule is increased in SLE patients, especially those with active disease, and also appears on some SLE B-lymphocytes (167). The latter observation may account for a relative T-independence of some SLE antibody formation. Treatment of NZB X SWR F1 mice with antibody to CD40L prevents autoimmune disease (168). MRL/lpr mice genetically deficient in CD40L, in contrast, develop autoantibodies to nuclear antigens, but these are skewed toward the IgM isotype, suggesting impairment of class switching (169). Renal disease appears to be diminished in such mice.

An interesting T-cell defect recently reported in AND T-cell transgenic MRL mice may help explain autoreactive T cells in this strain. These TCR-anticytochrome-C transgenic mice showed greater apparent intrinsic T-cell reactivity to peptide-MHC complexes, suggesting a lower signaling threshold (170). Parallel observations have been made using T cells from patients with SLE (171).

Regulatory T-Cell Abnormalities

T cells can exert a controlling influence on the generation of autoantibodies and on the regulation of organ-specific autoimmunity, but their involvement in systemic autoimmunity is less well established (172). Thymectomy of normal animals, in some systems, results in autoimmunity, both systemic and organ specific (173). Nude mice develop autoantibodies and immune complex renal disease, a process reversible by adoptive transfer of T cells (174,175), implying that regulatory T cells control antinuclear antibody production. In SLE, there are multiple reports of in vitro abnormalities of regulatory T-cell function both in animals in humans (176). Much of the extensive literature on suppressor defects in systemic autoimmunity merits reexamination in the context of present thinking about helper and cytotoxic cell subsets based on their cytokine phenotype. Very likely much of previously observed phenomena represent the potent action of cytokines derived from these T-helper subsets.

CYTOKINES IN SYSTEMIC AUTOIMMUNE DISEASE

A multiplicity of cytokine abnormalities has been associated with systemic autoimmune diseases and models. Some occur late in illness and are probably not causal, while others may be actively involved in regulation and dysregulation of immune responses. In general, IL-2 levels and the expression of IL-2 receptors are diminished both in human and murine SLE (177), and in several related autoimmune disorders. Circulating IL-2 receptors may be increased, however, in parallel with other circulating receptors (178), although assays for these receptors are difficult. Efforts to characterize SLE as a TH1 or TH2 disease based on the phenotype of helper cells have met with difficulty, but IL-10 seems to be increased in human and murine SLE, along with IL-6. The ratio of IL-10 to IFN-γ–secreting cells in SLE peripheral blood is increased, implying a predominance of TH2 cells in the circulation (179). Supporting the importance of TH2 cells in promoting systemic autoimmunity is the observation that some IL-4 transgenic mice develop SLE-like antinuclear antibodies, hemolytic anemia, and immune-mediated renal disease (180).

Interferons may be especially important for the pathogenesis of SLE. Interferon-producing cells are significantly more abundant among circulating T cells in patients with SLE (181); it is particularly noteworthy that they are found both in the circulation and within renal lesions in patients with diffuse proliferative glomerulonephritis (182). The importance of interferon-γ in SLE may reflect a more fundamental role in inflammation and autoimmunity than what would be expected merely from predominance of TH1 cells (183). Interferon-α may also play a special role in the pathogenesis of autoimmunity. This cytokine may be produced in response to immune complexes and apoptotic cells, and then serve to activate proinflammatory dendritic cells (184). It has recently been reported that SLE serum, due to its interferon-α content, exerts such an action on dendritic cells (185), although others have shown decreased dendritic cell function in this disease (186). Finally, a microarray approach has implicated an interferon-inducible gene contributed by NZB in the pathogenesis of disease in NZB/NZW mice (125).

For murine SLE models in general, cytokine patterns are variable. In both NZB/NZW and MRL/lpr, a complex pattern not fitting either TH1 or TH2 is seen, with increases in IL-6, IL-4, and IL-10 (187). TNF-α may also be increased, and evidence has been published that allelic polymorphisms at this locus predispose to SLE (188,189). For autoimmunity due to chronic GVH disease, a TH2 profile has been observed (190).

The newly discovered TNF family cytokine Blys (also known as TALL-1, BAFF, THANK, and zTNF4) is derived from monocyte-macrophages and has an important role in B-cell homeostasis. Mice overexpressing this molecule or its receptor develop hyperglobulinemia and systemic autoimmunity (191) and elevated levels of Blys have been observed in patients with SLE (192). This molecule presents a potential target for therapeutic intervention.

ENVIRONMENTAL INFLUENCES ON SYSTEMIC AUTOIMMUNITY

Limited and at times idiosyncratic forms of systemic autoimmune disease may be provoked or exacerbated by a variety of environmental agents, including drugs, infections, and toxins (193,194). Definition of environmental links to pathogenesis of SLE and other autoimmune disorders has been difficult (195). Mechanisms that have been invoked include adjuvant effects of silica (196), environmental estrogens (197), molecular mimicry induced by viral or bacterial antigens (198), or the immunostimulatory properties of their DNA.

The ingestion of certain drugs is clearly linked to development of an SLE-like syndrome (199). Unlike spontaneous SLE, renal and CNS involvement are rare, and the syndrome resolves after discontinuing the drug. Procainamide, used extensively for treatment of ventricular arrhythmias, is the best-studied agent provoking drug-induced SLE, but hydralazine, chlorpromazine, diphenylhydantoin, and many other drugs can also cause the SLE-like syndrome, characterized mainly by pleuropericarditis, arthritis, pulmonary infiltrates, and fever. Only about 10% of patients given procainamide develop clinically evident disease, but fluorescent antinuclear antibodies appear in the vast majority of patients taking the drug for prolonged periods. Antibodies are directed mostly against histones, and a distinct specificity and isotype pattern have been reported (200). No relationship to procainamide acetylator frequency governs SLE development. It has been proposed that procainamide exerts its action by hypomethylation of DNA, with consequent overexpression of LFA-1 on T-lymphocytes, leading to enhanced autoreactive T-cell help (201). An active metabolite of procainamide has been found to impair thymic tolerance to low-affinity self-antigens during positive selection, leading to emergence of autoreactive T cells and SLE-like autoimmunity (42).

The contribution of infectious agents to systemic autoimmunity remains an active area of investigation. It is clear that systemic autoimmunity can arise as an immediate consequence of infection with EBV and mycoplasma, and probably other viral infections (202). While antinuclear antibodies arising immediately after infectious mononucleosis are short-lived and probably are harmless, a remarkable statistical association of increased SLE prevalence with early EBV seroconversion has reawakened interest in the importance of this agent in precipitating SLE, possibly through molecular mimicry followed by epitope spreading (73).

Systemic autoimmunity may arise during the course of severe microbial infections, such as endocarditis and osteomyelitis. Occasionally, skin and kidney lesions are seen, probably representing deposits of immune complexes, possibly associated with rheumatoid factor (203).

Vasculitis, discussed below, accompanies meningococcal, rickettsial, spirochetal, and many other bacterial infections. Systemic autoimmunity is also a sometime feature of HIV infection, and may reflect imbalance of helper cell subsets (204). Various bacterial superantigens have been implicated in autoimmune phenomena, including vasculitis, associated with infections (205). Kawasaki disease, caused by an unknown agent, causes a serious vasculitis and alterations in Vβ expression suggesting the role of a superantigen (206).

The influence of infection on the development of murine SLE is controversial. NZB mice maintained germ free still develop antierythrocyte autoantibodies (207); however, NZB mice in a germ-free environment develop lower levels of IgG and antinuclear antibodies and less renal disease (208), and immunization of NZB/NZW mice with bacterial DNA accelerates development of renal disease (81). MRL/lpr mice, in contrast, develop similar levels of autoantibodies when raised in germ-free compared to conventional environments (209). Antigen-free animals develop milder renal disease, but this may reflect lipid intake changes necessitated by the antigen-free diet.

Certain toxins are capable of inducing systemic autoimmune disease. Mercuric chloride is the best-studied heavy metal associated with autoimmunity. Animals given HgCl$_2$ develop antinuclear antibodies and immune-complex nephritis. T cells are required, and background genes as well as MHC class II haplotype are important determinants of autoantibody specificity (210,211).

Systemic sclerosis and related fibrotic diseases believed to be of autoimmune origin may rarely be provoked by toxins. Workers exposed to polyvinyl chloride are at risk for a scleroderma-like syndrome (212), and an inflammatory and fibrotic scleroderma-like illness has been linked to the ingestion of rapeseed oil (213). An eosinophilic infiltrative disease is caused by a contaminant of L-tryptophan preparations (214). An area of great controversy has been the relationship between silicone breast implants and the development of scleroderma or other rheumatic diseases. Several studies have failed to find a true association (215,216) despite anecdotal reports.

APOPTOSIS ABNORMALITIES IN SYSTEMIC AUTOIMMUNE DISEASE

The realization that the autoimmune and lymphoproliferative syndromes of lpr and gld mice were due to mutations in the Fas apoptosis receptor and its ligand, together with the implication of apoptotic cells as possible sources of nuclear autoantigens, led to great interest in apoptosis in autoimmune diseases. ALPS (autoimmune lymphoproliferative syndrome), a rare illness resulting in lymphoid enlargement and immune cytopenias (217,218), results from a dominant nonfunctional Fas molecule or, in some cases, defective caspase signaling. Like lpr and gld mice, affected children develop "double-negative" T cells and hypergammaglobulinemia. Unlike the murine mutations, however, patients rarely develop antinuclear antibodies or lupus-like renal pathology.

The apoptosis resistance imparted by the mutant Fas molecule in lpr mice has been intensively studied. Thymic selection, as reflected by deletion of I-E and mammary tumor virus–reactive T cells, is normal in lpr mice although peripheral T-cell tolerance is impaired (219). The delayed development of autoimmunity in lpr mice probably reflects the gradual appearance and clonal expansion of such autoreactive T cells.

Chimeric (220) and tetraparental (221) experiments in which lpr T or B cells coexist with cells of normal origin have shown that B cells must also express the Fas defect in order for autoimmunity to occur, and B cells in both lpr and gld mice are resistant to apoptosis in vitro (222). In vivo studies of tolerance in mice expressing transgenic self-reactive antibodies have shown surprisingly little difference between lpr and normal mice. In the HEL–anti-HEL system, most B6/lpr mice maintain tolerance through early life. A significant minority, however, break through and generate autoantibodies at 5 months and beyond (46). These findings imply that other mechanisms can substitute effectively for the Fas/FasL system for maintenance of tolerance. Parallel results are reported for mice with an anti–H-2^k transgene: in a conventional facility, most lpr mice maintain tolerance as well as mice with a normal Fas gene, but a few develop anti–H-2^k autoantibodies (223). When housed in a specific pathogen-free colony, however, tolerance is intact, suggesting an important role for microbial influences.

Systemic autoimmune disease has been observed in animals with other impairments of apoptosis. Mice transgenic for the antiapoptosis Bcl-2 proto-oncogene develop antinuclear antibodies and immune-mediated renal disease (224). Animals lacking the related but proapoptotic protein Bim also develop autoimmunity late in life (225), reinforcing the idea that apoptosis regulation at multiple steps is required to prevent autoimmunity. In this regard, lupus-like autoimmunity also occurs in mice lacking IEX-1 (immediate-early response gene X-1). This gene targets NFκB and blocks apoptosis early in immune responses. In its absence, there is abnormal persistence of immune responses, including apparently self-responses. Mice with a partial deficiency in the PTEN tumor suppressor develop autoimmune disease similar to that seen in Fas-deficient mice, apparently because of defective up-regulation of Fas (226).

Bcl-2 expression has generally been found elevated in peripheral blood cells from SLE patients (227) and may be selectively expressed in T cells (228). Dramatic differences in apoptosis susceptibility seem unlikely to be uncovered in SLE patients (229,230), but it is likely that apoptosis abnormalities may be among the multiple genetic factors contributing to SLE susceptibility. This appears to be the case for several models, and apoptosis resistance is emerging as a contributing trait to the lupus phenotype (231).

A major direction in apoptosis research related to autoimmunity concerns aberrations in the disposition of apoptotic debris. Very large numbers of apoptotic cells are generated continuously and are efficiently engulfed by macrophages that recognize them via a battery of receptors including CD36/vitronectin receptor, a receptor for phosphatidylserine, complement receptors, CD14, mannose receptors, scavenger receptors A and B, and the membrane tyrosine kinase mer. Immunization of normal mice with large amounts of apoptotic cells leads to mild and short-lived autoimmunity, indicating the potential immunogenicity of apoptotic debris (69).

Complement is important in the clearance of apoptotic debris (232). The absence of CR2 converts the mildly autoimmune B6/lpr strain to a strain with severe lupus-like disease, probably reflecting impaired handling of apoptotic debris (233), as do B6/lpr mice lacking C4 (234). Humans with C1q deficiency develop SLE almost uniformly, as do mice in which the C1q gene is deleted (235). The well-known association between SLE and complement deficiency may reflect the role of the classical pathway in disposing of apoptotic corpses (236).

Other proteins participate in the removal of apoptotic bodies. SLE-like disease has been seen in mice lacking the acute phase reactant serum amyloid protein, which binds to chromatin and apparently facilitates the removal of nuclear debris (237). Lupus in mice lacking Dnase I may be due to the delayed clearance of nuclear debris in the absence of this enzyme (238).

Mice lacking the cytoplasmic domain of mer (239) develop SLE-like autoimmunity; in the absence of Axl and Tyro-3, two related membrane tyrosine kinases, disease is more severe and is accompanied by lymphoproliferation (240). Autoimmunity in mer–deficient mice probably is also due to the altered, proinflammatory pattern of cytokine production by their macrophages (241). Recently, it has been reported that lymph nodes from human SLE patients, compared to controls, contain greater numbers of apoptotic bodies located outside of macrophages, lending support to the notion that apoptotic debris might be of significance in human autoimmune disease (242).

AUTOIMMUNITY AND MALIGNANCY

Individuals with certain forms of systemic autoimmunity are at increased risk for development of malignancies, particularly those of the lymphoid system. While patients with SLE, rheumatoid arthritis, and most other connective tissue diseases are perhaps two or three times more likely to develop lymphoma, in Sjögren's syndrome the risk is over 40-fold increased (243). In NZB mice, there is also a marked increased incidence of lymphomas (244), and plasmacytoid tumors have been found to develop in MRL/lpr mice (245). Human lymphomas tend to be of the B-cell variety, sometimes secreting IgM paraproteins with rheumatoid factor activity, and may derive from cells producing the rheumatoid factors

of restricted clonality produced in this illness (246). In this regard, it has been proposed that rheumatoid factor–specific B cells from patients with Sjögren's syndrome may be particularly susceptible to infection with oncogenic viruses because of the specificity of their surface IgM for IgG (247). Others have viewed chronic stimulation of autoantibody-producing cells as the first stage of a process involving chromosome breaks and oncogene activation leading to lymphoma (248). Patients with ALPS have recently been reported to have a high incidence of lymphomas, implying an important role for Fas–Fas ligand interactions in immune surveillance (249).

Autoimmunity is a feature of certain malignancies, particularly tumors of the lymphoid system. Cold agglutinins, rheumatoid factors, anti-DNA antibodies, and other self-reactive antibodies are produced by certain lymphomas and show remarkably restricted use of certain VH genes, usually in unmutated form (250). For example, VH4-21 is frequently used in antierythrocyte autoantibodies associated with lymphomas, and may reflect the location of tumor origin as well as environmental factors promoting tumorigenesis (251). Lymphoma- and chronic lymphocyte leukemia–related autoantibodies usually arrive from germline V genes expressed in CD5 B cells (252). These B1 cells may be particularly susceptible to malignant transformation, and after that event, may be able to produce their autoreactive antibodies and cause pathology (253).

A wide variety of autoantibodies have been reported in lymphoid and nonlymphoid tumors, causing clotting and platelet abnormalities (254); neurologic paraneoplastic syndrome (255); pemphigus (256); and myasthenia gravis (257). The relationship of thymoma with myasthenia gravis is intriguing, and may reflect export of autoreactive T cells from the thymus into the periphery (257). Patients with malignancies not infrequently develop antibodies against oncogenes such as C-myc and C-myb, against p53, against proliferation-associated antigens such as cyclins, and against antigens expressed by their tumor (e.g., MAGE in melanoma) (258). The extent to which they contribute to tumor suppression is unclear, as is their mechanism of generation.

FEATURES OF HUMAN SYSTEMIC AUTOIMMUNE DISORDERS

Systemic Lupus Erythematosus

SLE is a multisystem disorder most frequently affecting young women. Arthritis, skin rash, CNS dysfunction, and renal disease are the most common clinical manifestations (259). The severity of illness has a remarkable tendency to fluctuate over time, confounding studies of drug treatment. Long-term survival is the rule, although there remains considerable morbidity and mortality, chiefly from renal disease.

Immunologic interest in SLE dates back to the 1940s, when elevated gamma globulin levels were noted, and attention was called to marrow tart cells. The realization that the spontaneous neutrophil phagocytosis of nuclear material observed *in vivo* could also be seen in buffy coat preparations from patients, and could be induced in normal buffy coat cells by addition of patient serum, gave rise to the notion that antibodies to nuclear material were of key importance. This led to many investigations of SLE antinuclear factors, demonstrated to be IgG, and to the development of a universal highly sensitive test for SLE, the fluorescent antinuclear antibody test (FANA) (260). More than 95% of SLE patients have positive FANAs; further, that the pattern of fluorescence staining was related to the antinuclear antibodies present in individual SLE serum (261). Diffuse staining, for example, was shown to be due to antibodies to histones and other DNA-binding proteins, rim staining to be due to antinative DNA, and a speckled pattern to reflect antibodies to components of the splicing apparatus such as snRNPs. Some antibodies, detected by more specific methods such as double immunodiffusion or ELISA, are quite specific for SLE (e.g., anti-Sm, anti-Su, anti-Ro, anti-La, and antinative DNA). Fig. 3 illustrates the variable clinical and laboratory findings in a typical SLE patient.

Although SLE is best known for its array of antinuclear antibodies (Table 1), antibodies to many other self-components are well described. With the exception of IgG, the antigens tend to be cell bound—for example, antibodies to lymphocytes, platelets, erythrocytes, neutrophils, and basement membranes. In the case of IgG and clotting factors, it is possible that the true autoantibody target is cell bound in the form of immune complexes or of activated clotting factors.

Despite the wealth of information regarding SLE autoantibodies, it is useful to realize that only a few are implicated in disease pathogenesis. SLE renal disease has been attributed to DNA–anti-DNA complexes trapped in glomerular endothelium and epithelium, presumably triggering complement-mediated vascular injury and inflammation, although the pathogenesis of renal disease involves other pathways (262). Although concentrated DNA–anti-DNA complexes are found in eluates from SLE glomeruli (263), other antigen–antibody systems may be as important (264).

Although presumably nonrenal manifestations of SLE are autoantibody mediated, little mechanistic data exist except for the various cytopenias, for which an immune basis is well supported. Inflammatory skin disease (Fig. 4) appears to be T-cell mediated, although antibodies to Ro and La may be of importance (265). Infants born to SLE patients occasionally have thrombocytopenia and lesions typical of subacute cutaneous SLE, together with the Ro and La antibodies typical of this condition and sometimes congenital heart block (266). Transplacental passage of IgG autoantibodies from mother to fetus explains the infant disease, as well as its spontaneous resolution, which is coincident with the disappearance of maternal antibody. Presumably the nonreversible heart block often seen in infants born to anti-Ro–positive mothers is also mediated by antibody, which damages the developing cardiac conduction system.

Several other SLE manifestations have been difficult to relate to immune processes. CNS involvement can lead to psychosis, seizures, and debilitating neurologic deficits (267). Nervous system tissue from affected patients is usually devoid of immunoglobulin deposition or evidence of cellular infiltration, the only usual finding being microvascular changes. The recent finding of autoantibodies to the NMDA receptor in SLE patients is provocative and may lead to a better understanding of the perplexing CNS findings in this disease (268). Immunologic studies of arthritis and of pleural and pericardial inflammation in SLE are few, and an immune basis can only be presumed.

Rheumatoid Arthritis

Rheumatoid arthritis (RA) is a common chronic inflammatory polyarthritis of worldwide distribution, with a female

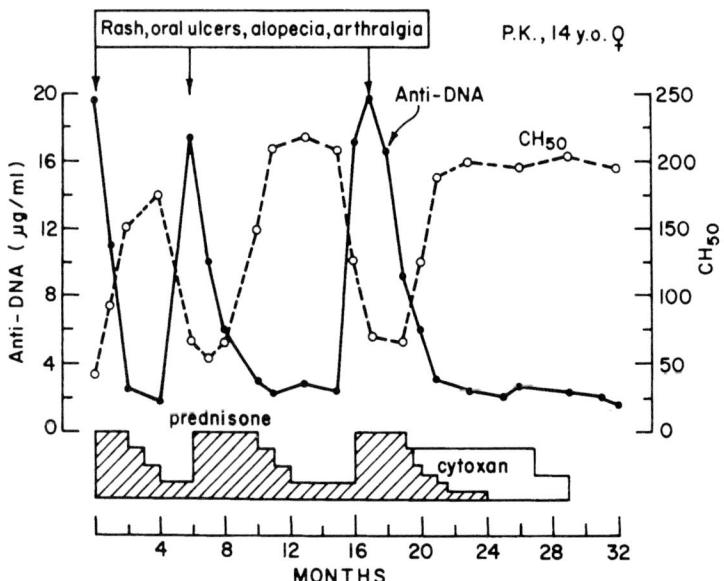

FIG. 3. Clinical course of a patient with systemic lupus erythematosus. Note the "mirror image" pattern of levels of anti-DNA antibodies and hemolytic complement (CH50) in the serum. Exacerbations of the disease (vertical arrows) coincide in this patient with increased levels of anti-DNA antibodies; this is not always the case.

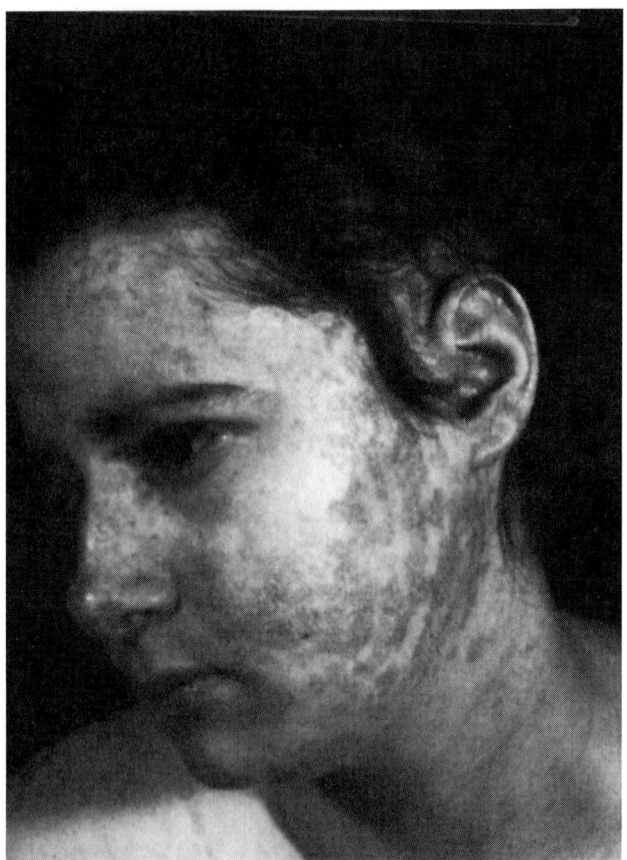

FIG. 4. Photosensitive rash in a patient with SLE. Note the erythematous and scaly quality of the rash, which crosses the bridge of the nose and gives rise to a "butterfly" pattern. No skin rash was noted in areas of the skin usually covered by clothing.

predominance of 3:1 and a peak onset in the fourth decade of life. Intense inflammation occurs in synovial joints, so that the normally delicate synovial "membrane" becomes infiltrated with mononuclear phagocytes, lymphocytes, and neutrophils (269). An inflammatory fluid is usually exuded by the inflamed synovium. In addition to pain and loss of mobility of joints, patients frequently develop systemic manifestations, such as anemia, subcutaneous nodules, pleurisy, pericarditis, interstitial lung disease, and manifestations of vasculitis such as nerve infarction, skin lesions, and inflammation of the ocular sclera. The course of RA is variable, but usually patients undergo progressive loss of cartilage and bone around joints with resulting diminished mobility.

Although the cause of RA remains unknown, a number of its features are suggestive of an autoimmune etiology. The pathology of arthritic joints suggests a T-cell–mediated chronic inflammatory reaction (270). Susceptibility to RA is significantly greater in individuals with the DR4 haplotype, owing to the QKRAA motif in the hypervariable region, thereby suggesting a role for autoantigen presentation (271). Most patients (over 80%) develop RF (20), mostly produced in the marrow, but with significant production by the inflamed synovium (272). The presence of intrasynovial

immune complexes, together with diminished levels of complement components, implies an involvement of RF in some of the local pathology (273). In recent years, however, much interest has focused on the T cells and mononuclear phagocytes infiltrating the joint. T cells are probably polyclonal (274), although evidence for selective expansion of certain $V\beta$ subsets exists and has led some investigators to propose a role for superantigens (275). Depletion of T cells by thoracic duct drainage (276), or by immunosuppressive drugs such as cyclosporine, has resulted in improvement, implying an important role for T cells in the inflammatory process (277). Much work on intrasynovial cytokines, however, has pointed toward mononuclear phagocytes as the prime driving force of the inflammatory process (278).

The synovial fluid in RA contains primarily cytokines of mononuclear origin, including IL-1, IL-6, and TNF-α. IL-1 receptor antagonist can also be demonstrated in most fluids. In contrast, IL-2, IFN-γ, and other T-cell cytokines are usually present in only small quantities, with the possible exception of IL-17. Efforts to treat RA with T-cell–depleting monoclonal antibodies have yielded disappointing results (279). In contrast, administration of monoclonal antibodies to TNF-α has resulted in marked reduction of inflammation (280). Modest improvement has also been reported for antibodies to IL-6 and with administration of IL-1 receptor antagonist.

Efforts to define the underlying etiology of RA have met with frustration. Numerous reports of isolation of viruses, mycoplasmas, and other infectious agents have not been confirmed. Because experimental anticollagen immunity in rodents results in an RA-like syndrome (281), it is possible that similar autoimmunity might be at work in RA. Although low levels of anticollagen antibodies and reactive T cells have been reported in RA, there is little to support the involvement of anticollagen immunity in this disorder (282).

The mechanism whereby joint inflammation results in crippling cartilage and bone erosion in RA is incompletely understood (283). It seems unlikely that leakage into cartilage of neutrophil or mononuclear phagocyte-derived proteolytic enzymes is responsible. The diffusion through the cartilage matrix of cytokines probably stimulates breakdown of cartilage and bone through an action on chondrocytes and osteoclasts. In this regard, the TNF-family cytokine RANK ligand (RANKL) appears to be of particular importance, as overexpression of RANKL and its receptor predispose to erosive arthritis in the collagen model, and lack of RANKL allows induction of arthritis yet prevents cartilaginous and bony destruction (284).

Reactive Arthritis and Spondyarthitides

An important group of rheumatic diseases is characterized by inflammation mostly of large joints, with a predilection for the sacroiliac joints in chronic cases, often associated with infection by certain organisms, or with psoriasis or inflammatory bowel disease (285). These illnesses share a tendency for inflammation to heal with brisk fibroblastic proliferation, together with the formation of new bone. They are unlike RA in that periarticular cartilage loss and osteopenia are uncharacteristic. A remarkable feature of these illnesses is their association with the HLA-B27 class I MHC allele. Reactive arthritis often involves genitourinary, oral mucosal, uveal tract, and skin inflammation. In most studies, about 90% of afflicted individuals have the B27 haplotype, compared to 7% of the normal population (286). Numerous outbreaks of reactive arthritis have been observed in HLA-B27 positive individuals following epidemic infections with diarrhea-causing bacteria (see below), as shown in Fig. 5.

Whether autoimmunity is operative in the pathogenesis of these forms of chronic arthritis is unclear (287). Autoantibodies to IgG are absent, as are antinuclear antibodies, and other autoantibodies are not described. There is some evidence that infection with inciting organisms (which include Chlamydia, Yersinia, Salmonella, and Shigella) may elicit antibodies or cell-mediated immunity which is cross reactive with self-antigen, but the pathogenesis of these illnesses is quite unclear (288). The class I association has given rise to the speculation that CD8 T cells are important in mediating self-reactivity, and this contention is supported by the

occurrence of joint inflammation and other features of reactive arthritis, often severe, in HIV-infected individuals with severely depressed CD4 counts yet relative preservation of CD8$^+$ T cells (289).

Rats expressing a human HLA-B27 transgene in high copy number develop arthritis, inflammatory bowel disease, and skin lesions (290). These are less severe in animals raised under germ-free conditions, implying a role for microbial flora. T cells are required for development of disease. In mice, imposition of the HLA-B27 transgene in mice lacking endogenous class I MHC molecules also gives rise to an arthritic and inflammatory syndrome (291). The predilection in humans for illness in B27-positive individuals may reflect different responses to bacterial antigens and differential clearance of bacteria (292).

Systemic Vasculitis

The susceptibility of the vascular system to injury from deposition within vessel walls of immune complexes or from intravascular cell-mediated lesions is the basis of a large group of disorders with multiple manifestations that depend on the

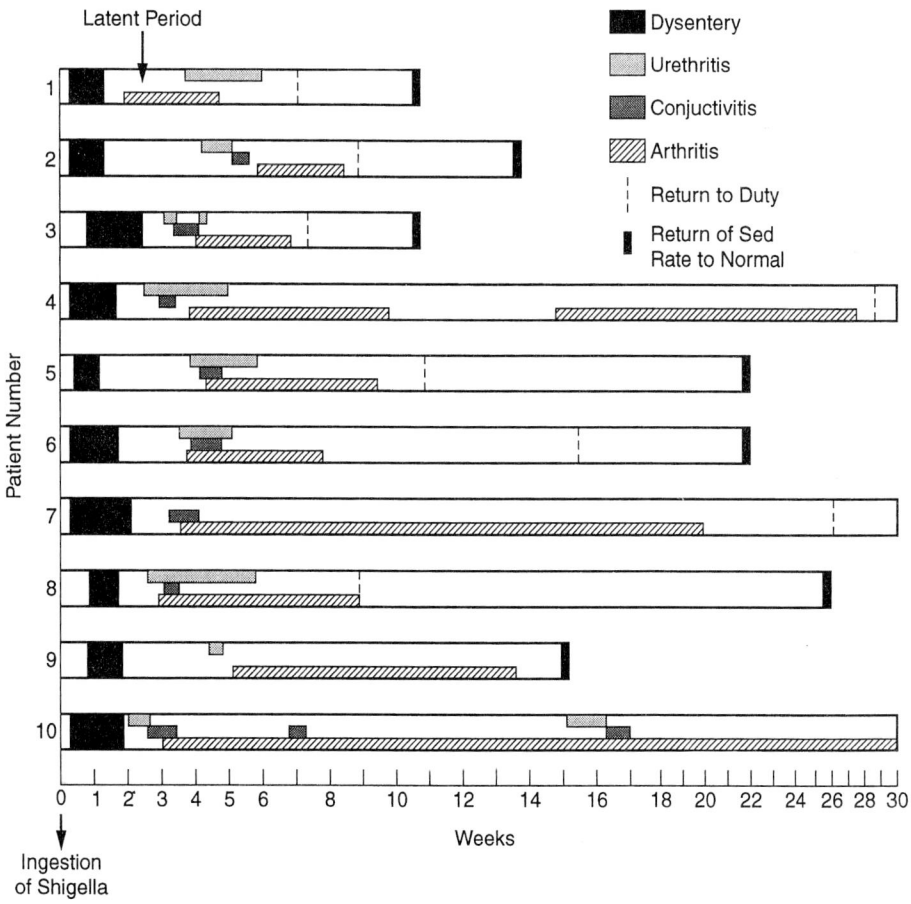

FIG. 5. The evolution of an outbreak of reactive arthritis among the crew of a naval vessel following an epidemic of Shigella dysentery is shown. Of over 600 crew members who developed diarrhea, only 11 developed features of reactive arthritis. Five of these sailors were traced 10 years later, and four were found to be HLA-B27 positive. From Noer (359), with permission.

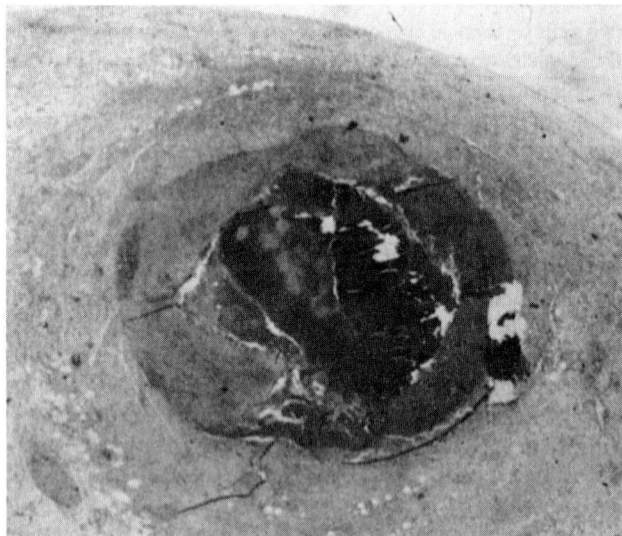

FIG. 6. Systemic necrotizing arteritis. Shown is a section of a subsegmental mesenteric artery of a 65-year-old man with severe abdominal pain and a bowel infarction. Note the disruption of the internal elastic lamina of the vessel, the intramural thrombus, and the leukocytic infiltrate. The patient had an excellent response to corticosteroids and cyclophosphamide.

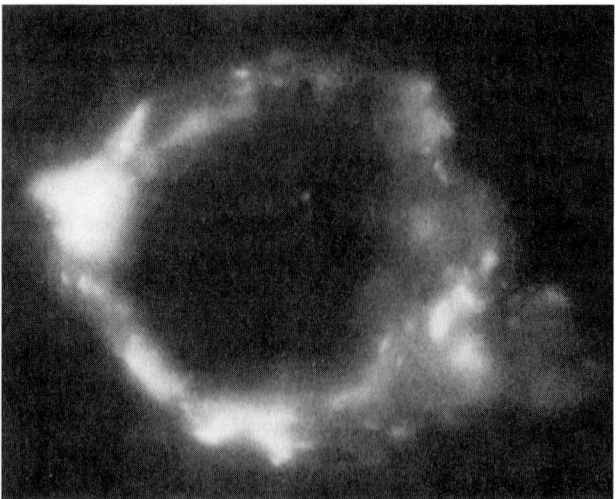

FIG. 7. Vasculitis in a patient with SLE. Note the presence of complement demonstrated using antihuman C3 in the wall of this artery.

severity of involvement and the nature of the affected blood vessel (293). Fig. 6 shows typical involvement of a medium-sized artery. In some cases, the mechanism is immune complexes formed in response to exogenous antigens, such as viruses (especially hepatitis B and C) (294) or drugs (295), while in other instances, autoantibodies or antibodies to as yet uncharacterized environmental agents are responsible. In still other instances, the injury to blood vessel is initiated by obscure causes, and is abetted by local expression of adhesion molecules, cytokines, chemokines, and activated clotting factors (296).

Autoimmune vasculitis can be seen alone or together with SLE or other rheumatic diseases. Fig. 7 demonstrates the deposition of C3 in the lumen of an inflamed small artery from an SLE patient with vasculitis. There is evidence for deposition of complexes of DNA–anti-DNA and IgG rheumatoid factor, with subsequent injury involving the complement system (297). On occasion, clinical disease correlates with cryoprecipitation of complexes in serum cooled below body temperature. A special example of vasculitis is that of mixed cryoglobulinemia (298), in which a monoclonal IgM (the product of a single aberrant B-cell clone) with autoantibody activity against IgG (i.e., rheumatoid factor activity) forms large circulating complexes that deposit in the walls of small and medium sized arteries, causing ischemia and infarction of skin, nerves, and kidney. There is a striking association between this illness and chronic infection with hepatitis C virus, yet the underlying etiology of the cryoglobulinemia remains unknown.

Vasculitis manifestations can range from skin lesions alone (small-vessel vasculitis) to ischemia of vital organs such as kidney, heart, brain, and liver. Attempts have been made to classify vasculitis based on known versus unknown etiology and rheumatic versus nonrheumatic. Fig. 8 schematizes the type of involvement that results from inflammation of blood vessels of differing caliber.

Wegener's granulomatosis is a rare form of vasculitis featuring the formation of granulomas around blood vessels with typical severe involvement of lung and kidney (299). The presence of antibodies to proteinase 3 or myeloperoxidase in most patients with this disorder has led to the hypothesis that antineutrophil cytoplasmic autoantibody (ANCA)–induced neutrophil activation is central to a chain of events leading to T-cell activation and a cellular immune response involving macrophage activation (300).

Sjögren's Syndrome

This lymphoproliferative and autoimmune disorder occurs in a primary form, not associated with a rheumatic disease, and as a complication of rheumatoid arthritis, SLE, or scleroderma. Patients develop infiltration of exocrine glands, mostly salivary and lacrimal glands, with activated polyclonal CD4+ T cells, together with hypergammaglobulinemia, autoantibodies, and sometimes vasculitis (301). Lymphocyte infiltration may extend beyond the exocrine glands to involve lungs, liver, and other viscera. Primary Sjögren's syndrome is associated with HLA-DR3, and with antibodies to Ro and La. There is an increased susceptibility to lymphoid malignancy, mostly B-cell lymphomas. An entity resembling Sjögren's syndrome has been described in HIV infection, with CD8- rather than CD4-bearing cells infiltrating exocrine glands (302).

Chronic Graft versus Host Disease

In animals undergoing chronic graft versus host disease (GVH) against class II determinants, a systemic autoimmune

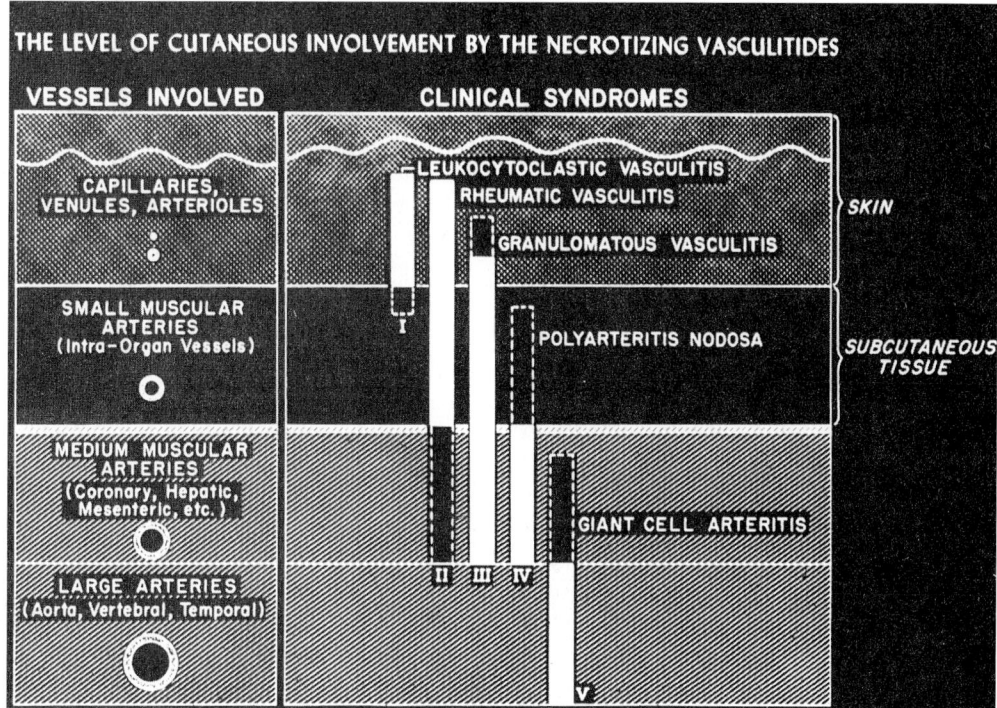

FIG. 8. The spectrum of vasculitis. The manifestations of vasculitis are dependent on the caliber of the involved vessel, which may in turn reflect the size, charge, or other physical properties of deposited immune complexes. Note that the resulting disease is dependent on the size of the inflamed vessel. Courtesy of the late James A. Gilliam, M.D.

syndrome with SLE-like features produces antinuclear antibodies, immune complex renal disease, and immune hemolytic anemia (303). Clinical manifestations vary according to background genes and according to the genetic barrier between strains; I-E differences generate higher levels of antinuclear antibodies, yet I-A differences result in more renal disease. In murine chronic GVH, induced across an MHC class II barrier, T and B cells interact in a cognate MHC-restricted fashion, implying a specific form of T-cell help rather than the nonspecific effect on B cells of excessive cytokines (304).

"Homologous disease" occurs in rats subjected to chronic GVH. Extensive sclerotic visceral lesions very like scleroderma occur (305). In human recipients of bone marrow, a chronic GVH syndrome is a major clinical problem, leading to fibrosis, skin pathology, and autoantibodies. The syndrome even occurs in recipients of autologous marrow, although in a milder form (306).

Scleroderma (Systemic Sclerosis)

This disease is marked by inflammation, followed by generation of increased amounts of collagen in skin and viscera, accompanied by certain antinuclear antibodies (307). Early lesions contain T-lymphocytes, and there is evidence of bias of the T-cell repertoire (308). Antibodies to topoisomerase I (Scl-70) correlate with visceral damage, while antibodies to centromere antigens connote a more benign

course (309). Scleroderma is characterized by marked vascular abnormalities, the most dramatic of which is the episodic reduction in peripheral arterial perfusion (often provoked by cold temperatures) known as Raynaud's phenomenon. Impairment of circulation can lead to pain, infections, and frequent ischemic amputation of the distal fingertips. Considerable disability can result from this and from the loss of hand mobility due to thickening of the overlying skin.

Patients with the severe form of scleroderma known as progressive systemic sclerosis develop serious injury to the skin, kidney, lung, and gastrointestinal tract. Therapy is usually ineffective. Despite the clear-cut evidence of serologic autoimmunity, the autoimmunity underlying the visceral and skin damage in the illness is only presumed, and nothing is known of the underlying mechanism. A strain of chickens develops an illness with marked scleroderma-like features (310).

The finding of increased numbers of cells of fetal origin in women with scleroderma has led to the proposal that this disorder might be due to persistent microchimerism and resulting chronic GVH disease (311). The occurrence of scleroderma in men and in nulliparous women might reflect the persistence of maternal cells transferred to patients during fetal life or parturition. While an attractive hypothesis, microchimerism as a cause of autoimmune disease must explain how such minute numbers of cells can exert powerful effects *in vivo*.

COMMONLY USED ANIMAL MODELS OF SYSTEMIC AUTOIMMUNE DISEASE

Several spontaneous murine models have been widely used to address SLE pathogenesis and treatment.

lpr and gld Mice

The autosomal recessive lpr mutation of the Fas apoptosis gene causes progressive, spectacular lymphadenopathy (Fig. 9), multiple SLE-like autoantibodies, and hypergammaglobulinemia (312). As is also true for the other murine SLE models, expression of laboratory and clinical manifestations of disease is highly dependent on other, poorly understood background genes (313). Thus, MRL/lpr mice, which are the best-studied strain, develop severe glomerulonephritis and vasculitis and have a markedly shortened lifespan; C57BL6/lpr (B6/lpr) manifest a milder syndrome with nearly normal longevity. The gld mutation is a single base substitution resulting in a nonfunctional Fas ligand protein. This defect leads to essentially the same syndrome caused by the lpr Fas mutation.

The failure of the Fas–Fas ligand system to delete autoreactive extrathymic T cells accounts for the accumulation of vast numbers of CD4⁻CD8⁻ anergic T cells, the unusual phenotype of which apparently represents a secondary mechanism for down-regulating function, in the absence of deletion. The Fas mutation is also expressed in B cells, leading to a failure to delete autoantibody-forming cells but not to lymphoproliferation analogous to T cells (220).

T cells are required for development of both lymphadenopathy and autoantibodies. In lpr mice with deletion of MHC class II genes (314) or lacking CD4 molecules (315), autoantibodies fail to develop, yet lymphadenopathy occurs; conversely, the absence of CD8 or β2 microglobulin (316) results in little change in autoantibody levels, but a marked decrease in lymphadenopathy. These and other studies

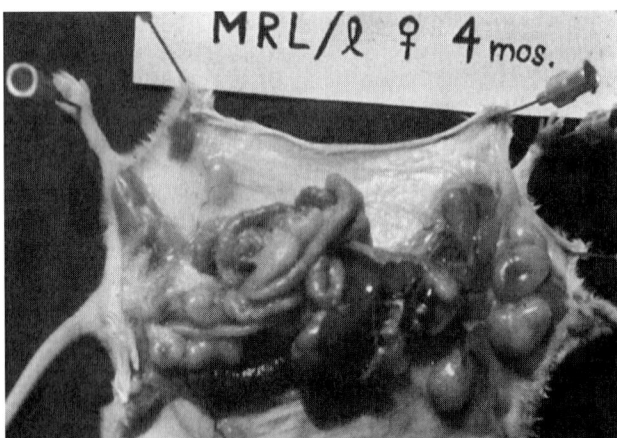

FIG. 9. MRL/lpr mouse (formerly called MRL/l), age 4 months. Note massive lymph node and spleen enlargement, due to CD4⁻ CD8⁻ T-cell infiltration. Courtesy of Robert Eisenberg, M.D.

support the idea that the abnormal "double-negative" T cells of lpr are descended primarily from CD8 precursors, which lose their CD8 as part of their evolution into anergic cells. The T cells that provide help for autoantibodies, on the other hand, are primarily CD4-bearing cells that recognize antigens (and presumably autoantigens) in the context of self–class II MHC. In MRL/lpr mice, immunopathology, including the abnormal accumulation of double-negative T cells, depends on B-lymphocytes, indicating their importance not only as antibody producing cells but also as antigen-presenting cells and perhaps in other roles in the development of autoimmunity (317).

NZB and NZB/NZW F1 Mice

NZB mice develop autoimmune hemolytic anemia, antinuclear antibodies, and late-life lymphoreticular neoplasms (318). The F1 offspring of this strain and near-normal NZW mice suffer from a much more fulminant and SLE-like syndrome leading to diffuse proliferative glomerulonephritis, high-titer antinuclear antibodies, and early death (especially in females). NZBxSWR F1 mice are another well-studied model that develops renal disease, offering the additional advantage that the SWR parents are free of endogenous retroviruses and without apparent additional immunopathology (319). The genetics of SLE in NZB crosses is complex and is discussed elsewhere. The SLE-like disease is characterized by both B- and T-cell defects, notably B-cell hyperactivity even in fetal life and a requirement for T cells for development of autoantibodies and disease (320).

BXSB Mice

These animals develop an age-dependent SLE-like syndrome that is much more severe in males because it is due to a mutation of a Y-chromosome gene (Yaa) (321). Unlike the lpr mutation, which provokes at least some degree of autoimmune disease regardless of genetic background, Yaa results in acceleration of autoimmunity only when bred onto the genomes of autoimmune mice. High-titer antinuclear antibodies and immune-complex nephritis lead to early mortality in males. Chimera studies using B6-Yaa mice have shown that it is largely the T-lymphocytes that are responsible for the autoimmune disease, as their elimination but not elimination of B cells reduces disease in chimeras. It has been suggested that the basic defect in this strain involves enhanced T-B interaction, possibly through abnormal adherence. The presence of a functional I-E molecule reduces serologic and clinical disease, possibly through presentation of peptide fragments of I-E by the I-A element (322).

Induction of Systemic Lupus-like Syndrome in Mice through Injection of Pristane

Pristane, a branched alkane, is widely used to produce peritoneal inflammation that primes mice for subsequent hybridoma implantation. It was fortuitously observed that mice receiving pristane alone developed a progressive autoimmune syndrome marked by development of SLE-like autoantibodies including anti-Sm and other highly characteristic specificities (323). SLE-like glomerular changes are observed, together with deposition of immunoglobulin and complement. Serologic features of the syndrome are dependent on the genetic background of the mouse, with H-2 playing a prominent role. For instance H-2s mice develop antiribosomal protein autoantibodies, while autoantibodies appear only in low titer in C57BL mice (324).

Systemic Autoimmunity Induced by Idiotype Infusion

A syndrome characterized by antinuclear antibodies, cytopenias, and immune-mediated renal disease occurs in mice given antibodies expressing the human 16/6 idiotype, which is found on certain human IgM monoclonal anti-DNA antibodies (325). Disease is preceded by antibodies to the 16/6 idiotype, and may represent precipitation of a cascade of aberrant idiotype–anti-idiotype network interactions involving T cells, as SLE manifestations can also be induced by T-cell lines from idiotype-immunized mice (326). These mice have also been reported to have anticardiolipin antibodies and abnormalities of hemostasis.

Viable Moth-eaten Mouse

Recent work has shown that the moth-eaten (Me) and viable moth-eaten (Me^v) phenotypes, which results in a severe neonatal autoimmune syndrome with hypergammaglobulinemia and autoantibodies to DNA and erythrocytes, are due to mutations in the SHP-1 tyrosine phosphatase expressed in hematopoietic cells (327). Virtually all of the mouse B cells are of the B1 subset. Death of Me mice occurs at about age 3 weeks, while Me^v mice, which have a partially functional SHP-1, live to about 9 weeks. In both strains, there is hypergammaglobulinemia, multiple autoantibodies, and severe interstitial pneumonitis. The mechanism whereby the phosphatase deficiency results in autoreactivity is unclear, but presumably reflects fundamental mechanisms controlling B-cell differentiation.

SEVERE AUTOIMMUNE DISEASE IN KNOCKOUT AND TRANSGENIC STRAINS

Mice homozygous for deletion of the TGFβ gene suffer a severe and fulminant autoimmune disorder characterized by multiorgan inflammatory disease and death by 3 weeks. The disorder is mediated by T-lymphocytes and can be adoptively transferred to MHC-compatible normal mice (328). Apparently the absence of the immunosuppressive and anti-inflammatory effects of TGFβ permits unregulated spontaneous inflammatory disease. A parallel situation occurs in mice without functional CTLA-4. The absence of negative regulation of T cells normally mediated by this molecule

also leads to a severe neonatal autoimmune and inflammatory disease (329).

Striking autoimmune disease, especially involving the intestinal tract but with hematologic and other systemic manifestations as well, occurs in mice with deleted IL-2 (330), IL-10 (331), and TCR genes (332). To some extent, the inflammatory disease is dependent on the microbiological environment of the mice, as well as the background strain, and has been attributed to the consequences of cytokine imbalances.

Mice transgenic for the Bcl-2 oncogene expressed in B cells develop certain SLE-like autoantibodies (333). The combination of the Bcl-2 apoptosis defect and the lpr Fas mutation results in mice with even further lymphoid hyperplasia, but no further increase in autoantibodies, suggesting that the apoptosis impairment resulting from the lpr mutation is maximal in terms of autoantibody production and cannot be further exacerbated (334).

TIGHT-SKIN MOUSE

The Tsk mutation is a dominant mutation on chromosome 2 which is lethal in its homozygous form (335). The mutant gene encodes a defective form of fibrillin-1, which apparently causes diffuse fibrosis (336). The mice develop progressive skin tightening, together with pulmonary fibrosis and cardiomyopathy. Antibodies to topoisomerase I (337) and RNA polymerase I have been detected. Mice lacking CD4 cells fail to develop skin lesions, but develop visceral abnormalities; lack of CD8 cells has little influence on the disease, and disease develops in RAG-deficient mice (338).

MODELS OF RHEUMATOID ARTHRITIS

Several rodent models of RA have been widely used (339). A chronic polyarthritis results from the injection of peptidoglycan-polysaccharide in rats, with extensive joint destruction (340). It is dependent on the genetic background of the rat (Lewis is the prototype susceptible strain, Buffalo is resistant), partly due to MHC genes, and requires T-lymphocytes. Considerable evidence suggests that the inflammatory disease is due to the persistence of bacterial debris. A relapsing form of the disease can be induced by intra-articular bacterial lipopolysaccharide in animals that have had an earlier injection of peptidoglycan-polysaccharide (341).

A chronic inflammatory arthritis model also in general use is induced by immunization with type II collagen in adjuvant (342). Collagen arthritis is mainly due to T-cell immunity to type II collagen, although antibody is also demonstrable and may provoke some of the injury. MHC influences and T-cell oligoclonality are important in this illness (343). A single injection of complete Freund's adjuvant alone causes a chronic arthritis in rats, but not in mice (344). It has been used as a way of evaluating anti-inflammatory drugs.

Inflammatory arthritis develops in mice transgenic for human T-cell leukemia virus type I (HTLV-I) tax (345). Such animals develop chronic erosive arthritis with synovial proliferation and pathologic changes resembling RA. They produce anticollagen antibodies, RF, and anti–heat-shock proteins and also manifest T-cell immunity to collagen and heat-shock proteins. A Sjögren's-like autoimmune exocrinopathy has also been reported in these animals (346). These findings are of special interest because humans with HTLV infection may also develop inflammatory arthritis, alone or in the presence of myelopathy (347).

A remarkable model of inflammatory and erosive arthritis was serendipitously discovered in mice expressing a ribonuclease-specific TCR transgene and the NOD class II MHC allele Ia^{g7}. These KRN mice develop RA-like synovial inflammation and subsequent deformity (348). Disease can be transferred with purified immunoglobulin, and the responsible antibody is directed against glucose-6-phosphate isomerase. Antibodies to this enzyme are found in some RA patient sera, and both antibody and antigen have been demonstrated in RA synovial tissue. How this antibody arises and the nature of its relation to RA pathogenesis are unanswered and timely questions. It is hypothesized that injury comes about through immune-complex deposition.

Mice transgenic for TNF-α also develop a spontaneous erosive arthritis, presumably due to the proinflammatory action of this cytokine (349). These studies support the proposed key role of TNF-α in RA.

IMMUNE INJURY IN SYSTEMIC AUTOIMMUNE DISEASE

The classification scheme of Gell and Coombs is still a useful way of subdividing injury mechanisms in systemic autoimmunity. Type I injury, mediated by IgE, is not important in these disorders. By contrast, tissue damage initiated by binding of autoantibody directly to target tissues (type II injury) is of importance, particularly in organ-specific autoimmune disease, but to a great extent also in systemic autoimmune disease where antibodies to cell and basement membranes, fibronectin, collagen, and other fixed components of tissue may exist. Binding of antibody to self-tissue leads to inflammation through a complex series of events involving the complement and coagulation pathways, leading to chemotaxis of neutrophils and monocytes, and their phagocytosis and release of local inflammatory mediators. Platelet aggregation, dilatation of vascular smooth muscle, and activation of mast cells are all part of the series of events triggered by autoantibody binding to tissue in type II injury; these topics are discussed in detail elsewhere in this textbook. Examples of autoantibodies provoking these changes probably include anticollagen antibodies and antiglomerular basement antibodies. Fig. 10 depicts the pathologic changes in Goodpastures' syndrome, a disorder causing hemorrhagic lung and kidney lesions due to antibodies directed against basement membrane proteins common to both organs.

Type III injury, mediated by immune complexes, is believed to account for much of the pathology of systemic autoimmune diseases, particularly SLE and vasculitis. In NZB/NZW mice, blocking of C5 using monoclonal antibody reduces nephritis and increases survival, supporting a role for classical pathway activation in the immune complex disease of this strain (350). The protean nature of immune complexes, which can range from just a few molecules of antigen and antibody to huge complexes involving whole cells coated or cross-linked by antibody, accounts for the great variety of pathology encountered in type III injury. Much interest has focused on defining the offending antigens that are present in injurious immune complexes in SLE and related diseases, with mixed success. SLE exacerbations are frequently preceded or accompanied by a fall in hemolytic complement, together with a rise in levels of antibodies to native (double-stranded) DNA. These antibodies are concentrated in the glomeruli of

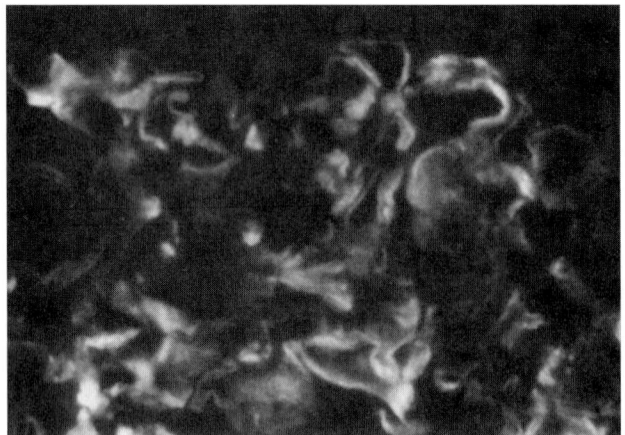
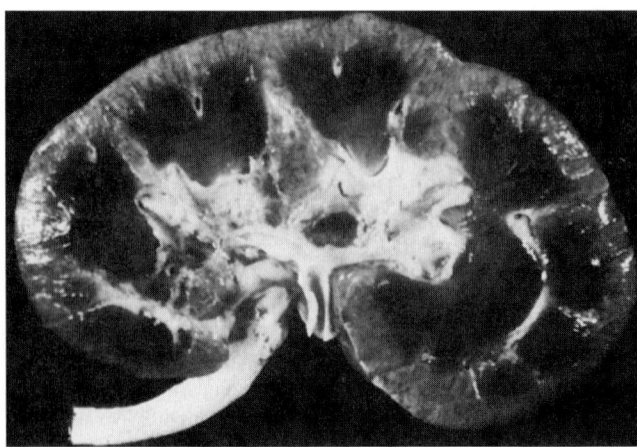

A   B

FIG. 10. Type II immune-mediated injury. **A:** Linear deposition of IgG against antigens present on the glomerular basement membrane of a patient with Goodpasture syndrome is illustrated using fluoresceinated antihuman IgG. Similar changes were seen in the lung. **B:** Hemorrhagic changes are visible in the gross pathology specimen from this patient, who came to autopsy. Courtesy of William J. Yount, M.D.

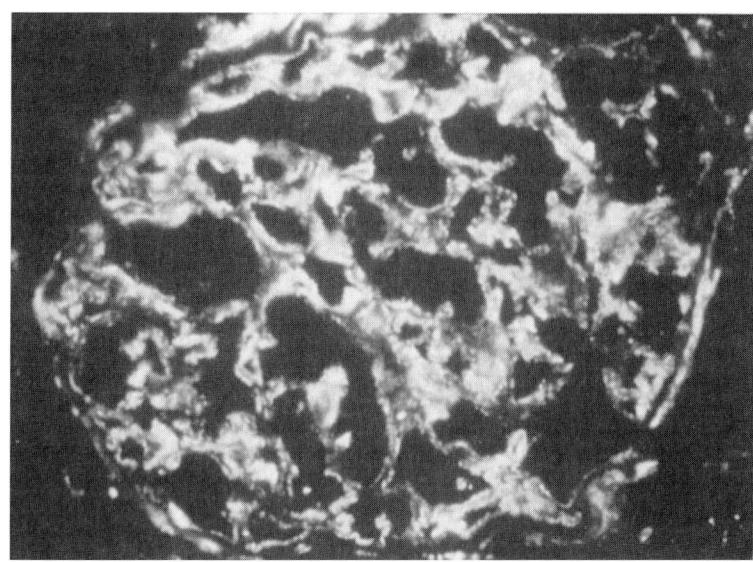

FIG. 11. Type III (immune complex) injury in an SLE renal biopsy specimen. This patient had proteinuria and red blood cells in her urine. Note the granular (sometimes called "lumpy-bumpy") distribution of the immune deposits in this section stained with antibody to human C3.

patients with SLE renal disease (Fig. 11), consistent with the idea that DNA–anti-DNA complexes may deposit in SLE kidneys and provoke inflammation. Although it seems likely that DNA–anti-DNA is an important antibody system in SLE renal disease, it is very likely that other kinds of autoantibodies also contribute in important ways to glomerular injury (351). Antichromatin, for example, forms immune complexes that may localize on the glomerular basement membrane. Current studies focus on the charge, size, and antigenic characteristics of such antibodies in relation to their ability to bind and to injury glomeruli.

Type IV injury is due to T-lymphocytes, macrophages, and perhaps other cells that infiltrate tissues, sometimes causing granulomas. Some systemic autoimmune diseases are dominated by type IV injury, for instance, Wegener's granulomatosis; yet it is more common for type IV mechanisms to coexist with types II and III. SLE, for instance, is frequently accompanied by destructive and inflammatory skin lesions dominated by T-lymphocytes; similarly, the destructive inflammatory muscle lesions of polymyositis occur together with antisynthetase antibodies and other serologic autoimmunity. There may be some contribution of cell-mediated immunity to SLE renal disease, but expression of MHC class I or class II molecules is unnecessary for development of nephritis in MRL/lpr mice (352).

Autoantibodies may also exert damage through their effects on the coagulation system. The antiphospholipid syndrome is marked by arterial and venous thromboses that may cause stroke, myocardial infarction, and thromboembolism. It is seen alone or as a feature of SLE, and is due not to true antiphospholipid antibodies, but rather to antibodies to phospholipid-binding proteins, mainly $\beta 2$ glycoprotein I (353). By an imperfectly understood mechanism, these antibodies enhance platelet aggregation and activation, and promote thrombus formation while paradoxically prolonging the *in vitro* partial thromboplastin time, an indicator of coagulation. This *in vitro* phenomenon is termed the lupus anticoagulant, and is present in a substantial minority of SLE patients as well as in many individuals with no other recognized illness. It is a major cause of early spontaneous abortion, and may be an important cause of thrombotic disease in the general population.

Tissue damage may also be mediated through antibodies to neutrophil cytoplasmic antigens (ANCA). These IgG antibodies, initially detected by immunofluorescence, have been divided by staining patterns into perinuclear (p-ANCA) and cytoplasmic (c-ANCA). p-ANCA are directed against myeloperoxidase, while c-ANCA are specific for proteinase 3 (354). These autoantibodies are useful markers for vasculitis, including Wegener's granulomatosis, pauci–immune necrotizing and crescentic "pauci-immune" glomerulonephritis, and polyarteritis nodosa, and their titers correlate with disease severity. The mechanism by which antibodies to these cytoplasmic antigens leads to blood vessel damage and inflammation is incompletely understood, but may involve expression on activated neutrophils of proteinase 3 and myeloperoxidase, and possibly release of free proteinase 3. Antibodies to these molecules may provoke enhanced neutrophil chemotaxis and adhesion, together with triggering of the respiratory burst. This may lead to a series of events culminating in activation of T cells and macrophages and the formation of necrotizing granulomas.

APPROACHES TO TREATMENT OF SYSTEMIC AUTOIMMUNE DISEASE

In general, the management of human systemic autoimmune disease is empirical and unsatisfactory. For the most part, broadly immunosuppressive drugs like corticosteroids are used in a wide variety of severe autoimmune and inflammatory disorders; in milder conditions anti-inflammatory agents acting on eicosanoid metabolism are often sufficient.

In addition to corticosteroids, other immunosuppressive agents are used in management of the systemic autoimmune diseases. Cyclophosphamide is an alkylating agent that causes profound depletion of both T- and B-lymphocytes and impairment of cell-mediated immunity. It is used in SLE nephritis, and is particularly effective in granulomatous vasculitis and polyarteritis nodosa. Its use entails the risks of immunosuppression, along with an increased incidence of lymphoreticular malignancies. Azathioprine and the closely related 6-mercaptopurine are used in parallel situations and are somewhat less effective but are less toxic.

Cyclosporine, tacrolimus, and mycophenolate mofetil are natural products with specific properties of T-lymphocyte suppression, and have been used with success in SLE, RA, and to a limited extent in vasculitis and myositis. They have significant renal toxicity in addition to their immunosuppressive effects.

Methotrexate is widely used as a "remittive" agent in rheumatoid arthritis, with the goal of reducing disease progression. It is also useful in polymyositis and other connective tissue diseases. Its mechanism of action here is controversial and may relate to its action on adenosine receptors rather than to its more familiar role as an antimetabolite (355).

There is optimism that more specific treatment for autoimmune disorders can be devised when their mechanisms become better understood. Oral tolerance holds promise as a means of attracting immunosuppressive T-lymphocytes to sites of active autoimmune pathology and suppressing inflammation by a bystander effect, probably involving TGF-β (356). Other approaches under development are monoclonal antibodies intended to block the action of cytokines or to deplete lymphocytes (279). With the exception of anti–TNF-α in RA (280), these have been disappointing so far.

CONCLUSIONS

The mechanisms of systemic autoimmune disease are diverse and incompletely understood. Several points are worthy of emphasis. The rules and restrictions governing ordinary immune responses seem to apply to autoimmune responses: there is little that is extraordinary about the immunoglobulin or T-cell receptor genes used nor in their rearrangements or process of diversification; antigen is required to initiate responses. Production of and response to cytokines and other mediators are similar to what is seen for responses to exogenous antigens, and T and B cells probably collaborate in MHC-restricted fashion. The recent availability of transgenic and knockout mice and the continuing progress in the understanding of the genome seem likely to open novel and fruitful approaches to the challenge of understanding the important disorders of systemic autoimmunity.

REFERENCES

1. Whitacre CC. Sex differences in autoimmune disease. *Nat Immunol* 2001;2:777–780.
2. Cervera R, Khamashta MA, Font J, et al. Systemic lupus erythematosus: clinical and immunologic patterns of disease expression in a cohort of 1,000 patients. *Medicine* 1993;72:113–124.
3. Lahita RG. Low plasma androgens in women with systemic lupus erythematosus. *Arthritis Rheum* 1987;30:241–248.
4. Peeva E, Grimaldi C, Spatz L, et al. Bromocriptine restores tolerance in estrogen-treated mice. *J Clin Invest* 2000;106:1373–1379.
5. Lorber M, Gershwin ME, Shoenfeld Y. The coexistence of SLE with other autoimmune diseases: the kaleidoscope of autoimmunity. *Semin Arthritis Rheum* 1994;24:105–113.
6. Sharp GC, Irvin WS, Tan EM, et al. Mixed connective tissue disease-an apparently distinct rheumatic disease syndrome associated with a specific antibody to an extractable nuclear antigen (ENA). *Am J Med* 1972;52:148–159.
7. Gottlieb AB, Lahita RG, Chiorazzi N, et al. Immune function in systemic lupus erythematosus: Impairment of in vitro T-cell proliferation and in vivo antibody response to exogenous antigen. *J Clin Invest* 1979; 63:885–892.
8. Hahn BH, Bagby MK, Osterland CK. Abnormalities of delayed hypersensitivity in systemic lupus erythematosus. *Am J Med* 1973;55:25–31.
9. Mirzayan MJ, Schmidt RE, Witte T. Prognostic parameters for flare in systemic lupus erythematosus. *Rheumatology (Oxford)* 2000;39:1316–1319.
10. Zonana-Nacach A, Camargo-Coronel A, Yanez P, et al. Infections in outpatients with systemic lupus erythematosus: a prospective study. *Lupus* 2001;10:505–510.
11. Ehrlich P, Morgenroth J. On haemolysis: third communication. In: *The Collected Papers of Paul Ehrlich,* vol. 2. London: Pergamon, 1957: 178–206.
12. Harrington WJ, Minnich V, Hollingsworth JW, et al. Demonstration of a thrombocytopenic factor in the blood of patients with thrombocytopenic purpura. *J Lab Clin Med* 1951;115:636–645.
13. Rose NR, Witebsky E. Studies on organ specificity. V. Changes in the thyroid glands of rabbits following acute immunization with rabbit thyroid extracts. *J Immunol* 1956;76:417–423.
14. Burnet FM. A modification of Jerne's theory of antibody production using the concept of clonal selection. *Austrian J Sci* 1957;20:67–69.
15. Kakkanaiah VN, Seth A, Nagarkatti M, et al. Autoreactive T cell clones isolated from normal and autoimmune-susceptible mice exhibit lymphokine secretory and functional properties of both Th1 and Th2 cells. *Clin Immunol Immunopathol* 1990;57:148–162.
16. Grabar P. Autoantibodies and the physiological role of immunoglobulins. *Immunol Today* 1983;4:337–339.
17. Hooper B, Whittingham S, Mathews JD, et al. Autoimmunity in a rural community. *Clin Exp Immunol* 1972;12:79–87.
18. Hawkins BR, O'Connor KJ, Dawkins RL, et al. Autoantibodies in an Australian population. I. Prevalence and persistence. *J Clin Lab Immunol* 1979;2:211–215.
19. Sutton B, Corper A, Bonagura V, et al. The structure and origin of rheumatoid factors. *Immunol Today* 2000;21:177–183.
20. Chen PP, Fong S, Carson DA. Rheumatoid factor. *Rheum Dis Clin North Am* 1987;13:545–568.
21. Nemazee DA, Sato VL. Induction of rheumatoid antibodies in the mouse: regulated production of autoantibody in the secondary humoral response. *J Exp Med* 1983;158:529–545.
22. Welch MJ, Fong S, Vaughan J, et al. Increased frequency of rheumatoid factor precursor B lymphocytes after immunization of normal adults with tetanus toxoid. *Clin Exp Immunol* 1983;51:299–304.
23. Bonfa E, Llovet R, Scheinberg M, et al. Comparison between autoantibodies in malaria and leprosy with lupus. *Clin Exp Immunol* 1987;70:529–537.
24. Sasso EH. The rheumatoid factor response in the etiology of mixed cryoglobulins associated with hepatitis C virus infection. *Ann Med Interne (Paris)* 2000;151:30–40.
25. Roosnek E, Lanzavecchia A. Efficient and selective presentation of antigen-antibody complexes by rheumatoid factor B cells. *J Exp Med* 1991;173:487–489.
26. Tighe H, Heaphy P, Baird S, et al. Human immunoglobulin (IgG) induced deletion of IgM rheumatoid factor B cells in transgenic mice. *J Exp Med* 1995;181:599–606.
27. Hartman AB, Mallett CP, Srinivasappa J, et al. Organ reactive autoantibodies from non-immunized adult BALB/c mice are polyreactive and express non-biased VH gene usage. *Mol Immunol* 1989;26:359–370.

28. Klinman DM, Banks S, Hartman A, et al. Natural murine autoantibodies and conventional antibodies exhibit similar degrees of antigenic cross-reactivity. *J Clin Invest* 1988;82:652–657.

29. Chen PP. From human autoantibodies to the fetal antibody repertoire to B cell malignancy: it's a small world after all. *Int Rev Immunol* 1990;5:239–251.

30. Koenig-Marrony S, Soulas P, Julien S, et al. Natural autoreactive B cells in transgenic mice reproduce an apparent paradox to the clonal tolerance theory. *J Immunol* 2001;166:1463–1470.

31. Casali P, Notkins AL. CD5+ B lymphocytes, polyreactive antibodies and the human B-cell repertoire. *Immunol Today* 1989;10:364–368.

32. Fagarasan S, Watanabe N, Honjo T. Generation, expansion, migration and activation of mouse B1 cells. *Immunol Rev* 2000;176:205–215.

33. Reap EA, Sobel ES, Cohen PL, et al. Conventional B cells, not B-1 cells, are responsible for producing autoantibodies in lpr mice. *J Exp Med* 1993;177:69–78.

34. Reap EA, Sobel ES, Jennette JC, et al. Conventional B cells, not B1 cells, are the source of autoantibodies in chronic graft versus host disease. *J Immunol* 1993;151:7316–7323.

35. Casali P. Polyclonal B cell activation and antigen-driven antibody response as mechanisms of autoantibody production in SLE. *Autoimmunity* 1990;5:147–150.

36. Dorner T, Foster SF, Farner NL, et al. Immunoglobulin kappa chain receptor editing in systemic lupus erythematosus. *J Clin Invest* 1998;102:688–694.

37. Dorner T, Farner NL, Lipsky PE. Ig lambda and heavy chain gene usage in early untreated systemic lupus erythematosus suggests intensive B cell stimulation. *J Immunol* 1999;163:1027–1036.

38. Rajewsky K, Takemori T. Genetics, expression, and function of idiotypes. *Annu Rev Immunol* 1983;1:569–607.

39. Gavalchin J, Seder RA, Datta SK. The NZB × SWR model of lupus nephritis. I. Cross-reactive idiotypes of monoclonal anti-DNA antibodies in relation to antigenic specificity, charge, and allotype. Identification of interconnected idiotype families inherited from the normal SWR and the autoimmune NZB parents. *J Immunol* 1987;138:128–137.

40. Zhang W, Winkler T, Kalden JR, et al. Isolation of human anti-idiotypes broadly cross reactive with anti-dsDNA antibodies from patients with systemic lupus erythematosus. *Scand J Immunol* 2001;53:192–197.

41. Sun H, Lu B, Li RQ, et al. Defective T cell activation and autoimmune disorder in Stra13-deficient mice. *Nat Immunol* 2001;2:1040–1047.

42. Kretz-Rommel A, Rubin RL. Disruption of positive selection of thymocytes causes autoimmunity. *Nat Med* 2000;6:298–305.

43. Oukka ME, Colucci-Guyon PL, Tran M, et al. CD4 T cell tolerance to nuclear proteins induced by medullary thymic epithelium. *Immunity* 1996;4:545–553.

44. Laufer TM, Fan L, Glimcher LH. Self-reactive T cells selected on thymic cortical epithelium are polyclonal and are pathogenic in vivo. *J Immunol* 1999;162:5078–5084.

45. Goldings EA, Cohen PL, McFadden SF, et al. Defective B cell tolerance in adult (NZB × NZW)F1 mice. *J Exp Med* 1980;152:730–735.

46. Rathmell JC, Goodnow CC. Effects of the lpr mutation on elimination and inactivation of self-reactive B cells. *J Exp Med* 1994;153:2831–2842.

47. Wither J, Vukusic B. T-cell tolerance induction is normal in the (NZB × NZW)F1 murine model of systemic lupus erythematosus. *Immunology* 2000;99:345–351.

48. Sato S, Ono N, Steeber DA, et al. CD19 regulates B lymphocyte signaling thresholds critical for the development of B-1 lineage cells and autoimmunity. *J Immunol* 1996;157:4371–4378.

49. Nishizumi H, Taniuchi I, Yamanashi Y, et al. Impaired proliferation of peripheral B cells and indication of autoimmune disease in lyn-deficient mice. *Immunity* 1995;3:549–560.

50. Nishimura H, Nose M, Hiai H, et al. Development of lupus-like autoimmune diseases by disruption of the PD-1 gene encoding an ITIM motif-carrying immunoreceptor. *Immunity* 1999;11:141–151.

51. O'Keefe TL, Williams GT, Batista FD, et al. Deficiency in CD22, a B cell specific inhibitory receptor, is sufficient to predispose to development of high affinity autoantibodies. *J Exp Med* 1999;189:1307–1313.

52. Dang H, Geiser AG, Letterio JJ, et al. SLE-like autoantibodies and Sjogren's syndrome-like lymphoproliferation in TGF-beta knockout mice. *J Immunol* 1995;155:3205–3212.

53. Majeti R, Xu Z, Parslow TG, et al. An inactivating point mutation in the inhibitory wedge of CD45 causes lymphoproliferation and autoimmunity. *Cell* 2000;103:1059–1070.

54. Bolland S, Ravetch V. Spontaneous autoimmune disease in Fc(gamma)RIIB-deficient mice results from strain-specific epistasis. *Immunity* 2000;13:277–285.

55. Tsui FW, Tsui HW. Molecular basis of the motheaten phenotype. *Immunol Rev* 1994;138:185–206.

56. Huck S, Le Corre R, Youinou P, et al. Expression of B cell receptor-associated signaling molecules in human lupus. *Autoimmunity* 2001;33:213–224.

57. Tan EM. Antinuclear antibodies: diagnostic markers for autoimmune diseases and probes for cell biology. *Adv Immunol* 1989;44:93–151.

58. Doyle HA, Yan J, Liang B, et al. Lupus autoantigens: their origins, forms, and presentation. *Immunol Res* 2001;24:131–147.

59. Dziarski R. Autoimmunity: polyclonal activation or antigen induction? *Immunol Today* 1988;9:340–342.

60. Fisher DE, Reeves WH, Conner GE, et al. Pulse labeling of small nuclear ribonucleoproteins in vivo reveals distinct patterns of antigen recognition by human autoimmune antibodies. *Proc Natl Acad Sci U S A* 1984;81:3185–3189.

61. Rokeach LA, Jannatipour M, Haselby JA, et al. Mapping of the immunoreactive domains of a small nuclear ribonucleoprotein-associated Sm-D autoantigen. *Clin Immunol Immunopathol* 1992;65:315–324.

62. Reeves WH, Pierani A, Chou CH, et al. Epitopes of the p70 and p80 (Ku) lupus autoantigens. *J Immunol* 1991;146:2678–2686.

63. Riemekasten G, Kawald A, Weiss C, et al. Strong acceleration of murine lupus by injection of the SmD1(83–119) peptide. *Arthritis Rheum* 2001;44:2435–2445.

64. Doyle HA, Mamula MJ. Post-translational protein modifications in antigen recognition and autoimmunity. *Trends Immunol* 2001;22:443–449.

65. Baeten D, Peene I, Union A, et al. Specific presence of intracellular citrullinated proteins in rheumatoid arthritis synovium: relevance to antifilaggrin autoantibodies. *Arthritis Rheum* 2001;44:2255–2262.

66. Utz PJ, Gensler TJ, Anderson P. Death, autoantigen modifications, and tolerance. *Arthritis Res* 2000;2:101–114.

67. Rosen A, Casciola-Rosen L. Autoantigens as substrates for apoptotic proteases: implications for the pathogenesis of systemic autoimmune disease. *Cell Death Differ* 1999;6:6–12.

68. Rosario MO, Fox OF, Koren E, et al. Anti-Ro (SS-A) antibodies from Ro (SS-A)-immunized mice. *Arthritis Rheum* 1988;31:227–237.

69. Mevorach D. The immune response to apoptotic cells. *Ann N Y Acad Sci* 1999;887:191–198.

70. James JA, Gross T, Scofield RH, et al. Immunoglobulin epitope spreading and autoimmune disease after peptide immunization: Sm B/B'–derived PPPGMRPP and PPPGIRGP induce spliceosome autoimmunity. *J Exp Med* 1995;181:453–461.

71. Mason LJ, Timothy LM, Isenberg DA, et al. Immunization with a peptide of Sm B/B' results in limited epitope spreading but not autoimmune disease. *J Immunol* 1999;162:5099–5105.

72. Vlachoyiannopoulos PG, Petrovas C, Tzioufas AG, et al. No evidence of epitope spreading after immunization with the major Sm epitope P-P-G-M-R-P-P anchored to sequential oligopeptide carriers (SOCs). *J Autoimmun* 2000;14:53–61.

73. James JA, Neas BR, Moser KL, et al. Systemic lupus erythematosus in adults is associated with previous Epstein–Barr virus exposure. *Arthritis Rheum* 2001;44:1122–1126.

74. Bockenstedt L, Gee R, Mamula M. Self-peptides in the initiation of lupus autoimmunity. *J Immunol* 1995;154:3516–3524.

75. Slobbe RL, Pruijn GJM, van Venrooij WJ. Ro (SS-A) and La (SS-B) ribonucleoprotein complexes: structure, function and antigenicity. *Ann Med Interne* 1991;142:592–600.

76. Deshmukh US, Lewis JE, Gaskin F, et al. Ro60 peptides induce antibodies to similar epitopes shared among lupus-related autoantigens. *J Immunol* 2000;164:6655–6661.

77. Reynolds P, Gordon TP, Purcell AW, et al. Hierarchical self-tolerance to T cell determinants within the ubiquitous nuclear self-antigen La (SS-B) permits induction of systemic autoimmunity in normal mice. *J Exp Med* 1996;184:1857–1870.

78. Fuchs S, Mozes E, Stollar BD. The nature of murine immune response to nucleic acids. *J Immunol* 1975;114:1287–1291.

79. Cooke MS, Mistry N, Wood C, et al. Immunogenicity of DNA damaged by reactive oxygen species—implications for anti-DNA antibodies in lupus. *Free Radic Biol Med* 1997;22:151–159.

80. Krieg AM, Yi AK, Matson S, et al. CpG motifs in bacterial DNA trigger direct B-cell activation. *Nature* 1995;374:546–549.

81. Gilkeson GS, Ruiz P, Pippen AM, et al. Modulation of renal disease in autoimmune NZB/NZW mice by immunization with bacterial DNA. *J Exp Med* 1996;183:1389–1397.

82. Rumore PM, Steinman CR. Endogenous circulating DNA in systemic lupus erythematosus. Occurrence as multimeric complexes bound to histone. *J Clin Invest* 1990;86:69–74.

83. Li JZ, Steinman CR. Plasma DNA in systemic lupus erythematosus. Characterizationof cloned base sequences. *Arthritis Rheum* 1989; 32:726–733.

84. Casciola-Rosen L, Rosen A, Petri M, et al. Surface blebs on apoptotic cells are sites of enhanced procoagulant activity: implications for coagulation events and antigenic spread in systemic lupus erythematosus. *Proc Natl Acad Sci U S A* 1996;93:1624–1629.

85. Larsson M, Fonteneau JF, Bhardwaj N. Dendritic cells resurrect antigens from dead cells. *Trends Immunol* 2001;22:141–148.

86. Fadok VA, McDonald PP, Bratton DL, et al. Regulation of macrophage cytokine production by phagocytosis of apoptotic and post-apoptotic cells. *Biochem Soc Trans* 1998;26:653–656.

87. Gallucci S, Matzinger P. Danger signals: SOS to the immune system. *Curr Opin Immunol* 2001;13:114–119.

88. Gallucci S, Lolkema M, Matzinger P. Natural adjuvants: endogenous activators of dendritic cells. *Nat Med* 1999;5:1249–1255.

89. Rudensky AY, Preston-Hurlburt P, Hong SC, et al. Sequence analysis of peptides bound to MHC class II molecules. *Nature* 1991;353:622–627.

90. Nygard NR, Bono C, Brown LR, et al. Antibody recognition of an immunogenic influenza hemagglutinin–human leukocyte antigen class II complex. *J Exp Med* 1991;174:243–251.

91. Freed JH, Marrs A, VanderWall J, et al. MHC class II-bound self peptides from autoimmune MRL/lpr mice reveal potential T cell epitopes for autoantibody production in murine systemic lupus erythematosus. *J Immunol* 2000;164:4697–4705.

92. Rothfield NF, Stollar BD. The relation of immunoglobulin class, pattern of anti-nuclear antibody, and complement-fixing antibodies to DNA in sera from patients with systemic lupus erythematosus. *J Clin Invest* 1967;46:1785–1794.

93. Radic MZ, Weigert M. Origins of anti-DNA antibodies and their implications for B-cell tolerance. *Ann N Y Acad Sci* 1995;764:384–396.

94. Schlomchik M, Mascelli M, Shan H, et al. Anti-DNA antibodies from autoimmune mice arise by clonal expansion and somatic mutation. *J Exp Med* 1990;171:265–298.

95. Bloom DD, Davignon JL, Cohen PL, et al. Overlap of the anti-Sm and anti-DNA responses of MRL/Mp– lpr/lpr mice. *J Immunol* 1993; 150:1579–1590.

96. Ibrahim SM, Weigert M, Basu C, et al. Light chain contribution to specificity in anti-DNA antibodies. *J Immunol* 1995;155:3223–3233.

97. Bloom DD, Davignon J-L, Retter MW, et al. V region gene analysis of anti-Sm hybridomas from MRL/Mp– lpr/lpr mice. *J Immunol* 1993;150:1591–1610.

98. Yang P-M, Olsen NJ, Siminovitch KA, et al. Possible deletion of a developmentally regulated heavy-chain variable region gene in autoimmune diseases. *Proc Natl Acad Sci U S A* 1990;87:7907–7911.

99. Pugh-Bernard AE, Silverman GJ, Cappione AJ, et al. Regulation of inherently autoreactive VH4-34 B cells in the maintenance of human B cell tolerance. *J Clin Invest* 2001;108:1061–1070.

100. Diamond B, Scharff MD. Somatic mutation of the T15 heavy chain gives rise to antibody with autoantibody specificity. *Proc Natl Acad Sci U S A* 1984;81:5841–5844.

101. Miller FW, Twitty SA, Biswas T, et al. Origin and regulation of a disease-specific autoantibody response. Antigenic epitopes, spectrotype stability, and isotype restriction of anti–Jo-1 autoantibodies. *J Clin Invest* 1990;85:468–475.

102. Huff JP, Roos G, Peebles CL, et al. Insights into native epitopes of proliferating cell nuclear antigen using recombinant DNA protein products. *J Exp Med* 1990;172:419–429.

103. Patton JR, Habets W, van Venrooij WJ, et al. U1 small nuclear ribonucleoprotein particle-specific proteins interact with the first and second stem-loops of U1 RNA, with the A protein binding directly to the RNA independently of the 70K and Sm proteins. *Mol Cell Biol* 1989;9:3360–3368.

104. von Muhlen CA, Tan EM. Autoantibodies in the diagnosis of systemic rheumatic diseases. *Semin Arthritis Rheum* 1995;24:323–358.

105. Papoian R, Pillarisetty R, Talal N. Immunological regulation of spon-

taneous antibodies to DNA and RNA. II. Sequential switch from IgM to IgG in NZB/NZW F1 mice. *Immunology* 1977;32:75–79.

106. Rubin RL, Tang F-L, Chan EK, et al. IgG subclasses of autoantibodies in systemic lupus erythematosus, Sjogren's syndrome, and drug-induced autoimmunity. *J Immunol* 1986;137:2528–2534.

107. Eisenberg RA, Winfield JB, Cohen PL. Subclass restriction of anti-Sm antibodies in MRL mice. *J Immunol* 1982;129:2146–2149.

108. Habets WJ, Sillekens PTH, Hoet MH, et al. Small nuclear RNA-associated proteins are immunologically related as revealed by mapping of autoimmune reactive B-cell epitopes. *Proc Natl Acad Sci U S A* 1989;86:4674–4678.

109. Targoff IN, Johnson AE, Miller FW. Antibody to signal recognition particle in polymyositis. *Arthritis Rheum* 1990;33:1361–1370.

110. Landberg G, Tan EM. Characterization of a DNA-binding nuclear autoantigen mainly associated with S phase and G2 cells. *Exp Cell Res* 1994;212:255–261.

111. Maddison PJ, Reichlin M. Quantitation of precipitating antibodies to certain soluble nuclear antigens in SLE. *Arthritis Rheum* 1977;20:819–824.

112. Budman DR, Merchant EB, Steinberg AD, et al. Increased spontaneous activity of antibody-forming cells in the peripheral blood of patients with active SLE. *Arthritis Rheum* 1977;20:829–833.

113. Hollinger FB, Sharp JT, Lidsky MD, et al. Antibodies to viral antigens in systemic lupus erythematosus. *Arthritis Rheum* 1971;14:1–10.

114. Maul GG, French BT, van Venrooij WJ, et al. Topoisomerase I identified by scleroderma 70 antisera: enrichment of topoisomerase I at the centromere in mouse mitotic cells before anaphase. *Proc Natl Acad Sci U S A* 1986;83:5145–5149.

115. Mathews MB, Bernstein RM. Myositis autoantibody inhibits histidyl-tRNA synthetase: a model for autoimmunity. *Nature* 1983;304:177–179.

116. Harley JB, Alexander EL, Bias WB, et al. Anti-Ro (SS-A) and anti-La (SS-B) in patients with Sjogren's syndrome. *Arthritis Rheum* 1986;29:196–206.

117. Mamula MJ, Fox OF, Yamagata H, et al. The Ro/SSA autoantigen as an immunogen. Some anti-Ro/SSA antibody binds IgG. *J Exp Med* 1986;164:1889–1901.

118. Eisenberg RA, Craven SY, Warren RW, et al. Stochastic control of anti-Sm autoantibodies in MRL/Mp– lpr/lpr mice. *J Clin Invest* 1987; 80:691–697.

119. Leslie RD, Hawa M. Twin studies in auto-immune disease. *Acta Genet Med Gemellol (Roma)* 1994;43:71–81.

120. Block SR, Winfield JB, Lockshin MD, et al. Studies of twins with systemic lupus erythematosus. A review of the literature and presentation of 12 additional sets. *Am J Med* 1975;59:533–552.

121. Wakeland EK, Liu K, Graham RR, et al. Delineating the genetic basis of systemic lupus erythematosus. *Immunity* 2001;15:397–408.

122. Morel L, Croker BP, Blenman KR, et al. Genetic reconstitution of systemic lupus erythematosus immunopathology with polycongenic murine strains. *Proc Natl Acad Sci U S A* 2000;97:6670–6675.

123. Boackle SA, Holers VM, Chen X, et al. Cr2, a candidate gene in the murine Sle1c lupus susceptibility locus, encodes a dysfunctional protein. *Immunity* 2001;15:775–785.

124. Vyse TJ, Drake CG, Rozzo SJ, et al. Genetic linkage of IgG autoantibody production in relation to lupus nephritis in New Zealand hybrid mice. *J Clin Invest* 1996;98:1762–1772.

125. Rozzo SJ, Allard JD, Choubey D, et al. Evidence for an interferon-inducible gene, Ifi202, in the susceptibility to systemic lupus. *Immunity* 2001;15:435–443.

126. Tsao BP, Cantor TM, Kalunian KC, et al. Evidence for linkage of a candidate chromosome 1 region to human systemic lupus erythematosus. *J Clin Invest* 1997;99:725–731.

127. Arnett FC. Genetic studies of human lupus in families. *Int Rev Immunol* 2000;19:297–317.

128. Ruddy S. Rheumatic diseases and inherited complement deficiencies. *Bull Rheum Dis* 1996;45:6–8.

129. Turner MW, Hamvas RM. Mannose-binding lectin: structure, function, genetics and disease associations. *Rev Immunogenet* 2000;2:305–322.

130. Wofsy D, Ledbetter JA, Hendler PL, et al. Treatment of murine lupus with monoclonal anti-T cell antibody. *J Immunol* 1985;134:852–857.

131. Wofsy D, Seaman WE. Successful treatment of autoimmunity in NZB/NZW F1 mice with monoclonal antibody to L3T4. *J Exp Med* 1985; 161:378–391.

132. Finck BK, Linsley PS, Wofsy D. Treatment of murine lupus with CTLA4Ig. *Science* 1994;265:1225–1227.

133. Craft J, Peng S, Fujii T, et al. Autoreactive T cells in murine lupus: origins and roles in autoantibody production. *Immunol Res* 1999;19:245–257.

134. Zandman-Goddard G, Lorber M, Shoenfeld Y. Systemic lupus erythematosus and thymoma—a double-edged sword. *Int Arch Allergy Immunol* 1995;108:99–102.

135. Byrd VM, Sergent JS. Suppression of systemic lupus erythematosus by the human immunodeficiency virus. *J Rheumatol* 1996;23:1295–1296.

136. Molina JF, Citera G, Rosler D, et al. Coexistence of human immunodeficiency virus infection and systemic lupus erythematosus. *J Rheumatol* 1995;22:347–350.

137. Jonsson R, Brokstad KA, Lipsky PE, et al. B-lymphocyte selection and autoimmunity. *Trends Immunol* 2001;22:653–654.

138. Nagarkatti PS, Snow EC, Kaplan AM. Characterization and function of autoreactive T-lymphocyte clones isolated from normal, unprimed mice. *Cell Immunol* 1985;94:32–48.

139. Sakane T, Steinberg AD, Arnett FC, et al. Studies of immune functions of patients with systemic lupus erythematosus. *Arthritis Rheum* 1979;22:770–776.

140. Saito K, Tamura A, Narimatsu H, et al. Cloned auto-Ia-reactive T cells elicit lichen planus–like lesion in the skin of syngeneic mice. *J Immunol* 1985;137:2485–2495.

141. Weston KM, Yeh ET, Sy MS. Autoreactivity accelerates the development of autoimmunity and lymphoproliferation in MRL/Mp-lpr/lpr mice. *J Immunol* 1987;139:734–742.

142. Deeg HJ. Graft-versus-host disease: host and donor views. *Sem Hematol* 1993;30:110–117.

143. Erkeller-Yusel F, Hulstaart F, Hannet I, et al. Lymphocyte subsets in a large cohort of patients with systemic lupus erythematosus. *Lupus* 1993;2:227–231.

144. Sfikakis PP, Via CS. Expression of CD28, CTLA4, CD80, and CD86 molecules in patients with autoimmune rheumatic diseases: implications for immunotherapy. *Clin Immunol Immunopathol* 1997;83:195–198.

145. Furukawa F, Tokura Y, Matsushita K, et al. Selective expansions of T cells expressing V beta 8 and V beta 13 in skin lesions of patients with chonic cutaneous lupus erythematosus. *J Dermatol* 1996;23:670–676.

146. Groen H, Aslander M, Bootsma H, et al. Bronchoalvelolar lavage cell analysis and lung function impairment in patients with systemic lupus erythematosus (SLE). *Clin Exp Immunol* 1993;94:127–133.

147. Alcocer-Varela J, Aleman-Hoey D, Alarcon-Segovia D. Interleukin-1 and interleukin-6 activities are increased in the cerebrospinal fluid of patients with CNS lupus erythematosus and correlate with local late T-cell activation markers. *Lupus* 1992;1:111–117.

148. Okubo M, Yamamoto K, Kato T, et al. Detection and epitope analysis of autoantigen-reactive T cells to the U1-small nuclear ribonucleoprotein A protein in autoimmune disease patients. *J Immunol* 1993;151:1108–1115.

149. Crow MK, DelGiudice-Asch G, Zehetbauer JB, et al. Autoantigen-specific T cell proliferation induced by the ribosomal P2 protein in patients with systemic lupus erythematosus. *J Clin Invest* 1994;94:345–352.

150. Davies ML, Taylor EJ, Gordon C, et al. Candidate T cell epitopes of the human La/SSB autoantigen. *Arthritis Rheum* 2002;46:209–214.

151. Desai-Mehta A, Mao C, Rajagopalan S, et al. Structure and specificity of T cell receptors expressed by potentially pathogenic anti-DNA antibody–inducing T cells in human lupus. *J Clin Invest* 1995;95:531–541.

152. Seaman WE, Wofsy D, Greenspan JS, et al. Treatment of autoimmune MRL/lpr mice with monoclonal antibody to Thy-1.2: a single injection has sustained effects on lymphoproliferation and renal disease. *J Immunol* 1983;130:1713–1718.

153. Roubinian JR, Papoian R, Talal N. Effects of neonatal thymectomy and splenectomy on survival and regulation of autoantibody formation in NZB/NZW F1 mice. *J Immunol* 1977;118:1524–1529.

154. Hang L, Theofilopoulos AN, Balderas RS, et al. The effect of thymectomy on lupus-prone mice. *J Immunol* 1984;132:1809–1813.

155. Steinberg AD, Roths JB, Murphy ED, et al. Effects of thymectomy or androgen administration upon the autoimmune disease of MRL/Mp-lpr/lpr mice. *J Immunol* 1980;125:871–873.

156. Rozzo SJ, Drake CG, Chiang B-L, et al. Evidence for polyclonal T cell activation in murine models of systemic lupus erythematosus. *J Immunol* 1994;153:1340–1351.

157. Sobel ES, Cohen PL, Eisenberg RA. lpr T cells are necessary for autoantibody production in lpr mice. *J Immunol* 1993;150:4160–4167.

158. Mountz JD, Zhou T, Eldridge J, et al. Transgenic rearranged T cell receptor gene inhibits lymphadenopathy and accumulation of CD4−CD8−B220+ T cells in lpr/lpr mice. *J Exp Med* 1990;172:1805–1817.

159. Peng SL, Fatenejad S, Craft J. Induction of nonpathologic, humoral autoimmunity in lupus-prone mice by a class II-restricted, transgenic alpha beta T cell. Separation of autoantigen-specific and -nonspecific help. *J Immunol* 1996;157:5225–5230.

160. Sobel ES, Kakkanaiah VN, Kakkanaiah M, et al. T-B collaboration for autoantibody production in lpr mice is cognate and MHC-restricted. *J Immunol* 1994;152:6011–6016.

161. Peng SL, Madaio MP, Hughes DPM, et al. Murine lupus in the absence of alpha-beta T cells. *J Immunol* 1996;156:4041–4049.

162. Bernard NF, Eisenberg RA, Cohen PL. Response of MRL/Mp−+/+ mice to mouse Sm: non-H-2–linked genes determine T cell recognition. *J Immunol* 1985;134:1422–1425.

163. Bernard NF, Eisenberg RA, Cohen PL. H-2–linked Ir gene control of T cell recognition of the Sm nuclear autoantigen and the aberrant response of autoimmune MRL/Mp−+/+ mice. *J Immunol* 1985;134:3812–3818.

164. Mohan C, Adams S, Stanik V, MRL/Mp−+/+ mice. Nucleosome: a major immunogen for pathogenic autoantibody-inducing T cells of lupus. *J Exp Med* 1993;177:1367–1381.

165. Kretz-Rommel A, Rubin RL. Early cellular events in systemic autoimmunity driven by chromatin-reactive T cells. *Cell Immunol* 2001;208:125–136.

166. Ebling FM, Tsao BP, Singh RR, et al. A peptide derived from an autoantibody can stimulate T cells in the (NZB × NZW)F1 mouse model of systemic lupus erythematosus. *Arthritis Rheum* 1993;36:355–364.

167. Desai-Mehta A, Lu L, Ramsey-Goldman R, et al. Hyperexpression of CD40 ligand by B and T cells in human lupus and its role in pathogenic autoantibody formation. *J Clin Invest* 1996;97:2063–2073.

168. Mohan C, Shi Y, Laman JD, et al. The interaction between CD40 and its ligand gp39 in the development of murine lupus nephritis. *J Immunol* 1995;154:1470–1480.

169. Ma J, Xu J, Madaio MP, et al. Autoimmune lpr/lpr mice deficient in CD40 ligand: spontaneous Ig class switching with dichotomy of autoantibody responses. *J Immunol* 1996;157:417–426.

170. Vratsanos GS, Jung S, Park YM, et al. CD4(+) T cells from lupus-prone mice are hyperresponsive to T cell receptor engagement with low and high affinity peptide antigens: a model to explain spontaneous T cell activation in lupus. *J Exp Med* 2001;193:329–337.

171. Vassilopoulos D, Kovacs B, Tsokos GC. TCR/CD3 complex-mediated signal transduction pathway in T cells and T cell lines from patients with systemic lupus erythematosus. *J Immunol* 1995;155:2269–2281.

172. Chatenoud L, Salomon B, Bluestone JA. Suppressor T cells—they're back and critical for regulation of autoimmunity! *Immunol Rev* 2001;182:149–163.

173. Bonomo A, Kehn PJ, Shevach EM. Post-thymectomy autoimmunity: abnormal T-cell homeostasis. *Immunol Today* 1995;16:61–67.

174. Monier JC, Costa O, Souweine G, et al. Lupus-like syndrome in some strains of nude mice. *Thymus* 1980;1:241–255.

175. Morse HC III, Steinberg AD, Schur PH, et al. Spontaneous "autoimmune disease" in nude mice. *J Immunol* 1974;113:688–696.

176. Tomer Y, Shoenfeld Y. The significance of T suppressor cells in the development of autoimmunity. *J Autoimmun* 1989;2:739–758.

177. Alcocer-Varela J, Alarcon-Segovia A. Longitudinal study on the production of and cellular response to interleukin-2 in patients with systemic lupus erythematosus. *Rheumatol Int* 1995;15:57–63.

178. Spronk PE, ter Borg EJ, Huitema MG, et al. Changes in levels of soluble T-cell activation markers, sIL-2R, sCD4 and sCD8, in relation to disease exacerbations in patients with systemic lupus erythematosus: a prospective study. *Ann Rheum Dis* 1994;53:235–239.

179. Hagiwara E, Gourley MF, Lee S, et al. Disease severity in patients with systemic lupus erythematosus correlates with an increased ratio of interleukin-10–interferon-gamma–secreting cells in the peripheral blood. *Arthritis Rheum* 1996;39:379–385.

180. Erb KJ, Rueger B, von Brevern M, et al. Constitutive expression of

interleukin (IL)-4 in vivo causes autoimmune-type disorders in mice. *J Exp Med* 1997;185:329–339.

181. Csiszar A, Nagy H, Gergely P, et al. Increased interferon-gamma (IFN-gamma), IL-10 and decreased IL-4 mRNA expression in peripheral blood mononuclear cells (PBMC) from patients with systemic lupus erythematosus (SLE). *Clin Exp Immunol* 2000;122:464–470.

182. Masutani K, Akahoshi M, Tsuruya K, et al. Predominance of Th1 immune response in diffuse proliferative lupus nephritis. *Arthritis Rheum* 2001;44:2097–2106.

183. Theofilopoulos AN, Koundouris S, Kono DH, et al. The role of IFN-gamma in systemic lupus erythematosus: a challenge to the Th1/Th2 paradigm in autoimmunity. *Arthritis Res* 2001;3:136–141.

184. Ronnblom L, Alm GV. An etiopathogenic role for the type I IFN system in SLE. *Trends Immunol* 2001;22:427–431.

185. Blanco P, Palucka AK, Gill M, et al. Induction of dendritic cell differentiation by IFN-alpha in systemic lupus erythematosus. *Science* 2001;294:1540–1543.

186. Scheinecker C, Zwolfer B, Koller M, et al. Alterations of dendritic cells in systemic lupus erythematosus: phenotypic and functional deficiencies. *Arthritis Rheum* 2001;44:856–865.

187. Handwerger BS, Rus V, da Silva L, et al. The role of cytokines in the immunopathogenesis of lupus. *Springer Semin Immunopathol* 1994;16:153–180.

188. Jacob CO, Fronek Z, Lewis GD, et al. Heritable major histocompatibility complex class II–associated differences in production of tumor necrosis factor alpha: relevance to genetic predisposition to systemic lupus erythematosus. *Proc Natl Acad Sci U S A* 1990;87:1233–1237.

189. Jacob CO, Hwang F. Definition of microsatellite size variants for TNFa and Hsp70 in autoimmune and nonautoimmune mouse strains. *Immunogenetics* 1995;36:182–188.

190. Rus V, Svetic A, Nguyen P, et al. Kinetics of Th1 and Th2 cytokine production during the early course of acute and chronic murine graft-versus-host disease. Regulatory role of donor CD8+ T cells. *J Immunol* 1995;155:2396–2406.

191. Do RK, Chen-Kiang S. Mechanism of BLyS action in B cell immunity. *Cytokine Growth Factor Rev* 2002;13:19–25.

192. Zhang J, Roschke V, Baker KP, et al. Cutting edge: a role for B lymphocyte stimulator in systemic lupus erythematosus. *J Immunol* 2001;166:6–10.

193. Maddison PJ. Nature and nurture in systemic lupus erythematosus. *Adv Exp Med Biol* 1999;455:7–13.

194. Heimer H. Outer causes inner conflicts: environment and autoimmunity. *Environ Health Perspect* 1999;107:A504–A509.

195. Cooper GS, Dooley MA, Treadwell EL, et al. Hormonal, environmental, and infectious risk factors for developing systemic lupus erythematosus. *Arthritis Rheum* 1998;41:1714–1724.

196. Parks CG, Conrad K, Cooper GS. Occupational exposure to crystalline silica and autoimmune disease. *Environ Health Perspect* 1999;107(suppl 5):793–802.

197. Lahita RG. Sex hormones and systemic lupus erythematosus. *Rheum Dis Clin North Am* 2000;26:951–968.

198. Pisetsky DS. Immune responses to DNA in normal and aberrant immunity. *Immunol Res* 2001;22:119–126.

199. Yung RL, Richardson BL. Drug-induced lupus. *Rheum Dis Clin North Am* 1994;20:61–86.

200. Rubin RL, McNally EM, Nusinow SR, et al. IgG antibodies to the histone complex H2A-H2B characterize procainamide-induced lupus. *Clin Immunol Immunopathol* 1985;36:49–59.

201. Yung RL, Johnson KJ, Richardson BC. New concepts in the pathogenesis of drug-induced lupus. *Lab Invest* 1995;73:746–759.

202. Sutton RNP, Emond RT, Thomas DB, et al. The occurrence of autoantibodies in infectious mononucleosis. *Clin Exp Immunol* 1974;17:427–436.

203. Maisch B. Autoreactive mechanisms in infective endocarditis. *Springer Semin Immunopathol* 1989;11:439–456.

204. Itescu S. Rheumatic aspects of acquired immunodeficiency syndrome. *Curr Opin Rheumatol* 1996;8:346–353.

205. Johnson HM, Torres BA, Soos JM. Superantigens: structure and relevance to human disease. *Proc Soc Exp Biol Med* 1996;212:99–109.

206. de Inocencio J, Hirsch R. The role of T cells in Kawasaki disease. *Crit Rev Immunol* 1995;15:349–357.

207. East J, Branca M. Autoimmune reactions and malignant changes in germ-free New Zealand Black mice. *Clin Exp Immunol* 1969;4:621–635.

208. Unni KK, Holley KE, McDuffie FC, et al. Comparative study of NZB mice under germfree and conventional conditions. *J Rheumatol* 1975;2:36–44.

209. Maldonado MA, Kakkanaiah V, MacDonald GC, et al. The role of environmental antigens in the spontaneous development of autoimmunity in MRL-lpr mice. *J Immunol* 1999;162:6322–6330.

210. Jiang Y, Moller G. In vitro effects of HgCl2 on murine lymphocytes. I. Selective activation of T cells expressing certain V beta TCR. *Int Immunol* 1996;8:1729–1736.

211. Bagenstose LM, Salgame P, Monestier M. Murine mercury-induced autoimmunity: a model of chemically related autoimmunity in humans. *Immunol Res* 1999;20:67–78.

212. Black C, Pereira S, McWhirter A, et al. Genetic susceptibility to scleroderma-like syndrome in symptomatic and asymptomatic workers exposed to vinyl chloride. *J Rheumatol* 1986;13:1059–1062.

213. Yoshida SH, German JB, Fletcher MP, et al. The toxic oil syndrome: a perspective on immunotoxicological mechanisms. *Regul Toxicol Pharmacol* 1994;19:60–79.

214. Kaufman LD. The eosinophilia-myalgia syndrome: current concepts and future directions. *Clin Exp Rheumatol* 1992;10:87–91.

215. Hochberg MC, Perlmutter DL, Medsger TA Jr, et al. Lack of association between augmentation mammaplasty and systemic sclerosis. *Arthritis Rheum* 1996;39:1125–1131.

216. Wong O. A critical assessment of the relationship between silicone breast implants and connective tissue diseases. *Regul Toxicol Pharmacol* 1996;23:74–85.

217. Fleisher TA, Puck JM, Strober W, et al. The autoimmune lymphoproliferative syndrome. A disorder of human lymphocyte apoptosis. *Clin Rev Allergy Immunol* 2001;20:109–120.

218. Vaishnaw AK, Toubi E, Ohsako S, et al. The spectrum of apoptotic defects and clinical manifestations, including systemic lupus erythematosus, in humans with CD95 (Fas/APO-1) mutations. *Arthritis Rheum* 1999;42:1833–1842.

219. Singer GG, Abbas AK. The Fas antigen is involved in peripheral but not thymic deletion of T lymphocytes in T cell receptor transgenic mice. *Immunity* 1994;1:365–371.

220. Perkins DL, Glaser RM, Mahon CA, et al. Evidence for an intrinsic B cell defect in lpr/lpr mice apparent in neonatal chimeras. *J Immunol* 1990;145:549–555.

221. Katagiri T, Azuma S, Toyoda Y, et al. Tetraparental mice reveal complex cellular interactions of the mutant, autoimmunity-inducing lpr gene. *J Immunol* 1992;148:430–438.

222. Reap EA, Leslie D, Abrahams M, et al. Apoptosis abnormalities of splenic lymphocytes in autoimmune lpr and gld mice. *J Immunol* 1995;154:936–943.

223. Rubio CF, Kench J, Russell DM, et al. Analysis of central B cell tolerance in autoimmune-prone MRL/lpr mice bearing autoantibody transgenes. *J Immunol* 1996;157:65–71.

224. Lopez-Hoyos M, Carrio T, Merino T, et al. Constitutive expression of Bcl-2 in B cells causes a lethal form of lupuslike autoimmune disease after induction of neonatal tolerance to H-2b alloantigens. *J Exp Med* 1996;183:2523–2531.

225. Bouillet P, Metcalf D, Huang DC, et al. Proapoptotic Bcl-2 relative Bim required for certain apoptotic responses, leukocyte homeostasis, and to preclude autoimmunity. *Science* 1999;286:1735–1738.

226. Di Cristofano A, Kotsi P, Peng YF, et al. Impaired Fas response and autoimmunity in Pten+/- mice. *Science* 1999;285:2122–2125.

227. Gatenby PA, Irvine M. The Bcl-2 proto-oncogene is overexpressed in systemic lupus erythematosus. *J Autoimmun* 1994;7:623–631.

228. Aringer M, Wintersberger W, Steiner CW, et al. High levels of Bcl-2 protein in circulating T lymphocytes, but not B lymphocytes, of patients with systemic lupus erythematosus. *Arthritis Rheum* 1994;37:1423–1430.

229. Lorenz HM, Grunke M, Hieronymus T, et al. In vitro apoptosis and expression of apoptosis-related molecules in lymphocytes from patients with systemic lupus erythematosus and other autoimmune diseases. *Arthritis Rheum* 1997;40:306–317.

230. Caricchio R, Cohen PL. Spontaneous and induced apoptosis in systemic lupus erythematosus: multiple assays fail to reveal consistent abnormalities. *Cell Immunol* 1999;198:54–60.

231. Mohan C. Murine lupus genetics: lessons learned. *Curr Opin Rheumatol* 2001;13:352–360.

232. Navratil JS, Ahearn JM. Apoptosis and autoimmunity: complement

deficiency and systemic lupus erythematosus revisited. *Curr Rheumatol Rep* 2000;2:32–38.

233. Prodeus AP, Goerg S, Shen LM, et al. A critical role for complement in maintenance of self-tolerance. *Immunity* 1998;9:721–731.

234. Einav S, Pozdnyakova OO, Ma M, et al. Complement C4 is protective for lupus disease independent of C3. *J Immunol* 2002;168:1036–1041.

235. Botto M. Links between complement deficiency and apoptosis. *Arthritis Res* 2001;3:207–210.

236. Walport MJ. Complement. *N Engl J Med* 2001;344:1140–1144.

237. Paul E, Carroll MC. SAP-less chromatin triggers systemic lupus erythematosus. *Nat Med* 1999;5:607–608.

238. Walport MJ. Lupus, DNase and defective disposal of cellular debris. *Nat Genet* 2000;25:135–136.

239. Scott RS, McMahon EJ, Pop SM, et al. Phagocytosis and clearance of apoptotic cells is mediated by MER. *Nature* 2001;411:207–211.

240. Lu Q, Lemke G. Homeostatic regulation of the immune system by receptor tyrosine kinases of the Tyro 3 family. *Science* 2001;293:306–311.

241. Camenisch TD, Koller BH, Earp HS, et al. A novel receptor tyrosine kinase, Mer, inhibits TNF-alpha production and lipopolysaccharide-induced endotoxic shock. *J Immunol* 1999;162:3498–3503.

242. Baumann I, Kolowos W, Voll RE, et al. Impaired uptake of apoptotic cells into tingible body macrophages in germinal centers of patients with systemic lupus erythematosus. *Arthritis Rheum* 2002;46:191–201.

243. Dighiero G. Autoimmunity and B-cell malignancies. *Hematol Cell Ther* 1998;40:1–9.

244. Talal N. Autoimmunity and lymphoid malignancy in New Zealand black mice. *Prog Clin Immunol* 1974;2:101–120.

245. Davidson WF, Giese T, Fredrickson TN. Spontaneous development of plasmacytoid tumors in mice with defective Fas–Fas ligand interactions. *J Exp Med* 1998;187:1825–1838.

246. Kipps TJ, Tomhave E, Chen PP, et al. Molecular characterization of a major autoantibody-associated cross-reactive idiotype in Sjogren's syndrome. *J Immunol* 1989;142:4261–4268.

247. Martin T, Weber TC, Levallois H, et al. Salivary gland lymphomas in patients with Sjogren's syndrome may frequently develop from rheumatoid factor B cells. *Arthritis Rheum* 2000;43:908–916.

248. Mariette X. Lymphomas complicating Sjogren's syndrome and hepatitis C virus infection may share a common pathogenesis: chronic stimulation of rheumatoid factor B cells. *Ann Rheum Dis* 2001;60:1007–1010.

249. Straus SE, Jaffe ES, Puck JM, et al. The development of lymphomas in families with autoimmune lymphoproliferative syndrome with germline Fas mutations and defective lymphocyte apoptosis. *Blood* 2001;98:194–200.

250. Kurosu K, Yumoto N, Furukawa M, et al. Low-grade pulmonary mucosa–associated lymphoid tissue lymphoma with or without intraclonal variation. *Am J Respir Crit Care Med* 1998;158:1613–1619.

251. Stevenson FK, Spellerberg MB, Chapman CJ, et al. Differential usage of an autoantibody-associated VH gene, VH4-21, by human B-cell tumors. *Leuk Lymphoma* 1995;16:379–384.

252. Ramsland PA, Brock CR, Moses J, et al. Structural aspects of human IgM antibodies expressed in chronic B lymphocytic leukemia. *Immunotechnology* 1999;4:217–229.

253. Lydyard PM, Jewell AP, Jamin C, et al. CD5 B cells and B-cell malignancies. *Curr Opin Hematol* 1999;6:30–36.

254. Michiels JJ, Budde U, van der Planken M, et al. Acquired von Willebrand syndromes: clinical features, aetiology, pathophysiology, classification and management. *Best Pract Res Clin Haematol* 2001;14:401–436.

255. Antoine JC. Immunological mechanisms in paraneoplastic peripheral neuropathy. *Clin Rev Allergy Immunol* 2000;19:61–72.

256. Bouloc A, Joly P, Saint-Leger E, et al. Paraneoplastic pemphigus with circulating antibodies directed exclusively against the pemphigus vulgaris antigen desmoglein 3. *J Am Acad Dermatol* 2000;43:714–717.

257. Buckley C, Douek D, Newsom-Davis J, et al. Mature, long-lived CD4+ and CD8+ T cells are generated by the thymoma in myasthenia gravis. *Ann Neurol* 2001;50:64–72.

258. Abu-Shakra M, Buskila D, Ehrenfeld M, et al. Cancer and autoimmunity: autoimmune and rheumatic features in patients with malignancies. *Ann Rheum Dis* 2001;60:433–441.

259. Hochberg MC, Boyd RE, Ahearn JM, et al. Systemic lupus erythematosus: a review of clinico-laboratory features and immunogenetic markers in 150 patients with emphasis on demographic subsets. *Medicine* 1985;64:285–295.

260. Friou GJ. Setting the scene: a historical and personal view of immunologic diseases, autoimmunity, and ANA. *Clin Exp Rheumatol* 1994;12(suppl 11):S23–S25.

261. Friou GJ. Antinuclear antibodies: diagnostic significance and methods. *Arthritis Rheum* 1967;10:151–159.

262. Mohan C, Datta SK. Lupus: key pathogenic mechanisms and contributing factors. *Clin Immunol Immunopathol* 1995;77:209–220.

263. Koffler D, Agnello V, Kunkel HG. Polynucleotide immune complexes in serum and glomeruli of patients with systemic lupus erythematosus. *Am J Pathol* 1974;74:109–124.

264. Mostoslavsky G, Fischel R, Yachimovich N, et al. Lupus anti-DNA autoantibodies cross-react with a glomerular structural protein: a case for tissue injury by molecular mimicry. *Eur J Immunol* 2001;31:1221–1227.

265. Lee LA, Gaither KK, Coulter SN, et al. Pattern of cutaneous immunoglobulin G deposition in subacute cutaneous lupus erythematosus is reproduced by infusing purified anti-Ro (SSA) autoantibodies into human skin–grafted mice. *J Clin Invest* 1989;83:1556–1562.

266. Buyon JP, Ben-Chetrit E, Karp S, et al. Acquired congenital heart block: pattern of maternal antibody response to biochemically defined antigens of the SSA/Ro–SSB/La system in neonatal lupus. *J Clin Invest* 1989;84:627–634.

267. Elkon K, Weissbach H, Brot N. Central nervous system function in systemic lupus erythematosus. *Neurochem Res* 1990;15:401–406.

268. DeGiorgio LA, Konstantinov KN, Lee SC, et al. A subset of lupus anti-DNA antibodies cross-reacts with the NR2 glutamate receptor in systemic lupus erythematosus. *Nat Med* 2001;7:1189–1193.

269. Palmer DG. The anatomy of the rheumatoid lesion. *Br Med Bull* 1995;51:286–295.

270. DeKeyser F, Elewaut D, Vermeesch J, et al. The role of T cells in rheumatoid arthritis. *Clin Rheumatol* 1995;14(suppl 2):5–9.

271. Winchester RJ, Gregersen PK. The molecular basis of susceptibility to rheumatoid arthritis: the conformational equivalence hypothesis. *Springer Semin Immunopathol* 1988;10:119–139.

272. Smiley JD, Hoffman WL, Moore SE, et al. The humoral immune response of the rheumatoid synovium. *Semin Arthritis Rheum* 1985;14:151–162.

273. Winchester RJ, Agnello V, Kunkel HG. Gamma globulin complexes in synovial fluids of patients with rheumatoid arthritis. Partial characterization and relationship to lowered complement levels. *Clin Exp Immunol* 1970;6:689–706.

274. Duby AD, Sinclair AK, Osborneo-Lawrence SL, et al. Clonal heterogeneity of synovial fluid T lymphocytes from patients with rheumatoid arthritis. *Proc Natl Acad Sci U S A* 1989;86:6206–6210.

275. Paliard X, West SG, Lafferty JA, et al. Evidence for the effects of a superantigen in rheumatoid arthritis. *Science* 1991;253:325–329.

276. Vaughan JH, Fox RI, Abresch RJ, et al. Thoracic duct drainage in rheumatoid arthritis. *Clin Exp Immunol* 1984;58:645–653.

277. Sany J. Immunological treatment of rheumatoid arthritis. *Clin Exp Rheumatol* 1990;8(suppl 5):81–88.

278. Feldmann M, Brennan FM, Maini RN. Role of cytokines in rheumatoid arthritis. *Annu Rev Immunol* 1996;14:397–440.

279. Fox DA. Biological therapies: a novel approach to the treatment of autoimmune disease. *Am J Med* 1995;99:82–88.

280. Elliott MJ, Maini RN, Feldmann M, et al. Randomised double-blind comparison of chimeric monoclonal antibody to tumour necrosis factor alpha (cA2) versus placebo in rheumatoid arthritis. *Lancet* 1997;344:1105–1110.

281. Nabozny GH, David CS. The immunogenetic basis of collagen induced arthritis in mice: an experimental model for the rational design of immunomodulatory treatments of rheumatoid arthritis. *Adv Exp Med Biol* 1994;347:55–63.

282. Ronnelid J, Klareskog L. Local versus systemic immunoreactivity to collagen and the collagen-like region of C1q in rheumatoid arthritis and SLE. *Scand J Rheumatol* 1995;101(suppl):57–61.

283. Zvaifler NJ, Firestein GS. Pannus and pannocytes. Alternative models of joint destruction in rheumatoid arthritis. *Arthritis Rheum* 1994;37:783–789.

284. Haynes DR, Crotti TN, Loric M, et al. Osteoprotegerin and receptor activator of nuclear factor kappaB ligand (RANKL) regulate osteoclast

formation by cells in the human rheumatoid arthritic joint. *Rheumatology (Oxford)* 2001;40:623–630.

285. Hughes RA, Keat AC. Reiter's syndrome and reactive arthritis: a current view. *Semin Arthritis Rheum* 1994;24:190–210.

286. Lopez-Larrea C, Gonzalez-Roces S, Alvarez V. HLA-B27 structure, function, and disease association. *Curr Opin Rheumatol* 1996;8:296–308.

287. Careless DJ, Inman RD. Etiopathogenesis of reactive arthritis and ankylosing spondylitis. *Curr Opin Rheumatol* 1995;7:290–294.

288. Hyrich KL, Inman RD. Infectious agents in chronic rheumatic diseases. *Curr Opin Rheumatol* 2001;13:300–304.

289. Cuellar ML. HIV infection-associated inflammatory musculoskeletal disorders. *Rheum Dis Clin North Am* 1998;24:403–421.

290. Taurog JD, Hammer RE. Experimental spondyloarthropathy in HLA-B27 transgenic rats. *Clin Rheumatol* 1996;15(suppl 1):22–27.

291. Khare SD, Luthra HS, David CS. Spontaneous inflammatory arthritis in HLA-B27 transgeni mice lacking beta 2–microglobulin: a model of human spondyloarthropathies. *J Exp Med* 1995;182:1153–1158.

292. Ebringer A, Wilson C. HLA molecules, bacteria and autoimmunity. *J Med Microbiol* 2000;49:305–311.

293. Cuchacovich R. Immunopathogenesis of vasculitis. *Curr Rheumatol Rep* 2002;4:9–17.

294. Mader R, Keystone EC. Infections that cause vasculitis. *Curr Opin Rheumatol* 1992;4:35–38.

295. Cuellar ML. Drug-induced vasculitis. *Curr Rheumatol Rep* 2002;4:55–59.

296. Langford CA. Systemic vasculitis: new insights and emerging issues. *Curr Opin Rheumatol* 2002;14:1–2.

297. Sunday JS, Haynes BF. Pathogenic mechanisms of vessel damage in vasculitis syndromes. *Rheum Dis Clin North Am* 1995;21:861–881.

298. Ramos-Casals M, Trejo O, Garcia-Carrasco M, et al. Mixed cryoglobulinemia: new concepts. *Lupus* 2000;9:83–91.

299. Hoffman GS, Kerr GS, Leavitt RY. Wegener's granulomatosis: an analysis of 158 patients. *Ann Intern Med* 1992;116:488–498.

300. Savige J, Davies D, Falk RJ, et al. Antineutrophil cytoplasmic antibodies and associated diseases: a review of the clinical and laboratory features. *Kidney Int* 2000;57:846–862.

301. Price EJ, Venables PJ. The etiopathogenesis of Sjogren's syndrome. *Semin Arthritis Rheum* 1995;25:117–133.

302. Itescu S, Brancato LJ, Winchester R. A sicca syndrome in HIV infection: association with HLA-DR5 and CD8 lymphocytosis. *Lancet* 1989;2:466–468.

303. Van Rappard-Van der Veen FM, Kiesel U, Poels L, et al. Further evidence against random polyclonal antibody formation in mice with lupus-like graft-vs-host disease. *J Immunol* 1984;132:1814–1820.

304. Morris SC, Cheek RL, Cohen PL, et al. Autoantibodies in chronic graft versus host result from cognate T–B interactions. *J Exp Med* 1990;171:503–517.

305. Stastny P, Stembridge VA, Ziff M. Homologous disease in the adult rat, a model for autommune disease. I. General features and cutaneous lesions. *J Exp Med* 1963;118:635–648.

306. Kennedy MJ, Hess AD. Autologous graft-versus-host disease. *Med Oncol* 1995;12:149–156.

307. Clements PJ. Systemic sclerosis (scleroderma) and related disorders: clinical aspects. *Baillieres Best Pract Res Clin Rheumatol* 2000;14:1–16.

308. White B. Immunologic aspects of scleroderma. *Curr Opin Rheumatol* 1995;7:541–545.

309. Weiner ES, Earnshaw WC, Senecal J-L, et al. Clinical associations of anticentromere antibodies and antibodies to topoisomerase I: a study of 355 patients. *Arthritis Rheum* 1988;31:378–385.

310. Gershwin ME, Abplanalp H, Castles JJ, et al. Characterization of a spontaneous disease of white leghorn chickens resembling progressive systemic sclerosis. *J Exp Med* 1981;153:1640–1659.

311. Nelson JL. Microchimerism and scleroderma. *Curr Rheumatol Rep* 1999;1:15–21.

312. Cohen PL, Eisenberg RA. Lpr and gld: single gene models of systemic autoimmunity and lymphoproliferative disease. *Annu Rev Immunol* 1991;9:243–269.

313. Izui S, Kelley VA, Masuda K, et al. Induction of various autoantibodies by mutant gene lpr in several strains of mice. *J Immunol* 1984;133:227–233.

314. Jevnikar AM, Grusby JJ, Glimcher JH. Prevention of nephritis in major

histocompatibility complex class II–deficient MRL-lpr mice. *J Exp Med* 1994;179:1137–1143.

315. Koh DR, Ho A, Rahemtulla A, et al. Murine lupus in MRL/lpr mice lacking CD4 or CD8 T cells. *Eur J Immunol* 1995;25:2558–2562.

316. Maldonado MA, Eisenberg RA, Roper E, et al. Greatly reduced lymphoproliferation in lpr mice lacking major histocompatibility complex class I. *J Exp Med* 1995;181:641–648.

317. Chan OT, Madaio MP, Shlomchik MJ. The central and multiple roles of B cells in lupus pathogenesis. *Immunol Rev* 1999;169:107–121.

318. Theofilopoulos AN, Dixon FJ. Murine models of systemic lupus erythematosus. *Adv Immunol* 1985;37:269–390.

319. Datta SK. A search for the underlying mechanisms of systemic autoimmune disease in the NZB × SWR model. *Clin Immunol Immunopathol* 1989;51:141–156.

320. Reininger L, Winkler TH, Kalbere CP, et al. Intrinsic B cell defects in NZB and NZW mice contribute to systemic lupus erythematosis in (NZB × NZW)F1 mice. *J Exp Med* 1996;184:853–861.

321. Izui S, Iwamoto M, Fossati L, et al. The Yaa gene model of systemic lupus erythematosus. *Immunol Rev* 1995;144:137–156.

322. Merino R, Fossati L, Lacour M, et al. H-2–linked control of the Yaa gene–induced acceleration of lupus-like autoimmune disease in BXSB mice. *Eur J Immunol* 1992;22:295–299.

323. Satoh M, Kumar A, Kanwar YS, et al. Anti-nuclear antibody production and immune-complex glomerulonephritis in BALB/c mice treated with pristane. *Proc Natl Acad Sci U S A* 1995;92:10934–10938.

324. Satoh M, Richards HB, Shaheen VM, et al. Widespread susceptibility among inbred mouse strains to the induction of lupus autoantibodies by pristane. *Clin Exp Immunol* 2000;121:399–405.

325. Shoenfeld Y, Mozes E. Pathogenic idiotypes of autoantibodies in autoimmunity: lessons from new experimental models of SLE. *FASEB J* 1990;4:2646–2651.

326. Fricke H, Mendlovic S, Blank M, et al. Idiotype specific T-cell lines inducing experimental systemic lupus erythematosus in mice. *Immunology* 1991;73:421–427.

327. Kozlowski M, Mlinaric-Rascan I, Feng GS, et al. Expression and catalyatic activity of the tyrosine phosphatase PTP1C is severely impaired in motheaten and viable motheaten mice. *J Exp Med* 1993;178:2157–2163.

328. Letterio JJ, Geiser AG, Kulkarni AB, et al. Autoimmunity associated with TGF-beta1–deficiency in mice is dependent on MHC class II antigen expression. *J Clin Invest* 1996;98:2109–2119.

329. Marengere LE, Waterhouse P, Duncan GS, et al. Regulation of T cell receptor signaling by tyrosine phosphatase SYP association with CTLA-4. *Science* 1996;272:1170–1173.

330. Sadlack B, Merz H, Schorle H, et al. Ulcerative colitis-like disease in mice with a disrupted interleukin-2 gene. *Cell* 1993;75:203–205.

331. Kuhn R, Lohler J, Rennick D, et al. Interleukin-10–deficient mice develop chronic enterocolitis. *Cell* 1993;75:263–274.

332. Mombaerts P, Mizoguchi E, Grusby MJ, et al. Spontaneous development of inflammatory bowel disease in T cell receptor mutants. *Cell* 1993;75:203–205.

333. Strasser A, Whittingham S, Vaux DL, et al. Enforced BCL2 expression in B-lymphoid cells prolongs antibody responses and elicits autoimmune disease. *Proc Natl Acad Sci U S A* 1991;88:8661–8665.

334. Reap EA, Felix NJ, Wolthusen PA, et al. Bcl-2 transgenic Lpr mice show profound enhancement of lymphadenopathy. *J Immunol* 1995;155:5455–5462.

335. Green MD, Sweet HO, Bunker LE. Tight-skin, a new mutation of the mouse causing excessive growth of connective tissue and skeleton. *Am J Pathol* 1976;892:493–512.

336. Bona CA, Murai C, Casares S, et al. Structure of the mutant fibrillin-1 gene in the tight skin (TSK) mouse. *DNA Res* 1997;4:267–271.

337. Hatakeyama A, Kasturi KN, Wolf I, et al. Correlation between the concentration onf serum anti–topoisomerase I autoantibodies and histological and biochemical alterations in the skin of tight skin mice. *Cell Immunol* 1996;167:135–140.

338. Siracusa LD, McGrath R, Fisher JK, et al. The mouse tight skin (Tsk) phenotype is not dependent on the presence of mature T and B lymphocytes. *Mamm Genome* 1998;9:907–909.

339. Houri JM, O'Sullivan FX. Animal models in rheumatoid arthritis. *Curr Opin Rheumatol* 1995;7:201–205.

340. Cromartie WJ, Craddock JG, Schwab JH, et al. Arthritis in rats after systemic injection of streptococcal cells or cell walls. *J Exp Med* 1977;146:1585–1602.

341. Stimpson SA, Esser RE, Carter PB, et al. Lipopolysaccharide induces recurrence of arthritis in rat joints previously injured by peptidoglycan-polysaccharide. *J Exp Med* 1987;165:1688–1702.
342. Taneja V, David CS. Lessons from animal models for human autoimmune diseases. *Nat Immunol* 2001;2:781–784.
343. Brand DD, Marion TN, Myers LK, et al. Autoantibodies to murine type II collagen in collagen-induced arthritis: a comparison of susceptible and nonsusceptible strains. *J Immunol* 1996;157:5178–5184.
344. Wilder RL, Remmers EF, Kawahito Y, et al. Genetic factors regulating experimental arthritis in mice and rats. *Curr Dir Autoimmun* 1999;1:121–165.
345. Yamamoto H, Sekiguchi T, Itagaki K, et al. Inflammatory polyarthritis in mice transgenic for human T cell leukemia virus type I. *Arthritis Rheum* 1993;36:1612–1620.
346. Green JE, Hinrich SH, Vogel J, et al. Exocrinopathy resembling Sjogren's syndrome in HTLV-1 tax transgenic mice. *Nature* 1989;341:72–74.
347. Nishioka K, Maruyama I, Sato K, et al. Chronic inflammatory arthopathy associated with HTLV-1. *Lancet* 1989;i(8635):441.
348. Kouskoff V, Korganow AS, Duchatelle V, et al. Organ-specific disease provoked by systemic autoimmunity. *Cell* 1996;87:811–822.
349. Brennan FM. Transgenic models for arthritis: useful clues to be gained? *Ann Med* 1996;28:271–274.
350. Wang Y, Hu Q, Madri JA, et al. Amelioration of lupus-like autoimmune disease in NZB/W F1 mice after treatment with a blocking monoclonal antibody specific for complement component C5. *Proc Natl Acad Sci U S A* 1996;93:8563–8568.
351. Lefkowith JB, Gilkeson GS. Nephritogenic autoantibodies in lupus. *Arthritis Rheum* 1996;39:894–903.
352. Mukherjee R, Zhang Z, Zhong R, et al. Lupus nephritis in the absence of renal major histocompatibility complex class I and class II molecules. *J Am Soc Nephrol* 1996;7:2445–2452.
353. Roubey RAS. Immunology of the antiphospholipid antibody syndrome. *Arthritis Rheum* 1996;39:1444–1454.
354. Wiik A. What you should know about PR3-ANCA. An introduction. *Arthritis Res* 2000;2:252–254.
355. Cronstein BN. The mechanism of action of methotrexate. *Rheum Dis Clin North Am* 1997;23:739–755.
356. Kagnoff MF. Oral tolerance: mechanisms and possible role in inflammatory joint diseases. *Baillieres Clin Rheumatol* 1996;10:41–54.
357. Souroujon M, White-Scharff ME, Andre-Schwartz J, et al. Preferential autoantibody reactivity of the preimmune B cell repertoire in normal mice. *J Immunol* 1988;140:4173–4179.
358. Eisenberg RA, Cohen PL. Mechanisms of autoantibody production in systemic lupus erythematosus. *Clin Aspects Autoimmun* 1988;2:11.
359. Noer HR. An "experimental" epidemic of Reiter's syndrome. *JAMA* 1966;198:693–698.

CHAPTER 45

Organ-Specific Autoimmunity

Matthias G. von Herrath and Dirk Homann

General Concepts in Organ-Specific Autoimmunity
    Immunity and Autoimmunity · The Burden of Autoimmune Diseases · Central and Peripheral Tolerance: Implementing an Operational Concept · Initiating Autoimmunity: Antigens, Genes, and Environment · Regulatory Circuits in Autoimmune Processes · Therapeutic Considerations
Organ-Specific Autoimmune Disorders
    Type 1 Diabetes · Multiple Sclerosis · Autoimmune Liver Diseases · Autoimmune Uveoretinitis · Rheumatoid Arthritis · Autoimmune Thyroiditis · Autoimmune Skin Disorders · Autoimmune Gut Disorders · Autoimmune Diseases of the Heart
Closing Remarks
References

GENERAL CONCEPTS IN ORGAN-SPECIFIC AUTOIMMUNITY

Immunity and Autoimmunity

The other side of immunity is autoimmunity. Indeed, in true dialectical fashion, immunity's inception as a scientific discipline centered around this conceptual problem that significantly shaped immunologic debates in the first 15 and last 50 years of the past century. As much as the prefix *auto* assigns a specific role for *auto* immunity apart from *proper* immunity, the idea of immunity is not conceivable, for better or worse, without the notion of the *self*. Immunity has always exhibited distinct association with the individual self, beginning with its etymologic roots in the Roman legal concept of an *individual's* exemption from duty, service, or tax, to its official introduction into the canon of medical terminology, where the 1878 edition of Emile Littré's *Dictionnaire de Médecine* (1) defined it as *"idio* syncratic condition." However, with the dawn of the 20th century following the seminal discoveries of protective immunity induced by active immunization with attenuated pathogens (2) or passive transfer of convalescent serum (2a) and the seemingly unstoppable success of the "New Immunology," the notion of the immunologic *self* underwent a dramatic reconfiguration. The price for immunity, it appeared, was autoimmunity, a concept so problematic that its existence had to be relegated to the realm of the almost unspeakable, that is, the Greco-Latin neologism of a "horror autotoxicus" (3). Paradoxically, the time that witnessed the "horror autotoxicus" acquired the status of "law of immunity research" (4) also became what Arthur Silverstein has termed the "classical period" of

autoimmunity research (5). Though declared anathema, autoimmune phenomena were reported in a quick succession of widely publicized observations. In 1902, Portier and Richet (6) reported the phenomenon of anaphylaxis (as linguistically opposed to prophylaxis); in 1903 Arthus (7) characterized the local inflammatory response that was to bear his name; Donath and Landsteiner (8) described the first human autoimmune disease (paroxysmal cold hemoglobinuria) in 1904; and the term allergy ("altered reactivity") was coined by von Pirquet and Schick (9) in their analysis of serum sickness in 1905. The idea that tissue destruction may lead to expanded immunopathology (currently referred to as "determinant spreading") was proposed by Weil and Braun (10) in 1909: In the course of an infectious disease, "tissue alterations lead to generation of complement binding factors that, [. . .] based on their affinity to bodily cells, themselves attack and damage the cells of the organism." Even the concepts of organ specificity (11), immunoprivilege, and a breakdown of regulatory mechanisms as a cause for autoimmunity (4) were developed in the early days of autoimmunity research.

This period of extraordinary productivity was followed by an almost 40-year hiatus, "the dark ages" of autoimmunity research (5). The reasons for such a generalized disinterest in autoimmune phenomena were manifold and include political reconfigurations after World War I, the death of both Ehrlich (1915) and Metchnikoff (1916), a misconception of "horror autotoxicus" that immune responses against "self" are *impossible* rather than *improbable,* and a paradigm shift in the field of immunology in favor of immunochemical approaches (5). The renaissance of autoimmunity research had to await observations about immunologic tolerance of mice congenitally infected with lymphocytic choriomeningitis virus (LCMV) (12), description of tolerance in chimeric cattle twins (13), and Medawar's work on skin transplant rejection (14–17), as well as the integration of these findings into a conceptual framework of self and non-self as determinants for immunologic reactivity (18). Burnet subsequently developed and extended these ideas into the "clonal selection theory of antibody formation" (19), thereby establishing the conceptual centrality of self, non-self, and immunologic tolerance. Although the dogmatic reading of "horror autotoxicus" was still prevalent (Ernest Witebsky delayed his publication about thyroid antibodies [20] for several years assuming an experimental error [5]), Ehrlich's original conception of "regulatory contrivances" that prevent autoimmunity was now validated within the context of the clonal selection theory.

Again, however, the usefulness of self and non-self as distinguishing parameters was questioned at the very time that they began their rise to prominence. Ludwik Fleck, in his singular study *Genesis and Development of a Scientific Fact* (21), questioned the capacity of an immune system that only interacts with structures that are strictly non-self: "[I]t is very doubtful whether an invasion in the old sense is possible, involving as it does an inference by completely foreign organisms in natural conditions. A completely foreign organism could find no receptors capable of reaction and thus could not generate a biological process." This view is echoed and elaborated on in the work of Jerne (22) and Coutinho et al. (23) and the possibility of a physiologic role for autoimmune processes was postulated by concepts such as "physiologic" (24), "positive" (25) or "protective" autoimmunity (25a). The importance of autoreactivity as an integral aspect of immunity is further demonstrated by the phenomenon of positive T-cell selection in the thymus or the T cell-mediated destruction of transformed or infected tissues that is based on the recognition of "foreign" (eg. viral peptides or even "self" as in the case of some tumor-derived antigens) in the context of "self" (major histocompatibility complexes). In fact, events associated with "danger" or the preservation of "tissue integrity" rather than the discrimination between "self/non-self" have been postulated as a primary driving force that engages the immune system (26,27).

While evolutionary constraints have favored the development of an immune system that indeed can be successfully conceptualized, to a certain extent, with the notions of "self/non-self distinction", "danger" and "tissue integrity", a utilitarian view of auto/immunity should emphasize a balanced perspective between practical consequences and ideational comprehensiveness.

While the notion of autoimmunity as an aberrant phenomenon has formed much of our understanding about the immune system and its functions, there appears to be a growing awareness that immunity and autoimmunity are historically and conceptually inextricably intertwined. An emerging consensus indicates that the anthropomorphisms of self and non-self should be overcome (e.g., as suggested in the respective forewords to two leading textbooks on autoimmunity [28,29]) and that autoimmunity is likely to be a universal phenomenon in the evolution of the vertebrate immune system. As part of the evolving organism, the immune system processes antigen stimuli in a deterministic fashion restricted by genetics, previous antigenic experience of the host, nature of the antigen and the conditions of its presentation (28). However, imbuing the immune system's function with an overriding purpose, no matter how important for our conceptualization and experimentation, has to consider that evolution is ignorant to teleology. In this respect, the remark by the Darwinist Paul Ehrlich (3) that production of autoantibodies is "dysteleological in the extreme" may be extended to the functionality of the immune system as a whole: there is no teleology in autoimmunity nor immunity, just the workings of a complex system under evolutionary constraints. The rules that inform immunity are the same ones that govern autoimmunity.

The Burden of Autoimmune Diseases

The existence of autoimmune diseases in humans has been known for almost 100 years. By now, autoimmune pathogenesis has been attributed to more than 40 human diseases (30), yet it is still far from clear which features can conclusively prove an underlying autoimmune pathogenesis. It has been suggested, somewhat provocatively, that with knowledge about an infectious origin, diseases are called immunopathologically mediated, whereas lack of such knowledge results in reference to such diseases as autoimmune (31). While this argument is akin to the medical taxonomy where diseases of unknown origin are assigned to the domain of the "endogenous," "idiotypic," "essential," or "primary," a "positive" definition for autoimmune diseases is very much needed to provide a specific diagnostic framework that allows for unequivocal identification of distinct autoimmune disorders, yet remains flexible enough to accommodate new insights into etiologic and symptomatologic processes. A first attempt to provide such a basis for the establishment of the autoimmune origin of human diseases was formulated by Witebsky et al. (32) who modeled their postulates on those of Koch: recognition of an autoimmune response (autoantibody or cell mediated) and identification of a corresponding autoantigen, as well as induction of an analogous autoimmune response and disease in experimental animals (32). A timely update for these criteria has been proposed by Rose and Bona (30) who suggested a combination of direct evidence (transfer of pathogenic antibodies or T cells), indirect evidence (reproduction of disease in experimental animals), and circumstantial evidence (clinical clues) to determine an underlying autoimmune etiology for human diseases. However, it is important to note that ultimately guidelines must be tailored to individual autoimmune disorders. An example for a catalog of diagnostic criteria to be evaluated in a scoring system for identification of patients with a specific autoimmune disease is the report of the International Autoimmune Hepatitis Group (33). This report also illustrates the importance of distinguishing between an autoimmune and infectious origin for hepatitis (33). Immunosuppressive therapy has a beneficial effect on the course of autoimmune hepatitis (AIH); responsiveness to such therapy is in fact one of the diagnostic criteria for AIH but may be detrimental when employed for treatment of virus-induced hepatitis.

In a first of its kind, a meta-study providing a comprehensive evaluation of the prevalence and incidence studies conducted for 24 autoimmune diseases since 1965 was published in 1997 (34). Overall, 1 in 31 Americans or ~8.5 million people were estimated to be afflicted by autoimmune diseases. The most prevalent disorders, divided into organ-specific and systemic conditions, and ranked in order of prevalence, are listed in Table 1. The study by Jacobson et al. (34) has documented some striking, if not entirely unexpected results. The number of studies conducted has not necessarily been related to the public health burden. Many autoimmune conditions are clearly understudied, and some of the most frequently epidemiologically studied diseases do not contribute a comparatively high number of cases per year. The specific reasons for this balance remain to be elucidated, but will likely include the presence or absence of effective therapy. Pernicious anemia, the sixth most common autoimmune disease in the United States, can be effectively managed, and therefore apparently attracts only limited epidemiologic interest. Other significantly less frequent conditions pose a pronounced health burden on afflicted individuals and thus warrant continued attention and efforts to provide amelioration or even cure. On the other hand, the availability of certain models for autoimmune diseases, again not necessarily a reflection of the epidemiologic importance of the corresponding human autoimmune disease, will have an impact on choices made by researchers charting their field of study. Finally,

as in other areas of research or clinical medicine, the funds and resources available are the result of multiple factors that may or may not include the public health burden a particular autoimmune disease poses. Balancing these aspects to appropriately appreciate the burden of autoimmune diseases, based on both the population and the afflicted individual, is a great challenge requiring our continued efforts to identify, investigate, inform, and, hopefully, improve the therapies for many autoimmune diseases.

Central and Peripheral Tolerance: Implementing an Operational Concept

A historical discussion of the concept of tolerance is beyond the scope of this chapter, but some aspects of the usage of the term require clarification at the outset. Tolerance in adaptive immunity, *strictu sensu,* is the absence of specific lymphocyte activity. This may be achieved by physical deletion or functional silencing of specific T and B cells. Some researchers refer to these tolerance mechanisms as "passive" or "recessive" tolerance to explicitly distinguish them from "active" or "dominant" tolerance. While the latter mechanisms constitute *bona fide* immune responses (therefore, other researchers do not categorize them as a mode of tolerance), their particular nature results in a phenotype that is comparable to that achieved by means of passive/recessive tolerance. Distinct effector mechanisms (e.g., immunosuppressive cytokines) and possibly dedicated classes of immune cells (e.g., "T-regulatory cells") ensure that local or systemic autoimmunity is avoided. The concept of T-cell suppressors, first proposed in the early 1970s by Gershon and Kondo (35), has

TABLE 1. *Prevalence and incidence of autoimmune diseases in United States (1996)*

Autoimmune disease	Weighted mean prevalence rate/100,000	Weighted mean incidence rate/100,000
Thyroiditis/hypothyroidism	1323.8	21.8
Grave's disease/hyperthyroidism	1151.5	13.9
→Rheumatoid arthritis	860.0	23.7
Vitiligo	400.2	
Type 1 diabetes	192.0	12.2
Pernicious anemia	150.9	—[a]
Multiple sclerosis	58.3	3.2
Glomerulonephritis (primary)	40.0	3.6
→Systemic lupus erythematosus	23.8	7.3
Glomerulonephritis (IgA)	23.2	2.4
→Sjogren's syndrome	14.4	—[a]
Addison's disease	5.0	—[a]
Myasthenia gravis	5.1	0.4
→Polymyositis/dermatomyositis	5.1	1.8
→Scleroderma	4.4	0.8
Primary biliary cirrhosis	3.5	0.9
Uveitis	1.7	18.9
Chronic active hepatitis	0.4	0.7

[a]No studies on disease incidence available.
Note: The prevalence/incidence rate from each study within a disease category contributed proportionally to the mean prevalence/incidence rate based on the population size of that study. The proportion or weight was calculated by dividing the study population denominator by the total of all study population denominators for each disease. From Jacobson et al. (34), with permission.
Systemic autoimmune disorders are marked by an arrow (→).

recently been resurrected in the form of CD25$^+$CD4$^+$ regulatory T cells and has attracted considerable attention. However, while there is indeed a CD25$^+$ lineage of T cells committed to regulatory activity in naïve, nonimmunized mice, we wish to underscore that regulatory functions, including those that limit autoimmunity, are a feature of the immune system as a whole and can be exercised by other classes of immune cells as well (e.g., CD8$^+$ T cells, $\gamma\delta$TCR T cells, NKT cells, etc.). Thus, while CD25$^+$CD4$^+$ regulatory T cells occupy a distinct and important niche in the complex dynamic network of immune functions, not all T-cell regulators are CD25$^+$CD4$^+$, nor do all CD25$^+$CD4$^+$ T cells function as suppressors. The multiplicity of current efforts to understand the nature of CD25$^+$CD4$^+$ regulatory T cells has been expertly reviewed elsewhere (36,37 and Chapter 30).

T-Cell Tolerance

Autoreactivity, by definition, designates a specific immune response to self-antigens. Antigen-nonspecific responses such as inflammatory and innate immune processes should not be considered autoimmune in the strict sense, although they may accompany, enhance, or even trigger autoimmune processes proper. Thus, antigen-specific T- or B-cell immunity will have to underlie a genuine autoimmune disorder. Furthermore, for organ-specific autoimmune diseases, antigen-specificity of primary effector lymphocytes must be largely restricted to autoantigens derived from defined organs or tissues. Once initiated, organ-specific responses that precipitate or "drive" the localized autoimmune reaction may diversify to comprise additional specificities ("determinant spreading") and pathogenic mechanisms.

How does the adaptive immune system restrict generation and activation of autoreactive lymphocytes? The central process by which the generation of T-cell receptor diversity is limited is called thymic selection. Thymic selection is a developmental process that selects T cells with a biased repertoire for export into the periphery (38–42). T cells that interact at least weakly with self-peptides presented in the context of MHC molecules are chosen in the course of positive selection (43,44), while those that do not effectively interact with MHC–peptide complexes die "by neglect." However, interactions above a certain avidity threshold result in elimination by negative selection and constitute the basis for "central tolerance" (38,42). Thus, central tolerance prevents widespread autoimmunity as a function of lymphocyte/antigen-complex avidity and preferentially selects T cells with specificity for antigens not expressed in thymic epithelium for export into the periphery. However, central tolerance is not complete and a sizable pool of T cells with intermediate avidity can escape negative selection and constitutes the majority of autoreactive T-cells found in the peripheral immune system. While the presence of these autoreactive T cells is to be considered physiologic, they are usually not activated and exhibit a "naïve" phenotype. Only an encounter under appropriate stimulatory conditions (i.e., presentation of autoantigen-derived peptides presented in the context of MHC class I or II molecules accompanied by antigen-nonspecific co-stimulatory interactions) can lead to their full activation in the periphery. As "armed effectors," autoreactive T cells are now potentially very dangerous and may initiate organ-specific autoimmunity, if they recognize the same or closely related autoantigen in a defined tissue. It is thought that a few autoaggressive "driver clones" with highly detrimental effector function can sustain a localized autoimmune process, and it is likely that high receptor/MHC/self-peptide avidity predisposes to this phenotype (45). However, not all self-reactive lymphocytes need to necessarily exhibit an aggressive phenotype. Depending on their specific effector functions, autoreactive T cells may exhibit regulatory functions and may critically modulate or even abort local autoimmune processes. Such autoreactive regulators might occur physiologically and constitute the majority of autoimmune responses present in healthy individuals.

The presence of autoreactive T cells in the periphery might suggest that detrimental autoimmunity should occur quite frequently if organ-specific autoantigens are not expressed in the thymus, or alternatively or in addition, such physiologically occurring autoimmunity is of a regulatory nature. Yet, there are several mechanisms that maintain tolerance in the periphery. Peripheral tolerance involves a set of mechanisms which ensures that autoreactive T-lymphocytes are not activated in the periphery. It should be noted that these mechanisms pertain to both autoreactive and "heteroreactive" T cells and involve the following pathways. First, it has been observed that naïve T cells triggered by a strong signal through the T-cell receptor alone may lose the ability to proliferate, and some but not all effector functions become "anergic" (46–48). Presence of certain cytokines or co-stimulatory interactions can avoid the induction of anergy or may reverse an anergic state. Second, highly activated T cells will eventually undergo activation-induced cell death (AICD) (49). AICD is thought to be essential for the down-modulation of immune responses and the reestablishment of immune homeostasis. Impairment of AICD may lead to continued immune activation and generalized autoreactivity. For CD4 lymphocytes, AICD is Fas/Fas-L dependent (50,51); it is not clear which interactions precisely control AICD in CD8 cells. Third, molecules that can deliver specific negative signals, such as the B7-binding CTLA-4 are involved in "turning off" of antigen-specific T cells (52,53). Finally, other factors such as regulatory lymphocytes and antigen-presenting cells (APC) might play important roles in maintaining peripheral tolerance (35,36,54).

B-Cell Tolerance

Although they are not selected in the thymus, similar paradigms apply to autoreactive B-lymphocytes. B cells mature independently of antigens in the bone marrow and clonally expand after recognizing antigens in the periphery. T-helper lymphocytes are needed for this process in response to most protein antigens, and these B-cell responses are therefore termed "thymus dependent" or, in other words, require

T cells with specificity linked to an epitope on the antigen that they are reacting with. T helper–cell independent B-cell responses occur mostly to bacterial and lipid antigens—for example, to lipopolysaccharide (LPS)—and are therefore rarely autoaggressive.

In conclusion, central (thymic) and peripheral tolerance mechanisms will effectively control the vast majority of autoreactive lymphocytes, which assures that autoaggressive immune responses are relatively rare (<5% overall population). Some of the considerations described in this paragraph are illustrated in Fig. 1.

Organ-Specific Tuning—Regulatory and Destructive Autoimmunity

As indicated above, while autoimmune disorders must conform to a set of general criteria, organ-specific autoimmunity must be considered in addition to the specific context of the target organ affected. Certain effector functions exerted by autoreactive lymphocytes will be detrimental only to particular cells or tissues. For example, the pancreatic β cells are more sensitive to the damaging effect of inflammatory cytokines than neighboring α cells (both cell types are part of the islets of Langerhans) and other cells in their vicinity (e.g., fibroblasts or acinar tissue of the pancreas) (55). On the other hand, some organs provide a microenvironment that suppresses inflammatory responses. For example, both the gut and the central nervous system (CNS) contain relatively large amounts of TGF-β, which is known to have direct anti-inflammatory effector functions on APCs (56–58). Also, certain large organs such as the liver may better tolerize lymphocyte responses direct toward them, because they contain a high number of cells that are incapable of co-stimulation (e.g.,

hepatocytes) and will, therefore, shut down naïve autoreactive lymphocytes that recognize them (26). Finally, the precise activation state, phenotype, and effector function of an autoreactive cell are critical in determining its impact on tissues expressing its cognate antigen. Some molecules will exert beneficial functions, such as interleukin-4 (IL-4) and probably IL-10 and TGFβ in type 1 diabetes (59–61). Antigen-specific regulatory cells are likely present in every local autoimmune process and are essential for delay or prevention of clinical disease altogether. While their induction is clearly a therapeutic goal, phenotype and mechanistic aspects essential for regulatory function are not yet understood in detail. Autoreactive regulatory cells may exert their function by targeted alteration of APC function. They may act as true bystander processors if their suppressive action via APC modulation is extended to aggressive immune responses regardless of specificity found in the microenvironment of the affected organ (Fig. 2). Indeed, such cells have been found in several animal models (60,62–64), but their existence and function in humans are not well defined. Alternatively, regulatory lymphocytes may directly affect activated or naïve aggressive lymphocytes and induce anergy or apoptosis. Finally, by changing the overall cytokine milieu of a given inflammatory process, the number and function of aggressive cells and cytokines/chemokines may be dampened in a localized area (65). Probably the best-understood balancing circuit employed by autoreactive regulatory cells is the T_H1/T_H2 paradigm (66–68). In light of these observations, autoreactivity is not necessarily detrimental. Furthermore, it is unlikely to identify a "typical" phenotype of autoaggressive lymphocytes that will cause damage at any site or organ. Rather, autoaggression has to be defined in relation to the target organ or cell that is under attack, lymphocytes detrimental in one organ/disease will not necessarily

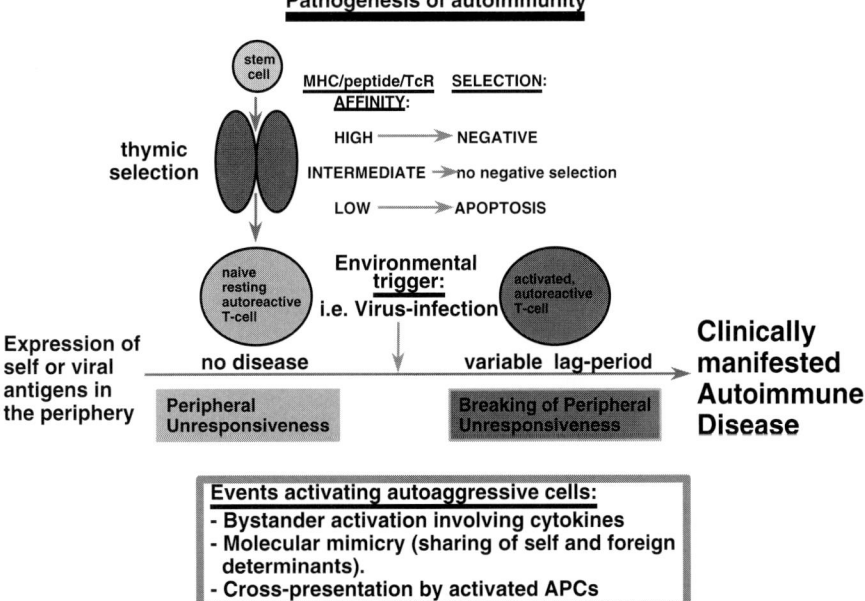

FIG. 1. Potentially autoreactive lymphocytes can escape thymic negative selection and escape into the periphery. Such initially naïve cells can be activated via several mechanisms involving cytokines, inflammation, and possibly external triggers such as viral infections.

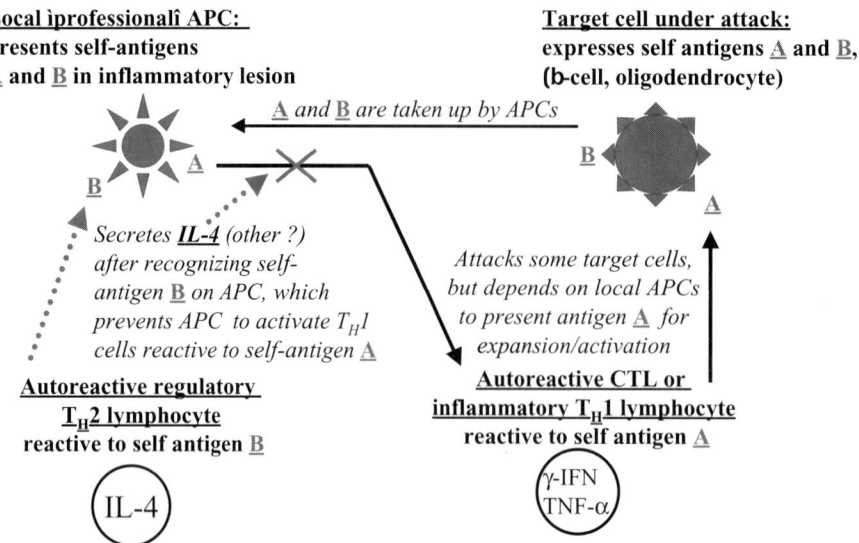

FIG. 2. The concept of bystander suppression via APCs. Organ (cell)-specific autoantigens are taken up and presented by APCs locally, for example in the draining lymph node. These will activate both aggressive lymphocytes directed to antigen A and regulatory lymphocytes directed to antigen B. Effector molecules secreted by autoreactive regulatory cells, such as IL-4 in type 1 diabetes, will dampen the aggressive response via APC modulation.

be detrimental to other organs, and ubiquitous autoimmunity will therefore occur very rarely.

Initiating Autoimmunity: Antigens, Genes, and Environment

Antigens

A central challenge in most human autoimmune disorders is the identification of an initiating autoantigen or autoantigens. Several candidate autoantigens have been identified in type 1 diabetes; however, whether any are actually involved in initiation of the disease remains unclear and controversial. A similar situation exists for multiple sclerosis (MS) and arthritis. Thus, distinguishing features that constitute an ideal candidate autoantigen and parameters by which potential candidates can be searched for and identified as the initiating autoantigen antigen for a given organ-specific disease must be determined with much greater precision to yield insights applicable to preventive or therapeutic interventions.

The concept that "processing of antigens determines the self" has been introduced by Sercarz (69,70). Autoantigens that are not expressed in the thymus or are of cryptic nature (69,71,72) may encounter a more extensive T-cell repertoire that is likely of higher avidity. Such antigens appear to be better targets. Low levels of thymic antigen expression or limited numbers of thymic medullary cells may lead to partial tolerance (58). In addition, the precise timing of antigen expression during embryonic development may play a major role for the establishment of tolerance. Antigens that are cryptic or not expressed during early embryonic development might become better targets later, because more autoreactive

T cells will be present in the periphery. It should be considered that certain "embryonic antigens" are involved in initiating autoimmune diseases.

Another parameter of importance is the constraints with which particular antigens can be presented to the immune system in a given target organ. Exogenous uptake of soluble antigens usually results in processing via the MHC class II presentation pathway.

Such antigens may also be processed through the MHC class I pathway by dendritic cells, a mechanism termed cross-presentation if the antigen itself was originally expressed by a cell different from the APC (73,74). Cross-presentation appears to be less efficient than direct endogenous presentation of antigens through the MHC class I pathway. At this point it is not clear which properties will make an antigen a more efficient candidate for cross-presentation. The class I pathway may be very important in the effector phase for many autoimmune disorders because CD8$^+$ T cells with cytotoxic function (CTL) can be induced in this fashion, and CTL have profound detrimental effector functions (interferon-γ [IFNγ] and TNF-α secretion, lysis of target cells) (75). Clearly, recent observations have shown that cross-presentation can lead to immunity, as well as tolerance, and in this way propagate or alternatively, halt autoimmune disease (73,76). It is unlikely that autoantigens that are not presented by professional APCs or within lymphoid organs after their release from target cells/organs can initiate autoimmunity. Only under extraneous circumstances (i.e., extremely high-density presentation of an antigen on a target cell) would this appear possible. However, experienced or primed autoaggressive lymphocytes will be capable of becoming activated after seeing antigen in the absence of co-stimulation.

The type of autoantigen will define its own potential "candidacy" in an autoimmune process. Autoantigens that are not expressed during development, or were cryptic for an extended period of time, as well as antigens secreted and cross-presented in lymphoid organs by APCs, appear to be better suited for assuming the role as primary culprits.

Genes

An abundance of empiric evidence indicates the association of many organ-specific autoimmune diseases with certain HLA haplotypes, as well as with other susceptibility or protective genes. The principal specific genetic linkages are discussed separately for each condition below. In general, MHC class I (such as HLA B 27) (77,78) or class II (such as DR4) genes might predispose to a certain disease by enhanced presentation of pathogenic peptides in the periphery or inefficacious presentation of autoantigen-derived peptides in the thymus. For example, the human HLA-DQ8 molecule has a striking structural similarity to the mouse I-A^{g7} class II that predisposes NOD mice to spontaneous autoimmune diabetes (79,80). However, the link to disease appears not to be as simple as reasoned above, and more complex mechanisms might be in place. Presentation of the pathogenic peptide in gluten-induced celiac disease involves acidic modification of the protein to generate the peptide ultimately presented by MHC class II (81) and other chemical modifications can be expected to alter peptide binding to MHC and the resulting conformation.

Other genes that encode immunoregulatory or inflammatory proteins may be involved in the disease process and, finally, genes that support tissue or wound repair (e.g., islet cell regeneration in type 1 diabetes) may be of help to prevent disease development (82). For most organ-specific autoimmune disorders, the genetic links are complex, not absolute, and many susceptibility and resistance genes act in concert to modulate the clinical phenotype. Still largely unexplored are genes responsible for transcriptional control of other proteins. Experimental models indicate that transcription factors can have profound effects on the development of autoimmune disease and variations in expression and activity levels may be found between susceptible and protected individuals. In summary, a complex interplay of many genes will predispose for a certain autoimmune disease, but the concordance of clinical manifestation is frequently not higher than 30% to 40% in monozygotic twins (83–88). For this reason, other factors are to be considered in triggering or propagating the organ-specific disease process.

Environment

Viral Infections

For many years viral infections have been discussed as potential candidates to trigger autoimmunity in susceptible individuals because of their capacity to directly infect target tissues and induce strong inflammatory responses and immune activation. While the association between viral infections and organ-specific autoimmune disorders is a very intriguing possibility, it has been exceedingly difficult to demonstrate a causative role for specific viruses in human autoimmune diseases. Some of the many obstacles follow: (a) all individuals undergo a multitude of viral infections during their lifetime; (b) one has to assume that viruses are frequently cleared at the time of diagnosis and viral footprints can be difficult to find in individuals affected by an autoimmune disease ("hit and run" event); (c) the precise viral strain, infection kinetics, and number of T cells and type of effector functions induced may play an instrumental role in determining its effect in an individual genetically at risk, necessitating a very detailed immunologic profiling (89); (d) due to MHC polymorphism, there is a significant variation in specificity of the antiviral response; and (e) viral infections might not, per se, trigger autoimmunity, but affect an ongoing autoimmune process in a detrimental way. Thus, a successful approach should be to first explore the underlying mechanisms in virally induced autoimmunity and then apply the precise insight and paradigms developed specifically to the human situation.

The most important mechanisms to be considered are summarized below and in Fig. 3.

1. Molecular mimicry, which implies the cross-reactivity between viral and self-determinants as a principal cause or mechanism to enhance autoimmunity (90,91).
2. Bystander activation, which postulates that APCs and autoreactive lymphocytes will become activated indirectly as a consequence of the cytokine/chemokine by virus infection of a particular organ (92).
3. Virally induced determinant spreading, which involves the presentation of autoantigens (possibly previously cryptic) by virus-activated APCs (93–95).

Experimental evidence is good for all of the above scenarios in various mouse models *in vivo*. However, none of these have been proven for any human autoimmune disorder due to the large size of human trials and the invasive nature of *in vivo* diagnostics required at the present stage. Thus, in the near future we will continue to depend on animal models until noninvasive human *in vivo* diagnostic strategies have advanced and allow for imaging of trafficking of antigen-specific lymphocytes and high-resolution definition of the immune process present in a specific organ. A final remark must be made for the existence of a negative association between viral infections and autoimmune disease found in several experimental models (96). These observations are in support of epidemiologic findings that the incidence of many autoimmune disorders is decreased in equatorial countries, where the presence of certain infectious diseases is significantly increased. However, no firm associations have been established to date.

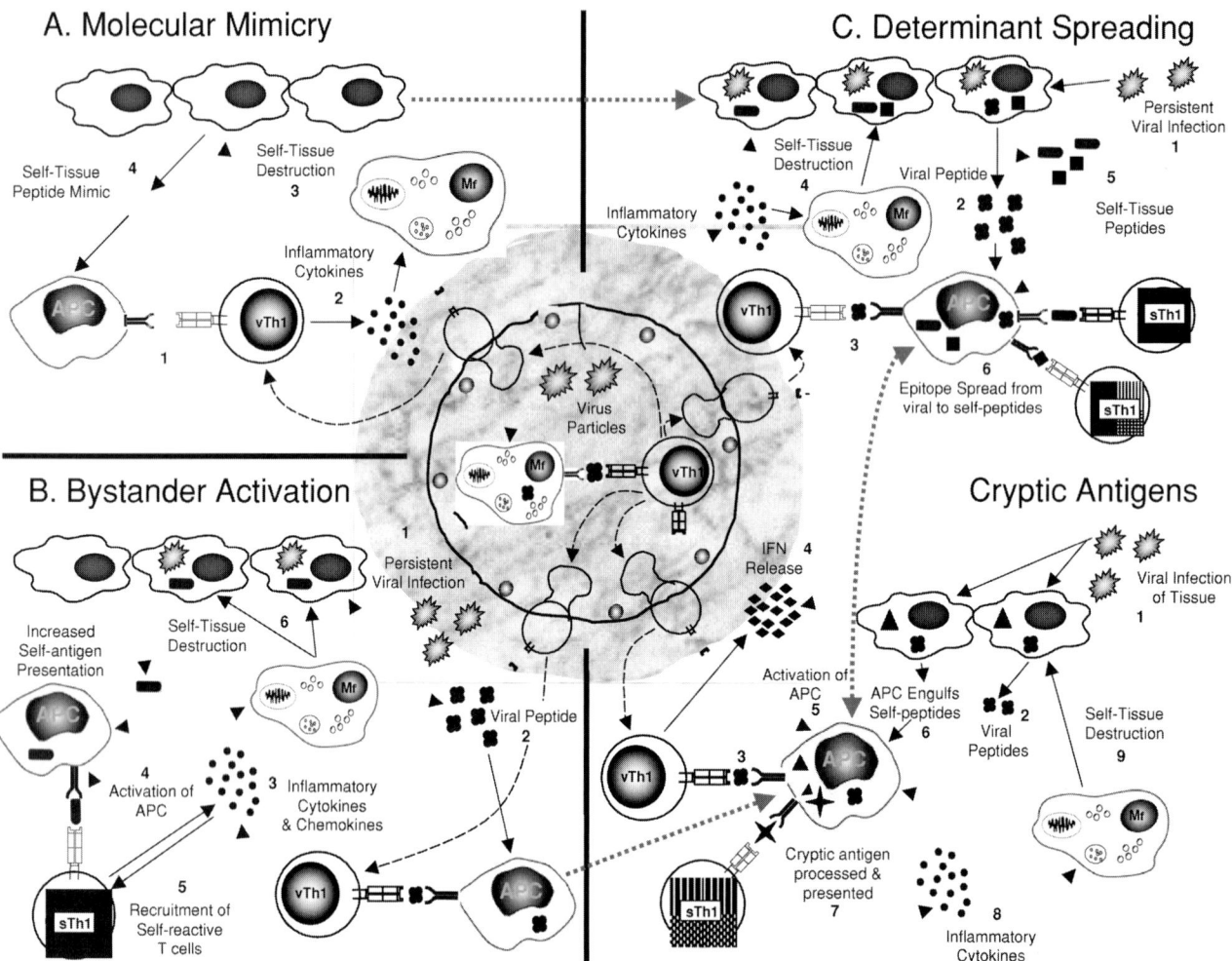

FIG. 3. Potential mechanisms of autoimmune disease induction. After a viral infection, activated virus–specific T helper (vTH1) cells migrate through a blood-tissue barrier to the infected organ. Molecular mimicry **(A)** describes the activation of cross-reactive TH1 cells that recognize both the viral epitope and the self-epitope (*1*). Activation of the cross-reactive T cells results in the release of cytokines and chemokines (*2*) that recruit and activate resident and peripheral monocyte/macrophage cells that can mediate self-tissue damage (*3*). The subsequent release of self-tissue antigens and their uptake by antigen-presenting cells (APCs) perpetuates the autoimmune disease (*4*). In the epitope spread model **(B),** persistent viral infection (*1*) results in the activation of virus-specific Th1 cells (*2, 3*), which mediate self-tissue damage (*4*) resulting in the release of self-peptides (*5*), which are engulfed by APCs and presented to self-reactive T-helper cells (sTH1) (*6*). Continual damage and release of self-peptides results in the spread of the self-reactive immune response to multiple self-epitopes (*6*). The bystander activation model **(C)** describes the nonspecific activation of self-reactive Th1 cells. Activation of virus-specific Th1 cells (*1, 2*) and the up-regulation of immune functions throughout the tissue (*3, 4*) results in the increased infiltration of T cells to the site of infection and the activation of self-reactive Th1 cells by T-cell receptor (TCR)–dependent and TCR-independent mechanisms (*5*). Self-reactive T cells activated in this manner can then mediate self-tissue damage and further perpetuate the autoimmune response (*6*). The cryptic antigen model describes the initiation of the autoimmune response by differential processing of self-peptides. After viral infection (*1*) interferons to (IFNs) are secreted both by activated virus-specific TH1 cells (*2, 3*) and virus-infected cells (*4*). This up-regulates the immune functions of APCs (*5*) and can lead to APC engulfing self-peptides (*6*) (*triangle*). Cytokine activation of APC can induce increased protease production and different processing of captured self-epitopes (*triangle*) resulting in "cryptic" epitopes (*star*). The presentation of these "cryptic" epitopes can activate self-reactive Th1 cells (*7*) and lead to self-tissue destruction (*8, 9*). Of course, the above-displayed mechanisms are not mutually exclusive and the *dotted arrows* indicate some of the mechanistic intersection points that are possible. Courtesy of Steve Miller and Ludovich Croxford, Northwestern University, Chicago, IL.

Other Environmental Causes

Similar to viral infections, other inflammatory stimuli may trigger or enhance autoimmunity. The gut deserves particular attention in this respect. At this site each individual harbors thousands of different bacterial strains and viral infections are common. Furthermore, the mucosal lining is permeable for nutrients and constitutes a very large interactive surface with the environment. Again, the complete absence of all bacteria results in severe immune dysfunction and possibly autoimmunity. However, it would be incorrect to conclude that infections are therefore always protective. Indeed, the commensal flora appears crucial in maintaining proper immune activation and function, but certain pathogens could definitely elicit strong gut immune responses that lead to autoimmune disease (97,98).

Regulatory Circuits in Autoimmune Processes

Cytokines

Cytokines and chemokines are essential regulators of cellular and humoral immune responses and lymphocyte trafficking (99–101). They play a central role in orchestrating autoimmune processes and constitute a multitude of positive, as well as negative feedback loops (102). Certain cytokines can negatively or positively influence the production of other cytokines (i.e., the T_H1/T_H2 paradigm) (66) and thus determine the balance between pro- and anti-inflammatory factors in the local environment. Furthermore, autocrine production feedback can augment or shut down production of a given cytokine by one cell. Cytokine networks operate with a fair amount of redundancy, and cytokines and chemokines share common receptors. They are the most likely mediators of "bystander activation" processes and also offer an effective and versatile therapeutic target *via* the temporally restricted use of cytokine- or chemokine-blocking antibodies. Their precise function can vary quite dramatically with respect to the autoimmune disease under investigation, and are discussed below. Further, their level and timing of expression during an ongoing disease process will determine whether they have a positive or negative effect (or any at all).

Apoptosis

It appears to be a general paradigm of great functional consequence that activation of the immune system is followed by a process that reverses the activation and reestablishes homeostatic baseline levels of immunity (49,51). In the absence of such regulatory mechanisms, immune responses will overshoot their goals and excessive immunopathology will occur. Thus, activation-induced cell death is believed to play an important role in regulating autoimmunity. Apoptotic lymphocytes, for example, are easily detected in islet infiltrates in type 1 diabetes (103) and targeted induction of limited apoptosis may even prevent onset of autoimmune disease

(104). While increased apoptosis of aggressive lymphocytes that exceeds the "supply" of newly activated cells may directly limit an ongoing autoimmune process, limited apoptosis of target tissues may indirectly facilitate induction of protective regulatory responses. On the other hand, while apoptosis of target cells should at best be limited, decreased apoptosis of autoreactive aggressive lymphocytes will propagate autoimmunity. It is important to consider precisely which cells undergo apoptosis in order to predict the possible outcome.

- If too many target cells die by apoptosis, organ destruction occurs more rapidly. However, at the same time, antigens released from apoptotic cells appear to propagate tolerance rather than immunity (90).
- If regulatory T cells die by apoptosis, autoimmunity will be enhanced (105).
- If aggressive lymphocytes die by apoptosis, this should in general ameliorate disease. However, since they have to first be activated, they might induce organ damage during their activation phase.

Thus, an ongoing autoimmune process can be viewed as a rather fine-tuned and fragile equilibrium of aggressive and regulatory components and the precise activation kinetics and survival times of all lymphocyte types implicated in the process will determine the outcome. We are, at present, unable to delineate the precise *in vivo* cellular kinetics and a more thorough understanding will require improved noninvasive diagnostic techniques.

Kinetics

One of the most important emerging areas for an improved understanding of the pathogenesis of autoimmunity is concerned with the kinetics of immune responses. The pathophysiologic or therapeutic effect of a given lymphocyte population depends not only on specificity, activation state, and effector functions, but is also a function of the timing, that is, the phase of an ongoing disease process in which it is present. Indeed, inflammatory cytokines such as IFNγ or TNF-α exhibit opposing effects in type 1 diabetes depending on the precise time point of generation (106). Early expression enhances islet destruction and disease development, whereas late expression ameliorates disease by inducing apoptosis of autoaggressive cells. These kinetic issues constitute a major obstacle for successful immune intervention because they preclude the use of specific blocking agents or administration of cytokines without precise knowledge of their kinetically differential role in the disease process. Figure 4 illustrates these kinetic considerations in relation to target cell destruction. A better understanding of the underlying "autoimmune kinetics" is essential, and treatments will likely have to be individualized, in particular for antigen-specific immune-based interventions.

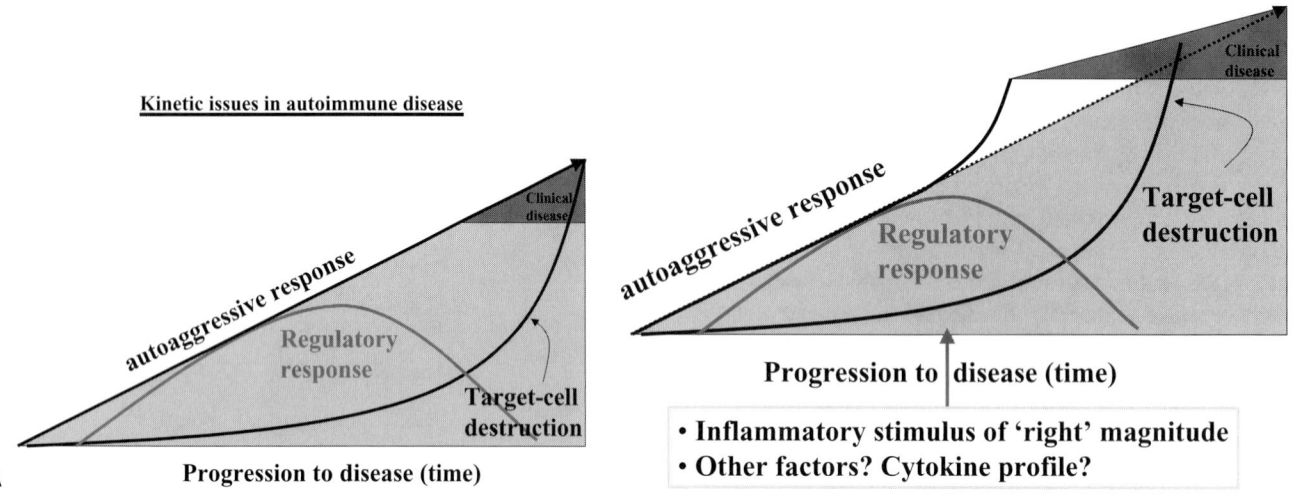

Kinetic issues in autoimmune disease

Inflammation can enhance autoimmunity

Increased regulation abrogates autoimmunity

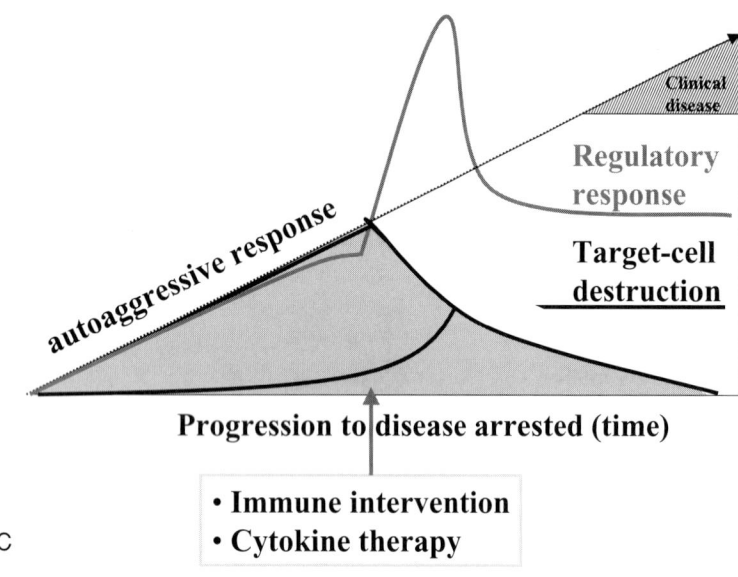

- Immune intervention
- Cytokine therapy

- Inflammatory stimulus of 'right' magnitude
- Other factors? Cytokine profile?

FIG. 4. A: Clinically manifested autoimmune disease is a result of a fine-tuned balance between autoreactive aggressive and regulatory responses. An important consideration is that usually target cell destruction will somewhat lag behind the aggressive response, thus allowing for counter-regulation to occur. **B:** Inflammatory stimuli of a certain magnitude are likely augmenting the aggressive response and will enhance disease progression. **C:** In contrast, enhancing the regulatory response will abrogate disease.

Therapeutic Considerations

Efficacy, Specificity, and Undesired Effects

Treatment of autoimmune disorders is not that different conceptually from cancer therapy. A fine balance must be found between efficacy of the intervention and acceptable undesired effects. The main goal of autoimmune disorder therapy is suppression of the pathologic autoimmune response. Therapeutic options range in principle from continuous immunosuppression of the entire immune system to specific, targeted, temporally limited, and local immunosuppression. Systemic immunomodulation or anti-inflammatory therapy will affect the entire immune system and may compromise the immune status of the individual. One of the more recent examples for effective systemic treatments is the blockade of TNF-α to ameliorate rheumatoid arthritis (RA) (107,108). While undesired effects are relatively low, systemic lupus

erythematosus(SLE)–like symptoms have been observed in a few patients, as has the enhanced susceptibility to tuberculosis. This is especially encouraging because blockade of TNF affects inflammatory pathways distinct from the targets of conventional anti-inflammatory therapy with corticosteroids or nonsteroidal anti-inflammatory drugs.

Autoantigen-specific immune interventions, in contrast, bear the promise of lower systemic side effects, since they can be targeted to antigens that are exclusively expressed in the diseased organ (109,110). However, the efficacy might be lower and suitable target antigens have to be chosen carefully, because enhancement of autoimmunity is an important concern. The goal is either deletion of aggressive autoreactive T cells or induction of regulatory cells (111). To achieve the latter, response modifiers are probably required at the time of immunization in order to skew the resulting immune response to exert regulatory effector functions. Deletion of

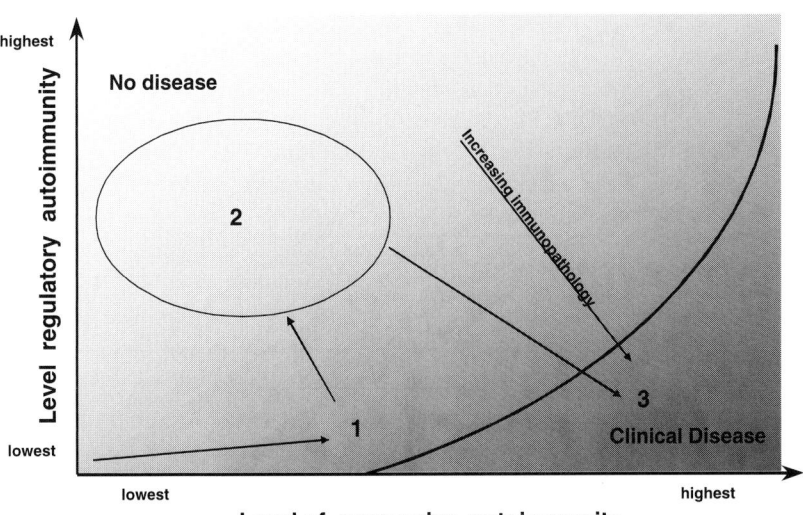

1 = Induction of disease (environmental trigger)

2 = Counter-regulation, epitope spreading (genetic factors)

3 = Progression to clinical disease (rapid or slow)

FIG. 5. Each inflammatory insult that might trigger autoimmunity (*1*) is met by a regulatory response (*2*) that attempts to reestablish homeo-static baseline levels. If this is not successful (or not therapeutically supported), the aggressive response will eventually win and disease will occur (*3*).

autoaggressive lymphocytes or anergy induction is even more risky, since only suboptimal immunization (i.e., in the absence of co-stimulators) will result in this outcome. To control this *in vivo* is rather difficult. Ultimately, antigen-specific therapy will likely have to be individualized due to MHC polymorphism and distinct T-cell repertoires among patients and should be combined with other systemically acting agents, such as antibodies against CD3 or CD4 or co-stimulation blockade.

Promising Targets

For anti-inflammatory interventions, the factor to be targeted should be as disease specific as possible. Therefore, blockade of TNF works well for RA but not for diabetes or MS (112). Experimental evidence supports this observation, because TNF is a crucial mediator found to be elevated in affected joints (108), but has clearly positive, as well as negative effector functions in murine models for MS and diabetes (113,114). Targeting ubiquitously present chemokines or cytokines will likely not bear much success, because of the resultant generalized immune modulation or suppression.

For antigen-specific interventions, antigens that are already targeted by regulatory autoreactivity are likely to constitute good targets to augment such a preexisting response (115). In contrast, these antigens should not be selected to delete autoreactive cells, which results in a loss of regulation. For anergy or apoptosis, induction antigens targeted by a primarily aggressive response will be better suited. The fact that autoantigenic and epitope spreading occurs during each ongoing autoreactive process makes such interventions difficult to design and individualization will likely be necessary.

Organ-Specific Issues: Reestablishment of Immune Regulation

One of the factors that pose a challenge to understanding the pathogenesis of distinct autoimmune diseases may also hold a clue to developing effective and specific treatment strategies. Each target cell, tissue, or organ exhibits specific features that distinguish it from other sites of the body. These site-specific features of autoimmunity will likely offer unique target sites for interventions with lower systemic side effects. However, one concern is that reestablishing proper immune homeostasis and regulation in one organ may still affect homeostasis systemically or at another site. Therefore, thorough preclinical evaluation and careful monitoring of undesired effects is urgently needed. Ideally, treatments have to be administered before complete organ destruction has occurred in patients identified by genetic or other screening to be at risk to develop full-blown clinical disease. During the preclinical state, frequently regulatory autoreactive responses are still strong and their augmentation can result in protection (Fig. 5). The goal to reestablish homeostasis and proper regulation after an initial insult that caused organ-specific inflammation appears to be a natural countermeasure to which the specific immune system may be successfully harnessed.

ORGAN-SPECIFIC AUTOIMMUNE DISORDERS

Type 1 Diabetes

Introduction

While the distinct symptoms of diabetes mellitus have been known since antiquity, the underlying pathophysiologic processes were only identified in the late 19th and early 20th centuries. The proof of the involvement of the pancreas in diabetes etiology was conducted by von Mering and Minkowski (1890), who demonstrated in 1890 that extirpation of the canine pancreas results in the classic symptomatology of hyperglycemia, abnormal hunger, increased thirst, polyuria, and glycosuria (116). Subsequently, inflammatory changes in the endocrine pancreas, that is, the islets of Langerhans, were correlated with diabetes by Schmidt in 1902 (117) and two decades later, Banting and Best (118) identified insulin as a pancreatic hormone, thereby providing the basis for insulin substitution therapy, which remains to this day the cornerstone for type 1 diabetes (T1D) management. In a classic 1965 paper, Gepts (119) noted the histopathologic similarity between thyroiditis and insulitis and suggested an immune basis for the disease. By 1974, the concept that T1D is an autoimmune syndrome was firmly established by the discovery of islet cell antibodies and an association between T1D and certain HLA genes (120–122).

Today, nearly 30 years later, the possible autoimmune origin of T1D is understood in much greater detail. However, the lymphocytic infiltration of the islets of Langerhans (Fig. 6) and the presence of antibodies specific for β cell antigens associated with the progressive destruction of insulin-producing β cells (123,124) still constitute the cardinal evidence for an autoimmune etiology. While there is a reasonably strong genetic linkage to certain HLA molecules, the disease has to be considered polygenic in nature (83) and a significant discordance of disease among monozygotic twins suggests that environmental factors contribute to trigger and/or exacerbate the disease. Furthermore, it remains unclear which islet antigens are the primary targets. The earliest islet-cell–specific antibodies in human individuals at risk are directed to insulin (125,126), and evidence from relevant animal models points toward insulin (127) or glutamic acid decarboxylase (GAD) (128), but definitive proof for a pathogenic role has not yet been obtained. The cellular

infiltrates found in the islets contain both CD4+ and CD8+ T-lymphocytes, and their irreducible role in β cell destruction has been documented in several animal models (129–131). CD8+ T cells can exert direct cytotoxic effects toward MHC class I–expressing β cells, while CD4+ T cells secrete inflammatory cytokines and can provide help to CD8+ T cells as well as B cells. Ultimately, it is important to consider that β cells constitute about 60% of the islets, which in turn contribute only ~2% to the pancreas mass and demonstrate, unlike many other tissues targeted in autoimmune disorders, an exquisite sensitivity to cytokines such as IL-1, TNF, and interferons that will result in their apoptotic cell death after prolonged exposure (55).

Despite intensive research, no effective prophylaxis, therapy, or cure of T1D is available to date. Even under optimal disease management with insulin-substitution therapy, T1D significantly shortens life expectancy due to eventual vascular complications in multiple organs. The most promising recent therapeutic advance was made by developing a specific protocol for gentle isolation and purification of human islets ("Edmonton protocol") that appear less prone to rejection after intraportal implantation into diabetic subjects (132). However, continued immune suppressive treatment is still necessary in recipients of such transplants to prevent renewed autoimmune destruction of islet transplants, which emphasizes the need for effective immune-based strategies of T1D prevention.

Immunology of T1D

Animal Models for T1D

Since the pancreas and its draining lymphoid organs are notoriously difficult to access, many important insights about diabetes immunology have been gained from suitable animal

Human Insulitis

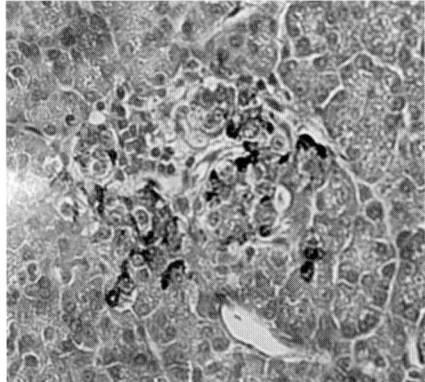

specific staining is for T-cells (CD45RO)

Mouse Insulitis

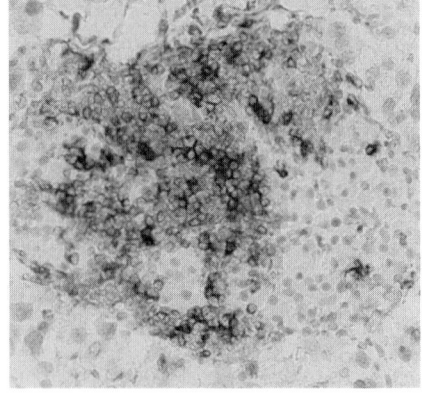

specific staining is for CD8 lymphocytes

FIG. 6. Comparison of human insulitis (*left*), courtesy of Francesco Dotta, University 'La Sapienzia', Rome, Italy, and mouse insulitis (*right*), RIP-LCMV mouse 14 days postviral infection with LCMV virus (trigger). Courtesy of La Jolla Institute for Allergy and Immunology, von Herrath Laboratory, San Diego, CA.

models that continue to refine our understanding of the pathogenesis and the development of potential prophylactic and therapeutic strategies. There are many animal models for T1D. The most commonly employed models take advantage of natural mutations that give rise to spontaneous diabetes onset or antigen-specific induction of disease using transgenic technology. Other models make use of β cell damage initiated by treatment with specific chemicals (e.g., streptozodozin) or virus infection. Encephalomyocarditis virus is diabetogeneic in mice and the incidence of disease is dependent on both virus and mouse strains used (91,133–140). Similarly, Coxsackie virus, associated with diabetes development in humans, causes extensive pancreatic tissue damage and release of sequestered autoantigens that lead to rapid diabetes development in some mouse strains (141).

Models of Spontaneous Diabetes Onset

There are several animal models of spontaneous T1D (142). The two most extensively used are the biobreeding (BB) rat, introduced in 1974 at the Bio Breeding Laboratories in Canada, and the nonobese diabetic mouse strain (NOD) established in 1974 in Osaka, Japan (142). Because the BB rat is associated with leucopenia and other abnormalities (142), the NOD mouse has been the model of choice due to its genetic linkages that are reminiscent of human T1D (142). In both models, adoptive transfer of T cells can induce disease (143). Interestingly, administration of viral infections, first shown with LCMV, can prevent insulin-dependent diabetes mellitus (IDDM) in both BB rats and NOD mice (144,145). This occurs in the absence of general immune suppression. While the mechanism involved is unclear, the generation of suppresser T cells has been suggested (145,146).

Models of Antigen-Specific Diabetes Induction

Expression of influenza virus hemagluttinin (HA) under control of the rat insulin promoter (RIP) resulted in a low incidence (10% to 20%) of spontaneous T1D, but no significant enhancement of disease occurred after infection of such RIP-HA mice with influenza virus. However, in RIP-HA mice expressing a transgenic T-cell receptor (TCR) specific for a determinant of the influenza virus HA, the incidence of spontaneous T1D increased to 100% (147). These studies clearly demonstrate the importance of autoreactive T cells present at sufficient numbers for induction of autoimmune disease. Thus, the inability of influenza strain PR8 to cause T1D in RIP-HA mice likely reflects the low precursor frequency of self-reactive CD8+ T cells. Interestingly, recent studies from the Sherman laboratory have demonstrated that spontaneous disease in this model is associated with cross-presentation of HA. It has been postulated that cross-presentation constitutes an important mechanism for unmasking of islet-specific antigens to autoaggressive CD8+ T cells. When the model antigen ovalbumin (OVA) was expressed as a self-antigen in β cells using the RIP, similar observations were made, underscoring the likely importance of cross-presentation in autoimmune

diabetes. These studies also demonstrated that the clinical outcome correlated with the number of autoreactive CD4+ and CD8+ cells generated and determined a "cut-off level" below which the autoimmune reaction would not take hold of the pancreas (148–150).

Similar to RIP-HA and RIP-OVA mice, the rat insulin promoter was also used to express the nucleoprotein (NP) or glycoprotein (GP) of LCMV in the insulin-producing beta cells (129,151,152). Diabetes develops 2 to 4 weeks after infection with LCMV due to a strong CD8+ or combined CD8+/CD4+ T-cell response directed to the viral/self GP or NP in the β cells. Insulitis is initiated only at a time when the systemic antiviral response reaches its peak and continues well after the LCMV infection has been eliminated (83,153). Therefore, the localized, islet-specific autoimmune process, although initiated by a response to the viral/self-transgene, can be regarded as an autoimmune process that follows kinetics distinctly different from systemic antiviral immunity. Indeed, antigenic spreading to insulin and GAD is observed during the prediabetic phase (154). Destruction of β cells requires activation of antigen-presenting cells (155) in the islets and is mediated by both perforin and inflammatory cytokines, predominantly IFN-γ (156). Thus, the RIP-LCMV model reproduces many features found in human diabetes as well as other mouse models. A distinct advantage of RIP-LCMV mice is that the time point for induction of the autoaggressive, LCMV NP–specific response can be chosen experimentally and that virus-specific, destructive CD4+ and CD8+ T cells can be enumerated, functionally evaluated, and localized using limiting dilution analyses, MHC tetramers, or intracellular cytokine stains (157,158). These aspects constituted an advantage in a recently published study, where we could demonstrate that feeding of insulin during the prediabetic period induces insulin B-chain–specific CD4+ regulatory lymphocytes that act as bystander suppressors and can locally down-regulate the autoaggressive diabetogeneic response in the pancreatic draining lymph node and the islets (158). Other studies in the RIP-LCMV model have underlined the role of thymic selection in allowing sufficient numbers of low-avidity autoaggressive T cells to emerge in the periphery (159), the role of non–MHC-linked genes in influencing the kinetics and severity of T1D even in the presence of high numbers of autoaggressive T cells (158), and the importance of antigen-presenting cells (APC) in breaking tolerance and sustaining autoaggressive T-cell responses (160–162).

Under some conditions, CD4+ or CD8+ T cells can induce T1D by adoptive immunization (143,163). In general, T1D develops slower or not at all in the absence of CD8+ CTL, MHC I, or perforin (55,164). Similar considerations are true for MHC class II and co-stimulatory molecules, unless their elimination affects the generation of regulatory lymphocytes (165,166). Cytokines, however, frequently play dual roles in T1D pathogenesis in animal models. IFN-γ, in general known as a proinflammatory mediator that up-regulates MHC molecules, can "unmask" β cells for immune-recognition by induction of MHC class I expression, but also exert direct antiviral effects and might be beneficial by increasing apoptosis of aggressive T-lymphocytes later in the disease (55). A similar dual role is true for TNF-α, which appears to enhance early disease (possibly by directly causing β cell death in conjunction with other cytokines) but ameliorates advanced autoimmunity just prior to onset of clinical disease (106,167). For these reasons, blockade of such inflammatory mediators might be problematic in T1D. Dual roles were also described for INF-α (168–170), IL-2 (171), and IL-10 (172,173). In some of these studies, the level of the cytokine might play as important a role as the precise timing of expression. The only cytokine with largely beneficial effects has been IL-4, which ameliorates the disease and therefore might be a good candidate for treating or preventing T1D (174). In general, those chemokines attract lymphocytes to the islets and activate macrophages that worsen the course of autoimmune diabetes. Figure 7 illustrates the pathogenetic hypotheses generated through research in multiple animal models.

Human Immunology of T1D

The detection of islet antigen–specific antibodies remains an essential tool in identifying prediabetic subjects and monitoring the progression of subclinical and clinical disease. Procedures for autoantibody determination have been substantially refined and standardized worldwide. Emerging data from clinical studies support the notion that with progression of the prediabetic phase generation of islet antibodies also is increased (154,175,176). Usually, antibodies to insulin become discernible first, followed by GAD, and then insulinoma antigen 2 (IA2). Individuals with islet antibodies to three or more distinct antigens have a greater than 90% risk of developing T1D. Thus, islet antibodies are an excellent marker for disease risk. However, they appear not to play a role pathogenetically, since transfer of antibodies from mothers to children does not increase the risk for T1D and B cells are not needed for human diabetes (177–179). In this crucial respect the NOD mouse appears to provide a paradigm that might not be applicable to human diabetes, since maternal antibodies are an essential factor for diabetes development in NOD offspring (180).

Human T-cell responses to islet antigens are not yet standardized and can vary considerably among laboratories. One reason for this may be the source of T cells that are generally subjected to specificity analyses: blood-borne CD4+ or CD8+ T cells may not reflect the specificity distribution and frequencies of islet-specific T cells found in the target organ, that is, the pancreas and its draining lymph nodes. Even the study of spleen-derived islet-specific T cells readily obtained

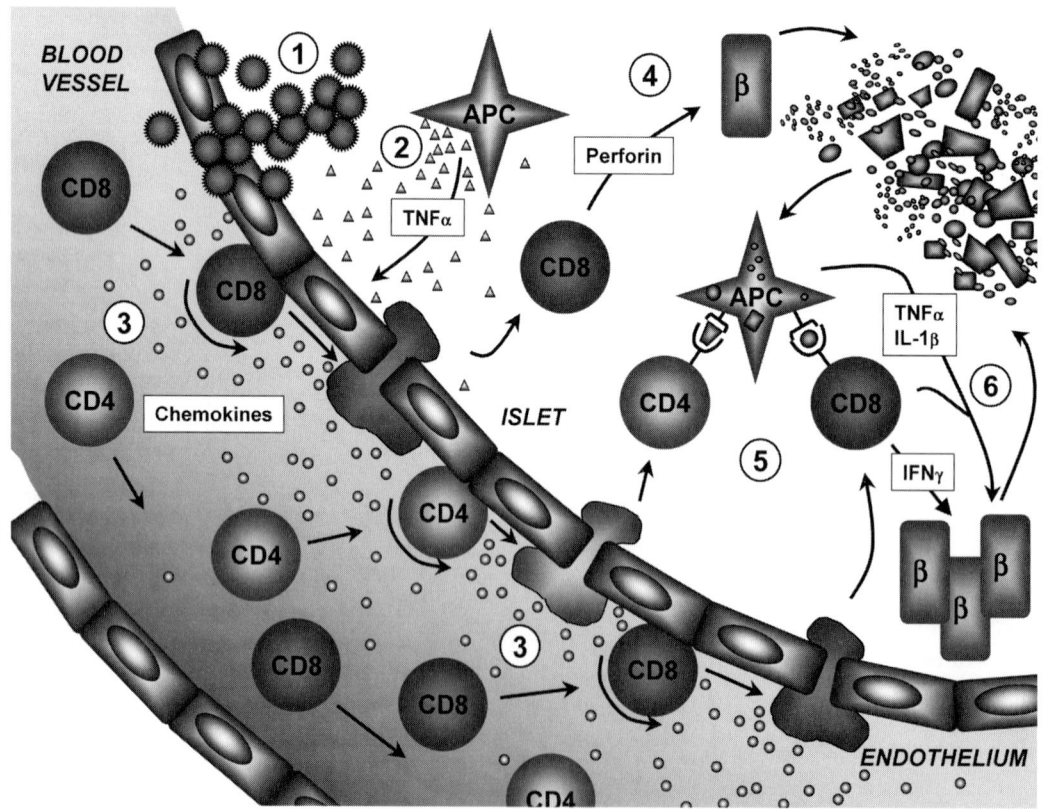

FIG. 7. Immunopathogenesis of T1D. Viral infections or other inflammatory stimuli (1) will activate APCs (2) that secrete mediators that attract lymphocytes to "rolling" and entry into the pancreatic tissue (3). Some beta cells might be directly destroyed via cytotoxicity (4) and others by cytokines secreted from lymphocytes (5) or activated APCs (6). Courtesy of Urs Christen, La Jolla Institute for Allergy and Immunology, San Diego, CA.

from NOD mice and analyzed in standardized proliferation assays has shown variations between different NOD colonies (181). Therefore, measurement of multiple effector functions (e.g., cytokine production) in highly standardized assays will likely be required to assess T-cell autoreactivity on a routine basis. Even under those circumstances, T-cell responses among individuals are expected to vary and depend on the HLA haplotype and individual trigger(s) that precipitate T1D.

Etiology

Genes

Since the discordance of T1D is significant in monozygotic twins (concordance rate approximately 35%), environmental factors have to act in concert with diabetes susceptibility genes to orchestrate the autoimmune destruction of β cells. The initial hope that only a few genes would contribute to disease pathogenesis and that genetic links would help to directly understand the mechanistic aspects of T1D pathogenesis has been progressively eroded. Instead, a complex network of susceptibility and resistance genes in both humans and animals (e.g., the NOD mouse) has slowly taken shape. Human T1D-associated loci (IDDM1-15) comprise MHC class II genes (IDDM1); insulin (IDDM2); IGF1 (IDDM3); immune-related proteins (IDDM4, ICAM, and CD3; IDDM7, HOXD8, and IDDM12, CTLA4); and other candidate genes that do not have an apparent link to immune functions and/or β cells. Additionally, certain maintenance, developmental, or growth factors may be involved (85). Many of these genes exhibit direct parallels to NOD diabetes susceptibility genes (182).

The association between particular HLA/MHC class II haplotypes and the occurrence of human diabetes has been of particular interest. DRB1/04-DQA1/0301/B1 and DRB1/03-DQA1/0501/0201 strongly predispose to T1D and more than 80% of patients carry either one or both alleles (183). In contrast, other MHC class II haplotypes can protect from disease, as evidenced by the six-fold reduced risk to T1D in DRB1/15-DQA1/B1/0602–bearing individuals.

An intriguing mechanistic hypothesis was put forth by McDevitt's observation that predisposing HLA class II alleles appear to express small neutral amino acids at position 57 of the DQ allele of Caucasoid populations, whereas an aspartic acid is found in resistant alleles at the same position (183a). Since position 57 is part of the peptide-anchoring pocket, amino acid substitutions in this area will affect peptide binding. Indeed, the susceptibility alleles prefer different peptides, but the contribution to T1D development is not yet clear and a mechanistic link has to be established. Both central and peripheral tolerance mechanisms have been implicated but no direct proof has been obtained. It is important to realize that the human-susceptibility MHC class II alleles share amino acids at position 57 with the I-A^{g7} alleles expressed in the NOD mouse and are required for NOD T1D predisposition. However, as previously mentioned, polymorphisms in the MHC class II coding region alone cannot explain diabetes pathogenesis. The amount of complexity involved in the immunogenetics of T1D has been well described by Serreze (184,185): "Many genes contributing to T1D may contribute to dysregulation of different biochemical steps in a common developmental or metabolic pathway. For example, sequential expression of hundreds, if not thousands, of genes would be expected in the developmental and functional maturation of a macrophage or dendritic cell from stem cell precursors. This process does not occur in a vacuum, but is contingent on cues provided by the physical environment. In the case for APC development, the microfloral and dietary environments are crucial." Thus, diabetes susceptibility and resistance genes contribute to disease in a polygenetic/multifactorial fashion that appears to gain in complexity as it is being unraveled. The link to environmental factors will be defined to shape gene expression and disease development. Major contributors in this respect appear to be the gut and viral infections.

Environment

With more than 400m^2 of mucosal epithelium, the gut constitutes the largest interactive surface area of the human body that connects us with the environment and its pathogens (97). Therefore, exposure to antigens or pathogens through the gut, mediated by the largest outpost of the immune system, the gut-associated lymphoid tissue (GALT), will strongly affect specific and general immune functions. It is intriguing that immune tolerance to the numerous foreign protein antigens found in food, as well as bacterial antigens derived from the commensal flora, is generally well maintained (186). This may be attributable to the high levels of IgA and TGF-β in the gut and to the phenomenon of "oral tolerance" (OT) (187). OT has been observed in animal models and humans and is characterized by tolerance induction to protein antigens present in the gut. It occurs via two principal mechanisms. Low amounts of antigens will induce a nonaggressive immune-regulatory response, while high amounts of antigen can lead to lymphocyte anergy or deletion (188–190) that is likely achieved via APC modulation. In addition, the profound immune dysregulation found in the absence of a bacterial flora in both animals and humans points to an important physiologic role that foreign antigens play in immune homeostasis in the gut (191). Furthermore, NOD mice only exhibit high levels of autoimmunity when kept in a clean, specific pathogen-free environment, and do not develop T1D when housed under "dirty" conditions (192). It currently remains unclear whether a baseline level of immune stimulation is needed for proper development and "tuning" of the immune system and which types and numbers of gut-derived or gut-induced regulatory cells are involved in the maintenance of immune tolerance, but CD4$^+$ T$_H$2–like regulators as well as $\gamma\delta$ intraepithelial lymphocytes (30% in mice, 15% in humans) (193) have been associated through various lines of evidence with active mucosal tolerance. Thus, changes in mucosal functions, infections of the gut, or certain dietary components may play a role in T1D pathogenesis.

Several reports and studies have attempted to establish a link between the introduction of cow's milk and development of T1D in young infants. This link was not observed in the German, Australian, and U.S. baby diabetes studies, but in a Finish epidemiologic study (194,195). The Finish study differed from most of the others by an extended observation time involving infant as well as childhood consumption of cow's milk. Therefore, a dietary link between milk feeding and T1D can be considered unlikely but not excluded after long-term exposure to cow albumin or other milk proteins. Similarly, wheat-derived gluten and milk-derived insulin have been implicated as a cause for childhood diabetes. The evidence, however, is not convincing at this point and no firm links have been established. Some intriguing observations have been published more recently supporting the concept of a viral etiology for T1D. The mechanistic links between viral infections and autoimmunity can be manifold and have been discussed in detail in the introductory section of this chapter. A significant association between rotavirus infection in young infants and the first occurrence of islet autoantibodies was established by Harrison's group in Australia (196). Rotavirus is a double-stranded RNA virus, infects the intestinal mucosa and is a common cause for seasonal childhood diarrhea. It can polyclonally activate T- and B-lymphocytes and might possibly harbor antigens that could immunologically mimic islet cell–derived self-proteins. However, it is not clear whether it infects the pancreas or islets directly. Another case can be made for enteroviruses. Coxsackie B4 virus has been isolated from islets of a child with acute-onset T1D (137,140,197), and Coxsackie B3 and 4 strains commonly infect the gut, pancreas, and heart (198). They lead to profound pancreatitis if they replicate at high enough titers and might harbor a mimicry antigen (P2C protein) (124) cross-reactive on the T-cell level with a human GAD epitope. However, this evidence could not be replicated by other laboratories and is still controversial. Similar to Coxsackie, other enteroviruses such as polio or echoviruses have been detected in the pancreas and might therefore at least have enhancing effects on ongoing islet destruction in prediabetic individuals at risk (197). The establishment of a firm association between viral infections and T1D is difficult, because the underlying mechanistic links established in several animal models allow for the virus to be cleared before autoimmunity develops (i.e., in the RIP-LCMV) and need not necessarily directly induce islet-reactive T-cell responses.

Therapeutic Concepts

Currently, there is no effective prevention for T1D and all strategies that look promising have either been evaluated in animal models or are in early clinical trials in humans. Part of the problem in devising such prophylactic or interventive immune-based approaches is that that the only endpoints in human trials are disease prevention and insulin require-

ments, as well as remaining insulin production (C peptide levels). No precise interim staging is possible, which makes efficient clinical evaluation very difficult compared to MS or RA, where access to the target organ either visually by MRI or directly by sampling fluids is much easier to achieve. Animal models have provided interesting ideas and evidence for a variety of antigen-specific and systemic interventions that bear promise for human diabetes.

Antigen-Specific Immunoregulation

Immunization with DNA plasmids that express islet self-antigens, with or without cytokines, that act as response modifiers can induce autoreactive regulatory CD4+ T cells. These cells are able to suppress autoaggressive CD4 and CD8 cells locally in the pancreatic draining lymph node, where they act as bystander suppressors. Phenotypically, they behave very similar to the T_H2-like regulators (115,199–202) induced after oral antigen administration. In treated mice (using several distinct diabetes models), insulitis is permanently reduced and progression to clinical diabetes can be prevented in 50% to 80% of the animals (110,115,199,200). To bring this approach to the clinic as a preventive therapy, a suitable marker will be needed that can predict early outcome—for example, levels and isotypes of autoantibodies. Like other antigen-specific interventions, this strategy will not likely be effective in late stages of the prediabetic phase and should therefore be thought of and tested as an early preventive therapy. The important advantage of this and other antigen-specific approaches is that the risk for systemic side effects is low, since the effector cells will act antigen specifically only in the area where autoimmune destruction is ongoing and their cognate antigen (e.g., GAD, insulin, or heat-shock protein) is presented. Cytokine response modifiers will be needed to avoid deleterious augmentation of aggressive responses.

Altered Peptide Ligands

Modified insulin peptides that favor a T_H2-like deviation of responder cells have been developed by Neurocrine (San Diego, CA) and showed great promise in the NOD mouse model. These are now being tested in preclinical safety studies and will soon go into clinical trials (203–205).

Anergy-Inducing Compounds

This strategy is based on the observation that immunization with antigen in the absence of proper ("professional") co-stimulation by B7 molecules will lead to incomplete T-cell activation and may result in anergy. *In vitro* and animal studies show much promise in that antigen-specific cells can be selectively deleted.

Modulatory Dendritic Cells

A few recent studies have shown that dendritic cells can be modulated in such a way that they can induce tolerance in an antigen-specific fashion. This is an emerging area and not much is yet understood as to how these modulations occur and what the precise *in vivo* effector mechanisms are (183).

Therapeutic Concepts under Clinical Evaluation

Anti-CD3. One of the more recent promising ongoing trials evaluates systemic administration of noncomplement-binding anti-CD3/Fab′$_2$ (206) in human diabetes and recipients of transplants. The effector mechanism is systemic and is likely relying on the induction of antigen-nonspecific regulators (165) that are CD62L^{hi} and CD25^{hi}, as well as anergy or deletion of activated aggressive lymphocytes. From data in animal models and initial data in humans, systemic immune suppression is not too profound, indicating good feasibility for this strategy. The recent completion of a randomized controlled trial confirms the effectiveness of this approach for treatment of individuals recently diagnosed with T1D (207).

Oral Tolerance. As for MS and RA, oral antigen trials have failed so far for T1D. The reasons for these failures after initially very promising animal data have become increasingly clear from follow-up animal experimentation. Likely, the dose of antigen was significantly too low (presumably by a factor of 100). This problem may be overcome by coupling the orally administered proteins to gut-response modifiers such as the cholera toxin B subunit. Second, the choice of antigen is very important and even minor amino acid changes can modify the dose–response curves. Without a reliable preclinical marker, it will be very difficult to tune this treatment to the human situation (191).

Heat-Shock Proteins. The first very promising diabetes prevention trial has recently been published and indicates a very good reduction of insulin requirements in patients that were treated with a heat-shock protein peptide derived from an islet heat-shock protein putative autoantigen. The precise mechanism still needs to be evaluated and long-term beneficial effects are still uncertain (208).

Immunization with Insulin B Peptides and Incomplete Freund's Adjuvant. This intervention, again evaluated and developed in the NOD mouse, were scheduled to enter into clinical phase 1 trials in 2003. The mechanism might involve immune deviation; however, the use of adjuvant might preclude long-term administrations due to local side effects at the immunization site.

Conclusions and Future Directions

One has to keep in mind that no known animal model will accurately reflect human diabetes, the individual treatment parameters might need to be adjusted, and some "mouse-interventions" will not work at all in humans, as is evident from failures in recent clinical trials. For example, to date we have more that 140 ways to prevent T1D in the NOD mouse (123), but not a single one that is as effective in humans. To improve this situation there is a dire need for preclinical

markers that accurately predict the potential success of an intervention being evaluated by a clinical trial. Better tracking reagents for blood autoreactive T cells such as tetramers, noninvasive high-resolution *in vivo* imaging systems, and perhaps isotype profiles of islet antigen autoantibodies and changes in them after a given preclinical intervention are good candidates (209). Similar considerations apply to the maintenance of long-term tolerance after islet transplantation, where prolonged systemic immunosuppression might not be feasible (210–213).

Multiple Sclerosis

Introduction

MS is the most predominant human demyelinating disease of the CNS. An autoimmune etiology is suggested by elevated frequencies of myelin basic protein (MBP)–specific T cells documented in several independent studies of individuals diagnosed with MS (214–217). Further, demonstrations that adoptive transfer of T cells specific for myelin or other CNS antigens can cause a CNS autoimmune syndrome in experimental animals resembling human MS support the concept of a direct T-cell–mediated pathogenesis. In addition, myelin-specific antibodies have been found in MS cerebrospinal fluid (218). These antibodies are able to complement-fix and induce antibody-dependent cellular cytotoxicity and may be involved in the demyelinating process. In spite of these clues, the etiology of MS remains unclear and a complex interplay of genetic and environmental factors (similar to T1D etiology) has to be postulated.

MS is a rather heterogeneous disease. However, we are only beginning to understand how clinical and pathologic differences may point toward distinct etiologies and, potentially, treatment strategies of differential applicability and efficacy. Different subtypes of MS are somewhat better histologically defined (e.g., the distinction between T-cell–rich and macrophage-rich lesions as well as the balance between demyelination and remyelination, which can vary dramatically) than those of T1 since many tissues from patients with clinically active disease are available *post mortem,* whereas pancreatic islets are mostly destroyed in type 1 diabetics and no immunologic correlates can be established at the end stage (219,220). MS predominantly affects younger women and its frequency, dependent on geographic location, may approach up to 3/1,000 (221). Clinically, the disease can take a mild or very debilitating course and, intriguingly, neuritis of the optical nerve is frequently the first sign for a beginning MS. Diagnosis is usually obtained by EEG and direct imaging that allows for identification of individual lesions, their development over time, and the success of therapeutic interventions. Immune-based approaches such as the use of interferon-β or Copaxone® combined with systemic immunomodulatory agents has brought some limited success for certain forms of MS. Thus, a cure for MS appears possibly a little closer than for T1D.

Immunology of MS

Animal Models for MS

Experimental allergic encephalitis (EAE) is one of the oldest and most widely studied animal models for a human autoimmune disease (70,222,223). EAE, a primarily CD4$^+$ T-cell–mediated disease, can be induced in susceptible mouse strains (SJL, PL/J) by immunization with MBP, PLP, MOG, or respective MHC class II–restricted epitopes together with complete Freund's adjuvant and pertussis toxin. More recently, a role for CD8$^+$ T cells has also been documented. The clinical picture resembles that of a relapsing/remitting disease with profound neurologic symptoms. CNS histologic findings include T-cell infiltration (mainly CD4$^+$ T-lymphocytes) (Fig. 8), APC, and microglia activation, as well as disruption of the blood–brain barrier. Some demyelination occurs and histologic changes can undergo periods of remission that are accompanied by remyelination. The predominant cytokine profile is T$_H$1-like, and T$_H$2 cytokines have a protective function (224). Epitope spreading occurs and activated APC takes a central role as "drivers" of the autoimmune process (225). A shortcoming of this model is the major extent of external manipulation required to break tolerance (adjuvant, pertussis). These might be necessary to affect the blood–brain barrier, skew the systemic cytokine profile to T$_H$1 phenotype, and support prolonged inflammation.

A lesser degree of additional nonspecific inflammatory conditions is required for some virus-induced animal models for MS. Infection with Theiler's murine encephalitis virus (TMEV), which replicates predominantly in neurons (particularly motor neurons during initial stages of infection), results in a poliomyelitis-like syndrome including flaccid paralysis. Certain strains of mice that survive the primary infection become persistently infected and develop a chronic progressive inflammatory demyelinating disease (225). Demyelination is the consequence of the CD4$^+$ T-cell response to persisting TMEV and involves determinant spreading as a consequence of infection and local inflammatory processes (225).

Studies from S. Miller's laboratory (226) have recently shown that APCs in the CNS are crucial for diversification/epitope-spreading of the initiating anti-TMEV response to other brain self-antigens such as MBP and PLP. Furthermore, when recombinant TMEV expressing PLP epitopes or modified mimic epitopes were employed, infection resulted in enhanced disease. These experiments provided *in vivo* evidence for a possible role of molecular mimicry in CNS autoimmune disease.

Somewhat similar to TMEV, infection with neurotropic strains of mouse hepatitis virus (MHV) induces neurologic disease accompanied by demyelination (227). An interesting difference is that MHV will not persist, and therefore allows for easier differentiation between the antiviral and the autoimmune response. CD4$^+$ as well as CD8$^+$ lymphocytes accompanied by inflammatory cytokines are needed for destruction. These virus-induced models of demyelination suggest that a transient or persisting presence of virus in the CNS may be needed in conjunction with a nontolerized antiviral response for disease induction and/or propagation (227). Indeed, another animal model of virally induced CNS disease, the transgenic MBP-LCMV model developed in analogy to the RIP-LCMV model for T1D only exhibits mild motor dysfunction despite good lymphocytic infiltration (228). It is possible that activation of APCs is insufficient in this model to locally propagate systemically induced autoaggressive lymphocytes once they have entered the parenchyma of the CNS. These considerations are depicted in Fig. 9.

Human Immunology of MS

Although myelin basic protein (MBP)–specific and proteolipoprotein (PLP)–specific T cells have been documented in patients with MS, some follow-up studies have reported similar frequencies in normal individuals (229). More recent studies have found increased numbers of MBP-specific T cells in MS patients reactive to six different MBP epitopes, supporting the concept of determinant spreading as a

Induction of EAE in SJL (H-2^s) mice by with PLP peptide aa 139-151

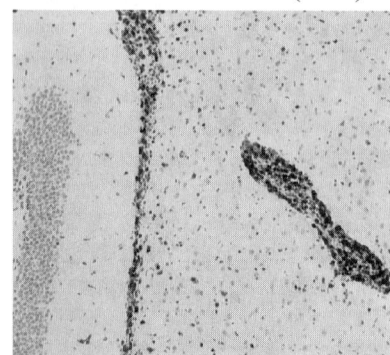 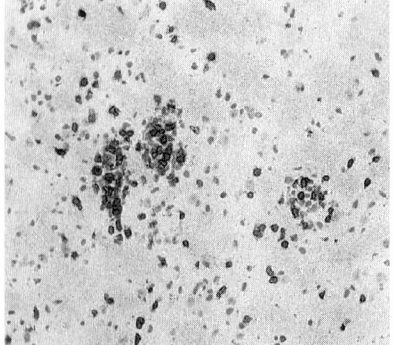

CD4 infiltrate, hippocampus   CD4 infiltrate, brain stem

FIG. 8. Induction of EAE in SJL mice with PLP peptide 139-151 and adjuvant. Courtesy of Andreas Holz, Max Plauclx Institute for Neurobiology, Munich, Germany.

Induction of profound autoimmune disease of the islets but only mild auto-immune infiltration in the CNS in RIP versus MBP-LCMV transgenic mice

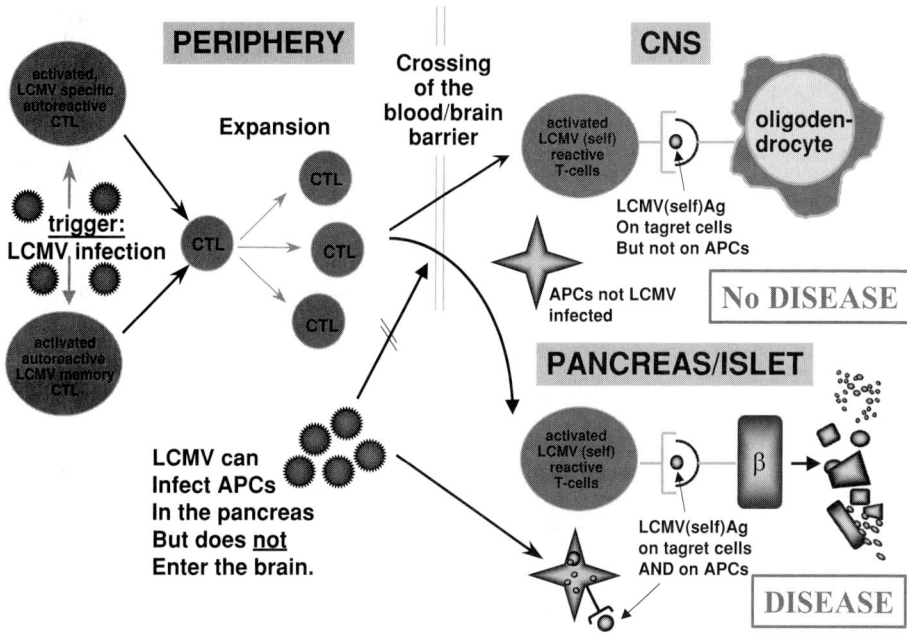

FIG. 9. APCs might be a crucial local driver to propagate an autoimmune process once initiated. This paradigm is illustrated when comparing the LCMV transgenic brain and islet models. Acute LCMV infection that functions as the trigger for self-transgene–directed organ-specific autoimmunity will only infect the pancreas but not the brain. As a consequence, clinical disease evolves in the islets (diabetes), but CNS clinical disease is extremely mild although autoaggressive lymphocytes can enter the brain parenchyma.

potential pathogenetic factor. Furthermore, their activation appears to be increased selectively in MS patients. Thus, it appears plausible that resting T cells specific for CNS antigens are present in both, healthy and affected individuals, but their activation is selectively increased under conditions of disease (memory/experienced phenotype) and their epitope/antigen recognition repertoire is different and appears to be expanded. In addition to cellular infiltrations, MS is usually marked by edema and inflammatory signs such as MHC up-regulation and cytokine and chemokine induction. A breakdown of the blood–brain barrier facilitates antibody access to the CNS. Antibodies specific for myelin structures are commonly found in MS patients and some studies indicate fluctuations, similar to T-cell responses of antibody titers in parallel to exacerbations and remissions of disease. These findings still await confirmation in larger patient cohorts. It is important to note that such antibodies can be directed to MBP, myelin oligodendrocyte associated protein (MOG) and other myelin constituents (230). The fact that they can fix complement and enhance complement-mediated cytotoxicity implicates them as possible agents of demyelination.

Etiology

There is a definite genetic link between progressive (HLA-DR3) as well as remitting/relapsing MS (DR2) and human

MHC class II alleles. However, similar to T1D, there is a significant discordance among monozygotic twins (>55%). A pronounced geographic gradient (higher incidence in northern as compared to southern regions) argues for additional environmental triggers or modulators (221). Many viruses have been implicated in the pathogenesis of MS, but a causal link has not been established. For example, human herpes virus 6 was discovered around MS lesions, but follow-up studies did not discover any differences comparing healthy, Alzheimer's, or Parkinson's tissues with MS lesions (231). Furthermore, antibodies to corona virus have been detected in serum of MS patients, which indicates that demyelination might occur similar to the mouse hepatitis virus model. Mechanistically, the same paradigms as for diabetes might apply (described in the introductory section), but a persistent viral infection might be more likely the culprit, based on similar observations in some mouse models (e.g., see the TMEV model). The difficulty in establishing conclusive proof is the multiplicity of infections during the course of a lifetime and the manifold viral traces that can usually be detected in healthy, as well as diseased individuals. Even if the same levels of viral antigen, RNA, or DNA are found comparing healthy patients with MS patients, this still does not rule out the possibility that a certain virus will only induce CNS disease in conjunction with a distinct MHC haplotype. Indeed, animal models indicate that this is in fact the case. With the advent of improved vaccination and antiviral treatment protocols for multiple infectious agents, we may be able to infer a causal relationship if the incidence of MS should recede after introduction of such an intervention.

Therapeutic Concepts

In Animal Models or under Clinical Evaluation

Similar to observations in the diabetes models (201), DNA vaccines that aim to skew the autoreactive response to MBP or PLP from a TH1 to a Th2 phenotype have shown some success in the EAE model. However, it remains to be seen, whether these findings can be directly translated to humans. At least for MS there are preclinical markers that can noninvasively and continuously track the size and appearance of current lesions and in this way indicate success or failure of a given therapy in a more immediate way as compared to T1D (232,233). Oral tolerance induction had shown much promise in EAE models, but recently failed in a human trial (234). Strong placebo effects were observed after feeding irrelevant protein versus MBP and the outcome was therefore not conclusive, leaving a smaller read-out window. Blockade of TNF-α has shown promise in animal models but not humans (112). The antidepressive agent Rolipram® is currently under clinical evaluation, after it exhibited anti-TNF effects in animal models for MS.

Current Treatment Strategies

Treatment of MS is, from the immunologic point of view, further advanced than treatment of T1D. It should be noted that life expectancy in MS is more reduced because no therapy comparable to insulin substitution is possible. Of the current regimens, interferon-β has shown very promising results in phase 3 clinical trials (235). Interestingly, interferon-γ, in contrast, has aggravated MS (236). Furthermore, Copaxone® has shown promise for certain forms of early MS in that it might act as a mixture of altered peptide ligands (as a polymer MBP analog) and in this way may skew immune responses systemically to a less aggressive phenotype (237). Lastly, phosphodiesterase inhibitors might induce TH2 skewing, as recently demonstrated in a small-scale trial (238). Finally, generalized immunosuppressive therapy with corticosteroids that are given in conjunction with relapses, and thereafter slowly phased out, still remain an important backbone for MS treatment. Not effective are azathioprine, cyclophosphamide, or plasmapheresis. Cyclosporine A is helpful but has profound side effects. Altered peptide ligands (APL) to human MBP epitopes have shown strong allergic side effects and have worsened disease in one study, indicating that APLs might activate *in vivo* aggressive, as well as regulatory lymphocytes, and that the success can therefore vary from individual to individual (239,240).

Conclusions and Future Directions

Therapeutic interventions in MS are becoming more effective, but will likely have to be individualized and fine-tuned with respect to the subtype of MS in a given patient. Antigen-specific therapy is in development but better understanding of the role of T cells in MS will be needed to translate experimental findings into clinical applications.

Autoimmune Liver Diseases

Introduction

Autoimmune liver diseases comprise a variety of immune system–mediated disorders, including autoimmune hepatitis (AIH), primary biliary cirrhosis (PBC), and primary sclerosing cholangitis (PSC) (241–243). Their respective syndromes partially overlap and a definite diagnosis is sometimes difficult to achieve. An important distinction needs to be made between AIH, which frequently evolves after chronic active hepatitis, and PBC, which constitutes the end stage of chronic destructive cholangitis. The primary targets in AIH are hepatocytes, whereas the autoimmune process in PBC is directed toward epithelial structures in the small intrahepatic cholangic ducts. Sometimes a mixed form of hepatic autoimmunopathy occurs that exhibits features of both disorders. In our discussion of autoimmune liver diseases, we have included "halothane hepatitis" as a paradigm for an immune-mediated adverse drug reaction (244).

Autoimmune Hepatitis

Autoimmunity had been invoked as a cause for hepatitis in the early 1950s (245–247), and based on the association of autoimmune hepatitis and antinuclear antibodies (ANA) the term "lupoid hepatitis" was proposed (248). Today, AIH contributes an estimated 10% to 20% to all cases of chronic hepatitis (which for the most part are due to infections with hepatitis viruses B, C, and D). While both liver damage and chronic course of viral hepatitis are due to immune functions, the etiology of autoimmune hepatitis (AIH) remains unclear (249) and an otherwise unspecified breakdown of tolerance to autologous liver tissue has to be assumed. A diagnostic scoring system has been defined by the International Autoimmune Hepatitis Group (33,250) and requires the inclusion (e.g., ANA), as well as exclusion (e.g., viral antigens) of certain criteria. Although AIH is not a uniform syndrome, and at least three subtypes have been classified, the following features are frequently shared by all AIH forms. Autoantibodies to certain hepatocytes antigens (especially mitochondrial) are present, as well as genetic linkage to HLAB8 and DR3, histologic "piecemeal" appearance, a higher prevalence among women, and frequent association with other autoimmune conditions. The etiology is unclear and additional environmental factors likely add to the genetic predisposition. It is possible that as of today unidentified hepatitis viruses or other chronic viral infections contribute to some AIH cases (241,251).

Immunology in Animal Models

To date only a handful of animal models for autoimmune hepatitis have been described.

1. In the HBsAg-transgenic mouse model, the hepatitis B–virus surface antigen (HBsAg) was expressed in hepatocytes under control of the mouse albumin promoter. Induction of transient hepatitis was possible after adoptive transfer of activated T cells from HBsAg-primed donor mice (252,253). This model has been extraordinarily helpful in understanding the role of interferons in inducing liver damage, as well as clearing HBV from the liver. Results have shown that interferons, in the absence of cytotoxicity, can purge virus from infected hepatocytes. Furthermore, induction of HBV-specific CD4$^+$ and CD8$^+$ T-cell responses can be evaluated in this model. The transgenic mice exhibit profound liver damage and infiltration after transfer of HBV-specific T-lymphocytes.

2. In another model system, the MHC class I molecule H-2K^b was transgenically expressed in the liver of mice that were additionally generating T-cells with a transgenic TcR specific for H-2K^b. Hepatitis induction was only successful when such mice were infected with a liver-specific pathogen, indicating that bystander activation within the liver microenvironment can be very potent in causing autoimmune damage (254).

3. More recently, H. Pircher's group (255) demonstrated that breaking of T-cell ignorance to a viral (transgene) antigen in the liver could induce hepatitis. Transgenic mice expressing the immunodominant LCMV glycoprotein epitope (GP$_{33}$) under the control of the albumin promoter exclusively in the liver did not develop spontaneous hepatitis nor did the adoptive transfer of TCR-transgenic, GP$_{33}$-specific T cells cause disease. However, when these mice were infected with LCMV and received adoptive transfer of TcR-transgenic cells, a transient form of hepatitis developed that became evident by elevated serum aminotransferase levels (255). Importantly, this model was used to evaluate the numbers of T cells needed to cause liver damage and illustrated that liver autoimmune processes are, similar to CNS and pancreatic autoimmunity, dependent on the "aggressiveness" and numbers of autoreactive T-lymphocytes.

4. Lastly, adenoviral infection with recombinant expressing the 2D6 antigen can lead to focal and confluent liver necrosis in mice resembling that of autoimmune hepatitis (Fig. 10).

In summary, the success of most mouse models has only been partial, since hepatitis was transient and induction of chronic disease appeared difficult to achieve. Figure 11 illustrates the possible pathogenetic mechanisms implicated in autoimmune hepatitis.

Immunology in Humans

Autoimmune hepatitis (AIH) is a severe form of adverse immune reaction afflicting the liver resulting in the progressive destruction of the hepatic parenchyma. One of the criteria to define subtypes of AIH is the pattern of patient autoantibodies. There are three classical subtypes of hepatitis virus antigen-negative autoimmune hepatitis that exhibit distinctive immunologic features.

1. The lupoid form exhibits a strong genetic linkage and usually is associated with antinuclear (ANA) and anti–liver membrane antigen (LMA) antibodies.

2. AIH type 2 exhibits a similar genetic linkage, but is characterized by antibodies to a liver (and kidney) mitochondrial antigen (LMK-1) that has recently been identified as the cytochrome P450 2D6 protein (256).

3. Lastly, type 3 AIH has no clear genetic linkage, but antibodies against a soluble liver antigen (SLA) are present.

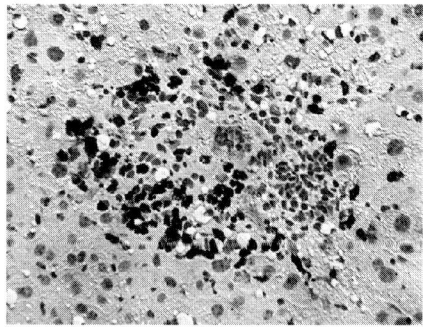

Confluent necrosis with infiltrating CD8 cells

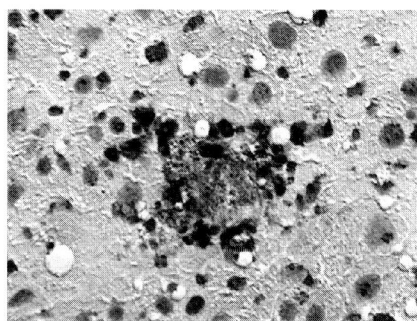

Focal necrosis with infiltrating CD8 cells

FIG. 10. Liver necrosis in 2D6 transgenic mice infected with an adenoviral recombinant expressing 2D6.

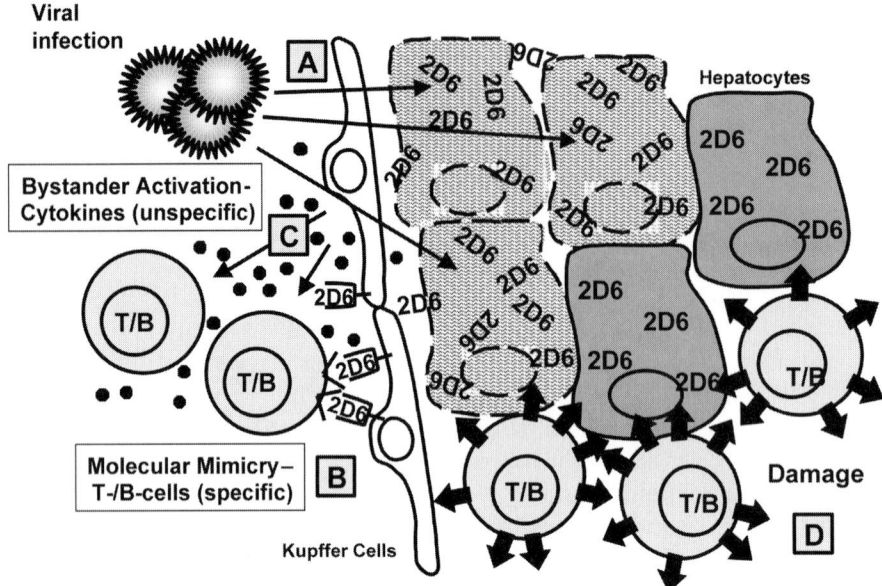

FIG. 11. Infection with a virus leads to high levels of expression of cytokines **(A).** This infection will most likely activate liver resident macrophages (Kupffer cells) **(B).** Specific anti-"viral" lymphocytes are activated and react against cells infected with the virus. In parallel, infection causes local inflammation and direct damage to some hepatocytes resulting in release of "self-antigens" such as cytochrome P450 IID6. Chemokines and cytokines most probably released by Kupffer cells **(C)** attract and activate infiltrating lymphocytes (bystander activation). Later on, activated lymphocytes migrate deeper into the liver parenchyma and cause further damage to hepatocytes expressing IID6 **(D).**

Other autoantibodies that are prominently present in AIH patients, such as antibodies to the asialoglycoprotein receptor present in up to 88% of individuals, are found in patients with chronic hepatitis B and C, alcoholic liver disease, and PBC, and thus may only be used as a general marker for liver autoimmunity. In addition, liver-kidney microsomal (LKM) antibodies are present in about 10% of cases of hepatitis C virus and 2% of hepatitis D virus infections. Clearly the vast majority of AIH cases are characterized by the breaking of tolerance to several liver-specific (and for type 2 also kidney-specific) autoantigens. Since the generation of such autoantibodies are T-helper cell dependent, it is not surprising that loss of tolerance also occurs on the T-cell level and lymphocytes isolated from livers of patients with AIH type 2 can react *in vitro* and expand after exposure to P4502D6 antigen. This finding supports the concept of a lymphocyte-driven autoaggression and might underlie pathogenesis. Furthermore, histologically mononuclear infiltration of the periportal areas is present that usually penetrates into the liver parenchyma when the disease progresses and causes the AIH-typical "piecemeal" appearance of the liver. Although evidence from animal models and human studies gives some indication that cytotoxic killing of hepatocytes could play a role, further analysis is still hampered by the fact that intrahepatic lymphocytes are difficult to access in humans.

Cytokines appear to play an essential role for human AIH. Importantly, administration of INF-α led to strong exacerbation of AIH, showing that it likely plays a central role in liver destruction (257). Interferons up-regulate MHC class I

and II molecules, enhance inflammation, and have strong antiviral effects. The outcome of IFN-α administration therefore argues against a role of an ongoing chronic (or acute) viral infection in patients with AIH who test negative for hepatitis virus antigen or antibodies. A negative regulatory role can possibly be attributed to IL-6 and TNF-α. These two cytokines are reduced in livers of AIH patients and have a negative effect on cytochrome P450 regulation (256). As a consequence, the lower levels of IL-6 and TNF might enhance IID6 antigen expression and in this way support autoimmunity directed to IID6 in patients with type 2 AIH. Lastly, AIH pathogenesis is not necessarily controlled by the T_H1/T_H2 paradigm: Interestingly, helper T-lymphocytes expressing T_H1 cytokines are elevated in type 1 AIH, whereas T_H2 cytokines are augmented in type 2 AIH in agreement with the high levels of IID6-directed antibodies present in these patients.

Is production of autoantibodies important for AIH pathogenesis or is it just an epiphenomenon signifying the breaking of tolerance to self-antigens? Evidence suggests that autoantibodies in AIH play a role that can be situated somewhere in between T1D, where autoantibodies and B-lymphocytes likely play no pathogenetically important role in humans, and SLE, where autoantibodies are complement fixing and enhance organ destruction. LKM antibodies found in AIH, for example, can inhibit cytochrome P450 function *in vitro* but not *in vivo,* and may participate in hepatocyte dysfunction or destruction. The major antigen component specifically recognized by LKM-1 antibodies was identified as the

2D6 isoform of the large cytochrome P450 enzyme family (CYP2D6). Epitope mapping revealed two immunodominant regions spanning aa 256–269 and aa 181–245 that are recognized by most of the AIH type 2 patient's sera. Since there is a significant genetic polymorphism in humans for the 2D6 antigen, it is possible that patients with AIH target IID6 protein selectively (LKM-1 antibodies), whereas cytochrome P4502D9 (LKM-2) is targeted in patients with drug-induced hepatitis, disulfide isomerase in halothane-induced hepatitis, or UDP-glycosyltransferases in hepatitis D virus–associated autoimmunity. Although the major target antigens have been identified down to the level of specific epitopes, the etiology of AIH is poorly understood. One major reason for this lack of comprehension is that there is no reliable animal model that would allow answers to the central questions of how tolerance to self-components, such as CYP2D6 and other molecules, is broken and of what mechanisms are involved in the immunopathogenesis of AIH.

The association with hepatitis C, D, and E virus–induced hepatitis and autoimmunity remains very intriguing. However, at this point, the prevalence of hepatitis C virus (HCV) for example, exhibits drastic variations between studies performed in different countries, and autoantibody titers appear much higher in patients with HCV-negative AIH. In a more recent study, it was found that sera of 38% of chronic hepatitis C patients reacted specifically with CYP2D6, whereas none of the sera obtained from patients with chronic hepatitis B showed CYP2D6 reactivity (257). Furthermore, it was found that HCV has the potential to induce autoreactive $CD8^+$ T cells that cross-reactively recognize the cytochrome P450 isoforms 2A6 and 2A7 that contain sequence homology to HCV aa 178–187. Such a phenomenon of cross-reactivity on the level of T-cell or antibody recognition is commonly referred to as "molecular mimicry." In this context it may be important to emphasize that molecular mimicry seems to be an important factor in other immune-mediated diseases of the liver. Hence, trifluoroacetyl (TFA)-protein adducts as generated during the metabolism of halothane by CYP2E1 confer molecular mimicry to the lipoic acid prosthetic group of the pyruvate dehydrogenase complex (PDC) and other members of the 2-oxoacid dehydrogenase family (45,129,152,258), which in turn are major autoantigens in primary biliary cirrhosis (PBC) (259). Consequently, halothane hepatitis and PBC may be linked on the level of cross-reactive autoantibodies that recognize similar target antigens.

It remains to be seen whether novel subtypes of hepatitis viruses can be found in AIH patients and whether further studies will corroborate such an association. It is likely, however, that viruses play a mutifactorial role in AIH pathogenesis (similar to type 1 diabetes) and that not one distinctive virus will be responsible for causing liver autoimmunity.

Primary Biliary Cirrhosis (PBC)

Similar to AIH, PBC, or chronic destructive cholangitis is characterized by autoantibodies to mitochondrial antigens.

However, although the disease is associated with other autoimmune-like syndromes and is more prevalent in females than in males, it is not ameliorated by immunosuppressive therapy, which argues against an autoimmune etiology or pathogenesis. The antimitochondrial antibodies (AMA) are directed against enzymes involved in ketone metabolism, such as pyruvate dehydrogenase. Several antigenic subtypes have been identified (M1 to M9) and the autoantibodies are complement binding. The clinical hallmark of PBC is a cholestatic syndrome and the nonbacterial resulting cholangitis. There is no effective causative treatment and immunosuppression has worsened PBC in several studies; therefore, liver transplantation is often the last resort for cases with terminal progressive PBC.

Halothane Hepatitis

Halothane hepatitis is a severe, life-threatening form of hepatic damage that affects a small subset of individuals exposed to the anesthetic agent halothane (260) and is thought to have an immunologic basis. Sera of afflicted individuals contain autoantibodies directed against the native and the trifluoroacetylated form of hepatic proteins. Trifluoroacteylated (TFA) proteins are generated during the oxidative metabolism of halothane (2-bromo-2-chloro-1,1,1-trifluoroethane) and include cytochrome P450, protein disulfide isomerase, microsomal carboxlesterase, calreticulin, Erp72, GRP78 (BiP), and GRP94. Current evidence suggests that such TFA proteins arise in all individuals exposed to halothane. However, the vast majority of individuals appear to tolerate this covalent protein modification. The lack of immunologic responsiveness was suggested to occur due to tolerance induced through the presence of structures in the repertoire of self-determinants, which immunochemically and structurally mimic TFA-proteins very closely. In fact, lipoic acid, the prosthetic group of the constitutively expressed E2 subunits of members of the 2-oxoacid dehydrogenase complex family was demonstrated by immunochemical and molecular modeling analysis to perfectly mimic N^6-trifluoroacteyl-L-lysine, the major haptenic group of TFA proteins. Interestingly, a fraction of patients with halothane hepatitis exhibit irregularities in the hepatic expression levels of these cross-reactive proteins. Thus, molecular mimicry of TFA lysine by lipoic acid, or the impairment thereof, can be considered a susceptibility factor of individuals for the development of halothane hepatitis (261). A small animal model for chemically induced liver diseases has recently been described (262).

Therapeutic Concepts

Immunosuppression is the therapy of choice for AIH. Since their introduction in 1968 (263), predinisolone and azathioprine have become part of standard treatment regimens (264). Immunosuppressive therapy improves survival of patients with severe AIH (265), but no guidelines are available for individuals with minimal symptoms. End-stage AIH is an important indication for liver transplantation (266). Recurrence of AIH has been reported after liver transplantation (267), but interestingly, is not as frequent as observed for islet transplants in T1D patients. Therapeutic use of interferons, effective for treatment of viral hepatitis, can worsen autoimmune liver disease (257) and challenges the assumption that unknown chronic viral infections of the liver, while possible initiators, maintain the active disease process. The effect of immunosuppression on the natural course of PBC and PSC is less pronounced and may in fact, as in the case of PBC, have a negative impact. Clinical symptoms, histology, and biochemistry of PBC are improved with use of ursodeoxycholic acid (UDCA), but the most effective treatment remains, just as for PSC, liver transplantation (268,269).

Conclusions and Future Directions

The presence of disease-specific autoantibodies in AIH, PBC, and PSC is indicative of autoimmune processes but none of the antibodies described is liver specific and their contribution to pathogenesis remains unclear. While the complex role of T cells is subject to current investigations, the same caveats of specificity and pathogenicity discussed earlier apply for autoimmune liver diseases (249). Although the success of immunosuppressive therapy, in fact a criterion for the diagnostic scoring system for AIH (33,250), further supports autoimmune etiology for AIH it is conceivable that a viral infection might initiate disease as a "hit-and-run" event. Following elimination of viral antigens, disease may be perpetuated by immune-mediated processes and preclude the identification of a particular virus as causative agent at the time

of liver disease diagnosis. Again, the role of "foreign" and "self" antigens becomes blurred and their interactions with the immune system in terms of immunity or autoimmunity conceptually problematic. Future investigations should seek to improve animal models, and focus on human autoantigens and the application of contemporary tools for identification and isolation of specific lymphocytes. On the basis of such developments, future *in vivo* tracking of autoaggressive lymphocytes with noninvasive methods should substantially improve our insight into disease pathogenesis.

Autoimmune Uveoretinitis

Various inflammatory diseases of the eye accompany other systemic or organ-specific autoimmune disorders and are displayed in Fig. 12. Some of these diseases are discussed very briefly since they are described in Chapter 44.

Introduction/Other Diseases Associated with Inflammatory Eye Disorders

M. Bechterew/Spondylarthoropathies

Iridocyclitis is frequently associated with Bechterew's disease (ankylosing spondylitis) that is characterized by a chronic spondylarthrosis of the ileosacral joints resulting in profound kyphosis, and is associated in 30% to 50% of cases with the HLA B27 allele (270–272). Interestingly, mucosal inflammation, ulcers, and vasculitis are frequently associated with this disease group. The immunologic pathogenesis is not clearly known, but cross-reactive antibodies to

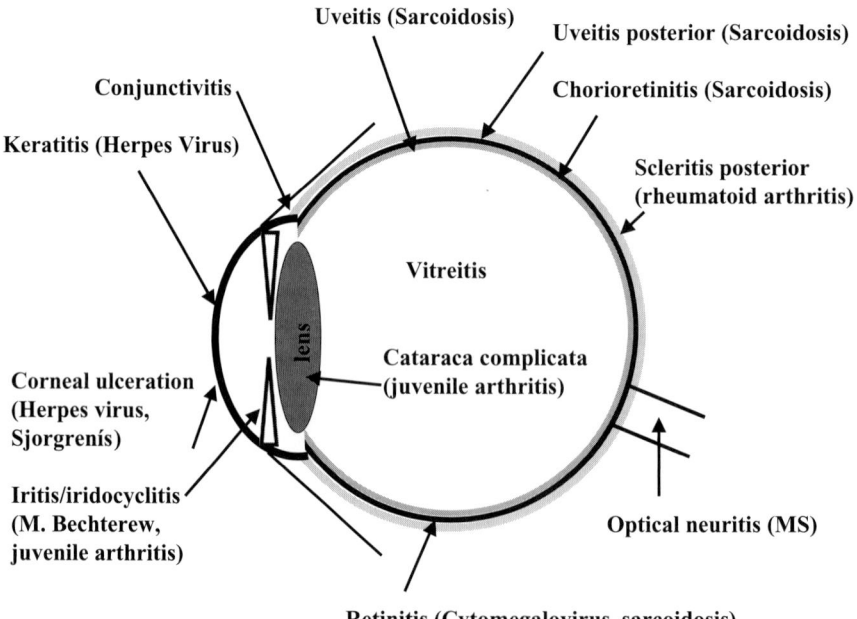

FIG. 12. Overview of the structures of the eye and the inflammatory diseases and their association with other systemic disorders (not comprehensive). No causative cure is available and usually, corticosteroids are the drug of choice.

bacterial proteins are frequently found in sera of patients with spondarthopathies such as Bechterew's disease, Reiter's syndrome, psoriasis, Crohn's disease, or ulcerative colitis. Therefore, molecular mimicry has been hypothesized as a cause for these disorders, but proof has been difficult to obtain. Several animal models have been developed, the most intriguing of which is probably a HLA-B27–transgenic rat that develops joint diseases, genital ulcers, and eye disease. Systemic immunosuppressive interventions are not effective and the treatment of choice is nonsteroidal anti-inflammatory drugs. Local steroids are frequently administered for symptoms affecting the eye.

Rheumatoid Arthritis

RA is an autoimmune joint disease (see below) that is frequently associated with scleritis and episcleritis. Inflammatory infiltrates can be found in the peripheral cornea leading to ulcerations. Local treatments are usually without effect and symptoms are ameliorated in conjunction with systemic immunosuppressive therapy. In contrast, juvenile arthritis is accompanied in about 20% of patients with cataracts and iridocyclitis, and ocular symptoms are often sensitive to local and systemic immunosuppression.

Sarcoidosis

Sarcoidosis is a chronic, systemic granulomatous inflammatory disease that involves the eye (uveitis in 20% of cases) and constitutes the cause for uveitis in about 10% of patients. Affected are multiple organs, particularly the lungs. The etiology is unclear and an autoimmune pathogenesis is suspected and multiple other inflammatory changes can occur in the eye (Fig. 12). Local therapy with steroids is usually helpful, and systemic immunosuppression can be considered.

Idiopathic Uveitis

About half of the cases of uveitis are not associated with a known primary syndrome and in young adults the association (50%) with HLA B27 is striking. Only a few of these patients will ultimately develop Bechterew's disease. Again, the etiology is quite unclear, but some evidence suggests that molecular mimicry between ocular and viral antigens (e.g., herpes virus) could play a role. Peptide therapy is currently being evaluated; otherwise steroids are the only effective choice. A summary of the eye structures and some of the systemic diseases that are associated with a putative autoimmune affectation of the eye are listed in Fig. 12.

Immunology in Animal Models

Small rodent models for autoimmune uveitis and herpes virus keratitis have been very useful for understanding the underlying immunopathology of inflammatory eye disorders.

Experimental Autoimmune Uveoretinitis

Experimental autoimmune uveoretinitis (EAU) is induced, similar to EAE, by immunizing susceptible rodent strains with retinal proteins such as the receptor retinoid binding protein (IRBP) (273). Extensive studies by R. Caspi and colleagues have revealed that EAU follows very similar autoimmune paradigms as other experimental autoimmune diseases including EAE and induced forms of diabetes. For example, a T_H1-like response drives the aggressive EAU process (274), whereas IL-10 in synergy with IL-4 has a pronounced protective function (275–277). Similarly, disease-resistant mice exhibit a predominantly T_H2-like response to IRBP. Experimental evidence indicates that sequestration and local immune privilege of IRBP and possibly other retinal antigens leads to a lack of systemic tolerance to these proteins and, as a consequence, destructive autoimmune responses can be readily induced. Conversely, tolerance can be reestablished by application of tolerizing retinal-Ag/Ig fusion proteins or by inducing peripheral tolerance by systemic expression under an MHC class II promoter in transgenic mice. Interestingly, peptide therapy using an HLA B27–restricted peptide appears to be effective in humans. The immunopathology of this EAU model in comparison to human uveitis, as found in sarcoidosis, is displayed in Fig. 13.

Herpesvirus-Induced Keratitis

Herpesvirus-induced keratitis has been explored in several animal models. The most intriguing studies come have come from the laboratory of H. Cantor. Inoculation of a genetically susceptible mouse strain with HSV-1 results in a viral infection of the eye and cornea that is accompanied by an immune response to HSV-1 (90). Interestingly, damage to the eye is only initiated by the virus and strongly depends on CD4 T cells that can cross-react with a self-protein. This animal model is one of the few that strongly indicate a direct immunopathologic role for molecular mimicry in an in vivo model for autoimmune disease. Studies by Rouse and colleagues have focused on the role of inflammatory bystander effects in the HSV-keratitis model (278,279). In these studies, inflammatory cytokines were shown to play a major role in mediating local damage and administration of DNA vaccine constructs expressing certain beneficial cytokines such as IL-10 ameliorated disease (280). It is important to point out that these studies were performed using a different HSV strain, and that the precise immunopathogenic process (mimicry versus bystander effects) indeed depends on the strain of HSV used (281). Additional observations have underscored the importance of regulatory cells in down-modulating a virally induced autoimmune disease. It is worthwhile mentioning that Streilein and colleagues have previously demonstrated regulatory cells in ocular autoimmune disease and found an important role for tolerizing antigen-presenting cells (282,283).

Mouse versus human uveitis - histopathology

Normal retina, mouse

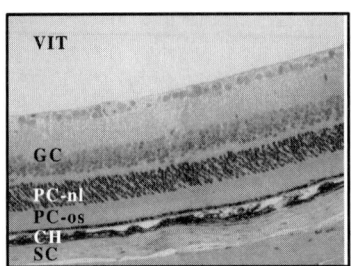

VIT: vitreous; GC: ganglion cells;
PO-nl: photoreceptor nuclear layer;
PO-os: photoreceptor outer segments;
CH: choroid; SC: sclera

EAU, mouse

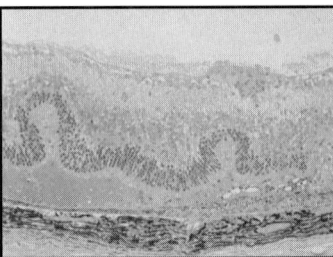

Ocular Sarcoidosis, human

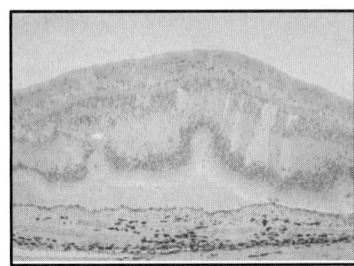

FIG. 13. Comparison of human versus mouse uveitis immunohistopathology. Courtesy of Rachel Caspi, National Eye Institute, Bethesda, MD.

Therapeutic Concepts in Humans

Due to the associated side effects, it is desirable to avoid systemic immunosuppressive interventions, as well as the local application of corticosteroids. Recently, a Munich group has identified an HLA B27–derived peptide that can function as a mimic to the retinal S antigen and induce EAU in Lewis rats (284). Using this mimic peptide as an orally administered antigen has produced very promising results in two human pilot trials in Germany. Thus, antigen-specific immunomodulation using retinal self-antigens or their peptide mimics may be developed as an effective therapeutic choice. It remains to be seen whether combination of such a treatment with cytokine-DNA vaccines, as demonstrated by Rouse's group for HSV keratitis or by Caspi's group for EAU, both in mouse models, might enhance efficacy.

Rheumatoid Arthritis

Introduction

RA is a severe debilitating disease with unknown etiology. Epidemiologically, the prevalence is about 1% in the overall population, women are affected three times more frequently than men, and the peak of incidence is within the fourth and sixth decade of life (108,285). Diagnostic criteria are the typical morning stiffness, joint swelling with fluid accumulation, defined radiologic changes, subcutaneous rheumatic nodes, and positive rheumatoid factor (autoantibodies) (Fig. 14). The prognosis is worse in HLA-DR4–positive patients and, similar to diabetes and MS, there is genetic linkage with certain MHC haplotypes. Without systemic immunosuppressive or anti-inflammatory therapy, the disease will eventually result

in destruction of many major joints and immobilize the patient. The major cause of death is infections that easily take a more severe course in immobile individuals (108).

The etiology is unclear. Since there is some possible overlap between infection-associated arthropathies (e.g., Reiter's syndrome), bacteria have always been good candidates as a cause for arthritis and molecular mimicry has been suggested as a cause, since cross-reactivities of autoantibodies between self and bacterial proteins have been detected (78). However, while it is quite possible to demonstrate cross-reactive antibodies and T cells in human blood, proof of their pathogenetic involvement is exceedingly difficult to obtain. The immune

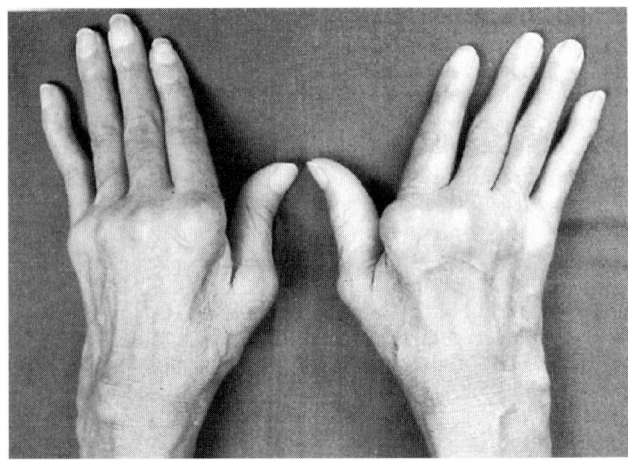

Typical ulnar deviation and swanís neck deformation of the hands in rheumatoid arthritis

FIG. 14. Rheumatoid arthritis.

system is likely to have developed to tolerate a low-level cross-reactivity, which might even be necessary for its proper function, and it remains very difficult to prove a mechanistic link between autoreactive cells and pathologic autoimmunity in humans.

Immunology

The evidence that RA is an autoimmune disease stems, as for MS and T1D, from the observation that T-lymphocytes in a patient's blood can react with joint-derived autoantigens and IgM autoantibodies, as well as antinuclear antibodies, are readily found in humans (286). Inflammatory signs in the serum include complement activation and increased erythrocyte sedimentation rate, which indicates that the antibodies could possibly play a role in the disease process. Similarly, immunization with collagen can induce arthritis in susceptible mouse strains. Figure 15 summarizes the major pathogenetic pathways leading to progressive joint destruction. As in many other autoimmune-disease animal models, collagen-induced arthritis models require strong immunization with autoantigens and adjuvant, supporting the concept that breaking of self-tolerance, even on a genetically susceptible background, requires a rather pronounced inflammatory stimulus. In contrast, how disease is initiated in humans is unclear.

Therapeutic Concepts and Conclusions

Treatment of RA is a difficult task, because the medications that adequately suppress joint inflammation also have strong systemic side effects. Therefore, a delicate balance between different therapeutic approaches that target different stages of the inflammatory process needs to be established. Corticosteroids and nonsteroidal anti-inflammatory drugs can provide some baseline relief but are not able to halt progressive joint destruction. Gold compounds, methotrexate, and cyclophosphamide are more effective but also have profound systemic side effects. For this reason, progress with novel immunomodulatory interventions is of important benefit for RA patients.

Application of cyclosporin A was shown to be effective by suppressing proliferation and activation of T-lymphocytes. More recently, a more selective intervention has been established based on research by M. Feldman's group (107). TNF-α was found to play a key role in an *in vitro* model of synovial destruction using human cells and TNF-α blocking agents to be applied *in vivo* were subsequently developed. After promising preclinical results in animal models, this intervention was tested in clinical trials and is now licensed for treatment of RA. Although side effects do occur, as expected, they appear tolerable and clinical improvement of disease is pronounced. In some patients, SLE-like symptoms were observed, indicating that blocking a cytokine beneficial for one autoimmune disorder might be detrimental for another one. Indeed, TNF blockade is not helpful in MS and T1D, because this cytokine exhibits complex dual functions depending on the disease stage. Based on the encouraging results with TNF blockade in RA, it may be possible to find similar key cytokines for T1D or MS treatment. It should be stressed that the successful intervention was developed based on human cell cultures and not animal models, underlining

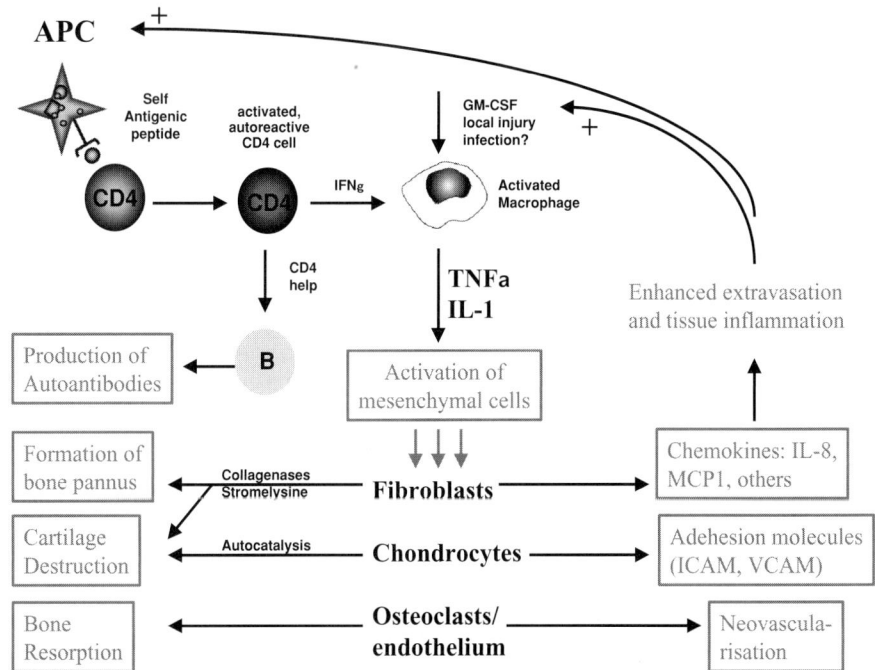

FIG. 15. Pathogenetic pathways leading to joint destruction in RA. Note the central role of TNF-α that is supported by the fact that TNF blockade ameliorates RA in humans.

the need for direct research on human materials, if and when possible.

Autoimmune Thyroiditis

Introduction

The year 1956 was seminal for the field of human autoimmunity given the discoveries of Hashimoto's thyroiditis as an autoimmune disease and of Graves' disease as caused by an autoantibody. These discoveries have prompted some straightforward and relatively uncomplicated treatments (287,288).

Interestingly, numerous viruses have been implicated in the pathogenesis of different thyroid diseases, but firm evidence for a direct involvement of viruses or virus-induced immune responses leading to clinically manifest disease is scarce. Subacute thyroiditis is a clinical and pathologic form of thyroid involvement that appears after infection with viruses such as measles, influenza, adenovirus, Epstein–Barr virus and Coxsackie virus (289). Again, however, a causative role *in vivo* has not been shown for any single infectious agent (290). Presence of viral material in the thyroid and elevated virus-specific antibody titers were found to correlate with subacute thyroiditis. In other instances, direct virally induced thyroiditis has been documented epidemiologically with thyroid or parathyroid disease.

Retroviruses, in particular HIV infections, have generated much interest. Although HIV infection and AIDS may affect multiple endocrine organ systems (291–294), thyroid dysfunction usually reflects weight loss, anorexia, and cachexia of advanced HIV disease, rather than a direct viral effect on the thyroid (295,296). Thus, direct involvement of the thyroid by HIV or by opportunistic infections is uncommon and may include subclinical hypothyroidism and "euthyroid sick syndrome." The clinical relevance is probably limited, since overt hyper- or hypo-thyroidism does not occur with greater frequency in HIV-infected and AIDS patients, as compared to patients with other nonthyroidal illnesses (HIV and the thyroid gland have been reviewed in Heufelder and Hofbauer [295]). Involvement of the parathyroid in patients with AIDS could be shown by reduced basal and maximal PTH levels, but the mechanisms underlying these findings have not yet been elucidated (297). To account for a possible role of HIV in thyroid autoimmunity, a 66% homology between the HIV-1 Nef protein and the human TSH receptor has been noted. However, reactivity of sera of Graves' patients against a Nef peptide showed no significant differences as compared to normal controls (298). This does not rule out the presence conformationally shared T- or B-cell epitopes with HIV proteins. In analyzing mechanisms of molecular mimicry, studies of potential antigenic surfaces have emerged as an important supplement to analysis of sequence similarity (299).

In addition, antibodies from a Graves' patient showed reactivity to the Gag proteins of another retrovirus, human foamy virus (HFV) (299). The association of HFV with Graves'

disease or subacute thyroiditis is controversial. Whereas one study demonstrated HFV-related sequences in the DNA of peripheral blood in two-thirds of the Graves' patients but none in normal controls (300), another study could not confirm these findings (301).

In other studies, an association between HTLV I and II and the occurrence of autoimmune thyroiditis or Graves' disease was reported (301–304). Further, as in the case of HIV, hepatitis C virus was shown to lead to a wide variety of autoimmune disorders including involvement of the thyroid gland (241,305–308). Moreover, treatment of chronic hepatitis B and C with INF-α lead to induction or enhancement of autoimmune disease (309–311). For congenital rubella infection, which has been associated with diabetes mellitus, Addison's disease, and growth hormone deficiencies, as well as thyroid disorders (312), it is not clear whether thyroid involvement is the result of a direct viral effect or a more generalized dysfunction of the immune system (290).

Animal models in mice and chicken have been used to study virus-induced thyroiditis (reviewed in Tomer and Davies [290]). Mice persistently infected with lymphocytic choriomeningitis virus (LCMV) showed reductions of thyroglobulin mRNA and circulating thyroid hormones in the absence of thyroid cell destruction (313). Thyroiditis characterized by focal destruction of the follicular structures, inflammatory infiltration, and generation of antibodies against thyroglobulin and thyroid peroxidase was observed in a reovirus type 1 mouse model of thyroiditis (314). The reovirus gene responsible for autoantibody induction was identified and the encoded polypeptide shown to bind to tissue-specific surface receptors (315). Spontaneous lymphocytic infiltration of the thyroid is observed in the obese strain of chickens. Such chickens express an endogenous retrovirus, avian leukosis virus (ev22), not found in healthy normal inbred strains (316). Although ev22 appears to be a genetic marker rather than cause for thyroiditis, infection of normal chicken embryos with avian leukosis virus can cause hypothyroidism (317). Moreover, aberrant MHC class II expression is demonstrated in obese-strain chickens and elevated levels of 2,5-oligoadenylate synthetase as well as 2,5-oligoadenylate polymer levels in the cytosol of thyroid epithelial cells occur, suggesting viral involvement (318). Again, not all cross-reactivities with self-ligands need to increase autoimmunity (319), and regulatory cells also play a major role in modulating autoimmune thyroiditis (320).

Immunology

Autoantigens targeted in thyroiditis are thyroid peroxidase, a cell-surface protein, and the thyrotropin receptor. Autoimmune responses to thyroglobulin are mainly seen in animal models but appear to play a lesser role in the human disease. The B-cell epitopes to these autoantigens have been mapped relatively well; however, as it is the case for other human autoimmune disorders, T-cell responses, their tracking and specificity, as well as their eliciting antigens in humans, have remained largely elusive (287). An interesting link has been established to the CTLA-4 gene region, which is supported by the finding that NOD mice exhibiting a link to this gene as well also present with thyroiditis. The usual suspects, including APC dysfunction, autoaggressive lymphocytes, and links to viral infections, have been examined, but no conclusive etiologic or mechanistic evidence has been obtained to date. It is noteworthy that a role for regulatory T cells has been established in D. Mason's animal model for thyroiditis (321).

Autoimmune Skin Disorders

Frequently, inflammation of the skin such as urticaria, vasculitis and erythema can accompany systemic autoimmune disorders, particularly Crohn's disease, ulcerative colitis, or SLE. Where applicable and relevant, these are discussed in the sections for the respective disease. Here we focus on "skin-only" autoimmune disorders, which include pemphigus, herpetiform dermatitis, and IgA dermatoses. While there is a relative paucity of animal models for human autoimmune skin disorders, the skin is one of the few organs that offer us direct access to T cells and proteins expressed in a human target organ; therefore, human data are detailed and mechanistic insight into the human diseases is good.

Pemphigus

Pemphigus is a serious bullous disease of the skin and mucous membranes. The cause for blister formation is the loss of cohesion between epidermal cells, epidermis, and the basal membrane and corium leading to the accumulation of fluid (322,323). A hallmark of pemphigus is the formation of autoantibodies directed to desmosomes and anchor fibrils that usually literally hold the skin together and in place. Figure 16 summarizes the targeted structures with respect to skin layer or location in various forms of pemphigus disease. Due to the appearance of these IgG antibodies (close to 100% of patients during the acute clinical phase) that are complement binding and because of their pathogenetic importance, pemphigus can be considered an autoimmune disease; as a matter of fact, it is the only one where the pathogenetic importance of one defined autoantigen is clearly established in humans (323,324). It is associated with HLA-DR4 and certain variations of the DQ beta chain (325); however, the milder form, bullous pemphigoid, does not exhibit any HLA linkage. The etiology is unclear, however; in some cases, a putative initiation through certain drugs has been observed. While pemphigus may be associated with other autoimmune diseases (323), its occurrence with certain malignant diseases has been defined as a separate entity (326). Other forms of pemphigus-like manifestations include the gestational pemphigus, the penicillamin-induced mucosal pemphigus, and bullous epidermolysis that sometimes accompanies SLE, Crohn's disease, or diabetes.

Despite the good response to glucocorticoid treatments, pemphigus remains a very serious clinical disease that frequently requires long-term immunosuppression that may result in severe systemic side effects. A causative intervention is not yet possible despite the fact that the autoantigens are quite well known and characterized. The disease is very painful and the clinical implications are similar to those seen with major burns. Larger scars will remain after the affected areas have healed.

Dermatitis Herpetiformis

This is a relatively rare, HLA B8/DR3–linked disorder that is characterized by string itching and is of unknown etiology. There are some IgA deposits in the skin and the disease is treated with sulfones that have significant side effects (327).

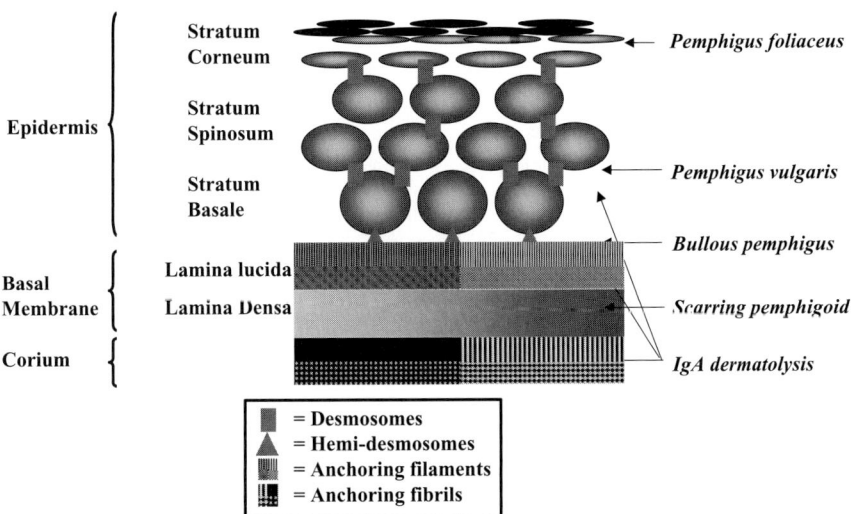

FIG. 16. Different skin layers and their affectation in autoimmune skin syndromes.

IgA Dermatoses

This is a bullous affectation of the skin that can comprise several layers depending on the subtype (Fig. 16). It is linked to HLA-B8/DR3 and is characterized by IgA deposition in the skin that leads to formation of tears and blisters. The treatment with sulfonamides and corticosteroids is usually effective; the etiology is unclear (328).

Autoimmune Gut Disorders

The gut constitutes a unique immunologic environment given its large interactive mucosal surface area and the need to maintain tolerance toward food antigens and bacteria normally present within the gut flora. The gut-associated immune system has an important regulatory and barrier function. Immune responses are usually initiated within the Peyer's patches that obtain a significant amount of antigens via the M cells located within the mucosa and specialized in antigen uptake and transport (98,329,330). Lymphocytes from the bone marrow will circulate through the Peyer's patches, where B- or T-cell responses can be initiated. Interestingly, the B-cell responses are characteristically IgA high. After antigen encounter, these cells will circulate to the mesenteric lymph nodes and enter the systemic circulation from there. Specifically for the gut, there are other extralymphoid locations, where immune cells are found and where immune responses (aggressive or regulatory) can be initiated. One is the intestinal lamina propria, where MHC class II is expressed and bacterial products can be presented. Predominantly CD4$^+$ T and B cells may assume regulatory functions and IgA is secreted with the mucus into the gut lumen. The second are intraepithelial lymphocytes (IELs). A significant proportion of IELs expresses the $\gamma\delta$ T-cell receptor and they have cytotoxic as well as immunoregulatory functions (331,332). Certain studies after oral or intranasal feeding of autoantigens have attributed regulatory function to $\gamma\delta$ lymphocytes. Overall, the hypothesis that the gut environment is ideally suited to induce a tolerizing or regulatory immune response to antigens present in the gut lumen is of high interest and well supported by evidence from animal models (e.g., "oral tolerance") (333). The rationale is that the immune system must have evolved to put some unique mechanisms into place to deal with the multitude of "foreign" antigens present in the gut and needed as nutrients and for digestive purposes. Indeed, mice housed within a sterile environment have a shorter life span and multiple immune defects, indicating that the gut's immune system is vital for regular immune development and functions.

Gastritis

Pernicious anemia is the end stage of autoimmune gastritis observed in about 10% to 20% of patients (334) and represents the most common cause of vitamin B$_{12}$ deficiency (335). Autoimmune gastritis is associated with autoantibody production to parietal cells and to its secreted product, intrinsic factor. In addition, a role for CD8 and CD4 T cells has been demonstrated (336). Animal models have been developed (337). Standard therapy is paternal B$_{12}$ administration. Interestingly, this disease also develops in mice after thymectomy and is characterized by a relative lack of CD25$^+$ regulatory CD4$^+$ T cells (111,338,339).

Ulcerative Colitis

Ulcerative colitis is a chronic inflammatory disease of the gut that affects men somewhat more frequently than women. It usually begins in the distal colon and rectum and will spread proximally resulting in severe cases in pancolitis. The hallmark is bloody mucoid diarrhea. The etiology is unclear, evidence points toward a certain genetic predisposition that has to meet triggering environmental factors. Unlike Crohn's disease, the inflammatory foci are not granulomatous and not discontinuous. Overall, inflammatory mediators are increased, but systemic symptoms are rare. Treatment is usually achieved by corticosteroids, in severe cases, ulcerative colitis may require removal of the colon.

Crohn's Disease

As opposed to ulcerative colitis, Crohn's disease begins as a discontinuous, granulomatous inflammation of the proximal ileum. Ulcerations are frequent and the disease is more severe than ulcerative colitis. The permeability of the mucosal epithelium is enhanced, which leads to a local breakdown of barrier functions and up-regulation of TNF, IL-1, IL-6, and other cytokines. The immune reaction involves the whole mucosa and regional lymph nodes. Interestingly, in addition to standard immunosuppressive treatments, blockade of TNF appears to be promising in recent clinical trials, similar to the situation in RA (340).

Autoimmune Diseases of the Heart

The etiology for primary myocarditis is unclear and an autoimmune cause has to be taken into account. The heart muscle is infiltrated mainly by CD4$^+$ T cells and macrophages and the infiltrates are usually diffuse and nonfocal. The infiltrating cells produce considerable amounts of INF-γ and TNF-α. As a consequence of the inflammation, heart muscle cells can swell, the heart can dilate and severe disturbances of the electrical conduction can occur. It is noteworthy that myocarditis can also occur in conjunction with certain systemic autoimmune diseases such as SLE, scleroderma, RA, polymyositis, and polyarteriitis nodosa.

CLOSING REMARKS

A common trait among diverse animal models for autoimmune diseases and the human conditions they aim to model appears to be the difficulty with which experimental autoimmunity is achieved. Breaking of tolerance to self-antigens requires in most instances strong inflammatory (e.g., pertussis toxin and adjuvant in EAE or collagen-induced arthritis) or infectious (e.g., RIP-LCMV model for T1D, or TMEV/MHV models for MS) stimuli. In addition, many animal models require a genetically susceptible background or have to rely on artificial autoantigen expression by means of transgenic technology. In contrast to the relatively easy detection of autoreactive lymphocytes in antigen-induced animal models, it has been a daunting endeavor in humans (as well as spontaneous disease models such as the NOD mouse) and data obtained frequently vary considerably between different patients as well as laboratories. What are the implications for our understanding of autoimmune diseases in humans given these challenges? First, it is unlikely that strong inflammatory stimuli can be provided under natural conditions in the absence of infectious disease. Thus, viral and bacterial infections remain prime candidates for causing secondary autoimmunity (see Miller's TMEV model of APC-mediated determinant spreading to autoantigens). Infectious pathogens can provide the "danger signals" (Matzinger) needed for propagation of extended inflammation leading to clinical disease. Nevertheless, proof of a causal relationship is exquisitely difficult (if not impossible), since traces of pathogens detected may have no relation to the underlying disease process, or may be cleared from the system by the time of secondary clinical disease. In addition, disease is likely dependent on individual pathogen strains, making a very detailed immunologic profiling in prospective clinical trials necessary. It is possible that the introduction of new antivirals might unmask such an association in the future. Second, a genetically susceptible background will likely be required to provide a "fertile field" for initiating a chronic inflammation involving autoantigens. This probably occurs via a multifaceted network of multiple susceptibility and protective genes, and it will be impossible to treat a respective disease just by analyzing the background genes involved. Last, autoreactive lymphocytes might predominantly be present in the affected organ or site and not in the peripheral blood, which makes their identification and characterization in humans rather difficult.

One last word of caution should be devoted to our interpretation of specific findings obtained in individual animal models. Animal models should serve to teach us paradigms of how a disease *could* develop kinetically *in vivo*. The precise parameters, targeted antigens, susceptibility genes and effector molecules may be considerably different in humans. Thus, for example, if there is indication that GAD is a primary antigen in the NOD mouse, this may or may not have direct relevance to the human disease. However, what Yoon's observations in the NOD mouse can teach us is that there may be a crucial primary yet-to-be-discovered antigen in human diabetes. Indeed, GAD appears to be targeted in humans in a more systemic disorder, stiff man's syndrome (SMS) (341), and study of the NOD mouse may facilitate our understanding of SMS. The opportunities as well as limits of each animal model have to be delineated. Again, the NOD mouse appears to be prone toward multiorgan autoimmunity (induction of EAE [342], neuritis [343], arthritis and hepatitis have all been observed in NOD or NOD-congenic mouse strains) and exhibits, in addition to diabetes, thyroiditis, sialitis, and orchitis. Thus, diabetes in the NOD mouse is clearly different from typical human type 1 diabetes. Therefore, treatments capable of correcting the systemic immune dysregulation that predominates in the NOD model may not directly apply to human T1D where no such pronounced systemic dysregulation is present. Based on these considerations it is not surprising that out of the more than 140 therapeutic strategies that prevent diabetes in the NOD mouse, only a handful have made it to phase 1 human trials. Experiments with human cells or materials should be undertaken in order to solidify the choice of molecules or target antigens. The successful story with respect to blockade of TNF-α to treat RA underlines the importance of this step. Employment of a multiplicity of models thus becomes imperative to evaluate potential candidate interventions, as does a careful proceeding, objective evaluation, and avoidance of premature conclusions. In addition to the researchers and clinicians, publishers as well as the news media will have to share this responsibility. Continued research will undoubtedly provide us eventually with sufficient insight into the complexities of organ-specific autoimmunity, but patience and perseverance coupled with experimental objectivity will be required.

REFERENCES

1. Littré E, Robin CH. *Dictionnaire de médecine, de chirugie, de pharmacie et de l'art veterinaire.* Paris: Baillière, 14th edition 1878.
2. Pasteur L. De l'atténuation du virus choléra des poules. *Compt Rend Acad Sci* 1880;91:673–680.
2a. von Behring E, Kitasato S. Über das Zustandekommen der Diphtherie-Immunität und der Tetanus-Immunität bei Thieren. *Dtsch Med Wochenschr* 1890;16:1113–1114.
3. Ehrlich P, Morgenroth J. Zytotoxine als Antikörper. *Berl Klin Wochenschr* 1901;38:251–260.
4. Römer P, Gebb H. *Albrecht von Graefes Arch Ophthalmol.* 1912;81:367–402.
5. Silverstein A. *A history of immunology.* San Diego: Academic Press, 1989.
6. Portier P, Richet C. De l'action anaphylactique de certain venins. *CR Soc Biol (Paris)* 1902;54:170–172.
7. Arthus M. Injections repétées de serum du cheval chez le lapin. *Compt Rend Soc Biol* (Paris) 1903;55:817–820.
8. Donath J, Landsteiner K. Über paroxysmale Hämoglobinurie. *Münch Med Wochenschr* 1904;51:1590–1601.
9. von Pirquet C, Schick B. *Die Serumkrankheit.* Leipzig: Deuticke, 1905.
10. Weil E, Braun H. Über das Wesen der luetischen Erkrankung auf Grund der neueren Forschungen. *Wien Klin Wochenschr* 1909;22:372–374.
11. Uhlenhuth P. *Festschrift zum 60. Geburtstag von Robert Koch.* Jena: Fisher, 1903.
12. Traub E. Persistence of Lymphocytic choriomeningitis virus in immune animals and its relation to immunity. *J Exp Med* 1936;63:847–861.
13. Owen RD. Immunogenetic consequences of vascular anastomoses between bovine cattle twins. *Science* 1945;102:400–401.
14. Medawar PB. The behaviour and fate of skin autografts and skin homografts in rabbits. *J Anat* 1944;78:176–199.

15. Medawar PB. A second study of the behaviour and fate of skin homografts in rabbits. *J Anat* 1945;79:157–176.

16. Medawar PB. Immunity to homologous grafted skin. I. The suppression of cell division in grafts transplanted to immunized animals. *Br J Exp Pathol* 1946;27:9–14.

17. Medawar PB. Immunity to homologous grafted skin. II. The immunity relationship between the antigens of blood and skin. *Br J Exp Pathol* 1946;27:15–24.

18. Burnet FM, Fenner F. *The production of antibodies.* New York: Macmillan, 1949.

19. Burnet FM. *The clonal selection theory of acquired immunity.* Cambridge: Cambridge University Press, 1957.

20. Witebsky E, Rose NR. Studies on organ specificity. V. Changes in the thyroid glands of rabbits following active immunization with rabbit thyroid extracts. *J Immunol* 1956;76:417–427.

21. Fleck L. *Entstehung und Entwicklung einer wissenschaftlichen Tatsache. Einführung in die Lehre vom Denkstil und Denkkollektiv.* B. Schwabe und Co., Verlagsbuchhandlung, Basel, 1935.

22. Jerne NK. Towards a network theory of the immune system. *Ann Immunol* 1974;373–389.

23. Coutinho A, Forni L, Holmberg D, et al. From an antigen-centered, clonal perspective of immune responses to an organism-centered, network perspective of autonomous activity in a self-referential immune system. *Immunol Rev* 1984;79:151–168.

24. Grabar P. Hypothesis. Auto-antibodies and immunological theories: an analytical review. *Clin Immunol Immunopathol* 1975;4:453–466.

25. Wigzell H. Positive autoimmunity. In: Talal N, ed. *Autoimmunity: genetic, immunologic, virologic and clinical aspects.* New York: Academic Press, 1997.

25a. Schwartz M, Cohen IR. Autoimmunity can benefit self-maintenance. *Immunol Today* 2000;21:265–268.

26. Matzinger P. Tolerance, danger, and the extended family. *Ann Rev Immunol* 1994;12:991–1045.

27. Dembic Z. Immune system protects integrity of tissues. *Mol Immunol* 2000;37:563–569.

28. Rose NR, Mackay IR. Prelude. In: Rose NR, Mackay IR, eds. *The autoimmune diseases.* San Diego: Academic Press, 1998.

29. Schwartz R. Foreword. In: Lahita RG, Chiorazzi N, Reeves WH, eds. *Textbook of the autoimmune diseases.* Philadelphia: Lippincott Williams & Wilkins, 2000.

30. Rose NR, Bona C. Defining criteria for autoimmune disease (Witebsky's postulates revisited). *Immunol Today* 1993;114:426–430.

31. Zinkernagel RM. Anti-infection immunity and autoimmunity. *Ann NY Acad Sci* 2002;958:3–6.

32. Witebsky E, Rose NR, Terplan K, et al. Chronic thyroiditis and autoimmunization. *J Am Med Assoc* 1957;164:1439–1447.

33. Alvarez F, Berg PA, Bianchi FB, et al. International Autoimmune Hepatitis Group Report: review of criteria for diagnosis of autoimmune hepatitis. *J Hepatol* 1999;31:929–938.

34. Jacobson DL, Gange SJ, Rose NR, et al. Epidemiology and estimated population burden of selected autoimmune diseases in the United States. *Clin Immunol Immunopathol* 1997;84:223–243.

35. Gershon RK, Kondo K. Infectious immunological tolerance. *Immunology* 1971;21:903–914.

36. Shevach EM. Regulatory T cells in autoimmmunity. *Annu Rev Immunol* 2000;18:423–449.

37. Shevach EM. CD4+ CD25+ suppressor T cells: more questions than answers. *Nat Rev Immunol* 2002;2:389–400.

38. Ashton-Rickardt PG, Bandeira A, Delaney J, et al. Evidence for a differential avidity model of T-cell selection in the thymus. *Cell* 1994;76:651–663.

39. Hoffmann MW, Heath WR, Ruschmeyer D, et al. Deletion of high-avidity T cells by thymic epithelium. *Proc Natl Acad Sci U S A* 1995;92:9851–9855.

40. Jameson SC, Bevan MJ. T-cell selection. *Curr Opin Immunol* 1998;10:214–219.

41. Sebzda E, Mariathasan S, Ohteki T, et al. Selection of the T cell repertoire. *Annu Rev Immunol* 1999;17:829–874.

42. Kishimoto H, Sprent J. The thymus and negative selection. *Immunol Res* 2000;21:315–323.

43. Nikolic-Zugic J, Bevan MJ. Role of self-peptides in positively selecting the T-cell repertoire. *Nature* 1990;344:65–67.

44. Surh CD, Lee DS, Fung-Leung WP, et al. Thymic selection by a single MHC/peptide ligand produces a semidiverse repertoire of CD4+ T cells. *Immunity* 1997;7:209–219.

45. Steinman L. A few autoreactive cells in an autoimmune infiltrate control a vast population of nonspecific cells: a tale of smart bombs and the infantry. *Proc Natl Acad Sci USA* 1996;93:2253–2256.

46. Allison JP. CD28–B7 interactions in T-cell activation. *Curr Opin Immunol* 1994;6:414–419.

47. Harding FA, Allison JP. CD28–B7 interactions allow the induction of CD8+ cytotoxic T-lymphocytes in the absence of exogenous help. *J Exp Med* 1993;177:1791–1796.

48. Schwartz RH. A cell culture model for T lymphocyte clonal anergy. *Science* 1990;248:1349–1356.

49. Lenardo M, Chan KM, Hornung F, et al. Mature T lymphocyte apoptosis—immune regulation in a dynamic and unpredictable antigenic environment. *Annu Rev Immunol* 1999;17:221–253.

50. Abbas AK. Die and let live: eliminating dangerous lymphocytes. *Cell* 1996;84:655–657.

51. Van Parijs L, Abbas AK. Homeostasis and self-tolerance in the immune system: turning lymphocytes off. *Science* 1998;280:243–248.

52. Chambers CA, Kuhns MS, Egen JG, et al. CTLA-4–mediated inhibition in regulation of T cell responses: mechanisms and manipulation in tumor immunotherapy. *Annu Rev Immunol* 2001;19:565–594.

53. Salomon B, Bluestone JA. Complexities of CD28/B7: CTLA-4 costimulatory pathways in autoimmunity and transplantation. *Annu Rev Immunol* 2001;19:225–252.

54. Weiner HL, Friedman A, Miller A, et al. Oral tolerance: immunologic mechanisms and treatment of animal and human organ-specific autoimmune diseases by oral administration of autoantigens. *Annu Rev Immunol* 1994;12:809–837.

55. Seewaldt S, Thomas HE, Ejrnaes M, et al. Virus-induced autoimmune diabetes: most beta-cells die through inflammatory cytokines and not perforin from autoreactive (anti-viral) cytotoxic T-lymphocytes. *Diabetes* 2000;49:1801–1809.

56. Marth T, Strober W, Seder RA, et al. Regulation of transforming growth factor-beta production by interleukin-12. *Eur J Immunol* 1997;27:1213–1220.

57. Seder RA, Marth T, Sieve MC, et al. Factors involved in the differentiation of TGF-b–producing cells from naive CD4+ T cells: IL-4 and IFN-g have opposing effects, while TGF-b positively regulates its own production. *J Immunol* 1998;160:5719–5728.

58. King C, Davies J, Mueller R, et al. TGF-b1 alters APC preference, polarizing islet antigen responses toward a Th2 phenotype. *Immunity* 1998;8:601–613.

59. Rizzo LV, Morawetz RA, Miller-Rivero NE, et al. IL-4 and IL-10 are both required for the induction of oral tolerance. *J Immunol* 1999;162:2613–2622.

60. Homann D, Holz A, Bot A, et al. Autoreactive CD4+ lymphocytes protect from autoimmune diabetes via bystander suppression using the IL-4/STAT6 pathway. *Immunity* 1999;11:463–472.

61. King C, Hoenger RM, Cleary MM, et al. Interleukin-4 acts at the locus of the antigen-presenting dendritic cell to counter-regulate cytotoxic CD8+ T-cell responses. *Nat Med* 2001;7:206–214.

62. Zhang ZY, Lee CS, Lider O, et al. Suppression of adjuvant arthritis in Lewis rats by oral administration of type II collagen. *J Immunol* 1990;145:2489–2493.

63. Maron R, Blogg NS, Polanski M, et al. Oral tolerance to insulin and the insulin B-chain: cell lines and cytokine patterns. *Ann NY Acad Sci* 1996;778:357.

64. Hancock WW, Polanski M, Zhang J, et al. Suppression of insulitis in non-obese diabetic (NOD) mice by oral insulin administration is associated with selective expression of interleukin-4 and -10, transforming growth factor-beta, and prostaglandin-E. *Am J Pathol* 1995;147:1193–1199.

65. Bergerot I, Arreaza GA, Cameron MJ, et al. Insulin B-chain reactive CD4+ regulatory T-cells induced by oral insulin treatment protect from type 1 diabetes by blocking the cytokine secretion and pancreatic infiltration of diabetogenic effector T-cells. *Diabetes* 1999;48:1720–1729.

66. Charlton B, Lafferty KJ. The Th1/Th2 balance in autoimmunity. *Curr Opin Immunol* 1995;7:793–798.

67. Paul WE. Interleukin-4: a prototypic immunoregulatory lymphokine. *Blood* 1991;77:1859–1870.

68. Lepault F, Gagnerault MC. Characterization of peripheral regulatory

CD4+ T cells that prevent diabetes onset in nonobese diabetic mice. *J Immunol* 2000;164:240–247.

69. Sercarz EE. Processing creates the self. *Nat Immunol* 2002;3:110–112.

70. Anderton SM, Viner NJ, Matharu P, et al. Influence of a dominant cryptic epitope on autoimmune T cell tolerance. *Nat Immunol* 2002;3:175–181.

71. Moudgil KD, Sekiguchi D, Kim SY, et al. Immunodominance is independent of structural constraints: each region within hen eggwhite lysozyme is potentially available upon processing of native antigen. *J Immunol* 1997;159:2574–2579.

72. Bhardwaj V, Kumar V, Geysen HM, et al. Degenerate recognition of a dissimilar antigenic peptide by myelin basic protein-reactive T cells. *J Immunol* 1993;151:5000–5010.

73. Carbone FR, Kurts C, Bennett SRM, et al. Cross-presentation: a general mechanism for CTL immunity and tolerance. *Immunol Today* 1998;19:368–373.

74. van Stipdonk MJ, Lemmens EE, Schoenberger SP. Naive CTLs require a single brief period of antigenic stimulation for clonal expansion and differentiation. *Nat Immunol* 2001;2:423–429.

75. Blattman JN, Sourdive DJ, Murali-Krishna K, et al. Evolution of the T cell repertoire during primary, memory, and recall responses to viral infection. *J Immunol* 2000;165:6081–6090.

76. Heath WR, Kurts C, Miller JFAP, et al. Cross-tolerance: a pathway for inducing tolerance to peripheral tissue antigens. *J Exp Med* 1998;187:1549–1553.

77. Taurog JD, Maika SD, Satumtira N, et al. Inflammatory disease in HLA-B27 transgenic rats. *Immunol Rev* 1999;169:209–223.

78. Schwimmbeck P, Yu DT, Oldstone MBA. Autoantibodies to HLA-B27 in sera of patients with ankylosing spondylitis and Reiter's syndrome. *J Exp Med* 1987;166:173–181.

79. McDevitt HO. The role of MHC class II molecules in susceptibility and resistance to autoimmunity. *Curr Opin Immunol* 1998;10:677–681.

80. Sonderstrup G, McDevitt HO. DR, DQ, and you: MHC alleles and autoimmunity. *J Clin Invest* 2001;107:795–796.

81. Molberg O, Kett K, Scott H, et al. Gliadin specific, HLA DQ2–restricted T cells are commonly found in small intestine biopsies from coeliac disease patients, but not from controls. *Scand J Immunol* 1997;46:103–108.

82. von Herrath M, Wolfe T, Mohrle U, et al. Protection from type 1 diabetes in the face of high levels of activated, auto-aggressive lymphocytes in a viral transgenic mouse model crossed to the SV129 strain. *Diabetes,* 2001;50:2700–2708.

83. Bach J-F. Organ-specific autoimmunity. *Immunol Today* 1995;16:353–355.

84. Bach J-F. Insulin dependent diabetes mellitus as an autoimmune disease. *Endocr Rev* 1994;15:516–542.

85. Bach J-F. Predictive medicine in autoimmune diseases: from the identification of genetic predisposition and environmental influence to precocious immunotherapy. *Clin Immunol Immunopathol* 1994;72:156–161.

86. Todd JA. The role of MHC class II genes in susceptibility to insulin-dependent diabetes mellitus. *Curr Top Microbiol Immunol* 1990;164:17–40.

87. Vyse TJ, Todd JA. Genetic analysis of autoimmune disease. *Cell* 1996;85:311–318.

88. Redondo MJ, Rewers M, Yu L, et al. Genetic determination of islet cell autoimmunity in monozygotic twin, dizygotic twin, and non-twin siblings of patients with type 1 diabetes: prospective twin study. *BMJ* 1999;318:698–702.

89. Sevilla N, Homann D, von Herrath MG, et al. Virus-induced diabetes in a transgenic model: role of cross-reacting viruses and quantitation of effector T cells needed to cause disease. *J Virol* 2000;74:3284–3292.

90. Zhao ZS, Granucci F, Yeh L, et al. Molecular mimicry by herpes simplex virus-type 1: autoimmune disease after viral infection. *Science* 1998;279:1344–1347.

91. Oldstone MBA. Molecular mimicry and autoimmune disease. *Cell* 1987;50:819–820.

92. Horwitz MS, Bradley LM, Harbertson J, et al. Diabetes induced by Coxsackie virus: initiation by bystander damage and not molecular mimicry. *Nat Med* 1998;4:781–785.

93. Olson JK, Girvin AM, Miller SD. Direct activation of innate and

94. Miller SD, Vanderlugt CL, Begolka WS, et al. Persistent infection with Theiler's virus leads to CNS autoimmunity via epitope spreading. *Nat Med* 1997;3:1133–1136.

95. Katz-Levy Y, Neville KL, Girvin AM, et al. Endogenous presentation of self myelin epitopes by CNS-resident APCs in Theiler's virus-infected mice. *J Clin Invest* 1999;104:599–610.

96. Oldstone MB. Prevention of type I diabetes in nonobese diabetic mice by virus infection. *Science* 1988;239:500–502.

97. Blumberg RS, Saubermann LJ, Strober W. Animal models of mucosal inflammation and their relation to human inflammatory bowel disease. *Cur Opin Immunol* 1999;11:648–656.

98. Kelsall BL, Strober W. Dendritic cells of the gastrointestinal tract. *Springer Semin Immunopathol* 1997;18:409–420.

99. La Cava A, Sarvetnick N. The role of cytokines in autoimmunity. *Curr Dir Autoimmun* 1999;1:56–71.

100. von Andrian UH, Mackay CR. T-cell function and migration. Two sides of the same coin. *N Engl J Med* 2000;343:1020–1034.

101. Godessart N, Kunkel SL. Chemokines in autoimmune disease. *Curr Opin Immunol* 2001;13:670–675.

102. O'Shea JJ, Ma A, Lipsky P. Cytokines and autoimmunity. *Nat Rev Immunol* 2002;2:37–45.

103. Kim S, Kim KA, Hwang DY, et al. Inhibition of autoimmune diabetes by Fas ligand: the paradox is solved. *J Immunol* 2000;164:2931–2936.

104. Hugues S, Mougneau E, Ferlin W, et al. Tolerance to islet antigens and prevention from diabetes induced by limited apoptosis of pancreatic beta cells. *Immunity* 2002;16:169–181.

105. Delovitch TL, Singh B. The nonobese diabetic mouse as a model of autoimmune diabetes: immune dysregulation gets the NOD. *Immunity* 1997;7:727–738.

106. Christen U, Wolfe T, Mohrle U, et al. A dual role for TNF-alpha in type 1 diabetes: islet-specific expression abrogates the ongoing autoimmune process when induced late but not early during pathogenesis. *J Immunol* 2001;166:7023–7032.

107. Maini RN, Elliott M, Brennan FM, et al. TNF blockade in rheumatoid arthritis: implications for therapy and pathogenesis. *APMIS* 1997;105:257–263.

108. Feldmann M, Brennan FM, Maini RN. Rheumatoid arthritis. *Cell* 1996;85:307–310.

109. Tisch R, McDevitt H. Antigen specific immunotherapy: is it a real possibility to combat T-cell medicated autoimmunity? *Proc Natl Acad Sci USA* 1994;91:437–438.

110. Tisch R, Wang B, Weaver DJ, et al. Antigen-specific mediated suppression of beta cell autoimmunity by plasmid DNA vaccination. *J Immunol* 2001;166:2122–2132.

111. Shevach EM, McHugh RS, Piccirillo CA, et al. Control of T-cell activation by CD4+ CD25+ suppressor T cells. *Immunol Rev* 2001;182:58–67.

112. Sicotte NL, Voskuhl RR. Onset of multiple sclerosis associated with anti-TNF therapy. *Neurology* 2001;57:1885–1888.

113. Riminton DS, Korner H, Strickland DH, et al. Challenging cytokine redundance: inflammatory cell movement and clinical course of experimental autoimmune encephalomyelitis are normal in lymphotoxin-deficient, but not tumor necrosis factor-deficient, mice. *J Exp Med* 1998;187:1517–1528.

114. Sedgwick JD, Riminton DS, Cyster JG, et al. Tumor necrosis factor: a master-regulator of leukocyte movement. *Immunol Today* 2000;21:110–113.

115. Coon B, An L-L, Whitton JL, et al. DNA immunization to prevent autoimmune diabetes. *J Clin Invest* 1999;104:189–194.

116. von Mering J, Minkowski O. Diabetes mellitus nach Pankreasextirpation. *Arch Exp Pathol Pharmakol* 1890;26:371–374.

117. Schmidt MB. Über die Beziehung der Langerhansschen Inseln des Pankreas zum Diabetes mellitus. *Münch Med Wochenschr* 1902;49:51–59.

118. Banting FG, Best CH. The internal secretion of the pancreas. *J Lab Clin Med* 1922;7:251–266.

119. Gepts W. Pathologic anatomy of the pancreas in juvenile diabetes mellitus. *Diabetes* 1965;14:619–633.

120. Bottazzo GF, Florin-Christensen A, Doniach D. Islet cell antibodies in diabetes mellitus with autoimmune polyendocrine deficiencies. *Lancet* 1974;2:1279–1281.

121. MacCuish AC, Irvine WJ, Barnes EW, et al. Antibodies to pancreatic islet cells in insulin-dependent diabetics with coexistent autoimmune disease. *Lancet* 1974;2:1529–1531.

122. Nerup J, Platz P, Andersen OO, et al. HL-A antigens and diabetes mellitus. *Lancet* 1974;2:864–866.

123. Atkinson MA, Eisenbarth GS. Type 1 diabetes: new perspectives on disease pathogenesis and treatment. *Lancet* 2001;358:221–229.

124. Atkinson MA, Maclaren NK. The pathogenesis of insulin-dependent diabetes mellitus. *N Engl J Med* 1994;331:1428–1436.

125. Jackson RA, Soeldner JS, Eisenbarth GS. Predicting insulin-dependent diabetes. *Lancet* 1988;10:627–628.

126. Eisenbarth GS, Gianani R, Yu L, et al. Dual-parameter model for prediction of type i diabetes mellitus. *Proc Assoc Am Phys* 1998;110:126–135.

127. Wong FS, Karttunen J, Dumont C, et al. Identification of an MHC class I-restricted autoantigen in type 1 diabetes by screening an organ-specific cDNA library. *Nature Med* 1999;5:1026–1031.

128. Yoon J-W, Yoon C-S, Lim H-W, et al. Control of autoimmune diabetes in NOD mice by GAD expression or suppression in beta cells. *Science* 1999;284:1183–1187.

129. von Herrath MG, Dockter J, Oldstone MBA. How virus induces a rapid or slow onset insulin-dependent diabetes mellitus in a transgenic model. *Immunity* 1994;1:231–242.

130. DiLorenzo TP, Graser RT, Ono T, et al. Major histocompatibility complex class I–restricted T cells are required for all but the end stages of diabetes development in nonobese diabetic mice and use a prevalent T cell receptor alpha chain gene rearrangement. *Proc Natl Acad Sci USA* 1998;95:12538–12543.

131. Graser RT, DiLorenzo TP, Wang F, et al. Identification of a CD8 T cell that can independently mediate autoimmune diabetes development in the complete absence of CD4 T cell helper functions. *J Immunol* 2000;164:3913–3918.

132. Shapiro AM, Lakey JR, Ryan EA, et al. Islet transplantation in seven patients with type 1 diabetes mellitus using a glucocorticoid-free immunosuppressive regimen. *N Engl J Med* 2000;343:230–238.

133. Babu PG, Huber SA, Craighead JE. Contrasting features of T-lymphocyte–mediated diabetes in encephalomyocarditis virus–infected Balb/cBy and Balb/cCum mice. *Am J Pathol* 1986;124:193–198.

134. Baum H. Mitochondrial antigens, molecular mimicry and autoimmune disease. *Biochim Biophys Acta* 1995;1271:111–121.

135. Gianani R, Sarvetnick N. Viruses, cytokines, antigens, and autoimmunity. *Proc Natl Acad Sci U S A* 1996;93:2257–2259.

136. Foulis AK, McGill M, Farquharson MA, et al. A search for evidence of viral infection in pancreases of newly diagnosed patients with IDDM. *Diabetologia* 1997;40:53–61.

137. Jenson AB, Rosenberg HS, Notkins AL. Pancreatic islet cell damage in children with fatal viral infections. *Lancet* 1980;2:354–358.

138. Shrinivasappa J, Saegusa J, Prabhakar B, et al. Frequency of reactivity of monoclonal antiviral antibodies with normal tissues. *J Virol* 1986;57:397–401.

139. Oldstone MBA. Molecular mimicry as a mechanism for the cause and as a probe uncovering etiologic agent(s) of autoimmune disease. *Curr Top Microbiol Immunol* 1989;145:127–135.

140. Notkins AL, Yoon JW. Virus-induced diabetes mellitus. In: Notkins AL, Oldstone MBA, eds. *Concepts in viral pathogenesis.* New York: Springer-Verlag, 1984:241–247.

141. Horwitz MS, Sarvetnick N. Viruses, host responses, and autoimmunity. *Immunol Rev* 1999;169:241–253.

142. Buschard K. Diabetic animal models. *APMIS* 1996;104:609–614.

143. Katz J, Benoist C, Mathis DX. T helper cell subsets in IDDM. *Science* 1995;268:1185–1188.

144. Wilberz S, Partke HJ, Dagnaes-Hansen F, et al. Persistent MHV (mouse hepatitis virus) infection reduces the incidence of diabetes mellitus in non-obese diabetic mice. *Diabetologia* 1991;34:2–5.

145. Oldstone MBA. Viruses as therapeutic agents. I. Treatment of nonobese insulin-dependent diabetes mice with virus prevents insulin-dependent diabetes mellitus while maintaining general immune competence. *J Exp Med* 1990;171:2077–2089.

146. Toshiyuki M, Ogawa M, Kobayashi F, et al. Electron microscope studies on the interaction of pancreatic islet cells and splenic lymphocytes in non-obese diabetic (NOD) mice. *Res* 1988;9:67–73.

147. Morgan D, Liblau R, Scott B, et al. CD8+ T cell–mediated spontaneous diabetes in neonatal mice. *J Immunol* 1996;157:978–984.

148. Kurts C, Cannarile M, Klebba I, et al. Cutting edge: dendritic cells are sufficient to cross-present self-antigens to CD8 T cells in vivo. *J Immunol* 2001;166:1439–1442.

149. Kurts C, Heath WR, Carbone FR, et al. Cross-presentation of self antigens to CD8+ T cells: the balance between tolerance and autoimmunity. In: *Proceedings of Novartis Foundation Symposium.* Chichester, UK: John Wiley and Sons, 1998:172–181, 181–190.

150. Kurts C, Heath WR, Kosaka H, et al. The peripheral deletion of autoreactive CD8+ T cells induced by cross-presentation of self-antigens involves signaling through CD95 (Fas, Apo-1). *J Exp Med* 1998;188:415–420.

151. Oldstone MBA, Nerenberg M, Southern P, et al. Virus infection triggers insulin-dependent diabetes mellitus in a transgenic model: role of anti-self (virus) immune response. *Cell* 1991;65:319–331.

152. Ohashi P, Oehen S, Buerki K, et al. Ablation of "tolerance" and induction of diabetes by virus infection in viral antigen transgenic mice. *Cell* 1991;65:305–317.

153. Berdanier CD. Diet, autoimmunity, and insulin-dependent diabetes mellitus: a controversy. *Proc Soc Exp Biol Med* 1995;209:223–230.

154. Eisenbarth GA. Type 1 diabetes mellitus. A chronic autoimmune disease. *N Engl J Med* 1986;314:1360–1368.

155. Hiltunen M, Hyoty H, Knip M, et al. Islet cell antibody seroconversion in children is temporally associated with enterovirus infections. Childhood Diabetes in Finland (DiMe) Study Group. *J Infect Dis* 1997;175:554–560.

156. Peterson JS, Dyrberg T, Karlsen AE, et al. Glutamic acid decarboxylase (GAD$_{65}$) autoantibodies in prediction of b-cell function and remission in recent onset IDDM after cyclosporin treatment. *Diabetes* 1994;43:1291–1296.

157. Peterson JS, Hejnaes KR, Moody A, et al. Detection of GAD$_{65}$ antibodies in diabetes and other autoimmune diseases using a simple radioligand assay. *Diabetes* 1994;43:459–467.

158. Wucherpfennig KW, Strominger JL. Molecular mimicry in T-cell mediated autoimmunity: viral peptides activate human T-cell clones specific for myelin basic protein. *Cell* 1995;80:695–705.

159. von Herrath MG, Dockter J, Oldstone MB. How virus induces a rapid or slow onset insulin-dependent diabetes mellitus in a transgenic model. *Immunity* 1994;1:231–242.

160. Ludewig B, Odermatt B, Landmann S, et al. Dendritic cells induce autoimmune diabetes and maintain disease via de novo formation of local lymphoid tissue. *J Exp Med* 1998;188:1493–1501.

161. Ludewig B, Odermatt B, Ochsenbein AF, et al. Role of dendritic cells in the induction and maintenance of autoimmune diseases. *Immunol Rev* 1999;169:45–54.

162. Ludewig B, Junt T, Hengartner H, et al. Dendritic cells in autoimmune diseases. *Curr Opin Immunol* 2001;13:657–662.

163. von Herrath MG, Guerder S, Lewicki H, et al. Coexpression of B7-1 and viral ("self") transgenes in pancreatic beta cells can break peripheral ignorance and lead to spontaneous autoimmune diabetes. *Immunity* 1995;3:727–738.

164. Kagi D, Odermatt B, Ohashi PS, et al. Development of insulitis without diabetes in transgenic mice lacking perforin-dependent cytotoxicity. *J Exp Med* 1996;183:2143–2152.

165. Chatenoud L, Salomon B, Bluestone JA. Suppressor T cells—they're back and critical for regulation of autoimmunity! *Immunol Rev* 2001; 182:149–163.

166. Herold KG, Lenschow DJ, Bluestone JA. CD28/B7 regulation of autoimmune diabetes. *Immunol Res* 1997;16:71–84.

167. Green EA, Flavell RA. The temporal importance of TNF alpha expression in the development of diabetes. *Immunity* 2000;12:459–469.

168. Brod SA, Atkinson M, Lavis VR, et al. Ingested IFN-alpha preserves residual beta cell function in type 1 diabetes. *J Interferon Cytokine Res* 2001;21:1021–1030.

169. Stauffer Y, Marguerat S, Meylan F, et al. Interferon-alpha–induced endogenous superantigen: a model linking environment and autoimmunity. *Immunity* 2001;15:591–601.

170. Bosi E, Minelli R, Bazzigaluppi E, et al. Fulminant autoimmune Type 1 diabetes during interferon-alpha therapy: a case of Th1-mediated disease? *Diabet Med* 2001;18:329–332.

171. von Herrath MG, Allison J, Miller JF, et al. Focal expression of interleukin-2 does not break unresponsiveness to "self" (viral) antigen expressed in beta cells but enhances development of autoimmune disease (diabetes) after initiation of an anti-self immune response. *J Clin Invest* 1995;95:477–485.

172. Lee MS, Wogensen L, Shizuru J, et al. Pancreatic islet production of murine interleukin-10 does not inhibit immune-mediated tissue destruction. *J Clin Invest* 1994;93:1332–1338.

173. Lee M-S, Mueller R, Wicker LS, et al. IL-10 is necessary and sufficient for autoimmune diabetes in conjunction with NOD MHC homozygosity. *J Exp Med* 1996;183:2663–2668.

174. King C, Mueller Hoenger R, Malo Cleary M, et al. Interleukin-4 acts at the locus of the antigen-presenting dendritic cell to counter-regulate cytotoxic CD8+ T-cell responses. *Nat Med* 2001;7:206–214.

175. Durinovic-Bello I, Hummel M, Ziegler AG. Cellular immune response to diverse islet cell antigens in IDDM. *Diabetes* 1996;45:795–800.

176. Fuchtenbusch M, Kredel K, Bonifacio E, et al. Exposure to exogenous insulin promotes IgG1 and the T-helper 2–associated IgG4 responses to insulin but not to other islet autoantigens. *Diabetes* 2000;49:918–925.

177. Roep BO, Stobbe I, Duinkerken G, et al. Auto- and alloimmune reactivity to human islet allografts transplanted into type 1 diabetic patients. *Diabetes* 1999;48:484–490.

178. Martin S, Wolf-Eichbaum D, Duinkerken G, et al. Development of type 1 diabetes despite severe hereditary B-lymphocyte deficiency. *N Engl J Med* 2001;345:1036–1040.

179. Hiemstra HS, Drijfhout JW, Roep BO. Antigen arrays in T cell immunology. *Curr Opin Immunol* 2000;12:80–84.

180. Noorchashm H, Lieu YK, Noorchashm N, et al. I-Ag7–mediated antigen presentation by B lymphocytes is critical in overcoming a checkpoint in T cell tolerance to islet beta cells of nonobese diabetic mice. *J Immunol* 1999;163:743–750.

181. Kaufman DL, Tisch R, Sarvetnick N, et al. Report from the 1st International NOD Mouse T-Cell Workshop and the follow-up miniworkshop. *Diabetes* 2001;50:2459–2463.

182. Wicker LS, Todd JA, Peterson LB. Genetic control of autoimmune diabetes in the NOD mouse. *Annu Rev Immunol* 1995;13:179–200.

183. McDevitt H, Singer S, Tisch R. The role of MHC class II genes in susceptibility and resistance to type I diabetes mellitus in the NOD mouse. *Horm Metab Res* 1996;28:287–288.

183a. Morel PA, Dorman JS, Todd JA, et al. Aspartic acid at position 57 of the HLA-DQ beta chain protects against type I diabetes: a family study. *Proc Natl Acad Sci USA* 1988;85:8111–8115.

184. Serreze DV, Leiter EH. Genes and cellular requirements for autoimmune diabetes susceptibility in nonobese diabetic mice. *Curr Dir Autoimmun* 2001;4:31–67.

185. von Herrath MG. *Molecular pathology of type 1 diabetes mellitus.* Basel: S. Karger AG, 2001.

186. Van Houten N, Blake SF. Direct measurement of anergy of antigen-specific T cells following oral tolerance induction. *J Immunol* 1996;157:1337–1341.

187. Weiner HL. Oral tolerance: mobilizing the gut. *Hosp Pract (Off Ed)* 1995;30:53–58.

188. Benson JM, Whitacre CC. The role of clonal deletion and anergy in oral tolerance. *Res Immunol* 1997;148:533–541.

189. Strobel S, Mc Mowat A. Immune responses to dietary antigens: oral tolerance. *Immunol Today* 1998;19:173–181.

190. Viney JL, Mowat AM, O'Malley JM, et al. Expanding dendritic cells in vivo enhances the induction of oral tolerance. *J Immunol* 1998;160:5815–5825.

191. Maeda Y, Noda S, Tanaka K, et al. The failure of oral tolerance induction is functionally coupled to the absence of T cells in Peyer's patches under germfree conditions. *Immunobiology* 2001;204:442–457.

192. Atkinson MA, Maclaren NK. The pathogenesis of insulin-dependent diabetes mellitus. *N Engl J Med* 1994;331:1428–1436.

193. Boismenu R, Feng L, Xia YY, et al. Chemokine expression by intraepithelial gamma delta T cells. Implications for the recruitment of inflammatory cells to damaged epithelia. *J Immunol* 1996;157:985–992.

194. Paronen J, Knip M, Savilahti E, et al. Effect of cow's milk exposure and maternal type 1 diabetes on cellular and humoral immunization to dietary insulin in infants at genetic risk for type 1 diabetes. Finnish trial to reduce IDDM in the Genetically at Risk Study Group. *Diabetes* 2000;49:1657–1665.

195. Karjalainen J, Martin JM, Knip M, et al. A bovine albumin peptide as a possible trigger of insulin-dependent diabetes mellitus. *N Engl J Med* 1992;327:302–307.

196. Honeyman MC, Coulson BS, Stone NL, et al. Association between rotavirus infection and pancreatic islet autoimmunity in children at risk of developing type 1 diabetes. *Diabetes* 2000;49:1319–1324.

197. Lonnrot M, Korpela K, Knip M, et al. Enterovirus infection as a risk factor for beta-cell autoimmunity in a prospectively observed birth cohort: the Finnish Diabetes Prediction and Prevention Study. *Diabetes* 2000;49:1314–1318.

198. Mena I, Fischer C, Gebhard JR, et al. Coxsackievirus infection of the pancreas: evaluation of receptor expression, pathogenesis, and immunopathology. *Virology* 2000;271:276–288.

199. von Herrath MG, Whitton JL. DNA vaccination to treat autoimmune diabetes. *Ann Med* 2000;32:285–292.

200. Bot A, Smith D, Bot S, et al. Plasmid vaccination with insulin b chain prevents autoimmune diabetes in nonobese diabetic mice. *J Immunol* 2001;167:2950–2955.

201. Garren H, Ruiz PJ, Watkins TA, et al. Combination of gene delivery and DNA vaccination to protect from and reverse Th1 autoimmune disease via deviation to the Th2 pathway. *Immunity* 2001;15:15–22.

202. Tisch R, Wang B, Atkinson MA, et al. A glutamic acid decarboxylase 65–specific Th2 cell clone immunoregulates autoimmune diabetes in nonobese diabetic mice. *J Immunol* 2001;166:6925–6936.

203. Gaur A, Boehme SA, Chalmers D, et al. Amelioration of relapsing experimental autoimmune encephalomyelitis with altered myelin basic protein peptides involves different cellular mechanisms. *J Neuroimmunol* 1997;74:149–158.

204. Pedotti R, Mitchell D, Wedemeyer J, et al. An unexpected version of horror autotoxicus: anaphylactic shock to a self-peptide. *Nat Immunol* 2001;2:216–222.

205. Kappos L, Comi G, Panitch H, et al. Induction of a non-encephalitogenic type 2 T helper–cell autoimmune response in multiple sclerosis after administration of an altered peptide ligand in a placebo-controlled, randomized phase II trial. The Altered Peptide Ligand in Relapsing MS Study Group. *Nat Med* 2000;6:1176–1182.

206. Chatenoud L, Thervet E, Primo J, et al. Anti-CD3 antibody induces long-term remission of overt autoimmunity in nonobese diabetic mice. *Proc Natl Acad Sci USA* 1994;91:123–127.

207. Herold KC, Hagopian W, Auger JA, et al. Anti-CD3 monoclonal antibody in new-onset type 1 diabetes mellitus. *N Engl J Med* 2002;346:1692–1698.

208. Raz I, Elias D, Avron A, et al. beta-cell function in new-onset type 1 diabetes and immunomodulation with a heat-shock protein peptide (DiaPep277): a randomised, double-blind, phase II trial. *Lancet* 2001;358:1749–1753.

209. Ettinger RA, Nepom GT. Molecular aspects of HLA class II alphabeta heterodimers associated with IDDM susceptibility and protection. *Rev Immunogenet* 2000;2:88–94.

210. Coulombe M, Yang H, Wolf LA, et al. Tolerance to antigen-presenting cell-depleted islet allografts is CD4 T cell dependent. *J Immunol* 1999;162:2503–2510.

211. Parker DC, Greiner DL, Phillips NE, et al. Survival of mouse pancreatic islet allografts in recipients treated with allogeneic small lymphocytes and antibody to CD40 ligand. *Proc Natl Acad Sci USA* 1995;92:9560–9564.

212. Rossini AA, Greiner DL, Mordes JP. Induction of immunologic tolerance for transplantation. *Physiological Reviews* 1999;79:99–141.

213. Welsh RM, Markees TG, Woda BA, et al. Virus-induced abrogation of transplantation tolerance induced by donor-specific transfusion and anti-CD154 antibody. *J Virol* 2000;74:2210–2218.

214. Wilson SB, Kent SC, Patton KT, et al. Extreme Th1 bias of invariant Valpha24JalphaQ T cells in type 1 diabetes. *Nature* 1998;391:177–181.

215. Utz U, Biddison WE, McFarland HF, et al. Skewed T-cell receptor repertoire in genetically identical twins correlates with MS. *Nature* 1993;364:243–247.

216. Muraro PA, Vergelli M, Kalbus M, et al. Immunodominance of a low-affinity major histocompatibility complex-binding myelin basic protein epitope (residues 111–129) in HLA-DR4 (B1*0401) subjects is associated with a restricted T cell receptor repertoire. *J Clin Invest* 1997;100:339–349.

217. Scholz C, Patton KT, Anderson DE, et al. Expansion of autoreactive T cells in multiple sclerosis is independent of exogenous B7 costimulation1. *J Immunol* 1998;160:1532–1538.

218. de Seze J, Dubucquoi S, Lefranc D, et al. IgG reactivity against citrullinated myelin basic protein in multiple sclerosis. *J Neuroimmunol* 2001;117:149–155.

219. Mason JL, Suzuki K, Chaplin DD, et al. Interleukin-1beta promotes repair of the CNS. *J Neurosci* 2001;21:7046–7052.

220. Arnett HA, Mason J, Marino M, et al. TNF alpha promotes proliferation of oligodendrocyte progenitors and remyelination. *Nat Neurosci* 2001;4:1116–1122.

221. Ebers G, Bulman D, Sadovnik A, et al. A population based study of multiple sclerosis in twins. *New Engl J Med* 1987;315:1638–1642.

222. Miller S, Karpus WJ. The immune pathogenesis and regulation of T-cell mediated demyelinating diseases. *Immunol Today* 1994;15:358–362.

223. Neumann H, Schmidt H, Cavalie A, et al. Major histocompatibility complex (MHC) class 1 gene expression in single neurons of the central nervous system: differential regulation by interferon (IFN-gamma) and tumor necrosis factor (TNF)-a. *J Exp Med* 1997;185:305–316.

224. Ruiz PJ, Garren H, Ruiz IU, et al. Suppressive immunization with DNA encoding a self-peptide prevents autoimmune disease: modulation of T cell costimulation. *J Immunol* 1999;162:3336–3341.

225. Katz-Levy Y, Neville KL, Girvin AM, et al. Endogenous presentation of self myelin epitopes by CNS-resident APCs in Theiler's virus-infected mice. *J Clin Invest* 1999;104:599–610.

226. Olson JK, Croxford JL, Calenoff MA, et al. A virus-induced molecular mimicry model of multiple sclerosis. *J Clin Invest* 2001;108:311–318.

227. Buchmeier MJ, Lane TE. Viral-induced neurodegenerative disease. *Curr Opin Microbiol* 1999;2:398–402.

228. Evans CF, Horwitz MS, Hobbs MV, et al. Viral infection of transgenic mice expressing a viral protein in oligodendrocytes leads to chronic central nervous system autoimmune disease. *J Exp Med* 1996;184:2371–2384.

229. Vergelli M, Mazzanti B, Traggiai E, et al. Short-term evolution of autoreactive T cell repertoire in multiple sclerosis. *J Neurosci Res* 2001;66:517–524.

230. Iglesias A, Bauer J, Litzenburger T, et al. T- and B-cell responses to myelin oligodendrocyte glycoprotein in experimental autoimmune encephalomyelitis and multiple sclerosis. *Glia* 2001;36:220–234.

231. Challoner PB, Smith KT, Parker JD, et al. Plaque-associated expression of human herpes virus 6 in multiple sclerosis. *Proc Natl Acad Sci USA* 1995;92:7440–7444.

232. Martin R, Sturzebecher CS, McFarland HF. Immunotherapy of multiple sclerosis: where are we? Where should we go? *Nat Immunol* 2001;2:785–788.

233. McFarland HF. Complexities in the treatment of autoimmune disease. *Science* 1996;274:2037–2038.

234. Weiner HL, Mackin GA, Matsui M, et al. Double-blind pilot trial of oral tolerization with myelin antigens in multiple sclerosis. *Science* 1993;259:1321–1324.

235. Jacobs LD, Beck RW, Simon JH, et al. Intramuscular interferon beta-1a therapy initiated during a first demyelinating event in multiple sclerosis. CHAMPS Study Group. *N Engl J Med* 2000;343:898–904.

236. Rice GP, Woelfel EL, Talbot PJ, et al. Immunological complications in multiple sclerosis patients receiving interferon. *Ann Neurol* 1985;18:439–442.

237. Chen M, Gran B, Costello K, et al. Glatiramer acetate induces a Th2-biased response and crossreactivity with myelin basic protein in patients with MS. *Mult Scler* 2001;7:209–219.

238. Bielekova B, Lincoln A, McFarland H, et al. Therapeutic potential of phosphodiesterase-4 and -3 inhibitors in Th1-mediated autoimmune diseases. *J Immunol* 2000;164:1117–1124.

239. Bielekova B, Goodwin B, Richert N, et al. Encephalitogenic potential of the myelin basic protein peptide (amino acids 83–99) in multiple sclerosis: results of a phase II clinical trial with an altered peptide ligand. *Nat Med* 2000;6:1167–1175.

240. Kappos L, Comi G, Panitch H, et al. Induction of a non-encephalitogenic type 2 T helper-cell autoimmune response in multiple sclerosis after administration of an altered peptide ligand in a placebo-controlled, randomized phase II trial. *Nat Med* 2000;6:1176–1182.

241. Manns MP, Rambusch EG. Autoimmunity and extrahepatic manifestations in hepatitis C virus infection. *J Hepatol* 1999;1:39–42.

242. Czaja AJ, Manns MP. The validity and importance of subtypes in autoimmune hepatitis: a point of view. *Am J Gastroenterol* 1995;90:1206–1211.

243. Desmet VJ, Gerber M, Hoofnagle JH, et al. Classification of chronic hepatitis: diagnosis, grading and staging. *Hepatology* 1994;19:1513–1520.

244. Neuberger J. Halothane hepatitis. *Eur J Gastroenterol Hepatol* 1998;10:631–633.

245. Waldenström J. Leber, Blutproteine und Nahrungseiweiss. *Dtsch Z Verdau Stoffwechselkrankh* 1950;2:113–119.

246. Kunkel HG, Ahrens EH, Eisenmemger WJ, et al. Extreme hyper-gammaglobulinemia in young women with liver disease of unknown etiology. *J Clin Invest* 1951;30:654(abst).

247. Bearn AG, Kunkel HG, Slater R. The problem of chronic liver disease in young women. *Am J Med* 1956;21:3–15.

248. Mackay IR, Taft CO, Cowling DS. Lupoid hepatitis. *Lancet* 1956;2:1323–1326.

249. Kita H, Mackay IR, Van De Water J, et al. The lymphoid liver: considerations on pathways to autoimmune injury. *Gastroenterology* 2001;120:1485–1501.

250. Johnson PJ, McFarlane IG. Meeting report: International Autoimmune Hepatitis Group. *Hepatology* 1993;18:998–1005.

251. Manns MP, Obermayer-Straub P. Viral induction of autoimmunity: mechanisms and examples in hepatology. *J Viral Hepat* 1997;4:42–47.

252. Guidotti LG, Ishikawa T, Hobbs MV, et al. Intracellular inactivation of the hepatitis B virus by cytotoxic T lymphocytes. *Immunity* 1996;4:25–36.

253. Chisari FV, Ferrari C. Hepatitis B virus immunopathogenesis. *Annu Rev Immunol* 1995;13:29–60.

254. Alferink J, Aigner S, Reibke R, et al. Peripheral T-cell tolerance: the contribution of permissive T-cell migration into parenchymal tissues of the neonate. *Immunol Rev* 1999;169:255–261.

255. Voehringer D, Blaser C, Grawitz AB, et al. Break of T cell ignorance to a viral antigen in the liver induces hepatitis. *J Immunol* 2000;165:2415–2422.

256. Obermayer-Straub P, Strassburg CP, Manns MP. Target proteins in human autoimmunity: cytochromes P450 and UDP-glucuronosyl-transferases. *Can J Gastroenterol* 2000;14:429–439.

257. Ruiz-Moreno M, Rua MJ, Carreno V, et al. Autoimmune chronic hepatitis type 2 manifested during interferon therapy in children. *J Hepatol* 1991;12:265–266.

258. Cerasoli DM, McGrath J, Carding SR, et al. Low avidity recognition of a class II–restricted neo-self peptide by virus-specific T cells. *Intl Immunol* 1995;7:935–945.

259. Ashton-Rickardt PG, Bandeira A, Delaney JR, et al. Evidence for a differential avidity model of T cell selection in the thymus. *Cell* 1994;76:651–663.

260. Lo SK, Wendon J, Mieli-Vergani G, et al. Halothane-induced acute liver failure: continuing occurrence and use of liver transplantation. *Eur J Gastroenterol Hepatol* 1998;10:635–639.

261. Gut J, Christen U, Frey N, et al. Molecular mimicry in halothane hepatitis: biochemical and structural characterization of lipoylated autoantigens. *Toxicology* 1995;97:199–224.

262. Kosuda LL, Bigazzi PE. Chemical-induced autoimmunity. In: Smialowicz RJ, Holsapple MP, eds. *Experimental immunotoxicology.* Boca Raton, FL: CRC Press, 1996:419–465.

263. Mackay IR. Chronic hepatitis: effect of prolonged suppressive treatment and comparison of azathioprine with prednisolone. *Q J Med* 1968;37:379–392.

264. Al-Khalidi JA, Czaja AJ. Current concepts in the diagnosis, pathogenesis, and treatment of autoimmune hepatitis. *Mayo Clin Proc* 2001;76:1237–1252.

265. Kirk AP, Jain S, Pocock S, et al. Late results of the Royal Free Hospital prospective controlled trial of prednisolone therapy in hepatitis B surface antigen negative chronic active hepatitis. *Gut* 1980;21:78–83.

266. Sanchez-Urdazpal L, Czaja AJ, van Hoek B, et al. Prognostic features and role of liver transplantation in severe corticosteroid-treated autoimmune chronic active hepatitis. *Hepatology* 1992;15:215–221.

267. Neuberger J, Portmann B, Calne R, et al. Recurrence of autoimmune chronic active hepatitis following orthotopic liver grafting. *Transplantation* 1984;37:363–365.

268. Markus BH, Dickson ER, Grambsch PM, et al. Efficiency of liver transplantation in patients with primary biliary cirrhosis. *N Engl J Med* 1989;320:1709–1713.

269. Nashan B, Schlitt HJ, Tusch G, et al. Biliary malignancies in primary sclerosing cholangitis: timing for liver transplantation. *Hepatology* 1996;23:1105–1111.

270. Lopez de Castro JA. The pathogentic role of HLA-B27 in chronic arthritis. *Cur Opin Immunol* 1998;10:59–66.

271. Wildner G, Diedrichs-Mohring M, Thurau SR. Induction of arthritis and uveitis in Lewis rats by antigenic mimicry of peptides from HLA-B27 and cytokeratin. *Eur J Immunol* 2002;32:299–306.

272. Lee SJ, Im HY, Schueller WC. HLA-B27 positive juvenile arthritis with cardiac involvement preceding sacroiliac joint changes. *Heart* 2001;86:E19–E25.

273. Sun B, Rizzo LV, Sun S-H, et al. Genetic susceptibility to experimental autoimmune uveitis involves more than a predisposition to generate a T helper-1–like or a T helper-2–like response. *J Immunol* 1997;159:1004–1011.

274. Tarrant TK, Silver PB, Chan CC, et al. Endogenous IL-12 is required for induction and expression of experimental autoimmune uveitis. *J Immunol* 1998;161:122–127.

275. Rizzo LV, Morawetz RA, Miller-Rivero NE, et al. IL-4 and IL-10 are both required for the induction of oral tolerance. *J Immunol* 1999; 162:2613–2622.

276. Wildner G, Thurau SR. Orally induced bystander suppression in experimental autoimmune uveoretinitis occurs only in the periphery and not in the eye. *Euro J Immunol* 1995;25:1292–1297.

277. Wildner G, Thurau SR. Orally induced bystander suppression in experimental autoimmune uveoretinitis occurs only in the periphery and not in the eye. *Eur J Immunol* 1995;25:1292–1297.

278. Gangappa S, Sam Babu J, Thomas J, et al. Virus-induced immunoinflammatory lesions in the absence of viral antigen recognition. *J Immunol* 1998;161:4289–4300.

279. Thomas J, Rouse BT. Immunopathology of herpetic stromal keratitis: discordance in CD4+ T cell function between euthymic host and reconstituted SCID recipients. *J Immunol* 1998;160:3965–3970.

280. Chun S, Daheshia M, Lee S, et al. Immune modulation by IL-10 gene transfer via viral vector and plasmid DNA: implication for gene therapy. *Cell Immunol* 1999;194:194–204.

281. Panoutsakopoulou V, Sanchirico ME, Huster KM, et al. Analysis of the relationship between viral infection and autoimmune disease. *Immunity* 2001;15:137–147.

282. Kosiewicz MM, Alard P, Streilein JW. Alterations in cytokine production following intraocular injection of soluble protein antigen: impairment in IFN-g and induction of TGF-b and IL-4 production. *J Immunol* 1998;161:5382–5390.

283. Takeuchi M, Alard P, Streilein JW. TGF-b promotes immune deviation by altering accessory signals of antigen-presenting cells. *J Immunol* 1998;160:1589–1597.

284. Thurau SR, Diedrichs-Mohring M, Fricke H, et al. Oral tolerance with an HLA-peptide mimicking retinal autoantigen as a treatment of autoimmune uveitis. *Immunol Lett* 1999;68:205–212.

285. Wicks I, McColl G, Harrison L. New perspectives on rheumatoid arthritis. *Immunol Today* 1994;15:553–556.

286. Rudolphi U, Hohlbaum A, Lang B, et al. The B cell repertoire of patients with rheumatoid arthritis. Frequencies and specificities of peripheral blood B cells reacting with human IgG, human collagens, a mycobacterial heat shock protein and other antigens. *Clin Exp Immunol* 1993;92:404–411.

287. Dayan CM, Daniels GH. Chronic autoimmune thyroiditis. *N Engl J Med* 1996;335:99–107.

288. Weetman AP. Graves' disease. *N Engl J Med* 2000;343:1236–1248.

289. Vrbikova J, Janatkova I, Zamrazil V, et al. Epstein–Barr virus serology in patients with autoimmune thyroiditis. *Exp Clin Endocrinol Diabetes* 1996;104:89–92.

290. Tomer Y, Davies TF. Infections and autoimmune endocrine disease. *Baillieres Clin Endocrinol Metab* 1995;9:47–70.

291. Sellmeyer DE, Grunfeld C. Endocrine and metabolic disturbances in human immunodeficiency virus infection and the acquired immune deficiency syndrome. *Endocr Rev* 1996;17:518–532.

292. Grinspoon SK, Bilezikian JP. HIV disease and the endocrine system. *N Engl J Med* 1992;327:1360–1365.

293. Hellerstein MK. Endocrinology abnormalities. In: Cohen PT, Sande M, Volberding P, eds. *The AIDS knowledge base.* Boston: Massachusetts Medical Society, 1995:1–10.

294. Dluhy RG. The growing spectrum of HIV-related endocrine abnormalities. *J Clin Endocrinol Metab* 1990;70:563–565.

295. Heufelder AH, Hofbauer LC. Human immunodeficiency virus infection and the thyroid gland. *Eur J Endocrin* 1996;134:669–674.

296. Friedman ND, Spelman DW. Subacute thyroiditis presenting as pyrexia of unknown origin in a patient with human immunodeficiency virus infection. *Clin Infect Dis* 1999;29:1352–1353.

297. Jaeger P, Otto S, Speck RF, et al. Altered parathyroid gland function in severely immunocompromised patients infected with human immunodeficiency virus. *J Clin Endocrinol Metab* 1994;79:1701–1705.

298. Burch HB, Nagy EV, Lukes YG, et al. Nucleotide and amino acid homology between the human thyrotropin receptor and HIV-1 nef protein: identification and functional analysis. *Biochem Biophys Res Comm* 1991;181:498–505.

299. Wick G, Trieb K, Aguzzi A, et al. Possible role of human foamy virus in Graves' disease. *Intervirology* 1993;35:101–107.

300. Lagaye S, Vexiau P, Morozov V, et al. Human spumaretrovirus-related sequences in the DNA of leukocytes from patients with Graves disease. *Proc Natl Acad Sci USA* 1992;89:10070–10074.

301. Mine H, Kawai H, Yokoi K, et al. High frequencies of human T-lymphotropic virus type I (HTLV-I) infection and presence of HTLV-II proviral DNA in blood donors with anti-thyroid antibodies. *J Mol Med* 1996;74:471–477.

302. Yokoi K, Kawai H, Akaike M, et al. Presence of human T-lymphotropic virus type II-related genes in DNA of peripheral leukocytes from patients with autoimmune thyroid diseases. *J Med Virol* 1995;45:392–398.

303. Mizokami T, Okamura K, Ikenoue H, et al. A high prevalence of human T-lymphotropic virus type I carriers in patients with antithyroid antibodies. *Thyroid* 1994;4:415–419.

304. Akamine H, Takasu N, Komiya I, et al. Association of HTLV-1 with autoimmune thyroiditis in patients with adult T-cell leukemia (ATL) and in HTLV-I carriers. *Clin Endocrinol (Oxf)* 1996;45:461–466.

305. McMurray RW, Elbourne K. Hepatitis C virus infection and autoimmunity. *Semin Arthritus Rheum* 1997;26:689–701.

306. Cosserat J, Cacoub P, Bletry O. Immunological disorders in C virus chronic hepatitis. *Nephrol Dial Transplant* 1996;11:31–35.

307. Degos F. Natural history of hepatitis C virus infection. *Nephrol Dial Transplant* 1996;4:16–18.

308. Ganne-Carrie N, Medini A, Coderc E, et al. Latent autoimmune thyroiditis in untreated patients with HCV chronic hepatitis: a case-control study. *J Autoimmun* 2000;14:189–193.

309. Preziati D, La Rosa L, Covini G, et al. Autoimmunity and thyroid function in patients with chronic active hepatitis treated with recombinant interferon alpha-2a. *Eur J Endocrinol* 1995;132:587–593.

310. Gregorio GV, Jones H, Choudhuri K, et al. Autoantibody prevalence in chronic hepatitis B virus infection: effect in interferon alfa. *Hepatology* 1996;24:520–523.

311. Fernandez-Soto L, Gonzalez A, Escobar-Jimenez F, et al. Increased risk of autoimmune thyroid disease in hepatitis C vs Hepatitis B before, during, and after discontinuing interferon therapy. *Arch Intern Med* 1998;158:1445–1448.

312. Sever JL, South MA, Shaver KA. Delayed manifestations of congenital rubella. *Rev Infect Dis* 1985;7:S164–S169.

313. Klavinskis LS, Notkins AL, Oldstone MBA. Persistent viral infection of the thyroid gland: alteration of thyroid function in the absence of tissue injury. *Endocrinology* 1988;122:567–575.

314. Srinivassapa J, Gazelli C, Onodera T, et al. Virus-induced thyroiditis. *Endocrinology* 1988;122:563–566.

315. Onodera T, Awaya A. Anti-thyroglobulin antibodies induced with recombinant reovirus infection in BALB/c mice. *Immunology* 1990;71:581–585.

316. Ziemiecki A, Kromer G, Muller RG, et al. ev 22, a new endogenous avian leukosis virus locus found in chickens with spontaneous autoimmune thyroiditis. *Arch Virol* 1988;100:267–271.

317. Carter JK, Smith RE. Rapid induction of hypothyroidism by an avian leukosis virus. *Infect Immun* 1983;40:795–805.

318. Kuhr T, Hala K, Dietrich H, et al. Genetically determined target organ susceptibility in the pathogenesis of spontaneous autoimmune thyroiditis: aberrant expression of HMC-class II antigens and the possible role of virus. *J Autoimmun* 1994;7:13–25.

319. Mason LJ, Timothy LM, Isenberg DA, et al. Immunization with a paptide of Sm B/B' results in limited epitope spreading but not autoimmune disease. *J Immunol* 1999;162:5099–5105.

320. Seddon B, Mason D. Peripheral autoantigen induces regulatory T cells that prevent autoimmunity. *J Exp Med* 1999;189:877–882.

321. Seddon B, Mason D. Peripheral autoantigen induces regulatory T cells that prevent autoimmunity. *J Exp Med* 1999;189:877–881.

322. Humbert P, Dupond JL, Vuitton D, et al. Dermatological autoimmune diseases and the multiple autoimmune syndromes. *Acta Derm Venereol Suppl (Stockh)* 1989;148:1–8.

323. Korman N. Pemphigus. *J Am Acad Dermatol* 1988;18:1219–1238.

324. Kawana S, Geoghegan WD, Jordon RE, et al. Deposition of the membrane attack complex of complement in pemphigus vulgaris and pemphigus foliaceus skin. *J Invest Dermatol* 1989;92:588–592.

325. Sinha AA, Brautbar C, Szafer F, et al. A newly characterized HLA DQ beta allele associated with pemphigus vulgaris. *Science* 1988; 239:1026–1029.

326. Camisa C, Helm TN. Paraneoplastic pemphigus is a distinct neoplasia-induced autoimmune disease. *Arch Dermatol* 1993;129:883–886.

327. Hall RP, 3rd. Dermatitis herpetiformis. *J Invest Dermatol* 1992;99: 873–881.

328. Collier PM, Wojnarowska F, Welsh K, et al. Adult linear IgA disease and chronic bullous disease of childhood: the association with human lymphocyte antigens Cw7, B8, DR3 and tumour necrosis factor influences disease expression. *Br J Dermatol* 1999;141:867–875.

329. Yamanaka T, Straumfors A, Morton H, et al. M cell pockets of human Peyer's patches are specialized extensions of germinal centers. *Eur J Immunol* 2001;31:107–117.

330. Iwasaki A, Kelsall BL. Localization of distinct Peyer's patch dendritic cell subsets and their recruitment by chemokines macrophage inflammatory protein (MIP)-3alpha, MIP-3beta, and secondary lymphoid organ chemokine. *J Exp Med* 2000;191:1381–1394.

331. Harrison LC, Dempsey-Collier M, Kramer DR, et al. Aerosol insulin induces regulatory CD8 gamma delta T cells that prevent murine insulin-dependent diabetes. *J Exp Med* 1996;184:2167–2174.

332. Hanninen A, Harrison LC. gd T cells as mediators of mucosal tolerance: the autoimmune diabetes model. *Immunol Rev* 2000;173:109–119.

333. Chen Y, Inobe J, Kuchroo VK, et al. Oral tolerance in myelin basic protein T-cell receptor transgenic mice: suppression of autoimmune encephalomyelitis and dose-dependent induction of regulatory cells. *Proc Natl Acad Sci U S A* 1996;93:388–391.

334. Strickland RG, Mackay IR. A reappraisal of the nature and significance of chronic atrophic gastritis. *Am J Dig Dis* 1973;18:426–440.

335. Carmel R. Prevalence of undiagnosed pernicious anemia in the elderly. *Arch Intern Med* 1996;156:1097–1100.

336. Toh BH, van Driel IR, Gleeson PA. Pernicious anemia. *N Engl J Med* 1997;337:1441–1448.

337. Alderuccio F, Sentry JW, Marshall AC, et al. Animal models of human disease: experimental autoimmune gastritis—a model for autoimmune gastritis and pernicious anemia. *Clin Immunol* 2002;102:48–58.

338. Thornton AM, Shevach EM. Suppressor effector function of CD4+CD25+ immunoregulatory T cells is antigen nonspecific. *J Immunol* 2000;164:183–190.

339. Itoh M, Takahashi T, Sakaguchi N, et al. Thymus and autoimmunity: production of CD25+CD4+ naturally anergic and suppressive T cells as a key function of the thymus in maintaining immunologic self-tolerance. *J Immunol* 1999;162:5317–5326.

340. Hanauer SB. Inflammatory bowel disease. *N Engl J Med* 1996;334: 841–848.

341. Powers AC, Bavik K, Tremble J, et al. Comparative analysis of epitope recognition of glutamic acid decarboxylase (GAD) by autoantibodies from different autoimmune disorders. *Clin Exp Immunol* 1999;118:349–356.

342. Winer S, Astsaturov I, Cheung RK, et al. Type I diabetes and multiple sclerosis patients target islet plus central nervous system autoantigens; nonimmunized nonobese diabetic mice can develop autoimmune encephalitis. *J Immunol* 2001;166:2831–2841.

343. Salomon B, Rhee L, Bour-Jordan H, et al. Development of spontaneous autoimmune peripheral polyneuropathy in B7-2–deficient NOD mice. *J Exp Med* 2001;194:677–684.

CHAPTER 46

Immunological Mechanisms of Allergic Disorders

Marsha Wills-Karp and Gurjit K. Khurana Hershey

Historical Perspective
General Features of Atopic Disorders
Allergens
 Definitions and General Characteristics of Allergens · Specific Allergens
CD4$^+$ Th2 Polarized Immune Responses in Atopy
Factors Contributing to Th2 Cell Development in Atopic Individuals
 Overview · Genetic Influences on Allergen Sensitization · Environmental Influences on Allergen Sensitization · Antigen Presentation in Atopic Individuals
Cytokine Regulation of Th2 Differentiation in Atopy
 Potential Dysregulation of Th2 Differentiation Factors in Atopy · Altered Interleukin-12 Production in Atopic Disorders
Th2 Cytokine Regulation of Allergic Inflammation
Regulation of Immunoglobulin E Synthesis
 Isotype Class Switching to Immunoglobulin E Production · Deletional Switch Recombination · Immunoglobulin E Receptors · Crystallized Fragment ε Receptor I–Mediated Signal Transduction · Regulation of Crystallized Fragment ε Receptor I Surface Expression · Crystallized Fragment ε Receptor II (CD23)
Effector Cells of the Allergic Response
 Overview · Development of Mast Cells and Basophils · Eosinophil Biology · Th2 Cells as Effector Cells
Characteristics of Specific Atopic Disorders
 Anaphylaxis · Allergic Rhinitis · Food Allergy · Atopic Dermatitis · Asthma
Acknowledgments
References

This chapter provides an overview of the current understanding of diseases under the nosological rubric of "allergy." The diverse diseases so gathered (anaphylaxis, asthma, allergic rhinitis, atopic dermatitis, food allergy) are united at least superficially by the facts that (a) all these conditions result from the expression of harmful immune responses; (b) all the implicated immune responses are associated with the generation of immunoglobulin E (IgE) (whether IgE is integral to pathogenesis or not); and (c) the antigens driving such immune responses are not derived from infectious pathogens (a criterion honored in the breach in such conditions as anaphylaxis caused by spillage of the contents of echinococcal cysts). The basic cellular and molecular mechanisms that underlie the pathogenesis of allergic disorders, as well as the environmental and genetic substrates for their generation, are closely considered. Although much of the current understanding of mechanism in allergic disease has been derived from the study of animal models, mechanistic data on human disease are discussed wherever possible. The chapter finishes with a brief survey of the clinical and therapeutic characteristics of the

major human allergic disorders. Readers are referred to clinically oriented texts for a fuller discussion of such issues.

HISTORICAL PERSPECTIVE

The term *allergy* was coined in 1906 by the astute pediatrician Clemens von Pirquet, who argued that antigenic stimuli led to two distinct categories or patterns of response: immunity and allergy (1). The former, an old concept, referred to responses leading to protection from infectious challenge. The latter, a novel theoretical construct, referred to "altered reactivity" that itself led to host damage. This idea of allergy—that is, the notion that the immune response itself can be a cause of disease—was a powerful conceptual advance that led to novel insights into the pathogenesis of a variety of diseases. Quite naturally, this concept of allergy initially included autoimmune diseases, in addition to conditions that are classified as allergic diseases today. As noted previously, current usage largely restricts the term *allergy* to diseases caused by the subset of harmful immune responses (to pathogen-unrelated antigens) that is associated with the generation of IgE. There is some artificiality to this. Very similar patterns of immune response can drive pathological processes in response to infectious pathogens such as tissue helminths. Furthermore, IgE may be more a marker of an underlying pattern of immune response than a mechanistic participant in the immunopathogenesis of at least some subtypes of allergic disease. As long as these caveats are kept in mind, however, this concept of allergic disease long enshrined by clinical subspecialists has considerable theoretical and practical utility.

The trail leading to the specific identification of IgE began with demonstration by Prausnitz and Kuster (2) in 1921 that hypersensitivity to an antigen could be passively transferred in serum from one individual to another. The instigating antigens (*allergens,* in contemporary parlance) were known as *atopens,* and the mysterious plasma factor that conferred sensitivity was called *atopic reagin.* It was not until 1966 that Ishizaka et al. (3–5) demonstrated that reaginic activity was carried by a novel class of immunoglobulin, IgE. The word *atopy* has since come to denote the propensity for developing allergic reactions to common environmental antigens (allergens), a propensity defined operationally by elevations in serum levels of IgE reactive with, or by skin test reactivity to, such antigens. Definitions of other key terms are given in Table 1.

TABLE 1. *Definitions of key terms*

Allergen	An environmental antigen that typically elicits allergic responses in susceptible individuals. These antigens ordinarily have little or no intrinsic toxicity.
Allergy	Clinically adverse reactions to environmental antigens reflecting acquired immune responses that are marked phenotypically by the presence of allergen-specific IgE, along with mast cell and eosinophil recruitment and/or activation. CD4+ T cells that produce a Th2 profile of cytokines (IL-4, IL-5, and IL-13) are thought to be central to the development of allergic responses.
Atopy	The propensity for developing immediate hypersensitivity reactions to common environmental allergens, defined operationally by elevations in serum levels of IgE reactive with allergens or by skin-test reactivity to allergens.
Allergic diseases	The group of clinical disorders [such as allergic asthma, allergic rhinitis (hay fever), and atopic dermatitis] in which IgE-associated immune responses, typically directed against otherwise innocuous environmental allergens, are thought to have a pathogenic role.

IgE, immunoglobulin E; IL, interleukin; Th2, T helper cell type 2.

Before proceeding to a direct focus on allergic diseases, it is useful to consider the classification scheme for harmful immune responses, or hypersensitivity reactions, initially outlined by Coombs and Gell (6). This widely used formulation, modified by Janeway and Travers (7) and Kay et al. (8), systematizes the major mechanisms initiating injurious processes that are mediated by the adaptive (as opposed to the innate) immune system (Table 2). The scheme delineates four classes of hypersensitivity: (a) type I, or immediate hypersensitivity, in which allergens interact with specific IgE [or, in the mouse, immunoglobulin G1 (IgG1)] on the surface of mast cells or basophils, which leads to the release of a variety of pharmacoactive inflammatory mediators; (b) type II hypersensitivity, or cytotoxic reactions, in which antibodies react with cell surface–associated antigens or receptors, which leads to tissue injury, altered receptor function, or both; (c) type III hypersensitivity, or immune complex reactions, in which damage is mediated by immune complexes generated by antibody in the presence of antigen excess; and (d) type IV, or delayed-type hypersensitivity, in which harmful T cell–driven inflammatory processes proceed without any necessary role for antibodies.

In light of this classification scheme, beloved of generations of immunologists and medical students alike, allergic reactions seem to fall squarely into the category of type I hypersensitivity responses. Enhanced mechanistic understanding of allergic processes has inevitably complicated matters, however. Most allergic responses are multiphasic, combining elements of diverse hypersensitivity types into one "allergic cascade." For example, the initial phase of the clinical asthmatic response to an aeroallergen is often caused by immediate (type I) hypersensitivity. However, this is frequently followed by late-phase responses more characteristic of delayed-type (type IV) hypersensitivity reactions.

GENERAL FEATURES OF ATOPIC DISORDERS

Allergic disorders are categorized by the anatomical site where disease is manifested: atopic dermatitis (skin), atopic rhinitis (nasal passages), atopic asthma (lung), food allergy (gut), and anaphylaxis (systemic) (Table 3). All these clinical entities involve a similar allergic effector cascade, at least superficially; differences in presentation probably reflect variation in the physiochemical characteristics of the allergen, the site of initial sensitization to the allergen, the route and dose of allergen exposure, and the programmed response of resident cells (e.g., epithelial cells) to injury and inflammation. Anaphylaxis aside, there is often a stereotypical sequence in the development of allergic manifestations of disease in patients with atopy, with early expression of food sensitivities or atopic dermatitis, and the subsequent development of either atopic rhinitis or asthma. Many individuals have all three of the latter clinical entities, which form the "atopic triad."

Atopic disorders represent a major health problem worldwide, affecting 5% to 30% of the population. The incidence of atopic diseases, including asthma, atopic rhinitis, and atopic

TABLE 2. *Modified coombs–gell classification of the four major types of initiating mechanisms of immunologically mediated adverse ("hypersensitivity") reactions*

Immunological specificity	Type 1: IgE antibody (+ IgG1 n mouse)	Type II: IgG antibody		Type III: IgG antibody	Type IV: T cells		
		a	b		a1 Th1 cells	a2 Th2 cells	B cytolytic T cells
Antigen	Soluble antigen "allergen"	Cell- or matrix-associated antigen	Cell surface receptors	Soluble antigen	Soluble antigen	Soluble antigen	Cell-associated antigen
Effector mechanism	FcεRI or FcγRIII-dependent mast cell/basophil activation, with release of mediators/cytokines	Complement, FcγR+ professional phagocytes, NK cells	Antibody alters signaling	FcγR+ cells, complement	Th1-associated effectors (e.g., macrophages)	Th2-associated effectors (e.g., eosinophils, basophils)	Direct cytotoxicity
Initial consequences	Rapidly developing (seconds to minutes) effects of mediators on target cells (usually not involving direct cytotoxicity)	Cell death and/or tissue injury	Pathology due to increased or diminished receptor-dependent cell function	Inflammation associated with recruitment and activation of neutrophils and other leukocytes	Chronic inflammation Reactions develop slowly (hours to days) and can persist for long periods	Chronic inflammation	Death of target cells
Examples and notes	IgE (or, in mouse, IgG1)–dependent anaphylaxis (potentially fatal systemic reaction) or passive cutaneous anaphylaxis (a local reaction)	Certain drug reactions and reactions to incompatible blood transfusions	Graves' disease (thyroid-stimulating agonist antibody); myasthenia gravis (antagonist antibody to acetylcholine receptor)	(Including mast cells in the mouse); Arthus reaction and other "immune complex"–mediated reactions	Contact dermatitis, tuberculin reaction	Chronic allergic inflammation (type I reactions may also contribute to chronic allergic inflammation)	Reactions to certain viral infected cells, certain forms of graft rejection

FcεRI, crystallized fragment ε receptor type I; FcγRIII, crystallized fragment γ receptor type III; IgE, immunoglobulin E; IgG1, immunoglobulin G1; NK, natural killer; Th1, Th2, T helper cell type 1, type 2.

TABLE 3. *Major features of allergic immune responses*

1. Responses are elicited by certain groups of environmental allergens such as foods, drugs, and proteins derived from pollens, insects (house dust mite), and animal dander.
2. In susceptible individuals, allergens are presented to naive T cells by dendritic cells residing in the mucosa of the skin, GI tract, or respiratory tract. For reasons that are not well understood, T cells of atopic individuals undergo differentiation to a Th2 cytokine–producing pattern.
3. Elaboration of Th2 cytokines (IL-4, IL-5, IL-3, IL-9) initiates the allergic cascade through their combined ability to regulate IgE production, FcεRI expression, mast cell phenotype and development, recruitment, and activation of eosinophils.
4. Under the control of Th2 cell–derived signals (IL-4, IL-13, and CD40L), B cells undergo class switching to production of the IgE subclass.
5. Upon reexposure to the offending allergen, acute responses occurring within minutes of allergen exposure result from release of preformed mediators (histamine, tryptase) from FcεRI-bearing cells via the cross-linking of allergen and IgE on their surface. Cells activated during the acute phase also release cytokines and mediators, which perpetuate the Th2-driven response.
6. Late-phase responses result from the combined effects of inflammatory cells (eosinophils and T cells) recruited to the tissues within 6–24 hours after the initial allergen exposure.
7. Repeated allergen exposures in the context of an already inflamed tissue results in structural changes (remodeling), such as smooth muscle thickening, tissue fibrosis, and mucous cell hyperplasia.

FcεRI, crystallized fragment ε receptor type I; GI, gastrointestinal; IgE, immunoglobulin E; IL, interleukin; Th2, T helper cell type 2.

dermatitis, has increased dramatically since the 1990s in industrialized countries (9–11). In such countries, 30% of the population manifest some form of atopic disease at some time in their lives. The widespread prevalence and morbidity of atopic diseases impose a heavy burden on society. The economic impact of allergic diseases in the United States, including health care costs and lost productivity, were estimated at $6.4 billion in 1990 alone.

The defining feature of atopy is the production of IgE in response to exposure (through mucosae or the skin) to a variety of ubiquitous, and otherwise innocuous, antigens. Such IgE production is a tightly regulated process, part of a complex network of cellular and molecular events necessary for the development of the allergic response. Initiation of this response appears to occur with presentation of the allergen by antigen-presenting cells (APCs) to CD4$^+$ T cells residing in mucosae (a process referred to as *sensitization*). In atopic individuals, responding allergen-specific T cells polarize to a type 2 T helper (Th2) pattern of production, with the elaboration of cytokines such as interleukin (IL)–4, IL-13, IL-5, and IL-9 (*vide infra*). Although T cells from nonatopic individuals clearly recognize these same environmental antigens, the expansion and differentiation of such T cells does not involve Th2

deviation. The mechanisms controlling allergen-associated Th2 polarization in atopic individuals are not completely understood. It appears likely that genetic and environmental factors affecting the antigen-presenting process play a key role.

The elaboration of Th2 cytokines sets into motion a complex series of events leading to IgE production: the development, recruitment, and activation of effector cells such as mast cells, basophils, eosinophils, and effector T cells and a variety of downstream effector cascades.

Once an atopic individual is sensitized, the manifestations of allergy are readily induced upon reexposure to the allergen (the elicitation phase). Although the effector phases of IgE-associated atopic disorders generally appear as a continuum, it is useful to define three temporal patterns: (a) acute reactions (developing within seconds to minutes of allergen exposure); (b) delayed or late reactions (developing hours after allergen exposure); and (c) chronic reactions (developing over days to years). Acute reactions result from cross-linking of high-affinity crystallized fragment ε receptor I (FcεRI) on the surface of mast cells/basophils, induced by the interaction of allergen with cell-bound IgE. Such cross-linking results in the release of vasoactive mediators, chemotactic factors, and cytokines, which initiate the so-called allergic cascade. This early reaction may resolve within minutes but is often followed by late-phase responses that begin 3 to 6 hours after antigen challenge and may persist for days in the absence of therapy. The pathophysiological consequences of chronic reactions are associated with the migration of eosinophils and lymphocytes from the blood into affected tissues.

ALLERGENS

Definition and General Characteristics of Allergens

Allergens are, by definition, antigens that can elicit specific IgE responses in genetically susceptible individuals. The list of structures that have been identified as allergens represents a tiny subset of the antigenic universe to which humans are routinely exposed. Allergens are generally subdivided by route of exposure and source. Such allergens include aeroallergens (pollens, mold spores, animal dander, fecal material excreted by mites and cockroaches), food allergens, allergens transmitted by stinging insects, pharmaceuticals, and latex.

Allergen Classification

Purified allergens are named in accordance with guidelines published in 1994 by the World Health Organization International Union of Immunologic Societies Allergen Nomenclature Sub-Committee, on the basis of their source and the order in which they were discovered (12). The names incorporate the first three letters of the genus and the first letter of the species from which the allergen is derived, plus an Arabic numeral that is used to denote structurally homologous allergens from the same species. For example, the two major species of dust mite (*Dermatophagoides pteronyssinus* and *Dermatophagoides farinae*) are designated as Der p (Der p 1, Der p 2) and Der f (Der f 1, Der f 2). Other major allergens include Fel d 1 from the cat, Bet v 1 from birch pollen, Amb a 1 from ragweed pollen, and Phl p 1 from the pollen of timothy grass.

Biological Properties of Allergens

The major allergens are a diverse group of proteins in which no one biological property appears to be dominant. However, recent studies indicate that a number of allergens from diverse sources have enzymatic activity that may bias the immune response toward a Th2 phenotype. For example, Der p 1 is a 25-kDa cysteine protease that has been shown to cleave CD25, the 55-kDa α subunit of the IL-2 receptor (13,14). As a result of cleavage of CD25, peripheral blood T cells show markedly diminished proliferation and interferon (IFN)-γ secretion in response to potent stimulation by anti-CD3 monoclonal antibody. These findings suggest that Der p 1 decreases the growth and expansion of antigen-specific Th1 cells, augmenting expansion of the antigen-specific Th2 cells that favor a proallergic response. Der p 1 may also contribute to the allergic phenotype by cleaving CD23 on murine B cells that would normally serve to inhibit IgE synthesis, thereby disrupting an important negative regulator of IgE production (15). Yet another potential mechanism by which proteolytic allergens such as Der p 1 may alter the immune response is through cleavage of complement components into their active components at the mucosal surface (16). Moreover, through its ability to disrupt epithelial architecture, Der p 1 may also facilitate its own passage across the mucosal surface epithelium, thus enhancing its own access to immune cells. Although allergens such as Der p 1 can potentially create a microenvironment conducive to Th2 cell expansion, normal individuals do not mount Th2 responses when exposed to these allergens, which suggests that despite the nature of these antigens, other factors are necessary for the development of allergic outcomes in susceptible individuals.

Specific Allergens

Aeroallergens

Aeroallergens are airborne proteins or glycoproteins derived from a variety of sources, including pollinating trees and grasses, mold spores, animal dander (cat, dog, and rodent), and particulates secreted by dust mites and cockroaches. Factors that affect the growth or accumulation of these latter organisms (high humidity, well-insulated homes, fitted carpets) increase the levels of these allergens in the indoor environment. Exposure to such indoor allergens is also dependent on a variety of geographical, climatic, and socioeconomic factors. Interestingly, whereas indoor allergens are more closely associated with development of asthma, outdoor allergens (e.g., ragweed pollen) appear to be more important in the

development of allergic rhinitis. The mechanisms underlying such associations remain obscure. Speculation has focused on the physiochemical nature (size, chemical structure) and pattern of exposure (acute vs. chronic).

Food Allergens

Although hundreds of different foods are ingested, only a small number account for most food allergies. The most common foods responsible for childhood food allergy are milk, eggs, peanuts, soy, and wheat. Responses to food allergens are relatively common in children younger than two years but usually disappear as the children age. In contrast, in adult food allergy, the most common offending foods are peanuts, tree nuts, fish, and shellfish. Most food allergens have been found to be water-soluble glycoproteins ranging in size from 10 to 40 kDa that are heat and acid stable and resistant to proteolytic degradation. Exceptions to these are fruit and vegetable allergens. Reactions to food allergens can be fatal; one of the most severe food reactions occurs in response to peanut allergens.

Latex Allergens

A new class of antigens associated with immediate hypersensitivity reactions to latex rubber has been identified in the last few years. Latex allergy is frequently seen in health care workers, rubber industry workers, and patients undergoing multiple surgical procedures in early infancy (17,18). Symptoms manifest as contact urticaria, rhinoconjunctivitis, asthma, and mucosal swelling. However, severe reactions and death have occurred upon exposure to latex balloons on the rectal mucosa, especially in children with spina bifida. Multiple individual latex allergens have been identified, of which eight have received an international nomenclature designation. These include Hev b 1, rubber elongation factor; Hev b 2, β-1,3-glucanase; Hev b 3, which is homologous to Hev b 1; Hev b 4, a microhelix component; Hev b 6, prohevein/hevein; and Hev b7, a patatin-like protein (19). It has been appreciated that individuals with allergies to certain fruits such as banana, avocado, kiwi, and chestnut develop clinical symptoms upon initial contact with latex (20). This phenomenon has been coined "the latex-fruit syndrome." It is thought to occur as a result of the presence of IgE reactive to enzymes such as β-glucanase and chitinases that are present in both fruits and rubber.

Pharmaceuticals

Adverse drug reactions are relatively common clinical problems. Most conventional pharmaceutical agents are relatively low-molecular-weight compounds that become allergens only after their haptenization to endogenous proteins. The penicillins are classic instigators of allergic reactions. Penicillin is associated with a relatively high incidence of allergic reactions because of the chemical reactivity of penicillin and its metabolites. Although penicillin itself is the major allergen, its metabolic products, penicilloate and penilloate, are minor allergens but are responsible for a disproportionate share of severe, life-threatening reactions. Moreover, the drug is often administered parenterally, which greatly increases the probability that an adverse IgE-associated response will be fatal. Cephalosporin drugs are structurally similar to penicillin, and penicillin-allergic individuals may have IgE antibodies that cross-react with cephalosporin. Other agents, such as quaternary ammonium compounds (neuromuscular blocking agents) and sulfonamides (antibiotics) are relatively common stimuli of allergic reactions.

Insect Venom Allergens

Hypersensitivity to venom of stinging insects develops in both nonatopic and atopic individuals. Individuals are sensitized when relatively high levels of proteins (approximately 50 μg) in venom are injected subcutaneously during a sting. The venom-associated allergens of several vespids (yellow jacket, wasp, fire ant, and white-faced hornet) are cross-reactive and include antigen 5, phospholipase, and hyaluronidase. The honeybee venom contains distinct allergens, including two major ones, phospholipase A_2 and hyaluronidase, and a less important one, melittin. Many of these allergens have proteolytic activity.

CD4+ Th2 POLARIZED IMMUNE RESPONSES IN ATOPY

As the primary orchestrators of specific immune responses to foreign antigens, the T-lymphocyte has been implicated in the pathogenesis of allergic diseases. Several lines of evidence support a causal role for T-lymphocytes in allergic disorders. Increased numbers of T-lymphocytes are found in the bronchial mucosa, nasal mucosa, and skin of patients with allergic asthma, rhinitis, and dermatitis, respectively, in comparison with nonatopic controls (21–23). In asthma and allergic rhinitis, CD4+ T cells predominate. In atopic dermatitis, however, excess CD4+ and CD8+ T populations are present in skin lesions (18). Furthermore, there is a generalized increase in T-cell activation in allergic individuals both at the site of disease and systemically. Increased cell-surface expression of T-cell activation markers such as the IL-2 receptor (IL-2R), class II major histocompatibility complex (MHC) antigens [human leukocyte antigen (HLA)–DR], and very late activation antigen (VLA)–1 have been observed in all disorders in the atopic triad (22,23).

As has been covered in detail in other sections of this text, functional subsets of CD4+ T cells have been distinguished at both clonal and population levels by the unique profiles of cytokines that they produce (24,25). The differential presence of these cytokine phenotypes in a variety of allergic and infectious diseases both in mice and in humans has provided descriptive power and theoretical insight into disease pathogenesis (25–27). Th1 cells producing tumor necrosis

factor (TNF) β and IFN-γ are critical in the development of cell-mediated immunity, macrophage activation, and the production of complement-fixing antibody isotypes (24,25). Th2 cells producing IL-4, IL-13, IL-5, IL-9, and IL-6 are important in the stimulation of IgE production, mucosal mastocytosis, eosinophilia, and macrophage deactivation (24,25).

An immunopathogenic role for Th2 cells in allergy was initially sought on the basis of the importance of these cytokines in IgE synthesis, along with eosinophil and mast cell regulation. Several lines of evidence support the involvement of these cytokines in the pathogenesis of allergic disorders. First, T cells at the site of disease in allergic individuals exhibit Th2 deviation (28–30). Specifically, T cells from both the bronchoalveolar lavage (BAL) fluids and bronchial biopsy specimens of allergic asthmatic patients express elevated levels of messenger ribonucleic acid (RNA) for IL-4, IL-13, granulocyte-macrophage colony-stimulating factor (GM-CSF), and IL-5. A similar T-cell phenotype is observed in the nasal mucosa of patients with atopic rhinitis (31). In patients with atopic dermatitis, elevated Th2 cytokines (IL-4, IL-13, IL-5) and their receptors (IL-4R, IL-5 receptor) are found in skin lesions in acute disease (32), whereas cytokine patterns in chronic lesions are mixed, both Th2 cytokines (IL-5 and IL-13) and Th1 cytokines (IFN-γ), being expressed (33,34). Second, it has been shown that successful therapeutic treatment of these disorders is associated with shifting of the cytokine phenotype from a Th2 to a Th1 pattern. For example, steroid treatment decreases IL-4 and IL-5 levels, while simultaneously increasing IFN-γ levels in the BAL of asthmatic patients (35). Both steroid treatment and immunotherapeutic regimens result in reductions in Th2 cytokine levels in the nasal mucosa (36) and allergen-stimulated peripheral blood mononuclear cells (PBMCs) (37) of patients with allergic rhinitis. Third, the increased numbers of activated T cells seen in these disorders correlate directly with both the numbers of activated eosinophils and the severity of each type of allergic disorder (23,38).

Although there is considerable descriptive evidence that CD4+ T-lymphocytes and Th2 cytokines are important in the pathogenesis of atopic disorders in humans, definitive proof is, of course, difficult to obtain. As a result, experimental animal models have been extremely useful in mechanistic delineation of the role of CD4+ T cells and T cell–derived cytokines in the pathogenesis of allergic disorders. Murine models of antigen-driven asthma have consistently revealed a causal role for CD4+ T cells in the development of the signs of allergic airway disease (39,40). In these models, sensitization with various allergens (ovalbumin, house dust mite, ragweed, Aspergillus species) by either intraperitoneal injections or airway challenge, followed by direct airway challenge, induces a phenotype closely resembling that observed in asthmatic humans (39,40). Specifically, allergen sensitization and challenge result in airway hyperresponsiveness, eosinophilic inflammation, elevations in allergen-specific IgE levels, and mucus hypersecretion. Regardless of mouse strains or exposure protocols, an absolute requirement for CD4$^+$ T cells for the development of allergic responses is clear in such models (39). A lack of CD4$^+$ T cells, achieved by either antibody depletion (39) or gene targeting (41), is associated with prevention of the development of allergen-induced airway responses. Conversely, depletion of CD8$^+$ cells does not affect airway responses to allergen challenge in mice (42). Furthermore, adoptive transfer of Th2 clones into the mouse lung can induce allergic airway symptoms (43). The involvement of each of the specific Th2 cytokines in atopic airway responses has been demonstrated in studies in which IL-4, IL-5, IL-13, and IL-9 have been manipulated through either antibody blockade (43,44) or gene targeting (45–48). Specifically, IL-4, through its critical role in Th2 differentiation, has been shown to be essential in the initiation of allergic airway responses (49,50). Collectively, the Th2 cytokines orchestrate the elicitation of the allergic response through their ability to regulate IgE production and recruitment and activation of various effector cells (e.g., mast cells, eosinophils). On the other hand, studies have shown that the administration of agents such as IL-12 and IFN-γ that inhibit Th2 cytokine production and stimulate Th1 pathways prevent the development of allergen-induced airway hyperresponsiveness and eosinophilic inflammation in murine models (51–53). Conversely, mice deficient in T-bet, a transcription factor important in IFN-γ secretion, spontaneously develop Th2-mediated allergic airway responses (54). Along these lines, prior infection of sensitized mice with bacille Calmette-Guérin (BCG) (55) or administration of CpG oligonucleotides (56) has resulted in suppression of eosinophilic airway inflammation, concomitant with a shift in cytokine production to a protective type-1 profile.

Similar mouse models have been used to study the pathogenesis of atopic rhinitis (57,58), food allergy (59), and atopic dermatitis (48). Although not as many laboratories have examined the effects of respiratory antigen exposure on the nasal mucosa, a role for CD4$^+$ T cells has also been established in a murine model of nasal allergy (60). Specifically, blockade of CD4$^+$ T cells before sensitization prevented the development of nasal symptoms and eosinophilia.

Oral exposure of mice to antigens such as ovalbumin and peanuts has been shown to induce responses similar to those observed in food-allergic individuals with infiltration of the large intestine with eosinophils, T cells, and mast cells. Functionally, these exposures are associated with diarrhea and, in some cases, with anaphylactic reactions. Adoptive transfer of primed CD4$^+$ T cells has been shown to simulate antigen responses in the gut, whereas blockade of IL-4 (61) has been shown to inhibit both the cellular response and the intestinal symptoms. Conversely, administration of recombinant IL-12 decreased anaphylactic responses to peanut antigens (59).

One of the most commonly used animal models of atopic dermatitis is one in which the NC/Nga strain of mice spontaneously develops an eczematous atopic dermatitis–like skin lesion when kept in conventional but not pathogen-free surroundings (62). The skin lesions in NC/Nga mice are characterized by infiltration with lymphocytes, eosinophils, and macrophages and with mast cell degranulation. The lesions develop concomitantly with elevations in serum IgE levels. Findings consistent with the mixed cytokine pattern observed in the skin of humans with atopic dermatitis are IL-4 and IL-5 in the lesions earlier on; IFN-γ is detected in the later stages. A role for CD4$^+$ T cells in development of these lesions has been demonstrated in that mice without recombination activating gene type 2 (RAG2$^{-/-}$) do not develop lesions (63). Interestingly, treatment of mice with IFN-γ, IL-12, and IL-18 early during their lives inhibits development of lesions and elevations in IgE levels (64). Moreover, treatment of NC/Nga mice with tacrolimus hydrate (FK506) suppresses skin infiltration and suppresses IL-4 and IL-5 production as well as IgE production (65).

FACTORS CONTRIBUTING TO Th2 CELL DEVELOPMENT IN ATOPIC INDIVIDUALS

Overview

Very little is known conclusively about the underlying causes of the aberrant expansion of Th2 cells in atopic humans. Naïve T helper cells have the ability to differentiate into either Th1 or Th2 cells, regardless of the specific T-cell receptor epitope. Although many immune responses are likely to retain a balanced (Th0) phenotype, responses may be polarized to either the Th1 or Th2 type. This process may be influenced by many factors, including (a) the genetic background of the host, (b) the antigen dose, (c) environmental factors, (d) the type and function of APCs involved in the interaction with naïve T cells, and (e) the polarizing cytokine microenvironment during antigen presentation. There are supportive data for each of these determinants in atopic diseases (Fig. 1).

Genetic Influences on Allergen Sensitization

The production of a Th2 pattern of cytokines appears to be genetically controlled and established early during childhood (66,67). In an elegant longitudinal study of children, Martinez et al. (66) and Prescott et al. (67) showed that the propensity for developing allergic asthma is associated with low stimulated levels of IFN-γ in children at 9 months of age, which suggests that a type 1 response is a protective factor. Furthermore, low stimulated levels of IL-2 and IFN-γ at 9 months of age were positively correlated with parental immediate skin test reactivity. In this regard, familial aggregation and twin studies have confirmed a fundamental contribution of genetic factors to the development of atopy and specific clinical atopic phenotypes (68). Specifically, individuals with a first-degree relative with atopy are at a significantly greater risk of developing atopy. Moreover, individuals with two atopic parents are at greater risk of developing an allergic disease than are those with only one atopic parent. Further support for this contention is the fact that there is a greater concordance for atopic disease between monozygotic twins than between dizygotic twins (69–71), although the concordance

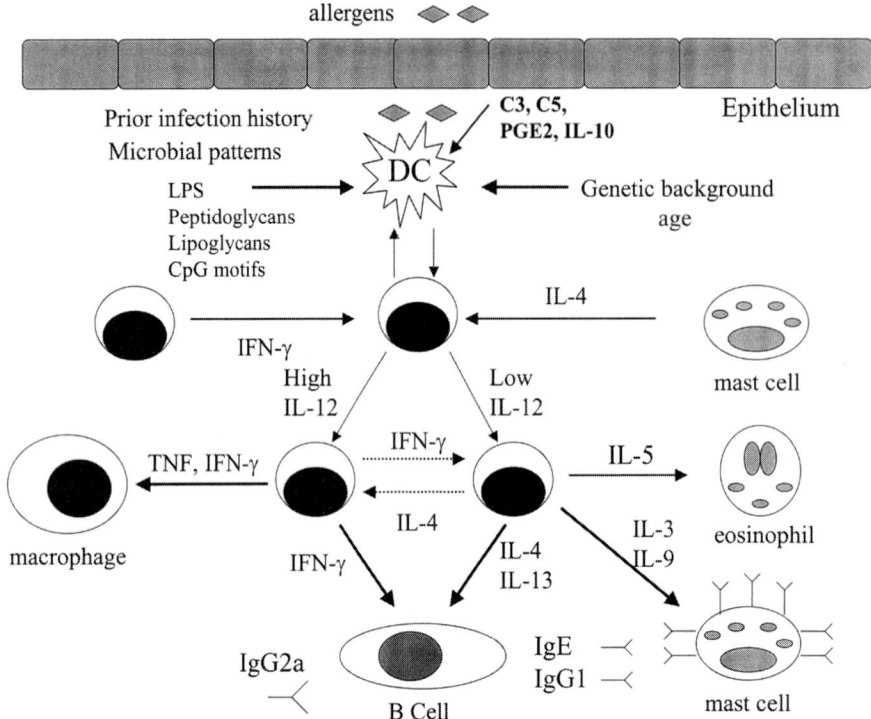

FIG. 1. Factors influencing antigen presentation and T-cell differentiation in atopy. Allergen presentation by dendritic cells to naïve T cells is influenced by release of mediators [C3, C5, prostaglandin E_2 (PGE$_2$), IL-10] from local cells such as epithelial cells, by the genetic background and microbial exposure of the individual. Under these influences, T cells differentiate along a type 2 T helper (Th2) pattern in atopic individuals. Elaboration of interleukin (IL)–4, IL-13, and IL-5 collectively results in immunoglobulin E (IgE) production and recruitment of eosinophils to the site of inflammation.

rates are not 100%. Thus, although atopy clearly has a genetic underpinning, it is also clearly a complex multigenic trait.

Multiple genome-wide screens have been conducted for indices of atopy and specific atopic disorders (Table 4). As shown in Table 4, when linkage to nonspecific indices of atopy (e.g., skin prick test positivity or serum IgE levels) have been examined, reproducible linkages have been found between the atopic phenotype and five primary chromosomal loci: (a) the Th2 cytokine gene cluster on 5q31–q33; (b) the HLA-D region on 6p21; (c) the region that contains the high-affinity IgE receptor gene (Fc∈RIb) on 11q13; (d) a large region on 12q14 that spans several candidate genes [signal transducer and activator of transcription protein 6 (STAT6), IFN-γ, stem cell factor, nitric oxide synthase 1]; and (e) a region of 14q11.2–q13 containing the TCRA/D gene. It is hypothesized that inheritance of these loci, either independently or in combination, may form a common genetic basis for all of the specific clinical atopic diseases. The strongest evidence in support of this hypothesis is the coexistence of atopic diseases in the same individual: 60% to 80% of allergic asthmatic patients have coexisting rhinitis (72), and about 40% of infants with atopic dermatitis develop asthma by the age of 4 years. Furthermore, the chromosomal regions and candidate genes [e.g., IL-4 receptor α (IL-4Rα), IL-13, CD14, IL-10] linked to atopy are the same regions that have been linked with all three clinical phenotypes, which supports

the concept that a common genetic basis is responsible for atopy, independent of specific clinical manifestations (72). Specific candidate genes implicated in atopic diseases are addressed in relevant sections throughout the text.

Environmental Influences on Allergen Sensitization

It is likely that multiple environmental factors influence the development of allergic diseases and that there may be complex interactions between these individual factors. The spectrum of antigens to which an atopic individual is sensitized is dependent on the person's environment in early life. This tenet is based on the positive correlations observed between allergen exposures present during the month of birth and the development of sensitization to the same allergens later in childhood (e.g., birch, grass, and dust mite allergens) (73,74). For example, Scandinavian babies born in late winter or early spring are more likely to develop IgE antibody to birch pollen, which is prevalent during the spring, than are those born at other times of the year (73). In addition, avoidance or withholding certain allergenic foods during the first few months of life, tends to prevent sensitization and subsequent allergic responses to these particular foods.

Numerous studies have demonstrated the relationship between sensitization risk and the level of allergen exposure (75,76). This has been best studied in relationship to dust

TABLE 4. *Summary of shared linkage regions for atopy, asthma, atopic dermatitis, and allergic rhinitis*

Locus	Candidate genes	Atopy[a]	Asthma[b]	Atopic dermatitis	Allergic rhinitis
2pter	Unknown	Wjst et al. (141)	Wjst et al. (325)		—
4q35	IRF-2	Daniels et al. (326)	—		—
5q23–q33	IL-3, IL-4, IL-5, IL-13, IL-9, CSF-2, GRL-1, ADR-B2, CD14	Marsh et al. (71) Meyers et al. (327) Doull et al. (328) Noguchi et al. (329) Hizawa et al. (330)	Postma et al. (127) CSGA (142) Noguchi et al. (329) Ober et al. (140)	Kawashima et al. (109)	—
6p21.1–p23	HLAD, TNF-α	Caraballo and Hernandez (331) Wjst et al. (325) Daniels et al. (326) Hizawa et al. (330)	CSGA (142) Wjst et al. (141)	—	—
7p15.2	TCR-G, IL-6	Daniels et al. (326)	Daniels et al. (326)		—
9q31.1	TMOD	Wjst et al. (141)	Wjst et al. (141)		—
11q13	FcER1B, CC16/CC10	Young et al. (332) Shirakawa et al. (335, 336) Hizawa et al. (337) Daniels et al. (326) Doull et al. (328) Palmer et al. (338) Cookson et al. (69)	van Herwerden et al. (333)	Folster-Holst et al. (334)	—
12q14–q24.33	STAT6, IFN SCF, IGF-1 LTA4H, NFγB BTG1	Barnes et al. (339) Nickel et al. (340) Wjst et al. (141)	Barnes et al. (339) CSGA (142) Ober et al. (140) Wilkinson et al. (341) Barnes (342) Wjst et al. (141)	— —	Barnes (339)
13q14.3	TPTI	Daniels et al. (326) Hizawa et al. (330) Leaves et al. (344)	CSGA (142) Kimura et al. (343)	—	—
14q11.2–q13	TCR-A/D, MCC	Moffatt et al. (345) Mansur et al. (347)	CSGA (142)	Mao et al. (346)	—

ADR-B2, adrenergic receptor B2; BTG1, B-cell translocation gene; CC, C-C chemokine; CD, cell differentiation antigen; CSF-2, colony-stimulating factor; GRL-2, glucocorticoid receptor 2; HLAD, human leukocyte antigen D; IFN, interferon; IGF-1, insulin-like growth factor 1; IL, interleukin; IRF, interferon regulatory factor; LTA4H, leukotriene A4 hydrolase; MCC, mast cell chymase; NFγB, B subunit of nuclear factor γ; SCF, Sertoli cell factor; STAT6, signal transducer and activator of transcription 6; TMOD, tropomyosin-binding protein; TNF-α, tumor necrosis factor α; TPTI, tumor protein, translationally controlled 1.

[a]The definition of atopy includes individual measurements or a composite measurement of total IgE, spIgE(RAST or skin prick test).

[b]In general asthma was defined as a qualitative trait in most studies, the definition of asthma included bronchial hyperresponsiveness as either a qualitative or a quantitative trait.

Adapted from Barnes, JACI, 2000;106:S192–200.

mite and cat antigens in early life. Among infants with two atopic parents, dust mite sensitization occurred with less than 1% prevalence when the infants were exposed to less than 0.1 μg of house dust mite allergen per gram of dust, but this value increased to 6% with allergen levels higher than 10 μg per gram of dust (75). Although antigen dose is positively correlated with sensitization, studies suggest that the relationship may be more complex. Specifically, high exposure to animal dander early in life has been shown to be protective against manifestations of asthma (77). Whether this represents immune tolerance as a result of high antigen dose or concomitant exposure to other factors such as endotoxin as a result of living with a pet is unknown.

More important than the actual dose of allergen is the age at which exposure occurs. The immune systems of neonatal mice and humans are thought to have a Th2 bias (67,78). Studies of human infants indicate that this Th2 skew gradually diminishes during the first 2 years of life in nonallergic individuals (67,79). In allergic infants, the reverse occurs: the strength of neonatal Th2 responses increases over a similar period (67,79). The persistence of this neonatal bias and the failure to produce Th1-type responses may be an important feature of the atopic disease state (80). The redirection of Th2 responses can be considered to occur simultaneously with childhood bacterial or viral infections. This relationship has been capsulated in the "hygiene hypothesis," according to which early childhood infections inhibit the tendency to develop allergic disease (81). In support of this hypothesis, at the population level, Shirakawa et al. (82) found that, among Japanese schoolchildren, there was a strong inverse association between delayed-type hypersensitivity to BCG and atopy. Positive tuberculin responses were predictive of a lower incidence of asthma, lower serum IgE levels, and cytokine profile biases toward a type 1 profile. These results suggest that exposure and response to BCG may, by modification of immune cytokines profiles, inhibit atopic disorders. Further epidemiological support for this hypothesis comes from studies demonstrating an inverse relationship between (a) farm living, pet ownership, or daycare attendance in early life and (b) atopy. In each case, the protective effect is thought to be a reflection of microbial exposure. Further support for this hypothesis is the striking association between a polymorphism in the CD14 gene and increased levels of soluble CD14 and decreased levels of IgE, which reflects the importance of bacterial lipopolysaccharide (LPS) in down-regulating Th2 responses (83).

In accordance with this assumption, bacterial exposures have been shown to reduce sensitization to inhaled antigens in mice. Specifically, sensitization to ovalbumin can be inhibited by previous or concurrent infection with *Mycobacterium vaccae* or *Mycobacterium bovis* (84,85) or by simultaneous administration of LPS and bacterial unmethylated CpG motifs (56). Although the hygiene hypothesis is probably oversimplified, it is theoretically possible that dendritic cells (DCs) at mucosal surfaces in atopic individuals receive less microbial stimuli (LPS, peptidoglycans, mycobacterial antigens)

to up-regulate IL-12 production and therefore fail to redirect weak Th2 responses into protective Th1 responses. Causes for reduced microbial exposures in industrialized societies probably include widespread use of broad-spectrum antibiotics, immunizations, and migration from farms to cities. This hypothesis may provide a plausible explanation for the rising prevalence of these disorders in industrialized countries.

Exposure to other environmental agents such as diesel particles, ozone, second-hand tobacco smoke, and rhinoviruses can also enhance sensitization to allergens in young children (86). Numerous epidemiological studies illustrate clear associations between exposure to these agents and enhanced antigenic sensitization and worsening of disease. Ozone can alter both immediate and late-phase responses of patients with asthma and those with allergic rhinitis to inhaled allergen. Nasal challenge with diesel alone increased IgE production in both atopic and nonatopic individuals, which suggests that, indeed, diesel may be a sensitizer (87). When evaluated together with allergen, diesel exposure of ragweed-sensitive subjects resulted in a significant increase in allergen-specific IgE with an increase in Th2 cytokine production. In summary, the complex interplay between genetic and environmental factors probably governs susceptibility to development of atopic disorders.

Antigen Presentation in Atopic Individuals

A pivotal step in induction of a T cell–mediated immune response is the uptake, processing, and presentation of antigen to naïve T cells by professional APCs. After exposure to antigens, APCs capture antigen and process it into small peptides of defined length for presentation on MHC molecules and presentation to the T-cell receptor on naïve T cells. Moreover, APCs express co-stimulatory molecules such as CD80, CD86, and intercellular adhesion molecule (ICAM)–1, which provide a second signal for optimal induction of T-cell activation, division, and differentiation. A number of professional APCs such as DCs, Langerhans cells, B cells, and macrophages are present at mucosal surfaces and have the cellular specialization to capture and process antigen for presentation to T cells. Early studies focused on the accessory cell capacity of macrophages, but numerous studies have shown that macrophages are poor accessory cells (88).

Epithelial cells lining the mucosal surfaces of the respiratory tract, gastrointestinal tract, and skin have also been thought to have antigen-presenting capabilities. Because epithelial cells line the mucosa surfaces, they are ideally situated to encounter antigens and present them to T cells. A role for airway epithelial cells as APCs has been suggested by the observation that epithelial cells express many of the co-stimulatory molecules important in antigen presentation, such as class II MHC molecules, CD40, B7 molecules, and ICAM-1 (89). However, to date, there is no definite evidence of their role in antigen presentation. These cells may instead be important in providing second signals for activation and recruitment of T cells and effector cells.

It has become increasingly clear that DCs or Langerhans cells are the most important professional APCs at mucosal surfaces. They are particularly important for inducing the primary immune response to antigen exposure in the mucosa that eventually leads to sensitization. DCs are located at sites of the body where maximal allergen encounter occurs, such as the skin, gut, and respiratory tract. At these sites, they form an extensive network of cells, extending cell projections in between resident cell types that ensure accessibility to allergens. DCs that reside in the periphery have an immature phenotype, specialized for uptake and recognition of antigens but not yet capable of stimulating naïve T cells, because they lack co-stimulatory molecules on their surface (CD80, CD86). When antigen is encountered in an inflammatory context (microbial, reactive oxygen species) or in the presence of inflammatory mediators such as GM-CSF, IL-1β, TNF-α, or IL-6 (probably produced by epithelial cells), DCs undergo maturation. Upon recognition of foreign antigens in the peripheral tissues, they migrate to T-cell areas of draining lymph nodes and present their antigen cargo to naïve T cells, at the same time providing essential co-stimulatory molecules for inducing the primary immune response. During this interaction with naïve T cells in the lymph nodes, DCs have an opportunity to influence the initial pattern of cytokines produced by T cells, a process termed *primary polarization.* Thus, DCs, by being such potent stimulators of T cells, are believed to play a key role in the initiation and orchestration of memory T cell–mediated immune responses within the respiratory tract, skin, and intestinal tract. Indeed, Lambrecht (90) demonstrated the importance of DCs in development of allergic responses. Lambrecht demonstrated that infusion of antigen pulsed bone marrow–derived DCs into the respiratory tract of mice primed them for development of Th2-mediated immune responses upon subsequent antigen challenge. Further evidence of a critical role for DC in generation of allergic responses is the demonstration that regular use of budesonide and fluticasone, which are associated with improvement in lung function, is associated with a reduction in the number of CD1a$^+$ HLA-DR$^+$ DCs in the airways of asthmatic patients (91).

It has been hypothesized that, in addition to presenting antigen to T cells, DCs probably play a pivotal role in instruction of T cells to become either Th1 or Th2 cells. It is proposed that DCs themselves can be subdivided into two groups, DC1 and DC2, on the basis of their ability to facilitate T cells to produce either Th1 or Th2 cytokines, respectively. In mice, Th1-inducing DC1s are of lymphoid origin, express CD8a$^+$, and produce large amounts of IL-12, whereas DC2s are myeloid derived and express CD11b (92). The opposite is observed in humans: CD11c$^+$ DC1s are monocyte-derived cells and express many myeloid markers, whereas CD11c$^+$ CD2s are probably of lymphoid origin, expressing CD4 and lacking myeloid markers. However, it has been shown that freshly isolated myeloid DCs from mice induce Th2 responses and that bone marrow–derived myeloid DCs can clearly be switched to IL-12 production and Th1

induction. Likewise, human monocyte-derived DCs can induce Th2 responses. Thus, it is clear that much remains to be learned about DC populations and their role in directing T-cell immune responses.

Several lines of evidence suggest that DC function may be altered in atopic individuals in a way that promotes Th2 immune responses. First, HLA-DR-expressing DCs are more numerous in the mucosal tissues of patients with asthma, allergic rhinitis, and atopic dermatitis, in comparison with the low level of DCs found in specimens from normal controls (91,93–96). In both humans and mice, DCs are not constitutively present in the tracheal-bronchial mucosa in the first year of life; their occurrence appears to be dependent on exposure to inhaled inflammatory stimuli (97,98). Exposure to certain irritants and infectious agents, such as cigarette smoke, and certain oxidants increase the number of DCs present in the respiratory tract. This relationship may explain the adjuvant effect of these irritants in induction of allergic responses referred to previously. Together, these studies suggest that exposure to certain pathogens and environmental irritants may either enhance or inhibit early sensitization to allergens by affecting DC recruitment and maturation.

Second, although detailed characterization of subpopulations of DCs have not been conducted in atopic individuals, several studies suggest that DCs from atopic individuals may be intrinsically different from those of nonatopic individuals (99–101). In one such study, Der p 1 stimulation of monocyte-derived DCs from Der p 1–sensitive patients resulted in preferential up-regulation of CD86 expression and proinflammatory cytokine production (IL-1β, TNF-α, IL-6) in comparison with cells from nonallergic patients or pollen-sensitive subjects (100). Purified T cells from house dust mite–sensitive patients stimulated by autologous Der p 1 pulsed DCs preferentially produced IL-4. Interestingly, DCs from nonatopic individuals stimulated with Der p 1 expressed CD80, produced IL-12, and stimulated IFN-γ production in T cells. Another intriguing finding of this study was that the effects of Der p 1 on co-stimulatory molecule expression in DCs from allergic patients were dependent on the enzymatic activity of Der p 1, inasmuch as a cysteine protease inhibitor prevented these effects. A similar phenomenon (role for antigen protease activity in directing T-cell activity) has also been observed in a murine model of leishmaniasis. In this model, infection of mice with mutant strains of *Leishmania* lacking the cysteine protease gene preferentially induced a shift from the type 2 phenotype associated with infection in the wild-type strain to a type 1 response (102). Alteration in responses of DCs from atopic individuals to proteolytic activity of common allergens provides an attractive hypothesis for their aberrant immune response to allergen exposure; however, it is not known whether this altered response is caused by differences in DC phenotypes or by a disrupted protease–antiprotease balance in atopic individuals.

In addition to their contribution to the primary immune response that leads to sensitization, DCs are likely to contribute to secondary immune responses in atopic individuals.

Several lines of evidence support the absolute requirement of these cells in the secondary response, despite the previously held view that memory/effector T cells are less dependent on co-stimulation and, in theory, respond to any APCs such as B cells, macrophages, and even eosinophils. First, during secondary immune responses, both human and rodent DCs are rapidly recruited to mucosal surfaces (103). Second, depletion of DCs in allergen-primed mice completely prevented the development of Th2-mediated allergic inflammation (104). Last, Hammad et al. (100) showed that adoptive transfer of myeloid DCs into PBMC-reconstituted hu-SCID mice boosted the production of house dust mite–specific IgE, which illustrates that DCs stimulate memory Th2 cells to enhance secondary immune responses. These results provide strong evidence that DCs play a pivotal role in the primary as well as secondary response to allergens, although the mechanisms remain obscure.

DCs may play a role in secondary immune responses through their surface expression of the high-affinity IgE receptor. Indeed, CD1a$^+$ airway DCs express the α chain of the high-affinity IgE receptor. When allergen is recognized through the FcϵRI on DCs, it is very efficiently targeted to the class II MHC–rich endocytic compartment, the site of peptide loading onto class II MHC molecules. It has been suggested that the presence of IgE on DCs lowers the threshold for allergen recognition, boosting the secondary immune response by efficiently stimulating memory T cells. In support of this concept, Coyle et al. (105) showed that when allergen-specific IgE was captured by a nonanaphylactogenic anti-IgE antibody in sensitized mice, they failed to produce Th2 cytokines upon reexposure to the sensitizing allergen. This perpetuation of the allergic response may indeed occur in atopic patients in that the proportion of DCs expressing the α subunit of the high-affinity IgE receptor is significantly increased in patients with asthma and atopic dermatitis, in comparison with nonatopic controls (106). This increase in FcϵRI on DCs may also be the result of higher endogenous levels of IL-4, a known modulator of immunoglobulin crystallized fragment receptors.

Collectively, these studies suggest that altered DC function may underlie the propensity of atopic individuals for mounting Th2-biased immune responses to environmental allergens. More detailed information regarding the exact mechanisms is awaited with further study of DC biology.

CYTOKINE REGULATION OF Th2 DIFFERENTIATION IN ATOPY

One of the most important variables in instruction of T-cell differentiation comes from the local cytokine milieu at the time of antigen presentation. Specifically, IL-12 directly primes CD4$^+$ T cells for Th1 differentiation (107), whereas Th2 differentiation is critically dependent on IL-4. Because IL-4 and IL-12 are known regulators of T-cell differentiation, alterations in either production of or responsiveness to these cytokines could result in the polarization of T-cell responses to allergens observed in atopic individuals.

Potential Dysregulation of Th2 Differentiation Factors in Atopy

The exact mechanisms regulating differentiation of uncommitted T cell responses into Th2 cells remain obscure. The presence of IL-4 at the site of antigen presentation is the most dominant factor in determining the likelihood for Th2 polarization of the naïve T helper cell in both mice and humans. In support of a central role for IL-4 in Th2 polarization in atopic disorders, the results of several studies suggest that genes regulating IL-4 production may be altered in atopic diseases, particularly in asthma. First, a specific polymorphism in the IL-4 gene itself has been shown to be correlated with high serum IgE levels and enhanced IL-4 gene expression (108). A similar association has been reported between the T allele of the −590C/T polymorphism of the IL-4 gene promoter region and atopic dermatitis (109). Moreover, Hershey et al. (110) demonstrated that expression of a mutant form of the IL-4Rα chain in allergic patients is associated with increased IL-4 signaling. Furthermore, strong support for the role of IL-4 signaling in Th2 polarization in atopic disorders is the demonstration of the importance of the STAT6 in development of Th2 differentiation and development of allergic responses in mice (111). Indeed, elevations in STAT6 expression in asthmatic tissues have been reported (112). Moreover, a GT repeat polymorphism in the first exon of the STAT6 gene has been found to be associated with increased prevalence of several atopic disorders (bronchial asthma, atopic dermatitis, food allergies) (113).

Another factor expressed in Th2 cells that appears to function as a potent coactivator of IL-4 gene transcription is nuclear factor of activated T cells (NF-AT). Studies in mice have shown that alterations in a number of the family members of the NF-AT protein family may result in altered IL-4 gene expression and polarization of T-cell responses toward the type 2 pattern. NF-AT proteins are expressed on T cells, B cells, and mast cells and control the transcription of a number of genes relevant to allergic disorders, including IL-4. Tamura et al. (114) demonstrated that NF-AT C2-deficient mice have an increased number of eosinophils in the bone marrow and blood, concomitant with increased production of Th2 cytokines. It has also been shown that other NF-AT family members, including NF-AT C1, are important in differentiation of T cells. Several groups have now shown that loss of NF-AT C1 activity results in impaired T lymphocyte activity and secretion of IL-4 in mice (115,116). Furthermore, strains of mice that are susceptible to development of Th2-driven immune responses to allergen have enhanced T-cell expression of NF-AT C1, in comparison with expression in resistant strains of mice (117). These experiments suggest that deficiencies in this transcription factor may lead to the development of the allergic phenotype.

A transcription factor that may be more widely involved in the induction and maintenance of the Th2 pattern of cytokine secretion is GATA-3. GATA-3 belongs to a subfamily of zinc finger transcription factors that interact with specific deoxyribonucleic acid (DNA) binding sequences in the regulatory regions of genes encoding Th2-like cytokines. GATA-3 has been shown to be differentially expressed in Th2 and Th1 cells, and expression of this gene is sufficient to drive Th2 differentiation (118). Altered regulation of GATA-3 expression may be important in atopy, inasmuch as GATA-3 expression has been shown to be elevated in BAL fluids and bronchial biopsy specimens of asthmatic patients in comparison with normal controls (112,119). Furthermore, blockade of this gene with a dominant negative mutant of GATA-3 inhibits allergic inflammation in mice (120).

Several other genes or chromosomal regions have been shown to be important in susceptibility to mounting Th2-driven immune responses in murine models; these include CNS-1 and T-cell immunoglobulin and mucin domain–containing molecule (TIM). It has been shown that deletion of a noncoding segment, CNS-1, on murine chromosome 11 (human 5q), which is in the intergenic region between the IL-4 and IL-13 genes, results in the loss of Th2 cytokine production in T cells (121). Similarly, a member of the TIM family of genes, also located on murine chromosome 11, has been shown to confer susceptibility to asthma in mice (122). Although it is not currently known whether inheritance of a single gene variant or a combination of genetic variants is required to drive Th2 cell commitment in atopic individuals, considerable evidence is mounting to suggest that genetic differences in factors important in Th2 cell commitment may underlie susceptibility to development of atopic disorders.

Altered Interleukin-12 Production in Atopic Disorders

Although Th2 cell polarization in atopic disorders can clearly arise as a result of aberrant expression of the genes important in Th2 differentiation, alterations in factors controlling expansion of the opposing Th1 pathways may also play an important role. In this regard, IL-12, a product of monocytes and DCs, is the primary determinant of T-cell differentiation to a Th1 pattern (107). Impaired IL-12 production has been reported in each of the atopic disorders (123,124). However, it is not known whether this is a primary or secondary event. Naseer et al. (124) demonstrated that the number of cells positive for IL-12 p40 messenger RNA is significantly lower in asthmatic patients than in normal controls. Furthermore, successful steroid treatment was characterized by a significant increase in the numbers of cells expressing IL-12 messenger RNA, whereas steroid therapy in steroid-resistant patients did not result in an increase in IL-12–expressing cells. In addition, another group has shown that *Staphylococcus aureus*–induced production of IL-12 p70 in whole blood cultures from asthmatic patients was significantly less than in nonatopic control subjects (125). Further support for the

importance of IL-12 in prevention of antigen-induced allergic airway responses has been provided by the observation that blockade of endogenous production of IL-12 in naturally resistant murine strains (C3H/HeJ) renders them susceptible to the development of allergen-induced airway hyperreactivity (AHR) and eosinophilic inflammation (126). Together, these studies suggest that dysregulation of endogenous IL-12 levels may be an important mechanism governing the pathogenesis of allergic disorders.

The mechanisms that give rise to alterations in IL-12 production are currently unclear; however, there exist several potential mechanisms, such as altered expression of the genes encoding either one or both of the individual subunits of the functional cytokine or alterations in receptor signaling pathways. The gene encoding the p40 subunit of the functional heterodimer is located in the region of human chromosome 5q that was previously linked to human atopic diseases (71,127). Although polymorphisms have been identified in the p40 gene, they have not been examined in the context of atopic disorders (128). Studies in mice have implied that loss of IL-12 responsiveness and subsequent inability of mice to mount Th1 responses are caused by altered expression of the IL-12 receptor B2 subunit (129). IL-12–dependent signaling in human Th1 cells was shown to correlate with the selective expression of the transcripts encoding the signaling component of the IL-12 receptor B2 and with the presence of high-affinity IL-12 binding sites selectively located on Th1 cells (130). Thus, it is proposed that not only is IL-12 receptor B2 (IL-12RB2) a marker of Th1 cells but also lack of expression of this receptor subunit may lead to a Th2-polarized immune response. Indeed, IL-12RB2–expressing cells have been shown to be reduced in tissues of persons with atopic asthma and rhinitis (131,132). Several polymorphisms in the IL-12RB2 gene have been reported (1188A→C, −4475-4insG, Glu186Asp, Ser226Asn). However, these polymorphisms were shown not to be associated with atopic diseases (133). Together with the demonstration that IL-12RB2 levels are increased in atopic patients after steroid treatment, these results suggest that the reduced expression of IL-12RB2 is probably not a result of a primary defect in the IL-12RB2 gene but that they occur as a consequence of reduced IL-12 production or elevated Th2 cytokine expression (132). Further support for the lack of a primary defect in IL-12RB2 gene expression is provided by the observation that, when reconstituted with IL-12, cells from atopic individuals produce normal amounts of IFN-γ (125).

Alternatively, the deficient production of IL-12 in atopic disorders may occur as a result of altered regulation of IL-12 production by mediators and cytokines, which either positively (IFN-γ, C5a), or negatively [IL-4, prostaglandin E$_2$ (PGE$_2$), IL-10, C3a] regulate its production. Clearly, IL-4 and PGE$_2$ levels are elevated in allergic diseases (134,135), whereas IFN-γ levels are reduced. PGE$_2$ has also been shown to cause early development of immature DC1s into Th2-promoting cells.

Studies suggest that perhaps complement components produced by cells in the mucosa, such as epithelial cells, may regulate IL-12 production (136). It is postulated that C5a and C3a play a reciprocal role in regulating IL-12 production, whereby C5a induces and C3a inhibits production of IL-12 (136). Interestingly, allergens such as house dust mite feces contain proteases that cleave both C5 and C3 into their active fragments, which suggests that allergens may directly activate complement and thereby regulate the type of immune response elicited at the mucosal surface (16). In accordance with a potential role for complement, several studies have now demonstrated that animals deficient in either C3a or C3 do not develop allergic airway responses and have reduced Th2 cytokine production, in comparison with wild-type mice (137,138). Conversely, lack of a functional C5 gene renders mice susceptible to development of allergen-driven Th2 immune responses (139). Support for a role for complement in human atopic diseases is provided by studies demonstrating enhanced expression of complement components in airway tissues from asthmatic patients (137). Further support for a primary role for complement in atopic disorders comes from several genetic studies showing linkage of asthma and related traits to chromosomal regions containing the C5 (140,141) and C5aR genes (142).

The role of IL-10 in IL-12 regulation and Th2-mediated immune responses is complex. First, although IL-10 has been shown *in vitro* to inhibit IL-12 production by APCs, the impaired IL-12 production in blood cultures from atopic individuals does not appear to be caused by elevated IL-10 levels, inasmuch as blockade of IL-10 did not restore IL-12 levels to normal (125). Although altered levels of IL-10 have been observed in atopic disorders, the relationship is not straightforward. For example, there are conflicting reports about the levels of IL-10 in atopic patients: Some studies demonstrated elevations in IL-10 levels in bronchial biopsies (143), PBMCs (144), BAL fluids (145), and the gut mucosa of asthmatic patients (146), whereas others reported diminished IL-10 production in sputum from asthmatic patients (147) and in isolated T cells from children with asthma or atopic dermatitis (148). Results from animal studies show similar disparities. IL-10 knockout mice have been shown to have both reduced allergic responses (149) and enhanced responses to allergen challenge (150). Investigators have suggested that the discrepancies in the results of studies with IL-10–deficient mice may be dependent on the genetic background of the strain (150). In contrast, studies in which animals have been treated with recombinant IL-10 (151) or overexpress the IL-10 gene (152) uniformly demonstrate that IL-10 suppresses inflammation and decreases development of Th2-mediated immune responses. Moreover, adoptive transfer of IL-10–expressing DCs induced tolerance to allergen exposure (153). The variability in the results may reflect the pleiotropic actions of IL-10 during the course of allergic reactions. IL-10 can clearly influence T-cell differentiation through its inhibitory actions on IL-12 and through its ability to reduce antigen presentation to T cells by limiting class II MHC, CD80, and CD86 expression on APCs. On the other hand, it is a potent anti-inflammatory cytokine, which can serve to dampen inflammation once initiated (154). The fact that steroids (155), *Lactobacillus* species (156), and standard immunotherapy regimens (157), all of which successfully resolve symptoms in atopic diseases, induce IL-10 production suggests that perhaps IL-10 is protective and that IL-10 production may be impaired in atopic individuals. Diminished IL-10 production may lead both to loss of tolerance to environmental antigens and to inability to control inflammation once initiated. The elevations in IL-10 tissue levels observed during challenge with allergens may reflect compensatory mechanisms designed to suppress harmful inflammatory responses. In this regard, genetic polymorphisms in the promoter of the IL-10 gene (C to A change at position 571) have been associated with asthma and elevated serum IgE levels (158).

Th2 CYTOKINE REGULATION OF ALLERGIC INFLAMMATION

The dependence of the immunopathogenic consequences of allergic immune responses on Th2 cells probably stems from their pivotal role in regulating the primary effectors of both the acute- and late-phase reactions: IgE and eosinophils. In addition, as discussed in a later section, Th2 cell–derived cytokines themselves also serve as effector cells of the allergic response.

One of the major roles of IL-4 in allergic inflammation is as the primary inducer of immunoglobulin-class switching in B cells that leads to the synthesis and secretion of IgE (159). The importance of IL-4 to IgE synthesis has been demonstrated by the fact that neither IL-4 nor STAT6-deficient mice produce IgE (111). The exact mechanisms by which IL-4 regulates IgE class switching is discussed later. IL-13 is also able to regulate IgE synthesis in humans, but its role in IgE synthesis in mice is controversial. The combination of IL-4's effects on IgE synthesis and mast cell growth suggests a primary role for IL-4 in the development of the early-phase response. As discussed in greater detail in a later section, IgE activation of mast cells leads to the synthesis and release of a number of inflammatory mediators that may contribute to the vascular, smooth muscle, and mucus changes observed in the early-phase response to allergen challenge.

Through their unique and overlapping actions, IL-4, IL-13, and IL-5 coordinately regulate the development, recruitment, and activation of eosinophils. Both IL-4 and IL-13 have been shown to contribute to the recruitment of eosinophils into sites of inflammation, as evidenced by the fact that gene deletion and inhibition of either IL-4 or IL-13 by antibody blockade eliminate allergen-driven increases in tissue eosinophils (50,160). Conversely, overexpression of these cytokine genes in mice results in tissue eosinophilia (46,161). The requirement for IL-4 probably stems from two mechanisms. First, IL-4 may mediate eosinophilia through its role in Th2 cell expansion and the subsequent production of IL-5. In addition, either IL-4 or IL-13 or both may regulate eosinophil influx by regulating vascular cell adhesion molecule 1 (VCAM-1) expression on the endothelium or by stimulating release of specific chemokines from resident airway cells or by both actions. In support of a role for IL-4– and IL-13–mediated VCAM-1 in pulmonary eosinophilia, numerous studies have shown that VCAM-1 is necessary for eosinophil recruitment into tissues in response to allergen provocation in mice (162).

Because IL-5 has been shown to be the primary determinant of eosinophil differentiation, activation, and survival, it is a likely candidate in eosinophil regulation in allergic responses. In bone marrow, IL-5 is important for stimulation of eosinophilopoiesis and promotion of the terminal differentiation of myeloid precursors into eosinophils. IL-5 also increases eosinophil adhesion to vascular endothelial cells, promotes the migration of eosinophils from the blood into tissues, prolongs eosinophil survival in tissues, and augments the cytotoxic activity of eosinophils. Furthermore, IL-5 may activate pulmonary eosinophils and cause them to release cytotoxic products. The importance of IL-5 in antigen-induced eosinophilia has been examined in numerous animal studies (163). For example, blockade of endogenous IL-5 levels in antigen-sensitized guinea pigs (163) and in mice (44) has resulted in significant suppression of both BAL and tissue eosinophilia. Consistent with these observations is the demonstration that intratracheal administration of IL-5 induces eosinophil accumulation in the guinea pig lung *in vivo*. More definitively, mice in which the IL-5 gene has been disrupted do not develop eosinophilic inflammation (45). Reconstitution of these mice with IL-5 completely restored aeroallergen-induced eosinophilia. Although these studies support the primary role of IL-5 in controlling circulating levels of eosinophils, other factors such as chemokine gradients (discussed in the section on eosinophils) probably also contribute to the regulation of tissue levels of eosinophils.

On the basis of the independent and overlapping roles of IL-4, IL-13, and IL-5 just discussed, we envision the following paradigm for regulation of allergen-induced tissue eosinophilia. After allergen-specific induction of Th2 cytokine production, IL-5 would rapidly induce differentiation of eosinophils from myeloid precursors in the bone marrow and stimulate their release into the bloodstream. IL-4 or IL-13 or both would promote eosinophil egress from the vascular compartment by up-regulating VCAM-1 expression on vascular endothelial cells. Once the cells accumulate in tissues, locally produced IL-5 along with other mediators would promote their actions by prolonging their survival in tissues. Within this paradigm, allergen driven eosinophil recruitment into tissues is coordinately regulated by the Th2 cytokines, IL-4, IL-13, and IL-5. Thus, through the coordinate regulation of IgE and eosinophilia, Th2 cytokines orchestrate the elicitation phase of allergic immune responses. In the next

section, we discuss in more detail the steps involved in IgE regulation.

REGULATION OF IMMUNOGLOBULIN E SYNTHESIS

Ishizaka et al. (4,164) purified immunoglobulin E in 1966. IgE has the shortest half-life (2.5 days) of all classes of immunoglobulins. In addition, it is present in serum at levels considerably lower than other immunoglobulin classes, such as IgG. There is considerable heterogeneity in the levels of IgE among individuals. For example, levels of less than 100 ng/mL are observed in most normals, whereas in parasitized or atopic individuals, IgE levels can reach as high as 1,000 ng/mL. The high variability in serum levels is in striking contrast to that of other immunoglobulin isotypes and suggests that tight control of IgE may therefore be important to prevent the potentially lethal consequences of IgE-mediated inflammation. Indeed, synthesis of IgE and its receptor expression appear to be regulated by a series of steps involving both cell–cell contact with CD4[+] Th2 cells and activation by cytokines secreted by these cells. In this section, we discuss the current knowledge of the complex steps involved in regulation of IgE synthesis and expression of its receptors.

Isotype Class Switching to Immunoglobulin E Production

The production of IgE antibodies by B cells is triggered by a complex series of secreted signals and cell surface interactions, followed by molecular genetic rearrangements at the immunoglobulin heavy chain locus (Fig. 2). The first step in IgE production is the binding of allergen to allergen-specific B cells through their membrane-bound immunoglobulin receptor. The B cells then internalize and process the allergen and present the processed allergen to T cells as peptide fragments in association with class II MHC molecules. The class II MHC/peptide complex is then recognized by the T-cell receptor on Th2 cells. Initially, all B cells produce immunoglobulin M (IgM) antibodies. At this point, a VH(D)JH cassette of sequences encoding the variable domain is immediately adjacent to the $C\mu$ exons, which encode the IgM constant regions at the 5' end of the immunoglobulin heavy chain locus. Further downstream in the immunoglobulin heavy chain are several widely spaced clusters of exons. C regions encode the constant region domains of the IgG, IgE, and immunoglobulin A (IgA) heavy chain isotypes. Upon stimulation by cytokines, along with critical cell–cell interactions with CD4[+] T-cell surface accessory molecules, B cells can change the isotype of the antibodies (or effector functions) that they produce while retaining their original antigenic specificity. This process requires that genomic DNA be spliced and rejoined to move the VDJ elements from their location proximal to $C\mu$ to a position many kilobases downstream next to the C-region exons encoding the heavy chains of other isotypes.

Regulation of IgE Synthesis

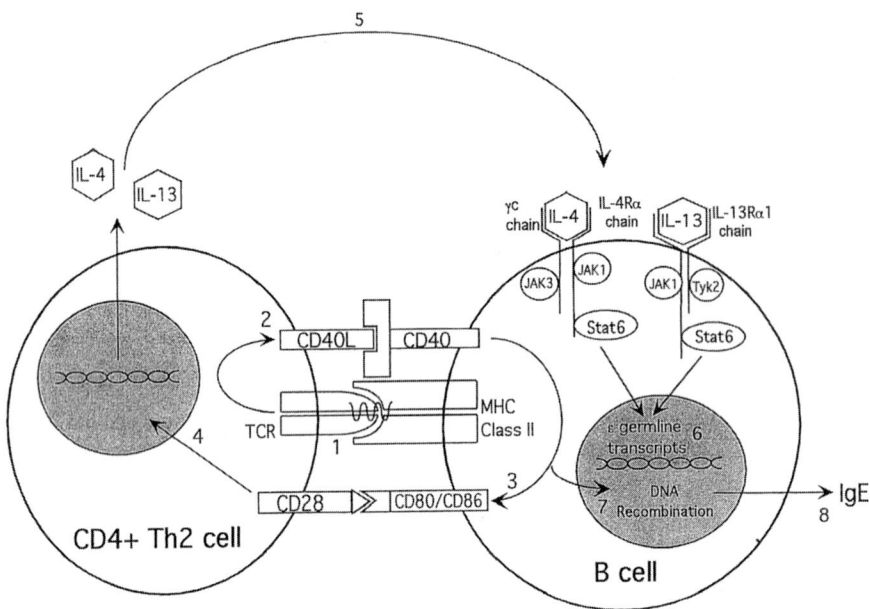

FIG. 2. The regulation of immunoglobulin E (IgE) synthesis involves many sequential steps: 1) recognition of antigen/major histocompatibility complex (MHC) class II by the T-cell receptor (TCR); 2) TCR activation leads to the induction of CD40 ligand (CD40L) on the T cell, which is then recognized by CD40 on the B cell; 3) CD40–CD40L cognate interaction leads to induction of CD80/CD86 on the B cell, which can then interact with CD28; 4) the type 2 T helper (Th2) cell secretes interleukin (IL)–4 and IL-13; 5) IL-4 and IL-13 bind their cognate receptors on B cells, which results in activation of signal transducer and activator of transcription protein 6 (STAT6); 6) IL-4 and IL-13 signaling events result in initiation of transcription at the Iε promotor and the production of immature germline ε transcripts; 7) the CD40–CD40L interaction provides the necessary second signal required for recombination of the germline locus; and 8) transcription of mature ε transcripts from the rearranged locus followed by translation and secretion of IgE.

A large amount of intervening DNA is excised and discarded in this irreversible process, and the mechanism is therefore referred to as *deletional switch recombination.*

Isotype switching to IgE production requires two signals (165). The first signal is provided by the Th2 cytokines IL-4 and IL-13 and is IgE isotype specific. IL-4 and IL-13 stimulate transcription at the Cε gene locus, which contains the exons encoding the constant-region domains of the IgE ε heavy chain. The second signal is a B-cell activating signal provided through CD40–CD40 ligand (CD40L) interactions. Together, these interactions result in induction of the necessary deletional switch recombination that brings into proximity all of the elements of a functional ε heavy chain.

The first signal for IgE class switching is provided by the T cell–derived cytokines IL-4 and IL-13. IL-4 induces RNA transcription at the Cε locus by stimulation of STAT6 through binding the type I IL-4 receptor composed of the IL-4Rα chain and the γ c chain. IL-13 has also been shown to regulate IgE class switching in humans through binding the type II IL-4 receptor composed of the IL-4Rα and IL-13 receptor α1 chains. However, there is considerable controversy about the role of IL-13 in IgE class switching in mice. After either IL-4 or IL-13 binding to its respective receptor complex,

Janus kinases phosphorylate tyrosine residues in the intracellular domains of the receptor chains, providing docking sites for STAT6. These STAT6 molecules become phosphorylated and then form homodimers that translocate to the nucleus. In the nucleus, they bind to specific sequences [TTCN(N)GAA] in the promoter of IL-4/IL-13 responsive genes, including Iε. The importance of STAT6 in IL-4–induced isotype switching is supported by the fact that germline transcription and IgE class switching are markedly impaired in STAT6-deficient mice (166). Other transcription factors are also important in induction of germline transcription of Cε locus. The importance of NFκB for the induction of germline transcripts has been confirmed by the finding that expression of germline transcripts for IgE is severely impaired in NFκB p50 knockout mice (167).

IL-4 or IL-13–induced transcription factor binding of the Cε locus results in germline transcription of the Cε locus. Germline transcripts originate from a 5′ promoter of the Iε exon, which is located just upstream of the four Cε exons. IL-4 induces the appearance of 1.7- to 1.9-kb germline Cε transcripts that contain an Iε exon, located 2 kb upstream of Sε, spliced to the Cε1 to Cε4 exons. After processing, the mature germline messenger RNAs include the 140-bp Iε exon and exons Cϵ1 to Cϵ4. These transcripts have been referred to as "sterile," because of the presence of stop codons in each of the three reading frames of Iϵ. Although the transcripts are "sterile," the process of transcription itself appears to facilitate the deletional switch recombination event. For example, Harriman et al. (168) analyzed IgA switching, using mice retaining a normal Iα promoter in which the Iα exon was replaced by an hypoxanthine phosphoribosyltransferase mini-gene and found that switching can occur to the locus despite the absence of complete Iα-containing transcripts. This has been demonstrated at the Cϵ locus in that switch recombination occurred at the Cϵ locus when the Iϵ exon and promoter were intact but Cϵ exons were absent (169).

The second signal for IgE class switching is dependent on cell-to-cell contact between T and B cells. Specifically, the interaction between CD40 on the surface of B cells with CD40L on the T-cell surface is critical for driving the IgE switch to completion and leading to IgE production. CD40 is a 50-kDa surface glycoprotein that is constitutively expressed on all human B-lymphocytes. CD40L is transiently induced on T cells after stimulation of the T-cell receptor by antigen/MHC complexes. Binding of newly expressed CD40L with CD40 on B cells provides the second signal for induction of deletional switch recombination to IgE.

Several lines of evidence support a critical role for CD40–CD40L interactions in isotype switching. First, it had been shown by numerous groups that isotype switching required the presence and contact with T cells. After an extensive search for the T-cell contact signal, it was discovered that CD40–CD40L interactions were responsible for the T-cell dependency of this process. Proof of this was provided by the observation that activation of CD40L could completely substitute for T-cell help (170). Furthermore, a soluble form of CD40 inhibits its interactions with CD40L, blocking IL-4–driven IgE synthesis in human B cells (171). Last, genetic deficiencies in CD40L or CD40 in humans and mice, respectively, disrupt IgE synthesis. In humans, CD40L is encoded on the X chromosome, and individuals with the X-linked hyper-IgM syndrome are deficient in CD40L. Their B cells are unable to produce IgG, IgA, or IgE (172). Mice deficient in either the CD40L or CD40 genes have the same defect in antibody production (173,174).

CD40–CD40L interactions are thought to provide a second signal through stimulation of a number of signaling pathways, which probably synergize with those initiated by IL-4 and IL-13 to achieve ϵ-germline transcription. Specifically, after interaction with CD40L on the B cell surface, CD40 aggregation triggers signal transduction through four intracellular proteins, which belong to the family of TNF receptor-associated factors (TRAFs). TRAF-2, TRAF-5, and TRAF-6 are known to associate with the intracytoplasmic domain of CD40 after its multimerization by interaction with CD40L. TRAF-2, TRAF-5, and TRAF-6 promote the dissociation of NFκB from its inhibitor, IκB. In turn, NFκB can synergize with STAT6 induced by IL-4/IL-13 signaling to activate the Iϵ promoter, as described previously. In addition to triggering

TRAF associations, engagement of CD40 activates protein tyrosine kinases, such as Janus kinases.

Another mechanism by which cytokine and CD40L activation may induce class switching is through induction of expression of proteins required in deletional recombination. Specifically, both cytokine and CD40L induction of class switching has been shown to require the synthesis of new proteins. One of these proteins has been identified as activation-induced deaminase (AID) (175). AID is expressed in activated B cells and in germinal centers of lymph nodes. Mice deficient in AID have a dramatic impairment in isotype switching, with elevated IgM levels and low or absent IgE, IgG, and IgA isotypes (176). Interestingly, a rare autosomal form of hyper-IgM syndrome has been attributed to mutations in this gene (177). Although these studies suggest that this protein is critical to isotype switching, the mechanisms by which it participates in switch recombination remain obscure at present. AID has homology to the RNA editing enzyme APOBEC, which modifies specific sites in apoB precursor RNA to give rise to a transcript encoding the functional apoB48 protein. AID might execute a similar RNA-editing function in B cells, processing pre–RNA-encoding proteins involved in the mechanisms of switch recombination and hypermutation. Alternatively, AID might mediate the construction of ribozymes and complex RNA structures with nuclease activity, or it could act directly on DNA substrates in the heavy chain locus.

Deletional Switch Recombination

After the delivery of both IL-4 and CD40/CD40L signals, deletional switch recombination occurs through a series of molecular events that are not yet fully understood (169,178). However, the current data are consistent with a model in which IL-4/IL-13-driven transcription originating at the Iϵ promoter alters the ϵ heavy chain locus in a way that permits isotype switch recombination (Fig. 3). However, because the ϵ-germline transcripts do not encode a functional protein, their precise role in isotype switching has long eluded investigators. A number of reports have begun to shed light on this subject. It appears that germline transcripts participate in the assembly of complex DNA-RNA hybrid structures, which then target nucleases to the ϵ locus for the initial DNA cleavage in the cut-and-paste reaction of deletional switch recombination. In deletional switch recombination at the ϵ locus, DNA cleavage and ligation are carried out within the switch (Sϵ) cassette, which contains repeats of GAGCT and GGGGT and is located between the Iϵ and Cϵ exons. ϵ-Germline transcripts, originating at the Iϵ promoter, pass through the Sϵ region and then on into the Cϵ exons. Transcription experiments have shown that the S region containing RNA does not separate from its genomic template but rather remains associated to form a DNA-RNA hybrid. Another group has shown that these hybrids create R-loops, in which the S transcript hybridizes to the template DNA, leaving the opposite strand as single-strand DNA. Two endogenous excision

Mechanism of IgE Class Switching

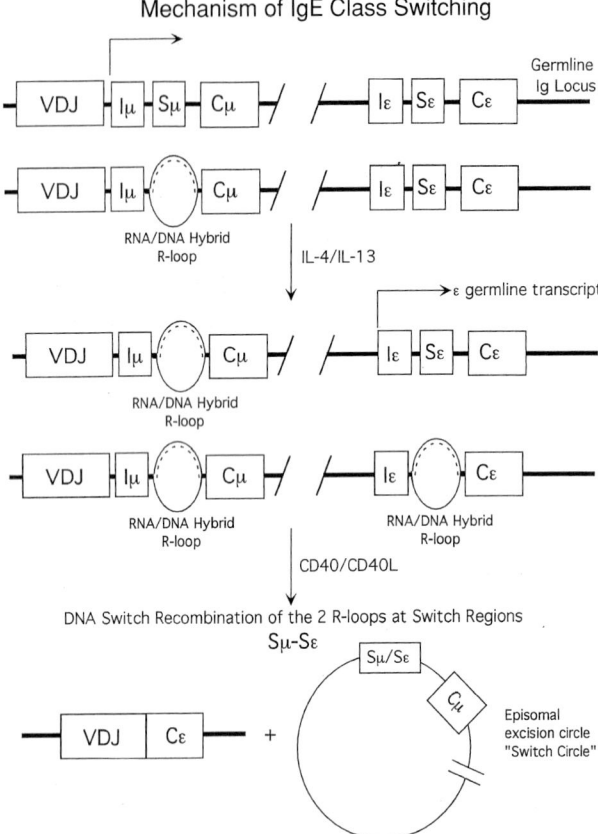

FIG. 3. Schematic representation of the molecular steps involved in immunoglobulin E (IgE) class switching. In naïve resting B cells, the VDJ sequences encoding the variable region are located at the 5′ end of the immunoglobulin locus. After stimulation by interleukin (IL)–4 or IL-13, transcription is initiated at the Iε promotor to produce ε germline transcripts. Sε ribonucleic acid (RNA) remains hybridized to the Sε deoxyribonucleic acid (DNA), forming an RNA–DNA hybrid structure, called an R-loop. The R-loop serves as a substrate for nucleases that result in double-strand DNA breaks. Switch recombination and joining is dependent on a second signal provided by the CD40–CD40 ligand (CD40L) interaction. This process results in the formation of an episomal excision circle that is eventually lost during cell division.

repair nucleases, XPF-ERCC1 and XPG, previously known to target duplex–single-strand junctions, have been shown to be capable of cleaving these R-loops. These new observations have given rise to a model in which R-loops formed by the association of Sε RNA with its Sε genomic template serve as substrates for nucleases that generate double-strand DNA breaks in the first step of deletional switching. In later steps, these breaks can be annealed by DNA end joining to analogous breaks in Sμ, located between VH(D)JH and the Cμ exons. This rearrangement brings the VH(D)JH segments encoding the antigen binding site into the immediate proximity of the Cε exons encoding the constant domains. The product of this recombination is the *de novo* generation of a complete multiexon gene that can be transcribed as a single message encoding the full ε heavy chain. Although these

new reports establish the existence of R-loops and demonstrate that these two nucleases can cleave these structures, it has not been definitively shown that these enzymes are the nucleases relevant to the deletional isotype switch mechanism. The specific nucleases used by B cells still need to be identified. These proteins may be constitutively expressed in B cells; however, as discussed previously, proteins such as AID may be induced as a result of either IL-4–IL-13 or CD40–CD40L interactions.

Negative Regulation of Immunoglobulin E Synthesis

IFN-γ can inhibit IL-4–dependent IgE synthesis in both mice (179) and humans (180). IFN-γ suppresses the expression of ε-germline transcripts in murine B cells stimulated with IL-4 and LPS. IFN-γ may affect recombination events without affecting the expression of ε-germline transcripts.

Immunoglobulin E Receptors

The two major crystallized fragment receptors for IgE are called FcεRI and FcεRII (CD23) (181). They are distinguished by their structure and their relative affinities for IgE. The high-affinity IgE receptor FcεRI binds monomeric IgE with an affinity constant of 10^{10} M^{-1}, whereas CD23 binds with a much lower affinity (Ka = 10^8 M^{-1}). The high-affinity receptors are constitutively expressed at high levels on mast cells and basophils. They are also found, albeit at lower levels, on peripheral blood DCs, monocytes, and human Langerhans cells. The low-affinity receptor is expressed on a wide variety of cells, including B cells, T cells, Langerhans cells, monocytes, macrophages, platelets, and eosinophils.

Crystallized Fragment ε Receptor I–Mediated Signal Transduction

The FcεRI is a member of the multisubunit immune response receptor family of cell surface receptors that lack intrinsic enzymatic activity but transduce intracellular signals through association with cytoplasmic tyrosine kinases (181). In rodents, FcεRI is expressed on mast cells and basophils as a heterotetramer consisting of a single IgE-binding α subunit, a β subunit and two disulfide-linked γ subunits. The α chain consists of two extracellular immunoglobulin-like loops, a single transmembrane region containing an aspartic acid residue, and a short cytoplasmic domain that lacks signal transduction motifs. The charged amino acid within the transmembrane domain mediates the association of the α subunit with the signaling component of the γ subunit. The β subunit consists of four membrane-spanning domains and a cytoplasmic tail capable of transducing intracellular signals that amplify γ-mediated signaling events. In rodents, all three subunits are required for the cell surface expression of FcεRI (181,182). In contrast, in humans, the receptor can be expressed as two different isoforms: a tetramer (αβγ2) or a trimer (αγ2). The tetrameric complex (αβγ2) is expressed on mast cells and basophils, whereas the trimer is expressed on Langerhans cells, DCs, monocytes and macrophages, and eosinophils.

FcεRI signaling occurs upon IgE binding to the receptor. This requires two sequential events: (a) binding of IgE antibody to the FcεRI and (b) cross-linking of IgE antibody by bivalent or multivalent antigen. Cross-linking of the receptor initiates a coordinated sequence of biochemical and morphological events that result in (a) exocytosis of secretory granules containing histamine and other preformed mediators; (b) synthesis and secretion of newly formed lipid mediators, such as prostaglandins and leukotrienes; and (c) synthesis and secretion of cytokines. Although the exact signaling pathways governing each of these functions are not known, the following model has been proposed. The β and γ subunits each contain a conserved immunoreceptor tyrosine-based activation motif (ITAM) within their cytoplasmic tails that is rapidly phosphorylated on tyrosine after FcεRI aggregation (182,183). Tyrosine phosphorylation of the β and γ ITAMs is mediated by Lyn, which is constitutively associated with the β subunit and activated after antigen-mediated FcεRI aggregation. FcεRI cross-linking leads to recruitment and activation of the tyrosine kinase Syk, which binds to the tyrosine-phosphorylated γ ITAMs through its tandem SH2 domains (181). Recruitment of Syk occurs upstream of several signal transduction pathways. The importance of Syk is demonstrated by the fact that Syk-deficient mast cells fail to degranulate, synthesize leukotrienes, or secrete cytokines after FcεRI stimulation (184). Ultimately, this pathway leads to the activation of mitogen-activated protein (MAP) kinases, and activation of protein kinase C pathways. Protein kinase C pathways are thought to be important in exocytosis and in granule content release and gene expression. Activation of MAP kinase also regulates the enzymatic activity of phospholipase A_2, leading to generation of a variety of lipid mediators [platelet-activating factor (PAF), prostaglandin D_2 (PGD$_2$), and leukotriene C_4 (LTC$_4$)]. Antigen-mediated aggregation of FcεRI also stimulates the recruitment and activation of p21ras, which has been implicated in FcεRI-induced cytokine transcription and secretion (181).

Regulation of Crystallized Fragment ε Receptor I Surface Expression

Although the expression of FcεRI on the surface of mast cells appears to occur early in their differentiation or maturation *in vivo*, their levels are known to be regulated by several factors after maturation. Studies in both mice and humans have revealed that the levels of FcεRI on mast cells can be regulated by IgE itself, as well as by Th2 cytokines. Indeed, atopic individuals with high serum IgE levels show markedly up-regulated mast cell and basophil FcεRI levels (185,186). Moreover, anti-IgE treatment of atopic individuals results in down-regulation of FcεRI expression on human basophils (187). Further evidence is provided by murine studies in which IgE-deficient mice exhibit dramatically reduced

levels of receptors on mast cells and basophils. Because IgE-deficient mice nonetheless express receptors, albeit at lower levels, other mechanisms of regulation are thought to exist. In fact, cytokines such as IL-4 and IL-13 have been shown to up-regulate FcεRIα expression on mast cells, basophils, and monocytes. Glucocorticoids have been shown to inhibit IL-4– and IL-13–induced up-regulation of the FcεRIα chain on monocytes (188). Together, these results suggest that, through a multistep positive feedback process, Th2 cytokines enhance both the production of IgE and the expression of its receptor, which leads to further mast cell activation and release of Th2 cytokines in the local microenvironment, serving to perpetuate the allergic response.

Mast cell activation is subject to negative regulation by a growing family of structurally and functionally related inhibitory receptors. These include FcγRIIB, cytotoxic T-lymphocyte–associated antigen 4 (CTLA-4), killer cell inhibitory receptors killer cell immunoglobulin-like receptors (KIR), and gp49B1 on mast cells. Indeed, gp49B1-deficient mice exhibit more severe anaphylactic reactions than do their normal counterparts (189). Each of these receptors possesses an immunoreceptor tyrosine-based inhibitory motif (ITIM). Coaggregation of FcεRI and these inhibitory receptors on the surface of mast cells results in transinhibition of FcεRI-induced mast cell activation (190,191). In general, inhibitory receptors are thought to inhibit the actions of activation receptors containing ITAMs by recruiting phosphatases through an ITIM (192).

Crystallized Fragment ε Receptor II (CD23)

In humans, CD23 (FcεRII, B cell differentiation antigen) is a Ca^{2+}-dependent C-type lectin of 45 kDa. It has wide distribution among hematopoietic and structural cells and exists in two forms, CD23a and CD23b, which result from alternative splicing at the N-terminal and differ by five amino acids in the cytoplasmic domain. The isoforms of CD23 are found on B cells; one is constitutively expressed (CD23a), whereas the other (CD23b) is induced by factors such as IL-4 (193), and CD40L in conjunction with IL-4. CD23b is also found on non–B cells such as T cells, Langerhans cells, monocytes, macrophages, platelets, and eosinophils (194,195), and it mediates different biological functions. CD23b has been shown to be associated with phagocytosis of soluble IgE complexes, whereas CD23a is associated with endocytosis of IgE-coated particulates (196).

Structurally, CD23 presents a single membrane-spanning domain, followed by an extracellular domain that consists of three regions: the α helical coiled-coil stalk region, which mediates the formation of trimers; the lectin head, which binds IgE; and, at the C-terminal, a short tail containing an inverse Arg-Gly-Asp sequence, a common recognition site of integrins (197,198). CD23 is cleaved at the membrane to yield a series of soluble fragments. Soluble CD23s of varying molecular weights arise by an autocatalytic process involving matrix metalloproteinase cleavage of membrane-bound CD23.

The endogenous proteases that participate in CD23 shedding have not been identified. However, interestingly, Der p 1, the major house dust mite antigen, has been shown to selectively cleave CD23 and to promote IgE synthesis (15). CD23 expression is up-regulated by several factors, including its ligand, IgE (199), and IL-4 (193). On the other hand, IFN-γ counteracts the inducing effect of IL-4 on CD23 expression.

CD23 is thought to mediate a number of effects, including regulation of IgE synthesis, antigen presentation, proliferation and differentiation of B cells, and activation of monocytes, effects that can be ascribed to the membrane and soluble forms of CD23 (198,200). Binding of IgE to the membrane-bound form of the receptor transduces an inhibitory signal that prevents further IgE synthesis (201). In contrast, the soluble forms described previously up-regulate IgE production, and their release has been found to be inhibited by IgE binding (202). Soluble CD23 also ligates CD11b/CD11c to promote release of proinflammatory mediators such as IL-1β, IL-6, and TNF-α (203).

CD23 expression on B cells and monocytes and soluble CD23 production is markedly increased in allergic disorders (32,204,205). Moreover, reduction of allergen-induced CD23 expression on B cells has been observed after successful desensitization therapy (206). Dysregulation of the CD23 pathway in atopic patients might be part of their propensity for developing IgE antibodies and part of an enhancement of the inflammatory reaction, through the action of soluble CD23 and through IgE-dependent triggering of CD23 on non–B cells.

EFFECTOR CELLS OF THE ALLERGIC RESPONSE

Overview

Once a genetically susceptible individual is sensitized to a given allergen and IgE antibody has been formed, subsequent exposure to allergens readily induces the manifestations of atopic disease. Although these responses are generally on a continuum, they have been categorized into three types on the basis of their temporal sequence: (a) acute or immediate responses; (b) late-phase reactions; and (c) chronic allergic inflammation.

Exposure of a sensitized individual to allergens results in immediate reactions, the characteristics of which are dependent on the site of entry of the allergen. In the nasal mucosa, allergen provocation of sensitized individuals results in sneezing, nasal itching, and nasal discharge. Acute allergic reactions elicited in the skin at the sites of allergen injection are characterized by intense itching, redness, and edema. In asthmatic patients subjected to allergen inhalation, these mediators rapidly elicit bronchial mucosa edema, mucus production, and smooth muscle constriction. Acute or immediate responses are thought to be caused by the release of preformed mediators released by antigen interaction with crystallized fragment receptors and IgE on IgE-bearing cells (mast cells and basophils). The release of mast cell products produces multiple local effects, including enhanced local vascular permeability (leading to leakage of plasma proteins, including fibrogen, and resulting in local deposition of cross-linked fibrin and tissue swelling), increased cutaneous blood flow (with intravascular fluid from postcapillary venules, producing erythema), and other effects, such as itching, caused by the stimulation of cutaneous sensory nerves by histamine. Typically, these reactions are detectable within a few minutes of allergen challenge, reach a maximum in 30 to 60 minutes, and then rapidly wane.

In many individuals, the acute phase is followed by what has been termed a late-phase reaction, which occurs within 6 to 48 hours after allergen exposure and can persist for several days without therapy. The characteristic signs and symptoms of late-phase reactions are reddening and swelling of the skin, sneezing and nasal discharge, and wheezing and cough upon lower airways challenge. Late-phase reactions are thought to occur as a result of recruitment of circulating leukocytes to the site of allergen exposure after antigen presentation to T cells. Both eosinophils and T cells are assumed to mediate the late-phase response. However, mast cells may also contribute to the late-phase response. The importance of leukocyte recruitment is supported by the fact that a variety of treatments, which are associated with a reduction in leukocyte recruitment that is elicited at sites of late-phase reactions, can also reduce the signs and symptoms of these responses.

In naturally occurring allergic diseases, patients typically experience repeated exposure to the offending allergens over a period of weeks to years. Although the specific features of pathological processes of each of these diseases vary according to the anatomical site affected, it has been generally recognized that the structural changes that occur in each tissue are caused by the persistence of inflammation. These tissue changes range from thickening of the skin and fibrotic papules to extensive remodeling of the airway wall with smooth muscle hypertrophy, subepithelial fibrosis, and mucus cell hypertrophy. In each case, these structural changes are associated with significant alterations in their function.

Development of Mast Cells and Basophils

History and Overview

Mast cells and basophils were discovered by Paul Ehrlich in the late 1800s from staining of their cytoplasmic granules with aniline and basophilic dyes, respectively (207). It was once thought that basophils might be circulating precursors of mast cells or that mast cells were "tissue basophils," but current evidence suggest that they are indeed distinct cell types. Although these cell types have unique functions and release a unique profile of mediators, they also produce an overlapping array of mediators that are known to contribute to the allergic diathesis. It is hypothesized that IgE produced by allergen-reactive B cells binds to Fcϵ receptors present on the surface of mast cells and basophils and that, when challenged with allergen, these cells release vasoactive mediators as well as chemotactic factors and cytokines that promote leukocyte infiltration and exacerbate the inflammatory response. Through the production and release of these proinflammatory molecules, mast cells and basophils set into motion a series of events that result in immediate responses to allergens in the skin, lungs, and nose of an atopic individual and may also contribute to the late-phase response.

Basophils

Basophils are a small population of peripheral blood leukocytes containing cytoplasmic granules that stain with basophilic dyes (Fig. 4). They typically exhibit a segmented nucleus with marked condensation of nuclear chromatin and contain round or oval cytoplasmic granules. Basophils are thought to arise from pluripotent CD34$^+$ progenitors found in cord blood, peripheral blood, and bone marrow. They have been suggested to evolve from CD34$^+$/IL-3 receptor α^+/IL-5$^+$ eosinophil/basophil progenitors, which is by the occurrence of granulocytes with a hybrid eosinophil/basophil phenotype in patients with chronic or acute myelogenous leukemia or in cell culture (208–210). Unlike mast cells, basophils differentiate and mature in the bone marrow and then circulate in the blood, in which they constitute fewer than 1% of circulating leukocytes. IL-3 appears to be an important developmental factor for basophils (211), although many other growth factors, such as IL-5, GM-CSF, TGF-α, and nerve growth factor, probably influence their development

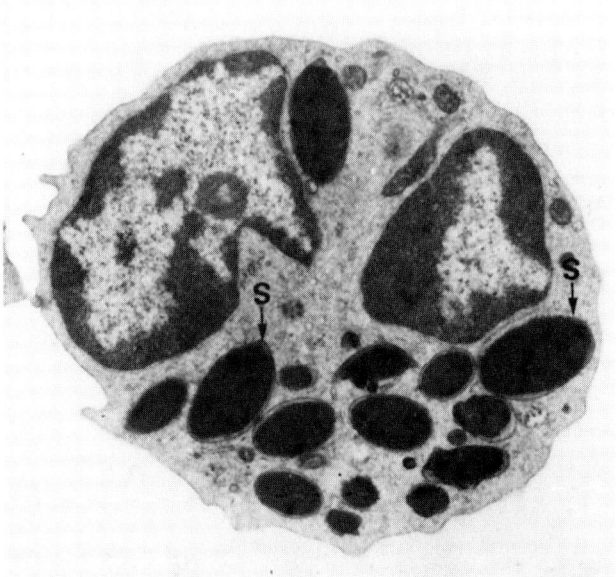

FIG. 4. Electron micrograph of a human basophil (10,500× magnification). Note the characteristic bilobed nucleus and the membrane-bound specific granules (S) filled with a closely packed, electron-dense material that contains mediators such as histamine and leukotrienes. From Wheater PR, Burkitt HG, Daniels VG. *Functional histology.* Edinburgh: Churchill Livingstone, 1979, with permission.

(212–214). Like mast cells, basophils possess high-affinity IgE receptors (FcεRI) that are cross-linked upon engagement of receptor-bound IgE with corresponding antigens, which results in release of a number of mediators that are, in part, common for both cell types.

Because of the lack of specific markers for detection of basophils in tissues and the inability to isolate significant numbers of these cells from peripheral blood, the study of basophil biology has been severely hampered. Participation of basophils in allergic reactions has traditionally been documented by indirect means, such as by determining the pattern of mast cell– or basophil-specific mediators such as histamine (derived from both), PGD$_2$ (mast cells only), and LTC$_4$ (primarily from basophils). Despite the difficulties in studying basophils, studies suggest that they rapidly produce large amounts of the immunoregulatory cytokines IL-4 and IL-13 and constitutively express CD40L and CCR3 on their surface. These findings, together with the demonstration that they are rapidly recruited to the skin (215), lungs (216), and nose (217) after allergen challenge, suggests that these cells probably play an important role in allergic diseases. However, because much more is known about the role of mast cells in the immune response, we confine our discussion to mast cells, except for situations in which specific information about basophils is available.

Mast Cells

Mast cells typically appear as round or elongated cells with a nonsegmented or occasionally binucleated or multinucleated nucleus (Fig. 5). Their intracellular granules become purple when stained with aniline blue dyes. This change in color represents the interaction of the dyes with the highly acidic heparin contained in the mast cell granules. Mast cells, like other granulocytes, are derived from CD34$^+$ hematopoietic progenitor cells; however, they are distinct from other granulocytes in that they mature in the periphery. Several lines of evidence suggest that interactions between the tyrosine kinase receptor c-kit, which is expressed on the surface of mast cells, and the c-kit ligand, stem cell factor (SCF), are essential for normal mast cell development and survival. For example, mice with mutations that result in either markedly impaired c-kit function or a reduction in c-kit virtually lack mast cells. Reconstitution with recombinant SCF can induce mast cell hyperplasia *in vivo* in mice, rats, nonhuman primates, and humans (218).

Mast cells are distributed throughout normal connective tissues, in which they often lie adjacent to blood and lymphatic vessels, near or within nerves, beneath epithelial surfaces that are exposed to the external environment, such as those of the respiratory tract, gastrointestinal tract, and skin. At these locations, they are ideally situated to encounter foreign antigens and to release their products close to their respective target cells (i.e., epithelial cells, vascular endothelium, smooth muscle, and fibroblasts). In humans and mice, the number of mast cells in a tissue varies markedly,

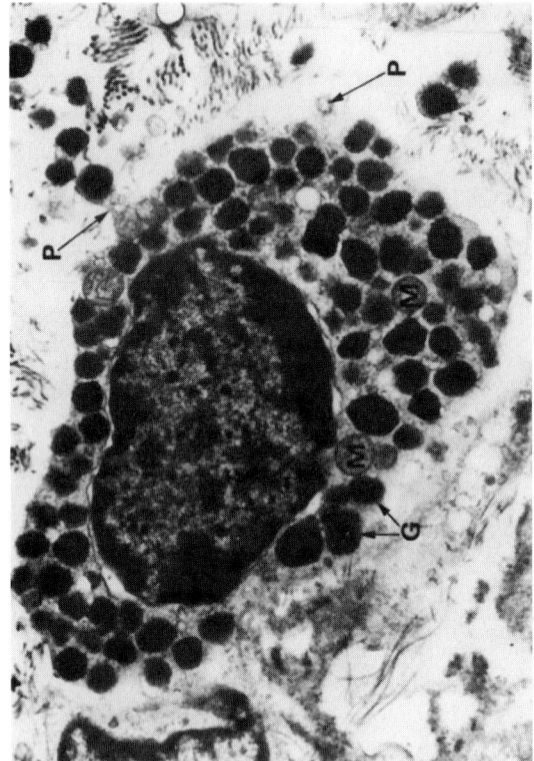

FIG. 5. Electron micrograph of a human mast cell (10,500× magnification). Mast cells contain a large, nonsegmented nucleus with multiple membrane-bound granules (G) containing a dense amorphous material. Upon activation, mediators and cytokines are released from the granules. Variable numbers of cytoplasmic processes (P) extend into the surrounding connective tissue matrix. The cytoplasm contains several rounded mitochondria (M) but little rough endoplasmic reticulum. From Wheater PR, Burkitt HG, Daniels VG. *Functional histology.* Edinburgh: Churchill Livingstone, 1979, with permission.

depending on the anatomical site and the immunological status of the host.

The mast cell population is composed of a group of cells heterogeneous with regard to their structure and function (219). On the basis of their content of neutral serine proteases, they had previously been divided into two phenotypes. One subset, designated MC_{TC}, contains tryptase, chymase, cathepsin G, and carboxypeptidase, whereas the other phenotype, designated MC_T, contains only tryptase. MC_{TC} is found predominantly in skin and at subepithelial locations in the bronchial, nasal, and gastrointestinal mucosa, whereas MC_T is located predominantly in alveolar walls, intestinal epithelium, and airway epithelium in patients with allergic disease. However, more recent studies in both humans and animal models suggest that mast cells in different anatomical sites and even within a single site can vary in several aspects of their phenotype, including morphology, responsiveness to various stimuli, and activation and mediator content.

The tissue levels of mast cells and their specific phenotypes are probably controlled by a complex interplay among

SCF, other growth factors, and cytokines. SCF is necessary to elicit the c-kit–mediated signaling that ensures the expansion of cells of the mast cell lineage, whereas the development of different phenotypes appears to be determined by their responsiveness to signals from T cells. Specifically, MC_T cell expansion appears to be T-cell dependent, whereas expansion of the MC_{TC} population is T-cell independent. This contention is supported by the fact that humans with T-cell deficiencies lack intraepithelial intestinal mast cells, while maintaining submucosal mast cell populations (220). Similarly, athymic mice lack intraepithelial cells and are unable to expand this population in the gastrointestinal tract in response to helminthic infections (221). IL-3, IL-4, and IL-9, in particular, are among the T cell–derived cytokines known to influence mast cell development and phenotypic characteristics. A role for IL-3 in mast cell hyperplasia has been demonstrated in intestinal helminthic infections, in which IL-3 depletion inhibits the intraepithelial mast cell hyperplasia normally observed in the jejunum of infected mice (222). A similar case can be made for IL-9, because IL-9 transgenic mice spontaneously develop intraepithelial mast cell hyperplasia in the jejunum (223). The action of IL-9 can be blocked by depletion of SCF. Moreover, IL-9 and IL-10 reversibly induce expression of mouse mast cell proteases 1 and 2 in mast cells through transcript stabilization, which suggests that T cell–derived cytokines can influence the spectrum of mediators produced by a given mast cell. Together, these studies suggest that the regulation of mast cell phenotype in the microenvironment is dynamic and that T cell–derived cytokines are major determinants of the numbers, distribution, and phenotype of mast cells in tissues.

Mast Cell–Derived Mediators

Mast cells and basophils release a wide array of potent biologically active mediators that have both unique and overlapping activities on various target cells (Table 5). Some of these products are stored preformed in the cytoplasmic granules, whereas others are synthesized upon activation of the cell by IgE-dependent processes or non–IgE-dependent stimuli. These mediators can be categorized into three main groups: (a) preformed secretory granule–associated mediators, (b) lipid-derived mediators, and (c) cytokines (Table 5).

Preformed Mediators

The secretory granules of human mast cells contain a crystalline complex of preformed inflammatory mediators ionically bound to a matrix of proteoglycan. When mast cell activation occurs, the granules swell and lose their crystalline nature, and the individual mediators are released by exocytosis. The mediators stored in mast cells include histamine, proteoglycans, serine proteases, carboxypeptidase A, and small amounts of sulfatases. In mouse and rat mast cells, the granules also contain serotonin (224–226).

TABLE 5. *Products of mast cells and basophils*

Mediators	Actions
Preformed mediators	
Histamine	Increase vascular permeability, smooth muscle contraction
Neutral proteases	
Tryptase, chymase	Physiologic function uncertain (different mast cell
Cathepsin G	populations express different combinations of
Carboxypeptidase	proteases)
Lipid Mediators	
PGD$_2$	Smooth muscle contraction
LTC$_4$	Increase vascular permeability, smooth muscle contraction, increase mucus production
LTB$_4$	Neutrophil chemotaxis
TXA$_2$	Vasoconstrictor, platelet aggregation, smooth muscle contraction
PAF	Vasoconstrictor, platelet aggregation, smooth muscle contraction, chemotactic for neutrophils and eosinophils
Cytokines	
TNF-α, IL-6, IL-8, IL-1α	Numerous proinflammatory actions
IL-4, IL-13	Switch factor for IgE, VCAM-1 expression
IL-5	Regulation of eosinophils
Chemokines	
MIP-1α, MCP-1, MIP-1b, RANTES	Chemotactic for monocyte/macrophages
Growth factors	
FGF, VEGF	Induce growth of fibroblasts and endothelial cells, respectively

FGF, fibroblast growth factor; IL, interleukin; LTB$_4$, leukotriene B$_4$; LTC$_4$, leukotriene C$_4$; MCP-1, monocyte chemotactic protein 1; MIP, macrophage inflammatory protein; PAF, platelet-activating factor; PGD$_2$, prostaglandin D$_2$; RANTES, regulated upon activation, normal T-cell expressed, presumably secreted; TNF-α, tumor necrosis factor α; TXA$_2$, thromboxane A$_2$; VEGF, vascular endothelial growth factor.

The mediator most associated with the mast cell is histamine. Histamine is a biogenic amine formed in mast cells and basophils by the decarboxylation of histidine. It is present in the granules at a level of approximately 100 mmol/L, or 1 pg/cell. Histamine has many potent activities that are pertinent to the early phase of the allergic response, including vasodilatation, increased vasopermeability, smooth muscle contraction, and increased mucus production. Histamine exerts its biological and pathological effects through specific receptors on various cells such as smooth muscle, endothelial cells, and nerves. At least three types of histamine receptors have been identified: H$_1$, H$_2$, and H$_3$. Histamine is very rapidly metabolized, with a half-life of about 1 minute by histamine N-methyltransferase and histaminase. Increased levels of histamine have been found in BAL fluids of patients with asthma, atopic dermatitis, and allergic rhinitis (227). Interestingly, although antihistamines inhibit the immediate allergic responses, they do not seem to inhibit late-phase responses.

Heparin is the predominant proteoglycan in human mast cells. It constitutes about 75% of the total. The remainder is composed of chondroitin sulfates. The proteoglycan is the storage matrix inside the granule, and the acid sulfate groups of the glycosaminoglycans provide binding sights for the other preformed mediators. Proteoglycans also have anticoagulant, anticomplement, and antikallikrein effects. In

addition to regulating the kinetics of release of mediators from the granule matrices, proteoglycans can also regulate the activity of some of the associated mediators.

The major mast cell protease that is present in all mast cells is tryptase. Tryptase is a serine protease, and it is stored fully active in the granule. There are two distinct forms of tryptase with 90% amino acid sequence homology: α-tryptase and β-tryptase (228,229). The β-tryptase form is a useful clinical biomarker for anaphylaxis. Tryptase level measurements obtained within 4 hours of a presumed anaphylactic reaction are more sensitive than serum or urine histamine measurements in implicating mast cell activation and degranulation (230–232). By weight, tryptase is the major enzyme stored in the cytoplasmic granules of human mast cells and occurs in all human mast cell populations. It has many activities, including cleavage of peptides such as vasoactive intestinal peptide, bronchodilator peptides, and calcitonin gene–related peptide, but not substance P; sensitization of smooth muscle; cleavage of type IV collagen, fibronectin, and type VI collagen; up-regulation of ICAM-1 on epithelial cells; and mitogenic activity for fibroblasts and epithelial cells (226). Some of these activities have led to speculation that mast cells may be involved in chronic inflammation and tissue remodeling (233).

The other major neutral protease in mast cells is chymase. It, too, is a serine protease that is stored in the active form in the granules of some human mast cells. Unlike tryptase, chymase is present in only a subset of mast cells. Chymase can cleave angiotensin I and neurotensin, but has no activities on vasoactive intestinal peptide or substance P. Of importance is that it can degrade IL-4. Some subsets of mast cells also contain other proteinases, such as carboxypeptidase and cathepsin G.

Newly Synthesized Mediators

Lipid Mediators

Activation of mast cells not only results in release of preformed granule-associated mediators but can also initiate the *de novo* synthesis of certain lipid-derived substances. Of particular importance are the cyclooxygenase and lipoxygenase metabolites of arachidonic acid, because these products possess potent inflammatory activity. Lipoxygenases generate leukotrienes, hydroperoxyeicosatetraenoic acids (HPETEs) and the reduced products of HPETES, hydroxyeicosatrenoic acids, whereas cyclooxygenase products include prostaglandins and thromboxanes.

Leukotrienes are produced by the activity of 5-lipoxygenase on arachidonic acid. Arachidonic acid is converted to 5-HPETE, which can then be converted to leukotriene B_4 (LTB_4) through the action of the leukotriene A_4 (LTA_4) hydrolase or to LTC_4 through LTC_4 synthase. LTC_4 can then be converted to leukotrienes D_4 and E_4 (LTD_4 and LTE_4). Human mast cells generally produce more LTC_4 than LTB_4. The leukotrienes were originally discovered in 1938 and were referred to as the slow-reacting substance of anaphylaxis until their structural elucidation in 1979 (234,235). In 1983, Samuelsson identified the slow-reacting substance of anaphylaxis as the cysteinyl leukotrienes LTC_4, LTD_4, and LTE_4 (235a).

Leukotrienes induce a prolonged cutaneous wheal-and-flare response, stimulate prolonged bronchoconstriction (10 to 1,000 times more potent than histamine), enhance vascular permeability, promote bronchial mucus secretion (236), and induce constriction of arterial and intestinal smooth muscle (237–240). Cysteinyl leukotrienes have been detected in the BAL fluid of asthmatic patients and in the urine of patients after inhaled allergen challenge or, in sensitive individuals, aspirin challenge. Cysteinyl leukotriene receptor antagonists and leukotriene synthesis blockers have been introduced into clinical practice as novel therapies for asthma. In asthmatic patients, clinical trials have demonstrated that approximately 80% of the early bronchoconstrictor response can be eliminated with cysteinyl leukotriene antagonists (241–243). These blockers also block 50% of the late-phase response to inhaled allergen, which supports the importance of cysteinyl leukotrienes in the late phase of the allergic response (241–243). However, the fact that PGD_2 and tryptase are not found in the BAL fluid during the late-phase reaction suggests that the cysteinyl leukotrienes noted in the late phase are the product of basophils or eosinophils and not mast cells.

In contrast to the cysteinyl leukotrienes, mast cells produce very little LTB_4. LTB_4 is a potent chemotactic factor for neutrophils and, to a lesser extent, for eosinophils (244). Certain mast cell types, including bone marrow–derived murine mast cells and human lung mast cells, may also secrete PAF (245,246). PAF has several actions that suggest that it is an important mediator of anaphylaxis, including: (a) its ability to induce aggregation and degranulation of platelets, (b) its induction of wheal-and-flare reactions in human skin, (c) its ability to increase lung resistance, and (d) induction of systemic hypotension.

The major cyclooxygenase-derived product in mast cells is PGD_2, which is a potent bronchoconstrictor. PGD_2 is rapidly degraded to $9\alpha,11\beta$-PGF_2, producing another potent bronchoconstrictor. Maximal activation of mast cells yields 50 to 100 ng of PGD_2 per 10^6 mast cells (247). Although PGD_2 is 100-fold less potent than cysteinyl leukotrienes, it is released in larger molar amounts and thus, is important in the early bronchoconstrictor response to airway allergen challenge (248). PGD_2 exerts its effects by interacting with the thromboxane receptor on airway smooth muscle (249). PGD_2 is also chemotactic for neutrophils and is an inhibitor of platelet aggregation. There is considerable evidence that prostanoids are generated during allergic reactions *in vivo*. PGD_2 is elevated in the BAL of asthmatic subjects following inhaled allergen challenge (250). Furthermore, the metabolite of PGD_2, $9\alpha,11\beta$–prostaglandin F_2 (PGF_2), rises markedly in the urine after allergen or aspirin challenge of sensitive asthmatic patients (251). Significantly raised $PGF_{2\alpha}$ and PGE_2 levels are reported in the serum of asthmatic patients (252,253). These findings are confused by the facts that there is no therapeutic benefit from cyclooxygenase inhibitors and that, in fact, cyclooxygenase inhibitors often exacerbate underlying asthma (254,255).

Mast Cell–Derived Cytokines

Mast cells may be important initiators of both the early- and late-phase allergic reaction because of their ability to synthesize and secrete cytokines. Mast cells express message for a number of cytokines, including (a) proinflammatory cytokines, (b) immunoregulatory cytokines, and (c) chemokines (Table 5).

Mast cells contain preformed stores of several proinflammatory cytokines, including TNF-α, IL-8, IL-6, and IL-1α. Release of these cytokines early in the immune response probably contributes to the recruitment of leukocytes during the late-phase response through their ability to increase expression of adhesion molecules such as P- and E-selectin, VCAM-1, and ICAM-1 on vascular endothelial cells. Mast cells appear to be an important initial source of TNF-α during allergic responses. Mast cells produce a number of immunoregulatory cytokines such as IL-3, IL-4, IL-5, GM-CSF, IL-13, and IL-16. In the human bronchial mucosa, IL-4 immunoreactivity is seen in approximately 80% of mast cells (256,257). Indeed, it has been suggested that mast cells are the primary source of IL-4 protein in inflamed airways. Although cytokine production by basophils has not been as extensively studied as that by mast cells, mast cells have been shown to produce large quantities of IL-4 and IL-13. The rapid and perhaps sustained production of cytokines by these cells at sites of allergic inflammation may intensify or perpetuate IgE production and Th2 cell differentiation. Mast cells have also been shown to produce a number of chemokines such as monocyte chemotactic protein (MCP)–1, macrophage inflammatory protein (MIP)–1β, MIP-1α, and regulated upon activation, normal T-cell expressed, presumably secreted (RANTES). Elaboration of these chemokines may contribute to the cellular component of the late-phase response.

Mast Cell Activation

Mast cell activation may be initiated upon interaction of a multivalent antigen with its specific IgE antibody attached to the cell membrane through its high-affinity receptor, FcϵRI. Cross-linking of IgE by the interaction of allergen with specific determinants on the antigen-binding fragment portion of the molecule brings the receptors into juxtaposition and initiates mast cell activation and mediator generation and release. Mast cells may also be activated by non–IgE-mediated stimuli such as neuropeptides, by complement components, and by certain drugs such as opiates. In addition to IgE-dependent stimuli, several non–IgE-dependent stimuli activate mast cells and basophils. C5a, IL-3, N-formyl-methionyl-leucyl-phenylalanine, and certain chemokines (RANTES) are known to induce histamine and mediator release in mast cells and basophils. Hyperosmolarity itself also stimulates mediator secretion from these cells. Degranulation produced by IgE-dependent stimuli appears similar to that produced by non–IgE-dependent stimuli. However, the biochemical processes that lead to mediator release may differ.

Role of Mast Cells in Acute-Phase Responses

Several lines of evidence suggest that mast cells and basophils play a pivotal role in the generation of acute-phase responses. First, allergen provocation of atopic individuals is associated with extensive activation of mast cells, as judged by the detection of the release of mast cell–associated mediators (histamine, tryptase) at the site of allergen challenge. Second, therapeutic agents that inhibit either the release of these mediators (mast cell stabilizers) or their actions (antihistamines) effectively attenuate acute allergic responses. Despite this evidence in humans, the data in animal models are conflicting. Although most studies in mice suggest that acute responses are mast cell and IgE dependent, others suggest that these responses are IgE independent. For example, it has been shown that responses induced in mice by passive transfer of allergen-specific IgE antibodies and subsequent intravenous allergen challenge are inhibited in genetically mast cell–deficient Kit^W/Kit^{W-v} mice. When these mice were reconstituted with mast cells by adoptive transfer, their acute-phase responses were restored (258). In contrast, some investigators have reported that anaphylactic responses develop normally in IgE-deficient mice (259). Although these conflicting results may reflect inherent differences in mast cell biology between humans and mice, they imply that both mast cell– and IgE–dependent and –independent processes are probably involved in the expression of the physiological features of the acute-phase reaction.

Role of Mast Cells in Late-Phase Responses

Although it has long been thought that mast cells contribute only to the early acute response, there is evidence of their potential contribution to the late-phase response. First, through the elaboration of proinflammatory cytokines, chemokines, and immunoregulatory cytokines as discussed previously, mast cells may contribute to the cellular component of the late-phase response, as well as favor the acquisition of the Th2 phenotype, by providing a continuously high concentration of IL-4. Second, mast cell–derived mediators may also contribute to the chronic remodeling of mucosal tissues, inasmuch as many of the mediators that they release influence connective tissue turnover. Specifically, histamine and tryptase have been shown to stimulate fibroblast growth and collagen synthesis *in vitro* and *in vivo*. Last, studies in humans have shown that stabilization of mast cells with sodium nedocromil effectively inhibits both the early- and late-phase responses to allergen exposure (260). Furthermore, clinical trials utilizing a monoclonal antibody against IgE resulted in reductions in symptoms and improvement in lung function in asthmatic patients (261). Although these reports together support a role for mast cells in the late-phase response, studies of animal models of atopic dermatitis and asthma suggest that late-phase reactions are similar in wild-type and IgE-deficient mice (48,262), which in turn suggests that, although mast cells are capable of inducing late-phase responses, additional mast cell–independent processes also contribute to the development of late-phase responses.

Eosinophil Biology

Eosinophil blood and tissue levels are generally quite low in the absence of parasitic infection or atopy. One of the hallmarks of allergic disorders is heightened production of eosinophils in the bone marrow and the accumulation of eosinophils in tissues and blood. Eosinophil differentiation, recruitment, and activation are regulated by a series of molecular events orchestrated by Th2 cytokines. Although the exact role of eosinophils in the pathological processes of allergic responses is not known, eosinophils are known to release a myriad of mediators and cytokines that have the potential to induce the symptoms of allergy and to amplify the allergic response through the release of immunoregulatory and proin-flammatory cytokines.

Eosinophils are bone marrow–derived granulocytes that are characterized by their bilobed nuclei and their distinctive cytoplasmic granules (Fig. 6) (263,264). They contain three distinct types of cytoplasmic granules: (a) eosinophil specific granules, which contain electron-dense crystalloid cores; (b) primary granules, which lack a crystalloid core and develop early in eosinophil maturation; and (c) smaller granules, which contain arylsulfatase and other enzymes. Eosinophils also contain varying numbers of lipid bodies. Lipid bodies are non–membrane-bound, lipid-rich inclusions that are also found in macrophages and mast cells and are thought to contribute to the formation of eicosanoid mediators. Although there are currently no known cell-surface markers for eosinophils, they are generally identified in blood and tissues by the affinity of their cytoplasmic granules for acid aniline dyes such as eosin. As eosinophils are often difficult to detect in tissues after degranulation, immunostaining for eosinophil-specific proteins [in particular, major basic protein (MBP)] has been used as a means to determine the presence of activated eosinophils in tissues.

Eosinophil-Derived Mediators

Eosinophil-Specific Cationic Proteins

Eosinophils store four highly basic, low-molecular-weight proteins in their cytoplasmic granules: MBP, eosinophil-derived neurotoxin (EDN), eosinophil peroxidase (EPO), and eosinophil cationic protein (ECP). MBP, EPO, and ECP are potent toxins for helminths and bacteria, and they are strongly implicated as mediators of allergic diseases such as asthma, atopic dermatitis, and allergic rhinitis (Fig. 7). MBP is potently toxic in mammalian cells *in vitro,* and high levels of MBP are found in the body fluids of patients with asthma and other allergic disorders (265). Both MBP and ECP exert their toxicity by damaging target cell membranes through charge-mediated interactions. In addition to its toxic properties, MBP activates platelets, mast cells, and basophils, which in turn release histamine. Furthermore, MBP administration to primates induces airway hyperresponsiveness. MBP may induce AHR through its demonstrated ability to competitively inhibit binding of cholinergic muscarinic M2 receptors on parasympathetic nerves (266). These receptors normally function as autoreceptors that inhibit the release of acetylcholine from the nerve ending. Thus, inhibition of these receptors by MBP

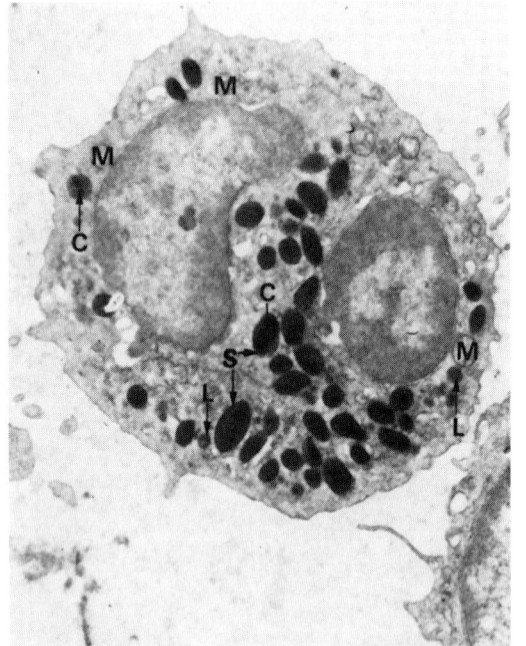
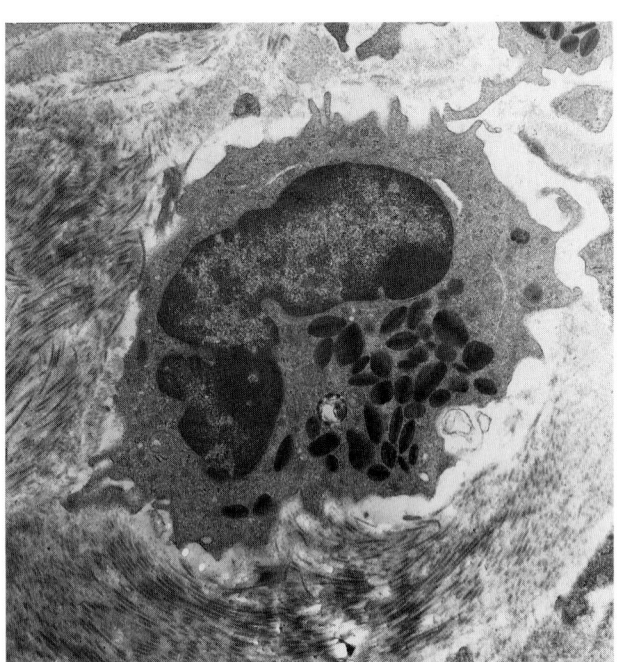

A   B

FIG. 6. Electron micrographs of human (**A**) and mouse (**B**) eosinophils (10,500× magnification). The most characteristic ultrastructural feature of eosinophils are the large, ovoid, specific granules (S), each containing a dense crystalloid (C) in the long axis of the granule; in humans, the crystalloids are irregular in form, but in many species, as in the mouse shown here, they have a regular, discoid shape. The specific granules are membrane-bound, and the matrix contains a variety of hydrolytic enzymes, including histaminase. The crystalloids are thought to be composed of basic proteins such as major basic protein (MBP), eosinophil peroxidase (EPO), and eosinophil cationic protein (ECP). Eosinophils also contain a small number of primary granules (L), which are less electron dense and lack crystalloids. Other cytoplasmic organelles such as mitochondria (M) are relatively sparse, and rough endoplasmic reticulum is absent. Note the characteristic bilobed nucleus. From Wheater PR, Burkitt HG, Daniels VG. *Functional histology.* Edinburgh: Churchill Livingstone, 1979, with permission. Micrograph of murine mast cell provided courtesy of Marc Rothenberg.

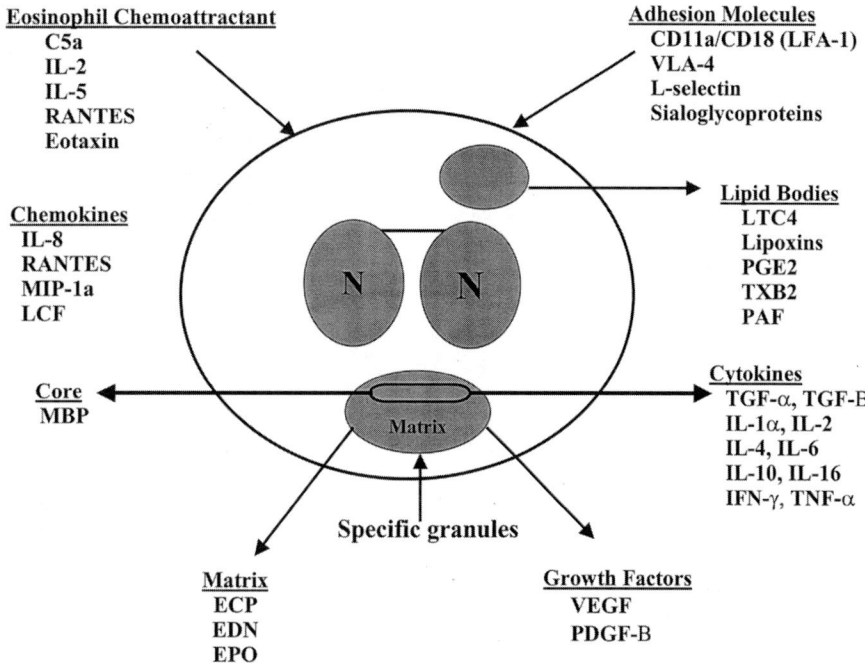

Eosinophil Chemoattractant
C5a
IL-2
IL-5
RANTES
Eotaxin

Chemokines
IL-8
RANTES
MIP-1a
LCF

Core
MBP

Matrix
ECP
EDN
EPO

Specific granules

Adhesion Molecules
CD11a/CD18 (LFA-1)
VLA-4
L-selectin
Sialoglycoproteins

Lipid Bodies
LTC4
Lipoxins
PGE2
TXB2
PAF

Cytokines
TGF-α, TGF-B
IL-1α, IL-2
IL-4, IL-6
IL-10, IL-16
IFN-γ, TNF-α

Growth Factors
VEGF
PDGF-B

FIG. 7. Eosinophils store and release a number of proteins in their specific granules. Specifically, major basic protein (MBP) is stored in the core of the granule, whereas eosinophil cationic protein (ECP), eosinophil-derived neurotoxin (EDN), and eosinophil peroxidase (EPO) are found in the matrix of the granules. Eosinophils also contain lipid bodies in which products of lipoxygenase and cyclooxygenase are formed. Eosinophils express a variety of adhesion molecules such as CD11α, very late activation antigen–4 (VLA-4), L-selectin, and sialoglycoproteins after activation. Eosinophils also release cytokines and chemokines, which are important in the allergic diathesis. Eosinophils are recruited to sites of inflammation in response to a number of chemoattractants, including C5α, interleukin (IL)–2, regulated upon activation, normal T-cell expressed, presumably secreted (RANTES), and eotaxin.

would enhance the release of acetylcholine in the airway wall, resulting in heightened contractile responses. Both ECP and EDN have partial sequence identity with pancreatic ribonucleases; however, EDN is more potent as a ribonuclease than is ECP.

EPO, which is distinct from the myeloperoxidase of neutrophils and monocytes, consists of two polypeptides of about 15 and 55 kDa. It catalyzes the formation of hypobromous acid from hydrogen peroxidase and halide ions (preferentially bromide). Hypobromous acid reacts with primary amines to form bromamines, and it converts tyrosine to 3-bromotyrosine. Increases in the levels of 3-bromotyrosine in BAL proteins have been observed in asthmatic patients after allergen provocation (267). Thus, the oxidative pathways induced in activated eosinophils may damage biomolecules *in vivo* (267).

Another prominent component of eosinophil primary granules are Charcot-Leyden crystals. This protein comprises up to 10% of the total cellular protein in human eosinophils. Although the Charcot-Leyden crystals protein possesses lysophospholipase activity, structural analysis suggest that the Charcot-Leyden crystal protein is similar to that of galectins 1 and 2, members of the "S-type" lectin superfamily (268). Studies in the mouse lung suggest that Charcot-Leyden crystals may contain a protein called YM-1 (T-lymphocyte–

derived eosinophil chemotactic factor), which has sequence homology to chitinase (269). Chitinase activity of these proteins may explain the strong association between eosinophilia and parasite infestations. These crystals are often found in sputum, feces, and tissues in patients with allergic asthma and other eosinophil-related diseases characterized by significant eosinophilia.

Lipid Mediators

Upon stimulation, eosinophils elaborate several bioactive lipids, including products of the 5- and 15-lipoxygenase pathway, products of the cyclooxygenase pathway, and PAF. Lipid bodies, or intracellular lipid-rich domains, are induced to develop in many activated eosinophils *in vivo* and are sites for enhanced synthesis of both lipoxygenase- and cyclooxygenase-derived eicosanoids. The activities of eosinophil-derived lipids, which are generally proinflammatory, are multiple and include potent smooth muscle contraction, vasoactivity, and mucus secretion activities.

Cytokines

It has been recognized that eosinophils are a major source of cytokines and appear to store some if not all of these cytokines in cytoplasmic specific granules. The cytokines reported to be made by eosinophils can be grouped into five major categories: (a) the myeloid-active and eosinophil-active growth factors (IL-3, IL-5, GM-CSF); other growth factors important in fibrosis and wound healing (TGF-β, TGF-α, vascular endothelial growth factor, platelet-derived growth factor β, heparin-binding epidermal growth factor); (c) immunoregulatory cytokines (IL-2, IL-4, IL-10, IL-12, IFN-γ); (d) proinflammatory cytokines (IL-1β, IL-6, IL-8, TNF-α); and (e) chemokines (RANTES, MIP-1α, eotaxin). Through the quick release of this diverse array of cytokines at the inflammatory loci, the eosinophil is poised to perpetuate and intensify the eosinophil-mediated inflammatory response, both by enhancing its own activation and through the release of Th2 cytokines.

Recruitment of Eosinophils to Sites of Inflammation

Preferential accumulation of eosinophils at sites of allergic inflammation involves multiple molecular events that are integrated and controlled by Th2 cytokines (270). These include (a) differentiation and release of mature eosinophils from the bone marrow into the bloodstream; (b) up-regulation of specific adhesion molecules on eosinophils and endothelium; (c) stimulation of C-C chemokine production and egress of eosinophils from the blood into the tissues; and (d) production of eosinophil-active cytokines that increase eosinophil survival in tissues.

Eosinophils are terminally differentiated granulocytes that develop from CD34$^+$ hematopoietic progenitor cells in the bone marrow. Under the influence of GM-CSF, IL-3, and IL-5, they differentiate into mature eosinophils. Each of these cytokines can promote eosinophilopoiesis *in vivo*, but the Th2 cytokine IL-5 has the most specific effects on eosinophil differentiation and production. In addition to its effects on eosinophil differentiation, IL-5 can rapidly induce the release of developed eosinophils from the bone marrow into the circulation. The importance of IL-5 in blood and tissue eosinophilia has been repeatedly shown in *in vitro* and *in vivo* studies of gene-targeted and gene-overexpressing mouse lines (45,271).

Circulating eosinophils are recruited to sites of inflammation by the combined actions of inflammatory mediators on adhesion molecule expression on the vascular endothelium and production of chemoattractants (Fig. 8). Several cell adhesion molecules have been implicated in eosinophil adherence to cytokine-stimulated vascular endothelium, including ICAM-1, E-selectin, L-selectin, and VLA-4/VCAM-1. The importance of VCAM-1 to eosinophil recruitment has been shown in primate and mouse studies in which blockade of

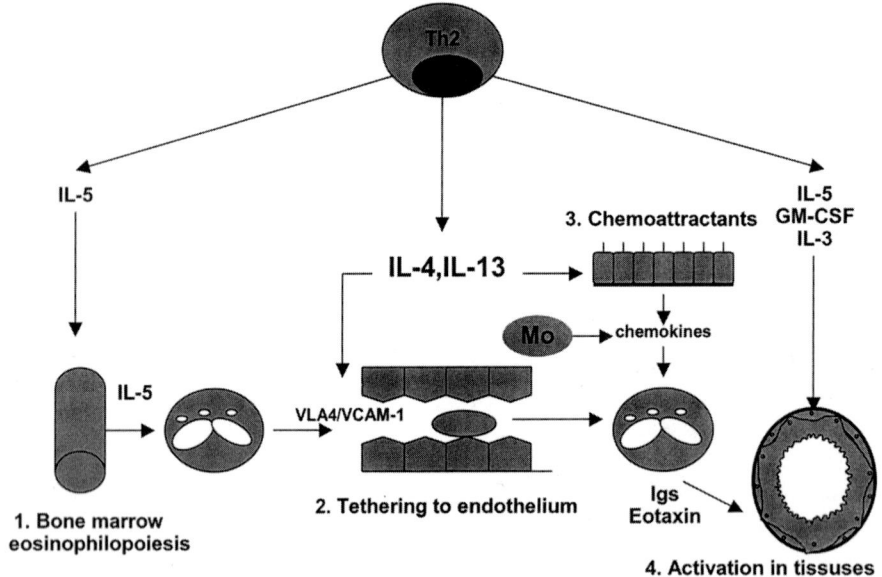

FIG. 8. Type 2 T helper (Th2) cytokine regulation of eosinophil recruitment and accumulation. Th2 cytokines coordinately regulate eosinophil recruitment, activation, and accumulation at the site of antigen exposure. After allergen-specific induction of Th2 cytokine production [interleukin (IL)–5, IL-4, IL-13, IL-3, granulocyte-macrophage colony-stimulating factor (GM-CSF)], IL-5 rapidly induces differentiation of eosinophils from myeloid precursors in the bone marrow to stimulate their release into the bloodstream. IL-4 or IL-13 or both promote eosinophil egress from the vascular compartment by up-regulating vascular cell adhesion molecule 1 (VCAM-1) expression on vascular endothelial cells. Subsequently, IL-4 and IL-13 guide eosinophils to the site of allergen exposure by regulating the production of various chemokines [e.g., regulated upon activation, normal T-cell expressed, presumably secreted (RANTES), eotaxin] by local cells such as macrophages and epithelial cells. Once these cells accumulate in tissues, locally produced IL-5 along with other cytokines, such as GM-CSF and IL-3, promote their actions by prolonging their survival in tissues.

VLA-4/VCAM-1 interactions inhibits eosinophil infiltration of tissues (272). IL-4 and IL-13 induce VCAM-1 expression on the surface of vascular endothelial cells, which leads to preferential recruitment of eosinophils into sites of allergic inflammation.

Eosinophil migration to the sites of inflammatory loci is mediated by a number of chemoattractants. Until the 1990s, mediators such as PAF, C5a, and LTB_4 were considered to be the most important eosinophil chemoattractants. Although potent chemoattractants, they do not show any specificity for eosinophils. In the 1990s, a family of chemotactic peptides (also known as chemokines) that control leukocyte migration and activation were identified. They have been divided into two main groups on the basis of their sequence homology and the position of the first two cysteine residues, C-X-C or C-C (273). Interestingly, a number of the C-C chemokines were identified as eosinophil active chemoattractants [RANTES, CCL5), eotaxin (CCL11), MCP-4 (CCL13), MCP-3 (CCl7), and MIP-α (CCL3)]. The levels of most of these chemokines have been shown to be up-regulated in the mucosal tissues of patients with asthma, atopic rhinitis, and atopic dermatitis. Although each of these chemokines is implicated in eosinophil chemotaxis, it was originally hypothesized that eotaxin would play a pivotal role in eosinophilic inflammation in that it binds specifically to the chemokine receptor 3 (CCR3), while the other C-C chemokines bind multiple receptors. The fact that CCR3 is highly expressed on eosinophils, basophils, and Th2 cells but not on neutrophils suggested that it plays an important role in Th2-mediated inflammatory responses (274,275). Surprisingly, however, eotaxin-deficient mice have shown only minor defects in eosinophil accumulation (276,277), which indicates that eotaxin alone is not sufficient for eosinophil accumulation. Along these lines, complete abrogation of eosinophil migration has not been observed by inhibition of any one chemokine (42,276,278–280), which suggests that multiple chemokines working in concert are necessary to direct leukocytes to specific sites of inflammation. Thus, it has been postulated that a panoply of chemokines may be necessary to establish the multiple chemical gradients required for eosinophils to migrate through several local compartments from the vascular spaces to the mucosal surfaces in the nose, airways, and skin. For example, in the airways, the eosinophil must emigrate from the vascular compartment through the interstitium and, finally, through and into the airways. Therefore, interstitial macrophage-derived chemokines might provide the chemotactic gradient for eosinophils to move from the vascular compartment into the interstitium, whereas airway epithelium-derived chemokines might provide a second gradient that localizes the cells around and into the airways (281). Further studies are needed to clarify the complex network of chemokines involved in regulation of these important effector cells of the allergic diathesis.

Last, eosinophils rapidly undergo apoptosis unless provided with signals from eosinophil growth factors such as IL-5, GM-CSF, and IL-3. As discussed previously, each of these mediators is found in increased levels in the tissues and fluids from allergic individuals. Prolonged survival of eosinophils under the influence of locally generated growth factors is thought to be an important mechanism for selective eosinophil accumulation in atopic diseases. Direct evidence for prolonged survival of eosinophils comes from a study in which anti-IL-5 monoclonal antibody caused rapid loss of eosinophils from cultured explants of nasal polyps. Interestingly, the number of apoptotic eosinophils in the airways of asthmatic individuals is increased in such patients treated with inhaled glucocorticoids (282). The effect of glucocorticoids on tissue eosinophils may result either from inhibition of T cell–derived growth factors or as a direct effect on eosinophil survival (283).

Mechanisms of Eosinophil Activation

The effector functions of eosinophils are mediated by stimuli that induce degranulation. Eosinophil degranulation can be regulated by multiple components, including those that primarily stimulate the cells (e.g., immunoglobulins, and lipid mediators), priming agents (e.g., cytokines), and chemokines. However, the precise mechanisms by which eosinophil degranulation occurs *in vivo* are still poorly understood.

Eosinophils express receptors for several immunoglobulins, including IgG, IgA, and IgE. Surfaces coated with IgG, IgA, and secretory IgA stimulate eosinophil degranulation *in vitro*. Of these immunoglobulins, secretory IgA is the best for inducing eosinophil degranulation and does not stimulate neutrophil degranulation. Because IgA is the most abundant immunoglobulin isotype in mucosal secretions of the respiratory and gastrointestinal tracts, it may be an important regulator of eosinophil activation at these sites. IgE may also be important for eosinophil activation, inasmuch as eosinophils can bind IgE through three distinct structures: the S-type lectin galectin-3, FcϵRII/CD23, and FcϵRI. It was initially shown that eosinophils isolated from patients with parasite-induced eosinophilia degranulate in response to IgE antibody or IgE-coated parasites (284,285). Subsequent studies showed that local allergen provocation induces expression of FcϵRI by eosinophils infiltrating the airways (286) and skin of patients with allergic diseases (287,288). In studies with sera from ragweed-allergic patients with hay fever, ragweed-specific IgG, but not IgE, induced allergen-dependent eosinophil degranulation *in vitro* (289,290). Thus, it remains to be determined whether IgE is an important regulator of eosinophil degranulation in atopy.

Eosinophil degranulation may also be induced by soluble stimuli alone. Cytokines, especially those with eosinophilopoietic activity, such as GM-CSF and IL-5, are potent inducers of eosinophil granule protein release. Interestingly, eosinophil granule proteins themselves, including MBP and EPO, stimulate eosinophils and cause degranulation, which suggests an autocrine mechanism of eosinophil degranulation (291). Other physiological stimuli for eosinophil degranulation include PAF, the complement fragments C5a and C3a, and the neuropeptide substance P (292). As discussed briefly earlier, chemokines may also activate eosinophils by binding CCR3. In this regard, eotaxin induces eosinophil degranulation and LTC_4 release.

Eosinophils as Effector Cells in Allergic Responses

Eosinophils are postulated to contribute to the clinical symptoms of the late phase of the allergic response through the actions of the eosinophil-specific basic proteins, as well as the lipid mediators on mucosal tissues. Circumstantial evidence for a causative role of eosinophils in allergic inflammation and the clinical symptoms of atopic disorders comes from a variety of studies (293). First, elevated levels of activated eosinophils and their protein products (MBP, ECP, EPO, and EDN) have been consistently demonstrated in BAL fluids and airway biopsy tissues from patients with asthma (293), in nasal specimens from patients with allergic rhinitis (nasal fluids and nasal biopsies) (294), and in skin lesions from patients with atopic dermatitis (295). Second, in each of these diseases, increased levels of eosinophils and of their proteins are correlated with disease severity. Last, successful steroid treatment is associated with a marked reduction in both blood and tissue eosinophil levels in patients with asthma and atopic rhinitis (296–298).

Despite the substantial body of circumstantial evidence that supports a causative role for eosinophils in the pathophysiological processes of atopic disorders, the results of studies designed to define a pathogenic role for eosinophils in atopic disorders are conflicting. Studies in IL-5 gene knockout (45) and transgenic mice (271) show that both eosinophilia and AHR are IL-5 dependent. In addition, anti–IL-5 treatment of cynomolgus monkeys inhibits allergen-induced airway reactivity and BAL eosinophilia (299). In contrast, other investigators have demonstrated that blockade of eosinophils by IL-5 ablation did not affect AHR (45,300). This dissociation between eosinophils and the late-phase response has been confirmed in a multiple-center study in asthmatic humans that demonstrated that, although anti–IL-5 treatment suppressed pulmonary eosinophils, it did not inhibit either early or late responses to inhaled allergens or improve lung function (301). Although multiple explanations for a lack of effect in this study can be made, including the small study size, dosing schedule, or acute nature of treatment, these studies suggest that blockade of eosinophils and IL-5 alone are not sufficient to inhibit clinical symptoms of atopic disease. One thing that should be stressed in interpreting these studies is that most studies have relied entirely on blockade of IL-5 to elucidate the role of eosinophils in allergic responses. Blockade of IL-5 does not completely eliminate eosinophils in either humans or mice. Because there are no currently known ways to completely and specifically deplete eosinophils, elucidation of the role of these cells in the pathophysiological consequences of atopic diseases awaits development of more specific tools. Nevertheless, it is possible to conclude from the combined data that multiple processes probably occur during the allergic response that work in concert to induce the clinical symptoms of atopic diseases.

Th2 Cells as Effector Cells

The updated understanding of the role of Th2 cells in the allergic diathesis suggests that they are important effector cells in the allergic response in addition to their well-accepted role as orchestrators of the inflammatory process. Specifically, the Th2 cytokine IL-13 has been implicated as an effector molecule in allergic disease. Evidence for this contention comes from studies in which blockade of endogenous levels of IL-13 in antigen-sensitized mice by administration of a soluble form of the IL-13 receptor $\alpha2$ (IL-13Rα2) chain, which binds only IL-13, completely reversed AHR and pulmonary mucus cell hyperplasia (40,302). Furthermore, it was shown that recombinant IL-13 was able to recreate the symptoms of asthma (airway hyperresponsiveness, mucus hypersecretion, eosinophilia) in the absence of functional T cells or B cells (40). These effects were shown to be independent from eosinophils as well (303). These results suggested that IL-13's effects were not ascribable to its known role in regulating IgE or eosinophil recruitment. Interestingly, despite the similarities in function between IL-13 and IL-4, IL-4 blockade at the time of antigen challenge does not ablate airway hyperresponsiveness (304). This was further supported by the finding that transfer of Th2 cells derived from IL-4–deficient mice was still able to confer airway hyperresponsiveness (305). Moreover, chronic expression of IL-13 in the murine lung results in development of these features, as well as subepithelial fibrosis and the formation of Charcot-Leyden crystals (161). In contrast, overexpression of the IL-4 gene in the murine lung does not result in AHR or subepithelial fibrosis (306).

IL-13 has several actions that implicate it as an effector in the allergic diathesis, such as its role in mucus production, fibrotic processes, and, perhaps, bronchoconstriction. First, it has been shown to play an important role in mucus hypersecretion. Mucus hypersecretion is a consistent feature of the allergic phenotype in both the upper and lower respiratory tract. In fact, extensive plugging of the airway lumen has been associated with fatal episodes of asthma. This response is a Th2 cell–dependent process, inasmuch as adoptive transfer of Th2 cells into the murine lung reconstitutes the effect of antigen challenge (305). Several lines of research suggest that mucus cell metaplasia is an IL-13–, not IL-4–, dependent process. For example, transfer of Th2 cells devoid of the IL-4 or IL-5 genes nonetheless induce extensive goblet cell metaplasia in the murine lung. However, blockade of the IL-4Rα chain or deficiency in STAT6 prevents the development of mucus cell metaplasia after allergen challenge, which suggests that IL-13 may be the ligand for the IL-4/STAT6 pathway in mucus cell changes (111). Indeed, administration of soluble IL-13Rα2 reversed the metaplastic response of goblet cells induced by allergen sensitization and challenge. Administration of recombinant IL-13 *in vivo* or overexpression of the IL-13 gene recapitulates antigen effects on mucus production. Conversely, allergen-induced goblet cell metaplasia is significantly reduced in IL-13–deficient mice (307). This metaplasia was not further reduced when IL-4 was blocked with neutralizing antibodies, which suggests that, indeed, IL-13 is the primary regulator *in vivo* of mucus cell hyperplasia.

Another feature of the chronic inflammatory response in both the skin and the airways is the presence of a fibrotic process. Data suggest that IL-13 is an important regulator of fibrotic processes. For example, overexpression of IL-13 in the murine lung induces a dramatic fibrotic response in the airway wall (161). Furthermore, IL-13 transgenic mice express matrix proteases such as matrix metalloproteases and cathepsins, which are thought to be important in the fibrotic response (308). A clear demarcation of function for IL-4 and IL-13 in fibrosis has been demonstrated in Th2-mediated pathological processes of *Schistosoma mansoni* infection in mice. Schistosome-induced collagen deposition is reduced in the lungs of STAT6-deficient animals but not in IL-4–deficient mice (309). Furthermore, secretory IL-13Rα2–immunoglobulin delivery completely prevented the fibrotic response in parasite-infected mice. Thus, in several models of Th2-mediated fibrosis, blockade of IL-13 selectively inhibited fibrotic remodeling processes, which suggests that this cytokine may be an important mediator of inflammation-induced tissue fibrosis.

Reports suggest that IL-13 may directly induce bronchoconstriction by means of its direct effects on airway smooth muscle. In this regard, Laporte et al. (310) reported that human airway smooth muscle cells express IL-4Rα, IL-13 receptor α1, and IL-13Rα2 chains. Moreover, they demonstrate that IL-13, but not IL-4, significantly reduces β-adrenoceptor–induced human airway smooth muscle cell stiffness through a MAP kinase–dependent pathway. Collectively, these results suggest that IL-13 may have direct effects on airway smooth muscle that contribute at least in part to the airway narrowing observed in asthmatic individuals. Because IL-13 receptors are expressed on resident cells in the mucosa such as epithelial cells, fibroblasts, macrophages, and smooth muscle cells, the effects of IL-13 are probably caused by direct stimulation of its receptor on each of these cells, although this remains to be determined.

The importance of IL-13 in allergic disorders in humans is supported by numerous reports of exaggerated IL-13 production in patients with asthma, atopic rhinitis, and allergic dermatitis (311). In asthma in particular, both message and protein levels of IL-13 are elevated in bronchial biopsy specimens and BAL cells from allergic individuals in comparison with those of control subjects (124). Conversely, IL-13 levels are reduced in patients with asthma and rhinitis undergoing allergen desensitization treatment regimens or steroid treatment (124). In support of the notion that IL-13 is a central effector of allergic immune responses, several groups have reported associations of polymorphisms in the IL-13 gene with various features of the asthmatic phenotype (312,313). Of particular interest is the Arg130/Gln substitution in the

coding region of IL-13 noted by two groups and detected across multiple ethnic populations. Molecular modeling suggests potential biological impacts of this change, including enhanced receptor binding and activation.

Unifying Hypothesis

The elicitation of allergic airway responses in a sensitized individual upon reexposure to offending allergens is probably the culmination of a complex network of cellular and molecular events (Fig. 9). After antigen challenge, cross-linking of antigen and IgE on IgE-bearing cells leads to the immediate release of substances such as histamine, leukotrienes, PGD$_2$, and tryptase. The actions of these mediators account for the immediate symptoms, such as smooth muscle constriction, vasodilation, and increased vascular permeability. It is possible that the release of IL-13 by either mast cells or basophils can also induce many of these same symptoms. Secretion of chemokines (eotaxin) and cytokines (IL-4, IL-5) by basophils and mast cells also serve to attract more T cells, APCs, and effector cells such as eosinophils to the site of insult. Simultaneously, DCs within the mucosa are presenting allergen to T cells, and within 6 to 48 hours, additional T cells are recruited to the area. The expression of FcεRI on the surface of DCs greatly facilitates their uptake, processing, and presentation of allergens to T cells during the elicitation phase of the response. Furthermore, the cytokine milieu created as a result of mast cell and basophil activation—namely, a Th2 cytokine environment—most likely drives a polarized Th2 response. Further production of Th2 cytokines at the local site augments the recruitment and activation of additional eosinophils and T cells. During the late phase, release of mediators from mast cells, basophils, eosinophils, and T cells act in concert to induce the vascular changes, bronchoconstriction, and mucus changes observed during the late-phase response. Many repetitions of this sequence lead to persistent inflammation, resulting in alterations in the structure and function of resident mucosal cells such as smooth muscle, fibroblasts, and epithelial cells. Because many of the actions of these effector cells are redundant, it is not surprising that depletion of neither mast cells nor eosinophils has been sufficient to significantly ablate the physiological consequences of allergen exposure. One point of convergence is the production of IL-13 by all of the likely suspects (e.g., basophil, mast cell, eosinophil, and T cells). With its newly described effector functions, IL-13 may not only provide a unifying explanation for the importance of multiple effector cells in allergic responses but may also provide an ideal target for therapy.

CHARACTERISTICS OF SPECIFIC ATOPIC DISORDERS

In this section, we briefly discuss the clinical manifestations, pathogenesis, and therapeutic strategies for the treatment of the classical atopic syndromes, including anaphylaxis,

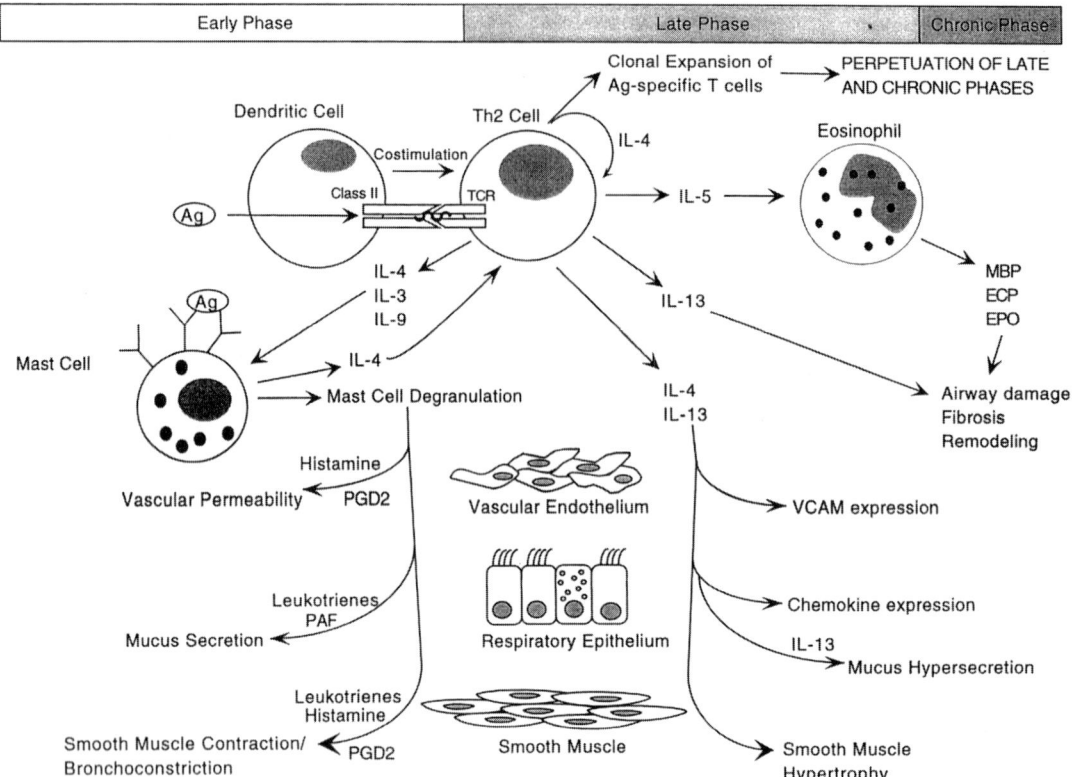

FIG. 9. Overview of the acute, late, and chronic phases of the allergic response. Cross-linking of surface immunoglobulin E (IgE) on sensitized mast cells by antigen results in mast cell degranulation and release of numerous mediators, including histamine, tryptase, prostaglandin G_2 (PDG$_2$), and cytokines. These mediators are largely responsible for the early phase of the allergic response. Antigen presentation by dendritic cells to type 2 T helper (Th2) cells results in activation and clonal expansion of antigen-specific T cells and the subsequent release of Th2 cytokines, interleukin (IL)–4, IL-5, and IL-13. These cytokines result in recruitment of eosinophils, chemokine expression, smooth muscle hypertrophy, and mucus hypersecretion. Ultimately, long-term exposure to IL-13 and eosinophilic effector molecules leads to the structural changes observed in tissues of individuals with chronic disease.

allergic rhinitis, atopic dermatitis, and asthma. Readers should consult clinical allergy textbooks for further details on these disorders.

Anaphylaxis

Anaphylaxis is a systemic, immediate hypersensitivity reaction that results from IgE-mediated release of vasoactive and inflammatory mediators from mast cells and basophils. Death from anaphylaxis is most often caused by respiratory obstruction or cardiovascular collapse. The initial experimental description of the phenomenon dates to a paper published in 1902, in which Portier and Richet (314) described the sensitization of dogs to sea anemone venom, a process with fatal sequelae upon subsequent exposure to nonlethal doses of the venom. In opposition to prophylaxis, this process was termed *anaphylaxis,* meaning against or without protection. Common causes of anaphylaxis in humans include exposure to antibiotics and other drugs, radiocontrast media, latex, venom, and foods. The cause of anaphylaxis remains unidentified in

up to two thirds of patients. Whereas anaphylactic reactions involve IgE-mediated mast cell and basophil degranulation by definition, anaphylactoid reactions result from mast cell and basophil degranulation by IgE-independent means. Underlying etiologies, when known, include drugs, biological agents, and physical factors (e.g., pressure, cold, sunlight); a substantial proportion of cases are idiopathic.

Allergic Rhinitis

In 1819, John Bostock first described *catarrus aestivus* or hay fever (315). In 1873, Charles Blackley recognized that pollen grains were the causative agents of hay fever. In the 1800s, hay fever was considered a rare disorder, restricted to the privileged class. This is certainly no longer the case. According to year 2000 estimates, up to 40% of children in the United States are affected by allergic rhinitis (316). Allergic rhinitis is an IgE-mediated disease characterized by sneezing, rhinorrhea, nasal congestion, and nasal pruritus (317,318). The seasonal form is caused by allergens released during tree, grass, or weed pollination; the perennial form is associated with allergies to animal dander, dust mites, or mold spores, or a combination of these. Skin testing—the experimental interrogation of the ability of a panel of antigen extracts to induce cutaneous immediate-type hypersensitivity responses—is often employed for diagnostic confirmation of atopy and to determine the allergens to which an individual is sensitized.

Treatment strategies include allergen avoidance, antihistamines, α-adrenergic agonists, intranasal steroids, topical ipratropium bromide, and immunotherapy regimens. Immunotherapy, introduced by Leonard Noon and John Freeman in 1911 as a method for protecting patients against the effects of "pollen toxin" (319), has been used since as a treatment for patients with allergic rhinitis and allergic asthma. Conventional allergen immunotherapy involves the subcutaneous injection of graded quantities of allergen. Although such immunotherapy has been associated with therapeutic benefit, the relevant immunological mechanisms remain obscure. In patients with venom anaphylaxis, allergen immunotherapy is the prophylactic treatment of choice.

Food Allergy

Food allergy must be carefully distinguished from the more common adverse reactions to ingested substances (e.g., food intolerance, dose-related toxic reactions) that are not immune mediated. True food allergy afflicts approximately 8% of children younger than 3 years and 2% of the adult population. Such food hypersensitivity comprises several disorders that vary in time of onset, severity, and persistence. The most common type of food allergy is immediate gastrointestinal hypersensitivity. Symptoms, which include nausea, abdominal pain, colic, vomiting, and diarrhea, develop within minutes to 2 hours of antigen exposure. Infants with this syndrome may present with intermittent vomiting and poor weight gain. The predominant response to orally induced antigens is the induction of tolerance. Food allergy represents an aberration of this process. Only a small number of foodstuffs account for most offending allergens. In childhood, the most common allergens are derived from milk, eggs, peanuts, soy, and wheat. In adults, the most common foods implicated are peanuts, tree nuts, fish, and shellfish. Most food allergens are relatively small, water-soluble, heat- and acid-stable glycoproteins that are resistant to proteolytic degradation. The higher incidence of disease in childhood is presumably related to factors regulating the ontogeny of the gut and immune system development (320,321). Therapy revolves around avoidance of the offending allergen. Interestingly, patients with atopic dermatitis commonly have subclinical food hypersensitivity; ingestion of the relevant allergen leads to worsening of the dermatitis.

Oral allergy syndrome represents a second type of food hypersensitivity. This is an immediate-type contact allergy that leads to pruritus and tingling and swelling of the lips, palate, and throat after ingestion of the offending allergen, which is usually in fruits or vegetables. Oral allergy syndrome

affects up to 40% of adults with defined pollen allergy, because of cross-reacting allergens. Therapy involves allergen avoidance.

The eosinophilic gastroenteritides (eosinophilic esophagitis, gastritis, gastroenteritis), although not thought in general to be caused by food allergy, deserve brief mention here. These syndromes are characterized pathologically by eosinophil infiltration and clinically by a variety of nonspecific symptoms, including abdominal pain, nausea, vomiting, and diarrhea, although the etiology and pathogenesis remain unclear in most cases. Some cases result from hypersensitivity reactions to antigens derived from *Ancylostoma caninum,* a common dog hookworm that is poorly adapted to and causes nonpatent infection in humans (322). Some cases may indeed be caused by food allergy.

Atopic Dermatitis

Atopic dermatitis is a common, chronic, relapsing, inflammatory skin disease characterized by dry skin, severe pruritus, secondary excoriation (which can lead to lichenification), and a heightened susceptibility to cutaneous infections. Atopic dermatitis can lead to significant suffering, both physical and psychological. The prevalence of atopic dermatitis has increased in the since the 1960s; currently, 10% are affected at some point during childhood in the United States. Both environmental and genetic factors seem to play a role in susceptibility. Because the heritability of atopy appears to be largely independent of disease type, it is notable that parental atopic dermatitis confers a higher risk for the development of atopic dermatitis than for either allergic asthma or allergic rhinitis in offspring, which suggests the likelihood of atopic dermatitis-specific genes (323). Disease generally manifests early in childhood and is associated with sensitivity to food or inhalant allergens or both. In adults, disease is associated primarily with sensitivity to inhalant allergens. Apart from exposure to specific food and inhalant allergens, environmental triggers such as irritating substances, emotional stress, climactic factors, hormones, and local infections are all known to be important in the expression of atopic dermatitis. Skin lesions generally display evidence of mast cell, eosinophil, and T-cell infiltration and activation. In contrast to other atopic disorders, a biphasic pattern of T-cell polarization or reactivity is present in atopic dermatitis: Th2 cytokines predominate in acute lesions, whereas chronic lesions express a mix of Th1 and Th2 cytokines.

Current treatment of atopic dermatitis is directed at symptomatic relief, skin hydration, the reduction of cutaneous inflammation, and avoidance of inciting antigens. Therapy includes antihistamines, topical immunosuppressive agents (glucocorticoids, FK506), moisturizers, environmental control measures for inhalant allergens, and food-elimination diets for food allergens. Phase I and II studies have supported the efficacy of short-term IFN-γ therapy in the treatment of severe atopic dermatitis (324), although the mechanism of action remains unclear.

Asthma

The term *asthma* was coined by Hippocrates to refer to attacks of breathlessness and wheezing. Asthma is a complex inflammatory disease of the lung, the prevalence, morbidity, and mortality of which have been increasing markedly since the 1960s. Asthma is a heterogeneous disorder with variations in the age at onset, severity of disease, and underlying pathogenesis. Although asthma is multifactorial in origin with both environmental and genetic influences, atopy is the strongest identifiable predisposing factor for the development of asthma. Most childhood asthma is allergic in nature and referred to as extrinsic or atopic asthma; however, asthma that develops in adulthood and some forms of childhood asthma are not associated with elevated IgE levels, and this form is referred to as intrinsic or nonatopic asthma. In the most common form of the disease, extrinsic asthma, the inflammatory process is thought to arise as a result of inappropriate immune responses to commonly inhaled antigens. The inflammatory response in the asthmatic lung is characterized by infiltration of the airway wall with lymphocytes, predominantly CD4+ T cells, eosinophils, and degranulated mast cells. Structurally, the airways of asthmatic patients are characterized by mucus cell hyperplasia, sub–basement membrane thickening, and loss of epithelial cell integrity. These cellular findings have consistently been associated with the main physiological abnormalities of the disease, including variable airflow obstruction and airway hyperresponsiveness. As discussed extensively in this chapter, the pathological consequences of this disease are thought to arise as a result of skewed T-cell responses to inhaled antigens, which, in turn, lead to activation and recruitment of the primary effector cells, mast cells, eosinophils, and T cells. Activation of these cells results in the release of a plethora of mediators that individually or in concert induce changes in airway geometry and produce the symptoms of the disease.

Current guidelines for asthma management emphasize environmental control measures, objective monitoring, and pharmacotherapy for comprehensive asthma management. The exact combination of pharmacotherapeutic agents is dependent on the severity of disease: Short-acting bronchodilators (β-adrenergic agonists) are recommended for mild, intermittent asthma, and the addition of anti-inflammatory medication, including inhaled or oral corticosteroids, cromolyn or nedocromil, or a leukotriene antagonist is indicated for more severe disease. Several novel therapies have been introduced since the 1990s, including a humanized monoclonal antibody directed against IgE, a soluble IL-4 receptor, and an anti–IL-5 antibody. Because clinical testing of these new therapies is in early stages, determination of their efficacy in asthma therapy awaits further study.

ACKNOWLEDGMENTS

The authors thank Christopher Karp for helpful discussions. The authors acknowledge the support of National Institutes of Health (NIH) grants HL65469, HL66623, PO1 ES09606, and HL10342 to Marsha Wills-Karp and NIH grants ES11170 and AI46652 and American Heart Association Grant 0060337B to Gurjit K. Khurana Hershey.

REFERENCES

1. von Pirquet C. Allergie. *Munch Med Wochenschr* (Prausnitz C, Trans). In Gell PHG, Coombs RRA, eds. *Clinical aspects of immunology.* vol 30. Oxford, UK: Blackwell Scientific Publications, 1906:1457.
2. Prausnitz C, Kustner H. Studies concerning sensitivity. *Zent bl Bakteriol I Orig* 1921;86:160–169.
3. Ishizaka K, Ishizaka T, Lee EH. Physiochemical properties of reaginic antibody. II. Characteristic properties of reaginic antibody different from human gamma-A- isohemagglutinin and gamma-D-globulin. *J Allergy* 1966;37:336–349.
4. Ishizaka K, Ishizaka T, Hornbrook MM. Physico-chemical properties of human reaginic antibody. IV. Presence of a unique immunoglobulin as a carrier of reaginic activity. *J Immunol* 1966;97:75–85.
5. Ishizaka K, Ishizaka T, Hornbrook MM. Physicochemical properties of reaginic antibody. V. Correlation of reaginic activity with gamma-E-globulin antibody. *J Immunol* 1966;97:840–853.
6. Galli SJ, Lantz CS. In: Paul WE, ed. *Allergy,* 4th ed. New York: Lippincott-Raven, 1999:1127–1174.
7. Janeway CA, Travers P. *Immunobiology: the immune system in health and disease,* vol. 11. New York: Garland, 1994.
8. Kay AB. Concepts of allergy and hypersensitivity. In: Kay AB, ed. *Allergy and allergic diseases,* vol 1. Oxford. Blackwell Science Ltd. 1997;23–35.
9. Holford-Strevens V, Warren P, Wong C, et al. Serum total immunoglobulin E levels in Canadian adults. *J Allergy Clin Immunol* 1984;73:516–522.
10. Peat JK, Britton WJ, Salome CM, et al. Bronchial hyperresponsiveness in two populations of Australian schoolchildren. III. Effect of exposure to environmental allergens. *Clin Allergy* 1987;17:291–300.
11. Cline MG, Burrows B. Distribution of allergy in a population sample residing in Tucson, Arizona. *Thorax* 1989;44:425–431.
12. Allergen nomenclature. IUIS/WHO Allergen Nomenclature Subcommittee. *Bull World Health Organ* 1994;72:797–806.
13. Thomas WR. Mite allergens groups I–VII. A catalogue of enzymes. *Clin Exp Allergy* 1993;23:350–353.
14. Schulz O, Sewell HF, Shakib F. Proteolytic cleavage of CD25, the alpha subunit of the human T cell interleukin 2 receptor, by Der p 1, a major mite allergen with cysteine protease activity. *J Exp Med* 1998;187:271–275.
15. Shakib F, Schulz O, Sewell H. A mite subversive: cleavage of CD23 and CD25 by Der p 1 enhances allergenicity. *Immunol Today* 1998;19:313–316.
16. Maruo K, Akaike T, Ono T, et al. Generation of anaphylatoxins through proteolytic processing of C3 and C5 by house dust mite protease. *J Allergy Clin Immunol* 1997;100:253–260.
17. Slater JE. Latex allergy. *J Allergy Clin Immunol* 1994;94:139–149.
18. Turjanmaa K, Alenius H, Makinen-Kiljunen S, et al. Natural rubber latex allergy. *Allergy* 1996;51:593–602.
19. Breiteneder H, Scheiner O. Molecular and immunological characteristics of latex allergens. *Int Arch Allergy Immunol* 1998;116:83–92.
20. Theissen U, Theissen JL, Mertes N, et al. IgE-mediated hypersensitivity to latex in childhood. *Allergy* 1997;52:665–669.
21. Karlsson MG, Davidsson A, Hellquist HB. Increase in CD4+ and CD45RO+ memory T cells in the nasal mucosa of allergic patients. *APMIS* 1994;102:753–758.
22. Azzawi M, Bradley B, Jeffery PK, et al. Identification of activated T lymphocytes and eosinophils in bronchial biopsies in stable atopic asthma. *Am Rev Respir Dis* 1990;142:1407–1413.
23. Corrigan CJ, Kay AB. CD4 T-lymphocyte activation in acute severe asthma. Relationship to disease severity and atopic status. *Am Rev Respir Dis* 1990;141:970–977.
24. Mosmann TR, Cherwinski H, Bond MW, et al. Two types of murine helper T cell clone. I. Definition according to profiles of lymphokine activities and secreted proteins. *J Immunol* 1986;136:2348–2357.
25. Street NE, Mosmann TR. Functional diversity of T lymphocytes due to secretion of different cytokine patterns. *FASEB J* 1991;5:171–177.

26. Kapsenberg ML, Wierenga EA, Bos JD, et al. Functional subsets of allergen-reactive human CD4+ T cells. *Immunol Today* 1991;12:392–395.

27. Del Prete GF, De Carli M, Mastromauro C, et al. Purified protein derivative of *Mycobacterium tuberculosis* and excretory-secretory antigen(s) of *Toxocara canis* expand *in vitro* human T cells with stable and opposite (type 1 T helper or type 2 T helper) profile of cytokine production. *J Clin Invest* 1991;88:346–350.

28. Walker C, Bode E, Boer L, et al. Allergic and nonallergic asthmatics have distinct patterns of T-cell activation and cytokine production in peripheral blood and bronchoalveolar lavage. *Am Rev Respir Dis* 1992;146:109–115.

29. Del Prete GF, De Carli M, D'Elios MM, et al. Allergen exposure induces the activation of allergen-specific Th2 cells in the airway mucosa of patients with allergic respiratory disorders. *Eur J Immunol* 1993;23:1445–1149.

30. Robinson DS, Hamid Q, Ying S, et al. Predominant TH2-like bronchoalveolar T-lymphocyte population in atopic asthma. *N Engl J Med* 1992;326:298–304.

31. Howarth PH, Salagean M, Dokic D. Allergic rhinitis: not purely a histamine-related disease. *Allergy* 2000;55(Suppl 64):7–16.

32. Akdis CA, Akdis M, Simon D, et al. T cells and T cell-derived cytokines as pathogenic factors in the nonallergic form of atopic dermatitis. *J Invest Dermatol* 1999;113:628–634.

33. Grewe M, Bruijnzeel-Koomen CA, Schopf E, et al. A role for Th1 and Th2 cells in the immunopathogenesis of atopic dermatitis. *Immunol Today* 1998;19:359–361.

34. Werfel T, Morita A, Grewe M, et al. Allergen specificity of skin-infiltrating T cells is not restricted to a type-2 cytokine pattern in chronic skin lesions of atopic dermatitis. *J Invest Dermatol* 1996;107:871–876.

35. Wilkinson JR, Lane SJ, Lee TH. Effects of corticosteroids on cytokine generation and expression of activation antigens by monocytes in bronchial asthma. *Int Arch Allergy Appl Immunol* 1991;94:220–221.

36. Fokkens WJ, Godthelp T, Holm AF, et al. Allergic rhinitis and inflammation: the effect of nasal corticosteroid therapy. *Allergy* 1997;52:29–32.

37. Secrist H, Chelen CJ, Wen Y, et al. Allergen immunotherapy decreases interleukin 4 production in CD4+ T cells from allergic individuals. *J Exp Med* 1993;178:2123–2130.

38. Wright ED, Christodoulopoulos P, Small P, et al. Th-2 type cytokine receptors in allergic rhinitis and in response to topical steroids. *Laryngoscope* 1999;109:551–556.

39. Gavett SH, Chen X, Finkelman F, et al. Depletion of murine CD4+ T lymphocytes prevents antigen-induced airway hyperreactivity and pulmonary eosinophilia. *Am J Respir Cell Mol Biol* 1994;10:587–593.

40. Grunig G, Warnock M, Wakil AE, et al. Requirement for IL-13 independently of IL-4 in experimental asthma. *Science* 1998;282:2261–2263.

41. Corry DB, Grunig G, Hadeiba H, et al. Requirements for allergen-induced airway hyperreactivity in T and B cell–deficient mice. *Mol Med* 1998;4:344–355.

42. Gonzalo JA, Lloyd CM, Kremer L, et al. Eosinophil recruitment to the lung in a murine model of allergic inflammation. The role of T cells, chemokines, and adhesion receptors. *J Clin Invest* 1996;98:2332–2345.

43. Cohn L, Homer RJ, Marinov A, et al. Induction of airway mucus production by T helper 2 (Th2) cells: a critical role for interleukin 4 in cell recruitment but not mucus production. *J Exp Med* 1997;186:1737–47.

44. Gavett SH, O'Hearn DJ, Karp CL, et al. Interleukin-4 receptor blockade prevents airway responses induced by antigen challenge in mice. *Am J Physiol* 1997;272:L253–L261.

45. Kung TT, Stelts DM, Zurcher JA, et al. Involvement of IL-5 in a murine model of allergic pulmonary inflammation: prophylactic and therapeutic effect of an anti–IL-5 antibody. *Am J Respir Cell Mol Biol* 1995;13:360–365.

46. Foster PS, Hogan SP, Ramsay AJ, et al. Interleukin 5 deficiency abolishes eosinophilia, airways hyperreactivity, and lung damage in a mouse asthma model. *J Exp Med* 1996;183:195–201.

47. Brusselle G, Kips J, Joos G, et al. Allergen-induced airway inflammation and bronchial responsiveness in wild-type and interleukin-4–deficient mice. *Am J Respir Cell Mol Biol* 1995;12:254–259.

48. Lukacs NW, Strieter RM, Chensue SW, et al. Interleukin-4–dependent pulmonary eosinophil infiltration in a murine model of asthma. *Am J Respir Cell Mol Biol* 1994;10:526–532.

49. Brusselle GG, Kips JC, Tavernier JH, et al. Attenuation of allergic airway inflammation in IL-4 deficient mice. *Clin Exp Allergy* 1994;24:73–80.

50. Coyle AJ, Le Gros G, Bertrand C, et al. Interleukin-4 is required for the induction of lung Th2 mucosal immunity. *Am J Respir Cell Mol Biol* 1995;13:54–59.

51. Gavett SH, O'Hearn DJ, Li X, et al. Interleukin 12 inhibits antigen-induced airway hyperresponsiveness, inflammation, and Th2 cytokine expression in mice. *J Exp Med* 1995;182:1527–1536.

52. Lack G, Bradley KL, Hamelmann E, et al. Nebulized IFN-gamma inhibits the development of secondary allergic responses in mice. *J Immunol* 1996;157:1432–1439.

53. Li XM, Chopra RK, Chou TY, et al. Mucosal IFN-gamma gene transfer inhibits pulmonary allergic responses in mice. *J Immunol* 1996;157:3216–3219.

54. Yin Z, Chen C, Szabo SJ, et al. T-Bet expression and failure of GATA-3 cross-regulation lead to default production of IFN-gamma by gammadelta T cells. *J Immunol* 2002;168:1566–1571.

55. Erb KJ, Holloway JW, Sobeck A, et al. Infection of mice with *Mycobacterium bovis*–bacillus Calmette-Guérin (BCG) suppresses allergen-induced airway eosinophilia. *J Exp Med* 1998;187:561–569.

56. Kline JN, Waldschmidt TJ, Businga TR, et al. Modulation of airway inflammation by CpG oligodeoxynucleotides in a murine model of asthma. *J Immunol* 1998;160:2555–2559.

57. Saito H, Howie K, Wattie J, et al. Allergen-induced murine upper airway inflammation: local and systemic changes in murine experimental allergic rhinitis. *Immunology* 2001;104:226–234.

58. Okano M, Azuma M, Yoshino T, et al. Differential role of CD80 and CD86 molecules in the induction and the effector phases of allergic rhinitis in mice. *Am J Respir Crit Care Med* 2001;164:1501–1507.

59. Lee SY, Huang CK, Zhang TF, et al. Oral administration of IL-12 suppresses anaphylactic reactions in a murine model of peanut hypersensitivity. *Clin Immunol* 2001;101:220–228.

60. Ogasawara H, Asakura K, Saito H, et al. Role of CD4-positive T cells in the pathogenesis of nasal allergy in the murine model. *Int Arch Allergy Immunol* 1999;118:37–43.

61. Kweon MN, Yamamoto M, Kajiki M, et al. Systemically derived large intestinal CD4(+) Th2 cells play a central role in STAT6-mediated allergic diarrhea. *J Clin Invest* 2000;106:199–206.

62. Kondo K, Nagami T, Tadokoro S. Differences in haematopoietic death among inbred strains of mice. In: Bond VP, Sugahara T, eds. *Comparative cellular and species radiosensitivity.* Tokyo: Igaku Shoin, 1969:20.

63. Woodward AL, Spergel JM, Alenius H, et al. An obligate role for T-cell receptor alphabeta+ T cells but not T-cell receptor gammadelta+ T cells, B cells, or CD40/CD40L interactions in a mouse model of atopic dermatitis. *J Allergy Clin Immunol* 2001;107:359–366.

64. Habu Y, Seki S, Takayama E, et al. The mechanism of a defective IFN-gamma response to bacterial toxins in an atopic dermatitis model, NC/Nga mice, and the therapeutic effect of IFN-gamma, IL-12, or IL-18 on dermatitis. *J Immunol* 2001;166:5439–5447.

65. Hiroi J, Sengoku T, Morita K, et al. Effect of tacrolimus hydrate (FK506) ointment on spontaneous dermatitis in NC/Nga mice. *Jpn J Pharmacol* 1998;76:175–183.

66. Martinez FD, Stern DA, Wright AL, et al. Association of interleukin-2 and interferon-gamma production by blood mononuclear cells in infancy with parental allergy skin tests and with subsequent development of atopy. *J Allergy Clin Immunol* 1995;96:652–660.

67. Prescott SL, Macaubas C, Holt BJ, et al. Transplacental priming of the human immune system to environmental allergens: universal skewing of initial T cell responses toward the Th2 cytokine profile. *J Immunol* 1998;160:4730–4737.

68. Ober C. Susceptibility genes in asthma and allergy. *Curr Allergy Asthma Rep* 2001;1:174–179.

69. Cookson WO, Sharp PA, Faux JA, et al. Linkage between immunoglobulin E responses underlying asthma and rhinitis and chromosome 11q. *Lancet* 1989;1:1292–1295.

70. Lympany P, Welsh K, MacCochrane G, et al. Genetic analysis using DNA polymorphism of the linkage between chromosome 11q13 and

atopy and bronchial hyperresponsiveness to methacholine. *J Allergy Clin Immunol* 1992;89:619–628.

71. Marsh DG, Neely JD, Breazeale DR, et al. Linkage analysis of IL4 and other chromosome 5q31.1 markers and total serum immunoglobulin E concentrations. *Science* 1994;264:1152–1156.

72. Barnes KC. Evidence for common genetic elements in allergic disease. *J Allergy Clin Immunol* 2000;106(5, Suppl):S192–S200.

73. Bjorksten F, Suoniemi I, Koski V. Neonatal birch-pollen contact and subsequent allergy to birch pollen. *Clin Allergy* 1980;10:585–591.

74. Carosso A, Ruffino C, Bugiani M. The effect of birth season on pollenosis. *Ann Allergy* 1986;56:300–303.

75. Wahn U, Lau S, Bergmann R, et al. Indoor allergen exposure is a risk factor for sensitization during the first three years of life. *J Allergy Clin Immunol* 1997;99:763–769.

76. Sporik R, Platts-Mills TAE. Allergen exposure and the development of asthma. *Thorax* 2001;56:1158–1163.

77. Remes ST, Castro-Rodriguez JA, Holberg CJ, et al. Dog exposure in infancy decreases the subsequent risk of frequent wheeze but not of atopy. *J Allergy Clin Immunol* 2001;108:509–515.

78. Barrios C, Brawand P, Berney M, et al. Neonatal and early life immune responses to various forms of vaccine antigens qualitatively differ from adult responses: predominance of a Th2-biased pattern which persists after adult boosting. *Eur J Immunol* 1996;26:1489–1496.

79. Prescott SL, Macaubas C, Smallacombe T, et al. Reciprocal age-related patterns of allergen-specific T-cell immunity in normal vs. atopic infants. *Clin Exp Allergy* 1998;28(Suppl 5):39–44.

80. Prescott SL, Macaubas C, Smallacombe T, et al. Development of allergen-specific T-cell memory in atopic and normal children. *Lancet* 1999;353:196–200.

81. Strachan DP. Hay fever, hygiene, and household size. *BMJ* 1989; 299:1259–1260.

82. Shirakawa T, Enomoto T, Shimazu S, et al. The inverse association between tuberculin responses and atopic disorder. *Science* 1997;275:77–79.

83. Gao PS, Mao XQ, Baldini M, et al. Serum total IgE levels and CD14 on chromosome 5q31 [Letter]. *Clin Genet* 1999;56:164–165.

84. Erb KJ, Kirman J, Delahunt B, et al. Infection of mice with *Mycobacterium bovis*–BCG induces both Th1 and Th2 immune responses in the absence of interferon-gamma signalling. *Eur Cytokine Netw* 1999;10:147–154.

85. Arkwright PD, David TJ. Intradermal administration of a killed *Mycobacterium vaccae* suspension (SRL 172) is associated with improvement in atopic dermatitis in children with moderate-to-severe disease. *J Allergy Clin Immunol* 2001;107:531–524.

86. Bjorksten B. The environmental influence on childhood asthma. *Allergy* 1999;54(Suppl 49):17–23.

87. Diaz-Sanchez D, Garcia MP, Wang M, et al. Nasal challenge with diesel exhaust particles can induce sensitization to a neoallergen in the human mucosa. *J Allergy Clin Immunol* 1999;104:1183–1188.

88. Lee TH, Lane SJ. The role of macrophages in the mechanisms of airway inflammation in asthma. *Am Rev Respir Dis* 1992;145:S27–S30.

89. Nakajima J, Ono M, Takeda M, et al. Role of costimulatory molecules on airway epithelial cells acting as alloantigen-presenting cells. *Transplant Proc* 1997;29:2297–2300.

90. Lambrecht BN. The dendritic cell in allergic airway diseases: a new player to the game. *Clin Exp Allergy* 2001;31:206–218.

91. Moller GM, Overbeek SE, Van Helden-Meeuwsen CG, et al. Increased numbers of dendritic cells in the bronchial mucosa of atopic asthmatic patients: downregulation by inhaled corticosteroids. *Clin Exp Allergy* 1996;26:517–524.

92. Moser M, Murphy KM. Dendritic cell regulation of TH1–TH2 development. *Nat Immunol* 2000;1:199–205.

93. Bellini A, Vittori E, Marini M, et al. Intraepithelial dendritic cells and selective activation of Th2-like lymphocytes in patients with atopic asthma. *Chest* 1993;103:997–1005.

94. Fokkens WJ, Vroom TM, Rijntjes E, et al. Fluctuation of the number of CD-1(T6)–positive dendritic cells, presumably Langerhans cells, in the nasal mucosa of patients with an isolated grass-pollen allergy before, during, and after the grass-pollen season. *J Allergy Clin Immunol* 1989;84:39–43.

95. Godthelp T, Fokkens WJ, Kleinjan A, et al. Antigen presenting cells in the nasal mucosa of patients with allergic rhinitis during allergen provocation. *Clin Exp Allergy* 1996;26:677–688.

96. Cerio R, Griffiths CE, Cooper KD, et al. Characterization of factor XIIIa positive dermal dendritic cells in normal and inflamed skin. *Br J Dermatol* 1989;121:421–431.

97. Tschernig T, Debertin AS, Paulsen F, et al. Dendritic cells in the mucosa of the human trachea are not regularly found in the first year of life. *Thorax* 2001;56:427–431.

98. Hamada K, Goldsmith CA, Goldman A, et al. Resistance of very young mice to inhaled allergen sensitization is overcome by coexposure to an air-pollutant aerosol. *Am J Respir Crit Care Med* 2000; 161:1285–1293.

99. Bellinghausen I, Brand U, Knop J, et al. Comparison of allergen-stimulated dendritic cells from atopic and nonatopic donors dissecting their effect on autologous naïve and memory T helper cells of such donors. *J Allergy Clin Immunol* 2000;105:988–996.

100. Hammad H, Charbonnier AS, Duez C, et al. Th2 polarization by Der p 1—pulsed monocyte-derived dendritic cells is due to the allergic status of the donors. *Blood* 2001;98:1135–1141.

101. van den Heuvel MM, Vanhee DD, Postmus PE, et al. Functional and phenotypic differences of monocyte-derived dendritic cells from allergic and nonallergic patients. *J Allergy Clin Immunol* 1998;101: 90–95.

102. Alexander J, Coombs GH, Mottram JC. *Leishmania mexicana* cysteine proteinase–deficient mutants have attenuated virulence for mice and potentiate a Th1 response. *J Immunol* 1998;161:6794–6801.

103. Jahnsen FL, Moloney ED, Hogan T, et al. Rapid dendritic cell recruitment to the bronchial mucosa of patients with atopic asthma in response to local allergen challenge. *Thorax* 2001;56:823–826.

104. Lambrecht BN, Salomon B, Klatzmann D, et al. Dendritic cells are required for the development of chronic eosinophilic airway inflammation in response to inhaled antigen in sensitized mice. *J Immunol* 1998;160:4090–4097.

105. Coyle AJ, Wagner K, Bertrand C, et al. Central role of immunoglobulin (Ig) E in the induction of lung eosinophil infiltration and T helper 2 cell cytokine production: inhibition by a non-anaphylactogenic anti-IgE antibody. *J Exp Med* 1996;183:1303–1310.

106. Tunon-De-Lara JM, Redington AE, Bradding P, et al. Dendritic cells in normal and asthmatic airways: expression of the alpha subunit of the high affinity immunoglobulin E receptor (Fc epsilon RI-alpha). *Clin Exp Allergy* 1996;26:648–655.

107. Hsieh CS, Macatonia SE, Tripp CS, et al. Development of TH1 CD4$^+$ T cells through IL-12 produced by *Listeria*-induced macrophages. *Science* 1993;260:547–549.

108. Rosenwasser LJ, Klemm DJ, Dresback JK, et al. Promoter polymorphisms in the chromosome 5 gene cluster in asthma and atopy. *Clin Exp Allergy* 1995;25(Suppl 2):74–78.

109. Kawashima T, Noguchi E, Arinami T, et al. Linkage and association of an interleukin 4 gene polymorphism with atopic dermatitis in Japanese families. *J Med Genet* 1998;35:502–504.

110. Hershey GK, Friedrich MF, Esswein LA, et al. The association of atopy with a gain-of-function mutation in the alpha subunit of the interleukin-4 receptor. *N Engl J Med* 1997;337:1720–1725.

111. Kuperman D, Schofield B, Wills-Karp M, et al. Signal transducer and activator of transcription factor 6 (Stat6)–deficient mice are protected from antigen-induced airway hyperresponsiveness and mucus production. *J Exp Med* 1998;187:939–948.

112. Christodoulopoulos P, Cameron L, Nakamura Y, et al. TH2 cytokine–associated transcription factors in atopic and nonatopic asthma: evidence for differential signal transducer and activator of transcription 6 expression. *J Allergy Clin Immunol* 2001;107:586–591.

113. Tamura K, Arakawa H, Suzuki M, et al. Novel dinucleotide repeat polymorphism in the first exon of the STAT-6 gene is associated with allergic diseases. *Clin Exp Allergy* 2001;31:1509–1514.

114. Viola JP, Kiani A, Bozza PT, et al. Regulation of allergic inflammation and eosinophil recruitment in mice lacking the transcription factor NFAT1: role of interleukin-4 (IL-4) and IL-5. *Blood* 1998;91:2223–2230.

115. Yoshida H, Nishina H, Takimoto H, et al. The transcription factor NF-ATc1 regulates lymphocyte proliferation and Th2 cytokine production. *Immunity* 1998;8:115–124.

116. Ranger AM, Hodge MR, Gravallese EM, et al. Delayed lymphoid repopulation with defects in IL-4–driven responses produced by inactivation of NF-ATc. *Immunity* 1998;8:125–134.

117. Keen JC, Sholl L, Wills-Karp M, et al. Preferential activation of nuclear factor of activated T cells c correlates with mouse strain

susceptibility to allergic responses and interleukin-4 gene expression. *Am J Respir Cell Mol Biol* 2001;24:58–65.

118. Macaubas C, Holt PG. Regulation of cytokine production in T-cell responses to inhalant allergen:GATA-3 expression distinguishes between Th1- and Th2-polarized immunity. *Int Arch Allergy Immunol* 2001;124:176–179.

119. Caramori G, Lim S, Ito K, et al. Expression of GATA family of transcription factors in T-cells, monocytes and bronchial biopsies. *Eur Respir J* 2001;18:466–473.

120. Zhang DH, Yang L, Cohn L, et al. Inhibition of allergic inflammation in a murine model of asthma by expression of a dominant-negative mutant of GATA-3. *Immunity* 1999;11:473–482.

121. Mohrs M, Blankespoor CM, Wang ZE, et al. Deletion of a coordinate regulator of type 2 cytokine expression in mice. *Nat Immunol* 2001;2:842–847.

122. McIntire JJ, Umetsu SE, Akbari O, et al. Identification of Tapr (an airway hyperreactivity regulatory locus) and the linked Tim gene family. *Nat Immunol* 2001;2:1109–1116.

123. Plummeridge MJ, Armstrong L, Birchall MA, et al. Reduced production of interleukin 12 by interferon gamma primed alveolar macrophages from atopic asthmatic subjects. *Thorax* 2000;55:842–847.

124. Naseer T, Minshall EM, Leung DY, et al. Expression of IL-12 and IL-13 mRNA in asthma and their modulation in response to steroid therapy. *Am J Respir Crit Care Med* 1997;155:845–851.

125. van der Pouw Kraan TC, Boeije LC, de Groot ER, et al. Reduced production of IL-12 and IL-12–dependent IFN-gamma release in patients with allergic asthma. *J Immunol* 1997;158:5560–5565.

126. Keane-Myers A, Wysocka M, Trinchieri G, et al. Resistance to antigen-induced airway hyperresponsiveness requires endogenous production of IL-12. *J Immunol* 1998;161:919–926.

127. Postma DS, Bleecker ER, Amelung PJ, et al. Genetic susceptibility to asthma—bronchial hyperresponsiveness coinherited with a major gene for atopy. *N Engl J Med* 1995;333:894–900.

128. Pravica V, Brogan IJ, Hutchinson IV. Rare polymorphisms in the promoter regions of the human interleukin-12 p35 and interleukin-12 p40 subunit genes. *Eur J Immunogenet* 2000;27:35–36.

129. Szabo SJ, Jacobson NG, Dighe AS, et al. Developmental commitment to the Th2 lineage by extinction of IL-12 signaling. *Immunity* 1995;2:665–675.

130. Rogge L, Barberis-Maino L, Biffi M, et al. Selective expression of an interleukin-12 receptor component by human T helper 1 cells. *J Exp Med* 1997;185:825–831.

131. Wright ED, Christodoulopoulos P, Frenkiel S, et al. Expression of interleukin (IL)–12 (p40) and IL-12 (beta 2) receptors in allergic rhinitis and chronic sinusitis. *Clin Exp Allergy* 1999;29:1320–1325.

132. Yokoe T, Suzuki N, Minoguchi K, et al. Analysis of IL-12 receptor beta 2 chain expression of circulating T lymphocytes in patients with atopic asthma. *Cell Immunol* 2001;208:34–42.

133. Noguchi E, Yokouchi Y, Shibasaki M, et al. Identification of missense mutation in the IL12B gene: lack of association between IL12B polymorphisms and asthma and allergic rhinitis in the Japanese population. *Genes Immun* 2001;2:401–403.

134. van der Pouw Kraan TC, Boeije LC, Smeenk RJ, et al. Prostaglandin-E2 is a potent inhibitor of human interleukin 12 production. *J Exp Med* 1995;181:775–779.

135. Snijders A, Van der Pouw Kraan TC, Engel M, et al. Enhanced prostaglandin E2 production by monocytes in atopic dermatitis (AD) is not accompanied by enhanced production of IL-6, IL-10 or IL-12. *Clin Exp Immunol* 1998;111:472–476.

136. Karp CL, Wills-Karp M. Complement and IL-12: yin and yang. *Microbes Infect* 2001;3:109–119.

137. Humbles AA, Lu B, Nilsson CA, et al. A role for the C3a anaphylatoxin receptor in the effector phase of asthma. *Nature* 2000;406:998–1001.

138. Drouin SM, Kildsgaard J, Haviland J, et al. Expression of the complement anaphylatoxin C3a and C5a receptors on bronchial epithelial and smooth muscle cells in models of sepsis and asthma. *J Immunol* 2001;166:2025–2032.

139. Karp CL, Grupe A, Schadt E, et al. Identification of complement factor 5 as a susceptibility locus for experimental allergic asthma. *Nat Immunol* 2000;1:221–226.

140. Ober C, Cox NJ, Abney M, et al. Genome-wide search for asthma susceptibility loci in a founder population. The Collaborative Study on the Genetics of Asthma. *Hum Mol Genet* 1998;7:1393–1398.

141. Wjst M, Fischer G, Immervoll T, et al. A genome-wide search for linkage to asthma. German Asthma Genetics Group. *Genomics* 1999;58:1–8.

142. A genome-wide search for asthma susceptibility loci in ethnically diverse populations. The Collaborative Study on the Genetics of Asthma (CSGA). *Nat Genet* 1997;15:389–392.

143. Robinson DS, Tsicopoulos A, Meng Q, et al. Increased interleukin-10 messenger RNA expression in atopic allergy and asthma. *Am J Respir Cell Mol Biol* 1996;14:113–117.

144. Moverare R, Elfman L, Stalenheim G, et al. Study of the Th1/Th2 balance, including IL-10 production, in cultures of peripheral blood mononuclear cells from birch-pollen–allergic patients. *Allergy* 2000;55:171–175.

145. Colavita AM, Hastie AT, Musani AI, et al. Kinetics of IL-10 production after segmental antigen challenge of atopic asthmatic subjects. *J Allergy Clin Immunol* 2000;106:880–886.

146. Lamblin C, Desreumaux P, Colombel JF, et al. Overexpression of IL-10 mRNA in gut mucosa of patients with allergic asthma. *J Allergy Clin Immunol* 2001;107:739–741.

147. Takanashi S, Hasegawa Y, Kanehira Y, et al. Interleukin-10 level in sputum is reduced in bronchial asthma, COPD and in smokers. *Eur Respir J* 1999;14:309–314.

148. Koning H, Neijens HJ, Baert MR, et al. T cells subsets and cytokines in allergic and non-allergic children. II. Analysis and IL-5 and IL-10 mRNA expression and protein production. *Cytokine* 1997;9:427–436.

149. Yang X, Wang S, Fan Y, et al. IL-10 deficiency prevents IL-5 overproduction and eosinophilic inflammation in a murine model of asthma-like reaction. *Eur J Immunol* 2000;30:382–391.

150. Grunig G, Corry DB, Leach MW, et al. Interleukin-10 is a natural suppressor of cytokine production and inflammation in a murine model of allergic bronchopulmonary aspergillosis. *J Exp Med* 1997;185:1089–1099.

151. Tournoy KG, Kips JC, Pauwels RA. Endogenous interleukin-10 suppresses allergen-induced airway inflammation and nonspecific airway responsiveness. *Clin Exp Allergy* 2000;30:775–783.

152. Stampfli MR, Cwiartka M, Gajewska BU, et al. Interleukin-10 gene transfer to the airway regulates allergic mucosal sensitization in mice. *Am J Respir Cell Mol Biol* 1999;21:586–596.

153. Akbari O, DeKruyff RH, Umetsu DT. Pulmonary dendritic cells producing IL-10 mediate tolerance induced by respiratory exposure to antigen. *Nat Immunol* 2001;2:725–731.

154. Read S, Powrie F. CD4(+) regulatory T cells. *Curr Opin Immunol* 2001;13:644–649.

155. Hodge S, Hodge G, Flower R, et al. Methyl-prednisolone up-regulates monocyte interleukin-10 production in stimulated whole blood. *Scand J Immunol* 1999;49:548–553.

156. Pessi T, Sutas Y, Hurme M, et al. Interleukin-10 generation in atopic children following oral *Lactobacillus rhamnosus* GG. *Clin Exp Allergy* 2000;30:1804–1808.

157. Bellinghausen I, Knop J, Saloga J. The role of interleukin 10 in the regulation of allergic immune responses. *Int Arch Allergy Immunol* 2001;126:97–101.

158. Hobbs K, Negri J, Klinnert M, et al. Interleukin-10 and transforming growth factor-beta promoter polymorphisms in allergies and asthma. *Am J Respir Crit Care Med* 1998;158:1958–1962.

159. Finkelman FD, Katona IM, Urban JF Jr, et al. IL-4 is required to generate and sustain *in vivo* IgE responses. *J Immunol* 1988;141:2335–2341.

160. Wills-Karp M. Interleukin-12 as a target for modulation of the inflammatory response in asthma. *Allergy* 1998;53:113–119.

161. Zhu Z, Homer RJ, Wang Z, et al. Pulmonary expression of interleukin-13 causes inflammation, mucus hypersecretion, subepithelial fibrosis, physiologic abnormalities, and eotaxin production. *J Clin Invest* 1999;103:779–788.

162. Yusuf-Makagiansar H, Anderson ME, Yakovleva TV, et al. Inhibition of LFA-1/ICAM-1 and VLA-4/VCAM-1 as a therapeutic approach to inflammation and autoimmune diseases. *Med Res Rev* 2002;22:146–167.

163. Mauser PJ, Pitman A, Witt A, et al. Inhibitory effect of the TRFK-5 anti-IL-5 antibody in a guinea pig model of asthma. *Am Rev Respir Dis* 1993;148:1623–1627.

164. Ishizaka K, Ishizaka T. Identification of γ-E-antibodies as a carrier of reaginic activity. *J Immunol* 1967;99:1187.

165. Vercelli D. The functional genomics of CD14 and its role in IgE responses: an integrated view. *J Allergy Clin Immunol* 2002;109:14–21.

166. Linehan LA, Warren WD, Thompson PA, et al. STAT6 is required for IL-4–induced germline Ig gene transcription and switch recombination. *J Immunol* 1998;161:302–310.

167. Snapper CM, Zelazowski P, Rosas FR, et al. B cells from p50/NF-kappa B knockout mice have selective defects in proliferation, differentiation, germ-line CH transcription, and Ig class switching. *J Immunol* 1996;156:183–191.

168. Harriman GR, Bradley A, Das S, et al. IgA class switch in I alpha exon–deficient mice. Role of germline transcription in class switch recombination. *J Clin Invest* 1996;97:477–485.

169. Oettgen HC, Geha RS. IgE in asthma and atopy: cellular and molecular connections. *J Clin Invest* 1999;104:829–835.

170. Jabara HH, Fu SM, Geha RS, et al. CD40 and IgE: synergism between anti-CD40 monoclonal antibody and interleukin 4 in the induction of IgE synthesis by highly purified human B cells. *J Exp Med* 1990;172:1861–1864.

171. Fanslow WC, Anderson DM, Grabstein KH, et al. Soluble forms of CD40 inhibit biologic responses of human B cells. *J Immunol* 1992;149:655–660.

172. Bacharier LB, Jabara H, Geha RS. Molecular mechanisms of immunoglobulin E regulation. *Int Arch Allergy Immunol* 1998;115:257–269.

173. Kawabe T, Naka T, Yoshida K, et al. The immune responses in CD40-deficient mice: impaired immunoglobulin class switching and germinal center formation. *Immunity* 1994;1:167–178.

174. Renshaw BR, Fanslow WC 3rd, Armitage RJ, et al. Humoral immune responses in CD40 ligand–deficient mice. *J Exp Med* 1994;180:1889–1900.

175. Honjo T, Kinoshita K, Muramatsu M. Molecular mechanism of class switch recombination: linkage with somatic hypermutation. *Annu Rev Immunol* 2002;20:165–196.

176. Muramatsu M, Kinoshita K, Fagarasan S, et al. Class switch recombination and hypermutation require activation-induced cytidine deaminase (AID), a potential RNA editing enzyme. *Cell* 2000;102:553–563.

177. Durandy A, Honjo T. Human genetic defects in class-switch recombination (hyper-IgM syndromes). *Curr Opin Immunol* 2001;13:543–548.

178. Shapira SK, Vercelli D, Jabara HH, et al. Molecular analysis of the induction of immunoglobulin E synthesis in human B cells by interleukin 4 and engagement of CD40 antigen. *J Exp Med* 1992;175:289–292.

179. Coffman RL, Carty J. A T cell activity that enhances polyclonal IgE production and its inhibition by interferon-gamma. *J Immunol* 1986;136:949–954.

180. Pene J, Rousset F, Briere F, et al. IgE production by normal human lymphocytes is induced by interleukin 4 and suppressed by interferons gamma and alpha and prostaglandin E$_2$. *Proc Natl Acad Sci U S A* 1988;85:6880–6884.

181. Kinet JP. The high-affinity IgE receptor (Fc epsilon RI): from physiology to pathology. *Annu Rev Immunol* 1999;17:931–972.

182. Reischl IG, Coward WR, Church MK. Molecular consequences of human mast cell activation following immunoglobulin E–high-affinity immunoglobulin E receptor (IgE-FcepsilonRI) interaction. *Biochem Pharmacol* 1999;58:1841–1850.

183. Turner H, Kinet JP. Signalling through the high-affinity IgE receptor Fc epsilonRI. *Nature* 1999;402(6760, Suppl):B24–B30.

184. Costello PS, Turner M, Walters AE, et al. Critical role for the tyrosine kinase Syk in signalling through the high affinity IgE receptor of mast cells. *Oncogene* 1996;13:2595–2605.

185. Malveaux FJ, Conroy MC, Adkinson NF Jr, et al. IgE receptors on human basophils. Relationship to serum IgE concentration. *J Clin Invest* 1978;62:176–181.

186. Conroy MC, Adkinson NF Jr, Lichtenstein LM. Measurement of IgE on human basophils: relation to serum IgE and anti-IgE–induced histamine release. *J Immunol* 1977;118:1317–1321.

187. MacGlashan DW Jr, Bochner BS, Adelman DC, et al. Down-regulation of Fc(epsilon)RI expression on human basophils during *in vivo* treatment of atopic patients with anti-IgE antibody. *J Immunol* 1997;158:1438–1445.

188. Gosset P, Lamblin-Degros C, Tillie-Leblond I, et al. Modulation of high-affinity IgE receptor expression in blood monocytes: opposite effect of IL-4 and glucocorticoids. *J Allergy Clin Immunol* 2001;107:114–122.

189. Daheshia M, Friend DS, Grusby MJ, et al. Increased severity of local and systemic anaphylactic reactions in gp49B1-deficient mice. *J Exp Med* 2001;194:227–34.

190. Kepley CL, Cambier JC, Morel PA, et al. Negative regulation of FcepsilonRI signaling by FcgammaRII costimulation in human blood basophils. *J Allergy Clin Immunol* 2000;106:337–348.

191. Katz HR, Vivier E, Castells MC, et al. Mouse mast cell gp49B1 contains two immunoreceptor tyrosine-based inhibition motifs and suppresses mast cell activation when coligated with the high-affinity Fc receptor for IgE. *Proc Natl Acad Sci U S A* 1996;93:10809–10814.

192. Long EO. Regulation of immune responses through inhibitory receptors. *Annu Rev Immunol* 1999;17:875–904.

193. Yokota A, Kikutani H, Tanaka T, et al. Two species of human Fc epsilon receptor II (Fc epsilon RII/CD23): tissue-specific and IL-4–specific regulation of gene expression. *Cell* 1988;55:611–618.

194. Delespesse G, Suter U, Mossalayi D, et al. Expression, structure, and function of the CD23 antigen. *Adv Immunol* 1991;49:149–191.

195. Abdelilah SG, Bouchaib L, Morita M, et al. Molecular characterization of the low-affinity IgE receptor Fc epsilonRII/CD23 expressed by human eosinophils. *Int Immunol* 1998;10:395–404.

196. Yokota A, Yukawa K, Yamamoto A, et al. Two forms of the low-affinity Fc receptor for IgE differentially mediate endocytosis and phagocytosis: identification of the critical cytoplasmic domains. *Proc Natl Acad Sci U S A* 1992;89:5030–5034.

197. Munoz O, Brignone C, Grenier-Brossette N, et al. Binding of anti-CD23 monoclonal antibody to the leucine zipper motif of Fcepsilon-RII/CD23 on B cell membrane promotes its proteolytic cleavage. Evidence for an effect on the oligomer/monomer equilibrium. *J Biol Chem* 1998;273:31795–31800.

198. Tsicopoulos A, Joseph M. The role of CD23 in allergic disease. *Clin Exp Allergy* 2000;30:602–605.

199. Kisselgof AB, Oettgen HC. The expression of murine B cell CD23, *in vivo,* is regulated by its ligand, IgE. *Int Immunol* 1998;10:1377–1384.

200. Bonnefoy JY, Lecoanet-Henchoz S, Gauchat JF, et al. Structure and functions of CD23. *Int Rev Immunol* 1997;16:113–128.

201. Sherr E, Macy E, Kimata H, et al. Binding the low affinity Fc epsilon R on B cells suppresses ongoing human IgE synthesis. *J Immunol* 1989;142:481–489.

202. Lee WT, Rao M, Conrad DH. The murine lymphocyte receptor for IgE. IV. The mechanism of ligand-specific receptor upregulation on B cells. *J Immunol* 1987;139:1191–1198.

203. Lecoanet-Henchoz S, Gauchat JF, Aubry JP, et al. CD23 regulates monocyte activation through a novel interaction with the adhesion molecules CD11b-CD18 and CD11c-CD18. *Immunity* 1995;3:119–125.

204. Gagro A, Rabatic S. Allergen-induced CD23 on CD4$^+$ T lymphocytes and CD21 on B lymphocytes in patients with allergic asthma: evidence and regulation. *Eur J Immunol* 1994;24:1109–1114.

205. Williams J, Johnson S, Mascali JJ, et al. Regulation of low affinity IgE receptor (CD23) expression on mononuclear phagocytes in normal and asthmatic subjects. *J Immunol* 1992;149:2823–2829.

206. Jung CM, Prinz JC, Rieber EP, et al. A reduction in allergen-induced Fc epsilon R2/CD23 expression on peripheral B cells correlates with successful hyposensitization in grass pollinosis. *J Allergy Clin Immunol* 1995;95:77–87.

207. Galli SJ. New concepts about the mast cell. *New Engl J Med* 1993;328:257–65.

208. Weil SC, Hrisinko MA. A hybrid eosinophilic-basophilic granulocyte in chronic granulocytic leukemia. *Am J Clin Pathol* 1987;87:66–70.

209. Denburg JA, Telizyn S, Messner H, et al. Heterogeneity of human peripheral blood eosinophil-type colonies: evidence for a common basophil-eosinophil progenitor. *Blood* 1985;66:312–318.

210. Leary AG, Ogawa M. Identification of pure and mixed basophil colonies in culture of human peripheral blood and marrow cells. *Blood* 1984;64:78–83.

211. Valent P, Schmidt G, Besemer J, et al. Interleukin-3 is a differentiation factor for human basophils. *Blood* 1989;73:1763–1769.

212. Denburg JA, Silver JE, Abrams JS. Interleukin-5 is a human basophilopoietin: induction of histamine content and basophilic

differentiation of HL-60 cells and of peripheral blood basophil-eosinophil progenitors. *Blood* 1991;77:1462–1468.

213. Yamaguchi M, Hirai K, Morita Y, et al. Hemopoietic growth factors regulate the survival of human basophils *in vitro*. *Int Arch Allergy Immunol* 1992;97:322–329.

214. Tsuda T, Wong D, Dolovich J, et al. Synergistic effects of nerve growth factor and granulocyte-macrophage colony-stimulating factor on human basophilic cell differentiation. *Blood* 1991;77:971–979.

215. Charlesworth EN, Hood AF, Soter NA, et al. Cutaneous late-phase response to allergen. Mediator release and inflammatory cell infiltration. *J Clin Invest* 1989;83:1519–1526.

216. Liu MC, Hubbard WC, Proud D, et al. Immediate and late inflammatory responses to ragweed antigen challenge of the peripheral airways in allergic asthmatics. Cellular, mediator, and permeability changes. *Am Rev Respir Dis* 1991;144:51–58.

217. Bascom R, Wachs M, Naclerio RM, et al. Basophil influx occurs after nasal antigen challenge: effects of topical corticosteroid pretreatment. *J Allergy Clin Immunol* 1988;81:580–589.

218. Wershil BK, Galli SJ. The analysis of mast cell function *in vivo* using mast cell–deficient mice. *Adv Exp Med Biol* 1994;347:39–54.

219. Austen KF, Boyce JA. Mast cell lineage development and phenotypic regulation. *Leuk Res* 2001;25:511–518.

220. Irani AM, Craig SS, DeBlois G, et al. Deficiency of the tryptase-positive, chymase-negative mast cell type in gastrointestinal mucosa of patients with defective T lymphocyte function. *J Immunol* 1987;138:4381–4386.

221. Ruitenberg EJ, Elgersma A. Absence of intestinal mast cell response in congenitally athymic mice during *Trichinella spiralis* infection. *Nature* 1976;264:258–260.

222. Lantz CS, Boesiger J, Song CH, et al. Role for interleukin-3 in mast-cell and basophil development and in immunity to parasites. *Nature* 1998;392:90–93.

223. Godfraind C, Louahed J, Faulkner H, et al. Intraepithelial infiltration by mast cells with both connective tissue–type and mucosal-type characteristics in gut, trachea, and kidneys of IL-9 transgenic mice. *J Immunol* 1998;160:3989–3996.

224. Stevens RL, Austen KF. Recent advances in the cellular and molecular biology of mast cells. *Immunol Today* 1989;10:381–386.

225. Huang C, Sali A, Stevens RL. Regulation and function of mast cell proteases in inflammation. *J Clin Immunol* 1998;18:169–183.

226. Church MK, Levi-Schaffer F. The human mast cell. *J Allergy Clin Immunol* 1997;99:155–160.

227. Casale TB, Wood D, Richerson HB, et al. Elevated bronchoalveolar lavage fluid histamine levels in allergic asthmatics are associated with methacholine bronchial hyperresponsiveness. *J Clin Invest* 1987;79:1197–1203.

228. Schwartz LB. Tryptase, a mediator of human mast cells. *J Allergy Clin Immunol* 1990;86:594–598.

229. Schwartz LB. Tryptase: a clinical indicator of mast cell-dependent events. *Allergy Proc* 1994;15:119–123.

230. Fisher MM, Baldo BA. The diagnosis of fatal anaphylactic reactions during anaesthesia: employment of immunoassays for mast cell tryptase and drug-reactive IgE antibodies. *Anaesth Intensive Care* 1993;21:353–357.

231. Schwartz LB, Bradford TR, Rouse C. Development of a new, more sensitive immunoassay for human tryptase: use in systemic anaphylaxis. *J Clin Immunol* 1994;14:190–194.

232. Schwartz LB, Yunginger JW, Miller J. Time course of appearance and disappearance of human mast cell tryptase in the circulation after anaphylaxis. *J Clin Invest* 1989;83:1551–1555.

233. Williams CMM, Galli SJ. The diverse potential effector and immunoregulatory roles of mast cells in allergic disease. *J Allergy Clin Immunol* 2000;105:847–859.

234. Peters SP, MacGlashan DW, Schleimer RP, et al. The pharmacologic modulation of the release of arachidonic acid metabolites from purified human lung mast cells. *Am Rev Respir Dis* 1985;132:367–373.

235. Hammarstrom S. Leukotrienes. *Annu Rev Biochem* 1983;52:355–377.

235a. Samuelsson B. Leukotrienes: mediators of immediate hypersensitivity reactions and inflammation. *Science* 1983;220:568–75.

236. Coles SJ, Neill KH, Reid LM, et al. Effects of leukotrienes C$_4$ and D$_4$ on glycoprotein and lysozyme by human bronchial mucosa. *Prostaglandins* 1983;25:155–170.

237. Weiss JW, Drazen JM, McFadden ERJ, et al. Airway constriction in normal humans produced by inhalation of leukotriene D. Potency, time course, and effect of aspirin therapy. *JAMA* 1983;249:2814–2817.

238. Barnes NC, Piper PJ, Costello JF. Comparative effects of inhaled leukotriene C$_4$, leukotriene D$_4$, and histamine in normal human subjects. *Thorax* 1984;39:500–504.

239. Hansson G, Bjorck T, Dahlen SE. Specific allergen induces contraction of bronchi and formation of leukotrienes C$_4$, D$_4$, and E$_4$ in human asthmatic lung. *Adv Prostaglandin Thromboxane Leukot Res* 1983;12:153–159.

240. Bjorck T, Dahlen SE. Leukotrienes and histamine mediate IgE-dependent contractions of human bronchi: pharmacological evidence obtained with tissues from asthmatic and non-asthmatic subjects. *Pulm Pharmacol* 1993;6:87–96.

241. Rasmussen JB. Leukotriene (LT) D$_4$ is involved in antigen=induced asthma: a study with the LTD$_4$ receptor antagonist, MK-571. *Ann N Y Acad Sci* 1991;629:436.

242. Findlay SR, Barden JM, Easley CB. Effect of the oral leukotriene antagonist, ICI 204,219 on antigen-induced bronchoconstriction in subjects with asthma. *J Allergy Clin Immunol* 1992;89:1040–1045.

243. Diamant Z, Timmers MC, van-der-Veen H, et al. The effect of MK-0591, a novel 5-lipoxygenase activating protein inhibitor, on leukotriene biosynthesis and allergen-induced airway responses in asthmatic subjects. *J Allergy Clin Immunol* 1995;95:42–51.

244. Middleton E, Reed CE, Ellis EF, et al. *Allergy: principles and practice*, 5th ed. St. Louis: Mosby, 1998.

245. Mencia-Huerta JM, Lewis RA, Razin E, et al. Antigen-initiated release of platelet-activating factor (PAF-acether) from mouse bone marrow–derived mast cells sensitized with monoclonal IgE. *J Immunol* 1983;131:2958–2964.

246. Triggiani M, Hubbard WC, Chilton FH. Synthesis of 1-acyl-2-acetyl-sn-glycero-3-phosphocholine by an enriched preparation of the human lung mast cell. *J Immunol* 1990;144:4773–4780.

247. Agius RM, Robinson C, Holgate ST. Release of histamine and newly generated mediators from human bronchoalveolar lavage cells. *Thorax* 1985;40:220.

248. Hardy CC, Robinson C, Tattersfield AE. The bronchoconstrictor effect of inhaled prostaglandin D2 in normal and asthmatic men. *N Engl J Med* 1984;311:209–213.

249. Featherstone RL, Robinson C, Holgate ST. Evidence for thromboxane receptor mediated contraction of guinea-pig and human airways *in vitro* by prostaglandin (PG) D$_2$, 9 alpha, 11 beta–PGF$_2$ and PGF$_2$ alpha. *Naunyn Schmiedebergs Arch Pharmacol* 1990;341:439–443.

250. Wensel SE, Fowler AA, Schwartz LB. Activation of pulmonary mast cells by bronchoalveolar allergen challenge. *In vivo* release of histamine and tryptase in atopic subjects with and without asthma. *Am Rev Respir Dis* 1988;137:1002–1008.

251. O'Sullivan S, Dahlen B, Dahlen S-E. Increased urinary excretion of the prostaglandin D$_2$ metabolite 9a, 11b–prostaglandin F$_2$ after aspirin challenge supports mast cell activation in aspirin-induced airway obstruction. *J Allergy Clin Immunol* 1996;98:421–432.

252. Hellewell PG, Jose PJ, Williams TJ. Inflammatory mechanisms in the passive cutaneous anaphylactic reaction in the rabbit: evidence that novel mediators are involved. *Br J Pharmacol* 1992;107:1163–1172.

253. Allegra J, Trautelein J, Demers L. Peripheral plasma determinations of prostaglandin E in asthmatics. *J Allergy Clin Immunol* 1976;58:546–550.

254. Szczeklik A. The cyclooxygenase theory of aspirin-induced asthma. *Eur Respir J* 1990;3:588–593.

255. Kowalski ML. Aspirin sensitive rhinosinusitis and asthma. *Allergy Proc* 1995;16:77–80.

256. Bradding P, Feather IH, Howarth PH, et al. Interleukin 4 is localized to and released by human mast cells. *J Exp Med* 1992;176:1381–1386.

257. Church MK, Okayama Y, Bradding P. The role of the mast cell in acute and chronic allergic inflammation. *Ann N Y Acad Sci* 1994;725:13–21.

258. Wershil BK, Mekori YA, Murakami T, et al. I-fibrin deposition in IgE-dependent immediate hypersensitivity reactions in mouse skin: demonstration of the role of mast cells using genetically mast cell–deficient mice locally reconstituted with cultured mast cells. *J Immunol* 1987;139:2605–2614.

259. Oettgen HC, Martin TR, Wynshaw-Boris A, et al. Active anaphylaxis in IgE-deficient mice. *Nature* 1994;370:367–370.

260. Konig P. The effects of cromolyn sodium and nedocromil sodium in early asthma prevention. *J Allergy Clin Immunol* 2000;105:S575–S581.

261. Fahy JV, Fleming HE, Wong HH, et al. The effect of an anti-IgE monoclonal antibody on the early- and late-phase responses to allergen inhalation in asthmatic subjects. *Am J Respir Crit Care Med* 1997;155:1828–1834.

262. Mehlhop PD, van de Rijn M, Goldberg AB, et al. Allergen-induced bronchial hyperreactivity and eosinophilic inflammation occur in the absence of IgE in a mouse model of asthma. *Proc Natl Acad Sci U S A* 1997;94:1344–1349.

263. Weller PF. Eosinophils: structure and functions. *Curr Opin Immunol* 1994;6:85–90.

264. Gleich GJ. Mechanisms of eosinophil-associated inflammation. *J Allergy Clin Immunol* 2000;105:651–663.

265. Weller PF, Lim K, Wan HC, et al. Role of the eosinophil in allergic reactions. *Eur Respir J Suppl* 1996;22:109s–115s.

266. Jacoby DB, Gleich GJ, Fryer AD. Human eosinophil major basic protein is an endogenous allosteric antagonist at the inhibitory muscarinic M2 receptor. *J Clin Invest* 1993;91:1314–1318.

267. Wu W, Samoszuk MK, Comhair SA, et al. Eosinophils generate brominating oxidants in allergen-induced asthma. *J Clin Invest* 2000;105:1455–1463.

268. Leonidas DD, Elbert BL, Zhou Z, et al. Crystal structure of human Charcot-Leyden crystal protein, an eosinophil lysophospholipase, identifies it as a new member of the carbohydrate-binding family of galectins. *Structure* 1995;3:1379–1393.

269. Guo L, Johnson RS, Schuh JC. Biochemical characterization of endogenously formed eosinophilic crystals in the lungs of mice. *J Biol Chem* 2000;275:8032–8037.

270. Wardlaw AJ. Molecular basis for selective eosinophil trafficking in asthma: a multistep paradigm. *J Allergy Clin Immunol* 1999;104:917–926.

271. Lee JJ, McGarry MP, Farmer SC, et al. Interleukin-5 expression in the lung epithelium of transgenic mice leads to pulmonary changes pathognomonic of asthma. *J Exp Med* 1997;185:2143–2156.

272. Lobb RR, Pepinsky B, Leone DR, et al. The role of alpha 4 integrins in lung pathophysiology. *Eur Respir J Suppl* 1996;22:104s–108s.

273. Rossi D, Zlotnik A. The biology of chemokines and their receptors. *Annu Rev Immunol* 2000;18:217–242.

274. Ponath PD, Qin S, Post TW, et al. Molecular cloning and characterization of a human eotaxin receptor expressed selectively on eosinophils. *J Exp Med* 1996;183:2437–2448.

275. Uguccioni M, Mackay CR, Ochensberger B, et al. High expression of the chemokine receptor CCR3 in human blood basophils. Role in activation by eotaxin, MCP-4, and other chemokines. *J Clin Invest* 1997;100:1137–1143.

276. Rothenberg ME, MacLean JA, Pearlman E, et al. Targeted disruption of the chemokine eotaxin partially reduces antigen-induced tissue eosinophilia. *J Exp Med* 1997;185:785–790.

277. Yang Y, Loy J, Ryseck RP, et al. Antigen-induced eosinophilic lung inflammation develops in mice deficient in chemokine eotaxin. *Blood* 1998;92:3912–3923.

278. Collins PD, Marleau S, Griffiths-Johnson DA, et al. Cooperation between interleukin-5 and the chemokine eotaxin to induce eosinophil accumulation *in vivo*. *J Exp Med* 1995;182:1169–1174.

279. Gonzalo JA, Lloyd CM, Wen D, et al. The coordinated action of CC chemokines in the lung orchestrates allergic inflammation and airway hyperresponsiveness. *J Exp Med* 1998;188:157–167.

280. Stafford S, Li H, Forsythe PA, et al. Monocyte chemotactic protein-3 (MCP-3)/fibroblast-induced cytokine (FIC) in eosinophilic inflammation of the airways and the inhibitory effects of an anti–MCP-3/FIC antibody. *J Immunol* 1997;158:4953–4960.

281. Lukacs NW. Role of chemokines in the pathogenesis of asthma. *Nat Rev Immunol* 2001;1:108–116.

282. Druilhe A, Wallaert B, Tsicopoulos A, et al. Apoptosis, proliferation, and expression of Bcl-2, Fas, and Fas ligand in bronchial biopsies from asthmatics. *Am J Respir Cell Mol Biol* 1998;19:747–757.

283. Meagher LC, Cousin JM, Seckl JR, et al. Opposing effects of glucocorticoids on the rate of apoptosis in neutrophilic and eosinophilic granulocytes. *J Immunol* 1996;156:4422–4428.

284. Gounni AS, Lamkhioued B, Ochiai K, et al. High-affinity IgE receptor on eosinophils is involved in defence against parasites. *Nature* 1994;367:183–186.

285. Tomassini M, Tsicopoulos A, Tai PC, et al. Release of granule proteins by eosinophils from allergic and nonallergic patients with eosinophilia on immunoglobulin-dependent activation. *J Allergy Clin Immunol* 1991;88:365–375.

286. Rajakulasingam K, Till S, Ying S, et al. Increased expression of high affinity IgE (FcepsilonRI) receptor-alpha chain mRNA and protein-bearing eosinophils in human allergen-induced atopic asthma. *Am J Respir Crit Care Med* 1998;158:233–240.

287. Barata LT, Ying S, Grant JA, et al. Allergen-induced recruitment of Fc epsilon RI+ eosinophils in human atopic skin. *Eur J Immunol* 1997;27:1236–1241.

288. Ying S, Barata LT, Meng Q, et al. High-affinity immunoglobulin E receptor (Fc epsilon RI)–bearing eosinophils, mast cells, macrophages and Langerhans' cells in allergen-induced late-phase cutaneous reactions in atopic subjects. *Immunology* 1998;93:281–288.

289. Kaneko M, Horie S, Kato M, et al. A crucial role for beta 2 integrin in the activation of eosinophils stimulated by IgG. *J Immunol* 1995;155:2631–2641.

290. Kita H, Kaneko M, Bartemes KR, et al. Does IgE bind to and activate eosinophils from patients with allergy? *J Immunol* 1999;162:6901–6911.

291. Kita H, Abu-Ghazaleh RI, Sur S, et al. Eosinophil major basic protein induces degranulation and IL-8 production by human eosinophils. *J Immunol* 1995;154:4749–4758.

292. Martin LB, Kita H, Leiferman KM, et al. Eosinophils in allergy: role in disease, degranulation, and cytokines. *Int Arch Allergy Immunol* 1996;109:207–215.

293. Seminario MC, Gleich GJ. The role of eosinophils in the pathogenesis of asthma. *Curr Opin Immunol* 1994;6:860–864.

294. Terada N, Konno A, Fukuda S, et al. Interleukin-5 gene expression in nasal mucosa and changes in amount of interleukin-5 in nasal lavage fluid after antigen challenge. *Acta Otolaryngol* 1994;114:203–208.

295. Kiehl P, Falkenberg K, Vogelbruch M, et al. Tissue eosinophilia in acute and chronic atopic dermatitis: a morphometric approach using quantitative image analysis of immunostaining. *Br J Dermatol* 2001;145:720–729.

296. Matsukura M, Yamada H, Yudate T, et al. Steroid-induced changes of eosinophils in atopic dermatitis. *Int Arch Allergy Immunol* 1997;114(Suppl 1):51–54.

297. Andersson M, Andersson P, Venge P, et al. Eosinophils and eosinophil cationic protein in nasal lavages in allergen-induced hyperresponsiveness: effects of topical glucocorticosteroid treatment. *Allergy* 1989;44:342–348.

298. Gauvreau GM, Doctor J, Watson RM, et al. Effects of inhaled budesonide on allergen-induced airway responses and airway inflammation. *Am J Respir Crit Care Med* 1996;154:1267–1271.

299. Mauser PJ, Pitman AM, Fernandez X, et al. Effects of an antibody to interleukin-5 in a monkey model of asthma. *Am J Respir Crit Care Med* 1995;152:467–472.

300. Corry DB, Folkesson HG, Warnock ML, et al. Interleukin 4, but not interleukin 5 or eosinophils, is required in a murine model of acute airway hyperreactivity [published erratum appears in *J Exp Med* 1997;185:1715]. *J Exp Med* 1996;183:109–117.

301. Leckie MJ, ten Brinke A, Khan J, et al. Effects of an interleukin-5 blocking monoclonal antibody on eosinophils, airway hyper-responsiveness, and the late asthmatic response. *Lancet* 2000;356:2144–2148.

302. Wills-Karp M, Luyimbazi J, Xu X, et al. Interleukin-13: central mediator of allergic asthma. *Science* 1998;282:2258–2261.

303. Yang, M, Hogan SP, Henry PJ, et al., Interleukin-13 mediates airways hyperreactivity through the IL-4 receptor-alpha chain and STAT-6 independently of IL-5 and eotaxin. *Am J Respir Cell Mol Biol* 2001;25:522–530.

304. Coyle AJ, Ackerman SJ, Burch R, et al. Human eosinophil-granule major basic protein and synthetic polycations induce airway hyper-responsiveness *in vivo* dependent on bradykinin generation. *J Clin Invest* 1995;95:1735–1740.

305. Cohn L, Tepper JS, Bottomly K. IL-4–independent induction of airway hyperresponsiveness by Th2, but not Th1, cells. *J Immunol* 1998;161:3813–3816.

306. Rankin JA, Picarella DE, Geba GP, et al. Phenotypic and physiologic characterization of transgenic mice expressing interleukin 4 in the lung: lymphocytic and eosinophilic inflammation without airway hyperreactivity. *Proc Natl Acad Sci U S A* 1996;93:7821–7825.

307. Webb DC, McKenzie AN, Koskinen AM, et al. Integrated signals between IL-13, IL-4, and IL-5 regulate airways hyperreactivity. *J Immunol* 2000;165:108–113.

308. Zheng T, Zhu Z, Wang Z, et al. Inducible targeting of IL-13 to the adult lung causes matrix metalloproteinase- and cathepsin-dependent emphysema. *J Clin Invest* 2000;106:1081–1093.

309. Chiaramonte MG, Donaldson DD, Cheever AW, et al. An IL-13 inhibitor blocks the development of hepatic fibrosis during a T-helper type 2–dominated inflammatory response. *J Clin Invest* 1999;104:777–785.

310. Laporte JC, Moore PE, Baraldo S, et al. Direct effects of interleukin-13 on signaling pathways for physiological responses in cultured human airway smooth muscle cells. *Am J Respir Crit Care Med* 2001;164:141–148.

311. Humbert M, Durham SR, Kimmitt P, et al. Elevated expression of messenger ribonucleic acid encoding IL-13 in the bronchial mucosa of atopic and nonatopic subjects with asthma. *J Allergy Clin Immunol* 1997;99:657–665.

312. Graves PE, Kabesch M, Halonen M, et al. A cluster of seven tightly linked polymorphisms in the IL-13 gene is associated with total serum IgE levels in three populations of white children. *J Allergy Clin Immunol* 2000;105:506–513.

313. Heinzmann A, Mao XQ, Akaiwa M, et al. Genetic variants of IL-13 signalling and human asthma and atopy. *Hum Mol Genet* 2000;9:549–559.

314. Portier P, Richet C. De l'action anaphylactique de certains venins. *C R Soc Biol* 1902;54:170.

315. Waite KJ. Blackley and the development of hay fever as a disease of civilization in the nineteenth century. *Med Hist* 1995;39:186–196.

316. American Academy of Allergy, Asthma, and Immunology. *The allergy report. Vol. 1. Overview of allergic diseases: diagnosis, management, and barriers to care.* Milwaukee, WI: American Academy of Allergy, Asthma, and Immunology, 2000.

317. Naclerio RM. Allergic rhinitis. *N Engl J Med* 1991;325:860–869.

318. Kaliner M, Eggleston PA, Mathews KP. Rhinitis and asthma. *JAMA* 1987;258:2851–2873.

319. Platts-Mills TA, Mueller GA, Wheatley LM. Future directions for allergen immunotherapy. *J Allergy Clin Immunol* 1998;102:335–343.

320. Sampson HA. Food allergy. Part 1: immunopathogenesis and clinical disorders. *J Allergy Clin Immunol* 1999;103:717–728.

321. Sampson HA. Food allergy. Part 2: Diagnosis and management. *J Allergy Clin Immunol* 1999;103:981–989.

322. Croese J, Loukas A, Opdebeeck J, et al. Human enteric infection with canine hookworms. *Ann Intern Med* 1994;120:369–374.

323. Lee YA, Wahn U, Kehrt R, et al. A major susceptibility locus for atopic dermatitis maps to chromosome 3q21. *Nat Genet* 2000;26:470–473.

324. Schneider LC, Baz Z, Zarcone C, et al. Long-term therapy with recombinant interferon-gamma (rIFN-γ) for atopic dermatitis. *Ann Allergy Asthma Immunol* 1998;80:263–268.

325. Wjst M, Heinrich J, Liu P, et al. Indoor factors and IgE levels in children. *Allergy* 1994;49:766–771.

326. Daniels SE, Bhattacharrya S, James A, et al. A genome-wide search for quantitative trait loci underlying asthma. *Nature* 1996;383:247–250.

327. Meyers DA, Postma DS, Panhuysen CI, et al. Evidence for a locus regulating total serum IgE levels mapping to chromosome 5. *Genomics* 1994;23:464–470.

328. Doull IJ, Lawrence S, Watson M, et al. Allelic association of gene markers on chromosomes 5q and 11q with atopy and bronchial hyperresponsiveness. *Am J Respir Crit Care Med* 1996;153:1280–1284.

329. Noguchi E, Shibasaki M, Arinami T, et al. Evidence for linkage between asthma/atopy in childhood and chromosome 5q31–q33 in a Japanese population. *Am J Respir Crit Care Med* 1997;156:1390–1393.

330. Hizawa N, Freidhoff LR, Chiu YF, et al. Genetic regulation of *Dermatophagoides pteronyssinus*–specific IgE responsiveness: a genome-wide multipoint linkage analysis in families recruited through 2 asthmatic sibs. Collaborative Study on the Genetics of Asthma (CSGA). *J Allergy Clin Immunol* 1998;102:436–442.

331. Caraballo LR, Hernandez M. HLA haplotype segregation in families with allergic asthma. *Tissue Antigens* 1990;35:182–186.

332. Young RP, Hart BJ, Merrett TG, et al. House dust mite allergy: interaction of genetic factors and dosage of allergen exposure. *Clin Exp Allergy* 1992;22:205–211.

333. van Herwerden L, Harrap SB, Wong ZY, et al. Linkage of high-affinity IgE receptor gene with bronchial hyperreactivity, even in absence of atopy. *Lancet* 1995;346:1262–1265.

334. Folster-Holst R, Moises HW, Yang L, et al. Linkage between atopy and the IgE high-affinity receptor gene at 11q13 in atopic dermatitis families. *Hum Genet* 1998;102:236–239.

335. Shirakawa T, Hashimoto T, Furuyama J, et al. Linkage between severe atopy and chromosome 11q13 in Japanese families. *Clin Genet* 1994;46:228–232.

336. Shirakawa T, Li A, Dubowitz M, et al. Association between atopy and variants of the beta subunit of the high-affinity immunoglobulin E receptor. *Nat Genet* 1994;7:125–129.

337. Hizawa N, Yamaguchi E, Furuya K, et al. Association between high serum total IgE levels and D11S97 on chromosome 11q13 in Japanese subjects. *J Med Genet* 1995;32:363–369.

338. Palmer LJ, Daniels SE, Rye PJ, et al. Linkage of chromosome 5q and 11q gene markers to asthma-associated quantitative traits in Australian children. *Am J Respir Crit Care Med* 1998;158:1825–1830.

339. Barnes KC, Neely JD, Duffy DL, et al. Linkage of asthma and total serum IgE concentration to markers on chromosome 12q: evidence from Afro-Caribbean and Caucasian populations. *Genomics* 1996;37:41–50.

340. Nickel R, Wahn U, Hizawa N, et al. Evidence for linkage of chromosome 12q15–q24.1 markers to high total serum IgE concentrations in children of the German Multicenter Allergy Study. *Genomics* 1997;46:159–162.

341. Wilkinson J, Grimley S, Collins A, et al. Linkage of asthma to markers on chromosome 12 in a sample of 240 families using quantitative phenotype scores. *Genomics* 1998;53:251–259.

342. Barnes PJ. Anti-IgE antibody therapy for asthma. *N Engl J Med* 1999; 341:2006–2008.

343. Kimura K, Noguchi E, Shibasaki M, et al. Linkage and association of atopic asthma to markers on chromosome 13 in the Japanese population. *Hum Mol Genet* 1999;8:1487–1490.

344. Leaves NI, Anderson GG, Bhattacharrya S, et al. A physical map of the atopy locus on human chromosome. *Am J Hum Genet* 1999; 65:A228.

345. Moffatt MF, Hill MR, Cornelis F, et al. Genetic linkage of T-cell receptor alpha/delta complex to specific IgE responses. *Lancet* 1994; 343:1597–1600.

346. Mao XQ, Shirakawa T, Yoshikawa T, et al. Association between genetic variants of mast-cell chymase and eczema. *Lancet* 1996; 348:581–583.

347. Mansur AH, Bishop DT, Markham AF, et al. Suggestive evidence for genetic linkage between IgE phenotypes and chromosome 14q markers. *Am J Respir Crit Care Med* 1999;159:1796–1802.

CHAPTER 47

Transplantation Immunology

Megan Sykes, Hugh Auchincloss Jr., and David H. Sachs

Introduction
Origins of Transplantation Immunology
Early History · History, Principles, and Discoveries of Immunogenetics
Donor Antigens Responsible for Graft Rejection
Major Histocompatibility Antigens · Minor Histocompatibility Antigens · Other Antigens of Potential Importance in Transplantation
Components of Immune System Involved in Graft Rejection
Antigen-Presenting Cells · B Cells and Antibodies · T Cells · Other Cells
Mechanisms of Graft Rejection
Rejection Caused by Preformed Antibodies (Hyperacute Rejection) · Early Rejection Caused by Induced Antibodies (Accelerated Rejection) · Rejection Caused by T Cells (Acute Rejection) · Chronic Rejection (B- and/or T-Cell–Mediated)
Physiologic Interactions Regulating Graft Rejection
Regulation of Sensitization · Communication between Helper and Effector Cells · Effector Cell Regulation
Manipulations to Prevent Graft Rejection
Nonspecific Techniques · Donor-Specific Tolerance Induction
Transplantation of Specific Organs and Tissues
Skin Grafting · Kidney Transplantation · Liver Transplantation · Heart and Lung Transplantation · Pancreas and Islet Transplantation · Hematopoietic Cell Transplantation · Xenogeneic Transplantation
Some Immunologic Issues in Clinical Transplantation
The Effect of Antigen Matching on Graft Survival and GVHD · Crossmatch · "Sensitized" Candidate for Organ Transplantation · The Diagnosis of Rejection · How Much Immunosuppression Is Enough?
Conclusion
Glossary of Terms and Abbreviations
References

INTRODUCTION*

The transplantation of organs and cells between individuals saves or prolongs thousands of lives each year. The growing list of organs transplanted includes corneas, kidneys, livers, hearts, lungs, small intestines, pancreata, and even hands. Currently, clinical cellular transplantation includes islets of Langerhans and hematopoietic cells, but the list is likely to expand in the future to include other cell types, such as hepatocytes and myoblasts, which are currently under investigation in experimental models. Success of all types of transplants depends on the ability to avoid rejection due to a host-versus-graft immune response. Hematopoietic cell transplantation is, in addition, associated with some special considerations, since the administration of a donor graft that contains mature

T cells to a conditioned, and consequently immunoincompetent recipient, is associated with the risk of rejection in the graft-versus-host (GVH) direction, that is, graft-versus-host disease (GVHD). Because all of these transplants are performed between different humans (i.e., members of the same species), they are referred to as allotransplants. However, improvements in immunosuppressive therapies have increased the success of allotransplantation to the point that a new limitation has been encountered—the insufficient supply of human organs. While this insufficiency can be partly overcome by the increasing use of living donors as sources of kidneys, liver, and lungs, such procedures are associated with significant risks to the donor, and some organs (e.g., the heart) can, obviously only be obtained from cadaveric donors. This organ shortage has led to considerable interest in alternative sources of organs, such as artificial organs, tissue grafts engineered *in vitro* from stem cells, and donors from other species. Transplants from other species, referred

---

*Note to the Reader: Due to space limitations, much of the referencing has been removed from the textbook version of this chapter. A more completely referenced chapter can be found on the CD version.

to as xenografts, are felt by many to be a promising solution to the organ shortage, but present even greater immunologic challenges than allografts, as well as potentially novel infectious risks, and these problems must be addressed before xenotransplantation can be effectively used in the clinic. This chapter presents an overview of the immunology of organ and cellular allotransplantation, as well as xenotransplantation.

Since the transplantation of tissues between members of a species or from other species does not occur in nature, an immunologic defense against transplantation provides no obvious advantage for the survival of the species. Thus, the allogeneic response (i.e., the immune response to the novel antigens of other members of the same species) and the xenogeneic response probably did not evolve for the purpose of graft rejection, and issues of fundamental immunology cannot be explained on the basis of their importance to allogeneic and xenogeneic immunity. Nevertheless, studies of transplantation biology have contributed significantly to our understanding of fundamental immunology by leading, for example, to the discovery of the major histocompatibility complex antigens and by providing the mixed lymphocyte response (MLR) assay for the study of T-cell activation. Now, however, the emphasis has shifted. With the increasing importance of clinical transplantation, the goal is to apply our knowledge of fundamental immunology to the problems of graft rejection and GVHD.

The common error in many summaries of transplantation immunology is to assume that the field can be understood simply by applying classical immunologic principles to describe the response to this particular set of foreign antigens. Allogeneic and xenogeneic responses, however, differ from other immunologic responses in at least two fundamental ways. First, they exhibit extraordinary strength and, probably for that reason, they include unusual types of responses that cannot be detected in classical immunology. Second, they can be stimulated by two different sets of antigen-presenting cells—those of the donor and those of the recipient. In this chapter, we emphasize these differences compared to classical immunology as we describe our current understanding of the several immune responses that cause graft rejection.

ORIGINS OF TRANSPLANTATION IMMUNOLOGY

Early History

The earliest known records of tissue transplantation are those of the Hindu surgeon Sushrutu who reported the use of a flap from a patient's forehead to repair an amputated nose. This procedure was probably practiced by Hindu surgeons as early as 700 B.C. In the 15th century, Italian surgeons began to practice rhinoplasty by means of flaps and extended the donor site to the patient's arm (1). In 1503, one such surgeon reported the first allograft—the grafting of skin from a slave for the reconstruction of the master's nose. A sizable legend grew out of such reports, although obviously unfounded in fact.

Skin grafting became an accepted practice in the late 1800s. Many workers, however, did not distinguish between auto-

grafts (donor and recipient the same individual) and allografts (donor and recipient of the same species) or even, sometimes, xenografts (donor and recipient of different species). The last of these formed the basis for an extensive practice known as zoografting in which patients were subjected to grafts from animals ranging from pigs to frogs (2). Billingham (3) points out that no one apparently cared whether the grafted skin "took" or merely promoted healing of the wound. The results of these efforts led to a period of confusion in transplantation. Without any clear understanding of the processes involved, surgeons embarked on all sorts of transplants, and a series of operations were reported that we know, from our present understanding of the laws of transplantation, could not possibly have been successful. Dr. Serge Voronoff, for example, attained considerable fame (and fortune) in Europe by developing an unusual grafting procedure in which testicles were transplanted from ape to human in order to restore men to youth and vitality.

The transplantation of internal organs awaited the development of techniques for vascular anastomosis. In 1908, Carrel, one of the pioneers of vascular surgery, reported the results of *en bloc* allotransplantation of both kidneys in a series of nine cats (4). He was able to obtain up to 25 days of urine output in some cats, but ultimately all of them died. Although other investigators repeated and modified Carrel's experiments, no major advances in prolonging the function of allografts or in understanding the cause for their failure were made for the following 3 decades.

During this same period, the closely related field of tumor transplantation gained momentum. In 1902, Jensen reported the transplantation of a mouse tumor through 19 successive generations of mice and was able to obtain tumor growth in some 50% of the mice he injected. Furthermore, he showed that mice in which the tumor grew for a while and then regressed were resistant to subsequent challenge with the same tumor. He was also able to prevent successful tumor grafting by prior treatment with grafts of normal tissues (3).

Although it seems obvious to us now that these experiments provided much of the information essential to an understanding of transplantation immunology, this was not clear at the time. Many workers still held to the "athrepsia theory" formulated by Erlich in 1906 (5). According to this hypothesis, living tissues required a vital substance specific for each species and provided only by the intact organism. Thus, a transplanted tumor might grow for a while until it used up its supply of this substance. Other workers who accepted a theory of immunity were nevertheless committed to the idea that they were studying an effect peculiar to tumor tissues. In his Harvey Lecture, Medawar summed up the confusion neatly by the statement, "Nearly everyone who supposed that he was using transplantation to study tumors was in fact using tumors to study transplantation."

In 1936, Voronoy, a Russian surgeon, reported the first clinical renal allograft (1). There was apparently a mismatch of blood types and the patient died having demonstrated only minimal renal function. The early postwar years saw reports of attempts at clinical renal homotransplantation from various locales around the world. In 1952, the first successful renal transplant was performed in Boston using the kidney of an identical twin (6).

One of the important contributions to the understanding of transplantation in this era was the work of Medawar. In 1943, Gibson and Medawar reported their experience with autologous and allogeneic skin grafts on a woman who had suffered extensive third-degree burns. The allografts in this case were taken from the patient's sibling, and for clinical reasons were transplanted in two different stages separated by about a week. The authors observed accelerated rejection of the second grafts. Appreciating the possible significance of these observations, Medawar followed them with a series of grafting experiments in rabbits and mice. By 1945, he was able to conclude that "resistance to homologous grafted skin therefore belongs to the general category of actively acquired immune reactions" (7), thereby establishing the relationship of clinical transplantation to the field of immunology.

History, Principles, and Discoveries of Immunogenetics

Inbred Strains

Rodents have provided an invaluable model for the study of the genetic basis for graft rejection. One of the main fea-

tures that has made them so valuable is the availability of a large number of inbred strains. Such strains consist of animals that have been produced by sequential pedigreed brother–sister matings for at least 20 generations and which are, therefore, essentially genetically identical. With the exception of the sex chromosomes, chromosomes in such strains are homozygous and therefore produce identical homozygous progeny.

The reason that sequential inbreeding leads to homozygosity is illustrated in Fig. 1. For the sake of simplicity, the first generation illustrated in this figure is indicated as a brother–sister mating in which for any given autosomal locus the alleles being bred will be of the form AB × AB. The more general case of AB × CD can also be analyzed statistically by a similar, although slightly more complicated, mathematical treatment. The ratio of genotypes of the offspring from this breeding is given by the binomial formula (AA:AB:BB = 1:2:1). Thus, as illustrated at the second generation, when a single brother–sister pair is chosen, the chance that both animals will have the genotype AA at the locus in question is 1/16. Similarly, the probability that the second-generation mating will take the form BB × BB is also 1/16. In either of these eventualities, all future generations will be fixed as homozygotes (either AA or BB) and therefore we speak of the locus as being fixed. Thus, the probability of fixation of a given autosomal locus at this generation is 1/8.

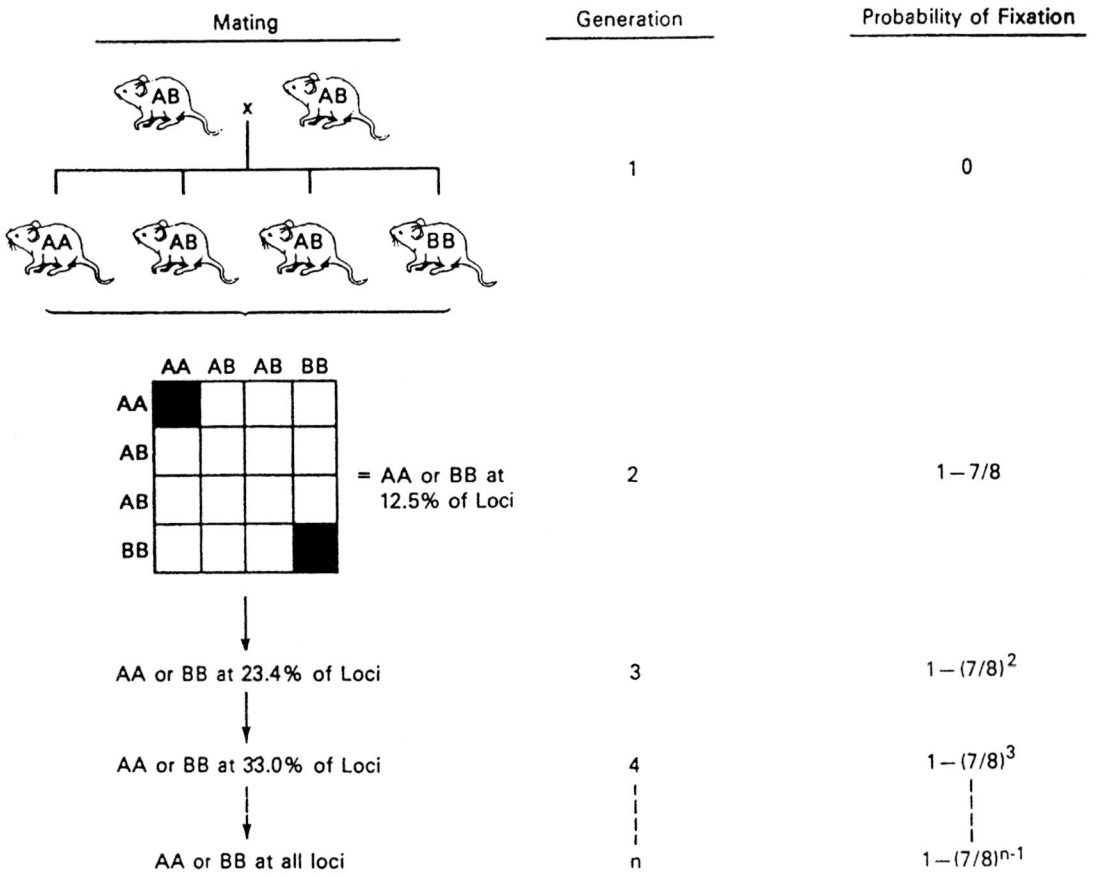

FIG. 1. Breeding scheme for inbred strains.

For segregation of a large number of independent loci, it is mathematically equivalent to state that the probability of fixing a given locus is 1/8, or that on the average 1/8 of the segregating loci will be fixed. If the locus in question is not fixed during this random breeding, then the chances that it will be fixed at the next breeding are still approximately 1/8 (actually a little higher). In other words, 1/8 of the loci would be expected to fix at the second inbreeding generation, 1/8 of the remaining unfixed loci would be expected to fix at the next generation, and so on. As indicated in Fig. 1, the probability of fixation (Pfix) is given by the formula

$$P_{fix} = 1 - \left(\frac{7}{8}\right)^{n-1}.$$

This equation describes a curve that rises asymptotically toward a probability of 100% fixation (Fig. 2). Since genes travel at meiosis in groups rather than individually, there is a finite number of units of genetic information that segregate. Therefore, for practical purposes, one can consider a strain inbred after 20 such brother–sister matings, since at this point there is a very small chance that any locus will not have reached homozygosity. All loci will be of the genotype either AA or BB, and there will no longer be any loci of the heterozygous form AB. The strain so derived is defined as an inbred strain. Hundreds of such well-characterized inbred strains are now available.

During the procedure of sequential brother–sister matings to produce such inbred strains there are, as expected, numerous cases in which lethal recessive genes become homozygous, leading to the loss of a particular line. However, since a very large number of sequential brother–sister pairs can be started and maintained from a single original breeding pair, it is generally possible to produce at least several inbred strains from the breeding of two outbred animals. If, for example, one sets up all possible brother–sister matings at the first two or three generations and then selects only a single brother–sister pair for all subsequent generations, one might easily obtain ten successful inbred strains, even if 90% of the lines

started were to succumb to lethal recessives. Since a large number of strains of mice can be housed in a small space, such a project is feasible in this species.

Inbred strains have also been produced in several other species including rats, guinea pigs, and rabbits. However, both space requirements and other genetic features, such as gestation times, age of sexual maturity, and litter size, make production of inbred strains in larger species much more difficult. Indeed, until recently, there were no inbred large animal species available. However, over the past 30 years, studies in one of our laboratories (D. Sachs) have produced highly inbred miniature swine (8). Swine were chosen for this purpose because they represent one of the few large animal species in which breeding characteristics make genetic experiments possible. Swine have a relatively large litter size (three to ten offspring) and a short gestation time (3 months). They reach sexual maturity at approximately 6 months of age, and sows have an estrous cycle every 3 weeks. These breeding characteristics made it possible to develop MHC homozygous lines of miniature swine in a relatively short time (8), to isolate new MHC recombinants and breed them to homozygosity, and to carry out short-term backcross experiments in order to identify and study the segregation of genetic characteristics. These miniature swine now represent the only large animal model in which MHC genetics can be reproducibly controlled. As such, these animals have been particularly useful in assessing the effects of MHC matching on rejection and/or tolerance induction (9).

At present, swine of three homozygous SLA haplotypes, SLA^a, SLA^c, SLA^d, and five lines bearing intra-SLA recombinant haplotypes are maintained, as illustrated in Fig. 3. All of these lines differ by minor histocompatibility loci, thus providing a model in which most of the transplantation combinations relevant to human transplantation can be mimicked. Thus, for example, transplants within an MHC homozygous herd simulate transplants between HLA identical siblings, while transplants between herds resemble cadaveric or non-matched sibling transplants. Likewise, transplants between pairs of heterozygotes can be chosen to resemble parent into offspring or one-haplotype mismatched sibling transplants. In addition, one subline of SLA^{dd} animals was selected for further inbreeding, in order to produce a fully inbred line of miniature swine. This subline has now reached a coefficient of inbreeding of >94%, and is now sufficiently inbred for histocompatibility, that is, reciprocal skin grafts among the offspring have not been rejected. These animals should be particularly useful in permitting adoptive transfer studies for the first time in a large animal model.

There are several factors that may mitigate against the obtaining of truly inbred animals. One such factor is known as forced heterozygosity. This situation arises when both possible alleles at a given locus are recessive lethals such that only heterozygotes are viable. In this case, the locus in question, as well as loci closely linked to this locus, will be maintained in a heterozygous state. This situation, although theoretically possible, has apparently been encountered only very rarely

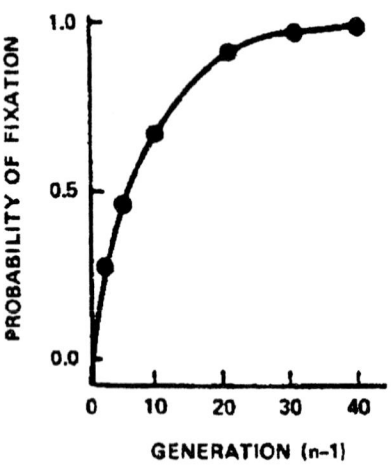

FIG. 2. Probability of fixation curve.

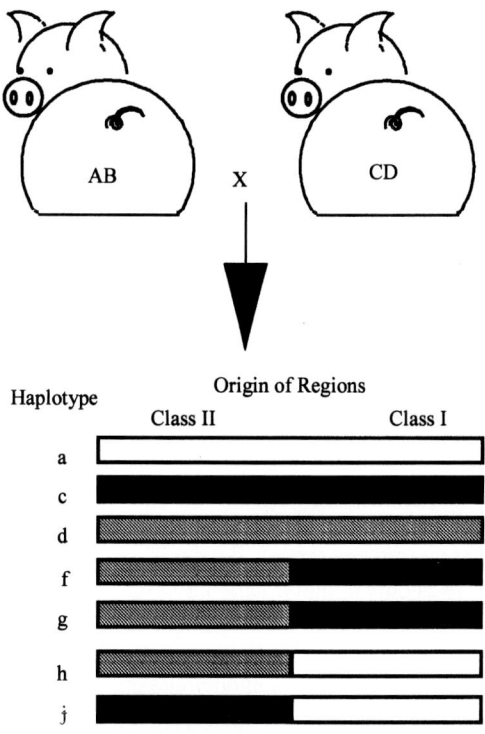

FIG. 3. Origin of minature swine haplotypes.

during the production of inbred strains. A more common problem in obtaining true homozygosity is that of mutation, which is of course a continuously occurring phenomenon that cannot be avoided. The average mutation frequency for mammalian genes has been estimated to be approximately 10^{-6} per base pair per meiosis. Since there are more than 10^6 genetic loci in mammalian organisms, one would expect at least one mutation to occur somewhere in the genome at every generation. While this source of reintroduction of heterozygosity cannot be avoided, one can ensure that such heterozygosity, once introduced, will not remain for very long by continuing to maintain a brother–sister pedigreed mating scheme for the reference line of any inbred strain. As indicated in Fig. 1, such a scheme will ensure that any mutation that occurs will either be lost or be fixed as a homozygous allele by this procedure. In order to ensure that inbred lines stay inbred, therefore, pedigreed reference lines for each inbred strain must be maintained. A single brother–sister mating is chosen at each generation and all other animals of the strain are bred from this pair or its progeny. Animals used for experiments in large numbers are bred in expansion and production colonies, but should not be more than a few generations away from the reference pedigreed line.

If a particular inbred strain is maintained in two different colonies, the pedigreed reference lines will accumulate different mutations. The lines will therefore be said to "drift" from each other. If proper sequential brother–sister mating is performed in both colonies, each line will remain truly inbred, although eventually the two lines will be distinct at

a number of genetic loci. Lines maintained separately are therefore called sublines and are designated by a series of letters following the strain designation that indicate the origin and location of the pedigreed reference line. Thus, for example, the C3H/HeJ and C3H/HeN lines are two different sublines of the C3H strain. Both were originally maintained by Heston (He), one subline then being maintained at Jackson Laboratory (C3H/HeJ) and the other at the National Instiues of Health (C3H/HeN). Although these strains are still quite similar for many properties, there are already several known differences between them, such as the responsiveness of their lymphocytes to LPS. Often differences between sublines are first detected when results from one laboratory are found difficult to reproduce in another.

Genetic Principles Governing Tissue Transplantation: The "Laws of Transplantation"

The earliest strains of inbred mice examined by geneticists had been produced for commercial rather than experimental purposes. Mouse fanciers in Europe and Japan had for many years attempted to maintain a variety of desirable characteristics in their mouse lines, such as coat color and behavioral patterns, and in selecting for such traits they had essentially inbred their mouse strains. In the early 1900s it was noted by tumor biologists that tumors arising in such animals could frequently be transplanted successfully to other animals of the same line, while this was usually impossible in outbred animals. Little (10) then studied this phenomenon systematically, and in the process produced and characterized a large number of inbred strains of mice.

In summarizing the results of these studies of tumor grafting in mice, Little described what have since been called the "five laws of transplantation" (see Table 1). These are not really laws but rather a set of apparently confusing observations in which the capacity for graft rejection exists in the parental generation, is lost in the F1 generation, but is regained in the F2 generation in most cases. For those attempting to identify the genetic basis for tumor (graft) acceptance, this pattern did not appear in keeping with Mendelian genetics. Little's remarkable insight was to reconcile these observations with the classical Mendelian principles by suggesting the true fundamental principle of graft rejection and

TABLE 1. *The laws of transplantation*

1. Transplants within inbred strains will succeed.
2. Transplants between inbred strains will fail.
3. Transplants from a member of an inbred parental strain to an F_1 offspring will succeed but those in the reverse direction will fail.
4. Transplants from F_2 and all subsequent generations to F_1 animals will succeed.
5. Transplants from inbred parental strains to the F_2 generation will usually, but not always, fail.

Adapted from Little CC. The genetics of tissue transplantation in mammals. *Cancer Res* 1924;8:75–95 by identifying the genetic basis for the unusual outcomes. His fundamental principle was that recipients would reject grafts if the donor expressed a product of any histocompatibility (tissue compatibility) locus that was not expressed by the recipient (a principle that is now second nature to any student of transplantation immunology). His explanation for the unusual inheritance pattern was to suggest, first, that there must be co-dominant expression of the histocompatibility genes, and second, that there must be a relatively large number of histocompatibility loci. Under these conditions, members of the F1 generation would express both parental alleles at all histocompatibility loci (and thus would fail to reject grafts from parental, F2, or subsequent generations) and members of the F2 generation would be unlikely to express all of the products of histocompatibility genes that are expressed by either parental generation (and thus would usually reject parental allografts).

Estimating the Number of Histocompatibility Genes

Given the availability of inbred strains and the genetic principles discussed above, one can experimentally determine the number of histocompatibility loci by which any two inbred strains differ. One breeds a large F2 population between these strains and then transplants tissues from one of the parental strains to all of the F2 offspring, measuring the fraction of grafts that survive. As illustrated in Fig. 4, if the two strains were to differ at only one histocompatibility locus, one would predict that 3/4 of the grafts would survive. If, however, the two strains differed by two independently segregating histocompatibility loci, then one would predict that $(3/4)^2$ or 9/16 of the grafts would survive since, of the 3/4 of animals accepting the graft due to histocompatibility at the first locus, only 3/4 would be expected to be histocompatible for the second locus. Similarly, if there were n loci by which these two strains differed, one would expect $(3/4)^n$ to be the fraction of surviving grafts.

When experiments designed to determine the number of histocompatibility loci were first performed, tumor grafts were employed. The number of loci detected was between four and ten, depending on the particular parental strains chosen and the tumor used for transplantation. Subsequently these experiments have been repeated, using skin grafts as the challenging transplant. In this case, numbers for n as high as 30 to 50 have been reported. Since there are only 20 chromosome pairs in the mouse genome, these larger numbers imply that many chromosomes carry more than one histocompatibility locus.

Producing Congenic Strains: Identifying the MHC

There are thus a very large number of histocompatibility loci, each encoding a cell protein capable of contributing to rejection of a graft. However, in addition to Little's insight that there were multiple histocompatibility loci, the genetic principles he identified also suggested the process for breeding mice that would generate strains differing from one another genetically at only a single histocompatibility locus. This process, pursued especially by Snell (11) at Jackson Laboratory, involved the production of congenic strains (inbred strains that differ from one another at only one independently segregating genetic locus) using the rejection of parental skin grafts as the trait used to select successive matings. The resulting congenic strains were therefore called "congenic-resistant" (CR) strains, since they resisted engraftment of tissues from one another. In the course of producing numerous CR strains, it became apparent that one histocompatibility locus could be distinguished from all the others by the speed with which it caused skin graft rejection. This is now called the major histocompatibility complex. All of the other 30 to 50 histocompatibility loci have since been called minor histocompatibility loci. There are now a very large number of H-2 CR strains of mice available (Table 2), as well as some that isolate minor histocompatibility loci and some rat CR strains.

One of the most useful breeding schemes to produce CR lines is illustrated in Fig. 5. Starting with two inbred strains, labeled for simplicity Strain A and Strain B, the objective is to obtain a strain that will share its entire genome with Strain A except for the major histocompatibility locus H-2, which will be derived from Strain B. The end product will be designated Strain A.B. According to the cross-intercross scheme illustrated in Fig. 4, the two inbred strains are first crossed to produce an F1 generation. Since, as described above, both inbred strains can be presumed to be homozygous at all autosomal loci, all loci of the F1 generation will be heterozygous (ab). These F1 animals are then intercrossed to produce an F2 generation. The distribution of alleles at all autosomal loci in this generation follows the binomial expansion. At any locus, 1/4 of the animals would be expected to be of genotype bb. A skin graft or tumor graft from Strain A is next placed onto all of the F2 offspring. Animals that reject the graft must be of genotype bb in at least one histocompatibility locus. Obviously, since there are many histocompatibility loci, most animals at this generation will reject the graft. However, if only animals rejecting vigorously are chosen, and if

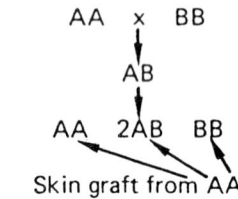

No. Loci	Expected Survivals
1	3/4
2	$(3/4)^2$
.	.
.	.
n	$(3/4)^n$

FIG. 4. Estimating the number of histocompatibility loci.

TABLE 2. *List of H-2 congenic resistant strains*

Strain	H-2 haplotype	Origin of background	MHC
A	a	A	—
A./BY	b	A	Brackyury
A./CA	f	A	Caracal
A./SW	s	A	Swiss
BALB/c	d	BALB/c	BALB/c
BALB.B	b	BALB/c	C57BL/10
BALB.K	k	BALB/c	C3H
B6.AKR-H-2^k	k	C57BL/6	AKR
B6.SJL	s	C57BL/6	SJL
B10	b	C57BL/10	C57BL/10
B10.A	a	C57BL/10	A
B10.D2	d	C57BL/10	DBA/2
B10.M	f	C57BL/10	Outbred
B10.BR	k	C57BL/10	C57BR
B10.SM	v	C57BL/10	SM
B10.RIII	r	C57BL/10	RIII
B10.PL	u	C57BL/10	PL/J
C3H	k	C3H	C3H
C3H.SW	b	C3H	Swiss
C3H.JK	j	C3H	JK
C3H.NB	p	C3H	NB
D1.C	d	DBA/1	BALB/c
D1.LP	b	DBA/1	LP
LP.RIII	r	LP	RIII

numerous such animals are selected, then one can be reasonably certain to have selected bb homozygotes at the H-2 locus by this procedure.

The process is next repeated by mating rejectors back to Strain A animals. For selected loci, therefore, the offspring once again are heterozygous. At all other nonselected loci, offspring will have a 50% probability of being homozygous for aa alleles or of being heterozygous ab. Obviously, therefore, approximately one-half of the nonselected genetic information is caused by this process to revert to the inbred Strain A type. Once again, these animals are intercrossed to produce the expected F2 distribution for selected loci. Another tissue graft from Strain A is performed, and again rejecting animals are selected. The fraction of animals rejecting grafts vigorously at this generation will be smaller than it was at the previous generation. Once again, by selecting only vigorous rejectors one will ensure the selection of the bb homozygote at the H-2 locus. A cross to Strain A is then again performed, once again producing the expected ab heterozygotes at the selected locus or loci. This time, however, the chances that any nonselected locus will still be heterozygous have fallen to 25%.

This process of crossing, intercrossing, and selecting by graft rejection is repeated sequentially. By the time nine cycles have been completed, one would expect only one histocompatibility locus to be segregating, so that only 25% of the intercross offspring should be capable of rejecting the graft. Assuming that vigorous rejection has been demanded throughout, one can be relatively certain that the selected locus will be H-2. In addition, the chances that any

other nonselected locus will still be heterozygous rather than having reverted to the homozygous aa genotype will have fallen to <0.2%. Stated another way, >99.8% of nonselected loci will be expected to be identical to their counterparts in Strain A. A male and a female homozygote from the final intercross are selected and used to establish a pedigreed inbred CR line A.B.

Because mammalian genes are transferred as linked units in chromosomes, this process will always lead to the retention of a variable amount of bb genetic information at genes closely linked to the locus being selected. However, as described below, the occurrence of recombination during intercrossing generations leads also to fixation of the aa genotype at loci on the same chromosome as the MHC (chromosome 17 in mice) but at a variable distance from H-2. For practical purposes, animals that have been through at least nine cycles of such selected breeding are considered to be congenic.

As indicated in Table 2, there are now a large number of H-2 congenic mouse strains available on a variety of backgrounds. In general, the names of each of these strains follow the rule A.B, with Strain A being the background strain used in the production of the congenic, and Strain B being the other parental strain from which the alternate allele at H-2 was selected. All of the early inbred mouse strains were assigned a small letter designation to represent the particular constellation of alleles that they possessed at genes in the MHC. This small letter designation is often called the haplotype designation, as indicated in Table 2. Thus, for example, Strain C57BL/10 is assigned the haplotype designation H-2b, and Strain DBA/2 the haplotype designation H-2d. The shorthand designation for C57BL/10 is B10 and that for DBA/2 is D2. Thus, the congenic strain B10.D2 represents a CR line in which the background is derived from the C57BL/10 and the MHC from the DBA/2. It thus resembles in almost every way the C57BL/10 congenic partner, except that it differs from this partner for all properties controlled by MHC-linked genes. Similarly, the C3H.B10 strain was derived from an initial cross between C3H (H-2k) and C57BL/10(H-2b).

The formal designation of a CR line also includes, in parentheses after the letters, a designation such as (18M), distinguishing different congenic lines derived from the same cross. Since a large number of CR lines have been developed in which histocompatibility loci other than H-2 have been transferred to the same background, these numbers are often included to distinguish different lines. However, for most purposes when one is describing an MHC congenic, one does not need to include its suffix. Thus, B10.D2 is a generally acceptable designation for the H-2 congenic between C57BL/10 and DBA/2.

Intra-MHC Recombinant Strains: Class I and II Antigens

As can be seen in Fig. 5, every alternate generation in this mating scheme involves the crossing of animals heterozygous at H-2. Whenever heterozygotes are bred, there is always a possibility of recombination between autosomal chromosomes

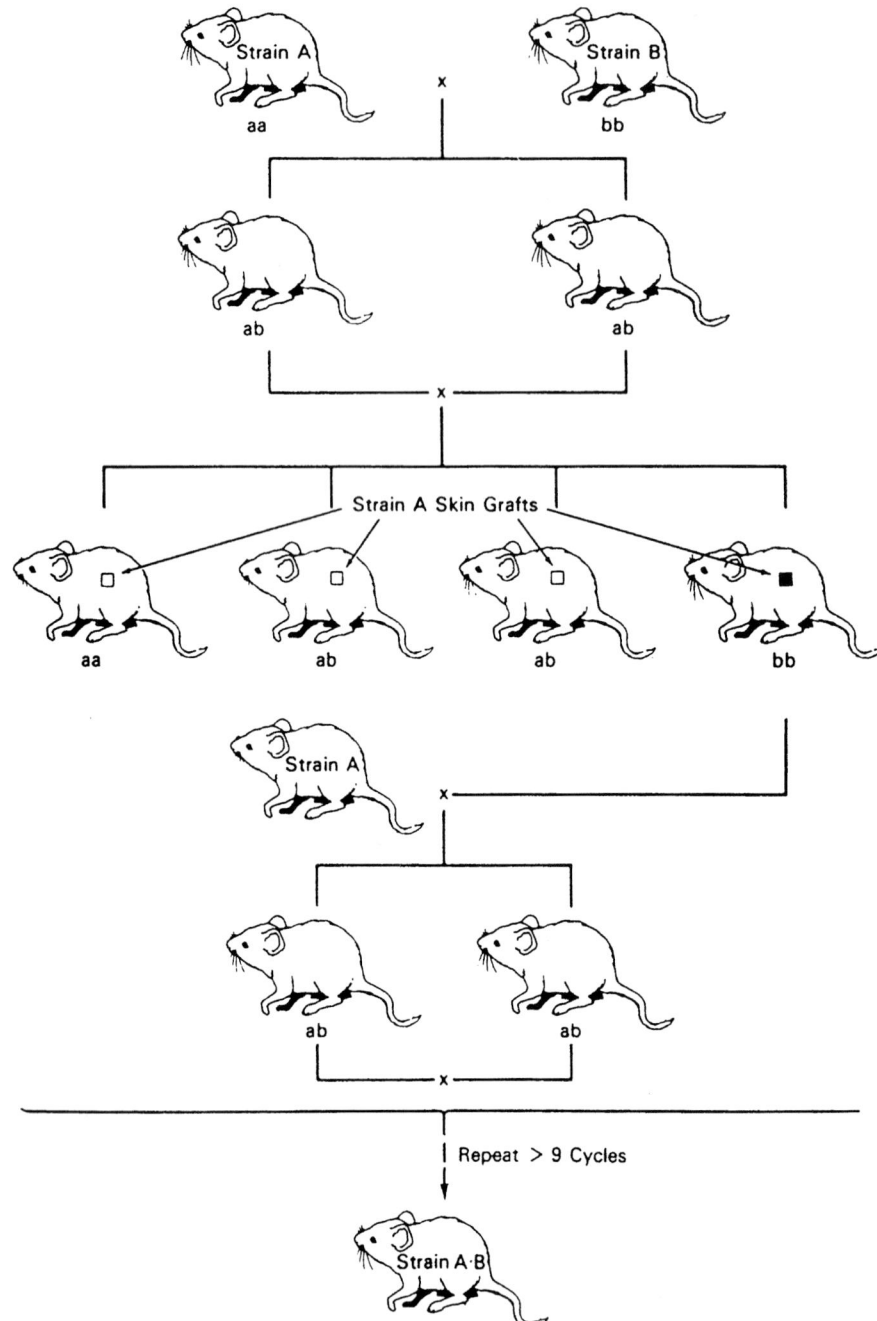

FIG. 5. Schematic representation for production of a congenic line.

at meiosis. During the production of congenic lines, such recombination will tend to decrease the amount of linked genetic information carried into the congenic from the H-2 source. Therefore, the more backcrosses a particular congenic line has been subjected to, the closer will be the boundaries on either side of H-2 at which the chromosome reverts to the background strain. Since it soon became apparent that the MHC was in fact made up of multiple loci, there was also the possibility for recombination within H-2 to occur during such crosses. Indeed, it was through the detection and characterization of such recombinants that the linkage map of H-2 was constructed. It is instructive to examine how such

recombinants would be detected and used in determining the genetic fine structure of the H-2 locus. In order to detect a recombination event, one must examine the intercross or backcross progeny for more than one of the distinguishing features of the MHC described in the previous section of this chapter. This is because one can only detect the occurrence of a recombination event if the two properties examined do not behave comparably in the progeny. Thus, during the production of the hypothetical CR strain A.B, a recombination such as that illustrated in Fig. 6 might occur. In this case, let us assume that progeny are being examined both for ability to reject vigorously a Strain A skin graft (i.e.,

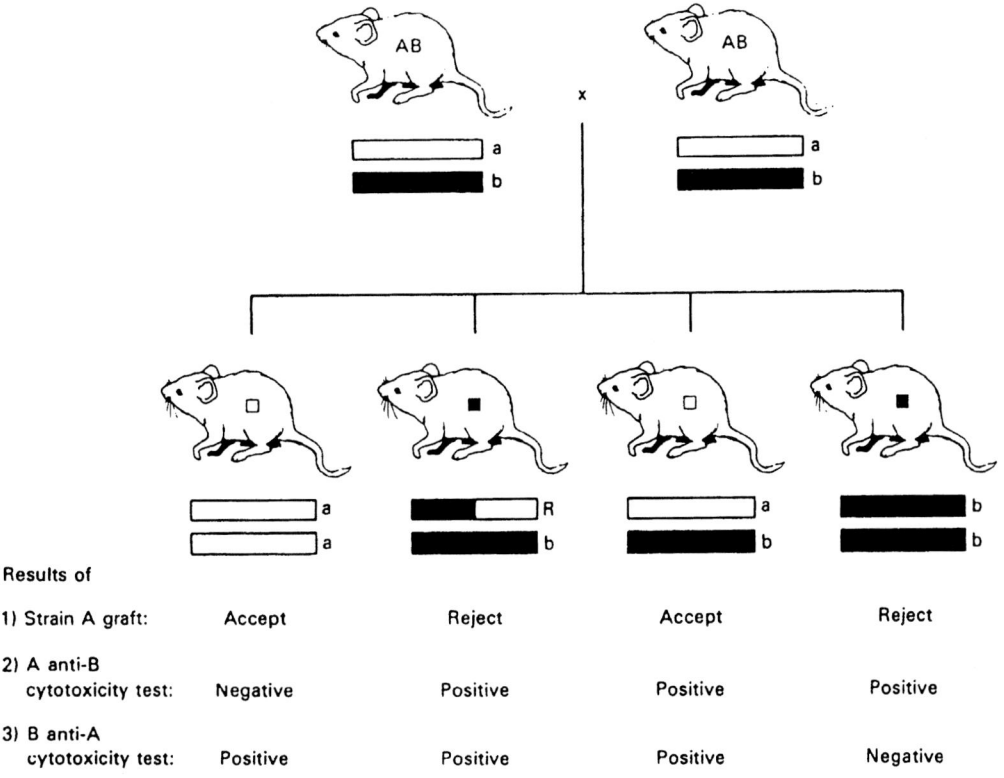

FIG. 6. Intra-MHC recombination.

genotype bb for a histocompatibility locus) and for presence of a or b gene products on lymphocyte surfaces as detected by a complement-mediated cytotoxic assay. The antisera used might be Strain A anti-Strain B (detecting products of bb) and Strain B anti-Strain A (detecting products of aa).

As seen in Fig. 6, an intra-H-2 recombinant event might lead to an animal which would type as bb by the skin graft analysis because it lacks a part of the H-2 complex that encodes products capable of causing skin graft rejection, but nevertheless type positively with both A anti-B and B anti-A antisera, suggesting an ab genotype. Such an animal would certainly not satisfy the requirement for an eventual A.B congenic line, so that other rejectors would be used for further crossing to produce the desired congenic. However, such an animal might be selected as a putative recombinant and back-crossed further to Strain A to produce a congenic recombinant line designated A.B(1R). The next such putative recombinant found would be called A.B(2R), and so on. In this way, a series of congenic lines might be obtained each differing from the background strain A at the MHC, and from each other by different points of recombination within the MHC.

Fortunately, mouse geneticists were aware of this possibility and saved numerous recombinants during the production of H-2 congenic lines. Thus, for example, there are now a series of recombinants between strain C57BL/10(H-2b) and A/WySn(H-2a) that were isolated by Stimpfling during production of the B10.A CR line and which have provided a great deal of information on the genetic fine structure of the H-2 complex. Strains B10.A(2R) and B10.A(4R), for example,

have been used to map a variety of immune response genes within the MHC. Table 3 presents a listing of many of the most useful congenic recombinant strains now available and their known or presumed points of recombination. Among the most important contributions that came from the study of intra-MHC recombinant strains was the progressive understanding that the loci within the MHC encoded two general types of MHC antigens, now referred to as class I and class II MHC antigens.

DONOR ANTIGENS RESPONSIBLE FOR GRAFT REJECTION

Major Histocompatibility Antigens

As discussed above, the genetic analysis of graft rejection indicated that the antigens encoded within the MHC are of particular importance in graft rejection. Table 4 summarizes important aspects of the MHC antigens that are worth emphasizing in this chapter on transplantation, while a much more detailed description of their structure and function can be found in Chapter 19.

Basic Features of MHC Antigens

Class I and Class II Antigens

Different loci within the complex encode two general types of MHC antigens, today called class I and class II antigens. Over the years the distinction between these two classes has

TABLE 3. *List of H-2 recombinant strains*

Recombinant interval haplotypes	Parental haplotypes	Haplotypes designation	KAESD	Presence of additional recombinant site	Strain bearing recombinant
K-A	b/m	bq1	b/k k k q	Yes	B10.MBR
	s/a1	t1	slk k k d	Yes	A.TL
A-E	a/b	h4	k klb b b	No	B10.A(4R)
	b/a	i5	b blk d d	Yes	B10.A(5R)
	b/a	i3	b blk d d	Yes	B10.A(3R)
E-S	k/d	a	k k kld d	No	A, B10.A
S-D	d/b	g	d d d dlb	No	HTG, B10.HTG
	d/k	o2	d d d dlk	No	C3H.OH
	a/b	h1,h2	k k k dlb	Yes	B10.A(2R)
	k/q	m	k k k klq	No	AKR.M, B10.AKM
	q/a	y2	q q q qld	No	B10.T(6R)
	s/A	t2	s s s sld	No	A.TH

Notes: Congenic recombinant haplotypes available from The Jackson Laboratory.

Note that many of the recombinants involve at least one haplotype already containing a point of recombination. These are indicated by "Yes" and are listed only under the recombinant interval representing the most recent recombination in the haplotype's history.

been based on several different criteria and thus the terminology applied to them has varied. Originally the class I antigens were identified most easily by serologic techniques, and they were therefore named SD, or serologically defined antigens. Class II antigens, however, were not originally detected by antibody responses, but by proliferative responses of allogeneic lymphocytes. Class II antigens were therefore called LD, or lymphocyte-defined antigens. Subsequently, serologic identification of class II antigens was accomplished and it was recognized that genes responsible for class II antigens were tightly linked to the I region of the mouse MHC. Thus, for a time, these antigens were called I region–associated or Ia antigens. Among other differences, class I and class II MHC antigens evoke allogeneic responses that differ in both character and magnitude, as will be discussed below.

Polymorphism

The MHC antigens exhibit extraordinary polymorphism. This polymorphism presumably provides an advantage to members of the species by ensuring a broad capacity to present the

TABLE 4. *Summary of features of MHC*

Class I antigens	Single polymorphic chain Three domains: alpha 1, 2, and 3 MW: 45,000 Associated with beta 2 microglobulin A, B, and C loci in humans Expressed on all tissues and cells
Class II antigens	Two polymorphic chains: alpha and beta Each with two domains: alpha 1 and 2, beta 1 and 2 MW: 33,000 and 28,000 DP, DQ, and DR loci in humans Expressed on macrophages, dendritic cells and B cells; vascular endothelium; activated human T cells

peptides of, and thus respond to, a large number of foreign antigens. In the human HLA complex, for example, there are currently at least 300 known alleles at each of the HLA-B and DRB1 loci (12). The high degree of polymorphism has important consequences for transplantation. Given that there are three class I loci (A, B, and C) and three to four class II loci (DQ, DP, DRB1, ± an expressed DRB 3, 4, or 5 locus present in some haplotypes) on each haplotype, the likelihood of achieving identity for MHC antigens in two unrelated humans is extremely small.

Tissue Distribution

The tissue distribution of the two types of MHC antigens is not identical. Class I antigens are present on all nucleated cells of the body, but may be sparsely represented on some types of cells, including certain antigen-presenting cells (APC) (13). Class II MHC antigens are more selective in their distribution. They are especially frequent on macrophages, dendritic cells (DC), and B-lymphocytes. They may be present on other lymphoid cells under some circumstances, and on vascular endothelium. Their expression on some tissues of the body is not constant and varies according to several stimuli (14). Finally, the tissue distribution of class II MHC antigens is not the same in all species. One of the important distinctions between rodents and many larger species is the lack of expression of class II antigens on the vascular endothelium and other cell populations in rodents, whereas pigs, monkeys, and humans do express class II antigens on these tissues (15).

Physiologic Function of MHC Antigens

MHC antigens are called "histocompatibility" antigens because of their powerful role in causing graft rejection; yet they did not evolve in nature to prevent tissue grafting. While the name serves to emphasize the historical importance of transplantation in the discovery of the MHC, the essential role of MHC antigens is now understood to involve the presentation of peptides of foreign antigens to responding T cells (see Chapters 19 and 20).

The Importance of MHC Antigens in Alloreactivity

Alloreactivity is the immune response to foreign antigens of other members of the same species. MHC antigens are exceptionally important in stimulating alloreactive responses, both *in vivo* and *in vitro*.

Vigorous Graft Rejection

Allogeneic MHC antigens are the most important antigens responsible for causing graft rejection. Their discovery depended largely on this feature, since early experiments showed that mouse skin grafts differing only in their MHC antigens were typically rejected in 8 to 10 days, whereas grafts differing by only a single minor histocompatibility antigen were typically rejected in 3 or more weeks. Subsequent experiments have confirmed the importance of MHC antigens for other types of grafts. In pigs, primarily vascularized organs, such as the kidney, may survive indefinitely in some cases, even without immunosuppression, if all MHC antigens are matched, whereas MHC-mismatched kidneys are always rejected within 2 weeks (15).

However, the clear evidence for the importance of MHC antigens in causing graft rejection generally depends on disparities of both class I and II antigens together. Thus, there are examples in mice of skin grafts that have only class I or only class II MHC antigen disparities that are not rejected at all. Furthermore, the importance of MHC antigen matching becomes harder to detect, especially for skin graft survival, when comparing MHC-antigen mismatched grafts with grafts differing in multiple minor histocompatibility antigens.

Primary In Vitro MLR and CML

Allogeneic MHC antigens also stimulate an extraordinarily strong T-cell response *in vitro*. This strength is manifested partly by the ability to achieve primary *in vitro* cell-mediated responses to allogeneic MHC antigens, whereas *in vitro* responses to "nominal" antigens, such as ovalbumin, generally require *in vivo* priming. The greater strength can also be measured by the higher precursor frequency of alloreactive T cells compared to that for other foreign antigens presented in association with self-MHC molecules. T cells reactive with an allogeneic MHC determinant may represent as many as 2% or more of the total T-cell population, while T cells reactive with an exogenous protein generally represent no more than one in 10,000 of the same T-cell pool (16). This high frequency of alloreactive cells is observed even when precursor frequencies are measured for a mutant MHC antigen varying from the responder by only a single amino acid.

Explanations for the Strong Response to Allogeneic MHC Antigens

Originally, efforts to explain the strength of the immune response stimulated by allogeneic MHC antigens focused on possible physiologic benefits of a strong alloreactive response. For example, some considered the possibility that alloreactivity might be helpful in terminating pregnancy at parturition or that it might help prevent the spread of infectious diseases between individuals. However, as the true physiologic function of MHC antigens has become better understood, most immunologists have concluded that the strong response to allogeneic MHC antigens is not physiologic, but rather an accidental occurrence that depends on two important features: first, that allogeneic MHC antigens are almost unique among foreign proteins in being able to stimulate an immune response without first being processed into peptides for presentation by self-MHC molecules, and second, that because of this feature they can be recognized on allogeneic rather than just on self-APC.

Direct Recognition of Allogeneic MHC Antigens

All theoretical explanations for the extraordinary strength of alloreactivity are based on the unusual feature that T cells can recognize allogeneic MHC antigens without the usual requirement that peptides of these antigens be processed and presented by self-MHC molecules. Transplantation immunologists refer to this special type of recognition as "direct" recognition of allogeneic MHC antigens. The capacity for direct recognition is believed to result from the similarity of the determinants formed by allo-MHC antigens with those created by the presentation of foreign peptides by self-MHC antigens. In shorthand terminology, this has been referred to as: "Allo = Self + X". The evidence supporting this cross-reactive property comes from studies of T-cell clones that are specific for peptide antigens presented by self-MHC molecules, but that also recognize allogeneic MHC antigens directly. Since the T-cell repertoire is selected in the thymus to recognize modified self-MHC antigens preferentially, it therefore also includes large numbers of receptors capable of recognizing allo-MHC antigens directly. The possible reasons for this extraordinarily high frequency of T cells that can respond directly to allo-MHC antigens are discussed below.

The Strength of Direct Alloreactivity

Three different, but not mutually exclusive hypotheses have been proposed to explain the high frequency of alloreactive T cells: (a) a genetic bias favoring T-cell receptor genes that are specific for MHC antigens, (b) a greater density of individual allogeneic MHC determinants on the surface of allogeneic APC, and (c) a greater frequency of different allogeneic MHC/peptide determinants on the donor APC.

Jerne was the first to propose that the genes that encode T-cell receptors might be maintained according to their ability to confer reactivity with the MHC antigens of the species (17). If so, then after the thymus deleted self-reactive T cells, the mature T-cell repertoire would include a high frequency of cells reactive with all other MHC antigens. Jerne's hypothesis was proposed before immunologists had learned about associative recognition and positive thymic selection, but his theory became even more attractive in light of these considerations. Since the thymus only selects T cells with some degree of MHC reactivity, a T-cell receptor gene pool that encodes a broad range of specificities (as is the case for B cells) would produce many useless precursors. A narrower pool of T-cell receptor genes, however, as suggested by Jerne's hypothesis, would allow for more efficient thymic selection. There is some evidence to support Jerne's hypothesis (18), although the selection of mature T cells within the thymus appears nonetheless to be extremely inefficient (19).

The second explanation for strong alloreactivity, sometimes called the "determinant density" hypothesis, considers the difference in the expression of nominal antigens, presented as peptides by self-MHC molecules on self-APC, and the expression of allogeneic MHC molecules on allogeneic APC (20). As illustrated in Fig. 7A, the density of nominal antigen determinants expressed by a self-APC would be quite low (since most MHC antigens present other peptides), whereas the density of an allogeneic MHC determinant on allogeneic APC would be very high (since every MHC antigen would represent a foreign determinant). According to this hypothesis there might not really be a higher precursor frequency of alloreactive T cells, but they would appear to exist in larger numbers since the more powerful stimulus of an allogeneic APC would activate many T cells with relatively low affinities.

The third explanation for alloreactivity, sometimes referred to as the "determinant frequency" hypothesis, was developed on the basis of the idea that T cells specific for allogeneic MHC antigens might be influenced by the peptides presented by these MHC molecules (21). If the MHC molecules on self-APC often present peptides of self-proteins (say, $X_{1,2...n}$), then allogeneic MHC antigens would also present peptides of allogeneic "self" proteins (e.g., "Allo + X_1, Allo + X_2, ... Allo + X_n") (Fig. 7B). In some cases, the self-peptides presented by self- or allogeneic MHC molecules might be identical, but these complexes would stimulate different TCR, since crystal structure data indicate that both peptide and MHC alpha helix residues contribute to the surface that is recognized by TCR (22–25). In addition, the peptides of self-proteins presented by allogeneic MHC might also differ from those presented on a self-APC. In either case, however, the set of determinants represented by "Self + $X_{1...n}$" would differ from that represented by "Allo + $X_{1...n}$." T cells responsive to self-peptides on self-APC (Self + X_1, Self + X_2, ..., etc.) are eliminated by the induction of self-tolerance, leaving only the rare self-MHC molecule, presenting a peptide of a nominal antigen, to stimulate an immune response. On the other hand, self-tolerance would not affect the response to the many self-peptides on allogeneic APC (Allo + X_1, Allo + X_2, ... etc.). Thus, the determinant frequency hypothesis suggests that alloreactive T cells really are more frequent, because each allogeneic MHC antigen generates a large number of different foreign determinants.

Choosing between the determinant density and frequency hypotheses depends on the degree to which alloreactive T cells are influenced by the peptides presented by allo-MHC molecules. There is some evidence that alloreactive T cells can recognize determinants that are not influenced by peptide presentation, and the CDR3 region of one crystallized alloreactive TCR was shown to only make contact with MHC, and not peptide residues (26). However, other evidence suggests that T cells generally see "Allo + X" (27). It has recently been shown that the degree of peptide dependency of alloreactive T cells varies inversely with the degree of disparity in the MHC between responder and stimulator cells (28). However, rejection of cardiac allografts from $DM^{-/-}$ mice, which lack the capacity to replace invariant chain–derived CLIP peptide with a more diverse array of peptides, is delayed to a similar extent as that of class II–deficient allografts (29). This result provides strong *in vivo* evidence for the importance of peptides in direct allorecognition. On the other hand, a new type of quantitative T-cell repertoire analysis that integrates the frequency of TCR mRNA specific for a particular $V\beta$ with the CDR3 length polymorphisms within that $V\beta$ family has revealed selective $V\beta$ expansions without CDR3 length

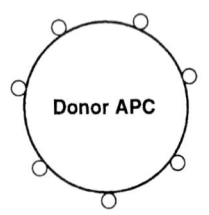

Donor APC with donor MHC antigens (O) all of which are foreign.

A

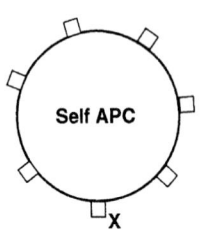

Self APC with self MHC molecules (□). The rare self MHC molecule presents a peptide (X) of an environmental pathogen.

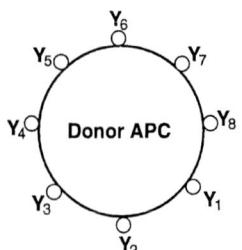

Donor MHC antigens (O). Each presents different "self peptides" generating different foreign determinants.

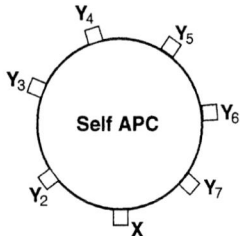

Self MHC molecules (□) also present self peptides ($Y_{1...N}$), but these are all self determinants.

B

FIG. 7. A: Determinant density hypothesis. **B:** Determinant frequency hypothesis.

skewing in MLR assays (30). This analysis agrees with crystallographic studies indicating that most of the binding energy of alloreactive TCR is dependent on TCR interactions with MHC α helices (31). Overall, the available information supports the inherent MHC-binding capacity of TCR, as well as the determinant frequency and the determinant-density hypothesis as explanations for the high frequency of T cells recognizing alloantigens through the direct pathway.

The finding that alloreactivity is so strong often generates confusion in light of the discussion of T-lymphocyte development in Chapter 9. There it was pointed out that the process of positive selection in the thymus generates a T-cell repertoire that is strongly biased toward recognition of peptides presented by self-MHC molecules rather than peptides presented by allogeneic MHC molecules. This would seem to suggest that the response to allogeneic MHC antigens ought to be weak, not strong. This confusion occurs, however, only if one forgets that the experiments demonstrating the principles of positive selection could only be performed after T-cell alloreactivity to a particular set of foreign MHC antigens was first eliminated. Under these circumstances, an individual "A" who was tolerant to self and tolerant to "B," whose T-cell repertoire developed in an "A" thymus, would develop T cells capable of recognizing "A + X" much more efficiently than "B + X." However, under ordinary circumstances, an individual "A" who was tolerant only to self, whose T-cell repertoire developed in an "A" thymus, would develop T cells capable of recognizing "A +X" and "B + X," but would also be capable of recognizing "B without X," even in the absence of *in vivo* priming. Thus, the recognition of "B + X" would be uninterpretable in these experiments. The phenomenon of thymocyte selection, therefore, represents the enrichment of T-cell receptors capable of seeing modified MHC antigens after those receptors with strong affinity for the same MHC antigens plus self-peptides have been removed. Alloreactivity can occur despite the influence of positive selection because negative selection never occurs for the vast majority of T cells recognizing allogeneic MHC antigens.

Minor Histocompatibility Antigens

The experimental process that initially defined the "major" histocompatibility complex similarly defined the "minor" loci by the slower rejection caused by their antigens. As understanding of MHC antigens increased, however, it became apparent that the separation between "major" and "minor" antigens could not depend on the speed of graft rejection alone. Class I or II MHC antigens alone, for example, do not necessarily cause rapid skin graft destruction in mice, whereas the combination of several "minor" histocompatibility discrepancies may bring about rejection as rapidly as a whole MHC difference. Thus, the identification of a major histocompatibility antigen depends in part on the location of the genes encoding the molecule and in part on the well-characterized structure of both class I and class II anti-

gens (see Chapter 19). For example, Qa and T1a antigens are generally considered class I–like products because of their structure, even though they are weak transplantation antigens in terms of rejection. Thus, minor histocompatibility antigens are those capable of causing cell-mediated graft rejection, but which lack the structural characteristics of MHC products. This definition of minor histocompatibility antigens does not include all non-MHC alloantigens, but rather focuses on those capable of eliciting a T-cell immune response. Other glycoproteins such as blood group antigens that can cause rejection through B-cell responses are considered elsewhere in this chapter.

For a long time investigators tended to assume that the minor histocompatibility antigens were other allelic cell-surface proteins, similar in nature if not in strength to the MHC antigens. We now recognize that this is not the case. The minor histocompatibility antigens, defined on the basis of cell-mediated rejection, are peptides of donor proteins that are presented by MHC molecules (32). Thus, the minor histocompatibility antigens are analogous to nominal foreign antigens, the peptide fragments of which are presented by MHC molecules to evoke a T-cell response. Of course, individuals are tolerant to the peptides derived from their own proteins, and can only respond to the peptides of another individual's proteins that have allelic variation, that is, polymorphism.

It has been estimated that there may be as many as 720 minor histocompatibility loci in mice (33), and at least 50 have been mapped to autosomes in the murine genome. Minor histocompatibility antigens can be expressed ubiquitously or in a tissue-selective or tissue-specific manner (see section below on tissue-specific antigens). During the past several years, some of the peptides representing minor histocompatibility antigens have been isolated in mice and humans, and, in many of these instances, the proteins from which they are derived have been identified (34–36). As expected, these proteins are not necessarily surface glycoproteins, and most are intracellular proteins such as nuclear transcription factors and myosin. One cell-surface glycoprotein that has polymorphic residues that function as minor histocompatibility antigens is CD31, and these polymorphisms may be of significance for GVHD risk in bone marrow transplant (BMT) recipients (37). Presumably any cellular protein with allelic variation could function as a minor histocompatibility antigen as long as it contains a peptide expressing that allelic variation that is capable of being presented by an MHC antigen in an immunogenic form. In mice, antigens derived from enzymes encoded by mitochondrial DNA are presented by nonclassical class I molecules and may function as maternally inherited minor histocompatibility antigens (38).

There are several ways in which minor histocompatibility alleles can be produced. Most minor antigens have been found to be diallelic peptides. Allelic variation in a particular peptide locus may result in allelic forms of the same peptide being presented by an MHC molecule. An example is the murine minor histocompatibility locus H13, in which recognition between congenic strains is bidirectional (39). Alternatively, allelic variation in the capacity of a peptide to bind to an MHC molecule can result in a situation in which one allele is presented and the other is not. An example is the human HA-1 minor antigen, in which only one of the two alleles resulting from a single amino acid polymorphism binds effectively to HLA-A2 and leads to an immune response (40). Another means by which minor antigenic determinants can be produced is the failure of one allele to be processed, as has been observed for allelic polymorphisms that make up the HLA-A2–restricted minor determinant HA-8. Although both alleles, when provided as peptides, can be recognized by HA-8–specific CTL, only one allele is naturally produced, apparently because the other allele is transported poorly by the TAP complex (41).

The notion that the minor antigens are peptides recognized in association with MHC molecules has explained many of the features of these antigens that were known, but poorly understood, for a long time (42). First, it is very difficult, if not impossible, to detect humoral responses to minor antigens. This is probably because minor histocompatibility antigens are presented as peptide/MHC complexes that may be too low in abundance on the cell surface to either stimulate an antibody response or be detectable on the cell surface with antibodies that may be induced. Second, minor antigens do not stimulate a primary *in vitro* cell-mediated response, whereas MHC antigens evoke a powerful primary response in both MLR and cell-mediated lympholysis (CML) assays. This is in keeping with the general difficulty in detecting *in vitro* T-cell responses to peptides of nominal antigens unless *in vivo* priming has occurred. Third, the recognition of minor antigens is MHC restricted, that is, secondary responses require that the minor antigens be presented in association with the same MHC molecules as during the primary exposure. This would be expected for any antigen that evokes a T-cell response by the presentation of its peptides in the cleft of an MHC molecule. Fourth, when multiple minor antigen discrepancies exist, the immune response to one of these antigens often predominates in a phenomenon known as "immunodominance." This is not due to weak recipient responsiveness to some of the minor antigens, since slight changes in the donor–recipient combination sometimes produce strong responses to antigens that evoked weak or no responses before. This phenomenon may be due to competition between peptides of different minor antigens for presentation by MHC molecules (33). Unfortunately, immunodominance of CTL responses measured *in vitro* does not necessarily reflect the immunodominance of the same antigens *in vivo*, as has been revealed by studies of GVHD in mice (33,43). This discrepancy may reflect the importance of helper T-cell responses to minor antigens in inducing GVHD (35).

While this discussion of minor histocompatibility antigens has emphasized general conclusions, it is based on studies of the responses to individual minor antigens. Several studies have been reported using a variety of CR mouse strains that were generated on the basis of weak rejection in order to isolate minor histocompatibility loci (e.g., H-1, H-3, H-41, or H-42). In addition, some of the most thoroughly studied minor antigens have been the H-Y antigens, encoded on the Y chromosome, that are therefore expressed only by males of a given species (44). Several different genes encoded on the Y chromosome have been identified as H-Y antigens in mice and humans (33,34,45). There is no reproducible antibody response to these antigens, primary *in vitro* cellular responses cannot be obtained, and secondary *in vitro* cell-mediated responses are MHC restricted. In addition, analysis of the anti–H-Y response has revealed that: (a) some strains are capable of generating this response while others are not; (b) the immune response genes determining responsiveness are encoded both within and outside the MHC; and (c) the rejection of grafts on the basis of the H-Y antigen alone requires that the antigen generate both helper determinants, recognized by CD4$^+$ cells in association with class II MHC antigens, and cytotoxic determinants, recognized by CD8$^+$ cells in association with class I antigens. This last feature suggests that to be identified as a minor histocompatibility antigen, a protein or perhaps a combination of proteins probably has to generate at least two different peptide fragments that show allelic variation (46). An exception to this rule is the capacity of transgenic CD4 T cells in female mice with a CD4 cell–derived TCR transgene specific for H-Y (bred to the Rag1$^{-/-}$ background so that there were no endogenously rearranged TCR and no CD8 T cells) to reject H-Y disparate skin grafts. This study demonstrated that either a Th1 or a Th2 response of sufficient magnitude is capable of such rejection in the absence of CTL (47).

The identification of minor histocompatibility antigens in humans has been achieved mainly in the setting of bone marrow transplantation, the vast majority of which has been performed in HLA-identical sibling pairs, thus permitting the analysis of responses to minor antigens. It is in the setting of GVHD and marrow graft rejection that CTL clones specific for certain minor antigens have been generated and used in the ultimate identification of these antigens (35,41,48). Immunodominance of CTL responses to particular H-Y and HA determinants has been detected in the setting of GVHD and marrow graft rejection, and certain HA incompatibilities (e.g., HA-1) in the GVH direction have been reported to be particularly associated with GVHD (49). Recently, tetrameric complexes of HLA molecules and autosomal (HA) and H-Y–derived minor antigenic peptides have been used to demonstrate the expansion of minor antigen-specific CTL in the setting of GVHD and graft rejection (50,51).

Most of the minor histocompatibility antigens that have been identified to date are determinants recognized by CTL. This largely reflects the relative ease with which CTL assays can be used to measure peptide-specific responses. Recently, a technique involving the use of DC to re-present peptides derived from COS cells transfected with genes encoding candidate Th minor histocompatibility determinants has allowed the molecular identification of two H-Y peptide epitopes recognized by CD4$^+$ Th (52).

Other Antigens of Potential Importance in Transplantation

The minor histocompatibility antigens, defined by their ability to evoke cell-mediated rejection, do not account for all of the non-MHC antigens that can elicit transplant rejection. Several other groups of antigens should also be considered.

Superantigens

Superantigens share the feature with MHC antigens that they can stimulate primary *in vitro* T-cell proliferative responses and activate an unusually high proportion of the T-cell repertoire. However, these antigens are not presented as peptides in the binding groove of MHC molecules, but instead bind to distinct regions of class II MHC molecules, and engage nonvariable portions of Vβ components of the T-cell receptor, rather than the hypervariable regions that recognize peptides. Furthermore, it does not appear that endogenous superantigens can serve as classical transplantation antigens, perhaps because they are not expressed by endothelial cells or parenchymal cells of most tissues (53). However, they have been implicated as antigens that contribute to GVH alloresponses and GVHD in mice (54).

Tissue-Specific Antigens

There is evidence that some peptides presented by MHC molecules may be derived from proteins with limited tissue distribution (55). For example, T-cell clones specific for allogeneic cells of one type do not always recognize cells of a different type from the same individual. The only well-described tissue-specific antigen that causes graft rejection is that for skin, referred to as the Sk antigen (56). Since it was identified on the basis of T-cell–mediated responses, this antigen most likely represents a peptide derived from a protein expressed only in skin that is presented by an MHC molecule.

The existence of tissue-specific antigens has importance in several ways. First, *in vitro* assays to measure T-cell responsiveness to donor antigens may be misleading when they use donor lymphohematopoietic cells as the stimulating population if the actual T-cell response is specific for donor tissue–specific antigens. Second, the need to develop self-tolerance to tissue-specific antigens emphasizes that the induction of tolerance might not be accomplished entirely in the thymus by a "central" process. Finally, the existence of tissue-specific antigens suggests that transplantation tolerance induced by one set of donor cells might not always induce complete tolerance to donor cells of a different sort. For example, induction of permanent hematopoietic chimerism and long-term tolerance via hematopoietic cell transplantation (HCT) may not necessarily lead to permanent tolerance to donor skin. This may be due to the existence of skin-specific antigens, which donor hematopoietic cells do not express. These tissue-specific proteins do not necessarily need to show allelic variation to be regarded as alloantigens in bone marrow chimeras,

since the determinant formed by "Allo + Xsk" (where Xsk is a peptide derived from the skin-specific protein) would be different from that formed by "Self + Xsk." Hence, T cells can be tolerant to the skin-specific antigen expressed on their own tissues, but responsive to this same antigen of a different individual. The tissue specificity of this antigen occurs because "Allo + Xsk" is expressed only by donor skin and not by other donor tissues.

In the field of HCT, interest has recently focused on the potential to use GVH-alloreactive donor T cells that recognize minor histocompatibility antigens expressed only on hematopoietic cells as a way of achieving graft-versus-leukemia (GVL) effects without GVHD. Several human minor histocompatibility antigens have demonstrated this pattern of expression, making this a promising approach to separating GVL from GVHD. However, GVH disparities for some of these same minor antigens (e.g., HA-1) have been associated with increased incidence of GVHD (49). Perhaps the presence of these immunodominant disparities helps to initiate an alloresponse that, by inducing APC activation and cytokine production, augments responses to additional minor histoincompatibilities that are shared by GVHD target organs.

Endothelial Glycoproteins

Blood Group Antigens

The blood group antigens do not evoke cell-mediated responses and hence are not classified as minor histocompatibility antigens. They are expressed on many types of cells and, importantly, are present on vascular endothelium where they may serve as the targets for an antibody-mediated attack on blood vessels.

Blood group antigens were identified because of their importance in transfusions. They represent the effects of glycosylation enzymes such that A and B individuals each express their respective antigen but O individuals have neither. The natural antibodies that develop against these antigens probably do so as a result of cross-reactions with common carbohydrate determinants of environmental microorganisms as long as the individual does not already express those determinants. Thus, O individuals will develop antibodies to the antigens of A and B donors, while A and B individuals will only develop antibodies reactive with antigens from each other, and AB individuals will develop responses to neither. Therefore, O recipients can only receive transfusions from O donors; A and B recipients can receive transfusions from O donors or from individuals sharing their blood type; and AB recipients can receive blood from donors of any blood type. The same rules apply to the transplantation of most primarily vascularized organs in humans, since the vascular endothelium expresses "ABO" antigens. In addition to the ABO locus, there are other loci-determining blood group antigens on erythrocytes, but these are irrelevant to organ transplantation because they are not expressed on vascular endothelium.

Other Allogeneic Endothelial Glycoproteins

In addition to the well-known blood group antigens, other glycoproteins expressed on the vascular endothelium may serve as targets for humoral responses. Very rarely, preformed antibodies to these antigens may give rise to hyperacute rejection of primarily vascularized organs. In addition, antibody responses to endothelial glycoproteins can be detected following kidney transplantation between MHC identical blood-group–matched individuals (57). However, these induced antibodies may not have any role in graft rejection.

Species-Specific Carbohydrate Determinants

Closely analogous to the blood group antigens are the carbohydrate determinants expressed on vascular endothelium that show species specificity. For example, pigs have a glycosyltransferase enzyme that is not expressed by humans, that glycosylates β-galactosyl N-acetyl glucosamine to form a Galα1-3Galβ1-4GlcNAc (αGal) determinant. In humans, a fucosyltransferase generates instead the H substance from the same substrate, leading to blood group O. Preformed or "natural" antibodies are present in human serum, which react to the novel pig determinant. Similarly, natural antibodies are present between all but the most closely related species combinations. Like the blood group antibodies, these natural antibodies probably arise from cross-reactions with environmental microorganisms (58), and they also cause hyperacute rejection of most primarily vascularized xenogeneic transplants. They may also be recognized by other components of the innate immune system, such as macrophages and NK cells.

The "Hh" Locus

In apparent violation of the laws of transplantation described above, a phenomenon has been described in mice whereby (AxB) F1 offspring are capable of rejecting bone marrow from parental donors. This phenomenon, as well as the phenomenon of rapid rejection of fully allogeneic marrow, was shown in studies by Kiessling et al. (59) to be mediated by natural killer (NK) cells. However, the identity of what appeared to be recessively inherited transplantation antigens responsible for this rejection could not be determined. Recently, it has become clear that the specificity of NK cell–mediated marrow rejection is due to the expression by NK cells of receptors such as Ly-49 molecules that recognize specific class I MHC ligands on target cells and transmit an inhibitory signal to the NK cell upon such recognition. These receptors are clonally distributed on NK cells, each of which may express one or more different inhibitory receptors. The only requirement for NK cells to be tolerant of "self" is that they express at least one inhibitory receptor for a "self" class I MHC molecule. Thus, as illustrated in Fig. 8, an AxB F1 recipient will have subsets of NK cells with inhibitory receptors that recognize

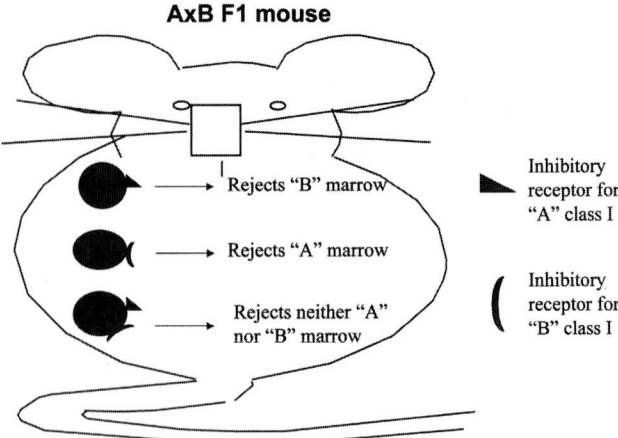

FIG. 8. An explanation for hybrid resistance. Each *solid circle* represents a subset of NK cells.

MHC of either the A parent, the B parent, or both. The absence of "B" class I molecules on, for example, AA parental hematopoietic cells, permits subsets of (AxB)F1 NK cells that have inhibitory receptors only for class I molecules from the B parent to destroy AA cells. Thus, the violation of the laws of transplantation that is observed in the phenomenon of hybrid resistance can be explained on the basis of "missing self" (60). NK cell–mediated resistance to fully allogeneic marrow grafts can also be explained by the absence of "self" class I molecules on allogeneic donors. The nature of NK cell recognition of class I MHC is discussed further below and in detail in Chapter 12.

COMPONENTS OF IMMUNE SYSTEM INVOLVED IN GRAFT REJECTION

Antigen-Presenting Cells

Types of APC

The role of specialized APC in the process of immune activation is discussed elsewhere in this textbook (see Chapter 20). The critical role of APC in graft rejection is best exemplified by the prolonged survival of some types of grafts when APC of the donor have been eliminated (61).

Several types of cells have antigen-presenting capability, including DC, macrophages, and activated B cells (62,63). In addition, several organ-specific cell populations, such as Kuppfer cells in the liver and Langerhans cells in the skin are probably subpopulations of DC. Not all APC are equally effective and those of the dendritic lineage are the most potent on a per cell basis (64). All of the "professional" APC are derived from bone marrow progenitors. In recent years it has become clear that there are multiple subpopulations of DC distinguished by their degree of maturation, their derivation from myeloid versus lymphoid lineages, and whether they express the CD8α chain, CD11c, IL-3 receptor, and a variety of other markers. These subpopulations have different functions and in some cases have been used in efforts to induce tolerance rather than activation of alloreactive T cells (65).

Mature APC express MHC class II antigens constitutively, and the level of class II antigen expression can be further increased by various cytokines, including IFN-γ and TNFα. Some APC may express relatively low levels of MHC class I antigens, which might serve to protect these crucial cells from destruction by the activated immune response before they can provide their full helper function (13).

An important feature of transplantation immunology is that the APC responsible for T-cell activation may potentially originate from either the donor graft or from the recipient. The types of APC in each case are unlikely to be the same, since those from the donor will generally be tissue-specific APC (such as Langerhans cells), while those from the recipient will generally be associated with lymphoid tissues. Furthermore, the MHC antigens expressed by the two different sets of APC will often be different and, thus, the specificities of the T cells stimulated by the two different sets of APC will generally differ. Unless there is matching of MHC antigens between donor and recipient, only the determinants expressed on donor APC will also be expressed by parenchymal cells of the graft.

Direct versus Indirect Antigen Presentation

Because the distinction between the two potential sets of APC is so important in describing and understanding the mechanisms of graft rejection, transplantation immunologists have developed a terminology to describe the two potential processes of T-cell sensitization. The "direct" pathway refers to antigen presentation by APC derived from the donor graft, while the "indirect" pathway refers to donor antigen presentation by recipient APC. Of course, indirect recognition corresponds to the form of presentation used in classical immunology and, thus, the terminology has the weakness that the term "indirect" seems to suggest that this is not the physiologic process for stimulating an immune response. Actually, direct recognition is the nonphysiologic pathway.

The use of the terms "direct" and "indirect" presentation is sometimes confusing for several reasons. The first problem is that not all investigators define the terms in the same way. The definition used in this chapter is based on which set of APC (donor vs. recipient) is involved in T-cell activation, not on whether peptide presentation is involved. This is because, while indirect presentation clearly involves peptide presentation (donor peptides by recipient APC), direct presentation may also do so. For example, if peptides of donor MHC class I molecules are presented by donor class II antigens (or by other donor class I antigens), this would still represent direct presentation, even though it involves antigen processing and peptide presentation. Thus, we have defined indirect responses as those occurring when T cells are stimulated by recipient APC and direct responses as those occurring when

they are stimulated by donor APC. A second source of confusion regarding direct and indirect presentation occurs when the donor and recipient share some MHC antigens. Under these circumstances, the determinants formed by direct and indirect presentation may be identical. For example, in the case of class II–matched allografts, the determinant formed by presentation of a donor class I peptide by class II molecules would be the same on both the donor and recipient APC. Nonetheless, the responses evoked by the two different sets of APC may not be the same, making it useful to use the terms "direct" and "indirect" to distinguish between the two separate pathways. A third source of confusion regarding the indirect pathway is that there are other terms that refer to the same process. For example, "cross-priming" is a term that was introduced into the literature well before discussion of indirect responses became popular. It was used to describe the observation that CD8$^+$ T cells can become sensitized to donor peptides presented by recipient class I molecules during allograft rejection (66). The term "cross-priming" is still used in the literature, always in reference to CD8$^+$ responses. Thus, it should be thought of as referring to one subset of responses involving an indirect pathway of antigen presentation. A fourth element of confusion is that the term "indirect" can be used in reference to two different stages during graft rejection: the sensitization of donor-specific T cells and the T-cell effector function that leads to graft destruction. Evidence that graft rejection could occur with the help of T cells sensitized through the indirect pathway was obtained some years ago. Only much more recently has evidence also been obtained to suggest that, under some circumstances, graft destruction can occur on the basis of effector T cells with indirect specificity (67). Finally, the use of the term "indirect" presentation in transplantation immunology is confusing because it suggests that this type of response is unusual or abnormal. Actually, the indirect pathway involves the normal process of generating an immune response: the recognition of foreign peptides presented by self-MHC molecules on self-APC. It is the direct response that is the unusual pathway during graft rejection.

Trafficking of APC after Transplantation

Since APC are the critical element in stimulating immune responses, an important issue in the regulation of transplant rejection and tolerance is which APC are available and where they are located. Studies in mice show that changes in the location of both donor and recipient APC take place almost immediately after transplantation. Donor APC begin to migrate from the graft to the recipient lymphoid compartments, finding their way to both draining lymph nodes and the spleen of the recipient (64). Simultaneously, bone marrow–derived APC from the recipient begin entering the graft and gradually replace the donor APC. The time required for this change probably varies for different organs. In the case of murine skin grafts, the replacement of donor by recipient APC seems to require many months, whereas the shift may occur over weeks in the case of pig kidney and human liver grafts.

Anatomic Sites of Sensitization

Although activation of T cells generally involves contact with APC and allogeneic APC are especially powerful stimulators, it does not necessarily follow that cell sensitization occurs within the donor graft. Since donor APC migrate to recipient lymphoid compartments, sensitization may occur primarily in these locations. Experiments by Barker (68), among others, have suggested that draining lymph nodes are the primary site of sensitization for skin graft rejection. They showed that skin grafts on vascular pedicles that had been deprived of lymphatic drainage failed to undergo rejection and failed to prime the recipient against donor antigens. These grafts, however, were susceptible to rejection if the recipient was sensitized by normal skin grafts placed concurrently. Recently, similar experiments using mice that lack secondary lymphoid organs as a result of a genetic defect have shown similar results (69).

The notion that allogeneic sensitization occurs primarily in draining lymph nodes is in keeping with the principles of fundamental immunology. Naïve T cells generally traffic in the lymphoid circulation, waiting for foreign antigens to be concentrated there. Only T cells that have been previously activated are allowed to migrate into the nonlymphoid tissues, seeking the source of the antigen challenge (70). On the other hand, some memory T cells that were previously activated by "Self + X" determinants may cross-react with allogeneic determinants of a new graft. Thus, it is not surprising that there is also evidence suggesting that activation, or perhaps reactivation, of alloreactive T cells can occur within grafts, especially when they are primarily vascularized and express donor endothelial cells (71).

B Cells and Antibodies

Preformed Antibodies

Antidonor antibodies that are present before transplantation are extremely important in causing rejection of many types of primarily vascularized organ transplants. If they are present in sufficient quantity, and recognize determinants expressed on vascular endothelium, preformed antibodies can cause hyperacute rejection. The preformed antibodies that do this are of two general types: natural antibodies and antibodies generated by previous exposure to transplantation antigens.

Natural Antibodies

Natural antibodies include those directed at blood group antigens and species-specific carbohydrate determinants. Their existence does not require previous exposure to transplanted tissues, since they are probably generated in response to carbohydrate determinants on microorganisms. They tend to be of the IgM class, although IgG isotypes may also occur. Their presence is generally thought to be T-cell independent and

their receptors are often in, or near, germline configuration. Studies in mice have shown that IgM natural antibodies are produced primarily by a CD5-negative and Mac1-negative, but otherwise B1b-like B-cell population in the spleen (72). Although large numbers of Mac1-positive B1 cells are present in the peritoneal cavity of mice, the peritoneal cavity B cells do not produce antibody unless stimulated with LPS for several days *in vitro*, at which point they lose Mac1 expression (72).

Preformed Antibodies from Prior Sensitization

Recipients may also express antidonor antibodies if they have been previously exposed to cells expressing the donor antigens. This can occur by prior blood transfusion, as a result of pregnancy, or from previous organ transplantation. The antibodies formed in this way are usually IgG in isotype, are directed at protein rather than carbohydrate determinants (usually against MHC antigens), and have much higher binding affinities than the natural antibodies. Probably because of the density of MHC antigen expression and high affinity of the antibodies, lower titers of these antibodies cause organ damage more consistently than even higher titers of natural antibodies.

Induced Antibodies

After transplantation, new antibodies may be formed to the novel determinants expressed on donor tissue. Often this antibody response is directed at MHC antigens, although antibody responses to other molecules with allelic variation may also occur, especially if the recipient is repeatedly immunized. Induced antibody responses start with IgM antibody formation and then convert to IgG production in a T-cell–dependent fashion.

In most cases induced antibodies are not responsible for acute graft rejection, either because they appear too late, after T-cell responses have already caused rejection, or because they appear so slowly, in the face of immunosuppression, that they fail to cause acute graft destruction. However, there are exceptions to this rule that are best demonstrated by primarily vascularized xenotransplants between closely related species (73–75). In these cases, the induced antibody response occurs especially rapidly and causes an accelerated form of rejection targeted at the vascular endothelium. A similar form of rejection occurs only rarely in allogeneic combinations, when antidonor antibodies appear unusually early, probably reflecting prior sensitization. Induced antibodies after transplantation may play a role in chronic graft rejection. This process also involves injury primarily to the donor vessels, but occurs over a much longer period of time.

T Cells

Most allograft rejection involves T-cell–mediated responses. The particular importance of T cells has been confirmed experimentally by the demonstration that athymic mice accept tissue grafts indefinitely from other members of the same species, and often from members of other species as well. Furthermore, repopulation of these mice with purified T cells reconstitutes their ability to reject grafts. In human beings, the use of reagents that specifically block T-cell responses, and the correlation of their effectiveness with their ability to eliminate T cells, supports the central role of T cells in graft rejection.

Because there is no phenotypic marker that correlates precisely with the function of particular T-cell subsets, it has been difficult to determine the exact role of the various subsets that participate in graft rejection. Nonetheless, a distinction between helper and effector functions can be made, and is important in understanding the process. In the case of T-dependent B-cell responses, the role of T cells as helper cells for B cells that produce alloantibodies has been demonstrated well (76). There have also been *in vivo* experiments that indicate a distinction between helper and effector T-cell functions for cell-mediated rejection. For example, there are particular cases of skin grafts that are not rejected unless simultaneous grafts that express both the antigenic determinants of the first graft and additional determinants as well, are placed elsewhere on the same recipient. The rejection of both grafts under these circumstances indicates that a T-cell effector mechanism was potentially available for the rejection of the first graft, but that it required an additional T-cell helper function to allow the effector response to occur. These types of experiments have defined the distinction between helper and effector T-cell functions for graft rejection *in vivo,* and they have suggested the terms "helper" and "effector" determinants based on which determinants were expressed on the first or second grafts. Because in these types of experiments, the effector determinants have usually been presented by class I antigens, which are likely to stimulate CD8$^+$ cells, while the helper determinants have usually been presented by class II antigens, which stimulate CD4$^+$ cells, the results of these experiments have supported the idea that CD4$^+$ T cells often provide help for CD8$^+$ cells, at least in those cases where the two functions reside in separate cell populations.

Other Cells

Natural Killer Cells

NK cells are large granular lymphocytes that lack T-cell receptors, and that have the ability to mediate cytolysis against certain tumor targets and hematopoietic cells. NK cells also produce a number of proinflammatory cytokines, including TNFα and IFNγ, as well as the hematopoietic cytokine GM-CSF. Recently, human NK cell subsets grown in IL-12 or IL-4 have, like Th, been shown to produce differing sets of cytokines, resulting in the designation of NK1 (IL-10– and IFN-γ–producing) and NK2 (IL-5– and IL-13–producing) subsets, respectively (77). NK cells can be activated and triggered to kill through a number of different cell-surface receptors, some of which may still be undefined, and they represent a first line of defense against a variety of microorganisms. NK cells of both humans and mice express clonally distributed inhibitory cell-surface receptors that are capable of recognizing specific class I MHC molecules. These class I receptors are type II C lectins (Ly49 family) or dimers of CD94 with NKG2 lectins in the mouse, and are either sIg family members (p58/p70) or dimers of CD94 with NKG2 lectins in humans. Recognition by an inhibitory receptor of a class I ligand results in intracellular transmission of an inhibitory signal via an immune receptor tyrosine–based inhibitory motif (ITIM) that interacts with a tyrosine phosphatase and counteracts activating signals transmitted from other cell-surface molecules. Recognition of "self" class I inhibitory ligands is believed to be important in preventing the NK cell from killing normal autologous cells (60). Molecules belonging to the same families as the above inhibitory receptors, but lacking an intracellular ITIM motif, are capable of associating with molecules that contain tyrosine-based activating motifs (DAP-10 and DAP-12) that activate cytolytic activity by NK cells (see Chapter 12).

Although the role of NK cells in mediating hybrid resistance and allogeneic marrow rejection is well established in mice, the amount of resistance mediated by NK cells to allogeneic pluripotent hematopoietic stem cells (PHSC) is limited, and can be readily overcome by increasing the dose of donor stem cells administered (78). Furthermore, despite the fact that human NK cells, like those of mice, have class I–dependent recognition mechanisms that inhibit lysis of targets expressing those class I molecules, a role for NK cells in resisting human allogeneic marrow engraftment has not been clearly demonstrated in heavily conditioned recipients. Antidonor NK reactivity was not demonstrable during the time of rejection in a patient receiving marrow from a donor whose HLA class I alleles would be incapable of triggering recipient KIRs recognizing class I alleles (79). While a role for NK cells in mediating marrow allograft rejection has not been demonstrated in heavily conditioned hosts, their role may become more significant if mismatched transplants are attempted with less toxic, nonmyeloablative regimens. Consistent with this possibility, patients with severe combined (T- and B-cell) immunodeficiency (SCID) who have functional NK cells require cytotoxic conditioning to permit engraftment of haplo-identical marrow. In contrast, those lacking NK cells have a low incidence of rejection in the absence of any such treatment (80).

Inhibitory receptors on NK cells are quite broad in their class I specificity (81), and recognition of even fully allogeneic class I molecules can confer some protection from NK-mediated marrow destruction compared to that observed for cells deficient in class I expression (82). Because of the increased disparity of xenogeneic compared to allogeneic MHC molecules, a greater role might be expected for NK cells in rejecting xenografts than allografts. Indeed, NK cells play a greater role in resisting xenogeneic marrow than allogeneic marrow engraftment (83,84).

A role for NK cells in the rejection of solid organ allografts is even less well defined than it is for marrow allografts. NK cells are prominent in infiltrates found in rejecting allogeneic organs and sponge allografts. However, evidence suggests that NK cells do not make an important contribution to solid organ allograft rejection under normal circumstances (85). If they do, NK cells must be dependent on T cells, since mice lacking T cells are unable to reject nonhematopoietic allografts. Furthermore, whereas bone marrow allografts from class I–deficient donors (β2m$^{-/-}$) are subject to potent NK-mediated rejection (because these cells cannot trigger inhibitory receptors on host NK cells [86]), β2m$^{-/-}$ skin grafts are not rejected by β2m$^+$ recipients (87). These results are consistent with the likelihood that NK cells do not reject solid tissue allografts. However, cells expressing NK cell markers (either NK cells or NK/T cells) have recently been reported to play a critical role in cardiac allograft rejection in CD28 knockout mice (88). NK cells are a prominent cell type infiltrating xenografts undergoing "delayed vascular rejection" (see below) and, for reasons discussed later in the chapter, may play a more significant role in solid organ xenograft rejection than allograft rejection (83).

Consistent with the hypothesis that NK cells are poorly inhibited by xenogeneic compared to allogeneic MHC molecules, NK cells have also been implicated in the accelerated rejection (89) that can destroy solid organ xenografts that have escaped hyperacute rejection (see below). Since one mechanism by which NK cells mediate cytolysis is via antibody-dependent cell-mediated cytotoxicity (ADCC), it is possible that IgG natural antibodies play a significant role in initiating NK cell–mediated rejection. NK cells also release cytokines such as IFN-γ and TNFα, which activate macrophages and endothelial cells and induce inflammation (89). In addition to failing to receive inhibitory signals from xenogeneic MHC molecules, NK cells may also be activated by direct recognition of xenogeneic determinants. For example, it has recently been suggested that lectins on the surface of human NK cells can activate cytolysis when xenogeneic carbohydrate determinants such as αGal are recognized (90).

T Cells That Express NK Cell–Associated Markers

In recent years, a subset of murine T cells that expresses NK cell–associated phenotypic surface markers has been defined. It appears that some of these cells are thymus dependent and others thymus independent. They produce a variety of cytokines, the most prominent of which are IFN-γ and IL-4, and also have cytolytic activity. They are often autoreactive, and can also produce the inhibitory cytokines IL-10 and TGF-β (91). These cells recognize and are positively selected by the nonclassical class I molecule CD1d, and many express an invariant Vα14/Jα281 chain with a restricted subset of β chains (Vβ8.2, Vβ7 or Vβ2). They recognize glycolipid antigens presented by CD1, and may provide an important link between innate and adaptive immunity (92). Most NK/T

cells are either CD4$^+$CD8$^-$, or CD4$^-$CD8$^-$. Humans have a parallel subset of cells that use a similar invariant α chain with restricted Vβ gene usage in their TCR (93). Studies in mice have associated a defect in this cell subset with diabetes in NOD mice (94), and studies in humans have linked abnormally high Th1 cytokines produced by NK/T cells with type 1 diabetes (95). Studies in mice have also shown that this subset of cells can inhibit GVHD via an IL-4–dependent mechanism (96). NK/T cells have also been reported to be required for tolerance induction to cardiac allografts with co-stimulatory blockade or blockade of LFA-1/ICAM interactions (97), and to be responsible for immune deviation induced by antigens placed in the anterior chamber of the eye (98). Despite these apparent inhibitory effects on immune responses, NK/T cells have also been suggested to play an important augmenting role in the elimination of tumors (99). In one study, this T-cell subset was also implicated in the phenomenon of hybrid resistance in mice, but this conclusion has been challenged by results of more recent studies.

Monocytes/Macrophages

A role in graft rejection for other "nonspecific" cellular effectors such as monocytes has been suggested (89), especially in xenograft rejection. It is likely that proinflammatory cytokines produced by activated monocytes and macrophages, such as IL-1 and TNFα, play a role in endothelial cell activation. Chemoattractants produced by the inflammatory process may partially explain monocyte recruitment.

MECHANISMS OF GRAFT REJECTION

There are at least four distinct mechanisms that can cause graft rejection that have been identified at this time and it is likely that additional mechanisms will be characterized in the future. It is convenient to describe these mechanisms according to the time frame in which they tend to occur in clinical practice, especially as their names (hyperacute rejection, accelerated rejection, acute rejection, and chronic rejection) have a clear temporal distinction. However, it is increasingly possible to characterize these mechanisms according to the cell types and processes involved and, in some cases, they may occur at uncharacteristic times.

Rejection Caused by Preformed Antibodies (Hyperacute Rejection)

Hyperacute rejection is said to occur when a vascularized organ suffers from rejection within minutes to hours after transplantation. The phenomenon is visible and dramatic. Transplanted kidneys that have initially perfused well turn blue and mottled shortly after vascularization is established. Urine output ceases and recovery does not occur. Microscopically, organs show evidence of extensive vascular thrombosis and hemorrhage with little evidence of a mononuclear cell infiltrate.

There are several important components involved in the mechanism of hyperacute rejection. First, there are donor endothelial MHC antigens or carbohydrate determinants as described above. Second, there are preformed antibodies that can bind these antigens. Third, the complement and coagulation cascades are activated by the binding of preformed antibodies to the donor antigens. Finally, there are complement regulatory proteins that can modify complement activation, and anticoagulants that can modify the coagulation pathway. The target of the hyperacute rejection process is the donor vascular endothelium.

The interaction of these components leading to hyperacute rejection is diagrammed in Fig. 9. The crucial event in the process is the formation of the membrane attack complex (MAC) made up of C5-9 of the complement cascade. In allogeneic combinations, this is always initiated by antibody/antigen binding, which activates complement through the classical pathway. In some xenogeneic combinations, complement activation can also occur through the alternative pathway, and thus does not require antibody binding. Complement activation is controlled by several regulatory molecules, including complement receptor 1, decay accelerating factor (DAF, CD55), membrane cofactor protein (MCP, CD46), and CD59, which act at different stages along the cascade (see Chapter 34). Many of these molecules are produced by the vascular endothelial cells. Since these regulatory proteins prevent unwanted complement activation in the face of low levels of perturbation to the system, the initial stimulus for activation must be strong enough to overcome these down-regulating molecules. Thus, the titer and avidity of the preformed antibodies must be relatively high. Preformed antibodies directed at MHC antigens almost always accomplish this activation, whereas the lower-affinity blood group antibodies lead to hyperacute rejection in only about 25% of cases. One of the reasons that hyperacute rejection is such an important feature in xenogeneic transplantation is that the complement regulatory proteins produced by the donor vascular endothelium of one species do not always function effectively with complement molecules derived from a different species.

Because of this homologous restriction, lower levels of an initial triggering signal lead to explosive complement activation.

Although the membrane attack complex is often thought of as a lytic molecule, its effect on the donor vascular endothelium, even before cell lysis, is to cause endothelial activation. This occurs rapidly, before there is time for new gene transcription or protein synthesis, and has been referred to as type I endothelial activation. The two principal manifestations of this activation are cell retraction, leading to gaps between endothelial cells, and the loss of antithrombotic molecules from the endothelium (100). Thus, type I endothelial activation is responsible for the two principal pathologic findings in hyperacute rejection: extravascular hemorrhage and edema, and intravascular thrombosis.

There are no known treatments that can stop the process of hyperacute rejection once it has started and, thus, it is essential to avoid the circumstances that initiate it. Experimentally, this can be accomplished for relatively short periods of time by administration of cobra venom factor, which depletes complement. In clinical practice, this is accomplished by avoiding transplantation in the face of preformed antibodies, both by avoiding blood-group antigen disparities and by testing recipients before transplantation to determine whether they have preformed anti-MHC antibodies that react with the donor's MHC antigens. This test is referred to as a "crossmatch," and is usually performed by adding recipient serum to a suspension of donor lymphocytes and measuring cell lysis in the presence of an exogenous source of complement. In a small number of cases, allogeneic transplantation in the face of preformed antibodies has been attempted after first removing antidonor antibodies by plasmapheresis. This has been successful in some cases involving blood group disparities, but rarely in cases involving preformed anti-MHC antibodies. Discordant xenogeneic transplantation always involves preformed antibodies, and thus cannot be accomplished without initial efforts to modify the process of hyperacute rejection.

Not all organs and tissues are equally susceptible to hyperacute rejection. Most primarily vascularized organs, such

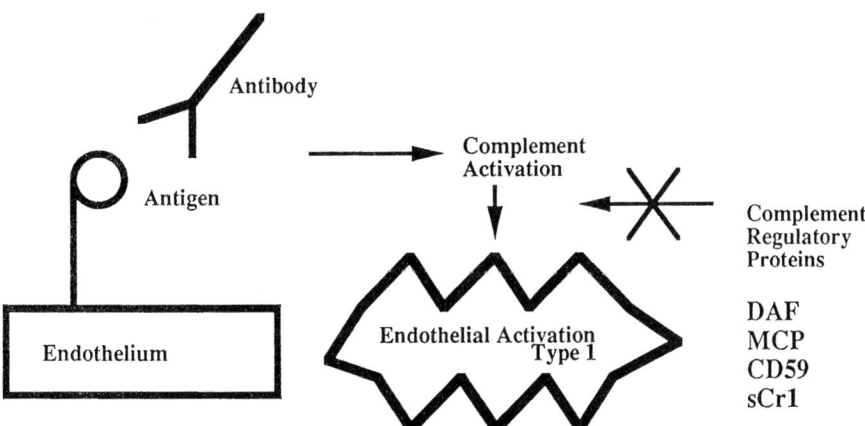

FIG. 9. Schematic representation of hyperacute rejection.

as kidneys and hearts, are very susceptible, but the liver can often survive without hyperacute rejection despite preexisting antidonor antibodies (101). It is not clear whether this unusual feature of the liver reflects the large surface area of its vascular endothelium or an intrinsic property of liver endothelial cells. It is possible that because of its anatomic position in the portal circulation, the liver has more powerful mechanisms to prevent endothelial activation resulting from antigen/antibody complexes. Nonetheless, hyperacute rejection of the liver has occurred in some cases, especially involving xenogeneic transplantation, indicating that its resistance to hyperacute rejection is not absolute. The other types of transplants that are resistant to hyperacute rejection are those that do not immediately expose donor vascular endothelium to the recipient's circulation. For example, skin grafts do not suffer hyperacute rejection because their blood vessels are not in communication with those of the recipient until about a week after transplantation. After this, large doses of exogenously administered antidonor antibodies can destroy skin grafts through a complement-dependent mechanism (102). Nonetheless, long-term survival of xenogeneic skin grafts has been achieved despite the presence of natural antibodies, suggesting that the threshold for initiating this late antibody-mediated rejection is hard to achieve. Fresh pancreatic islets appear to behave like skin grafts, but cultured pancreatic islets (which lose their endothelial components in culture) are probably never susceptible to hyperacute rejection. Free cellular transplants, such as bone marrow cells or hepatocytes, do not have an endothelium and thus are not susceptible to the mechanisms of hyperacute rejection. However, in many cases these cell transplants do express some of the antigens recognized by preformed antibodies, and there is evidence indicating that the presence of these antibodies can lead to resistance to engraftment (103). While in the case of HCT, this resistance can be overcome by transplanting larger numbers of cells (103–105), this finding suggests that preformed antibodies can cause cellular graft rejection by mechanisms that are distinct from hyperacute rejection. Additionally, antibody-independent complement activation has been shown to be a significant factor diminishing the engraftment of porcine bone marrow in mice (106).

Although hyperacute rejection is a dramatic and powerful mechanism of graft rejection, it is rarely encountered in clinical practice. The understanding of its causes, and the use of standard immunologic assays to detect preformed antidonor antibodies, has largely eliminated its occurrence. This is one of the best examples where an understanding of immunology has had an important impact on clinical transplantation.

Early Rejection Caused by Induced Antibodies (Accelerated Rejection)

A second mechanism of rejection, usually caused by antibodies, is almost as infrequent as hyperacute rejection. It occurs as a result of antibodies that are induced very rapidly after a transplant is performed. This type of rejection has sometimes been called "accelerated" rejection because it typically occurs within the first 5 days, but there is no consensus regarding this name. The process is characterized by fibrinoid necrosis of donor arterioles with intravascular thrombosis (107).

Accelerated rejection is rare in allogeneic combinations because it requires that an antibody response occur before the T-cell response that is typically responsible for early rejection episodes. Indeed, in allogeneic combinations, accelerated rejection is sufficiently rare that some investigators have questioned its existence. Others, who have studied this mechanism of rejection in xenogeneic combinations, have given it several different names, such as "acute vascular rejection" or "delayed xenograft rejection," thereby generating confusion about what may be a single process involving endothelial activation occurring later than the type I activation described above. In some xenogeneic cases, accelerated rejection may occur even without an antibody response, and may result from endothelial activation by NK cells or other components of the innate immune system.

There are several causes for the difficulty in characterizing accelerated rejection. First, the clinical circumstances are rare in which induced antibodies appear before T-cell–mediated rejection. Second, some patients develop antidonor alloantibodies weeks or months after their transplant, but without suffering an acute rejection episode. Finally, it is very difficult experimentally to induce a B-cell response in the absence of T-cell immunity. Thus, it has been hard to prove that an induced B-cell response, rather than an especially vigorous T-cell response, is responsible for a unique rejection mechanism.

Given these difficulties, the best characterization of accelerated rejection has been achieved using primarily vascularized organ transplants from closely related xenogeneic species. In these cases, the levels of preformed antibodies are not sufficient to cause hyperacute rejection, but antidonor antibodies appear rapidly (within 3 to 4 days) in association with the onset of rejection. Vigorous anti–T-cell immunosuppression has little effect on this early rejection, whereas immunosuppression with reagents that affect B-cell responses, such as cyclophosphamide, delays its onset until more typical T-cell–mediated rejection occurs (73). The two types of immunosuppression together can lead to prolonged graft survival, unless release of the B-cell suppression allows the appearance of antidonor antibodies and the concurrent initiation of rejection (73). The pathology in these cases reveals a paucity of lymphocytes infiltrating the donor graft, antibody binding to donor vascular endothelium, and fibrinoid necrosis of the donor vessels.

These studies of concordant xenograft rejection have indicated that the most important feature in "accelerated" rejection is the early appearance of antidonor antibodies. In fact, these antibodies appear so early, and despite the presence of anti–T-cell immunosuppression, that they probably do not represent a primary response to the donor's antigens in most cases. For xenografts, they may represent a rapid increase in the levels of natural antibodies that were present before transplantation, but at undetectable levels. In the case of allografts, low levels of preformed antibodies also exist occasionally as a result of previous exposure to donor MHC antigens, but with the levels having fallen to a point where they are not detected in the standard crossmatch. Thus, it is probably the unusual rapidity and perhaps the especially high levels of the antibody response that are critical in causing "accelerated" rejection.

As in hyperacute rejection, the process of "accelerated" rejection is usually initiated by antibody binding to antigens on the donor vascular endothelium. In this case, however, the subsequent endothelial changes occur more slowly, allowing time for gene transcription and new protein synthesis. This later form of activation has been called type II endothelial activation (108). Many of its features appear to be mediated by the transcription factor NFκB, which generates many of the responses associated with inflammation, including the secretion of inflammatory cytokines such as IL-1 and IL-8 and the expression of adhesion molecules such as E-selectin and ICAM-1 (109). In addition, type II endothelial activation causes the loss of thrombomodulin and other prothrombotic changes (110). Thus, the events following type II endothelial activation are associated with the pathologic changes that occur with "accelerated" rejection, including the tendency toward intravascular thrombosis and the inflammatory destruction of donor vessels that occurs in the absence of infiltrating lymphocytes.

Just as there are regulatory processes for complement activation, there are regulatory molecules that counter the tendency toward intravascular coagulation and the process of type II endothelial activation. For example, the expression of tissue factor protein inhibitor by vascular endothelium tends to inhibit factor Xa of the clotting cascade. In addition, the tendency toward type II endothelial activation is inhibited by the expression of a number of protective molecules, including Bcl-x_L, Bcl-2, and A20 (108). Although these are often thought of as antiapoptotic molecules, they also tend to inhibit activation mediated by NFκB. Just as the regulatory molecules of complement may not function across species differences, so too some of the regulatory molecules involved in type II endothelial activation may show homologous restriction (111). Thus, in addition to the more rapid appearance of antidonor antibodies, loss of regulation may also be responsible for the finding that accelerated rejection is an important aspect of xenogeneic graft rejection (once hyperacute rejection is avoided), whereas it is rarely seen in allografts.

Although vigorous early antibody responses generate type II endothelial activation and accelerated rejection, later antibody responses usually fail to do so. The process that enables transplanted organs to survive in the face of circulating antibodies that can bind endothelial antigens has been called "accommodation." In xenogeneic combinations, and some allogeneic combinations with preformed blood group antibodies, accommodation has been achieved by the removal of preformed antibodies for a period of 1 to 2 weeks and the allowance of their slow return after this time. Similarly, resistance to type II endothelial activation has been achieved in vitro by pretreatment with low levels of antiendothelial antibodies that are insufficient to trigger activation (112). The achievement of accommodation is associated with increased expression of the antiapoptotic genes described above and with changes in the isotype of the recipient's antibody responses (108,113). However, accommodation has not been convincingly demonstrated in a pig-to-primate xenograft model.

Although both hyperacute rejection and accelerated rejection occur early after transplantation and depend on antidonor antibodies, there are a number of important differences between the two. One of these is that while hyperacute rejection is primarily mediated by complement activation, accelerated rejection can occur in the absence of complement. On the other hand, accelerated graft rejection may involve different secondary mediators, such as monocytes and macrophages. In xenogeneic combinations (where the inhibition of NK cells by class I molecules is lost), NK cells may also participate in accelerated rejection using antibodies to generate an ADCC response. NK cells alone may cause type II endothelial activation in xenogeneic combinations, even in the absence of antidonor antibodies, perhaps by triggering adhesion and activation through lectin molecules that recognize xenogeneic carbohydrate moieties, and/or due to a lack of NK cell inhibitory ligands on the porcine cells (114).

Another important difference between the two early forms of antibody-mediated rejection involves treatment. Once hyperacute rejection is initiated, there is no known therapy that can stop graft destruction, whereas accelerated rejection can sometimes be reversed by vigorous therapy. This has usually included plasmapheresis to remove antidonor antibodies and treatment with anti–B-cell reagents, such as cyclophosphamide (73). These reagents may also have a direct effect on the donor endothelium, blocking the process of type II endothelial activation. Although treatment of accelerated rejection is possible, it is not always successful. In current clinical practice, this form of humoral rejection may be responsible for many of the relatively few cases in which immunologically mediated graft loss occurs during the first several months after transplantation.

Rejection Caused by T Cells (Acute Rejection)

Although in clinical practice few allogeneic organs suffer either hyperacute or accelerated rejection after careful crossmatching, rejection episodes occurring toward the end of the first week after transplantation are not infrequent, despite the use of immunosuppression. These episodes are separable from the humoral rejection processes by the later timing of their occurrence, by the absence in many cases of antidonor antibodies in the recipient, and by the cellular infiltrate usually present in the biopsy. Called "acute rejection" episodes, most rejection treated by clinicians is of this type. Acute rejection occurs with decreasing frequency after the first 3 months, but rejection by apparently similar mechanisms may occur much later after transplantation, especially if immunosuppressive medication is withdrawn.

Acute rejection of organ allografts is T-cell–mediated. Therefore, treatment is usually with increased doses of standard immunosuppressive drugs or with antilymphocyte antibodies. These strategies are so likely to be successful that the diagnosis of acute rejection is doubtful if they are not.

Because T-cell–mediated acute allograft rejection plays such an important role in clinical transplantation, there has been considerable study of the mechanisms involved. Nonetheless, the following discussion indicates that many important issues regarding this rejection process remain to be resolved. On the other hand, despite the absence of a thorough understanding of cell-mediated rejection, most current clinical therapies have still been extremely effective in controlling it. Whereas 30 years ago the majority of transplant recipients suffered one, or several, rejection episodes, and only about half of the recipients were able to keep their transplanted organ for a full year, the use of newer immunosuppressive drugs and monoclonal anti–T-cell antibodies has changed these numbers considerably. Currently, as many as 80% of kidney transplant recipients never experience an episode of acute rejection, and it is now quite rare to lose a transplanted organ to cell-mediated rejection during the first year after transplantation. However, the use of these highly effective immunosuppressive treatments is associated with significant morbidity. It is hoped that an improved understanding of cell-mediated rejection might lead to more specific, less broadly immunosuppressive, approaches to preventing and treating acute rejection, and possibly to specific, noninvasive approaches to diagnosing rejection.

The study of cell-mediated rejection *in vivo* has used four types of experiments. First, there have been the studies of clinical transplants, which are obviously highly relevant, but that are always performed in the presence of immunosuppression and without the capacity to control and manipulate important variables. Second, there have been studies of skin grafts or islet transplants in rodents, which provide large amounts of controlled data on highly immunogenic grafts, but that may

not accurately reflect the processes of rejection for primarily vascularized organs. Third, there have been studies of heart and other types of primarily vascularized organ transplants in rodents, but these types of transplants are more tolerogenic and hence more easily accepted than similar transplants in large animals and human beings. Finally, there have been studies of primarily vascularized organ transplants performed in large animals, such as monkeys or pigs, which have obvious clinical relevance. Unfortunately, these studies are expensive, difficult to perform in large numbers, and are limited by the lack of monitoring and support at the same level that is possible in humans. The conclusions suggested by these different approaches have not always been the same, and thus, the description of the general mechanisms of T-cell–mediated rejection is complicated by the need to identify exceptions and features that occur only in special cases.

Pathways of T-Cell–Mediated Rejection

T-cell–mediated rejection can, like all adaptive immune responses, be considered in terms of the afferent, or sensitization phase, and the efferent, or effector phase. The location and pathways of T-cell sensitization by allografts were discussed above. Figure 10A depicts a model whereby the direct pathway of CD4 T-cell sensitization may both generate CD4+ effector cells and provide help for the activation, differentiation, and proliferation of cytotoxic CD8+ cells. This model emphasizes the importance of direct recognition of donor class II–MHC antigens by recipient CD4+ T cells, which then serve as helper cells for recipient CD8+ cells that are sensitized by direct recognition of donor class I–MHC antigens. The CD4 help for CD8 cells consists of both cytokine (e.g., IL-2) production and "conditioning" of the APC, for example by interactions of CD40 on the APC with CD40L on the activated CD4 cell, to make it a more effective APC for CD8 cells. The CD8+ and CD4+ T cells then provide the effector mechanisms for graft rejection based on the direct recognition of parenchymal cells that express class I or II antigens throughout the donor graft.

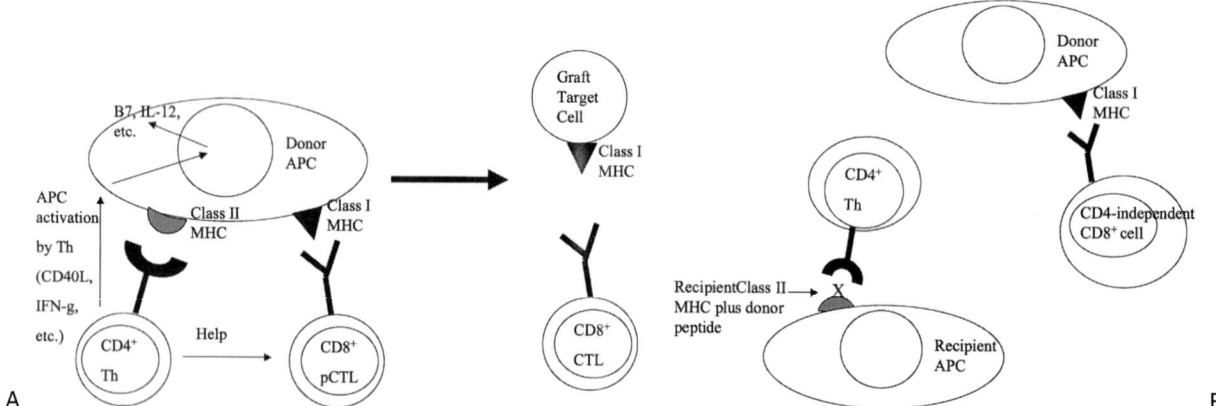

FIG. 10. Model of T-cell–mediated rejection. **A:** Interactions between CD4+ Th, donor APC, and CD8+ CTL. **B:** Additional pathways of T-cell sensitization that can lead to rejection.

As shown in Fig. 10B, there are additional pathways that have been implicated in some of the studies described below, including (a) direct activation of CD4-independent (so-called "helper-independent") CD8 T cells by donor APC; and (b) CD4$^+$ T-cell sensitization by recipient APC presenting reprocessed donor antigens (the indirect pathway of sensitization), resulting in the development of CD4$^+$ effector cells that can contribute to graft destruction via indirect effector mechanisms (discussed below). Not all of these pathways are available in every case, however, and their availability may change over time, especially as donor APC in a graft are replaced by recipient APC.

An additional pathway, the sensitization of CD8$^+$ T cells recognizing processed donor antigen presented by class I molecules on recipient APC, is not included in Fig. 10. This type of sensitization violates the original observation that peptides of exogenous antigens tend to be presented by MHC class II antigens while those of endogenous antigens are generally presented by MHC class I molecules (115). However, numerous exceptions to this principle have been reported, and several pathways have now been delineated for the processing and presentation of exogenous antigens by class I molecules (116). The phenomenon, termed "cross-priming," was originally demonstrated in a transplantation model by Bevan (117), who showed that when minor antigen-disparate grafts with MHC antigens of type A were placed on MHC (A × B) F1 recipients, the CD8$^+$ cells of these recipients became sensitized to the minor antigens presented by both A and B types of class I MHC molecules. A role for CD8$^+$ T cells sensitized in this manner has not yet been demonstrated in graft rejection. This is not to say that this pathway does not play a role, and indeed, the importance of this pathway in sensitizing CTL to viral antigens (116) makes it seem likely to play a significant role in the sensitization of CD8 T cells to donor minor histocompatibility antigens and MHC-derived peptides when there is sharing of class I alleles between the donor and recipient. Without class I sharing, indirect CD8$^+$ cell sensitization is unlikely to be important as a helper mechanism, since the help generated by CD8$^+$ cells has been found to be useful only for the CD8$^+$ cells themselves. Additionally, in this setting CD8$^+$ effectors sensitized indirectly would not recognize determinants expressed in the graft. However, these might contribute to graft rejection via indirect effector mechanisms or by producing cytokines that contribute to the overall regulation of the immune response. Thus, the question of how CD8$^+$ indirect sensitization might affect graft rejection remains one of the open issues in transplantation immunology.

The multiplicity of T-cell sensitization and effector pathways involved in graft rejection is demonstrated by the failure of elimination of either CD4$^+$ or CD8$^+$ T cells from the recipient to prevent graft rejection under many circumstances. As a result of the high precursor frequency of T cells that respond to allogeneic MHC antigens directly, populations of T cells that ordinarily have minimal significance become functionally important. A number of experimental systems

have been devised to investigate graft rejection that depends on the indirect pathway alone or that depends on direct recognition by CD8$^+$ cells in the absence of CD4$^+$ cells, and their results are summarized in the ensuing sections.

Helper Responses

Alloreactive Helper Activation Measurements

The standard *in vitro* assay of helper function in cellular immunity is the mixed lymphocyte response (MLR). This assay uses uptake of radio-labeled thymidine or loss of a fluorescent intracellular dye upon successive cell divisions to measure proliferation of T cells after allogeneic stimulation. Such analyses have led to frequency estimates of approximately 1% to 7% of T cells proliferating in a particular alloresponse. The helper response can also be quantified and characterized by measuring the production of particular cytokines such as IL-2 using biologic assays, ELISA, and ELISpot assays, intracellular cytokine staining with flow cytometry (118), and PCR. Extensive investigation of the pathways of alloreactive helper activation has been undertaken using these *in vitro* techniques (119). A summary of the experimental results is shown in Table 5, which indicates the magnitude of the helper response for each T-cell subpopulation in response to each type of antigenic challenge. It should be noted that in some cases where the response is shown in Table 5 to be absent (based on bulk culture experiments), there have been T-cell clones derived (presumably exceptional cases) that demonstrate this specificity.

The results summarized suggest that there are three main pathways of alloreactive helper activation *in vitro*: CD4$^+$ lymphocytes responding directly to allogeneic class II stimulation, CD4$^+$ lymphocytes responding to peptides of alloantigens presented in association with responder-type class II MHC molecules, and CD8$^+$ lymphocytes responding directly to class I alloantigens. The CD4$^+$ direct response is easily measured. The ability to measure the CD4$^+$ indirect response usually requires *in vivo* priming, although there is an unexpected, weak primary response to peptides of allogeneic MHC antigens presented by self-MHC molecules. The ability to measure the CD8$^+$ direct response is often enhanced if IL-2 production rather than just proliferation is measured, especially if an anti–IL-2 receptor antibody is used to prevent IL-2 consumption. In addition, detection of the CD8$^+$ direct response requires depletion of the CD4$^+$

TABLE 5. In vitro *pathways of alloreactivity*

| | Helper pathways | | | | Cytotoxic pathways | |
| | Direct | | Indirect | | | |
	I	II	I	II	I	II
CD4$^+$	−	++++	−	+++	−	++
CD8$^+$	++	−	+/−	−	++++	++

population or stimulation with just a class I–antigen disparity, since helper responses generated by whole MHC differences are generally dominated by CD4$^+$ cells. The CD8$^+$ cells that have helper function in allogeneic responses have been found to have particularly high affinity for class I alloantigens (120).

Recently, an *in vivo* assay, termed the "*trans-vivo* delayed-type hypersensitivity (DTH)" response, has been developed to assess tolerance and alloreactivity in humans (121). In this assay, peripheral blood lymphocytes are transferred from the patient to an immunodeficient mouse, with or without donor antigen and/or an irrelevant recall antigen. Using this assay, specific tolerance to donor antigens, along with the ability to actively down-regulate reactivity to irrelevant antigens, has been detected for PBMC of patients who have discontinued immunosuppression following organ allografting and not rejected the organ. In contrast, reactivity to the donor was detected for PBMC of a patient who rejected his donor graft after discontinuing immunosuppression. These studies provided evidence for an active regulatory mechanism that is dependent on TGF-β or IL-10 in tolerant patients (121). Because this assay permits dissection of *in vivo* mechanisms of alloreactivity and tolerance, and appears to provide different results from purely *in vitro* assays of such reactivity (122), it will be of considerable interest to see whether the *trans vivo* assay can be validated in large animals and larger groups of patients.

Two basic approaches have been used to study the pathways of alloreactive T-cell recognition in graft rejection. First, selected T-cell subpopulations have been depleted *in vivo* and, second, selected T-cell subpopulations have been transferred into immunodeficient (nude, SCID, or RAG$^{-/-}$) recipients that themselves lack the T-cell components of graft rejection (123). In both cases, the approach has been modified by placing grafts with narrow antigenic disparities or by using different types of tissues for transplantation. The results of these studies suggest that all three alloreactive helper pathways detected *in vitro* can also be detected *in vivo,* and that both direct and indirect effector mechanisms can contribute to rejection.

CD4$^+$ T Helper (Th) Cells in Graft Rejection

CD4$^+$ T cells alone can cause rejection of many types of grafts, including those with full MHC disparities (124), class II–antigen disparities alone, and multiple minor antigen disparities alone (123), and they seem to play a critical role in the rejection of fully MHC mismatched cardiac allografts in rodents (124). In BMT recipients, they can induce GVHD in the absence of CD8 cells in the setting of class II, full MHC, or multiple minor histoincompatibilities (125). In addition, CD4$^+$ cells have been shown to contribute to rejection of bone marrow grafts differing only at class I MHC loci (126,127). However, CD4$^+$ cells alone have been shown to be incapable of rejecting some types of class I–only disparate murine skin

grafts (123) or inducing GVHD across certain isolated class I and minor histocompatibility barriers (128).

Numerous studies have demonstrated that depletion of donor APC can prolong graft survival (61), illustrating the importance of direct allorecognition in causing graft rejection. The role of the direct pathway in stimulating CD4$^+$ cells has been demonstrated using genetically engineered, class II knockout mice as recipients after reconstitution of their CD4$^+$ T-cell population. These mice lack class II antigens on their own APC and, therefore, cannot generate an indirect response. Thus, CD4-dependent rejection of grafts by these recipients must reflect direct sensitization of CD4$^+$ cells *in vivo*. Recent studies of this nature have clearly shown that direct allorecognition by recipient CD4 T cells is both necessary and sufficient to induce cardiac allograft rejection in mice (129). This is somewhat surprising, since class II is far from ubiquitously expressed in cardiac grafts, and suggests that mechanisms directed at vascular endothelial cells that up-regulate class II under inflammatory conditions, and/or indirect effector mechanisms, may induce rejection.

There is also considerable evidence for a role for the indirect pathway of CD4 cell–mediated allorecognition in graft rejection. Indeed, over the past several years there has been an increasing tendency to stress the importance of indirect recognition (130). Evidence for its role includes the contribution of CD4$^+$ T cells to the rejection of class I–only disparate marrow (126,127). Furthermore, antibody blocking of recipient class II antigens *in vivo* can sometimes prevent rejection, and immunization of recipients with peptides of donor antigens before transplantation can accelerate subsequent graft rejection.

Some manipulations that alter the immune response to peptides of donor MHC antigens have been found to prevent rejection of grafts expressing the intact MHC antigens, suggesting that the indirect response to these antigens may induce tolerance that is dominant over the direct response in graft rejection (131,132). For example, miniature swine kidney allograft acceptance in animals receiving transduced autologous bone marrow expressing donor class II peptides through the indirect pathway (133) suggests that a dominant (regulatory) type of tolerance spreads from the indirect to the direct pathway of allorecognition. Likewise, expression of class II by recipient APC has been shown to be essential for the induction of hyporesponsiveness to fully MHC-mismatched allografts with co-stimulatory blockade, suggesting an important role for indirect recognition in this process (134).

Rejection of some grafts lacking class II antigen expression has been shown to be dependent on CD4$^+$ T cells, which were, therefore, presumably stimulated by modified class II antigens of the recipient (135). These studies in class II knockout mice have shown rejection through the indirect pathway to be a powerful event, and that it is often as difficult to control as rejection depending on direct recognition. Rejection of xenografts from highly disparate species in mice is very dependent on CD4$^+$ function, even though CD4$^+$ direct activation measured *in vitro* is very weak (136), suggesting a dominant role for the indirect pathway in this setting. Clinically, sensitization of indirect CD4 responses to donor MHC–derived peptides has been demonstrated in patients undergoing graft rejection, and some studies have suggested that an increase in the precursor frequency of T cells responding through the indirect pathway provides the best correlation with clinical events. A major role for indirect allorecognition has been suggested in the setting of chronic rejection, because this pathway is critical for the induction of antibody responses, which have been implicated in the pathogenesis of chronic rejection, and because the eventual replacement of donor APC by recipient APC would imply that the latter are responsible for fueling the immune response on a long-term basis. Indeed, direct alloresponses tend to subside over time in patients with heart or kidney allografts (137). Experimental and clinical evidence has supported this hypothesis. Th2 CD4 responses have been hypothesized to play a particularly important role in chronic rejection through indirect recognition and induction of antibody responses (138). However, a recent study has shown an association of Th2 clones recognizing donor peptides indirectly with stable graft function, whereas Th1 clones with similar specificity were associated with chronic renal allograft rejection in patients (139).

In view of the apparent importance of the indirect pathway of allorecognition in graft rejection, it is not obvious why donor APC depletion or the lack of donor class II MHC expression should be effective in preventing rejection in some situations (61,129). An essential role for indirect allorecognition has been easier to demonstrate in chronic rejection than acute rejection (138), and the indirect pathway alone may simply be insufficiently powerful to induce acute rejection. Long-term survival of APC-depleted endocrine allografts, which are not primarily vascularized, may reflect resistance to chronic rejection of tissues lacking donor-derived blood vessels. In the case of renal and cardiac allografts, APC depletion may allow the inherent tolerogenicity of the parenchymal tissue to prevail and spread to the indirect pathway. Initial sensitization through the direct pathway may be essential in producing the inflammatory conditions necessary to promote indirect pathway sensitization, so that the latter does not occur or is tolerogenic in the absence of the former. An alternative explanation might be that donor APC are essential for the sensitization of the effector cells responsible for graft rejection, while indirect presentation is available for the sensitization of helper cells. In the absence of donor APC, potential effector cells might undergo anergy as a result of encountering donor antigens directly only on parenchymal cells of a graft.

The indirect pathway of allorecognition also has implications regarding the potential effectiveness of some strategies to achieve donor-specific nonresponsiveness. Many of these strategies seek to present donor antigens to immunocompetent recipients in a manner that leads to T-cell downregulation rather than activation. If these strategies only involve manipulations of donor APC, they may be ineffective

in preventing indirect immune responses, since these depend on recipient APC.

Role of CD8⁺ Th in Graft Rejection

Depletion of $CD8^+$ T cells leads to a delay in the rejection of fully MHC-mismatched skin allografts, demonstrating that they play a role, but are not absolutely required, for rejection. $CD8^+$ T cells alone can reject skin grafts that express an MHC class I antigen disparity (123). They can reject bone marrow differing at isolated class I or minor histocompatibility loci (126,127), and can induce GVHD in the absence of CD4 T cells in the setting of full MHC, class I only, and minor antigen histoincompatibility (125). These results suggest that $CD8^+$ Th direct activation can also contribute to graft rejection and GVHD.

Direct $CD8^+$ cell activation does not appear to be as powerful as direct $CD4^+$ T cell activation, since grafts expressing only class I antigen disparities are usually rejected more slowly than class II disparate grafts, and responses dependent on $CD8^+$ helper responses are more easily suppressed by cyclosporine (CsA). Many primarily vascularized grafts that express only a class I antigen disparity still require $CD4^+$ cells to initiate rejection. Probably as a result of this weakness, rejection that depends on $CD8^+$ T cell direct activation is influenced by several factors that do not seem to be as important for $CD4^+$ T cell direct activation. First, $CD8^+$ direct activation is very dependent on the relative number of donor APC in a graft (140). Second, $CD8^+$ helper cells recognize modified self-class I antigens very poorly. Therefore, $CD8^+$ direct activation fails to initiate rejection of grafts with only a small number of minor antigen disparities and provides only a weak helper response even when there are a large number of foreign minor antigens.

$CD8^+$ helper cells also differ from $CD4^+$ helper cells in being unable to provide help for other cell populations. Apparently the IL-2 produced by these cells is used by the cells themselves as they develop effector function. Therefore, $CD8^+$ helper cells cannot provide help for $CD8^+$ cells with a different specificity. For a number of reasons, they cannot provide help for B-cell antibody responses. $CD4^+$ cells alone but not $CD8^+$ cells alone can reject skin grafts with only class II antigen disparities (123). This result correlates with the *in vitro* experiments showing that both $CD4^+$ and $CD8^+$ cells contain precursors of cytotoxic cells specific for allogeneic class II antigens, but that only the $CD4^+$ population has a helper pathway to generate mature class II–specific CTLs.

Some experimental evidence raises the possibility that CD4 helper cells sensitized by antigen presented on recipient APC might provide help for $CD8^+$ effector cells recognizing antigen presented by donor APC. This is a special feature of alloreactivity compared to ordinary immunology, in which two different populations of APC expressing different MHC antigens may collaborate in the process. The absence of a physical linkage afforded by the expression of different determinants on a single APC may limit the availability of help from one subpopulation during the sensitization of another subpopulation. This issue is discussed in more detail below, in the section on regulation of graft rejection.

Pathways of Alloreactivity: Effector Mechanisms

While there are many controversial aspects of helper T-cell function, there is even more uncertainty about the effector mechanisms of cell-mediated graft rejection. While cytotoxic T-cell function has attracted attention because it could account for the precise selectivity of graft destruction that is sometimes observed, the role of additional tissue-destructive mechanisms, and particularly of indirect effector mechanisms initiated by T cells specific for modified self-MHC antigens, has not been fully elucidated. A brief review of the available data on these issues is provided here.

In Vitro *Studies of Effector Mechanisms*

A standard assay measuring an alloreactive effector function is the CTL or CML assay measuring T-cell–mediated cytotoxicity against allogeneic targets. Alloreactive CTLs can easily be generated from naïve T cells after about 5 to 7 days of *in vitro* stimulation with MHC-disparate cells. Generation of CTLs to peptides of minor antigens presented by self-MHC molecules, however, requires that the T cells first be primed *in vivo*. The amount of cytotoxicity measured *in vitro* is a function of both the helper activation and the number of precursor CTLs available at the start of the *in vitro* culture. Therefore, to focus on just the cytotoxic effector function the assay is often performed with the addition of exogenous helper factors, such as IL-2, in order to provide excessive help. The assay can also be quantified by measuring precursor frequencies of cytotoxic T cells using limiting dilution cultures, but this assay has been shown to severely underestimate the number of CD8 T cells that proliferate or produce cytokines in an immune response.

Since alloreactive T cells to foreign MHC antigens can be measured even in naïve animals, the standard CML assay is inadequate to determine whether CTLs have been primed in recipients that have rejected MHC-disparate grafts. Therefore, efforts have been made to modify the assay to measure the effect of *in vivo* events. The presence of T cells that can kill donor targets without the period of *in vitro* sensitization (direct cytolytic activity), an increased precursor frequency of alloreactive T cells, and development of CTL under modified conditions have been used to demonstrate *in vivo* activation by alloantigens. More recently developed techniques, including ELISpot and intracellular cytokine staining, have considerably enhanced the ability to detect nonproliferating or noncytolytic CD8 T cells that have been sensitized *in vivo* (118). MHC-peptide tetramers containing minor histocompatibility antigenic peptides and their known class I MHC–presenting molecule have been very useful in detecting expansions of CTL recognizing minor histocompatibility antigens in the setting of GVHD and rejection of HLA-identical

hematopoietic cell grafts. However, the broad diversity of MHC alloantigen–specific T cells and undefined peptides recognized by such cells currently precludes the use of this approach to identify MHC-alloreactive T cells.

The *in vitro* CML assay has been used to determine the pathways of alloreactive T-cell cytotoxic function. The results of these assays are summarized in Table 5. CD8+ cytotoxic T cells reactive with donor class I antigens are the most frequent effectors *in vitro,* and CD8+ cytotoxic cells specific for self-class I antigens modified by allogeneic peptides can also be detected after *in vivo* priming (141). In addition, CD8+ cytotoxic cells specific for allogeneic class II antigens can be detected, although they would not be predicted in classical immunology. CD4+ cytotoxic cells specific for allogeneic class II antigens can also be measured *in vitro*. Thus, as for helper cells, there are multiple pathways for generating alloreactive cytotoxic T cells *in vitro*.

In Vivo *Analysis of Effector Mechanisms of Rejection and GVHD*

Selectivity of Allograft Rejection. A critical feature when considering *in vivo* effector mechanisms of graft rejection is the selectivity by which the process destroys foreign but not self tissues. When syngeneic skin is grafted adjacent to allogeneic skin on a single bed, the inflammation of rejection shows a perfect demarcation at the division between the two grafts (142). Results of grafting skin from tetraparental (allophenic) donors, which are mosaic animals produced by fusing embryonic cells of two parental pairs, also indicate a high degree of selectivity of rejection for cells expressing the allogeneic antigens, but these results are open to alternative interpretations. For example, the syngeneic elements that eventually survived from the tetraparental grafts might actually represent the product of epithelial seeding by a few syngeneic cells that remained as the tissue around them died. When syngeneic skin from bone marrow chimeras in which the APC of the skin had been replaced by cells derived from an allogeneic donor bone marrow was transplanted, the entire graft was rejected (143). Thus, entire skin grafts can be rejected when only the APC are foreign, indicating that nonselective destruction of grafted tissue can occur, especially if the inflammatory response is sufficiently vigorous. Skin grafts from class II knockout mice have been placed on SCID or nude recipients reconstituted with CD4+ but not CD8+ T cells. These experiments have shown that the class II–deficient grafts can be rejected by CD4+ cells alone, but much more slowly than when CD8+ cells are also present (144). The rejection of pancreatic islets is diminished substantially by the reduced expression of donor MHC antigens, unless the MHC-deficient islets are placed in xenogeneic recipients. In the case of bone marrow transplantation, donor CD4+ T cells destroy only class II–expressing recipient hematopoietic cells, with no evidence of damage to the hematopoietic microenvironment or of hematopoietic cells not expressing recipient class II (145). Together, these results suggest that indirect CD4 cell–mediated effector mechanisms can destroy transplanted tissue under some circumstances, but much less efficiently than direct mechanisms.

Rejection of class I–only disparate grafts has frequently been demonstrated in recipients depleted of CD8$^+$ T cells (123), even though *in vitro* assays have generally failed to reveal cytotoxic CD4$^+$ cells specific for class I alloantigens. These results appear to violate the correlation between graft rejection and the ability to measure *in vitro* cytotoxicity. Rosenberg et al. (146) and McCarthy et al. (147), however, demonstrated that mice depleted of CD8$^+$ T cells by antibody treatment still have a population of cytotoxic precursors (apparently of the CD8$^+$ lineage despite the absence of the CD8 antigen) that require *in vivo* priming and help from CD4$^+$ T cells for their activation. These investigators have demonstrated the presence of CD4$^-$, CD8$^-$, $\alpha\beta^+$ cytotoxic T cells after graft rejection in the mice that were treated with anti-CD8 antibodies. These results suggest that depletion of CD8$^+$ cells *in vivo* may not always eliminate all cytotoxic cells of this lineage and that the rejection of class I–disparate skin grafts apparently by CD4$^+$ cells alone is not actually a violation of the correlation between *in vitro* CTL activity and *in vivo* graft rejection. However, this conclusion is controversial, and other investigators have suggested that they apply only to the very limited antigenic disparities generated by the Bm strains of class I mutant mice. These other studies suggest that the larger number of foreign peptides generated by more disparate class I antigens are sufficient to generate an effector mechanism mediated by CD4$^+$ cells specific for class I peptides presented by class II molecules. These results do not distinguish a direct from an indirect effector mechanism, since the class II molecules of the donor and recipient are identical in these experiments, but they do suggest a lack of correlation between *in vivo* rejection and *in vitro* cytotoxicity, since CD4$^+$ cytotoxic T cells have not been detected after rejection in these experiments.

Since CTL activity to minor histocompatibility antigens can only be measured *in vitro* after *in vivo* priming, minor disparate graft rejection provides an opportunity to test whether every case of rejection is associated with the development of CTL activity. A particularly good model to test this correlation is the rejection of murine skin grafts that differ by only the H-Y antigen since some strains, but not others, can reject skin grafts with only this single minor antigen disparity. Experiments have indicated that the rejection of H-Y disparate grafts is not always associated with measurable *in vitro* cytotoxicity, while in other cases the development of CTLs *in vitro* occurs despite the absence of graft rejection. This may reflect the prevalence of non–CTL-mediated mechanisms of graft rejection in this system, or may simply reflect the failure of the *in vitro* conditions chosen for CTL assays to reflect the activity of CTL that indeed play an active role in rejection *in vivo*.

Solid organ graft rejection can be correlated with the presence in the graft of proteins and mRNA encoding perforin, granzymes, and proteases associated with cell-mediated cytotoxicity (148,149). The presence in urine of cell-derived RNA encoding perforin and granzyme B has been associated with renal allograft rejection (150). A functional analysis of the role of CTL in graft rejection and GVHD has been facilitated by the use of mice deficient in one or more effector proteins involved in CTL activity—particularly perforin, granzyme, and Fas/Fas ligand (FasL). Although the perforin/granzyme pathway of CTL activity is the major cytolytic pathway for CD8 T cells and CD4 cells tend to utilize the Fas/FasL pathway, both subsets are capable of both types of cytolytic activity, and the perforin pathway is available to both T-cell subsets mediating GVHD (151). Overall, these studies have shown all of these proteins to play contributory roles, but no single protein has been found to play a critical role in the induction of solid organ graft rejection, GVHD, or bone marrow graft rejection in the presence of clinically relevant mismatches. Critical cytotoxic interactions have been identified in a few special situations. For example, GVHD directed at isolated class II MHC disparities is markedly reduced in the absence of Fas/FasL interactions (152), and the survival of K^b mutant class I–only mismatched heart allografts is markedly prolonged in perforin-deficient recipients (153). Another interesting observation is the requirement for donor heart allografts to express IFN-γ receptor in order to be rejected by CD4$^+$ cells (154), raising the possibility that IFN-γ may itself be an effector molecule of graft destruction. Thus, direct cytotoxicity by T cells may, perhaps, represent one of several mechanisms for graft destruction and GVHD. Other, less direct cytotoxic mechanisms (e.g., TNFα–mediated cytotoxicity) and cytokine-mediated activation of accessory cell populations may play redundant roles in most settings.

Analysis of Cells Invading Allografts. Studies using sponge matrix allografts and rejecting allogeneic organs have revealed that many types of cells are present during graft rejection, including CD4$^+$ and CD8$^+$ T cells, NK cells, and macrophages (155). There are, however, relatively few B cells. Not surprisingly, L-selectin$^+$ T cells, which migrate through the lymph nodes via receptors on high endothelial vessels and do not circulate through parenchymal tissues, are absent from rejecting grafts. Further analysis of the invading cells within rejecting allografts has been undertaken by *in vitro* propagation of the T cells derived from rejecting organs. Most reports of such efforts have indicated that these T cells are polyclonal and that both cytotoxic and IL-2–producing lymphocytes of both CD4$^+$ and CD8$^+$ lineages can be obtained. Many T cells seem to be recruited nonspecifically into rejecting grafts, as only a fraction of them recognize donor antigens, but only the donor-reactive CTL show evidence of having been activated *in vivo,* as indicated by their ability to respond to donor antigens in limiting dilution analyses without further antigen-specific stimulation (156). Despite some early reports suggesting that an oligoclonal T-cell response occurs during allograft rejection, these studies may be subject to *in vitro* culturing artifacts and sampling error. Most analyses of the T-cell repertoire of T cells recognizing allogeneic MHC molecules have, as expected, revealed a broad, polyclonal repertoire utilizing many different $V\beta$. Nevertheless, CDR3 spectratype analysis has shown that, even in the setting of MHC disparity, graft-infiltrating cells of long-term rejected human kidneys and of acutely rejecting rat heart allografts show a markedly skewed repertoire. However, a similar type of skewing has not been evident among T cells infiltrating rejecting xenografts (157,158), suggesting that the larger number of histoincompatibilities between xenogeneic donors and recipients may result in a broader repertoire of responding T cells. Analyses of T cells mediating GVHD in the setting of multiple minor histoincompatibilities have revealed a markedly skewed repertoire, but still with the involvement of several different $V\beta$ families, each exhibiting an oligoclonal response (159).

The number of invading T cells in a graft is not necessarily related to the speed of the resulting rejection. Whole MHC and class II disparate grafts generally elicit dense cellular infiltrates, while class I disparate grafts are generally sparsely infiltrated, and only to a similar extent as syngeneic grafts (160). This finding has suggested that certain critical elements of the graft, such as its blood vessels, are the actual site of graft destruction and, indeed, endothelialitis is an important hallmark of clinically significant rejection activity (161). The number of cells within minor antigen disparate grafts is generally far greater than the number invading grafts with class I only differences, even when the rejection of the class I grafts is faster (160).

Cytokines as Mediators of Graft Rejection and GVHD. In recent years, numerous studies have been performed correlating the onset of graft rejection with the presence of immunologically active cytokines or mRNA encoding them in the graft and, in the case of renal transplantation, in the urine (150). RT-PCR and protein measurements have revealed high levels of both Th1 (IL-2, IFN-γ) and Th2 (IL-4, IL-5, IL-10) cytokines in rejecting allografts. As is discussed below in the section on tolerance, the finding of Th2-type cytokines in association with rejection does not support the hypothesis that Th2 cytokines are purely anti-inflammatory and prevent rejection. Indeed, under certain conditions, when Th1 cytokines are not available (e.g., in various knockout mice), Th2 have been shown to be capable of inducing allograft rejection, often with a prominent infiltration of eosinophils and mast cells. Furthermore, mice with induced mutations of signal transducers and activators of transduction (STAT) molecules critical for either Th1 or Th2 differentiation are both capable of rejecting cardiac allografts (162). Consistent with the multiplicity of cytokines associated with rejection, the use of knockout mice as recipients lacking various cytokines (e.g., IFN-γ, IL-2, IL-4) has failed to reveal any single molecule that is essential for graft destruction or GVHD. One exception is the rejection of established islet allografts in a SCID mouse model, in which rejection by adoptively transferred CD8 T cells is critically dependent on IFN-γ (163). IFN-γ is apparently also critical for the rejection of skin allografts mismatched only at class II MHC loci (164). Additionally, membrane-bound lymphotoxin (TNFβ) has been shown to play a critical role in CD8 cell–mediated rejection of intestinal allografts in the presence of co-stimulatory blockade, perhaps by inducing the production of critical chemokines (165). Paradoxically, the Th1 cytokine IFN-γ, and the cytokine that induces it, IL-12, have been shown to play inhibitory roles in graft rejection (166) and GVHD (167) under certain conditions, and Th2 responses have been clearly shown to contribute to graft rejection and GVHD. Nonetheless, a predominance of Th2 cytokines has been observed in some rodent models in which solid organ grafts, in the presence of certain immunologic manipulations, induce tolerance, and these cytokines have been implicated in tolerance induction. These cytokines have been shown to be present and to play an active role in tolerance induced by neonatal injection of allogeneic lymphocytes (168). Immune deviation to Th2 has been shown to be capable of inducing cardiac allograft acceptance in the setting of minor only, but not major histoincompatibilities, suggesting that this strategy may lead to tolerance only when the number of alloreactive T-cell clones is relatively small (169). In a paradox similar to that observed for allograft rejection, Th2 cytokines have been implicated in both acute and chronic GVHD, but have also been suggested to play a role in inhibiting acute GVHD. A reader new to the transplantation field may justifiably be confused by the above discussion, as the role of cytokines in graft rejection, GVHD, and tolerance is extraordinarily complex, and is far from being completely understood.

Final Mediators of T-Cell–Dependent Effector Mechanisms

The final mediators of cell-mediated graft rejection and GVHD may not be T cells themselves, but rather other components of the immune system that depend on helper T cells. There are several candidate mediators of graft destruction. Classical DTH responses are thought to depend on the activation of macrophages by helper T cells through production of IFN-γ. In turn, the destruction of tissues by activated macrophages may often involve the production of toxic molecules such as nitric oxide. Although an effector mechanism involving macrophages would appear to lack selectivity, the process might still cause limited tissue destruction if the donor cells (such as pancreatic islets) are especially sensitive to these inflammatory mediators, or if donor blood vessels in the immediate vicinity of the activated cells are especially likely to be injured by the inflammatory response. Cytokines are clearly involved in the mechanisms of graft rejection. However, most of the obvious examples of their participation involve their role in the helper mechanisms of T-cell sensitization. It is likely, however, that some cytokines, such as TNFα, may themselves be toxic to allogeneic tissues.

A similar situation prevails in the setting of GVHD. Cytokines such as TNFα and IFN-γ have been shown to play a role in the inflammatory cascade involving macrophage activation by LPS from the damaged gut epithelium and by IFN-γ to release TNFα, nitric oxide, and other mediators that may contribute to tissue injury. Studies on the relative roles of various cytolytic mechanisms in GVHD pathology have been performed in a variety of models, including irradiated and nonirradiated (parent to F1) recipients, various MHC disparities, and models that do and do not include a source of donor hematopoietic cells that should be exempt from cytolytic effects of donor T cells, and hence can protect the mice from death due to hematopoietic failure. It is unwise to extrapolate results from one such system to other GVHD models without direct evaluation. Bearing these limitations in mind, in certain models, TNFα had been shown to play a critical role in wasting disease and intestinal GVHD, and FasL to play a critical role in lymphoid hypoplasia and skin and liver GVHD. The perforin-granzyme pathway contributes to GVHD in undefined target organs. Overall, the Fas-mediated cytotoxic pathway appears to be of greater importance than the perforin pathway in the induction of GVHD. In contrast the perforin/granzyme pathway plays a predominant role in antileukemic effects, especially of CD8 cells, and selective blockade of the Fas/FasL pathway may ameliorate CD8-mediated GVHD without eliminating GVL effects. While the relative contribution of cytokine-dependent mechanisms versus direct cell-mediated cytotoxicity to GVHD is still a matter of debate, the capacity to induce GVHD with T cells lacking both the perforin-mediated and the Fas-mediated pathways of cytotoxicity, even in mice lacking TNFR1-mediated signaling pathways, demonstrates the capacity of cytokines alone to mediate significant end-organ damage.

Chronic Rejection (B- and/or T-Cell–Mediated)

Most experimental studies of rejection are performed without immunosuppression and, therefore, graft destruction usually occurs within the first several weeks by one of the mechanisms described above. In clinical practice, however, the use of immunosuppression usually allows graft survival for much longer periods of time. Nonetheless, clinical survival statistics reveal that even when 1-year graft survival has been achieved, the loss of transplanted organs continues to occur at a rate of about 3% to 5% per year and a significant portion of this loss appears to be due to immunologic mechanisms. The term "chronic rejection" has been used to describe this late process of graft destruction. As immunosuppressive reagents have become more effective at controlling acute rejection, chronic rejection has emerged as one of the most important problems in clinical practice. Indeed, Fig. 11 shows that while there has been ongoing improvement over the past 30 years in the 1-year graft survival rates for kidney transplants, the half-life for organs that have survived for 1 year has not changed significantly over that entire period of time. As a result of this ongoing loss, only about 50% of transplants are still functioning 10 years later.

Although almost every type of organ transplant suffers from chronic rejection, the pathologic manifestations are different in each case. Kidney biopsies tend to show interstitial fibrosis along with arterial narrowing from hyalinization of the vessels. In the heart, the process is manifested principally as a diffuse myointimal hyperplasia proceeding to fibrosis of the coronary arteries that has often been referred to as "accelerated atherosclerosis." Chronic rejection in lung transplants primarily affects the bronchioles with progressive narrowing of these structures, and is referred to as "bronchiolitis obliterans." The liver may be the one type of organ transplant that is relatively resistant to chronic rejection, but the progressive destruction of bile ducts referred to as the "vanishing bile duct syndrome" may be another manifestation of this process.

Some of the causes of chronic graft destruction may not be immunologic in origin. Potential factors that have been considered include the initial ischemic insult, the reduced mass of transplanted tissue (especially in the case of kidney transplants leading to hyperfiltration injury), the denervation of

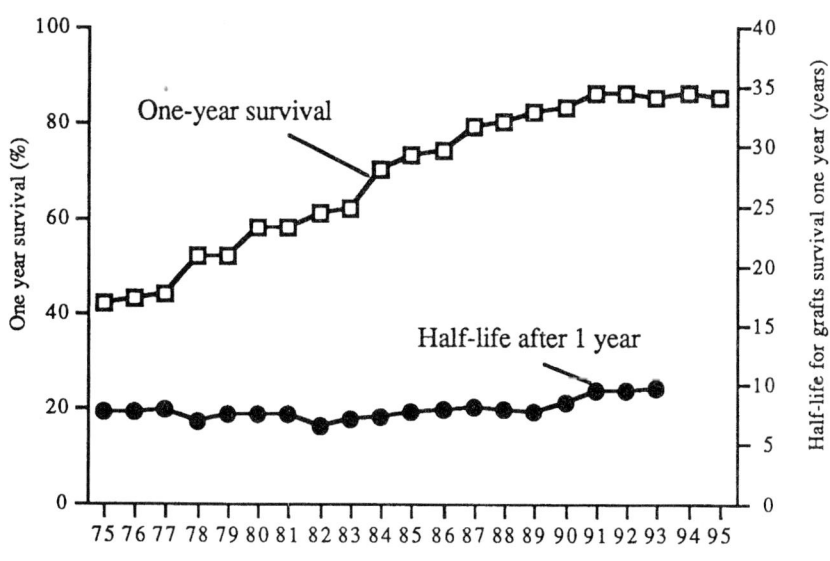

FIG. 11. One-year graft survival and chronic half-life over time.

the transplanted organ, the hyperlipidemia and hypertension associated with immunosuppressive drugs, the immunosuppressive drugs themselves, and chronic viral injury. Nonetheless, while these factors undoubtedly contribute to the process, there is a marked difference in survival between syngeneic and allogeneic transplants in experimental models. In addition, native hearts in kidney transplant recipients do not show manifestations of chronic rejection and vice versa. Thus, there is almost certainly an important immunologic component in most cases of chronic rejection.

Several important observations regarding chronic rejection have emerged from clinical practice. First, the process is frequently associated with the presence of antidonor antibodies. This was first recognized in the case of kidney transplants when a high correlation was found between the presence of alloantibodies and the hyalinization of renal arteries on late biopsy specimens. The same correlation has been found for other organs as well. Second, the process of chronic rejection is usually refractory to increases in immunosuppressive therapy, in contrast to acute rejection episodes that almost always respond to treatment. Third, there is a high correlation between the onset of chronic rejection and a history of early acute rejection episodes. Together, these clinical observations have suggested to some that chronic rejection is the result of chronic B-cell alloantibody production. They have suggested to others that chronic rejection requires the early sensitization of the immune system to donor antigens. Both suggestions may be correct, but neither the logic nor the evidence fully supports these conclusions. In the first place, alloantibody production often reflects indirect T-cell sensitization (see below), and hence it might equally well be a marker for other rejection mechanisms as opposed to a cause of chronic rejection. In addition, early rejection episodes probably reflect primarily the degree of antidonor immunoreactivity, and may not themselves be required for chronic rejection. Therefore, even if sufficient immunosuppression were given to prevent acute rejection, chronic rejection might still occur when the suppression was reduced to levels tolerable over the long term, even if acute rejection had never occurred. Finally, experimental studies have suggested that the mechanisms of chronic rejection are not absolutely dependent on either antibody formation or on the occurrence of acute rejection episodes.

The uncertainties that arise from the interpretation of the clinical data make it important to develop experimental models for studying the mechanisms of chronic rejection. It is difficult in the laboratory, however, to mimic a process that may take 5 or 10 years to develop in patients treated with immunosuppressive drugs. Thus, the effort to study chronic rejection experimentally has depended on surrogate short-term pathologic markers that are thought to predict the long-term changes of chronic rejection. In particular, these studies have concentrated on the development of the myointimal proliferation that is thought to be the precursor of the chronic vascular changes typically observed in patients. Both in rodents and in pigs, this has often been done with heart transplants after an initial period of immunosuppression that prevents acute

rejection. All of these experimental studies are subject to the caveat that the surrogate pathologic lesion occurs much earlier than the typical changes of chronic rejection in clinical patients. Thus, the process being studied experimentally may not be the same as the clinical process.

Pathologic Manifestations of Experimental Chronic Rejection

The typical pathologic features of the experimental lesion associated with chronic rejection are shown in Fig. 12. The marked narrowing of the vascular lumen is caused by the substantial proliferation of endothelial and then smooth muscle cells. Associated with this proliferation is progressive destruction of the media. In time, the cellular proliferation becomes less pronounced and is replaced by concentric fibrosis that narrows the vascular lumen. Immunohistologic staining indicates that there is increased expression of several adhesion molecules during the early manifestations of this process and easily detectable levels of several cytokines and factors, including nitric oxide synthase, acidic fibroblast growth factor, insulin-like growth factor, and endothelin. Ultimately, the ischemia resulting from vascular occlusion results in fibrosis in the parenchyma of the organ, and consequent organ dysfunction (170). In the case of the lung or the liver, chronic injury may cause changes most prominently in the bronchioles or the bile ducts, but this is also associated with arterial lumen loss, which may be the primary lesion causing bronchiolitis obliterans or bile duct fibrosis, respectively (170).

Immunologic Mechanisms of Chronic Rejection

Because it is assumed that stimulation of direct immune responses is likely to diminish over time as donor APC are replaced by recipient APC, it is commonly assumed that the predominant immune response that causes chronic rejection

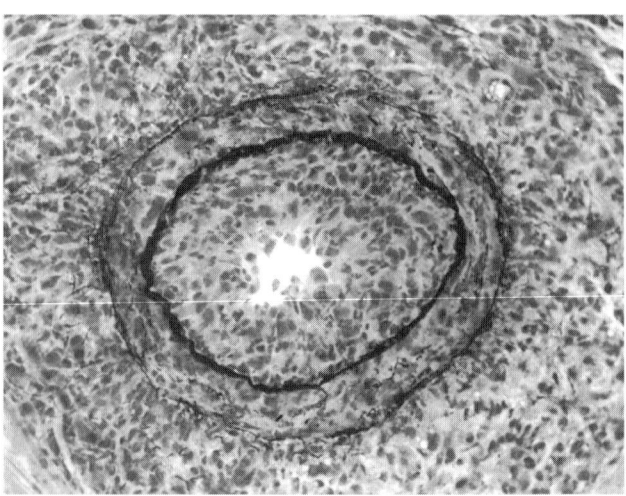

FIG. 12. Histology of chronic rejection.

occurs through the indirect pathway. The evidence supporting this hypothesis was discussed above.

Studies in pigs have suggested that the vascular changes of chronic rejection are more apt to develop when there are class I antigenic disparities than when there are only class II disparities and have suggested that the lesion depends especially on CD8$^+$ T cells (171). Mouse studies, however, have indicated that either CD4$^+$ or CD8$^+$ T cells can produce the lesion and that either class I or class II antigenic disparities are sufficient to stimulate chronic rejection (172). The finding that class II antigenic disparities are themselves sufficient to induce this pathology is consistent with the observation of class II MHC expression on the vascular endothelium and medial smooth muscle cells of mouse cardiac allografts with these vascular lesions (173). Since class II MHC is not constitutively expressed by murine vascular endothelial cells (174), indirect recognition of donor class II transferred from passenger leukocytes may be responsible for inducing an inflammatory response that leads to subsequent up-regulation of class II on the donor vascular endothelium. In keeping with the prediction of many clinical studies, adoptive transfer experiments into SCID mice have shown that alloantibodies in the absence of T cells can induce the typical pathologic vascular changes, and lesions can develop in T-cell–deficient mice (175). However, T cells without B cells have also been shown to cause the lesion, although there may be somewhat less tendency to progress to end-stage fibrosis. Several studies have indicated that the induction of donor-specific tolerance can prevent the development of the vascular changes of chronic rejection, although not all of the short-term manipulations that have been effective in preventing acute rejection have necessarily prevented the later onset of chronic rejection. Remarkably, mice rendered tolerant by neonatal injection of donor splenocytes, or by the induction of high levels of lasting, multilineage mixed chimerism with demonstrated central deletion of donor-reactive T cells and permanent acceptance of donor-specific skin grafts, demonstrate graft vasculopathy in donor cardiac allografts (176). In the same study, immunodeficient SCID mice and Rag1$^{-/-}$ mice were also shown to be capable of developing lesions. Such lesions do not develop in isografts, indicating that recognition of allogeneic differences are essential for their development. Together, these studies suggest that, in the complete absence of antidonor T-cell reactivity, other cell types (possibly NK cells) may induce these types of lesions in cardiac allografts (176). In addition, T-cell recognition of cardiac-specific antigens presented by donor MHC and not shared by donor hematopoietic cells could play a possible role in the development of these lesions in immunocompetent, tolerant mice.

From these data, it seems likely that multiple immunologic mechanisms may be capable of creating the graft arteriosclerotic lesions that are characteristic of chronic rejection, and that T-cell alloreactivity is not essential for their induction. Whether there is a critical final common mediator involved in all of these pathways is not currently known. However, IFN-γ has been shown to play an important role in the development of lesions in several models, and STAT4-deficient mice, which do not respond to IL-12 and therefore cannot generate Th1 responses, show markedly reduced severity of graft vasculopathy compared to wild-type mice (177). Additional data have implicated Th1 responses in these lesions, and Th2 responses have been associated with a reduction in them (139). However, Th2 CD4 responses have been hypothesized to play a particularly important role in chronic rejection through indirect recognition and induction of antibody responses (138). TGF-β has been shown to attenuate the lesions, but has also been detected within the lesions and implicated in the development of fibrosis. Th1 and Th2 responses are both profibrotic when they become chronic (170). Thus, the interplay between Th1 and Th2 cytokines in the pathogenesis of chronic rejection is incompletely understood.

Nonimmunologic factors, such as ischemic/reperfusion injury are believed to play a significant role in the ultimate development of chronic rejection (170), and the interaction of injury and immunologic factors deserves further study. A new twist in our understanding of this phenomenon has recently arisen from the observation that most of the proliferating intimal smooth muscle cells in vessels with graft arteriosclerosis are actually recipient-derived (178).

PHYSIOLOGIC INTERACTIONS REGULATING GRAFT REJECTION

The preceding sections described the interactions between donor antigens and the recipient immune system that lead to graft rejection. This section deals with the regulatory elements that control this process. Since the regulation of complement and endothelial activation was described in the sections on humoral mechanisms of rejection, this discussion concentrates on the regulation of T-cell responses. First, we consider the process of T-cell sensitization, and then we consider the interactions required between sensitized helper and effector cells, and finally, we consider the regulation of effector cell activity.

Regulation of Sensitization

Tissue Damage and Inflammatory Signals

Antigen-presenting cells require activation and/or maturation before they gain full APC function. These processes, as well as changes in chemokine and adhesion molecule expression and hence T-cell trafficking to target organs, are controlled by inflammatory cytokines, such as TNFα, IFN-γ, and IL-1. IFN-γ has a potent ability to activate macrophages to become effective APC and release chemokines (179). Tissue injury from any source is an important stimulus for releasing such cytokines and thus, the concept that a "danger" signal helps regulate graft rejection is important in transplantation immunology. All forms of transplantation involve ischemic and traumatic injury to the donor tissue, which may be one of the reasons that rejection episodes occur most frequently early after transplantation. In addition, later inflammation, either occurring in the transplanted organ or perhaps elsewhere in the body, may trigger late rejection episodes. On the other hand, it would be wrong to picture the role of nonspecific danger signals as the dominant feature controlling graft rejection. For example, skin or heart transplants placed on RAG1$^{-/-}$ recipients can be allowed to heal for long periods before immunologic reconstitution of the recipients, but rejection always occurs when this is done (180). Similarly, even achieving organ transplant survival for many years in clinical practice is rarely sufficient to allow the cessation of immunosuppression. Thus, it is better to picture the antigenic disparity and the recipient's immunoresponsiveness as the dominant features controlling graft rejection, while danger signals may influence the timing, intensity, or character of the rejection response. In the setting of allogeneic HCT, production of an inflammatory environment in GVHD target tissues by conditioning therapy probably plays a very significant role in increasing susceptibility to GVHD (see below).

Co-stimulatory Signals Involved in T-Cell Activation

The special features of APC involve not only their ability to present foreign antigens on their surface but also to provide additional signals for T-cell activation. This second component of T-cell activation is often referred to as the "second signal," although it more likely involves several different elements (181). The likely components of the "second signal" include the cytokines secreted by APC, including IL-12 and IL-1, and signals transmitted after binding of T-cell accessory molecules with their ligands on APC. These include the interaction of CD4 or CD8 with monomorphic determinants on MHC antigens; LFA-1 with ICAM-1, 2, or 3; CD2 with LFA-3 (CD48); CD40 with CD40 ligand; CD28 with B7.1 and B7.2; and the function of 4-1BB, ICOS, OX40, and other newly discovered co-stimulatory molecules (182). In addition, cytokines secreted by T cells and other cells, such as IL-2 and IL-15, may further contribute to the "second signal" for other T cells.

An important feature of the "second signal" is that in the absence of some or all of its components, T cells stimulated though their antigen receptor may be anergized (as discussed below in the section on tolerance induction). Since many of the cells of a transplanted organ are not APC, the induction of anergy would seem likely to be initiated after every organ transplant, a process, of course, in competition with the activation events stimulated by APC. Soon after transplantation, this competition probably favors APC activation since allograft rejection is almost universal, but the stimuli may be more evenly balanced months or years after transplantation when the donor APC have mostly been replaced by the recipient.

Down-Regulating Signals after T-Cell Activation

It has become increasingly apparent in recent years that cell-mediated immune responses are controlled by down-regulating interactions, such as by the ligation of CTLA-4 and by the interaction between Fas and FasL (183). In transplantation, there is evidence that high levels of expression of FasL on some or all donor tissue cells may prevent rejection and that FasL may be partly responsible for lack of rejection when tissues are transplanted to some "privileged sites," such as the testis or the anterior chamber of the eye (184). However, the overexpression of FasL has been shown to lead to a nonspecific inflammatory syndrome associated with prominent neutrophil infiltration (185). Thus, overexpression of FasL in pancreatic islets has tended to make them more susceptible to destruction rather than protect them from rejection. If the mechanisms by which FasL recruits neutrophils can be delineated and this complication avoided, overexpression of FasL alone might still not be successful as a strategy for inducing tolerance. FasL expression on donor tissues or cells would not eliminate recipient T cells recognizing donor antigens through the indirect pathway and, as is discussed above, there are significant indirect effector mechanisms for graft rejection.

CTLA4 is clearly important in the maintenance of self-tolerance, as evidenced by the T-cell lymphoproliferative autoimmune syndrome that develops in CTLA4 knockout mice. While CTLA4 has been shown to play a role in T-cell tolerance in several models (166), direct stimulation of this pathway has not been attempted as an approach to down-regulating alloimmunity. CD28 knockout mice have been found to reject allografts, despite unopposed signaling through CTLA-4 (186), indicating that the absence of CD28 signaling alone is insufficient to prevent rejection. Recently, PD1 has been identified as an additional down-regulatory molecule expressed by activated T cells, whose ligand is also a member of the B7 family. These findings suggest that an approach to preventing rejection might be to manipulate these molecular interactions, and it seems likely that a better understanding of the down-regulating events controlling immune responses will provide new approaches for preventing graft rejection in years to come.

Regulatory Cytokines

Many cytokines play a role in the regulation of graft rejection. However, since almost none of the cytokine or cytokine-receptor knockout mice have demonstrated a defective phenotype for graft rejection, it is impossible to describe more precisely that cytokines provide particular regulatory functions. It is usually assumed that IL-2 is important as a helper cytokine for effector T cells, but its role can apparently be replaced by other molecules, such as IL-15, which has the stimulatory activities of IL-2, but lacks the capacity to promote activation-induced cell death. IFN-γ is thought to play a role in activating other cells in the process of graft destruction and in up-regulating the expression of antigens, especially on donor vascular endothelium. However, graft rejection also occurs rapidly in IFN-γ knockout mice and IFN-γ has been shown to play a down-regulatory role in some models of GVHD and solid organ graft prolongation. While the mechanism by which IFN-γ inhibits graft rejection is not fully understood, this cytokine has been shown to have antiproliferative effects on CD4 T and CD8 cells (166), to up-regulate nitric oxide production, which has immunomodulatory properties, and to increase T-cell apoptosis via the Fas/FasL pathway. Studies in a GVHD model have shown that IFN-γ inhibits both CD4- and CD8-mediated GVHD, and mitigates the expansion of both T-cell subsets (167).

Several studies with anti-inflammatory cytokines, such as IL-10 or TGF-β, given either exogenously or via gene transfer, suggest that these may modify the process of graft destruction, while proinflammatory cytokines such as TNFα are thought to enhance the process (187). On the other hand, IL-10 can enhance cytolytic mechanisms of islet graft rejection (188). Both IL-10 and TGF-β have been suggested to be mediators of suppression mediated by regulatory CD4 T cells (see below). Studies of tolerance induction have suggested that in some cases shifts in the balance of Th1 and Th2 cytokines may be important in determining graft rejection versus acceptance. However, the difference in outcome based on Th1 versus Th2 production is far from clear, as has already been discussed. Thus, while cytokines are undoubtedly of enormous importance in causing and regulating the processes of graft rejection, our understanding of their role is quite limited at this time.

Presence of the Transplanted Organ

While early rejection episodes occur with most types of organ transplants, there are some exceptions to this rule. Kidney and liver transplants in mice can survive for long periods without immunosuppression even with MHC disparities, and there have been cases of prolonged liver transplant survival in pigs without immunosuppression. In addition, many types of rodent transplants, such as mouse heart transplants, require only a short course of immunosuppression to achieve prolonged survival. Furthermore, in the experimental animal studies, the long survival of these transplanted organs often diminishes, or even prevents, the subsequent rejection of antigenically identical skin grafts that would have been rejected rapidly by naïve animals. Even in clinical transplantation it appears that the long survival of a transplanted organ may diminish the rejection response, since much less immunosuppression is required late after transplantation than in the early period. Thus, there is substantial evidence that the mere survival of a transplanted organ generates a powerful regulating force that inhibits the specific antidonor immune response.

As discussed below, the induction of anergy, as donor grafts lose their APC, is one possible mechanism by which this might occur. However, it is also possible that down-regulating signals from the allograft, even potentially from allogeneic APC, or that changes in cytokine production contribute to the inhibition of graft rejection caused by the persistent survival of the organ.

There are two important features to emphasize regarding the capacity of transplanted organs to regulate their own survival. First, their capacity to do so often confuses the results of experimental studies designed to test tolerance-inducing strategies. For example, it is frequently reported that a particular form of immunosuppression induces tolerance when provided at the time of murine cardiac transplantation. While the result may be accurate, the conclusion that the form of immunosuppression employed leads to tolerance is not justified. The long survival of the transplanted heart, rather than the immunosuppression that achieved it, may be responsible for the tolerant condition. This issue can be tested by removing the transplanted organ to see if tolerance persists, or by testing the particular form of immunosuppression with other types of antigenic challenge from the donor. Second, it is important to understand that the processes that down-regulate graft rejection as a result of long-term graft survival may be inhibited by the standard forms of immunosuppression that are used clinically to achieve excellent graft survival. This is probably because many of the standard immunosuppressive drugs inhibit T-cell signaling and therefore inhibit active processes of tolerance induction. In other words, if T cells never learn that they have encountered donor antigens, they may not generate donor-specific mechanisms that inhibit graft rejection.

Communication between Helper and Effector Cells

APC play a role in regulating immune responses by serving as the focus for the interaction between helper and effector cells.

A Three-Cell Model of Helper and Effector Cell Interactions

An important tenet of fundamental immunology is that the cell–cell interactions that generate an immune response generally require intimate contact between the individual cells involved. Mitchison (189) demonstrated this principle in studies of the T–B collaborations leading to antibody production. He showed that T cells, B cells, and the APC that stimulate them must join together in a "three-cell cluster" to achieve effective collaboration between the helper T cells and effector B cells. Findings such as these have led to the concept that the cytokines involved in helper function tend to function like neurotransmitters, working only between two closely spaced cells, rather than as hormones acting over large distances.

In addition to Mitchison, others have performed experiments suggesting that the "three-cell cluster" model also applies to the interactions between helper T cells, effector T cells, and APC involved in graft rejection. For example, tail skin grafts from class I mutant mice (Bm7) placed on B6 recipients are not rejected, apparently because of a lack of helper stimulation. On the other hand, grafts from (Bm12 × Bm7)F1 mice, which express an additional class II–antigen disparity, are rejected. A Bm12 graft on one side of a B6 mouse, although itself rejected, does not induce the rejection of a Bm7 graft on the other side of the same animal, whereas a (Bm12 × Bm7)F1 graft on one side of a recipient does induce rejection of a Bm7 graft on the other side. These results suggest that the helper factors elicited during rejection of a Bm12 graft cannot function elsewhere in the body to assist potential effector cells specific for the Bm7 graft. On the other hand, when both the Bm12 and Bm7 antigens are expressed on the same graft, and therefore on the same APC, effector cells are generated that can function elsewhere in the body. As diagrammed in Fig. 13, it appears that the helper cells, effector cells, and the stimulating APC must join together in a "three-cell cluster" to allow efficient helper function for graft rejection. An attractive feature of the "three-cell model" is that it provides a mechanism for regulating the availability of help. Responses occurring elsewhere in the body, perhaps stimulated by environmental pathogens, will not generally initiate an immune response to the donor graft.

T-Cell Help for B-Cell Alloantibody Production

T-cell help for B-cell alloantibody production is an example in which several cell populations need to interact to achieve an immune response. Although it is commonly assumed that the B-cell production of antibodies to protein (usually MHC) antigens involves first the production of IgM antibodies, in a T-cell–independent process, and later the conversion to IgG antibodies, requiring T-cell help, studies of alloantibody production, at least after skin graft rejection, have actually suggested that even the initial IgM response also depends on CD4+ T cells (76). However, there are two potential pathways by which CD4+ T cells might provide help for alloreactive B cells (190). First, as diagrammed in Fig. 14, recipient CD4+ helper cells might recognize donor class II antigens directly while recipient B cells recognize donor class I MHC antigens. Alternatively, recipient CD4+ cells might recognize donor peptides presented by recipient APC through the indirect pathway, and then provide help to recipient B cells that recognize donor antigens directly. In the first case, the T and B cells would be in close physical association, but in the second case the T cells would interact with the B cells even more intimately, through their recognition of the B-cell's class II antigens presenting donor peptides. Experiments to examine these two possibilities have been performed using class II knockout mice as either donors or recipients and then testing alloantibody production. The results have indicated that there are two levels of help that can be provided by CD4+ T cells for B cells. First, the help provided by T cells brought into physical association with B cells through the direct pathway

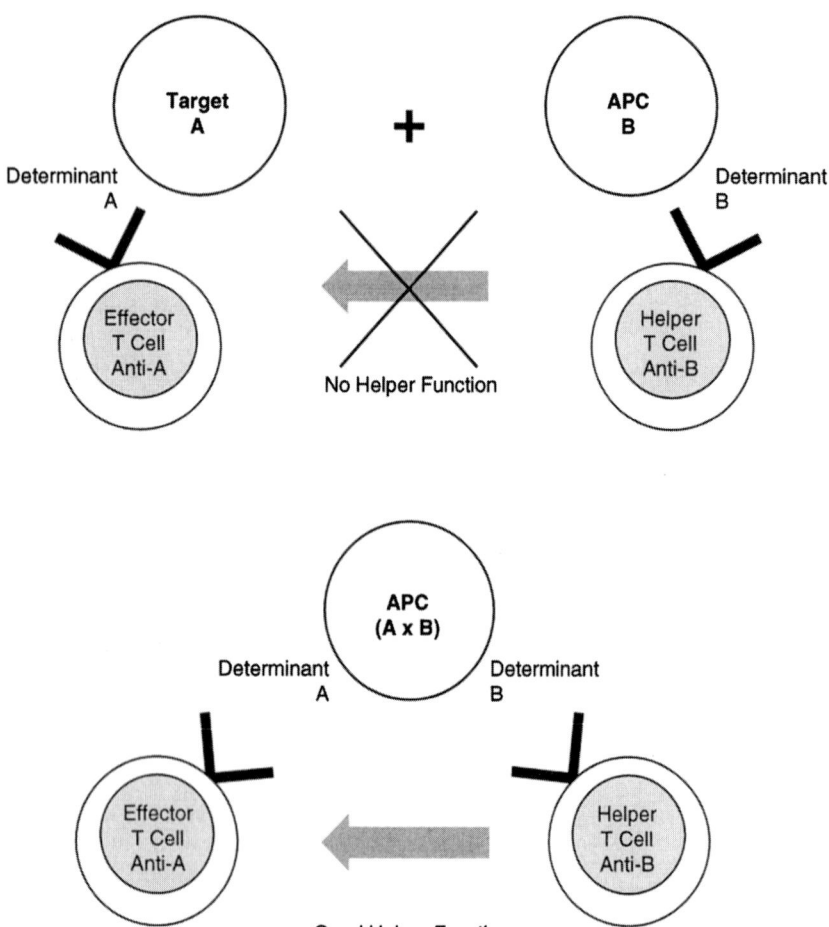

FIG. 13. Three-cell model of helper–effector interactions.

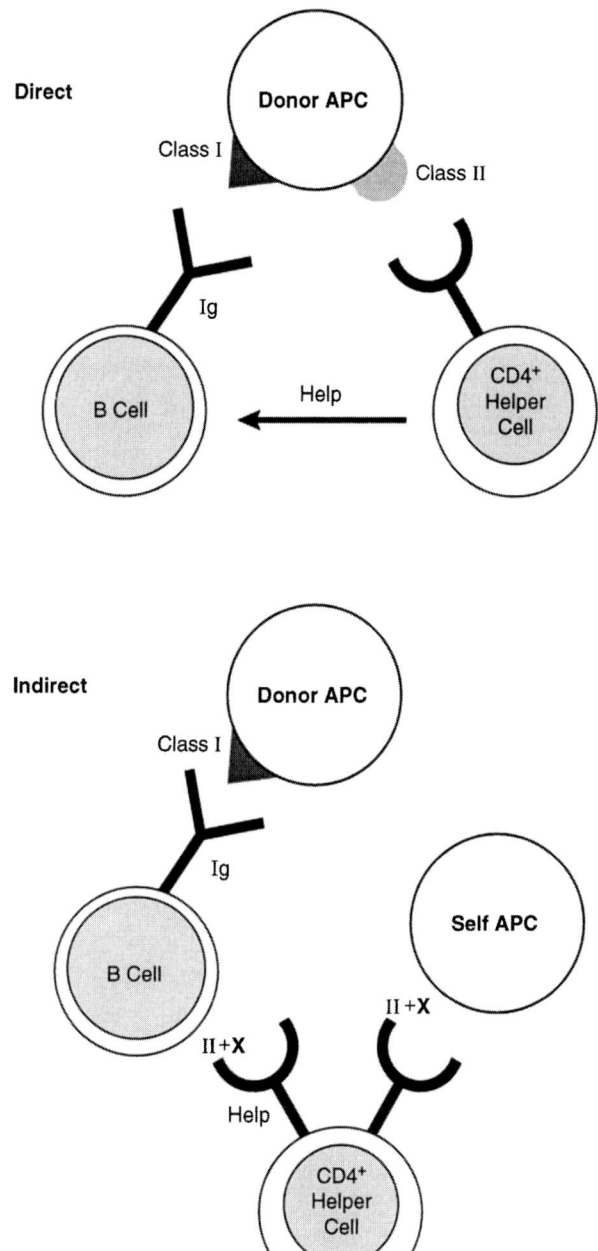

FIG. 14. T-cell help for B-cell alloantibody production.

allows B-cell IgM production. Second, the help provided by T cells sensitized indirectly allows B cells to produce IgM antibodies and to convert from IgM to IgG production. This class switching requires cognate help, which involves interactions between CD40L on the CD4 T-cell and CD40 on the B cell (191), as well as recognition by the CD4 cell of peptide antigen presented by class II molecules on the surface of the B-cell. B cells with Ig receptors specific for the donor antigen can most effectively focus the antigen for presentation to T cells recognizing peptides derived from these alloantigens. In addition to indicating the importance of the indirect pathway in this form of T-cell helper sensitization, these results also suggest that the conversion to IgG alloantibody produc-

tion can be used as a marker to demonstrate that indirect sensitization of CD4$^+$ T cells has occurred.

Can a "Four-Cell Cluster" Activate Effector T Cells?

It is easy to picture how donor APC, stimulating T-cell responses through direct presentation, provide the focus for a three-cell interaction during T-cell–mediated graft rejection, since donor APC can express both the helper determinants and the effector determinants necessary to bring the two T-cell populations together. On the other hand, when the indirect pathway for helper sensitization is considered, recipient APC will not necessarily express donor MHC antigens, and therefore will not generally express the same effector determinants that are present in the graft. Therefore, if an indirect helper response is to generate effector cells that recognize donor antigens directly, CD4$^+$ cells stimulated by recipient APC would have to provide help for CD8$^+$ cells that would be sensitized by donor APC. The "three-cell model" would not predict that productive helper–effector communication would occur under these circumstances. Nonetheless, while the evidence is clear that APC from one graft and APC from a second graft cannot work together, there is evidence that APC from a graft and APC from the recipient can join in a "four-cell cluster" with helper and effector cells to initiate graft rejection (135).

Effector Cell Regulation

The third level of regulatory interactions in graft rejection involves the effector cells after they have been sensitized by contact with donor antigens and been augmented by activated helper cells. Once activated, the effector cells appear capable of functioning anywhere in a recipient where they encounter donor antigens, in contrast to the limited range of helper function. Nonetheless, the function of effector T cells is controlled by regulation of the trafficking of effector cells and by the accessory molecules involved in the interaction of effector cells with their target cells.

Adhesion Molecules Regulate Effector Cell Trafficking

The regulation of lymphoid cell trafficking by adhesion molecules is one of the expanding areas of fundamental immunology (see Chapters 10, 14, and 26). A key feature of this regulation is that naïve T cells are kept within lymphatic tissues and that only activated or memory T cells are allowed to circulate into peripheral tissues. This pattern is controlled through the expression of L-selectin and its binding to the high endothelial venule (HEV) receptor PNAd on lymph node vessels, leading to rolling adhesion. Binding of the chemokine SLC to its receptor, CCR7, which is expressed on naïve T cells, then provides an inside-out signal that activates the T-cell's β2 integrin LFA-1 to mediate tight adhesion to the HEV, allowing egress into the lymph node and entry into the lymphatic circulation (192,193). In contrast to naïve T cells, activated/memory T cells lose L-selectin expression and a subset of memory cells (termed "effector memory" cells) do not express CCR7 (192,193). These cells do not enter the lymphoid tissue, and may enter nonlymphoid tissues, especially sites of inflammation, via expression of other adhesion molecules, such as VLA-4, cutaneous lymphocyte antigen (CLA), $\alpha 4\beta 7$ integrin, the functional form of PSGL1, and chemokine receptors such as CCR4, CCR5, CCR2, and CCR3 (192,193).

Expression of adhesion molecules and chemokines at the sites of inflammation controls the entry of cells into foreign tissues. Inflammation alters the trafficking patterns of lymphoid cells through the expression of P- and E-selectin, ICAM-1, ELAM, VCAM-1, and perhaps other adhesion molecules expressed on vascular endothelium (194,195). These molecules bind lymphoid cells, polymorphonuclear lymphocytes, and macrophages to sites of inflammation by halting their passage within vessels and stimulating the transmigration of these cells across the vascular endothelium. The expression of these adhesion molecules changes over time in response to various cytokines and other factors (194).

The cellular infiltrate associated with graft rejection is a special case of inflammation, and recent studies have investigated the unique features associated with allogeneic compared to syngeneic grafts. Both types of grafts show a cellular infiltrate during the first several days following transplantation, and both types express ICAM and ELAM adhesion molecules. By about the fourth day after transplantation, however, allografts can be distinguished from syngeneic grafts by the expression of VCAM-1 and the appearance of IL-2, IL-4, and IFN-γ. Further studies of this type may help to elucidate the regulatory elements of effector cell function in graft rejection. The pattern of adhesion molecule up-regulation in response to conditioning and BMT has not been well studied. Recently, up-regulation of ICAM-1 was demonstrated in the lungs following allogeneic BMT, along with a critical role for this adhesion molecule in the induction of post-BMT idiopathic pneumonia syndrome (196).

Role of Chemokines in Regulating T-Cell Trafficking in Graft Rejection and GVHD

The probable role of chemokines in controlling T-cell migration to grafted organs has been alluded to above. In the last few years, investigators have begun to examine the expression of chemokines in rejecting allografts (179) and in GVHD. These descriptive studies are consistent with a major role for this class of molecules in these processes. While there has been, to date, limited analysis of rejection and GVHD when specific chemokines or their receptors are blocked or in knockout mice, the few studies published to date are consistent with a major role for these molecules (196). Blockade of interactions of the chemokine macrophage inflammatory protein 1α (MIP1α) with its receptor, CCR5, on murine CD8$^+$ T cells, inhibited liver GVHD in one model (197). CCR5 expression on CD8 cells, but not on CD4 cells, appears to be important for their ability to

migrate into liver, lung, and spleen in murine GVHD (198). Of particular interest are studies involving mice deficient in the chemokine interferon gamma–inducible protein of 10 kD (IP-10), monokine induced by IFN-γ (Mig), or their receptor, CXCR3. These chemokine–receptor interactions appear to play a significant role in cardiac allograft rejection in mice, as donors deficient in the chemokines and recipients deficient in its receptor show graft prolongation or acceptance with minimal or no immunosuppressive therapy (199). In addition, CCR1 receptor–ligand interactions appear to play an important role in both acute and chronic rejection of cardiac allografts in mice (200). The chemokine fractalkine and/or its receptor CX(3)CR1 seem to also play a significant role in cardiac allograft rejection in rodents (201), and blockade of CCR5/ligand (MIP-1α and RANTES) interactions has led to significant prolongation of cardiac allografts in mice.

Target Cell Accessory Molecules and Effector Cell Function

In addition to altering cell trafficking, cell-surface molecules are important in controlling the interaction of effector T cells with their targets. The T-cell antigen receptor and CD3 proteins are naturally critical in this interaction. In addition, the CD4 and CD8 co-receptors, which bind to monomorphic determinants on MHC antigens, are important, as is the interaction of ICAM-1 with LFA-1. Of course these same molecules are also involved in the early stages of T-cell sensitization, but their additional role at the effector stage suggests that interruption of these interactions may alter graft rejection even after T cells have been activated.

MANIPULATIONS TO PREVENT GRAFT REJECTION

The importance of transplantation immunology lies ultimately in the application of its principles to clinical transplantation. Thus, the critical issue is to determine how the components and regulatory interactions involved in graft rejection might be manipulated to allow graft acceptance. One level of immunosuppression involves nonspecific approaches, reducing the overall immunocompetence of the recipient to all foreign antigens, and the second level seeks to prevent responses only to the antigens of a particular donor. Ultimately the goal is to achieve tolerance, which is lasting donor-specific nonresponsiveness.

Nonspecific Techniques

Standard Drugs

Reviewing the pharmacology of the nonspecific immunosuppressive drugs commonly used in clinical transplantation is beyond the scope of this chapter. It is important to realize, however, which the major advances in clinical transplantation have been made possible largely because of such agents. Most recipients of allogeneic organs receive exogenous immunosuppression in the form of combinations of several drugs, such as steroids, azathioprine, mycophenolate, cyclosporine, tacrolimus, or sirolimus. In general terms, both standard and experimental immunosuppressive drugs suppress immune responses by inhibiting lymphocyte gene transcription (e.g., cyclosporine, tacrolimus); cytokine signal transduction (e.g., rapamycin, leflunomide); nucleotide synthesis (e.g., azathioprine, mycophenolate mofetil); or differentiation (15-deoxyspergualin).

Corticosteroids have pleiotropic effects, including inhibition of T-cell proliferation and cytokine gene transcription (202). Azathioprine is an analog of 6-mercaptopurine that acts by inhibiting purine metabolism so as to block cell division. Mycophenolate mofetil is a prodrug of the active metabolite mycophenolic acid, which is related to azathioprine in its inhibition of purine synthesis. Its effect is limited, however, to the enzymatic pathways involved in lymphocyte proliferation, theoretically allowing normal development of other hematopoietic elements. However, significant side effects, including leukopenia, were observed in double-blind randomized trials comparing mycophenolate to azathioprine in renal allograft recipients. A significant reduction in rejection episodes, without any overall effect on early graft survival, was observed in the mycophenolate groups in these trials. CsA blocks the generation of IL-2 and other cytokines by T cells and thereby prevents sensitization (203). The discovery of cyclosporine played a major role in making cardiac and liver allotransplantation feasible, and it has become a mainstay of many immunosuppressive regimes. The complex of cyclosporine and its cytoplasmic receptor cyclophilin binds to and blocks the phosphatase activity of calcineurin, which is an intracellular signaling protein that is essential for transcriptional activation of the IL-2 gene. Tacrolimus is a macrolide that binds to a member of the intracellular FK506-binding protein (FKBP) family of intracellular receptors. The FK506-FKBP12 complex binds to and inactivates calcineurin, and thus has effects quite similar to those of cyclosporine. Sirolimus is a macrocyclic triene antibiotic somewhat analogous to FK506 (204). Despite binding to the same intracellular binding protein, FKBP12, as FK506, the FKBP12/rapamycin complex does not block calcineurin activity. Instead, sirolimus has a different ultimate target protein known as the mammalian target of rapamycin (mTOR), and it inhibits T-cell proliferation by blocking signal transduction mediated by IL-2 and other cytokines, not by inhibiting IL-2 production (204). Sirolimus has recently been approved for use as an immunosuppressive drug in combination with other agents.

In addition to the standard drugs for clinical transplantation, several other drugs are sometimes used. Cyclophosphamide is roughly equivalent to azathioprine in its effects at the doses used in transplantation. It is sometimes substituted for azathioprine to avoid particular side effects or with the hope of controlling B-cell responses. Prostaglandin E1 has been found to be immunosuppressive in some experimental models and it may reduce some of the toxicities associated with other agents. Actinomycin D inhibits bone marrow function and is used occasionally.

Experimental Drugs

The list of standard drugs will almost certainly be modified in the near future by the addition of drugs that are now considered experimental. 15-Deoxyspergualin is a distinctly different agent that has no effect on IL-2 production or utilization. It appears to prevent activated T and B cells from differentiating into mature effector cells. It is currently under clinical evaluation for rejection crises and for prophylaxis in highly sensitized patients. Leflunomide is an orally bioavailable prodrug that is converted to the active metabolite A77 1726, which has shown promise in treating acute and chronic rejection in animal models. It prevents lymphocyte proliferation both by inhibiting de novo pyrimidine synthesis and by inhibiting the activity of tyrosine kinases associated with cytokine receptors. Leflunomide can also prevent smooth muscle proliferation, and hence may be beneficial in preventing graft vasculopathy. Leflunomide has not only prolonged allo- and xeno-graft survival, but has also prevented the production of antidonor antibodies in animal models. Clinical trials are also in progress using a new immunosuppressive agent called FTY720. This drug has the unusual effect of altering T-cell trafficking, apparently in ways that prevent entry of the cells into donor grafts (205).

Anti–T-Cell Antibodies

Another form of nonspecific immunosuppressive therapy used both clinically and experimentally is that achieved with antibodies specific for T cells of the recipient. Originally, anti–T-cell antibodies were obtained from heterologous antisera prepared against lymphocytes or thymocytes of the recipient species. These powerful immunosuppressants are still used in some induction regimens and for the treatment of rejection episodes. Their major side effects include serum sickness and infectious complications. More recently, monoclonal antibodies such as OKT3, a mouse antibody directed against the CD3 antigen of humans, has been used in clinical transplantation. Like polyclonal sera, OKT3 is highly efficacious in reversing rejection episodes, and is also used in many centers in the first week or two post-transplant to prevent rejection episodes. Other pan–T-cell antibodies have been used in clinical trials, including CAMPATH-1, which causes prolonged and quite profound depletion of recipient T cells. The use of this antibody in combination with very low doses of other drugs has led some investigators to suggest that it allows the development of near-tolerance in transplant recipients.

Numerous experimental studies and a few clinical trials have explored the use of monoclonal anti–T-cell antibodies that are more selective for subpopulations of T cells. Subset-specific antibodies such as those recognizing CD4 or CD8 have helped define the pathways of alloreactivity in animal models, but it is unclear whether knowledge of these pathways could be used to predict accurately that antibodies will be effective clinically and under what circumstances. Monoclonal antibodies to the α chain of the IL-2 receptor (CD25) have been used in an effort to achieve greater antigen specificity with anti–T-cell antibodies. Because CD25 is only transiently expressed when T cells are activated, such therapy might selectively eliminate only those T cells activated at the time of allogeneic challenge. Clinical results using humanized versions of anti-CD25 antibodies have demonstrated that they are immunosuppressive, but they have not shown evidence of tolerance induction (206).

Monoclonal antibodies have also been used to block the effector mechanism of graft rejection. Anti-ICAM antibodies are immunosuppressive in monkeys and may function at the effector stage, and antitumor-necrosis-factor antibodies have also been tested experimentally. Agents that suppress T-cell co-stimulation via CD28 and/or CD40-ligand, and anti–CD2 mAbs have shown promise, particularly when given in combination, in animal models, and are undergoing clinical evaluation in some cases.

While monoclonal antibody therapy has been extremely effective (207), several problems still exist. First, the interaction of the monoclonal antibody OKT3 with the CD3 antigen initially activates T cells, stimulating release of several cytokines, before the target cells are depleted. Some of these cytokines, including TNFα, can cause significant clinical side effects, including fever, chills, and pulmonary edema. These side effects can usually be well controlled, and are seldom life threatening. Second, OKT3 and many of the monoclonal antibodies that have been evaluated in humans are mouse proteins. When these are injected, human recipients generally respond in time with antibody production against both constant region and idiotypic determinants of the monoclonal antibody (207). These antibody responses may hinder both repeated courses of therapy with the original antibody and treatment with other monoclonal antibodies of different specificity, although higher dose therapy can usually overcome a recipient's antibody response. Third, monoclonal antibody therapy may not always eliminate the target T-cell population. For example, during OKT3 treatment, cells of T-cell lineage expressing CD4 and CD8 antigens, but without the CD3 antigen, usually return to the circulation. This phenomenon is referred to as "modulation" of the target antigen (208). In the case of OKT3, the absence of the CD3 surface structure renders T cells immunologically incompetent. The loss of other surface antigens, however, may not be as immunosuppressive. Finally, OKT3 provides broad, nonspecific immunosuppression that renders the recipient significantly immunoincompetent. Although OKT3 does not cause permanent nonresponsiveness to environmental antigens, it unfortunately does not achieve permanent tolerance to the antigens of the graft either.

Many of the difficulties associated with monoclonal antibody therapy are associated with the constant region of the antibody. For example, T-cell activation does not occur when F(ab)'2 antibodies are used, and antiantibody responses by the recipient are much weaker in the absence of the constant region. Considerable effort has, therefore, been devoted to engineering ideal therapeutic antibodies. One approach has been to construct chimeric mouse antibodies with human Fc portions, or to graft the hypervariable (CDR3) component of a murine antibody to an otherwise human molecule. This latter process is known as "humanizing" a monoclonal antibody from another species. Another promising approach has been to couple toxic elements, such as ricin or diphtheria toxin, to the antibody (209).

Donor-Specific Tolerance Induction

The Need for Tolerance-Inducing Regimens

Specific immunosuppression in transplantation immunology involves suppression of the immune response to donor allo- or xeno-antigens but not to other antigens. The ultimate form of specific unresponsiveness is tolerance, in which donor-specific nonresponsiveness is maintained permanently without further treatment. Different workers define the state of tolerance differently: for some, a state in which a donor organ is accepted without immunosuppression, regardless of whether the immune system will accept other organs and tissues from the same donor (i.e., whether or not tolerance is "systemic" throughout the immune system), qualifies as tolerance; others define tolerance as a systemic state of immune nonresponsiveness to the donor. In both definitions, the recipient is capable of rejecting organs from a third-party donor, that is, the absence of rejection is specific to the donor. For the purpose of this discussion, we will define tolerance as specific acceptance of a donor organ, and will qualify the term as "systemic" when it applies to the entire immune system. Systemic tolerance is considered by some to be more reliable, since it seems less likely to be perturbed and cause graft rejection when environmental conditions change in the recipient, such as when a viral infection involves the donor organ.

The achievement of transplantation tolerance has been the goal of transplantation immunology for over 40 years, for three major reasons. First, while improvements in immunosuppressive therapy have dramatically increased the success of clinical organ transplantation, these drugs are associated with lifelong increased risks of infection and malignancy. Chronic drug treatment would not be required in tolerant recipients. Second, despite improved immunosuppression, chronic rejection is still a major problem, and leads to constantly down-sloping long-term survival curves for organ allografts. Chronic rejection is less likely to occur in tolerant recipients. Third, a critical shortage of allogeneic organs has increased interest in the use of other species as xenogeneic donors. However, immune barriers to xenografts may be even greater than those to allografts (210), and the induction of both B-cell and T-cell tolerance may be essential to the ultimate success of xenotransplantation.

Central and Peripheral Tolerance

The mechanisms by which tolerance to self-antigens is achieved are described in Chapter 29. For many developing T cells, these processes take place in the thymus, which is the central organ for T-cell development. Induction of deletional tolerance or anergy among developing thymocytes is referred to as "central," as distinguished from the "peripheral" tolerance that may develop among already mature T cells when they encounter antigen in the peripheral tissues. Peripheral tolerance may ensue as a consequence of the action of regulatory T cells recognizing the same antigen, or by other regulatory mechanisms, or by deletion or anergy. Peripheral tolerance mechanisms play an important role in tolerizing T cells that recognize tissue-specific self-antigens that may not be encountered in the thymus during T-cell development. However, a surprising number of antigens previously thought to be "tissue specific" and present only in the periphery have recently been found to be expressed in the thymus and to play a role in the induction of central tolerance.

B cells are also susceptible to tolerance induction by several mechanisms during development in the marrow. However, unlike T cells, the term "central" tolerance is not generally used in this context, largely because the marrow, the major organ for B lymphopoiesis in mammals, is not dedicated exclusively to this activity. B cells can also be rendered tolerant upon encounter with antigens in the periphery, as is discussed below.

Mechanisms of Transplantation Tolerance

The known mechanisms for inducing T- and B-cell tolerance can be grouped into the categories deletion, anergy, and suppression. In addition, a graft may simply be ignored by recipient lymphocytes. Each of these mechanisms is described briefly below, and a discussion of our current understanding of the role of the various mechanisms involved in particular strategies to induce transplantation tolerance follows.

Clonal Deletion

B Cells. Studies using Ig receptor transgenic mice suggest that B cells are susceptible to deletion at particular stages of development upon recognition of membrane-bound antigen (211). Antigen expression on either radio-resistant host cells or on a small population of hematopoietic cells appears to be sufficient to delete immature B cells specific for that antigen. However, more recent studies have indicated that receptor editing is an alternative mechanism that can result in a similar outcome without deleting the B cells. In this case, developing B cells with Ig receptors specific for self-antigens undergo further rearrangements of their receptors so that they no longer recognize self-antigens. Cells of the B1 subset, which are related to the subset of B cells that make the natural antibodies responsible for xenograft hyperacute rejection, can be deleted by an apoptotic process in mice when their surface Ig is cross-linked by cell-bound antigen.

T Cells. Most central T-cell tolerance occurs via a deletional mechanism due to recognition of self-antigens presented by hematopoietic cells and thymic epithelial cells (212,213). In addition, T cells recognizing self-antigens presented only by nonhematopoietic thymic stromal cells may be rendered anergic to such antigens. Antigens presented by thymic epithelium may also lead to the development of regulatory cells that recognize them and tolerize other T cells in the periphery (214,215). Deletion of self-reactive T cells is believed to occur when the avidity of an interaction between an immature thymocyte and an APC in the thymus is sufficiently high to induce apoptotic cell death (216,217). This high avidity is often due, at least in part, to a relatively high-affinity interaction between a rearranged TCR and a self-peptide/MHC complex presented in the thymus. TCR with lower affinity for such complexes are more likely to survive this process, and other mechanisms are required to prevent their activation in the periphery under conditions of, for example, inflammation and antigen up-regulation on normal tissues. Several hematopoietic cell types, including DC, B cells, and thymocytes, as well as nonhematopoietic cells of the thymic stroma (218), have the capacity to induce intrathymic tolerance by both deletional and nondeletional mechanisms. Transplantation tolerance induced by intrathymic deletion should be very reliable, since the absence of lymphocytes with reactivity to the donor would ensure that a specific response to donor antigens could not be induced under any circumstances.

Peripheral deletion has also been described for mature T cells upon exposure to antigen *in vivo*. Tolerance, with or without deletion, has been shown to occur following CD8 T-cell recognition of antigen expressed only in peripheral tissues in several models, and seems to be the natural consequence, under noninflammatory conditions, of re-presentation (i.e., cross-presentation) by lymph node DC of self-antigen expressed in parenchymal tissues to CD8+ CTL (219). Peripheral tolerization of CD4+ T cells recognizing antigens presented by parenchymal cells has also been reported to require re-presentation by hematopoietic cells (220). In this instance, the tolerance was due to anergy rather than deletion. Peripheral deletion of donor-reactive T cells has been demonstrated in a transplantation model involving BMT under cover of co-stimulatory blockade (221), or donor-specific transfusion with anti-CD154 mAb (222), and peripheral T-cell apoptosis has been implicated in a model involving tolerance induction with anti–CD154 mAb and rapamycin (223). Two distinct types of deletion have been reported to affect activated T cells: one, termed activation-induced cell death (AICD), is Fas dependent and promoted by IL-2; the second, termed passive cell death, occurs following IL-2 withdrawal, is Fas independent, and is blocked by Bcl-x_L expression (224). Early peripheral T-cell deletion in the model of BMT with co-stimulatory blockade has been shown to have features of both AICD and passive cell death (225), but passive cell death appears to play a more important role. AICD seems to play a critical role in tolerance induction with anti–CD154 mAb plus rapamycin (226). In addition, veto cells (see below) can delete alloreactive CTL precursors. Recently, a non-veto mechanism mediated by CD4⁻CD8⁻ cytotoxic regulatory cells has been reported to lead to the deletion of alloreactive CD8⁺ T cells with the same specificity as the regulatory cells (227).

Anergy

Anergy is a state that may result when T cells recognize peptide/MHC complexes, but without receiving adequate accessory or co-stimulatory signals. A lymphocyte is considered to be "anergic" if it cannot proliferate in response to the antigen for which it is specific. T-cell anergy has been associated with altered signaling and tyrosine phosphorylation patterns. Frequently, in the case of T cells, the anergic state is associated with a lack of IL-2 production, and can be overcome by providing exogenous IL-2 (181). However, a form of T-cell anergy has been described that is not overcome by exogenous IL-2 (228). Numerous methods of inducing T- and B-cell anergy have been described (181,211,229). In some cases anergy has been associated with TCR or Ig receptor down-regulation (211,230). In the case of B-cell tolerance, the induction of anergy versus activation may be dependent on antigen concentration (211). Anergy can also ensue upon recognition of autoantigen during B-cell development. Anergy may be the nondeletional mechanism responsible for the rapid tolerance of natural antibody-producing B cells in mice rendered mixed chimeric with bone marrow cells expressing an antigen for which natural antibody-producing cells preexist in the recipient (231).

T cells typically becomes anergic if they encounter antigen without co-stimulation, but they may also undergo anergy if they encounter peptide ligands for which they have low affinity (216,217). It appears that thymocytes (in addition to mature peripheral T cells) are also susceptible to anergy induction, and this can be induced by antigens presented on both hematopoietic and nonhematopoietic stromal cells. Anergy is generally reversible *in vivo* and can be overcome by infection or by removal of antigen, and therefore may not be as robust a form of transplantation tolerance as deletion. While deletion has been reported to ensue following the induction of anergy of T cells in the continued presence of antigen, this is not a universal outcome of anergy, and anergic T cells have been shown to persist for long periods of time in some systems. Anergic T cells have also been shown to have the capacity to down-regulate the activity of other T cells, so that they function as "suppressor" or "regulatory" T cells. This regulation may occur via conditioning of an antigen-presenting cell by an anergic T cell so that naïve T cells recognizing the same or different antigens on the same APC are also tolerized. This important effect may also explain the phenomenon known as "infectious tolerance" (see below).

Suppression

Various mechanisms suppressing T-cell and antibody responses have been described. Suppression mediated by antibodies and a number of different cell types has been described.

Idiotypes are unique antigenic determinants that characterize the binding sites of antibody or T-cell receptors. These determinants can be antigenic and induce the production of anti-idiotypic antibodies (232). Antibody-mediated suppression could theoretically occur through the recognition of idiotypes of antidonor Ig receptors. Anti-idiotypic antibodies can suppress antibody reactivity by directly binding to the antigen-binding site of the antibody, and the development of such antibodies has been suggested as one of the possible benefits of pre–kidney transplant blood transfusions. Such antibodies have also been suggested to contribute to the apparent hyporesponsiveness to noninherited maternal antigens in renal allograft recipients. In the past, it was also considered possible that anti-idiotypic antibodies might inhibit T-cell recognition of antigen, but this now seems unlikely, given that T cells recognize peptide/MHC complexes, whereas antibodies recognize epitopes of intact molecules. It continues to be an intriguing question whether normal regulatory mechanisms for B-cell responses might include anti-idiotypes, as suggested by Jerne. However, efforts to control transplantation using exogenous anti-idiotypic antibodies to either T- or B-cell receptors have been disappointing (233).

Antibodies can also induce tolerance through a process known as enhancement. Enhancement is defined as prolongation of graft survival achieved by the presence of antigraft antibodies (234). This phenomenon was first described in experiments involving allogeneic tumor growth. Subsequently, Stuart and colleagues and Batchelor (235) demonstrated that enhancing regimens using anti-MHC antibodies and/or soluble antigen could produce long-term tolerance for rodent allogeneic kidney transplants. The simple interpretation was that anti-MHC antibodies bind to the antigen and thereby block the immune response, but this explanation has not turned out to be sufficient. For example, tolerance following enhancement can be transferred by cells and not serum from enhanced recipients. Apparently, the administered antibody sets up a host reaction that leads to specific immunosuppression. An idiotype/anti-idiotype network would be an attractive explanation for this phenomenon. Unfortunately, the spectacular success obtained using enhancement for kidney graft survival in rats has not been observed for grafts in other species.

Cell populations may also mediate suppression. Suppression of T-cell responses has been attributed to both T cells and non–T cells, and may show varying degrees of specificity. In some instances, nonspecific suppressive effector molecules may be secreted in response to a specific antigenic stimulus, thus conferring apparent specificity. In the ensuing discussion, we categorize mechanisms of suppression in terms of the degree of specificity of their ability to suppress immune responses.

Nonspecific Suppression. Nonspecific suppression can result from secretion by cells, in a non–antigen-specific manner, of soluble molecules that down-modulate immune function. Such molecules include cytokines, nitric oxide, and prostaglandins. Nonspecific suppressive cell populations such as "natural suppressor" (NS) cells (236) have been reported to suppress mitogen responses, antibody responses, and T-cell alloresponses. NS cells have a "null" surface phenotype (i.e., do not express surface markers of T-cells, B-cells, or macrophages). CD4⁻CD8⁻ ("double-negative") T-cells expressing NK cell markers (NK/T cells) that have nonspecific suppressive activity fit into the "NS" cell definition. Activated NK cells have also been reported to have NS activity. Thus, it appears that several different cell types may mediate this activity. Soluble factors with widely varying physical characteristics have been reported to mediate NS activity. One of these has been identified as TGF-β. NS cells have been detected in normal bone marrow of several species, including humans, and are present in the setting of GVHD, in neonatal spleens and in the spleens of rodents treated with total lymphoid irradiation (TLI). Obviously, nonspecific suppressive mechanisms would only be of interest for tolerance induction if they could be induced temporarily during a critical period when alloreactivity was present. In the absence of mechanisms for ensuring specific tolerance, nonspecific suppressive cells offer no advantage over other nonspecific immunosuppressive therapies. Facilitation of specific suppressor cell development by natural suppressor cells has been described.

Veto Activity. "Veto" activity, which is the ability to inactivate CTLp reacting against alloantigens expressed on the surface of the veto cell (237), confers suppression of CTL responses directed against any antigens shared by the veto cell. CTL themselves, as well as activated NK cells and other hematopoietic cells, including CD34⁺ cells, have been found to have veto activity. While the mechanism of vetoing is poorly understood, in some instances it may involve signaling through the MHC class I molecule of the CTLp upon ligation by CD8 expressed on the veto cells. However, not all veto cells express CD8, so this mechanism cannot explain all veto phenomena. Veto activity has been suggested to involve the immunosuppressive cytokine TGF-β.

Antigen-Specific Suppression. The concept that regulatory T cells could suppress the reactivity of other T cells originated from the studies in the 1970s by Gershon (238), among others, who demonstrated the existence of complex regulatory networks involving several levels of T-cell–mediated suppression. Suppressor T cells were found to be CD8⁺, but the failure to identify additional markers, the failure to identify at the molecular level the I-J MHC locus reported to restrict suppressive activity, and the failure to discern clear-cut mechanisms of antigen recognition and presentation and of suppression itself, led to general disillusionment with the concept in the 1980s. During this period, however, functional evidence for the existence of alloantigen-specific suppressor cells was obtained in several transplantation models, and suppressive cells, including natural suppressor cells, NK/T cells, and CD8 cells were cloned in a few instances. In several instances, anti-idiotypic T-cell recognition by other T cells was implicated in mediating specific suppression of graft rejection, GVH responses (239,240) or autoimmunity.

In the last few years, the concept that regulatory T cells can suppress graft rejection and autoimmunity has undergone a renaissance. This began with the description of the T helper 1 (Th1) and T helper 2 (Th2) dichotomy of T-helper cell function (241). A shift to the IL-4– and IL-10–producing T-helper type 2 (Th2) type of response from a proinflammatory Th1 (IL-2– and IFN-γ–producing) response has been associated with allograft acceptance (242). Since Th1 and Th2 responses mutually down-regulate one another, these observations led to the hypothesis that Th2 responses are tolerogenic. Th2 responses may influence APC in a manner that prevents them from providing co-stimulation that could cause naïve T cells to differentiate into Th1 cells. Thus, the APC might serve as an important intermediary for this and other "infectious" forms of tolerance. For practical purposes, an immune response that is nondestructive and inhibits the development of destructive responses could provide a powerful means of ensuring graft acceptance. However, most of the data merely demonstrate an association of Th2-dominant responses with graft acceptance, and only limited data exist to implicate an active role for Th2 cells in tolerance induction. It is clear that Th2 responses are not always benign, as Th2 cells and Th2-associated cytokines can mediate or contribute to allograft rejection and GVHD. It has recently been suggested that the xenograft reaction in at least one species combination is associated with a predominant Th2-type response. However, Th2-associated cytokines have also been detected in accepted xenografts in which "accommodation" had occurred. Furthermore, the Th1/Th2 dichotomy of cytokine production is not always clear cut, and future studies are needed to better clarify the role of individual cytokines in inducing graft acceptance and rejection.

More recently, additional subsets of T cells have been described that produce cytokines which mediate a suppressive effect on other T cells. In fact, there are now so many partially characterized suppressive T-cell populations that it is difficult to deny the importance of regulatory phenomena in self-tolerance and regulation of autoimmunity, and in certain transplantation models. In contrast to the original description of suppressor cells as being CD8⁺, many of the recently described suppressive cell populations are CD4⁺. A subset of murine and human CD4⁺ cells (T regulatory cells 1, Tr1) that produces IL-10 but not IL-4 has been reported to suppress *in vitro* responses as well as inflammatory bowel disease *in vivo* (243). Production of TGF-β and IL-10 by T cells has been associated with suppression of autoimmune diseases induced by oral feeding of antigens (244). A population of human, mouse, and rat CD4 T cells that constitutively expresses CD25 and CTLA4 has been described and shown to regulate the development of inflammatory colitis, a variety of autoimmune phenomena, and *in vitro* alloresponses (243,245,246). Immature DC can support the *in vitro* development of IL-10–producing CD4⁺ regulatory T cells (247). The regulatory cells are themselves hyporesponsive to TCR-mediated stimulation, but, like "Tr1," can be grown slowly *in vitro* in the presence of certain cytokines, including IL-2. Unlike Tr1 cells, the *in vitro* suppressive function of CD4⁺CD25⁺ "Treg" may not be mediated by IL-10 and TGF-β, and the relationship, if any, between these cell types, is unclear. CD25⁺CD4⁺ cells generated by *in vitro* culture with alloantigen and anti-CD40L have been shown to be able to down-regulate GVHD, and CD25⁺CD4⁺ cells play a role in tolerance induced by a combination of donor-specific transfusion, depleting anti-CD4 mAb, and allogeneic heart transplantation in mice. The roles of CTLA4 and of the cytokines IL-4, IL-10 and TGF-β in mediating suppression by Treg are somewhat controversial, but there seems to be consensus that suppression requires cell-to-cell contact (245). In one murine system, the *in vitro* cell contact–dependent suppressive activity of Treg was reported to be mediated by cell-surface TGF-β expression. Both memory and naïve T-cell responses can be suppressed by these cells, which are themselves "memory" type on the basis of CD45 isoform expression. Although CD4 cells have been the most well-studied targets of this suppressive activity, these regulatory cells can also suppress CD8 T-cell reactivity. While the regulatory T cells show specificity for the antigen to which they are inducing suppression, the final effector mechanism of suppression appears to be non–antigen-specific. T-cell signaling through the cell fate determination receptor "Notch" has been reported to induce specific regulatory cell activity (248).

Treg are generated postnatally in the thymus (245,246), and their presence in insufficient numbers in neonatally thymectomized mice appears to be responsible for the development of multiorgan autoimmune disease in susceptible strains. CD4⁺ regulatory cells seem to be responsible for the tolerance induced by allogeneic thymic epithelial grafts placed in nude mice (249). One study suggests that Treg require an intermediate affinity ligand (too low for negative selection) expressed on nonhematopoietic cells of the thymus for their positive selection (245). Cortical thymic epithelium has been found to be the site of MHC class II expression required for the development of functional Treg (214).

NK/T cells are another subset of T cells with regulatory activity, possibly due to the production of Th2-type cytokines. The role of these cells in various transplantation models is discussed above in the section on NK/T cells. A double-negative, NK1.1-negative T-cell population that suppresses skin graft rejection by CD8 T cells with the same TCR has also been described in a TCR transgenic model (227), and the importance of this cell population in the setting of polyclonal T-cell responses remains to be determined. Human CD8⁺CD28⁻ T cells have been reported to suppress alloresponses and xenoresponses *in vitro*. The role of anergic CD4 T cells as suppressor cells has been discussed above. Thus, while multiple phenotypes and mechanisms of suppression have been described in recent years, much remains to be learned about their mechanisms, the conditions under that they are generated *in vivo*, and the relationships between the various cell populations.

Lymphocytes Ignoring Graft Antigens ("Ignorance")

Experimental situations have been described in which antigens are ignored by T cells (230) or B cells (211) that can recognize them. This may be due to the presentation of these antigens by "nonprofessional APC" that are unable to activate T cells, or it may reflect a failure of recipient T cells to migrate to the antigen-bearing tissue. The level of peripheral antigen expression, how recently the responding T-cell has emerged from the thymus (230), and the presence of proinflammatory cytokines and up-regulated co-stimulatory molecules within peripheral tissues may all influence the decision of a T-cell to ignore or respond to peripheral antigens. However, in contrast to a state of systemic tolerance, "ignorance" may be a more precarious state that can be upset by additional immunologic stimuli provoked by inflammation that may be induced, for example, by infections or by presentation of antigen on professional APC, as has been described for endocrine allografts that are depleted of APC prior to transplantation (61).

Strategies for Inducing Transplantation Tolerance

Strategies to Achieve Central Tolerance

Mixed Chimerism. The pioneering work of Owen, Medawar, and others, beginning more than 50 years ago, led to the observation that hematopoietic chimerism can be associated with a state of donor-specific tolerance (reviewed in Charlton et al. [250]). The capacity of hematopoietic cells to induce tolerance results largely from their ability to induce intrathymic clonal deletion of thymocytes specific for antigens expressed by the hematopoietic cells. Thus, bone marrow engraftment can reliably induce tolerance to the most immunogenic allografts, such as fully MHC-mismatched skin grafts and small bowel grafts. In view of this powerful tolerance-inducing capacity, it may seem surprising that hematopoietic cell transplantation has not yet been routinely applied to the induction of tolerance in man. However, bone marrow transplantation for tolerance induction in rodents has typically involved recipient treatment with lethal whole-body irradiation to eliminate mature recipient T cells and to make hematopoietic "space" for the marrow allograft. Removal of mature donor T cells before transplantation can prevent GVHD. Under these circumstances, a new immune system can develop that is tolerant to both donor and recipient antigens. While this approach has been successful in rodents, MHC-mismatched allogeneic bone marrow transplantation in larger animals, including humans, has proved to be less successful and more dangerous because of the high toxicity associated with myeloablative conditioning, and the inordinately high risks of GVHD and engraftment failure (251). Therefore, it will be essential to develop more specific and effective methods of overcoming the barriers to marrow engraftment with minimal GVHD risk before this highly effective approach to tolerance induction can be routinely used in patients. Achievement of this goal will require an understanding of the immunologic and physiologic obstacles to the engraftment and function of allogeneic and xenogeneic hematopoietic cells.

Cadaveric organ transplantation is often performed in the setting of complete or near-complete HLA disparity. It would be most desirable to achieve a state of mixed hematopoietic chimerism rather than full donor reconstitution in completely MHC-mismatched combinations. Three advantages of mixed chimerism over full chimerism are described below.

First, mixed chimerism can be achieved with less toxic (nonmyeloablative) conditioning regimens than those that lead to full donor chimerism. In addition to being less toxic, nonmyeloablative regimens allow recovery of host hematopoiesis, so that life-threatening marrow failure does not occur, even in the event that rejection of donor marrow occurs.

Second, compared to fully allogeneic chimeras, improved immunocompetence has been observed in mixed chimeras, which contain host-type APC in the peripheral tissues, presumably because these allow optimal antigen presentation to T cells that have developed in the host thymus, and that therefore preferentially recognize peptide antigens presented by host-type MHC molecules. Although the premise that hematopoietic cells do not participate in positive selection is controversial and has recently been challenged (252), studies of antiviral CTL responses in mixed chimeras showed exquisite specificity for recipient-derived MHC restricting elements (253).

In mixed chimeras, hematopoietic cells from both the recipient and the donor locate to the thymus and hence delete both host-reactive and donor-reactive T cells, resulting in a peripheral T-cell repertoire that is deleted of cells that recognize the donor or the host. Although nonhematopoietic thymic stromal cells have some capacity to induce deletional tolerance, the capacity of hematopoietic cells, especially DC, to do so, is particularly powerful. Thus, because there are host- as well as donor-derived hematopoietic APC in the thymi of mixed (but not full) chimeras, intrathymic deletion of host-reactive cells in addition to donor-reactive cells occurs in mixed chimeras to a greater extent than in full chimeras. While there are clearly other mechanisms by which host-reactive T cells can be tolerized in this setting, tolerance due to T-cell anergy can be broken under certain conditions, whereas T cells deleted in the thymus stand no chance of causing pathology under any circumstance. As might be expected, tolerance induced by intrathymic deletional mechanisms is systemic, as shown by both *in vivo* and *in vitro* studies (213).

In mixed chimeras prepared with a nonmyeloablative regimen consisting of low dose (3 Gy) TBI, T-cell depleting mAbs and thymic irradiation, systemic tolerance is reliably achieved (254). While anergy may play a role in tolerizing the few peripheral T cells that escape depletion with mAbs in this model, long-term tolerance appears to be maintained purely by a deletional mechanism. Administration of donor MHC-specific antibody to eliminate donor chimerism from established mixed chimeras leads to a loss of tolerance, and to the de novo appearance in the periphery of T cells with Vβ that recognize superantigens presented by the donor. However, if the recipient thymus is removed prior to elimination

of chimerism with antibody, specific tolerance to the donor is preserved, and donor-reactive TCR do not appear in the periphery (255). Thus, chimerism is needed *only* in the thymus and not in the periphery in order to ensure persistent tolerance. This is consistent with a purely deletional mechanism, since anergy and suppression generally require the relevant antigen to maintain the tolerance. The result also demonstrates that the thymus is sufficiently functional in senescent mice to generate donor-reactive T cells if donor antigen is not continuously present in the thymus. Since thymic APC are continually turning over, this emphasizes the need for true hematopoietic stem cell engraftment at sufficient levels in order to ensure an uninterrupted supply of donor APC in the recipient thymus for the life of the mixed chimera. The absence of suppressive tolerance mechanisms makes these animals particularly vulnerable to breaking of tolerance when nontolerant T cells emerge from the thymus after intentional depletion of donor antigen, or after exogenous administration of nontolerant host-type T cells (255).

Several approaches have been developed to permit the use of bone marrow transplantation to achieve mixed chimerism and specific tolerance. The use of total lymphoid irradiation (TLI) plus bone marrow transplantation has been studied extensively in rodents. The long bones are shielded during the radiation preparative regimen, so that bone marrow transplantation results in mixed chimerism rather than full donor reconstitution. While organ allograft tolerance has sometimes been achieved, TLI as the sole conditioning modality for BMT has only variably permitted the induction of mixed chimerism and tolerance in large animals, and this has often been associated with considerable toxicity (257). A trial of donor BMT with fractionated TLI in high-risk patients receiving renal allografts was not associated with chimerism, and significant toxicity was also observed (258). Mice treated in this way have been shown to be both resistant to GVHD and tolerant to skin grafts from donor but not third-party animals. The mechanism by which TLI induces this tolerance is incompletely understood and its success varies depending on the species involved. In rodent models, Th2-type responses appear to predominate when antigens are introduced following TLI, and this Th1 to Th2 shift may play a role in permitting graft acceptance. This cytokine shift may be facilitated by the predominance of NK/T cells (previously referred to as natural suppressor cells) detected in the lymphoid tissues of TLI-treated mice (236,259).

Mixed chimerism can also be achieved in rodents by administering a combination of T-cell–depleted syngeneic and allogeneic bone marrow cells to lethally irradiated recipients. Mixed bone marrow chimeras are fully immunocompetent (260) and are specifically tolerant to subsequent skin grafts from the donor (261).

In recent years, an evolving understanding of the minimal requirements for achievement of lasting chimerism have moved the mixed chimerism approach to tolerance induction toward clinical application. These requirements are summarized in Fig. 15, and their delineation began with the

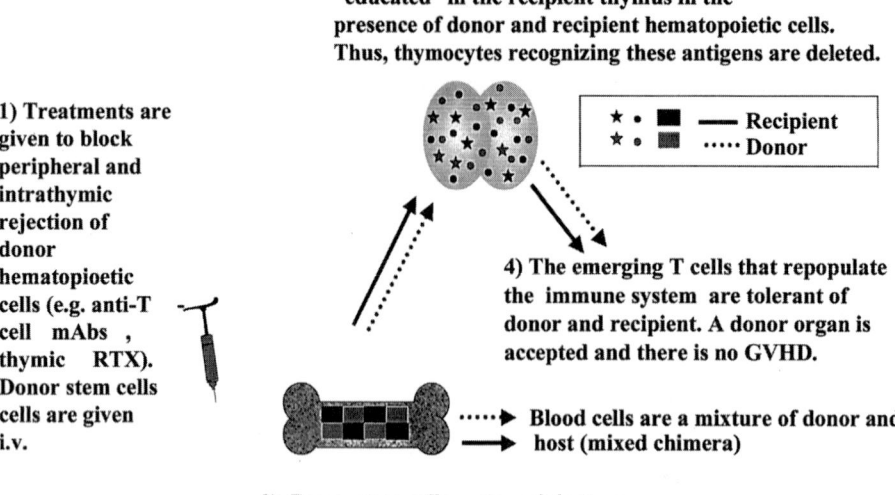

FIG. 15. Requirements for induction of long-term mixed hematopoietic chimerism.

demonstration that fully MHC-mismatched marrow engraftment and specific tolerance could be achieved by pretreating recipients with depleting doses of anti-CD4 and anti-CD8 mAbs along with a sublethal dose (6 Gy) of total body irradiation (TBI) (262) or even with a minimally myelosuppressive dose of TBI (3 Gy), if additional selective irradiation was given to the thymic area (referred to as "thymic irradiation" [TI]) (254). TI is needed to overcome residual alloreactivity that persists in the thymus, since mAb doses that effectively deplete peripheral T cells are insufficient to deplete alloreactive thymocytes (263). TI also creates some hematopoietic "space," leading to increased donor pluripotent stem cell engraftment, and additionally increases the intrathymic engraftment of donor thymocyte progenitors, which appears to be under separate regulation from hematopoietic "space." Because the conditioning regimen does not ablate the recipient's hematopoietic system, and hence is referred to as "nonmyeloablative," a state of mixed hematopoietic chimerism is achieved when allogeneic marrow engrafts. Recently, a number of modifications have made these conditioning regimens even less toxic. These include the replacement of TI with a second injection of depleting anti–T-cell mAbs, with pretransplant CsA treatment, or with a co-stimulatory blocker. Both TI and host T-cell depleting mAbs can be omitted by using co-stimulatory blockade. TBI can be omitted by administering very high marrow doses, and all preconditioning can be eliminated by giving a high dose of fully MHC-mismatched donor marrow followed by a single injection of each of two co-stimulatory blockers or repeated injections of anti-CD40 ligand. Apparently, the administration of very large hematopoietic cell doses can overcome the requirement to create "space" with myelosuppressive treatment in order to achieve marrow engraftment (264).

Several other regimens involving various combinations of anti–T-cell antibodies, irradiation, and immunosuppressive drugs, have also permitted the achievement of mixed chimerism in both large and small (264,265) animals. The successful induction of tolerance in a primate model using nonmyeloablative induction of mixed chimerism (265), combined with murine studies demonstrating the utility of mixed chimerism followed by delayed donor lymphocyte infusions (DLI) as an approach to achieving graft-versus-leukemia effects without GVHD (264) has been used as the basis for a clinical trial of mixed chimerism induction followed by DLI for the treatment of patients with hematologic malignancies (266). Success with this approach led to a pilot evaluation of combined kidney and bone marrow transplantation with this nonmyeloablative regimen in patients with renal failure due to multiple myeloma, which provided the first demonstration that transplantation tolerance could be achieved using nonmyeloablative allogeneic BMT (267).

The ability to replace recipient T-cell depletion with co-stimulatory blockade in the murine models is encouraging for several reasons. First, it has been difficult to achieve T-cell depletion with antibodies in large animals and humans that is as exhaustive as that achieved in the above rodent models, perhaps due to the use of inadequate doses or suboptimal reagents. A second concern is that, if sufficiently exhaustive T-cell depletion could be achieved in humans, T-cell recovery from the thymus might be dangerously slow, especially in older individuals. With increasing age, the adult human thymus becomes progressively more sluggish in achieving immune reconstitution after ablative treatments or with antiretroviral therapy in patients with HIV infection (reviewed in Haynes et al. [268]). However, it is also clear that normal adults do have thymic function, even in old age (268), and the capacity for regeneration and "rebound" thymopoiesis in an individual whose thymus has not been subjected to injury by the above agents is largely unknown. Nevertheless, it would clearly be desirable to minimize the degree and duration of T-cell depletion used in protocols for the induction of mixed chimerism. The ability to do this by replacing some or all (264) of the T-cell–depleting antibodies with a single injection of co-stimulatory blockers is therefore of considerable interest.

While long-term tolerance is maintained by intrathymic deletion in mixed chimeras prepared with co-stimulatory blockade (264), the mechanisms of initial tolerance in animals receiving BMT under cover of co-stimulatory blockade instead of T-cell depletion are not fully understood. Large numbers of alloreactive T cells present in the peripheral lymphoid tissues of these animals must be tolerized. Peripheral deletion of donor-reactive cells through a combination of activation-induced cell death and "passive cell death" appears to play a role. However, donor-specific tolerance is complete in mixed lymphocyte reactions by 1 week posttransplant, when deletion of donor-reactive CD4 cells is only partial (264), suggesting that mechanisms in addition to deletion are involved in the early tolerization of peripheral CD4 cells by donor bone marrow in the presence of co-stimulatory blockade.

Although attractive because they do not require host T-cell depletion, one limitation to the use of co-stimulatory blockade in place of peripheral T-cell depletion to achieve allogeneic bone marrow engraftment is that it is not 100% successful, that is, a fraction of animals fails to achieve permanent chimerism or donor-specific skin graft acceptance. Either CTLA4Ig or anti-CD154 mAb overcame the requirement for thymic irradiation in mice receiving a T-cell depletion regimen that was in itself insufficient to permit induction of lasting chimerism. In fact, a single injection of anti-CD40L mAb is sufficient to allow BMT to induce tolerance of CD4 cells in mice receiving an injection of depleting anti-CD8 mAb. The anti-CD40L mAb is required only to block the interaction between CD40L and CD40, and not to target activated T cells for depletion or to signal to the CD4 cell (264). These results indicate that CD4 cell–mediated alloresistance to bone marrow grafts is exquisitely dependent on CD40-CD40L interactions. This is somewhat surprising, since CD40-independent pathways can activate APC to induce antiviral CD4 cell responses. Much remains to be learned about the mechanisms by which CD4 T cells are tolerized to alloantigens when APC activation via CD40 is blocked.

GVHD does not occur in the rodent models discussed above, despite the use of unseparated donor bone marrow cells (BMC). This is most readily explained by the continued presence of the T-cell–depleting or co-stimulatory blocking antibodies in the serum of the hosts at the time of BMT (269). These levels are sufficient to prevent alloreactivity by the relatively small number of mature T cells in the donor marrow.

Gene Therapy of Autologous Marrow for Induction of Tolerance. An alternative to using allogeneic hematopoietic engraftment to achieve tolerance is to reconstitute recipients with autologous bone marrow cells that have been transduced with genes encoding foreign transplantation antigens. This approach has permitted markedly prolonged survival of class I–disparate skin grafts bearing the class I gene that was introduced into the autologous marrow. If the genes selected encode particularly important antigens (such as those determining class II antigens), then tolerance to these antigens may have a significant effect on the rejection of subsequent grafts expressing these and other transplantation antigens, and may lead to transplantation tolerance (270). In fact, fully MHC-mismatched allogeneic kidneys are accepted with a 12-day course of cyclosporine in miniature swine that have been lethally irradiated and reconstituted with autologous marrow transduced with a donor class II molecule.

Extension of Mixed Chimerism Approach to Xenotransplantation. Host treatment with mAbs to T cells and NK cells along with sublethal irradiation has also permitted rat marrow engraftment in mice, resulting in mixed xenogeneic chimerism and donor-specific tolerance. Both $\gamma\delta$ T cells and NK cells play a very significant role in rejecting rat marrow, but not allogeneic marrow, in mice (218). Once mixed chimerism is achieved in the rat-to-mouse species combination, donor-specific tolerance is observed at the level of both T cells and B cells (104,271). Despite this complete T- and B-cell tolerance, the levels of donor chimerism decline gradually over time. One explanation for this decline is the competitive advantage of autologous marrow over xenogeneic marrow in nonmyeloablated hosts. A competitive advantage of recipient mouse marrow over xenogeneic rat marrow has been demonstrated and shown to become increasingly evident as recovery of the host from low-dose TBI occurs. Species specificity or selectivity of cytokines, adhesion molecules, and other signaling molecules probably account for this advantage.

Although chronic host NK cell depletion did not mitigate the gradual decline in rat chimerism in mice (271), this does not prove that host NK cells are tolerized to the xenogeneic donor, since the competitive disadvantage of rat marrow discussed above may overshadow the effect of chronic NK cell–mediated rejection. The question of whether newly developing NK cells are tolerized by induction of mixed chimerism is especially relevant to xenotransplantation. Although this question has not been addressed in xenogeneic chimeras, it is relevant to discuss what has been observed in mixed allogeneic chimeras. NK cell tolerance in mixed allogeneic chimeras might require that each individual NK cell express inhibitory receptors for two completely disparate sets of MHC molecules on donor and host cells. However, observed changes in the expression of Ly-49 receptors among donor and host NK cells of mixed allogeneic chimeras are not consistent with such a mechanism. The presence of the MHC ligand (on hematopoietic or nonhematopoietic cells) for a given Ly-49 receptor leads to an antigen dose–related reduction in the level of that receptor on donor and host NK cells (83,264), suggesting that Ly-49 receptors are down-modulated by interactions with their ligand, rather than being calibrated to a specific level, as has been suggested (272). *In vitro* cytolytic assays showed a lack of tolerance of donor and host NK cells from mixed chimeras to the host and donor, respectively, but these results are at variance with *in vivo* studies demonstrating NK cell tolerance in mixed chimeras (272a), irradiation chimeras, and mice with mosaic expression of an MHC transgene (Tg) (82,83). *In vitro* studies of NK cells from mice with mosaic expression of a class I MHC transgene showed that the continued presence of cells lacking the transgenic MHC antigen was essential for the maintenance of this *in vitro* unresponsiveness (82). Thus, a better understanding of the level and nature of NK cell tolerance in mixed allogeneic and xenogeneic chimeras is needed.

Achievement of xenogeneic hematopoietic repopulation has proved to be an even more formidable challenge in highly disparate (discordant) species combinations. Hematopoietic function depends on interactions between adhesion molecules and their ligands, and on a number of specific molecular interactions between the stroma and hematopoietic cells. Human and pig progenitor cells have been shown to be capable of repopulating murine recipients at low levels, but the species specificity of critical regulatory molecules may be limiting. Administration of exogenous donor species–specific cytokines can partially overcome this barrier, and high levels of porcine hematopoietic stem cell engraftment have been achieved in immunodeficient mice transgenically expressing the porcine hematopoietic cytokines IL-3, stem cell factor, and GM-CSF (273). Macrophages also play a significant role in resisting engraftment of xenogeneic marrow from highly disparate species (274,275), and it seems likely that these and other cellular components of the innate system recognize foreign lipids and carbohydrates on highly disparate xenogeneic cells via specific receptors.

Pigs are widely believed to be the most suitable xenogeneic donor species for transplantation to humans, but transplantation from this species is impeded by the presence in human sera of Nab that cause hyperacute rejection of porcine vascularized xenografts. In humans, the major specificity recognized by Nab on porcine tissues is a ubiquitous carbohydrate epitope, αGal. Humans lack a functional α1-3Gal transferase (GalT) enzyme, as do GalT knockout mice, which also make anti-αGal Nab. Both preexisting and newly developing B cells producing anti-αGal antibodies are tolerized by the induction of mixed chimerism in GalT knockout mice receiving αGal-expressing allogeneic or xenogeneic marrow (264). The induction of mixed xenogeneic chimerism prevents hyperacute rejection, acute vascular rejection, and cell-mediated rejection of primarily vascularized cardiac xenografts (104). Long-term mixed xenogeneic chimeras produced in GalT knockout mice lack anti-αGal

surface-Ig–bearing cells in the spleen, and show tolerance in ELISPOT assays (264,276). Thus, mixed xenogeneic chimerism has the capacity to tolerize xenoreactive T cells, antibody-producing cells, and possibly NK cells.

Xenogeneic Thymic Transplantation. Because of the difficulties encountered in inducing xenogeneic hematopoietic cells to migrate to a recipient thymus and induce central tolerance, an alternative approach might involve replacement of the recipient thymus with a xenogeneic donor thymus after host T-cell depletion and thymectomy. Immunocompetent mice treated in this way demonstrate recovery of CD4$^+$ T cells in xenogeneic porcine thymic grafts (277). These cells repopulate the periphery, are competent to resist infection (278), and are tolerant of donor antigens in MLR, and even by the stringent measure of xenogeneic porcine skin grafting. Tolerance to both donor and host develops, at least in part, by intrathymic deletional mechanisms in these animals, and this reflects the presence of class II high cells from both species within the thymic graft (278). Since MHC restriction is determined by the MHC of the thymus, it is surprising that T cells which differentiated in a xenogeneic thymus are able to respond to peptide antigens presented by host MHC. Using TCR transgenic mice on selecting and nonselecting MHC backgrounds, it has been demonstrated in mice receiving porcine thymic transplants that positive selection is mediated only by porcine thymic MHC, with no influence of the murine class II$^+$ cells that are detectable in the grafts (279). However, the excellent immune function achieved in these mice and in humans receiving HLA-mismatched allogeneic thymic transplantation for the treatment of congenital thymic aplasia (DiGeorge syndrome) (280), suggests that "restriction incompatibility" may not be a major obstacle to the achievement of adequate immune function. Perhaps this high level of cross-reactivity, even between species, reflects the fact that MHC reactivity is inherent in unselected TCR sequences (281). Recently, it has been demonstrated that human T cells can be rendered specifically tolerant of the porcine donor during development in xenogeneic porcine thymus tissue grafted to immunodeficient mice (282). Thus, xenogeneic thymic transplantation has promise as an approach for the induction of T-cell tolerance across species barriers, and efforts to extend this approach to a pig-to-primate model are underway (see below).

Transplantation of allogeneic and concordant xenogeneic thymic tissue obtained from fetuses before the time that hematopoietic cells have seeded the organ can also induce a form of tolerance that permits skin graft acceptance. However, the mechanism of tolerance in such animals is unlikely to be deletional, as donor-specific mixed lymphocyte reactions are preserved. Active suppression has been implicated in the allogeneic model (283), and studies in the pig to mouse thymic transplantation model described above also suggest a possible role for suppression. Transplantation of xenogeneic thymic tissue into congenitally athymic recipients has frequently resulted in the development of a multiorgan autoimmune syndrome, possibly due to the lack of recipient-type thymic epithelium needed for the development of regulatory cells with specificity for certain antigens (214). This complication occurs much less frequently in thymectomized, T-cell–depleted mice receiving porcine thymic transplants (278), possibly due to the persistence of regulatory cells derived from the host thymus prior to thymectomy and T-cell depletion.

Development of Chimerism and Tolerance without T-Cell–Depleting or Myelosuppressive Treatment

Developmentally immunoincompetent recipients. In theory, fetuses might be permissive for engraftment of allogeneic hematopoietic stem cells, not only because of their immunologic immaturity, but because "space" might be available in their hematopoietic systems, so that engraftment could be achieved without host conditioning. Since prenatal diagnosis of a number of congenital diseases has become possible, there is renewed interest in the possibility of injecting allogeneic or xenogeneic PHSC to preimmune fetuses. Intrauterine injection of allogeneic hematopoietic stem cells has been used successfully to correct immunodeficiency diseases diagnosed in utero in human fetuses (284). However, chimerism was only detected in the T-cell compartment afflicted by the congenital deficiency, and not in other hematopoietic lineages. In view of this result and the observation of only low levels of chimerism in preimmune normal mouse fetuses and sheep receiving in utero transplants (285), the concept that hematopoietic "space" is present in preimmune fetuses is open to question. Co-administration of donor stromal cells may enhance xenogeneic hematopoiesis induced by such injections (286). In a large animal model, successful engraftment of enriched human PHSC populations has been successfully achieved without GVHD (287), raising hopes that this approach could be used for a broader spectrum of disorders in human fetuses. However, the ability of in utero HCT to induce transplantation tolerance has been somewhat unpredictable (288).

Untreated neonatal rodents can be rendered tolerant of alloantigens by the administration of allogeneic hematopoietic cells shortly after birth. The mechanisms responsible for this phenomenon of "neonatal tolerance" are slowly being unraveled. Lasting microchimerism and even sufficient levels of chimerism for flow cytometric detection have been observed in some neonatally tolerized mice, and evidence to support both intrathymic and extrathymic deletional mechanisms has been obtained in some, but not other, strain combinations (289). Furthermore, the presence of microchimerism does not always predict skin graft tolerance in recipients of allogeneic lymphocytes perinatally, and nontolerant animals can still maintain microchimerism following rejection of donor skin grafts. Thus, it is not surprising that several additional mechanisms have been implicated in rodents in which neonatal tolerance has been induced. First, tolerance cannot be easily broken by the infusion of nontolerant host-type lymphocytes in neonatally tolerized animals (239,289), and this has been attributed to the presence of suppressive T-cell populations (239). The ability of neonates to mount

host-anti-graft responses may be essential for the induction of these suppressive cell populations when donor antigen is given. In contrast, when deletional tolerance is induced in animals in which the preexisting peripheral T-cell response has been fully ablated (e.g., mixed chimeras prepared with the myeloablative or nonmyeloablative regimens described above), the absence of suppressive cell populations makes it easy to abolish tolerance by the infusion of nontolerant host-type lymphocytes (290). Second, neonatal mice have a tendency to produce Th2 responses, and these have been implicated in donor-specific skin graft acceptance (168). However, neonatal mice are capable of mounting CTL and Th1 responses under certain conditions. Third, the ability of allogeneic spleen cell infusions to induce tolerance has been suggested to reflect the high ratio of non–co-stimulatory APC (T and B cells) in donor inocula to recipient T cells in the neonate, rather than to any unique susceptibility to tolerance induction (291).

Adult recipients. Based on the recent observation that microchimerism can exist for many years in the tissues of human recipients of solid organ allografts recipients who did not receive hematopoietic cells transplants, it has been hypothesized that microchimerism, resulting from emigration of passenger leukocytes from the graft to recipient tissues, leads to a state of donor-specific tolerance (292). However, this hypothesis is controversial (293), and it is currently unclear whether microchimerism induces tolerance or is even an epiphenomenon that reflects either tolerance or adequate immunosuppressive pharmacotherapy. "Microchimerism," which requires highly sensitive techniques for its detection, should be distinguished from the mixed chimerism discussed above, in which multilineage chimerism is readily measurable by flow cytometry.

There are several mechanisms by which microchimerism might, in theory, induce peripheral T-cell tolerance. These include nonprofessional APC function of donor-derived B or T cells that can tolerize responding T cells. In addition, veto activity of T cells, NK cells, and other cell types eliminates CTL reactive against antigens expressed on the veto cells (294). In addition to these mechanisms by which chimerism might induce peripheral tolerance, donor leukocytes migrating to recipient thymi might induce central tolerance among T cells that develop subsequent to the time of donor engraftment. Recent evidence shows that adult rodent liver grafts contain self-renewing hematopoietic stem cells (295), and DC progenitors have been detected in the marrow of mice that spontaneously accept mouse liver allografts.

Numerous attempts have been made to demonstrate a relationship between microchimerism and tolerance. However, lasting microchimerism does not appear to play a role in several animal models of tolerance in which the issue has been carefully examined, and tolerance is by no means ensured in the presence of microchimerism. It has also become increasingly clear in humans that microchimerism neither denotes a state of tolerance nor is required to maintain an allograft under all circumstances (293).

Recently, several groups have evaluated the ability of donor bone marrow cell infusions given without recipient myelosuppression or T-cell depletion to enhance graft survival. Such transplants can be associated with significant risks from possible immunosuppressive effects of the transplant and from GVHD. The administration of donor marrow with solid organ allografts with standard chronic immunosuppressive therapy has augmented microchimerism. While no significant impact on acute rejection episodes or immunosuppressive medication doses were observed, the incidence of chronic renal allograft rejection was significantly reduced upon longer follow-up in one of these series (296). Of note, the level of donor chimerism, while low, increased over time following the transplant in patients who did not have rejection episodes (296).

These studies did not include intentional peripheral T-cell depletion of the hosts. In a primate model that includes recipient pretreatment with antilymphocyte serum for T-cell depletion, and, for optimal results, total lymphoid irradiation, veto cells in donor bone marrow that inactivate recipient CTLp may promote graft acceptance. However, only a fraction of recipients show long-term graft acceptance, with the best results obtained when the donor and recipient share a DR class II MHC allele (297).

In the primate bone-marrow transplantation model described in the preceding paragraph, no myelosuppressive treatment was included in the host-conditioning regimen, and, not surprisingly, only very low levels of chimerism were detected. In contrast, macroscopically detectable, though transient, chimerism has been observed in an otherwise similar primate model that includes a sublethal dose of host irradiation (265). The concept that myelosuppression must be used to create "space" in the hematopoietic compartment in order to allow donor hematopoietic cells to engraft has long been widely accepted. The mechanism by which myelosuppression promotes marrow engraftment is not fully understood, and could include both the creation of physical niches due to the destruction of host hematopoietic cells, and the up-regulation of cytokines that promote hematopoiesis. In syngeneic BMT recipients, a low dose of total body irradiation is required to make physiologic "space" for engraftment of syngeneic marrow cells given in numbers similar to those that could be obtained from marrow of living human allogeneic marrow donors. However, this requirement can be overcome by the administration of very high doses of syngeneic marrow. Furthermore, engraftment of high doses of allogeneic marrow can be achieved without myelosuppressive treatment in mice that receive T-cell–depleting mAbs or co-stimulatory blockade. This approach has been successfully extended to a full haplotype-mismatched porcine model (264). Importantly, these studies demonstrate that multilineage mixed chimerism and lasting, systemic deletional tolerance can be achieved without requiring recipient T-cell depletion or myelosuppression. Greatly increased stem cell doses can be obtained clinically following repeated phereses of G-CSF–treated donors. However, additional measures, such as

techniques for *in vitro* expansion of PHSC, might be necessary to practically allow administration of PHSC doses of the same magnitude as those used in the animal studies that exclude chemotherapy and irradiation.

Strategies to Achieve Peripheral Tolerance

There are numerous animal models in which peripheral T-cell tolerance has been induced, generally by mechanisms that are not fully understood. Evidence for anergy has been obtained in a few models, and recently, a role for regulatory cells has been found in many (see below). Some of these models were discussed above in the descriptions of the various mechanisms of tolerance induction. In the following, we discuss some of the strategies being evaluated for the induction of peripheral tolerance, and consider what is known about the mechanisms involved. The discussion is by no means inclusive of all approaches to achieving graft acceptance. It should be borne in mind by the reader that many of the strategies for inducing "tolerance" to primarily vascularized rodent allografts such as hearts and kidneys rely heavily on the capacity of the organ graft itself to induce tolerance, and that the tolerance thereby achieved is not systemic. Most of these tolerant states do not extend to the more stringent test of primary skin allografting. Since there are major differences between rodents and large animals in the biology of such grafts, perhaps due in part to the constitutive expression of class II MHC on endothelia of large animals but not rodents, many of the strategies that are effective for primarily vascularized allografts in rodents do not translate readily into tolerance in large animals and humans. Thus, a thorough understanding of the mechanisms involved in tolerance induction and successful extension to large animal models are important criteria to fulfill before these approaches can be attempted in humans as a substitute for chronic immunosuppressive therapy.

Donor-Specific Transfusion (DST) or Administration of Autologous Cells Transduced with Allogeneic MHC Genes. DST and donor antigen-transduced recipient cells have a limited capacity to induce tolerance across certain histocompatibility barriers in rodents. Numerous mechanisms have been implicated in this phenomenon, some of which were discussed above. DST and donor MHC gene-transduced recipient cells (298) used in combination with partially depleting anti-CD4 mAb and cardiac allografting more effectively induce tolerance to donor hearts. Administration of autologous bone marrow transduced with a single donor MHC antigen appears to allow induction of tolerance to other antigens expressed by the cardiac allograft donor in untreated and anti-CD4 mAb–treated mice (299), and similar observations have been made in lethally irradiated miniature swine receiving donor kidneys after reconstitution with autologous marrow transduced with a donor class II gene (133). The mechanisms of tolerance in the murine DST recipients have been shown to involve regulatory CD4 cell populations that are also capable of suppressing donor-specific indirect alloresponses *in vitro* (300). The Th2 cytokine IL-4 has been shown to play a limited role in the T-cell–mediated regulation in this model, but IL-10 appears to be critical for the function of the CD4$^+$CD45RB^{low} regulatory cell population (300). The fact that transduced autologous marrow is superior to donor-type marrow at inducing tolerance in the murine model (133) may reflect the power of regulatory mechanisms to tolerize T cells recognizing donor antigens through the indirect pathway when donor and recipient antigens are expressed on the same APC. Linked suppression from T cells recognizing donor antigens directly to those recognizing them indirectly may likewise explain the ability of haplo-identical, but not fully mismatched, allogeneic APC-depleted kidney grafts to induce tolerance in rats (301).

Co-stimulatory Blockade, With or Without Infusion of Donor Cells. Attempts to induce tolerance in transplantation models have included the introduction of alloantigen on non–co-stimulatory APC, such as cells whose antigen-presenting activity has been impaired by ultraviolet irradiation. It is possible that donor-specific transfusions facilitate tolerance induction (298) because of their resting B-cell and T-cell contents, both of which may be non–co-stimulatory, and can present antigen in a manner that induces tolerance. Efforts to induce tolerance by blocking the B7/CD28 co-stimulatory pathway have enjoyed success in animals receiving vascularized allografts or pancreatic islet xenografts under cover of CTLA4Ig, a synthetic soluble molecule that contains the B7-binding portion of CTLA4, one of the T-cell ligands of B7. CTLA4Ig blocks CD28 binding to both B7 molecules, B7-1 and B7-2. This appears to combine with the tolerogenic capacity of primarily vascularized organ allografts in rodents. The ability of differential blocking of B7-1 or B7-2 with specific mAbs to selectively drive Th1-type or Th2-type T-cell responses is controversial, and the distinct functions of each of these B7 molecules have not been clearly defined. Evidence in a rat renal allograft model suggests that CTLA4Ig may favor the development of Th2 responses, rather than inducing anergy (302).

Recent studies have demonstrated the importance of interactions between CD40 ligand (CD40L) on T cells and CD40, which is expressed not only on activated B cells, but also on a variety of APC. Signaling through the interaction of CD40 on APC with its T-cell ligand (CD40L, CD154, which is expressed transiently on activated CD4$^+$ cells) is necessary for the conversion of certain nonprofessional APC, such as resting B cells, to functional APC. In addition to being necessary for Ig class switching by B cells (191), signaling through CD40 leads to up-regulation by B cells and other APC of B7 expression, as well as other co-stimulatory molecules, class II MHC, and cytokines such as IL-12 (303). Thus, the CD40–CD40L interaction augments the provision of cognate help for B-cell activation and also plays an important role in activating APC so that they can optimally co-stimulate T-cell activation. This APC activation is a major facet of CD4 T-cell–mediated "help" for CTL generation (303). Administration of DST under cover of blocking anti-CD40L mAb leads to prevention of islet allograft rejection. In thymectomized mice, the combination of DST and anti-CD40L leads to long-term skin graft survival in fully MHC-mismatched recipients. In euthymic mice, only a small fraction of animals achieve long-term skin graft survival with this treatment. DST in this model seems to be important in allowing the deletion of donor-reactive CD8 T cells to occur (222), and can be replaced by CD8 depletion with mAb. CD4 cell depletion led to rapid rejection of donor skin grafts, suggesting that a CD4$^+$ regulatory population may be important in inducing and maintaining tolerance. However, adoptively transferred lymphocytes from "tolerant" mice slowly rejected donor-type skin grafts in secondary recipients, and did not suppress rejection by naïve T cells (304). Xenogeneic skin graft prolongation is also observed with DST and anti-CD40L (305). Even without DST, cardiac allograft survival is markedly prolonged in the absence of CD40 signaling (306). However, anti-CD40L more effectively and reliably blocks CD4-mediated than CD8-mediated rejection (307,308), and does not prevent chronic graft arteriosclerosis (309). Graft prolongation in association with CD40L–CD40 blockade or CD28 blockade has been associated with a Th2-dominant immune response (302), which may play a role in the development of graft arteriosclerosis.

The combination of CTLA4Ig and anti-CD40L antibody seems to provide particularly potent immunosuppression, with the ability to markedly prolong the survival of primary skin allografts and xenografts, without inducing tolerance. When performed in extensively MHC-mismatched combinations in euthymic recipients, these studies have achieved functional tolerance only in rodent models of cardiac or islet allografts (310) or islet xenografts (311), and not in the more stringent models of primary skin grafting or large-animal vascularized organ or islet allografts, in which prolongation has been seen without long-term tolerance (307,312). The extent to which skin graft survival is prolonged by co-stimulatory blockade appears to depend on genetic factors determining the extent to which CD8-mediated alloreactivity is suppressed, with considerable variation among recipient strains (313), an observation that is of considerable relevance to the application of this approach in outbred humans. One exception is the use of a short course of rapamycin with anti-CD40L and CTLA4Ig, which allows long-term acceptance of primary skin allografts across full MHC barriers in mice (314). However, unlike mixed chimeras induced with co-stimulatory blockade or T-cell depletion, in which the systemic nature of tolerance can be readily seen in MLR or CML assays (264), none of these other approaches have been shown to lead to systemic tolerance.

Co-stimulatory blockers have also proved beneficial in inhibiting GVHD in BMT recipients. This has been achieved with *in vivo* mAb treatment, in which B7/CD28 blockade or anti-CD40L mAb inhibits GVHD (315). Anti-CD40L mAb allows achievement of engraftment in sublethally irradiated NOD mice without GVHD (316), and pre-BMT exposure of donor T cells to recipient alloantigens in the presence of anti-CD40L inhibits GVHD via a mechanism involving CD25$^+$

regulatory CD4 cells (317). Clinically, a reduced incidence of acute GVHD has been observed in leukemic patients receiving HLA-mismatched BMT that had been exposed to recipient alloantigens in the presence of CD28 blockade with CTLA4Ig (318). The 4-1BB/4-1BBL co-stimulatory interaction has also been shown to play a role in GVH reactions and GVL effects of alloreactive CD4 and CD8 T cells (319).

The mechanisms of tolerance induced by organ transplantation with co-stimulatory blockade are only partly understood. Calcineurin inhibitors such as cyclosporine and FK506, which block priming for AICD by IL-2, have been shown to block graft prolongation induced by co-stimulatory blockade and rapamycin, apparently due to the prevention of IL-2–induced priming for AICD (314). Consistently, IL-2 has been shown to play an essential role in the induction of tolerance with CTLA4Ig and cardiac allografts (166). Somewhat surprisingly, however, Fas and TNFα receptors do not appear to be required for tolerance induction with this method (166,314). In the model involving BMT with co-stimulatory blockade (221), CsA only partially inhibits deletion of donor-reactive T cells in the periphery, and does not block induction of lasting chimerism and CD4 cell tolerance (264). In models involving co-stimulatory blockade with or without BMT, passive (associated with cytokine withdrawal) cell death (320) appears to play a critical role in peripheral deletion and tolerance induction (264,314).

Despite the observation that Th1-associated cytokines are associated with graft rejection, IFN-γ plays a critical role in graft prolongation induced with combined CD40–CD28 costimulatory blockade, DST with CD28 blockade (166) and DST with CD40 blockade (304). As mentioned above, IFN-γ has several known mechanisms for down-modulating T-cell responses, but the relevant mechanisms in the co-stimulatory blockade models are unclear.

Linked suppression and "infectious tolerance" have been demonstrated in mice receiving minor histocompatibility antigen-mismatched, MHC-identical skin grafts under cover of anti-CD40L and CD8 cell depletion, and in mice accepting islet allografts after treatment with CTLA4Ig (321). CD8 T cells are not tolerized by this method, and tolerance is not achieved in euthymic mice. Such mechanisms seem unlikely to be sufficiently powerful to maintain primary skin allograft tolerance in the MHC-mismatched setting. They do not appear to play a major role in maintaining the long-term tolerance induced by co-stimulatory blockade with BMT, since tolerance and chimerism are obliterated by the infusion of relatively small numbers of nontolerant recipient-type spleen cells in this model (321a). Since hematopoietic stem cell engraftment ensures complete central deletional tolerance in these long-term chimeras and peripheral deletion is also complete over time (264), there may be insufficient donor-reactive T cells present to maintain suppressive mechanisms, even if they are involved in the initial peripheral tolerance induction.

The donor-specific transfusion (DST) model alluded to above is of particular interest for comparison to the mixed chimerism model, since both models involve the use of hematopoietic cells in the presence of co-stimulatory blockade, but only the mixed chimerism model allows engraftment of hematopoietic stem cells and intrathymic deletion as a mechanism maintaining tolerance in the long term (264). Indeed, DST and anti-CD40L allow long-term skin graft survival in the majority of animals only if they are thymectomized prior to transplant (304). The inability to maintain tolerance in the presence of a thymus indicates the failure to establish central tolerance in the absence of substantial hematopoietic chimerism. In addition, the inability to resist breaking of tolerance by new thymic emigrants in this model argues that powerful peripheral regulatory mechanisms (suppression) are not operative in these animals. However, regulatory mechanisms may play a role in the initial suppression of CD4-mediated alloresponses, since depletion of CD4 cells abrogated skin graft acceptance (304), and both CTLA4 and IFN-γ have been shown to play an important role in the induction of tolerance in this model (166,264,304). Antibody to CTLA4 accelerates allograft rejection in CD28-deficient mice (322), and increases GVHD, GVL, and marrow rejection (323), indicating that this molecule is involved in down-modulating alloresponses in vivo. It is currently unclear whether tolerance inhibition by anti–CTLA4 mAb is due to depletion of regulatory cells and/or to blockade of the CTLA4 molecule itself. CTLA4 signaling stimulates several pathways that may be associated with tolerance, such as antiproliferative and anergy-inducing signals, T-cell apoptosis, and production of TGF-β.

Antibodies to T Cells and Adhesion Molecules. Combined treatment with mAbs against LFA-1 and its ligand ICAM-1 has been reported to induce profound tolerance in murine recipients of fully mismatched cardiac and islet allografts. Success with primary skin allografts has only been achieved with isolated class I or II mismatches (324). The mechanisms include anergy of donor-reactive CD8+ T cells, with preserved antidonor CD4 responses. Th2 cytokines have also been implicated in this long-term graft survival (324). While primary heart graft tolerance is induced with this approach, simultaneous grafting of primary skin and heart grafts from the same donor results in rapid rejection of both. Bone marrow rejection and GVHD have also been inhibited by anti–LFA-1 mAbs. The LFA-1–ICAM interaction appears to have co-stimulatory in addition to adhesive activity, making it difficult to discern the mechanisms of these in vivo effects. Blockade of VLA-4–VCAM-1 interactions has been reported to lead to cardiac allograft prolongation and, in some cases, long-term acceptance (325), and combinations of LFA-1/ICAM and VLA-4–VCAM blockade have also been evaluated.

Tolerance to MHC-matched, minor antigen–disparate skin allografts can be achieved by treatment with nondepleting anti–T-cell mAbs. This leads to "infectious tolerance," in which CD4+ T cells, rendered incapable of rejecting the allograft in the original recipients, can render naïve T cells unresponsive in secondary recipients. These tolerant T cells can, in turn, tolerize naïve T cells in tertiary recipients.

CD4$^+$ regulatory cells were shown to be capable of inhibiting rejection by presensitized CD4$^+$ and CD8$^+$ cells in this model. While Th2 may play a role in this infectious tolerance, a Th1 to Th2 shift may not fully account for the tolerance in the above model (321,326).

Anti-CD2 and anti-CD3 mAbs have also been used in combination to induce tolerance to nonvascularized heart allografts. IL-4 has been shown to play an important role in this tolerance, and IL-10 has been implicated as well (327). Tolerance has also been achieved with anti-CD2 alone in rats receiving vascularized heart allografts, and anti-CD2 plus anti-CD28 has shown efficacy in mouse heart allograft recipients. Nonmitogenic anti-CD3 mAbs have been shown to inhibit GVHD in mice and to reverse autoimmunity in NOD mice.

Anti-CD45RB antibodies, given alone or especially when used in combination with anti-CD40L, provide a powerful means of achieving skin graft prolongation and tolerance to islet allografts (328). Tolerated islet allografts show reduced expression of Th1 cytokines and increased Th2 cytokines, and T cells show an apparent conversion from the CD45RB^{high} to the CD45RB^{low} phenotype (328). Since the Treg described above are CD45RB^{low}, it is tempting to speculate that this conversion in phenotype may be related to the acquisition of suppressive T-cell function.

Total Lymphoid Irradiation. The use of TLI in conjunction with BMT, and the potential mechanisms of tolerance induced by TLI, were discussed above. TLI has also been evaluated as immunosuppression for organ transplantation without BMT, and has been successful in about one-third of baboons. In clinical transplantation, TLI has been reported to be beneficial, although it is cumbersome and toxic, especially in the case of cadaver–donor transplantation (258,329). Donor-specific tolerance has been demonstrated in a small number of patients in whom immunosuppressive therapy was terminated following kidney transplantation under cover of TLI (330). One of these patients was studied 12 years after immunosuppression withdrawal, and shown to have active antidonor MLR and no evidence for microchimerism (330). TLI used in conjunction with antithymocyte globulin has been shown to induce tolerance to kidneys and hearts, respectively, in a portion of monkeys and dogs.

The Use of Dendritic Cells for Tolerance Induction. Considerable interest has been focused on the potential of immature or genetically modified DC to induce T-cell tolerance. Examples of DC inducing deletion and anergy have been discussed above. As has already been discussed in the section on regulatory cells, stimulation with immature DC, or with DC expressing a ligand for Notch, can lead to the development of regulatory T cells (331). Attempts to intentionally immunize with "tolerogenic" DC have been associated with prolonged survival of heart, islet, and kidney allograft survival in rodent models, usually without permanent survival (331). The strategies used involved the administration of immature DC lacking co-stimulatory molecule expression, DC genetically engineered to inhibit NFκB activity, viral IL-10– and TGF-β–transfected DC, CTLA4Ig-transfected DC, and administration of CD8α^+ "lymphoid" DC. While success with these approaches has thus far been limited, future developments in the ability to generate large numbers of DC and in understanding their homing and other aspects of their biology may lead to further improvement. The combination of DC administration with co-stimulatory blockade may be particularly promising.

A Large Animal Model of Peripheral Tolerance Induction. MHC-defined, partially inbred miniature swine have provided a very instructive model allowing delineation of the role of various histoincompatibilities in tolerance and rejection in large animals. Studies of pig renal transplantation have demonstrated that spontaneous tolerance can be induced by organ grafts in large animals, provided that MHC antigens are matched. The ability to achieve such tolerance is dependent on one or possibly two non–MHC-linked genetic loci in the recipient animals. The presence of the "acceptor" phenotype also permits the spontaneous acceptance of single haplotype class I–mismatched kidney grafts (9). Graft acceptance is associated with donor-specific CTL unresponsiveness, apparently due to a deficiency in help for these CTL, and not due to a deletional mechanism. The requirement that class II antigens be matched between donor and recipient in order for this tolerance to be achieved may reflect the influence of a major difference in class II antigen expression that exists between large and small animals. Unlike large animals and man, in which class II antigens are expressed constitutively on vascular endothelial cells, the corresponding endothelial cells of rodent species do not express MHC class II molecules. Consistent with this interpretation, the use of a short course of CsA can facilitate the ability of renal allografts to induce tolerance in rodents across fully MHC-mismatched barriers, but tolerance induction in swine requires class II matching between donor and recipient for uniform success. Thus, in class II–matched, class I–mismatched porcine donor–recipient pairs, a 12-day course of high-dose (10 mg/kg/day) CsA permits long-term renal allograft acceptance in 100% of cases (9). Animals accepting such allografts are systemically tolerant to the donor's class I and minor antigens, as indicated by the fact that the accepted graft can be removed and replaced by a second donor-matched graft, which is accepted without immunosuppressive therapy. This ability of CsA to facilitate tolerance induction, and the ability of exogenous IL-2 to prevent the induction of tolerance in this model (9), are consistent with the interpretation that induction of tolerance of donor class I–reactive CTL is due, at least in part, to the absence of adequate T-cell "help" during the time of initial exposure to antigen. A selective decrease of expression of the Th1-associated cytokine IFN-γ relative to the Th2-associated cytokine IL-10 has been observed in these accepted grafts (332). The thymus appears to play a role in the induction of tolerance among preexisting peripheral T cells in this model, as removal of the host thymus prior to kidney allotransplantation leads to rejection (333). The possible mechanisms responsible for this role of the thymus in inducing peripheral tolerance phenomena are discussed elsewhere in this chapter.

The kidney allograft itself clearly plays an important role in the tolerance induced in this model. Class II–matched cardiac allografts are not accepted after a similar short course of CsA, but they are accepted if grafted to animals that are tolerized in this manner to kidney allografts bearing the same mismatched class I alleles as the donor heart (334). While the mechanisms of this regulation are incompletely understood, cells that specifically suppress antidonor CTL responses have been detected in the blood of tolerant, but not naïve, animals (335).

Relationship between Peripheral T-Cell Tolerance and Central Tolerance

The distinction between central and peripheral tolerance may not always be clear. In some systems, passenger leukocytes might emigrate from the graft to the host thymus and tolerize subsequently developing thymocytes. In addition, however, the thymus may be capable of tolerizing T cells that were already in the periphery at the time of organ grafting. In the pig model described above, the thymus appears to play a role in the induction of tolerance among preexisting peripheral T cells (333). It is possible that T cells that are activated in the periphery by the organ allograft recirculate to the thymus, as has been described (336), and encounter donor antigen there in ways that inactivate the T cells. This could be a mechanism for ensuring that T cells activated in the periphery of an animal are switched off if the same antigens are present on intrathymic leukocytes. Additionally, the migration of donor antigen to the thymus may result in the development of T cells that specifically recognize the donor antigen and down-regulate the activity of destructive alloreactive T cells when they enter the periphery. The role of the thymus in the development of Treg has already been discussed above. Finally, it is possible that recent thymic emigrants are required for the development of regulatory cells. However, this possibility is somewhat inconsistent with the observation in mice, rats, and humans that Treg express a phenotype associated with memory cells rather than naïve T cells.

A second situation in which the boundary between central and peripheral tolerance is blurred arises when donor antigens are injected intrathymically in order to induce tolerance. The initial idea underlying this approach was to use antibody treatment to deplete peripheral T cells and to induce central tolerance among recovering T cells by direct introduction of antigen into the thymus. However, more recent studies have shown that tolerance can be induced by intrathymic injection of soluble alloantigens without peripheral T-cell depletion (337). Since removal of the thymus before or within the first few days of allografting results in rejection of the allograft (131), the thymus must play an active role in tolerizing preexisting peripheral T cells, possibly by one of the mechanisms proposed in the preceding paragraph. In fact, evidence has been obtained to suggest that donor-reactive T cells must recirculate to the recipient thymus to induce tolerance in this model (338). Active regulatory cell populations have been reported in rats receiving intrathymic injections of allogeneic BMC (339). These results are consistent with the role of suppressive cell populations in tolerance induced by thymic allografts or xenografts.

There is an important role for the allograft in inducing tolerance in animals receiving intrathymic injection, and in other models in which a preexisting peripheral T-cell repertoire must be rendered tolerant. Transferable tolerance is not induced by intrathymic marrow injection alone without an organ allograft in rats (339), suggesting that the graft itself helps to tolerize the preexisting T-cell repertoire. In contrast, pure intrathymic deletional tolerance is not dependent on the continued presence of antigen in the periphery (255). Donor tissue can be grafted at any time, and tolerance is ensured. The intrathymic injection approach has not been successful in "high-responder" rat strain combinations and may even induce allosensitization, and has not successfully allowed xenotolerance induction. Furthermore, chronic rejection of cardiac allografts was not prevented by intrathymic injection of donor spleen cells in rats treated with antilymphocyte serum (340). While one attempt to use this approach in nonhuman primates was discouraging (341), another report described donor-specific skin graft prolongation in three animals receiving allogeneic or xenogeneic (human) CD34+ cells intrathymically (342). None of these studies have included a specific strategy for inactivating preexisting alloreactive thymocytes, and these cells may limit the success of this approach, as they do in mice receiving allogeneic BMT with nonmyeloablative conditioning that does not include measures to overcome intrathymic alloresistance (264).

Which Strategy to Achieve Transplantation Tolerance?

Although clinical trials have already begun in which tolerance-inducing strategies are combined with conventional pharmacologic immunosuppression, none of the strategies for achieving transplantation tolerance has been used to replace such chronic therapy in a large clinical series. In general, short-term results of most organ allograft transplants are excellent, making it essential to have extremely reliable methods of inducing tolerance in order to ethically justify their use in place of conventional chronic immunosuppressive therapies. While induction of central deletional tolerance with hematopoietic cell grafts is a reliable and durable approach to achieving permanent graft survival, earlier techniques for achieving central tolerance have involved more vigorous ablation of the lymphohematopoietic system than can be safely achieved in larger animals. Thus, the major challenge in bringing the mixed chimerism/central tolerance approach to clinical application is to develop highly specific, nontoxic methods of conditioning the host for acceptance of a hematopoietic allograft or xenograft. Regarding peripheral tolerance, most techniques to achieve peripheral tolerance in larger animals have not been as effective as in rodent models. Furthermore, peripheral mechanisms alone have not been sufficient to reliably overcome the most stringent transplantation barrier imposed by fully MHC-mismatched primary skin allografts in rodents. Conceptually, one major problem with peripheral tolerance strategies is that they cannot prevent the generation of new T cells in the recipient capable of recognizing donor antigens. While effector cells might be persistently driven toward anergy or deletion by the nonstimulating cells of the graft, potential stimulation of helper cells by professional APC through the indirect pathway might make this a precarious state of tolerance. The indirect pathway might potentially be tolerized through central deletion of thymocytes recognizing peptides of donor antigens presented in the thymus in association with host MHC antigens. Although thymic APC appear to be incapable of picking up and representing antigens from lymphoid cells to induce tolerance of T cells that recognize these antigens through the indirect pathway, mixed chimerism appears to tolerize the indirect (in addition to the direct) pathway of allorecognition, perhaps due to the presence of additional donor-derived cell types that more effectively provide antigens for this pathway. Since superantigens have been shown to be capable of inducing deletional tolerance in the thymus when presented by APC other than those that produced them (343), further definition of the circumstances under which indirect presentation of hematopoietic cell–derived antigens leads to intrathymic deletion is needed. Most importantly, large animal models achieving sustained mixed chimerism with nonmyeloablative conditioning are needed to document the safety and feasibility of this approach. Recent advances in primate and porcine models are encouraging in this regard (265,344). The "infectious" nature of suppressive mechanisms of tolerance makes them potentially attractive as a means of inducing robust and durable tolerance. However, it will be difficult to control the development of such mechanisms until they are better understood. It seems likely that the optimal approach to achieving clinical transplantation tolerance might require combinations of both central and peripheral strategies.

Mixed chimerism can be achieved with reduced toxicity using nonmyeloablative conditioning in patients with hematologic malignancies (345), and lymphohematopoietic GVH reactions induced by DLI can be used to achieve graft-versus-tumor effects (266). These observations provided an opportunity to evaluate the potential of this approach to induce transplantation tolerance in patients with a hematologic malignancy, multiple myeloma, and consequent renal failure. Several patients have received a simultaneous nonmyeloablative BMT and renal allograft from HLA-identical siblings, and have accepted their kidney graft without any immunosuppression for more than 4.5 years in the earliest case, while enjoying marked tumor regressions (267). Similar to the primate model described above, in which BMT has been shown to be essential for tolerance induction, chimerism in these patients was only transient (267), suggesting that the kidney graft itself may participate in tolerance induction and/or maintenance after chimerism has played its initial role. Because T-cell depletion is only partial in these models, it is clear that the pure central, deletional tolerance described above in

murine models has not yet been achieved with nonmyeloablative conditioning in large animals or humans. Nevertheless, the promising results obtained in these patients have provided an important proof of principle, which has led to initiation of a phase I/II trial of tolerance induction with this approach in patients with renal failure due to multiple myeloma.

TRANSPLANTATION OF SPECIFIC ORGANS AND TISSUES

Skin Grafting

Although allogeneic skin grafting represents a frequently used experimental model, its application in humans is unusual. Most skin transplantation in humans is done with autologous tissue. Recently, however, "artificial" skin grafts have been created that consist of stromal elements and cultured cells of allogeneic and even xenogeneic origin. Evidence suggests that these grafts are not rejected, although some of their components may be replaced by recipient tissues over time.

Skin grafts are frequently used experimentally on small animals to examine rejection because they can be performed rapidly in large numbers. On the one hand, the use of skin grafts has the disadvantage that they are not primarily vascularized and, thus, may not be susceptible to precisely the same mechanisms of rejection as are solid organs. On the other hand, the difficulty in prolonging skin graft survival in rodents more accurately reflects the difficulty in prolonging transplantation of solid organ survival in larger animals than does the transplantation of solid organs in rodents.

Kidney Transplantation

Kidneys have been the most frequently transplanted organs for many years. At present, approximately 10,000 kidney transplants are performed annually in the United States. The likelihood that a renal allograft will survive with good function for at least 1 year has slowly been rising. Patient survival after 1 year is expected to be better than 90% and the current likelihood of graft function, at 1 year, now exceeds 85% in many units, even when organs from totally unrelated donors are used.

Nonetheless, even well-matched recipients of renal transplants must, for the most part, continue to take immunosuppressive medications for the rest of their lives. These patients are susceptible to the complications of their immunosuppressive medications, including increased risks of infection, cancer, hypertension, and metabolic bone disease. Thus, they pay a price for their new organ stemming from our inability to provide specific immunosuppression. The success of clinical transplantation is a double-edged sword. With such good patient and graft survival rates initially, it is difficult to justify risky clinical trials of new approaches to immunosuppression which, by achieving antigen-specific tolerance, might avoid the long-term need for immunosuppression altogether.

Because of the success of modern nonspecific immunosuppression, the major obstacle to achieving a successful kidney transplant is no longer the early rejection of the organ after transplantation. Instead, the three major obstacles are now the shortage of organs, the problem of sensitization, and the chronic rejection of kidneys that may occur after many years. Partly because of the increasing success of renal transplantation, the number of candidates for the procedure has continued to grow and now far exceeds the supply of available organs. Unlike hearts and livers, where an inadequate supply of organs leads to the death of many candidates, those waiting for renal transplants are instead faced with long periods on dialysis. This waiting time is often 4 or more years even for unsensitized candidates seeking kidneys from cadaver donors. The second major obstacle in obtaining a successful renal transplant stems from the problem of sensitized candidates with broadly reactive antibodies resulting from prior antigen exposure. These highly sensitized individuals may wait many years to obtain a kidney that is crossmatch negative, and some never receive a transplant at all.

The late failure of kidney transplants many years after the procedure probably involves a component of immunologic rejection but may also be due to other factors, including the effects of the early ischemic injury and the ongoing effects of drugs and metabolic abnormalities in the recipient. Although the 1-year survival rate for kidney transplants has improved from roughly 40% to nearly 90% over the past 40 years, the conditional half-life for kidney transplants (defined as the number of years at that half of the kidneys have been lost among those recipients who had functioning kidneys at 1 year) has barely increased during that time period and is still less than 10 years.

One of the important changes in clinical kidney transplantation in recent years is the greater use of living unrelated donors. In the past, living-donor kidney transplantation was performed almost only when a related donor was available to the recipient with some, or complete, matching of the HLA antigens. The use of better immunosuppressive drugs has reduced the importance of genetic matching (see below) and the growing waiting list for cadaver donors has made the importance of finding a living donor much greater. Thus, it is now common for the living donor for a kidney transplant to be a completely unrelated and genetically unmatched individual, such as a spouse or best friend. The results of transplants from unrelated donors have been better than those from cadaver donors and as good as those from all but the most closely matched living related donors.

Liver Transplantation

Transplantation of the liver represents a major technical challenge. For this reason the organ and patient survival rates are less good than those for renal transplantation. However, successful liver transplantation can now be achieved with survival of about three-quarters of recipients at 1 year (346).

From an immunologist's point of view, liver transplantation is of interest first because the organ is apparently quite resistant to immediate antibody-mediated rejection. Transplantation across blood group barriers and in the face of a positive crossmatch (by retrospective analysis) has generally been successful in the short term (347). There is evidence, however, that long-term organ survival is diminished in blood-group incompatible patients (348). Second, the long-term survival of liver transplants has never seemed to depend on better HLA matching between donor and recipient, even before the use of new immunosuppressive agents. In fact, some data have suggested the opposite correlation. The possibility that poorly matched livers may survive better than well-matched ones might be due to an inability of recipient T cells, sensitized to viral pathogens in association with self-MHC antigens, to recognize those pathogens in the donor liver presented in association with donor HLA antigens. Thus, poorly matched livers might escape injury caused by immunologic responses to hepatotrophic viruses. Third, transplantation of the liver carries with it large numbers of donor lymphoid cells, thus creating the setting for GVHD. Donor lymphocytes can mediate an antibody-dependent hemolysis of recipient red blood cells in the case of recipient blood-group incompatibility with the donor. Thus, "A" or "B" recipients of "O" livers have been subject to an immune hemolytic anemia during the early posttransplant period. There may also be other manifestations of GVH disease even in blood-group compatible recipients.

Heart and Lung Transplantation

Heart transplantation is also a relatively recent component of standard clinical transplantation, with survival rates frequently in excess of 80% at 1 year. One of the immunologic issues of particular importance in heart transplantation is the high rate of new atherosclerotic disease in the coronary arteries of the donor organ. This atherosclerotic disease is a manifestation of chronic "rejection," but the causes appear to include more than just immunologic responses.

Lung transplantation, either in conjunction with heart transplantation or alone, is a still more recent addition to clinical transplantation. Recipients of lung transplants have demonstrated a tendency to develop pathologic changes of "bronchiolitis obliterans" that is also thought to be a manifestation of chronic rejection.

Pancreas and Islet Transplantation

Transplantation of the whole pancreas was almost without success until about 1980, largely for technical reasons. More recently, successful pancreas transplantation to treat diabetes mellitus has been achieved using new technical approaches, and with success rates approaching those for kidney transplantation, as long as the two organs are transplanted together. The lower survival rates achieved when pancreas transplantation is performed alone probably reflect the difficulty in diagnosing rejection episodes involving this organ. By the time blood sugar levels begin to rise, destruction of the pancreas is generally so far advanced that it cannot be reversed by immunotherapy. Measurement of the serum creatinine, reflecting early dysfunction of a simultaneous kidney transplant, allows much earlier detection of rejection activity and, thus, better outcomes. On the other hand, simultaneous transplantation of both a kidney and a pancreas from a single donor has demonstrated the interesting phenomenon that rejection activity in one organ is not always associated with rejection activity in the other. It is not known whether this occasional dichotomy reflects tissue-specific antigens or localized inflammatory events in one, but not the other organ.

Transplantation of the whole pancreas provides, of course, more tissue than is needed to treat diabetes mellitus. The intriguing aspect of pancreas transplantation, therefore, is the potential that useful results might be accomplished by transplantation of insulin-producing islet cells alone. Although islet cell transplants have been very successful in animal models, success in humans was unusual until very recently. According to the 1999 report of the Islet Transplant Registry, only 8% of over 200 type 1 diabetic patients had achieved insulin independence after an islet transplant. These dismal outcomes appear to be changing recently based on the use of the "Edmonton protocol." Investigators at that site used a combination of several new immunosuppressive agents (an anti-IL2R antibody, plus sirolimus and tacrolimus), avoided the use of steroids, and provided a larger number (more than 10,000 IEQ/kg) of carefully prepared islets. These investigators have reported that about 80% of islet transplants can be successful using this protocol (349).

However, even if islet transplantation could be performed routinely with current immunosuppressive drugs, it would not dramatically change the course of diabetes for these patients. This is because the primary goal of islet transplantation is to prevent the secondary neurologic, vascular, and retinal complications of diabetes that take many years to develop. However, performance of islet transplantation early in the course of the disease, when it might really affects these processes, would require exchanging insulin therapy for immunosuppressive drugs. Over 20 to 30 years, the latter is at least as damaging to human beings. Thus, even more than for other forms of transplantation, realization of the full potential of islet transplantation will require tolerance induction.

Hematopoietic Cell Transplantation

Bone marrow transplants, and more recently, transplants of hematopoietic stem cells and progenitors mobilized from the marrow into peripheral blood by treatment with G-CSF, are used most commonly for the treatment of otherwise incurable leukemias and lymphomas, aplastic anemia, and congenital immunodeficiency states. Additional applications include hemoglobinopathies and inborn errors of metabolism. Autologous hematopoietic cell transplants have been used quite widely for hematologic rescue following high-dose chemo/radiotherapy for the treatment of malignancies.

Additionally, autologous hematopoietic cell transplants (HCT) are currently being explored as a treatment for autoimmune diseases. However, autologous HCT will not be considered further here because it does not involve the broaching of any immunologic barriers.

One fundamental difference between hematopoietic cell transplantation and the transplantation of all other organs is that the recipient's treatment for his or her malignancy usually results in ablation of the immune and hematopoietic systems prior to transplantation—that is, the "conditioning" for transplantation is myeloablative. Originally, hematopoietic cell allografts were administered only as a means of replacing these ablated host functions. However, clinical experience soon showed that one of the main therapeutic benefits of allogeneic HCT is due to the graft-versus-leukemia (GVL) effect of donor lymphocytes (350). Thus, allogeneic bone marrow transplantation may also be thought of as immunotherapy leading to an attack on the residual leukemic cells that remain in cytoablated hosts. In view of this information, clinicians have recently begun to evaluate approaches using less toxic, nonmyeloablative conditioning as a means of allowing allogeneic marrow to engraft so that donor lymphocytes can mediate GVL effects. In contrast to HCT for malignancies and other indications in immunocompetent recipients, transplantation for immunodeficiency states does not require myeloablation or immunoablation in order to achieve engraftment of allogeneic marrow grafts, which often reconstitute only the deficient immune system and not other hematopoietic lineages.

Another major difference between HCT and solid organ transplantation is that the recovering immune system in HCT recipients is tolerant to the donor alloantigens, so there is no requirement for immunosuppressive therapy to prevent allograft rejection once the initial immune resistance to the allograft has been overcome.

A third unique feature of HCT (as well as transplants of other organs that are rich in lymphoid tissue, such as small intestinal grafts and, to a lesser extent, liver grafts) is the ability of T cells in the allograft to mount an immunologic attack on the recipient's tissues, resulting in GVHD. While GVHD rates can be reduced to acceptable levels using prophylaxis with a course of nonspecific immunosuppressive therapy when the donor and recipient are HLA-matched siblings, the frequency and severity of the GVHD that develops when extensive HLA barriers are traversed has essentially precluded the routine performance of such transplants, making bone marrow transplantation unavailable to many for whom no other curative treatment exists. The establishment of large marrow donor registries has permitted the performance of closely matched transplants from unrelated donors in a significant fraction of patients, but these transplants are also associated with a high incidence of severe GVHD, due in large part to the existence of HLA mismatches that went undetected by conventional serologic HLA-typing techniques (351), which are now being replaced by more specific molecular typing techniques (see section on HLA matching).

As is mentioned above, one of the major benefits of HCT in patients with hematologic malignancies has proven to be the GVL effect of allogeneic lymphocytes, especially T cells, within the donor graft. This GVL effect is due in large part to recognition by donor T cells of host alloantigens, which are also expressed on leukemic cells. Therefore, T-cell depletion of the donor graft has not proved to be an optimal solution to the GVHD problem, because the decreased incidence of GVHD is offset by an increased incidence of relapse of some leukemias (352). In addition, an increased risk of failure of engraftment is observed with the administration of T-cell–depleted stem cell grafts. This, however, can be offset by the use of increased host conditioning and high doses of donor hematopoietic stem cells, an approach that has recently permitted the engraftment of extensively (one haplotype) HLA-mismatched stem cell grafts without GVHD (353). A major and elusive goal in the HCT field has been to separate the graft-versus-leukemia (GVL) effect of donor T cells from GVHD.

Recently, several new approaches for inhibiting GVHD have been attempted. The use of co-stimulatory blockade was discussed above. Peptides containing the CDR3 portion of the mouse CD4 molecule have been shown to be capable of inhibiting both GVHD and resistance to allogeneic marrow engraftment. Since these approaches might be expected to block donor-anti-host responses nonspecifically, including those that eliminate residual leukemia in the host, it seems quite likely that they would also impair graft-versus-leukemia responses and might have their greatest utility in the treatment of nonmalignant diseases. Alternative approaches involve immunostimulatory cytokines such as IL-2, IFN-γ, or IL-12, all of which, paradoxically, inhibit GVHD in mouse models. These cytokines are of interest because they have been shown to preserve or enhance GVL effects while GVHD is inhibited. The inhibitory effect of IL-12 on GVHD is mediated by IFN-γ, which is also largely responsible for the GVL effect of CD8 T cells. Despite the ability of exogenously administered IL-10 to exacerbate GVHD under some conditions, ex vivo treatment of donor marrow with IL-10 or TGF-β can inhibit GVHD. A surprising approach to achieving immune deviation and GVHD inhibition involved the use of exogenously administered IL-11, which also preserved perforin-dependent GVL effects of CD4 and CD8 cells. Administration of keratinocyte growth factor (KGF) also appears to inhibit GVHD, while preserving GVL and promoting alloengraftment, through mechanisms that are not fully understood. Blockade of Fas/FasL, perforin, TNFα, and IL-1 pathways have shown some efficacy in animal models and the latter two have entered clinical trials (315). Synthetic random polymers of four amino acids, with promiscuous class II binding, block TCR–MHC interactions and inhibit GVHD in an MHC-matched combination in mice. The use of nondepleting anti-CD3 F(ab)′2 fragments in vivo has also shown promise in a mouse model for the ability to maintain GVL effects while attenuating GVHD. Many other strategies, such as immune deviation and the use of NK/T cells were discussed elsewhere in the chapter.

Another approach to separating the GVL potential from the GVHD-inducing capacity of MHC-directed alloreactivity is to separate the hematopoietic cell transplant and the administration of donor T cells in time, so that the T cells are given after some host recovery from the initial conditioning regimen has occurred. Established mixed hematopoietic chimeras produced with either lethal TBI or nonmyeloablative regimens are immunologically tolerant of their original marrow donor's antigens. As expected, a GVH reaction occurs after administration of nontolerant, donor lymphocyte infusions (DLI), resulting in conversion of the state of mixed hematopoietic chimerism to a state of full donor chimerism. Remarkably, this powerful GVH alloreaction against lymphohematopoietic cells is not associated with any clinically significant GVHD in mice, even though donor T cells are given in numbers that would cause rapidly lethal GVHD in freshly conditioned recipients (354,355). This demonstration that GVH reactions can be confined to the lymphohematopoietic system suggested a novel approach to separating GVHD from GVL reactions. Since hematologic malignancies reside largely in the lymphohematopoietic system, GVH reactions might be confined to this system and eliminate tumor cells without entering the epithelial GVHD target tissues. Apparently, host recovery from the injury associated with conditioning confers greater resistance to the induction of GVHD at late time points after BMT compared to the time of conditioning. A similar outcome has been seen in some patients receiving nonmyeloablative BMT with in vivo T-cell depletion of the donor and recipient, followed by delayed donor leukocyte infusions for the treatment of lymphomas (266). Improved T-cell depletion of the initial donor stem-cell inoculum to avoid subclinical GVHD before DLI, along with a better understanding of the factors induced by host conditioning that convert a beneficial lymphohematpoietic GVH alloresponse to GVHD in the epithelial tissues, should allow better control of this approach to separating GVHD and GVL. In addition to recovery of epithelial GVHD target tissues from conditioning-induced injury, increasing resistance to GVHD with time may be conferred by recovering T-cell populations that down-regulate GVH reactions. This has been demonstrated in models involving lethally irradiated mice receiving MHC-matched bone marrow (356,357), which enjoy GVL effects from delayed DLI without developing GVHD (358). Eradication of relapsed chronic myelogenous leukemia following delayed DLI is somewhat variably associated with GVHD, but generally to a lesser degree than would be expected in freshly conditioned recipients of similar cell numbers (350).

Several groups have investigated the possibility that CD4$^+$ or CD8$^+$ T-cell subsets could be identified that promote engraftment and GVL effects but do not cause GVHD (251). Clinical studies involving selective CD8 depletion in HLA-identical sibling transplantation have shown a higher incidence of engraftment failure than is observed for unmanipulated BMT, but the rate was lower than that observed for pan-T-cell–depleted transplants, and evidence for an antileukemic effect against chronic myelogenous leukemia was obtained. The relative importance of each T-cell subset in inducing GVHD and GVL is likely to vary in the setting of HLA-mismatched transplants and different types of leukemias.

Additional strategies for separating GVHD from allogeneic graft-versus-tumor effects include the transduction of donor T cells with suicide genes so that the alloresponse can be turned off at will, hopefully after residual tumor has been eradicated. Another approach is to avoid the GVH alloresponse, and try to target the donor immune response to tumor-specific antigens. This approach has been explored by numerous groups, and early reports of some success are starting to emerge (359). One class of leukemia-specific antigens that seems promising is the idiotypic determinants associated with unique Ig receptors and T-cell receptors on the surface of B- and T-cell malignancies, respectively, that may trigger an immune response when presented by professional APC such as DC (360). However, limitations to this approach include the low frequency of tumor antigen-specific T cells preexisting in a given T-cell repertoire. These frequencies are even lower than those against minor histocompatibility antigens, and the generation of meaningful tumor-specific responses is likely to necessitate donor presensitization along with *in vitro* expansion of tumor-specific effector cells, a process that can limit the homing capacity of injected cells. Such prolonged cultures may be impractical for use in the setting of BMT, in which leukemia-reactive cells must eliminate exponentially expanding leukemic cells. Immunization of HCT donors with tumor antigens could potentially overcome these limitations. Minor histocompatibility alloantigens expressed by lymphohematopoietic cells (including leukemias and lymphomas) but not by the epithelial GVHD target tissues may also be targeted using *in vitro* expanded CTL. Such antigens have recently been identified (361). Recently, it was shown that administration of primed T cells specific for a single immunodominant class I–restricted minor histocompatibility antigen could mediate GVL without GVHD. Avoidance of GVHD was dependent on the absence of GVH-reactive T cells with additional specificities in the donor inoculum (362). In theory, the less risky strategy of generating tumor-specific responses from autologous T cells could achieve similar outcomes. However, T-cell immunity may be markedly impaired in the tumor-bearing host, and the use of immunologically unimpaired allogeneic donors is therefore appealing.

Xenogeneic Transplantation

The increasing shortage of cadaver donor organs has evoked a worldwide resurgence of interest in xenotransplantation, that is, the replacement of human organs or tissues with those from a donor of a different species. Routine clinical application of this therapeutic modality is still in the future. However, recent progress, which is reviewed briefly here, offers cause for optimism.

Concordant versus Discordant Xenotransplantation

Xenotransplants have been classified into two groups—"concordant" and "discordant"—on the basis of phylogenetic distance between the species combination, speed of the rejection, and levels of detectable preformed antibodies. Animals that are evolutionarily closely related and that have minimal or no preformed natural antibodies specific for each other are called "concordant," while animals that belong to evolutionarily distant species and reject organs in a hyperacute manner are termed "discordant." There are, of course, many gradations between these extremes, and there are also a variety of known exceptions to the rule, making this nomenclature less than ideal.

Choice of Donor Species for Clinical Xenotransplantation

From a phylogenetic viewpoint, nonhuman primates would undoubtedly be the most similar to allotransplants immunologically. However, due to considerations of size, availability, and likelihood of transmission of infectious disease, most investigators have decided against the use of primates as a future source of xenogeneic organs. Instead, the discordant species, swine, has been chosen by many as the most suitable xenograft donor. The pig has essentially unlimited availability, as well as favorable breeding characteristics, and many of its organ systems are similar to those of humans. Partially inbred miniature swine are a particularly attractive choice, because of their size (adult weights of approximately 120 kilograms), their physiology (also similar to humans for many organ systems), and their breeding characteristics, which have permitted inbreeding and genetic manipulation (363).

Mechanisms of Xenograft Rejection

Xenografts are subject to all four of the rejection mechanisms described earlier in this chapter and give rise to more powerful immune responses than allografts, probably for each type of rejection. There are two fundamental reasons for this finding. First, xenografts offer more foreign antigens as targets for an immune response. Second, there are frequently molecular incompatibilities between members of different species that prevent the normal function of receptor–ligand interactions. Since in many cases the occurrence of "homologous restriction" for receptor–ligand pairs has been found to impair the regulatory processes that normally control immune and inflammatory responses, the result is that rejection mechanisms that may be relatively weak in allogeneic combinations become explosive following xenogeneic transplantation.

The well-recognized susceptibility of xenografts to hyperacute rejection demonstrates both of these fundamental problems. As described earlier, pigs express an endothelial carbohydrate determinant, αGal, which is not expressed by humans (276). As a result of this additional foreign antigen, pigs, in effect, express a new blood group antigen relative to all human recipients and thus their organs are subject to hyperacute rejection, initiated by the binding of preformed natural antibodies. However, the hyperacute rejection that occurs with pig-to-primate transplantation is more vigorous than in the case of allogeneic blood group disparities. This is true, at least in part, because the complement regulatory proteins expressed by pig endothelium are less efficient in controlling human complement activation than are the human regulatory proteins expressed by human organs. Thus, these molecular incompatibilities contribute to the increased intensity of the hyperacute rejection mechanism.

Similarly, the factors responsible for accelerated graft rejection are more prominent in xenogeneic than in allogeneic transplantation. The rapid induction of an antibody response against xenografts probably reflects the expression of additional foreign antigens, and the existence of preformed antibodies to these antigens, although at levels too low to initiate hyperacute rejection. In addition, the process of accelerated rejection is magnified considerably in xenografts by the failure of such regulatory molecules as tissue-factor protein inhibitor to function effectively with human factor Xa, thus increasing the tendency toward intravascular thrombosis (276). The likely participation of NK cells in this form of xenograft rejection probably also reflects both the presence of additional antigens and the importance of molecular incompatibilities in xenotransplantation, since novel carbohydrate determinants on pig endothelium may contribute to NK cell activation, while the molecular incompatibilities between human NK inhibitory receptors and swine class I molecules allows this activation to proceed without inhibition (364).

The available evidence also suggests that cell-mediated immune responses to xenografts are more powerful than those directed to allografts (210). Initially, there was some uncertainty about this point since cell-mediated immune responses to xenogeneic stimulating cells were first studied using mouse T cells, for which molecular incompatibilities with human cells lead to weaker direct recognition of xenogeneic than allogeneic stimulators in vitro. In this case, the incompatibilities turned out to involve the accessory molecules that are required for T-cell activation rather than a lack of molecules that stimulate a T-cell response. Thus, it seemed that cell-mediated rejection in vivo might also be weak. However, cell-mediated xenograft rejection, even by mice, has consistently been found to be extremely powerful in vivo, apparently initiated by CD4$^+$ T cells responding to the many additional antigenic peptides through the indirect pathway.

More recently, attention has been directed at investigation of the clinically relevant human-anti-pig cellular response. In contrast to the murine studies, direct responses by human CD4 and CD8 T cells to pig stimulators can be readily measured in vitro. In addition, the cell-mediated reaction in vitro has been found to include a significant contribution by NK cells that can lyse pig targets. Thus, in the human-anti-pig combination, an important molecular incompatibility is the failure of human NK inhibitory receptors to interact with pig class I molecules. Numerous other molecular interactions that might be important in human-anti-pig T-cell responses have been examined (see Table 6). With the exception of an apparently lower affinity of human CD8 for its binding site on pig class I molecules (which diminishes the direct human CD8$^+$ helper response to pig stimulators), and the failure of human IFN-γ to stimulate pig endothelium, the other molecular interactions appear to be at least partially functional.

The results of these studies have suggested that human-anti-pig T-cell responses are likely to be as great or greater than those in allogeneic combinations. Some investigators have identified a stronger indirect response by human T cells to pig stimulators than to allogeneic stimulators (365). This stronger indirect proliferation may indicate that human cell-mediated rejection of pig organs, both acutely and chronically, will indeed be more difficult to control than for allografts. Presumably, the source of this stronger indirect response lies partly in the larger number of foreign antigenic peptides generated by the disparate proteins of xenogeneic donors.

Therapeutic Strategies for Xenotransplantation

There are three main strategies that have been pursued to achieve long-term survival of xenogeneic transplants. The first has been to seek nonspecific immunosuppressive drugs that might prove especially effective for xenotransplantation. This approach was used very successfully to achieve the excellent survival of allografts in current clinical practice. However, each new drug that has contributed to better outcomes

TABLE 6. *Molecular Interactions between human and Pig*

Molecular interactions that are at least partially functional	
Human	Pig
TCR	SLA
CD4	SLA Class II
CD8	SLA Class I (+/−)
CD2	LFA-3 (+/−)
LFA-1	ICAM
CD28	B7
VLA-4	VCAM
Fas	FasL
FasL	Fas
CD40L	CD40

Molecular interactions that are significantly impaired	
Human	Pig
KIRs	SLA Class I
CD8	SLA Class I
IFN-γ	IFN-γ R

for allografts has been tested experimentally for xenografts, and none has so far proven to be the magic bullet that might make xenografting possible. Based on our scientific understanding of the immunologic barriers to xenotransplantation, it is unlikely that any such drug exists. Furthermore, the heightened immune response to xenografts compared to allografts suggests that larger amounts of exogenous immunosuppression would be required to achieve xenograft survival comparable to that of allografts. Given the narrow therapeutic window that already exists in allogeneic transplantation, most investigators believe that more than just immunosuppressive drugs will be needed to accomplish widespread clinical application of xenogeneic transplantation.

The second therapeutic approach has been to use genetic engineering of donor animals to lessen the immunologic barriers to xenografts. Since the two features that distinguish xenografts from allografts are the larger number of antigens and the molecular incompatibilities between species, these genetic modifications have been aimed primarily at correcting these two disadvantages of xenografts (Fig. 16). The first transgenic pigs produced by genetic engineering for xenotransplantation attempted to make use of the species specificity of complement regulatory proteins. Transgenic pigs were produced that expressed human genes for several of these proteins. Organs from animals expressing one of these molecules (hDAF) have been studied extensively, and appear to be significantly less susceptible to hyperacute rejection than are those from wild-type pigs (366). Numerous other potential transgenes are currently being examined experimentally, including genes encoding the human fucosyltransferase that produces the human blood group O determinant from the same substrate used by the pig galactosyltransferase, and genes encoding a glycosidase that might remove the αGal determinant. Additional transgenes are likely to be tested in attempts to alter the host response to xenografts. These may include genes that affect homing of human immune cells to the grafts, genes that affect the homing and function of pig hematopoietic cells in a human hematopoietic microenvironment, genes that regulate coagulation, and/or genes that may affect cell-mediated mechanisms of graft destruction (such

as expression of human class I analogs to inhibit NK cells or expression of down-regulating molecules for T cells, such as FasL).

The other genetic engineering technique being exploited for xenotransplantation involves knockout technology. In mice, homologous recombination has made it possible to eliminate the expression of some genes. For example, knockout mice have been generated that do not express the galactosyltransferase that is responsible for generating the $\alpha(1,3)$Gal determinant. Until recently this technology was not available in larger animals, including pigs, since homologous recombination was performed in embryonic stem cells (ES cells), which have only been derived in certain strains of mice. However, another means of generating knockout animals utilizes homologous recombination following nuclear transfer, a procedure that has recently been shown to be effective in several large animal species, including pigs. There has been a major effort devoted to knocking out a-1,3-galactosyltransferase from pigs by this technology, and the knockout of one copy of this gene has recently been reported (367). More recently, pigs in which both alleles of the galactosyltransferase are knocked out have been generated. The animals are viable, and ongoing studies will reveal their utility in experimental animals. In principle, the full knockout phenotype should eliminate one of the major problems remaining in the field of xenotransplantation.

The third strategy to achieve successful xenotransplantation is the induction of tolerance to donor antigens. Potential applications of this strategy have been described earlier in this chapter, with reference mainly to transplantation in rodent models (see above). Approaches attempting to utilize either mixed chimerism or thymic transplantation to induce tolerance across xenogeneic barriers in primates have also been reported (276). So far, long-term success by the mixed chimerism approach has been attained only for concordant cynomolgus monkey to baboon renal transplants. Both mixed chimerism and thymic transplantation approaches have been attempted for the discordant pig to baboon combination. Both of these approaches have had limited success, showing specific reduction of cell-mediated responses and inhibition

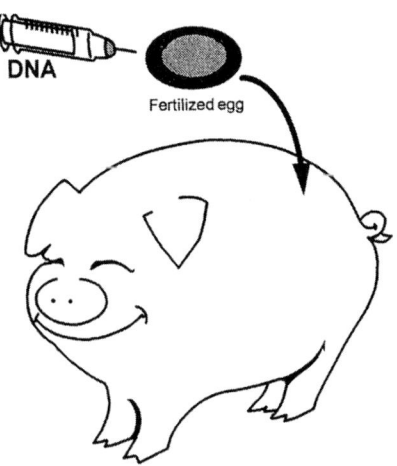

DNA

Fertilized egg

- **Complement inhibition**
  - **DAF**
  - **CD46**
  - **CD59**
- **Antibody binding**
  - **Galactosidase**
  - **Fucosyl transferase**
- **Growth factors**
  - **pIL-3, pSCF**
  - **Human GF receptors**
- **MHC genes**
  - **Class I (NK inhibition)**

FIG. 16. Transgenic pigs as xenograft donors.

of the induction of T-cell–dependent antibody responses to xenogeneic determinants. However, renal allograft survivals appeared to nevertheless be curtailed by the return of natural antibodies to αGal. Investigators are currently hopeful that a combination of these approaches, using tolerance induction and tissues and organs from the knockout animals described above, may extend these survivals in the near future. Indeed, it is possible that elimination of the natural antibody problem along with tolerance induction could make discordant xenotransplantation as successful as allogeneic transplantation in providing a long-term solution for patients waiting for transplants. Of course, it is possible that when these barriers are overcome, other obstacles, not yet apparent, will still limit the survival of xenogeneic transplants, and additional measures will be required to achieve success.

Nonimmunologic Barriers to Xenotransplantation

In addition to the immunologic mechanisms that prevent successful xenografting, there are two other potentially important obstacles to clinical application. First, the same kinds of molecular incompatibilities between species that alter immune responses may cause physiologic dysfunction of xenogeneic organs. For example, it appears that erythropoietin produced by pig kidneys may not function well in primates, causing progressive anemia in recipients with long-surviving pig kidney transplants. Presumably, there are many other such examples that will become apparent when long survival of metabolically complex organs, such as the liver, can be accomplished using discordant donors. On the other hand, there are also many examples where physiologic function remains intact across species differences, such as the ability of pig insulin to regulate human glucose appropriately. In addition, selective problems of physiologic dysfunction are likely to be correctable using transgenic technology. Thus, the physiologic dysfunction of xenogeneic organs is unlikely to be an insurmountable barrier to all forms of xenotransplantation, although it may impair the function of certain types of xenogeneic organs or tissues, at least until appropriate genetic engineering is possible.

The other nonimmunologic barrier to xenotransplantation is the risk of cross-species transfer of infectious agents, potentially creating a health hazard, not only for the recipient, but also for society as a whole. This possibility has gained significant attention, both in the scientific literature and in the lay press, and the issue has become confused by enormous uncertainties about the true risks that are involved.

"Zoonosis" is a term that has been used for some time to describe the general process of cross-species infection. More recently, the term "xeno-zoonosis" has been developed to describe infection transmission that might occur as a result of xenotransplantation. It is important to realize that from the point of view of the individual recipient, the risk of transmitting infection by xenotransplantation is likely to be less than by current clinical allotransplantation, both because of the natural resistance to cross-species transmission of infectious

diseases and because of the much longer time available to screen prospective donors. It is also important to point out that the risk of infectious transmission is unlikely to come from known pathogens, since if the agent is known, it is generally possible to screen for and eliminate its presence.

The major concern, therefore, regarding infections resulting from xenotransplantation is that endogenous retroviral sequences from donor cells might infect the recipient's cells, giving rise themselves, or after recombination with human endogenous retroviral sequences, to previously unrecognized pathogenic viruses. Such new viruses might prove hazardous to other human beings in addition to the xenograft recipient. While it has seemed to some that cross-species transmission of retroviruses would probably have occurred already in nature if it were likely to happen at all, others have pointed out that the circumstances of xenotransplantation may create unique conditions favoring this event. In particular, the prolonged coexistence of cells from two different species in patients who are taking immunosuppressive drugs or who have been rendered tolerant to their donors may be especially permissive for cross-species transfer of endogenous retroviruses. This concern has increased as a result of *in vitro* studies showing that pig proviruses can infect human cells when cells from both species are cultured together (368). At this time, however, there is no evidence that such cross-species transfer after a pig-to-human transplant would generate a virus that would be infectious or pathogenic. Indeed, a study of humans known to have been exposed to pig tissues did not reveal any cases of viremia nor of detectable pig endogenous retroviruses (PERV) in serum samples from over 160 people (369). Nevertheless, the concern about infections from xenotransplantation involves fear of the unknown, for which it is impossible to assign an accurate level of risk. At this time, therefore, public health agencies and members of the transplant community are attempting to design rational approaches for identifying the true risks of xenotransplantation and detecting untoward events rapidly, while at the same time allowing further progress in this potentially enormously important field of transplantation.

Clinical Progress in Xenotransplantation

Early clinical efforts in xenotransplantation took place in the 1960s, and involved organ transplants from nonhuman primates (276). One of the patients survived for 9 months with normal renal function provided by the kidney of a chimpanzee (370). Additional clinical trials thereafter, using baboon hearts and livers were considerably less successful. The most recent clinical trials have involved fetal pig cells transplanted into the brains of patients with Parkinson's or Huntington's diseases. Survival of pig tissue 8 months after the transplant was documented in a patient taking only moderate doses of immunosuppression (371). These studies suggest that cellular xenotransplantation may be achieved more easily, and thus may be performed sooner, than solid organ transplants, especially because free cellular transplants lack the vascular endothelium that is the target for both hyperacute and accelerated rejection. For organ xenotransplantation, many investigators (including us) believe that no further clinical testing should be performed until there is a reasonable expectation of success on the basis of pig-to-nonhuman-primate experimental studies.

SOME IMMUNOLOGIC ISSUES IN CLINICAL TRANSPLANTATION

The Effect of Antigen Matching on Graft Survival and GVHD

Organ Transplantation: Clinical Data

Transplantation antigens are defined by their ability to cause graft rejection and, in the absence of transplantation antigen disparities, graft rejection does not occur. Thus, there can be no argument with the statement that antigen matching improves graft survival. Contrary to this simple conclusion, however, the importance of antigen matching is one of the more controversial issues in clinical transplantation. The debate is frequently confused by failure to focus on the relevant quantitative issue of whether improved, but incomplete, antigen matching influences the outcome of organ transplantation sufficiently under current clinical circumstances to warrant its logistical difficulties. Further complicating the issue is variability in HLA typing techniques used. Until the recent development of molecular typing techniques, these analyses relied on serological and other techniques with relatively poor specificity. As an example of the degree to which molecular mismatches have been missed with serological typing, the DRB1 locus has more than 300 known alleles, yet only 17 specificities can be distinguished serologically (12). Furthermore, serological typing, which depends on human sera obtained from multiparous females or repeatedly transfused individuals, is relatively error prone in comparison to DNA-based typing, which utilizes standard reagents.

The evidence from transplantation of kidneys using living related donors provides a clinical demonstration of the importance of antigen matching in subsequent graft survival. Two siblings may share all of their HLA antigens (25% likelihood); half of their HLA antigens (50% likelihood); or none of their HLA antigens (25% likelihood). Identical twins share all of their transplantation antigens, but siblings are generally matched for only about half of the minor antigens that distinguish their parents, even if they are HLA identical. Table 7 shows one institution's survival rates for kidney grafts after 1 year for HLA-identical and one-haplotype–matched living related donors. Similar differences have been reported in the University of California-Los Angeles kidney transplant registry (372). Data from a large international database on kidney allograft survival from 1985 to 1999 showed a survival half-life of HLA-identical sibling allografts of 23.4 years, as compared to 12.8 years for haplo-identical related allografts (12). These data support the basic concept that antigen matching

TABLE 7. *One year kidney graft survival*

	1996 (%)	1986 (%)	1976 (%)
HLA-identical grafts (living-related)	100	100	90
One-haplotype matched grafts (living-related)	94	92	78
Cadaver-donor grafts	86	83	58

Data from the Transplantation Unit, Massachusetts General Hospital, Boston, MA.

matters, and for related donors, MHC antigen matching is widely agreed to be advantageous.

In the absence of a living related donor, transplantation is performed with organs from unrelated donors, usually from cadaveric sources. Because of the extensive polymorphism of MHC antigens, unrelated donors selected in a random fashion would not be expected to share many HLA antigens with the recipient. Similarly, there would only be sporadic matching of the minor histocompatibility antigens. Correspondingly, the survival of organs from cadaveric donors (half-life 11.1 years in the large registry referred to above [12]) has generally been shorter than that of HLA-identical or one-haplotype–mismatched related transplants. While longer ischemic time of cadaveric compared to living donor kidney transplants could account for some of this difference, a significant inverse correlation between graft survival and number of (serologically determined) HLA mismatches was evident among cadaveric donor recipients, and was still evident among the subgroup with short ischemic times. A similar effect could also be seen in recipients of living unrelated donor transplants with various mismatches (12). A long-term benefit for increased HLA matching could also be seen in recipients of cardiac, but not liver, allografts (12). Since all of the above analyses are retrospective, an unanswered question is whether the potential added ischemic time required for nonrandom distribution of cadaveric organs to achieve a larger number of matched antigens would achieve better results.

A second question for all unrelated transplants is whether the more specific typing information provided by molecular typing confers a graft survival advantage over serologic typing. It appears that the typing for loci that cannot be typed serologically, such as HLA-DP, as well as DNA typing within a serotype, can benefit the survival of cadaveric transplants in heavily presensitized recipients (12). However, in cadaveric transplant recipients as a group, improved graft survival was observed when molecular typing was used at a level of resolution that was not much greater than that of the serologic technique used in the same study, suggesting that improved accuracy of molecular typing may be the major source of benefit when compared to serologic typing in nonpresensitized recipients (12). High-resolution molecular typing would reduce the likelihood that a matched donor could be found by these more stringent criteria, and might increase the time required to perform HLA typing. Thus, it remains unclear that the distribution of organs to achieve such matching is worth the incumbent effort, expense, and increased ischemic time, which may also affect outcome.

Over the years, the controversy about the impact of antigen matching has focused on several specific issues. Some investigators have suggested that matching for particular alleles of the HLA antigens is especially important and others have suggested that matching for some loci is more important than for others. A major question is whether matching for class II antigens might be more important than matching for class I antigens. There are clinical data suggesting that class II antigen matching is of particular benefit to the outcome of transplantation.

Organ Transplantation: Experimental Data

As is discussed above, a particularly useful large animal model has been developed to test experimentally the importance of antigen matching. Over the past 20 years, three herds of partially inbred miniature swine have been developed for studies of transplantation biology (Fig. 3). Each herd has been bred to homozygosity for a different allele at the MHC (termed SLA in swine). Subsequent breeding has been intentionally randomized within herds in order to maintain a variety of segregating minor histocompatibility loci. Transplants among these animals thus resemble the situation within human families, that is, HLA identical versus nonidentical siblings.

Studies of skin and renal allografts between these animals produced the results shown in Table 8. The difference observed for skin graft survival between SLA-matched and-mismatched animals was modest. Matching had a much more profound effect on kidney graft survival. One-third of the grafts between SLA matched animals survived indefinitely without immunosuppression, despite the existence of multiple minor histoincompatibilities. The ability to reject renal allografts across minor differences was found to depend on an Ir gene, inherited in an autosomal dominant fashion and not linked to the MHC (9).

Using intra-MHC recombinants between minipig haplotypes, the relative importance of class I versus class II matching on renal allograft survival was examined in these large animals (9). The survival of renal allografts with class I–only differences and with class II–only differences is shown in Table 8. As in the mouse, both class I and class II differences appeared sufficient to cause prompt skin graft rejection.

However, for kidney allografts, class II matching was of particular importance in determining the outcome. In fact, the results for minor plus class I differences were indistinguishable from those for minor histocompatibility antigen differences alone.

These experimental data were obtained without the exogenous immunosuppression always administered in clinical studies. They demonstrate the biological principle that antigen matching is important to graft survival and further indicate that class II antigen matching is likely to be particularly important. No experimental system is likely to settle the empirical issue in clinical medicine, however, of how much benefit will be obtained under the conditions of current practice.

Hematopoietic Cell Transplantation: Clinical Data

In contrast to the results described above for solid organ transplants, the importance of HLA matching for unrelated hematopoietic cell transplantation is unquestioned. Until quite recently, HCT was performed almost exclusively in HLA-identical (or single HLA antigen–mismatched) sibling pairs. Although this restriction has severely limited the use of HCT (only 25% of individuals have an HLA-identical sibling; another 5% has a single antigen-mismatched related donor), the complications of HLA-mismatched transplantation have prohibited its widespread use. Among these complications, GVHD is the most prevalent and severe, with a severe form of the disease occurring in 75% to 80% of recipients of related donor transplants differing at one to three HLA-A, -B, or -DR loci (373). Additionally, the incidence of marrow graft rejection increases in the presence of HLA disparity: while only 2% of HLA-identical related donor grafts are rejected, the figure increases to approximately 12% in recipients of unmodified haplo-identical related donor grafts (351).

Similar to solid organ graft rejection, GVHD appears to be a particularly severe problem in the setting of class II MHC mismatching, as evidenced by its higher incidence in single antigen–mismatched related donor transplants with a class II compared to a class I disparity (351). This was confirmed for unrelated transplants in a study from Seattle (374), but the opposite appeared to be the case (i.e., class I mismatching conferred a greater GVHD risk than class II mismatching) in a Japanese study of unrelated donor transplants. Although HLA-DP disparity, which is commonly present in the unrelated donor setting, was originally found not to be associated

TABLE 8. *Graft survival and antigen matching in minipigs*

	Mismatch			
Graft	Minors only	Major and minors	Class I[a]	Class II[a]
Skin	11.8 ± 0.9	7.0 ± 0.4	10.8 ± 2.3	7.8 ± 1.0
Kidney	30.0 ± 15.0 (2/3) >120 (1/3)	12 ± 1.9	19.5 ± 6.8(2/3) >120 (1/3)	21.8 ± 10.4

[a]Single haplotype mismatch.

with increased GVHD risk, more recent studies suggest that a two-locus mismatch in the GVH direction is associated with significantly greater risk of severe GVHD (351). A recent analysis from Seattle (351) has confirmed the greater overall importance of class II mismatching compared to class I mismatching alone in GVHD, but also demonstrates synergy between mismatches at both class I and II loci in increasing GVHD risk.

With respect to marrow graft rejection, class I (including HLA-A, -B, and -C) disparities have been most strongly associated with increased risk, which increases in proportion to the number of such disparities (12,351,375). Although the importance of class I mismatching, and particularly that of HLA-C, might suggest a role for NK cell–mediated rejection, antidonor NK reactivity was not demonstrable during the time of rejection in a patient receiving marrow from a donor whose HLA class I alleles would be incapable of triggering recipient KIRs recognizing recipient class I alleles (79). Thus far, a role for NK cells in mediating marrow allograft rejection has not been demonstrated in heavily conditioned hosts, but their role may become more significant if mismatched transplants are attempted with less toxic, nonmyeloablative regimens. In contrast, a role for classical CTL is well established in the rejection of even HLA-identical donor marrow following myeloablative conditioning. Rejection of HLA-identical HCT is rare unless the donor product is T-cell depleted, but occurs quite frequently in the setting of HLA-mismatched transplants, even without T-cell depletion, and increases even further with T-cell depletion (251). Antidonor CTL specific for the mismatched donor class I allele have been associated with marrow rejection following unrelated donor transplantation (376). Class II disparities may also play a role in unrelated donor stem-cell graft rejection (351). Recently, $CD4^+$ CTL recognizing the only mismatched donor HLA allele, HLA-DP, were identified in the blood of a patient undergoing rejection following unrelated donor HCT (377).

High-resolution, PCR-based HLA typing methods have increased the capacity to avoid HLA disparities that would have previously (when only serological HLA typing was available) gone unrecognized. However, higher-resolution HLA typing will obviously reduce the chance of finding a fully matched unrelated donor, even with the availability of large registries such as the National Marrow Donor Program in the United States, which currently contains more than 4.5 million volunteer registrants. Already, many patients do not succeed in finding an unrelated donor, and thus the identification of "acceptable" mismatches in the unrelated donor setting is of the utmost importance.

Crossmatch

There are several means of detecting preexisting antibodies in the serum of potential recipients that have specificity for donor antigens. First, it is necessary to determine blood type since clinical transplantation across blood group barriers is never knowingly attempted for those organs susceptible to hy-

peracute rejection. One exception is the ability to transplant organs from donors of the A_2 blood group to recipients of other blood groups. Secondly, immediate pretransplant sera from prospective recipients are tested against lymphocytes of potential donors. This test is called a crossmatch and it is not the same as the "antigen matching" discussed above. An individual can have a "negative" crossmatch (meaning that they do not have antibodies reactive with donor antigens), but still be completely unmatched with respect to HLA antigens. On the other hand, matching for some HLA antigens may improve the chances of obtaining a negative crossmatch for prospective recipients who have developed antibodies reactive with many foreign HLA antigens. The crossmatch is generally performed by a two-step, antibody-mediated, complement-dependent cytotoxicity assay. In many centers, the test is augmented by the intermediate addition of antihuman immunoglobulin to increase the sensitivity for detecting lysis. More recently, flow cytometry has been used to detect preexisting recipient antibodies with still additional sensitivity, although the data from flow cytometric analysis may be too sensitive to be clinically applicable.

"Sensitized" Candidate for Organ Transplantation

Since kidneys and many other vascularized organs cannot currently be transplanted into recipients with preexisting antibodies, the clinical goal is to avoid the formation of antibodies reactive with donor antigens or to find organs that do not express the particular HLA antigens against which the recipient has been sensitized. Except for blood group antibodies, recipient sensitization to transplantation antigens always occurs by prior exposure to allogeneic tissue. This may occur as a result of blood transfusion, as a result of previous organ transplantation, or, in women, by exposure to paternal antigens during or just after pregnancy. The degree of sensitization of a potential kidney recipient is measured regularly by testing sera on a panel of lymphocytes selected from individuals who collectively express a broad representation of the HLA antigens. Transplantation candidates whose sera react with a high percentage of the cells in this panel (panel reactive antibody [PRA]) are said to be "highly sensitized." The term may be confusing to immunologists, since in the clinical setting it refers only to B-cell sensitization and does not necessarily imply sensitization of cell-mediated effector mechanisms. Highly sensitized candidates may wait years to receive a kidney transplant and some may never receive one.

If a recipient has detectable antibodies to HLA antigens, she or he cannot receive an organ bearing these HLA antigens. Prior screening of potential recipients against the panel of HLA antigens can predict some of the determinants against which antibodies already exist. Most highly sensitized individuals actually produce antibodies of relatively limited heterogeneity that are reactive with public epitopes of HLA antigens. Thus, the HLA phenotype of unsuitable donors for any given recipient can be predicted with some precision. In this case, HLA tissue typing has value in identifying kidneys that may have a negative crossmatch for highly sensitized individuals.

The level of sensitization manifested by transplantation candidates fluctuates over time. As a result, it is possible for recipients to have a negative crossmatch with a donor's cells using recently obtained serum, but a positive crossmatch using previously collected sera. Transplantation in the face of this "historical positive crossmatch" has been performed successfully.

Obtaining crossmatch-negative donors by locating well-matched organs or waiting for a decline in the level of sensitization represent the primary solutions currently available for sensitized patients. Despite numerous trials, no widespread protocol for the active treatment of sensitized individuals to remove antibody has been adopted.

The Diagnosis of Rejection

In clinical organ transplantation, the most obvious manifestation of the rejection process is diminished function of the transplanted organ. Other causes of graft dysfunction exist, however, and it is obviously important to confirm the immunologic origin of the event before increasing immunosuppression. The clinical pattern of dysfunction often helps to suggest the diagnosis of rejection. However, no clinical sign can definitively diagnose rejection. It would be useful, therefore, to determine a means of identifying rejection episodes based on systemic manifestations of the immunologic mechanisms involved. Unfortunately, a well-established assay to measure rejection activity does not yet exist. Two approaches include the measurement of antidonor antibody production and the sequential measurement of cell-mediated responses to donor antigens. Antibody responses have frequently been documented following graft rejection, but they tend to appear after rejection is complete. *In vitro* cell-mediated responses, both proliferative and cytotoxic, may or may not be present while a graft is in place and are not well correlated with clinical rejection episodes. Assays of humoral and cellular responses to donor antigens both suffer from the possibility that donor-specific elements of the response may be absorbed by the antigens of the graft, at least until the late stages of rejection. Furthermore, the existence of tissue-specific peptides may allow T-cell responses to occur *in vivo* that cannot be measured *in vitro* when donor lymphocytes are used as stimulators. A recent report (150) suggests that urinary perforin and granzyme B levels may be useful in the diagnosis of renal allograft rejection, but did not rule out the possibility that other conditions associated with renal allograft dysfunction, such as CMV infection, might produce a similar profile.

The "gold standard" in the diagnosis of allograft rejection has always been the biopsy of the transplanted organ itself. Pathologists have been able to identify the abnormal lymphocytic infiltrate within grafts, to grade the intensity of the infiltrate, and, for some organs, to describe histologic findings characterizing the effects of immunologic injury (378). Some pathologic changes, including a lymphocytic infiltrate of the vascular wall, seem to be well correlated with rejection activity (378). In addition, pathologic changes suggesting nonimmunologic causes of renal dysfunction may be helpful in patient management.

Despite the widespread reliance on the biopsy to define episodes of rejection, however, differentiation of rejection from its absence is often difficult, particularly when cyclosporine immunosuppression has been used. Since most clinical allograft biopsies are performed when the organ is not functioning well, and only after mechanical causes of dysfunction have been excluded, most organs that are biopsied, by selection, are undergoing rejection. Therefore, inability to detect nonrejection events in a few cases pathologically will still leave an excellent correlation between the diagnosis of rejection and the response to therapy. When routine biopsies of transplanted organs have been done, regardless of organ dysfunction, they have revealed a poor correlation between histologic findings and clinical evidence of rejection. Experimental studies of skin grafts, as discussed above, have found that the degree of lymphocytic infiltrate in an allograft correlated better with the nature of the antigenic disparity than with the intensity of the rejection process. Furthermore, several experimental models of tolerance induction have shown intense lymphocytic infiltrates in organs that go on to survive indefinitely in recipients who develop tolerance to the donor antigens. These studies suggest that the amount of lymphocytic infiltrate detected pathologically may not be helpful in diagnosing rejection episodes and determining the need for treatment.

How Much Immunosuppression Is Enough?

While the majority of transplant recipients respond immunologically to their new organ despite immunosuppression, some patients seem never to generate any rejection activity and maintain their transplanted organ with very small doses of immunosuppressive drugs. Indeed, a few patients have been known to stop all medications but have kept their transplant for years without rejection. On the other hand, some patients seem to require and tolerate very high doses of exogenous immunosuppression, while others seem to be severely immunocompromised by low doses of these drugs. These observations make it clear that the amount of immunosuppression that is required or that is safe is not the same for every individual or for all grafts. Unfortunately, there is no well-established assay to determine the amount of immunosuppression an individual requires and can safely tolerate for his or her particular transplant.

CONCLUSION

The great danger in any textbook chapter is that the need to summarize what we think is known will obscure the much greater amount still left to be learned. In recent years enormous progress has been made in the study of the major histocompatibility antigens, yet we still know too little about the products of the numerous other histocompatibility loci that encode the minor histocompatibility antigens. Recently we have gained important insight into the role of APC in T-cell sensitization; but we still have not explored adequately the role that indirect presentation of alloantigens plays in graft rejection. During the past 2 decades we have learned much about the generation and function of cytotoxic T-lymphocytes and about their likely role in some mechanisms of graft rejection and GVHD; however, our understanding of noncytolytic mechanisms of rejection and GVHD, which clearly exist, is much more limited. Finally, this chapter has outlined several techniques for the generation of immunologic tolerance to alloantigens in experimental systems; however, as is described above, the first human beings have only recently been transplanted with a tolerance-inducing regimen (nonmyeloablative allogeneic BMT with simultaneous donor kidney transplantation) that allows the early discontinuation of nonspecific immunosuppression. The encouraging initial results achieved with this approach raise hopes that routine tolerance induction may soon become a clinical reality. New insights into basic immunologic issues will likely have important consequences for clinical transplantation in the future.

GLOSSARY OF TERMS AND ABBREVIATIONS

αGal	Galα1-3Galβ1-4GlcNAc
ADCC	Antibody-dependent cell-mediated cytotoxicity
AICD	Activation-induced cell death
Allo	Allogeneic
APC	Antigen-presenting cell
β2m$^{-/-}$	β2 microglobulin
BMC	Bone marrow cells
BMT	Bone marrow transplant
CCR7	CC chemokine receptor 7
CD40L	CD40 ligand
CDR3	Complementarity-determining region 3
CML	Cell-mediated lympholysis
CMV	Cytomegalovirus
CsA	Cyclosporine
CTL	Cytotoxic T-lymphocyte
CTLp	Cytotoxic T-lymphocyte precursor
CXCR3	CXC chemokine receptor 3
DAF	Decay-accelerating factor
DC	Dendritic cell
DLI	Donor lymphocyte infusions
DST	Donor-specific transfusion
DTH	Delayed-type hypersensitivity
ELISA	Enzyme-linked immunosorbent assay
ELISpot	Enzyme-linked immunosorbent spot
ES cells	Embryonic stem cells
FasL	Fas ligand
FKBP	FK506-binding protein
GalT	α1-3Gal transferase
GVH	Graft versus host
GVHD	Graft-versus-host disease

GVL	Graft versus leukemia
H-2	Mouse MHC
HA	Histocompatibility antigen
HCT	Hematopoietic cell transplantation
HDAF	Human decay-accelerating factor
HEV	High endothelial venule
HLA	Human leukocyte antigen
IP-10	Interferon gamma-induciple protein of 10 kD
ITIM	Immune receptor tyrosine–based inhibitory motif
KGF	Keratinocyte growth factor
KIR	Killer inhibitory receptor
MAC	Membrane attack complex
Mac1	Myeloid cell-surface marker CD11b
MCP	Membrane cofactor protein
MHC	Major histocompatibility complex
Mig	Monokine induced by IFN-γ
MIP1α	Macrophage inflammatory protein 1α
MLR	Mixed lymphocyte response
NK	Natural killer
NS	Natural suppressor
PBMC	Peripheral blood mononuclear cell
PERV	Pig endogenous retrovirus
PHSC	Pluripotent hematopoietic stem cell
PRA	Panel reactive antibody
Rag	Recombinase-activating gene
SCID	Severe combined immunodeficiency
SLA	Swine leukocyte antigen
STAT	Signal transducers and activators of transduction
TBI	Total body irradiation
TC R	T-cell receptor
TI	Thymic irradiation
TLI	Total lymphoid irradiation
TNFR1	Tumor necrosis factor receptor 1
Tr1	T-regulatory cells 1
Treg	Regulatory T cells

REFERENCES

1. Woodruff MFA. *The transplantation of tissues and organs.* Springfield, IL: Charles C. Thomas, 1960.
2. Gibson T. Zoografting: a curious chapter in the history of plastic surgery. *Br J Plast Surg* 1955;8:234.
3. Billingham RE. Transplantation: past, present and future. *J Invest Dermatol* 1963;41:165.
4. Carrel A. *Transplantation in mass of the kidneys. J Exp Med* 1908; 10:98.
5. Converse JM, Casson PR. The historical background of transplantation. In: Rapaport FT, Dausset J, eds. *Human transplantation.* New York: Grune and Stratton, 1968:7.
6. Groth CG. Landmarks in clinical renal transplantation. *Surg Gynecol Obstetrics* 1972;134:327–328.
7. Medawar PB. Second study of behaviour and fate of skin homografts in rabbits. *J Anat* 1945;79:157.
8. Sachs DH. MHC-homozygous miniature swine. In: Swindle MM, Moody DC, Phillips LD, eds. *Swine as models in biomedical research.* Ames: Iowa State University Press 1992:3–15.
9. Gianello P, Fishbein JM, Sachs DH. Tolerance to primarily vascularized allografts in miniature swine. *Immunol Rev* 1993;133:19–44.
10. Little CC. The genetics of tissue transplantation in mammals. *Cancer Res* 1924;8:75–95.

11. Little CC. The genetics of tumor transplantation. In: Snell GD, ed. *Biology of the laboratory mouse.* New York: Dover Publications, 1941:279–309.

12. Erlich HA, Opelz G, Hansen J. HLA DNA typing and transplantation. *Immunity* 2001;14:447–356.

13. Caughman SW, Sharrow SO, Shimad S, et al. Ia+ murine epidermal Langerhans cells are deficient in surface expression of class I MHC. *Proc Natl Acad Sci U S A* 1986;83:7438–7442.

14. Glimcher LH, Kara CJ. Sequences and factors: a guide to MHC class-II transcription. *Annu Rev Immunol* 1992;10:13–49.

15. Pescovitz MD, Sachs DH, Lunney JK, et al. Localization of class II MHC antigens on porcine renal vascular endothelium. *Transplantation* 1984;37:627–630.

16. Suchin EJ, Langmuir PB, Palmer E, et al. Quantifying the frequency of alloreactive T cells in vivo: new answers to an old question. *J Immunol* 2001;166:973–981.

17. Jerne NK. The somatic generation of immune recognition. *Eur J Immunol* 1971;1:1–9.

18. Bevan MJ. In thymic selection, peptide diversity gives and takes away. *Immunity* 1997;7:175–178.

19. Sprent J, Lo D, Gao E-K, et al. T cell selection in the thymus. *Immunol Rev* 1988;101:174–190.

20. Bevan MJ. High determinant density may explain the phenomenon of alloreactivity. *Immunol Today* 1984;5:128–130.

21. Matzinger P, Bevan MJ. Hypothesis: why do so many lymphocytes respond to major histocompatibility complex antigens? *Cell Immunol* 1977;29:1–5.

22. Garboczi D, Ghosh P, Utz U, et al. Structure of the complex between human T-cell receptor, viral peptide and HLA-A2. *Nature* 1996;384:134–141.

23. Reinherz EL, Tan K, Tang L, et al. The crystal structure of a T cell receptor in complex with peptide and MHC class II. *Science* 1999;286:1913–1921.

24. Speir JA, Garcia KC, Brunmark A, et al. Structural basis of 2C TCR allorecognition of H-2Ld peptide complexes. *Immunity* 1998;8:553–562.

25. Rudolph MG, Speir JA, Brunmark A, et al. The crystal structures of K(bm1) and K(bm8) reveal that subtle changes in the peptide environment impact thermostability and alloreactivity. *Immunity* 2001;14:231–242.

26. Reiser JB, Darnault C, Guimezanes A, et al. Crystal structure of a T cell receptor bound to an allogeneic MHC molecule. *Nat Immunol* 2000;1:291–297.

27. Roetzschke O, Falk K, Faath S, et al. On the nature of peptides involved in T cell alloreactivity. *J Exp Med* 1991;174:1059–1071.

28. Obst R, Netuschil N, Klopfer K, et al. The role of peptides in T cell alloreactivity is determined by self–major histocompatibility complex molecules. *J Exp Med* 2000;191:805–812.

29. Felix NJ, Brickey WJ, Griffiths R, et al. H2-DMα(−/−) mice show the importance of major histocompatibility complex-bound peptide in cardiac allograft rejection. *J Exp Med* 2000;192:41–40.

30. Sebille F, Gagne K, Guillet M, et al. Direct recognition of foreign MHC determinants by naive T cells mobilizes specific Vβ families without skewing of the complementarity-determining region 3 length distribution. *J Immunol* 2001;167:4082–3088.

31. Garboczi DN, Biddison WE. Shapes of MHC restriction. *Immunity* 1999;10:1–7.

32. Elliott T, Townsend A, Cerundolo V. Naturally processed peptides. *Nature* 1990;348:195–197.

33. Perreault C, Roy DC, Fortin C. Immunodominant minor histocompatibility antigens: the major ones. *Immunol Today* 1998;19:69–74.

34. Simpson E, Roopenian D, Goulmy E. Much ado about minor histocompatibility antigens. *Immunol Today* 1998;19:108–111.

35. Goulmy E. Human minor histocompatibility antigens. *Curr Opin Immunol* 1996;8:75–81.

36. Malarkannan S, Horng T, Eden P, et al. Differences that matter: major cytotoxic T cell–stimulating minor histocompatibility antigens. *Immunity* 2000;13:433–344.

37. Grumet FC, Hiraki DD, Brown BWM, et al. CD31 mismatching affects marrow transplantation outcome. *Biol Blood Marrow Transplant* 2001;7:503–512.

38. Lindahl KF, Byers DE, Dabhi VM, et al. H2-M3, a full-service class Ib histocompatibility antigen. *Annu Rev Immunol* 1997;15:851–879.

39. Mendoza LM, Paz P, Zuberi A, et al. Minors held by major: the H13 minor histocompatibility locus defined as a peptide/MHC class I complex. *Immunity* 1997;7:461–472.

40. den Haan JMM, Meadows LM, Wang W, et al. The minor histocompatibility antigen HA-1: a diallelic gene with a single amino acid polymorphism. *Science* 1998;279:1054–1057.

41. Brickner AG, Warren EH, Caldwell JA, et al. The immunogenicity of a new human minor histocompatibility antigen results from differential antigen processing. *J Exp Med* 2001;193:195–206.

42. Roopenian DC. What are minor histocompatibility loci? A new look at an old question. *Immunol Today* 1992;13:7–10.

43. Korngold R, Wettstein PJ. Immunodominance in the graft-vs-host disease T cell response to minor histocompatibility antigens. *J Immunol* 1990;145:4079–4088.

44. Simpson E. The role of H-Y as a minor transplantation antigen. *Immunol Today* 1982;3:97–106.

45. Pierce RA, Field ED, den Haan JM, et al. Cutting edge: the HLA-A*0101–restricted HY minor histocompatibility antigen originates from DFFRY and contains a cysteinylated cysteine residue as identified by a novel mass spectrometric technique. *J Immunol* 1999;163:6360–6364.

46. Roopenian DC, David AP, Christianson GJ, et al. The functional basis of minor histocompatibility loci. *J Immunol* 1993;151:4595–4605.

47. Zelenika D, Adams E, Mellor A, et al. Rejection of H-Y disparate skin grafts by monospecific CD4+ Th1 and Th2 cells: no requirement for CD8+ T cells or B cells. *J Immunol* 1998;161:1868–1874.

48. Vogt MH, Goulmy E, Kloosterboer FM, et al. UTY gene codes for an HLA-B60–restricted human male-specific minor histocompatibility antigen involved in stem cell graft rejection: characterization of the critical polymorphic amino acid residues for T-cell recognition. *Blood* 2000;96:4126–3132.

49. Goulmy E, Schipper R, Pool J, et al. Mismatches of minor histocompatiblity antigens bwtween HLA-idnetical donors and recipients and the development of graft-versus-host disease after bone marrow transplantation. *N Engl J Med* 1996;334:281–285.

50. Mutis T, Gillespie G, Schrama E, et al. Tetrameric HLA class I-minor histocompatibility antigen peptide complexes demonstrate minor histocompatibility antigen-specific cytotoxic T lymphocytes in patients with graft-versus-host disesae. *Nat Med* 1999;5:839–842.

51. Vogt MH, de Paus RA, Voogt PJ, et al. DFFRY codes for a new human male-specific minor transplantation antigen involved in bone marrow graft rejection. *Blood* 2000;95:1100–1105.

52. Scott D, Addey C, Ellis P, et al. Dendritic cells permit identification of genes encoding MHC class II–restricted epitopes of transplantation antigens. *Immunity* 2000;12:711–720.

53. Jarvis CD, Germain RN, Hager GL, et al. Tissue-specific expression of messenger RNAs encoding endogenous viral superantigens. *J Immunol* 1994;152:1032–1038.

54. Jones MS, Riley H, Hamilton BL, et al. Endogenous superantigens in allogeneic bone marrow transplant recipients rapidly and selectively expand donor T cells which can produce IFN-gamma. *Bone Marrow Transplant* 1994;14:725–735.

55. Lorenz R, Allen PM. Processing and presentation of self proteins. *Immunol Rev* 1988;106:115–127.

56. Steinmuller D, Wachtel SS. Transplantation biology and immunogenetics of murine skin-specific antigens. *Transplant Proc* 1980;12[suppl 1]:100–106.

57. Joyce S, Mathew JM, Flye MW, et al. A polymorphic human kidney–specific non-MHC alloantigen. Its possible role in tissue-specific allograft immunity. *Transplant* 1992;53:1119–1127.

58. Platt JL, Bach FH. The barrier to xenotransplantation. *Transplant* 1991;52:937–947.

59. Kiessling R, Hochman PS, Haller O, et al. Evidence for a similar or common mechanism for natural killer activity and resistance to hemopoietic grafts. *Eur J Immunol* 1977;7:655–663.

60. Moretta L, Ciccone E, Moretta A, et al. Allorecognition by NK cells: nonself or no self? *Immunol Today* 1992;13:400–306.

61. Lafferty KJ, Bootes A, Dart G, et al. Effect of organ culture on the survival of thyroid allografts in mice. *Transplantation* 1976;22:138–149.

62. Janeway CA, Ron J, Katz ME. The B cell is the initiating antigen-presenting cell in peripheral lymph nodes. *J Immunol* 1987;138:1051–1055.

63. Ron Y, Sprent J. T cell priming in vivo: a major role for B cells in presenting antigen to T cells in lymph nodes. *J Immunol* 1987;138:2848–2856.

64. Steinman RM. The dendritic cell system and its role in immunogenicity. *Annu Rev Immunol* 1991;9:271–296.

65. Thomson AW, Lu L. Dendritic cells as regulators of immune reactivity: implications for transplantation. *Transplantation* 1999;68:1–8.

66. Bevan MJ. Minor antigens introduced on H-2 different stimulating cells cross-react at the cytotoxic T cell level during in vivo priming. *J Immunol* 1976;117:2233–2238.

67. Braun MY, Grandjean I, Feunou P, et al. Acute rejection in the absence of cognate recognition of allograft by T cells. *J Immunol* 2001; 166:4879–4883.

68. Barker CF, Billingham RE. The role of regional lymphatics in the skin homograft response. *Transplantation* 1967;5[suppl]:6.

69. Lakkis FG, Arakelov A, Konieczny BT, et al. Immunologic "ignorance" of vascularized organ transplants in the absence of secondary lymphoid tissue. *Nat Med* 2000;6:686–688.

70. Dustin ML, Springer TA. Role of lymphocyte adhesion receptors in transient interactions and cell locomotion. *Annu Rev Immunol* 1991; 9:27–66.

71. Kirby JA, Cunningham AC. Intragraft antigen presentation: the contribution of bone-marrow derived, epithelial and endothelial presenting cells. *Transplant Rev* 1997;11:127–140.

72. Ohdan H, Swenson KG, Kruger-Gray HW, et al. Mac-1–negative B-1b phenotype of natural antibody-producing cells, including those responding to Galα1,3Gal epitopes in α1,3-galactosyltransferase deficient mice. *J Immunol* 2000;165:5518–5529.

73. van den Bogaerde J, Aspinall R, Wang M-W, et al. Induction of long-term survival of hamster heart xenografts in rats. *Transplantation* 1991;52:15–20.

74. Cramer DV, Chapman FA, Jaffee BD, et al. The prolongation of concordant hamster-to-rat cardiac xenografts by brequinar sodium. *Transplantation* 1992;54:403–408.

75. Xiao F, Chong AS, Foster P, et al. Leflunomide controls rejection in hamster to rat cardiac xenografts. *Transplantation* 1994;58:828–834.

76. Auchincloss H Jr, Ghobrial RRM, Russell PS, et al. Anti-L3T4 in vivo prevents alloantibody formation after skin grafting without prolonging graft survival. *Transplantation* 1988;45:1118–1123.

77. Peritt D, Robertson S, Gri G, et al. Differentiation of human NK cells into NK1 and NK2 subsets. *J Immunol* 1998;161:5821–5824.

78. Lee LA, Sergio JJ, Sykes M. Natural killer cells weakly resist engraftment of allogeneic long-term multilineage-repopulating hematopoietic stem cells. *Transplantation* 1996;61:125–132.

79. Ruggeri L, Capanni M, Casucci M, et al. Role of natural killer cell alloreactivity in HLA-mismatched hematopoietic stem cell transplantation. *Blood* 1999;94:333–339.

80. O'Reilly RJ, Brochstein J, Collins N, et al. Evaluation of HLA-haplotype disparate parental marrow grafts depleted of T lymphocytes by differential agglutination with a soybean lectin and E-rosette depletion for the treatment of severe combined immunodeficiency. *Vox Sang* 1986;51[suppl 2]:81–86.

81. Renard V, Cambiaggi A, Vely F, et al. Transduction of cytotoxic signals in natural killer cells: a general model of fine tuning between activatory and inhibitory pathways in lymphocytes. *Immunol Rev* 1997;155:205–221.

82. Hoglund P, Sundback J, Olsson-Alheim MY, et al. Host MHC class I gene control of NK cell specificity in the mouse. *Immunol Rev* 1997; 155:11–28.

83. Manilay JO, Sykes M. Natural killer cells and their role in graft rejection. *Curr Opin Immunol* 1998;10:532–538.

84. Nikolic B, Cooke DT, Zhao G, et al. Both γδ T cells and NK cells inhibit the engraftment of xenogeneic rat bone marrow cells in mice. *J Immunol* 2001;166:1398–1404.

85. Heidecke CD, Araujo JL, Kupiec-Weglinski JW, et al. Lack of evidence for an active role for natural killer cells in acute rejection of organ allografts. *Transplantation* 1985;40:441–444.

86. Bix M, Liao N-S, Zijlstra M, et al. Rejection of class I MHC–deficient haemopoietic cells by irradiated MHC-matched mice. *Nature* 1991;349:429–331.

87. Zijlstra M, Auchincloss H Jr, Loring JM, et al. Skin graft rejection by β2–microglobulin–deficient mice. *J Exp Med* 1992;175:885–893.

88. Maier S, Tertilt C, Chambron N, et al. Inhibition of natural killer cells results in acceptance of cardiac allografts in CD28–/– mice. *Nat Med* 2001;7:557–562.

89. Goodman DJ, Millan MT, Ferran C, et al. Mechanisms of delayed xenograft rejection. In: Cooper DKC, Kemp E, Platt JL, et al, eds. *Xenotransplantation*. Heidelberg: Springer, 1997:77–94.

90. Inverardi L, Stolzer AL, Bender JR, et al. Human natural killer lymphocytes directly recognize evolutionarily conserved oligosaccharide ligands expressed by xenogeneic tissue. *Transplantation* 1997;63:1318–1330.

91. Hong S, Van Kaer L. Immune privilege: keeping an eye on natural killer T cells. *J Exp Med* 1999;190:1197–1200.

92. Park S-H, Bendelac A. CD1-restricted T-cell responses and microbial infection. *Nature* 2000;406:788–792.

93. Bendelac A. CD1: Presenting unusual antigens to unusual T lymphocytes. *Science* 1995;269:185–186.

94. Falcone M, Yeung B, Tucker L, et al. A defect in interleukin 12–induced activation and interferon γ secretion of peripheral natural killer T cells in nonobese diabetic mice suggests new pathogenic mechanisms for insulin-dependent diabetes mellitus. *J Exp Med* 1999; 190:963–972.

95. Wilson SB, Kent SC, Patton KT, et al. Extreme Th1 bias of invariant Vα24JαQ T cells in type 1 diabetes. *Nature* 1998;391:177–181.

96. Zeng D, Lewis D, Dejbakhsh-Jones S, et al. Bone marrow NK1.1– and NK1.1+ T cells reciprocally regulate acute graft versus host disease. *J Exp Med* 1999;189:1073–1081.

97. Seino KK, Fukao K, Muramoto K, et al. Requirement for natural killer T (NKT) cells in the induction of allograft tolerance. *Proc Natl Acad Sci U S A* 2001;98:2577–2581.

98. Sonoda K-H, Exley M, Snapper S, et al. CD1-reactive natural killer T cells are required for development of systemic tolerance through an immune-privileged site. *J Exp Med* 1999;190:1215–1225.

99. Cui J, Shin T, Kawano T, et al. Requirement for Vα14 NKT cells in IL-12–mediated rejection of tumors. *Science* 1998;278:1623–1626.

100. Platt JL, Vercellotti GM, Lindman BJ, et al. Release of heparan sulfate from endothelial cells: implications for pathogenesis of hyperacute rejection. *J Exp Med* 2002;171:1363–1368.

101. Doyle HR, Marino IR, Morelli F, et al. Assessing risk in liver transplantation: special reference to the significance of a positive cytotoxic crossmatch. *Ann Surg* 1996;224:168–177.

102. Baldamus CA, McKenzie IFC, Winn HJ, et al. Acute destruction by humoral antibody of rat skin grafted to mice. *J Immunol* 1973;110:1532–1541.

103. Aksentijevich I, Sachs DH, Sykes M. Natural antibodies can inhibit bone marrow engraftment in the rat→mouse species combination. *J Immunol* 1991;147:4140–4146.

104. Ohdan H, Yang Y-G, Swenson KG, et al. T cell and B cell tolerance to galα1,3gal-expressing heart xenografts is achieved in α1,3-galactosyltransferase-deficient mice by nonmyeloablative induction of mixed chimerism. *Transplantation* 2001;71:1532–1542.

105. Ohdan H, Swenson KG, Kitamura H, et al. Tolerization of Galα1,3Gal-reactive B cells in presensitized α1,3-galactosyltransferase-deficient mice by nonmyeloablative induction of mixed chimerism. *Xenotransplantation* 2001;8:227–238.

106. Yang Y-G, Chen AM, Sergio JJ, et al. Role of antibody-independent complement activation in rejection of porcine bone marrow cells in mice. *Transplantation* 1999;69:163–190.

107. Trpkov K, Campbell P, Pazderka F, et al. Pathologic features of acute renal allograft rejection associated with donor-specific antibody. Analysis using the Banff grading schema. *Transplantation* 1996; 61:1586–1592.

108. Bach FH, Ferran C, Hechenleitner P, et al. Accomodation of vascularized xenografts: expression of "protective genes" by donor endothelial cells in a host Th2 cytokine environment. *Nat Med* 1997;3:196–204.

109. Millan MT, Geczy C, Stuhlmeier KM, et al. Human monocytes activate porcine endothelial cells, resulting in increased E-selectin, interleukin-8, monocyte chemotactic protein-1, and plasminogen activator inhibitor-type-1 expression. *Transplantation* 1997;63:421–429.

110. Siegel JB, Grey ST, Lesnikoski B-A, et al. Xenogeneic endothelial cells activate human prothrombin. *Transplantation* 1997;64:888–896.

111. Lesnikoski B-A, Candinas D, Otsu I, et al. Thrombin inhibition in discordant xenograft rejection. *Xenotransplantation* 1997;4:140–146.

112. Dorling A, Stocker C, Tsao T, et al. In vitro accomodation of immortalized porcine endothelial cells. Resistance to complement mediated lysis and down-regulation of VCAM expression induced by low concentrations of polyclonal human IgG antipig antibodies. *Transplantation* 1996;62:1127–1136.

113. Dorling A, Jordan W, Brookes P, et al. "Accommodated" pig endothelial cells promote nitric oxide-dependent Th-2 cytokine responses from human T cells. *Transplantation* 2001;72:1597–1602.

114. Forte P, Pazmany L, Matter-Reissmann UB, et al HLA-G inhibits rolling adhesion of activated human NK cells on porcine endothelial cells. *J Immunol* 2001;167:6002–6008.

115. Monaco JJ. A molecular model of MHC class-I–restricted antigen processing. *Immunol Today* 1992;13:173–178.

116. den Haan JM, Bevan MJ. Antigen presentation to CD8+ T cells: cross-priming in infectious diseases. *Curr Opin Immunol* 2001;13:437–441.

117. Bevan MJ. Cross-priming for a secondary cytotoxic response to minor H antigens with H-2 congenic cells which do not cross-react in the cytotoxic assay. *J Exp Med* 1976;143:1283–1288.

118. Volk H-D, Kern F. Insights into the specificity and function of (allo)antigen-reactive T cells. *Am J Transplant* 2001;1:109–114.

119. Singer A, Munitz TI, Golding H, et al. Recognition requirements for the activation, differentiation, and function of T-helper cells specific for class I MHC alloantigens. *Immunol Rev* 1987;98:143–170.

120. Heath WR, Kjer-Nielsen L, Hoffman MW. Avidity of antigen can influence the helper dependence of CD8+ T lymphocytes. *J Immunol* 1993;151:5993–6001.

121. VanBuskirk AM, Burlingham WJ, Jankowska-Gan E, et al. Human allograft acceptance is associated with immune regulation. *J Clin Invest* 2000;106:145–155.

122. Geissler F, Jankowska-Gan E, DeVito-Haynes LD, et al. Human liver allograft acceptance and the "tolerance assay": in vitro anti-donor T cell assays show hyporeactivity to donor cells, but unlike DTH, fail to detect linked suppression. *Transplantation* 2001;72:571–580.

123. Rosenberg AS, Singer A. Cellular basis of skin allograft rejection: an in vivo model of immune-mediated tissue destruction. *Annu Rev Immunol* 1992;10:333–358.

124. Bishop DK, Chan S, Li W, et al. CD4+ helper T lymphocytes mediate mouse cardiac allograft rejection independent of donor alloantigen specific cytotoxic T lymphocytes. *Transplantation* 1993;56:892–897.

125. Korngold R, Sprent J. Purified T cell subsets and lethal graft-versus-host disease in mice. In: Gale RP, Champlin R, eds. *Progress in bone marrow transplantation.* New York: alan liss, 1987:213.

126. Sharabi Y, Sachs DH, Sykes M. T cell subsets resisting induction of mixed chimerism across various histocompatibility barriers. In: Gergely J, Benczur M, Falus A, et al, eds. *Progress in Immunology VIII. Proceedings of the Eighth International Congress of Immunology, Budapest 1992.* Heidelberg: Springer-Verlag, 1992:801–805.

127. Vallera DA, Taylor PA, Sprent J, et al. The role of host T cell subsets in bone marrow rejection directed to isolated major histocompatibility complex class I versus class II differences of bm1 and bm12 mutant mice. *Transplantation* 1994;57:249–256.

128. Korngold R, Sprent J. Variable capacity of L3T4+ T cells to cause lethal graft-versus-host disease across minor histocompatibility barriers in mice. *J Exp Med* 1987;165:1552–1564.

129. Pietra BA, Wiseman A, Bolwerk A, et al. CD4 T cell–mediated cardiac allograft rejection requires donor but not host MHC class II. *J Clin Invest* 2000;106:1003–1010.

130. Rogers NJ, Lechler RI. Allorecognition. *Am J Transplant* 2001;1:97–102.

131. Sayegh MH, Perico N, Gallon L, et al. Mechanisms of acquired thymic unresponsiveness to renal allografts. Thymic recognition of immunodominant allo-MHC peptides induces peripheral T cell anergy. *Transplantation* 1994;58:125–132.

132. Chowdhury NC, Murphy B, Sayegh MH, et al. Acquired systemic tolerance to rat cardiac allografts induced by intrathymic inoculation of synthetic polymorphic MHC class I allopeptides. *Transplantation* 1996;62:1878–1882.

133. Sonntag KC, Emery DW, Yasumoto A, et al. Tolerance to solid organ transplants through transfer of MHC class II genes. *J Clin Invest* 2001;107:65–71.

134. Yamada A, Chandraker A, Laufer TM, et al. Cutting edge: recipient MHC class II expression is required to achieve long-term survival of murine cardiac allografts after costimulatory blockade. *J Immunol* 2001;167:5522–5526.

135. Lee RS, Grusby MJ, Laufer TM, et al. CD8+ effector cells responding to residual class I antigens, with help from CD4+ cells stimulated indirectly, cause rejection of "major histocompatibility complex-deficient" skin grafts. *Transplantation* 1997;63:1123–1133.

136. Gill RG, Rosenberg AS, Lafferty KJ, et al. Characterization of primary T cell subsets mediating rejection of pancreatic islet grafts. *J Immunol* 1989;143:2176–2178.

137. Baker RJ, Hernandez-Fuentes MP, Brookes PA, et al. Loss of direct and maintenance of indirect alloresponses in renal allograft recipients: implications for the pathogenesis of chronic allograft nephropathy. *J Immunol* 2001;167:7199–7206.

138. Shirwan H. Chronic allograft rejection: do the Th2 cells preferentially induced by indirect alloantigen recognition play a predominant role? *Transplantation* 1999;68:715–726.

139. Waaga AM, Gasser M, Kist-van Holthe JE, et al. Regulatory functions of self-restricted MHC class II allopeptide–specific Th2 clones in vivo. *J Clin Invest* 2001;107:909–916.

140. Auchincloss Jr H, Lee R, Shea S, et al. The role of "indirect" recognition in initiating rejection of skin grafts from major histocompatibility complex class II–deficient mice. *Proc Natl Acad Sci U S A* 1993;90:4373–3377.

141. Swain SL. T cell subsets and the recognition of MHC class I. *Immunol Rev* 1983;74:129–142.

142. Rosenberg AS, Katz SI, Singer A. Rejection of skin allografts by CD4+ T cells is antigen-specific and requires expression of target alloantigen on Ia– epidermal cells. *J Immunol* 1989;143:2452–2456.

143. Doody DP, Stenger KS, Winn HJ. Immunologically nonspecific mechanisms of tissue destruction in the rejection of skin grafts. *J Exp Med* 1994;179:1645–1652.

144. Wecker H, Grusby MJ, Auchincloss Jr H. Effector cells must recognize antigens expressed in the graft to cause efficient skin graft rejection in SCID mice. *Transplantation* 1995;59:1223–1227.

145. Sprent J, Surh CD, Agus D, et al. Profound atrophy of the bone marrow reflecting major histocompatibility complex class II–restricted destruction of stem cells by CD4+ cells. *J Exp Med* 1994;180:307–317.

146. Rosenberg AS, Munitz TI, Maniero TG, et al. Cellular basis of skin allograft rejection across a class I major histocompatibility barrier in mice depleted of CD8+ T cells in vivo. *J Exp Med* 1991;173:1463–1471.

147. McCarthy SA, Kaldjian E, Singer A. Induction of anti–CD8 resistant cytotoxic T lymphocytes by anti-CD8 antibodies. Functional evidence for T cell signaling induced by multi-valent cross-linking of CD8 on precursor cells. *J Immunol* 1988;141:3737–3746.

148. Griffiths GM, Mueller C. Expression of perforin and granzymes in vivo: potential diagnostic markers for activated cytotoxic cells. *Immunol Today* 1991;12:415–418.

149. Sharma VK, Bologa RM, Li B, et al. Molecular executors of cell death—differential intrarenal expression of Fas ligand, Fas, granzyme B, and perforin during acute and/or chronic rejection of human renal allografts. *Transplantation* 1996;62:1860–1866.

150. Li B, Hartono C, Ding R, et al. Noninvasive diagnosis of renal-allograft rejection by measurement of messenger RNA for perforin and granzyme B in urine. *N Engl J Med* 2001;344:947–954.

151. Blazar BR, Taylor PA, Vallera DA. CD4+ and CD8+ T cells each can utilize a perforin-dependent pathway to mediate lethal graft-versus-host disease in major histocompatibiity complex-disparate recipients. *Transplantation* 1997;64:571–576.

152. Graubert TA, DiPersio JF, Russell JH, et al. Perforin/granzyme-dependent and independent mechanisms are both important for the development of graft-versus-host disease after murine bone marrow transplantation. *J Clin Invest* 1997;100:904–911.

153. Schulz M, Schuurman H-J, Joergensen J, et al. Acute rejection of vascular heart allografts by perforin-deficient mice. *Eur J Immunol* 1995;25:474–480.

154. Wiseman AC, Pietra BA, Kelly BP, et al. Donor IFN-gamma receptors are critical for acute CD4+ T cell–mediated cardiac allograft rejection. *J Immunol* 2001;167:5457–5463.

155. Bradley AJ, Bolton EM. The T-cell requirements for allograft rejection. *Transplant Rev* 1992;6:115–129.

156. Orosz CG, Horstemeyer B, Zinn NE, et al. Development and evaluation of a limiting dilution analysis technique that can discriminate in vivo alloactivated cytotoxic T lymphocytes from their naive CTL precursors. *Transplantation* 1989;47:189–194.

157. Brouard S, Sebille F, Vanhove B, et al. T cell repertoire alterations in allograft and xenograft rejection processes. *Transplant Proc* 2000;32:924–925.

158. Brouard S, Vanhove B, Gagne K, et al. T cell repertoire alterations of vascularized xenografts. *J Immunol* 1999;162:3367–3377.

159. Friedman TM, Statton D, Jones SC, et al. Vbeta spectratype analysis reveals heterogeneity of CD4+ T-cell responses to minor histocompatibility antigens involved in graft-versus-host disease: correlations with epithelial tissue infiltrate. *Biol Blood Marrow Transplant* 2001;7:2–13.

160. Mayer TG, Bhan AK, Winn HJ. Immunohistochemical analysis of skin graft rejection in mice: kinetics of lymphocyte infiltration in grafts of limited immunogenetic disparity. *Transplantation* 1988;46:890–999.

161. Colvin RB. The renal allograft biopsy. *Kidney Int* 1996;50:1069–1082.

162. Zhou P, Szot GL, Guo Z, et al. Role of STAT4 and STAT6 signaling in allograft rejection and CTLA4-Ig–mediated tolerance. *J Immunol* 2000;165:5580–5587.

163. Diamond AS, Gill RG. An essential contribution by IFN-gamma to CD8+ T cell–mediated rejection of pancreatic islet allografts. *J Immunol* 2000;165:247–255.

164. Ring GH, Saleem S, Dai Z, et al. Interferon-γ is necessary for initiating the acute rejection of major histocompatibility complex class II–disparate skin allografts. *Transplantation* 1999;67:1362–1383.

165. Guo Z, Wang J, Meng L, et al. Cutting edge: Membrane lymphotoxin regulates CD8+ T cell–mediated intestinal allograft rejection. *J Immunol* 2001;167:4796–4800.

166. Lakkis FG, Dai Z. The role of cytokines, CTLA-4 and costimulation in transplant tolerance and rejection. *Curr Opin Immunol* 1999;11:504–508.

167. Yang Y-G, Dey B, Sergio JJ, et al. Donor-derived Interferon γ is required for inhibition of acute GVHD by interleukin 12. *J Clin Invest* 1998;102:2126–2135.

168. Donckier V, Wissing M, Bruyns C, et al. Critical role of interleukin 4 in the induction of neonatal transplantation tolerance. *Transplantation* 1995;59:1571–1576.

169. Li XC, Zand MS, Li Y, et al. On histocompatibility barriers, Th1 to Th2 immune deviation, and the nature of the allograft response. *J Immunol* 1998;161:2241–2247.

170. Libby P, Pober JS. Chronic rejection. *Immunity* 2001;14:387–397.

171. Madsen JC, Sachs DH, Fallon JT, et al. Cardiac allograft vasculopathy in partially inbred miniature swine. *J Thorac Cardiovasc Surg* 1996;111:1230–1239.

172. Russell PS, Chase CM, Winn HJ, et al. Coronary atherosclerosis in transplanted mouse hearts. III. Effects of recipient treatment with a monoclonal antibody to interferon-gamma. *Transplantation* 1994;57:1367–1371.

173. Hasegawa S, Becker G, Nagano H, et al. Pattern of graft- and host-specific MHC class II expression in long-term murine cardiac allografts: origin of inflammatory and vascular wall cells. *Am J Pathol* 1998;153:69–79.

174. Choo JK, Seebach JD, Nickeleit V, et al. Species differences in the expression of major histocompatibility complex class II antigens on coronary artery endothelium: implications for cell-mediated xenoreactivity. *Transplantation* 1997;64:1315–1322.

175. Shi C, Lee WS, He Q, et al. Immunologic basis of transplant-associated arteriosclerosis. *Proc Natl Acad Sci U S A* 1996;93:4051–4056.

176. Russell PS, Chase CM, Sykes M, et al. Tolerance, mixed chimerism and chronic transplant arteriopathy. *J Immunol* 2001;167:5731–5740.

177. Koglin J, Glysing-Jensen T, Gadiraju S, et al. Attenuated cardiac allograft vasculopathy in mice with targeted deletion of the transcription factor STAT4. *Circulation* 2000;101:1034–1039.

178. Shimizu K, Sugiyama S, Aikawa M, et al. Host bone-marrow cells are a source of donor intimal smooth-muscle–like cells in murine aortic transplant arteriopathy. *Nat Med* 2001;7:738–741.

179. Hancock WW, Gao W, Faia KL, et al. Chemokines and their receptors in allograft rejection. *Curr Opin Immunol* 2000;12:511–516.

180. Bingaman AW, Ha J, Waitze S-Y, et al. Vigorous allograft rejection in the absence of danger. *J Immunol* 2000;164:3065–3071.

181. Schwartz RH. Costimulation of T lymphocytes: the role of CD28, CTLA-4, and B7/BB1 in interleukin-2 production and immunotherapy. *Cell* 1992;71:1065–1068.

182. Watts TH, DeBenedette MA. T cell co-stmulatory molecules other than CD28. *Curr Opin Immunol* 1999;11:286–293.

183. Bluestone JA. New perspectives of CD28–B7-mediated T cell costimulation. *Immunity* 1995;2:555–559.

184. Bellgrau D, Gold D, Selawry H, et al. A role for CD95 ligand in preventing graft rejection. *Nature* 1995;377:630–632.

185. Allison J, Georgiou HM, Strasser A, et al. Transgenic expression of CD95 ligand on islet beta cells induces a granulocytic infiltration but does not confer immune privilege upon islet allograft. *Proc Natl Acad Sci U S A* 1997;94:3943–3947.

186. Kawai K, Shahinian A, Mak TW, et al. Skin allograft rejection in CD28–deficient mice. *Transplantation* 1996;61:352–355.

187. Suthanthiran M. Molecular analyses of human renal allografts: differential intragraft gene expression during rejection. *Kidney Int* 1997;[suppl]58:15–21.

188. Zheng XX, Steele AW, Nickerson PW, et al. Administration of noncytolytic IL-10/Fc in murine models of lipopolysaccharide-induced septic shock and allogeneic islet transplantation. *J Immunol* 1995;154:5590–5600.

189. Mitchison NA. An exact comparison between the efficiency of two- and three-cell clusters in mediating helper activity. *Eur J Immunol* 1990;20:699–702.

190. Kelly CM, Benham AM, Sawyer GJ, et al. A three-cell cluster hypothesis for non cognate T-B collaboration via direct T cell recognition of allogenic dendritic cells. *Transplantation* 1996;61:1094–1099.

191. Durie FH, Foy TM, Masters SR, et al. The role of CD40 in the regulation of humoral and cell-mediated immunity. *Immunol Today* 1994;15:406–411.

192. Mackay CR. Dual personality of memory T cells. *Nature* 1999;401:659–660.

193. Campbell JJ, Butcher EC. Chemokines in tissue-specific and microenvironment-specific lymphocyte homing. *Curr Opin Immunol* 2000;12:336–341.

194. Hynes RO. Integrins: versatility, modulation, and signaling in cell adhesion. *Cell* 1992;69:11–25.

195. Shimizu Y, Newman W, Tanaka Y, et al. Lymphocyte interactions with endothelial cells. *Immunol Today* 1992;13:106–113.

196. Panoskaltsis-Mortari A, Hermanson JR, Haddad IY, et al. Intercellular adhesion molecule-I (ICAM-I, CD54) deficiency segregates the unique pathophysiological requirements for generating idiopathic pneumonia syndrome (IPS) versus graft-versus-host disease following allogeneic murine bone marrow transplantation. *Biol Blood Marrow Transplant* 2001;7:368–377.

197. Murai M, Yoneyama H, Harada A, et al. Active participation of CCR5+CD8+ T lymphocytes in the pathogenesis of liver injury in graft-versus-host disease. *J Clin Invest* 1999;104:49–57.

198. Serody JS, Burkett SE, Panoskaltsis-Mortari A, et al. T-lymphocyte production of macrophage inflammatory protein-1alpha is critical to the recruitment of CD8+ T cells to the liver, lung, and spleen during graft-versus-host disease. *Blood* 2000;96:2973–2980.

199. Hancock WW, Lu B, Gao W, et al. Requirement of the chemokine receptor CXCR3 for acute allograft rejection. *J Exp Med* 2000;192:1515–1520.

200. Gao W, Topham PS, King JA, et al. Targeting the chemokine receptor CCR1 suppresses development of acute and chronic cardiac allograft rejection. *J Clin Invest* 2000;105:45–44.

201. Robinson LA, Nataraj C, Thomas DW, et al. A role for fractalkine and its receptor (CX(3)CR1) in cardiac allograft rejection. *J Immunol* 2000;165:6067–6072.

202. Suthanthiran M, Morris RE, Strom TB. Immunosuppressants: cellular and molecular mechanisms of action. *Am J Kidney Dis* 1996;28:159.

203. Kahan BD. Cyclosporine. *N Engl J Med* 1989;321:1725–1738.

204. Abraham RT, Wiederrecht GJ. Immunopharmacology of rapamycin. *Annu Rev Immunol* 1996;14:483–510.

205. Brinkmann V, Pinschewer DD, Feng L, et al. FTY720: altered

lymphocyte traffic results in allograft protection. *Transplantation* 2001;72:764–769.

206. Vincenti F, Kirkman R, Light S, et al. Interleukin-2–receptor blockade with daclizumab to prevent acute rejection in renal transplantation. Daclizumab Triple Therapy Study Group. *N Engl J Med* 1998;338:161–165.

207. Russell PS, Colvin RB, Cosimi AB. Monoclonal antibodies for the diagnosis and treatment of transplant rejection. *Annu Rev Med* 1984;35:63–81.

208. Cosimi AB, Conti D, Delmonico FL, et al. In vivo effects of monoclonal antibody to ICAM-1 (CD54) in nonhuman primates with renal allografts. *J Immunol* 1990;144:4604–4612.

209. Vitetta ES, Uhr JW. The potential use of immunotoxins in transplantation, cancer therapy, and immunoregulation. *Transplantation* 1984;37:535–538.

210. Auchincloss HA. Why is cell-mediated xenograft rejection so strong? *Xenotransplantation* 1995;3:19–22.

211. Goodnow CC. Transgenic mice and analysis of B-cell tolerance. *Annu Rev Immunol* 1992;10:489–518.

212. Sykes M, Strober S. Mechanisms of tolerance. In: Thomas ED, Blume KG, Forman SJ, eds. *Hematopoietic cell transplantation*. Malden, MA: Blackwell Science, 1999:264–286.

213. Wekerle T, Sykes M. Mixed chimerism as an approach for the induction of transplantation tolerance. *Transplantation* 1999;68:459–467.

214. Bensinger SJ, Bandeira A, Jordan MS, et al. Major histocompatibility complex class II–positive cortical epithelium mediates the selection of CD4+25+ immunoregulatory T cells. *J Exp Med* 2001;194:427–438.

215. Jordan MS, Boesteanu A, Reed AJ, et al. Thymic selection of CD4+CD25+ regulatory T cells induced by an agonist self-peptide. *Nat Immunol* 2001;2:301–306.

216. Allen PM. Peptides in positive and negative selection: a delicate balance. *Cell* 1994;76:593–596.

217. Alam SM, Travers PJ, Wung JL, et al. T-cell-receptor affinity and thymocyte positive selection. *Nature* 1996;381:616–620.

218. Matzinger P. Tolerance, danger, and the extended family. *Annu Rev Immunol* 1994;12:991–1045.

219. Heath WR, Kurts C, Miller JFAP, et al. Cross-tolerance: a pathway for inducing tolerance to peripheral tissue antigens. *J Exp Med* 1998;187:1549–1553.

220. Adler AJ, Marsh DW, Yochum GS, et al. CD4+ T cell tolerance to parenchymal self-antigens requires presentation by bone marrow-derived antigen-presenting cells. *J Exp Med* 1998;187:1555–1564.

221. Wekerle T, Sayegh MH, Chandraker A, et al. Role of peripheral clonal deletion in tolerance induction with bone marrow transplantation and costimulatory blockade. *Transplant Proc* 1999;31:680.

222. Iwakoshi NN, Markees TG, Turgeon N, et al. Skin allograft maintenance in a new synchimeric model system of tolerance. *J Immunol* 2001;167:6623–6630.

223. Wells AD, Li XC, Li Y, et al. Requirement for T cell apoptosis in the induction of peripheral transplantation tolerance. *Nat Med* 1999;5:1303–1312.

224. Van Parijs L, Rafaeli Y, Lord JD, et al. Uncoupling IL-2 signals that regulate T cell proliferation, survival, and Fas-mediated activation-induced cell death. *Immunity* 1999;11:281–288.

225. Wekerle T, Kurtz J, Sayegh MH, et al. Peripheral deletion after bone marrow transplantation with costimulatory blockade has features of both activation-induced cell death and passive cell death. *J Immunol* 2001;166:2311–2316.

226. Li Y, Li XC, Zheng XX, et al. Blocking both signal 1 and signal 2 of T-cell activation prevents apoptosis of alloreactive T cells and induction of peripheral allograft tolerance. *Nat Med* 1999;5:1298–1302.

227. Zhang ZX, Yang L, Young KJ, et al. Identification of a previously unknown antigen-specific regulatory T cell and its mechanism of suppression. *Nat Med* 2000;6:782–789.

228. Bhandoola A, Cho EA, Yui K, et al. Reduced CD3-mediated protein tyrosine phosphorylation in anergic CD4+ and CD8+ T cells. *J Immunol* 1993;151:2355–2367.

229. Nossal GJV. Cellular mechanisms of immunologic tolerance. *Annu Rev Immunol* 1983;1:43–62.

230. Arnold B, Schonrich G, Hammerling GJ. Multiple levels of peripheral tolerance. *Immunol Today* 1993;14:12–14.

231. Ohdan H, Yang Y-G, Shimizu A, et al. Mixed bone marrow chimerism induced without lethal conditioning prevents T cell and anti-Galα1,3Gal antibody-mediated heart graft rejection. *J Clin Invest* 1999;104:281–290.

232. Kohler H. The immune network revisited. In: Kohler H, Urbain J, Cazenave P-A, eds. *Idiotypy in biology and medicine*. Orlando, FL: Academic Press, 1984:3–14.

233. Bluestone JA, Leo O, Epstein SL, et al. Idiotypic manipulation of the immune response to transplantation antigens. *Immunol Rev* 1986;90:5–27.

234. Carpenter CB, dice AJF, Abbas AK. The role of antibody in the rejection and enhancement of organ allografts. *Adv Immunol* 1976;22:1.

235. Batchelor JR. The riddle of kidney graft enhancement. *Transplantation* 1978;26:139–141.

236. Strober S. Natural suppressor (NS) cells, neonatal tolerance, and total lymphoid irradiation: exploring obscure relationships. *Annu Rev Immunol* 1984;2:219–237.

237. Miller RG. The veto phenomenon and T-cell regulation. *Immunol Today* 1986;7:112–114.

238. Gershon RK. A disquisition on suppressor T cells. *Transplant Rev* 1975;26:170–185.

239. Roser BJ. Cellular mechanisms in neonatal and adult tolerance. *Immunol Rev* 1989;107:179–202.

240. Wilson DB. Idiotypic regulation of T cells in graft-versus-host disease and autoimmunity. *Immunol Rev* 1989;107:159–176.

241. Mossman TR, Coffman RL. Th1 and Th2 cells: different patterns of lymphokine secretion lead to different functional properties. *Annu Rev Immunol* 1989;7:145–173.

242. Takeuchi T, Lowry RP, Konieczny B. Heart allografts in murine systems. The differential activation of Th2-like effector cells in peripheral tolerance. *Transplantation* 1992;53:1281–1294.

243. Groux H, Powrie F. Regulatory T cells and inflammatory bowel disease. *Immunol Today* 1999;20:442–446.

244. Weiner HL, Friedman A, Miller A, et al. Oral tolerance: immunologic mechanisms and treatment of animal and human organ–specific autoimmune diseases by oral administration of autoantigens. *Annu Rev Immunol* 1994;12:809–837.

245. Shevach EM. Certified professionals: CD4+CD25+ suppressor T cells. *J Exp Med* 2001;193:F41–F46.

246. Sedon B, Mason D. The third function of the thymus. *Immunol Today* 2000;21:95–99.

247. Jonuleit H, Schmitt E, Schuler G, et al. Induction of interleukin 10–producing, nonproliferating CD4+ T cells with regulatory properties by repetitive stimulation with allogeneic immature human dendritic cells. *J Exp Med* 2000;192:1213–1222.

248. Hoyne GF, Le Roux I, Corsin-Jimenez M, et al. Serrate1-induced notch signalling regulates the decision between immunity and tolerance made by peripheral CD4+ T cells. *Int Immunol* 2000;12:177–185.

249. Modigliani Y, Pereira P, Thomas-Vaslin V, et al. Regulatory T cells in thymic epithelium-induced tolerance. I. Suppression of mature peripheral non-tolerant T cells. *Eur J Immunol* 1995;25:2563–2571.

250. Charlton B, Auchincloss Jr H, Fathman CG. Mechanisms of transplantation tolerance. *Annu Rev Immunol* 1994;12:707–734.

251. Martin P. Overview of marrow transplantation immunology. In: Forman SJ, Blume KG, Thomas ED, eds. *Hematopoietic cell transplantation*. Cambridge: Blackwell Science, 1999:19–27.

252. Zinkernagel RM, Althage A. On the role of thymic epithelium vs. bone marrow-derived cells in repertoire selection of T cells. *Proc Natl Acad Sci U S A* 1999;96:8092–8097.

253. Ruedi E, Sykes M, Ildstad ST, et al. Antiviral T cell competence and restriction specificty of mixed allogeneic (P1+P2→P1) irradiation chimeras. *Cell Immunol* 1989;121:185–195.

254. Sharabi Y, Sachs DH. Mixed chimerism and permanent specific transplantation tolerance induced by a non-lethal preparative regimen. *J Exp Med* 1989;169:493–502.

255. Khan A, Tomita Y, Sykes M. Thymic dependence of loss of tolerance in mixed allogeneic bone marrow chimeras after depletion of donor antigen. Peripheral mechanisms do not contribute to maintenance of tolerance. *Transplantation* 1996;62:380–387.

256. Slavin S, Strober S, Fuks Z, et al. Induction of specific tissue transplantation tolerance using fractionated total lymphoid irradiation in adult mice: long-term survival of allogeneic bone marrow and skin grafts. *J Exp Med* 1977;146:44.

257. Myburgh JA, Smit JA, Browde S. Transplantation tolerance in the primate following total lymphoid irradiation (TLI) and bone marrow (BM) injection. *Transplant Proc* 1981;13:434–438.

258. Najarian JS, Ferguson RM, Sutherland DER, et al. Fractionated total lymphoid irradiation as preparative immunosuppression in high risk renal transplantation. *Ann Surg* 1982;196:442–451.

259. Lan F, Zeng D, Higuchi M, et al. Predominance of NK1.1+TCRαβ+ or DX5+TCRαβ+ T cells in mice conditioned with fractionated lymphoid irradiation protects against graft-versus-host-disease: "natural suppressor" cells. *J Immunol* 2001;167:2087–2096.

260. Singer A, Hathcock KS, Hodes RJ. Self recognition in allogeneic radiation chimeras. A radiation resistant host element dictates the self specificity and immune response gene phenotype of T-helper cells. *J Exp Med* 1981;153:1286–1301.

261. Ildstad ST, Sachs DH. Reconstitution with syngeneic plus allogeneic or xenogeneic bone marrow leads to specific acceptance of allografts or xenografts. *Nature* 1984;307:168–170.

262. Cobbold SP, Martin G, Qin S, et al. Monoclonal antibodies to promote marrow engraftment and tissue graft tolerance. *Nature* 1986;323:164–165.

263. Nikolic B, Khan A, Sykes M. Induction of tolerance by mixed chimerism with nonmyeloblative host conditioning: the importance of overcoming intrathymic alloresistance. *Biol Blood Marrow Transplant* 2001;7:144–153.

264. Sykes M. Mixed chimerism and transplant tolerance. *Immunity* 2001; 14:417–424.

265. Kawai T, Sachs DH, Cosimi AB. Tolerance to vascularized organ allografts in large animal models. *Curr Opin Immunol* 1999;11:516–526.

266. Spitzer TR, MCafee S, Sackstein R, et al. The intentional induction of mixed chimerism and achievement of anti-tumor responses following non-myeloablative conditioning therapy and HLA-matched and mismatched donor bone marrow transplantation for refractory hematologic malignancies. *Biol Blood Marrow Transplant* 1999;6:309–320.

267. Spitzer TR, Delmonico F, Tolkoff-Rubin N, et al. Combined HLA-matched donor bone marrow and renal transplantation for multiple myeloma with end stage renal disease: the induction of allograft tolerance through mixed lymphohematopoietic chimerism. *Transplantation* 1999;68:480–484.

268. Haynes BF, Markert ML, Sempowski GD, et al. The role of the thymus in immune reconstitutution in aging, bone marrow transplantion, and HIV-1 infection. *Annu Rev Immunol* 2000;18:529–560.

269. Tomita Y, Khan A, Sykes M. Mechanism by which additional monoclonal antibody injections overcome the requirement for thymic irradiation to achieve mixed chimerism in mice receiving bone marrow transplantation after conditioning with anti-T cell mAbs and 3 Gy whole body irradiation. *Transplantation* 1996;61:477–485.

270. Emery DW, Sablinski T, Shimada H, et al. Expression of an allogeneic MHC DRB transgene, through retroviral transduction of bone marrow, induces specific reduction of alloreactivity. *Transplantation* 1997;64:1414–1423.

271. Sykes M, Sachs DH. Xenogeneic tolerance through hematopoietic cell and thymic transplantation. In: Cooper DKC, Kemp E, Reemtsma K, et al., eds. *Xenotransplantation.* New York: Springer-Verlag, 1997: 496–518.

272. Kase A, Johannson MH, Olsson-Alheim MY, et al. External and internal calibration of the MHC class I–specific receptor Ly49A on murine natural killer cells. *J Immunol* 1998;161:6133–6138.

272a. Zhao Y, Ohdan H, Manilay JO, Sykes M. NK cell tolerance in mixed allogeneic chimeras. *J Immunol* 2003;170:In press.

273. Chen AM, Zhou Y, Swenson K, et al. Porcine stem cell engraftment and seeding of murine thymus with class II+ cells in mice expressing porcine cytokines: toward tolerance induction across discordant xenogeneic barriers. *Transplantation* 2000;69:2484–2490.

274. Terpstra W, Leenen PJ, van den Bos C, et al. Facilitated engraftment of human hematopoietic cells in severe combined immunodeficient mice following a single injection of Cl2MDP liposomes. *Leukemia* 1997;11:1049–1054.

275. Abe M, Cheng J, Qi J, et al. Elimination of porcine hematopoietic cells by macrophages in mice. *J Immunol* 2002;168:621–628.

276. Sachs DH, Sykes M, Robson S, et al. Xenotransplantation. *Adv Immunol* 2001;79:129–223.

277. Lee LA, Gritsch HA, Sergio JJ, et al. Specific tolerance across a discordant xenogeneic transplantation barrier. *Proc Natl Acad Sci U S A* 1994;91:10864–10867.

278. Zhao Y, Fishman JA, Sergio JJ, et al. Immune restoration by fetal pig thymus grafts in T cell-depleted, thymectomized mice. *J Immunol* 1997;158:1641–1649.

279. Zhao Y, Swenson K, Sergio JJ, et al. Pig MHC mediates positive selection of mouse CD4+ T cells with a mouse MHC-restricted TCR in pig thymus grafts. *J Immunol* 1998;161:1320–1326.

280. Markert ML, Boeck A, Hale LP, et al. Transplantation of thymus tissue in complete DiGeorge syndrome. *N Engl J Med* 1999;341:1180–1189.

281. Zerrahn J, Held W, Raulet DH. The MHC reactivity of the T cell repertoire prior to positive and negative selection. *Cell* 1997;88:627–636.

282. Nikolic B, Gardner JP, Scadden DT, et al. Normal development in porcine thymus grafts and specific tolerance of human T cells to porcine donor MHC. *J Immunol* 1999;162:3402–3407.

283. Modigliani Y, Tomas-Vaslin V, Bandeira A, et al. Lymphocytes selected in allogeneic thymic epithelium mediate dominant tolerance toward tissue grafts of the thymic epithelium haplotype. *Proc Natl Acad Sci U S A* 1995;92:7555–7559.

284. Touraine JL. Treatment of human fetuses and induction of immunological tolerance in humans by in utero transplantation of stem cells into fetal recipients. *Acta Haematol* 1996;96:115–119.

285. Carrier E, Lee TH, Busch MP, et al. Induction of tolerance in nondefective mice after in utero transplantation of major histocompatibility complex-mismatched fetal hematopoietic stem cells. *Blood* 1995;86:4681–4690.

286. Almeida-Porada G, Porada CD, Tran N, et al. Cotransplantation of human stromal cell progenitors into preimmune fetal sheep results in early apprearance of human donor cells in circulation and boosts cell levels in bone marrow at later time points after transplantation. *Blood* 2000;95:3620–3627.

287. Flake AW, Zanjani ED. In utero hematopoietic stem cell transplantation: ontogenic opportunities and biologic barriers. *Blood* 1999;94: 2179–2191.

288. Donahue J, Gilpin E, Lee TH, et al. Microchimerism does not induce tolerance and sustains immunity after in utero transplantation. *Transplantation* 2001;71:359–368.

289. Streilein JW. Neonatal tolerance of H-2 alloantigens. *Transplantation* 1991;52:1–10.

290. Sykes M, Sheard MA, Sachs DH. Effects of T cell depletion in radiation bone marrow chimeras. II. Requirement for allogeneic T cells in the reconstituting bone marrow inoculum for subsequent resistance to breaking of tolerance. *J Exp Med* 1988;168:661–673.

291. Ridge JP, Fuchs EJ, Matzinger P. Neonatal tolerance revisited: turning on newborn T cells with dendritic cells. *Science* 1996;271:1723–1726.

292. Starzl TE, Demetris AJ, Murase N, et al. The lost chord: microchimerism and allograft survival. *Immunol Today* 1996;17:577–584.

293. Wood K, Sachs DH. Chimerism and transplantation tolerance: cause and effect. *Immunol Today* 1996;17:584–588.

294. Burlingham WJ, Grailer AP, Fechner Jr JH, et al. Microchimerism linked to cytotoxic T lymphocyte functional unresponsiveness (clonal anergy) in a tolerant renal transplant recipient. *Transplantation* 1995; 59:1147–1155.

295. Murase N, Starzl TE, Ye Q, et al. Multilineage hematopoietic reconstitution of supralethally irradiated rats by syngeneic whole organ transplantation with particular reference to the liver. *Transplantation* 1996;61:1–4.

296. Ciancio G, Miller J, Garcia-Morales RO, et al. Six-year clinical effect of donor bone marrow infusions in renal transplant patients. *Transplantation* 2001;71:827–835.

297. Thomas JM, Verbanac KM, Smith JP, et al. The facilitating effect of one-DR antigen sharing in renal allograft tolerance induced by donor bone marrow in rhesus monkeys. *Transplantation* 1995;59:245–255.

298. Wood KJ. Transplantation tolerance with monoclonal antibodies. *Semin Immunol* 1990;2:389–399.

299. Wong W, Morris PJ, Wood KJ. Syngeneic bone marrow expressing a single donor class I MHC molecule permits acceptance of a fully allogeneic cardiac allograft. *Transplantation* 1996;62:1462–1468.

300. Hara M, Kingsley CI, Niimi M, et al. IL-10 is required for regulatory T cells to mediate tolerance to alloantigens in vivo. *J Immunol* 2001;166:3789–3796.

301. Lechler RI, Batchelor JR. Restoration of immunogenicity to passenger cell-depleted kidney allografts by the addition of donor strain dendritic cells. *J Exp Med* 1982;155:31–41.

302. Sayegh MH, Akalin E, Hancock WW, et al. CD28–B7 blockade after alloantigenic challenge in vivo inhibits Th1 cytokines but spares Th2. *J Exp Med* 1995;181:1869–1874.

303. Lanzavecchia A. Licence to kill. *Nature* 1998;393:413–414.

304. Markees TG, Phillips NE, Gordon EJ, et al. Long-term survival of skin allografts induced by donor splenocytes and anti-CD154 antibody in thymectomized mice requires CD4+ T cells, Interferon-γ, and CTLA4. *J Clin Invest* 1998;101:2446–2455.

305. Gordon EJ, Woda BA, Shultz LD, et al. Rat xenograft survival in mice treated with donor-specific transfusion and anti-CD154 antibody is enhanced by elimination of host CD4+ cells. *Transplantation* 2001;71:319–327.

306. Larsen CP, Alexander DZ, Hendrix R, et al. Fas-mediated cytotoxicity. An immunoeffector or immunoregulatory pathway in T cell–mediated immune responses? *Transplantation* 1995;60:221–224.

307. Tramblay J, Bingaman AW, Lin A, et al. Asialo GM1+ CD8+ T cells play a critical role in costimulation blockade-resistant allograft rejection. *J Clin Invest* 1999;104:1715–1722.

308. Ito H, Kurtz J, Shaffer J, et al. CD4 T cell–mediated alloresistance to fully MHC-mismatched allogeneic bone marrow engraftment is dependent on CD40–CD40L interactions, and lasting T cell tolerance is induced by bone marrow transplantation with initial blockade of this pathway. *J Immunol* 2001;166:2981.

309. Ensminger SM, Spriewald BM, Witzke O, et al. Intragraft interleukin-4 mRNA expression after short-term CD154 blockade may trigger delayed development of transplant arteriosclerosis in the absence of CD8+ T cells. *Transplantation* 2000;70:955–963.

310. Li Y, Zheng XX, Li XC, et al. Combined costimulation blockade plus rapamycin but not cyclosporine produces permanent engraftment. *Transplantation* 1998;66:1387–1388.

311. Lehnert AM, Yi S, Burgess JS, et al. Pancreatic islet xenograft tolerance after short-term costimulation blockade is associated with increased CD4+ T cell apoptosis but not immune deviation. *Transplantation* 2000;69:1176–1185.

312. Kirk AD, Burkly LC, Batty DS, et al. Treatment with humanized monoclonal antibody against CD154 prevents acute renal allograft rejection in nonhuman primates. *Nat Med* 1999;5:686–693.

313. Williams MA, Trambley J, Ha J, et al. Genetic characterization of strain differences in the ability to mediate CD40/CD28–independent rejection of skin allografts. *J Immunol* 2000;165:6849–6857.

314. Li XC, Wells AD, Strom TB, et al. The role of T cell apoptosis in transplantation tolerance. *Curr Opin Immunol* 2000;12:522–527.

315. Murphy WJ, Blazar BR. New strategies for preventing graft-versus-host disease. *Curr Opin Immunol* 1999;11:509–515.

316. Seung E, Iwakoshi N, Woda BA, et al. Allogeneic hematopoietic chimerism in mice treated with sublethal myeloablation and anti-CD154 antibody: absence of graft-versus-host disease, induction of skin allograft tolerance, and prevention of recurrent autoimmunity in islet-allografted NOD/Lt mice. *Blood* 2000;95:2175–2182.

317. Taylor PA, Noelle RJ, Blazar BR. CD4+CD25+ immune regulatory cells are required for induction of tolerance to alloantigen via costimulatory blockade. *J Exp Med* 2001;193:1311–1318.

318. Guinan EC, Boussiotis VA, Neuberg D, et al. Transplantation of anergic histoincompatible bone marrow allografts. *N Engl J Med* 1999;340:1704–1714.

319. Blazar BR, Kwon BS, Panoskaltsis-Mortari A, et al. Ligation of 4-1BB (CDw137) regulates graft-versus-host disease, graft-versus-leukemia, and graft rejection in allogeneic bone marrow transplant recipients. *J Immunol* 2001;166:3174–3183.

320. Grillot DAM, Merino R, Nunez G. Bcl-xL displays restricted distribution during T cell development and inhibits multiple forms of apoptosis but not clonal deletion in transgenic mice. *J Exp Med* 1995;182:1973–1983.

321. Waldmann H, Cobbold S. The use of monoclonal antibodies to achieve immunological tolerance. *Immunol Today* 1993;14:247–251.

321a. Kurtz J, Shaffer J, Anosova N, et al. Mechanisms of early peripheral CD4 cell tolerance induction by anti-CD154 monoclonal antibody and allogeneic bone marrow transplantation: Evidence for anergy and deletion, but not regulatory cells. Submitted 4.25.03.

322. Lin H, Rathmell JC, Gray GS, et al. Cytotoxic T lymphocyte antigen 4 (CTLA4) blockade accelerates the acute rejection of cardiac allografts in CD28-deficient mice: CTLA4 can function independently of CD28. *J Exp Med* 1998;188:199–204.

323. Blazar BR, Taylor PA, Panoskaltsis-Mortari A, et al. Opposing roles of CD28:B7 and CTLA-4:B7 pathways in regulating in vivo alloresponses in murine recipients of MHC disparate T cells. *J Immunol* 1999;162:6368–6377.

324. Isobe M, Suzuki J-I, Yamazaki S, et al. Acceptance of primary skin graft after treatment with anti-intercellular adhesion molecule-1 and anti-leukocyte function-associated antigen-1 monoclonal antibodies in mice. *Transplantation* 1996;62:411–413.

325. Isobe M, Suzuki J, Yagita H, et al. Immunosuppression to cardiac allografts and soluble antigens by anti-vascular cellular adhesion molecule-1 and anti–very late antigen-4 monoclonal antibodies. *J Immunol* 1994;153:5810–5818.

326. Cobbold SP, Adams E, Marshall SE, et al. Mechanisms of peripheral tolerance and suppression induced by monoclonal antibodies to CD4 and CD8. *Immunol Rev* 1996;149:5–34.

327. Punch JD, Tono T, Qin L, et al. Tolerance induction by anti-CD2 plus anti-CD3 monoclonal antibodies: evidence for an IL-4 requirement. *J Immunol* 1998;161:1156–1162.

328. Rothstein DM, Livak MF, Kishimoto K, et al. Targeting signal 1 through CD45RB synergizes with CD40 ligand blockade and promotes long term engraftment and tolerance in stringent transplant models. *J Immunol* 2001;166:322–329.

329. Myburgh JA, Meyers AM, Thomson PD, et al. Total lymphoid irradiation—current status. *Transplant Proc* 1989;21:826–828.

330. Strober S, Benike C, Krishnaswamy S, et al. Clinical transplantation tolerance twelve years after prospective withdrawal of immunosuppressive drugs: studies of chimerism and anti-donor reactivity. *Transplantation* 2000;69:1549–1554.

331. Hackstein H, Morelli AE, Thomson AW. Designer dendritic cells for tolerance induction: guided not misguided missiles. *Trends Immunol* 2001;22:437–442.

332. Blancho G, Gianello PR, Lorf T, et al. Molecular and cellular events implicated in local tolerance to kidney allografts in miniature swine. *Transplantation* 1997;63:26–33.

333. Yamada K, Gianello PR, Ierino FL, et al. Role of the thymus in transplantation tolerance in miniature swine. I. Requirement of the thymus for rapid and stable induction of tolerance to class I-mismatched renal allografts. *J Exp Med* 1997;186:497–506.

334. Madsen JC, Yamada K, Allan JS, et al. Transplantation tolerance prevents cardiac graft vasculopathy in major histocompatiblity complex class I–disparate miniature swine. *Transplantation* 1998;65:304–313.

335. Ierino FL, Yamada K, Hatch T, et al. Peripheral tolerance to class I mismatched renal allografts in miniature swine: donor acntigen-activated peripheral blood lymphocytes from tolerant swine inhibit antidonor CTL reactivity. *J Immunol* 1999;162:550–559.

336. Agus DB, Surh CD, Sprent J. Reentry of T cells to the adult thymus is restricted to activated T cells. *J Exp Med* 1991;173:1039–1046.

337. Oluwole SF, Jin M-X, Chowdhury NC, et al. Effectiveness of intrathymic inoculation of soluble antigens in the induction of specific unresponsiveness to rat islet allografts without transient recipient immunosuppression. *Transplantation* 1994;58:1077–1081.

338. Gopinathan R, DePaz HA, Oluwole OO, et al. Role of reentry of in vivo alloMHC peptide–activated T cells into the adult thymus in acquired systemic tolerance. *Transplantation* 2001;72:1533–1541.

339. Odorico JS, Onnor T, Campos L, et al. Examination of the mechanisms responsible for tolerance induction after intrathymic inoculation of allogeneic bone marrow. *Ann Surg* 1993;218:525–531.

340. Hillebrands JL, Raue HP, Klatter FA, et al. Intrathymic immune modulation prevents acute rejection but not the development of graft arteriosclerosis (chronic rejection). *Transplantation* 2001;71:914–924.

341. Jonker M, van Den HY, Noort RC, et al. Immunomodulation by intrathymic injection of donor leukocytes in rhesus monkeys1. *Transplantation* 2001;72:1432–1436.

342. Allen MD, Weyhrich J, Gaur L, et al. Prolonged allogeneic and xenogeneic microchimerism in unmatched primates without immunosuppression by intrathymic implantation of CD34+ donor marrow cells. *Cell Immunol* 1997;181:127–138.

343. Speiser DE, Schneider R, Hengartner H, et al. Clonal deletion of self-reactive T cells in irradiation bone marrow chimeras and neonatally

syngeneic animals became (and still is) a diagnostic criterion for the malignant phenotype of an experimental tumor. This criterion was especially useful because many rodent tumors are cancers of nonepithelial origin (sarcomas), for which a clear histological demonstration of local invasive growth can be especially difficult. Furthermore, these tumors are rarely metastatic, a characteristic that is shared by many other experimentally induced tumors in rodents. As outlined later, it is now known from studies of experimental tumors that strong, truly tumor-specific rejection antigens indeed exist and that they are caused by somatic tumor-specific mutations. For human tumors, for which rejection antigens in the real sense are very difficult to define, autologous tumor-reactive T cells have been used extensively for tumor antigen discovery (8). Serological methods, particularly serological analyses of recombinant complementary deoxyribonucleic acid (DNA) expression libraries of human tumors (SEREX), have become an important tool for discovering new tumor antigens (9).

Evidence of Tumor-Specific Rejection of Transplanted Cancers

The modern era of tumor immunology began with the discovery that inbred mice could be immunized against sarcomas induced by the chemical carcinogen methylcholanthrene (MCA). The first such demonstration of induced immunity to transplanted MCA-induced sarcomas, by Gross (10), was in 1943; however, it was not until the 1950s that more complete experiments provided unequivocal evidence for tumor-specific rejection of transplanted cancers (11–14). In particular, the experiments of Prehn and Main (12) in 1957 showed that the rejection antigens on the MCA-induced sarcomas probably were functionally tumor-specific, because transplantation assays could not detect these antigens in normal tissue of the mice used. These investigators showed that the tumor cells did not immunize against normal skin grafts from the mouse of tumor origin and that normal tissue of this mouse did not immunize against the tumor (Fig. 1). These results showed that it was highly unlikely that residual heterozygosity (22), if it existed in these inbred mice, was responsible for the immunogenicity of the transplanted tumors. The notion of tumor antigenicity was confirmed by further experiments demonstrating that tumor-specific resistance against MCA-induced tumors could be elicited in the autochthonous host (i.e., in the mouse in which the tumor had originated), if the tumors were first removed completely and then immunized with irradiated tumor cells (13). In subsequent years, it was demonstrated that the induction of tumor-specific transplantation resistance was not restricted to tumors induced by MCA, because such resistance could also be induced by tumors that resulted from other chemical or physical [e.g., ultraviolet (UV)] carcinogens or by spontaneous tumors (15,16).

Because protective immunity against the growth of transplanted tumors was used as the criterion for antigenicity, these antigens are also commonly referred to as *transplantation antigens* or *rejection antigens*. Unfortunately, several papers and reviews have been written on the subject of tumor rejection antigens without presenting evidence that the antigens described actually lead to tumor rejection. For example, the term *rejection antigen* is often improperly used for any antigen that is expressed on tumors and recognized by cytolytic T cells. However, tumors may grow very aggressively, even when tumor antigen–specific cytolytic T cells can be isolated from such tumors or the peripheral blood of the tumor-bearing hosts (mouse or human). Furthermore, there are remarkable differences in the potency of rejection antigens: Some elicit tumor rejection at any testable challenge dose, even in the absence of known co-stimulatory molecules on the tumor cells, whereas others antigens succeed only in delaying tumor outgrowth or cause rejection only at a threshold tumorigenic dose of tumor cells (17).

Antigens Are Unique for an Individual Cancer or Are Shared by Other Cancers

An early objective of the experiments with MCA-induced murine tumors was to search for tumor-specific antigens that were shared by different independently induced tumors. Such shared antigens might be used for either diagnosis or therapy of cancers occurring in different individuals. However, transplantation experiments (12,13,18,19) revealed that the strongest immunological protection against challenge with cancer cells was individually tumor specific. Immunization with one tumor protected effectively only against challenge with the same tumor but not against challenge with many other tumors tested (Table 1); that is, each cancer was unique, even though the cancers were of the same histological type and were induced by the same carcinogen in the same organ system in genetically identical individuals. The unique specificity indicated that each tumor had a unique transplantation antigen, expressed a unique combination of shared antigens, or both. In fact, careful studies suggested that the antigenic repertoire of these tumors is very large. Because of the impractical prospect of immunizing each patient against the unique antigen of the individual's tumor, studies were undertaken many years ago to identify shared antigens that could elicit effective and repeatable tumor rejection. The result of those studies was that no wide cross-protection was observed (18). Thus, in the search for antigens shared among ten MCA-induced tumors, no reproducible cross-protection (Fig. 2) was found in 90 tests with mice first immunized with one and then challenged with other syngeneic tumors (18). In addition to MCA, a number of other chemical or physical (15) carcinogens, such as 3,4-benzopyrene or UV light, also induce tumors that elicit strong transplantation immunity that is unique (i.e., individually tumor specific). Unique as well as shared tumor antigens have also been found to be *in vitro* targets of human autologous T cells. However, even when a shared antigen is recognized by cytolytic T cells, transplantation immunity may be individually tumor specific. For example, the shared antigen P1A is expressed by multiple lineages of

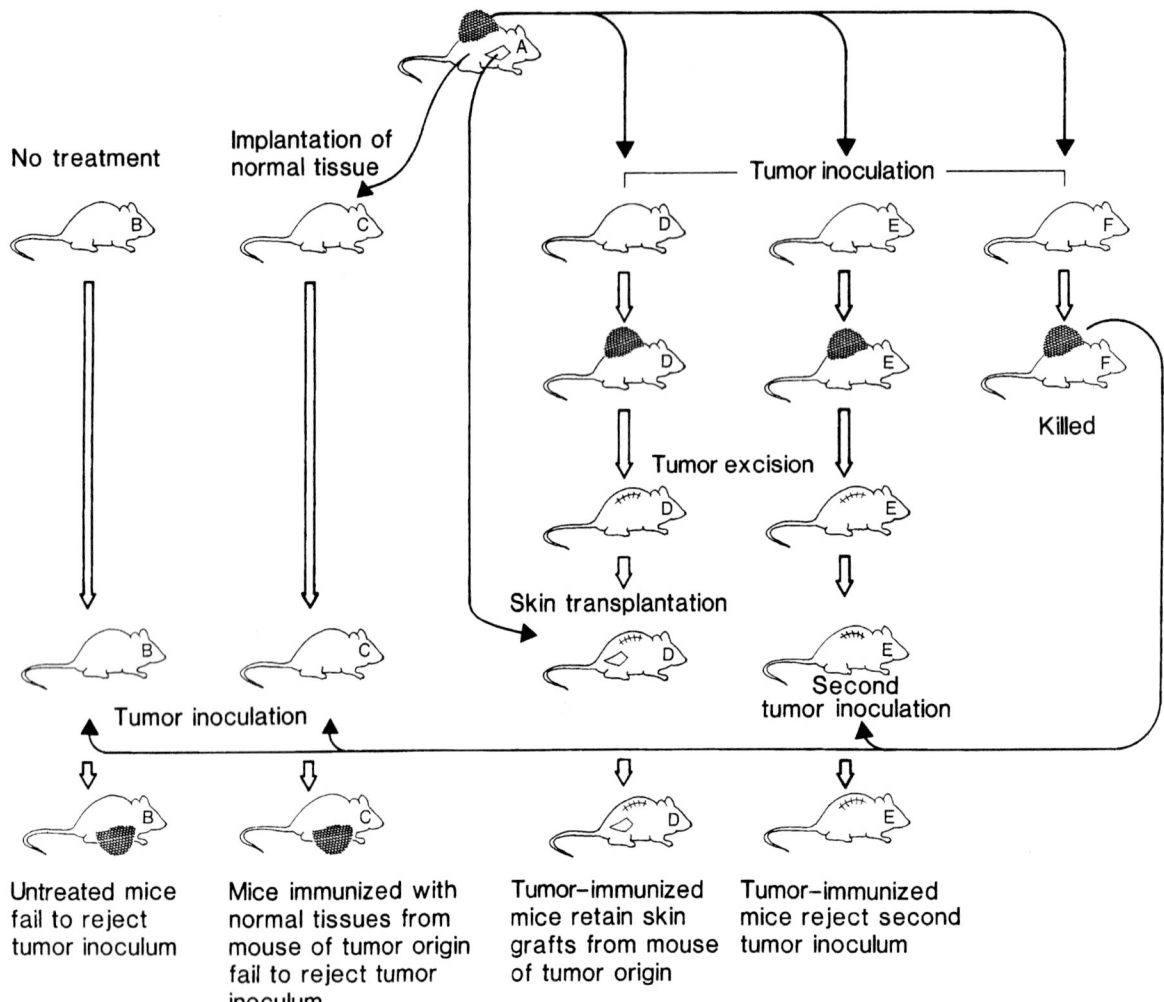

FIG. 1. Transplantation experiments demonstrating the existence of rejection antigens on methylcholanthrene (MCA)-induced murine sarcomas (12). Only the mice that had been immunized by previous tumor inoculation and removal (E) rejected the tumor upon second tumor inoculation. Tumor-immunized mice (D), however, still accepted normal tissue (skin grafts) of the mouse of tumor origin (A), and normal tissues of this mouse (A) did not protect other mice (C) against tumor challenge. Animal F was used simply to "store" the tumor from mouse A for the period required to immunize other mice (C, D, and E) with normal and malignant tissues. In similar experiments (13) (not shown), the original tumor was removed completely without killing the animal; after an interim period, during which the mouse was immunized repeatedly with irradiated tumor cells, viable tumor cells were reimplanted into this original mouse that now rejected the tumor that once originated from itself. This suggested that a mouse can be made immune to its autochthonous tumor after it has been removed completely from the animal.

tumors, as determined by Northern blots and sensitivity to lysis by P1A-specific cytolytic T-cell lymphocytes (CTLs), and P1A can induce cross-reactive T cells that are cytolytic for multiple tumor lineages (20). Despite this cross-reactivity, immunological protection was found to be mediated by unique antigens because there was no cross-protection (20).

Shared antigens might lead to cross-protection between independently induced tumors, and, indeed, cross-protection between independently derived tumors is regularly found

among murine melanomas induced by UV light or chemicals. Under selected experimental conditions, cross-protection is also found in the model of MCA or UV light–induced murine tumors (12,13,21). For example, hyperimmunization with a highly immunogenic regressor tumor led to protective immunity against challenge with several other less immunogenic progressor tumors. The finding of cross-protection has been taken as suggesting that the size of the antigenic repertoire may be limited or that common, yet tumor-specific, antigens

TABLE 1. *Characteristics of unique individually distinct rejection antigens on tumors*

Specific for each tumor and different from other tumors
    even when
    Of the same histological type
    Induced in the same organ system
    Induced by the same carcinogen
    In the same strain of mice or in the same mouse
Not detected on normal syngeneic cells
Defined by transplantation assays (not possible in humans)
Found predominantly on chemically and physically induced
    tumors but also on some spontaneous experimental
    tumors
Seemingly endless variety
Caused by somatic tumor-specific mutations

exist. Although this is possible, it is also important to note that the resistance induced by immunization with unrelated tumors is usually weak, rather short-lived, and sensitive to gamma radiation or requires hyperimmunization; in contrast, resistance induced by immunization with unique antigens is usually long-lived and, like other specific immune responses, becomes relatively radioresistant once immunization has occurred (22). Furthermore, weak resistance against challenge with living tumor cells has sometimes been induced with normal tissue (13). The weak cross-protective effects induced by hyperimmunization with unrelated tumors or normal tissues may therefore be caused by a nonspecific bolstering of immune responses to specific antigens (13). Alternatively, cross-protection among independently derived tumors could

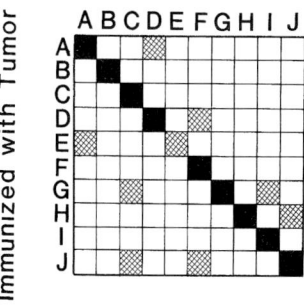

FIG. 2. Demonstration of the individual (unique) specificity of transplantation antigens on independently derived methylcholanthrene (MCA)–induced tumors in transplantation experiments (18). Mice were immunized by injecting nontumorigenic doses of viable cells. One to three weeks later, mice were challenged by injection with tumorigenic doses of the same tumor and nine other syngeneic tumors that had been induced independently in syngeneic mice. Protection was specific for the tumor used for immunization, because no repeatable cross-protection was found. The *solid black square* represents rejection of the tumor inoculum; the *cross-hatched square* represents unrepeatable rejections; the *white squares* represent combinations that showed no rejection. Adapted from Basombrio (18), with permission.

be caused by oncofetal, oncospermatogonal, viral, or differentiation antigens (see later discussion) that may be shared by many tumors, but these antigens may not be tumor-specific because they are also found on certain nonmalignant adult tissues or cells. Molecules that are tumor specific and are shared among independently induced human cancers do exist, however. Examples are the tumor-specific mutant proteins found in certain types of human cancers (see later discussion), but it remains uncertain how effectively shared tumor antigens on human tumors can be used as targets for immunotherapy to achieve rejection.

Transplantation Immunity Is Primarily T-Cell Mediated

Transplantation immunity elicited by immunization with cancer cells is primarily T-cell mediated (14). UV light–induced regressor tumors are rejected regularly by normal mice but grow progressively in T cell–deficient mice (23). Cloned CTLs that represent stable transferable and highly specific probes for rejection antigens can be generated. Through the use of such probes, it has sometimes been possible to demonstrate that tumors induced by chemical or physical carcinogens express unique, individually distinct antigenic epitopes (Fig. 3) (24). It is also possible to investigate whether an antigen recognized by a CTL clone in vitro acts as a rejection antigen in vivo (43). This was done by selecting antigen loss variants of regressor tumors in vitro for resistance to specific CTLs (Fig. 4). Results of injection of the variants derived in vitro into mice suggested that antigen loss caused a change from a regressor to a progressor phenotype in vivo (23). Thus, by isolating tumor variants with selective resistance to a CTL clone, the relative importance of single or several combined antigens or epitopes on the tumor cell in tumor rejection can be indicated. However, there have been no experiments to show that reexpression of the lost tumor-specific antigen alone suffices to restore the highly immunogenic regressor phenotype fully.

Multiplicity of Unique Tumor Antigens Expressed on a Single Cancer Cell

CTL clones can also be used to determine whether the antigenicity of a given tumor is attributable to single or multiple independent components. Such dissection of the antigenic complexity of a tumor can be done by selecting resistant tumor variants and by determining whether these variants have retained any other CTL-recognized antigen or epitopes (25). The results from such studies (24,26,27) suggest that CTL-defined antigenicity of murine and human tumor cells may be composed of multiple independent, unique epitopes. Thus, the diversity of unique tumor-specific antigens may be even larger than previously anticipated. Whether these multiple CTL-defined epitopes expressed by a single tumor cell reside on one or on different molecules is often unclear; in

ANTI–UV–6138 CYTOLYTIC T CELL CLONE

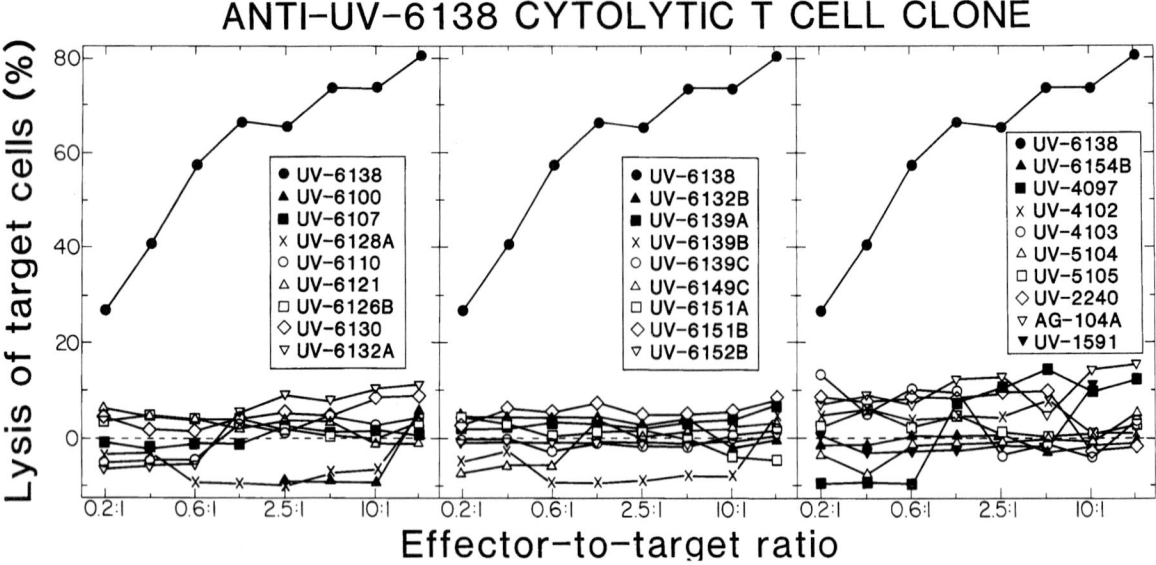

FIG. 3. Example of the unique specificity and strength with which cytolytic T-cell (CTL) clones can lyse cells of a particular ultraviolet light–induced tumor that had been used for immunization—in this case, UV-6138. None of the 25 other syngeneic C3H tumor cell lines shown in the three panels lysed, which demonstrates the uniqueness of the CTL-defined antigen. Effector cells were incubated with chromium-51–labeled target cells for 4.5 hours, and the amount of the radioisotope released from damaged tumor cells into the supernatant was used to determine the percentage of target cells lysed. Adapted from Ward (24), with permission.

any case, these epitopes appear to be functionally independent because CTL clones always selected for variants that had lost only the recognized epitope. This functional independence of epitopes makes this multiplicity important for understanding immune escape and for allowing combination immunotherapy (see section on selection of antigen loss or epitope loss variants).

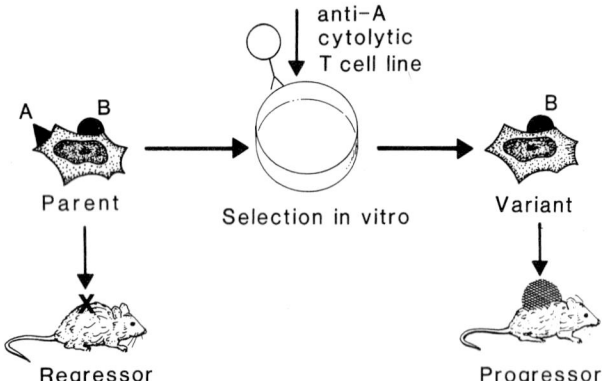

FIG. 4. Scheme of an experiment to test the relevance of a cytolytic T cell (CTL)–defined antigen for tumor rejection *in vivo*. Rare antigen loss variants can be selected by exposing the parental tumor cells *in vitro* to a CTL clone. In the example shown here, loss of the A antigen leads to variants that show progressive tumor growth in normal mice, whereas variants selected for loss of the B antigen (not shown) are still rejected by the normal host, like the parental ultraviolet light–induced regressor tumor. From Koeppen (27a), with permission.

TUMOR ANTIGENS ENCODED BY MUTANT CELLULAR GENES (TUMOR-SPECIFIC ANTIGENS)

Mutations Discovered by Immunological Analyses

Although unique tumor antigens (Table 1) were discovered in the 1960s, researchers have begun to learn about the molecular basis of the diversity of these antigens only since 1995 (28). In principle, there are three possible mechanisms that may lead to the appearance of these antigens: clonal amplification, mutation, and gene activation. Most chemical or physical carcinogens are mutagens. Therefore, it is generally assumed that unique tumor antigens on tumors induced by these carcinogens are products of mutated genes, possibly single genes with "hot spots" for mutations. However, Burnet proposed that the uniqueness of carcinogen-induced transplantation antigens on tumors may also result from clonal amplification of single cells expressing a particular normal antigen. According to this hypothesis, normal precursor cells in the host contain different antigens; these antigens, however, are not sufficient in amount to be recognized by the immune system until amplified by clonal expansion of the cancer cells. [An analogous situation may occur with clonal antigens (see later discussion) when an individual develops a malignancy of B- or T-cell origin; the idiotype, present on relatively few normal cells, may not be sufficient in amount to elicit a response in the normal host, but it may serve as target antigen for tumor cells bearing the same idiotype.] This possibility has been addressed experimentally. In one study, a nonmalignant fibroblast line was cloned *in vitro* and then expanded;

subclones, all derived from the same precursor cell, were malignantly transformed by MCA in diffusion chambers implanted into mice. Transplantation experiments showed that all the developing tumors had individually distinct antigens, even though all tumors had been derived from the same precursor cell. These results seemed to indicate the appearance of new antigens (neoantigens) after carcinogen exposure and that the unique antigens were not already expressed on the precursor cell. However, normal cells can generate considerable diversity of surface molecules during clonal expansion from a single precursor, and the transformation event caused by the carcinogen may simply fix a particular antigenic phenotype of the cell, giving rise to the malignant clone. Alternatively, normal genes that were previously silent may be activated by the carcinogen. Both mechanisms involving normal genes could produce considerable antigenic diversity of tumors. Therefore, previous experiments have not answered whether the appearance of the individually distinct (unique) antigens was caused by carcinogen-induced somatic mutations of structural DNA sequences or whether these antigens are encoded by normal genes. It was also not clear in what way unique rejection antigens caused by mutagen exposure of cancer cells in vitro may serve as a paradigm for individually distinct rejection antigens. Furthermore, several unique tumor antigens, claimed to be "tumor-specific" and encoded by "mutations," may be encoded by heterozygous germline genes, giving rise to unique, seemingly tumor-specific antigens. This uncertainty arises from the facts that residual germline heterozygosity and antigenic drift are commonly observed in inbred mouse strains and tumors derived from them and that absence of the described mutational changes from autologous normal DNA from the host of tumor origin was not demonstrated. Finally, although it is generally assumed that the appearance of unique tumor antigens is a

direct result of the exposure to carcinogen, there is no direct evidence for this, except when the antigens are encoded by the transforming genes of oncogenic viruses. Even the fact that unique tumor antigens are often shared by a majority (or all) of the cells in a given tumor implies only that the cells in the tumor arose from a single precursor cell. It is still possible that a precursor expressing the unique tumor antigen arose in a pretransformational or posttransformational cell population in which the other cells not expressing this antigen were eliminated or overgrown during the continuous evolution of the cancer.

Since 1995, the genetic origins of several T cell–recognized unique antigens from murine and human cancers have been identified, and in every case, the antigen was caused by a somatic mutation (i.e., by a genetic change absent from autologous normal DNA) and thus found to be truly tumor-specific (28–33). Table 2 shows that these antigens do not seem to involve a single gene family but rather involve multiple different unrelated genes and that the same mutation may be selected only rarely in another patient (30). The second fascinating finding was that many of these mutations do not appear to be located in random sites but rather occur in genes that code for functionally important parts of the expressed protein. For example, the mutation in the cyclin E–dependent kinase 4 reduces the binding to its inhibitor and tumor-suppressor protein, p16INK4a (30), and the same mutation is found in cases of familial melanoma. Also, the mutation in the β-catenin appears to prevent the degradation of this oncogene, and the mutation in the helicase protein p68 resulted in an amino acid substitution in a functionally important domain of this gene (33). The third fascinating finding was that several of these unique tumor-specific antigens are excellent targets because they cannot be lost by immune selection. These antigens are encoded by essential but mutant

TABLE 2. *Unique tumor antigens recognized by syngeneic or autologous T cells and caused by somatic mutations*

Mutant protein recognized	Recognizing T-cell subset	Tumor of origin	Somatic mutation/ tumor specificity	Reference
Mouse				
Ribosomal protein L9	CD4+	UV-induced sarcoma	Yes	(28)
Ribosomal protein L26	CD4+	UV-induced sarcoma	Yes	(34)
RNA helicase protein	CD8+	UV-induced sarcoma	Yes	(33)
Human				
CDC27 (cell cycle)	CD4+	Melanoma	Yes	(146)
RNA helicase protein	CD8+	Melanoma	Yes	(147)
Elongation factor 2	CD8+	Squamous cell carcinoma (lung)	Yes	(148)
Caspase-8	CD8+	Squamous cell carcinoma (head and neck)	Yes	(149)
MUM-1	CD8+	Melanoma	Yes	(29)
Cdk4 (cell cycle)	CD8+	Melanoma	Yes	(30)
β-catenin	CD8+	Melanoma	Yes	(31)
HLA-A2	CD8+	Renal cell carcinoma	Yes	(32)

Excluded are unique antigens that lack evidence for somatic mutation and thus tumor specificity because the analyzed genes were from tumors for which nonmalignant control cells were not available to distinguish between germline polymorphism or somatic mutation. These genes include connexin 37, c-akt, activated gag, or the mitogen-activated protein kinase ERK2 or the ribosomal protein L7(150).

HLA-A2, human leukocyte antigen A2; MUM-1, melanoma ubiquitous mutated protein; RNA, ribonucleic acid; UV, ultraviolet light.

household genes for which the tumor cell lacks the normal allele as a result of Knudson-type loss or mutation of the second allele (29,34). It is likely that only a fraction of the genetic changes needed to cause the different stages of different types of cancers is understood. Therefore, it is important to note that T cells against unique tumor antigens can identify novel, functionally important tumor-specific mutations that would probably not have been detected by other available technology.

Mutations Discovered by Functional or Genetic Analyses: "Reverse Immunology"

Many human cancers in industrialized countries are probably not induced by viruses but rather result from mutations caused by physical or chemical carcinogens (2). Some of these mutations may be the immediate result of the initial mutational damage to normal target cells and randomly affect many genes. However, most mutational changes are probably a disadvantage to the cancer cell, so that the mutations that are found when cancers eventually arise are highly selected, probably throughout the long process of carcinogenesis and tumor progression. These selected mutations occur preferentially in certain genes and often in highly selected locations in these genes; many of these mutations are causally related to, and specific for, the malignant process. These mutations were originally discovered because the mutant gene was found (a) to be overexpressed, (b) to cause transformation in transfection assays, or (c) to be involved in a cancer-specific chromosomal translocation. Several of the mutations affect DNA sequences that encode proteins and therefore result in the appearance of tumor-specific mutant proteins. These novel proteins may be the result of point mutations, internal deletions, or other gene rearrangements, including fusion of genes. The original reason for discovering these mutations was not the antigenicity of the encoded mutant proteins; therefore, these mutant proteins may not necessarily encode tumor-specific antigens. Computerized algorithms have been used [in a process called *reverse immunology* (8)] to predict the likelihood that a particular mutation will result in a strong antigen, and several of the mutant proteins and peptides have been used to explore the possibility of inducing tumor-specific immunity. It is interesting that antigens recognized by the host when immunized with tumor cells (direct immunology) have, so far, always been found to be encoded by different mutations (see previous section). Therefore, an important question is this: How commonly are mutant proteins that have been identified initially by nonimmunological methods effective targets for immunological rejection of cancer cells? Some examples (Table 3) are given as follows.

Mutant Ras Oncogene–Encoded Proteins

The tumorigenic potential of the Ras proto-oncogene can be acquired by *activating mutations,* which occur at selected predictable sites and affect amino acid residue 12 or 61 and,

less frequently, residue 13 of the p21 Ras protein (69). Mutant Ras can elicit specific antibody (71,72) but the protein is located at the inner tumor cell membrane, not at the cell surface. However, mutant Ras peptides elicit CD4$^+$ or CD8$^+$ T-cell responses (35,36). For example, human CD4$^+$ T cells have been shown to recognize a valine for glycine substitution at position 12 of Ras, which is one of the most common mutations in human cancers (35). The region of the mutant Ras protein from which the peptide was derived is identical for all the three members of the Ras proto-oncogene family, namely, H-Ras, K-Ras, and N-Ras, which have different prevalence in different cancers. Ras mutations occur in premalignant or malignant cells after thymic deletion of self-reactive clones, and most individuals should therefore have clones that respond to the mutant proteins. In all instances, the T cells have been induced with the purified Ras peptide or protein rather than tumor cells. A potential problem is that, in only some tumor cells, the peptide/MHC complexes may have sufficient density to be recognized by Ras-specific T cells. Also, the presentation of Ras peptides on MHC molecules has been found to be unconventional, and the antigenic specificity of the weak immunity that was found against transplanted tumor cells after immunization with a semipurified mutant Ras protein remains unclear. Furthermore, immunization of cancer-prone mice against the mutant region of transgenic Ras caused enhanced growth of primary tumors (37). Thus, at present, it remains uncertain whether mutant Ras can serve as an effective target for tumor rejection. For example, no immunological cross-reactivity in tumor protection assays was observed between chemically induced fibrosarcomas that shared the same Ras mutation (38). Nevertheless, clinical trials have been developed.

Mutant p53 Suppressor Gene–Encoded Proteins

Mutations in the p53 suppressor gene are among the most common mutations found in human and experimental cancers. The p53 gene was originally discovered by antibody raised against a murine sarcoma or against preparations of simian virus 40 (SV40) T antigen. The protein was found in a large variety of cancers (including those of no known viral etiology) but was not detected in nonmalignant embryonic or adult cells; this finding implies a possible central role for p53 in the malignant process. It is now understood that normal p53 protein, which acts as a suppressor of cell growth, is expressed little in normal cells and therefore is generally not detected, whereas the high levels of p53 commonly detected in malignant cells usually represent a mutant p53 protein. The mutations in p53 tend to cluster in evolutionarily conserved regions of the gene, but the exact locations of mutations in the p53 gene are highly diverse. Different mutations appear to cause common conformational changes (and possibly similar dysfunction), as evidenced by preferential reactivity of different mutant p53 proteins with certain anti-p53 monoclonal antibodies. Patients appear to mount an antibody response to mutant p53 proteins, particularly those that associate with

TABLE 3. Origin, distribution, and antigenicity of different categories of tumor antigens represented by examples

Category/type of antigen	Example	Mechanism of expression in cancer	Contributes to malignant behavior	Normal adult tissue distribution	Cancer specific	Normal precursor lineage	Occurrence: Type of cancer	Occurrence: Shared versus unique	Recognition by: T cells	Recognition by: B cells	Rejection antigen
Normal cellular gene products											
Oncospermatogonal antigen (cancer-testis antigens)	MAGE-1	Ectopic expression	?	Testis	–	–	Several	Shared	+	+	
	MAGE-3	Ectopic expression	?	Testis/trophoblast	–	–	Several	Shared	+	+	
Oncofetal antigen	P1A	Ectopic expression	?	Testis/trophoblast	–	–	Mastocytoma	Shared	+	–	Weak
	CEA	Amplification of regenerative cell	?	Colon/lactating breast	–	+	Several	Shared	–	+	Weak
Differentiation antigen	EpCam	Normal surface glycoprotein	–	Broad	–	+	Several	Shared	–	+	Passive
	PSA	Normal intracellular enzyme	–	Prostate	–	+	Prostate	Shared	–	–	
	Tyrosinase	Normal intracellular enzyme	–	Melanocytes	–	+	Melanoma	Shared	+	+	Passive
	Lewis (carbohydrate)	Aberrant glycosylation	?	Broad	–	+	Several	Shared	–	+	
	HER-2/neu (oncoprotein)	Overexpression	+(?)	Breast/ovary	–	+	Several	Shared	–	+	
	GD2/GD3 ganglioside	Overexpression	?	Broad	–	+	Several	Shared	–	+	Passive
Clonal antigen	Immunoglobulin idiotype	Clonal amplification	+	B-cell clone	–	+	B-cell malignancy	Unique	(+)	+	Weak
Mutant cellular gene products											
Primary detection as antigen											
Ribosomal protein	Mut L9	Point mutation	LOH +	–	+	–	Fibrosarcoma	Unique	+	+	?
Cyclin	Mut cdk4	Point mutation	+	–	+	–	Melanoma	Highly restricted	+	?	?
Primary detection as oncogene											
Oncogene product	Mut ras	Point mutation	+	–	+[a]	–	Several	Shared	+	+	?
Suppressor gene product	Mut p53	Point mutation	+	–	+[b]	–	Several	Unique	?	+	?
Internal fusion protein	Mut EGFR	Internal deletion	+(?)	–	+	–	Ganglioma	Shared	?	+	?
Chimeric fusion protein	BCR-ABL gene	Translocation	+	–	+	–	CML	Shared	+	+	?
Viral gene product											
Nuclear protein	E6/E7 of HPV16 or HPV18	Transforming viral gene	+	–	[a]	–	Cervical	Shared	+	+	+(?)

CEA, carcinogenic embryonic antigen; CML, chronic myelogenous leukemia; EGFR, epidermal growth factor receptor; EpCAM, epithelial cellular adhesion molecule; HER-2, human epidermal growth factor receptor 2; HPV, human papilloma virus; LOH, loss of heterozygosity; MCA, methylcholanthrene; Mut, mutant; PSA, prostate-specific antigen.

[a] Can also occur in carcinogen-induced benign premalignant lesions (e.g., papillomas).

[b] Also found as germline mutations in the dominantly inherited Li-Fraumeni familiar cancer syndrome.

heat-shock proteins, and the presence of these antibodies are correlated with a poor prognosis. Unlike antibodies, T cells recognize unique short mutant peptides in which common conformational changes are absent. Exploring mutant p53 proteins as a potential immunological target for therapy is attractive because T cells with unique specificity appear to mediate the strongest antitumor immunity, and p53-specific T cells have been induced. However, as with mutant Ras, immunization with tumor cells has generally not induced T cells specific for mutant p53 peptides, which suggests that other unique antigens may usually dominate the response. Nevertheless, tumor immunity *in vivo* has been induced by vaccination against mutant p53 peptides if given with interleukin (IL)–12. Because p53 is commonly overexpressed in cancer cells, T cells directed against normal p53 might preferentially destroy tumor cells. Vaccines designed to immunize against normal p53 would also not require tailoring the vaccines for the individual, highly diverse p53 mutations. However, normal p53 is a self-antigen of which individuals are tolerant. Because murine and human normal p53 sequences are not fully conserved, murine T cells specific for human normal p53 peptides that lyse human tumor cells have been induced. Furthermore, p53 knockout mice generate T cells specific for normal murine p53 that, on adoptive transfer into p53 wild-type mice, can eradicate murine p53-overexpressing tumors without signs of autoimmunity to the host. Nevertheless, it remains uncertain to what extent p53 can serve as an effective target for tumor rejection.

Fusion Proteins Resulting from Internal Deletions or Chromosomal Translocations

New antigenic determinants can arise from the juxtaposition of previously distant amino acid sequences, resulting in a new peptide sequence and possibly a change in conformational structure. Such fusion proteins can result from internal deletions within the coding sequence of a single gene. For example, about 40% of malignant glioblastomas, the most common primary brain malignancy in humans, have an internal deletion of the epidermal growth factor receptor gene, which results in a fusion protein. About half of the patients with this tumor have the same deletion, which generates a new amino acid at the fusion point. The new antigenic determinants on the surface of the cancer cells can be recognized specifically by a monoclonal antibody. Such truly tumor-specific antibody may be therapeutically useful against this cancer, which is untreatable by conventional therapy. Fusion proteins may also result from chromosomal translocations found in a variety of human cancers. The resulting fusion proteins are chimeric because parts of the same protein are encoded by sequences of two distinct genes. Remarkably, similar translocations and recombinational events may occur in a given type of cancer, which may result in the juxtaposition of exactly the same coding sequences from the two involved chromosomes. These highly conserved chromoso-

mal breakpoints may therefore give rise to the same fusion proteins in the same cancers from different individuals. The best examples are the chimeric BCR/ABL fusion proteins found in patients with chronic myelogenous leukemia. The fusion proteins can be recognized specifically by antibody (39) and human CD4+ T cells, and peptides spanning the fusion point of the BCR/ABL fusion protein can be presented by the class I MHC surface molecules of chronic myelogenous leukemia cells as targets to CD8+ human cytolytic T cells. Of importance is that many of these fusion proteins are essential for maintaining the malignant state of the cell, and tumor cells may not easily escape therapy by losing expression of fusion proteins. It is still uncertain, however, whether these fusion proteins can serve as effective targets for active or passive immunotherapy.

TUMOR ANTIGENS ENCODED BY NORMAL CELLULAR GENES (TUMOR-ASSOCIATED ANTIGENS)

All the antigens listed in this section are encoded by non-mutant cellular genes that are expressed not only by certain cancer cells but also by at least one subset of normal adult cells. Therefore, these antigens are not tumor specific, and they are commonly referred to as tumor-associated antigens. The extent to which these antigens are expressed by normal cells and tissues can vary from widespread expression to extreme restriction to a small population of normal cells. Furthermore, the time during development or differentiation when these markers are expressed on normal cells can vary considerably. Some of these antigens have been found only in spermatogonia, spermatocytes, and certain cancer cells (oncospermatogonal antigens) but not in normal cells of the tissue of tumor origin; that is, these antigens are expressed in a non–lineage-specific manner. Most tumor-associated antigens, however, are expressed at least at some level on the cell type from which the tumor developed; that is, these antigens are lineage specific and represent differentiation antigens. Some of these differentiation antigens are found in only a small clone of normal cells from which the malignancy originated (clonal antigens), whereas other differentiation antigens are also found prominently expressed in embryonic or fetal precursor cells and are, therefore, called *carcinoembryonic* or *oncofetal* antigens.

Even though none of the antigens discussed in this section are truly tumor specific, several mechanisms for an operational relative tumor specificity have been invoked for several tumor-associated antigens: (a) Malignant cells may express a given antigen at much higher levels (e.g., 10- to 100-fold), and some studies suggest that such differences in expression levels between normal and malignant cells can be exploited therapeutically. (b) Relative tumor specificity may also be attained because of better access of the antigen-specific effector cells to the malignant cells than to normal cells [e.g., the epithelial adhesion molecule (EPCAM) is expressed on individual colon cancer cells but only on the luminal surface of the normal colon cells]. (c) For certain antigens, the expression of the epitopes on the normal cells is hidden from the immune system by more complete glycosylation of the target molecule in the normal cells (in the case of epithelial mucins). (d) In the case of oncospermatogonal antigens, lack of expression of MHC molecules by the normal cells may prevent these cells from becoming a direct target for T cells. However, indirect presentation of antigens can occur for all antibody as well as T cell–recognized antigen, and a large body of experimental evidence supports the concept that the induction of protective T cell–mediated responses to tumor-specific antigens by active immunization is much more effective than inducing immune responses to target structures that lack tumor specificity (20,40). Nevertheless, passive immunization with monoclonal antibodies directed against human tumor-associated differentiation antigens have been described to be effective (41–43) (see later discussion), and the possibility of achieving therapeutic effects of active immunization against oncospermatogonal antigens is currently being explored.

Oncospermatogonal Antigens ("Cancer-Testis" Antigens)

It has been postulated repeatedly that certain normal genes that are completely silent in all nonmalignant cells may be activated exclusively in malignant cells. Alternatively, it has been postulated that cancer cells may express proteins (or immature forms of a protein) that are expressed only in fetal but not in nonmalignant adult cells [e.g., Coggin et al. (44)]. However, several previous similar claims of selective activation of normal genes (or selective expression of immature forms of proteins) in cancer cells leading to tumor-specific antigens have not been substantiated. Usually, at least transient expression of the same antigen by at least one normal cell type was later discovered. For example, the thymic leukemia (TL) antigen is encoded by a normal cellular gene in the MHC locus (45). Initially, it was found that the TL gene was not expressed in normal thymocytes of TL-negative mice, but it could be activated specifically in leukemias developing in these strains. However, much later studies demonstrated that the TL antigen was expressed by normal gut epithelium of TL-negative strains. As another example, certain CTL-recognized antigens on human melanomas and several other cancers [e.g., melanoma antigen-encoding gene (MAGE)–1, MAGE-2, MAGE-3] were reported to be encoded by normal genes that were found to be expressed only in the malignant cells (46). However, further research revealed that these antigens were also expressed by normal spermatogonia and primary spermatocytes in the testis (47) and possibly other normal cells. Therefore, these antigens are also referred to as "cancer-testis" antigens. Similar oncospermatogonal antigens have also been defined through the use of autologous sera of cancer patients as probes (48). Oncospermatogonal antigens may

also be found in murine tumor models, and a murine homolog of MAGE is expressed in postmeiotic spermatids. Furthermore, a CTL-recognized antigen on mouse mastocytoma P1A was reported to be expressed by a normal gene not expressed by normal cells; later work, however, revealed expression of the antigen in normal spermatogonia and trophoblast cells. Thus, there is a lack of convincing evidence that normally completely silent genes are specifically activated in cancer cells and can encode truly tumor-specific antigens.

The selective appearance of antigens in cancer cells as well as in spermatogonia and spermatocytes is very interesting, because it may be related to demethylation of genes. Such demethylation takes place rather selectively during spermatogenesis and cancer development and may lead to expression of a large number of genes. These genes either may be completely silent in other cells or, more likely, are expressed at some selective stage of cellular development, possibly in a cell type that has escaped observation. Consistent with this explanation is the finding that some tumor-associated antigen, such as P1A, MAGE-3, and MAGE-4, are found not only in spermatogonia but also in trophoblast cells and thus represent carcinoembryonic antigens (CEAs). In any case, unlike differentiation antigens, oncospermatogonal antigens are observantly expressed in cancer cells in a highly selective, non–lineage-specific manner. Because of their relative tumor specificity, the oncospermatogonal antigens may represent important targets for diagnosis of, as well as immunotherapy for, cancer.

Differentiation Antigens

Some antigens expressed on tumor cells are also expressed during at least some stage of differentiation on nonmalignant cells of the cell lineage from which the tumor developed. These lineage-specific antigens can therefore be considered differentiation markers. They represent a very diverse group of proteins, glycoproteins (including mucins), and glycolipids (carbohydrate or peptide epitopes); several are being explored as potential immunotherapeutic targets (41). Other lines of evidence support the idea that effectors and target structures may not need to have absolute specificity. For example, several chemotherapeutic agents are used successfully against cancer despite potential severe side effects on normal cells. Furthermore, an antibody to a normal surface glycoprotein expressed at similar levels on normal and malignant colonic epithelial cells has been found to be effective in inhibiting the growth of colorectal carcinoma cells in nude mice when given shortly after tumor cell injection (42). The same antibody appears to be effective in reducing the incidence of metastatic disease and in increasing long-term survival in humans when given shortly after surgery to patients with colorectal carcinoma (at which stage the seeded cancer cells may still be singular and the target antigen more accessible to the antibody) who have undergone tumor resection with curative intent (41). Similarly, passive antibodies against melanocyte-specific differentiation antigens are effective against metastatic spread of melanoma cells in mice when given at the time of seeding of the malignant cells (49), and similar antibodies may have analogous beneficial effects in human patients with melanoma (50).

Differentiation markers are found on cancer cells because malignant cells usually express at least some of the genes that are characteristic of normal cell types from which the tumor cell originated. The presence of these normal differentiation antigens can therefore help restrict the cytocidal effects of the therapeutic antibody to a single cell lineage. For example, CD20 is a signature B-cell differentiation antigen targeted by a genetically engineered monoclonal antibody that is relatively effective in the treatment of B-cell lymphoma (43). Differentiation antigens may also help determine the organ or cell type of origin (lineage) of a cancer. For example, B-cell tumors express surface immunoglobulin, and T-cell leukemias can be distinguished as helper and suppressor cell leukemias through the use of T-cell subset-specific monoclonal antibodies. Careful diagnostic delineation of different subtypes of cancer is important because different tumor subtypes may carry different prognoses and may be susceptible to different therapies. Although lineage-specific markers have been particularly useful for subclassifying hematopoietic cancers, relatively few cell type- or lineage-specific antigens have been found for cells outside the hematopoietic and melanocyte lineage. Instead, some of the other cell types can be characterized by distinct patterns of expression of antigenic markers that have a wider distribution. Tumors often acquire a less differentiated appearance with progression. In fact, metastatic lesions of tumors of quite different tissue origin are often morphologically so much alike that the retention of a cell type–specific antigen by the metastatic cells may give an important diagnostic clue as to the organ from which the cancer originated. However, the use of differentiation markers for histological or cytological tumor classification has pitfalls. First, cancer cells occasionally express differentiation antigens normally not expressed in the cell lineage from which the tumor originated (aberrant expression). Second, differentiation markers can be lost during tumor progression, leaving no clue as to the cancer's tissue of origin. Some tissue-specific antigens are detected only cytochemically or histochemically, whereas other tissue-specific antigens can be used as serum markers; for example, the prostate-specific antigen, a chymotrypsin-like protease, which is selectively expressed by the normal or malignant epithelial cells of the prostate gland, is elevated in benign hypertrophy of the prostate as well as in prostatic cancer. Therefore, detection of any prostate-specific antigen after complete surgical removal of the prostate indicates residual tumor cells, recurrence, or both. However, there are no immunological serum markers currently available that are specific for cancer, because levels of currently available serological markers are also elevated in a variety of nonmalignant diseases and conditions.

Several differentiation antigens (such as tyrosinase, the related brown locus protein, gp100, and Melan-A/MART-1) appear to be restricted to melanocytes, and all of them are being explored as possible immunotherapeutic targets (40,56). Immune recognition of the melanocyte differentiation antigens can lead to rejection of a tumor challenge (49), but this antigen-specific immunotherapy targets not only the tumor cells but also normal cells expressing the shared antigens (49,51), which results in the depigmentation of normal skin called vitiligo. Another useful target may be gangliosides GD2 and GD3, which are not only overexpressed in melanoma but also found in other cells of neural crest origin and in other tissues. Pancreatic, breast, and colon cancers express mucins that can be recognized on cancer cells by MHC-unrestricted cytolytic T cells that react specifically with repeated epitopes on the protein core of the mucin molecules exposed because of deficient glycosylation in the malignant cells (52). Finally, overexpression of the human epidermal growth factor receptor 2 (HER-2/neu) is observed in some breast and ovarian cancers and other adenocarcinomas, and high levels of expression correlate with a more aggressive clinical course. Monoclonal HER-2/neu–specific antibodies have shown effectiveness in adjuvant therapy of some patients with metastatic breast cancers that express elevated levels of the antigen (53). These antibodies may be effective at least in part by interfering with the function of the growth factor receptor.

Oncofetal and Carcinoembryonic Antigens

In 1932, human cancer cells were found to express antigens that serologically cross-react with normal embryonic tissue (54). There appear to be two different mechanisms for the appearance of such antigens. In the first mechanism, expression of embryonic or fetal antigens appears to occur as a result of malignant transformation, tumor progression, or both. This expression appears to result from an aberrant activation or "depression" of genes that are supposedly completely silent in adult nonmalignant cells of the lineage of tumor cell origin (e.g., caused by methylation) but are normally active in certain fetal and embryonic cells (e.g., trophoblast cells). Examples are non–lineage-specific tumor antigens such as the human MAGE-3 in humans and the murine P1A antigens that are expressed in cancer cells as a result of demethylation. In the second mechanism, the antigens are lineage-specific and expressed not only in fetal or embryonic cells but also already in the normal stem cells of the adult tissue from which the tumor originated. The more mature nonmalignant cells usually do not express these antigens, at least not at high levels, but these antigens are expressed in less mature nonmalignant adult cells, especially after various types of injury or disease. Tumors seem to represent an amplification and immortalization of such stem cells. An example is one of the best-studied embryonic tumor markers, CEA.

CEA was discovered as a tumor-specific antigen in human colon carcinoma (55) and as a fetal antigen restricted to fetal gut, pancreas, and liver in the first two trimesters of gestation (55). Now it is realized that CEA is also present in low levels in nonmalignant, nonfetal adult tissues such as normal colonic mucosa, lung, and lactating breast tissue. Therefore, the term *embryonic* or *fetal antigen* for these molecules that are also found in adult cells is confusing. CEA is a 200-kDa membrane-associated glycoprotein that is released into surrounding fluids. At one time, it was hoped that CEA could be used as a marker for early diagnosis of gastrointestinal malignancies; however, elevated serum levels of CEA are found not only in gastrointestinal malignancy but also in a number of other malignant diseases outside the gastrointestinal tract, such as cancers of the lung and breast. Furthermore, elevated levels of CEA are also found in the absence of malignancy (e.g., in smokers and in patients with inflammatory bowel diseases, such as ulcerative colitis). Although serum levels of CEA are not useful for detecting early cancer, the level of CEA in the blood can be used to monitor the effects of therapy to indicate whether a cancer has been successfully eradicated or has recurred. The possibility of using CEA as an immunotherapeutic target is also being explored. In addition, the usefulness of another oncofetal antigen, the immature laminin receptor protein, for cancer diagnosis and therapy needs further study (44).

α-Fetoprotein (AFP) was the first defined oncofetal protein (56). Although produced by fetal liver and yolk sac cells, it is also present in small amounts in the serum of normal adults. The amount of this protein is elevated in some patients with cancer of the liver or testis and in some patients with various nonmalignant liver diseases. Therefore, like CEA, AFP is not necessarily useful as a marker for the early diagnosis of cancer. Nevertheless, assays of AFP can detect primary liver cancer at a time when the cancer is treatable, and AFP assays are also used for monitoring patients after therapy. The fact that fetal and embryonic antigens are often found on nonmalignant adult tissue serum poses particular problems for using these antigens as targets for active or passive immunotherapy and may account for why using such developmental antigens as targets for immunotherapy has so far been unsuccessful or only modestly successful.

Clonal Antigens

Clonal antigens, in contrast to the other differentiation antigens just described, are expressed only on a few normal adult cells—that is, only on the clone of cells from which the tumor originated: for example, the idiotype of surface immunoglobulin-positive B-cell malignancies. In this particular case, it is interesting that immunization of mice against the idiotype induces an idiotype-specific transplantation immunity against the growth of the tumors (myeloma, lymphoma) expressing the idiotype (57). Human CTLs that express the specific receptor for the idiotype of immunoglobulin on autologous B-cell tumors have been generated. Furthermore, idiotype-specific antibodies prevented the growth of idiotype-positive murine myeloma cells *in vivo* or *in vitro*. Idiotype-specific antibodies have also been used in the therapy of murine or guinea pig idiotype-positive

B-cell leukemias. Finally, idiotype-specific monoclonal antibodies have caused several partial remissions and one complete remission in patients with B-cell lymphoma, and active idiotype-specific immunizations are also in clinical trials (58). It is necessary to generate different monoclonal antibodies or idiotypic vaccines for each individual cancer to be treated, but the advantage of using such clonal antigens over a less restricted tumor-associated antigen is that only a few normal cells bear the same antigen. For example, normal B-cell clone expressing the idiotype probably does not interfere with the use of the anti-idiotypic antibody; nor is it likely that the loss of a normal B-cell clone as a result of therapy would adversely affect the patient. Except for idiotypes on B-cell and T-cell malignancies, there are currently no candidates for other clonal antigens.

TUMOR ANTIGENS ENCODED BY VIRAL GENES

DNA Tumor Viruses

SV40 and polyoma viruses are cancer-inducing DNA viruses that encode functionally similar but antigenically distinct proteins required for the induction and maintenance of malignant transformation. As would be expected, these virally encoded proteins are shared by all tumors induced by the same virus regardless of tissue origin or animal species. These proteins appear intracellularly as predominantly nuclear antigens, but the same genes that encode these proteins are also required for the expression of the CTL-recognized, virus-specific, MHC-presented peptides acting as transplantation antigens on the tumor cell surface. The rejection antigens are tumor-specific in the sense that they are not expressed by normal host cells and are not encoded by genes of the host or presented on the virion particles themselves, which carry viral capsid antigens. In the early 1980s, extensive studies analyzed how the SV40-specific CTL could recognize the nuclear T antigen on the surface of tumor cells. By transfection of truncated nontransforming portions of the gene encoding the T-antigen epitopes, these studies provided an early hint that class I MHC antigen–restricted CTLs can recognize on the cell surface processed fragments of proteins that are primarily located intracellularly. Similar to the T antigens of SV40 and polyoma virus, adenoviruses and human papillomavirus (HPV) also have so-called early region genes, designated E1A/E1B and E6/E7, respectively, which are transcribed not only during early stages of viral replication but also in transformed cells, and expression of these antigens is required for maintenance of the transformed phenotype. Thus, DNA viruses, such as SV40, polyoma virus, HPV, and adenovirus, show stable but random integration of at least the early-region genes of the virus into the genome of the cells they transform. It is the protein product of the early region rather than the site of integration of the virus into the genome that seems to be important for inducing and maintaining the transformed phenotype. Thus, the early-region proteins are virally encoded, tumor-specific antigens that are clearly related to the transformed phenotype and the establishment of malignant behavior. Several of these antigens induce class I MHC–restricted CTLs. Infection with several types of DNA viruses have been associated with human cancer: certain subtypes of HPVs, with cervical cancer and certain other cancers; hepatitis B virus, with primary liver cancer; Epstein-Barr virus (EBV), with immunoblastic lymphomas in immunocompromised individuals, possibly with the endemic (African) Burkitt's lymphoma, and with nasopharyngeal carcinoma; and human herpesvirus 8, with Kaposi's sarcoma. In addition, SV40 may contribute to the development mesotheliomas, bone tumors, ependymomas, and chorion plexus tumors. The viral genes involved in the malignant transformation by EBV are largely unknown, but the lymphoma cells usually have integrated viral sequences. EBV can encode a number of CTL-recognized antigens that have been carefully mapped. Of particular importance are several EBV-encoded nuclear antigens and latent membrane proteins that are expressed in EBV-transformed cells. There is strong suggestive evidence that adoptive T-cell immunotherapy in immunosuppressed patients may be effective in eradicating more advanced EBV-associated lymphomas that express the full array of target antigens. HPV-associated cervical cancers regularly express the transforming proteins E6 and E7 but often at very low levels, but in mice, active immunization against E6/E7 can lead to rejection of transplanted tumor cells transfected to express E6/E7 antigens (168).

RNA Tumor Viruses

Ribonucleic acid (RNA) tumor viruses, which can be of exogenous or endogenous type, integrate into host cell DNA; however, for most of the viral life cycle, exogenous viruses exist and replicate as infectious particles capable of infecting other cells. In contrast, endogenous viruses remain, most of the time, as proviruses integrated into the host's genome and produce infectious particles only when "induced" by ionizing radiation, chemical carcinogens, mutagens, or protein synthesis inhibitors. Genomic DNA of inbred mice contains about 50 copies of normal murine leukemia virus (MuLV)–related proviral sequences. These proviruses can be categorized into three major groups, which are determined by the range of the host cells that can be infected by the infectious particles derived from these proviruses: ecotropic viruses, which replicate in mouse cells but not in nonmouse cells; xenotropic viruses, which replicate in nonmouse cells but not in mouse cells; and polytropic (amphotropic or dual-tropic) viruses, which replicate in both types of cells. The differences in host range of the viruses are determined by differences in their viral envelope (env) genes, which encode a 70-kDa glycoprotein (gp70). Thus, oligonucleotide probes specific for the three types of env genes or antibody probes specific for the three antigenic types of gp70 viral envelope proteins (45) can be used to group these proviruses into one of the three categories just listed. Apparently, all RNA tumor viruses share a number of antigenic determinants of envelope proteins, even when isolated from different species. This is consistent with the notion that RNA tumor viruses are rather closely related, which is supported by the similar genomic structure of these viruses.

Human T-lymphotropic virus 1 (HTLV-1) is the only RNA virus currently known to be associated with a human cancer, an endemic adult T-cell leukemia. However, expression of a human endogenous retroviral gene product has been reported in several human cancers, and RNA viruses are associated with several cancers in animals. Viral antigens found in these tumors include the virus envelope glycoproteins encoded by the env gene, several viral core proteins encoded by the viral gag gene, and superantigens encoded by an open reading frame (ORF) in the long terminal repeat of murine mammary tumor virus (Mtv) or by the gag gene of MuLV. Thus, proteins encoded by RNA tumor viruses are found in the virus particles as well as on the surface of virus-infected or virus-transformed cells. In contrast, proteins encoded by DNA tumor viruses are expressed not on the virus particles but only by the transformed or infected cells. There is strong evidence that certain proviral genes, such as the env genes encoding gp70 surface glycoproteins of MuLV, can be expressed on normal murine cells and on chemically induced or UV light–induced tumors without activation of the provirus to produce infectious particles (45). Therefore, expression of gp70 is commonly observed on normal cells, in which the appearance of these glycoproteins is regulated by the stage of cellular differentiation.

Injection of MuLV or murine sarcoma virus (MSV) into newborn animals induces cancer (59). Although antibodies to gp70 can apparently prevent viral infection, rejection of RNA tumor virus–transformed cells depends on MHC-restricted T cells specific for the viral antigens. These T cells detect both viral envelope (e.g., gp70) and viral core proteins (e.g., gag) of the MuLV- or MSV-induced tumor cells (60,61). Such proteins can also be recognized by T cells on chemically induced or spontaneously arising murine cancer cells. These experimental studies have shown that activation of endogenous retroviral sequences can lead to the expression of tumor antigens that are shared or appear to be unique; however, because of the lack of normal control cells from the mouse of tumor origin, it is not clear whether the transcriptional activation was tumor specific or caused by rearrangements already present in germline genes. Some RNA tumor viruses, such as the Mtv, are vertically transmitted (e.g., during nursing of the neonate), but neonatal exposure to antigens encoded by endogenous Mtv long terminal repeat sequences can prevent infection by exogenous Mtv [resulting from deletion of reactive T cells that act as carriers for the virus (62)] and result in a lower mammary tumor incidence. Transforming genes of DNA tumor viruses are not closely related to normal cellular genes; therefore, the products encoded by these genes may elicit a vigorous immune response. In contrast, transforming genes of RNA tumor viruses (also called *viral oncogenes*) are closely related to, and in some cases identical to, cellular oncogenes; their products, therefore, may elicit no or only weak responses. Thus, self-tolerance may account for why it is more difficult to induce CTLs specific for oncogene products of RNA tumor viruses than for proteins of SV40, EBV, and adenoviruses.

IMMUNOLOGICAL FACTORS INFLUENCING THE INCIDENCE OF CANCER

Immunosurveillance of Tumor Development

Early in the twentieth century, it was suggested by Paul Ehrlich (5) that cancer would occur at an "incredible frequency" if host defenses did not prevent the outgrowth of cancers from latent precursors that arise continuously. Ehrlich proposed that adaptive as well as natural (innate) defenses play a role.

Adaptive T Cell–Mediated Immunosurveillance

Ehrlich's eloquent hypothesis of immunological resistance of the host to the outgrowth of primary cancer did not receive major attention until the late 1950s (63) and 1960s, when the problem was restated and redefined. The extended hypothesis (63) suggested that the primary reason for development of T cell–mediated immunity during the evolution of vertebrates was defense against altered self-cells or neoplastic cells. Furthermore, the term *immunosurveillance* was coined to describe the concept of an immunological host resistance against the development of cancer. The concept of surveillance by adaptive immunity was especially attractive in the 1950s and 1960s because it provided evolutionary significance to T cell–mediated cellular immunity, which previously seemed to have no use other than to cause rejection of experimental allografts. It is now known that T cell–mediated immunity is necessary for resistance to many viral and other infections. For example, mice that lack adoptive T-cell immunity are highly susceptible to viral infections; however, an increased incidence or a shortened latency of chemically induced cancers has been found only in some experiments and not in others (64–68), although the incidence of lymphoreticular tumors is regularly increased among these mice. Similarly, beige mice that have defective granule formation

in several lymphocyte lineages develop lymphomas (akin to the human Chédiak-Higashi syndrome). Patients with certain congenital immunodeficiency diseases may also have a markedly (several thousand–fold) increased incidence of cancer (69) but mostly of lymphopoietic and reticuloendothelial origin. Most common forms of cancer do not occur earlier or at a significantly higher rate in the individuals than in the general immunocompetent population. It is therefore quite possible that the congenital abnormality in these tissues contributed significantly to the high incidence of these particular types of cancers. Most common forms of cancer are also not increased in patients with acquired immunodeficiency syndrome (AIDS) or in individuals who have been immunosuppressed by drug treatment because of transplantation or other conditions. However, patients with immunodeficiency are usually highly susceptible to viral infections, and Table 4 shows that these individuals have an increased incidence of cancers caused by virus [or UV light (see later discussion)].

In principle, adaptive T cell–mediated immunity may protect against the development of primary virus-associated cancers by either preventing or shortening the duration of infection with the oncogenic viruses or by eliminating virally transformed cells expressing the virus-encoded tumor antigens. Cells transformed by certain DNA or RNA viruses can be very immunogenic (70). For example, SV40 and polyoma viruses usually do not induce tumors in adult animals because the viruses induce rejection antigens on the transformed cells that are immunogenic enough to elicit rejection without prior immunization. Therefore, the use of immunoincompetent animals, such as very young or newborn animals or nude mice, is required for tumor induction, a finding that led to a breakthrough in studying the tumorigenicity of viruses and of cells transformed by viruses *in vitro*. Tumors induced by these viruses may nevertheless be serially passaged in adult mice, but only when very large numbers of tumor cells are used for transfer. It is important to note that this immunological resistance of the natural host is directed against virally transformed cells, not against the virus itself. Cells malignantly transformed by oncogenic DNA viruses do not (in contrast to oncogenic RNA viruses) produce viruses, and only the

TABLE 4. *Malignant neoplasms with an increased incidence in patients with immunodeficiency*

Type of immunodeficiency	Cancer	Carcinogen
Primary (inherited)	B-cell lymphoma	EBV
	Hepatocellular carcinoma	HBV
	Hematological malignancies	Germline
Secondary, drug-induced (patients with or without allograft)	B-cell lymphoma	EBV
	Squamous cell carcinoma (skin)	HPV, UV
	Hepatocellular carcinoma	HBV
	Cervical carcinoma	HPV
Acquired immunodeficiency syndrome	B-cell lymphoma	EBV
	Cloagenic or oral carcinoma	HPV
	Hepatocellular carcinoma	HBV

EBV, Epstein-Barr virus; HBV, hepatitis B virus; HPV, human papilloma virus; UV, ultraviolet light.

tumor formation, not infection by these viruses, may be prevented by the immune system. Such a resistance to tumor induction by DNA tumor viruses, for example, is consistent with the fact that polyoma virus is a common harmless passenger virus in adult mice and is commonly found in wild mice without inducing malignancies. In contrast, in the case of HPV, T cell–mediated responses may prevent or at least shorten the duration of viral infection, thereby reducing the chance that the initially mostly episomal virus integrates its oncogenic E6/E7 sequences into the host's epithelial cells; integration is needed for transformation. At present, it is uncertain how effectively T-cell immunity eliminates premalignant cells that have integrated E6/E7 but no longer produce the virus, particularly because the premalignant lesions may express less of the E6/E7 oncoprotein than the fully malignant cancers.

The resistance to tumor induction by oncogenic viruses is genetically determined, as illustrated by the example of the lymphotropic herpesvirus saimiri. In its natural host, the Old World squirrel monkey, the virus is an innocuous inhabitant. However, in some New World monkeys (such as the marmoset or owl monkey) that do not harbor the virus, inoculation of the virus regularly causes malignant lymphomas. It has been found that susceptible monkeys respond to the virally encoded antigens but too late and only at a time when lymphoma development has already occurred. To some extent, these results suggest that viruses with oncogenic potential select natural hosts that can effectively destroy cells transformed by such viruses, because lethal tumors would eliminate the virus along with the host. A further example of this is the lymphotropic EBV (70), which causes a self-limiting lymphoproliferative disease called mononucleosis in humans, the natural host of EBV. Thereafter, the EBV becomes latent, and although about 90% of adults are latently infected, only immunosuppressed individuals or patients with malaria appear to develop EBV-associated malignant lymphomas. EBV-encoded CTL-recognized antigens must be important for host recognition and tumor rejection, because lymphomas expressing these antigens in immunocompetent individuals have not been found. Instead, EBV-associated lymphomas express the full array of CTL-recognized antigens only in immunosuppressed patients, whereas Burkitt's lymphomas, which tend to appear before any obvious impairment of immune function, express only the EBV-encoded nuclear antigen 1, which is a poor target for CTL. Both types of EBV-associated lymphomas, however, share the same translocation involving the myc and the immunoglobulin loci. In conclusion, immunosurveillance by adoptive T-cell immunity is effective against the development of several virally induced cancers, but it is still uncertain how effectively adoptive T-cell immunity prevents the development of forms of cancers that are induced by chemical or physical carcinogens. For example, transporter associated with antigen processing (TAP) knockout mice do not have an increased or accelerated incidence of chemically induced cancers, regardless of whether these mice are also nullizygous for p53, even though TAP-deficient mice are deficient in presenting intracellular mutant peptides (the key targets of adaptive immunity to nonviral cancers) to $\alpha\beta$ receptor-bearing T cells, the key effectors of adaptive T-cell immunity.

Innate Immunosurveillance

The innate immune system uses nonrearranging germline receptors to trigger responses of cellular effectors that can recognize and kill cancer cells or normal cells lacking self-MHC antigens. These effectors also can produce large amounts of interferon (IFN)–γ. IFN-γ induces the transcriptional activator interferon regulatory factor 1 (IRF-1), which functions as a tumor suppressor. Loss of this factor increases spontaneous tumor susceptibility in mice carrying an overexpressed human c-Ha-Ras transgene or nullizygosity for p53 (71). Furthermore, fibroblasts from IRF-1 and p53 double-deficient mice are more susceptible to induced mutations, which suggests that IRF-1 may be involved in DNA repair in combination with p53. Similarly, animals with a defective IFN-γ signaling pathway [mice deficient in IFN-γ receptor or signal transducer and activator of transcription 1 (STAT1)] have an increased incidence of MCA-induced tumors, and the spontaneous tumor incidence was found to be increased when these mice also lacked p53 (68,72). Thus, the IFN-γ pathway may help the elimination of somatic cells harboring DNA damage. Finally, stimulation of the IFN-γ pathway by IL-12 may prevent spontaneous tumorigeneses (73). This surveillance effect of IFN-γ may be complemented by cytolytic $\gamma\delta$ T cells or natural killer T (NKT) cells that may use their NKG2d receptor to eliminate somatic cells exposed to the initiating chemical carcinogen followed by the tumor promoter TPA (67). The NKG2d ligands seem to be up-regulated by these agents, and mice lacking $\gamma\delta$ T cells and NKT cells are more prone to develop tumors induced in this way. Lymphocytes may use perforin for the elimination, inasmuch as perforin-deficient mice have a decreased surveillance of chemically induced tumors (74) and an accelerated spontaneous tumor development when one or both p53 alleles are also lacking (75). Renal transplant recipients also show a highly significant increase in skin cancers, preferentially on UV light–exposed sites of the body; this increase is independent of which immunosuppressive agent is being used (76). Thus, even treatment with the immunosuppressive drug cyclosporine (which has not been found to be mutagenic) caused a similar increase. Therefore, the restricted localization of these skin cancers to UV light–exposed sites argues against co-carcinogenic effects of the systemic drug treatment; rather, this observation supports the concept that indirect effects of the drug-induced suppression of the host's immune defenses can increase the development of primary skin cancers caused by UV light. In this regard, it is interesting that cyclosporine slightly reduced the latency period of UV light–induced skin cancers in mice, and it suppressed the rejection of transplanted UV light–induced regressor tumors by mice. At present, it is not known whether suppression of adoptive immunity [with the use of clonal T-cell receptor (TCR)–class I MHC/peptide interaction] or innate immunity with nonrearranging receptor-ligand pairs (e.g., NKG2D–NKG2D ligand) or suppression of another homeostatic surveillance mechanism results in the development of highly antigenic tumors. In any case, regulatory NKT cells can be induced by UV light irradiation (77). Together, protection against chemical- or radiation-induced cancers may be provided by various types of innate immune surveillance mechanisms that repair genetic damage, eliminate damaged cells from which cancers may arise, or eliminate premalignant cells expressing ligands that stimulate innate immunity.

Transplantation Studies

The term *immunosurveillance* should probably be reserved for description of effective host resistance to original (i.e., primary) tumors (e.g., certain virus-induced malignancies). Transplantation studies with tumor cells or cells transformed *in vitro* cannot adequately test the concept of immunosurveillance in the strict sense. Nevertheless, it is important to know that, for most tumors, a considerable number of tumor cells must be inoculated into a genetically identical animal or into a nude mouse before tumors develop; that is, whatever means of immune suppression is being used, a threshold number of tumor cells is usually needed. Therefore, this barrier to transplantation may well be caused by nonadaptive immunity or may be of a nonimmunological nature. Certainly, numerous nonimmunological homeostatic control mechanisms could be responsible for preventing the outgrowth of these transplanted tumor cells.

Numerous studies have demonstrated that primary tumors that develop in immunodeficient mice have slower growth rates than those developing in immunocompetent hosts (66,68,78,79). In addition, many of these tumors are "regressors," which means that they are rejected after initial growth when transplanted into immunocompetent mice. Progressor variants occasionally arise after nearly complete rejection of regressor tumors by normal mice. Some of these progressor variants have lost expression of the T cell–recognized antigens or of MHC molecules. Most progressor variants however, seem to retain their antigenicity but instead significantly increase their rapidity of growth and thus establish themselves faster as solid tumors when being transplanted. Tumors may not lose some of the tumor-specific antigens, because these antigens may be essential for tumor cell survival or may be causally related to the malignant phenotype. Rapid establishment may provide a protective microenvironment that allows the variants to escape destruction while retaining the antigens. Once established, the tumor may still stimulate immune responses in the tumor-bearing host, even though this response fails to prevent established cancer from continuing to grow. NKT cells may have been found to help or suppress (77,80) the rejection of transplanted tumor cells, but the relevance of these findings to immune surveillance of primary tumors is uncertain.

Stimulation of Tumor Development

As early as 1863, Virchow (81) suggested a possible functional relationship between inflammatory infiltrates and malignant growth. It is now known that such infiltrates can contribute to either the regression or the development (and progression) of cancer. However, these differences cannot be readily predicted from the histological appearance of the infiltrates, because inflammatory cellular reactions resulting from tumor destruction may not be easily distinguished histologically from inflammatory infiltrates causing tumor destruction. Furthermore, inflammatory cells, such as macrophages, may look morphologically identical, even though they may secrete different cytokines that have opposite effects on tumor growth. Despite continuous other claims, measurements of the inflammatory infiltration into tumors appear to remain a histopathological variable of unproven prognostic significance. This also applies to the finding of histologically "regressive" areas of progressive primary melanoma lesions, even when such a lesion is associated with an oligoclonal T-cell infiltrate or vitiligo (a depigmentation of normal skin). Destruction of parts of a malignant lesion may sometimes simply be the result of the infiltrative growth of the cancer cells into the surrounding tissue, which may destroy part of the tumor's blood supply. Thus, tumors have been compared with "wounds that do not heal" (82). Depending on the antigens, cell, and cytokine involvement, the result may be either inhibition or stimulation of the growth of the premalignant or malignant cells by acquired or innate immunity or both (Fig. 5). There is a strong association between chronic inflammatory conditions and eventual cancer development (83,84): The three types of conditions include (a) chronic infections (e.g., hepatitis C virus and hepatocellular carcinoma, *Helicobacter pylori* and gastric cancer, and schistosomiasis and bladder cancer), (b) chronic tissue damage by physical or chemical agents (e.g., reflux esophagitis and esophageal cancer; chronic pancreatitis and pancreatic carcinoma), and (c) inflammatory disorders of yet-unknown etiology (e.g., ulcerative colitis or Crohn's disease and colon cancer).

These conditions appear to help the early induction and promotion phase of cancer. Damaged, infected, and antigenic tissues produce cytokines as well attract inflammatory cells that produce further cytokines. For example, the macrophage migration inhibitory factory released by T cells and macrophages functionally inactivates p53, thereby creating a deficient response to genetic damage and allowing the accumulation of oncogenic mutations (85). The mechanisms of the tumor-promoting effects of stromal inflammation have become clearer in experiments with transgenic and knockout mice. Earlier studies already had shown that the effectiveness of promotion of skin tumor development by chemical

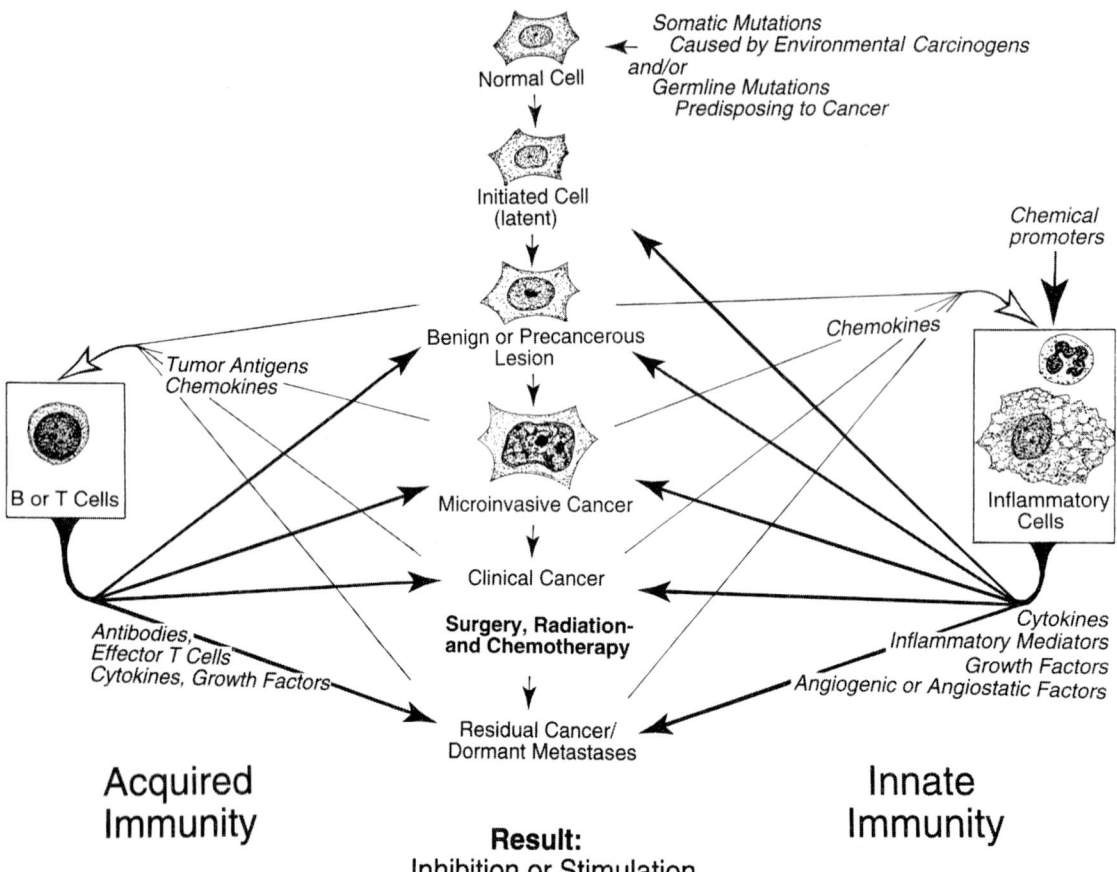

Somatic Mutations
Caused by Environmental Carcinogens
and/or
Germline Mutations
Predisposing to Cancer

Normal Cell

Initiated Cell
(latent)

Benign or Precancerous
Lesion

Microinvasive Cancer

Clinical Cancer

**Surgery, Radiation-
and Chemotherapy**

Residual Cancer/
Dormant Metastases

*Tumor Antigens
Chemokines*

B or T Cells

*Antibodies,
Effector T Cells
Cytokines, Growth Factors*

**Acquired
Immunity**

*Chemical
promoters*

Chemokines

Inflammatory
Cells

*Cytokines
Inflammatory Mediators
Growth Factors
Angiogenic or Angiostatic Factors*

**Innate
Immunity**

Result:
Inhibition or Stimulation

FIG. 5. Both acquired and innate immunity can have significant influence on tumor development and growth by exerting selective pressures. For example, specific T-cell immunity prevents the development of Epstein-Barr virus (EBV)–induced lymphomas in humans, whereas the presence of particular T-cell subsets helps the development of murine mammary tumor virus (Mtv)–associated tumors in mice. Innate immunity may also either stimulate or inhibit cancer development. For example, bacille Calmette-Guérin (BCG)–induced inflammation prevents recurrence of bladder cancers in humans, whereas prostaglandin H synthase 2–dependent inflammation seems to promote the development of certain skin and colon tumors. In principle, the two areas of the immune system can inhibit or stimulate tumor cells in any stage of the multistep process of cancer development and growth.

(phorbol esters) or physical (wounding) methods correlates directly with the degree of inflammation induced. Thus, strains of mice that have low or poor inflammatory reactions to wounding or phorbol esters are more resistant to tumor development after promotion. The induction of prostaglandin H synthase 2 encoded by the gene cyclooxygenase-2 is of central importance. Certain cytokines or chemical promoters induce the transcription of this gene in macrophages and other inflammatory cells, resulting in the local production of prostaglandin E_2 and other substances, such as reactive oxygen intermediates. Prostaglandin E_2 can (a) directly stimulate the growth of certain neoplastic cells (including colonic epithelial cells), (b) induce angiogenesis, and (c) block IL-12 and thus IFN-γ production. (Both cytokines may reduce the induction of primary cancers by chemical carcinogens.) In addition, the reactive oxygen intermediates can cause additional mutations in the initiated cells and thereby help tumors develop. The activity of the prostaglandin synthase–2

is not constitutive but induced in cells such as monocytes and macrophages, which are found as interstitial cells in epithelial tumors. Inhibition of the cyclooxygenase-2–encoded enzyme, by either specific chemicals or genetic knockout, significantly reduces the formation of intestinal tumors in mice prone to develop such neoplasms. Similarly, inhibition of prostaglandin production by nonsteroidal anti-inflammatory drugs can inhibit the development of skin papillomas and intestinal neoplasias. Thus, the ability to mount an inflammatory reaction can be essential for tumors to develop. As another example, a functioning TNF signaling pathway is required for induction of skin tumors by carcinogen followed by chemical promoters (86,87).

Whereas nonmalignant cells, under physiological conditions, produce cytokines only transiently for short-term signaling between cells, cancer cells can produce considerable and sustained amounts of various cytokines and chemokines, such as IL-8, transforming growth factor β (TGF-β), macrophage migration inhibitory factor, colony-stimulating factor 1 (CSF-1), and macrophage chemotactic proteins. These cytokines and chemokines may prevent the protective action of tumor suppressor genes, attract nonmalignant host cells and/or induce such cells to produce additional cytokines. For example, macrophage chemotactic proteins released from tumor cells attract macrophages to the site of tumor growth, and these tumor-associated macrophages are essential for angiogenesis and thus for any tumor to grow beyond a few millimeters in diameter. Tumor-associated leukocytes can also release other cytokines and growth factors, such as platelet-derived growth factor, to stimulate tumor growth. Similarly, latent TGF-β produced continuously by tumor cells can be activated by infiltrating inflammatory cells, such as macrophages, and active TGF-β may induce angiogenesis and the production of extracellular matrix and other cytokines by fibroblasts and endothelial cells. These infiltrating and sessile nonmalignant host cells and the extracellular matrix provide the stroma (literally, "bed") in which the tumor grows. Therefore, developing approaches to destroy the stroma of tumors may be of central importance for successful therapy for established solid tumors (88).

Not only early but also later stages of cancer development and tumor progression are dependent on leukocyte infiltrates, although these infiltrates may not contain many polymorphonuclear cells and therefore may not appear to be inflammatory. Certainly, continued growth of solid tumors requires neoangiogenesis, which depends on macrophages. Second, the surrounding stroma usually must provide some of the growth factors needed for continued tumor growth. In experimental skin carcinogenesis, tumor progression appears to depend on a continued inflammatory reaction, because regression of some papillomas is observed when the application of chemical promoters is stopped. Only promoter-independent tumors persist, and these tumors attract the stroma needed for vascularization and provision of growth factor. Thus, these later stages of tumor progression may also be influenced significantly by inflammatory cells. Cancer cells can acquire much more aggressive growth *in vivo* by acquisition of a paracrine stimulatory loop (78,89) by producing chemokines that attract leukocytes; these leukocyte cells in turn may produce cytokines and growth factors that stimulate tumor angiogenesis or the growth of the tumor cells directly. For example, there is a causal relationship between CSF-1 and breast cancer progression (90,91). The cytokine is prevalent in invasive cancer, as opposed to intraductal preinvasive cancer, and its presence is correlated with high-grade malignancy and poor prognosis. CSF-1 in an important regulator of macrophage proliferation, differentiation, and survival, and CSF-1 expression correlates with intense leukocyte infiltration (90,91). The autocrine production of CSF-1, a growth factor that acts on the proto-oncogene–encoded receptor cfms, causes proliferation, differentiation, and survival of macrophages and the production of matrix metalloproteinase–9. This matrix is a key factor that is released by leukocytes and mediates tumor progression by allowing the spread of tumor cells through

matrix basement membrane and into circulation. Another example is the production of viral IL-6 by nonmalignant stromal cells infected with Kaposi's sarcoma–associated herpesvirus. Viral IL-6 may play an essential role in the development of multiple myeloma (the second most frequent human malignancy of blood cells). This malignancy of plasma cells develops in about 25% of patients with a premalignant condition called *monoclonal gammopathy*. Other experiments have shown that cancer cells can switch during tumor progression from being inhibited to being stimulated by certain cytokines (e.g., TGF-β or IL-6). At the final stages of tumor progression in the most aggressive cancers, paracrine stimulation may also switch to autocrine stimulation when the cancer cells themselves begin to produce the stimulatory factors. This process of selection of autocrine variants may be hastened by incomplete therapy aimed at destroying the tumor stroma, which provides the paracrine growth factors. Finally, the homing of metastatic cells may be determined by the expression of chemokine receptors by cancer cells and the specific ligand at the sites of metastasis (92).

It has been postulated that, in general, T cell–mediated immune responses to tumor antigens stimulate tumor growth when "weak" and suppress tumor growth when "strong" (93). Because the original studies that were used to support this concept did not identify the antigens involved, it remained unclear whether antigen-specific or innate immunity played the significant role. More recent studies, however, provided the interesting example that the presence of a certain T-cell subset can result in a higher incidence of virally induced mammary tumors in mice. Mtv can be transmitted as milk-borne infection through the nursing mother to the offspring, resulting in mammary carcinoma later in the offspring in adulthood (94). A protein, the superantigen ORF, encoded in the ORF of the long terminal repeat of the Mtv genome, mediates the minor lymphocyte-stimulating response and stimulates or deletes particular T-cell subsets: for example, the Vb14 subset in the C3H/He mice. Dividing cells are more readily infected with retrovirus, and the T cells that are stimulated by ORF are preferentially infected. These T cells appear to be the primary carrier of virus to the mammary gland. The importance of this T-cell subset for the development of mammary tumors is demonstrated by the finding that transgenic mice expressing high levels of the ORF superantigen at birth delete the Vb14 subset and do not become infected with the milk-borne virus. Thus, those mice have a lower incidence of mammary tumors, whereas mice expressing lower levels of the same antigen did not delete this T-cell subset and remained susceptible (62). These results are consistent with earlier findings that neonatal thymectomy of mice greatly diminishes the incidence of mammary carcinomas. Interestingly, the incidence of breast cancer is reportedly decreased slightly among women who are chronically immunosuppressed after organ transplantation. Other studies have also supported the notion that adaptive T-cell immunity may, at least in some tumor systems, stimulate rather than suppress the development of primary cancers. For example, antigen-specific immune reactions against viral or mutant oncoproteins can be accompanied by an acceleration of tumor development (37). Furthermore, FVB/n mice lacking the $\alpha\beta$ TCR were found to be less susceptible to tumor development by chemical carcinogen and chemical promotion than were wild-type mice (67).

Certain bacterial substances, such as bacille Calmette-Guérin (BCG), and certain cytokines, when produced by transfected cancer cells, have significant antitumor effects (see later section on immunotherapy) that are associated with inflammatory responses, but at present, it is not known what determines whether a given inflammatory response suppresses rather than stimulates tumor growth. Once the differences in effector mechanisms and regulatory circuits of inflammatory responses are better understood, powerful new approaches to prevent as well as treat malignant diseases may be developed.

FACTORS INFLUENCING TUMOR IMMUNOGENICITY

Differences in Immunogenicity between Spontaneous and Induced Cancers

There is a widely held misconception that human cancers are usually less immunogenic than are murine tumors. However, convincing evidence indicates that many human cancers are antigenic, even when growth is progressive. Similarly, even the most antigenic murine "regressor" tumors grow progressively in, and invariably kill, the primary host (Fig. 6). Only transplantation of primary murine tumors into young, syngeneic, immunocompetent recipients reveals the immunogenicity that either can be so strong that the transplanted tumor fragments are rejected at any testable dose without prior immunization (i.e., the tumor is a regressor) or can be weaker so that the transplant will grow progressively (and the tumor thus represents a progressor). Therefore, it is quite possible that some human primary tumors are as immunogenic as murine regressor tumors, because only transplantation (not possible in humans) could reveal such immunogenicity.

The mode of tumor induction greatly influences the immunogenicity of the tumor induced, as measured by transplantation experiments. "Spontaneous" murine cancers that develop without any known exposure to carcinogens tend to be less immunogenic than cancers induced by DNA tumor viruses or by deliberate exposure to carcinogens (11,95). (Unfortunately, serially transplanted tumors were used for most of these comparisons, and transplantation may have been selected for less immunogenic variants, thereby confusing the results.) If spontaneous murine cancers more closely resembled human cancers, this could suggest that human cancers are poorly immunogenic. However, most human cancers are not "spontaneous" but induced by environmental carcinogens, and, as already mentioned, the immunogenicity of human tumors cannot be measured in transplantation experiments.

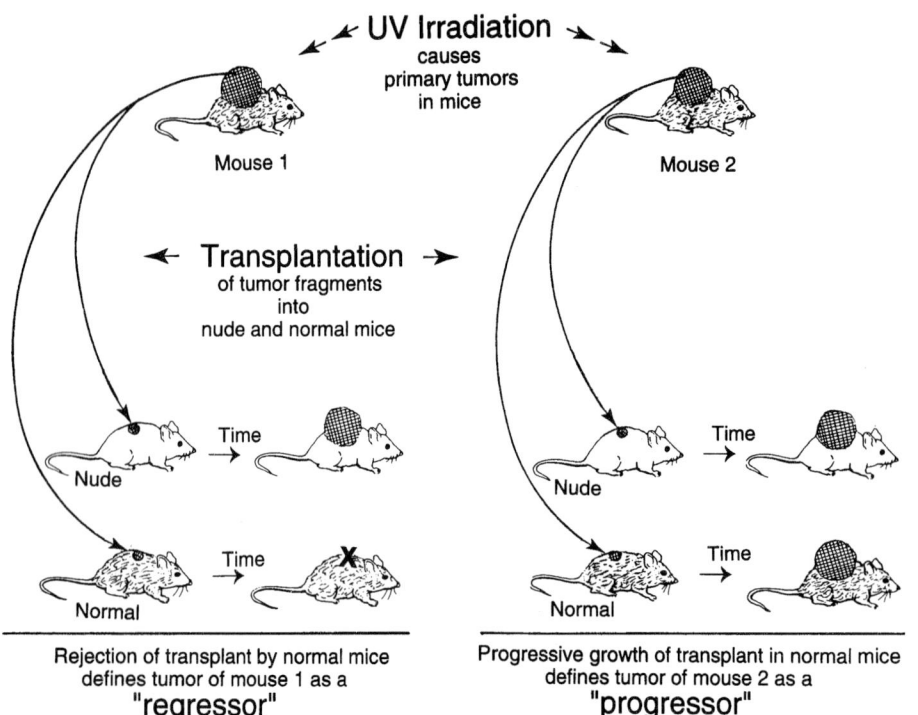

FIG. 6. Primary ultraviolet light–induced skin cancers are indistinguishable in the primary host regardless of whether the tumors are highly immunogenic or not. Only subsequent transplantations into normal young syngeneic mice define tumors as either regressors or progressors. Growth of the transplanted fragments in nude mice serves as control for the viability of the transplanted tumor fragments and for determining the T-cell dependence of the regressor phenotype.

Some UV light–induced tumors are among the most immunogenic cancers; transplantation resistance to these so-called regressor tumors appears to be absolute rather than relative. Rejection by normal syngeneic mice is observed without prior immunization of the mice, even when the largest testable doses of tumor cells or fragments are used (15); these tumor transplants grow for about a week and then disappear, although small numbers of the same tumor cells grow and kill athymic nude mice. Most MCA-induced fibrosarcomas display an intermediate degree of immunogenicity (12,13,21). This is shown by the fact that induction of immunological resistance to most chemically induced tumors requires prior immunization, because the initial graft of the tumor generally produces progressive lethal growth (12). Immunization can be induced either by administration of a small, nontumorigenic dose of tumor cells or by a complete surgical removal (excision or ligation) of an initial tumor transplant after the tumor has grown for several days or weeks. Immunological resistance induced by these chemically induced tumors is usually relative rather than absolute and breaks down when the number of tumor cells used for challenge is high.

Effect of Carcinogen Dose, Immunocompetence, and Tumor Latency

Most, if not all, carcinogens are mutagens (2), and mutations leading to cancer may also cause the expression of tumor-specific antigens. It therefore seems logical to postulate that the immunogenicity of a tumor is proportional to the dose of carcinogen used for induction; this might account for the usually low or absent immunogenicity of "spontaneous" tumors presumably induced by undetectable levels of environmental carcinogens. By analogy, tumors induced with larger doses of physical or chemical carcinogens, like experimentally induced tumors, would be immunogenic. However, it is not clear why tumors induced with the same dose of chemical or physical carcinogen may exhibit quite different degrees of immunogenicity (12,96). One reason might be that the actual local dose of carcinogen that is delivered to a particular target cell or target tissue may vary greatly from animal to animal. Another reason might be that the selected mutations favor malignant behavior irrespective of the degree of immunogenicity that a resultant mutant protein may have. This might occur because the autochthonous host may not respond to its own tumor unless it is immunized after tumor removal (14). This is consistent with the observation that considerable differences in immunogenicity of primary UV light–induced tumors become apparent only *after* transplantation into secondary hosts (24,96) (Fig. 6).

Immunocompetence of the host during cancer induction and development may sometimes allow the host to select for variants that have lost antigens. Conversely, immunosuppression or immune deficiency of the host during carcinogenesis should allow growth of highly immunogenic tumors (e.g., the appearance of highly antigenic EBV-associated lymphomas in immunosuppressed transplant recipients). Thus, it may be highly relevant that some carcinogens are immunosuppressive. In the mouse, for example, repeated exposures to UV light induce immunosuppression, which would allow the development of highly immunogenic regressor tumors. In contrast, the single injection of MCA required to induce tumors in 100% of mice induces only a short-lived state of immune suppression, thus allowing the host to select for less immunogenic variants during tumor development. This concept, that immunocompetence of a host influences the degree of immunogenicity of the developing tumor, has been tested experimentally by comparing the immunogenicity of MCA-induced tumors occurring in immunodeficient [nude, severe combined immunodeficiency (SCID), recombination activating gene knockout (RAG$^{-/-}$), UV light–irradiated] versus normal mice (66,68,79). Indeed, tumors induced with MCA in immunosuppressed mice were more frequently highly immunogenic regressor tumors than were tumors induced with MCA in immunocompetent mice.

There is no consistent correlation between the length of the latency period and the degree of immunogenicity in comparisons of different tumor models. For example, the length of the latency period correlates inversely with the degree of immunogenicity in MCA-induced tumors (14), but there is no such correlation in UV light–induced tumors (15). The reasons for this inconsistency may be that, as the latency period increases, so does the age of the host and that an age-related decrease in immunocompetence may prevent the host from selecting against highly immunogenic tumor cells. Therefore, cancers developing in old individuals after a long latency period are sometimes very immunogenic.

EFFECTOR MECHANISMS IN CANCER IMMUNITY

Because cancer is not a single disease, it is not surprising that findings with one tumor model may not apply to other tumor models. Considering the antigenic diversity found in tumors, it is also not surprising that the different components of humoral and cell-mediated immunity have been shown to play different roles in the destruction of malignant cells in one or another of the numerous tumor models.

Assays to Study the Importance of Effector Mechanisms *In Vivo*

In principle, four assays have been used to evaluate the importance of different effector mechanisms *in vivo*. The first type of assay involves transfer of effector cells, cytokines, or antibodies into sublethally irradiated, cyclophosphamide-pretreated, or normal animals challenged with tumor cells. There are certain limitations of this assay. Effector cells may not reach or localize in the tumor unless both the effector cells and cancer cells are injected intravenously and unless both are trapped in the lungs. Furthermore, if transferred cells or reagents are effective, the assay does not rule out the possibility that other effector mechanisms of the host may have been activated by the procedure. In a second procedure, the

Winn assay (13,14), tumor cells are mixed with effector cells or serum *in vitro,* and then the mixture is injected subcutaneously into an animal to determine whether tumor growth *in vivo* is prevented. Tumor cells may be killed within minutes before or shortly after the injection, although the readout takes much longer. Therefore, the Winn assay is, in part, an *in vitro* cytotoxicity assay, even though the host is used as a receptacle for tumor growth. A third method involves elimination of specific lymphocyte subsets or cytokines *in vivo* by treatment with antibodies specific for different lymphocyte subsets or cytokines [e.g., see Ward et al. (23)]. Failure of the host to resist a tumor challenge indicates that the particular subsets or cytokines are an essential component of the host resistance. An analysis of tumor variants that have escaped tumor destruction by the host provides the fourth way for determining the importance of immunological effectors *in vivo* (23). The phenotypic changes observed in these variants may indicate which effector mechanism was responsible for the selection. Therefore, the type of phenotypic change may give insight into the importance of a naturally occurring defense mechanism that may function in immunocompetent mice (analogous to deducing the action of an antibiotic from the type of change found in the bacterium that has become drug-resistant). This approach is illustrated with UV light–induced tumors. These cancers have strong tumor-specific antigens and are rejected regularly by syngeneic mice without prior immunization, although these regressor tumors do grow in immunodeficient (e.g., nude or anti–CD8 antibody–treated) mice. In rare cases, usually in fewer than 1% of the normal recipients, these tumors escape rejection by undergoing some heritable change. These escape variants, which grow progressively upon reimplantation into normal mice (progressor variants), were tested *in vitro* for changes in sensitivity to T cells, activated macrophages, or NK cells (23). Some of the progressor variants showed resistance to cytolytic T cells caused by the loss of a unique tumor antigen (23) and the increased resistance to activated macrophages and TNF *in vitro,* which suggests that cytolytic T cells and activated macrophages can have tumoricidal activity *in vivo* in this tumor system. However, at least some of the observed changes could be coincidental, and a failure to observe a change in resistance to an effector mechanism does not imply that such effector mechanism was unimportant. For example, the majority of the progressor variants retained the CD8$^+$ and the CD4$^+$ T cell–recognized antigens (23), and other heritable changes, such as establishment of a paracrine stimulatory loop, apparently enabled these variants to escape destruction by T cells (78,89).

Antibodies and B Cells

The role of B cells in regulating tumor immunity is poorly understood: In a tumor model in which CD4$^+$ helper T cells are required for tumor rejection, B cells appear to be necessary for efficient T-cell priming and tumor resistance. Conversely, in other tumor models, elimination of CD4$^+$ T cells promoted tumor rejection by CD8$^+$ cells, and an absence of B cells improved CTL responses and tumor rejection (97,98).

Human antisera and monoclonal antibodies reactive with autologous tumors have been isolated (45). However, a strong humoral response to tumor antigens does not seem to be correlated with demonstrable resistance of the host to the tumors. For example, an experimentally induced humoral immune response to MCA-induced sarcomas does not provide protective immunity against a tumor transplant. In another example, TL$^+$ leukemias induce high titers of TL-specific antibodies that are cytotoxic to TL$^+$ leukemia cells *in vitro* in the presence of heterologous complement (45), but TL$^+$ leukemias grow equally well in immunized mice that have high titers of TL antigen–specific antibody and in nonimmunized mice. Obviously, the presence of antibodies for these kinds of tumors has no relevance in predicting whether the host will reject the tumor. Normal or malignant cells of hematopoietic origin are generally lysed quite effectively by antibody and heterologous complement *in vitro;* however, certain normal or malignant cells derived from solid tissues may be much less affected, even when expressing high levels of antigen. The reasons for this striking difference are still unclear, but differences depending on the source of complement, the antigen distribution, or repair of complement-mediated lesions may be involved. *In vitro,* some tumor cells are killed by a process involving coating with antibody, opsonization, and subsequent phagocytosis by macrophages; this process may be enhanced by the presence of complement. Alternatively, antibody-coated tumor cells may be killed in the absence of phagocytosis by antibody-dependent cell-mediated cytotoxicity when cocultured with macrophages, NK cells, or neutrophils. The general relevance of these mechanisms for killing tumor cells *in vivo* is unclear. Passive transfer of monoclonal antibodies against B-cell lineage–specific differentiation antigens can destroy even larger established B-cell lymphomas (43). There are also therapeutic effects of monoclonal antibodies against differentiation antigens on colon cancer, but these effects seem to be restricted to the elimination of early microdisseminated cancer cells (41). It is unclear whether this restriction results from lack of accessibility of the antibody to the tumor antigen once the single disseminated cells form solid tumors. Down-regulation of growth factor receptor signaling may be the mechanism of the beneficial effects of anti–HER-2 antibody combined with chemotherapy against breast and other cancers overexpressing HER-2 (53).

T-Lymphocytes

It has been demonstrated convincingly that T cell–mediated immunity is of critical importance for the rejection of virally and chemically induced tumors (13,14) by immunized mice or for the rejection of allogeneic (287) and UV light–induced (15,23) tumors by normal mice. For example, in the model of murine MCA-induced tumors, it was shown that intravenous injection of immune cells, but not of immune serum, could transfer systemic tumor-specific immunity into sublethally x-irradiated mice (14). In another study, transfer of immunity to a plasma-cell tumor was abolished by pretreatment of the immune cells by anti–T cell antibodies and complement. These results are consistent with studies showing that immune cells, but not immune serum, when mixed with tumor cells *in vitro* and then injected subcutaneously, could prevent outgrowth of the tumor; this procedure is a local adoptive transfer assay (the Winn assay). Similarly, T cells are also required for the rejection of UV light–induced regressor tumors by nonimmunized (normal) mice (15,23). The relative importance of various T-cell subsets in tumor rejection has been the subject of repeated, and probably unnecessary, controversies. Different tumors are dissimilar enough that differences would be expected in the T-cell subsets required for rejection. For certain tumors, such as UV light–induced tumors, the CD8+ cytolytic T-cell subset appears to be regularly required for rejection (23). $\gamma\delta$ T cells may use their NKG2D receptor to counteract cutaneous carcinogenesis and to kill skin carcinoma cells *in vitro* (67). Relatively little is known about how the CD4+ T-cell subsets can influence antitumor immunity, but truly tumor-specific CD4+ T cell–recognized tumor antigens exist (28). CD4+ T cells seem to be critical for the development of CD8+ T-cell memory and for the survival of adoptively transferred CD8+ T cells. Certain CD4+ subsets may also negatively influence tumor rejection, because elimination of the CD4+ T-cell subset may increase tumor resistance in certain tumor models (99). Murine CTLs that kill tumor targets in a 4- to 5-hour chromium-51 (^{51}Cr) release assay can be freshly isolated from mice after repeated intraperitoneal injection of antigenic tumor cells or generated *in vitro* in a 7-day mixed lymphocyte–tumor cell culture. In most experimental tumor models, specific T cells were generated from tumor-free syngeneic mice. Because this approach is not feasible in humans, T-lymphocytes from cancer patients have been isolated from peripheral blood (100) or from the tumor (tumor-infiltrating lymphocytes). Such T cells can react *in vitro* with autologous cancer cells. When freshly isolated from the patient, these lymphocytes usually require 16 to 48 hours of incubation with the tumor target before a significant level of lysis or growth inhibition of the tumor cells can be observed, whereas lymphocytes that have been grown and restimulated in culture often lyse the tumor cells in a 4- to 5-hour ^{51}Cr release assay.

Natural Killer Cells and Lymphokine-Activated Killer Cells

NK cells (297–302) are distinct subpopulations of lymphocytes that, without prior sensitization and without the requirement for MHC restriction, can kill some cancer cells as well as nonmalignant nonself cells (for review, see Chapter 12). Furthermore, cancer cells that fail to express at least one of the class I MHC alleles of the host are more effectively rejected (101,102) (for review, see Chapter 12) by a mechanism involving NK cells (103). Conversely, expression of an

MHC allele by cancer cells can protect tumor cells from lysis by NK cells. It is now known that ligation of receptors on NK cells that recognize MHC molecules exerts an inhibitory signal to prevent the activation of NK cells for lysis. The cytotoxicity of murine and human NK cells against malignant cells has been most fully characterized *in vitro* through the use of highly sensitive cell lines, such as the murine T-cell leukemia line yeast artificial chromosome (YAC) and the human erythroleukemia cell line K562. Studies *in vivo* suggest that NK cells may help reduce metastatic dissemination of intravenously injected cancer cells.

Activation of peripheral blood cells *in vitro* with high doses of IL-2 induce lymphokine-activated killer (LAK) cells (104). Cancer cells, even when resistant to NK cells, are usually susceptible to killing by LAK cells *in vitro*, whereas most nonmalignant target cells have been reported to be resistant to killing by LAK cells. However, fetal and placental cells and occasionally normal peripheral blood cells (104) have been reported to be susceptible to killing by LAK cells. Intravenous injection of LAK cells early after intravenous seeding of cancer cells into mice reduces the metastatic tumor-cell growth in the lungs, but with this procedure, both LAK and cancer cells are trapped in the lungs. Antitumor responses have also been reported in humans after adoptive transfer of LAK cells in patients with renal cell carcinoma and melanoma. This selectivity is difficult to explain, in view of the general susceptibility of cancer cells to LAK cells *in vitro*. The cells that mediate the killing *in vitro* of a broad range of malignant cells are more than 90% activated CD16+/CD3− NK cells, but which cells have antitumor activity *in vivo* is not fully established. Even though murine LAK cells can be generated from nude mouse spleen cells, it has not been demonstrated that LAK cells from nude mice and normal mice have similar therapeutic effects against tumor cells *in vivo*. Other cell types, such as CD3+ lymphocytes, which are regularly present in every preparation of LAK cells, may contribute significantly to the killing of tumor cells *in vivo*, particularly because activated CD8+ T cells express the stimulatory lectin-like NKG2D receptor and can kill tumor cells expressing the ligands for the receptor.

Macrophages and Neutrophils

Macrophages and neutrophils from normal donors are generally not cytotoxic to tumor cells or normal cells *in vitro*; however, macrophages and neutrophil granulocytes can be activated by bacterial products *in vitro* to cause selective cytolysis or cytostasis of malignant cells (105–108). Such tumoricidal activation of macrophages and neutrophils does not seem to occur when using tumor cells that are uncontaminated by bacteria or their products. Apparently, cancer cells lack the "danger signal" necessary for such direct activation of these effector cells of innate immunity. With fully activated macrophages, long-term (16- to 72-hour) assays are necessary to demonstrate *in vitro* tumoricidal activity in isotope-release assays or cytostatic activity in growth-inhibition assays. Some of the cytolytic or cytostatic effects of macrophages on tumor cells involve cell contact or the secretion of various cytotoxic substances or both, but phagocytosis may also play an important role.

TNF (109) produced by activated macrophages can account for all of the classical tumoricidal effects against some tumors *in vitro*. For example, variants that were resistant to TNF were also completely resistant to activated macrophages; in the converse experiment, variants for resistant-to-activated macrophages were completely resistant to TNF. Furthermore, macrophage cytotoxicity could be inhibited completely with antibodies to recombinant TNF. TNF also seems to be an important effector molecule in the killing of certain tumor cells by human peripheral blood monocytes. As might be expected because of the plethora of cytotoxic molecules that can be released by macrophages (110), mechanisms not involving TNF are also involved in the killing of some tumor cells. For example, activated macrophages synthesize nitrogen oxides from L-arginine, and these reactive nitrogen intermediates also appear to be important mediators of killing of tumor cells by activated macrophages.

Because of the rather selective cytotoxicity of activated macrophages against malignant cells, numerous studies have considered the potential role of this cell type in immunosurveillance and immunotherapy. It is known that the normal host can select for variant cancer cells resistant to the effects of TNF and activated macrophages *in vitro*. However, this selection appears to be dependent on T cells, which are known to produce large amounts of TNF on antigenic stimulation. Therefore, there is, at present, no critical evidence to establish or refute the idea that activated macrophages destroy nascent tumors and therefore play a role in immune surveillance. The more important question may be whether activated macrophages can be useful in cancer therapy. Experimental evidence indicates that activation of macrophages *in vivo* or adoptive transfer of macrophages activated *in vitro* can eliminate or reduce metastasis in some experimental models.

Cytokines

The possible stimulatory effects of cytokines produced by the tumor cells or by the nonmalignant host cells in the tumor stroma on tumor growth were discussed earlier in this chapter (see section on stimulation of tumor growth). The effects of locally sustained high levels of various cytokines have been studied by using tumor cells transfected to produce large amounts of certain cytokines. Some cytokines, such as granulocyte colony-stimulating factor (G-CSF), IL-2, IL-4, IFN-γ, and TNF, when secreted in sufficiently large amounts by the transfected tumor cells, may lead to significant growth inhibition, even in the absence of T cells, but, with certain cytokines or smaller amounts of secretion, inhibition can be dependent on the presence of T cells. Researchers are only beginning to understand the mechanisms leading to this growth inhibition, and such mechanisms are likely to be quite different for different cytokines.

TNF provides example of the difficulties in analyzing the mechanism involved the inhibition of tumor growth *in vivo* by a particular cytokine. Variant tumor cells, which are heritably stable and completely macrophage- and TNF-resistant *in vitro*, nonetheless form tumors *in vivo* that remain as highly susceptible as the TNF-sensitive parental tumor to hemorrhagic necrosis after injections of TNF. Thus, sensitivity of tumor cells to the direct cytotoxicity of TNF *in vitro* may not be important *in vivo* for the effects of passive TNF treatment. Tumor products may sensitize the vascular bed of the tumor to become susceptible to hemorrhagic necrosis by TNF. This notion is supported by the finding that tumor cells can produce tissue factors that enhance the procoagulant response to TNF, but the precise nature of this signal remains elusive. Tumor cells transfected to produce TNF are also completely resistant to TNF *in vitro* but are arrested by the produced TNF *in vivo*, even in the absence of T-cell immunity. Interestingly, the mechanism of this TNF-mediated growth arrest does not involve hemorrhagic necrosis.

Some tumor cells produce a given cytokine constitutively, whereas other tumor cells can be stimulated to produce cytokines by various agents, such as other cytokines, bacterial products (such as lipopolysaccharide), irradiation, or drugs. Thus, treatments could be aimed at eliciting the release of an inhibitory cytokine from the tumors themselves. Such an approach may be advantageous *in vivo*, because targeting every cell with a therapeutic gene seems unrealistic and also because systemic applications of recombinant cytokines may cause major systemic toxicity, insufficient local cytokine concentrations, or both at the site of tumor growth.

FACTORS LIMITING EFFECTIVE TUMOR IMMUNITY

As might be expected from the diversity of tumors, tumor cells can escape or fail to elicit tumor-specific immune responses by various mechanisms (Table 5). Cancer cells are genetically and phenotypically less stable than normal cells and can rapidly change to escape immune destruction. The following sections detail examples of some of the ways tumors escape or host resistance fails.

Major Histocompatibility Complex Haplotype

Tumor cells may express mutant proteins that are tumor specific, but these mutant proteins may not serve as an antigen if they lack mutant peptides that can be presented by the MHC molecules or by a TCR that recognizes the peptide/MHC complex. For example, depending on the genetic MHC background, only some mouse strains recognize a particular mutant Ras protein as an antigen, whereas others do not (36). MHC genes may also regulate immune responses to antigens on cancer cells or to cancer-causing viruses; since the discovery that the MHC profoundly influences the susceptibility of mice to leukemia, investigators have searched

TABLE 5. *Mechanisms of tumor escape from immunological destruction*

Tumor-related

Failure of the tumor to provide a suitable target (defective immunosensitivity)

    Tumor cells

        Lack of antigenic epitope

        Lack of MHC class I molecule

        Deficient antigen processing by tumor cell

        Antigenic modulation

        Antigenic masking of the tumor cell

        Resistance of tumor cell to tumoricidal effector pathway

    Tumor Stroma

        Stromal barrier hindering T cell access

Failure of the tumor to induce an effective immune response (defective immunogenicity)

    Tumor cells

        Lack of antigenic epitope (see above)

        Decreased MHC or antigen expression by the tumor cell (see above)

        Lack of costimulatory signal

        Production of inhibitory substances (e.g., cytokines) by the tumor cell

        Shedding of antigen and tolerance induction

        Induction of apoptosis in T cells by expression of Fas ligand by cancer cells

        Induction of T cell signaling defects by tumor cells

    Tumor stroma

        Stromal barrier hindering antigen release

Development of a stromal barrier before an immune response is induced (e.g., rapid establishment due to a paracrine stimulatory loop)

Host-related

Failure of the host to respond to an antigenic tumor

    Immune suppression of deficiency of host including apoptosis and signaling defects of T cells due to carcinogen (physical, chemical), infections, or age

    Deficient presentation of tumor antigens by host antigen-presenting cells

Failure of host to kill variant tumor cells because of an immunodominant response to antigens on parental tumor cells

MHC, major histocompatibility complex.

for a possible association between MHC type and cancer susceptibility in humans and mice. So far, however, no firm association between human leukocyte antigen (HLA) haplotype and the occurrence of any major human cancer has been established except for certain types of leukemias.

Tolerance versus Ignorance

Even when cancer cells express a potentially antigenic molecule, the host may not respond to the tumor because of tolerance or clonal ignorance. Tolerance to self may explain why oncofetal and carcinoembryonic or oncospermatogonal antigens that are expressed on some normal adult cells induce weaker protection than is usually found in animals immunized with unique (i.e., mutant-self) tumor antigens (20,22,40). It is possible that only the T cells that react with self-antigens at low avidity can escape deletion and tolerance. One approach to overcome this tolerance is to generate allo-MHC–restricted T cells against tumor-associated peptides preferentially expressed as malignant cells (111). Another approach is to use mutant peptides to elicit T cells with higher affinity. However, a critical problem of low-affinity interaction with the original tumor-derived peptides at the site of tumor growth probably remains. Nevertheless, at least certain cancers do not follow the rules that prevent immune recognition of normal self-tissues. Thus, some tumor-bearing host may readily recognize normal differentiation antigens on certain cancers such as melanomas. In this type of cancer, it appears to be possible to uncouple the mechanisms of autoimmunity from tumor immunity (112,113) even though adoptively transferred cells may rapidly become anergic and then fail to control tumor growth (114). Tolerance may also be readily induced to xenogeneic or viral antigens expressed by cancer cells that rapidly disseminate in the host (lymphomas or leukemias) (115).

Injected cell suspensions are not ignored, regardless of whether they are rejected or grow. However, tumor cells embedded in stroma are much more tumorigenic, and stroma may sequester solid tumor cells from immune recognition by the host, thereby favoring tumor growth (88). It has also been suggested that nonmetastatic solid tumors grow because they fail to release tumor cells to draining lymph nodes and therefore fail to induce immunity and are "ignored" (116,117). However, solid UV light–induced regressor tumors are not ignored but very efficiently rejected as fragment by naïve hosts without being metastatic (24). It is also unlikely that the T cells in the tumor-bearing host simply "ignore" the tumor antigen, because complete removal of a tumor sometimes results in specific immunity to rechallenge with the tumor, even without additional immunization. Thus, these T cells have been exposed to antigen but are anergic either systemically or just locally. Passive treatment of tumor-bearing mice with monoclonal antibodies to the regulatory molecule cytotoxic T-lymphocyte–associated antigen 4 has counteracted tolerance in some but not other tumor models (118,119). Passive antibody to the activation molecule 4-1BB on T cells has also been found to be effective against the problem of induced tolerance (119). It is not clear whether, under some conditions, the host may ignore completely the presence of antigens on tumors.

Tumor Microenvironment: Tumor Stroma and Other Local Factors

Experiments have shown that stroma is critical for preventing or permitting the immunological destruction of tumor cells (88), and it is also likely that tumor stroma is an important factor in the rapidly developing resistance of solid tumors to systemic immunity, even at relatively early stages of tumor establishment. Local factors must explain why tumor-bearing mice fail to reject their primary implants of tumors, even though the animals may be resistant to later implants of small numbers of tumor cells at second sites; this phenomenon is called *concomitant immunity* (120). Local factors particular to the tumor environment may also explain why mice bearing malignant grafts fail to reject the established tumors but do reject nonmalignant grafts that express, through gene transfer, the same rejection antigen (121). This seems to occur even in TCR transgenic mice, in which both the tumor and the nonmalignant graft are recognized by a single type of TCR (122). Thus, T cells in these tumor-bearing mice that fail to reject the tumor are not clonally exhausted, systemically anergic, or ignorant (122). The disparity in response to normal and malignant grafts is also not explained by the expression of weaker rejection antigens on the tumor, because tumor and normal grafts express the same antigen. The difference may result from the fact that the stroma of tumors is nonantigenic and interferes as a physical barrier with the rejection of the cancer cells (88), whereas the presence of an antigenic stroma, as it exists in nonmalignant allografts, can help T cells to destroy also the tumor cells (88). For example, T cell–mediated destruction of allogeneic stroma not only may destroy the vascular support for the tumor and allow T cells to reach the cancer cells by breaking a physical barrier but also may generate local help for T cells and other leukocytes needed for tumor rejection. Lack of "help" at the site of tumor growth may be an important reason for the failure to reject solid tumor. The situation might be somewhat analogous to that of transgenic mice that express class I allo-MHC molecules as self-antigen on islet cells and also have autoreactive T cells that infiltrate the islets (123): Even after priming, these autoreactive cells fail to destroy the islet cells unless local help is provided in the form of IL-2 (123). Antigen-specific T cells can infiltrate even tumors growing in immunologically privileged sites, but proper differentiation of the infiltrating T cells is prevented. In fact, it appears that the growing tumor itself can create an immunologically privileged site (124). Lack of co-stimulatory molecules on the malignant cells or expression of Fas ligand by these cells may lead to peripheral anergy. Indirect presentation by host antigen-presenting cells (APCs) of antigens released from tumor cells can play a significant role (125). Direct presentation may be hindered by tumor stroma; however, under certain conditions, direct presentation may be more efficient than indirect presentation in inducing a response (116,117) and may be required for a full cytolytic activation (385). In addition, transfecting tumor cells to express one of several cytokines or co-stimulatory molecules (such as B7) can make tumor cells more effective inducers of immune responses. However, the effectiveness of any induced response is limited by the wild-type (i.e., the untransfected) tumor cells, and the environment surrounding these tumor cells may still counteract tumor destruction for the reasons mentioned previously (122). Thus, the critical unresolved problem may be to provide local help and co-stimulation at the site of tumor growth to accomplish effective tumor destruction. Finally, as mentioned earlier, the stroma can provide factors essential for the development of certain cancers, and the stroma is the site for paracrine stimulatory loops that cause rapid malignant growth and thereby impede immunological rejection (89).

Changes in Expression of Class I Major Histocompatibility Complex Antigens

In some cancers, changes in class I MHC expression result from a total or selective loss or down-regulation of class I MHC molecules (126). In other cancers, such changes may result from mutations in the gene coding for β_2-microglobulin. These mechanisms for escape from host immunity may occur especially in cancer cells in which the tumor-specific antigen cannot be lost because expression is required for the maintenance of the malignant phenotype (e.g., cancer cells that express E6 and E7 of HPV). Changes in the expression of class I MHC antigens are particularly frequent in metastatic cancer cells (127). Thus, studies on class I MHC expression with tissue sections of human metastatic melanoma, metastatic breast cancer, colon cancer, or cervical cancer have commonly detected changes in HLA expression; in these studies, loss of a single class I HLA allele was found more commonly than loss of all class I alleles. Oncogenes such as myc may cause locus-specific suppression of class I MHC antigen expression, and results of clinical studies have thus far not proved the concept that down-regulation of class I MHC expression is the result of escape from T-cell attack and leads to a poorer clinical prognosis. Nevertheless, defective antigen presentation by tumor cells is definitely a major problem for cell-mediated immune therapy, because an effective direct immune attack by effector T cells is prevented (128). Even worse, an antigen that no longer serves as a target for destruction, because of loss of the MHC allele, may prevent an effective immune response to the cancer cells. This may occur because this antigen can still be presented indirectly by host APCs and induce an immunodominant response (see next section) that excludes a response to possible target antigens on the cancer cells (125).

Selection of Antigen Loss or Epitope Loss Variants

During the slow, stepwise development of cancer from the original target cell, host selection should clearly favor the emergence of nonimmunogenic, nonrejectable tumor cell variants. However, demonstrating such a mechanism by clinical studies is difficult, if not impossible, because the antigenicity cannot be known for the original single cancer cell or its premalignant precursor, and there are no probes for the putative antigens. Nevertheless, a possible example of sequential changes consistent with immune selection in a patient at later stages of malignancy has been reported.

Loss of immunogenicity of tumors can be the result of serial transplantation, and heritable tumor variants showing increased malignant growth can be isolated from mice transplanted with immunogenic tumors. Some of these variants escaped immune destruction by having lost a CTL-recognized target antigen (23). The finding of such variants is consistent with the notion that selection for antigen loss variants may also occur naturally during tumor progression. However, loss of the antigenicity of the target molecule, rather than loss of its expression, may sometimes be the mechanism of escape. Cytolytic T cells usually recognize only a few discrete epitopes on even a large protein antigen, and point mutations leading to amino acid replacements in the peptide sequence of these epitopes may lead to loss of antigenicity. An example of such a mechanism was demonstrated by SV40 T gene–transformed cancer cells that have escaped destruction by CTLs *in vitro*. Analysis of such variants revealed point mutations in the amino acid sequences representing the CTL-recognized epitopes of the T antigen. This mechanism allowed the cancer cells not only to escape T-cell destruction but also to continue to express a gene essential for maintaining malignant transformation. At present, it is uncertain whether this mechanism of escape is being used for other virus-associated cancers. For example, mutational changes in the transforming genes E6 and E7 of HPV have not been observed in cervical cancer cells, whereas total or allelic loss of class I HLA expression is commonly observed in this cancer.

As mentioned earlier, experimental and human tumors have multiple tumor-specific CTL-recognized epitopes that are lost independently by selection with T cells *in vitro* (24,25). However, the host fails to recognize all antigens simultaneously on a tumor cell; recognition of the second antigen occurred only after the first antigen was lost by most of the tumor cells. This suggested that an immunodominant antigen by a tumor cell could prevent sensitization to other tumor antigens and in this way prevent immune attack on variants, thereby leading to sequential loss of the antigens from the tumor cells. A hierarchy in the immune response to multiple independent antigens has also been described in the study of immune responses to multiple minor histocompatibility antigens expressed on a single cell. The mechanism for this hierarchy is unclear in either system, and understanding how to break the hierarchy could help prevent immune selection and tumor escape. For example, studies *in vitro* with CTL clones suggest that the rate of mutation resulting in the loss of a single antigen from the tumor cells is less than 10^{-6}. Even if the frequency were as high as 10^{-4}, only one tumor cell that had lost four independent antigens would be expected in 10^{16} tumor cells (i.e., in a tumor larger than the human body). Thus, if the immune response of the host could be manipulated so that all four antigens were attacked simultaneously, no escape of tumors should occur. Experimental evidence suggests that immunization with *in vitro* selected tumor cell variants expressing selective antigenic components can overcome immunodominance and prevent tumor escape. Alternatively, immunization with dendritic cells can break immunodominance (129).

Partial immune suppression may lead to the rapid selection and outgrowth of antigen loss variants. It was found that fully immunocompetent mice regularly rejected highly immunogenic regressor tumors with only very rare exceptions,

whereas mice lacking T cell–mediated immunity (e.g., nude or x-irradiated thymectomized mice) did not select for antigen loss variants. In contrast, the tumors grew in UV light–irradiated mice at a very high frequency, but all of the tumors were found to consist of heritably stable variants that had lost the CTL-defined rejection antigen. This was apparently because UV light–irradiated mice show a partial immunocompetence, so that the generation of cytolytic T cells was delayed until the tumor had reached a size that contained a sufficient number of antigen loss variants so that the tumor could escape. (Incomplete therapy of bacterial infections with antibiotic drugs also favors the outgrowth of variant bacterial strains that show heritable resistance to these drugs, so that, by analogy, partial or incomplete immunotherapy of cancer-bearing individuals may lead to selection of antigen loss variants.)

Antigenic Modulation

The phenomenon of antigenic modulation represents a reversible antibody-induced, complement-independent loss of an antigen from the surface of a cell. This phenomenon was first demonstrated with leukemia cells expressing the TL antigen. Mice expressing the TL antigen at a very low level (TL mice) and immunized with TL$^+$ leukemia cells developed high titers of anti-TL antibodies that lysed TL$^+$ leukemia cells *in vitro;* nevertheless, the leukemia cells grew *in vivo* equally well in immunized and nonimmunized mice. Loss of sensitivity to anti-TL antibody and complement occurred because the antibody caused patching, capping, and disappearance of the TL antigen from the cell surface. Surface immunoglobulin is another cell surface protein that modulates upon exposure to specific antibody; however, several other cell surface antigens do not modulate, and it is not known why certain surface molecules are more susceptible to antigenic modulation than are others.

Immunological Enhancement Blocking Factors and Suppressor T Cells

In the early days of transplantation immunology, it was found that mice preimmunized with disrupted cells of certain allogeneic tumors failed to reject challenge with the viable tumor, whereas normal mice rejected the same tumor after initial brief growth. Injecting immune serum into nonimmunized hosts also sometimes enhanced tumor allografts, and this was effective when given at the time of challenge or up to 1 week before or after tumor grafting. Furthermore, alloimmune antisera were found to protect target cells from lysis by allosensitized lymphocytes *in vitro*, which suggests a possible mechanism for enhancement *in vivo*. Although the phenomenon of enhancement has clearly been demonstrated in allogeneic tumor systems, its relevance for immune responses to syngeneic tumors has remained uncertain (130). Antibody, complexes of tumor antigen and antibody (130), and shed antigen have all been implicated in this phenomenon of blocking. Complexes of tumor antigen and antibody can induce suppressor T cells (131), which may play a role in the mechanism by which blocking factors function. There is evidence that CD4$^+$ NKT cells may be important in UV light–induced immune suppression as well as play an essential role in preventing mice from effectively rejecting inoculated tumor cells (77,80).

Immune Suppression or Immunodeficiency

In the earlier section, on immunosurveillance of tumor development, it was mentioned that patients with immune suppression and immune deficiencies [primary (inherited), secondary (drug-induced), or AIDS] have an increased incidence of virally associated cancers.

Carcinogens

Many chemical and physical carcinogens used in experimental animals are immunosuppressive; for example, immune suppression by UV light irradiation may in part be responsible for the outgrowth of highly immunogenic tumors (132). UV light irradiation damages DNA, which leads to impaired function of APCs. Possibly as a result of this dysfunction, suppressor cells are induced in mice. Suppression can be demonstrated by adoptive transfer assays (132) and appears to be mediated by CD4$^+$ NKT cells (77). Thus, it was found that lethally x-irradiated mice rejected UV light–induced regressor tumors when reconstituted by intravenous injection of spleen and lymph node cells from normal mice; however, transferring a mixture of lymphoid cells from UV light–irradiated and normal mice prevented the rejection of the regressor tumors by the recipients. Moreover, adoptive transfer of spleen cells from UV light–irradiated mice also appeared to shorten the latency period of development of primary UV light–induced tumors in the recipients. The UV light–induced suppressor cells were not specific for an individual tumor; instead, they suppressed immune responses to all syngeneic UV light–induced tumors; however, the suppressor cells did not affect the capability of the reconstituted mice to reject allogeneic tumors.

Gamma radiation or certain chemotherapeutic drugs are carcinogenic as well as immunosuppressive in mice and humans. However, it is not clear whether immune suppression induced by chemical or physical carcinogens is important for tumor escape in humans. In most instances, humans are probably exposed to much lower doses of these carcinogens than are commonly given to experimental animals, and this may result in less immune suppression. However, the immunosuppressive effects of carcinogens may differ from species to species. This makes interpretation difficult, because cancer that develops after exposure to these agents could result from carcinogenic action, from suppression of immune responses to transformed cells, or from both types of actions.

Oncogenic viruses represent another interesting example of how the immunosuppressive component of a carcinogen can help tumor induction by preventing effective host immunity. For example, the E1A gene of the adenovirus (Ad) strain Ad12 suppresses class I MHC expression, which may permit escape from destruction by CTLs and lead to the formation of a tumor. However, reduced levels of class I MHC antigens may not be sufficient to explain the higher oncogenicity of the E1A gene of Ad12. For example, no correlation between the level of class I MHC expression and differences in tumorigenicity of Ad2 and Ad5 in immunocompetent syngeneic adult animals was found when mouse and hamster cells transformed with these viruses were examined. Another viral protein, P15E, that is encoded in murine RNA tumor viruses has been studied extensively for its immunosuppressive properties, and a P15E-related immunosuppressive antigen was found in human malignant cells.

Tumor Burden

In a number of different experimental tumor models and in humans, it has been well documented that many tumor-bearing hosts have suppressed immune functions. Sometimes, the tumor cells themselves appear to release substances that are immunosuppressive: for example, prostaglandins, TGF-β, P15E, and probably several other yet-unidentified substances, which may suppress the immune system directly or indirectly. In other cases, tumors can invade the lymphoid tissue and thereby interfere with the immune responses. The mechanisms, magnitude, and specificity of tumor-induced suppression probably differ widely among different cancers and at different stages of the cancers. The degree of immune suppression caused by a tumor burden can be profound; for example, it was found that mice bearing UV light–induced or MCA-induced progressor tumors fail to reject most immunogenic regressor tumors that are regularly rejected by normal mice. The capability of these mice to mount humoral immune responses to conventional antigen or to reject allogeneic tumors or normal skin grafts remained intact. Thus, as in UV light–induced immune suppression, immune responses to a number of independently derived tumors were affected, but other responses in these animals were not.

Tumor-bearing mice and humans can have alterations in the signal-transduction machinery of systemic or tumor-associated T cells, beginning with a decrease in the NFκB p65 and followed, after continued tumor growth, by loss of TCR ζ chain and p56 Lck (133), and activated macrophages can secrete substances that induce these structural abnormalities. The induction of suppressor T cells was mentioned earlier. Maintenance of the suppression requires a continuous presence of the cancer, but residual tumor tissues remaining after incomplete tumor removal can be sufficient for continuing the suppression. However, suppression is short-lived after complete tumor removal and may give way to specific immunity without further immunization.

It has been shown convincingly by adoptive transfer experiments that in some animal models, the induction and maintenance of suppression require T cells. In other tumor models, the suppressor cells had the phenotype of B cells or macrophages. As might be expected from the diversity of tumors, there also appears to be a large degree of variability in the specificity of the suppression. In some tumor models, immune suppression appeared to be selective for the tumor that induced suppression, whereas in other instances, the responses to a broad range of other tumors were suppressed. Even responses to conventional antigens can be suppressed, especially in instances in which the tumor originated from or invaded the immune system; for example, in patients with Hodgkin's disease, immune suppression often results in depressed delayed-type hypersensitivity to a wide variety of antigens and increased susceptibility to various types of infections. In certain tumor models, it has been shown that immune suppression by tumor burden may also prevent effective adoptive immunotherapy by immune T cells (134). Therefore, ionizing radiation, cyclophosphamide, or other agents have been used to pretreat animals before adoptive immunotherapy (134).

Radiation or Chemotherapeutic Agents

Treatment of patients with anticancer agents, such as chemotherapeutic radiomimetic drugs or ionizing radiation, can be very immunosuppressive. Lymphocytes are highly sensitive to destruction by many chemotherapeutic drugs and ionizing radiation; therefore, these agents (e.g., cyclophosphamide) are also used to deliberately suppress immune responses for organ transplantation. As expected, the immunosuppression caused by these agents often leads to increased susceptibility to infection. In addition, many anticancer agents, such as cyclophosphamide, are mutagenic and carcinogenic. Induction of a second malignancy may therefore follow successful therapy of the first cancer as a late complication of successful chemotherapy or radiation therapy. Most second malignancies originate from the hematopoietic, lymphopoietic, and reticuloendothelial systems, which are the most sensitive direct targets of the immunosuppressive anticancer agents; similar types of malignancies are commonly seen in organ transplant recipients who are treated with immunosuppressive drugs. The development of these secondary malignancies is related to direct carcinogenic effects of the anticancer agents on the lymphoreticular system or to immune suppression, which permits development of virally associated cancers.

Age

Some immune responses gradually decline with age, whereas the incidence of malignancy increases considerably with age. Thus, the increased incidence of cancer in old individuals could result from ineffective immunosurveillance. However, carcinogenesis requires multiple steps, and the length of the latency period of a tumor is usually inversely proportional to the dose of carcinogen. Many cancers may occur late in life simply because they were induced by a very low dose of carcinogens, which is associated with a long latency period, or because exposure is cumulative over many years. Experimentally, there is a decrease in immune responses to transplanted cancer with age. For example, murine UV light–induced regressor tumors that are rejected by young syngeneic mice may grow progressively in untreated old mice. The defective immune responses in old individuals may prevent immune selection and allow tumors developing in old individuals to retain tumor antigens that can serve as targets for therapy. However, the development of effective immunotherapy of cancer in older individuals may also require rescuing the age-dependent immune deficiencies.

IMMUNOPREVENTION

Because there is convincing evidence that immunosurveillance can prevent or reduce the incidence of cancers associated with certain viruses, active immunization against the viral capsid proteins may prevent infection and hence cancer induction. In addition, elimination of certain bacterial or parasitic infections may prevent tumor promotion. DNA-free viruslike particles containing the coat proteins are being tested as immunogens against HPV-associated diseases and against hepatitis B virus in an attempt to reduce the incidence of cervical and hepatocellular carcinoma. Other cancers, such as that arising from Kaposi's sarcoma–associated herpesvirus and human T-cell leukemia associated with HTLV-1, offer additional opportunities. Once infected, an animal or human may still be able to prevent the development of premalignant and malignant cells by immunizing against the viral transforming proteins, if they are expressed by the premalignant and malignant cells. Among hamsters, for example, that receive a single inoculation of polyoma or SV40 virus at birth, there was a high incidence of primary tumors that developed several months later; however, tumor incidence was reduced if a second dose of the virus, or irradiated tumor cells transformed by this virus, were given during the latency period. The neonatally inoculated hamsters were obviously not tolerant because they generated a protective response when exposed to the same antigen later. With a single inoculation of virus, the neoplastic clones apparently escaped unnoticed by the immune system. Additional immunization with a sufficient dose of antigens during the latency period between virus inoculation and tumor development could prevent this problem and reduce the tumor incidence. It has not yet been shown in HPV-infected humans that cervical cancers can be prevented by inducing immunity to T cell–recognized epitopes on the transforming HPV proteins E6 and E7, expressed by the virus-induced premalignant lesions in patients at early stages of the disease (dysplasia) before carcinoma in situ or invasive cancer occurs. Passive or active immunization against an overexpressed growth factor receptor, HER-2/hen, induces antibody and markedly delays the development of primary mammary tumors in mice, possibly by down-regulating the activity of the receptor (135). It is also important to determine whether cancer may also be prevented by active immunization of cancer-prone individuals carrying a predisposing mutation. An ever-increasing number of such mutations that encode tumor-specific proteins in cells in these individuals are being identified. However, inducing immune responses against them may be problematic because these proteins are self. For example, active immunization against an oncogenic viral protein encoded by a transgene became ineffective in preventing cancer development in the cancer-prone mice when the immunization was begun after the oncogenic protein was expressed in premalignant host tissues, which is suggestive of induction of peripheral tolerance. Finally, researchers need to determine how to predictively achieve immunological prevention and avoid stimulation of cancer development (37). In any case, premalignant lesions often persist for a very long time before developing into cancer, and using this time to effectively destroy these lesions would be expected to prevent cancer development.

IMMUNOTHERAPY

Multiple immunotherapeutic strategies involving innate or acquired immunity have been developed to control cancer; they include (a) local application of a live bacterial vaccine, BCG; (b) use of cytokines; (c) active immunization; (d) passive therapy with antibodies; and (e) adoptive transfer of effector cells. Very few immunotherapeutic approaches are clearly effective or the treatment of choice. One example is the topical use of BCG for treating patients with residual superficial bladder cancer, which typically recurs after surgery (136). Repeated instillation of the live mycobacteria into the bladder by way of a catheter after surgery has become the treatment of choice for superficial bladder cancer. The local infection with BCG leads to a prolonged inflammatory response in the bladder wall, which reduces significantly the risk of cancer recurrence (136). Interestingly, the first attempts at nonspecific immunotherapy by intratumoral injection of bacteria were conducted more than 100 years ago in Germany and the United States (137–139).

Immunotherapy that involves acquired immunity (i.e., tumor antigens or effector cells and molecules specific for them) can, in principle, be divided into (a) active therapeutic immunization, (b) adoptive transfer of T cells, and (c) passive therapy with antibodies. It is important to know that, by attempting active therapeutic vaccination, tumor immunologists have taken an approach that has been completely abandoned in the clinical management of infectious diseases, except for rabies, which has a particularly long incubation period. Cancer cells have a slower generation time than do most infectious organisms, and most of the bulk of the tumor load can often be removed by other therapy (e.g., surgery). At the time when the antigen load is the lowest, the suppressive environment may be removed, and active immunization may lead to an effective therapeutic immune response. The critical question, therefore, is whether residual and dormant cancers can be treated effectively by active immunization.

In considering immunotherapy of cancer, the distinction between immunogenicity and immunosensitivity of cancer cells is important. Certain cancer cells may be fully sensitive to tumor-specific T cells or antibodies but, for various reasons, fail to induce an immune response. Experimental studies suggest that such cancers may still be rejected if specific effector T cells or antibodies can be induced. This requires effective immunization against the relevant target antigen on the tumor cells. The reasons for a poor immunogenicity of the target antigen on the tumor cells may vary; therefore, different methods must be used for different cancers to immunize effectively against it. Also, either T cells or antibodies might be most effective therapeutically; therefore, different methods of immunization may have to be used to preferentially induce one or the other. Immunization with viable tumor cells may cause cancer and kill the host, but dead and disrupted tumor cells, membrane fractions, or cell extracts are usually poor immunogens and may enhance the growth of the cancer. One way to circumvent this problem is to destroy the proliferative potential of the tumor cells while leaving the cells viable and metabolically active, at least temporarily. For example, this can be done by exposing the cells to gamma radiation or certain cytostatic chemicals, such as mitomycin C. These methods alone are often insufficient to elicit a cytolytic T-cell response to cancer cells. Many strategies have been designed to increase the immunogenicity of the tumor cell inoculum (Fig. 7). One approach is to increase the antigenicity of the tumor cell by (a) heterogenization of the tumor cells by infection with certain viruses, somatic cell fusion with various nontumorigenic cells (including syngeneic or allogeneic dendritic cells), transfection of self or foreign class I or class II MHC molecules, hapten conjugation, or exposure to mutagens; (b) transfection of tumor cells to express the B7 ligand that can provide a co-stimulating signal to T cells (140); (c) co-injection of tumor cells with killed bacteria, such as *Corynebacterium parvum* (141,142); and (d) transfection of tumor cells to produce certain cytokines (143), such as IL-2, IFN-γ, IL-4, IL-6, IL-7, G-CSF, granulocyte-macrophage colony-stimulating factor (GM-CSF), or TNF. At present, GM-CSF appears to be particularly attractive, because this cytokine leads to the recruitment and activation of dendritic cells, which are powerful APCs. Finally, tumor cells have been transfected to express antisense RNA of a required growth factor. This transfection resulted in terminal differentiation in the cancer cells and increased immunogenicity for unknown reasons. In fact, irrespective of which particular genetic engineering of the tumor cells is used to decrease their growth potential *in vivo*, rejection of the modified tumor cells is often followed by T cell–mediated immunity against the unmodified tumor cells. It is possible that the growth arrest and ultimate rejection of the altered but metabolically viable cancer cells result in a prolonged exposure to the antigen that allows T-cell immunity to develop.

Pure antigens are often ineffective in inducing an acquired (i.e., antigen-specific) immune response unless certain "adjuvants" are used to stimulate innate immunity, which in turn

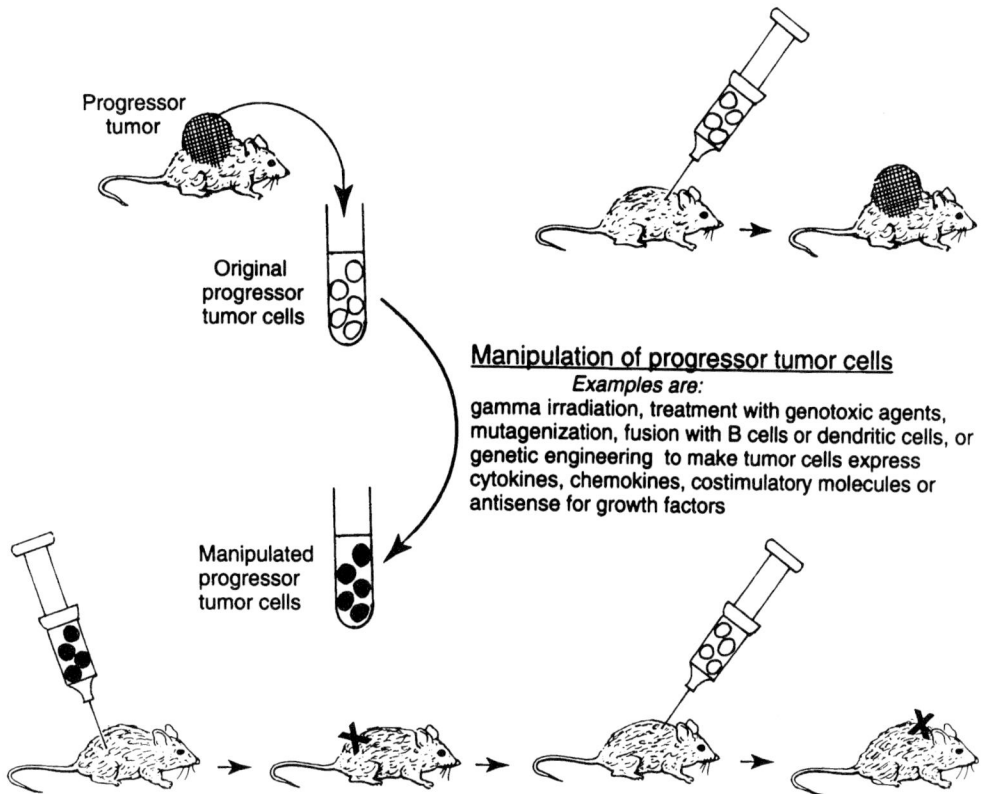

FIG. 7. Many different methods can be used to increase the immunogenicity of spontaneous or experimentally induced tumor cells. Poorly immunogenic tumor cells kill normal syngeneic hosts when transplanted (progressor tumors). All the various manipulations listed in the text and the illustration result in metabolically active tumor cells that fail to form tumors when injected into normal syngeneic mice [i.e., the inocula are rejected (x)]. In addition, these mice are often protected against subsequent challenge with the unmodified tumor cells. Thus, the manipulated tumor cells can serve as a preventive vaccine. However, the use of such manipulated cells for therapeutic vaccination (not shown here) seems to be restricted almost invariably to very early stages of tumor growth, usually a few days to less than 2 weeks of tumor growth. For longer established tumors (which may be more comparable with human cancers when they are clinically detected in the patients), the efficiency of the active therapeutic vaccination through these methods is usually reduced dramatically.

helps the generation of an antigen-specific response. Therefore, numerous approaches are designed to stimulate innate immunity at the site of vaccinations by the use of chemical or bacterial agents or both. Synthetic peptides used in vaccines have to be designed for particular MHC haplotypes and may be ineffective or even "tolerize" the host; delivering antigenic peptides after loading to heat-shock protein (or as recombinant viruslike particles) can increase the efficacy of immunization. Effective induction of an immune response requires antigen presentation in an environment that provides appropriate help or secondary signals. Therefore, several experimental designs involve the use of dendritic cells pulsed with virus-specific or tumor-associated peptides to induce tumor-reactive T cells and rejection of transplanted tumor cells. Dendritic cells can be loaded with either synthetic antigenic peptides or recombinant proteins. Dendritic cells can also be loaded (a) with native peptides stripped from tumor cell surfaces; (b) with tumor-derived, peptide-loaded heat-shock proteins; (c) with tumor-derived messenger RNA; or

(d) by fusion of tumor cells. One advantage of the latter three strategies is that powerful immunity to (unique) individually distinct tumor antigens, as well as tumor-associated antigen, can be induced without having to identify the antigens. The limitation of these customized approaches that use molecularly unidentified antigens is that the antigen dose cannot be standardized.

For tumor antigens that are identified molecularly, recombinant vaccines have been developed with vaccinia, *Listeria,* or viruslike particles. Other strategies of active immunization include genetic vaccination—for example, by injecting naked DNA plasmid constructs, thereby intramuscularly encoding the tumor antigen [whereby the gene for GM-CSF may also be used to improve the presentation of the antigen by dendritic cells at the site of injection]—and vaccination with anti-idiotypic antibodies, which bear the internal image of a tumor antigen. It is hoped that some of these novel ways of active immunization will be effective against cancers, particularly in patients with clinically undetectable (residual or

1588 / CHAPTER 48

dormant) cancers or premalignant lesions. Whether any of these procedures will be effective against longer established or advanced stages of cancer is questionable because therapeutic effects of active immunization in experimental tumor transplant models are usually limited to early stages of malignant growth.

The major alternative to active immunization is passive antibody therapy or adoptive transfer of tumor-specific T cells. In certain experimental tumor models, passive immunization with antibody can protect against challenge with tumor cells and can be therapeutic when given soon after challenge with the cancer cells [e.g., see Herlyn et al. (42)]. Thus, the antibody is usually given simultaneously or only a few hours or days after tumor-cell challenge. Passive immunization of patients with a murine monoclonal antibody against a tumor-associated antigen on human colon cancer has been found to reduce the incidence of metastatic spread significantly and to increase long-term survival when treatment is begun shortly after surgery in patients with no clinically detectable metastatic spread or residual disease (41). Passively given antibodies against B cell–lineage differentiation antigens CD20 or CD22 can also be highly effective, even against already advanced non-Hodgkin's B-cell lymphomas (43). Previously, anti-idiotypic antibody treatment of an experimental B-cell leukemia was also found to be effective occasionally in inducing the cancer cells to go into a long-lasting dormant state, and anti-idiotypic antibodies have been used in the treatment of patients with B-cell lymphoma (also see section on clonal antigens). Some therapeutic effects have also been observed in patients treated with other murine monoclonal antibodies. However, the therapeutic effectiveness of monoclonal antibody in treating advanced solid human cancers that are not of hematopoietic origin is uncertain. It is therefore important to determine the conditions under which antibody therapy can be successful and which of a large number of possible mechanisms are responsible for tumor escape from the therapeutic effects of antibodies. Because antibody-induced tumor regression may occur weeks after treatment, direct antibody-mediated tumor-cell lysis may sometimes not be the mechanism of the antitumor effect. Other approaches have involved the use of antibodies to growth factor receptors on cancer cells for inhibiting cancer growth. For example, the oncogene neu-1/HER-2 encodes a growth factor receptor that is overexpressed on certain cancers, and monoclonal antibodies to this antigen have been found to inhibit tumor growth, possibly by inducing differentiation. Similarly, antibodies to the IL-2 receptors can cause tumor regression in patients with cutaneous T-cell lymphoma. Considerable technological efforts are being made to enhance the ability of antibodies to kill tumor cells by using them as carriers for cytokines or cytotoxic agents, such as radiochemicals or natural toxins. The recombinant antibody-cytokine or antibody-toxin fusion proteins may be useful for concentrating these agents in the stroma surrounding the tumor cells, but some of these coupled antibodies may have serious toxicity unless selective delivery of the conjugates to the tumor is achieved. An alter-native, possibly fruitful approach is the engineering of bispecific monoclonal antibodies that bind effector cells as well as tumor antigens on the cancer cells. Murine monoclonal antibodies have also been "humanized" to reduce the stimulation of neutralizing antimurine antibodies by the patients. The clinical usefulness of these various engineered antibody molecules will remain unknown until necessary clinical trials in patients have been carried out. Alternative immunotherapeutic approaches that are being developed involve the use of monoclonal antibodies specific for regulatory and activation molecules expressed on T cells (118,119) to increase their antitumor activity.

With most currently available immunotherapeutic procedures tested in animal experiments, therapeutic efficiency occurs in relatively early stages after tumor transplantation; unfortunately, there have been no experimental studies that tested the therapeutic efficacy in mice with small tumor loads of long-established cancer that is dormant or remains after surgery or chemotherapy. Adoptive transfer of T cells may be more effective with longer established tumor loads (144). It is uncertain, however, which antigens will be the most effective target molecules on human cancers and in which way specific T cells should be generated *in vitro* so that they are effective *in vivo* upon adoptive transfer. T cells that have been isolated from the patients can be expanded *in vitro* with IL-2 and then infused into patients who receive IL-2 as well. In a selected group of patients with melanoma, favorable responses were observed in several patients, and an apparent cure was seen in one patient (145). It is not clear whether insufficient specificity of the T cells or failure of these cells to localize specifically is responsible for the difficulty in achieving permanent therapeutic effects. Early evidence suggests that adoptive transfer of T cells may be effective against the development of EBV-associated lymphomas in immunocompromised patients, but much more work remains before this approach is applicable to other tumors.

CONCLUSIONS

Cancer immunology is at the interphase of two extraordinarily complex fields of research. Cancers generally harbor (and are caused by) multiple cancer-specific mutations, many of which have not been defined but may be detected by T cells. Cancer-specific mutations that can be functionally important are the basis for individually distinct (unique) tumor antigens, and it is now certain that truly tumor-specific antigens indeed exist. There are also tumor-nonspecific, nonmutant antigens to which the host can respond. Some of these normal-self antigens are not found on normal cells of the lineage of tumor origin; instead, the expression of these antigens on normal cells appears to be highly restricted to spermatogonia and trophoblast cells. These antigens may therefore have a particular diagnostic and therapeutic potential. Immunity to other normal self-antigens may be also effective against cancers for which deleterious autoimmunity and tolerance can be avoided.

Surveillance by adaptive immunity protects humans from many infectious agents and prevents, or at least reduces, the incidence of certain cancers caused by viruses such as EBV or HPV. Therefore, researchers are currently trying to prevent infection or the growth of the virally transformed cells by active immunization. However, preventive vaccination, which is extensively used for protecting against infectious diseases, may not be feasible for most cancers. Investigators have identified a great diversity of mechanisms that may contribute to the failure of antigenic cancers to be destroyed by the host's immune system. This understanding of basic regulatory mechanisms and molecules offers hope for finding new ways to counteract tumor escape. Much evidence suggests that the local environment surrounding tumor cells may prevent the effective immunity against established solid tumors, cause dormancy of metastatic cells, or promote recurrence, but the critical mechanisms still need to be defined. In particular, researchers need a better understanding of the mechanisms whereby inflammation or regulatory T cells can lead to tumor promotion or tumor inhibition. The availability of genetically engineered tumor cells and mouse strains offers many important new models for examining fundamental issues of surveillance, self–nonself discrimination, and inflammation and for elucidating the mechanisms of tumor escape, promotion, and progression, but there still is a lack of models for tumor dormancy and recurrence.

With the rapid advances in biotechnology and in the understanding of cancer and of the immune system, numerous new immunotherapeutic strategies for cancer are being developed and must be examined in preclinical models for their potential usefulness. Even though therapeutic active vaccination has been all but abandoned in the clinical management of infectious disease, numerous novel methods of active immunization that may prove to be effective in cancer are being developed. In addition, passive antibody therapy and adoptive T-cell therapy offer important alternative approaches. Together, these lines of research offer great promise that tumor immunology can be exploited not only to increase further the understanding of cancer biology and immunology but eventually also to significantly improve the diagnosis and therapy of cancer.

REFERENCES

1. Cotran R, Kumar V, Robbins S. Neoplasia. In: *Robbins pathologic basis of disease.* Philadelphia: WB Saunders, 1994:241–303.
2. Schottenfeld D, Fraumeni JF Jr. *Cancer epidemiology and prevention,* 2nd ed. Oxford, UK: Oxford University Press, 1996.
3. Rous P, Beard JW. The progression to carcinoma of virus-induced rabbit papillomas (Shope). *J Exp Med* 1935;62:523–528.
4. Foulds L. The experimental study of tumor progression. A review. *Cancer Res* 1954;14:327–339.
5. Ehrlich P. Über den jetzigen Stand der Karzinomforschung. *Ned Tijdschr Geneeskd* 1909;5:273–290.
6. Woglom WH. Immunity to transplantable tumors. *Cancer Rev* 1929;4:129–214.
7. Gorer PA. Some recent work on tumor immunity. *Adv Cancer Res* 1956;4:149–186.
8. Boon T, van der Bruggen P. Human tumor antigens recognized by T lymphocytes. *J Exp Med* 1996;183:725–729.
9. Old LJ, Chen YT. New paths in human cancer serology. *J Exp Med* 1998;187:1163–1167.
10. Gross L. Intradermal immunization of C3H mice against a sarcoma that originated in an animal of the same line. *Cancer Res* 1943;3:326–333.
11. Foley EJ. Antigenic properties of methylcholanthrene-induced tumors in mice of the strain of origin. *Cancer Res* 1953;13:835–837.
12. Prehn RT, Main JM. Immunity to methylcholanthrene-induced sarcomas. *J Natl Cancer Inst* 1957;18:769–778.
13. Klein G, Sjögren HO, Klein E, et al. Demonstration of resistance against methylcholanthrene-induced sarcomas in the primary autochthonous host. *Cancer Res* 1960;20:1561–1572.
14. Old LJ, Boyse EA, Clarke DA, et al. Antigenic properties of chemically induced tumors. *Ann N Y Acad Sci* 1962;101:80–106.
15. Kripke ML. Antigenicity of murine skin tumors induced by ultraviolet light. *J Natl Cancer Inst* 1974;53:1333–1336.
16. Vaage J. Nonvirus-associated antigens in virus-induced mouse mammary tumors. *Cancer Res* 1968;28:2477–2483.
17. Brandle D, Bilsborough J, Rulicke T, et al. The shared tumor-specific antigen encoded by mouse gene P1A is a target not only for cytolytic T lymphocytes but also for tumor rejection. *Eur J Immunol* 1998;28:4010–4019.
18. Basombrio MA. Search for common antigenicities among twenty-five sarcomas induced by methylcholanthrene. *Cancer Res* 1970;30:2458–2462.
19. Basombrio MA, Prehn RT. Studies on the basis for diversity and time of appearance of antigens in chemically induced tumors. *Natl Cancer Inst Monogr* 1972;35:117–124.
20. Ramarathinam L, Sarma S, Maric M, et al. Multiple lineages of tumors express a common tumor antigen, P1A, but they are not cross-protected. *J Immunol* 1995;155:5323–5329.
21. Leffell MS, Coggin JH Jr. Common transplantation antigens on methylcholanthrene-induced murine sarcomas detected by three assays of tumor rejection. *Cancer Res* 1977;37:4112–4119.
22. Brent L, Medawar P. Quantitative studies on tissue transplantation immunity. 8. The effects of irradiation. *Proc R Soc Lond B Biol Sci* 1966;165:413–423.
23. Ward PL, Koeppen HK, Hurteau T, et al. Major histocompatibility complex class I and unique antigen expression by murine tumors that escaped from CD8$^+$ T-cell–dependent surveillance. *Cancer Res* 1990;50:3851–3858.
24. Ward PL, Koeppen H, Hurteau T, et al. Tumor antigens defined by cloned immunological probes are highly polymorphic and are not detected on autologous normal cells. *J Exp Med* 1989;170:217–232.
25. Wortzel RD, Philipps C, Schreiber H. Multiple tumour-specific antigens expressed on a single tumour cell. *Nature* 1983;304:165–167.
26. Knuth A, Wölfel T, Klehmann E, et al. Cytolytic T-cell clones against an autologous human melanoma: specificity study and definition of three antigens by immunoselection. *Proc Natl Acad Sci U S A* 1989;86:2804–2808.
27. Van den Eynde B, Hainaut P, Herin M, et al. Presence on a human melanoma of multiple antigens recognized by autologous CTL. *Int J Cancer* 1989;44:634–640.
27a. Koeppen H, Rowley DA, Schreiber H. Tumor-specific antigens and immunological resistance to cancer. In: Steinman RM, North RJ, eds. *Mechanisms of host resistance for infectious agents, tumors and allografts.* New York: Rockefeller University Press, 1986:359–386.
28. Monach PA, Meredith SC, Siegel CT, et al. A unique tumor antigen produced by a single amino acid substitution. *Immunity* 1995;2:45–59.
29. Coulie PG, Lehmann F, Lethe B, et al. A mutated intron sequence codes for an antigenic peptide recognized by cytolytic T lymphocytes on a human melanoma. *Proc Natl Acad Sci U S A* 1995.92:7976–7980.
30. Wölfel T, Hauer M, Schneider J, et al. A p16INK4a-insensitive CDK4 mutant targeted by cytolytic T lymphocytes in a human melanoma. *Science* 1995;269:1281–1284.
31. Robbins PF, El-Gamil M, Li YF, et al. A mutated beta-catenin gene encodes a melanoma-specific antigen recognized by tumor infiltrating lymphocytes. *J Exp Med* 1996;183:1185–1192.
32. Brändle D, Brasseur F, Weynants P, et al. A mutated HLA-A2 molecule recognized by autologous cytotoxic T lymphocytes on a human renal cell carcinoma. *J Exp Med* 1996;183:2501–2508.
33. Dubey P, Hendrickson RC, Meredith SC, et al. The immunodominant

antigen of an ultraviolet-induced regressor tumor is generated by a somatic point mutation in the DEAD box helicase p68. *J Exp Med* 1997; 185:695–705.

34. Beck-Engeser GB, Monach PA, Mumberg D, et al. Point mutation in essential genes with loss or mutation of the second allele: relevance to the retention of tumor-specific antigens. *J Exp Med* 2001;194:285–300.

35. Jung S, Schluesener HJ. Human T lymphocytes recognize a peptide of single point-mutated, oncogenic ras proteins. *J Exp Med* 1991; 173:273–276.

36. Peace DJ, Chen W, Nelson H, et al. T cell recognition of transforming proteins encoded by mutated ras proto-oncogenes. *J Immunol* 1991; 146:2059–2065.

37. Siegel CT, Schreiber K, Meredith SC, et al. Enhanced growth of primary tumors in cancer-prone mice after immunization against the mutation region of an inherited oncoprotein. *J Exp Med* 2000;191:1945–1956.

38. Carbone G, Borrello MG, Molla A, et al. Activation of ras oncogenes and expression of tumor-specific transplantation antigens in methylcholanthrene-induced murine fibrosarcomas. *Int J Cancer* 1991; 47:619–625.

39. van Denderen J, Hermans A, Meeuwsen T, et al. Antibody recognition of the tumor-specific bcr-abl joining region in chronic myeloid leukemia. *J Exp Med* 1989;169:87–98.

40. Colella TA, Bullock TN, Russell LB, et al. Self-tolerance to the murine homologue of a tyrosinase-derived melanoma antigen: implications for tumor immunotherapy. *J Exp Med* 2000;191:1221–1232.

41. Riethmuller G, Holz E, Schlimok G, et al. Monoclonal antibody therapy for resected Dukes' C colorectal cancer: seven-year outcome of a multicenter randomized trial. *J Clin Oncol* 1998;16:1788–1794.

42. Herlyn DM, Steplewski Z, Herlyn MF, et al. Inhibition of growth of colorectal carcinoma in nude mice by monoclonal antibody. *Cancer Res* 1980;40:717–721.

43. Grillo-Lopez AJ, White CA, Dallaire BK, et al. Rituximab: the first monoclonal antibody approved for the treatment of lymphoma. *Curr Pharm Biotechnol* 2000;1:1–9.

44. Coggin JH Jr, Barsoum AL, Rohrer JW. Tumors express both unique TSTA and crossprotective 44 kDa oncofetal antigen. *Immunol Today* 1998;19:405–408.

45. Old LJ. Cancer immunology: the search for specificity—G. H. A. Clowes Memorial lecture. *Cancer Res* 1981;41:361–375.

46. van der Bruggen P, Traversari C, Chomez P, et al. A gene encoding an antigen recognized by cytolytic T lymphocytes on a human melanoma. *Science* 1991;254:1643–1647.

47. Takahashi K, Shichijo S, Noguchi M, et al. Identification of MAGE-1 and MAGE-4 proteins in spermatogonia and primary spermatocytes of testis. *Cancer Res* 1995;55:3478–3482.

48. Chen YT, Scanlan MJ, Sahin U, et al. A testicular antigen aberrantly expressed in human cancers detected by autologous antibody screening. *Proc Natl Acad Sci U S A* 1997;94:1914–1918.

49. Hara I, Takechi Y, Houghton AN. Implicating a role for immune recognition of self in tumor rejection: passive immunization against the brown locus protein. *J Exp Med* 1995;182:1609–1614.

50. Livingston PO. Approaches to augmenting the immunogenicity of melanoma gangliosides: from whole melanoma cells to ganglioside-KLH conjugate vaccines. *Immunol Rev* 1995;145:147–166.

51. Yee C, Thompson JA, Roche P, et al. Melanocyte destruction after antigen-specific immunotherapy of melanoma: direct evidence of T cell–mediated vitiligo. *J Exp Med* 2000;192:1637–1644.

52. Finn OJ, Jerome KR, Henderson RA, et al. MUC-1 epithelial tumor mucin-based immunity and cancer vaccines. *Immunol Rev* 1995; 145:61–89.

53. Slamon DJ, Leyland-Jones B, Shak S, et al. Use of chemotherapy plus a monoclonal antibody against HER2 for metastatic breast cancer that overexpresses HER2. *N Engl J Med* 2001;344:783–792.

54. Hirszfeld L, Halber W, Rosenblat J. Untersuchungen über Verwandtschaftsreaktionen zwischen Embryonal- und Krebsgewebe. II. Menschenembryo und Menschenkrebs. *Z Immunitätsforsch* 1932;75: 209–216.

55. Gold P, Freedman SO. Specific carcinoembryonic antigens of the human digestive system. *J Exp Med* 1965;122:467–481.

56. Abelev GI, Perova SD, Khramkov NI, et al. Production of embryonal α-globulin by transplantable mouse hepatomas. *Transplantation* 1963;1:174–180.

57. Lynch RG, Graff RJ, Sirisinha S, et al. Myeloma proteins as tumor-specific transplantation antigens. *Proc Natl Acad Sci U S A* 1972;69: 1540–1544.

58. Hsu FJ, Benike C, Fagnoni F, et al. Vaccination of patients with B-cell lymphoma using autologous antigen-pulsed dendritic cells. *Nat Med* 1996;2:52–58.

59. Fefer A, McCoy JL, Glynn JP. Induction and regression of primary Moloney sarcoma virus–induced tumors in mice. *Cancer Res* 1967; 27:1626–1631.

60. Plata F, Langlade-Demoyen P, Abastado JP, et al. Retrovirus antigens recognized by cytolytic T lymphocytes activate tumor rejection *in vivo*. *Cell* 1987;48:231–240.

61. Klarnet JP, Kern DE, Okuno K, et al. FBL-reactive CD8$^+$ cytotoxic and CD4$^+$ helper T lymphocytes recognize distinct Friend murine leukemia virus–encoded antigens. *J Exp Med* 1989;169:457–467.

62. Golovkina TV, Chervonsky A, Dudley JP, et al. Transgenic mouse mammary tumor virus superantigen expression prevents viral infection. *Cell* 1992;69:637–645.

63. Thomas L. Discussion of cellular and humoral aspects of the hypersensitive states. In: Lawrence HS, ed. *Cellular and humoral aspects of hypersensitivity states.* New York: Hoeber-Harper, 1959:529–532.

64. Stutman O. Tumor development after 3-methylcholanthrene in immunologically deficient athymic nude mice. *Science* 1979;183:534–536.

65. Engel AM, Svane IM, Mouritsen S, et al. Methylcholanthrene-induced sarcomas in nude mice have short induction times and relatively low levels of surface MHC class I expression. *APMIS* 1996;104:629–639.

66. Engel AM, Svane IM, Rygaard J, et al. MCA sarcomas induced in scid mice are more immunogenic than MCA sarcomas induced in congenic, immunocompetent mice. *Scand J Immunol* 1997;45:463–470.

67. Girardi M, Oppenheim DE, Steele CR, et al. Regulation of cutaneous malignancy by gamma delta T cells. *Science* 2001;294:605–609.

68. Shankaran V, Ikeda H, Bruce AT, et al. IFN gamma and lymphocytes prevent primary tumour development and shape tumour immunogenicity. *Nature* 2001;410:1107–1111.

69. Good R. Relations between immunity and malignancy. *Proc Natl Acad Sci U S A* 1972;69:1026–1030.

70. Klein G. Immunological surveillance against neoplasia. *Harvey Lect* 1975;69:71–102.

71. Nozawa H, Oda E, Nakao K, et al. Loss of transcription factor IRF-1 affects tumor susceptibility in mice carrying the Ha-ras transgene or nullizygosity for p53. *Genes Dev* 1999;13:1240–1245.

72. Kaplan DH, Shankaran V, Dighe AS, et al. Demonstration of an interferon gamma–dependent tumor surveillance system in immunocompetent mice. *Proc Natl Acad Sci U S A* 1998;95:7556–7561.

73. Boggio K, Nicoletti G, Di Carlo E, et al. Interleukin 12–mediated prevention of spontaneous mammary adenocarcinomas in two lines of Her-2/neu transgenic mice. *J Exp Med* 1998;188:589–596.

74. van den Broek ME, Kagi D, Ossendorp F, et al. Decreased tumor surveillance in perforin-deficient mice. *J Exp Med* 1996;184:1781–1790.

75. Smyth MJ, Thia KY, Street SE, et al. Perforin-mediated cytotoxicity is critical for surveillance of spontaneous lymphoma. *J Exp Med* 2000; 192:755–760.

76. Bouwes Bavinck JN, Hardie DR, Green A, et al. The risk of skin cancer in renal transplant recipients in Queensland, Australia. A follow-up study. *Transplantation* 1996;61:715–721.

77. Moodycliffe AM, Nghiem D, Clydesdale G, et al. Immune suppression and skin cancer development: regulation by NKT cells. *Nat Immunol* 2000;1:521–525.

78. Seung LP, Seung SK, Schreiber H. Antigenic cancer cells that escape immune destruction are stimulated by host cells. *Cancer Res* 1995; 55:5094–5100.

79. Svane IM, Engel AM, Nielsen MB, et al. Chemically induced sarcomas from nude mice are more immunogenic than similar sarcomas from congenic normal mice. *Eur J Immunol* 1996;26:1844–1850.

80. Terabe M, Matsui S, Noben-Trauth N, et al. NKT cell–mediated repression of tumor immunosurveillance by IL-13 and the IL-4R–STAT6 pathway. *Nat Immunol* 2000;1:515–520.

81. Virchow R. Aetiologie der neoplastischen Geschwülste/Pathogenie der neoplastischen Geschwülste. In: *Die Krankhaften Geschwülste.* Berlin: Verlag von August Hirschwald, 1863:57–101.

82. Dvorak HF. Tumors: wounds that do not heal. Similarities between

tumor stroma generation and wound healing. *N Engl J Med* 1986; 315:1650–1659.

83. Schreiber H, Rowley DA. Inflammation and cancer. In: Gallin JI, Snyderman R, eds. *Inflammation: basic principles and clinical correlates.* Philadelphia: Lippincott Williams & Wilkins, 1999:1117–1129.

84. Cordon-Cardo C, Prives C. At the crossroads of inflammation and tumorigenesis. *J Exp Med* 1999;190:1367–1370.

85. Hudson JD, Shoaibi MA, Maestro R, et al. A proinflammatory cytokine inhibits p53 tumor suppressor activity. *J Exp Med* 1999;190:1375–1382.

86. Suganuma M, Okabe S, Marino MW, et al. Essential role of tumor necrosis factor alpha (TNF-alpha) in tumor promotion as revealed by TNF-alpha–deficient mice. *Cancer Res* 1999;59:4516–4518.

87. Moore RJ, Owens DM, Stamp G, et al. Mice deficient in tumor necrosis factor–alpha are resistant to skin carcinogenesis. *Nat Med* 1999;5:828–831.

88. Singh S, Ross SR, Acena M, et al. Stroma is critical for preventing or permitting immunological destruction of antigenic cancer cells. *J Exp Med* 1992;175:139–146.

89. Seung LP, Rowley DA, Dubey P, et al. Synergy between T-cell immunity and inhibition of paracrine stimulation causes tumor rejection. *Proc Natl Acad Sci U S A* 1995;92:6254–6258.

90. Lin EY, Nguyen AV, Russell RG, et al. Colony-stimulating factor 1 promotes progression of mammary tumors to malignancy. *J Exp Med* 2001;193:727–740.

91. Coussens LM, Werb Z. Inflammatory cells and cancer: think different! *J Exp Med* 2001;193:F23–F26.

92. Strieter RM. Chemokines: not just leukocyte chemoattractants in the promotion of cancer. *Nat Immunol* 2001;2:285–286.

93. Prehn RT. The immune reaction as a stimulator of tumor growth. *Science* 1972;176:170–171.

94. Bittner JJ. Some possible effects of nursing on the mammary gland tumor incidence in mice. *Am J Cancer* 1936;25:162.

95. Hewitt HB, Blake ER, Walder AS. A critique of the evidence for active host defence against cancer, based on personal studies of 27 murine tumours of spontaneous origin. *Br J Cancer* 1976;33:241–259.

96. Kripke ML. Latency, histology, and antigenicity of tumors induced by ultraviolet light in three inbred mouse strains. *Cancer Res* 1977; 37:1395–1400.

97. Monach PA, Schreiber H, Rowley DA. CD4+ and B lymphocytes in transplantation immunity. II. Augmented rejection of tumor allografts by mice lacking B cells. *Transplantation* 1993;55:1356–1361.

98. Qin Z, Richter G, Schuler L, et al. B cells inhibit induction of T cell–dependent tumor immunity. *Nat Med* 1998;4:627–630.

99. Awwad M, North RJ. Immunologically mediated regression of a murine lymphoma after treatment with anti-L3T4 antibody. A consequence of removing L3T4+ suppressor T cells from a host generating predominantly Lyt-2+ T cell–mediated immunity. *J Exp Med* 1988;168:2193–2206.

100. Mukherji B, MacAlister TJ. Clonal analysis of cytotoxic T cell response against human melanoma. *J Exp Med* 1983;158:240–245.

101. Snell GD. Histocompatibility genes of the mouse. II. Production and analysis of isogenic resistant lines. *J Natl Cancer Inst* 1958;21:843–877.

102. Cudkowicz G, Cosgrove GE. Immunologically competent cells in adult mouse liver: studies with parent-to-hybrid radiation chimeras (26113). *Proc Soc Exp Biol Med* 1960;105:366–371.

103. Karre K, Ljunggren HG, Piontek G, et al. Selective rejection of H-2–deficient lymphoma variants suggests alternative immune defence strategy. *Nature* 1986;319:675–678.

104. Grimm EA, Rosenberg SA. The human lymphokine-activated killer cell phenomenon. *Lymphokines* 1984;9:279–311.

105. Hibbs JB Jr, Lambert LH Jr, Remington JS. Possible role of macrophage mediated nonspecific cytotoxicity in tumour resistance. *Nat New Biol* 1972;235:48–50.

106. Evans R, Alexander P. Mechanism of immunologically specific killing of tumour cells by macrophages. *Nature* 1972;236:168–170.

107. Nathan CF, Karnovsky ML, David JR. Alterations of macrophage functions by mediators from lymphocytes. *J Exp Med* 1971;133:1356–1376.

108. Lichtenstein A. Granulocytes as possible effectors of tumor immunity. *Immunol Allergy Clin North Am* 1990;10:731–746.

109. Carswell EA, Old LJ, Kassel RL, et al. An endotoxin-induced serum factor that causes necrosis of tumors. *Proc Natl Acad Sci U S A* 1975; 72:3666–3670.

110. Nathan CF, Murray HW, Cohn ZA. The macrophage as an effector cell. *N Engl J Med* 1980;303:622–626.

111. Stauss HJ. Immunotherapy with CTLs restricted by nonself MHC. *Immunol Today* 1999;20:180–183.

112. Bowne WB, Srinivasan R, Wolchok JD, et al. Coupling and uncoupling of tumor immunity and autoimmunity. *J Exp Med* 1999;190:1717–1722.

113. Clynes R, Takechi Y, Moroi Y, et al. Fc receptors are required in passive and active immunity to melanoma. *Proc Natl Acad Sci U S A* 1998;95:652–656.

114. Lee PP, Yee C, Savage PA, et al. Characterization of circulating T cells specific for tumor-associated antigens in melanoma patients. *Nat Med* 1999;5:677–685.

115. Staveley-O'Carroll K, Sotomayor E, Montgomery J, et al. Induction of antigen-specific T cell anergy: an early event in the course of tumor progression. *Proc Natl Acad Sci U S A* 1998;95:1178–1183.

116. Ochsenbein AF, Klenerman P, Karrer U, et al. Immune surveillance against a solid tumor fails because of immunological ignorance. *Proc Natl Acad Sci U S A* 1999;96:2233–2238.

117. Ochsenbein AF, Sierro S, Odermatt B, et al. Roles of tumour localization, second signals and cross priming in cytotoxic T-cell induction. *Nature* 2001;411:1058–1064.

118. Leach DR, Krummel MF, Allison JP. Enhancement of antitumor immunity by CTLA-4 blockade. *Science* 1996;271:1734–1736.

119. Melero I, Shuford WW, Newby SA, et al. Monoclonal antibodies against the 4-1BB T-cell activation molecule eradicate established tumors. *Nat Med* 1997;3:682–685.

120. Gorelik E. Concomitant tumor immunity and the resistance to a second tumor challenge. *Adv Cancer Res* 1983;93:71–120.

121. Perdrizet GA, Ross SR, Stauss HJ, et al. Animals bearing malignant grafts reject normal grafts that express through gene transfer the same antigen. *J Exp Med* 1990;171:1205–1220.

122. Wick M, Dubey P, Koeppen H, et al. Antigenic cancer cells can grow progressively in immune hosts without evidence for T cell exhaustion or systemic anergy. *J Exp Med* 1997;186:229–237.

123. Heath WR, Allison J, Hoffmann MW, et al. Autoimmune diabetes as a consequence of locally produced interleukin-2. *Nature* 1992;359:547–549.

124. Ksander BR, Acevedo J, Streilein JW. Local T helper cell signals by lymphocytes infiltrating intraocular tumors. *J Immunol* 1992;148:1955–1963.

125. Seung S, Urban JL, Schreiber H. A tumor escape variant that has lost one major histocompatibility complex class I restriction element induces specific CD8+ T cells to an antigen that no longer serves as a target. *J Exp Med* 1993;178:933–940.

126. Marincola FM, Jaffee EM, Hicklin DJ, et al. Escape of human solid tumors from T-cell recognition: molecular mechanisms and functional significance. *Adv Immunol* 2000;74:181–273.

127. Garcia-Lora A, Algarra I, Gaforio JJ, et al. Immunoselection by T lymphocytes generates repeated MHC class I–deficient metastatic tumor variants. *Int J Cancer* 2001;91:109–119.

128. Benitez R, Godelaine D, Lopez-Nevot MA, et al. Mutations of the beta2-microglobulin gene result in a lack of HLA class I molecules on melanoma cells of two patients immunized with MAGE peptides. *Tissue Antigens* 1998;52:520–529.

129. Grufman P, Sandberg JK, Wolpert EZ, et al. Immunization with dendritic cells breaks immunodominance in CTL responses against minor histocompatibility and synthetic peptide antigens. *J Leukoc Biol* 1999;66:268–271.

130. Hellström KE, Hellström I. Lymphocyte-mediated cytotoxicity and blocking serum activity to tumor antigens. *Adv Immunol* 1974;18:209–277.

131. Gershon RK, Mokyr MB, Mitchell MS. Activation of suppressor T cells by tumour cells and specific antibody. *Nature* 1974;250:594–596.

132. Fisher MS, Kripke ML. Systemic alteration induced in mice by ultraviolet light irradiation and its relationship to ultraviolet carcinogenesis. *Proc Natl Acad Sci U S A* 1977;74:1688–1692.

133. Rabinowich H, Suminami Y, Reichert TE, et al. Expression of cytokine genes or proteins and signaling molecules in lymphocytes associated with human ovarian carcinoma. *Int J Cancer* 1996;68:276–284.

134. North RJ. Cyclophosphamide-facilitated adoptive immunotherapy of an established tumor depends on elimination of tumor-induced suppressor T cells. *J Exp Med* 1982;155:1063–1074.

135. Katsumata M, Okudaira T, Samanta A, et al. Prevention of breast tumour development *in vivo* by downregulation of the p185neu receptor. *Nat Med* 1995;1:644–648.

136. Morales A, Eidinger D, Bruce AW. Intracavitary bacillus Calmette-Guérin in the treatment of superficial bladder tumors. *J Urol* 1976; 116:180–183.

137. Fehleisen F. Über die Züchtung der Erysipel-Kokken auf künstlichen Nährböden und die Übertragbarkeit auf den Menschen. *Deutsche Med Wschr* 1882;8:553–554.

138. Bruns P. Die Heilwirkung des Erysipels auf Geschwülste. *Beitr Klin Chir* 1887–1888;3:443–466.

139. Coley WB. The treatment of malignant tumors by repeated inoculations of erysipelas: with a report of ten original cases. *Am J Med Sci* 1893;105:487–511.

140. Chen L, Ashe S, Brady WA, et al. Costimulation of antitumor immunity by the B7 counter-receptor for the T lymphocyte molecules CD28 and CTLA-4. *Cell* 1992;71:1093–1102.

141. Woodruff MF, Boak JL. Inhibitory effect of injection of *Corynebacterium parvum* on the growth of tumour transplants in isogenic hosts. *Br J Cancer* 1966;20:345–355.

142. Dye ES, North RJ, Mills CD. Mechanisms of anti-tumor action of *Corynebacterium parvum*. I. Potentiated tumor-specific immunity and its therapeutic limitations. *J Exp Med* 1981;154:609–620.

143. Blankenstein T, Cayeux S, Qin Z. Genetic approaches to cancer immunotherapy. *Rev Physiol Biochem Pharmacol* 1996;129:1–49.

144. Yee C, Riddell SR, Greenberg PD. Prospects for adoptive T cell therapy. *Curr Opin Immunol* 1997;9:702–708.

145. Rosenberg SA, Packard BS, Aebersold PM, et al. Use of tumor-infiltrating lymphocytes and interleukin-2 in the immunotherapy of patients with metastatic melanoma. A preliminary report. *N Engl J Med* 1988;319:1676–1680.

146. Housseau F, Moorthy A, Langer DA, et al. N-linked carbohydrates in tyrosinase are required for its recognition by human MHC class II–restricted CD4(+) T cells. *Eur J Immunol* 2001;31:2690–2701.

147. Baurain JF, Colau D, van Baren N, et al. High frequency of autologous anti-melanoma CTL directed against an antigen generated by a point mutation in a new helicase gene. *J Immunol* 2000;164:6057–6066.

148. Hogan KT, Eisinger DP, Cupp SB, et al. The peptide recognized by HLA-A68.2–restricted, squamous cell carcinoma of the lung-specific cytotoxic T lymphocytes is derived from a mutated elongation factor 2 gene. *Cancer Res* 1998;58:5144–5150.

149. Mandruzzato S, Brasseur F, Andry G, et al. A CASP-8 mutation recognized by cytolytic T lymphocytes on a human head and neck carcinoma. *J Exp Med* 1997;186:785–793.

150. Matsutake T, Srivastava PK. The immunoprotective MHC II epitope of a chemically induced tumor harbors a unique mutation in a ribosomal protein. *Proc Natl Acad Sci U S A* 2001;98:3992–3997.

CHAPTER 49

Primary Immunodeficiency Diseases

Rebecca H. Buckley

Introduction
Molecular Genetics of Primary Immunodeficiency
  Human Immunodeficiency Diseases
Defects Characterized by Antibody Deficiency
  X-Linked Agammaglobulinemia · Autosomal Recessive Agammaglobulinemia · Immunodeficiency with Elevated IgM (Hyper IgM) · Autosomal Recessive Hyper IgM · X-Linked Lymphoproliferative Disease · Common Variable Immunodeficiency · Selective IgA Deficiency · Immunodeficiency with Thymoma · IgG Subclass Deficiencies
Cellular Immunodeficiency
  Thymic Hypoplasia (DiGeorge's Syndrome)
Combined Immunodeficiency Disorders
  Severe Combined Immunodeficiency · Combined Immunodeficiency
T-Cell Activation Defects
  CD8 Lymphocytopenia Resulting from ζ-Chain–Associated Protein (ZAP70) Deficiency · CD8 Deficiency Resulting from a Mutation in the CD8α Gene · Defective Expression of the T-Cell Receptor–CD3 Complex (Ti-CD3) · Defective Cytokine Production
Hyperimmunoglobulinemia E (Hyper IgE) Syndrome
  STAT4 Knockout Mice
Conclusions
References

INTRODUCTION

Recognition of the first human primary immunodeficiency diseases in the early 1950s (1,2) set the stage for an exponential increase in information about the functions of the various components of the immune system. Since then, more than 100 human primary immunodeficiency disorders have been recognized (3–5). These discoveries, together with several naturally occurring immune defects in animal species, and the ability to create "knockout mice" have seemingly opened the door to the ultimate dissection of the immune system (6).

Primary, or genetically determined, immunodeficiency disorders may affect one or more components of the immune system, including T, B, and natural killer (NK) lymphocytes, phagocytic cells, and complement proteins. This chapter focuses on the currently understood genetic bases of and faulty immunologic mechanisms underlying some of the most important human immunodeficiency diseases involving lymphocytes (Table 1).

Immunodeficiency diseases are characterized by undue susceptibility to infection. Paradoxically, many immunodeficiency syndromes are also characterized by autoimmune diseases and excessive production of immunoglobulin E (IgE) antibodies. Because of the ability of antibiotics to control many types of infections, autoimmune diseases now account for significant morbidity among patients with immunodeficiency. Finally, there is an increased incidence of malignant disease in patients with immunodeficiency diseases (7). Whether the latter is the result of increased susceptibility to infection with agents predisposing to malignancy or defective tumor immunosurveillance is unknown.

With the exception of selective IgA deficiency (A Def), genetically determined immunodeficiency is rare (4). B-cell defects far outnumber those affecting T cells, phagocytic cells, or complement proteins. Although general population statistics are not available in the United States, it has been estimated that agammaglobulinemia occurs with a frequency of 1:50,000 and severe combined immunodeficiency (SCID) with a frequency of 1:100,000 to 1:500,000 live births. Selective absence of serum and secretory IgA is the most common defect, with reported incidences ranging from 1:333 to 1:700 (8,9). Primary immunodeficiency is seen more often in infants and children than in adults. During childhood, there is a 5:1 male-to-female sex predominance for these disorders.

TABLE 1. *Abnormal genes known to cause primary immunodeficiency*

Chromosome	Disease
1q21	MHC class II antigen deficiency caused by RFX5 mutation*
1q25	Chronic granulomatous disease (CGD) caused by gp67^{phox} deficiency*
1q42–43	Chédiak-Higashi syndrome*
2p11	κ chain deficiency*
2q12	CD8 lymphocytopenia caused by ZAP70 deficiency*
5p13	SCID due to IL-7 receptor α chain deficiency*
6p21.3	MHC class I antigen defect caused by mutations in *TAP1* or *TAP2**
6p21.3	(?) Common variable immunodeficiency and selective IgA deficiency
6q22–q23	Interferon-γ receptor 1 mutations*
7q11.23	CGD caused by p47^{phox} deficiency*
8q21	Nijmegen breakage syndrome due to mutations in *Nibrin**
9p13	Cartilage hair hypoplasia due to mutations in endoribonuclease *RMRP**
10p13	SCID (Athabascan, radiation sensitive) due to mutations in the *Artemis* gene*
10p13	DiGeorge's syndrome/velocardiofacial syndrome
11p13	Il-2 receptor α chain deficiency*
11p13	SCID caused by RAG1 or RAG2 deficiencies*
11q22.3	Ataxia-telangiectasia (AT), attributable to AT mutation, causing deficiency of DNA-dependent kinase*
11q23	CD3 γ or ϵ chain deficiency*
12p13	Autosomal recessive hyper-IgM caused by mutations in the activation-induced cytidine deaminase (*AID*) gene*
13q	MHC class II antigen deficiency caused by *RFXAP* mutation*
14q13.1	Purine nucleoside phosphorylase (PNP) deficiency*
14q32.3	Immunoglobulin heavy-chain deletion*
16p13	MHC class II antigen deficiency caused by *CIITA* mutation*
16q24	CGD caused by gp22^{phox} deficiency*
17	Human nude defect*
19p13.1	SCID caused by Janus kinase 3 (Jak3) deficiency*
19p13.2	Agammaglobulinemia caused by mutations in Ig α gene*
20q13.11	SCID caused by adenosine deaminase (ADA) deficiency*
21q22.3	Leukocyte adhesion deficiency, type 1 (LAD-1), caused by CD18 deficiency*
22q11.2	Agammaglobulinemia caused by mutations in λ5 surrugate light chain gene*
22q11.2	DiGeorge's syndrome
Xp21.1	CGD caused by gp91^{phox} deficiency*
Xp11.23	Wiskott-Aldrich syndrome (WAS) caused by WAS protein (WASP) deficiency*
Xp11.3–p21.1	Properdin deficiency*
Xq13.1	X-linked SCID caused by γ_c deficiency*
Xq22	X-linked agammaglobulinemia caused by Bruton tyrosine kinase (Btk) deficiency*
Xq24–26	X-linked lymphoproliferative syndrome caused by mutations in the *SH2D1A* gene*
Xq26	Immunodeficiency with hyper-IgM caused by CD154 (CD40 ligand) deficiency*
Xq28	Anhidrotic ectodermal dysplasia with immunodeficiency caused by mutations in the nuclear factor kappa B essential modulator (NEMO)*

*Gene cloned and sequenced; gene product known.

DNA, deoxyribonucleic acid; IgA and IgM, immunoglobulins A and M; IL-7, interleukin-7; MHC, major histocompatibility complex; RAG1 and RAG2, recombinase activating genes 1 and 2; SCID, severe combined immunodeficiency disease.

This later reverses, so there is a slight predominance (1:1.4) in women.

MOLECULAR GENETICS OF PRIMARY IMMUNODEFICIENCY

Human Immunodeficiency Diseases

Until the 1990s, there was little insight into the fundamental problems underlying most of these conditions. It is impressive that the underlying genetic defects have now been identified in more than 40 of these diseases (Table 1) (3,5). Since the mid-1990s, the molecular bases of six X-linked immunodeficiency disorders have been discovered: X-linked agammaglobulinemia (XLA), X-linked immunodeficiency with hyper IgM (XHIM), Wiskott-Aldrich syndrome (WAS), X-linked SCID (SCID-X1), X-linked lymphoproliferative disease (XLP), and nuclear factor of κB (NFκB) essential modulator (NEMO) deficiency (Fig. 1, Table 1) (3). The abnormal gene in X-linked chronic granulomatous disease was identified in 1987 (10), and the gene encoding properdin (mutated in properdin deficiency) has also been cloned (11). An X-linked recessive immunologic disorder characterized by multisystem autoimmunity, particularly early-onset type 1

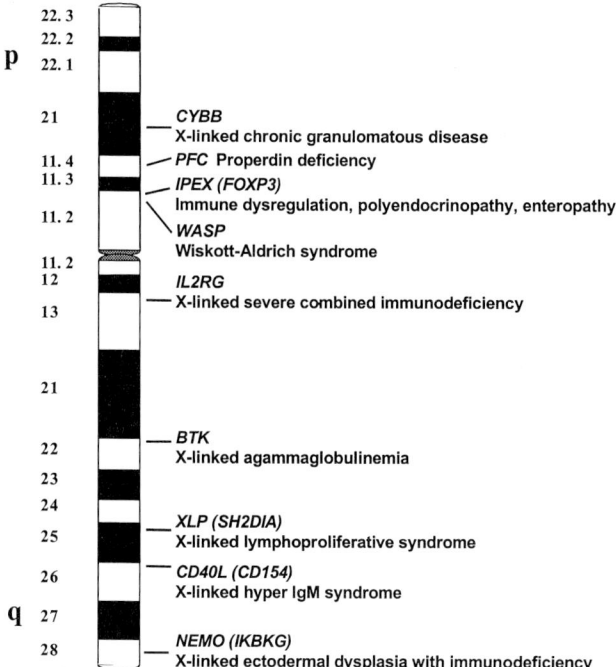

FIG. 1. Location of the X-linked immunodeficiency disease loci. Correspondence with the cytogenetic map of the X chromosome is indicated on the left. Most of these defects have been discovered since the early 1990s.

diabetes mellitus, associated with manifestations of severe atopy and eosinophilic inflammation was found to result from mutations in a gene (*IPEX*) on Xp11.23 that encodes a forkhead domain–containing protein. The findings suggest a role for IPEX in self-tolerance and T helper (Th) cell differentiation (12,13). In addition to these X-linked defects, the underlying bases for nearly three dozen autosomal recessive immunodeficiencies have also been identified (Table 1) (3,5). The discovery and cloning of the genes for these diseases have obvious implications for the potential of gene therapy. The rapidity of these advances suggests that there will soon be many more to come. A committee of the World Health Organization has published several versions of a classification of primary immunodeficiency diseases since 1970, most recently in 1999 (4). Table 1 lists the conditions for which the molecular bases are currently known. Table 2 is my attempt to classify these diseases according to the type of molecular defect present. As the fundamental causes of more of these disorders are identified, it is likely that future classifications will be based on mutations.

DEFECTS CHARACTERIZED BY ANTIBODY DEFICIENCY

X-Linked Agammaglobulinemia

Most boys afflicted with XLA, also known as Bruton's agammaglobulinemia (2) remain well during the first 6 to 9 months of life by virtue of maternally transmitted IgG antibodies (14).

Thereafter, they repeatedly acquire infections with extracellular pyogenic organisms such as pneumococci, streptococci, and *Haemophilus* unless they are given prophylactic antibiotics or gamma globulin therapy. Chronic fungal infections are not usually present, and *Pneumocystis carinii* pneumonia rarely occurs unless there is an associated neutropenia (15). Viral infections are also usually handled normally, with the notable exceptions of the hepatitis viruses and the enteroviruses (16,17). In addition to septic arthritis, patients with this condition may have joint inflammation similar to that seen in rheumatoid arthritis. Infections with *Ureaplasma urealyticum* (18,19) and viral agents such as echoviruses, coxsackieviruses, and adenovirus have been identified from joint fluid cultures of patients, even those receiving intravenous immunoglobulin (IVIG) replacement therapy. These observations suggest a primary role for antibody, particularly secretory IgA, in host defense against this group of viruses, because normal T-cell numbers and function have been present in all patients with XLA and persistent enterovirus infections reported thus far. Concentrations of immunoglobulins of all isotypes are very low, and circulating B cells are usually absent. Pre–B cells are present in reduced numbers in the bone marrow. Tonsils are usually very small, and lymph nodes are rarely palpable because of absence of germinal centers from these lymphoid tissues. Thymus architecture, including Hassall's corpuscles, is normal, as are the thymus-dependent areas of spleen and lymph nodes. In 1993, two groups of investigators independently and almost simultaneously discovered the mutated gene in XLA. Because XLA had been precisely mapped to position Xq22 (Fig. 1), one group successfully used the technique of positional cloning to identify an abnormal gene in patients with this defect (Table 1) (20). For other reasons, the second group had sought and found a B-cell–specific tyrosine kinase important in murine B-lymphocyte signaling (21); the kinase was found to be encoded by a gene on the mouse X chromosome. When the human gene counterpart was cloned, it was found to reside at Xq22, and the gene product was identical to that found by the first group. This intracellular signaling tyrosine kinase was named Bruton tyrosine kinase (or Btk) in honor of Dr. Bruton. Btk is a member of the Tec family of cytoplasmic protein tyrosine kinases (22). It is expressed at high levels in all B-lineage cells, including pre–B cells. This kinase appears to be necessary for pre–B-cell expansion and maturation into surface immunoglobulin-expressing B cells, but it probably has a role at all stages of B-cell development (23). It has not been detected in any cells of T lineage, but it has been found in cells of the myeloid series (21). Thus far, all males with known XLA (by family history) have had low or undetectable Btk mRNA and kinase activity (24). To date, more than 250 different mutations in the human *Btk* gene have been recognized (24–26). These have encompassed most parts of the coding portions of the gene, and there has not been any clear correlation between the location of the mutation and the clinical phenotype (24–27).

TABLE 2. *Classification of known molecular defects causing human primary immunodeficiency*

Deficiencies of signaling molecules
Tyrosine kinases or phosphatases
  Bruton tyrosine kinase (btk) deficiency. Disease: X-linked agammaglobulinemia
  ζ-associated protein 70 (ZAP70) deficiency. Disease: CD8 lymphocytopenia
  Janus kinase 3 (Jak3) deficiency. Disease: autosomal recessive SCID
  CD45 deficiency. Disease: SCID
Other intracellular molecules
  Igα (B-cell antigen receptor signaling molecule) deficiency. Disease: autosomal recessive, B cell–negative
    agammaglobulinemia
  B-cell linker (*BLNK*) adaptor protein gene mutations. Disease: autosomal recessive, B cell–negative
    agammaglobulinemia
  Vesicle membrane component deficiency. Disease: Chédiak-Higashi syndrome
  Proline-rich protein deficiency. Disease: Wiskott-Aldrich syndrome protein
  DNA-dependent protein kinase deficiency. Disease: ataxia telangiectasia
  Recombinase activating gene (RAG1, RAG2) product deficiencies. Disease: T-B-NK+SCID
  Artemis deficiency. Disease: T-B-NK+SCID
  Transporter protein (*TAP1* and *TAP2*) deficiency. Disease: class I MHC deficiency
Transcription factor deficiencies
X-box binding protein (RFX5) deficiency. Disease: class II MHC deficiency
Class II transactivator (CIITA) deficiency. Disease: class II MHC deficiency
RFXAP deficiency. Disease: class II MHC deficiency
RFANK deficiency. Disease: class II MHC deficiency
Deficiencies of cytokine receptor chains
Common cytokine receptor γ chain deficiency. Disease: X-linked SCID
IL-7 receptor α chain deficiency. Disease: autosomal recessive SCID
IL-2 receptor α chain (CD25) deficiency. Disease: lymphoproliferative T cell deficiency
IFN-γ receptor chain 1 and chain 2 (IFN-γ R) deficiencies. Disease: disseminated mycobacterial disease
IL-12 receptor β1 deficiency. Disease: disseminated mycobacterial disease
Deficiencies of cytokines
IL-12 deficiency. Disease: disseminated bacille Calmette-Guérin and *Salmonella* infections
Deficiencies of adhesion molecules or member of ligand pairs
CD18 deficiency. Disease: leukocyte adhesion deficiency, type I (LAD1)
CD154 deficiency. Disease: X-linked hyper-IgM
Structural gene deficiencies
λ5/14.1 (surrogate light-chain) deficiency. Disease: B cell–negative agammaglobulinemia
Immunoglobulin heavy-chain gene deficiency. Disease: B cell–negative agammaglobulinemia due to μ chain
    mutations; other chain deficiencies lead to absence of the isotype
κ chain deficiency. Disease: All immunoglobulins bear λ chains
CD3 γ or ϵ chain deficiency. Disease: CD3 deficiency
Metabolic defects
Adenosine deaminase (ADA) deficiency. Disease: SCID
Purine nucleoside phosphorylase deficiency. Disease: Combined immunodeficiency

DNA, deoxyribonucleic acid; IFN-γ, interferon γ; IgM, immunoglobulin M; IL-12, interleukin-12; MHC, major histocompatibility complex; SCID, severe combined immunodeficiency disease; T-B-NK+, T-cell and B-cell deficiency with normal NK cells.

Female carriers of XLA can be identified by the finding of nonrandom X chromosome inactivation in their B cells or by the detection of the mutated gene (if known in the family) (28,29). Prenatal diagnosis of affected or nonaffected male fetuses has also been accomplished by detection of the mutated gene in chorionic villous or amniocentesis samples. Studies of Btk protein, enzymatic activity, or mRNA have also permitted identification of X-linked inheritance in some agammaglobulinemic boys with no family history. The finding that Btk is also expressed in cells of myeloid lineage is of interest in light of the well-known occurrence of intermittent neutropenia in boys with XLA, particularly at the onset of an acute infection (15,30). It is conceivable that Btk is only one of several signaling molecules participating in myeloid

maturation and that neutropenia would be observed in XLA only when rapid production of such cells is needed. XLA was also reported in association with growth hormone deficiency in nine cases (31–34).

X-Linked Immunodeficiency (Xid) in Mice

The animal model for human XLA is the X-linked immunodeficiency (Xid) mutation in CBA/N mice (35). Xid mice have normal numbers of pre–B cells in their bone marrow but abnormally low numbers of B cells in their lymphoid tissues (35). These animals have low serum IgG and IgM concentrations and fail to produce antipolysaccharide antibodies to thymus-independent (TI) antigens type 2 (TI-2). Unlike most humans with XLA, Xid mice have some B cells of mature phenotype, and they produce some antibodies to TI-1 antigens. However, B cells from Xid mice do not proliferate after ligation of CD40, even in the presence of interleukin-4 (IL-4) or anti-Ig reagents (36). A mutation at position 28 of the murine *btk* gene has been shown to be the basis for the B-cell defect in CBA/N mice (37,38). Because such mice have a much milder antibody deficiency than boys with XLA, speculation had been that humans with mutations in the non–kinase-encoding part of the *Btk* gene may have a less severe immunodeficiency. However, humans with classic XLA have been identified with mutations affecting the same residue as in CBA/N mice (39). Again, as in female carriers of human XLA, female mice heterozygous for Xid display nonrandom X-chromosome inactivation in their B cells.

Autosomal Recessive Agammaglobulinemia

Conditions that resemble XLA phenotypically occur in some agammaglobulinemic females (40). These diseases are caused by mutations in the genes that encode immunoglobulin heavy or light chains or their associated signaling molecules, leading to agammaglobulinemia or hypogammaglobulinemia (41). In μ-chain, λ5/14.1 (surrogate light-chain), Igα (B-cell antigen receptor signaling molecule), and B-cell linker (*BLNK*) gene mutations, circulating B cells are also absent (42–46). In the case of other heavy-chain gene mutations, deficiencies of individual immunoglobulin classes or subclasses are seen, and circulating B cells are present (47). Mutations in the κ chain gene result in molecules with only λ light chains.

Immunodeficiency with Elevated IgM (Hyper IgM)

The hyper IgM syndrome is characterized by very low serum IgG, IgA, and IgE levels but either a normal or a markedly elevated concentration of polyclonal IgM. It is now known that the hyper IgM syndrome includes at least four distinct genetic diseases. Patients with this rare primary immunodeficiency syndrome resemble those with agammaglobulinemia in their susceptibility to encapsulated bacterial infections (48–50). However, patients with one of the X-linked forms of hyper IgM also frequently present in infancy with *Pneumocystis carinii* pneumonia. The finding that many also have coexistent neutropenia was formerly considered a possible explanation for the susceptibility of some such patients to opportunistic infection; however, it is now known that one X-linked disease resulting in this syndrome is actually a T-cell defect, more likely accounting for that susceptibility. Thus far, two X-linked and two autosomal recessive diseases have been found to cause this syndrome, and there are likely to be more. Distinctive clinical features permit presumptive recognition of the type of mutation in these patients, thereby aiding proper choice of therapy. However, all such patients should undergo molecular analysis to ascertain the affected gene for purposes of genetic counseling, carrier detection, and definitive therapy.

CD154 (CD40 Ligand) Deficiency

Like boys with XLA, those with XHIM syndrome may become symptomatic during the first or second year of life with recurrent pyogenic infections. However, they also are highly prone to have *Pneumocystis carinii* pneumonia and to have profound neutropenia (4,48,49). They have very small tonsils and a paucity of palpable lymph nodes. Normal numbers of B lymphocytes are usually present in the circulation of these patients.

Until the early 1990s, this condition was classified as a B-cell defect because only IgM is produced. However, in 1986, B cells from patients with XHIM syndrome were shown to have the capacity to synthesize IgM, IgA, and IgG normally when these cells were cocultured with a "switch" T-cell line, a finding suggesting that in those patients the defect lay in T-lineage cells (51). This was puzzling, because routine tests of T-cell function were usually normal in such patients. In 1993, the abnormal gene in XHIM syndrome was localized to Xq26 (52) and was identified by five groups almost simultaneously (53–56). The gene product is a surface molecule known as CD154 (or CD40 ligand) on the surfaces of activated helper T cells (57) that interacts with CD40 molecules on B cells(53). Cross-linking of CD40 on either normal or XHIM B cells with a monoclonal antibody to CD40 or with soluble CD154 in the presence of cytokines (IL-2, IL-4, or IL-10) causes the B cells (which are intrinsically normal in XHIM syndrome) to undergo proliferation and isotype switching and to secrete various types of immunoglobulins. CD154 is a type II integral membrane glycoprotein with significant sequence homology to tumor necrosis factor (TNF); it is found only on activated T cells, primarily of the CD4 phenotype (Fig. 2) (57). Mutations in the gene encoding CD154 on XHIM patients' T cells result in a lack of signaling of their normal B cells when their T cells are activated. Therefore, XHIM B cells fail to undergo isotype switching and produce only IgM; there is an absence of CD27[+] memory B cells (58). Lymph node histology shows only abortive germinal center formation and a severe depletion and phenotypic abnormalities of follicular dendritic cells (59). Of further importance to effective immune responses, the lack of stimulation of CD40 also causes these patients' B cells not to up-regulate CD80 and CD86. The latter are important co-stimulatory molecules that interact with CD28/cytotoxic T-lymphocyte–associated antigen 4 (CTLA-4) on T cells (60). The failure of interaction of the molecules of those pathways results in a propensity for tolerogenic T-cell signaling and defective recognition of tumor cells.

More than 73 distinct point mutations or deletions in the gene encoding CD154 have been identified in 87 unrelated XHIM families, giving rise to frameshifts, premature stop codons, and single amino acid substitutions, most of which were clustered in the TNF homology domain located

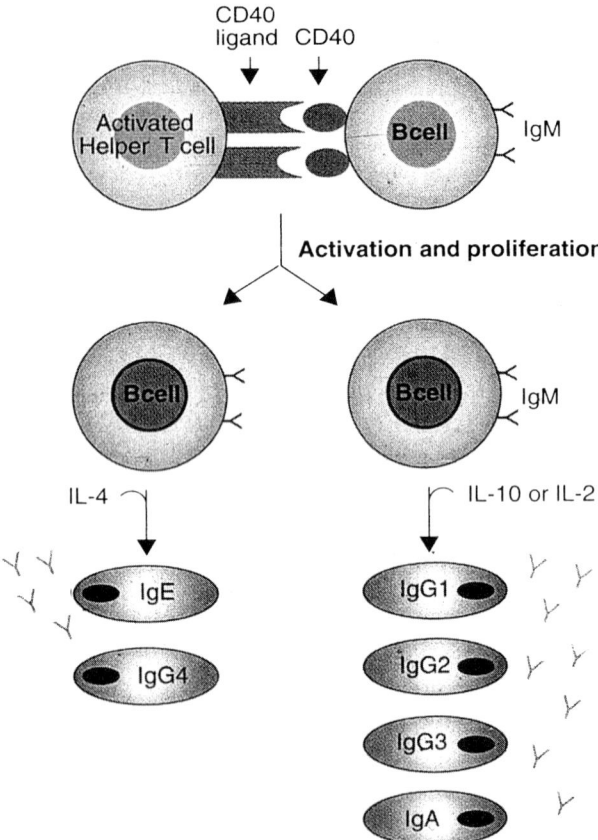

FIG. 2. Cartoon showing the role of the CD40 ligand (CD154) in B-cell class switching. The *CD154* gene is mutated in X-linked hyper IgM. Thus, this is a T-cell, not a B-cell, defect. From Allen RC, Armitage RJ, Conley ME, et al. (53), with permission.

in the carboxy-terminal region (50). A highly polymorphic microsatellite dinucleotide (CA) repeat region in the 3' untranslated end of the gene for CD154 is useful for detecting carriers of XHIM and for making a prenatal diagnosis of this condition (61).

In a retrospective study of 56 patients with XHIM syndrome, 13 (23.3%) had died, and the mean age at death was 11.7 years (49). In addition to opportunistic infections such as *Pneumocystis carinii* pneumonia, there is an increased incidence of cryptosporidial enteritis and subsequent liver disease in this syndrome. There is also an increased risk of malignancy. Because of the poor prognosis, the treatment of choice is a human leukocyte antigen (HLA)–identical sibling bone marrow transplant at an early age (62,63). Treatment for this condition also includes monthly IVIG infusions (64). In some patients with severe neutropenia, the use of granulocyte colony-stimulating factor has been beneficial (65).

Nuclear Factor κB Essential Modulator (NEMO or Iκκγ) Deficiency

This is a newly recognized syndrome characterized most often clinically as anhidrotic ectodermal dysplasia with associated immunodeficiency (EDA-ID) in males and incontinentia pigmenti in females (66,67). The condition results from mutations in the *IKBKG* gene at position 28q on the X chromosome that encodes NEMO. NEMO is a regulatory protein that serves as a scaffold for two kinases necessary for activation of the transcription factor NFκB. Activation of NFκB by proinflammatory stimuli normally leads to increased expression of genes involved in inflammation, such as TNF-α and IL-12. B cells from patients with NEMO deficiency fail to undergo class switch recombination, and their antigen-presenting cells fail to produce TNF-α and IL-12 (67). Germline loss-of-function mutations cause the X-linked dominant condition incontinentia pigmenti and are lethal in male fetuses. Mutations in the coding region of *IKBKG* are associated with EDA-ID.

The immunodeficiency has been variable; most patients with EDA-ID have shown impaired antibody responses to polysaccharide antigens (66). However, two patients with EDA-ID presented with hyper IgM syndrome (67). Pharmacologic inhibitors of NFκB activation have been shown to down-regulate CD154 mRNA and protein levels, a finding suggesting the mechanism of hyper IgM in this condition (68). Stop codon mutations in *IKBKG* are associated with osteopetrosis, lymphedema, EDA, and immunodeficiency (OL-EDA-ID). Neither type of mutation abolishes NFκB signaling entirely. The immune cells of patients with OL-EDA-ID respond poorly to lipopolysaccharide, IL-1β, IL-18, TNF-α, and CD154, a finding accounting for the seriousness of their infections. Patients with hyper IgM syndrome who have this defect should be easily recognizable because of the presence of EDA.

Autosomal Recessive Hyper IgM

Activation-Induced Cytidine Deaminase Deficiency

It has been known for some time now that not all males with hyper IgM have a mutation in the gene encoding CD154 (69), and there are many examples in females (70), a finding indicating that this condition has more than one genetic cause. As in XHIM, concentrations of serum IgG, IgA, and IgE are very low in this autosomal recessive form of hyper IgM. However, in contrast to X-linked CD40L deficiency, in which the IgM level is normal or only slightly elevated, the serum IgM concentration in patients with autosomal recessive hyper IgM is often markedly elevated and polyclonal (71). Patients with autosomal recessive hyper IgM are generally older at age of onset of infections, do not have susceptibility to *Pneumocystis carinii* pneumonia, often do have isohemagglutinins, and are less likely to have anemia, neutropenia, or thrombocytopenia (71). Normal numbers of B lymphocytes are usually present in the circulation of these patients. However, in further contrast to patients with XHIM, B cells from patients with autosomal hyper IgM are not able to switch from IgM-secreting to IgG-, IgA-, or IgE-secreting cells, even when the cells are cocultured with monoclonal antibodies to CD40 and various cytokines (69). Thus, in these patients, the condition truly is a B-cell defect.

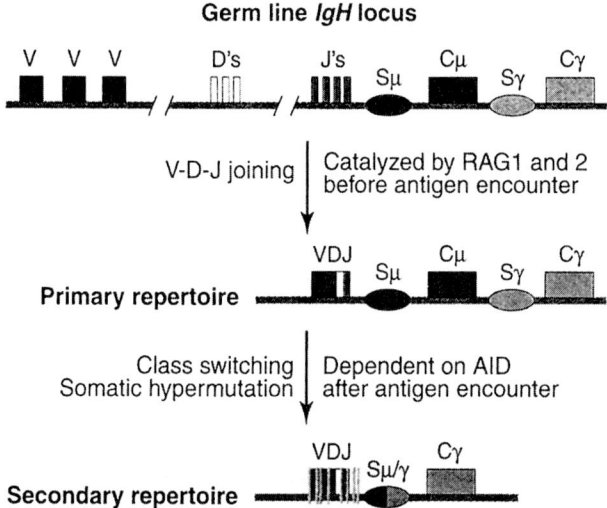

Germ line *IgH* locus

FIG. 3. Schematic representation of the generation of antibody repertoires. Rearrangement of antigen receptor genes from their germline configuration occurs through the actions of the products of recombinase activating genes 1 and 2 without antigen encounter to generate a primary antibody repertoire composed of IgM antibodies. However, class switch recombination and somatic hypermutation require the action of activation-induced cytidine deaminase (AID) after antigen encounter. The *A/D* gene is mutated in one autosomal recessive form of hyper IgM. Thus, this is truly a B-cell defect because the B cells are unable to generate a secondary repertoire. From Neuberger MS, Scott J. *Science* 2000;289:1705, with permission.

The defect in many patients with autosomal recessive hyper IgM has been identified as mutations in a gene on chromosome 12p13 that encodes an activation-dependent cytidine deaminase (AID), an RNA-editing enzyme specifically expressed in germinal center B cells (71,72). A deficiency of AID results in impaired terminal differentiation of B cells and a failure of isotype switching, and there is a lack of immunoglobulin gene somatic hypermutation (Fig. 3). Unlike patients with XHIM, who have minimal lymphoid tissue, patients with this defect have lymphoid hyperplasia because they have enhanced germinal center formation, even though they are defective germinal centers. Nearly all such patients have markedly elevated polyclonal serum IgM levels, and, when their B cells are cultured *in vitro,* they spontaneously secrete large amounts of IgM. This IgM secretion is not further augmented by the addition of IL-4 or anti-CD40 with IL-4 or other cytokines. Their B cells are positive for CD27 (72). With early diagnosis and treatment with IVIG, as well as good management of infections with antibiotics, patients with AID mutations generally have a more benign course than do those with XHIM.

Mutations in CD40

CD40 is a type I integral membrane glycoprotein encoded by a gene on chromosome 20 and belonging to the TNF and nerve growth factor receptor superfamily. It is expressed on B cells, macrophages, dendritic cells, and a few other types of cells (Fig. 2). Three patients with autosomal recessive hyper IgM syndrome were identified who failed to express CD40 on their B-cell surfaces (73). Their clinical presentations were similar to those with XHIM resulting from CD40L deficiency. Sequence analysis of their CD40 genomic DNA showed that one patient carried a homozygous silent mutation at the fifth base pair position of exon 5, involving an exonic splicing enhancer and leading to exon skipping and premature termination; the other two patients showed a homozygous point mutation in exon 3, resulting in a cysteine-to-arginine substitution. These findings show that mutations of the CD40 gene can also cause an autosomal recessive form of hyper IgM, which is immunologically and clinically indistinguishable from XHIM caused by CD40L deficiency (73).

X-Linked Lymphoproliferative Disease

XLP, also referred to as Duncan's disease (after the original kindred in which it was described), is a recessive trait characterized by an inadequate immune response to infection with Epstein-Barr virus (EBV) (74,75). Affected boys are apparently healthy until they experience infectious mononucleosis (74,75). The mean age of presentation is less than 5 years. There are three major clinical phenotypes: (a) fulminant, often fatal, infectious mononucleosis (50% of cases); (b) lymphomas, predominantly involving B-lineage cells (25%); and (c) acquired hypogammaglobulinemia (25%). Unless there is a family history of XLP, diagnosis before the onset of complications is often difficult. There is a marked impairment in production of antibodies to the EBV nuclear antigen (EBNA), whereas titers of antibodies to the viral capsid antigen have ranged from zero to markedly elevated. There is also a deficiency in long-lived T-cell immunity to EBV. Studies of lymphocyte subpopulations with monoclonal antibodies have frequently revealed elevated percentages of CD8$^+$ T-cells. Antibody-dependent cell-mediated cytotoxicity against EBV-infected cells has been low in many of these cells; there is a failure to control cytotoxic T-cell proliferation, and there is defective NK cell function.

The defective gene in XLP was localized to the Xq26-q27 region, cloned and initially named *SAP* (for SLAM-associated protein); it is now known officially as *SH2D1A* (Fig. 1, Table 1) (76–78). The human and mouse *SH2D1A* gene consist of four exons and three introns spanning approximately 25kb (76,79). In the mouse, *SH2D1A* is highly expressed in thymocytes and peripheral T cells with a prevalent expression on Th1 cells (79). Although SH2D1A is also expressed by NK cells (80–82), its presence in B lymphocytes is unclear.

The SH2D1A protein consists of 128 amino acids comprising an SH2 domain and a 24-amino acid tail. The SH2D1A protein has been shown to bind to the SLAM family of surface immune receptors (76,78,81). An SH2D1A-like molecule named EAT-2 (83) interacts with the same SLAM-family members as SH2D1A in non-T hematopoietic cells (84,85).

SH2D1A competes with SHP-2 for binding and as such is a regulatory molecule. In patients with XLP, the lack of SH2D1A may lead to an uncontrolled cytotoxic T-cell immune response to EBV. The SH2D1A protein permissively associates with 2B4 on NK cells; thus, selective impairment of 2B4-mediated NK-cell activation may also contribute to the immunopathology of XLP.

Two pedigrees have been reported in which boys in one arm of each pedigree had been diagnosed with common variable immunodeficiency (CVID), whereas those in the other arms had fulminant infectious mononucleosis (Fig. 4) (86). The family members with CVID never gave a history of infectious mononucleosis. However, all affected members of each pedigree had the same distinct SH2D1A mutation despite the different clinical phenotypes. Because the SH2D1A mutation was the same but the phenotype varied in these families, XLP should be considered in all males with a diagnosis of CVID, particularly if there is more than one male family member with this phenotype.

XLP overall has an unfavorable prognosis, because 70% of affected boys die by age 10. Only two patients with XLP are known to have survived beyond 40 years. Approximately half of the limited number of patients with XLP given HLA-identical related or unrelated unfractionated bone marrow transplants are currently surviving without signs of the disease (62).

Common Variable Immunodeficiency

CVID is a syndrome characterized by hypogammaglobulinemia with B cells. Most, if not all, patients have no known molecular diagnosis. It is highly likely that this syndrome consists of several different molecular defects. Also known as acquired hypogammaglobulinemia because of generally a later age of onset of infections, the patients may appear similar clinically to those with XLA in the kinds of infections experienced and the bacterial etiologic agents involved (4,87). Fortunately, however, for unknown reasons, echovirus meningoencephalitis does not occur as frequently in patients with CVID (17). In comparing the two defects further, in CVID there is an almost equal sex distribution, a tendency to autoantibody formation, normal-sized or enlarged tonsils and lymph nodes, and splenomegaly in approximately 25% of those affected. Lymphoid interstitial pneumonia, pseudolymphoma, amyloidosis, and noncaseating granulomata of the lungs, spleen, skin, and liver have also been seen. There is a 438-fold increase in lymphomas in affected women in the fifth and sixth decades (88).

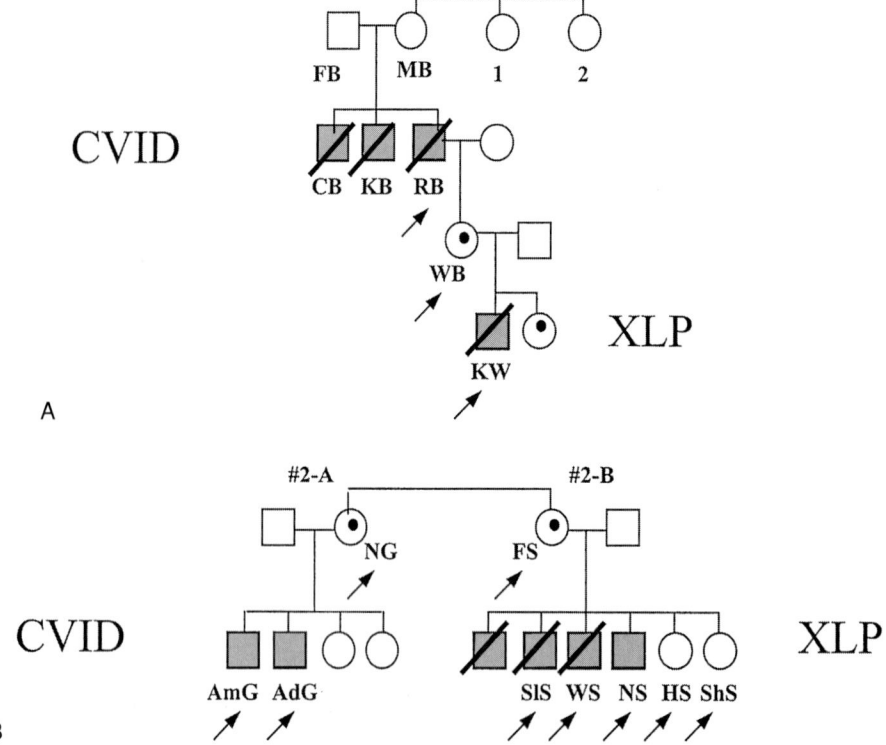

FIG. 4. Two pedigrees (**A** and **B**) in which boys in one arm of each had the clinical phenotype of common variable immunodeficiency (CVID) and in the other fulminating infectious mononucleosis, leading to a diagnosis of X-linked lymphoproliferative disease (XLP). The pedigree unique mutations in *SH2D1A* were the same in those with CVID as in those with XLP. Thus, boys with CVID should be screened for this mutation. From Morra M, Silander O, Calpe-Klores S, et al. (86), with permission.

The serum immunoglobulin and antibody deficiencies in CVID may be as profound as in XLA. Despite normal numbers of circulating immunoglobulin-bearing B lymphocytes and the presence of lymphoid cortical follicles, blood B lymphocytes from patients with CVID do not differentiate into immunoglobulin-producing cells when these lymphocytes are stimulated with PWM *in vitro,* even when they are cocultured with normal T cells (87). From these observations, it was thought that the defects in this syndrome are intrinsic to the B cell. However, CVID B cells can be stimulated to isotype-switch and to synthesize and secrete immunoglobulin when they are stimulated with anti-CD40 plus IL-4 or IL-10 (89,90).

T cells and T-cell subsets are usually present in normal percentages, but a dominance of $\gamma\delta$ T cells has been observed in some patients (91), and depressed T-cell function has been reported in others (92,93). In addition, decreased numbers and function of antigen-specific T cells were noted in patients with CVID who were immunized with keyhole limpet hemocyanin (94,95). Tonsils and lymph nodes are either normal in size or enlarged, and splenomegaly occurs in approximately 25% of patients with CVID. In addition, there is a tendency to autoantibody formation, and several cases of lupus erythematosus have converted to CVID (96). Rarely, CVID has been reported to resolve transiently or permanently when some such patients acquired human immunodeficiency virus infection (97).

Because this disorder occurs in first-degree relatives of patients with A Def and some patients with A Def later became panhypogammaglobulinemic (98), it has long been suspected that these diseases have a common genetic basis (99,100). The high incidences of abnormal immunoglobulin concentrations, autoantibodies, autoimmune disease, and malignancy in families of both types of patients also suggested a shared hereditary influence. This concept is supported by the finding of a high incidence of C4-A gene deletions and C2 rare gene alleles in the class III major histocompatibility complex (MHC) region in individuals with either A Def (101) or CVID (102), a finding suggesting that there is a susceptibility gene in this region on chromosome 6. However, the abnormal gene has not yet been identified. These studies also have shown that a few HLA haplotypes are shared by individuals affected with CVID and A Def, with at least one of two particular haplotypes present in 77% of those affected (102). In one large family with 13 members, two had A Def and three had CVID (99). All the immunodeficient patients in the family had at least one copy of an MHC haplotype shown to be abnormally frequent in A Def and CVID: HLA-DQB1 *0201, HLA-DR3, C4B-Sf, C4A-deleted, G11-15, Bf-0.4, C2a, HSP70-7.5, TNF-α5, HLA-B8, and HLA-A1 (103). However, four immunologically normal members of the pedigree also possessed this haplotype, a finding indicating that its presence alone is not sufficient for expression of the defects (99). Environmental factors, particularly drugs such as phenytoin, have been suspected as providing the triggers for disease expression in persons with the permissive

genetic background. The prognosis for patients with CVID is reasonably good unless severe autoimmune disease or malignancy develops (88).

As noted earlier, two pedigrees have been reported in which boys in one arm of each pedigree had CVID, whereas those in the other had fulminant infectious mononucleosis (Fig. 4) (86). Thus, there is evidence that some boys with what appears clinically to be CVID may actually have XLP. In addition, four patients with CVID have been found to have homozygous loss of the "inducible co-stimulator" (ICOS) on activated T cells (100a). T cells were otherwise normal but there was a deficiency of naive, switched and memory B cells. These findings further emphasize the known heterogeneity of CVID. As the molecular bases of more and more primary immunodeficiency syndromes are being identified, it will be important to consider various genetic mutations that can lead to the hypogammaglobulinemia seen in CVID. These include mutations in *BTK, SH2D1A, CD40L, CD40, ICOS,* and *AID* genes.

Selective IgA Deficiency

An isolated absence or near absence (i.e., <10 mg/dL) of serum and secretory IgA is thought to be the most common well-defined immunodeficiency disorder; a frequency of 1:333 is reported among some blood donors (8,9,101). Although this disorder has been observed in apparently healthy persons (8), it is commonly associated with ill health. As would be expected when there is a deficiency of the major immunoglobulin of external secretions, infections occur predominantly in the respiratory, gastrointestinal, and urogenital tracts (9). Bacterial agents responsible are essentially the same as in other types of antibody deficiency syndromes. There is no clear evidence that patients with this disorder have an undue susceptibility to viral agents. Similar to CVID, there is a frequent association of A Def with collagen-vascular and autoimmune diseases. In further similarity to patients with CVID, there is an increased incidence of malignancy.

Serum concentrations of other immunoglobulins are usually normal in patients with A Def, although IgG2 subclass deficiency has been reported (104), and IgM (usually elevated) may be monomeric. Children with A Def who were vaccinated with killed poliovirus intranasally produced local IgM and IgG antibodies. Of possible etiologic and great clinical significance is the presence of antibodies to IgA in the sera of as many as 44% of patients with A Def (8). IgG anti-IgA antibodies can fix complement and can remove IgA from the circulation four to 20 times faster than the normal catabolic rate for IgA. Some patients with A Def have had severe or fatal anaphylactic reactions after intravenous administration of blood products containing IgA, and anti-IgA antibodies, particularly IgE anti-IgA antibodies(105), have been implicated. For this reason, only five times washed (in 200-mL volumes) normal donor erythrocytes or blood products from other IgA-absent persons should be administered to these patients. Patients with A Def also frequently have

IgG antibodies against cow milk and ruminant serum proteins (106). These antiruminant antibodies often falsely detect "IgA" in immunoassays that employ goat (but not rabbit) antisera (9). A high incidence of autoantibodies has also been noted (107).

The basic defect leading to A Def is unknown. *In vitro* cultures of B cells from some IgA-deficient patients could be stimulated to produce IgA by the combination of anti-CD40 and IL-10; those whose B cells did not produce IgA with these treatments appeared to be more prone to infection (108,109). Treatment with phenytoin, sulfasalazine (110), D-penicillamine, or gold has been suspected as being the cause of A Def; the condition has also been known to remit after discontinuation of phenytoin therapy or spontaneously (111,112). Usually, when this happens, the remission is permanent. The occurrence of A Def in both males and females and in families is consistent with autosomal inheritance; in most families, this appears to be dominant with variable expressivity (99). As already noted, this defect occurs in pedigrees with patients with CVID; some patients with A Def have gone on to develop CVID (98), and studies suggest that the susceptibility genes for these two defects may reside in the MHC class III region as an allelic condition on chromosome 6 (Table 1) (99,100,102,103).

Immunodeficiency with Thymoma

Patients with immunodeficiency with thymoma are adults who almost simultaneously develop recurrent infections, panhypogammaglobulinemia, deficits in cell-mediated immunity, and benign thymoma (4). They may also have eosinophilia or eosinopenia, aregenerative or hemolytic anemia, agranulocytosis, thrombocytopenia, or pancytopenia. Antibody formation is poor, and progressive lymphopenia develops, although percentages of Ig-bearing B lymphocytes are usually normal. The thymomas are predominantly of the spindle cell variety, although other types of benign and malignant thymic tumors have also been seen.

IgG Subclass Deficiencies

Some patients have been reported to have deficiencies of one or more subclasses of IgG, despite normal or elevated total IgG serum concentrations (113–115). IgG2 deficiency would be suspected if patients have repeated problems with encapsulated bacterial pathogens, because most of the antipolysaccharide antibody molecules are of the IgG2 isotype. Most persons with absent or very low concentrations of IgG2 have been patients with A Def (104,114). However, not all patients with A Def who have recurrent infections have IgG2 deficiency, and some patients with A Def have defective antipolysaccharide antibody responses despite normal levels of IgG2. Similarly, patients with WAS, who have a profound antipolysaccharide antibody deficiency, have normal levels of IgG2. Marked deficiencies of antipolysaccharide antibodies have also been noted in other children and adults who do not have WAS but who have recurrent infections and normal con-

centrations of IgG2, as well as normal concentrations of all the other immunoglobulin isotypes (116). Conversely, some healthy children have been described who had low levels of IgG2 but normal responses to polysaccharide antigens when they were immunized (117). In other patients with IgG2 deficiency, continued follow-up revealed an evolving pattern of immunodeficiency (e.g., into CVID), a finding suggesting that the presence of IgG subclass deficiency may be a marker for more general immune dysfunction (118). Thus, the more relevant question to ask is "What is the capacity of the patient to make specific antibodies to protein and polysaccharide antigens?" It is therefore difficult to know the biologic significance of the multiple moderate deficiencies of IgG subclasses that have been reported, particularly when completely asymptomatic persons have been described who totally lacked IgG1, IgG2, IgG4, and IgG1 as a result of gene deletion (Table 1) (47).

CELLULAR IMMUNODEFICIENCY

In general, patients with partial or absolute defects in T-cell function have infections or other clinical problems for which there is no effective treatment or that are more severe than those in patients with antibody deficiency disorders. It is also rare that such persons survive beyond infancy or childhood.

Thymic Hypoplasia (DiGeorge's Syndrome)

Thymic hypoplasia results from dysmorphogenesis of the third and fourth pharyngeal pouches during early embryogenesis that leads to hypoplasia or aplasia of the thymus and parathyroid glands (119,120). Other structures forming at the same age are also frequently affected, resulting in anomalies of the great vessels (right-sided aortic arch), esophageal atresia, bifid uvula, upper limb malformations, congenital heart disease (conotruncal, atrial, and ventricular septal defects), a short philtrum of the upper lip, hypertelorism, an antimongoloid slant to the eyes, mandibular hypoplasia, and low-set, often notched ears (121). A variable degree of hypoplasia of the thymus and parathyroid glands (partial DiGeorge's syndrome) is more frequent than total aplasia (122). Patients with complete DiGeorge's syndrome are susceptible to infections with opportunistic pathogens and to graft-versus-host disease (GVHD) from nonirradiated blood transfusions. There are many clinical similarities among DiGeorge's syndrome, the velocardiofacial syndrome, fetal alcohol syndrome, and retinoic acid toxicity (119,120).

Patients with DiGeorge's syndrome are usually only mildly lymphopenic (122,123). However, the percentage of CD3$^+$ T cells is variably decreased. Immunoglobulin concentrations are usually normal, although sometimes IgE is elevated, and IgA may be low (122,123). Responses of blood lymphocytes after mitogen stimulation have been absent, reduced, or normal, depending on the degree of thymic deficiency (122). Thymic tissue, when found, does contain Hassall's corpuscles and a normal density of thymocytes; corticomedullary distinction is present. Lymphoid follicles are usually present, but lymph node paracortical areas and thymus-dependent regions of the spleen show variable degrees of depletion.

DiGeorge's syndrome has occurred in both male and female patients. It is rarely familial, but cases of apparent autosomal dominant inheritance have been reported (120). Microdeletions of specific DNA sequences from chromosome 22q11.2 (the DiGeorge chromosomal region) have been shown in most patients (124–126), and several candidate genes have been identified in this region (120,124,127–129). There appears to be an excess of 22q11.2 deletions of maternal origin (130). Another deletion associated with DiGeorge's and velocardiofacial syndromes has been identified on chromosome 10p13 (131–133).

No immunologic treatment is needed for the partial form of this disorder. If patients with partial DiGeorge's syndrome do not have a severe cardiac lesion, they will have few clinical problems, except some patients experience seizures and developmental delay. Three patients with complete DiGeorge's syndrome have experienced immunologic reconstitution after unfractionated HLA-identical bone marrow transplantation (134). Transplantation of cultured, mature thymic epithelial explants has successfully reconstituted the immune function of several infants with complete DiGeorge's syndrome (135).

COMBINED IMMUNODEFICIENCY DISORDERS

Severe Combined Immunodeficiency

SCID is a fatal syndrome of diverse genetic cause characterized by profound deficiencies of T- and B-cell (and sometimes NK cell) function (4,5,136,137). Affected infants present during the first few months of life with frequent episodes of diarrhea, pneumonia, otitis, sepsis, and cutaneous infections. Persistent infections with opportunistic organisms such as *Candida albicans, Pneumocystis carinii,* varicella-zoster virus, parainfluenzae 3 virus, respiratory syncytial virus, adenovirus, cytomegalovirus, EBV, and bacillus Calmette-Guérin (BCG) lead to death. These infants also lack the ability to reject foreign tissue and are therefore at risk of GVHD from maternal T cells that cross into the fetal circulation while the SCID infant is *in utero* or from T lymphocytes in nonirradiated blood products or allogeneic bone marrow (62).

Infants with SCID are lymphopenic (136,138). They have an absence of lymphocyte proliferative responses to mitogens, antigens, and allogeneic cells *in vitro,* even on samples collected *in utero* or from the cord blood (139). Therefore, physicians caring for newborns need to be aware of the normal range for the cord blood absolute lymphocyte count (2,000 to 11,000/mm^3) and arrange for T-cell phenotypic and functional studies to be performed on blood from neonates with values lower than this range (136,138,139). The normal absolute lymphocyte count is much higher at 6 to 7 months of age, when most SCIDs are diagnosed, so any count lower than 4,000/mm^3 at that age is lymphopenic (140). Serum immunoglobulin concentrations are diminished to

absent, and no antibody formation occurs after immunization. Typically, all patients with SCID have a very small thymus (usually <1 g), which fails to descend from the neck, contains no thymocytes, and lacks corticomedullary distinction and Hassall's corpuscles. However, the thymic epithelium is normal, and results of bone marrow stem cell transplantation have shown that the tiny thymus is capable of supporting normal T-cell development (141). Thymus-dependent areas of the spleen are depleted of lymphocytes in patients with SCID, and lymph nodes, tonsils, adenoids, and Peyer's patches are absent or extremely underdeveloped.

In the many years since the initial description of SCID (1), it has become evident that the genetic origins of this condition are quite diverse (5,137,142). X-linked SCID (SCID-X1) is the most common form, accounting for approximately 44% of cases in the United States (137,138). Mutated genes on autosomal chromosomes have been identified in six genetic types of SCID: adenosine deaminase (ADA) deficiency, Janus kinase 3 (Jak3) deficiency, IL-7 receptor α-chain (IL-7Rα) deficiency, recombinase-activating gene (*RAG1* or *RAG2*) deficiencies, *Artemis* deficiency, and CD45 deficiency; there are likely other causes yet to be discovered (Table 1) (137).

X-Linked Recessive Severe Combined Immunodeficiency Disease

Despite the uniformly profound lack of T- or B-cell function, patients with SCID-X1 usually have few or no T or NK cells but normal or elevated number of B cells (Table 2) (136,138,143,144). However, SCID-X1 B cells do not produce immunoglobulin normally, even after T-cell reconstitution by bone marrow transplantation (136,138). The abnormal gene in SCID-X1 was mapped to the Xq13 region (145) and was identified as the gene encoding a common γ (γ_c) chain shared by several cytokine receptors, including those for IL-2, IL-4, IL-7, IL-9, IL-15, and IL-21 (Figs. 1 and 5) (146–148). Of the first 136 patients studied, 95 distinct mutations spanning all eight *IL2RG* exons were identified, most of them consisting of small changes at the level of one to a few nucleotides (Fig. 6) (149). These mutations resulted in abnormal γ_c chains in two-thirds of the cases and absent γ_c protein in the remainder. The finding that the mutated gene results in faulty signaling through several cytokine receptors explains how multiple cell types can be affected by a mutation in a single gene (148,150,151).

Autosomal Recessive Severe Combined Immunodeficiency Disease

Adenosine Deaminase Deficiency

An absence of the enzyme ADA has been observed in approximately 15% of patients with SCID (136–138,152). The gene encoding ADA is on chromosome 20q13-ter and was cloned and sequenced in 1986 (152). There are certain distinguishing features of ADA deficiency, including the presence of multiple skeletal abnormalities of chondro-osseous

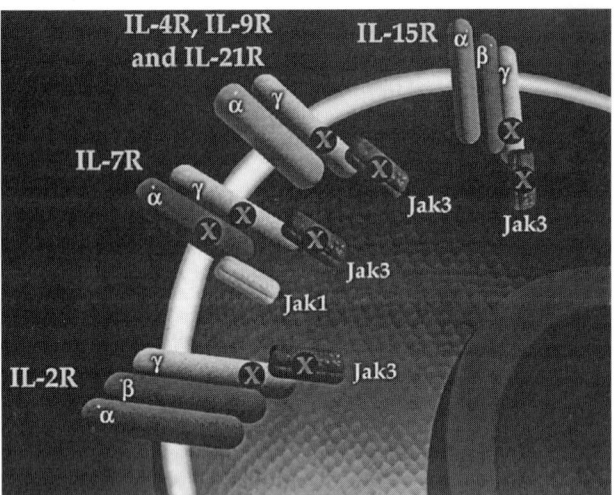

FIG. 5. Diagram showing that Janus kinase 3 (Jak3) is the major signal transducer for the γ_c chain shared by multiple cytokine receptors. Mutations in the *IL2RG* gene cause X-linked severe combined immunodeficiency (SCID), whereas mutations in the *JAK3* gene result in a form of autosomal recessive SCID that mimics X-SCID in lymphocyte phenotype (i.e., T−, B+, NK−). Mutations in the α chain of the interleukein-7 (IL-7) receptor also cause SCID, but unlike X-linked and Jak3-deficient SCID, IL-7Rα-chain–deficient SCID infants have both B and NK cells (i.e., are T−, B+, NK+). From Buckley RH. *J Allerg Clin Immunol* 2002;109:747, with permission.

dysplasia on radiographic examination; these occur predominantly at the costochondral junctions, at the apophyses of the iliac bones, and in the vertebral bodies (causing a "bone-in-bone" effect) (153). ADA-deficient infants usually have a much more profound lymphopenia than those with other types of SCID, with mean absolute lymphocyte counts of less than 500/mm^3. ADA deficiency results in pronounced accumulations of adenosine, 2′-deoxyadenosine, and 2′-O-methyladenosine (152). The latter metabolites directly or indirectly lead to apoptosis of thymocytes and circulating lymphocytes and thus cause the immunodeficiency. As with other types of SCID, ADA deficiency can be cured by HLA-identical or haploidentical T-cell–depleted bone marrow transplantation, which remains the treatment of choice (62,138). Enzyme replacement therapy with polyethylene glycol–modified bovine ADA (PEG-ADA) administered subcutaneously once weekly, has resulted in both clinical and immunologic improvement in more than 100 ADA-deficient patients (154–156). However, the immunocompetence achieved is not nearly so great as with bone marrow transplantation (138). In view of this result, PEG-ADA therapy should not be initiated if bone marrow transplantation is contemplated, because it will confer graft-rejection capability on the infant. After T-cell function is effected by bone marrow transplantation (without pretransplantation chemotherapy), infants with ADA deficiency generally have B-cell function.

IL2RG MUTATIONS IN 87 FAMILIES WITH X-LINKED SCID

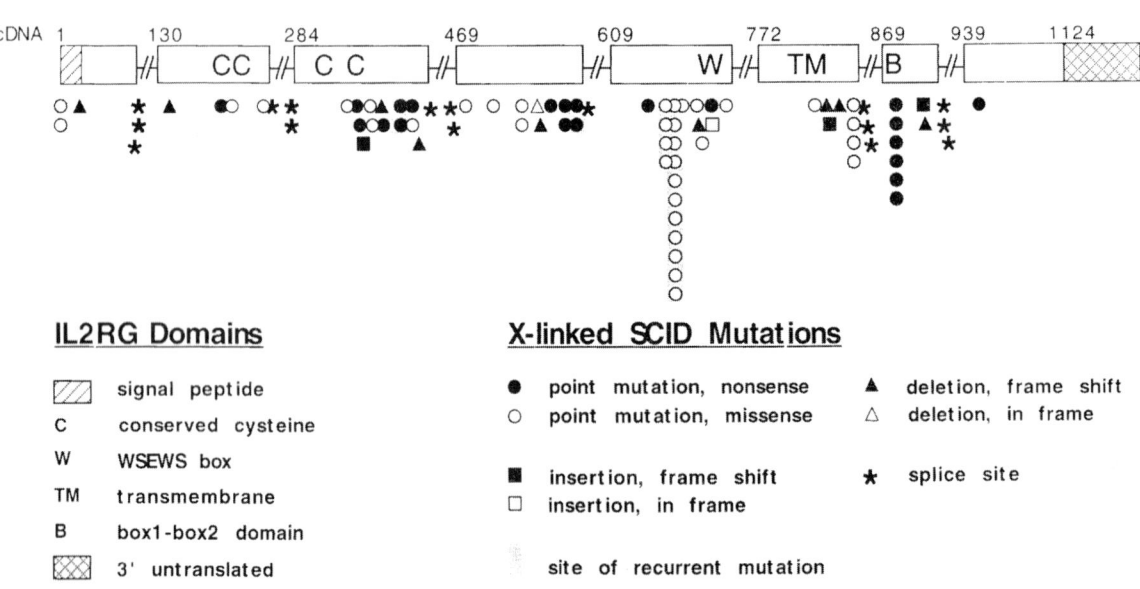

FIG. 6. *IL2RG* cDNA map showing exons, cDNA numbers corresponding to the first coding nucleotide of each exon, protein domains, and sites of mutations found in 87 unrelated families with X-linked severe combined immunodeficiency (X-SCID). Identical mutations found in unrelated patients are surrounded by *shaded boxes*. From Puck JM, Pepper AE, Henthorn PS, et al. (149), with permission.

Janus Kinase 3 Deficiency

Patients with autosomal recessive SCID caused by Jak3 deficiency resemble patients with all other types in their susceptibility to infection and to GVHD from allogeneic T cells. However, they have lymphocyte characteristics most closely resembling those of patients with SCID-X1, including an elevated percentage of B cells and very low percentages of T and NK cells (Table 1) (136,138). Because Jak3 is the only signaling molecule known to be associated with γ_c, it was a candidate gene for mutations leading to autosomal recessive SCID of unknown molecular type (Fig. 6) (157–159). Thus far, more than 20 patients who lack Jak3 have been identified (Fig. 6) (138,160–162). Even after successful T-cell reconstitution by transplantation of haploidentical stem cells, Jak3-deficient infants with SCID fail to have persistent development of NK cells (62). Moreover, in further similarity to patients with SCID-X1, these infants often fail to develop normal B-cell function after transplantation despite their high numbers of B cells. Their failure to develop NK cells or B-cell function is believed to result from the host cells' abnormal cytokine receptors.

Interleukin-7 Receptor α-Chain Deficiency

Because mice whose genes for either the α chain of the IL-7 receptor or of IL-7 itself have been mutated are profoundly deficient in T- and B-cell function but have normal NK-cell function (6), naturally occurring mutations in these genes were sought in some of my patients who had $T^-B^+NK^+$ SCID and who had previously been shown not to have either γ_c or Jak3 deficiency. Mutations in the gene for IL-7Rα on chromosome 5p13 have thus far been found in 16 of my patients (138,163). These findings imply that the T-cell defect, but not the NK-cell defect, in SCID-X1 and Jak3-deficient SCID results from an inability to signal through the IL-7 receptor (Fig. 6). The finding that these patients have developed normal B-cell function after nonablative haploidentical bone marrow stem cell transplantation despite lacking donor B cells also suggests that the B-cell defect in SCID-X1 is not the result of failure of IL-7 signaling.

Recombinase-Activating Gene (RAG1 or RAG2) Deficiencies

Infants with autosomal recessive SCID caused by mutations in recombinase activating genes, *RAG1* and *RAG2,* resemble all others in their infection susceptibility and complete absence of T- or B-cell function. However, their lymphocyte phenotype differs from those of patients with SCID caused by γ_c, Jak3, IL-7Rα, or ADA deficiencies in that they lack both B and T lymphocytes and have primarily NK cells in their circulation ($T^-B^-NK^+$ SCID; Table 1). This particular phenotype suggested a possible problem with their antigen receptor genes and led to the discovery of mutations in *RAG1* and *RAG2* in some (but not all) such infants with SCID (164–166). These genes, on chromosome 11p13, encode proteins necessary for somatic rearrangement of antigen receptor genes on T and B cells. The proteins recognize recombination signal sequences and introduce a DNA double-stranded break, permitting V, D, and J gene rearrangements. *RAG1* or *RAG2* mutations result in a functional inability to form antigen receptors through genetic recombination.

Patients with Omenn syndrome also have mutations in *RAG1* or *RAG2* genes, resulting in partial and impaired V(D)J recombinational activity (166,167). Omenn syndrome is characterized by the development soon after birth of generalized erythroderma and desquamation, diarrhea, hepatosplenomegaly, hypereosinophilia, and markedly elevated serum IgE levels. This last feature is caused by circulating activated, oligoclonal T lymphocytes that do not respond normally to mitogens or antigens *in vitro* (168,169). Circulating B cells are not found, and lymph node architecture is abnormal resulting from a lack of germinal centers (170). The condition is fatal unless it is corrected by bone marrow transplantation (62).

Deficiencies of the Artemis Gene

The most recently discovered cause of human SCID is a deficiency of a novel V(D)J recombination/DNA repair factor that belongs to the metallo-β-lactamase superfamily. It is encoded by a gene on chromosome 10p called *Artemis* (171). A deficiency of this factor results in an inability to repair DNA after double-stranded cuts have been made by *RAG1* or *RAG2* gene products in rearranging antigen receptor genes from their germline configuration. Similar to *RAG1*- and *RAG2*-deficient SCID, this defect results in another form of $T^-B^-NK^+$ SCID, also called Athabascan SCID (Table 1). In addition, there is increased radiation sensitivity of both skin fibroblasts and bone marrow cells of persons affected with this type of SCID.

CD45 Deficiency

Another recently discovered molecular defect causing SCID is a mutation in the gene encoding the common leukocyte surface protein CD45 (172,173). This hematopoietic cell–specific transmembrane protein tyrosine phosphatase functions to regulate Src kinases required for T- and B-cell antigen receptor signal transduction. A 2-month-old male infant presented with a clinical picture of SCID and was found to have a very low number of T cells but a normal number of B cells. The T cells failed to respond to mitogens, and serum immunoglobulins diminished with time. He was found to have a large deletion at one *CD45* allele and a point mutation causing an alteration of the intervening sequence 13 donor splice site at the other (172). A second case of SCID resulting from CD45 deficiency has been reported (173). Figure 7 shows the frequency of the various genetic forms of SCID evaluated by me over the past 3.5 decades (173).

Treatment and Prognosis

SCID is a pediatric emergency (136,138). Replacement therapy with IVIG fails to halt the progressively downhill

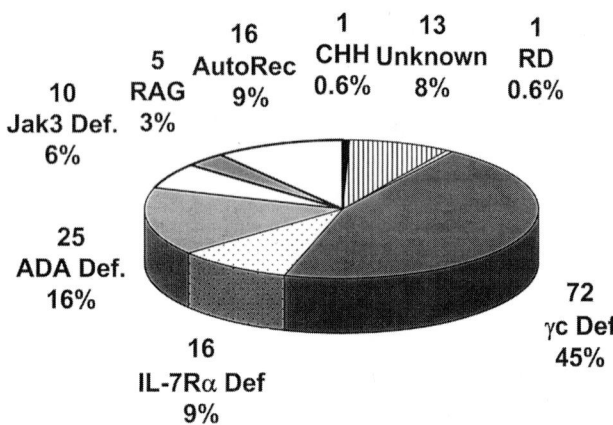

FIG. 7. Relative frequencies of the different genetic types of severe combined immunodeficiency (SCID) among 160 of my patients seen consecutively by over 3.5 decades.

course (64). Unless bone marrow transplantation from HLA-identical or haploidentical donors can be performed, death usually occurs before the patient's first birthday and almost invariably before the second. Conversely, transplantation in the first 3.5 months of life offers a greater than 97% chance of survival (138). Therefore, early diagnosis is essential. Studies have shown that the immune reconstitution effected by stem cell transplants results from thymic education of the transplanted allogeneic stem cells (141). The thymic output appears to occur sooner and to a greater degree in those infants who undergo transplantation in the neonatal period as opposed to those who undergo transplantation procedures later (139,174). Currently, there are more than 400 patients with SCID who are surviving worldwide as a result of successful bone marrow transplantation (62).

ADA deficiency was the first genetic defect in which gene therapy was attempted; these early efforts were unsuccessful (175–177). However, within the past few years, a normal γ_c cDNA was successfully transduced into autologous marrow cells of nine infants with SCID-X1 by retroviral gene transfer, with subsequent full correction of their T-cell and NK-cell defects (178). This offered hope that gene therapy would become the treatment of choice for all patients with SCID or other genetically determined immunodeficiency diseases for whom the molecular basis is known. However, serious adverse events (in the form of leukemia) developed in two of these XSCID children at approximately 3 years after gene therapy, due to insertional mutagenesis. Therefore, all retroviral gene therapy has been halted.

The *Bosma SCID mouse* defect is now known to result from a nonsense mutation in the gene on murine chromosome 16 encoding the catalytic subunit of a DNA-dependent protein kinase, p350 or the Ku protein (179,180). A human gene encoding a similar protein has been assigned to human chromosome 8p12øq22, but thus far no human SCID has been identified with this type of mutation (181). *Arabian horses* have long been known to carry a recessive gene for SCID, and more recently the mode of inheritance has been confirmed as autosomal recessive (182). Studies suggest that the

same gene may be mutated in the Arabian horse as is mutated in the Bosma SCID mouse (see earlier). *Reticular dysgenesis* was first described in 1959 in identical twin male infants who exhibited a total lack of both lymphocytes and granulocytes in their peripheral blood and bone marrow. Seven of the eight infants thus far reported with this defect died between 3 and 119 days of age from overwhelming infections; the eighth underwent complete immunologic reconstitution from a bone marrow transplant (4). Mature, normal-appearing granulocytes (although markedly reduced in number) were noted in three patients and a normal percentage of E-rosetting T cells was seen in the cord blood of a fourth patient, findings arguing against a total failure of stem cell differentiation in this defect. However, despite the normal percentage of T cells in the last patient's cord blood, the cells failed to give an *in vitro* proliferative response to mitogens. The thymus glands have all weighed less than 1 g, no Hassall's corpuscles have been present, and few or no thymocytes have been seen. The molecular basis of this autosomal recessive disorder is unknown.

Combined Immunodeficiency

Combined immunodeficiency, or CID, is a syndrome characterized by low but not absent T-cell function. Patients with CID present during infancy with recurrent or chronic pulmonary infections, failure to thrive, oral or cutaneous candidiasis, chronic diarrhea, recurrent skin infections, gram-negative sepsis, urinary tract infections, or severe varicella (4). Serum immunoglobulins may be normal or elevated for all classes, but A Def, marked elevation of IgE, and elevated IgD levels have been found in some cases. Although antibody-forming capacity has been impaired in a few patients, it has not been absent and has been apparently normal in roughly one-third of the reported cases. Studies of cellular immune function have shown lymphopenia, deficiencies of CD3[+] T cells, and extremely low but not absent lymphocyte proliferative responses to mitogens and allogeneic cells *in vitro*. Peripheral lymphoid tissues demonstrate paracortical lymphocyte depletion. The thymus of such patients is very small and has a paucity of thymocytes and usually no Hassall's corpuscles. An autosomal recessive pattern of inheritance is usually seen.

Patients with CID usually survive longer than do infants with SCID, but they fail to thrive and die early in life. Some have been successfully reconstituted by unfractionated matched sibling or unrelated adult donor bone marrow transplants or cord blood transplants, but T-cell–depleted haploidentical marrow stem cell transplants have not been very successful because they require chemoablation before transplantation to achieve graft acceptance, and there is resistance to engraftment.

Purine Nucleoside Phosphorylase Deficiency

More than 40 patients with CID have been found to have purine nucleoside phosphorylase (PNP) deficiency (183). Deaths have occurred from generalized vaccinia, varicella, lymphosarcoma, and GVHD mediated by T cells from non-irradiated allogeneic blood or bone marrow. Two-thirds of patients have had neurologic abnormalities ranging from spasticity to mental retardation. One-third of patients developed autoimmune diseases, the most common of which is autoimmune hemolytic anemia. Most patients have normal or elevated concentrations of all serum immunoglobulins. PNP-deficient patients are as profoundly lymphopenic as those with ADA deficiency, with absolute lymphocyte counts usually less than 500/mm³. T-cell function is low but not absent and is variable with time. The gene encoding PNP is on chromosome 14q13.1, and it has been cloned and sequenced. Various mutations have been found in the PNP gene in patients with PNP deficiency (184). Unlike ADA deficiency, serum and urinary uric acid are deficient because PNP is needed to form the urate precursors hypoxanthine and xanthine. Prenatal diagnosis is possible. PNP deficiency is invariably fatal in childhood unless immunologic reconstitution can be achieved. Bone marrow transplantation is the treatment of choice but has thus far been successful in only three such patients (62,185).

Ataxia-Telangiectasia

Ataxia-telangiectasia (AT) is a complex combined immunodeficiency syndrome with associated neurologic, endocrinologic, hepatic, and cutaneous abnormalities (4,186). The most prominent features are progressive cerebellar ataxia, oculocutaneous telangiectasias, chronic sinopulmonary disease, a high incidence of malignancy (187), and variable humoral and cellular immunodeficiency. The ataxia typically becomes evident shortly after the child begins to walk and progresses until he or she is confined to a wheelchair, usually by 10 to 12 years of age. The telangiectasias develop at between 3 and 6 years of age. Recurrent, usually bacterial, sinopulmonary infections occur in roughly 80% of these patients. Fatal varicella occurred in one patient, and transfusion-associated GVHD has also been reported (188). A Def is found in 50% to 80% of those affected (189). IgE concentrations are usually low, and IgG2 or total IgG may be decreased. Specific antibody titers may be decreased or normal. The percentages of CD3⁺ and CD4⁺ T cells are only modestly low, and *in vitro* tests of lymphocyte function have generally shown moderately depressed proliferative responses to T- and B-cell mitogens. The thymus is hypoplastic, exhibits poor organization, and is lacking in Hassall's corpuscles. Cells from patients as well as those of heterozygous carriers have increased sensitivity to ionizing radiation, defective DNA repair, and frequent chromosomal abnormalities (189,190). The malignancies reported in this condition usually have been of the lymphoreticular type, but adenocarcinoma and other forms also have been seen; there is also an increased incidence of malignant disease in unaffected relatives.

Inheritance of AT follows an autosomal recessive pattern. The mutated gene (*ATM*) responsible for this defect was mapped by restriction fragment length polymorphism analysis to the long arm of chromosome 11 (11q22–23) and was cloned (189,191,192). The gene product is a DNA-dependent protein kinase localized predominantly to the nucleus and believed to be involved in mitogenic signal transduction, meiotic recombination, and cell-cycle control (186,193–195). No satisfactory definitive treatment has been found (189).

Immunodeficiency with Thrombocytopenia and Eczema (Wiskott-Aldrich Syndrome)

WAS is an X-linked recessive syndrome characterized by eczema, thrombocytopenic purpura with normal-appearing megakaryocytes but small defective platelets, and undue susceptibility to infection (4,5). Patients usually present during infancy with prolonged bleeding from the circumcision site, bloody diarrhea, or excessive bruising. Atopic dermatitis and recurrent infections usually also develop during the first year of life. Infections are usually those produced by pneumococci and other encapsulated bacteria, and they result in otitis media, pneumonia, meningitis, or sepsis. Later, infections with opportunistic agents such as *Pneumocystis carinii* and the herpesviruses become more problematic. Autoimmune cytopenias and vasculitis are common in patients who live beyond infancy. Survival beyond the teens is rare. Infections, vasculitis, and bleeding are major causes of death, but the most common cause of death in patients with WAS currently is EBV-induced lymphoreticular malignancy (196).

Patients with WAS have an impaired humoral immune response to polysaccharide antigens, as evidenced by absent or greatly diminished isohemagglutinins and poor or absent antibody responses to polysaccharide antigens (4,197,198). In addition, antibody titers to protein antigens fall with time. Most often, there is a low serum IgM, elevated IgA and IgE, and a normal or slightly low IgG concentration. Flow cytometry of blood lymphocytes has shown a moderately reduced percentage of T cells, and lymphocyte responses to mitogens are moderately depressed (196).

The mutated gene responsible for this defect was mapped to Xp11.22–11.23(199) and was isolated in 1994 by Derry and colleagues (200). It was found to be limited in expression to lymphocytic and megakaryocytic lineages (200). The gene product, a 501-amino acid proline-rich protein that lacks a hydrophobic transmembrane domain, was designated WASP (WAS protein). It has been shown to bind CDC42H2 and rac, members of the Rho family of GTPases, which are important in actin polymerization (201–204). A large and varied number of mutations in the *WASP* gene have been identified in patients with WAS (205–207), with some correlation to the site of the mutation with severity of infection susceptibility or other problems in one series(208), but not in others (209,210). Isolated X-linked thrombocytopenia is also caused by mutations in the *WASP* gene (211). Carriers can be detected by the finding of nonrandom X-chromosome inactivation in several hematopoietic cell lineages or by detection of the mutated gene (if known in the family) (212–214). Prenatal diagnosis of WAS can also be made by chorionic villous sampling or amniocentesis if the mutation is known in that family. Two families with apparent autosomal inheritance of a clinical phenotype similar to WAS have been reported (215,216), and, in one case, a girl was shown to have this as an X-linked defect (217).

Numerous patients with WAS have had complete corrections of both the platelet and the immunologic abnormalities by HLA-identical sibling bone marrow transplants after conditioning with irradiation or busulfan and cyclophosphamide (62). Success has been minimal with T-cell–depleted haploidentical stem cell transplants in WAS, primarily because of resistance to engraftment (62,218). Some success has been achieved in the treatment of WAS with matched-unrelated donor transplants in children less than 5 years of age (218,219). It is likely that matched cord blood transplants will be similarly successful because, in both cases, T cells can be left in the donor cell suspension. Several patients who required splenectomy for uncontrollable bleeding had impressive rises in their platelet counts and have done well clinically while being administered prophylactic antibiotics and IVIG (220,221).

Cartilage-Hair Hypoplasia

In 1965, an unusual form of short-limbed dwarfism with frequent and severe infections was reported among the Pennsylvania Amish population; non-Amish cases have since been described (4,222). These patients have short and pudgy hands with redundant skin, metaphyseal chondrodysplasia, hyperextensible joints of hands and feet but an inability to extend the elbows completely, and fine, sparse light hair and eyebrows. These features led to the name cartilage-hair hypoplasia (CHH). Radiographically, the bones show scalloping and sclerotic or cystic changes in the metaphyses. In contrast to ADA deficiency, in which the predominant changes are in the apophyses of the iliac bones, the ribs and vertebral bodies, the chondrodysplasia in CHH principally affects the limbs. Severe and often fatal varicella infections, progressive vaccinia, and vaccine-associated poliomyelitis have been observed. Associated conditions include deficient erythrogenesis, Hirschsprung's disease, and an increased risk of malignant disease.

Three patterns of immune dysfunction have emerged: defective antibody-mediated immunity, defective cellular immunity (most common form), and SCID. NK cells, however, are increased in number and function.

CHH is an autosomal recessive condition, and the defective gene has been mapped to chromosome 9p21–p13 in Amish and Finnish families (Table 1) (223). The endoribonuclease RNAse MRP consists of an RNA molecule bound to several proteins. It has at least two functions, namely, cleavage of RNA in mitochondrial DNA synthesis and nucleolar cleaving of pre-RNA. Numerous mutations were found in the untranslated *RMRP* gene that co-segregate with the CHH phenotype (224). The authors concluded that mutations in *RMRP* cause CHH by disrupting a function of RNAse MRP RNA that affects multiple organ systems. Bone marrow transplantation has resulted in immunologic reconstitution in some patients with CHH and the SCID phenotype (138). Those with milder

types of immune deficiency have lived to adulthood, some even to old age.

Nijmegen Breakage Syndrome

This is a rare autosomal recessive condition in which the immunologic, cytogenetic, and radiation-sensitivity findings are almost identical to those in AT (225–227). However, the patients are quite distinct from AT clinically in that they have short stature, "birdlike" facies, and microcephaly from birth. They lack the classic clinical features of AT, including ataxia and telangiectasia, and they have normal serum α-fetoprotein levels. Intelligence can vary from normal findings to moderate mental retardation. The immunodeficiency appears to be more severe than in AT. Most patients have recurrent respiratory infections. The tendency to express rearrangements of chromosomes 7 and 14 and to develop malignant disease is much higher than in AT. More than 40 patients from approximately 30 families have been reported, and most are of Eastern European origin (225,227). Complementation studies have indicated that patients with this syndrome are genetically distinct from those with AT. The abnormal gene in this condition has been mapped to chromosome 8q21 (Table 1) (228).

Defective Expression of Major Histocompatibility Complex Antigens

There are two main forms: (a) class I MHC antigen deficiency (bare lymphocyte syndrome) and (b) class II MHC antigen deficiency.

MHC Class I Antigen Deficiency

An isolated deficiency of MHC class I antigens is rare, and the resulting immunodeficiency is milder than that in SCID, contributing to a later age of presentation. Sera from affected persons contain normal quantities of class I MHC antigens and β_2-microglobulin, but class I MHC antigens are not detected on any cells in the body. There is a deficiency of CD8$^+$ but not of CD4$^+$ T cells. Mutations have been found in two genes within the MHC locus on chromosome 6 that encode the peptide transporter proteins, TAP1 and TAP2 (Table 1) (229–233). TAP proteins function to transport peptide antigens from the cytoplasm across the Golgi apparatus membrane to join the α chain of MHC class I molecules and β_2 microglobulin. The complex can then move to the cell surface; when the assembly of the complex cannot be completed because there is no peptide antigen, the MHC class I complex is destroyed in the cytoplasm (234). MHC class I antigen deficiency can also be caused by a mutation in the gene encoding tapasin, another component of this complex that links TAP to the class I heavy chain (234a).

MHC Class II Antigen Deficiency

Many persons affected with this autosomal recessive syndrome are of North African descent (235). More than

70 patients have been identified. They present in infancy with persistent diarrhea, often associated with cryptosporidiosis, as well as with bacterial pneumonia, pneumocystis, septicemia, and viral or monilial infections. Nevertheless, their immunodeficiency is not as severe as in SCID, as evidenced by their failure to develop BCG-induced disease or GVHD from nonirradiated blood transfusions (235). MHC class II–deficient patients have a very low number of CD4+ T cells but normal or elevated numbers of CD8+ T cells. Lymphopenia is only moderate. The MHC class II antigens, HLA-DP, DQ, and DR, are undetectable on blood B cells and monocytes. Patients have impaired antigen-specific responses caused by the absence of these antigen-presenting molecules. In addition, MHC antigen-deficient B cells fail to stimulate allogeneic cells in mixed leukocyte culture. Lymphocytes respond normally to mitogens but not to antigens. The thymus and other lymphoid organs are severely hypoplastic. The lack of class II molecules results in abnormal thymic selection, because recognition of HLA molecules by thymocytes is central to both positive and negative selection. The latter results in circulating CD4+ T cells that have altered CDR3 profiles (236). The associated defects of both B- and T-cell immunity and of HLA expression emphasize the important biologic role for HLA determinants in effective immune cell cooperation.

Four different molecular defects resulting in impaired expression of MHC class II antigens have been identified (Table 1) (235). In one, there is a mutation in the gene on chromosome 1q that encodes a protein called RFX5, a subunit of RFX, a multiprotein complex that binds the X box motif of MHC class II promoters (237). A second form is caused by mutations in a gene on chromosome 13q that encodes a second 36-kDa subunit of the RFX complex, called RFX-associated protein (RFXAP) (238). The most recently discovered and most common causes of MHC class II defects are mutations in *RFXANK,* the gene encoding a third subunit of RFX (239). In a fourth type, there is a mutation in the gene on chromosome 16p13 that encodes a novel MHC class II transactivator (CIITA), a non-DNA-binding co-activator that controls the cell-type specificity and inducibility of MHC class II expression (240). All these defects cause impairment in the coordinate expression of MHC class II molecules on the surface of B cells and macrophages.

Leukocyte Adhesion Deficiency

Leukocyte Adhesion Deficiency-1

Leukocyte adhesion deficiency-1 (LAD-1) is attributable to mutations in the gene on chromosome 21 at position q22.3 encoding CD18, a 95-kDa β subunit shared by three adhesive heterodimers: leukocyte function–associated antigen-1 (LFA-1) on B, T, and NK lymphocytes; complement receptor type 3 (CR3) on neutrophils, monocytes, macrophages, eosinophils, and NK cells; and p150,95 (another complement receptor) (Table 1) (241–243). The α chains of these three molecules (encoded by genes on chromosome 16) are not

expressed because of the abnormal β chain. Those so affected have histories of delayed separation of the umbilical cord, omphalitis, gingivitis, recurrent skin infections, repeated otitis media, pneumonia, septicemia, ileocolitis (244,245), peritonitis, perianal abscesses, and impaired wound healing. Life-threatening bacterial and fungal infections account for the high mortality. Affected people do not have increased susceptibility to viral infections or malignant disease. Blood neutrophil counts are usually significantly elevated even when no infection is present because of an inability of the cells to adhere to vascular endothelium and migrate out of the intravascular compartment. All cytotoxic lymphocyte functions are considerably impaired because of a lack of the adhesion protein LFA-1; deficiency of LFA-1 also interferes with immune cell interaction and immune recognition. CR3 binds fixed iC3b fragments of C3 and β-glucans; its absence causes abnormal phagocytic cell adherence and chemotaxis and a reduced respiratory burst with phagocytosis. Deficiencies of these glycoproteins can be screened for by flow cytometry with monoclonal antibodies to CD18 or to CD11a, b, or c. Because the CD18 gene has been cloned and sequenced, this disorder is another potential candidate for gene therapy (177).

Leukocyte Adhesion Deficiency-2

LAD-2 is attributable to the absence of neutrophil Sialyl-Lewis^x, a ligand of E-selectin on vascular endothelium (246). This disorder was discovered in two unrelated Israeli boys, 3 and 5 years of age, each the child of consanguineous parents (247). Both had severe mental retardation, short stature, a distinctive facial appearance, and the Bombay (hh) blood phenotype, and both were secretor negative and Lewis negative. They both had had recurrent severe bacterial infections similar to those seen in patients with LAD-1, including pneumonia, peridontitis, otitis media, and localized cellulitis. As in patients with LAD-1, their infections were accompanied by pronounced leukocytosis (30,000 to 150,000/mm^3), but without pus formation at sites of recurrent cellulitis. *In vitro* studies revealed a pronounced defect in neutrophil motility. Because the genes for the red blood cell H antigen and for the secretor status encode for distinct $\alpha_{1,2}$-fucosyltransferases and the synthesis of Sialyl-Lewis^x requires an α1,3-fucosyltransferase, Etzioni and associates postulated a general defect in fucose metabolism as the basis for this disorder (247). These same researchers found that GDP-L-fucose transport into Golgi vesicles was specifically impaired (248) and then discovered missense mutations in the GDP-fucose transporter cDNA of three patients with LAD-2. Thus, GDP-fucose transporter deficiency is a cause of LAD-2 (249).

Interleukin-2 Receptor α-Chain (CD25) Mutation

A male infant born of a consanguineous union presented at 6 months of age with cytomegalovirus pneumonia, persistent oral and esophageal candidiasis, adenoviral gastroenteritis, and failure to thrive. He developed lymphadenopathy, hepatosplenomegaly, and chronic inflammation of his lungs and mandible. Biopsies revealed extensive lymphocytic infiltration of his lung, liver, gut, and bone. Serum IgG and IgM were elevated, but IgA was low. He had T-cell lymphocytopenia, with an even CD4:CD8 ratio. The T cells responded poorly to anti-CD3, to PHA and other mitogens, and to IL-2. He was found to have a truncated mutation of IL-2Rα (CD25) (Table 1) (250). He could not reject an allogeneic skin graft. He was given a successful allogeneic bone marrow transplant after cytoreduction.

Young mutant mice lacking IL-2Rα have phenotypically normal T- and B-cell development (251). However, as adults, they develop massive lymphoid organ enlargement and polyclonal T- and B-cell expansion attributed to defective apoptosis. They also develop autoimmune disorders, including hemolytic anemia and inflammatory bowel disease. Similarly, gene targeted mice lacking IL-2Rβ developed exhaustive differentiation of B cells into plasma cells, elevated IgG1 and IgE, and autoantibodies that caused hemolytic anemia (252). T cells did not respond to polyclonal or antigen-specific activators. It is known that IL-2 programs murine αβ T lymphocytes for apoptosis (253). From these observations, it is deduced that both IL-2Rα and IL-2Rβ play an important role in influencing the activation programs of T cells, the balance between clonal expansion and cell death after lymphocyte activation, and the prevention of autoimmunity.

Interferon-γ Receptor-1 and Receptor-2 Mutations

Disseminated BCG infections occur in infants with SCID or with other severe T-cell defects. However, in approximately half the cases, no specific host defect has been found. One possible explanation for this predilection was found in a 2.5-month-old Tunisian female infant who had fatal idiopathic disseminated BCG infection(254) and in four children from Malta who had disseminated atypical mycobacterial infection in the absence of a recognized immunodeficiency (255). In the case of all five children, there was consanguinity in their pedigrees. All affected children were found to have a functional defect in the up-regulation of TNF-α production by their blood macrophages in response to stimulation with interferon-γ (IFN-γ). Further, all lacked expression of IFN-γ receptors on their blood monocytes or lymphocytes, and each was found to have a mutation in the gene on chromosome 6q22–q23 that encodes IFN-γ receptor-1. These children did not appear to be susceptible to infection with agents other than mycobacteria. T helper cell (Th1) responses appeared to be normal in these patients. The susceptibility of these children to mycobacterial infections thus apparently results from an intrinsic impairment of the IFN-γ pathway response to these particular intracellular pathogens, a finding showing that IFN-γ is obligatory for efficient macrophage antimycobacterial activity (254,255). Since the previously described initial discoveries of IFN-γ receptor-1–deficient

humans, many more examples have been found, and IFN-γ R-2–deficient persons have been found as well (256).

Interleukin-12 and Interleukin-12 Receptor β1 Mutations

IL-12 is produced by activated antigen-presenting cells (dendritic cells, macrophages) (256). It promotes the development of Th1 responses and is a powerful inducer of IFN-γ production by T and NK cells. A child with BCG and *Salmonella enteritidis* infection was found to have a large homozygous deletion within the IL-12 p40 subunit gene, precluding expression of functional IL-12 p70 cytokine by activated dendritic cells and phagocytes. As a result, IFN-γ production by the child's lymphocytes was markedly impaired (257). This finding suggested that IL-12 is essential for protective immunity to intracellular bacteria such as mycobacteria and *Salmonella*. In further support of this concept, T and NK cells from seven unrelated patients who had severe idiopathic mycobacterial and *Salmonella* infections failed to produce IFN-γ when these cells were stimulated with IL-12. The patients were otherwise healthy. They were found to have mutations in the IL-12 receptor β1 chain resulting in premature stop codons in the extracellular domain, leading to unresponsiveness to this cytokine, again demonstrating the crucial role of IL-12 in host defense (258,259).

Germline STAT1 Mutation

IFNs induce the formation of two transcriptional activators: γ-activating factor (GAF) and IFN-stimulated γ factor 3 (ISGF3). A natural heterozygous germline signal transducer and activator of transcription-1 (STAT1) mutation associated with susceptibility to mycobacterial but not viral disease was found in two unrelated patients with unexplained mycobacterial disease (260). This mutation caused a loss of GAF and ISGF3 activation but was dominant for one cellular phenotype and recessive for the other. It impaired the nuclear accumulation of GAF, but not of ISGF3, in cells stimulated by IFNs, a finding implying that the antimycobacterial, but not the antiviral, effects of human IFNs are mediated by GAF.

Chédiak-Higashi Syndrome

This rare disease is characterized by oculocutaneous albinism and susceptibility to recurrent respiratory tract and other types of infections (261). The hallmark of the disease is giant lyosomal granules, not only in neutrophils, but also in most of the other cells of the body, including melanocytes (262), neural Schwann cells, renal tubular cells, gastric mucosa, pneumatocytes, hepatocytes, Langerhans cells of the skin, and adrenal cells (263). The granules in neutrophils are positive for peroxidase, acid phosphatase, and esterase. The abnormal lysosomes are unable to fuse with phagosomes, so ingested bacteria cannot be lysed normally. In addition, there is nearly complete absence of cytotoxic T-lymphocyte and NK-cell activity as a result of abnormal lysosomal granule function (264,265). Abnormal chemotaxis has also been reported, and there is evidence of a profound alteration of the cytoskeleton of the neutrophils. There are reports of a decreased number of centriole-associated microtubules and abnormalities in tubulin tyrosinolation.

The fundamental defect in this autosomal recessive disorder was found to be caused by mutations in a gene on human chromosome 1 at position q42–43 (Table 1) (266,267). This gene is similar to the one mutated in the murine beige defect (268–270). The gene product is postulated to function with other proteins as components of a vesicle membrane-associated signal transduction complex that regulates intracellular protein trafficking (266).

Approximately 85% of these patients develop an "accelerated phase" of the disease, with fever, jaundice, hepatosplenomegaly, lymphadenopathy, pancytopenia, bleeding diathesis, and neurologic changes (271). Once the accelerated phase occurs, the disease is usually fatal within 30 months unless successful treatment with an unfractionated HLA-identical bone marrow transplant after cytoreductive conditioning can be accomplished (62,272).

T-CELL ACTIVATION DEFECTS

These conditions are characterized by the presence of normal or elevated numbers of blood T cells that appear phenotypically normal but that fail to proliferate or produce cytokines in response to stimulation with mitogens, antigens, or other signals delivered to the T-cell antigen receptor resulting from defective signal transduction from the T-cell receptor to intracellular metabolic pathways (Fig. 8) (273). These patients have problems similar to those of other T-cell–deficient persons, and some with severe T-cell activation defects may clinically resemble patients with SCID.

CD8 Lymphocytopenia Resulting from ζ-Chain–Associated Protein (ZAP70) Deficiency

Patients with CD8 lymphocytopenia caused by ζ-chain–associated protein 70 (ZAP70) deficiency present during infancy with severe, recurrent, sometimes fatal infections similar to those in SCID patients; however, they often live longer and present later than patients with SCID. More than eight cases have been reported, and most were Mennonites

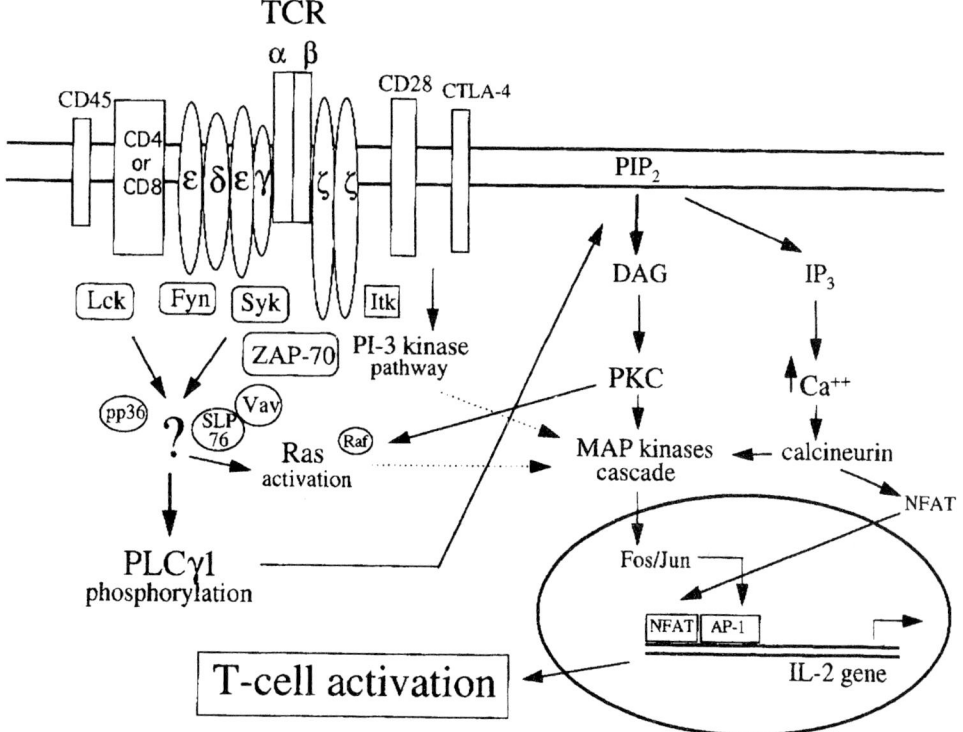

FIG. 8. T-cell signal transduction pathway. The T-cell receptor (TCR) spans the plasma membrane in association with CD3 and ζ, CD4 or CD8, CD28 and CD45. Cytoplasmic protein tyrosine kinases (PTKs) associated with the TCR are activated on antigen binding to the TCR. These PTKs include Lck, Fyn, ZAP70, and Syk. PTK activation results in the phosphorylation of phospholipase Cγ1 and the activation of other signaling molecules. Distal signaling events, including PKC activation and Ca²⁺ mobilization, result in the transcription of genes encoding interleukin-2 (IL-2) and other proteins, culminating in T-cell activation, differentiation, and proliferation. Ionomycin and phorbol myristate acetate (PMA) can be used to mimic distal signaling events. Mutations in the gene encoding ZAP70 result in markedly impaired T-cell activation, in addition to abnormal thymic selection resulting in CD8 deficiency. (Modified from Elder ME: *Pediatric Research* 39: 744, 1996, courtesy of Dr. Melissa Elder.)

(274–276). These patients have normal, low, or elevated serum immunoglobulin concentrations and normal or elevated numbers of circulating CD4$^+$ T lymphocytes but essentially no CD8$^+$ cells. These CD4$^+$ T cells fail to respond to mitogens or to allogeneic cells *in vitro* or to generate cytotoxic T lymphocytes. By contrast, NK activity is normal. The thymus of one patient exhibited normal architecture; there were normal numbers of CD4:CD8 double-positive thymocytes but an absence of CD8 single-positive thymocytes. This condition has been attributed to mutations in the gene encoding ZAP70, a non-src family protein tyrosine kinase important in T-cell signaling (Fig. 8) (274,275). The gene is on chromosome 2 at position q12. ZAP70 has been shown to have an essential role in both positive and negative selection in the thymus (Table 1) (277). The hypothesis to explain why there are normal numbers of CD4$^+$ T cells is that thymocytes can use the other member of the same tyrosine kinase family, Syk, to facilitate positive selection of CD4$^+$ cells. In addition, there is a stronger association of Lck with CD4$^+$ than with CD8$^+$ cells. Syk is present at fourfold higher levels in thymocytes than in peripheral T cells, possibly accounting for the lack of normal responses by the CD4$^+$ blood T cells.

CD8 Deficiency Resulting from a Mutation in the CD8α Gene

A new cause of CD8 deficiency (in addition to ZAP70 deficiency and MHC class I antigen deficiency) was discovered in a 25-year-old Spanish man with a history of recurrent respiratory infections since childhood. Immunoglobulins and antibodies were normal, as were T-cell proliferation studies and NK-cell function. However, he was found to have a complete absence of CD8$^+$ T cells. Molecular studies revealed a missense mutation in both alleles of the immunoglobulin domain of the CD8a gene in the patient and in two of his sisters (278).

Defective Expression of the T-Cell Receptor–CD3 Complex (Ti-CD3)

The first type of this disorder was found in two male siblings in a Spanish family (279). The proband presented with severe infections and died at 31 months of age with autoimmune hemolytic anemia and viral pneumonia. His lymphocytes had responded poorly to mitogens and to anti-CD3 *in vitro* and could not be stimulated to develop cytotoxic T cells. However, his antibody responses to protein antigens had been normal, indicating normal Th cell function. His 12-year-old brother was healthy but had almost no CD3-bearing T cells and IgG2 deficiency similar to that of his sibling. The defect in this family was shown to result from mutations in the CD3 γ chain (Table 1) (279). The second phenotype of CD3 deficiency was found in a 4-year-old French boy who had recurrent *Haemophilus influenzae* pneumonia and otitis media in early life but then remained healthy. He had a partial defect in expression of CD3-Ti, resulting in an about half-normal percentage of CD3$^+$ cells, all with very low CD3 staining on flow cytometry. His T cells did not proliferate in response to anti-CD3 or anti-CD2, nor did they express the IL-2 receptor or have normal calcium influx after these treatments. However, they did respond normally to co-stimulation with anti-CD28 or antigens, such as tetanus toxoid (280). The defect was shown to result from two independent CD3ϵ gene mutations, leading to defective CD3 ϵ-chain synthesis and preventing normal association and membrane expression of the T-cell receptor/CD3ϵ complex (Table 1) (281).

Defective Cytokine Production

Other than IL-12 deficiency, only a few human patients have been reported with defects in cytokine production. A selective inability to produce IL-2 was reported in two infants who had severe recurrent infections (282,283). The IL-2 gene was present in both, but no IL-2 message or protein was produced. Other T-cell cytokines were produced normally. Defective transcription of several lymphokine genes, including IL-2, IL-3, IL-4, and IL-5, attributed to abnormal binding of nuclear factor of activated T cells (NF-AT) to response element in IL-2 and IL-4 enhancer was reported in a single patient who also presented during infancy with severe recurrent infections and failure to thrive (284). Two male infants born to consanguineous parents had SCID-like infection susceptibility despite phenotypically normal blood lymphocytes, but their T cells were unable to produce IL-2, IFN-γ, IL-4, or TNF-α. Electrophoretic mobility shift assays revealed that the binding of NF-AT to its IL-2 promoter response element was barely detectable before and after T-cell stimulation (285). The findings in the latter two reports suggest that defective NF-AT/DNA binding was responsible for the multiple cytokine deficiencies in these cases. The molecular defects have not been identified in any of these patients.

HYPERIMMUNOGLOBULINEMIA E (HYPER IgE) SYNDROME

The hyperimmunoglobulinemia E (hyper IgE) syndrome is a relatively rare primary immunodeficiency syndrome characterized by recurrent severe staphylococcal abscesses of the skin, lungs, and viscera and greatly elevated levels of serum IgE (286,287). The disorder was first reported by the author in two young boys in 1972 (286); since then, I have evaluated more than 40 patients with the condition, and many other examples have been reported (287). These patients all have histories of staphylococcal abscesses involving the skin, lungs, joints, and other sites from infancy; persistent pneumatoceles develop as a result of their recurrent pneumonias. The pruritic dermatitis that occurs is not typical atopic eczema, and it does not always persist; respiratory allergic symptoms are usually absent. I noted coarse facial features in the first two patients (286), and this has been a consistent feature of all the patients I have evaluated with this syndrome. Patients with hyper IgE syndrome look very different from their nonaffected family members. Distinctive facial characteristics were again pointed out by Grimbacher and his associates (288). Among the findings reported were a prominent forehead, deep-set eyes, a broad nasal bridge, a wide fleshy nasal tip, mild prognathism, facial asymmetry, and hemihypertrophy. These investigators also found that the mean nasal interalar distance in these patients was greater than the 98th percentile ($p < .001$). These findings were present in all patients in that study by age 16 years (288). High incidences of scoliosis and hyperextensible joints were also noted. An interesting observation in that group of patients that had not been previously reported was a 72% incidence of failure or delayed shedding of the primary teeth, owing to lack of root resorption (288). Unexplained osteopenia is also present in most patients with the hyper IgE syndrome, many of whom have problems with recurrent fractures from even minor trauma (288,289).

Laboratory features include the following: exceptionally high serum IgE; elevated serum IgD; usually normal concentrations of IgG, IgA, and IgM; pronounced blood and sputum eosinophilia; abnormally low anamnestic antibody responses to booster immunizations; and poor antibody-mediated and cell-mediated responses to neoantigens. *In vitro* studies have shown normal percentages of CD2$^+$, CD3$^+$, CD4$^+$, and CD8$^+$ lymphocytes, and there is no increase in the percentage of IgE-bearing B lymphocytes. Most patients have normal lymphocyte-proliferative responses to mitogens but very low or absent responses to antigens or allogeneic cells from family members. Blood, sputum, and histologic sections of lymph nodes, spleen, and lung cysts show striking eosinophilia. Hassall's corpuscles and normal thymic architecture were observed at postmortem examination of one patient. Phagocytic cell ingestion, metabolism, killing, and total hemolytic complement activity have been normal in all patients. Variable defects of mononuclear or polymorphonuclear chemotaxis have been present in some but not all patients and hence are not the basic problem in these patients (287).

The fundamental problem in this condition is unknown despite intense study. I have observed a decreased percentage of T cells with the memory (CD45RO) phenotype in the blood of these patients, and such a decrease possibly is related to these patients' impaired anamnestic antibody responses, impaired antigen-specific T-cell responses, and abnormal mixed leukocyte responses. Paradoxically, B cells from these patients do not produce as much IgE as normal or atopic B cells do when they are cultured with IL-4 and anti-CD40 *in vitro* (290). The latter indicates that the B cells may have already been exposed to IL-4 *in vivo* and were no longer sensitive to it because they had already isotype-switched *in vivo*. Because of the very short half-life of IL-4, serum levels cannot be detected; therefore, it has been difficult to prove that the condition is caused by excessive IL-4 production. The presence of increased numbers of eosinophils in blood, sputum, and tissues is suggestive that some of the pathologic features seen may be eosinophil mediated. The finding that both men and women have been affected, as have members of succeeding generations, is suggestive of an autosomal dominant form of inheritance with incomplete penetrance. The hyper IgE syndrome has been mapped to chromosome 4, but a candidate gene has not yet been identified (291).

The most effective management for this condition is long-term therapy with a penicillinase-resistant penicillin or cephalosporin, with the addition of other antibiotics or antifungal agents as required for specific infections, and appropriate thoracic surgery for superinfected pneumatoceles or those persisting beyond 6 months. IFN-γ therapy has been tried but has had no clinical benefit (292). If the diagnosis is made early and antistaphylococcal antibiotic therapy is rendered in treatment doses continuously, the prognosis is good. The prognosis is poor, primarily because of progressive lung disease, in patients who are not so treated. Three patients are known to have died of lymphoreticular malignant disease, and three have experienced cryptococcal meningitis.

STAT4 Knockout Mice

Of potential relevance to the fundamental problem in patients with the hyper IgE syndrome are mice that were made deficient in the STAT4 protein by gene targeting. This protein is tyrosine phosphorylated only after stimulation of T cells with IL-12. STAT4-deficient mice were found have a disruption of all IL-12 functions, including the induction of IFN-γ, mitogenesis, enhancement of NK cytolytic function, and Th1 differentiation. As a consequence, they have a Th2 dominance because of their failure to produce IFN-γ in response to IL-12 (293,294). STAT4 deficiency could thus be one potential fundamental cause of human diseases characterized by Th2 dominance, such as the hyper IgE syndrome. Alternately, some other component of the signaling pathway for IL-12 could be at fault.

CONCLUSIONS

Since the discovery of XLA in 1952, more than 100 genetically determined immunodeficiencies have been identified, and the list is rapidly growing. Research has led to major breakthroughs in the definition of the molecular bases of many of these disorders and, undoubtedly, this will soon be the case for many others. This information will obviously be of great value in clarifying variant forms of these diseases, in carrier detection, in prenatal diagnosis, and, one hopes, eventually in permitting gene therapy for many of these conditions (177).

In addition to the knowledge gained about the immune system from studying the clinical and immunologic features of these rare patients, even greater information about the functioning of the immune system should come from the integrated and comparative study of immune abnormalities in patients and from studies of gene-targeted mutant mice. In addition, these studies should lead to the design of more specific and effective therapies.

Although treatment of these rare defects has not advanced quite as rapidly as the discovery of newer primary immunodeficiency diseases and the fundamental causes of many of them, major therapeutic advances have been made since the early 1980s. These include (a) the development of safe intravenous forms of human immunoglobulin that make it possible to deliver high quantities of missing antibodies to antibody-deficient patients, (b) the development of T-cell–depletion techniques that permit the use of half-matched parents as donors of corrective stem cells for human infants with SCID, and (c) the outstanding success in gene therapy in human SCID-X1. However, the problem of insertional mutagenesis is a major obstacle to the further application of retroviral gene transfer therapy. The creation of human chimeras by nonablative allogeneic bone marrow stem cell transplantation has made it possible to study early human T-, B-, and NK-cell ontogeny, tolerance induction, and MHC restriction mechanisms (i.e. "thymic education") in a manner heretofore not possible. In the next few years, human patients with genetically determined immunodeficiency diseases, as well as artificially created immunodeficient animals, will undoubtedly provide many more insights into the normal workings of the immune system.

REFERENCES

1. Glanzmann E, Riniker P. Essentielle Lymphocytophtose: ein neues Krankeitsbild aus der Sauglingspathologie. *Ann Paediatr* 1950;174:1–5.
2. Bruton OC. Agammaglobulinemia. *Pediatrics* 1952;9:722–728.
3. Ochs HD, Smith CIE, Puck JM, eds. *Primary immunodeficiency diseases: a molecular and genetic approach.* New York: Oxford University Press, 1999.
4. International Union of Immunological Societies. Primary immunodeficiency diseases: report of an IUIS Scientific Committee. *Clin Exp Immunol* 1999;118[Suppl 1]:1–28.
5. Buckley RH. Primary immunodeficiency diseases due to defects in lymphocytes. *N Engl J Med* 2000;343:1313–1324.
6. Kokron CM, Bonilla FA, Oettgen HC, et al. Searching for genes involved in the pathogenesis of primary immunodeficiency diseases: lessons from mouse knockouts. *J Clin Immunol* 1997;17:109–126.
7. Elenitoba-Johnson KSJ, Jaffe ES. Lymphoproliferative disorders associated with congenital immunodeficiencies. *Semin Diagn Pathol* 1997;14:35–47.
8. Clark JA, Callicoat PA, Brenner NA. Selective IgA deficiency in blood donors. *Am J Clin Pathol* 1983;80:210–213.
9. Buckley RH. Clinical and immunologic features of selective IgA deficiency. In: Bergsma D, Good RA, Finstad J, et al, eds. *Immunodeficiency in man and animals.* Stamford, CT: Sinauer Associates, 1975:134–142.
10. Dinauer MC, Orkin SH, Brown R. The glycoprotein encoded by the X-linked chronic granulomatous disease locus is a component of the neutrophil cytochrome b complex. *Nature* 1987;327:717.
11. Westberg J, Fredrikson GN, Truedsson L, et al. Sequence-based analysis of properdin deficiency: identification of point mutations in two phenotypic forms of an X-linked immunodeficiency. *Genomics* 1995;29:1–8.
12. Bennett CL, Ochs HD. IPEX is a unique X-linked syndrome characterized by immune dysfunction, polyendocrinopathy, enteropathy, and a variety of autoimmune phenomena. *Curr Opin Pediatr* 2001;13:533–538.
13. Chatila TA, Blaeser F, Ho N, et al. JM2, encoding a fork head-related protein, is mutated in X-linked autoimmunity-allergic disregulation syndrome. *J Clin Invest* 2000;106:R75–R81.
14. Conley ME, Rohrer J, Minegishi Y. X-linked agammaglobulinemia. *Clin Rev Allergy Immunol* 2000;19:183–204.
15. Buckley RH, Rowlands DR. Allergy rounds: agammaglobulinemia, neutropenia, fever and abdominal pain. *J Allergy Clin Immunol* 1973;51:308–318.
16. Wilfert CM, Buckley RH, Mohanakumar T, et al. Persistent and fatal central nervous system echovirus infections in patients with agammaglobulinemia. *N Engl J Med* 1977;296:1485–1489.
17. McKinney RE, Katz SL, Wilfert CM. Chronic enteroviral meningoencephalitis in agammaglobulinemic patients. *Rev Infect Dis* 1987;9:334–356.
18. Roberts D, Murray AE, Pratt BC, et al. Mycoplasma hominis as a respiratory pathogen in X-linked hypogammaglobulinemia. *J Infect* 1989;18:175–177.
19. Mohiuddin AA, Corren J, Harbeck RJ, et al. Ureaplasma urealyticum chronic osteomyelitis in a patient with hypogammaglobulinemia. *J Allergy Clin Immunol* 1991;87:104–107.
20. Vetrie D, Vorechovsky I, Sideras P, et al. The gene involved in X-linked agammaglobulinaemia is a member of the src family of protein-tyrosine kinases. *Nature* 1993;361:226–233.
21. Tsukada S, Saffran DC, Rawlings DJ, et al. Deficient expression of a B cell cytoplasmic tyrosine kinase in human X-linked agammaglobulinemia. *Cell* 1993;72:279–290.
22. Kitanaka A, Mano H, Conley ME, et al. Expression and activation of the nonreceptor tyrosine kinase Tec in human B cells. *Blood* 1998;91:940–948.
23. de Weers M, Verschuren MCM, Kraakman MEM, et al. The Bruton's tyrosine kinase gene is expressed throughout B cell differentiation, from early precursor B cell stages preceding immunoglobulin gene rearrangement up to mature B cell stages. *Eur J Immunol* 1993;23:3109–3114.
24. Conley ME, Rohrer J, Minegishi Y. X-linked agammaglobulinemia. *Clin Rev Allergy Immunol* 2000;19:183–204.
25. Haire RN, Ohta Y, Strong SJ, et al. Unusual patterns of exon skipping in Bruton tyrosine kinase are associated with mutations involving the intron 17 3′ splice site. *Am J Hum Genet* 1997;60:798–807.
26. Vihinen M, Arredondo-Vega FX, Casanova JL, et al. Primary immunodeficiency mutation databases. *Adv Genet* 2001;43:103–188.
27. Vihinen M, Kwan SP, Lester T, et al. Mutations of the human BTK gene coding for bruton tyrosine kinase in X-linked agammaglobulinemia. *Hum Mutat* 1999;13:280–285.
28. Puck JM. Molecular and genetic basis of X-linked immunodeficiency disorders. *J Clin Immunol* 1994;14:81–89.
29. Sideras P, Smith CIE. Molecular and cellular aspects of X-linked agammaglobulinemia. *Adv Immunol* 1995;59:135–223.
30. Farrar JE, Rohrer J, Conley ME. Neutropenia in X-linked agammaglobulinemia. *Clin Immunol Immunopathol* 1996;81:271–276.
31. Conley ME, Burks AW, Herrod HG, et al. Molecular analysis of X-linked agammaglobulinemia with growth hormone deficiency. *J Pediatr* 1991;119:392–397.
32. Fleisher TA, White RM, Broder S, et al. X-linked hypogammaglobulinemia and isolated growth hormone deficiency. *N Engl J Med* 1980;302:1429–1434.
33. Sitz KV, Burks AW, Williams LW, et al. Confirmation of X-linked hypogammaglobulinemia with isolated growth hormone deficiency as a disease entity. *J Pediatr* 1990;116:292–294.
34. Monafo V, Maghnie M, Terracciano L, et al. X-linked agammaglobulinemia and isolated growth hormone deficiency. *Acta Paediatr Scand* 1991;80:563–566.
35. Scher I. The CBA/N mouse strain: an experimental model illustrating the influence of X-chromosome on immunity. *Adv Immunol* 1982;33:1.
36. Hasbold J, Klaus GG. B cells from CBA/N mice do not proliferate following ligation of CD40. *Eur J Immunol* 1997;24:152–157.
37. Thomas JD, Sideras P, Smith CIE, et al. Colocalization of X-linked agammaglobulinemia and X-linked immunodeficiency genes. *Science* 1993;261:355–361.
38. Rawlings DJ, Saffran DC, Tsudaka S, et al. Mutation of unique region of Bruton's tyrosine kinase in immunodeficient XID mice. *Science* 1993;261:358.
39. de Weers M, Mensink RGJ, Kraakman MEM, et al. Mutation analysis of the Bruton's tyrosine kinase gene in X-linked agammaglobulinemia: identification of a mutation which affects the same codon as is

altered in immunodeficient xid mice. *Hum Mol Genet* 1994;3:161–166.

40. Conley ME, Sweinberg SK. Females with a disorder phenotypically identical to X-linked agammaglobulinemia. *J Clin Immunol* 1992;12:139–143.

41. Gaspar HB, Conley ME. Early B cell defects. *Clin Exp Immunol* 2000;119:383–389.

42. Meffre E, LeDeist F, de Saint Basile G, et al. A human non-XLA immunodeficiency disease characterized by blockage of B cell development at an early proB cell stage. *J Clin Invest* 1996;98:1519–1526.

43. Yel L, Minegishi Y, Coustan-Smith E, et al. Mutations in the mu heavy chain gene in patients with agammaglobulinemia. *N Engl J Med* 1996;335:1486–1493.

44. Minegishi Y, Coustan-Smith E, Wang YH, et al. Mutations in the human lambda 5/14.1 gene result in B cell deficiency and agammaglobulinemia. *J Exp Med* 1998;187:71–77.

45. Minegishi Y, Coustan-Smith E, Rapalus L, et al. Mutations in Ig alpha (CD79a) result in a complete block in B-cell development. *J Clin Invest* 1999;104:1115–1121.

46. Minegishi Y, Rohrer J, Coustan-Smith E, et al. An essential role for BLNK in human B cell development. *Science* 1999;286:1954–1957.

47. Lefranc MP, Hammarstrom L, Smith CIE, et al. Gene deletions in the human immunoglobulin heavy chain constant region locus: molecular and immunological analysis. *Immunol Rev* 1991;2:265–281.

48. Notarangelo LD, Duse M, Ugazio AG. Immunodeficiency with hyper-IgM (HIM). *Immunodef Rev* 1992;3:101–121.

49. Levy J, Espanol-Boren T, Thomas C, et al. Clinical spectrum of X-linked hyper IgM syndrome. *J Pediatr* 1997;131:47–54.

50. Ramesh N, Geha RS, Notarangelo LD. CD40 ligand and the hyper IgM syndrome. In: Ochs HD, Smith CIE, Puck JM, eds. *Primary immunodeficiency diseases: a molecular and genetic approach.* New York: Oxford University Press, 1999:233–249.

51. Mayer L, Swan SP, Thompson C. Evidence for a defect in "switch" T cells in patients with immunodeficiency and hyperimmunoglobulinemia M. *N Engl J Med* 1986;314:409–413.

52. Padayachee M, Feighery C, Finn A, et al. Mapping of the X-linked form of hyper IgM syndrome (HIGM1) to Xq26 by close linkage to HPRT. *Genomics* 1992;14:551–553.

53. Allen RC, Armitage RJ, Conley ME, et al. CD40 ligand gene defects responsible for X-linked hyper IgM syndrome. *Science* 1993;259:990–993.

54. Korthauer U, Graf D, Mages HW. Defective expression of T cell CD40 ligand causes X-linked immunodeficiency with hyper IgM. *Nature* 1993;361:539–541.

55. Di Santo JP, Bonnefoy JY, Gauchat JF, et al. CD40 ligand mutations in X-linked immunodeficiency with hyper IgM. *Nature* 1993;361:541–543.

56. Aruffo A, Farrington M, Hollenbaugh D, et al. The CD40 ligand, gp39, is defective in activated T cells from patients with X-linked hyper IgM syndrome. *Cell* 1993;72:291–300.

57. Noelle RJ, Roy M, Shepherd DM, et al. A 39–kDa protein on activated helper T cells binds CD40 and transduces the signal for cognate activation of B cells. *Proc Natl Acad Sci USA* 1992;89:6550–6554.

58. Agematsu K, Nagumo H, Shinozaki K, et al. Absence of IgD-CD27(+) memory B cell population in X-linked hyper-IgM syndrome. *J Clin Invest* 1998;102:853–860.

59. Facchetti F, Appiani C, Salvi L, et al. Immunohistologic analysis of ineffective CD40–CD40 ligand interaction in lymphoid tissues from patients with X-linked immunodeficiency with hyper IgM. *J Immunol* 1995;154:6624–6633.

60. Yang Y, Wilson JM. CD40 ligand-dependent T cell activation: requirement of B7–CD28 signaling through CD40. *Science* 1996;273:1862–1864.

61. Disanto JP, Markiewicz S, Gauchat JF, et al. Brief report: prenatal diagnosis of X-linked hyper-IgM syndrome. *N Engl J Med* 1994;330:969–973.

62. Buckley RH, Fischer A. Bone marrow transplantation for primary immunodeficiency diseases. In: Ochs HD, Smith CIE, Puck JM, eds. *Primary immunodeficiency diseases: a molecular and genetic approach.* New York: Oxford University Press, 1999:459–475.

63. Khawaja K, Gennery AR, Flood TJ, et al. Bone marrow transplantation for CD40 ligand deficiency: a single centre experience. *Arch Dis Child* 2001;84:508–511.

64. Buckley RH, Schiff RI. The use of intravenous immunoglobulin in immunodeficiency diseases. *N Engl J Med* 1991;325:110–117.

65. Wang WC, Cordoba J, Infante AJ, et al. Successful treatment of neutropenia in the hyper-immunoglobulin M syndrome with granulocyte colony-stimulating factor. *Am J Pediatr Hematol Oncol* 1994;16:160–163.

66. Doffinger R, Smahi A, Bessia C, et al. X-linked anhidrotic ectodermal dysplasia with immunodeficiency is caused by impaired NF-kappaB signaling. *Nat Genet* 2001;27:277–285.

67. Jain A, Ma CA, Liu S, et al. Specific missense mutations in NEMO result in hyper-IgM syndrome with hypohydrotic ectodermal dysplasia. *Nat Immunol* 2001;2:223–228.

68. Srahna M, Remacle JE, Annamalai K, et al. NF-kappaB is involved in the regulation of CD154 (CD40 ligand) expression in primary human T cells. *Clin Exp Immunol* 2001;125:229–236.

69. Conley ME, Larche M, Bonagura VR, et al. Hyper IgM syndrome associated with defective CD40–mediated B cell activation. *J Clin Invest* 1994;94:1404–1409.

70. Oliva A, Quinti I, Scala E, et al. Immunodeficiency with hyperimmunoglobulinemia M in two female patients is not associated with abnormalities of CD40 or CD40 ligand expression. *J Allergy Clin Immunol* 1995;96:403–410.

71. Minegishi Y, Lavoie A, Cunningham-Rundles C, et al. Mutations in activation-induced cytidine deaminase in patients with hyper IgM syndrome. *Clin Immunol* 2000;97:203–210.

72. Revy P, Muto T, Levy Y, et al. Activation-induced cytidine deaminase (AID) deficiency causes the autosomal recessive form of the Hyper-IgM syndrome (HIGM2). *Cell* 2000;102:565–575.

73. Ferrari S, Giliani S, Insalaco A, et al. Mutations of CD40 gene cause an autosomal recessive form of immunodeficiency with hyper IgM. *Proc Natl Acad Sci USA* 2001;98:12614–12619.

74. Sullivan JL, Woda BA. X-linked lymphoproliferative syndrome. *Immunodef Rev* 1989;1:325–347.

75. Grierson HL, Skare J, Hawk J, et al. Immunoglobulin class and subclass deficiencies prior to Epstein-Barr virus infection in males with X-linked lymphoproliferative disease. *Am J Med Genet* 1991;40:294–297.

76. Coffey AJ, Brooksbank RA, Brandau O, et al. Host response to EBV infection in X-linked lymphoproliferative disease results from mutations in an SH2–domain encoding gene. *Nat Genet* 1998;20:129–135.

77. Nichols KE, Harkin DP, Levitz S, et al. Inactivating mutations in an SH2 domain-encoding gene in X-linked lymphoproliferative syndrome. *Proc Natl Acad Sci USA* 1998;95:13765–13770.

78. Sayos J, Wu C, Morra M, et al. The X-linked lymphoproliferative-disease gene product SAP regulates signals induced through the co-receptor SLAM. *Nature* 1998;395:462–469.

79. Wu C, Sayos J, Wang N, et al. Genomic organization and characterization of mouse SAP, the gene that is altered in X-linked lymphoproliferative disease. *Immunogenetics* 2000;51:805–815.

80. Nagy N, Cerboni C, Mattsson K, et al E. SH2D1A and SLAM protein expression in human lymphocytes and derived cell lines. *Int J Cancer* 2000;88:439–447.

81. Sayos J, Martin M, Chen A, et al. Cell surface receptors Ly-9 and CD84 recruit the X-linked lymphoproliferative disease gene product SAP. *Blood* 2001;97:3867–3874.

82. Tangye SG, Lazetic S, Woollatt E, et al. Cutting edge: human 2B4, an activating NK cell receptor, recruits the protein tyrosine phosphatase SHP-2 and the adaptor signaling protein SAP. *J Immunol* 1999;162:6981–6985.

83. Thompson AD, Braun BS, Arvand A, et al. EAT-2 is a novel SH2 domain containing protein that is up regulated by Ewing's sarcoma EWS/FLI1 fusion gene. *Oncogene* 1996;13:2649–2658.

84. Howie D, Sayos J, Terhorst C, et al. The gene defective in X-linked lymphoproliferative disease controls T cell dependent immune surveillance against Epstein-Barr virus. *Curr Opin Immunol* 2000;12:474–478.

85. Morra M, Howie D, Grande MS, et al. X-linked lymphoproliferative disease: a progressive immunodeficiency. *Annu Rev Immunol* 2001;19:657–682.

86. Morra M, Silander O, Calpe-Flores S, et al. Alterations of the X-linked lymphoproliferative disease gene *SH2D1A* in common variable immunodeficiency syndrome. *Blood* 2001;98:1321–1325.

87. Cunningham-Rundles C, Bodian C. Common variable immunodeficiency: clinical and immunological features of 248 patients. *Clin Immunol* 1999;92:34–48.

88. Cunningham-Rundles C, Siegal FP, Cunningham-Rundles S, et al. Incidence of cancer in 98 patients with common varied immunodeficiency. *J Clin Immunol* 1987;7:294–298.

89. Nonoyama S, Farrington M, Ochs HM. Activated B cells from patients with common variable immunodeficiency proliferate and synthesize immunoglobulin. *J Clin Invest* 1993;92:1281–1287.

90. Punnonen J, Kainulainen L, Ruuskanen O, et al. IL-4 synergizes with IL-10 and anti-CD40 MoAbs to induce B cell differentiation in patients with common variable immunodeficiency. *Scand J Immunol* 1997;45:203–212.

91. Katial RK, Lieberman MM, Muehlbauer SL, et al. $\gamma\delta$ T lymphocytosis associated with common variable immunodeficiency. *J Clin Immunol* 1997;17:34–42.

92. Fischer MB, Wolf HM, Hauber I, et al. Activation via the antigen receptor is impaired in T cells, but not in B cells from patients with common variable immunodeficiency. *Eur J Immunol* 1996;26:231–237.

93. Eisenstein EM, Jaffe JS, Strober W. Reduced interleukin-2 (IL-2) production in common variable immunodeficiency is due to a primary abnormality of CD4+ T cell differentiation. *J Clin Immunol* 1993;13:247–258.

94. Kondratenko I, Amlot PL, Webster ADB, et al. Lack of specific antibody response in common variable immunodeficiency (CVID) associated with failure in production of antigen-specific memory T cells. *Clin Exp Immunol* 1997;108:9–13.

95. Farrington M, Grosmaire LS, Nonoyama S, et al. CD40 ligand expression is defective in a subset of patients with common variable immunodeficiency. *Proc Natl Acad Sci USA* 1994;91:1099–1103.

96. Baum CG, Chiorazzi N, Frankel S, et al. Conversion of systemic lupus erythematosus to common variable hypogammaglobulinemia. *Am J Med* 1989;87:449–456.

97. Wright JJ, Birx DL, Wagner DK, et al. Normalization of antibody responsiveness in a patient with common variable hypogammaglobulinemia and HIV infection. *N Engl J Med* 1987;317:1516–1519.

98. Slyper AH, Pietryga D. Conversion of selective IgA deficiency to common variable immunodeficiency in an adolescent female with 18q deletion syndrome. *Eur J Pediatr* 1997;155:155–159.

99. Ashman RF, Schaffer FM, Kemp JD, et al. Genetic and immunologic analysis of a family containing five patients with common variable immune deficiency or selective IgA deficiency. *J Clin Immunol* 1992;12:406–414.

100. Truedsson L, Baskin B, Pan Q, et al. Genetics of IgA deficiency. *APMIS* 1995;103:833–842.

100a. Grimbacher B, Hutloff A, Schlesier M, Glocker E, Warnatz K, Drager R, Eibel H, Fischer B, Schaffer AA, Mages HW, Kroczek RA, Peter HH. Homozygous loss of ICOS is associated with adult-onset common variable immunodeficiency. *Nat Immunol* 2003;4:261–268.

101. Schaffer FM, Monteiro RC, Volanakis JE, et al. IgA deficiency. *Immunodef Rev* 1991;3:15–44.

102. Volanakis JE, Zhu Z-B, Schaffer FM, et al. Major histocompatibility complex class III genes and susceptibility to immunoglobulin A deficiency and common variable immunodeficiency. *J Clin Invest* 1992;89:1914–1922.

103. Fiore M, Pera C, Delfino L, et al. DNA typing of DQ and DR alleles in IgA deficient subjects. *Eur J Immunogenet* 1995;22:403–411.

104. Oxelius VA, Laurell AB, Lindquist B. IgG subclasses in selective IgA deficiency. *N Engl J Med* 1981;304:1476–1477.

105. Burks AW, Sampson HA, Buckley RH. Anaphylactic reactions after gamma globulin administration in patients with hypogammaglobulinemia. *N Engl J Med* 1986;314:560–564.

106. Buckley RH, Dees SC. The correlation of milk precipitins with IgA deficiency. *N Engl J Med* 1969;281:465–469.

107. Goshen E, Livne A, Krupp M, et al. Antinuclear and related autoantibodies in sera of healthy subjects with IgA deficiency. *J Autoimmun* 1989;2:51–60.

108. Briere F, Bridon JM, Chevet D, et al. Interleukin 10 induces B lymphocytes from IgA-deficient patients to secrete IgA. *J Clin Invest* 1994;94:97–104.

109. Friman V, Hanson LA, Bridon JM, et al. IL-10–driven immunoglobulin production by B lymphocytes from IgA-deficient individuals correlates to infection proneness. *Clin Exp Immunol* 1996;104:432–438.

110. Leickly FE, Buckley RH. Development of IgA and IgG2 subclass deficiency after sulfasalazine therapy. *J Pediatr* 1986;108:481–482.

111. Plebani A, Monafo V, Ugazio AG, et al. Clinical heterogeneity and reversibility of selective immunoglobulin A deficiency in 80 children. *Lancet* 1986;1:829–831.

112. DeLaat PCJ, Weemaes CMR, Bakkeren JAJM. Immunoglobulin levels during follow-up of children with selective IgA deficiency. *Scand J Immunol* 1992;35:719–725.

113. Preud'Homme JL, Hanson LA. IgG subclass deficiency. *Immunodef Rev* 1990;2:129–149.

114. Cunningham-Rundles C, Fotino M, Rosina O, et al. Selective IgA deficiency, IgG subclass deficiency, and the major histocompatibility complex. *Clin Immunol Immunopathol* 1991;61:S61–S69.

115. Shield JPH, Strobel S, Levinsky RJ, et al. Immunodeficiency presenting as hypergammaglobulinaemia with IgG2 subclass deficiency. *Lancet* 1992;340:448–450.

116. Ambrosino DM, Umetsu DT, Siber GR, et al. Selective defect in the antibody response to *Haemophilus influenzae* type b in children with recurrent infections and normal IgG subclass levels. *J Allergy Clin Immunol* 1988;81:1175–1179.

117. Shackelford PG. IgG subclasses: Importance in pediatric practice. *Pediatr Rev* 1993;14:291–296.

118. Shackelford PG, Granoff DM, Polmar SH, et al. Subnormal serum concentrations of IgG2 in children with frequent infections associated with varied patters of immunologic dysfunction. *J Pediatr* 1990;116:529–538.

119. Hong R. The DiGeorge anomaly. *Immunodef Rev* 1991;3:1–14.

120. Demczuk S, Aurias A. DiGeorge syndrome and related syndromes associated with 22q11.2 deletions: a review. *Ann Genet* 1995;38:59–76.

121. Cormier-Daire V, Iserin L, Theophile D, et al. Upper limb malformations in DiGeorge syndrome. *Am J Med Genet* 1995;56:39–41.

122. Junker AK, Driscoll DA. Humoral immunity in DiGeorge syndrome. *J Pediatr* 1995;127:231–237.

123. Jawad AF, McDonald-McGinn DM, Zackai E, et al. Immunologic features of chromosome 22q11.2 deletion syndrome (DiGeorge syndrome/velocardiofacial syndrome). *J Pediatr* 2001;139:715–723.

124. Gong W, Emanuel BS, Collins J, et al. A transcription map of the DiGeorge and velo-cardio-facial syndrome minimal critical region on 22q11. *Hum Mol Genet* 1996;5:789–800.

125. Driscoll DA, Sullivan KE. DiGeorge syndrome: a chromosome 22q11.2 deletion syndrome. In: Ochs HD, Smith CIE, Puck JM, eds. *Primary immunodeficiency diseases: a molecular and genetic approach.* New York: Oxford University Press, 1999:198–208.

126. Webber SA, Hatchwell E, Barber JCK, et al. Importance of microdeletions of chromosomal region 22q11 as a cause of selected malformations of the ventricular outflow tracts and aortic arch: a three year prospective study. *J Pediatr* 1996;129:26–32.

127. Budarf ML, Collins J, Gong W, et al. Cloning a balanced translocation associated with DiGeorge syndrome and identification of a disrupted candidate gene. *Nat Genet* 1995;10:269–278.

128. Kkurahashi H, Akagi K, Inazawa J, et al. Isolation and characterization of a novel gene deleted in DiGeorge syndrome. *Hum Mol Genet* 1995;4:541–549.

129. Llevadot R, Scambler P, Estivill X, et al. Genomic organization of TUPLE1/HIRA: a gene implicated in DiGeorge syndrome. *Mamm Genome* 1996;7:911–914.

130. Demczuk SLA, Aubry M, Croquette M, et al. Excess of deletions of maternal origin in the DiGeorge/velo-cardio-facial syndromes: a study of 22 new patients and review of the literature. *Hum Genet* 1995;96:9–13.

131. Daw SC, Taylor C, Kraman M, et al. A common region of 10p deleted in DiGeorge and velocardiofacial syndromes. *Nat Genet* 1996;13:458–460.

132. Schuffenhauer S, Seidel H, Oechsler H, et al. DiGeorge syndrome and partial monosomy 10p: case report and review. *Ann Genet* 1995;38:162–167.

133. Lipson A, Fagan K, Colley A, et al. Velo-cardio-facial and partial DiGeorge phenotype in a child with interstitial deletion at 10p13: implications for cytogenetics and molecular biology. *Am J Med Genet* 1996;65:304–306.

134. Goldsobel AB, Haas A, Stiehm ER. Bone marrow transplantation in DiGeorge syndrome. *J Pediatr* 1987;111:40–44.

135. Markert ML, Boeck A, Hale LP, et al. Thymus transplantation in complete DiGeorge syndrome. *N Engl J Med* 1999;341:1180–1189.

136. Buckley RH, Schiff RI, Schiff SE, et al. Human severe combined immunodeficiency (SCID): genetic, phenotypic and functional diversity in 108 infants. *J Pediatr* 1997;130:378–387.

137. Buckley RH. Advances in the understanding and treatment of human severe combined immunodeficiency. *Immunol Res* 2001;22:237–251.

138. Buckley RH, Schiff SE, Schiff RI, et al. Hematopoietic stem cell transplantation for the treatment of severe combined immunodeficiency. *N Engl J Med* 1999;340:508–516.

139. Myers LA, Patel DD, Puck JM, et al. Hematopoietic stem cell transplantation for severe combined immunodeficiency in the neonatal period leads to superior thymic output and improved survival. *Blood* 2002;99:872–878.

140. Altman PL. Blood leukocyte values: man. In: Dittmer DS, ed. *Blood and other body fluids.* Washington, DC: Federation of American Societies for Experimental Biology, 1961:125–126.

141. Patel DD, Gooding ME, Parrott RE, et al. Thymic function after hematopoietic stem-cell transplantation for the treatment of severe combined immunodeficiency. *N Engl J Med* 2000;342:1325–1332.

142. Fischer A. Severe combined immunodeficiencies (SCID). *Clin Exp Immunol* 2000;122:143–149.

143. Stephan JL, Vlekova V, Le Deist F, et al. Severe combined immunodeficiency: a retrospective single-center study of clinical presentation and outcome in 117 cases. *J Pediatr* 1993;123:564–572.

144. Conley ME, Buckley RH, Hong R, et al. X-linked severe combined immunodeficiency: diagnosis in males with sporadic severe combined immunodeficiency and clarification of clinical findings. *J Clin Invest* 1990;85:1548–1554.

145. Puck JM, Conley ME, Bailey LC. Refinement of linkage of human severe combined immunodeficiency (SCIDX1) to polymorphic markers in Xq13. *Am J Hum Genet* 1993;53:176–184.

146. Puck JM, Deschenes SM, Porter JC, et al. The interleukin-2 receptor gamma chain maps to Xq13.1 and is mutated in X-linked severe combined immunodeficiency, SCIDX1. *Hum Mol Genet* 1993;2:1099–1104.

147. Noguchi M, Yi H, Rosenblatt HM, et al. Interleukin-2 receptor gamma chain mutation results in X-linked severe combined immunodeficiency in humans. *Cell* 1993;73:147–157.

148. Vosshenrich CA, Di Santo JP. Cytokines: IL-21 joins the gamma(c)-dependent network? *Curr Biol* 2001;11:R175–R177.

149. Puck JM, Pepper AE, Henthorn PS, et al. Mutation analysis of IL2RG in human X-linked severe combined immunodeficiency. *Blood* 1997;89:1968–1977.

150. Russell SM, Keegan AD, Harada N, et al. Interleukin-2 receptor gamma chain: a functional component of the interleukin-4 receptor. *Science* 1993;262:1880–1883.

151. Noguchi M, Nakamura Y, Russell SM, et al. Interleukin-2 receptor gamma chain: a functional component of the interleukin-7 receptor. *Science* 1993;262:1977–1980.

152. Hirschhorn R. Immunodeficiency diseases due to deficiency of adenosine deaminase. In: Ochs HD, Smith CIE, Puck JM, eds. *Primary immunodeficiency diseases: a molecular and genetic approach.* New York: Oxford University Press, 1999:121–139.

153. Yin EZ, Frush DP, Donnelly LF, et al. Primary immunodeficiency disorders in pediatric patients: clinical features and imaging findings. *AJR Am J Roentgenol* 2001;176:1541–1552.

154. Hershfield MS, Buckley RH, Greenberg ML, et al. Treatment of adenosine deaminase deficiency with polyethylene glycol-modified adenosine deaminase (PEG-ADA). *N Engl J Med* 1987;316:589–596.

155. Hershfield MS. PEG-ADA: an alternative to haploidentical bone marrow transplantation and an adjunct to gene therapy for adenosine deaminase deficiency. *Hum Mutat* 1995;5:107–112.

156. Hershfield MS. PEG-ADA replacement therapy for adenosine deaminase deficiency: an update after 8.5 years. *Clin Immunol Immunopathol* 1995;76:S228–S232.

157. Kawamura M, McVicar DW, Johnston JA, et al. Molecular cloning of L-Jak, a Janus family protein tyrosine kinase expressed in natural killer cells and activated leukocytes. *Proc Natl Acad Sci USA* 1994;91:6374–6378.

158. Johnston JA, Kawamura M, Kirken RA, et al. Phosphorylation and

159. Russell SM, Johnston JA, Noguchi M, et al. Interaction of IL-2R beta and gamma c chains with Jak1 and Jak3: implications for XSCID and XCID. *Science* 1994;266:1042–1045.

160. Russell SM, Tayebi N, Nakajima H, et al. Mutation of Jak3 in a patient with SCID: essential role of Jak3 in lymphoid development. *Science* 1995;270:797–800.

161. Macchi P, Villa A, Gillani S, et al. Mutations of Jak-3 gene in patients with autosomal severe combined immune deficiency (SCID). *Nature* 1995;377:65–68.

162. Candotti F, Villa A, Notarangelo L. Severe combined immunodeficiency due to defects of JAK3 tyrosine kinase. In: Ochs HD, Smith CIE, Puck JM, eds. *Primary immunodeficiency diseases: a molecular and genetic approach.* New York: Oxford University Press, 1999:111–120.

163. Puel A, Ziegler SF, Buckley RH, et al. Defective IL7R expression in T(−)B(+)NK(+) severe combined immunodeficiency. *Nat Genet* 1998;20:394–397.

164. Schwarz K, Gauss GH, Ludwig L, et al. RAG mutations in human B cell-negative SCID. *Science* 1996;274:97–99.

165. Schwarz K, Notarangelo L, Spanopoulou E, et al. Recombination defects. In: Ochs HD, Smith CIE, Puck JM, eds. *Primary immunodeficiency diseases: a molecular and genetic approach.* New York: Oxford University Press, 1999:155–166.

166. Corneo B, Moshous D, Gungor T, et al. Identical mutations in RAG1 or RAG2 genes leading to defective V(D)J recombinase activity can cause either T-B-severe combined immune deficiency or Omenn syndrome. *Blood* 2001;97:2772–2776.

167. Villa A, Santagata S, Bozzi F, et al. Partial V(D)J recombination activity leads to Omenn syndrome. *Cell* 1998;93:885–896.

168. Rieux-Laucat F, Bahadoran P, Brousse N, et al. Highly restricted human T cell repertoire in peripheral blood and tissue-infiltrating lymphocytes in Omenn's syndrome. *J Clin Invest* 1998;102:312–321.

169. Brooks EG, Filipovich AH, Padgett JW, et al. T-cell receptor analysis in Omenn's syndrome: evidence for defects in gene rearrangement and assembly. *Blood* 1999;93:242–250.

170. Martin JV, Willoughby PB, Giusti V, et al. The lymph node pathology of Omenn's syndrome. *Am J Surg Pathol* 1995;19:1082–1087.

171. Nicolas N, Moshous D, Cavazzana-Calvo M, et al. A human severe combined immunodeficiency (SCID) condition with increased sensitivity to ionizing radiations and impaired V(D)J rearrangements defines a new DNA recombination/repair deficiency. *J Exp Med* 1998;188:627–634.

172. Kung C, Pingel JT, Heikinheimo M, et al. Mutations in the tyrosine phosphatase CD45 gene in a child with severe combined immunodeficiency disease. *Nat Med* 2000;6:343–345.

173. Tchilian EZ, Wallace DL, Wells RS, et al. A deletion in the gene encoding the CD45 antigen in a patient with SCID. *J Immunol* 2001;166:1308–1313.

174. Kane L, Gennery AR, Crooks BN, et al. Neonatal bone marrow transplantation for severe combined immunodeficiency. *Arch Dis Child* 2001;85:F110–F113.

175. Candotti F. Gene therapy for immunodeficiency. *Curr Allergy Asthma Rep* 2001;1:407–415.

176. Candotti F. The potential for therapy of immune disorders with gene therapy. *Pediatr Clin North Am* 2000;47:1389–1407.

177. Fischer A, Hacein-Bey S, Le Deist F, et al. Gene therapy for human severe combined immunodeficiencies. *Immunity* 2001;15:1–4.

178. Cavazzana-Calvo M, Hacein-Bey S, deSaint Basile G, et al. Gene therapy of human severe combined immunodeficiency (SCID)-X1 disease. *Science* 2000;288:669–672.

179. Miller RD, Hogg J, Ozaki JH, et al. Gene for catalytic subunit of mouse DNA-dependent protein kinase maps to the scid locus. *Proc Natl Acad Sci USA* 1995;92:10792–10795.

180. Araki R, Fujimori A, Hamatani K, et al. Nonsense mutation at Tyr-4046 in the DNA-dependent protein kinase catalytic subunit of severe combined immune deficiency mice. *Proc Natl Acad Sci USA* 1997;94:2438–2443.

181. Itoh M, Hamatani K, Komatsu K, et al. Human chromosome 8(p12 - q22) complements radiosensitivity in the severe combined immune deficiency (SCID) mouse. *Radiat Res* 1993;134:364–368.

182. Felsburg PJ, Somberg RL, Perryman LE. Domestic animal models of severe combined immunodeficiency: canine X-linked severe

combined immunodeficiency and severe combined immunodeficiency in horses. *Immunodef Rev* 1992;3:277–303.

183. Markert ML. Purine nucleoside phosphorylase deficiency. *Immunodef Rev* 1991;3:45–81.

184. Pannicke U, Tuchschmid P, Friedrich W, et al. Two novel missense and frameshift mutations in exons 5 and 6 of the purine nucleoside phosphorylase (PNP) gene in a severe combined immunodeficiency (SCID) patient. *Hum Genet* 1996;98:706–709.

185. Broome CB, Graham ML, Saulsbury FT, et al. Correction of purine nucleoside phosphorylase deficiency by transplantation of allogeneic bone marrow from a sibling. *J Pediatr* 1996;128:373–376.

186. Gilad S, Chessa L, Khosravi R, et al. Genotype-phenotype relationships in ataxia telangiectasia and variants. *Am J Hum Genet* 1998; 62:551–561.

187. Taylor AMR, Metcalfe JA, Thick J, et al. Leukemia and lymphoma in ataxia telangiectasia. *Blood* 1996;87:423–438.

188. Watson HG, McLaren KM, Todd A, et al. Transfusion associated graft-versus-host disease in ataxia telangiectasia. *Lancet* 1997;349: 179.

189. Gatti RA, Boder E, Vinters HV, et al. Ataxia-telangiectasia: an interdisciplinary approach to pathogenesis. *Medicine (Baltimore)* 1991; 70:99–117.

190. Beamish H, Williams R, Chen P, et al. Defect in multiple cell cycle checkpoints in ataxia telangiectasia postirradiation. *J Biol Chem* 1996; 271:20486–20493.

191. Savitsky K, Bar-Shira A, Gilad S, et al. A single ataxia telangiectasia gene with a product similar to PI-3 kinase. *Science* 1995;268:1749–1753.

192. Lavin MF, Shiloh Y. Ataxia telangiectasia. In: Ochs HD, Smith CIE, Puck JM, eds. *Primary immunodeficiency diseases: a molecular and genetic approach.* New York: Oxford University Press, 1999:306–323.

193. Hartley KO, Gell D, Smith GC, et al. DNA-dependent protein kinase catalytic subunit: a relative of phosphatidylinositol 3–kinase and the ataxia telangiectasia gene product. *Cell* 1995;82:849–856.

194. Xu Y, Baltimore D. Dual roles of ATM in the cellular response to radiation and in cell growth control. *Genes Dev* 1996;10:2401–2410.

195. Heintz N. Ataxia telangiectasia: cell signaling, cell death and the cell cycle. *Curr Opin Neurol* 1996;9:137–140.

196. Sullivan KE, Mullen CA, Blaese RM, et al. A multiinstitutional survey of the Wiskott-Aldrich syndrome. *J Pediatr* 1994;125:876–885.

197. Conley ME, Notarangelo LD, Etzioni A. Diagnostic criteria for primary immunodeficiencies: representing PAGID (Pan-American Group for Immunodeficiency) and ESID (European Society for Immunodeficiencies). *Clin Immunol* 1999;93:190–197.

198. Inoue R, Kondo N, Kuwabara N, et al. Aberrant patterns of immunoglobulin levels in Wiskott-Aldrich syndrome. *Scand J Immunol* 1995;41:188–193.

199. de Saint Basile G, Fraser NJ, Craig IW, et al. Close linkage of hypervariable marker DXS255 to disease locus of Wiskott-Aldrich syndrome. *Lancet* 1989;2:1319–1320.

200. Derry JMJ, Ochs HD, Francke U. Isolation of a novel gene mutated in Wiskott-Aldrich syndrome [published erratum appears in *Cell* 1994;79:922a]. *Cell* 1994;78:635–644.

201. Symons M, Derry JMJ, Karlak B, et al. Wiskott-Aldrich syndrome protein, a novel effector for the GTPase CDC42H2, is implicated in actin polymerization. *Cell* 1996;84:723–734.

202. Aspenstrom P, Lindberg U, Hall A. Two GTPases, cdc42 and rac, bind directly to a protein implicated in the immunodeficiency disorder Wiskott-Aldrich syndrome. *Curr Biol* 1996;6:70.

203. Haddad E, Zugaza JL, Louache F, et al. The interaction between Cdc42 and WASP is required for SDF-1–induced T- lymphocyte chemotaxis. *Blood* 2001;97:33–38.

204. Finan PM, Soames CJ, Wilson L, et al. Identification of regions of the Wiskott-Aldrich syndrome protein responsible for association with selected Src homology 3 domains. *J Biol Chem* 1996;271:25646–25656.

205. Schwarz K. WASPbase: a database of WAS- and XLT-causing mutations. *Immunol Today* 1996;17:496–502.

206. Schwartz M, Bekassy A, Donner M, et al. Mutation spectrum in patients with Wiskott-Aldrich syndrome and X-linked thrombocytopenia: identification of twelve different mutations in the WASP gene. *Thromb Haemost* 1996;75:546–550.

207. Rong SB, Vihinen M. Structural basis of Wiskott-Aldrich syndrome causing mutations in the WH1 domain. *J Mol Med* 2000;78:530–537.

208. Ochs HD, Rosen FS. The Wiskott-Aldrich syndrome. In: Ochs HD, Smith CIE, Puck JM, eds. *Primary immunodeficiency diseases: a molecular and genetic approach.* New York: Oxford University Press, 1999:292–305.

209. Schindelhauer D, Weiss M, Hellebrand H, et al. Wiskott-Aldrich syndrome: no strict genotype-phenotype correlations but clustering of missense mutations in the amino-terminal part of the WASP gene product. *Hum Genet* 1996;98:68–76.

210. Greer WL, Shehabeldin A, Schulman J, et al. Identification of WASP mutations, mutation hotspots and genotype-phenotype disparities in 24 patients with Wiskott-Aldrich syndrome. *Hum Genet* 1996;98:685–690.

211. de Saint Basile G, Lagelouse RD, Lambert N, et al. Isolated X-linked thrombocytopenia in two unrelated families is associated with point mutations in the Wiskott-Aldrich syndrome gene. *J Pediatr* 1996; 129:56–62.

212. Wengler G, Gorlin JB, Williamson JM, et al. Non-random inactivation of the X chromosome in early lineage hematopoietic cells in carriers of Wiskott-Aldrich syndrome. *Blood* 1995;85:2471–2477.

213. Kwan SP, Hagemann TL, Radtke BE, et al. Identification of mutations in the Wiskott-Aldrich syndrome gene and characterization of a polymorphic dinucleotide repeat at the DXS6940, adjacent to the disease gene. *Proc Natl Acad Sci USA* 1995;92:4706–4710.

214. Ariga T, Yamada M, Sakiyama Y. Mutation analysis of five Japanese families with Wiskott-Aldrich syndrome and determination of the family members' carrier status using three different methods. *Pediatr Res* 1997;41:535–540.

215. Kondoh T, Hayashi K, Matsumoto T, et al. Two sisters with clinical diagnosis of Wiskott-Aldrich syndrome: is the condition in the family autosomal recessive? *Am J Med Genet* 1995;60:364–369.

216. Rocca B, Bellacosa A, de Cristofaro R, et al. Wiskott-Aldrich syndrome: report of an autosomal dominant variant. *Blood* 1996;87: 4538–4543.

217. Parolini O, Ressmann G, Haas OA, et al. X-linked Wiskott-Aldrich syndrome in a girl. *N Engl J Med* 1998;338:291–295.

218. Filipovich AH, Pelz C, Sobocinski K, et al. Allogeneic bone marrow transplantation (BMT) for Wiskott Aldrich syndrome (WAS): comparison of outcomes by donor type. *J Allergy Clin Immunol* 1997;99S: 102.

219. Filipovich AH, Stone JV, Tomany SC, et al. Impact of donor type on outcome of bone marrow transplantation for Wiskott-Aldrich syndrome: collaborative study of the International Bone Marrow Transplant Registry and the National Marrow Donor Program. *Blood* 2001; 97:1598–1603.

220. Mullen CA, Anderson KD, Blaese RM. Splenectomy and/or bone marrow transplantation in the management of the Wiskott-Aldrich syndrome: long-term follow-up of 62 cases. *Blood* 1993;82:2961–2966.

221. Litzman J, Jones A, Hann I, et al. Intravenous immunoglobulin, splenectomy, and antibiotic prophylaxis in Wiskott-Aldrich syndrome. *Arch Dis Child* 1996;75:436–439.

222. Polmar SH, Pierce GF. Cartilage hair hypoplasia: immunological aspects and their clinical implications. *Clin Immunol Immunopathol* 1986;40:87–93.

223. Sulisalo T, van der Burgt I, Rimoin DL, et al. Genetic homogeneity of cartilage-hair hypoplasia. *Hum Genet* 1995;95:157–160.

224. Ridanpaa M, van Eenennaam H, Pelin K, et al. Mutations in the RNA component of RNase MRP cause a pleiotropic human disease, cartilage-hair hypoplasia. *Cell* 2001;104:195–203.

225. Weemaes CMR, Smeets DFCM, van der Burgt CJAM. Nijmegen breakage syndrome: a progress report. *Int J Radiat Biol* 1994;66: S185–S188.

226. Kleijer WJ, van der Kraan M, Los FJ, et al. Prenatal diagnosis of ataxia telangiectasia and Nijmegen breakage syndrome by the assay of radioresistant DNA synthesis. *Int J Radiat Biol* 1994;66:S167–S174.

227. Chrzanowska KH, Kleijer WJ, Krajewska-Walasek M, et al. Eleven Polish patients with microcephaly, immunodeficiency, and chromosomal instability: the Nijmegen breakage syndrome. *Am J Med Genet* 1995;57:462–471.

228. Saar K, Chrzanowska KH, Stumm M, et al. The gene for the ataxia-telangiectasia variant, Nijmegen breakage syndrome, maps to a 1-cM interval on chromosome 8q21. *Am J Hum Genet* 1997;60:605–610.

229. Furukawa H, Murata S, Yabe T, et al. Splice acceptor site mutation of the transporter associated with antigen processing-1 gene in human bare lymphocyte syndrome. *J Clin Invest* 1999;103:755–758.

230. de la Salle H, Zimmer J, Fricker D, et al. HLA class I deficiencies due to mutations in subunit 1 of the peptide transporter TAP1. *J Clin Invest* 1999;103:R9–R13.

231. de la Salle H, Hanau D, Fricker D. Homozygous human TAP peptide transporter mutation in HLA class I deficiency. *Science* 1994; 265:237–241.

232. Teisserenc H, Schmitt W, Blake N, et al. A case of primary immunodeficiency due to a defect of the major histocompatibility gene complex class I processing and presentation pathway. *Immunol Lett* 1997;57:183–187.

233. Donato L, de la Salle H, Hanau D, et al. Association of HLA class I antigen deficiency related to a TAP2 gene mutation with familial bronchiectasis. *J Pediatr* 1995;127:895–900.

234. Grandea AG, Androlewicz MJ, Athwal RS, et al. Dependence of peptide binding by MHC class I molecules on their interaction with TAP. *Science* 1995;270:105–108.

234a. Yabe T, Kawamura S, Sato M, Kashiwase K, Tanaka H, Ishikawa Y, Asao Y, Oyama J, Tsuruta K, Tokunaga K, Tadokoro K, Juji T. A subject with a novel type I bare lymphocyte syndrome has tapasin deficiency due to deletion of 4 exons by Alu-mediated recombination. *Blood* 2002;100:1496–1498.

235. Reith W, Mach B. The bare lymphocyte syndrome and the regulation of MHC expression. *Annu Rev Immunol* 2001;19:331–373.

236. Henwood J, van Eggermond MC, van Boxel-Dezaire AN, et al. Human T cell repertoire generation in the absence of MHC class II expression results in a circulating CD4+CD8–population with altered physicochemical properties of complementarity-determining region 3. *J Immunol* 1996;156:895–906.

237. Steimle V, Durand B, Barras E, et al. A novel DNA-binding regulatory factor is mutated in primary MHC class II deficiency (bare lymphocyte syndrome). *Genes Dev* 1995;9:1021–1032.

238. Durand B, Sperisen P, Emery P, et al. RFXAP, a novel subunit of the RFX DNA binding complex is mutated in MHC class II deficiency. *EMBO J* 1997;16:1045–1055.

239. Masternak K, Barras E, Zufferey M, et al. A gene encoding a novel RFX-associated transactivator is mutated in the majority of MHC class II deficiency patients. *Nat Genet* 1998;20:273–277.

240. Zhou H, Glimcher LH. Human MHC class II gene transcription directed by the carboxyl terminus of CIITA, one of the defective genes in type II MHC combined immune deficiency. *Immunity* 1995;2:545–553.

241. Fischer A, Lisowska-Grospierre B, Anderson DC, et al. Leukocyte adhesion deficiency: molecular basis and functional consequences. *Immunodef Rev* 1988;1:39–54.

242. Etzioni A. Adhesion molecule deficiencies and their clinical significance. *Cell Adhes Commun* 1994;2:257–260.

243. Kishimoto TK, Springer TA. Human leukocyte adhesion deficiency: molecular basis for a defective immune response to infections of the skin. *Curr Probl Dermatol* 1989;18:106.

244. D'Agata ID, Paradis K, Chad Z, et al. Leucocyte adhesion deficiency presenting as a chronic ileocolitis. *Gut* 1996;39:605–608.

245. Rivera-Matos IR, Rakita RM, Mariscalco MM, et al. Leukocyte adhesion deficiency mimicking Hirschprung disease. *J Pediatr* 1995; 127:755–757.

246. Etzioni A, Tonetti M. Leukocyte adhesion deficiency II: from A to almost Z. *Immunol Rev* 2000;178:138–147.

247. Etzioni A, Frydman M, Pollack S, et al. Brief report: recurrent severe infections caused by a novel leukocyte adhesion deficiency. *N Engl J Med* 1992;327:1789–1792.

248. Sturla L, Puglielli L, Tonetti M, et al. Impairment of the Golgi GDP-L-fucose transport and unresponsiveness to fucose replacement therapy in LAD II patients. *Pediatr Res* 2001;49:537–542.

249. Lubke T, Marquardt T, Etzioni A, et al. Complementation cloning identifies CDG-IIc, a new type of congenital disorders of glycosylation, as a GDP-fucose transporter deficiency. *Nat Genet* 2001;28: 73–76.

250. Sharfe N, Dadi HK, Shahar M, et al. Human immune disorder arising from mutation of the alpha chain of the interleukin-2 receptor. *Proc Natl Acad Sci USA* 1997;94:3168–3171.

251. Willerford DM, Chem J, Ferry JA, et al. Interleukin-2 receptor α chain regulates the size and content of the peripheral lymphoid compartment. *Immunity* 1995;3:521–530.

252. Suzuki H, Kundig TM, Furlonger C, et al. Deregulated T cell activation and autoimmunity in mice lacking interleukin-2 receptor β. *Science* 1995;268:1472–1476.

253. Lenardo MJ. Interleukin-2 programs mouse αβ T lymphocytes for apoptosis. *Nature* 1991;353:858–861.

254. Jouanguy E, Altare F, Lamhamedi S, et al. Interferon-gamma-receptor deficiency in an infant with fatal bacille Calmette-Guerin infection. *N Engl J Med* 1996;335:1956–1961.

255. Newport MJ, Huxley CM, Huston S, et al. A mutation in the interferon-gamma-receptor gene and susceptibility to mycobacterial infection. *N Engl J Med* 1996;335:1941–1949.

256. Dorman SE, Holland SM. Interferon-gamma and interleukin-12 pathway defects and human disease. *Cytokine Growth Factor Rev* 2000; 11:321–333.

257. Altare F, Lammas D, Revy P, et al. Inherited interleukin 12 deficiency in a child with bacille Calmette-Guerin and *Salmonella enteritidis* disseminated infection. *J Clin Invest* 1998;102:2035–2040.

258. Altare F, Durandy A, Lammas D, et al. Impairment of mycobacterial immunity in human interleukin-12 receptor deficiency. *Science* 1998;280:1432–1435.

259. de Jong R, Altare F, Haagen I, et al. Severe mycobacterial and *Salmonella* infections in interleukin-12 receptor-deficient patients. *Science* 1998;280:1435–1438.

260. Dupuis S, Dargemont C, Fieschi C, et al. Impairment of mycobacterial but not viral immunity by a germline human STAT1 mutation. *Science* 2001;293:300–303.

261. Stolz W, Graubner U, Gerstmeier J, et al. Chediak syndrome: approaches to diagnosis and treatment. *Curr Probl Dermatol* 1989;18: 93.

262. Zhao H, Boissy YL, Abdel-Malek Z, et al. On the analysis of the pathophysiology of Chediak-Higashi syndrome: defects expressed by cultured melanocytes. *Lab Invest* 1994;71:25–34.

263. Holcombe RF, Jones KL, Stewart RM. Lysosomal enzyme activities in Chediak-Higashi syndrome: evaluation of lymphoblastoid cell lines and review of the literature. *Immunodeficiency* 1994;5:131–140.

264. Merino F, Esparza B, Sabino E. Chediak-Higashi syndrome natural killer cells: a protein kinase C defective activation/regulation defect? *Eur J Pediatr* 1996;155:254–258.

265. Baetz K, Isaaz S, Griffiths GM. Loss of cytotoxic T lymphocyte function in Chediak-Higashi syndrome arises from a secretory defect that prevents lytic granule exocytosis. *J Immunol* 1995;154:6122–6131.

266. Nagle DL, Karim MA, Woolf EA, et al. Identification and mutation analysis of the complete gene for Chediak-Higashi syndrome. *Nat Genet* 1996;14:307–311.

267. Barrat FJ, Auloge L, Pastural E, et al. Genetic and physical mapping of the Chediak-Higashi syndrome on chromosome 1q42–43. *Am J Hum Genet* 1996;59:625–632.

268. Perou CM, Moore KJ, Nagle DL, et al. Identification of the murine beige gene by YAC complementation and positional cloning. *Nat Genet* 1996;13:303–308.

269. Barbosa MDFS, Nguyen QA, Tchernev VT, et al. Identification of the homologous beige and Chediak-Higashi syndrome genes. *Nature* 382, 262–265. 1996.

270. Fukai K, Oh J, Karim MA, et al. Homozygosity mapping of the gene for Chediak-Higashi syndrome to chromosome 1q42–q44 in a segment of conserved synteny that includes the mouse beige locus (bg). *Am J Hum Genet* 1996;59:620–624.

271. Aslan Y, Erduran E, Gedik Y, et al. The role of high dose methyl-prednisolone and splenectomy in the accelerated phase of Chediak-Higashi syndrome. *Acta Haematol* 1996;96:105–107.

272. Haddad E, Le Deist F, Blanche S, et al. Treatment of Chediak-Higashi syndrome by allogenic bone marrow transplantation: report of 10 cases. *Blood* 1995;85:3328–3333.

273. Chatila T, Wong R, Young M, et al. An immunodeficiency characterized by defective signal transduction in T lymphocytes. *N Engl J Med* 1989;320:696–702.

274. Elder ME, Lin D, Clever J, et al. Human severe combined immunodeficiency due to a defect in ZAP-70, a T cell tyrosine kinase. *Science* 1994;264:1596–1599.

275. Arpaia E, Shahar M, Dadi H, et al. Defective T cell receptor signaling and CD8+ thymic selection in humans lacking zap-70 kinase. *Cell* 1994;76:947–958.

276. Elder ME. Severe combined immunodeficiency due to a defect in the tyrosine kinase ZAP-70. *Pediatr Res* 1996;39:743–748.

277. Negishi I, Motoyama N, Nakayama K, et al. Essential role for ZAP-70 in both positive and negative selection of thymocytes. *Nature* 1995;376:435–438.

278. Calle-Martin O, Hernandez M, Ordi J, et al. Familial CD8 deficiency due to a mutation in the CD8 alpha gene. *J Clin Invest* 2001;108:117–123.

279. Arnaiz-Villena A, Timon M, Corell A, et al. Brief report: primary immunodeficiency caused by mutations in the gene encoding the CD3–γ subunit of the T lymphocyte receptor. *N Engl J Med* 1992;327:529–533.

280. Thoenes G, Soudais C, Le Deist F, et al. Structural analysis of low TCR-CD3 complex expression in T cells of an immunodeficient patient. *J Biol Chem* 1992;267:487–493.

281. Soudais C, de Villartay J-P, Le Deist F, et al. Independent mutations of the human CD3–ϵ gene resulting in a T cell receptor/CD3 complex immunodeficiency. *Nat Genet* 1993;3:77–81.

282. Weinberg K, Parkman R. Severe combined immunodeficiency due to a specific defect in the production of interleukin-2. *N Engl J Med* 1990; 322:1718–1723.

283. Disanto JP, Keever CA, Small TN, et al. Absence of interleukin 2 production in a severe combined immunodeficiency disease syndrome with T cells. *J Exp Med* 1990;171:1697–1704.

284. Castigli E, Pahwa R, Good RA, et al. Molecular basis of a multiple lymphokine deficiency in a patient with severe combined immunodeficiency. *Proc Natl Acad Sci USA* 1993;90:4728–4732.

285. Feske S, Muller JM, Graf D, et al. Severe combined immunodeficiency due to defective binding of the nuclear factor of activated T cells in T lymphocytes of two male siblings. *Eur J Immunol* 1996;26:2119–2126.

286. Buckley RH, Wray BB, Belmaker EZ. Extreme hyperimmunoglobulinemia E and undue susceptibility to infection. *Pediatrics* 1972; 49:59–70.

287. Buckley RH. The hyper-IgE syndrome. *Clin Rev Allergy Immunol* 2001;20:139–154.

288. Grimbacher B, Holland SM, Gallin JI, et al. Hyper-IgE syndrome with recurrent infections: an autosomal dominant multisystem disorder. *N Engl J Med* 1999;340:692–702.

289. Kirchner SG, Sivit CJ, Wright PF. Hyperimmunoglobulinemia E syndrome: association with osteoporosis and recurrent fractures. *Radiology* 1985;156:362.

290. Claassen JL, Levine AD, Schiff SE, et al. Mononuclear cells from patients with the hyper IgE syndrome produce little IgE when stimulated with recombinant interleukin 4 in vitro. *J Allergy Clin Immunol* 1991;88:713–721.

291. Grimbacher B, Schaffer AA, Holland SM, et al. Genetic linkage of hyper-IgE syndrome to chromosome 4. *Am J Hum Genet* 1999; 65:735–744.

292. King CL, Gallin JI, Malech HL, et al. Regulation of immunoglobulin production in hyperimmunoglobulin E recurrent infection syndrome by interferon. *Proc Natl Acad Sci USA* 1989;86:10085–10089.

293. Kaplan MH, Sun YL, Hoey T, et al. Impaired IL-12 responses and enhanced development of Th2 cells in stat4–deficient mice. *Nature* 1996;382:174–177.

294. Thierfelder WE, van Deursen JM, Yamamoto K, et al. Requirement for stat4 in interleukin-12–mediated responses of natural killer and T cells. *Nature* 1996;382:171–173.

CHAPTER 50

Immunotherapy

Ellen S. Vitetta, Elaine Coleman, Maria-Ana Ghetie, Victor Ghetie, Jaroslav Michálek, Laurentiu M. Pop, Joan E. Smallshaw, and Camelia Spiridon

Introduction
    Immunotherapy of Cancer
Immunomodulators
    Intact Microbes: Bacillus Calmette-Guérin and *Corynebacterium parvum* • *Streptococcus pyogenes* and *Propionibacterium avidum* • Bacteriolytic Therapy of Tumors • Other Immunostimulatory Bacterial Agents • Thymic Hormones and Analogs • Cytokines • Soluble Co-Stimulatory Molecules
Antibodies
    History • Clinical Considerations • Affinity • Persistence and Size • Effector Functions • Immunogenicity • How Monoclonal Antibodies Work • Engineering Monoclonal Antibodies with Enhanced or Decreased Activities • Immunoglobulin G and Monoclonal Antibodies in Clinical Practice • Bispecific Monoclonal Antibodies
Immunoconjugates
    Introduction • Immunotoxins • Monoclonal Antibody–Drug Conjugates (Chemoconjugates) • Antibody-Directed Enzyme Prodrug Therapy (ADEPT) • Radioimmunoconjugates • Immunoliposomes • Other Emerging Imunoconjugate Strategies • Conclusions
Cellular Strategies
    Nonspecific Cellular Therapy • Lymphokine-Activated Killer cells • Natural Killer Cells • Dendritic Cells • Macrophage-Activated Killer Cells • Specific Cellular Transfer • Genetically Engineered Cells • Graft-Versus-Leukemia T Cells and Graft-Versus-Tumor Effects • Regulatory T Cells
Vaccination
    Strategies • Vaccination with Defined Antigens • Id Vaccines • Anticytokine Vaccines • Synthetic Carbohydrate Antigen Vaccines • Recombinant Bacterial Vaccines • Recombinant Viral Vector Vaccines • DNA Vaccines • Dendritic Cell Vaccines • Vaccination with Unidentified Antigens • Immunoprevention of Cancer • Conclusions
Concluding Remarks
Acknowledgments
References

INTRODUCTION

Immunotherapy refers to the use of cells, molecules, and genes of the immune system for the therapy of infectious disease, autoimmunity, neoplastic diseases, and graft-versus-host disease (GVHD), and to prevent the rejection of organ transplants. Immunotherapy can be passive, involving the administration of immunoglobulin (Ig), antibodies, cells, and immunoconjugates (ICs), for example, which home to the target tissue and generate a therapeutic effect *in situ*. Immunotherapy can also be active, involving mobilization of the immune system by the administration of vaccines or immunomodulators, which increase the immunogenicity of endogenous or exogenous antigens. Both passive and active immunotherapies are interrelated because the administration of any agent will have downstream effects on various immunologic circuits. In this chapter, we describe the various modalities that have been developed over the past several decades.

Since 1980, the field of immunotherapy has undergone an explosion as new technologies for generating recombinant molecules and purified cells have been perfected and as our understanding of the immune system has continued to evolve. Despite these advances, the translation of novel techniques into clinical practice has been a slow and difficult process, not only because of the costs and complexities of conducting clinical trials in humans, but also because the animal models in which many agents have shown efficacy do not always translate well into humans. For example, in cancer, spontaneous tumors and prior therapies can render the outcome of a new therapy in humans quite different from that achieved using well-defined experimental animal models. In addition, many therapies tested in mice rely on using large doses with very little regard for toxicity. In humans, the situation is reversed; toxicities can frequently lead to the demise of a new reagent that could have clinical benefits if it were administered using a different dose regimen or in a different setting. Because of the expense and the time required to test all the variables in humans, many of these agents have been shelved. Despite this, some immunotherapies have achieved success in humans and several immunopharmaceuticals have been approved or are being evaluated in advanced clinical trials.

Immunotherapy of Cancer

It has long been postulated that the use of cells or molecules of the immune system or the active mobilization of the immune system should provide specific clinical benefits that would be difficult to achieve by the administration of broadly reactive cytotoxic agents. In the case of cancer, this goal has been difficult to attain because of the impediments to treating cancer *per se*. For a long time, there was significant controversy about whether there was *any* immune response against cancer cells or whether the immune system played any role in either preventing or containing neoplasia. More recently, cancer has been viewed as the *failure* of the immune system either to respond robustly enough or to keep up with the extraordinary rates of tumor cell growth and mutation. The general problems that make cancer difficult to treat by immunologic approaches are as follows: (a) the similarity in antigens between tumor cells and normal cells and the finding that most tumors are not strongly immunogenic because they are recognized as self-tissue; (b) the finding that antigens or tumor cells mutate at a high rate and hence circumvent ongoing immune responses; and (c) the finding that many tumors down-regulate major histocompatibility (MHC) antigens and make poor targets for cytotoxic T cells (CTLs); moreover, many tumors interfere with the immune system and are able to dampen or avoid the immune response by suppressing it or by killing effector cells.

As we unravel the steps in antigen recognition, presentation, and stimulation of the appropriate subsets of T and B cells, strategies for enhancing these processes to achieve therapeutic effects in the setting of neoplasia will continue to evolve. Clearly, the passive administration of antibodies, ICs, cells, and cytokines requires a great deal of information concerning the immune system, because it is sometimes necessary to suppress the immune response against therapeutic molecules without enhancing tumor growth at the same time. In the case of active immunotherapies, enhancing immunogenicity without inducing autoimmunity is the goal.

At present, conventional wisdom suggests that if targets on tumors could be identified, and if the host immune response against these targets could be used (either actively or passively) to destroy tumor cells, it could be possible to use immunotherapy in conjunction with conventional therapies to prolong remissions or, in some cases, achieve cures. For example, passive therapies could be followed by vaccination to arm the host with the appropriate endogenous immune response to prevent relapses. Therefore, it will be critical to optimize appropriate combination regimens. Combination therapy is particularly attractive when these pharmaceuticals

have different mechanisms of action and different side effects. Although much will depend on trial and error, many questions can be addressed in animal models.

Early detection is key in the success of any therapy for cancer. However, with respect to immunotherapy, many immunologists initially postulated that immunotherapies would work best in an adjuvant setting. Studies conducted since the late 1990s have, however, suggested that this may not always be the case. Thus, certain immunotherapies may actually render tumor cells more sensitive to other conventional therapeutic agents, a finding suggesting that they should be given first or concomitantly. In addition, because cancer cells undergo high rates of mutation, tumor antigens also change during the course of the disease, and in an adjuvant setting, there may be more mutant clones to destroy than in early disease. These mutant clones will be difficult to target using single immunotherapeutic agents. Finally, as noted, cytotoxic therapies as well as advanced neoplasia can often immunosuppress the host such that active immunotherapies will be less effective in advanced disease.

In this chapter, we discuss the various immunotherapies that have been developed to date. In each instance, we review the immunologic basis for each therapy, some of the *in vitro* and *in vivo* effects in experimental models, and, finally, their current status with regard to human clinical trials. Although some immunotherapies have received approval in the United States or Europe, many others are in development. There is no doubt that immunotherapies have made their debut in clinical medicine.

IMMUNOMODULATORS

Agents that enhance the immune response of the host against cancer, infectious diseases, or immunologic disorders are referred to as "immunomodulators." Immunomodulators belong to a highly heterogeneous group of molecules with different mechanisms of action. Immunomodulators can be co-administered with antigens to increase their local retention (depot effect) and thereby facilitate their slow release into the body (1,2). Immunomodulators can also alert the immune system to "danger" by inducing changes in antigen-presenting cells (APCs), particularly dendritic cells (DCs). For example, one of the most potent immunomodulators, complete Freund's adjuvant, contains a water/oil emulsion of the antigen, which is responsible for its local retention, and a bacterial component (from mycobacterial cells), which induces both cellular and humoral immunity by activating APCs.

This section emphasizes primarily those immunomodulators that have been used clinically to enhance immunoreactivity against infections and cancer, even though the success of immunomodulators in cancer immunotherapy has been limited. The agents that exert antitumor activity do so only if they are administered directly into the tumor site or systemically under conditions leading to their localization in tumor metastases, usually after the resection of a primary tumor (3).

This most likely reason is the need to activate APCs in and near the tumor site.

The immunomodulators discussed in this chapter and currently in use include intact microbes and bacterial derivatives (e.g., muramylpeptide and trehalose mycolate derivatives), bacterial DNA fractions, thymic hormones and their analogs, and cytokines.

Intact Microbes: Bacillus Calmette-Guérin and *Corynebacterium parvum*

Mechanism of Action

Mycobacterial immunomodulators can enhance the uptake of antigens by APCs such as macrophages and DCs. These cells respond to foreign antigens by migrating into lymphoid tissues, up-regulating their co-stimulatory molecules, and presenting peptides to T cells through both class I and class II pathways. They stimulate T helper (Th) cells and CTLs. The Th cells can then interact with B cells, which eventually make antibodies.

Applications in Cancer

Viable mycobacteria, and in particular the attenuated vaccine strain *bacillus Calmette-Guérin* (BCG), and heat-killed or formalin-inactivated *Corynebacterium parvum* were employed as first-generation microbial immunomodulators to enhance the resistance of the host to neoplasms and to several infections (4). Preparations containing formalinized *C. parvum* are licensed in Europe but not in the United States. Numerous studies suggest that, under certain circumstances, BCG may be effective in reducing tumor growth. For example, the effectiveness of BCG in superficial cancers of the bladder was assessed in 3,000 patients (5), in whom repeated injections of BCG into the lumen of the bladder resulted in the recruitment of activated lymphocytes into the bladder wall, increased levels of interleukins in the urine, and generated systemic immunity to BCG. As compared with chemotherapy, this regimen temporarily eradicated residual disease after surgery, prevented local recurrence, increased survival from 68% to 86%, and decreased treatment failures by 20% (5). Treatment with BCG is prolonged, expensive, and associated with side effects, however. In another study, patients with advanced gastric carcinomas received chemotherapy and BCG. The antitumor response in these patients was superior to that observed in patients receiving chemotherapy alone (6). BCG injected directly into melanoma nodules in patients with tuberculin sensitivity caused regression of some tumor nodules (7), probably by inducing secondary inflammatory immune responses. Similar results have been reported in metastatic breast cancer, basal cell tumors of the skin, and other solid tumor nodules (8). Recombinant BCG strains have been engineered to secrete cytokines such as interleukin-2 (IL-2), interferon-γ (IFN-γ), or granulocyte-monocyte colony-stimulating factor (GM-CSF), which

further enhance immune responses (9). In summary, bacterial stimulants can exert therapeutic effects in terms of improved durations of remission and percentage of survival, and their greatest antitumor activities are achieved when they are administered by intralesional injection and in combination with other forms of immunotherapy or chemotherapy. They are likely to work by providing a "danger signal" to DCs, which then migrate to lymphoid tissues and present weakly antigenic epitopes to T cells.

Streptococcus pyogenes and *Propionibacterium avidum*

Mechanism of Action

Picibanil or OK-432 is a lyophilized preparation of inactivated *Streptococcus pyogenes* that augments nonspecific T-cell cytotoxicity, lymphokine-activated killer cell (LAK) activity, and macrophage activation.

Applications in Cancer

In two phase III studies in 467 patients with gastric carcinomas, administration of OK-432 after standard surgery and chemotherapy increased 5-year survivals from 24% to 29% to 45%. Forty-eight patients with resected high-risk melanoma who participated in a phase IB clinical trial with OK-432 showed a significant increase in IL-1, tumor necrosis factor (TNF-α), and IFN-γ secretion, as well as suppression of superoxide production by mononuclear cells (10).

Similarly, preoperative administration of *Propionibacterium avidum* to patients with stage I and II colorectal carcinomas increased survival, decreased disease recurrence and metastasis, and improved the quality of life. A possible explanation for this last effect is the nonspecific immune stimulation that counteracted the immunosuppressive effect of major surgical trauma, as well as the prevention of microbial infections associated with the perioperative period (10).

Bacteriolytic Therapy of Tumors

Since the 1950s, nonpathogenic bacteria that preferentially localize in tumors have been investigated for their ability to induce regression of human and mouse tumors (11). The organisms studied in greatest detail are various strains of *Clostridium*. Results have been variable (11). More recently, however, engineered spores of *C. novyi* devoid of their lethal toxin were used to treat colon carcinoma and melanoma xenografts in nude mice (12). The spores localized and germinated in the avascular regions of the tumors and thereby increased necrosis of the viable tumor cells adjacent to the original regions of necrosis. When nonlethal *C. novyi* was administered together with chemotherapeutic and antivascular agents, impressive regressions of most tumors and even complete responses (CR) in a significant percentage of treated mice were observed (12). This strategy, which is based on the finding that regions of necrosis in tumors are sites for the growth of certain anaerobic bacteria, should be useful for treating large tumors but not micrometastatic disease.

Other Immunostimulatory Bacterial Agents

Bacterial Derivatives

Muramyldipeptide Derivatives

The cell wall fraction of mycobacteria (especially the *Mycobacterium bovis* strain) and related bacteria (e.g., *Nocardia, Corynebacteria,* or *Listeria*) is the major active immunomodulatory components of bacterial cells (13). The minimal glycopeptide subunit of bacterial cell walls essential for the mycobacterial immunostimulatory activity is muramyldipeptide (MDP) (14).

Mechanism of Action. Bacterial immunomodulators serve as ligands for various receptors on immune cells and, once bound, induce cellular responses. DCs and macrophages express two types of receptors recognized by bacterial immunomodulators. These include Toll-like receptors (TLR-2 and TLR-4) and receptors recognizing a unique motif in the cell wall fraction of BCG. Both receptors engage signaling pathways leading to activation of the innate immune system. This, in turn, activates APCs.

Applications in Cancer and Other Diseases. Clinical trials using a BCG cell wall fraction have been carried out in patients with lung cancer, acute myeloblastic leukemia, acute lymphoblastic leukemia, and gastric carcinomas. In these patients, prolonged survival has been reported (13). Several synthetic MDP analogs enhanced nonspecific resistance against viral infections such as human immunodeficiency virus (HIV), influenza, herpes simplex, Sendai, vaccinia, and murine hepatitis viruses, as well as bacterial infections (9). Synthetic MDP analogs are potent inducers of the secretion of cytokines such as IL-1, IL-6, TNF-α, and IFN-γ (14). One such analog, MDP-Lys (Romurtide), has been licensed in Japan. This drug is effective in restoring decreased neutrophils and platelets in patients with cancer (14). Liposomes containing MDP have entered clinical trials in patients with advanced osteosarcoma and have resulted in longer remissions (13).

Trehalose Dimycolate Derivatives

Mycolic acids in bacterial cell walls belong to the cord factor–like glycolipid family, and they are found not only in mycobacteria but also in the lipid fractions of related bacteria such as *Nocardia* and *Corynebacterium*. Their synthetic analog, trehalose dimycolate (TDM), has various biologic activities, including stimulation of the human immune response against mycobacteria (13).

Mechanism of Action. TDM stimulates host resistance against infections with bacteria, fungi, viruses, and parasites.

It also has antitumor activity in mice. TDM can synergize with monophosphoryl lipid A to enhance the immune response against both tumors and infectious agents (13).

Applications in Cancer. TDM was used in combination with a nonviable mycobacterial vaccine in 34 patients with metastatic malignant melanoma and metastatic lung cancer (15). In seven of 17 patients with malignant melanoma and in one of seven patients with lung cancer, clinical improvements were observed, suggesting that mycolic acids and their derivatives can mobilize the immune response against weakly immunogenic tumors.

Bacterial DNA Fractions

Role of the CpG Motif

After binding to TLR-9, bacterial DNA can exert antitumor activity that is dependent on natural killer (NK) cell activation (13). The minimal sequence required for NK-cell activation, and found exclusively in bacterial DNA, is a nonmethylated 6-bp motif (13). The nonmethylated CpG motif also stimulates IgG production (13).

Mechanism of Action. CpG DNA exerts direct and indirect effects on all major cellular elements of both the innate and acquired immune response. CpG DNA enhances the cytotoxic activity of NK cells, stimulates macrophage responses leading to the release of inflammatory mediators, enhances functions of APCs, and activates DCs by up-regulating MHC class II molecules and the co-stimulatory molecule, CD40 (16). CpG DNA is mitogenic for T and B cells and can induce polyclonal B-cell activation and antibody production. In addition, the same motif can induce the secretion of the Th1-associated cytokines, IL-12, IFN-α, TNF-α, and other proinflammatory mediators such as IL-6 and IL-10, produced by B cells, as well IFN-γ produced by NK cells. These cytokines influence cellular immune responses (17). The DNA from *Mycobacterium bovis* and *Escherichia coli* have the most marked activity for the induction of IFN-γ and NK-cell activity (13). Taken together, the CpG DNA from bacteria promotes immune responses of Th1 cells through direct effects on APCs and B cells as well as indirect effects on other cytokines, most notably IFN-γ.

Applications in Cancer and Other Diseases. CpG DNA, either alone as an adjuvant or as a component of a DNA vaccine, has broad applications in both tumor immunotherapy and the eradication of infections. As a single agent, it decreases disease severity in some autoimmune models of renal diseases, encephalomyelitis, and inflammatory arthritis. CpG DNA has potent immunostimulatory activity against hepatitis B, HIV-1, influenza, malaria, leishmaniasis, and *Listeria monocytogenes* (18). However, CpG can promote the development of autoimmune disease when it is used as an adjuvant for the administration of self-antigens.

Phase I clinical trials in patients with non-Hodgkin's lymphoma (NHL), melanoma, and renal carcinoma have been initiated. In addition, nearly 200 normal human volunteers have been injected intramuscularly or subcutaneously with CpG vaccines for infectious disease and for the immunotherapy of allergy. Thus far, CpG DNA has been well tolerated and devoid of serious adverse effects. Preliminary efficacy has been observed at surprisingly low doses (19).

Thymic Hormones and Analogs

Thymic hormones isolated and purified from crude bovine thymic extracts include thymopoietin, thymulin, thymic humoral factor, and thymosin. Thymopentin is a synthetic pentapeptide containing the active site of thymopoietin. This preparation, along with other synthetic peptides of thymic hormones, can induce the expression of differentiation markers on T cells and on prothymocytes, can modulate T-cell proliferation, and can enhance the function of Th cells, T suppressor cells (A.K.A. T regulatory cells), and CTLs. These substances also enhance the production of cytokines (14).

Applications

Preparations containing thymic extracts are used as immunostimulatory therapy for infectious diseases and can enhance the host immune defense during viral diseases and persistent bacterial infections. Therapy with thymus extract preparations such as thymostimulin or thymopentin reduces the frequency and intensity of recurrences of acute respiratory infections. Administration of thymopentin to zidovudine-treated HIV-positive patients has decreased the rates of progression to acquired immunodeficiency syndrome (AIDS) in some patients (9).

Analogs

Methylinosine monophosphate is a thymomimetic immunomodulator capable of inducing the expression of T-lymphocyte differentiation markers on human prothymocytes.

Applications

Methylinosine monophosphate enhances mitogen-induced proliferation of lymphocytes, augments IgM production, induces delayed-type hypersensitivity, and normalizes an impaired response to IL-2. Depressed phytohemagglutinin responses of lymphocytes from patients with AIDS can be restored by methylinosine monophosphate (9).

Summary

Immunomodulators of natural, synthetic, and recombinant origin, along with bacterial DNA fractions, can stimulate host defense mechanisms for the prophylaxis and treatment

of some microbial infections and cancer in both experimental animals and in humans. Several immunomodulators are already licensed for use in patients with specific diseases, and numerous others are being extensively investigated in preclinical and clinical studies. These agents may work by activating DCs, which subsequently migrate to lymphoid tissue and present weakly immunogenic antigens to T cells. More clinical trials must be carried out before we know how broadly applicable these agents will be and why they work in some, but not all, patients. Although the enthusiasm for many of these agents has decreased, there has been a resurgence in approaches using engineered bacteria.

Cytokines

General Properties and Functions

Cytokines are soluble mediators secreted by virtually all nucleated cells in the body and particularly by the cells of the immune system (20). They are relatively small proteins that influence the behavior of other cells expressing appropriate receptors. Cytokines have both autocrine and paracrine activities, and virtually all act on multiple cellular targets. The 160 cytokines thus far described have been grouped into several families based on their structure (20,21). These consist of the type I cytokines, including IL-6 family members, IFNs, TNF family members, Ig supergene family members, and chemokines. Other classifications are described in the literature (21).

Most cytokines are also functionally pleiotropic (21) and can enhance or suppress local immune responses. Depending on the particular cytokine and the local environment, they may promote or inhibit the growth and differentiation of tumor cells (22). Cytokines regulate many fundamental biologic processes including hematopoiesis, immune and inflammatory responses, the development and maturation of cells, and tissue repair. They bind to cell-surface receptors and activate intracellular signal transduction cascades.

Cells that participate in the immune response become polarized in their production of cytokines. As the cells migrate, they alter the cytokine levels of surrounding microenvironments. Changing the cytokine balance of an organ or of the entire body has major immunologic consequences (23). The manipulation of this balance is becoming an increasingly important strategy in immunotherapy. Recombinant cytokines are used for the adjuvant therapy of infectious disease, cancer, and other inflammatory disorders (21).

Clinical Applications

Table 1 summarizes the current status of cytokines in clinical trials for the treatment of cancer and other diseases (24). In general, there have been many obstacles to the development of cytokines as immunotherapeutic agents because they are so pleiotropic and can act on many normal tissues. Nevertheless,

TABLE 1. *Cytokines approved for clinical use*

Drug	Cytokine	Clinical setting or effect
Actimmune	IFN-γ	Chronic granulomatous disease
Alferon N	IFN-α	Condyloma acuminatum (genital warts)
Avonex	IFN-β1a	Multiple sclerosis
Betaseron	IFN-β1b	Multiple sclerosis
Epogen (Procrit)	Erythropoietin	Anemia in patients with cancer, AIDS, or chronic kidney failure
Humalog	Insulin	Diabetes
Humatrope (variant of Protropin)	HGH	Growth hormone deficiency
Infergen	IFN-α-con-1	Chronic hepatitis C
Intron A, Roferon A	IFN-α	Hairy cell leukemia, Kaposi's sarcoma, genital warts, chronic hepatitis C
Intron A and Rebeto	IFN-α2b	Hepatitis B, melanoma, hepatitis C, follicular lymphoma
Leukine	GM-CSF	Neutropenia, BMT, AML, PBSC mobilization
Neumega	IL-11	Thrombocytopenia after high-dose chemotherapy
Neupogen (Filgrastim)	G-CSF	Infections in cancer patients, neutropenia, PBSC mobilization, AML
PEG-Intron	IFN-α2b	Chronic hepatitis C
Proleukin	IL-2	Kidney cancer, melanoma, renal cell carcinoma
Protropin	HGH	Growth hormone deficiency
Somatropin		Treatment of wasting and cachexia in AIDS
Wellferon	IFN-αn1	Chronic hepatitis C

AIDS, acquired immunodeficiency syndrome; AML, acute myeloblastic leukemia; BMT, bone marrow transplantation; G-CSF, granulocyte colony-stimulating factor; GM-CSF, granulocyte-macrophage colony-stimulating factor; HGH, human growth hormone; IFN, interferon; IL, interleukin; PBSC, peripheral blood stem cell.

From Gillis and Williams (24), with permission.

there have been several successes using this approach in the therapy of both neoplastic and non-neoplastic diseases.

Cancer Therapy

Cytokines are involved in both the growth and the death of malignant cells. Antiapoptotic signals generated by cytokines can promote cell survival and signal transduction pathways involved in the pathogenesis of neoplasia. Conversely, cytokines are crucial for the activation and development of immune responses *against* tumor cells. Therefore, these two effects must be manipulated in a manner that will be therapeutically useful (25).

IL-2. IL-2 was the first cytokine to be molecularly characterized. It is a molecule whose functions are highly pleiotropic. It is involved in the activation of antigen-specific T and B cells, and it also triggers innate immunity by stimulating several functions of NK cells and macrophages. IL-2 can circumvent defective or suboptimal antigen-mediated activation and thus overcome tolerance. This finding suggests that IL-2 may be useful in tumor immunotherapy by enhancing the activity of NK cells or by activating tolerant or poorly responsive antitumor T cells (26,27).

In several animal models, systemic administration of IL-2 induces antitumor responses that can result in the partial or complete destruction of the tumor. Based on these observations, clinical trials were designed to evaluate the antitumor activity of IL-2 in patients with cancer (27). In patients with renal carcinoma, IL-2 had antitumor activity in 20% of patients; 7% to 10% achieved durable CRs, and 8% to 10% achieved objective partial responses (PRs) (28). Although

these clinical responses were limited, this was the first convincing evidence that manipulation of the immune system could result in regression of metastatic lesions. This led to the approval of IL-2 by the United States Food and Drug Administration (FDA) and by several European regulatory agencies for the treatment of metastatic renal cell carcinoma. The FDA also approved IL-2 for the treatment of metastatic melanoma (10,27). Several combination regimens have been evaluated to determine the optimal way to use IL-2. In patients with renal cancer, a combination of recombinant (r)IL-2 and IFN-γ induced higher response rates than those achieved using either cytokine alone. However, there was no apparent survival advantage. Combinations of IL-2 and chemotherapy increased toxicity and had no proven benefits. When rIL-2 was combined with LAKs or tumor-infiltrating lymphocytes (TILs), responses were comparable to those achieved with rIL-2 alone. In malignant melanoma, the antitumor activity of combinations of rIL-2, chemotherapy, and IFN-γ have been promising and randomized trials are under way. rIL-2 is also being evaluated in hematologic malignancies. rIL-2 initiates cytokine-mediated proinflammatory events leading to adverse effects. It has been suggested that rIL-2–related toxicity is mediated through the release of secondary cytokines, including TNF, IFN-γ, IL-6, and IL-1. The administration of selective antagonists of these cytokines may reduce the toxicity associated with rIL-2 without interfering with its therapeutic activity (29).

Early trials using rIL-2 as adjuvant therapy for DC-based vaccine therapy yielded promising results (29). There is evidence to suggest that DC-based vaccines, in combination with IL-2 or other cytokines, will become an adjunct to current treatments for human cancers, such as colorectal carcinoma (30). Tumor vaccines, in conjunction with cytokine gene therapy, have also been investigated. Clinical responses in patients with advanced prostate cancer have been limited but promising (31).

IFN-α. IFN-α therapy has had the greatest efficacy in the treatment of hematologic malignant diseases such as hairy cell leukemia, lymphoma, and chronic myelogenous leukemia. IFN-α inhibits cell growth by inducing G1 arrest. The success of IFN-α therapy is greater when it is combined with other anticancer agents. IFN-α has prolonged the survival of patients with renal cell carcinoma (32) and has increased survival and relapse-free intervals in node-positive melanoma patients (33). However, the latter results have not been confirmed in other trials (34). Studies in patients with stage II melanoma treated with lower doses of this cytokine have resulted in an increase in disease-free, but not overall, survival (10).

IFN-γ. IFN-γ is best known for its ability to augment the cytotoxic activity of CTLs and NK cells and to increase the expression of MHC molecules on various cells. IFN-γ also activates monocytes and macrophages. IFN-γ has been used in patients with metastatic renal cell cancer, and although the response rate was only 15%, some responses were durable. In patients with advanced colorectal cancer, IFN-γ had no proven benefits (10,35).

TNF-α. TNF-α has demonstrated immunologic activity in phase I studies in patients with various types of tumors, but clinical responses have been virtually absent (10,36). However, TNF-α used in combination with cytotoxic drugs during locoregional perfusion gave encouraging results in metastatic melanoma, soft tissue sarcoma, and metastatic colorectal cancer (10).

IL-6, GM-CSF, and IL-12. IL-6 (37) and GM-CSF (38) have demonstrated modest antitumor activity in patients with metastatic renal cell carcinoma. IL-12 had some activity in patients with advanced renal cell carcinoma and melanoma, but further studies are warranted before its effectiveness can be determined (39). Like IL-2 and TNF, IL-12 may further potentiate the immunomodulatory effects of chemotherapeutic agents. The effectiveness of such treatment combinations has been documented in animal models (40). However, efficacy in humans has not yet been extensively investigated (40).

The effect of cytokines on tumor growth versus inhibition of growth by enhancing a cellular immune response is a complex issue. It has been suggested that the inflammatory cells and cytokines localized in tumors are more likely to contribute to tumor growth and to immunosuppression of the host. An examination of the role of cytokines in the pathogenesis and management of AIDS-related NHL suggested that the activation of subsets of T cells that produce one cytokine versus another may lead to a different prognosis (41). Present goals are to reduce side effects, possibly by targeting cytokines to tumors, and to determine which cytokines may work in combination with conventional therapies.

Therapy of Other Diseases

In addition to their use in cancer, cytokines represent an effective strategy for treating infectious diseases, acute or chronic inflammation, autoimmune disorders, and imbalances in angiogenesis. Indeed, this may be the area in which cytokine therapy will prove to be most useful. These conditions can be treated in three ways: (a) by adding cytokines to the "environment"; (b) by administering their respective receptors to compete for binding; or (c) by using antibodies to block the function of the cytokines in the disease environment.

Fibroblast Growth Factor (FGF), IFN-α, IL-10, IL-11, and IL-12, Vascular Endothelial Growth Factor (VEGF), and GM-CSF. Recombinant human (rh)IL-11 has been evaluated in phase I/II clinical trials in patients with active rheumatoid arthritis. rhIL-11 was safe and well tolerated, and it induced a 20% response rate. The only adverse event was a reaction at the injection site (42). Anti-inflammatory cytokines (IL-10) and cytokines that inhibit Th2 cells (IL-12 and IFN-γ) have been used in the treatment of asthma and allergy (43–45). VEGF has shown promising results in the repair of ischemic myocardia, and FGF has accelerated the rate of healing of second-degree burns (21). rGM-CSF has been used successfully to heal cutaneous wounds and ulcers (21).

Cytokine Receptors

Cytokine receptors are excellent targets for the treatment of many diseases (24). The number of small molecule inhibitors of cytokine receptors is growing rapidly, and some receptors have demonstrated efficacy in inflammatory disease. For example, soluble TNF receptor Enbrel™ has completed safety testing and has shown efficacy in clinical trials for the therapy of rheumatoid arthritis (46).

Soluble cytokine receptors participate in the control of cytokine activity *in vivo* by inhibiting the ability of cytokines to bind to their receptors. Many soluble cytokine receptors are effective *in vitro* and in experimental therapy models. Soluble cytokine receptors are sometimes modified or are given in combination with other agents to increase their therapeutic efficacy. Soluble cytokine receptors have significant potential for the treatment of many different human diseases (47,48).

Conclusions

Cytokines and their antagonists are being evaluated in numerous clinical settings, and several have been FDA-approved. However, side effects remain a problem. Because cytokine production is under the homeostatic control of the host, targeted activation of cytokine genes may yield better safety profiles than administration of their protein counterparts, which act on so many tissues, often with high morbidity. Some improvements have been made in both the formulation and delivery of cytokines. However, specific targeting of cytokines or activation of cytokines *in situ* will be necessary before cytokine therapy will show more impressive effects. In addition, combination therapy with other agents must be explored in animal models. When some of these problems are solved, cytokines will probably find a niche in the treatment of infectious diseases and immunologic disorders. Cancer represents a more difficult challenge.

Soluble Co-Stimulatory Molecules

Since the early 1990s, the importance of co-stimulatory molecules on APCs, T cells, and B cells in the elaboration of a normal thymus-dependent immune response has been well established (49,50). These molecules include CTL-associated antigen 4 (CTLA-4; CD152), CD28, B7.1 (CD80), B7.2 (CD86), and CD154. Pairs of co-stimulatory molecules on interacting cells must be engaged for cell activation. This insight has led to strategies to inhibit these interactions to induce immunosuppression in the setting of autoimmuity (51) and graft rejection. The most effective inhibitors are soluble forms of these molecules (52).

CD152

CD152 on APCs interacts with CD28 on T cells. Soluble CD152-Ig binds to CD80 and CD86 and thereby inhibits interactions between APCs and T cells. This leads to suppression of both cellular and humoral immune responses (53). At doses 50-fold higher than those required to inhibit an antibody response, there has been no evidence of CD152-Ig–mediated toxicity in primates. CD152-Ig is being evaluated in phase I trials both in patients with autoimmunity and in patients in whom the induction of tolerance against certain proteins is of clinical importance (54). CD152-Ig is also being tested for its ability to induce tolerance against allografts and to enhance the uptake of antigens by APCs to improve the immunogenicity of DNA vaccines (55).

Anti-CD40L (CD154)

CD154 on T cells is the ligand for CD40 on B cells and APCs. Once these two molecules interact, the APCs or B cells express CD80/CD86, which can then interact with CD28 on T cells. Both CD40 and CD154 belong to the TNF family of receptors that play an important role in the effector function of fully differentiated T cells. They also play an important role in the activation of macrophages and B cells.

ANTIBODIES

History

Unlike the pleiotropic cytokines and immunomodulators, antibodies are much more specific. There has therefore been enormous interest in using them to target disease-causing cells.

First-generation therapeutic antibodies were described at the end of the 19th century. These were polyclonal antibodies that were used to neutralize bacterial toxins (e.g., diphtheria, tetanus) and to treat rabies, varicella, and other infectious diseases (56). Advances in the study of vaccines and the successful use of antibiotic therapy have decreased the use of polyclonal antibodies, except in the case of some antitoxins against snake and spider venoms.

More complete characterization of the antibody molecule (57), as well as the development of the newer procedures to isolate and purify gamma globulins from normal pooled sera (58), paved the way for the introduction of second-generation therapeutic antibodies, in the form of intravenous immunoglobulin (IVIG). IVIG is used for the prophylaxis of infectious and autoimmune diseases and as replacement therapy for primary and secondary immunodeficiencies (59). Treatment with IVIG is well tolerated by patients and is becoming widely used (Table 2).

Monoclonal antibodies (mAbs) were first described in 1975 (60). mAbs directed against numerous cellular targets have been generated (61). However, because of their immunogenicity, murine mAbs had limited success in the therapy of human cancers and other diseases (62). Of the 49 murine mAbs entering clinical trials, only one has reached

TABLE 2. *IVIG for autoimmune disorders*

Cytopenias
  Idiopathic thrombocytopenia
  Autoimmune hemolytic anemia
  Immune neutropenia
Coagulopathies
  Antihemophilic factor VIII inhibitor
  Antiphospholipid antibody syndrome
Vasculitides
  Kawasaki syndrome
  ANCA-associated disease
Collagen disorders
  Systemic lupus erythematosus
  Rheumatoid arthritis
  Polymyositis
Dermatological diseases
  Bullous pemphigoid
Neurological diseases
  Myasthenia gravis
  Multiple sclerosis
  Guillain-Barré syndrome
  Chronic polyneuropathy
  Amyotrophic lateral sclerosis (Lou Gehrig's disease)
Inflammatory bowel disease
  Crohn's disease
  Ulcerative colitis
Organ-specific disorders
  Insulin-dependent diabetes
  Autoimmune thyroiditis
  Graves' ophthalmopathy
Other disorders
  Chronic fatigue syndrome

ANCA, anti-neutrophil cytoplasmic antibody.
From Strand (114), with permission.

the market. This is Muromonab-CD3, approved by FDA in 1986 to prevent the rejection of kidney transplants (63).

Because of immunogenicity, research in the 1980s focused on creating less immunogenic mAbs by combining mAb technology with recombinant DNA technology. The result was the production of chimeric (1984) and humanized (1986) mAbs (64–66). Chimeric mAbs contain mouse heavy-chain and light-chain variable regions joined to human heavy-chain and light-chain constant regions. Humanized mAbs contain only the six mouse complementarity-determining regions (CDRs) grafted into the human variable region. These fourth-generation "nonimmunogenic" mAbs entered clinical trials in 1987 (63). At present, more than 70 chimeric and humanized mAbs are undergoing evaluation in clinical trials (63). Most of these mAbs are not immunogenic in humans and persist in the circulation. Because they have a human Fc, they mediate effector functions, thus leading to a higher success rate in humans (63).

Fully humanized mAbs with higher affinities were subsequently created by the selection of human variable regions from phage display libraries (67). Transgenic mice with human Ig genes produce human antibodies after immunization (68) At present, two human mAbs are being evaluated in clinical trials (Table 3), and their approval is imminent (63).

Clinical Considerations

The preferred isotype for therapeutic human mAbs is IgG, which, in comparison with IgM and IgA, has a lower molecular mass (150 kDa), is more stable in vivo, and is easier to prepare. To be effective as a therapeutic molecule, an IgG antibody should have both specificity for the corresponding antigen and the ability to recruit Fc receptor (FcR)–bearing cells and complement components after binding to the antigen. In addition to conventional effector function, some antitumor mAbs can also induce neoplastic cells to undergo cell cycle arrest or apoptosis (69). These signaling functions may be critical for an effective antitumor response, although this remains to be proven.

Other important characteristics of mAbs are their persistence in the circulation and their immunogenicity. For example, increased persistence of IgG is desirable because it creates an increased concentration gradient across the interstitium leading to better penetration of the targeted tissue. The persistence of IgG antibody is controlled by its size and by the presence of the Fc portion of the molecule (70). Smaller fragments lacking Fc regions (e.g., Fab or Fv fragments) have shorter half-lives in the circulation but, because of their smaller size, penetrate targeted tumors more effectively even if they do not persist. Thus, the relative efficacy of each is still a matter of contention and may depend on the setting in which each is used.

Depending on the immune status of the host, IgG mAbs can often elicit an immune response. Immunogenicity depends on the form of the molecule used (e.g., aggregated versus disaggregated or intact versus fragments). If the mAb is immunogenic, the anti-antibodies facilitate rapid removal of the therapeutic mAb from the circulation and therefore decrease its ability to reach and penetrate targeted tissue.

Affinity

The affinity of an mAb can affect its ability to localize in a tumor. However, there is controversy concerning the role of affinity in the successful targeting and retention of mAbs in tumors. One theory postulates that high-affinity mAbs cannot penetrate deeply into the tumors because of the blocking effect of the "first" antigen on tumor cells encountered near the vasculature, which then blocks further diffusion of the mAb into the tumor (71). Another theory postulates that the most effective tumor targeting is achieved using mAbs with high affinities because low dissociation rates will prolong the retention of the mAb in the tumor site (72). Biodistribution studies of radioiodinated single chain (sc) Fv fragments of anti-Her-2 antibody in mice with severe combined immunodeficiency that were xenografted with human ovarian carcinoma tumors have shown that the degree and specificity of tumor localization increases with increasing affinity. However, tumor retention did not significantly increase beyond an affinity of more than 10^{-9}M (72). These results were interpreted to support the existence of a "binding barrier" effect, as postulated by the first theory (71).

TABLE 3. Selective list of unconjugated chimeric, humanized, and human antibody used in clinical trials for cancer

Monoclonal antibody	Targeted antigen	Human immunoglobulin G	Cancer
Rituximab (Rituxan)[a]	CD20	Chimeric	Low-grade and follicular NHL
Trastuzumab (Herceptin)[a]	Her-2/neu	Humanized	MBC overexpressing Her-2
Alemtuzumab (Campath)	CD52	Humanized	B-cell CLL
Epratuzumab (Lymphocide)	CD22	Humanized	NHL
Cetuximab (IMC-C225)	EGFR	Chimeric	Colorectal and advanced head and neck
Bevacizumab (Avastin)	VEGF	Human	Metastatic non–small cell lung and colorectal
Zamyl	CD33	Human	AML

AML, acute myeloblastic leukemia; CLL, chronic lymphocytic leukemia; EGFR, epidermal growth factor receptor; MBC, metastatic breast cancer; NHL, non-Hodgkin's lymphoma; VEGF, vascular endothelial growth factor.
[a]Approved by the U.S. Food and Drug Administration.
From Reichert (63) and Glennie and Johnson (84), with permission.

Persistence and Size

The persistence of IgG antibodies in the circulation is a function of their molecular size and their ability to interact with the neonatal Fc receptor (FcRn) (70). FcRn is expressed on endothelial cells of the microvasculature (70), and binding of IgG to the FcRn protects the IgG from destruction within these cells and recycles it back to the circulation. The FcRn recognizes some amino acid residues in the Fc region of IgG. Therefore, removing the Fc region from a molecule of IgG considerably shortens its half-life because it cannot bind to "salvaging" FcRns. In addition, there is rapid renal elimination because of its smaller size. The ability of mAbs to penetrate tumors is impaired by their larger size and the high interstitial pressure of tumors (73), both of which decrease the diffusion of IgG into the tumor. Thus, smaller Fab/Fv fragments will be superior at penetrating tumors, but their short half-life will decrease their ability to reach an effective concentration gradient in the tumor. The rate of diffusion is proportional to the concentration of the mAb in the circulation and is inversely proportional to its size. Therefore, antibody size, half-life, and tumor penetration are interrelated. In terms of efficacy, it is possible that the longer persistence accompanying larger size may predominate over better penetration by smaller molecules of higher affinity. The lack of persistence of murine mAbs in the circulation of humans is at least partially responsible for the modest efficacy of therapeutic mouse mAbs. The reason is that the human FcRs do not bind murine IgG (74), so that it is rapidly eliminated from the circulation.

Effector Functions

Therapeutic mAbs can act either by recruiting FcR-bearing effector cells (e.g., macrophages, NK cells) or by activating the complement cascade. In both cases, the end result is the removal or destruction of the target cells. The species of origin and isotype of IgG affect the capacity of the mAb to harness host effector mechanisms (75). Thus, mouse IgGs have inferior effector function as compared with human IgGs when tested *in vitro* using human effector cells or human complement (75,76). Several studies have shown that human IgG1 is the isotype of choice for chimeric and humanized mAbs when the activation of effector functions is desired (64). When effector functions are not desirable, human IgG4, which has little or no effector activity, is the best choice. It has been suggested that antibody-dependent cellular cytotoxicity (ADCC) is a more general mechanism of lysis of nucleated cells than complement-dependent cytotoxicity (CDC) (77), because CDC is down-regulated by the presence of regulatory proteins (e.g., CD59) expressed on cells. Some of these proteins protect normal and tumor cells from lysis by mAbs and complement (78).

Immunogenicity

As mentioned previously, the major impediment to therapy with mouse mAbs is that patients rapidly develop human antimouse antibodies (HAMA). HAMA can neutralize the therapeutic mAb or result in its rapid elimination from the circulation. The antibody response to infused mouse mAbs can be divided into an anti-isotype (Fc fragment) response and an anti-idiotype (Id) (Fab fragment) response. It has been reported that the presence of the murine Fc region may make mAbs more immunogenic, whereas the Fab fragments are much less immunogenic (79). Using murine anti-CD4 mAbs in rhesus monkeys, it has been possible to obtain therapeutic effects in the presence of host antimouse IgG antibodies only if no anti-Id antibodies are present (80). The presence of anti-Fc region antibodies increased the efficacy of the anti-CD4 antibodies. This improvement has also been observed in patients with colorectal cancer treated with a mouse mAb, edrecolomab (Panorex) (81). However it remains to be proven in ongoing clinical trials whether human mAbs will have less immunogenicity in patients than humanized or chimeric mAbs because the antihuman antibody response (HAHA) elicited in patients is directed against the Id of the therapeutic antibody, which is "foreign" in both human and humanized mAbs (82). Hence, HAHA could be dependent on the presence of immunodominant epitopes in a given Id and not on humanization versus chimerization *per se*.

In various clinical trials using chimeric or humanized mAbs, only very low frequencies and titers of anti-Id antibodies have been reported (83). With regard to the development of HAHA, two distinct types have been observed: (a) type I (49% of patients) is characterized by an early onset and the lack of infusion-related adverse effects; (b) type II (17% of patients) is characterized by a later onset and adverse events requiring the discontinuation of treatment. The presence or absence of HAHA in the serum of patients with various diseases may also depend not only on the immune status of the patients but also the nature and stage of the disease, as well as on the dose regimen. These variables may explain the differences in the frequencies and titers of HAHA reported by different groups.

How Monoclonal Antibodies Work

There are three major mechanisms involved in the action of therapeutic mAbs. These include blocking, targeting, and signaling (84). Blocking prevents the interaction among various ligands and their receptors as well as the "cross-talk" among cells. Targeting involves binding to specific cells, which are then removed or destroyed by ADCC or CDC. Signaling, leading to the arrest of cell growth or the induction of apoptosis, occurs after cross-linking of neighboring receptors. Any given therapeutic mAb may work by one or more of these mechanisms.

Blocking

mAbs can block cytokines or receptor-ligand interactions that play key roles in immune responses. Therefore, most blocking mAbs are used for the treatment of autoimmune diseases or for immunosuppression. One example is the use of a chimeric mAb against TNF-α, infliximab (Remicade), which is a key cytokine in the pathogenesis of inflammation. Anti–TNF-α neutralizes its activity and reduces the tissue injury caused by autoimmune responses and is used in the treatment of rheumatoid arthritis (85) and Crohn's disease (86). Other mAbs block IL-2Rs (daclizumab and basiliximab) by binding to their α (CD25) subunit. High-affinity CD25-containing IL-2Rs are present on the surface of activated, but not resting, T and B lymphocytes. These mAbs thereby inhibit IL-2–mediated cell growth. Such mAbs are recommended for the prophylaxis of acute organ rejection. Short-term blockade of T-cell function may lead to long-term tolerance of the transplanted organs (87).

Targeting

Because most mAbs are not cytotoxic *per se,* cooperation with FcR-bearing effector cells is required. This was demonstrated by using either FcγRI and FcγRIII knockout mice or mutant mAbs devoid of the ability to interact with FcRs (88). In both cases, the antitumor activity of the mAbs was completely abolished. Conversely, the antitumor activity of some mAbs was increased in FcγRIIb knockout mice, a finding suggesting that this is an inhibitory receptor endowed with a check-and-balance role in ADCC (88). The efficacy of the mAb also depends on the nature of the targeted antigen and its behavior after binding of the mAb. Some membrane antigens are internalized rapidly after the binding of antibody (e.g., CD3, CD19), whereas others are not (e.g., CD20, CD52). For clinical responses requiring the lysis of target cells by a particular mAb, a nonmodulating antigen may be preferable. Studies in patients treated with alemtuzumab (Campath-1H; chimerized anti-CD52) have shown the importance of both the isotype of the mAb and the expression and stability of CD52 on the surface of the targeted cells (75). However, despite the consensus that ADCC is of critical importance in determining clinical outcome, this has not been formally proven in humans. This lack of data emphasizes the importance of *in vivo* models for studying the effector functions of mAbs, because some mAbs that have performed very well *in vitro* have failed in clinical trials (89). The role of cell-mediated cytotoxicity (CMC) in the therapeutic activity of mAb both in mice and in patients with cancer remains controversial (84).

Signaling

A signaling role for mAbs was first demonstrated using anti-Fas (CD95) antibody, which induced apoptosis in all CD95+ cells (90). Similarly, clinical studies demonstrated a correlation between the ability of therapeutic mAbs to induce transmembrane signaling in lymphoma cells and clinical responses in patients (91). Many mAbs that have been candidates for the treatment of lymphoma are capable of negatively signaling neoplastic B cells. Thus, both anti-CD19 and anti-CD22 mAbs can induce cell-cycle arrest in targeted cells both

in vitro and in mice xenografted with human tumors (92,93). In the case of CD20+ lymphoma cells, cross-linking CD20 with various mAbs, including the chimerized anti-CD20 mAb, rituximab (Rituxan), induces certain signaling events such as increased protein tyrosine phosphorylation, activation of protein kinase C, and up-regulation of Myc (94). The binding of anti-CD20 mAbs to some neoplastic B-cell lines can induce apoptosis, but the induction of apoptosis is clearly dependent upon cross-linking and, more accurately, on hyper–cross-linking by the mAb (95,96). Signaling through CD20 may be related to the rapid movement of this antigen and Src kinases into lipid rafts (97). Similarly, in the murine BCL₁ (B lymphoma) tumor model, anti-Id can induce tumor dormancy (98). Tumor cells that eventually escape anti-Id–mediated dormancy often show alterations in their levels of critical signaling proteins such as Syk, HS-1, and Lyn (98).

Another example of a signaling antibody is anti–CD152, which enhances the activity of T cells that recognize tumor antigens. The treatment of mice with some, but not other, tumors is highly effective (99). The same antibody can induce autoimmunity in other situations, so its use must be carefully evaluated. Clinical trials with anti-CD152 are ongoing (99).

Engineering Monoclonal Antibodies with Enhanced or Decreased Activities

It is often desirable to change the affinity, specificity, and effector functions and to decrease the immunogenicity of mAbs for clinical use. These changes can be achieved by engineering the CDRs (involved in antigen binding) or the amino acid residues in the Fc region of the molecule (involved in the binding of FcR or C1q) and the epitopes responsible for immunogenicity. The generation of human mAbs with high affinity and specificity for the targeted antigen can be achieved by phage display using various procedures such as the shuffling of heavy- and light-chain genes and random or directed mutagenesis of CDRs. These techniques, followed by selection of the desired mutants, has resulted in mAbs with affinities in the nanomolar or even picomolar ranges (75). In addition, it is sometimes desirable to modify the effector function and pharmacokinetics of an mAb to improve or decrease binding to FcR-bearing cells and complement components or to prolong or shorten persistence in the circulation. MAbs lacking the ability to mediate effector functions are used when local inflammation is undesirable. For example, one may want to prevent allograft rejection but not generate a massive inflammatory response *in situ.* Aglycosylated antibody obtained by a single mutation in the Asn-297 residue has greatly reduced binding to FcR and C1q, and an aglycosylated humanized mAb against CD3 is being evaluated in clinical trials to prevent allograft rejection (100). Modifications in residues 233 to 236 (in the lower hinge region) (101) or a single mutation of the residue Asp-265 (102) considerably decreased the activity of an mAb both *in vitro* (101) and *in vivo* (102).

Conversely, when effector functions and an inflammatory response are highly desirable, the goal is to improve CDC and ADCC. In this regard, high-resolution mapping of the binding site of human IgG1 for $Fc\gamma RI$, II, and III has led to the design of IgG1 variants with improved binding to all three FcRs (103). MAbs with increased binding to C1q have been obtained by modifying only two amino acid residues (Lys-326 and Glu-333) in the CH2 domain of the chimeric mAb, rituximab (104).

As noted previously, the persistence of IgG antibody in the circulation depends on its interactions with FcRn (70). By mapping the binding site on mouse IgG for FcRn, it has been demonstrated that a few amino acid residues localized at the interface of the CH2 (Ile-253, His-310) and CH3 (His-435, His-436) domains are responsible for the persistence of mouse IgG in the circulation (70). By modifying these or nearby amino acid residues, various mutants with increased or decreased affinities for FcRns have been generated (103). These have prolonged (105) or shortened (106) half-lives in mice. Increasing the persistence of antibody in the circulation facilitates tumor penetration by increasing the concentration gradient across the interstitium. Decreasing the persistence is desirable for delivering a toxic payload in which rapid clearance of the unbound toxic conjugate may diminish its harmful side effects.

As mentioned, immunogenicity of mAbs has been decreased by chimerization or humanization of mouse mAbs or by generating human mAbs. Prophylactic induction of tolerance against therapeutic mAbs is also an attractive approach. For example, when injected into mice expressing CD52, modified alemtuzumab (Campath-1H, which cannot bind to cells) induced tolerance against the wild-type cell-binding mAb (75).

Immunoglobulin G and Monoclonal Antibodies in Clinical Practice

Intravenous Immunoglobulin

The criteria for an optimal IVIG preparation are as follows: (a) the use of IgGs with native structure and function; (b) isolation of these IgGs from a large pool of plasma (15,000 to 30,000 donors) containing the entire spectrum of IgG antibodies; (c) the presence of all four isotypes in physiologic ratios; and (d) the lack of infectious agents, large aggregates, or any toxic material. The FDA has approved the use of IVIG in three clinical situations: (a) replacement therapy for immunodeficiencies, (b) prevention and treatment of infectious diseases; and (c) therapy of autoimmune disorders.

Replacement Therapy in Immunodeficiencies

Gamma globulins were first used to treat the primary immunodeficiency, Bruton's X-linked agammaglobulinemia (107). Many other defects in antibody formation have been identified, and in all cases IVIG therapy has been used successfully.

The most prominent clinical manifestation of antibody deficiency syndromes is infection by a wide variety of bacteria, viruses, protozoa, and fungi. Noninfectious complications are also common in patients with antibody deficiencies including malignant diseases (e.g., lymphomas, adenocarcinomas) and autoimmune diseases (e.g., idiopathic thrombocytopenic purpura, hemolytic anemia). IVIG therapy has been used with some degree of success in secondary or acquired immunodeficiencies such as those induced by protein loss through the kidney (nephrotic syndrome), bowel (ulcerative colitis), and skin (burned patients). IVIG has also shown promise in patients with bone marrow transplants.

Prevention and Treatment of Infectious Diseases

IVIG contains antibodies against a wide variety of bacterial and viral pathogens. Therefore, administration of IVIG provides passive protection against many infectious diseases.

The benefits of IVIG therapy have been attributed to the neutralization of common infectious agents such as *Pseudomonas aeruginosa*, varicella virus, *Streptococcus pneumoniae*, *Haemophilus influenzae*, cytomegalovirus (CMV), respiratory syncytial virus, hepatitis A and B viruses, and many other pathogens. Because only certain antiviral antibodies are present in sufficient amounts in standard IVIG preparations, hyperimmune preparations have been obtained from selected high-titer plasma donors or from immunized or vaccinated subjects. HYPERIVIG is commercially available for intravenous or intramuscular administration in cases of infections with CMV, *P. aeruginosa*, and hepatitis B virus and in Rh incompatibility (107).

Therapy of Autoimmune Disorders

The surprising efficacy of IVIG in increasing platelet counts in patients with idiopathic thrombocytopenic purpura (ITP) (108) led to the empiric and often successful use of IVIG therapy in a large number of autoimmune diseases (Table 2). In almost all these diseases, treatment with IVIG has proven to be more beneficial than conventional therapy. Thus, in the treatment of patients with Guillain-Barré syndrome (109) or myasthenia gravis (110), the infusion of IVIG gave a more favorable outcome than plasmapheresis. Studies comparing the efficacy of IVIG versus aspirin in the treatment of Kawasaki's syndrome demonstrated that IVIG was superior with regard to both the duration and the outcome of the disease (111).

Mechanism of Action of Intravenous Immunoglobulin

The mechanism of action of high doses of IVIG in the treatment of autoimmune disorders is not well understood, and none of the numerous mechanisms proposed can satisfactorily explain the clinical results. Several hypotheses have been proposed. The first is the involvement of the Id–anti-Id network; that is, IVIG passively transfers autoanti-Ids and actively alters the endogenous regulation of autoantibody production through Id–anti-Id interactions (112). IVIG contains a vast assortment of anti-Id autoantibodies able to neutralize the autoantibodies in the circulation. Clinical observations in anti–factor VIII autoimmune disease, myasthenia gravis, systemic lupus erythematosus, Guillain-Barré syndrome, and other autoimmune diseases have indicated that patients responding to IVIG treatment develop anti-Id antibodies directed against the implicated autoantibodies. Thus, patients with myasthenia gravis have received lasting benefits after IVIG treatment with a significant decrease in autoantibody titers against the acetylcholine receptor resulting from the development of anti-Id (113). Second, it has been proposed that the Id–anti-Id immune complexes present in the IVIG preparation as dimers may down-regulate autoantibody production by cross-bridging FcRs and antigen receptors on B cells or by interacting with other cell surface receptors that may alter the secretion of cytokines that modulate T- and B-cell functions (114). FcR blockade emphasizes the role of the Fc region in the therapeutic effect of IVIG. Decreased binding of autoantibody-coated target cells (e.g., platelets, red blood cells) to FcR-bearing effector cells of the reticuloendothelial system (mainly macrophages) is considered to be the predominant mechanism involved in the efficacy of the IVIG treatment in various cytopenias (115). IVIG blocks the binding of autoantibody-coated platelets and prevents their destruction by macrophages expressing the $Fc\gamma RIII$ activation receptor. The blockade of $Fc\gamma RIII$ by IVIG is suggested by studies showing that the same clinical effects were obtained in the treatment of ITP with anti-$Fc\gamma RIII$ mAb (116) or with the Fc fragment of IVIG (117). Another explanation for the role of FcR has been presented using a mouse model of ITP (118). It has been shown that injected IVIG induces the increased expression of inhibitory $Fc\gamma RIIb$ on splenic macrophages. Cross-linking the newly expressed $Fc\gamma RIIb$ and the $Fc\gamma RIII$ by the platelet-antiplatelet antibody immune complexes abolishes the activation signal induced by $Fc\gamma RIII$ and results in abrogation of phagocytosis and platelet depletion. In addition, the Fc region of IVIG can also bind to the C3b and C4b components of complement and thereby can both inhibit their binding to target cells and solubilize the harmful circulating immune complexes (119). Consistent with this explanation, decreased C3 binding and prolongation of red blood cell survival in the circulation were observed after treatment of patients with autoimmune hemolytic anemia (119). Finally, hypercatabolism of autoantibody induced by high doses of IVIG (120,121) results from an IgG concentration effect on catabolism (122) and the role of FcRn in the regulation of the rate of IgG catabolism. The increased catabolism of endogenous IgG (including autoantibodies) by the administration of high doses of IVIG could be the result of the saturation of FcRn in the patient and the random destruction of excess IgG molecules.

Alterations in IgG catabolism, the blockade of the function of FcR-bearing effector cells, and the Id–anti-Id network may all contribute to the effects of IVIG therapy in autoimmune diseases. However, the relative contribution of each mechanism may differ from one disease to another.

Monoclonal Antibodies

The desired criteria for an optimal therapeutic mAb are as follows: (a) the choice of IgG1 or IgG4, depending on whether effector function is desirable (IgG1) or not (IgG4); (b) lack of cross-reactivity (or expression of) antigens on life-sustaining tissues or organs; and (c) low rates of endocytosis after interaction of the target antigen with the mAb. The mAbs currently approved by the FDA are used in the treatment of malignant disease, some inflammatory diseases, and toxic shock.

Cancer

Treatment of B-Cell Lymphomas with Rituximab. In 1997, the first mAb to treat cancer was approved by the FDA, a chimeric IgG1 antihuman CD20 (rituximab) (Table 3). The CD20 antigen is an appropriate target for mAb therapy because it is expressed on 90% of malignant B cells. Although CD20 is also expressed on normal B cells, it is not expressed on B-cell precursors, plasma cells, or stem cells. Patients treated with rituximab recover their B-cell population in 3 to 12 months without any significant increase in the incidence of infections. CD20 is not shed and does not undergo modulation after binding to rituximab. The mechanism of action may involve ADCC/CMC, as suggested by *in vitro* experiments using this mAb constructed with a human IgG4 instead of IgG1. Treatment of patients with indolent NHL led to a response rate of 48% with a median duration of 12 months, with 10% to 15% of patients sustaining remissions for more than 24 months in the absence of additional therapy. The adverse events were minor, and HAMA was detected in only 1% of treated patients (123). The low frequency of immune responses is probably related to previous immunosuppressive treatments or to the immunosuppressive nature of the disease. Rituximab was also combined with chemotherapy in patients with diffuse large cell B-cell lymphoma, and responses were significantly better than with chemotherapy alone (124). Rituximab has also been used as a first-line treatment of indolent NHL. Responses were higher in patients with fewer previous treatments (125). Finally, rituximab can be administered with various chemotherapeutic regimens without increased toxicity.

Another mAb used for the treatment of NHL, but not yet approved by the FDA, is epratuzumab (LymphoCide) (Table 3), a humanized IgG1 anti-CD22 antibody. This mAb is being evaluated in advanced clinical trials. In contrast to CD20, the CD22 antigen is internalized after binding to the mAb. In a phase I clinical trial involving 51 patients with indolent and diffuse B-cell lymphomas, responses were lower than those achieved using rituximab. A possible explanation for the lower efficacy is the internalization of the CD22 antigen, which may shorten its persistence on tumor cells and hence may decrease ADCC/CMC. Treatment was well tolerated, and HAHA was rare. Further studies to evaluate the therapeutic role of this mAb are warranted (126).

Treatment of Breast Cancer with Trastuzumab (Herceptin). Overexpression of Her-2 occurs on primary breast cancers in 20% to 25% of patients and is associated with a poor prognosis (127). Because Her-2 is involved in the pathogenesis of breast cancer, it became an important target for mAb therapy. Her-2 belongs to the family of epidermal growth factor (EGF) receptors. Therefore, anti–Her-2 (trastuzumab) may inhibit cell growth either by preventing the soluble growth factor from binding to its cognate receptor or by inducing an antimitogenic signal. The presence of mAb on the surface of tumor cells may also trigger the lysis of target cells by ADCC or CMC. However, Her-2 is internalized to a significant degree, and the extracellular domain of the molecule can also be cleaved from the cell surface (127). The function of this soluble receptor is not known, but it has been demonstrated that, in patients with circulating soluble Her-2, the anti–Her-2 mAb has a decreased half-life (127). Anti–Her-2 also appears to prevent the release of some angiogenic cytokines from tumor cells (128,129), and this should decrease their metastatic potential.

Trastuzumab has been evaluated in several clinical trials in women with metastatic breast cancer overexpressing Her-2. In a pivotal trial, 15% of the 222 women with metastatic breast cancer who were previously treated with chemotherapy had an objective response (OR). The response was even higher (31%) in patients with the highest levels of Her-2 expression on their tumors (130). The addition of trastuzumab to a chemotherapy regimen resulted in more ORs, and the best synergy was observed using the taxanes. In the case of trastuzumab plus doxorubicin or cyclophosphamide, the incidence of cardiotoxicity was increased when trastuzumab was used. The basis for this increase in cardiotoxicity is unclear, but the finding that Her-2 is expressed at low levels in the myocardium may play a role in the increased cardiotoxicity

of the combined treatment. Not every patient responds, and the reasons for this are currently unclear. Many other mAbs are presently being tested in clinical trials as single agents or in combination with chemotherapy (Table 3).

Non-neoplastic Disease

Many mAbs are currently being evaluated in clinical trials for their activity in inflammatory diseases (e.g., rheumatoid arthritis, Crohn's disease) and allograft rejection. A partial list of such mAbs is presented in Table 4, and one mAb is FDA approved.

Rheumatoid Arthritis and Crohn's Disease. The first mAb to be used in clinical trials for non-neoplastic disease was infliximab (Remicade), a chimerized human IgG1 mAb which binds to and neutralizes TNF-α (a potent proinflammatory cytokine). Rapid clinical improvements (lasting 1 to 2 months) were observed in patients with rheumatoid arthritis, and the duration of the responses was related to the concentration of the mAb in the circulation. Repeated treatments were necessary to maintain a therapeutic effect, but the duration was progressively shortened after repeated treatments (131). Half of the patients receiving retreatment cycles developed HAMA, and this may account for treatment failures. To decrease HAMA, methotrexate was administered (131). To decrease immunogenicity, other versions of anti–TNF-α were constructed. These include humanized and fully human (D2E7) mAbs (Table 4). Infliximab has also been used for the treatment of Crohn's disease. About two-thirds of the patients responded to a single infusion of this mAb, a finding indicating that retreatment cycles may be necessary. Of major clinical interest is the beneficial effect of this mAb on the healing of fistulae in Crohn's disease for which no optimal therapy is available (86). The adverse effects of infliximab include infections and autoimmune reactions. Because TNF-α plays a significant role in tumor surveillance, long-term or extended treatment risks may include lymphoproliferative disorders.

TABLE 4. *Selective list of unconjugated chimeric, humanized, and human antibody used in clinical trials for diseases other than cancer*

Drug	Targeted antigen	Immunoglobulin antibody type	Disease
D2E7	TNF-γ	Human	Rheumatoid arthritis
Infliximab (Remicade)	TNF-γ	Chimeric	Crohn's disease and rheumatoid arthritis
Basiliximab (SIMULECT)	CD25	Chimeric	Allograft rejection
Daclizumab (ZENAPAX)	CD25	Humanized	Allograft rejection
IDEC-131	CD40 ligand	Humanized	Multiple sclerosis and systemic lupus erythematosus
Natalizumab (ANTEGREN)	CD49[a]	Humanized	Multiple sclerosis
ABX-IL8	IL-8	Human	Psoriasis
Siplizumab (MEDI-507)	CD2	Humanized	GVHD
rhuMAb-E25	IgE	Humanized	Asthma and allergy

GVHD, graft-versus-host disease; IgE, immunoglobulin E; IL-8, interleukin-8; TNF-γ, tumor necrosis factor γ.

[a]VLA-4, alpha-4 integrin.

From Reichert (63) and Glennie and Johnson (84), with permission.

Organ Transplantation

A murine mAb against human CD3 on T cells was the first mAb to enter clinical trials to prevent organ rejection. The original mouse mAb (OKT3) is FDA approved and is still used to reverse corticosteroid-resistant transplant rejection episodes. To decrease both the immunogenicity and the cytokine release syndrome/cytokine storm associated with the use of OKT3 treatment, humanized mAbs were generated. These mAbs had decreased immunogenicity, and because they were IgG4s and did not bind to FcR-bearing effector cells, they functionally blocked the targeted $CD3^+$ T cells without lysing them (132). Clinical trials using the humanized anti-CD3 mAb confirmed its ability to reverse the acute rejection of renal allografts in the absence of cytokine storm. Current combination therapies for the prophylaxis of acute organ rejection in adult patients include either chimeric (basiliximab [Simulect]) or humanized (daclizumab [Zenapax]) mAbs, both of which are directed against CD25 on activated T cells. No cytokine storm or significant decreases in circulating lymphocytes have been observed. Importantly, there have been fewer opportunistic infections or lymphoproliferative disorders as compared with the use of other immunosuppressive agents. The efficacy of these anti-CD3, CD4, CD25, and other anti–T-cell mAbs in allograft rejection still falls short of the expectation generated by the results obtained in animal models, in which such treatments may induce tolerance to the graft. Nevertheless, mAbs are highly beneficial in human patients. Anti-CD4 and anti-CD25 are under intensive study.

Conclusions

IVIG and mAbs are rapidly becoming standard care in many diseases. In some cases, their mechanisms of action are well defined, but in others they are not. Problems such as immunogenicity, serum half-life, and tumor penetration have been addressed and in many cases solved by genetic engineering. For some applications, IVIG and mAbs can be used as stand-alone therapy, whereas in others, they are more effective in combination with other conventional or experimental therapies.

Bispecific Monoclonal Antibodies

Basic Considerations

Bispecific mAbs (BsmAbs) are mAbs with dual specificities: one arm recognizes the target cell, and the other recognizes an effector cell or a toxic molecule (Fig. 1A and B). Most BsmAbs are being developed to treat cancer. The three major approaches for creating BsmAbs (Fig. 1C) are as follows: (a) chemical cross-linking of two mAbs to create a tetravalent molecule with two intact immunoglobulins, each with two binding sites for a specific antigen; (b) fusion of two hybridomas, to generate quadroma cell lines (133), which produce divalent immunoglobulins in which each VH-VL pair has one of two different specificities; and (c) genetic

engineering (134), to create chimeric proteins that are multivalent and consist of two recombinant mAb fragments linked genetically or by a conventional chemical cross-linker or a single-chain chimeric protein.

BsmAbs have been used to deliver cytotoxic drugs or toxins to tumor cells. These include toxins, such as saporin, ricin A chain (RTA), and vinca alkaloids, as well as radioisotopes (Fig. 1A). One arm of the BsmAb binds to a surface molecule on the targeted cell, and the other arm is preloaded with the agent to be delivered (135,136). It is critical that both arms retain binding affinity *in vivo* and that favorable pharmacokinetics and biodistribution are achieved. BsmAbs have also been used successfully in animals (137) to activate different effector cells (e.g., phagocytic cells, NK cells, and T lymphocytes) *in situ* after cross-linking them to target cells (Fig. 1B). Generally, T cells are targeted through CD3, which is an integral part of the antigen-specific T-cell receptor (TCR), NK cells are targeted through $Fc\gamma RIII$ (CD16), and phagocytic cells are targeted through $Fc\gamma RI$ (CD64) (136). These targeted effector cells become cytotoxic when they are bound to the tumor cell, and the killing of normal bystander cells is avoided.

The lytic machinery of the cytotoxic cell depends on whether it is a T cell, an NK cell, or a macrophage. Hence, T and NK cells release cytotoxic granules or cytokines or induce receptor-mediated apoptosis, whereas phagocytic cells (e.g., granulocytes, neutrophils, and macrophages) induce ADCC through their $Fc\gamma$ receptors. In addition, other FcRs (138) and adhesion molecules (139) have been identified as alternative signaling molecules on effector cells. The effector cells can be adoptively transferred after *in vitro* treatment with BsmAbs, or the patient's own cells can be targeted *in vivo*. However, preactivation of the effector cells is almost always required (140), and the presence of co-stimulatory molecules, such as CD28, IL-2, lymphocyte function–associated antigen-1 (LFA-1), CD2, and GM-CSF, is often necessary to achieve activation. Recently designed BsmAbs (BiLu, which is a mouse IgG2a x rat IgG2b) (141) redirect not only T cells but also FcR-positive $(FcR)^+$ (accessory) cells to the tumor site (142). This trifunctional BsmAb can kill tumor cells very efficiently without any additional co-stimulation of effector cells *in vitro*. Long-lasting antitumor immunity is induced in mice (142).

There are two major limitations to using BsmAbs. These include their large size (twice the size of mAbs), which decreases their ability to penetrate tumors and, in the case of mouse mAbs, the generation of HAMA. The first drawback can be improved by preparing recombinant Fvs (134,143), whereas the second problem can be solved by using humanized and chimeric BsmAbs.

Clinical Applications

BsmAbs for delivering immune effector cells and, to a lesser extent, for delivering radionuclides, drugs, and toxins to tumors have been evaluated in clinical trials (83). The most extensively used target molecules are CD3 on T cells,

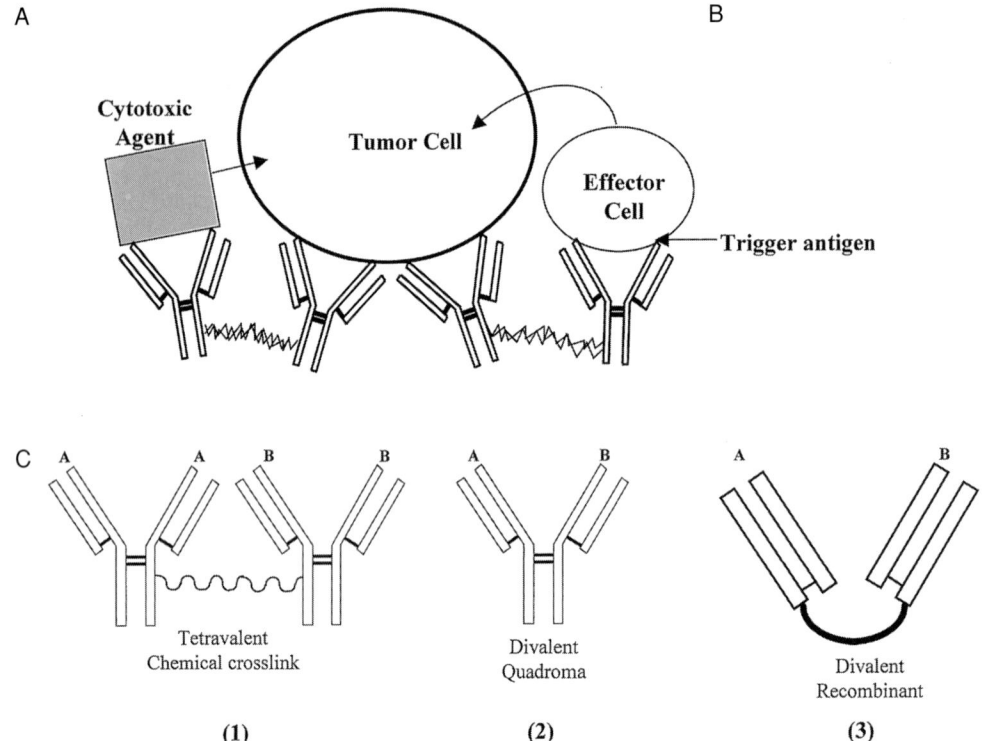

FIG. 1. How BsMAbs kill cells. (A) One arm of the BsMAb binds to the targeted tumor cell and the other arm binds to a drug, toxin, or isotope. (B) Effector cells are brought into contact with a tumor cell *via* a BsMAb, where one arm binds to the tumor cell and the other to a surface antigen on the effector cell (T cell, NK cell, macrophage, granulocyte, or neutrophil). MAb binding triggers lytic activity or the release of damaging cytokines from the cytotoxic cell. (C) Bispecific MAbs. (1) These are tetravalent, chemically cross-linked molecules. Two MAbs are held together covalently by a chemical cross-linker. This construct has four binding sites: two for antigen A, and two for antigen B. (2) Divalent quadromas are obtained from the secretions of hybrid hybridomas (quadromas). The quadroma receives one set of heavy and light chains from each parent hybridoma, creating one binding site for antigen A and one for antigen B. (3) Divalent recombinant molecules are single-chain fusion proteins with one binding site for antigen A and one for antigen B (153). "Reprinted with permission from R. Farah, B. Clinchy, L. Herrera and E. S. Vitetta. *Critical Reviews in Eukaryotic Gene Expression,* 1998;8(3&4): 321–356."

FcγRIII (CD16) on NK cells, and FcγRI (CD64) on granulocytes and macrophages. More recently, FcαRI (CD89) on macrophages has been targeted (144). Clinical trials in B-cell malignancies have been initiated (145), and several phase I/II trials for Hodgkin's disease (HD) have been conducted (146). Some small-scale trials involving intracavitary administration of BsmAbs to treat ovarian cancer have produced encouraging results (147), but treatment failures occurred because of the presence of metastatic cells, which were refractory to intracavitary administration of the BsmAbs (83). Promising early results have been obtained in trials for neurocarcinomas (148), colorectal cancer (149), renal cancer (150), and lung cancer (151). However, a common clinical problem associated with BsmAb therapy is the systemic activation of effector cells that cause cytokine storm, leading to serious side effects. Moreover, the pharmaceutical development of BsmAbs is costly because of the difficulty of producing them in sufficient quantities and purity for clinical trials (83). Despite proof of principle, a major challenge in this field is to develop technologies to produce larger quantities of better BsmAbs for human use.

IMMUNOCONJUGATES

Introduction

ICs are cell-targeting molecules, such as mAbs, cytokines, or soluble receptors that have been genetically or biochemically coupled to cytotoxic moieties (152). Thus, the cell-targeting portion of an IC is used as a delivery system for toxins, radioisotopes, drugs, enzymes that can activate prodrugs, liposomes, or effector cell-recruiting structures (Fig. 2) (153). From the multitude of ICs, three types have entered clinical trials in humans: immunotoxins (ITs), radiolabeled mAbs, and antibody-directed enzyme prodrug therapy (ADEPT) (152). The following sections describe some of these constructs, the rationale for their development, and their clinical evaluation (153).

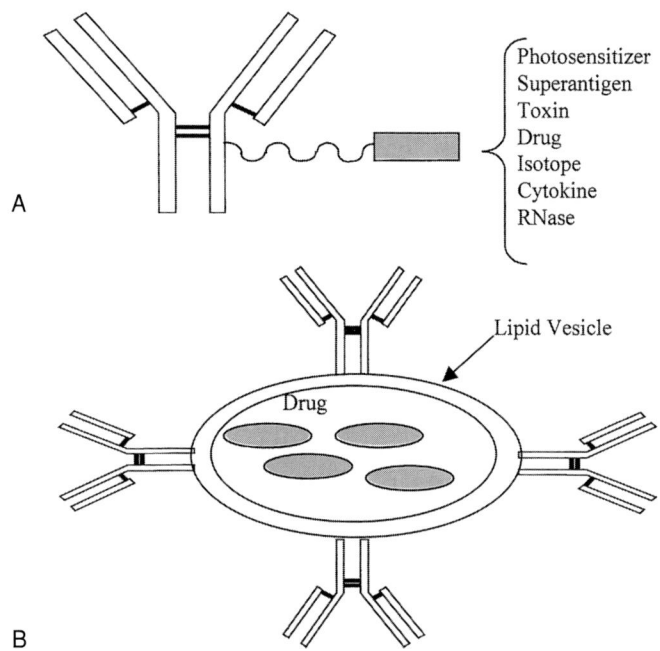

A

Photosensitizer
Superantigen
Toxin
Drug
Isotope
Cytokine
RNase

Lipid Vesicle

Drug

B

FIG. 2. (A) ICs are MAbs linked to a variety of toxic agents or effector molecules. The linkage can be chemical or the IC can be generated by genetic engineering. (B) Immunoliposomes consist of a toxic agent encapsulated within a lipid vesicle with multiple MAbs attached to the vesicle as targeting moieties (153). "Reprinted with permission from R. Farah, B. Clinchy, L. Herrera and E. S. Vitetta. *Critical Reviews in Eukaryotic Gene Expression*, 1998;8(3&4):321–356."

Immunotoxins

Development

The conjugates referred to as ITs are hybrid molecules consisting of mAbs linked to powerful toxins (or toxin subunits) purified from plants, fungi, or bacteria (154–156) (Fig. 2A). These toxins inhibit protein synthesis after the IT is inter-

nalized and lead to death of the targeted cell. mAbs that are unable to signal cells negatively or to elicit effector functions can still be useful as ITs as long as they are cycled into target cells. There are several advantages in using ITs. First, very small quantities of ITs are required for effective killing of target cells (e.g., a single toxin molecule in the cytosol can kill a cell), whereas significantly larger amounts of unconjugated mAbs are used with comparable or often inferior effects. Second, ITs kill both resting and dividing cells. Therefore, as compared with chemotherapeutic agents, they can also be effective against dormant, noncycling tumor cells (153). ITs do, however, induce more systemic toxicity because of their toxic moieties.

Characteristics of Toxins

ITs were first described in the late 1970s (153). Since that time, the numbers of ITs, as well as the toxins used to construct them, have increased significantly (Table 5) (153). The most frequently used toxins are modified RTA and a portion of *Pseudomonas* exotoxin (PE). Despite their different origins and mechanisms of action, both inhibit protein synthesis. After binding to the target through the mAb portion (specific for antigens present on the cell surface), the toxic moiety must be internalized and eventually translocated into the cytosol, to block protein synthesis.

Plant toxins are ribosome-inactivating proteins (RIPs). Based on their structure, RIPs can be divided into types I and II. Both inactivate the 60S ribosomal subunit by cleaving the 28S rRNA, thus preventing its interaction with elongation factor 2. Type I RIPs have a single enzymatically active protein A chain, whereas type II RIPs holotoxins consist of two chains, A and B, linked together by disulfide bonds (157). The A chain contains the enzymatic activity, and the B chain is responsible for cell binding and entry. To prepare an IT, the B chain has to be removed or modified because its galactose-binding domains can bind nonspecifically

TABLE 5. *Toxins used for the preparation of immunotoxins*

Source	Ribosome-inactivating protein type	Toxin	Enzymatic activity
Plant	I	Pokeweed antiviral protein (PAP) Saporin (SAP) Gelonin Momordin Trichosanthin Barley toxin	N-glycosidase for 28s ribosomal RNA
	II	Abrin Ricin Viscumin	
Bacteria		Diphtheria toxin *Pseudomonas* exotoxin	ADP ribosylation of EF2
Fungi		Sarcin Restrictocin	Ribonuclease for 28s RNA

ADP, adenosine diphosphate; EF2, elongation factor 2; RNA, ribonucleic acid.
From Farah et al. (153), with permission.

to galactose-containing glycoproteins and glycolipids expressed on all normal mammalian cells. The galactose-binding sites in the B chain of ricin have been specifically modified to generate blocked ricin (158). This is not a problem for type I RIPs, because they lack B chains or their equivalents.

The bacterial toxins, PE and diphtheria toxin (DT) are single polypeptides, with enzymatic activity, cell binding, and entry functions located in different domains of the protein (159,160). DT is cleaved extracellularly, resulting in two fragments held together by a disulfide bond. Both DT and PE inhibit protein synthesis by catalyzing the ADP-ribosylation of elongation factor 2, thus leading to its inactivation (160).

Characteristics of Cross-Linkers

The most important characteristic of the cross-linker used to link the toxin or toxin subunit to the cell-binding moiety is to create a bond that, although stable extracellularly in the blood and tissues, is labile inside the target cell, thus allowing the toxin to enter the cytosol of the target cell. The cross-linkers may vary depending on whether the toxin is a holotoxin (containing A and B chains) or a single-chain toxin or RIP. In the first case, the disulfide bond between the A and B chains is present for release intracellularly, whereas in the second case, it is necessary to introduce a disulfide bond between the mAb and toxin or toxin subunit, because this is the only linkage that will release the toxin inside the cell. Various heterobifunctional cross-linkers have been used to introduce disulfide bonds into mAbs (161,162). To prevent *in vivo* attack by thiols, which can destabilize the disulfide bond, extracellular, hindered disulfide bonds have been developed (163). In the case of type I RIPs, thiol-containing groups cross-linkers can be introduced, but this can decrease toxicity. Thioether bonds are more stable in the blood, but they can be used only in holotoxins or fragments that already contain intrachain disulfide bonds or proteolytic cleavage sites, because cleavage of these bonds is critical for the translocation of the active A chain from the endosome into the cytosol of the cell (153).

Characteristics of Target Antigens

The most important features of the antigens used as targets for ITs are their ability to be internalized after binding to the IT and the subsequent intracellular routing pathway used. The IT is effective only when it binds to a cell membrane antigen (e.g., growth factor receptors), which can be internalized into nonlysosomal compartments (e.g., endosomes or other acidic vesicles). It has also been reported that ITs directed against antigenic epitopes that are proximal to the plasma membrane are more effective than those directed against epitopes that are more distal (164). Moreover, every target cell must express the antigen recognized by the IT because there is no bystander effect on antigen-negative cells. Because such uniformity in antigen expression rarely happens, mixtures of ITs will eventually be necessary.

Fusion Toxins

ITs have also been prepared by genetic engineering and expressed as single-chain chimeric fusion toxins. PE and DT have been successfully expressed as recombinant toxins containing domains responsible for enzymatic activity and lacking domains with cell-binding activity (165). Fusion proteins with RTA have also been prepared, but their potency is suboptimal (166). Recombinant ITs offer advantages over conventionally constructed ITs. They are smaller and can penetrate tissues more efficiently. However, their half-life in the circulation is shorter, so continuous infusion regimens may be necessary (167).

The toxin molecule can be altered through genetic engineering. There are several ways to modify toxins (153): (a) by introducing sequences that can provide better intracellular routing, (b) by introducing residues that simplify coupling to the toxin, and (3) by eliminating or altering sequences that induce side effects such as hepatotoxicity or vascular leak syndrome. To date, several toxins have been modified. With respect to the single-chain ITs, there is a major technical problem owing to the instability of the Fv portion of the mAb, but this problem can be overcome by constructing fusion proteins in which a disulfide bond is used to link the Fv to the toxin. Such molecules are more stable *in vivo* (168,169).

Limitations

Major limitations to IT therapy include immunogenicity and systemic toxicity. The immunogenicity of some ITs can be decreased by derivatizing them with polyethylene glycol (PEG) or by concomitant administration of immunosuppressive agents (53,170). With respect to toxicity, clinical trials have shown two major dose-limiting side effects of IT therapy: hepatotoxicity (for PE-based ITs) and vascular leak syndrome (VLS) (for RTA-based and DT-based ITs) (171,172). Hepatotoxicity is probably the result of the interactions between sequences in the PE or DT-molecule and liver cells. With regard to vascular leak syndrome, type I and II RIPs damage vascular endothelial cells (173) and increase vascular permeability, which can cause edema, hypoxia, and even organ failure. These limitations are being addressed by modifying the structure of the toxins. With regard to RTA-mediated VLS, effort to generate RTA mutants lacking this activity appear to be encouraging (170a).

Clinical Applications

Experimental results with ITs in animal models are not available for all ITs that have been used in clinical trials. However, when animal models have been developed, the data from several studies demonstrated that cocktails of ITs targeting more than one surface antigen had better therapeutic activity than single ITs (174,175). When ITs were combined with conventional chemotherapy, the animals were cured (176–179).

TABLE 6. *Immunotoxins used in clinical trials for cancer*

Toxin	Disease targeted	Reference
Ricin or ricin A chain	Leukemia	(213,366,367,
	Lymphoma	368–375)
	Colon cancer	(376)
	Breast cancer	(377)
	Melanoma	(378,378)
	Lung cancer	(380)
	CNS tumors	(381)
Pseudomonas exotoxin	Leukemia/ lymphoma	(382–384)
	Ovarian cancer	(385)
	Colorectal cancer	(386)
	Breast cancer	(386)
Saporin	Leukemia	(387)
	Lymphoma	
Diphtheria toxin	Lymphoma	(172)
	CTCL, PTCL	(172)
	AML	
	Brain tumors	
	Glioma	

AML, acute myelocytic leukemia; CNS, central nervous system; CTCL, cutaneous T-cell lymphoma; PTCL, peripheral T-cell lymphoma.

The first clinical trials with ITs commenced in the 1980s, using chemically conjugated ITs, followed by recombinant mAb fusion proteins in 1990, as summarized in Table 6 (153,172). ITs showed very encouraging results in phase I trials designed to treat patients with lymphoma and leukemia or the *ex vivo* purging of bone marrow. In contrast, treatment of large bulky solid carcinomas (e.g., ovarian, breast, and colon tumors) was less successful, most likely because of poor penetration of ITs into solid tumors. ITs should, however, be useful in treating metastases of solid tumors, provided the cells are accessible to the circulation. There are ongoing and planned clinical trials using DT conjugates and recombinant ITs. The DT-based IT, DAB$_{389}$-IL-2 (ONTAK), was approved in 1999 by the FDA for the treatment of cutaneous T-cell lymphoma (Table 7) (169,172). Long-term

therapy with ITs is usually not possible because of their immunogenicity and systemic toxicity. Thus, it is envisioned that ITs will be suited for transient adjuvant therapy in the treatment of micrometastasis and minimal residual disease.

Monoclonal Antibody–Drug Conjugates (Chemoconjugates)

Development

Conventional cytotoxic drugs have been conjugated to tumor-binding mAbs (180,181) (Fig. 2A). The first chemoconjugate was obtained by binding chlorambucil to Ig by a noncovalent linkage simply by mixing the two (182). Since then, various chemotherapeutic agents such as doxorubicin, idarubicin, bleomycin, methotrexate, cytosine arabinoside, chlorambucil, cisplatin, vinca alkaloids, maytansine, calicheamicin, and mitomycin C have been conjugated to various mAbs. Chemoconjugates can be prepared by covalently coupling the drugs directly to mAbs (183) or indirectly through an intermediate carrier such as dextran (184), human serum albumin (185), polyglutamic acid (186), carboxymethyl dextran (187), or amino-dextran (188). An indirect linkage has the advantage of allowing the linkage of more drug molecules to each carrier and thus resulting in an increased delivery of drugs to the tumor. The mAb-chemoconjugates have different mechanisms of actions: they can act as antimetabolites (e.g., methotrexate), alkylating agents (e.g., chlorambucil, mitomycin C, cisplatin), anthracyclines (e.g., doxorubicin), antimitotic agents (e.g., vinca alkaloids), or through other mechanisms (e.g., calicheamicin).

Clinical Applications

The chemoconjugates have the following advantages: (a) they improve the therapeutic index by increasing drug uptake by tumor cells, (b) they reduce toxicity to normal cells, and

TABLE 7. *Status of ongoing clinical trials*

Immunotoxin	Targeted antigen	Disease
Tf-CRM107	Transferrin receptor	Glioma
DAB$_{389}$–IL-2	IL-2	CLL, NHL, PTCL, CD25$^+$ CTCL
DT$_{388}$–GM-CSF	GM-CSF	AML
A-dmDT$_{390}$–bisFv		T-ALL
LMB-2-PE	CD25(Tac)	T- and B-cell leukemia and lymphoma
RFT5-dgA	CD25	T- and B-cell tumors, GVHD
BLL22-P38	CD22	B-cell leukemia and lymphoma
LMB-9	Le^Y	Colon, breast, other epithelial
SS1P	Mesothelin	Ovarian, cervical, mesothelioma
TGF-α–PE38	EGF receptor	Glioblastoma

AML, acute myelocytic leukemia; CLL, chronic lymphocytic leukemia; CTCL, cutaneous T-cell lymphoma; GM-CSF, granulocyte-macrophage colony-stimulating factor; GVHD, graft-versus-host disease; IL-2, interleukin-2; Le^Y, Lewis antigen Y; NHL, non-Hodgkin's lymphoma; PE, *Pseudomonas* exotoxin; PTCL, peripheral T-cell lymphoma; T-ALL, T-cell acute lymphoblastic leukemia; TGF-α, transforming growth factor α.
From Pastan (169) and Frankel (172), with permission.

(c) they prolong the bioavailability of the drug for more extensive exposure to tumor cells (189). The disadvantage of chemoconjugates is that both the mAb and the drug can be damaged by chemical conjugation (190). Despite technical difficulties, mAb-chemoconjugates have shown efficacy both *in vitro* and *in vivo* in animals and humans. Several preclinical and clinical studies have been conducted to treat lung cancer, colon cancer, leukemia and lymphoma, melanoma, ovarian carcinoma, hepatoma, breast cancer, and neuroblastoma. Most preclinical studies have been performed in mice with human tumor xenografts. Results have been impressive (191,192), although the eradication of larger tumors has not been reported. Antitumor activity has also been observed in phase I clinical studies (190). A novel anti-CD33 antibody-calicheamicin conjugate, gemtuzumab-ozogamicin (Mylotarg), was reported to be safe and effective for the treatment of acute myeloblastic leukemia (193). In a phase II trial in patients with acute myeloblastic leukemia, veno-occlusive disease was associated with the treatment in 4% of patients (193), and 12% of patients developed veno-occlusive disease in trials using multiple regimens (194). Mylotarg was recently approved by the FDA. Further studies incorporating humanized mAbs and improved conjugation methods are in progress.

Antibody-Directed Enzyme Prodrug Therapy (ADEPT)

Development

The ADEPT approach (195,196) involves the use of mAb-enzyme conjugates directed against tumor-associated antigens that achieve *in situ* activation of subsequently administered prodrugs (Fig. 2A). Prodrugs are toxicologically and pharmacodynamically inert or less active than the corresponding drug until they are converted by tumor cell-bound mAb-enzyme conjugates into active products (197). An ideal prodrug would (a) be a good substrate for the enzyme under physiologic conditions, (b) display significant differential cytotoxicity between drug and prodrug, (c) kill both proliferating and dormant cells, and (d) have a very short half-life, to limit the possibility of escape of active drug into the circulation where it can reach healthy tissues. The enzyme should (a) have high specific activity under physiologic conditions, (b) have low immunogenicity, (c) lack a mammalian homolog capable of performing the same reaction in normal tissues, (d) have enzymatic activity that is not affected by mAb binding, (e) be joined by a stable linker to the mAb, and (f) not be internalized by the target cell because a period of up to 72 hours can elapse between the administration of the mAb-enzyme conjugate and the administration of prodrug (198). The advantages of ADEPT are as follows: (a) it allows the use of extremely toxic agents that cannot readily be used in conventional chemotherapy; (b) a single enzyme molecule has the potential of cleaving many prodrug molecules, resulting in an amplification effect within the tumor site; and (c) the mAb enzyme need not bind to every tumor cell because the converted prodrug can diffuse into the tumor site (198). Limitations of ADEPT include (a) suboptimal tumor uptake resulting from heterogeneity in antigen expression, (b) development of immune responses against the enzyme component, (c) the risk of diffusion of the active drug away from the tumor site, and (d) the complexity of dosing schedules.

Clinical Applications

Various enzyme-prodrug combinations have been described, and they are categorized by the class of enzyme used. To date, only the carboxypeptidase G2 system has been evaluated in humans (199,200). In a phase I clinical trial, ADEPT was administered to ten patients with nonresectable metastatic or locally recurrent colorectal carcinoma. Carboxypeptidase G2 activity was found in metastatic tumor biopsies but not in normal tissues. Although the prodrug was converted successfully to active drug, leakage into the bloodstream did occur (200). Treatment was well tolerated, and clinical responses were observed in four patients (201).

A variation of this therapy is to use methyloxypolyethylene glycol (MPEG) conjugated to carboxypeptidase G2. This polymer has been substituted for mAbs to reduce immunogenicity (202). These polymers selectively accumulate in tumors (203). There have been attempts to improve ADEPT by generating mAb-enzyme conjugates that localize in tumors and are cleared more rapidly from the blood (202).

Tumors have also been targeted with the genes encoding prodrug-activating enzymes. This approach has been called virus-directed enzyme prodrug therapy (VDEPT) or, more generally, gene-directed enzyme prodrug therapy (GDEPT) (202,204).

Radioimmunoconjugates

Development

Radioimmunoconjugates are therapeutic agents obtained by coupling mAbs to radionuclides (Fig. 2A). They have many advantages in the treatment of cancer. Cell killing does not rely on the host's immune system and occurs by the ionizing effects of emitted radioactive particles (205,206). These radioactive cytotoxic particles are effective over several cell diameters, thus allowing eradication of antigen-negative cells by "crossfire" from adjacent antigen-positive tumor cells (205). This is very useful considering the heterogeneity of antigen expression in tumors. Finally, the amount of radioactive mAb delivered to a tumor can be measured noninvasively by imaging (181). The most important factors for therapeutic efficacy with radioimmunoconjugates are good penetration, favorable biodistribution, a reasonable half-life, and a long residence time in the tumor (207).

Choice of Radionuclides

Several radionuclides have been used for radioimmunotherapy: (a) beta-emitters (iodine-131, yttrium-90, rhenium-188, rhenium-186, and copper-67); (b) alpha-emitters (bismuth-211 and astatine-211); and (c) electron capture radionuclides (iodine-125) (208). Most preclinical and clinical investigations have used beta-emitting radionuclides, which are long-range emitters suitable for large tumors. Iodine-131 has been the most popular radiolabel, followed by yttrium-90, which has been promising because of its higher-energy beta emissions and lack of gamma emissions. However, it concentrates in bones, resulting in significant hematopoietic toxicity (209). Therapy with alpha-emitters has been more difficult because of their short half-lives (210). Often, a test dose of mAb, trace-labeled with the radionuclide to be used for treatment, is infused to provide information about the biodistribution of the mAb in tumor sites versus normal organs. Dosimetric information allows the determination of the amount of radioactivity to administer in subsequent therapeutic infusions to achieve maximal efficacy while avoiding serious toxicity.

Clinical Applications

The earliest clinical trials evaluated iodine-131–labeled polyclonal antiferritin antibodies to treat ferritin-rich tumors such as HD and hepatomas. This therapy provided symptomatic relief to 77% of patients with refractory HD and produced tumor regressions in 40% of patients (211). Subsequent studies using yttrium-90–labeled antiferritin showed ORs of 60%, including 31% CRs (212). More recent trials favored the use of mAbs instead of polyclonal antibodies and reported higher response rates in patients with hematologic malignancies (205,213,214), compared with patients with solid tumors (215,216). Myelosuppression has been the dose-limiting toxicity and has resulted in both "low-dose" nonmyeloablative treatment regimens (217–219) and "high-dose" myeloablative regimens (220,221). The most impressive results with nonmyeloablative regimens documented ORs in 70% to 80% of patients, CRs in 30% to 50% of patients, minimal toxicity, and a median response duration of 12 months (218). In trials with myeloablative regimens, performed in conjunction with autologous hematopoietic bone marrow or stem cell transplantation (SCT), ORs were achieved in 95% of patients and CRs in 85% of patients, with a progression-free survival of 62% and an overall survival of 93% with a median follow-up of more than 5 years (222). These results are impressive and should soon lead to approval of a 131-labeled anti-CD20 by the FDA.

Despite extremely encouraging results, considerable controversy concerning the optimal mAb, radionuclide, dose of mAb, and schedule of administration still exists. Several clinical trials with iodine 131–labeled anti-CD20 (tositumomab [Bexxar] and yttrium-90–labeled anti-CD20 (ibritumomab [Zevalin]) were been undertaken to compare different radionuclides for the therapy of low-grade and transformed low-grade NHL. Ibritumomab gave CR rates of between 27% and 75% and ORs of 48% to 80%. Zevalin has recently been approved by the FDA for use in patients with NHL. Three phase I/II clinical trials and one phase I trial with

tositumomab in patients with relapsed lymphomas gave CR rates of 17% to 80% and ORs of 65% to 90% (222–224). Ongoing clinical trials for the treatment of relapsed low-grade or transformed low-grade NHL (with >25% marrow involvement) or relapsed chronic lymphocytic leukemia are in progress. A phase II multicenter trial for consolidation after cyclophosphamide-hydroxydaunomycin-vincristine-prednisone (CHOP) therapy for diffuse low-grade NHL (222), and other ongoing trials using tositumomab combined with fludarabine, showed ORs of 93% in low-grade NHL, with only minor nonhematologic toxicity (225). Future research in this area will focus on the combination of radioimmunotherapy and other treatment modalities to achieve cures.

Immunoliposomes

Development

Immunoliposomes are small (<100 nm in diameter) unilamellar or multilamellar lipid vesicles used as drug delivery systems (226) (Fig. 2B). The usual composition is phosphatidylcholine, cholesterol, and sometimes PEG. An advantage of immunoliposomes over other mAb-drug formulations is that liposomes can accommodate a very wide range of drugs and agents, regardless of size or solubility, and they can carry a much larger drug load per vesicle. Liposomal encapsulation of a drug significantly increases its in vivo half-life. For example, in rats, liposome-encapsulated doxorubicin has an estimated serum half-life of 10 hours as compared with 5 minutes for free doxorubicin (227). Drug encapsulation also reduces systemic toxicity. Liposomes can be targeted to the desired cells or tissues with mAbs that are coupled to their surface using either a noncovalent avidin-biotin method or a covalent thioether or hydrazide bond at the N-terminal of PEG (228). When bound to the target cell, the lipid vesicles fuse with the cell membrane, and their contents are delivered into the cytosol. Target cell binding and internalization depend on the number of mAb molecules conjugated to each liposome. Under optimal conditions, up to 25,000 liposomes can be taken up successfully by a single cell. A problem with immunoliposome therapy in vivo has been the uptake by liver cells, with resulting hepatotoxicity. Many of the problems originally encountered with liposomes have been resolved by altering the composition of the lipid bilayers. Improvements in mAb-targeted liposomal-encapsulated drugs have led to (a) the use of "stealth" liposomes sterically stabilized with PEG that have longer circulation times in vivo (229,230) and (b) new coupling techniques resulting in more stable attachment of the mAb, less hepatotoxicity, and improved target cell recognition (228).

In Vivo Use

Immunoliposomes have been used to deliver chemotherapeutic drugs to tumor cells in animals with squamous cell carcinoma, ovarian cancer, B-cell lymphoma (231), lung cancer (232), and breast cancer (208). Because immunoliposomes are too large to extravasate (40 to 100 nm), only tumor cells within the blood, bone marrow, lymph, or peritoneal cavity are easily accessible targets. Thus, hematologic disorders or metastases in the marrow represent promising applications. Anti–Her-2-coated liposomes loaded with doxorubicin have been developed for clinical use (233,234), and a phase I study using liposome-encapsulated paclitaxel is ongoing in patients with solid tumors (235).

Other Emerging Immunoconjugate Strategies

mAbs have also been conjugated to various compounds, such as photosensitizers, cytokines, superantigens, and RNAses (Fig. 2A).

Monoclonal Antibody–Photosensitizer Conjugates

Photodynamic therapy is based on the administration of tumor-localizing photosensitizers, followed by the exposure of the neoplastic area to light absorbed by the photosensitizer (236,237). The toxicity to the tumor tissue is induced by the local activation of the photosensitizer, so normal tissues are spared. Many delivery systems have been used for photosensitizers. These include liposomes, microspheres, and lipoproteins. More recently, mAb-photosensitizer conjugates have been used to increase their selectivity. This approach is called antibody-targeted photolysis or photoimmunotherapy. The first report of this strategy, dating back to the early 1980s (238), showed that hematoporphyrin coupled to an antimyosarcoma mAb had selective in vitro and in vivo phototoxicity. Similar results have been achieved with other conjugates used on various types of tumor cells (236). Targeted photodestruction of human colon carcinoma cells using charged 17.1 A-chlorine e6 ICs has been reported (239). Despite the excellent selectivity of mAb-photosensitizer conjugates in vitro, the limited numbers of studies on their biodistribution in tumor-bearing animals are not encouraging because of the high photosensitizer levels found in some normal tissues (237). However, these ICs may be beneficial in ex vivo purging of tumor cells from bone marrow.

Monoclonal Antibody–Cytokine Conjugates

Recombinant mAb-cytokine fusion proteins combine the targeting abilities of mAbs with the biologic activities of cytokines (240). They have been used to achieve sufficient local concentrations of cytokines. An example is IL-2, which has been used to recruit T cells and to induce T-cell–mediated antitumor responses in animals (241–243). Other cytokine-mAb conjugates, containing IFN-α or lymphotoxin, have targeted growth-inhibitory cytokines directly to tumors (244,245). An anti-Id/GM-CSF fusion protein has also been used as a vaccine against B-cell lymphoma (240). mAb-cytokine fusion proteins offer the advantage of avoiding the dose-limiting toxicities associated with systemic delivery of cytokines. Furthermore, the antigen need not be present on every cell in the tumor lesion, because a bystander effect can

occur. A potential disadvantage of these molecules is that they rely entirely on the T-cell immunity of the host, which, in the case of patients with cancer, may be suppressed.

Monoclonal Antibody–Superantigen Conjugates

The bacterial enterotoxins are powerful toxins that cause food poisoning and toxic shock in humans. The bacterial superantigen *Staphylococcus* enterotoxin A (SEA) binds to MHC class II antigens on APCs and on T cells expressing certain TCR Vβ chains. SEA can thereby act as a powerful nonspecific stimulator of T-cell activity (246). Fusion proteins constructed with mutated SEA molecules that have a low affinity for MHC class II molecules but can still bind to T cells can be targeted to tumors by coupling them to specific mAbs (247). Hence, these hybrid molecules direct SEA-responsive T cells into tumor sites and induce responses. Mechanisms of T-cell killing may involve the release of growth-inhibiting cytokines (IFN-γ and TNF-α), as well as direct cellular cytotoxicity. Theoretically, this is an attractive method for focusing killer cells onto target cells because a comparatively large portion of the T-cell population can be recruited. Although mutated SEA molecules appear to have less systemic toxicity (248), safety issues remain to be addressed.

Colon carcinoma (249–252), chronic B-lymphocytic leukemia (253), and neuroblastoma have been treated with mAb-SEA conjugates *in vitro* and in mice (254). They have also been used in patients with pancreatic and colorectal carcinoma, with some encouraging results (255).

Monoclonal Antibody—RNAse Conjugates

mAbs have also been coupled to RNAses isolated from various sources (256). RNAses inhibit protein synthesis by degrading ribosomal RNA. In addition, some RNAses destroy transfer RNA (257). Antitransferrin mAbs coupled to RNAse, either chemically or as recombinant fusion proteins, have shown specific cytotoxic activity against several tumors both *in vitro* and *in vivo* (258–260). The advantages of mAb-RNAse constructs over conventional ITs include less systemic toxicity and perhaps lower immunogenicity (although this has not yet been documented), because the RNAse is derived from mammalian sources rather than from plants or bacteria. Furthermore, a greater degree of humanization has been possible with recombinant constructs using human genes encoding homologs of pancreatic RNAse and humanized antitransferrin mAbs (261–263). A potential problem in using mAb-RNAse–conjugates therapeutically is the presence of RNAse inhibitors in the blood and tissues. For this reason, RNAses that are resistant to these inhibitors are being explored (264).

Conclusions

mAb-based constructs, as we know them today, represent a heterogeneous class of antitumor agents that possess remarkable efficacy in the treatment of experimental cancers in animals. Several of these constructs have been evaluated in patients with cancer, and some have activity at safe doses. Although issues of systemic toxicity and immunogenicity remain to be addressed in more detail, several ICs have been FDA approved.

CELLULAR STRATEGIES

The cellular arm of the immune system plays a key role in maintaining antitumor immunity. In cellular therapy, immune cells with antitumor activity are transferred to a tumor-bearing host. Cellular immunotherapeutic strategies can be aimed directly or indirectly at the tumor cells. Successful cellular therapy depends on the types of cells transferred and their effector functions, the ability of the cells to reach the tumor site, and their ability to overcome tolerance or immunosuppression in the host (265). Although most studies have been carried out in mice, several cellular therapies have demonstrated therapeutic efficacy in human patients.

Nonspecific Cellular Therapy

The objective of nonspecific cellular therapy is to enhance the antitumor effector mechanisms that are not dependent on a specific tumor antigen. The concept of nonspecific therapy originates from Coley, who found that solid tumors regressed after patients were injected with bacterial toxins to stimulate their immune system (10). Nonspecific cellular therapy employs effector cells that have been isolated from patients and cultured *ex vivo* with agents that activate or enhance their antitumor activity.

There are several advantages of nonspecific cellular therapy: (a) effector cells respond to a wide range of tumor types; (b) activating agents that would be toxic to the host *in vivo* can activate the cells *in vitro,* thus circumventing immunoregulation and immunosuppression by the host; and (c) host effector cells can be activated and reinjected into autologous donors (266). The last feature provides a readily available source of cells, and it avoids complications of host rejection.

Lymphokine-Activated Killer Cells

LAK cells are peripheral blood mononuclear cells that have been expanded *ex vivo* with IL-2 and then reinfused along with IL-2. In animal studies with B16 melanomas, LAK cells prolonged the survival of tumor-bearing mice. This effect was independent of prior treatment regimens, as well as whether the LAK cells were obtained from tumor-bearing or naïve mice (267). In clinical trials, LAK cell therapy was most successful in renal cell carcinoma and melanoma, although further studies indicated that LAK cells did not significantly improve the therapeutic efficacy of IL-2 alone (10). It has been postulated that LAK cells may enhance the activity of macrophages or may induce the release of cytokines such as IFN-γ, TNF-α, and macrophage-CSF (7).

Natural Killer Cells

NK cells are important in antitumor immunity and graft rejection because of their ability to target and destroy cells in the body that fail to express significant levels of MHC class I antigens. This role in immunosurveillance was demonstrated by studies showing that, as the NK-cell activity decreased, the number of spontaneous tumors increased. In addition, nude mice, which have few or no T cells, rejected tumors as a result of their NK cells (268).

Activation of NK cells with IL-2 can produce antileukemic effects. Hence, *in vitro* activated NK cells can kill leukemic cells from bone marrow before autologous transplants. *In vivo* studies in mice have shown that NK cells may reduce metastatic dissemination of cancer cells (268). NK cells can also be activated with IFN-α, but the clinical outcome of this maneuver remains to be determined (8).

Hematopoietic SCT is being used for the treatment of various cancers. However, GVHD and the risk of tumor relapse continue to result in significant complications. Immunosuppressive drugs that decrease the risk of GVHD increase the rate of relapse of the cancer and *vice versa.* Immunotherapy with host-derived cells provides an attractive opportunity to treat the cancer without stimulating further GVHD. Studies in animals have shown that activated NK cells can promote hematopoietic engraftment after syngeneic or allogeneic SCT. In addition, NK cells can inhibit GVHD through the action of the immunosuppressive cytokine transforming growth factor-β (TGF-β), and they can still protect and promote engraftment while retaining antitumor activity. This NK-cell activity is only observed when cells are administered within 3 days after SCT (269).

Dendritic Cells

DCs are the most potent APCs because they present antigen through both class I and class II pathways. In addition, they can be activated with very little antigen, and they are the only APCs that can activate naïve T cells. Because DCs generate efficient primary immune responses, they may play an important role in natural tumor immunity (270). DCs may be ineffective in inducing tumor immunity for several reasons: (a) DCs may not have access to the tumor because low levels of cytokines produced by tumors may decrease the migration of DCs into tumor sites; (b) the tumor cells may secrete factors that prevent DCs from migrating to the regional lymph node, so that activation of T cells does not occur; (c) the tumor cells may not send "danger signals" to DCs, thereby preventing effective antigen presentation; and (d) tumors may secrete immunosuppressive cytokines or may down-regulate co-stimulatory molecules. In addition, current cancer therapies often employ agents that are immunosuppressive, such as steroids (271).

Despite the foregoing caveats, the unique antigen-presenting function of DCs makes them excellent candidates for inducing tumor immunity. Much of the current work on immunotherapy with DCs involves specific stimulation with tumor antigens, as discussed in detail later. DCs can be stimulated nonspecifically to induce their *in vivo* expansion, activation, and migration to tumor sites. In *in vivo* studies, DCs have been stimulated by local administration of a BCG adjuvant into the tumor site and through the systemic administration of factors that can promote expansion (GM-CSF and Flt3-L), and activation of DCs (CD154 and RANK-L). In addition, tumor cells have been removed and transfected *ex vivo* with activation-encoding genes or co-stimulatory molecules such as CD80 or the TNF/TNF receptor family or with MHC II and then readministered to the patient. These approaches are effective in preclinical animal models, and initial clinical trials are under way (271). A major challenge, however, is to regulate the activation of the DCs and the loading of tumor peptides effectively. For example, presentation of antigens by immature DCs can induce immune tolerance (272). In contrast, mature DCs are especially beneficial because they up-regulate MHC class I and II molecules and co-stimulatory molecules, thus enhancing T-cell activity (271). Targeting DCs for cancer immunotherapy appears promising, and current clinical trials will reveal the therapeutic potential of these cells as immunotherapeutic adjuvants or vaccines.

Macrophage-Activated Killer Cells

Immunotherapy with macrophages is based on early studies demonstrating that macrophages activated *in vitro* with IFN-γ could induce the regression of subcutaneous tumors in nude mice (8). This created the opportunity for various applications because macrophages from patients are readily available, and they are rarely affected by tumor-induced immunosuppression.

Macrophage-activated killer (MAK) cells are a well-tolerated form of therapy. No dose-limiting toxicity has been observed, and only low-grade fever and chills have occurred (273). Although clinical trials using MAK therapy in various cancers have not demonstrated PRs or CRs, several studies have shown that MAK cells can induce tumor stabilization or necrosis, cause a reduction in ascitic fluid, and alter chemoresistance (8,273,274). Several mechanisms have been proposed to explain MAK cell activity, but no conclusions have been drawn. TNF-α is thought to be the major cytokine responsible for MAK cell activity (268).

Other studies using macrophages have been designed to improve their therapeutic activity. Attempts have been made to increase their killing capacity by activating them with IFN-γ and endotoxin. In addition, researchers have attempted to increase the specificity of MAK cells by incubating them with tumor antigens, to enhance antigen presentation before the cells are reinjected into their autologous donors (274). These attempts have not significantly improved their overall therapeutic activity, but continued studies in MAK cell immunotherapy are being pursued because MAK cells are so well tolerated.

Specific Cellular Transfer

Adoptive immunotherapy by specific cellular transfer presents new possibilities for the targeted therapy of many human diseases, including cancer. The transfer of immune cells with antitumor activity can be divided into at least two categories: TILs and antigen-specific or tumor-specific CTLs.

Tumor-Infiltrating Lymphocytes

TILs are lymphocytes that have been obtained from tumor tissue by mechanical and enzymatic digestion of a tumor specimen. The resulting single-cell suspension is cultured for several weeks before the TILs can be harvested (265). TILs cultured in the presence of IL-2 produce tumor-specific cytotoxic effects in mouse sarcoma, melanoma, colon carcinoma, and bladder carcinoma (267).

The success of several *in vitro* and *in vivo* studies in animals led researchers to examine the possibilities of TIL therapy in humans. TILs have been difficult to use clinically. Attempts to obtain TIL cell lines have met with limited success, and when obtained, many lines are not specifically reactive *in vivo* (275). However, patients with melanoma or renal cell carcinoma have benefited from TIL therapy, possibly because these tumors are more immunogenic (265,267).

In metastatic melanoma, a 34% to 38% response rate was achieved, and this response was independent of prior chemotherapy. The effect lasted for several months (10,267,275,276). Further studies with melanoma-specific TILs have sought to identify their respective tumor antigens and test the appropriate T-cell clones on other tumors. One study demonstrated that a melanoma-reactive T-cell clone cross-reacted with a breast cancer tumor antigen (267).

Depending on the treatment protocol used to treat renal cell carcinoma, there have been variable responses. When TILs were primed with various cytokines *in vivo* and were then expanded *in vitro*, the infused cells induced an overall response rates of 34% to 38%, with a 14-month median duration. The OR rate dropped to 25% when the TILs were both activated and expanded *in vitro*, and the OR rate increased to 43.5% when only CD8$^+$ TILs were used (265). TILs appear to be a promising therapeutic strategy, but further studies are needed to optimize treatment protocols.

Adoptive Antigen-Specific Cytotoxic Lymphocyte Therapy

General Strategy

Studies since the early 1990s have provided evidence that the augmentation of immune effector functions by the infusion of virus-reactive or tumor-reactive T lymphocytes represents a potentially highly specific modality for the treatment of viral diseases and cancer. It has been demonstrated that infusions of donor T lymphocytes into patients with relapsed leukemia after allogeneic hematopoietic SCT induces remissions in the majority of patients (277). Since the establishment of methods to isolate genes encoding antigens recognized by

CTLs, many antigens have been identified and characterized for their suitability as immunotherapeutic targets. Van der Bruggen and colleagues (278) pioneered techniques that used tumor-reactive CTL clones, isolated from patients with cancer, as reagents to screen target cells that had been transfected with a cDNA library derived from autologous tumor cells. Alternatively, tumor antigens can be identified by serologic analysis of proteins generated from recombinant cDNA expression libraries (SEREX) (279). Serum from patients with cancer is used to detect prokaryotically expressed proteins encoded by cDNA libraries prepared from tumors. Antigenic epitopes recognized by tumor-specific CTLs are derived from proteins encoded by tumor-associated viruses, mutated cytosolic proteins, and proteins that exhibit selective expression or overexpression (Table 8).

The identification of target antigens expressed by tumor cells from different individuals has facilitated the development of T-cell immunotherapy protocols with broad applicability. Patients could be sensitized *in vivo* by immunization. Then, peripheral blood lymphocytes or cells from vaccine-draining lymph nodes could be boosted *in vitro* using the same antigen. To improve tumor reactivity, T-cell clones with appropriate antigen specificity could be identified. Once isolated from bulk cultures, these clones could be expanded *in vitro* and infused into the patient. Cloned T cells should be highly effective for adoptive immunotherapy, because they can eliminate established tumors in several mouse models, and the phenotype of transferred cells can be manipulated by selecting a clone with specific characteristics (280,281). Conversely, there are many reasons that *in vitro*–derived tumor-reactive T cells could fail to eradicate tumor cells *in vivo*, such as the following: (a) the lack of uniformity of antigen or MHC expression on tumor cells could influence the efficacy of T-cell therapy as the outgrowth of tumor antigen-loss variants arise; (b) tumor antigens can be masked by other proteins; (c) tumor cells produce immunosuppressive cytokines such as IL-10, TGF-β, or prostaglandins that interfere with the activation of T cells; (d) modulation of tumor vasculature results in poor infiltration of lymphocytes into the tumor mass; (e) processing and presentation of tumor antigens by APCs are not optimal, or co-stimulation is absent; and (f) induction of anergy, apoptosis, or elimination of infused tumor-reactive T cells can occur (282–286).

Genetically Engineered Cells

The application of efficient gene-transfer techniques to lymphocyte populations may overcome some of the limitations of specific cellular transfer in the therapy of cancer. Approaches to the gene therapy of neoplastic disease include, but are not limited to, genetically modified tumor cells or APCs as vaccines, introduction of wild-type tumor suppressor genes into tumors with mutated nonfunctional or lost tumor suppressor genes, other mutated host genes, introduction of oncogene antisense into tumors, and gene-modified effector cells. In this section, we discuss the gene-modified effector cells. Other vaccine strategies are reviewed later in this chapter and elsewhere (287).

Genetically engineered lymphocytes possess unique functional characteristics that can be exploited in novel treatment protocols. The first transfers into humans were performed by Rosenberg and associates in 1990 (288), who demonstrated the feasibility and safety of using retrovirally mediated gene transduction of the gene encoding neomycin resistance

TABLE 8. *Antigens expressed by cancer cells that can be potentially recognized by T lymphocytes*

Tumor antigen group	Name	Cancer type
Virus-associated tumor antigens	HPV E6 and E7	Cervical carcinoma (389)
	EBV LMP-1, EBNA-1	HD, nasopharyngeal carcinoma (390)
Product of mutated gene or chromosomal rearrangement	BCR/ABL	Chronic myeloid leukemia (391)
	PML/RARA	Acute promyelocytic leukemia (392)
	TEL/AML1	Precursor B acute lymphoblastic leukemia (393)
	β-catenin	Melanoma (394)
	MUM-1, MUM-2, MUM-3, CD4	Melanoma (395)
Product of overexpressed normal gene	hTERT[c]	~90% of tumors (396)
	CEA	Epithelial tumors (397)
	Her-2/neu	Breast and other epithelial tumors (397)
	WT-1	Leukemia and epithelial tumors (398)
Tissue-specific differentiation antigens	Tyrosinase, melan A, gp 100, TRP-1, TRP-2	Melanoma (399)
	PSA	Prostate cancer (400)
Embryonic proteins	MAGE, BAGE, GAGE, NY-ESO proteins	Melanoma and other epithelial tumors (399,401)
Idiotypic proteins	Immunoglobulin chains	NHL, multiple myeloma (402)

CEA, carcinogenic embryonic antigen; EBV, Epstein Barr virus; EBNA-1, EBV-associated nuclear antigen 1; gp100, glycoprotein 100; HD, Hodgkin's disease; HPV, human papilloma virus; hTERT[c], human telomerase c; LMP-1, latent membrane protein 1; MUM-1, melanoma ubiquitous mutated protein; NHL, non-Hodgkin's lymphoma; PML/RARA, promyelocyte/retinoic acid receptor α; PSA, prostate-specific antigen; TEL/AML1, translocation ets leukemia/acute myeloid leukemia; TRP-1 and TRP-2, tyrosinase-related proteins 1 and 2; WT-1, Wilms' tumor 1.

into human TILs before their infusion into patients with metastatic melanoma. The infusion of genetically engineered neomycin-marked T cells has been used to assess transfer of immunity, persistence in the peripheral blood, and the migration of these cells to lymph nodes or tissues (289–293). The ability of lymphocytes to traffic to tumors can be harnessed to deliver therapeutically active molecules to the tumor environment. Hence, such cells can be transfected with cytokine or other genes. Specific changes in the local milieu may augment the host immune response, while avoiding the toxicity associated with high-dose systematic administration of cytokines such as IL-2. IL-2 can prolong the life span of transferred cells, and TNF-α can mediate the regression of tumors. In addition to the few examples mentioned earlier, the construction of chimeric TCRs has led to the direct coupling of the recognition and effector phases of the immune response. Stancovski and associates (294) transfected CTLs with a gene encoding a single-chain chimeric TCR gene with specificity for Her-2, a known breast carcinoma–associated antigen. These modified CTLs demonstrated specific recognition and lysis of target cells expressing Her-2. Similar examples of chimeric TCR constructs for other cancers have been reported (287). Genetically modified lymphocytes show great promise as therapeutic vehicles in the gene therapy of cancer, and several ongoing clinical trials are testing the safety and efficacy of such approaches.

Applications

Viral Disease

In persistent viral infections such as Epstein-Barr virus (EBV) and CMV, in which viral replication is controlled by specific CTLs, adoptive transfer of CTLs generated from the original marrow donor into immunosuppressed patients after allogeneic SCT has been beneficial in reducing the incidence of serious viral disease (289–292). EBV causes potentially lethal immunoblastic lymphoma in patients receiving T-cell–depleted allogeneic SCTs. Donor-derived EBV-specific T lymphocytes were used for prophylaxis of posttransplant immunoblastic lymphoma in 39 children considered to be at high risk of developing EBV-induced lymphoma. EBV-specific CTL cell lines persisted in recipients for as long as 18 weeks and prevented the development of lymphoma in all patients. In addition, two patients with already established immunoblastic lymphoma responded fully to the infusion of EBV-specific CTLs (289). These positive results in transplant recipients suggest that T-cell therapy may be applicable to other malignant diseases that contain EBV genomes, such as nasopharyngeal carcinoma and a subset of HD. In one study, three patients with multiply relapsed HD were treated with autologous EBV-specific CTLs. The CTLs persisted for more than 13 weeks after infusion and retained their potent antiviral effects *in vivo*, thereby enhancing the immune response of the patients against EBV (290).

The occurrence of life-threatening CMV disease after allogeneic SCT correlates with the absence of CMV-specific CD8$^+$ T-cell responses. Thus, adoptive transfer of CMV-specific CTL clones isolated from the SCT donor can restore protective immunity against CMV. Up to 10^9 CD8$^+$ CTL/m^2 were infused into 14 patients at risk of posttransplant CMV disease. Therapy did not cause any toxicity, and the CMV-specific CTLs persisted for more than 12 weeks. None of the patients developed CMV disease after therapy (291). Another demonstration of the potential of adoptive cellular therapy emerged from studies with HIV-positive patients. Brodie and associates (293) transferred HIV-1–specific CTLs to three HIV-positive patients and demonstrated that the infused CTLs retained lytic function, accumulated in areas adjacent to HIV-infected cells in lymph nodes, and transiently reduced the levels of productively infected circulating CD4$^+$ cells. These studies provide direct evidence that virus-specific CTLs mediate strong antiviral activity and indicate that the development of immunotherapeutic approaches to sustain a strong CTL response against target antigens may be useful in other diseases, such as cancer.

Cancer

The discovery of tumor-specific genes that encode tumor antigens recognized by T cells has provided opportunities for adoptive transfer therapy. CTLs could be sensitized *in vivo* or *in vitro* by immunization with cells or peptides. Selection of individual T-cell clones with a high degree of antigen specificity and tumor reactivity may improve the outcome of treatment, as shown in several preclinical studies (280,281). The ability to select specific T-cell phenotypes for adoptive transfer led to the initiation of clinical trials with glycoprotein (gp)100 peptide–specific T-cell clones for the treatment of patients with metastatic melanoma. Using defined antigens in mouse tumor models, several studies demonstrated a correlation between T-cell avidity *in vitro* and the efficacy of adoptive transfer *in vivo* (295,296). Dudley and colleagues (296) also demonstrated the safety and feasibility of infusing cloned T cells, even though these cells lacked clinical effectiveness; these investigators reported one minor response and one mixed response in 13 patients with metastatic melanoma. These data suggested that successful therapy required the transfer of different or additional cell types. In addition, in contrast to transferred and long-lived virus-specific CTLs (289–292), transferred T cells in this study were undetectable 2 weeks after infusion. The generation of sufficient numbers of CTLs from nonimmunized individuals for adoptive immunotherapy presents additional technical challenges.

Immunodeficiency

One of the successful examples of cellular transfer therapy is the use of allogeneic hematopoietic SCT (297) in patients with primary T-cell or combined T- and B-cell immunodeficiency syndromes. The development of techniques to deplete donor T cells permits the safe use of even haploidentical hematopoietic SCT for the correction of severe combined immunodeficiency and other fatal immunodeficiency syndromes with a success rate of 70% to 80%. Patients with less severe forms of cellular immunodeficiency, such as combined immunodeficiency, Wiscott-Aldrich syndrome, cytokine deficiency, or MHC antigen deficiency, require chemoablative treatment before transplantation to avoid allograft rejection. Patients with these conditions have also been treated successfully with human leukocyte antigen (HLA)–identical SCT after appropriate conditioning (298).

Graft-Versus-Leukemia T Cells and Graft-Versus-Tumor Effects

The graft-versus-leukemia (GVL) effect achieved after allogeneic hematopoietic SCT for human malignant diseases represents the clearest example of the power of the human immune system to eradicate cancer. Barnes and associates first suggested the existence of a GVL effect in 1956, when they noted eradication of leukemia in irradiated mice receiving allogeneic bone marrow transplants (299). The evidence for such an effect in humans emerged from studies reporting that relapse rates after allogeneic transplantation were markedly lower in patients who developed GVHD compared with those who did not (300). Subsequent studies demonstrated that posttransplant relapse rates were higher in patients receiving T-cell–depleted grafts in an attempt to alleviate GVHD. Thus, donor T cells play a major role in GVL responses. Further verification of the GVL effect was generated from efforts to treat patients for posttransplant leukemic relapse by infusing donor lymphocytes. Sustained CRs were achieved in more than 70% of patients with chronic myelogenous leukemia and in some patients with other hematologic malignant diseases (301). With increased evidence of the GVL effect and development of methods to better exploit it, clinical research is beginning to focus on allogeneic hematopoietic SCT as an immunotherapeutic approach, rather than solely as a way to rescue patients from high-dose myeloablative therapy.

Regulatory T Cells

Studies in both rodents and humans have demonstrated the presence of a subpopulation (5% to 10%) of $CD4^+$ peripheral blood T cells that are $CD25^+$ and that markedly suppress the expansion of T cells after antigenic stimulation in a contact-dependent manner (302,303). $CD4^+CD25^+$ regulatory T cells in humans express CD45RO, the histocompatibility leukocyte antigen DR, and CD152. They are in G1/G0 cell-cycle arrest and do not produce IL-2, IL-4, or IFN-γ. The anergic state of $CD4^+CD25^+$ T cells is not reversible by stimulation with anti-CD28 or anti-CD3 (303). These regulatory T cells may have the potential of controlling autoimmune diseases. However, definitive evidence is lacking that these cells represent a functionally unique population of T cells rather than populations of $CD4^+$ cells that were previously activated, yet remain $CD25^+$ but anergic. The manipulation of these cells for therapeutic purposes is an exciting ongoing effort.

VACCINATION

Strategies

With the exception of immunomodulators and some cellular therapies, most of the immunotherapeutic strategies described in the preceding sections of this chapter are passive therapies, particularly those using IVIG, mAbs, and ICs. It would be highly desirable to induce an *active* immune response against various tumor antigens with one of several vaccination strategies. Because vaccines against infectious agents are discussed elsewhere, we confine our discussion to cancer vaccines. In this setting, vaccination involves targeting antigenic differences between tumor cells and normal cells. For historical reasons, these antigens are known as tumor-specific transplantation antigens or tumor-associated antigens (TAAs) (Table 9). Ideally, these target antigens should

TABLE 9. *Select examples of tumor-associated antigens of different types*

Category	Antigen	Source tumor
Unique antigens	bcr-abl	CML
	Mutated β-catenin	Colon
Oncogenes	Mutated ras	Pancreatic, lung, colon
Mutated tumor suppressors	p53	Breast, colon, others
	BRCA-1 and BRCA-2	Familial breast cancer
Viral antigens	human papilloma	Cervical, uterine
	hepatitis	Hepatic
Cancer testis antigens	MAGE, CAGE, BAGE families	Breast, melanoma, bladder, head and neck
Differentiation antigens	CEA	Colon, breast, pancreas, others
	MART-1	Melanoma
	Glycoprotein 100	Melanoma
	Tyrosinase	Melanoma
Abnormally glycosylated	MUC-1	Pancreatic, breast
	M-TAAS	Melanoma
Glycolipids	Blood groups (T, Tn, sialosyl-Tn)	Carcinoma
	Gangliosides (GM2, GD2, GD3)	Melanoma, sarcoma, neuroblastoma, glioblastoma
Aberrantly expressed	Her-2/neu	Breast, ovary, others

CEA, carcinogenic embryonic antigen; CML, chronic myelogenous leukemia; MART-1, melanoma antigen recognized by T cells 1; M-TAAS, melanoma tumor–associated antigen; MUC-1, mucin-1.
From Bremers and Parmiani (10), Bremers et al. (304), and Chamberlain (332), with permission.

be unique to the tumor, arising from mutations or chromosomal translocations, including altered oncogenes and tumor suppressor proteins. Transcriptionally reactivated antigens or oncofetal antigens can also be tumor-specific antigens, as can viral antigens, in the case of virally induced tumors. In B- and T-cell malignancies, Ids are tumor-specific antigens in B-cell receptors or TCRs. Differentiation antigens are unique to the tissue from which the tumor arose but are not expressed in other tumors or tissues, thereby making them only relatively tumor-specific. Increased levels of expression or alterations in glycosylation patterns can also distinguish antigens on a tumor from those on normal tissue (10).

In the case of existing disease, the goal of cancer vaccination is to reintroduce one or more of these targets to the immune system in a more immunogenic form, so the host can raise tumor-specific antibodies or T cells. Tumor cells, with all their various antigenic differences from normal tissue, have evaded detection by the immune system or have simply grown too rapidly to be contained by an immune response (304). Escape variants that express lower levels of the immunogenic antigen or little or no MHC antigens are prevalent (305). Hence, tumor antigens are not presented to T cells. In addition, TAAs from dead tumor cells presented by DCs lacking co-stimulatory molecules tend to induce tolerance, as demonstrated by the presence of TAA-reactive anergic T cells in patients. Other strategies that tumors use to evade immune surveillance include the release of inhibitory cytokines such as TGF-β or IL-2 (306) or the expression of the CD95 ligand on the tumor cells (307). Whatever the mechanism used by the tumor to evade an immune response, an effective vaccination strategy must break immune tolerance or enhance the immunogenicity of weakly immunogenic antigens by priming naïve lymphocytes or by activating existing TAA-specific lymphocytes. The target antigens listed in Table 9 can be used as vaccines, and many have been tested experimentally with varying degrees of success.

Vaccination with Defined Antigens

Peptides and Proteins

Vaccination using one or more of the proteins listed in Table 9 can often generate strong humoral responses against tumors. Promising target proteins are those involved in cell transformation, such as *ras* or p53. However, proteins can also induce autoimmune responses because they are present in normal tissues. Proteins can potentially induce or maintain tolerance in normal tissues. Conversely, the goal of tumor vaccines is to break tolerance against self peptides (308). Peptide vaccines that are restricted to specific HLA serotypes for presentation to the immune system by APCs are being developed. These vaccines consist of one or more peptides expressed or synthesized as a single chain that are HLA matched to individuals or groups of individuals (10).

Peptide vaccine candidates have been identified by analyzing the sequences of target proteins for stretches of amino acids capable of being bound in the grooves of MHC class I or class II molecules and then further testing them for their ability to induce an immune response *in vivo* (309). Another approach is to elute and purify individual peptides from the grooves of MHC molecules expressed on tumor cells (310). These peptides can be loaded directly onto autologous or MHC-matched allogeneic DCs, or they can also be screened for their ability to elicit a response and then individually sequenced and synthesized.

Peptide vaccines have been tested in many clinical trials, with mixed results. Two studies used mutant *ras* peptides administered in Detox adjuvant to treat colon, lung, and pancreatic carcinomas. Although specific T-cell responses were detected, there were no clinical responses (311,312). Another study used a peptide derived from gp100 to treat patients with metastatic melanoma (313). The peptide was administered in incomplete Freund's adjuvant either in its native form or a mutant form designed to bind to HLA (314), and the mutant peptide was administered with or without IL-2. The modified peptide was more immunogenic to T cells and, in conjunction with the administration of IL-2, induced some clinical responses.

Peptide therapy that can inhibit Th1 responses is also being used experimentally to treat numerous autoimmune disorders (315). A subset of Th2 cells responds to regions of the TCR on Th1 cells and down-regulates them. Peptides derived from Th1 TCR V genes, which are responsible for this inflammatory response and the resulting disease, are being used to induce regulatory Th2 cells to secrete IL-10, which inhibits Th1 responses. Several trials investigating this approach have been conducted, specifically to treat multiple sclerosis, rheumatoid arthritis, and psoriasis. These vaccines appear to be safe and well tolerated, and some can induce a clinical response.

Id Vaccines

Id proteins are another specialized example of protein vaccines. B-cell receptors and TCRs have clonal sequences, which make them unique tumor targets for lymphomas, leukemias, and myelomas (316,317). However, a significant disadvantage of this type of vaccine is the laborious and time-consuming task of purifying the Id proteins and their use in a relatively restricted group of patients.

Nevertheless, vaccination with Id protein induces humoral and occasionally cellular anti-Id responses that correlate with increased relapse-free and overall survival of patients with lymphoma. In animal models, protection or prophylaxis against subsequent tumor challenge has been demonstrated. The first experimental animal models used to test this type of treatment included the BCL$_1$ lymphoma (316), L2C leukemia (318), 141 lymphoma (319), and MPC-11 myeloma (320) models. In an effort to boost the therapeutic effect, numerous different strategies were used, including the use of keyhole limpet hemocyanin (KLH) as an immunologic carrier or the inclusion of complete Freund's adjuvant or Syntex adjuvant formulation (SAF-1). There is indirect evidence to suggest that the effector mechanisms responsible for Id-specific immunity against tumors involves ADCC mediated by anti-Id antibody bound to NK cells, especially LAK cells, and to TNF-secreting macrophages (321). IFN-γ secreted by T cells or macrophages has also been implicated in the BCL_1 tumor model (322).

In the 1990s, the first clinical trials using Id vaccines were initiated in patients with follicular lymphoma. Some of these trials included GM-CSF as an immunologic adjuvant (240). Clinical trials using this or any protein vaccine induce primarily humoral rather than cellular responses, and this may not be optimal because CTLs are probably critical for the long-term effectiveness of these vaccines.

Anticytokine Vaccines

The main aim of this type of vaccination is to generate neutralizing antibodies to block the accumulation of an overproduced cytokine. To break immunologic tolerance, a cytokine is coupled to a foreign carrier such as tetanus toxoid, purified protein derivative of tuberculosis, or KLH, to induce a T-dependent B-cell response (323). This technique was the starting point for vaccines against TNF-α (324), IL-1 (325), IL-9 (326), and epidermal growth factor (327). It is too early to predict how well these vaccines will perform in humans.

Synthetic Carbohydrate Antigen Vaccines

Carbohydrate antigens overexpressed on the surface of malignant cells are potential targets for immunotherapy. These include gangliosides (GM2, GM3, GD2, GD3, and 9-0-acetyl-GD3) expressed on most melanomas, sarcomas, and tumors of neuroectodermal origin, glycoproteins (Thomsen Friedenreich antigen, Tn, sTn) and neutral glycolipids and glycoproteins (Lewis^y and globo-H) overexpressed on epithelial cancers such as breast, ovarian, prostate, and lung carcinomas (328). Because carbohydrate antigens are poor (T-independent) immunogens, they have been coupled to carrier proteins (e.g., KLH) and used with a saporin adjuvant (QS-21). With rare exceptions (329,330), immunizations with these types of antigens do not induce cellular immune responses. Hapten-carrier conjugate vaccines induce a high level of IgM antibodies and some class-switching to IgG (331). For example, studies with GM2-KLH conjugates mixed with the QS-21 adjuvant induced a high-titer of IgM anti-GM2 antibodies and sustained IgG titers in all patients (332). In a clinical study in patients with metastatic breast cancer, a fully synthetic globo-H-KLH conjugate plus QS-21 generated globo-H-specific antibodies that mediated CDC and ADCC (333).

Recombinant Bacterial Vaccines

Bacteria, such as *Salmonella* (334), BCG (335), and *Listeria monocytogenes* (336), can be engineered to express TAAs or peptides. These vaccines can be administered orally to elicit strong antitumor responses. In model systems, recombinant strains bearing tumor antigens are used to infect animals and to induce specific CTL responses. These responses protect against tumor challenge and, in some cases, reduce tumor burdens in established disease (337).

Recombinant Viral Vector Vaccines

Because of the induction of inflammatory responses, viral infections elicit strong immune responses, which result in both specific and nonspecific immunity. Recombinant DNA technologies are used to incorporate additional genes encoding one or more complete or partial TAAs or peptide epitopes (332). These are expressed by infected cells and are presented in the context of MHC class I antigens. They are taken up by DCs at the site of the infection and are presented by both MHC class I and class II molecules to Th cells and CTLs (cross-priming) (332).

Most viral vectors used experimentally and clinically are poxvirus based, although retrovirus, adenovirus, adenovirus-associated virus, and herpesvirus vectors are also being investigated. Clinical trials targeting carcinoembryonic antigens, mucin-1, prostate-specific antigen, human papillomavirus, melanoma antigen recognized by T cells, and gp100, and in some cases with the addition of genes encoding costimulatory factors (e.g., CD80) or cytokines (e.g., IL-2), have been initiated. Although immune responses have been achieved, clinical improvements have been rare in these advanced cases (338).

DNA Vaccines

A simpler and perhaps safer method than viral vectors to introduce TAA-encoding DNA into patients is to use "naked" DNA. In an attempt to induce anti-DNA antibodies, it was discovered that DNA injected intramuscularly was taken up by cells in the muscle, and an immune response specific for the encoded genes was induced, indicating the genes were expressed in self-tissue (339). Both MHC class I and II restricted responses have been observed, suggesting that DCs either directly take up the DNA and present peptides in MHC molecules or "indirectly" present myocyte-expressed proteins as peptides to cross-prime T cells. DNA vaccines can also be administered intradermally using a gene gun. The DNA is taken up by resident Langerhans cells, transported to lymph nodes, and presented to T cells. Both routes ensure a long-lasting depot of antigen to stimulate an immune response continuously (340,341).

DNA vaccines are usually based on bacterial vectors, so they do not replicate *in vivo*. The gene of interest is placed under the control of a strong viral promoter for expression. Bacterial DNA contains immunostimulatory sequences that stimulate an innate immune response. Bacterial DNA is rarely incorporated into the host genome, nor is it especially immunogenic, so it is unlikely to elicit an anti-DNA immune response. DNA vaccination can break tolerance in experimental animals (340,341).

Numerous DNA vaccines are entering clinical trials in patients with cancer. These include patients with adenocarcinoma of the breast and colon, B- and T-cell lymphomas, and prostate carcinomas. Emerging data attest to safety and the ability of these vaccines to induce immune responses (342). This treatment is also being evaluated in various infectious diseases, such as HIV infection, hepatitis B, herpes simplex, influenza, and malaria (343). Problems with inducing only weak immune responses are being addressed by linking adjuvant sequences to DNA sequences encoding epitopes on tumor antigens (344).

Dendritic Cell Vaccines

DCs have the unique ability to initiate primary immune responses by means of their ability to present antigen, with concomitant co-stimulation, to virgin and memory T cells. DCs are powerful APCs that have been used either to prime or boost tumor immunity or to break tolerance by various different mechanisms. Autologous DCs can be harvested directly from the patient, propagated *ex vivo* from CD34$^+$ DC progenitors or by *ex vivo*–induced differentiation of CD14$^+$ monocytes. Alternatively, MHC-matched allogeneic DCs, obtained by any of these methods, can be used (271,345).

As with other cancer vaccine strategies, there are many choices and sources of TAAs. There are also numerous ways to introduce TAAs into DCs for presentation to T cells *in vivo* (272,345). Individual tumor peptides or peptide mixtures, whole proteins, tumor lysates or apoptotic tumor cells can be used to pulse DC *ex vivo*. Alternatively, tumor cells can be cocultured with DCs so they incorporate low levels of TAAs. These DCs can then be reintroduced into the patient. DCs can also be transfected with genes encoding tumor proteins or peptides, or with isolated tumor mRNA *ex vivo,* for subsequent antigen presentation *in vivo*. Transfection of DCs has also been accomplished *in vivo* by oral administration of recombinant bacterial vectors, such as *Salmonella,* or by liposomal delivery.

Hybrid cell vaccines are made by fusing a patient's tumor cells to allogeneic MHC-matched MHC class II$^+$ cells, especially DCs (346). This approach has been used in several animal models including hepatocarcinoma (347), thymoma (348), and adenocarcionoma of different origins (349). At least one animal study demonstrated the contribution of both CD4$^+$ Th cells and CD8$^+$ T cells in the immune response (348).

A clinical trial in patients with melanoma using freshly isolated tumor cells fused to activated allogeneic B cells has been initiated. Results have been encouraging (346). In another clinical trial, 17 patients with metastatic renal cell carcinoma were treated with hybrids of autologous tumor cells and allogeneic DCs. After a mean follow-up time of 13 months, four patients had rejected all metastatic lesions, two had PRs, and one a mixed response (350).

Vaccination with Unidentified Antigens
Autologous or Allogeneic Tumor Cells

Identifying highly immunogenic target antigens in a tumor can be difficult and time-consuming, and, for optimal results, vaccines will require more than one target antigen to avoid the escape of antigen-negative mutants. To obviate this search, preparations of live autologous or allogeneic tumor cells that are irradiated or lysed are administered with or without adjuvants, in an attempt to induce immune responses to the most immunogenic epitopes on the tumor without actually identifying them (351). Although autologous cells may be the best choice, they can be difficult to obtain. Many tumors contain shared antigens, common to many tumor types or at least to tumors of a given type isolated from many individuals. Thus, allogeneic vaccines prepared from a multitude of cell lines, expressing a range of HLA serotypes, can be used to vaccinate many different patients. These vaccines are more immunogenic and therapeutic than those containing autologous cells.

Whole cell vaccines and their lysates have been tested for the treatment of a wide variety of cancers, including breast and colorectal carcinomas, glioblastoma, gynecologic tumors, lung tumors, leukemias, melanomas, renal tumors, and sarcomas (351). These trials have resulted in many different outcomes, ranging from no clinical benefit to 98% survival at 2 years for patients with advanced-stage colorectal carcinoma after tumor resection (352).

Genetically Modified Autologous or Allogeneic Tumor Cells

Tumor cells are often ineffective at either priming DCs or acting as effective targets for CTLs, and hence they grow despite an intact immune system. To improve their immunogenicity, tumor tissues have been transduced *in vivo* or *ex vivo* to express various molecules, including MHC class I, for improved presentation, co-stimulatory molecules, such as CD80/86, and cytokines, such as GM-CSF, IL-2, IL-4, IL-7, IL-12, IFN-γ, and TNF-α (353). Various methods have been used for gene transfer, including transfection with viral vectors (retroviral, adenoviral), lipofection, and ballistic delivery of gene-coated particles. Small clinical trials conducted to treat a range of malignant diseases have yielded some promising results, such as PRs and stable disease, but this approach awaits further study and testing in larger numbers of patients for a critical evaluation (354).

Heat-Shock Proteins

Heat-shock proteins (Hsps), ubiquitously expressed in all cells, serve as chaperones for cytosolic peptides and are important components of immune function, by serving to transfer cytosolic peptides onto MHC class I molecules in the endoplasmic reticulum and possibly the MHC class II as well

(355). Isolates of Hsp, in particular gp96, Hsp90, and Hsp70, with accompanying peptides from tumor cells, contain the entire repertoire of peptides from these cells (356). When administered to mice, they protect them from challenge only with the tumor of origin. Tumor cells often express low levels of MHC molecules on their surface, but this approach relies on cross-priming DCs and thus circumvents this problem. Because the peptides associated with the Hsps are not MHC-restricted, they serve to cross-prime many individuals in outbred species such as humans (19).

Safety

After preclinical studies in mice are completed, the efficacy and safety of tumor-specific vaccination strategies must be evaluated in patients with cancer (357). Vaccines must be safe, especially if they are given prophylactically. Safety can be difficult to demonstrate, because clinical trials are conducted in patients with significant disease who often have impaired or immature immune systems. In addition, in immunologically normal persons, the follow-up time is very long, and large groups of patients must be used. The first wave of clinical trials has shown that most vaccination strategies are safe. However, examples of clinical responses are still rare (341,358).

Additional considerations are related to potential side effects of DNA vaccines. DNA has the potential to (a) integrate into the host genome and cause malignancy, (b) induce systemic or organ-specific autoimmune disease, (c) induce tolerance rather than immunity, or (d) stimulate the production of cytokines that affect the capacity of the host to respond to other types of vaccines and thus suppress immune function (358).

The frequency with which carcinogenic chromosomal insertions can occur is difficult to predict because DNA can linger for long periods in some cell types. However, based on *in vitro* and *in vivo* studies, it is estimated that such an event would likely occur with a probability several orders of magnitude lower than the rate of spontaneous mutations that lead to cancer (359,360).

Immunoprevention of Cancer

The immunoprevention of cancer represents a new goal for cancer treatment. This involves eliminating the cellular disorders that can appear in the early stages of carcinogenesis (361). Altered gene products that will become TAAs represent the main targets (362). Many new tumor vaccines, which can induce protection against subsequent tumor challenge, particularly in the setting of multidrug resistance, are currently being evaluated in clinical trials.

About 50% and 15% of human malignant diseases have mutations in p53 and *ras,* respectively (362). Mutant p53-specific CTLs can lyse such cells (363). Various studies in animals are under way to develop immunization strategies using p53 peptides and specific CTLs. In one study, IL-12

administered with the p53 peptide vaccine resulted in the regression of a p53-expressing Meth A sarcomas in mice (364).

Many tumors are characterized by the overexpression of certain proteins that make them good candidate immunogens for vaccination. Proteins with limited tissue distribution, such as Her-2/neu, are being targeted, with excellent results (365).

Conclusions

Although vaccinating humans against all cancers remains a long-term goal, tumor vaccines are currently used primarily to treat existing cancers in mice and, to some extent, in humans. Many obstacles must be overcome, including the weak immunogenicity of tumors and their ability to evade the immune response. Nevertheless, vaccines based on DCs, peptides, and DNA are providing new solutions.

CONCLUDING REMARKS

There is no shortage of immunotherapeutic agents or strategies that work successfully in mice. However, translation into humans is difficult, costly, and not always predictable. Furthermore, strategies that are highly effective in one disease may be a total failure in another, and the reasons for this are not always obvious. Despite these problems, several immunotherapeutic agents have been approved in the United States and Europe.

Many issues and challenges remain in this field. For example we must (a) optimize each individual strategy for the disease setting in which it is used, (b) determine which combinations of immunotherapies and immunotherapies plus conventional therapies are useful, (c) understand the differences in treating early versus advanced disease, (d) address mechanisms underlying toxicity, and (e) identify new targets. As new insights from basic immunology emerge, immunotherapies will continue to be refined further. For this reason, interactions among basic scientists, translational scientists, and clinicians will be critical for the future success of this field. At this time, there is every reason for optimism.

ACKNOWLEDGMENTS

We thank Ms. Linda Owens and Ms. Shannon Flowers for excellent administrative assistance. We thank Dr. Jonathan Uhr for his critical evaluation of the chapter.

REFERENCES

1. Gupta RK, Siber GR. Adjuvants for human vaccines-current status, problems and future prospects. *Vaccine* 1995;13:1263–1276.
2. Audibert FM, Lise LD. Adjuvants: current status, clinical perspectives and future prospects. *Immunol Today* 1993;14:281–284.
3. Baldwin RW, Beyers VS. Immuno-regulation by bacterial organisms and their role in the immunotherapy of cancer. *Springer Semin Immunopathol* 1979;2:79–100.
4. Bast RC, Zbar B, Borsos T, et al. BCG and cancer. *N Engl J Med* 1974;290:1458–1469.

5. Friberg S. BCG in the treatment of superficial cancer of the bladder: a review. *Med Oncol Tumor Pharmacother* 1993;10:31–36.

6. Nakazato H, Koike A, Ichihashi H. A controlled clinical trial with an extract from tubercle bacilli of human type (SSM) for a advanced gastric carcinoma. *Saishin Geka* 1980;1:1–37.

7. Sell S, Berkower I, Max EE. Immunology, immunopathology and immunity. In: 5th. 1996:943–968.

8. Ben-Efraim S. One hundred years of cancer immunotherapy a critical appraisal. *Tumor Biol* 1999;20:1–24.

9. Masihi KN. Immunomodulatory agents for prophylaxis and therapy of infections. *Int J Antimicrob Agents* 2000;14:181–191.

10. Bremers AJA, Parmiani G. Immunology and immunotherapy of human cancer: present concepts and clinical developments. *Crit Rev Oncol Hematol* 2000;34:1–25.

11. Jain RK, Forbes NS. Can engineered bacteria help control cancer? *Proc Natl Acad Sci USA* 2001;98:14748–14750.

12. Dang LH, Bettegowda C, Huso DL, et al. Combination bacteriolytic therapy for the treatment of experimental tumors. *Proc Natl Acad Sci USA* 2001;98:15155–15160.

13. Azuma I, Seya T. Development of immunoadjuvants of immunotherapy of cancer. *Int Immunopharmacol* 2001;1:1249–1259.

14. Masihi KN. Immunomodulators in infectious diseases: panoply of possibilites. *Int J Immunopharmacol* 2000;22:1083–1091.

15. Vosika G, Schmidtke J, Goldman A, et al. Phase I-II study of intralesional immunotherapy with attached *Mycobacterium smegmatis* cell wall skeleton and trehalose dimycolate. *Cancer Immunol Immunother* 1979;6:135–142.

16. Hartmann G, Weiner GJ, Krieg AM. CpG DNA: a potent signal for growth, activation, and maturation of human dendritic cells. *Proc Natl Acad Sci USA* 1999;96:9305–9310.

17. Pisetsky DS. Mechanism of immune stimulation by bacterial DNA. *Springer Semin Immunopathol* 2000;22:21–33.

18. Krieg AM, Wagner HP. Causing a commotion in the blood: immunotherapy progress from bacteria to bacterial DNA. *Immunol Today* 2000;10:521–527.

19. Davis ID. An overview of cancer immunotherapy. *Immunol Cell Biol* 2000;78:179–195.

20. Thomson AW. *The cytokine handbook.* San Diego: Academic Press, 1998.

21. Xing Z, Wang J. Consideration of cytokines as therapeutics agents or targets. *Curr Pharm Design* 2000;6:599–611.

22. Lillehei KO, Liu Y, Kong Q. Current perspectives in immunotherapy. *Ann Thorac Surg* 1999;68:S28–33.

23. Kourilsky P, Paolo TB. Cytokine fields and the polarization of the immune response. *Trends Immunol* 2001;22:502–509.

24. Gillis S, Williams DE. Cytokine therapy: lessons learned and future challenges. *Curr Opin Immunol* 1998;10:501–503.

25. White MK, McCubrey JA. Suppression of apoptosis: role in cell growth and neoplasia. *Leukemia* 2001;15:1011–1021.

26. Foster JR. The function of cytokines and their uses in toxicology. *Int J Exp Pathol* 2001;82:171–192.

27. Parmiani G, Rivoltini L, Reola G, et al. Cytokines in cancer therapy. *Immunol Lett* 2000;74:41–44.

28. Rosenberg SA, Yang JC, White DE, et al. Durability of complete responses in patients with metastatic cancer treated with high-dose interleukin-2: identification of the antigens mediating response. *Ann Surg* 1998;228:307–319.

29. Mekhail T, Wood L, Bukowski R. Interleukin-2 in cancer therapy: uses and optimum management of adverse effects. *Biodrugs* 2000;14:299–318.

30. Chen WX, Rains N, Young D, et al. Dendritic cell-based cancer immunotherapy: potential for treatment of colorectal cancer? *J Gastroenterol Hepatol* 2000;15:698–705.

31. Kurataukuri K, Nishisaka N, Jones RF, et al. Clinical trials of immunotherapy for advanced prostate cancer. *Urol Oncol* 2000;5:265–276.

32. Tagawa M. Cytokine therapy for cancer. *Curr Pharm Design* 2000;6:681–699.

33. Kirkwood JM, Strawderman MH, Ernstoff MS, et al. Interferon α-2β adjuvant therapy of high-risk resected cutaneous melanoma: the Eastern Cooperative Oncology Group Trial EST: 1648. *J Clin Oncol* 1996;14:7–17.

34. Kirkwood JM, Ibrahim J, Sondak VK. Preliminary analysis of the E1690/C9190 Intergroup Postsperative Adjuvant Trial of high- and

35. low-dose IFN-α 2B (HDI and LDI) in high-risk primary of lymph node metastatic melanoma. *Proc Am Soc Clin Oncol* 1999;18:537a.

36. Brown TD, Goodman PJ, Fleming T, et al. Phase II trial of recombinant DNA gamma-interferon in advanced colorectal cancer: a Southwest Oncology Group study. *J Immunother* 1991;10:379–382.

37. Schiller JH, Storer BE, Witt PL, et al. Biological and clinical effects of intravenous tumor necrosis factor-α administered three times weekly. *Cancer Res* 1991;51:1651–1658.

38. Stouthard JM, Goey H, de Vries EG, et al. Recombinant human interleukin 6 in metastatic renal cell cancer: a phase II trial. *Br J Cancer* 1996;73:789–793.

39. Rini BI, Stadler WM, Spielberger RT, et al. Granulocyte-macrophage-colony stimulating factor in metastatic renal cell carcinoma: a phase II trial. *Cancer* 1998;82:1352–1358.

40. Atkins MB, Robertson MJ, Gordon M, et al. Phase I evaluation of intravenous recombinant human interleukin 12 in patients with advanced malignancies. *Clin Cancer Res* 1997;3:409–417.

41. Zagozdzon R, Golab J. Immunomodulation by anticancer chemotherapy: more is not always better. *Int J Oncol* 2001;18:417–424.

42. Fassone L, Gaidano G, Ariatti C, et al. The role of cytokines in the pathogenesis and management of AIDS-related lymphomas. *Leuk Lymphoma* 2000;38:481–488.

43. Moreland L, Gugliotti R, King K, et al. Results of phase-I/II randomized, masked, placebo-controlled trial of recombinant human interleukin-11 (rhIL-11) in the treatment of subjects with active rheumatoid arthritis. *Arthritis Res* 2001;3:247–252.

44. Rolland JM, Douglass J, O'Hehir RE. Allergen immunotherapy: current and new therapeutic stratagies. *Expert Opin Invest Drugs* 2000;9:515–527.

45. Chung F. Anti-imflammatory cytokines in asthma and allergy: interleukin-10, interleukin-12, interferon-gamma. *Mediators Inflamm* 2001;10:51–59.

46. Renauld JC. New insights into the role of cytokines in asthma. *J Clin Pathol* 2001;54:577–589.

47. Balkwill F, Mantovani A. Inflammation and cancer: back to Virchow? *Lancet* 2001;357:539–545.

48. Fernandez-Botran R. Soluble cytokine receptors: novel immunotherapeutic agents. *Expert Opin Invest Drugs* 2000;9:497–514.

49. Miossec P. Cytokines in rheumatoid arthritis: is it all TNF-alpha? *Cell Mol Biol* 2001;47:675–678.

50. Lenschow DJ, Zeng Y, Thistlethwaite JR, et al. Long-term survival of xenogeneic pancreatic islet grafts induced by CTLA4Ig. *Science* 1992;257:789–792.

51. Linsley PS, Wallace PM, Johnson J, et al. A. Immunosuppression *in vivo* by a soluble form of the CTLA-4 T cell activation molecule. *Science* 1992;257:792–795.

52. Linsley PS, Wallace PM, Johnson J, et al. A. CTLA4Ig (BMS-188667)–mediated blockade of T cell costimulation in patients with psoriasis vulgaris. *J Invest Dermatol* 1992;108:570–575.

53. Shyu WC, Srinivas NR, Weiner RS, et al. Pharmacokinetics of intravenous CTLA4Ig (BMS-1888667) in cynomolgus monkeys following single and multiple doses. *Science* 1996;108:570–575.

54. Siegall CB, Haggerty HG, Warner GL, et al. Prevention of immunotoxin-induced immunogenicity by coadministration with CTLA4Ig enhances antitumor efficacy. *J Immunol* 1997;159:5168–5173.

55. Zheng XX, Markees TG, Hancock WW, et al. CTLA4 signals are required to optimally induce allograft tolerance with combined donor-specific transfusion and anti-CD154 monoclonal antibody treatment. *J Immunol* 1999;162:4983–4990.

56. Janeway CA, Travers P, Walport M, et al. CD40 ligand (CD40L). In: Immunobiology: The immune system in health and disease. Austin P, Lawrence E, eds. 5th edition. New York: Garland Publishing (Taylor & Francis Group), 2001:304–560.

57. Browning CN. Emil Behring and Paul Ehrlich: their contribution to science. *Nature* 1995;175:570–575.

58. Tiselius A, Kabat EA. Electrophoresis of immune serum. *Science* 1938;87:416–417.

59. Edsal JT. The plasma protein and their fractionation. *Adv Prot Chem* 1947;3:383–479.

60. Janeway CA. The development of clinical uses of immunoglobulins: a review. In: Merler E, ed. *Immunoglobulins: biologic aspects and clinical uses* Washington, DC: National Academy Press, 1970: 3–23.

60. Kohler G, Milstein C. Continuous cultures of fused cells secreting antibody of predefined specificity. *Nature* 1975;256:495–497.

61. Miller RA. Treatment of B-cell lymphoma with monoclonal anti-idiotype antibody. *N Engl J Med* 1982;306:517–522.

62. Schroff RW, Foon KA, Beatty SM, et al. Human anti-murine responses in patients recieiving monoclonal antibody therapy. *Cancer Res* 1985;45:879–885.

63. Reichert JM. Monoclonal antibodies in the clinic. *Nat Biotechnol* 2001;19:819–822.

64. Morrison SL, Johnson MJ, Herzenberg LA, et al. Chimeric human antibody molecules: mouse antigen-binding domains with human contact regions. *Proc Natl Acad Sci USA* 1984;81:6851–6855.

65. Boulianne GL, Hozumi N, Shulman MJ. Production of functional chimeric mouse/human antibody. *Nature* 1984;312:643–646.

66. Riechmann L, Clark M, Waldmann H, et al. Reshaping human antibodies for therapy. *Nature* 1988;332:323–327.

67. Winter G, Griffiths AD, Hawkins RE, et al. Making antibodies by phage-display technology. *Annu Rev Immunol* 1994;12:433–435.

68. Bruggemann M, Spicer C, Buluwela L, et al. Human antibody expression in transgenic mice: expression from 100 kb of the human IgG locus. *Eur J Immunol* 1991;21:1323–1326.

69. Vitetta ES, Uhr JW. Monoclonal antibodies as agonists: an expanded role for their use in cancer therapy. *Cancer Res* 1994;54:5301–5309.

70. Ghetie V, Ward ES. Multiple roles for the major histocompatibility complex class I-related receptor FcRn. *Annu Rev Immunol* 2000; 18:739–760.

71. Fujimori K, Covel DG, Fletcher JE, et al. A modeling analysis of monoclonal antibody percolation through tumors: a binding site barrier. *J Nucl Med* 1990;31:1191–1198.

72. Adams GP, Schier R, McCall AM, et al. High affinity restricts the localization and tumor penetration of single-chain Fv antibody molecules. *Cancer Res* 2001;61:4750–4755.

73. Jain RK. Physiological barrier to delivery of monoclonal antibodies and other macromolecules in tumors. *Cancer Res* 1990;50:815–819.

74. Ober RJ, Radu CG, Ghetie V, et al. Differences in promiscuity for antibody-FcRn interactions across species: implications for therapeutic antibodies. *Int Immunol* 2001;13:1250–1255.

75. Waldman H, Gilliland CK, Cobbold SP, et al. Immunotherapy. In: Paul WE, ed. *Fundamental immunology*. New York: Raven Press, 1999.

76. Ward ES, Ghetie V. The effector functions of immunoglobulins: implications for therapy. *Ther Immunol* 1995;2:77–94.

77. Isaacs JD, Clark MR, Greenwood J, et al. Therapy with monoclonal antibodies: an *in vivo* model for the assessment of therapeutic potential. *J Immunol* 1992;148:3062–3071.

78. Morgan BP. Regulation of the complement membrane attack. *Crit Rev Immunol* 1999;19:173–178.

79. Kuus-Reichel K, Grauer LS, Karavodin LM, et al. Will immunogenicity limit the use, efficacy and further development of therapeutic monoclonal antibodies? *Clin Diagn Lab Immunol* 1994;1:305–372.

80. Jonker M, DenBrok JHAM. Idiotype switching of CD4 specific monoclonal antibodies can prolong the therapeutic effectiveness in spite of host anti-mouse IgG antibody. *Eur J Immunol* 1987;17:1547–1553.

81. Reithmuller G. Monoclonal antibody therapy for resected Dukes' colorectal cancer: seven year outcome of a multi-center randomized trial. *J Clin Oncol* 1998;16:1788–1794.

82. Clark M. Antibody humanization: a case of the "emperor's new clothes" *Immunol Today* 2000;21:397–402.

83. Carter P. Improving the efficacy of antibody-based cancer therapies. *Nature* 2001;1:118–129.

84. Glennie MJ, Johnson PNM. Clinical trials of antibody therapy. *Immunol Today* 2000;21:403–410.

85. Feldman M, Elliott MJ, Woody JN, et al. Anti–tumor necrois factor-α therapy of rheumatoid arthritis. *Adv Immunol* 1997;64:283–350.

86. Present DH, Rutgeerts P, Targan S, et al. Infliximab for the treatment of fistulas in patients with Crohn's disease. *N Engl J Med* 1999; 340:1398–1405.

87. Waldmann H, Cobbold S. How do monoclonal antibodies induce tolerance? A role for infectious tolerance? *Annu Rev Immunol* 1999;16:619–644.

88. Ravetech JV, Lanier LL. Immune inhibitory receptors. *Science* 2000; 290:84–89.

89. Tutt AL, French R, Illidge TM, et al. Monoclonal antibody therapy of B cell lymphoma: signaling activity on tumor cells appears more important than recruitment of effector. *J Immunol* 1998;161:3176–3185.

90. Debatin KM, Krammer PH. Resistance to APO-1 (CD95) induced apoptosis in T-ALL is determined by a BCL-2 independent anti-apoptotic program. *Leukemia* 1995;9:815–821.

91. Vuist WMJ, Levy R, Maloney DG. Lymphoma regression induced by monoclonal anti-idiotypic antibodies correlates with their ability to induce Ig signal transduction and is not prevented by tumor expression of high levels of Bcl-2 protein. *Blood* 1994;83:899–906.

92. Ghetie MA, Picker LJ, Richardson JA, et al. Anti-CD19 inhibits the growth of human B-cell tumor lines *in vitro* and of Daudi cells in SCID mice by inducing cell cycle arrest. *Blood* 1994;83:1329–1336.

93. Chaouchi N, Vazquez A, Galanaud P, et al. B cell antigen receptor-mediated apoptosis: Importance of accessory molecules CD19 and CD22 and of surface IgM cross-linking. *Immunology* 1995;154:3096–3104.

94. Cragg MS, French RR, Glennie MJ. Signaling antibodies in cancer therapy. *Curr Opin Immunol* 1999;11:541–547.

95. Shan D, Ledbetter JA, Press OW. Apoptosis of malignant human B cells by ligation of CD20 with monoclonal antibodies. *Blood* 1998;91:1644–1652.

96. Ghetie MA, Podar EM, Ilgen A, et al. Homodimerization of tumor-reactive monoclonal antibodies markedly increases their ability to induce growth arrest or apoptosis of tumor cells. *Proc Natl Acad Sci USA* 1997;94:7509–7514.

97. Deans JP, Robbins SM, Polyak MJ, et al. Rapid redistribution of CD20 to a low density detergent-insoluble membrane compartment. *J Biol Chem* 1998;273:344–348.

98. Vitetta ES, Tucker TF, Racila E, et al. Tumor dormancy and cell signaling. V. Regrowth of the BCL₁ tumor after dormancy is established. *Blood* 1997;89:4425–4436.

99. Chambers CA, Kuhns MS, Egen JG, et al. CTLA-4–Mediated inhibition in regulation of t cell responses: mechanisms and manipulation in tumor immunotherapy. *Annu Rev Immunol* 2002;19:565–595.

100. Bolt S, Routledge EG, Lloyd IS, et al. The generation of humanized, non-mitogenic CD3 monoclonal antibody which retains *in vitro* immunosuppresive properties. *Eur J Immunol* 1993;23:403–411.

101. Armour K, Clark M, Hadley A, et al. Recombinant human IgG molecules lacking Fc γ receptor I binding and monocyte triggering activities. *Eur J Immunol* 1999;29:2613–2624.

102. Clynes RA, Towers TL, Presta LG, et al. Inhibitory Fc receptors modulate *in vivo* cytoxicity against tumor targets. *Nat Med* 2000;6:443–446.

103. Shields RL, Namenuk AK, Hong K, et al. High resolution mapping of the binding site on human IgG1 for FcγRI, FcγRII, FcγRIII and FcRn and design of IgG1 variants with improved binding to FcγR. *J Biol Chem* 2001;276:6591–6604.

104. Idusogie EE, Wong PY, Presta LG, et al. Engineered antibody with increased activity to recruit complement. *J Immunol* 2001;166:2571–2575.

105. Ghetie V, Popov S, Borvak J, et al. Increasing the serum persistence of an IgG fragment by random mutagenesis. *Nat Biotech* 1997;15:637–640.

106. Medesan C, Matesoi D, Radu C, et al. Delineation of the amino acid residues involved in transcytosis and catabolism of mouse IgG. *J Immunol* 1997;158:2211–2217.

107. Schiff RI. Treatment of primary immunodeficiency diseases with gammaglobulin. In: Lee ML, Strand V, eds. *Intravenous immunoglobulins in clinical practice*. New York: Marcel Dekker, 1997:175–190.

108. Imbach P, Wagner HP, Berchtold W, et al. Intravenous immunoglobulin versus oral corticosteroids in acute immune thrombocytopenic purpura in childhood. *Lancet* 1985;2:495–498.

109. Van der Meche FGA, Van Dorn PA. Guillain-Barre syndrome. In: Lee ML, Strand V, eds. *Intravenous immunoglobulins in clinical practice*. New York: Marcel Dekker, 1997:337–348.

110. Grob D. Intravenous immunogloblin in the management of myasthenia gravis. In: Lee ML, Strand V, eds. *Intravenous immunoglobulins in clinical practice*. New York: Marcel Dekker, 1997:362–380.

111. Melish ME. Use of IVIG in Kawasaki syndrome. In: Lee ML, Strand V, eds. *Intravenous immunoglobulins in clinical practice*. New York: Marcel Dekker, 1997:293–308.

112. Kaveri S, Dietrich G, Kazatchkine M. Intravenous immune globulin

in the treatment of autoimmune diseases. *Clin Exp Immunol* 1991; 86:192–198.

113. Arsura EL. Experience with intravenous immunoglobulin in myastenia gravis. *Clin Immunol Immunopathol* 1989;53:5170–5179.

114. Strand V. Proposed mechanisms for the efficacy of intravenous immunoglobulin treatment. In: Lee ML, Strand V, eds. *Intravenous immunoglobulins in clinical practice.* New York: Marcel Dekker, 1997: 23–36.

115. Ballow M. Mechanisms of action of intravenous immune serum globulin therapy. *Pediatr Infect Dis J* 1994;13:806–811.

116. Clarkson SB, Bussel JB, Kimberly RP, et al. Treatment of refractory immune thrombocytopenic purpura with an anti-Fc receptor antibody. *N Engl J Med* 1986;314:1236–1239.

117. Debre M, Bonnet MC, Fridman WH, et al. Infusion of Fcγ fragments for the treatment of children with acute immune thrombocytopenic purpura. *Lancet* 1993;342:945–946.

118. Samuelson A, Towers TL, Ravetch JV. Anti-inflammatory activity of IVIG mediated through the inhibitory Fc receptor. *Science* 2001; 291:484–486.

119. Frank M, Basta M, Fries L. The effect of IVIG on complement-dependent immune damage of cells and tissues. *Clin Immunol Immunopathol* 1992;62:582–586.

120. Masson PL. Elimination of infectious antigens and increase of IgG catabolism as possible modes of action of IVIG. *J Autoimmun* 1993; 6:683–689.

121. Yu Z, Lennon VA. Mechanism of intravenous immune gloublin therapy in antibody-mediated autoimmune diseases. *N Engl J Med* 1999; 340:227–228.

122. Sell S, Fahey JL. Relationship between gamma-globulin metabolism and low serum gamma-globulin in germ free mice. *J Immunol* 1963; 93:81–87.

123. Multani PS, Grossbard ML. Monoclonal antibody based therapies for hematologic malignancies. *J Clin Oncol* 1998;16:3691–3710.

124. Maloney D. Rituximab in agressive NHL: standard of care? *First International Congress on Monoclonal Antibodies in Cancer, Banff (Canada), August 30–September 2, 2001.*

125. Hainsworth J. Recommendations regarding use of rituximab in low grade NHL: data from recent trials. *First International Congress on Monoclonal Antibodies in Cancer, Banff (Canada), August 30–September 2, 2001.*

126. Leonard J. Targeting CD22 in patients with relapsed NHL. *First International Congress on Monoclonal Antibodies in Cancer, Banff (Canada), August 30–September 2, 2001.*

127. Pegram M, Slamon D. Biological rationale for Her2/neu (c-erbB2) as a target for monoclonal antibody therapy. *Semin Oncol* 2000;27:13–19.

128. Viloria-Petit AM, Rak J, Hung MC, et al. Neutralizing antibodies against epidermal growth factor and ErbB-2/neu receptor tyrosine kinases down-regulate vascular endothelial growth factor production by tumor cells *in vitro* and *in vivo*. *Am J Pathol* 1997;151:1523–1530.

129. Kerbel RS, Viloria-Petit A, Okada F, et al. Establishing a link between oncogenes and tumor angiogenesis. *Mol Med* 1998;4:286–295.

130. Baselga J. Clinical trials of single-agent trastuzumab (Herceptin). *Semin Oncol* 2000;27:20–26.

131. Taylor PC. Antibodies in inflammatory diseases: cytokines. In: George AJT, Urch CE, eds. *Diagnostic and therapeutic antibody.* Totowa, NJ: Humana Press, 2000:115–140.

132. Wise M, Zelenika D. Monoclonal antibody therapy in organ transplantation. In: Shepherd P, Dean C, eds. *Monoclonal antibody.* New York: Oxford University Press, 2000;431–448.

133. Staerz UD, Kanagawa O, Bevan MJ. Hybrid antibodies can target sites for attack by T cells. *Nature* 1985;314:628–631.

134. Pluckthun A, Pack P. New protein engineering approaches to multivalent and bispecific antibody fragments. *Immunotechnology* 1997; 3:83–105.

135. Brissinck J, Demanet C, Moser M, et al. Bispecific antibodies in lymphoma. *Int Rev Immunol* 1993;10:187–194.

136. de Gast GC, van de Winkel JGJ, Bast EJ. Clinical perspectives of bispecific antibodies in cancer. *Cancer Immunother* 1997;45:121–123.

137. Schmidt M, Wels W. Targeted inhibition of tumour cell growth by a bispecific single-chain toxin containing an antibody domain and TGF alpha. *Br J Cancer* 1996;74:853–862.

138. Valerius T, Stockmeyer B, van Spriel AB, et al. Fc alpha RI (CD89)

as a novel trigger molecule for bispecific antibody therapy. *Blood* 1997;90:4485–4492.

139. Segal DM, Sconocchia G, Titus JA, et al. Alternative triggering molecules and single chain bispecific antibodies. *J Hematother* 1995;4:377–382.

140. Haagen IA. Performance of CD3xCD19 bispecific monoclonal antibodies in B cell malignancy. *Leuk Lymphoma* 1995;19:381–393.

141. Lindhofer H, Mocikat R, Steipe B, et al. Preferential species-restricted heavy/light chain pairing in rat/mouse quadromas: implications for a single-step purification of bispecific antibodies. *J Immunol* 1995;155:219–225.

142. Ruf P, Lindhofer H. Induction of a long-lasting antitumor immunity by a trifunctional bispecific antibody. *Blood* 2001;98:2526–2534.

143. DeJonge J, Heirman C, DeVeerman M, et al. Bispecific antibody treatment of murine B cell lymphoma. *Cancer Immunol Immunother* 1997;45:162–165.

144. van Spriel AB, van Ojik HH, van de Winkel JG. Immunotherapeutic perspective for bispecific antibodies. *Immunol Today* 2000;21:391–397.

145. de Gast GC, Haagen IA, van Houten AA, et al. CD8 T cell activation after intravenous administration of CD3 x CD19 bispecific antibody in patients with non-Hodgkin lymphoma. *Cancer Immunol Immunother* 1995;40:390–396.

146. Hartmann F, Renner C, Jung W, et al. Treatment of Hodgkinisease with bispecific antibodies. *Ann Oncol* 1996;7:143–146.

147. Lamers CH, Bolhuis RL, Warnaar SO, et al. Local but no systemic immunodulation by intraperitoneal treatment of advanced ovarian cancer with autologous T lymphocytes retargeted by a bispecific monoclonal antibody. *Int J Cancer* 1997;73:211–219.

148. Nitta T, Sato K, Yagita H, et al. Preliminary trial of specific targeting therapy against malignant glioma. *Lancet* 1990;335:368–371.

149. Riethmuller G, Schneider-Gadicke E, Schlimok G, et al. Randomized trial of monoclonal antibody for adjuvant therapy of resected Dukescolorectal carcinoma. *Lancet* 1994;343:1177–1183.

150. Kroesen BJ, Buter J, Sleijfer DT, et al. Phase I study of intravenously applied bispecific antibody in renal cell cancer patients receiving subcutaneous interleukin-2. *Br J Cancer* 1994;70:652–661.

151. Kroesen BJ, Nieken J, Sleijfer DT, et al. Approaches to lung cancer treatment using the CD3 x EGP-2–directed bispecific monoclonal antibody BIS-1. *Cancer Immunol Immunother* 1997;45:203–206.

152. Ghetie MA, Ghetie V, Vitetta ES. The use of immunoconjugates in cancer therapy. *Expert Opin Invest Drugs* 1996;5:309–321.

153. Farah RA, Clinchy B, Herrera L, et al. The development of monoclonal antibodies for the therapy of cancer. *Crit Rev Eukaryot Gene Expr* 1998;8:321–356.

154. Ghetie V, Vitetta ES. Immunotoxins in the therapy of cancer: from bench to clinic. *Pharmacol Ther* 1994;63:209–234.

155. Siegall CB. Targeted toxins as anticancer agents. *Cancer* 1994;74: 1006–1012.

156. Thrush GR, Lark LR, Clinchy BC, et al. Immunotoxins: an update. *Annu Rev Immunol* 1996;14:49–71.

157. Barbieri L, Battelli MG, Stirpe F. Ribosome-inactivating proteins from plants. *Biochim Biophys Acta* 1993;154:237–282.

158. Multani PS, Grossbard ML. Immunotoxin therapy of lymphoma: studies with anti-B4–blocked ricin. In: Grossbard ML, ed. *Monoclonal-based therapy of cancer.* New York: Marcel Dekker, Inc. 1998:91–112.

159. Brinkmann U, Pastan I. Immunotoxins against cancer. *Biochim Biophys Acta* 1994;1198:27–45.

160. Middlebrook JL, Dorland RB. Bacterial toxins: cellular mechanisms of action. *Microbiol Rev* 1984;48:199–221.

161. Cumber JA, Forrester JA, Foxwell BMJ, et al. Preparation of antibody-toxin conjugates. *Methods Enzymol* 1985;112:207–225.

162. Thorpe PE, Ross WC. The preparation and cytotoxic properties of antibody-toxin conjugates. *Immunol Rev* 1982;62:119–158.

163. Thorpe PE, Wallace PM, Knowles PP, et al. New coupling agents for the synthesis of immunotoxins containing a hindered disulfide bond with improved stability *in vivo*. *Cancer Res* 1987;47:5924–5931.

164. May RD, Finkelman FD, Uhr JW, et al. Evaluation of ricin A chain-containing immunotoxins directed against different epitopes on the delta-chain of cell surface-associated IgD on murine B cells. *J Immunol* 1990;144:3637–3642.

165. Pastan I. Targeted therapy of cancer with recombinant immunotoxins. *Biochim Biophys Acta* 1997;1333:C1–C6.

166. Ore M, Brown AN, Hussain K, et al. Cytotoxicity of a recombinant ricin–A-chain fusion protein containing a proteolytically-cleavable spacer sequence. *FEBS Lett* 1990;273:200–204.

167. Benhar I, Reiter Y, Pai LH, et al. Administration of disulfide-stabilized Fv-immunotoxins B1 (dsFv)-PE38 and B3 (dsFv) -PE38 by continuous infusion increases their efficacy in curing large tumor xenografts in nude mice. *Int J Cancer* 1995;62:351–355.

168. Reiter Y, Pastan I. Antibody engineering of recombinant Fv immunotoxins for Improved targeting of cancer: disulfide-stabilized Fv immunotoxins. *Clin Cancer Res* 1996;2:245–252.

169. Pastan I. Immunotoxins: current status and future prospects. *First International Congress on Monoclonal Antibodies in Cancer, Banff (Canada), August 30–September 2,* 2001.

170. Gelber EE, Vitetta ES. Effect of immunosuppressive agents on the immunogenicity and efficacy of an immunotoxin in mice. *Clin Cancer Res* 1998;4:1297–1304.

170a. Smallshaw JE, Ghetie V, Rizo J, et al. Genetic engineering of an immunotoxin to eliminate pulmonary vascular leak in mice. *Nat Biotechnol* 2003;21:387–391.

171. Baluna R, Vitetta ES. Vascular leak syndrome: a side effect of immunotherapy. *Immunopharmacology* 1996;37:117–132.

172. Frankel A. Diptheria toxin conjugate therapy of cancer. *First International Congress on Monoclonal Antibodies in Cancer, Banff (Canada), August 30–September 2,* 2001.

173. Soler-Rodriguez AM, Ghetie MA, Oppenheimer-Marks N, et al. Ricin A-chain and ricin A-chain immunotoxins rapidly damage human endothelial cells: implications for vascular leak syndrome. *Exp Cell Res* 1993;206:227–234.

174. Ghetie MA, Tucker K, Richardson J, et al. The anti-tumor activity of an anti-CD22 immunotoxin in SCID mice with disseminated Daudi lymphoma is enhanced by either an anti- CD19 antibody or an anti-CD19 immunotoxin. *Blood* 1992;80:2315–2320.

175. Flavell DJ, Boehm DA, Emery L, et al. Therapy of human B-cell lymphoma bearing SCID mice is more effective with anti-CD19 and anti-CD38 saporin immunotoxins used in combination than with either immunotoxin used alone. *Int J Cancer* 1995;62:1–8.

176. Jansen B, Kersey JH, Jaszcz WB, et al. Effective immunochemotherapy of human t(4;11) leukemia in mice with severe combined immunodeficiency (SCID) using B43 (anti-CD19)-pokeweed antiviral protein immunotoxin plus cyclophosphamide. *Leukemia* 1993;7:290–297.

177. Uckun FM, Chelstrom LM, Finnegan D, et al. Effective immunochemotherapy of CALLA$^+$Cμ^+ human pre-B acute lymphoblastic leukemia in mice with severe combined immunodeficiency using B43 (anti-CD19) pokeweed antiviral protein immunotoxin plus cyclophosphamide. *Blood* 1992;79:3116–3129.

178. Ghetie MA, Tucker K, Richardson J, et al. Eradication of minimal disease in severe combined immunodeficient mice with disseminated Daudi lymphoma using chemotherapy and an immunotoxin cocktail. *Blood* 1994;84:702–707.

179. O'Connor R, Liu C, Ferris CA, et al. Anti-B4–blocked ricin synergizes with doxorubicin and etoposide on multidrug-resistant and drug-sensitive tumors. *Blood* 1995;86:4286–4294.

180. Dillman RO, Johnson DE, Ogden J, et al. Significance of antigen, drug, and tumor cell targets in the preclinical evaluation of doxorubicin, daunorubicin, methotrexate, and mitomycin-C monoclonal antibody immunoconjugates. *Mol Biother* 1989;1:250–255.

181. Goldenberg DM. Monoclonal antibodies in cancer detection and therapy. *Am J Med* 1993;94:297–312.

182. Ghose T, Norvell ST, Guclu A, et al. Immunochemotherapy of cancer with chlorambucil-carrying antibody. *BMJ* 1972;3:495–499.

183. Hurwitz E, Levy R, Maron R, et al. The covalent binding of daunomycin and Adriamycin to antibodies, with retention of both drug and antibody activities. *Cancer Res* 1975;35:1175–1181.

184. Bernstein A, Hurwitz E, Maron R, et al. Higher antitumor efficacy of daunomycin when linked to dextran:*in vivo* and *in vitro* studies. *J Natl Cancer Inst* 1978;60:379–384.

185. Garnett MC, Embleton MJ, Jacobs E, et al. Preparation and properties of a drug-carrier-antibody conjugate showing selective antibody-directed cytotoxicity *in vitro. Int J Cancer* 1983;31:661–670.

186. Tsukada Y, Kato Y, Umemoto N, et al. An antialpha-fetoprotein-daunomycin conjugate with a novel poly-L-glutamic acid derivative as intermediate drug carrier. *J Natl Cancer Inst* 1984;73:721–729.

187. Schechter B, Pauzner R, Arnon R, et al. Selective cytotoxicity against tumor cells by cisplatin complexed to antitumor antibodies *via* carboxymethyl dextran. *Cancer Immunol Immunother* 1987;25:225–230.

188. Shih LB, Sharkey RM, Primus FJ, et al. Site-specific linkage of methotrexate to monoclonal antibodies using an intermediate carrier. *Int J Cancer* 1988;41:832–839.

189. Dillman RO, Johnson DE, Shawler DL, et al. A. Superiority of an acid-labile daunorubicin-monoclonal antibody immunoconjugate compared to free drug. *Cancer Res* 1988;48:6097–6102.

190. Pietersz GA, Krauer K. Antibody-targeted drugs for the therapy of cancer. *J Drug Targeting* 1994;2:183–215.

191. Liu C, Tadayoni BM, Bourret LA, et al. Eradication of large colon tumor xenografts by targeted delivery of maytansinoids. *Proc Natl Acad Sci USA* 1996;93:8618–8623.

192. Trail PA, Willner D, Lasch SJ, et al. Cure of xenografted human carcinomas by BR96–doxorubicin immunoconjugates. *Science* 1993;261:212–215.

193. Sievers EL, Larson RA, Stadtmauer EA, et al. Efficacy and safety of gemtuzumab ozogamicin in patients with CD33-positive acute myeloid leukemia in first relapse. *J Clin Oncol* 2001;19:3244–3254.

194. Tallman MS. Single Agent Gemtuzumab Ozogamicin in relapsed AML. *First International Congress on Monoclonal Antibodies in Cancer, Banff (Canada), August 30–September 2,* 2001.

195. Bagshawe KD. Antibody directed enzymes revive anti-cancer prodrugs concept. *Br J Cancer* 1987;56:531–532.

196. Senter PD, Saulnier MG, Schreiber GJ, et al. Anti-tumor effects of antibody-alkaline phosphatase conjugates in combination with etoposide phosphate. *Proc Natl Acad Sci USA* 1988;85:4842–4846.

197. Connors TA, Knox RJ. Prodrugs in cancer chemotherapy. *Stem Cells* 1995;13:501–511.

198. Deonarain MP, Epenetos AA. Targeting enzymes for cancer therapy: old enzymes in new roles. *Br J Cancer* 1994;70:786–794.

199. Bagshawe KD, Sharma SK, Springer CJ, et al. Antibody directed enzyme prodrug therapy (ADEPT): clinical report. *Dis Markers* 1991;9:233–238.

200. Martin J, Stribbling SM, Poon GK, et al. Antibody-directed enzyme prodrug therapy: pharmacokinetics and plasma levels of prodrug and drug in a phase I clinical trial. *Cancer Chemother Pharmacol* 1997;40:189–201.

201. Bagshawe KD, Begent RHJ. First clinical experience with ADEPT. *Adv Drug Deliv Rev* 1996;22:365–367.

202. Bagshawe KD, Sharma, SK, Burke PJ, et al. Developments with targeted enzymes in cancer therapy. *Curr Opin Immunol* 1999;11:579–583.

203. Seymour LW. Passive tumor targeting of soluble macromolecule and drug conjugates. *Crit Rev Ther Drug Carrier Syst* 1992;9:135–187.

204. Niculescu-Duvaz I, Spooner R, Marais R, et al. Gene-directed enzyme prodrug therapy. *Bioconjug Chem* 1998;9:4–22.

205. Press OW, Appelbaum FR, Eary JF, et al. Radiolabeled antibody therapy of lymphomas. In: DeVita VT, Hellman S, Rosenberg SA, eds. *Important Advances in Oncology.* Philadelphia: JB Lippincott, 1995:157–171.

206. Wilder RB, DeNardo GL, DeNardo SJ. Radioimmunotherapy: recent results and future directions. *J Clin Oncol* 1996;14:1383–1400.

207. Stigbrand T, Ullen A, Sandstrom P, et al. Twenty years with monoclonal antibodies. *Acta Oncol* 1996;35:259–265.

208. Park CH. The role of radioisotopes in radiation oncology. *Semin Oncol* 1997;24:639–654.

209. Jurcic JG, Scheinberg DA, Houghton AN. Monoclonal antibody therapy of cancer. In: Pinedo HM, Longo DL, Chabner BA, eds. *Cancer Chemotherapy and Biological Response Modifiers, 16.* Elsevier Science, 1996:168–188.

210. Zalutsky MR, Bigner DD. Radioimmunotherapy with α-particle emitting radioimmunoconjugates. *Acta Oncol* 1996;35:373–379.

211. Lenhard RE Jr, Order SE, Spunberg JJ,et al. Isotopic immunoglobulin: a new systemic therapy for advanced Hodgkin's disease. *J Clin Oncol* 1985;3:1296–1300.

212. Vriesendorp HM, Herpst JM, Germack MA, et al. Phase I-II studies of yttrium-labeled antiferritin treatment for end-stage Hodgkin's disease, including Radiation Therapy Oncology Group, 87–01. *J Clin Oncol* 1991;9:918–928.

213. Grossbard ML, Freedman AS, Ritz J, et al. Serotherapy of B-cell neoplasms with anti-B4–blocked ricin: a phase 1 trial of daily bolus infusion. *Blood* 1992;79:576–585.

214. Corcoran MC, Eary J, Bernstein I, et al. Radioimmunotherapy strategies for non-Hodgkin's lymphomas. *Ann Oncol* 1997;8:133–138.

215. Behr TM, Goldenberg DM, Becker WS. Radioimmunotherapy of solid tumors: a review "of mice and men." *Hybridoma* 1997;16:101–107.

216. Bombardieri E, Ferrari L, Spinelli A, et al. Radioimmunotherapy of ovarian cancer with radiolabelled monoclonal antibodies: biological basis, present status and future perspectives. *Anticancer Res* 1997;17:1719–1730.

217. Kaminski MS, Fig LM, Zasadny KR, et al. Imaging, dosimetry, and radioimmunotherapy with iodine 131–labeled anti-CD37 antibody in B-cell lymphoma. *J Clin Oncol* 1992;10:1696–1711.

218. Kaminski MS, Zasadny KR, Francis IR, et al. Iodine-131–anti-B1 radioimmunotherapy for B-cell lymphoma. *J Clin Oncol* 1996;14:1974–1981.

219. Knox SJ, Goris ML, Trisler K, et al. Yttrium-90–labeled anti-CD20 monoclonal antibody therapy of recurrent B-cell lymphoma. *Clin Cancer Res* 1996;2:457–470.

220. Press OW, Eary JF, Appelbaum FR, Bernstein, I. D. Myeloablative radiolabeled antibody therapy with autologous bone marrow transplantation for relapsed B cell lymphomas. *Cancer Treat Res* 1995;76:281–297.

221. Press OW, Eary JF, Appelbaum FR, et al. Phase II trial of ^{131}I-B1(anti-CD20) antibody therapy with autologous stem cell transplantation for relapsed B cell lymphomas. *Lancet* 1995;346:336–340.

222. Kaminski MS. ^{131}I-Tositumomab (Bexxar) in relapsed and transformed lymphoma. *First International Congress on Monoclonal Antibodies in Cancer, Banff (Canada), August 30–September 2, 2001.*

223. DeNardo G. Radiolabeled monoclonal antibodies: basic science and current prospects. *First International Congress on Monoclonal Antibodies in Cancer, Banff (Canada), August 30–September 2, 2001.*

224. Witzig TE. ^{90}Y-ibritumomab (Zevelin): current data in low grade NHL. *First International Congress on Monoclonal Antibodies in Cancer, Banff (Canada), August 30–September 2, 2001.*

225. Zelentz A. Newer data with ^{131}I-tositumomab (Bexxar). *First International Congress on Monoclonal Antibodies in Cancer, Banff (Canada), August 30–September 2, 2001.*

226. Gregoriadis G. Engineering liposomes for drug delivery: progress and problems. *Trends Biotechnol* 1995;13:527–537.

227. Park JW, Hong K, Carter P, et al. Development of anti-p185[HER2] immunoliposomes fo cancer therapy. *Proc Natl Acad Sci USA* 1995;92:1327–1331.

228. Hansen CB, Kao GY, Moase EH, et al. Attachment of antibodies to sterically stabilized liposomes: evaluation, comparison and optimization of coupling procedures. *Biochim Biophys Acta* 1995;1239:133–144.

229. Blume G, Cevc G. Liposomes for the sustained drug release *in vivo*. *Biochim Biophys Acta* 1990;1029:91–97.

230. Senior J, Delgado C, Fisher D, et al. Influence of surface hydrophilicity of liposomes on their interaction with plasma protein and clearance from the circulation: studies with poly (ethylene glycol)-coated vesicles. *Biochim Biophys Acta* 1991;1062:77–82.

231. Allen TM, Ahmad I, Lopes de Menezes DE, et al. Immunoliposome-mediated targeting of anti-cancer drugs *in vivo*. *Biochem Soc Trans* 1995;23:1073–1079.

232. Ahmad I, Longenecker M, Samuel J, et al. Antibody-targeted delivery of doxorubicin entrapped in sterically stabilized liposomes can eradicate lung cancer in mice. *Cancer Res* 1993;53:1484–1488.

233. Park JW, Hong K, Kirpotin DB, et al. Anti-HER2 immunoliposomes for targeted therapy of human tumors. *Cancer Lett* 1997;118:153–160.

234. Park JW, Kirpotin DB, Hong K, et al. Applications of immunoliposome technology for targeted drug delivery. *Clin Cancer Res* 2001;7:784S.

235. Soepenberg O, Sparreboom A, de Jonge MJ, et al. Phase I and pharmacologic study of a weekly schedule of LEP (liposome encapsulated paclitaxel) in patients with solid tumors. *Clin Cancer Res* 2001;7:785S.

236. Yarmush ML, Thorpe WP, Strong L, et al. Antibody targeted photolysis. *Crit Rev Ther Drug Carrier Syst* 1993;10:197–252.

237. Reddi E. New trends in photobiology: role of delivery vehicles for photosensitizers in the photodynamic therapy of tumors. *J Photochem Photobiol B* 1997;37:189–195.

238. Mew D, Wat CK, Towers GHN, et al. Photoimmunotherapy: treatment of animal tumors with tumor-specific monoclonal antibody hematoporphyrin conjugates. *J Immunol* 1983;130:1473–1477.

239. Del Governatore M, Hamblin MR, Piccinni EE, et al. Targeted photodestruction of human colon cancer cells using charged 17.1 A chlorin e6 immunoconjugates. *Cancer* 2000;82:56–64.

240. Tao MH, Levy R. Idiotype/granulocyte-macrophage colony-stimulating factor fusion protein as a vaccine for B-cell lymphoma. *Nature* 1993;362:755–758.

241. Gillies SD, Reilly EB, Reisfeld RA. Antibody-targeted interleukin-2 stimulates T-cell killing of autologous tumor cells. *Proc Natl Acad Sci USA* 1992;89:1428–1432.

242. Becker JC, Pancook JD, Gillies SD, et al. T cell-mediated eradication of murine metastatic melanoma induced by targeted interleukin 2 therapy. *J Exp Med* 1996;183:2361–2366.

243. Xiang R, Lode HN, Dolman CS, et al. Elimination of established murine colon carcinoma metastases by antibody interleukin-2 fusion protein therapy. *Cancer Res* 1997;57:4948–4955.

244. Ozzello L, De Rosa CM, Blank EW, et al. The use of natural interferon alpha conjugated to a monoclonal antibody antimammary epithelial mucin (Mc5) for the treatment of human breast cancer xenografts. *Breast Cancer Res Treat* 1993;25:265–276.

245. Reisfeld RA, Gillies SD, Mendelson J, et al. Involvement of B lymphocytes in the growth inhibition of human pulmonary melanoma metastases in athymic nu/nu mice by an antibody-lymphotoxin fusion protein. *Cancer Res* 1996;56:1707–1712.

246. Marrack P, Kappler J. The staphylococcal enterotoxins and their relatives. *Science* 1990;248:705–711.

247. Kalland T, Dohlsten M, Abrahmsen L, et al. Targeting of superantigens. *Cell Biophys* 1993;22:147–164.

248. Hansson J, Ohlsson L, Persson R, et al. Genetically engineered superantigens as tolerable antitumor agents. *Proc Natl Acad Sci USA* 1997;94:2489–2494.

249. Dohlsten M, Abrahmsen L, Björk P, et al. Monoclonal antibody-superantigen fusion proteins: tumor-specific agents for T-cell-based tumor therapy. *Proc Natl Acad Sci USA* 1994;91:8945–8949.

250. Kuge S, Miura Y, Nakamura Y, et al. Superantigen-induced human CD4+ helper/killer T cell phenomenon: selective induction of the Th1 helper/killer T cells and application to tumor immunotherapy. *J Immunol* 1995;154:1777–1785.

251. Lando PA, Dohlsten M, Hedlund G, et al. T cell killing of human colon carcinomas by monoclonal-antibody-targeted superantigens. *Cancer Immunol Immunother* 1993;36:223–228.

252. Lando PA, Dohlsten M, Ohlsson L, et al. Tumor-reactive superantigens suppress tumor growth in humanized SCID mice. *Int J Cancer* 1995;62:466–471.

253. Gidlof C, Dohlsten M, Lando PA, et al. A superantigen-antibody fusion protein for T cell immunotherapy of human B-lineage malignancies. *Blood* 1997;89:2089–2097.

254. Holzer U, Bethge W, Krull F, et al. Superantigen *Staphylococcal enterotoxin* A–dependent and antibody-targeted lysis of GD2-positive neuroblastoma cells. *Cancer Immunol Immunother* 1995;41:129–136.

255. Giantonio BJ, Alpaugh RK, Schultz J, et al. Superantigen-based immunotherapy: a phase I trial of PNU-214565, a monoclonal antibody staphylococcal enterotoxin A recombinant fusion protein, in advanced pancreatic and colorectal cancer. *J Clin Oncol* 1997;15:1994–2007.

256. Youle RJ, Newton D, Wu YN, et al. Cytotoxic ribonucleases and chimeras in cancer therapy. *Crit Rev Ther Drug Carrier Syst* 1993;10:1–28.

257. Lin JJ, Newton DL, Mikulski SM, et al. Characterization of the mechanism of cellular and cell free protein synthesis inhibition by an antitumor ribonuclease. *Biochem Biophys Res Commun* 1994;204:156–162.

258. Rybak SM, Saxena SK, Ackerman EJ, et al. Cytotoxic potential of ribonuclease and ribonuclease hybrid proteins. *J Biol Chem* 1991;266:21202–21207.

259. Newton DL, Ilercil O, Laske DW, et al. Cytotoxic ribonuclease chimeras: targeted tumoricidal activity *in vitro* and *in vivo*. *J Biol Chem* 1992;267:19572–19578.

260. Deonarain MP, Epenetos AA. Design, characterization and antitumour cytotoxicity of a panel of recombinant, mammalian ribonuclease-based immunotoxins. *Br J Cancer* 1998;77:537–546.

261. Newton DL, Nicholls PJ, Rybak SM, et al. Expression and characterization of recombinant human eosinophil-derived neurotoxin and

eosinophil-derived neurotoxin-anti-transferrin receptor sFv. *J Biol Chem* 1994;269:26739–26745.

262. Rybak SM, Hoogenboom HR, Meade HM, et al. Humanization of immunotoxins. *Proc Natl Acad Sci USA* 1992;89:3165–3169.

263. Rybak SM, Hoogenboom HR, Newton DL, et al. Rational immunotherapy with ribonuclease chimeras: an approach toward humanizing immunotoxins. *Cell Biophys* 1992;21:121–138.

264. Wu Y, Mikulski SM, Ardelt W, et al. A cytotoxic ribonuclease: study of the mechanism of onconase cytotoxicity. *J Biol Chem* 1993; 268:10686–10693.

265. Rosenberg SA. Cell transfer therapy: clinical applications. In: *Melanoma,* 3rd ed. Philadelphia: Lippincott Williams & Wilkins, 2001:322–345.

266. Ben-Efraim S. Cancer immunotherapy: hopes and pitfall. *Anticancer Res* 1996;16:3235–3240.

267. Dudley ME. Cell transfer therapy: basic principles and preclinical studies. In: *Biologic therapy of cancer.* 2001:305–321.

268. Schreiber H. In: Paul WE, ed. *Tumor immunology,* 2nd ed. New York: Raven Press, 1989:923–955.

269. Murphy WJ, Longo DL. The potential role of NK cells in the separation of graft-versus-host disease after allogeneic bone marrow transplantation. *Immunol Rev* 1997;157:167–176.

270. Meidenbauer N, Reesen R, Mackensen A. Dendritic cells for specific cancer immunotherapy. *Biol Chem* 2001;382:507–520.

271. Gunzer M, Janich S, Varga G, et al. Dendritic cells and tumor immunity. *Semin Immunol* 2001;13:291–302.

272. Gunzer M, Grabbe S. Dendritic cells in cancer immunotherapy. *Crit Rev Immunol* 2001;21:133–145.

273. Hennemann B, Beckmann G, Eichelmann A, et al. Phase I trial of adoptive immunotherapy of cancer patients using monocyte-derived macrophages activated with interferon gamma and lipopolysaccharide. *Cancer Immunol Immunother* 1998;45:250–256.

274. Bartoleyns J, Romet-Lemonne JL, Chokri M, et al. Immune therapy with macrophages: present status and critical requirements for implementation. *Immunobiology* 1996;195:550–562.

275. Kammula US, Marincola FM. Cancer immunotherapy: is there real progress at last? *Biodrugs* 1999;11:249–260.

276. Rosenberg SA, Yannelli JR, Yang JC, et al. Treatment of patients with metastatic melanoma with autologous tumor-infiltrating lymphocytes and interleukin-2. *J Natl Cancer Inst* 1994;86:1159–1166.

277. Peggs KS, MacKinnon S. Cellular therapy: donor lymphocytes infusion. *Curr Opin Hematol* 2001;8:349–354.

278. Van der Bruggen P, Traversari C, Chomez P, et al. A gene encoding an antigen recognized by cytotoxic T lymphocytes on a human melanoma. *Science* 1991;254:1643–1647.

279. Sahin U, Tureci O, Schmitt H, et al. Human neoplasms elicit multiple specific immune responses in the autologous host. *Proc Natl Acad Sci USA* 1995;92:11810–11813.

280. Hanson HL, Donermeyer DL, Ikeda H, et al. Eradication of established tumors by CD8$^+$ T cell adoptive immunotherapy. *Immunity* 2000;13:265–276.

281. Shilyansky J, Yang JC, Custer MC, et al. Identification of a T cell receptor from a therapeutic murine T-cell clone. *J Immunother* 1997; 20:247–255.

282. Jager E, Ringhoffer M, Altmannsberger M, et al. Immunoselection *in vivo*: independent loss of MHC class I and melanocyte differentiation antigen expression in metastatic melanoma. *Int J Cancer* 1997; 71:142–147.

283. Theobald M, Ruppert T, Kuckelkorn U, et al. The sequence alteration associated with a mutational hotspot in p 53 protects cells from lysis by cytotoxic T lymphocytes specific for a flanking peptide epitope. *J Exp Med* 1998;188:1017–1028.

284. Musiani P, Modesti A, Giovarelli M, et al. Cytokines, tumor-cell death and immunogenicity: a question of choice. *Immunol Today* 1997;18:32–36.

285. Staveley-O'Caroll K, Sotomayer E, Montgomery J, et al. Introduction of antigen-specific T cell anergy: an early event in the course of tumor progression. *Proc Natl Acad Sci USA* 1998;95:1178–1183.

286. Cohen PA, Peng L, Kjaergaard J, et al. T cell adoptive therapy of tumors: mechanisms of improved therapeutic performance. *Crit.Rev.Immunol* 2001;21:215–248.

287. Geraghty PJ, Mule JJ. Genetically modified lymphocytes and hematopoietic stem cells as therapeutic vehicles. In: Huber BE, Margrath I, eds. *Gene therapy in the treatment of cancer.* 1998:137–148.

288. Rosenberg SA, Aebersold P, Cornetta K, et al. Gene transfer into humans: immunotherapy of patients with advanced melanoma, using tumor-infiltrating lymphocytes modified by retroviral gene transduction. *N Engl J Med* 1990;323:570–578.

289. Rooney CM, Smith CA, Ng CYC, et al. Infusion of cytotoxic T cells for the prevention and treatment of Epstein-Barr virus–induced lymphoma in allogeneic transplant recipients. *Blood* 1998;92:1549–1555.

290. Roskow MA, Suzuki N, Gan Y, et al. Epstein-Barr (EBV)-specific cytotoxic T lymphocytes for the treatment of patients with EBV-positive relapsed Hodgkinisease. *Blood* 1998;91:2925–2934.

291. Walter EA, Greenberg PD, Gilbert MJ, et al. Reconstitution of cellular immunity against cytomegalovirus in recipients of allogeneic bone marrow by transfer of T cell clones from the donor. *N Engl J Med* 1995; 333:1038–1044.

292. Riddell SR, Greenberg PD. T cell therapy of cytomegalovirus and human immunodeficiency virus infection. *J Antimicrob Chemother* 2000;45:35–43.

293. Brodie SR, Lewinsohn DA, Patterson BK, et al. *In vivo* migration and function of transferred HIV-1–specific cytotoxic T cells. *Nat Med* 1999;5:34–41.

294. Stancovski I, Schindler DG, Waks T, et al. Targeting of T lymphocytes to Neu/HER2-expressing cells using chimeric single chain Fv receptors. *J Immunol* 1993;151:6577–6582.

295. Alexander-Miller MA, Leggatt GR, Berzofsky JA. Selective expansion of high-or low- avidity cytotoxic T lymphocytes and efficacy for adoptive immunotherapy. *Proc Natl Acad Sci USA* 1996;93:4102–4107.

296. Dudley ME, Wunderlich J, Nishimura MI, et al. Adoptive transfer of cloned melanoma-reactive T lymphocytes for the treatment of patients with metastatic melanoma. *J Immunother* 2001;24:363–373.

297. Filipovich AH, Shapiro RS, Ramsay NK, et al. Unrelated donor bone marrow transplantation for correction of lethal congenital immunodeficiencies. *Blood* 1992;80:270–276.

298. Lenarsky C, Parkman R. Bone marrow transplantation for the treatment of immune deficiency states. *Bone Marrow Transplant* 1990; 6:361–369.

299. Barnes DWH, Corp MJ, Loutit JF, et al. Treatment of murine leukemia with x-rays and homologous bone marrow: preliminary communication. *BMJ* 1956;2:626–627.

300. Weiden PL, Flournoy N, Thomas ED, et al. Antileukemic effect of graft-versus-host disease in human recipients of allogeneic-marrow grafts. *N Engl J Med* 1979;300:1068–1073.

301. Kolb HJ, Schattenberg A, Goldman JM, et al. Graft-versus-leukemia effect of donor lymphocyte transfusion in marrow grafted patients: European Group for Blood and Marrow Transplantation Working Party Chronic Leukemia. *Blood* 1995;86:2041–2050.

302. Zhang ZX, Yang L, Young KJ, et al. Identification of a previously unknown antigen-specific regulatory T cell and its mechanism of suppression. *Nat Med* 2000;6:782–789.

303. Jonuleit H, Schmitt E, Stassen M, et al. Identification and functional characterization of human CD4+ CD25+ T cells with regulatory properties isolated from peripheral blood. *J Exp Med* 2001;193:1285–1294.

304. Bremers AJA, Kuppen PJK, Parmiani G. Tumor immunotherapy: the adjuvant treatment of the 21st century? *Eur J Surg Oncol* 2000; 26:418–424.

305. Garrido F, Algarra I. MHC antigens and tumor escape from immune surveillance. *Adv Cancer Res* 2001;83:117–158.

306. Dorigo O, Shawler DL, Royston I, et al. Combination of transforming growth factor beta antisense and interleukin-2 gene therapy in the murine ovarian teratoma model. *Gynecol Oncol* 1998;71:204–210.

307. Winter H, Hu HM, Urba WJ, et al. Tumor regression after adoptive transfer of effector T cells is independent of perforin or Fas ligand (APO-1L/CD95L). *J Immunol* 1999;163:4462–4472.

308. Renner C, Kubuschok B, Trumper L, et al. Clinical approaches to vaccination in oncology. *Ann Hematol* 2001;80:255–266.

309. Schultze JL, Vonderheide RH. From cancer genomics to cancer immunotherapy: toward second-generation tumor antigens. *Trends Immunol* 2001;22:516–523.

310. Bellone M, Giandomenica I, Imro MA, et al. Cancer Immunotherapy: synthetic and natural peptides in the balance. *Immunol Today* 1999;20:457–462.

311. Abrams SI, Khleif SN, Bergmann-Leitner E, et al. Generation of stable CD4(+) and CD8(+) T cell lines from patients immunized with ras oncogene-derived peptides reflecting codon 12 mutations. *Cell Immunol* 1997;182:137–151.

312. Khleif SN, Abrams SI, Hamilton JM, et al. A phase I vaccine trial with peptides reflecting ras oncogene mutations of solid tumors. *J Immunother* 1999;22:155–165.

313. Rosenberg SA, Yang JC, Schwartzentruber DJ, et al. Immunologic and therapeutic evaluation of a synthetic peptide vaccine for the treatment of patients with metastatic melanoma. *Nat Med* 1998;4:321–327.

314. Parkhurst MR, Salgaller ML, Southwood S, et al. Improved induction of melanoma-reactive CTL with peptides from the melanoma antigen gp100 modified at HLA-A-asterisk-0201–binding residues. *J Immunol* 1996;157:2539–2548.

315. Vandenbark AA, Morgan E, Bartholomew R, et al. TCR peptide therapy in human autoimmune diseases. *Neurochem Res* 2001;26:713–730.

316. Krolick KA, Isakson PC, Uhr JW, et al. BCL$_1$, a murine model for chronic lymphocytic leukemia: use of the surface immunoglobulin idiotype for the detection and treatment of tumor. *Immunol Rev* 1979;48:81–106.

317. Greenspan NS, Bona CA. Idiotypes: structure and immunogenicity. *FASEB J* 1993;7:437–444.

318. Stevenson FK, Gordon J. Immunization with idiotypic immunoglobulin protects against development of B lymphocytic leukemia, but emerging tumor cells can evade antibody attack by modulation. *J Immunol* 1983;130:970–973.

319. Suga, S, Palmer DW, Talal N, et al. Protective and cellular immune responses to idiotypic determinants on cells from a spontaneous lymphoma of NZB-NZW F1 mice. *J Exp Med* 1974;140:1547–1558.

320. Freedman PM, Autry JR, Tokuda S, et al. Tumor immunity induced by preimmunization with BALB/c mouse myeloma protien. *J Natl Cancer Inst* 1976;56:735–740.

321. Abbas AK, Lichtman AH, Pober JS. Immunity to tumors. In: *Cellular and molecular immunology,* 3rd ed. Philadelphia: WB Saunders, 1997:382–405.

322. Farrar JD, Katz KH, Windsor J, et al. Cancer dormancy. VII. A regulatory role of CD8$^+$ T cells and IFN-γ in establishing and maintaining the tumor-dormant state. *J Immunol* 1999;162:2842–2849.

323. Zagury D, Burny A, Gallo RC. Toward a new generation of vaccines: the anti-cytokine therapeutic vaccines. *Proc Natl Acad Sci USA* 2001;98:8024–8029.

324. Dalum I, Butler DM, Jensen MR, et al. Therapeutic antibodies elicited by immunization against TNF-α. *Nat Biotechnol* 1999;17:666–669.

325. Svenson M, Hansen MB, Thomsen AR, et al. Cytokine vaccination: neutralising IL-1 alpha autoantibodies induced by immunisation with homologous IL-1alpha. *J Immunol Methods* 2000;236:1–8.

326. Richard M, Grencis RK, Humphreys NE, et al. Anti-IL-9 vaccination prevents worm expulsion and blood eosinophilia in *Trichuris muris*–infected mice. *Proc Natl Acad Sci USA* 2000;97:767–772.

327. Gonzalez G, Crombet T, Catala M, et al. A novel cancer vaccine composed of human-recombinant epidermal growth factor linked to a carrier protein: report of a pilot clinical trial. *Ann Oncol* 1998;9:431–435.

328. Ragupathi G. Carbohydrate antigens as targets for active specific immunotherapy. *Cancer Immunol Immunother* 1996;43:152–157.

329. Michaelsson E, Malmstrom V Reis S, et al. T cell recognition of carbohydrates on type II collagen. *J Exp Med* 1994;180:745–749.

330. Haurum JS, Arsequell G, Lellouch AC, et al. Recognition of carbohydrate by major histocompatibility complex class I-restricted, glycopeptide-specific cytotoxic T lymphocytes. *J Exp Med* 1994;180:739–744.

331. Livingston PO, Ragupathi G. Carbohydrate vaccines that induce antibodies against cancer. II. Previous experience and future plans. *Cancer Immunol Immunother* 1997;45:1–9.

332. Chamberlain RS. Prospects for the therapeutic use of anticancer vaccines. *Drugs* 1999;57:309–325.

333. Gilewski T, Ragupathi G, Bhuta S, et al. Immunization of metastatic breast cancer patients with a fully synthetic globo H conjugate: a phase I trial. *Proc Natl Acad Sci USA* 2001;98:3270–3275.

334. Paglia P, Medina E, Arioli I, et al. Gene transfer in dendritic cells, induced by oral DNA vaccination with *Salmonella typhimurium*, re-

sults in protective immunity against a murine fibrosarcoma. *Blood* 1998;92:3172–3176.

335. Gicquel B. BCG as a vector for the construction of multivalent recombinant vaccines. *Biologicals* 1995;23:113–118.

336. Weiskirch LM, Pan ZK, Paterson, Y. The tumor recall response of antitumor immunity primed by a live, recombinant *Listeria monocytogenes* vaccine comprises multiple effector mechanisms. *Clin Immunol* 2001;98:346–357.

337. Mollenkopf H, Dietrich G, Kaufmann SHE. Intracellular bacteria as targets and carriers for vaccination. *Biol Chem* 2001;382:521–532.

338. Schlom J, Panicali D. Cancer vaccines: clinical applications. Recombinant poxvirus vaccines. In: Rosenberg SA, ed. *Principles and practice of the biologic therapy of cancer,* 3rd ed. Philadelphia: Lippincott Williams & Wilkins, 2000:686–694.

339. Wolff JA, Malone RW, Williams P, et al. Direct gene transfer into mouse muscle *in vivo*. *Science* 1990;247:1465–1468.

340. Shedlock DJ, Weiner DB. DNA vaccination: antigen presentation and the induction of immunity. *J Leukoc Biol* 2000;68:793–806.

341. Gurunathan S, Klinman DM, Seder RA. DNA vaccines: immunology, application, and optimization. *Annu Rev Immunol* 2000;18:927–974.

342. Koide Y, Nagata T, Yoshida A, et al. DNA vaccines. *Jpn J Pharmacol* 2000;83:167–174.

343. Robinson HL, Pertman TM. DNA Vaccines for viral infections: basic studies and applications. *Adv Virus Res* 2000;55:1–74.

344. King CA, Spellerberg MB, Zhu D, et al. DNA vaccines with single-chain Fv fused to fragment C of tetanus toxin induce protective immunity against lymphoma and myeloma. *Nat Med* 1998;4:1281–1286.

345. Sprinzi GM, Grabbe S, Sprinzi GM, et al. Dendritic cell vaccines for cancer therapy. *Cancer Treat Rev* 2001;27:247–255.

346. Trefzer U, Weingart G, Chen Y, et al. Hybrid cell vaccination for cancer immune therapy: first clinical trial with metastatic melanoma. *Int J Cancer* 2000;85:618–626.

347. Guo Y, Wu M, Chen H, et al. Effective tumor vaccine generated by fusion of hepatoma cells with activated B cells. *Science* 1994;263:518–520.

348. Stuhler G, Walden P. Recruitment of helper T cells for induction of tumour rejection by cytolytic T lymphocytes. *Cancer Immunol Immunother* 1994;39:342–345.

349. Gong J, Chen D, Kashiwaba M, et al. Induction of antitumor activity by immunization with fusions of dendritic and carcinoma cells. *Nat Med* 1997;3:558–561.

350. Kugler A, Stuhler G, Walden P, et al. Regression of human metastatic renal cell carcinoma after vaccination with tumor cell-dendritic cell hybrids. *Nat Med* 2000;6:332–336.

351. Sivanandham M, Stavropoulos CI, Wallack MK. Cancer vaccines: clinical applications. Whole cell and lysate vaccines. In: Rosenberg SA, ed. *Principles and practice of the biologic therapy of cancer,* 3rd ed. Philadelphia: Lippincott Williams & Wilkins, 2000:632–647.

352. Ockert D, Schirrmacher V, Beck N, et al. Newcastle disease virus–infected intact autologous tumor cell vaccine for adjuvant active specific immunotherapy of resected colorectal carcinoma. *Clin Cancer Res* 1996;2:21–28.

353. Nawrocki S, Wysocki PJ, Mackiewicz A. Genetically modified tumor vaccines: an obstacle race to break host tolerance to cancer. *Expert Opin Biol Ther* 2001;1:193–204.

354. Pardoll DM, Jaffee EM. Cancer vaccines: clinical applications. Genetically modified tumor vaccines. In: Rosenberg SA, ed. *Principles and practice of the biologic therapy of cancer,* 3rd ed. Philadelphia: Lippincott Williams & Wilkins, 2000:647–662.

355. Menoret A, Chandawarkar R. Heat-shock protein-based anticancer immunotherapy: An idea whose time has come. *Semin Oncol* 1998;25:654–660.

356. Graner M, Raymond A, Romney D, et al. Immunoprotective activities of multiple chaperone proteins isolated from murine B-cell leukemia/lymphoma. *Clin Cancer Res* 2000;6:909–915.

357. Offringa R, van der Burg SH, Ossendorp F, et al. Design and evaluation of antigen-specific vaccination strategies against cancer. *Curr Opin Immunol* 2000;12:576–582.

358. Klinman DM, Takeno M, Ichino M, et al. DNA vaccines: safety and efficacy issues. *Springer Semin Immunopathol* 1997;19:245–256.

359. Kurth R. Risk potential of the chromosomal insertion of foreign DNA. *Ann NY Acad Sci* 1995;772:140–151.

360. Martin T, Parker SE, Hedstrom R, et al. Plasmid DNA malaria vaccine:

the potential for genomic integration after intramuscular injection. *Hum Gene Ther* 1999;10:759–768.

361. Hrelia P, Tanneberger S. Immunoprevention of cancer poses a challenge to pharmacological research. *Pharmacol Res* 1997;35:391–401.

362. Disis ML, Cheever MA. Oncogenic proteins as tumor antigens. *Curr Opin Immunol* 1996;8:637–642.

363. Yanuck M, Carbone DP, Pendleton CD, et al. A mutant p53 tumor suppressor protein is a target for peptide-induced CD8+ cytotoxic T-cells. *Cancer Res* 1993;53:3257–3261.

364. Noguchi Y, Richards EC, Chen YT, et al. Influence of interleukin 12 on p53 peptide vaccination against established Meth A sarcoma. *Proc Natl Acad Sci USA* 1995;92:2219–2223.

365. Cefai D, Morrison BW, Sckell A, et al. Targeting HER-2/neu for active-specific immunotherapy in a mouse model of spontaneous breast cancer. *Int J Cancer* 1999;83:393–400.

366. Hertler AA, Schlossman DM, Borowitz MJ. A phase I study of T101-ricin A chain immunotoxin in refractory chronic lymphocytic leukemia. *J Biol Resp Modif* 1988;7:97–113.

367. LeMaistre CF, Rosen, S, Frankel A, et al. Phase I trial of H65-RTA immunoconjugate in patients with cutaneous T-cell lymphoma. *Blood* 1991;78:1173–1182.

368. Spitler LE. In: Frankel AE, ed. *Clinical studies: solid tumors.* Norwell, MA: Kluwer Academic, 1988:493–515.

369. Vitetta ES, Stone M, Amlot P, et al. A phase I immunotoxin trial in patients with B-cell lymphoma. *Cancer Res* 1991;51:4052–4058.

370. Conry RM, Khazaeli MB, Saleh MN, et al. F. Phase I trial of an anti-CD19 deglycosylated ricin A chain immunotoxin in non-Hodgkin's lymphoma: effect of an intensive schedule of administration. *J Immunother* 1995;18:231–241.

371. Grossbard ML, Lambert JM, Goldmacher VS, et al. Anti-B4-blocked ricin: a phase I trial of 7-day continuous infusion in patients with B-cell neoplasms. *J Clin Oncol* 1993;11:726–737.

372. Sausville EA, Headlee D, Stetler-Stevenson M, et al. Continuous infusion of the anti-CD22 immunotoxin IgG-RFB4-SMPT-dgA in patients with B-cell lymphoma: a phase I study. *Blood* 1995;85:3457–3465.

373. Stone MJ, Sausville EA, Fay JW, et al. A phase I study of bolus versus continuous infusion of the anti-CD19 immunotoxin, IgG-HD37-dgA, in patients with B-cell lymphoma. *Blood* 1996;88:1188–1197.

374. Engert A, Diehl V, Schnell R, et al. A Phase-I study of an anti-CD25 ricin A-chain immunotoxin (RFT5-SMPT-dgA) in patients with refractory Hodgkin's lymphoma. *Blood* 1997;89:403–410.

375. Frankel AE, Laver JH, Willingham MC, et al. Therapy of patients with T-cell lymphomas and leukemias using an anti-CD7 monoclonal antibody ricin A chain immunotoxin. *Leuk Lymphoma* 1997;26:287–298.

376. Byers VS, Rodvien R, Grant K, et al. Phase I study of monoclonal antibody-ricin A chain immunotoxin XomaZyme-791 in patients with metastatic colon cancer. *Cancer Res* 1989;49:6153–6160.

377. Weiner LM, O'Dwyer J, Kitson J, et al. Phase I evaluation of an anti-breast carcinoma monoclonal antibody 260F9-recombinant ricin A chain immunoconjugate. *Cancer Res* 1989;49:4062–4067.

378. Oratz R, Speyer JL, Wernz JC, et al. Antimelanoma monoclonal antibody-ricin A chain immunoconjugate (XMMME-001-RTA) plus cyclophosphamide in the treatment of metastatic malignant melanoma: results of a phase II trial. *J Biol Resp Modif* 1990;9:345–354.

379. Selvaggi K, Saria EA, Schwartz R, et al. Phase I/II study of murine monoclonal antibody-ricin A chain (XOMAZYME-mel) immunoconjugate plus cyclosporine A in patients with metastatic melanoma. *J Immunother* 1993;13:201–207.

380. Lynch TJ Jr, Lambert JM, Coral F, et al. Immunotoxin therapy of small-cell lung cancer: A phase I study of N901-blocked ricin. *J Clin Oncol* 1997;15:723–734.

381. Laske DW, Muraszko KM, Oldfield EH, et al. Intraventricular immunotoxin therapy for leptomeningeal neoplasia. *Neurosurgery* 1997;41:1039–1049.

382. Kreitman RJ, Pastan I. Targeting *Pseudomonas* exotoxin to hematologic malignancies. *Cancer Biol* 1995;6:297–306.

383. Kreitman RJ. Immunotoxins. *Expert Opin Pharmacother* 2000;1:1117–1129.

384. Kreitman RJ, Wilson WH, Bergeron K, et al. Efficacy of the anti-CD22 recombinant immunotoxin BL22 in classic or variant hairy-cell leukemia resistant to chemotherapy. *N Engl J Med* 2001;345:241–247.

385. Pai LH, Bookman MA, Ozols RF, et al. Clinical evaluation of intraperitoneal Pseudomonas exotoxin immunoconjugate OVB3-PE in patients with ovarian cancer. *J Clin Oncol.* 1991;9:2095–2103.

386. Pai LH, Wittes R, Setser A, et al. Treatment of advanced solid tumors with immunotoxin LMB-1: an antibody linked to *Pseudomonas* exotoxin. *Nat Med* 1996;2:350–353.

387. Falini B, Bolognesi A, Flenghi L, et al. Response of refractory Hodgkin's disease to monoclonal anti-CD30 immunotoxin. *Lancet* 1992;339:1195–1196.

388. Frankel A, Man S, Elliott P, et al. Lack of multicellular drug resistance observed in human ovarian and prostate carcinoma treated with the proteasome inhibitor PS-341. *Clin Cancer Res* 2000;6:3719–3728.

389. Rudolf MP, Man S, Melief CJM, et al. Human T-cell responses to HLA-A–restricted high binding affinity peptides of human papillomavirus type 18 proteins E6 and E7. *Clin Cancer Res* 2001;7[Suppl]:788s–795s.

390. Murray RJ, Kurilla MG, Brooks JM, et al. B. Identification of target antigens for the human cytotoxic T cell response to Epstein-Barr virus (EBV): implications for the immune control of EBV-positive malignancies. *J Exp Med* 1992;176:157–168.

391. den Bosch GJA, Joosten AM, Kessler JH, et al. Recognition of BCR-ABL positive leukemic blasts by human CD4+ T cells elicited by primary *in vitro* immunization with a BCR-ABL breakpoint peptide. *Blood* 1995;88:3522–3527.

392. Gambacorti-Passerini C, Grignani F, Arienti F, et al. Human CD4 lymphocytes specifically recognize a peptide representing the fusion region of the hybrid protein pml/RAR alpha present in acute promyelocytic leukemia cells. *Blood* 1993;81:1369–1375.

393. Yun C, Senju S, Fujita H, et al. Augmentation of immune response by altered peptide ligands of the antigenic peptide in a human CD4+ T cell clone reacting to TEL/AML1 fusion protein. *Tissue Antigens* 1999;54:153–161.

394. Robbins PF, El-Gamil M, Li YF, et al. A. A mutated beta-catenin gene encodes a melanoma-specific antigen recognized by tumor infiltrating lymphocytes. *J Exp Med* 1996;183:1185–1192.

395. Renkvist N, Chiara C, Paul FR, et al. A listing of human tumor antigens recognized by T cells. *Cancer Immunol Immunother* 2000;50:3–15.

396. Minev B, Hipp J, Friat H, et al. Cytotoxic T cell immunity against telomerase reverse transcriptase in humans. *Proc Natl Acad Sci USA* 2000;97:4796–4801.

397. Kawashima I, Tsai V, Southwood S, et al. Identification of HLA-A3–restricted cytotoxic T lymphocyte epitopes from carcinoembryonic antigen and HER-2/neu by primary *in vitro* immunization with peptide-pulsed dendritic cells. *Cancer Res* 1999;59:431–435.

398. Oka Y, Elisseeva OA, Tsuboi A, et al. Human cytotoxic T-lymphocyte responses specific for peptides of the wild-type Wilms' tumor gene (WT1) product. *Immunogenetics* 2000;51:99–107.

399. Van den Eynde BJ, Van der Bruggen PT cell defined tumor antigens. *Curr Opin Immunol* 1997;9:684–693.

400. Correale P, Walmsley K, Nieroda C, et al. *In vitro* generation of human cytotoxic T lymphocytes specific for peptides derived from prostate-specific antigen. *J Natl Cancer Inst* 1997;89:293–300.

401. Romero P, Dutoit V, Rubio-Godoy V, et al. CD8+ T-cell response to NY-ESO-1: relative antigenicity and *in vitro* immunogenicity of natural and analogue sequences. *Clin Cancer Res* 2001;7[Suppl]:766s–772s.

402. Cull G, Durrant L, Stainer C, et al. Generation of anti-idiotype immune responses following vaccination with idiotype-protein pulsed dendritic cells in myeloma. *Br J Haematol* 1999;107:648–655.

Subject Index

A

α chains
   mucosal immunity, 971–972
$\alpha\beta$ lineage, *versus* $\epsilon\delta$ lineage, commitment
      to, T-cell receptor, 237
$\alpha\beta$ T-cell receptor
   ligand interactions, 237–241
      CD4, role of, 241
   structure, 229–231
   superantigens, 245–246
α/δ locus, T-cell receptor, 234–235
Abelson murine leukemia virus, in
      transformation of pre-B-cells,
      119–120
Abnormality in apoptosis, with systemic
      autoimmunity, 1381–1382
Accessory molecules, 393–417. *See also*
      Dendritic cells
   B7-1, structure, expression, 395–396
   B7-1/B7-2, therapeutic manipulation of,
      397
   B7-1/B7-2:CD28/cytotoxic T lymphocyte-
      associated antigen 4 pathway,
      394–396
   B7-2, structure, expression, 395–396
   B7:CD28 superfamily, 393–405
   CD28, function, biochemical basis for,
      397–398
   CD28/CTLA-4
      pathway, 397
      structure, expression, 395
   CD40:CD154 pathway, 401–404, 409
      4-1BB:4-IBBL pathway, 405
      in autoimmunity, 403–404
      blockade of, in transplantation, 404
      CD2 superfamily, 405–409
      CD27:CD70 pathway, 404–405
      CD40, 401–402
      CD40:CD154 interactions, in germinal
         center, 402–403
      CD84, 409
      CD134-CD134L pathway, 404
      CD150, 408
      CD154, 402
      CD244, 408–409
      hyper-immunoglobulin M syndrome,
         403
      in infection, 403
      signaling through CD40, 402
   CTLA-4

function, biochemical basis for, 397–398
   in regulating peripheral T-cell tolerance,
      396–397
ICOS:ICOSL pathway, 399–400
inducible co-stimulator ligand-inducible
      co-stimulator pathway, 398–401
PD-1
   function, biochemical basis for, 401
   structure, expression of, 400
   PD-L1/Pd-L2, interactions, 400–401
   PD-ligand/PD-1 pathway, 400–401
   tumor necrosis factor receptor pathways,
      with co-stimulatory function, 404–405
Acellular pertussis vaccine, 1329, 1342
   history of, 1342–1343
Acidification, with intracellular bacteria,
      1236–1237
Acquired immune response
   antigen presentation, 1243–1244
   β 2 microglobulin, 1244–1245
   bacterial infection, 1240–1245
   CD1 molecules, 1243–1244
   $\epsilon\delta$ T-cells, 1245
   T-cell subpopulations, 1241–1243
Acquired immunodeficiency syndrome, 2–3,
      41–42, 1203, 1285–1318. *See also*
      Human immunodeficiency virus
   bacterial infection, 1229, 1241
   historical overview of, 41–42
Actin polymerization
   phagocytosis, 1116
   in phagocytosis, 1116
Activation, in inflammation, 1157–1158
Acute inflammatory response, 1151–1169
   allergy and, 1160–1161
   blister fluid, soluble mediators in, temporal
      analysis of, 1161
   cellular mediators, acute inflammatory
      response, 1156–1160
      endothelial cells, 1160
      eosinophils, 1160
      monocytes, 1160
      neutrophils, 1156–1160
      platelets, 1160
   chronic inflammation, 1162–1163
   historical overview, 1151–1152
   human model systems of, 1161
   initiation of, 1152–1153
   molecular mediators, acute inflammatory
      response, 1153–1156

acute-phase reactants, 1155
   leptin, 1156
   lipid, 1154–1155
   nitric oxide, 1155
   peptides, 1155
   plasma proteases, 1153–1154
   proinflammatory cytokines, 1155–1156
murine models of, 1161
neutrophil recruitment, activation, 1153
novel anti-inflammatory therapies, 1163
resolution of
   angiogenesis, 1162
   apoptosis, 1162
   vasodilation, 1153
Acute-phase reactants, inflammation, 1155
ADA. *See* Adenosine deaminase
Adaptive immune system, components of,
      521–553
Adaptive immunity
   age-related changes in, 1055–1064
   agnathia, 546–547
   chemokines, 816–819
      afferent trafficking to secondary
         lymphoid tissue, 816–817
      CD4+ T-cell differentiation, 818
      efferent trafficking, 817–818
      positioning within lymph node, 817–818
      tissue-specific lymphocyte homing,
         818–819
   innate immune system, control of, 512–513
   origins of, 561–565
Adenosine, extracellular, cytotoxic
      T-lymphocytes, 1141
Adenosine deaminase deficiency, 1603–1605
Adenoviruses, 1202, 1214
ADEPT. *See* Antibody-directed enzyme
      prodrug therapy
Adherence, in inflammation, 1158
Adhesion
   intracellular bacteria, 1234
   as response to chemokines, 808
   strengthening, cytotoxic T-lymphocytes,
      1134–1135
Adjuvants
   aluminum compounds, as adjuvants, 1337
   antigens
      microencapsulation of, 1339–1340
      molecular targeting of, 1341
   cytokines as adjuvants, 1340–1341
   design of, principles, 1336

1661

Adjuvants (*contd.*)
  emulsions, as adjuvants, 1337–1338
  in immunotherapy, 1335–1342
    antigen-presenting cell activation,
      1335–1336
    microparticles, 1338
    mucosal adjuvants, 1341–1342
    oligonucleotides, 1339
Adoptive antigen-specific cytotoxic
    lymphocyte therapy, in
    immunotherapy, 1644–1645
Aeroallergens, 1443
Affinity, 71–80
  chemical equilibrium in solution, 70–71
  free energy, 71
  maturation, 70–80, 306–309, 1629–1630.
    See also Germinal center;
    Hypermutation
    B lymphocytes, 10–11
  monovalent ligand, interaction in solution
    with, 73–79
    average affinities, 76
    B/F, plot, 77–78
    heterogeneity of affinity, 75–76
    indices of heterogeneity, 76–77
    intrinsic affinity, 78
    monogamous bivalency, 79
    multivalent ligands, interaction with, 78
    Scatchard analysis, 74–75
  Sips plot, 76–77
  two-phase systems, 79–80
African trypanosomiasis, 1172
Aϵglobulinemia
  autosomal recessive, 1597
  X-linked, 1595–1596
Aging. *See also* Elderly
  cytokine production, changes in, 1053
  immune response, with cancer, 1585
  immunology of, 1043–1075
    adaptive immunity, age-related changes
      in, 1055–1064
    antigen presentation, age-related
      changes in, 1064
    autoimmune disease, increases in,
      1045–1046
    barriers, age-related changes in,
      1049–1050
    B-cell immunity, age-related changes in,
      1062–1064
    cancer, increases in, 1044–1045
    complement, age-related changes in,
      1050
    graft-*versus*-host disease, increase in
      with age, 1047
    hematopoiesis, age-related changes in,
      1064–1065
    immune dysfunction, 1043–1049
    infectious diseases, increase in,
      1043–1044
    innate immunity, age-related changes in,
      1049–1055
    interventions, 1065–1066
      exercise, 1065

hormones, 1066
    immunotherapy, 1066
    nutrition, 1065–1066
    vaccination, 1065
  longevity, immunity, 1047–1048
  T-cells
    age-related changes in, 1055–1060
    cell biology of, age-related changes
      in, 1060–1062
    vaccination, decline in response to, with
      age, 1046–1047
  local, systemic innate immunity with, 1050
  local innate immunity, changes in, 1050
  macrophage function, 1051
  in neutrophil function, 1051
  in NK cells, 1052
  systemic innate immunity, changes with,
    1050
  T-cells, 1055
Agnathia, adaptive immune responses,
    546–547
AIDS. *See* Acquired immunodeficiency
    syndrome
Allelic exclusion
  T-cell receptor, 237
  V gene assembly recombination, 128–130
Allergens, 1442–1444
  biological properties of, 1443
  classification, 1442–1443
  venom, 1444
Allergic immune responses, major features
    of, 1442
Allergic rhinitis, linkage regions, 1447
Allergy, 29–30, 1439–1479. *See also under*
    specific disorder
  aeroallergens, 1443
  allergens, 1442–1444
    biological properties of, 1443
    classification, 1442–1443
  allergic inflammation, Th2 cytokine
    regulation of, 1452–1453
  anaphylaxis, 1470
  antigen presentation, 1448–1450
  asthma, 1472
  atopic dermatitis, 1471–1472
  atopic disorders, general features of,
    1440–1442
  basophils, 1459
    development of, 1458–1463
  CD4+ Th2 polarized immune responses,
    1444–1445
  crystallized fragment ϵ receptor I, surface
    expression, regulation of, 1457
  crystallized fragment ϵ receptor II,
    1457–1458
  crystallized fragment ϵ receptor I-mediated
    signal transduction, 1456–1457
  cytokine regulation, Th2 differentiation,
    1450–1452
  disorders, 1469–1472
  effector cells, allergic response, 1458–1459
  environmental influences, 1446–1448
  eosinophils, 1463–1468

activation, 1467–1468
    as effector cells, 1468
    eosinophil-derived mediators,
      1464–1466
    cytokines, 1465–1466
    eosinophil-specific cationic proteins,
      1464–1465
    lipid mediators, 1465
    recruitment to sites of inflammation,
      1466–1467
  food allergens, 1443, 1471
  genetics in, 1445–1446
  historical overview, 1439–1440
  immunoglobulin E receptors, 1456
  immunoglobulin E synthesis, 1453–1458
    deletional switch recombination,
      1455–1456
    isotype class switching, 1453–1455
    negative regulation of, 1456
  inflammation in, 1160–1161
    Th2 cytokine regulation of, 1452–1453
  insect venom allergens, 1444
  interleukin-12 production, 1451–1452
  latex allergens, 1443
  lipid mediators, 1462
  mast cell activation, 1463
  mast cell-derived cytokines, 1462–1463
  mast cell-derived mediators, 1460
  mast cells, 1459–1460
    in acute-phase responses, 1463
    development of, 1458–1463
    in late-phase responses, 1463
  mucosal, 1008–1009
  newly synthesized mediators, 1462
  pharmaceuticals, 1443–1444
  preformed mediators, 1460–1462
  rhinitis, allergic, 1470–1471
  Th2 cells
    development, factors contributing to,
      1445–1450
    as effector cells, 1468–1469
  Th2 differentiation, potential dysregulation
    of, 1450–1451
Allison, James, 41
Allograft rejection, regulatory T-cells, control
    of, 953–954
Alloreactivity, *in vitro* pathways of, 1505
Allorecognition, in evolution of immune
    response, 560–561
Altered peptide ligands, in organ-specific
    autoimmunity, 1416
Alternative pathway of complement
    activation, 21–22
Amino acid sequences, major
    histocompatibility complex, 592–593
    primary structure, 592–593
Amino acid substitution, effects of altered
    peptide ligands, 666–668
Amphibians
  evolution of immune response, 548–549
  evolution of lymphocyte differentiation,
    545
Analogs, in immunotherapy, 1625

Anaphylatoxin receptors, 1091
Anaphylaxis, 1470
Anatomical path of T-cell development,
    264–265
Anergy-inducing compounds, in
    organ-specific autoimmunity, 1416
Ankylosing spondylitis, human leukocyte
    antigen associations, 588
Anthrax
    bioterrorism and, 1363
    vaccine, 1329
Antibacterial immunity
    conventional T-cells in, 1241
    T cytokines in, 1244
    unconventional T-cells in, 1241
Antibodies. See also Monoclonal antibodies
    antigenic determinants recognized by,
        631–637
        carbohydrate antigens, 632–637
            blood group antigens, 634–635
            dextran-binding myeloma proteins,
                635–637
            immunochemistry of salmonella O
                antigens, 632–634
            haptens, 631–632
    cancer immunity and, 1578
    in immunotherapy, 1628–1636
        affinity, 1629–1630
        bispecific monoclonal antibodies,
            1635–1636
        clinical considerations, 1629
        effector functions, 1630
        historical overview, 1628–1629
        immunogenicity, 1630
        immunoglobulin G, 1632–1635
        intravenous immunoglobulin,
            1632–1633
            mechanism of action, 1632–1633
            monoclonal antibodies, 1632–1635
            organ transplantation, 1635
        size, 1630
    monoclonal, 38–39
    mucosal, 971–976
        function, 973–974
        immunoglobulin isotypes, distribution
            of, 971
        mucosal immunoglobulins, origin,
            transport of, 974–976
        secretory immunoglobulin A, structure
            of, 971–973
    production, 26–27
        template theory, 27–29
    unconjugated, for cancer, 1629
Antibody globulins, chemistry of, 31–34
    myeloma proteins, 34
Antibody-directed enzyme prodrug therapy,
    in immunotherapy, 1640
Anti-CD40L, immunotherapy and, 1628
Anticytokine vaccine, 1649
Antidisease vaccine, 1360
Antigen matching
    in minipigs, 1544
    in transplantation, 1543–1545

Antigen-antibody interactions, 69–105
    affinity, 71–80
        chemical equilibrium in solution, 70–71
        free energy, 71
        monovalent ligand, interaction in
            solution with, 73–79
            average affinities, 76
            B/F, plot, 77–78
            heterogeneity of affinity, 75–76
            indices of heterogeneity, 76–77
            intrinsic affinity, 78
            monogamous bivalency, 79
            multivalent ligands, interaction with,
                78
            Scatchard analysis, 74–75
            Sips plot, 76–77
            two-phase systems, 79–80
    cross-reactivity, 86–89
    hemagglutination, 94
        inhibition, 94
    immunoblot, 94–95
    immunodiffusion, 91–92
    immunoelectrophoresis, 92–94
    kinetics, 70–73
    Ouchterlony method, 91–92
    quantitative precipitin, 90–91
    radioimmunoassay, 81–86
        analysis of data, 82–84
            corrections for B, F, T, 83–84
        bound, free antigen, separation of, 81–82
            solid-phase methods, 81–82
            solution methods, 81
        data analysis, 82–84
            corrections for B, F, T, 83–84
        enzyme-linked immunosorbent assay,
            84–85
        enzyme-linked immunospot assay,
            85–86
        graphic representation, 82–84
        nonequilibrium radioimmunoassay, 84
        numerical representation, 82–84
        tracer concentrations, optimization of,
            82
    specificity, 86–89
        multispecificity, 89
    surface plasmon resonance, 95–96
    thermodynamics, 70–73
        acidity, effects of, 71–72
        chemical equilibrium in solution, 70–71
        free energy, 71
        salt concentration, effects of, 71–72
        temperature, effects of, 71–72
Antigen-driven selection, glucocorticoid Th
    cells, 218–219
Antigenic modulation, tumor formation and,
    1583
Antigenic structures, mapping, 646–648
    monoclonal T-cells, 647–648
    polyclonal T-cell response, 646–647
Antigen-independent clustering, dendritic
    cells, 467
Antigen-nonspecific deleterious response,
    extracellular bacteria, 1276–1277

Antigen-nonspecific host defense response,
    extracellular bacteria, 1271–1273
    local response, 1271–1272
    mucosal defense, 1271
    systemic response, 1272–1273
Antigen-presenting cells
    major histocompatibility complex, 19.
        See also Dendritic cells
    parasites and, 1175–1177
    T-lymphocyte activation, 323–324
Antigen-primed B-cells, T-cell help to,
    214–217
    immune synapse II, 214–216
Antigens. See also Superantigen; specific
        antigens, types
    in autoimmune disease, 1406–1407
    delivery systems, mucosal immunity,
        999–1000
    encoded by normal cellular genes,
        1566–1569
        carcinoembryonic antigens, 1568–1569
        clonal antigens, 1569
        differentiation antigens, 1567–1568
        oncofetal antigens, 1568–1569
        oncospermatogonal antigens, 1567
    encoded by viral genes, 1569–1571
        DNA tumor viruses, 1569–1570
        RNA tumor viruses, 1570–1571
    expressed by cancer cells, 1645
    expressed on cancer cell, 1561–1562
    loss, tumor formation and, 1582–1583
    major histocompatibility complex class I,
        changes in expression of, 1582
        tumor formation and, 1582
    presentation
        age-related changes in, 1064
        in allergic disorders, 1448–1450
        inhibition, through class I major
            histocompatibility complex
            pathway, 1218
    processing, 613–629, 649–654
    dendritic cells, 462–464
        class II major histocompatibility
            complex-restricted presentation,
            462–464
        endoplasmic reticulum
            class II assembly of major
                histocompatibility complex
                molecules in, 618–620
            peptide transport into, 615–616
        influence on expressed T-cell repertoire,
            649–651
        inhibition of transporter associated with,
            viral, 1219
        invariant chain, endocytic processing of,
            620–622
        major histocompatibility complex, 578
        major histocompatibility complex class I
            associated peptides, source of, 617
            peptide complexes, assembly of,
                616–617
            release of molecules from
                endoplasmic reticulum, 617–618

Antigens (*contd.*)
    restricted antigen presentation,
        613–618
    restricted presentation of extracellular
        proteins, 618
    major histocompatibility complex
        class II
        peptide loading, molecules, 622–624
        restricted antigen presentation,
            618–625
    major histocompatibility complex
        molecules delivery to cell surface,
        624
    peptide generation, 613–629
    presentation, major histocompatibility
        complex, 16–19, 613–629
    proteins, endocytosis of, 624–625
    T-cell receptors, antigen recognition by,
        6123
    processing of
        T-cells restricted to major
            histocompatibility complex
            molecule class I, 651–653
        T-cells restricted to major
            histocompatibility complex
            molecule class II, 651–653
    recognition, $\epsilon\delta$-CD3, 247–249
    rejection
        tumor, individually distinct,
            characteristics of, 1561
        on tumors, 1558–1562
    structure, immunogenicity, 631–683
        antigen processing, 649–654
            influence on expressed T-cell
                repertoire, 649–651
        antigenic determinants recognized by
            antibodies, 631–637
            carbohydrate antigens, 632–637
                blood group antigens, 634–635
                dextran-binding myeloma proteins,
                    635–637
                immunochemistry of salmonella O
                    antigens, 632–634
            haptens, 631–632
        antigenic structures, mapping, 646–
            648
            monoclonal T-cells, 647–648
            polyclonal T-cell response, 646–647
        helper T-cell epitopes, B-cell epitopes,
            relationship between, 671–673
        immunodominant determinants, steps
            focusing T-cell response on,
            648–668
        major histocompatibility complex
            class II
            T-cells restricted to, 651–653
            transport pathways leading to
                presentation, 657–658
            molecules, antigen interaction with,
                658–664
        major histocompatibility complex
            binding, 658–664
        major histocompatibility complex class I

    molecules, T-cells restricted to,
        processing of antigen, 653–654
    transport pathways leading to
        presentation, 654–657
    polysaccharide immunogenicity,
        637–646
        epitopes, mapping of, 638–641
        native proteins, antipeptide antibodies
            binding, at specific site, 642–643
        peptides, immunogenicity of, 643–646
        protein
            peptide antigenic determinants,
                conformational equilibria,
                641–642
            polypeptide antigenic determinants,
                637–646
        proteins, immunogenicity of, 643–646
    stable major histocompatibility
        complex/peptide complex,
        assembly of, 658–664
    T-cell epitopes, prediction of, 668–671
    T-cell receptor recognition, 664–668
        amino acid substitution
            altered peptide ligands, effects of,
                666–668
            mapping by, 666–668
        epitope mapping, 665–666
    T-cells, antigenic determinants
        recognized by, 646–671
    tumor, 1559–1561
        antigenicity, 1565
    tumor-associated, 1566–1569
        examples, 1647
    tumor-specific, 1562–1566
    uptake, dendritic cells, 461–462
Antigen-specific deleterious response,
    extracellular bacteria, 1277
Antigen-specific host defense response
    B-cells, 1273–1274
    extracellular bacteria, 1273–1276
        antibodies, protective mechanisms of,
            1274–1276
        responses of host, 1273–1274
        T-cell immune system, 1276
Antigen-specific immune mechanism
    effector functions of, viruses, 1210–1211
    induction of, viruses, 1206–1210
    in organ-specific autoimmunity, 1416
Antigen-specific T-cell
    activation of innate immune system,
        212–213
    immune synapse 1, 213
    naive antigen-specific B-cells, 214
    Th-cell differentiation, 213–214
Antihapten antibodies, specificity of, 632
Anti-inflammatory cytokines, human
    immunodeficiency virus, 1310
Antiretroviral therapy, human
    immunodeficiency virus, 1288
Antitumor cytotoxic T-lymphocyte activity,
    cellular cytotoxicity pathways, 1142
Antiviral effector mechanisms, innate
    immune system, 512

APAF proteins, programmed cell death,
    856
Apoptosis
    abnormalities, in systemic autoimmunity,
        1381–1382
    in autoimmune disease, 1409
    cell cycle arrest, 1030
    intracellular bacteria, 1239–1240
APRIL, 766–768
Arber, Werner, 40
Arenaviruses, 1202
Arita, Isao, 1323
Arrhenius, Svante, 27
Artemis
    deficiencies of gene, 1605
    role in switch recombination, 124–125
Arthritis
    reactive, 1384–1385
    rheumatoid, 1383–1384, 1426–1428
        human leukocyte antigen associations,
            588
        immunology, 1427
        interleukin-1 receptor antagonist, 794
        models of, 1389–1390
Asthma, 1472
    chemokines, 821
    linkage regions, 1447
    mucosal immunity, 1008–1009
Ataxia-telangiectasia, 1607
Atherosclerosis, chemokines, 821
Atopic dermatitis, 1471–1472
    linkage regions, 1447
Atopic disorders, 1439–1480
Atopy, linkage regions, 1447
Autoantibody, characteristics of, 1375–1377
Autoimmune disorders
    burden of, 1402–1403
    features of, 1382–1387
    gastritis, regulatory T-cells, 950
    immunotherapy, 1632
    increases in, with aging, 1045–1046
    intravenous immunoglobulin for, 1628
    organ-specific, causes of, 938
    prevalence, incidence of, in United States,
        1403
    systemic, 1371–1399
        autoantibodies to nuclear proteins in,
            1377
    thyroiditis, regulatory T-cells, 951
Autoimmunity
    after virus infections, 1216
    chemokines, 820–821
    crystallized fragment receptors, 697
    cytotoxic T-lymphocytes, 1143
    organ-specific, 1401–1438
        B-cell tolerance, 1404–1405
        burden of autoimmune diseases,
            1402–1403
        diabetes, type 1, 1411–1417
            etiology, 1415–1416
            immunology of, 1412–1415
            therapeutic concepts, 1416–1417
        disorders, 1411–1430

eye disorders, inflammatory
    in animal models, 1425–1426
        diseases associated with, 1424–1425
    in human, 1426
gut disorders, 1430
heart, autoimmune diseases of, 1430
immune regulation, reestablishment,
    1411
initiation of, 1406–1409
    antigens, 1406–1407
    environment, 1407–1409
    genes, 1407
liver disease, 1420–1424
    in animal models, 1421
    halothane hepatitis, 1423
    hepatitis, 1420–1421
    in human, 1421–1423
    primary biliary cirrhosis, 1423
    therapeutic concepts, 1423–1424
multiple sclerosis, 1417–1420
    etiology, 1419–1420
    immunology of, 1418–1419
    therapeutic concepts, 1420
organ-specific tuning, 1405–1406
oveoretinitis, 1424–1426
promising targets, 1411
regulatory circuits in, 1409–1410
    apoptosis, 1409
    cytokines, 1409
    kinetics, 1409–1410
rheumatoid arthritis, 1426–1428
    immunology, 1427
skin disorders, 1429–1430
    dermatitis herpetiformis, 1429–1430
    pemphigus, 1429
T-cell tolerance, 1404
therapeutic considerations, 1410–1411
    efficacy, 1410–1411
    specificity, 1410–1411
    undesired effects, 1410–1411
thyroiditis, 1428–1429
    immunology, 1428–1429
tolerance
    central, 1403–1406
    peripheral, 1403–1406
Autologous T-cells, tumor antigens,
    recognized by syngeneic, somatic
    mutation, 1563
Autonomic innervation, immune organs, 1035
Autonomic nervous system, immune system
    interactions, 1034–1037
Autonomic neurotransmitter receptors,
    immune cells, 1035
Autosomal recessive aϵglobulinemia, 1597

B
B1 B cells, 7, 160, 164, 165, 172, 174–177,
    179, 182, 183, 209–210
B7-1, structure, expression, 395–396
B7-1/B7-2
    CD28/cytotoxic T lymphocyte-associated
        antigen 4 pathway, 394–396
    therapeutic manipulation of, 397

B7-2, structure, expression, 395–396
B7:CD28 superfamily, 393–405
β chain, cytokine receptors sharing, 711–712
β locus, T-cell receptor, 235
β_c, cytokine receptors sharing, 711–712
    features of, 712
β-glucan receptor, 505
β-selection, T-cell development, 270–276
    constituent events in, 273–275
    death mechanisms, 275
    later T-cell differentiation and, 275–276
    T-cell receptor-independent, to T-cell
        receptor-dependent T-cell
        development, transition, 270–271
    triggering requirements for, 271–273
Bacillus Calmette-Guérin, 1321, 1329, 1623
Bacteria
    extracellular, 1263–1283
        antigen-nonspecific deleterious
            response, 1276–1277
        antigen-nonspecific host defense
            response, 1271–1273
            local response, 1271–1272
            mucosal defense, 1271
            systemic response, 1272–1273
        antigen-specific deleterious response,
            1277
        antigen-specific host defense response,
            1273–1276
            antibodies, protective mechanisms of,
                1274–1276
            responses of host, 1273–1274
            T-cell immune system, 1276
        deleterious host response, 1276–1277
        gram-positive
            bacterial surface structure of,
                1265–1267
            gram-negative bacteria, bacterial
                surface structure of, 1265–1267
        invasion of host, 1269–1271
        virulence factors, 1267–1269
    intracellular, 1229–1262. *See also* specific
        pathogen
        acidification, 1236–1237
        acquired immune response, 1240–1245
            antigen presentation, 1243–1244
            β 2 microglobulin, 1244–1245
            CD1 molecules, 1243–1244
            dendritic cells, 1241
            $\epsilon\delta$ T-cells, 1245
            T-cell subpopulations, 1241–1243
        adhesion, 1234
        antibacterial immunity, conventional
            T-cells in, 1241
        apoptosis, 1239–1240
        cell-to-cell spreading, 1239
        cytokines, 1248–1251
            down-regulation, antibacterial host
                response, 1250–1251
            granuloma formation, 1248–1249
            leukocyte recruitment, 1248
            macrophage activation, 1249–1250
            protective T-cell response, 1250

cytoplasm, evasion into, 1239
delayed-type hypersensitivity, 1255
DN cells, group 1 CD1-restricted, 1244
experimental listeriosis, 1255
facultative, 1231–1232
facultative intracellular bacteria, major
    infections of humans caused by,
    1231
features of, 1230
genetic control, resistance against
    intracellular bacteria, 1255–1256
granulomatous lesion, 1253–1255
    granuloma formation, 1254
    leukocyte extravasation, 1253–1254
    tuberculosis, 1254–1255
hallmarks of, 1230–1231
hallmarks of infections, 1230
host cells, 1233–1240
immunity to, 1229–1261
infected cells, death of, 1252–1253
intracellular iron, 1237–1238
invasion, 1234
leprosy, 1255
Listeria monocytogenes, 1233
listeriosis, 1233
major histocompatibility complex class
    Ib-restricted CD8 T-cells, 1243
microbes, recognition receptors for,
    1234–1236
Mycobacterium tuberculosis, 1232–1233
natural killer T-cells, with specificity for
    group 2 CD1 molecules, 1244
Nramp 1 gene, 1256
obligate intracellular, 1231–1232
    major infections of humans caused by,
    1232
pattern recognition receptors
    mediating microbial binding, uptake,
    1236
    mediating signaling, 1235
    recognizing host molecules, 1236
phagocytes, nonprofessional, invasion
    of, 1236
phagosome maturation, 1236–1237
phagosome-lysosome fusion, 1236–1237
professional phagocytes, 1240
    mononuclear phagocytes, 1240
    polymorphonuclear granulocytes,
    1240
Salmonella enterica, 1233
salmonellosis, 1233
T cytokines, in antibacterial immunity,
    1244
T-cell functions, during infection,
    1245–1248
Th1 cell activities, 1251–1252
toxic effector molecules, 1238–1239
trigger mechanisms, entry by, 1234
tryptophan degradation, 1238
tuberculosis, 1232–1233
vaccine design, 1246
virulence, intracellular bacteria,
    1230–1232

Bacteria (*contd.*)
  vitamin D receptor, 1256
  zipper mechanisms, entry by, 1234
Bacterial DNA fractions, immunotherapy,
    1624–1625
Bacterial enterotoxins, mucosal immunity,
    998–999
Bacterial pathogen, 1232
Bacterial vaccine, 1342–1349
  early, 1321–1322
Bacteriolytic immunotherapy
  muramyldipeptide derivatives, 1624
  trehalose dimycolate derivatives, 1624
  tumors, 1623–1624
Basophils, 20
  in allergic disorders, 1458–1463
  development of, in allergic disorders,
      1458–1463
  as effector cells, 1459
  immune system mediation, 1029–1030
  products of, 1461
BCAP, in B-cell activation, role for adaptor
    molecules, 200–202
B-cell activation, 195–225
  antigen-primed B-cells, T-cell help to,
      214–217
    immune synapse II, 214–216
    isotype switch recombination, 216
    short-lived plasma cells, development of,
        216–217
  antigen-specific T-cell help, recruitment of
    activation of innate immune system,
        212–213
    immune synapse 1, 213
    naive antigen-specific B-cells, 214
    Th-cell differentiation, 213–214
  BCAP, role for adaptor molecules, 200–202
  B-cell memory response, 219–221
    immune synapse IV, response to antigen
        recall, 220–221
    memory B-cell maintenance, 220
    memory B-cell subsets, 219–220
  B-cell subsets, mature, 209–210
    B-1 B-cells, 209–210
    marginal zone B-cells, 210
  BLNK, role for adaptor molecules,
      200–202
  Btk recruitment, activation, 202
  capacitative calcium entry, 203–205
  defects in
    age-related changes, 1064
    aging and, 1064
  dendritic cells, 472–473
  early intracellular activation cascades,
      198–203
  effector cells, signaling pathways, 203–207
  germinal center reaction, 217–219
    antigen-driven selection, glucocorticoid
        Th cells, 218–219
    germinal center microenvironment,
        formation of, 217–218
    somatic hypermutation, BCR
        diversification, 218

helper T-regulated B-cell responses,
    211–221
  intracellular calcium stores, mobilization
      of, 203
  NF-ATc activation, calcium-mediated
      regulation of, 205
  NF-κB activation, regulation of, 206
  Pas/MAPK signaling pathways, 207
  PI-3K recruitment to membrane, 202
  PI-3K/Akt signaling pathway, 206–207
  PKC pathway, 206
  PL-Cc-ε2 activation, 202–203
  SFK recruitment, activation, 198–200
  surface-expressed modulators, BCR
      signaling, 207–209
    CD19, 208
    CD22, 208
    CD45, 207–208
    FcεRIIb, 208–209
  Syk recruitment, activation, 200
  T-cell-independent B-cell responses,
      210–211
    regulation of TI-2 B-cell responses, 211
    type 1 T-independent B-cell responses,
        210
    type 2 T-Independent B-cell responses,
        210–211
B-cell compartment, mucosal immune
    system, 981–983
B-cell development
  age-related changes in, 1062–1063
  age-related changes in, 1062–1063
B-cell follicles, lymph nodes, 432–433
B-cell homeostasis, 846–847
B-cell immunity, age-related changes in,
    1062–1064
B-cell malignancies, treatment of, 181–182
B-cell maturation, B-cell receptor regulation
    of, 130
B-cell memory
  generation of, 874–878
  identification of, 880–881
  life span of, 885
  maintenance of, 888
  response, 219–221
B-cell migration, maintenance, 174
B-cell repertoire, age-related changes in,
    1063–1064
B-cell signal transduction, defects in,
    age-related changes, 1064
B-cell signaling mechanisms, 195–225
  BCR proximal signaling mechanisms,
      196–198
  BCR signaling complex, 196
  membrane microdomains, 196–198
  receptor aggregation, 198
B-cell subsets, age-related changes in,
    1063–1064
B-cell tolerance, 178–179
  in autoimmune diseases, 1404–1405
  in systemic autoimmunity, 1374
B-cell turnover, 174–175
B-cell vaccine

parasites, 1190–1192
parasitic pathogens, 1190–1192
B-cell-specific heavy-chain switch, 142
Bcl-2
  family, programmed cell death, 853–856
  homology structures, programmed cell
      death, 857–858
Bedson, H.S., 1323
Berg, Paul, 40
Bernoulli, Daniel, 24
Bernstein, Felix, 30
Besredka, Alexandre, 25
Bifunctional antibodies, 98–99
Biliary cirrhosis, primary, 1423
Bill and Melinda Gates Foundation,
    1326–1327, 1348–1349, 1361
Billingham, Rupert E., 35
Bioterrorism
  vaccination and, 1363
Birds, evolution of immune response,
    549–550
Bishop, Ruth, 1352
Bispecific antibodies, 98–99, 1635–1636
Bjorkman, Pamela, 40
Black Death, 42
Blister fluid, soluble mediators in, temporal
    analysis of, 1161
B lymphocytes, 3–11
  activation, 5–6, 195–225, 472–473, 1064,
      1209–1210
    viruses, 1209–1210
  affinity maturation, 10–11
  B1 B, 7, 160, 164, 165, 172, 174–177, 179,
      182, 183, 209–210
  biology of, 159–194
  cancer immunity, 1578
  CD5+ B, 7, 160, 164, 175–177, 179, 183
  development, 3–5, 126–127, 159–195
    abnormalities, 181
    B-cell malignancies, treatment of,
        181–182
    chicken, 182–183
    developmental pathways, 183–184
    fetal development, 180
    germinal center differentiation, 181
    humans, mice, compared, 180–184
    in mouse, 159–180
      B-1 B-cells, 176–177
      B-cell migration, maintenance, 174
      B-cell tolerance, 178–179
      B-cell turnover, 174–175
      bone marrow developmental stages,
          164–172
        culture systems, 165–168
        functional definition, 164
        microenvironmental interactions,
            165–168
        phenotypic definition, 164–165
      CD5, 179–180
      chemokines, in migration of B-cell
          precursors, 168
      complement, in B-cell tolerance,
          response, 179–180

early development, 160–164
  bone marrow, early B-cell
    progenitors in, 160
  follicular B-cells, 174
  gene expression, 168–169
  germinal center B-cells, 175
  growth of early B-lineage cells,
    regulators of, 166
  immature B-cells, generation of, 172
  immunoglobulin
    heavy chain, 169–172
    rearrangement, 168–169
    light-chain rearrangement, 172
  marginal zone B-cells, 177–178
  memory B-cells, 175–176
  ontogeny, sites of B lymphopoiesis
    during, 160
  peripheral maturation stages,
    functional subsets, 172–180
  Pre-BCR, 169–172
  receptor editing, 178–179
  serum antibody, in B-cell tolerance,
    response, 179–180
  stem cells, 160
  transcription factors, 162–164
  transgenic models, B-cell tolerance,
    178
  transitional B-cells, 172–174
  rabbit, 183
differentiation, 6–7
human immunodeficiency virus,
  1297–1298
lymphopoiesis environment, 812–813
signaling, 195–227
somatic hypermutation, 10–11. See also
  Hypermutation; Somatic
  hypermutation
suppression, crystallized fragment
  receptors, 691
tolerance, 7–8, 906–909, 918–919,
  921–925, 928–929
Blood dendritic cells, human
  immunodeficiency virus, 1291
Blood group antigens, 634–635
Blood groups, 30–31
Blood-brain barrier, active transport of
  cytokines across, 1023–1024
BLyS, 766–768
Bone marrow, 419–422
  cell rejection, mediated by natural killer
    cells, 369
  developmental stages
    B lymphocyte development, 164–172,
      180
    culture systems, 165–168
    phenotypic definition, 164–165
    microenvironmental interactions,
      165–168
  function
    apoptosis in, 422
    normal, apoptosis in, 422
  hematopoietic stem cells, 419–420
  inflammation, 1156–1157

stromal cells, microenvironment created
  by, 420–421
structure, function, 420–422
transplantation, major histocompatibility
  complex, 585
Bony fish
  evolution of immune response, 547–548
  evolution of lymphocyte differentiation,
    544–545
Bordet, Jules, 27, 30
Bordetella pertussis, infections, 1264
Botulinum, bioterrorism and, 1363
Bound, free antigen, separation of, 81–82
  solid-phase methods, 81–82
  solution methods, 81
Bowel disease, inflammatory. See
  Inflammatory bowel disease
Breinl, Friedrich, 29
Brent, Leslie, 35, 39, 41
Brucella species, 1231, 1270, 1273
Brucellosis, bacterial pathogen, 1231
Brugia, 1178, 1181
Brundtland, Gro Harlem, 1327
Bunyaviruses, 1202
Burnet, Frank Macfarlane, 25–26, 35–37,
  40, 41
BXSB mice, systemic autoimmunity, 1388

C
C1q, 1091–1092
  triggering phagocytosis, 1091
C3, 1088–1091
  complement activation, role of, 1081–1082
C3/α^2 complement, macroglobulin
  superfamily, 1080
C3b, 1085
C5, 1086–1087
Calcium stores, intracellular, B-cell activation
  and, 203
Calprotectin, 511
Calreticulin, 1091–1092, 1134
Campylobacter jejuni, 1277
Cancer, 1557–1592. See also Tumors
  age, immune response and, 1585
  antigens, 1559–1561, 1583
    encoded by normal cellular genes,
      1566–1569
    carcinoembryonic antigens,
      1568–1569
    clonal antigens, 1569
    differentiation antigens, 1567–1568
    oncofetal antigens, 1568–1569
    oncospermatogonal antigens, 1567
    encoded by viral genes, 1569–1571
      DNA tumor viruses, 1569–1570
      RNA tumor viruses, 1570–1571
    expressed on cancer cell, 1561–1562
    loss, 1582–1583
    tumor-associated, 1566–1569
    tumor-specific, 1562–1566
  cancer-testis antigens, 1567
  cells, antigens expressed by, 1645
  chemokines, 821–822

dendritic cell-based immunotherapy for,
  474–475
epitope loss, 1582–1583
escape from immunological destruction,
  mechanisms of, 1581
  immune suppression vs.
    immunodeficiency, 1584–1585
    carcinogens, 1584
    tumor burden, 1584–1585
immunity, effector mechanisms in,
  1577–1580
  antibodies, 1578
  B-cells, 1578
  cytokines, 1580
  lymphokine-activated killer cells,
    1579
  macrophages, 1579–1580
  natural killer cells, 1579
  neutrophils, 1579–1580
  T-lymphocytes, 1578–1579
  in vivo, assays, 1577–1578
immunodeficiency, 1584–1585
immunogenicity
  carcinogen dose, 1577
  factors influencing, 1576–1577
  immunocompetence, 1577
  spontaneous, induced cancers,
    contrasted, 1576–1577
  tumor latency, 1577
immunological enhancement blocking
  factors, 1583–1584
immunological factors influencing,
  1571–1576
immunoprevention, 1585–1586, 1651
immunosurveillance, tumor development,
  1571–1573
  adaptive T-cell-mediated, 1571–1572
  innate, 1572–1573
immunotherapy, 1586–1588. See also
  Immunotherapy
immunotoxins in clinical trials for, 1639
increases in, with aging, 1044–1045
major histocompatibility complex class I,
  antigens, changes in expression of,
  1582
major histocompatibility complex
  haplotype, 1580–1581
microenvironment of, 1581–1582
mutations
  chromosomal translocations, fusion
    proteins resulting from, 1566
  discovered by functional, genetic
    analyses, 1564–1566
    fusion proteins, 1566
    mutant p53 suppressor gene-encoded
      proteins, 1564–1566
    mutant ras oncogene-encoded
      proteins, 1564
  discovered by immunological analyses,
    1562–1564
  internal deletions, fusion proteins
    resulting from, 1566
natural killer cells, 383–384

Cancer (*contd.*)
 radiation *vs.* chemotherapeutic agents,
  1585
 rejection antigens on, 1558–1562
 spontaneous, induced, contrasted,
  1576–1577
 T-cells
  suppressor, 1583–1584
  in transplantation immunity mediation,
   1561
 transplantation, 1573
  immunity, T-cell mediation, 1561
  tumor-specific rejection, 1559
 tumor development stimulation,
  1573–1576
 tumor immunity, factors limiting,
  1580–1585
 tumor stroma, 1581–1582
 tumor-specific rejection, transplanted
  cancers, 1559
Cancer-testis antigens, 1567
Capacitative calcium, 203–205
Carbohydrate antigens, antigenic determinant
  recognition, 632–637
Carbohydrate vaccine, 1330
Carcinoembryonic antigens, 1568–1569
Carcinogen dose, 1577
 immunogenicity and, 1577
 tumor formation and, 1577
Cartilage-hair hypoplasia, 1608
Cartilaginous fish
 evolution of immune response, 547
 evolution of lymphocyte differentiation,
  544
Caspase-dependent, independent pathways,
  granule exocytosis cytotoxic
  mechanism, target death, 1139
Caspases
 apoptosis initiation mediated by, 848–849
 programmed cell death, 851–853
 structure, programmed cell death, 858
Catalytic antibodies, 98
Cathelicidins, 511
Cathepsin C, 1132
C chemokines
 family, 804, 805
 properties of, 835–837
CD1, major histocompatibility complex,
  598–599
 class Ib, 598–599
CD2, superfamily, 405–409
 structure, expression of, 406
CD3, polypeptides, 231–234
 intracellular assembly, 233–234
 sequence, 232–233
 structure, 234
CD4
 $\alpha\beta$ T-cell receptor-ligand interactions, 241
  role of, 241
 CD8 co-receptors, T-lymphocyte
  activation, 328–329
 CD8 T-cells, group 1 CD1-restricted,
  1244

helper T-cell *versus* CD8 cytotoxic T-cell
  lineage commitment, 284–292
CD4+, suppressor function, TGF-β and, 942
CD4+ CD25-immunoregulatory T-cells,
  958–959
 mucosal immune system, 985
 role in mucosal immunity, 985
CD4+ T-cells
 activated, suppressor effector function, 941
 depletion
  human immunodeficiency virus,
   1293–1296
  potential mechanisms of, 1293
 depletion of, augments immune response to
  tumor vaccine, 955
 genes selectively activated in, 945
 human immunodeficiency virus, 1291,
  1293–1296
  mechanisms of depletion, 1293–1296
 in mucosal tolerance, 1002–1003
 responses, human immunodeficiency virus,
  1302
CD4+ Th2 polarized immune responses,
  1444–1445
CD4/CD8 lineage
 divergence, models for, 287–288
 molecules implicated in, 288–290
 positive selection, negative selection,
  relationships between, 291–292
CD4+CD25+, suppressor T-cells
 cytokine requirements, 944–945
 gene expression by, molecular analysis of,
  945
 naturally occurring, 939–946
 thymic origin of, 943–944
CD4+CD25+-like T-cells, generation in
  periphery, 949–950
CD5, 179–180
CD5+ B-lymphocytes, 7, 160, 164, 175–179,
  183
CD8
 $\alpha\beta$ T-cell receptor-ligand interactions, role
  of, 241
 single-positive thymocytes, maturation,
  export of, 290–291
CD8+ T-cells, 957–958
 antigen processing for activation of,
  viruses, 1209
 human immunodeficiency virus, 1296
 secreted factors, human immunodeficiency
  virus, 1301–1302
CD8 T-cells, group 1 CD1-restricted, 1244
CD19, BCR signaling, 208
CD22, BCR signaling, 208
CD25+, suppressor function, TGF-β and, 942
CD25+ T-cells
 activated, suppressor effector function, 941
 depletion of, augments immune response to
  tumor vaccine, 955
 genes selectively activated in, 945
CD27, 404–405, 764–765
CD28
 biochemical basis for function, 397–398

family of receptors, comparison of, 394
 function, biochemical basis for, 397–398
CD28/CTLA-4 structure, expression, 395
CD30, 764, 765
CD40, 401–404, 408–409
 CD84, 409
 isotype switching by, 139–140
 mutations in, 1599
CD40:CD154 interactions, in germinal
  center, 402–403
CD45
 BCR signaling, 207–208
 deficiency, 1605
 protein-tyrosine phosphatase, 339–340
CD70, 404–405
CD80. *See* B7-1
CD84, 409
CD134, 404
CD150, 408
CD154, 401–404
 deficiency, with primary
  immunodeficiency, 1597–1598
CD244, 408–409
Celiac disease, human leukocyte antigen
  associations, 588
Cell antigen receptors. *See* T-cell receptors
Cell death, programmed, 841–864
 APAF proteins, 856
 B-cell homeostasis, 846–847
 caspase complexes, apoptosis initiation
  mediated by, 848–849
 cellular homeostasis, in multicellular
  organisms, 841–842
 cellular mechanisms, 848–850
 dendritic cell homeostasis, 847
 as immune effector mechanism, 847
 immune regulation, 842–847
 as immune therapy, 858
 mitochondrion, role of, 849–850
 necrosis, programmed, 850
 peripheral T-cells, homeostasis of, 843–844
 regulation of, 851–856
  Bcl-2 gene family, 853–856
  caspases, 851–853
  TNF-receptor superfamily members, 853
 structural regulation of, 856–859
  Bcl-2 homology structures, 857–858
  caspase structure, 858
  hexahelical bundle, 858
  lymphoid malignancy, 858–859
  TNF-TNFR structure, 856–857
 T-cell death, passive, lymphokine
  withdrawal, 845–846
 T-cell memory, 846
 thymic deletion, 843
 T-lymphocyte death, active,
  antigen-stimulated, 844–845
Cell surface Ly49 receptors, 381
Cell-to-cell spreading, intracellular bacteria,
  1239
Cellular homeostasis, in multicellular
  organisms, 841–842
Cellular immunodeficiency, 1602–1603

Cellular immunology, 34–39
  clonal selection theory, 36–38
  graft rejection, 35–36
  lymphocytes, 38
  monoclonal antibodies, 38–39
  thymus, biology of, 38
  tolerance, graft, 35–36
Cellular mechanisms, parasites, 1174–1175
Cellular mediators, acute inflammatory
      response, 1156–1160
  epithelial cells, 1160
  lymphocytes, 1160
  macrophages, 1160
Cellular strategies in immunotherapy,
      1643–1647
  cellular transfer, 1644–1645
    adoptive antigen-specific cytotoxic
        lymphocyte therapy, 1644–1645
    tumor-infiltrating lymphocytes, 1644
  dendritic cells, 1643–1644
  genetically engineered cells, 1645–1647
  graft-versus-leukemia T-cells, 1647
  graft-versus-tumor effects, 1647
  lymphokine-activated killer cells, 1643
  macrophage-active killer cells, 1644
  natural killer cells, 1643
  nonspecific cellular therapy, 1643
  regulatory T-cells, 1647
Cellular transfer, in immunotherapy,
      1644–1645
Central nervous system, human
      immunodeficiency virus, 1292
  cytokine network in, 1312
Central tolerance, in autoimmune diseases,
      1403–1406
Chagas' disease, 1172
Chang, Timothy, 38
Chase, Merrill W., 35
Chediak-Higashi syndrome, 1610–1611
Chemokine fold, 806–807
Chemokine knockout mice, phenotypes of,
      840
Chemokine system, pathogenetic factors in
      human disease, 819
Chemokines, 16, 801–840, 1134
  7TM-chemokine receptors, 833
  adaptive immunity, 816–819
    afferent trafficking to secondary
        lymphoid tissue, 816–817
    CD4+ T-cell differentiation, 818
    efferent trafficking, 817–818
    positioning within lymph node, 817–818
    tissue-specific lymphocyte homing,
        818–819
  B lymphopoiesis, 812–813
  C chemokines, properties of, 835
  CC chemokines, properties of, 836–837
  cell responses to, 808–809
    adhesion, 808
    apoptosis, 809
    cytotoxicity, 808–809
    migration, 808
    proliferation, 809

CX3C chemokines, properties of, 835
CXC, properties of, 835
cytotoxic T-lymphocyte, 1134
disease, 819–822
  acute neutrophil-mediated inflammatory
      disorders, 820
  asthma, 821
  atherosclerosis, 821
  autoimmunity, 820–821
  cancer, 821–822
  immunodeficiency/infectious diseases,
      819–820
  transplant rejection, 820
in evolution of immune response, 550–552
hematopoiesis regulation, 812–814
  CXCL12, in myelopoiesis, 812–813
  myelopoiesis, 812–813
  myelosuppressive chemokines, 813
  phagocyte positioning in peripheral
      tissue, 814
  T-lymphopoiesis, 814
history of, 802
human immunodeficiency virus, 824–826,
      1307–1312
immune response, chemokine regulation
      of, 814–816
  innate immunity, 814–816
    CXCL8, 814–815
    mononuclear phagocytes, 815–816
    neutrophil-targeted chemokines,
        814–815
    NK cells, 815
    transition to adaptive immune
        response, 815–816
knockout mice, phenotypes of, 840
malaria, 826
in migration of B-cell precursors, 168
mimicry in infectious disease, 822–824
  herpesvirus, 822–824
  poxvirus, 822–824
molecular organization, 802–806
  chemokine redundancy, 806
  genes, evolution and, 805–806
  immunologic classification, 804–805
  structural classification, 802–804
presentation mechanisms, 808
production, changes in, with age, 1053
receptor
  knockout mice, phenotypes of, 838–839
  for resting human leukocyte subsets, 834
  structure, 807–808
  viral chemokines, 823
regulation of action, 811–812
  expression, 811–812
  processing, 812
  receptor deactivation, 812
  targeting, 812
signaling pathways, 809–811
  cross talk, 811
  Gi-dependent effectors, 809–811
  Gi-independent effectors, 811
  G-protein signaling, 809
  mechanisms of gradient sensing, 811

structural biology, 806–808
  chemokine fold, 806–807
  chemokine presentation mechanisms,
      808
  chemokine receptor structure, 807–808
therapeutic applications, 826–827
  biological response modifiers, 827
  drug development, 826–827
Chemotaxis
  in, inflammation, 1158
  in inflammation, 1158
Chemotherapeutic agents, vs. radiation, tumor
      formation and, 1585
Chicken
  B lymphocyte development, 182–183
  evolution of lymphocyte differentiation,
      545–546
Chitinases, 510
Chlamydia pneumoniae, 1232
Chlamydia psittaci, 1232, 1236, 1237, 1238
Chlamydia trachomatis, 1232, 1237
Cholera vaccine, 1329, 1343–1345
Cholinergic autonomic nervous system
      responses, immune-mediated
      diseases, 1036–1037
Chromosomal translocations, fusion proteins
      resulting from, 1566
Chronic inflammation, 1162–1163
Chronic stress, immune system-mediated
      disease, 1034
Circumventricular organ, passive transport of
      cytokines across, 1023
Cirrhosis, biliary, primary, 1423
CIS/SOCS/JAB/SSI family, inhibitory
      adapter proteins, 734
Class switching, 10, 138–144
Clinical transplantation, major
      histocompatibility complex, 584–586
Clonal selection theory, 36–38
Clostridium difficile, 1270
Clostridium perfringens, infections, 1264
Clostridium tetani, infections, 1264
Clotting, in inflammation, 1154
CMV. See Cytomegalovirus
Coca, Arthur, 29
Cohn, Edwin, 32
Colitis, ulcerative, 1430
Collagen C1q receptor, 1091–1092
Collectins
  innate immune system, 505–506
  in phagocytosis, 1112–1113
  receptor, 1091–1092, 1112–1113
Colloid chemistry, 27–29
Colony-stimulating factors, human
      immunodeficiency virus, 1310
Combination vaccine, 1330
Combined immunodeficiency, 1603–1611.
      See also Severe combined
      immunodeficiency
  autosomal recessive, 1603–1605
  severe combined immunodeficiency,
      1603–1606
  X-linked recessive, 1603

Common variable immunodeficiency, 1600–1601
Complement, 21–22, 1077–1103
  activation, 1081–1082
    C3, role of, 1081–1082
    control of, 1099
    inhibition of, 1098, 1221
    via classical pathway, 1082–1083
    viral inhibition of, 1221
  age-related changes in, 1050
  alternative pathway, 21–22
    activation via, 1085–1086
  anaphylatoxin receptors, 1091
  in B-cell tolerance, response, 179–180
  biosynthesis, 1080
  C1q receptor, 1091–1092
    triggering phagocytosis, 1091
  C3aR, C5aR, 1091
  C3b, 1085, 1086
  C5aR, 1091
  calreticulin, 1091–1092
  classical pathway, 21
    activation, 1082–1083
    regulation, 1083
  collagen C1q receptor, 1091–1092
  collectin receptor, 1091–1092
  contribution, to pathogenesis and/or
      perpetuation, human disease with,
      1092
  control proteins, mode of action of, 1083
  defense against infection, 1093–1095
  deficiencies, 1096–1097
  in disease, 1092–1093
  drug therapy and, 1097–1099
  as functional system, 1077–1079
  genetics, 1095–1096
  globular head C1q receptor, 1092
  historical overview, 1079
  in inflammation, 1153–1154
  lectin pathway
    activation of, 1084
    regulation of, 1084–1085
  mimicry of, by microorganisms,
      1094–1095
  in neurologic disease, 1093
  nomenclature, 1080
  as pathogenic factor in disease, 1092–1093
  phylogenetic aspects, 1079–1080
  protein families, 1080–1081
    complement C3/α^2 macroglobulin
        superfamily, 1080
    serine protease module, proteins with,
        1081
    short consensus repeat units, proteins
        with, 1080–1081
    terminal pathway components, protein
        motifs found in, 1081
  receptor phagocytosis, signaling events in,
      1115
  receptors, 1088–1092, 1111–1112
    C3 receptors, 1088–1091
      complement receptor type 1,
          1088–1090

  complement receptor type 2, 1090
  complement receptor type 3, 1090
  complement receptor type 4, 1091
  in phagocytosis, 1111–1112
    complement receptor type 1, 1111
    integrin complement receptors,
        1111–1112
  type 1, 1088–1090, 1111
  type 2, 1090
  type 3, 1090
  type 4, 1091
  in renal disease, 1092–1093
  as target in drug therapy, 1097–1099
    monoclonal antibodies, derivatives of,
        1099
    native, modified complement regulators,
        1097–1099
    synthetic molecules, 1099
  terminal, 22
    biological properties of, 1088
    formation of, 1087
    pathway, 1086–1088
      C5, 1086–1087
      control of, 1088
      terminal complement complex, 1087
        biological properties of, 1088
Complementarity-determining region 3
    diversification, 251–252
Conjugate vaccine, 1330
Conjunctivitis, bacterial pathogen, 1232
Cooke, Robert, 29
Coombs-Gell classification, initiating
    mechanisms, 1441
Co-receptor interactions, major
    histocompatibility complex, 600
Corner, George, 29
Coronary heart disease, bacterial pathogen,
    1232
Corynebacterium diphtheria, infections,
    1264
Coxiella burnetii, 1232
Coxsackie adenovirus, 1204, 1216
CpG motif, in immunotherapy, 1339,
    1624–1625
C-reactive protein, 506
Crick, Francis, 34
Crile, George, 31
Crohn's disease, 1430
Crossmatch, transplantation immunology,
    1545
Cross-reactivity
  antigen-antibody interactions, 86–89
  monoclonal antibodies, 101
Cryptosporidium parasite, 1171, 1179
Cryptosporidium parvum, 1174, 1179
Crystallized fragment
  complement receptor phagocytosis,
      morphological differences between, in
      phagocytosis, 1113–1114
  ϵ receptor I, surface expression, regulation
      of, in allergic disorders, 1457
  ϵ receptor II, in allergic disorders,
      1457–1458

  ϵ receptor I-mediated signal transduction,
      in allergic disorders, 1456–1457
  ϵ receptor-mediated phagocytosis,
      signaling events in, 1114–1115
  receptors, 685–700
    disease, 697–698
      autoimmunity, 697
      inflammation, 697–698
      tolerance, 697
    expression, 688–689
    historical overview, 685–686
    mimetics, viruses, 1222
    molecular genetics, 686–688
      gene organization, 688
      linkage, 688
      polymorphisms, 688
      species comparisons, 688
      subunit composition, 686–688
    signaling, 691–693
      immunoreceptor tyrosine-based
          activation motif pathways,
          691–692
      immunoreceptor tyrosine-based
          inhibitor motif pathways,
          692–693
    structure, 686–690
      three-dimensional structure, 689–690
    in vitro activity, 690–691
      B lymphocyte suppression, 691
      binding properties, 690
      effector cell activation, 691
    in vivo activity, 693–697
      cytotoxic immunoglobulin G,
          695–696
      efferent response, 694–697
      ϵ receptors in afferent response,
          693–694
      hypersensitivity, immediate, 695
      immune complex-mediated
          inflammation, 696–697
CTLA-4
  biochemical basis for function, 397–398
  in regulating peripheral T-cell tolerance,
      396–397
CTLs. See Cytotoxic T-lymphocytes
CVID. See Common variable
    immunodeficiency
CX3C chemokine family, 804, 835
CXC chemokine family, 804, 835
Cyanoacrylates, 1340
Cyclic nucleotides, fluxes in, T-lymphocyte
    activation, 348–349
Cyclospora parasite, 1171
Cytidine deaminase deficiency,
    activation-induced, 1598–1599
Cytokine-related molecules, with regulatory
    effects on human immunodeficiency
    virus replication, 1309
Cytokines, 16, 702–706, 718–721, 732–733,
    1248–1251, 1307–1312, 1380. See
    also specific cytokines
  approved for clinical use, 1626
  in autoimmune disease, 1409

cancer immunity and, 1580
dendritic cell-derived, polarizing, 468–469
in evolution of immune response, 550–552
helical-bundle, 703
human immunodeficiency virus,
    1307–1312
in immunotherapy, 1625–1628
inducing switches to immunoglobulin A,
    986–987
inhibition of, 1221
    viral, 1221
interleukin-6 family of, composition of
    receptors for, 714
intracellular bacteria, 1248–1251
    down-regulation, antibacterial host
        response, 1250–1251
    granuloma formation, 1248–1249
    leukocyte recruitment, 1248
    macrophage activation, 1249–1250
    protective T-cell response, 1250
Jaks activated, 722
mast cell-derived, in allergic disorders,
    1462–1463
mimetics
    viral, 1221
    viruses, 1221
mucosal immunity, 968
in mucosal immunity, 968
in pathogenesis, treatment of inflammatory
    bowel disease, 950
peripherally produced, central nervous
    system functions induced by,
    1024–1026
production
    changes in, with age, 1053
    secondary, within CNS, 1
receptor
    diseases associated with, 736
    diseases of, 735–736
    ϵ chain, cytokines sharing, 706–711
    immunotherapy and, 1627
    interferon, 721
    mucosal immunity, 968
    mycobacterial infections, 736
    redundancy, 717–718
    severe combined immunodeficiency
        disease, 735–736
    sharing β_c, features of, 712
    sharing gp130, 713
    soluble, 718
    type I, 701–747
        common β chain, β_c, cytokine
            receptors sharing, 711–712
        common cytokine receptor ϵ chain,
            cytokines sharing, 706–711
        cytokine pleiotropy,
            717–718
        cytokine receptor pleiotropy, 717–718
        cytokine receptor redundancy,
            717–718
        cytokine redundancy, 717–718
        families of, 706–717
        features common to, 704

G-CSF receptor, receptors with
    similarities to, 715–716
glycoprotein 130, receptors with
    similarities to, 715–716
heterodimers, 705–706
higher order receptor oligomers,
    705–706
homodimers, 705–706
IL-2, 716–717
IL-4, 716
IL-7, 716
IL-12, 715–716
IL-23, 715
IL-27, 715–716
leptin, 715
nomenclature, 702
obesity receptor, receptors with
    similarities to, 715–716
receptor chains, sharing of,
    significance of, 715
thymic stromal lymphopoietin, 716
type I cytokines, 702–706
    structure, 702–704
X-linked severe combined
    immunodeficiency disease, ϵ_c
    mutations, 709–711
WZSX-1/TCCR type I receptor,
    mutations in, 736
redundancy, 717–718
regulation
    immunoglobulin A production, mucosal
        immune system, 988–989
    Th2 differentiation, in allergic disorders,
        1450–1452
with regulatory effects on human immuno-
    deficiency virus replication, 1309
release, dendritic cells, 465–466
    interferon-α, 465–466
    interleukin-2, 466
    interleukin-12, 465
signaling molecules, 732–733
signals, down-modulation, 733–734
species specificity of, 721
STATs activated, 723
systemic autoimmunity, 1380
type I, phenotypes of mice deficiency in,
    726–727
type II, 719
    phenotypes of mice deficiency in,
        726–727
viral interference, 1221–1222
Cytolysin. See Perforin
Cytomegalovirus, 1215
    mouse, natural killer cells, 385–386
Cytopathic viruses, 1214
Cytoplasm, intracellular bacteria evasion into,
    1239
Cytoplasmic protein-tyrosine kinases, TCR
    ITAMs and, 334
Cytoplasmic-to-nuclear signaling, latent
    transcription factors, 732
Cytoskeletal changes, T-lymphocyte
    activation, 349–350

Cytoskeleton in phagocytosis,
    1115–1117
Cytotoxic immunoglobulin G, 695–696
Cytotoxic mediators, differentiation-
    dependent expression of, 1140–1141
Cytotoxic T-lymphocyte-associated antigen 4,
    942
Cytotoxic T-lymphocyte-mediated induction,
    target Fas, 1140
Cytotoxic T-lymphocytes, 15–16,
    1127–1150
    adenosine, extracellular, 1141
    adhesion strengthening, 1134–1135
    antitumor cytotoxic T-lymphocyte activity,
        cellular cytotoxicity pathways,
        1142
    autoimmunity, 1143
    calreticulin, 1134
    chemokines, 1134
    in control of viral infections, 1142–1143
    cytotoxic mediators, differentiation-
        dependent expression of, 1140–1141
    dipeptidyl peptidase I, 1132
    in disease pathogenesis, 1143
    effector functions, therapeutic modulation,
        1144–1145
    Fas ligand, 1133
    graft-versus-host disease, 1143–1144
    granule exocytosis cytotoxic mechanism,
        1134–1140
        adhesion, 1134–1135
        caspase-dependent, independent
            pathways, target death, 1139
        detachment, 1139
        effector polarization, 1135–1136
        exocytosis, 1137
        granzymes, in target death,
            1137–1138
        perforin-mediated granzyme entry,
            1138–1139
        self-protection, 1139–1140
        signaling exocytosis, 1137
    granule membrane proteins, 1133–1134
    granules, properties, 1129–1130
    granulysin, 1133
    granzymes, 1131–1132
    homeostasis, immune system, 1141–1142
    as host defense, 1142
    human immunodeficiency virus,
        1299–1301
    hypersensitivity, cytotoxic mediators in
        contact, 1144
    liver carcinogenesis, 1144–1145
    lymphocyte granzymes, 1132
    lymphocyte-mediated cytotoxicity
        mechanisms of, distinguishing,
            1128–1129
        properties of, 1128
    lysosomal enzymes, 1133
    membrane mixing, 1134–1135
    mucosal, 989–990
    perforin, 1130–1131, 1141–1142
    proteoglycan, 1132–1133

Cytotoxic T-lymphocytes (*contd.*)
  secretory granules, 1129–1134
  secretory pathways, 1129
  target Fas, cytotoxic T-lymphocyte-
      mediated induction of,
      1140
  in vitro functional activity, 1127–1128
  in vivo localization, 1145
  in vivo studies, *in vitro* studies, contrasted,
      cytotoxicity, 1140–1141
Cytotoxicity, as response to chemokines,
      808–809

D
Dale, Henry, 29
Darwin, Charles, 35
Davis, Mark, 41
DCs. *See* Dendritic cells
Defensins, 510–511
  in evolution of immune response, 555–556
Degranulation, in inflammation,
      1158–1159
Delayed-type hypersensitivity, 1255
Deletional switch recombination,
      immunoglobulin E synthesis, in
      allergic disorders, 1455–1456
Dendritic cells, 305–306, 455–480, 509
  antigen processing, 462–464
    class II major histocompatibility
        complex-restricted presentation,
        462–464
  antigen uptake, 461–462
  antigen-independent clustering, 467
  antigen-presenting cells, 468
  B-cell activation, 472–473
  cancer, dendritic cell-based
      immunotherapy for, 474–475
  cells from dendritic family, hallmarks of,
      459–466
  class II/peptide combinations,
      sequestration of, 463
  co-stimulation, adhesion, 460–461
  cytokine release, 465–466
    interferon-α, 465–466
    interleukin-2, 466
    interleukin-12, 465
  cytokines, dendritic cell-derived,
      polarizing, 468–469
  discovery of, 455–456
  homeostasis, 847
  human immunodeficiency virus,
      1296–1297
  immune escape, 468
  in immunotherapy, 1643–1644
  interstitial dendritic cells, 457–458
  intracellular bacteria, 1241
  Langerhans cells, 456–457
  lineages, phenotypes in mouse, humans,
      458
  major histocompatibility
      complex-restricted class I,
      presentation, 464
  maturation process, 461

  migratory properties, 464–465
    migration in situ, 465
  modulatory, in organ-specific
      autoimmunity, 1416–1417
  monocyte-derived dendritic cells, 458
  natural killer cells, 473–474
  plasmacytoid-derived dendritic cells, 459
  polarization, mechanisms of, 469–470
  polarization of immune response, 468–470
  precursors, 458
  shift in class II half-life, mature, immature,
      contrasted, 462–463
  subsets presenting peptide-major
      histocompatibility complex ligands
      in vivo, 307
  T-cell tolerance, 470–472
    central tolerance, 470
    interleukin-10, 472
    peripheral tolerance, 470–472
      immature dendritic cells, 471
      specialized subsets of, 471–472
  T-cell/dendritic cell synapses, 467
  T-cell-mediated immunity, 466–468
    adoptive transfer, 466
    immunostimulatory properties *in vitro*,
        466
    as physiological adjuvant, 466–467
  vaccine, 1650
    in immunotherapy, 1650
  veiled cells, 458
  in vivo distribution, 456–459
d'Entrecolles, Father, 23
Deoxyribonucleic acid vaccine, 1360
Dermatitis
  atopic, 1471–1472
  herpetiformis, 1429–1430
Destruction of immune cells, human
      cytomegalovirus, 1217
Dextran-binding myeloma proteins,
      635–637
Diabetes
  antigen-specific induction of, 1413–1414
  insulin-dependent
    human leukocyte antigen associations,
        588
    regulatory T-cells, 951–952
  spontaneous onset, models of, 1413
  type 1, 1411–1417
    etiology, 1415–1416
    immunology of, 1412–1415
    therapeutic concepts, 1416–1417
Diarrheal disease vaccine, 1343–1345
Differentiation antigens, encoded by normal
      cellular genes, 1567–1568
DiGeorge's syndrome, 1602–1603
Dipeptidyl peptidase I, 1132
Diphtheria
  history of vaccination, 1342–1343
  vaccine, 1329, 1342–1343
DN cells, group 1 CD1-restricted, 1244
DNA breaks in V regions, 147–148
DNA tumor viruses, 1569–1570
DNA vaccine, 1649–1650

DNA-PK, 123–124
Double negative suppressor T-cells, 958
Double positive thymocyte stage, T-cell
      development, 280–281
Dubos, René, 29
Duesberg, Peter, 42
Dunn, Thelma, 34

E
Early development, bone marrow, early
      B-cell progenitors in, 160
Early replication, viruses, obstacles to,
      1203–1204
Ebola virus, 1205
  transmission of, 1203
Ectodysplasin, 768
Eczema, immunodeficiency with, 1607–
      1608
EDAR, 768
Edelmann, Gerald, 34
Edible vaccine, 1334
Effector activity, continued expression of,
      immunological memory and, 881–882
Effector cells. *See also specific cells; specific
      types*
  in allergic response, 1458–1459
  signaling pathways, 203–207
Effector mechanisms, 19–22
  basophils, 20
  in cancer immunity, 1577–1580
    B-cells, 1578
    cytokines, 1580
    macrophages, 1579–1580
    natural killer cells, 1579
    T-lymphocytes, 1578–1579
    in vivo, assays, 1577–1578
  eosinophils, 21
  granulocytes, 20
  innate immune system, 510–512
    antiviral effector mechanisms of,
        512
    BPI, 510
    calprotectin, 511
    cathelicidins, 511
    chitinases, 510
    defensins, 510–511
    lactoferrin, 511
    lysozyme, 510
    myeloperoxidase, 511–512
    nitric oxide synthase, 511–512
    NRAMP, 511
    oxidase, 511–512
    phagocyte, 511–512
    phospholipase A2, 510
    serprocedins, 511
  macrophages, 20
  mast cells, 20
  monocytes, 20
  natural killer cells, 20
Effector sites, mucosal immune system,
      980–981
Ehrlich, Paul, 26, 40, 1321
Eimeria, 1179

Elderly. *See also* Aging
  immunologic dysfunction in, clinical
    evidence, 1044
  vaccination of, 1365–1366
ELISA test, 42
  development of, 30
Encapsulated organisms, vaccine against,
    1347–1348
Endemic typhus, bacterial pathogen, 1232
Endoplasmic reticulum
  class II assembly of major
    histocompatibility complex molecules
    in, 618–620
  peptide transport into, antigen processing
    and, 615–616
Endothelial cells, in inflammation, 1160
Entamoeba histolytica, 1173, 1190
Environment, effect on allergic disorders,
    1446–1448
Environmental influences, on systemic
    autoimmunity, 1380–1381
Enzyme-linked immunosorbent assay,
    84–85
Enzyme-linked immunospot assay, 85–86
Eosinophils, 21, 509, 1029–1030
  activation of, in allergic disorders,
    1467–1468
  in allergic disorders, 1463–1468
    eosinophil-derived mediators,
      1464–1466
      cytokines, 1465–1466
      eosinophil-specific cationic proteins,
        1464–1465
      lipid mediators, 1465
  as effector cells, in allergic disorders, 1468
  in inflammation, 1160
  recruitment to sites of inflammation,
    1466–1467
Epithelial cells, in mucosal immunity,
    966–970
  adaptive immune functions of, 968–970
  cytokines, 968
  epithelium, innate functions of, 966–968
  transcellular transport functions of, 968
Epithelium
  adaptive immune functions of, 968–970
  functions of, mucosal immune system,
    966–968
  innate functions of, 966–968
  molecules associated with adaptive
    immunity, 969
  transcellular transport functions of, 968
Epitope loss, tumor formation and,
    1582–1583
Epstein-Barr virus, 1204
ER. *See* Endoplasmic reticulum
Error-prone polymerases, 148–149
Escherichia coli, 1267, 1270, 1273
  infections, 1264
Evasion
  of immune recognition, parasites,
    1183–1184
  by immune suppression, parasites, 1184

Evolution of immune system, 519–570
  adaptive immune responses, 546–550
    agnathia, 546–547
    amphibians, 548–549
    birds, 549–550
    bony fish, 547–548
    cartilaginous fish, 547
    mammals, 549–550
    reptiles, 549
  adaptive immunity, origins of, 561–565
  allorecognition, 560–561
  chemokines, 550–552
  components, adaptive immune system,
    521–553
  cytokines, 550–552
  defensins, 555–556
  hematopoiesis, 552–553
  IL-1, 550
  IL-8, 550
  IMD pathways, 559
  immunoglobulin superfamily, 555
  immunoglobulins, 526–532
    gene organization, 532
      chondrichthyan germline-joined
        genes, 532
      organization of rearranging genes,
        532
    immunoglobulin D homologues, 527
    immunoglobulin heavy-chain isotypes,
      526
    immunoglobulin light chains, 531
    immunoglobulin M, 526
    immunoglobulin NAR, 526
    immunoglobulin R/immunoglobulin
      NARC/immunoglobulin
      W/immunoglobulin X, 527
    J chain, 531–532
    V_H regions, 528–429
      D segments, 528
      J segments, 528
      V_H evolution, 528–531
  inflammatory cytokines, 550
  innate immunity, evolution of, 553–561
  interferons, 551
  interleukin 2, 550–551
  invertebrate cells, 553–554
  lectins, 555
  lymphocyte differentiation
    amphibians, 545
    bony fish, 544–545
    cartilaginous fish, 544
    chickens, 545–546
    mammals, 546
    rearrangement, diversification of TCR,
      immunoglobulin genes, 544–546
  lymphoid tissues, 541–544
    amphibians, 542–543
    birds, 543–544
    bony fish, 541–542
    cartilaginous fish, 541
    reptiles, 543–544
  major histocompatibility complex,
    532–541, 583

  class I/II expression, 540–541
  class I/II structure, 532–535
  classical, nonclassical class I, chain II,
    535
  disease associations, 537–538
  gene organization, 539–540
  locus complexity, selection on, 539
  mating preferences, 538–539
  origins, 561–562
  polymorphism, genes, 535–537
  parasites, recognition of, 559–560
  pentraxins, 555
  phagocytosis, 558
  proteolytic cascades, 556–558
  RAG, 553
  rearranging receptors
    antigen receptor, 563
    C1 domain, 563
    hypermutation and, 562–563
    origins of, 562–565
    rearranging machinery, 562
    V, VC1 segments, 563–565
    V domain, 563
    V segment, 563–565
    VC1 segment, 563–565
  signaling, 558–560
  T-cell receptors, 521–526
    α/β constant domains, 523–524
    α/β variable domains, 524–525
    CD3 complex, 525–526
    ϵ/δ TCR, 525
  TdT, 553
  TNF, 550
  toll, pathways, 559
  transforming growth factor β, 551–552
Exercise, aging and, 1065
Exonuclease, in V gene assembly
    recombination, 125–126
External secretions, immunoglobulins, 971
Extracellular bacteria, 1263–1283
  antigen-nonspecific deleterious response,
    1276–1277
  antigen-nonspecific host defense response,
    1271–1273
    local response, 1271–1272
    mucosal defense, 1271
    systemic response, 1272–1273
  antigen-specific deleterious response,
    1277
  antigen-specific host defense response,
    1273–1276
    antibodies, protective mechanisms of,
      1274–1276
    responses of host, 1273–1274
    T-cell immune system, 1276
  deleterious host response, 1276–1277
  gram-positive, bacterial surface structure
    of, 1265–1267
  infections, susceptibility to, T genes
    associated with, 1273
  invasion of host, 1269–1271
  virulence factors, 1267–1269
Extracellular parasites, 1180–1182

Eye disorders, inflammatory
  in animal models, 1425–1426
  diseases associated with, 1424–1425
  in human, 1426

F

FAB, structure, function, 51–55
F-actin
  association with phagosome membrane,
    1116–1117
  phagosome membrane, 1116–1117
F-actin nucleation, 1116
  in phagocytosis, 1116
F-actin organization, regulation of, 1117
  in phagocytosis, 1117
Facultative intracellular bacteria, 1231–1232
  infections of humans caused by,
    1231
  major infections of humans caused by,
    1231
Fas ligand, 759–760, 1133
  cytotoxic T-lymphocytes, 1133, 1140
Fas-mediated cytotoxicity, 1141–1142
Fc receptors, 63
FcεRIIb, BCR signaling, 208–209
FcRn, major histocompatibility complex
    molecules class Ib, 599
Fenner, Frank, 35
Fetal development, B lymphocytes, 180
Fetal liver, macrophages, 485
Fibrinolytic proteins, in inflammation, 1154
Filoviruses, 1202
Find T-cell, changes in, subsets with age,
    1058–1059
Fish
  bony
    evolution of immune response, 547–548
    lymphocyte differentiation, in evolution
      of immune response, 544–545
  cartilaginous
    evolution of immune response, 547
    lymphocyte differentiation, in evolution
      of immune response, 544
Flaviviruses, 1202
Fleming, Alexander, 25
Follicular B-cells, 174
Food allergens, 1443, 1471
Fragment receptors, crystallized, 685–700
  disease, 697–698
    autoimmunity, 697
    inflammation, 697–698
  expression, 688–689
  historical overview, 685–686
  molecular genetics, 686–688
    gene organization, 688
    species comparisons, 688
    subunit composition, 686–688
  signaling, 691–693
    immunoreceptor tyrosine-based
      activation motif pathways, 691–692
    immunoreceptor tyrosine-based inhibitor
      motif pathways, 692–693
  structure, 686–690

three-dimensional structure, 689–690
  in vitro activity, 690–691
    B lymphocyte suppression, 691
    binding properties, 690
    effector cell activation, 691
  in vivo functions, 693–697
    cytotoxic immunoglobulin G, 695–696
    efferent response, 694–697
    ε receptors in afferent response, 693–694
    hypersensitivity, immediate, 695
    immune complex-mediated
      inflammation, 696–697
Francisella tularensis, 1231
Free energy, affinity, 71
Fusion proteins
  chromosomal translocations, resulting
    from, 1566
  internal deletions, resulting from, 1566
  tumor formation and, 1566
Fusion toxins, in immunotherapy, 1638
Fyn PTK, 334–335

G

ε locus, T-cell receptor, 235–236
ε receptors in afferent response, 693–694
εδ lineage choice, 278–280
εδ T-cells, 249–250
  complementarity-determining region 3
    length distribution analysis, 250
  ligands, multivalence of, 250–251
εδ-CD3, 246–251
  antigen recognition, 247–249
  identification of, 246–247
  immune defense, αβ T-cells, contrasted,
    247
  nonpeptide antigens, stimulation by, 249
  T22 tetramers, 248–249
ε-interferon-activated sequence motifs,
    732
Gastritis, 1430
  autoimmune, regulatory T-cells, 950
Gastrointestinal tract
  allergy, mucosal immunity, 1009
  lymphocyte homing in, 993–994
Gates, Vaccine Initiative, 1326–1327,
    1348–1349, 1361
Gaudillière, Jean-Paul, 38
GC1qR, 1092
G-CSF receptor, receptors with similarities
    to, 715–716
Gene activation events, T-lymphocyte
    activation, 350–354
  cell surface molecules, expression of,
    353–354
  early gene activation events, 351
  lymphokine genes, activation of, 351–353
Gene alterations, immunoglobulins, in
    germinal centers, 137–149
  heavy-chain switch, 138–144
    assaying switch recombination, 139
    isotype switching by CD40, 139–140
    isotype-specific regulation of germline
      transcripts, 140–141

non-"standard" isotype switching,
    143–144
  sterile transcription in class switch
    recombination, 141
  switch junctions, 138–139
  targeting class switch recombination to
    switch regions, 141–142
somatic mutation, 144–149
  cellular context of, 145
  early evidence for, 144
  hypermutation, role of, 144–145
  molecular mechanism of hypermutation,
    147–149
    DNA breaks in V regions, 147–148
    error-prone polymerases, 148–149
  targeting, distribution of mutations,
    145–147
Gene cloning, V gene assembly,
    immunoglobulins, 108–109
Gene expression
  B lymphocyte development, 168–169
  immunoglobulins, regulation of, 135–137
Gene libraries, to derive monoclonal
    antibodies, 97–98
Gene loci, immunoglobulins, 111–116
  heavy chain genes, 111–114
    membrane versus secreted
      immunoglobulin, 112–113
    organization of CH gene loci, 113–114
  κ-light-chain genes, 114
  λ light-chain genes, 114–116
    human λ locus, 115–116
    murine λ locus, 114–115
  λ-related "surrogate" light chains, 116
Genes, cancer mutations, discovered by
    functional, genetic analyses, mutant
    ras oncogene-encoded proteins, 1564
Genetic maps, major histocompatibility
    complex, 579–582
Genetic requirements, T-cell development,
    T-lineage specification, 268–270
Genetically engineered cells, in
    immunotherapy, 1645–1647
Genetics
  in allergic disorders, 1445–1446
  autoimmune disease, 1407
  complements, 1095–1096
  human immunodeficiency virus,
    1302–1303
  molecular, immunoglobulins, 107–158
  in organ-specific autoimmunity, 1415
  phagocytosis, 1106–1107
  systemic autoimmunity, 1377–1378
Genital tract, immune responses in,
    997–998
Germinal center
  B-cells, 175
  differentiation, B lymphocytes, 181
  gene alterations in, immunoglobulins,
    137–149
    heavy-chain switch, 138–144
      assaying switch recombination, 139
      isotype switching by CD40, 139–140

isotype-specific regulation of germline transcripts, 140–141
sterile transcription in class switch recombination, 141
switch junctions, 138–139
targeting class switch recombination to switch regions, 141–142
immunoglobulin gene alterations in, heavy-chain switch, B-cell-specific, *versus* ubiquitously expressed components of class switch recombination machinery, 142
Germline diversity, immunoglobulins, 132–135
combinatorial diversity estimates, 135
human germline VH locus, 134
human germline V_κ locus, 134–135
human JH, DH regions, 134
mouse germline JH, DH regions, 132–133
murine germline V_κ locus, 133–134
of murine VH locus, 132
Germline STAT1 mutation, primary immunodeficiency and, 1610
Gerontology. *See* Aging
Giardia parasite, 1171, 1182, 1190
Gi-dependent effectors, chemokines, 809–811
Gi-independent effectors, chemokines, 811
Gld mice, systemic autoimmunity, 1388
Glick, Bruce, 38
Global Alliance for Vaccines and Immunization, 1327–1328, 1330
Global impact of parasitic disease, 1172
Globular head C1q receptor, 1092
Glucocorticoids
dysregulation, immune-mediated diseases, 1030–1037
effect on adhesion molecule, 1027
effect on apoptosis, 1030
effect on basophils, 1029
effect on cell cycle arrest, 1030
effect on cell migration, 1029
effect on chemoattractants, 1029
effect on eosinophils, 1029
effect on inflammatory mediator production, 1029
effect on mast cells, 1029
effect on monocytes, 1029
effect on neutrophils, 1029
effect on resident tissue immune cells, 1030
effect on thymic regulation of T-cell selection, 1030
lymphocyte selection, 1030
molecular mechanisms of action, 1026–1027
resistance, inflammatory/autoimmune disease, 1033
Th cells, antigen-driven selection, 218–219
Glycophosphatidylinositol toxin, 1360
vaccine, 1360
Glycoprotein 130, receptors with similarities to, 715–716

Good, Robert, 38
Goodman, Howard, 33
Goodpasture, Ernest, 1322
gp130, cytokines, receptors sharing, 713
G-protein signaling, chemokines, 809
Gradient sensing, mechanisms of, chemokines, 811
Graft rejection, 35–36
components of immune system in, 1496–1500
antibodies, 1498
antigen-presenting cells, 1496–1498
B-cells, 1498
T-cells, 1498–1499
diagnosis of, 1546
donor antigens, 1489–1496
major histocompatibility antigens, 1489–1493
minor histocompatibility antigens, 1493–1494
mechanisms of, 1500–1513
accelerated rejection, 1502–1503
acute rejection, 1503–1511
chronic rejection, 1511–1513
hyperacute rejection, 1500–1502
induced antibodies, 1502–1503
preformed antibodies, 1500–1502
T-cells, 1503–1511
physiologic interactions, 1513–1518
effector cell regulation, 1517–1518
helper, effector cells, communication between, 1515–1517
sensitization, regulation of, 1513–1515
prevention of, 1518–1535
donor-specific tolerance induction, 1520–1535
nonspecific techniques, 1518–1520
Graft survival, minipigs, antigen matching in, 1544
Graft tolerance, 35–36
Graft *versus* host disease, chronic, 1386–1387
Graft-*versus*-host disease
cytotoxic T-lymphocytes, 1143–1144
increase in with age, 1047
Graft-*versus*-leukemia T-cells, in immunotherapy, 1647
Graft-*versus*-tumor effects, in immunotherapy, 1647
Gram-negative extracellular bacteria, bacterial surface structure of, 1265–1267
Gram-positive extracellular bacteria, bacterial surface structure of, 1265–1267
Grant, James, 1324
Granule exocytosis, cytotoxic mechanism, 1134–1140
adhesion, 1134–1135
caspase-dependent, independent pathways, target death, 1139
detachment, 1139
effector polarization, 1135–1136
exocytosis, 1137

granzymes, in target death, 1137–1138
perforin-mediated granzyme entry, 1138–1139
self-protection, 1139–1140
signaling exocytosis, 1137
Granule membrane proteins, cytotoxic T-lymphocytes, 1133–1134
Granulomatous lesion, intracellular bacteria, 1253–1255
granuloma formation, 1254
leukocyte extravasation, 1253–1254
tuberculosis, 1254–1255
Granulysin, 1133
Granzymes, 1131–1132
lymphocyte, 1132
Group A streptococci vaccine, 1349
Gut disorders, autoimmune, 1430
Gut-associated lymphoepithelial tissue, 977–978
mucosal immunity, 977–978
GVHD. *See* Graft-*versus*-host disease
GVP, Global Programme for Vaccines and Immunization

H

H-2 complex
locus, major histocompatibility complex, mutations at, 589–590
recombinant strains, 1490
H-2^b haplotype mutants, sequence changes, major histocompatibility complex, 589
H2-M3, major histocompatibility complex, 598
class Ib, 598
Haemophilus ducreyi, 1267, 1277
infections, 1264
Haemophilus influenzae, 1267, 1268, 1269, 1277
infections, 1264
type B, 1267
vaccine, 1322–1323, 1329, 1342, 1347–1348
Hairpins, V gene assembly recombination, 120–121
Halothane hepatitis, 1423
Hantavirus, 1201–1203
Haptens
antigenic determinant recognition, 631–632
inhibition, analysis of salmonella O-antigen structure by, 634
Haurowitz, Felix, 23, 29, 33, 34
HcRn, histocompatibility complex molecules, 599
Heart, autoimmune diseases of, 1430
Heart transplantation, 1536
Heat-shock proteins
in immunotherapy, 1650–1651
Heavy chain genes, 111–114
membrane *versus* secreted immunoglobulin, 112–113
organization of CH gene loci, 113–114

Heavy-chain switch
  assaying switch recombination, 139
  B-cell-specific, *versus* ubiquitously
      expressed components of class switch
      recombination machinery, 142
  germinal centers, switch regions, 138–139
  isotype switching by CD40, 139–140
  isotype-specific regulation of germline
      transcripts, 140–141
  non-"standard" isotype switching, 143–144
  sterile transcription in class switch
      recombination, 141
  targeting class switch recombination to
      switch regions, 141–142
Hedrick, Steve, 41
Heidelberger, Michael, 34
Hektoen, Ludwig, 31
Helical-bundle cytokines, 703
Helicobacter pylori, 1267, 1273
  infections, 1264
  vaccine, 1345–1347
Heligomosoides polygyrus, 1181, 1182
Helminths, vaccination, 1193–1194
Helper T-cells, 14–15
  cell differentiation, antigen-specific T-cell
      help, recruitment of, 213–214
  clones, mucosal, 983–984
  epitopes, B-cell epitopes, relationship
      between, 671–673
  mucosal, CD4+, 983–984
  subsets, regulation of mucosal immunity
      by, 987–988
  Th cells, glucocorticoid, 218–219
  Th1, 734–735, 1027
    activities, intracellular bacteria,
        1251–1252
    glucocorticoid effect on, 1027
    imbalanced, cell-cytokine network, 1002
    responses, chronic, pathogenesis of,
        1186–1188
    role in mucosally-induced tolerance, 983
    subsets, 983
  Th2, 734–735, 1027
    cell development, factors contributing to,
        allergic disorders, 1445–1450
    cells, as effector cells, in allergic
        disorders, 1468–1469
    cytokine regulation of allergic
        inflammation, 1452–1453
    differentiation
      cytokine regulation, in allergic
          disorders, 1450–1452
      potential dysregulation of, allergic
          disorders, 1450–1451
    glucocorticoid effect on, 1027
    imbalanced, cell-cytokine network, 1002
    responses, chronic, pathogenesis of,
        1188–1190
    role in mucosally-induced tolerance, 983
    subsets, 983
  Th3
    mucosal immune system, 984–985
    role in mucosal immunity, 984–985

Helper T-regulated B-cell responses,
    211–221
Hemagglutination, 94
  antigen-antibody inhibition, 94
  antigen-antibody interactions, 94
Hematopoiesis
  age-related changes in, 1064–1065
  chemokine regulation, 812–814
    CXCL12, in myelopoiesis, 812–813
    myelosuppressive chemokines,
        813
    phagocyte positioning in peripheral
        tissue, 814
    T-lymphopoiesis, 814
  in evolution of immune response, 552–553
  regulation, myelopoiesis, 812–813
Hematopoietic cell transplantation,
    1537–1539
Hemochromatosis, human leukocyte antigen
    associations, 588
Henderson
  D.A., 1323, 1324
  R.H., 1324
Hepadnaviruses, 1202
Hepatitis
  autoimmune, 1420–1421
  halothane, 1423
Hepatitis A, 1214
  transmission of, 1203
  vaccine, 1329, 1350–1351
Hepatitis B
  transmission of, 1203
  vaccine, 1322–1323, 1329, 1342,
      1350–1351
Hepatitis c, 1215
Hepatitis C, vaccine, 1350–1351
Herpes simplex virus, 1215, 1219
Herpesviruses, 1202, 1204, 1215
  keratitis, 1425
Heterodimers, 705–706
Hib. *See Haemophilus influenzae,* type b
High-affinity foreign peptide-major
    histocompatibility complex ligands
  particulate antigens, 307–308
  presentation of, 307–309
  skin-surface antigens, 308
  soluble antigens, 308–309
Hill, A.V.S., 1360
Hinge, immunoglobulin, 56–58
Hinges
  immunoglobulin, 56–58
  immunoglobulin A, properties of, 57
  immunoglobulin D, properties of, 57
  immunoglobulin G, properties of, 57
Hirszfeld
  Hanna, 30
  Ludwik, 30
Histamine
  inflammation, 1155
  in inflammation, 1155
Histocompatibility, 39–41
Histocompatibility testing
  family studies, 586–587

major histocompatibility complex, family
    studies in, 586–587
History of immunology, 23–46
  acquired immunodeficiency syndrome,
      41–42
  allergy, 29–30
  antibody globulins, chemistry of, 31–34
    myeloma proteins, 34
  antibody production, 26–27
    template theory, 27–29
  blood groups, 30–31
  cellular immunology, 34–39
    clonal selection theory, 36–38
    graft rejection, 35–36
    lymphocytes, 38
    monoclonal antibodies, 38–39
    thymus, biology of, 38
    tolerance, graft, 35–36
  colloid chemistry, 27–29
  graft rejection, 35–36
  histocompatibility, 39–41
  League of Nations, 30
  molecular immunology, 39–41
  selection theories, 34–39
  serology, age of, 25–31
  side-chain theory, 26–27
  T-cell receptor, 39–41
  template theory, antibody production,
      27–29
  transfusion, 30–31
  vaccination, 23–25
HIV. *See* Human immunodeficiency virus
HLA. *See* Human leukocyte antigen
HLA-DM, effect of, on peptide on rates, off
    rates for binding to HLA-DR1, 658
Hodgkin's disease, human leukocyte antigen
    associations, 588
Hoffman, S.L., 1360
Homeostasis
  cellular, in multicellular organisms,
      841–842
  immune system, cytotoxic T-lymphocytes,
      1141–1142
Homodimers, 705–706
Hood, Leroy, 40
Hormonal stress response, 1031
Hormones, aging and, 1066
Host cells, intracellular bacteria, 1233–
    1240
HPV. *See* Human papillomavirus
HSPs. *See* Heat-shock proteins
Human autoimmune disorders, features of,
    1382–1387
Human cytomegalovirus, 1217
Human external secretions,
    immunoglobulins, 971
Human immunodeficiency virus, 1285–1318.
    See also Acquired immunodeficiency
    syndrome
  antiretroviral therapy, 1288
  B lymphocytes, 1297–1298
  CD4+ T-cells, 1293–1296
    mechanisms of depletion, 1293–1296

CD8+ T-cells, 1296
cellular activation, role of, 1307
cellular immune responses, 1299–1302
  CD4+ T-cell responses, 1302
  cytotoxic T-lymphocytes, 1299–1301
  soluble CD8+ T-cell secreted factors,
    1301–1302
central nervous system, cytokine network
  in, 1312
chemokines, 824–826, 1307–1312
cytokines, 1307–1312
  anti-inflammatory cytokines, 1310
  chemokines, 1310–13112
  colony-stimulating factors, 1310
  interferons, 1310
  proinflammatory cytokines, 1309–1310
dendritic cells, 1296–1297
effect on cytokine production, 1311–1312
epidemiology, 1286
genetic factors, 1302–1303
historical overview of, 42
humoral immune responses, 1299
immune dysfunction caused by, 1292–
  1298
immune responses, 1298–1302
long-term nonprogressors, 1303–1305
  host genetic factors, 1303–1304
  host immune-response factors,
    1304–1305
  virologic factors, 1305
macrophages, 1298
monocytes, 1298
natural killer cells, 1298
nonprogression with, possible mechanisms
  of, 1303
polymorphonuclear leukocytes, 1298
potential reservoirs of, 1289
prophylactic vaccine against, 1354–1357
reservoirs of, 1288–1292
  central nervous system, 1292
  lymphoid tissue, 1290–1291
  macrophages, 1291–1292
  monocytes, 1291–1292
  peripheral blood dendritic cells, 1291
  reproductive tract, 1292
  resting CD4+ T-cells, 1291
spectrum of, 1286–1288
  advanced, 1287–1288
  chronic/persistent infection, 1287
  long-term nonprogression, 1288
  primary infection, 1286–1287
therapeutic vaccine, 1357
type 1, 1005, 1203
vaccine, 1305–1307
virus replication, immune system-mediated
  restriction of, evasion of, proposed
  mechanisms, 1300
Human leukocyte antigen. See also Major
  histocompatibility complex
class I alleles, 574–575
genetic basis of structural variation on,
  582
nomenclature, 573

Human leukocyte antigen alleles
  class I, listing of, 574
  class II, listing of, 575
Human leukocyte antigen compatibility,
  major histocompatibility complex,
  587
  functional tests of, 587
Human leukocyte antigen gene products,
  major histocompatibility complex,
  codominant expression, 590
Human leukocyte subsets, resting, chemokine
  receptors, 834
Human monoclonal antibodies, production
  of, 99–100
Human papillomaviruses, 1214
Human primary immunodeficiency,
  molecular defects causing, 1596
Human T-cell leukemia viruses, 1214
Humanized monoclonal antibodies, 99–100
Humoral mechanisms, parasites, 1173–1174
Humphrey, John, 38
HVEM ligand, 759
Hybridomas, derivation of, 96–98
  gene libraries to derive monoclonal
    antibodies, 97–98
  from species other than mice, 97
Hyper immunoglobulin M, 1597–1598
Hyper-immunoglobulin M syndrome, 403
Hyperimmunoglobulinemia E syndrome,
  1612–1613
  STAT4 knockout mice, 1613
Hypermutation, 562–563
  BCR diversification and, 218
  mismatch repair in, 149
  molecular mechanism, 147–149
    DNA breaks in V regions, 147–148
    error-prone polymerases, 148–149
  role of, 144–145
  somatic, role of, 144–145
Hypersensitivity
  cytotoxic mediators, cytotoxic
    T-lymphocytes, 1144
  delayed type, stress effects on, 1034
Hypothalamic pituitary adrenal axis,
  1030–1031
autoimmune inflammatory disease,
  1032
blunted, genetic animal models, 1032
glucocorticoid dysregulation, immune-
  mediated diseases, 1030–1037
interruption
  immune-mediated diseases, 1037
  surgical, pharmacologic, effects on
    autoimmune/inflammatory disease,
    1032–1033
pathologic conditions associated with
  dysregulation of, 1031–1034
pathophysiologic role, 1030–1037
regulation of immune responses by, 1031
role of, in inflammation, 1035–1036
in septic shock, 1035–1036
surgical interruption of, effects on
  autoimmune disease, 1032–1044

I
IBD. See Inflammatory bowel disease
ICOS:ICOSL, pathway, therapeutic
  manipulation of, 399–400
Id vaccine, 1648–1649
IDDM. See Insulin-dependent diabetes
  mellitus
IELs. See Intraepithelial lymphocytes
IFN. See Interferon
IgA. See Immunoglobulin A
IgD. See Immunoglobulin D
IgE. See Immunoglobulin E
IgM. See Immunoglobulin M
IL-1. See Interleukin-1
IL-2. See Interleukin-2
IL-4, 716
IL-6. See Interleukin-6
IL-7, 716
IL-8. See Interleukin-8
IL-10. See Interleukin-10
IL-12. See Interleukin-12
IL-19, 720
IL-20, 720
IL-22, 720
IL-23, 715
IL-24, 720
IL-26, 720
IL-27, 715–716
IMD, pathways, in evolution of immune
  response, 559
Idiotype infusion, systemic autoimmunity
  induced by, 1389
Immature B-cells, generation of, 172
Immune complex-mediated inflammation,
  696–697
Immune effector mechanism, programmed
  cell death as, 847
Immune escape, dendritic cells, 468
Immune evasion, parasites, mechanisms of,
  1183–1185
Immune injury, 1390–1391
Immune regulation, programmed cell death,
  842–847
Immune response
  chemokines, chemokine regulation of,
    814–816
    innate immunity, 814–816
    CXCL8, 814–815
    mononuclear phagocytes, 815–816
    NK cells, 815
  macrophages, 481–495
    activation, modulation of, in vitro,
      492–493
    activation in vivo, 489–490
    differentiation, 483–484
    fetal liver, 485
    gene expression, secretion, 492
    lymph nodes, 488
    nonlymphoid organs, 488–489
    Peyer's patch, 488
    phagocytic recognition, 490–492
    properties, 483–493
    research landmarks, 481–483

Immune response (*contd.*)
spleen, 486–488
marginal zone macrophages, 487–488
red pulp macrophages, 488
white pulp macrophages, 488
thymus, 485–486
tissue distribution, 484–489
mucosal, 995–1000
antigen-delivery systems, 998–1000
genital tract, immune responses in, 997–998
intestinal infections, 995–996
mucosal adjuvants, 998–1000
nasal immunization, 996–997
Immune suppression *vs.* immunodeficiency, tumor formation and, 1584–1585
carcinogens, 1584
tumor burden, 1584–1585
Immune synapse II, antigen-primed B-cells, 214–216
Immune synapse IV, response to antigen recall, 220–221
Immune system, 1–22
B lymphocytes, 3–11
activation, 5–6, 195–225, 472–473, 1064, 1209–1210
affinity maturation, 10–11
B1 B, 7, 160, 164, 165, 172, 174–177, 179, 182, 183, 209–210
development, 3–5, 159–195
differentiation, 6–7
signaling, 195–227
somatic hypermutation, 10–11. *See also* Hypermutation; Somatic hypermutation
tolerance, 7–8, 906–909, 918–919, 921–929
cells of, 3. *See also under* specific cell
chemokines, 16, 801–840
class switching, 10, 138–144
complement system, 21–22, 1077–1103
cytokines, 16, 702–706, 718–721, 732–733, 1248–1251, 1307–1312, 1380
deficiency of. *See* Immunodeficiency
effector mechanisms, 19–22
basophils, 20
eosinophils, 21
granulocytes, 20
macrophages, 20
mast cells, 20
monocytes, 20
natural killer cells, 20
evolution of, 519–570
adaptive immune responses, 546–550
agnathia, 546–547
amphibians, 548–549
birds, 549–550
bony fish, 547–548
cartilaginous fish, 547
mammals, 549–550
reptiles, 549

adaptive immune system, components of, 521–553
adaptive immunity, origins of, 561–565
allorecognition, 560–561
chemokines, 550–552
cytokines, 550–552
defensins, 555–556
hematopoiesis, 552–553
IL-1, 550
IL-8, 550
IMD pathways, 559
immunoglobulin superfamily, 555
immunoglobulins, 526–532
gene organization, 532
chondrichthyan germline-joined genes, 532
organization of rearranging genes, 532
immunoglobulin D homologues, 527
immunoglobulin heavy-chain isotypes, 526
immunoglobulin light chains, 531
immunoglobulin M, 526
immunoglobulin NAR, 526
immunoglobulin R/immunoglobulin NARC/immunoglobulin W/immunoglobulin X, 527
J chain, 531–532
V_H regions, 528–429
D segments, 528
J segments, 528
V_H evolution, 528–531
inflammatory cytokines, 550
innate immunity, evolution of, 553–561
interferons, 551
interleukin 2, 550–551
invertebrate cells, 553–554
lectins, 555
lymphocyte differentiation
amphibians, 545
bony fish, 544–545
cartilaginous fish, 544
chickens, 545–546
mammals, 546
rearrangement, diversification of TCR, immunoglobulin genes, 544–546
lymphoid tissues, 541–544
amphibians, 542–543
birds, 543–544
bony fish, 541–542
cartilaginous fish, 541
reptiles, 543–544
major histocompatibility complex, 532–541
class I/II expression, 540–541
class I/II structure, 532–535
classical, nonclassical class I, chain II, 535
disease associations, 537–538
gene organization, 539–540

locus complexity, selection on, 539
mating preferences, 538–539
polymorphism, genes, 535–537
major histocompatibility complex origins, 561–562
parasites, recognition of, 559–560
parasitoids, recognition of, 559–560
pentraxins, 555
phagocytosis, 558
proteolytic cascades, 556–558
RAG, 553
rearranging receptors
antigen receptor, 563
C1 domain, 563
hypermutation and, 562–563
origins of, 562–565
rearranging machinery, 562
V, VC1 segments, 563–565
V domain, 563
V segment, 563–565
VC1 segment, 563–565
signaling, 558–560
T-cell receptors, 521–526
α/β constant domains, 523–524
α/β variable domains, 524–525
CD3 complex, 525–526
ϵ/δ TCR, 525
TdT, 553
TNF, 550
toll, pathways, 559
transforming growth factor β, 551–552
immunity, principles of, 3
immunoglobulins
genetics, 9, 107–158
structure, 8–9, 47–68
innate immunity, 1–2, 497–517, 814–816. *See also* Innate immunity
aging and, 1050–1053
immunosurveillance, 1572–1573
intracellular bacterial infection, 1251–1252
recognition, viral, 1204–1205
major histocompatibility complex, 16–19, 571–612
antigen processing, 16–19, 613–629
antigen-presenting cells, 19. *See also* Dendritic cells
class I molecules, 16–17, 571–612
class II molecules, 17–18, 571–612
presentation, 18–19
T-lymphocyte recognition of, restricted recognition, 18–19
mucosal, 965–1020
response characteristics, 1–3. *See also* Immune response
acquired immunodeficiency syndrome, 2–3, 1285–1318
autoimmune disease
organ-specific autoimmunity, 1401–1438
systemic autoimmunity, 1371–1399
immunologic memory, 2, 865–899, 1211–1212. *See also* Memory

factors contributing to, 881
longevity of, 865–866
primary, 2. *See also* B lymphocyte
    development; Lymphoid tissues;
    Peripheral T-lymphocytes
secondary, 2. *See also* B lymphocyte
    development; Immunologic
    memory; Lymphoid tissues;
    Peripheral T-lymphocytes
self-antigen tolerance, 2, 901–934
specificity of, 2
suppression of. *See* Immunosuppression
T lymphocytes, 11–16
    activation, 13, 321–363
    antigen recognition, 11, 571–629
    cytotoxic, 15–16, 1127–1150
    development, 13–14, 259–301
    functions, 14, 303–319
    helpers, 14–15
    receptors, 11–13, 227–258
    regulatory, 15, 935–963
Immune therapy, programmed cell death as,
    858
Immunization
    expanded program on, 1324–1325.
        See also Vaccination
    "prime-boost" strategies, 1334
    schedule, standard, 1342
Immunoblot, 94–95
Immunocompetence, immunogenicity and,
    1577
Immunoconjugates, 1636–1643
    antibody-directed enzyme prodrug therapy,
        1640
    immunoliposomes, 1641–1642
    immunotoxins, 1637–1638
        fusion toxins, 1638
    monoclonal antibody-cytokine conjugates,
        1642
    monoclonal antibody-drug conjugates,
        1639–1640
    monoclonal antibody-photosensitizer
        conjugates, 1642
    monoclonal antibody-RNAse conjugates,
        1642
    monoclonal antibody-superantigen
        conjugates, 1642
    radioimmunoconjugates, 1640–1641
Immunodeficiency
    with cancer, 1584–1585
    malignant neoplasms, with increased
        incidence with, 1571
    primary, molecular defects causing, 1596
    replacement therapy in, 1632
    vs. immune suppression, tumor formation
        and, 1584–1585
        carcinogens, 1584
        tumor burden, 1584–1585
Immunodeficiency disease, primary,
    1593–1620
    ataxia-telangiectasia, 1607
    autosomal recessive aϵglobulinemia, 1597
    cartilage-hair hypoplasia, 1608

CD40, mutations in, 1599
CD154 deficiency, 1597–1598
cellular immunodeficiency, 1602–1603
Chediak-Higashi syndrome, 1610–1611
combined immunodeficiency, 1603–1611,
    1606–1611
    autosomal recessive, 1603–1605
    severe combined immunodeficiency,
        1603–1606
    X-linked recessive, 1603
common variable immunodeficiency,
    1600–1601
cytidine deaminase deficiency,
    activation-induced, 1598–1599
eczema, immunodeficiency with,
    1607–1608
germline STAT1 mutation,
    1610
hyper immunoglobulin M, 1597–1598
hyperimmunoglobulinemia E syndrome,
    1612–1613
    STAT4 knockout mice, 1613
immunoglobulin A deficiency, selective,
    1601–1602
immunoglobulin G subclass deficiencies,
    1602
interferon-ϵ receptor mutations, 1610
interleukin-2 receptor α-chain mutation,
    1609–1610
interleukin-12, 1610
    receptor β1 mutations, 1610
leukocyte adhesion deficiency, 1609
lymphoproliferative disease, X-linked,
    1599–1600
major histocompatibility complex antigens,
    defective expression of, 1608–1609
molecular genetics, 1594–1595
    human immunodeficiency diseases,
        1594–1595
Nijmegen breakage syndrome, 1608
nuclear factor κB essential modulator
    deficiency, 1598
purine nucleoside phosphorylase
    deficiency, 1606–1607
T-cell activation defects, 1611–1612
    CD8 deficiency, from CD8α gene
        mutation, 2612
    CD8 lymphocytopenia, from
        ζ-chain-associated protein
        deficiency, 1611–1612
    defective cytokine production, 1612
    T-cell receptor-CD3 complex, defective
        expression of, 1612
thrombocytopenia, immunodeficiency
    with, 1607–1608
thymoma, immunodeficiency with,
    1602
X-linked
    aϵglobulinemia, 1595–1596
    in mice, 1596–1597
Immunodiffusion, 91–92
Immunodominant determinants, steps
    focusing T-cell response on, 648–668

Immunodominant T-cell epitopes, major
    histocompatibility complex class II,
    molecules, examples of, 648
Immunoelectrophoresis, 92–94
Immunogenetics, discoveries of, 1483–1489
Immunogenicity
    antigen structure, 631–683
    antigen processing, 649–654
        influence on expressed T-cell
            repertoire, 649–651
    antigenic determinants recognized by
        antibodies, 631–637
        carbohydrate antigens, 632–637
            blood group antigens, 634–635
            dextran-binding myeloma proteins,
                635–637
            immunochemistry of salmonella O
                antigens, 632–634
        haptens, 631–632
    antigenic structures, mapping, 646–648
        monoclonal T-cells, 647–648
        polyclonal T-cell response, 646–647
    class II major histocompatibility
        complex, transport pathways
        leading to presentation, 657–658
    class II major histocompatibility
        complex molecules, processing of
        antigen for T-cells restricted to,
        651–653
    helper T-cell epitopes, B-cell epitopes,
        relationship between, 671–673
    immunodominant determinants, steps
        focusing T-cell response on,
        648–668
    major histocompatibility complex
        binding, 658–664
    major histocompatibility complex
        class I, transport pathways leading
        to presentation, 654–657
    major histocompatibility complex class I
        molecules, T-cells restricted to,
        processing of antigen, 653–654
    major histocompatibility complex
        molecules, antigen interaction with,
        658–664
    polysaccharide immunogenicity,
        637–646
        epitopes, mapping of, 638–641
        native proteins, antipeptide antibodies
        binding, at specific site,
        642–643
        peptides, immunogenicity of,
        643–646
        protein
            peptide antigenic determinants,
                conformational equilibria,
                641–642
            polypeptide antigenic determinants,
                637–646
        proteins, immunogenicity of, 643–646
    stable major histocompatibility
        complex/peptide complex,
        assembly of, 658–664

Immunogenicity (*contd.*)
  T-cell epitopes, prediction of, 668–671
  T-cell receptor recognition, 664–668
    amino acid substitution
      altered peptide ligands, effects of, 666–668
      mapping by, 666–668
    epitope mapping, 665–666
    T-cells, antigenic determinants recognized by, 646–671
  carcinogen dose, 1577
  factors influencing, 1576–1577
  immunocompetence, 1577
  spontaneous, induced cancers, contrasted, 1576–1577
  tumor latency, 1577
Immunoglobulin, intravenous
  for autoimmune disorders, 1628
  in immunotherapy, 1632–1633
Immunoglobulin A, 60–61
  biological properties of, 973
  cytokines inducing switches to, 986–987
  functions/biological properties of, 973
  hinges in, properties of, 57
  mucosal
    α chains, 971–972
    assembly of, 972–973
    J chain, 972
    origin, 974–976
    polymeric, receptor expression, 975–976
    secretory component, 972
    structure of, 971–973
    transport, cellular interactions, 975
  mucosal immune system, 986–987
  secretory, structure of, secretory components, 972
  transport, 974–976
Immunoglobulin A deficiency
  mucosal immune system, 1004–1005
  selective, 1601–1602
Immunoglobulin A dermatoses, 1430
Immunoglobulin A isotype switching, mucosal immune system, 985–987
Immunoglobulin A production, cytokine regulation of, mucosal immune system, 988–989
Immunoglobulin A receptors, mucosal immune system, 976
Immunoglobulin class switching, 10, 138–144
Immunoglobulin crystallized fragment receptors, 1109–1111
Immunoglobulin D, 60
  hinges in, properties of, 57
Immunoglobulin domain, immunoglobulins, 49–51
Immunoglobulin E, 61
Immunoglobulin E receptors, in allergic disorders, 1456
Immunoglobulin E synthesis, in allergic disorders, 1453–1458
  deletional switch recombination, 1455–1456

isotype class switching, 1453–1455
  negative regulation of, 1456
Immunoglobulin G, 61–63
  hinges in, properties of, 57
  in immunotherapy, 1632–1635
Immunoglobulin G subclass deficiencies, 1602
Immunoglobulin H chain
Immunoglobulin heavy chain, 169–172
Immunoglobulin isotypes
  distribution of, mucosal immune system, 981
  mucosal, distribution of, 971
Immunoglobulin M, 58–60
Immunoglobulin rearrangement, 168–169
Immunoglobulin superfamily, in evolution of immune response, 555
Immunoglobulins, 47–68
  antigen-antibody interactions, 55–56
  CDR regions, immunoglobulin chains, residues defining framework, 53
  evolution and, 64
  in evolution of immune response, 526–532
    gene organization, 532
      chondrichthyan germline-joined genes, 532
      organization of rearranging genes, 532
    immunoglobulin D homologues, 527
    immunoglobulin heavy-chain isotypes, 526
    immunoglobulin light chains, 531
    immunoglobulin M, 526
    immunoglobulin NAR, 526
    immunoglobulin R/immunoglobulin NARC/immunoglobulin W/immunoglobulin X, 527
    J chain, 531–532
    V_H regions, 528–429
      D segments, 528
      J segments, 528
      V_H evolution, 528–531
  FAB, structure, function, 51–55
  Fc, structure, 58
  Fc receptors, 63
  genetics, 9, 107–158
  higher-order structure, 63–64
  historical perspective, 48
  in human external secretions, 971
  immunoglobulin A, 60–61
    hinges in, properties of, 57
  immunoglobulin D, 60
    hinges in, properties of, 57
  immunoglobulin domain, 49–51
  immunoglobulin E, 61
  immunoglobulin G, 61–63
    hinges in, properties of, 57
  immunoglobulin hinge, 56–58
  immunoglobulin isotypes, properties of, 59
  immunoglobulin M, 58–60
  levels of, in human external secretions, 971
  molecular genetics, 107–158
    gene alterations, in germinal centers, 137–149

heavy-chain switch, 138–144
  assaying switch recombination, 139
  isotype switching by CD40, 139–140
  isotype-specific regulation of germline transcripts, 140–141
  non-"standard" isotype switching, 143–144
  sterile transcription in class switch recombination, 141
  switch junctions, 138–139
  switch regions, 138–139
  targeting class switch recombination to switch regions, 141–142
  somatic mutation, 144–149
    cellular context of, 145
    early evidence for, 144
    hypermutation, role of, 144–145
    molecular mechanism of hypermutation, 147–149
      DNA breaks in V regions, 147–148
      error-prone polymerases, 148–149
    targeting, distribution of mutations, 145–147
  gene expression, regulation of, 135–137
  gene loci, 111–116
    heavy chain genes, 111–114
      membrane *versus* secreted immunoglobulin, 112–113
      organization of CH gene loci, 113–114
    κ-light-chain genes, 114
    λ light-chain genes, 114–116
      human λ locus, 115–116
      murine λ locus, 114–115
    λ-related "surrogate" light chains, 116
  germline diversity, 132–135
    combinatorial diversity estimates, 135
    human germline VH locus, 134
    human germline V_κ locus, 134–135
    human JH, DH regions, 134
    mouse germline JH, DH regions, 132–133
    murine germline V_κ locus, 133–134
    of murine VH locus, 132
  somatic mutation, molecular mechanism of hypermutation, mismatch repair in somatic hypermutation, 149
  V gene assembly
    overview, 108–111
    recombination
      diversity and, 109–111
      signal elements, 111
    Southern blot tests, gene cloning, 108–109
  V gene assembly recombination, 116–132
    allelic exclusion, 128–130
    B lymphocyte development, 126–127

B-cell maturation, B-cell receptor
    regulation of, 130
hairpins, 120–121
late recombination activating gene
    expression, 130–132
mechanisms, 119–126
P nucleotides, 120–121
receptor editing, 130–132
receptor revision, 130–132
recombination activating gene
    proteins, V-D-J recombination,
    121–123
recombination intermediates, 120–121
recombination model, 119
recombinational accessibility,
    127–128
regulated V(D)J recombination,
    128–130
regulation, 126–132
substrates, experiments, 119–120
topology, 116–117
    deletion versus inversion, 116–117
    secondary recombinations,
        117–118
transcription, 127–128
V-D-J recombination
    artemis, 124–125
    DNA breaks, proteins binding to,
        125
    DNA-PK, 123–124
    exonuclease, 125–126
    Ku, 123–124
    N regions, 125
    terminal deoxynucleotide
        transferase, 125
    XRCC4, 123–124
nomenclature, 48–49
structure, 8–9, 47–68
Immunoliposomes, in immunotherapy,
    1641–1642
Immunologic memory, 865–899. See also
    Memory
B-cell memory, maintenance of, 888
factors contributing to, 881
factors contributing to memory, 881–884
    effector activity, continued expression
        of, 881–882
    memory cells, altered properties of,
        883–884
    naive state, memory, systemic
        differences between, 882–883
generation of memory, 866–878
longevity of, 865–866
    after virus infection, 866
maintenance of memory, 885–888
memory B-cells
    generation of, 874–878
    identification of, 880–881
    life span of, 885
memory cells
    identifying, 878–881
    life span, turnover of, 884–885
memory T-cells

generation of, 867–874
identification of, 878–880
life span of, 884–885
T-cell memory, maintenance of, 885–888
viruses, 1211–1212
Immunologic tolerance, 901–934. See also
    Tolerance
activation, versus tolerance thresholds, 905
activation thresholds, T-cell tuning of,
    905–906
as adaptive process, 901–902
antigen-presenting cell
    role of, 915–921
B-cell compartment, negative selection,
    906–907
B-cells, mature, tolerance induction,
    921–925
    B-cell anergy, 922–924
        clonal deletion, 924
        thymic-independent antigens, 924–925
    receptor blockade, 921–922
bone marrow, mechanisms of negative
    selection in, 907
CD4+CD25+ suppressor T-cells, 914–915
CD8+ cytotoxic T-cells, 920–921
CD28/B7, CD40/CD40L co-stimulation,
    918–919
CTLA-4, PD-1 coinhibition, T-cell
    activation, 919–920
fetal-maternal relationship, 929–931
heat-shock proteins, 916–917
immature B-cells, 908–909
immune-privileged sites, 929
immunoregulation, 926–929
    antibody-mediated immunoregulation,
        928
    anti-idiotypic B-cell regulation, 928–929
    anti-idiotypic T-cell regulation, 929
    CD4+ T-regulatory 1 cells, 926–927
    CD8+ suppressor T-cells, 927–928
    CD8+ veto cells, 928
    immune deviation, 926
    nasal tolerance, 927
    oral tolerance, 927
negative selection
    antigen-presenting cells for, 903–904
    during B-cell development, 906–909
    B-cells, antigen characteristics required
        for, 907–908
Nods, receptors, 916–917
OX40/OX40L, ICOS/ICOSL
    co-stimulation, 919
peripheral antigens, tolerance to, 909–921
T-cell activation, "two-signal" model of,
    917–918
T-cell anergy, 912–914
T-cell development
    negative selection during, 902–906
    stages at which negative selection
        occurs, 903
thymocyte clonal detection, biochemical
    events in, 904–905
tissue-specific peptide antigens, 909–910

Immunological enhancement blocking
    factors, tumor formation and,
    1583–1584
Immunological function, major
    histocompatibility complex, 577–579
Immunology, history of, 23–46
    acquired immunodeficiency syndrome,
        41–42
    allergy, 29–30
    antibody globulins, chemistry of, 31–34
        myeloma proteins, 34
    antibody production, 26–27
        template theory, 27–29
    blood groups, 30–31
    cellular immunology, 34–39
        clonal selection theory, 36–38
        graft rejection, 35–36
        lymphocytes, 38
        monoclonal antibodies, 38–39
        thymus, biology of, 38
        tolerance, graft, 35–36
    colloid chemistry, 27–29
    histocompatibility, 39–41
    League of Nations, 30
    molecular immunology, 39–41
    selection theories, 34–39
    serology, age of, 25–31
    side-chain theory, 26–27
    T-cell receptor, 39–41
    template theory, antibody production,
        27–29
    transfusion, 30–31
    vaccination, 23–25
Immunology of aging, 1043–1075
Immunomodulators, 2622–1623
    bacillus Calmette-Guérin,
        Corynebacterium parvum, 1623
    Propionibacterium avidum, 1623
    Streptococcus pyogenes, 1623
Immunopathology, mucosal, 1004–1009
    human immunodeficiency virus type 1
        infection, 1005
    immunoglobulin A deficiency,
        1004–1005
    inflammatory bowel disease, 1005–1008
    mucosal allergies, 1008–1009
Immunoprevention. See also Vaccination
    cancer, 1585–1586, 1651
Immunoreceptor tyrosine-based activation
    motif pathways, 691–692
Immunoreceptor tyrosine-based inhibitor
    motif pathways, 692–693
Immunostimulatory complexes
    in vaccination, 1338
Immunostimulatory DNA sequences,
    microbial, mucosal immune system,
    999
Immunosuppression, in transplantation,
    1546
Immunosurveillance, tumor development,
    1571–1573
    adaptive T-cell-mediated, 1571–1572
    innate, 1572–1573

Immunotherapy, 1621–1659
  antibodies, 1628–1636
    affinity, 1629–1630
    bispecific monoclonal antibodies,
        1635–1636
    clinical considerations, 1629
    effector functions, 1630
    historical overview, 1628–1629
    immunogenicity, 1630
    immunoglobulin G, 1632–1635
    intravenous immunoglobulin,
        1632–1633
      mechanism of action, 1632–1633
    monoclonal antibodies, 1632–1635
      organ transplantation, 1635
    size, 1630
  bacteriolytic therapy
    muramyldipeptide derivatives, 1624
    trehalose dimycolate derivatives, 1624
    tumors, 1623–1624
  cancer, 1586–1588
  cellular strategies, 1643–1647
    cellular transfer, 1644–1645
      adoptive antigen-specific cytotoxic
          lymphocyte therapy, 1644–1645
      tumor-infiltrating lymphocytes, 1644
    dendritic cells, 1643–1644
    genetically engineered cells, 1645–1647
    graft-versus-leukemia T-cells, 1647
    graft-versus-tumor effects, 1647
    lymphokine-activated killer cells, 1643
    macrophage-active killer cells, 1644
    natural killer cells, 1643
    nonspecific cellular therapy, 1643
    regulatory T-cells, 1647
  cytokines, 1625–1628
  immunoconjugates, 1636–1643
    antibody-directed enzyme prodrug
        therapy, 1640
    immunoliposomes, 1641–1642
    immunotoxins, 1637–1638
      fusion toxins, 1638
    monoclonal antibody-cytokine
        conjugates, 1642
    monoclonal antibody-drug conjugates,
        1639–1640
    monoclonal antibody-photosensitizer
        conjugates, 1642
    monoclonal antibody-RNAse
        conjugates, 1642
    monoclonal antibody-superantigen
        conjugates, 1642
    radioimmunoconjugates, 1640–1641
  immunomodulators, 2622–1623
    bacillus Calmette-Guérin,
        Corynebacterium parvum, 1623
    Propionibacterium avidum, 1623
    Streptococcus pyogenes, 1623
  immunoprevention of cancer, 1651
  soluble co-stimulatory molecules, 1628
    anti-CD40L, 1628
  thymic hormones, analogs, 1625
  vaccination, 1647–1651

    anticytokine, 1649
    with defined antigens, 1648
      peptides, 1648
      proteins, 1648
    dendritic cell, 1650
    DNA, 1649–1650
    Id, 1648–1649
    recombinant bacterial, 1649
    recombinant viral vector, 1649
    synthetic carbohydrate antigen, 1649
    with unidentified antigens, 1650–1651
      autologous, allogeneic tumor cells,
          1650
      heat-shock proteins, 1650–1651
Immunotoxins, 1637–1638
  in clinical trials for cancer, 1639
  fusion toxins, 1638
  toxins used for preparation of, 1637
In autoimmunity, 403–404
In infection, 403
In inflammation, 1151–1170
In vivo studies, in vitro studies, contrasted,
    cytotoxicity, 1140–1141
Induced regulatory T-cells, 946–950
  anergic T-cell clones, regulatory function,
      949
  CD4+CD25+-like T-cells, generation in
      periphery, 949–950
  oral tolerance, 946–947
  pharmacological induction, 948–949
  T regulatory 1 cells, 947–948
Inductive sites, mucosal immune system,
    977–980
Inert microparticles
  mucosal immune system, 999–1000
  mucosal immunity, 999–1000
Infections, 1264. See also specific infections
Inflammation, 1151–1169
  acute inflammatory response, initiation of,
      1152–1153
  allergy and, 1160–1161
  blister fluid, soluble mediators in, temporal
      analysis of, 1161
  bone marrow, 1156–1157
  cellular mediators, acute inflammatory
      response, 1156–1160
    endothelial cells, 1160
    eosinophils, 1160
    monocytes, 1160
    neutrophils, 1156–1160
    platelets, 1160
  chronic inflammation, 1162–1163
  historical overview, 1151–1152
  human model systems of, 1161
  molecular mediators, acute inflammatory
      response, 1153–1156
    acute-phase reactants, 1155
    leptin, 1156
    lipid mediators, 1154–1155
    nitric oxide, 1155
    peptides, 1155
    plasma proteases, 1153–1154
    proinflammatory cytokines, 1155–1156

  murine models of, 1161
  neutrophil recruitment, activation, 1153
  novel anti-inflammatory therapies, 1163
  resolution of, 1162
    angiogenesis, 1162
    anti-inflammatory mediators, 1162
    apoptosis, 1162
    cell senescence, 1162
    hypothalamic-pituitary-adrenocortical
        axis, 1162
    wound repair, 1162
  sympathetic nervous system, 1035–1036
  vascular permeability, increased, 1153
  vasodilation, 1153
Inflammatory bowel disease
  animal models, 1006
  cytokines in treatment of, 950
  mucosal immune system, 1005–1008
  regulatory T-cells, 950–951
Inflammatory cytokines, in evolution of
    immune response, 550
Influenza vaccine, 1322, 1329, 1353–1354
Influenza virus, 1204, 1214
  transmission of, 1203
Inhibitors of complement activation, 1098
Inhibitory receptor expression during, NKC
    differentiation, 379
Innate immune recognition, 497–498
  strategies of, 497
  targets of, 498
Innate immune system, 497–517
  adaptive immunity, control of, 512–513
  cells of, 508–510
    dendritic cells, 509
    eosinophils, 509
    macrophages, 508–509
    mast cells, 509
    neutrophils, 509
    surface epithelium, 509–510
  effector mechanisms of, 510–512
    antiviral effector mechanisms of, 512
    BPI, 510
    calprotectin, 511
    cathelicidins, 511
    chitinases, 510
    defensins, 510–511
    lactoferrin, 511
    lysozyme, 510
    myeloperoxidase, 511–512
    nitric oxide synthase, 511–512
    NRAMP, 511
    oxidase, 511–512
    phagocyte, 511–512
    phospholipase A2, 510
    serprocedins, 511
  innate immune recognition, 497–498
    strategies of, 497
    targets of, 498
  intracellular recognition systems, 506–508
    2'-5'-oligoadenylate synthase, 507–508
    NOD family, 508
    PKR, 507
    RNaseL, 507–508

phagocytic receptors, 504–505
  β-glucan receptor, 505
  macrophage mannose receptor, 504–505
  scavenger receptors, 504
receptors of, 498–508
secreted pattern-recognition molecules,
    505–506
  BPI, 506
  collectins, 505–506
  C-reactive protein, 506
  LBP, 506
  PGRPs, 506
  serum amyloid A, 506
toll-like receptors, 499–504
  TKR4, 500–501
  TLR signaling pathways, 502–504
  TLR1, 501
  TLR2, 501
  TLR3, 501–502
  TLR5, 502
  TLR6, 501
  TLR9, 502
Innate immunity
  activation of, 212–213
  adaptive immunity, control of, 512–513
  age-related changes in, 1049–1055
  aging and, 1050–1053
  antiviral effector mechanisms of, 512
  cells of, 508–510
  effector mechanisms of, 510–512
  evolution of, 553–561
  immunosurveillance, 1572–1573
  intracellular bacterial infection, 1251–1252
  receptors, 498–508
  recognition, 497–498
    targets of, 498
    viral, 1204–1205
Insect venom allergens, 1444
Insulin receptor-substrate proteins, 733
Insulin-dependent diabetes mellitus
  human leukocyte antigen associations, 588
  regulatory T-cells, 951–952
Integrin complement receptors, 1111–1112
Interferon, 718–720, 1205
  cytokine receptors, 721
  in evolution of immune response, 551
  human immunodeficiency virus, 1310
  inhibition of, viral, 1222
Interferon-α, dendritic cells, 465–466
Interferon-ϵ receptor mutations, 1610
Interleukin-1, 775–799
  blocking in disease, 788–790
  cells producing interleukin-1 family
      members, 778
  cleavage, inhibition of
    viral, 1221–1222
    virus, 1221–1222
  in evolution of immune response, 550
  historical overview, 776
  interleukin-1 knockouts, effects in, 781
  interleukin-1 receptor family, 782–785
  interleukin-1 receptor type I, 783–785
    gene, surface regulation of, 785

interleukin-1 receptor type II, 785
interleukin-1 receptor type-I, deficient
    mice, 781–782
interleukin-1α
  autoantibodies to, 781
  autocrine growth factor, 780
interleukin-1α-, interleukin-1β-deficient
    mice, contrasted, 781
interleukin-1α-deficient mice, studies in,
    781
interleukin-1β, 780
interleukin-1β converting enzyme,
    779–780
interleukin-1β-deficient mice, 782
interleukin-18, 780
  binding protein, 785–786
membrane interleukin-1α, 780
P2X-7 receptor, 780
receptor antagonist, 790–794
  in animals, humans, 790–794
  interleukin-1 receptor antagonist,
      rheumatoid arthritis, 794
receptor type I, blocking in disease,
    788–789
signal transduction, 786–788
  cytoplasmic signaling cascades,
      786–787
  interleukin-1 receptor binding, activation
      of mitogen-activating protein
      kinases, 788
  interleukin-1 receptor type I
    cytoplasmic domain of, 787
    human abnormalities in expression,
        788
  kinases, 786
  MyD88, recruitment of, 787–788
  p38 mitogen-activating protein kinase
      activation, 788
    inhibition of, 788
  soluble receptor type I, effect in humans,
      789
  structures, 777–778
  transcriptional regulation, 778–779
Interleukin-1 knockouts, effects in,
    781
Interleukin-1 receptor binding, activation of
    mitogen-activating protein kinases,
    788
Interleukin-1 receptor type I, 783–785
  blocking in disease, 788–789
  cytoplasmic domain of, 787
  gene, surface regulation of, 785
  human abnormalities in expression, 788
  receptor antagonist, 790–794
    in animals, humans, 790–794
    interleukin-1 receptor antagonist,
        rheumatoid arthritis, 794
  soluble receptor type I, effect in humans,
      789
Interleukin-1 receptor type II, 785
Interleukin-1 receptor type-I-deficient mice,
    781–782
Interleukin-1 superfamily members, 777

Interleukin-1α
  autoantibodies to, 781
  autocrine growth factor, 780
Interleukin-1α-deficient mice
  interleukin-1β-deficient mice, contrasted,
      781
  studies in, 781
Interleukin-1β, 780
Interleukin-1β converting enzyme, 779–780
Interleukin-1β-deficient mice, 782
  effects in, 782
Interleukin-1R family, nomenclature of, 783
Interleukin-1Ra, effects of, 792–793
Interleukin-2
  classes of, 716–717
  dendritic cells, 466
  in evolution of immune response, 550–551
  production, proliferation, T-cell activation,
      310–311
Interleukin-2 receptor α-chain mutation,
    1609–1610
Interleukin-2 receptors
  classes of, 717
  soluble, in human disease, 719
Interleukin-4, 716
Interleukin-6 family of cytokines,
    composition of receptors for, 714
Interleukin-7, 716
Interleukin-7 receptor α-chain deficiency,
    1605
Interleukin-8, 814–815
  in evolution of immune response, 550
Interleukin-10, 720
  type II cytokines and, 720
Interleukin-12, 715
  dendritic cells, 465
  production, in allergic disorders,
      1451–1452
  receptors with similarities to, 715–716
Interleukin-12 receptor β1 mutations, 1610
  with primary immunodeficiency, 1610
  in primary immunodeficiency disease, 1610
Interleukin-18, 780
  binding protein, 785–786
  inhibition of
    viral, 1222
    viruses, 1222
Internal deletions, fusion proteins resulting
    from, 1566
Interstitial dendritic cells, 457–458
Intestinal epithelial cells, mucosal immunity,
    991–992
Intestinal infections, mucosal immune
    system, 995–996
Intestinal protozoa, vaccination, 1190
Intracellular bacteria, 1229–1262. See also
    specific pathogen
  acidification, 1236–1237
  acquired immune response, 1240–1245
    antigen presentation, 1243–1244
    β2 microglobulin, 1244–1245
    CD1 molecules, 1243–1244
    dendritic cells, 1241

Intracellular bacteria (*contd.*)
 ϵδ T-cells, 1245
 T-cell subpopulations, 1241–1243
 adhesion, 1234
 antibacterial immunity, conventional
  T-cells in, 1241
 apoptosis, 1239–1240
 cell-to-cell spreading, 1239
 cytokines, 1248–1251
  down-regulation, antibacterial host
   response, 1250–1251
  granuloma formation, 1248–1249
  leukocyte recruitment, 1248
  macrophage activation, 1249–1250
  protective T-cell response, 1250
 cytoplasm, evasion into, 1239
 delayed-type hypersensitivity, 1255
 DN cells, group 1 CD1-restricted, 1244
 experimental listeriosis, 1255
 facultative, 1231–1232
  major infections of humans caused by,
   1231
 facultative intracellular bacteria, major
  infections of humans caused by, 1231
 features of, 1230
 genetic control, resistance against
  intracellular bacteria, 1255–1256
 granulomatous lesion, 1253–1255
  granuloma formation, 1254
  leukocyte extravasation, 1253–1254
  tuberculosis, 1254–1255
 hallmarks of, 1230–1231
 host cells, 1233–1240
 immunity to, 1229–1261
 infected cells, death of, 1252–1253
 intracellular iron, 1237–1238
 invasion, 1234
 leprosy, 1255
 Listeria monocytogenes, 1233
 listeriosis, 1233
 major histocompatibility complex class
  Ib-restricted CD8 T-cells, 1243
 microbes, recognition receptors for,
  1234–1236
 Mycobacterium tuberculosis, 1232–1233
 natural killer T-cells, with specificity for
  group 2 CD1 molecules, 1244
 Nramp 1 gene, 1256
 obligate, major infections of humans
  caused by, 1232
 obligate intracellular, 1231–1232
  major infections of humans caused by,
   1232
 pattern recognition receptors
  mediating microbial binding, uptake,
   1236
  mediating signaling, 1235
  recognizing host molecules, 1236
 phagocytes, nonprofessional, invasion of,
  1236
 phagosome maturation, 1236–1237
 phagosome-lysosome fusion, 1236–1237
 professional phagocytes, 1240
  mononuclear phagocytes, 1240
  polymorphonuclear granulocytes, 1240
 Salmonella enterica, 1233
 salmonellosis, 1233
 T cytokines, in antibacterial immunity,
  1244
 T-cell functions, during infection,
  1245–1248
 Th1, activities, 1251–1252
 toxic effector molecules, 1238–1239
 trigger mechanisms, entry by, 1234
 tryptophan degradation, 1238
 tuberculosis, 1232–1233
 vaccine design, 1246
 virulence, intracellular bacteria, 1230–1232
 vitamin D receptor, 1256
 zipper mechanisms, entry by, 1234
Intracellular iron, intracellular bacteria,
 1237–1238
Intracellular microbes, natural killer cells,
 382–383
Intracellular parasites, 1178–1180
Intracellular pathogens
 vaccination, 1348–1349
Intracellular recognition systems
 innate immune system, 506–508
  2'-5'-oligoadenylate synthase, 507–508
  NOD family, 508
  PKR, 507
  RNaseL, 507–508
Intraepithelial lymphocytes
 development of, 990–991
 in mucosal defense, 992
 mucosal immunity, 991–992
 in mucosal tolerance, 1003
Intrathymic precursors, T-cell development,
 developmental potential of, 266–267
Intravenous immunoglobulin
 for autoimmune disorders, 1628
 in immunotherapy, 1632–1633
  mechanism of action, 1632–1633
  mechanism of action of, 1632–1633
Invertebrate cells, in evolution of immune
 response, 553–554
Iron, intracellular, intracellular bacteria,
 1237–1238
Islet transplantation, 1536–1537
Isotype class switching, immunoglobulin E
 synthesis, in allergic disorders,
 1453–1455
Isotype switch recombination,
 antigen-primed B-cells, 216
Isotypes, immunoglobulin, properties of, 59

J
J chain, mucosal immunity, 972
Jak3. *See* Janus kinase 3
Jaks
 cytokine activation, 722
 substrate for. *See* STATS
Janus family tyrosine kinases. *See* Jaks
Janus kinase 3 deficiency, 1605
Janus kinase 3 mutations, 723

Janus kinases, 721–722
 activation of, 723–725
 signaling, 722–723
 substrates, 732
Jenner, Edward, 24, 1320–1321
Jennerian era, 1320–1321
Jerne, Niels, 36, 39, 40
Jurin, James, 24

K
κ-light-chain genes, 114
Kabat, Elvin, 32
Kabat-Wu variability plots, major
 histocompatibility complex class I,
 597
Kahn, Rudolf, 30
Kahn test, development of, 30
Kappler, John, 41
Köhler, Georges, 38–39
Küstner, Hans, 29
Keratitis, herpesvirus-induced, 1425
Kidney graft survival, one year, 1543
Kidney transplantation, 1535–1536
Killed microorganisms, vaccine consisting of,
 1329
Kinetics, 72–73
 antigen-antibody interactions, 70–73
 in autoimmune disease, 1409–1410
Kinins, in inflammation, 1154
Kitasato, Shibasaburo, 26, 1321
Klebsiella pneumonia, 1267
Koch, Robert, 24, 35, 1321
Kolle, Wilhelm, 24
Koprowski, Hilary, 39
Ku, role in switch recombination, 123–124

L
la Force, Mark, 1348
λ light-chain genes, 114–116
 human λ locus, 115–116
 murine λ locus, 114–115
λ-related "surrogate" light chains, 116
Lactoferrin, 511
Landsteiner, Karl, 27–31, 40
Langerhans cells, 456–457
Lassa fever virus, transmission of, 1203
Latency
 parasites, 1184–1185
  mechanisms of, 1183–1185
 viral, 1217
Latex allergens, 1443
Löwy, Ilana, 38
Lawrence, Sherwood, 35
LBP, 506
Lck
 dynamic regulation of, 340
 in signal transduction by T-cell antigen
  receptor, dynamic regulation of, 340
Lck PTK, 335–336
League of Nations, 30
Lectin pathway, complement, 1084–1085
Lectins
 in evolution of immune response, 555

T-lymphocyte activation, 324–325
Legionella pneumophila species, 1230, 1231, 1236, 1237, 1238
Legionella species, 1231
Legionnaire's disease, bacterial pathogen, 1231
Leishman, Sir William, 24
Leishmania major, 1251
Leishmania mexicana, 1175
Leishmania parasite, 1171, 1172, 1173, 1174, 1177, 1178, 1179, 1183, 1274
Leishmaniasis, 1172
    vaccination, 1192, 1361
Leporipoxvirus species, 1221
Leprosy, 1255
    bacterial pathogen, 1231
    vaccine, 1329, 1348–1349
Leptin, 715
    in inflammation, 1156
Leukocyte adhesion deficiency, 1609
Leukocyte adhesion deficiency-1, 1609
Leukocyte adhesion deficiency-2, 1609
Leukotrienes, in inflammation, 1154
Levine, Philip, 30
Ligands, major histocompatibility complex, complexes with, 599–602
Light chains, λ-related "surrogate," 116
Light-chain rearrangement, B lymphocyte development, 172
Lipid mediators
    in allergic disorders, 1462
    in inflammation, 1154–1155
Liposomes
    in immunotherapy, 1338
Lister, John, 23
Listeria donovani, 1256
Listeria monocytogenes, 1230, 1231, 1232, 1233, 1235, 1236, 1237, 1239, 1240, 1242, 1243, 1245, 1246, 1247, 1250, 1252, 1255
Listeriosis, 1233
    bacterial pathogen, 1231
    experimental, 1255
    intracellular bacteria, 1255
Live attenuated vaccine, 1329–1329
Live microbial vectors, mucosal immunity, 1000
Liver
    carcinogenesis, cytotoxic T-lymphocytes, 1144–1145
    fetal, macrophages, 485
    transplantation, 1536
Liver disease, 1420–1424
    in animal models, 1421
    halothane hepatitis, 1423
    hepatitis, autoimmune, 1420–1421
    in human, 1421–1423
    primary biliary cirrhosis, 1423
    therapeutic concepts, 1423–1424
Liver stages
    malaria, vaccination, 1192–1193
    in malaria, vaccination against, 1192–1193
Longevity, immunity and, 1047–1048

Long-term nonprogression, human immunodeficiency virus, 1288, 1303–1305
    host genetic factors, 1303–1304
    host immune-response factors, 1304–1305
    virologic factors, 1305
Low hormonal stress response, 1031
Low-affinity self-peptide-major histocompatibility complex ligands, presentation of, 306–307
Lpr mice, systemic autoimmunity, 1388
Lung transplantation, 1536
Lung-associated lymphoepithelial lymphocyte homing, 994–995
Lupus erythematosus, systemic, 1382–1383
Lupus-like syndrome, induction of, 1388–1389
Ly-1/CD5+ B-cells. *See* CD5+ B-lymphocytes
Ly49 gene, monoallelic expression of, 379–380
Ly49 receptors, cell surface, 381
Lymph nodes, 429–433
    B-cell follicles, 432–433
    immune response, macrophages, 488
    structure, organization of, 429–432
Lymphatic filariasis, 1172
Lymphocyte differentiation, rearrangement, diversification of TCR, immunoglobulin genes, 544–546
Lymphocyte granzymes, 1132
Lymphocyte homeostasis, regulatory T-cells, autoimmunity and, 952–953
Lymphocyte homing, in nasal-associated lymphoepithelial, lung-associated tissues, 994–995
Lymphocyte-mediated cytotoxicity
    mechanisms of, distinguishing, 1128–1129
    properties of, 1128
Lymphocytes, 38. *See also* B lymphocytes; Cytotoxic T-lymphocytes; T lymphocytes
    intraepithelial
        development of, 990–991
        mucosal immunity, 990–992
Lymphogranuloma, bacterial pathogen, 1232
Lymphoid malignancy, programmed cell death, 858–859
Lymphoid organs, 419–429
    bone marrow, 419–422
        function, apoptosis in, 422
        hematopoietic stem cells, 419–420
        stromal cells, microenvironment created by, 420–421
        structure, function, 420–422
    cell lineages signaling, 441
    chronic inflammation, 442–443
    lymph nodes, 429–433
        B-cell follicles, 432–433
        structure, organization of, 429–432
    lymphocyte recruitment, 443–444
    lymphopoiesis, stromal cell cultures, 421–422

lymphotoxin, in lymphoid organ formation, 438–440
mucosal-associated lymphoid tissues, 433–435
NK cell differentiation, stromal cells contributing to, 422
organogenesis, 442–443
Peyer's patches, structural features of, 434–435
respiratory tract-associated lymphoid tissues, 435
spleen
    spontaneous mouse mutations affecting development, 436–438
    structure, function, 435–436
thymus, 422–428
    embryologic development, 423–425
    mature architecture, 425–427
    nonlymphoid bone marrow-derived cells, 427
    normal anatomy, 422–423
    T-lymphopoiesis, thymic compartments, relationship, 427–428
Lymphoid tissues, 428–444
    in evolution of immune response, 541–544
        amphibians, 542–543
        birds, 543–544
        bony fish, 541–542
        cartilaginous fish, 541
        reptiles, 543–544
    human immunodeficiency virus, 1290–1291
Lymphokine-activated killer cells
    cancer immunity and, 1579
    in immunotherapy, 1643
Lymphopenia, causes of, 938
Lymphopoiesis, stromal cell cultures, 421–422
Lymphoproliferative disease, X-linked, 1599–1600
Lymphotoxin, 758–759
    in lymphoid organ formation, 438–440
Lysosomal enzymes, cytotoxic T-lymphocytes, 1133
Lysozyme, 510
Lyssavirus species, 1201, 1207

M
Macrophage function, age-related changes, 1051
Macrophage mannose receptor, 504–505
Macrophage-active killer cells, in immunotherapy, 1644
Macrophages, 20, 508–509
    age-related changes in, 1050–1051
    cancer immunity and, 1579–1580
    human immunodeficiency virus, 1291–1292, 1298
    immune response, 481–495
        activation, modulation of, *in vitro,* 492–493
        activation *in vivo,* 489–490
        differentiation, 483–484

Macrophages (contd.)
  fetal liver, 485
  gene expression, secretion, 492
  lymph nodes, 488
  nonlymphoid organs, 488–489
  Peyer's patch, 488
  phagocytic recognition, 490–492
  properties, 483–493
  research landmarks, 481–483
  spleen, 486–488
    marginal zone macrophages, 487–488
    red pulp macrophages, 488
    white pulp macrophages, 488
  thymus, 485–486
  tissue distribution, 484–489
Macropinocytosis, 1115
Madsen, Thorvald, 30
Major histocompatibility complex, 16–19,
    571–613
  amino acid sequences, primary structure,
    592–593
  antigen presenting, 19. See also Dendritic
    cells
  antigen processing, 16–19, 578, 613–629
  antigens, defective expression of, with
    primary immunodeficiency,
    1608–1609
  binding, 658–664
    antigen structure and, 658–664
    assembly of stable major
      histocompatibility complex/peptide
      complex, 658–664
  bone marrow transplantation, 585
  class I
    antigen deficiency, 1608
    antigens, changes in expression of,
      tumor formation and, 1582
    dislocation into cytoplasm, viral, 1219
    dislocation of molecules into lysosomes,
      viral, 1219
    gene, 579–582
    Kabat-Wu variability plots, 597
    molecule, 16–17, 571–612
      associated molecules, 580
      in endoplasmic reticulum, retention
        of, viral, 1219
      genetics, 580
      molecular structure, 580
      motifs for peptides binding to, 662
      natural killer cell recognition, 580
      nature of peptides bound, 580
      peptide binding rules, 580
      peptide-binding motifs, 594
      polymorphism, 580
      site of peptide acquisition, 580
      T-cell recognition, 580
      T-cells restricted to, processing of
        antigen, 651–654
      tissue specific expression, 580
    pathway, 1218
      viral, 1218
    peptide complexes
      assembly of, 616–617

  surface-expressed, interference with,
    viral, 1219
  in pre-Golgi/Golgi compartment,
    retention of, 1219
    viral, 1219
  presentation, 654–657
  release of molecules from endoplasmic
    reticulum, 617–618
  restricted presentation
    antigen, 613–618
    extracellular proteins, 618
  synthesis, inhibition, viral, 1217
  transport pathways leading to
    presentation, 654–657
class Ib, 598–599
  CD1, 598–599
  FcRn, 599
  H2-M3, 598
  molecule, 598–599
class Ib-restricted CD8 T-cells, 1243
class II
  antigen deficiency, 1608–1609
  gene, 579–582
  molecule, 17–18, 571–612
    associated molecules, 580
    genetics, 580
    immunodominant T-cell epitopes,
      association with, 648
    molecular structure, 580
    motifs for peptides binding to, 662
    natural killer cell recognition, 580
    nature of peptides bound, 580
    peptide binding rules, 580
    peptide-binding motifs, 595
    polymorphism, 580
    processing of antigen for T-cells
      restricted to, 651–653
    site of peptide acquisition, 580
    T-cell recognition, 580
    T-cells restricted to, processing of
      antigen for, 651–653
    tissue specific expression, 580
  peptide-binding motifs, 595
  presentation, transport pathways leading
    to, 654–657
  restricted antigen presentation, 618–625
  structures, 596–598
  superantigen, 600–602
  transport pathways leading to
    presentation, 657–658
co-receptor interactions, 600
disease, 587–589
in evolution of immune response, 532–541
  class I/II expression, 540–541
  class I/II structure, 532–535
  classical, nonclassical class I, chain II,
    535
  disease associations, 537–538
  gene organization, 539–540
  locus complexity, selection on, 539
  mating preferences, 538–539
  polymorphism, genes, 535–537
evolutionary mechanism, 583

features of, 1490
genetic maps, 579–582
haplotype, tumor formation and,
  1580–1581
histocompatibility testing, family studies,
  586–587
human leukocyte antigen
  class I alleles, 574–575
  compatibility, 587
  gene products, codominant expression,
    590
  genetic basis of structural variation on,
    582
  nomenclature, 573
immunological function of, 577–579
molecule, 590–591
  antigen interaction with, 658–664
  complexes with ligands, 599–602
  delivery to cell surface, 624
  interactions of, 602
    multivalent major histocompatibility
      complex/peptide complexes, 602
    physical assays, 602
mouse strains, H2 haplotypes, major
  histocompatibility complex, 576
mutations at H2 locus, 589
natural killer cell interactions, 600–601
nomenclature, 572–577
origins, 561–562
peptides bound by, identification of,
  593–594
polymorphism, 582–583
receptors, 370–375
  CD94/NKG2 receptors, 372
  class I down-regulation, 373–374
  expression patterns, 373
  killer cell immunoglobulin-like
    receptors, 371
  Lag-3 receptors, 372–373
  leukocyte immunoglobulin-like
    receptors, 372
  Ly49 receptors, 370–371
  natural killer cells through inhibition,
    viral evasion, 374–375
  stimulatory complex-specific natural
    killer cell receptors, 375
renal graft survival, 585
residues conserved in factor, 533
  functions of, 534
restricted presentation class I, dendritic
  cells, 464
restricted presentation class II, dendritic
  cells, 462–464
restriction
  binding to, 660
  CD4, CD8 lineage differentiation,
    285–287
  sequence changes, H-2^b haplotype
    mutants, 589
structure, 591–602
T-cell
  receptor interactions, 600
  receptor-peptide, 241–245

T-lymphocyte recognition of, restricted
recognition, 18–19
transplantation, 583–584
clinical, 584–586
Mak, Tak, 41
Makgoba, Malegapuru, 42
Malaria, 1172
chemokines, 826
extracellular stages of, vaccine targeting,
1190–1192
liver stages
targeting extracellular stages of,
1190–1192
vaccination, 1190–1192, 1357–1358
liver stages, 1192–1193
as vaccine molecule, 1360
Malaria plasmodia, 1244
Malignancy
B-cell, treatment of, 181–182
lymphoid, programmed cell death,
858–859
in systemic autoimmunity, 1382
Malignant neoplasms, with increased
incidence, with immunodeficiency,
1571
Mammals
evolution of immune response, 549–550
evolution of lymphocyte differentiation,
546
Marburg virus, 1201
Marginal zone B-cells, 177–178, 210
Marginal zone macrophages, spleen,
487–488
Marrack
J.R., 29, 41
P., 41
Martin, A.J.P., 33
Mast cell activation, in allergic disorders,
1463
Mast cell-derived cytokines, in allergic
disorders, 1462–1463
Mast cell-derived mediators, in allergic
disorders, 1460
Mast cells, 20, 509
in allergic disorders, 1459–1460
acute-phase responses, 1463
late-phase responses, 1463
development of, in allergic disorders,
1458–1463
immune system mediation, 1029–1030
products of, 1461
Measles, 1209, 1214
eradication of, 1327
transmission of, 1203
vaccine, 1322, 1329, 1342
Medawar, Sir Peter, 35
Membrane mixing, cytotoxic T-lymphocytes,
1134–1135
Memory
effect of peripheral cytokines on, 1025
immunologic, 865–899
B-cell memory, maintenance of, 888
factors contributing to, 881–884

effector activity, continued expression
of, 881–882
memory cells, altered properties of,
883–884
naive state, memory, systemic
differences between, 882–883
generation of memory, 866–878
longevity of, 865–866
after virus infection, 866
maintenance of memory, 885–888
memory B-cells
generation of, 874–878
identification of, 880–881
life span of, 885
memory cells
identifying, 878–881
life span, turnover of, 884–885
memory T-cells
generation of, 867–874
identification of, 878–880
life span of, 884–885
T-cell memory, maintenance of, 885–888
Memory B-cell, 175–176
maintenance, 220
subsets, 219–220
Memory CD4 T-cell, 313–314
Memory CD8 T-cell, 313
Memory consolidation, effect of peripheral
cytokines on, 1025
Meningococci vaccine, 1329, 1347–1348
Metchnikov, Elie, 25
MHC. *See* Major histocompatibility complex
Mice. *See* Mouse
Microbes
phagocytosis, 1121–1123
recognition receptors for, intracellular
bacteria, 1234–1236
Microbial vectors, live, mucosal immune
system, 1000
Migratory properties, dendritic cells, 464–465
migration in situ, 465
Miller, Jacques, 38
Milstein, César, 38–39
Mimicry in infectious disease
chemokines, 822–824
herpesvirus, 822–824
poxvirus, 822–824
Minipigs, graft survival, 1544
Mitochondrion, programmed cell death, role
in, 849–850
Molecular genetics, immunoglobulins,
107–158
gene alterations, in germinal centers,
137–149
heavy-chain switch, 138–144
assaying switch recombination, 139
isotype switching by CD40, 139–140
isotype-specific regulation of
germline transcripts, 140–141
non-"standard" isotype switching,
143–144
sterile transcription in class switch
recombination, 141

switch junctions, 138–139
switch regions, 138–139
targeting class switch recombination
to switch regions, 141–142
somatic mutation, 144–149
cellular context of, 145
early evidence for, 144
hypermutation, role of, 144–145
molecular mechanism of
hypermutation, 147–149
DNA breaks in V regions, 147–148
error-prone polymerases, 148–149
targeting, distribution of mutations,
145–147
gene expression, regulation of, 135–137
gene loci, 111–116
heavy chain genes, 111–114
membrane *versus* secreted
immunoglobulin, 112–113
organization of CH gene loci,
113–114
κ-light-chain genes, 114
λ light-chain genes, 114–116
human λ locus, 115–116
murine λ locus, 114–115
λ-related "surrogate" light chains, 116
germline diversity, 132–135
combinatorial diversity estimates, 135
human germline VH locus, 134
human germline V_κ locus, 134–135
human JH, DH regions, 134
mouse germline JH, DH regions,
132–133
murine germline V_κ locus, 133–134
of murine VH locus, 132
V gene assembly
overview, 108–111
recombination, diversity and, 109–111
recombination signal elements,
111
Southern blot tests, gene cloning,
108–109
V gene assembly recombination, 116–132
allelic exclusion, 128–130
B lymphocyte development, 126–127
B-cell maturation, B-cell receptor
regulation of, 130
hairpins, 120–121
late recombination activating gene
expression, 130–132
mechanisms, 119–126
P nucleotides, 120–121
receptor editing, 130–132
receptor revision, 130–132
recombination activating gene proteins,
V-D-J recombination, 121–123
recombination intermediates, 120–121
recombination model, 119
recombinational accessibility, 127–128
regulated V(D)J recombination,
128–130
regulation, 126–132
substrates, experiments, 119–120

Molecular genetics, (contd.)
  topology, 116–117
    deletion versus inversion, 116–117
    secondary recombinations, 117–118
  transcription, 127–128
  V-D-J recombination
    artemis, 124–125
    DNA breaks, proteins binding to, 125
    DNA-PK, 123–124
    exonuclease, 125–126
    Ku, 123–124
    N regions, 125
    terminal deoxynucleotide transferase, 125
    XRCC4, 123–124
Molecular immunology, 39–41
Molecular mediators, acute inflammatory response, 1153–1156
  amines, 1155
  lipcalins, 1156
Molecular vaccine, 1330
Molecule expression, major histocompatibility complex, 590–591
Molecule structure, major histocompatibility complex, 591–602
Monoallelic expression, ly49 gene, 379–380
Monoclonal antibodies, 38–39, 96–101
  alternative to, 100
  applications, 98–100
    bifunctional antibodies, 98–99
    bispecific antibodies, 98–99
    catalytic antibodies, 98
    clinical applications, 99
    human monoclonal antibodies, production of, 99–100
    humanized monoclonal antibodies, 99–100
    nucleotide aptamers, 100
  cross-reactions of, 101
  derivatives of, 1099
  hybridomas, derivation of, 96–98
    gene libraries to derive monoclonal antibodies, 97–98
    from species other than mice, 97
  in immunotherapy, 1632–1635
  organ transplantation, 1635
  polyclonal, versus monoclonal antibodies, 101
  specificity of, 100–101
  T-lymphocyte activation, 325
Monoclonal antibody-cytokine conjugates, 1642
  in immunotherapy, 1642
Monoclonal antibody-drug conjugates, in immunotherapy, 1639–1640
Monoclonal antibody-photosensitizer conjugates, 1642
  in immunotherapy, 1642
Monoclonal antibody-RNAse conjugates, 1642
  in immunotherapy, 1642

Monoclonal antibody-superantigen conjugates, 1642
  in immunotherapy, 1642
Monocyte-derived dendritic cells, 458
Monocytes, 20
  age-related changes in, 1050–1051
  human immunodeficiency virus, 1291–1292, 1298
  in inflammation, 1160
Monomeric immunoglobulin A-producing cells, distribution of, mucosal immune system, 981–983
Mononuclear phagocytes, intracellular bacteria, 1240
Monovalent ligand, antigen-antibody interactions, interaction in solution with, 73–79
  affinity, 76–77
  average affinities, 76
  B/F, plot, 77–78
  heterogeneity of affinity, 75–76
  intrinsic affinity, 78
  monogamous bivalency, 79
  multivalent ligands, interaction with, 78
  Scatchard analysis, 74–75
Montagu, Lady Mary, 24, 1320
Mood, 1025
  effect of peripheral cytokines on, 1025
Moore, Stanford, 33
Moss, Bernard, 1330
Mouse. See also under Murine
  B lymphocyte development, 159–180
    B-1 B-cells, 176–177
    B-cell migration, maintenance, 174
    B-cell tolerance, 178–179
    B-cell turnover, 174–175
    bone marrow developmental stages, 164–172
      culture systems, 165–168
      functional definition, 164
      microenvironmental interactions, 165–168
      phenotypic definition, 164–165
    CD5, 179–180
    chemokines, in migration of B-cell precursors, 168
    complement, in B-cell tolerance, response, 179–180
    early development, 160–164
      bone marrow, early B-cell progenitors in, 160
    follicular B-cells, 174
    gene expression, 168–169
    germinal center B-cells, 175
    growth of early B-lineage cells, regulators of, 166
    immature B-cells, generation of, 172
    immunoglobulin
      heavy chain, 169–172
      rearrangement, 168–169
    light-chain rearrangement, 172
    marginal zone B-cells, 177–178
    memory B-cells, 175–176

    ontogeny, sites of B lymphopoiesis during, 160
    peripheral maturation stages, functional subsets, 172–180
    Pre-BCR, 169–172
    receptor editing, 178–179
    serum antibody, in B-cell tolerance, response, 179–180
    stem cells, 160
    transcription factors, 162–164
    transgenic models, B-cell tolerance, 178
    transitional B-cells, 172–174
  cytomegalovirus infection, natural killer cells in, 385–386
  humans, B lymphocyte development, compared, 180–184
  strains, H2 haplotypes, major histocompatibility complex, 576
MPs. See Mononuclear phagocytes
mRNA levels, OPG steady-state, expression of, in stromal cells, osteoblast-like cells, 761
MS. See Multiple sclerosis
Mu-α switching, T-cells for, 986
Mucosal adjuvants, 998–1000
Mucosal allergies, 1008–1009
Mucosal barrier, 966–970
  epithelial cells, 966–970
    cytokine receptors, 968
    mucosal microbiota, 970
Mucosal CD4+ T helper cells, 983–984
Mucosal cell trafficking, homing, 992–995
Mucosal cytokines, mucosal immunity, 999
Mucosal helper T-cell clones, 983–984
Mucosal immune system, 965–1020
  B-cell compartment, 981–983
  effector sites, 980–981
  gastrointestinal allergy, 1009
  immune responses, 995–1000
    antigen-delivery systems, 998–1000
    genital tract, immune responses in, 997–998
    intestinal infections, 995–996
    mucosal adjuvants, 998–1000
    nasal immunization, 996–997
    upper respiratory tract immunization, 996–997
  inductive sites, 976–995
    gut-associated lymphoepithelial tissue, 977–978
    nasal-associated lymphoepithelial tissue, 979–980
    organization of, 976–977
  intraepithelial lymphocytes, 990–992
  mouse lymphocyte subpopulations associated with, 979
  mucosal antibodies, 971–976
    function, 973–974
    IgA
      α chains, 971–972
      assembly of, 972–973
      J chain, 972
      origin, 974–976

polymeric, receptor expression, 975–976
secretory component, 972
structure of, 971–973
transport, cellular interactions, 975
immunoglobulin isotypes, distribution of, 971
mucosal immunoglobulins, origin, transport of, 974–976
secretory immunoglobulin A, structure of, 971–973
mucosal barrier, 966–970
epithelial cells, 966–970
adaptive immune functions of, 968–970
cytokines, 968
epithelium, innate functions of, 966–968
transcellular transport functions of, 968
mucosal microbiota, 970
quantitative data, 970
mucosal cell trafficking, homing, 992–995
mucosal cytotoxic T-cells, 989–990
mucosal immunopathology, 1004–1009
human immunodeficiency virus type 1 infection, 1005
immunoglobulin A deficiency, 1004–1005
inflammatory bowel disease, 1005–1008
mucosal allergies, 1008–1009
mucosal tolerance, 1000–1004
mechanisms for, 1000–1004
organization of, 976–977
regulatory T-cells, 983
T-cell compartment, 983–989
viruses, 1212–1213
Mucosal microbiota, quantitative, qualitative aspects of, 970
Mucosal regulatory T-cells, 984–985
Mucosal vaccine, 1332–1333
Mucosal-associated lymphoid tissues, 433–435
Multiple sclerosis, 1417–1420
etiology, 1419–1420
human immunology of, 1418–1419
human leukocyte antigen associations, 588
immunology of, 1418–1419
therapeutic concepts, 1420
Multispecificity, antigen-antibody interactions, 89
Multivalent major histocompatibility complex/peptide complexes, 602
Mumps, 1214
transmission of, 1203
vaccine, 1329, 1342
Muramyldipeptide derivatives, immunotherapy, 1624
Murine macrophage heterogeneity, differentiation antigens used to study, 485
Murine models of inflammation, 1161

Murine VH locus, germline diversity, immunoglobulins, 132
Murray, Joseph, 35
Mutant p53 suppressor gene-encoded proteins, 1564–1566
Mutant ras oncogene-encoded proteins, 1564
Mutation, viral, 1216–1217
Mycobacterial infections, 736
Mycobacterium avium, 1236, 1256
Mycobacterium bovis, 1231
Mycobacterium intracellulare, 1256
Mycobacterium leprae, 1231, 1236, 1239, 1255
Mycobacterium lepraemurium, 1256
Mycobacterium tuberculosis, 1230–1233, 1235–1250, 1254–1255
MyD88, recruitment of, 787–788
Myeloma proteins, 34
Myeloperoxidase, 511–512
Myelopoiesis, 812–813

N
NADPH oxidase, 1159–1160
in inflammation, 1159–1160
Naive antigen-specific B-cells, antigen-specific T-cell help, recruitment of, 214
Naive T-cells, 304–305
generation, 304
recirculation, 304
survival, 304–305
Narcolepsy, human leukocyte antigen associations, 588
Nasal immunization, 996–997
Nasal tolerance
immunoregulation and, 927
mucosal immune system, 1003
Nasal-associated lymphoepithelial lymphocyte homing, 994–995
Nasal-associated lymphoepithelial tissue, 979–980
Native proteins, antipeptide antibodies binding, at specific site, 642–643
Natural immunity. See Innate immunity
Natural killer cells, 20, 365–391, 958
2B4, 378
activation, 384–385
age-related changes, 1052
age-related changes in, 1052–1053
cancer immunity and, 1579
cell surface Ly49 receptors, 381
dendritic cells, 473–474
development, 378–379
differentiation, 378–379
inhibitory receptor expression during, 379
discovery of, 365–366
in disease, 381–384
cancer, 383–384
effector functions, 381–382
intracellular microbes, 382–383
viral infections, 382

human immunodeficiency virus, 1298
in immunotherapy, 1643
interactions, major histocompatibility complex, 600–601
Ly49 gene, monoallelic expression of, 379–380
major histocompatibility complex-specific receptors, 370–375
CD94/NKG2 receptors, 372
class I down-regulation, 373–374
expression patterns, 373
killer cell immunoglobulin-like receptors, 371
Lag-3 receptors, 372–373
leukocyte immunoglobulin-like receptors, 372
Ly49 receptors, 370–371
natural killer cells through inhibition, viral evasion, 374–375
stimulatory major histocompatibility complex-specific natural killer cell receptors, 375
missing self hypothesis, 369–370
in mouse cytomegalovirus infection, 385–386
NKG2A gene, monoallelic expression of, 379–380
NKG2D, 376–377
NKp30, 377
NKp44, 377
NKp46, 377
NKR-P1, 377–378
phenotype, 366–367
receptors, general properties of, 367–369
self-tolerance, 379–381
with specificity for group 2 CD1 molecules, 1244
stimulatory, inhibitory signaling, integration of, 378
stimulatory receptors, specific for non-major histocompatibility complex ligands, 376–378
target cell recognition by, 367–378
T-cell development, 293–294
T-cell surface markers of, 366
viral inhibition of, 1220–1221
Natural killer-lysin/519, 1133
Necrosis, programmed, 850. See also Programmed cell death
Negative selection
in T-cell development, 280–284
time windows, T-cell development, 281–282
Neisseria gonorrhoeae, 1267, 1268, 1269, 1270, 1277
infections, 1264
Neisseria meningitidis, 1264, 1265, 1267, 1269, 1270, 1273, 1277
Neisseria organisms, 1267
Neoplasms. See also Tumors
malignant, with increased incidence, with immunodeficiency, 1571

Neural immune interactions, 1021–1042
  central nervous system
    effects of immune factors on, 1021–1026
    effects of peripheral immune factors on, 1022–1026
    immune factors expressed within, 1021–1022
  central nervous system regulation, immune system, 1026–1037
  glucocorticoid dysregulation, immune-mediated diseases, 1030–1037
  hypothalamic pituitary adrenal axis, immune-mediated diseases, 1030–1037
  neuroendocrine regulation, immune system, glucocorticoid effects, 1026–1030
  neuroendocrine stress response, activation of, 1025–1026
  sleep, central nervous system effects, 1024–1026
  stress, hypersensitivity, delayed type, effects on, 1034
  therapeutic implications, 1037–1038
Neuroendocrine stress response
  activation of, 1025–1026
  effect of peripheral cytokines on, 1025
Neurologic disease, complement in, 1093
Neuropeptides
  inflammation, 1155
  in inflammation, 1155
Neutrophil granules, major components of, 1158
Neutrophil primary granules
  components of, 1158
  in inflammation, 1158
Neutrophil-mediated inflammatory disorders, chemokines, 820
Neutrophils, 509, 1029
  activation, agents promoting, 1157
    in inflammation, 1157
  age-related changes in, 1051–1052
  cancer immunity and, 1579–1580
  function, age-related changes, 1051
  in inflammation, 1156–1160
  recruitment, activation, in inflammation, 1153
Neutrophil-targeted chemokines, 814–815
NF-AT, 732
NF-ATc activation, calcium-mediated regulation of, 205
NFκB, 732
NF-κB activation, regulation of, 206
Nijmegen breakage syndrome, 1608
Nippostrongylus brasiliensis, 1177, 1181, 1182
Nirenberg, Marshall, 34
Nitric oxide
  in inflammation, 1155
  synthase, 511–512
NK cells. *See* Natural killer cells

NKG2A gene, monoallelic expression of, 379–380
NKG2D, 376–377
NK-lysin/519, 1133
NKp30, 377
NKp44, 377
NKp46, 377
NKR-P1, 377–378
NOD family, 508
Nods, receptors, tolerance and, 916–917
Non-antigen-specific antiviral defense mechanisms, viruses, 1205–1206
Nonequilibrium radioimmunoassay, 84
Nonlymphoid organs, immune response, macrophages, 488–489
Nonopsonic recognition, in phagocytosis, 1108–1109
Nonpathologic systemic autoimmunity, 1372–1373
Nonprogression, long-term, human immunodeficiency virus, 1288, 1303–1305
Non-"standard" isotype switching, 143–144
Nossal, Sir Gus, 35
NRAMP, 511
Nramp 1 gene, intracellular bacteria, 1256
Nuclear factor κB essential modulator deficiency, 1598
Nuclear proteins, autoantibodies to, in systemic autoimmune disease, 1377
Nucleic acid vaccine, 1331–1332
Nucleotide aptamers, 100
Nucleotides, cyclic, fluxes in, T-lymphocyte activation, 348–349
Nutrition, with aging, 1065–1066
NZB mice, systemic autoimmunity, 1388
NZB/NZW F1 mice, 1388
  systemic autoimmunity, 1388

O

Obesity receptor, receptors with similarities to, 715–716
Obligate intracellular bacteria, major infections of humans caused by, 1232
Obligate intracellular intracellular bacteria, 1231–1232
Oligomers, higher order receptor, 705–706
Onchocerciasis, 1172
Oncofetal antigens, encoded by normal cellular genes, 1568–1569
Oncogenes. *See* Genes
Oncospermatogonal antigens, 1567
Opsonin receptors, 1109–1111
  in phagocytosis, 1109–1111
    immunoglobulin crystallized fragment receptors, 1109–1111
Oral tolerance
  in humans, mucosal immune system, 1003–1004
  regulatory T-cell in, 1002–1003
Organ transplantation
  immunotherapy, 1635
  monoclonal antibodies, 1635

Organ-specific autoimmunity, 1401–1438. *See also specific diseases*
  B-cell tolerance, 1404–1405
  burden of autoimmune diseases, 1402–1403
  causes of, 938
  diabetes, type 1, 1411–1417
    etiology, 1415–1416
    immunology of, 1412–1415
    therapeutic concepts, 1416–1417
  disorders, 1411–1430
  eye disorders, inflammatory
    in animal models, 1425–1426
    diseases associated with, 1424–1425
    in human, 1426
  gut disorders, 1430
  heart, autoimmune diseases of, 1430
  immune regulation, reestablishment, 1411
  initiation of, 1406–1409
    antigens, 1406–1407
    environment, 1407–1409
    genes, 1407
  liver disease, 1420–1424
    in animal models, 1421
    halothane hepatitis, 1423
    hepatitis, 1420–1421
    in human, 1421–1423
    primary biliary cirrhosis, 1423
    therapeutic concepts, 1423–1424
  multiple sclerosis, 1417–1420
    etiology, 1419–1420
    immunology of, 1418–1419
    therapeutic concepts, 1420
  organ-specific tuning, 1405–1406
  oveoretinitis, 1424–1426
  promising targets, 1411
  regulatory circuits in, 1409–1410
    apoptosis, 1409
    cytokines, 1409
    kinetics, 1409–1410
  rheumatoid arthritis, 1426–1428
    immunology, 1427
  skin disorders, 1429–1430
    dermatitis herpetiformis, 1429–1430
    pemphigus, 1429
  T-cell tolerance, 1404
  therapeutic considerations, 1410–1411
    efficacy, 1410–1411
    specificity, 1410–1411
    undesired effects, 1410–1411
  thyroiditis, 1428–1429
    immunology, 1428–1429
  tolerance
    central, 1403–1406
    peripheral, 1403–1406
Organ-specific tuning, in autoimmune diseases, 1405–1406
Orthomyxoviruses, 1202, 1214
Orthopoxvirus species, 1221–1222
Osteoprotegerin, 760–761
Ouchterlony method, antigen-antibody interactions, 91–92

Oveoretinitis, autoimmune, 1424–1426
  experimental, 1425
OX40 ligand, 764, 766
Oxidase, 511–512
Oxygen, role in cytotoxicity, 1140–1141

P

P nucleotides, V gene assembly
      recombination, 120–121
P2X-7 receptor, 780
P38 mitogen-activating protein kinase
      activation, 788
  inhibition of, 788
P53 suppressor gene-encoded proteins, tumor
      formation and, 1564–1566
PAF. See Platelet-activating factor
Pancreas transplantation, 1536–1537
Paoletti, Enzo, 1330
Paramyxovirus, 1202, 1204, 1214
Parasites, 1171–1200
  antigen-presenting cells, 1175–1177
  B-cell vaccine, 1190–1192
  cellular mechanisms, 1174–1175
  evasion by immune suppression, 1184
  evasion of immune recognition, 1183–1184
  extracellular parasites, 1180–1182
  global health importance, parasitic
      pathogens, 1171–1172
  global impact of disease, 1172
  helminths, vaccination, 1193–1194
  homeostasis, in anti-infective immune
      response, 1186
  humoral mechanisms, 1173–1174
  immune evasion, mechanisms of, 1183–1185
  immune response, 1171–1200
      hallmarks of, 1172–1173
  immune suppression, 1184–1185
  immunopathologic mechanisms,
      1185–1190
  intestinal protozoa, vaccination, 1190
  intracellular parasites, 1178–1180
  latency, 1184–1185
      mechanisms of, 1183–1185
  leishmaniasis, vaccination, 1192
  malaria
      liver stages, vaccination, 1192–1193
      vaccination, 1190–1192
  recognition of, in evolution of immune
      response, 559–560
  T-cell vaccine, 1192–1194
  Th1 responses, chronic, pathogenesis of,
      1186–1188
  Th2 responses, chronic, pathogenesis of,
      1188–1190
  vaccination, 1190–1194, 1357–1362
      helminths, 1193–1194
      intestinal protozoa, 1190
      leishmaniasis, 1192
      malaria
          extracellular stages of, 1190–1192
          liver stages, 1192–1193
          to prevent pathology, 1193
      strategies, 1190–1194

Parasitoids, recognition of, in evolution of
      immune response, 559–560
Parasympathetic nervous system, 1034
Parrott, Delphine, 38
Pas/MAPK signaling pathways, 207
Pasteur, Louis, 24, 25, 1321
Pattern-recognition molecules, secreted,
      innate immune system
  BPI, 506
  serum amyloid A, 506
Pauli, Wolfgang, 32
Pauling, Linus, 33, 34
PD-1, structure, expression of, 400
PD-1 function
  biochemical basis, 401
  PD-L1/Pd-L2 interactions, 400–401
  PD-ligand/PD-1 pathway, 400–401
Pemphigus, 1429
Pentraxins
  in evolution of immune response, 555
  in phagocytosis, 1113
  receptors, 1113
Peptidases, inhibition of
  viral, 1217–1219
Peptide-binding motifs, major
      histocompatibility complex
  class I, molecules, 594
  class II, molecules, 595
Peptide-major histocompatibility complex
      ligands, in vivo presentation of,
      306–309
Peptides
  antigenic determinants, conformational
      equilibria, 641–642
  bound by major histocompatibility
      complex, molecule identification,
      593–594
  complex antigens, T-lymphocyte
      activation, 324
  generation, antigen processing, 613–615,
      624–625
  in inflammation, 1155
  T-lymphocyte activation, 324
  vaccination with, in immunotherapy,
      1648
  vaccine, 1332
Perforin, 1130–1131, 1141–1142
Peripheral nervous system, regulation of
      immunity, 1037
Peripheral T-lymphocytes, 303–319
  dendritic cells, 305–306
  high-affinity foreign peptide-major
      histocompatibility complex ligands
      particulate antigens, 307–308
      presentation of, 307–309
      skin-surface antigens, 308
      soluble antigens, 308–309
  homeostasis of, 843–844
  low-affinity self-peptide-major
      histocompatibility complex ligands,
      presentation of, 306–307
  naive T-cells, 304–305
      generation, 304

  recirculation, 304
  survival, 304–305
  peptide-major histocompatibility complex
      ligands, in vivo presentation of,
      306–309
  T-cell activation, 309–314
      effector cells, 311–313
      IL-2 production, 310–311
      memory cells, 313–314
          memory CD4 T-cells, 313–314
          memory CD8 T-cells, 313
      signal transduction, 309–310
Peripheral tolerance, in autoimmune disease,
      1403–1406
Persistent virus infections, 1213–1216
Pertussis, vaccine, 1329
  acellular, 1342–1343
Peterson, P.A., 40
Petrov, Rem Viktorovich, 38
Peyer's patches
  immune response, macrophages, 488
  in oral tolerance, 1001–1002
  structural features of, 434–435
Pfeiffer, Richard, 24
PGRPs, 506
Phagocytes, 511–512
  intracellular bacteria, 1240
  nonprofessional, invasion of, intracellular
      bacteria, 1236
Phagocytic receptors, innate immune system,
      504–505
  β-glucan receptor, 505
  macrophage mannose receptor, 504–505
  scavenger receptors, 504
Phagocytic recognition, macrophages,
      490–492
Phagocytosis, 1105–1126
  actin polymerization, 1116
  activation of, 1112
      complement receptors for, 1112
  C1q receptor triggering, 1091
  cell biology of, 1108–1121
  collectins, 1112–1113
  complement receptors, 1111–1112
      complement receptor type 1, 1111
      integrin complement receptors,
          1111–1112
      phagocytosis, signaling events in, 1115
      signaling events in, 1115
  consequences of, 1118–1120
  crystallized fragment
      complement receptor phagocytosis,
          morphological differences between,
          1113–1114
      ϵ receptor-mediated phagocytosis,
          signaling events in, 1114–1115
  cytoskeleton in, 1115–1117
  derivations of, 1107–1108
  in evolution of immune response, 558
  F-actin
      association with phagosome membrane,
          1116–1117
      nucleation, 1116

Phagocytosis (contd.)
  organization, regulation of, 1117
  genetics, 1106–1107
  in inflammation, 1158
  macropinocytosis, 1115
  mechanisms of, 1113–1114
  microbes, 1121–1123
  negative regulation, 1121
  nonopsonic recognition, 1108–1109
  opsonin receptors, 1109–1111
    immunoglobulin crystallized fragment
      receptors, 1109–1111
  pentraxins, 1113
  phagocytic target, recognition of,
    1108–1113
  phagolysosome, 1117–1118
  phagosome, 1117–1118
  phosphatidylinositols, in crystallized
    fragment receptor-mediated
    phagocytosis, 1114–1115
  positive regulation, 1120–1121
  regulation of, 1120–1121
  signaling proteins to phagosome,
    localization of, 1117
  zipper hypothesis, 1113
Phagosome, 1117–1118
  localization of signaling proteins to, 1117
  maturation, intracellular bacteria,
    1236–1237
  signaling proteins to, localization of, 1117
Phagosome-lysosome fusion, with
    intracellular bacteria, 1236–1237
Phipps, James, 1321
Phosphatidylinositol, 1114–1115
  3-kinase, 733
  in crystallized fragment receptor-mediated
    phagocytosis, phagocytosis,
    1114–1115
Phospholipase A2, 510
PI-3K recruitment to membrane, in B-cell
    activation, 202
PI-3K/Akt signaling pathway, 206–207
PIAS proteins, 734
Pick, Ernst Peter, 27
Picornaviruses, 1202, 1214
Pig, human, molecular interactions between,
    1540
PKC pathway, 206
PKR, 507
Plasma cells, short-lived, development of,
    216–217
Plasma proteases, in inflammation,
    1153–1154
Plasmacytoid-derived dendritic cells, 459
Plasmodium berghei, 1180, 1187
Plasmodium chabaudi, 1174, 1187
Plasmodium falciparum, 1175, 1179, 1184,
    1186, 1187, 1190, 1193
  life cycle of, 1358–1361
Plasmodium knowles, 1180
Plasmodium malariae, 1185
Plasmodium species, 1179
Plasmodium vivax, 1185

Plasmodium yoelii, 1180
Plasticity, T-cell receptor, 242–245
Platelet-activating factor, in inflammation,
    1155
Platelets, in inflammation, 1160
PL-Cc-ε2 activation, 202–203
Pleiotropy
  cytokine receptor, 717–718
Pneumococci vaccine, 1322–1323, 1329,
    1347–1348
Pneumonia, bacterial pathogen, 1232
Polarization
  dendritic cells, mechanisms of, 469–470
  immune response, dendritic cells, 468–470
Poliomyelitis
  eradication, 1325–1327
  transmission of, 1203
  vaccine, 1322, 1329, 1342
Polyclonal antibodies, versus monoclonal
    antibodies, 101
Polymerases, error-prone, 148–149
Polymeric immunoglobulin A-producing
    cells, distribution of, mucosal immune
    system, 981–983
Polymeric immunoglobulin receptor
    expression, regulation of, 975–976
Polymorphism, major histocompatibility
    complex, 582–583
Polymorphonuclear granulocytes,
    intracellular bacteria, 1240
Polymorphonuclear leukocytes, human
    immunodeficiency virus, 1298
Polyoma viruses, 1202
Polypeptide
  antigenic determinants, 637–646
  T-cell receptors, 228
Polysaccharide immunogenicity, 637–646
  epitopes, mapping of, 638–641
  native proteins, antipeptide antibodies
    binding, at specific site, 642–643
  peptides, immunogenicity of, 643–646
  protein
    peptide antigenic determinants,
      conformational equilibria, 641–642
    polypeptide antigenic determinants,
      637–646
    proteins, immunogenicity of, 643–646
Porath, Jerker, 33
Porphyromonas gingivalis, 1270
Porter, Rodney, 33–34
Positive selection
  in T-cell development, 280–284
  time windows, T-cell development,
    281–282
  triggering, results of, 282
Potter, Michael, 34, 39
Poulik, M.D., 34
Poxviruses, 1202, 1214, 1220
PP. See Peyer's patches
Prausnitz, Carl, 29
Pre-BCR, 169–172
Preformed mediators, in allergic disorders,
    1460–1462

Primary biliary cirrhosis, 1423
Primary immunodeficiency, 1593–1620
  adenosine deaminase deficiency,
    1603–1605
  artemis gene, deficiencies of, 1605
  ataxia-telangiectasia, 1607
  autosomal recessive aεglobulinemia, 1597
  cartilage-hair hypoplasia, 1608
  CD40, mutations in, 1599
  CD45 deficiency, 1605
  CD154 deficiency, 1597–1598
  cellular immunodeficiency, 1602–1603
  Chediak-Higashi syndrome, 1610–1611
  combined immunodeficiency, 1603–1611
    autosomal recessive, 1603–1605
    severe combined immunodeficiency,
      1603–1606
    X-linked recessive, 1603
  common variable immunodeficiency,
    1600–1601
  cytidine deaminase deficiency,
    activation-induced, 1598–1599
  eczema, immunodeficiency with,
    1607–1608
  germline STAT1 mutation, 1610
  hyper immunoglobulin M, 1597–1598
  hyperimmunoglobulinemia E syndrome,
    1612–1613
    STAT4 knockout mice, 1613
  immunoglobulin A deficiency, selective,
    1601–1602
  immunoglobulin G subclass deficiencies,
    1602
  interferon-ε receptor mutations, 1610
  interleukin-2 receptor α-chain mutation,
    1609–1610
  interleukin-7 receptor a-chain deficiency,
    1605
  interleukin-12, 1610
  interleukin-12 receptor β1 mutations, 1610
  Janus kinase 3 deficiency, 1605
  leukocyte adhesion deficiency, 1609
  leukocyte adhesion deficiency-1, 1609
  leukocyte adhesion deficiency-2, 1609
  lymphoproliferative disease, X-linked,
    1599–1600
  major histocompatibility complex
    antigens, defective expression of,
      1608–1609
    class I, antigen deficiency, 1608
    class II, antigen deficiency, 1608–1609
  molecular defects causing, 1596
  molecular genetics, 1594–1595
    human immunodeficiency diseases,
      1594–1595
  Nijmegen breakage syndrome, 1608
  nuclear factor κB essential modulator
    deficiency, 1598
  purine nucleoside phosphorylase
    deficiency, 1606–1607
  recombinase-activating gene deficiencies,
    1605
  T-cell activation defects, 1611–1612

CD8 deficiency, from CD8α gene mutation, 2612
CD8 lymphocytopenia, from ζ-chain-associated protein deficiency, 1611–1612
defective cytokine production, 1612
T-cell receptor-CD3 complex, defective expression of, 1612
thrombocytopenia, immunodeficiency with, 1607–1608
thymoma, immunodeficiency with, 1602
X-linked
    aϵglobulinemia, 1595–1596
    in mice, 1596–1597
Prime-boost strategies of immunization, 1334–1335
Priming, in inflammation, 1157–1158
Pristane, systemic lupus-like syndrome, 1388–1389
Programmed cell death, 841–864
    APAF proteins, 856
    B-cell homeostasis, 846–847
    caspase complexes, apoptosis initiation mediated by, 848–849
    cellular homeostasis, in multicellular organisms, 841–842
    cellular mechanisms, 848–850
    dendritic cell homeostasis, 847
    as immune effector mechanism, 847
    immune regulation, 842–847
    as immune therapy, 858
    mitochondrion, role of, 849–850
    necrosis, programmed, 850
    peripheral T-cells, homeostasis of, 843–844
    regulation of, 851–856
        Bcl-2 gene family, 853–856
        caspases, 851–853
        TNF-receptor superfamily members, 853
    structural regulation of, 856–859
        Bcl-2 homology structures, 857–858
        caspase structure, 858
        hexahelical bundle, 858
        lymphoid malignancy, 858–859
        TNF-TNFR structure, 856–857
    T-cell death, passive, lymphokine withdrawal, 845–846
    T-cell memory, 846
    thymic deletion, 843
    T-lymphocyte death, active, antigen-stimulated, 844–845
Proinflammatory cytokines
    human immunodeficiency virus, 1309–1310
    in inflammation, 1155–1156
Proliferation, as response to chemokines, 809
Propionibacterium avidum, immunotherapy, 1623
Prostaglandins
    inflammation, 1154
    in inflammation, 1154
Protein biosynthesis, inflammation, 1160
Protein vaccine, 1330
Proteins, endocytosis of, antigen processing and, 624–625

Protein-tyrosine phosphatase, CD45, 339–340
Proteoglycan, 1132–1133
Proteolytic cascades, in evolution of immune response, 556–558
Protozoa, intestinal, vaccination, 1190
Pseudomonas aeruginosa, 1273
    infections, 1264
Psittacosis, bacterial pathogen, 1232
Psoriasis, human leukocyte antigen associations, 588
PTK activation, TCR-mediated, consequences of, 340–348
Purine nucleoside phosphorylase deficiency, 1606–1607
Putnam, Frank, 34

Q
Q-fever, bacterial pathogen, 1232
Quantitative precipitin, 90–91

R
Rabbit, B lymphocyte development, 183
Rabies
    transmission of, 1203
    vaccine, 1329
Rabinovich, Regina, 1361
Radiation vs. chemotherapeutic agents, tumor formation and, 1585
Radioimmunoassay, antigen-antibody interactions, 81–86
    analysis of data, 82–84
        corrections for B, F, T, 83–84
    bound, free antigen, separation of, 81–82
        solid-phase methods, 81–82
        solution methods, 81
    data analysis, 82–84
        corrections for B, F, T, 83–84
    enzyme-linked immunosorbent assay, 84–85
    enzyme-linked immunospot assay, 85–86
    graphic representation, 82–84
    nonequilibrium radioimmunoassay, 84
    numerical representation, 82–84
    tracer concentrations, optimization of, 82
Radioimmunoconjugates, in immunotherapy, 1640–1641
Radionuclides, choice of, 1640–1641
RAG, in evolution of immune response, 553
Ramon, Gaston, 1322
RANK ligand, 760–761
    expression of, in stromal cells, osteoblast-like cells, 761
Ras oncogene-encoded proteins, mutant, 1564
Ras pathway, in signal transduction by T-cell antigen receptor, activation of, 347–348
Rask-Nielsen, Ragna, 34
Ras/mitogen-activated protein kinase pathway, 733
Rearranging receptors
    antigen receptor, in evolution of immune response, 563

C1 domain, in evolution of immune response, 563
hypermutation, in evolution of immune response, 562–563
machinery, in evolution of immune response, 562
origins of, in evolution of immune response, 562–565
V domain, in evolution of immune response, 563
V segment, in evolution of immune response, 563–565
VC1 segment, in evolution of immune response, 563–565
Receptors, 3. See also specific type
    chains, sharing of, significance of, 715
    collectin, phagocytosis, 1091–1092, 1112–1113
    editing
        B lymphocyte development, 178–179
        V gene assembly recombination, 130–132
    immunoglobulin crystallized fragment, phagocytosis, 1109–1111
    innate immune system, 498–508
    integrin complement, phagocytosis, 1111–1112
    mimetics, viral, 1221
    opsonin, phagocytosis, 1109–1111
    revision, V gene assembly recombination, 130–132
    T lymphocytes, 11–13, 227–258. See also specific type
Recognition of viruses, by innate immune system, 1204–1205
Recombinant bacterial vaccine, 1649
Recombinant viral vector vaccine, 1649
Recombinase-activating gene deficiencies, 1605
Red pulp macrophages, spleen, 488
Regulated proliferation in T-cell development, 263–264
Regulatory T-cells, 935–963
    abnormalities, in systemic autoimmunity, 1379–1380
    allograft rejection, control of, 953–954
    control of autoimmune disease by, 950–953
        autoimmune gastritis, 950
        autoimmune thyroiditis, 951
        autoimmunity, antigenic specificity in, 952
        inflammatory bowel disease, 950–951
        insulin-dependent diabetes mellitus, 951–952
        lymphocyte homeostasis, autoimmunity and, 952–953
    function, enhancement of, 960
    graft-versus-host disease, control of, 953–954
    in immunotherapy, 1647
    induced, 946–950
    infectious agents, control of immunity to, 955–957

Regulatory T-cells (*contd.*)
  oral tolerance, 1002–1003
  in oral tolerance, 1002–1003
  in T-cell development, 294
  therapeutic manipulation of function,
      959–960
  tumor immunity, 954–955
Reinherz, Ellis, 41
Reiter's disease, human leukocyte antigen
      associations, 588
Rejection
  antigens, tumor, 1558–1562
    individually distinct, characteristics of,
        1561
  graft, 35–36
    chemokines, 820
    components of immune system in,
        1496–1500
      antibodies, 1498
      antigen-presenting cells, 1496–1498
      B-cells, 1498
      T-cells, 1498–1499
    donor antigens, 1489–1496
      major histocompatibility antigens,
          1489–1493
      minor histocompatibility antigens,
          1493–1494
    mechanisms of, 1500–1513
      accelerated rejection, 1502–1503
      acute rejection, 1503–1511
      chronic rejection, 1511–1513
      hyperacute rejection, 1500–1502
      induced antibodies, 1502–1503
      preformed antibodies, 1500–1502
      T-cells, 1503–1511
    prevention of, 1518–1535
      donor-specific tolerance induction,
          1520–1535
      nonspecific techniques, 1518–1520
    regulatory T-cells, control of, 953–954
Renal disease, complement in, 1092–1093
Renal graft survival, major histocompatibility
      complex, 585
Reoviruses, 1202, 1214
Replication, viruses, obstacles to, 1203–1204
Reproductive tract, human immunodeficiency
      virus, 1292
Reptiles, evolution of immune response, 549
Reservoirs, human immunodeficiency virus,
      1288–1292
Residues, framework of immunoglobulin
      chains, 53
Respiratory syncytial virus, 1214
  vaccine, 1352–1353
Respiratory tract-associated lymphoid tissues,
      435
Response characteristics
  autoimmune diseases, organ-specific
      autoimmunity, 1401–1438
  diversity of, 2
  immune system, 1–3
    acquired immunodeficiency syndrome,
        2–3, 1285–1318

autoimmune diseases, systemic
      autoimmunity, 1371–1399
  primary, 2
  secondary, 2
  self-antigen tolerance, 2, 901–934
  specificity of, 2
immunologic memory, 2
secondary, 2
Resting CD4+ T-cells, human
      immunodeficiency virus, 1291
Retroviruses, 1202
Rhabdoviruses, 1202
Rhesus antigen, development of, 39
Rheumatoid arthritis, 1383–1384, 1425–1428
  human leukocyte antigen associations, 588
  immunology, 1427
  interleukin-1 receptor antagonist, 794
  models of, 1389–1390
Rhinitis, allergic, 1470–1471
  linkage regions, 1447
Rhinovirus species, 1201
Rhinoviruses, 1214
Richet, Charles, 29
Rickettsia species, 1230, 1231, 1232, 1242
RNA tumor viruses, 1570–1571
RNaseL, 507–508
Robertson
  Bruce, 31
  Oswald, 31
Rocky Mountain fever, bacterial pathogen,
      1232
Ross, George, 25
Rotavirus, 1214
  transmission of, 1203
  vaccine, 1351–1352
Roux, ÁEmile, 1321
RSV. *See* Respiratory syncytial virus
Rubella. *See also* Measles
  transmission of virus, 1203
  vaccine, 1322, 1329, 1342

S
Sabin, Albert, 1322, 1329
Salk, Jonas, 1322, 1329
Salmonella enterica, 1230–39, 1242, 1245,
      1246, 1250, 1252, 1256, 1267
Salmonella O antigens, immunochemistry of,
      632–634
Salmonellosis, 1233
Salt concentration, thermodynamics and,
      antigen-antibody interactions, effects
      of, 71–72
Sarcoidosis, 1425
Söderqvist, Thomas, 36
Scavenger receptors, 504
Schedule, immunization, standard, 1342
Schick, Béa, 29
Schistosoma, 1178
Schistosoma haematobium, 1188
Schistosoma japonicum, 1188
Schistosomiasis, 1172
  vaccine, 1361–1362
Schlossman, Stuart, 41

Scleroderma, 1387
Scrub typhus, bacterial pathogen, 1232
Secreted pattern-recognition molecules,
      innate immune system, 505–506
  collectins, 505–506
  C-reactive protein, 506
  LBP, 506
  PGRPs, 506
Secretory immunoglobulin A
  assembly of, mucosal immune system,
      972–973
  structure of, 972
Selection theories, 34–39
Self-antigen tolerance, 2, 901–934
Sendai virus, 1204
Septic shock
  hypothalamic pituitary adrenal axis, role
      of, 1035–1036
  sympathetic nervous system, 1035–1036
Sequella Global Tuberculosis Foundation,
      1349
Serine protease module, proteins with,
      1081
Serology, age of, 25–31
Serotonin, inflammation, 1155
Serprocedins, 511
Serum amyloid A, 506
Serum antibody, in B-cell tolerance, response,
      179–180
Severe combined immunodeficiency disease,
      735–736
Sexual stage vaccine, 1360
SFK recruitment, in B-cell activation,
      activation, 198–200
SH2 domains, in signal transduction
      pathways, 338–339
Shigella species, 1239, 1270
Shigellosis vaccine, 1343–1345
Shock, septic
  hypothalamic pituitary adrenal axis, role
      of, 1035–1036
  sympathetic nervous system, 1035–1036
Shope fibroma virus, 1220
Short-lived plasma cells, development of,
      216–217
Sickness behavior, effect of peripheral
      cytokines on, 1025
Side-chain theory, 26–27
Signal transduction
  defects in, aging and, 1064
  by T-cell antigen receptor, 343–344
Signaling mechanisms, B-cell, 195–225
  BCR signaling, 196–198
  membrane microdomains, 196–198
  receptor aggregation, 198
Sips plot, 76–77
Sjögren's syndrome, 1386
Skin disorders, autoimmune, 1429–1430
  dermatitis herpetiformis, 1429–1430
  pemphigus, 1429
Skin grafting, 1535
Sloane, Hans, 1320
SMADs, 732

Smallpox, 1202, 1203
    bioterrorism and, 1363
    eradication of, 1320–1321, 1323–1324
Smithies, Oliver, 33
Sober, Herbert, 33
Soluble CD8+ T-cell secreted factors, human
        immunodeficiency virus, 1301–1302
Soluble co-stimulatory molecules, in
        immunotherapy, 1628
    anti-CD40L, 1628
Soluble cytokine receptors, 718
Soluble interleukin-2 receptors, in human
        disease, 719
Somatic hypermutation
    B lymphocytes, 10–11. See also
        Hypermutation; Somatic
        hypermutation
    BCR diversification, 218
Somatic mutation, 144–149
    cellular context of, 145
    early evidence for, 144
    hypermutation, role of, 144–145
    molecular mechanism of hypermutation,
        147–149
        DNA breaks in V regions, 147–148
        error-prone polymerases, 148–149
    targeting, distribution of mutations,
        145–147
Southern blot tests, V gene assembly,
        immunoglobulins, 108–109
Specificity
    antigen-antibody interactions, 86–89
    multispecificity, 89
    monoclonal antibodies, 100–101
Spleen
    macrophages, 486–488
        marginal zone macrophages, 487–488
        red pulp macrophages, 488
        white pulp macrophages, 488
    spontaneous mouse mutations affecting
        development, 436–438
    structure, function, 435–436
Spondylarthitides, 1384–1385
Spondylarthoropathies, 1424–1425
Src
    homology-2 domains, with T-cell
        activation, 339
    PTKs
        immunologic synapse, generation of,
            343–344
        in signal transduction by T-cell antigen
            receptor, 334–338
            Ca2+, increases in, 346–347
            Fyn PTK, 334–335
            immunologic synapse, generation of,
                343–344
            Lck PTK, 335–336
            phosphatidylinositol
                second-messenger pathway,
                344–346
            protein signaling complexes, 341–342
            protein-tyrosine phosphatase, CD45,
                339–340

PTK activation, TCR-mediated,
        consequences of, 340–348
    Ras pathway, activation of, 347–348
    second messengers of pathway,
        344–346
    SH2 domains in signal transduction
        pathways, 338–339
    signaling molecules formed upon
        TCR activation, 343–344
    Src, Syk PTKs, interaction of,
        337–338
    substrate phosphorylation, 341–342
    Syk family PTKs, 336–337
    Syk PTKs, interaction of, 337–338
Stable major histocompatibility
        complex/peptide complex, assembly
        of, 658–664
Staphylococcus aureus, 1269
    infections, 1264
Staphylococcus epidermidis, 1269
STATs, 725–732
    cytokine activation, 723
    evolution, 731
    functions of, 731–732
    specificity of, 730–731
    transcriptional activation by, 730
Stähelin, Hartmann, 36
Stein, William, 33
Stem cells, B lymphocyte development, 160
Streptococcus agalactiae, infections, 1264
Streptococcus pneumoniae, 1265, 1266,
        1267, 1269, 1270, 1273
    infections, 1264
Streptococcus pyogenes, 1268, 1269, 1270
    immunotherapy, 1623
    infections, 1264
    mechanism of action, 1623
Stress
    chronic disease and, 1034
    effects on bacterial infection, 1033
    effects on delayed type hypersensitivity,
        1034
    effects on immune-mediated disease,
        1033–1034
    effects on viral infection, 1033
    immune system-mediated disease, 1034
Stromal cell
    bone marrow, microenvironment created
        by, 420–421
    contributing to natural killer cell
        differentiation, 422
    cultures supporting lymphopoiesis,
        421–422
Stromal factors supporting lymphopoiesis,
        421–422
Strominger, J.L., 40
Strongyloides stercoralis, 1174, 1181
Substrate phosphorylation, signal
        transduction by T-cell antigen
        receptor, 341–342
Summerlin, William, 36
Superantigens
    αβ T-cell receptor, 245–246

    endogenous, 245
    T-lymphocyte activation, 324
Suppressor T-cells, 935–963
    in cancer, 1583–1584
    CD4+CD25+ naturally occurring, 939–946
    CD8+, 957–958
    double negative, 958
    therapeutic down-regulation of function,
        959–960
Surface epithelium, innate immune system,
        509–510
Surface plasmon resonance, 95–96
Surface-expressed modulators, BCR
        signaling, 207–209
    CD22, 208
    CD45, 207–208
Svedberg, Theodor, 31–32
Switch, heavy chain. See Immunoglobulin
        class switching
Syk, Src PTKs, interaction of, 336–338
Syk recruitment, in B-cell activation,
        activation, 200
Sympathetic nervous system
    immune disease, 1034, 1037
        interruptions, 1035
        inflammation, 1035–1036
Synthetic carbohydrate antigen vaccine, 1649
Synthetic molecules, complements, 1099
Syphilis, Wasserman test for, 39
Systemic autoimmunity, 1371–1399. See also
        under specific disease
    animal models, 1388–1389
        BXSB mice, 1388
        gld mice, 1388
        idiotype infusion, systemic
            autoimmunity induced by, 1389
        lpr mice, 1388
        lupus-like syndrome, induction of,
            1388–1389
        NZB mice, 1388
    apoptosis abnormalities, 1381–1382
    arthritis, reactive, 1384–1385
    autoantibodies
        characteristics of, 1375–1377
        to nuclear proteins in, 1377
    autoantigens, nature of, 1374–1375
    autoimmune diseases, 1371–1399
    B-cell tolerance in, 1374
    cytokines, 1380
    environmental influences, 1380–1381
    genetics, 1377–1378
    graft versus host disease, chronic,
        1386–1387
    historical overview, 1372
    human autoimmune disorders, features of,
        1382–1387
    immune injury, 1390–1391
    knockout strains, 1389
    lupus erythematosus, systemic, 1382–1383
    malignancy, 1382
    nonpathologic systemic autoimmunity,
        1372–1373
    regulatory T-cell abnormalities, 1379–1380

Systemic autoimmunity (*contd.*)
rheumatoid arthritis, 1383–1384
models of, 1389–1390
scleroderma, 1387
Sjögren's syndrome, 1386
spondyalrthitides, 1384–1385
T-cells, 1378–1380
autoantibody formation, 1378–1379
tolerance, 1373–1374
tight-skin mouse, 1389
tolerance, 1373–1374
transgenic strains, 1389
treatment of, 1391–1392
vasculitis, 1385–1386
Systemic lupus-like syndrome, pristane, 1388–1389
Systemic sclerosis. *See* Scleroderma

T
T cytokines
antibacterial immunity, 1244
T extracellular bacteria, associated with diseases, 1264
T helper cells. *See* Helper T-cells
T lymphocyte-mediated immunity, dendritic cells, 466–468
adoptive transfer, 466
immunostimulatory properties *in vitro*, 466
as physiological adjuvant, 466–467
T lymphocytes, 11–16. *See also* Cytotoxic T-lymphocytes; Helper T-cells
activation, 13, 309–314, 321–363
acidity, changes in, 348
antigen-presenting cells, 323–324
cellular responses, 349–350
complex antigens, peptides, 324
cyclic nucleotides, fluxes in, 348–349
cytolytic mechanism, activation of, 350
cytoskeletal changes, 349–350
defects, with primary immunodeficiency, 1611–1612
CD8 deficiency, from CD8α gene mutation, 2612
CD8 lymphocytopenia, from ζ-chain-associated protein deficiency, 1611–1612
defective cytokine production, 1612
T-cell receptor-CD3 complex, defective expression of, 1612
early biochemical events, 348–349
early signal transduction events, consequences of, 348–354
effector cells, 311–313
experimental models, 323–326
gene activation events, 350–354
cell surface molecules, expression of, 353–354
early gene activation events, 351
lymphokine genes, activation of, 351–353
inhibitors used to study, 325
lectins, 324–325
major events in, 356

membrane potential, changes in, 349
monoclonal antibodies, 325
requirements for initiation of, 326–331
accessory molecules, 329
CD4, CD8 co-receptors contribute, 328–329
co-stimulatory signal, 329–331
primary signal for T-cell activation, 326–328
signal transduction, 309–310
antigen receptor, 331–348
cytoplasmic protein-tyrosine kinases, TCR ITAMs and, 334
Lck, dynamic regulation of, 340
Src PTKs, 334–338
Ca²⁺, increases in, 346–347
Fyn PTK, 334–335
Lck PTK, 335–336
phosphatidylinositol second-messenger pathway, 344–346
plasma membrane heterogeneity, 342–343
protein-tyrosine phosphatase, CD45, 339–340
PTK activation, TCR-mediated, consequences of, 340–348
Ras pathway, activation of, 347–348
SH2 domains in signal transduction pathways, 338–339
Src, Syk PTKs, interaction of, 337–338
substrate phosphorylation, 341–342
Syk family PTKs, 336–337
structure, 331–334
superantigens, 324
T-cell inactivation, 355–356
terminating T-cell responses, 354–355
age-related changes, 1055–1060
anergy
mucosal immune system, 1002
in antibacterial immunity, 1241
antigen recognition, 11, 571–629
antigenic determinants recognized by, 646–671
autoantibody formation, 1378–1379
cancer immunity and, 1578–1579
CD4+, in mucosal tolerance, 1002–1003
CD4+ CD25- immunoregulatory, 958–959
cell biology of, age-related changes in, 1060–1062
cell death, passive, lymphokine withdrawal, 845–846
compartment, mucosal immune system, 983–989
cytotoxic, 15–16, 1127–1150
adhesion strengthening, 1134–1135
calreticulin, 1134
chemokines, 1134
dipeptidyl peptidase I, 1132

Fas ligand, 1133
granulysin, 1133
granzymes, 1131–1132
human immunodeficiency virus, 1299–1301
lymphocyte granzymes, 1132
mucosal, 989–990
perforin, 1130–1131
proteoglycan, 1132–1133
target Fas, cytotoxic T-lymphocyte-mediated induction of, 1140
death, active, antigen-stimulated, 844–845
dendritic cell synapses, dendritic cells, 467
development, 13–14, 259–301
age-related changes in, 1055–1058
anatomical path of, 264–265
CD4 single-positive thymocytes, maturation, export of, 290–291
CD8 single-positive thymocytes, maturation, export of, 290–291
cell stage markers, 260
changes with age, 1055–1058
developmental overview, 259–266
early lineage choices, 266–270
intrathymic precursors, developmental potential of, 266–267
ontogeny, variations in thymocyte development in, 265
regulated proliferation in, 263–264
regulatory T-cells, 294
stage markers, mouse-human comparison, 266
T-cell receptor genes, 260
thymocyte development, species other than mouse, 265–266
epitopes, prediction of, 668–671
function, 14, 303–319
age-related changes in, 1062
intracellular bacteria, 1245–1248
helpers, 14–15
inactivation, 355–356
independent B-cell responses, 210–211
mediated target cell lysis, inhibition of, viral, 1219–1220
memory
generation of, 867–874
identification of, 878–880
life span of, 884–885
maintenance of, 885–888
programmed cell death, 846
for mu-α switching, 986
natural killer, 958
peripheral, 303–319
dendritic cells, 305–306
high-affinity foreign peptide-major histocompatibility complex ligands
particulate antigens, 307–308
presentation of, 307–309
skin-surface antigens, 308
soluble antigens, 308–309

low-affinity self-peptide-major
  histocompatibility complex ligands,
  presentation of, 306–307
naive T-cells, 304–305
  generation, 304
  recirculation, 304
  survival, 304–305
peptide-major histocompatibility
  complex ligands, *in vivo*
  presentation of, 306–309
T-cell activation, 309–314
  effector cells, 311–313
  IL-2 production, 310–311
  memory cells, 313–314
    memory CD4 T-cells, 313–314
    memory CD8 T-cells, 313
  signal transduction, 309–310
recognition, major histocompatibility
  complex, restricted recognition, 18–19
regulatory, 15, 935–963
  allograft rejection, control of, 953–954
  function, enhancement of, 960
  induced, 946–950
  infectious agents, control of immunity
    to, 955–957
  in oral tolerance, 1002–1003
  therapeutic manipulation of function,
    959–960
  tumor immunity, 954–955
selection, thymic regulation of, 1030
subsets, changes with age, 1058–1059
suppressor, 935–963
  in cancer, 1583–1584
  CD4+CD25+, naturally occurring,
    939–946
  CD8+, 957–958
  double negative, 958
systemic autoimmunity, 1378–1380
tolerance
  in autoimmune diseases, 1404
  dendritic cells, 470–472
    central tolerance, 470
    interleukin-10, 472
    peripheral tolerance, 470–472
      immature dendritic cells, 471
    specialized subsets of, 471–472
  in systemic autoimmunity, 1373–1374
transplantation immunity, 1561
vaccine, parasites, 1192–1194
T regulatory 1 cells, 947–948
mucosal immune system, 985
T22 tetramers, $\epsilon\delta$-CD3, 248–249
Talmage, David, 36–37
Tat-associated protein, 1092
T-cell activation, memory cells and, 313–314
T-cell antigen receptors. *See* T-cell receptors
T-cell receptors, 39–41, 227–258
  $\alpha\beta$
    genetic regulation of, *versus* T-cell
      receptor $\epsilon\delta$ cell production,
      277–278
    T-cell receptor $\epsilon\delta$ lineage cells,
      divergence of, 276–280

$\alpha\beta$ T-cell receptor, superantigens, 245–246
$\alpha\beta$ T-cell receptor structure, 229–231
$\alpha\beta$ T-cell receptor-ligand interactions,
  237–241
  CD4, role of, 241
  CD8, role of, 241
antigen processing, antigen recognition by,
  6123
CD3 polypeptides, 231–234
  intracellular assembly, 233–234
  sequence, 232–233
  structure, 234
changes with age, 1059–1060
complementarity-determining region 3
  diversification, 251–252
in evolution of immune response, 521–526
  α/β constant domains, 523–524
  α/β variable domains, 524–525
  CD3 complex, 525–526
  ϵ/δ TCR, 525
$\epsilon\delta$ cells, generation of, 277
$\epsilon\delta$ T-cells, 249–250
  complementarity-determining region 3
    length distribution analysis, 250
  ligands, multivalence of, 250–251
$\epsilon\delta$-CD3, 246–251
  antigen recognition, 247–249
  identification of, 246–247
  immune defense, $\alpha\beta$ T-cells, contrasted,
    247
  nonpeptide antigens, stimulation by, 249
  T22 tetramers, 248–249
genes, 234–237
  α/δ locus, 234–235
  allelic exclusion, 237
  β locus, 235
  commitment to $\alpha\beta$ lineage *versus* $\epsilon\delta$
    lineage, 237
  ϵ locus, 235–236
  transcriptional control, 236
  translocations associated with disease,
    236–237
immunoglobulin, in mouse, human,
  chromosomal locations of, 236
interactions, major histocompatibility
  complex, 600
ligand binding, 238
lymphocytes, 11–13, 227–258
plasticity, 242–245
polypeptides, 228
recognition, 664–668
  amino acid substitution
    altered peptide ligands, effects of,
      666–668
    mapping by, 666–668
      effects of altered peptide ligands,
        666–668
  epitope mapping, 665–666
repertoire, changes in with age, 1059–1060
structure, 228–231
T-cell receptor-peptide/major
  histocompatibility complex, 241–245
T-cells. *See* T lymphocytes

TCRs. *See* T-cell receptors
TdT, in evolution of immune response, 553
Template theory
  antibody production, 27–29
  of Felix Haurowitz, 23
Terminal complement complex, 1087
  biological properties of, 1088
Terminal components of complement system,
  22
Terminal deoxynucleotide transferase, 125
Tetanus
  vaccine, 1329, 1342–1343
Th1 cells. *See* Helper T-cells
Th2 cells. *See* Helper T-cells
Theiler, Max, 1322
Thermodynamics
  in antigen-antibody interactions, 70–73
    acidity, effects of, 71–72
    chemical equilibrium in solution, 70–71
    free energy, 71
    salt concentration, effects of, 71–72
    temperature, effects of, 71–72
Thrombocytopenia, immunodeficiency with,
  1607–1608
Thymic cortex, autoreactivity in, 284
Thymic deletion, programmed cell death, 843
Thymic hormones, analogs, in
  immunotherapy, 1625
Thymic regulation, T-cell selection, 1030
Thymic stromal lymphopoietin, 716
Thymocyte development
  ontogeny in, 265
  species other than mouse, 265–266
Thymoma, immunodeficiency with, 1602
Thymus, 422–428
  biology of, 38
  embryologic development, 423–425
  macrophages, 485–486
  mature architecture, 425–427
  nonlymphoid bone marrow-derived cells,
    427
  normal anatomy, 422–423
  T-lymphopoiesis, thymic compartments,
    relationship, 427–428
Thyroiditis, autoimmune, 1428–1429
  immunology, 1428–1429
  regulatory T-cells, 951
TI-2 B-cell responses, regulation of, 211
Timoni, Emmannuel, 23
Tiselius, Arne, 32
TKR4, 500–501
T-lineage specification, T-cell development,
  molecular indices of, 267–268
TLR signaling pathways, 502–504
TLR1, 501
TLR2, 501
TLR3, 501–502
TLR5, 502
TLR6, 501
TLR9, 502
T-lymphopoiesis, thymic compartments,
  relationship, 427–428
TNF. *See* Tumor necrosis factor

Togaviruses, 1202
Tolerance
    antigen-presenting cell, 917
        role of, 915–921
    B-cell
        in autoimmune diseases, 1404–1405
        compartment, negative selection,
            906–907
        mature, tolerance induction, 921–925
            B-cell anergy, 922–924
                clonal deletion, 924
                thymic-independent antigens,
                    924–925
            receptor blockade, 921–922
    bone marrow, mechanisms of negative
        selection in, 907
    CD4+CD25+ suppressor T-cells, 914–915
    CD8+ cytotoxic T-cells, 920–921
    CD28/B7, CD40/CD40L co-stimulation,
        918–919
    central, in autoimmune diseases,
        1403–1406
    CTLA-4, PD-1 coinhibition, T-cell
        activation, 919–920
    fetal-maternal relationship, 929–931
    graft, 35–36
    heat-shock proteins, 916–917
    immature B-cells, 908–909
    immune-privileged sites, 929
    immunoregulation, 926–929
        antibody-mediated immunoregulation,
            928
        anti-idiotypic B-cell regulation, 928–929
        anti-idiotypic T-cell regulation, 929
        CD4+ T-regulatory 1 cells, 926–927
        CD8+ suppressor T-cells, 927–928
        CD8+ veto cells, 928
        immune deviation, 926
        nasal tolerance, 927
        oral tolerance, 927
    mucosal, 1000–1004
        mechanisms for, 1000–1004
    negative selection, B-cells, antigen
        characteristics required for, 907–908
    Nods, receptors, 916–917
    OX40/OX40L, ICOS/ICOSL
        co-stimulation, 919
    peripheral
        antigens, tolerance to, 909–921
        in autoimmune disease, 1403–1406
    in systemic autoimmunity, 1373–1374
    T-cell
        activation, "two-signal" model of,
            917–918
        anergy, 912–914
        in autoimmune diseases, 1404
        tissue-specific peptide antigens, 909–910
Toll pathways, in evolution of immune
    response, 559
Toll-like receptors, 491
    innate immune system, 499–504
    TKR4, 500–501
    TLR signaling pathways, 502–504

TLR1, 501
TLR2, 501
TLR3, 501–502
TLR5, 502
TLR6, 501
TLR9, 502
Tonegawa, Susumu, 40
Toxic effector molecules, intracellular
    bacteria, 1238–1239
Toxins, in vaccination, 1321–1322
Toxoids, in vaccination, 1321–1322,
    1329–1330
Toxoplasma cruzi, 1174, 1175, 1179, 1185,
    1186
Toxoplasma gondii, 1171, 1174, 1175, 1178,
    1179, 1185, 1186, 1187, 1238
Toxoplasma species, 1171, 1172, 1174
Tracer concentrations, antigen-antibody
    interactions, optimization of, 82
Trachoma, bacterial pathogen, 1232
Transcription factors, B lymphocyte
    development, 162–164
Transcriptional control, T-cell receptor, 236
Transdermal vaccine, 1334
Transforming growth factor β, in evolution of
    immune response, 551–552
Transfusion, 30–31
Transgenic models, B-cell tolerance, 178
Transgenic plants, mucosal immunity and, 999
Transitional B-cells, 172–174
Translocations associated with disease, T-cell
    receptor, 236–237
Transplantation, 1481–1555
    antigen matching, 1543–1545
    cancer and, 1573
    chemokines, in rejection, 820
    crossmatch, 1545
    donor antigens, graft rejection, 1489–1496
        major histocompatibility antigens,
            1489–1493
        minor histocompatibility antigens,
            1493–1494
    graft rejection
        components of immune system in,
            1496–1500
            antibodies, 1498
            antigen-presenting cells, 1496–1498
            B-cells, 1498
            T-cells, 1498–1499
        mechanisms of, 1500–1513
            chronic rejection, 1511–1513
            induced antibodies, 1502–1503
            preformed antibodies, 1500–1502
            T-cells, 1503–1511
    heart, 1536
    hematopoietic cell transplantation,
        1537–1539
    immunity, T-cell mediation, 1561
    immunogenetics, discoveries of,
        1483–1489
    immunologic issues, 1543–1546
    immunology, 1481–1555
        origins of, 1482–1489

    immunosuppression, 1546
    immunotherapy, 1635
    islet, 1536–1537
    kidney transplantation, 1535–1536
    laws of, 1485
    liver transplantation, 1536
    lung, 1536
    major histocompatibility complex,
        583–584
        clinical, 584–586
    origins of, 1482–1489
    pancreas, 1536–1537
    physiologic interactions, graft rejection,
        1513–1518
        effector cell regulation, 1517–1518
        helper, effector cells, communication
            between, 1515–1517
        sensitization, regulation of, 1513–1515
    prevention of graft rejection, 1518–1535
        donor-specific tolerance induction,
            1520–1535
        nonspecific techniques, 1518–1520
    rejection, diagnosis of, 1546
    "sensitized" candidate, 1545–1546
    skin grafting, 1535
    xenogeneic transplantation, 1539–1543
Transplanted cancers, tumor-specific
    rejection, 1559
Trehalose dimycolate derivatives, in
    immunotherapy, 1624
Treponema pallidum, 1264, 1267
Trichinella species, 1183
Trichinella spiralis, 1181
Trigger mechanism entry, intracellular
    bacteria, 1234
Trypanosome brucei gambiense, 1173
Trypanosome brucei rhodesiense,
    1173
Trypanosome brucei species, 1173, 1175,
    1183
Tryptophan degradation, intracellular
    bacteria, 1238
Tswett, M., 33
Tuberculosis, 1232–1233
    bacterial pathogen, 1231
    vaccine, 1329, 1348–1349
Tularemia, bacterial pathogen, 1231
Tumor antigens
    antigenicity, 1565
    recognized by syngeneic, autologous
        T-cells, somatic mutation, 1563
Tumor cell types, treated with tumor necrosis
    factor-related apoptosis-inducing
    ligand, with chemotherapeutics,
    762
Tumor necrosis factor
    apoptosis-inducing ligand, 761–764
        as cancer chemotherapeutic, 763–764
        receptors, 762–763
        tumor cell types treated with, with
            chemotherapeutics, 762
    in evolution of immune response, 550
    ligands, classification of, 752

programmed cell death, 856–857
receptor pathways, with co-stimulatory
    function, 404–405
signaling, inflammatory properties
    associated with, 757
superfamily, 749–773
    4-1BB, 765–766
    apoptosis-inducing ligand, 761–764
        as cancer chemotherapeutic, 763–764
        receptors, 762–763
    APRIL, 766–768
    BLyS, 766–768
    CD27, 764–765
    CD30, 765
    ectodysplasin, 768
    EDAR, 768
    expression, chromosome location of, 402
    FAS, 759–760
    Fas ligand, 759–760
    HVEM ligand, 759
    lymphotoxin, 758–759
    osteoprotegerin, 760–761
    OX40, 766
    OX40 ligand, 766
    programmed cell death, 853
    RANK, 760–761
    RANK ligand, 760–761
    receptors, 750
    structure-function relationships,
        751–753
    TNF-α
        biological functions of, 754–755
        expression, regulation of, 753–754
        signaling, 755–758
    TWEAK, 764
Tumor necrosis factor-α
    biological functions of, 754–755
    expression, regulation of, 753–754
    signaling, 755–758
Tumor stroma, tumor formation and,
    1581–1582
Tumor-associated antigens, examples, 1647
Tumor-infiltrating lymphocytes, in
    immunotherapy, 1644
Tumors, 1557–1592
    age, immune response and, 1585
    antigen loss, 1582–1583
    antigenic modulation, 1583
    antigens, 1559–1561
        encoded by normal cellular genes,
            1566–1569
            carcinoembryonic antigens,
                1568–1569
            clonal antigens, 1569
            differentiation antigens, 1567–1568
            oncofetal antigens, 1568–1569
            oncospermatogonal antigens, 1567
        encoded by viral genes, 1569–1571
            DNA tumor viruses, 1569–1570
            RNA tumor viruses, 1570–1571
        expressed on cancer cell, 1561–1562
        tumor-associated, 1566–1569
        tumor-specific, 1562–1566

cancer
    immunity, effector mechanisms in,
        1577–1580
        antibodies, 1578
        B-cells, 1578
        cytokines, 1580
        lymphokine-activated killer cells,
            1579
        macrophages, 1579–1580
        natural killer cells, 1579
        neutrophils, 1579–1580
        T-lymphocytes, 1578–1579
        in vivo, assays, 1577–1578
    immunological factors influencing,
        1571–1576
cancer-testis antigens, 1567
development stimulation, 1573–1576
epitope loss, 1582–1583
escape from immunological destruction,
    mechanisms of, 1581
immune suppression vs.
        immunodeficiency, 1584–1585
    carcinogens, 1584
    tumor burden, 1584–1585
immunity, factors limiting, 1580–1585
immunodeficiency, 1584–1585
immunogenicity
    carcinogen dose, 1577
    factors influencing, 1576–1577
    immunocompetence, 1577
    spontaneous, induced cancers,
        contrasted, 1576–1577
    tumor latency, 1577
immunological enhancement blocking
    factors, 1583–1584
immunoprevention, 1585–1586
immunosurveillance, tumor development,
    1571–1573
    adaptive T-cell-mediated, 1571–1572
    innate, 1572–1573
immunotherapy, 1586–1588
latency, immunogenicity and, 1577
major histocompatibility complex
    class I, antigens, changes in expression
        of, 1582
    haplotype, 1580–1581
microenvironment of, 1581–1582
mutations
    chromosomal translocations, fusion
        proteins resulting from, 1566
    discovered by functional, genetic
        analyses, 1564–1566
        fusion proteins, 1566
        mutant p53 suppressor gene-encoded
            proteins, 1564–1566
        mutant ras oncogene-encoded
            proteins, 1564
    discovered by immunological analyses,
        1562–1564
    internal deletions, fusion proteins
        resulting from, 1566
radiation vs. chemotherapeutic agents,
    1585

rejection antigens, individually distinct,
    characteristics of, 1561
rejection antigens on, 1558–1562
stroma, 1581–1582
T-cells
    suppressor, 1583–1584
    in transplantation immunity mediation,
        1561
transplantation, 1573
    T-cell mediation, 1561
tumor-specific rejection, transplanted
    cancers, 1559
Tumor-specific antigens, 1562–1566
Tumor-specific rejection, transplanted
    cancers, 1559
TWEAK, 764
Two-phase systems, antigen-antibody
    interactions, affinity, 79–80
Type 1 T-independent B-cell responses, 210
Type 2 T-Independent B-cell responses,
    210–211
Type I cytokine receptors, 701–747
    common β chain, β_c, cytokine receptors
        sharing, 711–712
    common cytokine receptor ϵ chain,
        cytokines sharing, 706–711
    cytokine pleiotropy, 717–718
    cytokine receptor
        pleiotropy, 717–718
        redundancy, 717–718
    cytokine redundancy, 717–718
    families of, 706–717
    features common to, 704
    G-CSF receptor, receptors with similarities
        to, 715–716
    glycoprotein 130, receptors with
        similarities to, 715–716
    heterodimers, 705–706
    higher order receptor oligomers, 705–706
    homodimers, 705–706
    IL-2, 716–717
    IL-4, 716
    IL-7, 716
    IL-12, 715–716
    IL-23, 715
    IL-27, 715–716
    leptin, 715
    nomenclature, 702
    obesity receptor, receptors with similarities
        to, 715–716
    receptor chains, sharing of, significance of,
        715
    thymic stromal lymphopoietin, 716
    type I cytokines, 702–706
        structure, 702–704
    X-linked severe combined
        immunodeficiency disease, ϵ_c
        mutations, 709–711
Type I cytokines, phenotypes of mice
    deficiency in, 726–727
Type II cytokines, 718–720
    interleukin-10, 720
    phenotypes of mice deficiency in, 726–727

Typhoid fever, bacterial pathogen, 1231
Typhoid vaccine, 1329, 1343–1345
Typhus, bacterial pathogen, 1232
Tyrosine kinase, 732–733
  syk
    initiation of phagocytosis, 1114
    phagocytosis, 1114
Tyrosine phosphorylated, following TCR
  stimulation, 341
Tyrosine-based activation motif pathways,
  691–692
Tyrosine-based inhibitor motif pathways,
  692–693

U

Ulcerative colitis, 1430
Unconjugated antibodies
  for cancer, 1629
  for diseases other than cancer, 1634
Uveitis, idiopathic, 1425

V

V gene assembly
  immunoglobulins
    overview, 108–111
    recombination, diversity and, 109–111
    recombination signal elements, 111
    Southern blot tests, gene cloning,
      108–109
  recombination, immunoglobulins, 116–132
    allelic exclusion, 128–130
    B lymphocyte development, 126–127
    B-cell maturation, B-cell receptor
      regulation of, 130
    hairpins, 120–121
    late recombination activating gene
      expression, 130–132
    mechanisms, 119–126
    P nucleotides, 120–121
    receptor editing, 130–132
    receptor revision, 130–132
    recombination activating gene proteins,
      V-D-J recombination, 121–123
    recombination intermediates, 120–121
    recombination model, 119
    recombinational accessibility, 127–128
    regulated V(D)J recombination, 128–130
    regulation, 126–132
    substrates, experiments, 119–120
    topology, 116–117
      deletion *versus* inversion, 116–117
      secondary recombinations, 117–118
    transcription, 127–128
    V-D-J recombination
      artemis, 124–125
      DNA breaks, proteins binding to, 125
      DNA-PK, 123–124
      exonuclease, 125–126
      Ku, 123–124
      N regions, 125
      terminal deoxynucleotide transferase,
        125
      XRCC4, 123–124

Vaccination, 1319–1369, 1647–1651.
  See also Immunization
  acellular pertussis, 1329, 1342
    history of vaccination, 1342–1343
  adjuvants, 1335–1342
    aluminum compounds, 1337
    antigen-presenting cell activation,
      1335–1336
    antigens
      microencapsulation of, 1339–1340
      molecular targeting of, 1341
    cytokines as adjuvants, 1340–1341
    emulsions, as adjuvants, 1337–1338
    microparticles, 1338
    mucosal adjuvants, 1341–1342
    oligonucleotides, 1339
  adverse effects of, 1363–1365
  aging and, 1065
  anthrax, 1329
  anticytokine, 1649
  antidisease, 1360
  bacterial, 1342–1349
  bioterrorism, 1363
  carbohydrate, 1330
  cholera, 1329, 1343–1345
  classification of, 1328–1330
  combination, 1330
  conjugate, 1330
  CpG motifs, 1339
  dendritic cell, 1650
  deoxyribonucleic acid, 1360
  diarrheal disease, 1343–1345
  diphtheria, 1329, 1342–1343
  DNA, 1649–1650
  early bacterial, 1321–1322
  early toxins, 1321–1322
  early viral, 1322
  edible, 1334
  Ehrlich, Paul, 1321
  for elderly, 1365–1366
  encapsulated organisms, 1347–1348
  Gates Malaria Vaccine Initiative,
    1361
  Global Alliance for Vaccines and
    Immunization, 1327–1328, 1330
  glycophosphatidylinositol toxin, 1360
  group A streptococci, 1349
  Haemophilus influenzae type B,
    1322–1323, 1329, 1342,
    1347–1348
  Helicobacter pylori, 1345–1347
  helminths, 1193–1194
  hepatitis A, 1329, 1350–1351
  hepatitis B, 1322–1323, 1329, 1342,
    1350–1351
  hepatitis C, 1350–1351
  historical perspectives, 1320–1323
  history of, 23–25
  human immunodeficiency virus,
    1305–1307
    prophylactic, 1354–1357
    therapeutic vaccine, 1357
  Id, 1648–1649

  immunization, expanded program on,
    1324–1325
  immunization schedules, 1342
  immunostimulatory complexes, 1338
  influenza, 1322, 1329, 1353–1354
  intestinal protozoa, 1190
  intracellular pathogens, 1348–1349
    in vaccination, 1348–1349
  Jennerian era, 1320–1321
  killed microorganisms, 1329
  leishmaniasis, 1192, 1361
  leprosy, 1329, 1348–1349
  liposomes, 1338
  live attenuated, 1329–1329
  malaria, 1190–1192, 1357–1358
    extracellular stages, 1190–1192
    liver stages, 1192–1193
    as vaccine molecule, 1360
  measles, 1322, 1327, 1329, 1342
  meningococci, 1329, 1347–1348
  molecular, 1330
  molecular era, 1322–1323
  mucosal, 1332–1333
  mumps, 1329, 1342
  new approaches, 1330–1335
  nucleic acid, 1331–1332
  parasitic diseases, 1357–1362
  parasitic pathogens, 1190–1194
  peptide, 1332
  pertussis, 1329
  Plasmodium falciparum, life cycle of,
    1358–1361
  pneumococcus, 1322–1323, 1329, 1342,
    1347–1348
  poliomyelitis, 1322, 1325–1327, 1329,
    1342
  to prevent pathology, 1193
  prime-boost strategies, 1334–1335
  protein, 1330, 1648
  public health triumphs, 1323–1328
  rabies, 1329
  recombinant bacterial, 1649
  recombinant viral vector, 1649
  respiratory syncytial virus, 1352–1353
  rotavirus, 1351–1352
  rubella, 1322, 1329, 1342
  schistosomiasis, 1361–1362
  sexual stage, 1360
  shigellosis, 1343–1345
  smallpox, 1323–1324
  synthetic carbohydrate antigen, 1649
  tetanus, 1329, 1342
    history of vaccination, 1342–1343
  tissue culture revolution, 1322
  toxins, 1321–1322
  toxoids, 1321–1322, 1329–1330
  transdermal, 1334
  tuberculosis, 1329, 1348–1349
  typhoid, 1329, 1343–1345
  with unidentified antigens, 1650–1651
    autologous or allogeneic tumor cells,
      1650
    heat-shock proteins, 1650–1651

varicella, 1329, 1342
vectored, 1330–1331
viral, 1349–1357
virosomes, 1338
viruslike particles, 1338
yellow fever, 1322, 1329
for young, 1365–1366
Vaccine design
approaches to, 1329
intracellular bacteria, 1246
Vaccinia virus, 1222
Vagus nerve stimulation, 1024
Varicella vaccine, 1329, 1342
Vasculitis, 1385–1386
Vasodilation, in inflammation, 1153
Vβ specificity of exogenous, 245
V-D-J recombination
immunoglobulins
artemis, 124–125
DNA breaks, proteins binding to, 125
exonuclease, 125–126
Ku, 123–124
N regions, 125
V gene assembly recombination
DNA-PK, 123–124
terminal deoxynucleotide transferase,
125
XRCC4, 123–124
Vectored vaccine, 1330–1331
Veiled cells, dendritic, 458
Venom allergens, 1444
Vibrio cholera, infections, 1264
Vibrio fischeri, 1270
Viral chemokines, chemokine receptors,
823
Viral entry, early replication, obstacles to,
1203–1204
Viral genes, antigens encoded by, 1569–1571
Viral immunology, 1201–1228
antigen processing, inhibition of
transporter associated with, 1219
antigen-specific immune mechanisms,
effector functions of, 1210–1211
antigen-specific immune responses,
induction of, 1206–1210
autoimmunity, after virus infections, 1216
B-cells, activation of, 1209–1210
CD8+ T-cells, antigen processing for
activation of, 1209
complement activation, inhibition of, 1221
crystallized fragment receptor mimetics,
1222
cytokine mimetics, 1221
cytokines
inhibition of, 1221
interference of, 1221–1222

escape
by destruction of immune cells, 1217
by hiding, 1217
by latency, 1217
by mutations, 1216–1217
by subverting antigen processing,
antigen presentation, 1217–1219
humans, viruses pathogenic in, 1203
immunologic memory, 1211–1212
interferons, inhibition of, 1222
interleukin-1 cleavage, inhibition of,
1221–1222
interleukin-18, inhibition of, 1222
major histocompatibility complex class I
dislocation into cytoplasm, 1219
dislocation of molecules into lysosomes,
1219
molecules, in endoplasmic reticulum,
retention of, 1219
pathway, inhibition of antigen
presentation through, 1218
peptide complexes, surface-expressed,
interference with, 1219
in pre-Golgi/Golgi compartment,
retention of, 1219
synthesis, inhibition, 1217
major histocompatibility complex class II
molecules, in endoplasmic reticulum,
retention of, 1219
synthesis, inhibition, 1217
mucosal immune system, 1212–1213
natural killer cell activity, inhibition of,
1220–1221
non-antigen-specific antiviral defense
mechanisms, 1205–1206
peptidases, inhibition of, 1217–1219
persistent virus infections, 1213–1216
receptor mimetics, 1221
recognition of viruses, by innate immune
system, 1204–1205
taxonomy of viruses, 1202
T-cell-mediated target cell lysis, inhibition
of, 1219–1220
viral entry, early replication, obstacles to,
1203–1204
viral subversion of immune responses,
1216–1222
viral superantigens, 1216
Viral infections, natural killer cells, 382
Viral superantigens, 1216
Viral vaccine, 1349–1357
early, 1322
Virosomes
in immunotherapy, 1338
vaccine, 1338
Virulence, intracellular bacteria, 1230–1232

Virus
interferon, 1205–1206
in organ-specific autoimmunity, 1407–1409
pathogenic in humans, 1203
replication, human immunodeficiency
virus, immune system-mediated
restriction of, 1300
taxonomy of, 1202
Viruslike particles, 1338
in immunotherapy, 1338
Vitamin D receptor, intracellular bacteria,
1256
von Behring, Emil, 26, 1321
von Pirquet, Clemens, 29, 35

W
Waksman, Byron, 36, 38
WAS. See Wiskott-Aldrich syndrome
Wasserman test, 30, 39
Watson, James, 34
Week agonist-antagonist binding, 240
West Nile virus, 1201
transmission of, 1203
Western blot, antigen-antibody interactions,
94–95
White pulp macrophages, spleen,
488
Wiener, Alexander, 30, 39
Wiley, Don, 40
Wiskott-Aldrich syndrome, 1607–1608
Wright, Sir Almroth, 24, 25, 29
Wucheria bancrofti, 1181
WZSX-1/TCCR type I receptor, mutations in,
736

X
Xenogeneic transplantation, 1539–1543
Xenograft rejection. See Rejection
X-linked aεglobulinemia, 1595–1596
X-linked immunodeficiency, in mice,
1596–1597
X-linked severe combined immunodeficiency,
εc mutations, 709–711
XRCC4, 123–124
XSCID, features of, 709

Y
Yellow fever vaccine, 1322, 1329
Yersin, Alexandre, 1321
Young persons, vaccination of,
1365–1366

Z
Zipper mechanism
intracellular bacteria entry, 1234
phagocytosis, 1113

42. Blackman MA, Tigges MA, Minie ME, et al. A model system for peptide hormone action in differentiation: interleukin 2 induces a B lymphoma to transcribe the J chain gene. *Cell* 1986;47:609.

43. Siegel JP, Sharon M, Smith PL, et al. The IL-2 receptor β chain (p70): role in mediating signals for LAK, NK, and proliferative activities. *Science* 1987;238:75.

44. Lanier LL, Phillips JH. Natural killer cells. *Curr Opin Immunol* 1992; 4:38.

45. Janssen RAJ, Mulder NH, The TH, et al. The immunobiological effects of interleukin-2 *in vivo*. *Cancer Immunol Immunother* 1994; 39:207.

46. Lenardo M, Chan KM, Hornung F, et al. Mature T lymphocyte apoptosis–immune regulation in a dynamic and unpredictable antigenic environment. *Annu Rev Immunol* 1999;17:221.

47. Lin J-X, Leonard WJ. Interleukin-2. In: Thomson A, Lotze MT, eds. *The cytokine handbook,* 4th ed. New York: Academic Press, in press.

48. Taniguchi T, Matsui H, Fujita T, et al. Structure and expression of a cloned cDNA for human interleukin-2. *Nature* 1983;302:305.

49. Leonard WJ, Depper JM, Crabtree GR, et al. Molecular cloning and expression of cDNAs for the human interleukin-2 receptor. *Nature* 1984;311:625.

50. Nikaido T, Shimizu A, Ishida N, et al. Molecular cloning of cDNA encoding human interleukin-2 receptor. *Nature* 1984;311:631.

51. Lin J-X, Leonard WJ. Signaling from the IL-2 receptor to the nucleus. *Cytokine Growth Factor Rev* 1997;8:313.

52. Siegel LJ, Harper ME, Wong-Staal F, et al. Gene for T-cell growth factor: location on human chromosome 4q and feline chromosome B1. *Science* 1984;223:175.

53. Leonard WJ, Depper JM, Uchiyama T, et al. A monoclonal antibody that appears to recognize the receptor for human T-cell growth factor; partial characterization of the receptor. *Nature* 1982;300:267.

54. Sharon M, Klausner RD, Cullen BR, et al. Novel interleukin-2 receptor subunit detected by cross-linking under high affinity conditions. *Science* 1986;234:859.

55. Tsudo M, Kozak RW, Goldman CK, et al. Demonstration of a non-Tac peptide that binds interleukin-2: a potential participant in a multichain interleukin-2 receptor complex. *Proc Natl Acad Sci U S A* 1986;83:9694.

56. Teshigawara K, Wang HM, Kata K, et al. Interleukin-2 high affinity receptor expression requires two distinct binding proteins. *J Exp Med* 1987;165:223.

57. Hatakeyama M, Tsudo M, Minamoto S, et al. Interleukin-2 receptor β chain gene; generation of three receptor forms by cloned human α and β cDNAs. *Science* 1989;244:551.

58. Paul WE. Interleukin-4: a prototypic immunoregulatory lymphokine. *Blood* 1991;77:1859.

59. Nelms K, Keegan AD, Zamorano J, et al. The IL-4 receptor: signaling mechanisms and biologic functions. *Annu Rev Immunol* 1999; 17:701.

60. Yoshimoto T, Bendelac A, Watson C, et al. Role of NK1.1+ T cells in a TH2 response and in immunoglobulin E production. *Science* 1995;270:1845.

61. Paul WE. The role of IL-4 in the regulation of B cell development, growth, and differentiation. In: Spits H, ed. *IL-4: structure and function.* Boca Raton, FL: CRC Press, 1992:57.

62. Boulay J-L, Paul WE: Hematopoietin sub-family classification based on size, gene organization and sequence homology, *Curr Biol* 1993; 3:573.

63. Mosley B, Beckmann MP, March CJ, et al. The murine interleukin-4 receptor: molecular cloning and characterization of secreted and membrane bound forms. *Cell* 1989;59:335.

64. Idzerda RL, March CJ, Mosley B, et al. Human interleukin 4 receptor confers biological responsiveness and defines a novel receptor superfamily. *J Exp Med* 1990;171:861.

65. Galizzi J-P, Zuber CE, Harada N, et al. Molecular cloning of a cDNA encoding the human interleukin 4 receptor. *Int Immunol* 1990;2: 669.

66. Namen AE, Lupton S, Hjerrild K, et al. Stimulation of B-cell progenitors by cloned murine interleukin-7. *Nature* 1988;333:571.

67. Goodwin RG, Lupton S, Schmierer A, et al. Human interleukin-7: molecular cloning and growth factor activity on human and murine B-lineage cells. *Cell* 1990;60:940.

68. Watson JD, Morrissey PJ, Namen AE, et al. Effect of IL-7 on the growth of fetal thymocytes in culture. *J Immunol* 1989;143:1215.

69. Murray R, Suda T, Wrighton N, et al. IL-7 is a growth and maintenance factor for mature and immature thymocyte subsets. *Int Immunol* 1989;1:526.

70. Peschon J, Morrissey PJ, Grabstein KH, et al. Early lymphocyte expansion is severely impaired in interleukin 7 receptor—deficient mice. *J Exp Med* 1994;180:1955.

71. von Freeden-Jeffry U, Vieira P, Lucian LA, et al. Lymphopenia in interleukin (IL)–7 gene–deleted mice identifies IL-7 as a nonredundant cytokine. *J Exp Med* 1995;181:1519.

72. Fry TJ, Mackall CL. Interleukin-7: from bench to clinic. *Blood* 2002;99:3892.

73. Tan JT, Dudl E, LeRoy E, et al. IL-7 is critical for homeostatic proliferation and survival of naive T cells. *Proc Natl Acad Sci U S A* 2001;98:8732.

74. Schluns KS, Kieper WC, Jameson SC, et al. Interleukin-7 mediates the homeostasis of naive and memory CD8 T cells in *vivo*. *Nat Immunol* 2000;1:426.

75. Chazen GD, Pereira GMB, LeGros G, et al. Interleukin 7 is a T-cell growth factor. *Proc Natl Acad Sci U S A* 1989;86:5923.

76. Morrissey PJ, Goodwin RG, Nordan RP, et al. Recombinant interleukin 7, pre–B cell growth factor, has costimulatory activity on purified mature T cells. *J Exp Med* 1989;169:707.

77. Leonard WJ. The defective gene in X-linked severe combined immunodeficiency encodes a shared interleukin receptor subunit: implications for cytokine pleiotropy and redundancy. *Curr Opin Immunol* 1994;6:631.

78. Brunton LL, Lupton SD. An STS in the human IL7 gene located at 8p12–13. *Nucl Acids Res* 1990;18:1315.

79. Goodwin RG, Friend D, Ziegler SF, et al. Cloning of the human and murine interleukin-7 receptors: demonstration of a soluble form and homology to a new receptor superfamily. *Cell* 1990;60:940.

80. Van Snick J, Goethals A, Renauld J-C, et al. Cloning and characterization of a cDNA for a new mouse T cell growth factor (P40). *J Exp Med* 1989;169:363.

81. Yang Y, Ricciardi S, Ciarletta A, et al. Expression cloning of a cDNA encoding a novel human hematopoietic growth factor: human homologue of murine T-cell growth factor P40. *Blood* 1989;74: 1880.

82. Demoulin JB, Renauld JC. Interleukin 9 and its receptor: an overview of structure and function. *Int Rev Immunol* 1998;16:345.

83. Hultner L, Moeller J, Schmitt E, et al. Thiol-sensitive mast cell lines derived from mouse bone marrow respond to a mast cell growth-enhancing activity different from both IL-3 and IL-4. *J Immunol* 1989;142:3440.

84. Renauld J-C, Vink A, Louahed J, et al. Interleukin-9 is a major anti-apoptotic factor for thymic lymphomas. *Blood* 1995;85:1300.

85. Townsend JM, Fallon GP, Matthews JD, et al. IL-9–deficient mice establish fundamental roles for IL-9 in pulmonary mastocytosis and goblet cell hyperplasia but not T cell development. *Immunity* 2000; 13:573.

86. Temann UA, Geba GP, Rankin JA, et al. Expression of interleukin 9 in the lungs of transgenic mice causes airway inflammation, mast cell hyperplasia, and bronchial hyperresponsiveness. *J Exp Med* 1998; 188:1307.

87. McMillan SJ, Bishop B, Townsend MJ, et al. The absence of interleukin 9 does not affect the development of allergen-induced pulmonary inflammation nor airway hyperreactivity. *J Exp Med* 2002;195:51–7.

88. Renauld JC. New insights into the role of cytokines in asthma. *J Clin Pathol* 2001;54:577.

89. Modi WS, Pollock DD, Mock BA, et al. Regional localization of the human glutaminase (GLS) and interleukin-9 (IL9) genes by in *situ* hybridization. *Cytogenet Cell Genet* 1991;57:114.

90. Renauld J-C, Druez C, Kermouni A, et al. Expression cloning of the murine and human interleukin 9 receptor cDNAs. *Proc Natl Acad Sci U S A* 1992;89:5690.

91. Grabstein KH, Eisenman J, Shanebeck K, et al. Cloning of a T cell growth factor that interacts with the β chain of the interleukin-2 receptor. *Science* 1994;264:965.

92. Burton JD, Famford RN, Peters C, et al. A lymphokine, provisionally designated interleukin T and produced by a human adult T-cell leukemia line, stimulates T-cell proliferation and the induction of lymphokine-activated killer cells. *Proc Natl Acad Sci U S A* 1994;91:4935.